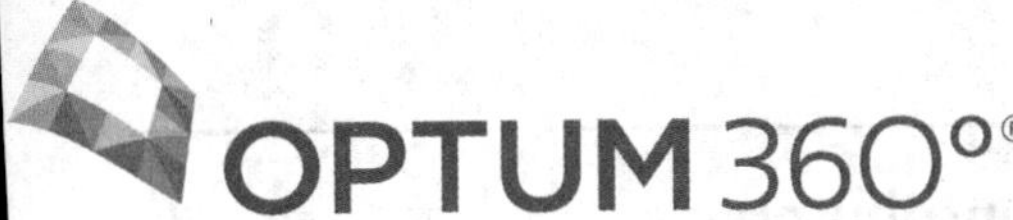

EXPERT

Current Procedural Coding Expert

CPT® codes with Medicare essentials for enhanced accuracy

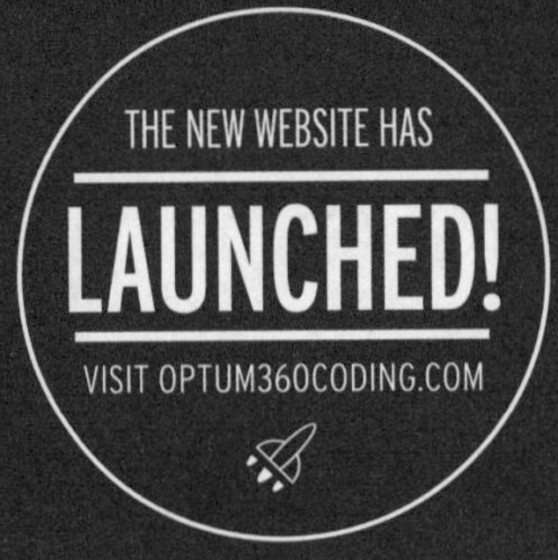

2020

Notice

The *2020 Current Procedural Coding Expert* is designed to be an accurate and authoritative source of information about the CPT® coding system. Every effort has been made to verify the accuracy of the listings, and all information is believed reliable at the time of publication. Absolute accuracy cannot be guaranteed, however. This publication is made available with the understanding that the publisher is not engaged in rendering legal or other services that require a professional license.

American Medical Association Notice

Fee schedules, relative value units, conversion factors and/or related components are not assigned by the AMA, are not part of CPT, and the AMA is not recommending their use. The AMA does not directly or indirectly practice medicine or dispense medical services. The AMA assumes no liability for data contained or not contained herein.

CPT is a registered trademark of the American Medical Association.

Our Commitment to Accuracy

Optum360 is committed to producing accurate and reliable materials.

To report corrections, please email accuracy@optum.com. You can also reach customer service by calling 1.800.464.3649, option 1.

Copyright

Made in the USA

ISBN 978-1-62254-550-6

Acknowledgments

Gregory A. Kemp, MA, *Product Manager*
Karen Schmidt, BSN, *Technical Director*
Stacy Perry, *Manager, Desktop Publishing*
Lisa Singley, *Project Manager*
Karen Krawzik, RHIT, CCS, AHIMA, AHIMA-approved ICD-10-CM/PCS Trainer, *Clinical/Technical Editor*
Elizabeth Leibold, RHIT, *Clinical/Technical Editor*
Anita Schmidt, BS, RHIA, AHIMA-approved ICD-10-CM/PCS Trainer, *Clinical/Technical Editor*
LaJuana Green, RHIA, CCS, *Clinical/Technical Editor*
Tracy Betzler, *Senior Desktop Publishing Specialist*
Hope M. Dunn, *Senior Desktop Publishing Specialist*
Katie Russell, *Desktop Publishing Specialist*
Kate Holden, *Editor*

About the Contributors

Karen Krawzik, RHIT, CCS, AHIMA, AHIMA-approved ICD-10-CM/PCS Trainer

Ms. Krawzik has expertise in ICD-10-CM, ICD-9-CM, CPT/HCPCS, DRG, and data quality and analytics, with more than 30 years' experience coding in multiple settings, including inpatient, observation, ambulatory surgery, ancillary, and emergency room. She has served as a DRG analyst and auditor of commercial and government payer claims, as a contract administrator, and worked on a team providing enterprise-wide conversion of the ICD-9-CM code set to ICD-10. More recently, she has been developing print and electronic content related to ICD-10-CM and ICD-10-PCS coding systems, MS-DRGs, and HCCs. Ms. Krawzik is credentialed by the American Health Information Management Association (AHIMA) as a Registered Health Information Technician (RHIT) and a Certified Coding Specialist (CCS) and is an AHIMA-approved ICD-10-CM/PCS trainer. She is an active member of AHIMA and the Missouri Health Information Management Association.

Elizabeth Leibold, RHIT

Ms. Leibold has more than 25 years of experience in the health care profession. She has served in a variety of roles, ranging from patient registration to billing and collections, and has an extensive background in both physician and hospital outpatient coding and compliance. She has worked for large health care systems and health information management services companies, and has wide-ranging experience in facility and professional component coding, along with CPT expertise in interventional procedures, infusion services, emergency department, observation, and ambulatory surgery coding. Her areas of expertise include chart-to-claim coding audits and providing staff education to both tenured and new coding staff. She is an active member of the American Health Information Management Association (AHIMA).

Anita Schmidt, BS, RHIA, AHIMA-approved ICD-10-CM/PCS Trainer

Ms. Schmidt has expertise in ICD-10-CM/PCS, DRG, and CPT with more than 15 years' experience in coding in multiple settings, including inpatient, observation, and same-day surgery. Her experience includes analysis of medical record documentation, assignment of ICD-10-CM and PCS codes, and DRG validation. She has conducted training for ICD-10-CM/PCS and electronic health record. She has also collaborated with clinical documentation specialists to identify documentation needs and potential areas for physician education. Most recently she has been developing content for resource and educational products related to ICD-10-CM, ICD-10-PCS, DRG, and CPT. Ms. Schmidt is an AHIMA-approved ICD-10-CM/PCS trainer and is an active member of the American Health Information Management Association (AHIMA) and the Minnesota Health Information Management Association.

LaJuana Green, RHIA, CCS

Ms. Green is a Registered Health Information Administrator with over 35 years of experience in multiple areas of information management. She has proven expertise in the analysis of medical record documentation, assignment of ICD-10-CM and PCS codes, DRG validation, and CPT code assignment in ambulatory surgery units and the hospital outpatient setting. Her experience includes serving as a director of a health information management department, clinical technical editing, new technology research and writing, medical record management, utilization review activities, quality assurance, tumor registry, medical library services, and chargemaster maintenance. Ms. Green is an active member of the American Health Information Management Association (AHIMA).

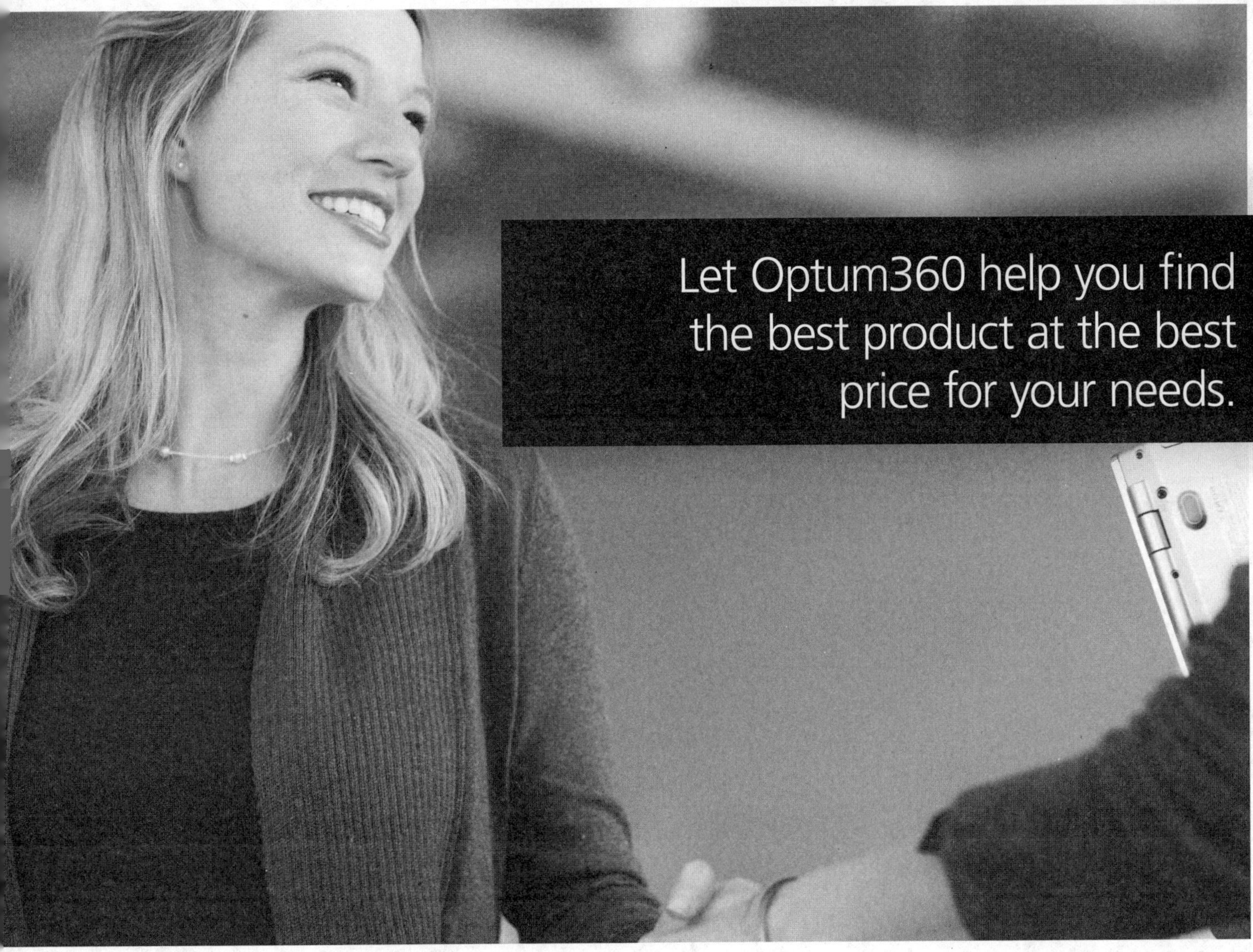

Contents

Introduction

Welcome to Optum360's *Current Procedural Coding Expert*, an exciting Medicare coding and reimbursement tool and definitive procedure coding source that combines the work of the Centers for Medicare and Medicaid Services, American Medical Association, and Optum360 experts with the technical components you need for proper reimbursement and coding accuracy. Handy snap in tabs are included to indicate those sections used most often for easy reference.

This approach to CPT® Medicare coding utilizes innovative and intuitive ways of communicating the information you need to code claims accurately and efficiently. *Includes* and *Excludes* notes, similar to those found in the ICD-10-CM manual, help determine what services are related to the codes you are reporting. Icons help you crosswalk the code you are reporting to laboratory and radiology procedures necessary for proper reimbursement. CMS-mandated icons and relative value units (RVUs) help you determine which codes are most appropriate for the service you are reporting. Add to that additional information identifying age and sex edits, ambulatory surgery center (ASC) and ambulatory payment classification (APC) indicators, and Medicare coverage and payment rule citations, and *Current Procedural Coding Expert* provides the best in Medicare procedure reporting.

Current Procedural Coding Expert includes the information needed to submit claims to federal contractors and most commercial payers, and is correct at the time of printing. However, CMS, federal contractors, and commercial payers may change payment rules at any time throughout the year. *Current Procedural Coding Expert* includes effective codes that will not be published in the AMA's Physicians' Current Procedural Terminology (CPT) book until the following year. Commercial payers will announce changes through monthly news or information posted on their websites. CMS will post changes in policy on its website at http://www.cms.gov/transmittals. National and local coverage determinations (NCDs and LCDs) provide universal and individual contractor guidelines for specific services. The existence of a procedure code does not imply coverage under any given insurance plan.

Current Procedural Coding Expert is based on the AMA's Physicians' Current Procedural Terminology coding system, which is copyrighted and owned by the physician organization. The CPT codes are the nation's official, Health Information Portability and Accountability Act (HIPAA) compliant code set for procedures and services provided by physicians, ambulatory surgery centers (ASCs), and hospital outpatient services, as well as laboratories, imaging centers, physical therapy clinics, urgent care centers, and others.

Getting Started with *Current Procedural Coding Expert*

Current Procedural Coding Expert is an exciting tool combining the most current material at the time of our publication from the AMA's CPT 2020, CMS's online manual system, the Correct Coding initiative, CMS fee schedules, official Medicare guidelines for reimbursement and coverage, the Integrated outpatient coding Editor (I/OCE), and Optum360's own coding expertise.

These coding rules and guidelines are incorporated into more specific section notes and code notes. Section notes are listed under a range of codes and apply to all codes in that range. Code notes are found under individual codes and apply to the single code.

Material is presented in a logical fashion for those billing Medicare, Medicaid, and many private payers. The format, based on customer comments, better addresses what customers tell us they need in a comprehensive Medicare procedure coding guide.

Designed to be easy to use and full of information, this product is an excellent companion to your AMA CPT manual, and other Optum360 and Medicare resources.

For mid-year code updates, official errata changes, correction notices, and any other changes pertinent to the information in *Current Procedural Coding Expert*, see our product update page at https://www.optum360coding.com/ProductUpdates/. The password for 2020 is PROCEDURE2020.

Note: The AMA releases code changes quarterly as well as errata or corrections to CPT codes and guidelines and posts them on their web site. Some of these changes may not appear in the AMA's CPT book until the following year. *Current Procedural Coding Expert* incorporates the most recent errata or release notes found on the AMA's web site at our publication time, including new, revised and deleted codes. *Current Procedural Coding Expert* identifies these new or revised codes from the AMA website errata or release notes with an icon similar to the AMA's current new ● and revised ▲ icons. For purposes of this publication, new CPT codes and revisions that won't be in the AMA book until the next edition are indicated with a ● and a ▲ icon. For the next year's edition of *Current Procedural Coding Expert*, these codes will appear with standard black new or revised icons, as appropriate, to correspond with those changes as indicated in the AMA CPT book. CPT codes that were new for 2019 and appeared in the 2019 *Current Procedural Coding Expert* but did not appear in the CPT code book until 2020 are identified in appendix B as "Web Release New and Revised Codes."

General Conventions

Many of the sources of information in this book can be determined by color.

- All CPT codes and descriptions and the Evaluation and Management guidelines from the American Medical Association are in **black text**.
- Includes, Excludes, and other notes appear in **blue text**. The resources used for this information are a variety of Medicare policy manuals, the *National Correct Coding Initiative Policy Manual* (NCCI), AMA resources and guidelines, and specialty association resources and our Optum360 clinical experts.

Resequencing of CPT Codes

The American Medical Association (AMA) uses a numbering methodology of resequencing, which is the practice of displaying codes outside of their numerical order according to the description relationship. According to the AMA, there are instances in which a new code is needed within an existing grouping of codes but an unused code number is not available. In these situations, the AMA will resequence the codes. In other words, it will assign a code that is not in numeric sequence with the related codes. However, the code and description will appear in the CPT manual with the other related codes.

An example of resequencing from *Current Procedural Coding Expert* follows:

	21555	**Excision, tumor, soft tissue of neck or anterior thorax, subcutaneous; less than 3 cm**
#	**21552**	**3 cm or greater**
	21556	**Excision, tumor, soft tissue of neck or anterior thorax, subfascial (eg, intramuscular); less than 5 cm**
#	**21554**	**5 cm or greater**

In *Current Procedural Coding Expert* the resequenced codes are listed twice. They appear in their resequenced position as shown above as well as in their original numeric position with a note indicating that the code is out of numerical sequence and where it can be found. (See example below.)

21554 **Resequenced code. See code following 21556.**

This differs from the AMA CPT book, in which the coder is directed to a code range that contains the resequenced code and description, rather than to a specific location.

Introduction

Resequenced codes will appear in brackets in the headers, section notes, and code ranges. For example:

27327-27329 [27337, 27339] Excision Soft Tissue Tumors Femur/Knee. Codes [27337, 27339] are included in section 27327-27329 in their resequenced positions.

Code also toxoid/vaccine (90476-90749 [90620, 90621, 90625, 90630, 90644, 90672, 90673, 90674, 90750, 90756])

This shows codes 90620, 90621, 90625, 90630, 90644, 90672, 90673, 90674, 90750, and 90756 are resequenced in this range of codes.

Code Ranges for Medicare Billing

Appendix E identifies all resequenced CPT codes. Optum360 will display the resequenced coding as assigned by the AMA in its CPT products so that the user may understand the code description relationships.

Each particular group of CPT codes in *Current Procedural Coding Expert* is organized in a more intuitive fashion for Medicare billing, being grouped by the Medicare rules and regulations as found in the official CMS online manuals that govern payment of these particular procedures and services, as in this example:

99221-99233 Inpatient Hospital Visits: Initial and Subsequent

CMS: 100-4,11,40.1.3 Independent Attending Physician Services; 100-4,12,100.1.1 Teaching Physicians E/M Services; 100-4,12,30.6.10 Consultation Services; 100-4,12,30.6.15.1 Prolonged Services With Direct Face-to-Face Patient Contact; 100-4,12,30.6.4 Services Furnished Incident to Physician's Service; 100-4,12,30.6.9 Hospital Visit and Critical Care on Same Day

Icons

● **New Codes**
Codes that have been added since the last edition of the AMA CPT book was printed.

▲ **Revised Codes**
Codes that have been revised since the last edition of the AMA CPT book was printed.

● **New Web Release**
Codes that are new for the current year but will not be in the AMA CPT book until 2021.

▲ **Revised Web Release**
Codes that have been revised for the current year, but will not be in the AMA CPT book until 2021.

Resequenced Codes
Codes that are out of numeric order but apply to the appropriate category.

★ **Telemedicine Services**
Codes that may be reported for telemedicine services. Modifier 95 must be appended to code.

❍ **Reinstated Code**
Codes that have been reinstated since the last edition of the book was printed.

Pink Color Bar—Not Covered by Medicare
Services and procedures identified by this color bar are never covered benefits under Medicare. Services and procedures that are not covered may be billed directly to the patient at the time of the service.

Gray Color Bar—Unlisted Procedure
Unlisted CPT codes report procedures that have not been assigned a specific code number. An unlisted code delays payment due to the extra time necessary for review.

Green Color Bar—Resequenced Codes
Resequenced codes are codes that are out of numeric sequence—they are indicated with a green color bar. They are listed twice, in their resequenced position as well as in their original numeric position with a note that the code is out of numerical sequence and where the resequenced code and description can be found.

INCLUDES **Includes notes**
Includes notes identify procedures and services that would be bundled in the procedure code. These are derived from AMA, CMS, NCCI, and Optum360 coding guidelines. This is not meant to be an all-inclusive list.

EXCLUDES **Excludes notes**
Excludes notes may lead the user to other codes. They may identify services that are not bundled and may be separately reported, OR may lead the user to another more appropriate code. These are derived from AMA, CMS, NCCI, and Optum360 coding guidelines. This is not meant to be an all-inclusive list.

Code Also This note identifies an additional code that should be reported with the service and may relate to another CPT code or an appropriate HCPCS code(s) that should be reported along with the CPT code when appropriate.

Code First Found under add-on codes, this note identifies codes for primary procedures that should be reported first, with the add-on code reported as a secondary code.

Laboratory/Pathology Crosswalk
This icon denotes CPT codes in the laboratory and pathology section of CPT that may be reported separately with the primary CPT code.

Radiology Crosswalk
This icon denotes codes in the radiology section that may be used with the primary CPT code being reported.

TC **Technical Component Only**
Codes with this icon represent only the technical component (staff and equipment costs) of a procedure or service. Do not use either modifier 26 (professional component) or TC (technical component) with these codes.

26 **Professional Component**
Only codes with this icon represent the physician's work or professional component of a procedure or service. Do not use either modifier 26 (professional component) or TC (technical component) with these codes.

50 **Bilateral Procedure**
This icon identifies codes that can be reported bilaterally when the same surgeon provides the service for the same patient on the same date. Medicare allows payment for both procedures at 150 percent of the usual amount for one procedure. The modifier does not apply to bilateral procedures inclusive to one code.

80 **Assist-at-Surgery Allowed**
Services noted by this icon are allowed an assistant at surgery with a Medicare payment equal to 16 percent of the allowed amount for the global surgery for that procedure. No documentation is required.

80 **Assist-at-Surgery Allowed with Documentation**
Services noted by this icon are allowed an assistant at surgery with a Medicare payment equal to 16 percent of the allowed amount for the global surgery for that procedure. Documentation is required.

+ **Add-on Codes**
This icon identifies procedures reported in addition to the primary procedure. The icon "**+**" denotes add-on codes. An add-on code is neither a stand-alone code nor subject to multiple procedure rules since it describes work in addition to the primary procedure.

According to Medicare guidelines, add-on codes may be identified in the following ways:

- The code is found on Change Request (CR) 7501 or successive CRs as a Type I, Type II, or Type III add-on code.

- The add-on code most often has a global period of "ZZZ" in the Medicare Physician Fee Schedule Database.
- The code is found in the CPT book with the icon "+" appended. Add-on code descriptors typically include the phrases "each additional" or "(List separately in addition to primary procedure)."

⑤⓪ **Optum Modifier 50 Exempt**
Codes identified by this icon indicate that the procedure should not be reported with modifier 50 (Bilateral procedures).

⊘ **Modifier 51 Exempt**
Codes identified by this icon indicate that the procedure should not be reported with modifier 51 (Multiple procedures).

⑤① **Optum Modifier 51 Exempt**
Codes identified by this Optum360 icon indicate that the procedure should not be reported with modifier 51 (Multiple procedures). Any code with this icon is backed by official AMA guidelines but was not identified by the AMA with their modifier 51 exempt icon.

Correct Coding Initiative (CCI)
Current Procedural Coding Expert identifies those codes with corresponding CCI edits. The CCI edits define correct coding practices that serve as the basis of the national Medicare policy for paying claims. The code noted is the major service/procedure. The code may represent a column 1 code within the column 1/column 2 correct coding edits table or a code pair that is mutually exclusive of each other.

CLIA Waived Test
This symbol is used to distinguish those laboratory tests that can be performed using test systems that are waived from regulatory oversight established by the Clinical Laboratory Improvement Amendments of 1988 (CLIA). The applicable CPT code for a CLIA waived test may be reported by providers who perform the testing but do not hold a CLIA license.

⑥③ **Modifier 63 Exempt**
This icon identifies procedures performed on infants that weigh less than 4 kg. Due to the complexity of performing procedures on infants less than 4 kg, modifier 63 may be added to the surgery codes to inform the payers of the special circumstances involved.

A2–Z3 **ASC Payment Indicators**
This icon identifies ASC status payment indicators. They indicate how the ASC payment rate was derived and/or how the procedure, item, or service is treated under the revised ASC payment system. For more information about these indicators and how they affect billing, consult Optum360's *Outpatient Billing Editor*.

A2 Surgical procedure on ASC list in 2007; payment based on OPPS relative payment weight.

B5 Alternative code may be available; no payment made.

D5 Deleted/discontinued code; no payment made.

F4 Corneal tissue acquisition; hepatitis B vaccine; paid at reasonable cost.

G2 Non-office-based surgical procedure added in CY 2008 or later; payment based on OPPS relative payment weight.

H2 Brachytherapy source paid separately when provided integral to a surgical procedure on ASC list; payment based on OPPS rate.

J7 OPPS pass-through device paid separately when provided integral to a surgical procedure on ASC list; payment contractor-priced.

J8 Device-intensive procedure; paid at adjusted rate.

K2 Drugs and biologicals paid separately when provided integral to a surgical procedure on ASC list; payment based on OPPS rate.

K7 Unclassified drugs and biologicals; payment contractor-priced.

L1 Influenza vaccine; pneumococcal vaccine. Packaged item/service; no separate payment made.

L6 New technology intraocular lens (NTIOL); special payment.

N1 Packaged service/item; no separate payment made.

P2 Office-based surgical procedure added to ASC list in CY 2008 or later with MPFS nonfacility practice expense (PE) RVUs; payment based on OPPS relative payment weight.

P3 Office-based surgical procedure added to ASC list in CY 2008 or later with MPFS nonfacility PE RVUs; payment based on MPFS nonfacility PE RVUs.

R2 Office-based surgical procedure added to ASC list in CY 2008 or later without MPFS nonfacility PE RVUs; payment based on OPPS relative payment weight.

Z2 Radiology or diagnostic service paid separately when provided integral to a surgical procedure on ASC list; payment based on OPPS relative payment weight.

Z3 Radiology or diagnostic service paid separately when provided integral to a surgical procedure on ASC list; payment based on MPFS nonfacility PE RVUs.

A **Age Edit**
This icon denotes codes intended for use with a specific age group, such as neonate, newborn, pediatric, and adult. This edit is based on age specifications in the CPT code descriptors or the product/service represented by the code *MAY* have age restrictions. Carefully review the code description to ensure the code you report most appropriately reflects the patient's age.

M **Maternity**
This icon identifies procedures that by definition should be used only for maternity patients generally between 12 and 55 years of age based on CMS I/OCE designations.

♀ **Female Only**
This icon identifies procedures designated by CMS for females only based on CMS I/OCE designations.

♂ **Male Only**
This icon identifies procedures designated by CMS for males only based on CMS I/OCE designations.

Facility RVU
This icon precedes the facility RVU from CMS's 2018 physician fee schedule (PFS). It can be found under the code description.

New codes include no RVU information.

Nonfacility RVU
This icon precedes the nonfacility RVU from CMS's 2018 PFS. It can be found under the code description.

New codes include no RVU information.

FUD: Global days are sometimes referred to as "follow-up days" or FUDs. The global period is the time following surgery during which routine care by the physician is considered postoperative and included in the surgical fee. Office visits or other routine care related to the original surgery cannot be separately reported if provided during the global period. The statuses are:

- 000 No follow-up care included in this procedure
- 010 Normal postoperative care is included in this procedure for ten days
- 090 Normal postoperative care is included in the procedure for 90 days
- MMM Maternity codes; usual global period does not apply
- XXX The global concept does not apply to the code

Introduction

YYY The carrier is to determine whether the global concept applies and establishes postoperative period, if appropriate, at time of pricing

ZZZ The code is related to another service and is always included in the global period of the other service

CMS: This notation indicates that there is a specific CMS guideline pertaining to this code in the CMS Online Manual System which includes the internet-only manual (IOM) *National Coverage Determinations Manual* (NCD). These CMS sources present the rules for submitting these services to the federal government or its contractors and are included in appendix G of this book.

AMA: This indicates discussion of the code in the American Medical Association's *CPT Assistant* newsletter. Use the citation to find the correct issue. This includes citations for the current year and the preceding six years. In the event no citations can be found during this time period, the most recent citations that can be found are used.

Drug Not Approved by FDA
The AMA CPT Editorial Panel is publishing new vaccine product codes prior to Food and Drug Administration approval. This symbol indicates which of these codes are pending FDA approval at press time.

[A]–[Y] **OPPS Status Indicators (OPSI)**
Status indicators identify how individual CPT codes are paid or not paid under the latest available hospital outpatient prospective payment system (OPPS). The same status indicator is assigned to all the codes within an ambulatory payment classification (APC). Consult your payer or other resource to learn which CPT codes fall within various APCs.

[A] Services furnished to a hospital outpatient that are paid under a fee schedule or payment system other than OPPS. For example:
- Ambulance services
- Separately payable clinical diagnostic laboratory services
- Separately payable non-implantable prosthetics and orthotics
- Physical, occupational, and speech therapy
- Diagnostic mammography
- Screening mammography

[B] Codes that are not recognized by OPPS when submitted on an outpatient hospital Part B bill type (12x and 13x)

[C] Inpatient procedures

[D] Discontinued codes

[E1] Items, codes, and services:
- Not covered by any Medicare outpatient benefit category
- Statutorily excluded by Medicare
- Not reasonable and necessary

[E2] Items, codes, and services for which pricing information and claims data are not available

[F] Corneal tissue acquisition; certain CRNA services and hepatitis B vaccines

[G] Pass-through drugs and biologicals

[H] Pass-through device categories

[J1] Hospital Part B services paid through a comprehensive APC

[J2] Hospital Part B services that may be paid through a comprehensive APC

[K] Nonpass-through drugs and nonimplantable biologicals, including therapeutic radiopharmaceuticals

[L] Influenza vaccine; pneumococcal pneumonia vaccine

[M] Items and services not billable to the MAC

[N] Items and services packaged into APC rates

[P] Partial hospitalization

[Q1] STV-packaged codes

[Q2] T-packaged codes

[Q3] Codes that may be paid through a composite APC

[Q4] Conditionally packaged laboratory tests

[R] Blood and blood products

[S] Procedure or service, not discounted when multiple

[T] Procedure or service, multiple procedure reduction applies

[U] Brachytherapy sources

[V] Clinic or emergency department visit

[Y] Nonimplantable durable medical equipment

Appendixes

Appendix A: Modifiers—This appendix identifies modifiers. A modifier is a two-position alpha or numeric code that is appended to a CPT or HCPCS code to clarify the services being billed. Modifiers provide a means by which a service can be altered without changing the procedure code. They add more information, such as anatomical site, to the code. In addition, they help eliminate the appearance of duplicate billing and unbundling. Modifiers are used to increase the accuracy in reimbursement and coding consistency, ease editing, and capture payment data.

Appendix B: New, Revised, and Deleted Codes—This is a list of new, revised, and deleted CPT codes for the current year. This appendix also includes a list of web release new and revised codes, which indicate official code changes in *Current Procedural Coding Expert* that will not be in the CPT code book until the following year.

Appendix C: Evaluation and Management Extended Guidelines—This appendix presents an overview of evaluation and management (E/M) services that augment the official AMA CPT E/M services. It includes tables that distinguish documentation components of each E/M code and the federal documentation guidelines (1995 and 1997) currently in use by the Centers for Medicare and Medicaid Services (CMS).

Appendix D: Crosswalk of Deleted Codes—This appendix is a cross-reference from a deleted CPT code to an active code when one is available. The deleted code cross-reference will also appear under the deleted code description in the tabular section of the book.

Appendix E: Resequenced Codes—This appendix contains a list of codes that are not in numeric order in the book. AMA resequenced some of the code numbers to relocate codes in the same category but not in numeric sequence.

Appendix F: Add-on, Optum Modifier 50 Exempt, Modifier 51 Exempt, Optum Modifier 51 Exempt, Modifier 63 Exempt, and Modifier 95 Telemedicine Services—This list includes add-on codes that cannot be reported alone, codes that are exempt from modifiers 50 and 51, codes that should not be reported with modifier 63, and codes identified by the ★ icon to which modifier 95 may be appended when the service is provided as a synchronous telemedicine service.

Appendix G: Medicare Internet-only Manual (IOMs)—This appendix contains a verbatim printout of the Medicare Internet Only Manual references that pertain to specific codes. The reference, when available, is listed after the header in the CPT section. For example:

93784-93790 Ambulatory Blood Pressure Monitoring
CMS: 100-3,20.19 Ambulatory Blood Pressure Monitoring (20.19); 100-4,32,10.1 Ambulatory Blood Pressure Monitoring Billing Requirements

Since appendix G contains these references from the *Medicare National Coverage Determinations (NCD) Manual*, Pub 100-3, chapter 20, section 20.19, and the *Medicare Claims Processing Manual*, Pub 100-4, chapter 32, section 10.1, there is no need to search the Medicare website for the applicable reference.

Appendix H: Quality Payment Program (QPP)—Previously, this appendix contained lists of the numerators and denominators applicable to the Medicare PQRS. However, with the implementation of the Quality Payment Program (QPP) mandated by passage of the Medicare Access and Chip Reauthorization Act (MACRA) of 2015, the PQRS system will be obsolete. This appendix now contains information pertinent to that legislation as well as a comprehensive overview of the QPP.

Appendix I: Medically Unlikely Edits—This appendix contains the published medically unlikely edits (MUEs). These edits establish maximum daily allowable units of service. The edits will be applied to the services provided to the same patient, for the same CPT code, on the same date of service when billed by the same provider. Included are the physician and facility edits.

Appendix J: Inpatient-Only Procedures—This appendix identifies services with the status indicator "C." Medicare will not pay an OPPS hospital or ASC when these procedures are performed on a Medicare patient as an outpatient. Physicians should refer to this list when scheduling Medicare patients for surgical procedures. CMS updates this list quarterly.

Appendix K: Place of Service and Type of Service—This appendix contains lists of place-of-service codes that should be used on professional claims and type-of-service codes used by the Medicare Common Working File.

Appendix L: Multianalyte Assays with Algorithmic Analyses —This appendix lists the administrative codes for multianalyte assays with algorithmic analyses. The AMA updates this list three times a year.

Appendix M: Glossary—This appendix contains general terms and definitions as well as those that would apply to or be helpful for billing and reimbursement.

Appendix N: Listing of Sensory, Motor, and Mixed Nerves—This appendix lists a summary of each sensory, motor, and mixed nerve with its appropriate nerve conduction study code.

Appendix O: Vascular Families—Appendix O contains a table of vascular families starting with the aorta. Additional information can be found in the interventional radiology illustrations located behind the index.

Appendix P: Interventional Radiology Illustrations—This appendix contains illustrations specific to interventional radiology procedures.

Note: All data current as of November 11, 2019.

Anatomical Illustrations

Body Planes and Movements

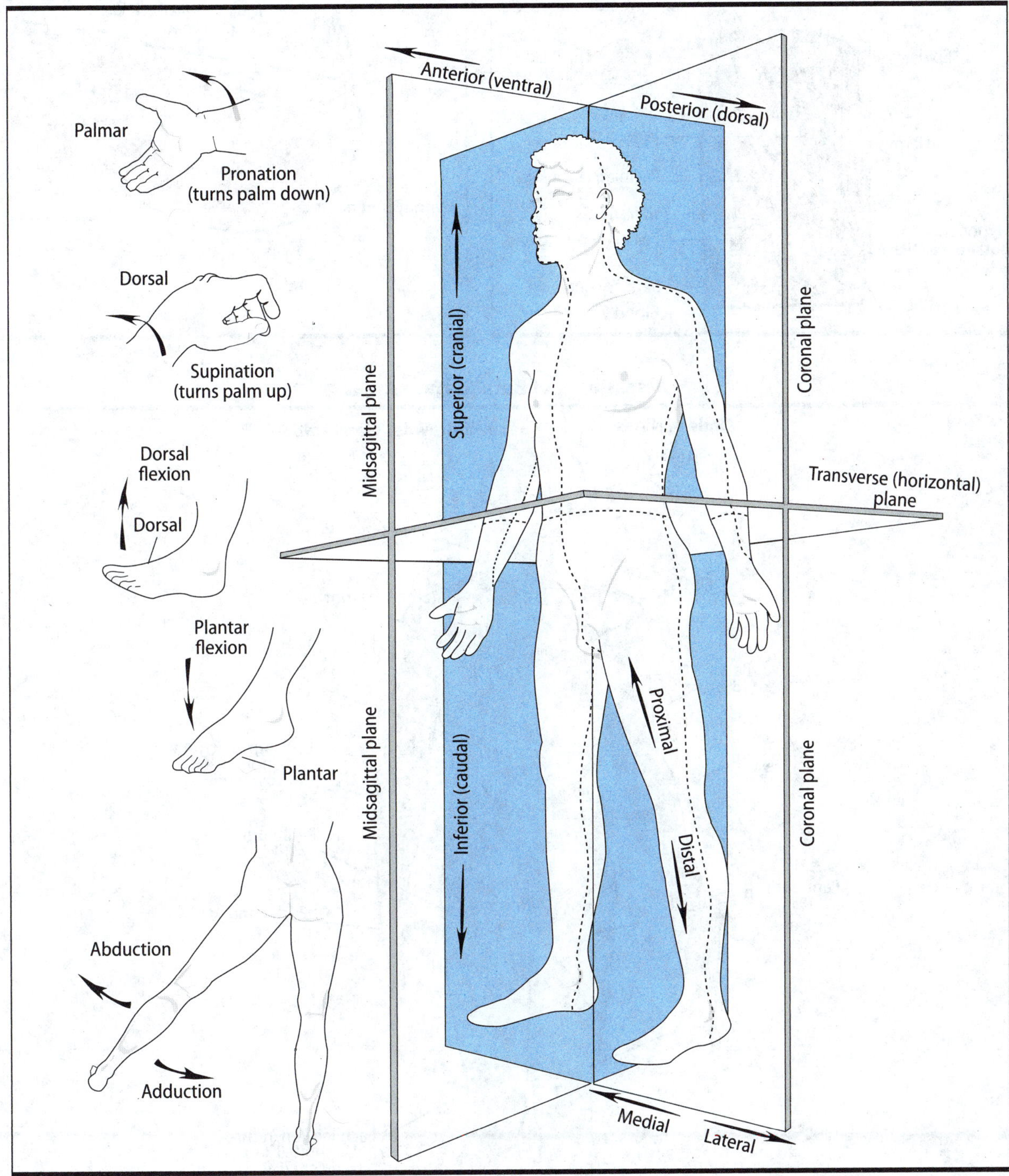

Integumentary System

Skin and Subcutaneous Tissue

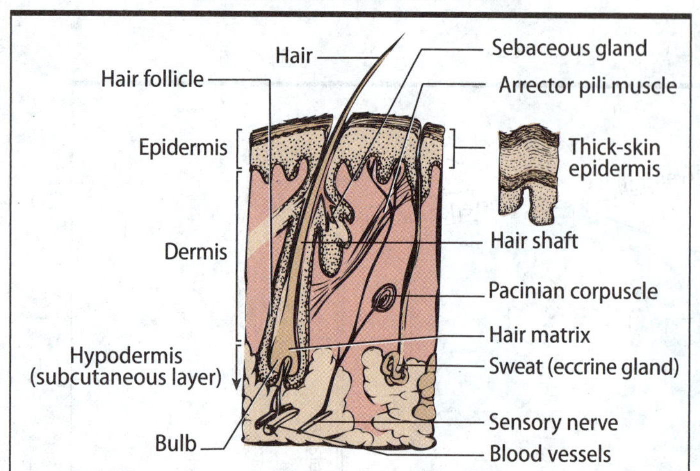

Nail Anatomy

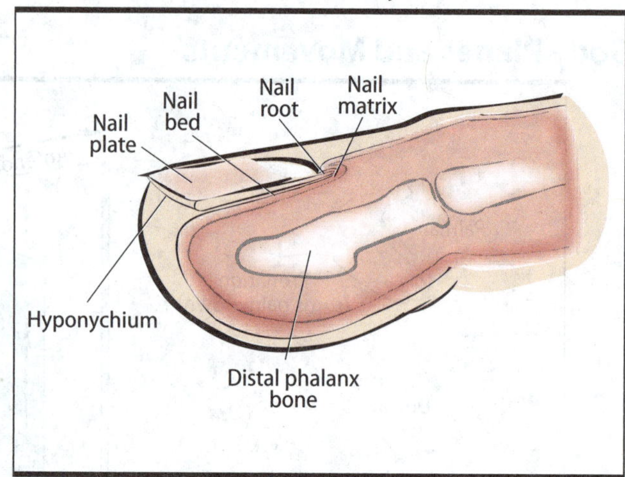

Assessment of Burn Surface Area

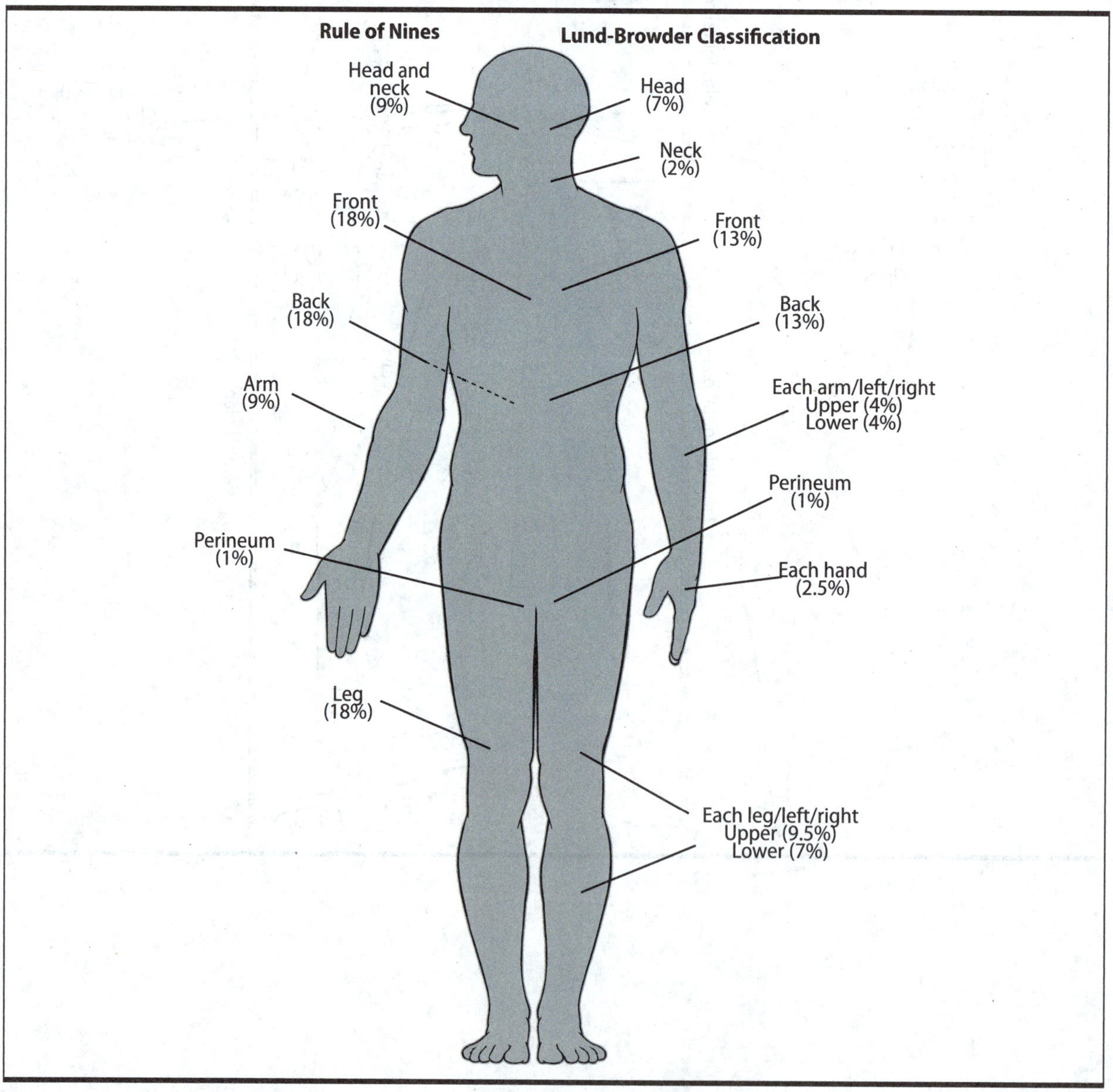

Rule of Nines

Head and neck (9%)

Front (18%)

Back (18%)

Arm (9%)

Perineum (1%)

Leg (18%)

Lund-Browder Classification

Head (7%)

Neck (2%)

Front (13%)

Back (13%)

Each arm/left/right
Upper (4%)
Lower (4%)

Perineum (1%)

Each hand (2.5%)

Each leg/left/right
Upper (9.5%)
Lower (7%)

Musculoskeletal System

Bones and Joints

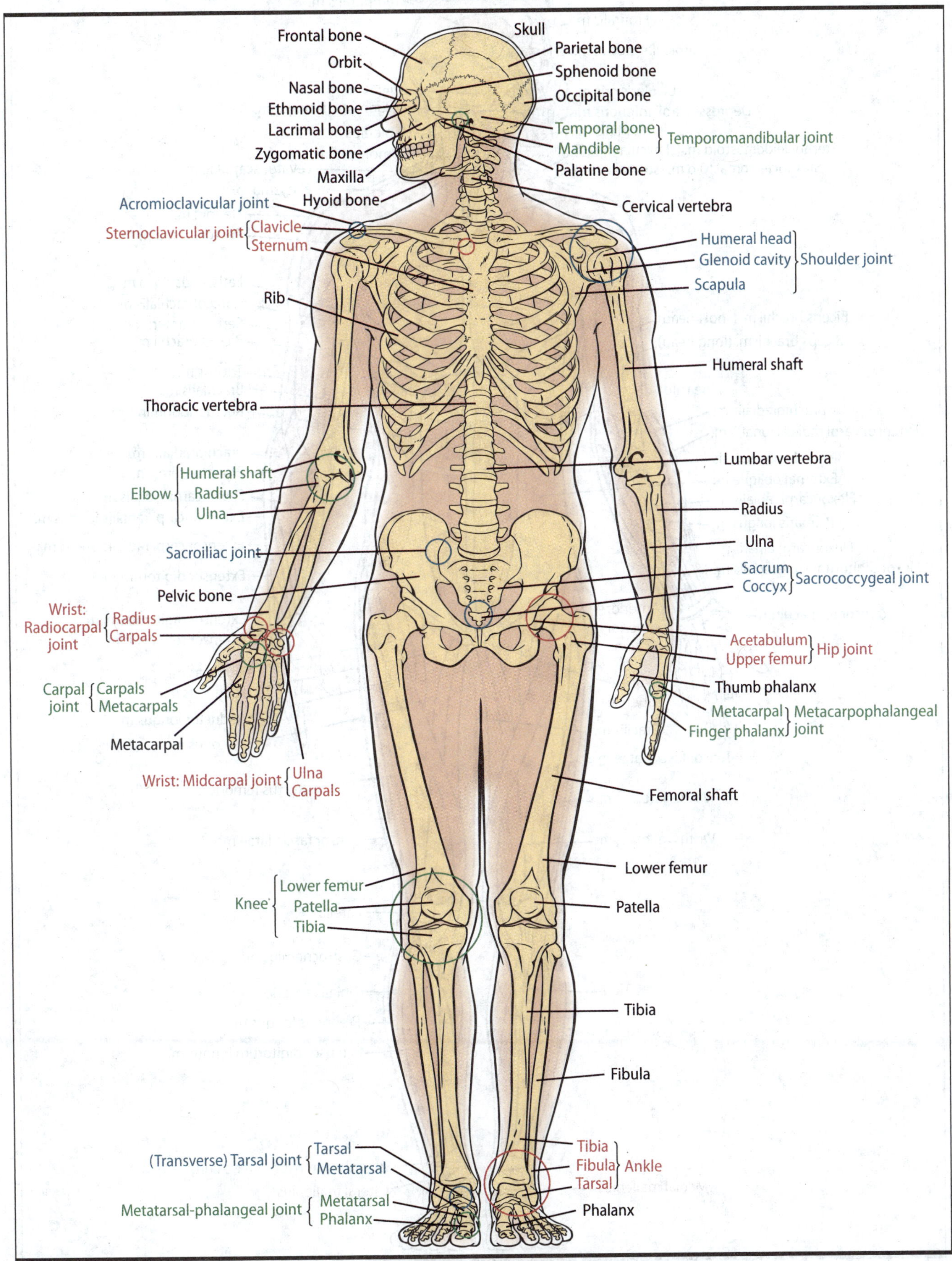

Muscles

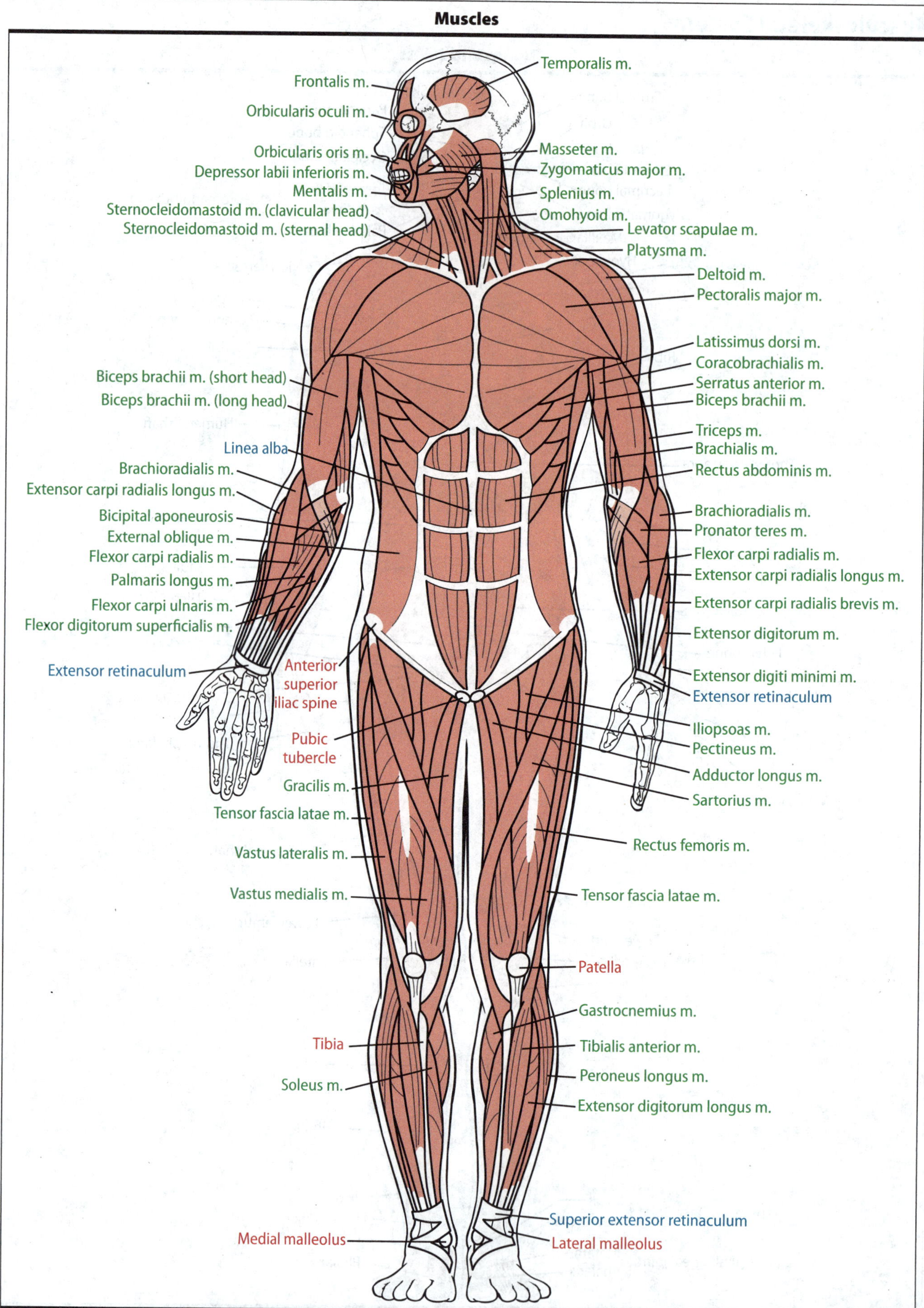

Temporalis m.
Frontalis m.
Orbicularis oculi m.
Orbicularis oris m.
Depressor labii inferioris m.
Mentalis m.
Sternocleidomastoid m. (clavicular head)
Sternocleidomastoid m. (sternal head)
Masseter m.
Zygomaticus major m.
Splenius m.
Omohyoid m.
Levator scapulae m.
Platysma m.
Deltoid m.
Pectoralis major m.
Latissimus dorsi m.
Coracobrachialis m.
Serratus anterior m.
Biceps brachii m.
Biceps brachii m. (short head)
Biceps brachii m. (long head)
Triceps m.
Brachialis m.
Linea alba
Rectus abdominis m.
Brachioradialis m.
Extensor carpi radialis longus m.
Bicipital aponeurosis
External oblique m.
Flexor carpi radialis m.
Palmaris longus m.
Flexor carpi ulnaris m.
Flexor digitorum superficialis m.
Brachioradialis m.
Pronator teres m.
Flexor carpi radialis m.
Extensor carpi radialis longus m.
Extensor carpi radialis brevis m.
Extensor digitorum m.
Extensor retinaculum
Anterior superior iliac spine
Extensor digiti minimi m.
Extensor retinaculum
Pubic tubercle
Iliopsoas m.
Pectineus m.
Adductor longus m.
Gracilis m.
Sartorius m.
Tensor fascia latae m.
Rectus femoris m.
Vastus lateralis m.
Vastus medialis m.
Tensor fascia latae m.
Patella
Gastrocnemius m.
Tibia
Tibialis anterior m.
Peroneus longus m.
Soleus m.
Extensor digitorum longus m.
Superior extensor retinaculum
Medial malleolus
Lateral malleolus

Head and Facial Bones

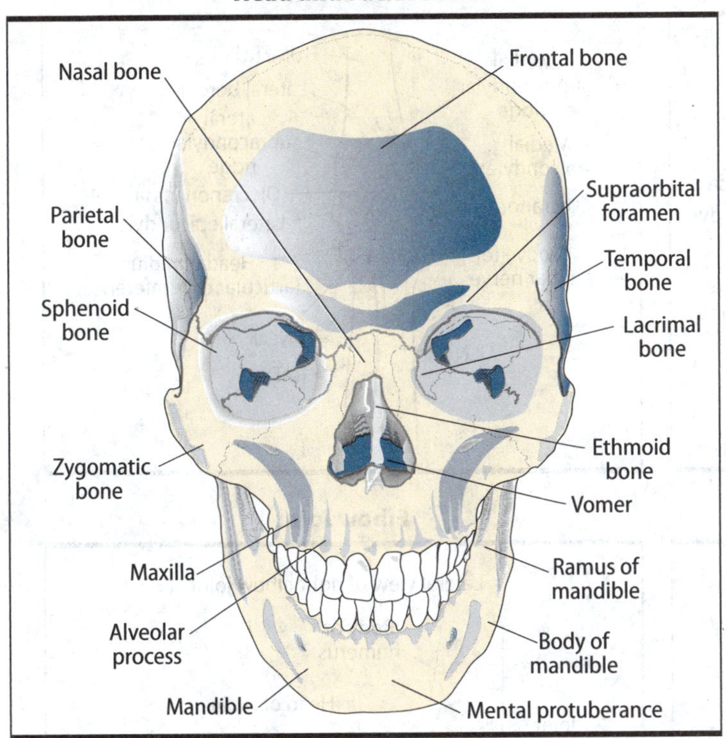

Nose

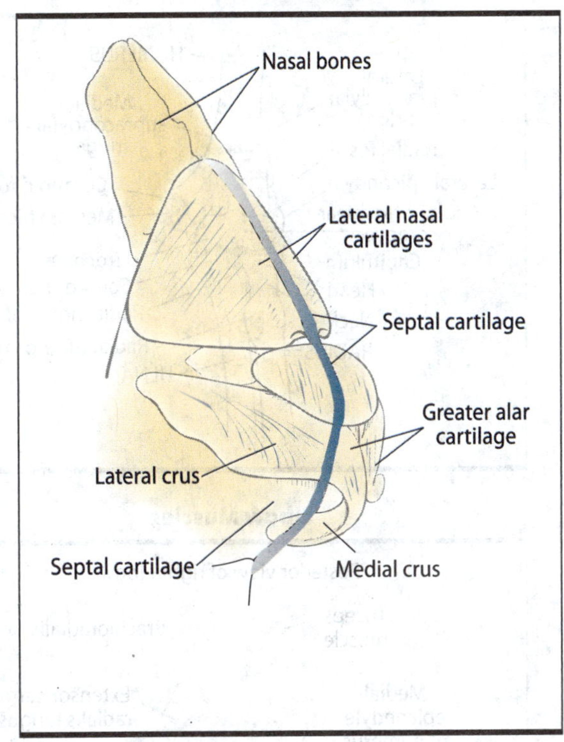

Shoulder (Anterior View)

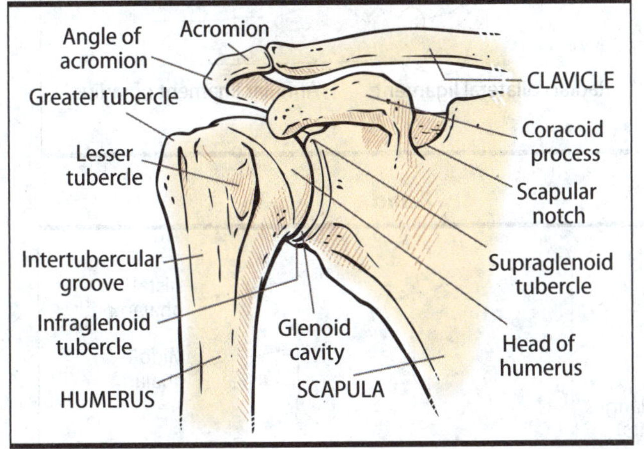

Shoulder (Posterior View)

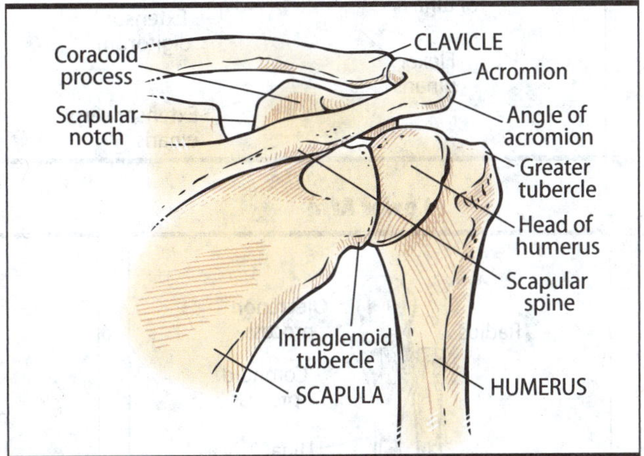

Shoulder Muscles

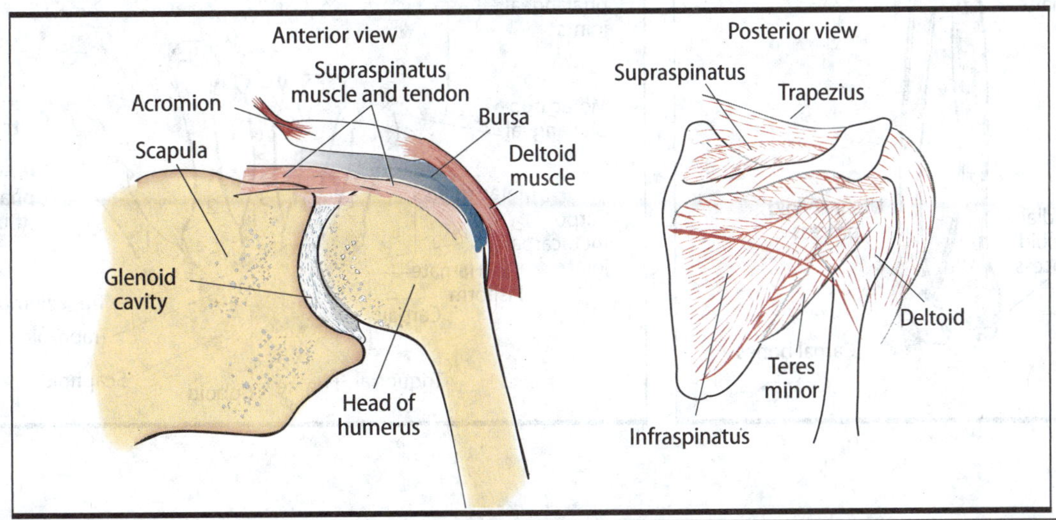

Elbow (Anterior View)

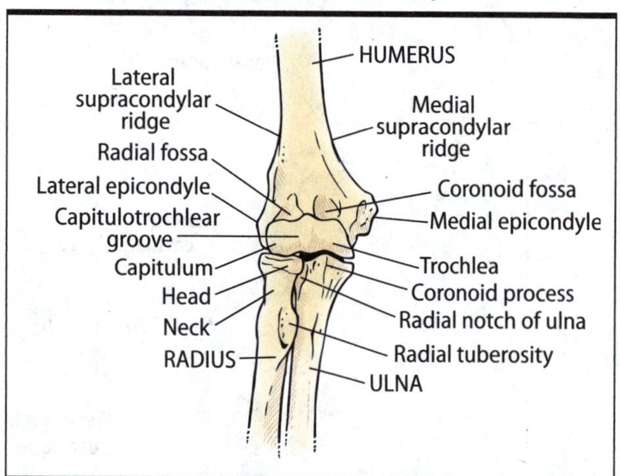

Elbow (Posterior View)

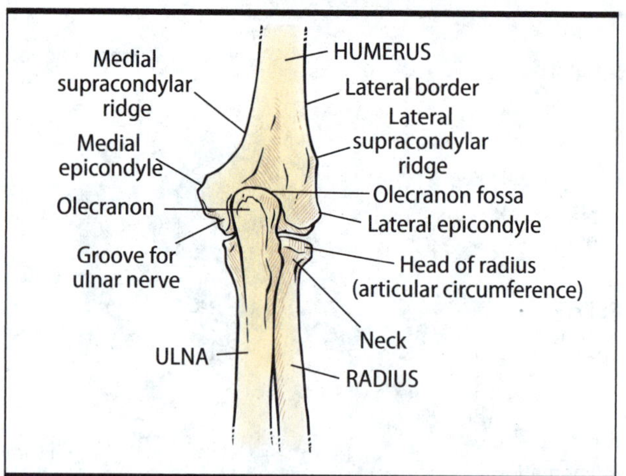

Elbow Muscles

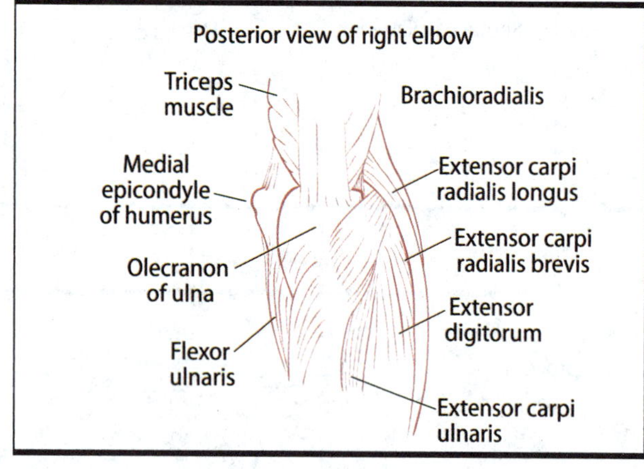

Elbow Joint

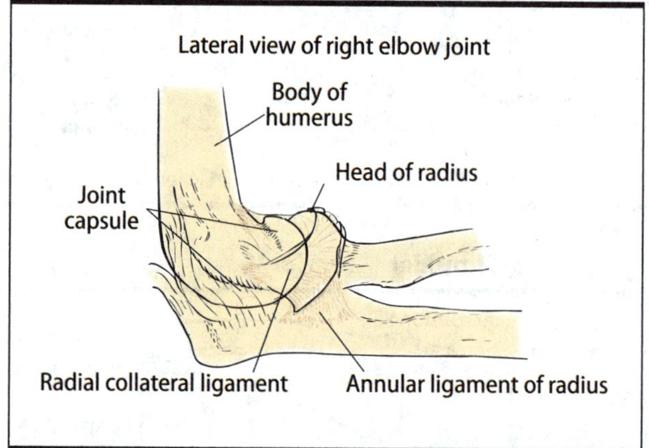

Lower Arm

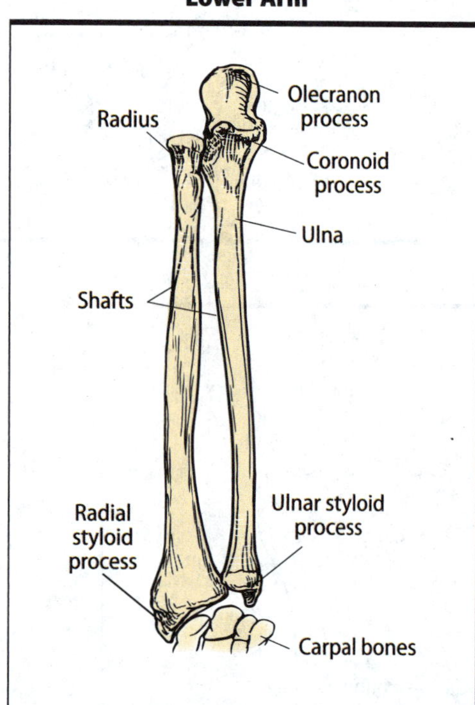

Hand

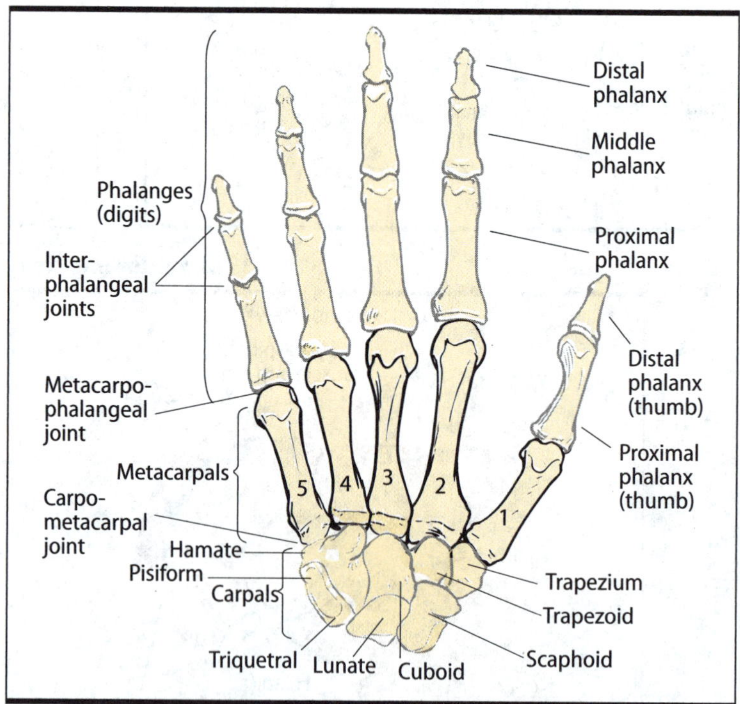

Hip (Anterior View)

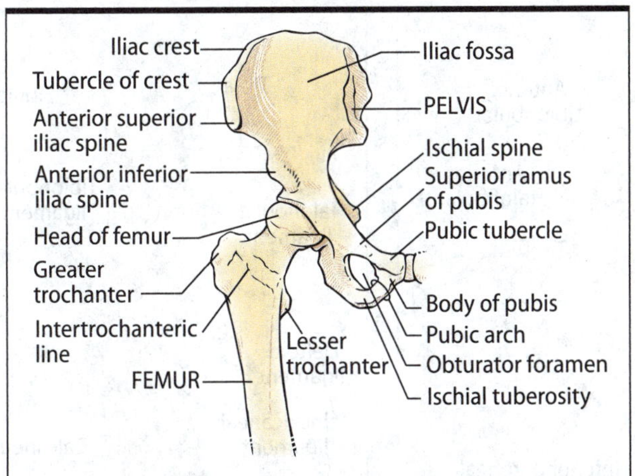

Hip (Posterior View)

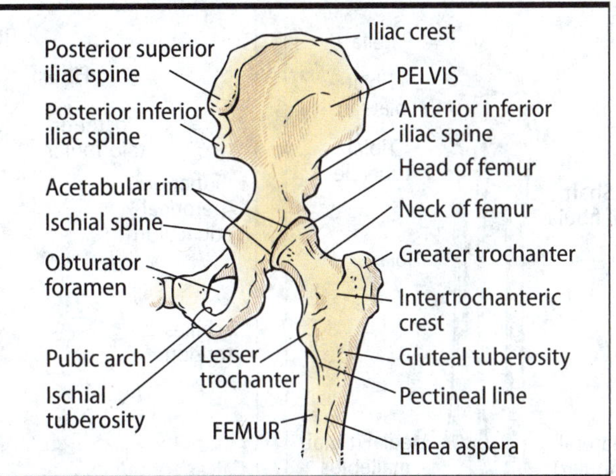

Knee (Anterior View)

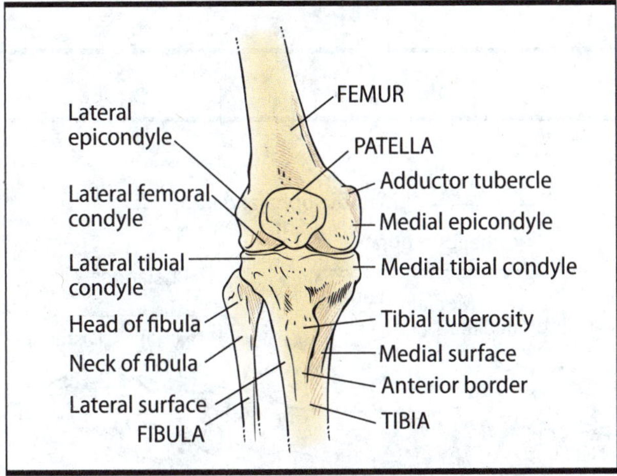

Knee (Posterior View)

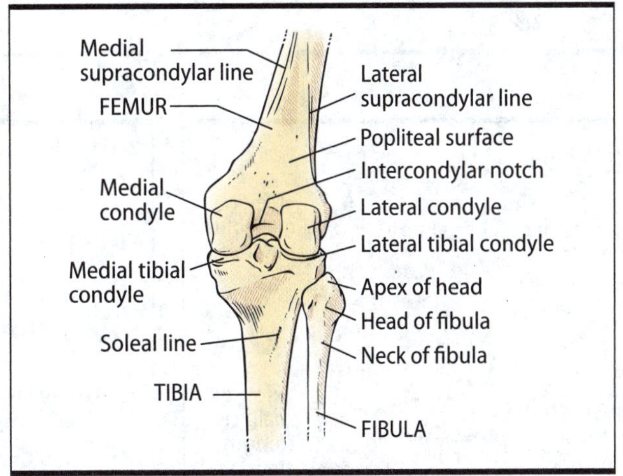

Knee Joint (Anterior View)

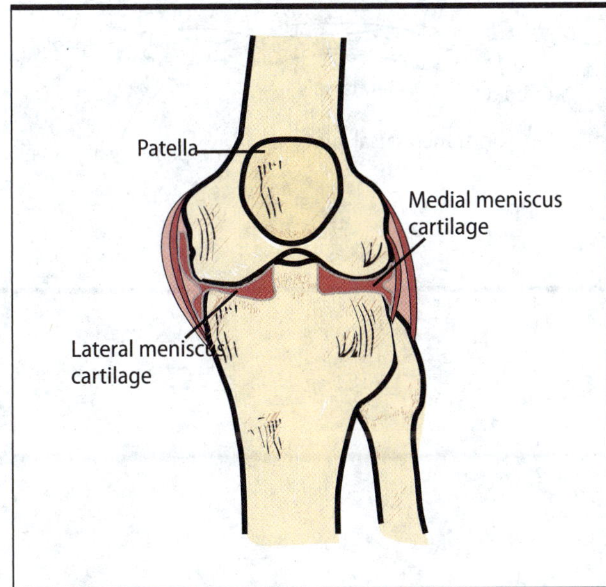

Knee Joint (Lateral View)

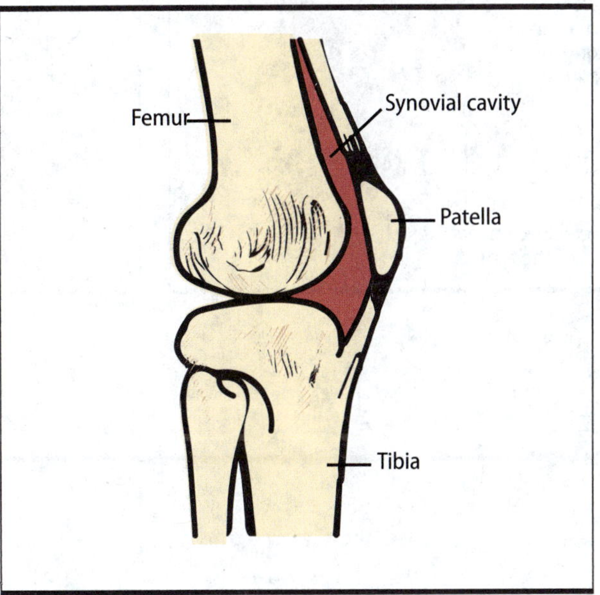

Lower Leg

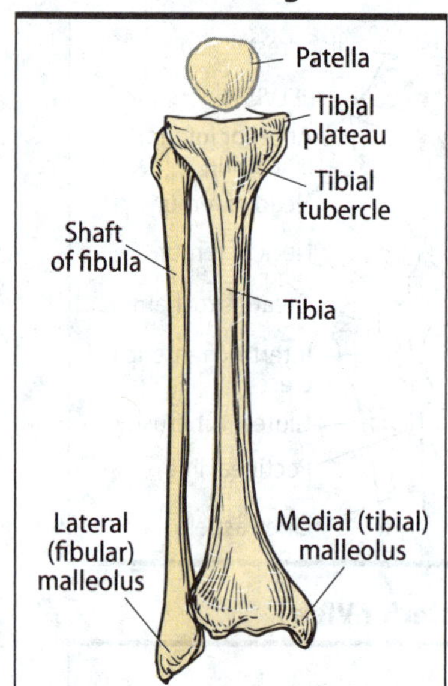

Ankle Ligament (Lateral View)

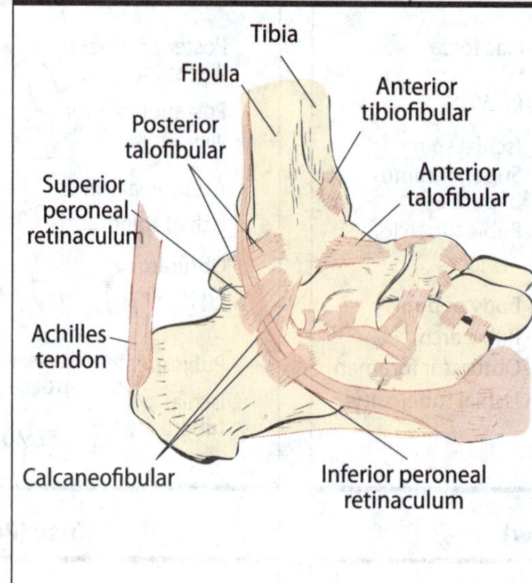

Ankle Ligament (Posterior View)

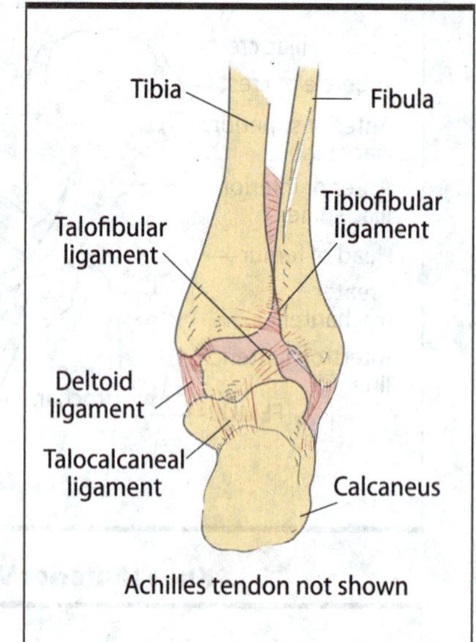

Achilles tendon not shown

Foot Tendons

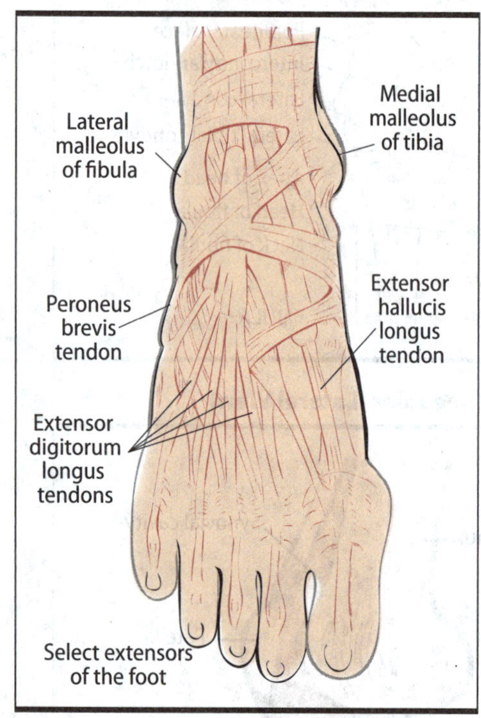

Foot Bones

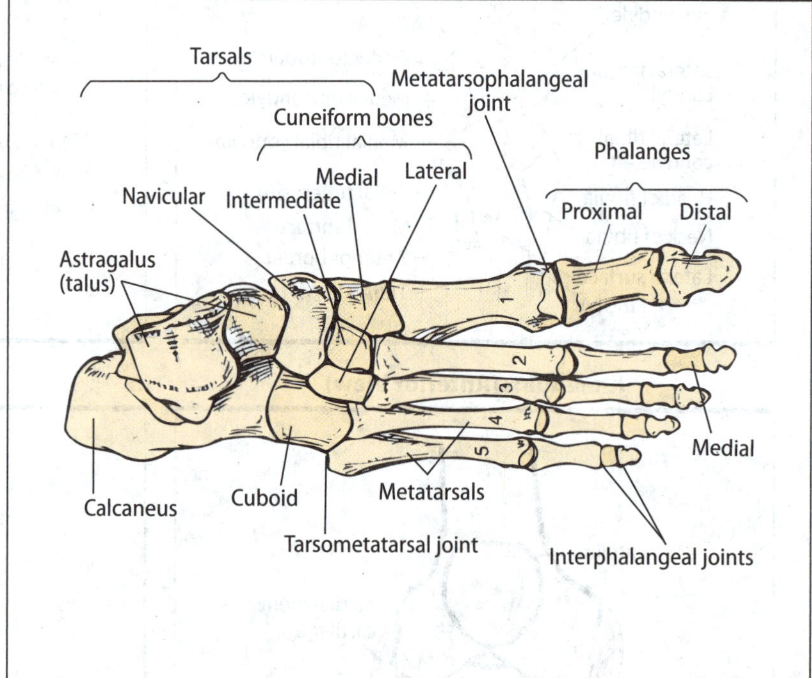

Respiratory System

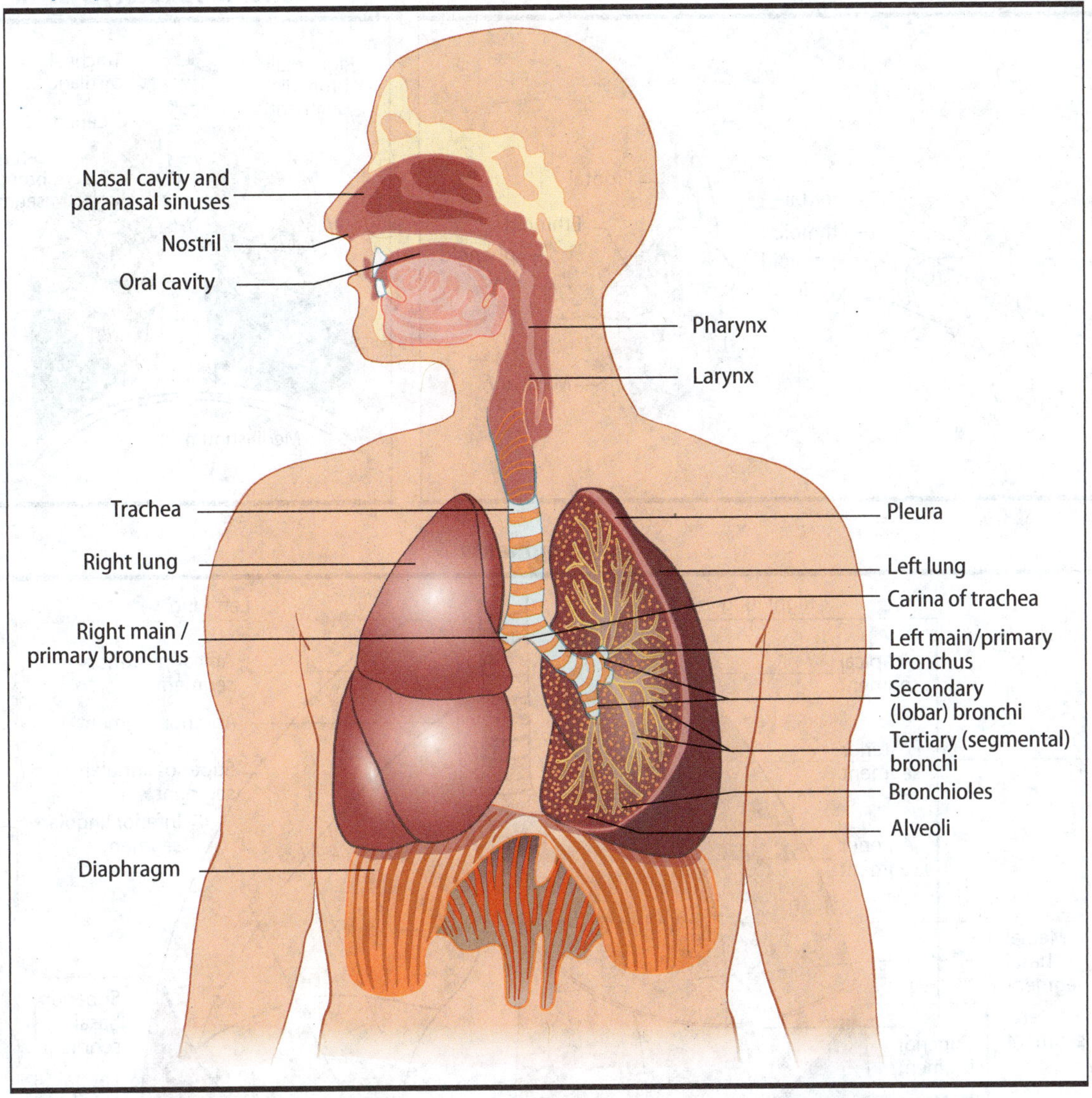

Nasal cavity and paranasal sinuses
Nostril
Oral cavity
Pharynx
Larynx
Trachea
Right lung
Right main / primary bronchus
Diaphragm
Pleura
Left lung
Carina of trachea
Left main/primary bronchus
Secondary (lobar) bronchi
Tertiary (segmental) bronchi
Bronchioles
Alveoli

Upper Respiratory System

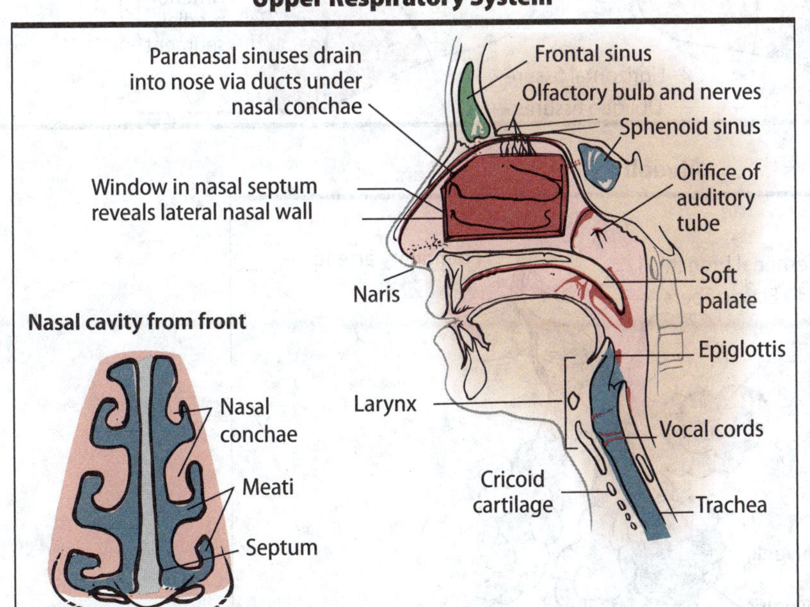

Nasal Turbinates

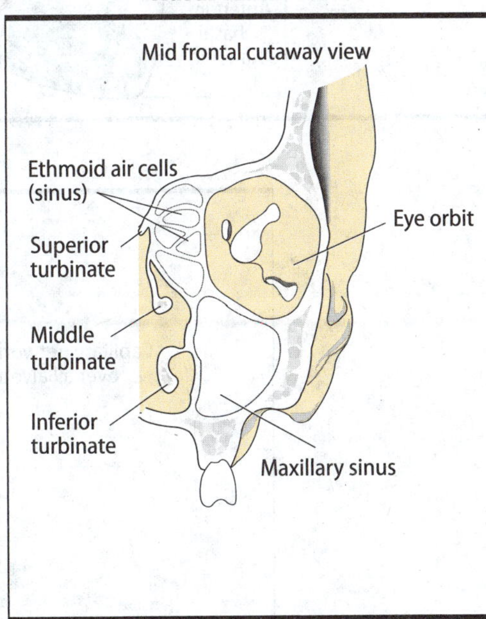

Paranasal Sinuses

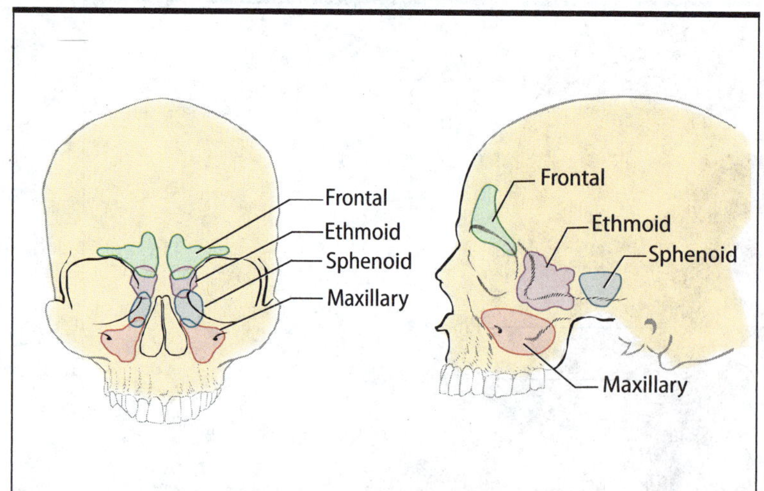

Lower Respiratory System

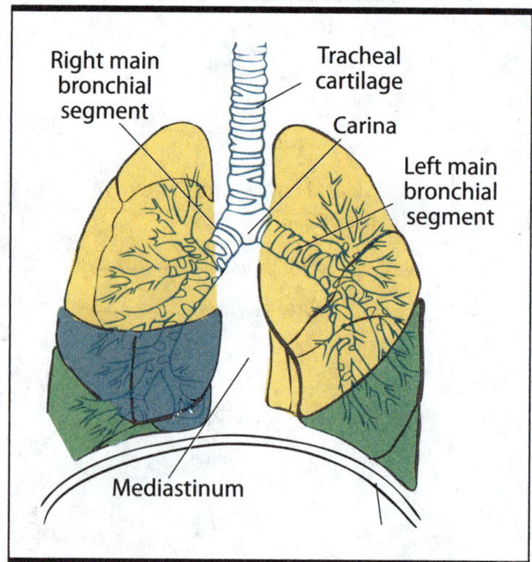

Lung Segments

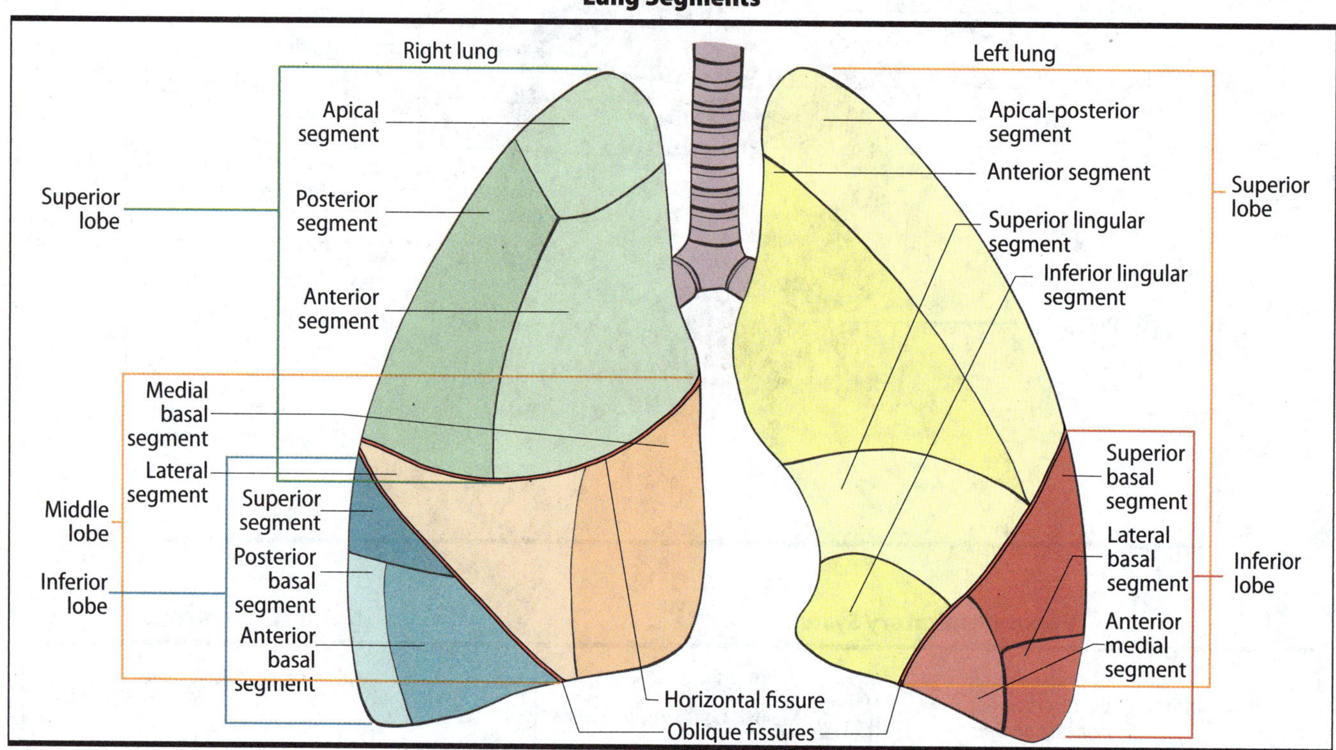

Alveoli

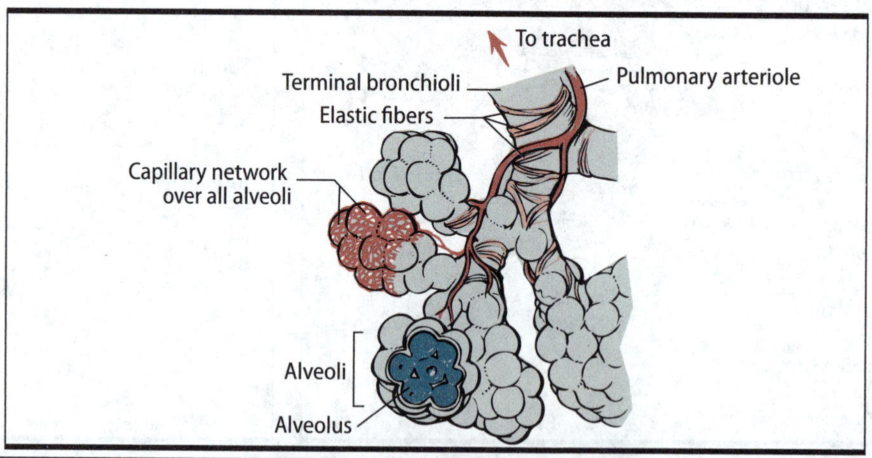

Arterial System

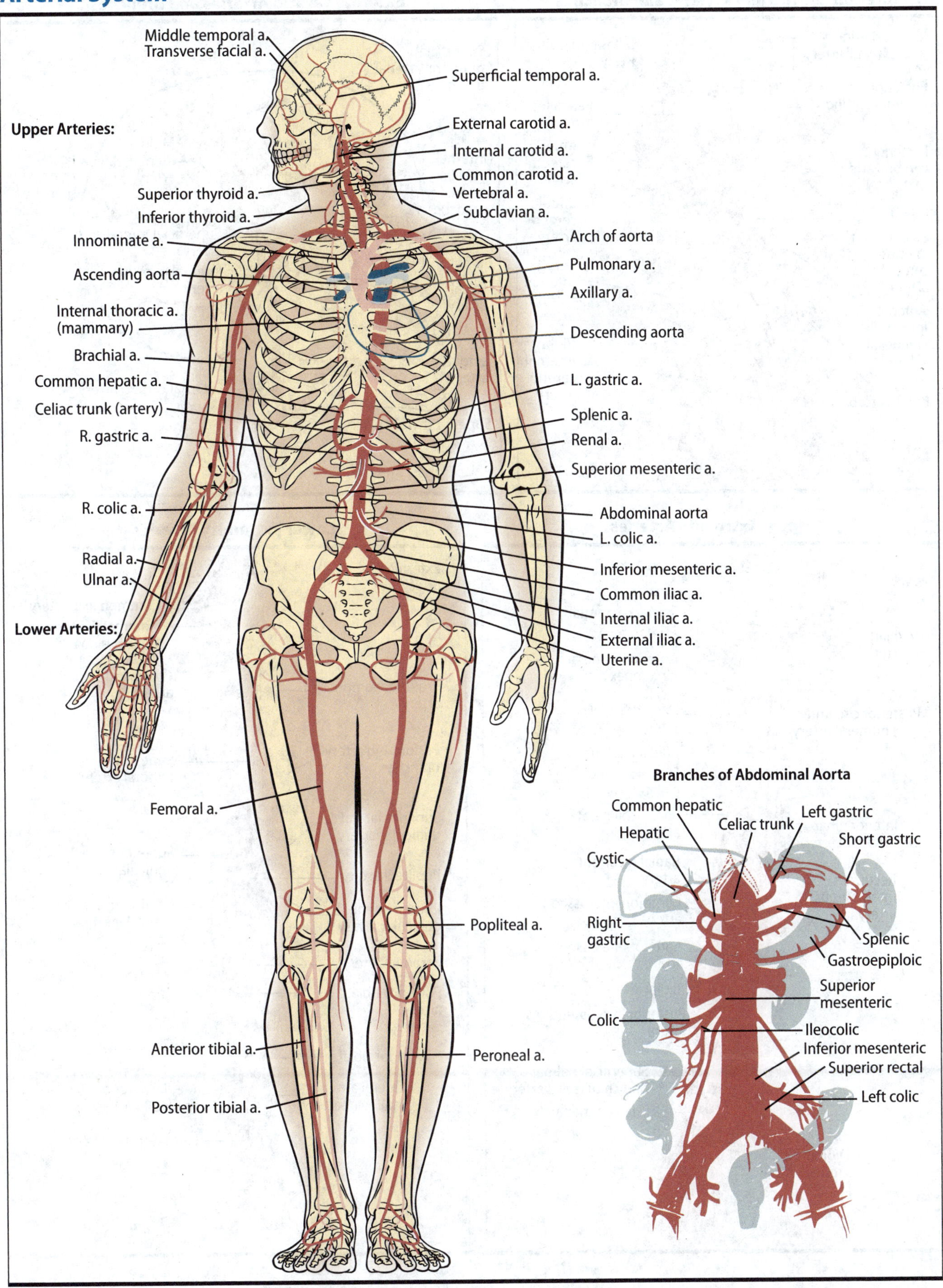

Internal Carotid and Arteries and Branches

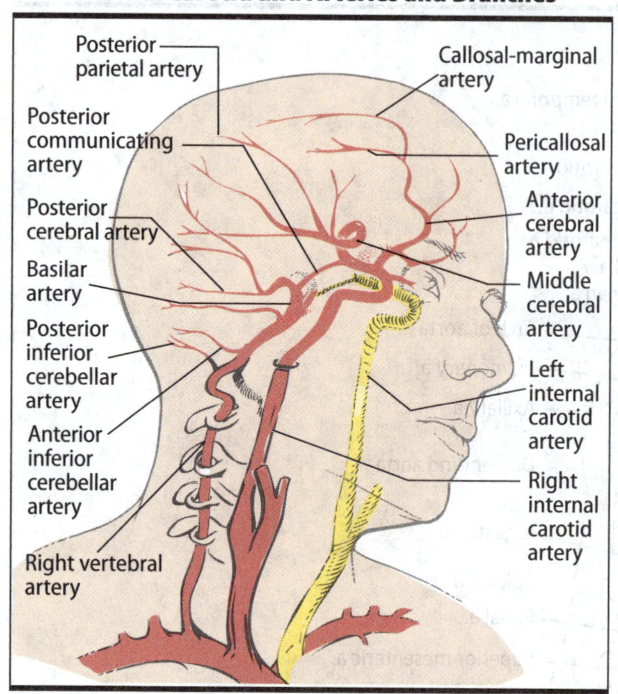

External Carotid Arteries and Branches

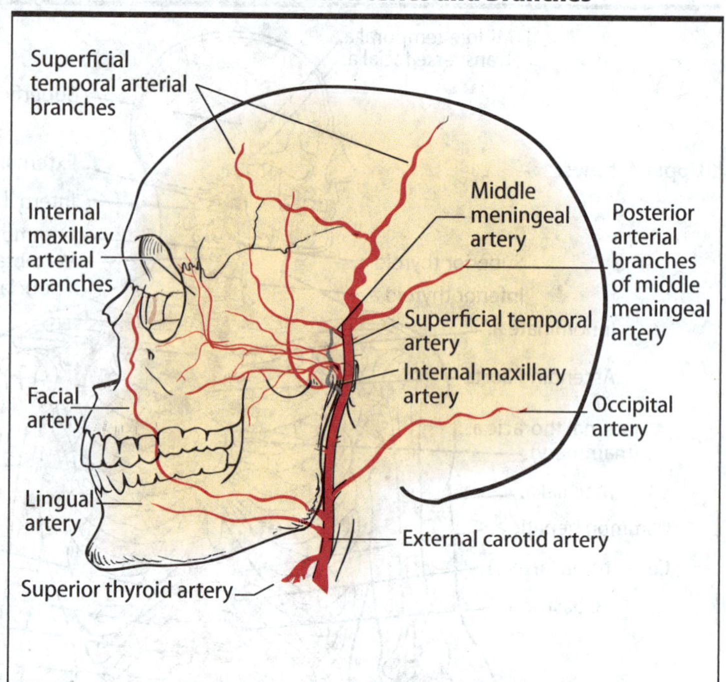

Upper Extremity Arteries

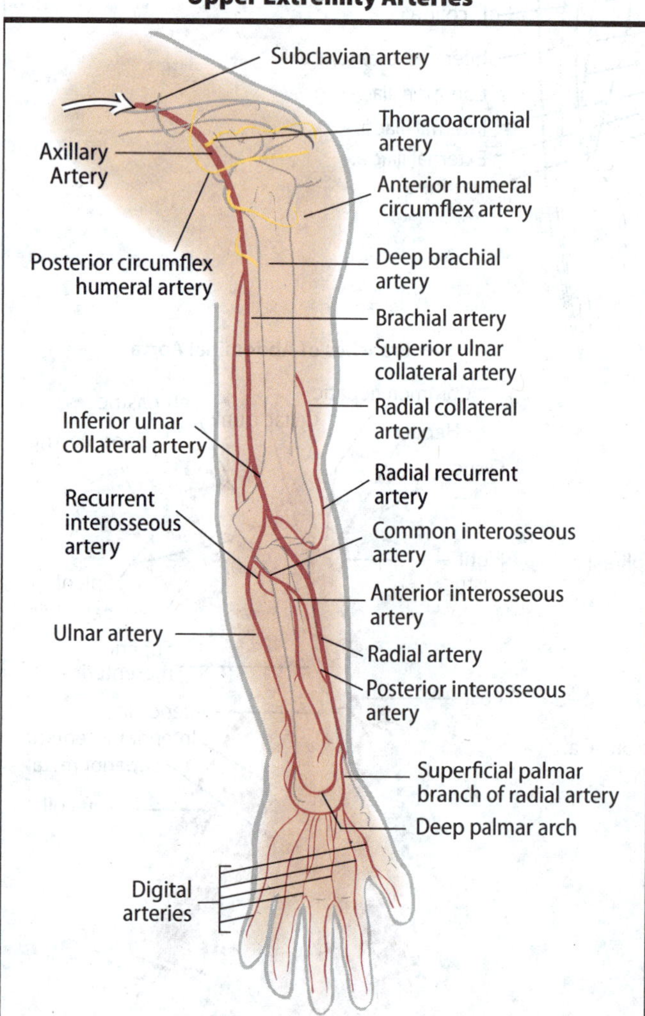

Lower Extremity Arteries

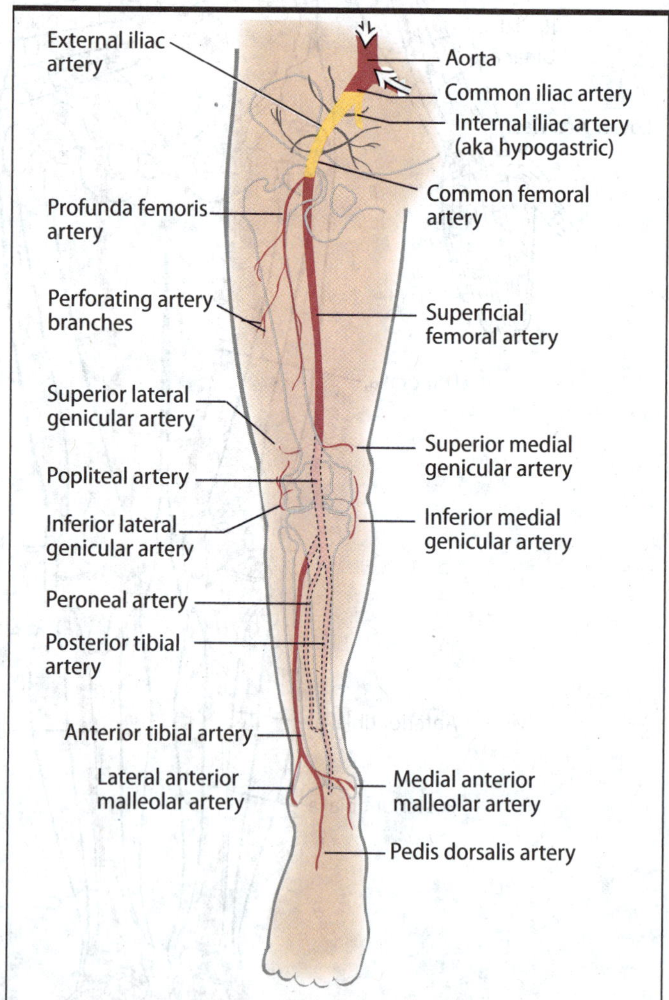

Venous System

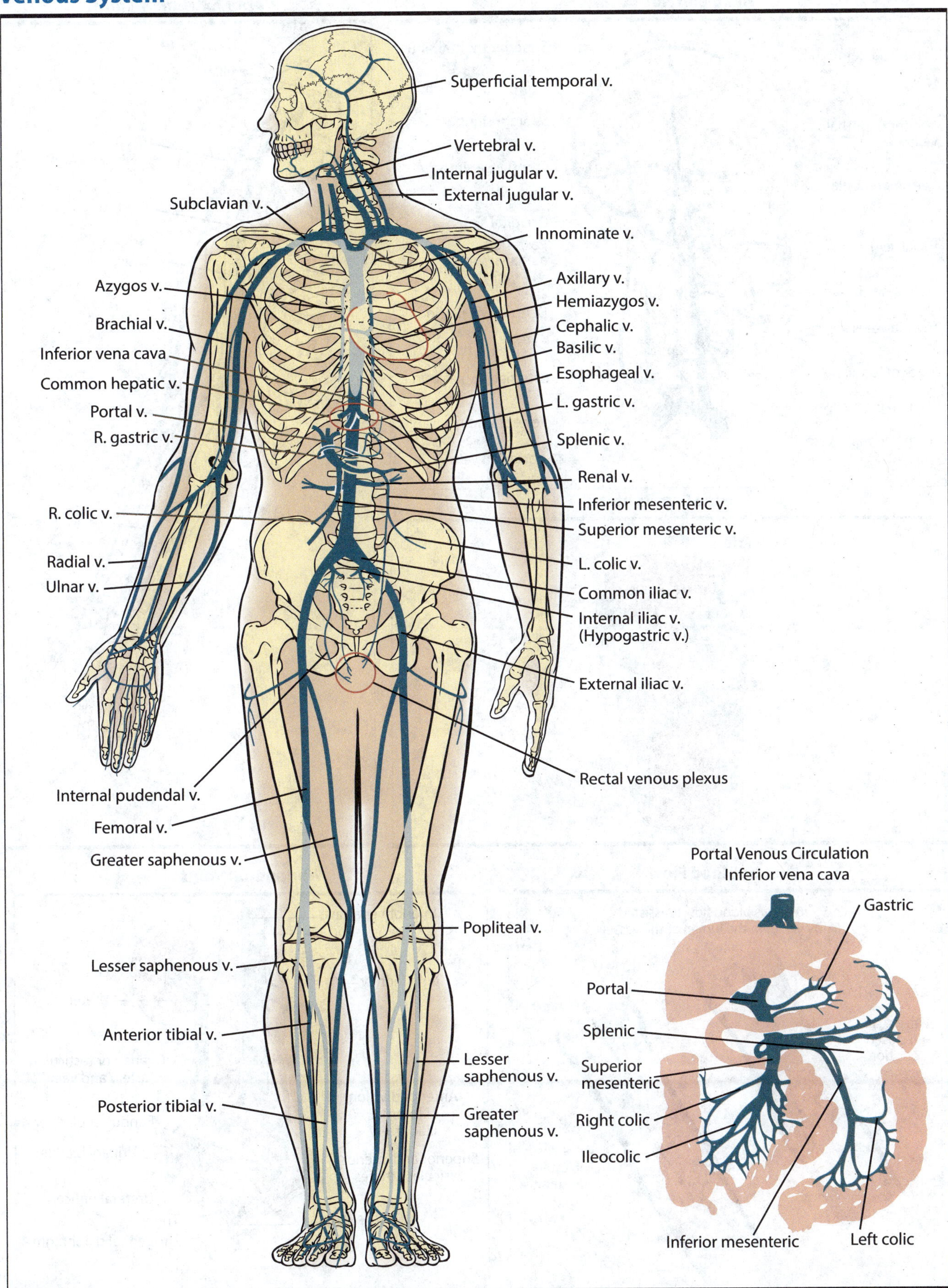

Head and Neck Veins

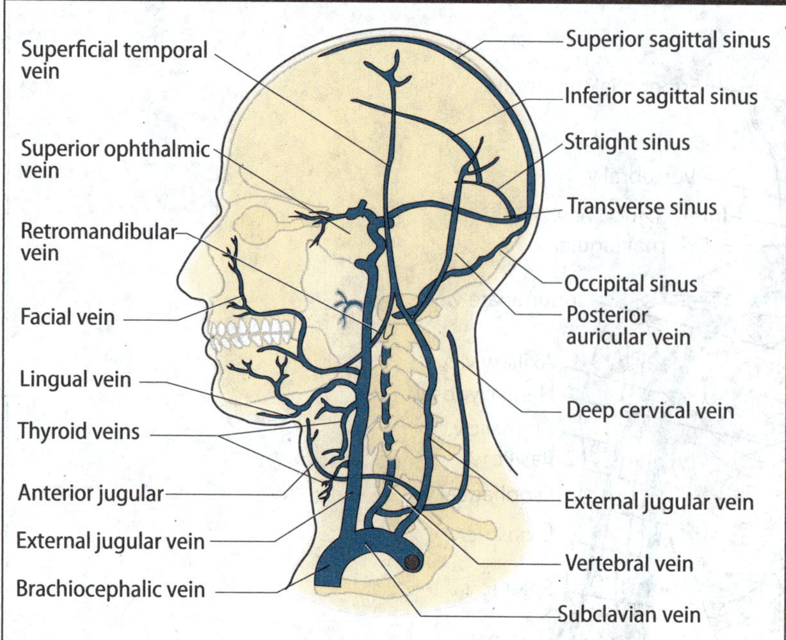

Upper Extremity Veins

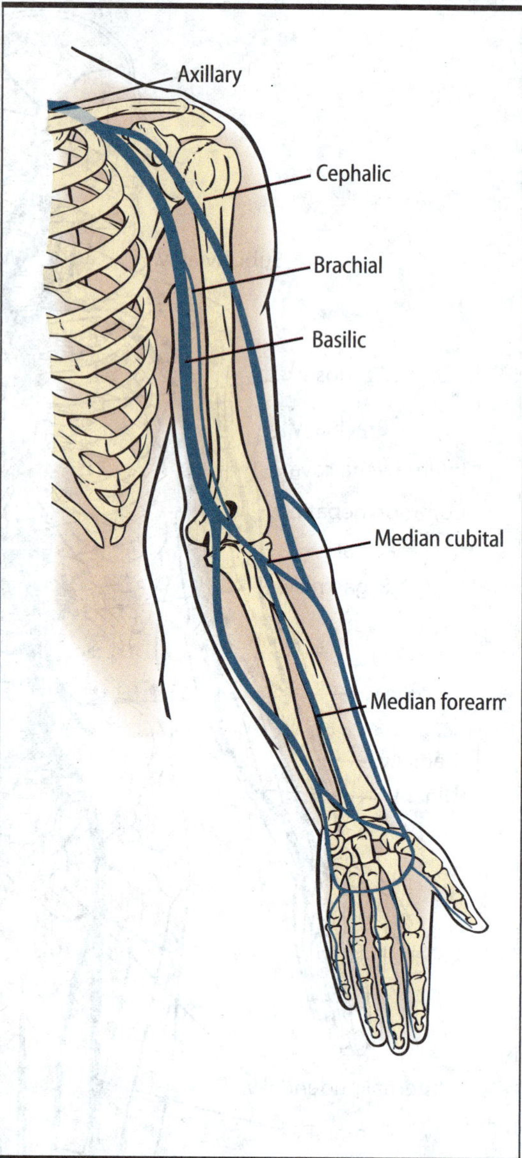

Venae Comitantes

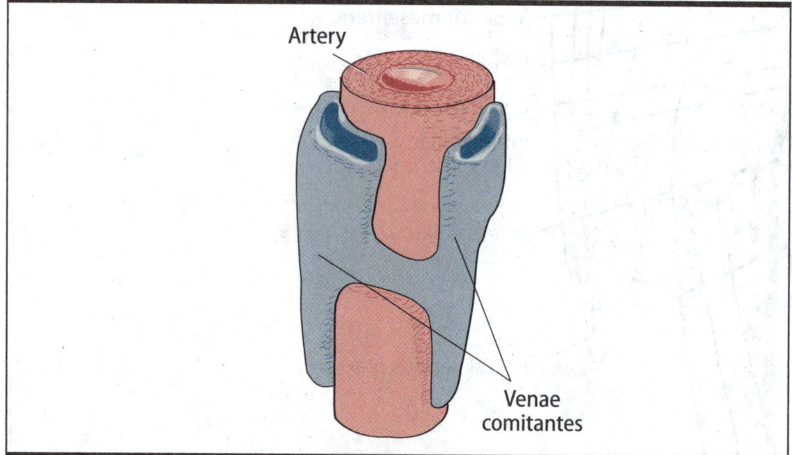

Venous Blood Flow

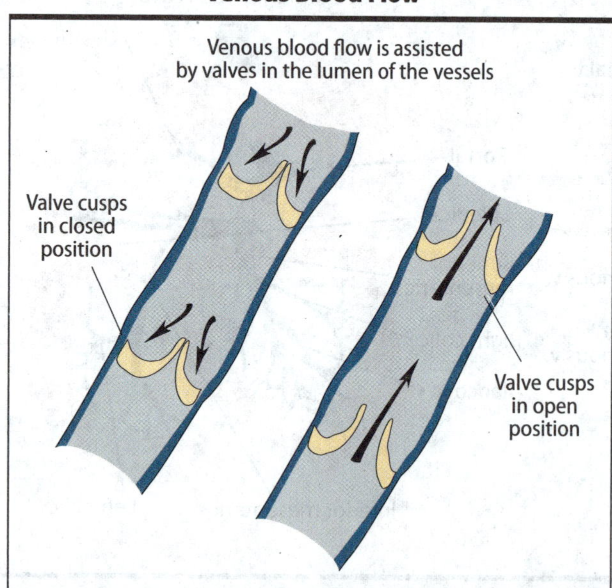

Abdominal Veins

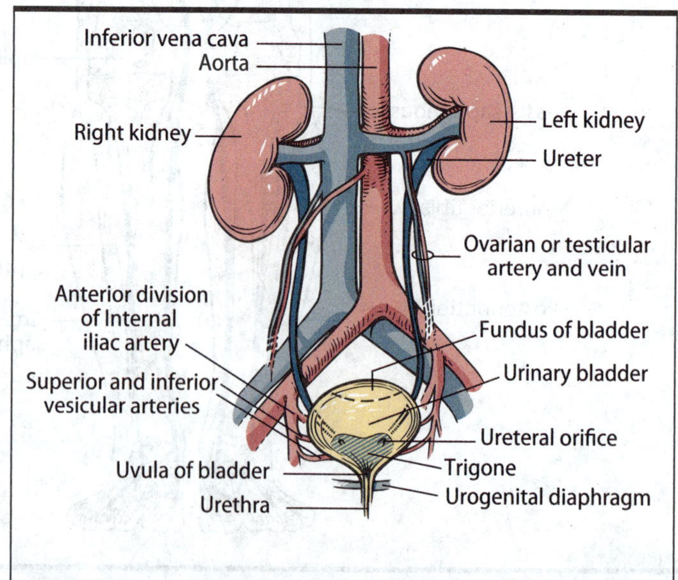

Cardiovascular System

Coronary Veins

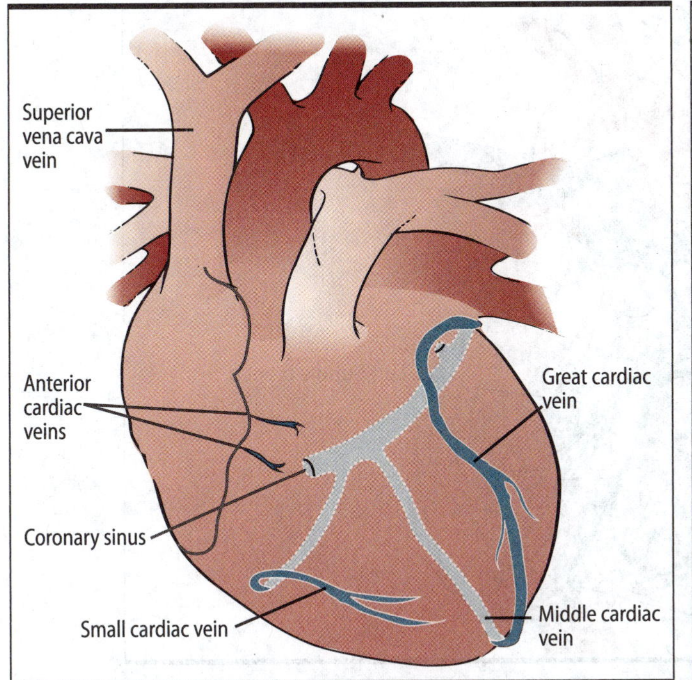

Anatomy of the Heart

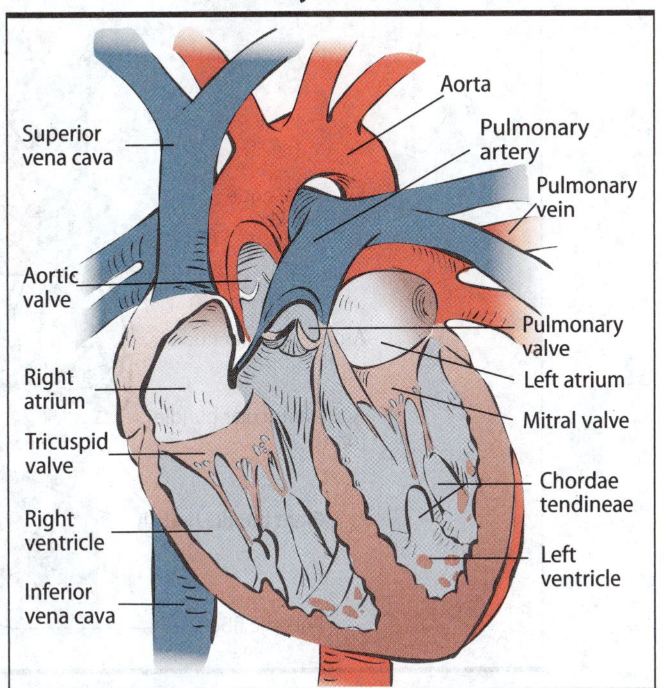

Heart Cross Section

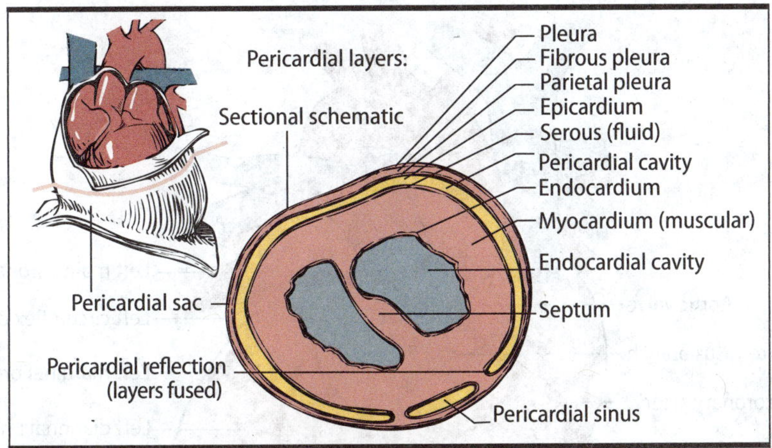

Heart Valves

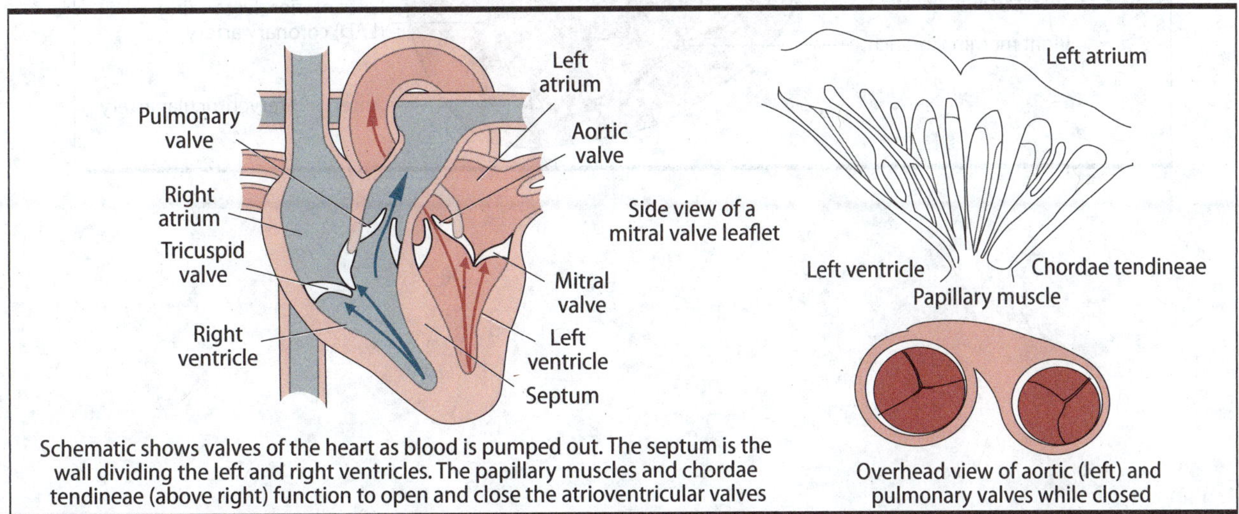

Schematic shows valves of the heart as blood is pumped out. The septum is the wall dividing the left and right ventricles. The papillary muscles and chordae tendineae (above right) function to open and close the atrioventricular valves

Overhead view of aortic (left) and pulmonary valves while closed

Heart Conduction System

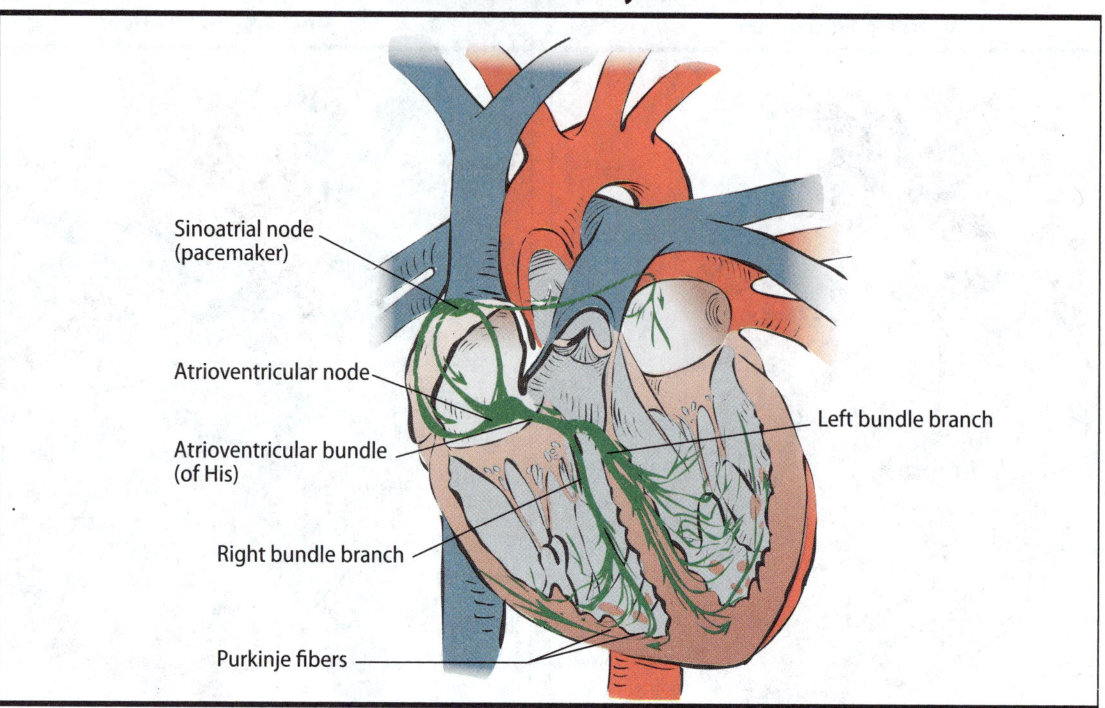

Coronary Arteries

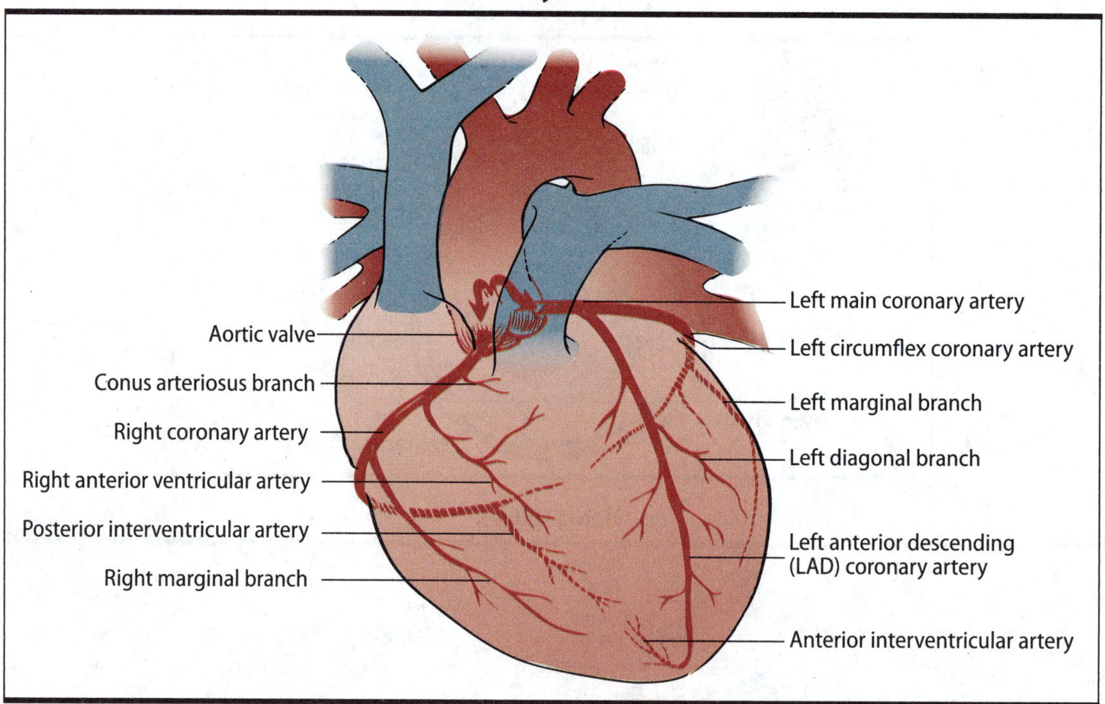

Lymphatic System

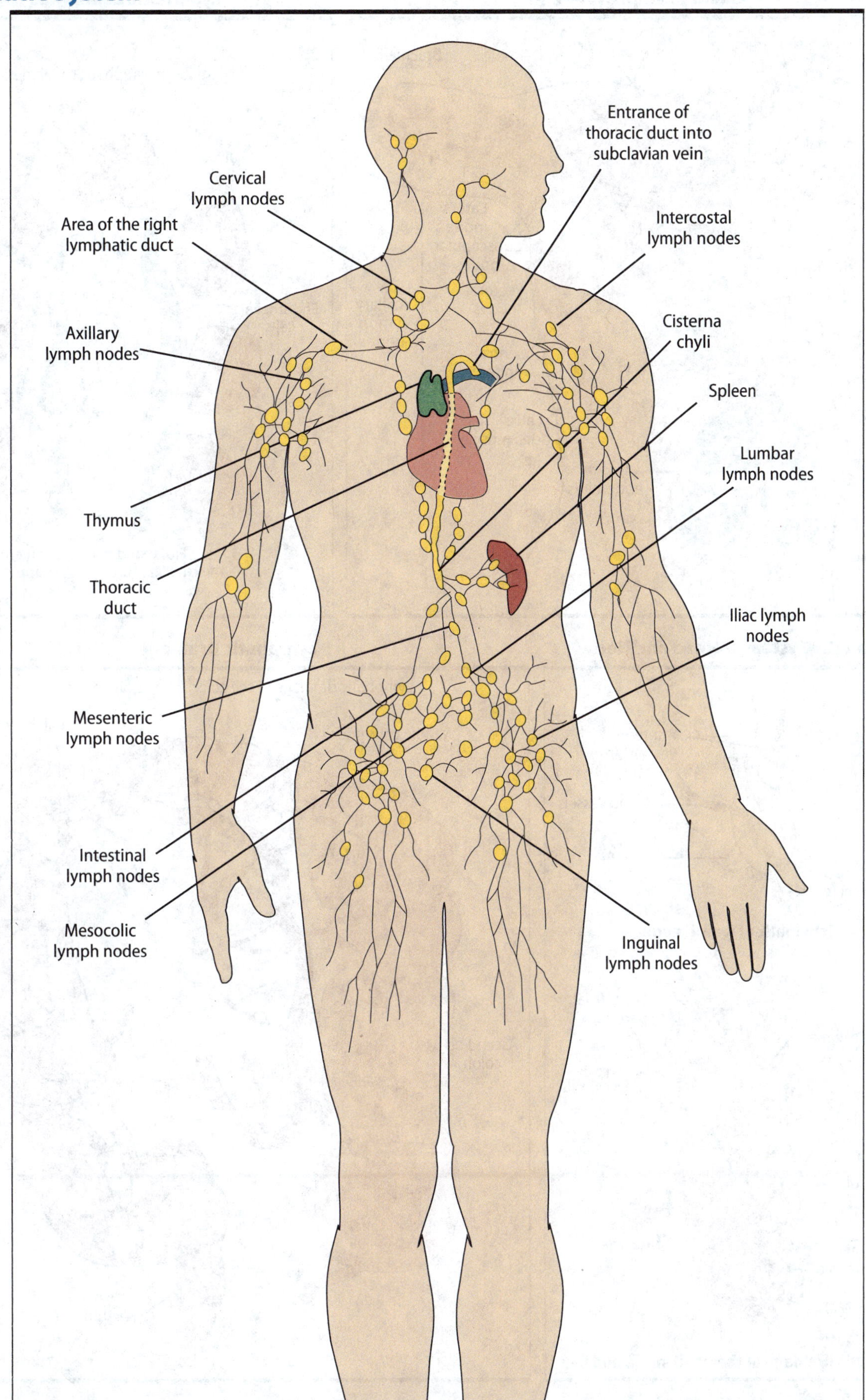

Axillary Lymph Nodes

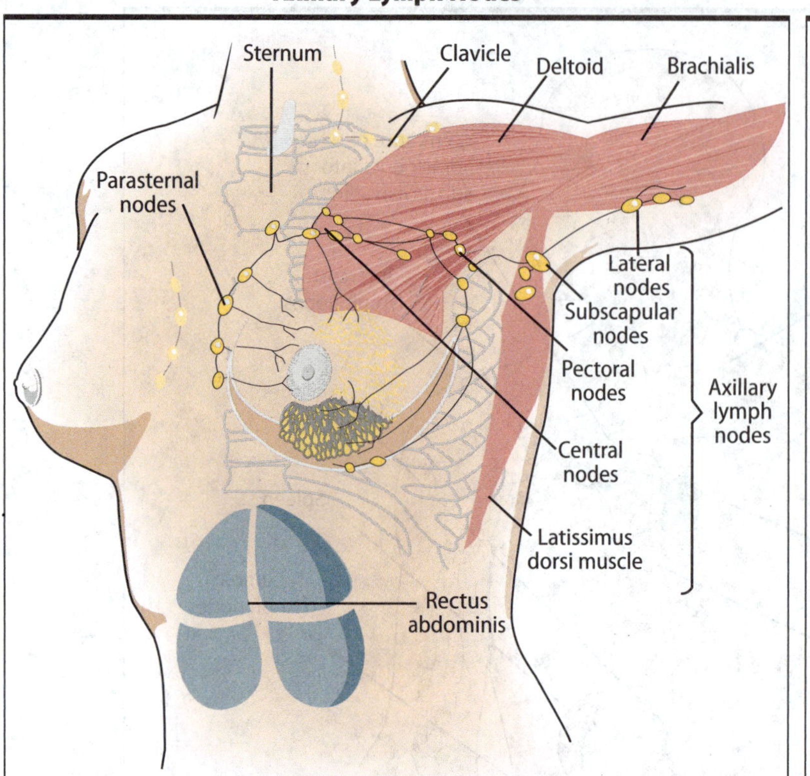

Lymphatic Capillaries

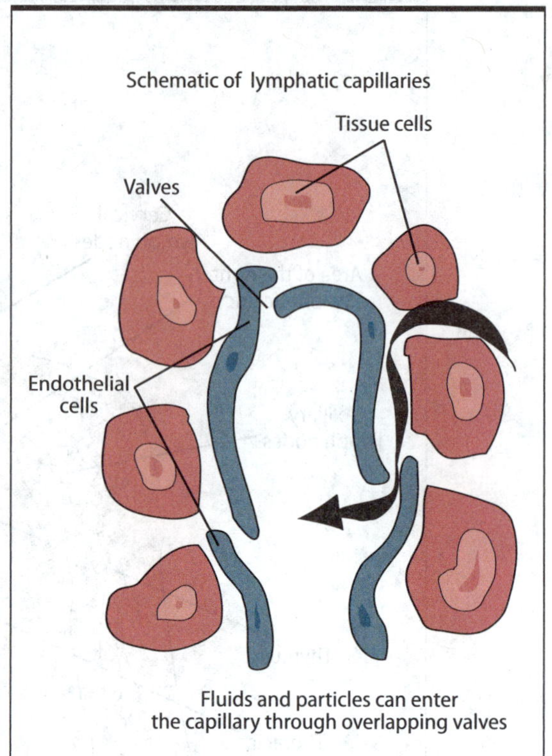

Lymphatic System of Head and Neck

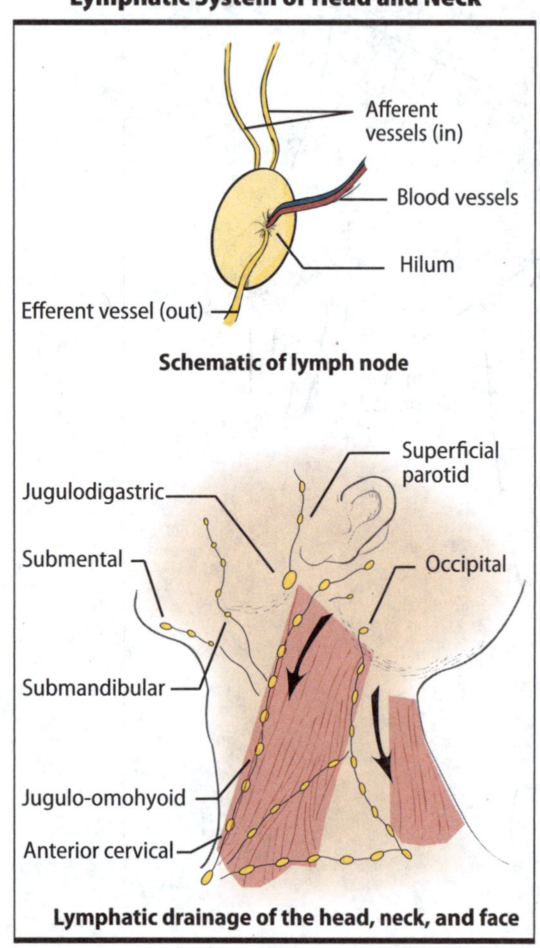

Schematic of lymph node

Lymphatic drainage of the head, neck, and face

Lymphatic Drainage

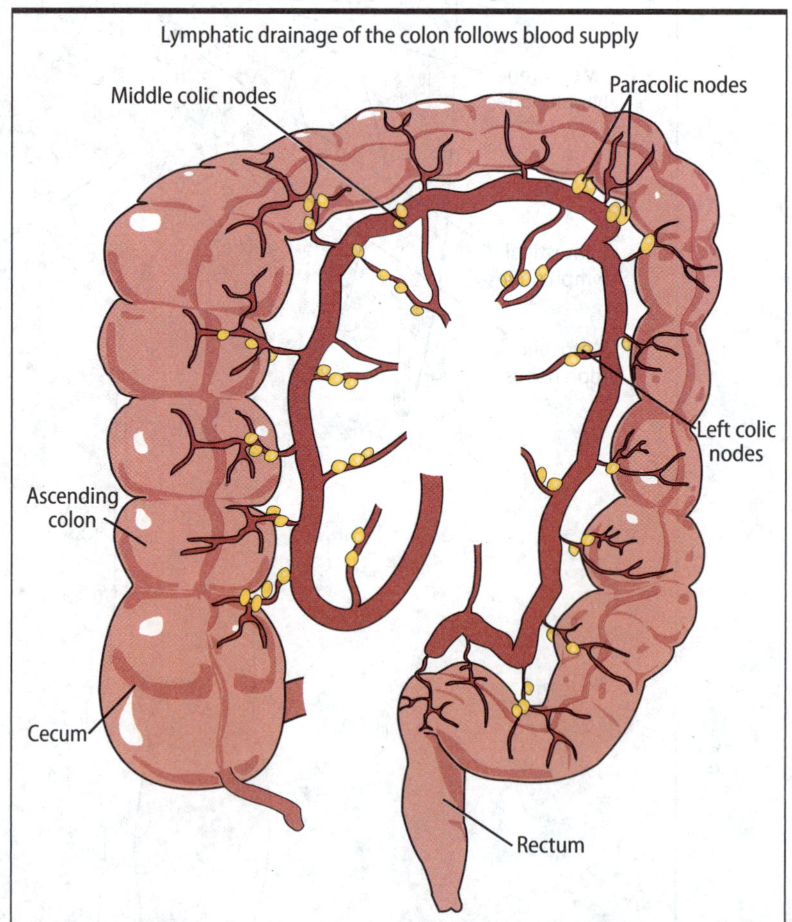

Spleen Internal Structures

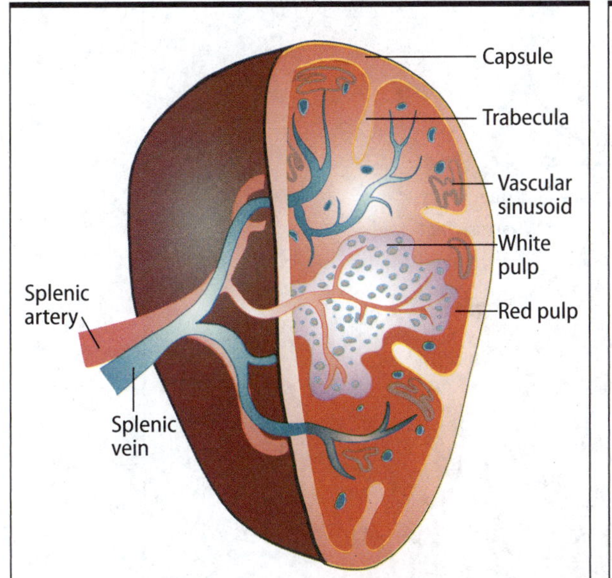

Spleen External Structures

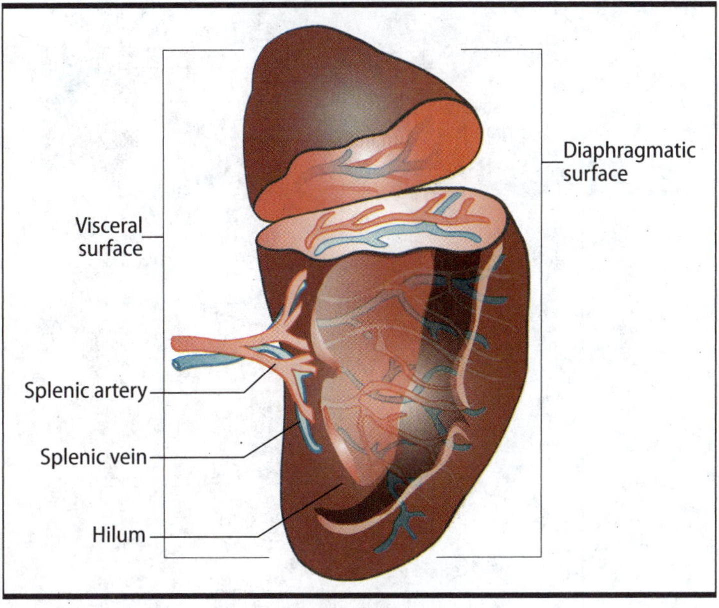

Digestive System

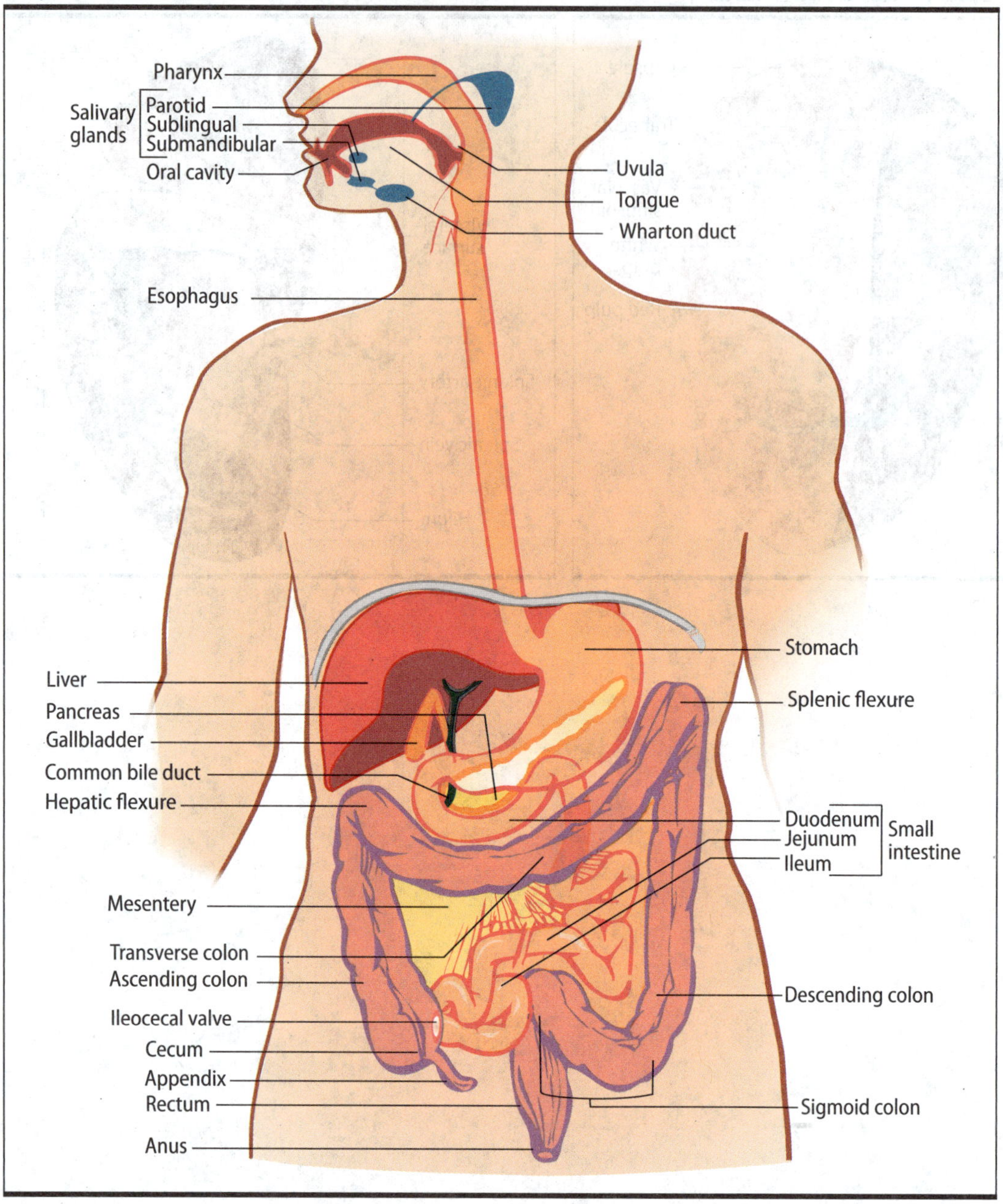

Pharynx
Salivary glands
Parotid
Sublingual
Submandibular
Oral cavity
Uvula
Tongue
Wharton duct
Esophagus
Stomach
Liver
Splenic flexure
Pancreas
Gallbladder
Common bile duct
Hepatic flexure
Duodenum
Jejunum
Ileum
Small intestine
Mesentery
Transverse colon
Ascending colon
Descending colon
Ileocecal valve
Cecum
Appendix
Rectum
Sigmoid colon
Anus

Gallbladder

Right and left bile ducts
Right hepatic artery
Cystic artery
Triangle of Calot
Common hepatic artery
Cystic duct
Portal vein
Gallstone in fundus
Hartmann's pouch (infundibulum
Common bile duct empties into Duodenum

Stomach

Distal esophagus
Diaphragm
Inferior esophageal sphincter
Fundus of stomach
Pyloric sphincter
Pylorus
Inner stomach

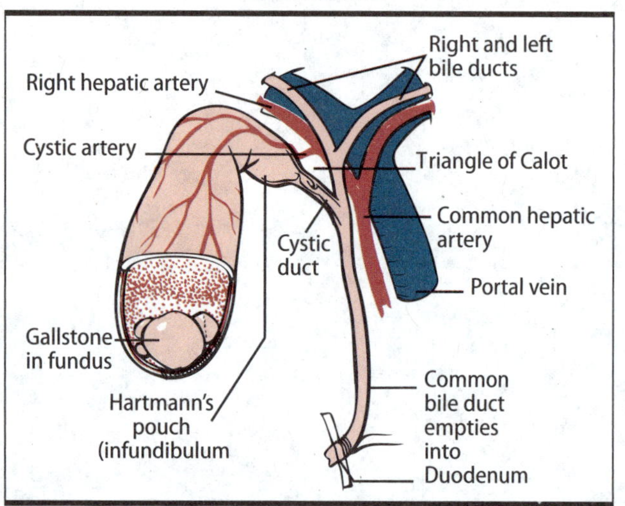

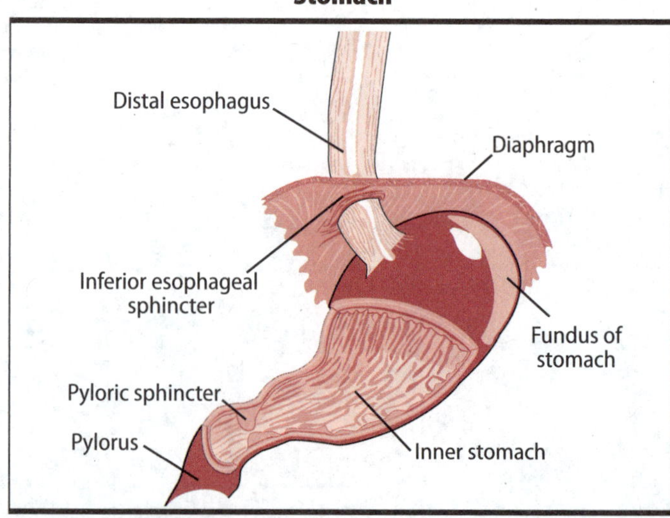

Mouth (Upper)

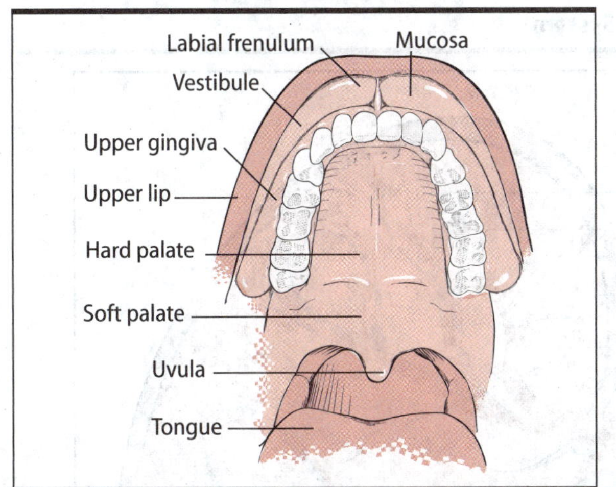

Mouth (Lower)

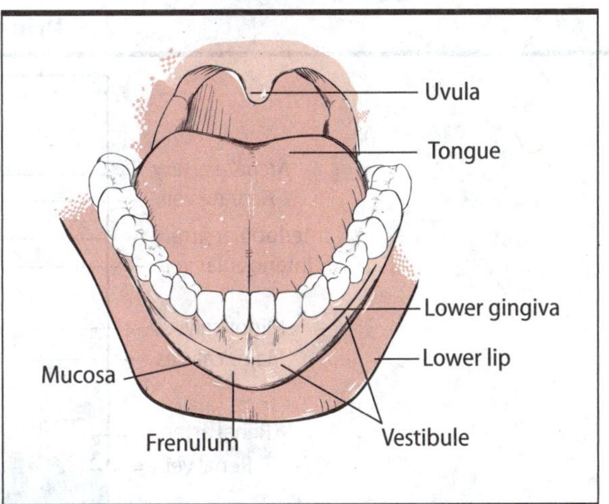

Pancreas

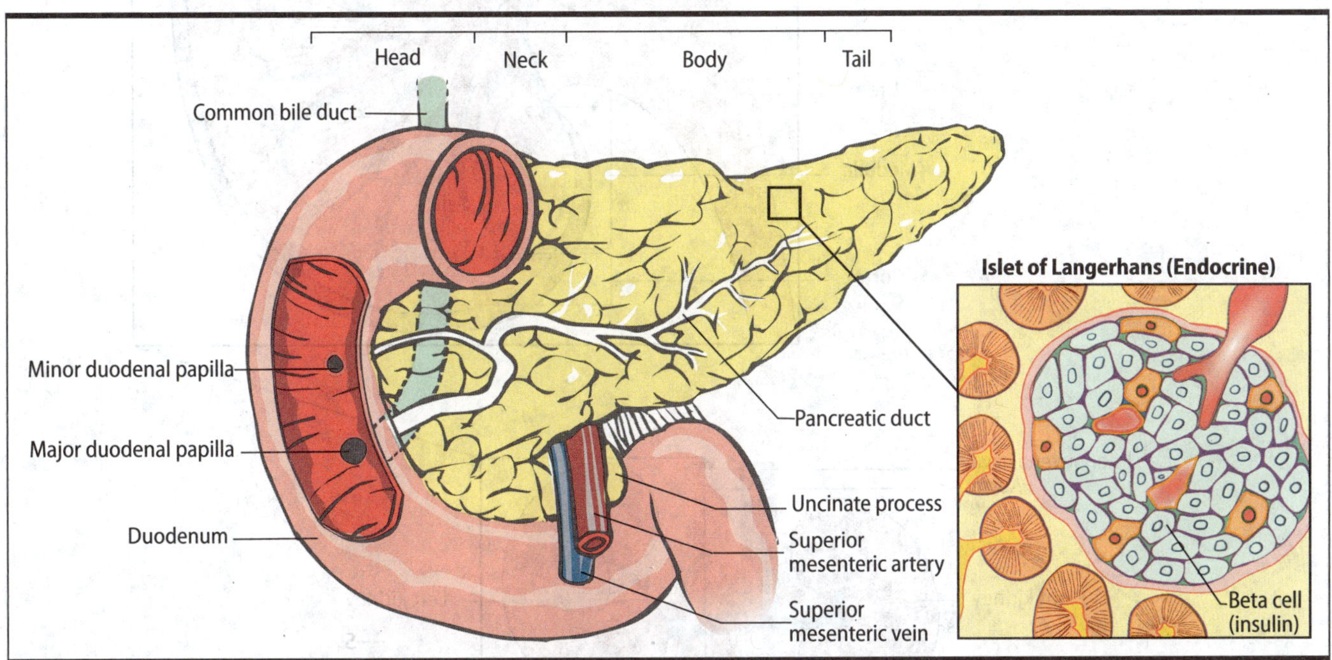

Liver

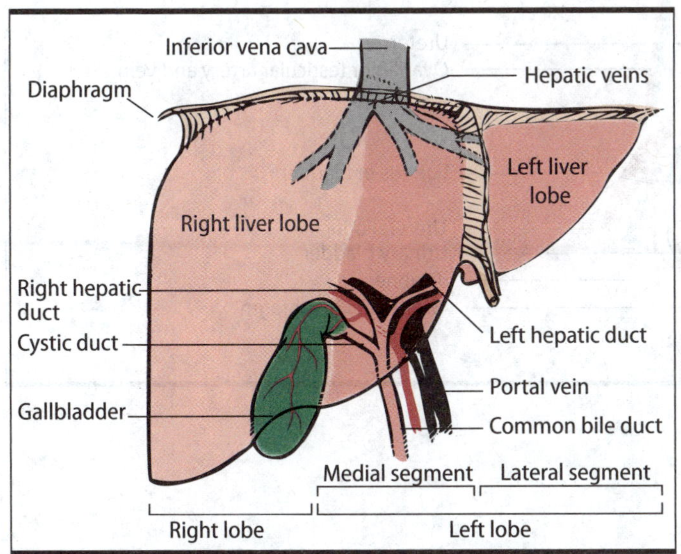

Anus

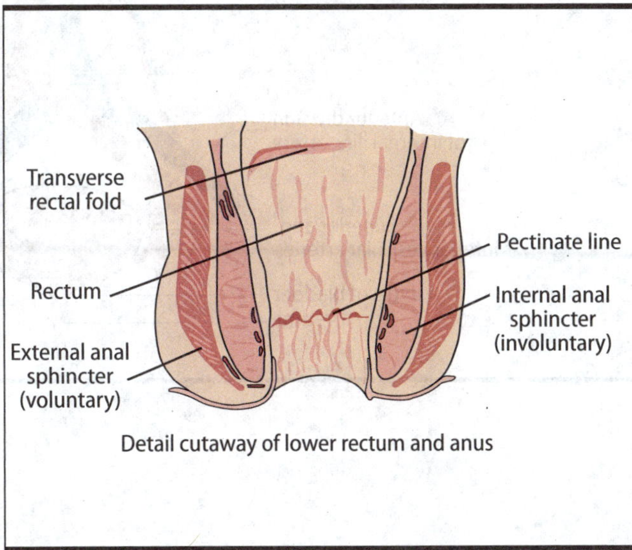

Detail cutaway of lower rectum and anus

Genitourinary System

Urinary System

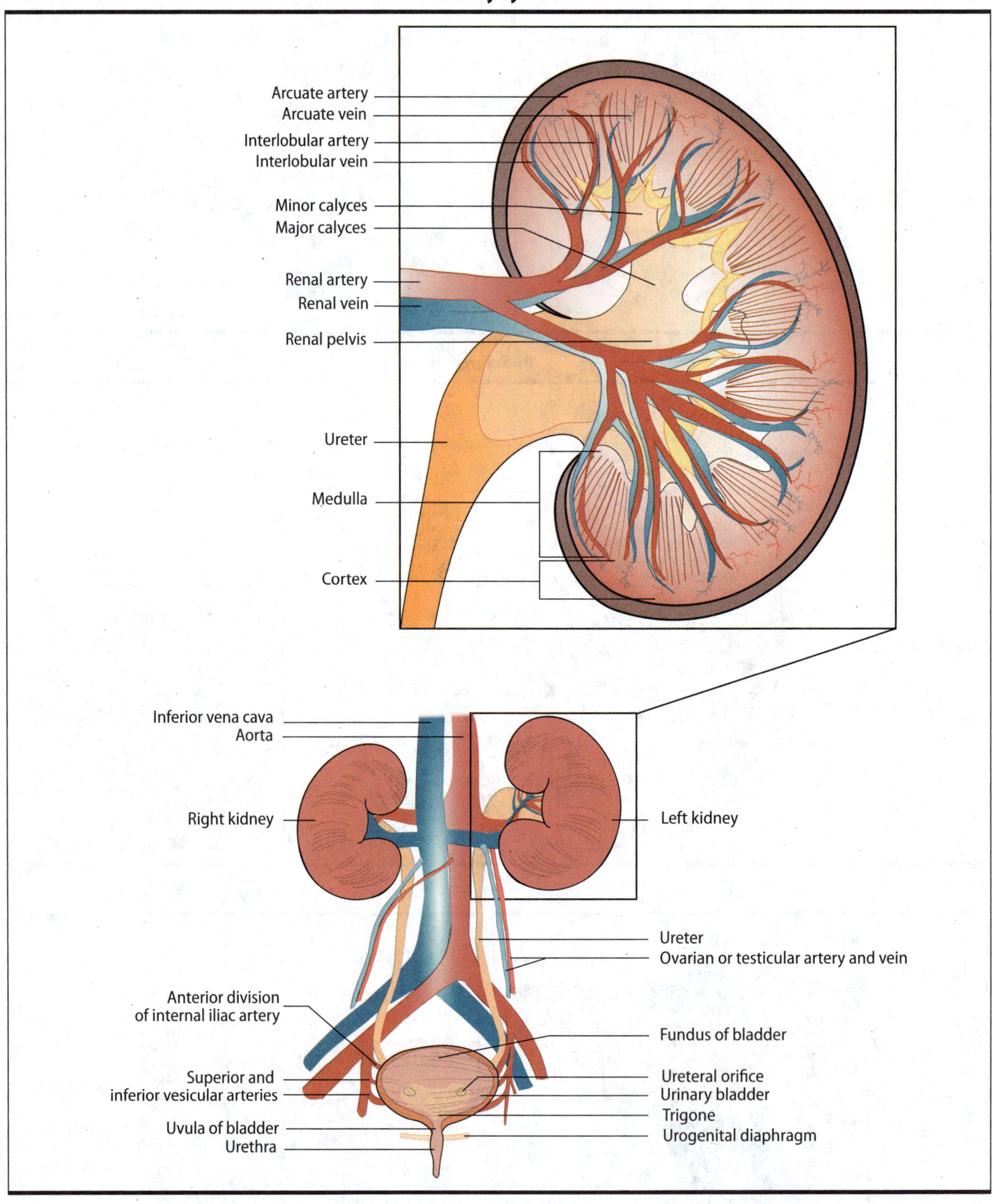

Nephron

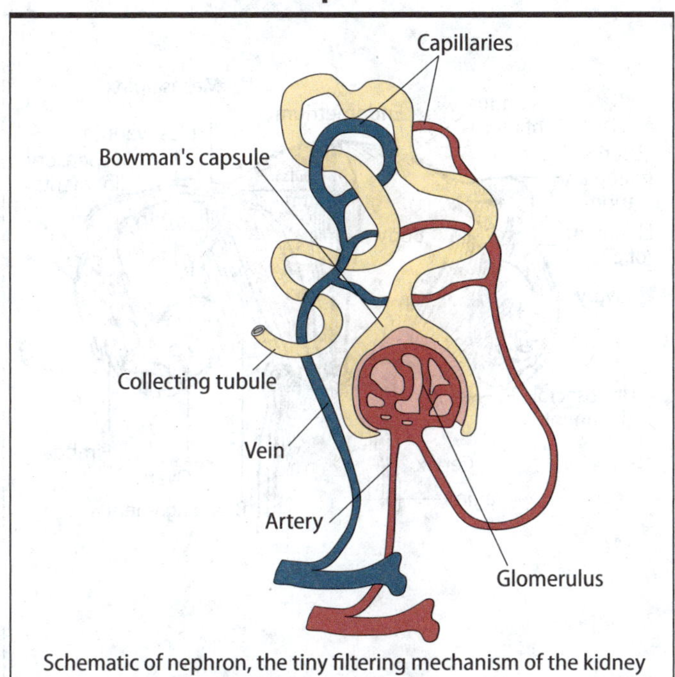

Schematic of nephron, the tiny filtering mechanism of the kidney

Male Genitourinary

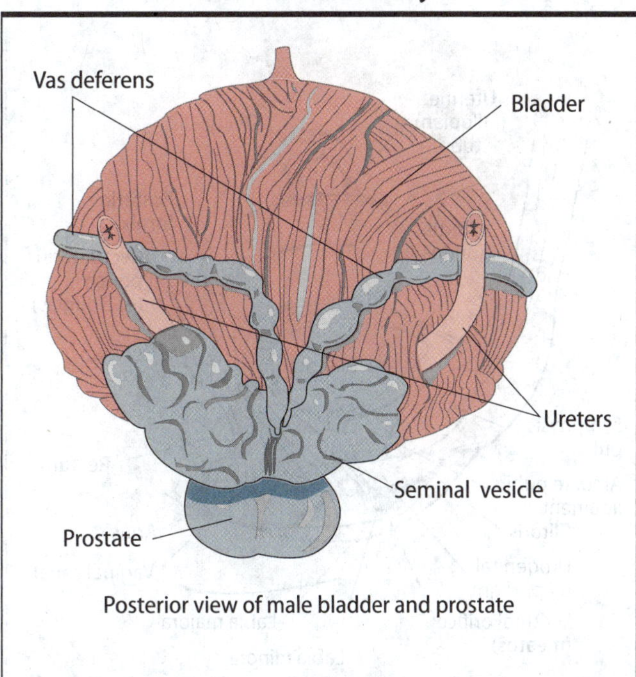

Posterior view of male bladder and prostate

Testis and Associate Structures

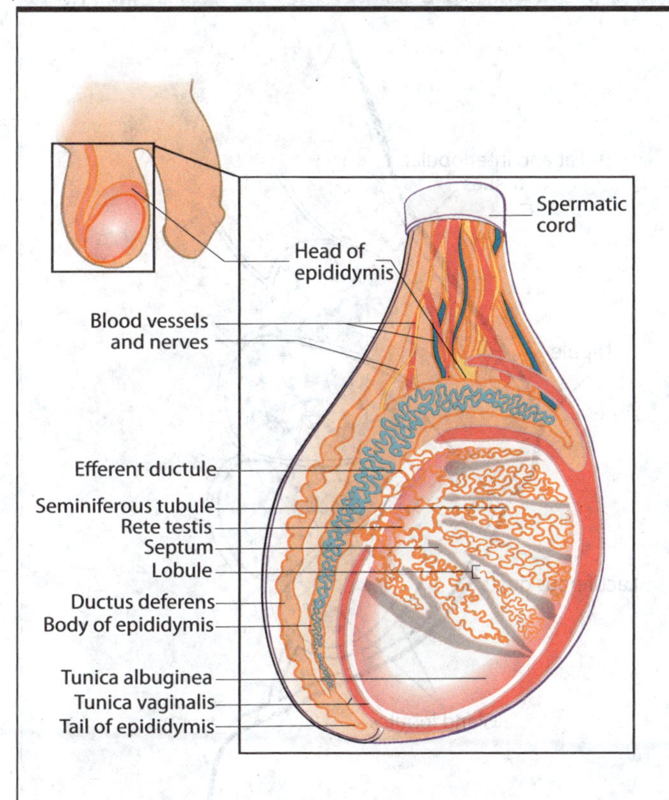

Male Genitourinary System

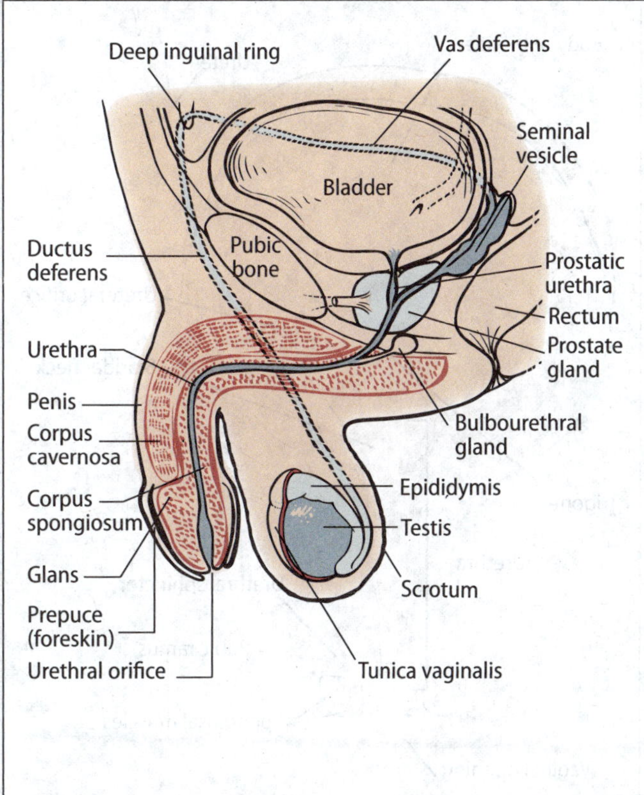

Female Genitourinary

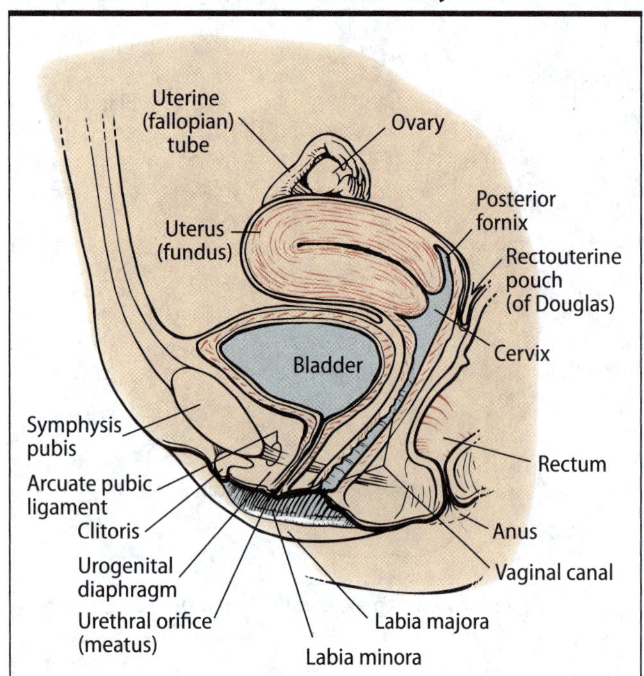

Female Reproductive System

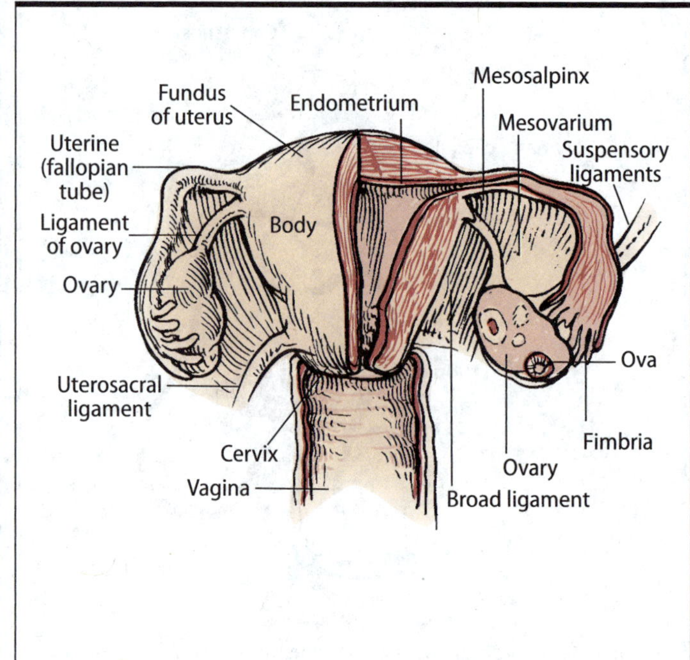

Female Bladder

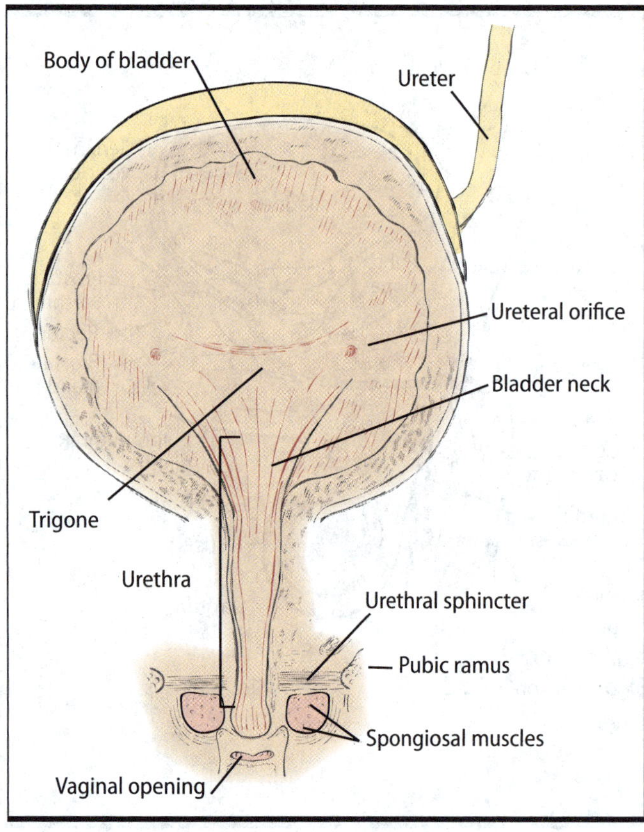

Female Breast

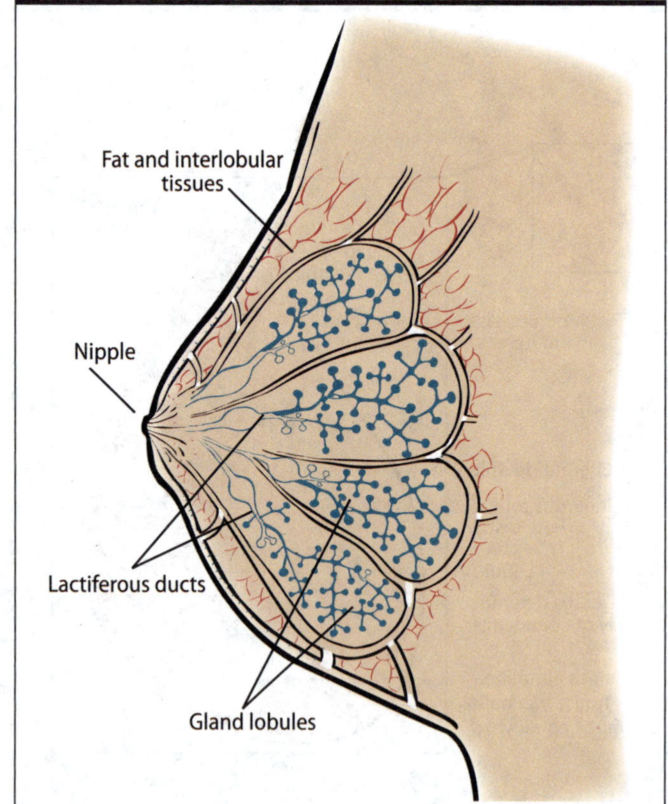

Endocrine System

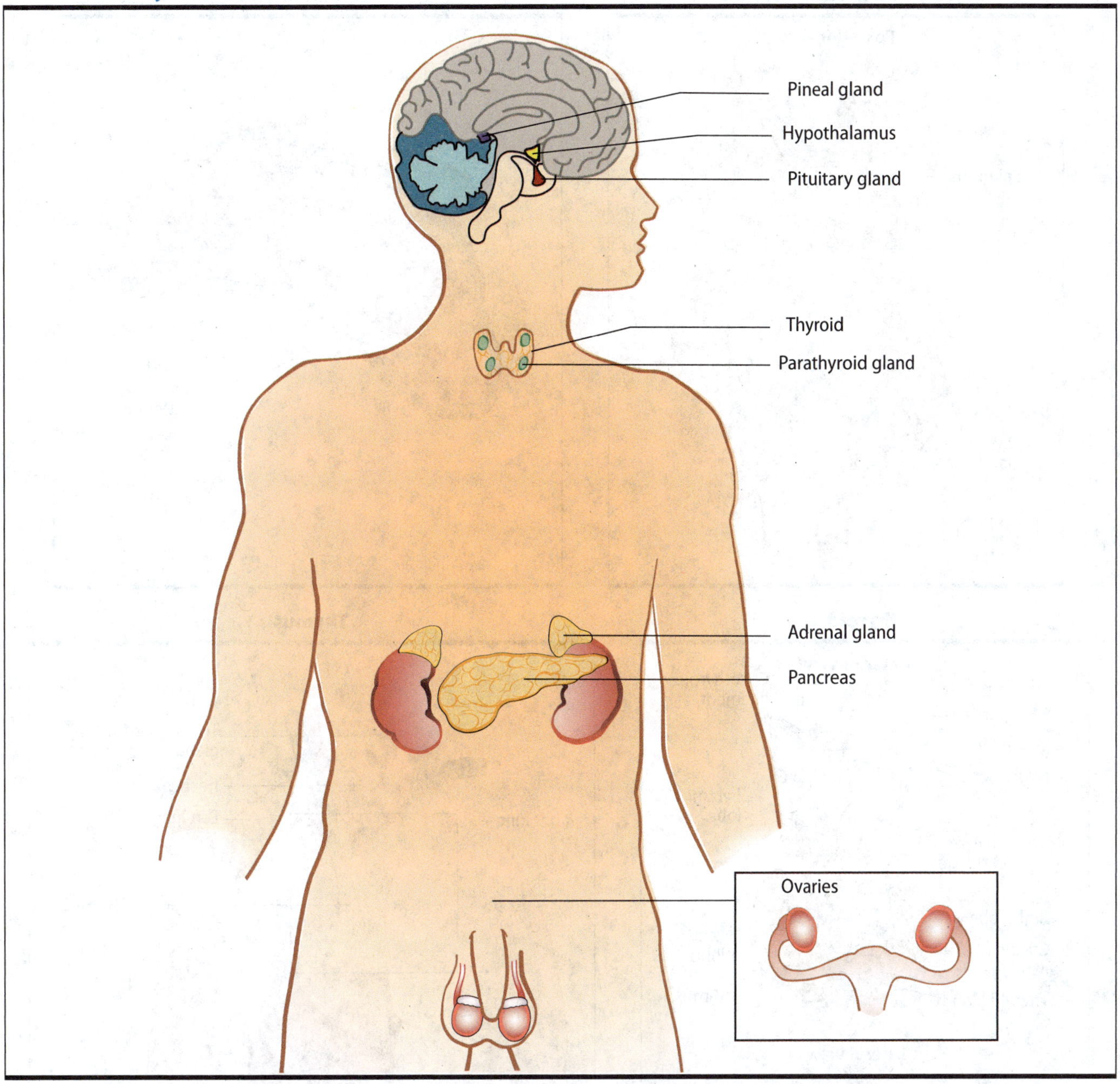

Pineal gland

Hypothalamus

Pituitary gland

Thyroid

Parathyroid gland

Adrenal gland

Pancreas

Ovaries

Structure of an Ovary

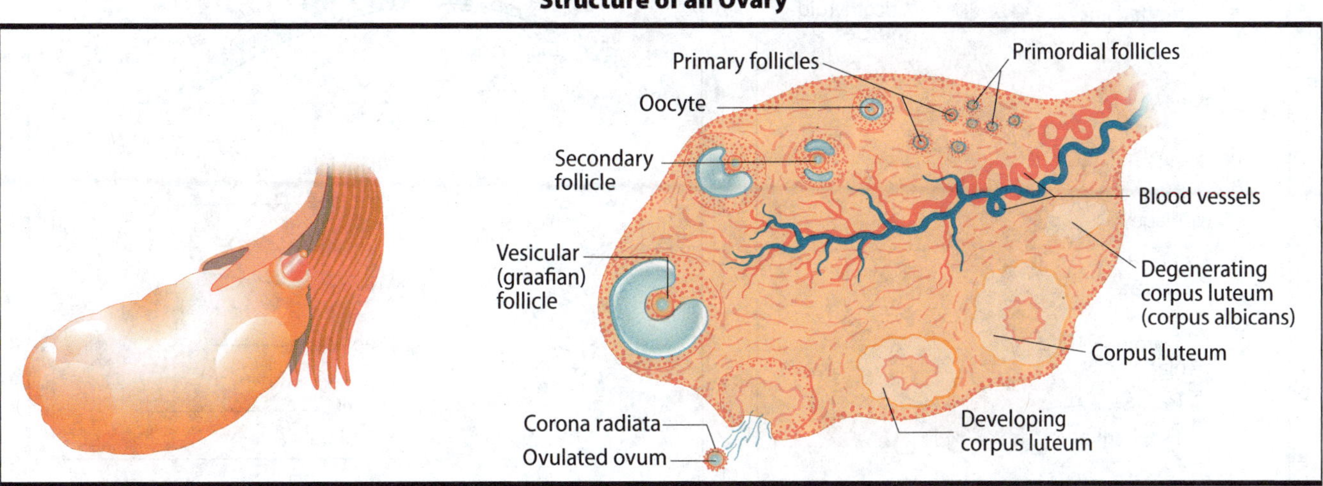

Thyroid and Parathyroid Glands

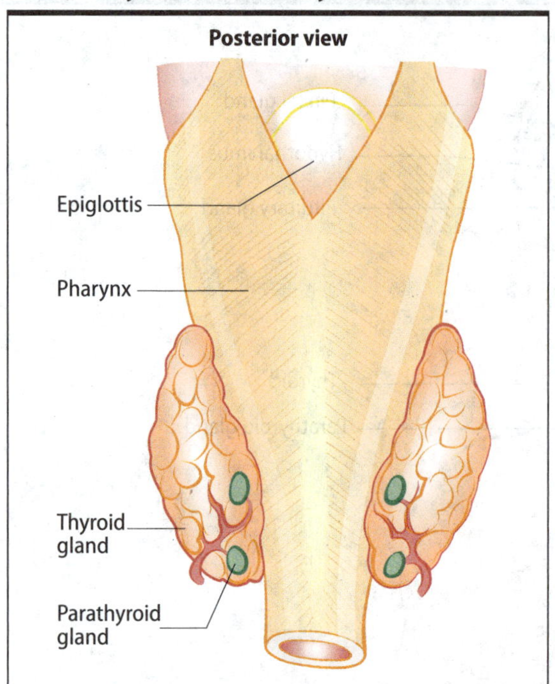

Adrenal Gland

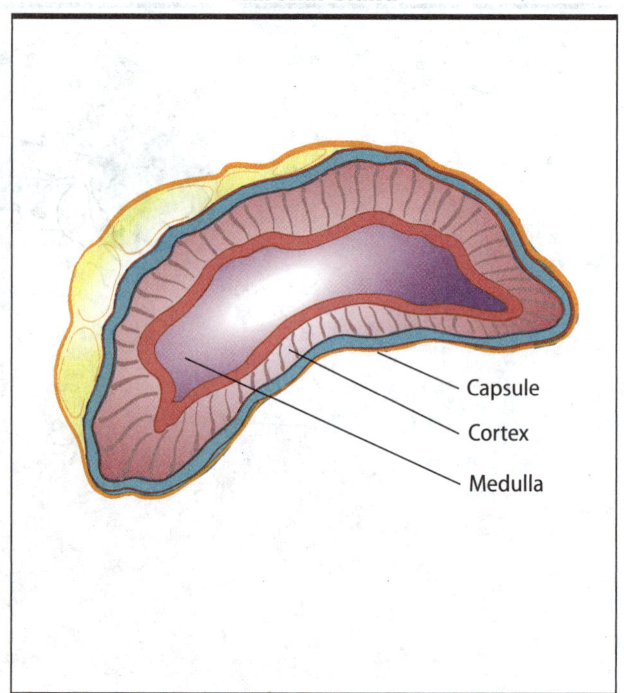

Thyroid

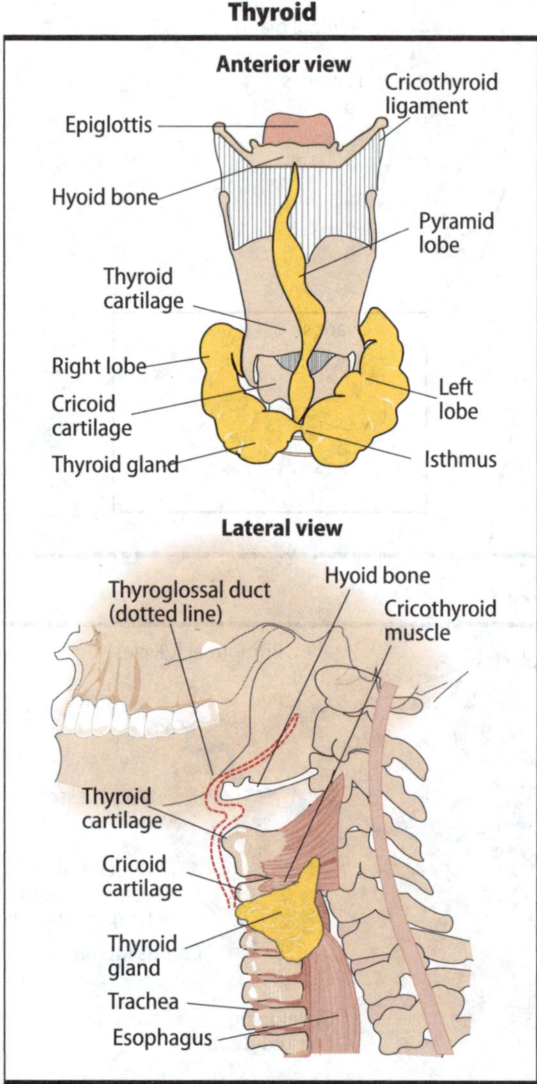

Thymus

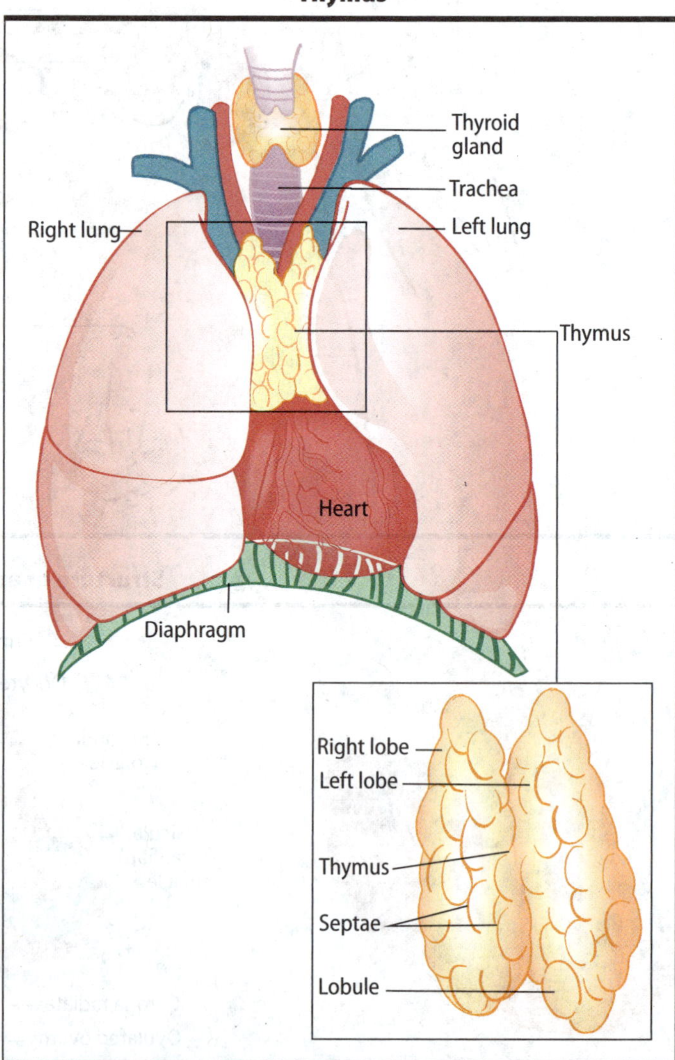

Nervous System

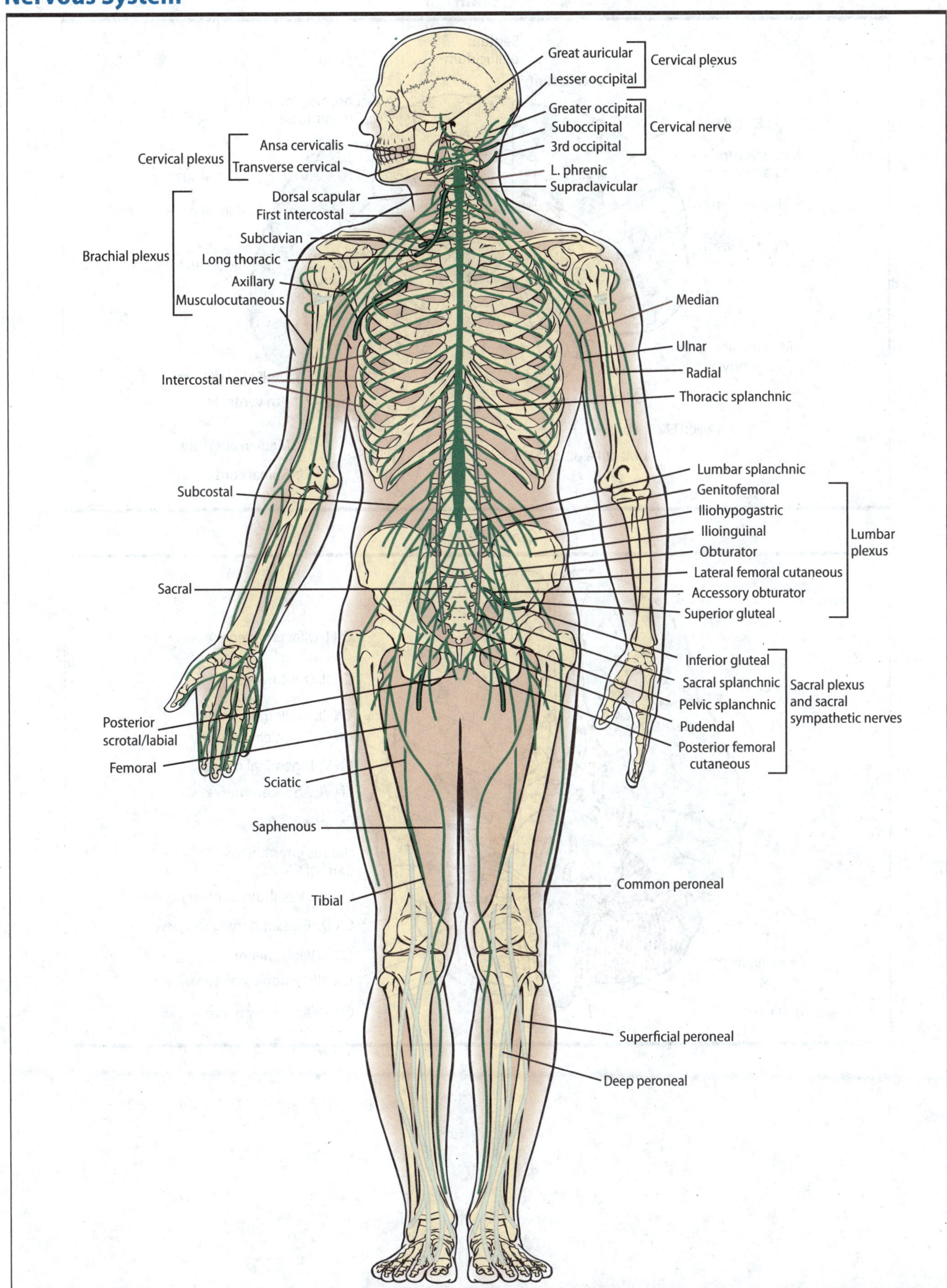

Brain

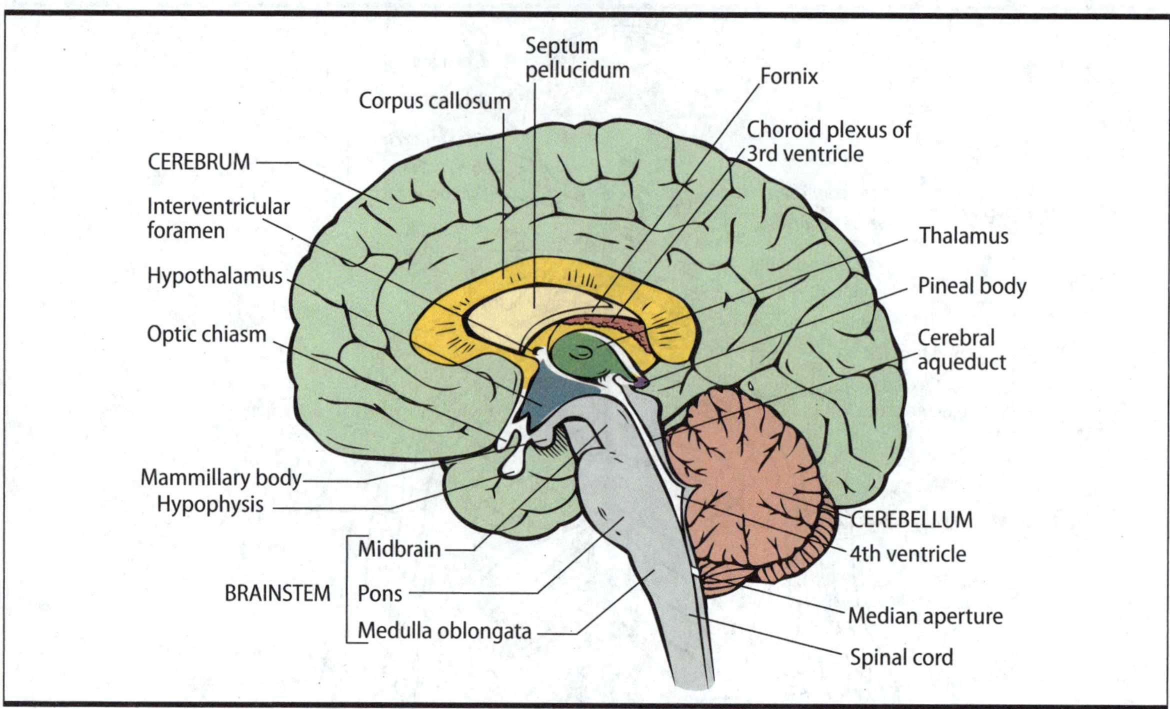

Cranial Nerves

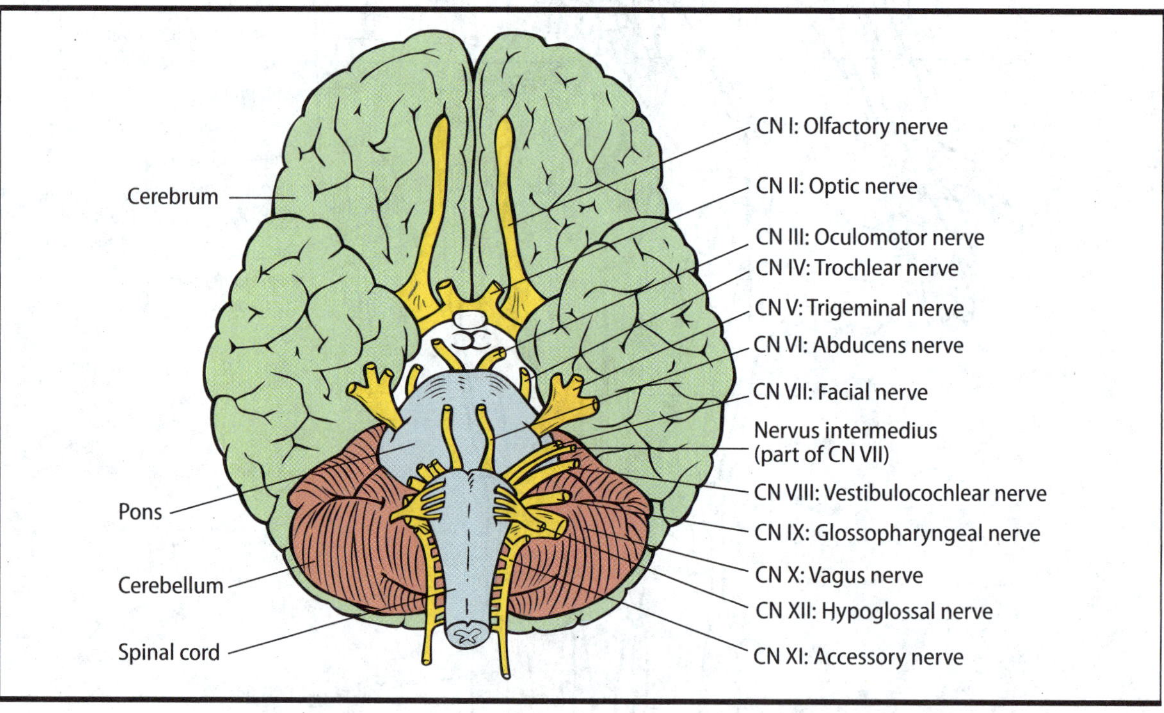

Spinal Cord and Spinal Nerves

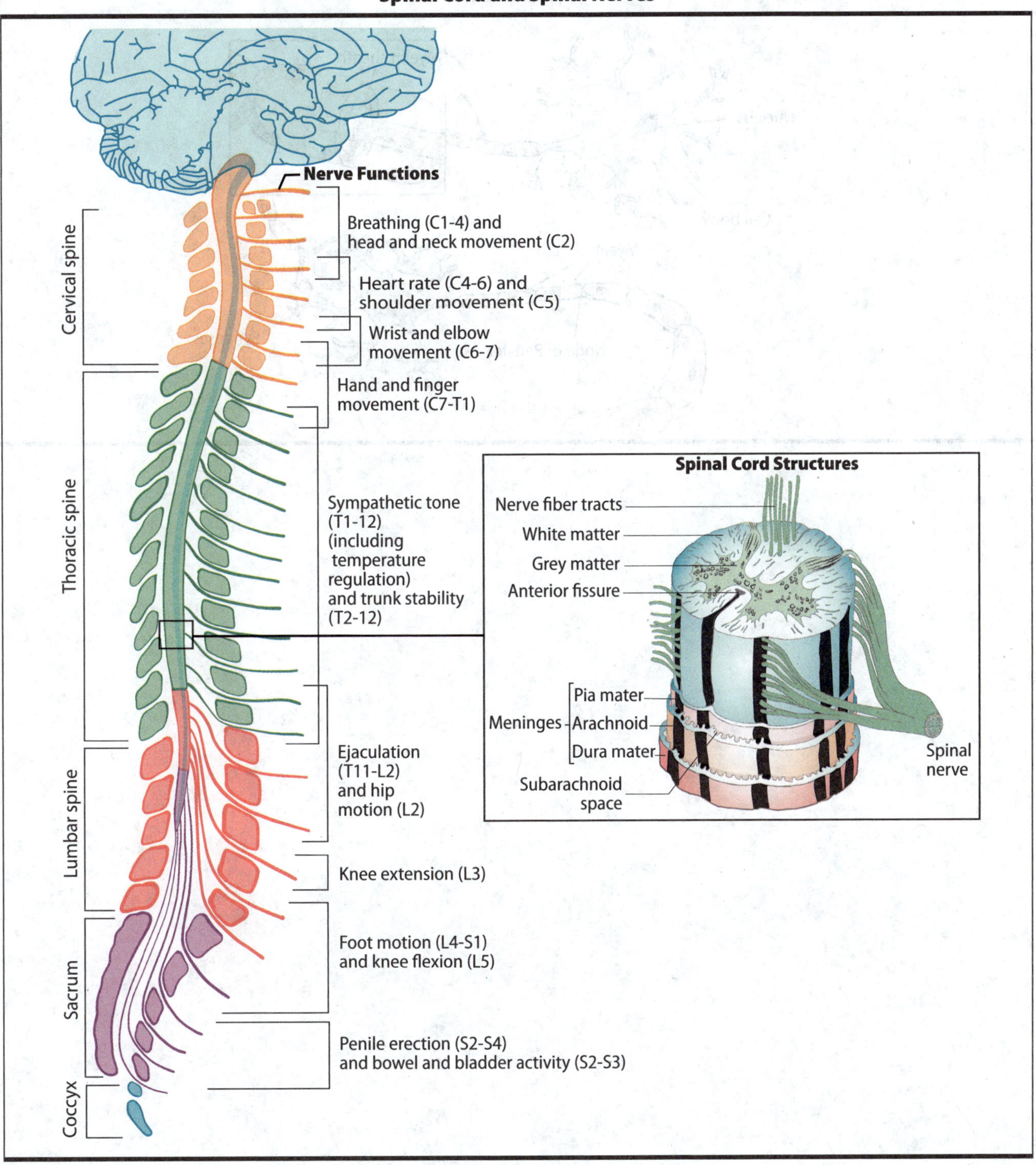

Nerve Cell

Myelin sheath
Nucleus
Axon
Cell body
Myelin sheath
Node of Ranvier
Synapses

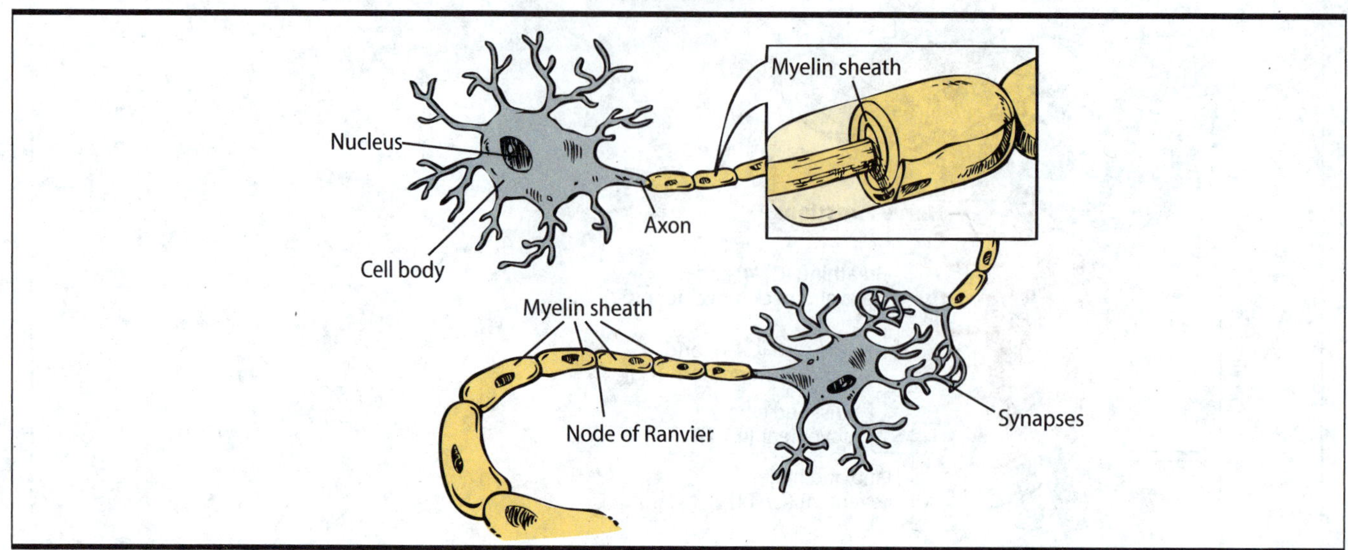

Eye

Eye Structure

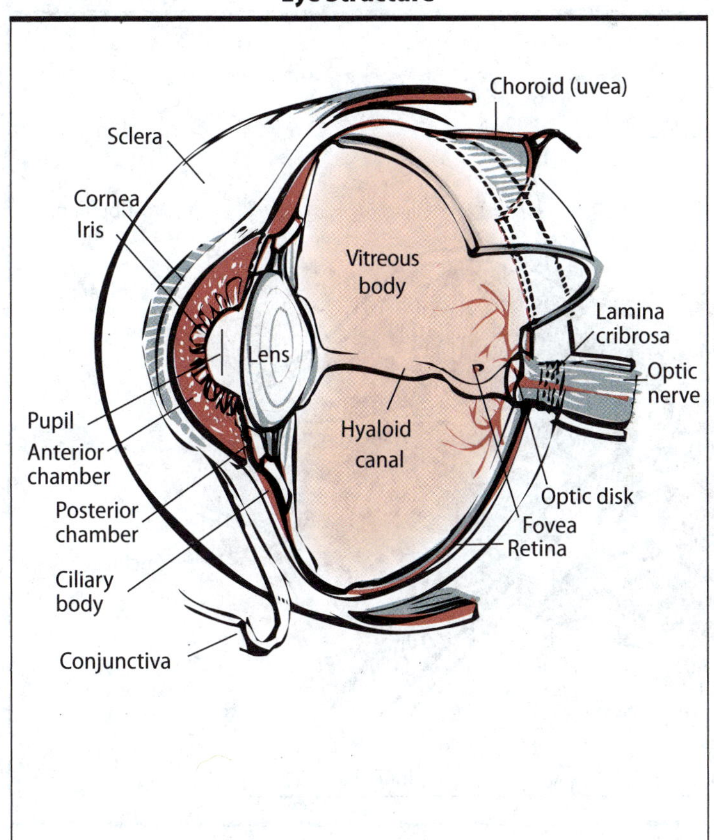

Posterior Pole of Globe/Flow of Aqueous Humor

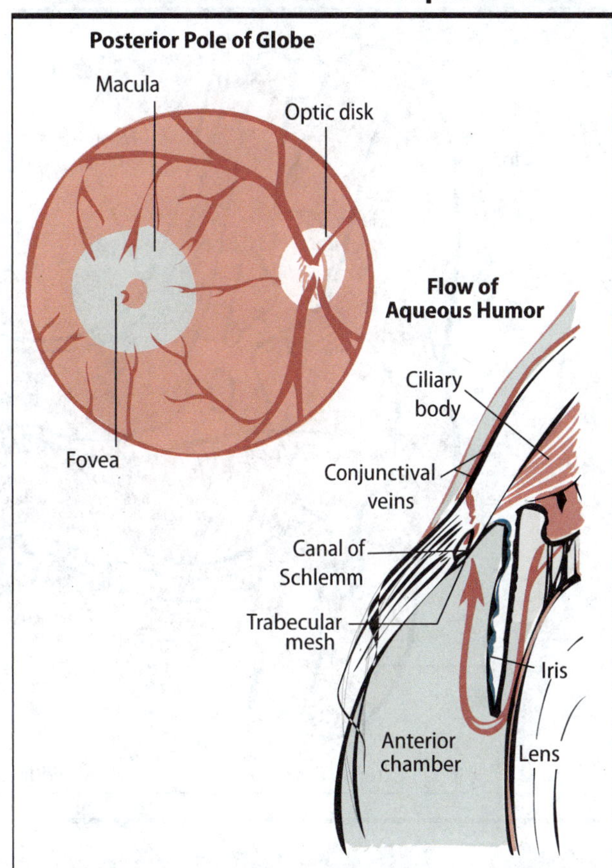

Eye Musculature

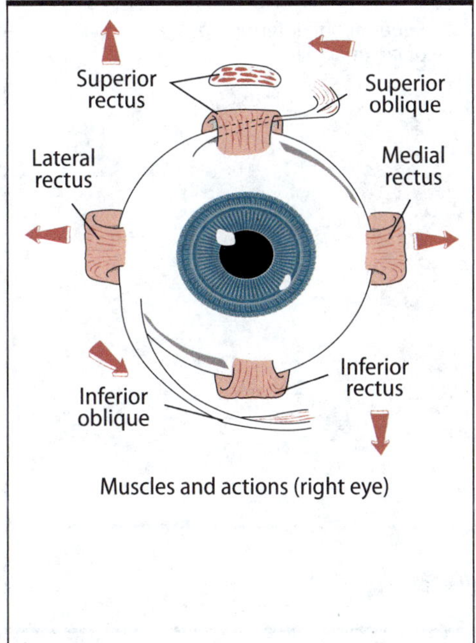

Muscles and actions (right eye)

Eyelid Structures

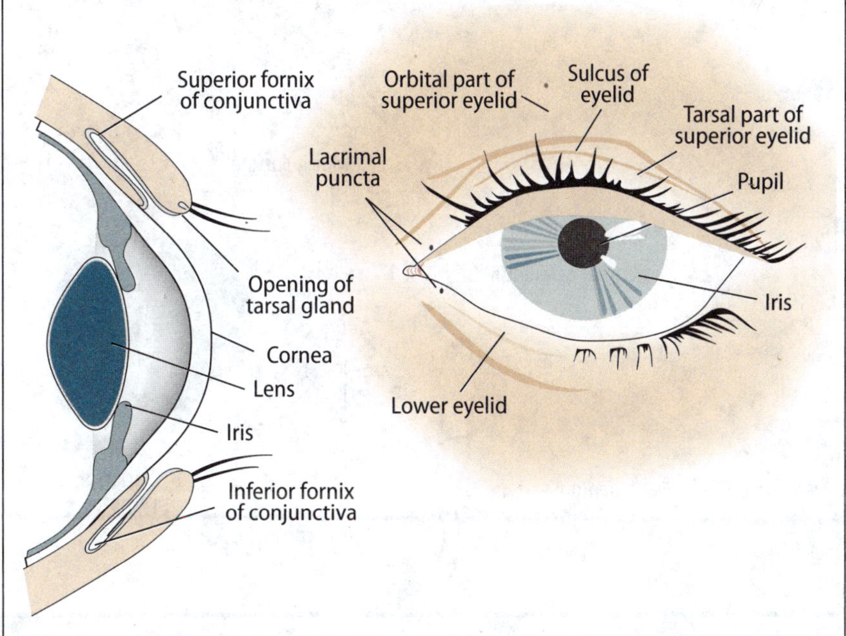

Ear and Lacrimal System

Ear Anatomy

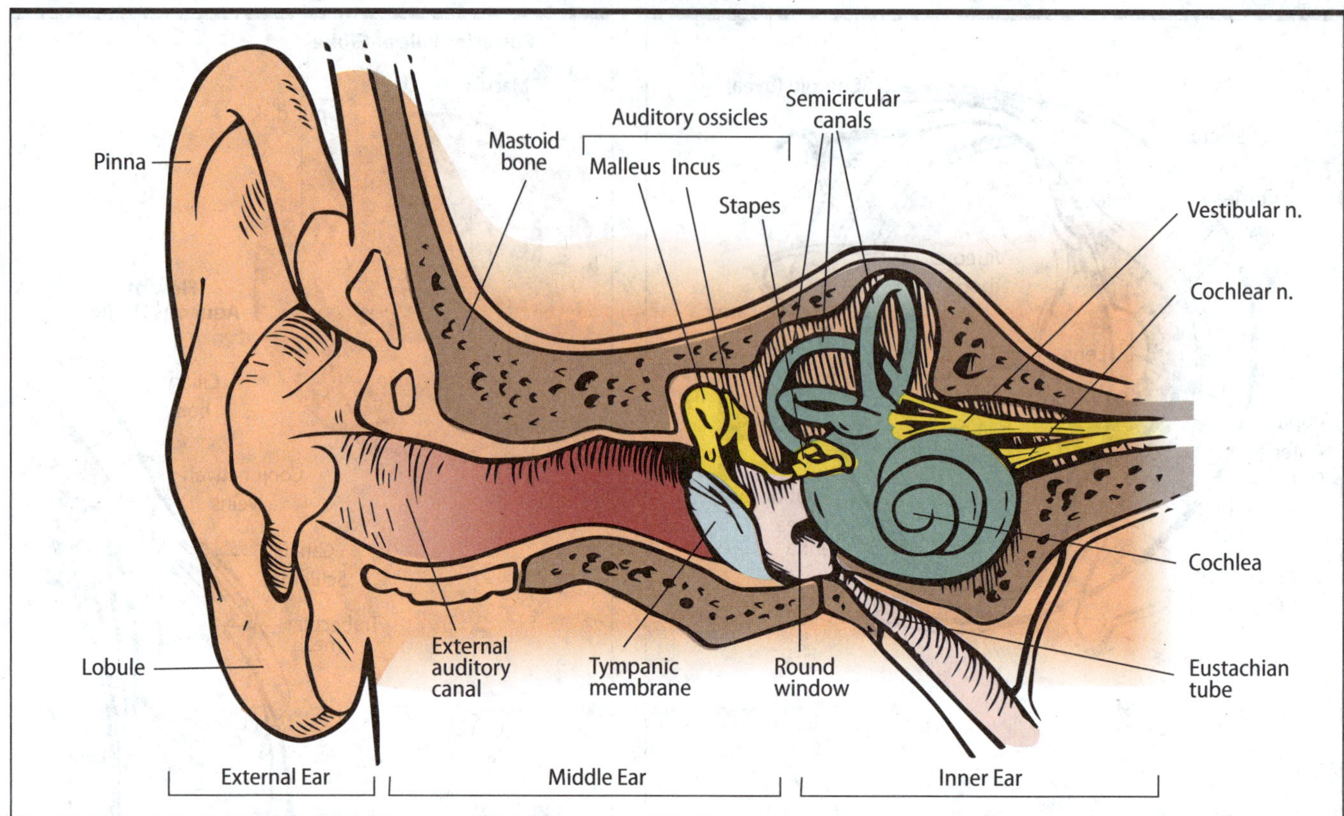

Lacrimal System

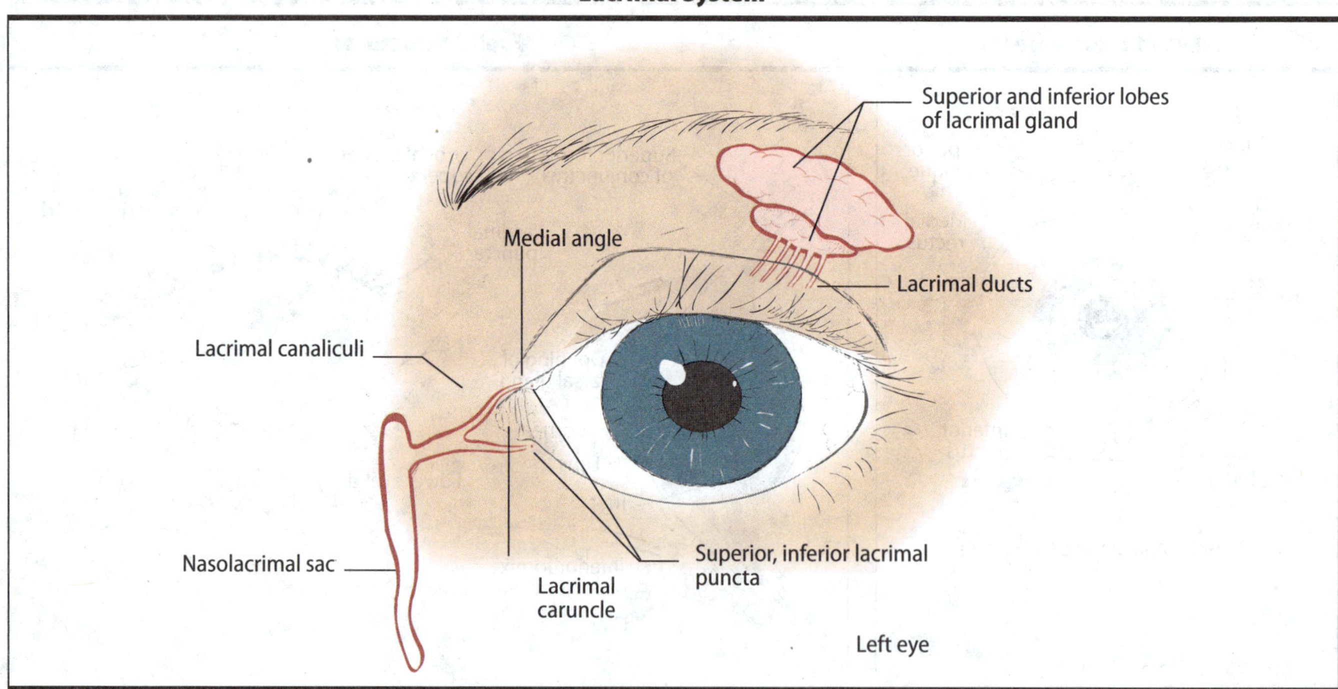

0-Numeric

A

 [Resequenced]

 [Resequenced]

 [Resequenced]

B

C

[Resequenced]

 [Resequenced]

 [Resequenced]

 [Resequenced]

 [Resequenced]

F

 [Resequenced]

[Resequenced]

[Resequenced]

Index

Intramuscular Autologous Bone Marrow Cell Therapy — Joint

 [Resequenced]

P

[Resequenced]

 [Resequenced]

[Resequenced]

R

 [Resequenced]

[Resequenced]

Index
Repair — Repair

 [Resequenced]

 [Resequenced]

[Resequenced]

[Resequenced]

T

 [Resequenced]

 [Resequenced]

W

X

Y

Z

00100-00126 Anesthesia for Cleft Lip, Ear, ECT, Eyelid, and Salivary Gland Procedures

CMS: 100-04,12,140.1 Qualified Nonphysician Anesthetists; 100-04,12,140.3 Payment for Qualified Nonphysician Anesthetists; 100-04,12,140.3.3 Billing Modifiers; 100-04,12,140.3.4 General Billing Instructions; 100-04,12,140.4.1 Anesthesiologist/Qualified Nonphysican Anesthetist; 100-04,12,140.4.2 Anesthetist and Anesthesiologist in a Single Procedure; 100-04,12,140.4.3 Payment for Medical /Surgical Services by CRNAs; 100-04,12,140.4.4 Conversion Factors for Anesthesia Services; 100-04,12,140.5 Payment for Anesthesia Services Furnished by a Teaching CRNA; 100-04,4,250.3.2 Anesthesia in a Hospital Outpatient Setting

00100 **Anesthesia for procedures on salivary glands, including biopsy**
0.00 0.00 FUD XXX N
AMA: 2018,Jan,8; 2017,Dec,8; 2017,Jan,8; 2016,Jan,13; 2015,Jan,16; 2014,Aug,5; 2014,Jan,11

00102 **Anesthesia for procedures involving plastic repair of cleft lip**
0.00 0.00 FUD XXX N
AMA: 2018,Jan,8; 2017,Dec,8; 2017,Jan,8; 2016,Jan,13; 2015,Jan,16; 2014,Aug,5; 2014,Jan,11

00103 **Anesthesia for reconstructive procedures of eyelid (eg, blepharoplasty, ptosis surgery)**
0.00 0.00 FUD XXX N
AMA: 2018,Jan,8; 2017,Dec,8; 2017,Jan,8; 2016,Jan,13; 2015,Jan,16; 2014,Aug,5; 2014,Jan,11

00104 **Anesthesia for electroconvulsive therapy**
0.00 0.00 FUD XXX N
AMA: 2018,Jan,8; 2017,Dec,8; 2017,Jan,8; 2016,Jan,13; 2015,Jan,16; 2014,Aug,5; 2014,Jan,11

00120 **Anesthesia for procedures on external, middle, and inner ear including biopsy; not otherwise specified**
0.00 0.00 FUD XXX N
AMA: 2018,Jan,8; 2017,Dec,8; 2017,Jan,8; 2016,Jan,13; 2015,Jan,16; 2014,Aug,5; 2014,Jan,11

00124 **otoscopy**
0.00 0.00 FUD XXX N
AMA: 2018,Jan,8; 2017,Dec,8; 2017,Jan,8; 2016,Jan,13; 2015,Jan,16; 2014,Aug,5; 2014,Jan,11

00126 **tympanotomy**
0.00 0.00 FUD XXX N
AMA: 2018,Jan,8; 2017,Dec,8; 2017,Jan,8; 2016,Jan,13; 2015,Jan,16; 2014,Aug,5; 2014,Jan,11

00140-00148 Anesthesia for Eye Procedures

CMS: 100-04,12,140.1 Qualified Nonphysician Anesthetists; 100-04,12,140.3 Payment for Qualified Nonphysician Anesthetists; 100-04,12,140.3.3 Billing Modifiers; 100-04,12,140.3.4 General Billing Instructions; 100-04,12,140.4.1 Anesthesiologist/Qualified Nonphysican Anesthetist; 100-04,12,140.4.2 Anesthetist and Anesthesiologist in a Single Procedure; 100-04,12,140.4.3 Payment for Medical /Surgical Services by CRNAs; 100-04,12,140.4.4 Conversion Factors for Anesthesia Services; 100-04,12,140.5 Payment for Anesthesia Services Furnished by a Teaching CRNA; 100-04,4,250.3.2 Anesthesia in a Hospital Outpatient Setting

00140 **Anesthesia for procedures on eye; not otherwise specified**
0.00 0.00 FUD XXX N
AMA: 2018,Jan,8; 2017,Dec,8; 2017,Jan,8; 2016,Jan,13; 2015,Jan,16; 2014,Aug,5; 2014,Jan,11

00142 **lens surgery**
0.00 0.00 FUD XXX N
AMA: 2018,Jan,8; 2017,Dec,8; 2017,Jan,8; 2016,Jan,13; 2015,Jan,16; 2014,Aug,5; 2014,Jan,11

00144 **corneal transplant**
0.00 0.00 FUD XXX N
AMA: 2018,Jan,8; 2017,Dec,8; 2017,Jan,8; 2016,Jan,13; 2015,Jan,16; 2014,Aug,5; 2014,Jan,11

00145 **vitreoretinal surgery**
0.00 0.00 FUD XXX N
AMA: 2018,Jan,8; 2017,Dec,8; 2017,Jan,8; 2016,Jan,13; 2015,Jan,16; 2014,Aug,5; 2014,Jan,11

00147 **iridectomy**
0.00 0.00 FUD XXX N
AMA: 2018,Jan,8; 2017,Dec,8; 2017,Jan,8; 2016,Jan,13; 2015,Jan,16; 2014,Aug,5; 2014,Jan,11

00148 **ophthalmoscopy**
0.00 0.00 FUD XXX N
AMA: 2018,Jan,8; 2017,Dec,8; 2017,Jan,8; 2016,Jan,13; 2015,Jan,16; 2014,Aug,5; 2014,Jan,11

00160-00326 Anesthesia for Face and Head Procedures

CMS: 100-04,12,140.1 Qualified Nonphysician Anesthetists; 100-04,12,140.3 Payment for Qualified Nonphysician Anesthetists; 100-04,12,140.3.3 Billing Modifiers; 100-04,12,140.3.4 General Billing Instructions; 100-04,12,140.4.1 Anesthesiologist/Qualified Nonphysican Anesthetist; 100-04,12,140.4.2 Anesthetist and Anesthesiologist in a Single Procedure; 100-04,12,140.4.4 Conversion Factors for Anesthesia Services; 100-04,12,140.5 Payment for Anesthesia Services Furnished by a Teaching CRNA; 100-04,4,250.3.2 Anesthesia in a Hospital Outpatient Setting

00160 **Anesthesia for procedures on nose and accessory sinuses; not otherwise specified**
0.00 0.00 FUD XXX N
AMA: 2018,Jan,8; 2017,Dec,8; 2017,Jan,8; 2016,Jan,13; 2015,Jan,16; 2014,Aug,5; 2014,Jan,11

00162 **radical surgery**
0.00 0.00 FUD XXX N
AMA: 2018,Jan,8; 2017,Dec,8; 2017,Jan,8; 2016,Jan,13; 2015,Jan,16; 2014,Aug,5; 2014,Jan,11

00164 **biopsy, soft tissue**
0.00 0.00 FUD XXX N
AMA: 2018,Jan,8; 2017,Dec,8; 2017,Jan,8; 2016,Jan,13; 2015,Jan,16; 2014,Aug,5; 2014,Jan,11

00170 **Anesthesia for intraoral procedures, including biopsy; not otherwise specified**
0.00 0.00 FUD XXX N
AMA: 2018,Jan,8; 2017,Dec,8; 2017,Jan,8; 2016,Jan,13; 2015,Jan,16; 2014,Aug,5; 2014,Jan,11

00172 **repair of cleft palate**
0.00 0.00 FUD XXX N
AMA: 2018,Jan,8; 2017,Dec,8; 2017,Jan,8; 2016,Jan,13; 2015,Jan,16; 2014,Aug,5; 2014,Jan,11

00174 **excision of retropharyngeal tumor**
0.00 0.00 FUD XXX N
AMA: 2018,Jan,8; 2017,Dec,8; 2017,Jan,8; 2016,Jan,13; 2015,Jan,16; 2014,Aug,5; 2014,Jan,11

00176 **radical surgery**
0.00 0.00 FUD XXX C
AMA: 2018,Jan,8; 2017,Dec,8; 2017,Jan,8; 2016,Jan,13; 2015,Jan,16; 2014,Aug,5; 2014,Jan,11

00190 **Anesthesia for procedures on facial bones or skull; not otherwise specified**
0.00 0.00 FUD XXX N
AMA: 2018,Jan,8; 2017,Dec,8; 2017,Jan,8; 2016,Jan,13; 2015,Jan,16; 2014,Aug,5; 2014,Jan,11

00192 **radical surgery (including prognathism)**
0.00 0.00 FUD XXX C
AMA: 2018,Jan,8; 2017,Dec,8; 2017,Jan,8; 2016,Jan,13; 2015,Jan,16; 2014,Aug,5; 2014,Jan,11

00210 **Anesthesia for intracranial procedures; not otherwise specified**
0.00 0.00 FUD XXX N
AMA: 2018,Jan,8; 2017,Dec,8; 2017,Jan,8; 2016,Jan,13; 2015,Jan,16; 2014,Aug,5; 2014,Jan,11

00211 **craniotomy or craniectomy for evacuation of hematoma**
0.00 0.00 FUD XXX C
AMA: 2018,Jan,8; 2017,Dec,8; 2017,Jan,8; 2016,Jan,13; 2015,Jan,16; 2014,Aug,5; 2014,Jan,11

00212 **subdural taps**
0.00 0.00 FUD XXX N
AMA: 2018,Jan,8; 2017,Dec,8; 2017,Jan,8; 2016,Jan,13; 2015,Jan,16; 2014,Aug,5; 2014,Jan,11

00214 **burr holes, including ventriculography**
0.00 0.00 FUD XXX C
AMA: 2018,Jan,8; 2017,Dec,8; 2017,Jan,8; 2016,Jan,13; 2015,Jan,16; 2014,Aug,5; 2014,Jan,11

00215 cranioplasty or elevation of depressed skull fracture, extradural (simple or compound)
0.00 0.00 FUD XXX C
AMA: 2018,Jan,8; 2017,Dec,8; 2017,Jan,8; 2016,Jan,13; 2015,Jan,16; 2014,Aug,5; 2014,Jan,11

00216 vascular procedures
0.00 0.00 FUD XXX N
AMA: 2018,Jan,8; 2017,Dec,8; 2017,Jan,8; 2016,Jan,13; 2015,Jan,16; 2014,Aug,5; 2014,Jan,11

00218 procedures in sitting position
0.00 0.00 FUD XXX N
AMA: 2018,Jan,8; 2017,Dec,8; 2017,Jan,8; 2016,Jan,13; 2015,Jan,16; 2014,Aug,5; 2014,Jan,11

00220 cerebrospinal fluid shunting procedures
0.00 0.00 FUD XXX N
AMA: 2018,Jan,8; 2017,Dec,8; 2017,Jan,8; 2016,Jan,13; 2015,Jan,16; 2014,Aug,5; 2014,Jan,11

00222 electrocoagulation of intracranial nerve
0.00 0.00 FUD XXX N
AMA: 2018,Jan,8; 2017,Dec,8; 2017,Jan,8; 2016,Jan,13; 2015,Jan,16; 2014,Aug,5; 2014,Jan,11

00300 Anesthesia for all procedures on the integumentary system, muscles and nerves of head, neck, and posterior trunk, not otherwise specified
0.00 0.00 FUD XXX N
AMA: 2018,Jan,8; 2017,Dec,8; 2017,Jan,8; 2016,Jan,13; 2015,Jan,16; 2014,Aug,5; 2014,Jan,11

00320 Anesthesia for all procedures on esophagus, thyroid, larynx, trachea and lymphatic system of neck; not otherwise specified, age 1 year or older
0.00 0.00 FUD XXX N
AMA: 2018,Jan,8; 2017,Dec,8; 2017,Jan,8; 2016,Jan,13; 2015,Jan,16; 2014,Aug,5; 2014,Jan,11

00322 needle biopsy of thyroid
EXCLUDES *Cervical spine and spinal cord procedures (00600, 00604, 00670)*
0.00 0.00 FUD XXX N
AMA: 2018,Jan,8; 2017,Dec,8; 2017,Jan,8; 2016,Jan,13; 2015,Jan,16; 2014,Aug,5; 2014,Jan,11

00326 Anesthesia for all procedures on the larynx and trachea in children younger than 1 year of age A
INCLUDES Anesthesia for patient of extreme age, younger than 1 year and older than 70 (99100)
0.00 0.00 FUD XXX N
AMA: 2018,Jan,8; 2017,Dec,8; 2017,Jan,8; 2016,Jan,13; 2015,Jan,16; 2014,Aug,5; 2014,Jan,11

00350-00352 Anesthesia for Neck Vessel Procedures

CMS: 100-04,12,140.1 Qualified Nonphysician Anesthetists; 100-04,12,140.3 Payment for Qualified Nonphysician Anesthetists; 100-04,12,140.3.3 Billing Modifiers; 100-04,12,140.3.4 General Billing Instructions; 100-04,12,140.4.1 Anesthesiologist/Qualified Nonphysican Anesthetist; 100-04,12,140.4.2 Anesthetist and Anesthesiologist in a Single Procedure; 100-04,12,140.4.3 Payment for Medical /Surgical Services by CRNAs; 100-04,12,140.4.4 Conversion Factors for Anesthesia Services; 100-04,12,140.5 Payment for Anesthesia Services Furnished by a Teaching CRNA; 100-04,4,250.3.2 Anesthesia in a Hospital Outpatient Setting

EXCLUDES *Arteriography (01916)*

00350 Anesthesia for procedures on major vessels of neck; not otherwise specified
0.00 0.00 FUD XXX N
AMA: 2018,Jan,8; 2017,Dec,8; 2017,Jan,8; 2016,Jan,13; 2015,Jan,16; 2014,Aug,5; 2014,Jan,11

00352 simple ligation
0.00 0.00 FUD XXX N
AMA: 2018,Jan,8; 2017,Dec,8; 2017,Jan,8; 2016,Jan,13; 2015,Jan,16; 2014,Aug,5; 2014,Jan,11

00400-00529 Anesthesia for Chest/Pectoral Girdle Procedures

CMS: 100-04,12,140.1 Qualified Nonphysician Anesthetists; 100-04,12,140.3 Payment for Qualified Nonphysician Anesthetists; 100-04,12,140.3.3 Billing Modifiers; 100-04,12,140.3.4 General Billing Instructions; 100-04,12,140.4.1 Anesthesiologist/Qualified Nonphysican Anesthetist; 100-04,12,140.4.2 Anesthetist and Anesthesiologist in a Single Procedure; 100-04,12,140.4.3 Payment for Medical /Surgical Services by CRNAs; 100-04,12,140.4.4 Conversion Factors for Anesthesia Services; 100-04,12,140.5 Payment for Anesthesia Services Furnished by a Teaching CRNA; 100-04,4,250.3.2 Anesthesia in a Hospital Outpatient Setting

00400 Anesthesia for procedures on the integumentary system on the extremities, anterior trunk and perineum; not otherwise specified
0.00 0.00 FUD XXX N
AMA: 2018,Jan,8; 2017,Dec,8; 2017,Jan,8; 2016,Jan,13; 2015,Jan,16; 2014,Aug,5; 2014,Jan,11

00402 reconstructive procedures on breast (eg, reduction or augmentation mammoplasty, muscle flaps)
0.00 0.00 FUD XXX N
AMA: 2018,Jan,8; 2017,Dec,8; 2017,Jan,8; 2016,Jan,13; 2015,Jan,16; 2014,Aug,5; 2014,Jan,11

00404 radical or modified radical procedures on breast
0.00 0.00 FUD XXX N
AMA: 2018,Jan,8; 2017,Dec,8; 2017,Jan,8; 2016,Jan,13; 2015,Jan,16; 2014,Aug,5; 2014,Jan,11

00406 radical or modified radical procedures on breast with internal mammary node dissection
0.00 0.00 FUD XXX N
AMA: 2018,Jan,8; 2017,Dec,8; 2017,Jan,8; 2016,Jan,13; 2015,Jan,16; 2014,Aug,5; 2014,Jan,11

00410 electrical conversion of arrhythmias
0.00 0.00 FUD XXX N
AMA: 2018,Jan,8; 2017,Dec,8; 2017,Jan,8; 2016,Jan,13; 2015,Jan,16; 2014,Aug,5; 2014,Jan,11

00450 Anesthesia for procedures on clavicle and scapula; not otherwise specified
0.00 0.00 FUD XXX N
AMA: 2018,Jan,8; 2017,Dec,8; 2017,Jan,8; 2016,Jan,13; 2015,Jan,16; 2014,Aug,5; 2014,Jan,11

00454 biopsy of clavicle
0.00 0.00 FUD XXX N
AMA: 2018,Jan,8; 2017,Dec,8; 2017,Jan,8; 2016,Jan,13; 2015,Jan,16; 2014,Aug,5; 2014,Jan,11

00470 Anesthesia for partial rib resection; not otherwise specified
0.00 0.00 FUD XXX N
AMA: 2018,Jan,8; 2017,Dec,8; 2017,Jan,8; 2016,Jan,13; 2015,Jan,16; 2014,Aug,5; 2014,Jan,11

00472 thoracoplasty (any type)
0.00 0.00 FUD XXX N
AMA: 2018,Jan,8; 2017,Dec,8; 2017,Jan,8; 2016,Jan,13; 2015,Jan,16; 2014,Aug,5; 2014,Jan,11

00474 radical procedures (eg, pectus excavatum)
0.00 0.00 FUD XXX C
AMA: 2018,Jan,8; 2017,Dec,8; 2017,Jan,8; 2016,Jan,13; 2015,Jan,16; 2014,Aug,5; 2014,Jan,11

00500 Anesthesia for all procedures on esophagus
0.00 0.00 FUD XXX N
AMA: 2018,Jan,8; 2017,Dec,8; 2017,Jan,8; 2016,Jan,13; 2015,Jan,16; 2014,Aug,5; 2014,Jan,11

00520 Anesthesia for closed chest procedures; (including bronchoscopy) not otherwise specified
0.00 0.00 FUD XXX N
AMA: 2018,Jan,8; 2017,Dec,8; 2017,Jan,8; 2016,Jan,13; 2015,Jan,16; 2014,Aug,5; 2014,Jan,11

00522 needle biopsy of pleura
0.00 0.00 FUD XXX N
AMA: 2018,Jan,8; 2017,Dec,8; 2017,Jan,8; 2016,Jan,13; 2015,Jan,16; 2014,Aug,5; 2014,Jan,11

00524 **pneumocentesis**
0.00 0.00 FUD XXX C
AMA: 2018,Jan,8; 2017,Dec,8; 2017,Jan,8; 2016,Jan,13; 2015,Jan,16; 2014,Aug,5; 2014,Jan,11

00528 **mediastinoscopy and diagnostic thoracoscopy not utilizing 1 lung ventilation**
EXCLUDES *Tracheobronchial reconstruction (00539)*
0.00 0.00 FUD XXX N
AMA: 2018,Jan,8; 2017,Dec,8; 2017,Jan,8; 2016,Jan,13; 2015,Jan,16; 2014,Aug,5; 2014,Jan,11

00529 **mediastinoscopy and diagnostic thoracoscopy utilizing 1 lung ventilation**
0.00 0.00 FUD XXX N
AMA: 2018,Jan,8; 2017,Dec,8; 2017,Jan,8; 2016,Jan,13; 2015,Jan,16; 2014,Aug,5; 2014,Jan,11

00530 Anesthesia for Cardiac Pacemaker Procedure

CMS: 100-03,10.6 Anesthesia in Cardiac Pacemaker Surgery; 100-04,12,140.1 Qualified Nonphysician Anesthetists; 100-04,12,140.3 Payment for Qualified Nonphysician Anesthetists; 100-04,12,140.3.3 Billing Modifiers; 100-04,12,140.3.4 General Billing Instructions; 100-04,12,140.4.1 Anesthesiologist/Qualified Nonphysican Anesthetist; 100-04,12,140.4.2 Anesthetist and Anesthesiologist in a Single Procedure; 100-04,12,140.4.3 Payment for Medical /Surgical Services by CRNAs; 100-04,12,140.4.4 Conversion Factors for Anesthesia Services; 100-04,12,140.5 Payment for Anesthesia Services Furnished by a Teaching CRNA; 100-04,4,250.3.2 Anesthesia in a Hospital Outpatient Setting

00530 **Anesthesia for permanent transvenous pacemaker insertion**
0.00 0.00 FUD XXX N
AMA: 2018,Jan,8; 2017,Dec,8; 2017,Jan,8; 2016,Jan,13; 2015,Jan,16; 2014,Aug,5; 2014,Jan,11

00532-00550 Anesthesia for Heart and Lung Procedures

CMS: 100-04,12,140.1 Qualified Nonphysician Anesthetists; 100-04,12,140.3 Payment for Qualified Nonphysician Anesthetists; 100-04,12,140.3.3 Billing Modifiers; 100-04,12,140.3.4 General Billing Instructions; 100-04,12,140.4.1 Anesthesiologist/Qualified Nonphysican Anesthetist; 100-04,12,140.4.2 Anesthetist and Anesthesiologist in a Single Procedure; 100-04,12,140.4.3 Payment for Medical /Surgical Services by CRNAs; 100-04,12,140.4.4 Conversion Factors for Anesthesia Services; 100-04,12,140.5 Payment for Anesthesia Services Furnished by a Teaching CRNA; 100-04,4,250.3.2 Anesthesia in a Hospital Outpatient Setting

00532 **Anesthesia for access to central venous circulation**
0.00 0.00 FUD XXX N
AMA: 2018,Jan,8; 2017,Dec,8; 2017,Jan,8; 2016,Jan,13; 2015,Jan,16; 2014,Aug,5; 2014,Jan,11

00534 **Anesthesia for transvenous insertion or replacement of pacing cardioverter-defibrillator**
EXCLUDES *Transthoracic approach (00560)*
0.00 0.00 FUD XXX N
AMA: 2018,Jan,8; 2017,Dec,8; 2017,Jan,8; 2016,Jan,13; 2015,Jan,16; 2014,Aug,5; 2014,Jan,11

00537 **Anesthesia for cardiac electrophysiologic procedures including radiofrequency ablation**
0.00 0.00 FUD XXX N
AMA: 2018,Jan,8; 2017,Dec,8; 2017,Jan,8; 2016,Jan,13; 2015,Jan,16; 2014,Aug,5; 2014,Jan,11

00539 **Anesthesia for tracheobronchial reconstruction**
0.00 0.00 FUD XXX N
AMA: 2018,Jan,8; 2017,Dec,8; 2017,Jan,8; 2016,Jan,13; 2015,Jan,16; 2014,Aug,5; 2014,Jan,11

00540 **Anesthesia for thoracotomy procedures involving lungs, pleura, diaphragm, and mediastinum (including surgical thoracoscopy); not otherwise specified**
EXCLUDES *Thoracic spine and spinal cord procedures via anterior transthoracic approach (00625-00626)*
0.00 0.00 FUD XXX C
AMA: 2018,Jan,8; 2017,Dec,8; 2017,Jan,8; 2016,Jan,13; 2015,Jan,16; 2014,Aug,5; 2014,Jan,11

00541 **utilizing 1 lung ventilation**
EXCLUDES *Thoracic spine and spinal cord procedures via anterior transthoracic approach (00625-00626)*
0.00 0.00 FUD XXX N
AMA: 2018,Jan,8; 2017,Dec,8; 2017,Jan,8; 2016,Jan,13; 2015,Jan,16; 2014,Aug,5; 2014,Jan,11

00542 **decortication**
0.00 0.00 FUD XXX C
AMA: 2018,Jan,8; 2017,Dec,8; 2017,Jan,8; 2016,Jan,13; 2015,Jan,16; 2014,Aug,5; 2014,Jan,11

00546 **pulmonary resection with thoracoplasty**
0.00 0.00 FUD XXX C
AMA: 2018,Jan,8; 2017,Dec,8; 2017,Jan,8; 2016,Jan,13; 2015,Jan,16; 2014,Aug,5; 2014,Jan,11

00548 **intrathoracic procedures on the trachea and bronchi**
0.00 0.00 FUD XXX N
AMA: 2018,Jan,8; 2017,Dec,8; 2017,Jan,8; 2016,Jan,13; 2015,Jan,16; 2014,Aug,5; 2014,Jan,11

00550 **Anesthesia for sternal debridement**
0.00 0.00 FUD XXX N
AMA: 2018,Jan,8; 2017,Dec,8; 2017,Jan,8; 2016,Jan,13; 2015,Jan,16; 2014,Aug,5; 2014,Jan,11

00560-00580 Anesthesia for Open Heart Procedures

CMS: 100-04,12,140.1 Qualified Nonphysician Anesthetists; 100-04,12,140.3 Payment for Qualified Nonphysician Anesthetists; 100-04,12,140.3.3 Billing Modifiers; 100-04,12,140.3.4 General Billing Instructions; 100-04,12,140.4.1 Anesthesiologist/Qualified Nonphysican Anesthetist; 100-04,12,140.4.2 Anesthetist and Anesthesiologist in a Single Procedure; 100-04,12,140.4.3 Payment for Medical /Surgical Services by CRNAs; 100-04,12,140.4.4 Conversion Factors for Anesthesia Services; 100-04,12,140.5 Payment for Anesthesia Services Furnished by a Teaching CRNA; 100-04,4,250.3.2 Anesthesia in a Hospital Outpatient Setting

00560 **Anesthesia for procedures on heart, pericardial sac, and great vessels of chest; without pump oxygenator**
0.00 0.00 FUD XXX C
AMA: 2018,Jan,8; 2017,Dec,8; 2017,Jan,8; 2016,Jan,13; 2015,Jan,16; 2014,Aug,5; 2014,Jan,11

00561 **with pump oxygenator, younger than 1 year of age** A
INCLUDES Anesthesia complicated by utilization of controlled hypotension (99135)
Anesthesia complicated by utilization of total body hypothermia (99116)
Anesthesia for patient of extreme age, younger than 1 year and older than 70 (99100)
0.00 0.00 FUD XXX C
AMA: 2018,Jan,8; 2017,Dec,8; 2017,Jan,8; 2016,Jan,13; 2015,Jan,16; 2014,Aug,5; 2014,Jan,11

00562 **with pump oxygenator, age 1 year or older, for all noncoronary bypass procedures (eg, valve procedures) or for re-operation for coronary bypass more than 1 month after original operation** A
0.00 0.00 FUD XXX C
AMA: 2018,Jan,8; 2017,Dec,8; 2017,Jan,8; 2016,Jan,13; 2015,Jan,16; 2014,Aug,5; 2014,Jan,11

00563 **with pump oxygenator with hypothermic circulatory arrest**
0.00 0.00 FUD XXX N
AMA: 2018,Jan,8; 2017,Dec,8; 2017,Jan,8; 2016,Jan,13; 2015,Jan,16; 2014,Aug,5; 2014,Jan,11

00566 **Anesthesia for direct coronary artery bypass grafting; without pump oxygenator**
0.00 0.00 FUD XXX N
AMA: 2018,Jan,8; 2017,Dec,8; 2017,Jan,8; 2016,Jan,13; 2015,Jan,16; 2014,Aug,5; 2014,Jan,11

00567 **with pump oxygenator**
0.00 0.00 FUD XXX C
AMA: 2018,Jan,8; 2017,Dec,8; 2017,Jan,8; 2016,Jan,13; 2015,Jan,16; 2014,Aug,5; 2014,Jan,11

00580 **Anesthesia for heart transplant or heart/lung transplant**
0.00 0.00 FUD XXX C
AMA: 2018,Jan,8; 2017,Dec,8; 2017,Jan,8; 2016,Jan,13; 2015,Jan,16; 2014,Aug,5; 2014,Jan,11

00600-00670 Anesthesia for Spinal Procedures

CMS: 100-04,12,140.1 Qualified Nonphysician Anesthetists; 100-04,12,140.3 Payment for Qualified Nonphysician Anesthetists; 100-04,12,140.3.3 Billing Modifiers; 100-04,12,140.3.4 General Billing Instructions; 100-04,12,140.4.1 Anesthesiologist/Qualified Nonphysican Anesthetist; 100-04,12,140.4.2 Anesthetist and Anesthesiologist in a Single Procedure; 100-04,12,140.4.3 Payment for Medical /Surgical Services by CRNAs; 100-04,12,140.4.4 Conversion Factors for Anesthesia Services; 100-04,12,140.5 Payment for Anesthesia Services Furnished by a Teaching CRNA; 100-04,4,250.3.2 Anesthesia in a Hospital Outpatient Setting

00600 **Anesthesia for procedures on cervical spine and cord; not otherwise specified**

EXCLUDES *Percutaneous image-guided spine and spinal cord anesthesia services (01935-01936)*

0.00 0.00 **FUD** XXX N

AMA: 2018,Jan,8; 2017,Dec,8; 2017,Jan,8; 2016,Jan,13; 2015,Jan,16; 2014,Aug,5; 2014,Jan,11

00604 **procedures with patient in the sitting position**

0.00 0.00 **FUD** XXX C

AMA: 2018,Jan,8; 2017,Dec,8; 2017,Jan,8; 2016,Jan,13; 2015,Jan,16; 2014,Aug,5; 2014,Jan,11

00620 **Anesthesia for procedures on thoracic spine and cord, not otherwise specified**

0.00 0.00 **FUD** XXX N

AMA: 2018,Jan,8; 2017,Dec,8; 2017,Jan,8; 2016,Jan,13; 2015,Jan,16; 2014,Aug,5; 2014,Jan,11

00625 **Anesthesia for procedures on the thoracic spine and cord, via an anterior transthoracic approach; not utilizing 1 lung ventilation**

EXCLUDES *Anesthesia services for thoracotomy procedures other than spine (00540-00541)*

0.00 0.00 **FUD** XXX N

AMA: 2018,Jan,8; 2017,Dec,8; 2017,Jan,8; 2016,Jan,13; 2015,Jan,16; 2014,Aug,5; 2014,Jan,11

00626 **utilizing 1 lung ventilation**

EXCLUDES *Anesthesia services for thoracotomy procedures other than spine (00540-00541)*

0.00 0.00 **FUD** XXX N

AMA: 2018,Jan,8; 2017,Dec,8; 2017,Jan,8; 2016,Jan,13; 2015,Jan,16; 2014,Aug,5; 2014,Jan,11

00630 **Anesthesia for procedures in lumbar region; not otherwise specified**

0.00 0.00 **FUD** XXX N

AMA: 2018,Jan,8; 2017,Dec,8; 2017,Jan,8; 2016,Jan,13; 2015,Jan,16; 2014,Aug,5; 2014,Jan,11

00632 **lumbar sympathectomy**

0.00 0.00 **FUD** XXX C

AMA: 2018,Jan,8; 2017,Dec,8; 2017,Jan,8; 2016,Jan,13; 2015,Jan,16; 2014,Aug,5; 2014,Jan,11

00635 **diagnostic or therapeutic lumbar puncture**

0.00 0.00 **FUD** XXX N

AMA: 2018,Jan,8; 2017,Dec,8; 2017,Jan,8; 2016,Jan,13; 2015,Jan,16; 2014,Aug,5; 2014,Jan,11

00640 **Anesthesia for manipulation of the spine or for closed procedures on the cervical, thoracic or lumbar spine**

0.00 0.00 **FUD** XXX N

AMA: 2018,Jan,8; 2017,Dec,8; 2017,Jan,8; 2016,Jan,13; 2015,Jan,16; 2014,Aug,5; 2014,Jan,11

00670 **Anesthesia for extensive spine and spinal cord procedures (eg, spinal instrumentation or vascular procedures)**

0.00 0.00 **FUD** XXX C

AMA: 2018,Jan,8; 2017,Dec,8; 2017,Jan,8; 2016,Jan,13; 2015,Jan,16; 2014,Aug,5; 2014,Jan,11

00700-00882 Anesthesia for Abdominal Procedures

CMS: 100-04,12,140.1 Qualified Nonphysician Anesthetists; 100-04,12,140.3 Payment for Qualified Nonphysician Anesthetists; 100-04,12,140.3.3 Billing Modifiers; 100-04,12,140.3.4 General Billing Instructions; 100-04,12,140.4.1 Anesthesiologist/Qualified Nonphysican Anesthetist; 100-04,12,140.4.2 Anesthetist and Anesthesiologist in a Single Procedure; 100-04,12,140.4.3 Payment for Medical /Surgical Services by CRNAs; 100-04,12,140.4.4 Conversion Factors for Anesthesia Services; 100-04,12,140.5 Payment for Anesthesia Services Furnished by a Teaching CRNA; 100-04,4,250.3.2 Anesthesia in a Hospital Outpatient Setting

00700 **Anesthesia for procedures on upper anterior abdominal wall; not otherwise specified**

0.00 0.00 **FUD** XXX N

AMA: 2018,Jan,8; 2017,Dec,8; 2017,Jan,8; 2016,Jan,13; 2015,Jan,16; 2014,Aug,5; 2014,Jan,11

00702 **percutaneous liver biopsy**

0.00 0.00 **FUD** XXX N

AMA: 2018,Jan,8; 2017,Dec,8; 2017,Jan,8; 2016,Jan,13; 2015,Jan,16; 2014,Aug,5; 2014,Jan,11

00730 **Anesthesia for procedures on upper posterior abdominal wall**

0.00 0.00 **FUD** XXX N

AMA: 2018,Jan,8; 2017,Dec,8; 2017,Jan,8; 2016,Jan,13; 2015,Jan,16; 2014,Aug,5; 2014,Jan,11

00731 **Anesthesia for upper gastrointestinal endoscopic procedures, endoscope introduced proximal to duodenum; not otherwise specified**

EXCLUDES *Combination of upper and lower endoscopic gastrointestinal procedures (00813)*

0.00 0.00 **FUD** XXX N

AMA: 2018,Jan,8; 2017,Dec,8

00732 **endoscopic retrograde cholangiopancreatography (ERCP)**

EXCLUDES *Combination of upper and lower endoscopic gastrointestinal procedures (00813)*

0.00 0.00 **FUD** XXX N

AMA: 2018,Jan,8; 2017,Dec,8

00750 **Anesthesia for hernia repairs in upper abdomen; not otherwise specified**

0.00 0.00 **FUD** XXX N

AMA: 2018,Jan,8; 2017,Dec,8; 2017,Jan,8; 2016,Jan,13; 2015,Jan,16; 2014,Aug,5; 2014,Jan,11

00752 **lumbar and ventral (incisional) hernias and/or wound dehiscence**

0.00 0.00 **FUD** XXX N

AMA: 2018,Jan,8; 2017,Dec,8; 2017,Jan,8; 2016,Jan,13; 2015,Jan,16; 2014,Aug,5; 2014,Jan,11

00754 **omphalocele**

0.00 0.00 **FUD** XXX N

AMA: 2018,Jan,8; 2017,Dec,8; 2017,Jan,8; 2016,Jan,13; 2015,Jan,16; 2014,Aug,5; 2014,Jan,11

00756 **transabdominal repair of diaphragmatic hernia**

0.00 0.00 **FUD** XXX N

AMA: 2018,Jan,8; 2017,Dec,8; 2017,Jan,8; 2016,Jan,13; 2015,Jan,16; 2014,Aug,5; 2014,Jan,11

00770 **Anesthesia for all procedures on major abdominal blood vessels**

0.00 0.00 **FUD** XXX N

AMA: 2018,Jan,8; 2017,Dec,8; 2017,Jan,8; 2016,Jan,13; 2015,Jan,16; 2014,Aug,5; 2014,Jan,11

00790 **Anesthesia for intraperitoneal procedures in upper abdomen including laparoscopy; not otherwise specified**

0.00 0.00 **FUD** XXX N

AMA: 2018,Jan,8; 2017,Dec,8; 2017,Jan,8; 2016,Jan,13; 2015,Jan,16; 2014,Aug,5; 2014,Jan,11

00792 **partial hepatectomy or management of liver hemorrhage (excluding liver biopsy)**

0.00 0.00 **FUD** XXX C

AMA: 2018,Jan,8; 2017,Dec,8; 2017,Jan,8; 2016,Jan,13; 2015,Jan,16; 2014,Aug,5; 2014,Jan,11

00794 pancreatectomy, partial or total (eg, Whipple procedure)
0.00 0.00 FUD XXX C
AMA: 2018,Jan,8; 2017,Dec,8; 2017,Jan,8; 2016,Jan,13; 2015,Jan,16; 2014,Aug,5; 2014,Jan,11

00796 liver transplant (recipient)
EXCLUDES *Physiological support during liver harvest (01990)*
0.00 0.00 FUD XXX C
AMA: 2018,Jan,8; 2017,Dec,8; 2017,Jan,8; 2016,Jan,13; 2015,Jan,16; 2014,Aug,5; 2014,Jan,11

00797 gastric restrictive procedure for morbid obesity
0.00 0.00 FUD XXX N
AMA: 2018,Jan,8; 2017,Dec,8; 2017,Jan,8; 2016,Jan,13; 2015,Jan,16; 2014,Aug,5; 2014,Jan,11

00800 Anesthesia for procedures on lower anterior abdominal wall; not otherwise specified
0.00 0.00 FUD XXX N
AMA: 2018,Jan,8; 2017,Dec,8; 2017,Jan,8; 2016,Jan,13; 2015,Jan,16; 2014,Aug,5; 2014,Jan,11

00802 panniculectomy
0.00 0.00 FUD XXX C
AMA: 2018,Jan,8; 2017,Dec,8; 2017,Jan,8; 2016,Jan,13; 2015,Jan,16; 2014,Aug,5; 2014,Jan,11

00811 Anesthesia for lower intestinal endoscopic procedures, endoscope introduced distal to duodenum; not otherwise specified
0.00 0.00 FUD XXX N
AMA: 2018,Jan,8; 2017,Dec,8

00812 screening colonoscopy
INCLUDES Anesthesia services for all screening colonoscopy irrespective of findings
0.00 0.00 FUD XXX N
AMA: 2018,Jan,8; 2017,Dec,8

00813 Anesthesia for combined upper and lower gastrointestinal endoscopic procedures, endoscope introduced both proximal to and distal to the duodenum
0.00 0.00 FUD XXX N
AMA: 2018,Jan,8; 2017,Dec,8

00820 Anesthesia for procedures on lower posterior abdominal wall
0.00 0.00 FUD XXX N
AMA: 2018,Jan,8; 2017,Dec,8; 2017,Jan,8; 2016,Jan,13; 2015,Jan,16; 2014,Aug,5; 2014,Jan,11

00830 Anesthesia for hernia repairs in lower abdomen; not otherwise specified
EXCLUDES *Anesthesia for hernia repairs on infants one year old or less (00834, 00836)*
0.00 0.00 FUD XXX N
AMA: 2018,Jan,8; 2017,Dec,8; 2017,Jan,8; 2016,Jan,13; 2015,Jan,16; 2014,Aug,5; 2014,Jan,11

00832 ventral and incisional hernias
EXCLUDES *Anesthesia for hernia repairs on infants one year old or less (00834, 00836)*
0.00 0.00 FUD XXX N
AMA: 2018,Jan,8; 2017,Dec,8; 2017,Jan,8; 2016,Jan,13; 2015,Jan,16; 2014,Aug,5; 2014,Jan,11

00834 Anesthesia for hernia repairs in the lower abdomen not otherwise specified, younger than 1 year of age A
INCLUDES Anesthesia for patient of extreme age, younger than 1 year and older than 70 (99100)
0.00 0.00 FUD XXX N
AMA: 2018,Jan,8; 2017,Dec,8; 2017,Jan,8; 2016,Jan,13; 2015,Jan,16; 2014,Aug,5; 2014,Jan,11

00836 Anesthesia for hernia repairs in the lower abdomen not otherwise specified, infants younger than 37 weeks gestational age at birth and younger than 50 weeks gestational age at time of surgery A
INCLUDES Anesthesia for patient of extreme age, younger than 1 year and older than 70 (99100)
0.00 0.00 FUD XXX N
AMA: 2018,Jan,8; 2017,Dec,8; 2017,Jan,8; 2016,Jan,13; 2015,Jan,16; 2014,Aug,5; 2014,Jan,11

00840 Anesthesia for intraperitoneal procedures in lower abdomen including laparoscopy; not otherwise specified
0.00 0.00 FUD XXX N
AMA: 2018,Jan,8; 2017,Dec,8; 2017,Jan,8; 2016,Jan,13; 2015,Jan,16; 2014,Aug,5; 2014,Jan,11

00842 amniocentesis M ♀
0.00 0.00 FUD XXX N
AMA: 2018,Jan,8; 2017,Dec,8; 2017,Jan,8; 2016,Jan,13; 2015,Jan,16; 2014,Aug,5; 2014,Jan,11

00844 abdominoperineal resection
0.00 0.00 FUD XXX C
AMA: 2018,Jan,8; 2017,Dec,8; 2017,Jan,8; 2016,Jan,13; 2015,Jan,16; 2014,Aug,5; 2014,Jan,11

00846 radical hysterectomy ♀
0.00 0.00 FUD XXX C
AMA: 2018,Jan,8; 2017,Dec,8; 2017,Jan,8; 2016,Jan,13; 2015,Jan,16; 2014,Aug,5; 2014,Jan,11

00848 pelvic exenteration
0.00 0.00 FUD XXX C
AMA: 2018,Jan,8; 2017,Dec,8; 2017,Jan,8; 2016,Jan,13; 2015,Jan,16; 2014,Aug,5; 2014,Jan,11

00851 tubal ligation/transection ♀
0.00 0.00 FUD XXX N
AMA: 2018,Jan,8; 2017,Dec,8; 2017,Jan,8; 2016,Jan,13; 2015,Jan,16; 2014,Oct,14; 2014,Aug,5; 2014,Jan,11

00860 Anesthesia for extraperitoneal procedures in lower abdomen, including urinary tract; not otherwise specified
0.00 0.00 FUD XXX N
AMA: 2018,Jan,8; 2017,Dec,8; 2017,Jan,8; 2016,Jan,13; 2015,Jan,16; 2014,Aug,5; 2014,Jan,11

00862 renal procedures, including upper one-third of ureter, or donor nephrectomy
0.00 0.00 FUD XXX N
AMA: 2018,Jan,8; 2017,Dec,8; 2017,Jan,8; 2016,Jan,13; 2015,Jan,16; 2014,Aug,5; 2014,Jan,11

00864 total cystectomy
0.00 0.00 FUD XXX C
AMA: 2018,Jan,8; 2017,Dec,8; 2017,Jan,8; 2016,Jan,13; 2015,Jan,16; 2014,Aug,5; 2014,Jan,11

00865 radical prostatectomy (suprapubic, retropubic) ♂
0.00 0.00 FUD XXX C
AMA: 2018,Jan,8; 2017,Dec,8; 2017,Jan,8; 2016,Jan,13; 2015,Jan,16; 2014,Aug,5; 2014,Jan,11

00866 adrenalectomy
0.00 0.00 FUD XXX C
AMA: 2018,Jan,8; 2017,Dec,8; 2017,Jan,8; 2016,Jan,13; 2015,Jan,16; 2014,Aug,5; 2014,Jan,11

00868 renal transplant (recipient)
EXCLUDES *Anesthesia for donor nephrectomy (00862)*
Physiological support during kidney harvest (01990)
0.00 0.00 FUD XXX C
AMA: 2018,Jan,8; 2017,Dec,8; 2017,Jan,8; 2016,Jan,13; 2015,Jan,16; 2014,Aug,5; 2014,Jan,11

00870 cystolithotomy
0.00 0.00 FUD XXX N
AMA: 2018,Jan,8; 2017,Dec,8; 2017,Jan,8; 2016,Jan,13; 2015,Jan,16; 2014,Aug,5; 2014,Jan,11

00872 Anesthesia for lithotripsy, extracorporeal shock wave; with water bath
0.00 0.00 FUD XXX N
AMA: 2018,Jan,8; 2017,Dec,8; 2017,Jan,8; 2016,Jan,13; 2015,Jan,16; 2014,Aug,5; 2014,Jan,11

00873 without water bath
0.00 0.00 FUD XXX N
AMA: 2018,Jan,8; 2017,Dec,8; 2017,Jan,8; 2016,Jan,13; 2015,Jan,16; 2014,Aug,5; 2014,Jan,11

00880 Anesthesia for procedures on major lower abdominal vessels; not otherwise specified
0.00 0.00 FUD XXX N
AMA: 2018,Jan,8; 2017,Dec,8; 2017,Jan,8; 2016,Jan,13; 2015,Jan,16; 2014,Aug,5; 2014,Jan,11

00882 inferior vena cava ligation
0.00 0.00 FUD XXX C
AMA: 2018,Jan,8; 2017,Dec,8; 2017,Jan,8; 2016,Jan,13; 2015,Jan,16; 2014,Aug,5; 2014,Jan,11

00902-00952 Anesthesia for Genitourinary Procedures

CMS: 100-04,12,140.1 Qualified Nonphysician Anesthetists; 100-04,12,140.3 Payment for Qualified Nonphysician Anesthetists; 100-04,12,140.3.3 Billing Modifiers; 100-04,12,140.3.4 General Billing Instructions; 100-04,12,140.4.1 Anesthesiologist/Qualified Nonphysican Anesthetist; 100-04,12,140.4.2 Anesthetist and Anesthesiologist in a Single Procedure; 100-04,12,140.4.3 Payment for Medical /Surgical Services by CRNAs; 100-04,12,140.4.4 Conversion Factors for Anesthesia Services; 100-04,12,140.5 Payment for Anesthesia Services Furnished by a Teaching CRNA; 100-04,4,250.3.2 Anesthesia in a Hospital Outpatient Setting

EXCLUDES *Procedures on perineal skin, muscles, and nerves (00300, 00400)*

00902 Anesthesia for; anorectal procedure
0.00 0.00 FUD XXX N
AMA: 2018,Jan,8; 2017,Dec,8; 2017,Jan,8; 2016,Jan,13; 2015,Jan,16; 2014,Aug,5; 2014,Jan,11

00904 radical perineal procedure
0.00 0.00 FUD XXX C
AMA: 2018,Jan,8; 2017,Dec,8; 2017,Jan,8; 2016,Jan,13; 2015,Jan,16; 2014,Aug,5; 2014,Jan,11

00906 vulvectomy ♀
0.00 0.00 FUD XXX N
AMA: 2018,Jan,8; 2017,Dec,8; 2017,Jan,8; 2016,Jan,13; 2015,Jan,16; 2014,Aug,5; 2014,Jan,11

00908 perineal prostatectomy ♂
0.00 0.00 FUD XXX C
AMA: 2018,Jan,8; 2017,Dec,8; 2017,Jan,8; 2016,Jan,13; 2015,Jan,16; 2014,Aug,5; 2014,Jan,11

00910 Anesthesia for transurethral procedures (including urethrocystoscopy); not otherwise specified
0.00 0.00 FUD XXX N
AMA: 2018,Jan,8; 2017,Dec,8; 2017,Jan,8; 2016,Jan,13; 2015,Jan,16; 2014,Aug,5; 2014,Jan,11

00912 transurethral resection of bladder tumor(s)
0.00 0.00 FUD XXX N
AMA: 2018,Jan,8; 2017,Dec,8; 2017,Jan,8; 2016,Jan,13; 2015,Jan,16; 2014,Aug,5; 2014,Jan,11

00914 transurethral resection of prostate ♂
0.00 0.00 FUD XXX N
AMA: 2018,Jan,8; 2017,Dec,8; 2017,Jan,8; 2016,Jan,13; 2015,Jan,16; 2014,Aug,5; 2014,Jan,11

00916 post-transurethral resection bleeding
0.00 0.00 FUD XXX N
AMA: 2018,Jan,8; 2017,Dec,8; 2017,Jan,8; 2016,Jan,13; 2015,Jan,16; 2014,Aug,5; 2014,Jan,11

00918 with fragmentation, manipulation and/or removal of ureteral calculus
0.00 0.00 FUD XXX N
AMA: 2018,Jan,8; 2017,Dec,8; 2017,Jan,8; 2016,Jan,13; 2015,Jan,16; 2014,Aug,5; 2014,Jan,11

00920 Anesthesia for procedures on male genitalia (including open urethral procedures); not otherwise specified ♂
0.00 0.00 FUD XXX N
AMA: 2018,Jan,8; 2017,Dec,8; 2017,Jan,8; 2016,Jan,13; 2015,Jan,16; 2014,Aug,5; 2014,Jan,11

00921 vasectomy, unilateral or bilateral ♂
0.00 0.00 FUD XXX N
AMA: 2018,Jan,8; 2017,Dec,8; 2017,Jan,8; 2016,Jan,13; 2015,Jan,16; 2014,Aug,5; 2014,Jan,11

00922 seminal vesicles ♂
0.00 0.00 FUD XXX N
AMA: 2018,Jan,8; 2017,Dec,8; 2017,Jan,8; 2016,Jan,13; 2015,Jan,16; 2014,Aug,5; 2014,Jan,11

00924 undescended testis, unilateral or bilateral ♂
0.00 0.00 FUD XXX N
AMA: 2018,Jan,8; 2017,Dec,8; 2017,Jan,8; 2016,Jan,13; 2015,Jan,16; 2014,Aug,5; 2014,Jan,11

00926 radical orchiectomy, inguinal ♂
0.00 0.00 FUD XXX N
AMA: 2018,Jan,8; 2017,Dec,8; 2017,Jan,8; 2016,Jan,13; 2015,Jan,16; 2014,Aug,5; 2014,Jan,11

00928 radical orchiectomy, abdominal ♂
0.00 0.00 FUD XXX N
AMA: 2018,Jan,8; 2017,Dec,8; 2017,Jan,8; 2016,Jan,13; 2015,Jan,16; 2014,Aug,5; 2014,Jan,11

00930 orchiopexy, unilateral or bilateral ♂
0.00 0.00 FUD XXX N
AMA: 2018,Jan,8; 2017,Dec,8; 2017,Jan,8; 2016,Jan,13; 2015,Jan,16; 2014,Aug,5; 2014,Jan,11

00932 complete amputation of penis ♂
0.00 0.00 FUD XXX C
AMA: 2018,Jan,8; 2017,Dec,8; 2017,Jan,8; 2016,Jan,13; 2015,Jan,16; 2014,Aug,5; 2014,Jan,11

00934 radical amputation of penis with bilateral inguinal lymphadenectomy ♂
0.00 0.00 FUD XXX C
AMA: 2018,Jan,8; 2017,Dec,8; 2017,Jan,8; 2016,Jan,13; 2015,Jan,16; 2014,Aug,5; 2014,Jan,11

00936 radical amputation of penis with bilateral inguinal and iliac lymphadenectomy ♂
0.00 0.00 FUD XXX C
AMA: 2018,Jan,8; 2017,Dec,8; 2017,Jan,8; 2016,Jan,13; 2015,Jan,16; 2014,Aug,5; 2014,Jan,11

00938 insertion of penile prosthesis (perineal approach) ♂
0.00 0.00 FUD XXX N
AMA: 2018,Jan,8; 2017,Dec,8; 2017,Jan,8; 2016,Jan,13; 2015,Jan,16; 2014,Aug,5; 2014,Jan,11

00940 Anesthesia for vaginal procedures (including biopsy of labia, vagina, cervix or endometrium); not otherwise specified ♀
0.00 0.00 FUD XXX N
AMA: 2018,Jan,8; 2017,Dec,8; 2017,Jan,8; 2016,Jan,13; 2015,Jan,16; 2014,Aug,5; 2014,Jan,11

00942 colpotomy, vaginectomy, colporrhaphy, and open urethral procedures ♀
0.00 0.00 FUD XXX N
AMA: 2018,Jan,8; 2017,Dec,8; 2017,Jan,8; 2016,Jan,13; 2015,Jan,16; 2014,Aug,5; 2014,Jan,11

00944 vaginal hysterectomy ♀
0.00 0.00 FUD XXX C
AMA: 2018,Jan,8; 2017,Dec,8; 2017,Jan,8; 2016,Jan,13; 2015,Jan,16; 2014,Aug,5; 2014,Jan,11

00948 cervical cerclage ♀
0.00 0.00 FUD XXX N
AMA: 2018,Jan,8; 2017,Dec,8; 2017,Jan,8; 2016,Jan,13; 2015,Jan,16; 2014,Aug,5; 2014,Jan,11

00950 **culdoscopy** ♀ N
0.00 0.00 FUD XXX
AMA: 2018,Jan,8; 2017,Dec,8; 2017,Jan,8; 2016,Jan,13; 2015,Jan,16; 2014,Aug,5; 2014,Jan,11

00952 **hysteroscopy and/or hysterosalpingography** ♀ N
0.00 0.00 FUD XXX
AMA: 2018,Jan,8; 2017,Dec,8; 2017,Jan,8; 2016,Jan,13; 2015,Jan,16; 2014,Aug,5; 2014,Jan,11

01112-01522 Anesthesia for Lower Extremity Procedures

CMS: 100-04,12,140.1 Qualified Nonphysician Anesthetists; 100-04,12,140.3 Payment for Qualified Nonphysician Anesthetists; 100-04,12,140.3.3 Billing Modifiers; 100-04,12,140.3.4 General Billing Instructions; 100-04,12,140.4.1 Anesthesiologist/Qualified Nonphysican Anesthetist; 100-04,12,140.4.2 Anesthetist and Anesthesiologist in a Single Procedure; 100-04,12,140.4.3 Payment for Medical /Surgical Services by CRNAs; 100-04,12,140.4.4 Conversion Factors for Anesthesia Services; 100-04,12,140.5 Payment for Anesthesia Services Furnished by a Teaching CRNA; 100-04,4,250.3.2 Anesthesia in a Hospital Outpatient Setting

01112 **Anesthesia for bone marrow aspiration and/or biopsy, anterior or posterior iliac crest** N
0.00 0.00 FUD XXX
AMA: 2018,Jan,8; 2017,Dec,8; 2017,Jan,8; 2016,Jan,13; 2015,Jan,16; 2014,Aug,5; 2014,Jan,11

01120 **Anesthesia for procedures on bony pelvis** N
0.00 0.00 FUD XXX
AMA: 2018,Jan,8; 2017,Dec,8; 2017,Jan,8; 2016,Jan,13; 2015,Jan,16; 2014,Aug,5; 2014,Jan,11

01130 **Anesthesia for body cast application or revision** N
0.00 0.00 FUD XXX
AMA: 2018,Jan,8; 2017,Dec,8; 2017,Jan,8; 2016,Jan,13; 2015,Jan,16; 2014,Aug,5; 2014,Jan,11

01140 **Anesthesia for interpelviabdominal (hindquarter) amputation** C
0.00 0.00 FUD XXX
AMA: 2018,Jan,8; 2017,Dec,8; 2017,Jan,8; 2016,Jan,13; 2015,Jan,16; 2014,Aug,5; 2014,Jan,11

01150 **Anesthesia for radical procedures for tumor of pelvis, except hindquarter amputation** C
0.00 0.00 FUD XXX
AMA: 2018,Jan,8; 2017,Dec,8; 2017,Jan,8; 2016,Jan,13; 2015,Jan,16; 2014,Aug,5; 2014,Jan,11

01160 **Anesthesia for closed procedures involving symphysis pubis or sacroiliac joint** N
0.00 0.00 FUD XXX
AMA: 2018,Jan,8; 2017,Dec,8; 2017,Jan,8; 2016,Jan,13; 2015,Jan,16; 2014,Aug,5; 2014,Jan,11

01170 **Anesthesia for open procedures involving symphysis pubis or sacroiliac joint** N
0.00 0.00 FUD XXX
AMA: 2018,Jan,8; 2017,Dec,8; 2017,Jan,8; 2016,Jan,13; 2015,Jan,16; 2014,Aug,5; 2014,Jan,11

01173 **Anesthesia for open repair of fracture disruption of pelvis or column fracture involving acetabulum** N
0.00 0.00 FUD XXX
AMA: 2018,Jan,8; 2017,Dec,8; 2017,Jan,8; 2016,Jan,13; 2015,Jan,16; 2014,Aug,5; 2014,Jan,11

01200 **Anesthesia for all closed procedures involving hip joint** N
0.00 0.00 FUD XXX
AMA: 2018,Jan,8; 2017,Dec,8; 2017,Jan,8; 2016,Jan,13; 2015,Jan,16; 2014,Aug,5; 2014,Jan,11

01202 **Anesthesia for arthroscopic procedures of hip joint** N
0.00 0.00 FUD XXX
AMA: 2018,Jan,8; 2017,Dec,8; 2017,Jan,8; 2016,Jan,13; 2015,Jan,16; 2014,Aug,5; 2014,Jan,11

01210 **Anesthesia for open procedures involving hip joint; not otherwise specified** N
0.00 0.00 FUD XXX
AMA: 2018,Jan,8; 2017,Dec,8; 2017,Jan,8; 2016,Jan,13; 2015,Jan,16; 2014,Aug,5; 2014,Jan,11

01212 **hip disarticulation** C
0.00 0.00 FUD XXX
AMA: 2018,Jan,8; 2017,Dec,8; 2017,Jan,8; 2016,Jan,13; 2015,Jan,16; 2014,Aug,5; 2014,Jan,11

01214 **total hip arthroplasty** C
0.00 0.00 FUD XXX
AMA: 2018,Jan,8; 2017,Dec,8; 2017,Jan,8; 2016,Jan,13; 2015,Jan,16; 2014,Aug,5; 2014,Jan,11

01215 **revision of total hip arthroplasty** N
0.00 0.00 FUD XXX
AMA: 2018,Jan,8; 2017,Dec,8; 2017,Jan,8; 2016,Jan,13; 2015,Jan,16; 2014,Aug,5; 2014,Jan,11

01220 **Anesthesia for all closed procedures involving upper two-thirds of femur** N
0.00 0.00 FUD XXX
AMA: 2018,Jan,8; 2017,Dec,8; 2017,Jan,8; 2016,Jan,13; 2015,Jan,16; 2014,Aug,5; 2014,Jan,11

01230 **Anesthesia for open procedures involving upper two-thirds of femur; not otherwise specified** N
0.00 0.00 FUD XXX
AMA: 2018,Jan,8; 2017,Dec,8; 2017,Jan,8; 2016,Jan,13; 2015,Jan,16; 2014,Aug,5; 2014,Jan,11

01232 **amputation** C
0.00 0.00 FUD XXX
AMA: 2018,Jan,8; 2017,Dec,8; 2017,Jan,8; 2016,Jan,13; 2015,Jan,16; 2014,Aug,5; 2014,Jan,11

01234 **radical resection** C
0.00 0.00 FUD XXX
AMA: 2018,Jan,8; 2017,Dec,8; 2017,Jan,8; 2016,Jan,13; 2015,Jan,16; 2014,Aug,5; 2014,Jan,11

01250 **Anesthesia for all procedures on nerves, muscles, tendons, fascia, and bursae of upper leg** N
0.00 0.00 FUD XXX
AMA: 2018,Jan,8; 2017,Dec,8; 2017,Jan,8; 2016,Jan,13; 2015,Jan,16; 2014,Aug,5; 2014,Jan,11

01260 **Anesthesia for all procedures involving veins of upper leg, including exploration** N
0.00 0.00 FUD XXX
AMA: 2018,Jan,8; 2017,Dec,8; 2017,Jan,8; 2016,Jan,13; 2015,Jan,16; 2014,Aug,5; 2014,Jan,11

01270 **Anesthesia for procedures involving arteries of upper leg, including bypass graft; not otherwise specified** N
0.00 0.00 FUD XXX
AMA: 2018,Jan,8; 2017,Dec,8; 2017,Jan,8; 2016,Jan,13; 2015,Jan,16; 2014,Aug,5; 2014,Jan,11

01272 **femoral artery ligation** C
0.00 0.00 FUD XXX
AMA: 2018,Jan,8; 2017,Dec,8; 2017,Jan,8; 2016,Jan,13; 2015,Jan,16; 2014,Aug,5; 2014,Jan,11

01274 **femoral artery embolectomy** C
0.00 0.00 FUD XXX
AMA: 2018,Jan,8; 2017,Dec,8; 2017,Jan,8; 2016,Jan,13; 2015,Jan,16; 2014,Aug,5; 2014,Jan,11

01320 **Anesthesia for all procedures on nerves, muscles, tendons, fascia, and bursae of knee and/or popliteal area** N
0.00 0.00 FUD XXX
AMA: 2018,Jan,8; 2017,Dec,8; 2017,Jan,8; 2016,Jan,13; 2015,Jan,16; 2014,Aug,5; 2014,Jan,11

01340 **Anesthesia for all closed procedures on lower one-third of femur** N
0.00 0.00 FUD XXX
AMA: 2018,Jan,8; 2017,Dec,8; 2017,Jan,8; 2016,Jan,13; 2015,Jan,16; 2014,Aug,5; 2014,Jan,11

01360 **Anesthesia for all open procedures on lower one-third of femur** N
0.00 0.00 FUD XXX
AMA: 2018,Jan,8; 2017,Dec,8; 2017,Jan,8; 2016,Jan,13; 2015,Jan,16; 2014,Aug,5; 2014,Jan,11

01380 **Anesthesia for all closed procedures on knee joint**
0.00 0.00 **FUD** XXX N
AMA: 2018,Jan,8; 2017,Dec,8; 2017,Jan,8; 2016,Jan,13; 2015,Jan,16; 2014,Aug,5; 2014,Jan,11

01382 **Anesthesia for diagnostic arthroscopic procedures of knee joint**
0.00 0.00 **FUD** XXX N
AMA: 2018,Jan,8; 2017,Dec,8; 2017,Jan,8; 2016,Jan,13; 2015,Jan,16; 2014,Aug,5; 2014,Jan,11

01390 **Anesthesia for all closed procedures on upper ends of tibia, fibula, and/or patella**
0.00 0.00 **FUD** XXX N
AMA: 2018,Jan,8; 2017,Dec,8; 2017,Jan,8; 2016,Jan,13; 2015,Jan,16; 2014,Aug,5; 2014,Jan,11

01392 **Anesthesia for all open procedures on upper ends of tibia, fibula, and/or patella**
0.00 0.00 **FUD** XXX N
AMA: 2018,Jan,8; 2017,Dec,8; 2017,Jan,8; 2016,Jan,13; 2015,Jan,16; 2014,Aug,5; 2014,Jan,11

01400 **Anesthesia for open or surgical arthroscopic procedures on knee joint; not otherwise specified**
0.00 0.00 **FUD** XXX N
AMA: 2018,Jan,8; 2017,Dec,8; 2017,Jan,8; 2016,Jan,13; 2015,Jan,16; 2014,Aug,5; 2014,Jan,11

01402 **total knee arthroplasty**
0.00 0.00 **FUD** XXX C
AMA: 2018,Jan,8; 2017,Dec,8; 2017,Jan,8; 2016,Jan,13; 2015,Jan,16; 2014,Aug,5; 2014,Jan,11

01404 **disarticulation at knee**
0.00 0.00 **FUD** XXX C
AMA: 2018,Jan,8; 2017,Dec,8; 2017,Jan,8; 2016,Jan,13; 2015,Jan,16; 2014,Aug,5; 2014,Jan,11

01420 **Anesthesia for all cast applications, removal, or repair involving knee joint**
0.00 0.00 **FUD** XXX N
AMA: 2018,Jan,8; 2017,Dec,8; 2017,Jan,8; 2016,Jan,13; 2015,Jan,16; 2014,Aug,5; 2014,Jan,11

01430 **Anesthesia for procedures on veins of knee and popliteal area; not otherwise specified**
0.00 0.00 **FUD** XXX N
AMA: 2018,Jan,8; 2017,Dec,8; 2017,Jan,8; 2016,Jan,13; 2015,Jan,16; 2014,Aug,5; 2014,Jan,11

01432 **arteriovenous fistula**
0.00 0.00 **FUD** XXX N
AMA: 2018,Jan,8; 2017,Dec,8; 2017,Jan,8; 2016,Jan,13; 2015,Jan,16; 2014,Aug,5; 2014,Jan,11

01440 **Anesthesia for procedures on arteries of knee and popliteal area; not otherwise specified**
0.00 0.00 **FUD** XXX N
AMA: 2018,Jan,8; 2017,Dec,8; 2017,Jan,8; 2016,Jan,13; 2015,Jan,16; 2014,Aug,5; 2014,Jan,11

01442 **popliteal thromboendarterectomy, with or without patch graft**
0.00 0.00 **FUD** XXX C
AMA: 2018,Jan,8; 2017,Dec,8; 2017,Jan,8; 2016,Jan,13; 2015,Jan,16; 2014,Aug,5; 2014,Jan,11

01444 **popliteal excision and graft or repair for occlusion or aneurysm**
0.00 0.00 **FUD** XXX C
AMA: 2018,Jan,8; 2017,Dec,8; 2017,Jan,8; 2016,Jan,13; 2015,Jan,16; 2014,Aug,5; 2014,Jan,11

01462 **Anesthesia for all closed procedures on lower leg, ankle, and foot**
0.00 0.00 **FUD** XXX N
AMA: 2018,Jan,8; 2017,Dec,8; 2017,Jan,8; 2016,Jan,13; 2015,Jan,16; 2014,Aug,5; 2014,Jan,11

01464 **Anesthesia for arthroscopic procedures of ankle and/or foot**
0.00 0.00 **FUD** XXX N
AMA: 2018,Jan,8; 2017,Dec,8; 2017,Jan,8; 2016,Jan,13; 2015,Jan,16; 2014,Aug,5; 2014,Jan,11

01470 **Anesthesia for procedures on nerves, muscles, tendons, and fascia of lower leg, ankle, and foot; not otherwise specified**
0.00 0.00 **FUD** XXX N
AMA: 2018,Jan,8; 2017,Dec,8; 2017,Jan,8; 2016,Jan,13; 2015,Jan,16; 2014,Aug,5; 2014,Jan,11

01472 **repair of ruptured Achilles tendon, with or without graft**
0.00 0.00 **FUD** XXX N
AMA: 2018,Jan,8; 2017,Dec,8; 2017,Jan,8; 2016,Jan,13; 2015,Jan,16; 2014,Aug,5; 2014,Jan,11

01474 **gastrocnemius recession (eg, Strayer procedure)**
0.00 0.00 **FUD** XXX N
AMA: 2018,Jan,8; 2017,Dec,8; 2017,Jan,8; 2016,Jan,13; 2015,Jan,16; 2014,Aug,5; 2014,Jan,11

01480 **Anesthesia for open procedures on bones of lower leg, ankle, and foot; not otherwise specified**
0.00 0.00 **FUD** XXX N
AMA: 2018,Jan,8; 2017,Dec,8; 2017,Jan,8; 2016,Jan,13; 2015,Jan,16; 2014,Aug,5; 2014,Jan,11

01482 **radical resection (including below knee amputation)**
0.00 0.00 **FUD** XXX N
AMA: 2018,Jan,8; 2017,Dec,8; 2017,Jan,8; 2016,Jan,13; 2015,Jan,16; 2014,Aug,5; 2014,Jan,11

01484 **osteotomy or osteoplasty of tibia and/or fibula**
0.00 0.00 **FUD** XXX N
AMA: 2018,Jan,8; 2017,Dec,8; 2017,Jan,8; 2016,Jan,13; 2015,Jan,16; 2014,Aug,5; 2014,Jan,11

01486 **total ankle replacement**
0.00 0.00 **FUD** XXX C
AMA: 2018,Jan,8; 2017,Dec,8; 2017,Jan,8; 2016,Jan,13; 2015,Jan,16; 2014,Aug,5; 2014,Jan,11

01490 **Anesthesia for lower leg cast application, removal, or repair**
0.00 0.00 **FUD** XXX N
AMA: 2018,Jan,8; 2017,Dec,8; 2017,Jan,8; 2016,Jan,13; 2015,Jan,16; 2014,Aug,5; 2014,Jan,11

01500 **Anesthesia for procedures on arteries of lower leg, including bypass graft; not otherwise specified**
0.00 0.00 **FUD** XXX N
AMA: 2018,Jan,8; 2017,Dec,8; 2017,Jan,8; 2016,Jan,13; 2015,Jan,16; 2014,Aug,5; 2014,Jan,11

01502 **embolectomy, direct or with catheter**
0.00 0.00 **FUD** XXX C
AMA: 2018,Jan,8; 2017,Dec,8; 2017,Jan,8; 2016,Jan,13; 2015,Jan,16; 2014,Aug,5; 2014,Jan,11

01520 **Anesthesia for procedures on veins of lower leg; not otherwise specified**
0.00 0.00 **FUD** XXX N
AMA: 2018,Jan,8; 2017,Dec,8; 2017,Jan,8; 2016,Jan,13; 2015,Jan,16; 2014,Aug,5; 2014,Jan,11

01522 **venous thrombectomy, direct or with catheter**
0.00 0.00 **FUD** XXX N
AMA: 2018,Jan,8; 2017,Dec,8; 2017,Jan,8; 2016,Jan,13; 2015,Jan,16; 2014,Aug,5; 2014,Jan,11

01610-01680 Anesthesia for Shoulder Procedures

CMS: 100-04,12,140.1 Qualified Nonphysician Anesthetists; 100-04,12,140.3 Payment for Qualified Nonphysician Anesthetists; 100-04,12,140.3.3 Billing Modifiers; 100-04,12,140.3.4 General Billing Instructions; 100-04,12,140.4.1 Anesthesiologist/Qualified Nonphysican Anesthetist; 100-04,12,140.4.2 Anesthetist and Anesthesiologist in a Single Procedure; 100-04,12,140.4.3 Payment for Medical /Surgical Services by CRNAs; 100-04,12,140.4.4 Conversion Factors for Anesthesia Services; 100-04,12,140.5 Payment for Anesthesia Services Furnished by a Teaching CRNA; 100-04,4,250.3.2 Anesthesia in a Hospital Outpatient Setting

INCLUDES Acromioclavicular joint
Humeral head and neck
Shoulder joint
Sternoclavicular joint

01610 Anesthesia for all procedures on nerves, muscles, tendons, fascia, and bursae of shoulder and axilla
0.00 0.00 FUD XXX N
AMA: 2018,Jan,8; 2017,Dec,8; 2017,Jan,8; 2016,Jan,13; 2015,Jan,16; 2014,Aug,5; 2014,Jan,11

01620 Anesthesia for all closed procedures on humeral head and neck, sternoclavicular joint, acromioclavicular joint, and shoulder joint
0.00 0.00 FUD XXX N
AMA: 2018,Jan,8; 2017,Dec,8; 2017,Jan,8; 2016,Jan,13; 2015,Jan,16; 2014,Aug,5; 2014,Jan,11

01622 Anesthesia for diagnostic arthroscopic procedures of shoulder joint
0.00 0.00 FUD XXX N
AMA: 2018,Jan,8; 2017,Dec,8; 2017,Jan,8; 2016,Jan,13; 2015,Jan,16; 2014,Aug,5; 2014,Jan,11

01630 Anesthesia for open or surgical arthroscopic procedures on humeral head and neck, sternoclavicular joint, acromioclavicular joint, and shoulder joint; not otherwise specified
0.00 0.00 FUD XXX N
AMA: 2018,Jan,8; 2017,Dec,8; 2017,Jan,8; 2016,Jan,13; 2015,Jan,16; 2014,Aug,5; 2014,Jan,11

01634 shoulder disarticulation
0.00 0.00 FUD XXX C
AMA: 2018,Jan,8; 2017,Dec,8; 2017,Jan,8; 2016,Jan,13; 2015,Jan,16; 2014,Aug,5; 2014,Jan,11

01636 interthoracoscapular (forequarter) amputation
0.00 0.00 FUD XXX C
AMA: 2018,Jan,8; 2017,Dec,8; 2017,Jan,8; 2016,Jan,13; 2015,Jan,16; 2014,Aug,5; 2014,Jan,11

01638 total shoulder replacement
0.00 0.00 FUD XXX C
AMA: 2018,Jan,8; 2017,Dec,8; 2017,Jan,8; 2016,Jan,13; 2015,Jan,16; 2014,Aug,5; 2014,Jan,11

01650 Anesthesia for procedures on arteries of shoulder and axilla; not otherwise specified
0.00 0.00 FUD XXX N
AMA: 2018,Jan,8; 2017,Dec,8; 2017,Jan,8; 2016,Jan,13; 2015,Jan,16; 2014,Aug,5; 2014,Jan,11

01652 axillary-brachial aneurysm
0.00 0.00 FUD XXX C
AMA: 2018,Jan,8; 2017,Dec,8; 2017,Jan,8; 2016,Jan,13; 2015,Jan,16; 2014,Aug,5; 2014,Jan,11

01654 bypass graft
0.00 0.00 FUD XXX C
AMA: 2018,Jan,8; 2017,Dec,8; 2017,Jan,8; 2016,Jan,13; 2015,Jan,16; 2014,Aug,5; 2014,Jan,11

01656 axillary-femoral bypass graft
0.00 0.00 FUD XXX C
AMA: 2018,Jan,8; 2017,Dec,8; 2017,Jan,8; 2016,Jan,13; 2015,Jan,16; 2014,Aug,5; 2014,Jan,11

01670 Anesthesia for all procedures on veins of shoulder and axilla
0.00 0.00 FUD XXX N
AMA: 2018,Jan,8; 2017,Dec,8; 2017,Jan,8; 2016,Jan,13; 2015,Jan,16; 2014,Aug,5; 2014,Jan,11

01680 Anesthesia for shoulder cast application, removal or repair, not otherwise specified
0.00 0.00 FUD XXX N
AMA: 2018,Jan,8; 2017,Dec,8; 2017,Jan,8; 2016,Jan,13; 2015,Jan,16; 2014,Aug,5; 2014,Jan,11

01710-01860 Anesthesia for Upper Extremity Procedures

CMS: 100-04,12,140.1 Qualified Nonphysician Anesthetists; 100-04,12,140.3 Payment for Qualified Nonphysician Anesthetists; 100-04,12,140.3.3 Billing Modifiers; 100-04,12,140.3.4 General Billing Instructions; 100-04,12,140.4.1 Anesthesiologist/Qualified Nonphysican Anesthetist; 100-04,12,140.4.2 Anesthetist and Anesthesiologist in a Single Procedure; 100-04,12,140.4.3 Payment for Medical /Surgical Services by CRNAs; 100-04,12,140.4.4 Conversion Factors for Anesthesia Services; 100-04,12,140.5 Payment for Anesthesia Services Furnished by a Teaching CRNA; 100-04,4,250.3.2 Anesthesia in a Hospital Outpatient Setting

01710 Anesthesia for procedures on nerves, muscles, tendons, fascia, and bursae of upper arm and elbow; not otherwise specified
0.00 0.00 FUD XXX N
AMA: 2018,Jan,8; 2017,Dec,8; 2017,Jan,8; 2016,Jan,13; 2015,Jan,16; 2014,Aug,5; 2014,Jan,11

01712 tenotomy, elbow to shoulder, open
0.00 0.00 FUD XXX N
AMA: 2018,Jan,8; 2017,Dec,8; 2017,Jan,8; 2016,Jan,13; 2015,Jan,16; 2014,Aug,5; 2014,Jan,11

01714 tenoplasty, elbow to shoulder
0.00 0.00 FUD XXX N
AMA: 2018,Jan,8; 2017,Dec,8; 2017,Jan,8; 2016,Jan,13; 2015,Jan,16; 2014,Aug,5; 2014,Jan,11

01716 tenodesis, rupture of long tendon of biceps
0.00 0.00 FUD XXX N
AMA: 2018,Jan,8; 2017,Dec,8; 2017,Jan,8; 2016,Jan,13; 2015,Jan,16; 2014,Aug,5; 2014,Jan,11

01730 Anesthesia for all closed procedures on humerus and elbow
0.00 0.00 FUD XXX N
AMA: 2018,Jan,8; 2017,Dec,8; 2017,Jan,8; 2016,Jan,13; 2015,Jan,16; 2014,Aug,5; 2014,Jan,11

01732 Anesthesia for diagnostic arthroscopic procedures of elbow joint
0.00 0.00 FUD XXX N
AMA: 2018,Jan,8; 2017,Dec,8; 2017,Jan,8; 2016,Jan,13; 2015,Jan,16; 2014,Aug,5; 2014,Jan,11

01740 Anesthesia for open or surgical arthroscopic procedures of the elbow; not otherwise specified
0.00 0.00 FUD XXX N
AMA: 2018,Jan,8; 2017,Dec,8; 2017,Jan,8; 2016,Jan,13; 2015,Jan,16; 2014,Aug,5; 2014,Jan,11

01742 osteotomy of humerus
0.00 0.00 FUD XXX N
AMA: 2018,Jan,8; 2017,Dec,8; 2017,Jan,8; 2016,Jan,13; 2015,Jan,16; 2014,Aug,5; 2014,Jan,11

01744 repair of nonunion or malunion of humerus
0.00 0.00 FUD XXX N
AMA: 2018,Jan,8; 2017,Dec,8; 2017,Jan,8; 2016,Jan,13; 2015,Jan,16; 2014,Aug,5; 2014,Jan,11

01756 radical procedures
0.00 0.00 FUD XXX C
AMA: 2018,Jan,8; 2017,Dec,8; 2017,Jan,8; 2016,Jan,13; 2015,Jan,16; 2014,Aug,5; 2014,Jan,11

01758 excision of cyst or tumor of humerus
0.00 0.00 FUD XXX N
AMA: 2018,Jan,8; 2017,Dec,8; 2017,Jan,8; 2016,Jan,13; 2015,Jan,16; 2014,Aug,5; 2014,Jan,11

01760 total elbow replacement
0.00 0.00 FUD XXX N
AMA: 2018,Jan,8; 2017,Dec,8; 2017,Jan,8; 2016,Jan,13; 2015,Jan,16; 2014,Aug,5; 2014,Jan,11

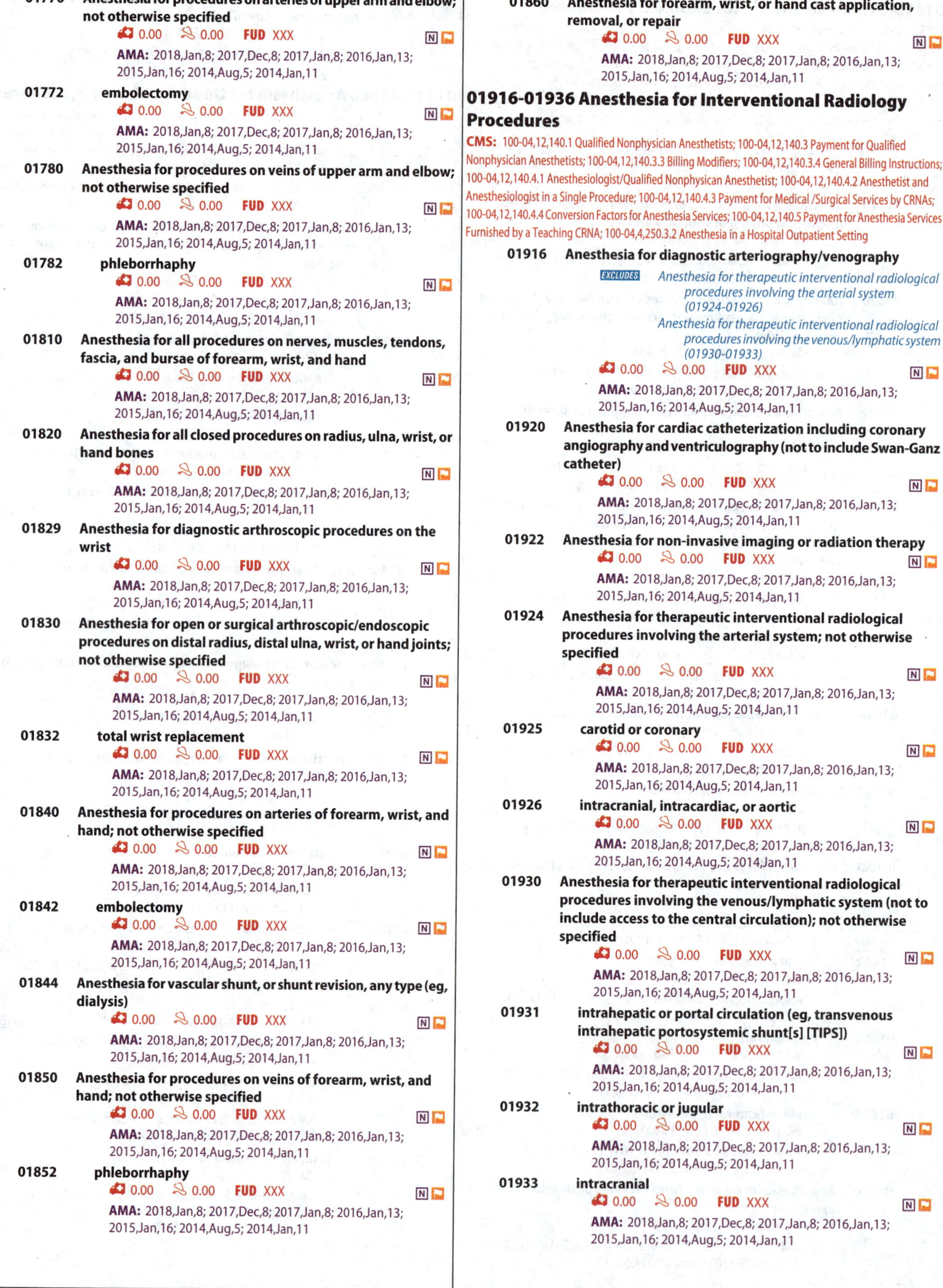

01770 **Anesthesia for procedures on arteries of upper arm and elbow; not otherwise specified**
0.00 0.00 FUD XXX
AMA: 2018,Jan,8; 2017,Dec,8; 2017,Jan,8; 2016,Jan,13; 2015,Jan,16; 2014,Aug,5; 2014,Jan,11

01772 **embolectomy**
0.00 0.00 FUD XXX
AMA: 2018,Jan,8; 2017,Dec,8; 2017,Jan,8; 2016,Jan,13; 2015,Jan,16; 2014,Aug,5; 2014,Jan,11

01780 **Anesthesia for procedures on veins of upper arm and elbow; not otherwise specified**
0.00 0.00 FUD XXX
AMA: 2018,Jan,8; 2017,Dec,8; 2017,Jan,8; 2016,Jan,13; 2015,Jan,16; 2014,Aug,5; 2014,Jan,11

01782 **phleborrhaphy**
0.00 0.00 FUD XXX
AMA: 2018,Jan,8; 2017,Dec,8; 2017,Jan,8; 2016,Jan,13; 2015,Jan,16; 2014,Aug,5; 2014,Jan,11

01810 **Anesthesia for all procedures on nerves, muscles, tendons, fascia, and bursae of forearm, wrist, and hand**
0.00 0.00 FUD XXX
AMA: 2018,Jan,8; 2017,Dec,8; 2017,Jan,8; 2016,Jan,13; 2015,Jan,16; 2014,Aug,5; 2014,Jan,11

01820 **Anesthesia for all closed procedures on radius, ulna, wrist, or hand bones**
0.00 0.00 FUD XXX
AMA: 2018,Jan,8; 2017,Dec,8; 2017,Jan,8; 2016,Jan,13; 2015,Jan,16; 2014,Aug,5; 2014,Jan,11

01829 **Anesthesia for diagnostic arthroscopic procedures on the wrist**
0.00 0.00 FUD XXX
AMA: 2018,Jan,8; 2017,Dec,8; 2017,Jan,8; 2016,Jan,13; 2015,Jan,16; 2014,Aug,5; 2014,Jan,11

01830 **Anesthesia for open or surgical arthroscopic/endoscopic procedures on distal radius, distal ulna, wrist, or hand joints; not otherwise specified**
0.00 0.00 FUD XXX
AMA: 2018,Jan,8; 2017,Dec,8; 2017,Jan,8; 2016,Jan,13; 2015,Jan,16; 2014,Aug,5; 2014,Jan,11

01832 **total wrist replacement**
0.00 0.00 FUD XXX
AMA: 2018,Jan,8; 2017,Dec,8; 2017,Jan,8; 2016,Jan,13; 2015,Jan,16; 2014,Aug,5; 2014,Jan,11

01840 **Anesthesia for procedures on arteries of forearm, wrist, and hand; not otherwise specified**
0.00 0.00 FUD XXX
AMA: 2018,Jan,8; 2017,Dec,8; 2017,Jan,8; 2016,Jan,13; 2015,Jan,16; 2014,Aug,5; 2014,Jan,11

01842 **embolectomy**
0.00 0.00 FUD XXX
AMA: 2018,Jan,8; 2017,Dec,8; 2017,Jan,8; 2016,Jan,13; 2015,Jan,16; 2014,Aug,5; 2014,Jan,11

01844 **Anesthesia for vascular shunt, or shunt revision, any type (eg, dialysis)**
0.00 0.00 FUD XXX
AMA: 2018,Jan,8; 2017,Dec,8; 2017,Jan,8; 2016,Jan,13; 2015,Jan,16; 2014,Aug,5; 2014,Jan,11

01850 **Anesthesia for procedures on veins of forearm, wrist, and hand; not otherwise specified**
0.00 0.00 FUD XXX
AMA: 2018,Jan,8; 2017,Dec,8; 2017,Jan,8; 2016,Jan,13; 2015,Jan,16; 2014,Aug,5; 2014,Jan,11

01852 **phleborrhaphy**
0.00 0.00 FUD XXX
AMA: 2018,Jan,8; 2017,Dec,8; 2017,Jan,8; 2016,Jan,13; 2015,Jan,16; 2014,Aug,5; 2014,Jan,11

01860 **Anesthesia for forearm, wrist, or hand cast application, removal, or repair**
0.00 0.00 FUD XXX
AMA: 2018,Jan,8; 2017,Dec,8; 2017,Jan,8; 2016,Jan,13; 2015,Jan,16; 2014,Aug,5; 2014,Jan,11

01916-01936 Anesthesia for Interventional Radiology Procedures

CMS: 100-04,12,140.1 Qualified Nonphysician Anesthetists; 100-04,12,140.3 Payment for Qualified Nonphysician Anesthetists; 100-04,12,140.3.3 Billing Modifiers; 100-04,12,140.3.4 General Billing Instructions; 100-04,12,140.4.1 Anesthesiologist/Qualified Nonphysican Anesthetist; 100-04,12,140.4.2 Anesthetist and Anesthesiologist in a Single Procedure; 100-04,12,140.4.3 Payment for Medical /Surgical Services by CRNAs; 100-04,12,140.4.4 Conversion Factors for Anesthesia Services; 100-04,12,140.5 Payment for Anesthesia Services Furnished by a Teaching CRNA; 100-04,4,250.3.2 Anesthesia in a Hospital Outpatient Setting

01916 **Anesthesia for diagnostic arteriography/venography**
EXCLUDES *Anesthesia for therapeutic interventional radiological procedures involving the arterial system (01924-01926)*
Anesthesia for therapeutic interventional radiological procedures involving the venous/lymphatic system (01930-01933)
0.00 0.00 FUD XXX
AMA: 2018,Jan,8; 2017,Dec,8; 2017,Jan,8; 2016,Jan,13; 2015,Jan,16; 2014,Aug,5; 2014,Jan,11

01920 **Anesthesia for cardiac catheterization including coronary angiography and ventriculography (not to include Swan-Ganz catheter)**
0.00 0.00 FUD XXX
AMA: 2018,Jan,8; 2017,Dec,8; 2017,Jan,8; 2016,Jan,13; 2015,Jan,16; 2014,Aug,5; 2014,Jan,11

01922 **Anesthesia for non-invasive imaging or radiation therapy**
0.00 0.00 FUD XXX
AMA: 2018,Jan,8; 2017,Dec,8; 2017,Jan,8; 2016,Jan,13; 2015,Jan,16; 2014,Aug,5; 2014,Jan,11

01924 **Anesthesia for therapeutic interventional radiological procedures involving the arterial system; not otherwise specified**
0.00 0.00 FUD XXX
AMA: 2018,Jan,8; 2017,Dec,8; 2017,Jan,8; 2016,Jan,13; 2015,Jan,16; 2014,Aug,5; 2014,Jan,11

01925 **carotid or coronary**
0.00 0.00 FUD XXX
AMA: 2018,Jan,8; 2017,Dec,8; 2017,Jan,8; 2016,Jan,13; 2015,Jan,16; 2014,Aug,5; 2014,Jan,11

01926 **intracranial, intracardiac, or aortic**
0.00 0.00 FUD XXX
AMA: 2018,Jan,8; 2017,Dec,8; 2017,Jan,8; 2016,Jan,13; 2015,Jan,16; 2014,Aug,5; 2014,Jan,11

01930 **Anesthesia for therapeutic interventional radiological procedures involving the venous/lymphatic system (not to include access to the central circulation); not otherwise specified**
0.00 0.00 FUD XXX
AMA: 2018,Jan,8; 2017,Dec,8; 2017,Jan,8; 2016,Jan,13; 2015,Jan,16; 2014,Aug,5; 2014,Jan,11

01931 **intrahepatic or portal circulation (eg, transvenous intrahepatic portosystemic shunt[s] [TIPS])**
0.00 0.00 FUD XXX
AMA: 2018,Jan,8; 2017,Dec,8; 2017,Jan,8; 2016,Jan,13; 2015,Jan,16; 2014,Aug,5; 2014,Jan,11

01932 **intrathoracic or jugular**
0.00 0.00 FUD XXX
AMA: 2018,Jan,8; 2017,Dec,8; 2017,Jan,8; 2016,Jan,13; 2015,Jan,16; 2014,Aug,5; 2014,Jan,11

01933 **intracranial**
0.00 0.00 FUD XXX
AMA: 2018,Jan,8; 2017,Dec,8; 2017,Jan,8; 2016,Jan,13; 2015,Jan,16; 2014,Aug,5; 2014,Jan,11

01935 **Anesthesia for percutaneous image guided procedures on the spine and spinal cord; diagnostic**
0.00 0.00 FUD XXX N
AMA: 2018,Jan,8; 2017,Dec,8; 2017,Jan,8; 2016,Jan,13; 2015,Jan,16; 2014,Aug,5; 2014,Jan,11

01936 **therapeutic**
0.00 0.00 FUD XXX N
AMA: 2018,Jan,8; 2017,Dec,8; 2017,Jan,8; 2016,Jan,13; 2015,Jan,16; 2014,Aug,5; 2014,Jan,11

01951-01953 Anesthesia for Burn Procedures

CMS: 100-04,12,140.1 Qualified Nonphysician Anesthetists; 100-04,12,140.3 Payment for Qualified Nonphysician Anesthetists; 100-04,12,140.3.3 Billing Modifiers; 100-04,12,140.3.4 General Billing Instructions; 100-04,12,140.4.1 Anesthesiologist/Qualified Nonphysican Anesthetist; 100-04,12,140.4.2 Anesthetist and Anesthesiologist in a Single Procedure; 100-04,12,140.4.3 Payment for Medical /Surgical Services by CRNAs; 100-04,12,140.4.4 Conversion Factors for Anesthesia Services; 100-04,12,140.5 Payment for Anesthesia Services Furnished by a Teaching CRNA; 100-04,4,250.3.2 Anesthesia in a Hospital Outpatient Setting

01951 **Anesthesia for second- and third-degree burn excision or debridement with or without skin grafting, any site, for total body surface area (TBSA) treated during anesthesia and surgery; less than 4% total body surface area**
0.00 0.00 FUD XXX N
AMA: 2018,Jan,8; 2017,Dec,8; 2017,Jan,8; 2016,Jan,13; 2015,Jan,16; 2014,Aug,5; 2014,Jan,11

01952 **between 4% and 9% of total body surface area**
0.00 0.00 FUD XXX N
AMA: 2018,Jan,8; 2017,Dec,8; 2017,Jan,8; 2016,Jan,13; 2015,Jan,16; 2014,Aug,5; 2014,Jan,11

\+ 01953 **each additional 9% total body surface area or part thereof (List separately in addition to code for primary procedure)**
Code first (01952)
0.00 0.00 FUD XXX N
AMA: 2018,Jan,8; 2017,Dec,8; 2017,Jan,8; 2016,Jan,13; 2015,Jan,16; 2014,Aug,5; 2014,Jan,11

01958-01969 Anesthesia for Obstetric Procedures

CMS: 100-04,12,140.1 Qualified Nonphysician Anesthetists; 100-04,12,140.3 Payment for Qualified Nonphysician Anesthetists; 100-04,12,140.3.3 Billing Modifiers; 100-04,12,140.3.4 General Billing Instructions; 100-04,12,140.4.1 Anesthesiologist/Qualified Nonphysican Anesthetist; 100-04,12,140.4.2 Anesthetist and Anesthesiologist in a Single Procedure; 100-04,12,140.4.3 Payment for Medical /Surgical Services by CRNAs; 100-04,12,140.4.4 Conversion Factors for Anesthesia Services; 100-04,12,140.5 Payment for Anesthesia Services Furnished by a Teaching CRNA; 100-04,4,250.3.2 Anesthesia in a Hospital Outpatient Setting

01958 **Anesthesia for external cephalic version procedure** M
0.00 0.00 FUD XXX N
AMA: 2018,Jan,8; 2017,Dec,8; 2017,Jan,8; 2016,Jan,13; 2015,Jan,16; 2014,Aug,5; 2014,Jan,11

01960 **Anesthesia for vaginal delivery only** M ♀
0.00 0.00 FUD XXX N
AMA: 2018,Jan,8; 2017,Dec,8; 2017,Jan,8; 2016,Jan,13; 2015,Jan,16; 2014,Aug,5; 2014,Jan,11

01961 **Anesthesia for cesarean delivery only** M ♀
0.00 0.00 FUD XXX N
AMA: 2018,Jan,8; 2017,Dec,8; 2017,Jan,8; 2016,Jan,13; 2015,Jan,16; 2014,Aug,5; 2014,Jan,11

01962 **Anesthesia for urgent hysterectomy following delivery** M ♀
0.00 0.00 FUD XXX N
AMA: 2018,Jan,8; 2017,Dec,8; 2017,Jan,8; 2016,Jan,13; 2015,Jan,16; 2014,Aug,5; 2014,Jan,11

01963 **Anesthesia for cesarean hysterectomy without any labor analgesia/anesthesia care** M ♀
0.00 0.00 FUD XXX N
AMA: 2018,Jan,8; 2017,Dec,8; 2017,Jan,8; 2016,Jan,13; 2015,Jan,16; 2014,Aug,5; 2014,Jan,11

01965 **Anesthesia for incomplete or missed abortion procedures** M ♀
0.00 0.00 FUD XXX N
AMA: 2018,Jan,8; 2017,Dec,8; 2017,Jan,8; 2016,Jan,13; 2015,Jan,16; 2014,Aug,5; 2014,Jan,11

01966 **Anesthesia for induced abortion procedures** M ♀
0.00 0.00 FUD XXX N
AMA: 2018,Jan,8; 2017,Dec,8; 2017,Jan,8; 2016,Jan,13; 2015,Jan,16; 2014,Aug,5; 2014,Jan,11

01967 **Neuraxial labor analgesia/anesthesia for planned vaginal delivery (this includes any repeat subarachnoid needle placement and drug injection and/or any necessary replacement of an epidural catheter during labor)** M ♀
0.00 0.00 FUD XXX N
AMA: 2018,Jan,8; 2017,Dec,8; 2017,Jan,8; 2016,Jan,13; 2015,Jan,16; 2014,Oct,14; 2014,Aug,5; 2014,Jan,11

\+ 01968 **Anesthesia for cesarean delivery following neuraxial labor analgesia/anesthesia (List separately in addition to code for primary procedure performed)** M ♀
Code first (01967)
0.00 0.00 FUD XXX N
AMA: 2018,Jan,8; 2017,Dec,8; 2017,Jan,8; 2016,Jan,13; 2015,Jan,16; 2014,Oct,14; 2014,Aug,5; 2014,Jan,11

\+ 01969 **Anesthesia for cesarean hysterectomy following neuraxial labor analgesia/anesthesia (List separately in addition to code for primary procedure performed)** M ♀
Code first (01967)
0.00 0.00 FUD XXX N
AMA: 2018,Jan,8; 2017,Dec,8; 2017,Jan,8; 2016,Jan,13; 2015,Jan,16; 2014,Aug,5; 2014,Jan,11

01990-01999 Anesthesia Miscellaneous

CMS: 100-04,12,140.1 Qualified Nonphysician Anesthetists; 100-04,12,140.3 Payment for Qualified Nonphysician Anesthetists; 100-04,12,140.3.3 Billing Modifiers; 100-04,12,140.3.4 General Billing Instructions; 100-04,12,140.4.1 Anesthesiologist/Qualified Nonphysican Anesthetist; 100-04,12,140.4.2 Anesthetist and Anesthesiologist in a Single Procedure; 100-04,12,140.4.3 Payment for Medical /Surgical Services by CRNAs; 100-04,12,140.4.4 Conversion Factors for Anesthesia Services; 100-04,12,140.5 Payment for Anesthesia Services Furnished by a Teaching CRNA; 100-04,4,250.3.2 Anesthesia in a Hospital Outpatient Setting

01990 **Physiological support for harvesting of organ(s) from brain-dead patient**
0.00 0.00 FUD XXX C
AMA: 2018,Jan,8; 2017,Dec,8; 2017,Jan,8; 2016,Jan,13; 2015,Jan,16; 2014,Aug,5; 2014,Jan,11

01991 **Anesthesia for diagnostic or therapeutic nerve blocks and injections (when block or injection is performed by a different physician or other qualified health care professional); other than the prone position**
EXCLUDES *Bier block for pain management (64999)*
Moderate Sedation (99151-99153, 99155-99157)
Pain management via intra-arterial or IV therapy (96373-96374)
Regional or local anesthesia of arms or legs for surgical procedure
0.00 0.00 FUD XXX N
AMA: 2018,Jan,8; 2017,Dec,8; 2017,Jan,8; 2016,Jan,13; 2015,Jan,16; 2014,Aug,5; 2014,Jan,11

01992 **prone position**
EXCLUDES *Bier block for pain management (64999)*
Moderate sedation (99151-99153, 99155-99157)
Pain management via intra-arterial or IV therapy (96373-96374)
Regional or local anesthesia of arms or legs for surgical procedure
0.00 0.00 FUD XXX N
AMA: 2018,Jan,8; 2017,Dec,8; 2017,Jan,8; 2016,Jan,13; 2015,Jan,16; 2014,Aug,5; 2014,Jan,11

01996 Daily hospital management of epidural or subarachnoid continuous drug administration

INCLUDES Continuous epidural or subarachnoid drug services performed after insertion of an epidural or subarachnoid catheter

0.00 0.00 FUD XXX N

AMA: 2018,Jan,8; 2017,Dec,8; 2017,Sep,6; 2017,Jan,8; 2016,Jan,13; 2015,May,10; 2015,Jan,16; 2014,Aug,5; 2014,Jan,11

01999 Unlisted anesthesia procedure(s)

0.00 0.00 FUD XXX N

AMA: 2018,Jan,8; 2017,Dec,8; 2017,Jan,8; 2016,Jan,13; 2015,May,10; 2015,Jan,16; 2014,Aug,5; 2014,Aug,14; 2014,Jan,11

10004-10012 [10004, 10005, 10006, 10007, 10008, 10009, 10010, 10011, 10012] Fine Needle Aspiration

EXCLUDES *Percutaneous localization clip placement during breast biopsy (19081-19086)*
Percutaneous needle biopsy of:
Abdominal or retroperitoneal mass (49180)
Bone (20220, 20225)
Bone marrow (38220-38222)
Epididymis (54800)
Kidney (50200)
Liver (47000)
Lung or mediastinum (32405)
Lymph node (38505)
Muscle (20206)
Nucleus pulposus, paravertebral tissue, intervertebral disc (62267)
Pancreas (48102)
Pleura (32400)
Prostate (55700, 55706)
Salivary gland (42400)
Spinal cord (62269)
Testis (54500)
Thyroid (60100)
Soft tissue percutaneous fluid drainage by catheter using image guidance (10030)
Thyroid cyst (60300)

Code also multiple biopsies on same date of service:
FNA biopsies using same imaging guidance: report imaging add-on code for second and successive procedures
FNA biopsies separate lesions, different imaging guidance: append modifier 59 to codes for additional imaging modality used
FNA and core needle biopsy same lesion, same imaging guidance, procedure includes imaging guidance for core needle procedure
FNA and core needle biopsies separate lesions, same or different imaging guidance, append modifier 59 to code for core needle biopsy and imaging guidance

10004 **Resequenced code. See code following 10021.**
10005 **Resequenced code. See code following 10021.**
10006 **Resequenced code. See code following 10021.**
10007 **Resequenced code. See code following 10021.**
10008 **Resequenced code. See code following 10021.**
10009 **Resequenced code. See code following 10021.**
10010 **Resequenced code. See code following 10021.**
10011 **Resequenced code. See code following 10021.**
10012 **Resequenced code. See code following 10021.**

10021 **Fine needle aspiration biopsy, without imaging guidance; first lesion**
(88172-88173)
1.61 2.78 FUD XXX T P3 80
AMA: 2019,May,10; 2019,Apr,4; 2019,Feb,8; 2018,Jan,8; 2017,Jan,8; 2016,Jan,13; 2015,Jan,16; 2014,Jan,11

\+ # **10004** **each additional lesion (List separately in addition to code for primary procedure)**
EXCLUDES *Fine needle biopsy using other imaging methods for same lesion ([10005, 10006, 10007, 10008, 10009, 10010, 10011, 10012])*
(88172-88173, [88177])
Code first (10021)
1.25 1.49 FUD ZZZ N1 80
AMA: 2019,Apr,4; 2019,Feb,8

10005 **Fine needle aspiration biopsy, including ultrasound guidance; first lesion**
INCLUDES Imaging guidance (76942)
(88172-88173, [88177])
2.10 3.59 FUD XXX P3 80
AMA: 2019,May,10; 2019,Feb,8; 2019,Apr,4

\+ # **10006** **each additional lesion (List separately in addition to code for primary procedure)**
INCLUDES Imaging guidance (76942)
(88172-88173, [88177])
Code first ([10005])
1.43 1.71 FUD ZZZ N1 80
AMA: 2019,Apr,4; 2019,Feb,8

10007 **Fine needle aspiration biopsy, including fluoroscopic guidance; first lesion**
INCLUDES Imaging guidance (77002)
(88172-88173, [88177])
2.70 8.09 FUD XXX P3 80
AMA: 2019,Apr,4; 2019,Feb,8

\+ # **10008** **each additional lesion (List separately in addition to code for primary procedure)**
INCLUDES Imaging guidance (77002)
(88172-88173, [88177])
Code first ([10007])
1.76 4.56 FUD ZZZ N1 80
AMA: 2019,Apr,4; 2019,Feb,8

10009 **Fine needle aspiration biopsy, including CT guidance; first lesion**
INCLUDES Imaging guidance (77012)
(88172-88173, [88177])
3.27 13.2 FUD XXX P2 80
AMA: 2019,Apr,4; 2019,Feb,8

\+ # **10010** **each additional lesion (List separately in addition to code for primary procedure)**
INCLUDES Imaging guidance (77012)
(88172-88173, [88177])
Code first ([10009])
2.39 7.98 FUD ZZZ N1 80
AMA: 2019,Apr,4; 2019,Feb,8

10011 **Fine needle aspiration biopsy, including MR guidance; first lesion**
INCLUDES Imaging guidance (77021)
(88172-88173, [88177])
0.00 0.00 FUD XXX R2 80
AMA: 2019,Apr,4; 2019,Feb,8

\+ # **10012** **each additional lesion (List separately in addition to code for primary procedure)**
INCLUDES Imaging guidance (77021)
(88172-88173, [88177])
Code first ([10011])
0.00 0.00 FUD ZZZ N1 80
AMA: 2019,Apr,4; 2019,Feb,8

10030-10180 Treatment of Lesions: Skin and Subcutaneous Tissues

EXCLUDES *Excision benign lesion (11400-11471)*

10030 **Image-guided fluid collection drainage by catheter (eg, abscess, hematoma, seroma, lymphocele, cyst), soft tissue (eg, extremity, abdominal wall, neck), percutaneous**
INCLUDES Radiologic guidance (75989, 76942, 77002-77003, 77012, 77021)
EXCLUDES *Percutaneous drainage with imaging guidance of:*
Peritoneal or retroperitoneal collections (49406)
Visceral collections (49405)
Transvaginal or transrectal drainage with imaging guidance of:
Peritoneal or retroperitoneal collections (49407)
Code also every instance of fluid collection drained using a separate catheter (10030)
3.97 16.2 FUD 000 T G2 80
AMA: 2019,Apr,4; 2018,Jan,8; 2017,Aug,9; 2017,Jan,8; 2016,Jan,13; 2015,Jan,16; 2014,May,3; 2014,May,9

Integumentary System

10035 — 11004

10035 **Placement of soft tissue localization device(s) (eg, clip, metallic pellet, wire/needle, radioactive seeds), percutaneous, including imaging guidance; first lesion**

INCLUDES Radiologic guidance (76942, 77002-77003, 77012, 77021)

EXCLUDES *Sites with a more specific code descriptor, such as the breast*

Use of code more than one time per site, regardless of the number of markers used

Code also each additional target on the same or opposite side (10036)

2.48   13.6   **FUD** 000   T N1 80 50

AMA: 2018,Jan,8; 2017,Jan,8; 2016,Jun,3

\+ **10036** **each additional lesion (List separately in addition to code for primary procedure)**

INCLUDES Radiologic guidance (76942, 77002, 77012, 77021)

EXCLUDES *Sites with a more specific code descriptor, such as the breast*

Use of code more than one time per site, regardless of the number of markers used

Code first (10035)

1.25   11.7   **FUD** ZZZ   N N1 80

AMA: 2018,Jan,8; 2017,Jan,8; 2016,Jun,3

10040 **Acne surgery (eg, marsupialization, opening or removal of multiple milia, comedones, cysts, pustules)**

1.66   3.09   **FUD** 010   Q1 N1

AMA: 2018,Jan,8; 2017,Jan,8; 2016,Jan,13; 2015,Jan,16; 2014,Jan,11

10060 **Incision and drainage of abscess (eg, carbuncle, suppurative hidradenitis, cutaneous or subcutaneous abscess, cyst, furuncle, or paronychia); simple or single**

2.81   3.37   **FUD** 010   T P3

AMA: 2018,Jan,8; 2017,Jan,8; 2016,Jan,13; 2015,Jan,16; 2014,Jan,11

10061 **complicated or multiple**

5.16   5.87   **FUD** 010   T P3

AMA: 2018,Jan,8; 2017,Jan,8; 2016,Jan,13; 2015,Jan,16; 2014,Jan,11

10080 **Incision and drainage of pilonidal cyst; simple**

2.93   5.23   **FUD** 010   T P3

AMA: 2018,Jan,8; 2017,Jan,8; 2016,Jan,13; 2015,Jan,16; 2014,Jan,11

10081 **complicated**

EXCLUDES *Excision of pilonidal cyst (11770-11772)*

4.87   7.84   **FUD** 010   T P3

AMA: 2018,Jan,8; 2017,Jan,8; 2016,Jan,13; 2015,Jan,16; 2014,Jan,11

10120 **Incision and removal of foreign body, subcutaneous tissues; simple**

2.96   4.32   **FUD** 010   T P3

AMA: 2018,Jan,8; 2017,Jan,8; 2016,Jan,13; 2015,Jan,16; 2014,Jan,11

10121 **complicated**

EXCLUDES *Debridement associated with a fracture or dislocation (11010-11012)*

Exploration penetrating wound (20100-20103)

5.32   7.77   **FUD** 010   J A2

AMA: 2018,Jan,8; 2017,Jan,8; 2016,Jan,13; 2015,Jan,16; 2014,Jan,11

10140 **Incision and drainage of hematoma, seroma or fluid collection**

(76942, 77002, 77012, 77021)

3.40   4.77   **FUD** 010   J P3

AMA: 2018,Jan,8; 2017,Jan,8; 2016,Jan,13; 2015,Jan,16; 2014,Nov,5; 2014,Jan,11

Hematoma may be decompressed with a hemostat

Drain may be placed to allow further drainage

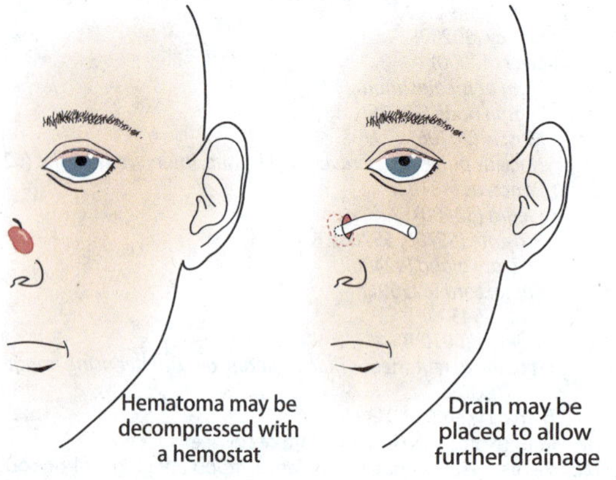

10160 **Puncture aspiration of abscess, hematoma, bulla, or cyst**

(76942, 77002, 77012, 77021)

2.72   3.70   **FUD** 010   T P3

AMA: 2018,Jan,8; 2017,Aug,9; 2017,Jan,8; 2016,Jan,13; 2015,Jan,16; 2014,Jan,11

10180 **Incision and drainage, complex, postoperative wound infection**

EXCLUDES *Wound dehiscence (12020-12021, 13160)*

5.10   7.12   **FUD** 010   J A2

AMA: 2018,Jan,8; 2017,Jan,8; 2016,Jan,13; 2015,Jan,16; 2014,Nov,5; 2014,Jan,11

11000-11012 Removal of Foreign Substances and Infected/Devitalized Tissue

EXCLUDES *Debridement of:*

Burns (16000-16030)

Deeper tissue (11042-11047 [11045, 11046])

Nails (11720-11721)

Skin only (97597-97598)

Wounds (11042-11047 [11045, 11046])

Dermabrasions (15780-15783)

Pressure ulcer excision (15920-15999)

11000 **Debridement of extensive eczematous or infected skin; up to 10% of body surface**

EXCLUDES *Necrotizing soft tissue infection of:*

Abdominal wall (11005-11006)

External genitalia and perineum (11004, 11006)

0.82   1.57   **FUD** 000   T P3

AMA: 2018,Feb,10; 2018,Jan,8; 2017,Jan,8; 2016,Jan,13; 2015,Jan,16; 2014,Jan,11

\+ **11001** **each additional 10% of the body surface, or part thereof (List separately in addition to code for primary procedure)**

EXCLUDES *Necrotizing soft tissue infection of:*

Abdominal wall (11005-11006)

External genitalia and perineum (11004, 11006)

Code first (11000)

0.41   0.62   **FUD** ZZZ   N N1

AMA: 2018,Feb,10; 2018,Jan,8; 2017,Jan,8; 2016,Jan,13; 2015,Jan,16; 2014,Jan,11

11004 **Debridement of skin, subcutaneous tissue, muscle and fascia for necrotizing soft tissue infection; external genitalia and perineum**

EXCLUDES *Skin grafts or flaps (14000-14350, 15040-15770)*

16.6   16.6   **FUD** 000   C

AMA: 2018,Feb,10; 2018,Jan,8; 2017,Jan,8; 2016,Jan,13; 2015,Jan,16; 2014,Jan,11

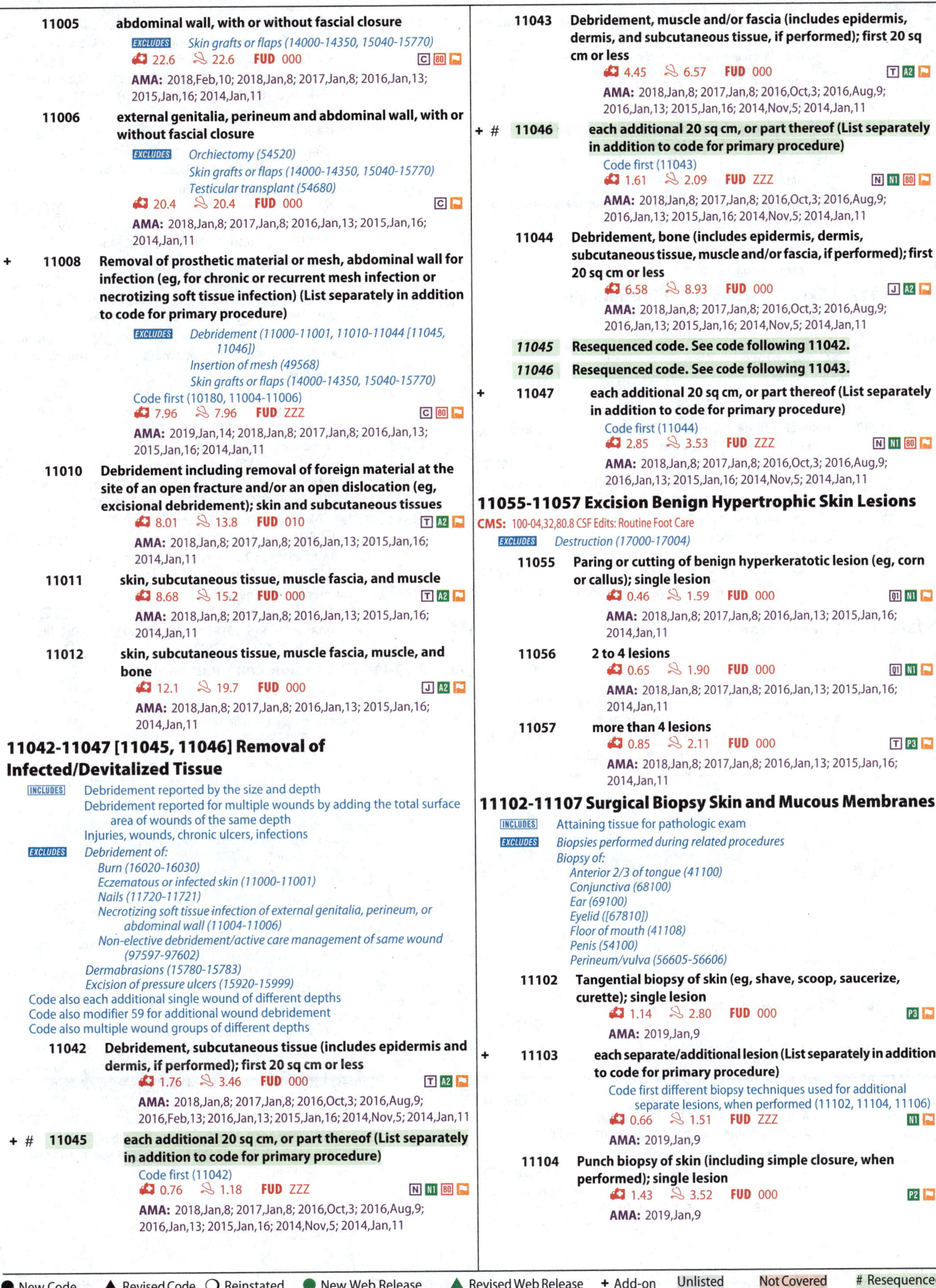

11005 **abdominal wall, with or without fascial closure**

EXCLUDES *Skin grafts or flaps (14000-14350, 15040-15770)*

22.6 22.6 FUD 000 C 80

AMA: 2018,Feb,10; 2018,Jan,8; 2017,Jan,8; 2016,Jan,13; 2015,Jan,16; 2014,Jan,11

11006 **external genitalia, perineum and abdominal wall, with or without fascial closure**

EXCLUDES *Orchiectomy (54520)*
Skin grafts or flaps (14000-14350, 15040-15770)
Testicular transplant (54680)

20.4 20.4 FUD 000 C

AMA: 2018,Jan,8; 2017,Jan,8; 2016,Jan,13; 2015,Jan,16; 2014,Jan,11

\+ **11008** **Removal of prosthetic material or mesh, abdominal wall for infection (eg, for chronic or recurrent mesh infection or necrotizing soft tissue infection) (List separately in addition to code for primary procedure)**

EXCLUDES *Debridement (11000-11001, 11010-11044 [11045, 11046])*
Insertion of mesh (49568)
Skin grafts or flaps (14000-14350, 15040-15770)

Code first (10180, 11004-11006)

7.96 7.96 FUD ZZZ C 80

AMA: 2019,Jan,14; 2018,Jan,8; 2017,Jan,8; 2016,Jan,13; 2015,Jan,16; 2014,Jan,11

11010 **Debridement including removal of foreign material at the site of an open fracture and/or an open dislocation (eg, excisional debridement); skin and subcutaneous tissues**

8.01 13.8 FUD 010 T A2

AMA: 2018,Jan,8; 2017,Jan,8; 2016,Jan,13; 2015,Jan,16; 2014,Jan,11

11011 **skin, subcutaneous tissue, muscle fascia, and muscle**

8.68 15.2 FUD 000 T A2

AMA: 2018,Jan,8; 2017,Jan,8; 2016,Jan,13; 2015,Jan,16; 2014,Jan,11

11012 **skin, subcutaneous tissue, muscle fascia, muscle, and bone**

12.1 19.7 FUD 000 J A2

AMA: 2018,Jan,8; 2017,Jan,8; 2016,Jan,13; 2015,Jan,16; 2014,Jan,11

11042-11047 [11045, 11046] Removal of Infected/Devitalized Tissue

INCLUDES Debridement reported by the size and depth
Debridement reported for multiple wounds by adding the total surface area of wounds of the same depth
Injuries, wounds, chronic ulcers, infections

EXCLUDES *Debridement of:*
Burn (16020-16030)
Eczematous or infected skin (11000-11001)
Nails (11720-11721)
Necrotizing soft tissue infection of external genitalia, perineum, or abdominal wall (11004-11006)
Non-elective debridement/active care management of same wound (97597-97602)
Dermabrasions (15780-15783)
Excision of pressure ulcers (15920-15999)

Code also each additional single wound of different depths
Code also modifier 59 for additional wound debridement
Code also multiple wound groups of different depths

11042 **Debridement, subcutaneous tissue (includes epidermis and dermis, if performed); first 20 sq cm or less**

1.76 3.46 FUD 000 T A2

AMA: 2018,Jan,8; 2017,Jan,8; 2016,Oct,3; 2016,Aug,9; 2016,Feb,13; 2016,Jan,13; 2015,Jan,16; 2014,Nov,5; 2014,Jan,11

\+ # **11045** **each additional 20 sq cm, or part thereof (List separately in addition to code for primary procedure)**

Code first (11042)

0.76 1.18 FUD ZZZ N N1 80

AMA: 2018,Jan,8; 2017,Jan,8; 2016,Oct,3; 2016,Aug,9; 2016,Jan,13; 2015,Jan,16; 2014,Nov,5; 2014,Jan,11

11043 **Debridement, muscle and/or fascia (includes epidermis, dermis, and subcutaneous tissue, if performed); first 20 sq cm or less**

4.45 6.57 FUD 000 T A2

AMA: 2018,Jan,8; 2017,Jan,8; 2016,Oct,3; 2016,Aug,9; 2016,Jan,13; 2015,Jan,16; 2014,Nov,5; 2014,Jan,11

\+ # **11046** **each additional 20 sq cm, or part thereof (List separately in addition to code for primary procedure)**

Code first (11043)

1.61 2.09 FUD ZZZ N N1 80

AMA: 2018,Jan,8; 2017,Jan,8; 2016,Oct,3; 2016,Aug,9; 2016,Jan,13; 2015,Jan,16; 2014,Nov,5; 2014,Jan,11

11044 **Debridement, bone (includes epidermis, dermis, subcutaneous tissue, muscle and/or fascia, if performed); first 20 sq cm or less**

6.58 8.93 FUD 000 J A2

AMA: 2018,Jan,8; 2017,Jan,8; 2016,Oct,3; 2016,Aug,9; 2016,Jan,13; 2015,Jan,16; 2014,Nov,5; 2014,Jan,11

11045 **Resequenced code. See code following 11042.**

11046 **Resequenced code. See code following 11043.**

\+ **11047** **each additional 20 sq cm, or part thereof (List separately in addition to code for primary procedure)**

Code first (11044)

2.85 3.53 FUD ZZZ N N1 80

AMA: 2018,Jan,8; 2017,Jan,8; 2016,Oct,3; 2016,Aug,9; 2016,Jan,13; 2015,Jan,16; 2014,Nov,5; 2014,Jan,11

11055-11057 Excision Benign Hypertrophic Skin Lesions

CMS: 100-04,32,80.8 CSF Edits: Routine Foot Care

EXCLUDES *Destruction (17000-17004)*

11055 **Paring or cutting of benign hyperkeratotic lesion (eg, corn or callus); single lesion**

0.46 1.59 FUD 000 Q1 N1

AMA: 2018,Jan,8; 2017,Jan,8; 2016,Jan,13; 2015,Jan,16; 2014,Jan,11

11056 **2 to 4 lesions**

0.65 1.90 FUD 000 Q1 N1

AMA: 2018,Jan,8; 2017,Jan,8; 2016,Jan,13; 2015,Jan,16; 2014,Jan,11

11057 **more than 4 lesions**

0.85 2.11 FUD 000 T P3

AMA: 2018,Jan,8; 2017,Jan,8; 2016,Jan,13; 2015,Jan,16; 2014,Jan,11

11102-11107 Surgical Biopsy Skin and Mucous Membranes

INCLUDES Attaining tissue for pathologic exam

EXCLUDES *Biopsies performed during related procedures*
Biopsy of:
Anterior 2/3 of tongue (41100)
Conjunctiva (68100)
Ear (69100)
Eyelid ([67810])
Floor of mouth (41108)
Penis (54100)
Perineum/vulva (56605-56606)

11102 **Tangential biopsy of skin (eg, shave, scoop, saucerize, curette); single lesion**

1.14 2.80 FUD 000 P3

AMA: 2019,Jan,9

\+ **11103** **each separate/additional lesion (List separately in addition to code for primary procedure)**

Code first different biopsy techniques used for additional separate lesions, when performed (11102, 11104, 11106)

0.66 1.51 FUD ZZZ N1

AMA: 2019,Jan,9

11104 **Punch biopsy of skin (including simple closure, when performed); single lesion**

1.43 3.52 FUD 000 P2

AMA: 2019,Jan,9

\+ **11105** **each separate/additional lesion (List separately in addition to code for primary procedure)**

Code first different biopsy techniques used for additional separate lesions, when performed (11104, 11106)

0.78 1.73 FUD ZZZ N1

AMA: 2019,Jan,9

11106 **Incisional biopsy of skin (eg, wedge) (including simple closure, when performed); single lesion**

1.74 4.26 FUD 000 P3

AMA: 2019,Jan,9

\+ **11107** **each separate/additional lesion (List separately in addition to code for primary procedure)**

Code first (11106)

0.93 2.04 FUD ZZZ N1

AMA: 2019,Jan,9

11200-11201 Skin Tag Removal - All Techniques

INCLUDES Chemical destruction
Electrocauterization
Electrosurgical destruction
Ligature strangulation
Removal with or without local anesthesia
Sharp excision or scissoring

EXCLUDES *Extensive or complicated secondary wound closure (13160)*

11200 **Removal of skin tags, multiple fibrocutaneous tags, any area; up to and including 15 lesions**

2.10 2.51 FUD 010 Q1 N1

AMA: 2018,Jan,8; 2017,Jan,8; 2016,Jan,13; 2015,Jan,16; 2014,Jan,11

\+ **11201** **each additional 10 lesions, or part thereof (List separately in addition to code for primary procedure)**

Code first (11200)

0.48 0.54 FUD ZZZ N N1

AMA: 2018,Jan,8; 2017,Jan,8; 2016,Jan,13; 2015,Jan,16; 2014,Jan,11

11300-11313 Skin Lesion Removal: Shaving

INCLUDES Local anesthesia
Partial thickness excision by horizontal slicing
Wound cauterization

11300 **Shaving of epidermal or dermal lesion, single lesion, trunk, arms or legs; lesion diameter 0.5 cm or less**

1.01 2.77 FUD 000 Q1 N1 80

AMA: 2019,Jan,9; 2018,Feb,10; 2018,Jan,8; 2017,Dec,14; 2017,Jan,8; 2016,Jan,13; 2015,Jan,16; 2014,Jan,11

Shave excision of an elevated lesion; technique also used to biopsy

Elliptical excision is often used when tissue removal is larger than 4 mm or when deep pathology is suspected

A punch biopsy cuts a core of tissue as the tool is twisted downward

11301 **lesion diameter 0.6 to 1.0 cm**

1.53 3.40 FUD 000 Q1 N1 80

AMA: 2019,Jan,9; 2018,Feb,10; 2018,Jan,8; 2017,Dec,14; 2017,Jan,8; 2016,Jan,13; 2015,Jan,16; 2014,Jan,11

11302 **lesion diameter 1.1 to 2.0 cm**

1.80 3.98 FUD 000 Q1 N1 80

AMA: 2019,Jan,9; 2018,Feb,10; 2018,Jan,8; 2017,Dec,14; 2017,Jan,8; 2016,Jan,13; 2015,Jan,16; 2014,Jan,11

11303 **lesion diameter over 2.0 cm**

2.13 4.39 FUD 000 Q1 N1 80

AMA: 2019,Jan,9; 2018,Feb,10; 2018,Jan,8; 2017,Dec,14; 2017,Jan,8; 2016,Jan,13; 2015,Jan,16; 2014,Jan,11

11305 **Shaving of epidermal or dermal lesion, single lesion, scalp, neck, hands, feet, genitalia; lesion diameter 0.5 cm or less**

1.12 2.90 FUD 000 Q1 N1 80

AMA: 2019,Jan,9; 2018,Feb,10; 2018,Jan,8; 2017,Dec,14; 2017,Jan,8; 2016,Jan,13; 2015,Jan,16; 2014,Jan,11

11306 **lesion diameter 0.6 to 1.0 cm**

1.49 3.45 FUD 000 Q1 N1 80

AMA: 2019,Jan,9; 2018,Feb,10; 2018,Jan,8; 2017,Dec,14; 2017,Jan,8; 2016,Jan,13; 2015,Jan,16; 2014,Jan,11

11307 **lesion diameter 1.1 to 2.0 cm**

1.92 4.09 FUD 000 T P2 80

AMA: 2019,Jan,9; 2018,Feb,10; 2018,Jan,8; 2017,Dec,14; 2017,Jan,8; 2016,Jan,13; 2015,Jan,16; 2014,Jan,11

11308 **lesion diameter over 2.0 cm**

2.14 4.34 FUD 000 Q1 N1 80

AMA: 2019,Jan,9; 2018,Feb,10; 2018,Jan,8; 2017,Dec,14; 2017,Jan,8; 2016,Jan,13; 2015,Jan,16; 2014,Jan,11

11310 **Shaving of epidermal or dermal lesion, single lesion, face, ears, eyelids, nose, lips, mucous membrane; lesion diameter 0.5 cm or less**

1.36 3.23 FUD 000 T P3 80

AMA: 2019,Jan,9; 2018,Feb,10; 2018,Jan,8; 2017,Dec,14; 2017,Jan,8; 2016,Jan,13; 2015,Jan,16; 2014,Jan,11

11311 **lesion diameter 0.6 to 1.0 cm**

1.88 3.86 FUD 000 T P2 80

AMA: 2019,Jan,9; 2018,Feb,10; 2018,Jan,8; 2017,Dec,14; 2017,Jan,8; 2016,Jan,13; 2015,Jan,16; 2014,Jan,11

11312 **lesion diameter 1.1 to 2.0 cm**

2.23 4.52 FUD 000 T P3 80

AMA: 2019,Jan,9; 2018,Feb,10; 2018,Jan,8; 2017,Dec,14; 2017,Jan,8; 2016,Jan,13; 2015,Jan,16; 2014,Jan,11

11313 **lesion diameter over 2.0 cm**

2.89 5.30 FUD 000 T P3 80

AMA: 2019,Jan,9; 2018,Feb,10; 2018,Jan,8; 2017,Dec,14; 2017,Jan,8; 2016,Jan,13; 2015,Jan,16; 2014,Jan,11

11400-11446 Skin Lesion Removal: Benign

INCLUDES Biopsy on same lesion
Cicatricial lesion excision
Full thickness removal including margins
Lesion measurement before excision at largest diameter plus margin
Local anesthesia
Simple, nonlayered closure

EXCLUDES *Adjacent tissue transfer: report only adjacent tissue transfer (14000-14302)*
Biopsy of eyelid ([67810])
Destruction:
Benign lesions, any method (17110-17111)
Cutaneous vascular proliferative lesions (17106-17108)
Destruction of eyelid lesion (67850)
Malignant lesions (17260-17286)
Premalignant lesions (17000, 17003-17004)
Escharotomy (16035-16036)
Excision and reconstruction of eyelid (67961-67975)
Excision of chalazion (67800-67808)
Eyelid procedures involving more than skin (67800 and subsequent codes)
Laser fenestration for scars (0479T-0480T)
Shave removal (11300-11313)

Code also complex closure (13100-13153)
Code also each separate lesion
Code also intermediate closure (12031-12057)
Code also modifier 22 if excision is complicated or unusual
Code also reconstruction (15002-15261, 15570-15770)

11400 **Excision, benign lesion including margins, except skin tag (unless listed elsewhere), trunk, arms or legs; excised diameter 0.5 cm or less**

2.33 3.53 FUD 010 T P3

AMA: 2018,Sep,7; 2018,Feb,10; 2018,Jan,8; 2017,Jan,8; 2016,Apr,3; 2016,Jan,13; 2015,Jan,16; 2014,Mar,4; 2014,Mar,12; 2014,Jan,11

11401 excised diameter 0.6 to 1.0 cm
2.99 4.30 FUD 010 T P3
AMA: 2018,Sep,7; 2018,Feb,10; 2018,Jan,8; 2017,Jan,8; 2016,Apr,3; 2016,Jan,13; 2015,Jan,16; 2014,Mar,4; 2014,Mar,12; 2014,Jan,11

11402 excised diameter 1.1 to 2.0 cm
3.29 4.78 FUD 010 T P3
AMA: 2018,Sep,7; 2018,Feb,10; 2018,Jan,8; 2017,Jan,8; 2016,Apr,3; 2016,Jan,13; 2015,Jan,16; 2014,Mar,12; 2014,Mar,4; 2014,Jan,11

11403 excised diameter 2.1 to 3.0 cm
4.25 5.53 FUD 010 T P3
AMA: 2018,Sep,7; 2018,Feb,10; 2018,Jan,8; 2017,Jan,8; 2016,Apr,3; 2016,Jan,13; 2015,Jan,16; 2014,Mar,12; 2014,Mar,4; 2014,Jan,11

11404 excised diameter 3.1 to 4.0 cm
4.67 6.27 FUD 010 J A2
AMA: 2018,Sep,7; 2018,Feb,10; 2018,Jan,8; 2017,Jan,8; 2016,Apr,3; 2016,Jan,13; 2015,Jan,16; 2014,Mar,12; 2014,Mar,4; 2014,Jan,11

11406 excised diameter over 4.0 cm
7.11 9.02 FUD 010 J A2
AMA: 2018,Sep,7; 2018,Feb,10; 2018,Jan,8; 2017,Jan,8; 2016,Apr,3; 2016,Jan,13; 2015,Jan,16; 2014,Mar,4; 2014,Mar,12; 2014,Jan,11

11420 Excision, benign lesion including margins, except skin tag (unless listed elsewhere), scalp, neck, hands, feet, genitalia; excised diameter 0.5 cm or less
2.33 3.53 FUD 010 J P3
AMA: 2018,Sep,7; 2018,Feb,10; 2018,Jan,8; 2017,Jan,8; 2016,Apr,3; 2016,Jan,13; 2015,Jan,16; 2014,Mar,4; 2014,Mar,12; 2014,Jan,11

11421 excised diameter 0.6 to 1.0 cm
3.15 4.49 FUD 010 T P3
AMA: 2018,Sep,7; 2018,Feb,10; 2018,Jan,8; 2017,Jan,8; 2016,Apr,3; 2016,Jan,13; 2015,Jan,16; 2014,Mar,12; 2014,Mar,4; 2014,Jan,11

11422 excised diameter 1.1 to 2.0 cm
3.90 5.06 FUD 010 J P3
AMA: 2018,Sep,7; 2018,Feb,10; 2018,Jan,8; 2017,Jan,8; 2016,Apr,3; 2016,Jan,13; 2015,Jan,16; 2014,Mar,12; 2014,Mar,4; 2014,Jan,11

11423 excised diameter 2.1 to 3.0 cm
4.48 5.77 FUD 010 J P3
AMA: 2018,Sep,7; 2018,Feb,10; 2018,Jan,8; 2017,Jan,8; 2016,Apr,3; 2016,Jan,13; 2015,Jan,16; 2014,Mar,12; 2014,Mar,4; 2014,Jan,11

11424 excised diameter 3.1 to 4.0 cm
5.16 6.69 FUD 010 J A2
AMA: 2018,Sep,7; 2018,Feb,10; 2018,Jan,8; 2017,Jan,8; 2016,Apr,3; 2016,Jan,13; 2015,Jan,16; 2014,Mar,12; 2014,Mar,4; 2014,Jan,11

11426 excised diameter over 4.0 cm
7.93 9.59 FUD 010 J A2
AMA: 2018,Sep,7; 2018,Feb,10; 2018,Jan,8; 2017,Jan,8; 2016,Apr,3; 2016,Jan,13; 2015,Jan,16; 2014,Mar,12; 2014,Mar,4; 2014,Jan,11

11440 Excision, other benign lesion including margins, except skin tag (unless listed elsewhere), face, ears, eyelids, nose, lips, mucous membrane; excised diameter 0.5 cm or less
2.96 3.91 FUD 010 T P3
AMA: 2019,Jan,14; 2018,Sep,7; 2018,Feb,10; 2018,Jan,8; 2017,Jan,8; 2016,Apr,3; 2016,Jan,13; 2015,Jan,16; 2014,Mar,12; 2014,Mar,4; 2014,Jan,11

The physician removes a benign lesion from the external ear, nose, or mucous membranes

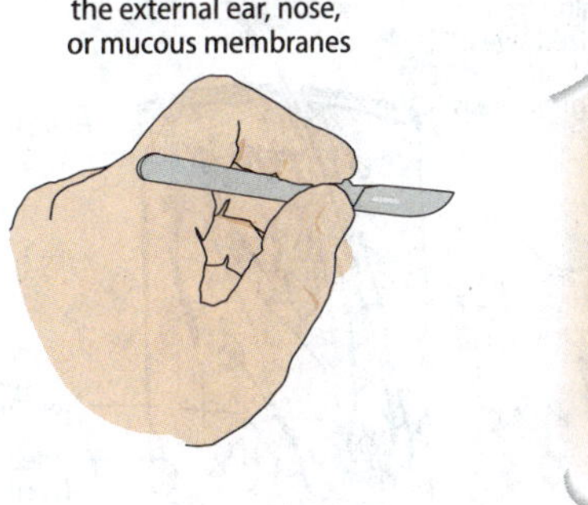
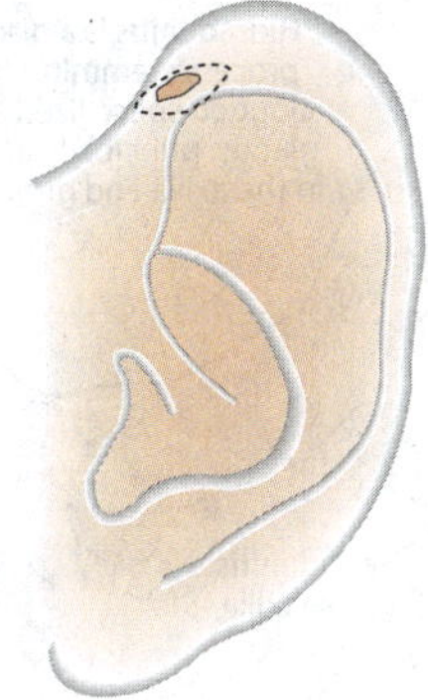

11441 excised diameter 0.6 to 1.0 cm
3.76 4.83 FUD 010 T P3
AMA: 2019,Jan,14; 2018,Sep,7; 2018,Feb,10; 2018,Jan,8; 2017,Jan,8; 2016,Apr,3; 2016,Jan,13; 2015,Jan,16; 2014,Mar,12; 2014,Mar,4; 2014,Jan,11

11442 excised diameter 1.1 to 2.0 cm
4.16 5.39 FUD 010 T P3
AMA: 2019,Jan,14; 2018,Sep,7; 2018,Feb,10; 2018,Jan,8; 2017,Jan,8; 2016,Apr,3; 2016,Jan,13; 2015,Jan,16; 2014,Mar,12; 2014,Mar,4; 2014,Jan,11

11443 excised diameter 2.1 to 3.0 cm
5.11 6.42 FUD 010 J P3
AMA: 2019,Jan,14; 2018,Sep,7; 2018,Feb,10; 2018,Jan,8; 2017,Jan,8; 2016,Apr,3; 2016,Jan,13; 2015,Jan,16; 2014,Mar,12; 2014,Mar,4; 2014,Jan,11

11444 excised diameter 3.1 to 4.0 cm
6.51 8.05 FUD 010 J A2
AMA: 2019,Jan,14; 2018,Sep,7; 2018,Feb,10; 2018,Jan,8; 2017,Jan,8; 2016,Apr,3; 2016,Jan,13; 2015,Jan,16; 2014,Mar,12; 2014,Mar,4; 2014,Jan,11

11446 excised diameter over 4.0 cm
9.33 11.1 FUD 010 J A2
AMA: 2019,Jan,14; 2018,Sep,7; 2018,Feb,10; 2018,Jan,8; 2017,Jan,8; 2016,Apr,3; 2016,Jan,13; 2015,Jan,16; 2014,Mar,12; 2014,Mar,4; 2014,Jan,11

11450-11471 Treatment of Hidradenitis: Excision and Repair

Code also closure by skin graft or flap (14000-14350, 15040-15770)

11450 **Excision of skin and subcutaneous tissue for hidradenitis, axillary; with simple or intermediate repair**
7.33   11.2   **FUD** 090   J A2 50
AMA: 2018,Sep,7; 2018,Feb,10; 2018,Jan,8; 2017,Jan,8; 2016,Aug,9; 2016,Jan,13; 2015,Jan,16; 2014,Jan,11

Hidradenitis is a disease process stemming from clogged specialized sweat glands, principally located in the axilla and groin areas

Hair shaft
Hair matrix
Sweat (eccrine gland)
Hidradenitis of the axilla

11451 **with complex repair**
9.37   14.1   **FUD** 090   J A2 80 50
AMA: 2018,Sep,7; 2018,Feb,10; 2018,Jan,8; 2017,Jan,8; 2016,Aug,9; 2016,Jan,13; 2015,Jan,16; 2014,Jan,11

11462 **Excision of skin and subcutaneous tissue for hidradenitis, inguinal; with simple or intermediate repair**
6.98   10.9   **FUD** 090   J A2 80 50
AMA: 2018,Sep,7; 2018,Feb,10; 2018,Jan,8; 2017,Jan,8; 2016,Aug,9; 2016,Jan,13; 2015,Jan,16; 2014,Jan,11

11463 **with complex repair**
9.42   14.3   **FUD** 090   J A2 80 50
AMA: 2018,Sep,7; 2018,Feb,10; 2018,Jan,8; 2017,Jan,8; 2016,Aug,9; 2016,Jan,13; 2015,Jan,16; 2014,Jan,11

11470 **Excision of skin and subcutaneous tissue for hidradenitis, perianal, perineal, or umbilical; with simple or intermediate repair**
8.08   12.0   **FUD** 090   J A2
AMA: 2018,Sep,7; 2018,Feb,10; 2018,Jan,8; 2017,Jan,8; 2016,Aug,9; 2016,Jan,13; 2015,Jan,16; 2014,Jan,11

11471 **with complex repair**
9.99   14.7   **FUD** 090   J A2 80
AMA: 2018,Sep,7; 2018,Feb,10; 2018,Jan,8; 2017,Jan,8; 2016,Aug,9; 2016,Jan,13; 2015,Jan,16; 2014,Jan,11

11600-11646 Skin Lesion Removal: Malignant

INCLUDES Biopsy on same lesion
Excision of additional margin at same operative session
Full thickness removal including margins
Lesion measurement before excision at largest diameter plus margin
Local anesthesia
Simple, nonlayered closure

EXCLUDES *Adjacent tissue transfer. Report only adjacent tissue transfer (14000-14302)*
Destruction (17260-17286)
Excision of additional margin at subsequent operative session (11600-11646)

Code also complex closure (13100-13153)
Code also each separate lesion
Code also intermediate closure (12031-12057)
Code also modifier 58 if re-excision is performed during postoperative period
Code also reconstruction (15002-15261, 15570-15770)

11600 **Excision, malignant lesion including margins, trunk, arms, or legs; excised diameter 0.5 cm or less**
3.45   5.53   **FUD** 010   T P3
AMA: 2018,Sep,7; 2018,Jan,8; 2017,Jan,8; 2016,Jan,13; 2015,Jan,16; 2014,Mar,4; 2014,Mar,12; 2014,Jan,11

11601 **excised diameter 0.6 to 1.0 cm**
4.29   6.52   **FUD** 010   T P3
AMA: 2018,Sep,7; 2018,Jan,8; 2017,Jan,8; 2016,Jan,13; 2015,Jan,16; 2014,Mar,4; 2014,Mar,12; 2014,Jan,11

11602 **excised diameter 1.1 to 2.0 cm**
4.70   7.06   **FUD** 010   T P3
AMA: 2018,Sep,7; 2018,Jan,8; 2017,Jan,8; 2016,Jan,13; 2015,Jan,16; 2014,Mar,4; 2014,Mar,12; 2014,Jan,11

11603 **excised diameter 2.1 to 3.0 cm**
5.63   8.07   **FUD** 010   T P3
AMA: 2018,Sep,7; 2018,Jan,8; 2017,Jan,8; 2016,Jan,13; 2015,Jan,16; 2014,Mar,4; 2014,Mar,12; 2014,Jan,11

11604 **excised diameter 3.1 to 4.0 cm**
6.19   8.95   **FUD** 010   T A2
AMA: 2018,Sep,7; 2018,Jan,8; 2017,Jan,8; 2016,Jan,13; 2015,Jan,16; 2014,Mar,4; 2014,Mar,12; 2014,Jan,11

11606 **excised diameter over 4.0 cm**
9.24   12.8   **FUD** 010   J A2
AMA: 2018,Sep,7; 2018,Jan,8; 2017,Jan,8; 2016,Jan,13; 2015,Jan,16; 2014,Mar,4; 2014,Mar,12; 2014,Jan,11

11620 **Excision, malignant lesion including margins, scalp, neck, hands, feet, genitalia; excised diameter 0.5 cm or less**
3.49   5.57   **FUD** 010   J P3
AMA: 2018,Sep,7; 2018,Jan,8; 2017,Jan,8; 2016,Jan,13; 2015,Jan,16; 2014,Mar,4; 2014,Mar,12; 2014,Jan,11

11621 **excised diameter 0.6 to 1.0 cm**
4.32   6.55   **FUD** 010   T P3
AMA: 2018,Sep,7; 2018,Jan,8; 2017,Jan,8; 2016,Jan,13; 2015,Jan,16; 2014,Mar,4; 2014,Mar,12; 2014,Jan,11

11622 **excised diameter 1.1 to 2.0 cm**
4.93   7.30   **FUD** 010   T P3
AMA: 2018,Sep,7; 2018,Jan,8; 2017,Jan,8; 2016,Jan,13; 2015,Jan,16; 2014,Mar,4; 2014,Mar,12; 2014,Jan,11

11623 **excised diameter 2.1 to 3.0 cm**
6.10   8.55   **FUD** 010   J P3
AMA: 2018,Sep,7; 2018,Jan,8; 2017,Jan,8; 2016,Jan,13; 2015,Jan,16; 2014,Mar,4; 2014,Mar,12; 2014,Jan,11

11624 **excised diameter 3.1 to 4.0 cm**
6.92   9.67   **FUD** 010   J A2
AMA: 2018,Sep,7; 2018,Jan,8; 2017,Jan,8; 2016,Jan,13; 2015,Jan,16; 2014,Mar,4; 2014,Mar,12; 2014,Jan,11

11626 **excised diameter over 4.0 cm**
8.48   11.6   **FUD** 010   J A2
AMA: 2018,Sep,7; 2018,Jan,8; 2017,Jan,8; 2016,Jan,13; 2015,Jan,16; 2014,Mar,4; 2014,Mar,12; 2014,Jan,11

11640 **Excision, malignant lesion including margins, face, ears, eyelids, nose, lips; excised diameter 0.5 cm or less**
EXCLUDES *Eyelid excision involving more than skin (67800-67808, 67840-67850, 67961-67966)*
3.61   5.74   **FUD** 010   T P3
AMA: 2018,Sep,7; 2018,Jan,8; 2017,Jan,8; 2016,Jan,13; 2015,Jan,16; 2014,Mar,4; 2014,Mar,12; 2014,Jan,11

11641 **excised diameter 0.6 to 1.0 cm**
EXCLUDES *Eyelid excision involving more than skin (67800-67808, 67840-67850, 67961-67966)*
4.50   6.78   **FUD** 010   T P3
AMA: 2018,Sep,7; 2018,Jan,8; 2017,Jan,8; 2016,Jan,13; 2015,Jan,16; 2014,Mar,4; 2014,Mar,12; 2014,Jan,11

11642 **excised diameter 1.1 to 2.0 cm**
EXCLUDES *Eyelid excision involving more than skin (67800-67808, 67840-67850, 67961-67966)*
5.30   7.73   **FUD** 010   T P3
AMA: 2018,Sep,7; 2018,Jan,8; 2017,Jan,8; 2016,Jan,13; 2015,Jan,16; 2014,Mar,4; 2014,Mar,12; 2014,Jan,11

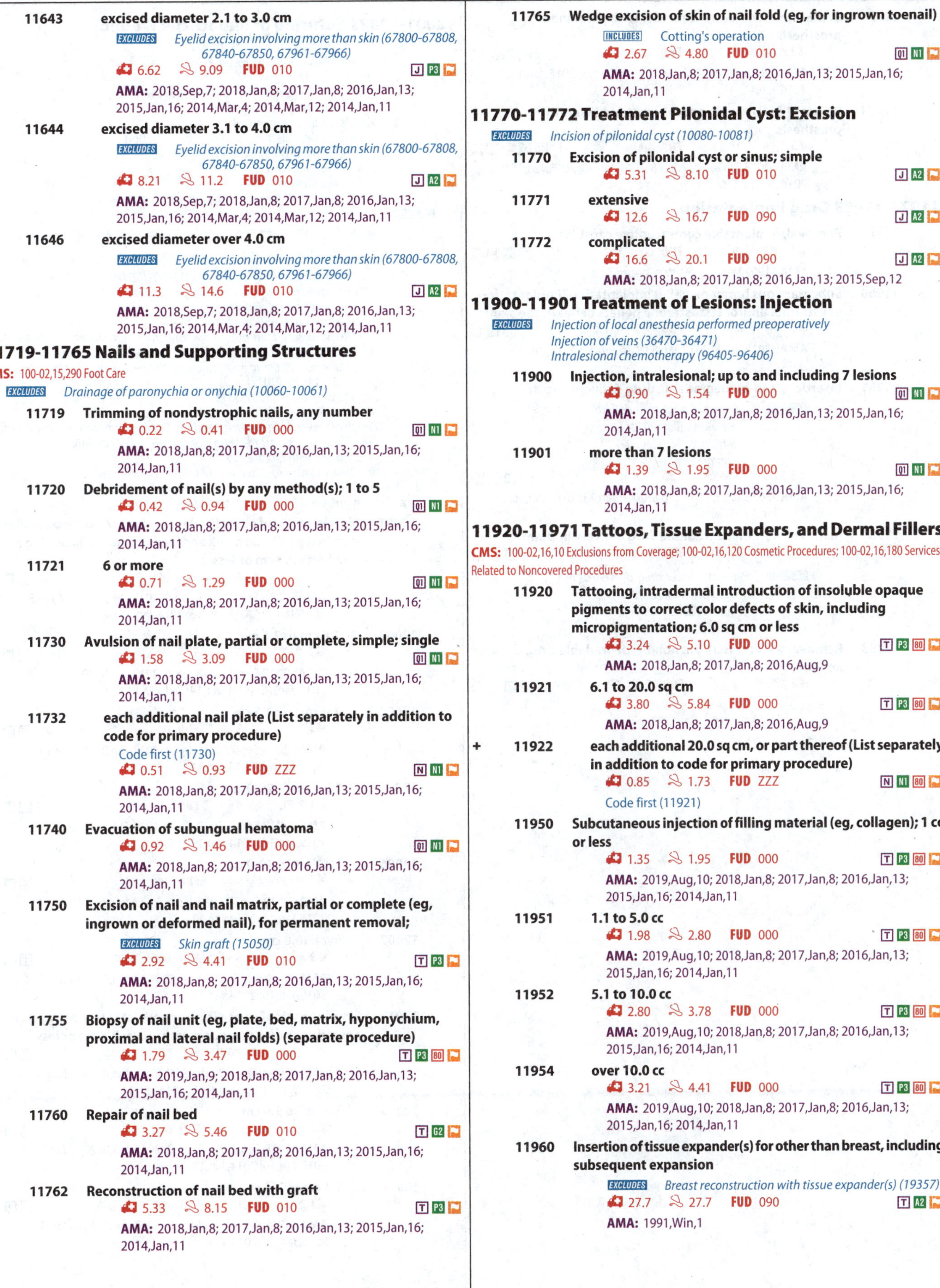

11643 excised diameter 2.1 to 3.0 cm
EXCLUDES *Eyelid excision involving more than skin (67800-67808, 67840-67850, 67961-67966)*
6.62 | 9.09 | FUD 010 | J P3
AMA: 2018,Sep,7; 2018,Jan,8; 2017,Jan,8; 2016,Jan,13; 2015,Jan,16; 2014,Mar,4; 2014,Mar,12; 2014,Jan,11

11644 excised diameter 3.1 to 4.0 cm
EXCLUDES *Eyelid excision involving more than skin (67800-67808, 67840-67850, 67961-67966)*
8.21 | 11.2 | FUD 010 | J A2
AMA: 2018,Sep,7; 2018,Jan,8; 2017,Jan,8; 2016,Jan,13; 2015,Jan,16; 2014,Mar,4; 2014,Mar,12; 2014,Jan,11

11646 excised diameter over 4.0 cm
EXCLUDES *Eyelid excision involving more than skin (67800-67808, 67840-67850, 67961-67966)*
11.3 | 14.6 | FUD 010 | J A2
AMA: 2018,Sep,7; 2018,Jan,8; 2017,Jan,8; 2016,Jan,13; 2015,Jan,16; 2014,Mar,4; 2014,Mar,12; 2014,Jan,11

11719-11765 Nails and Supporting Structures

CMS: 100-02,15,290 Foot Care
EXCLUDES *Drainage of paronychia or onychia (10060-10061)*

11719 Trimming of nondystrophic nails, any number
0.22 | 0.41 | FUD 000 | Q1 N1
AMA: 2018,Jan,8; 2017,Jan,8; 2016,Jan,13; 2015,Jan,16; 2014,Jan,11

11720 Debridement of nail(s) by any method(s); 1 to 5
0.42 | 0.94 | FUD 000 | Q1 N1
AMA: 2018,Jan,8; 2017,Jan,8; 2016,Jan,13; 2015,Jan,16; 2014,Jan,11

11721 6 or more
0.71 | 1.29 | FUD 000 | Q1 N1
AMA: 2018,Jan,8; 2017,Jan,8; 2016,Jan,13; 2015,Jan,16; 2014,Jan,11

11730 Avulsion of nail plate, partial or complete, simple; single
1.58 | 3.09 | FUD 000 | Q1 N1
AMA: 2018,Jan,8; 2017,Jan,8; 2016,Jan,13; 2015,Jan,16; 2014,Jan,11

+ **11732** each additional nail plate (List separately in addition to code for primary procedure)
Code first (11730)
0.51 | 0.93 | FUD ZZZ | N N1
AMA: 2018,Jan,8; 2017,Jan,8; 2016,Jan,13; 2015,Jan,16; 2014,Jan,11

11740 Evacuation of subungual hematoma
0.92 | 1.46 | FUD 000 | Q1 N1
AMA: 2018,Jan,8; 2017,Jan,8; 2016,Jan,13; 2015,Jan,16; 2014,Jan,11

11750 Excision of nail and nail matrix, partial or complete (eg, ingrown or deformed nail), for permanent removal;
EXCLUDES *Skin graft (15050)*
2.92 | 4.41 | FUD 010 | T P3
AMA: 2018,Jan,8; 2017,Jan,8; 2016,Jan,13; 2015,Jan,16; 2014,Jan,11

11755 Biopsy of nail unit (eg, plate, bed, matrix, hyponychium, proximal and lateral nail folds) (separate procedure)
1.79 | 3.47 | FUD 000 | T P3 80
AMA: 2019,Jan,9; 2018,Jan,8; 2017,Jan,8; 2016,Jan,13; 2015,Jan,16; 2014,Jan,11

11760 Repair of nail bed
3.27 | 5.46 | FUD 010 | T G2
AMA: 2018,Jan,8; 2017,Jan,8; 2016,Jan,13; 2015,Jan,16; 2014,Jan,11

11762 Reconstruction of nail bed with graft
5.33 | 8.15 | FUD 010 | T P3
AMA: 2018,Jan,8; 2017,Jan,8; 2016,Jan,13; 2015,Jan,16; 2014,Jan,11

11765 Wedge excision of skin of nail fold (eg, for ingrown toenail)
INCLUDES Cotting's operation
2.67 | 4.80 | FUD 010 | Q1 N1
AMA: 2018,Jan,8; 2017,Jan,8; 2016,Jan,13; 2015,Jan,16; 2014,Jan,11

11770-11772 Treatment Pilonidal Cyst: Excision

EXCLUDES *Incision of pilonidal cyst (10080-10081)*

11770 Excision of pilonidal cyst or sinus; simple
5.31 | 8.10 | FUD 010 | J A2

11771 extensive
12.6 | 16.7 | FUD 090 | J A2

11772 complicated
16.6 | 20.1 | FUD 090 | J A2
AMA: 2018,Jan,8; 2017,Jan,8; 2016,Jan,13; 2015,Sep,12

11900-11901 Treatment of Lesions: Injection

EXCLUDES *Injection of local anesthesia performed preoperatively*
Injection of veins (36470-36471)
Intralesional chemotherapy (96405-96406)

11900 Injection, intralesional; up to and including 7 lesions
0.90 | 1.54 | FUD 000 | Q1 N1
AMA: 2018,Jan,8; 2017,Jan,8; 2016,Jan,13; 2015,Jan,16; 2014,Jan,11

11901 more than 7 lesions
1.39 | 1.95 | FUD 000 | Q1 N1
AMA: 2018,Jan,8; 2017,Jan,8; 2016,Jan,13; 2015,Jan,16; 2014,Jan,11

11920-11971 Tattoos, Tissue Expanders, and Dermal Fillers

CMS: 100-02,16,10 Exclusions from Coverage; 100-02,16,120 Cosmetic Procedures; 100-02,16,180 Services Related to Noncovered Procedures

11920 Tattooing, intradermal introduction of insoluble opaque pigments to correct color defects of skin, including micropigmentation; 6.0 sq cm or less
3.24 | 5.10 | FUD 000 | T P3 80
AMA: 2018,Jan,8; 2017,Jan,8; 2016,Aug,9

11921 6.1 to 20.0 sq cm
3.80 | 5.84 | FUD 000 | T P3 80
AMA: 2018,Jan,8; 2017,Jan,8; 2016,Aug,9

+ **11922** each additional 20.0 sq cm, or part thereof (List separately in addition to code for primary procedure)
0.85 | 1.73 | FUD ZZZ | N N1 80
Code first (11921)

11950 Subcutaneous injection of filling material (eg, collagen); 1 cc or less
1.35 | 1.95 | FUD 000 | T P3 80
AMA: 2019,Aug,10; 2018,Jan,8; 2017,Jan,8; 2016,Jan,13; 2015,Jan,16; 2014,Jan,11

11951 1.1 to 5.0 cc
1.98 | 2.80 | FUD 000 | T P3 80
AMA: 2019,Aug,10; 2018,Jan,8; 2017,Jan,8; 2016,Jan,13; 2015,Jan,16; 2014,Jan,11

11952 5.1 to 10.0 cc
2.80 | 3.78 | FUD 000 | T P3 80
AMA: 2019,Aug,10; 2018,Jan,8; 2017,Jan,8; 2016,Jan,13; 2015,Jan,16; 2014,Jan,11

11954 over 10.0 cc
3.21 | 4.41 | FUD 000 | T P3 80
AMA: 2019,Aug,10; 2018,Jan,8; 2017,Jan,8; 2016,Jan,13; 2015,Jan,16; 2014,Jan,11

11960 Insertion of tissue expander(s) for other than breast, including subsequent expansion
EXCLUDES *Breast reconstruction with tissue expander(s) (19357)*
27.7 | 27.7 | FUD 090 | T A2
AMA: 1991,Win,1

11970 **Replacement of tissue expander with permanent prosthesis**
17.4 17.4 **FUD** 090 J A2 50
AMA: 2018,Jan,8; 2017,Jan,8; 2016,Jan,13; 2015,Jan,16; 2014,Jan,11

11971 **Removal of tissue expander(s) without insertion of prosthesis**
9.16 13.5 **FUD** 090 Q2 A2 80 50
AMA: 2018,Jan,8; 2017,Jan,8; 2016,Jan,13; 2015,Jan,16; 2014,Jan,11

11976-11983 Drug Implantation

11976 **Removal, implantable contraceptive capsules** ♀
2.68 4.13 **FUD** 000 Q2 P3 80
AMA: 1992,Win,1; 1991,Win,1

11980 **Subcutaneous hormone pellet implantation (implantation of estradiol and/or testosterone pellets beneath the skin)**
1.61 2.69 **FUD** 000 Q1 N1
AMA: 2018,Jan,8; 2017,Jan,8; 2016,Jan,13; 2015,Jan,16; 2014,Jan,11

11981 **Insertion, non-biodegradable drug delivery implant**
EXCLUDES *Insertion of deep drug-delivery device:*
Intra-articular (20704)
Intramedullary (20702)
Subfascial (20700)
2.40 4.05 **FUD** XXX Q1 N1 80
AMA: 2018,Jan,8; 2017,Jan,8; 2016,Jan,13; 2015,Jan,16; 2014,Jan,11

11982 **Removal, non-biodegradable drug delivery implant**
2.87 4.49 **FUD** XXX Q1 N1 80
EXCLUDES *Removal of deep drug-delivery device:*
Intra-articular (20705)
Intramedullary (20703)
Subfascial (20701)

11983 **Removal with reinsertion, non-biodegradable drug delivery implant**
5.12 6.56 **FUD** XXX Q1 N1 80

12001-12021 Suturing of Superficial Wounds

INCLUDES Administration of local anesthesia
Cauterization without closure
Simple:
Exploration nerves, blood vessels, tendons
Vessel ligation, in wound
Simple repair that involves:
Routine debridement and decontamination
Simple one layer closure
Superficial tissues
Sutures, staples, tissue adhesives
Total length of several repairs in same code category

EXCLUDES *Adhesive strips only, see appropriate E&M service*
Complex repair nerves, blood vessels, tendons (see appropriate anatomical section)
Debridement:
Performed separately, no closure (11042-11047 [11045, 11046])
That requires:
Comprehensive cleaning
Removal of significant tissue
Removal soft tissue and/or bone, no fracture/dislocation (11042-11047 [11045, 11046])
Removal soft tissue and/or bone with open fracture/dislocation (11010-11012)
Deep tissue repair (12031-13153)
Major exploration (20100-20103)
Repair of nerves, blood vessels, tendons (See appropriate anatomical section. These repairs include simple and intermediate closure. Report complex closure with modifier 59.)
Secondary closure/dehiscence (13160)

Code also modifier 59 added to the less complicated procedure code if reporting more than one classification of wound repair

12001 **Simple repair of superficial wounds of scalp, neck, axillae, external genitalia, trunk and/or extremities (including hands and feet); 2.5 cm or less**
1.27 2.53 **FUD** 000 Q1 N1
AMA: 2018,Sep,7; 2018,Jan,8; 2017,Dec,14; 2017,Jan,8; 2016,Jan,13; 2015,Jan,16; 2014,Jan,11

12002 **2.6 cm to 7.5 cm**
1.67 3.08 **FUD** 000 Q1 N1
AMA: 2018,Sep,7; 2018,Jan,8; 2017,Jan,8; 2016,Jan,13; 2015,Jan,16; 2014,Oct,14; 2014,Jan,11

12004 **7.6 cm to 12.5 cm**
2.09 3.61 **FUD** 000 Q1 N1
AMA: 2018,Sep,7; 2018,Jan,8; 2017,Jan,8; 2016,Jan,13; 2015,Jan,16; 2014,Jan,11

12005 **12.6 cm to 20.0 cm**
2.71 4.69 **FUD** 000 Q1 A2
AMA: 2018,Sep,7; 2018,Jan,8; 2017,Jan,8; 2016,Jan,13; 2015,Jan,16; 2014,Jan,11

12006 **20.1 cm to 30.0 cm**
3.33 5.54 **FUD** 000 Q2 A2
AMA: 2018,Sep,7; 2018,Jan,8; 2017,Jan,8; 2016,Jan,13; 2015,Jan,16; 2014,Jan,11

12007 **over 30.0 cm**
4.15 6.37 **FUD** 000 T A2
AMA: 2018,Sep,7; 2018,Jan,8; 2017,Jan,8; 2016,Jan,13; 2015,Jan,16; 2014,Jan,11

12011 **Simple repair of superficial wounds of face, ears, eyelids, nose, lips and/or mucous membranes; 2.5 cm or less**
1.57 3.09 **FUD** 000 Q1 N1
AMA: 2018,Sep,7; 2018,Jan,8; 2017,Jan,8; 2016,Nov,7; 2016,Jan,13; 2015,Jan,16; 2014,Jan,11

12013 **2.6 cm to 5.0 cm**
1.66 3.23 **FUD** 000 Q1 N1
AMA: 2018,Sep,7; 2018,Jan,8; 2017,Jan,8; 2016,Jan,13; 2015,Jan,16; 2014,Jan,11

12014 **5.1 cm to 7.5 cm**
2.14 3.88 **FUD** 000 Q1 N1
AMA: 2018,Sep,7; 2018,Jan,8; 2017,Jan,8; 2016,Jan,13; 2015,Jan,16; 2014,Jan,11

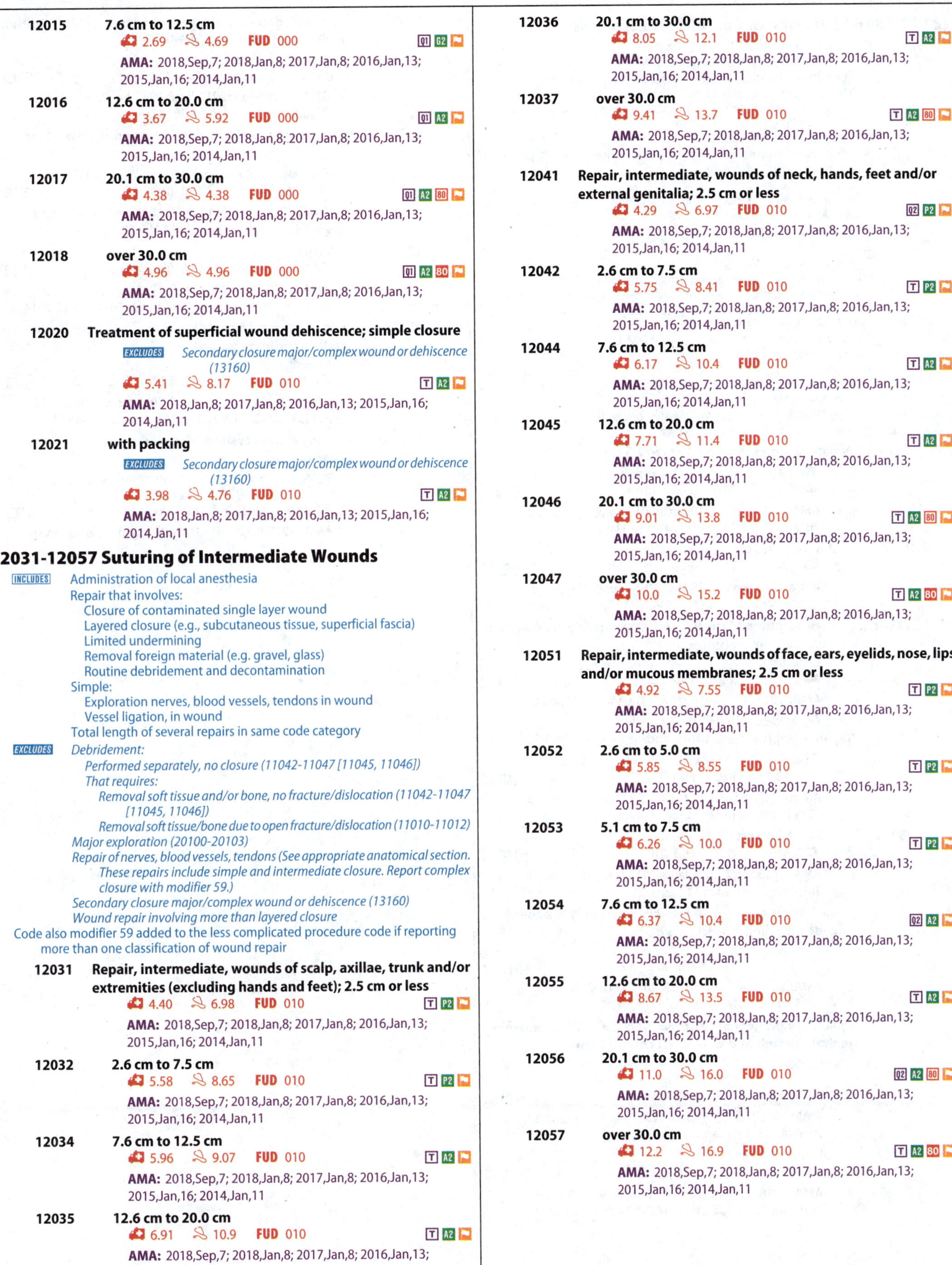

12015 **7.6 cm to 12.5 cm**
2.69 4.69 **FUD** 000 Q1 G2
AMA: 2018,Sep,7; 2018,Jan,8; 2017,Jan,8; 2016,Jan,13; 2015,Jan,16; 2014,Jan,11

12016 **12.6 cm to 20.0 cm**
3.67 5.92 **FUD** 000 Q1 A2
AMA: 2018,Sep,7; 2018,Jan,8; 2017,Jan,8; 2016,Jan,13; 2015,Jan,16; 2014,Jan,11

12017 **20.1 cm to 30.0 cm**
4.38 4.38 **FUD** 000 Q1 A2 80
AMA: 2018,Sep,7; 2018,Jan,8; 2017,Jan,8; 2016,Jan,13; 2015,Jan,16; 2014,Jan,11

12018 **over 30.0 cm**
4.96 4.96 **FUD** 000 Q1 A2 80
AMA: 2018,Sep,7; 2018,Jan,8; 2017,Jan,8; 2016,Jan,13; 2015,Jan,16; 2014,Jan,11

12020 **Treatment of superficial wound dehiscence; simple closure**
EXCLUDES *Secondary closure major/complex wound or dehiscence (13160)*
5.41 8.17 **FUD** 010 T A2
AMA: 2018,Jan,8; 2017,Jan,8; 2016,Jan,13; 2015,Jan,16; 2014,Jan,11

12021 **with packing**
EXCLUDES *Secondary closure major/complex wound or dehiscence (13160)*
3.98 4.76 **FUD** 010 T A2
AMA: 2018,Jan,8; 2017,Jan,8; 2016,Jan,13; 2015,Jan,16; 2014,Jan,11

12031-12057 Suturing of Intermediate Wounds

INCLUDES Administration of local anesthesia
Repair that involves:
- Closure of contaminated single layer wound
- Layered closure (e.g., subcutaneous tissue, superficial fascia)
- Limited undermining
- Removal foreign material (e.g. gravel, glass)
- Routine debridement and decontamination

Simple:
- Exploration nerves, blood vessels, tendons in wound
- Vessel ligation, in wound

Total length of several repairs in same code category

EXCLUDES *Debridement:*
- *Performed separately, no closure (11042-11047 [11045, 11046])*
- *That requires:*
  - *Removal soft tissue and/or bone, no fracture/dislocation (11042-11047 [11045, 11046])*
  - *Removal soft tissue/bone due to open fracture/dislocation (11010-11012)*

Major exploration (20100-20103)
Repair of nerves, blood vessels, tendons (See appropriate anatomical section. These repairs include simple and intermediate closure. Report complex closure with modifier 59.)
Secondary closure major/complex wound or dehiscence (13160)
Wound repair involving more than layered closure

Code also modifier 59 added to the less complicated procedure code if reporting more than one classification of wound repair

12031 **Repair, intermediate, wounds of scalp, axillae, trunk and/or extremities (excluding hands and feet); 2.5 cm or less**
4.40 6.98 **FUD** 010 T P2
AMA: 2018,Sep,7; 2018,Jan,8; 2017,Jan,8; 2016,Jan,13; 2015,Jan,16; 2014,Jan,11

12032 **2.6 cm to 7.5 cm**
5.58 8.65 **FUD** 010 T P2
AMA: 2018,Sep,7; 2018,Jan,8; 2017,Jan,8; 2016,Jan,13; 2015,Jan,16; 2014,Jan,11

12034 **7.6 cm to 12.5 cm**
5.96 9.07 **FUD** 010 T A2
AMA: 2018,Sep,7; 2018,Jan,8; 2017,Jan,8; 2016,Jan,13; 2015,Jan,16; 2014,Jan,11

12035 **12.6 cm to 20.0 cm**
6.91 10.9 **FUD** 010 T A2
AMA: 2018,Sep,7; 2018,Jan,8; 2017,Jan,8; 2016,Jan,13; 2015,Jan,16; 2014,Jan,11

12036 **20.1 cm to 30.0 cm**
8.05 12.1 **FUD** 010 T A2
AMA: 2018,Sep,7; 2018,Jan,8; 2017,Jan,8; 2016,Jan,13; 2015,Jan,16; 2014,Jan,11

12037 **over 30.0 cm**
9.41 13.7 **FUD** 010 T A2 80
AMA: 2018,Sep,7; 2018,Jan,8; 2017,Jan,8; 2016,Jan,13; 2015,Jan,16; 2014,Jan,11

12041 **Repair, intermediate, wounds of neck, hands, feet and/or external genitalia; 2.5 cm or less**
4.29 6.97 **FUD** 010 Q2 P2
AMA: 2018,Sep,7; 2018,Jan,8; 2017,Jan,8; 2016,Jan,13; 2015,Jan,16; 2014,Jan,11

12042 **2.6 cm to 7.5 cm**
5.75 8.41 **FUD** 010 T P2
AMA: 2018,Sep,7; 2018,Jan,8; 2017,Jan,8; 2016,Jan,13; 2015,Jan,16; 2014,Jan,11

12044 **7.6 cm to 12.5 cm**
6.17 10.4 **FUD** 010 T A2
AMA: 2018,Sep,7; 2018,Jan,8; 2017,Jan,8; 2016,Jan,13; 2015,Jan,16; 2014,Jan,11

12045 **12.6 cm to 20.0 cm**
7.71 11.4 **FUD** 010 T A2
AMA: 2018,Sep,7; 2018,Jan,8; 2017,Jan,8; 2016,Jan,13; 2015,Jan,16; 2014,Jan,11

12046 **20.1 cm to 30.0 cm**
9.01 13.8 **FUD** 010 T A2 80
AMA: 2018,Sep,7; 2018,Jan,8; 2017,Jan,8; 2016,Jan,13; 2015,Jan,16; 2014,Jan,11

12047 **over 30.0 cm**
10.0 15.2 **FUD** 010 T A2 80
AMA: 2018,Sep,7; 2018,Jan,8; 2017,Jan,8; 2016,Jan,13; 2015,Jan,16; 2014,Jan,11

12051 **Repair, intermediate, wounds of face, ears, eyelids, nose, lips and/or mucous membranes; 2.5 cm or less**
4.92 7.55 **FUD** 010 T P2
AMA: 2018,Sep,7; 2018,Jan,8; 2017,Jan,8; 2016,Jan,13; 2015,Jan,16; 2014,Jan,11

12052 **2.6 cm to 5.0 cm**
5.85 8.55 **FUD** 010 T P2
AMA: 2018,Sep,7; 2018,Jan,8; 2017,Jan,8; 2016,Jan,13; 2015,Jan,16; 2014,Jan,11

12053 **5.1 cm to 7.5 cm**
6.26 10.0 **FUD** 010 T P2
AMA: 2018,Sep,7; 2018,Jan,8; 2017,Jan,8; 2016,Jan,13; 2015,Jan,16; 2014,Jan,11

12054 **7.6 cm to 12.5 cm**
6.37 10.4 **FUD** 010 Q2 A2
AMA: 2018,Sep,7; 2018,Jan,8; 2017,Jan,8; 2016,Jan,13; 2015,Jan,16; 2014,Jan,11

12055 **12.6 cm to 20.0 cm**
8.67 13.5 **FUD** 010 T A2
AMA: 2018,Sep,7; 2018,Jan,8; 2017,Jan,8; 2016,Jan,13; 2015,Jan,16; 2014,Jan,11

12056 **20.1 cm to 30.0 cm**
11.0 16.0 **FUD** 010 Q2 A2 80
AMA: 2018,Sep,7; 2018,Jan,8; 2017,Jan,8; 2016,Jan,13; 2015,Jan,16; 2014,Jan,11

12057 **over 30.0 cm**
12.2 16.9 **FUD** 010 T A2 80
AMA: 2018,Sep,7; 2018,Jan,8; 2017,Jan,8; 2016,Jan,13; 2015,Jan,16; 2014,Jan,11

13100-13160 Suturing of Complicated Wounds

INCLUDES Creation of a limited defect for repair
Debridement complicated wounds/avulsions
Repair with layered closure that involves at least one of the following:
- Debridement of wound edges
- Exposure of underlying structures, such as bone, cartilage, tendon, or named neovascular structure
- Extensive undermining
- Free margin involvement of helical or nostril rim or vermillion border
- Retention suture placement

Simple:
- Exploration nerves, vessels, tendons in wound
- Vessel ligation in wound

Total length of several repairs in same code category

EXCLUDES *Excision (of or for):*
- *Benign lesions (11400-11446)*
- *Extensive debridement of open fracture/dislocation (11010-11012)*
- *Extensive debridement of penetrating or blunt trauma not associated with open fracture/dislocation (11042-11047 [11045, 11046])*
- *Malignant lesions (11600-11646)*
- *Surgical preparation of a wound bed (15002-15005)*

Extensive exploration (20100-20103)
Repair of nerves, blood vessel, tendons (See appropriate anatomical section. These repairs include simple and intermediate closure. Report complex closure with modifier 59.)

Code also modifier 59 added to the less complicated procedure code if reporting more than one classification of wound repair

13100 Repair, complex, trunk; 1.1 cm to 2.5 cm
EXCLUDES *Complex repair 1.0 cm or less (12001, 12031)*
5.90 9.66 **FUD** 010 T A2
AMA: 2018,Sep,7; 2018,Jan,8; 2017,Apr,9; 2017,Jan,8; 2016,Jan,13; 2015,Jan,16; 2014,Jan,11

13101 2.6 cm to 7.5 cm
7.27 11.3 **FUD** 010 T A2
AMA: 2018,Sep,7; 2018,Jan,8; 2017,Apr,9; 2017,Jan,8; 2016,Jan,13; 2015,Jan,16; 2014,Jan,11

\+ **13102 each additional 5 cm or less (List separately in addition to code for primary procedure)**
Code first (13101)
2.14 3.46 **FUD** ZZZ N N1
AMA: 2018,Sep,7; 2018,Jan,8; 2017,Apr,9; 2017,Jan,8; 2016,Jan,13; 2015,Jan,16; 2014,Jan,11

13120 Repair, complex, scalp, arms, and/or legs; 1.1 cm to 2.5 cm
EXCLUDES *Complex repair 1.0 cm or less (12001, 12031)*
6.78 10.0 **FUD** 010 T A2
AMA: 2018,Sep,7; 2018,Jan,8; 2017,Jan,8; 2016,Jan,13; 2015,Jan,16; 2014,Jan,11

13121 2.6 cm to 7.5 cm
7.67 12.2 **FUD** 010 T A2
AMA: 2018,Sep,7; 2018,Jan,8; 2017,Jan,8; 2016,Jan,13; 2015,Jan,16; 2014,Jan,11

\+ **13122 each additional 5 cm or less (List separately in addition to code for primary procedure)**
Code first (13121)
2.47 3.78 **FUD** ZZZ N N1
AMA: 2018,Sep,7; 2018,Jan,8; 2017,Jan,8; 2016,Jan,13; 2015,Jan,16; 2014,Jan,11

13131 Repair, complex, forehead, cheeks, chin, mouth, neck, axillae, genitalia, hands and/or feet; 1.1 cm to 2.5 cm
EXCLUDES *Complex repair 1.0 cm or less (12001, 12011, 12031, 12041, 12051)*
7.17 11.0 **FUD** 010 T A2
AMA: 2018,Sep,7; 2018,Jan,8; 2017,Apr,9; 2017,Jan,8; 2016,Jan,13; 2015,Jan,16; 2014,Jan,11

13132 2.6 cm to 7.5 cm
9.03 13.6 **FUD** 010 T A2
AMA: 2018,Sep,7; 2018,Jan,8; 2017,Apr,9; 2017,Jan,8; 2016,Jan,13; 2015,Jan,16; 2014,Oct,14; 2014,Jan,11

\+ **13133 each additional 5 cm or less (List separately in addition to code for primary procedure)**
Code first (13132)
3.77 5.06 **FUD** ZZZ N N1
AMA: 2018,Sep,7; 2018,Jan,8; 2017,Apr,9; 2017,Jan,8; 2016,Jan,13; 2015,Jan,16; 2014,Jan,11

13151 Repair, complex, eyelids, nose, ears and/or lips; 1.1 cm to 2.5 cm
EXCLUDES *Complex repair 1.0 cm or less (12011, 12051)*
8.25 12.1 **FUD** 010 T A2
AMA: 2018,Sep,7; 2018,Jan,8; 2017,Jan,8; 2016,Jan,13; 2015,Jan,16; 2014,May,3; 2014,Mar,12; 2014,Jan,11

13152 2.6 cm to 7.5 cm
9.99 14.4 **FUD** 010 T A2
AMA: 2018,Sep,7; 2018,Jan,8; 2017,Jan,8; 2016,Jan,13; 2015,Jan,16; 2014,Oct,14; 2014,May,3; 2014,Mar,12; 2014,Jan,11

\+ **13153 each additional 5 cm or less (List separately in addition to code for primary procedure)**
Code first (13152)
4.07 5.50 **FUD** ZZZ N N1
AMA: 2018,Sep,7; 2018,Jan,8; 2017,Jan,8; 2016,Jan,13; 2015,Jan,16; 2014,May,3; 2014,Mar,12; 2014,Jan,11

13160 Secondary closure of surgical wound or dehiscence, extensive or complicated
EXCLUDES *Packing or simple secondary wound closure (12020-12021)*
22.9 22.9 **FUD** 090 T A2
AMA: 2018,Jan,8; 2017,Jan,8; 2016,Jan,13; 2015,Jan,16; 2014,Jan,11

14000-14350 Reposition Contiguous Tissue

INCLUDES Excision (with or without lesion) with repair by adjacent tissue transfer or tissue rearrangement
Size of defect includes primary (due to excision) and secondary (due to flap design)
Z-plasty, W-plasty, VY-plasty, rotation flap, advancement flap, double pedicle flap, random island flap

EXCLUDES *Closure of wounds by undermining surrounding tissue without additional incisions (13100-13160)*
Full thickness closure of:
Eyelid (67930-67935, 67961-67975)
Lip (40650-40654)

Code also skin graft necessary to repair secondary defect (15040-15731)

14000 Adjacent tissue transfer or rearrangement, trunk; defect 10 sq cm or less

INCLUDES Burrow's operation

EXCLUDES *Excision of lesion with repair by adjacent tissue transfer or tissue rearrangement (11400-11446, 11600-11646)*

14.3 17.8 **FUD** 090 T A2

AMA: 2018,Jan,8; 2017,Oct,9; 2017,Jan,8; 2016,Jan,13; 2015,Sep,12; 2015,Feb,10; 2015,Jan,16; 2014,Apr,10; 2014,Jan,11

Example of common Z-plasty. Lesion is removed with oval-shaped incision

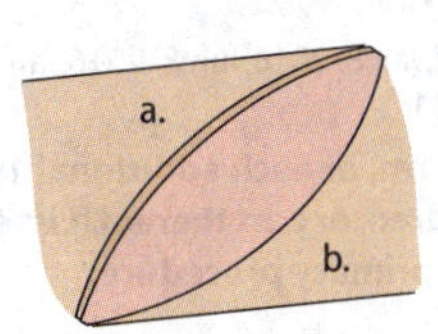

Two additional incisions (a. and b.) intersect the area

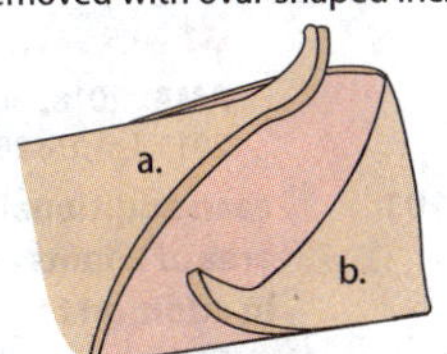

Skin of each incision is reflected back

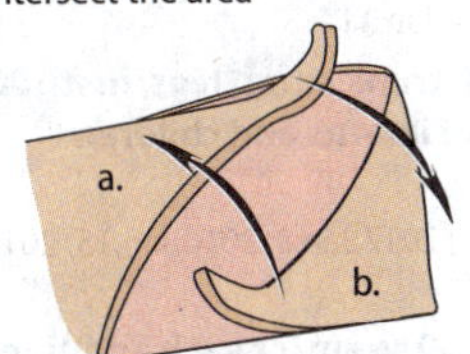

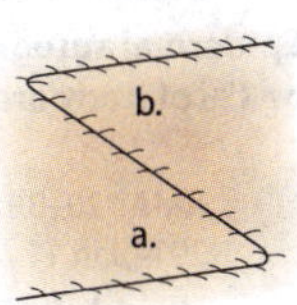

The flaps are then transposed and the repair is closed

An adjacent flap, or other rearrangement flap, is performed to repair a defect

14001 defect 10.1 sq cm to 30.0 sq cm

EXCLUDES *Excision of lesion with repair by adjacent tissue transfer or tissue rearrangement (11400-11446, 11600-11646)*

18.7 22.8 **FUD** 090 T A2

AMA: 2018,Jan,8; 2017,Oct,9; 2017,Jan,8; 2016,Jan,13; 2015,Feb,10; 2015,Jan,16; 2014,Apr,10; 2014,Jan,11

14020 Adjacent tissue transfer or rearrangement, scalp, arms and/or legs; defect 10 sq cm or less

EXCLUDES *Excision of lesion with repair by adjacent tissue transfer or tissue rearrangement (11400-11446, 11600-11646)*

16.2 19.8 **FUD** 090 T A2

AMA: 2018,Jan,8; 2017,Jan,8; 2016,Jan,13; 2015,Jan,16; 2014,Jan,11

14021 defect 10.1 sq cm to 30.0 sq cm

EXCLUDES *Excision of lesion with repair by adjacent tissue transfer or tissue rearrangement (11400-11446, 11600-11646)*

20.5 24.7 **FUD** 090 T A2

AMA: 2018,Jan,8; 2017,Jan,8; 2016,Jan,13; 2015,Jan,16; 2014,Jan,11

14040 Adjacent tissue transfer or rearrangement, forehead, cheeks, chin, mouth, neck, axillae, genitalia, hands and/or feet; defect 10 sq cm or less

INCLUDES Krimer's palatoplasty

EXCLUDES *Excision of lesion with repair by adjacent tissue transfer or tissue rearrangement (11400-11446, 11600-11646)*

18.1 21.7 **FUD** 090 T A2

AMA: 2018,Jan,8; 2017,Nov,6; 2017,Jan,8; 2016,Jan,13; 2015,Jan,16; 2014,Jan,11

14041 defect 10.1 sq cm to 30.0 sq cm

EXCLUDES *Excision of lesion with repair by adjacent tissue transfer or tissue rearrangement (11400-11446, 11600-11646)*

22.3 26.7 **FUD** 090 T A2

AMA: 2018,Jan,8; 2017,Nov,6; 2017,Jan,8; 2016,Jan,13; 2015,Jan,16; 2014,Jan,11

14060 Adjacent tissue transfer or rearrangement, eyelids, nose, ears and/or lips; defect 10 sq cm or less

INCLUDES Denonvillier's operation

EXCLUDES *Excision of lesion with repair by adjacent tissue transfer or tissue rearrangement (11400-11446, 11600-11646)*
Eyelid, full thickness (67961-67966)

19.3 22.1 **FUD** 090 T A2

AMA: 2018,Jan,8; 2017,Nov,6; 2017,Jan,8; 2016,Jan,13; 2015,Jan,16; 2014,Jan,11

14061 defect 10.1 sq cm to 30.0 sq cm

EXCLUDES *Excision of lesion with repair by adjacent tissue transfer or tissue rearrangement (11400-11446, 11600-11646)*
Eyelid, full thickness (67961 and subsequent codes)

23.8 28.7 **FUD** 090 T A2

AMA: 2018,Jan,8; 2017,Nov,6; 2017,Jan,8; 2016,Jan,13; 2015,Jan,16; 2014,Jan,11

14301 Adjacent tissue transfer or rearrangement, any area; defect 30.1 sq cm to 60.0 sq cm

EXCLUDES *Excision of lesion with repair by adjacent tissue transfer or tissue rearrangement (11400-11446, 11600-11646)*

25.2 30.7 **FUD** 090 T G2 80

AMA: 2018,Jan,8; 2017,Nov,6; 2017,Apr,9; 2017,Jan,8; 2016,Jan,13; 2015,Jan,16; 2014,Jan,11

\+ **14302 each additional 30.0 sq cm, or part thereof (List separately in addition to code for primary procedure)**

EXCLUDES *Excision of lesion with repair by adjacent tissue transfer or tissue rearrangement (11400-11446, 11600-11646)*

Code first (14301)

6.34 6.34 **FUD** ZZZ N N1 80

AMA: 2018,Jan,8; 2017,Nov,6; 2017,Jan,8; 2016,Jan,13; 2015,Jan,16; 2014,Jan,11

14350 Filleted finger or toe flap, including preparation of recipient site

19.6 19.6 **FUD** 090 T A2 80

AMA: 2018,Jan,8; 2017,Jan,8; 2016,Jan,13; 2015,Jan,16; 2014,Jan,11

15002-15005 Development of Base for Tissue Grafting

INCLUDES Add together the surface area of multiple wounds in the same anatomical locations as indicated in the code descriptor groups, such as face and scalp. Do not add together multiple wounds at different anatomical site groups such as trunk and face
Ankle or wrist if code description describes leg or arm
Cleaning and preparing a viable wound surface for grafting or negative pressure wound therapy used to heal the wound primarily
Code selection based on the defect size and location
Percentage applies to children younger than age 10
Removal of nonviable tissue in nonchronic wounds for primary healing
Square centimeters applies to children and adults age 10 or older

EXCLUDES *Chronic wound management on wounds left to heal by secondary intention (11042-11047 [11045, 11046], 97597-97598)*
Necrotizing soft tissue infections for specific anatomical locations (11004-11008)

15002 **Surgical preparation or creation of recipient site by excision of open wounds, burn eschar, or scar (including subcutaneous tissues), or incisional release of scar contracture, trunk, arms, legs; first 100 sq cm or 1% of body area of infants and children**
EXCLUDES *Linear scar revision (13100-13153)*
Facility RVU 6.47 Non-Facility RVU 9.94 FUD 000 T A2 80
AMA: 2018,Jan,8; 2017,Jan,8; 2016,Jan,13; 2015,Jan,16; 2014,Mar,12; 2014,Jan,11

\+ **15003** **each additional 100 sq cm, or part thereof, or each additional 1% of body area of infants and children (List separately in addition to code for primary procedure)**
Code first (15002)
Facility RVU 1.32 Non-Facility RVU 2.11 FUD ZZZ N N1 80
AMA: 2018,Jan,8; 2017,Jan,8; 2016,Jan,13; 2015,Jan,16; 2014,Mar,12; 2014,Jan,11

15004 **Surgical preparation or creation of recipient site by excision of open wounds, burn eschar, or scar (including subcutaneous tissues), or incisional release of scar contracture, face, scalp, eyelids, mouth, neck, ears, orbits, genitalia, hands, feet and/or multiple digits; first 100 sq cm or 1% of body area of infants and children**
Facility RVU 7.68 Non-Facility RVU 11.3 FUD 000 T A2 80
AMA: 2018,Jan,8; 2017,Jan,8; 2016,Jan,13; 2015,Jan,16; 2014,Mar,12; 2014,Jan,11

\+ **15005** **each additional 100 sq cm, or part thereof, or each additional 1% of body area of infants and children (List separately in addition to code for primary procedure)**
Code first (15004)
Facility RVU 2.64 Non-Facility RVU 3.52 FUD ZZZ N N1 80
AMA: 2018,Jan,8; 2017,Jan,8; 2016,Jan,13; 2015,Jan,16; 2014,Mar,12; 2014,Jan,11

15040 Obtain Autograft

INCLUDES Ankle or wrist if code description describes leg or arm
Percentage applies to children younger than age 10
Square centimeters applies to children and adults age 10 or older

15040 **Harvest of skin for tissue cultured skin autograft, 100 sq cm or less**
Facility RVU 3.62 Non-Facility RVU 7.29 FUD 000 T A2
AMA: 2018,Jan,8; 2017,Jan,8; 2016,Jan,13; 2015,Jan,16; 2014,Jan,11

15050 Pinch Graft

INCLUDES Autologous skin graft harvest and application
Current graft removal
Fixation and anchoring skin graft
Simple cleaning

EXCLUDES *Removal of devitalized tissue from wound(s), non-selective debridement, without anesthesia (97602)*

Code also graft or flap necessary to repair donor site

15050 **Pinch graft, single or multiple, to cover small ulcer, tip of digit, or other minimal open area (except on face), up to defect size 2 cm diameter**
Facility RVU 12.7 Non-Facility RVU 16.1 FUD 090 T A2
AMA: 2018,Jan,8; 2017,Jan,8; 2016,Jun,8; 2016,Jan,13; 2015,Jan,16; 2014,Jan,11

15100-15261 Skin Grafts and Replacements

INCLUDES Add together the surface area of multiple wounds in the same anatomical locations as indicated in the code description groups, such as face and scalp. Do not add together multiple wounds at different anatomical site groups such as trunk and face.
Ankle or wrist if code description describes leg or arm
Autologous skin graft harvest and application
Code selection based on recipient site location and size and type of graft
Current graft removal
Fixation and anchoring skin graft
Percentage applies to children younger than age 10
Simple cleaning
Simple tissue debridement
Square centimeters applies to children and adults age 10 or older

EXCLUDES *Debridement without immediate primary closure, when wound is grossly contaminated and extensive cleaning is needed, or when necrotic or contaminated tissue is removed (11042-11047 [11045, 11046], 97597-97598)*
Removal of devitalized tissue from wound(s), non-selective debridement, without anesthesia (97602)

Code also graft or flap necessary to repair donor site
Code also primary procedure requiring skin graft for definitive closure

15100 **Split-thickness autograft, trunk, arms, legs; first 100 sq cm or less, or 1% of body area of infants and children (except 15050)**
Facility RVU 20.5 Non-Facility RVU 24.5 FUD 090 T A2
AMA: 2018,Jan,8; 2017,Jan,8; 2016,Jun,8; 2016,Jan,13; 2015,Jan,16; 2014,Jan,11

\+ **15101** **each additional 100 sq cm, or each additional 1% of body area of infants and children, or part thereof (List separately in addition to code for primary procedure)**
Code first (15100)
Facility RVU 3.22 Non-Facility RVU 5.31 FUD ZZZ N N1
AMA: 2018,Jan,8; 2017,Jan,8; 2016,Jun,8; 2016,Jan,13; 2015,Jan,16; 2014,Jan,11

15110 **Epidermal autograft, trunk, arms, legs; first 100 sq cm or less, or 1% of body area of infants and children**
Facility RVU 19.8 Non-Facility RVU 22.8 FUD 090 T A2
AMA: 2018,Jan,8; 2017,Jan,8; 2016,Jan,13; 2015,Jan,16; 2014,Jan,11

\+ **15111** **each additional 100 sq cm, or each additional 1% of body area of infants and children, or part thereof (List separately in addition to code for primary procedure)**
Code first (15110)
Facility RVU 3.00 Non-Facility RVU 3.32 FUD ZZZ N N1
AMA: 2018,Jan,8; 2017,Jan,8; 2016,Jan,13; 2015,Jan,16; 2014,Jan,11

15115 **Epidermal autograft, face, scalp, eyelids, mouth, neck, ears, orbits, genitalia, hands, feet, and/or multiple digits; first 100 sq cm or less, or 1% of body area of infants and children**
Facility RVU 19.6 Non-Facility RVU 22.6 FUD 090 T A2
AMA: 2018,Jan,8; 2017,Jan,8; 2016,Jan,13; 2015,Jan,16; 2014,Jan,11

\+ **15116** **each additional 100 sq cm, or each additional 1% of body area of infants and children, or part thereof (List separately in addition to code for primary procedure)**
Code first (15115)
Facility RVU 4.38 Non-Facility RVU 4.80 FUD ZZZ N N1
AMA: 2018,Jan,8; 2017,Jan,8; 2016,Jan,13; 2015,Jan,16; 2014,Jan,11

15120 **Split-thickness autograft, face, scalp, eyelids, mouth, neck, ears, orbits, genitalia, hands, feet, and/or multiple digits; first 100 sq cm or less, or 1% of body area of infants and children (except 15050)**
EXCLUDES *Other eyelid repair (67961-67975)*
Facility RVU 20.0 Non-Facility RVU 24.2 FUD 090 T A2
AMA: 2018,Jan,8; 2017,Jan,8; 2016,Jun,8; 2016,Jan,13; 2015,Jan,16; 2014,Jan,11

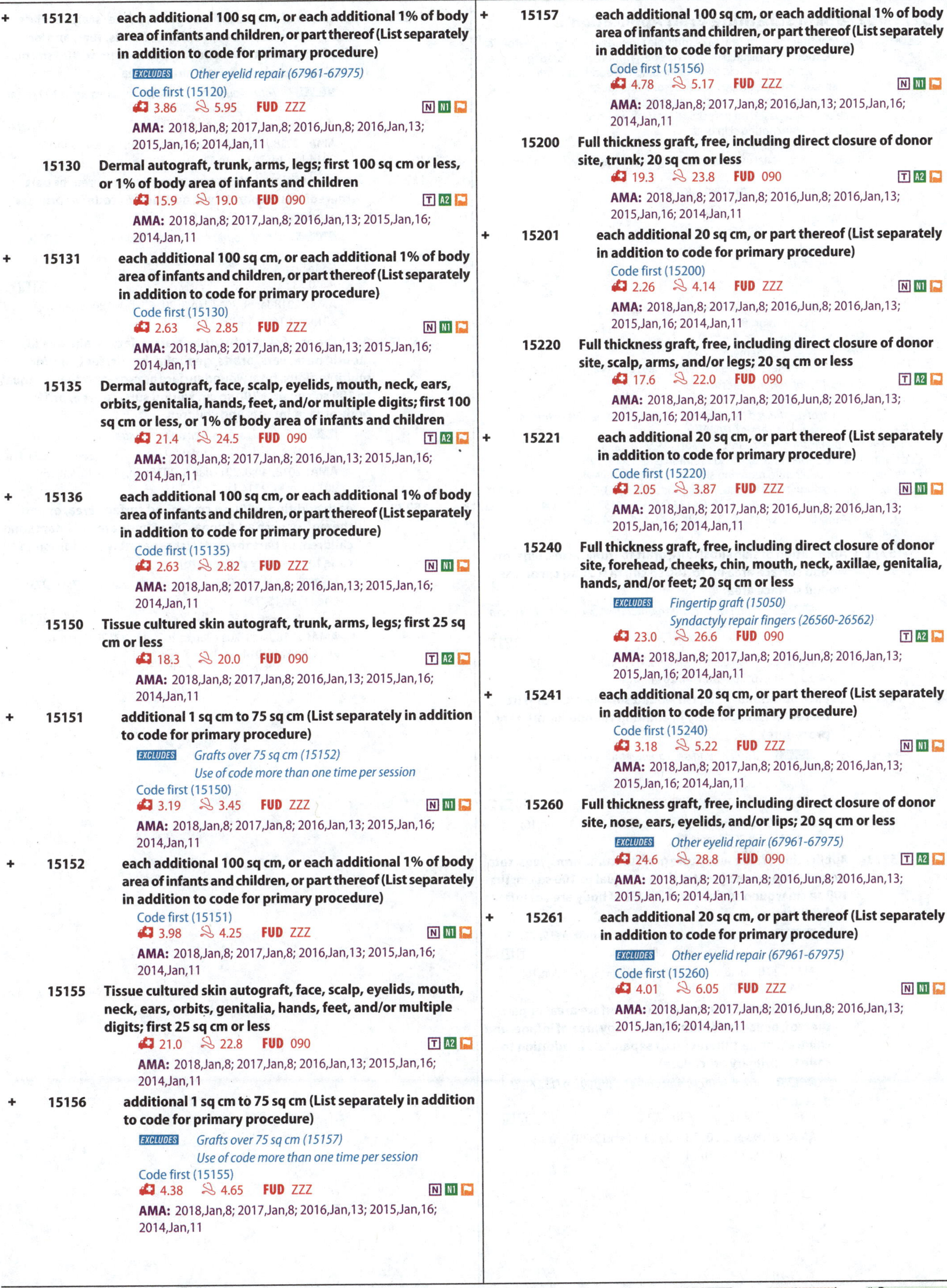

\+ 15121 **each additional 100 sq cm, or each additional 1% of body area of infants and children, or part thereof (List separately in addition to code for primary procedure)**

EXCLUDES *Other eyelid repair (67961-67975)*

Code first (15120)

3.86 5.95 FUD ZZZ N N1

AMA: 2018,Jan,8; 2017,Jan,8; 2016,Jun,8; 2016,Jan,13; 2015,Jan,16; 2014,Jan,11

15130 **Dermal autograft, trunk, arms, legs; first 100 sq cm or less, or 1% of body area of infants and children**

15.9 19.0 FUD 090 T A2

AMA: 2018,Jan,8; 2017,Jan,8; 2016,Jan,13; 2015,Jan,16; 2014,Jan,11

\+ 15131 **each additional 100 sq cm, or each additional 1% of body area of infants and children, or part thereof (List separately in addition to code for primary procedure)**

Code first (15130)

2.63 2.85 FUD ZZZ N N1

AMA: 2018,Jan,8; 2017,Jan,8; 2016,Jan,13; 2015,Jan,16; 2014,Jan,11

15135 **Dermal autograft, face, scalp, eyelids, mouth, neck, ears, orbits, genitalia, hands, feet, and/or multiple digits; first 100 sq cm or less, or 1% of body area of infants and children**

21.4 24.5 FUD 090 T A2

AMA: 2018,Jan,8; 2017,Jan,8; 2016,Jan,13; 2015,Jan,16; 2014,Jan,11

\+ 15136 **each additional 100 sq cm, or each additional 1% of body area of infants and children, or part thereof (List separately in addition to code for primary procedure)**

Code first (15135)

2.63 2.82 FUD ZZZ N N1

AMA: 2018,Jan,8; 2017,Jan,8; 2016,Jan,13; 2015,Jan,16; 2014,Jan,11

15150 **Tissue cultured skin autograft, trunk, arms, legs; first 25 sq cm or less**

18.3 20.0 FUD 090 T A2

AMA: 2018,Jan,8; 2017,Jan,8; 2016,Jan,13; 2015,Jan,16; 2014,Jan,11

\+ 15151 **additional 1 sq cm to 75 sq cm (List separately in addition to code for primary procedure)**

EXCLUDES *Grafts over 75 sq cm (15152)*
Use of code more than one time per session

Code first (15150)

3.19 3.45 FUD ZZZ N N1

AMA: 2018,Jan,8; 2017,Jan,8; 2016,Jan,13; 2015,Jan,16; 2014,Jan,11

\+ 15152 **each additional 100 sq cm, or each additional 1% of body area of infants and children, or part thereof (List separately in addition to code for primary procedure)**

Code first (15151)

3.98 4.25 FUD ZZZ N N1

AMA: 2018,Jan,8; 2017,Jan,8; 2016,Jan,13; 2015,Jan,16; 2014,Jan,11

15155 **Tissue cultured skin autograft, face, scalp, eyelids, mouth, neck, ears, orbits, genitalia, hands, feet, and/or multiple digits; first 25 sq cm or less**

21.0 22.8 FUD 090 T A2

AMA: 2018,Jan,8; 2017,Jan,8; 2016,Jan,13; 2015,Jan,16; 2014,Jan,11

\+ 15156 **additional 1 sq cm to 75 sq cm (List separately in addition to code for primary procedure)**

EXCLUDES *Grafts over 75 sq cm (15157)*
Use of code more than one time per session

Code first (15155)

4.38 4.65 FUD ZZZ N N1

AMA: 2018,Jan,8; 2017,Jan,8; 2016,Jan,13; 2015,Jan,16; 2014,Jan,11

\+ 15157 **each additional 100 sq cm, or each additional 1% of body area of infants and children, or part thereof (List separately in addition to code for primary procedure)**

Code first (15156)

4.78 5.17 FUD ZZZ N N1

AMA: 2018,Jan,8; 2017,Jan,8; 2016,Jan,13; 2015,Jan,16; 2014,Jan,11

15200 **Full thickness graft, free, including direct closure of donor site, trunk; 20 sq cm or less**

19.3 23.8 FUD 090 T A2

AMA: 2018,Jan,8; 2017,Jan,8; 2016,Jun,8; 2016,Jan,13; 2015,Jan,16; 2014,Jan,11

\+ 15201 **each additional 20 sq cm, or part thereof (List separately in addition to code for primary procedure)**

Code first (15200)

2.26 4.14 FUD ZZZ N N1

AMA: 2018,Jan,8; 2017,Jan,8; 2016,Jun,8; 2016,Jan,13; 2015,Jan,16; 2014,Jan,11

15220 **Full thickness graft, free, including direct closure of donor site, scalp, arms, and/or legs; 20 sq cm or less**

17.6 22.0 FUD 090 T A2

AMA: 2018,Jan,8; 2017,Jan,8; 2016,Jun,8; 2016,Jan,13; 2015,Jan,16; 2014,Jan,11

\+ 15221 **each additional 20 sq cm, or part thereof (List separately in addition to code for primary procedure)**

Code first (15220)

2.05 3.87 FUD ZZZ N N1

AMA: 2018,Jan,8; 2017,Jan,8; 2016,Jun,8; 2016,Jan,13; 2015,Jan,16; 2014,Jan,11

15240 **Full thickness graft, free, including direct closure of donor site, forehead, cheeks, chin, mouth, neck, axillae, genitalia, hands, and/or feet; 20 sq cm or less**

EXCLUDES *Fingertip graft (15050)*
Syndactyly repair fingers (26560-26562)

23.0 26.6 FUD 090 T A2

AMA: 2018,Jan,8; 2017,Jan,8; 2016,Jun,8; 2016,Jan,13; 2015,Jan,16; 2014,Jan,11

\+ 15241 **each additional 20 sq cm, or part thereof (List separately in addition to code for primary procedure)**

Code first (15240)

3.18 5.22 FUD ZZZ N N1

AMA: 2018,Jan,8; 2017,Jan,8; 2016,Jun,8; 2016,Jan,13; 2015,Jan,16; 2014,Jan,11

15260 **Full thickness graft, free, including direct closure of donor site, nose, ears, eyelids, and/or lips; 20 sq cm or less**

EXCLUDES *Other eyelid repair (67961-67975)*

24.6 28.8 FUD 090 T A2

AMA: 2018,Jan,8; 2017,Jan,8; 2016,Jun,8; 2016,Jan,13; 2015,Jan,16; 2014,Jan,11

\+ 15261 **each additional 20 sq cm, or part thereof (List separately in addition to code for primary procedure)**

EXCLUDES *Other eyelid repair (67961-67975)*

Code first (15260)

4.01 6.05 FUD ZZZ N N1

AMA: 2018,Jan,8; 2017,Jan,8; 2016,Jun,8; 2016,Jan,13; 2015,Jan,16; 2014,Jan,11

15271-15278 Skin Substitute Graft Application

INCLUDES Add together the surface area of multiple wounds in the same anatomical locations as indicated in the code description groups, such as face and scalp. Do not add together multiple wounds at different anatomical site groups such as trunk and face.
Ankle or wrist if code description describes leg or arm
Code selection based on defect site location and size
Fixation and anchoring skin graft
Graft types include:
Biological material used for tissue engineering (e.g.,scaffold) for growing skin
Nonautologous human skin such as:
Acellular
Allograft
Cellular
Dermal
Epidermal
Homograft
Nonhuman grafts
Percentage applies to children younger than age 10
Removing current graft
Simple cleaning
Simple tissue debridement
Square centimeters applies to children and adults age 10 or older

EXCLUDES *Application of nongraft dressing*
Injected skin substitutes
Removal of devitalized tissue from wound(s), non-selective debridement, without anesthesia (97602)
Skin application procedures, low cost (C5271-C5278)

Code also biologic implant for soft tissue reinforcement (15777)
Code also primary procedure requiring skin graft for definitive closure
Code also supply of high cost skin substitute product (C9363, Q4101, Q4103-Q4110, Q4116, Q4121-Q4123, Q4126-Q4128, Q4132-Q4133, Q4137-Q4138, Q4140-Q4141, Q4143, Q4146-Q4148, Q4150-Q4161, Q4163-Q4164, Q4169, Q4173, Q4175, Q4178)

15271 Application of skin substitute graft to trunk, arms, legs, total wound surface area up to 100 sq cm; first 25 sq cm or less wound surface area

EXCLUDES *Total wound area greater than or equal to 100 sq cm (15273-15274)*

2.42 4.14 FUD 000 T G2

AMA: 2018,Jan,8; 2017,Oct,9; 2017,Jan,8; 2016,Jan,13; 2015,Jan,16; 2014,Jun,14; 2014,Jan,11

+ 15272 each additional 25 sq cm wound surface area, or part thereof (List separately in addition to code for primary procedure)

EXCLUDES *Total wound area greater than or equal to 100 sq cm (15273-15274)*

Code first (15271)

0.50 0.76 FUD ZZZ N N1

AMA: 2018,Jan,8; 2017,Jan,8; 2016,Jan,13; 2015,Jan,16; 2014,Jun,14; 2014,Jan,11

15273 Application of skin substitute graft to trunk, arms, legs, total wound surface area greater than or equal to 100 sq cm; first 100 sq cm wound surface area, or 1% of body area of infants and children

EXCLUDES *Total wound surface area up to 100 cm (15271-15272)*

5.84 8.73 FUD 000 T G2

AMA: 2018,Jan,8; 2017,Jan,8; 2016,Jan,13; 2015,Jan,16; 2014,Jun,14; 2014,Jan,11

+ 15274 each additional 100 sq cm wound surface area, or part thereof, or each additional 1% of body area of infants and children, or part thereof (List separately in addition to code for primary procedure)

EXCLUDES *Total wound surface area up to 100 cm (15271-15272)*

Code first (15273)

1.33 2.15 FUD ZZZ N N1

AMA: 2018,Jan,8; 2017,Jan,8; 2016,Jan,13; 2015,Jan,16; 2014,Jun,14; 2014,Jan,11

15275 Application of skin substitute graft to face, scalp, eyelids, mouth, neck, ears, orbits, genitalia, hands, feet, and/or multiple digits, total wound surface area up to 100 sq cm; first 25 sq cm or less wound surface area

EXCLUDES *Total wound area greater than or equal to 100 sq cm (15277-15278)*

2.74 4.37 FUD 000 T G2

AMA: 2018,Jan,8; 2017,Jan,8; 2016,Jan,13; 2015,Jan,16; 2014,Jun,14; 2014,Jan,11

+ 15276 each additional 25 sq cm wound surface area, or part thereof (List separately in addition to code for primary procedure)

EXCLUDES *Total wound area greater than or equal to 100 sq cm (15277-15278)*

Code first (15275)

0.73 0.98 FUD ZZZ N N1

AMA: 2018,Jan,8; 2017,Jan,8; 2016,Jan,13; 2015,Jan,16; 2014,Jun,14; 2014,Jan,11

15277 Application of skin substitute graft to face, scalp, eyelids, mouth, neck, ears, orbits, genitalia, hands, feet, and/or multiple digits, total wound surface area greater than or equal to 100 sq cm; first 100 sq cm wound surface area, or 1% of body area of infants and children

EXCLUDES *Total surface area up to 100 sq cm (15275-15276)*

6.60 9.55 FUD 000 T G2

AMA: 2018,Jan,8; 2017,Jan,8; 2016,Jan,13; 2015,Jan,16; 2014,Jun,14; 2014,Jan,11

+ 15278 each additional 100 sq cm wound surface area, or part thereof, or each additional 1% of body area of infants and children, or part thereof (List separately in addition to code for primary procedure)

EXCLUDES *Total surface area up to 100 sq cm (15275-15276)*

Code first (15277)

1.66 2.54 FUD ZZZ N N1

AMA: 2018,Jan,8; 2017,Jan,8; 2016,Jan,13; 2015,Jan,16; 2014,Jun,14; 2014,Jan,11

15570-15731 Wound Reconstruction: Skin Flaps

INCLUDES Ankle or wrist if code description describes leg or arm
Code based on recipient site when the flap is attached in the transfer or to a final site and is based on donor site when a tube is created for transfer later or when the flap is delayed prior to transfer
Fixation and anchoring skin graft
Simple tissue debridement
Tube formation for later transfer

EXCLUDES *Contiguous tissue transfer flaps (14040-14041, 14060-14061, 14301-14302)*
Debridement without immediate primary closure (11042-11047 [11045, 11046], 97597-97598)
Excision of:
Benign lesion (11400-11471)
Burn eschar or scar (15002-15005)
Malignant lesion (11600-11646)
Microvascular repair (15756-15758)
Primary procedure--see appropriate anatomical site

Code also application of extensive immobilization apparatus
Code also repair of donor site with skin grafts or flaps

15570 **Formation of direct or tubed pedicle, with or without transfer; trunk**

INCLUDES Flaps without a vascular pedicle
21.0 26.0 FUD 090 T A2
AMA: 2018,Jan,8; 2017,Jan,8; 2016,Jan,13; 2015,Jan,16; 2014,Jan,11

Pedicle flap

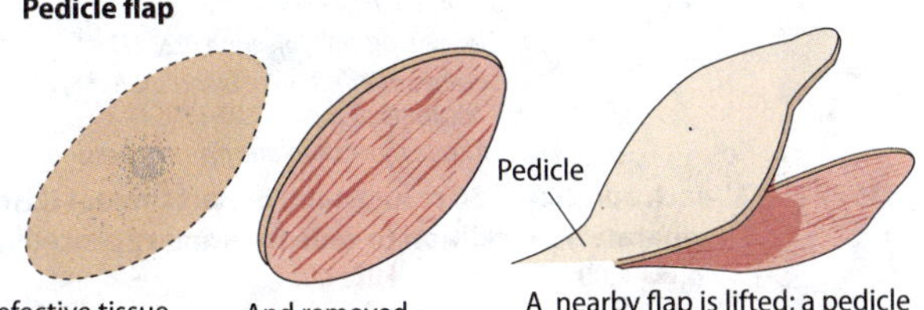

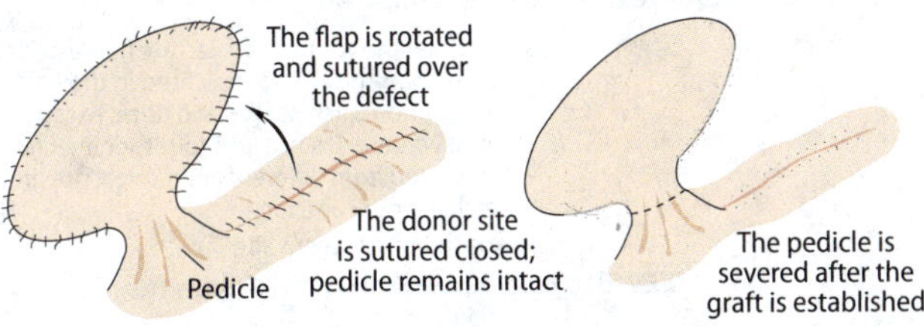

15572 **scalp, arms, or legs**

INCLUDES Flaps without a vascular pedicle
21.3 25.3 FUD 090 T A2
AMA: 2018,Jan,8; 2017,Jan,8; 2016,Jan,13; 2015,Jan,16; 2014,Jan,11

15574 **forehead, cheeks, chin, mouth, neck, axillae, genitalia, hands or feet**

INCLUDES Flaps without a vascular pedicle
21.7 25.8 FUD 090 T A2
AMA: 2018,Jan,8; 2017,Jan,8; 2016,Jan,13; 2015,Jan,16; 2014,Jan,11

15576 **eyelids, nose, ears, lips, or intraoral**

INCLUDES Flaps without a vascular pedicle
19.1 22.9 FUD 090 T A2
AMA: 2018,Jan,8; 2017,Jan,8; 2016,Jan,13; 2015,Jan,16; 2014,Jan,11

15600 **Delay of flap or sectioning of flap (division and inset); at trunk**

5.91 9.30 FUD 090 T A2 80
AMA: 2019,Jun,14; 2018,Jan,8; 2017,Jan,8; 2016,Jan,13; 2015,Jan,16; 2014,Jan,11

15610 **at scalp, arms, or legs**

6.86 10.1 FUD 090 T A2 80
AMA: 2018,Jan,8; 2017,Jan,8; 2016,Jan,13; 2015,Jan,16; 2014,Jan,11

15620 **at forehead, cheeks, chin, neck, axillae, genitalia, hands, or feet**

9.27 12.5 FUD 090 T A2
AMA: 2018,Jan,8; 2017,Jan,8; 2016,Jan,13; 2015,Jan,16; 2014,Jan,11

15630 **at eyelids, nose, ears, or lips**

9.87 13.0 FUD 090 T A2
AMA: 2018,Jan,8; 2017,Jan,8; 2016,Jan,13; 2015,Jan,16; 2014,Jan,11

15650 **Transfer, intermediate, of any pedicle flap (eg, abdomen to wrist, Walking tube), any location**

EXCLUDES *Defatting, revision, or rearranging of transferred pedicle flap or skin graft (13100-14302)*
Eyelids, ears, lips, and nose - refer to anatomical area
11.0 14.5 FUD 090 T A2 80
AMA: 2018,Jan,8; 2017,Jan,8; 2016,Jan,13; 2015,Jan,16; 2014,Jan,11

15730 **Midface flap (ie, zygomaticofacial flap) with preservation of vascular pedicle(s)**

26.4 43.6 FUD 090 T G2
AMA: 2018,Apr,10; 2018,Jan,8; 2017,Nov,6

15731 **Forehead flap with preservation of vascular pedicle (eg, axial pattern flap, paramedian forehead flap)**

EXCLUDES *Muscle, myocutaneous, or fasciocutaneous flap of the head or neck (15733)*
28.7 32.0 FUD 090 T A2 80
AMA: 2018,Jan,8; 2017,Nov,6; 2017,Jan,8; 2016,Jan,13; 2015,Jan,16; 2014,Jan,11

15733-15738 Wound Reconstruction: Muscle Flaps

INCLUDES Code based on donor site

EXCLUDES *Contiguous tissue transfer flaps (14040-14041, 14060-14061, 14301-14302)*
Microvascular repair (15756-15758)

Code also application of extensive immobilization apparatus
Code also repair of donor site with skin grafts or flaps

15733 **Muscle, myocutaneous, or fasciocutaneous flap; head and neck with named vascular pedicle (ie, buccinators, genioglossus, temporalis, masseter, sternocleidomastoid, levator scapulae)**

INCLUDES Repair of extracranial defect by anterior pericranial flap on vascular pedicle (15731)
30.1 30.1 FUD 090 T A2
AMA: 2018,Apr,10; 2018,Jan,8; 2017,Nov,6

15734 **trunk**

43.4 43.4 FUD 090 T A2 80
AMA: 2018,Aug,10; 2018,Jan,8; 2017,Nov,6; 2017,Jan,8; 2016,Jan,13; 2015,Jan,16; 2014,Apr,10; 2014,Jan,11

15736 **upper extremity**

35.3 35.3 FUD 090 T A2
AMA: 2018,Jan,8; 2017,Nov,6; 2017,Jan,8; 2016,Jan,13; 2015,Jan,16; 2014,Jan,11

15738 **lower extremity**

37.6 37.6 FUD 090 T A2 80
AMA: 2018,Jan,8; 2017,Nov,6; 2017,Jan,8; 2016,Jan,13; 2015,Jan,16; 2014,Jan,11

15740-15758 Wound Reconstruction: Other

INCLUDES Fixation and anchoring skin graft
Routine dressing
Simple tissue debridement

EXCLUDES *Adjacent tissue transfer (14000-14302)*
Excision of:
Benign lesion (11400-11471)
Burn eschar or scar (15002-15005)
Malignant lesion (11600-11646)
Flaps without addition of a vascular pedicle (15570-15576)
Primary procedure--see appropriate anatomical section
Skin graft for repair of donor site (15050-15278)

Code also repair of donor site with skin grafts or flaps (14000-14350, 15050-15278)

15740 Flap; island pedicle requiring identification and dissection of an anatomically named axial vessel

EXCLUDES *V-Y subcutaneous flaps, random island flaps, and other flaps from adjacent areas (14000-14302)*

24.2 28.8 FUD 090 T A2

AMA: 2018,Jan,8; 2017,Dec,14; 2017,Jan,8; 2016,Jan,13; 2015,Jan,16; 2014,Jan,11

15750 neurovascular pedicle

EXCLUDES *V-Y subcutaneous flaps, random island flaps, and other flaps from adjacent areas (14000-14302)*

26.3 26.3 FUD 090 T A2 80

AMA: 2018,Jan,8; 2017,Dec,14

15756 Free muscle or myocutaneous flap with microvascular anastomosis

INCLUDES Operating microscope (69990)

66.2 66.2 FUD 090 C 80

AMA: 2018,Jan,8; 2017,Jan,8; 2016,Feb,12; 2016,Jan,13; 2015,Jan,16; 2014,Jan,11

15757 Free skin flap with microvascular anastomosis

INCLUDES Operating microscope (69990)

65.5 65.5 FUD 090 C 80

AMA: 2018,Jan,8; 2017,Jan,8; 2016,Apr,8; 2016,Feb,12; 2016,Jan,13; 2015,Jan,16; 2014,Jan,11

15758 Free fascial flap with microvascular anastomosis

INCLUDES Operating microscope (69990)

66.0 66.0 FUD 090 C 80

AMA: 2018,Jan,8; 2017,Jan,8; 2016,Feb,12; 2016,Jan,13; 2015,Jan,16; 2014,Jan,11

15760-15774 [15769] Other Grafts

EXCLUDES *Adjacent tissue transfer (14000-14302)*
Excision of:
Benign lesion (11400-11471)
Burn eschar or scar (15002-15005)
Malignant lesion (11600-11646)
Flaps without addition of vascular pedicle (15570-15576)
Microvascular repair (15756-15758)
Primary procedure (see appropriate anatomical site)
Repair of donor site with skin grafts or flaps (14000-14350, 15050-15278)

15760 Graft; composite (eg, full thickness of external ear or nasal ala), including primary closure, donor area

INCLUDES Fixation and anchoring skin graft
Routine dressing
Simple tissue debridement

20.2 24.2 FUD 090 T A2

AMA: 2018,Jan,8; 2017,Jan,8; 2016,Jan,13; 2015,Jan,16; 2014,Jan,11

15769 **Resequenced code. See code following 15770.**

15770 derma-fat-fascia

INCLUDES Fixation and anchoring skin graft
Routine dressing
Simple tissue debridement

19.0 19.0 FUD 090 T A2 80

AMA: 2018,Jan,8; 2017,Jan,8; 2016,Jan,13; 2015,Jan,16; 2014,Jan,11

● # **15769 Grafting of autologous soft tissue, other, harvested by direct excision (eg, fat, dermis, fascia)**

0.00 0.00 FUD 000

INCLUDES Excisional graft harvest and recipient site placement

EXCLUDES *Autologous grafts of specific tissue types, such as skin, bone, nerve, tendon, fascia lata, or vessels*
Autologous white blood cell concentrate injection (0481T)
Harvesting of adipose tissue for adipose-derived regenerative cell therapy (0489T-0490T)
Platelet-rich plasma injection (0232T)
Suction assisted lipectomy (15876-15879)

● **15771 Grafting of autologous fat harvested by liposuction technique to trunk, breasts, scalp, arms, and/or legs; 50 cc or less injectate**

INCLUDES Add together the volume of injectate harvested from each anatomical area indicated in the code description, such as face and neck, to report the total volume. Do not add together injectate harvested from different anatomical site groups, such as trunk and face
Code based on recipient site

EXCLUDES *Autologous white blood cell concentrate injection (0481T)*
Liposuction not for grafting purposes (15876-15879)
Obtaining tissue for adipose-derived regenerative cell therapy (0489T-0490T)
Platelet-rich plasma injection (0232T)
Subcutaneous injection of filling material, at same anatomical site (11950-11954)
Use of code more than one time per session

● + **15772 each additional 50 cc injectate, or part thereof (List separately in addition to code for primary procedure)**

0.00 0.00 FUD 000

Code first (15771)

● **15773 Grafting of autologous fat harvested by liposuction technique to face, eyelids, mouth, neck, ears, orbits, genitalia, hands, and/or feet; 25 cc or less injectate**

INCLUDES Add together the volume of injectate harvested from each anatomical area indicated in the code description, such as face and neck, to report the total volume. Do not add together injectate harvested from different anatomical site groups, such as trunk and face
Code based on recipient site

EXCLUDES *Autologous white blood cell concentrate injection (0481T)*
Liposuction not for grafting purposes (15876-15879)
Obtaining tissue for adipose-derived regenerative cell therapy (0489T-0490T)
Platelet-rich plasma injection (0232T)
Subcutaneous injection of filling material, at same anatomical site (11950-11954)
Use of code more than one time per session

● + **15774 each additional 25 cc injectate, or part thereof (List separately in addition to code for primary procedure)**

0.00 0.00 FUD 000

Code first (15773)

15775-15839 Plastic, Reconstructive, and Aesthetic Surgery

CMS: 100-02,16,10 Exclusions from Coverage; 100-02,16,120 Cosmetic Procedures; 100-02,16,180 Services Related to Noncovered Procedures

15775 Punch graft for hair transplant; 1 to 15 punch grafts

EXCLUDES *Strip transplant (15220)*

6.42 | 8.74 | FUD 000 | T A2 80

AMA: 2018,Jan,8; 2017,Jan,8; 2016,Jan,13; 2015,Jan,16; 2014,Jan,11

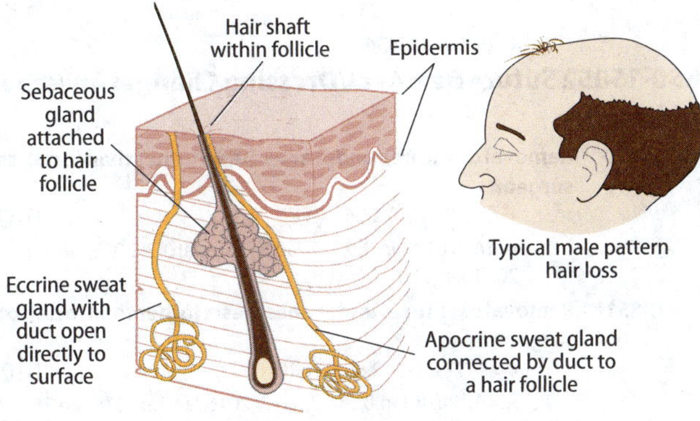

15776 more than 15 punch grafts

EXCLUDES *Strip transplant (15220)*

9.12 | 12.5 | FUD 000 | T A2 80

AMA: 2018,Jan,8; 2017,Jan,8; 2016,Jan,13; 2015,Jan,16; 2014,Jan,11

+ **15777 Implantation of biologic implant (eg, acellular dermal matrix) for soft tissue reinforcement (ie, breast, trunk) (List separately in addition to code for primary procedure)**

EXCLUDES *Application of skin substitute (high cost) to an external wound (15271-15278)*
Application of skin substitute (low cost) to an external wound (C5271-C5278)
Mesh implantation for:
Open repair of ventral or incisional hernia (49560-49566) and (49568)
Repair of devitalized soft tissue infection (11004-11006) and (49568)
Repair of pelvic floor (57267)
Repair anorectal fistula with plug (46707)
Reporting with modifier 50. Report once for each side when performed bilaterally
Soft tissue reinforcement with biologic implants other than in the breast or trunk (17999)

Code also supply of biologic implant

Code also synthetic or non-biological implant to reinforce abdominal wall (0437T)

Code first primary procedure

6.25 | 6.25 | FUD ZZZ | 50 N N1

AMA: 2019,Jan,14; 2018,Jan,8; 2017,Jan,8; 2016,Jan,13; 2015,Jan,16; 2014,Jan,11

15780 Dermabrasion; total face (eg, for acne scarring, fine wrinkling, rhytids, general keratosis)

20.1 | 26.1 | FUD 090 | J P3 80

AMA: 2018,Jan,8; 2017,Jan,8; 2016,Jan,13; 2015,Jan,16; 2014,Jan,11

15781 segmental, face

12.3 | 15.7 | FUD 090 | T P2

AMA: 1997,Nov,1

15782 regional, other than face

11.9 | 16.3 | FUD 090 | J P3 80

AMA: 1997,Nov,1

15783 superficial, any site (eg, tattoo removal)

10.6 | 13.6 | FUD 090 | T P2 80

AMA: 2018,Jan,8; 2017,Jan,8; 2016,Jan,13; 2015,Jan,16; 2014,Jan,11

15786 Abrasion; single lesion (eg, keratosis, scar)

3.91 | 6.98 | FUD 010 | Q1 N1

AMA: 1997,Nov,1

+ **15787 each additional 4 lesions or less (List separately in addition to code for primary procedure)**

Code first (15786)

0.50 | 1.27 | FUD ZZZ | N N1

AMA: 1997,Nov,1

15788 Chemical peel, facial; epidermal

6.81 | 12.7 | FUD 090 | Q1 N1

AMA: 1997,Nov,1; 1993,Win,1

15789 dermal

11.8 | 15.7 | FUD 090 | T P2

AMA: 1997,Nov,1; 1993,Win,1

15792 Chemical peel, nonfacial; epidermal

7.02 | 11.8 | FUD 090 | Q1 N1 80

AMA: 1997,Nov,1; 1993,Win,1

15793 dermal

10.3 | 14.0 | FUD 090 | Q1 N1 80

AMA: 1997,Nov,1; 1993,Win,1

15819 Cervicoplasty

22.7 | 22.7 | FUD 090 | T G2 80

AMA: 1997,Nov,1

15820 Blepharoplasty, lower eyelid;

14.5 | 16.2 | FUD 090 | T A2 80 50

AMA: 2018,Jan,8; 2017,Jan,8; 2016,Jan,13; 2015,Jan,16; 2014,Jan,11

15821 with extensive herniated fat pad

15.5 | 17.3 | FUD 090 | T A2 80 50

AMA: 2018,Jan,8; 2017,Jan,8; 2016,Jan,13; 2015,Jan,16; 2014,Jan,11

15822 Blepharoplasty, upper eyelid;

11.1 | 12.7 | FUD 090 | T A2 50

AMA: 2018,Jan,8; 2017,Jan,8; 2016,Jan,13; 2015,Jan,16; 2014,Jan,11

15823 with excessive skin weighting down lid

15.5 | 17.3 | FUD 090 | T A2 50

AMA: 2018,Jan,8; 2017,Jan,8; 2016,Jan,13; 2015,Jan,16; 2014,Jan,11

15824 Rhytidectomy; forehead

EXCLUDES *Repair of brow ptosis (67900)*

0.00 | 0.00 | FUD 000 | T A2 80 50

AMA: 2018,Jan,8; 2017,Apr,9

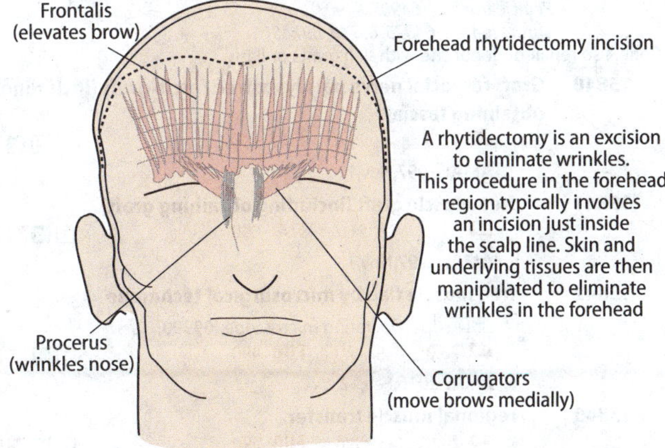

15825 neck with platysmal tightening (platysmal flap, P-flap)

0.00 | 0.00 | FUD 000 | T A2 80 50

AMA: 2018,Jan,8; 2017,Apr,9

15826 glabellar frown lines

0.00 | 0.00 | FUD 000 | T A2 80 50

AMA: 1997,Nov,1

15828 cheek, chin, and neck
0.00 0.00 **FUD** 000 T A2 80 50
AMA: 1997,Nov,1

15829 superficial musculoaponeurotic system (SMAS) flap
0.00 0.00 **FUD** 000 T A2 80 50
AMA: 1997,Nov,1

15830 Excision, excessive skin and subcutaneous tissue (includes lipectomy); abdomen, infraumbilical panniculectomy
33.7 33.7 **FUD** 090 J A2 80
EXCLUDES *Adjacent tissue transfer, trunk (14000-14001, 14302)*
Complex wound repair, trunk (13100-13102)
Intermediate wound repair, trunk (12031-12032, 12034-12037)
Other abdominoplasty (17999)
Code also (15847)

15832 thigh
26.4 26.4 **FUD** 090 J A2 80 50
AMA: 1997,Nov,1

15833 leg
25.0 25.0 **FUD** 090 J A2 80 50
AMA: 1997,Nov,1

15834 hip
25.5 25.5 **FUD** 090 J A2 80 50
AMA: 1997,Nov,1

15835 buttock
26.8 26.8 **FUD** 090 J A2 80
AMA: 1997,Nov,1

15836 arm
22.6 22.6 **FUD** 090 J A2 80 50
AMA: 1997,Nov,1

15837 forearm or hand
20.6 24.7 **FUD** 090 J G2 80
AMA: 1997,Nov,1

15838 submental fat pad
18.3 18.3 **FUD** 090 J G2 80
AMA: 1998,Feb,1; 1997,Nov,1

15839 other area
21.1 25.2 **FUD** 090 J A2 80
AMA: 1997,Nov,1

15840-15845 Reanimation of the Paralyzed Face

INCLUDES Routine dressing and supplies
EXCLUDES *Intravenous fluorescein evaluation of blood flow in graft or flap (15860)*
Nerve:
Decompression (69720, 69725, 69955)
Pedicle transfer (64905, 64907)
Suture (64831-64876, 69740, 69745)
Code also repair of donor site with skin grafts or flaps

15840 Graft for facial nerve paralysis; free fascia graft (including obtaining fascia)
28.8 28.8 **FUD** 090 T A2
AMA: 1997,Nov,1

15841 free muscle graft (including obtaining graft)
51.2 51.2 **FUD** 090 T A2 80
AMA: 1997,Nov,1

15842 free muscle flap by microsurgical technique
INCLUDES Operating microscope (69990)
78.0 78.0 **FUD** 090 T G2 80
AMA: 2016,Feb,12

15845 regional muscle transfer
28.8 28.8 **FUD** 090 T A2 80
AMA: 1998,Feb,1; 1997,Nov,1

15847 Removal of Excess Abdominal Tissue Add-on

CMS: 100-02,16,10 Exclusions from Coverage; 100-02,16,120 Cosmetic Procedures; 100-02,16,180 Services Related to Noncovered Procedures

\+ **15847** Excision, excessive skin and subcutaneous tissue (includes lipectomy), abdomen (eg, abdominoplasty) (includes umbilical transposition and fascial plication) (List separately in addition to code for primary procedure)
0.00 0.00 **FUD** YYY N N1 80
EXCLUDES *Abdominal wall hernia repair (49491-49587)*
Other abdominoplasty (17999)
Code first (15830)

15850-15852 Suture Removal/Dressing Change: Anesthesia Required

15850 Removal of sutures under anesthesia (other than local), same surgeon
1.19 2.56 **FUD** XXX T G2
AMA: 2018,Jan,8; 2017,Jan,8; 2016,Jan,13; 2015,Jan,16; 2014,Jan,11

15851 Removal of sutures under anesthesia (other than local), other surgeon
1.31 2.85 **FUD** 000 T P3
AMA: 2018,Jan,8; 2017,Jan,8; 2016,Jan,13; 2015,Jan,16; 2014,Jan,11

15852 Dressing change (for other than burns) under anesthesia (other than local)
EXCLUDES *Dressing change for burns (16020-16030)*
1.33 1.33 **FUD** 000 Q1 N1
AMA: 1997,Nov,1

15860 Injection for Vascular Flow Determination

15860 Intravenous injection of agent (eg, fluorescein) to test vascular flow in flap or graft
3.10 3.10 **FUD** 000 Q1 N1 80
AMA: 2002,May,7; 1997,Nov,1

15876-15879 Liposuction

CMS: 100-02,16,10 Exclusions from Coverage; 100-02,16,120 Cosmetic Procedures; 100-02,16,180 Services Related to Noncovered Procedures

EXCLUDES *Liposuction for autologous fat grafting (15771-15774)*
Obtaining tissue for adipose-derived regenerative cell therapy (0489T-0490T)

15876 Suction assisted lipectomy; head and neck
0.00 0.00 **FUD** 000 T A2 80
AMA: 2019,Aug,10; 2018,Sep,12

Cannula typically inserted through incision in front of ear

15877 trunk
0.00 0.00 **FUD** 000 T A2 80
AMA: 2019,Aug,10; 2018,Sep,12; 2018,Jan,8; 2017,Jan,8; 2016,Jan,13; 2015,Jan,16; 2014,Jan,11

15878 upper extremity
0.00 0.00 **FUD** 000 T A2 80 50
AMA: 2019,Aug,10; 2018,Sep,12

15879 lower extremity
0.00 0.00 FUD 000 T A2 80 50
AMA: 2019,Aug,10; 2018,Sep,12

15920-15999 Treatment of Decubitus Ulcers

Code also free skin graft to repair ulcer or donor site

15920 **Excision, coccygeal pressure ulcer, with coccygectomy; with primary suture**
17.8 17.8 FUD 090 J A2 80
AMA: 2011,May,3-5; 1997,Nov,1

15922 **with flap closure**
22.5 22.5 FUD 090 T A2 80
AMA: 2011,May,3-5; 1997,Nov,1

15931 **Excision, sacral pressure ulcer, with primary suture;**
19.9 19.9 FUD 090 J A2
AMA: 2011,May,3-5; 1997,Nov,1

15933 **with ostectomy**
24.5 24.5 FUD 090 J A2 80
AMA: 2011,May,3-5; 1997,Nov,1

15934 **Excision, sacral pressure ulcer, with skin flap closure;**
27.1 27.1 FUD 090 T A2
AMA: 2011,May,3-5; 1997,Nov,1

15935 **with ostectomy**
31.6 31.6 FUD 090 T A2 80
AMA: 2011,May,3-5; 1997,Nov,1

15936 **Excision, sacral pressure ulcer, in preparation for muscle or myocutaneous flap or skin graft closure;**
Code also any defect repair with:
Muscle or myocutaneous flap (15734, 15738)
Split skin graft (15100-15101)
25.7 25.7 FUD 090 T A2
AMA: 2011,May,3-5; 1998,Nov,1

15937 **with ostectomy**
Code also any defect repair with:
Muscle or myocutaneous flap (15734, 15738)
Split skin graft (15100-15101)
29.8 29.8 FUD 090 T A2
AMA: 2011,May,3-5; 1998,Nov,1

15940 **Excision, ischial pressure ulcer, with primary suture;**
20.1 20.1 FUD 090 J A2
AMA: 2011,May,3-5; 1997,Nov,1

15941 **with ostectomy (ischiectomy)**
26.0 26.0 FUD 090 J A2 80
AMA: 2011,May,3-5; 1997,Nov,1

15944 **Excision, ischial pressure ulcer, with skin flap closure;**
25.8 25.8 FUD 090 T A2 80
AMA: 2011,May,3-5; 1997,Nov,1

15945 **with ostectomy**
28.4 28.4 FUD 090 T A2 80
AMA: 2011,May,3-5; 1997,Nov,1

15946 **Excision, ischial pressure ulcer, with ostectomy, in preparation for muscle or myocutaneous flap or skin graft closure**
Code also any defect repair with:
Muscle or myocutaneous flap (15734, 15738)
Split skin graft (15100-15101)
46.8 46.8 FUD 090 T A2
AMA: 2018,Jan,8; 2017,Jan,8; 2016,Jan,13; 2015,Jan,16; 2014,Jan,11

15950 **Excision, trochanteric pressure ulcer, with primary suture;**
17.3 17.3 FUD 090 J A2
AMA: 2011,May,3-5; 1997,Nov,1

15951 **with ostectomy**
25.3 25.3 FUD 090 J A2 80
AMA: 2011,May,3-5; 1997,Nov,1

15952 **Excision, trochanteric pressure ulcer, with skin flap closure;**
26.0 26.0 FUD 090 T A2 80
AMA: 2011,May,3-5; 1997,Nov,1

15953 **with ostectomy**
28.6 28.6 FUD 090 T A2
AMA: 2011,May,3-5; 1997,Nov,1

15956 **Excision, trochanteric pressure ulcer, in preparation for muscle or myocutaneous flap or skin graft closure;**
Code also any defect repair with:
Muscle or myocutaneous flap (15734, 15738)
Split skin graft (15100-15101)
33.3 33.3 FUD 090 T A2
AMA: 2011,May,3-5; 1998,Nov,1

15958 **with ostectomy**
Code also any defect repair with:
Muscle or myocutaneous flap (15734-15738)
Split skin graft (15100-15101)
34.0 34.0 FUD 090 T A2
AMA: 2011,May,3-5; 1998,Nov,1

15999 **Unlisted procedure, excision pressure ulcer**
0.00 0.00 FUD YYY T 80
AMA: 2011,May,3-5; 1997,Nov,1

16000-16036 Burn Care

INCLUDES Local care of burn surface only
EXCLUDES *Application of skin grafts including all services described in the following codes (15100-15777)*
E&M services
Flaps (15570-15650)
Laser fenestration for scars (0479T-0480T)

16000 **Initial treatment, first degree burn, when no more than local treatment is required**
1.32 2.00 FUD 000 Q1 N1
AMA: 2018,Jan,8; 2017,Jan,8; 2016,Jan,13; 2015,Jan,16; 2014,Jan,11

16020 **Dressings and/or debridement of partial-thickness burns, initial or subsequent; small (less than 5% total body surface area)**
INCLUDES Wound coverage other than skin graft
1.55 2.32 FUD 000 Q1 N1
AMA: 2018,Jan,8; 2017,Jan,8; 2016,Jan,13; 2015,Jan,16; 2014,Jan,11

16025 **medium (eg, whole face or whole extremity, or 5% to 10% total body surface area)**
INCLUDES Wound coverage other than skin graft
3.16 4.26 FUD 000 T A2
AMA: 2018,Jan,8; 2017,Jan,8; 2016,Jan,13; 2015,Jan,16; 2014,Jan,11

16030 **large (eg, more than 1 extremity, or greater than 10% total body surface area)**
INCLUDES Wound coverage other than skin graft
3.82 5.40 FUD 000 T A2
AMA: 2018,Jan,8; 2017,Jan,8; 2016,Jan,13; 2015,Jan,16; 2014,Jan,11

16035 **Escharotomy; initial incision**
EXCLUDES *Debridement or scraping of burn (16020-16030)*
5.65 5.65 FUD 000 T G2
AMA: 2018,Jan,8; 2017,Jan,8; 2016,Jan,13; 2015,Jan,16; 2014,Jan,11

+ **16036** **each additional incision (List separately in addition to code for primary procedure)**
EXCLUDES *Debridement or scraping of burn (16020-16030)*
Code first (16035)
2.36 2.36 FUD ZZZ C
AMA: 2018,Jan,8; 2017,Jan,8; 2016,Jan,13; 2015,Jan,16; 2014,Jan,11

Integumentary System

17000 — 17270

17000-17004 Destruction Any Method: Premalignant Lesion

CMS: 100-03,140.5 Laser Procedures

EXCLUDES *Cryotherapy acne (17340)*
Destruction of:
Benign lesions other than cutaneous vascular proliferative lesions (17110-17111)
Cutaneous vascular proliferative lesions (17106-17108)
Malignant lesions (17260-17286)
Plantar warts (17110-17111)
Destruction of lesion of:
Anus (46900-46917, 46924)
Conjunctiva (68135)
Eyelid (67850)
Penis (54050-54057, 54065)
Vagina (57061, 57065)
Vestibule of mouth (40820)
Vulva (56501, 56515)
Destruction or excision of skin tags (11200-11201)
Escharotomy (16035-16036)
Excision benign lesion (11400-11446)
Laser fenestration for scars (0479T-0480T)
Localized chemotherapy treatment see appropriate office visit service code
Paring or excision of benign hyperkeratotic lesion (11055-11057)
Shaving skin lesions (11300-11313)
Treatment of inflammatory skin disease via laser (96920-96922)

17000 **Destruction (eg, laser surgery, electrosurgery, cryosurgery, chemosurgery, surgical curettement), premalignant lesions (eg, actinic keratoses); first lesion**
1.53 1.85 **FUD** 010 Q1 N1
AMA: 2018,Jan,8; 2017,Dec,14; 2017,Jan,8; 2016,Apr,3; 2016,Jan,13; 2015,Jan,16; 2014,Jan,11

\+ **17003** **second through 14 lesions, each (List separately in addition to code for first lesion)**
Code first (17000)
0.07 0.16 **FUD** ZZZ N N1
AMA: 2018,Jan,8; 2017,Dec,14; 2017,Jan,8; 2016,Apr,3; 2016,Jan,13; 2015,Jan,16; 2014,Jan,11

17004 **Destruction (eg, laser surgery, electrosurgery, cryosurgery, chemosurgery, surgical curettement), premalignant lesions (eg, actinic keratoses), 15 or more lesions**
EXCLUDES *Use of code for destruction of less than 15 lesions (17000-17003)*
2.85 4.31 **FUD** 010 T P3
AMA: 2018,Jan,8; 2017,Dec,14; 2017,Jan,8; 2016,Apr,3; 2016,Jan,13; 2015,Jan,16; 2014,Jan,11

17106-17250 Destruction Any Method: Vascular Proliferative Lesion

CMS: 100-02,16,10 Exclusions from Coverage; 100-02,16,120 Cosmetic Procedures

EXCLUDES *Destruction of lesion of:*
Anus (46900-46917, 46924)
Conjunctiva (68135)
Eyelid (67850)
Penis (54050-54057, 54065)
Vagina (57061, 57065)
Vestibule of mouth (40820)
Vulva (56501, 56515)
Treatment of inflammatory skin disease via laser (96920-96922)

17106 **Destruction of cutaneous vascular proliferative lesions (eg, laser technique); less than 10 sq cm**
7.93 9.78 **FUD** 090 T P2
AMA: 2019,Sep,10; 2018,Jan,8; 2017,Dec,14; 2017,Jan,8; 2016,Apr,3; 2016,Jan,13; 2015,Jan,16; 2014,Jan,11

17107 **10.0 to 50.0 sq cm**
10.1 12.6 **FUD** 090 T P2
AMA: 2018,Jan,8; 2017,Dec,14; 2017,Jan,8; 2016,Apr,3; 2016,Jan,13; 2015,Jan,16; 2014,Jan,11

17108 **over 50.0 sq cm**
15.2 18.3 **FUD** 090 T P3 80
AMA: 2018,Jan,8; 2017,Dec,14; 2017,Jan,8; 2016,Apr,3; 2016,Jan,13; 2015,Jan,16; 2014,Jan,11

17110 **Destruction (eg, laser surgery, electrosurgery, cryosurgery, chemosurgery, surgical curettement), of benign lesions other than skin tags or cutaneous vascular proliferative lesions; up to 14 lesions**
1.96 3.13 **FUD** 010 Q1 N1
AMA: 2018,Jan,8; 2017,Dec,14; 2017,Jan,8; 2016,Apr,3; 2016,Jan,13; 2015,Jan,16; 2014,Jan,11

17111 **15 or more lesions**
EXCLUDES *Destruction of neurofibromas, 50-100 lesions (0419T-0420T)*
2.41 3.71 **FUD** 010 Q1 N1
AMA: 2018,Jan,8; 2017,Dec,14; 2017,Jan,8; 2016,Apr,3; 2016,Jan,13; 2015,Jan,16; 2014,Jan,11

17250 **Chemical cauterization of granulation tissue (ie, proud flesh)**
EXCLUDES *Excision/removal codes for the same lesion*
Chemical cauterization when applied for hemostasis of wound
Wound care management (97597-97598, 97602)
1.05 2.31 **FUD** 000 Q1 N1
AMA: 2018,Jan,8; 2017,Dec,14; 2017,Jan,8; 2016,Jan,13; 2015,Jan,16; 2014,Jan,11

17260-17286 Destruction, Any Method: Malignant Lesion

CMS: 100-03,140.5 Laser Procedures

EXCLUDES *Destruction of lesion of:*
Anus (46900-46917, 46924)
Conjunctiva (68135)
Eyelid (67850)
Penis (54050-54057, 54065)
Vestibule of mouth (40820)
Vulva (56501-56515)
Localized chemotherapy treatment see appropriate office visit service code
Shaving skin lesion (11300-11313)
Treatment of inflammatory skin disease via laser (96920-96922)

17260 **Destruction, malignant lesion (eg, laser surgery, electrosurgery, cryosurgery, chemosurgery, surgical curettement), trunk, arms or legs; lesion diameter 0.5 cm or less**
2.03 2.71 **FUD** 010 Q1 N1
AMA: 2018,Jan,8; 2017,Dec,14; 2017,Jan,8; 2016,Jan,13; 2015,Jan,16; 2014,Jan,11

17261 **lesion diameter 0.6 to 1.0 cm**
2.58 4.11 **FUD** 010 Q1 N1
AMA: 2018,Jan,8; 2017,Dec,14; 2017,Jan,8; 2016,Jan,13; 2015,Jan,16; 2014,Jan,11

17262 **lesion diameter 1.1 to 2.0 cm**
3.30 5.01 **FUD** 010 Q1 N1
AMA: 2018,Jan,8; 2017,Dec,14; 2017,Jan,8; 2016,Jan,13; 2015,Jan,16; 2014,Jan,11

17263 **lesion diameter 2.1 to 3.0 cm**
3.66 5.47 **FUD** 010 Q1 N1
AMA: 2018,Jan,8; 2017,Dec,14; 2017,Jan,8; 2016,Jan,13; 2015,Jan,16; 2014,Jan,11

17264 **lesion diameter 3.1 to 4.0 cm**
3.90 5.85 **FUD** 010 T P3
AMA: 2018,Jan,8; 2017,Dec,14; 2017,Jan,8; 2016,Jan,13; 2015,Jan,16; 2014,Jan,11

17266 **lesion diameter over 4.0 cm**
4.60 6.66 **FUD** 010 T P3
AMA: 2018,Jan,8; 2017,Dec,14; 2017,Jan,8; 2016,Jan,13; 2015,Jan,16; 2014,Jan,11

17270 **Destruction, malignant lesion (eg, laser surgery, electrosurgery, cryosurgery, chemosurgery, surgical curettement), scalp, neck, hands, feet, genitalia; lesion diameter 0.5 cm or less**
2.84 4.24 **FUD** 010 T P2
AMA: 2018,Jan,8; 2017,Dec,14; 2017,Jan,8; 2016,Jan,13; 2015,Jan,16; 2014,Jan,11

17271 **lesion diameter 0.6 to 1.0 cm**
3.14 4.67 FUD 010 T P2
AMA: 2018,Jan,8; 2017,Dec,14; 2017,Jan,8; 2016,Jan,13; 2015,Jan,16; 2014,Jan,11

17272 **lesion diameter 1.1 to 2.0 cm**
3.63 5.33 FUD 010 Q1 N1
AMA: 2018,Jan,8; 2017,Dec,14; 2017,Jan,8; 2016,Jan,13; 2015,Jan,16; 2014,Jan,11

17273 **lesion diameter 2.1 to 3.0 cm**
4.11 5.94 FUD 010 T P3
AMA: 2018,Jan,8; 2017,Dec,14; 2017,Jan,8; 2016,Jan,13; 2015,Jan,16; 2014,Jan,11

17274 **lesion diameter 3.1 to 4.0 cm**
5.04 7.01 FUD 010 T P3
AMA: 2018,Jan,8; 2017,Dec,14; 2017,Jan,8; 2016,Jan,13; 2015,Jan,16; 2014,Jan,11

17276 **lesion diameter over 4.0 cm**
6.02 8.11 FUD 010 T P3
AMA: 2018,Jan,8; 2017,Dec,14; 2017,Jan,8; 2016,Jan,13; 2015,Jan,16; 2014,Jan,11

17280 **Destruction, malignant lesion (eg, laser surgery, electrosurgery, cryosurgery, chemosurgery, surgical curettement), face, ears, eyelids, nose, lips, mucous membrane; lesion diameter 0.5 cm or less**
2.58 3.97 FUD 010 Q1 N1
AMA: 2018,Jan,8; 2017,Dec,14; 2017,Jan,8; 2016,Jan,13; 2015,Jan,16; 2014,Jan,11

17281 **lesion diameter 0.6 to 1.0 cm**
3.54 5.09 FUD 010 T P3
AMA: 2018,Jan,8; 2017,Dec,14; 2017,Jan,8; 2016,Jan,13; 2015,Jan,16; 2014,Jan,11

17282 **lesion diameter 1.1 to 2.0 cm**
4.10 5.84 FUD 010 T P3
AMA: 2018,Jan,8; 2017,Dec,14; 2017,Jan,8; 2016,Jan,13; 2015,Jan,16; 2014,Jan,11

17283 **lesion diameter 2.1 to 3.0 cm**
5.13 6.99 FUD 010 T P3
AMA: 2018,Jan,8; 2017,Dec,14; 2017,Jan,8; 2016,Jan,13; 2015,Jan,16; 2014,Jan,11

17284 **lesion diameter 3.1 to 4.0 cm**
5.97 7.97 FUD 010 T P3
AMA: 2018,Jan,8; 2017,Dec,14; 2017,Jan,8; 2016,Jan,13; 2015,Jan,16; 2014,Jan,11

17286 **lesion diameter over 4.0 cm**
8.03 10.2 FUD 010 T P3
AMA: 2018,Jan,8; 2017,Dec,14; 2017,Jan,8; 2016,Jan,13; 2015,Jan,16; 2014,Jan,11

17311-17315 Mohs Surgery

INCLUDES The following surgical/pathology services performed by the same physician or other qualified health care provider:
- Evaluation of skin margins by surgeon
- Pathology exam on Mohs surgery specimen (by Mohs surgeon) (88302-88309)
- Routine frozen section stain (88314)
- Tumor removal, mapping, preparation, and examination of lesion

EXCLUDES *Frozen section if no prior diagnosis determination has been performed (88331)*

Code also any special histochemical stain on a frozen section, nonroutine (with modifier 59) (88311-88314, 88342)
Code also biopsy (with modifier 59) if no prior diagnosis determination has been performed, if biopsy is indeterminate, or performed more than 90 days preoperatively (11102, 11104, 11106)
Code also complex repair (13100-13160)
Code also flaps or grafts (14000-14350, 15050-15770)
Code also intermediate repair (12031-12057)
Code also simple repair (12001-12021)

17311 **Mohs micrographic technique, including removal of all gross tumor, surgical excision of tissue specimens, mapping, color coding of specimens, microscopic examination of specimens by the surgeon, and histopathologic preparation including routine stain(s) (eg, hematoxylin and eosin, toluidine blue), head, neck, hands, feet, genitalia, or any location with surgery directly involving muscle, cartilage, bone, tendon, major nerves, or vessels; first stage, up to 5 tissue blocks**
10.8 18.9 FUD 000 T P2
AMA: 2018,Jan,8; 2017,Jan,8; 2016,Jan,13; 2015,Jan,16; 2014,Oct,14; 2014,Feb,10

+ **17312** **each additional stage after the first stage, up to 5 tissue blocks (List separately in addition to code for primary procedure)**
Code first (17311)
5.76 11.2 FUD ZZZ N N1
AMA: 2018,Jan,8; 2017,Jan,8; 2016,Jan,13; 2015,Jan,16; 2014,Oct,14; 2014,Feb,10

17313 **Mohs micrographic technique, including removal of all gross tumor, surgical excision of tissue specimens, mapping, color coding of specimens, microscopic examination of specimens by the surgeon, and histopathologic preparation including routine stain(s) (eg, hematoxylin and eosin, toluidine blue), of the trunk, arms, or legs; first stage, up to 5 tissue blocks**
9.70 17.7 FUD 000 T P2
AMA: 2018,Jan,8; 2017,Jan,8; 2016,Jan,13; 2015,Jan,16; 2014,Oct,14; 2014,Feb,10

+ **17314** **each additional stage after the first stage, up to 5 tissue blocks (List separately in addition to code for primary procedure)**
Code first (17313)
5.34 10.7 FUD ZZZ N N1
AMA: 2018,Jan,8; 2017,Jan,8; 2016,Jan,13; 2015,Jan,16; 2014,Oct,14; 2014,Feb,10

+ **17315** **Mohs micrographic technique, including removal of all gross tumor, surgical excision of tissue specimens, mapping, color coding of specimens, microscopic examination of specimens by the surgeon, and histopathologic preparation including routine stain(s) (eg, hematoxylin and eosin, toluidine blue), each additional block after the first 5 tissue blocks, any stage (List separately in addition to code for primary procedure)**
Code first (17311-17314)
1.52 2.26 FUD ZZZ N N1
AMA: 2018,Jan,8; 2017,Jan,8; 2016,Jan,13; 2015,Jan,16; 2014,Oct,14; 2014,Feb,10; 2014,Jan,11

17340-17999 Treatment for Active Acne and Permanent Hair Removal

CMS: 100-02,16,10 Exclusions from Coverage; 100-02,16,120 Cosmetic Procedures

17340 **Cryotherapy (CO_2 slush, liquid N_2) for acne**
1.40 1.49 FUD 010 Q1 N1
AMA: 2018,Jan,8; 2017,Jan,8; 2016,Jan,13; 2015,Jan,16; 2014,Jan,11

17360 **Chemical exfoliation for acne (eg, acne paste, acid)**
2.77 3.61 FUD 010 Q1 N1
AMA: 2018,Jan,8; 2017,Jan,8; 2016,Jan,13; 2015,Jan,16; 2014,Jan,11

17380 **Electrolysis epilation, each 30 minutes**
EXCLUDES *Actinotherapy (96900)*
0.00 0.00 FUD 000 T R2 80
AMA: 2018,Jan,8; 2017,Jan,8; 2016,Jan,13; 2015,Jan,16; 2014,Jan,11

17999 **Unlisted procedure, skin, mucous membrane and subcutaneous tissue**
0.00 0.00 FUD YYY Q1 80
AMA: 2019,Sep,10; 2019,Mar,10; 2019,Jan,14; 2018,Jan,8; 2017,Dec,13; 2017,Jan,8; 2016,May,13; 2016,Jan,13; 2015,Jan,16; 2014,Jan,11

19000-19030 Treatment of Breast Abscess and Cyst with Injection, Aspiration, Incision

19000 **Puncture aspiration of cyst of breast;**
(76942, 77021)
1.26 3.12 FUD 000 T P3
AMA: 2018,Jan,8; 2017,Jan,8; 2016,Jan,13; 2015,Jan,16; 2014,Jan,11

\+ **19001** **each additional cyst (List separately in addition to code for primary procedure)**
Code first (19000)
(76942, 77021)
0.62 0.77 FUD ZZZ N N1
AMA: 2018,Jan,8; 2017,Jan,8; 2016,Jan,13; 2015,Jan,16; 2014,Jan,11

19020 **Mastotomy with exploration or drainage of abscess, deep**
8.84 13.5 FUD 090 J A2 50
AMA: 2018,Jan,8; 2017,Jan,8; 2016,Jan,13; 2015,Jan,16; 2014,Dec,16; 2014,Dec,16; 2014,Jan,11

19030 **Injection procedure only for mammary ductogram or galactogram**
(77053-77054)
2.23 4.74 FUD 000 N N1 50
AMA: 2018,Jan,8; 2017,Jan,8; 2016,Jan,13; 2015,Jan,16; 2014,Jan,11

19081-19086 Breast Biopsy with Imaging Guidance

CMS: 100-03,220.13 Percutaneous Image-guided Breast Biopsy; 100-04,12,40.7 Bilateral Procedures; 100-04,13,80.1 Physician Presence; 100-04,13,80.2 S&I Multiple Procedure Reduction

INCLUDES Breast biopsy with placement of localization devices
Fluoroscopic guidance for needle placement (77002)
Magnetic resonance guidance for needle placement (77021)
Radiological examination, surgical specimen (76098)
Ultrasonic guidance for needle placement (76942)

EXCLUDES *Biopsy of breast without imaging guidance (19100-19101)*
Lesion removal without concentration on surgical margins (19110-19126)
Open biopsy after placement of localization device (19101)
Partial mastectomy (19301-19302)
Placement of localization devices only (19281-19288)
Total mastectomy (19303-19307)

Code also additional biopsies performed with different imaging modalities

19081 **Biopsy, breast, with placement of breast localization device(s) (eg, clip, metallic pellet), when performed, and imaging of the biopsy specimen, when performed, percutaneous; first lesion, including stereotactic guidance**
4.85 18.4 FUD 000 J G2 80 50
AMA: 2019,Apr,4; 2018,Jan,8; 2017,Jan,8; 2016,Jun,3; 2016,Jan,13; 2015,May,8; 2015,Mar,5; 2015,Jan,16; 2014,Jun,14; 2014,May,3

\+ **19082** **each additional lesion, including stereotactic guidance (List separately in addition to code for primary procedure)**
Code first (19081)
2.44 15.0 FUD ZZZ N N1 80
AMA: 2019,Apr,4; 2018,Jan,8; 2017,Jan,8; 2016,Jun,3; 2016,Jan,13; 2015,May,8; 2015,Mar,5; 2015,Jan,16; 2014,Jun,14; 2014,May,3

19083 **Biopsy, breast, with placement of breast localization device(s) (eg, clip, metallic pellet), when performed, and imaging of the biopsy specimen, when performed, percutaneous; first lesion, including ultrasound guidance**
4.57 18.0 FUD 000 J G2 80 50
AMA: 2019,Apr,4; 2018,Jan,8; 2017,Jan,8; 2016,Jun,3; 2016,Jan,13; 2015,May,8; 2015,Mar,5; 2015,Jan,16; 2014,Jun,14; 2014,May,3

\+ **19084** **each additional lesion, including ultrasound guidance (List separately in addition to code for primary procedure)**
Code first (19083)
2.28 14.4 FUD ZZZ N N1 80
AMA: 2019,Apr,4; 2018,Jan,8; 2017,Jan,8; 2016,Jun,3; 2016,Jan,13; 2015,May,8; 2015,Mar,5; 2015,Jan,16; 2014,Jun,14; 2014,May,3

19085 **Biopsy, breast, with placement of breast localization device(s) (eg, clip, metallic pellet), when performed, and imaging of the biopsy specimen, when performed, percutaneous; first lesion, including magnetic resonance guidance**
5.30 27.3 FUD 000 J G2 80 50
AMA: 2019,Apr,4; 2018,Jan,8; 2017,Jan,8; 2016,Jun,3; 2016,Jan,13; 2015,May,8; 2015,Mar,5; 2015,Jan,16; 2014,Jun,14; 2014,May,3

\+ **19086** **each additional lesion, including magnetic resonance guidance (List separately in addition to code for primary procedure)**
Code first (19085)
2.65 21.9 FUD ZZZ N N1 80
AMA: 2019,Apr,4; 2018,Jan,8; 2017,Jan,8; 2016,Jun,3; 2016,Jan,13; 2015,May,8; 2015,Mar,5; 2015,Jan,16; 2014,Jun,14; 2014,May,3

19100-19101 Breast Biopsy Without Imaging Guidance

EXCLUDES *Biopsy of breast with imaging guidance (19081-19086)*
Lesion removal without concentration on surgical margins (19110-19126)
Partial mastectomy (19301-19302)
Total mastectomy (19303-19307)

19100 **Biopsy of breast; percutaneous, needle core, not using imaging guidance (separate procedure)**
EXCLUDES *Fine needle aspiration:*
With imaging guidance ([10005, 10006, 10007, 10008, 10009, 10010, 10011, 10012])
Without imaging guidance (10021, [10004])
2.03 4.32 FUD 000 J A2 50
AMA: 2018,Jan,8; 2017,Jan,8; 2016,Jan,13; 2015,Jan,16; 2014,May,3; 2014,Jan,11

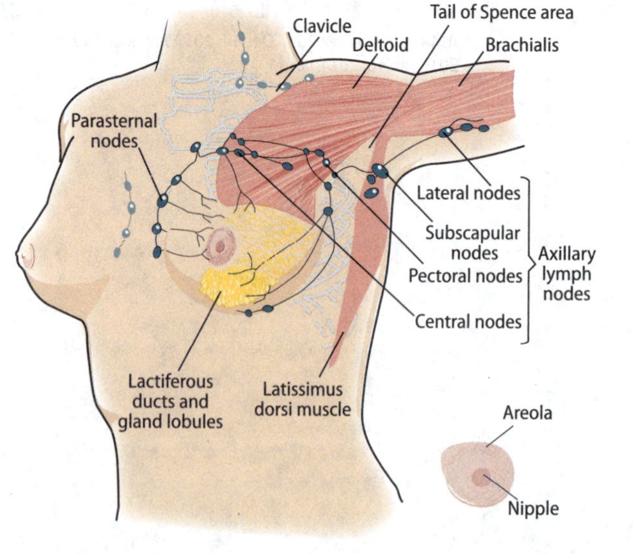

19101 open, incisional

Code also placement of localization device with imaging guidance (19281-19288)

6.39 9.64 FUD 010 J A2 50

AMA: 2018,Jan,8; 2017,Jan,8; 2016,Jan,13; 2015,Jan,16; 2014,May,3; 2014,Jan,11

19105 Treatment of Fibroadenoma: Cryoablation

CMS: 100-04,13,80.1 Physician Presence; 100-04,13,80.2 S&I Multiple Procedure Reduction

INCLUDES Adjacent lesions treated with one cryoprobe
Ultrasound guidance (76940, 76942)

EXCLUDES *Cryoablation of malignant breast tumors (0581T)*

19105 **Ablation, cryosurgical, of fibroadenoma, including ultrasound guidance, each fibroadenoma**

6.13 80.5 FUD 000 J J8 50

AMA: 2007,Mar,7-8

19110-19126 Excisional Procedures: Breast

INCLUDES Open removal of breast mass without concentration on surgical margins

Code also placement of localization device with imaging guidance (19281-19288)

19110 **Nipple exploration, with or without excision of a solitary lactiferous duct or a papilloma lactiferous duct**

9.94 13.9 FUD 090 J A2 50

AMA: 2018,Jan,8; 2017,Jan,8; 2016,Jan,13; 2015,Jan,16; 2014,Jan,11

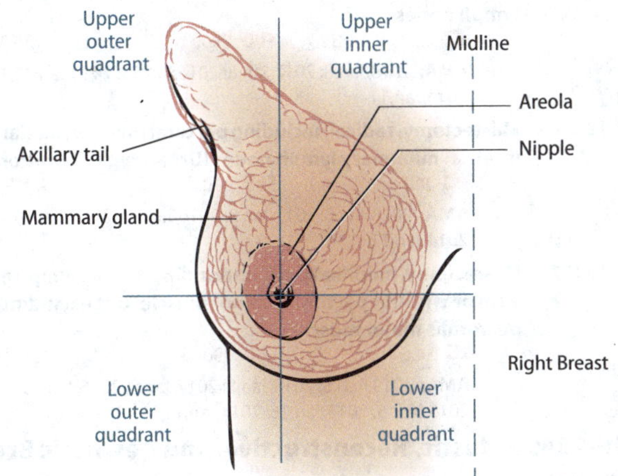

19112 **Excision of lactiferous duct fistula**

9.04 13.1 FUD 090 J A2 80 50

AMA: 2018,Jan,8; 2017,Jan,8; 2016,Jan,13; 2015,Jan,16; 2014,Jan,11

19120 **Excision of cyst, fibroadenoma, or other benign or malignant tumor, aberrant breast tissue, duct lesion, nipple or areolar lesion (except 19300), open, male or female, 1 or more lesions**

11.9 14.3 FUD 090 J A2 50

AMA: 2018,Jan,8; 2017,Jan,8; 2016,Jan,13; 2015,Mar,5; 2015,Jan,16; 2014,Mar,13; 2014,Jan,11

19125 **Excision of breast lesion identified by preoperative placement of radiological marker, open; single lesion**

INCLUDES Intraoperative clip placement

13.2 15.8 FUD 090 J A2 50

AMA: 2018,Jan,8; 2017,Jan,8; 2016,Jan,13; 2015,Mar,5; 2015,Jan,16; 2014,Jan,11

+ **19126** **each additional lesion separately identified by a preoperative radiological marker (List separately in addition to code for primary procedure)**

INCLUDES Intraoperative clip placement

Code first (19125)

4.68 4.68 FUD ZZZ N N1

AMA: 2018,Jan,8; 2017,Jan,8; 2016,Jan,13; 2015,Jan,16; 2014,Jan,11

19260-19272 Excisional Procedures: Chest Wall

~~**19260**~~ ~~**Excision of chest wall tumor including ribs**~~

To report, see (21601)

~~**19271**~~ ~~**Excision of chest wall tumor involving ribs, with plastic reconstruction; without mediastinal lymphadenectomy**~~

To report, see (21602)

~~**19272**~~ ~~**with mediastinal lymphadenectomy**~~

To report, see (21603)

19281-19288 Placement of Localization Markers

INCLUDES Placement of localization devices only

EXCLUDES *Biopsy of breast without imaging guidance (19100-19101)*
Fluoroscopic guidance for needle placement (77002)
Localization device placement with biopsy of breast (19081-19086)
Magnetic resonance guidance for needle placement (77021)
Ultrasonic guidance for needle placement (76942)

Code also open excision of breast lesion when performed after localization device placement (19110-19126)

Code also open incisional breast biopsy when performed after localization device placement (19101)

Code also radiography of surgical specimen (76098)

19281 **Placement of breast localization device(s) (eg, clip, metallic pellet, wire/needle, radioactive seeds), percutaneous; first lesion, including mammographic guidance**

2.91 6.90 FUD 000 Q1 N1 80 50

AMA: 2018,Jan,8; 2017,Jan,8; 2016,Jun,3; 2016,Jan,13; 2015,May,8; 2015,Jan,16; 2014,Jun,14; 2014,May,3

+ **19282** **each additional lesion, including mammographic guidance (List separately in addition to code for primary procedure)**

Code first (19281)

1.46 4.82 FUD ZZZ N N1 80

AMA: 2018,Jan,8; 2017,Jan,8; 2016,Jun,3; 2016,Jan,13; 2015,May,8; 2015,Jan,16; 2014,Jun,14; 2014,May,3

19283 **Placement of breast localization device(s) (eg, clip, metallic pellet, wire/needle, radioactive seeds), percutaneous; first lesion, including stereotactic guidance**

2.93 7.73 FUD 000 Q1 N1 80 50

AMA: 2018,Jan,8; 2017,Jan,8; 2016,Jun,3; 2016,May,13; 2016,Jan,13; 2015,May,8; 2015,Jan,16; 2014,May,3

+ **19284** **each additional lesion, including stereotactic guidance (List separately in addition to code for primary procedure)**

Code first (19283)

1.50 5.87 FUD ZZZ N N1 80

AMA: 2018,Jan,8; 2017,Jan,8; 2016,Jun,3; 2016,May,13; 2016,Jan,13; 2015,May,8; 2015,Jan,16; 2014,May,3

19285 **Placement of breast localization device(s) (eg, clip, metallic pellet, wire/needle, radioactive seeds), percutaneous; first lesion, including ultrasound guidance**

2.50 13.7 FUD 000 Q1 N1 80 50

AMA: 2018,Jan,8; 2017,Jan,8; 2016,Jun,3; 2016,May,13; 2016,Jan,13; 2015,May,8; 2015,Jan,16; 2014,May,3

+ **19286** **each additional lesion, including ultrasound guidance (List separately in addition to code for primary procedure)**

Code first (19285)

1.25 11.9 FUD ZZZ N N1 80

AMA: 2018,Jan,8; 2017,Jan,8; 2016,Jun,3; 2016,May,13; 2016,Jan,13; 2015,May,8; 2015,Jan,16; 2014,May,3

19287 **Placement of breast localization device(s) (eg clip, metallic pellet, wire/needle, radioactive seeds), percutaneous; first lesion, including magnetic resonance guidance**

3.72 23.3 FUD 000 Q1 N1 80 50

AMA: 2018,Jan,8; 2017,Jan,8; 2016,Jun,3; 2016,May,13; 2016,Jan,13; 2015,Jan,16; 2014,May,3

\+ **19288** **each additional lesion, including magnetic resonance guidance (List separately in addition to code for primary procedure)**

Code first (19287)

1.87 18.6 FUD ZZZ N N1 80

AMA: 2018,Jan,8; 2017,Jan,8; 2016,Jun,3; 2016,May,13; 2016,Jan,13; 2015,Jan,16; 2014,May,3

19294-19298 Radioelement Application

\+ **19294** **Preparation of tumor cavity, with placement of a radiation therapy applicator for intraoperative radiation therapy (IORT) concurrent with partial mastectomy (List separately in addition to code for primary procedure)**

4.71 4.71 FUD ZZZ N N1 80

Code first (19301-19302)

19296 **Placement of radiotherapy afterloading expandable catheter (single or multichannel) into the breast for interstitial radioelement application following partial mastectomy, includes imaging guidance; on date separate from partial mastectomy**

6.09 113. FUD 000 J J8 80 50

AMA: 2018,Jan,8; 2017,Jan,8; 2016,Jan,13; 2015,Jan,16; 2014,Jan,11

\+ **19297** **concurrent with partial mastectomy (List separately in addition to code for primary procedure)**

Code first (19301-19302)

2.75 2.75 FUD ZZZ N N1 80

AMA: 2019,Apr,10; 2018,Jan,8; 2017,Jan,8; 2016,Jan,13; 2015,Jan,16; 2014,Jan,11

19298 **Placement of radiotherapy after loading brachytherapy catheters (multiple tube and button type) into the breast for interstitial radioelement application following (at the time of or subsequent to) partial mastectomy, includes imaging guidance**

9.17 28.2 FUD 000 J G2 80 50

AMA: 2018,Jan,8; 2017,Jan,8; 2016,Jan,13; 2015,Jan,16; 2014,Jan,11

19300-19307 Mastectomies: Partial, Simple, Radical

CMS: 100-04,12,40.7 Bilateral Procedures

INCLUDES Intraoperative clip placement

EXCLUDES *Insertion of prosthesis (19340, 19342)*

19300 **Mastectomy for gynecomastia** ♂

EXCLUDES *Removal of breast tissue for:*

Other than gynecomastia (19318)

Treatment or prevention of breast cancer (19301-19307)

11.9 15.3 FUD 090 J A2 50

AMA: 2018,Jan,8; 2017,Jan,8; 2016,Jan,13; 2015,Jan,16; 2014,Mar,13; 2014,Jan,11

19301 **Mastectomy, partial (eg, lumpectomy, tylectomy, quadrantectomy, segmentectomy);**

EXCLUDES *Insertion of radiotherapy afterloading balloon during separate encounter (19296)*

Code also intraoperative radiofrequency spectroscopy margin assessment and report (0546T)

Code also insertion of radiotherapy afterloading balloon catheter, when performed at same time (19297)

Code also insertion of radiotherapy afterloading brachytherapy catheter, when performed at same time (19298)

Code also tumor cavity preparation with intraoperative radiation therapy applicator, when performed (19294)

18.8 18.8 FUD 090 J A2 80 50

AMA: 2018,Jan,8; 2017,Oct,9; 2017,Jan,8; 2016,Jan,13; 2015,Mar,5; 2015,Jan,16; 2014,Jan,11

19302 **with axillary lymphadenectomy**

EXCLUDES *Insertion of radiotherapy afterloading balloon during separate encounter (19296)*

Code also intraoperative radiofrequency spectroscopy margin assessment and report (0546T)

Code also insertion of radiotherapy afterloading balloon catheter, when performed at same time (19297)

Code also insertion of radiotherapy afterloading brachytherapy catheter, when performed at same time (19298)

Code also tumor cavity preparation with intraoperative radiation therapy applicator, when performed (19294)

25.9 25.9 FUD 090 J A2 80 50

AMA: 2019,Feb,8; 2018,Jan,8; 2017,Jan,8; 2016,Jan,13; 2015,Mar,5; 2015,Jan,16; 2014,Jan,11

19303 **Mastectomy, simple, complete**

EXCLUDES *Excision of pectoral muscles and axillary or internal mammary lymph nodes*

Removal of breast tissue for:

Gynecomastia (19300)

Other than gynecomastia (19318)

27.6 27.6 FUD 090 J A2 80 50

AMA: 2018,Jan,8; 2017,Jan,8; 2016,Jan,13; 2015,Mar,5; 2015,Jan,16; 2014,Jan,11

~~**19304** **Mastectomy, subcutaneous**~~

19305 **Mastectomy, radical, including pectoral muscles, axillary lymph nodes**

32.7 32.7 FUD 090 C 80 50

AMA: 2018,Jan,8; 2017,Jan,8; 2016,Jan,13; 2015,Jan,16; 2014,Jan,11

19306 **Mastectomy, radical, including pectoral muscles, axillary and internal mammary lymph nodes (Urban type operation)**

34.7 34.7 FUD 090 C 80 50

AMA: 2018,Jan,8; 2017,Jan,8; 2016,Jan,13; 2015,Jan,16; 2014,Jan,11

19307 **Mastectomy, modified radical, including axillary lymph nodes, with or without pectoralis minor muscle, but excluding pectoralis major muscle**

34.6 34.6 FUD 090 J 80 50

AMA: 2019,Feb,8; 2018,Jan,8; 2017,Jan,8; 2016,Jan,13; 2015,Mar,5; 2015,Jan,16; 2014,Jan,11

19316-19499 Plastic, Reconstructive, and Aesthetic Breast Procedures

CMS: 100-03,140.2 Breast Reconstruction Following Mastectomy; 100-04,12,40.7 Bilateral Procedures

Code also biologic implant for tissue reinforcement (15777)

19316 **Mastopexy**

22.1 22.1 FUD 090 J A2 80 50

AMA: 2018,Jan,8; 2017,Jan,8; 2016,Jan,13; 2015,Jan,16; 2014,Jan,11

19318 **Reduction mammaplasty**

INCLUDES Aries-Pitanguy mammaplasty

Biesenberger mammaplasty

31.5 31.5 FUD 090 J A2 80 50

AMA: 2018,Jan,8; 2017,Jan,8; 2016,Jan,13; 2015,Jan,16; 2014,Apr,10; 2014,Jan,11

19324 **Mammaplasty, augmentation; without prosthetic implant**

15.2 15.2 FUD 090 J A2 80 50

AMA: 2018,Jan,8; 2017,Jan,8; 2016,Jan,13; 2015,Jan,16; 2014,Jan,11

19325 **with prosthetic implant**

EXCLUDES *Flap or graft (15100-15650)*

18.4 18.4 FUD 090 J G2 80 50

AMA: 2018,Jan,8; 2017,Jan,8; 2016,Jan,13; 2015,Jan,16; 2014,Jan,11

19328 **Removal of intact mammary implant**

14.2 14.2 FUD 090 Q2 A2 50

AMA: 2018,Jan,8; 2017,Jan,8; 2016,Jan,13; 2015,Jan,16; 2014,Jan,11

19330 **Removal of mammary implant material**
18.1 18.1 **FUD** 090 Q2 A2 50
AMA: 2018,Jan,8; 2017,Jan,8; 2016,Jan,13; 2015,Jan,16; 2014,Jan,11

19340 **Immediate insertion of breast prosthesis following mastopexy, mastectomy or in reconstruction**
EXCLUDES *Supply of prosthetic implant (99070, L8030, L8039, L8600)*
28.6 28.6 **FUD** 090 J A2 50
AMA: 2018,Jan,8; 2017,Jan,8; 2016,Jan,13; 2015,Dec,18; 2015,Jan,16; 2014,Jan,11

19342 **Delayed insertion of breast prosthesis following mastopexy, mastectomy or in reconstruction**
EXCLUDES *Preparation of moulage for custom breast implant (19396)*
26.5 26.5 **FUD** 090 J A2 80 50
AMA: 2018,Jan,8; 2017,Jan,8; 2016,Jan,13; 2015,Nov,10; 2015,Jan,16; 2014,Jan,11

19350 **Nipple/areola reconstruction**
19.3 23.6 **FUD** 090 J A2 50
AMA: 2018,Jan,8; 2017,Jan,8; 2016,Aug,9; 2016,Jan,13; 2015,Jan,16; 2014,Jan,11

19355 **Correction of inverted nipples**
17.7 21.5 **FUD** 090 J A2 80 50
AMA: 2018,Jan,8; 2017,Jan,8; 2016,Jan,13; 2015,Jan,16; 2014,Jan,11

19357 **Breast reconstruction, immediate or delayed, with tissue expander, including subsequent expansion**
43.1 43.1 **FUD** 090 J J8 80 50
AMA: 2018,Jan,8; 2017,Jan,8; 2016,Jan,13; 2015,Feb,10; 2015,Jan,16; 2014,Jan,11

19361 **Breast reconstruction with latissimus dorsi flap, without prosthetic implant**
EXCLUDES *Implant of prosthesis (19340)*
45.2 45.2 **FUD** 090 C 80 50
AMA: 2018,Jan,8; 2017,Jan,8; 2016,Jan,13; 2015,Feb,10; 2015,Jan,16; 2014,Jan,11

19364 **Breast reconstruction with free flap**
INCLUDES Closure of donor site
Harvesting of skin graft
Inset shaping of flap into breast
Microvascular repair
Operating microscope (69990)
79.2 79.2 **FUD** 090 C 80 50
AMA: 2018,Jan,8; 2017,Jan,8; 2016,Feb,12; 2016,Jan,13; 2015,Feb,10; 2015,Jan,16; 2014,Apr,10; 2014,Jan,11

19366 **Breast reconstruction with other technique**
INCLUDES Operating microscope (69990)
Code also implant of prosthesis if appropriate (19340, 19342)
40.3 40.3 **FUD** 090 J A2 80 50
AMA: 2018,Jan,8; 2017,Jan,8; 2016,Jan,13; 2015,Feb,10; 2015,Jan,16; 2014,Apr,10; 2014,Jan,11

19367 **Breast reconstruction with transverse rectus abdominis myocutaneous flap (TRAM), single pedicle, including closure of donor site;**
51.3 51.3 **FUD** 090 C 80 50
AMA: 2018,Jan,8; 2017,Jan,8; 2016,Jan,13; 2015,Feb,10; 2015,Jan,16; 2014,Jan,11

19368 **with microvascular anastomosis (supercharging)**
INCLUDES Operating microscope (69990)
63.2 63.2 **FUD** 090 C 80 50
AMA: 2018,Jan,8; 2017,Jan,8; 2016,Feb,12; 2016,Jan,13; 2015,Feb,10; 2015,Jan,16; 2014,Jan,11

19369 **Breast reconstruction with transverse rectus abdominis myocutaneous flap (TRAM), double pedicle, including closure of donor site**
58.6 58.6 **FUD** 090 C 80 50
AMA: 2018,Jan,8; 2017,Jan,8; 2016,Jan,13; 2015,Feb,10; 2015,Jan,16; 2014,Jan,11

19370 **Open periprosthetic capsulotomy, breast**
19.7 19.7 **FUD** 090 J A2 50
AMA: 2018,Jan,8; 2017,Jan,8; 2016,Jan,13; 2015,Dec,18; 2015,Jan,16; 2014,Jan,11

19371 **Periprosthetic capsulectomy, breast**
22.5 22.5 **FUD** 090 J A2 50
AMA: 2018,Jan,8; 2017,Jan,8; 2016,Jan,13; 2015,Jan,16; 2014,Jan,11

19380 **Revision of reconstructed breast**
22.2 22.2 **FUD** 090 J A2 50
AMA: 2018,Jan,8; 2017,Dec,13; 2017,Jan,8; 2016,Jan,13; 2015,Dec,18; 2015,Jan,16; 2014,Jan,11

19396 **Preparation of moulage for custom breast implant**
4.17 8.23 **FUD** 000 J G2 80 50
AMA: 2018,Jan,8; 2017,Jan,8; 2016,Jan,13; 2015,Jan,16; 2014,Jan,11

19499 **Unlisted procedure, breast**
0.00 0.00 **FUD** YYY J 80 50
AMA: 2019,Aug,10; 2019,Apr,10; 2018,Jan,8; 2017,Jan,8; 2016,Dec,16; 2016,Jan,13; 2015,Mar,5; 2015,Jan,16; 2014,Dec,16; 2014,Dec,16; 2014,Jan,11

20100-20103 Exploratory Surgery of Traumatic Wound

INCLUDES Debridement
Expanded dissection of wound for exploration
Extraction of foreign material
Open examination
Tying or coagulation of small vessels

EXCLUDES *Cutaneous/subcutaneous incision and drainage procedures (10060-10061)*
Laparotomy (49000-49010)
Repair of major vessels of:
Abdomen (35221, 35251, 35281)
Chest (35211, 35216, 35241, 35246, 35271, 35276)
Extremity (35206-35207, 35226, 35236, 35256, 35266, 35286)
Neck (35201, 35231, 35261)
Thoracotomy (32100-32160)

20100 Exploration of penetrating wound (separate procedure); neck
17.5 17.5 FUD 010 T 80 50
AMA: 2018,Jan,8; 2017,Jan,8; 2016,Jan,13; 2015,Jan,16; 2014,Jan,11

20101 chest
6.05 12.9 FUD 010 T
AMA: 2018,Jan,8; 2017,Jan,8; 2016,Jan,13; 2015,Jan,16; 2014,Jan,11

20102 abdomen/flank/back
7.39 14.0 FUD 010 T
AMA: 2018,Jan,8; 2017,Jan,8; 2016,Jan,13; 2015,Jan,16; 2014,Jan,11

20103 extremity
9.99 16.6 FUD 010 T G2 80
AMA: 2018,Jan,8; 2017,Jan,8; 2016,Jan,13; 2015,Jan,16; 2014,Jan,11

20150 Epiphyseal Bar Resection

20150 Excision of epiphyseal bar, with or without autogenous soft tissue graft obtained through same fascial incision
29.0 29.0 FUD 090 J G2 80 50
AMA: 1996,Nov,1

20200-20206 Muscle Biopsy

EXCLUDES *Removal of muscle tumor (see appropriate anatomic section)*

20200 Biopsy, muscle; superficial
2.73 5.95 FUD 000 J A2

20205 deep
4.48 8.35 FUD 000 J A2

20206 Biopsy, muscle, percutaneous needle
EXCLUDES *Fine needle aspiration (10021, [10004, 10005, 10006, 10007, 10008, 10009, 10010, 10011, 10012])*
(76942, 77002, 77012, 77021)
(88172-88173)
1.68 6.71 FUD 000 J A2
AMA: 2019,Apr,4

20220-20225 Percutaneous Bone Biopsy

EXCLUDES *Bone marrow aspiration(s) or biopsy(ies) (38220-38222)*

20220 Biopsy, bone, trocar, or needle; superficial (eg, ilium, sternum, spinous process, ribs)
(77002, 77012, 77021)
2.06 4.79 FUD 000 J A2
AMA: 2018,Jan,8; 2017,Jan,8; 2016,Jan,13; 2015,Jan,16; 2014,Jan,11

20225 deep (eg, vertebral body, femur)
EXCLUDES *Percutaneous vertebroplasty (22510-22515)*
Percutaneous sacral augmentation (sacroplasty) (0200T-0201T)
(77002, 77012, 77021)
3.07 14.7 FUD 000 J A2
AMA: 2018,Jan,8; 2017,Jan,8; 2016,Jan,13; 2015,Jan,8; 2015,Jan,16; 2014,Jan,11

20240-20251 Open Bone Biopsy

EXCLUDES *Sequestrectomy or incision and drainage of bone abscess of:*
Calcaneus (28120)
Carpal bone (25145)
Clavicle (23170)
Humeral head (23174)
Humerus (24134)
Olecranon process (24138)
Radius (24136, 25145)
Scapula (23172)
Skull (61501)
Talus (28120)
Ulna (24138, 24145)

20240 Biopsy, bone, open; superficial (eg, sternum, spinous process, rib, patella, olecranon process, calcaneus, tarsal, metatarsal, carpal, metacarpal, phalanx)
4.31 4.31 FUD 000 J A2
AMA: 2018,Jan,8; 2017,Jan,8; 2016,Jan,13; 2015,Jan,16; 2014,Jan,11

20245 deep (eg, humeral shaft, ischium, femoral shaft)
10.1 10.1 FUD 000 J A2
AMA: 2018,Jan,8; 2017,Jan,8; 2016,Jan,13; 2015,Jan,16; 2014,Jan,11

20250 Biopsy, vertebral body, open; thoracic
11.5 11.5 FUD 010 J A2
AMA: 2018,Jan,8; 2017,Jan,8; 2016,Jan,13; 2015,Jan,16; 2014,Jan,11

20251 lumbar or cervical
12.4 12.4 FUD 010 J A2 80
AMA: 2018,Jan,8; 2017,Jan,8; 2016,Jan,13; 2015,Jan,16; 2014,Jan,11

20500-20501 Injection Fistula/Sinus Tract

EXCLUDES *Arthrography injection of:*
Ankle (27648)
Elbow (24220)
Hip (27093, 27095)
Sacroiliac joint (27096)
Shoulder (23350)
Temporomandibular joint (TMJ) (21116)
Wrist (25246)
Autologous adipose-derived regenerative cells injection (0490T)

20500 Injection of sinus tract; therapeutic (separate procedure)
2.45 3.09 FUD 010 T P3
(76080)

20501 diagnostic (sinogram)
1.09 3.62 FUD 000 N N1
EXCLUDES *Contrast injection or injections for radiological evaluation of existing gastrostomy, duodenostomy, jejunostomy, gastro-jejunostomy, or cecostomy (or other colonic) tube from percutaneous approach (49465)*
(76080)

20520-20525 Foreign Body Removal

20520 Removal of foreign body in muscle or tendon sheath; simple
4.20 5.87 FUD 010 J P3

20525 deep or complicated
7.11 13.6 FUD 010 J A2

20526-20561 [20560, 20561] Therapeutic Injections: Tendons, Trigger Points

EXCLUDES *Autologous adipose-derived regenerative cells injection (0489T-0490T)*
Platelet rich plasma (PRP) injections (0232T)

20526 Injection, therapeutic (eg, local anesthetic, corticosteroid), carpal tunnel
1.66 2.20 FUD 000 T P3 50
AMA: 2018,Jan,8; 2017,Jan,8; 2016,Jan,13; 2015,Jan,16; 2014,Jan,11

20527 **Injection, enzyme (eg, collagenase), palmar fascial cord (ie, Dupuytren's contracture)**

EXCLUDES *Postinjection palmar fascial cord manipulation (26341)*

1.90 2.39 FUD 000 T P3 50

AMA: 2018,Jan,8; 2017,Jan,8; 2016,Jan,13; 2015,Jan,16; 2014,Jan,11

20550 **Injection(s); single tendon sheath, or ligament, aponeurosis (eg, plantar "fascia")**

EXCLUDES *Autologous WBC injection (0481T)*
Platelet rich plasma injection (0232T)
Morton's neuroma (64455, 64632)

(76942, 77002, 77021)

1.13 1.51 FUD 000 T P3 50

AMA: 2018,Jan,8; 2017,Jan,8; 2016,Jan,13; 2015,Jan,16; 2014,Oct,9; 2014,Jan,11

20551 **single tendon origin/insertion**

EXCLUDES *Autologous WBC injection (0481T)*
Platelet rich plasma injection (0232T)

(76942, 77002, 77021)

1.15 1.53 FUD 000 T P3

AMA: 2018,Jan,8; 2017,Dec,13; 2017,Jan,8; 2016,Jan,13; 2015,Jan,16; 2014,Oct,9; 2014,Jan,11

20552 **Injection(s); single or multiple trigger point(s), 1 or 2 muscle(s)**

EXCLUDES *Autologous WBC injection (0481T)*
Needle insertion(s) without injection(s) for the same muscle(s) ([20560, 20561])
Platelet rich plasma injection (0232T)

(76942, 77002, 77021)

1.09 1.57 FUD 000 T P3

AMA: 2018,Jan,8; 2017,Dec,13; 2017,Jun,10; 2017,Jan,8; 2016,Jan,13; 2015,Jan,16; 2014,Oct,9; 2014,Jan,11

20553 **single or multiple trigger point(s), 3 or more muscles**

EXCLUDES *Needle insertion(s) without injection(s) for the same muscle(s) ([20560, 20561])*

(76942, 77002, 77021)

1.24 1.81 FUD 000 T P3

AMA: 2018,Dec,8; 2018,Dec,8; 2018,Jan,8; 2017,Jun,10; 2017,Jan,8; 2016,Jan,13; 2015,Jan,16; 2014,Oct,9; 2014,Jan,11

● # **20560** **Needle insertion(s) without injection(s); 1 or 2 muscle(s)**

0.00 0.00 FUD 000

INCLUDES Dry needling and trigger-point acupuncture

● # **20561** **3 or more muscles**

0.00 0.00 FUD 000

INCLUDES Dry needling and trigger-point acupuncture

20555-20561 Placement of Catheters/Needles for Brachytherapy

Code also interstitial radioelement application (77770-77772, 77778)

20555 **Placement of needles or catheters into muscle and/or soft tissue for subsequent interstitial radioelement application (at the time of or subsequent to the procedure)**

EXCLUDES *Interstitial radioelement:*
Devices placed into the breast (19296-19298)
Placement of needle, catheters, or devices into muscle or soft tissue of the head and neck (41019)
Placement of needles or catheters into pelvic organs or genitalia (55920)
Placement of needles or catheters into prostate (55875)

(76942, 77002, 77012, 77021)

9.49 9.49 FUD 000 J R2 80

AMA: 2018,Jan,8; 2017,Jan,8; 2016,Jan,13; 2015,Jan,16; 2014,Jan,11

20560 **Resequenced code. See code following 20553.**

20561 **Resequenced code. See code before 20555.**

20600-20611 Aspiration and/or Injection of Joint

CMS: 100-03,150.7 Prolotherapy, Joint Sclerotherapy, and Ligamentous Injections with Sclerosing Agents

EXCLUDES *Autologous adipose-derived regenerative cells injection (0489T-0490T)*
Ultrasonic guidance for needle placement (76942)

20600 **Arthrocentesis, aspiration and/or injection, small joint or bursa (eg, fingers, toes); without ultrasound guidance**

(77002, 77012, 77021)

1.03 1.38 FUD 000 T P3 50

AMA: 2018,Sep,12; 2018,Jan,8; 2017,Aug,9; 2017,Jan,8; 2016,Jan,13; 2015,Nov,10; 2015,Feb,6; 2015,Jan,16; 2014,Jan,11

20604 **with ultrasound guidance, with permanent recording and reporting**

EXCLUDES *Autologous adipose-derived regenerative cells injection (0489T-0490T)*

(77002, 77012, 77021)

1.34 2.10 FUD 000 T P3 50

AMA: 2018,Sep,12; 2018,Jan,8; 2017,Jan,8; 2016,Jan,13; 2015,Jul,10; 2015,Feb,6

20605 **Arthrocentesis, aspiration and/or injection, intermediate joint or bursa (eg, temporomandibular, acromioclavicular, wrist, elbow or ankle, olecranon bursa); without ultrasound guidance**

(77002, 77012, 77021)

1.07 1.44 FUD 000 T P3 50

AMA: 2018,Jan,8; 2017,Aug,9; 2017,Jan,8; 2016,Jan,13; 2015,Nov,10; 2015,Feb,6; 2015,Jan,16; 2014,Jan,11

20606 **with ultrasound guidance, with permanent recording and reporting**

(77002, 77012, 77021)

1.53 2.32 FUD 000 T P3 50

AMA: 2018,Jan,8; 2017,Jan,8; 2016,Jan,13; 2015,Jul,10; 2015,Feb,6

20610 **Arthrocentesis, aspiration and/or injection, major joint or bursa (eg, shoulder, hip, knee, subacromial bursa); without ultrasound guidance**

EXCLUDES *Injection of contrast for knee arthrography (27369)*

(77002, 77012, 77021)

1.32 1.71 FUD 000 T P3 50

AMA: 2019,Aug,7; 2018,Jan,8; 2017,Apr,9; 2017,Jan,8; 2016,Jan,13; 2015,Nov,10; 2015,Aug,6; 2015,Feb,6; 2015,Jan,16; 2014,Dec,18; 2014,Jan,11

20611 **with ultrasound guidance, with permanent recording and reporting**

EXCLUDES *Injection of contrast for knee arthrography (27369)*

(77002, 77012, 77021)

1.75 2.61 FUD 000 T P3 50

AMA: 2019,Aug,7; 2018,Jan,8; 2017,Jan,8; 2016,Jan,13; 2015,Nov,10; 2015,Aug,6; 2015,Jul,10; 2015,Feb,6

20612-20615 Aspiration and/or Injection of Cyst

EXCLUDES *Autologous adipose-derived regenerative cells injection (0489T-0490T)*

20612 **Aspiration and/or injection of ganglion cyst(s) any location**

1.20 1.71 FUD 000 T P3

Code also modifier 59 for multiple major joint aspirations or injections

20615 **Aspiration and injection for treatment of bone cyst**

4.63 6.95 FUD 010 T P3

20650-20697 Procedures Related to Bony Fixation

20650 **Insertion of wire or pin with application of skeletal traction, including removal (separate procedure)**

4.58 6.07 FUD 010 J A2

20660 **Application of cranial tongs, caliper, or stereotactic frame, including removal (separate procedure)**

7.07 7.07 FUD 000 Q2

AMA: 2018,Jan,8; 2017,Jan,8; 2016,Jan,13; 2015,Jan,16; 2014,Jan,11

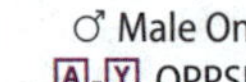
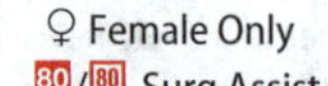
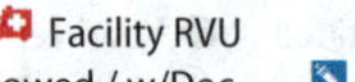
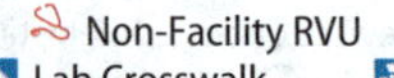
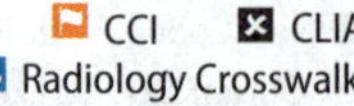

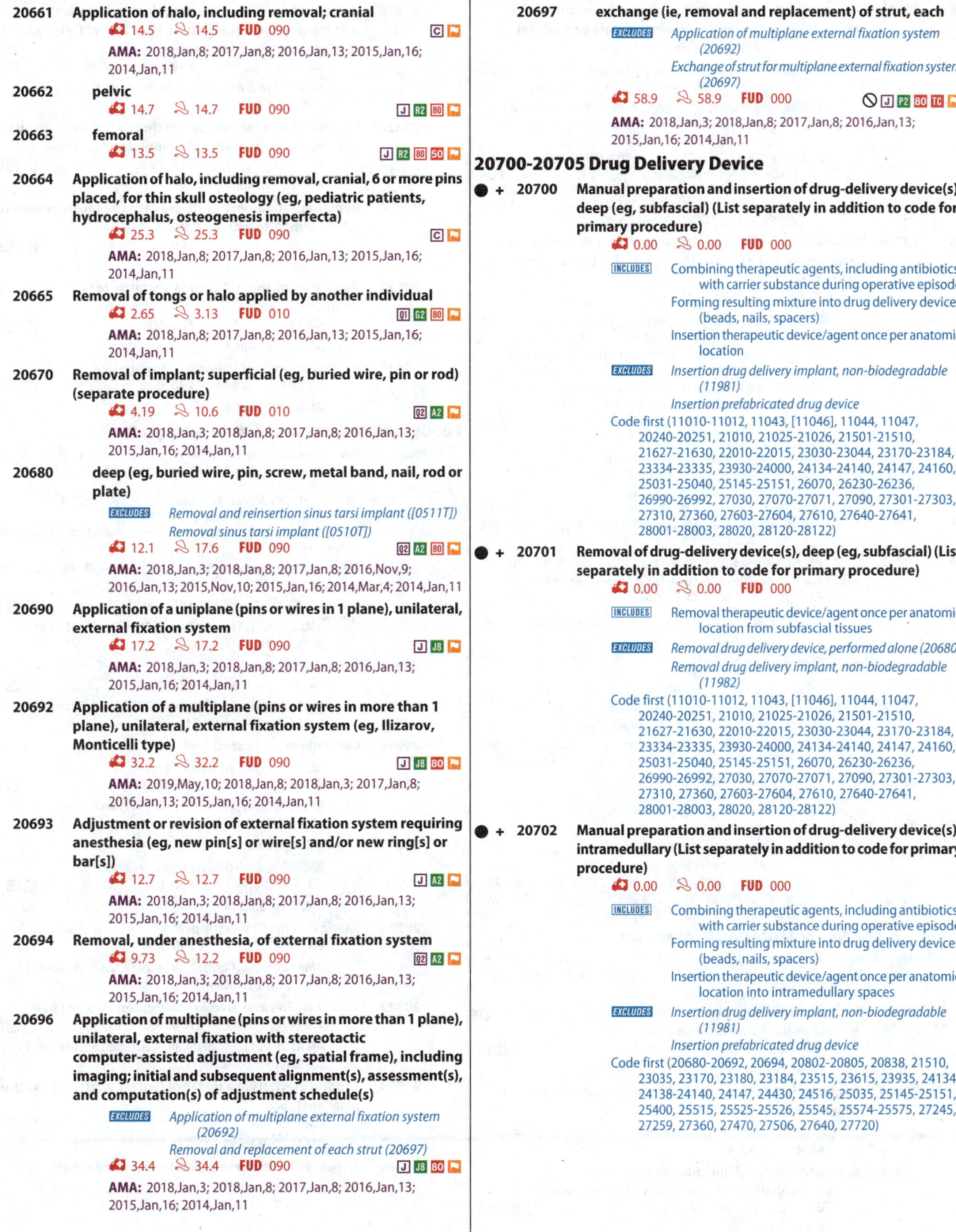

20661 Application of halo, including removal; cranial
14.5 14.5 FUD 090 C
AMA: 2018,Jan,8; 2017,Jan,8; 2016,Jan,13; 2015,Jan,16; 2014,Jan,11

20662 pelvic
14.7 14.7 FUD 090 J R2 80

20663 femoral
13.5 13.5 FUD 090 J R2 80 50

20664 Application of halo, including removal, cranial, 6 or more pins placed, for thin skull osteology (eg, pediatric patients, hydrocephalus, osteogenesis imperfecta)
25.3 25.3 FUD 090 C
AMA: 2018,Jan,8; 2017,Jan,8; 2016,Jan,13; 2015,Jan,16; 2014,Jan,11

20665 Removal of tongs or halo applied by another individual
2.65 3.13 FUD 010 Q1 G2 80
AMA: 2018,Jan,8; 2017,Jan,8; 2016,Jan,13; 2015,Jan,16; 2014,Jan,11

20670 Removal of implant; superficial (eg, buried wire, pin or rod) (separate procedure)
4.19 10.6 FUD 010 Q2 A2
AMA: 2018,Jan,3; 2018,Jan,8; 2017,Jan,8; 2016,Jan,13; 2015,Jan,16; 2014,Jan,11

20680 deep (eg, buried wire, pin, screw, metal band, nail, rod or plate)
EXCLUDES *Removal and reinsertion sinus tarsi implant ([0511T])*
Removal sinus tarsi implant ([0510T])
12.1 17.6 FUD 090 Q2 A2 80
AMA: 2018,Jan,3; 2018,Jan,8; 2017,Jan,8; 2016,Nov,9; 2016,Jan,13; 2015,Nov,10; 2015,Jan,16; 2014,Mar,4; 2014,Jan,11

20690 Application of a uniplane (pins or wires in 1 plane), unilateral, external fixation system
17.2 17.2 FUD 090 J J8
AMA: 2018,Jan,3; 2018,Jan,8; 2017,Jan,8; 2016,Jan,13; 2015,Jan,16; 2014,Jan,11

20692 Application of a multiplane (pins or wires in more than 1 plane), unilateral, external fixation system (eg, Ilizarov, Monticelli type)
32.2 32.2 FUD 090 J J8 80
AMA: 2019,May,10; 2018,Jan,8; 2018,Jan,3; 2017,Jan,8; 2016,Jan,13; 2015,Jan,16; 2014,Jan,11

20693 Adjustment or revision of external fixation system requiring anesthesia (eg, new pin[s] or wire[s] and/or new ring[s] or bar[s])
12.7 12.7 FUD 090 J A2
AMA: 2018,Jan,3; 2018,Jan,8; 2017,Jan,8; 2016,Jan,13; 2015,Jan,16; 2014,Jan,11

20694 Removal, under anesthesia, of external fixation system
9.73 12.2 FUD 090 Q2 A2
AMA: 2018,Jan,3; 2018,Jan,8; 2017,Jan,8; 2016,Jan,13; 2015,Jan,16; 2014,Jan,11

20696 Application of multiplane (pins or wires in more than 1 plane), unilateral, external fixation with stereotactic computer-assisted adjustment (eg, spatial frame), including imaging; initial and subsequent alignment(s), assessment(s), and computation(s) of adjustment schedule(s)
EXCLUDES *Application of multiplane external fixation system (20692)*
Removal and replacement of each strut (20697)
34.4 34.4 FUD 090 J J8 80
AMA: 2018,Jan,3; 2018,Jan,8; 2017,Jan,8; 2016,Jan,13; 2015,Jan,16; 2014,Jan,11

20697 exchange (ie, removal and replacement) of strut, each
EXCLUDES *Application of multiplane external fixation system (20692)*
Exchange of strut for multiplane external fixation system (20697)
58.9 58.9 FUD 000 J P2 80 TC
AMA: 2018,Jan,3; 2018,Jan,8; 2017,Jan,8; 2016,Jan,13; 2015,Jan,16; 2014,Jan,11

20700-20705 Drug Delivery Device

● + **20700 Manual preparation and insertion of drug-delivery device(s), deep (eg, subfascial) (List separately in addition to code for primary procedure)**
0.00 0.00 FUD 000
INCLUDES Combining therapeutic agents, including antibiotics, with carrier substance during operative episode
Forming resulting mixture into drug delivery devices (beads, nails, spacers)
Insertion therapeutic device/agent once per anatomic location
EXCLUDES *Insertion drug delivery implant, non-biodegradable (11981)*
Insertion prefabricated drug device
Code first (11010-11012, 11043, [11046], 11044, 11047, 20240-20251, 21010, 21025-21026, 21501-21510, 21627-21630, 22010-22015, 23030-23044, 23170-23184, 23334-23335, 23930-24000, 24134-24140, 24147, 24160, 25031-25040, 25145-25151, 26070, 26230-26236, 26990-26992, 27030, 27070-27071, 27090, 27301-27303, 27310, 27360, 27603-27604, 27610, 27640-27641, 28001-28003, 28020, 28120-28122)

● + **20701 Removal of drug-delivery device(s), deep (eg, subfascial) (List separately in addition to code for primary procedure)**
0.00 0.00 FUD 000
INCLUDES Removal therapeutic device/agent once per anatomic location from subfascial tissues
EXCLUDES *Removal drug delivery device, performed alone (20680)*
Removal drug delivery implant, non-biodegradable (11982)
Code first (11010-11012, 11043, [11046], 11044, 11047, 20240-20251, 21010, 21025-21026, 21501-21510, 21627-21630, 22010-22015, 23030-23044, 23170-23184, 23334-23335, 23930-24000, 24134-24140, 24147, 24160, 25031-25040, 25145-25151, 26070, 26230-26236, 26990-26992, 27030, 27070-27071, 27090, 27301-27303, 27310, 27360, 27603-27604, 27610, 27640-27641, 28001-28003, 28020, 28120-28122)

● + **20702 Manual preparation and insertion of drug-delivery device(s), intramedullary (List separately in addition to code for primary procedure)**
0.00 0.00 FUD 000
INCLUDES Combining therapeutic agents, including antibiotics, with carrier substance during operative episode
Forming resulting mixture into drug delivery devices (beads, nails, spacers)
Insertion therapeutic device/agent once per anatomic location into intramedullary spaces
EXCLUDES *Insertion drug delivery implant, non-biodegradable (11981)*
Insertion prefabricated drug device
Code first (20680-20692, 20694, 20802-20805, 20838, 21510, 23035, 23170, 23180, 23184, 23515, 23615, 23935, 24134, 24138-24140, 24147, 24430, 24516, 25035, 25145-25151, 25400, 25515, 25525-25526, 25545, 25574-25575, 27245, 27259, 27360, 27470, 27506, 27640, 27720)

Musculoskeletal System 20661 — 20702

● New Code ▲ Revised Code ○ Reinstated ● New Web Release ▲ Revised Web Release + Add-on Unlisted Not Covered # Resequenced
⑤⓪ Optum Mod 50 Exempt ⊘ AMA Mod 51 Exempt ⑤ Optum Mod 51 Exempt ⑥③ Mod 63 Exempt Non-FDA Drug ★ Telemedicine M Maternity A Age Edit

● + **20703** **Removal of drug-delivery device(s), intramedullary (List separately in addition to code for primary procedure)**
0.00 0.00 FUD 000

INCLUDES Removal therapeutic device/agent once per anatomic location from intramedullary spaces

EXCLUDES *Removal drug delivery device, performed alone (20680)*
Removal drug delivery implant, non-biodegradable (11982)

Code first (20690-20692, 20694, 20802-20805, 20838, 21510, 23035, 23170, 23180, 23184, 23515, 23615, 23935, 24134, 24138-24140, 24147, 24430, 24516, 25035, 25145-25151, 25400, 25515, 25525-25526, 25545, 25574-25575, 27245, 27259, 27360, 27470, 27506, 27640, 27720)

● + **20704** **Manual preparation and insertion of drug-delivery device(s), intra-articular (List separately in addition to code for primary procedure)**
0.00 0.00 FUD 000

INCLUDES Combining therapeutic agents, including antibiotics, with carrier substance during operative episode
Forming resulting mixture into drug delivery devices (beads, nails, spacers)
Insertion therapeutic device/agent once per anatomic location into intra-articular spaces

EXCLUDES *Insertion drug delivery implant, non-biodegradable (11981)*
Insertion prefabricated drug device
Removal hip prosthesis (27091)
Removal knee prosthesis (27488)

Code first (22864-22865, 23040-23044, 23334, 24000, 24160, 25040, 25250-25251, 26070-26080, 26990, 27030, 27090, 27301, 27310, 27603, 27610, 28020)

● + **20705** **Removal of drug-delivery device(s), intra-articular (List separately in addition to code for primary procedure)**
0.00 0.00 FUD 000

INCLUDES Removal therapeutic device/agent once per anatomic location from intra-articular space(s)

EXCLUDES *Open treatment femoral neck fracture/internal fixation or prosthetic replacement (27236)*
Partial knee replacement (27446)
Partial or total hip replacement (27125-27130)
Patella arthroplasty with prosthesis (27438)
Removal drug delivery device, performed alone (20680)
Removal drug delivery implant, non-biodegradable (11982)
Removal hip prosthesis (27091)
Removal knee prosthesis (27488)
Removal shoulder prosthesis (23335)
Revision hip arthroplasty (27134-27138)
Revision knee arthroplasty (27486-27487)

Code first (22864-22865, 23040-23044, 23334, 24000, 24160, 25040, 25250-25251, 26070-26080, 26990, 27030, 27090, 27301, 27310, 27603, 27610, 28020)

20802-20838 Reimplantation Procedures

EXCLUDES *Repair of incomplete amputation (see individual repair codes for bone(s), ligament(s), tendon(s), nerve(s), or blood vessel(s) and append modifier 52)*

20802 **Replantation, arm (includes surgical neck of humerus through elbow joint), complete amputation**
79.6 79.6 FUD 090 C 80 50
AMA: 1997,Apr,4

20805 **Replantation, forearm (includes radius and ulna to radial carpal joint), complete amputation**
94.8 94.8 FUD 090 C 80 50
AMA: 1997,Apr,4

20808 **Replantation, hand (includes hand through metacarpophalangeal joints), complete amputation**
114. 114. FUD 090 C 80 50
AMA: 1997,Apr,4

20816 **Replantation, digit, excluding thumb (includes metacarpophalangeal joint to insertion of flexor sublimis tendon), complete amputation**
59.6 59.6 FUD 090 C 80
AMA: 2018,Jan,8; 2017,Jan,8; 2016,Jan,13; 2015,Jan,16; 2014,Jan,11

20822 **Replantation, digit, excluding thumb (includes distal tip to sublimis tendon insertion), complete amputation**
51.2 51.2 FUD 090 J G2 80
AMA: 1997,Apr,4

20824 **Replantation, thumb (includes carpometacarpal joint to MP joint), complete amputation**
59.7 59.7 FUD 090 C 80 50
AMA: 1997,Apr,4

20827 **Replantation, thumb (includes distal tip to MP joint), complete amputation**
52.6 52.6 FUD 090 C 80 50
AMA: 1997,Apr,4

20838 **Replantation, foot, complete amputation**
80.6 80.6 FUD 090 C 80 50
AMA: 1997,Apr,4

20900-20926 Bone and Tissue Autografts

EXCLUDES *Acquisition of autogenous bone, bone marrow, cartilage, tendon, fascia lata or other grafts through distinct incision unless included in the code description*
Autologous fat graft obtained by liposuction (15771-15774)
Bone graft procedures on the spine (20930-20938)
Other autologous soft tissue grafts (fat, dermis, fascia) harvested by direct excision ([15769])

20900 **Bone graft, any donor area; minor or small (eg, dowel or button)**
5.37 11.7 FUD 000 J A2 80
AMA: 2018,Jul,14; 2018,Jan,8; 2017,Jan,8; 2016,Jan,13; 2015,Jan,16; 2014,Jan,11

20902 **major or large**
8.20 8.20 FUD 000 J A2 80
AMA: 2018,Jul,14; 2018,Jan,8; 2017,Jan,8; 2016,Jan,13; 2015,Jan,16; 2014,Jan,11

20910 **Cartilage graft; costochondral**
EXCLUDES *Graft with ear cartilage (21235)*
13.4 13.4 FUD 090 T A2 80
AMA: 2018,Jul,14; 2018,Jan,8; 2017,Jan,8; 2016,Jan,13; 2015,Jan,16; 2014,Jan,11

20912 **nasal septum**
EXCLUDES *Graft with ear cartilage (21235)*
13.6 13.6 FUD 090 T A2 80
AMA: 2018,Jul,14

20920 **Fascia lata graft; by stripper**
11.5 11.5 FUD 090 T A2
AMA: 2018,Jul,14; 2018,Jan,8; 2017,Jan,8; 2016,Jan,13; 2015,Jan,16; 2014,Jan,11

20922 **by incision and area exposure, complex or sheet**
14.0 17.0 FUD 090 T A2 80
AMA: 2018,Jul,14; 2018,Jan,8; 2017,Jan,8; 2016,Jan,13; 2015,Jan,16; 2014,Jan,11

20924 **Tendon graft, from a distance (eg, palmaris, toe extensor, plantaris)**
14.5 14.5 FUD 090 J A2 80
AMA: 2018,Jul,14

~~**20926** **Tissue grafts, other (eg, paratenon, fat, dermis)**~~

20930-20939 Bone Allograft and Autograft of Spine

EXCLUDES *Acquisition of autogenous bone, bone marrow, cartilage, tendon, fascia lata, or other grafts through distinct incision unless included in the code description*
Autologous fat graft obtained by liposuction (15771-15774)
Other autologous soft tissue grafts (fat, dermis, fascia) harvested by direct excision ([15769])

\+ **20930** **Allograft, morselized, or placement of osteopromotive material, for spine surgery only (List separately in addition to code for primary procedure)**
Code first (22319, 22532-22533, 22548-22558, 22590-22612, 22630, 22633-22634, 22800-22812)
0.00 0.00 FUD XXX N N1
AMA: 2019,May,7; 2018,Jul,14; 2018,Jan,8; 2017,Mar,7; 2017,Jan,8; 2016,Jan,13; 2015,Jan,16; 2014,Jan,11

\+ **20931** **Allograft, structural, for spine surgery only (List separately in addition to code for primary procedure)**
Code first (22319, 22532-22533, 22548-22558, 22590-22612, 22630, 22633-22634, 22800-22812)
3.26 3.26 FUD ZZZ N N1
AMA: 2019,May,7; 2018,Jul,14; 2018,Jan,8; 2017,Mar,7; 2017,Jan,8; 2016,Jan,13; 2015,Jan,16; 2014,Jan,11

\+ **20932** **Allograft, includes templating, cutting, placement and internal fixation, when performed; osteoarticular, including articular surface and contiguous bone (List separately in addition to code for primary procedure)**
EXCLUDES *Allograft, intercalary (20933-20934)*
Injection of contrast for ankle arthrography (27648)
Osteotomy, femur (27448)
Radical resection tumor:
Clavicle (23200)
Fibula (27646)
Ischial tuberosity/greater trochanter femur (27078)
Radial head or neck (24152)
Talus or calcaneus (27647)
Removal hip prosthesis (27090-27091)
Code also insertion of joint prosthesis
Code first (23210, 23220, 24150, 25170, 27075-27077, 27365, 27645, 27704)
20.5 20.5 FUD ZZZ N1 80
AMA: 2019,May,7

\+ **20933** **hemicortical intercalary, partial (ie, hemicylindrical) (List separately in addition to code for primary procedure)**
EXCLUDES *Allograft, intercalary, complete (20934)*
Allograft, osteoarticular (20932)
Arthroplasty procedures, hip (27130, 27132, 27134, 27138)
Bone graft (20955-20957, 20962)
Excision of cyst with allograft (23146, 23156, 24116, 24126, 25126, 25136, 27356, 27638, 28103, 28107)
Injection of contrast for ankle arthrography (27648)
Open treatment femoral fractures (27236, 27244)
Osteotomy, femur (27448)
Radical resection tumor:
Clavicle (23200)
Fibula (27646)
Ischial tuberosity/greater trochanter femur (27078)
Radial head or neck (24152)
Talus or calcaneus (27647)
Removal hip prosthesis (27090-27091)
Code also insertion of joint prosthesis
Code first (23210, 23220, 24150, 25170, 27075-27077, 27365, 27645, 27704)
18.8 18.8 FUD ZZZ N1 80
AMA: 2019,May,7

\+ **20934** **intercalary, complete (ie, cylindrical) (List separately in addition to code for primary procedure)**
Allograft, intercalary, partial (20933)
Allograft, osteoarticular (20932)
Excision of cyst with allograft (23146, 23156)
Injection of contrast for ankle arthrography (27648)
Osteotomy, femur (27448)
Radical resection tumor:
Clavicle (23200)
Fibula (27646)
Ischial tuberosity/greater trochanter femur (27078)
Radial head or neck (24152)
Talus or calcaneus (27647)
Removal hip prosthesis (27090-27091)
Code also insertion of joint prosthesis
Code first (23210, 23220, 24150, 25170, 27075-27077, 27365, 27645, 27704)
20.5 20.5 FUD ZZZ N1 80
AMA: 2019,May,7

\+ **20936** **Autograft for spine surgery only (includes harvesting the graft); local (eg, ribs, spinous process, or laminar fragments) obtained from same incision (List separately in addition to code for primary procedure)**
Code first (22319, 22532-22533, 22548-22558, 22590-22612, 22630, 22633-22634, 22800-22812)
0.00 0.00 FUD XXX N N1
AMA: 2018,Jul,14; 2018,Jan,8; 2017,Mar,7; 2017,Jan,8; 2016,Jan,13; 2015,Jan,16; 2014,Jan,11

\+ **20937** **morselized (through separate skin or fascial incision) (List separately in addition to code for primary procedure)**
Code first (22319, 22532-22533, 22548-22558, 22590-22612, 22630, 22633-22634, 22800-22812)
4.88 4.88 FUD ZZZ N N1 80
AMA: 2018,Jul,14; 2018,Jan,8; 2017,Mar,7; 2017,Jan,8; 2016,Jan,13; 2015,Jan,16; 2014,Jan,11

\+ **20938** **structural, bicortical or tricortical (through separate skin or fascial incision) (List separately in addition to code for primary procedure)**
EXCLUDES *Bone marrow for bone grafting in spinal surgery (20939)*
Code first (22319, 22532-22533, 22548-22558, 22590-22612, 22630, 22633-22634, 22800-22812)
5.40 5.40 FUD ZZZ N N1 80
AMA: 2018,Jul,14; 2018,Jan,8; 2017,Mar,7; 2017,Jan,8; 2016,Jan,13; 2015,Jan,16; 2014,Jan,11

\+ **20939** **Bone marrow aspiration for bone grafting, spine surgery only, through separate skin or fascial incision (List separately in addition to code for primary procedure)**
EXCLUDES *Bone marrow aspiration for other than bone grafting in spinal surgery (20999)*
Diagnostic bone marrow aspiration (38220, 38222)
Platelet rich plasma injection (0232T)
Reporting with modifier 50. Report once for each side when performed bilaterally
Code first (22319, 22532-22534, 22548, 22551-22552, 22554, 22556, 22558, 22590, 22595, 22600, 22610, 22612, 22630, 22633-22634, 22800, 22802, 22804, 22808, 22810, 22812)
1.92 1.92 FUD ZZZ 50 N N1 80
AMA: 2018,May,3

20950 Measurement of Intracompartmental Pressure

20950 **Monitoring of interstitial fluid pressure (includes insertion of device, eg, wick catheter technique, needle manometer technique) in detection of muscle compartment syndrome**
2.60 7.41 FUD 000 T G2 80
AMA: 2018,Jan,8; 2017,Jan,8; 2016,Jan,13; 2015,Jan,16; 2014,Jan,11

20955-20973 Bone and Osteocutaneous Grafts

INCLUDES Operating microscope (69990)

20955 **Bone graft with microvascular anastomosis; fibula**
71.6 71.6 FUD 090 C 80
AMA: 2019,May,7; 2018,Jan,8; 2017,Jan,8; 2016,Feb,12; 2016,Jan,13; 2015,Jan,16; 2014,Jan,11

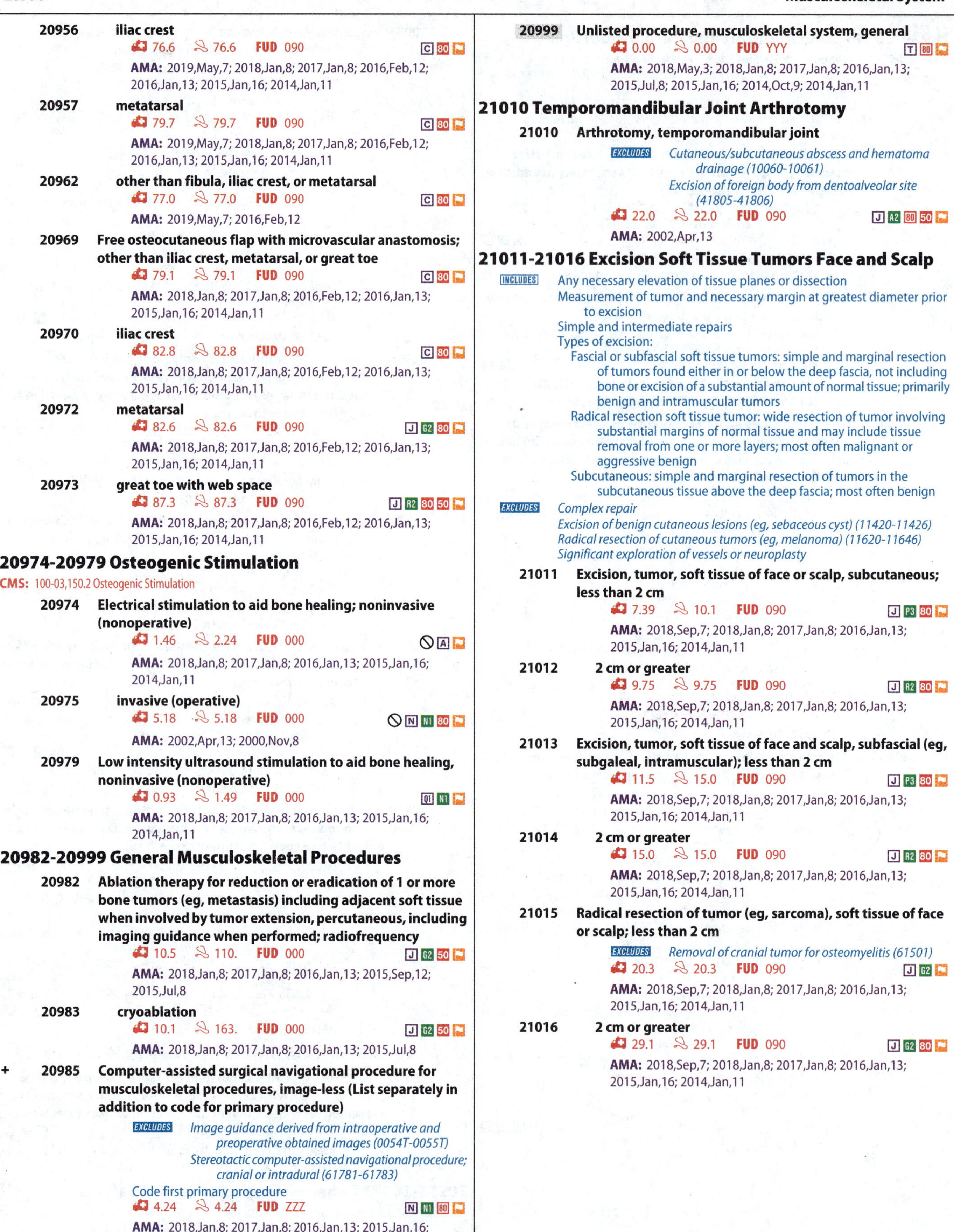

20956 **iliac crest**
76.6 76.6 **FUD** 090 C 80
AMA: 2019,May,7; 2018,Jan,8; 2017,Jan,8; 2016,Feb,12; 2016,Jan,13; 2015,Jan,16; 2014,Jan,11

20957 **metatarsal**
79.7 79.7 **FUD** 090 C 80
AMA: 2019,May,7; 2018,Jan,8; 2017,Jan,8; 2016,Feb,12; 2016,Jan,13; 2015,Jan,16; 2014,Jan,11

20962 **other than fibula, iliac crest, or metatarsal**
77.0 77.0 **FUD** 090 C 80
AMA: 2019,May,7; 2016,Feb,12

20969 **Free osteocutaneous flap with microvascular anastomosis; other than iliac crest, metatarsal, or great toe**
79.1 79.1 **FUD** 090 C 80
AMA: 2018,Jan,8; 2017,Jan,8; 2016,Feb,12; 2016,Jan,13; 2015,Jan,16; 2014,Jan,11

20970 **iliac crest**
82.8 82.8 **FUD** 090 C 80
AMA: 2018,Jan,8; 2017,Jan,8; 2016,Feb,12; 2016,Jan,13; 2015,Jan,16; 2014,Jan,11

20972 **metatarsal**
82.6 82.6 **FUD** 090 J G2 80
AMA: 2018,Jan,8; 2017,Jan,8; 2016,Feb,12; 2016,Jan,13; 2015,Jan,16; 2014,Jan,11

20973 **great toe with web space**
87.3 87.3 **FUD** 090 J R2 80 50
AMA: 2018,Jan,8; 2017,Jan,8; 2016,Feb,12; 2016,Jan,13; 2015,Jan,16; 2014,Jan,11

20974-20979 Osteogenic Stimulation

CMS: 100-03,150.2 Osteogenic Stimulation

20974 **Electrical stimulation to aid bone healing; noninvasive (nonoperative)**
1.46 2.24 **FUD** 000 A
AMA: 2018,Jan,8; 2017,Jan,8; 2016,Jan,13; 2015,Jan,16; 2014,Jan,11

20975 **invasive (operative)**
5.18 5.18 **FUD** 000 N N1 80
AMA: 2002,Apr,13; 2000,Nov,8

20979 **Low intensity ultrasound stimulation to aid bone healing, noninvasive (nonoperative)**
0.93 1.49 **FUD** 000 Q1 N1
AMA: 2018,Jan,8; 2017,Jan,8; 2016,Jan,13; 2015,Jan,16; 2014,Jan,11

20982-20999 General Musculoskeletal Procedures

20982 **Ablation therapy for reduction or eradication of 1 or more bone tumors (eg, metastasis) including adjacent soft tissue when involved by tumor extension, percutaneous, including imaging guidance when performed; radiofrequency**
10.5 110. **FUD** 000 J G2 50
AMA: 2018,Jan,8; 2017,Jan,8; 2016,Jan,13; 2015,Sep,12; 2015,Jul,8

20983 **cryoablation**
10.1 163. **FUD** 000 J G2 50
AMA: 2018,Jan,8; 2017,Jan,8; 2016,Jan,13; 2015,Jul,8

+ **20985** **Computer-assisted surgical navigational procedure for musculoskeletal procedures, image-less (List separately in addition to code for primary procedure)**

EXCLUDES *Image guidance derived from intraoperative and preoperative obtained images (0054T-0055T)*
Stereotactic computer-assisted navigational procedure; cranial or intradural (61781-61783)

Code first primary procedure
4.24 4.24 **FUD** ZZZ N N1 80
AMA: 2018,Jan,8; 2017,Jan,8; 2016,Jan,13; 2015,Jan,16; 2014,Jan,11

20999 **Unlisted procedure, musculoskeletal system, general**
0.00 0.00 **FUD** YYY T 80
AMA: 2018,May,3; 2018,Jan,8; 2017,Jan,8; 2016,Jan,13; 2015,Jul,8; 2015,Jan,16; 2014,Oct,9; 2014,Jan,11

21010 Temporomandibular Joint Arthrotomy

21010 **Arthrotomy, temporomandibular joint**

EXCLUDES *Cutaneous/subcutaneous abscess and hematoma drainage (10060-10061)*
Excision of foreign body from dentoalveolar site (41805-41806)

22.0 22.0 **FUD** 090 J A2 80 50
AMA: 2002,Apr,13

21011-21016 Excision Soft Tissue Tumors Face and Scalp

INCLUDES Any necessary elevation of tissue planes or dissection
Measurement of tumor and necessary margin at greatest diameter prior to excision
Simple and intermediate repairs
Types of excision:
- Fascial or subfascial soft tissue tumors: simple and marginal resection of tumors found either in or below the deep fascia, not including bone or excision of a substantial amount of normal tissue; primarily benign and intramuscular tumors
- Radical resection soft tissue tumor: wide resection of tumor involving substantial margins of normal tissue and may include tissue removal from one or more layers; most often malignant or aggressive benign
- Subcutaneous: simple and marginal resection of tumors in the subcutaneous tissue above the deep fascia; most often benign

EXCLUDES *Complex repair*
Excision of benign cutaneous lesions (eg, sebaceous cyst) (11420-11426)
Radical resection of cutaneous tumors (eg, melanoma) (11620-11646)
Significant exploration of vessels or neuroplasty

21011 **Excision, tumor, soft tissue of face or scalp, subcutaneous; less than 2 cm**
7.39 10.1 **FUD** 090 J P3 80
AMA: 2018,Sep,7; 2018,Jan,8; 2017,Jan,8; 2016,Jan,13; 2015,Jan,16; 2014,Jan,11

21012 **2 cm or greater**
9.75 9.75 **FUD** 090 J R2 80
AMA: 2018,Sep,7; 2018,Jan,8; 2017,Jan,8; 2016,Jan,13; 2015,Jan,16; 2014,Jan,11

21013 **Excision, tumor, soft tissue of face and scalp, subfascial (eg, subgaleal, intramuscular); less than 2 cm**
11.5 15.0 **FUD** 090 J P3 80
AMA: 2018,Sep,7; 2018,Jan,8; 2017,Jan,8; 2016,Jan,13; 2015,Jan,16; 2014,Jan,11

21014 **2 cm or greater**
15.0 15.0 **FUD** 090 J R2 80
AMA: 2018,Sep,7; 2018,Jan,8; 2017,Jan,8; 2016,Jan,13; 2015,Jan,16; 2014,Jan,11

21015 **Radical resection of tumor (eg, sarcoma), soft tissue of face or scalp; less than 2 cm**

EXCLUDES *Removal of cranial tumor for osteomyelitis (61501)*

20.3 20.3 **FUD** 090 J G2
AMA: 2018,Sep,7; 2018,Jan,8; 2017,Jan,8; 2016,Jan,13; 2015,Jan,16; 2014,Jan,11

21016 **2 cm or greater**
29.1 29.1 **FUD** 090 J G2 80
AMA: 2018,Sep,7; 2018,Jan,8; 2017,Jan,8; 2016,Jan,13; 2015,Jan,16; 2014,Jan,11

21025-21070 Procedures of Cranial and Facial Bones

INCLUDES Any necessary elevation of tissue planes or dissection
Measurement of tumor and necessary margins prior to excision
Radical resection of bone tumor involves resection of the tumor (may include entire bone) and wide margins of normal tissue primarily for malignant or aggressive benign tumors
Simple and intermediate repairs

EXCLUDES *Complex repair*
Excision of soft tissue tumors, face and scalp (21011-21016)
Radical resection of cutaneous tumors (e.g., melanoma) (11620-11646)
Significant exploration of vessels, neuroplasty, reconstruction, or complex bone repair

21025 **Excision of bone (eg, for osteomyelitis or bone abscess); mandible**
21.0 24.8 FUD 090 J A2
AMA: 2018,Sep,7; 2018,Jan,8; 2017,Jan,8; 2016,Jan,13; 2015,Jan,16; 2014,Jan,11

21026 **facial bone(s)**
13.8 17.0 FUD 090 J A2
AMA: 2018,Sep,7

21029 **Removal by contouring of benign tumor of facial bone (eg, fibrous dysplasia)**
18.2 22.0 FUD 090 J A2 80
AMA: 2018,Sep,7

Area of benign bone growth

Vestibular incision

Burrs, files, and osteotomes used to remove bone

21030 **Excision of benign tumor or cyst of maxilla or zygoma by enucleation and curettage**
11.7 14.6 FUD 090 J P3 50
AMA: 2018,Sep,7; 2018,Jan,8; 2017,Jan,8; 2016,Jan,13; 2015,Jan,16; 2014,Jan,11

21031 **Excision of torus mandibularis**
8.34 11.3 FUD 090 J P3 50
AMA: 2018,Sep,7

21032 **Excision of maxillary torus palatinus**
8.21 11.3 FUD 090 J P3
AMA: 2018,Sep,7

21034 **Excision of malignant tumor of maxilla or zygoma**
33.0 37.5 FUD 090 J A2 80
AMA: 2018,Sep,7; 2018,Jan,8; 2017,Jan,8; 2016,Jan,13; 2015,Jan,16; 2014,Jan,11

21040 **Excision of benign tumor or cyst of mandible, by enucleation and/or curettage**
INCLUDES Removal of benign tumor or cyst without osteotomy
EXCLUDES *Removal of benign tumor or cyst with osteotomy (21046-21047)*
11.7 14.7 FUD 090 J A2
AMA: 2018,Sep,7; 2018,Jan,8; 2017,Jan,8; 2016,Jan,13; 2015,Jan,16; 2014,Jan,11

21044 **Excision of malignant tumor of mandible;**
25.0 25.0 FUD 090 J A2 80
AMA: 2018,Sep,7

21045 **radical resection**
Code also bone graft procedure (21215)
35.1 35.1 FUD 090 C 80
AMA: 2018,Sep,7

21046 **Excision of benign tumor or cyst of mandible; requiring intra-oral osteotomy (eg, locally aggressive or destructive lesion[s])**
31.5 31.5 FUD 090 J A2 80
AMA: 2018,Sep,7; 2018,Jan,8; 2017,Jan,8; 2016,Jan,13; 2015,Jan,16; 2014,Jan,11

21047 **requiring extra-oral osteotomy and partial mandibulectomy (eg, locally aggressive or destructive lesion[s])**
37.6 37.6 FUD 090 J A2 80
AMA: 2018,Sep,7; 2018,Jan,8; 2017,Jan,8; 2016,Jan,13; 2015,Jan,16; 2014,Jan,11

21048 **Excision of benign tumor or cyst of maxilla; requiring intra-oral osteotomy (eg, locally aggressive or destructive lesion[s])**
32.0 32.0 FUD 090 J R2 80
AMA: 2018,Sep,7; 2018,Jan,8; 2017,Jan,8; 2016,Jan,13; 2015,Jan,16; 2014,Jan,11

21049 **requiring extra-oral osteotomy and partial maxillectomy (eg, locally aggressive or destructive lesion[s])**
34.7 34.7 FUD 090 J 80
AMA: 2018,Sep,7; 2018,Jan,8; 2017,Jan,8; 2016,Jan,13; 2015,Jan,16; 2014,Jan,11

21050 **Condylectomy, temporomandibular joint (separate procedure)**
25.9 25.9 FUD 090 J A2 80 50
AMA: 2018,Sep,7

21060 **Meniscectomy, partial or complete, temporomandibular joint (separate procedure)**
23.5 23.5 FUD 090 J A2 80 50
AMA: 2018,Sep,7

21070 **Coronoidectomy (separate procedure)**
18.3 18.3 FUD 090 J A2 80 50
AMA: 2018,Sep,7

21073 Temporomandibular Joint Manipulation with Anesthesia

21073 **Manipulation of temporomandibular joint(s) (TMJ), therapeutic, requiring an anesthesia service (ie, general or monitored anesthesia care)**
EXCLUDES *Closed treatment of TMJ dislocation (21480, 21485)*
Manipulation of TMJ without general or MAC anesthesia (97140, 98925-98929, 98943)
7.30 11.0 FUD 090 T P3 80 50
AMA: 2018,Sep,7; 2018,Jan,8; 2018,Jan,3; 2017,Jan,8; 2016,Jan,13; 2015,Jan,16; 2014,Jan,11

21076-21089 Medical Impressions for Fabrication Maxillofacial Prosthesis

INCLUDES Design, preparation, and professional services rendered by a physician or other qualified health care professional

EXCLUDES *Application or removal of caliper or tongs (20660, 20665)*
Professional services rendered for outside laboratory designed and prepared prosthesis

21076 **Impression and custom preparation; surgical obturator prosthesis**
23.1 27.6 FUD 010 T P3 80
AMA: 2018,Sep,7; 2018,Jan,8; 2017,Jan,8; 2016,Jan,13; 2015,Jan,16; 2014,Jan,11

21077 **orbital prosthesis**
57.9 68.8 **FUD** 090 J P3 80 50
AMA: 2018,Sep,7; 2018,Jan,8; 2017,Jan,8; 2016,Jan,13; 2015,Jan,16; 2014,Jan,11

21079 **interim obturator prosthesis**
38.8 46.6 **FUD** 090 J P3
AMA: 2018,Sep,7; 2018,Jan,8; 2017,Jan,8; 2016,Jan,13; 2015,Jan,16; 2014,Jan,11

21080 **definitive obturator prosthesis**
43.3 52.7 **FUD** 090 J P3
AMA: 2018,Sep,7; 2018,Jan,8; 2017,Jan,8; 2016,Jan,13; 2015,Jan,16; 2014,Jan,11

21081 **mandibular resection prosthesis**
39.8 48.5 **FUD** 090 J P3 80
AMA: 2018,Sep,7; 2018,Jan,8; 2017,Jan,8; 2016,Jan,13; 2015,Jan,16; 2014,Jan,11

21082 **palatal augmentation prosthesis**
36.8 45.3 **FUD** 090 J P3 80
AMA: 2018,Sep,7; 2018,Jan,8; 2017,Jan,8; 2016,Jan,13; 2015,Jan,16; 2014,Jan,11

21083 **palatal lift prosthesis**
34.3 43.2 **FUD** 090 J P3 80
AMA: 2018,Sep,7; 2018,Jan,8; 2017,Jan,8; 2016,Jan,13; 2015,Jan,16; 2014,Jan,11

21084 **speech aid prosthesis**
39.6 49.5 **FUD** 090 J P3 80
AMA: 2018,Sep,7; 2018,Jan,8; 2017,Jan,8; 2016,Jan,13; 2015,Jan,16; 2014,Jan,11

21085 **oral surgical splint**
15.7 21.0 **FUD** 010 T P2 80
AMA: 2018,Sep,7; 2018,Jan,8; 2017,Sep,14; 2017,Jan,8; 2016,Jan,13; 2015,Jan,16; 2014,Jan,11

21086 **auricular prosthesis**
42.7 51.1 **FUD** 090 J P3 80 50
AMA: 2018,Sep,7; 2018,Jan,8; 2017,Jan,8; 2016,Jan,13; 2015,Jan,16; 2014,Jan,11

21087 **nasal prosthesis**
42.7 51.1 **FUD** 090 J P3 80
AMA: 2018,Sep,7; 2018,Jan,8; 2017,Jan,8; 2016,Jan,13; 2015,Jan,16; 2014,Jan,11

21088 **facial prosthesis**
0.00 0.00 **FUD** 090 J R2 80
AMA: 2018,Sep,7; 2018,Jan,8; 2017,Jan,8; 2016,Jan,13; 2015,Jan,16; 2014,Jan,11

21089 **Unlisted maxillofacial prosthetic procedure**
0.00 0.00 **FUD** YYY T
AMA: 2018,Sep,7; 2018,Jan,8; 2017,Jan,8; 2016,Jan,13; 2015,Jan,16; 2014,Jan,11

21100-21110 Application Fixation Device

21100 **Application of halo type appliance for maxillofacial fixation, includes removal (separate procedure)**
11.3 19.8 **FUD** 090 J A2 80
AMA: 2018,Sep,7

21110 **Application of interdental fixation device for conditions other than fracture or dislocation, includes removal**
EXCLUDES *Interdental fixation device removal by different provider (20670-20680)*
19.5 23.3 **FUD** 090 Q2 P2
AMA: 2018,Sep,7; 2018,Jan,8; 2017,Jan,8; 2016,Jan,13; 2015,Jan,16; 2014,Jan,11

21116 Injection for TMJ Arthrogram

CMS: 100-02,15,150.1 Treatment of Temporomandibular Joint (TMJ) Syndrome; 100-04,13,80.1 Physician Presence; 100-04,13,80.2 S&I Multiple Procedure Reduction

21116 **Injection procedure for temporomandibular joint arthrography**
(70332)
1.38 5.08 **FUD** 000 N N1 50
AMA: 2018,Sep,7; 2018,Jan,8; 2017,Jan,8; 2016,May,13; 2016,Jan,13; 2015,Aug,6

21120-21299 Repair/Reconstruction Craniofacial Bones

EXCLUDES *Cranioplasty (21179-21180, 62120, 62140-62147)*

21120 **Genioplasty; augmentation (autograft, allograft, prosthetic material)**
15.2 19.3 **FUD** 090 J G2
AMA: 2018,Sep,7

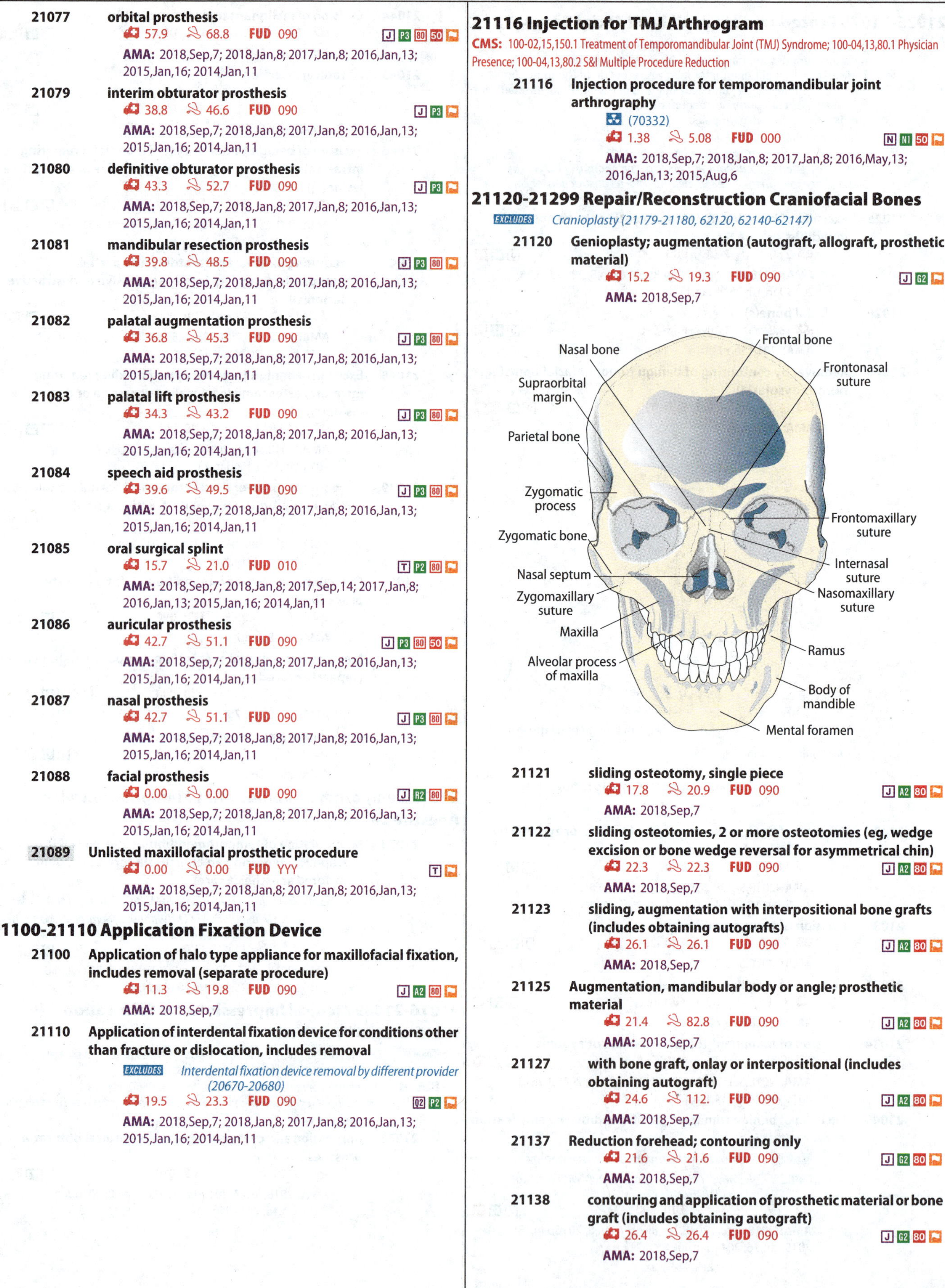

21121 **sliding osteotomy, single piece**
17.8 20.9 **FUD** 090 J A2 80
AMA: 2018,Sep,7

21122 **sliding osteotomies, 2 or more osteotomies (eg, wedge excision or bone wedge reversal for asymmetrical chin)**
22.3 22.3 **FUD** 090 J A2 80
AMA: 2018,Sep,7

21123 **sliding, augmentation with interpositional bone grafts (includes obtaining autografts)**
26.1 26.1 **FUD** 090 J A2 80
AMA: 2018,Sep,7

21125 **Augmentation, mandibular body or angle; prosthetic material**
21.4 82.8 **FUD** 090 J A2 80
AMA: 2018,Sep,7

21127 **with bone graft, onlay or interpositional (includes obtaining autograft)**
24.6 112. **FUD** 090 J A2 80
AMA: 2018,Sep,7

21137 **Reduction forehead; contouring only**
21.6 21.6 **FUD** 090 J G2 80
AMA: 2018,Sep,7

21138 **contouring and application of prosthetic material or bone graft (includes obtaining autograft)**
26.4 26.4 **FUD** 090 J G2 80
AMA: 2018,Sep,7

21139 **contouring and setback of anterior frontal sinus wall**
32.1 32.1 **FUD** 090 J G2 80
AMA: 2018,Sep,7

21141 **Reconstruction midface, LeFort I; single piece, segment movement in any direction (eg, for Long Face Syndrome), without bone graft**
39.4 39.4 **FUD** 090 C 80
AMA: 2018,Sep,7

21142 **2 pieces, segment movement in any direction, without bone graft**
40.5 40.5 **FUD** 090 C 80
AMA: 2018,Sep,7

21143 **3 or more pieces, segment movement in any direction, without bone graft**
42.3 42.3 **FUD** 090 C 80
AMA: 2018,Sep,7

21145 **single piece, segment movement in any direction, requiring bone grafts (includes obtaining autografts)**
46.2 46.2 **FUD** 090 C 80
AMA: 2018,Sep,7

21146 **2 pieces, segment movement in any direction, requiring bone grafts (includes obtaining autografts) (eg, ungrafted unilateral alveolar cleft)**
48.2 48.2 **FUD** 090 C 80
AMA: 2018,Sep,7

21147 **3 or more pieces, segment movement in any direction, requiring bone grafts (includes obtaining autografts) (eg, ungrafted bilateral alveolar cleft or multiple osteotomies)**
50.8 50.8 **FUD** 090 C 80
AMA: 2018,Sep,7

21150 **Reconstruction midface, LeFort II; anterior intrusion (eg, Treacher-Collins Syndrome)**
47.6 47.6 **FUD** 090 J G2 80
AMA: 2018,Sep,7

21151 **any direction, requiring bone grafts (includes obtaining autografts)**
52.4 52.4 **FUD** 090 C 80
AMA: 2018,Sep,7

21154 **Reconstruction midface, LeFort III (extracranial), any type, requiring bone grafts (includes obtaining autografts); without LeFort I**
56.4 56.4 **FUD** 090 C 80
AMA: 2018,Sep,7

21155 **with LeFort I**
62.6 62.6 **FUD** 090 C 80
AMA: 2018,Sep,7

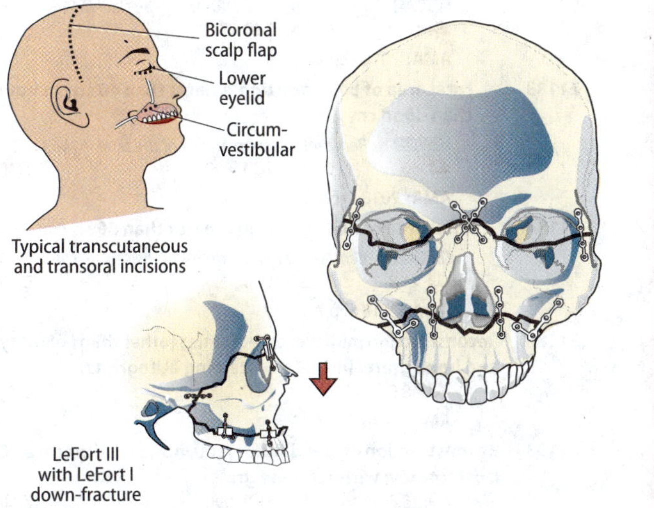

21159 **Reconstruction midface, LeFort III (extra and intracranial) with forehead advancement (eg, mono bloc), requiring bone grafts (includes obtaining autografts); without LeFort I**
75.0 75.0 **FUD** 090 C 80
AMA: 2018,Sep,7

21160 **with LeFort I**
81.4 81.4 **FUD** 090 C 80
AMA: 2018,Sep,7

21172 **Reconstruction superior-lateral orbital rim and lower forehead, advancement or alteration, with or without grafts (includes obtaining autografts)**
EXCLUDES *Frontal or parietal craniotomy for craniosynostosis (61556)*
60.8 60.8 **FUD** 090 J 80
AMA: 2018,Sep,7

21175 **Reconstruction, bifrontal, superior-lateral orbital rims and lower forehead, advancement or alteration (eg, plagiocephaly, trigonocephaly, brachycephaly), with or without grafts (includes obtaining autografts)**
EXCLUDES *Bifrontal craniotomy for craniosynostosis (61557)*
63.8 63.8 **FUD** 090 J 80
AMA: 2018,Sep,7

21179 **Reconstruction, entire or majority of forehead and/or supraorbital rims; with grafts (allograft or prosthetic material)**
EXCLUDES *Extensive craniotomy for numerous suture craniosynostosis (61558-61559)*
43.8 43.8 **FUD** 090 C 80
AMA: 2018,Sep,7

21180 **with autograft (includes obtaining grafts)**
EXCLUDES *Extensive craniotomy for numerous suture craniosynostosis (61558-61559)*
49.0 49.0 **FUD** 090 C 80
AMA: 2018,Sep,7

21181 **Reconstruction by contouring of benign tumor of cranial bones (eg, fibrous dysplasia), extracranial**
21.2 21.2 **FUD** 090 J A2 80
AMA: 2018,Sep,7

21182 **Reconstruction of orbital walls, rims, forehead, nasoethmoid complex following intra- and extracranial excision of benign tumor of cranial bone (eg, fibrous dysplasia), with multiple autografts (includes obtaining grafts); total area of bone grafting less than 40 sq cm**

EXCLUDES *Removal of benign tumor of the skull (61563-61564)*

61.2 61.2 FUD 090 C 80

AMA: 2018,Sep,7

21183 **total area of bone grafting greater than 40 sq cm but less than 80 sq cm**

EXCLUDES *Removal of benign tumor of the skull (61563-61564)*

66.7 66.7 FUD 090 C 80

AMA: 2018,Sep,7

21184 **total area of bone grafting greater than 80 sq cm**

EXCLUDES *Removal of benign tumor of the skull (61563-61564)*

71.8 71.8 FUD 090 C 80

AMA: 2018,Sep,7

21188 **Reconstruction midface, osteotomies (other than LeFort type) and bone grafts (includes obtaining autografts)**

48.0 48.0 FUD 090 C 80

AMA: 2018,Sep,7

21193 **Reconstruction of mandibular rami, horizontal, vertical, C, or L osteotomy; without bone graft**

36.8 36.8 FUD 090 J 80

AMA: 2018,Sep,7; 2018,Jan,8; 2017,Jan,8; 2016,Jan,13; 2015,Jan,16; 2014,Jan,11

21194 **with bone graft (includes obtaining graft)**

42.3 42.3 FUD 090 C 80

AMA: 2018,Sep,7; 2018,Jan,8; 2017,Jan,8; 2016,Jan,13; 2015,Jan,16; 2014,Jan,11

21195 **Reconstruction of mandibular rami and/or body, sagittal split; without internal rigid fixation**

41.0 41.0 FUD 090 J 80

AMA: 2018,Sep,7; 2018,Jan,8; 2017,Jan,8; 2016,Jan,13; 2015,Jan,16; 2014,Jan,11

21196 **with internal rigid fixation**

42.1 42.1 FUD 090 C 80

AMA: 2018,Sep,7; 2018,Jan,8; 2017,Jan,8; 2016,Jan,13; 2015,Jan,16; 2014,Jan,11

21198 **Osteotomy, mandible, segmental;**

EXCLUDES *Total maxillary osteotomy (21141-21160)*

33.0 33.0 FUD 090 J G2 80

AMA: 2018,Sep,7; 2018,Jan,8; 2017,Jan,8; 2016,Jan,13; 2015,Jan,16; 2014,Jan,11

21199 **with genioglossus advancement**

EXCLUDES *Total maxillary osteotomy (21141-21160)*

30.9 30.9 FUD 090 J G2 80

AMA: 2018,Sep,7; 2018,Jan,8; 2017,Jan,8; 2016,Jan,13; 2015,Jan,16; 2014,Jan,11

21206 **Osteotomy, maxilla, segmental (eg, Wassmund or Schuchard)**

34.1 34.1 FUD 090 J A2 80

AMA: 2018,Sep,7

21208 **Osteoplasty, facial bones; augmentation (autograft, allograft, or prosthetic implant)**

23.2 49.9 FUD 090 J A2 80

AMA: 2018,Sep,7

21209 **reduction**

19.3 25.7 FUD 090 J A2 80

AMA: 2018,Sep,7

21210 **Graft, bone; nasal, maxillary or malar areas (includes obtaining graft)**

EXCLUDES *Cleft palate procedures (42200-42225)*

23.9 60.2 FUD 090 J A2

AMA: 2018,Sep,7

21215 **mandible (includes obtaining graft)**

24.9 114. FUD 090 J A2

AMA: 2018,Sep,7

21230 **Graft; rib cartilage, autogenous, to face, chin, nose or ear (includes obtaining graft)**

EXCLUDES *Augmentation of facial bones (21208)*

21.3 21.3 FUD 090 J A2 80

AMA: 2018,Sep,7

21235 **ear cartilage, autogenous, to nose or ear (includes obtaining graft)**

EXCLUDES *Augmentation of facial bones (21208)*

16.2 20.7 FUD 090 J A2

AMA: 2018,Sep,7; 2018,Jan,8; 2017,Jan,8; 2016,Jan,13; 2015,Jan,16

21240 **Arthroplasty, temporomandibular joint, with or without autograft (includes obtaining graft)**

32.1 32.1 FUD 090 J A2 80 50

AMA: 2018,Sep,7

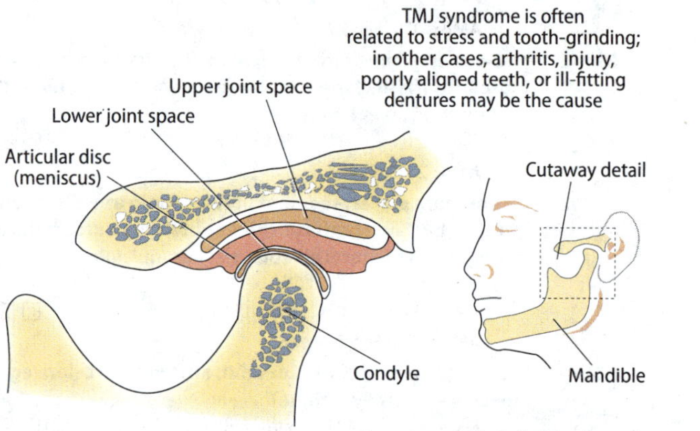

Cutaway view of temporomandibular joint (TMJ)

Symptoms include facial pain and chewing problems; TMJ syndrome occurs more frequently in women

21242 **Arthroplasty, temporomandibular joint, with allograft**

30.0 30.0 FUD 090 J A2 80 50

AMA: 2018,Sep,7

21243 **Arthroplasty, temporomandibular joint, with prosthetic joint replacement**

48.9 48.9 FUD 090 J J8 80 50

AMA: 2018,Sep,7

21244 **Reconstruction of mandible, extraoral, with transosteal bone plate (eg, mandibular staple bone plate)**

30.0 30.0 FUD 090 J J8 80

AMA: 2018,Sep,7

21245 **Reconstruction of mandible or maxilla, subperiosteal implant; partial**

27.5 34.9 FUD 090 J A2 80

AMA: 2018,Sep,7

21246 **complete**

25.4 25.4 FUD 090 J A2 80

AMA: 2018,Sep,7

21247 **Reconstruction of mandibular condyle with bone and cartilage autografts (includes obtaining grafts) (eg, for hemifacial microsomia)**

47.3 47.3 FUD 090 C 80 50

AMA: 2018,Sep,7

21248 **Reconstruction of mandible or maxilla, endosteal implant (eg, blade, cylinder); partial**

EXCLUDES *Midface reconstruction (21141-21160)*

25.3 31.1 FUD 090 J A2

AMA: 2018,Sep,7

21249 complete

EXCLUDES *Midface reconstruction (21141-21160)*

36.7 44.9 FUD 090 J A2 80

AMA: 2018,Sep,7

21255 **Reconstruction of zygomatic arch and glenoid fossa with bone and cartilage (includes obtaining autografts)**

40.6 40.6 FUD 090 C 80 50

AMA: 2018,Sep,7

21256 **Reconstruction of orbit with osteotomies (extracranial) and with bone grafts (includes obtaining autografts) (eg, micro-ophthalmia)**

35.7 35.7 FUD 090 J 80 50

AMA: 2018,Sep,7

21260 **Periorbital osteotomies for orbital hypertelorism, with bone grafts; extracranial approach**

40.1 40.1 FUD 090 J G2 80

AMA: 2018,Sep,7

21261 combined intra- and extracranial approach

71.1 71.1 FUD 090 J 80

AMA: 2018,Sep,7

21263 with forehead advancement

65.8 65.8 FUD 090 J 80

AMA: 2018,Sep,7

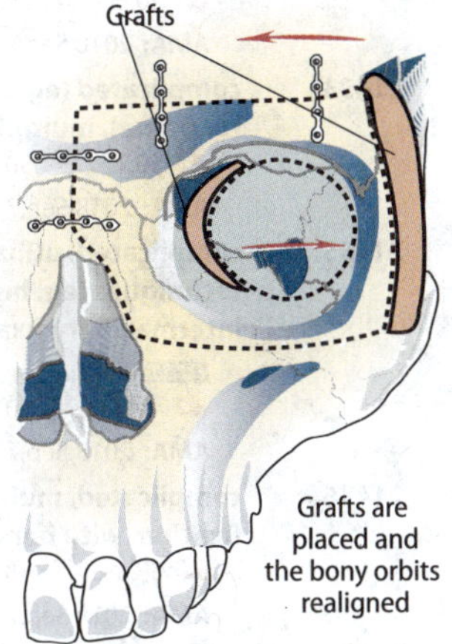

21267 **Orbital repositioning, periorbital osteotomies, unilateral, with bone grafts; extracranial approach**

47.0 47.0 FUD 090 J A2 80 50

AMA: 2018,Sep,7

21268 combined intra- and extracranial approach

58.9 58.9 FUD 090 C 80 50

AMA: 2018,Sep,7

21270 **Malar augmentation, prosthetic material**

EXCLUDES *Augmentation procedure with bone graft (21210)*

21.6 29.0 FUD 090 J A2 80 50

AMA: 2018,Sep,7

21275 **Secondary revision of orbitocraniofacial reconstruction**

24.1 24.1 FUD 090 J G2 80

AMA: 2018,Sep,7

21280 **Medial canthopexy (separate procedure)**

EXCLUDES *Reconstruction of canthus (67950)*

16.4 16.4 FUD 090 J A2 80 50

AMA: 2018,Sep,7

21282 **Lateral canthopexy**

11.0 11.0 FUD 090 J A2 50

AMA: 2018,Sep,7

21295 **Reduction of masseter muscle and bone (eg, for treatment of benign masseteric hypertrophy); extraoral approach**

5.37 5.37 FUD 090 T A2 80 50

AMA: 2018,Sep,7

21296 intraoral approach

11.7 11.7 FUD 090 J A2 80 50

AMA: 2018,Sep,7

21299 **Unlisted craniofacial and maxillofacial procedure**

0.00 0.00 FUD YYY T 80

AMA: 2018,Sep,7

21310-21499 Care of Fractures/Dislocations of the Cranial and Facial Bones

EXCLUDES *Closed treatment of skull fracture, report with appropriate E&M service*
Open treatment of skull fracture (62000-62010)

21310 **Closed treatment of nasal bone fracture without manipulation**

0.78 3.76 FUD 000 T A2

AMA: 2019,Sep,3; 2018,Sep,7; 2018,Jan,3

21315 **Closed treatment of nasal bone fracture; without stabilization**

4.32 7.84 FUD 010 T A2

AMA: 2019,Sep,3; 2018,Sep,7; 2018,Jan,3

21320 with stabilization

3.83 7.23 FUD 010 J A2

AMA: 2019,Sep,3; 2018,Sep,7

21325 **Open treatment of nasal fracture; uncomplicated**

13.3 13.3 FUD 090 J A2 80

AMA: 2018,Sep,7

21330 complicated, with internal and/or external skeletal fixation

16.1 16.1 FUD 090 J A2 80

AMA: 2018,Sep,7

21335 with concomitant open treatment of fractured septum

20.5 20.5 FUD 090 J A2

AMA: 2018,Sep,7

21336 **Open treatment of nasal septal fracture, with or without stabilization**

18.3 18.3 FUD 090 J A2 80

AMA: 2018,Sep,7

21337 **Closed treatment of nasal septal fracture, with or without stabilization**

8.42 11.6 FUD 090 J A2 80

AMA: 2019,Sep,3; 2018,Sep,7

21338 **Open treatment of nasoethmoid fracture; without external fixation**

18.8 18.8 FUD 090 J J8 80

AMA: 2018,Sep,7

21339 with external fixation

21.3 21.3 FUD 090 J A2 80

AMA: 2018,Sep,7

21340 **Percutaneous treatment of nasoethmoid complex fracture, with splint, wire or headcap fixation, including repair of canthal ligaments and/or the nasolacrimal apparatus**

21.3 21.3 FUD 090 J A2 80

AMA: 2018,Sep,7

21343 **Open treatment of depressed frontal sinus fracture**

30.8 30.8 FUD 090 C 80

AMA: 2018,Sep,7

21344 **Open treatment of complicated (eg, comminuted or involving posterior wall) frontal sinus fracture, via coronal or multiple approaches**

39.7 39.7 FUD 090 C 80

AMA: 2018,Sep,7

21345 **Closed treatment of nasomaxillary complex fracture (LeFort II type), with interdental wire fixation or fixation of denture or splint**
17.9 22.2 FUD 090 T A2 80
AMA: 2018,Sep,7

21346 **Open treatment of nasomaxillary complex fracture (LeFort II type); with wiring and/or local fixation**
26.6 26.6 FUD 090 J
AMA: 2018,Sep,7

21347 **requiring multiple open approaches**
29.0 29.0 FUD 090 C 80
AMA: 2018,Sep,7

21348 **with bone grafting (includes obtaining graft)**
31.0 31.0 FUD 090 C 80
AMA: 2018,Sep,7

21355 **Percutaneous treatment of fracture of malar area, including zygomatic arch and malar tripod, with manipulation**
9.17 12.1 FUD 010 J A2 80 50
AMA: 2018,Sep,7

21356 **Open treatment of depressed zygomatic arch fracture (eg, Gillies approach)**
10.8 14.3 FUD 010 J A2 80 50
AMA: 2018,Sep,7

21360 **Open treatment of depressed malar fracture, including zygomatic arch and malar tripod**
14.6 14.6 FUD 090 J G2 80 50
AMA: 2018,Sep,7

21365 **Open treatment of complicated (eg, comminuted or involving cranial nerve foramina) fracture(s) of malar area, including zygomatic arch and malar tripod; with internal fixation and multiple surgical approaches**
31.9 31.9 FUD 090 J 80 50
AMA: 2018,Sep,7

21366 **with bone grafting (includes obtaining graft)**
36.7 36.7 FUD 090 C 80 50
AMA: 2018,Sep,7

21385 **Open treatment of orbital floor blowout fracture; transantral approach (Caldwell-Luc type operation)**
21.6 21.6 FUD 090 J 80 50
AMA: 2018,Sep,7

21386 **periorbital approach**
19.9 19.9 FUD 090 J 80 50
AMA: 2018,Sep,7

21387 **combined approach**
22.6 22.6 FUD 090 J 80 50
AMA: 2018,Sep,7

21390 **periorbital approach, with alloplastic or other implant**
22.9 22.9 FUD 090 J G2 80 50
AMA: 2018,Sep,7

21395 **periorbital approach with bone graft (includes obtaining graft)**
29.0 29.0 FUD 090 J 80 50
AMA: 2018,Sep,7

21400 **Closed treatment of fracture of orbit, except blowout; without manipulation**
4.59 5.73 FUD 090 T A2 80 50
AMA: 2018,Sep,7

21401 **with manipulation**
9.23 14.7 FUD 090 T A2 80 50
AMA: 2018,Sep,7

21406 **Open treatment of fracture of orbit, except blowout; without implant**
16.5 16.5 FUD 090 J G2 80 50
AMA: 2018,Sep,7

21407 **with implant**
18.5 18.5 FUD 090 J G2 80 50
AMA: 2018,Sep,7

21408 **with bone grafting (includes obtaining graft)**
25.9 25.9 FUD 090 J 80 50
AMA: 2018,Sep,7

21421 **Closed treatment of palatal or maxillary fracture (LeFort I type), with interdental wire fixation or fixation of denture or splint**
17.2 20.3 FUD 090 J A2 80
AMA: 2018,Sep,7

21422 **Open treatment of palatal or maxillary fracture (LeFort I type);**
18.9 18.9 FUD 090 C 80
AMA: 2018,Sep,7

21423 **complicated (comminuted or involving cranial nerve foramina), multiple approaches**
22.2 22.2 FUD 090 C 80
AMA: 2018,Sep,7

21431 **Closed treatment of craniofacial separation (LeFort III type) using interdental wire fixation of denture or splint**
20.6 20.6 FUD 090 C 80
AMA: 2018,Sep,7

21432 **Open treatment of craniofacial separation (LeFort III type); with wiring and/or internal fixation**
20.6 20.6 FUD 090 C 80
AMA: 2018,Sep,7

21433 **complicated (eg, comminuted or involving cranial nerve foramina), multiple surgical approaches**
50.1 50.1 FUD 090 C 80
AMA: 2018,Sep,7

21435 **complicated, utilizing internal and/or external fixation techniques (eg, head cap, halo device, and/or intermaxillary fixation)**
EXCLUDES *Removal of internal or external fixation (20670)*
40.4 40.4 FUD 090 C 80
AMA: 2018,Sep,7

21436 **complicated, multiple surgical approaches, internal fixation, with bone grafting (includes obtaining graft)**
58.8 58.8 FUD 090 C 80
AMA: 2018,Sep,7

21440 **Closed treatment of mandibular or maxillary alveolar ridge fracture (separate procedure)**
14.0 17.3 FUD 090 J P3 80
AMA: 2018,Sep,7

21445 **Open treatment of mandibular or maxillary alveolar ridge fracture (separate procedure)**
18.0 22.2 FUD 090 J A2 80
AMA: 2018,Sep,7

21450 **Closed treatment of mandibular fracture; without manipulation**
13.4 16.4 FUD 090 T A2 80
AMA: 2018,Sep,7

21451 **with manipulation**
18.2 21.7 FUD 090 T A2 80
AMA: 2018,Sep,7

21452 **Percutaneous treatment of mandibular fracture, with external fixation**
11.4 19.1 FUD 090 J A2 80
AMA: 2018,Sep,7

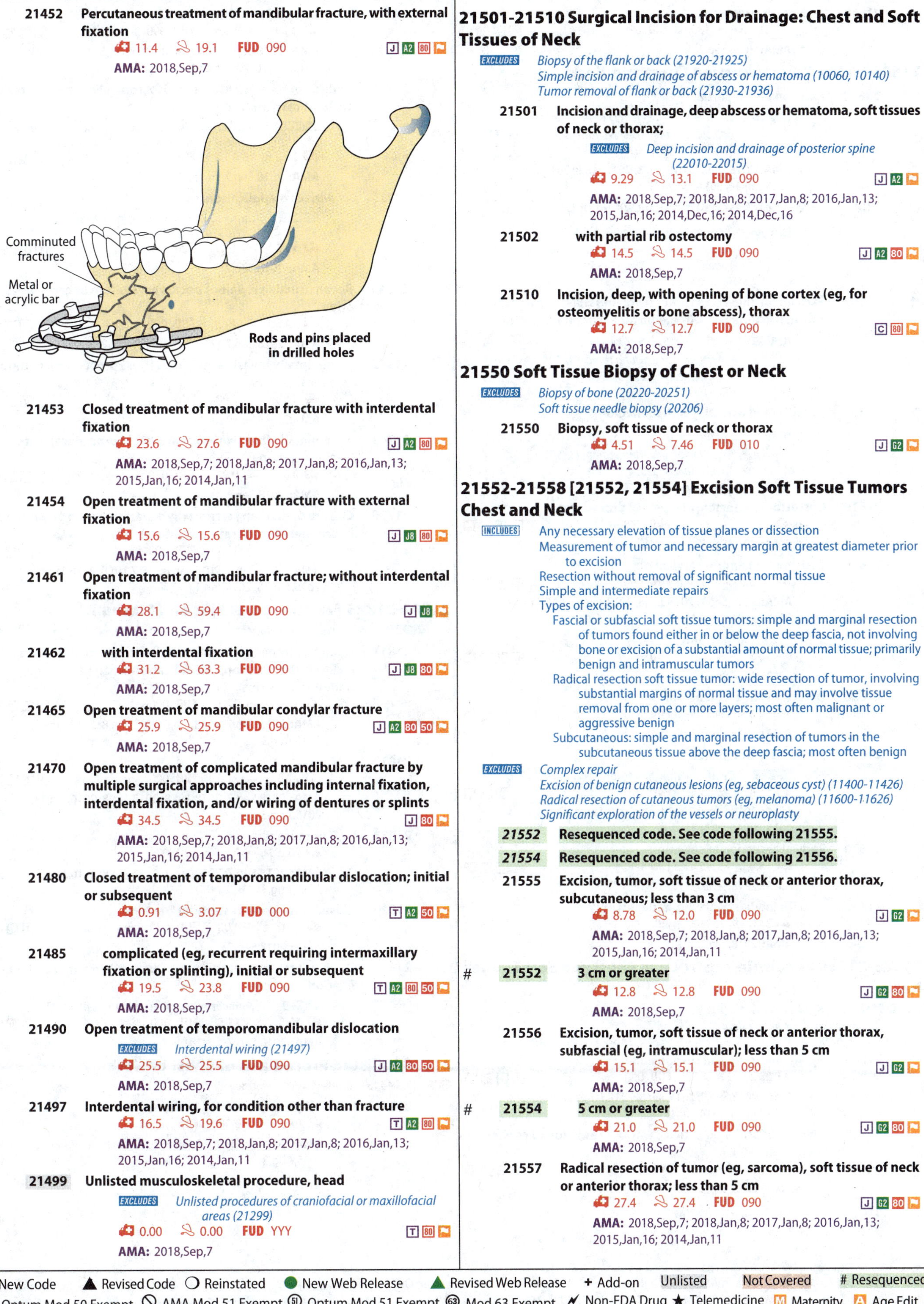

21453 **Closed treatment of mandibular fracture with interdental fixation**
23.6 27.6 FUD 090 J A2 80
AMA: 2018,Sep,7; 2018,Jan,8; 2017,Jan,8; 2016,Jan,13; 2015,Jan,16; 2014,Jan,11

21454 **Open treatment of mandibular fracture with external fixation**
15.6 15.6 FUD 090 J J8 80
AMA: 2018,Sep,7

21461 **Open treatment of mandibular fracture; without interdental fixation**
28.1 59.4 FUD 090 J J8
AMA: 2018,Sep,7

21462 **with interdental fixation**
31.2 63.3 FUD 090 J J8 80
AMA: 2018,Sep,7

21465 **Open treatment of mandibular condylar fracture**
25.9 25.9 FUD 090 J A2 80 50
AMA: 2018,Sep,7

21470 **Open treatment of complicated mandibular fracture by multiple surgical approaches including internal fixation, interdental fixation, and/or wiring of dentures or splints**
34.5 34.5 FUD 090 J 80
AMA: 2018,Sep,7; 2018,Jan,8; 2017,Jan,8; 2016,Jan,13; 2015,Jan,16; 2014,Jan,11

21480 **Closed treatment of temporomandibular dislocation; initial or subsequent**
0.91 3.07 FUD 000 T A2 50
AMA: 2018,Sep,7

21485 **complicated (eg, recurrent requiring intermaxillary fixation or splinting), initial or subsequent**
19.5 23.8 FUD 090 T A2 80 50
AMA: 2018,Sep,7

21490 **Open treatment of temporomandibular dislocation**
EXCLUDES *Interdental wiring (21497)*
25.5 25.5 FUD 090 J A2 80 50
AMA: 2018,Sep,7

21497 **Interdental wiring, for condition other than fracture**
16.5 19.6 FUD 090 T A2 80
AMA: 2018,Sep,7; 2018,Jan,8; 2017,Jan,8; 2016,Jan,13; 2015,Jan,16; 2014,Jan,11

21499 **Unlisted musculoskeletal procedure, head**
EXCLUDES *Unlisted procedures of craniofacial or maxillofacial areas (21299)*
0.00 0.00 FUD YYY T 80
AMA: 2018,Sep,7

21501-21510 Surgical Incision for Drainage: Chest and Soft Tissues of Neck

EXCLUDES *Biopsy of the flank or back (21920-21925)*
Simple incision and drainage of abscess or hematoma (10060, 10140)
Tumor removal of flank or back (21930-21936)

21501 **Incision and drainage, deep abscess or hematoma, soft tissues of neck or thorax;**
EXCLUDES *Deep incision and drainage of posterior spine (22010-22015)*
9.29 13.1 FUD 090 J A2
AMA: 2018,Sep,7; 2018,Jan,8; 2017,Jan,8; 2016,Jan,13; 2015,Jan,16; 2014,Dec,16; 2014,Dec,16

21502 **with partial rib ostectomy**
14.5 14.5 FUD 090 J A2 80
AMA: 2018,Sep,7

21510 **Incision, deep, with opening of bone cortex (eg, for osteomyelitis or bone abscess), thorax**
12.7 12.7 FUD 090 C 80
AMA: 2018,Sep,7

21550 Soft Tissue Biopsy of Chest or Neck

EXCLUDES *Biopsy of bone (20220-20251)*
Soft tissue needle biopsy (20206)

21550 **Biopsy, soft tissue of neck or thorax**
4.51 7.46 FUD 010 J G2
AMA: 2018,Sep,7

21552-21558 [21552, 21554] Excision Soft Tissue Tumors Chest and Neck

INCLUDES Any necessary elevation of tissue planes or dissection
Measurement of tumor and necessary margin at greatest diameter prior to excision
Resection without removal of significant normal tissue
Simple and intermediate repairs
Types of excision:
Fascial or subfascial soft tissue tumors: simple and marginal resection of tumors found either in or below the deep fascia, not involving bone or excision of a substantial amount of normal tissue; primarily benign and intramuscular tumors
Radical resection soft tissue tumor: wide resection of tumor, involving substantial margins of normal tissue and may involve tissue removal from one or more layers; most often malignant or aggressive benign
Subcutaneous: simple and marginal resection of tumors in the subcutaneous tissue above the deep fascia; most often benign

EXCLUDES *Complex repair*
Excision of benign cutaneous lesions (eg, sebaceous cyst) (11400-11426)
Radical resection of cutaneous tumors (eg, melanoma) (11600-11626)
Significant exploration of the vessels or neuroplasty

21552 **Resequenced code. See code following 21555.**

21554 **Resequenced code. See code following 21556.**

21555 **Excision, tumor, soft tissue of neck or anterior thorax, subcutaneous; less than 3 cm**
8.78 12.0 FUD 090 J G2
AMA: 2018,Sep,7; 2018,Jan,8; 2017,Jan,8; 2016,Jan,13; 2015,Jan,16; 2014,Jan,11

21552 **3 cm or greater**
12.8 12.8 FUD 090 J G2 80
AMA: 2018,Sep,7

21556 **Excision, tumor, soft tissue of neck or anterior thorax, subfascial (eg, intramuscular); less than 5 cm**
15.1 15.1 FUD 090 J G2
AMA: 2018,Sep,7

21554 **5 cm or greater**
21.0 21.0 FUD 090 J G2 80
AMA: 2018,Sep,7

21557 **Radical resection of tumor (eg, sarcoma), soft tissue of neck or anterior thorax; less than 5 cm**
27.4 27.4 FUD 090 J G2 80
AMA: 2018,Sep,7; 2018,Jan,8; 2017,Jan,8; 2016,Jan,13; 2015,Jan,16; 2014,Jan,11

21558 **5 cm or greater**
38.7 38.7 FUD 090 J G2 80
AMA: 2018,Sep,7

21600-21632 Bony Resection Chest and Neck

21600 **Excision of rib, partial**
EXCLUDES *Extensive debridement (11044, 11047)*
Radical resection, chest wall/rib cage for tumor (21601)
15.8 15.8 FUD 090 J A2 80
AMA: 2018,Sep,7; 2018,Jan,8; 2017,Jan,8; 2016,Jan,13; 2015,Jan,16; 2014,Jan,11

● **21601** **Excision of chest wall tumor including rib(s)**
EXCLUDES *Exploratory thoracotomy (32100)*
Resection of apical lung tumor (32503-32504)
Thoracentesis (32554-32555)
Tube thoracostomy (32551)

● **21602** **Excision of chest wall tumor involving rib(s), with plastic reconstruction; without mediastinal lymphadenectomy**
EXCLUDES *Exploratory thoracotomy (32100)*
Resection of apical lung tumor (32503-32504)
Thoracentesis (32554-32555)
Tube thoracostomy (32551)

● **21603** **with mediastinal lymphadenectomy**
EXCLUDES *Exploratory thoracotomy (32100)*
Resection of apical lung tumor (32503-32504)
Thoracentesis (32554-32555)
Tube thoracostomy (32551)

21610 **Costotransversectomy (separate procedure)**
35.1 35.1 FUD 090 J A2 80
AMA: 2018,Sep,7

21615 **Excision first and/or cervical rib;**
17.5 17.5 FUD 090 C 80 50
AMA: 2018,Sep,7; 2018,Jan,8; 2017,Jan,8; 2016,Jan,13; 2015,Jan,16; 2014,Mar,13

21616 **with sympathectomy**
20.5 20.5 FUD 090 C 80 50
AMA: 2018,Sep,7

21620 **Ostectomy of sternum, partial**
14.5 14.5 FUD 090 C 80
AMA: 2018,Sep,7

21627 **Sternal debridement**
EXCLUDES *Debridement with sternotomy closure (21750)*
15.4 15.4 FUD 090 C 80
AMA: 2018,Sep,7; 2018,Jan,8; 2017,Jan,8; 2016,Jan,13; 2015,Jan,16; 2014,Jan,11

21630 **Radical resection of sternum;**
35.4 35.4 FUD 090 C 80
AMA: 2018,Sep,7

21632 **with mediastinal lymphadenectomy**
34.8 34.8 FUD 090 C 80
AMA: 2018,Sep,7

21685-21750 Repair/Reconstruction Chest and Soft Tissues Neck

EXCLUDES *Biopsy of chest or neck (21550)*
Repair of simple wounds (12001-12007)
Tumor removal of chest or neck (21552-21558 [21552, 21554])

21685 **Hyoid myotomy and suspension**
28.2 28.2 FUD 090 J G2 80
AMA: 2018,Sep,7; 2018,Jan,8; 2017,Jan,8; 2016,Jan,13; 2015,Jan,16; 2014,Jan,11

21700 **Division of scalenus anticus; without resection of cervical rib**
10.3 10.3 FUD 090 J A2 80 50
AMA: 2018,Sep,7

21705 **with resection of cervical rib**
15.4 15.4 FUD 090 C 80 50
AMA: 2018,Sep,7; 2018,Jan,8; 2017,Jan,8; 2016,Jan,13; 2015,Jan,16; 2014,Mar,13

21720 **Division of sternocleidomastoid for torticollis, open operation; without cast application**
EXCLUDES *Transection of spinal accessory and cervical nerves (63191, 64722)*
15.2 15.2 FUD 090 J A2 80
AMA: 2018,Sep,7

21725 **with cast application**
EXCLUDES *Transection of spinal accessory and cervical nerves (63191, 64722)*
15.5 15.5 FUD 090 T A2 80
AMA: 2018,Sep,7

21740 **Reconstructive repair of pectus excavatum or carinatum; open**
29.8 29.8 FUD 090 C 80
AMA: 2018,Sep,7

21742 **minimally invasive approach (Nuss procedure), without thoracoscopy**
0.00 0.00 FUD 090 J 80
AMA: 2018,Sep,7

21743 **minimally invasive approach (Nuss procedure), with thoracoscopy**
0.00 0.00 FUD 090 J 80
AMA: 2018,Sep,7

21750 **Closure of median sternotomy separation with or without debridement (separate procedure)**
19.7 19.7 FUD 090 C 80
AMA: 2018,Sep,7; 2018,Jan,8; 2017,Jan,8; 2016,Jan,13; 2015,Jan,16; 2014,Jan,11

21811-21825 Fracture Care: Ribs and Sternum

EXCLUDES *E&M services for treatment of closed uncomplicated rib fractures*

21811 **Open treatment of rib fracture(s) with internal fixation, includes thoracoscopic visualization when performed, unilateral; 1-3 ribs**
17.1 17.1 FUD 000 J 80 50
AMA: 2018,Sep,7; 2018,Jan,8; 2017,Jan,8; 2016,Jan,13; 2015,Aug,3

21812 **4-6 ribs**
21.0 21.0 FUD 000 J 80 50
AMA: 2018,Sep,7; 2018,Jan,8; 2017,Jan,8; 2016,Jan,13; 2015,Aug,3

21813 **7 or more ribs**
28.6 28.6 FUD 000 J 80 50
AMA: 2018,Sep,7; 2018,Jan,8; 2017,Jan,8; 2016,Jan,13; 2015,Aug,3

21820 **Closed treatment of sternum fracture**
4.10 4.08 FUD 090 T A2
AMA: 2018,Sep,7

21825 **Open treatment of sternum fracture with or without skeletal fixation**
EXCLUDES *Treatment of sternoclavicular dislocation (23520-23532)*
15.5 15.5 FUD 090 C 80
AMA: 2018,Sep,7

21899 Unlisted Procedures of Chest or Neck

CMS: 100-04,4,180.3 Unlisted Service or Procedure

21899 **Unlisted procedure, neck or thorax**
0.00 0.00 FUD YYY T 80
AMA: 2018,Sep,7; 2018,Jan,8; 2017,Jan,8; 2016,Jan,13; 2015,Aug,3

21920-21925 Biopsy Soft Tissue of Back and Flank

EXCLUDES *Soft tissue needle biopsy (20206)*

21920 Biopsy, soft tissue of back or flank; superficial
4.55 7.30 FUD 010 J P3
AMA: 2018,Sep,7

21925 deep
10.3 13.1 FUD 090 J A2
AMA: 2018,Sep,7

21930-21936 Excision Soft Tissue Tumors Back or Flank

INCLUDES Any necessary elevation of tissue planes or dissection
Measurement of tumor and necessary margin at greatest diameter prior to excision
Simple and intermediate repairs
Types of excision:
Fascial or subfascial soft tissue tumors: simple and marginal resection of tumors found either in or below the deep fascia, not involving bone or excision of a substantial amount of normal tissue; most often benign and intramuscular tumors
Radical resection soft tissue tumor: wide resection of tumor, involving substantial margins of normal tissue and may include tissue removal from one or more layers; most often malignant or aggressive benign
Subcutaneous: simple and marginal resection of tumors in the subcutaneous tissue above the deep fascia; most often benign

EXCLUDES *Complex repair*
Excision of benign cutaneous lesions (eg, sebaceous cyst) (11400-11406)
Radical resection of cutaneous tumors (eg, melanoma) (11600-11606)
Significant exploration of the vessels or neuroplasty

21930 Excision, tumor, soft tissue of back or flank, subcutaneous; less than 3 cm
10.4 13.8 FUD 090 J G2
AMA: 2018,Sep,7; 2018,Jan,8; 2017,Jan,8; 2016,Jan,13; 2015,Jan,16; 2014,Jan,11

21931 3 cm or greater
13.5 13.5 FUD 090 J G2 80
AMA: 2018,Sep,7

21932 Excision, tumor, soft tissue of back or flank, subfascial (eg, intramuscular); less than 5 cm
19.0 19.0 FUD 090 J G2 80
AMA: 2018,Sep,7

21933 5 cm or greater
21.2 21.2 FUD 090 J G2 80
AMA: 2018,Sep,7

21935 Radical resection of tumor (eg, sarcoma), soft tissue of back or flank; less than 5 cm
29.6 29.6 FUD 090 J G2
AMA: 2018,Sep,7

21936 5 cm or greater
40.9 40.9 FUD 090 J G2 80
AMA: 2018,Sep,7

22010-22015 Incision for Drainage of Deep Spinal Abscess

EXCLUDES *Incision and drainage of hematoma (10060, 10140)*
Injection:
Chemonucleolysis (62292)
Discography (62290-62291)
Facet joint (64490-64495, [64633, 64634, 64635, 64636])
Myelography (62284)
Needle/trocar biopsy (20220-20225)

22010 Incision and drainage, open, of deep abscess (subfascial), posterior spine; cervical, thoracic, or cervicothoracic
27.7 27.7 FUD 090 C 80
AMA: 2018,Sep,7

22015 lumbar, sacral, or lumbosacral

EXCLUDES *Incision and drainage, complex, postoperative wound infection (10180)*
Incision and drainage, open, of deep abscess (subfascial), posterior spine; cervical, thoracic, or cervicothoracic (22010)
Removal of posterior nonsegmental instrumentation (eg, Harrington rod) (22850)
Removal of posterior segmental instrumentation (22852)

27.4 27.4 FUD 090 C
AMA: 2018,Sep,7

22100-22103 Partial Resection Vertebral Component

EXCLUDES *Back or flank biopsy (21920-21925)*
Bone biopsy (20220-20251)
Injection:
Chemonucleolysis (62292)
Discography (62290-62291)
Facet joint (64490-64495, [64633, 64634, 64635, 64636])
Myelography (62284)
Removal of tumor flank or back (21930)
Soft tissue needle biopsy (20206)
Spinal reconstruction with vertebral body prosthesis:
Cervical (20931, 20938, 22554, 63081)
Thoracic (20931, 20938, 22556, 63085, 63087)

22100 Partial excision of posterior vertebral component (eg, spinous process, lamina or facet) for intrinsic bony lesion, single vertebral segment; cervical
24.8 24.8 FUD 090 J 80
AMA: 2018,Sep,7; 2018,Jan,8; 2017,Mar,7; 2017,Jan,8; 2016,Jan,13; 2015,Jan,16

22101 thoracic
24.8 24.8 FUD 090 J 80
AMA: 2018,Sep,7; 2018,Jan,8; 2017,Mar,7; 2017,Jan,8; 2016,Jan,13; 2015,Jan,16

22102 lumbar
Code also posterior spinous process distraction device insertion, if applicable (22867-22870)
23.4 23.4 FUD 090 J G2 80
AMA: 2018,Sep,7; 2018,Jan,8; 2017,Mar,7; 2017,Jan,8; 2016,Jan,13; 2015,Jan,16

+ **22103 each additional segment (List separately in addition to code for primary procedure)**
Code first (22100-22102)
4.10 4.10 FUD ZZZ N N1 80
AMA: 2018,Sep,7

22110-22116 Partial Resection Vertebral Component without Decompression

EXCLUDES *Back or flank biopsy (21920-21925)*
Bone biopsy (20220-20251)
Bone grafting procedures (20930-20938)
Harvest bone graft (20931, 20938)
Injection:
Chemonucleolysis (62292)
Discography (62290-62291)
Facet joint (64490-64495, [64633, 64634, 64635, 64636])
Myelography (62284)
Osteotomy (22210-22226)
Removal of tumor flank or back (21930)
Restoration after vertebral body resection (22585, 63082, 63086, 63088, 63091)
Spinal restoration with graft:
Cervical (20931, 20938, 22554, 63081)
Lumbar (20931, 20938, 22558, 63087, 63090)
Thoracic (20931, 20938, 22556, 63085, 63087)
Spinal restoration with prosthesis:
Cervical (20931, 20938, 22554, 22853-22854 [22859], 63081)
Lumbar (20931, 20938, 22558, 22853-22854 [22859], 63087, 63090)
Thoracic (20931, 20938, 22556, 22853-22854 [22859], 63085, 63087)
Vertebral corpectomy (63081-63091)

22110 Partial excision of vertebral body, for intrinsic bony lesion, without decompression of spinal cord or nerve root(s), single vertebral segment; cervical
30.2 30.2 FUD 090 C 80
AMA: 2018,Sep,7; 2018,Jan,8; 2017,Mar,7; 2017,Jan,8; 2016,Jan,13; 2015,Jan,16

22112 **thoracic**
32.7 32.7 **FUD** 090 C 80
AMA: 2018,Sep,7; 2018,Jan,8; 2017,Mar,7; 2017,Jan,8; 2016,Jan,13; 2015,Jan,16

22114 **lumbar**
32.7 32.7 **FUD** 090 C 80
AMA: 2018,Sep,7; 2018,Jan,8; 2017,Mar,7; 2017,Jan,8; 2016,Jan,13; 2015,Jan,16

\+ **22116** **each additional vertebral segment (List separately in addition to code for primary procedure)**
Code first (22110-22114)
4.12 4.12 **FUD** ZZZ C 80
AMA: 2018,Sep,7

22206-22216 Spinal Osteotomy: Posterior/Posterolateral Approach

EXCLUDES *Decompression of the spinal cord and/or nerve roots (63001-63308)*
Injection:
Chemonucleolysis (62292)
Discography (62290-62292)
Facet joint (64490-64495, [64633, 64634, 64635, 64636])
Myelography (62284)
Repair of vertebral fracture by the anterior approach, see appropriate arthrodesis, bone graft, instrumentation codes, and (63081-63091)

Code also arthrodesis (22590-22632)
Code also bone grafting procedures (20930-20938)
Code also spinal instrumentation (22840-22855 [22859])

22206 **Osteotomy of spine, posterior or posterolateral approach, 3 columns, 1 vertebral segment (eg, pedicle/vertebral body subtraction); thoracic**
EXCLUDES *Osteotomy of spine, posterior or posterolateral approach, lumbar (22207)*
Procedures performed at same level (22210-22226, 22830, 63001-63048, 63055-63066, 63075-63091, 63101-63103)
71.3 71.3 **FUD** 090 C 80
AMA: 2018,Sep,7; 2018,Jan,8; 2017,Mar,7; 2017,Jan,8; 2016,Jan,13; 2015,Jan,16; 2014,Jan,11

22207 **lumbar**
EXCLUDES *Osteotomy of spine, posterior or posterolateral approach, thoracic (22206)*
Procedures performed at the same level (22210-22226, 22830, 63001-63048, 63055-63066, 63075-63091, 63101-63103)
69.8 69.8 **FUD** 090 C 80
AMA: 2018,Sep,7; 2018,Jan,8; 2017,Mar,7; 2017,Jan,8; 2016,Jan,13; 2015,Jan,16; 2014,Jan,11

\+ **22208** **each additional vertebral segment (List separately in addition to code for primary procedure)**
EXCLUDES *Procedures performed at the same level (22210-22226, 22830, 63001-63048, 63055-63066, 63075-63091, 63101-63103)*
Code first (22206, 22207)
17.2 17.2 **FUD** ZZZ C 80
AMA: 2018,Sep,7; 2018,Jan,8; 2017,Jan,8; 2016,Jan,13; 2015,Jan,16; 2014,Jan,11

22210 **Osteotomy of spine, posterior or posterolateral approach, 1 vertebral segment; cervical**
52.0 52.0 **FUD** 090 C 80
AMA: 2018,Sep,7; 2018,Jan,8; 2017,Mar,7; 2017,Jan,8; 2016,Jan,13; 2015,Jan,16

Patient is stabilized by halo and traction to correct cervical problem
Several sections may be removed
C-6
C-7
T-1

Physician removes spinous processes, lamina

22212 **thoracic**
43.2 43.2 **FUD** 090 C 80
AMA: 2018,Sep,7; 2018,Jan,8; 2017,Mar,7; 2017,Jan,8; 2016,Jan,13; 2015,Jan,16; 2014,Jan,11

22214 **lumbar**
43.4 43.4 **FUD** 090 C 80
AMA: 2018,Sep,7; 2018,Jan,8; 2017,Mar,7; 2017,Jan,8; 2016,Jan,13; 2015,Jan,16; 2014,Dec,16; 2014,Dec,16; 2014,Jan,11

\+ **22216** **each additional vertebral segment (List separately in addition to primary procedure)**
Code first (22210-22214)
10.6 10.6 **FUD** ZZZ C 80
AMA: 2018,Sep,7; 2018,Jan,8; 2017,Jan,8; 2016,Jan,13; 2015,Jan,16; 2014,Jan,11

22220-22226 Spinal Osteotomy: Anterior Approach

EXCLUDES *Corpectomy (63081-63091)*
Decompression of the spinal cord and/or nerve roots (63001-63308)
Injection:
Chemonucleolysis (62292)
Discography (62290-62291)
Facet joint (64490-64495, [64633], [64634], [64635], [64636])
Myelography (62284)
Needle/trocar biopsy (20220-20225)
Repair of vertebral fracture by the anterior approach, see appropriate arthrodesis, bone graft, instrumentation codes, and (63081-63091)

Code also arthrodesis (22590-22632)
Code also bone grafting procedures (20930-20938)
Code also spinal instrumentation (22840-22855 [22859])

22220 **Osteotomy of spine, including discectomy, anterior approach, single vertebral segment; cervical**
47.0 47.0 **FUD** 090 C 80
AMA: 2018,Sep,7; 2018,Jan,8; 2017,Mar,7; 2017,Jan,8; 2016,Jan,13; 2015,Jan,16

22222 **thoracic**
51.1 51.1 **FUD** 090 C 80
AMA: 2018,Sep,7; 2018,Jan,8; 2017,Mar,7; 2017,Jan,8; 2016,Jan,13; 2015,Jan,16; 2014,Jan,11

22224 **lumbar**
45.9 45.9 **FUD** 090 C 80
AMA: 2018,Sep,7; 2018,Jan,8; 2017,Mar,7; 2017,Jan,8; 2016,Jan,13; 2015,Jan,16

\+ **22226** **each additional vertebral segment (List separately in addition to code for primary procedure)**
Code first (22220-22224)
10.5 10.5 **FUD** ZZZ C 80
AMA: 2018,Sep,7

22310-22315 Closed Treatment Vertebral Fractures

EXCLUDES *Injection:*

Chemonucleolysis (62292)

Discography (62290-62291)

Facet joint (64490-64495, [64633], [64634], [64635], [64636])

Myelography (62284)

Percutaneous vertebroplasty at same level (22510-22515)

Code also arthrodesis (22590-22632)

Code also bone grafting procedures (20930-20938)

Code also spinal instrumentation (22840-22855 [22859])

22310 **Closed treatment of vertebral body fracture(s), without manipulation, requiring and including casting or bracing**

8.17 8.82 FUD 090 T A2

AMA: 2018,Sep,7; 2018,Jan,8; 2017,Mar,7; 2017,Jan,8; 2016,Jan,13; 2015,Jan,16; 2015,Jan,8; 2014,Jul,8; 2014,Jan,11

22315 **Closed treatment of vertebral fracture(s) and/or dislocation(s) requiring casting or bracing, with and including casting and/or bracing by manipulation or traction**

EXCLUDES *Spinal manipulation (97140)*

22.2 25.3 FUD 090 J A2

AMA: 2018,Sep,7; 2018,Jan,8; 2017,Mar,7; 2017,Jan,8; 2016,Jan,13; 2015,Jan,8; 2015,Jan,16; 2014,Jan,11

22318-22319 Open Treatment Odontoid Fracture: Anterior Approach

EXCLUDES *Injection:*

Chemonucleolysis (62292)

Discography (62290-62291)

Facet joint (64490-64495, [64633, 64634, 64635, 64636])

Myelography (62284)

Needle/trocar biopsy (20220-20225)

Code also arthrodesis (22590-22632)

Code also bone grafting procedures (20930-20938)

Code also spinal instrumentation (22840-22855 [22859])

22318 **Open treatment and/or reduction of odontoid fracture(s) and or dislocation(s) (including os odontoideum), anterior approach, including placement of internal fixation; without grafting**

47.6 47.6 FUD 090 C 80

AMA: 2018,Sep,7; 2018,Jan,8; 2017,Mar,7; 2017,Jan,8; 2016,Jan,13; 2015,Jan,16; 2014,Jan,11

22319 **with grafting**

53.6 53.6 FUD 090 C 80

AMA: 2018,Sep,7; 2018,May,3; 2018,Jan,8; 2017,Mar,7; 2017,Jan,8; 2016,Jan,13; 2015,Jan,16; 2014,Jan,11

22325-22328 Open Treatment Vertebral Fractures: Posterior Approach

EXCLUDES *Corpectomy (63081-63091)*

Injection:

Chemonucleolysis (62292)

Discography (62290-62291)

Facet joint (64490-64495, [64633], [64634], [64635], [64636])

Myelography (62284)

Needle/trocar biopsy (20220-20225)

Spine decompression (63001-63091)

Vertebral fracture care by arthrodesis (22548-22632)

Vertebral fracture care frontal approach (63081-63091)

Code also arthrodesis (22548-22632)

Code also bone grafting procedures (20930-20938)

Code also spinal instrumentation (22840-22855 [22859])

22325 **Open treatment and/or reduction of vertebral fracture(s) and/or dislocation(s), posterior approach, 1 fractured vertebra or dislocated segment; lumbar**

EXCLUDES *Percutaneous vertebral augmentation performed at same level (22514-22515)*

Percutaneous vertebroplasty performed at same level (22511-22512)

41.9 41.9 FUD 090 C 80

AMA: 2018,Sep,7; 2018,Jan,8; 2017,Aug,9; 2017,Mar,7; 2017,Jan,8; 2016,Jan,13; 2015,Jan,16; 2015,Jan,8; 2014,Jan,11

22326 **cervical**

EXCLUDES *Percutaneous vertebroplasty performed at same level (22510, 22512)*

43.4 43.4 FUD 090 C 80

AMA: 2018,Sep,7; 2018,Jan,8; 2017,Mar,7; 2017,Jan,8; 2016,Jan,13; 2015,Jan,16; 2014,Jan,11

22327 **thoracic**

EXCLUDES *Percutaneous vertebral augmentation performed at same level (22515)*

Percutaneous vertebroplasty performed at same level (22510, 22512-22513)

43.8 43.8 FUD 090 C 80

AMA: 2018,Sep,7; 2018,Jan,8; 2017,Mar,7; 2017,Jan,8; 2016,Jan,13; 2015,Jan,8; 2015,Jan,16; 2014,Jan,11

\+ **22328** **each additional fractured vertebra or dislocated segment (List separately in addition to code for primary procedure)**

Code first (22325-22327)

8.25 8.25 FUD ZZZ C 80

AMA: 2018,Sep,7

22505 Spinal Manipulation with Anesthesia

EXCLUDES *Manipulation not requiring anesthesia (97140)*

22505 **Manipulation of spine requiring anesthesia, any region**

3.79 3.79 FUD 010 J A2

AMA: 2018,Sep,7; 2018,Jan,8; 2017,Jan,8; 2016,Jan,13; 2015,Jan,16; 2014,Jan,11

22510-22515 Percutaneous Vertebroplasty/Kyphoplasty

INCLUDES Bone biopsy when applicable (20225)

Radiological guidance

EXCLUDES *Closed treatment vertebral fractures (22310, 22315)*

Open treatment/reduction vertebral fractures (22325, 22327)

Sacroplasty/augmentation (0200T-0201T)

22510 **Percutaneous vertebroplasty (bone biopsy included when performed), 1 vertebral body, unilateral or bilateral injection, inclusive of all imaging guidance; cervicothoracic**

12.5 49.8 FUD 010 J G2

AMA: 2018,Sep,7; 2018,Jan,8; 2017,Jan,8; 2016,Jan,13; 2015,Jan,8

22511 **lumbosacral**

11.7 49.3 FUD 010 J G2

AMA: 2018,Sep,7; 2018,Jan,8; 2017,Jan,8; 2016,Jan,13; 2015,Apr,8; 2015,Jan,8

\+ **22512** **each additional cervicothoracic or lumbosacral vertebral body (List separately in addition to code for primary procedure)**

Code first (22510-22511)

5.99 25.6 FUD ZZZ N N1

AMA: 2018,Sep,7; 2018,Jan,8; 2017,Jan,8; 2016,Jan,13; 2015,Jan,8

22513 **Percutaneous vertebral augmentation, including cavity creation (fracture reduction and bone biopsy included when performed) using mechanical device (eg, kyphoplasty), 1 vertebral body, unilateral or bilateral cannulation, inclusive of all imaging guidance; thoracic**

14.9 195. FUD 010 J G2

AMA: 2018,Sep,7; 2018,Jan,8; 2017,Jan,8; 2016,Jan,13; 2015,Jan,8

22514 **lumbar**

13.9 194. FUD 010 J G2

AMA: 2018,Sep,7; 2018,Jan,8; 2017,Jan,8; 2016,Jan,13; 2015,Jan,8

\+ **22515** **each additional thoracic or lumbar vertebral body (List separately in addition to code for primary procedure)**

Code first (22513-22514)

6.46 113. FUD ZZZ N N1

AMA: 2018,Sep,7; 2018,Jan,8; 2017,Jan,8; 2016,Jan,13; 2015,Jan,8

22526-22527 Percutaneous Annuloplasty

CMS: 100-04,32,220.1 Thermal Intradiscal Procedures (TIPS)

INCLUDES Fluoroscopic guidance (77002, 77003)

EXCLUDES *Needle/trocar biopsy (20220-20225)*
Injection:
Chemonucleolysis (62292)
Discography (62290-62291)
Facet joint (64490-64495, [64633], [64634], [64635], [64636])
Myelography (62284)
Procedure performed by other methods (22899)

22526 **Percutaneous intradiscal electrothermal annuloplasty, unilateral or bilateral including fluoroscopic guidance; single level**

9.76 | 65.0 | **FUD** 010 | E

AMA: 2018,Sep,7; 2018,Jan,8; 2017,Jan,8; 2016,Jan,13; 2015,Jan,8; 2015,Jan,16; 2014,Jan,11

\+ **22527** **1 or more additional levels (List separately in addition to code for primary procedure)**

Code first (22526)

4.61 | 54.6 | **FUD** ZZZ | E

AMA: 2018,Sep,7; 2018,Jan,8; 2017,Jan,8; 2016,Jan,13; 2015,Jan,8; 2015,Jan,16; 2014,Jan,11

22532-22534 Spinal Fusion: Lateral Extracavitary Approach

EXCLUDES *Corpectomy (63101-63103)*
Exploration of spinal fusion (22830)
Fracture care (22310-22328)
Injection:
Chemonucleolysis (62292)
Discography (62290-62291)
Facet joint (64490-64495, [64633], [64634], [64635], [64636])
Myelography (62284)
Laminectomy (63001-63017)
Needle/trocar biopsy (20220-20225)
Osteotomy (22206-22226)

Code also bone grafting procedures (20930-20938)
Code also spinal instrumentation (22840-22855 [22859])

22532 **Arthrodesis, lateral extracavitary technique, including minimal discectomy to prepare interspace (other than for decompression); thoracic**

52.4 | 52.4 | **FUD** 090 | C 80

AMA: 2018,Sep,7; 2018,May,3; 2018,Jan,8; 2017,Mar,7; 2017,Feb,9; 2017,Jan,8; 2016,Jan,13; 2015,Jan,16; 2014,Jan,11

22533 **lumbar**

48.1 | 48.1 | **FUD** 090 | C 80

AMA: 2018,Sep,7; 2018,May,3; 2018,Jan,8; 2017,Mar,7; 2017,Feb,9; 2017,Jan,8; 2016,Jan,13; 2015,Jan,16; 2014,Jan,11

\+ **22534** **thoracic or lumbar, each additional vertebral segment (List separately in addition to code for primary procedure)**

Code first (22532-22533)

10.5 | 10.5 | **FUD** ZZZ | C 80

AMA: 2018,Sep,7; 2018,May,3; 2017,Feb,9

22548-22634 Spinal Fusion: Anterior and Posterior Approach

EXCLUDES *Corpectomy (63081-63091)*
Exploration of spinal fusion (22830)
Fracture care (22310-22328)
Facet joint arthrodesis (0219T-0222T)
Injection:
Chemonucleolysis (62292)
Discography (62290-62291)
Facet joint (64490-64495, [64633], [64634], [64635], [64636])
Myelography (62284)
Laminectomy (63001-63017)
Needle/trocar biopsy (20220-20225)
Osteotomy (22206-22226)

Code also bone grafting procedures (20930-20938)
Code also spinal instrumentation (22840-22855 [22859])

22548 **Arthrodesis, anterior transoral or extraoral technique, clivus-C1-C2 (atlas-axis), with or without excision of odontoid process**

EXCLUDES *Laminectomy or laminotomy with disc removal (63020-63042)*

57.5 | 57.5 | **FUD** 090 | C 80

AMA: 2018,Sep,7; 2018,May,3; 2018,Jan,8; 2017,Mar,7; 2017,Jan,8; 2016,Jan,13; 2015,Jan,16; 2014,Jan,11

22551 **Arthrodesis, anterior interbody, including disc space preparation, discectomy, osteophytectomy and decompression of spinal cord and/or nerve roots; cervical below C2**

INCLUDES Operating microscope (69990)

49.6 | 49.6 | **FUD** 090 | J J8 80

AMA: 2018,Sep,7; 2018,Aug,10; 2018,May,3; 2018,Jan,8; 2017,Mar,7; 2017,Jan,8; 2016,May,13; 2016,Feb,12; 2016,Jan,13; 2015,Jan,13; 2015,Jan,16; 2014,Jan,11

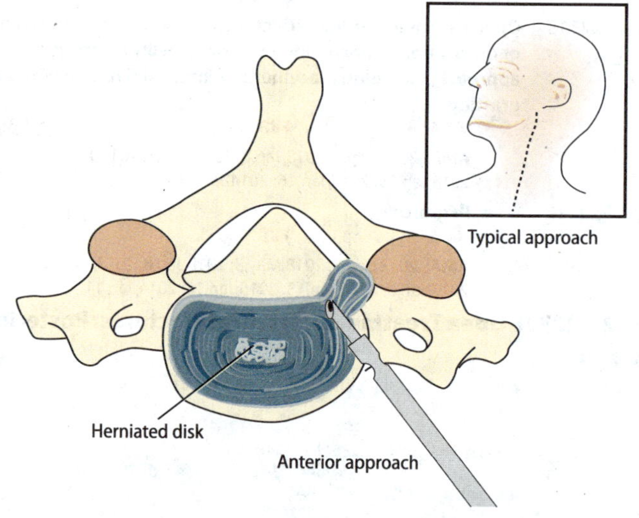

\+ **22552** **cervical below C2, each additional interspace (List separately in addition to code for separate procedure)**

INCLUDES Operating microscope (69990)

Code first (22551)

11.6 | 11.6 | **FUD** ZZZ | N N1 80

AMA: 2018,Sep,7; 2018,Aug,10; 2018,May,3; 2018,Jan,8; 2017,Mar,7; 2017,Jan,8; 2016,Feb,12; 2016,Jan,13; 2015,Jan,16; 2014,Jan,11

22554 **Arthrodesis, anterior interbody technique, including minimal discectomy to prepare interspace (other than for decompression); cervical below C2**

EXCLUDES *Anterior discectomy and interbody fusion during the same operative session (regardless if performed by multiple surgeons) (22551)*

Discectomy, anterior, with decompression of spinal cord and/or nerve root(s), cervical (even by separate individual) (63075-63076)

36.4 36.4 **FUD** 090 J J8 80

AMA: 2018,Sep,7; 2018,May,3; 2018,Jan,8; 2017,Mar,7; 2017,Jan,8; 2016,Jan,13; 2015,Apr,7; 2015,Jan,16; 2014,Jan,11

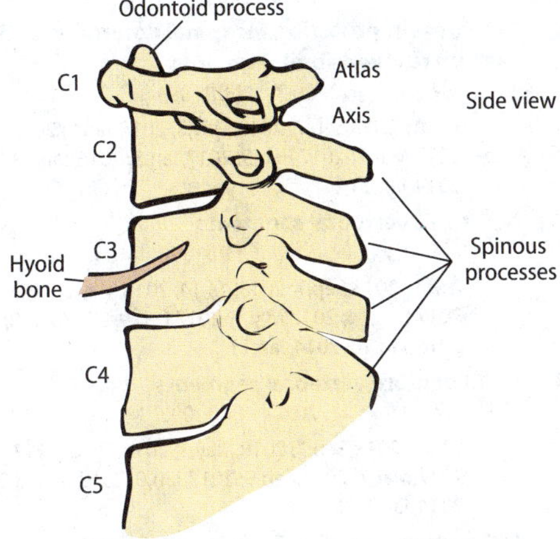

22556 **thoracic**

48.5 48.5 **FUD** 090 C 80

AMA: 2018,Sep,7; 2018,May,3; 2018,Jan,8; 2017,Mar,7; 2017,Jan,8; 2016,Jan,13; 2015,Jan,16; 2014,Jan,11

22558 **lumbar**

EXCLUDES *Arthrodesis using pre-sacral interbody technique (22586)*

44.4 44.4 **FUD** 090 C 80

AMA: 2018,Sep,7; 2018,May,3; 2018,Jan,8; 2017,Mar,7; 2017,Feb,9; 2017,Jan,8; 2016,Jan,13; 2015,Mar,9; 2015,Jan,16; 2014,Jan,11

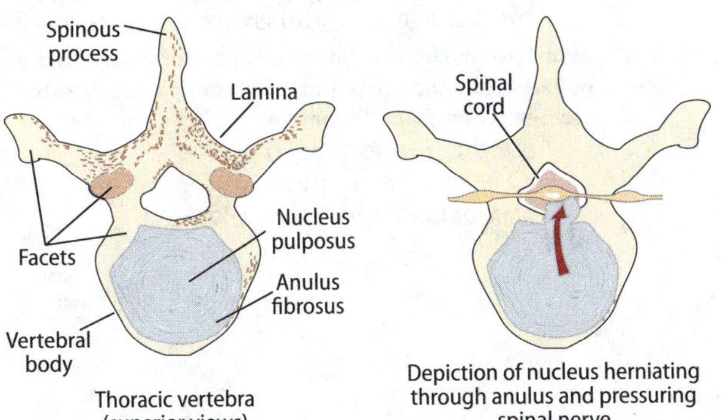

Thoracic vertebra (superior views)

Depiction of nucleus herniating through anulus and pressuring spinal nerve

\+ **22585** **each additional interspace (List separately in addition to code for primary procedure)**

EXCLUDES *Anterior discectomy and interbody fusion during the same operative session (regardless if performed by multiple surgeons) (22552)*

Discectomy, anterior, with decompression of spinal cord and/or nerve root(s), cervical (even by separate individual) (63075)

Code first (22554-22558)

9.55 9.55 **FUD** ZZZ N N1 80

AMA: 2018,Sep,7; 2018,Jan,8; 2017,Jan,8; 2016,Jan,13; 2015,Jan,16; 2014,Jan,11

22586 **Arthrodesis, pre-sacral interbody technique, including disc space preparation, discectomy, with posterior instrumentation, with image guidance, includes bone graft when performed, L5-S1 interspace**

INCLUDES Radiologic guidance (77002-77003, 77011-77012)

EXCLUDES *Allograft and autograft of spinal bone (20930-20938)*

Epidurography, radiological supervision and interpretation (72275)

Pelvic fixation, other than sacrum (22848)

Posterior non-segmental instrumentation (22840)

59.6 59.6 **FUD** 090 C 80

AMA: 2018,Sep,7

22590 **Arthrodesis, posterior technique, craniocervical (occiput-C2)**

EXCLUDES *Posterior intrafacet implant insertion (0219T-0222T)*

45.9 45.9 **FUD** 090 C 80

AMA: 2018,Sep,7; 2018,May,3; 2018,Jan,8; 2017,Mar,7; 2017,Jan,8; 2016,Jan,13; 2015,Jan,16; 2014,Jan,11

Skull and cervical vertebrae; posterior view

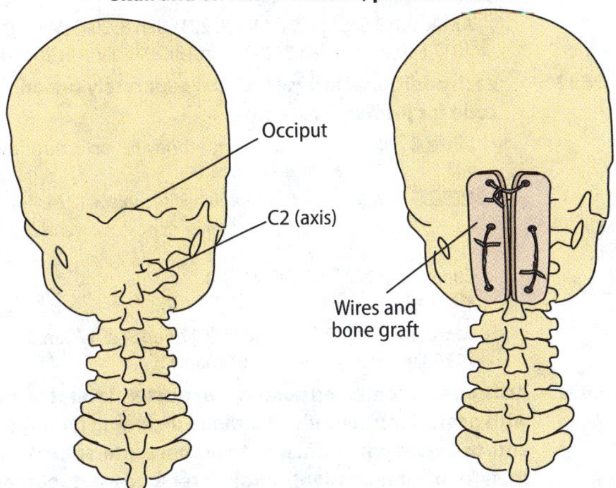

The physician fuses skull to C2 (axis) to stabilize cervical vertebrae; anchor holes are drilled in the occiput of the skull

22595 **Arthrodesis, posterior technique, atlas-axis (C1-C2)**

EXCLUDES *Posterior intrafacet implant insertion (0219T-0222T)*

43.8 43.8 **FUD** 090 C 80

AMA: 2018,Sep,7; 2018,May,3; 2018,Jan,8; 2017,Mar,7; 2017,Jan,8; 2016,Jan,13; 2015,Jan,16; 2014,Jan,11

22600 **Arthrodesis, posterior or posterolateral technique, single level; cervical below C2 segment**

EXCLUDES *Posterior intrafacet implant insertion (0219T-0222T)*

37.4 37.4 **FUD** 090 C 80

AMA: 2018,Sep,7; 2018,May,3; 2018,Jan,8; 2017,Mar,7; 2017,Jan,8; 2016,Jan,13; 2015,Jan,16; 2014,Jan,11

22610 **thoracic (with lateral transverse technique, when performed)**

EXCLUDES *Posterior intrafacet implant insertion (0219T-0222T)*

36.7 36.7 **FUD** 090 C 80

AMA: 2018,Sep,7; 2018,May,3; 2018,Jan,8; 2017,Mar,7; 2017,Jan,8; 2016,Jan,13; 2015,Jan,16; 2014,Jan,11

22612 **lumbar (with lateral transverse technique, when performed)**

EXCLUDES *Arthrodesis performed at same interspace and segment (22630)*

Combined technique at the same interspace and segment (22633)

Posterior intrafacet implant insertion (0219T-0222T)

46.0 46.0 **FUD** 090 J G2 80

AMA: 2018,Sep,7; 2018,May,3; 2018,Jan,8; 2017,Mar,7; 2017,Feb,9; 2017,Jan,8; 2016,Jan,13; 2015,Jan,16; 2014,Jan,11

+ **22614** **each additional vertebral segment (List separately in addition to code for primary procedure)**

INCLUDES Additional level fusion arthrodesis posterior or posterolateral interbody

EXCLUDES *Additional level interbody arthrodesis combined posterolateral or posterior with posterior interbody arthrodesis (22634)*

Additional level posterior interbody arthrodesis (22632)

Posterior intrafacet implant insertion (0219T-0222T)

Code first (22600, 22610, 22612, 22630, 22633)

11.4 11.4 **FUD** ZZZ N N1 80

AMA: 2018,Sep,7; 2018,Jan,8; 2017,Feb,9; 2017,Jan,8; 2016,Jan,13; 2015,Jan,16; 2014,Jan,11

22630 **Arthrodesis, posterior interbody technique, including laminectomy and/or discectomy to prepare interspace (other than for decompression), single interspace; lumbar**

EXCLUDES *Arthrodesis performed at same interspace and segment (22612)*

Combined technique (22612 and 22630) for same interspace and segment (22633)

45.8 45.8 **FUD** 090 C 80

AMA: 2018,Sep,7; 2018,May,3; 2018,Jan,8; 2017,Mar,7; 2017,Feb,9; 2017,Jan,8; 2016,Jan,13; 2015,Jan,16; 2014,Jan,11

+ **22632** **each additional interspace (List separately in addition to code for primary procedure)**

INCLUDES Includes posterior interbody fusion arthrodesis, additional level

EXCLUDES *Additional level combined technique (22634)*

Additional level posterior or posterolateral fusion (22614)

Code first (22612, 22630, 22633)

9.40 9.40 **FUD** ZZZ C 80

AMA: 2018,Sep,7; 2018,Jan,8; 2017,Feb,9; 2017,Jan,8; 2016,Jan,13; 2015,Jan,16; 2014,Jan,11

22633 **Arthrodesis, combined posterior or posterolateral technique with posterior interbody technique including laminectomy and/or discectomy sufficient to prepare interspace (other than for decompression), single interspace and segment; lumbar**

EXCLUDES *Arthrodesis performed at same interspace and segment (22612, 22630)*

53.8 53.8 **FUD** 090 C 80

AMA: 2018,Sep,7; 2018,Jul,14; 2018,May,9; 2018,May,3; 2018,Jan,8; 2017,Mar,7; 2017,Feb,9; 2017,Jan,8; 2016,Oct,11; 2016,Jan,13; 2015,Jan,16; 2014,Jan,11

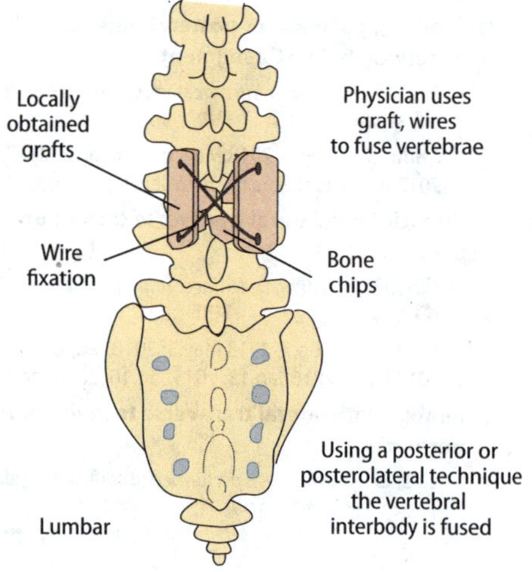

+ **22634** **each additional interspace and segment (List separately in addition to code for primary procedure)**

Code first (22633)

14.4 14.4 **FUD** ZZZ C 80

AMA: 2018,Sep,7; 2018,Jul,14; 2018,May,3; 2018,Jan,8; 2017,Mar,7; 2017,Feb,9; 2017,Jan,8; 2016,Jan,13; 2015,Jan,16; 2014,Jan,11

22800-22819 Procedures to Correct Anomalous Spinal Vertebrae

CMS: 100-03,150.2 Osteogenic Stimulation

EXCLUDES *Facet injection (64490-64495, [64633, 64634, 64635, 64636])*

Code also bone grafting procedures (20930-20938)

Code also spinal instrumentation (22840-22855 [22859])

22800 **Arthrodesis, posterior, for spinal deformity, with or without cast; up to 6 vertebral segments**

39.3 39.3 **FUD** 090 C 80

AMA: 2018,Sep,7; 2018,May,3; 2018,Jan,8; 2017,Sep,14; 2017,Mar,7; 2017,Feb,9; 2017,Jan,8; 2016,Jan,13; 2015,Jan,16; 2014,Jan,11

22802 **7 to 12 vertebral segments**

61.1 61.1 **FUD** 090 C 80

AMA: 2018,Sep,7; 2018,Jul,14; 2018,May,3; 2018,Jan,8; 2017,Sep,14; 2017,Mar,7; 2017,Feb,9; 2017,Jan,8; 2016,Jan,13; 2015,Jan,16; 2014,Jan,11

22804 **13 or more vertebral segments**

70.6 70.6 **FUD** 090 C 80

AMA: 2018,Sep,7; 2018,May,3; 2018,Jan,8; 2017,Sep,14; 2017,Mar,7; 2017,Feb,9; 2017,Jan,8; 2016,Jan,13; 2015,Jan,16; 2014,Jan,11

22808 **Arthrodesis, anterior, for spinal deformity, with or without cast; 2 to 3 vertebral segments**

INCLUDES Smith-Robinson arthrodesis

53.7 53.7 **FUD** 090 C 80

AMA: 2018,Sep,7; 2018,May,3; 2018,Jan,8; 2017,Sep,14; 2017,Mar,7; 2017,Jan,8; 2016,Jan,13; 2015,Jan,16; 2014,Jan,11

22810 **4 to 7 vertebral segments**

60.2 60.2 **FUD** 090 C 80

AMA: 2018,Sep,7; 2018,May,3; 2018,Jan,8; 2017,Sep,14; 2017,Mar,7; 2017,Jan,8; 2016,Jan,13; 2015,Jan,16; 2014,Jan,11

22812 **8 or more vertebral segments**

64.0 64.0 **FUD** 090 C 80

AMA: 2018,Sep,7; 2018,May,3; 2018,Jan,8; 2017,Sep,14; 2017,Mar,7; 2017,Jan,8; 2016,Jan,13; 2015,Jan,16; 2014,Jan,11

22818 **Kyphectomy, circumferential exposure of spine and resection of vertebral segment(s) (including body and posterior elements); single or 2 segments**

EXCLUDES *Arthrodesis (22800-22804)*

62.8 62.8 **FUD** 090 C 80

AMA: 2018,Sep,7; 2018,Jan,8; 2017,Sep,14

22819 **3 or more segments**

EXCLUDES *Arthrodesis (22800-22804)*

72.2 72.2 **FUD** 090 C 80

AMA: 2018,Sep,7; 2018,Jan,8; 2017,Sep,14

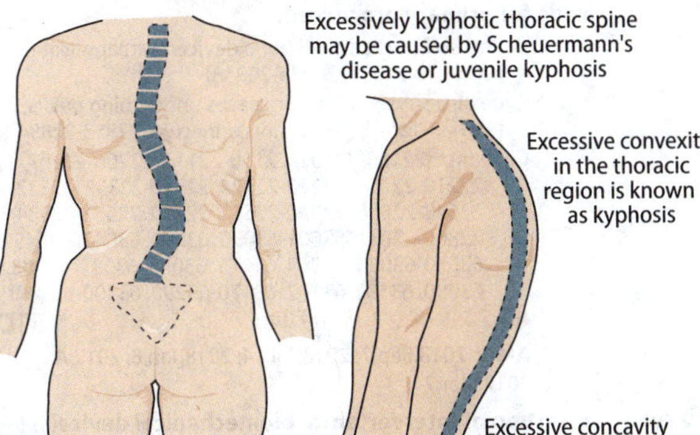

22830 Surgical Exploration Previous Spinal Fusion

CMS: 100-03,150.2 Osteogenic Stimulation

EXCLUDES *Arthrodesis (22532-22819)*
Bone grafting procedures (20930-20938)
Facet injection (64490-64495, [64633, 64634, 64635, 64636])
Instrumentation removal (22850, 22852, 22855)
Spinal decompression (63001-63103)

Code also spinal instrumentation (22840-22855 [22859])

22830 **Exploration of spinal fusion**

23.6 23.6 **FUD** 090 C 80

AMA: 2018,Sep,7; 2018,Jan,8; 2017,Jan,8; 2016,Jan,13; 2015,Jan,16; 2014,Jan,11

22840-22848 Posterior, Anterior, Pelvic Spinal Instrumentation

INCLUDES Removal or revision of previously placed spinal instrumentation during same session as insertion of new instrumentation at levels including all or part of previously instrumented segments (22849, 22850, 22852, 22855)

EXCLUDES *Arthrodesis (22532-22534, 22548-22812)*
Bone grafting procedures (20930-20938)
Exploration of spinal fusion (22830)
Fracture treatment (22325-22328)
Use of more than one instrumentation code per incision

\+ **22840** **Posterior non-segmental instrumentation (eg, Harrington rod technique, pedicle fixation across 1 interspace, atlantoaxial transarticular screw fixation, sublaminar wiring at C1, facet screw fixation) (List separately in addition to code for primary procedure)**

Code first (22100-22102, 22110-22114, 22206-22207, 22210-22214, 22220-22224, 22310-22327, 22532-22533, 22548-22558, 22590-22612, 22630, 22633-22634, 22800-22812, 63001-63030, 63040-63042, 63045-63047, 63050-63056, 63064, 63075, 63077, 63081, 63085, 63087, 63090, 63101-63102, 63170-63290, 63300-63307)

22.2 22.2 **FUD** ZZZ N N1 80

AMA: 2018,Sep,7; 2018,Jan,8; 2017,Jun,10; 2017,Feb,9; 2017,Jan,8; 2016,Jan,13; 2015,Jan,16; 2014,Oct,14; 2014,Jan,11

\+ **22841** **Internal spinal fixation by wiring of spinous processes (List separately in addition to code for primary procedure)**

Code first (22100-22102, 22110-22114, 22206-22207, 22210-22214, 22220-22224, 22310-22327, 22532-22533, 22548-22558, 22590-22612, 22630, 22633-22634, 22800-22812, 63001-63030, 63040-63042, 63045-63047, 63050-63056, 63064, 63075, 63077, 63081, 63085, 63087, 63090, 63101-63102, 63170-63290, 63300-63307)

0.00 0.00 **FUD** XXX C

AMA: 2018,Sep,7; 2018,Jan,8; 2017,Feb,9; 2017,Jan,8; 2016,Jan,13; 2015,Jan,16; 2014,Jan,11

\+ **22842** **Posterior segmental instrumentation (eg, pedicle fixation, dual rods with multiple hooks and sublaminar wires); 3 to 6 vertebral segments (List separately in addition to code for primary procedure)**

Code first (22100-22102, 22110-22114, 22206-22207, 22210-22214, 22220-22224, 22310-22327, 22532-22533, 22548-22558, 22590-22612, 22630, 22633-22634, 22800-22812, 63001-63030, 63040-63042, 63045-63047, 63050-63056, 63064, 63075, 63077, 63081, 63085, 63087, 63090, 63101-63102, 63170-63290, 63300-63307)

22.3 22.3 **FUD** ZZZ N N1 80

AMA: 2018,Sep,7; 2018,Jan,8; 2017,Feb,9; 2017,Jan,8; 2016,Jan,13; 2015,Jan,16; 2014,Jan,11

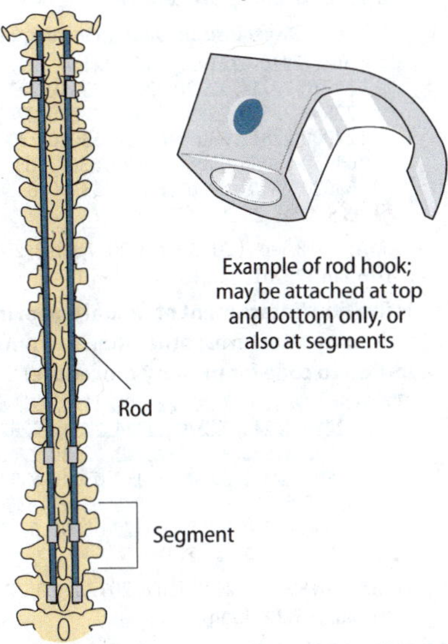

\+ **22843** **7 to 12 vertebral segments (List separately in addition to code for primary procedure)**

Code first (22100-22102, 22110-22114, 22206-22207, 22210-22214, 22220-22224, 22310-22327, 22532-22533, 22548-22558, 22590-22612, 22630, 22633-22634, 22800-22812, 63001-63030, 63040-63042, 63045-63047, 63050-63056, 63064, 63075, 63077, 63081, 63085, 63087, 63090, 63101-63102, 63170-63290, 63300-63307)

23.8 23.8 **FUD** ZZZ C 80

AMA: 2018,Sep,7; 2018,Jul,14; 2018,Jan,8; 2017,Jan,8; 2016,Jan,13; 2015,Jan,16; 2014,Jan,11

\+ **22844** **13 or more vertebral segments (List separately in addition to code for primary procedure)**

Code first (22100-22102, 22110-22114, 22206-22207, 22210-22214, 22220-22224, 22310-22327, 22532-22533, 22548-22558, 22590-22612, 22630, 22633-22634, 22800-22812, 63001-63030, 63040-63042, 63045-63047, 63050-63056, 63064, 63075, 63077, 63081, 63085, 63087, 63090, 63101-63102, 63170-63290, 63300-63307)

28.8 28.8 **FUD** ZZZ C 80

AMA: 2018,Sep,7; 2018,Jan,8; 2017,Jan,8; 2016,Jan,13; 2015,Jan,16; 2014,Jan,11

\+ **22845** **Anterior instrumentation; 2 to 3 vertebral segments (List separately in addition to code for primary procedure)**

INCLUDES Dwyer instrumentation technique

Code first (22100-22102, 22110-22114, 22206-22207, 22210-22214, 22220-22224, 22310-22327, 22532-22533, 22548-22558, 22590-22612, 22630, 22633-22634, 22800-22812, 63001-63030, 63040-63042, 63045-63047, 63050-63056, 63064, 63075, 63077, 63081, 63085, 63087, 63090, 63101-63102, 63170-63290, 63300-63307)

21.3 21.3 **FUD** ZZZ N N1 80

AMA: 2018,Sep,7; 2018,Jan,8; 2017,Mar,7; 2017,Jan,8; 2016,May,13; 2016,Jan,13; 2015,Apr,7; 2015,Mar,9; 2015,Jan,16; 2015,Jan,13; 2014,Nov,14; 2014,Jan,11

\+ **22846** **4 to 7 vertebral segments (List separately in addition to code for primary procedure)**

INCLUDES Dwyer instrumentation technique

Code first (22100-22102, 22110-22114, 22206-22207, 22210-22214, 22220-22224, 22310-22327, 22532-22533, 22548-22558, 22590-22612, 22630, 22633-22634, 22800-22812, 63001-63030, 63040-63042, 63045-63047, 63050-63056, 63064, 63075, 63077, 63081, 63085, 63087, 63090, 63101-63102, 63170-63290, 63300-63307)

22.1 22.1 FUD ZZZ C 80

AMA: 2018,Sep,7; 2018,Jan,8; 2017,Jan,8; 2016,May,13; 2016,Jan,13; 2015,Jan,16; 2014,Jan,11

\+ **22847** **8 or more vertebral segments (List separately in addition to code for primary procedure)**

INCLUDES Dwyer instrumentation technique

Code first (22100-22102, 22110-22114, 22206-22207, 22210-22214, 22220-22224, 22310-22327, 22532-22533, 22548-22558, 22590-22612, 22630, 22633-22634, 22800-22812, 63001-63030, 63040-63042, 63045-63047, 63050-63056, 63064, 63075, 63077, 63081, 63085, 63087, 63090, 63101-63102, 63170-63290, 63300-63307)

23.5 23.5 FUD ZZZ C 80

AMA: 2018,Sep,7; 2018,Jan,8; 2017,Jan,8; 2016,May,13; 2016,Jan,13; 2015,Jan,16; 2014,Jan,11

\+ **22848** **Pelvic fixation (attachment of caudal end of instrumentation to pelvic bony structures) other than sacrum (List separately in addition to code for primary procedure)**

Code first (22100-22102, 22110-22114, 22206-22207, 22210-22214, 22220-22224, 22310-22327, 22532-22533, 22548-22558, 22590-22612, 22630, 22633-22634, 22800-22812, 63001-63030, 63040-63042, 63045-63047, 63050-63056, 63064, 63075, 63077, 63081, 63085, 63087, 63090, 63101-63102, 63170-63290, 63300-63307)

10.5 10.5 FUD ZZZ C 80

AMA: 2018,Sep,7; 2018,Jan,8; 2017,Jan,8; 2016,Jan,13; 2015,Jan,16; 2014,Jan,11

22849-22855 [22859] Miscellaneous Spinal Instrumentation

EXCLUDES *Arthrodesis (22532-22534, 22548-22812)*
Bone grafting procedures (20930-20938)
Exploration of spinal fusion (22830)
Facet injection (64490-64495, [64633], [64634], [64635], [64636])
Fracture treatment (22325-22328)

22849 **Reinsertion of spinal fixation device**

INCLUDES Removal of instrumentation at the same level (22850, 22852, 22855)

37.7 37.7 FUD 090 C 80

AMA: 2018,Sep,7; 2018,Jan,8; 2017,Jun,10; 2017,Jan,8; 2016,May,13; 2016,Jan,13; 2015,Jan,16; 2014,Jan,11

22850 **Removal of posterior nonsegmental instrumentation (eg, Harrington rod)**

21.0 21.0 FUD 090 C 80

AMA: 2018,Sep,7; 2018,Jan,8; 2017,Jun,10; 2017,Jan,8; 2016,May,13; 2016,Jan,13; 2015,Jan,16; 2014,Jan,11

22852 **Removal of posterior segmental instrumentation**

20.2 20.2 FUD 090 C 80

AMA: 2018,Sep,7; 2018,Jan,8; 2017,Jun,10; 2017,Jan,8; 2016,Jan,13; 2015,Jan,16; 2014,Jan,11

\+ **22853** **Insertion of interbody biomechanical device(s) (eg, synthetic cage, mesh) with integral anterior instrumentation for device anchoring (eg, screws, flanges), when performed, to intervertebral disc space in conjunction with interbody arthrodesis, each interspace (List separately in addition to code for primary procedure)**

Code also intervertebral bone device/graft application (20930-20931, 20936-20938)

Code also subsequent disc spaces undergoing device insertion when disc spaces are not connected (22853-22854, [22859])

Code first (22100-22102, 22110-22114, 22206-22207, 22210-22214, 22220-22224, 22310-22327, 22532-22533, 22548-22558, 22590-22612, 22630, 22633-22634, 22800-22812, 63001-63030, 63040, 63042, 63045-63047, 63050-63056, 63064, 63075, 63077, 63081, 63085, 63087, 63090, 63101-63102, 63170-63290, 63300-63307)

7.55 7.55 FUD ZZZ N N1 80

AMA: 2018,Sep,7; 2018,Jul,14; 2018,Jan,8; 2017,Aug,9; 2017,Mar,7

\+ **22854** **Insertion of intervertebral biomechanical device(s) (eg, synthetic cage, mesh) with integral anterior instrumentation for device anchoring (eg, screws, flanges), when performed, to vertebral corpectomy(ies) (vertebral body resection, partial or complete) defect, in conjunction with interbody arthrodesis, each contiguous defect (List separately in addition to code for primary procedure)**

Code also intervertebral bone device/graft application (20930-20931, 20936-20938)

Code also subsequent disc spaces undergoing device insertion when disc spaces are not connected (22853-22854, [22859])

Code first (22100-22102, 22110-22114, 22206-22207, 22210-22214, 22220-22224, 22310-22327, 22532-22533, 22548-22558, 22590-22612, 22630, 22633-22634, 22800-22812, 63001-63030, 63040, 63042, 63045-63047, 63050-63056, 63064, 63075, 63077, 63081, 63085, 63087, 63090, 63101-63102, 63170-63290, 63300-63307)

9.78 9.78 FUD ZZZ N N1 80

AMA: 2018,Sep,7; 2018,Jan,8; 2017,Mar,7

\+ # **22859** **Insertion of intervertebral biomechanical device(s) (eg, synthetic cage, mesh, methylmethacrylate) to intervertebral disc space or vertebral body defect without interbody arthrodesis, each contiguous defect (List separately in addition to code for primary procedure)**

Code also intervertebral bone device/graft application (20930-20931, 20936-20938)

Code also subsequent disc spaces undergoing device insertion when disc spaces are not connected (22853-22854, 22854)

Code first (22100-22102, 22110-22114, 22206-22207, 22210-22214, 22220-22224, 22310-22327, 22532-22533, 22548-22558, 22590-22612, 22630, 22633-22634, 22800-22812, 63001-63030, 63040-63042, 63045-63047, 63050-63056, 63064, 63075, 63077, 63081, 63085, 63087, 63090, 63101-63102, 63170-63290, 63300-63307)

9.78 9.78 FUD ZZZ N N1 80

AMA: 2018,Sep,7; 2018,Jan,8; 2017,Mar,7

22855 **Removal of anterior instrumentation**

32.1 32.1 FUD 090 C 80

AMA: 2018,Sep,7; 2018,Jan,8; 2017,Jun,10; 2017,Jan,8; 2016,Jan,13; 2015,Jan,16; 2014,Jan,11

22856-22865 [22858] Artificial Disc Replacement

EXCLUDES *Fluoroscopy*
Spinal decompression (63001-63048)

22856 **Total disc arthroplasty (artificial disc), anterior approach, including discectomy with end plate preparation (includes osteophytectomy for nerve root or spinal cord decompression and microdissection); single interspace, cervical**

INCLUDES Operating microscope (69990)

EXCLUDES *Application of intervertebral biomechanical device(s) at the same level (22853-22854, [22859])*
Arthrodesis at the same level (22554)
Discectomy at the same level (63075)
Insertion of instrumentation at the same level (22845)

Code also arthroplasty more than one interspace, when performed ([22858])

47.6 47.6 FUD 090 J J8 80

AMA: 2018,Sep,7; 2018,Jan,8; 2017,Jan,8; 2016,Feb,12; 2016,Jan,13; 2015,Apr,7

+ # **22858** **second level, cervical (List separately in addition to code for primary procedure)**

Code first (22856)

14.9 14.9 FUD ZZZ N N1 80

AMA: 2018,Sep,7; 2018,Jan,8; 2017,Jan,8; 2016,Feb,12; 2016,Jan,13; 2015,Apr,7

22857 **Total disc arthroplasty (artificial disc), anterior approach, including discectomy to prepare interspace (other than for decompression), single interspace, lumbar**

INCLUDES Operating microscope (69990)

EXCLUDES *Application of intervertebral biomechanical device(s) at the same level (22853-22854, [22859])*
Arthrodesis at the same level (22558)
Insertion of instrumentation at the same level (22845)
Retroperitoneal exploration (49010)

Code also arthroplasty more than one interspace, when performed (0163T)

51.4 51.4 FUD 090 C 80

AMA: 2018,Sep,7; 2016,Feb,12

22858 **Resequenced code. See code following 22856.**

22859 **Resequenced code. See code following 22854.**

22861 **Revision including replacement of total disc arthroplasty (artificial disc), anterior approach, single interspace; cervical**

INCLUDES Operating microscope (69990)

EXCLUDES *Procedures performed at the same level (22845, 22853-22854, [22859], 22864, 63075)*
Revision of additional cervical arthroplasty (0098T)

68.4 68.4 FUD 090 C 80

AMA: 2018,Sep,7; 2016,Feb,12

22862 **lumbar**

EXCLUDES *Arthroplasty revision more than one interspace (0165T)*
Procedures performed at the same level (22558, 22845, 22853-22854, [22859], 22865, 49010)

54.9 54.9 FUD 090 C 80

AMA: 2018,Sep,7; 2018,Jan,8; 2017,Jan,8; 2016,Jan,13; 2015,Jan,16; 2014,Jan,11

22864 **Removal of total disc arthroplasty (artificial disc), anterior approach, single interspace; cervical**

INCLUDES Operating microscope (69990)

EXCLUDES *Cervical total disc arthroplasty with additional interspace removal (0095T)*
Revision of total disc arthroplasty (22861)

60.9 60.9 FUD 090 C 80

AMA: 2018,Sep,7

22865 **lumbar**

EXCLUDES *Arthroplasty more than one level (0164T)*
Exploration, retroperitoneal area with or without biopsy(s) (49010)

57.2 57.2 FUD 090 C 80

AMA: 2018,Sep,7; 2018,Jan,8; 2017,Jan,8; 2016,Jan,13; 2015,Jan,16; 2014,Jan,11

22867-22899 Spinal Distraction/Stabilization Device

22867 **Insertion of interlaminar/interspinous process stabilization/distraction device, without fusion, including image guidance when performed, with open decompression, lumbar; single level**

EXCLUDES *Interlaminar/interspinous stabilization/distraction device insertion (22869, 22870)*
Procedures at the same level (22532-22534, 22558, 22612, 22614, 22630, 22632-22634, 22800, 22802, 22804, 22840-22842, 22869-22870, 63005, 63012, 63017, 63030, 63035, 63042, 63044, 63047-63048, 77003)

28.2 28.2 FUD 090 J J8 80

AMA: 2018,Sep,7; 2018,Jan,8; 2017,Feb,9

+ **22868** **second level (List separately in addition to code for primary procedure)**

EXCLUDES *Interlaminar/interspinous stabilization/distraction device insertion (22869-22870)*
Procedures at the same level (22532-22534, 22558, 22612, 22614, 22630, 22632-22634, 22800, 22802, 22804, 22840-22842, 22869-22870, 63005, 63012, 63017, 63030, 63035, 63042, 63044, 63047-63048, 77003)

Code first (22867)

7.06 7.06 FUD ZZZ N N1 80

AMA: 2018,Sep,7; 2018,Jan,8; 2017,Feb,9

22869 **Insertion of interlaminar/interspinous process stabilization/distraction device, without open decompression or fusion, including image guidance when performed, lumbar; single level**

13.2 13.2 FUD 090 J J8 80

AMA: 2018,Sep,7; 2018,Jan,8; 2017,Feb,9

+ **22870** **second level (List separately in addition to code for primary procedure)**

EXCLUDES *Procedures at the same level (22532-22534, 22558, 22612, 22614, 22630, 22632-22634, 22800, 22802, 22804, 22840-22842, 63005, 63012, 63017, 63030, 63035, 63042, 63044, 63047-63048, 77003)*

Code first (22869)

3.96 3.96 FUD ZZZ N N1 80

AMA: 2018,Sep,7; 2018,Jan,8; 2017,Feb,9

22899 **Unlisted procedure, spine**

0.00 0.00 FUD YYY T 80

AMA: 2018,Sep,7; 2018,May,10; 2018,Jan,8; 2017,Feb,9; 2017,Jan,8; 2016,Jan,13; 2015,Jan,8; 2015,Jan,16; 2014,Oct,14; 2014,Jan,11

22900-22999 Musculoskeletal Procedures of Abdomen

INCLUDES Any necessary elevation of tissue planes or dissection
Measurement of tumor and necessary margin at greatest diameter prior to excision
Simple and intermediate repairs
Types of excision:
- Fascial or subfascial soft tissue tumors: simple and marginal resection of tumors found either in or below the deep fascia, not involving bone or excision of a substantial amount of normal tissue; primarily benign and intramuscular tumors
- Radical resection soft tissue tumor: wide resection of tumor involving substantial margins of normal tissue and may include tissue removal from one or more layers; most often malignant or aggressive benign
- Subcutaneous: simple and marginal resection of tumors in the subcutaneous tissue above the deep fascia; most often benign

EXCLUDES *Complex repair*
Excision of benign cutaneous lesions (eg, sebaceous cyst) (11400-11406)
Radical resection of cutaneous tumors (eg, melanoma) (11600-11606)
Significant exploration of the vessels or neuroplasty

22900 **Excision, tumor, soft tissue of abdominal wall, subfascial (eg, intramuscular); less than 5 cm**
16.2 16.2 **FUD** 090 J G2 80
AMA: 2018,Sep,7

22901 **5 cm or greater**
19.2 19.2 **FUD** 090 J G2 80
AMA: 2018,Sep,7

22902 **Excision, tumor, soft tissue of abdominal wall, subcutaneous; less than 3 cm**
9.53 12.8 **FUD** 090 J G2 80
AMA: 2018,Sep,7

22903 **3 cm or greater**
12.6 12.6 **FUD** 090 J G2 80
AMA: 2018,Sep,7

22904 **Radical resection of tumor (eg, sarcoma), soft tissue of abdominal wall; less than 5 cm**
30.4 30.4 **FUD** 090 J G2 80
AMA: 2018,Sep,7

22905 **5 cm or greater**
38.5 38.5 **FUD** 090 J G2 80
AMA: 2018,Sep,7

22999 **Unlisted procedure, abdomen, musculoskeletal system**
0.00 0.00 **FUD** YYY T 80
AMA: 2018,Sep,7

23000-23044 Surgical Incision Shoulder: Drainage, Foreign Body Removal, Contracture Release

23000 **Removal of subdeltoid calcareous deposits, open**
EXCLUDES *Arthroscopic removal calcium deposits of bursa (29999)*
10.3 16.0 **FUD** 090 J A2 80 50
AMA: 2018,Sep,7

23020 **Capsular contracture release (eg, Sever type procedure)**
EXCLUDES *Simple incision and drainage (10040-10160)*
19.8 19.8 **FUD** 090 J A2 80 50
AMA: 2018,Sep,7

23030 **Incision and drainage, shoulder area; deep abscess or hematoma**
7.20 12.4 **FUD** 010 J A2
AMA: 2018,Sep,7

23031 **infected bursa**
5.99 11.4 **FUD** 010 J A2 50
AMA: 2018,Sep,7

Section of left shoulder

The fibrous capsule enclosing the shoulder is thin and loose to allow freedom of movement; four rotator cuff muscles (supraspinatous, infraspinatous, teres minor, and scapularis) work together to hold the head of the humerus in the glenoid cavity

23035 **Incision, bone cortex (eg, osteomyelitis or bone abscess), shoulder area**
19.4 19.4 **FUD** 090 J A2 80 50
AMA: 2018,Sep,7

23040 **Arthrotomy, glenohumeral joint, including exploration, drainage, or removal of foreign body**
20.6 20.6 **FUD** 090 J A2 80 50
AMA: 2018,Sep,7

23044 **Arthrotomy, acromioclavicular, sternoclavicular joint, including exploration, drainage, or removal of foreign body**
16.3 16.3 **FUD** 090 J A2 50
AMA: 2018,Sep,7

23065-23066 Shoulder Biopsy

EXCLUDES *Soft tissue needle biopsy (20206)*

23065 **Biopsy, soft tissue of shoulder area; superficial**
4.81 6.34 **FUD** 010 J P3 50
AMA: 2018,Sep,7

23066 **deep**
10.4 16.1 **FUD** 090 J A2 50
AMA: 2018,Sep,7

23071-23078 [23071, 23073] Excision Soft Tissue Tumors of Shoulder

INCLUDES Any necessary elevation of tissue planes or dissection
Measurement of tumor and necessary margin at greatest diameter prior to excision
Simple and intermediate repairs
Types of excision:
- Fascial or subfascial soft tissue tumors: simple and marginal resection of tumors found either in or below the deep fascia, not involving bone or excision of a substantial amount of normal tissue; primarily benign and intramuscular tumors
- Radical resection soft tissue tumor: wide resection of tumor, involving substantial margins of normal tissue and may involve tissue removal from one or more layers; most often malignant or aggressive benign
- Subcutaneous: simple and marginal resection of tumors in the subcutaneous tissue above the deep fascia; most often benign

EXCLUDES *Complex repair*
Excision of benign cutaneous lesions (eg, sebaceous cyst) (11400-11406)
Radical resection of cutaneous tumors (eg, melanoma) (11600-11606)
Significant exploration of the vessels or neuroplasty

23071 **Resequenced code. See code following 23075.**

23073 **Resequenced code. See code following 23076.**

23075 **Excision, tumor, soft tissue of shoulder area, subcutaneous; less than 3 cm**
9.41 13.9 FUD 090 J G2 50
AMA: 2018,Sep,7; 2018,Jan,8; 2017,Jan,8; 2016,Jan,13; 2015,Jan,16; 2014,Jan,11

23071 **3 cm or greater**
12.0 12.0 FUD 090 J G2 80 50
AMA: 2018,Sep,7

23076 **Excision, tumor, soft tissue of shoulder area, subfascial (eg, intramuscular); less than 5 cm**
15.6 15.6 FUD 090 J G2 50
AMA: 2018,Sep,7; 2018,Jan,8; 2017,Jan,8; 2016,Jan,13; 2015,Jan,16; 2014,Jan,11

23073 **5 cm or greater**
20.0 20.0 FUD 090 J G2 80 50
AMA: 2018,Sep,7

23077 **Radical resection of tumor (eg, sarcoma), soft tissue of shoulder area; less than 5 cm**
32.8 32.8 FUD 090 J G2 80 50
AMA: 2018,Sep,7

23078 **5 cm or greater**
41.4 41.4 FUD 090 J G2 80 50
AMA: 2018,Sep,7

23100-23195 Bone and Joint Procedures of Shoulder

INCLUDES Acromioclavicular joint
Clavicle
Head and neck of humerus
Scapula
Shoulder joint
Sternoclavicular joint

23100 **Arthrotomy, glenohumeral joint, including biopsy**
14.4 14.4 FUD 090 J A2 80 50
AMA: 2018,Sep,7

23101 **Arthrotomy, acromioclavicular joint or sternoclavicular joint, including biopsy and/or excision of torn cartilage**
13.1 13.1 FUD 090 J A2 50
AMA: 2018,Sep,7

23105 **Arthrotomy; glenohumeral joint, with synovectomy, with or without biopsy**
18.3 18.3 FUD 090 J A2 80 50
AMA: 2018,Sep,7

23106 **sternoclavicular joint, with synovectomy, with or without biopsy**
14.3 14.3 FUD 090 J A2 50
AMA: 2018,Sep,7

23107 **Arthrotomy, glenohumeral joint, with joint exploration, with or without removal of loose or foreign body**
19.0 19.0 FUD 090 J A2 80 50
AMA: 2018,Sep,7

23120 **Claviculectomy; partial**
INCLUDES Mumford operation
EXCLUDES *Arthroscopic claviculectomy (29824)*
16.8 16.8 FUD 090 J A2 80 50
AMA: 2018,Sep,7; 2018,Jan,8; 2017,Jan,8; 2016,Jan,13; 2015,Jan,16; 2014,Jan,11

23125 **total**
20.4 20.4 FUD 090 J A2 80 50
AMA: 2018,Sep,7

23130 **Acromioplasty or acromionectomy, partial, with or without coracoacromial ligament release**
17.6 17.6 FUD 090 J A2 50
AMA: 2018,Sep,7; 2018,Jan,8; 2017,Jan,8; 2016,Jan,13; 2015,Mar,7; 2015,Feb,10; 2015,Jan,16; 2014,Jan,11

23140 **Excision or curettage of bone cyst or benign tumor of clavicle or scapula;**
15.9 15.9 FUD 090 J A2 50
AMA: 2018,Sep,7

23145 **with autograft (includes obtaining graft)**
20.0 20.0 FUD 090 J A2 80 50
AMA: 2018,Sep,7

23146 **with allograft**
17.9 17.9 FUD 090 J A2 80 50
AMA: 2019,May,7; 2018,Sep,7

23150 **Excision or curettage of bone cyst or benign tumor of proximal humerus;**
18.9 18.9 FUD 090 J A2 80 50
AMA: 2018,Sep,7

23155 **with autograft (includes obtaining graft)**
22.9 22.9 FUD 090 J A2 80 50
AMA: 2018,Sep,7

23156 **with allograft**
19.4 19.4 FUD 090 J A2 80 50
AMA: 2019,May,7; 2018,Sep,7

23170 **Sequestrectomy (eg, for osteomyelitis or bone abscess), clavicle**
16.1 16.1 FUD 090 J A2 50
AMA: 2018,Sep,7

23172 **Sequestrectomy (eg, for osteomyelitis or bone abscess), scapula**
16.3 16.3 FUD 090 J A2 80 50
AMA: 2018,Sep,7

23174 **Sequestrectomy (eg, for osteomyelitis or bone abscess), humeral head to surgical neck**
21.9 21.9 FUD 090 J A2 80 50
AMA: 2018,Sep,7

23180 **Partial excision (craterization, saucerization, or diaphysectomy) bone (eg, osteomyelitis), clavicle**
18.9 18.9 FUD 090 J A2 50
AMA: 2018,Sep,7

23182 **Partial excision (craterization, saucerization, or diaphysectomy) bone (eg, osteomyelitis), scapula**
18.9 18.9 FUD 090 J A2 80 50
AMA: 2018,Sep,7

23184 **Partial excision (craterization, saucerization, or diaphysectomy) bone (eg, osteomyelitis), proximal humerus**
21.1 21.1 FUD 090 J A2 80 50
AMA: 2018,Sep,7

23190 **Ostectomy of scapula, partial (eg, superior medial angle)**
16.5 16.5 FUD 090 J A2 80 50
AMA: 2018,Sep,7

23195 **Resection, humeral head**
EXCLUDES *Arthroplasty with replacement with implant (23470)*
21.4 21.4 FUD 090 J A2 80 50
AMA: 2018,Sep,7

23200-23220 Radical Resection of Bone Tumors of Shoulder

INCLUDES Any necessary elevation of tissue planes or dissection
Excision of adjacent soft tissue during bone tumor resection (23071-23078 [23071, 23073])
Measurement of tumor and necessary margin at greatest diameter prior to excision
Radical resection of cutaneous tumors (e.g., melanoma)
Resection of the tumor (may include entire bone) and wide margins of normal tissues primarily for malignant or aggressive benign tumors
Simple and intermediate repairs
EXCLUDES *Complex repair*
Significant exploration of vessels, neuroplasty, reconstruction, or complex bone repair

23200 **Radical resection of tumor; clavicle**
43.7 43.7 FUD 090 C 80 50
AMA: 2019,May,7; 2018,Sep,7

23210 **scapula**
51.4 51.4 FUD 090 C 80 50
AMA: 2019,May,7; 2018,Sep,7

23220 Radical resection of tumor, proximal humerus
56.3 56.3 FUD 090 C 80 50
AMA: 2019,May,7; 2018,Sep,7

23330-23335 Removal Implant/Foreign Body from Shoulder

EXCLUDES *Bursal arthrocentesis or needling (20610)*
K-wire or pin insertion (20650)
K-wire or pin removal (20670, 20680)

23330 Removal of foreign body, shoulder; subcutaneous
4.79 8.03 FUD 010 T A2 80 50
AMA: 2018,Sep,7; 2018,Jan,8; 2017,Jan,8; 2016,Jan,13; 2015,Jan,16; 2014,Mar,4; 2014,Jan,11

23333 deep (subfascial or intramuscular)
13.2 13.2 FUD 090 J G2 80 50
AMA: 2018,Sep,7; 2018,Jan,8; 2017,Jan,8; 2016,Jan,13; 2015,Jan,16; 2014,Mar,4

23334 Removal of prosthesis, includes debridement and synovectomy when performed; humeral or glenoid component
EXCLUDES *Foreign body removal (23330, 23333)*
Prosthesis removal and replacement in same shoulder (eg, glenoid and/or humeral components) (23473-23474)
30.8 30.8 FUD 090 J G2 50
AMA: 2018,Sep,7; 2018,Jan,8; 2017,Jan,8; 2016,Jan,13; 2015,Jan,16; 2014,Mar,4

23335 humeral and glenoid components (eg, total shoulder)
EXCLUDES *Foreign body removal (23330, 23333)*
Prosthesis removal and replacement in same shoulder (eg, glenoid and/or humeral components) (23473-23474)
36.8 36.8 FUD 090 C 50
AMA: 2018,Sep,7; 2018,Jan,8; 2017,Jan,8; 2016,Jan,13; 2015,Jan,16; 2014,Mar,4

23350 Injection for Shoulder Arthrogram

23350 Injection procedure for shoulder arthrography or enhanced CT/MRI shoulder arthrography
EXCLUDES *Shoulder biopsy (29805-29826)*
(73040, 73201-73202, 73222-73223, 77002)
1.47 3.97 FUD 000 N N1 50
AMA: 2018,Sep,7; 2018,Jan,8; 2017,Jan,8; 2016,May,13; 2016,Jan,13; 2015,Aug,6; 2015,Jan,16; 2014,Jan,11

23395-23491 Repair/Reconstruction of Shoulder

23395 Muscle transfer, any type, shoulder or upper arm; single
36.9 36.9 FUD 090 J A2 80
AMA: 2018,Sep,7

23397 multiple
32.6 32.6 FUD 090 J A2 80
AMA: 2018,Sep,7

23400 Scapulopexy (eg, Sprengels deformity or for paralysis)
28.0 28.0 FUD 090 J A2 80 50
AMA: 2018,Sep,7

23405 Tenotomy, shoulder area; single tendon
17.7 17.7 FUD 090 J A2 80
AMA: 2018,Sep,7

23406 multiple tendons through same incision
22.2 22.2 FUD 090 J A2 80
AMA: 2018,Sep,7

23410 Repair of ruptured musculotendinous cuff (eg, rotator cuff) open; acute
EXCLUDES *Arthroscopic repair (29827)*
23.6 23.6 FUD 090 J A2 80 50
AMA: 2018,Sep,7; 2018,Jan,8; 2017,Jan,8; 2016,Jan,13; 2015,Jan,16; 2014,Jan,11

23412 chronic
EXCLUDES *Arthroscopic repair (29827)*
24.5 24.5 FUD 090 J A2 80 50
AMA: 2018,Sep,7; 2018,Jan,8; 2017,Jan,8; 2016,Jan,13; 2015,Jun,10; 2015,Feb,10; 2015,Jan,16; 2014,Jan,11

23415 Coracoacromial ligament release, with or without acromioplasty
EXCLUDES *Arthroscopic repair (29826)*
20.1 20.1 FUD 090 J A2 50
AMA: 2018,Sep,7; 2018,Jan,8; 2017,Jan,8; 2016,Jan,13; 2015,Mar,7

23420 Reconstruction of complete shoulder (rotator) cuff avulsion, chronic (includes acromioplasty)
27.9 27.9 FUD 090 J A2 80 50
AMA: 2018,Sep,7; 2018,Jan,8; 2017,Jan,8; 2016,Jan,13; 2015,Jan,16; 2014,Jan,11

23430 Tenodesis of long tendon of biceps
EXCLUDES *Arthroscopic biceps tenodesis (29828)*
21.4 21.4 FUD 090 J A2 80 50
AMA: 2018,Sep,7

23440 Resection or transplantation of long tendon of biceps
21.7 21.7 FUD 090 J A2 80 50
AMA: 2018,Sep,7

23450 Capsulorrhaphy, anterior; Putti-Platt procedure or Magnuson type operation
EXCLUDES *Arthroscopic thermal capsulorrhaphy (29999)*
27.4 27.4 FUD 090 J A2 80 50
AMA: 2018,Sep,7

23455 with labral repair (eg, Bankart procedure)
EXCLUDES *Arthroscopic repair (29806)*
28.7 28.7 FUD 090 J A2 80 50
AMA: 2018,Sep,7

23460 Capsulorrhaphy, anterior, any type; with bone block
INCLUDES Bristow procedure
31.5 31.5 FUD 090 J A2 80 50
AMA: 2018,Sep,7

23462 with coracoid process transfer
EXCLUDES *Open thermal capsulorrhaphy (23929)*
30.3 30.3 FUD 090 J A2 80 50
AMA: 2018,Sep,7

23465 Capsulorrhaphy, glenohumeral joint, posterior, with or without bone block
EXCLUDES *Sternoclavicular and acromioclavicular joint repair (23530, 23550)*
32.3 32.3 FUD 090 J G2 80 50
AMA: 2018,Sep,7

23466 Capsulorrhaphy, glenohumeral joint, any type multi-directional instability
32.1 32.1 FUD 090 J A2 80 50
AMA: 2018,Sep,7

23470 Arthroplasty, glenohumeral joint; hemiarthroplasty
34.5 34.5 FUD 090 J 80 50
AMA: 2018,Sep,7; 2018,Jan,8; 2017,Jan,8; 2016,Jan,13; 2015,Jan,16; 2014,Mar,4

23472 total shoulder (glenoid and proximal humeral replacement (eg, total shoulder))
EXCLUDES *Proximal humerus osteotomy (24400)*
Removal of total shoulder components (23334-23335)
41.9 41.9 FUD 090 C 80 50
AMA: 2018,Sep,7; 2018,Jan,8; 2017,Jan,8; 2016,Jan,13; 2015,Jan,16; 2014,Mar,4; 2014,Jan,11

23473 **Revision of total shoulder arthroplasty, including allograft when performed; humeral or glenoid component**
EXCLUDES *Removal of prosthesis only (glenoid and/or humeral component) (23334-23335)*
46.7 46.7 FUD 090 J 80 50
AMA: 2018,Sep,7; 2018,Jan,8; 2017,Jan,8; 2016,Jan,13; 2015,Jan,16; 2014,Mar,4; 2014,Jan,11

23474 **humeral and glenoid component**
EXCLUDES *Removal of prosthesis only (glenoid and/or humeral component) (23334-23335)*
50.5 50.5 FUD 090 C 80 50
AMA: 2018,Sep,7; 2018,Jan,8; 2017,Jan,8; 2016,Jan,13; 2015,Jan,16; 2014,Mar,4; 2014,Jan,11

23480 **Osteotomy, clavicle, with or without internal fixation;**
23.7 23.7 FUD 090 J A2 50
AMA: 2018,Sep,7

23485 **with bone graft for nonunion or malunion (includes obtaining graft and/or necessary fixation)**
27.5 27.5 FUD 090 J J8 80 50
AMA: 2018,Sep,7

23490 **Prophylactic treatment (nailing, pinning, plating or wiring) with or without methylmethacrylate; clavicle**
24.6 24.6 FUD 090 J A2 80 50
AMA: 2018,Sep,7

23491 **proximal humerus**
29.3 29.3 FUD 090 J A2 80 50
AMA: 2018,Sep,7

23500-23680 Treatment of Shoulder Fracture/Dislocation

23500 **Closed treatment of clavicular fracture; without manipulation**
6.37 6.24 FUD 090 T A2 50
AMA: 2018,Sep,7

23505 **with manipulation**
9.51 10.1 FUD 090 J A2 50
AMA: 2018,Sep,7

23515 **Open treatment of clavicular fracture, includes internal fixation, when performed**
20.7 20.7 FUD 090 J J8 80 50
AMA: 2018,Sep,7; 2018,Jan,8; 2017,Jan,8; 2016,Jan,13; 2015,Jan,16; 2014,Jan,11

23520 **Closed treatment of sternoclavicular dislocation; without manipulation**
6.73 6.72 FUD 090 J A2 80 50
AMA: 2018,Sep,7

23525 **with manipulation**
10.2 11.1 FUD 090 T A2 80 50
AMA: 2018,Sep,7

23530 **Open treatment of sternoclavicular dislocation, acute or chronic;**
16.5 16.5 FUD 090 J A2 80 50
AMA: 2018,Sep,7

23532 **with fascial graft (includes obtaining graft)**
18.0 18.0 FUD 090 J A2 80 50
AMA: 2018,Sep,7

23540 **Closed treatment of acromioclavicular dislocation; without manipulation**
6.56 6.54 FUD 090 T A2 50
AMA: 2018,Sep,7

23545 **with manipulation**
8.93 9.91 FUD 090 T A2 80 50
AMA: 2018,Sep,7

23550 **Open treatment of acromioclavicular dislocation, acute or chronic;**
16.3 16.3 FUD 090 J A2 80 50
AMA: 2018,Sep,7

23552 **with fascial graft (includes obtaining graft)**
18.8 18.8 FUD 090 J J8 80 50
AMA: 2018,Sep,7

23570 **Closed treatment of scapular fracture; without manipulation**
6.83 6.62 FUD 090 T A2 50
AMA: 2018,Sep,7

23575 **with manipulation, with or without skeletal traction (with or without shoulder joint involvement)**
10.8 11.5 FUD 090 J A2 80 50
AMA: 2018,Sep,7

23585 **Open treatment of scapular fracture (body, glenoid or acromion) includes internal fixation, when performed**
28.2 28.2 FUD 090 J A2 80 50
AMA: 2018,Sep,7; 2018,Jan,8; 2017,Jan,8; 2016,Jan,13; 2015,Jan,16; 2014,Jan,11

23600 **Closed treatment of proximal humeral (surgical or anatomical neck) fracture; without manipulation**
8.82 9.37 FUD 090 T P2 50
AMA: 2018,Sep,7

23605 **with manipulation, with or without skeletal traction**
12.1 13.3 FUD 090 J A2 50
AMA: 2018,Sep,7

23615 **Open treatment of proximal humeral (surgical or anatomical neck) fracture, includes internal fixation, when performed, includes repair of tuberosity(s), when performed;**
25.4 25.4 FUD 090 J J8 80 50
AMA: 2018,Sep,7; 2018,Jan,8; 2017,Jan,8; 2016,Jan,13; 2015,Jan,16; 2014,Jan,11

23616 **with proximal humeral prosthetic replacement**
35.7 35.7 FUD 090 J J8 80 50
AMA: 2018,Sep,7

23620 **Closed treatment of greater humeral tuberosity fracture; without manipulation**
7.32 7.65 FUD 090 T P2 50
AMA: 2018,Sep,7

23625 **with manipulation**
10.0 10.9 FUD 090 J A2 50
AMA: 2018,Sep,7

23630 **Open treatment of greater humeral tuberosity fracture, includes internal fixation, when performed**
22.4 22.4 FUD 090 J A2 80 50
AMA: 2018,Sep,7

23650 **Closed treatment of shoulder dislocation, with manipulation; without anesthesia**
8.29 9.10 FUD 090 T A2 50
AMA: 2018,Sep,7

23655 **requiring anesthesia**
11.5 11.5 FUD 090 J A2 50
AMA: 2018,Sep,7

23660 **Open treatment of acute shoulder dislocation**
EXCLUDES *Chronic dislocation repair (23450-23466)*
16.7 16.7 FUD 090 J A2 80 50
AMA: 2018,Sep,7; 2018,Jan,8; 2017,Jan,8; 2016,Jan,13; 2015,Jan,16; 2014,Jan,11

23665 **Closed treatment of shoulder dislocation, with fracture of greater humeral tuberosity, with manipulation**
11.3 12.2 FUD 090 J A2 50
AMA: 2019,Feb,10; 2018,Sep,7

23670 **Open treatment of shoulder dislocation, with fracture of greater humeral tuberosity, includes internal fixation, when performed**
25.2 25.2 FUD 090 J A2 80 50
AMA: 2018,Sep,7

23675 **Closed treatment of shoulder dislocation, with surgical or anatomical neck fracture, with manipulation**
14.3 15.7 FUD 090 J A2 50
AMA: 2018,Sep,7

23680 **Open treatment of shoulder dislocation, with surgical or anatomical neck fracture, includes internal fixation, when performed**
26.7 26.7 FUD 090 J J8 80 50
AMA: 2018,Sep,7

23700-23929 Other/Unlisted Shoulder Procedures

23700 **Manipulation under anesthesia, shoulder joint, including application of fixation apparatus (dislocation excluded)**
5.64 5.64 FUD 010 J A2 50
AMA: 2018,Sep,7; 2018,Jan,8; 2017,Jan,8; 2016,Jan,13; 2015,Jun,10; 2015,Jan,16; 2014,Jan,11

23800 **Arthrodesis, glenohumeral joint;**
29.6 29.6 FUD 090 J G2 80 50
AMA: 2018,Sep,7

23802 **with autogenous graft (includes obtaining graft)**
37.0 37.0 FUD 090 J G2 80 50
AMA: 2018,Sep,7

23900 **Interthoracoscapular amputation (forequarter)**
40.1 40.1 FUD 090 C 80
AMA: 2018,Sep,7

23920 **Disarticulation of shoulder;**
32.5 32.5 FUD 090 C 80 50
AMA: 2018,Sep,7

23921 **secondary closure or scar revision**
13.4 13.4 FUD 090 T A2 50
AMA: 2018,Sep,7

23929 **Unlisted procedure, shoulder**
0.00 0.00 FUD YYY T 80
AMA: 2018,Sep,7

23930-24006 Surgical Incision Elbow/Upper Arm

EXCLUDES *Simple incision and drainage procedures (10040-10160)*

23930 **Incision and drainage, upper arm or elbow area; deep abscess or hematoma**
6.13 10.1 FUD 010 J A2 50
AMA: 2018,Sep,7

23931 **bursa**
4.48 8.19 FUD 010 J A2 50
AMA: 2018,Sep,7

23935 **Incision, deep, with opening of bone cortex (eg, for osteomyelitis or bone abscess), humerus or elbow**
14.6 14.6 FUD 090 J A2 80 50
AMA: 2018,Sep,7

24000 **Arthrotomy, elbow, including exploration, drainage, or removal of foreign body**
13.7 13.7 FUD 090 J A2 80 50
AMA: 2018,Sep,7

24006 **Arthrotomy of the elbow, with capsular excision for capsular release (separate procedure)**
20.5 20.5 FUD 090 J A2 80 50
AMA: 2018,Sep,7

24065-24066 Biopsy of Elbow/Upper Arm

EXCLUDES *Soft tissue needle biopsy (20206)*

24065 **Biopsy, soft tissue of upper arm or elbow area; superficial**
4.78 7.40 FUD 010 J P3 50
AMA: 2018,Sep,7

24066 **deep (subfascial or intramuscular)**
12.0 18.0 FUD 090 J A2 50
AMA: 2018,Sep,7

24071-24079 [24071, 24073] Excision Soft Tissue Tumors Elbow/Upper Arm

INCLUDES Any necessary elevation of tissue planes or dissection
Measurement of tumor and necessary margin at greatest diameter prior to excision
Types of excision:
Fascial or subfascial soft tissue tumors: simple and marginal resection of tumors found either in or below the deep fascia, not involving bone or excision of a substantial amount of normal tissue; primarily benign and intramuscular tumors
Radical resection of soft tissue tumor: wide resection of tumor involving substantial margins of normal tissue and may involve tissue removal from one or more layers; most often malignant or aggressive benign
Subcutaneous: simple and marginal resection of tumors found in the subcutaneous tissue above the deep fascia; most often benign

EXCLUDES *Complex repair*
Excision of benign cutaneous lesion (eg, sebaceous cyst) (11400-11406)
Radical resection of cutaneous tumors (eg, melanoma) (11600-11606)
Significant exploration of vessels or neuroplasty

24071 **Resequenced code. See code following 24075.**

24073 **Resequenced code. See code following 24076.**

24075 **Excision, tumor, soft tissue of upper arm or elbow area, subcutaneous; less than 3 cm**
9.48 14.4 FUD 090 J G2 50
AMA: 2018,Sep,7

24071 **3 cm or greater**
11.7 11.7 FUD 090 J G2 80 50
AMA: 2018,Sep,7

24076 **Excision, tumor, soft tissue of upper arm or elbow area, subfascial (eg, intramuscular); less than 5 cm**
15.6 15.6 FUD 090 J G2 50
AMA: 2018,Sep,7

24073 **5 cm or greater**
19.9 19.9 FUD 090 J G2 80 50
AMA: 2018,Sep,7

24077 **Radical resection of tumor (eg, sarcoma), soft tissue of upper arm or elbow area; less than 5 cm**
29.9 29.9 FUD 090 J G2 50
AMA: 2018,Sep,7

24079 **5 cm or greater**
38.2 38.2 FUD 090 J G2 80 50
AMA: 2018,Sep,7

24100-24149 Bone/Joint Procedures Upper Arm/Elbow

24100 **Arthrotomy, elbow; with synovial biopsy only**
12.0 12.0 FUD 090 J A2 80 50
AMA: 2018,Sep,7

24101 **with joint exploration, with or without biopsy, with or without removal of loose or foreign body**
14.3 14.3 FUD 090 J A2 80 50
AMA: 2018,Sep,7

24102 **with synovectomy**
17.7 17.7 FUD 090 J A2 80 50
AMA: 2018,Sep,7

24105 **Excision, olecranon bursa**
10.1 10.1 FUD 090 J A2 50
AMA: 2018,Sep,7

24110 **Excision or curettage of bone cyst or benign tumor, humerus;**
16.8 16.8 FUD 090 J A2 50
AMA: 2018,Sep,7

24115 **with autograft (includes obtaining graft)**
21.2 21.2 FUD 090 J J8 80 50
AMA: 2018,Sep,7

24116 **with allograft**
24.8 24.8 FUD 090 J A2 80 50
AMA: 2019,May,7; 2018,Sep,7

24120 **Excision or curettage of bone cyst or benign tumor of head or neck of radius or olecranon process;**
15.2 15.2 FUD 090 J A2 80 50
AMA: 2018,Sep,7

24125 **with autograft (includes obtaining graft)**
17.8 17.8 FUD 090 J A2 80 50
AMA: 2018,Sep,7

24126 **with allograft**
18.7 18.7 FUD 090 J J8 80 50
AMA: 2019,May,7; 2018,Sep,7

24130 **Excision, radial head**
EXCLUDES *Radial head arthroplasty with implant (24366)*
14.6 14.6 FUD 090 J A2 50
AMA: 2018,Sep,7

24134 **Sequestrectomy (eg, for osteomyelitis or bone abscess), shaft or distal humerus**
21.5 21.5 FUD 090 J A2 80 50
AMA: 2018,Sep,7

24136 **Sequestrectomy (eg, for osteomyelitis or bone abscess), radial head or neck**
18.1 18.1 FUD 090 J A2 50
AMA: 2018,Sep,7

24138 **Sequestrectomy (eg, for osteomyelitis or bone abscess), olecranon process**
19.5 19.5 FUD 090 J A2 80 50
AMA: 2018,Sep,7

24140 **Partial excision (craterization, saucerization, or diaphysectomy) bone (eg, osteomyelitis), humerus**
20.2 20.2 FUD 090 J A2 80 50
AMA: 2018,Sep,7

24145 **Partial excision (craterization, saucerization, or diaphysectomy) bone (eg, osteomyelitis), radial head or neck**
17.0 17.0 FUD 090 J A2 50
AMA: 2018,Sep,7

24147 **Partial excision (craterization, saucerization, or diaphysectomy) bone (eg, osteomyelitis), olecranon process**
17.9 17.9 FUD 090 J A2 50
AMA: 2018,Sep,7

24149 **Radical resection of capsule, soft tissue, and heterotopic bone, elbow, with contracture release (separate procedure)**
EXCLUDES *Capsular and soft tissue release (24006)*
33.8 33.8 FUD 090 J G2 80 50
AMA: 2018,Sep,7

24150-24152 Radical Resection Bone Tumor Upper Arm

INCLUDES Any necessary elevation of tissue planes or dissection
Excision of adjacent soft tissue during bone tumor resection (24071-24079 [24071, 24073])
Measurement of tumor and necessary margin at greatest diameter prior to excision
Resection of the tumor (may include entire bone) and wide margins of normal tissue primarily for malignant or aggressive benign tumors
Simple and intermediate repairs

EXCLUDES *Complex repair*
Significant exploration of vessels, neuroplasty, reconstruction, or complex bone repair

24150 **Radical resection of tumor, shaft or distal humerus**
44.9 44.9 FUD 090 J 80 50
AMA: 2019,May,7; 2018,Sep,7

24152 **Radical resection of tumor, radial head or neck**
39.0 39.0 FUD 090 J G2 80 50
AMA: 2019,May,7; 2018,Sep,7

24155 Elbow Arthrectomy

24155 **Resection of elbow joint (arthrectomy)**
24.6 24.6 FUD 090 J A2 80 50
AMA: 2018,Sep,7

24160-24201 Removal Implant/Foreign Body from Elbow/Upper Arm

EXCLUDES *Bursal or joint arthrocentesis or needling (20605)*
K-wire or pin insertion (20650)
K-wire or pin removal (20670, 20680)

24160 **Removal of prosthesis, includes debridement and synovectomy when performed; humeral and ulnar components**
INCLUDES Prosthesis removal and replacement in same elbow (eg, humeral and/or ulnar component(s)) (24370-24371)
EXCLUDES *Foreign body removal (24200-24201)*
Hardware removal other than prosthesis (20680)
36.4 36.4 FUD 090 Q2 A2 50
AMA: 2018,Sep,7; 2018,Jan,8; 2017,Jan,8; 2016,Jan,13; 2015,Jan,16; 2014,Mar,4; 2014,Jan,11

24164 **radial head**
EXCLUDES *Foreign body removal (24200-24201)*
Hardware removal other than prosthesis (20680)
20.8 20.8 FUD 090 Q2 A2 50
AMA: 2018,Sep,7; 2018,Jan,8; 2017,Jan,8; 2016,Jan,13; 2015,Jan,16; 2014,Mar,4

24200 **Removal of foreign body, upper arm or elbow area; subcutaneous**
3.99 6.02 FUD 010 J P3 80 50
AMA: 2018,Sep,7; 2018,Jan,8; 2017,Jan,8; 2016,Jan,13; 2015,Jan,16; 2014,Mar,4

24201 **deep (subfascial or intramuscular)**
10.4 15.8 FUD 090 J A2 50
AMA: 2018,Sep,7; 2018,Jan,8; 2017,Jan,8; 2016,Jan,13; 2015,Jan,16; 2014,Mar,4

24220 Injection for Elbow Arthrogram

24220 **Injection procedure for elbow arthrography**
EXCLUDES *Injection tennis elbow (20550)*
(73085)
1.95 4.71 FUD 000 N N1 80 50
AMA: 2018,Sep,7; 2018,Jan,8; 2017,Jan,8; 2016,May,13; 2016,Jan,13; 2015,Aug,6

24300-24498 Repair/Reconstruction of Elbow/Upper Arm

24300 **Manipulation, elbow, under anesthesia**
EXCLUDES *External fixation (20690, 20692)*
12.0 12.0 FUD 090 J G2 50
AMA: 2018,Sep,7

24301 **Muscle or tendon transfer, any type, upper arm or elbow, single (excluding 24320-24331)**
21.6 21.6 FUD 090 J A2 80
AMA: 2018,Sep,7

24305 **Tendon lengthening, upper arm or elbow, each tendon**
16.5 16.5 FUD 090 J A2 80
AMA: 2018,Sep,7

24310 **Tenotomy, open, elbow to shoulder, each tendon**
13.4 13.4 FUD 090 J A2 80
AMA: 2018,Sep,7

24320 **Tenoplasty, with muscle transfer, with or without free graft, elbow to shoulder, single (Seddon-Brookes type procedure)**
22.5 22.5 FUD 090 J A2 80
AMA: 2018,Sep,7

24330 **Flexor-plasty, elbow (eg, Steindler type advancement);**
20.7 20.7 FUD 090 J A2 80 50
AMA: 2018,Sep,7

24331 **with extensor advancement**
22.6 22.6 FUD 090 J A2 80 50
AMA: 2018,Sep,7

24332 **Tenolysis, triceps**
17.6 17.6 FUD 090 J G2 50
AMA: 2018,Sep,7

24340 **Tenodesis of biceps tendon at elbow (separate procedure)**
17.6 17.6 FUD 090 J A2 80 50
AMA: 2018,Sep,7

24341 **Repair, tendon or muscle, upper arm or elbow, each tendon or muscle, primary or secondary (excludes rotator cuff)**
21.4 21.4 FUD 090 J A2 80 50
AMA: 2018,Sep,7

24342 **Reinsertion of ruptured biceps or triceps tendon, distal, with or without tendon graft**
22.3 22.3 FUD 090 J A2 80 50
AMA: 2018,Sep,7; 2018,Jan,8; 2017,Apr,9

24343 **Repair lateral collateral ligament, elbow, with local tissue**
20.4 20.4 FUD 090 J G2 80 50
AMA: 2018,Sep,7

24344 **Reconstruction lateral collateral ligament, elbow, with tendon graft (includes harvesting of graft)**
31.4 31.4 FUD 090 J J8 80 50
AMA: 2018,Sep,7

24345 **Repair medial collateral ligament, elbow, with local tissue**
20.2 20.2 FUD 090 J A2 80 50
AMA: 2018,Sep,7

24346 **Reconstruction medial collateral ligament, elbow, with tendon graft (includes harvesting of graft)**
31.7 31.7 FUD 090 J G2 80 50
AMA: 2018,Sep,7

24357 **Tenotomy, elbow, lateral or medial (eg, epicondylitis, tennis elbow, golfer's elbow); percutaneous**
EXCLUDES *Arthroscopy, elbow, surgical; debridement (29837-29838)*
11.9 11.9 FUD 090 J G2 80 50
AMA: 2018,Sep,7; 2018,Jan,8; 2017,Jan,8; 2016,Jan,13; 2015,Jan,16; 2014,Jan,11

24358 **debridement, soft tissue and/or bone, open**
EXCLUDES *Arthroscopy, elbow, surgical; debridement (29837-29838)*
15.0 15.0 FUD 090 J G2 80 50
AMA: 2018,Sep,7; 2018,Jan,8; 2017,Jan,8; 2016,Jan,13; 2015,Jan,16; 2014,Jan,11

24359 **debridement, soft tissue and/or bone, open with tendon repair or reattachment**
EXCLUDES *Arthroscopy, elbow, surgical; debridement (29837-29838)*
19.0 19.0 FUD 090 J G2 80 50
AMA: 2018,Sep,7; 2018,Jan,8; 2017,Jan,8; 2016,Jan,13; 2015,Jan,16; 2014,Jan,11

24360 **Arthroplasty, elbow; with membrane (eg, fascial)**
26.0 26.0 FUD 090 J A2 80 50
AMA: 2018,Sep,7

24361 **with distal humeral prosthetic replacement**
29.0 29.0 FUD 090 J J8 80 50
AMA: 2018,Sep,7

24362 **with implant and fascia lata ligament reconstruction**
30.6 30.6 FUD 090 J J8 80 50
AMA: 2018,Sep,7

24363 **with distal humerus and proximal ulnar prosthetic replacement (eg, total elbow)**
EXCLUDES *Total elbow implant revision (24370-24371)*
41.9 41.9 FUD 090 J J8 80 50
AMA: 2018,Sep,7; 2018,Jan,8; 2017,Jan,8; 2016,Jan,13; 2015,Jan,16; 2014,Jan,11

24365 **Arthroplasty, radial head;**
18.4 18.4 FUD 090 J G2 80 50
AMA: 2018,Sep,7

24366 **with implant**
19.6 19.6 FUD 090 J J8 80 50
AMA: 2018,Sep,7

24370 **Revision of total elbow arthroplasty, including allograft when performed; humeral or ulnar component**
EXCLUDES *Prosthesis removal without replacement (eg, humeral and/or ulnar component/s) (24160)*
44.7 44.7 FUD 090 J J8 80 50
AMA: 2018,Sep,7; 2018,Jan,8; 2017,Jan,8; 2016,Jan,13; 2015,Jan,16; 2014,Mar,4

24371 **humeral and ulnar component**
EXCLUDES *Prosthesis removal without replacement (eg, humeral and/or ulnar component/s) (24160)*
51.3 51.3 FUD 090 J J8 80 50
AMA: 2018,Sep,7; 2018,Jan,8; 2017,Jan,8; 2016,Jan,13; 2015,Jan,16; 2014,Mar,4

24400 **Osteotomy, humerus, with or without internal fixation**
23.7 23.7 FUD 090 J A2 80 50
AMA: 2018,Sep,7; 2018,Jan,8; 2017,Jan,8; 2016,Jan,13; 2015,Jan,16; 2014,Mar,4

24410 **Multiple osteotomies with realignment on intramedullary rod, humeral shaft (Sofield type procedure)**
30.5 30.5 FUD 090 J G2 80 50
AMA: 2018,Sep,7

24420 **Osteoplasty, humerus (eg, shortening or lengthening) (excluding 64876)**
28.5 28.5 FUD 090 J A2 80 50
AMA: 2018,Sep,7

24430 **Repair of nonunion or malunion, humerus; without graft (eg, compression technique)**
30.4 30.4 FUD 090 J J8 80 50
AMA: 2018,Sep,7

24435 **with iliac or other autograft (includes obtaining graft)**
31.0 31.0 FUD 090 J J8 80 50
AMA: 2018,Sep,7

24470 **Hemiepiphyseal arrest (eg, cubitus varus or valgus, distal humerus)**
19.3 19.3 FUD 090 J A2 80 50
AMA: 2018,Sep,7

24495 **Decompression fasciotomy, forearm, with brachial artery exploration**
21.3 21.3 FUD 090 J A2 80 50
AMA: 2018,Sep,7

24498 **Prophylactic treatment (nailing, pinning, plating or wiring), with or without methylmethacrylate, humeral shaft**
24.9 24.9 FUD 090 J J8 80 50
AMA: 2018,Sep,7

24500-24685 Treatment of Fracture/Dislocation of Elbow/Upper Arm

INCLUDES Treatment for either closed or open fractures or dislocations

24500 **Closed treatment of humeral shaft fracture; without manipulation**
9.35 10.2 FUD 090 T A2 50
AMA: 2018,Sep,7

24505 **with manipulation, with or without skeletal traction**
12.8 14.2 FUD 090 J A2 50
AMA: 2018,Sep,7

24515 **Open treatment of humeral shaft fracture with plate/screws, with or without cerclage**
25.2 25.2 FUD 090 J J8 80 50
AMA: 2018,Sep,7

24516 **Treatment of humeral shaft fracture, with insertion of intramedullary implant, with or without cerclage and/or locking screws**
24.7 24.7 FUD 090 J J8 80 50
AMA: 2018,Sep,7; 2018,Jan,8; 2018,Jan,3; 2017,Jan,8; 2016,Jan,13; 2015,Jan,16; 2014,Jan,11

24530 **Closed treatment of supracondylar or transcondylar humeral fracture, with or without intercondylar extension; without manipulation**
9.89 10.8 FUD 090 T A2 50
AMA: 2018,Sep,7

24535 **with manipulation, with or without skin or skeletal traction**
16.3 17.6 FUD 090 J A2 50
AMA: 2018,Sep,7

24538 **Percutaneous skeletal fixation of supracondylar or transcondylar humeral fracture, with or without intercondylar extension**
21.5 21.5 FUD 090 J A2 50
AMA: 2018,Sep,7; 2018,Jan,8; 2017,Jan,8; 2016,Jan,13; 2015,Jan,16; 2014,Jan,11

24545 **Open treatment of humeral supracondylar or transcondylar fracture, includes internal fixation, when performed; without intercondylar extension**
26.7 26.7 FUD 090 J J8 80 50
AMA: 2018,Sep,7

24546 **with intercondylar extension**
29.9 29.9 FUD 090 J J8 80 50
AMA: 2018,Sep,7

24560 **Closed treatment of humeral epicondylar fracture, medial or lateral; without manipulation**
8.28 9.29 FUD 090 T A2 50
AMA: 2018,Sep,7

24565 **with manipulation**
14.1 15.3 FUD 090 J A2 50
AMA: 2018,Sep,7

24566 **Percutaneous skeletal fixation of humeral epicondylar fracture, medial or lateral, with manipulation**
20.6 20.6 FUD 090 J A2 50
AMA: 2018,Sep,7

24575 **Open treatment of humeral epicondylar fracture, medial or lateral, includes internal fixation, when performed**
21.0 21.0 FUD 090 J A2 80 50
AMA: 2018,Sep,7

24576 **Closed treatment of humeral condylar fracture, medial or lateral; without manipulation**
8.75 9.80 FUD 090 T A2 50
AMA: 2018,Sep,7

24577 **with manipulation**
14.4 15.8 FUD 090 J A2 50
AMA: 2018,Sep,7

24579 **Open treatment of humeral condylar fracture, medial or lateral, includes internal fixation, when performed**
EXCLUDES *Closed treatment without manipulation (24530, 24560, 24576, 24650, 24670)*
Repair with manipulation (24535, 24565, 24577, 24675)
24.0 24.0 FUD 090 J J8 80 50
AMA: 2018,Sep,7

24582 **Percutaneous skeletal fixation of humeral condylar fracture, medial or lateral, with manipulation**
23.3 23.3 FUD 090 J A2 50
AMA: 2018,Sep,7

24586 **Open treatment of periarticular fracture and/or dislocation of the elbow (fracture distal humerus and proximal ulna and/or proximal radius);**
31.2 31.2 FUD 090 J G2 80 50
AMA: 2018,Sep,7

24587 **with implant arthroplasty**
EXCLUDES *Distal humerus arthroplasty with implant (24361)*
31.4 31.4 FUD 090 J J8 80 50
AMA: 2018,Sep,7

24600 **Treatment of closed elbow dislocation; without anesthesia**
9.60 10.5 FUD 090 T A2 50
AMA: 2018,Sep,7

24605 **requiring anesthesia**
13.5 13.5 FUD 090 J A2 50
AMA: 2018,Sep,7

24615 **Open treatment of acute or chronic elbow dislocation**
20.5 20.5 FUD 090 J A2 80 50
AMA: 2018,Sep,7

24620 **Closed treatment of Monteggia type of fracture dislocation at elbow (fracture proximal end of ulna with dislocation of radial head), with manipulation**
15.8 15.8 FUD 090 J A2 80 50
AMA: 2018,Sep,7

24635 **Open treatment of Monteggia type of fracture dislocation at elbow (fracture proximal end of ulna with dislocation of radial head), includes internal fixation, when performed**
19.3 19.3 FUD 090 J J8 80 50
AMA: 2018,Sep,7

24640 **Closed treatment of radial head subluxation in child, nursemaid elbow, with manipulation** A
2.23 2.86 FUD 010 T P3 80 50
AMA: 2018,Sep,7

24650 **Closed treatment of radial head or neck fracture; without manipulation**
6.89 7.45 FUD 090 T P2 50
AMA: 2018,Sep,7

24655 **with manipulation**
11.4 12.6 FUD 090 J A2 50
AMA: 2018,Sep,7

24665 **Open treatment of radial head or neck fracture, includes internal fixation or radial head excision, when performed;**
18.7 18.7 FUD 090 J A2 80 50
AMA: 2018,Sep,7

24666 **with radial head prosthetic replacement**
21.0 21.0 FUD 090 J J8 80 50
AMA: 2018,Sep,7

24670 **Closed treatment of ulnar fracture, proximal end (eg, olecranon or coronoid process[es]); without manipulation**
7.53 8.28 FUD 090 T A2 50
AMA: 2018,Sep,7

24675 **with manipulation**
11.9 13.1 FUD 090 J A2 50
AMA: 2018,Sep,7

24685 **Open treatment of ulnar fracture, proximal end (eg, olecranon or coronoid process[es]), includes internal fixation, when performed**
EXCLUDES *Arthrotomy, elbow (24100-24102)*
18.8 18.8 FUD 090 J J8 80 50
AMA: 2018,Sep,7; 2018,Jan,3

24800-24999 Other/Unlisted Elbow/Upper Arm Procedures

24800 **Arthrodesis, elbow joint; local**
23.9 23.9 FUD 090 J A2 80 50
AMA: 2018,Sep,7

24802 **with autogenous graft (includes obtaining graft)**
28.9 28.9 FUD 090 J G2 80 50
AMA: 2018,Sep,7

24900 **Amputation, arm through humerus; with primary closure**
21.2 21.2 FUD 090 C 80 50
AMA: 2018,Sep,7

24920 open, circular (guillotine)
21.1 21.1 FUD 090 C 80 50
AMA: 2018,Sep,7

24925 secondary closure or scar revision
16.3 16.3 FUD 090 J A2 80 50
AMA: 2018,Sep,7

24930 re-amputation
22.3 22.3 FUD 090 C 80 50
AMA: 2018,Sep,7

24931 with implant
26.9 26.9 FUD 090 C 80 50
AMA: 2018,Sep,7

24935 Stump elongation, upper extremity
33.6 33.6 FUD 090 J 80 50
AMA: 2018,Sep,7

24940 Cineplasty, upper extremity, complete procedure
0.00 0.00 FUD 090 C 80 50
AMA: 2018,Sep,7

24999 Unlisted procedure, humerus or elbow
0.00 0.00 FUD YYY T 80 50
AMA: 2018,Sep,7

25000-25001 Incision Tendon Sheath of Wrist

25000 Incision, extensor tendon sheath, wrist (eg, deQuervains disease)
EXCLUDES *Carpal tunnel release (64721)*
9.70 9.70 FUD 090 J A2 50
AMA: 2018,Sep,7

25001 Incision, flexor tendon sheath, wrist (eg, flexor carpi radialis)
9.88 9.88 FUD 090 J G2 50
AMA: 2018,Sep,7

25020-25025 Decompression Fasciotomy Forearm/Wrist

25020 Decompression fasciotomy, forearm and/or wrist, flexor OR extensor compartment; without debridement of nonviable muscle and/or nerve
EXCLUDES *Brachial artery exploration (24495)*
Superficial incision and drainage (10060-10160)
16.4 16.4 FUD 090 J A2 50
AMA: 2018,Sep,7

25023 with debridement of nonviable muscle and/or nerve
EXCLUDES *Debridement (11000-11044 [11045, 11046])*
Decompression fasciotomy with exploration brachial artery exploration (24495)
Superficial incision and drainage (10060-10160)
31.8 31.8 FUD 090 J A2 80 50
AMA: 2018,Sep,7

25024 Decompression fasciotomy, forearm and/or wrist, flexor AND extensor compartment; without debridement of nonviable muscle and/or nerve
22.4 22.4 FUD 090 J A2 50
AMA: 2018,Sep,7

25025 with debridement of nonviable muscle and/or nerve
34.8 34.8 FUD 090 J A2 80 50
AMA: 2018,Sep,7

25028-25040 Incision for Drainage/Foreign Body Removal

25028 Incision and drainage, forearm and/or wrist; deep abscess or hematoma
15.1 15.1 FUD 090 J A2 50
AMA: 2018,Sep,7

25031 bursa
10.0 10.0 FUD 090 J A2 80 50
AMA: 2018,Sep,7

25035 Incision, deep, bone cortex, forearm and/or wrist (eg, osteomyelitis or bone abscess)
16.8 16.8 FUD 090 J A2 80 50
AMA: 2018,Sep,7

25040 Arthrotomy, radiocarpal or midcarpal joint, with exploration, drainage, or removal of foreign body
16.1 16.1 FUD 090 J A2 80 50
AMA: 2018,Sep,7

25065-25066 Biopsy Forearm/Wrist

EXCLUDES *Soft tissue needle biopsy (20206)*

25065 Biopsy, soft tissue of forearm and/or wrist; superficial
4.64 7.32 FUD 010 J P3 50
AMA: 2018,Sep,7

25066 deep (subfascial or intramuscular)
10.3 10.3 FUD 090 J A2 50
AMA: 2018,Sep,7

25071-25078 [25071, 25073] Excision Soft Tissue Tumors Forearm/Wrist

INCLUDES Any necessary elevation of tissue planes or dissection
Measurement of tumor and necessary margin at greatest diameter prior to excision
Simple and intermediate repairs
Types of excision:
Fascial or subfascial soft tissue tumors: simple and marginal resection of tumors found either in or below the deep fascia, not involving bone or excision of a substantial amount of normal tissue; primarily benign and intramuscular tumors
Radical resection soft tissue tumor: wide resection of tumor involving substantial margins of normal tissue and may include tissue removal from one or more layers; most often malignant or aggressive benign
Subcutaneous: simple and marginal resection of tumors in the subcutaneous tissue above the deep fascia; most often benign

EXCLUDES *Complex repair*
Excision of benign cutaneous lesions (eg, sebaceous cyst) (11400-11406)
Radical resection of cutaneous tumors (eg, melanoma) (11600-11606)
Significant exploration of vessels or neuroplasty

25071 **Resequenced code. See code following 25075.**

25073 **Resequenced code. See code following 25076.**

25075 Excision, tumor, soft tissue of forearm and/or wrist area, subcutaneous; less than 3 cm
9.09 14.0 FUD 090 J G2 50
AMA: 2018,Sep,7

\# 25071 3 cm or greater
12.2 12.2 FUD 090 J G2 80 50
AMA: 2018,Sep,7

25076 Excision, tumor, soft tissue of forearm and/or wrist area, subfascial (eg, intramuscular); less than 3 cm
14.8 14.8 FUD 090 J G2 50
AMA: 2018,Sep,7

\# 25073 3 cm or greater
15.3 15.3 FUD 090 J G2 80 50
AMA: 2018,Sep,7

25077 Radical resection of tumor (eg, sarcoma), soft tissue of forearm and/or wrist area; less than 3 cm
25.4 25.4 FUD 090 J G2 50
AMA: 2018,Sep,7

25078 3 cm or greater
33.6 33.6 FUD 090 J G2 80 50
AMA: 2018,Sep,7

25085-25240 Procedures of Bones/Joints Lower Arm/Wrist

25085 Capsulotomy, wrist (eg, contracture)
12.9 12.9 FUD 090 J A2 80 50
AMA: 2018,Sep,7

25100 Arthrotomy, wrist joint; with biopsy
9.96 9.96 FUD 090 J A2 80 50
AMA: 2018,Sep,7

25101 **with joint exploration, with or without biopsy, with or without removal of loose or foreign body**
11.6 11.6 FUD 090 J A2 80 50
AMA: 2018,Sep,7

25105 **with synovectomy**
13.8 13.8 FUD 090 J A2 80 50
AMA: 2018,Sep,7

25107 **Arthrotomy, distal radioulnar joint including repair of triangular cartilage, complex**
17.7 17.7 FUD 090 J A2 80 50
AMA: 2018,Sep,7

25109 **Excision of tendon, forearm and/or wrist, flexor or extensor, each**
15.4 15.4 FUD 090 J G2 50
AMA: 2018,Sep,7

25110 **Excision, lesion of tendon sheath, forearm and/or wrist**
9.82 9.82 FUD 090 J A2 50
AMA: 2018,Sep,7

25111 **Excision of ganglion, wrist (dorsal or volar); primary**
EXCLUDES *Excision of ganglion hand or finger (26160)*
9.21 9.21 FUD 090 J A2 50
AMA: 2018,Sep,7

25112 **recurrent**
EXCLUDES *Excision of ganglion hand or finger (26160)*
11.1 11.1 FUD 090 J A2 50
AMA: 2018,Sep,7

25115 **Radical excision of bursa, synovia of wrist, or forearm tendon sheaths (eg, tenosynovitis, fungus, Tbc, or other granulomas, rheumatoid arthritis); flexors**
EXCLUDES *Finger synovectomy (26145)*
21.8 21.8 FUD 090 J A2 50
AMA: 2018,Sep,7; 2018,Jan,8; 2017,Jan,8; 2016,Jan,13; 2015,Jan,16

25116 **extensors, with or without transposition of dorsal retinaculum**
EXCLUDES *Finger synovectomy (26145)*
17.2 17.2 FUD 090 J A2 80 50
AMA: 2018,Sep,7

25118 **Synovectomy, extensor tendon sheath, wrist, single compartment;**
EXCLUDES *Finger synovectomy (26145)*
10.9 10.9 FUD 090 J A2 50
AMA: 2018,Sep,7; 2018,Jan,8; 2017,Jan,8; 2016,Jan,13; 2015,Jun,10; 2015,Jan,16; 2014,Jan,11

25119 **with resection of distal ulna**
EXCLUDES *Finger synovectomy (26145)*
14.2 14.2 FUD 090 J A2 80 50
AMA: 2018,Sep,7

25120 **Excision or curettage of bone cyst or benign tumor of radius or ulna (excluding head or neck of radius and olecranon process);**
EXCLUDES *Removal of bone cyst or tumor of radial head, neck, or olecranon process (24120-24126)*
14.3 14.3 FUD 090 J A2 80 50
AMA: 2018,Sep,7

25125 **with autograft (includes obtaining graft)**
17.0 17.0 FUD 090 J A2 80 50
AMA: 2018,Sep,7

25126 **with allograft**
17.2 17.2 FUD 090 J J8 80 50
AMA: 2019,May,7; 2018,Sep,7

25130 **Excision or curettage of bone cyst or benign tumor of carpal bones;**
12.8 12.8 FUD 090 J A2 80 50
AMA: 2018,Sep,7

25135 **with autograft (includes obtaining graft)**
16.0 16.0 FUD 090 J A2 80 50
AMA: 2018,Sep,7

25136 **with allograft**
14.0 14.0 FUD 090 J A2 80 50
AMA: 2019,May,7; 2018,Sep,7

25145 **Sequestrectomy (eg, for osteomyelitis or bone abscess), forearm and/or wrist**
14.9 14.9 FUD 090 J A2 80 50
AMA: 2018,Sep,7

25150 **Partial excision (craterization, saucerization, or diaphysectomy) of bone (eg, for osteomyelitis); ulna**
16.2 16.2 FUD 090 J A2 50
AMA: 2018,Sep,7

25151 **radius**
EXCLUDES *Partial removal of radial head, neck, or olecranon process (24145, 24147)*
16.7 16.7 FUD 090 J A2 80 50
AMA: 2018,Sep,7

25170 **Radical resection of tumor, radius or ulna**
INCLUDES Any necessary elevation of tissue planes or dissection
Excision of adjacent soft tissue during bone tumor resection (25071-25078 [25071, 25073])
Measurement of tumor and necessary margin at greatest diameter prior to excision
Resection of the tumor (may include entire bone) and wide margins of normal tissue primarily for malignant or aggressive benign tumors
Resection without removal of significant normal tissue
Simple and intermediate repairs
EXCLUDES *Complex repair*
Excision of adjacent soft tissue during bone tumor resection (25076-25078 [25073])
Radical resection of cutaneous tumors (e.g., melanoma) (11600-11646)
Significant exploration of vessels, neuroplasty, reconstruction, or complex bone repair
42.7 42.7 FUD 090 J 80 50
AMA: 2019,May,7; 2018,Sep,7

25210 **Carpectomy; 1 bone**
EXCLUDES *Carpectomy with insertion of implant (25441-25445)*
14.0 14.0 FUD 090 J A2 80
AMA: 2018,Sep,7

25215 **all bones of proximal row**
17.7 17.7 FUD 090 J A2 80 50
AMA: 2019,Feb,10; 2018,Sep,7

25230 **Radial styloidectomy (separate procedure)**
12.4 12.4 FUD 090 J A2 50
AMA: 2018,Sep,7

25240 **Excision distal ulna partial or complete (eg, Darrach type or matched resection)**
EXCLUDES *Acquisition of fascia for interposition (20920, 20922)*
Implant replacement (25442)
12.3 12.3 FUD 090 J A2 80 50
AMA: 2018,Sep,7

25246 Injection for Wrist Arthrogram

25246 **Injection procedure for wrist arthrography**
EXCLUDES *Excision of superficial foreign body (20520)*
(73115)
2.16 4.88 FUD 000 N N1 50
AMA: 2018,Sep,7; 2018,Jan,8; 2017,Jan,8; 2016,Jan,13; 2015,Aug,6

25248-25251 Removal Foreign Body of Wrist

EXCLUDES *Excision of superficial foreign body (20520)*
K-wire, pin, or rod insertion (20650)
K-wire, pin, or rod removal (20670, 20680)

25248 **Exploration with removal of deep foreign body, forearm or wrist**
11.8 11.8 FUD 090 J A2 50
AMA: 2018,Sep,7

25250 **Removal of wrist prosthesis; (separate procedure)**
15.2 15.2 FUD 090 Q2 A2 80 50
AMA: 2018,Sep,7

25251 **complicated, including total wrist**
20.7 20.7 FUD 090 Q2 A2 80 50
AMA: 2018,Sep,7

25259 Manipulation of Wrist with Anesthesia

25259 **Manipulation, wrist, under anesthesia**
EXCLUDES *Application external fixation (20690, 20692)*
12.0 12.0 FUD 090 J G2 50
AMA: 2018,Sep,7; 2018,Jan,8; 2017,Jan,8; 2016,Jan,13; 2015,Jan,16; 2014,Jan,11

25260-25492 Repair/Reconstruction of Forearm/Wrist

25260 **Repair, tendon or muscle, flexor, forearm and/or wrist; primary, single, each tendon or muscle**
18.1 18.1 FUD 090 J A2
AMA: 2018,Sep,7

25263 **secondary, single, each tendon or muscle**
18.1 18.1 FUD 090 J A2 80
AMA: 2018,Sep,7

25265 **secondary, with free graft (includes obtaining graft), each tendon or muscle**
21.4 21.4 FUD 090 J A2 80
AMA: 2018,Sep,7

25270 **Repair, tendon or muscle, extensor, forearm and/or wrist; primary, single, each tendon or muscle**
14.0 14.0 FUD 090 J A2 80
AMA: 2018,Sep,7

25272 **secondary, single, each tendon or muscle**
15.9 15.9 FUD 090 J A2 80
AMA: 2018,Sep,7

25274 **secondary, with free graft (includes obtaining graft), each tendon or muscle**
19.1 19.1 FUD 090 J A2 80
AMA: 2018,Sep,7

25275 **Repair, tendon sheath, extensor, forearm and/or wrist, with free graft (includes obtaining graft) (eg, for extensor carpi ulnaris subluxation)**
19.2 19.2 FUD 090 J A2 80 50
AMA: 2018,Sep,7

25280 **Lengthening or shortening of flexor or extensor tendon, forearm and/or wrist, single, each tendon**
16.1 16.1 FUD 090 J A2 80
AMA: 2018,Sep,7

25290 **Tenotomy, open, flexor or extensor tendon, forearm and/or wrist, single, each tendon**
12.5 12.5 FUD 090 J A2
AMA: 2018,Sep,7

25295 **Tenolysis, flexor or extensor tendon, forearm and/or wrist, single, each tendon**
15.1 15.1 FUD 090 J A2
AMA: 2018,Sep,7; 2018,Jan,8; 2017,Jan,8; 2016,Jan,13; 2015,Jan,16; 2014,Jan,11

25300 **Tenodesis at wrist; flexors of fingers**
19.5 19.5 FUD 090 J A2 80 50
AMA: 2018,Sep,7

25301 **extensors of fingers**
18.4 18.4 FUD 090 J A2 80 50
AMA: 2018,Sep,7

25310 **Tendon transplantation or transfer, flexor or extensor, forearm and/or wrist, single; each tendon**
17.7 17.7 FUD 090 J A2 80
AMA: 2018,Sep,7; 2018,Jan,8; 2017,Jan,8; 2016,Jan,13; 2015,Jan,16; 2014,Jan,11

25312 **with tendon graft(s) (includes obtaining graft), each tendon**
20.6 20.6 FUD 090 J A2 80
AMA: 2018,Sep,7

25315 **Flexor origin slide (eg, for cerebral palsy, Volkmann contracture), forearm and/or wrist;**
22.2 22.2 FUD 090 J A2 80 50
AMA: 2018,Sep,7

25316 **with tendon(s) transfer**
26.4 26.4 FUD 090 J A2 80 50
AMA: 2018,Sep,7

25320 **Capsulorrhaphy or reconstruction, wrist, open (eg, capsulodesis, ligament repair, tendon transfer or graft) (includes synovectomy, capsulotomy and open reduction) for carpal instability**
28.3 28.3 FUD 090 J A2 80 50
AMA: 2018,Sep,7

25332 **Arthroplasty, wrist, with or without interposition, with or without external or internal fixation**
EXCLUDES *Acquiring fascia for interposition (20920, 20922)*
Arthroplasty with prosthesis (25441-25446)
24.2 24.2 FUD 090 J A2 80 50
AMA: 2019,Feb,10; 2018,Sep,7; 2018,Jan,8; 2017,Jan,8; 2016,Jan,13; 2015,Jan,16; 2014,Jan,11

25335 **Centralization of wrist on ulna (eg, radial club hand)**
27.2 27.2 FUD 090 J A2 80 50
AMA: 2018,Sep,7; 2018,May,10

25337 **Reconstruction for stabilization of unstable distal ulna or distal radioulnar joint, secondary by soft tissue stabilization (eg, tendon transfer, tendon graft or weave, or tenodesis) with or without open reduction of distal radioulnar joint**
EXCLUDES *Acquiring fascia lata graft (20920, 20922)*
25.6 25.6 FUD 090 J A2 50
AMA: 2018,Sep,7

25350 **Osteotomy, radius; distal third**
19.3 19.3 FUD 090 J A2 80 50
AMA: 2018,Sep,7

25355 **middle or proximal third**
22.0 22.0 FUD 090 J A2 80 50
AMA: 2018,Sep,7

25360 **Osteotomy; ulna**
18.8 18.8 FUD 090 J A2 80 50
AMA: 2018,Sep,7

25365 **radius AND ulna**
26.4 26.4 FUD 090 J A2 80 50
AMA: 2018,Sep,7

25370 **Multiple osteotomies, with realignment on intramedullary rod (Sofield type procedure); radius OR ulna**
29.0 29.0 FUD 090 J A2 80 50
AMA: 2018,Sep,7

25375 **radius AND ulna**
27.5 27.5 FUD 090 J A2 80 50
AMA: 2018,Sep,7

25390 **Osteoplasty, radius OR ulna; shortening**
22.1 22.1 FUD 090 J J8 80 50
AMA: 2018,Sep,7

25391 **lengthening with autograft**
28.7 28.7 FUD 090 J J8 80 50
AMA: 2018,Sep,7

25392 **Osteoplasty, radius AND ulna; shortening (excluding 64876)**
29.2 29.2 FUD 090 J A2 80 50
AMA: 2018,Sep,7

25393 **lengthening with autograft**
32.6 32.6 FUD 090 J A2 80 50
AMA: 2018,Sep,7

25394 **Osteoplasty, carpal bone, shortening**
22.6 22.6 FUD 090 J G2 80 50
AMA: 2018,Sep,7

25400 **Repair of nonunion or malunion, radius OR ulna; without graft (eg, compression technique)**
23.1 23.1 FUD 090 J J8 80 50
AMA: 2018,Sep,7

25405 **with autograft (includes obtaining graft)**
29.9 29.9 FUD 090 J J8 80 50
AMA: 2018,Sep,7

25415 **Repair of nonunion or malunion, radius AND ulna; without graft (eg, compression technique)**
27.9 27.9 FUD 090 J J8 80 50
AMA: 2018,Sep,7

25420 **with autograft (includes obtaining graft)**
33.7 33.7 FUD 090 J J8 80 50
AMA: 2018,Sep,7

25425 **Repair of defect with autograft; radius OR ulna**
27.8 27.8 FUD 090 J A2 80 50
AMA: 2018,Sep,7

25426 **radius AND ulna**
32.4 32.4 FUD 090 J G2 80 50
AMA: 2018,Sep,7

25430 **Insertion of vascular pedicle into carpal bone (eg, Hori procedure)**
21.0 21.0 FUD 090 J G2 50
AMA: 2018,Sep,7

25431 **Repair of nonunion of carpal bone (excluding carpal scaphoid (navicular)) (includes obtaining graft and necessary fixation), each bone**
22.7 22.7 FUD 090 J G2 80 50
AMA: 2018,Sep,7

25440 **Repair of nonunion, scaphoid carpal (navicular) bone, with or without radial styloidectomy (includes obtaining graft and necessary fixation)**
22.1 22.1 FUD 090 J A2 80 50
AMA: 2018,Sep,7

25441 **Arthroplasty with prosthetic replacement; distal radius**
27.0 27.0 FUD 090 J J8 80 50
AMA: 2018,Sep,7; 2018,Jan,8; 2017,Aug,9; 2017,Jan,8; 2016,Jan,13; 2015,Jan,16; 2014,Jan,11

25442 **distal ulna**
23.2 23.2 FUD 090 J J8 80 50
AMA: 2018,Sep,7; 2018,Jan,8; 2017,Aug,9; 2017,Jan,8; 2016,Jan,13; 2015,Jan,16; 2014,Jan,11

25443 **scaphoid carpal (navicular)**
22.5 22.5 FUD 090 J A2 80 50
AMA: 2018,Sep,7; 2018,Jan,8; 2017,Jan,8; 2016,Jan,13; 2015,Jan,16; 2014,Jan,11

25444 **lunate**
23.8 23.8 FUD 090 J J8 80 50
AMA: 2018,Sep,7; 2018,Jan,8; 2017,Jan,8; 2016,Jan,13; 2015,Jan,16; 2014,Jan,11

25445 **trapezium**
20.7 20.7 FUD 090 J J8 50
AMA: 2018,Sep,7; 2018,Jan,8; 2017,Jan,8; 2016,Jan,13; 2015,Jan,16; 2014,Jan,11

25446 **distal radius and partial or entire carpus (total wrist)**
33.8 33.8 FUD 090 J J8 80 50
AMA: 2018,Sep,7; 2018,Jan,8; 2017,Jan,8; 2016,Jan,13; 2015,Jan,16; 2014,Jan,11

25447 **Arthroplasty, interposition, intercarpal or carpometacarpal joints**
EXCLUDES *Wrist arthroplasty (25332)*
23.8 23.8 FUD 090 J A2 80 50
AMA: 2018,Sep,7; 2018,Jan,8; 2017,Jan,8; 2016,Jan,13; 2015,Jan,16; 2014,Jan,11

25449 **Revision of arthroplasty, including removal of implant, wrist joint**
29.7 29.7 FUD 090 J A2 80 50
AMA: 2018,Sep,7

25450 **Epiphyseal arrest by epiphysiodesis or stapling; distal radius OR ulna**
17.7 17.7 FUD 090 J A2 50
AMA: 2018,Sep,7

25455 **distal radius AND ulna**
20.9 20.9 FUD 090 J A2 50
AMA: 2018,Sep,7

25490 **Prophylactic treatment (nailing, pinning, plating or wiring) with or without methylmethacrylate; radius**
20.7 20.7 FUD 090 J A2 80 50
AMA: 2018,Sep,7

25491 **ulna**
21.3 21.3 FUD 090 J A2 80 50
AMA: 2018,Sep,7

25492 **radius AND ulna**
26.1 26.1 FUD 090 J A2 80 50
AMA: 2018,Sep,7

25500-25695 Treatment of Fracture/Dislocation of Forearm/Wrist

Code also external fixation (20690)

25500 **Closed treatment of radial shaft fracture; without manipulation**
7.16 7.87 FUD 090 T P2 50
AMA: 2018,Sep,7

25505 **with manipulation**
13.0 14.2 FUD 090 J A2 50
AMA: 2018,Sep,7

25515 **Open treatment of radial shaft fracture, includes internal fixation, when performed**
19.2 19.2 FUD 090 J J8 80 50
AMA: 2018,Sep,7

25520 **Closed treatment of radial shaft fracture and closed treatment of dislocation of distal radioulnar joint (Galeazzi fracture/dislocation)**
15.5 16.4 FUD 090 J A2 50
AMA: 2018,Sep,7

25525 **Open treatment of radial shaft fracture, includes internal fixation, when performed, and closed treatment of distal radioulnar joint dislocation (Galeazzi fracture/ dislocation), includes percutaneous skeletal fixation, when performed**
22.6 22.6 FUD 090 J J8 80 50
AMA: 2018,Sep,7

25526 **Open treatment of radial shaft fracture, includes internal fixation, when performed, and open treatment of distal radioulnar joint dislocation (Galeazzi fracture/ dislocation), includes internal fixation, when performed, includes repair of triangular fibrocartilage complex**
27.5 27.5 FUD 090 J A2 80 50
AMA: 2018,Sep,7

25530 **Closed treatment of ulnar shaft fracture; without manipulation**
6.80 7.46 FUD 090 T P2 50
AMA: 2018,Sep,7

25535 **with manipulation**
12.9 14.0 FUD 090 T A2 50
AMA: 2018,Sep,7

25545 **Open treatment of ulnar shaft fracture, includes internal fixation, when performed**
17.9 17.9 FUD 090 J A2 80 50
AMA: 2018,Sep,7; 2018,Jan,8; 2017,Jan,8; 2016,Jan,13; 2015,Jan,16; 2014,Jan,11

25560 **Closed treatment of radial and ulnar shaft fractures; without manipulation**
7.22 8.03 FUD 090 T P2 50
AMA: 2018,Sep,7

25565 **with manipulation**
13.2 14.7 FUD 090 J A2 50
AMA: 2018,Sep,7

25574 **Open treatment of radial AND ulnar shaft fractures, with internal fixation, when performed; of radius OR ulna**
19.3 19.3 FUD 090 J J8 80 50
AMA: 2018,Sep,7; 2018,Jan,8; 2017,Jan,8; 2016,Jan,13; 2015,Jan,16; 2014,Jan,11

25575 **of radius AND ulna**
25.9 25.9 FUD 090 J J8 80 50
AMA: 2018,Sep,7

25600 **Closed treatment of distal radial fracture (eg, Colles or Smith type) or epiphyseal separation, includes closed treatment of fracture of ulnar styloid, when performed; without manipulation**
INCLUDES Closed treatment of ulnar styloid fracture (25650)
8.93 9.40 FUD 090 T P2 50
AMA: 2018,Sep,7; 2018,Jan,8; 2017,Jan,8; 2016,Jan,13; 2015,Jan,16; 2014,Jan,11

25605 **with manipulation**
INCLUDES Closed treatment of ulnar styloid fracture (25650)
14.5 15.4 FUD 090 J A2 50
AMA: 2018,Sep,7; 2018,Jan,8; 2017,Jan,8; 2016,Jan,13; 2015,Jan,16; 2014,Jan,11

25606 **Percutaneous skeletal fixation of distal radial fracture or epiphyseal separation**
EXCLUDES *Closed treatment of ulnar styloid fracture (25650)*
Open repair of ulnar styloid fracture (25652)
Percutaneous repair of ulnar styloid fracture (25651)
19.0 19.0 FUD 090 J A2 50
AMA: 2018,Sep,7

25607 **Open treatment of distal radial extra-articular fracture or epiphyseal separation, with internal fixation**
EXCLUDES *Closed treatment of ulnar styloid fracture (25650)*
Open repair of ulnar styloid fracture (25652)
Percutaneous repair of ulnar styloid fracture (25651)
21.1 21.1 FUD 090 J J8 80 50
AMA: 2018,Sep,7; 2018,Jan,8; 2017,Jan,8; 2016,Jan,13; 2015,Jan,16; 2014,Jan,11

25608 **Open treatment of distal radial intra-articular fracture or epiphyseal separation; with internal fixation of 2 fragments**
EXCLUDES *Closed treatment of ulnar styloid fracture (25650)*
Open repair of ulnar styloid fracture (25652)
Open treatment of distal radial intra-articular fracture or epiphyseal separation; with internal fixation of 3 or more fragments (25609)
Percutaneous repair of ulnar styloid fracture (25651)
23.7 23.7 FUD 090 J J8 80 50
AMA: 2018,Sep,7; 2018,Jan,8; 2017,Jan,8; 2016,Jan,13; 2015,Jan,16; 2014,Jan,11

25609 **with internal fixation of 3 or more fragments**
EXCLUDES *Closed treatment of ulnar styloid fracture (25650)*
Open repair of ulnar styloid fracture (25652)
Percutaneous repair of ulnar styloid fracture (25651)
30.1 30.1 FUD 090 J J8 80 50
AMA: 2018,Sep,7; 2018,Jan,8; 2017,Jan,8; 2016,Jan,13; 2015,Jan,16; 2014,Jan,11

25622 **Closed treatment of carpal scaphoid (navicular) fracture; without manipulation**
7.98 8.70 FUD 090 T P2 50
AMA: 2018,Sep,7

25624 **with manipulation**
12.5 13.8 FUD 090 J A2 80 50
AMA: 2018,Sep,7

25628 **Open treatment of carpal scaphoid (navicular) fracture, includes internal fixation, when performed**
20.7 20.7 FUD 090 J A2 80 50
AMA: 2018,Sep,7

25630 **Closed treatment of carpal bone fracture (excluding carpal scaphoid [navicular]); without manipulation, each bone**
8.04 8.69 FUD 090 T P2 50
AMA: 2018,Sep,7

25635 **with manipulation, each bone**
11.9 13.1 FUD 090 J A2 80 50
AMA: 2018,Sep,7

25645 **Open treatment of carpal bone fracture (other than carpal scaphoid [navicular]), each bone**
16.4 16.4 FUD 090 J A2 80 50
AMA: 2018,Sep,7

25650 **Closed treatment of ulnar styloid fracture**
EXCLUDES *Closed treatment of distal radial fracture (25600, 25605)*
Open treatment of distal radial extra-articular fracture or epiphyseal separation, with internal fixation (25607-25609)
8.57 9.20 FUD 090 T P2 50
AMA: 2018,Sep,7; 2018,Jan,8; 2017,Jan,8; 2016,Jan,13; 2015,Jan,16; 2014,Jan,11

25651 **Percutaneous skeletal fixation of ulnar styloid fracture**
13.9 13.9 FUD 090 J G2 80 50
AMA: 2018,Sep,7

25652 **Open treatment of ulnar styloid fracture**
17.9 17.9 FUD 090 J G2 50
AMA: 2018,Sep,7; 2018,Jan,8; 2017,Jan,8; 2016,Jan,13; 2015,Jan,16; 2014,Jan,11

25660 **Closed treatment of radiocarpal or intercarpal dislocation, 1 or more bones, with manipulation**
11.8 11.8 FUD 090 T A2 80 50
AMA: 2018,Sep,7

25670 **Open treatment of radiocarpal or intercarpal dislocation, 1 or more bones**
17.4 17.4 FUD 090 J A2 80 50
AMA: 2018,Sep,7

25671 **Percutaneous skeletal fixation of distal radioulnar dislocation**
15.1 15.1 FUD 090 J A2 50
AMA: 2018,Sep,7

25675 **Closed treatment of distal radioulnar dislocation with manipulation**
11.3 12.5 FUD 090 T A2 80 50
AMA: 2018,Sep,7

25676 **Open treatment of distal radioulnar dislocation, acute or chronic**
18.0 18.0 FUD 090 J A2 80 50
AMA: 2018,Sep,7

25680 **Closed treatment of trans-scaphoperilunar type of fracture dislocation, with manipulation**
15.0 15.0 FUD 090 T A2 80 50
AMA: 2018,Sep,7

25685 **Open treatment of trans-scaphoperilunar type of fracture dislocation**
21.2 21.2 FUD 090 J A2 80 50
AMA: 2018,Sep,7

25690 **Closed treatment of lunate dislocation, with manipulation**
13.9 13.9 FUD 090 J A2 80 50
AMA: 2018,Sep,7

25695 **Open treatment of lunate dislocation**
18.2 18.2 FUD 090 J A2 80 50
AMA: 2018,Sep,7

25800-25830 Wrist Fusion

25800 **Arthrodesis, wrist; complete, without bone graft (includes radiocarpal and/or intercarpal and/or carpometacarpal joints)**
21.0 21.0 FUD 090 J G2 80 50
AMA: 2018,Sep,7

25805 **with sliding graft**
24.4 24.4 FUD 090 J J8 80 50
AMA: 2018,Sep,7

25810 **with iliac or other autograft (includes obtaining graft)**
24.9 24.9 FUD 090 J J8 80 50
AMA: 2018,Sep,7

25820 **Arthrodesis, wrist; limited, without bone graft (eg, intercarpal or radiocarpal)**
17.8 17.8 FUD 090 J J8 80 50
AMA: 2018,Sep,7

25825 **with autograft (includes obtaining graft)**
21.9 21.9 FUD 090 J J8 80 50
AMA: 2018,Sep,7; 2018,Jan,8; 2017,Jan,8; 2016,Jan,13; 2015,Jan,16; 2014,Jan,11

25830 **Arthrodesis, distal radioulnar joint with segmental resection of ulna, with or without bone graft (eg, Sauve-Kapandji procedure)**
27.0 27.0 FUD 090 J J8 80 50
AMA: 2018,Sep,7

25900-25999 Amputation Through Forearm/Wrist

25900 **Amputation, forearm, through radius and ulna;**
20.4 20.4 FUD 090 C 80 50
AMA: 2018,Sep,7

25905 **open, circular (guillotine)**
20.2 20.2 FUD 090 C 80 50
AMA: 2018,Sep,7

25907 **secondary closure or scar revision**
17.6 17.6 FUD 090 J A2 80 50
AMA: 2018,Sep,7

25909 **re-amputation**
19.7 19.7 FUD 090 J 80 50
AMA: 2018,Sep,7

25915 **Krukenberg procedure**
33.8 33.8 FUD 090 C 80 50
AMA: 2018,Sep,7

25920 **Disarticulation through wrist;**
20.2 20.2 FUD 090 C 80 50
AMA: 2018,Sep,7

25922 **secondary closure or scar revision**
17.7 17.7 FUD 090 J A2 80 50
AMA: 2018,Sep,7

25924 **re-amputation**
19.7 19.7 FUD 090 C 80 50
AMA: 2018,Sep,7

25927 **Transmetacarpal amputation;**
23.2 23.2 FUD 090 C 80 50
AMA: 2018,Sep,7

25929 **secondary closure or scar revision**
17.1 17.1 FUD 090 T A2 80 50
AMA: 2018,Sep,7

25931 **re-amputation**
21.3 21.3 FUD 090 J G2 50
AMA: 2018,Sep,7

25999 **Unlisted procedure, forearm or wrist**
0.00 0.00 FUD YYY T 80 50
AMA: 2019,Feb,10; 2018,Sep,7

26010-26037 Incision Hand/Fingers

26010 **Drainage of finger abscess; simple**
3.90 7.74 FUD 010 T P2
AMA: 2018,Sep,7

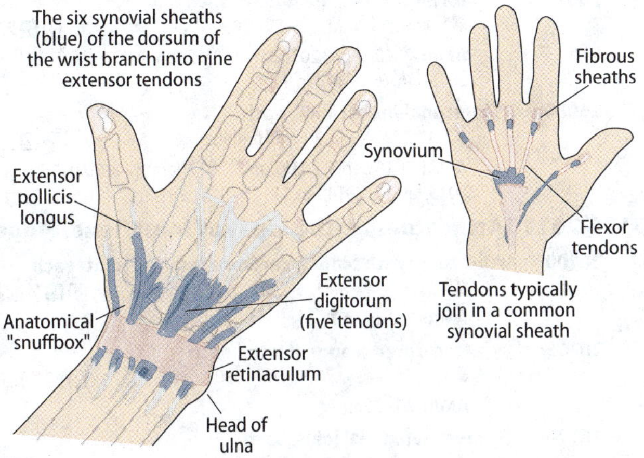

26011 **complicated (eg, felon)**
5.28 11.4 FUD 010 J A2
AMA: 2018,Sep,7

26020 **Drainage of tendon sheath, digit and/or palm, each**
12.4 12.4 FUD 090 J A2
AMA: 2018,Sep,7

26025 **Drainage of palmar bursa; single, bursa**
12.1 12.1 FUD 090 J A2 80 50
AMA: 2018,Sep,7

26030 **multiple bursa**
14.0 14.0 FUD 090 J A2 80 50
AMA: 2018,Sep,7

26034 **Incision, bone cortex, hand or finger (eg, osteomyelitis or bone abscess)**
15.6 15.6 FUD 090 J A2
AMA: 2018,Sep,7

26035 **Decompression fingers and/or hand, injection injury (eg, grease gun)**
24.7 24.7 FUD 090 J G2 80
AMA: 2018,Sep,7

26037 **Decompressive fasciotomy, hand (excludes 26035)**
EXCLUDES *Injection injury (26035)*
16.2 16.2 FUD 090 J G2 80 50
AMA: 2018,Sep,7

26040-26045 Incision Palmar Fascia

EXCLUDES *Enzyme injection fasciotomy (20527, 26341)*
Fasciectomy (26121, 26123, 26125)

26040 **Fasciotomy, palmar (eg, Dupuytren's contracture); percutaneous**
8.96 8.96 FUD 090 J A2 50
AMA: 2018,Sep,7; 2018,Jan,8; 2017,Jan,8; 2016,Jan,13; 2015,Jan,16; 2014,Jan,11

26045 **open, partial**
13.4 13.4 FUD 090 J A2 50
AMA: 2018,Sep,7; 2018,Jan,8; 2017,Jan,8; 2016,Jan,13; 2015,Jan,16; 2014,Jan,11

26055-26080 Incision Tendon/Joint of Fingers/Hand

26055 **Tendon sheath incision (eg, for trigger finger)**
8.91 16.1 FUD 090 J A2
AMA: 2018,Sep,7

26060 **Tenotomy, percutaneous, single, each digit**
EXCLUDES *Arthrocentesis (20610)*
7.36 7.36 FUD 090 J A2 80
AMA: 2018,Sep,7

26070 **Arthrotomy, with exploration, drainage, or removal of loose or foreign body; carpometacarpal joint**
9.19 9.19 FUD 090 J A2 50
AMA: 2018,Sep,7

26075 **metacarpophalangeal joint, each**
9.59 9.59 FUD 090 J A2 50
AMA: 2018,Sep,7; 2018,Jan,8; 2017,Jan,8; 2016,Jan,13; 2015,Jan,16; 2014,Jan,11

26080 **interphalangeal joint, each**
11.2 11.2 FUD 090 J A2
AMA: 2018,Sep,7; 2018,Jan,8; 2017,Jan,8; 2016,Jan,13; 2015,Jan,16; 2014,Jan,11

26100-26110 Arthrotomy with Biopsy of Joint Hand/Fingers

26100 **Arthrotomy with biopsy; carpometacarpal joint, each**
9.64 9.64 FUD 090 J A2 80 50
AMA: 2018,Sep,7

26105 **metacarpophalangeal joint, each**
9.71 9.71 FUD 090 J A2 80 50
AMA: 2018,Sep,7

26110 **interphalangeal joint, each**
9.25 9.25 FUD 090 J A2
AMA: 2018,Sep,7

26111-26118 [26111, 26113] Excision Soft Tissue Tumors Fingers and Hand

INCLUDES Any necessary elevation of tissue planes or dissection
Measurement of tumor and necessary margin at greatest diameter prior to excision
Simple and intermediate repairs
Types of excision:
- Fascial or subfascial soft tissue tumors: simple and marginal resection of tumors found either in or below the deep fascia, not involving bone or excision of a substantial amount of normal tissue; primarily benign and intramuscular tumors
  - Tumors of fingers and toes involving joint capsules, tendons and tendon sheaths
- Radical resection soft tissue tumor: wide resection of tumor, involving substantial margins of normal tissue and may include tissue removal from one or more layers; most often malignant or aggressive benign
  - Tumors of fingers and toes adjacent to joints, tendons and tendon sheaths
- Subcutaneous: simple and marginal resection of tumors found in the subcutaneous tissue above the deep fascia; most often benign

EXCLUDES *Complex repair*
Excision of benign cutaneous lesions (eg, sebaceous cyst) (11420-11426)
Radical resection of cutaneous tumors (eg, melanoma) (11620-11626)
Significant exploration of the vessels or neuroplasty

26111 **Resequenced code. See code following 26115.**

26113 **Resequenced code. See code following 26116.**

26115 **Excision, tumor or vascular malformation, soft tissue of hand or finger, subcutaneous; less than 1.5 cm**
9.54 14.8 FUD 090 J G2
AMA: 2018,Sep,7

\# **26111** **1.5 cm or greater**
11.9 11.9 FUD 090 J G2 80
AMA: 2018,Sep,7

26116 **Excision, tumor, soft tissue, or vascular malformation, of hand or finger, subfascial (eg, intramuscular); less than 1.5 cm**
15.1 15.1 FUD 090 J G2
AMA: 2018,Sep,7; 2018,Jan,8; 2017,Jan,8; 2016,Jan,13; 2015,Jan,16; 2014,Jan,11

\# **26113** **1.5 cm or greater**
15.7 15.7 FUD 090 J G2 80
AMA: 2018,Sep,7

26117 **Radical resection of tumor (eg, sarcoma), soft tissue of hand or finger; less than 3 cm**
21.3 21.3 FUD 090 J G2
AMA: 2018,Sep,7

26118 **3 cm or greater**
30.2 30.2 FUD 090 J G2 80
AMA: 2018,Sep,7

26121-26236 Procedures of Bones, Fascia, Joints and Tendons Hands and Fingers

26121 **Fasciectomy, palm only, with or without Z-plasty, other local tissue rearrangement, or skin grafting (includes obtaining graft)**
EXCLUDES *Enzyme injection fasciotomy (20527, 26341)*
Fasciotomy (26040, 26045)
17.1 17.1 FUD 090 J A2 50
AMA: 2018,Sep,7; 2018,Jan,8; 2017,Jan,8; 2016,Jan,13; 2015,Jan,16; 2014,Jan,11

26123 **Fasciectomy, partial palmar with release of single digit including proximal interphalangeal joint, with or without Z-plasty, other local tissue rearrangement, or skin grafting (includes obtaining graft);**
EXCLUDES *Enzyme injection fasciotomy (20527, 26341)*
Fasciotomy (26040, 26045)
24.0 24.0 FUD 090 J A2 50
AMA: 2018,Sep,7; 2018,Jan,8; 2017,Jan,8; 2016,Jan,13; 2015,Jan,16; 2014,Jan,11

+ **26125** **each additional digit (List separately in addition to code for primary procedure)**

EXCLUDES *Enzyme injection fasciotomy (20527, 26341)*
Fasciotomy (26040, 26045)

Code first (26123)

7.89 7.89 FUD ZZZ N N1

AMA: 2018,Sep,7; 2018,Jan,8; 2017,Jan,8; 2016,Jan,13; 2015,Jan,16; 2014,Jan,11

26130 **Synovectomy, carpometacarpal joint**

13.1 13.1 FUD 090 J A2 50

AMA: 2018,Sep,7

26135 **Synovectomy, metacarpophalangeal joint including intrinsic release and extensor hood reconstruction, each digit**

15.8 15.8 FUD 090 J A2 80

AMA: 2018,Sep,7

26140 **Synovectomy, proximal interphalangeal joint, including extensor reconstruction, each interphalangeal joint**

14.5 14.5 FUD 090 J A2

AMA: 2018,Sep,7

26145 **Synovectomy, tendon sheath, radical (tenosynovectomy), flexor tendon, palm and/or finger, each tendon**

EXCLUDES *Wrist synovectomy (25115-25116)*

14.7 14.7 FUD 090 J A2

AMA: 2018,Sep,7

26160 **Excision of lesion of tendon sheath or joint capsule (eg, cyst, mucous cyst, or ganglion), hand or finger**

EXCLUDES *Trigger finger (26055)*
Wrist ganglion removal (25111-25112)

9.59 16.6 FUD 090 J A2

AMA: 2019,Jul,10; 2018,Sep,7

26170 **Excision of tendon, palm, flexor or extensor, single, each tendon**

EXCLUDES *Excision extensor tendon, with implantation of synthetic rod for delayed tendon graft, hand or finger, each rod (26415)*
Excision flexor tendon, with implantation of synthetic rod for delayed tendon graft, hand or finger, each rod (26390)

11.6 11.6 FUD 090 J A2 80

AMA: 2018,Sep,7; 2018,Jan,8; 2017,Jan,8; 2016,Jan,13; 2015,Jan,16

26180 **Excision of tendon, finger, flexor or extensor, each tendon**

EXCLUDES *Excision extensor tendon, with implantation of synthetic rod for delayed tendon graft, hand or finger, each rod (26390)*
Excision flexor tendon, with implantation of synthetic rod for delayed tendon graft, hand or finger, each rod (26390)

12.7 12.7 FUD 090 J A2 80

AMA: 2018,Sep,7

26185 **Sesamoidectomy, thumb or finger (separate procedure)**

15.8 15.8 FUD 090 J A2 80 50

AMA: 2018,Sep,7

26200 **Excision or curettage of bone cyst or benign tumor of metacarpal;**

12.9 12.9 FUD 090 J A2 80

AMA: 2018,Sep,7

26205 **with autograft (includes obtaining graft)**

17.3 17.3 FUD 090 J A2

AMA: 2018,Sep,7

26210 **Excision or curettage of bone cyst or benign tumor of proximal, middle, or distal phalanx of finger;**

12.7 12.7 FUD 090 J A2

AMA: 2018,Sep,7

26215 **with autograft (includes obtaining graft)**

16.2 16.2 FUD 090 J A2

AMA: 2018,Sep,7

26230 **Partial excision (craterization, saucerization, or diaphysectomy) bone (eg, osteomyelitis); metacarpal**

14.3 14.3 FUD 090 J A2 80

AMA: 2018,Sep,7

26235 **proximal or middle phalanx of finger**

14.1 14.1 FUD 090 J A2 80

AMA: 2019,Jul,10; 2018,Sep,7

26236 **distal phalanx of finger**

12.6 12.6 FUD 090 J A2

AMA: 2019,Jul,10; 2018,Sep,7

26250-26262 Radical Resection Bone Tumor of Hand/Finger

INCLUDES Any necessary elevation of tissue planes or dissection
Excision of adjacent soft tissue during bone tumor resection (26111-26118 [26111, 26113])
Measurement of tumor and necessary margin at greatest diameter prior to excision
Resection of the tumor (may include entire bone) and wide margins of normal tissue primarily for malignant or aggressive benign tumors
Simple and intermediate repairs

EXCLUDES *Complex repair*
Significant exploration of vessels, neuroplasty, reconstruction, or complex bone repair

26250 **Radical resection of tumor, metacarpal**

30.8 30.8 FUD 090 J A2 80

AMA: 2018,Sep,7

26260 **Radical resection of tumor, proximal or middle phalanx of finger**

23.1 23.1 FUD 090 J A2 80

AMA: 2018,Sep,7

26262 **Radical resection of tumor, distal phalanx of finger**

18.2 18.2 FUD 090 J A2 80

AMA: 2018,Sep,7

26320 Implant Removal Hand/Finger

26320 **Removal of implant from finger or hand**

EXCLUDES *Excision of foreign body (20520, 20525)*

9.98 9.98 FUD 090 Q2 A2

AMA: 2018,Sep,7

26340-26548 Repair/Reconstruction of Fingers and Hand

26340 **Manipulation, finger joint, under anesthesia, each joint**

EXCLUDES *Application external fixation (20690, 20692)*

9.67 9.67 FUD 090 J G2 50

AMA: 2018,Sep,7; 2018,Jan,8; 2017,Jan,8; 2016,Jan,13; 2015,Jan,16; 2014,Jan,11

26341 **Manipulation, palmar fascial cord (ie, Dupuytren's cord), post enzyme injection (eg, collagenase), single cord**

EXCLUDES *Enzyme injection fasciotomy (20527)*

Code also custom orthotic fabrication and/or fitting

2.17 2.90 FUD 010 T P3 50

AMA: 2018,Sep,7; 2018,Jan,8; 2017,Jan,8; 2016,Jan,13; 2015,Jan,16; 2014,Jan,11

26350 **Repair or advancement, flexor tendon, not in zone 2 digital flexor tendon sheath (eg, no man's land); primary or secondary without free graft, each tendon**

20.0 20.0 FUD 090 J A2

AMA: 2018,Sep,7

26352 **secondary with free graft (includes obtaining graft), each tendon**

23.0 23.0 FUD 090 J A2 80

AMA: 2018,Sep,7

26356 **Repair or advancement, flexor tendon, in zone 2 digital flexor tendon sheath (eg, no man's land); primary, without free graft, each tendon**

22.8 22.8 FUD 090 J A2

AMA: 2018,Sep,7; 2018,Jan,8; 2017,Dec,14; 2017,Jan,8; 2016,Jan,13; 2015,Jan,16; 2014,Sep,13; 2014,Jan,11

26357 secondary, without free graft, each tendon
25.5 25.5 FUD 090 J A2 80
AMA: 2018,Sep,7

26358 secondary, with free graft (includes obtaining graft), each tendon
28.3 28.3 FUD 090 J A2 80
AMA: 2018,Sep,7

26370 Repair or advancement of profundus tendon, with intact superficialis tendon; primary, each tendon
21.2 21.2 FUD 090 J A2 80
AMA: 2018,Sep,7; 2018,Jan,8; 2017,Jan,8; 2016,Jan,13; 2015,Jan,16; 2014,Jan,11

26372 secondary with free graft (includes obtaining graft), each tendon
25.0 25.0 FUD 090 J A2 80
AMA: 2018,Sep,7

26373 secondary without free graft, each tendon
23.9 23.9 FUD 090 J A2 80
AMA: 2018,Sep,7

26390 Excision flexor tendon, with implantation of synthetic rod for delayed tendon graft, hand or finger, each rod
23.6 23.6 FUD 090 J A2 80
AMA: 2018,Sep,7

26392 Removal of synthetic rod and insertion of flexor tendon graft, hand or finger (includes obtaining graft), each rod
27.5 27.5 FUD 090 J A2 80
AMA: 2018,Sep,7

26410 Repair, extensor tendon, hand, primary or secondary; without free graft, each tendon
15.8 15.8 FUD 090 J A2
AMA: 2018,Sep,7

26412 with free graft (includes obtaining graft), each tendon
19.1 19.1 FUD 090 J A2 80
AMA: 2018,Sep,7

26415 Excision of extensor tendon, with implantation of synthetic rod for delayed tendon graft, hand or finger, each rod
23.0 23.0 FUD 090 J A2 80
AMA: 2018,Sep,7

26416 Removal of synthetic rod and insertion of extensor tendon graft (includes obtaining graft), hand or finger, each rod
25.0 25.0 FUD 090 J A2
AMA: 2018,Sep,7; 2018,Jan,8; 2017,Jan,8; 2016,Jan,13; 2015,Jan,16; 2014,Jan,11

26418 Repair, extensor tendon, finger, primary or secondary; without free graft, each tendon
16.2 16.2 FUD 090 J A2
AMA: 2018,Sep,7; 2018,Jan,8; 2017,Jan,8; 2016,Jan,13; 2015,Jan,16; 2014,Jan,11

26420 with free graft (includes obtaining graft) each tendon
19.9 19.9 FUD 090 J A2 80
AMA: 2018,Sep,7

26426 Repair of extensor tendon, central slip, secondary (eg, boutonniere deformity); using local tissue(s), including lateral band(s), each finger
14.4 14.4 FUD 090 J A2
AMA: 2018,Sep,7

26428 with free graft (includes obtaining graft), each finger
21.3 21.3 FUD 090 J A2 80
AMA: 2018,Sep,7

26432 Closed treatment of distal extensor tendon insertion, with or without percutaneous pinning (eg, mallet finger)
13.9 13.9 FUD 090 J A2
AMA: 2018,Sep,7

26433 Repair of extensor tendon, distal insertion, primary or secondary; without graft (eg, mallet finger)
EXCLUDES *Trigger finger (26055)*
14.8 14.8 FUD 090 J A2
AMA: 2018,Sep,7

26434 with free graft (includes obtaining graft)
EXCLUDES *Trigger finger (26055)*
18.2 18.2 FUD 090 J A2 80
AMA: 2018,Sep,7

26437 Realignment of extensor tendon, hand, each tendon
17.5 17.5 FUD 090 J A2
AMA: 2018,Sep,7

26440 Tenolysis, flexor tendon; palm OR finger, each tendon
17.4 17.4 FUD 090 J A2
AMA: 2018,Sep,7; 2018,Jan,8; 2017,Jan,8; 2016,Jan,13; 2015,Jun,10; 2015,Jan,16; 2014,Jan,11

26442 palm AND finger, each tendon
27.1 27.1 FUD 090 J A2
AMA: 2018,Sep,7

26445 Tenolysis, extensor tendon, hand OR finger, each tendon
16.1 16.1 FUD 090 J A2
AMA: 2018,Sep,7; 2018,Jan,8; 2017,Jan,8; 2016,Jan,13; 2015,Jan,16; 2014,Jan,11

26449 Tenolysis, complex, extensor tendon, finger, including forearm, each tendon
19.9 19.9 FUD 090 J A2 80
AMA: 2018,Sep,7

26450 Tenotomy, flexor, palm, open, each tendon
11.4 11.4 FUD 090 J A2 80
AMA: 2018,Sep,7

26455 Tenotomy, flexor, finger, open, each tendon
11.3 11.3 FUD 090 J A2 80
AMA: 2018,Sep,7

26460 Tenotomy, extensor, hand or finger, open, each tendon
11.1 11.1 FUD 090 J A2
AMA: 2018,Sep,7

26471 Tenodesis; of proximal interphalangeal joint, each joint
17.3 17.3 FUD 090 J A2 80
AMA: 2018,Sep,7

26474 of distal joint, each joint
16.9 16.9 FUD 090 J A2 80
AMA: 2018,Sep,7

26476 Lengthening of tendon, extensor, hand or finger, each tendon
16.7 16.7 FUD 090 J A2
AMA: 2018,Sep,7

26477 Shortening of tendon, extensor, hand or finger, each tendon
16.3 16.3 FUD 090 J A2
AMA: 2018,Sep,7

26478 Lengthening of tendon, flexor, hand or finger, each tendon
17.4 17.4 FUD 090 J A2 80
AMA: 2018,Sep,7; 2018,Jan,8; 2017,Jan,8; 2016,Jan,13; 2015,Jan,16; 2014,Jan,11

26479 Shortening of tendon, flexor, hand or finger, each tendon
17.6 17.6 FUD 090 J A2 80
AMA: 2018,Sep,7

26480 Transfer or transplant of tendon, carpometacarpal area or dorsum of hand; without free graft, each tendon
21.1 21.1 FUD 090 J A2 80
AMA: 2018,Sep,7; 2018,Jan,8; 2017,Jan,8; 2016,Jan,13; 2015,Jan,16; 2014,Jan,11

26483 with free tendon graft (includes obtaining graft), each tendon
23.7 23.7 FUD 090 J A2 80
AMA: 2018,Sep,7

26485 Transfer or transplant of tendon, palmar; without free tendon graft, each tendon
22.7 22.7 FUD 090 J A2 80
AMA: 2018,Sep,7

26489 with free tendon graft (includes obtaining graft), each tendon
26.4 26.4 FUD 090 J A2 80
AMA: 2018,Sep,7

26490 Opponensplasty; superficialis tendon transfer type, each tendon
EXCLUDES *Thumb fusion (26820)*
22.5 22.5 FUD 090 J A2 80
AMA: 2018,Sep,7

26492 tendon transfer with graft (includes obtaining graft), each tendon
EXCLUDES *Thumb fusion (26820)*
25.0 25.0 FUD 090 J A2 80
AMA: 2018,Sep,7

26494 hypothenar muscle transfer
EXCLUDES *Thumb fusion (26820)*
22.6 22.6 FUD 090 J A2 80
AMA: 2018,Sep,7

26496 other methods
EXCLUDES *Thumb fusion (26820)*
24.2 24.2 FUD 090 J A2 80
AMA: 2018,Sep,7

26497 Transfer of tendon to restore intrinsic function; ring and small finger
24.5 24.5 FUD 090 J A2 80
AMA: 2018,Sep,7

26498 all 4 fingers
32.5 32.5 FUD 090 J A2 80
AMA: 2018,Sep,7

26499 Correction claw finger, other methods
23.5 23.5 FUD 090 J A2 80
AMA: 2018,Sep,7

26500 Reconstruction of tendon pulley, each tendon; with local tissues (separate procedure)
17.4 17.4 FUD 090 J A2 80
AMA: 2018,Sep,7

26502 with tendon or fascial graft (includes obtaining graft) (separate procedure)
20.0 20.0 FUD 090 J A2 80
AMA: 2018,Sep,7

26508 Release of thenar muscle(s) (eg, thumb contracture)
17.7 17.7 FUD 090 J A2 80 50
AMA: 2018,Sep,7

26510 Cross intrinsic transfer, each tendon
16.7 16.7 FUD 090 J A2 80
AMA: 2018,Sep,7

26516 Capsulodesis, metacarpophalangeal joint; single digit
19.7 19.7 FUD 090 J A2 80 50
AMA: 2018,Sep,7

26517 2 digits
23.3 23.3 FUD 090 J A2 80 50
AMA: 2018,Sep,7

26518 3 or 4 digits
23.6 23.6 FUD 090 J A2 80 50
AMA: 2018,Sep,7

26520 Capsulectomy or capsulotomy; metacarpophalangeal joint, each joint
EXCLUDES *Carpometacarpal joint arthroplasty (25447)*
18.2 18.2 FUD 090 J A2
AMA: 2018,Sep,7

26525 interphalangeal joint, each joint
EXCLUDES *Carpometacarpal joint arthroplasty (25447)*
18.3 18.3 FUD 090 J A2
AMA: 2018,Sep,7; 2018,Jan,8; 2017,Jan,8; 2016,Jan,13; 2015,Jun,10; 2015,Jan,16; 2014,Jan,11

26530 Arthroplasty, metacarpophalangeal joint; each joint
EXCLUDES *Carpometacarpal joint arthroplasty (25447)*
15.4 15.4 FUD 090 J A2 80
AMA: 2018,Sep,7

26531 with prosthetic implant, each joint
EXCLUDES *Carpometacarpal joint arthroplasty (25447)*
17.9 17.9 FUD 090 J J8 80
AMA: 2018,Sep,7; 2018,Jan,8; 2017,Jan,8; 2016,Jan,13; 2015,Jan,16; 2014,Jan,11

26535 Arthroplasty, interphalangeal joint; each joint
EXCLUDES *Carpometacarpal joint arthroplasty (25447)*
12.3 12.3 FUD 090 J A2
AMA: 2018,Sep,7

26536 with prosthetic implant, each joint
EXCLUDES *Carpometacarpal joint arthroplasty (25447)*
20.0 20.0 FUD 090 J J8 80
AMA: 2018,Sep,7

26540 Repair of collateral ligament, metacarpophalangeal or interphalangeal joint
18.5 18.5 FUD 090 J A2 80
AMA: 2018,Sep,7

26541 Reconstruction, collateral ligament, metacarpophalangeal joint, single; with tendon or fascial graft (includes obtaining graft)
22.5 22.5 FUD 090 J A2 80
AMA: 2018,Sep,7; 2018,Jan,8; 2017,Jan,8; 2016,Jan,13; 2015,Jan,16; 2014,Jan,11

26542 with local tissue (eg, adductor advancement)
19.1 19.1 FUD 090 J A2 80
AMA: 2018,Sep,7; 2018,Jan,8; 2017,Jan,8; 2016,Jan,13; 2015,Jan,16; 2014,Jan,11

26545 Reconstruction, collateral ligament, interphalangeal joint, single, including graft, each joint
19.9 19.9 FUD 090 J A2 80
AMA: 2018,Sep,7

26546 Repair non-union, metacarpal or phalanx (includes obtaining bone graft with or without external or internal fixation)
28.1 28.1 FUD 090 J A2 80 50
AMA: 2018,Sep,7

26548 Repair and reconstruction, finger, volar plate, interphalangeal joint
21.4 21.4 FUD 090 J A2 80
AMA: 2018,Sep,7

26550-26556 Reconstruction Procedures with Finger and Toe Transplants

26550 Pollicization of a digit
46.8 46.8 FUD 090 J A2 80 50
AMA: 2018,Sep,7

26551 Transfer, toe-to-hand with microvascular anastomosis; great toe wrap-around with bone graft
INCLUDES Operating microscope (69990)
EXCLUDES *Big toe with web space (20973)*
94.6 94.6 FUD 090 C 80 50
AMA: 2018,Sep,7; 2018,Jan,8; 2017,Jan,8; 2016,Feb,12; 2016,Jan,13; 2015,Jan,16; 2014,Jan,11

26553 other than great toe, single
INCLUDES Operating microscope (69990)
93.9 93.9 FUD 090 C 80 50
AMA: 2018,Sep,7; 2018,Jan,8; 2017,Jan,8; 2016,Feb,12; 2016,Jan,13; 2015,Jan,16; 2014,Jan,11

26554 other than great toe, double
INCLUDES Operating microscope (69990)
109. 109. FUD 090 C 80 50
AMA: 2018,Sep,7; 2018,Jan,8; 2017,Jan,8; 2016,Feb,12; 2016,Jan,13; 2015,Jan,16; 2014,Jan,11

26555 Transfer, finger to another position without microvascular anastomosis
38.9 38.9 FUD 090 J A2 80
AMA: 2018,Sep,7

26556 Transfer, free toe joint, with microvascular anastomosis
INCLUDES Operating microscope (69990)
EXCLUDES *Big toe to hand transfer (20973)*
97.6 97.6 FUD 090 C 80
AMA: 2018,Sep,7; 2018,Jan,8; 2017,Jan,8; 2016,Feb,12; 2016,Jan,13; 2015,Jan,16; 2014,Jan,11

26560-26596 Repair of Other Deformities of the Fingers/Hand

26560 Repair of syndactyly (web finger) each web space; with skin flaps
16.5 16.5 FUD 090 J A2 80
AMA: 2018,Sep,7

26561 with skin flaps and grafts
26.8 26.8 FUD 090 J A2 80
AMA: 2018,Sep,7

26562 complex (eg, involving bone, nails)
38.1 38.1 FUD 090 J A2 80
AMA: 2018,Sep,7

26565 Osteotomy; metacarpal, each
19.0 19.0 FUD 090 J A2 80
AMA: 2018,Sep,7

26567 phalanx of finger, each
19.2 19.2 FUD 090 J A2 80
AMA: 2018,Sep,7; 2018,Jan,8; 2017,Jan,8; 2016,Jan,13; 2015,Jan,16; 2014,Jan,11

26568 Osteoplasty, lengthening, metacarpal or phalanx
25.4 25.4 FUD 090 J A2 80
AMA: 2018,Sep,7

26580 Repair cleft hand
INCLUDES Barsky's procedure
43.0 43.0 FUD 090 J A2 80 50
AMA: 2018,Sep,7

26587 Reconstruction of polydactylous digit, soft tissue and bone
EXCLUDES *Soft tissue removal only (11200)*
30.0 30.0 FUD 090 J A2 80
AMA: 2018,Sep,7; 2018,Jan,8; 2017,Jan,8; 2016,Jan,13; 2015,Jan,16; 2014,Jan,11

26590 Repair macrodactylia, each digit
40.0 40.0 FUD 090 J A2 80
AMA: 2018,Sep,7; 2018,Jan,8; 2017,Jan,8; 2016,Jan,13; 2015,Jan,16; 2014,Jan,11

26591 Repair, intrinsic muscles of hand, each muscle
12.3 12.3 FUD 090 J A2 80
AMA: 2018,Sep,7; 2018,Jan,8; 2017,Jan,8; 2016,Jan,13; 2015,Jan,16; 2014,Jan,11

26593 Release, intrinsic muscles of hand, each muscle
16.9 16.9 FUD 090 J A2
AMA: 2018,Sep,7

26596 Excision of constricting ring of finger, with multiple Z-plasties
EXCLUDES *Graft repair or scar contracture release (11042, 14040-14041, 15120, 15240)*
21.6 21.6 FUD 090 J A2 80
AMA: 2018,Sep,7

26600-26785 Treatment of Fracture/Dislocation of Fingers and Hand

INCLUDES Closed, percutaneous, and open treatment of fractures or dislocations

26600 Closed treatment of metacarpal fracture, single; without manipulation, each bone
7.94 8.39 FUD 090 T P2
AMA: 2018,Sep,7

26605 with manipulation, each bone
8.38 9.24 FUD 090 T A2
AMA: 2018,Sep,7

26607 Closed treatment of metacarpal fracture, with manipulation, with external fixation, each bone
13.4 13.4 FUD 090 J A2 80
AMA: 2018,Sep,7

26608 Percutaneous skeletal fixation of metacarpal fracture, each bone
13.7 13.7 FUD 090 J A2 80
AMA: 2018,Sep,7

26615 Open treatment of metacarpal fracture, single, includes internal fixation, when performed, each bone
16.5 16.5 FUD 090 J A2
AMA: 2018,Sep,7

26641 Closed treatment of carpometacarpal dislocation, thumb, with manipulation
9.72 10.7 FUD 090 T P2 80 50
AMA: 2018,Sep,7

26645 Closed treatment of carpometacarpal fracture dislocation, thumb (Bennett fracture), with manipulation
11.2 12.3 FUD 090 J A2 80 50
AMA: 2018,Sep,7

26650 Percutaneous skeletal fixation of carpometacarpal fracture dislocation, thumb (Bennett fracture), with manipulation
13.7 13.7 FUD 090 J A2 50
AMA: 2018,Sep,7

26665 Open treatment of carpometacarpal fracture dislocation, thumb (Bennett fracture), includes internal fixation, when performed
17.9 17.9 FUD 090 J A2 50
AMA: 2018,Sep,7

26670 Closed treatment of carpometacarpal dislocation, other than thumb, with manipulation, each joint; without anesthesia
8.86 9.86 FUD 090 T P2 80
AMA: 2018,Sep,7

26675 requiring anesthesia
12.0 13.1 FUD 090 J A2 80
AMA: 2018,Sep,7

26676 Percutaneous skeletal fixation of carpometacarpal dislocation, other than thumb, with manipulation, each joint
14.4 14.4 FUD 090 J A2
AMA: 2018,Sep,7

26685 Open treatment of carpometacarpal dislocation, other than thumb; includes internal fixation, when performed, each joint
16.4 16.4 FUD 090 J A2
AMA: 2018,Sep,7

26686 complex, multiple, or delayed reduction
17.9 17.9 FUD 090 J A2 80
AMA: 2018,Sep,7

26700 **Closed treatment of metacarpophalangeal dislocation, single, with manipulation; without anesthesia**
8.73 9.38 FUD 090 T P2
AMA: 2018,Sep,7

26705 **requiring anesthesia**
10.9 11.9 FUD 090 J A2 80
AMA: 2018,Sep,7

26706 **Percutaneous skeletal fixation of metacarpophalangeal dislocation, single, with manipulation**
12.6 12.6 FUD 090 J A2
AMA: 2018,Sep,7

26715 **Open treatment of metacarpophalangeal dislocation, single, includes internal fixation, when performed**
16.4 16.4 FUD 090 J A2 80
AMA: 2018,Sep,7

26720 **Closed treatment of phalangeal shaft fracture, proximal or middle phalanx, finger or thumb; without manipulation, each**
5.26 5.62 FUD 090 T P2
AMA: 2018,Sep,7

26725 **with manipulation, with or without skin or skeletal traction, each**
8.66 9.66 FUD 090 T P2
AMA: 2018,Sep,7

26727 **Percutaneous skeletal fixation of unstable phalangeal shaft fracture, proximal or middle phalanx, finger or thumb, with manipulation, each**
13.5 13.5 FUD 090 J A2
AMA: 2018,Sep,7

26735 **Open treatment of phalangeal shaft fracture, proximal or middle phalanx, finger or thumb, includes internal fixation, when performed, each**
17.1 17.1 FUD 090 J A2
AMA: 2018,Sep,7

26740 **Closed treatment of articular fracture, involving metacarpophalangeal or interphalangeal joint; without manipulation, each**
6.19 6.56 FUD 090 T P2
AMA: 2018,Sep,7

26742 **with manipulation, each**
9.57 10.6 FUD 090 J A2
AMA: 2018,Sep,7

26746 **Open treatment of articular fracture, involving metacarpophalangeal or interphalangeal joint, includes internal fixation, when performed, each**
21.3 21.3 FUD 090 J A2
AMA: 2018,Sep,7

26750 **Closed treatment of distal phalangeal fracture, finger or thumb; without manipulation, each**
5.28 5.25 FUD 090 T P3
AMA: 2018,Sep,7

26755 **with manipulation, each**
7.77 8.99 FUD 090 T G2
AMA: 2018,Sep,7

26756 **Percutaneous skeletal fixation of distal phalangeal fracture, finger or thumb, each**
11.9 11.9 FUD 090 J A2 80
AMA: 2018,Sep,7

26765 **Open treatment of distal phalangeal fracture, finger or thumb, includes internal fixation, when performed, each**
14.3 14.3 FUD 090 J A2
AMA: 2018,Sep,7

26770 **Closed treatment of interphalangeal joint dislocation, single, with manipulation; without anesthesia**
7.29 7.94 FUD 090 T G2
AMA: 2018,Sep,7

26775 **requiring anesthesia**
9.91 10.9 FUD 090 T P2
AMA: 2018,Sep,7

26776 **Percutaneous skeletal fixation of interphalangeal joint dislocation, single, with manipulation**
12.7 12.7 FUD 090 J A2
AMA: 2018,Sep,7

26785 **Open treatment of interphalangeal joint dislocation, includes internal fixation, when performed, single**
15.7 15.7 FUD 090 J A2
AMA: 2018,Sep,7

26820-26863 Fusion of Joint(s) of Fingers or Hand

26820 **Fusion in opposition, thumb, with autogenous graft (includes obtaining graft)**
22.2 22.2 FUD 090 J J8 80 50
AMA: 2018,Sep,7

26841 **Arthrodesis, carpometacarpal joint, thumb, with or without internal fixation;**
20.4 20.4 FUD 090 J A2 80 50
AMA: 2018,Sep,7

26842 **with autograft (includes obtaining graft)**
22.0 22.0 FUD 090 J A2 80 50
AMA: 2018,Sep,7

26843 **Arthrodesis, carpometacarpal joint, digit, other than thumb, each;**
20.8 20.8 FUD 090 J A2 80
AMA: 2018,Sep,7; 2018,Jan,8; 2017,Jan,8; 2016,Jan,13; 2015,Jan,16; 2014,Jan,11

26844 **with autograft (includes obtaining graft)**
23.1 23.1 FUD 090 J J8 80
AMA: 2018,Sep,7

26850 **Arthrodesis, metacarpophalangeal joint, with or without internal fixation;**
19.4 19.4 FUD 090 J A2 80
AMA: 2018,Sep,7

26852 **with autograft (includes obtaining graft)**
22.4 22.4 FUD 090 J A2 80
AMA: 2018,Sep,7

26860 **Arthrodesis, interphalangeal joint, with or without internal fixation;**
15.9 15.9 FUD 090 J A2
AMA: 2018,Sep,7; 2018,Jan,8; 2017,Jan,8; 2016,Jan,13; 2015,Jan,16; 2014,Jan,11

+ 26861 **each additional interphalangeal joint (List separately in addition to code for primary procedure)**
Code first (26860)
2.98 2.98 FUD ZZZ N N1
AMA: 2018,Sep,7; 2018,Jan,8; 2017,Jan,8; 2016,Jan,13; 2015,Jan,16; 2014,Jan,11

26862 **with autograft (includes obtaining graft)**
20.4 20.4 FUD 090 J A2 80
AMA: 2018,Sep,7

+ 26863 **with autograft (includes obtaining graft), each additional joint (List separately in addition to code for primary procedure)**
Code first (26862)
6.64 6.64 FUD ZZZ N N1 80
AMA: 2018,Sep,7

26910-26989 Amputations and Unlisted Procedures Finger/Hand

26910 **Amputation, metacarpal, with finger or thumb (ray amputation), single, with or without interosseous transfer**
EXCLUDES *Repositioning (26550, 26555)*
Transmetacarpal amputation of hand (25927)
20.4 20.4 FUD 090 J A2
AMA: 2018,Sep,7

26951 **Amputation, finger or thumb, primary or secondary, any joint or phalanx, single, including neurectomies; with direct closure**
EXCLUDES *Repair necessitating flaps or grafts (15050-15758)*
Transmetacarpal amputation of hand (25927)
18.4 18.4 FUD 090 J A2
AMA: 2018,Sep,7

26952 **with local advancement flaps (V-Y, hood)**
EXCLUDES *Repair necessitating flaps or grafts (15050-15758)*
Transmetacarpal amputation of hand (25927)
18.1 18.1 FUD 090 J A2
AMA: 2018,Sep,7

26989 **Unlisted procedure, hands or fingers**
0.00 0.00 FUD YYY T
AMA: 2018,Sep,7

26990-26992 Incision for Drainage of Pelvis or Hip

EXCLUDES *Simple incision and drainage procedures (10040-10160)*

26990 **Incision and drainage, pelvis or hip joint area; deep abscess or hematoma**
18.3 18.3 FUD 090 J A2
AMA: 2018,Sep,7

26991 **infected bursa**
15.0 20.2 FUD 090 J A2 80
AMA: 2018,Sep,7

26992 **Incision, bone cortex, pelvis and/or hip joint (eg, osteomyelitis or bone abscess)**
27.9 27.9 FUD 090 C 80
AMA: 2018,Sep,7; 2018,Jan,8; 2017,Jan,8; 2016,Jan,13; 2015,Jan,16; 2014,Jan,11

27000-27006 Tenotomy Procedures of Hip

27000 **Tenotomy, adductor of hip, percutaneous (separate procedure)**
11.6 11.6 FUD 090 J A2 50
AMA: 2018,Sep,7

27001 **Tenotomy, adductor of hip, open**
15.4 15.4 FUD 090 J A2 80 50
AMA: 2018,Sep,7

27003 **Tenotomy, adductor, subcutaneous, open, with obturator neurectomy**
17.0 17.0 FUD 090 J A2 80 50
AMA: 2018,Sep,7

27005 **Tenotomy, hip flexor(s), open (separate procedure)**
20.8 20.8 FUD 090 C 80 50
AMA: 2018,Sep,7

27006 **Tenotomy, abductors and/or extensor(s) of hip, open (separate procedure)**
20.7 20.7 FUD 090 J 80 50
AMA: 2018,Sep,7

27025-27036 Surgical Incision of Hip

27025 **Fasciotomy, hip or thigh, any type**
26.3 26.3 FUD 090 C 80 50
AMA: 2018,Sep,7

27027 **Decompression fasciotomy(ies), pelvic (buttock) compartment(s) (eg, gluteus medius-minimus, gluteus maximus, iliopsoas, and/or tensor fascia lata muscle), unilateral**
25.4 25.4 FUD 090 J 80 50
AMA: 2018,Sep,7

27030 **Arthrotomy, hip, with drainage (eg, infection)**
27.0 27.0 FUD 090 C 80 50
AMA: 2018,Sep,7

27033 **Arthrotomy, hip, including exploration or removal of loose or foreign body**
28.0 28.0 FUD 090 J A2 80 50
AMA: 2018,Sep,7; 2018,Jan,8; 2017,Jan,8; 2016,Jan,13; 2015,Jan,16; 2014,Jan,11

27035 **Denervation, hip joint, intrapelvic or extrapelvic intra-articular branches of sciatic, femoral, or obturator nerves**
EXCLUDES *Transection of obturator nerve (64763, 64766)*
32.8 32.8 FUD 090 J A2 80 50
AMA: 2018,Sep,7; 2018,Jan,8; 2017,Jan,8; 2016,Jan,13; 2015,Jan,16; 2014,Mar,13

27036 **Capsulectomy or capsulotomy, hip, with or without excision of heterotopic bone, with release of hip flexor muscles (ie, gluteus medius, gluteus minimus, tensor fascia latae, rectus femoris, sartorius, iliopsoas)**
29.1 29.1 FUD 090 C 80 50
AMA: 2018,Sep,7

27040-27041 Biopsy of Hip/Pelvis

EXCLUDES *Soft tissue needle biopsy (20206)*

27040 **Biopsy, soft tissue of pelvis and hip area; superficial**
5.70 9.83 FUD 010 J A2 50
AMA: 2018,Sep,7

27041 **deep, subfascial or intramuscular**
20.1 20.1 FUD 090 J A2 50
AMA: 2018,Sep,7

27043-27059 [27043, 27045, 27059] Excision Soft Tissue Tumors Hip/ Pelvis

INCLUDES Any necessary elevation of tissue planes or dissection
Measurement of tumor and necessary margin at greatest diameter prior to excision
Simple and intermediate repairs
Types of excision:
- Fascial or subfascial soft tissue tumors: simple and marginal resection of tumors found either in or below the deep fascia, not involving bone or excision of a substantial amount of normal tissue; primarily benign and intramuscular tumors
- Radical resection of soft tissue tumor: wide resection of tumor involving substantial margins of normal tissue and may involve tissue removal from one or more layers; mostly malignant or aggressive benign,
- Subcutaneous: simple and marginal resection of tumors found in the subcutaneous tissue above the deep fascia; most often benign

EXCLUDES *Complex repair*
Excision of benign cutaneous lesions (eg, sebaceous cyst) (11400-11406)
Radical resection of cutaneous tumors (eg, melanoma) (11600-11606)
Significant exploration of vessels, neuroplasty, reconstruction, or complex bone repair

27043 **Resequenced code. See code following 27047.**

27045 **Resequenced code. See code following 27048.**

27047 **Excision, tumor, soft tissue of pelvis and hip area, subcutaneous; less than 3 cm**
10.4 13.6 FUD 090 J G2 50
AMA: 2018,Sep,7

27043 **3 cm or greater**
13.5 13.5 FUD 090 J G2 50
AMA: 2018,Sep,7

27048 **Excision, tumor, soft tissue of pelvis and hip area, subfascial (eg, intramuscular); less than 5 cm**
17.6 17.6 FUD 090 J G2 80 50
AMA: 2018,Sep,7

27045 **5 cm or greater**
21.3 21.3 FUD 090 J G2 80 50
AMA: 2018,Sep,7

27049 **Radical resection of tumor (eg, sarcoma), soft tissue of pelvis and hip area; less than 5 cm**
38.6 38.6 FUD 090 J G2 80 50
AMA: 2018,Sep,7

27059 5 cm or greater
52.6 52.6 FUD 090 J G2 80 50
AMA: 2018,Sep,7

27050-27071 Procedures of Bones and Joints of Hip and Pelvis

27050 Arthrotomy, with biopsy; sacroiliac joint
11.5 11.5 FUD 090 J A2 80 50
AMA: 2018,Sep,7

27052 hip joint
16.6 16.6 FUD 090 J A2 80 50
AMA: 2018,Sep,7

27054 Arthrotomy with synovectomy, hip joint
19.7 19.7 FUD 090 C 80 50
AMA: 2018,Sep,7

27057 Decompression fasciotomy(ies), pelvic (buttock) compartment(s) (eg, gluteus medius-minimus, gluteus maximus, iliopsoas, and/or tensor fascia lata muscle) with debridement of nonviable muscle, unilateral
29.2 29.2 FUD 090 J 80 50
AMA: 2018,Sep,7

27059 Resequenced code. See code following 27049.

27060 Excision; ischial bursa
13.3 13.3 FUD 090 J A2 50
AMA: 2018,Sep,7

27062 trochanteric bursa or calcification
EXCLUDES *Arthrocentesis (20610)*
13.1 13.1 FUD 090 J A2 50
AMA: 2018,Sep,7

27065 Excision of bone cyst or benign tumor, wing of ilium, symphysis pubis, or greater trochanter of femur; superficial, includes autograft, when performed
14.9 14.9 FUD 090 J A2 80 50
AMA: 2018,Sep,7

27066 deep (subfascial), includes autograft, when performed
23.1 23.1 FUD 090 J A2 80 50
AMA: 2018,Sep,7

27067 with autograft requiring separate incision
29.8 29.8 FUD 090 J A2 80 50
AMA: 2018,Sep,7

27070 Partial excision, wing of ilium, symphysis pubis, or greater trochanter of femur, (craterization, saucerization) (eg, osteomyelitis or bone abscess); superficial
24.6 24.6 FUD 090 C 80 50
AMA: 2018,Sep,7

27071 deep (subfascial or intramuscular)
26.6 26.6 FUD 090 C 80 50
AMA: 2018,Sep,7

27075-27078 Radical Resection Bone Tumor of Hip/Pelvis

INCLUDES Any necessary elevation of tissue planes or dissection
Excision of adjacent soft tissue during bone tumor resection (27043-27049 [27043, 27045, 27059])
Measurement of tumor and necessary margin at greatest diameter prior to excision
Resection of the tumor (may include entire bone) and wide margins of normal tissue primarily for malignant or aggressive benign tumors
Simple and intermediate repairs

EXCLUDES *Complex repair*
Significant exploration of vessels, neuroplasty, reconstruction, or complex bone repair

27075 Radical resection of tumor; wing of ilium, 1 pubic or ischial ramus or symphysis pubis
60.7 60.7 FUD 090 C 80
AMA: 2019,May,7; 2018,Sep,7

27076 ilium, including acetabulum, both pubic rami, or ischium and acetabulum
73.5 73.5 FUD 090 C 80
AMA: 2019,May,7; 2018,Sep,7

27077 innominate bone, total
82.0 82.0 FUD 090 C 80
AMA: 2019,May,7; 2018,Sep,7

27078 ischial tuberosity and greater trochanter of femur
59.8 59.8 FUD 090 C 80 50
AMA: 2019,May,7; 2018,Sep,7

27080 Excision of Coccyx

EXCLUDES *Surgical excision of decubitus ulcers (15920, 15922, 15931-15958)*

27080 Coccygectomy, primary
14.7 14.7 FUD 090 J A2 80
AMA: 2018,Sep,7

27086-27091 Removal Foreign Body or Hip Prosthesis

27086 Removal of foreign body, pelvis or hip; subcutaneous tissue
4.83 8.63 FUD 010 J A2 80 50
AMA: 2018,Sep,7; 2018,Jan,8; 2017,Jan,8; 2016,Jan,13; 2015,Jan,16; 2014,Jan,11

27087 deep (subfascial or intramuscular)
17.6 17.6 FUD 090 J A2 80 50
AMA: 2018,Sep,7

A foreign body is removed from the pelvis or hip

27090 Removal of hip prosthesis; (separate procedure)
23.9 23.9 FUD 090 C 80 50
AMA: 2019,May,7; 2018,Sep,7

27091 complicated, including total hip prosthesis, methylmethacrylate with or without insertion of spacer
46.0 46.0 FUD 090 C 80 50
AMA: 2019,May,7; 2018,Sep,7; 2018,Jan,8; 2017,Jan,8; 2016,Jan,13; 2015,Jan,16; 2014,Jan,11

27093-27096 Injection for Arthrogram Hip/Sacroiliac Joint

27093 Injection procedure for hip arthrography; without anesthesia
(73525)
2.01 5.72 FUD 000 N N1 50
AMA: 2018,Sep,7; 2018,Jan,8; 2017,Jan,8; 2016,Jan,13; 2015,Aug,6; 2015,Jan,16; 2014,Jan,11

27095 with anesthesia
(73525)
2.41 7.62 FUD 000 N N1 50
AMA: 2018,Sep,7; 2018,Jan,8; 2017,Jan,8; 2016,Jan,13; 2016,Jan,11; 2015,Aug,6; 2015,Jan,16; 2014,Jan,11

27096 **Injection procedure for sacroiliac joint, anesthetic/steroid, with image guidance (fluoroscopy or CT) including arthrography when performed**

INCLUDES Confirmation of intra-articular needle placement with CT or fluoroscopy
Fluoroscopic guidance (77002-77003)

EXCLUDES *Procedure performed without fluoroscopy or CT guidance (20552)*

2.38 4.56 FUD 000 B 50

AMA: 2018,Sep,7; 2018,Jan,8; 2017,Jan,8; 2016,Jan,13; 2015,Aug,6; 2015,Jan,16; 2014,Jan,11

27097-27187 Revision/Reconstruction Hip and Pelvis

INCLUDES Closed, open and percutaneous treatment of fractures and dislocations

27097 **Release or recession, hamstring, proximal**

19.6 19.6 FUD 090 J A2 80 50

AMA: 2018,Sep,7

27098 **Transfer, adductor to ischium**

20.0 20.0 FUD 090 J A2 80 50

AMA: 2018,Sep,7

27100 **Transfer external oblique muscle to greater trochanter including fascial or tendon extension (graft)**

INCLUDES Eggers procedure

23.6 23.6 FUD 090 J A2 80 50

AMA: 2018,Sep,7

27105 **Transfer paraspinal muscle to hip (includes fascial or tendon extension graft)**

25.0 25.0 FUD 090 J A2 80 50

AMA: 2018,Sep,7

27110 **Transfer iliopsoas; to greater trochanter of femur**

28.0 28.0 FUD 090 J A2 80 50

AMA: 2018,Sep,7

27111 **to femoral neck**

25.9 25.9 FUD 090 J A2 80 50

AMA: 2018,Sep,7

27120 **Acetabuloplasty; (eg, Whitman, Colonna, Haygroves, or cup type)**

37.5 37.5 FUD 090 C 80 50

AMA: 2018,Sep,7

27122 **resection, femoral head (eg, Girdlestone procedure)**

31.7 31.7 FUD 090 C 80 50

AMA: 2018,Sep,7

27125 **Hemiarthroplasty, hip, partial (eg, femoral stem prosthesis, bipolar arthroplasty)**

EXCLUDES *Hip replacement following hip fracture (27236)*

32.7 32.7 FUD 090 C 80 50

AMA: 2018,Sep,7; 2018,Jan,8; 2017,Jan,8; 2016,Jan,13; 2015,Jan,16; 2014,Jan,11

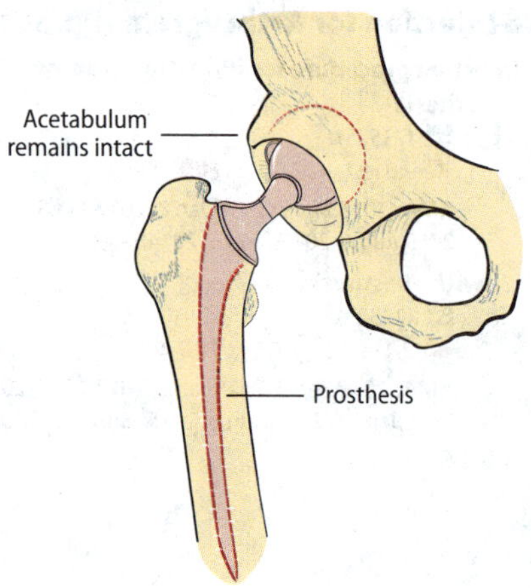

27130 **Arthroplasty, acetabular and proximal femoral prosthetic replacement (total hip arthroplasty), with or without autograft or allograft**

39.0 39.0 FUD 090 C 80 50

AMA: 2019,May,7; 2018,Sep,7; 2018,Jan,8; 2017,Jan,8; 2016,Jan,13; 2015,Jan,16; 2014,Jan,11

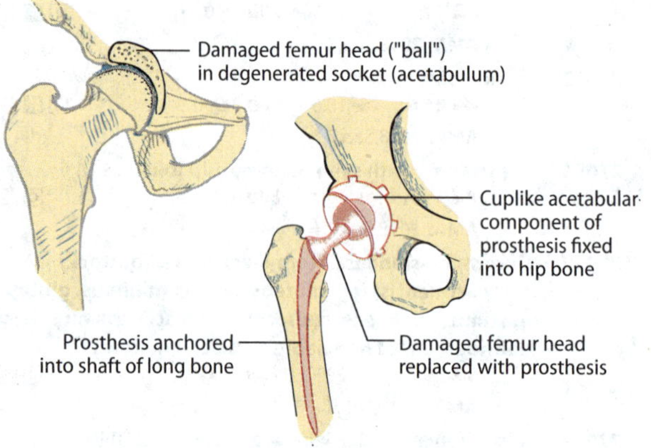

27132 **Conversion of previous hip surgery to total hip arthroplasty, with or without autograft or allograft**

48.3 48.3 FUD 090 C 80 50

AMA: 2019,May,7; 2018,Sep,7; 2018,Jan,8; 2017,Sep,14; 2017,Jan,8; 2016,Jan,13; 2015,Jan,16; 2014,Jan,11

27134 **Revision of total hip arthroplasty; both components, with or without autograft or allograft**

55.2 55.2 FUD 090 C 80 50

AMA: 2019,May,7; 2018,Sep,7; 2018,Jan,8; 2017,Jan,8; 2016,Jan,13; 2015,Jan,16; 2014,Jan,11

27137 **acetabular component only, with or without autograft or allograft**

42.4 42.4 FUD 090 C 80 50

AMA: 2018,Sep,7; 2018,Jan,8; 2017,Jan,8; 2016,Jan,13; 2015,Jan,16; 2014,Jan,11

27138 **femoral component only, with or without allograft**

44.1 44.1 FUD 090 C 80 50

AMA: 2019,May,7; 2018,Sep,7; 2018,Jan,8; 2017,Jan,8; 2016,Jan,13; 2015,Jan,16; 2014,Jan,11

27140 **Osteotomy and transfer of greater trochanter of femur (separate procedure)**

25.6 25.6 FUD 090 C 80 50

AMA: 2018,Sep,7

27146 **Osteotomy, iliac, acetabular or innominate bone;**

INCLUDES Salter osteotomy

36.8 36.8 FUD 090 C 80 50

AMA: 2018,Sep,7; 2018,Jan,8; 2017,Jan,8; 2016,Jan,13; 2015,Jan,16; 2014,Jan,11

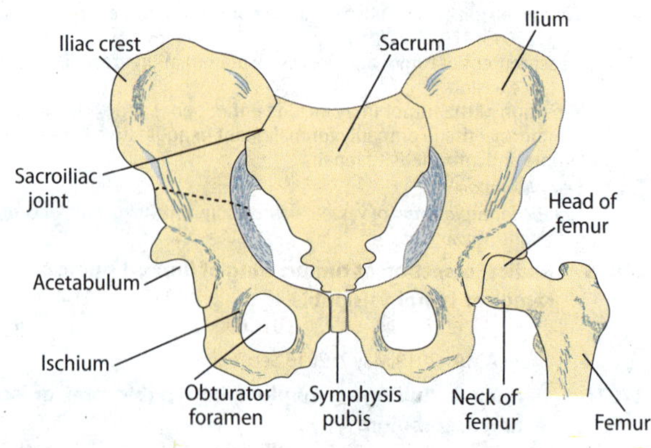

27147 with open reduction of hip

INCLUDES Pemberton osteotomy

42.4 42.4 FUD 090 C 80 50

AMA: 2018,Sep,7

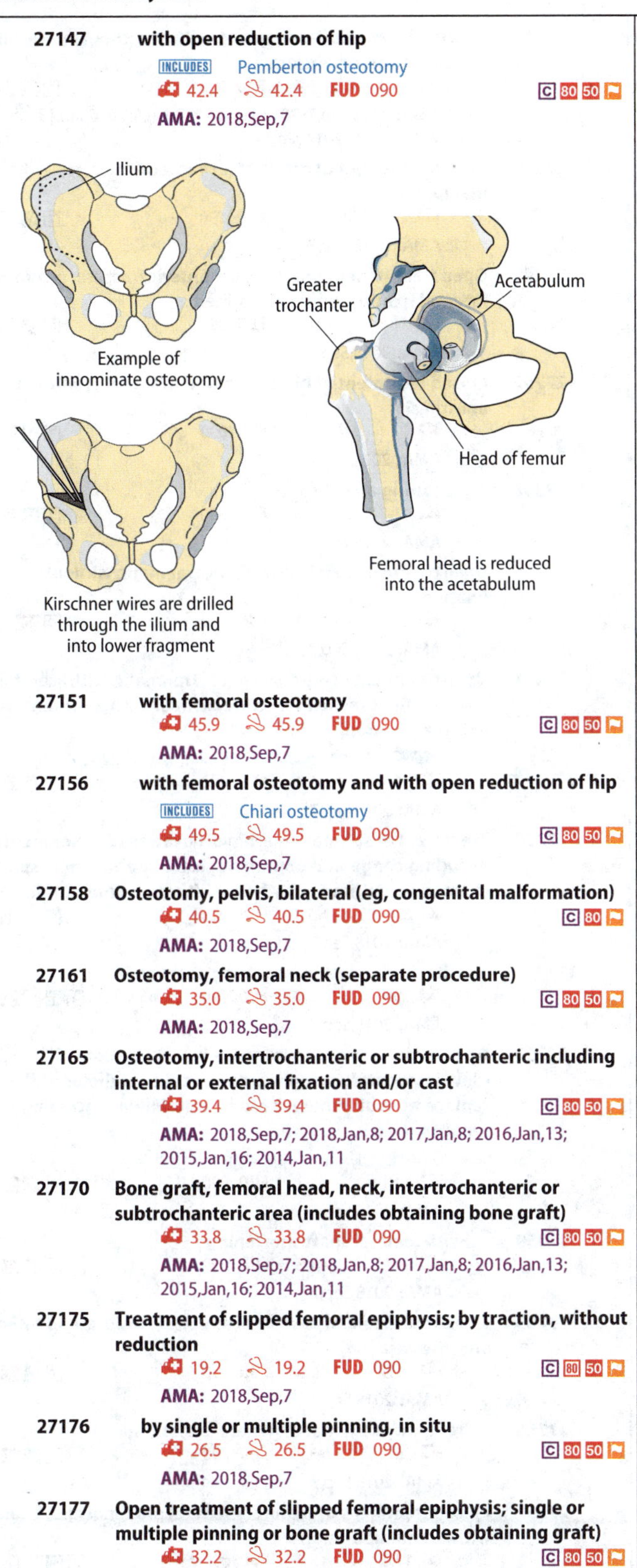

27151 with femoral osteotomy

45.9 45.9 FUD 090 C 80 50

AMA: 2018,Sep,7

27156 with femoral osteotomy and with open reduction of hip

INCLUDES Chiari osteotomy

49.5 49.5 FUD 090 C 80 50

AMA: 2018,Sep,7

27158 Osteotomy, pelvis, bilateral (eg, congenital malformation)

40.5 40.5 FUD 090 C 80

AMA: 2018,Sep,7

27161 Osteotomy, femoral neck (separate procedure)

35.0 35.0 FUD 090 C 80 50

AMA: 2018,Sep,7

27165 Osteotomy, intertrochanteric or subtrochanteric including internal or external fixation and/or cast

39.4 39.4 FUD 090 C 80 50

AMA: 2018,Sep,7; 2018,Jan,8; 2017,Jan,8; 2016,Jan,13; 2015,Jan,16; 2014,Jan,11

27170 Bone graft, femoral head, neck, intertrochanteric or subtrochanteric area (includes obtaining bone graft)

33.8 33.8 FUD 090 C 80 50

AMA: 2018,Sep,7; 2018,Jan,8; 2017,Jan,8; 2016,Jan,13; 2015,Jan,16; 2014,Jan,11

27175 Treatment of slipped femoral epiphysis; by traction, without reduction

19.2 19.2 FUD 090 C 80 50

AMA: 2018,Sep,7

27176 by single or multiple pinning, in situ

26.5 26.5 FUD 090 C 80 50

AMA: 2018,Sep,7

27177 Open treatment of slipped femoral epiphysis; single or multiple pinning or bone graft (includes obtaining graft)

32.2 32.2 FUD 090 C 80 50

AMA: 2018,Sep,7

27178 closed manipulation with single or multiple pinning

26.5 26.5 FUD 090 C 80 50

AMA: 2018,Sep,7

27179 osteoplasty of femoral neck (Heyman type procedure)

28.2 28.2 FUD 090 J 80 50

AMA: 2018,Sep,7

27181 osteotomy and internal fixation

32.4 32.4 FUD 090 C 80 50

AMA: 2018,Sep,7

27185 Epiphyseal arrest by epiphysiodesis or stapling, greater trochanter of femur

20.7 20.7 FUD 090 C 50

AMA: 2018,Sep,7

27187 Prophylactic treatment (nailing, pinning, plating or wiring) with or without methylmethacrylate, femoral neck and proximal femur

28.6 28.6 FUD 090 C 80 50

AMA: 2018,Sep,7; 2018,Jan,8; 2017,Jan,8; 2016,Jan,13; 2015,Jan,16; 2014,Jan,11

27197-27269 Treatment of Fracture/Dislocation Hip/Pelvis

27197 Closed treatment of posterior pelvic ring fracture(s), dislocation(s), diastasis or subluxation of the ilium, sacroiliac joint, and/or sacrum, with or without anterior pelvic ring fracture(s) and/or dislocation(s) of the pubic symphysis and/or superior/inferior rami, unilateral or bilateral; without manipulation

3.57 3.57 FUD 000 T G2

AMA: 2018,Sep,7; 2018,Jan,8; 2017,Jun,9

27198 with manipulation, requiring more than local anesthesia (ie, general anesthesia, moderate sedation, spinal/epidural)

EXCLUDES *Closed treatment anterior pelvic ring, pubic symphysis, inferior rami fracture/dislocation--see appropriate E&M codes*

8.67 8.67 FUD 000 T G2 80

AMA: 2018,Sep,7; 2018,Jan,3; 2018,Jan,8; 2017,Jun,9

27200 Closed treatment of coccygeal fracture

5.39 5.26 FUD 090 T P3

AMA: 2018,Sep,7

27202 Open treatment of coccygeal fracture

15.3 15.3 FUD 090 J A2 80

AMA: 2018,Sep,7

27215 Open treatment of iliac spine(s), tuberosity avulsion, or iliac wing fracture(s), unilateral, for pelvic bone fracture patterns that do not disrupt the pelvic ring, includes internal fixation, when performed

18.0 18.0 FUD 090 E

AMA: 2018,Sep,7

27216 Percutaneous skeletal fixation of posterior pelvic bone fracture and/or dislocation, for fracture patterns that disrupt the pelvic ring, unilateral (includes ipsilateral ilium, sacroiliac joint and/or sacrum)

EXCLUDES *Sacroiliac joint arthrodesis without fracture and/or dislocation, percutaneous or minimally invasive (27279)*

26.7 26.7 FUD 090 E

AMA: 2018,Sep,7; 2018,Jan,8; 2017,Jan,8; 2016,Jan,13; 2015,Jan,16; 2014,Mar,4

27217 Open treatment of anterior pelvic bone fracture and/or dislocation for fracture patterns that disrupt the pelvic ring, unilateral, includes internal fixation, when performed (includes pubic symphysis and/or ipsilateral superior/inferior rami)

25.0 25.0 FUD 090 E

AMA: 2018,Sep,7

27218 **Open treatment of posterior pelvic bone fracture and/or dislocation, for fracture patterns that disrupt the pelvic ring, unilateral, includes internal fixation, when performed (includes ipsilateral ilium, sacroiliac joint and/or sacrum)**

EXCLUDES *Sacroiliac joint arthrodesis without fracture and/or dislocation, percutaneous or minimally invasive (27279)*

34.6 34.6 FUD 090 E

AMA: 2018,Sep,7; 2018,Jan,8; 2017,Jan,8; 2016,Jan,13; 2015,Jan,16; 2014,Mar,4

27220 **Closed treatment of acetabulum (hip socket) fracture(s); without manipulation**

15.1 15.3 FUD 090 T G2 50

AMA: 2018,Sep,7

27222 **with manipulation, with or without skeletal traction**

28.0 28.0 FUD 090 C 50

AMA: 2018,Sep,7

27226 **Open treatment of posterior or anterior acetabular wall fracture, with internal fixation**

30.4 30.4 FUD 090 C 80 50

AMA: 2018,Sep,7

27227 **Open treatment of acetabular fracture(s) involving anterior or posterior (one) column, or a fracture running transversely across the acetabulum, with internal fixation**

47.9 47.9 FUD 090 C 80 50

AMA: 2018,Sep,7

27228 **Open treatment of acetabular fracture(s) involving anterior and posterior (two) columns, includes T-fracture and both column fracture with complete articular detachment, or single column or transverse fracture with associated acetabular wall fracture, with internal fixation**

54.3 54.3 FUD 090 C 80 50

AMA: 2018,Sep,7

27230 **Closed treatment of femoral fracture, proximal end, neck; without manipulation**

13.5 13.7 FUD 090 T A2 50

AMA: 2018,Sep,7

27232 **with manipulation, with or without skeletal traction**

21.4 21.4 FUD 090 C 50

AMA: 2018,Sep,7

27235 **Percutaneous skeletal fixation of femoral fracture, proximal end, neck**

26.2 26.2 FUD 090 J 50

AMA: 2018,Sep,7; 2018,Jan,8; 2017,Jan,8; 2016,Jan,13; 2015,Jan,16; 2014,Jan,11

27236 **Open treatment of femoral fracture, proximal end, neck, internal fixation or prosthetic replacement**

34.4 34.4 FUD 090 C 80 50

AMA: 2019,May,7; 2018,Sep,7; 2018,Jan,8; 2017,Jan,8; 2016,Nov,9; 2016,Jan,13; 2015,Jan,16; 2014,Jan,11

27238 **Closed treatment of intertrochanteric, peritrochanteric, or subtrochanteric femoral fracture; without manipulation**

13.2 13.2 FUD 090 J A2 50

AMA: 2018,Sep,7; 2018,Jan,8; 2017,Jan,8; 2016,Jan,13; 2015,Jan,16; 2014,Jan,11

27240 **with manipulation, with or without skin or skeletal traction**

27.6 27.6 FUD 090 C 50

AMA: 2018,Sep,7; 2018,Jan,8; 2017,Jan,8; 2016,Jan,13; 2015,Jan,16; 2014,Jan,11

27244 **Treatment of intertrochanteric, peritrochanteric, or subtrochanteric femoral fracture; with plate/screw type implant, with or without cerclage**

35.5 35.5 FUD 090 C 80 50

AMA: 2019,May,7; 2018,Sep,7; 2018,Jan,8; 2017,Jan,8; 2016,Jan,13; 2015,Jan,16; 2014,Jan,11

27245 **with intramedullary implant, with or without interlocking screws and/or cerclage**

35.4 35.4 FUD 090 C 80 50

AMA: 2018,Sep,7; 2018,Jan,8; 2017,Jan,8; 2016,Jan,13; 2015,Jan,16; 2014,Jan,11

27246 **Closed treatment of greater trochanteric fracture, without manipulation**

11.0 11.1 FUD 090 T A2 50

AMA: 2018,Sep,7

27248 **Open treatment of greater trochanteric fracture, includes internal fixation, when performed**

21.4 21.4 FUD 090 C 80 50

AMA: 2018,Sep,7

27250 **Closed treatment of hip dislocation, traumatic; without anesthesia**

5.17 5.17 FUD 000 T A2 50

AMA: 2018,Sep,7

27252 **requiring anesthesia**

21.8 21.8 FUD 090 J A2 50

AMA: 2018,Sep,7

27253 **Open treatment of hip dislocation, traumatic, without internal fixation**

27.1 27.1 FUD 090 C 80 50

AMA: 2018,Sep,7

27254 **Open treatment of hip dislocation, traumatic, with acetabular wall and femoral head fracture, with or without internal or external fixation**

EXCLUDES *Acetabular fracture treatment (27226-27227)*

36.4 36.4 FUD 090 C 80 50

AMA: 2018,Sep,7

27256 **Treatment of spontaneous hip dislocation (developmental, including congenital or pathological), by abduction, splint or traction; without anesthesia, without manipulation**

6.78 8.73 FUD 010 T G2 80 50

AMA: 2018,Sep,7

27257 **with manipulation, requiring anesthesia**

10.4 10.4 FUD 010 J A2 80 50

AMA: 2018,Sep,7

27258 **Open treatment of spontaneous hip dislocation (developmental, including congenital or pathological), replacement of femoral head in acetabulum (including tenotomy, etc);**

INCLUDES Lorenz's operation

32.1 32.1 FUD 090 C 80 50

AMA: 2018,Sep,7

27259 **with femoral shaft shortening**

44.8 44.8 FUD 090 C 80 50

AMA: 2018,Sep,7

27265 **Closed treatment of post hip arthroplasty dislocation; without anesthesia**

11.5 11.5 FUD 090 T A2 50

AMA: 2018,Sep,7

27266 **requiring regional or general anesthesia**

16.7 16.7 FUD 090 J A2 50

AMA: 2018,Sep,7

27267 **Closed treatment of femoral fracture, proximal end, head; without manipulation**

12.4 12.4 FUD 090 J G2 80 50

AMA: 2018,Sep,7; 2018,Jan,8; 2017,Jan,8; 2016,Jan,13; 2015,Jan,16; 2014,Jan,11

27268 **with manipulation**

15.5 15.5 FUD 090 C 80 50

AMA: 2018,Sep,7; 2018,Jan,8; 2017,Jan,8; 2016,Jan,13; 2015,Jan,16; 2014,Jan,11

26/TC PC/TC Only A2-Z3 ASC Payment 50 Bilateral ♂ Male Only ♀ Female Only Facility RVU Non-Facility RVU CCI CLIA
FUD Follow-up Days CMS: IOM AMA: CPT Asst A-Y OPPSI 80/80 Surg Assist Allowed / w/Doc Lab Crosswalk Radiology Crosswalk

27269 **Open treatment of femoral fracture, proximal end, head, includes internal fixation, when performed**

EXCLUDES *Arthrotomy, hip (27033)*
Open treatment of hip dislocation, traumatic, without internal fixation (27253)

35.8 35.8 FUD 090 C 80 50

AMA: 2018,Sep,7; 2018,Jan,8; 2017,Jan,8; 2016,Jan,13; 2015,Jan,16; 2014,Jan,11

27275 Hip Manipulation with Anesthesia

27275 **Manipulation, hip joint, requiring general anesthesia**

5.27 5.27 FUD 010 J A2

AMA: 2018,Sep,7; 2018,Jan,8; 2017,Jan,8; 2016,May,13; 2016,Jan,11; 2016,Jan,13; 2015,Jan,16; 2014,Jan,11

27279-27286 Arthrodesis of Hip and Pelvis

27279 **Arthrodesis, sacroiliac joint, percutaneous or minimally invasive (indirect visualization), with image guidance, includes obtaining bone graft when performed, and placement of transfixing device**

19.9 19.9 FUD 090 J J8 80 50

AMA: 2018,Sep,7

27280 **Arthrodesis, open, sacroiliac joint, including obtaining bone graft, including instrumentation, when performed**

EXCLUDES *Sacroiliac joint arthrodesis without fracture and/or dislocation, percutaneous or minimally invasive (27279)*

39.2 39.2 FUD 090 C 80 50

AMA: 2018,Sep,7; 2018,Jan,8; 2017,Jan,8; 2016,Jan,13; 2015,Jan,16; 2014,Mar,4; 2014,Jan,11

27282 **Arthrodesis, symphysis pubis (including obtaining graft)**

24.7 24.7 FUD 090 C 80

AMA: 2018,Sep,7

27284 **Arthrodesis, hip joint (including obtaining graft);**

46.7 46.7 FUD 090 C 80 50

AMA: 2018,Sep,7

27286 **with subtrochanteric osteotomy**

47.7 47.7 FUD 090 C 80 50

AMA: 2018,Sep,7; 2018,Jan,8; 2017,Jan,8; 2016,Jan,13; 2015,Jan,16; 2014,Jan,11

27290-27299 Amputations and Unlisted Procedures of Hip and Pelvis

27290 **Interpelviabdominal amputation (hindquarter amputation)**

INCLUDES Pean's amputation

47.0 47.0 FUD 090 C 80

AMA: 2018,Sep,7; 2018,Jan,8; 2017,Jan,8; 2016,Jan,13; 2015,Jan,16; 2014,Jan,11

27295 **Disarticulation of hip**

36.3 36.3 FUD 090 C 80 50

AMA: 2018,Sep,7; 2018,Jan,8; 2017,Jan,8; 2016,Jan,13; 2015,Jan,16; 2014,Jan,11

27299 **Unlisted procedure, pelvis or hip joint**

0.00 0.00 FUD YYY T 80 50

AMA: 2018,Sep,7; 2018,Jan,8; 2017,Jan,8; 2016,Jun,8; 2016,Jan,13; 2015,Jan,16; 2014,Mar,13; 2014,Jan,11

27301-27310 Incisional Procedures Femur or Knee

EXCLUDES *Superficial incision and drainage (10040-10160)*

27301 **Incision and drainage, deep abscess, bursa, or hematoma, thigh or knee region**

14.5 19.3 FUD 090 J A2 50

AMA: 2018,Sep,7; 2018,Jan,8; 2017,Jan,8; 2016,Jan,13; 2015,Jan,16; 2014,Jan,11

27303 **Incision, deep, with opening of bone cortex, femur or knee (eg, osteomyelitis or bone abscess)**

18.4 18.4 FUD 090 C 80 50

AMA: 2018,Sep,7

27305 **Fasciotomy, iliotibial (tenotomy), open**

EXCLUDES *Ober-Yount (gluteal-iliotibial) fasciotomy (27025)*

13.8 13.8 FUD 090 J A2 80 50

AMA: 2018,Sep,7

27306 **Tenotomy, percutaneous, adductor or hamstring; single tendon (separate procedure)**

9.89 9.89 FUD 090 J A2 80 50

AMA: 2018,Sep,7; 2018,Jan,8; 2017,Aug,9

27307 **multiple tendons**

13.8 13.8 FUD 090 J A2 80 50

AMA: 2018,Sep,7; 2018,Jan,8; 2017,Aug,9

27310 **Arthrotomy, knee, with exploration, drainage, or removal of foreign body (eg, infection)**

21.0 21.0 FUD 090 J A2 80 50

AMA: 2018,Sep,7; 2018,Jan,8; 2017,Jan,8; 2016,Jan,13; 2015,Jan,16; 2014,Jan,11

27323-27324 Biopsy Femur or Knee

EXCLUDES *Soft tissue needle biopsy (20206)*

27323 **Biopsy, soft tissue of thigh or knee area; superficial**

5.15 7.91 FUD 010 J A2 50

AMA: 2018,Sep,7; 2018,Jan,8; 2017,Jan,8; 2016,Jan,13; 2015,Jan,16; 2014,Jan,11

27324 **deep (subfascial or intramuscular)**

11.5 11.5 FUD 090 J A2 50

AMA: 2018,Sep,7; 2018,Jan,8; 2017,Jan,8; 2016,Jan,13; 2015,Jan,16; 2014,Jan,11

27325-27326 Neurectomy

27325 **Neurectomy, hamstring muscle**

16.1 16.1 FUD 090 J A2 80 50

AMA: 2018,Sep,7

27326 **Neurectomy, popliteal (gastrocnemius)**

14.8 14.8 FUD 090 J A2 80 50

AMA: 2018,Sep,7

27327-27329 [27337, 27339] Excision Soft Tissue Tumors Femur/ Knee

INCLUDES Any necessary elevation of tissue planes or dissection
Measurement of tumor and necessary margin at greatest diameter prior to excision
Simple and intermediate repairs
Types of excision:
- Fascial or subfascial soft tissue tumors: simple and marginal resection of tumors found either in or below the deep fascia, not including bone or excision of a substantial amount of normal tissue; primarily benign and intramuscular tumors
- Radical resection of soft tissue tumor: wide resection of tumor involving substantial margins of normal tissue and may involve tissue removal from one or more layers; most often malignant or aggressive benign
- Subcutaneous: simple and marginal resection of tumors in the subcutaneous tissue above the deep fascia; most often benign

EXCLUDES *Complex repair*
Excision of benign cutaneous lesions (eg, sebaceous cyst) (11400-11406)
Radical resection of cutaneous tumors (eg, melanoma) (11600-11606)
Significant exploration of vessels or neuroplasty

27327 **Excision, tumor, soft tissue of thigh or knee area, subcutaneous; less than 3 cm**

9.00 13.5 FUD 090 J G2 50

AMA: 2018,Sep,7

\# **27337** **3 cm or greater**

12.0 12.0 FUD 090 J G2 80 50

AMA: 2018,Sep,7

27328 **Excision, tumor, soft tissue of thigh or knee area, subfascial (eg, intramuscular); less than 5 cm**

17.9 17.9 FUD 090 J G2 50

AMA: 2018,Sep,7; 2018,Jan,8; 2017,Jan,8; 2016,Nov,9

27329 **Resequenced code. See code following 27360.**

27339 **5 cm or greater**
21.7 21.7 FUD 090 J G2 80 50
AMA: 2018,Sep,7

27330-27360 Resection Procedures Thigh/Knee

27330 **Arthrotomy, knee; with synovial biopsy only**
11.9 11.9 FUD 090 J A2 50
AMA: 2018,Sep,7; 2018,Jan,8; 2017,Jan,8; 2016,Jan,13; 2015,Jan,16; 2014,Jan,11

27331 **including joint exploration, biopsy, or removal of loose or foreign bodies**
13.6 13.6 FUD 090 J A2 80 50
AMA: 2018,Sep,7; 2018,Jan,8; 2017,Jan,8; 2016,Jan,13; 2015,Jan,16; 2014,Jan,11

27332 **Arthrotomy, with excision of semilunar cartilage (meniscectomy) knee; medial OR lateral**
18.5 18.5 FUD 090 J A2 80 50
AMA: 2018,Sep,7

Lateral meniscus
Posterior cruciate ligament
Medial meniscus
Anterior horns
Posterior horns
Patellar ligament
Anterior cruciate ligament
Bucket handle tear
Radial tear
Meniscus

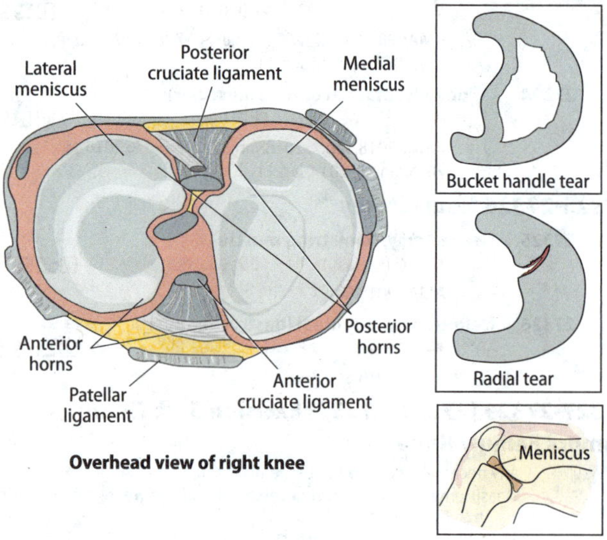

Overhead view of right knee

27333 **medial AND lateral**
16.8 16.8 FUD 090 J A2 80 50
AMA: 2018,Sep,7; 2018,Jan,8; 2017,Jan,8; 2016,Jan,13; 2015,Jan,16; 2014,Jan,11

27334 **Arthrotomy, with synovectomy, knee; anterior OR posterior**
19.7 19.7 FUD 090 J A2 80 50
AMA: 2018,Sep,7

27335 **anterior AND posterior including popliteal area**
21.9 21.9 FUD 090 J A2 80 50
AMA: 2018,Sep,7

27337 **Resequenced code. See code following 27327.**

27339 **Resequenced code. See code before 27330.**

27340 **Excision, prepatellar bursa**
10.6 10.6 FUD 090 J A2 50
AMA: 2018,Sep,7

27345 **Excision of synovial cyst of popliteal space (eg, Baker's cyst)**
13.8 13.8 FUD 090 J A2 80 50
AMA: 2018,Sep,7

27347 **Excision of lesion of meniscus or capsule (eg, cyst, ganglion), knee**
15.1 15.1 FUD 090 J A2 80 50
AMA: 2018,Sep,7

27350 **Patellectomy or hemipatellectomy**
18.7 18.7 FUD 090 J A2 80 50
AMA: 2018,Sep,7

27355 **Excision or curettage of bone cyst or benign tumor of femur;**
17.4 17.4 FUD 090 J A2 80 50
AMA: 2018,Sep,7

27356 **with allograft**
21.3 21.3 FUD 090 J G2 80 50
AMA: 2019,May,7; 2018,Sep,7

27357 **with autograft (includes obtaining graft)**
23.4 23.4 FUD 090 J A2 80 50
AMA: 2018,Sep,7; 2018,Jan,8; 2017,Jan,8; 2016,Jan,13; 2015,Jan,16; 2014,Jan,11

\+ 27358 **with internal fixation (List in addition to code for primary procedure)**
Code first (27355-27357)
8.07 8.07 FUD ZZZ N N1 80
AMA: 2018,Sep,7

27360 **Partial excision (craterization, saucerization, or diaphysectomy) bone, femur, proximal tibia and/or fibula (eg, osteomyelitis or bone abscess)**
24.7 24.7 FUD 090 J A2 80 50
AMA: 2018,Sep,7

27329-27365 [27329] Radical Resection Tumor Knee/Thigh

INCLUDES Any necessary elevation of tissue planes or dissection
Excision of adjacent soft tissue during bone tumor resection
Measurement of tumor and necessary margin at greatest diameter prior to excision
Radical resection of bone tumor: resection of the tumor (may include entire bone) and wide margins of normal tissue primarily for malignant or aggressive benign tumors
Radical resection of soft tissue tumor: wide resection of tumor involving substantial margins of normal tissue that may include tissue removal from one or more layers; most often malignant or aggressive benign
Simple and intermediate repairs

EXCLUDES *Complex repair*
Radical resection of cutaneous tumors (eg, melanoma) (11600-11606)
Significant exploration of vessels, neuroplasty, reconstruction, or complex bone repair

\# 27329 **Radical resection of tumor (eg, sarcoma), soft tissue of thigh or knee area; less than 5 cm**
29.9 29.9 FUD 090 J G2 80 50
AMA: 2018,Sep,7

27364 **5 cm or greater**
45.2 45.2 FUD 090 J G2 80 50
AMA: 2018,Sep,7

27365 **Radical resection of tumor, femur or knee**
EXCLUDES *Soft tissue tumor excision thigh or knee area (27329, 27364)*
59.6 59.6 FUD 090 C 80 50
AMA: 2019,May,7; 2018,Sep,7

27369 Injection for Arthrogram of Knee

EXCLUDES *Arthrocentesis, aspiration and/or injection, knee (20610-20611)*
Arthroscopy, knee (29871)

27369 **Injection procedure for contrast knee arthrography or contrast enhanced CT/MRI knee arthrography**
Code also fluoroscopic guidance, when performed for CT arthrography (73701-73702, 77002)
(73580, 73701-73702, 73722-73723)
1.17 4.06 FUD 000 N1 50
AMA: 2019,Aug,7

27372 Foreign Body Removal Femur or Knee

EXCLUDES *Arthroscopic procedures (29870-29887)*
Removal knee prosthesis (27488)

27372 **Removal of foreign body, deep, thigh region or knee area**
11.4 17.0 FUD 090 J A2 80 50
AMA: 2018,Sep,7

27380-27499 Repair/Reconstruction of Femur or Knee

27380 Suture of infrapatellar tendon; primary
17.1 17.1 FUD 090 J A2 80 50
AMA: 2018,Sep,7

27381 secondary reconstruction, including fascial or tendon graft
23.0 23.0 FUD 090 J A2 80 50
AMA: 2018,Sep,7

27385 Suture of quadriceps or hamstring muscle rupture; primary
16.6 16.6 FUD 090 J A2 80 50
AMA: 2018,Sep,7; 2018,Jan,8; 2017,Aug,9

27386 secondary reconstruction, including fascial or tendon graft
23.9 23.9 FUD 090 J A2 80 50
AMA: 2018,Sep,7

27390 Tenotomy, open, hamstring, knee to hip; single tendon
12.9 12.9 FUD 090 J A2 80 50
AMA: 2018,Sep,7

27391 multiple tendons, 1 leg
16.4 16.4 FUD 090 J A2 80
AMA: 2018,Sep,7

27392 multiple tendons, bilateral
20.5 20.5 FUD 090 J A2 80
AMA: 2018,Sep,7

27393 Lengthening of hamstring tendon; single tendon
14.6 14.6 FUD 090 J A2 80 50
AMA: 2018,Sep,7

27394 multiple tendons, 1 leg
18.5 18.5 FUD 090 J A2 80
AMA: 2018,Sep,7

27395 multiple tendons, bilateral
25.3 25.3 FUD 090 J A2 80
AMA: 2018,Sep,7

27396 Transplant or transfer (with muscle redirection or rerouting), thigh (eg, extensor to flexor); single tendon
17.7 17.7 FUD 090 J J8 80 50
AMA: 2018,Sep,7

27397 multiple tendons
26.4 26.4 FUD 090 J G2 80 50
AMA: 2018,Sep,7

27400 Transfer, tendon or muscle, hamstrings to femur (eg, Egger's type procedure)
20.0 20.0 FUD 090 J A2 80 50
AMA: 2018,Sep,7

27403 Arthrotomy with meniscus repair, knee
EXCLUDES *Arthroscopic treatment (29882)*
18.4 18.4 FUD 090 J J8 80 50
AMA: 2019,May,10; 2018,Sep,7

27405 Repair, primary, torn ligament and/or capsule, knee; collateral
19.4 19.4 FUD 090 J A2 80 50
AMA: 2018,Sep,7; 2018,Jan,8; 2017,Jan,8; 2016,Jan,13; 2015,Jan,16; 2014,Jan,11

27407 cruciate
EXCLUDES *Reconstruction (27427)*
22.9 22.9 FUD 090 J A2 80 50
AMA: 2018,Sep,7

27409 collateral and cruciate ligaments
EXCLUDES *Reconstruction (27427-27429)*
27.9 27.9 FUD 090 J A2 80 50
AMA: 2018,Sep,7

27412 Autologous chondrocyte implantation, knee
EXCLUDES *Arthrotomy, knee (27331)*
Autologous fat graft obtained by liposuction (15771-15774)
Manipulation of knee joint under general anesthesia (27570)
Obtaining chondrocytes (29870)
Other autologous soft tissue grafts (fat, dermis, fascia) harvested by direct excision ([15769])
47.8 47.8 FUD 090 J 80 50
AMA: 2018,Sep,7

27415 Osteochondral allograft, knee, open
EXCLUDES *Arthroscopic procedure (29867)*
Osteochondral autograft knee (27416)
38.9 38.9 FUD 090 J J8 80 50
AMA: 2019,Apr,10; 2018,Sep,7; 2018,Jan,8; 2017,Jan,8; 2016,Jan,13; 2015,Jan,16; 2014,Jan,11

27416 Osteochondral autograft(s), knee, open (eg, mosaicplasty) (includes harvesting of autograft[s])
EXCLUDES *Procedures in the same compartment (29874, 29877, 29879, 29885-29887)*
Procedures performed at the same surgical session (27415, 29870-29871, 29875, 29884)
Surgical arthroscopy of the knee with osteochondral autograft(s) (29866)
28.3 28.3 FUD 090 J J8 80 50
AMA: 2018,Sep,7; 2018,Jan,8; 2017,Jan,8; 2016,Jan,13; 2015,Jan,16; 2014,Jan,11

27418 Anterior tibial tubercleplasty (eg, Maquet type procedure)
23.8 23.8 FUD 090 J A2 80 50
AMA: 2018,Sep,7; 2018,Jan,8; 2017,Jan,8; 2016,Jan,13; 2015,Jan,16; 2014,Jan,11

27420 Reconstruction of dislocating patella; (eg, Hauser type procedure)
21.3 21.3 FUD 090 J A2 80 50
AMA: 2018,Sep,7; 2018,Jan,8; 2017,Jan,8; 2016,Jan,13; 2015,Jan,16; 2014,Jan,11

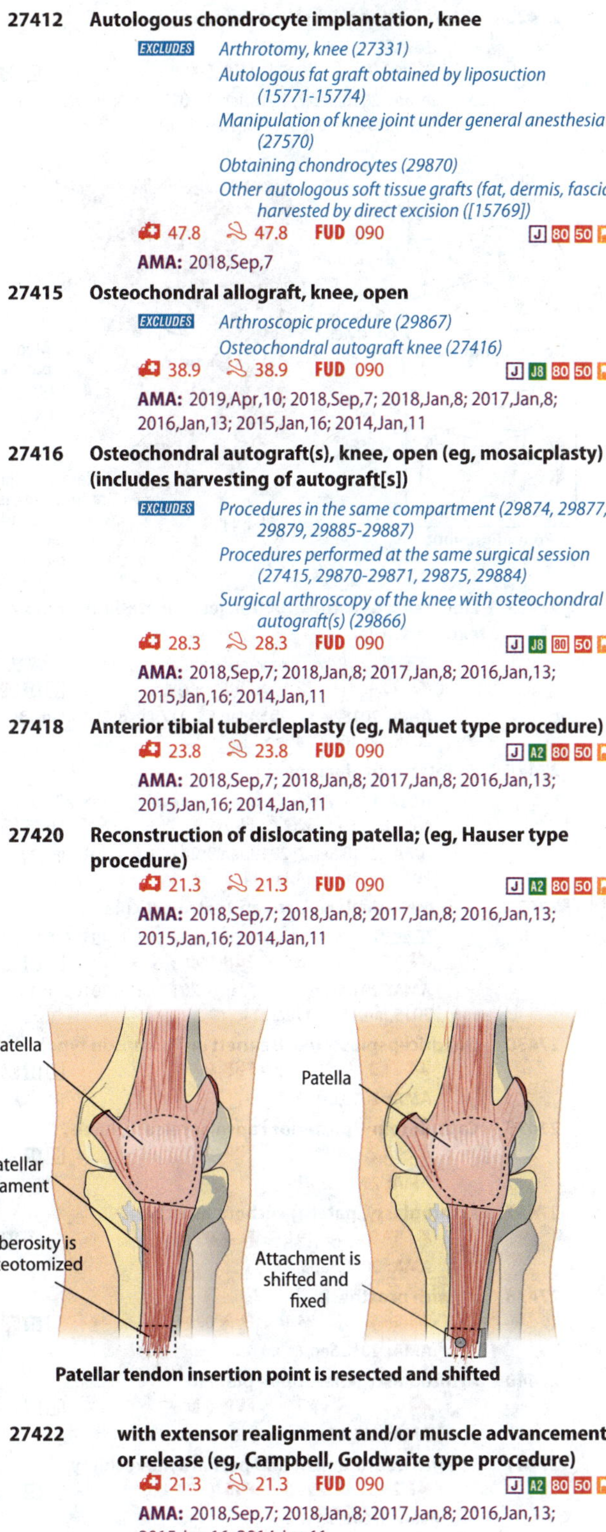

Patellar tendon insertion point is resected and shifted

27422 with extensor realignment and/or muscle advancement or release (eg, Campbell, Goldwaite type procedure)
21.3 21.3 FUD 090 J A2 80 50
AMA: 2018,Sep,7; 2018,Jan,8; 2017,Jan,8; 2016,Jan,13; 2015,Jan,16; 2014,Jan,11

27424 with patellectomy
21.5 21.5 FUD 090 J A2 80 50
AMA: 2018,Sep,7

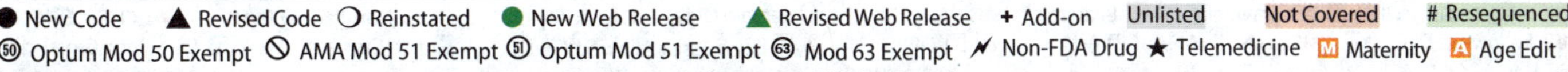

27425 Lateral retinacular release, open

EXCLUDES *Arthroscopic release (29873)*

12.9 12.9 FUD 090 J A2 50

AMA: 2018,Sep,7; 2018,Jan,8; 2017,Jan,8; 2016,Jan,13; 2015,Nov,7; 2015,Jan,16; 2014,Jan,11

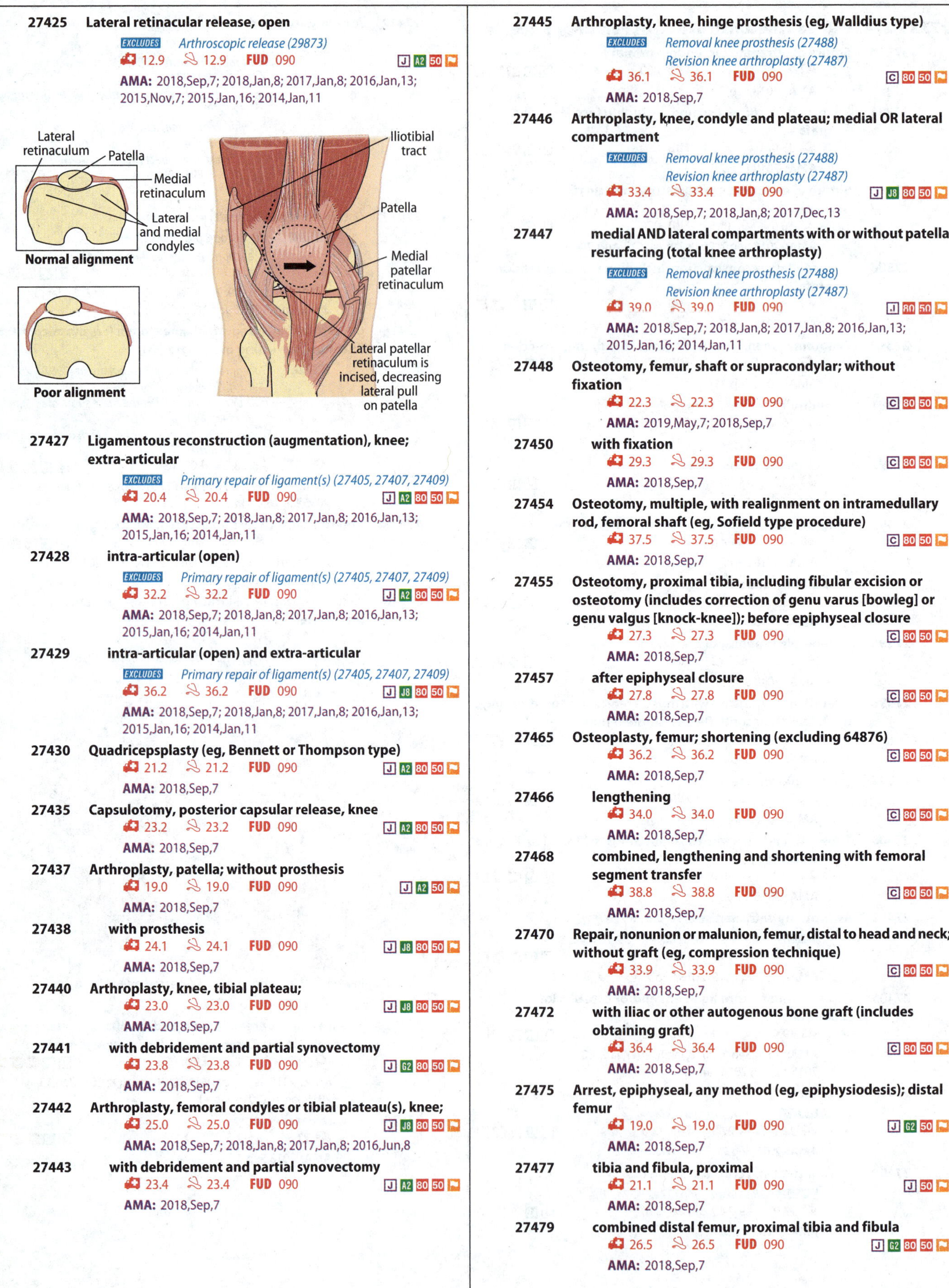

27427 Ligamentous reconstruction (augmentation), knee; extra-articular

EXCLUDES *Primary repair of ligament(s) (27405, 27407, 27409)*

20.4 20.4 FUD 090 J A2 80 50

AMA: 2018,Sep,7; 2018,Jan,8; 2017,Jan,8; 2016,Jan,13; 2015,Jan,16; 2014,Jan,11

27428 intra-articular (open)

EXCLUDES *Primary repair of ligament(s) (27405, 27407, 27409)*

32.2 32.2 FUD 090 J A2 80 50

AMA: 2018,Sep,7; 2018,Jan,8; 2017,Jan,8; 2016,Jan,13; 2015,Jan,16; 2014,Jan,11

27429 intra-articular (open) and extra-articular

EXCLUDES *Primary repair of ligament(s) (27405, 27407, 27409)*

36.2 36.2 FUD 090 J J8 80 50

AMA: 2018,Sep,7; 2018,Jan,8; 2017,Jan,8; 2016,Jan,13; 2015,Jan,16; 2014,Jan,11

27430 Quadricepsplasty (eg, Bennett or Thompson type)

21.2 21.2 FUD 090 J A2 80 50

AMA: 2018,Sep,7

27435 Capsulotomy, posterior capsular release, knee

23.2 23.2 FUD 090 J A2 80 50

AMA: 2018,Sep,7

27437 Arthroplasty, patella; without prosthesis

19.0 19.0 FUD 090 J A2 50

AMA: 2018,Sep,7

27438 with prosthesis

24.1 24.1 FUD 090 J J8 80 50

AMA: 2018,Sep,7

27440 Arthroplasty, knee, tibial plateau;

23.0 23.0 FUD 090 J J8 80 50

AMA: 2018,Sep,7

27441 with debridement and partial synovectomy

23.8 23.8 FUD 090 J G2 80 50

AMA: 2018,Sep,7

27442 Arthroplasty, femoral condyles or tibial plateau(s), knee;

25.0 25.0 FUD 090 J J8 80 50

AMA: 2018,Sep,7; 2018,Jan,8; 2017,Jan,8; 2016,Jun,8

27443 with debridement and partial synovectomy

23.4 23.4 FUD 090 J A2 80 50

AMA: 2018,Sep,7

27445 Arthroplasty, knee, hinge prosthesis (eg, Walldius type)

EXCLUDES *Removal knee prosthesis (27488)*
Revision knee arthroplasty (27487)

36.1 36.1 FUD 090 C 80 50

AMA: 2018,Sep,7

27446 Arthroplasty, knee, condyle and plateau; medial OR lateral compartment

EXCLUDES *Removal knee prosthesis (27488)*
Revision knee arthroplasty (27487)

33.4 33.4 FUD 090 J J8 80 50

AMA: 2018,Sep,7; 2018,Jan,8; 2017,Dec,13

27447 medial AND lateral compartments with or without patella resurfacing (total knee arthroplasty)

EXCLUDES *Removal knee prosthesis (27488)*
Revision knee arthroplasty (27487)

39.0 39.0 FUD 090 J 80 50

AMA: 2018,Sep,7; 2018,Jan,8; 2017,Jan,8; 2016,Jan,13; 2015,Jan,16; 2014,Jan,11

27448 Osteotomy, femur, shaft or supracondylar; without fixation

22.3 22.3 FUD 090 C 80 50

AMA: 2019,May,7; 2018,Sep,7

27450 with fixation

29.3 29.3 FUD 090 C 80 50

AMA: 2018,Sep,7

27454 Osteotomy, multiple, with realignment on intramedullary rod, femoral shaft (eg, Sofield type procedure)

37.5 37.5 FUD 090 C 80 50

AMA: 2018,Sep,7

27455 Osteotomy, proximal tibia, including fibular excision or osteotomy (includes correction of genu varus [bowleg] or genu valgus [knock-knee]); before epiphyseal closure

27.3 27.3 FUD 090 C 80 50

AMA: 2018,Sep,7

27457 after epiphyseal closure

27.8 27.8 FUD 090 C 80 50

AMA: 2018,Sep,7

27465 Osteoplasty, femur; shortening (excluding 64876)

36.2 36.2 FUD 090 C 80 50

AMA: 2018,Sep,7

27466 lengthening

34.0 34.0 FUD 090 C 80 50

AMA: 2018,Sep,7

27468 combined, lengthening and shortening with femoral segment transfer

38.8 38.8 FUD 090 C 80 50

AMA: 2018,Sep,7

27470 Repair, nonunion or malunion, femur, distal to head and neck; without graft (eg, compression technique)

33.9 33.9 FUD 090 C 80 50

AMA: 2018,Sep,7

27472 with iliac or other autogenous bone graft (includes obtaining graft)

36.4 36.4 FUD 090 C 80 50

AMA: 2018,Sep,7

27475 Arrest, epiphyseal, any method (eg, epiphysiodesis); distal femur

19.0 19.0 FUD 090 J G2 50

AMA: 2018,Sep,7

27477 tibia and fibula, proximal

21.1 21.1 FUD 090 J 50

AMA: 2018,Sep,7

27479 combined distal femur, proximal tibia and fibula

26.5 26.5 FUD 090 J G2 80 50

AMA: 2018,Sep,7

27485 **Arrest, hemiepiphyseal, distal femur or proximal tibia or fibula (eg, genu varus or valgus)**
19.3 19.3 FUD 090 J 50
AMA: 2018,Sep,7

27486 **Revision of total knee arthroplasty, with or without allograft; 1 component**
40.5 40.5 FUD 090 C 80 50
AMA: 2018,Sep,7; 2018,Apr,10; 2018,Jan,8; 2017,Jan,8; 2016,Jan,13; 2015,Jul,10; 2015,Jan,16; 2014,Jan,11

27487 **femoral and entire tibial component**
50.7 50.7 FUD 090 C 80 50
AMA: 2018,Sep,7; 2018,Jan,8; 2017,Jan,8; 2016,Jan,13; 2015,Jan,16

27488 **Removal of prosthesis, including total knee prosthesis, methylmethacrylate with or without insertion of spacer, knee**
34.6 34.6 FUD 090 C 80 50
AMA: 2018,Sep,7; 2018,Jan,8; 2017,Jan,8; 2016,Jan,13; 2015,Jan,16

27495 **Prophylactic treatment (nailing, pinning, plating, or wiring) with or without methylmethacrylate, femur**
32.5 32.5 FUD 090 C 80 50
AMA: 2018,Sep,7

27496 **Decompression fasciotomy, thigh and/or knee, 1 compartment (flexor or extensor or adductor);**
15.6 15.6 FUD 090 J A2 50
AMA: 2018,Sep,7

27497 **with debridement of nonviable muscle and/or nerve**
16.7 16.7 FUD 090 J A2 80 50
AMA: 2018,Sep,7

27498 **Decompression fasciotomy, thigh and/or knee, multiple compartments;**
18.8 18.8 FUD 090 J A2 80 50
AMA: 2018,Sep,7

27499 **with debridement of nonviable muscle and/or nerve**
20.1 20.1 FUD 090 J A2 80 50
AMA: 2018,Sep,7

27500-27566 Treatment of Fracture/Dislocation of Femur/Knee

INCLUDES Closed, percutaneous, and open treatment of fractures and dislocations

27500 **Closed treatment of femoral shaft fracture, without manipulation**
13.7 14.9 FUD 090 T A2 50
AMA: 2018,Sep,7

27501 **Closed treatment of supracondylar or transcondylar femoral fracture with or without intercondylar extension, without manipulation**
14.3 14.5 FUD 090 T A2 80 50
AMA: 2018,Sep,7

27502 **Closed treatment of femoral shaft fracture, with manipulation, with or without skin or skeletal traction**
21.8 21.8 FUD 090 J A2 50
AMA: 2018,Sep,7; 2018,Jan,8; 2017,Jan,8; 2016,Jan,13; 2015,Jan,16; 2014,Jan,11

27503 **Closed treatment of supracondylar or transcondylar femoral fracture with or without intercondylar extension, with manipulation, with or without skin or skeletal traction**
23.0 23.0 FUD 090 J A2 80 50
AMA: 2018,Sep,7

27506 **Open treatment of femoral shaft fracture, with or without external fixation, with insertion of intramedullary implant, with or without cerclage and/or locking screws**
38.6 38.6 FUD 090 C 80 50
AMA: 2018,Sep,7; 2018,Jan,8; 2017,Jan,8; 2016,Jan,13; 2015,Jan,16; 2014,Jan,11

27507 **Open treatment of femoral shaft fracture with plate/screws, with or without cerclage**
28.0 28.0 FUD 090 C 80 50
AMA: 2018,Sep,7

27508 **Closed treatment of femoral fracture, distal end, medial or lateral condyle, without manipulation**
14.1 15.0 FUD 090 T A2 50
AMA: 2018,Sep,7

27509 **Percutaneous skeletal fixation of femoral fracture, distal end, medial or lateral condyle, or supracondylar or transcondylar, with or without intercondylar extension, or distal femoral epiphyseal separation**
18.6 18.6 FUD 090 J J8 80 50
AMA: 2018,Dec,10; 2018,Dec,10; 2018,Sep,7

Pins are placed percutaneously

27510 **Closed treatment of femoral fracture, distal end, medial or lateral condyle, with manipulation**
19.6 19.6 FUD 090 J A2 50
AMA: 2018,Sep,7

27511 **Open treatment of femoral supracondylar or transcondylar fracture without intercondylar extension, includes internal fixation, when performed**
28.7 28.7 FUD 090 C 80 50
AMA: 2018,Sep,7

27513 **Open treatment of femoral supracondylar or transcondylar fracture with intercondylar extension, includes internal fixation, when performed**
35.8 35.8 FUD 090 C 80 50
AMA: 2018,Sep,7

27514 **Open treatment of femoral fracture, distal end, medial or lateral condyle, includes internal fixation, when performed**
27.9 27.9 FUD 090 C 80 50
AMA: 2018,Sep,7

27516 **Closed treatment of distal femoral epiphyseal separation; without manipulation**
13.7 14.6 FUD 090 T A2 50
AMA: 2018,Sep,7

27517 **with manipulation, with or without skin or skeletal traction**
19.7 19.7 FUD 090 J A2 80 50
AMA: 2018,Sep,7

27519 **Open treatment of distal femoral epiphyseal separation, includes internal fixation, when performed**
25.8 25.8 FUD 090 C 80 50
AMA: 2018,Sep,7

27520 **Closed treatment of patellar fracture, without manipulation**
8.46 9.21 FUD 090 T A2 50
AMA: 2018,Sep,7

27524 Open treatment of patellar fracture, with internal fixation and/or partial or complete patellectomy and soft tissue repair
21.6 21.6 FUD 090 J G2 80 50
AMA: 2018,Sep,7

27530 Closed treatment of tibial fracture, proximal (plateau); without manipulation
EXCLUDES *Arthroscopic repair (29855-29856)*
8.05 8.63 FUD 090 T A2 50
AMA: 2018,Sep,7

27532 with or without manipulation, with skeletal traction
EXCLUDES *Arthroscopic repair (29855-29856)*
16.5 17.7 FUD 090 J A2 50
AMA: 2018,Sep,7

27535 Open treatment of tibial fracture, proximal (plateau); unicondylar, includes internal fixation, when performed
EXCLUDES *Arthroscopic repair (29855-29856)*
25.9 25.9 FUD 090 C 80 50
AMA: 2018,Sep,7

27536 bicondylar, with or without internal fixation
EXCLUDES *Arthroscopic repair (29855-29856)*
34.2 34.2 FUD 090 C 80 50
AMA: 2018,Sep,7

27538 Closed treatment of intercondylar spine(s) and/or tuberosity fracture(s) of knee, with or without manipulation
EXCLUDES *Arthroscopic repair (29850-29851)*
12.7 13.6 FUD 090 T A2 80 50
AMA: 2018,Sep,7

27540 Open treatment of intercondylar spine(s) and/or tuberosity fracture(s) of the knee, includes internal fixation, when performed
23.4 23.4 FUD 090 C 80 50
AMA: 2018,Sep,7

27550 Closed treatment of knee dislocation; without anesthesia
13.8 14.9 FUD 090 T A2 80 50
AMA: 2018,Sep,7

27552 requiring anesthesia
18.0 18.0 FUD 090 J A2 80 50
AMA: 2018,Sep,7

27556 Open treatment of knee dislocation, includes internal fixation, when performed; without primary ligamentous repair or augmentation/reconstruction
25.3 25.3 FUD 090 C 80 50
AMA: 2018,Sep,7

27557 with primary ligamentous repair
30.3 30.3 FUD 090 C 80 50
AMA: 2018,Sep,7

27558 with primary ligamentous repair, with augmentation/reconstruction
34.5 34.5 FUD 090 C 80 50
AMA: 2018,Sep,7

27560 Closed treatment of patellar dislocation; without anesthesia
EXCLUDES *Recurrent dislocation (27420-27424)*
9.66 10.5 FUD 090 T A2 50
AMA: 2018,Sep,7

27562 requiring anesthesia
EXCLUDES *Recurrent dislocation (27420-27424)*
13.9 13.9 FUD 090 T A2 80 50
AMA: 2018,Sep,7

27566 Open treatment of patellar dislocation, with or without partial or total patellectomy
EXCLUDES *Recurrent dislocation (27420-27424)*
25.8 25.8 FUD 090 J A2 80 50
AMA: 2018,Sep,7

27570 Knee Manipulation with Anesthesia

27570 Manipulation of knee joint under general anesthesia (includes application of traction or other fixation devices)
4.34 4.34 FUD 010 J A2 50
AMA: 2018,Sep,7; 2018,Jan,8; 2017,Jan,8; 2016,Jan,13; 2015,Jan,16; 2014,Jan,11

27580 Knee Arthrodesis

27580 Arthrodesis, knee, any technique
INCLUDES Albert's operation
41.5 41.5 FUD 090 C 80 50
AMA: 2018,Sep,7

27590-27599 Amputations and Unlisted Procedures at Femur or Knee

27590 Amputation, thigh, through femur, any level;
22.9 22.9 FUD 090 C 80 50
AMA: 2018,Sep,7; 2018,Jan,8; 2017,Dec,13

27591 immediate fitting technique including first cast
27.9 27.9 FUD 090 C 80 50
AMA: 2018,Sep,7

27592 open, circular (guillotine)
19.6 19.6 FUD 090 C 80 50
AMA: 2018,Sep,7

27594 secondary closure or scar revision
14.6 14.6 FUD 090 J A2 50
AMA: 2018,Sep,7

27596 re-amputation
20.7 20.7 FUD 090 C 50
AMA: 2018,Sep,7

27598 Disarticulation at knee
INCLUDES Batch-Spittler-McFaddin operation
Callander knee disarticulation
Gritti amputation
20.5 20.5 FUD 090 C 80 50
AMA: 2018,Sep,7

27599 Unlisted procedure, femur or knee
0.00 0.00 FUD YYY T 80 50
AMA: 2019,Apr,10; 2018,Dec,10; 2018,Dec,10; 2018,Sep,7; 2018,Apr,10; 2018,Jan,8; 2017,Aug,9; 2017,Mar,10; 2017,Jan,8; 2016,Nov,9; 2016,Jun,8; 2016,Jan,13; 2015,Jan,13; 2015,Jan,16; 2014,Jan,11; 2014,Jan,9

27600-27602 Decompression Fasciotomy of Leg

EXCLUDES *Fasciotomy with debridement (27892-27894)*
Simple incision and drainage (10140-10160)

27600 Decompression fasciotomy, leg; anterior and/or lateral compartments only
11.6 11.6 FUD 090 J A2 50
AMA: 2018,Sep,7

27601 posterior compartment(s) only
12.8 12.8 FUD 090 J A2 50
AMA: 2018,Sep,7

27602 anterior and/or lateral, and posterior compartment(s)
13.9 13.9 FUD 090 J A2 80 50
AMA: 2018,Sep,7

27603-27612 Incisional Procedures Lower Leg and Ankle

27603 Incision and drainage, leg or ankle; deep abscess or hematoma
11.1 15.2 FUD 090 J A2 50
AMA: 2018,Sep,7

27604 infected bursa
9.61 13.6 FUD 090 J A2 80 50
AMA: 2018,Sep,7

27605 **Tenotomy, percutaneous, Achilles tendon (separate procedure); local anesthesia**
5.36 9.88 FUD 010 J A2 80 50
AMA: 2018,Sep,14; 2018,Sep,7

27606 **general anesthesia**
8.01 8.01 FUD 010 J A2 50
AMA: 2018,Sep,7; 2018,Sep,14

27607 **Incision (eg, osteomyelitis or bone abscess), leg or ankle**
17.5 17.5 FUD 090 J A2 50
AMA: 2018,Sep,7

27610 **Arthrotomy, ankle, including exploration, drainage, or removal of foreign body**
18.7 18.7 FUD 090 J A2 50
AMA: 2018,Sep,7

27612 **Arthrotomy, posterior capsular release, ankle, with or without Achilles tendon lengthening**
EXCLUDES *Lengthening or shortening tendon (27685)*
16.3 16.3 FUD 090 J A2 80 50
AMA: 2018,Sep,7

27613-27614 Biopsy Lower Leg and Ankle

EXCLUDES *Needle biopsy (20206)*

27613 **Biopsy, soft tissue of leg or ankle area; superficial**
4.62 7.19 FUD 010 J P3 50
AMA: 2018,Sep,7

27614 **deep (subfascial or intramuscular)**
11.6 16.5 FUD 090 J A2 50
AMA: 2018,Sep,7

27615-27634 [27632, 27634] Excision Soft Tissue Tumors Lower Leg/Ankle

INCLUDES Any necessary elevation of tissue planes or dissection
Measurement of tumor and necessary margin at greatest diameter prior to excision
Resection without removal of significant normal tissue
Simple and intermediate repairs
Types of excision:
Fascial or subfascial soft tissue tumors: simple and marginal resection of most often benign and intramuscular tumors found either in or below the deep fascia, not involving bone
Resection of the tumor (may include entire bone) and wide margins of normal tissue primarily for malignant or aggressive benign tumors
Subcutaneous: simple and marginal resection of most often benign tumors found in the subcutaneous tissue above the deep fascia

EXCLUDES *Complex repair*
Excision of benign cutaneous lesions (eg, sebaceous cyst) (11400-11406)
Radical resection of cutaneous tumors (eg, melanoma) (11600-11606)
Significant exploration of vessels or neuroplasty

27615 **Radical resection of tumor (eg, sarcoma), soft tissue of leg or ankle area; less than 5 cm**
29.5 29.5 FUD 090 J G2 80 50
AMA: 2018,Sep,7

27616 **5 cm or greater**
36.6 36.6 FUD 090 J G2 80 50
AMA: 2018,Sep,7

27618 **Excision, tumor, soft tissue of leg or ankle area, subcutaneous; less than 3 cm**
8.83 13.2 FUD 090 J G2 50
AMA: 2018,Sep,7; 2018,Jan,8; 2017,Jan,8; 2016,Jan,13; 2015,Jan,16; 2014,Jan,11

\# 27632 **3 cm or greater**
11.9 11.9 FUD 090 J G2 80 50
AMA: 2018,Sep,7

27619 **Excision, tumor, soft tissue of leg or ankle area, subfascial (eg, intramuscular); less than 5 cm**
13.3 13.3 FUD 090 J G2 50
AMA: 2018,Sep,7

\# 27634 **5 cm or greater**
19.5 19.5 FUD 090 J G2 80 50
AMA: 2018,Sep,7

27620-27641 Bone and Joint Procedures Ankle/Leg

27620 **Arthrotomy, ankle, with joint exploration, with or without biopsy, with or without removal of loose or foreign body**
13.0 13.0 FUD 090 J A2 80 50
AMA: 2018,Sep,7

27625 **Arthrotomy, with synovectomy, ankle;**
16.4 16.4 FUD 090 J A2 80 50
AMA: 2018,Sep,7

27626 **including tenosynovectomy**
17.5 17.5 FUD 090 J A2 80 50
AMA: 2018,Sep,7

27630 **Excision of lesion of tendon sheath or capsule (eg, cyst or ganglion), leg and/or ankle**
10.4 15.9 FUD 090 J A2 50
AMA: 2018,Sep,7

27632 **Resequenced code. See code following 27618.**

27634 **Resequenced code. See code following 27619.**

27635 **Excision or curettage of bone cyst or benign tumor, tibia or fibula;**
16.7 16.7 FUD 090 J A2 50
AMA: 2018,Sep,7; 2018,Jan,8; 2017,Jan,8; 2016,Jan,13; 2015,Jan,16; 2014,Jan,11

27637 **with autograft (includes obtaining graft)**
21.4 21.4 FUD 090 J A2 80 50
AMA: 2018,Sep,7

27638 **with allograft**
22.0 22.0 FUD 090 J A2 80 50
AMA: 2019,May,7; 2018,Sep,7

27640 **Partial excision (craterization, saucerization, or diaphysectomy), bone (eg, osteomyelitis); tibia**
EXCLUDES *Excision of exostosis (27635)*
23.9 23.9 FUD 090 J A2 50
AMA: 2018,Sep,7; 2018,Jan,8; 2017,Jan,8; 2016,Jan,13; 2015,Jan,16; 2014,Jan,11

27641 **fibula**
EXCLUDES *Excision of exostosis (27635)*
19.0 19.0 FUD 090 J A2 50
AMA: 2018,Sep,7

27645-27647 Radical Resection Bone Tumor Ankle/Leg

INCLUDES Any necessary elevation of tissue planes or dissection
Excision of adjacent soft tissue during bone tumor resection (27615-27619 [27632, 27634])
Measurement of tumor and necessary margin at greatest diameter prior to excision
Resection of the tumor (may include entire bone) and wide margins of normal tissue primarily for malignant or aggressive benign tumors
Simple and intermediate repairs

EXCLUDES *Complex repair*
Significant exploration of vessels, neuroplasty, reconstruction, or complex bone repair

27645 **Radical resection of tumor; tibia**
51.4 51.4 FUD 090 C 80 50
AMA: 2019,May,7; 2018,Sep,7

27646 **fibula**
44.6 44.6 FUD 090 C 80 50
AMA: 2019,May,7; 2018,Sep,7

27647 **talus or calcaneus**
29.3 29.3 FUD 090 J A2 80 50
AMA: 2019,May,7; 2018,Sep,7

● New Code ▲ Revised Code ○ Reinstated ● New Web Release ▲ Revised Web Release + Add-on Unlisted Not Covered # Resequenced
Optum Mod 50 Exempt AMA Mod 51 Exempt Optum Mod 51 Exempt Mod 63 Exempt Non-FDA Drug ★ Telemedicine Maternity Age Edit

27648 Injection for Ankle Arthrogram

EXCLUDES *Arthroscopy (29894-29898)*

27648 **Injection procedure for ankle arthrography**

(73615)

1.52 5.22 FUD 000 N N1 80 50

AMA: 2019,May,7; 2018,Sep,7; 2018,Jan,8; 2017,Jan,8; 2016,Jan,13; 2015,Aug,6

27650-27745 Repair/Reconstruction Lower Leg/Ankle

27650 **Repair, primary, open or percutaneous, ruptured Achilles tendon;**

18.9 18.9 FUD 090 J A2 80 50

AMA: 2018,Sep,7; 2018,Jan,8; 2017,Jan,8; 2016,Jan,13; 2015,Jan,16; 2014,Jul,5

27652 **with graft (includes obtaining graft)**

19.3 19.3 FUD 090 J A2 50

AMA: 2018,Sep,7; 2018,Jan,8; 2017,Jan,8; 2016,Jan,13; 2015,Jan,16; 2014,Jul,5

27654 **Repair, secondary, Achilles tendon, with or without graft**

20.4 20.4 FUD 090 J A2 80 50

AMA: 2018,Sep,7; 2018,Jan,8; 2017,Jan,8; 2016,Dec,16; 2016,Jan,13; 2015,Jan,16; 2014,Jul,5

27656 **Repair, fascial defect of leg**

11.4 18.2 FUD 090 J A2 80 50

AMA: 2018,Sep,7

27658 **Repair, flexor tendon, leg; primary, without graft, each tendon**

10.6 10.6 FUD 090 J A2 80

AMA: 2018,Sep,7

27659 **secondary, with or without graft, each tendon**

13.5 13.5 FUD 090 J A2 80

AMA: 2018,Sep,7; 2018,Jan,8; 2017,Jan,8; 2016,Jan,13; 2015,Jan,13

27664 **Repair, extensor tendon, leg; primary, without graft, each tendon**

10.4 10.4 FUD 090 J A2 80

AMA: 2018,Sep,7; 2018,Jan,8; 2017,Jan,8; 2016,Jan,13; 2015,Jan,13

27665 **secondary, with or without graft, each tendon**

11.9 11.9 FUD 090 J A2 80

AMA: 2018,Sep,7

27675 **Repair, dislocating peroneal tendons; without fibular osteotomy**

14.1 14.1 FUD 090 J A2 80 50

AMA: 2018,Sep,7

27676 **with fibular osteotomy**

17.2 17.2 FUD 090 J A2 80 50

AMA: 2018,Sep,7

27680 **Tenolysis, flexor or extensor tendon, leg and/or ankle; single, each tendon**

12.2 12.2 FUD 090 J A2

AMA: 2018,Sep,7; 2018,Jan,8; 2017,Jan,8; 2016,Jan,13; 2015,Jan,16; 2014,Jan,11

27681 **multiple tendons (through separate incision[s])**

15.7 15.7 FUD 090 J A2 50

AMA: 2018,Sep,7

27685 **Lengthening or shortening of tendon, leg or ankle; single tendon (separate procedure)**

13.3 19.0 FUD 090 J A2 80 50

AMA: 2018,Sep,7; 2018,Sep,14; 2018,Jan,8; 2017,Jan,8; 2016,Jan,13; 2015,Jan,16; 2014,Jan,11

27686 **multiple tendons (through same incision), each**

15.7 15.7 FUD 090 J A2 50

AMA: 2018,Sep,7; 2018,Jan,8; 2017,Jan,8; 2016,Jan,13; 2015,Jan,16; 2014,Jan,11

27687 **Gastrocnemius recession (eg, Strayer procedure)**

13.0 13.0 FUD 090 J A2 80 50

AMA: 2018,Sep,7

27690 **Transfer or transplant of single tendon (with muscle redirection or rerouting); superficial (eg, anterior tibial extensors into midfoot)**

INCLUDES Toe extensors considered a single tendon with transplant into midfoot

18.3 18.3 FUD 090 J A2 80 50

AMA: 2018,Sep,7

27691 **deep (eg, anterior tibial or posterior tibial through interosseous space, flexor digitorum longus, flexor hallucis longus, or peroneal tendon to midfoot or hindfoot)**

INCLUDES Barr procedure

Toe extensors considered a single tendon with transplant into midfoot

21.4 21.4 FUD 090 J A2 80 50

AMA: 2018,Sep,7

+ **27692** **each additional tendon (List separately in addition to code for primary procedure)**

INCLUDES Toe extensors considered a single tendon with transplant into midfoot

Code first (27690-27691)

3.02 3.02 FUD ZZZ N N1 80

AMA: 2018,Sep,7

27695 **Repair, primary, disrupted ligament, ankle; collateral**

13.6 13.6 FUD 090 J A2 50

AMA: 2018,Nov,11; 2018,Sep,7; 2018,Jan,8; 2017,Jan,8; 2016,Jan,13; 2015,Jan,16; 2014,Mar,13; 2014,Jan,11

Lateral view of right ankle showing components of the collateral ligament

Tibia
Fibula
Posterior talofibular
Anterior talofibular
Calcaneus
Calcaneofibular

27696 **both collateral ligaments**

15.9 15.9 FUD 090 J J8 50

AMA: 2018,Nov,11; 2018,Sep,7; 2018,Jan,8; 2017,Jan,8; 2016,Jan,13; 2015,Jan,16; 2014,Mar,13

27698 **Repair, secondary, disrupted ligament, ankle, collateral (eg, Watson-Jones procedure)**

18.3 18.3 FUD 090 J A2 80 50

AMA: 2018,Sep,7; 2018,Jan,8; 2017,Jan,8; 2016,Jan,13; 2015,Jan,16; 2014,Mar,13

27700 **Arthroplasty, ankle;**

17.5 17.5 FUD 090 J A2 80 50

AMA: 2018,Sep,7

27702 **with implant (total ankle)**

27.7 27.7 FUD 090 C 80 50

AMA: 2018,Sep,7

27703 **revision, total ankle**

31.9 31.9 FUD 090 C 80 50

AMA: 2018,Sep,7

27704 Removal of ankle implant
16.5 16.5 FUD 090 Q2 A2 50
AMA: 2019,May,7; 2018,Sep,7

27705 Osteotomy; tibia
EXCLUDES *Genu varus or genu valgus repair (27455-27457)*
21.8 21.8 FUD 090 J J8 80 50
AMA: 2018,Sep,7

27707 fibula
EXCLUDES *Genu varus or genu valgus repair (27455-27457)*
11.5 11.5 FUD 090 J A2 50
AMA: 2018,Sep,7

27709 tibia and fibula
EXCLUDES *Genu varus or genu valgus repair (27455-27457)*
33.6 33.6 FUD 090 J J8 80 50
AMA: 2018,Sep,7

27712 multiple, with realignment on intramedullary rod (eg, Sofield type procedure)
EXCLUDES *Genu varus or genu valgus repair (27455-27457)*
31.9 31.9 FUD 090 C 80 50
AMA: 2018,Sep,7

27715 Osteoplasty, tibia and fibula, lengthening or shortening
INCLUDES Anderson tibial lengthening
30.9 30.9 FUD 090 C 80 50
AMA: 2018,Sep,7

27720 Repair of nonunion or malunion, tibia; without graft, (eg, compression technique)
25.1 25.1 FUD 090 J J8 80 50
AMA: 2018,Sep,7

27722 with sliding graft
25.7 25.7 FUD 090 J 80 50
AMA: 2018,Sep,7

27724 with iliac or other autograft (includes obtaining graft)
36.4 36.4 FUD 090 C 80 50
AMA: 2018,Sep,7; 2018,Jan,8; 2017,Jan,8; 2016,Jan,13; 2015,Jan,16; 2014,Jan,11

27725 by synostosis, with fibula, any method
35.1 35.1 FUD 090 C 80 50
AMA: 2018,Sep,7

27726 Repair of fibula nonunion and/or malunion with internal fixation
INCLUDES Osteotomy; fibula (27707)
27.7 27.7 FUD 090 J J8 50
AMA: 2018,Sep,7; 2018,Jan,8; 2017,Jan,8; 2016,Jan,13; 2015,Jan,16; 2014,Jan,11

27727 Repair of congenital pseudarthrosis, tibia
29.9 29.9 FUD 090 C 80 50
AMA: 2018,Sep,7

27730 Arrest, epiphyseal (epiphysiodesis), open; distal tibia
16.9 16.9 FUD 090 J A2 50
AMA: 2018,Sep,7

27732 distal fibula
12.9 12.9 FUD 090 J A2 50
AMA: 2018,Sep,7

27734 distal tibia and fibula
18.9 18.9 FUD 090 J A2 50
AMA: 2018,Sep,7

27740 Arrest, epiphyseal (epiphysiodesis), any method, combined, proximal and distal tibia and fibula;
EXCLUDES *Epiphyseal arrest of proximal tibia and fibula (27477)*
20.4 20.4 FUD 090 J G2 80 50
AMA: 2018,Sep,7

27742 and distal femur
EXCLUDES *Epiphyseal arrest of proximal tibia and fibula (27477)*
22.4 22.4 FUD 090 J A2 80 50
AMA: 2018,Sep,7

27745 Prophylactic treatment (nailing, pinning, plating or wiring) with or without methylmethacrylate, tibia
21.7 21.7 FUD 090 J J8 80 50
AMA: 2018,Sep,7

27750-27848 Treatment of Fracture/Dislocation Lower Leg/Ankle

INCLUDES Treatment of open or closed fracture or dislocation

27750 Closed treatment of tibial shaft fracture (with or without fibular fracture); without manipulation
9.11 9.87 FUD 090 T A2 50
AMA: 2018,Sep,7; 2018,Jan,8; 2017,Jan,8; 2016,Jan,13; 2015,Jan,16; 2014,Jan,11

27752 with manipulation, with or without skeletal traction
14.1 15.3 FUD 090 J A2 50
AMA: 2018,Sep,7; 2018,Jan,8; 2018,Jan,3; 2017,Jan,8; 2016,Jan,13; 2015,Jan,16; 2014,Jan,11

27756 Percutaneous skeletal fixation of tibial shaft fracture (with or without fibular fracture) (eg, pins or screws)
16.6 16.6 FUD 090 J J8 80 50
AMA: 2018,Sep,7; 2018,Jan,8; 2017,Jan,8; 2016,Jan,13; 2015,Jan,16; 2014,Jan,11

27758 Open treatment of tibial shaft fracture (with or without fibular fracture), with plate/screws, with or without cerclage
25.7 25.7 FUD 090 J J8 80 50
AMA: 2018,Sep,7; 2018,Jan,8; 2017,Jan,8; 2016,Jan,13; 2015,Jan,16; 2014,Jan,11

27759 Treatment of tibial shaft fracture (with or without fibular fracture) by intramedullary implant, with or without interlocking screws and/or cerclage
28.8 28.8 FUD 090 J J8 80 50
AMA: 2018,Sep,7; 2018,Jan,8; 2017,Jan,8; 2016,Jan,13; 2015,Jan,16; 2014,Jan,11

27760 Closed treatment of medial malleolus fracture; without manipulation
8.72 9.50 FUD 090 T A2 50
AMA: 2018,Sep,7

27762 with manipulation, with or without skin or skeletal traction
12.3 13.6 FUD 090 J A2 50
AMA: 2018,Sep,7

27766 Open treatment of medial malleolus fracture, includes internal fixation, when performed
17.4 17.4 FUD 090 J A2 50
AMA: 2018,Sep,7

27767 Closed treatment of posterior malleolus fracture; without manipulation
EXCLUDES *Treatment of bimalleolar ankle fracture (27808-27814)*
Treatment of trimalleolar ankle fracture (27816-27823)
8.08 8.08 FUD 090 T P2 50
AMA: 2018,Sep,7

27768 with manipulation
EXCLUDES *Treatment of bimalleolar ankle fracture (27808-27814)*
Treatment of trimalleolar ankle fracture (27816-27823)
12.7 12.7 FUD 090 J G2 50
AMA: 2018,Sep,7

27769 Open treatment of posterior malleolus fracture, includes internal fixation, when performed
EXCLUDES *Treatment of bimalleolar ankle fracture (27808-27814)*
Treatment of trimalleolar ankle fracture (27816-27823)
21.0 21.0 FUD 090 J G2 50
AMA: 2018,Sep,7

27780 Closed treatment of proximal fibula or shaft fracture; without manipulation
7.98 8.71 FUD 090 T A2 50
AMA: 2018,Sep,7; 2018,Jan,8; 2017,Jan,8; 2016,Jan,13; 2015,Jan,16; 2014,Jan,11

Musculoskeletal System

27704 — 27780

27781 with manipulation
11.3 12.3 FUD 090 J A2 50
AMA: 2018,Sep,7

27784 Open treatment of proximal fibula or shaft fracture, includes internal fixation, when performed
20.6 20.6 FUD 090 J A2 50
AMA: 2018,Sep,7; 2018,Jan,8; 2017,Jan,8; 2016,Jan,13; 2015,Jan,16; 2014,Jan,11

27786 Closed treatment of distal fibular fracture (lateral malleolus); without manipulation
8.17 8.97 FUD 090 T A2 50
AMA: 2018,Sep,7

27788 with manipulation
11.0 12.1 FUD 090 T A2 50
AMA: 2018,Sep,7

27792 Open treatment of distal fibular fracture (lateral malleolus), includes internal fixation, when performed
EXCLUDES *Repair of tibia and fibula shaft fracture (27750-27759)*
18.6 18.6 FUD 090 J J8 50
AMA: 2018,Sep,7; 2018,Jan,8; 2017,Jan,8; 2016,Jan,13; 2015,Jan,16; 2014,Jan,11

27808 Closed treatment of bimalleolar ankle fracture (eg, lateral and medial malleoli, or lateral and posterior malleoli or medial and posterior malleoli); without manipulation
8.62 9.53 FUD 090 T A2 50
AMA: 2018,Sep,7

27810 with manipulation
12.1 13.3 FUD 090 J A2 50
AMA: 2018,Sep,7

27814 Open treatment of bimalleolar ankle fracture (eg, lateral and medial malleoli, or lateral and posterior malleoli, or medial and posterior malleoli), includes internal fixation, when performed
22.1 22.1 FUD 090 J J8 80 50
AMA: 2018,Sep,7; 2018,Jan,8; 2017,Jan,8; 2016,Feb,13

27816 Closed treatment of trimalleolar ankle fracture; without manipulation
8.28 9.27 FUD 090 T A2 50
AMA: 2018,Sep,7

27818 with manipulation
12.4 13.9 FUD 090 J A2 50
AMA: 2018,Sep,7

27822 Open treatment of trimalleolar ankle fracture, includes internal fixation, when performed, medial and/or lateral malleolus; without fixation of posterior lip
24.7 24.7 FUD 090 J J8 80 50
AMA: 2018,Sep,7

27823 with fixation of posterior lip
28.0 28.0 FUD 090 J J8 80 50
AMA: 2018,Sep,7

27824 Closed treatment of fracture of weight bearing articular portion of distal tibia (eg, pilon or tibial plafond), with or without anesthesia; without manipulation
8.71 9.02 FUD 090 T A2 50
AMA: 2018,Sep,7

27825 with skeletal traction and/or requiring manipulation
14.2 15.7 FUD 090 J A2 80 50
AMA: 2018,Sep,7

27826 Open treatment of fracture of weight bearing articular surface/portion of distal tibia (eg, pilon or tibial plafond), with internal fixation, when performed; of fibula only
24.2 24.2 FUD 090 J A2 80 50
AMA: 2018,Sep,7

27827 of tibia only
31.7 31.7 FUD 090 J J8 80 50
AMA: 2018,Sep,7

27828 of both tibia and fibula
37.8 37.8 FUD 090 J J8 80 50
AMA: 2018,Sep,7; 2018,Jan,8; 2017,Jan,8; 2016,Jan,13; 2015,Jan,16; 2014,Apr,10

27829 Open treatment of distal tibiofibular joint (syndesmosis) disruption, includes internal fixation, when performed
20.0 20.0 FUD 090 J A2 80 50
AMA: 2018,Sep,7; 2018,Jan,8; 2017,Jan,8; 2016,Feb,13; 2016,Jan,13; 2015,Jan,16; 2014,Jan,11

27830 Closed treatment of proximal tibiofibular joint dislocation; without anesthesia
10.2 11.0 FUD 090 T A2 80 50
AMA: 2018,Sep,7

27831 requiring anesthesia
11.5 11.5 FUD 090 J A2 80 50
AMA: 2018,Sep,7

27832 Open treatment of proximal tibiofibular joint dislocation, includes internal fixation, when performed, or with excision of proximal fibula
21.8 21.8 FUD 090 J A2 80 50
AMA: 2018,Sep,7

27840 Closed treatment of ankle dislocation; without anesthesia
10.7 10.7 FUD 090 T A2 50
AMA: 2018,Sep,7

27842 requiring anesthesia, with or without percutaneous skeletal fixation
14.0 14.0 FUD 090 J A2 50
AMA: 2018,Sep,7

27846 Open treatment of ankle dislocation, with or without percutaneous skeletal fixation; without repair or internal fixation
EXCLUDES *Arthroscopy (29894-29898)*
20.7 20.7 FUD 090 J A2 80 50
AMA: 2018,Sep,7

27848 with repair or internal or external fixation
EXCLUDES *Arthroscopy (29894-29898)*
23.0 23.0 FUD 090 J A2 80 50
AMA: 2018,Sep,7

27860 Ankle Manipulation with Anesthesia

27860 Manipulation of ankle under general anesthesia (includes application of traction or other fixation apparatus)
4.92 4.92 FUD 010 J A2 80 50
AMA: 2018,Sep,7

27870-27871 Arthrodesis Lower Leg/Ankle

27870 Arthrodesis, ankle, open
EXCLUDES *Arthroscopic arthrodesis of ankle (29899)*
29.5 29.5 FUD 090 J J8 80 50
AMA: 2018,Sep,7

27871 Arthrodesis, tibiofibular joint, proximal or distal
19.8 19.8 FUD 090 J J8 80 50
AMA: 2018,Sep,7

27880-27889 Amputations of Lower Leg/Ankle

27880 Amputation, leg, through tibia and fibula;
INCLUDES Burgess amputation
26.3 26.3 FUD 090 C 80 50
AMA: 2018,Sep,7

27881 with immediate fitting technique including application of first cast
24.9 24.9 FUD 090 C 80 50
AMA: 2018,Sep,7

27882 open, circular (guillotine)
17.2 17.2 FUD 090 C 80 50
AMA: 2018,Sep,7

27884 secondary closure or scar revision
16.4 16.4 FUD 090 J A2 50
AMA: 2018,Sep,7

27886 re-amputation
18.8 18.8 FUD 090 C 50
AMA: 2018,Sep,7

27888 **Amputation, ankle, through malleoli of tibia and fibula (eg, Syme, Pirogoff type procedures), with plastic closure and resection of nerves**
19.0 19.0 FUD 090 C 80 50
AMA: 2018,Sep,7

27889 **Ankle disarticulation**
18.6 18.6 FUD 090 J A2 50
AMA: 2018,Sep,7

27892-27899 Decompression Fasciotomy Lower Leg

EXCLUDES *Decompression fasciotomy without debridement (27600-27602)*

27892 **Decompression fasciotomy, leg; anterior and/or lateral compartments only, with debridement of nonviable muscle and/or nerve**
15.8 15.8 FUD 090 J A2 80 50
AMA: 2018,Sep,7

27893 posterior compartment(s) only, with debridement of nonviable muscle and/or nerve
17.5 17.5 FUD 090 J A2 80 50
AMA: 2018,Sep,7

27894 anterior and/or lateral, and posterior compartment(s), with debridement of nonviable muscle and/or nerve
24.3 24.3 FUD 090 J A2 80 50
AMA: 2018,Sep,7

27899 **Unlisted procedure, leg or ankle**
0.00 0.00 FUD YYY T 80 50
AMA: 2018,Sep,7; 2018,Jan,8; 2017,Jan,8; 2016,Dec,16; 2016,Jan,13; 2015,Jan,16; 2014,Jan,11

28001-28008 Surgical Incision Foot/Toe

EXCLUDES *Simple incision and drainage (10060-10160)*

28001 **Incision and drainage, bursa, foot**
4.90 8.03 FUD 010 J P3
AMA: 2018,Sep,7

28002 **Incision and drainage below fascia, with or without tendon sheath involvement, foot; single bursal space**
9.20 12.7 FUD 010 J A2
AMA: 2018,Sep,7

28003 multiple areas
16.0 20.1 FUD 090 J A2
AMA: 2018,Sep,7

28005 **Incision, bone cortex (eg, osteomyelitis or bone abscess), foot**
16.6 16.6 FUD 090 J A2
AMA: 2018,Sep,7

28008 **Fasciotomy, foot and/or toe**
EXCLUDES *Plantar fascia division (28250)*
Plantar fasciectomy (28060, 28062)
8.46 12.5 FUD 090 J A2 50
AMA: 2018,Sep,7

28010-28011 Tenotomy/Toe

EXCLUDES *Open tenotomy (28230-28234)*
Simple incision and drainage (10140-10160)

28010 **Tenotomy, percutaneous, toe; single tendon**
5.99 6.69 FUD 090 J P3
AMA: 2018,Sep,7

28011 multiple tendons
8.14 9.14 FUD 090 J A2
AMA: 2018,Sep,7

28020-28024 Arthrotomy Foot/Toe

EXCLUDES *Simple incision and drainage (10140-10160)*

28020 **Arthrotomy, including exploration, drainage, or removal of loose or foreign body; intertarsal or tarsometatarsal joint**
10.4 15.5 FUD 090 J A2
AMA: 2018,Sep,7

28022 metatarsophalangeal joint
9.32 14.0 FUD 090 J A2
AMA: 2018,Sep,7

28024 interphalangeal joint
8.67 13.1 FUD 090 J A2
AMA: 2018,Sep,7

28035 Tarsal Tunnel Release

EXCLUDES *Other nerve decompression (64722)*
Other neuroplasty (64704)

28035 **Release, tarsal tunnel (posterior tibial nerve decompression)**
10.2 15.2 FUD 090 J A2 50
AMA: 2018,Sep,7

28039-28047 [28039, 28041] Excision Soft Tissue Tumors Foot/Toe

INCLUDES Any necessary elevation of tissue planes or dissection
Measurement of tumor and necessary margin at greatest diameter prior to excision
Simple and intermediate repairs
Types of excision:
- Fascial or subfascial soft tissue tumors: simple and marginal resection of tumors found either in or below the deep fascia, not involving bone or excision of a substantial amount of normal tissue; primarily benign and intramuscular tumors
  - Tumors of fingers and toes involving joint capsules, tendons and tendon sheaths
- Radical resection soft tissue tumor: wide resection of tumor, involving substantial margins of normal tissue and may involve tissue removal from one or more layers; most often malignant or aggressive benign
  - Tumors of fingers and toes adjacent to joints, tendons and tendon sheaths
- Subcutaneous: simple and marginal resection of tumors in the subcutaneous tissue above the deep fascia; most often benign

EXCLUDES *Complex repair*
Excision of benign cutaneous lesions (eg, sebaceous cyst) (11420-11426)
Radical resection of cutaneous tumors (eg, melanoma) (11620-11626)
Significant exploration of vessels, neuroplasty, or reconstruction

28039 **Resequenced code. See code following 28043.**

28041 **Resequenced code. See code following 28045.**

28043 **Excision, tumor, soft tissue of foot or toe, subcutaneous; less than 1.5 cm**
7.56 11.4 FUD 090 J G2 50
AMA: 2018,Sep,7

28039 1.5 cm or greater
9.94 14.3 FUD 090 J G2 80 50
AMA: 2018,Sep,7

28045 **Excision, tumor, soft tissue of foot or toe, subfascial (eg, intramuscular); less than 1.5 cm**
10.0 14.2 FUD 090 J G2 80 50
AMA: 2018,Sep,7

28041 1.5 cm or greater
13.0 13.0 FUD 090 J G2 80 50
AMA: 2018,Sep,7

28046 **Radical resection of tumor (eg, sarcoma), soft tissue of foot or toe; less than 3 cm**
20.8 20.8 FUD 090 J G2 50
AMA: 2018,Sep,7

28047 3 cm or greater
30.1 30.1 FUD 090 J G2 80 50
AMA: 2018,Sep,7

28050-28160 Resection Procedures Foot/Toes

28050 Arthrotomy with biopsy; intertarsal or tarsometatarsal joint
8.05 12.2 FUD 090 J A2 50
AMA: 2002,Apr,13; 1998,Nov,1

28052 metatarsophalangeal joint
8.15 12.8 FUD 090 J A2 50
AMA: 2002,Apr,13

28054 interphalangeal joint
6.77 10.8 FUD 090 J A2 80 50
AMA: 2002,Apr,13

28055 Neurectomy, intrinsic musculature of foot
11.0 11.0 FUD 090 J A2 80 50

28060 Fasciectomy, plantar fascia; partial (separate procedure)
EXCLUDES *Plantar fasciotomy (28008, 28250)*
10.3 15.0 FUD 090 J A2 50
AMA: 2018,Jan,8; 2017,Jan,8; 2016,Jan,13; 2015,Jan,16; 2014,Jan,11

28062 radical (separate procedure)
EXCLUDES *Plantar fasciotomy (28008, 28250)*
11.7 16.8 FUD 090 J A2 50
AMA: 2002,Apr,13

28070 Synovectomy; intertarsal or tarsometatarsal joint, each
10.2 15.4 FUD 090 J A2
AMA: 2002,Apr,13

28072 metatarsophalangeal joint, each
9.26 14.1 FUD 090 J A2
AMA: 2002,Apr,13

28080 Excision, interdigital (Morton) neuroma, single, each
10.5 15.1 FUD 090 J A2 80
AMA: 2018,Jan,8; 2017,Jan,8; 2016,Jan,13; 2015,Jan,16; 2014,Jan,11

28086 Synovectomy, tendon sheath, foot; flexor
10.3 15.7 FUD 090 J A2 80 50
AMA: 2002,Apr,13

28088 extensor
8.22 13.0 FUD 090 J A2 80 50
AMA: 2002,Apr,13

28090 Excision of lesion, tendon, tendon sheath, or capsule (including synovectomy) (eg, cyst or ganglion); foot
8.86 13.5 FUD 090 J A2 50
AMA: 2002,Apr,13; 1998,Nov,1

28092 toe(s), each
7.79 12.3 FUD 090 J A2
AMA: 2002,Apr,13; 1998,Nov,1

28100 Excision or curettage of bone cyst or benign tumor, talus or calcaneus;
11.9 17.6 FUD 090 J A2 80 50
AMA: 2002,Apr,13

28102 with iliac or other autograft (includes obtaining graft)
17.5 17.5 FUD 090 J J8 80 50
AMA: 2002,Apr,13

28103 with allograft
11.2 11.2 FUD 090 J A2 80 50
AMA: 2019,May,7

28104 Excision or curettage of bone cyst or benign tumor, tarsal or metatarsal, except talus or calcaneus;
10.2 15.4 FUD 090 J A2 80
AMA: 2002,May,7; 2002,Apr,13

28106 with iliac or other autograft (includes obtaining graft)
12.3 12.3 FUD 090 J A2 80
AMA: 2002,May,7; 2002,Apr,13

28107 with allograft
10.0 14.8 FUD 090 J A2 80
AMA: 2019,May,7

28108 Excision or curettage of bone cyst or benign tumor, phalanges of foot
EXCLUDES *Partial excision bone, toe (28124)*
8.30 12.7 FUD 090 J A2
AMA: 2002,Apr,13

28110 Ostectomy, partial excision, fifth metatarsal head (bunionette) (separate procedure)
8.37 13.4 FUD 090 J A2 50
AMA: 2018,Jan,8; 2017,Jan,8; 2016,Jan,13; 2015,Jan,16; 2014,Jan,11

28111 Ostectomy, complete excision; first metatarsal head
9.32 14.1 FUD 090 J A2 50
AMA: 2002,Apr,13

28112 other metatarsal head (second, third or fourth)
8.99 14.1 FUD 090 J A2 50
AMA: 2002,Apr,13

28113 fifth metatarsal head
12.2 17.0 FUD 090 J A2 80 50
AMA: 2002,Apr,13

28114 all metatarsal heads, with partial proximal phalangectomy, excluding first metatarsal (eg, Clayton type procedure)
23.9 30.7 FUD 090 J A2 80 50
AMA: 2002,Apr,13; 1998,Nov,1

28116 Ostectomy, excision of tarsal coalition
16.6 22.0 FUD 090 J A2 50
AMA: 2002,Apr,13

28118 Ostectomy, calcaneus;
11.9 17.2 FUD 090 J A2 80 50
AMA: 2018,Jan,8; 2017,Jan,8; 2016,Jan,13; 2015,Jan,13; 2015,Jan,16; 2014,Jan,11

28119 for spur, with or without plantar fascial release
10.3 15.1 FUD 090 J A2 50
AMA: 2018,Jan,8; 2017,Jan,8; 2016,Jan,13; 2015,Jan,16; 2014,Jan,11

28120 Partial excision (craterization, saucerization, sequestrectomy, or diaphysectomy) bone (eg, osteomyelitis or bossing); talus or calcaneus
INCLUDES Barker operation
14.3 19.5 FUD 090 J A2 50
AMA: 2018,Jan,8; 2017,Jan,8; 2016,Jan,13; 2015,Jan,16; 2014,Jan,11

28122 tarsal or metatarsal bone, except talus or calcaneus
EXCLUDES *Hallux rigidus cheilectomy (28289)*
Partial removal of talus or calcaneus (28120)
12.6 17.2 FUD 090 J A2 80 50
AMA: 2002,Apr,13; 1998,Nov,1

28124 phalanx of toe
9.54 13.8 FUD 090 J P3 50
AMA: 2002,Apr,13

28126 Resection, partial or complete, phalangeal base, each toe
7.14 11.4 FUD 090 J A2
AMA: 2018,Jan,8; 2017,Jan,8; 2016,Jan,13; 2015,Mar,9

28130 Talectomy (astragalectomy)
INCLUDES Whitman astragalectomy
EXCLUDES *Calcanectomy (28118)*
18.3 18.3 FUD 090 J A2 80 50
AMA: 2002,Apr,13

28140 Metatarsectomy
12.5 17.1 FUD 090 J A2
AMA: 2002,Apr,13

28150 Phalangectomy, toe, each toe
8.04 12.2 FUD 090 J A2
AMA: 2002,Apr,13; 1998,Nov,1

28153 **Resection, condyle(s), distal end of phalanx, each toe**
7.63 11.9 FUD 090 J A2
AMA: 2018,Jan,8; 2017,Jan,8; 2016,Jan,13; 2015,Jan,16; 2014,Jan,11

28160 **Hemiphalangectomy or interphalangeal joint excision, toe, proximal end of phalanx, each**
7.70 12.0 FUD 090 J A2
AMA: 2002,Apr,13; 1998,Nov,1

28171-28175 Radical Resection Bone Tumor Foot/Toes

INCLUDES Any necessary elevation of tissue planes or dissection
Excision of adjacent soft tissue during bone tumor resection (28039-28047 [28039, 28041])
Measurement of tumor and necessary margin at greatest diameter prior to excision
Resection of the tumor (may include entire bone) and wide margins of normal tissue primarily for malignant or aggressive benign tumors
Simple and intermediate repairs

EXCLUDES *Complex repair*
Radical tumor resection calcaneus or talus (27647)
Significant exploration of vessels, neuroplasty, reconstruction, or complex bone repair

28171 **Radical resection of tumor; tarsal (except talus or calcaneus)**
32.2 32.2 FUD 090 J A2 80
AMA: 2002,Apr,13; 1994,Win,1

28173 **metatarsal**
21.3 21.3 FUD 090 J A2
AMA: 2002,Apr,13; 1994,Win,1

28175 **phalanx of toe**
13.7 13.7 FUD 090 J A2
AMA: 2002,Apr,13

28190-28193 Foreign Body Removal: Foot

28190 **Removal of foreign body, foot; subcutaneous**
3.85 7.35 FUD 010 T P3 50
AMA: 2018,Jan,8; 2017,Jan,8; 2016,Jan,13; 2015,Jan,16; 2014,Jan,11

28192 **deep**
8.99 13.5 FUD 090 J A2 50
AMA: 2018,Jan,8; 2017,Jan,8; 2016,Jan,13; 2015,Jan,16; 2014,Jan,11

28193 **complicated**
10.6 15.3 FUD 090 J A2 50
AMA: 2002,Apr,13

28200-28360 [28295] Repair/Reconstruction of Foot/Toe

INCLUDES Closed, open, and percutaneous treatment of fractures and dislocations

28200 **Repair, tendon, flexor, foot; primary or secondary, without free graft, each tendon**
9.32 14.2 FUD 090 J A2
AMA: 2018,Jan,8; 2017,Jan,8; 2016,Feb,15; 2016,Jan,13; 2015,Jan,16; 2014,Jul,5; 2014,Jan,11

28202 **secondary with free graft, each tendon (includes obtaining graft)**
12.4 17.5 FUD 090 J A2 80
AMA: 2002,Apr,13

28208 **Repair, tendon, extensor, foot; primary or secondary, each tendon**
9.09 13.9 FUD 090 J A2
AMA: 2002,Apr,13; 1998,Nov,1

28210 **secondary with free graft, each tendon (includes obtaining graft)**
12.0 17.0 FUD 090 J A2 80
AMA: 2002,Apr,13

28220 **Tenolysis, flexor, foot; single tendon**
8.73 13.0 FUD 090 J P3 50
AMA: 2002,Apr,13; 1998,Nov,1

28222 **multiple tendons**
10.2 14.9 FUD 090 J A2 50
AMA: 2002,Apr,13; 1998,Nov,1

28225 **Tenolysis, extensor, foot; single tendon**
7.65 12.1 FUD 090 J A2 50
AMA: 2002,Apr,13; 1998,Nov,1

28226 **multiple tendons**
11.3 17.6 FUD 090 J A2 50
AMA: 2002,Apr,13; 1998,Nov,1

28230 **Tenotomy, open, tendon flexor; foot, single or multiple tendon(s) (separate procedure)**
8.17 12.5 FUD 090 J P3 50
AMA: 2002,Apr,13; 1998,Nov,1

28232 **toe, single tendon (separate procedure)**
6.98 11.1 FUD 090 J P3
AMA: 2018,Jan,8; 2017,Jan,8; 2016,Jan,13; 2015,Mar,9

28234 **Tenotomy, open, extensor, foot or toe, each tendon**
EXCLUDES *Tendon transfer (27690-27691)*
7.59 11.8 FUD 090 J A2
AMA: 2018,Jan,8; 2017,Jan,8; 2016,Jan,13; 2015,Jan,16; 2014,Jan,11

28238 **Reconstruction (advancement), posterior tibial tendon with excision of accessory tarsal navicular bone (eg, Kidner type procedure)**
EXCLUDES *Extensor hallucis longus transfer with big toe fusion (28760)*
Jones procedure (28760)
Subcutaneous tenotomy (28010-28011)
Transfer or transplant of tendon with muscle redirection or rerouting (27690-27692)
14.0 19.3 FUD 090 J A2 80 50
AMA: 2002,Apr,13; 2002,May,7

28240 **Tenotomy, lengthening, or release, abductor hallucis muscle**
8.59 13.2 FUD 090 J A2 50
AMA: 2002,Apr,13

28250 **Division of plantar fascia and muscle (eg, Steindler stripping) (separate procedure)**
11.5 16.6 FUD 090 J A2 80 50
AMA: 2002,Apr,13; 1998,Nov,1

28260 **Capsulotomy, midfoot; medial release only (separate procedure)**
14.6 19.8 FUD 090 J A2 80 50
AMA: 2002,Apr,13

28261 **with tendon lengthening**
23.4 29.7 FUD 090 J A2 80 50
AMA: 2002,Apr,13

28262 **extensive, including posterior talotibial capsulotomy and tendon(s) lengthening (eg, resistant clubfoot deformity)**
32.5 40.4 FUD 090 J J8 80 50
AMA: 2002,Apr,13; 1998,Nov,1

28264 **Capsulotomy, midtarsal (eg, Heyman type procedure)**
22.1 29.1 FUD 090 J A2 80 50
AMA: 2002,Apr,13; 1998,Nov,1

28270 **Capsulotomy; metatarsophalangeal joint, with or without tenorrhaphy, each joint (separate procedure)**
9.64 14.2 FUD 090 J A2 50
AMA: 2018,Jan,8; 2017,Jan,8; 2016,Jan,13; 2015,Jan,16; 2014,Sep,13; 2014,Jan,11

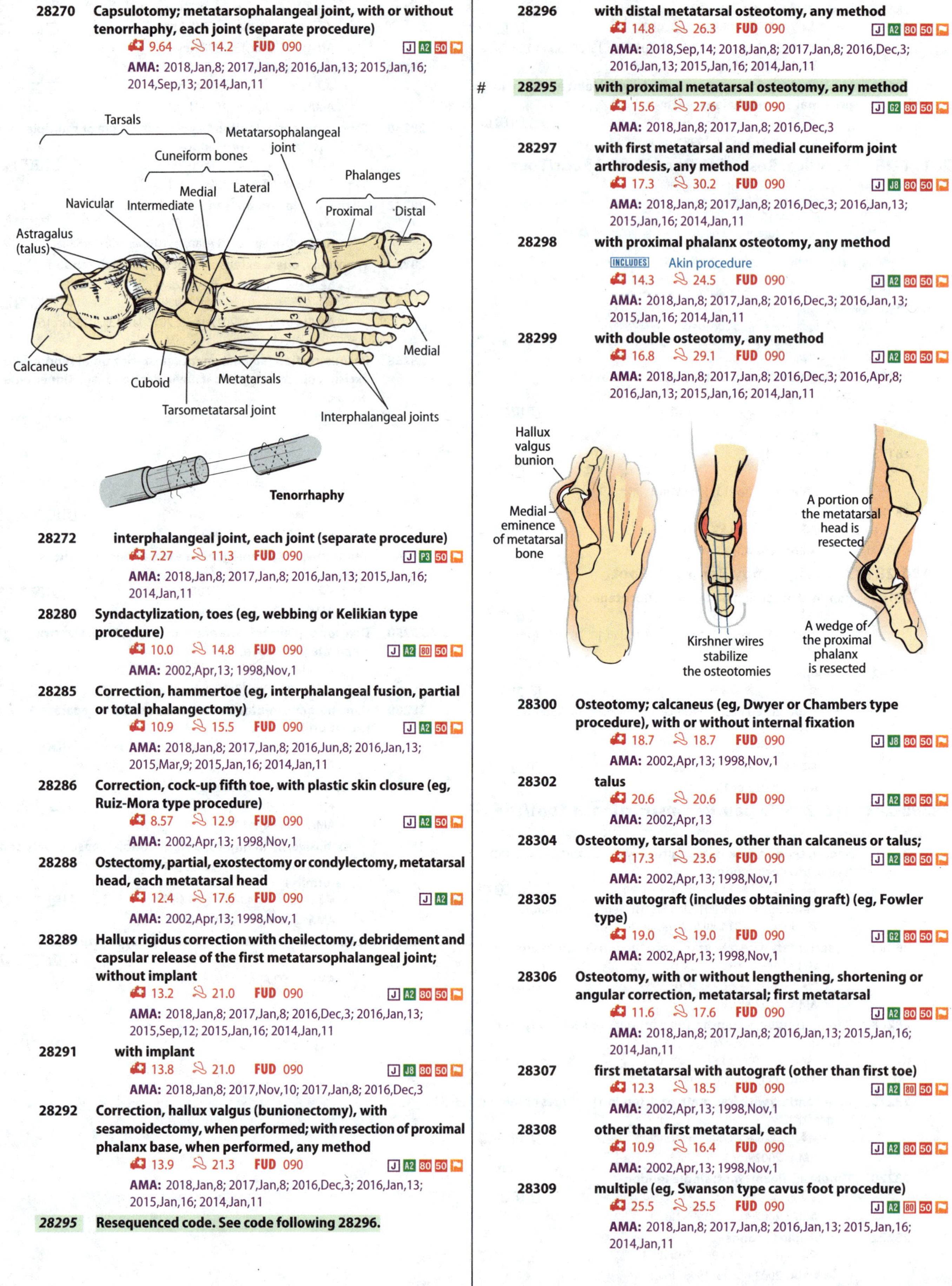

28272 **interphalangeal joint, each joint (separate procedure)**
7.27 11.3 FUD 090 J P3 50
AMA: 2018,Jan,8; 2017,Jan,8; 2016,Jan,13; 2015,Jan,16; 2014,Jan,11

28280 **Syndactylization, toes (eg, webbing or Kelikian type procedure)**
10.0 14.8 FUD 090 J A2 80 50
AMA: 2002,Apr,13; 1998,Nov,1

28285 **Correction, hammertoe (eg, interphalangeal fusion, partial or total phalangectomy)**
10.9 15.5 FUD 090 J A2 50
AMA: 2018,Jan,8; 2017,Jan,8; 2016,Jun,8; 2016,Jan,13; 2015,Mar,9; 2015,Jan,16; 2014,Jan,11

28286 **Correction, cock-up fifth toe, with plastic skin closure (eg, Ruiz-Mora type procedure)**
8.57 12.9 FUD 090 J A2 50
AMA: 2002,Apr,13; 1998,Nov,1

28288 **Ostectomy, partial, exostectomy or condylectomy, metatarsal head, each metatarsal head**
12.4 17.6 FUD 090 J A2
AMA: 2002,Apr,13; 1998,Nov,1

28289 **Hallux rigidus correction with cheilectomy, debridement and capsular release of the first metatarsophalangeal joint; without implant**
13.2 21.0 FUD 090 J A2 80 50
AMA: 2018,Jan,8; 2017,Jan,8; 2016,Dec,3; 2016,Jan,13; 2015,Sep,12; 2015,Jan,16; 2014,Jan,11

28291 **with implant**
13.8 21.0 FUD 090 J J8 80 50
AMA: 2018,Jan,8; 2017,Nov,10; 2017,Jan,8; 2016,Dec,3

28292 **Correction, hallux valgus (bunionectomy), with sesamoidectomy, when performed; with resection of proximal phalanx base, when performed, any method**
13.9 21.3 FUD 090 J A2 80 50
AMA: 2018,Jan,8; 2017,Jan,8; 2016,Dec,3; 2016,Jan,13; 2015,Jan,16; 2014,Jan,11

28295 **Resequenced code. See code following 28296.**

28296 **with distal metatarsal osteotomy, any method**
14.8 26.3 FUD 090 J A2 80 50
AMA: 2018,Sep,14; 2018,Jan,8; 2017,Jan,8; 2016,Dec,3; 2016,Jan,13; 2015,Jan,16; 2014,Jan,11

\# **28295** **with proximal metatarsal osteotomy, any method**
15.6 27.6 FUD 090 J G2 80 50
AMA: 2018,Jan,8; 2017,Jan,8; 2016,Dec,3

28297 **with first metatarsal and medial cuneiform joint arthrodesis, any method**
17.3 30.2 FUD 090 J J8 80 50
AMA: 2018,Jan,8; 2017,Jan,8; 2016,Dec,3; 2016,Jan,13; 2015,Jan,16; 2014,Jan,11

28298 **with proximal phalanx osteotomy, any method**
INCLUDES Akin procedure
14.3 24.5 FUD 090 J A2 80 50
AMA: 2018,Jan,8; 2017,Jan,8; 2016,Dec,3; 2016,Jan,13; 2015,Jan,16; 2014,Jan,11

28299 **with double osteotomy, any method**
16.8 29.1 FUD 090 J A2 80 50
AMA: 2018,Jan,8; 2017,Jan,8; 2016,Dec,3; 2016,Apr,8; 2016,Jan,13; 2015,Jan,16; 2014,Jan,11

28300 **Osteotomy; calcaneus (eg, Dwyer or Chambers type procedure), with or without internal fixation**
18.7 18.7 FUD 090 J J8 80 50
AMA: 2002,Apr,13; 1998,Nov,1

28302 **talus**
20.6 20.6 FUD 090 J A2 80 50
AMA: 2002,Apr,13

28304 **Osteotomy, tarsal bones, other than calcaneus or talus;**
17.3 23.6 FUD 090 J A2 80 50
AMA: 2002,Apr,13; 1998,Nov,1

28305 **with autograft (includes obtaining graft) (eg, Fowler type)**
19.0 19.0 FUD 090 J G2 80 50
AMA: 2002,Apr,13; 1998,Nov,1

28306 **Osteotomy, with or without lengthening, shortening or angular correction, metatarsal; first metatarsal**
11.6 17.6 FUD 090 J A2 80 50
AMA: 2018,Jan,8; 2017,Jan,8; 2016,Jan,13; 2015,Jan,16; 2014,Jan,11

28307 **first metatarsal with autograft (other than first toe)**
12.3 18.5 FUD 090 J A2 80 50
AMA: 2002,Apr,13; 1998,Nov,1

28308 **other than first metatarsal, each**
10.9 16.4 FUD 090 J A2 80 50
AMA: 2002,Apr,13; 1998,Nov,1

28309 **multiple (eg, Swanson type cavus foot procedure)**
25.5 25.5 FUD 090 J A2 80 50
AMA: 2018,Jan,8; 2017,Jan,8; 2016,Jan,13; 2015,Jan,16; 2014,Jan,11

26/TC PC/TC Only | A2-Z3 ASC Payment | 50 Bilateral | ♂ Male Only | ♀ Female Only | Facility RVU | Non-Facility RVU | CCI | CLIA
FUD Follow-up Days | CMS: IOM | AMA: CPT Asst | A-Y OPPSI | 80/80 Surg Assist Allowed / w/Doc | Lab Crosswalk | Radiology Crosswalk

28310 **Osteotomy, shortening, angular or rotational correction; proximal phalanx, first toe (separate procedure)**
10.2 15.7 FUD 090 J A2 50
AMA: 2018,Jan,8; 2017,Jan,8; 2016,Jan,13; 2015,Jan,16

28312 **other phalanges, any toe**
9.11 14.5 FUD 090 J A2
AMA: 2002,Apr,13

28313 **Reconstruction, angular deformity of toe, soft tissue procedures only (eg, overlapping second toe, fifth toe, curly toes)**
10.1 15.0 FUD 090 J A2
AMA: 2002,Apr,13; 1998,Nov,1

28315 **Sesamoidectomy, first toe (separate procedure)**
9.37 13.9 FUD 090 J A2 50
AMA: 2002,Apr,13

28320 **Repair, nonunion or malunion; tarsal bones**
17.5 17.5 FUD 090 J J8 80 50
AMA: 2002,Apr,13; 1998,Nov,1

28322 **metatarsal, with or without bone graft (includes obtaining graft)**
16.5 22.6 FUD 090 J J8 80
AMA: 2002,Apr,13

28340 **Reconstruction, toe, macrodactyly; soft tissue resection**
11.8 16.6 FUD 090 J A2
AMA: 2002,Apr,13

28341 **requiring bone resection**
14.1 19.3 FUD 090 J A2
AMA: 2002,Apr,13

28344 **Reconstruction, toe(s); polydactyly**
8.07 12.3 FUD 090 J A2 50
AMA: 2002,Apr,13

28345 **syndactyly, with or without skin graft(s), each web**
10.5 15.0 FUD 090 J A2 80
AMA: 2002,Apr,13

28360 **Reconstruction, cleft foot**
31.4 31.4 FUD 090 J 80 50
AMA: 2002,Apr,13

28400-28675 Treatment of Fracture/Dislocation of Foot/Toe

28400 **Closed treatment of calcaneal fracture; without manipulation**
6.52 7.09 FUD 090 T A2 50
AMA: 2002,Apr,13

28405 **with manipulation**
INCLUDES Bohler reduction
10.1 11.2 FUD 090 T A2 80 50
AMA: 2002,Apr,13

28406 **Percutaneous skeletal fixation of calcaneal fracture, with manipulation**
15.1 15.1 FUD 090 J A2 80 50
AMA: 2002,Apr,13

28415 **Open treatment of calcaneal fracture, includes internal fixation, when performed;**
32.1 32.1 FUD 090 J J8 80 50
AMA: 2002,Apr,13

28420 **with primary iliac or other autogenous bone graft (includes obtaining graft)**
36.8 36.8 FUD 090 J J8 80 50
AMA: 2002,Apr,13

28430 **Closed treatment of talus fracture; without manipulation**
6.01 6.81 FUD 090 T P2 50
AMA: 2002,Apr,13

28435 **with manipulation**
9.29 10.4 FUD 090 J A2 80 50
AMA: 2002,Apr,13

28436 **Percutaneous skeletal fixation of talus fracture, with manipulation**
12.9 12.9 FUD 090 J G2 50
AMA: 2002,Apr,13

28445 **Open treatment of talus fracture, includes internal fixation, when performed**
30.2 30.2 FUD 090 J A2 80 50
AMA: 2002,Apr,13

28446 **Open osteochondral autograft, talus (includes obtaining graft[s])**
INCLUDES Osteotomy; fibula (27707)
Osteotomy; tibia (27705)
EXCLUDES *Arthroscopically aided osteochondral talus graft (29892)*
Open osteochondral allograft or repairs with industrial grafts (28899)
35.3 35.3 FUD 090 J G2 80 50
AMA: 2018,Jan,8; 2017,Jan,8; 2016,Jan,13; 2015,Jan,16; 2014,Jan,11

28450 **Treatment of tarsal bone fracture (except talus and calcaneus); without manipulation, each**
5.47 6.09 FUD 090 T P2
AMA: 2018,Jan,8; 2017,Jan,8; 2016,Jan,13; 2015,Jan,16; 2014,Jan,11

28455 **with manipulation, each**
7.41 8.28 FUD 090 J P3 80
AMA: 2002,Apr,13

28456 **Percutaneous skeletal fixation of tarsal bone fracture (except talus and calcaneus), with manipulation, each**
9.25 9.25 FUD 090 J A2
AMA: 2002,Apr,13

28465 **Open treatment of tarsal bone fracture (except talus and calcaneus), includes internal fixation, when performed, each**
18.1 18.1 FUD 090 J J8
AMA: 2019,Aug,10

28470 **Closed treatment of metatarsal fracture; without manipulation, each**
5.83 6.26 FUD 090 T P2
AMA: 2002,Apr,13

28475 **with manipulation, each**
6.50 7.35 FUD 090 T P2
AMA: 2002,Apr,13

28476 **Percutaneous skeletal fixation of metatarsal fracture, with manipulation, each**
10.1 10.1 FUD 090 J A2 80
AMA: 2002,Apr,13

28485 **Open treatment of metatarsal fracture, includes internal fixation, when performed, each**
15.6 15.6 FUD 090 J J8
AMA: 2019,Aug,10

28490 **Closed treatment of fracture great toe, phalanx or phalanges; without manipulation**
3.57 4.12 FUD 090 T P3 50
AMA: 2002,Apr,13

28495 **with manipulation**
4.28 5.13 FUD 090 T P2 50
AMA: 2002,Apr,13

28496 **Percutaneous skeletal fixation of fracture great toe, phalanx or phalanges, with manipulation**
7.03 13.2 FUD 090 J A2 50
AMA: 2002,Apr,13

28505 **Open treatment of fracture, great toe, phalanx or phalanges, includes internal fixation, when performed**
14.3 19.1 FUD 090 J A2 50
AMA: 2002,Apr,13

28510 **Closed treatment of fracture, phalanx or phalanges, other than great toe; without manipulation, each**
3.43 3.51 FUD 090 T P3
AMA: 2002,Apr,13

28515 **with manipulation, each**
4.08 4.67 FUD 090 T P3
AMA: 2002,Apr,13

28525 **Open treatment of fracture, phalanx or phalanges, other than great toe, includes internal fixation, when performed, each**
11.5 16.4 FUD 090 J A2 80
AMA: 2002,Apr,13

28530 **Closed treatment of sesamoid fracture**
2.95 3.34 FUD 090 T P3 80 50
AMA: 2002,Apr,13

28531 **Open treatment of sesamoid fracture, with or without internal fixation**
5.23 9.85 FUD 090 J A2 50
AMA: 2002,Apr,13

28540 **Closed treatment of tarsal bone dislocation, other than talotarsal; without anesthesia**
5.00 5.56 FUD 090 T P2 80 50
AMA: 2002,Apr,13

28545 **requiring anesthesia**
7.58 8.60 FUD 090 J G2 80 50
AMA: 2002,Apr,13

28546 **Percutaneous skeletal fixation of tarsal bone dislocation, other than talotarsal, with manipulation**
9.82 16.7 FUD 090 J A2 80 50
AMA: 2002,Apr,13

28555 **Open treatment of tarsal bone dislocation, includes internal fixation, when performed**
18.9 24.9 FUD 090 J J8 80 50
AMA: 2002,Apr,13

28570 **Closed treatment of talotarsal joint dislocation; without anesthesia**
5.51 6.54 FUD 090 T P2 80 50
AMA: 2002,Apr,13

28575 **requiring anesthesia**
9.54 10.5 FUD 090 J A2 80 50
AMA: 2002,Apr,13

28576 **Percutaneous skeletal fixation of talotarsal joint dislocation, with manipulation**
11.2 11.2 FUD 090 J A2 80 50
AMA: 2002,Apr,13

28585 **Open treatment of talotarsal joint dislocation, includes internal fixation, when performed**
19.6 25.0 FUD 090 J J8 80 50
AMA: 2018,Jan,8; 2017,Jan,8; 2016,Jan,13; 2015,Jan,16; 2014,Jan,11

28600 **Closed treatment of tarsometatarsal joint dislocation; without anesthesia**
5.35 6.26 FUD 090 T P2 80
AMA: 2002,Apr,13

28605 **requiring anesthesia**
8.51 9.52 FUD 090 T A2 80
AMA: 2002,Apr,13

28606 **Percutaneous skeletal fixation of tarsometatarsal joint dislocation, with manipulation**
11.2 11.2 FUD 090 J A2
AMA: 2002,Apr,13

28615 **Open treatment of tarsometatarsal joint dislocation, includes internal fixation, when performed**
23.2 23.2 FUD 090 J J8 80
AMA: 2002,Apr,13

28630 **Closed treatment of metatarsophalangeal joint dislocation; without anesthesia**
3.15 4.49 FUD 010 T P3 80
AMA: 2002,Apr,13

28635 **requiring anesthesia**
3.82 5.08 FUD 010 J A2 80
AMA: 2002,Apr,13

28636 **Percutaneous skeletal fixation of metatarsophalangeal joint dislocation, with manipulation**
5.91 9.25 FUD 010 J A2
AMA: 2002,Apr,13

28645 **Open treatment of metatarsophalangeal joint dislocation, includes internal fixation, when performed**
13.9 18.9 FUD 090 J A2
AMA: 2018,Jan,8; 2017,Jan,8; 2016,Jan,13; 2015,Jan,16; 2014,Sep,13

28660 **Closed treatment of interphalangeal joint dislocation; without anesthesia**
2.56 3.38 FUD 010 T P3
AMA: 2002,Apr,13

28665 **requiring anesthesia**
3.76 4.45 FUD 010 T A2 80
AMA: 2002,Apr,13

28666 **Percutaneous skeletal fixation of interphalangeal joint dislocation, with manipulation**
4.53 4.53 FUD 010 J A2
AMA: 2002,Apr,13

28675 **Open treatment of interphalangeal joint dislocation, includes internal fixation, when performed**
11.5 16.4 FUD 090 J A2
AMA: 2002,Apr,13

28705-28760 Arthrodesis of Foot/Toe

28705 **Arthrodesis; pantalar**
35.5 35.5 FUD 090 J J8 80 50
AMA: 2002,Apr,13

28715 **triple**
27.1 27.1 FUD 090 J J8 80 50
AMA: 2002,Apr,13; 1998,Nov,1

28725 **subtalar**
INCLUDES Dunn arthrodesis
Grice arthrosis
22.4 22.4 FUD 090 J J8 80 50
AMA: 2018,Jan,8; 2017,Jan,8; 2016,Jan,13; 2015,Jan,16; 2014,Jan,11

28730 **Arthrodesis, midtarsal or tarsometatarsal, multiple or transverse;**
INCLUDES Lambrinudi arthrodesis
21.1 21.1 FUD 090 J J8 80 50
AMA: 2002,Apr,13

28735 **with osteotomy (eg, flatfoot correction)**
22.4 22.4 FUD 090 J J8 80 50
AMA: 2019,May,10

28737 **Arthrodesis, with tendon lengthening and advancement, midtarsal, tarsal navicular-cuneiform (eg, Miller type procedure)**
20.0 20.0 FUD 090 J J8 80 50
AMA: 2002,Apr,13; 2002,May,7

28740 **Arthrodesis, midtarsal or tarsometatarsal, single joint**
17.9 24.3 FUD 090 J J8 80 50
AMA: 2018,Jan,8; 2017,Jan,8; 2016,Jan,13; 2015,Jan,16; 2014,Jan,11

28750 **Arthrodesis, great toe; metatarsophalangeal joint**
16.8 23.1 FUD 090 J J8 80 50
AMA: 2018,Jan,8; 2017,Jan,8; 2016,Dec,3; 2016,Jan,13; 2015,Jan,16; 2014,Jan,11

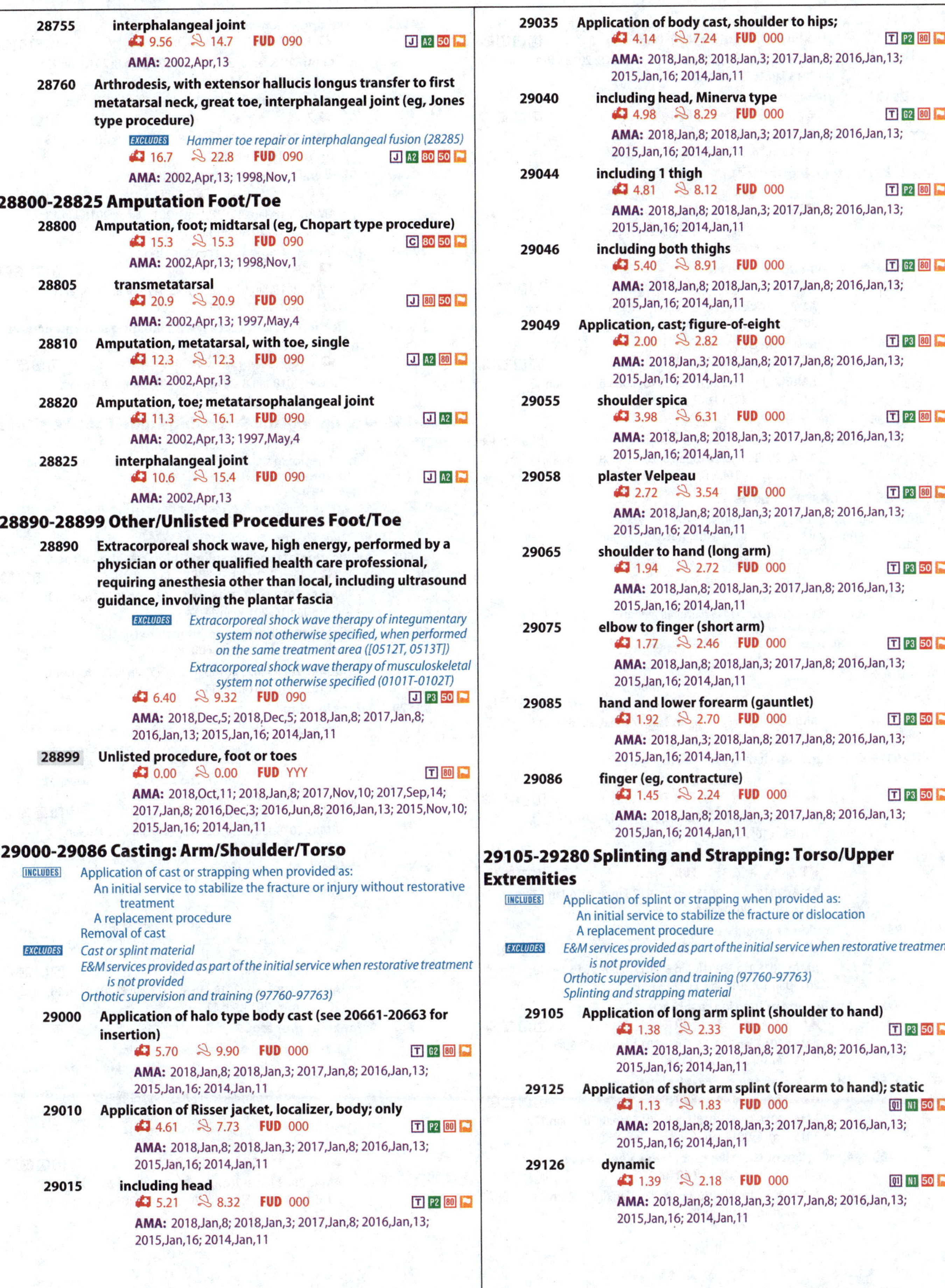

28755 **interphalangeal joint**
9.56 14.7 **FUD** 090 J A2 50
AMA: 2002,Apr,13

28760 **Arthrodesis, with extensor hallucis longus transfer to first metatarsal neck, great toe, interphalangeal joint (eg, Jones type procedure)**
EXCLUDES *Hammer toe repair or interphalangeal fusion (28285)*
16.7 22.8 **FUD** 090 J A2 80 50
AMA: 2002,Apr,13; 1998,Nov,1

28800-28825 Amputation Foot/Toe

28800 **Amputation, foot; midtarsal (eg, Chopart type procedure)**
15.3 15.3 **FUD** 090 C 80 50
AMA: 2002,Apr,13; 1998,Nov,1

28805 **transmetatarsal**
20.9 20.9 **FUD** 090 J 80 50
AMA: 2002,Apr,13; 1997,May,4

28810 **Amputation, metatarsal, with toe, single**
12.3 12.3 **FUD** 090 J A2 80
AMA: 2002,Apr,13

28820 **Amputation, toe; metatarsophalangeal joint**
11.3 16.1 **FUD** 090 J A2
AMA: 2002,Apr,13; 1997,May,4

28825 **interphalangeal joint**
10.6 15.4 **FUD** 090 J A2
AMA: 2002,Apr,13

28890-28899 Other/Unlisted Procedures Foot/Toe

28890 **Extracorporeal shock wave, high energy, performed by a physician or other qualified health care professional, requiring anesthesia other than local, including ultrasound guidance, involving the plantar fascia**
EXCLUDES *Extracorporeal shock wave therapy of integumentary system not otherwise specified, when performed on the same treatment area ([0512T, 0513T])*
Extracorporeal shock wave therapy of musculoskeletal system not otherwise specified (0101T-0102T)
6.40 9.32 **FUD** 090 J P3 50
AMA: 2018,Dec,5; 2018,Dec,5; 2018,Jan,8; 2017,Jan,8; 2016,Jan,13; 2015,Jan,16; 2014,Jan,11

28899 **Unlisted procedure, foot or toes**
0.00 0.00 **FUD** YYY T 80
AMA: 2018,Oct,11; 2018,Jan,8; 2017,Nov,10; 2017,Sep,14; 2017,Jan,8; 2016,Dec,3; 2016,Jun,8; 2016,Jan,13; 2015,Nov,10; 2015,Jan,16; 2014,Jan,11

29000-29086 Casting: Arm/Shoulder/Torso

INCLUDES Application of cast or strapping when provided as:
- An initial service to stabilize the fracture or injury without restorative treatment
- A replacement procedure

Removal of cast

EXCLUDES *Cast or splint material*
E&M services provided as part of the initial service when restorative treatment is not provided
Orthotic supervision and training (97760-97763)

29000 **Application of halo type body cast (see 20661-20663 for insertion)**
5.70 9.90 **FUD** 000 T G2 80
AMA: 2018,Jan,8; 2018,Jan,3; 2017,Jan,8; 2016,Jan,13; 2015,Jan,16; 2014,Jan,11

29010 **Application of Risser jacket, localizer, body; only**
4.61 7.73 **FUD** 000 T P2 80
AMA: 2018,Jan,8; 2018,Jan,3; 2017,Jan,8; 2016,Jan,13; 2015,Jan,16; 2014,Jan,11

29015 **including head**
5.21 8.32 **FUD** 000 T P2 80
AMA: 2018,Jan,8; 2018,Jan,3; 2017,Jan,8; 2016,Jan,13; 2015,Jan,16; 2014,Jan,11

29035 **Application of body cast, shoulder to hips;**
4.14 7.24 **FUD** 000 T P2 80
AMA: 2018,Jan,8; 2018,Jan,3; 2017,Jan,8; 2016,Jan,13; 2015,Jan,16; 2014,Jan,11

29040 **including head, Minerva type**
4.98 8.29 **FUD** 000 T G2 80
AMA: 2018,Jan,8; 2018,Jan,3; 2017,Jan,8; 2016,Jan,13; 2015,Jan,16; 2014,Jan,11

29044 **including 1 thigh**
4.81 8.12 **FUD** 000 T P2 80
AMA: 2018,Jan,8; 2018,Jan,3; 2017,Jan,8; 2016,Jan,13; 2015,Jan,16; 2014,Jan,11

29046 **including both thighs**
5.40 8.91 **FUD** 000 T G2 80
AMA: 2018,Jan,8; 2018,Jan,3; 2017,Jan,8; 2016,Jan,13; 2015,Jan,16; 2014,Jan,11

29049 **Application, cast; figure-of-eight**
2.00 2.82 **FUD** 000 T P3 80
AMA: 2018,Jan,3; 2018,Jan,8; 2017,Jan,8; 2016,Jan,13; 2015,Jan,16; 2014,Jan,11

29055 **shoulder spica**
3.98 6.31 **FUD** 000 T P2 80
AMA: 2018,Jan,8; 2018,Jan,3; 2017,Jan,8; 2016,Jan,13; 2015,Jan,16; 2014,Jan,11

29058 **plaster Velpeau**
2.72 3.54 **FUD** 000 T P3 80
AMA: 2018,Jan,8; 2018,Jan,3; 2017,Jan,8; 2016,Jan,13; 2015,Jan,16; 2014,Jan,11

29065 **shoulder to hand (long arm)**
1.94 2.72 **FUD** 000 T P3 50
AMA: 2018,Jan,8; 2018,Jan,3; 2017,Jan,8; 2016,Jan,13; 2015,Jan,16; 2014,Jan,11

29075 **elbow to finger (short arm)**
1.77 2.46 **FUD** 000 T P3 50
AMA: 2018,Jan,8; 2018,Jan,3; 2017,Jan,8; 2016,Jan,13; 2015,Jan,16; 2014,Jan,11

29085 **hand and lower forearm (gauntlet)**
1.92 2.70 **FUD** 000 T P3 50
AMA: 2018,Jan,3; 2018,Jan,8; 2017,Jan,8; 2016,Jan,13; 2015,Jan,16; 2014,Jan,11

29086 **finger (eg, contracture)**
1.45 2.24 **FUD** 000 T P3 50
AMA: 2018,Jan,8; 2018,Jan,3; 2017,Jan,8; 2016,Jan,13; 2015,Jan,16; 2014,Jan,11

29105-29280 Splinting and Strapping: Torso/Upper Extremities

INCLUDES Application of splint or strapping when provided as:
- An initial service to stabilize the fracture or dislocation
- A replacement procedure

EXCLUDES *E&M services provided as part of the initial service when restorative treatment is not provided*
Orthotic supervision and training (97760-97763)
Splinting and strapping material

29105 **Application of long arm splint (shoulder to hand)**
1.38 2.33 **FUD** 000 T P3 50
AMA: 2018,Jan,3; 2018,Jan,8; 2017,Jan,8; 2016,Jan,13; 2015,Jan,16; 2014,Jan,11

29125 **Application of short arm splint (forearm to hand); static**
1.13 1.83 **FUD** 000 01 N1 50
AMA: 2018,Jan,8; 2018,Jan,3; 2017,Jan,8; 2016,Jan,13; 2015,Jan,16; 2014,Jan,11

29126 **dynamic**
1.39 2.18 **FUD** 000 01 N1 50
AMA: 2018,Jan,8; 2018,Jan,3; 2017,Jan,8; 2016,Jan,13; 2015,Jan,16; 2014,Jan,11

29130 **Application of finger splint; static**
0.83 1.17 **FUD** 000 Q1 N1 50
AMA: 2018,Jan,8; 2018,Jan,3; 2017,Jan,8; 2016,Jan,13; 2015,Jan,16; 2014,Jan,11

29131 **dynamic**
0.96 1.46 **FUD** 000 Q1 N1 50
AMA: 2018,Jan,8; 2018,Jan,3; 2017,Jan,8; 2016,Jan,13; 2015,Jan,16; 2014,Jan,11

29200 **Strapping; thorax**
EXCLUDES *Strapping of low back (29799)*
0.54 0.91 **FUD** 000 T P3
AMA: 2018,Jan,8; 2018,Jan,3; 2017,Jan,8; 2016,Jan,13; 2015,Jan,16; 2014,Jan,11

29240 **shoulder (eg, Velpeau)**
0.54 0.87 **FUD** 000 Q1 N1 50
AMA: 2018,Jan,3; 2018,Jan,8; 2017,Jan,8; 2016,Jan,13; 2015,Jan,16; 2014,Jan,11

29260 **elbow or wrist**
0.56 0.85 **FUD** 000 Q1 N1 50
AMA: 2018,Jan,8; 2018,Jan,3; 2017,Jan,8; 2016,Jan,13; 2015,Jan,16; 2014,Jan,11

29280 **hand or finger**
0.58 0.87 **FUD** 000 Q1 N1 50
AMA: 2018,Jan,8; 2018,Jan,3; 2017,Jan,8; 2016,Jan,13; 2015,Jan,16; 2014,Jan,11

29305-29450 Casting: Legs

INCLUDES Application of cast when provided as:
An initial service to stabilize the fracture or injury without restorative treatment
A replacement procedure
Removal of cast

EXCLUDES *Cast or splint materials*
E&M services provided as part of the initial service when restorative treatment is not provided
Orthotic supervision and training (97760-97763)

29305 **Application of hip spica cast; 1 leg**
EXCLUDES *Hip spica cast thighs only (29046)*
4.57 7.02 **FUD** 000 T P2 80
AMA: 2018,Jan,8; 2018,Jan,3; 2017,Jan,8; 2016,Jan,13; 2015,Jan,16; 2014,Jan,11

29325 **1 and one-half spica or both legs**
EXCLUDES *Hip spica cast thighs only (29046)*
5.11 7.75 **FUD** 000 T P2 80
AMA: 2018,Jan,8; 2018,Jan,3; 2017,Jan,8; 2016,Jan,13; 2015,Jan,16; 2014,Jan,11

29345 **Application of long leg cast (thigh to toes);**
2.87 3.85 **FUD** 000 T P3 50
AMA: 2018,Jan,3; 2018,Jan,8; 2017,Jan,8; 2016,Jan,13; 2015,Jan,16; 2014,Jan,11

29355 **walker or ambulatory type**
3.06 4.03 **FUD** 000 T P3 50
AMA: 2018,Jan,3; 2018,Jan,8; 2017,Jan,8; 2016,Jan,13; 2015,Jan,16; 2014,Jan,11

29358 **Application of long leg cast brace**
2.99 4.57 **FUD** 000 T P3 50
AMA: 2018,Jan,3; 2018,Jan,8; 2017,Jan,8; 2016,Jan,13; 2015,Jan,16; 2014,Jan,11

29365 **Application of cylinder cast (thigh to ankle)**
2.51 3.49 **FUD** 000 T P3 50
AMA: 2018,Jan,3; 2018,Jan,8; 2017,Jan,8; 2016,Jan,13; 2015,Jan,16; 2014,Jan,11

29405 **Application of short leg cast (below knee to toes);**
1.70 2.30 **FUD** 000 T P3 50
AMA: 2018,Jan,3; 2018,Jan,8; 2017,Jan,8; 2016,Jan,13; 2015,Jan,16; 2014,Jan,11

29425 **walking or ambulatory type**
1.60 2.20 **FUD** 000 T P3 50
AMA: 2018,Jan,3; 2018,Jan,8; 2017,Jan,8; 2016,Jan,13; 2015,Jan,16; 2014,Jan,11

29435 **Application of patellar tendon bearing (PTB) cast**
2.38 3.35 **FUD** 000 T P3 50
AMA: 2018,Jan,3; 2018,Jan,8; 2017,Jan,8; 2016,Jan,13; 2015,Jan,16; 2014,Jan,11

29440 **Adding walker to previously applied cast**
0.82 1.24 **FUD** 000 T P3 50
AMA: 2018,Jan,8; 2018,Jan,3; 2017,Jan,8; 2016,Jan,13; 2015,Jan,16; 2014,Jan,11

29445 **Application of rigid total contact leg cast**
2.94 3.73 **FUD** 000 T P3 50
AMA: 2018,Jan,3; 2018,Jan,8; 2017,Jan,8; 2016,Jan,13; 2015,Jan,16; 2014,Jan,11

29450 **Application of clubfoot cast with molding or manipulation, long or short leg**
3.26 4.15 **FUD** 000 T P3 50
AMA: 2018,Jan,8; 2018,Jan,3; 2017,Jan,8; 2016,Jan,13; 2015,Jan,16; 2014,Jan,11

29505-29584 Splinting and Strapping Ankle/Foot/Leg/Toes

INCLUDES Application of splinting and strapping when provided as:
An initial service to stabilize the fracture or injury without restorative treatment
A replacement procedure

EXCLUDES *E&M services provided as part of the initial service when restorative treatment is not provided*
Orthotic supervision and training (97760-97763)

29505 **Application of long leg splint (thigh to ankle or toes)**
1.45 2.43 **FUD** 000 T P3 50
AMA: 2018,Jan,3; 2018,Jan,8; 2017,Jan,8; 2016,Jan,13; 2015,Jan,16; 2014,Jan,11

29515 **Application of short leg splint (calf to foot)**
1.42 2.03 **FUD** 000 T P3 50
AMA: 2018,Jan,8; 2018,Jan,3; 2017,Jan,8; 2016,Jan,13; 2015,Jan,16; 2014,Jan,11

29520 **Strapping; hip**
EXCLUDES *For treatment of the same extremity:*
Endovenous ablation therapy of incompetent vein (36473-36479, [36482], [36483])
Sclerosal injection for incompetent vein(s) ([36465], [36466], 36468-36471)
0.55 0.97 **FUD** 000 Q1 N1 80 50
AMA: 2018,Jan,8; 2018,Jan,3; 2017,Jan,8; 2016,Jan,13; 2015,Jan,16; 2014,Jan,11

29530 **knee**
EXCLUDES *For treatment of the same extremity:*
Endovenous ablation therapy of incompetent vein (36473-36479, [36482], [36483])
Sclerosal injection for incompetent vein(s) ([36465], [36466], 36468-36471)
0.54 0.86 **FUD** 000 Q1 N1 50
AMA: 2018,Jan,3; 2018,Jan,8; 2017,Jan,8; 2016,Jan,13; 2015,Jan,16; 2014,Jan,11

29540 **ankle and/or foot**
EXCLUDES *For treatment of the same extremity:*
Endovenous ablation therapy of incompetent vein (36473-36479, [36482, 36483])
Multi-layer compression system (29581)
Sclerosal injection for incompetent vein(s) ([36465], [36466], 36468-36471)
Unna boot (29580)
0.52 0.82 **FUD** 000 T P3 50
AMA: 2018,Jan,3; 2018,Jan,8; 2017,Jan,8; 2016,Aug,3; 2016,Jan,13; 2015,Jan,16; 2014,Mar,4; 2014,Jan,11

29550 **toes**

EXCLUDES *For treatment of the same extremity:*
Endovenous ablation therapy of incompetent vein (36473-36479, [36482, 36483])
Sclerosal injection for incompetent vein(s) ([36465], [36466], 36468-36471)

0.33 0.55 FUD 000 Q1 N1 50

AMA: 2018,Jan,8; 2018,Jan,3; 2017,Jan,8; 2016,Jan,13; 2015,Jan,16; 2014,Jan,11

29580 **Unna boot**

EXCLUDES *Application of multi-layer compression system (29581)*
For treatment of the same extremity:
Endovenous ablation therapy of incompetent vein (36473-36479, [36482, 36483])
Sclerosal injection for incompetent vein(s) ([36465], [36466], 36468-36471)
Strapping of ankle or foot (29540)

0.79 1.78 FUD 000 T P3 50

AMA: 2018,Jan,3; 2018,Jan,8; 2017,Jan,8; 2016,Aug,3; 2016,Jan,13; 2015,Jan,16; 2014,Mar,4; 2014,Jan,11

29581 **Application of multi-layer compression system; leg (below knee), including ankle and foot**

EXCLUDES *For treatment of the same extremity:*
Endovenous ablation therapy of incompetent vein (36473-36479, [36482, 36483])
Sclerosal injection for incompetent vein(s) ([36465], [36466], 36468-36471)
Strapping (29540, 29580)

0.80 2.47 FUD 000 T P3 80 50

AMA: 2018,Mar,3; 2018,Jan,8; 2018,Jan,3; 2017,Jan,8; 2016,Nov,3; 2016,Aug,3; 2016,Jan,13; 2015,Mar,9; 2015,Jan,16; 2014,Oct,6; 2014,Mar,4; 2014,Jan,11

29584 **upper arm, forearm, hand, and fingers**

EXCLUDES *For treatment of the same extremity:*
Endovenous ablation therapy of incompetent vein (36473-36479, [36482], [36483])
Sclerosal injection for incompetent vein(s) ([36465], [36466], 36468-36471)

0.47 2.29 FUD 000 T P2 80 50

AMA: 2018,Jan,3; 2018,Jan,8; 2017,Jan,8; 2016,Aug,3; 2016,Jan,13; 2015,Mar,9

29700-29799 Casting Services Other Than Application

INCLUDES Casts applied by treating individual
Removal of casts applied by treating individual

29700 **Removal or bivalving; gauntlet, boot or body cast**

0.96 1.82 FUD 000 T P3

AMA: 2018,Jan,3; 2018,Jan,8; 2017,Jan,8; 2016,Jan,13; 2015,Jan,16; 2014,Jan,11

29705 **full arm or full leg cast**

1.33 1.85 FUD 000 T P3 50

AMA: 2018,Jan,3; 2018,Jan,8; 2017,Jan,8; 2016,Jan,13; 2015,Jan,16; 2014,Jan,11

29710 **shoulder or hip spica, Minerva, or Risser jacket, etc.**

2.41 3.51 FUD 000 T P3 80 50

AMA: 2018,Jan,3; 2018,Jan,8; 2017,Jan,8; 2016,Jan,13; 2015,Jan,16; 2014,Jan,11

29720 **Repair of spica, body cast or jacket**

1.28 2.41 FUD 000 T P3

AMA: 2018,Jan,3; 2018,Jan,8; 2017,Jan,8; 2016,Jan,13; 2015,Jan,16; 2014,Jan,11

29730 **Windowing of cast**

1.27 1.79 FUD 000 T P3

AMA: 2018,Jan,3; 2018,Jan,8; 2017,Jan,8; 2016,Jan,13; 2015,Jan,16; 2014,Jan,11

29740 **Wedging of cast (except clubfoot casts)**

2.03 2.83 FUD 000 T P3

AMA: 2018,Jan,3; 2018,Jan,8; 2017,Jan,8; 2016,Jan,13; 2015,Jan,16; 2014,Jan,11

29750 **Wedging of clubfoot cast**

2.26 3.07 FUD 000 T P3 80 50

AMA: 2018,Jan,3; 2018,Jan,8; 2017,Jan,8; 2016,Jan,13; 2015,Jan,16; 2014,Jan,11

29799 **Unlisted procedure, casting or strapping**

0.00 0.00 FUD YYY T 80

AMA: 2018,Jan,3; 2018,Jan,8; 2017,Jan,8; 2016,Aug,3; 2016,Jan,13; 2015,Jan,16; 2014,Jan,11

29800-29999 [29914, 29915, 29916] Arthroscopic Procedures

INCLUDES Diagnostic arthroscopy with surgical arthroscopy
Code also modifier 51 if arthroscopy is performed with arthrotomy

29800 **Arthroscopy, temporomandibular joint, diagnostic, with or without synovial biopsy (separate procedure)**

15.2 15.2 FUD 090 J A2 80 50

AMA: 2018,Jan,8; 2017,Jan,8; 2016,Jan,13; 2015,Jan,16

29804 **Arthroscopy, temporomandibular joint, surgical**

EXCLUDES *Open surgery (21010)*

18.4 18.4 FUD 090 J A2 80 50

AMA: 2018,Jan,8; 2017,Jan,8; 2016,Jan,13; 2015,Jan,16

29805 **Arthroscopy, shoulder, diagnostic, with or without synovial biopsy (separate procedure)**

EXCLUDES *Open surgery (23065-23066, 23100-23101)*

13.5 13.5 FUD 090 J A2 50

AMA: 2018,Jan,8; 2017,Jan,8; 2016,Jan,13; 2015,Jun,10; 2015,Jan,16

29806 **Arthroscopy, shoulder, surgical; capsulorrhaphy**

EXCLUDES *Open surgery (23450-23466)*
Thermal capsulorrhaphy (29999)

30.5 30.5 FUD 090 J A2 50

AMA: 2018,Jun,11; 2018,Jan,8; 2017,Jan,8; 2016,Jan,13; 2015,Jul,10; 2015,Mar,7; 2015,Jan,16

29807 **repair of SLAP lesion**

29.8 29.8 FUD 090 J A2 50

AMA: 2018,Jan,8; 2017,Jan,8; 2016,Jan,13; 2015,Mar,7; 2015,Jan,16

29819 **with removal of loose body or foreign body**

EXCLUDES *Open surgery (23040-23044, 23107)*

16.8 16.8 FUD 090 J A2 50

AMA: 2018,Jun,11; 2018,Jan,8; 2017,Jan,8; 2016,Jan,13; 2015,Mar,7; 2015,Jan,16

29820 **synovectomy, partial**

EXCLUDES *Open surgery (23105)*

15.3 15.3 FUD 090 J A2 80 50

AMA: 2018,Jan,8; 2017,Jan,8; 2016,Jan,13; 2015,Mar,7; 2015,Jan,16

29821 **synovectomy, complete**

EXCLUDES *Open surgery (23105)*

16.8 16.8 FUD 090 J A2 80 50

AMA: 2018,Jan,8; 2017,Jan,8; 2016,Jan,13; 2015,Mar,7; 2015,Jan,16

29822 **debridement, limited**

EXCLUDES *Open surgery (see specific shoulder section)*

16.3 16.3 FUD 090 J A2 80 50

AMA: 2018,Jan,7; 2018,Jan,8; 2017,Jan,8; 2016,Jan,13; 2015,Mar,7; 2015,Jan,16; 2014,Jan,11

29823 **debridement, extensive**

EXCLUDES *Open surgery (see specific shoulder section)*

17.7 17.7 FUD 090 J A2 80 50

AMA: 2018,Jan,7; 2018,Jan,8; 2017,Jan,8; 2016,Dec,16; 2016,Jan,13; 2015,Mar,7; 2015,Jan,16; 2014,Jan,11

29824 **distal claviculectomy including distal articular surface (Mumford procedure)**

INCLUDES Mumford procedure

EXCLUDES *Open surgery (23120)*

19.1 19.1 FUD 090 J A2 80 50

AMA: 2018,Jan,8; 2017,Jan,8; 2016,Jan,13; 2015,Mar,7; 2015,Jan,16

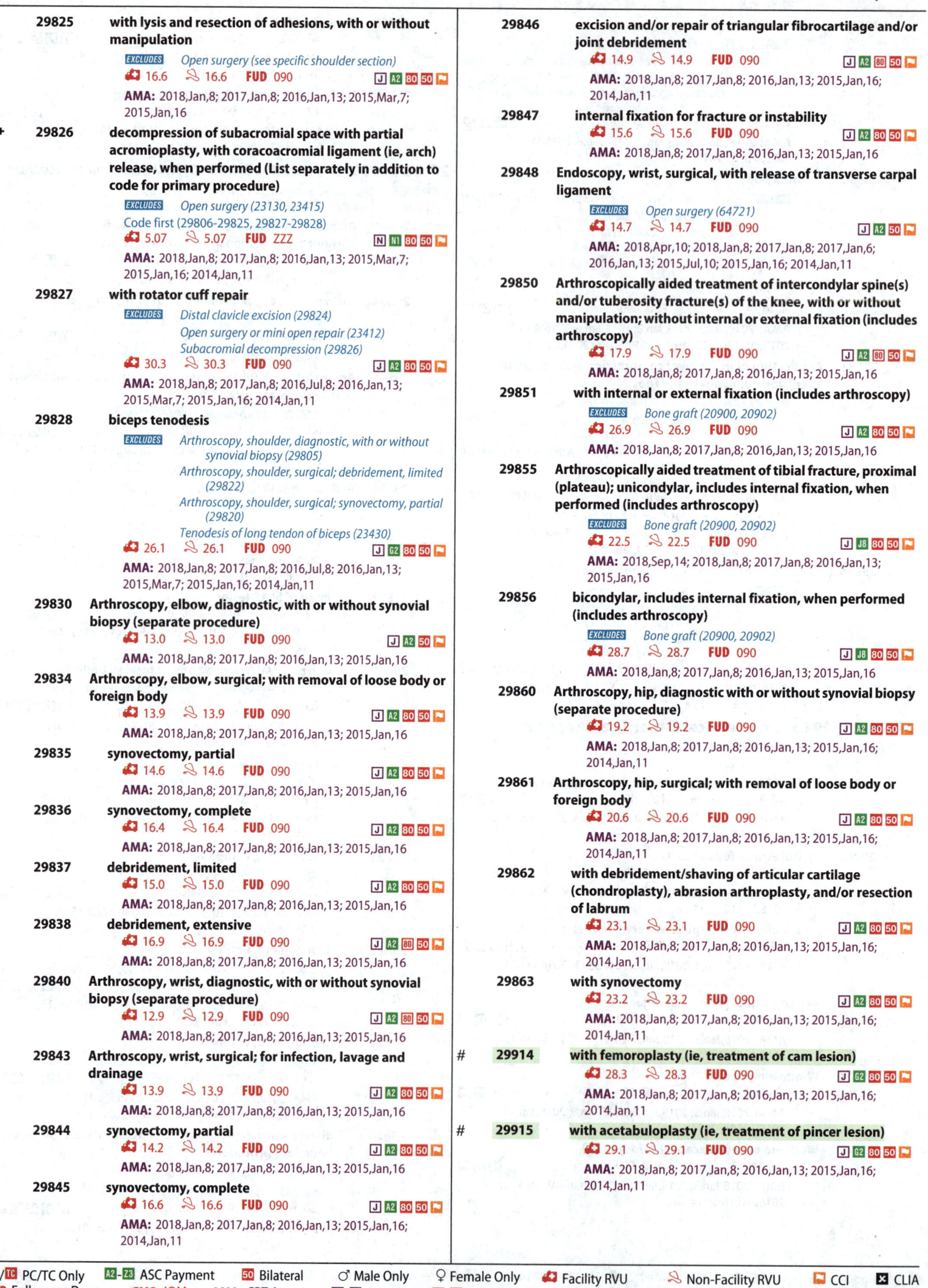

29825 **with lysis and resection of adhesions, with or without manipulation**
EXCLUDES *Open surgery (see specific shoulder section)*
16.6 16.6 FUD 090 J A2 80 50
AMA: 2018,Jan,8; 2017,Jan,8; 2016,Jan,13; 2015,Mar,7; 2015,Jan,16

\+ **29826** **decompression of subacromial space with partial acromioplasty, with coracoacromial ligament (ie, arch) release, when performed (List separately in addition to code for primary procedure)**
EXCLUDES *Open surgery (23130, 23415)*
Code first (29806-29825, 29827-29828)
5.07 5.07 FUD ZZZ N N1 80 50
AMA: 2018,Jan,8; 2017,Jan,8; 2016,Jan,13; 2015,Mar,7; 2015,Jan,16; 2014,Jan,11

29827 **with rotator cuff repair**
EXCLUDES *Distal clavicle excision (29824)*
Open surgery or mini open repair (23412)
Subacromial decompression (29826)
30.3 30.3 FUD 090 J A2 80 50
AMA: 2018,Jan,8; 2017,Jan,8; 2016,Jul,8; 2016,Jan,13; 2015,Mar,7; 2015,Jan,16; 2014,Jan,11

29828 **biceps tenodesis**
EXCLUDES *Arthroscopy, shoulder, diagnostic, with or without synovial biopsy (29805)*
Arthroscopy, shoulder, surgical; debridement, limited (29822)
Arthroscopy, shoulder, surgical; synovectomy, partial (29820)
Tenodesis of long tendon of biceps (23430)
26.1 26.1 FUD 090 J G2 80 50
AMA: 2018,Jan,8; 2017,Jan,8; 2016,Jul,8; 2016,Jan,13; 2015,Mar,7; 2015,Jan,16; 2014,Jan,11

29830 **Arthroscopy, elbow, diagnostic, with or without synovial biopsy (separate procedure)**
13.0 13.0 FUD 090 J A2 50
AMA: 2018,Jan,8; 2017,Jan,8; 2016,Jan,13; 2015,Jan,16

29834 **Arthroscopy, elbow, surgical; with removal of loose body or foreign body**
13.9 13.9 FUD 090 J A2 80 50
AMA: 2018,Jan,8; 2017,Jan,8; 2016,Jan,13; 2015,Jan,16

29835 **synovectomy, partial**
14.6 14.6 FUD 090 J A2 80 50
AMA: 2018,Jan,8; 2017,Jan,8; 2016,Jan,13; 2015,Jan,16

29836 **synovectomy, complete**
16.4 16.4 FUD 090 J A2 80 50
AMA: 2018,Jan,8; 2017,Jan,8; 2016,Jan,13; 2015,Jan,16

29837 **debridement, limited**
15.0 15.0 FUD 090 J A2 80 50
AMA: 2018,Jan,8; 2017,Jan,8; 2016,Jan,13; 2015,Jan,16

29838 **debridement, extensive**
16.9 16.9 FUD 090 J A2 80 50
AMA: 2018,Jan,8; 2017,Jan,8; 2016,Jan,13; 2015,Jan,16

29840 **Arthroscopy, wrist, diagnostic, with or without synovial biopsy (separate procedure)**
12.9 12.9 FUD 090 J A2 80 50
AMA: 2018,Jan,8; 2017,Jan,8; 2016,Jan,13; 2015,Jan,16

29843 **Arthroscopy, wrist, surgical; for infection, lavage and drainage**
13.9 13.9 FUD 090 J A2 80 50
AMA: 2018,Jan,8; 2017,Jan,8; 2016,Jan,13; 2015,Jan,16

29844 **synovectomy, partial**
14.2 14.2 FUD 090 J A2 80 50
AMA: 2018,Jan,8; 2017,Jan,8; 2016,Jan,13; 2015,Jan,16

29845 **synovectomy, complete**
16.6 16.6 FUD 090 J A2 80 50
AMA: 2018,Jan,8; 2017,Jan,8; 2016,Jan,13; 2015,Jan,16; 2014,Jan,11

29846 **excision and/or repair of triangular fibrocartilage and/or joint debridement**
14.9 14.9 FUD 090 J A2 80 50
AMA: 2018,Jan,8; 2017,Jan,8; 2016,Jan,13; 2015,Jan,16; 2014,Jan,11

29847 **internal fixation for fracture or instability**
15.6 15.6 FUD 090 J A2 80 50
AMA: 2018,Jan,8; 2017,Jan,8; 2016,Jan,13; 2015,Jan,16

29848 **Endoscopy, wrist, surgical, with release of transverse carpal ligament**
EXCLUDES *Open surgery (64721)*
14.7 14.7 FUD 090 J A2 50
AMA: 2018,Apr,10; 2018,Jan,8; 2017,Jan,8; 2017,Jan,6; 2016,Jan,13; 2015,Jul,10; 2015,Jan,16; 2014,Jan,11

29850 **Arthroscopically aided treatment of intercondylar spine(s) and/or tuberosity fracture(s) of the knee, with or without manipulation; without internal or external fixation (includes arthroscopy)**
17.9 17.9 FUD 090 J A2 80 50
AMA: 2018,Jan,8; 2017,Jan,8; 2016,Jan,13; 2015,Jan,16

29851 **with internal or external fixation (includes arthroscopy)**
EXCLUDES *Bone graft (20900, 20902)*
26.9 26.9 FUD 090 J A2 80 50
AMA: 2018,Jan,8; 2017,Jan,8; 2016,Jan,13; 2015,Jan,16

29855 **Arthroscopically aided treatment of tibial fracture, proximal (plateau); unicondylar, includes internal fixation, when performed (includes arthroscopy)**
EXCLUDES *Bone graft (20900, 20902)*
22.5 22.5 FUD 090 J J8 80 50
AMA: 2018,Sep,14; 2018,Jan,8; 2017,Jan,8; 2016,Jan,13; 2015,Jan,16

29856 **bicondylar, includes internal fixation, when performed (includes arthroscopy)**
EXCLUDES *Bone graft (20900, 20902)*
28.7 28.7 FUD 090 J J8 80 50
AMA: 2018,Jan,8; 2017,Jan,8; 2016,Jan,13; 2015,Jan,16

29860 **Arthroscopy, hip, diagnostic with or without synovial biopsy (separate procedure)**
19.2 19.2 FUD 090 J A2 80 50
AMA: 2018,Jan,8; 2017,Jan,8; 2016,Jan,13; 2015,Jan,16; 2014,Jan,11

29861 **Arthroscopy, hip, surgical; with removal of loose body or foreign body**
20.6 20.6 FUD 090 J A2 80 50
AMA: 2018,Jan,8; 2017,Jan,8; 2016,Jan,13; 2015,Jan,16; 2014,Jan,11

29862 **with debridement/shaving of articular cartilage (chondroplasty), abrasion arthroplasty, and/or resection of labrum**
23.1 23.1 FUD 090 J A2 80 50
AMA: 2018,Jan,8; 2017,Jan,8; 2016,Jan,13; 2015,Jan,16; 2014,Jan,11

29863 **with synovectomy**
23.2 23.2 FUD 090 J A2 80 50
AMA: 2018,Jan,8; 2017,Jan,8; 2016,Jan,13; 2015,Jan,16; 2014,Jan,11

\# **29914** **with femoroplasty (ie, treatment of cam lesion)**
28.3 28.3 FUD 090 J G2 80 50
AMA: 2018,Jan,8; 2017,Jan,8; 2016,Jan,13; 2015,Jan,16; 2014,Jan,11

\# **29915** **with acetabuloplasty (ie, treatment of pincer lesion)**
29.1 29.1 FUD 090 J G2 80 50
AMA: 2018,Jan,8; 2017,Jan,8; 2016,Jan,13; 2015,Jan,16; 2014,Jan,11

29916 **with labral repair**
29.1 29.1 FUD 090 J G2 80 50
AMA: 2018,Jan,8; 2017,Jan,8; 2016,Jan,13; 2015,Jan,16; 2014,Jan,11

29866 **Arthroscopy, knee, surgical; osteochondral autograft(s) (eg, mosaicplasty) (includes harvesting of the autograft[s])**
EXCLUDES *Open osteochondral autograft of the knee (27416)*
Procedures performed at the same surgical session (29870-29871, 29875, 29884)
Procedures performed in the same compartment (29874, 29877, 29879, 29885-29887)
30.3 30.3 FUD 090 J G2 80 50
AMA: 2018,Jan,8; 2017,Jan,8; 2016,Jan,13; 2015,Jan,16

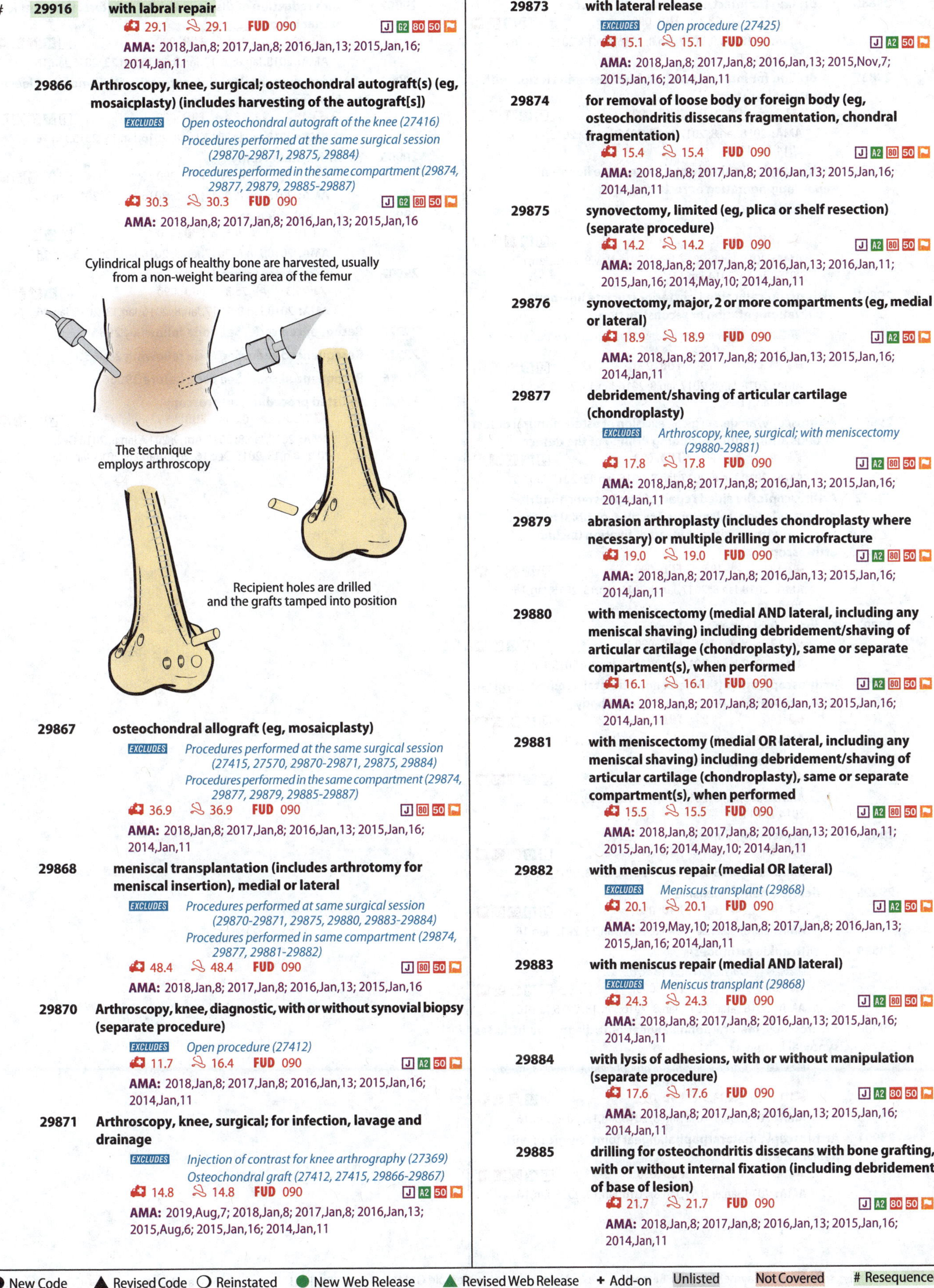

29867 **osteochondral allograft (eg, mosaicplasty)**
EXCLUDES *Procedures performed at the same surgical session (27415, 27570, 29870-29871, 29875, 29884)*
Procedures performed in the same compartment (29874, 29877, 29879, 29885-29887)
36.9 36.9 FUD 090 J 80 50
AMA: 2018,Jan,8; 2017,Jan,8; 2016,Jan,13; 2015,Jan,16; 2014,Jan,11

29868 **meniscal transplantation (includes arthrotomy for meniscal insertion), medial or lateral**
EXCLUDES *Procedures performed at same surgical session (29870-29871, 29875, 29880, 29883-29884)*
Procedures performed in same compartment (29874, 29877, 29881-29882)
48.4 48.4 FUD 090 J 80 50
AMA: 2018,Jan,8; 2017,Jan,8; 2016,Jan,13; 2015,Jan,16

29870 **Arthroscopy, knee, diagnostic, with or without synovial biopsy (separate procedure)**
EXCLUDES *Open procedure (27412)*
11.7 16.4 FUD 090 J A2 50
AMA: 2018,Jan,8; 2017,Jan,8; 2016,Jan,13; 2015,Jan,16; 2014,Jan,11

29871 **Arthroscopy, knee, surgical; for infection, lavage and drainage**
EXCLUDES *Injection of contrast for knee arthrography (27369)*
Osteochondral graft (27412, 27415, 29866-29867)
14.8 14.8 FUD 090 J A2 50
AMA: 2019,Aug,7; 2018,Jan,8; 2017,Jan,8; 2016,Jan,13; 2015,Aug,6; 2015,Jan,16; 2014,Jan,11

29873 **with lateral release**
EXCLUDES *Open procedure (27425)*
15.1 15.1 FUD 090 J A2 50
AMA: 2018,Jan,8; 2017,Jan,8; 2016,Jan,13; 2015,Nov,7; 2015,Jan,16; 2014,Jan,11

29874 **for removal of loose body or foreign body (eg, osteochondritis dissecans fragmentation, chondral fragmentation)**
15.4 15.4 FUD 090 J A2 80 50
AMA: 2018,Jan,8; 2017,Jan,8; 2016,Jan,13; 2015,Jan,16; 2014,Jan,11

29875 **synovectomy, limited (eg, plica or shelf resection) (separate procedure)**
14.2 14.2 FUD 090 J A2 80 50
AMA: 2018,Jan,8; 2017,Jan,8; 2016,Jan,13; 2016,Jan,11; 2015,Jan,16; 2014,May,10; 2014,Jan,11

29876 **synovectomy, major, 2 or more compartments (eg, medial or lateral)**
18.9 18.9 FUD 090 J A2 50
AMA: 2018,Jan,8; 2017,Jan,8; 2016,Jan,13; 2015,Jan,16; 2014,Jan,11

29877 **debridement/shaving of articular cartilage (chondroplasty)**
EXCLUDES *Arthroscopy, knee, surgical; with meniscectomy (29880-29881)*
17.8 17.8 FUD 090 J A2 80 50
AMA: 2018,Jan,8; 2017,Jan,8; 2016,Jan,13; 2015,Jan,16; 2014,Jan,11

29879 **abrasion arthroplasty (includes chondroplasty where necessary) or multiple drilling or microfracture**
19.0 19.0 FUD 090 J A2 80 50
AMA: 2018,Jan,8; 2017,Jan,8; 2016,Jan,13; 2015,Jan,16; 2014,Jan,11

29880 **with meniscectomy (medial AND lateral, including any meniscal shaving) including debridement/shaving of articular cartilage (chondroplasty), same or separate compartment(s), when performed**
16.1 16.1 FUD 090 J A2 80 50
AMA: 2018,Jan,8; 2017,Jan,8; 2016,Jan,13; 2015,Jan,16; 2014,Jan,11

29881 **with meniscectomy (medial OR lateral, including any meniscal shaving) including debridement/shaving of articular cartilage (chondroplasty), same or separate compartment(s), when performed**
15.5 15.5 FUD 090 J A2 80 50
AMA: 2018,Jan,8; 2017,Jan,8; 2016,Jan,13; 2016,Jan,11; 2015,Jan,16; 2014,May,10; 2014,Jan,11

29882 **with meniscus repair (medial OR lateral)**
EXCLUDES *Meniscus transplant (29868)*
20.1 20.1 FUD 090 J A2 50
AMA: 2019,May,10; 2018,Jan,8; 2017,Jan,8; 2016,Jan,13; 2015,Jan,16; 2014,Jan,11

29883 **with meniscus repair (medial AND lateral)**
EXCLUDES *Meniscus transplant (29868)*
24.3 24.3 FUD 090 J A2 80 50
AMA: 2018,Jan,8; 2017,Jan,8; 2016,Jan,13; 2015,Jan,16; 2014,Jan,11

29884 **with lysis of adhesions, with or without manipulation (separate procedure)**
17.6 17.6 FUD 090 J A2 80 50
AMA: 2018,Jan,8; 2017,Jan,8; 2016,Jan,13; 2015,Jan,16; 2014,Jan,11

29885 **drilling for osteochondritis dissecans with bone grafting, with or without internal fixation (including debridement of base of lesion)**
21.7 21.7 FUD 090 J A2 80 50
AMA: 2018,Jan,8; 2017,Jan,8; 2016,Jan,13; 2015,Jan,16; 2014,Jan,11

29886 **drilling for intact osteochondritis dissecans lesion**
18.3 18.3 FUD 090 J A2 50
AMA: 2018,Jan,8; 2017,Jan,8; 2016,Jan,13; 2015,Jan,16; 2014,Jan,11

29887 **drilling for intact osteochondritis dissecans lesion with internal fixation**
21.6 21.6 FUD 090 J A2 80 50
AMA: 2018,Jan,8; 2017,Jan,8; 2016,Jan,13; 2015,Jan,16; 2014,Jan,11

29888 **Arthroscopically aided anterior cruciate ligament repair/augmentation or reconstruction**
EXCLUDES *Ligamentous reconstruction (augmentation), knee (27427-27429)*
28.3 28.3 FUD 090 J J8 80 50
AMA: 2018,Jan,8; 2017,Jan,8; 2016,Nov,9; 2016,Jan,13; 2015,Jan,16; 2014,Jan,11

29889 **Arthroscopically aided posterior cruciate ligament repair/augmentation or reconstruction**
EXCLUDES *Ligamentous reconstruction (augmentation), knee (27427-27429)*
35.3 35.3 FUD 090 J A2 80 50
AMA: 2018,Jan,8; 2017,Jan,8; 2016,Jan,13; 2015,Jan,16; 2014,Jan,11

29891 **Arthroscopy, ankle, surgical, excision of osteochondral defect of talus and/or tibia, including drilling of the defect**
19.3 19.3 FUD 090 J A2 80 50
AMA: 2018,Jan,8; 2017,Jan,8; 2016,Jan,13; 2015,Jan,16

29892 **Arthroscopically aided repair of large osteochondritis dissecans lesion, talar dome fracture, or tibial plafond fracture, with or without internal fixation (includes arthroscopy)**
18.8 18.8 FUD 090 J A2 80 50
AMA: 2018,Jan,8; 2017,Jan,8; 2016,Jan,13; 2015,Jan,16; 2014,Jan,11

29893 **Endoscopic plantar fasciotomy**
12.3 17.8 FUD 090 J A2 50
AMA: 2018,Jan,8; 2017,Jan,8; 2016,Jan,13; 2015,Jan,16

29894 **Arthroscopy, ankle (tibiotalar and fibulotalar joints), surgical; with removal of loose body or foreign body**
14.2 14.2 FUD 090 J A2 80 50
AMA: 2018,Jan,8; 2017,Jan,8; 2016,Jan,13; 2015,Jan,16

29895 **synovectomy, partial**
13.4 13.4 FUD 090 J A2 80 50
AMA: 2018,Jan,8; 2017,Jan,8; 2016,Jan,13; 2015,Jan,16; 2014,Jan,11

29897 **debridement, limited**
14.4 14.4 FUD 090 J A2 80 50
AMA: 2018,Jan,8; 2017,Jan,8; 2016,Jan,13; 2015,Jan,16

29898 **debridement, extensive**
16.1 16.1 FUD 090 J A2 80 50
AMA: 2018,Jan,8; 2017,Jan,8; 2016,Jan,13; 2015,Jan,16

29899 **with ankle arthrodesis**
EXCLUDES *Open procedure (27870)*
29.8 29.8 FUD 090 J J8 80 50
AMA: 2018,Jan,8; 2017,Jan,8; 2016,Jan,13; 2015,Jan,16

29900 **Arthroscopy, metacarpophalangeal joint, diagnostic, includes synovial biopsy**
EXCLUDES *Arthroscopy, metacarpophalangeal joint, surgical (29901-29902)*
14.3 14.3 FUD 090 J A2 80 50
AMA: 2018,Jan,8; 2017,Jan,8; 2016,Jan,13; 2015,Jan,16

29901 **Arthroscopy, metacarpophalangeal joint, surgical; with debridement**
15.4 15.4 FUD 090 J A2 80 50
AMA: 2018,Jan,8; 2017,Jan,8; 2016,Jan,13; 2015,Jan,16

29902 **with reduction of displaced ulnar collateral ligament (eg, Stenar lesion)**
16.3 16.3 FUD 090 J A2 80 50
AMA: 2018,Jan,8; 2017,Jan,8; 2016,Jan,13; 2015,Jan,16

29904 **Arthroscopy, subtalar joint, surgical; with removal of loose body or foreign body**
18.4 18.4 FUD 090 J G2 80 50
AMA: 2018,Jan,8; 2017,Jan,8; 2016,Jan,13; 2015,Jan,16

29905 **with synovectomy**
14.9 14.9 FUD 090 J G2 80 50
AMA: 2018,Jan,8; 2017,Jan,8; 2016,Jan,13; 2015,Jan,16

29906 **with debridement**
19.5 19.5 FUD 090 J G2 80 50
AMA: 2018,Jan,8; 2017,Jan,8; 2016,Jan,13; 2015,Jan,16

29907 **with subtalar arthrodesis**
25.3 25.3 FUD 090 J J8 80 50
AMA: 2018,Jan,8; 2017,Jan,8; 2016,Jan,13; 2015,Jan,16

29914 **Resequenced code. See code following 29863.**

29915 **Resequenced code. See code following 29863.**

29916 **Resequenced code. See code before 29866.**

29999 **Unlisted procedure, arthroscopy**
0.00 0.00 FUD YYY T 80 50
AMA: 2018,Jan,8; 2017,Apr,9; 2017,Jan,8; 2016,Dec,16; 2016,Jan,13; 2015,Dec,16; 2015,Jan,16; 2014,Jan,11

26/TC PC/TC Only A2-Z3 ASC Payment 50 Bilateral ♂ Male Only ♀ Female Only Facility RVU Non-Facility RVU CCI CLIA
FUD Follow-up Days CMS: IOM AMA: CPT Asst A-Y OPPSI 80/80 Surg Assist Allowed / w/Doc Lab Crosswalk Radiology Crosswalk

30000-30115 I&D, Biopsy, Excision Procedures of the Nose

30000 Drainage abscess or hematoma, nasal, internal approach

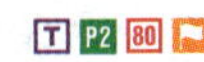 *Incision and drainage (10060, 10140)*

3.37 | 6.83 | FUD 010 | T P2 80

AMA: 2005,May,13-14; 1994,Spr,24

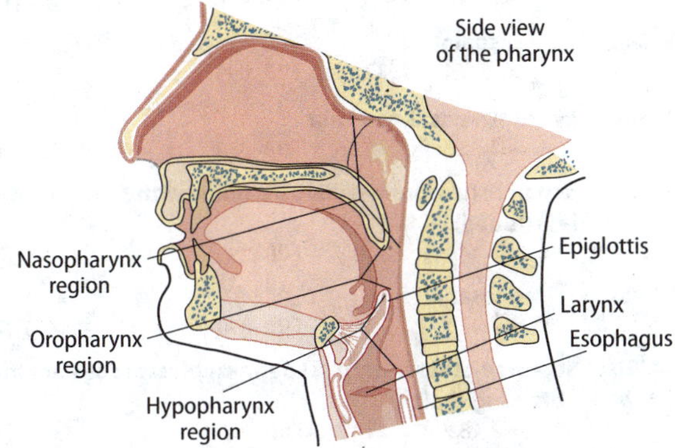

The nasopharynx is the membranous passage above the level of the soft palate; the oropharynx is the region between the soft palate and the upper edge of the epiglottis; the hypopharynx is the region of the epiglottis to the juncture of the larynx and esophagus; the three regions are collectively known as the pharynx

30020 Drainage abscess or hematoma, nasal septum

3.37 | 6.90 | FUD 010 | T P3

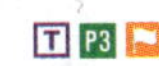 *Lateral rhinotomy incision (30118, 30320)*

30100 Biopsy, intranasal

EXCLUDES *Superficial biopsy of nose (11102-11107)*

1.93 | 4.00 | FUD 000 | T P3

AMA: 2019,Jan,9

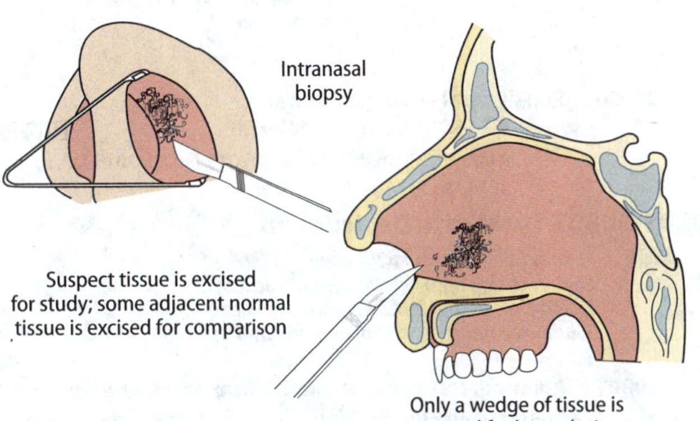

30110 Excision, nasal polyp(s), simple

3.69 | 6.65 | FUD 010 | T P3 50

30115 Excision, nasal polyp(s), extensive

12.4 | 12.4 | FUD 090 | J A2 50

30117-30118 Destruction Procedures Nose

CMS: 100-03,140.5 Laser Procedures

30117 Excision or destruction (eg, laser), intranasal lesion; internal approach

9.56 | 25.6 | FUD 090 | J A2

AMA: 2019,Jul,10

30118 external approach (lateral rhinotomy)

22.1 | 22.1 | FUD 090 | J A2

30120-30140 Excision Procedures Nose, Turbinate

30120 Excision or surgical planing of skin of nose for rhinophyma

12.3 | 14.6 | FUD 090 | J A2

AMA: 2018,Jan,8; 2017,Jan,8; 2016,Jan,13; 2015,Jan,16; 2014,Jan,11

30124 Excision dermoid cyst, nose; simple, skin, subcutaneous

8.19 | 8.19 | FUD 090 | T R2

30125 complex, under bone or cartilage

17.5 | 17.5 | FUD 090 | J A2 80

30130 Excision inferior turbinate, partial or complete, any method

EXCLUDES *Ablation, soft tissue of inferior turbinates, unilateral or bilateral, any method (30801-30802)*
Excision middle/superior turbinate(s) (30999)
Fracture nasal inferior turbinate(s), therapeutic (30930)

11.0 | 11.0 | FUD 090 | J A2 50

AMA: 2018,Jan,8; 2017,Jan,8; 2016,Jan,13; 2015,Jan,16; 2014,Jan,11

30140 Submucous resection inferior turbinate, partial or complete, any method

EXCLUDES *Ablation, soft tissue of inferior turbinates, unilateral or bilateral, any method (30801-30802)*
Endoscopic resection of concha bullosa of middle turbinate (31240)
Fracture nasal inferior turbinate(s), therapeutic (30930)
Submucous resection:
Nasal septum (30520)
Superior or middle turbinate (30999)

5.12 | 7.92 | FUD 000 | J A2 50

AMA: 2018,Jan,8; 2017,Jan,8; 2016,Jan,13; 2015,Jan,16; 2014,Jan,11

30150-30160 Surgical Removal: Nose

EXCLUDES *Reconstruction and/or closure (primary or delayed primary intention) (13151-13160, 14060-14302, 15120-15121, 15260-15261, 15760, 20900-20912)*

30150 Rhinectomy; partial

22.0 | 22.0 | FUD 090 | J A2

30160 total

22.2 | 22.2 | FUD 090 | J A2 80

30200-30320 Turbinate Injection, Removal Foreign Substance in the Nose

30200 Injection into turbinate(s), therapeutic

1.66 | 3.18 | FUD 000 | T P3

AMA: 2018,Jan,8; 2017,Jan,8; 2016,Jan,13; 2015,Jan,16; 2014,Jan,11

30210 Displacement therapy (Proetz type)

2.82 | 4.25 | FUD 010 | T P3

AMA: 2018,Jan,8; 2017,Jan,8; 2016,Jan,13; 2015,Jan,16; 2014,Jan,11

30220 Insertion, nasal septal prosthesis (button)

3.55 | 8.60 | FUD 010 | T A2

30300 Removal foreign body, intranasal; office type procedure

3.14 | 5.26 | FUD 010 | Q1 N1

AMA: 2018,Jan,8; 2017,Jan,8; 2016,Jan,13; 2015,Jan,16; 2014,Jan,11

30310 requiring general anesthesia

5.77 | 5.77 | FUD 010 | J A2 80

30320 by lateral rhinotomy

13.0 | 13.0 | FUD 090 | T A2 80

30400-30630 Reconstruction or Repair of Nose

EXCLUDES *Harvesting of bone/tissue/fat grafts ([15769], 15773-15774, 20900-20924, 21210)*
Liposuction for autologous fat grafting (15773-15774)

30400 **Rhinoplasty, primary; lateral and alar cartilages and/or elevation of nasal tip**
30.9 | 30.9 | FUD 090 | J A2 80
INCLUDES Carpue's operation
EXCLUDES *Reconstruction of columella (13151-13153)*

30410 **complete, external parts including bony pyramid, lateral and alar cartilages, and/or elevation of nasal tip**
35.8 | 35.8 | FUD 090 | J A2 80

30420 **including major septal repair**
39.4 | 39.4 | FUD 090 | J A2
AMA: 2018,Jan,8; 2017,Nov,11; 2017,Jan,8; 2016,Jul,8

30430 **Rhinoplasty, secondary; minor revision (small amount of nasal tip work)**
27.2 | 27.2 | FUD 090 | J A2 80

30435 **intermediate revision (bony work with osteotomies)**
33.7 | 33.7 | FUD 090 | J A2 80

30450 **major revision (nasal tip work and osteotomies)**
44.9 | 44.9 | FUD 090 | J A2 80

30460 **Rhinoplasty for nasal deformity secondary to congenital cleft lip and/or palate, including columellar lengthening; tip only**
23.5 | 23.5 | FUD 090 | J A2 80
AMA: 2018,Jan,8; 2017,Jan,8; 2016,Jan,13; 2015,Jan,16; 2014,Dec,18

Cleft lip and cleft palate are described according to length of cleft and whether bilateral or unilateral

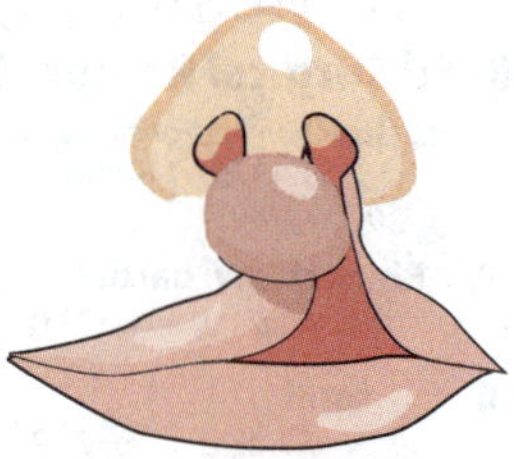

Complete unilateral cleft lip

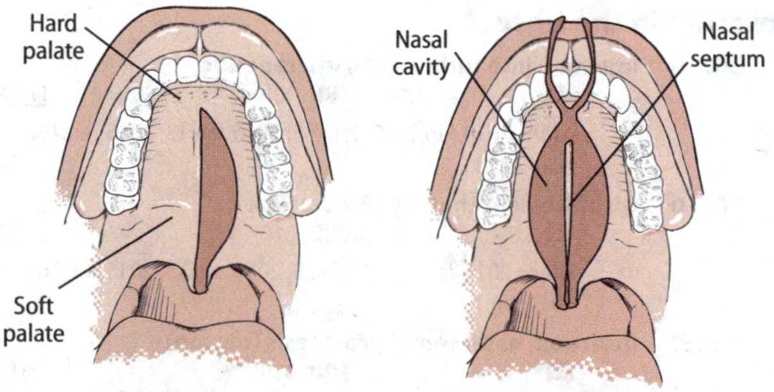

Hard palate
Soft palate
Nasal cavity
Nasal septum

Isolated unilateral complete cleft of palate

Bilateral complete cleft of lip and palate

30462 **tip, septum, osteotomies**
45.1 | 45.1 | FUD 090 | J A2 80
AMA: 2018,Jan,8; 2017,Jan,8; 2016,Jan,13; 2015,Jan,16; 2014,Dec,18

30465 **Repair of nasal vestibular stenosis (eg, spreader grafting, lateral nasal wall reconstruction)**
28.1 | 28.1 | FUD 090 | J A2 80
INCLUDES Bilateral procedure
Code also modifier 52 for unilateral procedure

30520 **Septoplasty or submucous resection, with or without cartilage scoring, contouring or replacement with graft**
EXCLUDES *Turbinate resection (30140)*
18.0 | 18.0 | FUD 090 | J A2
AMA: 2019,Jul,10; 2018,Jan,8; 2017,Jan,8; 2016,Jan,13; 2015,Jul,10; 2015,Jan,16; 2014,Jan,11

30540 **Repair choanal atresia; intranasal**
19.8 | 19.8 | FUD 090 | 63 J A2 80

30545 **transpalatine**
27.1 | 27.1 | FUD 090 | 63 J A2 80

30560 **Lysis intranasal synechia**
3.95 | 7.96 | FUD 010 | T A2

30580 **Repair fistula; oromaxillary (combine with 31030 if antrotomy is included)**
14.2 | 18.3 | FUD 090 | J A2

30600 **oronasal**
12.5 | 16.2 | FUD 090 | J A2 80

30620 **Septal or other intranasal dermatoplasty (does not include obtaining graft)**
18.2 | 18.2 | FUD 090 | J A2

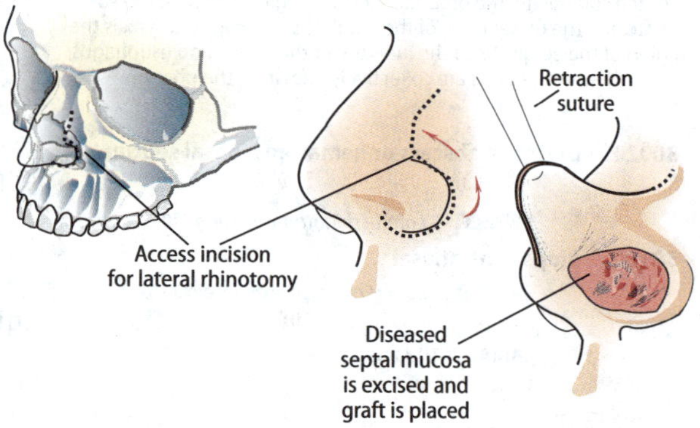

Retraction suture
Access incision for lateral rhinotomy
Diseased septal mucosa is excised and graft is placed

30630 **Repair nasal septal perforations**
18.0 | 18.0 | FUD 090 | J A2 80
AMA: 2018,Jan,8; 2017,Jan,8; 2016,Jan,13; 2015,Jan,16; 2014,Jan,11

30801-30802 Turbinate Destruction

EXCLUDES *Ablation middle/superior turbinates (30999)*
Cautery to stop nasal bleeding (30901-30906)
Excision inferior turbinate, partial or complete, any method (30130)
Submucous resection inferior turbinate, partial or complete, any method (30140)

30801 **Ablation, soft tissue of inferior turbinates, unilateral or bilateral, any method (eg, electrocautery, radiofrequency ablation, or tissue volume reduction); superficial**
EXCLUDES *Submucosal ablation inferior turbinates (30802)*
3.98 | 6.32 | FUD 010 | T A2
AMA: 2019,Jul,10

30802 **intramural (ie, submucosal)**
EXCLUDES *Superficial ablation inferior turbinates (30801)*
5.48 | 8.03 | FUD 010 | T A2
AMA: 2019,Jul,10; 2018,Jan,8; 2017,Jan,8; 2016,Jan,13; 2015,Jan,16; 2014,Jan,11

30901-30920 Control Nose Bleed

30901 **Control nasal hemorrhage, anterior, simple (limited cautery and/or packing) any method**
1.62 | 3.91 | FUD 000 | Q1 N1 50
AMA: 1990,Win,4

30903 **Control nasal hemorrhage, anterior, complex (extensive cautery and/or packing) any method**
2.25 6.16 FUD 000 T A2 50
AMA: 1990,Win,4

30905 **Control nasal hemorrhage, posterior, with posterior nasal packs and/or cautery, any method; initial**
3.01 9.36 FUD 000 T A2
AMA: 2018,Jan,8; 2017,Jan,8; 2016,Jan,13; 2015,Jan,16; 2014,Jan,11

30906 **subsequent**
3.90 9.79 FUD 000 T A2
AMA: 2002,May,7

30915 **Ligation arteries; ethmoidal**
16.5 16.5 FUD 090 T A2
EXCLUDES *External carotid artery (37600)*

30920 **internal maxillary artery, transantral**
24.0 24.0 FUD 090 T A2
EXCLUDES *External carotid artery (37600)*

30930-30999 Other and Unlisted Procedures of Nose

30930 **Fracture nasal inferior turbinate(s), therapeutic**
EXCLUDES *Excision inferior turbinate, partial or complete, any method (30130)*
Fracture of superior or middle turbinate(s) (30999)
Submucous resection inferior turbinate, partial or complete, any method (30140)
3.43 3.43 FUD 010 J A2 50
AMA: 2018,Jan,8; 2017,Nov,11; 2017,Jan,8; 2016,Jul,8; 2016,Jan,13; 2015,Jan,16; 2014,Jan,11

30999 **Unlisted procedure, nose**
0.00 0.00 FUD YYY T 80
AMA: 2018,Jan,8; 2017,Jan,8; 2016,Jan,13; 2015,Jan,16

31000-31230 Opening Sinuses

31000 **Lavage by cannulation; maxillary sinus (antrum puncture or natural ostium)**
3.02 5.17 FUD 010 T P2 50
AMA: 2018,Jan,8; 2017,Jan,8; 2016,Jan,13; 2015,Jan,16; 2014,Apr,10

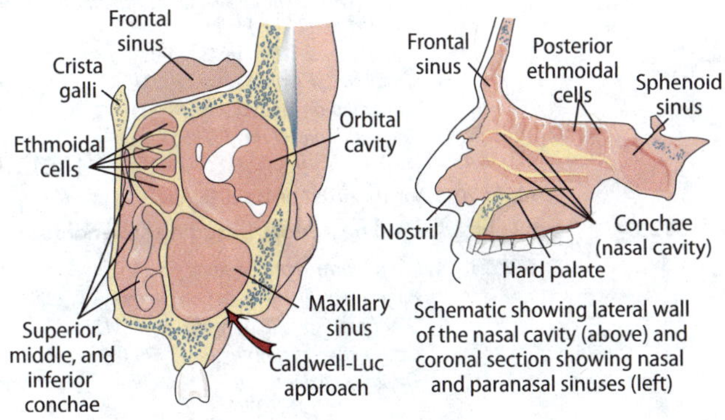

Frontal sinus
Crista galli
Ethmoidal cells
Orbital cavity
Superior, middle, and inferior conchae
Maxillary sinus
Caldwell-Luc approach
Frontal sinus
Posterior ethmoidal cells
Sphenoid sinus
Nostril
Conchae (nasal cavity)
Hard palate

Schematic showing lateral wall of the nasal cavity (above) and coronal section showing nasal and paranasal sinuses (left)

31002 **sphenoid sinus**
5.39 5.39 FUD 010 T R2 80 50

31020 **Sinusotomy, maxillary (antrotomy); intranasal**
10.4 13.6 FUD 090 J A2 50

31030 **radical (Caldwell-Luc) without removal of antrochoanal polyps**
15.0 19.1 FUD 090 J A2 50

31032 **radical (Caldwell-Luc) with removal of antrochoanal polyps**
16.5 16.5 FUD 090 J A2 50

31040 **Pterygomaxillary fossa surgery, any approach**
22.0 22.0 FUD 090 J R2 50
EXCLUDES *Transantral ligation internal maxillary artery (30920)*

31050 **Sinusotomy, sphenoid, with or without biopsy;**
13.9 13.9 FUD 090 J A2 50

31051 **with mucosal stripping or removal of polyp(s)**
18.6 18.6 FUD 090 J A2 50

31070 **Sinusotomy frontal; external, simple (trephine operation)**
12.6 12.6 FUD 090 J A2 50
INCLUDES Killian operation
EXCLUDES *Intranasal frontal sinusotomy (31276)*

31075 **transorbital, unilateral (for mucocele or osteoma, Lynch type)**
22.4 22.4 FUD 090 J A2 80 50

31080 **obliterative without osteoplastic flap, brow incision (includes ablation)**
29.6 29.6 FUD 090 J A2 80 50
INCLUDES Ridell sinusotomy

31081 **obliterative, without osteoplastic flap, coronal incision (includes ablation)**
31.9 31.9 FUD 090 J A2 80 50

31084 **obliterative, with osteoplastic flap, brow incision**
33.1 33.1 FUD 090 J A2 80 50

31085 **obliterative, with osteoplastic flap, coronal incision**
34.1 34.1 FUD 090 J A2 80 50

31086 **nonobliterative, with osteoplastic flap, brow incision**
32.1 32.1 FUD 090 J A2 80 50

31087 **nonobliterative, with osteoplastic flap, coronal incision**
30.9 30.9 FUD 090 J A2 80 50

31090 **Sinusotomy, unilateral, 3 or more paranasal sinuses (frontal, maxillary, ethmoid, sphenoid)**
29.6 29.6 FUD 090 J A2 50
AMA: 1998,Nov,1; 1997,Nov,1

31200 **Ethmoidectomy; intranasal, anterior**
16.7 16.7 FUD 090 J A2 50
AMA: 2018,Jan,8; 2017,Jan,8; 2016,Feb,10

31201 **intranasal, total**
21.4 21.4 FUD 090 J A2 50
AMA: 2018,Jan,8; 2017,Jan,8; 2016,Feb,10

31205 **extranasal, total**
26.1 26.1 FUD 090 J A2 80 50
AMA: 2018,Jan,8; 2017,Jan,8; 2016,Feb,10

31225 **Maxillectomy; without orbital exenteration**
52.8 52.8 FUD 090 C 80 50

31230 **with orbital exenteration (en bloc)**
58.3 58.3 FUD 090 C 80 50
EXCLUDES *Orbital exenteration without maxillectomy (65110-65114)*
Skin grafts (15120-15121)

31231-31235 Nasal Endoscopy, Diagnostic

INCLUDES Complete sinus exam (e.g., nasal cavity, turbinates, sphenoethmoidal recess)
Code also stereotactic navigation, if performed (61782)

31231 **Nasal endoscopy, diagnostic, unilateral or bilateral (separate procedure)**
1.86 5.69 FUD 000 T P2
AMA: 2018,Apr,3; 2018,Jan,8; 2017,Jul,7; 2017,Jan,8; 2017,Jan,6; 2016,Dec,13; 2016,Feb,10; 2016,Jan,13; 2015,Jan,16; 2014,Jan,11

▲ **31233** **Nasal/sinus endoscopy, diagnostic; with maxillary sinusoscopy (via inferior meatus or canine fossa puncture)**
EXCLUDES *Nasal/sinus endoscopy, surgical; with dilation of maxillary sinus ostium (31295)*
When performed on the same side:
Dilation of maxillary sinus ostium (31295)
Maxillary antrostomy (31256, 31267)
3.87 7.41 FUD 000 T A2 80 50
AMA: 2018,Apr,3; 2018,Jan,8; 2017,Jan,8; 2016,Jan,13; 2015,Jan,16; 2014,Jan,11

▲ **31235 with sphenoid sinusoscopy (via puncture of sphenoidal face or cannulation of ostium)**

EXCLUDES *Insertion of drug-eluting implant performed with biopsy, debridement, or polypectomy (31237)*
Insertion of drug-eluting implant without other nasal/sinus endoscopic procedure (31299)
When performed on the same side:
Sinus dilation (31297-31298)
Sphenoidotomy (31287-31288)
Total ethmoidectomy with sphenoidotomy ([31257, 31259])

4.58 8.47 FUD 000 J A2 80 50

AMA: 2018,Apr,3; 2018,Jan,8; 2017,Jan,8; 2016,Jan,13; 2015,Jan,16; 2014,Jan,11

31237-31253 Nasal Endoscopy, Surgical

INCLUDES Diagnostic nasal/sinus endoscopy
Unilateral procedure

EXCLUDES *Frontal sinus exploration (31276)*
Maxillary antrostomy (31256)
Osteomeatal complex (OMC) resection and/or partial (anterior) ethmoidectomy (31254)
Removal of maxillary sinus tissue (31267)
Total (anterior and posterior) ethmoidectomy (31255)

Code also stereotactic navigation, if performed (61782)

31237 Nasal/sinus endoscopy, surgical; with biopsy, polypectomy or debridement (separate procedure)

EXCLUDES *When performed on the same side:*
Frontal sinus exploration (31276)
Maxillary antrostomy (31256, 31267)
Nasal hemorrhage control (31238)
Optic nerve decompression (31294)
Orbital wall decompression, medial and/or inferior (31292-31293)
Other total ethmoidectomy procedures ([31253], 31255, [31257], [31259])
Partial ethmoidectomy (31254)
Repair of CSF leak (31290-31291)
Sphenoidotomy (31287-31288)

4.58 7.26 FUD 000 J A2 50

AMA: 2019,Jul,7; 2019,Apr,10; 2018,Apr,3; 2018,Jan,8; 2017,Jan,8; 2016,Feb,10; 2016,Jan,13; 2015,Jan,16; 2015,Jan,13; 2014,Jan,11

31238 with control of nasal hemorrhage

EXCLUDES *When performed on the same side:*
Biopsy, polypectomy, or debridement (31237)
Sphenopalatine artery ligation (31241)

4.80 7.17 FUD 000 J A2 80 50

AMA: 2018,Apr,3; 2018,Jan,8; 2017,Jan,8; 2016,Jan,13; 2015,Jan,16; 2014,Jan,11

31239 with dacryocystorhinostomy

17.5 17.5 FUD 010 J A2 80 50

AMA: 2018,Apr,3; 2018,Jan,8; 2017,Jan,8; 2016,Jan,13; 2015,Jan,16; 2014,Jan,11

31240 with concha bullosa resection

4.56 4.56 FUD 000 J A2 80 50

AMA: 2018,Apr,3; 2018,Jan,8; 2017,Jan,8; 2016,Feb,10; 2016,Jan,13; 2015,Jan,16; 2014,Jan,11

31241 with ligation of sphenopalatine artery

EXCLUDES *Nasal/sinus endoscopy, surgical; with control of nasal hemorrhage, on the same side (31238)*

12.8 12.8 FUD 000 C 80 50

AMA: 2018,Apr,3

31253 **Resequenced code. See code following 31255.**

31254-31259 [31253, 31257, 31259] Nasal Endoscopy with Ethmoid Removal

INCLUDES Diagnostic nasal/sinus endoscopy
Sinusotomy, when applicable

Code also stereotactic navigation, if performed (61782)

31254 Nasal/sinus endoscopy, surgical with ethmoidectomy; partial (anterior)

EXCLUDES *When performed on the same side:*
Biopsy, polypectomy, or debridement (31237)
Optic nerve decompression (31294)
Orbital wall decompression, medial and/or inferior (31292-31293)
Other total ethmoidectomy procedures (31253, 31255, [31257], [31259])
Repair of CSF leak (31290-31291)

7.01 11.7 FUD 000 J A2 50

AMA: 2019,Apr,10; 2018,Apr,3; 2018,Jan,8; 2017,Jan,8; 2016,Feb,10; 2016,Jan,13; 2015,Jan,16; 2014,Jan,11

31255 with ethmoidectomy, total (anterior and posterior)

EXCLUDES *When performed on the same side:*
Biopsy, polypectomy, or debridement (31237)
Frontal sinus exploration (31276)
Optic nerve decompression (31294)
Orbital wall decompression, medial and/or inferior (31292-31293)
Other total ethmoidectomy procedures (31253, [31257], [31259])
Partial ethmoidectomy (31254)
Repair of CSF leak (31290-31291)
Sphenoidotomy (31287-31288)

9.33 9.33 FUD 000 J A2 50

AMA: 2019,Apr,10; 2018,Apr,3; 2018,Apr,10; 2018,Jan,8; 2017,Jan,8; 2016,Feb,10; 2016,Jan,13; 2015,Jan,16; 2014,Jan,11

\# **31253 total (anterior and posterior), including frontal sinus exploration, with removal of tissue from frontal sinus, when performed**

EXCLUDES *When performed on the same side:*
Biopsy, debridement, or polypectomy (31237)
Dilation of sinus (31296, 31298)
Frontal sinus exploration (31276)
Optic nerve decompression (31294)
Orbital wall decompression, medial and/or inferior (31292-31293)
Partial ethmoidectomy (31254)
Repair of CSF leak (31290-31291)
Sinus dilation (31296, 31298)
Total ethmoidectomy (31255)

14.4 14.4 FUD 000 J G2 50

AMA: 2019,Apr,10; 2018,Apr,10; 2018,Apr,3

\# **31257 total (anterior and posterior), including sphenoidotomy**

EXCLUDES *When performed on the same side:*
Biopsy, debridement, or polypectomy (31237)
Diagnostic sphenoid sinusoscopy (31235)
Optic nerve decompression (31294)
Orbital wall decompression, medial and/or inferior (31292-31293)
Other total ethmoidectomy procedures (31255, [31259])
Partial ethmoidectomy (31254)
Repair of CSF leak (31290-31291)
Sinus dilation (31297-31298)
Sphenoidotomy (31287-31288)

12.8 12.8 FUD 000 J G2 50

AMA: 2019,Apr,10; 2018,Apr,10; 2018,Apr,3

\# **31259** **total (anterior and posterior), including sphenoidotomy, with removal of tissue from the sphenoid sinus**

EXCLUDES *When performed on the same side:*
Biopsy, debridement, or polypectomy (31237)
Diagnostic sphenoid sinusoscopy (31235)
Optic nerve decompression (31294)
Orbital wall decompression, medial and/or inferior (31292-31293)
Other total ethmoidectomy procedures (31255, [31257])
Partial ethmoidectomy (31254)
Repair of CSF leak (31290-31291)
Sinus dilation (31297-31298)
Sphenoidotomy (31287-31288)

13.6 13.6 FUD 000 J G2 50

AMA: 2019,Apr,10; 2018,Apr,3

31256-31267 Nasal Endoscopy with Maxillary Procedures

INCLUDES Diagnostic nasal/sinus endoscopy
Nasal/sinus endoscopy, surgical; with dilation of maxillary sinus ostium (31295)
Sinusotomy, when applicable

Code also stereotactic navigation, if performed (61782)

31256 **Nasal/sinus endoscopy, surgical, with maxillary antrostomy;**

EXCLUDES *When performed on the same side:*
Biopsy, polypectomy, or debridement (31237)
Dilation of maxillary sinus ostium (31295)
Maxillary antrostomy with removal of tissue (31267)
Maxillary sinusoscopy (31233)

5.19 5.19 FUD 000 J A2 50

AMA: 2019,Apr,10; 2018,Apr,3; 2018,Apr,10; 2018,Jan,8; 2017,Jan,8; 2016,Jan,13; 2015,Jan,16; 2014,Jan,11

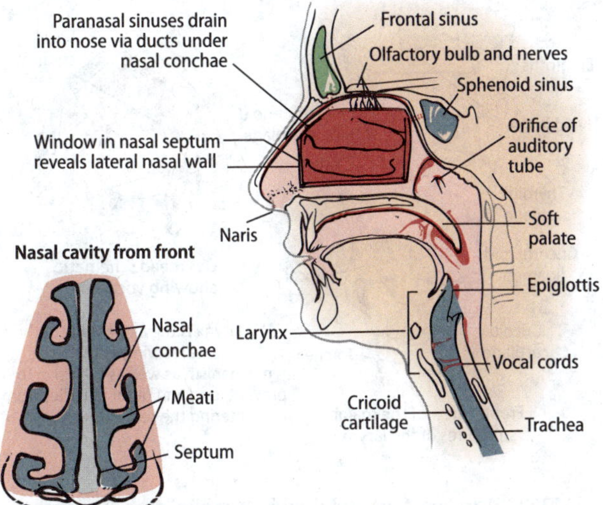

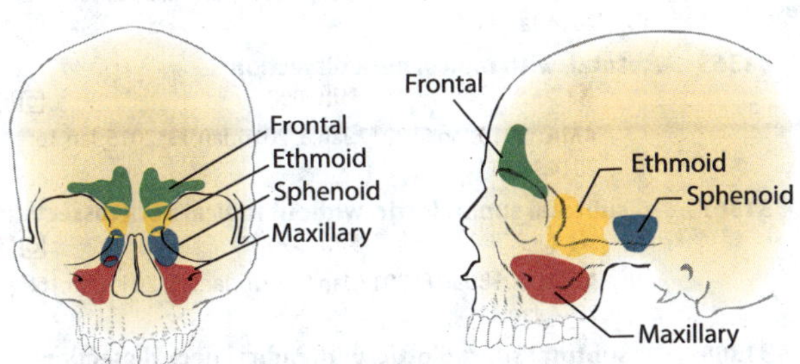

31257 **Resequenced code. See code following 31255.**

31259 **Resequenced code. See code following 31255.**

31267 **with removal of tissue from maxillary sinus**

EXCLUDES *When performed on the same side:*
Biopsy, polypectomy, or debridement (31237)
Dilation of maxillary sinus ostium (31295)
Maxillary antrostomy without tissue removal (31256)
Maxillary sinusoscopy (31233)

7.65 7.65 FUD 000 J A2 50

AMA: 2019,Apr,10; 2018,Apr,3; 2018,Jan,8; 2017,Jan,8; 2016,Jan,13; 2015,Jan,16; 2014,Jan,11

31276 Nasal Endoscopy with Frontal Sinus Examination

INCLUDES Diagnostic nasal/sinus endoscopy
Sinusotomy, when applicable
Unilateral procedure

EXCLUDES *When performed on the same side:*
Biopsy, polypectomy, or debridement (31237)
Dilation of frontal or frontal and sphenoid sinus (31296, 31298)
Other total ethmoidectomy procedures (31253, 31255)

Code also stereotactic navigation, if performed (61782)

31276 **Nasal/sinus endoscopy, surgical, with frontal sinus exploration, including removal of tissue from frontal sinus, when performed**

10.9 10.9 FUD 000 J A2 50

AMA: 2019,Apr,10; 2018,Apr,3; 2018,Apr,10; 2018,Jan,8; 2017,Jan,8; 2016,Jan,13; 2015,Jan,16; 2014,Jan,11

31287-31288 Nasal Endoscopy with Sphenoid Procedures

EXCLUDES *Other total ethmoidectomy procedures (31253, 31255, [31257], [31259])*
Sinus dilation (31297-31298)

Code also stereotactic navigation, if performed (61782)

31287 **Nasal/sinus endoscopy, surgical, with sphenoidotomy;**

EXCLUDES *When performed on the same side:*
Biopsy, polypectomy, or debridement (31237)
Diagnostic sphenoid sinusoscopy (31235)
Optic nerve decompression (31294)
Other total ethmoidectomy procedures (31255, [31257], [31259])
Repair of CSF leak (31291)
Sphenoidotomy with removal of tissue (31288)

5.80 5.80 FUD 000 J A2 80 50

AMA: 2019,Apr,10; 2018,Apr,3; 2018,Jan,8; 2017,Jan,8; 2016,Jan,13; 2015,Jan,16; 2014,Jan,11

31288 **with removal of tissue from the sphenoid sinus**

EXCLUDES *When performed on the same side:*
Biopsy, polypectomy, or debridement (31237)
Diagnostic sphenoid sinusoscopy (31235)
Optic nerve decompression (31294)
Other total ethmoidectomy procedures (31255, [31257], [31259])
Repair of CSF leak (31291)
Sphenoidotomy without removal of tissue (31287)

6.75 6.75 FUD 000 J A2 80 50

AMA: 2019,Apr,10; 2018,Apr,3; 2018,Jan,8; 2017,Jan,8; 2016,Feb,10; 2016,Jan,13; 2015,Jan,16; 2014,Jan,11

31290-31294 Nasal Endoscopy with Repair and Decompression

INCLUDES Diagnostic nasal/sinus endoscopy
Sinusotomy, when applicable

Code also stereotactic navigation, if performed (61782)

31290 **Nasal/sinus endoscopy, surgical, with repair of cerebrospinal fluid leak; ethmoid region**

EXCLUDES *When performed on the same side:*
Biopsy, polypectomy, or debridement (31237)
Other total ethmoidectomy procedures ([31253], 31255, [31257], [31259])
Partial ethmoidectomy (31254)

32.8 32.8 FUD 010 C 80 50

AMA: 2018,Apr,3; 2018,Jan,8; 2017,Jan,8; 2016,Feb,10; 2016,Jan,13; 2015,Jan,16; 2014,Jan,11

31291 **sphenoid region**

EXCLUDES *When performed on the same side:*
Biopsy, polypectomy, or debridement (31237)
Other total ethmoidectomy procedures ([31253], 31255, [31257], [31259])
Partial ethmoidectomy (31254)
Sphenoidotomy (31287-31288)

Facility RVU 34.9 Non-Facility RVU 34.9 FUD 010 C 80 50

AMA: 2018,Apr,3; 2018,Jan,8; 2017,Jan,8; 2016,Jan,13; 2015,Jan,16; 2014,Jan,11

▲ 31292 **Nasal/sinus endoscopy, surgical, with orbital decompression; medial or inferior wall**

EXCLUDES *When performed on the same side:*
Biopsy, polypectomy, or debridement (31237)
Dilation of frontal sinus only (31296)
Orbital wall decompression, medial and inferior (31293)
Other total ethmoidectomy procedures ([31253], 31255, [31257], [31259])
Partial ethmoidectomy (31254)

Facility RVU 28.3 Non-Facility RVU 28.3 FUD 010 J 80 50

AMA: 2018,Apr,3; 2018,Jan,8; 2017,Jan,8; 2016,Jan,13; 2015,Jan,16; 2014,Jan,11

▲ 31293 **medial and inferior wall**

EXCLUDES *When performed on the same side:*
Biopsy, polypectomy, or debridement (31237)
Orbital wall decompression, medial or inferior (31292)
Other total ethmoidectomy procedures ([31253], 31255, [31257], [31259])
Partial ethmoidectomy (31254)

Facility RVU 30.8 Non-Facility RVU 30.8 FUD 010 J 80 50

AMA: 2018,Apr,3; 2018,Jan,8; 2017,Jan,8; 2016,Jan,13; 2015,Jan,16; 2014,Jan,11

▲ 31294 **Nasal/sinus endoscopy, surgical, with optic nerve decompression**

EXCLUDES *When performed on the same side:*
Biopsy, polypectomy, or debridement (31237)
Other total ethmoidectomy procedures ([31253], 31255, [31257], [31259])
Partial ethmoidectomy (31254)
Sphenoidotomy (31287-31288)

Facility RVU 35.2 Non-Facility RVU 35.2 FUD 010 J 80 50

AMA: 2018,Apr,3; 2018,Jan,8; 2017,Jan,8; 2016,Jan,13; 2015,Jan,16; 2014,Jan,11

31295-31298 Nasal Endoscopy with Sinus Ostia Dilation

INCLUDES Any method of tissue displacement
Fluoroscopy, when performed

Code also stereotactic navigation, if performed (61782)

▲ 31295 **Nasal/sinus endoscopy, surgical, with dilation (eg, balloon dilation); maxillary sinus ostium, transnasal or via canine fossa**

EXCLUDES *When performed on the same side:*
Maxillary antrostomy (31256-31267)
Maxillary sinusoscopy (31233)

Facility RVU 4.55 Non-Facility RVU 55.6 FUD 000 J P2 80 50

AMA: 2018,Apr,3; 2018,Jan,8; 2017,Jan,8; 2016,Jan,13; 2015,Jan,16; 2014,Jan,11

▲ 31296 **frontal sinus ostium**

EXCLUDES *When performed on the same side:*
Frontal sinus exploration (31276)
Sinus dilation (31297-31298)
Total ethmoidectomy (31253)

Facility RVU 5.17 Non-Facility RVU 56.3 FUD 000 J P2 80 50

AMA: 2018,Apr,3; 2018,Jan,8; 2017,Jan,8; 2016,Jan,13; 2015,Jan,16; 2014,Jan,11

▲ 31297 **sphenoid sinus ostium**

EXCLUDES *When performed on the same side:*
Diagnostic sphenoid sinusoscopy (31235)
Sinus dilation (31296, 31298)
Sphenoidotomy (31287-31288)
Total ethmoidectomy procedures ([31257], [31259])

Facility RVU 4.14 Non-Facility RVU 55.2 FUD 000 J P2 80 50

AMA: 2018,Apr,3; 2018,Jan,8; 2017,Jan,8; 2016,Jan,13; 2015,Jan,16; 2014,Jan,11

▲ 31298 **frontal and sphenoid sinus ostia**

EXCLUDES *When performed on the same side:*
Diagnostic sphenoid sinusoscopy (31235)
Dilation of frontal sinus only (31296)
Dilation of sphenoid sinus only (31297)
Frontal sinus exploration (31276)
Other total ethmoidectomy procedures (31253, [31257], [31259])
Sphenoidotomy (31287-31288)

Facility RVU 7.37 Non-Facility RVU 106. FUD 000 J G2 80 50

AMA: 2018,Apr,3

31299 Unlisted Procedures of Accessory Sinuses

CMS: 100-04,4,180.3 Unlisted Service or Procedure

EXCLUDES *Hypophysectomy (61546, 61548)*

31299 **Unlisted procedure, accessory sinuses**

Facility RVU 0.00 Non-Facility RVU 0.00 FUD YYY T 80

AMA: 2019,Jul,7; 2019,Apr,10; 2018,Jan,8; 2017,Nov,11; 2017,Jan,8; 2016,Feb,10; 2016,Jan,13; 2015,Jul,10; 2015,Jan,16; 2014,Jan,11

31300-31502 Procedures of the Larynx

31300 **Laryngotomy (thyrotomy, laryngofissure), with removal of tumor or laryngocele, cordectomy**

Facility RVU 36.6 Non-Facility RVU 36.6 FUD 090 J A2 80

Epiglottis
Hyoid bone
Thyroid cartilage
Cricothyroid ligament
Cricoid cartilage
Trachea
Vocal cord
Arytenoid cartilage
Vocal cords

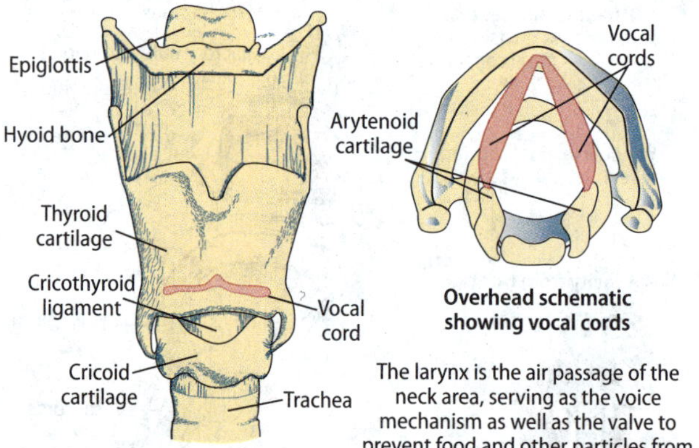

Frontal view of the major structures of the larynx

Overhead schematic showing vocal cords

The larynx is the air passage of the neck area, serving as the voice mechanism as well as the valve to prevent food and other particles from entering the respiratory tract

31360 **Laryngectomy; total, without radical neck dissection**

Facility RVU 59.8 Non-Facility RVU 59.8 FUD 090 C 80

AMA: 2018,Jan,8; 2017,Jan,8; 2016,Jan,13; 2015,Jan,16; 2014,Jan,11

31365 **total, with radical neck dissection**

Facility RVU 73.8 Non-Facility RVU 73.8 FUD 090 C 80

AMA: 2018,Jan,8; 2017,Jan,8; 2016,Jan,13; 2015,Jan,16; 2014,Jan,11

31367 **subtotal supraglottic, without radical neck dissection**

Facility RVU 63.2 Non-Facility RVU 63.2 FUD 090 C 80

AMA: 2018,Jan,8; 2017,Jan,8; 2016,Jan,13; 2015,Jan,16; 2014,Jan,11

31368 **subtotal supraglottic, with radical neck dissection**

Facility RVU 70.2 Non-Facility RVU 70.2 FUD 090 C 80

31370 **Partial laryngectomy (hemilaryngectomy); horizontal**

Facility RVU 59.4 Non-Facility RVU 59.4 FUD 090 C 80

31375 **laterovertical**
56.4 56.4 FUD 090 C 80

31380 **anterovertical**
55.6 55.6 FUD 090 C 80

31382 **antero-latero-vertical**
61.0 61.0 FUD 090 C 80

31390 **Pharyngolaryngectomy, with radical neck dissection; without reconstruction**
81.9 81.9 FUD 090 C 80

31395 **with reconstruction**
86.4 86.4 FUD 090 C 80

31400 **Arytenoidectomy or arytenoidopexy, external approach**
28.1 28.1 FUD 090 J A2 80
EXCLUDES *Endoscopic arytenoidectomy (31560)*

31420 **Epiglottidectomy**
23.5 23.5 FUD 090 J A2 80

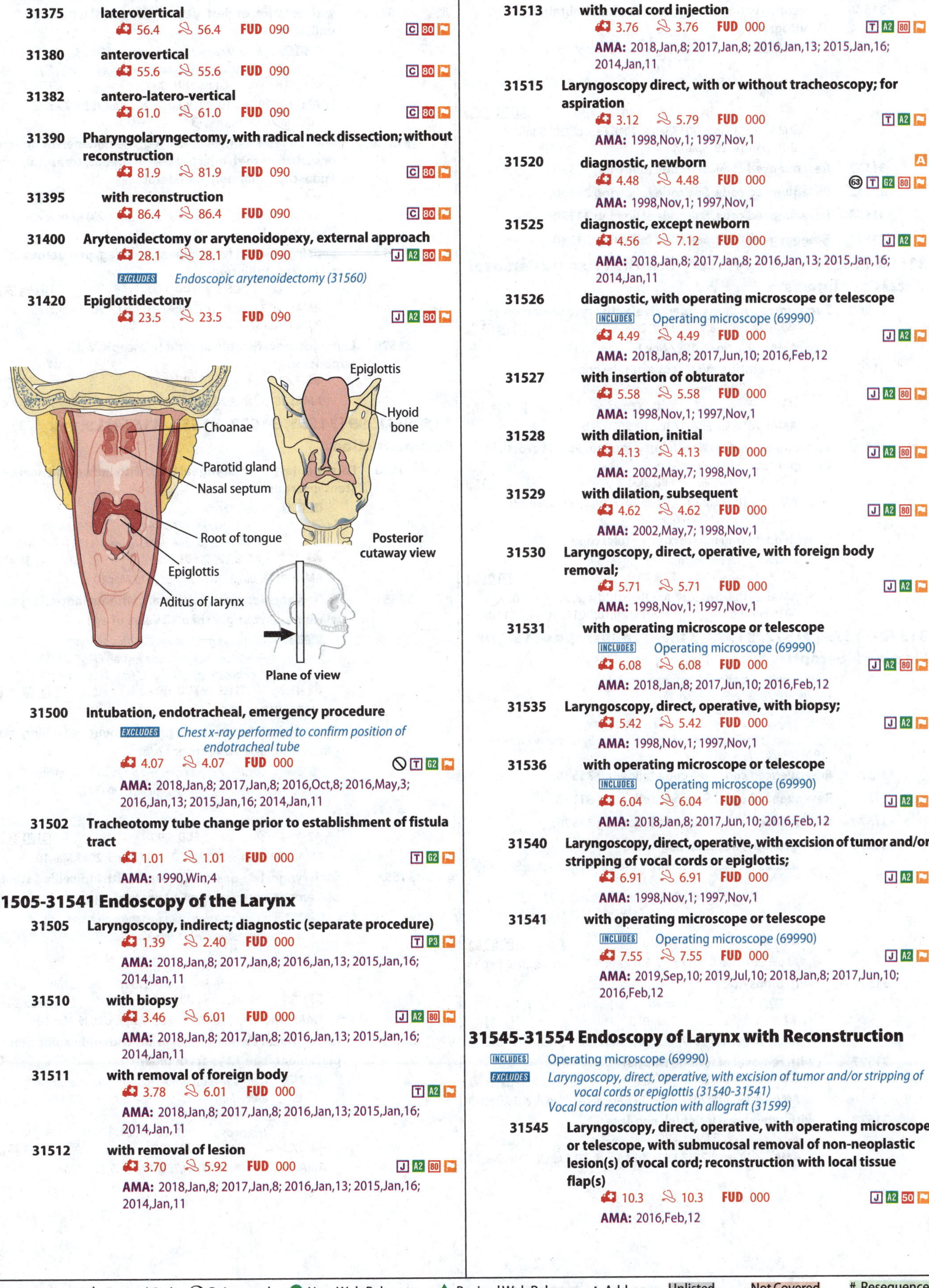

31500 **Intubation, endotracheal, emergency procedure**
EXCLUDES *Chest x-ray performed to confirm position of endotracheal tube*
4.07 4.07 FUD 000 ⃠ T G2
AMA: 2018,Jan,8; 2017,Jan,8; 2016,Oct,8; 2016,May,3; 2016,Jan,13; 2015,Jan,16; 2014,Jan,11

31502 **Tracheotomy tube change prior to establishment of fistula tract**
1.01 1.01 FUD 000 T G2
AMA: 1990,Win,4

31505-31541 Endoscopy of the Larynx

31505 **Laryngoscopy, indirect; diagnostic (separate procedure)**
1.39 2.40 FUD 000 T P3
AMA: 2018,Jan,8; 2017,Jan,8; 2016,Jan,13; 2015,Jan,16; 2014,Jan,11

31510 **with biopsy**
3.46 6.01 FUD 000 J A2 80
AMA: 2018,Jan,8; 2017,Jan,8; 2016,Jan,13; 2015,Jan,16; 2014,Jan,11

31511 **with removal of foreign body**
3.78 6.01 FUD 000 T A2
AMA: 2018,Jan,8; 2017,Jan,8; 2016,Jan,13; 2015,Jan,16; 2014,Jan,11

31512 **with removal of lesion**
3.70 5.92 FUD 000 J A2 80
AMA: 2018,Jan,8; 2017,Jan,8; 2016,Jan,13; 2015,Jan,16; 2014,Jan,11

31513 **with vocal cord injection**
3.76 3.76 FUD 000 T A2 80
AMA: 2018,Jan,8; 2017,Jan,8; 2016,Jan,13; 2015,Jan,16; 2014,Jan,11

31515 **Laryngoscopy direct, with or without tracheoscopy; for aspiration**
3.12 5.79 FUD 000 T A2
AMA: 1998,Nov,1; 1997,Nov,1

31520 **diagnostic, newborn** A
4.48 4.48 FUD 000 63 T G2 80
AMA: 1998,Nov,1; 1997,Nov,1

31525 **diagnostic, except newborn**
4.56 7.12 FUD 000 J A2
AMA: 2018,Jan,8; 2017,Jan,8; 2016,Jan,13; 2015,Jan,16; 2014,Jan,11

31526 **diagnostic, with operating microscope or telescope**
INCLUDES Operating microscope (69990)
4.49 4.49 FUD 000 J A2
AMA: 2018,Jan,8; 2017,Jun,10; 2016,Feb,12

31527 **with insertion of obturator**
5.58 5.58 FUD 000 J A2 80
AMA: 1998,Nov,1; 1997,Nov,1

31528 **with dilation, initial**
4.13 4.13 FUD 000 J A2 80
AMA: 2002,May,7; 1998,Nov,1

31529 **with dilation, subsequent**
4.62 4.62 FUD 000 J A2 80
AMA: 2002,May,7; 1998,Nov,1

31530 **Laryngoscopy, direct, operative, with foreign body removal;**
5.71 5.71 FUD 000 J A2
AMA: 1998,Nov,1; 1997,Nov,1

31531 **with operating microscope or telescope**
INCLUDES Operating microscope (69990)
6.08 6.08 FUD 000 J A2 80
AMA: 2018,Jan,8; 2017,Jun,10; 2016,Feb,12

31535 **Laryngoscopy, direct, operative, with biopsy;**
5.42 5.42 FUD 000 J A2
AMA: 1998,Nov,1; 1997,Nov,1

31536 **with operating microscope or telescope**
INCLUDES Operating microscope (69990)
6.04 6.04 FUD 000 J A2
AMA: 2018,Jan,8; 2017,Jun,10; 2016,Feb,12

31540 **Laryngoscopy, direct, operative, with excision of tumor and/or stripping of vocal cords or epiglottis;**
6.91 6.91 FUD 000 J A2
AMA: 1998,Nov,1; 1997,Nov,1

31541 **with operating microscope or telescope**
INCLUDES Operating microscope (69990)
7.55 7.55 FUD 000 J A2
AMA: 2019,Sep,10; 2019,Jul,10; 2018,Jan,8; 2017,Jun,10; 2016,Feb,12

31545-31554 Endoscopy of Larynx with Reconstruction

INCLUDES Operating microscope (69990)
EXCLUDES *Laryngoscopy, direct, operative, with excision of tumor and/or stripping of vocal cords or epiglottis (31540-31541)*
Vocal cord reconstruction with allograft (31599)

31545 **Laryngoscopy, direct, operative, with operating microscope or telescope, with submucosal removal of non-neoplastic lesion(s) of vocal cord; reconstruction with local tissue flap(s)**
10.3 10.3 FUD 000 J A2 50
AMA: 2016,Feb,12

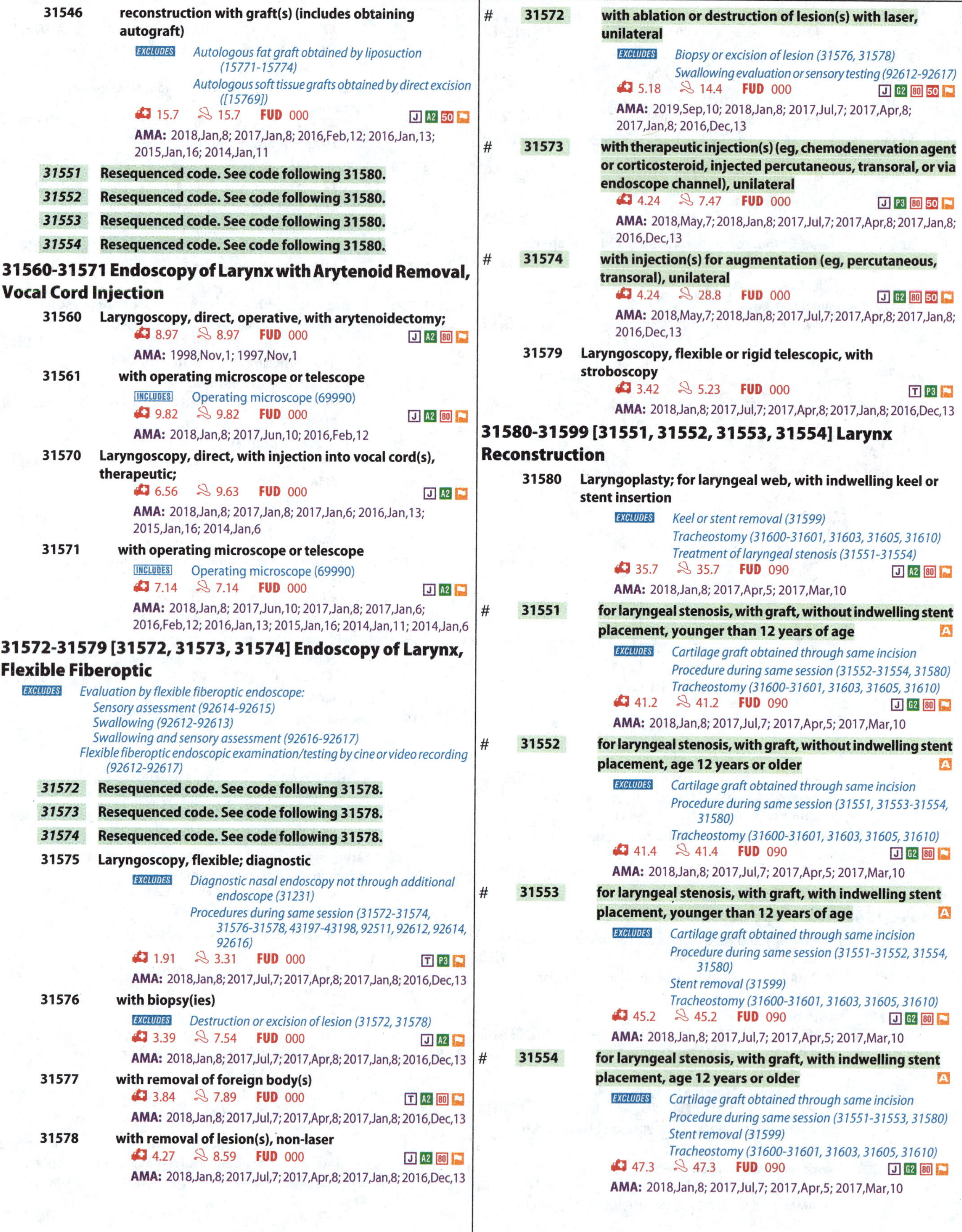

31546 reconstruction with graft(s) (includes obtaining autograft)

EXCLUDES *Autologous fat graft obtained by liposuction (15771-15774)*
Autologous soft tissue grafts obtained by direct excision ([15769])

15.7 15.7 FUD 000 J A2 50

AMA: 2018,Jan,8; 2017,Jan,8; 2016,Feb,12; 2016,Jan,13; 2015,Jan,16; 2014,Jan,11

31551 Resequenced code. See code following 31580.

31552 Resequenced code. See code following 31580.

31553 Resequenced code. See code following 31580.

31554 Resequenced code. See code following 31580.

31560-31571 Endoscopy of Larynx with Arytenoid Removal, Vocal Cord Injection

31560 Laryngoscopy, direct, operative, with arytenoidectomy;

8.97 8.97 FUD 000 J A2 80

AMA: 1998,Nov,1; 1997,Nov,1

31561 with operating microscope or telescope

INCLUDES Operating microscope (69990)

9.82 9.82 FUD 000 J A2 80

AMA: 2018,Jan,8; 2017,Jun,10; 2016,Feb,12

31570 Laryngoscopy, direct, with injection into vocal cord(s), therapeutic;

6.56 9.63 FUD 000 J A2

AMA: 2018,Jan,8; 2017,Jan,8; 2017,Jan,6; 2016,Jan,13; 2015,Jan,16; 2014,Jan,6

31571 with operating microscope or telescope

INCLUDES Operating microscope (69990)

7.14 7.14 FUD 000 J A2

AMA: 2018,Jan,8; 2017,Jun,10; 2017,Jan,8; 2017,Jan,6; 2016,Feb,12; 2016,Jan,13; 2015,Jan,16; 2014,Jan,11; 2014,Jan,6

31572-31579 [31572, 31573, 31574] Endoscopy of Larynx, Flexible Fiberoptic

EXCLUDES *Evaluation by flexible fiberoptic endoscope:*
Sensory assessment (92614-92615)
Swallowing (92612-92613)
Swallowing and sensory assessment (92616-92617)
Flexible fiberoptic endoscopic examination/testing by cine or video recording (92612-92617)

31572 Resequenced code. See code following 31578.

31573 Resequenced code. See code following 31578.

31574 Resequenced code. See code following 31578.

31575 Laryngoscopy, flexible; diagnostic

EXCLUDES *Diagnostic nasal endoscopy not through additional endoscope (31231)*
Procedures during same session (31572-31574, 31576-31578, 43197-43198, 92511, 92612, 92614, 92616)

1.91 3.31 FUD 000 T P3

AMA: 2018,Jan,8; 2017,Jul,7; 2017,Apr,8; 2017,Jan,8; 2016,Dec,13

31576 with biopsy(ies)

EXCLUDES *Destruction or excision of lesion (31572, 31578)*

3.39 7.54 FUD 000 J A2

AMA: 2018,Jan,8; 2017,Jul,7; 2017,Apr,8; 2017,Jan,8; 2016,Dec,13

31577 with removal of foreign body(s)

3.84 7.89 FUD 000 T A2 80

AMA: 2018,Jan,8; 2017,Jul,7; 2017,Apr,8; 2017,Jan,8; 2016,Dec,13

31578 with removal of lesion(s), non-laser

4.27 8.59 FUD 000 J A2 80

AMA: 2018,Jan,8; 2017,Jul,7; 2017,Apr,8; 2017,Jan,8; 2016,Dec,13

\# **31572** with ablation or destruction of lesion(s) with laser, unilateral

EXCLUDES *Biopsy or excision of lesion (31576, 31578)*
Swallowing evaluation or sensory testing (92612-92617)

5.18 14.4 FUD 000 J G2 80 50

AMA: 2019,Sep,10; 2018,Jan,8; 2017,Jul,7; 2017,Apr,8; 2017,Jan,8; 2016,Dec,13

\# **31573** with therapeutic injection(s) (eg, chemodenervation agent or corticosteroid, injected percutaneous, transoral, or via endoscope channel), unilateral

4.24 7.47 FUD 000 J P3 80 50

AMA: 2018,May,7; 2018,Jan,8; 2017,Jul,7; 2017,Apr,8; 2017,Jan,8; 2016,Dec,13

\# **31574** with injection(s) for augmentation (eg, percutaneous, transoral), unilateral

4.24 28.8 FUD 000 J G2 80 50

AMA: 2018,May,7; 2018,Jan,8; 2017,Jul,7; 2017,Apr,8; 2017,Jan,8; 2016,Dec,13

31579 Laryngoscopy, flexible or rigid telescopic, with stroboscopy

3.42 5.23 FUD 000 T P3

AMA: 2018,Jan,8; 2017,Jul,7; 2017,Apr,8; 2017,Jan,8; 2016,Dec,13

31580-31599 [31551, 31552, 31553, 31554] Larynx Reconstruction

31580 Laryngoplasty; for laryngeal web, with indwelling keel or stent insertion

EXCLUDES *Keel or stent removal (31599)*
Tracheostomy (31600-31601, 31603, 31605, 31610)
Treatment of laryngeal stenosis (31551-31554)

35.7 35.7 FUD 090 J A2 80

AMA: 2018,Jan,8; 2017,Apr,5; 2017,Mar,10

\# **31551** for laryngeal stenosis, with graft, without indwelling stent placement, younger than 12 years of age A

EXCLUDES *Cartilage graft obtained through same incision*
Procedure during same session (31552-31554, 31580)
Tracheostomy (31600-31601, 31603, 31605, 31610)

41.2 41.2 FUD 090 J G2 80

AMA: 2018,Jan,8; 2017,Jul,7; 2017,Apr,5; 2017,Mar,10

\# **31552** for laryngeal stenosis, with graft, without indwelling stent placement, age 12 years or older A

EXCLUDES *Cartilage graft obtained through same incision*
Procedure during same session (31551, 31553-31554, 31580)
Tracheostomy (31600-31601, 31603, 31605, 31610)

41.4 41.4 FUD 090 J G2 80

AMA: 2018,Jan,8; 2017,Jul,7; 2017,Apr,5; 2017,Mar,10

\# **31553** for laryngeal stenosis, with graft, with indwelling stent placement, younger than 12 years of age A

EXCLUDES *Cartilage graft obtained through same incision*
Procedure during same session (31551-31552, 31554, 31580)
Stent removal (31599)
Tracheostomy (31600-31601, 31603, 31605, 31610)

45.2 45.2 FUD 090 J G2 80

AMA: 2018,Jan,8; 2017,Jul,7; 2017,Apr,5; 2017,Mar,10

\# **31554** for laryngeal stenosis, with graft, with indwelling stent placement, age 12 years or older A

EXCLUDES *Cartilage graft obtained through same incision*
Procedure during same session (31551-31553, 31580)
Stent removal (31599)
Tracheostomy (31600-31601, 31603, 31605, 31610)

47.3 47.3 FUD 090 J G2 80

AMA: 2018,Jan,8; 2017,Jul,7; 2017,Apr,5; 2017,Mar,10

31584 **with open reduction and fixation of (eg, plating) fracture, includes tracheostomy, if performed**

EXCLUDES *Cartilage graft obtained through same incision*

39.6 39.6 FUD 090 J 80

AMA: 2018,Jan,8; 2017,Apr,5; 2017,Mar,10

31587 **Laryngoplasty, cricoid split, without graft placement**

EXCLUDES *Tracheostomy (31600-31601, 31603, 31605, 31610)*

33.2 33.2 FUD 090 J 80

AMA: 2018,Jan,8; 2017,Apr,5; 2017,Mar,10

31590 **Laryngeal reinnervation by neuromuscular pedicle**

25.0 25.0 FUD 090 J A2 80

AMA: 2018,Jan,8; 2017,Mar,10

31591 **Laryngoplasty, medialization, unilateral**

30.0 30.0 FUD 090 J G2 80

AMA: 2018,Jan,8; 2017,Jul,7; 2017,Apr,5; 2017,Mar,10

31592 **Cricotracheal resection**

EXCLUDES *Advancement or rotational flaps performed not requiring additional incision*
Cartilage graft obtained through same incision
Tracheal stenosis excision/anastomosis (31780-31781)
Tracheostomy (31600-31601, 31603, 31605, 31610)

49.2 49.2 FUD 090 J G2 80

AMA: 2018,Jan,8; 2017,Jul,7; 2017,Apr,5; 2017,Mar,10; 2017,Feb,14

31599 **Unlisted procedure, larynx**

0.00 0.00 FUD YYY T 80

AMA: 2018,Jan,8; 2017,Apr,5; 2017,Mar,10; 2017,Jan,8; 2017,Jan,6; 2016,Dec,13; 2016,Jan,13; 2015,Jan,16; 2014,Jan,11

31600-31610 Stoma Creation: Trachea

EXCLUDES *Aspiration of trachea, direct vision (31515)*
Endotracheal intubation (31500)

31600 **Tracheostomy, planned (separate procedure);**

8.91 8.91 FUD 000 J

AMA: 2019,Sep,10; 2017,Apr,5

31601 **younger than 2 years** A

12.9 12.9 FUD 000 J 80

AMA: 2017,Apr,5

31603 **Tracheostomy, emergency procedure; transtracheal**

9.31 9.31 FUD 000 T A2

AMA: 2017,Apr,5

31605 **cricothyroid membrane**

9.61 9.61 FUD 000 T G2

AMA: 2017,Apr,5

31610 **Tracheostomy, fenestration procedure with skin flaps**

27.2 27.2 FUD 090 J

AMA: 2017,Apr,5

31611-31614 Procedures of the Trachea

31611 **Construction of tracheoesophageal fistula and subsequent insertion of an alaryngeal speech prosthesis (eg, voice button, Blom-Singer prosthesis)**

15.2 15.2 FUD 090 J A2 80

31612 **Tracheal puncture, percutaneous with transtracheal aspiration and/or injection**

EXCLUDES *Tracheal aspiration under direct vision (31515)*

1.39 2.39 FUD 000 J A2 80

AMA: 1994,Win,1

31613 **Tracheostoma revision; simple, without flap rotation**

12.6 12.6 FUD 090 J A2

31614 **complex, with flap rotation**

21.0 21.0 FUD 090 J A2

31615 Endoscopy Through Tracheostomy

INCLUDES Diagnostic bronchoscopy

EXCLUDES *Endobronchial ultrasound [EBUS] guided biopsies of mediastinal or hilar lymph nodes (31652-31653)*
Tracheoscopy (31515-31578)

Code also endobronchial ultrasound [EBUS] during diagnostic/therapeutic peripheral lesion intervention (31654)

31615 **Tracheobronchoscopy through established tracheostomy incision**

3.29 4.83 FUD 000 T A2

AMA: 2018,Jan,8; 2017,Jan,8; 2016,Jan,13; 2015,Jan,16; 2014,Jan,11

31622-31654 [31651] Endoscopy of Lung

INCLUDES Diagnostic bronchoscopy with surgical bronchoscopy procedures
Fluoroscopic imaging guidance, when performed

31622 **Bronchoscopy, rigid or flexible, including fluoroscopic guidance, when performed; diagnostic, with cell washing, when performed (separate procedure)**

3.78 6.84 FUD 000 J A2

AMA: 2018,Jan,8; 2017,Jan,8; 2016,Apr,5; 2016,Jan,13; 2015,Jan,16; 2014,Jan,11

31623 **with brushing or protected brushings**

3.81 7.51 FUD 000 J A2

AMA: 2018,Jan,8; 2017,Jan,8; 2016,Apr,5; 2016,Jan,13; 2015,Jan,16; 2014,Jan,11

31624 **with bronchial alveolar lavage**

3.86 7.10 FUD 000 J A2

AMA: 2018,Jan,8; 2017,Jun,10; 2017,Jan,8; 2016,Apr,5; 2016,Jan,13; 2015,Jan,16; 2014,Jan,11

31625 **with bronchial or endobronchial biopsy(s), single or multiple sites**

4.49 9.59 FUD 000 J A2

AMA: 2018,Jan,8; 2017,Jan,8; 2016,Apr,5; 2016,Jan,13; 2015,Jan,16; 2014,Jan,11

31626 **with placement of fiducial markers, single or multiple**

Code also device

5.72 23.9 FUD 000 J G2 80

AMA: 2018,Jan,8; 2017,Jun,10; 2017,Jan,8; 2016,Apr,5; 2016,Jan,13; 2015,Jun,6; 2015,Jan,16; 2014,Jan,11

+ **31627** **with computer-assisted, image-guided navigation (List separately in addition to code for primary procedure[s])**

INCLUDES 3D reconstruction (76376-76377)

Code first (31615, 31622-31626, 31628-31631, 31635-31636, 31638-31643)

2.80 37.8 FUD ZZZ N N1 80

AMA: 2018,Jan,8; 2017,Jan,8; 2016,Jan,13; 2015,Jan,16; 2014,Jan,11

31628 **with transbronchial lung biopsy(s), single lobe**

INCLUDES All biopsies taken from lobe

EXCLUDES *Transbronchial biopsies by needle aspiration (31629, 31633)*

Code also transbronchial biopsies of additional lobe(s) (31632)

5.06 10.1 FUD 000 J A2

AMA: 2018,Jan,8; 2017,Jun,10; 2017,Jan,8; 2016,Apr,5; 2016,Jan,13; 2015,Jan,16; 2014,Jan,11

31629 **with transbronchial needle aspiration biopsy(s), trachea, main stem and/or lobar bronchus(i)**

INCLUDES All biopsies from same lobe or upper airway

EXCLUDES *Transbronchial biopsies of lung (31628, 31632)*

Code also transbronchial needle biopsies of additional lobe(s) (31633)

5.38 12.5 FUD 000 J A2

AMA: 2018,Jan,8; 2017,Jan,8; 2016,Apr,5; 2016,Jan,13; 2015,Jan,16; 2014,Jan,11

31630 **with tracheal/bronchial dilation or closed reduction of fracture**

5.71 5.71 FUD 000 J A2

AMA: 2018,Jan,8; 2017,Jan,8; 2016,Jan,13; 2015,Jan,16; 2014,Jan,11

31631 **with placement of tracheal stent(s) (includes tracheal/bronchial dilation as required)**

EXCLUDES *Bronchial stent placement (31636-31637)*
Revision bronchial or tracheal stent (31638)

6.58 6.58 FUD 000 J A2

AMA: 2018,Jan,8; 2017,Jan,8; 2016,Jan,13; 2015,Jan,16; 2014,Jan,11

\+ **31632** **with transbronchial lung biopsy(s), each additional lobe (List separately in addition to code for primary procedure)**

INCLUDES All biopsies of additional lobe of lung

Code first (31628)

1.41 1.81 FUD ZZZ N N1

AMA: 2018,Jan,8; 2017,Jan,8; 2016,Jan,13; 2015,Jan,16; 2014,Jan,11

\+ **31633** **with transbronchial needle aspiration biopsy(s), each additional lobe (List separately in addition to code for primary procedure)**

INCLUDES All needle biopsies from another lobe or from trachea

Code first (31629)

1.83 2.27 FUD ZZZ N N1

AMA: 2018,Jan,8; 2017,Jan,8; 2016,Jan,13; 2015,Jan,16; 2014,Jan,11

31634 **with balloon occlusion, with assessment of air leak, with administration of occlusive substance (eg, fibrin glue), if performed**

EXCLUDES *Bronchoscopy, rigid or flexible, including fluoroscopic guidance, when performed; with balloon occlusion, when performed, assessment of air leak, airway sizing, and insertion of bronchial valve(s), initial lobe (31647, [31651])*

5.53 49.4 FUD 000 J G2 80

AMA: 2018,Jan,8; 2017,Jan,8; 2016,Jan,13; 2015,Jan,16; 2014,Jan,11

31635 **with removal of foreign body**

EXCLUDES *Removal implanted bronchial valves (31648-31649)*

5.06 8.03 FUD 000 J A2

AMA: 2018,Jan,8; 2017,Jan,8; 2016,Jan,13; 2015,Jan,16; 2014,Jan,11

31636 **with placement of bronchial stent(s) (includes tracheal/bronchial dilation as required), initial bronchus**

6.35 6.35 FUD 000 J J8

AMA: 2018,Jan,8; 2017,Jan,8; 2016,Jan,13; 2015,Jan,16; 2014,Jan,11

\+ **31637** **each additional major bronchus stented (List separately in addition to code for primary procedure)**

Code first (31636)

2.22 2.22 FUD ZZZ N N1

AMA: 2018,Jan,8; 2017,Jan,8; 2016,Jan,13; 2015,Jan,16; 2014,Jan,11

31638 **with revision of tracheal or bronchial stent inserted at previous session (includes tracheal/bronchial dilation as required)**

7.21 7.21 FUD 000 J A2

AMA: 2018,Jan,8; 2017,Jan,8; 2016,Jan,13; 2015,Jan,16; 2014,Jan,11

31640 **with excision of tumor**

7.22 7.22 FUD 000 J A2

AMA: 2018,Jan,8; 2017,Jan,8; 2016,Apr,5; 2016,Jan,13; 2015,Jan,16; 2014,Jan,11

31641 **with destruction of tumor or relief of stenosis by any method other than excision (eg, laser therapy, cryotherapy)**

Code also any photodynamic therapy via bronchoscopy (96570-96571)

7.39 7.39 FUD 000 J A2

AMA: 2018,Jan,8; 2017,Jan,8; 2016,Jan,13; 2015,Jan,16; 2014,Jan,11

31643 **with placement of catheter(s) for intracavitary radioelement application**

Code also if appropriate (77761-77763, 77770-77772)

5.09 5.09 FUD 000 J A2

AMA: 2018,Jan,8; 2017,Jan,8; 2016,Apr,5; 2016,Jan,13; 2015,Jan,16; 2014,Jan,11

31645 **with therapeutic aspiration of tracheobronchial tree, initial (eg, drainage of lung abscess)**

EXCLUDES *Bedside aspiration of trachea, bronchi (31725)*

4.21 7.42 FUD 000 J A2

AMA: 2018,Jan,8; 2017,Jan,8; 2016,Apr,5; 2016,Jan,13; 2015,Jan,16; 2014,Jan,11

31646 **with therapeutic aspiration of tracheobronchial tree, subsequent**

EXCLUDES *Bedside aspiration of trachea, bronchi (31725)*

4.09 4.09 FUD 000 T A2

AMA: 2018,Sep,3; 2018,Jan,8; 2017,Jan,8; 2016,Apr,5; 2016,Jan,13; 2015,Jan,16; 2014,Jan,11

31647 **with balloon occlusion, when performed, assessment of air leak, airway sizing, and insertion of bronchial valve(s), initial lobe**

6.10 6.10 FUD 000 J G2

AMA: 2018,Sep,3; 2018,Jan,8; 2017,Jan,8; 2016,Jan,13; 2015,Jan,16; 2014,Jan,11

\+ # **31651** **with balloon occlusion, when performed, assessment of air leak, airway sizing, and insertion of bronchial valve(s), each additional lobe (List separately in addition to code for primary procedure[s])**

Code first (31647)

2.13 2.13 FUD ZZZ N N1

AMA: 2018,Sep,3; 2018,Jan,8; 2017,Jan,8; 2016,Jan,13; 2015,Jan,16; 2014,Jan,11

31648 **with removal of bronchial valve(s), initial lobe**

EXCLUDES *Removal with reinsertion bronchial valve during same session (31647 and 31648) and ([31651])*

5.80 5.80 FUD 000 J G2

AMA: 2018,Sep,3; 2018,Jan,8; 2017,Jan,8; 2016,Jan,13; 2015,Jan,16; 2014,Jan,11

\+ **31649** **with removal of bronchial valve(s), each additional lobe (List separately in addition to code for primary procedure)**

Code first (31648)

1.94 1.94 FUD ZZZ Q2 G2

AMA: 2018,Sep,3; 2018,Jan,8; 2017,Jan,8; 2016,Jan,13; 2015,Jan,16; 2014,Jan,11

31651 **Resequenced code. See code following 31647.**

31652 **with endobronchial ultrasound (EBUS) guided transtracheal and/or transbronchial sampling (eg, aspiration[s]/biopsy[ies]), one or two mediastinal and/or hilar lymph node stations or structures**

EXCLUDES *Procedures performed more than one time per session*

6.39 27.4 FUD 000 J G2

AMA: 2018,Jan,8; 2017,Jan,8; 2016,Apr,5

31653 **with endobronchial ultrasound (EBUS) guided transtracheal and/or transbronchial sampling (eg, aspiration[s]/biopsy[ies]), 3 or more mediastinal and/or hilar lymph node stations or structures**

EXCLUDES *Procedures performed more than one time per session*

7.08 28.7 FUD 000 J G2

AMA: 2018,Jan,8; 2017,Jan,8; 2016,Apr,5

+ **31654** **with transendoscopic endobronchial ultrasound (EBUS) during bronchoscopic diagnostic or therapeutic intervention(s) for peripheral lesion(s) (List separately in addition to code for primary procedure[s])**

EXCLUDES *Endobronchial ultrasound [EBUS] for mediastinal/hilar lymph node station/adjacent structure access (31652-31653)*

Procedures performed more than one time per session

Code first (31622-31626, 31628-31629, 31640, 31643-31646)

1.94 3.53 FUD ZZZ N N1

AMA: 2018,Jan,8; 2017,Jan,8; 2016,Apr,5

31660-31661 Bronchial Thermoplasty

INCLUDES Fluoroscopic imaging guidance, when performed

31660 **Bronchoscopy, rigid or flexible, including fluoroscopic guidance, when performed; with bronchial thermoplasty, 1 lobe**

5.62 5.62 FUD 000 J

AMA: 2018,Jan,8; 2017,Jan,8; 2016,Jan,13; 2015,Jan,16; 2014,Jan,11

31661 **with bronchial thermoplasty, 2 or more lobes**

5.93 5.93 FUD 000 J

AMA: 2018,Jan,8; 2017,Jan,8; 2016,Jan,13; 2015,Jan,16; 2014,Jan,11

31717-31899 Respiratory Procedures

EXCLUDES *Endotracheal intubation (31500)*

Tracheal aspiration under direct vision (31515)

31717 **Catheterization with bronchial brush biopsy**

3.18 7.98 FUD 000 T A2

AMA: 2018,Jan,8; 2017,Jan,8; 2016,Jan,13; 2015,Jan,16; 2014,Jan,11

31720 **Catheter aspiration (separate procedure); nasotracheal**

1.43 1.43 FUD 000 Q1 N1

AMA: 1994,Win,1

31725 **tracheobronchial with fiberscope, bedside**

2.29 2.29 FUD 000 C

31730 **Transtracheal (percutaneous) introduction of needle wire dilator/stent or indwelling tube for oxygen therapy**

4.32 34.2 FUD 000 J A2

AMA: 1992,Win,1

31750 **Tracheoplasty; cervical**

39.5 39.5 FUD 090 J A2 80

31755 **tracheopharyngeal fistulization, each stage**

49.9 49.9 FUD 090 J A2 80

31760 **intrathoracic**

39.6 39.6 FUD 090 C 80

31766 **Carinal reconstruction**

51.4 51.4 FUD 090 C 80

31770 **Bronchoplasty; graft repair**

38.5 38.5 FUD 090 C 80

EXCLUDES *Bronchoplasty done with lobectomy (32501)*

31775 **excision stenosis and anastomosis**

40.4 40.4 FUD 090 C 80

EXCLUDES *Bronchoplasty done with lobectomy (32501)*

31780 **Excision tracheal stenosis and anastomosis; cervical**

34.3 34.3 FUD 090 C 80

AMA: 2018,Jan,8; 2017,Apr,5; 2017,Feb,14

31781 **cervicothoracic**

40.1 40.1 FUD 090 C 80

AMA: 2018,Jan,8; 2017,Apr,5; 2017,Feb,14

31785 **Excision of tracheal tumor or carcinoma; cervical**

30.9 30.9 FUD 090 J 80

AMA: 2003,Jan,1

31786 **thoracic**

41.7 41.7 FUD 090 C 80

31800 **Suture of tracheal wound or injury; cervical**

20.6 20.6 FUD 090 C 80

AMA: 1994,Win,1

31805 **intrathoracic**

23.5 23.5 FUD 090 C 80

31820 **Surgical closure tracheostomy or fistula; without plastic repair**

9.35 12.3 FUD 090 J A2 80

EXCLUDES *Tracheoesophageal fistula repair (43305, 43312)*

31825 **with plastic repair**

13.7 17.1 FUD 090 J A2 80

EXCLUDES *Tracheoesophageal fistula repair (43305, 43312)*

31830 **Revision of tracheostomy scar**

9.87 12.7 FUD 090 J A2 80

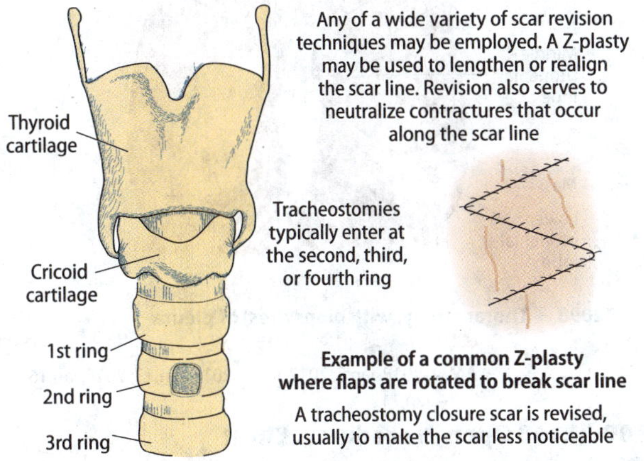

Thyroid cartilage

Cricoid cartilage

1st ring

2nd ring

3rd ring

Tracheostomies typically enter at the second, third, or fourth ring

Any of a wide variety of scar revision techniques may be employed. A Z-plasty may be used to lengthen or realign the scar line. Revision also serves to neutralize contractures that occur along the scar line

Example of a common Z-plasty where flaps are rotated to break scar line

A tracheostomy closure scar is revised, usually to make the scar less noticeable

31899 **Unlisted procedure, trachea, bronchi**

0.00 0.00 FUD YYY T 80

AMA: 2018,Jan,8; 2017,Jan,8; 2016,Jan,13; 2015,Jan,16; 2014,May,10; 2014,Jan,11

32035-32036 Procedures for Empyema

EXCLUDES *Wound exploration without thoracotomy for penetrating wound of chest (20101)*

32035 **Thoracostomy; with rib resection for empyema**

20.9 20.9 FUD 090 C 80 50

32036 **with open flap drainage for empyema**

22.3 22.3 FUD 090 C 80 50

32096-32098 Open Biopsy of Chest and Pleura

INCLUDES Varying amounts of lung tissue excised for analysis

Wedge technique with tissue obtained without precise consideration of margins

EXCLUDES *Percutaneous needle biopsy of pleura, lung, and mediastinum (32400, 32405)*

Thoracoscopy with biopsy (32607-32609)

Thoracoscopy with diagnostic wedge resection resulting in anatomic lung resection (32668)

Thoracotomy with diagnostic wedge resection resulting in anatomic lung resection (32507)

32096 **Thoracotomy, with diagnostic biopsy(ies) of lung infiltrate(s) (eg, wedge, incisional), unilateral**

EXCLUDES *Procedure performed more than one time per lung*

Removal of lung (32440-32445, 32488)

Code also appropriate add-on code for the more extensive procedure at the same location if diagnostic wedge resection results in the need for further surgery (32507, 32668)

23.2 23.2 FUD 090 C 80

AMA: 2018,Jan,8; 2017,Jan,8; 2016,Jan,13; 2015,Jan,16; 2014,Jan,11

32097 **Thoracotomy, with diagnostic biopsy(ies) of lung nodule(s) or mass(es) (eg, wedge, incisional), unilateral**

EXCLUDES *Procedure performed more than one time per lung*
Removal of lung (32440-32445, 32488)

Code also appropriate add-on code for the more extensive procedure in the same location if diagnostic wedge resection results in the need for further surgery (32507, 32668)

23.1 23.1 FUD 090 C 80

AMA: 2018,Jan,8; 2017,Jan,8; 2016,Jan,13; 2015,Jan,16; 2014,Jan,11

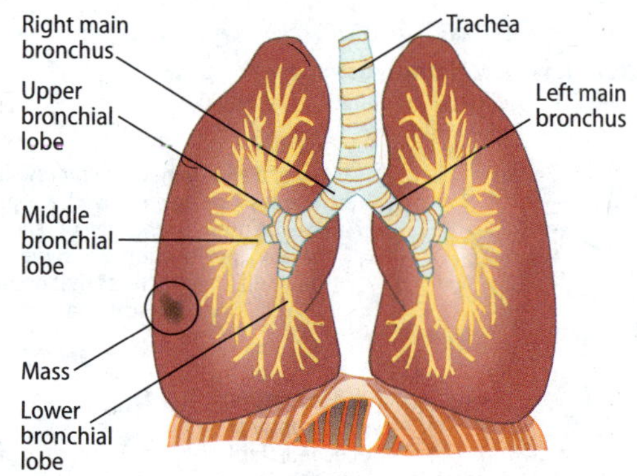

32098 **Thoracotomy, with biopsy(ies) of pleura**

21.9 21.9 FUD 090 C 80

AMA: 2018,Jan,8; 2017,Jan,8; 2016,Jan,13; 2015,Jan,16; 2014,Jan,11

32100-32160 Open Procedures: Chest

INCLUDES Exploration of penetrating wound of chest

EXCLUDES *Lung resection (32480-32504)*
Wound exploration without thoracotomy for penetrating wound of chest (20101)

32100 **Thoracotomy; with exploration**

EXCLUDES *Excision of chest wall tumor, when performed (21601-21603)*
Extracorporeal membrane oxygenation (ECMO)/extracorporeal life support (ECLS) (33955-33957, [33963, 33964])
Resection of apical lung tumor (32503-32504)

23.3 23.3 FUD 090 C 80

AMA: 2018,Jan,8; 2017,Jan,8; 2016,Jan,13; 2015,Jul,3; 2015,Jan,16; 2014,Jan,11

32110 **with control of traumatic hemorrhage and/or repair of lung tear**

42.4 42.4 FUD 090 C 80

AMA: 2018,Jan,8; 2017,Jan,8; 2016,Jan,13; 2015,Jan,16; 2014,Jan,11

32120 **for postoperative complications**

25.1 25.1 FUD 090 C 80

32124 **with open intrapleural pneumonolysis**

26.7 26.7 FUD 090 C 80

AMA: 2018,Jan,8; 2017,Jan,8; 2016,Jan,13; 2015,Jan,16; 2014,Jan,11

32140 **with cyst(s) removal, includes pleural procedure when performed**

28.6 28.6 FUD 090 C 80

AMA: 2018,Jan,8; 2017,Jan,8; 2016,Jan,13; 2015,Jan,16; 2014,Jan,11

32141 **with resection-plication of bullae, includes any pleural procedure when performed**

EXCLUDES *Lung volume reduction (32491)*

44.0 44.0 FUD 090 C 80

AMA: 2018,Jan,8; 2017,Jan,8; 2016,Jan,13; 2015,Jan,16; 2014,Jan,11

32150 **with removal of intrapleural foreign body or fibrin deposit**

28.9 28.9 FUD 090 C 80

AMA: 2018,Jan,8; 2017,Jan,8; 2016,Jan,13; 2015,Jan,16; 2014,Jan,11

32151 **with removal of intrapulmonary foreign body**

29.0 29.0 FUD 090 C 80

32160 **with cardiac massage**

22.9 22.9 FUD 090 C 80

32200-32320 Open Procedures: Lung

32200 **Pneumonostomy, with open drainage of abscess or cyst**

EXCLUDES *Image-guided, percutaneous drainage (eg, abscess, cyst) of lungs/mediastinum via catheter (49405)*

(75989)

32.8 32.8 FUD 090 C 80

AMA: 2013,Nov,9; 1997,Nov,1

32215 **Pleural scarification for repeat pneumothorax**

22.9 22.9 FUD 090 C 80 50

32220 **Decortication, pulmonary (separate procedure); total**

45.7 45.7 FUD 090 C 80 50

32225 **partial**

28.6 28.6 FUD 090 C 80 50

32310 **Pleurectomy, parietal (separate procedure)**

26.3 26.3 FUD 090 C 80

AMA: 1994,Win,1

32320 **Decortication and parietal pleurectomy**

46.1 46.1 FUD 090 C 80

AMA: 1994,Fall,1

32400-32405 Lung Biopsy

EXCLUDES *Fine needle aspiration (10004-10012, 10021)*
Open lung biopsy (32096-32097)
Open mediastinal biopsy (39000-39010)
Thoracoscopic (VATS) biopsy of lung, pericardium, pleural or mediastinal space (32604-32609)

32400 **Biopsy, pleura, percutaneous needle**

(76942, 77002, 77012, 77021)

2.50 4.41 FUD 000 J A2

AMA: 2019,Apr,4; 2018,Jan,8; 2017,Jan,8; 2016,Jan,13; 2015,Jan,16; 2014,Jan,11

32405 **Biopsy, lung or mediastinum, percutaneous needle**

(76942, 77002, 77012, 77021)

2.61 11.1 FUD 000 J A2

AMA: 2019,Apr,4; 2018,Jan,8; 2017,Jan,8; 2016,Jan,13; 2015,Jan,16; 2014,Jan,11

32440-32501 Lung Resection

32440 Removal of lung, pneumonectomy;

Code also excision of chest wall tumor, when performed (21601-21603)

45.1 45.1 FUD 090 C 80

AMA: 2018,Jan,8; 2017,Jan,8; 2016,Jan,13; 2015,Jan,16; 2014,Jan,11

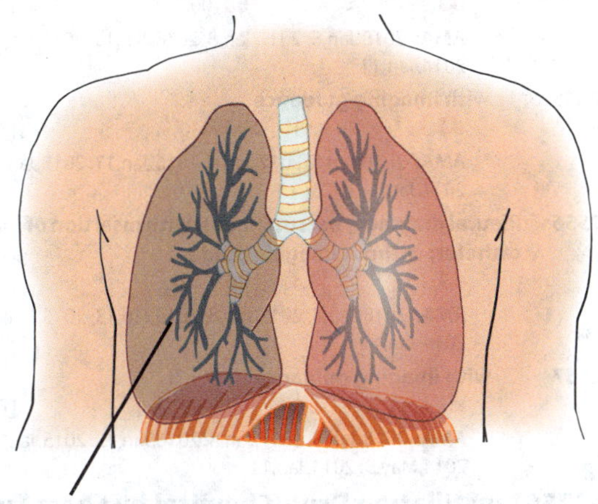

Removal of entire lung

32442 with resection of segment of trachea followed by broncho-tracheal anastomosis (sleeve pneumonectomy)

Code also excision of chest wall tumor, when performed (21601-21603)

88.9 88.9 FUD 090 C 80

AMA: 2018,Jan,8; 2017,Jun,10; 2017,Jan,8; 2016,Jan,13; 2015,Jan,16; 2014,Jan,11

32445 extrapleural

Code also empyemectomy with extrapleural pneumonectomy (32540)

Code also excision of chest wall tumor, when performed (21601-21603)

102. 102. FUD 090 C 80

AMA: 2018,Jan,8; 2017,Jan,8; 2016,Jan,13; 2015,Jan,16; 2014,Jan,11

32480 Removal of lung, other than pneumonectomy; single lobe (lobectomy)

EXCLUDES *Lung removal with bronchoplasty (32501)*

Code also decortication (32320)

Code also excision of chest wall tumor, when performed (21601-21603)

42.6 42.6 FUD 090 C 80

AMA: 2018,Jan,8; 2017,Jan,8; 2016,Jan,13; 2015,Jan,16; 2014,Jan,11

32482 2 lobes (bilobectomy)

EXCLUDES *Lung removal with bronchoplasty (32501)*

Code also decortication (32320)

Code also excision of chest wall tumor, when performed (21601-21603)

45.6 45.6 FUD 090 C 80

AMA: 2018,Jan,8; 2017,Jan,8; 2016,Jan,13; 2015,Jan,16; 2014,Jan,11

32484 single segment (segmentectomy)

EXCLUDES *Lung removal with bronchoplasty (32501)*

Code also decortication (32320)

Code also excision of chest wall tumor, when performed (21601-21603)

41.3 41.3 FUD 090 C 80

AMA: 2018,Jan,8; 2017,Jan,8; 2016,Jan,13; 2015,Jan,16; 2014,Jan,11

32486 with circumferential resection of segment of bronchus followed by broncho-bronchial anastomosis (sleeve lobectomy)

Code also decortication (32320)

Code also excision of chest wall tumor, when performed (21601-21603)

68.1 68.1 FUD 090 C 80

AMA: 2018,Jan,8; 2017,Jun,10; 2017,Jan,8; 2016,Jan,13; 2015,Jan,16; 2014,Jan,11

32488 with all remaining lung following previous removal of a portion of lung (completion pneumonectomy)

Code also decortication (32320)

Code also excision of chest wall tumor, when performed (21601-21603)

69.3 69.3 FUD 090 C 80

AMA: 2018,Jan,8; 2017,Jan,8; 2016,Jan,13; 2015,Jan,16; 2014,Jan,11

32491 with resection-plication of emphysematous lung(s) (bullous or non-bullous) for lung volume reduction, sternal split or transthoracic approach, includes any pleural procedure, when performed

42.6 42.6 FUD 090 C 80 50

AMA: 2018,Jan,8; 2017,Jan,8; 2016,Jan,13; 2015,Jan,16; 2014,Jan,11

\+ **32501 Resection and repair of portion of bronchus (bronchoplasty) when performed at time of lobectomy or segmentectomy (List separately in addition to code for primary procedure)**

INCLUDES Plastic closure of bronchus, not closure of a resected end of bronchus

Code first (32480-32484)

7.07 7.07 FUD ZZZ C 80

AMA: 1995,Win,1

32503-32504 Excision of Lung Neoplasm

EXCLUDES *Excision of chest wall tumor (21601-21603)*
Thoracentesis, needle or catheter, aspiration of the pleural space (32554-32555)
Thoracotomy; with exploration (32100)
Tube thoracostomy (32551)

32503 Resection of apical lung tumor (eg, Pancoast tumor), including chest wall resection, rib(s) resection(s), neurovascular dissection, when performed; without chest wall reconstruction(s)

52.0 52.0 FUD 090 C 80

AMA: 2012,Oct,9-11; 2012,Sep,3-8

32504 with chest wall reconstruction

59.3 59.3 FUD 090 C 80

AMA: 2012,Oct,9-11; 2012,Sep,3-8

32505-32507 Thoracotomy with Wedge Resection

INCLUDES Wedge technique with tissue obtained with precise consideration of margins and complete resection

Code also resection of chest wall tumor with lung resection, when performed (21601-21603)

32505 Thoracotomy; with therapeutic wedge resection (eg, mass, nodule), initial

EXCLUDES *Removal of lung (32440, 32442, 32445, 32488)*

Code also a more extensive procedure of the lung when performed on the contralateral lung or different lobe with modifier 59 regardless of intraoperative pathology consultation

26.8 26.8 FUD 090 C 80

AMA: 2018,Jan,8; 2017,Jan,8; 2016,Jan,13; 2015,Jan,16; 2014,Jan,11

+ 32506 **with therapeutic wedge resection (eg, mass or nodule), each additional resection, ipsilateral (List separately in addition to code for primary procedure)**

Code also a more extensive procedure of the lung when performed on the contralateral lung or different lobe with modifier 59

Code first (32505)

4.53 4.53 FUD ZZZ C 80

AMA: 2018,Jan,8; 2017,Jan,8; 2016,Jan,13; 2015,Jan,16; 2014,Jan,11

+ 32507 **with diagnostic wedge resection followed by anatomic lung resection (List separately in addition to code for primary procedure)**

INCLUDES Classification as a diagnostic wedge resection if intraoperative pathology consultation dictates more extensive resection in the same anatomical area

EXCLUDES *Diagnostic wedge resection by thoracoscopy (32668)*

Therapeutic wedge resection (32505-32506, 32666-32667)

Code first (32440, 32442, 32445, 32480-32488, 32503-32504)

4.52 4.52 FUD ZZZ C 80

AMA: 2018,Jan,8; 2017,Jan,8; 2016,Jan,13; 2015,Jan,16; 2014,Jan,11

32540 Removal of Empyema

32540 **Extrapleural enucleation of empyema (empyemectomy)**

EXCLUDES *Lung removal code when empyemectomy is performed with lobectomy (see appropriate lung removal code)*

Code also appropriate removal of lung code when done with lobectomy (32480-32488)

49.6 49.6 FUD 090 C 80

AMA: 1994,Fall,1

32550-32552 Chest Tube/Catheter

32550 **Insertion of indwelling tunneled pleural catheter with cuff**

EXCLUDES *Procedures performed on same side of chest with (32554-32557)*

(75989)

5.98 21.2 FUD 000 J G2

AMA: 2018,Jan,8; 2017,Jan,8; 2016,Jan,13; 2015,Jan,16; 2014,May,3; 2014,Mar,13; 2014,Jan,11

32551 **Tube thoracostomy, includes connection to drainage system (eg, water seal), when performed, open (separate procedure)**

EXCLUDES *Procedures performed on same side of chest with (33020, 33025)*

4.53 4.53 FUD 000 T 50

AMA: 2018,Jul,7; 2018,Jan,8; 2017,Jun,10; 2017,Jan,8; 2016,Jan,13; 2015,Jan,16; 2014,May,3; 2014,Jan,11

32552 **Removal of indwelling tunneled pleural catheter with cuff**

4.55 5.26 FUD 010 Q2 G2 80

AMA: 2018,Jan,8; 2017,Jan,8; 2016,Jan,13; 2015,Jan,16; 2014,Jan,11

32553 Intrathoracic Placement Radiation Therapy Devices

EXCLUDES *Percutaneous placement of interstitial device(s) for radiation therapy guidance: intra-abdominal, intrapelvic, and/or retroperitoneal (49411)*

Code also device

32553 **Placement of interstitial device(s) for radiation therapy guidance (eg, fiducial markers, dosimeter), percutaneous, intra-thoracic, single or multiple**

(76942, 77002, 77012, 77021)

5.18 14.8 FUD 000 S G2 80

AMA: 2018,Jan,8; 2017,Jan,8; 2016,Jun,3; 2016,Jan,13; 2015,Jun,6; 2015,Jan,16; 2014,Jan,11

32554-32557 Pleural Aspiration and Drainage

EXCLUDES *Chest x-ray performed to confirm position of chest tube, complications, adequacy of procedure*

Open tube thoracostomy (32551)

Placement of indwelling tunneled pleural drainage catheter (cuffed) (32550)

Radiologic guidance (75989, 76942, 77002, 77012, 77021)

32554 **Thoracentesis, needle or catheter, aspiration of the pleural space; without imaging guidance**

2.58 6.01 FUD 000 T G2 50

AMA: 2018,Jan,8; 2017,Jan,8; 2016,Jan,13; 2015,Jan,16; 2014,Jan,11

32555 **with imaging guidance**

3.22 8.51 FUD 000 T G2 50

AMA: 2018,Jan,8; 2017,Jan,8; 2016,Jan,13; 2015,Jan,16; 2014,Jan,11

32556 **Pleural drainage, percutaneous, with insertion of indwelling catheter; without imaging guidance**

3.55 17.4 FUD 000 J G2 50

AMA: 2018,Jan,8; 2017,Jan,8; 2016,Jan,13; 2015,Jan,16; 2014,Jan,11

32557 **with imaging guidance**

4.39 16.0 FUD 000 T G2 50

AMA: 2018,Jan,8; 2017,Jan,8; 2016,Jan,13; 2015,Jan,16; 2014,May,3; 2014,Jan,11

32560-32562 Instillation Drug/Chemical by Chest Tube

EXCLUDES *Insertion of chest tube (32551)*

32560 **Instillation, via chest tube/catheter, agent for pleurodesis (eg, talc for recurrent or persistent pneumothorax)**

2.25 7.17 FUD 000 T

AMA: 2018,Jan,8; 2017,Jan,8; 2016,Jan,13; 2015,Jan,16; 2014,Jan,11

32561 **Instillation(s), via chest tube/catheter, agent for fibrinolysis (eg, fibrinolytic agent for break up of multiloculated effusion); initial day**

EXCLUDES *Use of code more than one time on the date of initial treatment*

1.97 2.66 FUD 000 T 80

AMA: 2018,Jan,8; 2017,Jan,8; 2016,Jan,13; 2015,Jan,16; 2014,Jan,11

32562 **subsequent day**

EXCLUDES *Use of code more than one time on each day of subsequent treatment*

1.76 2.38 FUD 000 T 80

AMA: 2018,Jan,8; 2017,Jan,8; 2016,Jan,13; 2015,Jan,16; 2014,Jan,11

32601-32674 Thoracic Surgery: Video-Assisted (VATS)

INCLUDES Diagnostic thoracoscopy in surgical thoracoscopy

32601 **Thoracoscopy, diagnostic (separate procedure); lungs, pericardial sac, mediastinal or pleural space, without biopsy**

8.90 8.90 FUD 000 J 80

AMA: 2018,Jan,8; 2017,Jan,8; 2016,Jan,13; 2015,Jan,16; 2014,Jan,11

32604 **pericardial sac, with biopsy**

EXCLUDES *Open biopsy of pericardium (39010)*

13.9 13.9 FUD 000 J 80

AMA: 2018,Jan,8; 2017,Jan,8; 2016,Jan,13; 2015,Jan,16; 2014,Jan,11

32606 **mediastinal space, with biopsy**

13.3 13.3 FUD 000 J 80

AMA: 2018,Jan,8; 2017,Jan,8; 2016,Jan,13; 2015,Jan,16; 2014,Jan,11

32607 **Thoracoscopy; with diagnostic biopsy(ies) of lung infiltrate(s) (eg, wedge, incisional), unilateral**

EXCLUDES *Removal of lung (32440-32445, 32488)*
Thoracoscopy, surgical; with removal of lung (32671)
Use of code more than one time per lung

8.89 8.89 FUD 000 J 80

AMA: 2018,Jan,8; 2017,Jan,8; 2016,Jan,13; 2015,Jan,16; 2014,Jan,11

32608 **with diagnostic biopsy(ies) of lung nodule(s) or mass(es) (eg, wedge, incisional), unilateral**

EXCLUDES *Removal of lung (32440-32445, 32488)*
Thoracoscopy, surgical; with removal of lung (32671)
Use of code more than one time per lung

10.9 10.9 FUD 000 J 80

AMA: 2018,Jan,8; 2017,Jan,8; 2016,Jan,13; 2015,Jan,16; 2014,Jan,11

32609 **with biopsy(ies) of pleura**

7.45 7.45 FUD 000 J 80

AMA: 2018,Jan,8; 2017,Jan,8; 2016,Jan,13; 2015,Jan,16; 2014,Jan,11

32650 **Thoracoscopy, surgical; with pleurodesis (eg, mechanical or chemical)**

19.1 19.1 FUD 090 C 80 50

AMA: 2018,Jan,8; 2017,Jan,8; 2016,Jan,13; 2015,Jan,16; 2014,Jan,11

32651 **with partial pulmonary decortication**

31.6 31.6 FUD 090 C 80 50

AMA: 2018,Jan,8; 2017,Jan,8; 2016,Jan,13; 2015,Jan,16; 2014,Jan,11

32652 **with total pulmonary decortication, including intrapleural pneumonolysis**

47.9 47.9 FUD 090 C 80 50

AMA: 2018,Jan,8; 2017,Jan,8; 2016,Jan,13; 2015,Jan,16; 2014,Jan,11

32653 **with removal of intrapleural foreign body or fibrin deposit**

30.6 30.6 FUD 090 C 80

AMA: 2018,Jan,8; 2017,Jan,8; 2016,Jan,13; 2015,Jan,16; 2014,Jan,11

32654 **with control of traumatic hemorrhage**

33.2 33.2 FUD 090 C 80 50

AMA: 2018,Jan,8; 2017,Jan,8; 2016,Jan,13; 2015,Jan,16; 2014,Jan,11

32655 **with resection-plication of bullae, includes any pleural procedure when performed**

EXCLUDES *Thoracoscopic lung volume reduction surgery (32672)*

27.5 27.5 FUD 090 C 80 50

AMA: 2018,Jan,8; 2017,Jan,8; 2016,Jan,13; 2015,Jan,16; 2014,Jan,11

32656 **with parietal pleurectomy**

23.0 23.0 FUD 090 C 80 50

AMA: 2018,Jan,8; 2017,Jan,8; 2016,Jan,13; 2015,Jan,16; 2014,Jan,11

32658 **with removal of clot or foreign body from pericardial sac**

20.6 20.6 FUD 090 C 80

AMA: 2018,Jan,8; 2017,Jan,8; 2016,Jan,13; 2015,Jan,16; 2014,Jan,11

32659 **with creation of pericardial window or partial resection of pericardial sac for drainage**

21.1 21.1 FUD 090 C 80

AMA: 2018,Jan,8; 2017,Jan,8; 2016,Jan,13; 2015,Jan,16; 2014,Jan,11

32661 **with excision of pericardial cyst, tumor, or mass**

23.0 23.0 FUD 090 C 80

AMA: 2018,Jan,8; 2017,Jan,8; 2016,Jan,13; 2015,Jan,16; 2014,Jan,11

32662 **with excision of mediastinal cyst, tumor, or mass**

25.7 25.7 FUD 090 C 80

AMA: 2018,Jan,8; 2017,Jan,8; 2016,Jan,13; 2015,Jan,16; 2014,Jan,11

32663 **with lobectomy (single lobe)**

EXCLUDES *Thoracoscopic segmentectomy (32669)*

40.4 40.4 FUD 090 C 80

AMA: 2018,Jan,8; 2017,Jan,8; 2016,Jan,13; 2015,Jan,16; 2014,Jan,11

32664 **with thoracic sympathectomy**

24.5 24.5 FUD 090 C 80 50

AMA: 2018,Jan,8; 2017,Jan,8; 2016,Jan,13; 2015,Dec,16; 2015,Jan,16; 2014,Jan,11

32665 **with esophagomyotomy (Heller type)**

EXCLUDES *Exploratory thoracoscopy with and without biopsy (32601-32609)*

35.6 35.6 FUD 090 C 80

AMA: 2018,Jan,8; 2017,Jan,8; 2016,Jan,13; 2015,Jan,16; 2014,Jan,11

32666 **with therapeutic wedge resection (eg, mass, nodule), initial unilateral**

EXCLUDES *Removal of lung (32440-32445, 32488)*
Thoracoscopy, surgical; with removal of lung (32671)

Code also a more extensive procedure of the lung when performed on the contralateral lung or different lobe with modifier 59 regardless of pathology consultation

25.1 25.1 FUD 090 C 80 50

AMA: 2018,Jan,8; 2017,Jan,8; 2016,Jan,13; 2015,Jan,16; 2014,Jan,11

\+ 32667 **with therapeutic wedge resection (eg, mass or nodule), each additional resection, ipsilateral (List separately in addition to code for primary procedure)**

EXCLUDES *Removal of lung (32440-32445, 32488)*
Thoracoscopy, surgical; with removal of lung (32671)

Code also a more extensive procedure of the lung when performed on the contralateral lung or different lobe with modifier 59 regardless of intraoperative pathology consultation

Code first (32666)

4.54 4.54 FUD ZZZ C 80

AMA: 2018,Jan,8; 2017,Jan,8; 2016,Jan,13; 2015,Jan,16; 2014,Jan,11

\+ 32668 **with diagnostic wedge resection followed by anatomic lung resection (List separately in addition to code for primary procedure)**

INCLUDES Classification as a diagnostic wedge resection if intraoperative pathology consultation dictates more extensive resection in the same anatomical area

Code first (32440-32488, 32503-32504, 32663, 32669-32671)

4.54 4.54 FUD ZZZ C 80

AMA: 2018,Jan,8; 2017,Jan,8; 2016,Jan,13; 2015,Jan,16; 2014,Jan,11

32669 **with removal of a single lung segment (segmentectomy)**

38.7 38.7 FUD 090 C 80

AMA: 2018,Jan,8; 2017,Jan,8; 2016,Jan,13; 2015,Jan,16; 2014,Jan,11

32670 **with removal of two lobes (bilobectomy)**

46.2 46.2 FUD 090 C 80

AMA: 2018,Jan,8; 2017,Jan,8; 2016,Jan,13; 2015,Jan,16; 2014,Jan,11

32671 **with removal of lung (pneumonectomy)**

51.5 51.5 FUD 090 C 80

AMA: 2018,Jan,8; 2017,Jan,8; 2016,Jan,13; 2015,Jan,16; 2014,Jan,11

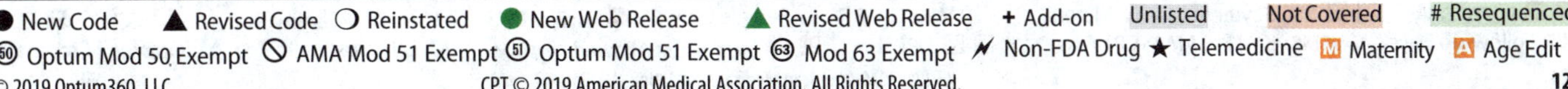

32672 **with resection-plication for emphysematous lung (bullous or non-bullous) for lung volume reduction (LVRS), unilateral includes any pleural procedure, when performed**

44.0 44.0 FUD 090 C 80

AMA: 2018,Jan,8; 2017,Jan,8; 2016,Jan,13; 2015,Jan,16; 2014,Jan,11

32673 **with resection of thymus, unilateral or bilateral**

EXCLUDES *Exploratory thoracoscopy with and without biopsy (32601-32609)*
Open excision mediastinal cyst (39200)
Open excision mediastinal tumor (39220)
Open thymectomy (60520-60522)

35.0 35.0 FUD 090 C 80

AMA: 2018,Jan,8; 2017,Jan,8; 2016,Jan,13; 2015,Jan,16; 2014,Jan,11

\+ **32674** **with mediastinal and regional lymphadenectomy (List separately in addition to code for primary procedure)**

INCLUDES Mediastinal lymph nodes:
- Left side:
  - Aortopulmonary window
  - Inferior pulmonary ligament
  - Paraesophageal
  - Subcarinal
- Right side:
  - Inferior pulmonary ligament
  - Paraesophageal
  - Paratracheal
  - Subcarinal

EXCLUDES *Mediastinal and regional lymphadenectomy by thoracotomy (38746)*

Code first (21601, 31760, 31766, 31786, 32096-32200, 32220-32320, 32440-32491, 32503-32505, 32601-32663, 32666, 32669-32673, 32815, 33025, 33030, 33050-33130, 39200-39220, 39560-39561, 43101, 43112, 43117-43118, 43122-43123, 43287-43288, 43351, 60270, 60505)

6.24 6.24 FUD ZZZ C 80

AMA: 2018,Jan,8; 2017,Jan,8; 2016,Jan,13; 2015,Jan,16; 2014,May,3; 2014,Jan,11

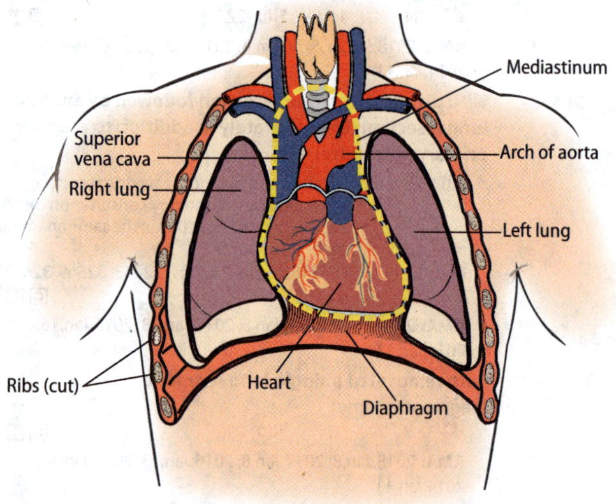

32701 Target Delineation for Stereotactic Radiation Therapy

INCLUDES Collaboration between the radiation oncologist and surgeon
Correlation of tumor and contiguous body structures
Determination of borders and volume of tumor
Identification of fiducial markers
Verification of target when fiducial markers are not used

EXCLUDES *Fiducial marker insertion (31626, 32553)*
Procedure performed by same physician as radiation treatment management (77427-77499)
Radiation oncology services (77295, 77331, 77370, 77373, 77435)
Therapeutic radiology (77261-77799 [77295, 77385, 77386, 77387, 77424, 77425])

32701 **Thoracic target(s) delineation for stereotactic body radiation therapy (SRS/SBRT), (photon or particle beam), entire course of treatment**

6.21 6.21 FUD XXX B 80 26

AMA: 2018,Jan,8; 2017,Jan,8; 2016,Jan,13; 2015,Jun,6

32800-32820 Chest Repair and Reconstruction Procedures

32800 **Repair lung hernia through chest wall**

27.0 27.0 FUD 090 C 80

32810 **Closure of chest wall following open flap drainage for empyema (Clagett type procedure)**

26.0 26.0 FUD 090 C 80

32815 **Open closure of major bronchial fistula**

81.0 81.0 FUD 090 C 80

32820 **Major reconstruction, chest wall (posttraumatic)**

38.4 38.4 FUD 090 C 80

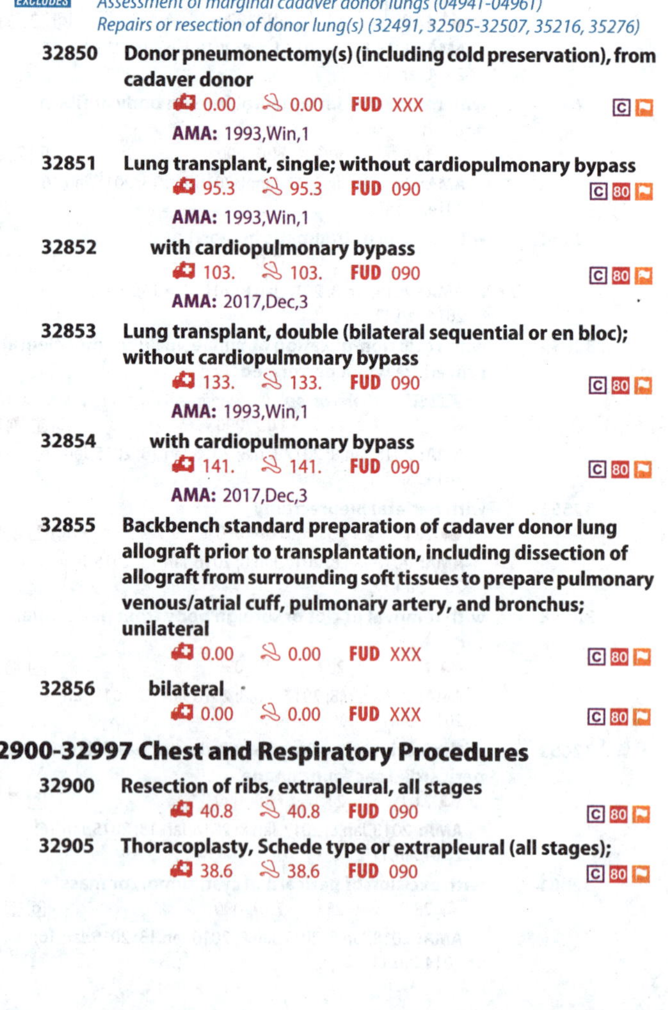

32850-32856 Lung Transplant Procedures

INCLUDES Harvesting donor lung(s), cold preservation, preparation of donor lung(s), transplantation into recipient

EXCLUDES *Assessment of marginal cadaver donor lungs (0494T-0496T)*
Repairs or resection of donor lung(s) (32491, 32505-32507, 35216, 35276)

32850 **Donor pneumonectomy(s) (including cold preservation), from cadaver donor**

0.00 0.00 FUD XXX C

AMA: 1993,Win,1

32851 **Lung transplant, single; without cardiopulmonary bypass**

95.3 95.3 FUD 090 C 80

AMA: 1993,Win,1

32852 **with cardiopulmonary bypass**

103. 103. FUD 090 C 80

AMA: 2017,Dec,3

32853 **Lung transplant, double (bilateral sequential or en bloc); without cardiopulmonary bypass**

133. 133. FUD 090 C 80

AMA: 1993,Win,1

32854 **with cardiopulmonary bypass**

141. 141. FUD 090 C 80

AMA: 2017,Dec,3

32855 **Backbench standard preparation of cadaver donor lung allograft prior to transplantation, including dissection of allograft from surrounding soft tissues to prepare pulmonary venous/atrial cuff, pulmonary artery, and bronchus; unilateral**

0.00 0.00 FUD XXX C 80

32856 **bilateral**

0.00 0.00 FUD XXX C 80

32900-32997 Chest and Respiratory Procedures

32900 **Resection of ribs, extrapleural, all stages**

40.8 40.8 FUD 090 C 80

32905 **Thoracoplasty, Schede type or extrapleural (all stages);**

38.6 38.6 FUD 090 C 80

32906 with closure of bronchopleural fistula
47.7 47.7 FUD 090 C 80

EXCLUDES *Open closure of bronchial fistula (32815)*
Resection first rib for thoracic compression (21615-21616)

32940 Pneumonolysis, extraperiosteal, including filling or packing procedures
35.7 35.7 FUD 090 C 80

32960 Pneumothorax, therapeutic, intrapleural injection of air
2.63 3.61 FUD 000 T G2

32994 **Resequenced code. See code following 32998.**

32997 Total lung lavage (unilateral)
EXCLUDES *Broncho-alveolar lavage by bronchoscopy (31624)*
9.84 9.84 FUD 000 C 50
AMA: 2018,Jan,8; 2017,Jan,8; 2016,Jan,13; 2015,Jan,16; 2014,Jan,11

32998-32999 [32994] Destruction of Lung Neoplasm

32998 Ablation therapy for reduction or eradication of 1 or more pulmonary tumor(s) including pleura or chest wall when involved by tumor extension, percutaneous, including imaging guidance when performed, unilateral; radiofrequency
12.8 100. FUD 000 J G2 80 50
AMA: 2018,Jan,8; 2017,Nov,8

32994 cryoablation
13.2 159. FUD 000 J G2 80 50
AMA: 2018,Jan,8; 2017,Nov,8

32999 Unlisted procedure, lungs and pleura
0.00 0.00 FUD YYY T
AMA: 2018,Jan,8; 2017,Jan,8; 2016,Jan,13; 2015,Dec,16; 2015,Jun,6; 2015,Jan,16; 2014,Jan,11

Respiratory System

32906 — 32999

33010-33050 Procedures of the Pericardial Sac

EXCLUDES *Surgical thoracoscopy (video-assisted thoracic surgery [VATS]) procedures of pericardium (32601, 32604, 32658-32659, 32661)*

~~33010~~ ~~Pericardiocentesis; initial~~

To report, see (33016-33019)

~~33011~~ ~~subsequent~~

To report, see (33016-33019)

~~33015~~ ~~Tube pericardiostomy~~

To report, see (33017-33019)

● **33016 Pericardiocentesis, including imaging guidance, when performed**

INCLUDES Imaging guidance for needle placement:
- Computed tomography (77012)
- Fluoroscopy (77002)
- Magnetic resonance (77021)
- Ultrasound (76942)

EXCLUDES *Echocardiography for pericardiocentesis guidance (93303-93325)*

● **33017 Pericardial drainage with insertion of indwelling catheter, percutaneous, including fluoroscopy and/or ultrasound guidance, when performed; 6 years and older without congenital cardiac anomaly**

INCLUDES Catheters that remain in the patient at the conclusion of the procedure

Imaging guidance for needle placement:
- Fluoroscopy (77002)
- Magnetic resonance (77021)
- Ultrasound (76942)

EXCLUDES *Echocardiography for pericardiocentesis guidance (93303-93325)*

Pericardial drainage for patients:
- *Any age with congenital cardiac anomaly (33018)*
- *Younger than 6 years of age (33018)*

Radiologically guided catheter placement for percutaneous drainage (75989)

● **33018 birth through 5 years of age or any age with congenital cardiac anomaly**

INCLUDES Catheters that remain in the patient at the conclusion of the procedure

Imaging guidance for needle placement:
- Fluoroscopy (77002)
- Magnetic resonance (77021)
- Ultrasound (76942)

Patient of age birth to 5 years without congenital cardiac anomaly

Patient of any age with congenital cardiac anomaly, such as heterotaxy, dextrocardia, mesocardia, or single ventricle anomaly, or 90 days following repair of congenital cardiac anomaly

EXCLUDES *CT guided pericardial drainage (33019)*

Echocardiography for pericardiocentesis guidance (93303-93325)

Radiologically guided catheter placement for percutaneous drainage (75989)

● **33019 Pericardial drainage with insertion of indwelling catheter, percutaneous, including CT guidance**

INCLUDES Catheters that remain in the patient at the conclusion of the procedure

Imaging guidance for needle placement:
- Computed tomography (77012)
- Fluoroscopy (77002)
- Magnetic resonance (77021)
- Ultrasound (76942)

EXCLUDES *Radiologically guided catheter placement for percutaneous drainage (75989)*

33020 Pericardiotomy for removal of clot or foreign body (primary procedure)

EXCLUDES *Tube thoracostomy if chest tube or pleural drain placed on same side (32551)*

25.3 25.3 FUD 090 C 80

AMA: 1997,Nov,1

33025 Creation of pericardial window or partial resection for drainage

INCLUDES Tube thoracostomy if chest tube or pleural drain placed on same side (32551)

EXCLUDES *Surgical thoracoscopy (video-assisted thoracic surgery [VATS]) creation of pericardial window (32659)*

23.0 23.0 FUD 090 C 80

AMA: 1997,Nov,1

33030 Pericardiectomy, subtotal or complete; without cardiopulmonary bypass

INCLUDES Delorme pericardiectomy

57.8 57.8 FUD 090 C 80

AMA: 1997,Nov,1; 1994,Win,1

33031 with cardiopulmonary bypass

71.5 71.5 FUD 090 C 80

AMA: 2017,Dec,3

33050 Resection of pericardial cyst or tumor

EXCLUDES *Open biopsy of pericardium (39010)*

Surgical thoracoscopy (video-assisted thoracic surgery [VATS]) resection of cyst, mass, or tumor of pericardium (32661)

29.1 29.1 FUD 090 C 80

AMA: 1997,Nov,1

33120-33130 Neoplasms of Heart

Code also removal of thrombus through a separate heart incision, when performed (33310-33315); append modifier 59 to (33315)

33120 Excision of intracardiac tumor, resection with cardiopulmonary bypass

60.6 60.6 FUD 090 C 80

AMA: 2018,Jan,8; 2017,Dec,3; 2017,Jan,8; 2016,Jan,13; 2015,Jan,16; 2014,Jan,11

33130 Resection of external cardiac tumor

39.8 39.8 FUD 090 C 80

AMA: 2018,Jan,8; 2017,Jan,8; 2016,Jan,13; 2015,Jan,16; 2014,Jan,11

33140-33141 Transmyocardial Revascularization

33140 Transmyocardial laser revascularization, by thoracotomy; (separate procedure)

45.5 45.5 FUD 090 C 80

AMA: 2018,Jan,8; 2017,Jan,8; 2016,Jan,13; 2015,Jan,16; 2014,Jan,11

\+ **33141 performed at the time of other open cardiac procedure(s) (List separately in addition to code for primary procedure)**

Code first (33390-33391, 33404-33496, 33510-33536, 33542)

3.80 3.80 FUD ZZZ C 80

AMA: 2018,Jan,8; 2017,Jan,8; 2016,Jan,13; 2015,Jan,16; 2014,Jan,11

33202-33203 Placement Epicardial Leads

INCLUDES Imaging guidance:
Fluoroscopy (76000)
Ultrasound (76942, 76998, 93318)
Temporary pacemaker (33210-33211)

Code also insertion of pulse generator when performed by same physician/same surgical session (33212-33213, [33221], 33230-33231, 33240)

33202 Insertion of epicardial electrode(s); open incision (eg, thoracotomy, median sternotomy, subxiphoid approach)

22.3 22.3 FUD 090 C

AMA: 2019,Mar,6; 2018,Jan,8; 2017,Jan,8; 2016,Aug,5; 2016,May,5; 2016,Jan,13; 2015,May,3; 2015,Jan,16; 2014,Nov,5; 2014,Jan,11

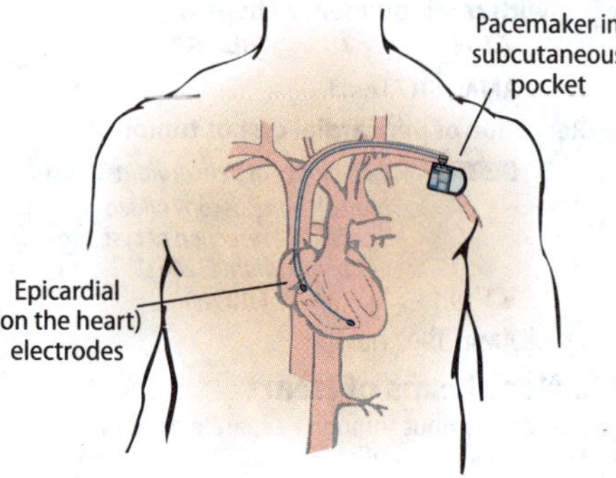

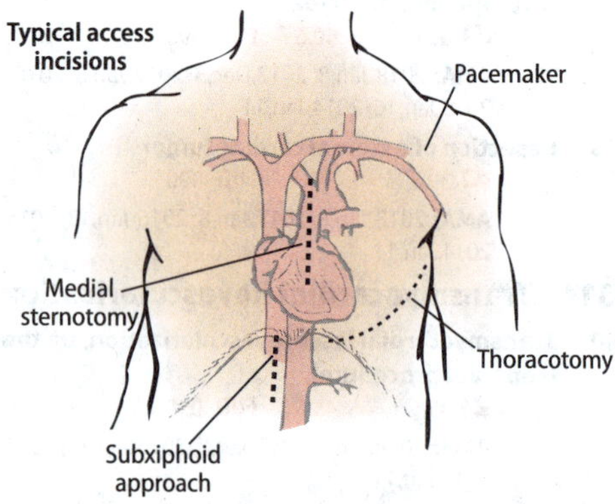

33203 endoscopic approach (eg, thoracoscopy, pericardioscopy)

23.4 23.4 FUD 090 C

AMA: 2019,Mar,6; 2018,Jan,8; 2017,Jan,8; 2016,Aug,5; 2016,May,5; 2016,Jan,13; 2015,May,3; 2015,Jan,16; 2014,Nov,5; 2014,Jan,11

33206-33214 [33221] Pacemakers

INCLUDES Device evaluation (93279-93298 [93260, 93261])
Dual lead: device that paces and senses in two heart chambers
Imaging guidance:
Fluoroscopy (76000)
Ultrasound (76942, 76998, 93318)
Multiple lead: device that paces and senses in three or more heart chambers
Radiological supervision and interpretation for pacemaker procedure
Single lead: device that paces and senses in one heart chamber
Skin pocket revision, when performed
If revision includes incision/drainage of a wound infection or hematoma code also (10140, 10180, 11042-11047 [11045, 11046])
Temporary pacemaker (33210-33211)

EXCLUDES *Electrode repositioning:*
Left ventricle (33226)
Pacemaker (33215)
Insertion of lead for left ventricular (biventricular) pacing (33224-33225)
Leadless pacemaker systems ([33274, 33275])

33206 Insertion of new or replacement of permanent pacemaker with transvenous electrode(s); atrial

INCLUDES Pulse generator insertion/single transvenous electrode placement

EXCLUDES *Insertion of transvenous electrode only (33216-33217)*
Removal with immediate replacement of pacemaker pulse generator only, single lead system ([33227])

Code also removal of old pacemaker pulse generator and electrode, when replacement of entire system is performed:
Electrode (33234)
Pulse generator (33233)

13.1 13.1 FUD 090 J J8

AMA: 2019,Mar,6; 2018,Jan,8; 2017,Jan,8; 2016,Aug,5; 2016,May,5; 2016,Jan,13; 2015,May,3; 2015,Jan,16; 2014,Nov,5; 2014,Jan,11

33207 ventricular

INCLUDES Pulse generator insertion/single transvenous electrode placement

EXCLUDES *Insertion of transvenous electrode only (33216-33217)*
Removal with immediate replacement of pacemaker pulse generator only, single lead system ([33227])

Code also removal of old pacemaker pulse generator and electrode, when replacement of entire system is performed:
Electrode (33234)
Pulse generator (33233)

13.9 13.9 FUD 090 J J8

AMA: 2019,Mar,6; 2018,Jan,8; 2017,Jan,8; 2016,Aug,5; 2016,May,5; 2016,Jan,13; 2015,May,3; 2015,Jan,16; 2014,Nov,5; 2014,Jan,11

33208 atrial and ventricular

INCLUDES Pulse generator insertion/dual transvenous electrode placement

EXCLUDES *Insertion of transvenous electrode(s) only (33216-33217)*
Removal with immediate replacement of pacemaker pulse generator only, dual or multiple lead system ([33228, 33229])

Code also removal of old pacemaker pulse generator and electrodes, when replacement of entire system is performed:
Electrodes (33235)
Pulse generator (33233)

15.1 15.1 FUD 090 J J8

AMA: 2019,Mar,6; 2018,Jan,8; 2017,Jan,8; 2016,Aug,5; 2016,May,5; 2016,Jan,13; 2015,May,3; 2015,Jan,16; 2014,Nov,5; 2014,Jan,11

33210 Insertion or replacement of temporary transvenous single chamber cardiac electrode or pacemaker catheter (separate procedure)

4.76 4.76 FUD 000 J G2

AMA: 2019,Mar,6; 2018,Jan,8; 2017,Jan,8; 2016,Aug,5; 2016,May,5; 2016,Jan,13; 2015,May,3; 2015,Jan,16; 2014,Nov,5; 2014,Jan,11

33211 Insertion or replacement of temporary transvenous dual chamber pacing electrodes (separate procedure)

4.95 4.95 FUD 000 J J8

AMA: 2019,Mar,6; 2018,Jan,8; 2017,Jan,8; 2016,Aug,5; 2016,May,5; 2016,Jan,13; 2015,May,3; 2015,Jan,16; 2014,Nov,5; 2014,Jan,11

33212 Insertion of pacemaker pulse generator only; with existing single lead

EXCLUDES *Insertion for replacement of single lead pacemaker pulse generator ([33227])*
Insertion of transvenous electrode(s) (33216-33217)
Removal of permanent pacemaker pulse generator only (33233)

Code also placement of epicardial leads by same physician/same surgical session (33202-33203)

9.31 9.31 FUD 090 J J8

AMA: 2019,Mar,6; 2018,Jan,8; 2017,Jan,8; 2016,Aug,5; 2016,May,5; 2016,Jan,13; 2015,May,3; 2015,Jan,16; 2014,Nov,5; 2014,Jan,11

33213 with existing dual leads

EXCLUDES *Insertion for replacement of dual lead pacemaker pulse generator ([33228])*
Insertion of transvenous electrode(s) (33216-33217)
Removal of permanent pacemaker pulse generator only (33233)

Code also placement of epicardial leads by same physician/same surgical session (33202-33203)

9.74 9.74 FUD 090 J J8

AMA: 2019,Mar,6; 2018,Jan,8; 2017,Jan,8; 2016,Aug,5; 2016,May,5; 2016,Jan,13; 2015,May,3; 2015,Jan,16; 2014,Nov,5; 2014,Jan,11

33221 with existing multiple leads

EXCLUDES *Insertion for replacement of multiple lead pacemaker pulse generator ([33229])*
Insertion of transvenous electrode(s) (33216-33217)
Removal of permanent pacemaker pulse generator only (33233)

Code also placement of epicardial leads by same physician/same surgical session (33202-33203)

10.4 10.4 FUD 090 J J8

AMA: 2019,Mar,6; 2018,Jan,8; 2017,Jan,8; 2016,Aug,5; 2016,May,5; 2016,Jan,13; 2015,May,3; 2015,Jan,16; 2014,Nov,5; 2014,Jan,11

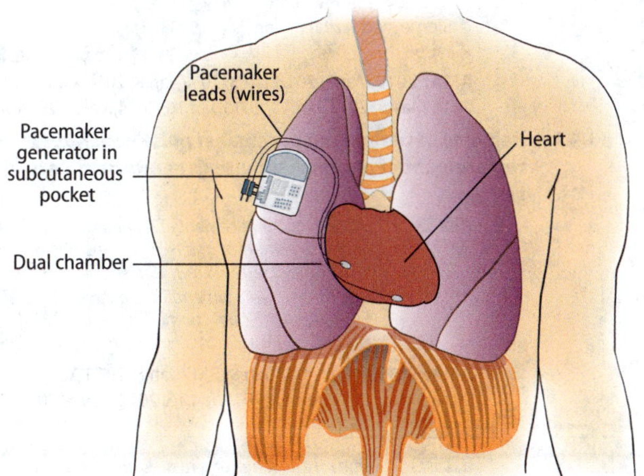

33214 Upgrade of implanted pacemaker system, conversion of single chamber system to dual chamber system (includes removal of previously placed pulse generator, testing of existing lead, insertion of new lead, insertion of new pulse generator)

EXCLUDES *Insertion of transvenous electrode(s) (33216-33217)*
Removal and replacement of pacemaker pulse generator (33227-33229)

13.9 13.9 FUD 090 J J8 80

AMA: 2019,Mar,6; 2018,Jan,8; 2017,Jan,8; 2016,Aug,5; 2016,May,5; 2016,Jan,13; 2015,May,3; 2015,Jan,16; 2014,Nov,5; 2014,Jan,11

33215-33249 [33227, 33228, 33229, 33230, 33231, 33262, 33263, 33264] Pacemakers/Implantable Defibrillator/ Electrode Insertion/Replacement/Revision/Repair

INCLUDES Device evaluation (93279-93298 [93260, 93261])
Dual lead: device that paces and senses in two heart chambers
Imaging guidance:
Fluoroscopy (76000)
Ultrasound (76942, 76998, 93318)
Multiple lead: device that paces and senses in three or more heart chambers
Radiological supervision and interpretation for pacemaker or pacing cardioverter-defibrillator procedure
Single lead: device that paces and senses in one heart chamber
Skin pocket revision, when performed
If revision includes incision/drainage of a wound infection or hematoma code also (10140, 10180, 11042-11047 [11045, 11046])
Temporary pacemaker (33210-33211)

EXCLUDES *Electrode repositioning:*
Left ventricle (33226)
Pacemaker or implantable defibrillator (33215)
Insertion of lead for left ventricular (biventricular) pacing (33224-33225)
Removal of leadless pacemaker system ([33275])
Removal of subcutaneous implantable defibrillator electrode ([33272])
Testing of defibrillator threshold (DFT) during follow-up evaluation (93642-93644)
Testing of defibrillator threshold (DFT) during insertion/replacement (93640-93641)

33215 Repositioning of previously implanted transvenous pacemaker or implantable defibrillator (right atrial or right ventricular) electrode

9.02 9.02 FUD 090 T G2

AMA: 2019,Mar,6; 2018,Jan,8; 2017,Jan,8; 2016,Aug,5; 2016,May,5; 2016,Jan,13; 2015,May,3; 2015,Jan,16; 2014,Nov,5; 2014,Jan,11

33216 Insertion of a single transvenous electrode, permanent pacemaker or implantable defibrillator

EXCLUDES *Insertion or replacement of a lead for a cardiac venous system (33224-33225)*
Insertion or replacement of permanent implantable defibrillator generator or system (33249)
Removal and replacement of permanent pacemaker or implantable defibrillator (33206-33208, 33212-33213, [33221], 33227-33229, 33230-33231, 33240, [33262, 33263, 33264])

10.7 10.7 FUD 090 J J8

AMA: 2019,Mar,6; 2018,Jan,8; 2017,Jan,8; 2016,Aug,5; 2016,May,5; 2016,Jan,13; 2015,May,3; 2015,Jan,16; 2014,Nov,5; 2014,Jan,11

33217 Insertion of 2 transvenous electrodes, permanent pacemaker or implantable defibrillator

EXCLUDES *Insertion or replacement of a lead for a cardiac venous system (33224-33225)*
Insertion or replacement of permanent implantable defibrillator generator or system (33249)
Removal and replacement of permanent pacemaker or implantable defibrillator (33206-33208, 33212-33213, [33221], 33227-33229, 33230-33231, 33240, [33262, 33263, 33264])

10.6 10.6 FUD 090 J J8

AMA: 2019,Mar,6; 2018,Jan,8; 2017,Jan,8; 2016,Aug,5; 2016,May,5; 2016,Jan,13; 2015,May,3; 2015,Jan,16; 2014,Nov,5; 2014,Jan,11

33218 Repair of single transvenous electrode, permanent pacemaker or implantable defibrillator

Code also removal of old generator with insertion of new generator replacement, when performed:
Implantable defibrillator ([33262, 33263, 33264])
Pacemaker ([33227, 33228, 33229])

11.2 11.2 FUD 090 T G2

AMA: 2019,Mar,6; 2018,Jan,8; 2017,Jan,8; 2016,Aug,5; 2016,May,5; 2016,Jan,13; 2015,May,3; 2015,Jan,16; 2014,Nov,5; 2014,Jan,11

33220 Repair of 2 transvenous electrodes for permanent pacemaker or implantable defibrillator

Code also modifier 52 Reduced services, when one electrode of a two-chamber system is repaired
Code also removal of old generator with insertion of new generator replacement, when performed:
Implantable defibrillator ([33263, 33264])
Pacemaker ([33228, 33229])

11.3 11.3 FUD 090 T G2

AMA: 2019,Mar,6; 2018,Jan,8; 2017,Jan,8; 2016,Aug,5; 2016,May,5; 2016,Jan,13; 2015,May,3; 2015,Jan,16; 2014,Nov,5; 2014,Jan,11

***33221* Resequenced code. See code following 33213.**

33222 Relocation of skin pocket for pacemaker

INCLUDES Formation of the new pocket
Procedures related to the existing pocket:
Accessing the pocket
Incision/drainage of any abscess or hematoma (10140, 10180)
Pocket closure (13100-13102)

EXCLUDES *Debridement, subcutaneous tissue (11042-11047 [11045, 11046])*

Code also removal and replacement of an existing generator

9.81 9.81 FUD 090 T A2

AMA: 2019,Mar,6; 2018,Jan,8; 2017,Jan,8; 2016,Aug,5; 2016,May,5; 2016,Jan,13; 2015,May,3; 2015,Jan,16; 2014,Nov,5; 2014,Jan,11

33223 Relocation of skin pocket for implantable defibrillator

INCLUDES Formation of the new pocket
Procedures related to the existing pocket:
Accessing the pocket
Incision/drainage of any abscess or hematoma (10140, 10180)
Pocket closure (13100-13102)

EXCLUDES *Debridement, subcutaneous tissue (11042-11047 [11045, 11046])*

Code also removal and replacement of an existing generator

11.8 11.8 FUD 090 T A2 80

AMA: 2019,Mar,6; 2018,Jan,8; 2017,Jan,8; 2016,Aug,5; 2016,Jan,13; 2015,Jan,16; 2014,Nov,5; 2014,Jan,11

33224 Insertion of pacing electrode, cardiac venous system, for left ventricular pacing, with attachment to previously placed pacemaker or implantable defibrillator pulse generator (including revision of pocket, removal, insertion, and/or replacement of existing generator)

Code also placement of epicardial electrode when appropriate (33202-33203)

15.0 15.0 FUD 000 J J8

AMA: 2019,Mar,6; 2018,Jan,8; 2017,Jan,8; 2016,Aug,5; 2016,May,5; 2016,Jan,13; 2015,May,3; 2015,Jan,16; 2014,Nov,5; 2014,Jan,11

\+ **33225 Insertion of pacing electrode, cardiac venous system, for left ventricular pacing, at time of insertion of implantable defibrillator or pacemaker pulse generator (eg, for upgrade to dual chamber system) (List separately in addition to code for primary procedure)**

Code first (33206-33208, 33212-33213, [33221], 33214, 33216-33217, 33223, 33228-33229, 33230-33231, 33233, 33234-33235, 33240, [33263, 33264], 33249)
Code first (33223) for relocation of pocket for implantable defibrillator
Code first (33222) for relocation of pocket for pacemaker pulse generator

13.6 13.6 FUD ZZZ N N1

AMA: 2019,Mar,6; 2018,Jan,8; 2017,Jan,8; 2016,Aug,5; 2016,May,5; 2016,Jan,13; 2015,May,3; 2015,Jan,16; 2014,Nov,5; 2014,Jan,11

33226 Repositioning of previously implanted cardiac venous system (left ventricular) electrode (including removal, insertion and/or replacement of existing generator)

14.4 14.4 FUD 000 T G2

AMA: 2019,Mar,6; 2018,Jan,8; 2017,Jan,8; 2016,Aug,5; 2016,May,5; 2016,Jan,13; 2015,May,3; 2015,Jan,16; 2014,Nov,5; 2014,Jan,11

***33227* Resequenced code. See code following 33233.**

***33228* Resequenced code. See code following 33233.**

***33229* Resequenced code. See code before 33234.**

***33230* Resequenced code. See code following 33240.**

***33231* Resequenced code. See code before 33241.**

33233 Removal of permanent pacemaker pulse generator only

EXCLUDES *Removal with immediate replacement of pacemaker pulse generator, without replacement of electrode(s):*
Dual lead system ([33228])
Multiple lead system ([33229])
Single lead system ([33227])

Code also insertion of replacement pacemaker pulse generator with transvenous electrode(s) (total system), when performed:
Pacemaker and dual leads (33208)
Pacemaker and single atrial lead (33206)
Pacemaker and single ventricular lead (33207)
Code also removal of electrode(s), when removal of total system without replacement is performed:
Dual leads (atrial and ventricular) (33235)
Single lead (atrial or ventricular) (33234)

6.68 6.68 FUD 090 Q2 G2

AMA: 2019,Mar,6; 2018,Jan,8; 2017,Jan,8; 2016,Aug,5; 2016,May,5; 2016,Jan,13; 2015,Jan,16; 2014,Nov,5; 2014,Jan,11

\# **33227 Removal of permanent pacemaker pulse generator with replacement of pacemaker pulse generator; single lead system**

EXCLUDES *Removal and replacement of entire system, pacemaker pulse generator and transvenous electrode, use (33206-33207, 33233, 33234)*
Removal and replacement for conversion from single chamber to dual chamber system (33214)

9.82 9.82 FUD 090 J J8

AMA: 2019,Mar,6; 2018,Jan,8; 2017,Jan,8; 2016,Aug,5; 2016,May,5; 2016,Jan,13; 2015,Jan,16; 2014,Nov,5; 2014,Jan,11

\# **33228 dual lead system**

EXCLUDES *Removal and replacement of entire system, pacemaker pulse generator and transvenous electrode(s), use (33208, 33233, 33235)*

10.2 10.2 FUD 090 J J8

AMA: 2019,Mar,6; 2018,Jan,8; 2017,Jan,8; 2016,Aug,5; 2016,May,5; 2016,Jan,13; 2015,Jan,16; 2014,Nov,5; 2014,Jan,11

33229 **multiple lead system**

EXCLUDES *Removal and replacement of entire system, pacemaker pulse generator and transvenous electrode(s), use (33208, 33233, 33235)*

10.8 10.8 FUD 090 J J8

AMA: 2019,Mar,6; 2018,Jan,8; 2017,Jan,8; 2016,Aug,5; 2016,May,5; 2016,Jan,13; 2015,Jan,16; 2014,Nov,5; 2014,Jan,11

33234 **Removal of transvenous pacemaker electrode(s); single lead system, atrial or ventricular**

EXCLUDES *Thoracotomy to remove electrode (33238)*

Code also pacing electrode insertion in cardiac venous system for pacing of left ventricle during insertion of pulse generator (pacemaker or implantable defibrillator) when performed (33225)

Code also removal of old pacemaker pulse generator and insertion of replacement pacemaker pulse generator with transvenous electrode (total system), when performed:

Insertion of pacemaker and atrial lead (33206) OR

Insertion of pacemaker and ventricular lead (33207) AND

Removal of generator (33233)

14.1 14.1 FUD 090 Q2 G2

AMA: 2019,Mar,6; 2018,Jan,8; 2017,Jan,8; 2016,Aug,5; 2016,May,5; 2016,Jan,13; 2015,Jan,16; 2014,Nov,5; 2014,Jan,11

33235 **dual lead system**

EXCLUDES *Thoracotomy to remove electrodes (33238)*

Code also pacing electrode insertion in cardiac venous system for pacing of left ventricle during insertion of pulse generator (pacemaker or implantable defibrillator) when performed (33225)

Code also removal of old pacemaker pulse generator and insertion of replacement pacemaker pulse generator with transvenous electrodes (total system), when performed:

Insertion of generator and dual leads (33208) AND

Removal of generator (33233)

18.5 18.5 FUD 090 Q2 G2

AMA: 2019,Mar,6; 2018,Jan,8; 2017,Jan,8; 2016,Aug,5; 2016,May,5; 2016,Jan,13; 2015,Jan,16; 2014,Nov,5; 2014,Jan,11

33236 **Removal of permanent epicardial pacemaker and electrodes by thoracotomy; single lead system, atrial or ventricular**

EXCLUDES *Removal of implantable defibrillator electrode(s) by thoracotomy (33243)*

Removal of transvenous electrodes by thoracotomy (33238)

Removal of transvenous pacemaker electrodes, single or dual lead system; without thoracotomy (33234, 33235)

22.6 22.6 FUD 090 C 80

AMA: 2019,Mar,6; 2018,Jan,8; 2017,Jan,8; 2016,Aug,5; 2016,May,5; 2016,Jan,13; 2015,Jan,16; 2014,Nov,5; 2014,Jan,11

33237 **dual lead system**

EXCLUDES *Removal of implantable defibrillator electrode(s) by thoracotomy (33243)*

Removal of transvenous electrodes by thoracotomy (33238)

Removal of transvenous pacemaker electrodes, single or dual lead system; without thoracotomy (33234, 33235)

24.3 24.3 FUD 090 C 80

AMA: 2019,Mar,6; 2018,Jan,8; 2017,Jan,8; 2016,Aug,5; 2016,May,5; 2016,Jan,13; 2015,Jan,16; 2014,Nov,5; 2014,Jan,11

33238 **Removal of permanent transvenous electrode(s) by thoracotomy**

EXCLUDES *Removal of implantable defibrillator electrode(s) by thoracotomy (33243)*

Removal of transvenous pacemaker electrodes, single or dual lead system; without thoracotomy (33234, 33235)

27.0 27.0 FUD 090 C 80

AMA: 2018,Jan,8; 2017,Jan,8; 2016,Aug,5; 2016,May,5; 2016,Jan,13; 2015,Jan,16; 2014,Nov,5; 2014,Jan,11

33240 **Insertion of implantable defibrillator pulse generator only; with existing single lead**

EXCLUDES *Insertion of electrode(s) (33216-33217, [33271])*

Removal and replacement of implantable defibrillator pulse generator only ([33262, 33263, 33264])

Code also placement of epicardial leads by same physician/same surgical session as generator insertion (33202-33203)

10.6 10.6 FUD 090 J J8

AMA: 2018,Jan,8; 2017,Jan,8; 2016,Aug,5; 2016,Jan,13; 2015,Jan,16; 2014,Nov,5; 2014,Jan,11

33230 **with existing dual leads**

EXCLUDES *Insertion of a single transvenous electrode, permanent pacemaker or implantable defibrillator (33216-33217)*

Removal and replacement of implantable defibrillator pulse generator only ([33262, 33263, 33264])

Code also placement of epicardial leads by same physician/same surgical session as generator insertion (33202-33203)

11.0 11.0 FUD 090 J J8

AMA: 2019,Mar,6; 2018,Jan,8; 2017,Jan,8; 2016,Aug,5; 2016,Jan,13; 2015,Jan,16; 2014,Nov,5; 2014,Jan,11

33231 **with existing multiple leads**

EXCLUDES *Insertion of a single transvenous electrode, permanent pacemaker or implantable defibrillator (33216-33217)*

Removal and replacement of implantable defibrillator pulse generator only ([33262, 33263, 33264])

Code also placement of epicardial leads by same physician/same surgical session as generator placement (33202-33203)

11.6 11.6 FUD 090 J J8

AMA: 2019,Mar,6; 2018,Jan,8; 2017,Jan,8; 2016,Aug,5; 2016,Jan,13; 2015,Jan,16; 2014,Nov,5; 2014,Jan,11

33241 **Removal of implantable defibrillator pulse generator only**

EXCLUDES *Removal with immediate replacement of implantable defibrillator pulse generator only ([33262, 33263, 33264])*

Removal of substernal implantable defibrillator pulse generator only (0580T)

Code also removal of electrode(s) and insertion of replacement defibrillator with electrode(s) (total system), when performed:

Removal of electrode(s) (33243-33244) AND

Insertion of defibrillator system, single or dual (33249) OR

Removal of subcutaneous electrode ([33272]) AND

Insertion of subcutaneous defibrillator system ([33270])

Code also removal of electrode(s), when total system is removed without replacement:

Subcutaneous electrode ([33272])

Transvenous electrode(s) (33243)

6.24 6.24 FUD 090 Q2 G2

AMA: 2018,Jan,8; 2017,Jan,8; 2016,Aug,5; 2016,Jan,13; 2015,Jan,16; 2014,Nov,5; 2014,Jan,11

33262 **Removal of implantable defibrillator pulse generator with replacement of implantable defibrillator pulse generator; single lead system**

EXCLUDES *Insertion of electrode(s) (33216-33217, [33271])*

Removal and replacement of implantable defibrillator pulse generator and electrode(s) (total system) (33241, 33243-33244, 33249)

Removal and replacement of subcutaneous defibrillator pulse generator and electrode(s) (total system) (33241, [33270], [33272])

Removal of implantable defibrillator pulse generator only (33241)

Repair of implantable defibrillator pulse generator and/or leads (33218, 33220)

Code also electrode(s) removal by thoracotomy (33243)

Code also subcutaneous electrode removal ([33272])

Code also transvenous removal of electrode(s) (33244)

10.8 10.8 FUD 090 J J8

AMA: 2018,Jan,8; 2017,Jan,8; 2016,Aug,5; 2016,Jan,13; 2015,Jan,16; 2014,Nov,5; 2014,Jan,11

\# **33263** **dual lead system**

EXCLUDES *Insertion of a single transvenous electrode, permanent pacemaker or implantable defibrillator (33216-33217)*
Removal and replacement of implantable defibrillator pulse generator and electrode(s) (total system) (33241, 33243-33244, 33249)
Removal and replacement of subcutaneous defibrillator pulse generator and electrode (total system) (33241, [33270], [33272])
Removal of implantable defibrillator pulse generator only (33241)
Repair of implantable defibrillator pulse generator and/or leads (33218, 33220)

Code also removal of electrodes by thoracotomy (33243)
Code also transvenous removal of electrodes (33244)

11.2 11.2 FUD 090 J J8

AMA: 2018,Jan,8; 2017,Jan,8; 2016,Aug,5; 2016,Jan,13; 2015,Jan,16; 2014,Nov,5; 2014,Jan,11

\# **33264** **multiple lead system**

EXCLUDES *Insertion of a single transvenous electrode, permanent pacemaker or implantable defibrillator (33216-33217)*
Removal and replacement of implantable defibrillator pulse generator and electrode(s) (total system) (33241, 33243-33244, 33249)
Removal and replacement of subcutaneous defibrillator pulse generator and electrode(s) (total system) (33241, [33270], [33272])
Removal of implantable defibrillator pulse generator only (33241)
Repair of implantable defibrillator pulse generator and/or leads (33218, 33220)

Code also removal of electrodes by thoracotomy (33243)
Code also transvenous removal of electrodes (33244)

11.7 11.7 FUD 090 J J8

AMA: 2018,Jan,8; 2017,Jan,8; 2016,Aug,5; 2016,Jan,13; 2015,Jan,16; 2014,Nov,5; 2014,Jan,11

33243 **Removal of single or dual chamber implantable defibrillator electrode(s); by thoracotomy**

EXCLUDES *Transvenous removal of defibrillator electrode(s) (33244)*

Code also removal of implantable defibrillator pulse generator and insertion of replacement defibrillator with electrodes (total system), when entire system is being replaced:
Insertion of defibrillator system, single or dual (33249)
Removal of generator (33241)
Code also removal of implantable defibrillator pulse generator, when entire system is removed without replacement (33241)
Code also replacement of implantable defibrillator pulse generator, when performed:
Dual lead system ([33263])
Multiple lead system ([33264])
Single lead system ([33262])

39.6 39.6 FUD 090 C 80

AMA: 2018,Jan,8; 2017,Jan,8; 2016,Aug,5; 2016,Jan,13; 2015,Jan,16; 2014,Nov,5; 2014,Jan,11

33244 **by transvenous extraction**

EXCLUDES *Thoracotomy to remove electrodes (33238, 33243)*

Code also removal of implantable defibrillator pulse generator and insertion of replacement defibrillator with electrodes (total system), when entire system is being replaced:
Insertion of defibrillator system, single or dual (33249)
Removal of generator (33241)
Code also removal of implantable defibrillator pulse generator, when entire system is removed without replacement (33241)
Code also replacement of implantable defibrillator pulse generator, when performed:
Dual lead system ([33263])
Multiple lead system ([33264])
Single lead system ([33262])

25.0 25.0 FUD 090 Q2

AMA: 2018,Jan,8; 2017,Jan,8; 2016,Aug,5; 2016,Jan,13; 2015,Jan,16; 2014,Nov,5; 2014,Jan,11

33249 **Insertion or replacement of permanent implantable defibrillator system, with transvenous lead(s), single or dual chamber**

EXCLUDES *Insertion of a single transvenous electrode, permanent pacemaker or implantable defibrillator (33216-33217)*

Code also removal of implantable defibrillator pulse generator and removal of electrode(s), when entire system is being replaced:
Removal of electrode(s) (33243-33244)
Removal of generator (33241)
Code also removal of defibrillator generator when upgrading from single to dual-chamber system (33241)

26.6 26.6 FUD 090 J J8

AMA: 2018,Jan,8; 2017,Jan,8; 2016,Aug,5; 2016,Jan,13; 2015,Jan,16; 2014,Nov,5; 2014,Jan,11

33270-33275 [33270, 33271, 33272, 33273, 33274, 33275] Subcutaneous Implantable Defibrillator

INCLUDES Programming and interrogation of:
Leadless pacemaker (93279, 93286, 93288, 93294, 93296)
Subcutaneous implantable defibrillator ([93260, 93261])

\# **33270** **Insertion or replacement of permanent subcutaneous implantable defibrillator system, with subcutaneous electrode, including defibrillation threshold evaluation, induction of arrhythmia, evaluation of sensing for arrhythmia termination, and programming or reprogramming of sensing or therapeutic parameters, when performed**

INCLUDES Electrophysiologic evaluation at time of initial insertion (93644)

EXCLUDES *Insertion of subcutaneous implantable defibrillator electrode only ([33271])*
Insertion/replacement of permanent implantable defibrillator system with substernal electrode (0571T)

Code also electrophysiologic evaluation following replacement of subcutaneous implantable defibrillator, when performed (93644)
Code also removal of subcutaneous implantable defibrillator and removal of subcutaneous electrode, when the entire system is being replaced:
Defibrillator (33241)
Electrode ([33272])

16.4 16.4 FUD 090 J J8

AMA: 2018,Jan,8; 2017,Jan,8; 2016,Aug,5; 2016,Jan,13; 2015,Jan,16; 2014,Nov,5

\# **33271** **Insertion of subcutaneous implantable defibrillator electrode**

EXCLUDES *Insertion of implantable defibrillator pulse generator only, other than subcutaneous:*
Initial insertion (33240)
Removal/replacement ([33262])
Insertion of subcutaneous implantable defibrillator and electrode (total system) ([33270])
Insertion of substernal defibrillator electrode (0572T)

13.2 13.2 FUD 090 J J8

AMA: 2018,Jan,8; 2017,Jan,8; 2016,Aug,5; 2016,Jan,13; 2015,Jan,16; 2014,Nov,5

\# **33272** **Removal of subcutaneous implantable defibrillator electrode**

EXCLUDES *Removal of substernal defibrillator electrode (0573T)*

Code also removal of subcutaneous implantable defibrillator and insertion of replacement implantable subcutaneous defibrillator with electrode (total system), when entire system is being replaced:
Insertion of total system ([33270])
Removal of defibrillator (33241)
Code also removal of implantable defibrillator, when performed:
Removal with replacement ([33262])
Removal without replacement (33241)

10.0 10.0 FUD 090 Q2

AMA: 2018,Jan,8; 2017,Jan,8; 2016,Aug,5; 2016,Jan,13; 2015,Jan,16; 2014,Nov,5

33273 **Repositioning of previously implanted subcutaneous implantable defibrillator electrode**

EXCLUDES *Repositioning of substernal defibrillator electrode (0574T)*

11.6 11.6 FUD 090 T G2

AMA: 2018,Jan,8; 2017,Jan,8; 2016,Aug,5; 2016,Jan,13; 2015,Jan,16; 2014,Nov,5

33274 **Transcatheter insertion or replacement of permanent leadless pacemaker, right ventricular, including imaging guidance (eg, fluoroscopy, venous ultrasound, ventriculography, femoral venography) and device evaluation (eg, interrogation or programming), when performed**

INCLUDES Cardiac catheterization for insertion leadless pacemaker (93451, 93453, 93456-93457, 93460-93461, 93530-93533)
Femoral venography (75820)
Imaging guidance (76000, 76937, 77002)
Right ventriculography (93566)

EXCLUDES *Removal permanent leadless pacemaker ([33275])*
Services for pacemakers with leads (33202-33203, 33206-33208, 33212-33214 [33221], 33215-33218, 33220, 33233-33237 [33227, 33228, 33229])

14.2 14.2 FUD 090 J8

AMA: 2019,Mar,6

▲ # 33275 **Transcatheter removal of permanent leadless pacemaker, right ventricular, including imaging guidance (eg, fluoroscopy, venous ultrasound, ventriculography, femoral venography), when performed**

INCLUDES Cardiac catheterization for insertion leadless pacemaker (93451, 93453, 93456-93457, 93460-93461, 93530-93533)
Femoral venography (75820)
Imaging guidance (76000, 76937, 77002)
Right ventriculography (93566)

EXCLUDES *Insertion/replacement leadless pacemaker ([33274])*
Services for pacemakers with leads (33202-33203, 33206-33208, 33212-33214 [33221], 33215-33218, 33220, 33233-33237 [33227, 33228, 33229])

15.1 15.1 FUD 090 G2

AMA: 2019,Mar,6

33250-33251 Surgical Ablation Arrhythmogenic Foci, Supraventricular

INCLUDES Procedures using cryotherapy, laser, microwave, radiofrequency, and ultrasound

33250 **Operative ablation of supraventricular arrhythmogenic focus or pathway (eg, Wolff-Parkinson-White, atrioventricular node re-entry), tract(s) and/or focus (foci); without cardiopulmonary bypass**

EXCLUDES *Pacing and mapping during surgery by other provider (93631)*

42.4 42.4 FUD 090 C 80

AMA: 2018,Jan,8; 2017,Jan,8; 2016,Jan,13; 2015,Jan,16; 2014,Jan,11

33251 **with cardiopulmonary bypass**

47.2 47.2 FUD 090 C 80

AMA: 2018,Jan,8; 2017,Dec,3; 2017,Jan,8; 2016,Jan,13; 2015,Jan,16; 2014,Jan,11

33254-33256 Surgical Ablation Arrhythmogenic Foci, Atrial (e.g., Maze)

INCLUDES Excision or isolation of the left atrial appendage
Procedures using cryotherapy, laser, microwave, radiofrequency, and ultrasound

EXCLUDES *Any procedure involving median sternotomy or cardiopulmonary bypass*
Aortic valve procedures (33390-33391, 33404-33415)
Aortoplasty (33417)
Ascending aorta graft (33858-33859, 33863-33864)
Coronary artery bypass (33510-33516, 33517-33523, 33533-33536)
Excision of intracardiac tumor, resection (33120)
Mitral valve procedures (33418-33430)
Outflow tract augmentation (33478)
Prosthetic valve repair (33496)
Pulmonary artery embolectomy (33910-33920)
Pulmonary valve procedures (33470-33477)
Repair aberrant coronary artery anatomy (33500-33507)
Repair aberrant heart anatomy (33600-33853)
Resection of external cardiac tumor (33130)
Temporary pacemaker (33210-33211)
Thoracotomy; with exploration (32100)
Tricuspid valve procedures (33460-33468)
Tube thoracostomy, includes connection to drainage system (32551)
Ventricular reconstruction (33542-33548)
Ventriculomyotomy (33416)

33254 **Operative tissue ablation and reconstruction of atria, limited (eg, modified maze procedure)**

39.4 39.4 FUD 090 C 80

AMA: 2018,Jan,8; 2017,Jan,8; 2016,Jan,13; 2015,Jan,16; 2014,Jan,11

33255 **Operative tissue ablation and reconstruction of atria, extensive (eg, maze procedure); without cardiopulmonary bypass**

47.3 47.3 FUD 090 C 80

AMA: 2018,Jan,8; 2017,Jan,8; 2016,Jan,13; 2015,Jan,16; 2014,Jan,11

33256 **with cardiopulmonary bypass**

56.1 56.1 FUD 090 C 80

AMA: 2018,Jan,8; 2017,Dec,3; 2017,Jan,8; 2016,Jan,13; 2015,Jan,16; 2014,Jan,11

33257-33259 Surgical Ablation Arrhythmogenic Foci, Atrial, with Other Heart Procedure(s)

EXCLUDES *Operative tissue ablation and reconstruction of atria (without other cardiac procedure), limited or extensive:*
Endoscopic (33265-33266)
Open (33254-33256)
Temporary pacemaker (33210-33211)
Tube thoracostomy, includes connection to drainage system (32551)

\+ 33257 **Operative tissue ablation and reconstruction of atria, performed at the time of other cardiac procedure(s), limited (eg, modified maze procedure) (List separately in addition to code for primary procedure)**

16.8 16.8 FUD ZZZ C 80

Code first (33120-33130, 33250-33251, 33261, 33300-33335, 33365, 33390-33391, 33404-33417 [33440], 33420-33430, 33460-33476, 33478, 33496, 33500-33507, 33510-33516, 33533-33548, 33600-33619, 33641-33697, 33702-33732, 33735-33767, 33770, 33877, 33910-33922, 33925-33926, 33975-33983)

\+ 33258 **Operative tissue ablation and reconstruction of atria, performed at the time of other cardiac procedure(s), extensive (eg, maze procedure), without cardiopulmonary bypass (List separately in addition to code for primary procedure)**

18.8 18.8 FUD ZZZ C 80

Code first, if performed without cardiopulmonary bypass (33130, 33250, 33300, 33310, 33320-33321, 33330, 33365, 33420, 33470-33471, 33501-33503, 33510-33516, 33533-33536, 33690, 33735, 33737, 33750-33766, 33800-33813, 33820-33824, 33840-33852, 33875, 33877, 33915, 33925, 33981, 33982)

+ **33259** **Operative tissue ablation and reconstruction of atria, performed at the time of other cardiac procedure(s), extensive (eg, maze procedure), with cardiopulmonary bypass (List separately in addition to code for primary procedure)**

Code first, if performed with cardiopulmonary bypass (33120, 33251, 33261, 33305, 33315, 33322, 33335, 33390-33391, 33404-33410, 33411-33417, 33422-33430, 33460-33468, 33474-33478, 33496, 33500, 33504-33507, 33510-33516, 33533-33548, 33600-33688, 33692-33726, 33730, 33732, 33736, 33767, 33770, 33783, 33786-33788, 33814, 33853, 33858-33877, 33910, 33916-33922, 33926, 33975-33980, 33983)

24.4 24.4 FUD ZZZ C 80

AMA: 2017,Dec,3

33261-33264 Surgical Ablation Arrhythmogenic Foci, Ventricular

33261 **Operative ablation of ventricular arrhythmogenic focus with cardiopulmonary bypass**

47.0 47.0 FUD 090 C 80

AMA: 2018,Jan,8; 2017,Dec,3; 2017,Jan,8; 2016,Jan,13; 2015,Jan,16; 2014,Jan,11

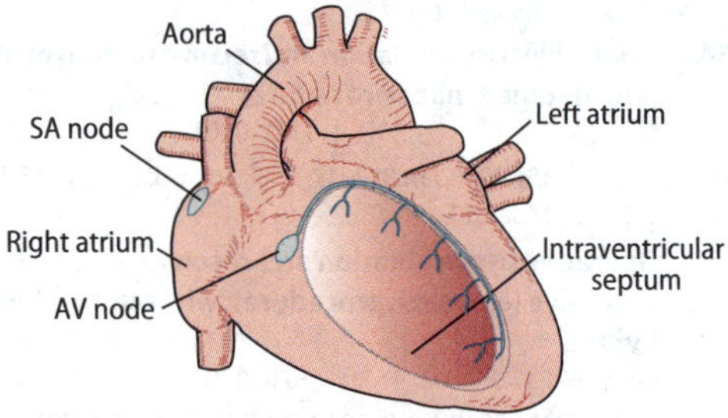

Impulse centers that are causing arrhythmia are treated with ablation

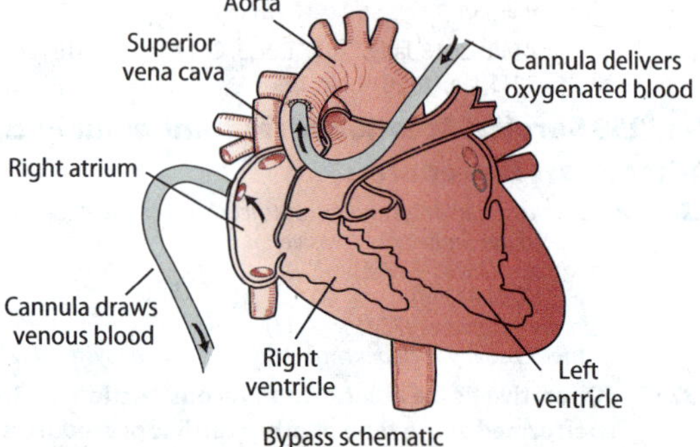

Bypass schematic

33262 **Resequenced code. See code following 33241.**

33263 **Resequenced code. See code following 33241.**

33264 **Resequenced code. See code before 33243.**

33265-33275 Surgical Ablation Arrhythmogenic Foci, Endoscopic

EXCLUDES *Insertion or replacement of temporary transvenous single chamber cardiac electrode or pacemaker catheter (separate procedure) (33210-33211)*
Tube thoracostomy, includes connection to drainage system (32551)

33265 **Endoscopy, surgical; operative tissue ablation and reconstruction of atria, limited (eg, modified maze procedure), without cardiopulmonary bypass**

39.3 39.3 FUD 090 C 80

AMA: 2018,Jan,8; 2017,Jan,8; 2016,Jan,13; 2015,Jan,16; 2014,Jan,11

33266 **operative tissue ablation and reconstruction of atria, extensive (eg, maze procedure), without cardiopulmonary bypass**

53.4 53.4 FUD 090 C 80

AMA: 2018,Jan,8; 2017,Jan,8; 2016,Jan,13; 2015,Jan,16; 2014,Jan,11

33270 **Resequenced code. See code following 33249.**

33271 **Resequenced code. See code following 33249.**

33272 **Resequenced code. See code following 33249.**

33273 **Resequenced code. See code following 33249.**

33274 **Resequenced code. See code following 33249.**

33275 **Resequenced code. See code following 33249.**

33285-33289 Cardiac Rhythm Monitor System

33285 **Insertion, subcutaneous cardiac rhythm monitor, including programming**

INCLUDES Implantation of device into subcutaneous prepectoral pocket
Initial programming

EXCLUDES *Successive analysis and/or reprogramming (93285, 93291, 93298)*

2.59 146. FUD 000 J8

AMA: 2019,Apr,3

33286 **Removal, subcutaneous cardiac rhythm monitor**

2.54 3.80 FUD 000 G2

AMA: 2019,Apr,3

33289 **Transcatheter implantation of wireless pulmonary artery pressure sensor for long-term hemodynamic monitoring, including deployment and calibration of the sensor, right heart catheterization, selective pulmonary catheterization, radiological supervision and interpretation, and pulmonary artery angiography, when performed**

INCLUDES Device implantation into subcutaneous pocket
Fluoroscopy (76000)
Pulmonary artery angiography/injection (75741, 75743, 75746, 93568)
Pulmonary artery catheterization (36013-36015)
Radiologic supervision and interpretation
Remote monitoring (93264)
Right heart catheterization (93451, 93453, 93456-93457, 93460-93461, 93530-93533)
Sensor deployment and calibration

9.51 9.51 FUD 000 80

AMA: 2019,Jun,3

33300-33315 Procedures for Injury of the Heart

INCLUDES Procedures with and without cardiopulmonary bypass

EXCLUDES *Cardiac assist services (33946-33949, 33967-33983, 33990-33993)*

33300 **Repair of cardiac wound; without bypass**

71.0 71.0 FUD 090 C 80

AMA: 1997,Nov,1

33305 **with cardiopulmonary bypass**

119. 119. FUD 090 C 80

AMA: 2017,Dec,3

33310 **Cardiotomy, exploratory (includes removal of foreign body, atrial or ventricular thrombus); without bypass**

EXCLUDES *Other cardiac procedures unless separate incision into heart is necessary in order to remove thrombus*

34.0 34.0 FUD 090 C 80

AMA: 1997,Nov,1

33315 **with cardiopulmonary bypass**

EXCLUDES *Other cardiac procedures unless separate incision into heart is necessary in order to remove thrombus*

Code also excision of thrombus with cardiopulmonary bypass and append modifier 59 if separate incision is required with (33120, 33130, 33420-33430, 33460-33468, 33496, 33542, 33545, 33641-33647, 33670, 33681, 33975-33980)

55.3 55.3 FUD 090 C 80

AMA: 2018,Jan,8; 2017,Dec,3; 2017,Jan,8; 2016,Jan,13; 2015,Jan,16; 2014,Jan,11

33320-33335 Procedures for Injury of the Aorta/Great Vessels

33320 **Suture repair of aorta or great vessels; without shunt or cardiopulmonary bypass**
30.5 30.5 **FUD** 090 C 80
AMA: 2018,Jun,11; 2018,Jan,8; 2017,Jan,8; 2016,Jan,13; 2015,Jan,16; 2014,Jan,11

33321 **with shunt bypass**
34.6 34.6 **FUD** 090 C 80
AMA: 2018,Jun,11

33322 **with cardiopulmonary bypass**
40.0 40.0 **FUD** 090 C 80
AMA: 2018,Jun,11; 2018,Jan,8; 2017,Dec,3; 2017,Jan,8; 2016,Jan,13; 2015,Jan,16; 2014,Jan,11

33330 **Insertion of graft, aorta or great vessels; without shunt, or cardiopulmonary bypass**
41.5 41.5 **FUD** 090 C 80
AMA: 2018,Jun,11

33335 **with cardiopulmonary bypass**
54.6 54.6 **FUD** 090 C 80
AMA: 2018,Jun,11; 2017,Dec,3

33340 Closure Left Atrial Appendage

EXCLUDES *Cardiac catheterization except for reasons other than closure left atrial appendage (93451-93453, 93456, 93458-93461, 93462, 93530-93533)*

33340 **Percutaneous transcatheter closure of the left atrial appendage with endocardial implant, including fluoroscopy, transseptal puncture, catheter placement(s), left atrial angiography, left atrial appendage angiography, when performed, and radiological supervision and interpretation**
23.0 23.0 **FUD** 000 C 80
AMA: 2018,Jan,8; 2017,Jul,3

33361-33369 Transcatheter Aortic Valve Replacement

CMS: 100-03,20.32 Transcatheter Aortic Valve Replacement (TAVR); 100-04,32,290.1.1 Coding Requirements for TAVR Services; 100-04,32,290.2 Claims Processing for TAVR/ Professional Claims; 100-04,32,290.3 Claims Processing TAVR Inpatient; 100-04,32,290.4 Payment of TAVR for MA Plan Participants

INCLUDES Access and implantation of the aortic valve (33361-33366)
Access sheath placement
Advancement of valve delivery system
Arteriotomy closure
Balloon aortic valvuloplasty
Cardiac or open arterial approach
Deployment of valve
Percutaneous access
Temporary pacemaker
Valve repositioning when necessary
Radiology procedures:
- Angiography during and after procedure
- Assessment of access site for closure
- Documentation of completion of the intervention
- Guidance for valve placement
- Supervision and interpretation

EXCLUDES *Cardiac catheterization procedures included in the TAVR/TAVI service (93452-93453, 93458-93461, 93567)*
Percutaneous coronary interventional procedures
Transvascular ventricular support (33967, 33970, 33973, 33975-33976, 33990-33993, 33999)

Code also cardiac catheterization services for purposes other than TAVR/TAVI
Code also diagnostic coronary angiography at a different session from the interventional procedure
Code also diagnostic coronary angiography at the same time as TAVR/TAVI when:
- A previous study is available, but documentation states the patient's condition has changed since the previous study, visualization of the anatomy/pathology is inadequate, or a change occurs during the procedure warranting additional evaluation of an area outside the current target area
- No previous catheter-based coronary angiography study is available, and a full diagnostic study is performed, with the decision to perform the intervention based on that study

Code also modifier 59 when diagnostic coronary angiography procedures are performed as separate and distinct procedural services on the same day or session as TAVR/TAVI
Code also modifier 62 as all TAVI/TAVR procedures require the work of two physicians

33361 **Transcatheter aortic valve replacement (TAVR/TAVI) with prosthetic valve; percutaneous femoral artery approach**
Code also cardiopulmonary bypass when performed (33367-33369)
39.4 39.4 **FUD** 000 C 80
AMA: 2018,Jan,8; 2017,Jan,8; 2016,Jan,13; 2015,Mar,9; 2015,Jan,16; 2014,Jul,8; 2014,Jan,5; 2014,Jan,11

33362 **open femoral artery approach**
Code also cardiopulmonary bypass when performed (33367-33369)
43.1 43.1 **FUD** 000 C 80
AMA: 2018,Jan,8; 2017,Dec,3; 2017,Jan,8; 2016,Jan,13; 2015,Mar,9; 2015,Jan,16; 2014,Jul,8; 2014,Jan,5; 2014,Jan,11

33363 **open axillary artery approach**
Code also cardiopulmonary bypass when performed (33367-33369)
44.6 44.6 **FUD** 000 C 80
AMA: 2018,Jan,8; 2017,Dec,3; 2017,Jan,8; 2016,Jan,13; 2015,Mar,9; 2015,Jan,16; 2014,Jul,8; 2014,Jan,5; 2014,Jan,11

33364 **open iliac artery approach**
Code also cardiopulmonary bypass when performed (33367-33369)
46.1 46.1 **FUD** 000 C 80
AMA: 2018,Jan,8; 2017,Dec,3; 2017,Jan,8; 2016,Jan,13; 2015,Mar,9; 2015,Jan,16; 2014,Jul,8; 2014,Jan,5; 2014,Jan,11

33365 **transaortic approach (eg, median sternotomy, mediastinotomy)**
Code also cardiopulmonary bypass when performed (33367-33369)
51.8 51.8 **FUD** 000 C 80
AMA: 2018,Jan,8; 2017,Jan,8; 2016,Jan,13; 2015,Mar,9; 2015,Jan,16; 2014,Jul,8; 2014,Jan,5; 2014,Jan,11

33366 **transapical exposure (eg, left thoracotomy)**

Code also cardiopulmonary bypass when performed (33367-33369)

56.0 56.0 FUD 000

AMA: 2018,Jan,8; 2017,Jan,8; 2016,Jan,13; 2015,Mar,9; 2015,Jan,16; 2014,Jul,8; 2014,Jan,5

\+ **33367** **cardiopulmonary bypass support with percutaneous peripheral arterial and venous cannulation (eg, femoral vessels) (List separately in addition to code for primary procedure)**

EXCLUDES *Cardiopulmonary bypass support with open or central arterial and venous cannulation (33368-33369)*

Code first (33361-33366, 33418, 33477, 0483T-0484T, 0544T, 0545T, 0569T-0570T)

18.2 18.2 FUD ZZZ

AMA: 2018,Jan,8; 2017,Jan,8; 2016,Mar,5; 2016,Jan,13; 2015,Sep,3; 2015,Jan,16

\+ **33368** **cardiopulmonary bypass support with open peripheral arterial and venous cannulation (eg, femoral, iliac, axillary vessels) (List separately in addition to code for primary procedure)**

EXCLUDES *Cardiopulmonary bypass support with percutaneous or central arterial and venous cannulation (33367, 33369)*

Code first (33361-33366, 33418, 33477, 0483T-0484T, 0544T, 0545T, 0569T-0570T)

21.7 21.7 FUD ZZZ

AMA: 2018,Jan,8; 2017,Jan,8; 2016,Mar,5; 2016,Jan,13; 2015,Sep,3; 2015,Jan,16

\+ **33369** **cardiopulmonary bypass support with central arterial and venous cannulation (eg, aorta, right atrium, pulmonary artery) (List separately in addition to code for primary procedure)**

EXCLUDES *Cardiopulmonary bypass support with percutaneous or open arterial and venous cannulation (33367-33368)*

Code first (33361-33366, 33418, 33477, 0483T-0484T, 0544T, 0545T, 0569T-0570T)

28.6 28.6 FUD ZZZ

AMA: 2018,Jan,8; 2017,Jan,8; 2016,Mar,5; 2016,Jan,13; 2015,Sep,3; 2015,Jan,16

33390-33415 [33440] Aortic Valve Procedures

33390 **Valvuloplasty, aortic valve, open, with cardiopulmonary bypass; simple (ie, valvotomy, debridement, debulking, and/or simple commissural resuspension)**

54.9 54.9 FUD 090

AMA: 2018,Jan,8; 2017,Dec,3

33391 **complex (eg, leaflet extension, leaflet resection, leaflet reconstruction, or annuloplasty)**

INCLUDES Simple aortic valvuloplasty (33390)

66.1 66.1 FUD 090

AMA: 2018,Jan,8; 2017,Dec,3

33404 **Construction of apical-aortic conduit**

51.0 51.0 FUD 090

AMA: 2018,Jan,8; 2017,Dec,3; 2017,Jan,8; 2016,Jan,13; 2015,Jan,16; 2014,Jan,11

33405 **Replacement, aortic valve, open, with cardiopulmonary bypass; with prosthetic valve other than homograft or stentless valve**

65.6 65.6 FUD 090

AMA: 2019,Apr,6; 2018,Jan,8; 2017,Dec,3; 2017,Jan,8; 2016,Jan,13; 2015,Jan,16; 2014,Jan,11

33406 **with allograft valve (freehand)**

83.2 83.2 FUD 090

AMA: 2019,Apr,6; 2018,Jan,8; 2017,Dec,3; 2017,Jan,8; 2016,Jan,13; 2015,Jan,16; 2014,Jan,11

33410 **with stentless tissue valve**

73.6 73.6 FUD 090

AMA: 2019,Apr,6; 2018,Jan,8; 2017,Dec,3; 2017,Jan,8; 2016,Jan,13; 2015,Jan,16; 2014,Jan,11

\# **33440** **Replacement, aortic valve; by translocation of autologous pulmonary valve and transventricular aortic annulus enlargement of the left ventricular outflow tract with valved conduit replacement of pulmonary valve (Ross-Konno procedure)**

INCLUDES Open replacement aortic valve with aortic annulus enlargement (33411-33412)

Open replacement aortic valve with translocation pulmonary valve (33413)

EXCLUDES *Aortoplasty for supravalvular stenosis (33417)*

Open replacement aortic valve (33405-33406, 33410)

Repair complex cardiac anomaly (except pulmonary atresia) (33608)

Repair left ventricular outlet obstruction (33414)

Repair pulmonary atresia (33920)

Replacement pulmonary valve (33475)

Resection/incision subvalvular tissue for aortic stenosis (33416)

98.1 98.1 FUD 090

AMA: 2019,Apr,6

33411 **Replacement, aortic valve; with aortic annulus enlargement, noncoronary sinus**

97.3 97.3 FUD 090

AMA: 2019,Apr,6; 2018,Jan,8; 2017,Dec,3; 2017,Jan,8; 2016,Jan,13; 2015,Jan,16; 2014,Jan,11

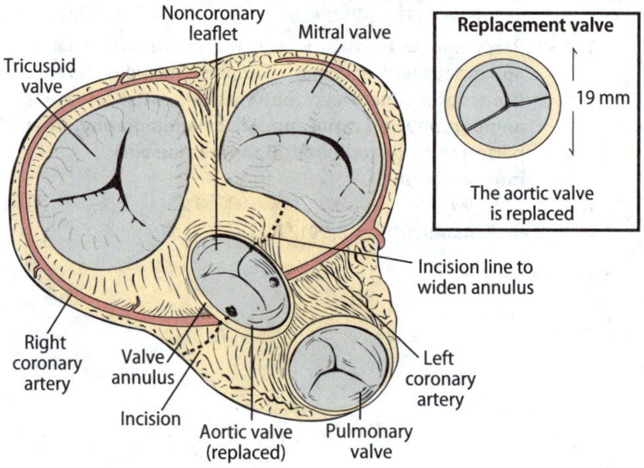

Overhead schematic of major heart valves

33412 **with transventricular aortic annulus enlargement (Konno procedure)**

EXCLUDES *Replacement aortic valve by translocation pulmonary valve, aortic annulus enlargement, valved conduit pulmonary valve replacement ([33440])*

Replacement aortic valve with translocation pulmonary valve (33413)

92.1 92.1 FUD 090

AMA: 2019,Apr,6; 2018,Jan,8; 2017,Dec,3; 2017,Jan,8; 2016,Jan,13; 2015,Jan,16; 2014,Jan,11

33413 **by translocation of autologous pulmonary valve with allograft replacement of pulmonary valve (Ross procedure)**

EXCLUDES *Replacement aortic valve by translocation pulmonary valve, aortic annulus enlargement, valved conduit pulmonary valve replacement ([33440])*

Replacement aortic valve with transventricular aortic annulus enlargement (33412)

94.3 94.3 FUD 090

AMA: 2019,Apr,6; 2018,Jan,8; 2017,Dec,3; 2017,Jan,8; 2016,Jan,13; 2015,Jan,16; 2014,Jan,11

33414 **Repair of left ventricular outflow tract obstruction by patch enlargement of the outflow tract**

62.0 62.0 FUD 090

AMA: 2019,Apr,6; 2018,Jan,8; 2017,Dec,3; 2017,Jan,8; 2016,Jan,13; 2015,Jan,16; 2014,Jan,11

33415 **Resection or incision of subvalvular tissue for discrete subvalvular aortic stenosis**
58.7 58.7 FUD 090 C 80
AMA: 2018,Jan,8; 2017,Dec,3; 2017,Jan,8; 2016,Jan,13; 2015,Jan,16; 2014,Jan,11

33416 Ventriculectomy

CMS: 100-03,20.26 Partial Ventriculectomy

EXCLUDES *Percutaneous transcatheter septal reduction therapy (93583)*

33416 **Ventriculomyotomy (-myectomy) for idiopathic hypertrophic subaortic stenosis (eg, asymmetric septal hypertrophy)**
58.6 58.6 FUD 090 C 80
AMA: 2019,Apr,6; 2018,Jan,8; 2017,Dec,3; 2017,Jan,8; 2016,Jan,13; 2015,Jan,16; 2014,Jan,11

33417 Repair of Supravalvular Stenosis by Aortoplasty

33417 **Aortoplasty (gusset) for supravalvular stenosis**
48.1 48.1 FUD 090 C 80
AMA: 2019,Apr,6; 2018,Jan,8; 2017,Dec,3; 2017,Jan,8; 2016,Jan,13; 2015,Jan,16; 2014,Jan,11

33418-33419 Transcatheter Mitral Valve Procedures

INCLUDES Access sheath placement
Advancement of valve delivery system
Deployment of valve
Radiology procedures:
Angiography during and after procedure
Documentation of completion of the intervention
Guidance for valve placement
Supervision and interpretation
Valve repositioning when necessary

EXCLUDES *Cardiac catheterization services for purposes other than TMVR*
Diagnostic angiography at different session from interventional procedure
Percutaneous approach through the coronary sinus for TMVR (0345T)
Percutaneous coronary interventional procedures
Transcatheter mitral valve annulus reconstruction (0544T)
Transcatheter TMVI by percutaneous or transthoracic approach (0483T-0484T)

Code also cardiopulmonary bypass:
Central (33369)
Open peripheral (33368)
Percutaneous peripheral (33367)

Code also diagnostic coronary angiography and cardiac catheterization procedures when:
No previous study available and full diagnostic study performed
Previous study inadequate or patient's clinical indication for the study changed prior to or during the procedure
Use modifier 59 with cardiac catheterization procedures when on same day or same session as TMVR

Code also transvascular ventricular support:
Balloon pump (33967, 33970, 33973)
Ventricular assist device (33990-33993)

33418 **Transcatheter mitral valve repair, percutaneous approach, including transseptal puncture when performed; initial prosthesis**
Code also left heart catheterization when performed by transapical puncture (93462)
52.3 52.3 FUD 090 C 80
AMA: 2018,Jan,8; 2017,Jan,8; 2016,Jan,13; 2015,Sep,3

+ 33419 **additional prosthesis(es) during same session (List separately in addition to code for primary procedure)**
EXCLUDES *Procedures performed more than one time per session*
Code first (33418)
12.3 12.3 FUD ZZZ N N1 80
AMA: 2018,Jan,8; 2017,Jan,8; 2016,Jan,13; 2015,Sep,3

33420-33440 Mitral Valve Procedures

Code also removal of thrombus through a separate heart incision, when performed (33310-33315); append modifier 59 to (33315)

33420 **Valvotomy, mitral valve; closed heart**
42.3 42.3 FUD 090 C
AMA: 2018,Jan,8; 2017,Jan,8; 2016,Jan,13; 2015,Sep,3; 2015,Jan,16; 2014,Jan,11

33422 **open heart, with cardiopulmonary bypass**
48.5 48.5 FUD 090 C 80
AMA: 2018,Jan,8; 2017,Dec,3; 2017,Jan,8; 2016,Jan,13; 2015,Sep,3; 2015,Jan,16; 2014,Jan,11

33425 **Valvuloplasty, mitral valve, with cardiopulmonary bypass;**
79.0 79.0 FUD 090 C 80
AMA: 2018,Jan,8; 2017,Dec,3; 2017,Jan,8; 2016,Jan,13; 2015,Sep,3; 2015,Jan,16; 2014,Jan,11

33426 **with prosthetic ring**
68.9 68.9 FUD 090 C 80
AMA: 2018,Jan,8; 2017,Dec,3; 2017,Jan,8; 2016,Jan,13; 2015,Sep,3; 2015,Jan,16; 2014,Jan,11

33427 **radical reconstruction, with or without ring**
70.8 70.8 FUD 090 C 80
AMA: 2018,Jan,8; 2017,Dec,3; 2017,Jan,8; 2016,Jan,13; 2015,Sep,3; 2015,Jan,16; 2014,Jan,11

33430 **Replacement, mitral valve, with cardiopulmonary bypass**
81.0 81.0 FUD 090 C 80
AMA: 2018,Jan,8; 2017,Dec,3; 2017,Jan,8; 2016,Jan,13; 2015,Sep,3; 2015,Jan,16; 2014,Jan,11

33440 **Resequenced code. See code following 33410.**

33460-33468 Tricuspid Valve Procedures

EXCLUDES *Transcatheter tricuspid valve annulus reconstruction (0545T)*
Transcatheter tricuspid valve repair (0569T-0570T)

Code also removal of thrombus through a separate heart incision, when performed (33310-33315); append modifier 59 to (33315)

33460 **Valvectomy, tricuspid valve, with cardiopulmonary bypass**
70.2 70.2 FUD 090 C 80
AMA: 2018,Jan,8; 2017,Dec,3; 2017,Jan,8; 2016,Jan,13; 2015,Jan,16; 2014,Jan,11

33463 **Valvuloplasty, tricuspid valve; without ring insertion**
89.5 89.5 FUD 090 C 80
AMA: 2018,Jan,8; 2017,Dec,3; 2017,Jan,8; 2016,Jan,13; 2015,Jan,16; 2014,Jan,11

33464 **with ring insertion**
70.7 70.7 FUD 090 C 80
AMA: 2018,Jan,8; 2017,Dec,3; 2017,Jan,8; 2016,Jan,13; 2015,Jan,16; 2014,Jan,11

33465 **Replacement, tricuspid valve, with cardiopulmonary bypass**
79.9 79.9 FUD 090 C 80
AMA: 2018,Jan,8; 2017,Dec,3; 2017,Jan,8; 2016,Jan,13; 2015,Jan,16; 2014,Jan,11

33468 **Tricuspid valve repositioning and plication for Ebstein anomaly**
71.2 71.2 FUD 090 C 80
AMA: 2018,Jan,8; 2017,Dec,3; 2017,Jan,8; 2016,Jan,13; 2015,Jan,16; 2014,Jan,11

33470-33474 Pulmonary Valvotomy

INCLUDES Brock's operation

Code also the concurrent ligation/takedown of a systemic-to-pulmonary artery shunt (33924)

33470 **Valvotomy, pulmonary valve, closed heart; transventricular**
35.9 35.9 FUD 090 63 C 80
AMA: 2018,Jan,8; 2017,Jan,8; 2016,Jan,13; 2015,Jan,16; 2014,Jan,11

33471 **via pulmonary artery**
EXCLUDES *Percutaneous valvuloplasty of pulmonary valve (92990)*
38.3 38.3 FUD 090 C 80
AMA: 2018,Jan,8; 2017,Jan,8; 2016,Jan,13; 2015,Jan,16; 2014,Jan,11

33474 **Valvotomy, pulmonary valve, open heart, with cardiopulmonary bypass**
63.2 63.2 FUD 090 C 80
AMA: 2017,Dec,3

33475-33476 Other Procedures Pulmonary Valve

Code also the concurrent ligation/takedown of a systemic-to-pulmonary artery shunt (33924)

33475 **Replacement, pulmonary valve**

67.6 67.6 FUD 090 C 80

AMA: 2019,Apr,6; 2018,Jan,8; 2017,Dec,3; 2017,Jan,8; 2016,Jan,13; 2015,Jan,16; 2014,Jan,11

33476 **Right ventricular resection for infundibular stenosis, with or without commissurotomy**

INCLUDES Brock's operation

44.1 44.1 FUD 090 C 80

AMA: 2018,Jan,8; 2017,Dec,3; 2017,Jan,8; 2016,Jan,13; 2015,Jan,16; 2014,Jan,11

33477 Transcatheter Pulmonary Valve Implantation

INCLUDES Cardiac catheterization, contrast injection, angiography, fluoroscopic guidance and the supervision and interpretation for device placement
Percutaneous balloon angioplasty within the treatment area
Pre-, intra-, and post-operative hemodynamic measurements
Valvuloplasty or stent insertion in pulmonary valve conduit (37236-37237, 92997-92998)

EXCLUDES *Balloon pump insertion (33967, 33970, 33973)*
Cardiopulmonary bypass performed in the same session (33367-33369)
Extracorporeal membrane oxygenation (ECMO) (33946-33959 [33962, 33963, 33964, 33965, 33966, 33969, 33984, 33985, 33986, 33987, 33988, 33989])
Fluoroscopy (76000)
Injection procedure during cardiac catheterization (93563, 93566-93568)
Percutaneous cardiac intervention procedures, when performed
Procedures performed more than one time per session
Right heart catheterization (93451, 93453-93461, 93530-93533)
Ventricular assist device (VAD) (33990-33993)

Code also the concurrent ligation/takedown of a systemic-to-pulmonary artery shunt (33924)

33477 **Transcatheter pulmonary valve implantation, percutaneous approach, including pre-stenting of the valve delivery site, when performed**

39.7 39.7 FUD 000 C 80

AMA: 2018,Jan,8; 2017,Jan,8; 2016,Aug,9; 2016,Mar,5

33478 Outflow Tract Augmentation

Code also for cavopulmonary anastomosis to a second superior vena cava (33768)
Code also the concurrent ligation/takedown of a systemic-to-pulmonary artery shunt (33924)

33478 **Outflow tract augmentation (gusset), with or without commissurotomy or infundibular resection**

45.6 45.6 FUD 090 C 80

AMA: 2018,Jan,8; 2017,Dec,3; 2017,Jan,8; 2016,Jan,13; 2015,Jan,16; 2014,Jan,11

33496 Prosthetic Valve Repair

Code also removal of thrombus through a separate heart incision, when performed (33310-33315); append modifier 59 to (33315)
Code also reoperation if performed (33530)

33496 **Repair of non-structural prosthetic valve dysfunction with cardiopulmonary bypass (separate procedure)**

48.5 48.5 FUD 090 C 80

AMA: 2018,Jan,8; 2017,Dec,3; 2017,Jan,8; 2016,Jan,13; 2015,Jan,16; 2014,Jan,11

33500-33507 Repair Aberrant Coronary Artery Anatomy

INCLUDES Angioplasty and/or endarterectomy

33500 **Repair of coronary arteriovenous or arteriocardiac chamber fistula; with cardiopulmonary bypass**

45.5 45.5 FUD 090 C 80

AMA: 2017,Dec,3

33501 **without cardiopulmonary bypass**

32.5 32.5 FUD 090 C 80

AMA: 2007,Mar,1-3; 1997,Nov,1

33502 **Repair of anomalous coronary artery from pulmonary artery origin; by ligation**

37.0 37.0 FUD 090 63 C 80

AMA: 2017,Dec,3

33503 **by graft, without cardiopulmonary bypass**

38.4 38.4 FUD 090 63 C 80

AMA: 2007,Mar,1-3; 1997,Nov,1

33504 **by graft, with cardiopulmonary bypass**

42.5 42.5 FUD 090 C 80

AMA: 2017,Dec,3

33505 **with construction of intrapulmonary artery tunnel (Takeuchi procedure)**

60.0 60.0 FUD 090 63 C 80

AMA: 2017,Dec,3

33506 **by translocation from pulmonary artery to aorta**

59.7 59.7 FUD 090 63 C 80

AMA: 2017,Dec,3

33507 **Repair of anomalous (eg, intramural) aortic origin of coronary artery by unroofing or translocation**

50.0 50.0 FUD 090 C 80

AMA: 2018,Jan,8; 2017,Dec,3; 2017,Jan,8; 2016,Jan,13; 2015,Jan,16; 2014,Jan,11

33508 Endoscopic Harvesting of Venous Graft

INCLUDES Diagnostic endoscopy

EXCLUDES *Harvesting of vein of upper extremity (35500)*

Code first (33510-33523)

\+ **33508** **Endoscopy, surgical, including video-assisted harvest of vein(s) for coronary artery bypass procedure (List separately in addition to code for primary procedure)**

0.47 0.47 FUD ZZZ N N1 80

AMA: 1997,Nov,1

33510-33516 Coronary Artery Bypass: Venous Grafts

INCLUDES Obtaining saphenous vein grafts
Venous bypass grafting only

EXCLUDES *Arterial bypass (33533-33536)*
Combined arterial-venous bypass (33517-33523, 33533-33536)
Obtaining vein graft:
Femoropopliteal vein (35572)
Upper extremity vein (35500)
Percutaneous ventricular assist devices (33990-33993)

Code also modifier 80 when assistant at surgery obtains grafts

33510 **Coronary artery bypass, vein only; single coronary venous graft**

55.9 55.9 FUD 090 C 80

AMA: 2018,Jan,8; 2017,Dec,3; 2017,Jan,8; 2016,Jan,13; 2015,Jan,16; 2014,Aug,14; 2014,Jan,11

33511 **2 coronary venous grafts**

61.4 61.4 FUD 090 C 80

AMA: 2018,Jan,8; 2017,Dec,3; 2017,Jan,8; 2016,Jan,13; 2015,Jan,16; 2014,Aug,14; 2014,Jan,11

33512 **3 coronary venous grafts**

69.9 69.9 FUD 090 C 80

AMA: 2018,Jan,8; 2017,Dec,3; 2017,Jan,8; 2016,Jan,13; 2015,Jan,16; 2014,Aug,14; 2014,Jan,11

33513 **4 coronary venous grafts**

72.0 72.0 FUD 090 C 80

AMA: 2018,Jan,8; 2017,Dec,3; 2017,Jan,8; 2016,Jan,13; 2015,Jan,16; 2014,Aug,14; 2014,Jan,11

33514 **5 coronary venous grafts**

75.7 75.7 FUD 090 C 80

AMA: 2018,Jan,8; 2017,Dec,3; 2017,Jan,8; 2016,Jan,13; 2015,Jan,16; 2014,Aug,14; 2014,Jan,11

33516 **6 or more coronary venous grafts**

78.9 78.9 FUD 090 C 80

AMA: 2018,Jan,8; 2017,Dec,3; 2017,Jan,8; 2016,Jan,13; 2015,Jan,16; 2014,Aug,14; 2014,Jan,11

33517-33523 Coronary Artery Bypass: Venous AND Arterial Grafts

INCLUDES Obtaining saphenous vein grafts

EXCLUDES *Obtaining arterial graft:*
Upper extremity (35600)
Obtaining vein graft:
Femoropopliteal vein graft (35572)
Upper extremity (35500)
Percutaneous ventricular assist devices (33990-33993)

Code also modifier 80 when assistant at surgery obtains grafts
Code first (33533-33536)

+ **33517** **Coronary artery bypass, using venous graft(s) and arterial graft(s); single vein graft (List separately in addition to code for primary procedure)**
5.41 5.41 FUD ZZZ C 80
AMA: 2018,Jan,8; 2017,Jan,8; 2016,Jan,13; 2015,Jan,16; 2014,Jan,11

+ **33518** **2 venous grafts (List separately in addition to code for primary procedure)**
11.9 11.9 FUD ZZZ C 80
AMA: 2018,Jan,8; 2017,Jan,8; 2016,Jan,13; 2015,Jan,16; 2014,Jan,11

+ **33519** **3 venous grafts (List separately in addition to code for primary procedure)**
15.7 15.7 FUD ZZZ C 80
AMA: 2018,Jan,8; 2017,Jan,8; 2016,Jan,13; 2015,Jan,16; 2014,Jan,11

+ **33521** **4 venous grafts (List separately in addition to code for primary procedure)**
18.9 18.9 FUD ZZZ C 80
AMA: 2018,Jan,8; 2017,Jan,8; 2016,Jan,13; 2015,Jan,16; 2014,Jan,11

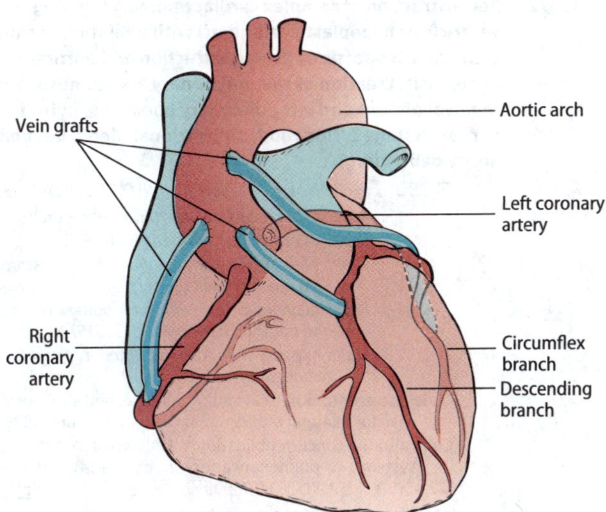

+ **33522** **5 venous grafts (List separately in addition to code for primary procedure)**
21.2 21.2 FUD ZZZ C 80
AMA: 2018,Jan,8; 2017,Jan,8; 2016,Jan,13; 2015,Jan,16; 2014,Jan,11

+ **33523** **6 or more venous grafts (List separately in addition to code for primary procedure)**
24.0 24.0 FUD ZZZ C 80
AMA: 2018,Jan,8; 2017,Jan,8; 2016,Jan,13; 2015,Jan,16; 2014,Jan,11

33530 Reoperative Coronary Artery Bypass Graft or Valve Procedure

EXCLUDES *Percutaneous ventricular assist devices (33990-33993)*

Code first (33390-33391, 33404-33496, 33510-33536, 33863)

+ **33530** **Reoperation, coronary artery bypass procedure or valve procedure, more than 1 month after original operation (List separately in addition to code for primary procedure)**
15.2 15.2 FUD ZZZ C 80
AMA: 2018,Jan,8; 2017,Jan,8; 2016,Jan,13; 2015,Jan,16; 2014,Jan,11

33533-33536 Coronary Artery Bypass: Arterial Grafts

INCLUDES Obtaining arterial graft (eg, epigastric, internal mammary, gastroepiploic and others)

EXCLUDES *Obtaining arterial graft:*
Upper extremity (35600)
Obtaining venous graft:
Femoropopliteal vein (35572)
Upper extremity (35500)
Percutaneous ventricular assist devices (33990-33993)
Venous bypass (33510-33516)

Code also for combined arterial venous grafts (33517-33523)
Code also modifier 80 when assistant at surgery obtains grafts

33533 **Coronary artery bypass, using arterial graft(s); single arterial graft**
54.0 54.0 FUD 090 C 80
AMA: 2018,Jan,8; 2017,Dec,3; 2017,Jan,8; 2016,Jan,13; 2015,Jan,16; 2014,Nov,14; 2014,Jan,11

33534 **2 coronary arterial grafts**
63.6 63.6 FUD 090 C 80
AMA: 2018,Jan,8; 2017,Dec,3; 2017,Jan,8; 2016,Jan,13; 2015,Jan,16; 2014,Jan,11

33535 **3 coronary arterial grafts**
70.9 70.9 FUD 090 C 80
AMA: 2018,Jan,8; 2017,Dec,3; 2017,Jan,8; 2016,Jan,13; 2015,Jan,16; 2014,Jan,11

33536 **4 or more coronary arterial grafts**
76.1 76.1 FUD 090 C 80
AMA: 2018,Jan,8; 2017,Dec,3; 2017,Jan,8; 2016,Jan,13; 2015,Jan,16; 2014,Nov,14; 2014,Jan,11

33542-33548 Ventricular Reconstruction

33542 **Myocardial resection (eg, ventricular aneurysmectomy)**
Code also removal of thrombus through a separate heart incision, when performed (33310-33315); append modifier 59 to (33315)
76.2 76.2 FUD 090 C 80
AMA: 2018,Jan,8; 2017,Dec,3; 2017,Jan,8; 2016,Jan,13; 2015,Jan,16; 2014,Jan,11

33545 **Repair of postinfarction ventricular septal defect, with or without myocardial resection**
Code also removal of thrombus through a separate heart incision, when performed (33310-33315); append modifier 59 to (33315)
89.7 89.7 FUD 090 C 80
AMA: 2018,Jan,8; 2017,Dec,3; 2017,Jan,8; 2016,Jan,13; 2015,Jan,16; 2014,Jan,11

33548 **Surgical ventricular restoration procedure, includes prosthetic patch, when performed (eg, ventricular remodeling, SVR, SAVER, Dor procedures)**
EXCLUDES *Batista procedure or pachopexy (33999)*
Cardiotomy, exploratory (33310, 33315)
Temporary pacemaker (33210-33211)
Tube thoracostomy (32551)
85.7 85.7 FUD 090 C 80
AMA: 2018,Jan,8; 2017,Dec,3; 2017,Jan,8; 2016,Jan,13; 2015,Jan,16; 2014,Jan,11

33572 Endarterectomy with CABG (LAD, RCA, Cx)

Code first (33510-33516, 33533-33536)

\+ **33572** **Coronary endarterectomy, open, any method, of left anterior descending, circumflex, or right coronary artery performed in conjunction with coronary artery bypass graft procedure, each vessel (List separately in addition to primary procedure)**

6.67 6.67 FUD ZZZ C 80

AMA: 1997,Nov,1; 1994,Win,1

33600-33622 Repair Aberrant Heart Anatomy

33600 **Closure of atrioventricular valve (mitral or tricuspid) by suture or patch**

49.8 49.8 FUD 090 C 80

AMA: 2018,Jan,8; 2017,Dec,3; 2017,Jan,8; 2016,Jan,13; 2015,Jan,16; 2014,Jan,11

33602 **Closure of semilunar valve (aortic or pulmonary) by suture or patch**

Code also the concurrent ligation/takedown of a systemic-to-pulmonary artery shunt (33924)

48.4 48.4 FUD 090 C 80

AMA: 2017,Dec,3

33606 **Anastomosis of pulmonary artery to aorta (Damus-Kaye-Stansel procedure)**

Code also the concurrent ligation/takedown of a systemic-to-pulmonary artery shunt (33924)

51.6 51.6 FUD 090 C 80

AMA: 2017,Dec,3

33608 **Repair of complex cardiac anomaly other than pulmonary atresia with ventricular septal defect by construction or replacement of conduit from right or left ventricle to pulmonary artery**

EXCLUDES *Unifocalization of arborization anomalies of pulmonary artery (33925, 33926)*

Code also the concurrent ligation/takedown of a systemic-to-pulmonary artery shunt (33924)

52.2 52.2 FUD 090 C 80

AMA: 2019,Apr,6; 2017,Dec,3

33610 **Repair of complex cardiac anomalies (eg, single ventricle with subaortic obstruction) by surgical enlargement of ventricular septal defect**

Code also the concurrent ligation/takedown of a systemic-to-pulmonary artery shunt (33924)

51.5 51.5 FUD 090 63 C 80

AMA: 2017,Dec,3

33611 **Repair of double outlet right ventricle with intraventricular tunnel repair;**

Code also the concurrent ligation/takedown of a systemic-to-pulmonary artery shunt (33924)

56.7 56.7 FUD 090 63 C 80

AMA: 2017,Dec,3

33612 **with repair of right ventricular outflow tract obstruction**

Code also the concurrent ligation/takedown of a systemic-to-pulmonary artery shunt (33924)

58.2 58.2 FUD 090 C 80

AMA: 2017,Dec,3

33615 **Repair of complex cardiac anomalies (eg, tricuspid atresia) by closure of atrial septal defect and anastomosis of atria or vena cava to pulmonary artery (simple Fontan procedure)**

Code also the concurrent ligation/takedown of a systemic-to-pulmonary artery shunt (33924)

58.0 58.0 FUD 090 C 80

AMA: 2017,Dec,3

33617 **Repair of complex cardiac anomalies (eg, single ventricle) by modified Fontan procedure**

Code also cavopulmonary anastomosis to a second superior vena cava (33768)

Code also the concurrent ligation/takedown of a systemic-to-pulmonary artery shunt (33924)

61.2 61.2 FUD 090 C 80

AMA: 2017,Dec,3

33619 **Repair of single ventricle with aortic outflow obstruction and aortic arch hypoplasia (hypoplastic left heart syndrome) (eg, Norwood procedure)**

79.3 79.3 FUD 090 63 C 80

AMA: 2018,Jan,8; 2017,Dec,3; 2017,Jan,8; 2016,Jul,3; 2016,Jan,13; 2015,Jan,16; 2014,Jan,11

33620 **Application of right and left pulmonary artery bands (eg, hybrid approach stage 1)**

EXCLUDES *Banding of main pulmonary artery related to septal defect (33690)*

Code also transthoracic insertion of catheter for stent placement with removal of catheter and closure when performed during same session (33621)

47.9 47.9 FUD 090 C 80

AMA: 2018,Jan,8; 2017,Dec,3; 2017,Jan,8; 2016,Jul,3; 2016,Jan,13; 2015,Jan,16; 2014,Jan,11

33621 **Transthoracic insertion of catheter for stent placement with catheter removal and closure (eg, hybrid approach stage 1)**

Code also application of right and left pulmonary artery bands when performed during same session (33620)

Code also stent placement (37236)

27.0 27.0 FUD 090 C 80

AMA: 2018,Jan,8; 2017,Dec,3; 2017,Jan,8; 2016,Jul,3; 2016,Jan,13; 2015,Jan,16; 2014,Jan,11

33622 **Reconstruction of complex cardiac anomaly (eg, single ventricle or hypoplastic left heart) with palliation of single ventricle with aortic outflow obstruction and aortic arch hypoplasia, creation of cavopulmonary anastomosis, and removal of right and left pulmonary bands (eg, hybrid approach stage 2, Norwood, bidirectional Glenn, pulmonary artery debanding)**

EXCLUDES *Excision of coarctation of aorta (33840, 33845, 33851)*
Repair of hypoplastic or interrupted aortic arch (33853)
Repair of patent ductus arteriosus (33822)
Repair of pulmonary artery stenosis by reconstruction with patch or graft (33917)
Repair of single ventricle with aortic outflow obstruction and aortic arch hypoplasia (33619)
Shunt; superior vena cava to pulmonary artery for flow to both lungs (33767)

Code also anastomosis, cavopulmonary, second superior vena cava for bilateral bidirectional Glenn procedure (33768)

Code also the concurrent ligation/takedown of a systemic-to-pulmonary artery shunt (33924)

100. 100. FUD 090 C 80

AMA: 2018,Jan,8; 2017,Dec,3; 2017,Jan,8; 2016,Jul,3; 2016,Jan,13; 2015,Jan,16; 2014,Jan,11

33641-33645 Closure of Defect: Atrium

Code also removal of thrombus through a separate heart incision, when performed (33310-33315); append modifier 59 to (33315)

33641 **Repair atrial septal defect, secundum, with cardiopulmonary bypass, with or without patch**

47.3 47.3 FUD 090 C 80

AMA: 2018,Jan,8; 2017,Dec,3; 2017,Jan,8; 2016,Jan,13; 2015,Jan,16; 2014,Jan,11

33645 **Direct or patch closure, sinus venosus, with or without anomalous pulmonary venous drainage**

EXCLUDES *Repair of isolated partial anomalous pulmonary venous return (33724)*
Repair of pulmonary venous stenosis (33726)

50.2 50.2 FUD 090 C 80

AMA: 2017,Dec,3

33647 Closure of Septal Defect: Atrium AND Ventricle

EXCLUDES *Tricuspid atresia repair procedures (33615)*

Code also removal of thrombus through a separate heart incision, when performed (33310-33315); append modifier 59 to (33315)

33647 **Repair of atrial septal defect and ventricular septal defect, with direct or patch closure**
52.8 52.8 FUD 090 63 C 80
AMA: 2017,Dec,3

33660-33670 Closure of Defect: Atrioventricular Canal

33660 **Repair of incomplete or partial atrioventricular canal (ostium primum atrial septal defect), with or without atrioventricular valve repair**
51.0 51.0 FUD 090 C 80
AMA: 2017,Dec,3

33665 **Repair of intermediate or transitional atrioventricular canal, with or without atrioventricular valve repair**
55.6 55.6 FUD 090 C 80
AMA: 2017,Dec,3

33670 **Repair of complete atrioventricular canal, with or without prosthetic valve**
Code also removal of thrombus through a separate heart incision, when performed (33310-33315); append modifier 59 to (33315)
57.4 57.4 FUD 090 63 C 80
AMA: 2017,Dec,3

33675-33677 Closure of Multiple Septal Defects: Ventricle

EXCLUDES *Closure of single ventricular septal defect (33681, 33684, 33688)*
Insertion or replacement of temporary transvenous single chamber cardiac electrode or pacemaker catheter (33210)
Percutaneous closure (93581)
Thoracentesis (32554-32555)
Thoracotomy (32100)
Tube thoracostomy (32551)

33675 **Closure of multiple ventricular septal defects;**
57.3 57.3 FUD 090 C 80
AMA: 2018,Jan,8; 2017,Dec,3; 2017,Jan,8; 2016,Jan,13; 2015,Jan,16; 2014,Jan,11

33676 **with pulmonary valvotomy or infundibular resection (acyanotic)**
58.8 58.8 FUD 090 C 80
AMA: 2018,Jan,8; 2017,Dec,3; 2017,Jan,8; 2016,Jan,13; 2015,Jan,16; 2014,Jan,11

33677 **with removal of pulmonary artery band, with or without gusset**
61.1 61.1 FUD 090 C 80
AMA: 2018,Jan,8; 2017,Dec,3; 2017,Jan,8; 2016,Jan,13; 2015,Jan,16; 2014,Jan,11

33681-33688 Closure of Septal Defect: Ventricle

EXCLUDES *Repair of pulmonary vein that requires creating an atrial septal defect (33724)*

33681 **Closure of single ventricular septal defect, with or without patch;**
Code also removal of thrombus through a separate heart incision, when performed (33310-33315); append modifier 59 to (33315)
53.0 53.0 FUD 090 C 80
AMA: 2018,Jan,8; 2017,Dec,3; 2017,Jan,8; 2016,Jan,13; 2015,Jan,16; 2014,Jan,11

33684 **with pulmonary valvotomy or infundibular resection (acyanotic)**
Code also concurrent ligation/takedown of a systemic-to-pulmonary artery shunt if performed (33924)
54.8 54.8 FUD 090 C 80
AMA: 2017,Dec,3

33688 **with removal of pulmonary artery band, with or without gusset**
Code also the concurrent ligation/takedown of a systemic-to-pulmonary artery shunt if performed (33924)
54.8 54.8 FUD 090 C 80
AMA: 2017,Dec,3

33690 Reduce Pulmonary Overcirculation in Septal Defects

EXCLUDES *Left and right pulmonary artery banding in a single ventricle (33620)*

33690 **Banding of pulmonary artery**
34.7 34.7 FUD 090 63 C 80
AMA: 2018,Jan,8; 2017,Jan,8; 2016,Jan,13; 2015,Jan,16; 2014,Jan,11

33692-33697 Repair of Defects of Tetralogy of Fallot

Code also the concurrent ligation/takedown of a systemic-to-pulmonary artery shunt (33924)

33692 **Complete repair tetralogy of Fallot without pulmonary atresia;**
56.9 56.9 FUD 090 C 80
AMA: 2017,Dec,3

33694 **with transannular patch**
56.7 56.7 FUD 090 63 C 80
AMA: 2017,Dec,3

33697 **Complete repair tetralogy of Fallot with pulmonary atresia including construction of conduit from right ventricle to pulmonary artery and closure of ventricular septal defect**
59.7 59.7 FUD 090 C 80
AMA: 2018,Jan,8; 2017,Dec,3; 2017,Jan,8; 2016,Jan,13; 2015,Jan,16; 2014,Jan,11

33702-33722 Repair Anomalies Sinus of Valsalva

33702 **Repair sinus of Valsalva fistula, with cardiopulmonary bypass;**
44.8 44.8 FUD 090 C 80
AMA: 2018,Jan,8; 2017,Dec,3; 2017,Jan,8; 2016,Jan,13; 2015,Jan,16; 2014,Jan,11

33710 **with repair of ventricular septal defect**
59.6 59.6 FUD 090 C 80
AMA: 2017,Dec,3

33720 **Repair sinus of Valsalva aneurysm, with cardiopulmonary bypass**
44.9 44.9 FUD 090 C 80
AMA: 2017,Dec,3

33722 **Closure of aortico-left ventricular tunnel**
47.2 47.2 FUD 090 C 80
AMA: 2018,Jan,8; 2017,Dec,3; 2017,Jan,8; 2016,Jan,13; 2015,Jan,16; 2014,Jan,11

33724-33732 Repair Aberrant Pulmonary Venous Connection

33724 **Repair of isolated partial anomalous pulmonary venous return (eg, Scimitar Syndrome)**
EXCLUDES *Temporary pacemaker (33210-33211)*
Tube thoracostomy (32551)
44.2 44.2 FUD 090 C 80
AMA: 2018,Jan,8; 2017,Dec,3; 2017,Jan,8; 2016,Jan,13; 2015,Jan,16; 2014,Jan,11

33726 **Repair of pulmonary venous stenosis**
EXCLUDES *Temporary pacemaker (33210-33211)*
Tube thoracostomy (32551)
59.1 59.1 FUD 090 C 80
AMA: 2018,Jan,8; 2017,Dec,3; 2017,Jan,8; 2016,Jan,13; 2015,Jan,16; 2014,Jan,11

33730 **Complete repair of anomalous pulmonary venous return (supracardiac, intracardiac, or infracardiac types)**
EXCLUDES *Partial anomalous pulmonary venous return (33724)*
Repair of pulmonary venous stenosis (33726)
58.2 58.2 FUD 090 63 C 80
AMA: 2018,Jan,8; 2017,Dec,3; 2017,Jan,8; 2016,Jan,13; 2015,Jan,16; 2014,Jan,11

33732 **Repair of cor triatriatum or supravalvular mitral ring by resection of left atrial membrane**
47.8 47.8 FUD 090 63 C 80
AMA: 2018,Jan,8; 2017,Dec,3; 2017,Jan,8; 2016,Jan,13; 2015,Jan,16; 2014,Jan,11

33735-33737 Creation of Atrial Septal Defect

Code also the concurrent ligation/takedown of a systemic-to-pulmonary artery shunt (33924)

33735 Atrial septectomy or septostomy; closed heart (Blalock-Hanlon type operation)
37.5 37.5 FUD 090
AMA: 2018,Jan,8; 2017,Jan,8; 2016,Jan,13; 2015,Jan,16; 2014,Jan,11

33736 open heart with cardiopulmonary bypass
39.6 39.6 FUD 090
AMA: 2017,Dec,3

33737 open heart, with inflow occlusion
EXCLUDES *Atrial septectomy/septostomy:*
Blade method (92993)
Transvenous balloon method (92992)
37.6 37.6 FUD 090
AMA: 2007,Mar,1-3; 1997,Nov,1

33750-33767 Systemic Vessel to Pulmonary Artery Shunts

Code also the concurrent ligation/takedown of a systemic-to-pulmonary artery shunt (33924)

33750 Shunt; subclavian to pulmonary artery (Blalock-Taussig type operation)
36.6 36.6 FUD 090
AMA: 2017,Dec,3

33755 ascending aorta to pulmonary artery (Waterston type operation)
38.1 38.1 FUD 090
AMA: 2017,Dec,3

33762 descending aorta to pulmonary artery (Potts-Smith type operation)
37.2 37.2 FUD 090
AMA: 2017,Dec,3

33764 central, with prosthetic graft
38.1 38.1 FUD 090
AMA: 2017,Dec,3

33766 superior vena cava to pulmonary artery for flow to 1 lung (classical Glenn procedure)
38.6 38.6 FUD 090
AMA: 2017,Dec,3

33767 superior vena cava to pulmonary artery for flow to both lungs (bidirectional Glenn procedure)
41.3 41.3 FUD 090
AMA: 2018,Jan,8; 2017,Dec,3; 2017,Jan,8; 2016,Jul,3

33768 Cavopulmonary Anastomosis to Decrease Volume Load

EXCLUDES *Temporary pacemaker (33210-33211)*
Tube thoracostomy (32551)

Code first (33478, 33617, 33622, 33767)

+ **33768 Anastomosis, cavopulmonary, second superior vena cava (List separately in addition to primary procedure)**
12.1 12.1 FUD ZZZ
AMA: 2018,Jan,8; 2017,Jan,8; 2016,Jul,3; 2016,Jan,13; 2015,Jan,16; 2014,Jan,11

33770-33783 Repair Aberrant Anatomy: Transposition Great Vessels

Code also the concurrent ligation/takedown of a systemic-to-pulmonary artery shunt (33924)

33770 Repair of transposition of the great arteries with ventricular septal defect and subpulmonary stenosis; without surgical enlargement of ventricular septal defect
61.5 61.5 FUD 090
AMA: 2018,Jan,8; 2017,Dec,3; 2017,Jan,8; 2016,Jan,13; 2015,Jan,16; 2014,Jan,11

33771 with surgical enlargement of ventricular septal defect
63.3 63.3 FUD 090
AMA: 2017,Dec,3

33774 Repair of transposition of the great arteries, atrial baffle procedure (eg, Mustard or Senning type) with cardiopulmonary bypass;
52.2 52.2 FUD 090
AMA: 2017,Dec,3

33775 with removal of pulmonary band
53.8 53.8 FUD 090
AMA: 2017,Dec,3

33776 with closure of ventricular septal defect
56.9 56.9 FUD 090
AMA: 2017,Dec,3

33777 with repair of subpulmonic obstruction
54.9 54.9 FUD 090
AMA: 2017,Dec,3

33778 Repair of transposition of the great arteries, aortic pulmonary artery reconstruction (eg, Jatene type);
68.3 68.3 FUD 090
AMA: 2017,Dec,3

33779 with removal of pulmonary band
67.6 67.6 FUD 090
AMA: 2017,Dec,3

33780 with closure of ventricular septal defect
68.9 68.9 FUD 090
AMA: 2017,Dec,3

33781 with repair of subpulmonic obstruction
67.3 67.3 FUD 090
AMA: 2018,Jan,8; 2017,Dec,3; 2017,Jan,8; 2016,Jan,13; 2015,Jan,16; 2014,Jan,11

33782 Aortic root translocation with ventricular septal defect and pulmonary stenosis repair (ie, Nikaidoh procedure); without coronary ostium reimplantation
EXCLUDES *Closure of single ventricular septal defect (33681)*
Repair of complex cardiac anomaly other than pulmonary atresia (33608)
Repair of pulmonary atresia with ventricular septal defect (33920)
Repair of transposition of the great arteries (33770-33771, 33778, 33780)
Replacement, aortic valve (33412-33413)
94.0 94.0 FUD 090
AMA: 2017,Dec,3

33783 with reimplantation of 1 or both coronary ostia
101. 101. FUD 090
AMA: 2017,Dec,3

33786-33788 Repair Aberrant Anatomy: Truncus Arteriosus

33786 Total repair, truncus arteriosus (Rastelli type operation)
Code also the concurrent ligation/takedown of a systemic-to-pulmonary artery shunt (33924)
66.2 66.2 FUD 090
AMA: 2018,Jan,8; 2017,Dec,3; 2017,Jan,8; 2016,Jan,13; 2015,Jan,16; 2014,Jan,11

33788 Reimplantation of an anomalous pulmonary artery
EXCLUDES *Pulmonary artery banding (33690)*
44.5 44.5 FUD 090
AMA: 2018,Jan,8; 2017,Dec,3; 2017,Jan,8; 2016,Jan,13; 2015,Jan,16; 2014,Jan,11

33800-33853 Repair Aberrant Anatomy: Aorta

33800 Aortic suspension (aortopexy) for tracheal decompression (eg, for tracheomalacia) (separate procedure)
28.6 28.6 FUD 090
AMA: 2018,Jan,8; 2017,Jan,8; 2016,Jan,13; 2015,Jan,16; 2014,Jan,11

33802 Division of aberrant vessel (vascular ring);
31.4 31.4 FUD 090
AMA: 2017,Dec,3

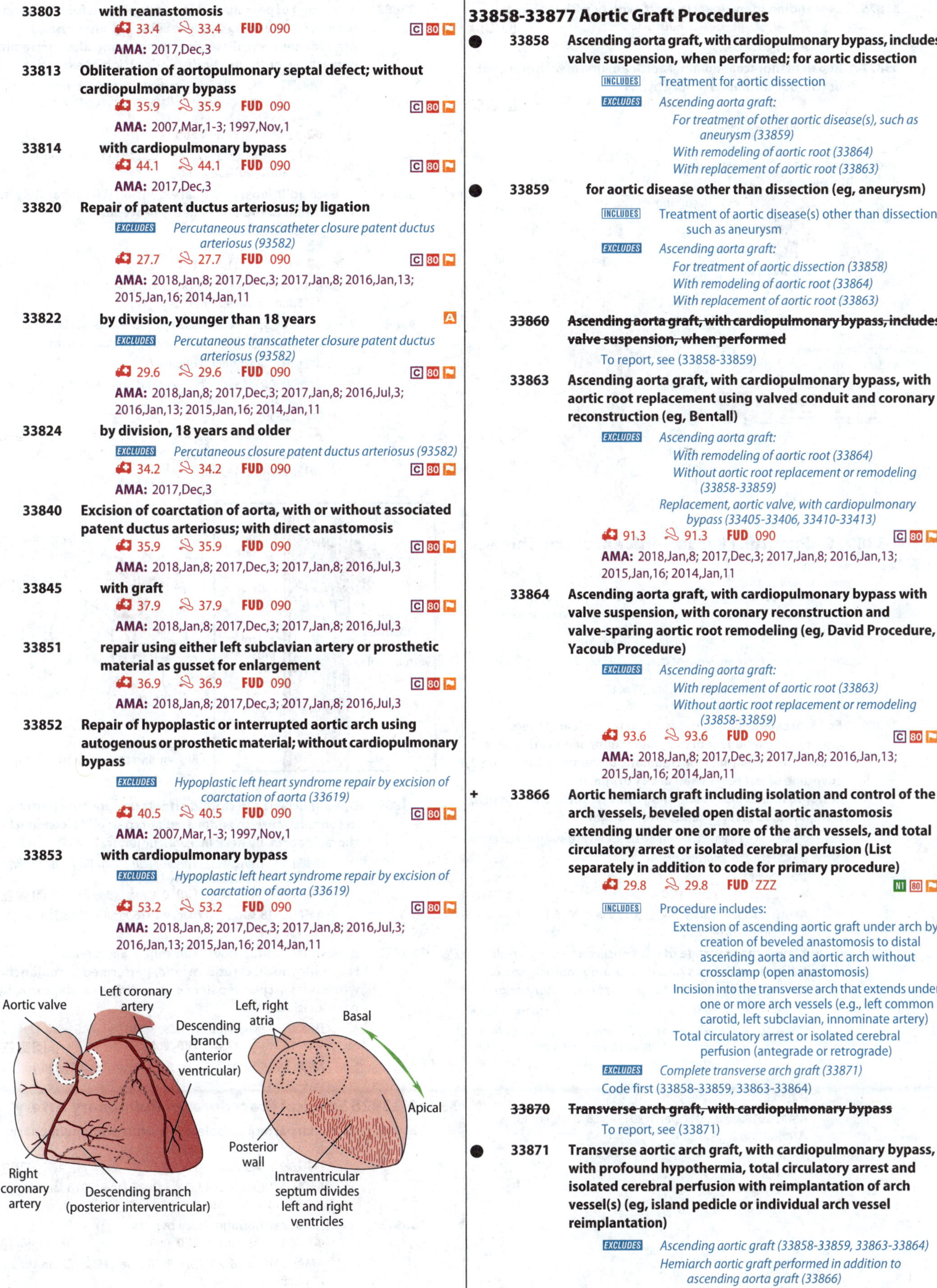

33803 **with reanastomosis**
33.4 33.4 **FUD** 090
AMA: 2017,Dec,3

33813 **Obliteration of aortopulmonary septal defect; without cardiopulmonary bypass**
35.9 35.9 **FUD** 090
AMA: 2007,Mar,1-3; 1997,Nov,1

33814 **with cardiopulmonary bypass**
44.1 44.1 **FUD** 090
AMA: 2017,Dec,3

33820 **Repair of patent ductus arteriosus; by ligation**
EXCLUDES *Percutaneous transcatheter closure patent ductus arteriosus (93582)*
27.7 27.7 **FUD** 090
AMA: 2018,Jan,8; 2017,Dec,3; 2017,Jan,8; 2016,Jan,13; 2015,Jan,16; 2014,Jan,11

33822 **by division, younger than 18 years**
EXCLUDES *Percutaneous transcatheter closure patent ductus arteriosus (93582)*
29.6 29.6 **FUD** 090
AMA: 2018,Jan,8; 2017,Dec,3; 2017,Jan,8; 2016,Jul,3; 2016,Jan,13; 2015,Jan,16; 2014,Jan,11

33824 **by division, 18 years and older**
EXCLUDES *Percutaneous closure patent ductus arteriosus (93582)*
34.2 34.2 **FUD** 090
AMA: 2017,Dec,3

33840 **Excision of coarctation of aorta, with or without associated patent ductus arteriosus; with direct anastomosis**
35.9 35.9 **FUD** 090
AMA: 2018,Jan,8; 2017,Dec,3; 2017,Jan,8; 2016,Jul,3

33845 **with graft**
37.9 37.9 **FUD** 090
AMA: 2018,Jan,8; 2017,Dec,3; 2017,Jan,8; 2016,Jul,3

33851 **repair using either left subclavian artery or prosthetic material as gusset for enlargement**
36.9 36.9 **FUD** 090
AMA: 2018,Jan,8; 2017,Dec,3; 2017,Jan,8; 2016,Jul,3

33852 **Repair of hypoplastic or interrupted aortic arch using autogenous or prosthetic material; without cardiopulmonary bypass**
EXCLUDES *Hypoplastic left heart syndrome repair by excision of coarctation of aorta (33619)*
40.5 40.5 **FUD** 090
AMA: 2007,Mar,1-3; 1997,Nov,1

33853 **with cardiopulmonary bypass**
EXCLUDES *Hypoplastic left heart syndrome repair by excision of coarctation of aorta (33619)*
53.2 53.2 **FUD** 090
AMA: 2018,Jan,8; 2017,Dec,3; 2017,Jan,8; 2016,Jul,3; 2016,Jan,13; 2015,Jan,16; 2014,Jan,11

33858-33877 Aortic Graft Procedures

● **33858** **Ascending aorta graft, with cardiopulmonary bypass, includes valve suspension, when performed; for aortic dissection**
INCLUDES Treatment for aortic dissection
EXCLUDES *Ascending aorta graft:*
For treatment of other aortic disease(s), such as aneurysm (33859)
With remodeling of aortic root (33864)
With replacement of aortic root (33863)

● **33859** **for aortic disease other than dissection (eg, aneurysm)**
INCLUDES Treatment of aortic disease(s) other than dissection, such as aneurysm
EXCLUDES *Ascending aorta graft:*
For treatment of aortic dissection (33858)
With remodeling of aortic root (33864)
With replacement of aortic root (33863)

33860 ~~**Ascending aorta graft, with cardiopulmonary bypass, includes valve suspension, when performed**~~
To report, see (33858-33859)

33863 **Ascending aorta graft, with cardiopulmonary bypass, with aortic root replacement using valved conduit and coronary reconstruction (eg, Bentall)**
EXCLUDES *Ascending aorta graft:*
With remodeling of aortic root (33864)
Without aortic root replacement or remodeling (33858-33859)
Replacement, aortic valve, with cardiopulmonary bypass (33405-33406, 33410-33413)
91.3 91.3 **FUD** 090
AMA: 2018,Jan,8; 2017,Dec,3; 2017,Jan,8; 2016,Jan,13; 2015,Jan,16; 2014,Jan,11

33864 **Ascending aorta graft, with cardiopulmonary bypass with valve suspension, with coronary reconstruction and valve-sparing aortic root remodeling (eg, David Procedure, Yacoub Procedure)**
EXCLUDES *Ascending aorta graft:*
With replacement of aortic root (33863)
Without aortic root replacement or remodeling (33858-33859)
93.6 93.6 **FUD** 090
AMA: 2018,Jan,8; 2017,Dec,3; 2017,Jan,8; 2016,Jan,13; 2015,Jan,16; 2014,Jan,11

+ **33866** **Aortic hemiarch graft including isolation and control of the arch vessels, beveled open distal aortic anastomosis extending under one or more of the arch vessels, and total circulatory arrest or isolated cerebral perfusion (List separately in addition to code for primary procedure)**
29.8 29.8 **FUD** ZZZ
INCLUDES Procedure includes:
Extension of ascending aortic graft under arch by creation of beveled anastomosis to distal ascending aorta and aortic arch without crossclamp (open anastomosis)
Incision into the transverse arch that extends under one or more arch vessels (e.g., left common carotid, left subclavian, innominate artery)
Total circulatory arrest or isolated cerebral perfusion (antegrade or retrograde)
EXCLUDES *Complete transverse arch graft (33871)*
Code first (33858-33859, 33863-33864)

33870 ~~**Transverse arch graft, with cardiopulmonary bypass**~~
To report, see (33871)

● **33871** **Transverse aortic arch graft, with cardiopulmonary bypass, with profound hypothermia, total circulatory arrest and isolated cerebral perfusion with reimplantation of arch vessel(s) (eg, island pedicle or individual arch vessel reimplantation)**
EXCLUDES *Ascending aortic graft (33858-33859, 33863-33864)*
Hemiarch aortic graft performed in addition to ascending aorta graft (33866)

33875 **Descending thoracic aorta graft, with or without bypass**
79.7 79.7 FUD 090 C 80
AMA: 2017,Dec,3

33877 **Repair of thoracoabdominal aortic aneurysm with graft, with or without cardiopulmonary bypass**
105. 105. FUD 090 C 80
AMA: 2017,Dec,3

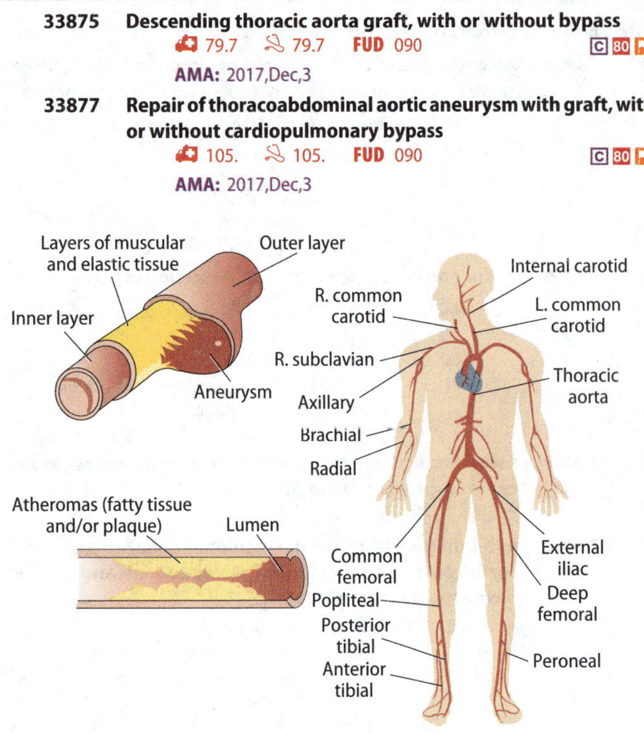

33880-33891 Endovascular Repair Aortic Aneurysm: Thoracic

INCLUDES Balloon angioplasty
Deployment of stent
Introduction, manipulation, placement, and deployment of the device

EXCLUDES *Additional interventional procedures provided during the endovascular repair*
Carotid-carotid bypass (33891)
Guidewire and catheter insertion (36140, 36200-36218)
Open exposure of artery/subsequent closure ([34812], 34714-34716 [34820, 34833, 34834])
Subclavian to carotid artery transposition (33889)
Substantial artery repair/replacement (35226, 35286)

33880 **Endovascular repair of descending thoracic aorta (eg, aneurysm, pseudoaneurysm, dissection, penetrating ulcer, intramural hematoma, or traumatic disruption); involving coverage of left subclavian artery origin, initial endoprosthesis plus descending thoracic aortic extension(s), if required, to level of celiac artery origin**
INCLUDES Placement of distal extensions in distal thoracic aorta
EXCLUDES *Proximal extensions*
(75956)
52.0 52.0 FUD 090 C 80
AMA: 2018,Jan,8; 2017,Dec,3; 2017,Jan,8; 2016,Jan,13; 2015,Jan,16; 2014,Jan,11

33881 **not involving coverage of left subclavian artery origin, initial endoprosthesis plus descending thoracic aortic extension(s), if required, to level of celiac artery origin**
INCLUDES Placement of distal extensions in distal thoracic aorta
EXCLUDES *Procedure where the placement of extension includes coverage of left subclavian artery origin (33880)*
Proximal extensions
(75957)
44.6 44.6 FUD 090 C 80
AMA: 2018,Jan,8; 2017,Dec,3; 2017,Jan,8; 2016,Jan,13; 2015,Jan,16; 2014,Jan,11

33883 **Placement of proximal extension prosthesis for endovascular repair of descending thoracic aorta (eg, aneurysm, pseudoaneurysm, dissection, penetrating ulcer, intramural hematoma, or traumatic disruption); initial extension**
EXCLUDES *Procedure where the placement of extension includes coverage of left subclavian artery origin (33880)*
(75958)
32.3 32.3 FUD 090 C 80
AMA: 2018,Jan,8; 2017,Dec,3; 2017,Jan,8; 2016,Jan,13; 2015,Jan,16; 2014,Jan,11

\+ **33884** **each additional proximal extension (List separately in addition to code for primary procedure)**
Code first (33883)
(75958)
11.4 11.4 FUD ZZZ C 80
AMA: 2018,Jan,8; 2017,Dec,3; 2017,Jan,8; 2016,Jan,13; 2015,Jan,16; 2014,Jan,11

33886 **Placement of distal extension prosthesis(s) delayed after endovascular repair of descending thoracic aorta**
INCLUDES All modules deployed
EXCLUDES *Endovascular repair of descending thoracic aorta (33880, 33881)*
(75959)
27.7 27.7 FUD 090 C 80
AMA: 2018,Jan,8; 2017,Dec,3; 2017,Jan,8; 2016,Jan,13; 2015,Jan,16; 2014,Jan,11

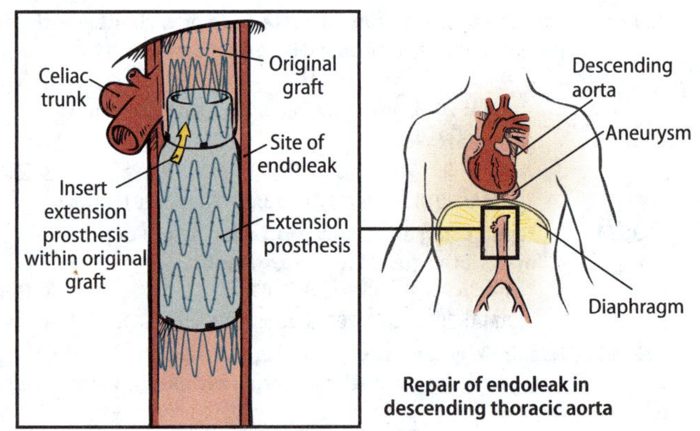

Repair of endoleak in descending thoracic aorta

33889 **Open subclavian to carotid artery transposition performed in conjunction with endovascular repair of descending thoracic aorta, by neck incision, unilateral**
EXCLUDES *Transposition and/or reimplantation; subclavian to carotid artery (35694)*
22.8 22.8 FUD 000 C 80 50
AMA: 2018,Jan,8; 2017,Jan,8; 2016,Jan,13; 2015,Jan,16; 2014,Jan,11

33891 **Bypass graft, with other than vein, transcervical retropharyngeal carotid-carotid, performed in conjunction with endovascular repair of descending thoracic aorta, by neck incision**
EXCLUDES *Bypass graft (35509, 35601)*
27.9 27.9 FUD 000 C 80 50
AMA: 2018,Jan,8; 2017,Jan,8; 2016,Jan,13; 2015,Jan,16; 2014,Jan,11

33910-33926 Surgical Procedures of Pulmonary Artery

33910 **Pulmonary artery embolectomy; with cardiopulmonary bypass**
76.2 76.2 FUD 090 C 80
AMA: 2018,Jan,8; 2017,Dec,3; 2017,Jan,8; 2016,Jan,13; 2015,Jan,16; 2014,Jan,11

33915 **without cardiopulmonary bypass**
40.1 40.1 FUD 090 C 80
AMA: 2018,Jan,8; 2017,Jan,8; 2016,Jan,13; 2015,Jan,16; 2014,Jan,11

33916 Pulmonary endarterectomy, with or without embolectomy, with cardiopulmonary bypass
123. 123. FUD 090 C 80
AMA: 2018,Jan,8; 2017,Dec,3; 2017,Jan,8; 2016,Jan,13; 2015,Jan,16; 2014,Jan,11

33917 Repair of pulmonary artery stenosis by reconstruction with patch or graft
Code also the concurrent ligation/takedown of a systemic-to-pulmonary artery shunt (33924)
42.2 42.2 FUD 090 C 80
AMA: 2018,Jan,8; 2017,Dec,3; 2017,Jan,8; 2016,Jul,3; 2016,Jan,13; 2015,Jan,16; 2014,Jan,11

33920 Repair of pulmonary atresia with ventricular septal defect, by construction or replacement of conduit from right or left ventricle to pulmonary artery
EXCLUDES *Repair of complicated cardiac anomalies by creating/replacing conduit from ventricle to pulmonary artery (33608)*
Code also the concurrent ligation/takedown of a systemic-to-pulmonary artery shunt (33924)
52.6 52.6 FUD 090 C 80
AMA: 2019,Apr,6; 2018,Jan,8; 2017,Dec,3; 2017,Jan,8; 2016,Jan,13; 2015,Jan,16; 2014,Jan,11

33922 Transection of pulmonary artery with cardiopulmonary bypass
Code also the concurrent ligation/takedown of a systemic-to-pulmonary artery shunt (33924)
40.2 40.2 FUD 090 63 C 80
AMA: 2017,Dec,3

\+ **33924 Ligation and takedown of a systemic-to-pulmonary artery shunt, performed in conjunction with a congenital heart procedure (List separately in addition to code for primary procedure)**
Code first (33470-33478, 33600-33617, 33622, 33684-33688, 33692-33697, 33735-33767, 33770-33783, 33786, 33917, 33920-33922, 33925-33926, 33935, 33945)
8.31 8.31 FUD ZZZ C 80
AMA: 1997,Nov,1; 1995,Win,1

33925 Repair of pulmonary artery arborization anomalies by unifocalization; without cardiopulmonary bypass
49.9 49.9 FUD 090 C 80
Code also the concurrent ligation/takedown of a systemic-to-pulmonary artery shunt (33924)

33926 with cardiopulmonary bypass
Code also the concurrent ligation/takedown of a systemic-to-pulmonary artery shunt (33924)
70.3 70.3 FUD 090 C 80
AMA: 2017,Dec,3

33927-33945 Heart and Heart-Lung Transplants

INCLUDES Backbench work to prepare the donor heart and/or lungs for transplantation (33933, 33944)
Harvesting of donor organs with cold preservation (33930, 33940)
Transplantation of heart and/or lungs into recipient (33935, 33945)

33927 Implantation of a total replacement heart system (artificial heart) with recipient cardiectomy
EXCLUDES *Implantation ventricular assist device:*
Extracorporeal (33975-33976)
Intracorporeal (33979)
Percutaneous (33990-33991)
74.2 74.2 FUD XXX C 80
AMA: 2018,Jun,3

33928 Removal and replacement of total replacement heart system (artificial heart)
EXCLUDES *Replacement or revision elements of artificial heart (33999)*
0.00 0.00 FUD XXX C 80
AMA: 2018,Jun,3

\+ **33929 Removal of a total replacement heart system (artificial heart) for heart transplantation (List separately in addition to code for primary procedure)**
Code first (33945)
0.00 0.00 FUD ZZZ C 80
AMA: 2018,Jun,3

33930 Donor cardiectomy-pneumonectomy (including cold preservation)
0.00 0.00 FUD XXX C
AMA: 1997,Nov,1

33933 Backbench standard preparation of cadaver donor heart/lung allograft prior to transplantation, including dissection of allograft from surrounding soft tissues to prepare aorta, superior vena cava, inferior vena cava, and trachea for implantation
0.00 0.00 FUD XXX C 80
AMA: 1997,Nov,1

33935 Heart-lung transplant with recipient cardiectomy-pneumonectomy
Code also the concurrent ligation/takedown of a systemic-to-pulmonary artery shunt (33924)
143. 143. FUD 090 C 80
AMA: 2017,Dec,3

33940 Donor cardiectomy (including cold preservation)
0.00 0.00 FUD XXX C
AMA: 2018,Jan,8; 2017,Jan,8; 2016,Jan,13; 2015,Jan,16; 2014,Jan,11

33944 Backbench standard preparation of cadaver donor heart allograft prior to transplantation, including dissection of allograft from surrounding soft tissues to prepare aorta, superior vena cava, inferior vena cava, pulmonary artery, and left atrium for implantation
EXCLUDES *Procedures performed on donor heart (33300, 33310, 33320, 33390, 33463-33464, 33510, 33641, 35216, 35276, 35685)*
0.00 0.00 FUD XXX C 80
AMA: 1997,Nov,1

33945 Heart transplant, with or without recipient cardiectomy
Code also the concurrent ligation/takedown of a systemic-to-pulmonary artery shunt (33924)
141. 141. FUD 090 C 80
AMA: 2018,Jun,3; 2017,Dec,3

33946-33989 [33962, 33963, 33964, 33965, 33966, 33969, 33984, 33985, 33986, 33987, 33988, 33989] Extracorporeal Circulatory and Respiratory Support

INCLUDES Cannula repositioning and cannula insertion performed during same procedure
Multiple physician and nonphysician team collaboration
Veno-arterial ECMO/ECLS for heart and lung support
Veno-venous ECMO/ECLS for lung support
Code also extensive arterial repair/replacement (35266, 35286, 35371, 35665)
Code also overall daily management services needed to manage a patient; report the appropriate observation, hospital inpatient, or critical care E/M codes

33946 Extracorporeal membrane oxygenation (ECMO)/extracorporeal life support (ECLS) provided by physician; initiation, veno-venous
EXCLUDES *Daily ECMO/ECLS veno-venous management on day of initial service (33948)*
Repositioning of ECMO/ECLS cannula on day of initial service (33957-33959 [33962, 33963, 33964])
Code also cannula insertion (33951-33956)
8.99 8.99 FUD XXX 63 C
AMA: 2018,Jan,8; 2017,Jan,8; 2016,Mar,5; 2016,Jan,13; 2015,Jul,3

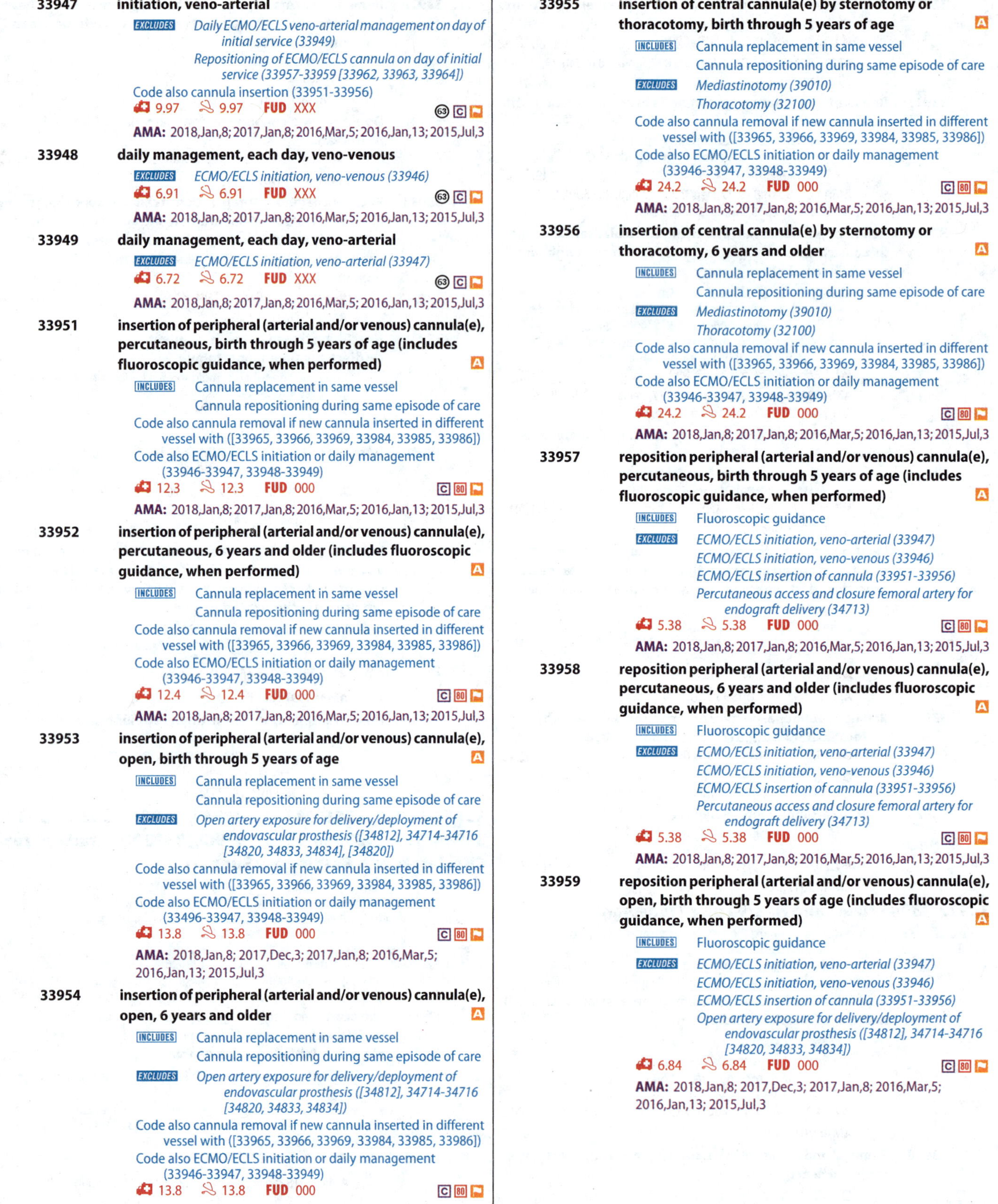

33947 **initiation, veno-arterial**

EXCLUDES *Daily ECMO/ECLS veno-arterial management on day of initial service (33949)*
Repositioning of ECMO/ECLS cannula on day of initial service (33957-33959 [33962, 33963, 33964])

Code also cannula insertion (33951-33956)

9.97 9.97 FUD XXX 63 C

AMA: 2018,Jan,8; 2017,Jan,8; 2016,Mar,5; 2016,Jan,13; 2015,Jul,3

33948 **daily management, each day, veno-venous**

EXCLUDES *ECMO/ECLS initiation, veno-venous (33946)*

6.91 6.91 FUD XXX 63 C

AMA: 2018,Jan,8; 2017,Jan,8; 2016,Mar,5; 2016,Jan,13; 2015,Jul,3

33949 **daily management, each day, veno-arterial**

EXCLUDES *ECMO/ECLS initiation, veno-arterial (33947)*

6.72 6.72 FUD XXX 63 C

AMA: 2018,Jan,8; 2017,Jan,8; 2016,Mar,5; 2016,Jan,13; 2015,Jul,3

33951 **insertion of peripheral (arterial and/or venous) cannula(e), percutaneous, birth through 5 years of age (includes fluoroscopic guidance, when performed)** A

INCLUDES Cannula replacement in same vessel
Cannula repositioning during same episode of care

Code also cannula removal if new cannula inserted in different vessel with ([33965, 33966, 33969, 33984, 33985, 33986])

Code also ECMO/ECLS initiation or daily management (33946-33947, 33948-33949)

12.3 12.3 FUD 000 C 80

AMA: 2018,Jan,8; 2017,Jan,8; 2016,Mar,5; 2016,Jan,13; 2015,Jul,3

33952 **insertion of peripheral (arterial and/or venous) cannula(e), percutaneous, 6 years and older (includes fluoroscopic guidance, when performed)** A

INCLUDES Cannula replacement in same vessel
Cannula repositioning during same episode of care

Code also cannula removal if new cannula inserted in different vessel with ([33965, 33966, 33969, 33984, 33985, 33986])

Code also ECMO/ECLS initiation or daily management (33946-33947, 33948-33949)

12.4 12.4 FUD 000 C 80

AMA: 2018,Jan,8; 2017,Jan,8; 2016,Mar,5; 2016,Jan,13; 2015,Jul,3

33953 **insertion of peripheral (arterial and/or venous) cannula(e), open, birth through 5 years of age** A

INCLUDES Cannula replacement in same vessel
Cannula repositioning during same episode of care

EXCLUDES *Open artery exposure for delivery/deployment of endovascular prosthesis ([34812], 34714-34716 [34820, 34833, 34834], [34820])*

Code also cannula removal if new cannula inserted in different vessel with ([33965, 33966, 33969, 33984, 33985, 33986])

Code also ECMO/ECLS initiation or daily management (33496-33947, 33948-33949)

13.8 13.8 FUD 000 C 80

AMA: 2018,Jan,8; 2017,Dec,3; 2017,Jan,8; 2016,Mar,5; 2016,Jan,13; 2015,Jul,3

33954 **insertion of peripheral (arterial and/or venous) cannula(e), open, 6 years and older** A

INCLUDES Cannula replacement in same vessel
Cannula repositioning during same episode of care

EXCLUDES *Open artery exposure for delivery/deployment of endovascular prosthesis ([34812], 34714-34716 [34820, 34833, 34834])*

Code also cannula removal if new cannula inserted in different vessel with ([33965, 33966, 33969, 33984, 33985, 33986])

Code also ECMO/ECLS initiation or daily management (33946-33947, 33948-33949)

13.8 13.8 FUD 000 C 80

AMA: 2018,Jan,8; 2017,Dec,3; 2017,Jan,8; 2016,Mar,5; 2016,Jan,13; 2015,Jul,3

33955 **insertion of central cannula(e) by sternotomy or thoracotomy, birth through 5 years of age** A

INCLUDES Cannula replacement in same vessel
Cannula repositioning during same episode of care

EXCLUDES *Mediastinotomy (39010)*
Thoracotomy (32100)

Code also cannula removal if new cannula inserted in different vessel with ([33965, 33966, 33969, 33984, 33985, 33986])

Code also ECMO/ECLS initiation or daily management (33946-33947, 33948-33949)

24.2 24.2 FUD 000 C 80

AMA: 2018,Jan,8; 2017,Jan,8; 2016,Mar,5; 2016,Jan,13; 2015,Jul,3

33956 **insertion of central cannula(e) by sternotomy or thoracotomy, 6 years and older** A

INCLUDES Cannula replacement in same vessel
Cannula repositioning during same episode of care

EXCLUDES *Mediastinotomy (39010)*
Thoracotomy (32100)

Code also cannula removal if new cannula inserted in different vessel with ([33965, 33966, 33969, 33984, 33985, 33986])

Code also ECMO/ECLS initiation or daily management (33946-33947, 33948-33949)

24.2 24.2 FUD 000 C 80

AMA: 2018,Jan,8; 2017,Jan,8; 2016,Mar,5; 2016,Jan,13; 2015,Jul,3

33957 **reposition peripheral (arterial and/or venous) cannula(e), percutaneous, birth through 5 years of age (includes fluoroscopic guidance, when performed)** A

INCLUDES Fluoroscopic guidance

EXCLUDES *ECMO/ECLS initiation, veno-arterial (33947)*
ECMO/ECLS initiation, veno-venous (33946)
ECMO/ECLS insertion of cannula (33951-33956)
Percutaneous access and closure femoral artery for endograft delivery (34713)

5.38 5.38 FUD 000 C 80

AMA: 2018,Jan,8; 2017,Jan,8; 2016,Mar,5; 2016,Jan,13; 2015,Jul,3

33958 **reposition peripheral (arterial and/or venous) cannula(e), percutaneous, 6 years and older (includes fluoroscopic guidance, when performed)** A

INCLUDES Fluoroscopic guidance

EXCLUDES *ECMO/ECLS initiation, veno-arterial (33947)*
ECMO/ECLS initiation, veno-venous (33946)
ECMO/ECLS insertion of cannula (33951-33956)
Percutaneous access and closure femoral artery for endograft delivery (34713)

5.38 5.38 FUD 000 C 80

AMA: 2018,Jan,8; 2017,Jan,8; 2016,Mar,5; 2016,Jan,13; 2015,Jul,3

33959 **reposition peripheral (arterial and/or venous) cannula(e), open, birth through 5 years of age (includes fluoroscopic guidance, when performed)** A

INCLUDES Fluoroscopic guidance

EXCLUDES *ECMO/ECLS initiation, veno-arterial (33947)*
ECMO/ECLS initiation, veno-venous (33946)
ECMO/ECLS insertion of cannula (33951-33956)
Open artery exposure for delivery/deployment of endovascular prosthesis ([34812], 34714-34716 [34820, 34833, 34834])

6.84 6.84 FUD 000 C 80

AMA: 2018,Jan,8; 2017,Dec,3; 2017,Jan,8; 2016,Mar,5; 2016,Jan,13; 2015,Jul,3

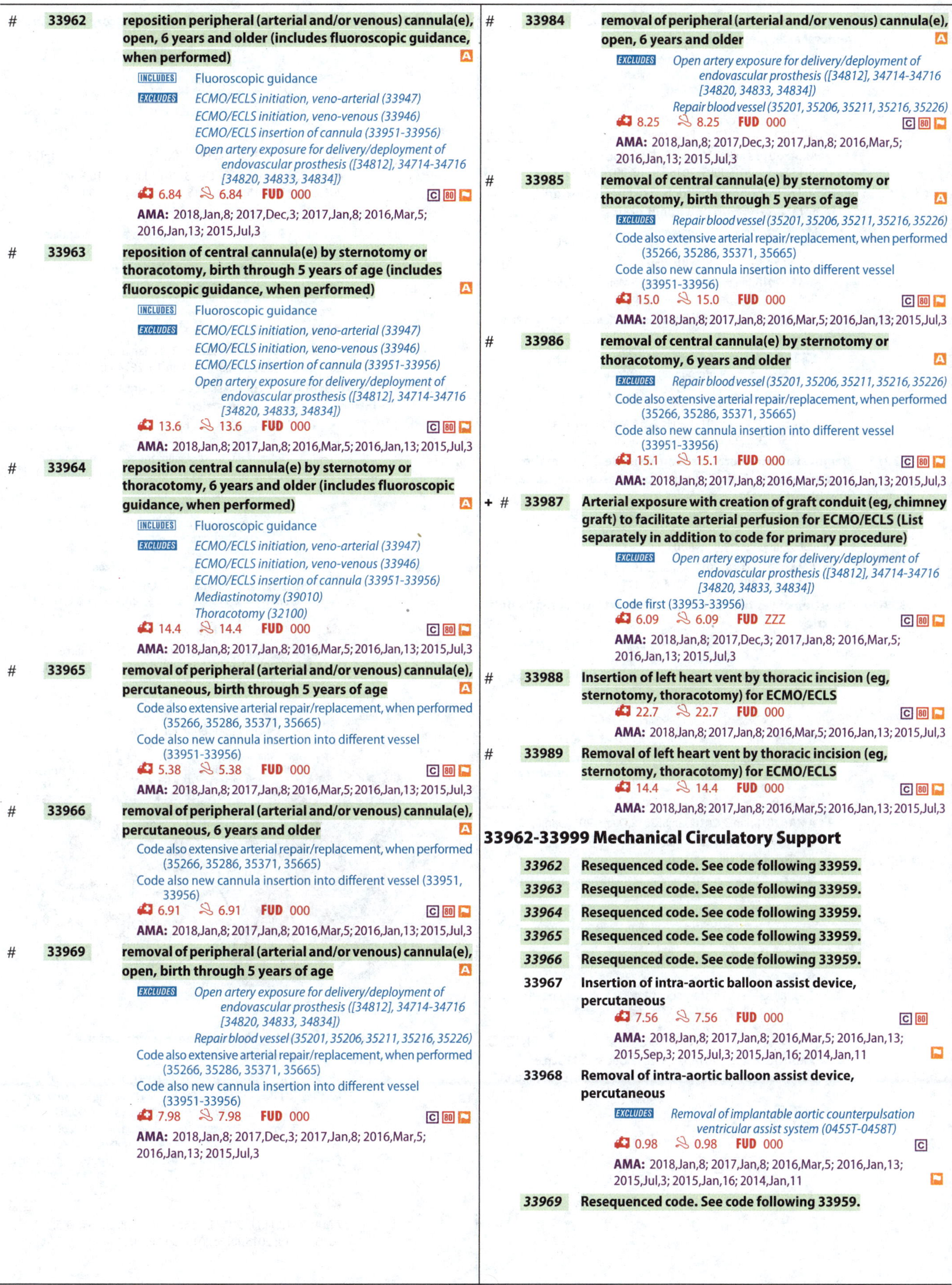

\# **33962** **reposition peripheral (arterial and/or venous) cannula(e), open, 6 years and older (includes fluoroscopic guidance, when performed)** A

INCLUDES Fluoroscopic guidance

EXCLUDES *ECMO/ECLS initiation, veno-arterial (33947)*
ECMO/ECLS initiation, veno-venous (33946)
ECMO/ECLS insertion of cannula (33951-33956)
Open artery exposure for delivery/deployment of endovascular prosthesis ([34812], 34714-34716 [34820, 34833, 34834])

6.84 6.84 FUD 000

AMA: 2018,Jan,8; 2017,Dec,3; 2017,Jan,8; 2016,Mar,5; 2016,Jan,13; 2015,Jul,3

\# **33963** **reposition of central cannula(e) by sternotomy or thoracotomy, birth through 5 years of age (includes fluoroscopic guidance, when performed)** A

INCLUDES Fluoroscopic guidance

EXCLUDES *ECMO/ECLS initiation, veno-arterial (33947)*
ECMO/ECLS initiation, veno-venous (33946)
ECMO/ECLS insertion of cannula (33951-33956)
Open artery exposure for delivery/deployment of endovascular prosthesis ([34812], 34714-34716 [34820, 34833, 34834])

13.6 13.6 FUD 000

AMA: 2018,Jan,8; 2017,Jan,8; 2016,Mar,5; 2016,Jan,13; 2015,Jul,3

\# **33964** **reposition central cannula(e) by sternotomy or thoracotomy, 6 years and older (includes fluoroscopic guidance, when performed)** A

INCLUDES Fluoroscopic guidance

EXCLUDES *ECMO/ECLS initiation, veno-arterial (33947)*
ECMO/ECLS initiation, veno-venous (33946)
ECMO/ECLS insertion of cannula (33951-33956)
Mediastinotomy (39010)
Thoracotomy (32100)

14.4 14.4 FUD 000

AMA: 2018,Jan,8; 2017,Jan,8; 2016,Mar,5; 2016,Jan,13; 2015,Jul,3

\# **33965** **removal of peripheral (arterial and/or venous) cannula(e), percutaneous, birth through 5 years of age** A

Code also extensive arterial repair/replacement, when performed (35266, 35286, 35371, 35665)
Code also new cannula insertion into different vessel (33951-33956)

5.38 5.38 FUD 000

AMA: 2018,Jan,8; 2017,Jan,8; 2016,Mar,5; 2016,Jan,13; 2015,Jul,3

\# **33966** **removal of peripheral (arterial and/or venous) cannula(e), percutaneous, 6 years and older** A

Code also extensive arterial repair/replacement, when performed (35266, 35286, 35371, 35665)
Code also new cannula insertion into different vessel (33951, 33956)

6.91 6.91 FUD 000

AMA: 2018,Jan,8; 2017,Jan,8; 2016,Mar,5; 2016,Jan,13; 2015,Jul,3

\# **33969** **removal of peripheral (arterial and/or venous) cannula(e), open, birth through 5 years of age** A

EXCLUDES *Open artery exposure for delivery/deployment of endovascular prosthesis ([34812], 34714-34716 [34820, 34833, 34834])*
Repair blood vessel (35201, 35206, 35211, 35216, 35226)

Code also extensive arterial repair/replacement, when performed (35266, 35286, 35371, 35665)
Code also new cannula insertion into different vessel (33951-33956)

7.98 7.98 FUD 000

AMA: 2018,Jan,8; 2017,Dec,3; 2017,Jan,8; 2016,Mar,5; 2016,Jan,13; 2015,Jul,3

\# **33984** **removal of peripheral (arterial and/or venous) cannula(e), open, 6 years and older** A

EXCLUDES *Open artery exposure for delivery/deployment of endovascular prosthesis ([34812], 34714-34716 [34820, 34833, 34834])*
Repair blood vessel (35201, 35206, 35211, 35216, 35226)

8.25 8.25 FUD 000

AMA: 2018,Jan,8; 2017,Dec,3; 2017,Jan,8; 2016,Mar,5; 2016,Jan,13; 2015,Jul,3

\# **33985** **removal of central cannula(e) by sternotomy or thoracotomy, birth through 5 years of age** A

EXCLUDES *Repair blood vessel (35201, 35206, 35211, 35216, 35226)*

Code also extensive arterial repair/replacement, when performed (35266, 35286, 35371, 35665)
Code also new cannula insertion into different vessel (33951-33956)

15.0 15.0 FUD 000

AMA: 2018,Jan,8; 2017,Jan,8; 2016,Mar,5; 2016,Jan,13; 2015,Jul,3

\# **33986** **removal of central cannula(e) by sternotomy or thoracotomy, 6 years and older** A

EXCLUDES *Repair blood vessel (35201, 35206, 35211, 35216, 35226)*

Code also extensive arterial repair/replacement, when performed (35266, 35286, 35371, 35665)
Code also new cannula insertion into different vessel (33951-33956)

15.1 15.1 FUD 000

AMA: 2018,Jan,8; 2017,Jan,8; 2016,Mar,5; 2016,Jan,13; 2015,Jul,3

\+ # **33987** **Arterial exposure with creation of graft conduit (eg, chimney graft) to facilitate arterial perfusion for ECMO/ECLS (List separately in addition to code for primary procedure)**

EXCLUDES *Open artery exposure for delivery/deployment of endovascular prosthesis ([34812], 34714-34716 [34820, 34833, 34834])*

Code first (33953-33956)

6.09 6.09 FUD ZZZ

AMA: 2018,Jan,8; 2017,Dec,3; 2017,Jan,8; 2016,Mar,5; 2016,Jan,13; 2015,Jul,3

\# **33988** **Insertion of left heart vent by thoracic incision (eg, sternotomy, thoracotomy) for ECMO/ECLS**

22.7 22.7 FUD 000

AMA: 2018,Jan,8; 2017,Jan,8; 2016,Mar,5; 2016,Jan,13; 2015,Jul,3

\# **33989** **Removal of left heart vent by thoracic incision (eg, sternotomy, thoracotomy) for ECMO/ECLS**

14.4 14.4 FUD 000

AMA: 2018,Jan,8; 2017,Jan,8; 2016,Mar,5; 2016,Jan,13; 2015,Jul,3

33962-33999 Mechanical Circulatory Support

33962 **Resequenced code. See code following 33959.**

33963 **Resequenced code. See code following 33959.**

33964 **Resequenced code. See code following 33959.**

33965 **Resequenced code. See code following 33959.**

33966 **Resequenced code. See code following 33959.**

33967 **Insertion of intra-aortic balloon assist device, percutaneous**

7.56 7.56 FUD 000

AMA: 2018,Jan,8; 2017,Jan,8; 2016,Mar,5; 2016,Jan,13; 2015,Sep,3; 2015,Jul,3; 2015,Jan,16; 2014,Jan,11

33968 **Removal of intra-aortic balloon assist device, percutaneous**

EXCLUDES *Removal of implantable aortic counterpulsation ventricular assist system (0455T-0458T)*

0.98 0.98 FUD 000

AMA: 2018,Jan,8; 2017,Jan,8; 2016,Mar,5; 2016,Jan,13; 2015,Jul,3; 2015,Jan,16; 2014,Jan,11

33969 **Resequenced code. See code following 33959.**

33970 Insertion of intra-aortic balloon assist device through the femoral artery, open approach

EXCLUDES *Insertion/replacement implantable aortic counterpulsation ventricular assist system (0451T-0454T)*

Percutaneous insertion of intra-aortic balloon assist device (33967)

10.2 10.2 FUD 000 C 80

AMA: 2018,Jan,8; 2017,Jan,8; 2016,Mar,5; 2016,Jan,13; 2015,Sep,3; 2015,Jul,3; 2015,Jan,16; 2014,Jan,11

33971 Removal of intra-aortic balloon assist device including repair of femoral artery, with or without graft

EXCLUDES *Removal of implantable aortic counterpulsation ventricular assist system (0455T-0458T)*

20.5 20.5 FUD 090 C

AMA: 2018,Jan,8; 2017,Jan,8; 2016,Mar,5; 2016,Jan,13; 2015,Jul,3; 2015,Jan,16; 2014,Jan,11

33973 Insertion of intra-aortic balloon assist device through the ascending aorta

EXCLUDES *Insertion/replacement of implantable aortic counterpulsation ventricular assist system (0451T-0454T)*

15.0 15.0 FUD 000 C 80

AMA: 2018,Jan,8; 2017,Jan,8; 2016,Mar,5; 2016,Jan,13; 2015,Sep,3; 2015,Jul,3; 2015,Jan,16; 2014,Jan,11

33974 Removal of intra-aortic balloon assist device from the ascending aorta, including repair of the ascending aorta, with or without graft

EXCLUDES *Removal of implantable aortic counterpulsation ventricular assist system (0455T-0458T)*

25.8 25.8 FUD 090 C

AMA: 2018,Jan,8; 2017,Jan,8; 2016,Mar,5; 2016,Jan,13; 2015,Jul,3; 2015,Jan,16; 2014,Jan,11

33975 Insertion of ventricular assist device; extracorporeal, single ventricle

INCLUDES Insertion of the new pump with de-airing, connection, and initiation

Removal of the old pump with replacement of the entire ventricular assist device system, including pump(s) and cannulas

Transthoracic approach

EXCLUDES *Percutaneous approach (33990-33991)*

Code also removal of thrombus through a separate heart incision, when performed (33310-33315); append modifier 59 to (33315)

37.9 37.9 FUD XXX C 80

AMA: 2018,Jun,3; 2018,Jan,8; 2017,Dec,3; 2017,Jan,8; 2016,Mar,5; 2016,Jan,13; 2015,Jul,3; 2015,Jan,16; 2014,Jan,11

33976 extracorporeal, biventricular

INCLUDES Insertion of the new pump with de-airing, connection, and initiation

Removal with replacement of the entire ventricular assist device system, including pump(s) and cannulas

Transthoracic approach

EXCLUDES *Percutaneous approach (33990-33991)*

Code also removal of thrombus through a separate heart incision, when performed (33310-33315); append modifier 59 to (33315)

46.4 46.4 FUD XXX C 80

AMA: 2018,Jun,3; 2018,Jan,8; 2017,Dec,3; 2017,Jan,8; 2016,Mar,5; 2016,Jan,13; 2015,Jul,3; 2015,Jan,16; 2014,Jan,11

33977 Removal of ventricular assist device; extracorporeal, single ventricle

INCLUDES Removal of the entire device and the cannulas

EXCLUDES *Removal of ventricular assist device when performed at the same time of insertion of a new device*

Code also removal of thrombus through a separate heart incision, when performed (33310-33315); append modifier 59 to (33315)

32.6 32.6 FUD XXX C 80

AMA: 2018,Jan,8; 2017,Dec,3; 2017,Jan,8; 2016,Mar,5; 2016,Jan,13; 2015,Jul,3; 2015,Jan,16; 2014,Jan,11

33978 extracorporeal, biventricular

INCLUDES Removal of the entire device and the cannulas

EXCLUDES *Removal of ventricular assist device when performed at the same time of insertion of a new device*

Code also removal of thrombus through a separate heart incision, when performed (33310-33315); append modifier 59 to (33315)

38.8 38.8 FUD XXX C 80

AMA: 2018,Jan,8; 2017,Dec,3; 2017,Jan,8; 2016,Mar,5; 2016,Jan,13; 2015,Jul,3; 2015,Jan,16; 2014,Jan,11

33979 Insertion of ventricular assist device, implantable intracorporeal, single ventricle

INCLUDES New pump insertion with connection, de-airing, and initiation

Removal with replacement of the entire ventricular assist device system, including pump(s) and cannulas

Transthoracic approach

EXCLUDES *Insertion/replacement of implantable aortic counterpulsation ventricular assist system (0451T-0454T)*

Percutaneous approach (33990-33991)

Code also removal of thrombus through a separate heart incision, when performed (33310-33315); append modifier 59 to (33315)

56.6 56.6 FUD XXX C 80

AMA: 2018,Jun,3; 2018,Jan,8; 2017,Dec,3; 2017,Jan,8; 2016,Mar,5; 2016,Jan,13; 2015,Jul,3; 2015,Jan,16; 2014,Jan,11

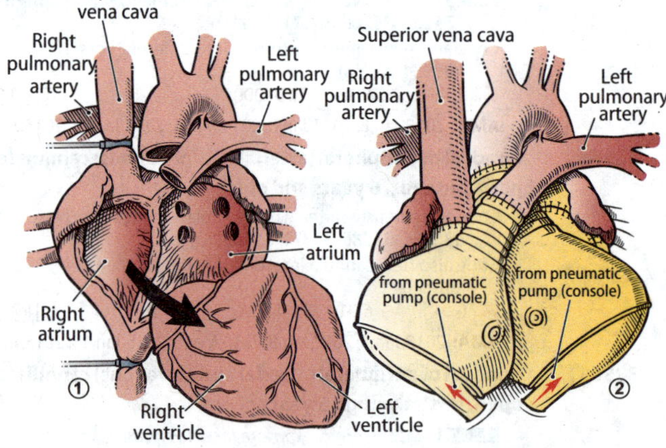

33980 Removal of ventricular assist device, implantable intracorporeal, single ventricle

INCLUDES Removal of the entire device and the cannulas

EXCLUDES *Removal of implantable aortic counterpulsation ventricular assist system (0455T-0458T)*

Removal of ventricular assist device when performed at the same time of insertion of a new device

Code also removal of thrombus through a separate heart incision, when performed (33310-33315); append modifier 59 to (33315)

51.8 51.8 FUD XXX C 80

AMA: 2018,Jan,8; 2017,Dec,3; 2017,Jan,8; 2016,Mar,5; 2016,Jan,13; 2015,Jul,3; 2015,Jan,16; 2014,Jan,11

33981 Replacement of extracorporeal ventricular assist device, single or biventricular, pump(s), single or each pump

INCLUDES Insertion of the new pump with de-airing, connection, and initiation
Removal of the old pump

24.3 24.3 FUD XXX C 80

AMA: 2018,Jan,8; 2017,Jan,8; 2016,Mar,5; 2016,Jan,13; 2015,Jul,3; 2015,Jan,16; 2014,Jan,11

33982 Replacement of ventricular assist device pump(s); implantable intracorporeal, single ventricle, without cardiopulmonary bypass

INCLUDES New pump insertion with connection, de-airing, and initiation
Removal of the old pump

57.1 57.1 FUD XXX C 80

AMA: 2018,Jan,8; 2017,Jan,8; 2016,Mar,5; 2016,Jan,13; 2015,Jul,3; 2015,Jan,16; 2014,Jan,11

33983 implantable intracorporeal, single ventricle, with cardiopulmonary bypass

INCLUDES Removal of the old pump

EXCLUDES *Insertion/replacement of implantable aortic counterpulsation ventricular assist system (0451T-0454T)*
Percutaneous transseptal approach (33999)

67.1 67.1 FUD XXX C 80

AMA: 2018,Jan,8; 2017,Dec,3; 2017,Jan,8; 2016,Mar,5; 2016,Jan,13; 2015,Jul,3; 2015,Jan,16; 2014,Jan,11

***33984* Resequenced code. See code following 33959.**

***33985* Resequenced code. See code following 33959.**

***33986* Resequenced code. See code following 33959.**

***33987* Resequenced code. See code following 33959.**

***33988* Resequenced code. See code following 33959.**

***33989* Resequenced code. See code following 33959.**

33990 Insertion of ventricular assist device, percutaneous including radiological supervision and interpretation; arterial access only

INCLUDES Initial insertion and replacement of percutaneous ventricular assist device

EXCLUDES *Extensive artery repair/replacement (35226, 35286)*
Insertion/replacement of implantable aortic counterpulsation ventricular assist system (0451T-0454T)
Open arterial approach to aid insertion of percutaneous ventricular assist device, when used ([34812], 34714-34716 [34820, 34833, 34834], [34820])
Removal of percutaneous ventricular assist device at time of replacement of the entire system (33992)
Transthoracic approach (33975-33976)

12.4 12.4 FUD XXX C 80

AMA: 2018,Jun,3; 2018,Jan,8; 2017,Dec,3; 2017,Jan,8; 2016,Mar,5; 2016,Jan,13; 2015,Sep,3; 2015,Jan,16; 2014,Oct,14; 2014,Jan,11

33991 both arterial and venous access, with transseptal puncture

INCLUDES Initial insertion as well as replacement of percutaneous ventricular assist device

EXCLUDES *Extensive artery repair/replacement (35226, 35286)*
Insertion/replacement of implantable aortic counterpulsation ventricular assist system (0451T-0454T)
Open arterial approach to aid with insertion of percutaneous ventricular assist device, when performed ([34812], 34714-34716 [34820, 34833, 34834])
Removal of percutaneous ventricular assist device at time of replacement of the entire system (33992)
Transthoracic approach (33975-33976)

18.1 18.1 FUD XXX C 80

AMA: 2018,Jun,3; 2018,Jan,8; 2017,Dec,3; 2017,Jan,8; 2016,Mar,5; 2016,Jan,13; 2015,Sep,3; 2015,Jan,16; 2014,Jan,11

33992 Removal of percutaneous ventricular assist device at separate and distinct session from insertion

INCLUDES Removal of device and cannulas

EXCLUDES *Removal of implantable aortic counterpulsation ventricular assist system (0455T-0458T)*

Code also modifier 59 when percutaneous ventricular assist device is removed on the same day as the insertion, but at a different session

5.80 5.80 FUD XXX C 80

AMA: 2018,Jan,8; 2017,Jan,8; 2016,Mar,5; 2016,Jan,13; 2015,Sep,3; 2015,Jan,16; 2014,Jan,11

33993 Repositioning of percutaneous ventricular assist device with imaging guidance at separate and distinct session from insertion

EXCLUDES *Repositioning of a percutaneous ventricular assist device without image guidance*
Repositioning of device/electrode (0460T-0461T)
Repositioning of the percutaneous ventricular assist device at the same session as the insertion (33990-33991)
Skin pocket relocation with replacement implantable aortic counterpulsation ventricular assist device and electrodes (0459T)

Code also modifier 59 when percutaneous ventricular assist device is repositioned using imaging guidance on the same day as the insertion, but at a different session

5.09 5.09 FUD XXX C 80

AMA: 2018,Jan,8; 2017,Jan,8; 2016,Mar,5; 2016,Jan,13; 2015,Sep,3; 2015,Jan,16; 2014,Jan,11

33999 Unlisted procedure, cardiac surgery

0.00 0.00 FUD YYY T 80

AMA: 2019,Apr,10; 2019,Jan,14; 2018,Jun,3; 2018,Jan,8; 2017,Jan,8; 2016,May,5; 2016,Jan,13; 2015,Jan,16; 2014,Dec,16; 2014,Dec,16; 2014,Jan,11

34001-34530 Surgical Revascularization: Veins and Arteries

INCLUDES Repair of blood vessel
Surgeon's component of operative arteriogram

34001 Embolectomy or thrombectomy, with or without catheter; carotid, subclavian or innominate artery, by neck incision

27.8 27.8 FUD 090 C 80 50

AMA: 1997,Nov,1

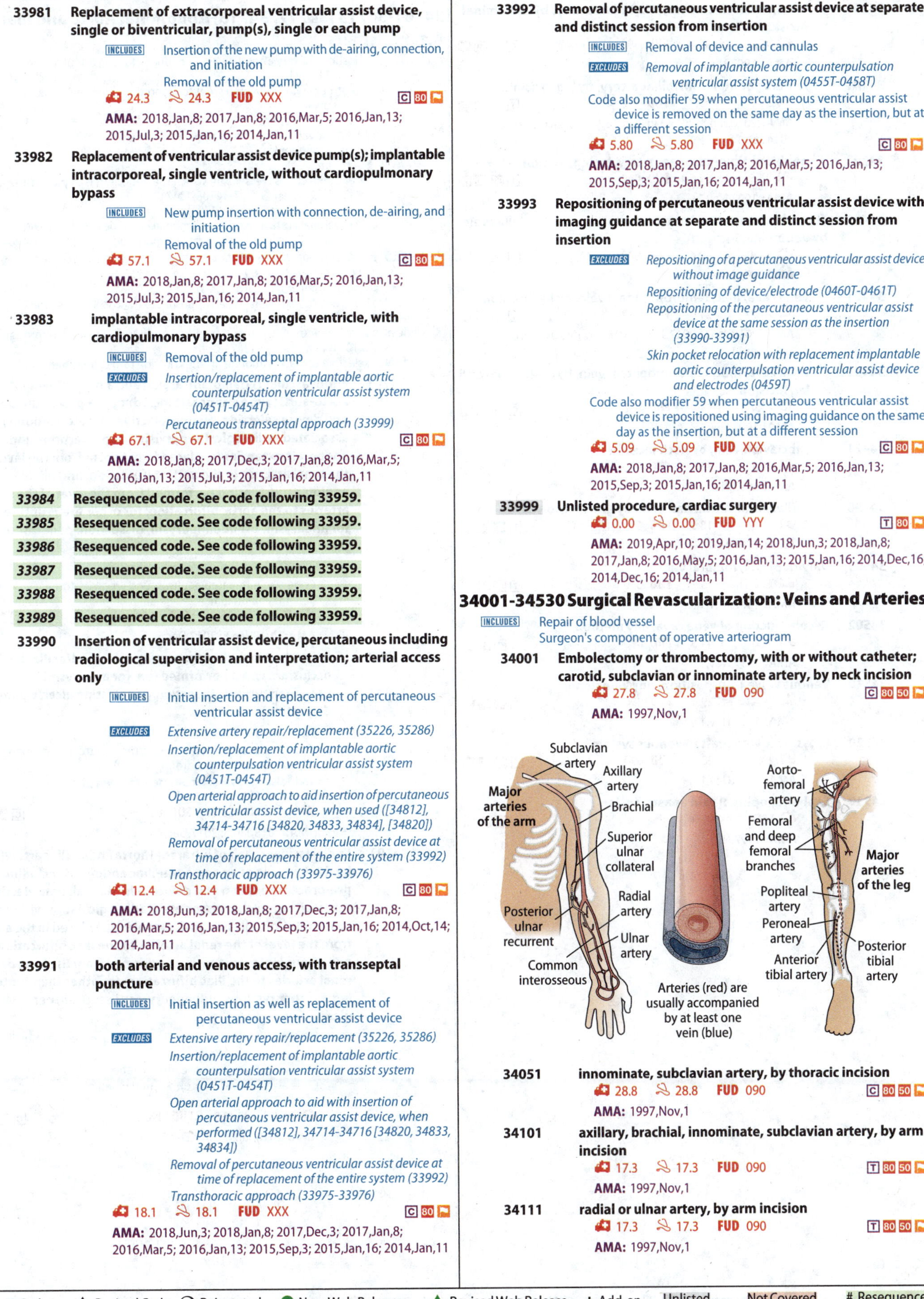

34051 innominate, subclavian artery, by thoracic incision

28.8 28.8 FUD 090 C 80 50

AMA: 1997,Nov,1

34101 axillary, brachial, innominate, subclavian artery, by arm incision

17.3 17.3 FUD 090 T 80 50

AMA: 1997,Nov,1

34111 radial or ulnar artery, by arm incision

17.3 17.3 FUD 090 T 80 50

AMA: 1997,Nov,1

● New Code ▲ Revised Code ○ Reinstated ● New Web Release ▲ Revised Web Release + Add-on Unlisted Not Covered # Resequenced
Optum Mod 50 Exempt AMA Mod 51 Exempt Optum Mod 51 Exempt Mod 63 Exempt Non-FDA Drug ★ Telemedicine M Maternity A Age Edit

34151 **renal, celiac, mesentery, aortoiliac artery, by abdominal incision**
40.4 40.4 FUD 090 C 80 50
AMA: 1997,Nov,1

34201 **femoropopliteal, aortoiliac artery, by leg incision**
29.7 29.7 FUD 090 T 80 50
AMA: 2018,Jan,8; 2017,Jan,8; 2016,Jan,13; 2015,Jan,16; 2014,Jan,11

34203 **popliteal-tibio-peroneal artery, by leg incision**
27.5 27.5 FUD 090 T 80 50
AMA: 1997,Nov,1

34401 **Thrombectomy, direct or with catheter; vena cava, iliac vein, by abdominal incision**
42.4 42.4 FUD 090 C 80 50
AMA: 1997,Nov,1

34421 **vena cava, iliac, femoropopliteal vein, by leg incision**
21.3 21.3 FUD 090 T 80 50
AMA: 2018,Jan,8; 2017,Jan,8; 2016,Jan,13; 2015,Jan,16; 2014,Jan,11

34451 **vena cava, iliac, femoropopliteal vein, by abdominal and leg incision**
41.4 41.4 FUD 090 C 80 50
AMA: 1997,Nov,1

34471 **subclavian vein, by neck incision**
31.1 31.1 FUD 090 T 50
AMA: 1997,Nov,1

34490 **axillary and subclavian vein, by arm incision**
18.5 18.5 FUD 090 T G2 50
AMA: 1997,Nov,1

34501 **Valvuloplasty, femoral vein**
25.7 25.7 FUD 090 T 80 50
AMA: 1997,Nov,1

34502 **Reconstruction of vena cava, any method**
44.6 44.6 FUD 090 C 80
AMA: 1997,Nov,1

34510 **Venous valve transposition, any vein donor**
29.4 29.4 FUD 090 T 80 50
AMA: 1997,Nov,1

34520 **Cross-over vein graft to venous system**
28.5 28.5 FUD 090 T 80 50
AMA: 1997,Nov,1

34530 **Saphenopopliteal vein anastomosis**
27.0 27.0 FUD 090 T 80 50
AMA: 1997,Nov,1

34701-34713 [34717, 34718] Abdominal Aorta and Iliac Artery Repairs

INCLUDES Closure of artery after delivery of endograft using a sheath size less than 12 French
Treatment with a covered stent for conditions such as:
- Aneurysm
- Aortic dissection
- Arteriovenous malformation
- Pseudoaneurysm
- Trauma

Treatment zones (vessel(s) in which the endograft is deployed):
- Iliac artery(ies) (34707-34708, [34717], [34718])
- Infrarenal aorta (34701-34702)
- Infrarenal aorta and both common iliac arteries (34705-34706)
- Infrarenal aorta and ipsilateral common iliac artery (34703-34704)

EXCLUDES *Treatment of atherosclerotic occlusive disease with covered stent:*
- *Aorta (37236-37237)*
- *Iliac artery(ies) (37221, 37223)*

Code also open arterial exposure, when appropriate ([34812], 34714 [34820, 34833, 34834], 34715-34716)
Code also percutaneous closure of artery when endograft is delivered through a sheath 12 French or larger (34713)
Code also selective catheterization of arteries outside target treatment zone

34701 **Endovascular repair of infrarenal aorta by deployment of an aorto-aortic tube endograft including pre-procedure sizing and device selection, all nonselective catheterization(s), all associated radiological supervision and interpretation, all endograft extension(s) placed in the aorta from the level of the renal arteries to the aortic bifurcation, and all angioplasty/stenting performed from the level of the renal arteries to the aortic bifurcation; for other than rupture (eg, for aneurysm, pseudoaneurysm, dissection, penetrating ulcer)**
INCLUDES Nonselective catheterization
Code also intravascular ultrasound when performed (37252-37253)
35.8 35.8 FUD 090 C 80
AMA: 2018,Jan,8; 2017,Dec,3

34702 **for rupture including temporary aortic and/or iliac balloon occlusion, when performed (eg, for aneurysm, pseudoaneurysm, dissection, penetrating ulcer, traumatic disruption)**
INCLUDES Nonselective catheterization
Code also decompressive laparotomy for treatment abdominal compartment syndrome (49000)
Code also intravascular ultrasound when performed (37252-37253)
53.5 53.5 FUD 090 C 80
AMA: 2018,Jan,8; 2017,Dec,3

34703 **Endovascular repair of infrarenal aorta and/or iliac artery(ies) by deployment of an aorto-uni-iliac endograft including pre-procedure sizing and device selection, all nonselective catheterization(s), all associated radiological supervision and interpretation, all endograft extension(s) placed in the aorta from the level of the renal arteries to the iliac bifurcation, and all angioplasty/stenting performed from the level of the renal arteries to the iliac bifurcation; for other than rupture (eg, for aneurysm, pseudoaneurysm, dissection, penetrating ulcer)**
INCLUDES Endograft extensions ending in the common iliac arteries
Nonselective catheterization
Code also intravascular ultrasound when performed (37252-37253)
40.3 40.3 FUD 090 C 80
AMA: 2018,Jan,8; 2017,Dec,3

34704 **for rupture including temporary aortic and/or iliac balloon occlusion, when performed (eg, for aneurysm, pseudoaneurysm, dissection, penetrating ulcer, traumatic disruption)**

INCLUDES Endograft extensions ending in the common iliac arteries
Nonselective catheterization

Code also decompressive laparotomy for treatment abdominal compartment syndrome (49000)

Code also intravascular ultrasound when performed (37252-37253)

67.2 67.2 FUD 090 C 80

AMA: 2018,Jan,8; 2017,Dec,3

34705 **Endovascular repair of infrarenal aorta and/or iliac artery(ies) by deployment of an aorto-bi-iliac endograft including pre-procedure sizing and device selection, all nonselective catheterization(s), all associated radiological supervision and interpretation, all endograft extension(s) placed in the aorta from the level of the renal arteries to the iliac bifurcation, and all angioplasty/stenting performed from the level of the renal arteries to the iliac bifurcation; for other than rupture (eg, for aneurysm, pseudoaneurysm, dissection, penetrating ulcer)**

INCLUDES Endograft extensions ending in the common iliac arteries
Nonselective catheterization

Code also intravascular ultrasound when performed (37252-37253)

44.3 44.3 FUD 090 C 80

AMA: 2018,Jan,8; 2017,Dec,3

34706 **for rupture including temporary aortic and/or iliac balloon occlusion, when performed (eg, for aneurysm, pseudoaneurysm, dissection, penetrating ulcer, traumatic disruption)**

INCLUDES Endograft extensions ending in the common iliac arteries
Nonselective catheterization

Code also decompressive laparotomy for treatment abdominal compartment syndrome (49000)

Code also intravascular ultrasound when performed (37252-37253)

66.8 66.8 FUD 090 C 80

AMA: 2018,Jan,8; 2017,Dec,3

34707 **Endovascular repair of iliac artery by deployment of an ilio-iliac tube endograft including pre-procedure sizing and device selection, all nonselective catheterization(s), all associated radiological supervision and interpretation, and all endograft extension(s) proximally to the aortic bifurcation and distally to the iliac bifurcation, and treatment zone angioplasty/stenting, when performed, unilateral; for other than rupture (eg, for aneurysm, pseudoaneurysm, dissection, arteriovenous malformation)**

INCLUDES Endograft extensions ending in the common iliac arteries
Nonselective catheterization

EXCLUDES *Deployment of iliac branched endograft:*
At the time of aorto-iliac graft placement ([34717])
Delayed/separate from aorto-iliac endograft deployment ([34718])

Code also intravascular ultrasound when performed (37252-37253)

33.4 33.4 FUD 090 C 80 50

AMA: 2018,Jan,8; 2017,Dec,3

34708 **for rupture including temporary aortic and/or iliac balloon occlusion, when performed (eg, for aneurysm, pseudoaneurysm, dissection, arteriovenous malformation, traumatic disruption)**

INCLUDES Endograft extensions ending in the common iliac arteries
Nonselective catheterization

EXCLUDES *Deployment of iliac branched endograft:*
At the time of aorto-iliac graft placement ([34717])
Delayed/separate from aorto-iliac endograft deployment ([34718])

Code also decompressive laparotomy for treatment abdominal compartment syndrome (49000)

Code also intravascular ultrasound when performed (37252-37253)

53.6 53.6 FUD 090 C 80 50

AMA: 2018,Jan,8; 2017,Dec,3

● + # **34717** **Endovascular repair of iliac artery at the time of aorto-iliac artery endograft placement by deployment of an iliac branched endograft including pre-procedure sizing and device selection, all ipsilateral selective iliac artery catheterization(s), all associated radiological supervision and interpretation, and all endograft extension(s) proximally to the aortic bifurcation and distally in the internal iliac, external iliac, and common femoral artery(ies), and treatment zone angioplasty/stenting, when performed, for rupture or other than rupture (eg, for aneurysm, pseudoaneurysm, dissection, arteriovenous malformation, penetrating ulcer, traumatic disruption), unilateral (List separately in addition to code for primary procedure)**

0.00 0.00 FUD 000 50

INCLUDES Endograft extensions into internal and external iliac, and/or common femoral arteries

EXCLUDES *Delayed deployment of branched iliac endograft, separate from aorto-iliac endograft placement ([34718])*
Placement of prosthesis extensions on same side (34709, 34710-34711)
Reporting with modifier 50. Report once for each side when performed bilaterally

Code first (34703-34706)

\+ **34709** **Placement of extension prosthesis(es) distal to the common iliac artery(ies) or proximal to the renal artery(ies) for endovascular repair of infrarenal abdominal aortic or iliac aneurysm, false aneurysm, dissection, penetrating ulcer, including pre-procedure sizing and device selection, all nonselective catheterization(s), all associated radiological supervision and interpretation, and treatment zone angioplasty/stenting, when performed, per vessel treated (List separately in addition to code for primary procedure)**

EXCLUDES *Placement of covered stent (37236-37237)*
Placement of iliac branched endograft ([34717], [34718])
Use of code more than one time for each vessel treated

Code first (34701-34708)

9.38 9.38 FUD ZZZ C 80

AMA: 2018,Jan,8; 2017,Dec,3

● # **34718** **Endovascular repair of iliac artery, not associated with placement of an aorto-iliac artery endograft at the same session, by deployment of an iliac branched endograft, including pre-procedure sizing and device selection, all ipsilateral selective iliac artery catheterization(s), all associated radiological supervision and interpretation, and all endograft extension(s) proximally to the aortic bifurcation and distally in the internal iliac, external iliac, and common femoral artery(ies), and treatment zone angioplasty/stenting, when performed, for other than rupture (eg, for aneurysm, pseudoaneurysm, dissection, arteriovenous malformation, penetrating ulcer), unilateral**

0.00 0.00 FUD 000

INCLUDES Endograft extensions into internal and external iliac, and/or common femoral arteries

EXCLUDES *Branched iliac endograft deployed at same session as aorto-iliac endograft placement (34703-34706, [34717])*

Placement of isolated iliac branched endograft, for rupture (37799)

Placement of prosthesis extensions on same side (34709, 34710-34711)

34710 **Delayed placement of distal or proximal extension prosthesis for endovascular repair of infrarenal abdominal aortic or iliac aneurysm, false aneurysm, dissection, endoleak, or endograft migration, including pre-procedure sizing and device selection, all nonselective catheterization(s), all associated radiological supervision and interpretation, and treatment zone angioplasty/stenting, when performed; initial vessel treated**

EXCLUDES *Fenestrated endograft repair (34841-34848)*

Initial endovascular repair by endograft (34701-34709)

Use of code more than one time per procedure

Code also decompressive laparotomy for treatment abdominal compartment syndrome (49000)

23.2 23.2 FUD 090 C 80

AMA: 2018,Jan,8; 2017,Dec,3

\+ **34711** **each additional vessel treated (List separately in addition to code for primary procedure)**

EXCLUDES *Fenestrated endograft repair (34841-34848)*

Initial endovascular repair by endograft (34701-34709)

Use of code more than one time per procedure

Code first (34710)

8.66 8.66 FUD ZZZ C 80

AMA: 2018,Jan,8; 2017,Dec,3

34712 **Transcatheter delivery of enhanced fixation device(s) to the endograft (eg, anchor, screw, tack) and all associated radiological supervision and interpretation**

EXCLUDES *Use of code more than one time per procedure*

19.8 19.8 FUD 090 C 80

AMA: 2018,Jan,8; 2017,Dec,3

\+ **34713** **Percutaneous access and closure of femoral artery for delivery of endograft through a large sheath (12 French or larger), including ultrasound guidance, when performed, unilateral (List separately in addition to code for primary procedure)**

INCLUDES Ultrasound imaging guidance

Unilateral procedure through large sheath of 12 French or larger

EXCLUDES *Reporting with modifier 50. Report once for each side when performed bilaterally*

Code first (33880-33881, 33883-33884, 33886, 34701-34708, [34718], 34710, 34712, 34841-34848)

3.73 3.73 FUD ZZZ 50 N N1 80

AMA: 2018,Jan,8; 2017,Dec,3

34812-34834 [34812, 34820, 34833, 34834] Open Exposure for Endovascular Prosthesis Delivery

INCLUDES Balloon angioplasty/stent deployment within the target treatment zone

Introduction, manipulation, placement, and deployment of the device

Open exposure of femoral or iliac artery/subsequent closure

Thromboendarterectomy at site of aneurysm

EXCLUDES *Additional interventional procedures outside of target treatment zone*

Guidewire and catheter insertion (36140, 36200, 36245-36248)

Substantial artery repair/replacement (35226, 35286)

\+ # **34812** **Open femoral artery exposure for delivery of endovascular prosthesis, by groin incision, unilateral (List separately in addition to code for primary procedure)**

INCLUDES Unilateral procedure

EXCLUDES *ECMO/ECLS insertion, removal or repositioning (33953-33954, 33959, [33962], [33969], [33984], [33987])*

Extensive repair of femoral artery (35226, 35286, 35371)

Reporting with modifier 50. Report once for each side when performed bilaterally

Code first (33880-33881, 33883-33884, 33886, 33990-33991, 34701-34708, [34718], 34710, 34712, 34841-34848)

6.00 6.00 FUD ZZZ 50 C 80

AMA: 2018,Jan,8; 2017,Dec,3; 2017,Jan,8; 2016,Jan,13; 2015,Jul,3; 2015,Jan,16; 2014,Jan,11

\+ **34714** **Open femoral artery exposure with creation of conduit for delivery of endovascular prosthesis or for establishment of cardiopulmonary bypass, by groin incision, unilateral (List separately in addition to code for primary procedure)**

INCLUDES Unilateral procedure

EXCLUDES *Delivery of endovascular prosthesis via open femoral artery ([34812])*

ECMO/ECLS insertion, removal or repositioning on same side (33953-33954, 33959, [33962], [33969], [33984])

Reporting with modifier 50. Report once for each side when performed bilaterally

Transcatheter aortic valve replacement via open axillary artery (33362)

Code first (32852, 32854, 33031, 33120, 33251, 33256, 33259, 33261, 33305, 33315, 33322, 33335, 33390-33391, 33404-33406, 33410, [33440], 33411-33417, 33422, 33425-33427, 33430, 33460, 33463-33465, 33468, 33474-33476, 33478, 33496, 33500, 33502, 33504-33507, 33510-33516, 33533-33536, 33542, 33545, 33548, 33600-33688, 33692, 33694, 33697, 33702, 33710, 33720, 33722, 33724, 33726, 33730, 33732, 33736, 33750, 33755, 33762, 33764, 33766-33767, 33770-33783, 33786, 33788, 33802-33803, 33814, 33820, 33822, 33824, 33840, 33845, 33851, 33853, 33858-33859, 33863-33864, 33871, 33875, 33877, 33880-33881, 33883-33884, 33886, 33910, 33916-33917, 33920, 33922, 33926, 33935, 33945, 33975-33980, 33983, 33990-33991, 34701-34708, [34718], 34710, 34712, 34841-34848)

7.84 7.84 FUD ZZZ 50 N N1 80

AMA: 2018,Jan,8; 2017,Dec,3

\+ # **34820** **Open iliac artery exposure for delivery of endovascular prosthesis or iliac occlusion during endovascular therapy, by abdominal or retroperitoneal incision, unilateral (List separately in addition to code for primary procedure)**

INCLUDES Unilateral procedure

EXCLUDES *ECMO/ECLS insertion, removal or repositioning (33953-33954, 33959, [33962], [33969], [33984])*

Reporting with modifier 50. Report once for each side when performed bilaterally

Code first (33880-33881, 33883-33884, 33886, 33990-33991, 34701-34708, [34718], 34710, 34712, 34841-34848)

10.0 10.0 FUD ZZZ 50 C 80

AMA: 2018,Jan,8; 2017,Dec,3; 2017,Jan,8; 2016,Jan,13; 2015,Jul,3; 2015,Jan,16; 2014,Jan,11

+ # 34833 Open iliac artery exposure with creation of conduit for delivery of endovascular prosthesis or for establishment of cardiopulmonary bypass, by abdominal or retroperitoneal incision, unilateral (List separately in addition to code for primary procedure)

INCLUDES Unilateral procedure

EXCLUDES *Delivery of endovascular prosthesis via open iliac artery ([34820])*

ECMO/ECLS insertion, removal or repositioning on same side (33953-33954, 33959, [33962], [33969], [33984])

Reporting with modifier 50. Report once for each side when performed bilaterally

Transcatheter aortic valve replacement via open iliac artery (33364)

Code first (32852, 32854, 33031, 33256, 33259, 33261, 33305, 33315, 33322, 33335, 33390-33391, 33404-33406, 33410, [33440], 33411-33417, 33422, 33425-33427, 33430, 33460, 33463-33465, 33468, 33474-33476, 33478, 33496, 33500, 33502, 33504-33514, 33516, 33533-33536, 33542, 33545, 33548, 33600-33688, 33692, 33694, 33697, 33702, 33710, 33720, 33722, 33724, 33726, 33730, 33732, 33736, 33750, 33755, 33762, 33764, 33766-33767, 33770-33783, 33786, 33788, 33802-33803, 33814, 33820, 33822, 33824, 33840, 33845, 33851, 33853, 33858-33859, 33863-33864, 33871, 33875, 33877, 33880-33881, 33883-33884, 33886, 33910, 33916-33917, 33920, 33922, 33926, 33935, 33945, 33975-33980, 33983, 33990-33991, 34701-34708, [34718], 34710, 34712, 34841-34848)

11.7 11.7 FUD ZZZ ⑩ C 80

AMA: 2018,Jan,8; 2017,Dec,3; 2017,Jan,8; 2016,Jan,13; 2015,Jul,3; 2015,Jan,16; 2014,Jan,11

+ # 34834 Open brachial artery exposure for delivery of endovascular prosthesis, unilateral (List separately in addition to code for primary procedure)

INCLUDES Unilateral procedure

EXCLUDES *ECMO/ECLS insertion, removal or repositioning (33953-33954, 33959, [33962], [33969], [33984])*

Reporting with modifier 50. Report once for each side when performed bilaterally

Code first (33880-33881, 33883-33884, 33886, 33990-33991, 34701-34708, [34718], 34710, 34712, 34841-34848)

3.75 3.75 FUD ZZZ ⑩ C 80

AMA: 2018,Jan,8; 2017,Dec,3; 2017,Jan,8; 2016,Jan,13; 2015,Jul,3; 2015,Jan,16; 2014,Jan,11

+ 34715 Open axillary/subclavian artery exposure for delivery of endovascular prosthesis by infraclavicular or supraclavicular incision, unilateral (List separately in addition to code for primary procedure)

INCLUDES Unilateral procedure

EXCLUDES *ECMO/ECLS insertion, removal or repositioning on same side (33953-33954, 33959, [33962], [33969], [33984])*

Implantation or replacement of aortic counterpulsation ventricular assist system (0451T-0452T, 0455T-0456T)

Reporting with modifier 50. Report once for each side when performed bilaterally

Transcatheter aortic valve replacement via open axillary artery (33363)

Code first (33880-33881, 33883-33884, 33886, 33990-33991, 34701-34708, [34718], 34710, 34712, 34841-34848)

8.79 8.79 FUD ZZZ ⑩ N N1 80

AMA: 2018,Jan,8; 2017,Dec,3

+ 34716 Open axillary/subclavian artery exposure with creation of conduit for delivery of endovascular prosthesis or for establishment of cardiopulmonary bypass, by infraclavicular or supraclavicular incision, unilateral (List separately in addition to code for primary procedure)

INCLUDES Unilateral procedure

EXCLUDES *ECMO/ECLS insertion, removal or repositioning on same side (33953-33954, 33959, [33962], [33969], [33984])*

Implantation or replacement of aortic counterpulsation ventricular assist system (0451T-0452T, 0455T-0456T)

Reporting with modifier 50. Report once for each side when performed bilaterally

Code first (32852, 32854, 33031, 33120, 33251, 33256, 33259, 33261, 33305, 33315, 33322, 33335, 33390-33391, 33404-33406, 33410, [33440], 33411-33417, 33422, 33425-33427, 33430, 33460, 33463-33465, 33468, 33474-33476, 33478, 33496, 33500, 33502, 33504-33514, 33516, 33533-33536, 33542, 33545, 33548, 33600-33688, 33692, 33694, 33697, 33702-33722, 33724, 33726, 33730, 33732, 33736, 33750, 33755, 33762, 33764, 33766-33767, 33770-33783, 33786, 33788, 33802-33803, 33814, 33820, 33822, 33824, 33840, 33845, 33851, 33853, 33858-33859, 33863-33864, 33871, 33875, 33877, 33880-33881, 33883-33884, 33886, 33910, 33916-33917, 33920, 33922, 33926, 33935, 33945, 33975-33980, 33983, 33990-33991, 34701-34708, [34718], 34710, 34712, 34841-34848)

10.8 10.8 FUD ZZZ ⑩ N N1 80

AMA: 2018,Jan,8; 2017,Dec,3

34717 **Resequenced code. See code following 34708.**

34718 **Resequenced code. See code following 34709.**

+ 34808 Endovascular placement of iliac artery occlusion device (List separately in addition to code for primary procedure)

Code first (34701-34704, 34707-34708, 34709, 34710, 34813, 34841-34844)

6.11 6.11 FUD ZZZ C 80

AMA: 2018,Jan,8; 2017,Jan,8; 2016,Jan,13; 2015,Jan,16; 2014,Jan,11

34812 **Resequenced code. See code following 34713.**

+ 34813 Placement of femoral-femoral prosthetic graft during endovascular aortic aneurysm repair (List separately in addition to code for primary procedure)

EXCLUDES *Grafting of femoral artery (35521, 35533, 35539, 35540, 35556, 35558, 35566, 35621, 35646, 35654-35661, 35666, 35700)*

Code first ([34812])

6.85 6.85 FUD ZZZ C 80

AMA: 2018,Jan,8; 2017,Jan,8; 2016,Jan,13; 2015,Jan,16; 2014,Jan,11

34820 **Resequenced code. See code following 34714.**

34830 Open repair of infrarenal aortic aneurysm or dissection, plus repair of associated arterial trauma, following unsuccessful endovascular repair; tube prosthesis

50.9 50.9 FUD 090 C 80

AMA: 2018,Jan,8; 2017,Jan,8; 2016,Jan,13; 2015,Jan,16; 2014,Jan,11

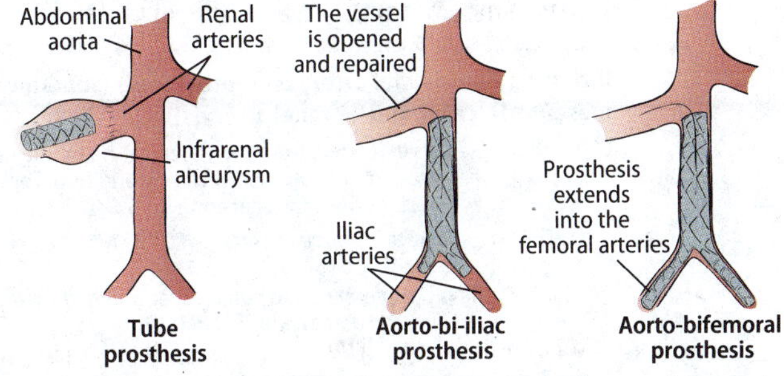

A tube prosthesis is placed and any associated arterial trauma is repaired

34831 **aorto-bi-iliac prosthesis**
55.9 55.9 FUD 090 C 80
AMA: 2018,Jan,8; 2017,Jan,8; 2016,Jan,13; 2015,Jan,16; 2014,Jan,11

34832 **aorto-bifemoral prosthesis**
54.7 54.7 FUD 090 C 80
AMA: 2018,Jan,8; 2017,Jan,8; 2016,Jan,13; 2015,Jan,16; 2014,Jan,11

34833 **Resequenced code. See code following 34714.**

34834 **Resequenced code. See code following 34714.**

34839-34848 Repair Visceral Aorta with Fenestrated Endovascular Grafts

INCLUDES Angiography
Balloon angioplasty before and after deployment of graft
Fluoroscopic guidance
Guidewire and catheter insertion of vessels in the target treatment zone
Radiologic supervision and interpretation
Visceral aorta (34841-34844)
Visceral aorta and associated infrarenal abdominal aorta (34845-34848)

EXCLUDES *Catheterization of:*
Arterial families outside treatment zone
Hypogastric arteries
Distal extension prosthesis terminating in the common femoral, external iliac, or internal iliac artery (34709-34711 [34718])
Insertion of bare metal or covered intravascular stents in visceral branches in the target treatment zone (37236-37237)
Interventional procedures outside treatment zone
Open exposure of access vessels (34713-34716 [34812, 34820, 34833, 34834])
Placement of distal extension prosthesis into internal/external iliac or common femoral artery (34709, [34718], 34710-34711)
Repair of abdominal aortic aneurysm without a fenestrated graft (34701-34708)
Substantial artery repair (35226, 35286)

Code also associated endovascular repair of descending thoracic aorta (33880-33886, 75956-75959)

34839 **Physician planning of a patient-specific fenestrated visceral aortic endograft requiring a minimum of 90 minutes of physician time**
0.00 0.00 FUD YYY B 80

EXCLUDES *3D rendering with interpretation and reporting of imaging (76376-76377)*
Endovascular repair procedure on day of or day after planning (34701-34706, 34841-34848)
Planning on day of or day before endovascular repair procedure
Total planning time of less than 90 minutes

34841 **Endovascular repair of visceral aorta (eg, aneurysm, pseudoaneurysm, dissection, penetrating ulcer, intramural hematoma, or traumatic disruption) by deployment of a fenestrated visceral aortic endograft and all associated radiological supervision and interpretation, including target zone angioplasty, when performed; including one visceral artery endoprosthesis (superior mesenteric, celiac or renal artery)**

EXCLUDES *Endovascular repair of aorta (34701-34706, 34845-34848)*
Physician planning of a patient-specific fenestrated visceral aortic endograft (34839)

0.00 0.00 FUD YYY C 80
AMA: 2018,Jan,8; 2017,Dec,3; 2017,Jul,3; 2017,Jan,8; 2016,Jan,13; 2015,Jan,16; 2014,Jan,11

34842 **including two visceral artery endoprostheses (superior mesenteric, celiac and/or renal artery[s])**

INCLUDES Repairs extending from the visceral aorta to one or more of the four visceral artery origins to the level of the infrarenal aorta

EXCLUDES *Endovascular repair of aorta (34701-34706, 34845-34848)*
Physician planning of a patient-specific fenestrated visceral aortic endograft (34839)

0.00 0.00 FUD YYY C 80
AMA: 2018,Jan,8; 2017,Dec,3; 2017,Jul,3; 2017,Jan,8; 2016,Jan,13; 2015,Jan,16; 2014,Jan,11

34843 **including three visceral artery endoprostheses (superior mesenteric, celiac and/or renal artery[s])**

INCLUDES Repairs extending from the visceral aorta to one or more of the four visceral artery origins to the level of the infrarenal aorta

EXCLUDES *Endovascular repair of aorta (34701-34706, 34845-34848)*
Physician planning of a patient-specific fenestrated visceral aortic endograft (34839)

0.00 0.00 FUD YYY C 80
AMA: 2018,Jan,8; 2017,Dec,3; 2017,Jul,3; 2017,Jan,8; 2016,Jan,13; 2015,Jan,16; 2014,Jan,11

34844 **including four or more visceral artery endoprostheses (superior mesenteric, celiac and/or renal artery[s])**

INCLUDES Repairs extending from the visceral aorta to one or more of the four visceral artery origins to the level of the infrarenal aorta

EXCLUDES *Endovascular repair of aorta (34701-34706, 34845-34848)*
Physician planning of a patient-specific fenestrated visceral aortic endograft (34839)

0.00 0.00 FUD YYY C 80
AMA: 2018,Jan,8; 2017,Dec,3; 2017,Jul,3; 2017,Jan,8; 2016,Jan,13; 2015,Jan,16; 2014,Jan,11

34845 **Endovascular repair of visceral aorta and infrarenal abdominal aorta (eg, aneurysm, pseudoaneurysm, dissection, penetrating ulcer, intramural hematoma, or traumatic disruption) with a fenestrated visceral aortic endograft and concomitant unibody or modular infrarenal aortic endograft and all associated radiological supervision and interpretation, including target zone angioplasty, when performed; including one visceral artery endoprosthesis (superior mesenteric, celiac or renal artery)**

INCLUDES Placement of device and extensions into the common iliac arteries
Repairs extending from the visceral aorta into the common iliac arteries

EXCLUDES *Direct repair aneurysm (35081, 35102)*
Endovascular repair of aorta (34701-34706, 34841-34844)
Physician planning of a patient-specific fenestrated visceral aortic endograft (34839)

Code also iliac artery revascularization when performed outside zone of target treatment (37220-37223)

0.00 0.00 FUD YYY C 80
AMA: 2018,Jan,8; 2017,Dec,3; 2017,Jul,3; 2017,Jan,8; 2016,Jan,13; 2015,Jan,16; 2014,Jan,11

34846 **including two visceral artery endoprostheses (superior mesenteric, celiac and/or renal artery[s])**

INCLUDES Placement of device and extensions into the common iliac arteries
Repairs extending from the visceral aorta into the common iliac arteries

EXCLUDES *Direct repair aneurysm (35081, 35102)*
Endovascular repair of aorta (34701-34706, 34841-34844)
Physician planning of a patient-specific fenestrated visceral aortic endograft (34839)

Code also iliac artery revascularization when performed outside zone of target treatment (37220-37223)

0.00 0.00 FUD YYY C 80
AMA: 2018,Jan,8; 2017,Dec,3; 2017,Jul,3; 2017,Jan,8; 2016,Jan,13; 2015,Jan,16; 2014,Jan,11

34847 **including three visceral artery endoprostheses (superior mesenteric, celiac and/or renal artery[s])**

INCLUDES Placement of device and extensions into the common iliac arteries
Repairs extending from the visceral aorta into the common iliac arteries

EXCLUDES *Direct repair aneurysm (35081, 35102)*
Endovascular repair of aorta (34701-34706, 34841-34844)
Physician planning of a patient-specific fenestrated visceral aortic endograft (34839)

Code also iliac artery revascularization when performed outside zone of target treatment (37220-37223)

0.00 0.00 FUD YYY C 80

AMA: 2018,Jan,8; 2017,Dec,3; 2017,Jul,3; 2017,Jan,8; 2016,Jan,13; 2015,Jan,16; 2014,Jan,11

34848 **including four or more visceral artery endoprostheses (superior mesenteric, celiac and/or renal artery[s])**

INCLUDES Placement of device and extensions into the common iliac arteries
Repairs extending from the visceral aorta into the common iliac arteries

EXCLUDES *Direct repair aneurysm (35081, 35102)*
Endovascular repair of aorta (34701-34706, 34841-34844)
Physician planning of a patient-specific fenestrated visceral aortic endograft (34839)

Code also iliac artery revascularization when performed outside zone of target treatment (37220-37223)

0.00 0.00 FUD YYY C 80

AMA: 2018,Jan,8; 2017,Dec,3; 2017,Aug,9; 2017,Jul,3; 2017,Jan,8; 2016,Jul,6; 2016,Jan,13; 2015,Jan,16; 2014,Jan,11

35001-35152 Repair Aneurysm, False Aneurysm, Related Arterial Disease

INCLUDES Endarterectomy procedures

EXCLUDES *Endovascular repairs of:*
Abdominal aortic aneurysm (34701-34716 [34717, 34718, 34812, 34820, 34833, 34834])
Thoracic aortic aneurysm (33858-33859, 33863-33875)
Intracranial aneurysms (61697-61710)
Repairs related to occlusive disease only (35201-35286)

35001 **Direct repair of aneurysm, pseudoaneurysm, or excision (partial or total) and graft insertion, with or without patch graft; for aneurysm and associated occlusive disease, carotid, subclavian artery, by neck incision**

32.2 32.2 FUD 090 C 80 50

AMA: 2002,May,7; 2000,Dec,1

35002 **for ruptured aneurysm, carotid, subclavian artery, by neck incision**

32.7 32.7 FUD 090 C 80 50

AMA: 2002,May,7; 1997,Nov,1

35005 **for aneurysm, pseudoaneurysm, and associated occlusive disease, vertebral artery**

28.6 28.6 FUD 090 C 80 50

AMA: 2002,May,7; 1997,Nov,1

An incision is made in the back of the neck to directly approach an aneurysm or false aneurysm of the vertebral artery. The artery is either repaired directly or excised with a graft

Graft repair
Vertebral artery
Subclavian artery

35011 **for aneurysm and associated occlusive disease, axillary-brachial artery, by arm incision**

29.0 29.0 FUD 090 T 80 50

AMA: 2002,May,7; 1997,Nov,1

35013 **for ruptured aneurysm, axillary-brachial artery, by arm incision**

36.3 36.3 FUD 090 C 80 50

AMA: 2002,May,7; 1997,Nov,1

35021 **for aneurysm, pseudoaneurysm, and associated occlusive disease, innominate, subclavian artery, by thoracic incision**

36.6 36.6 FUD 090 C 80 50

AMA: 2002,May,7; 1997,Nov,1

35022 **for ruptured aneurysm, innominate, subclavian artery, by thoracic incision**

40.6 40.6 FUD 090 C 80 50

AMA: 2002,May,7; 1997,Nov,1

35045 **for aneurysm, pseudoaneurysm, and associated occlusive disease, radial or ulnar artery**

28.4 28.4 FUD 090 T 80 50

AMA: 2002,May,7; 1997,Nov,1

35081 **for aneurysm, pseudoaneurysm, and associated occlusive disease, abdominal aorta**

50.2 50.2 FUD 090 C 80

AMA: 2018,Jan,8; 2017,Jan,8; 2016,Jan,13; 2015,Jan,16; 2014,Jan,11

35082 **for ruptured aneurysm, abdominal aorta**

63.3 63.3 FUD 090 C 80

AMA: 2002,May,7; 1997,Nov,1

35091 **for aneurysm, pseudoaneurysm, and associated occlusive disease, abdominal aorta involving visceral vessels (mesenteric, celiac, renal)**

51.8 51.8 FUD 090 C 80 50

AMA: 2018,Jan,8; 2017,Jan,8; 2016,Jan,13; 2015,Jan,16; 2014,Jan,11

35092 **for ruptured aneurysm, abdominal aorta involving visceral vessels (mesenteric, celiac, renal)**

75.5 75.5 FUD 090 C 80 50

AMA: 2002,May,7; 1997,Nov,1

35102 **for aneurysm, pseudoaneurysm, and associated occlusive disease, abdominal aorta involving iliac vessels (common, hypogastric, external)**
54.5 54.5 FUD 090 C 80 50
AMA: 2018,Jan,8; 2017,Jan,8; 2016,Jan,13; 2015,Jan,16; 2014,Jan,11

35103 **for ruptured aneurysm, abdominal aorta involving iliac vessels (common, hypogastric, external)**
64.9 64.9 FUD 090 C 80 50
AMA: 2002,May,7; 1997,Nov,1

35111 **for aneurysm, pseudoaneurysm, and associated occlusive disease, splenic artery**
38.3 38.3 FUD 090 C 80 50
AMA: 2002,May,7; 1997,Nov,1

35112 **for ruptured aneurysm, splenic artery**
47.2 47.2 FUD 090 C 80 50
AMA: 2002,May,7; 1997,Nov,1

35121 **for aneurysm, pseudoaneurysm, and associated occlusive disease, hepatic, celiac, renal, or mesenteric artery**
48.3 48.3 FUD 090 C 80 50
AMA: 2002,May,7; 1997,Nov,1

35122 **for ruptured aneurysm, hepatic, celiac, renal, or mesenteric artery**
54.6 54.6 FUD 090 C 80 50
AMA: 2002,May,7; 1997,Nov,1

35131 **for aneurysm, pseudoaneurysm, and associated occlusive disease, iliac artery (common, hypogastric, external)**
40.2 40.2 FUD 090 C 80 50
AMA: 2018,Jan,8; 2017,Jan,8; 2016,Jan,13; 2015,Jan,16; 2014,Jan,11

35132 **for ruptured aneurysm, iliac artery (common, hypogastric, external)**
47.2 47.2 FUD 090 C 80 50
AMA: 2002,May,7; 1997,Nov,1

35141 **for aneurysm, pseudoaneurysm, and associated occlusive disease, common femoral artery (profunda femoris, superficial femoral)**
31.9 31.9 FUD 090 C 80 50
AMA: 2002,May,7; 1997,Nov,1

35142 **for ruptured aneurysm, common femoral artery (profunda femoris, superficial femoral)**
38.5 38.5 FUD 090 C 80 50
AMA: 2002,May,7; 1997,Nov,1

35151 **for aneurysm, pseudoaneurysm, and associated occlusive disease, popliteal artery**
35.8 35.8 FUD 090 C 80 50
AMA: 2002,May,7; 1997,Nov,1

35152 **for ruptured aneurysm, popliteal artery**
40.3 40.3 FUD 090 C 80 50
AMA: 2002,May,7; 1997,Nov,1

35180-35190 Surgical Repair Arteriovenous Fistula

35180 **Repair, congenital arteriovenous fistula; head and neck**
25.4 25.4 FUD 090 T 80
AMA: 2018,Jan,8; 2017,Jan,8; 2016,Jan,13; 2015,Jan,16; 2014,Jan,11

35182 **thorax and abdomen**
51.9 51.9 FUD 090 C 80
AMA: 2018,Jan,8; 2017,Jan,8; 2016,Jan,13; 2015,Jan,16; 2014,Jan,11

35184 **extremities**
27.8 27.8 FUD 090 T 80
AMA: 2018,Jan,8; 2017,Jan,8; 2016,Jan,13; 2015,Jan,16; 2014,Jan,11

35188 **Repair, acquired or traumatic arteriovenous fistula; head and neck**
37.7 37.7 FUD 090 T A2 80
AMA: 2018,Jan,8; 2017,Jan,8; 2016,Jan,13; 2015,Jan,16; 2014,Jan,11

35189 **thorax and abdomen**
43.5 43.5 FUD 090 C 80
AMA: 2018,Jan,8; 2017,Jan,8; 2016,Jan,13; 2015,Jan,16; 2014,Jan,11

35190 **extremities**
22.0 22.0 FUD 090 T 80
AMA: 2018,Jan,8; 2017,Jan,8; 2016,Jan,13; 2015,Jan,16; 2014,Jan,11

35201-35286 Surgical Repair Artery or Vein

EXCLUDES *Arteriovenous fistula repair (35180-35190)*
Primary open vascular procedures

35201 **Repair blood vessel, direct; neck**
EXCLUDES *Removal ECMO/ECLS of cannula ([33969, 33984, 33985, 33986])*
27.2 27.2 FUD 090 T 80 50
AMA: 2018,Jan,8; 2017,Jan,8; 2016,Jan,13; 2015,Jul,3; 2015,Jan,16; 2014,Mar,8

35206 **upper extremity**
EXCLUDES *Removal ECMO/ECLS of cannula ([33969, 33984, 33985, 33986])*
22.6 22.6 FUD 090 T 80 50
AMA: 2018,Jan,8; 2017,Jan,8; 2016,Jan,13; 2015,Jul,3; 2015,Jan,16; 2014,Apr,10; 2014,Jan,11

35207 **hand, finger**
21.7 21.7 FUD 090 T A2 50
AMA: 2012,Apr,3-9; 2003,Feb,1

35211 **intrathoracic, with bypass**
EXCLUDES *Removal ECMO/ECLS of cannula ([33969, 33984, 33985, 33986])*
40.0 40.0 FUD 090 C 80 50
AMA: 2015,Jul,3

35216 **intrathoracic, without bypass**
EXCLUDES *Removal ECMO/ECLS of cannula ([33969, 33984, 33985, 33986])*
59.7 59.7 FUD 090 C 80 50
AMA: 2018,Jan,8; 2017,Jan,8; 2016,Jan,13; 2015,Jan,16; 2014,Jan,11

35221 **intra-abdominal**
42.4 42.4 FUD 090 C 80 50
AMA: 2012,Apr,3-9; 2003,Feb,1

35226 **lower extremity**
EXCLUDES *Removal ECMO/ECLS of cannula ([33969, 33984, 33985, 33986])*
24.1 24.1 FUD 090 T 80 50
AMA: 2019,Jul,10; 2018,Jan,8; 2017,Aug,10; 2017,Jul,3; 2017,Jan,8; 2016,Jul,6; 2016,Jan,13; 2015,Jul,3; 2015,Jan,16; 2014,Jan,11

35231 **Repair blood vessel with vein graft; neck**
35.7 35.7 FUD 090 T 80 50
AMA: 2012,Apr,3-9; 2003,Feb,1

35236 **upper extremity**
29.0 29.0 FUD 090 T 80 50
AMA: 2018,Jan,8; 2017,Jan,8; 2016,Jan,13; 2015,Jan,16; 2014,Jan,11

35241 **intrathoracic, with bypass**
41.8 41.8 FUD 090 C 80 50
AMA: 2012,Apr,3-9; 2003,Feb,1

35246 **intrathoracic, without bypass**
45.6 45.6 FUD 090 C 80 50
AMA: 2012,Apr,3-9; 2003,Feb,1

35251 **intra-abdominal**
50.4 50.4 FUD 090 C 80 50
AMA: 2012,Apr,3-9; 2003,Feb,1

35256 lower extremity
29.6 29.6 FUD 090 T 80 50
AMA: 2012,Apr,3-9; 2003,Feb,1

35261 Repair blood vessel with graft other than vein; neck
28.2 28.2 FUD 090 T 80 50
AMA: 2012,Apr,3-9; 2003,Feb,1

35266 upper extremity
25.1 25.1 FUD 090 T 80 50
AMA: 2018,Jan,8; 2017,Jan,8; 2016,Jan,13; 2015,Jan,16; 2014,Jan,11

35271 intrathoracic, with bypass
40.0 40.0 FUD 090 C 80 50
AMA: 2012,Apr,3-9; 2003,Feb,1

35276 intrathoracic, without bypass
42.4 42.4 FUD 090 C 80 50
AMA: 2012,Apr,3-9; 2003,Feb,1

35281 intra-abdominal
46.8 46.8 FUD 090 C 80 50
AMA: 2012,Apr,3-9; 2003,Feb,1

35286 lower extremity
26.9 26.9 FUD 090 T 80 50
AMA: 2019,Jul,10; 2018,Jan,8; 2017,Aug,10; 2017,Jul,3; 2017,Jan,8; 2016,Jul,6; 2016,Jan,13; 2015,Jan,16; 2014,Jan,11

35301-35372 Surgical Thromboendarterectomy Peripheral and Visceral Arteries

INCLUDES Obtaining saphenous or arm vein for graft
Thrombectomy/embolectomy

EXCLUDES *Coronary artery bypass procedures (33510-33536, 33572)*
Thromboendarterectomy for vascular occlusion on a different vessel during the same session

35301 Thromboendarterectomy, including patch graft, if performed; carotid, vertebral, subclavian, by neck incision
32.7 32.7 FUD 090 C 80 50
AMA: 2018,Jan,8; 2017,Jan,8; 2016,Jan,13; 2015,Jan,16; 2014,Jan,11

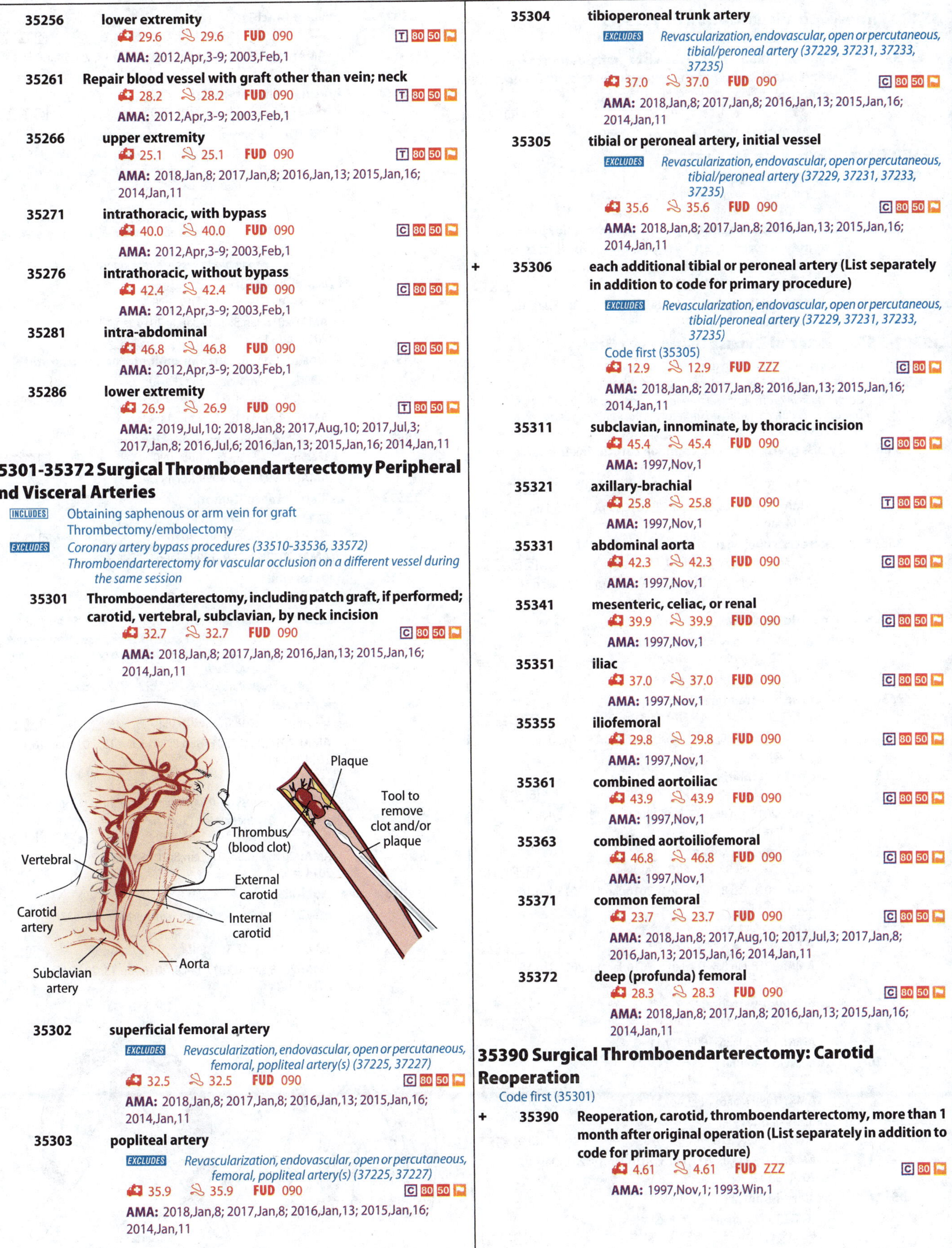

35302 superficial femoral artery
EXCLUDES *Revascularization, endovascular, open or percutaneous, femoral, popliteal artery(s) (37225, 37227)*
32.5 32.5 FUD 090 C 80 50
AMA: 2018,Jan,8; 2017,Jan,8; 2016,Jan,13; 2015,Jan,16; 2014,Jan,11

35303 popliteal artery
EXCLUDES *Revascularization, endovascular, open or percutaneous, femoral, popliteal artery(s) (37225, 37227)*
35.9 35.9 FUD 090 C 80 50
AMA: 2018,Jan,8; 2017,Jan,8; 2016,Jan,13; 2015,Jan,16; 2014,Jan,11

35304 tibioperoneal trunk artery
EXCLUDES *Revascularization, endovascular, open or percutaneous, tibial/peroneal artery (37229, 37231, 37233, 37235)*
37.0 37.0 FUD 090 C 80 50
AMA: 2018,Jan,8; 2017,Jan,8; 2016,Jan,13; 2015,Jan,16; 2014,Jan,11

35305 tibial or peroneal artery, initial vessel
EXCLUDES *Revascularization, endovascular, open or percutaneous, tibial/peroneal artery (37229, 37231, 37233, 37235)*
35.6 35.6 FUD 090 C 80 50
AMA: 2018,Jan,8; 2017,Jan,8; 2016,Jan,13; 2015,Jan,16; 2014,Jan,11

+ **35306** each additional tibial or peroneal artery (List separately in addition to code for primary procedure)
EXCLUDES *Revascularization, endovascular, open or percutaneous, tibial/peroneal artery (37229, 37231, 37233, 37235)*
Code first (35305)
12.9 12.9 FUD ZZZ C 80
AMA: 2018,Jan,8; 2017,Jan,8; 2016,Jan,13; 2015,Jan,16; 2014,Jan,11

35311 subclavian, innominate, by thoracic incision
45.4 45.4 FUD 090 C 80 50
AMA: 1997,Nov,1

35321 axillary-brachial
25.8 25.8 FUD 090 T 80 50
AMA: 1997,Nov,1

35331 abdominal aorta
42.3 42.3 FUD 090 C 80 50
AMA: 1997,Nov,1

35341 mesenteric, celiac, or renal
39.9 39.9 FUD 090 C 80 50
AMA: 1997,Nov,1

35351 iliac
37.0 37.0 FUD 090 C 80 50
AMA: 1997,Nov,1

35355 iliofemoral
29.8 29.8 FUD 090 C 80 50
AMA: 1997,Nov,1

35361 combined aortoiliac
43.9 43.9 FUD 090 C 80 50
AMA: 1997,Nov,1

35363 combined aortoiliofemoral
46.8 46.8 FUD 090 C 80 50
AMA: 1997,Nov,1

35371 common femoral
23.7 23.7 FUD 090 C 80 50
AMA: 2018,Jan,8; 2017,Aug,10; 2017,Jul,3; 2017,Jan,8; 2016,Jan,13; 2015,Jan,16; 2014,Jan,11

35372 deep (profunda) femoral
28.3 28.3 FUD 090 C 80 50
AMA: 2018,Jan,8; 2017,Jan,8; 2016,Jan,13; 2015,Jan,16; 2014,Jan,11

35390 Surgical Thromboendarterectomy: Carotid Reoperation

Code first (35301)

+ **35390** Reoperation, carotid, thromboendarterectomy, more than 1 month after original operation (List separately in addition to code for primary procedure)
4.61 4.61 FUD ZZZ C 80
AMA: 1997,Nov,1; 1993,Win,1

35400 Endoscopic Visualization of Vessels

Code first the therapeutic intervention

+ **35400** **Angioscopy (noncoronary vessels or grafts) during therapeutic intervention (List separately in addition to code for primary procedure)**
4.32 4.32 FUD ZZZ C 80
AMA: 1997,Dec,1; 1997,Nov,1

35500 Obtain Arm Vein for Graft

EXCLUDES *Endoscopic harvest (33508)*
Harvesting of multiple vein segments (35682, 35683)
Code first (33510-33536, 35556, 35566, 35570-35571, 35583-35587)

+ **35500** **Harvest of upper extremity vein, 1 segment, for lower extremity or coronary artery bypass procedure (List separately in addition to code for primary procedure)**
9.29 9.29 FUD ZZZ N 80
AMA: 2018,Jan,8; 2017,Jan,8; 2016,Jan,13; 2015,Jan,16; 2014,Jan,11

35501-35571 Arterial Bypass Using Vein Grafts

INCLUDES Obtaining saphenous vein grafts
EXCLUDES *Obtaining multiple vein segments (35682, 35683)*
Obtaining vein grafts, upper extremity or femoropopliteal (35500, 35572)
Treatment of different sites with different bypass procedures during the same operative session

35501 **Bypass graft, with vein; common carotid-ipsilateral internal carotid**
43.3 43.3 FUD 090 C 80 50
AMA: 2018,Jan,8; 2017,Jan,8; 2016,Jan,13; 2015,Jan,16; 2014,Jan,11

35506 **carotid-subclavian or subclavian-carotid**
36.7 36.7 FUD 090 C 80 50
AMA: 2018,Jan,8; 2017,Jan,8; 2016,Jan,13; 2015,Jan,16; 2014,Jan,11

35508 **carotid-vertebral**
INCLUDES Endoscopic procedure
38.3 38.3 FUD 090 C 80 50
AMA: 1999,Mar,6; 1999,Apr,11

35509 **carotid-contralateral carotid**
40.8 40.8 FUD 090 C 80 50
AMA: 2018,Jan,8; 2017,Jan,8; 2016,Jan,13; 2015,Jan,16; 2014,Jan,11

35510 **carotid-brachial**
35.5 35.5 FUD 090 C 80 50
AMA: 2018,Jan,8; 2017,Jan,8; 2016,Jan,13; 2015,Jan,16; 2014,Jan,11

35511 **subclavian-subclavian**
32.3 32.3 FUD 090 C 80 50
AMA: 2018,Jan,8; 2017,Jan,8; 2016,Jan,13; 2015,Jan,16; 2014,Jan,11

35512 **subclavian-brachial**
34.8 34.8 FUD 090 C 80 50
AMA: 2018,Jan,8; 2017,Jan,8; 2016,Jan,13; 2015,Jan,16; 2014,Jan,11

35515 **subclavian-vertebral**
38.3 38.3 FUD 090 C 80 50
AMA: 1999,Mar,6; 1999,Apr,11

35516 **subclavian-axillary**
35.2 35.2 FUD 090 C 80 50
AMA: 1999,Mar,6; 1999,Apr,11

35518 **axillary-axillary**
32.9 32.9 FUD 090 C 80 50
AMA: 2018,Jan,8; 2017,Jan,8; 2016,Jan,13; 2015,Jan,16; 2014,Jan,11

35521 **axillary-femoral**
EXCLUDES *Synthetic graft (35621)*
35.4 35.4 FUD 090 C 80 50
AMA: 2018,Jan,8; 2017,Jan,8; 2016,Jan,13; 2015,Jan,16; 2014,Jan,11

35522 **axillary-brachial**
34.9 34.9 FUD 090 C 80 50
AMA: 2018,Jan,8; 2017,Jan,8; 2016,Jan,13; 2015,Jan,16; 2014,Jan,11

35523 **brachial-ulnar or -radial**
37.1 37.1 FUD 090 C 80 50
EXCLUDES *Bypass graft using synthetic conduit (37799)*
Bypass graft, with vein; brachial-brachial (35525)
Distal revascularization and interval ligation (DRIL), upper extremity hemodialysis access (steal syndrome) (36838)
Harvest of upper extremity vein, 1 segment, for lower extremity or coronary artery bypass procedure (35500)
Repair blood vessel, direct; upper extremity (35206)

35525 **brachial-brachial**
33.0 33.0 FUD 090 C 80 50
AMA: 2018,Jan,8; 2017,Jan,8; 2016,Jan,13; 2015,Jan,16; 2014,Jan,11

35526 **aortosubclavian, aortoinnominate, or aortocarotid**
EXCLUDES *Synthetic graft (35626)*
50.5 50.5 FUD 090 C 80 50
AMA: 1999,Mar,6; 1999,Apr,11

35531 **aortoceliac or aortomesenteric**
56.3 56.3 FUD 090 C 80 50
AMA: 1999,Mar,6; 1999,Apr,11

35533 **axillary-femoral-femoral**
EXCLUDES *Synthetic graft (35654)*
43.4 43.4 FUD 090 C 80 50
AMA: 2012,Apr,3-9; 1999,Mar,6

35535 **hepatorenal**
54.9 54.9 FUD 090 C 80 50
EXCLUDES *Bypass graft (35536, 35560, 35631, 35636)*
Harvest of upper extremity vein, 1 segment, for lower extremity or coronary artery bypass procedure (35500)
Repair blood vessel (35221, 35251, 35281)

35536 **splenorenal**
48.8 48.8 FUD 090 C 80 50
AMA: 2018,Jan,8; 2017,Jan,8; 2016,Jan,13; 2015,Jan,16; 2014,Jan,11

35537 **aortoiliac**
EXCLUDES *Bypass graft, with vein; aortobi-iliac (35538)*
Synthetic graft (35637)
60.2 60.2 FUD 090 C 80
AMA: 2018,Jan,8; 2017,Jan,8; 2016,Jan,13; 2015,Jan,16; 2014,Jan,11

35538 **aortobi-iliac**
EXCLUDES *Bypass graft, with vein; aortoiliac (35537)*
Synthetic graft (35638)
67.5 67.5 FUD 090 C 80
AMA: 2018,Jan,8; 2017,Jan,8; 2016,Jan,13; 2015,Jan,16; 2014,Jan,11

35539 **aortofemoral**

EXCLUDES *Bypass graft, with vein; aortobifemoral (35540)*
Synthetic graft (35647)

63.3 63.3 FUD 090 C 80 50

AMA: 2018,Jan,8; 2017,Jan,8; 2016,Jan,13; 2015,Jan,16; 2014,Jan,11

35540 **aortobifemoral**

EXCLUDES *Bypass graft, with vein; aortofemoral (35539)*
Synthetic graft (35646)

70.6 70.6 FUD 090 C 50

AMA: 2018,Jan,8; 2017,Jan,8; 2016,Jan,13; 2015,Jan,16; 2014,Jan,11

35556 **femoral-popliteal**

40.5 40.5 FUD 090 C 80 50

AMA: 2018,Jan,8; 2017,Jan,8; 2016,Jan,13; 2015,Jan,16; 2014,Jan,11

35558 **femoral-femoral**

35.6 35.6 FUD 090 C 80 50

AMA: 2012,Apr,3-9; 1999,Mar,6

35560 **aortorenal**

49.2 49.2 FUD 090 C 80 50

AMA: 2018,Jan,8; 2017,Jan,8; 2016,Jan,13; 2015,Jan,16; 2014,Jan,11

35563 **ilioiliac**

38.2 38.2 FUD 090 C 80 50

AMA: 1999,Mar,6; 1999,Apr,11

35565 **iliofemoral**

38.1 38.1 FUD 090 C 80 50

AMA: 2012,Apr,3-9; 2004,Oct,6

35566 **femoral-anterior tibial, posterior tibial, peroneal artery or other distal vessels**

48.3 48.3 FUD 090 C 80 50

AMA: 2018,Jan,8; 2017,Jan,8; 2016,Jan,13; 2015,Jan,16; 2014,Jan,11

35570 **tibial-tibial, peroneal-tibial, or tibial/peroneal trunk-tibial**

EXCLUDES *Repair of blood vessel with graft (35256, 35286)*

43.7 43.7 FUD 090 C 80 50

AMA: 2018,Jan,8; 2017,Jan,8; 2016,Jan,13; 2015,Jan,16; 2014,Jan,11

35571 **popliteal-tibial, -peroneal artery or other distal vessels**

38.3 38.3 FUD 090 C 80 50

AMA: 2018,Jan,8; 2017,Jan,8; 2016,Jan,13; 2015,Jan,16; 2014,Jan,11

35572 Obtain Femoropopliteal Vein for Graft

EXCLUDES *Reporting with modifier 50. Report once for each side when performed bilaterally*

Code first (33510-33523, 33533-33536, 34502, 34520, 35001-35002, 35011-35022, 35102-35103, 35121-35152, 35231-35256, 35501-35587, 35879-35907)

\+ 35572 **Harvest of femoropopliteal vein, 1 segment, for vascular reconstruction procedure (eg, aortic, vena caval, coronary, peripheral artery) (List separately in addition to code for primary procedure)**

10.0 10.0 FUD ZZZ ⑩ N N1 80

AMA: 2018,Jan,8; 2017,Jan,8; 2016,Jan,13; 2015,Jan,16; 2014,Jan,11

35583-35587 Lower Extremity Revascularization: In-situ Vein Bypass

INCLUDES Obtaining saphenous vein grafts

EXCLUDES *Obtaining multiple vein segments (35682, 35683)*
Obtaining vein graft, upper extremity or femoropopliteal (35500, 35572)

35583 **In-situ vein bypass; femoral-popliteal**

Code also aortobifemoral bypass graft other than vein for aortobifemoral bypass using synthetic conduit and femoral-popliteal bypass with vein conduit in situ (35646)

Code also concurrent aortofemoral bypass for aortofemoral bypass graft with synthetic conduit and femoral-popliteal bypass with vein conduit in-situ (35647)

Code also concurrent aortofemoral bypass (vein) for an aortofemoral bypass using a vein conduit or a femoral-popliteal bypass with vein conduit in-situ (35539)

41.8 41.8 FUD 090 C 80 50

AMA: 2018,Jan,8; 2017,Jan,8; 2016,Jan,13; 2015,Jan,16; 2014,Jan,11

35585 **femoral-anterior tibial, posterior tibial, or peroneal artery**

48.4 48.4 FUD 090 C 80 50

AMA: 2018,Jan,8; 2017,Jan,8; 2016,Jan,13; 2015,Jan,16; 2014,Jan,11

35587 **popliteal-tibial, peroneal**

39.5 39.5 FUD 090 C 80 50

AMA: 2018,Jan,8; 2017,Jan,8; 2016,Jan,13; 2015,Jan,16; 2014,Jan,11

35600 Obtain Arm Artery for Coronary Bypass

EXCLUDES *Transposition and/or reimplantation of arteries (35691-35695)*

Code first (33533-33536)

\+ 35600 **Harvest of upper extremity artery, 1 segment, for coronary artery bypass procedure (List separately in addition to code for primary procedure)**

7.43 7.43 FUD ZZZ C 80

AMA: 2018,Jan,8; 2017,Jan,8; 2016,Jan,13; 2015,Jan,16; 2014,Jan,11

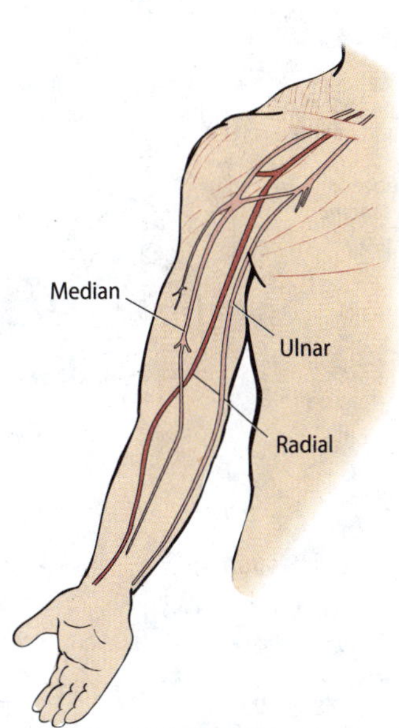

An upper extremity artery or segment is harvested for a coronary artery bypass procedure

35601-35671 Arterial Bypass: Grafts Other Than Veins

EXCLUDES *Transposition and/or reimplantation of arteries (35691-35695)*

35601 **Bypass graft, with other than vein; common carotid-ipsilateral internal carotid**

EXCLUDES *Open transcervical common carotid-common carotid bypass with endovascular repair of descending thoracic aorta (33891)*

40.4 40.4 **FUD** 090 C 80 50

AMA: 2018,Jan,8; 2017,Jan,8; 2016,Jan,13; 2015,Jan,16; 2014,Jan,11

35606 **carotid-subclavian**

EXCLUDES *Open subclavian to carotid artery transposition performed with endovascular thoracic aneurysm repair via neck incision (33889)*

34.0 34.0 **FUD** 090 C 80 50

AMA: 1997,Nov,1

35612 **subclavian-subclavian**

30.1 30.1 **FUD** 090 C 80 50

AMA: 1997,Nov,1

35616 **subclavian-axillary**

31.8 31.8 **FUD** 090 C 80 50

AMA: 1997,Nov,1

35621 **axillary-femoral**

31.7 31.7 **FUD** 090 C 80 50

AMA: 2018,Jan,8; 2017,Jan,8; 2016,Jan,13; 2015,Jan,16; 2014,Jan,11

35623 **axillary-popliteal or -tibial**

37.9 37.9 **FUD** 090 C 80 50

AMA: 2012,Apr,3-9; 1997,Nov,1

35626 **aortosubclavian, aortoinnominate, or aortocarotid**

46.0 46.0 **FUD** 090 C 80 50

AMA: 1997,Nov,1

35631 **aortoceliac, aortomesenteric, aortorenal**

53.7 53.7 **FUD** 090 C 80 50

AMA: 1997,Nov,1

Vena cava and renal veins
Celiac trunk
Abdominal aorta
Superior mesenteric
Renal
Abdominal aorta as it exits diaphragm
Synthetic graft
Blockage

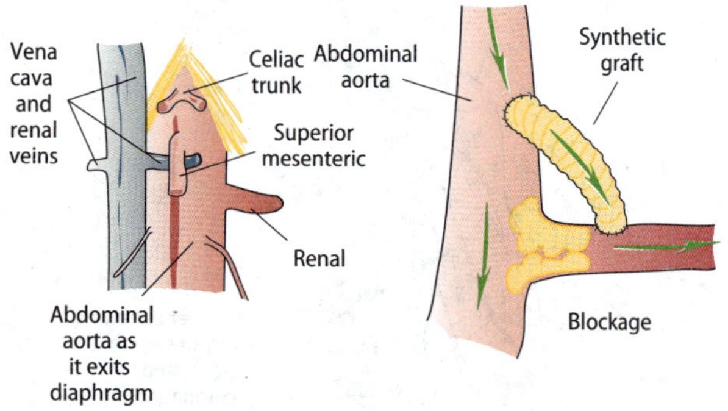

35632 **ilio-celiac**

52.2 52.2 **FUD** 090 C 80 50

EXCLUDES *Bypass graft (35531, 35631)*
Repair of blood vessel (35221, 35251, 35281)

35633 **ilio-mesenteric**

57.8 57.8 **FUD** 090 C 80 50

EXCLUDES *Bypass graft (35531, 35631)*
Repair of blood vessel (35221, 35251, 35281)

35634 **iliorenal**

51.0 51.0 **FUD** 090 C 80 50

EXCLUDES *Bypass graft (35536, 35560, 35631)*
Repair of blood vessel (35221, 35251, 35281)

35636 **splenorenal (splenic to renal arterial anastomosis)**

46.0 46.0 **FUD** 090 C 80 50

AMA: 1997,Nov,1; 1994,Win,1

35637 **aortoiliac**

EXCLUDES *Bypass graft (35638, 35646)*

47.9 47.9 **FUD** 090 C 80

AMA: 2018,Jan,8; 2017,Jan,8; 2016,Jan,13; 2015,Jan,16; 2014,Jan,11

35638 **aortobi-iliac**

EXCLUDES *Bypass graft (35637, 35646)*
Open placement of aorto-bi-iliac prosthesis after a failed endovascular repair (34831)

50.9 50.9 **FUD** 090 C 80

AMA: 2018,Jan,8; 2017,Jan,8; 2016,Jan,13; 2015,Jan,16; 2014,Jan,11

35642 **carotid-vertebral**

28.4 28.4 **FUD** 090 C 80 50

AMA: 1997,Nov,1

35645 **subclavian-vertebral**

27.3 27.3 **FUD** 090 C 80 50

AMA: 1997,Nov,1

35646 **aortobifemoral**

EXCLUDES *Bypass graft using vein graft (35540)*
Open placement of aortobifemoral prosthesis after a failed endovascular repair (34832)

49.7 49.7 **FUD** 090 C 80

AMA: 2018,Jan,8; 2017,Jan,8; 2016,Jan,13; 2015,Jan,16; 2014,Jan,11

35647 **aortofemoral**

EXCLUDES *Bypass graft using vein graft (35539)*

45.0 45.0 **FUD** 090 C 80 50

AMA: 2018,Jan,8; 2017,Jan,8; 2016,Jan,13; 2015,Jan,16; 2014,Jan,11

35650 **axillary-axillary**

31.3 31.3 **FUD** 090 C 80 50

AMA: 1997,Nov,1

35654 **axillary-femoral-femoral**

39.6 39.6 **FUD** 090 C 80

AMA: 2018,Jan,8; 2017,Jan,8; 2016,Jan,13; 2015,Jan,16; 2014,Jan,11

35656 **femoral-popliteal**

31.3 31.3 **FUD** 090 C 80 50

AMA: 2018,Jan,8; 2017,Jan,8; 2016,Jan,13; 2015,Jan,16; 2014,Jan,11

35661 **femoral-femoral**

31.4 31.4 **FUD** 090 C 80 50

AMA: 2018,Jan,8; 2017,Jan,8; 2016,Jan,13; 2015,Jan,16; 2014,Jan,11

35663 **ilioiliac**

35.1 35.1 **FUD** 090 C 80 50

AMA: 1997,Nov,1

35665 **iliofemoral**

34.0 34.0 **FUD** 090 C 80 50

AMA: 2018,Jan,8; 2017,Jan,8; 2016,Jan,13; 2015,Jan,16; 2014,Jan,11

35666 **femoral-anterior tibial, posterior tibial, or peroneal artery**

36.6 36.6 **FUD** 090 C 80 50

AMA: 2018,Jan,8; 2017,Jan,8; 2016,Jan,13; 2015,Jan,16; 2014,Jan,11

35671 **popliteal-tibial or -peroneal artery**

32.2 32.2 **FUD** 090 C 80 50

AMA: 2012,Apr,3-9; 1997,Nov,1

35681-35683 Arterial Bypass Using Combination Synthetic and Donor Graft

INCLUDES Acquiring multiple segments of vein from sites other than the extremity for which the arterial bypass is performed
Anastomosis of vein segments to create bypass graft conduits

+ **35681 Bypass graft; composite, prosthetic and vein (List separately in addition to code for primary procedure)**
EXCLUDES *Bypass graft (35682, 35683)*
Code first primary procedure
2.34 2.34 FUD ZZZ C 80
AMA: 2018,Jan,8; 2017,Jan,8; 2016,Jan,13; 2015,Jan,16; 2014,Jan,11

+ **35682 autogenous composite, 2 segments of veins from 2 locations (List separately in addition to code for primary procedure)**
EXCLUDES *Bypass graft (35681, 35683)*
Code first (35556, 35566, 35570-35571, 35583-35587)
10.2 10.2 FUD ZZZ C 80
AMA: 2018,Jan,8; 2017,Jan,8; 2016,Jan,13; 2015,Jan,16; 2014,Jan,11

+ **35683 autogenous composite, 3 or more segments of vein from 2 or more locations (List separately in addition to code for primary procedure)**
EXCLUDES *Bypass graft (35681-35682)*
Code first (35556, 35566, 35570-35571, 35583-35587)
11.8 11.8 FUD ZZZ C 80
AMA: 2018,Jan,8; 2017,Jan,8; 2016,Jan,13; 2015,Jan,16; 2014,Jan,11

35685-35686 Supplemental Procedures

INCLUDES Additional procedures that may be needed with a bypass graft to increase the patency of the graft
EXCLUDES *Composite grafts (35681-35683)*

+ **35685 Placement of vein patch or cuff at distal anastomosis of bypass graft, synthetic conduit (List separately in addition to code for primary procedure)**
INCLUDES Connection of a segment of vein (cuff or patch) between the distal portion of the synthetic graft and the native artery
Code first (35656, 35666, 35671)
5.76 5.76 FUD ZZZ N 80
AMA: 2018,Jan,8; 2017,Jan,8; 2016,Jan,13; 2015,Jan,16; 2014,Jan,11

+ **35686 Creation of distal arteriovenous fistula during lower extremity bypass surgery (non-hemodialysis) (List separately in addition to code for primary procedure)**
INCLUDES Creation of a fistula between the peroneal or tibial artery and vein at or past the site of the distal anastomosis
Code first (35556, 35566, 35570-35571, 35583-35587, 35623, 35656, 35666, 35671)
4.66 4.66 FUD ZZZ N 80
AMA: 2018,Jan,8; 2017,Jan,8; 2016,Jan,13; 2015,Jan,16; 2014,Jan,11

35691-35697 Arterial Translocation

CMS: 100-03,160.8 Electroencephalographic Monitoring During Cerebral Vasculature Surgery

35691 Transposition and/or reimplantation; vertebral to carotid artery
27.2 27.2 FUD 090 C 80 50
AMA: 1997,Nov,1; 1993,Win,1

35693 vertebral to subclavian artery
24.0 24.0 FUD 090 C 80 50
AMA: 1997,Nov,1; 1994,Sum,29

35694 subclavian to carotid artery
EXCLUDES *Subclavian to carotid artery transposition procedure (open) with concurrent repair of descending thoracic aorta (endovascular) (33889)*
28.5 28.5 FUD 090 C 80 50
AMA: 1997,Nov,1; 1993,Win,1

35695 carotid to subclavian artery
29.5 29.5 FUD 090 C 80 50
AMA: 1997,Nov,1; 1993,Win,1

+ **35697 Reimplantation, visceral artery to infrarenal aortic prosthesis, each artery (List separately in addition to code for primary procedure)**
EXCLUDES *Repair of thoracoabdominal aortic aneurysm with graft (33877)*
Code first primary procedure
4.30 4.30 FUD ZZZ C 80
AMA: 1997,Nov,1

35700 Reoperative Bypass Lower Extremities

Code first (35556, 35566, 35570-35571, 35583, 35585, 35587, 35656, 35666, 35671)

+ **35700 Reoperation, femoral-popliteal or femoral (popliteal)-anterior tibial, posterior tibial, peroneal artery, or other distal vessels, more than 1 month after original operation (List separately in addition to code for primary procedure)**
4.42 4.42 FUD ZZZ C 80
AMA: 2018,Jan,8; 2017,Jan,8; 2016,Jan,13; 2015,Jan,16; 2014,Jan,11

35701-35761 Arterial Exploration without Repair

EXCLUDES *Exploration to identify recipient artery for microvascular anastomosis of free graft/flap of:*
Bone (20955-20962)
Jejunum (43496)
Muscle, skin or fascia (15756-15758)
Omentum (49906)
Osteocutaneous (20969-20973)
Exploration without surgical repair of:
Abdominal artery (49000)
Chest artery (32100)
Other arteries not of the neck, upper or lower extremities, chest, abdomen or retroperitoneum (37799)
Retroperitoneal artery (49010)
Code also nonvascular surgical procedures performed in addition to exploration when the exploration is through a separate incision

▲ **35701 Exploration not followed by surgical repair, artery; neck (eg, carotid, subclavian)**
EXCLUDES *Exploration for postoperative hemorrhage, thrombosis or infection (35800)*
Repair of blood vessel on same side of neck (35201, 35231, 35261)
16.4 16.4 FUD 090 C 80 50
AMA: 1997,Nov,1

● **35702 upper extremity (eg, axillary, brachial, radial, ulnar)**
EXCLUDES *Exploration for postoperative hemorrhage, thrombosis or infection in same extremity (35860)*
Repair of blood vessel in same extremity (35206-35207, 35236, 35266)

● **35703 lower extremity (eg, common femoral, deep femoral, superficial femoral, popliteal, tibial, peroneal)**
EXCLUDES *Exploration for postoperative hemorrhage, thrombosis or infection in same extremity (35860)*
Repair of blood vessel in same extremity (35256, 35286)

~~35721 femoral artery~~

~~35741 popliteal artery~~

~~35761 other vessels~~

35800-35860 Arterial Exploration for Postoperative Complication

INCLUDES Return to the operating room for postoperative hemorrhage

35800 Exploration for postoperative hemorrhage, thrombosis or infection; neck
20.8 20.8 FUD 090 C 80
AMA: 1997,Nov,1

35820 chest
58.3 58.3 FUD 090 C 80
AMA: 1997,Nov,1

35840 **abdomen**
34.6 34.6 FUD 090
AMA: 1997,May,4; 1997,Nov,1

35860 **extremity**
24.2 24.2 FUD 090
AMA: 2018,Jan,8; 2017,Jan,8; 2016,Jan,13; 2015,Jan,16; 2014,Apr,10

35870 Repair Secondary Aortoenteric Fistula

35870 **Repair of graft-enteric fistula**
35.9 35.9 FUD 090
AMA: 1997,Nov,1

35875-35876 Removal of Thrombus from Graft

EXCLUDES *Thrombectomy dialysis fistula or graft (36831, 36833)*
Thrombectomy with blood vessel repair, lower extremity, vein graft (35256)
Thrombectomy with blood vessel repair, lower extremity, with/without patch angioplasty (35226)

35875 **Thrombectomy of arterial or venous graft (other than hemodialysis graft or fistula);**
17.2 17.2 FUD 090
AMA: 2018,Jan,8; 2017,Jan,8; 2016,Jan,13; 2015,Jan,16; 2014,Jan,11

35876 **with revision of arterial or venous graft**
27.4 27.4 FUD 090
AMA: 1999,Mar,6; 1999,Nov,1

35879-35884 Revision Lower Extremity Bypass Graft

EXCLUDES *Removal of infected graft (35901-35907)*
Revascularization following removal of infected graft(s)
Thrombectomy dialysis fistula or graft (36831, 36833)
Thrombectomy with blood vessel repair, lower extremity, vein graft (35256)
Thrombectomy with blood vessel repair, lower extremity, with/without patch angioplasty (35226)
Thrombectomy with graft revision (35876)

35879 **Revision, lower extremity arterial bypass, without thrombectomy, open; with vein patch angioplasty**
26.8 26.8 FUD 090
AMA: 2018,Jan,8; 2017,Jan,8; 2016,Jan,13; 2015,Jan,16; 2014,Jan,11

35881 **with segmental vein interposition**
EXCLUDES *Revision of femoral anastomosis of synthetic arterial bypass graft (35883-35884)*
29.4 29.4 FUD 090
AMA: 2018,Jan,8; 2017,Jan,8; 2016,Jan,13; 2015,Jan,16; 2014,Jan,11

35883 **Revision, femoral anastomosis of synthetic arterial bypass graft in groin, open; with nonautogenous patch graft (eg, Dacron, ePTFE, bovine pericardium)**
EXCLUDES *Reoperation, femoral-popliteal or femoral (popliteal)-anterior tibial, posterior tibial, peroneal artery, or other distal vessels (35700)*
Revision, femoral anastomosis of synthetic arterial bypass graft in groin, open; with autogenous vein patch graft (35884)
Thrombectomy of arterial or venous graft (35875)
34.8 34.8 FUD 090
AMA: 2018,Jan,8; 2017,Jan,8; 2016,Jan,13; 2015,Jan,16; 2014,Jan,11

35884 **with autogenous vein patch graft**
EXCLUDES *Reoperation, femoral-popliteal or femoral (popliteal)-anterior tibial, posterior tibial, peroneal artery, or other distal vessels (35700)*
Revision, femoral anastomosis of synthetic arterial bypass graft in groin, open; with autogenous vein patch graft (35883)
Thrombectomy of arterial or venous graft (35875-35876)
35.8 35.8 FUD 090
AMA: 2018,Jan,8; 2017,Jan,8; 2016,Jan,13; 2015,Jan,16; 2014,Jan,11

35901-35907 Removal of Infected Graft

35901 **Excision of infected graft; neck**
13.5 13.5 FUD 090
AMA: 1997,Nov,1; 1993,Win,1

Infected graft is removed
Internal jugular vein
Internal carotid
External carotid
Common carotid artery
Sternocleido-mastoid muscle

The physician removes an infected graft from the neck and repairs the blood vessel. If a new graft is placed, report the appropriate revascularization code

35903 **extremity**
16.3 16.3 FUD 090
AMA: 2018,Aug,10

35905 **thorax**
48.5 48.5 FUD 090
AMA: 1997,Nov,1; 1993,Win,1

35907 **abdomen**
55.2 55.2 FUD 090
AMA: 1997,Nov,1; 1993,Win,1

36000 Intravenous Access Established

INCLUDES Venous access for phlebotomy, prophylactic intravenous access, infusion therapy, chemotherapy, hydration, transfusion, drug administration, etc. which is included in the work value of the primary procedure

36000 **Introduction of needle or intracatheter, vein**
0.27 0.77 FUD XXX
AMA: 2019,Aug,8; 2018,Mar,3; 2018,Jan,8; 2017,Jan,8; 2016,Nov,3; 2016,Jan,13; 2015,Jan,16; 2014,Oct,6; 2014,Sep,13; 2014,May,4; 2014,Jan,11

36002 Injection Treatment of Pseudoaneurysm

INCLUDES Insertion of needle or catheter, local anesthesia, injection of contrast, power injections, and all pre- and postinjection care provided
EXCLUDES *Arteriotomy site sealant*
Compression repair pseudoaneurysm, ultrasound guided (76936)
Medications, contrast material, catheters

36002 **Injection procedures (eg, thrombin) for percutaneous treatment of extremity pseudoaneurysm**
(76942, 77002, 77012, 77021)
3.04 4.49 FUD 000
AMA: 2018,Mar,3; 2018,Jan,8; 2017,Jan,8; 2016,Nov,3; 2016,Jan,13; 2015,Jan,16; 2014,Oct,6; 2014,Jan,11

36005-36015 Insertion Needle or Intracatheter: Venous

INCLUDES Insertion of needle/catheter, local anesthesia, injection of contrast, power injections, all pre- and postinjection care
EXCLUDES *Medications, contrast materials, catheters*
Code also catheterization of second order vessels (or higher) supplied by the same first order branch, same vascular family (36012)
Code also each vascular family (e.g., bilateral procedures are separate vascular families)

36005 **Injection procedure for extremity venography (including introduction of needle or intracatheter)**
(75820, 75822)
1.40 8.76 FUD 000
AMA: 2018,Mar,3; 2018,Jan,8; 2017,Jan,8; 2016,Nov,3; 2016,Jul,6; 2016,Jan,13; 2015,Jan,16; 2014,Oct,6

36010 **Introduction of catheter, superior or inferior vena cava**
3.19 14.2 FUD XXX N N1 50
AMA: 2018,Jan,8; 2017,Feb,14; 2017,Jan,8; 2016,Jul,6; 2016,Jan,13; 2015,Jan,16; 2014,Jan,11

36011 **Selective catheter placement, venous system; first order branch (eg, renal vein, jugular vein)**
4.54 24.0 FUD XXX N N1 50
AMA: 2018,Jan,8; 2017,Jan,8; 2016,Jul,6; 2016,Jan,13; 2015,Jan,16; 2014,Jan,11

36012 **second order, or more selective, branch (eg, left adrenal vein, petrosal sinus)**
5.03 24.5 FUD XXX N N1 50
AMA: 2018,Oct,3; 2018,Jan,8; 2017,Jan,8; 2016,Jul,6; 2016,Jan,13; 2015,Jan,16; 2014,Jan,11

36013 **Introduction of catheter, right heart or main pulmonary artery**
3.52 21.8 FUD XXX N N1
AMA: 2019,Jun,3; 2018,Jan,8; 2017,Jan,8; 2016,Jul,6; 2016,Jan,13; 2015,Jan,16; 2014,Jan,11

36014 **Selective catheter placement, left or right pulmonary artery**
4.38 23.0 FUD XXX N N1 50
AMA: 2019,Jun,3; 2018,Jan,8; 2017,Jan,8; 2016,Jul,6; 2016,Jan,13; 2015,Jan,16; 2014,Jan,11

36015 **Selective catheter placement, segmental or subsegmental pulmonary artery**
EXCLUDES *Placement of Swan Ganz/other flow directed catheter for monitoring (93503)*
Selective blood sampling, specific organs (36500)
4.98 24.9 FUD XXX N N1 50
AMA: 2019,Jun,3; 2018,Jan,8; 2017,Jan,8; 2016,Jul,6; 2016,Jan,13; 2015,Jan,16; 2014,Jan,11

36100-36218 Insertion Needle or Intracatheter: Arterial

INCLUDES Introduction of the catheter and catheterization of all lesser order vessels used for the approach
Local anesthesia, placement of catheter/needle, injection of contrast, power injections, all pre- and postinjection care

EXCLUDES *Angiography (36222-36228, 75600-75774)*
Angioplasty ([37246, 37247])
Chemotherapy injections (96401-96549)
Injection procedures for cardiac catheterizations (93455, 93457, 93459, 93461, 93530-93533, 93564)
Internal mammary artery angiography without left heart catheterization (36216, 36217)
Medications, contrast, catheters
Transcatheter interventions (37200, 37211, 37213-37214, 37241-37244, 61624, 61626)

Code also additional first order or higher catheterization for vascular families if the vascular family is supplied by a first order vessel that is different from one already coded
Code also catheterization of second and third order vessels supplied by the same first order branch, same vascular family (36218, 36248)

36100 **Introduction of needle or intracatheter, carotid or vertebral artery**
4.54 14.8 FUD XXX N N1 50
AMA: 2000,Oct,4; 1998,Apr,1

36140 **Introduction of needle or intracatheter, upper or lower extremity artery**
EXCLUDES *Arteriovenous cannula insertion (36810-36821)*
2.62 12.7 FUD XXX N N1
AMA: 2018,Jan,8; 2017,Jan,8; 2016,Jan,13; 2015,Jan,16; 2014,Jan,11

36160 **Introduction of needle or intracatheter, aortic, translumbar**
3.59 14.6 FUD XXX N N1
AMA: 2018,Jan,8; 2017,Jan,8; 2016,Jan,13; 2015,Jan,16; 2014,Jan,11

36200 **Introduction of catheter, aorta**
EXCLUDES *Nonselective angiography of the extracranial carotid and/or cerebral vessels and cervicocerebral arch (36221)*
4.05 16.2 FUD 000 N N1 50
AMA: 2018,Jan,8; 2017,Mar,3; 2017,Jan,8; 2016,Jul,6; 2016,Jan,13; 2015,Jan,16; 2014,Jan,11

36215 **Selective catheter placement, arterial system; each first order thoracic or brachiocephalic branch, within a vascular family**
INCLUDES Introduction of catheter into the aorta (36200)
EXCLUDES *Placement of catheter for coronary angiography (93454-93461)*
6.16 29.4 FUD 000 N N1
AMA: 2018,Jan,8; 2017,Mar,3; 2017,Jan,8; 2016,Jul,6; 2016,Jan,13; 2015,Jan,16; 2014,Jan,11

36216 **initial second order thoracic or brachiocephalic branch, within a vascular family**
7.93 31.6 FUD 000 N N1
AMA: 2018,Jan,8; 2017,Jan,8; 2016,Jul,6; 2016,Jan,13; 2015,Jan,16; 2014,Jan,11

36217 **initial third order or more selective thoracic or brachiocephalic branch, within a vascular family**
9.51 53.1 FUD 000 N N1
AMA: 2018,Jan,8; 2017,Jan,8; 2016,Jul,6; 2016,Jan,13; 2015,Jan,16; 2014,Jan,11

+ **36218** **additional second order, third order, and beyond, thoracic or brachiocephalic branch, within a vascular family (List in addition to code for initial second or third order vessel as appropriate)**
Code also transcatheter therapy procedures (37200, 37211, 37213-37214, 37236-37239, 37241-37244, 61624, 61626)
Code first (36216-36217, 36225-36226)
1.51 6.89 FUD ZZZ N N1
AMA: 2018,Oct,3; 2018,Jan,8; 2017,Jan,8; 2016,Jul,6; 2016,Jan,13; 2015,Jan,16; 2014,Jan,11

36221-36228 Diagnostic Studies: Aortic Arch/Carotid/Vertebral Arteries

INCLUDES Accessing the vessel
Arterial contrast injection that includes arterial, capillary, and venous phase imaging, when performed
Arteriotomy closure (pressure or closure device)
Catheter placement
Radiologic supervision and interpretation
Reporting of selective catheter placement based on intensity of services in the following hierarchy:
36226>36225
36224>36223>36222

EXCLUDES *3D rendering when performed (76376-76377)*
Interventional procedures
Transcatheter intravascular stent placement of common carotid or innominate artery on the same side (37217)
Ultrasound guidance (76937)

Code also diagnostic angiography of upper extremities/other vascular beds during the same session, if performed (75774)

36221 **Non-selective catheter placement, thoracic aorta, with angiography of the extracranial carotid, vertebral, and/or intracranial vessels, unilateral or bilateral, and all associated radiological supervision and interpretation, includes angiography of the cervicocerebral arch, when performed**
EXCLUDES *Selective catheter placement, common carotid or innominate artery (36222-36226)*
Transcatheter intravascular stent placement of common carotid or innominate artery on the same side (37217)
5.80 29.3 FUD 000 Q2 N1
AMA: 2018,Jan,8; 2017,Jan,8; 2016,Mar,3; 2016,Jan,13; 2015,Nov,3; 2015,May,7; 2015,Jan,16; 2014,Mar,8; 2014,Jan,11

36222 **Selective catheter placement, common carotid or innominate artery, unilateral, any approach, with angiography of the ipsilateral extracranial carotid circulation and all associated radiological supervision and interpretation, includes angiography of the cervicocerebral arch, when performed**

INCLUDES Unilateral catheterization of artery

EXCLUDES *Transcatheter placement of intravascular stent(s) (37215-37218)*

Code also modifier 59 when different territories on both sides of the body are being studied

8.22 34.7 **FUD** 000 Q2 N1 50

AMA: 2018,Jan,8; 2017,Jan,8; 2016,Mar,3; 2016,Jan,13; 2015,Nov,3; 2015,Nov,10; 2015,May,7; 2015,Jan,16; 2014,Mar,8; 2014,Jan,11

36223 **Selective catheter placement, common carotid or innominate artery, unilateral, any approach, with angiography of the ipsilateral intracranial carotid circulation and all associated radiological supervision and interpretation, includes angiography of the extracranial carotid and cervicocerebral arch, when performed**

INCLUDES Unilateral catheterization of artery

EXCLUDES *Transcatheter placement of intravascular stent(s) (37215-37218)*

Code also modifier 59 when different territories on both sides of the body are being studied

9.18 43.9 **FUD** 000 Q2 N1 50

AMA: 2018,Jan,8; 2017,Jan,8; 2016,Mar,3; 2016,Jan,13; 2015,Nov,3; 2015,Jan,16; 2014,Mar,8; 2014,Jan,11

36224 **Selective catheter placement, internal carotid artery, unilateral, with angiography of the ipsilateral intracranial carotid circulation and all associated radiological supervision and interpretation, includes angiography of the extracranial carotid and cervicocerebral arch, when performed**

INCLUDES Unilateral catheterization of artery

EXCLUDES *Transcatheter placement of intravascular stent(s) (37215-37218)*

Code also modifier 59 when different territories on both sides of the body are being studied

10.4 56.8 **FUD** 000 Q2 N1 50

AMA: 2018,Jan,8; 2017,Jan,8; 2016,Mar,3; 2016,Jan,13; 2015,Nov,3; 2015,Jan,16; 2014,Mar,8; 2014,Jan,11

36225 **Selective catheter placement, subclavian or innominate artery, unilateral, with angiography of the ipsilateral vertebral circulation and all associated radiological supervision and interpretation, includes angiography of the cervicocerebral arch, when performed**

EXCLUDES *Transcatheter placement of intravascular stent(s) (37217)*

9.16 42.3 **FUD** 000 Q2 N1 50

AMA: 2018,Jan,8; 2017,Jan,8; 2016,Mar,3; 2016,Jan,13; 2015,Nov,3; 2015,Jan,16; 2014,Mar,8; 2014,Jan,11

36226 **Selective catheter placement, vertebral artery, unilateral, with angiography of the ipsilateral vertebral circulation and all associated radiological supervision and interpretation, includes angiography of the cervicocerebral arch, when performed**

EXCLUDES *Transcatheter placement of intravascular stent(s) (37217)*

10.3 53.7 **FUD** 000 Q2 N1 50

AMA: 2018,Jan,8; 2017,Jan,8; 2016,Mar,3; 2016,Jan,13; 2015,Nov,3; 2015,Jan,16; 2014,Mar,8

\+ **36227** **Selective catheter placement, external carotid artery, unilateral, with angiography of the ipsilateral external carotid circulation and all associated radiological supervision and interpretation (List separately in addition to code for primary procedure)**

INCLUDES Unilateral catheter placement/diagnostic imaging of ipsilateral external carotid circulation

EXCLUDES *Reporting with modifier 50. Report once for each side when performed bilaterally*

Transcatheter placement of intravascular stent(s) (37217)

Code first (36222-36224)

3.41 7.23 **FUD** ZZZ 50 N N1

AMA: 2018,Jan,8; 2017,Jan,8; 2016,Jan,13; 2015,Nov,10; 2015,Jan,16; 2014,Mar,8; 2014,Jan,11

\+ **36228** **Selective catheter placement, each intracranial branch of the internal carotid or vertebral arteries, unilateral, with angiography of the selected vessel circulation and all associated radiological supervision and interpretation (eg, middle cerebral artery, posterior inferior cerebellar artery) (List separately in addition to code for primary procedure)**

INCLUDES Unilateral catheter placement/imaging of initial and each additional intracranial branch of internal carotid or vertebral arteries

EXCLUDES *Procedure performed more than 2 times per side*

Reporting with modifier 50. Report once for each side when performed bilaterally

Code first (36223-36226)

7.03 37.6 **FUD** ZZZ 50 N N1

AMA: 2018,Jan,8; 2017,Jan,8; 2016,Jan,13; 2015,Nov,3; 2015,Jan,16; 2014,Jan,11

36245-36254 Catheter Placement: Arteries of the Lower Body

INCLUDES Introduction of the catheter and catheterization of all lesser order vessels used for the approach

Local anesthesia, placement of catheter/needle, injection of contrast, power injections

EXCLUDES *Angiography (36222-36228, 75600-75774)*

Chemotherapy injections (96401-96549)

Injection procedures for cardiac catheterizations (93455, 93457, 93459, 93461, 93530-93533, 93564)

Internal mammary artery angiography without left heart catheterization (36216-36217)

Medications, contrast, catheters

Transcatheter procedures (37200, 37211, 37213-37214, 37236-37239, 37241-37244, 61624, 61626)

Code also additional first order or higher catheterization for vascular families if the vascular family is supplied by a first order vessel that is different from one already coded

Code also catheterization of second and third order vessels supplied by the same first order branch, same vascular family (36218, 36248)

(75600-75774)

36245 **Selective catheter placement, arterial system; each first order abdominal, pelvic, or lower extremity artery branch, within a vascular family**

6.89 37.4 **FUD** XXX N N1 50

AMA: 2018,Jan,8; 2017,Jan,8; 2016,Jul,6; 2016,Jan,13; 2015,Jan,16; 2014,Jan,11

36246 **initial second order abdominal, pelvic, or lower extremity artery branch, within a vascular family**

7.39 23.8 **FUD** 000 N N1 50

AMA: 2018,Jan,8; 2017,Jan,8; 2016,Jul,6; 2016,Jan,13; 2015,Jan,16; 2014,Jan,11

36247 **initial third order or more selective abdominal, pelvic, or lower extremity artery branch, within a vascular family**

8.78 42.6 **FUD** 000 N N1 50

AMA: 2018,Jan,8; 2017,Jan,8; 2016,Jul,6; 2016,Jan,13; 2015,Jan,16; 2014,Jan,11

\+ 36248 additional second order, third order, and beyond, abdominal, pelvic, or lower extremity artery branch, within a vascular family (List in addition to code for initial second or third order vessel as appropriate)
Code first (36246, 36247)
1.42 4.11 FUD ZZZ N N1
AMA: 2018,Oct,3; 2018,Jan,8; 2017,Jan,8; 2016,Jul,6; 2016,Jan,13; 2015,Jan,16; 2014,Jan,11

36251 Selective catheter placement (first-order), main renal artery and any accessory renal artery(s) for renal angiography, including arterial puncture and catheter placement(s), fluoroscopy, contrast injection(s), image postprocessing, permanent recording of images, and radiological supervision and interpretation, including pressure gradient measurements when performed, and flush aortogram when performed; unilateral
INCLUDES Closure device placement at vascular access site
EXCLUDES *Transcatheter renal sympathetic denervation, percutaneous approach (0338T-0339T)*
7.55 39.2 FUD 000 Q2 N1
AMA: 2018,Jan,8; 2017,Jan,8; 2016,Jan,13; 2015,Jan,16; 2014,Jan,11

36252 bilateral
INCLUDES Closure device placement at vascular access site
EXCLUDES *Transcatheter renal sympathetic denervation, percutaneous approach (0338T-0339T)*
10.4 42.4 FUD 000 Q2 N1
AMA: 2018,Jan,8; 2017,Jan,8; 2016,Jan,13; 2015,Jan,16; 2014,Jan,11

36253 Superselective catheter placement (one or more second order or higher renal artery branches) renal artery and any accessory renal artery(s) for renal angiography, including arterial puncture, catheterization, fluoroscopy, contrast injection(s), image postprocessing, permanent recording of images, and radiological supervision and interpretation, including pressure gradient measurements when performed, and flush aortogram when performed; unilateral
INCLUDES Closure device placement at vascular access site
EXCLUDES *Procedure performed on same kidney with (36251)*
Transcatheter renal sympathetic denervation, percutaneous approach (0338T-0339T)
10.3 62.6 FUD 000 Q2 N1
AMA: 2018,Jan,8; 2017,Jan,8; 2016,Jan,13; 2015,Jan,16; 2014,Jan,11

36254 bilateral
INCLUDES Closure device placement at vascular access site
EXCLUDES *Selective catheter placement (first-order), main renal artery and any accessory renal artery(s) for renal angiography (36252)*
Transcatheter renal sympathetic denervation, percutaneous approach (0338T-0339T)
12.1 60.8 FUD 000 Q2 N1
AMA: 2018,Jan,8; 2017,Jan,8; 2016,Jan,13; 2015,Jan,16; 2014,Jan,11

36260-36299 Implanted Infusion Pumps: Intra-arterial

36260 Insertion of implantable intra-arterial infusion pump (eg, for chemotherapy of liver)
18.8 18.8 FUD 090 T J8
AMA: 2018,Jan,8; 2017,Jan,8; 2016,Jan,13; 2015,Jan,16; 2014,Jan,11

36261 Revision of implanted intra-arterial infusion pump
11.6 11.6 FUD 090 T J8 80
AMA: 2000,Oct,4; 1997,Nov,1

36262 Removal of implanted intra-arterial infusion pump
8.90 8.90 FUD 090 Q2 G2
AMA: 2000,Oct,4; 1997,Nov,1

36299 Unlisted procedure, vascular injection
0.00 0.00 FUD YYY N 80
AMA: 2000,Oct,4; 1997,Nov,1

36400-36425 Specimen Collection: Phlebotomy

EXCLUDES *Collection of specimen from:*
A completely implantable device (36591)
An established catheter (36592)

36400 Venipuncture, younger than age 3 years, necessitating the skill of a physician or other qualified health care professional, not to be used for routine venipuncture; femoral or jugular vein A
0.53 0.75 FUD XXX N N1
AMA: 2018,Jan,8; 2017,Jan,8; 2016,Jan,13; 2015,Jan,16; 2014,May,4; 2014,Jan,11

36405 scalp vein A
0.44 0.66 FUD XXX N N1
AMA: 2018,Jan,8; 2017,Jan,8; 2016,Jan,13; 2015,Jan,16; 2014,May,4; 2014,Jan,11

36406 other vein A
0.25 0.47 FUD XXX N N1
AMA: 2018,Jan,8; 2017,Jan,8; 2016,Jan,13; 2015,Jan,16; 2014,May,4; 2014,Jan,11

36410 Venipuncture, age 3 years or older, necessitating the skill of a physician or other qualified health care professional (separate procedure), for diagnostic or therapeutic purposes (not to be used for routine venipuncture) A
0.27 0.49 FUD XXX N N1
AMA: 2019,Aug,8; 2018,Mar,3; 2018,Jan,8; 2017,Jan,8; 2016,Nov,3; 2016,Jan,13; 2015,Jan,16; 2014,Oct,6; 2014,Jan,11

36415 Collection of venous blood by venipuncture
0.00 0.00 FUD XXX 63 Q
AMA: 2019,Aug,8; 2018,Jan,8; 2017,Jan,8; 2016,Jan,13; 2015,Jan,16; 2014,May,4; 2014,Jan,11

36416 Collection of capillary blood specimen (eg, finger, heel, ear stick)
0.00 0.00 FUD XXX N N1
AMA: 2008,Apr,-9; 2003,Feb,7

36420 Venipuncture, cutdown; younger than age 1 year A
1.35 1.35 FUD XXX 63 Q1 N1 80
AMA: 2018,Jan,8; 2017,Jan,8; 2016,Jan,13; 2015,Jan,16; 2014,Jan,11

36425 age 1 or over A
EXCLUDES *Endovenous ablation therapy of incompetent vein, extremity (36475-36476, 36478-36479)*
1.16 1.16 FUD XXX Q1 N1
AMA: 2018,Mar,3; 2018,Jan,8; 2017,Jan,8; 2016,Nov,3; 2016,Jan,13; 2015,Jan,16; 2014,Oct,6

36430-36460 Transfusions

CMS: 100-01,3,20.5 Blood Deductibles; 100-03,110.16 Transfusion in Kidney Transplants; 100-03,110.7 Blood Transfusions; 100-03,110.8 Blood Platelet Transfusions

36430 Transfusion, blood or blood components
EXCLUDES *Infant partial exchange transfusion (36456)*
0.99 0.99 FUD XXX S P3
AMA: 2019,Jun,5; 2018,Jan,8; 2017,Jul,3; 2017,Jan,8; 2016,Jan,13; 2015,Jan,16; 2014,Jan,11

36440 Push transfusion, blood, 2 years or younger A
EXCLUDES *Infant partial exchange transfusion (36456)*
1.46 1.46 FUD XXX S R2 80
AMA: 2018,Jan,8; 2017,Jul,3; 2017,Jan,8; 2016,Jan,13; 2015,Jan,16; 2014,Jan,11

36450 Exchange transfusion, blood; newborn A
EXCLUDES *Infant partial exchange transfusion (36456)*
4.94 4.94 FUD XXX 63 S R2 80
AMA: 2018,Jan,8; 2017,Jul,3

36455 other than newborn A
3.68 3.68 FUD XXX S G2
AMA: 2003,Apr,7; 1997,Nov,1

36456 **Partial exchange transfusion, blood, plasma or crystalloid necessitating the skill of a physician or other qualified health care professional, newborn** A

EXCLUDES *Transfusions of other types (36430-36450)*

3.03 3.03 FUD XXX 63 S 80

AMA: 2018,Jan,8; 2017,Jul,3

36460 **Transfusion, intrauterine, fetal** A ♀

(76941)

9.84 9.84 FUD XXX 63 S 80

AMA: 2003,Apr,7; 1997,Nov,1

36465-36466 [36465, 36466] Destruction Spider Veins

INCLUDES All supplies, equipment, compression stockings or bandages when performed in the physician office

EXCLUDES *Multi-layer compression system applied to leg (29581, 29584)*
Strapping of leg: ankle, foot, hip, knee, toes of same extremity (29520, 29530, 29540, 29550)
Unna boot (29580)
Use of code more than one time for each extremity treated
Vascular embolization and occlusion (37241-37244)
Vascular embolization vein in same operative field (37241)

36465 **Resequenced code. See code following 36471.**

36466 **Resequenced code. See code following 36471.**

36468 **Injection(s) of sclerosant for spider veins (telangiectasia), limb or trunk**

(76942)

0.00 0.00 FUD 000 01 N1 80

AMA: 2018,Mar,3; 2018,Jan,8; 2017,Jan,8; 2016,Nov,3; 2016,Jan,13; 2015,Apr,10; 2015,Jan,16; 2014,Oct,6; 2014,Aug,14

36470 **Injection of sclerosant; single incompetent vein (other than telangiectasia)**

EXCLUDES *Injection of foam sclerosant with ultrasound guidance for compression maneuvers (36465-36466)*

(76942)

1.11 3.02 FUD 000 T P3 50

AMA: 2018,Dec,10; 2018,Dec,10; 2018,Mar,3; 2018,Jan,8; 2017,Jan,8; 2016,Nov,3; 2016,Jan,13; 2015,Nov,10; 2015,Apr,10; 2015,Jan,16; 2014,Oct,6; 2014,Aug,14

36471 **multiple incompetent veins (other than telangiectasia), same leg**

EXCLUDES *Injection of foam sclerosant with ultrasound guidance for compression maneuvers (36465-36466)*

(76942)

2.21 5.47 FUD 000 T P3 50

AMA: 2018,Dec,10; 2018,Dec,10; 2018,Mar,3; 2018,Jan,8; 2017,Jan,8; 2016,Nov,3; 2016,Jan,13; 2015,Nov,10; 2015,Aug,8; 2015,Apr,10; 2015,Jan,16; 2014,Oct,6; 2014,Aug,14

36465 **Injection of non-compounded foam sclerosant with ultrasound compression maneuvers to guide dispersion of the injectate, inclusive of all imaging guidance and monitoring; single incompetent extremity truncal vein (eg, great saphenous vein, accessory saphenous vein)**

EXCLUDES *Ablation of vein using chemical adhesive ([36482, 36483])*
Injection of foam sclerosant without ultrasound guidance for compression maneuvers (36470-36471)

3.45 43.6 FUD 000 T G2 50

AMA: 2019,Feb,9; 2018,Dec,10; 2018,Dec,10; 2018,Mar,3

36466 **multiple incompetent truncal veins (eg, great saphenous vein, accessory saphenous vein), same leg**

EXCLUDES *Ablation of vein using chemical adhesive ([36482, 36483])*
Injection of foam sclerosant without ultrasound guidance for compression maneuvers (36470-36471)

4.39 45.8 FUD 000 T G2 50

AMA: 2019,Feb,9; 2018,Dec,10; 2018,Dec,10; 2018,Mar,3

36473-36483 [36482, 36483] Vein Ablation

INCLUDES Multi-layer compression system applied to leg (29581, 29584)
Patient monitoring
Radiological guidance (76000, 76937, 76942, 76998, 77002)
Venous access/injections (36000-36005, 36410, 36425)

EXCLUDES *Duplex scans (93970-93971)*
Strapping of leg: ankle, foot, hip, knee, toes of same extremity (29520, 29530, 29540, 29550)
Transcatheter embolization (75894)
Unna boot (29580)
Vascular embolization vein in same operative field (37241)

36473 **Endovenous ablation therapy of incompetent vein, extremity, inclusive of all imaging guidance and monitoring, percutaneous, mechanochemical; first vein treated**

INCLUDES Local anesthesia

EXCLUDES *Laser ablation incompetent vein (36478-36479)*
Radiofrequency ablation incompetent vein (36475-36476)

5.15 41.4 FUD 000 T P2 50

AMA: 2019,Feb,9; 2018,Mar,3; 2018,Jan,8; 2017,Jan,8; 2016,Nov,3

+ **36474** **subsequent vein(s) treated in a single extremity, each through separate access sites (List separately in addition to code for primary procedure)**

INCLUDES Local anesthesia

EXCLUDES *Laser ablation incompetent vein (36478-36479)*
Radiofrequency ablation incompetent vein (36475-36476)
Use of code more than one time per extremity

Code first (36473)

2.57 7.87 FUD ZZZ N N1 50

AMA: 2019,Feb,9; 2018,Mar,3; 2018,Jan,8; 2017,Jan,8; 2016,Nov,3

36475 **Endovenous ablation therapy of incompetent vein, extremity, inclusive of all imaging guidance and monitoring, percutaneous, radiofrequency; first vein treated**

INCLUDES Tumescent anesthesia

EXCLUDES *Ablation of vein using chemical adhesive ([36482, 36483])*
Endovenous ablation therapy of incompetent vein (36478-36479)

8.11 40.6 FUD 000 T A2 50

AMA: 2018,Mar,3; 2018,Jan,8; 2017,Jan,8; 2016,Nov,3; 2016,Aug,3; 2016,Jan,13; 2015,Apr,10; 2015,Jan,16; 2014,Oct,6; 2014,Aug,14; 2014,Mar,4; 2014,Jan,11

+ **36476** **subsequent vein(s) treated in a single extremity, each through separate access sites (List separately in addition to code for primary procedure)**

INCLUDES Tumescent anesthesia

EXCLUDES *Ablation of vein using chemical adhesive ([36482, 36483])*
Endovenous ablation therapy of incompetent vein (36478-36479)
Use of code more than one time per extremity
Vascular embolization or occlusion (37242-37244)

Code first (36475)

3.93 8.55 FUD ZZZ N N1 50

AMA: 2018,Mar,3; 2018,Jan,8; 2017,Jan,8; 2016,Nov,3; 2016,Aug,3; 2016,Jan,13; 2015,Apr,10; 2015,Jan,16; 2014,Oct,6; 2014,Aug,14; 2014,Mar,4; 2014,Jan,11

36478 **Endovenous ablation therapy of incompetent vein, extremity, inclusive of all imaging guidance and monitoring, percutaneous, laser; first vein treated**

INCLUDES Tumescent anesthesia

EXCLUDES *Ablation of vein using chemical adhesive ([36482, 36483])*
Endovenous ablation therapy of incompetent vein (36475-36476)

8.06 32.1 FUD 000 T A2 50

AMA: 2018,Mar,3; 2018,Jan,8; 2017,Jan,8; 2016,Nov,3; 2016,Aug,3; 2016,Jan,13; 2015,Apr,10; 2015,Jan,16; 2014,Oct,6; 2014,Aug,14; 2014,Mar,4; 2014,Jan,11

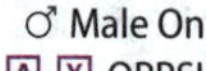
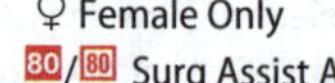
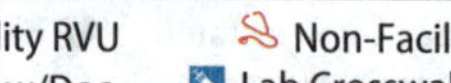
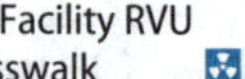

+ **36479** **subsequent vein(s) treated in a single extremity, each through separate access sites (List separately in addition to code for primary procedure)**

INCLUDES Tumescent anesthesia

EXCLUDES *Ablation of vein using chemical adhesive ([36482, 36483])*
Endovenous ablation therapy of incompetent vein (36475-36476)
Vascular embolization or occlusion (37241)

Code first (36478)

3.95 9.03 FUD ZZZ N N1 50

AMA: 2018,Mar,3; 2018,Jan,8; 2017,Jan,8; 2016,Nov,3; 2016,Aug,3; 2016,Jan,13; 2015,Apr,10; 2015,Jan,16; 2014,Oct,6; 2014,Aug,14; 2014,Mar,4; 2014,Jan,11

\# **36482** **Endovenous ablation therapy of incompetent vein, extremity, by transcatheter delivery of a chemical adhesive (eg, cyanoacrylate) remote from the access site, inclusive of all imaging guidance and monitoring, percutaneous; first vein treated**

INCLUDES Local anesthesia

EXCLUDES *Laser ablation incompetent vein (36478-36479)*
Radiofrequency ablation incompetent vein (36475-36476)

5.12 57.9 FUD 000 T G2 50

AMA: 2019,Feb,9; 2018,Mar,3

+ # **36483** **subsequent vein(s) treated in a single extremity, each through separate access sites (List separately in addition to code for primary procedure)**

INCLUDES Local anesthesia

EXCLUDES *Laser ablation incompetent vein (36478-36479)*
Radiofrequency ablation incompetent vein (36475-36476)
Use of code more than one time per extremity

Code first ([36482])

2.57 4.26 FUD ZZZ N N1 50

AMA: 2019,Feb,9; 2018,Mar,3

36481-36510 Other Venous Catheterization Procedures

EXCLUDES *Collection of a specimen from:*
A completely implantable device (36591)
An established catheter (36592)

36481 **Percutaneous portal vein catheterization by any method**

(75885, 75887)

9.67 55.4 FUD 000 N N1

AMA: 2018,Jan,8; 2017,Jan,8; 2016,Jan,13; 2015,Jan,16; 2014,Jan,11

36482 **Resequenced code. See code following 36479.**

36483 **Resequenced code. See code following 36479.**

36500 **Venous catheterization for selective organ blood sampling**

EXCLUDES *Inferior or superior vena cava catheterization (36010)*

(75893)

5.30 5.30 FUD 000 N N1

AMA: 2014,Jan,11

36510 **Catheterization of umbilical vein for diagnosis or therapy, newborn** A

EXCLUDES *Collection of a specimen from:*
Capillary blood (36416)
Venipuncture (36415)

1.54 2.34 FUD 000 63 N N1 80

AMA: 2018,Jan,8; 2017,Jan,8; 2016,May,3; 2016,Jan,13; 2015,Jan,16; 2014,Jan,11

36511-36516 Apheresis

CMS: 100-03,110.14 Apheresis (Therapeutic Pheresis); 100-04,4,231.9 Billing for Pheresis and Apheresis Services

EXCLUDES *Collection of a specimen for therapeutic treatment from:*
A completely implantable device (36591)
An established catheter (36592)

36511 **Therapeutic apheresis; for white blood cells**

3.10 3.10 FUD 000 S G2

AMA: 2018,Jan,8; 2017,Jan,8; 2016,Jan,13; 2015,Jan,16; 2014,Jan,11

36512 **for red blood cells**

3.11 3.11 FUD 000 S G2

AMA: 2018,Jan,8; 2017,Jan,8; 2016,Jan,13; 2015,Jan,16; 2014,Jan,11

36513 **for platelets**

EXCLUDES *Collection of platelets from donors*

3.16 3.16 FUD 000 S R2

AMA: 2018,Jan,8; 2017,Jan,8; 2016,Jan,13; 2015,Jan,16; 2014,Jan,11

36514 **for plasma pheresis**

2.76 20.5 FUD 000 S G2

AMA: 2018,May,10; 2018,Jan,8; 2017,Jan,8; 2016,Jan,13; 2015,Jan,16; 2014,Jan,11

36516 **with extracorporeal immunoadsorption, selective adsorption or selective filtration and plasma reinfusion**

Code also modifier 26 for professional evaluation

2.46 56.2 FUD 000 S P3

AMA: 2018,Jan,8; 2017,Jan,8; 2016,Jan,13; 2015,Jan,16; 2014,Jan,11

36522 Extracorporeal Photopheresis

CMS: 100-03,110.4 Extracorporeal Photopheresis; 100-04,32,190 Billing for Extracorporeal Photopheresis; 100-04,32,190.2 Extracorporeal Photopheresis; 100-04,32,190.3 Medicare Denial Codes; 100-04,4,231.9 Billing for Pheresis and Apheresis Services

36522 **Photopheresis, extracorporeal**

2.79 61.2 FUD 000 S G2

AMA: 2018,May,10; 2018,Jan,8; 2017,Jan,8; 2016,Jan,13; 2015,Jan,16; 2014,Jan,11

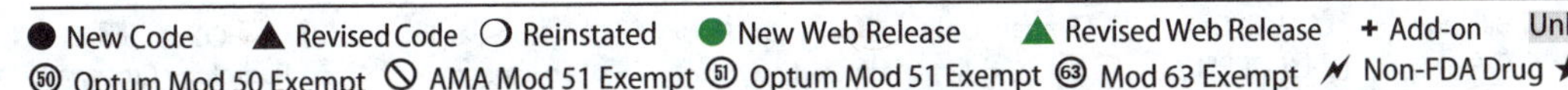

36555-36573 [36572, 36573] Placement of Implantable Venous Access Device

INCLUDES Devices accessed by an exposed catheter, or a subcutaneous port or pump
Devices inserted via cutdown or percutaneous access:
Centrally (eg, femoral, jugular, subclavian veins, or inferior vena cava)
Peripherally (e.g., basilic, cephalic, saphenous vein)
Devices terminating in the brachiocephalic (innominate), iliac, or subclavian veins, vena cava, or right atrium

EXCLUDES *Insertion midline catheter (36400, 36406, 36410)*
Maintenance/refilling of implantable pump/reservoir (96522)

Code also removal of central venous access device (if code available) when a new device is placed through a separate venous access

36555 **Insertion of non-tunneled centrally inserted central venous catheter; younger than 5 years of age** A

EXCLUDES *Peripheral insertion (36568)*
(76937, 77001)
2.46   5.33   **FUD** 000   T A2
AMA: 2019,May,3; 2018,Jan,8; 2017,Jan,8; 2016,Jan,13; 2015,Jan,16; 2014,Jan,11

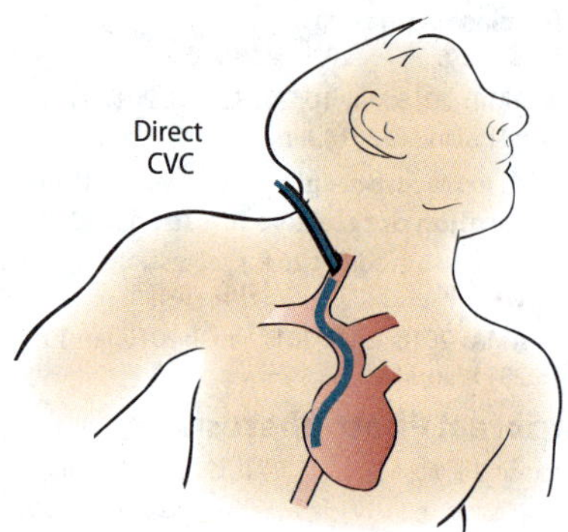

A non-tunneled centrally inserted CVC is inserted

36556 **age 5 years or older** A

EXCLUDES *Peripheral insertion (36569)*
(76937, 77001)
2.45   5.99   **FUD** 000   T A2
AMA: 2019,May,3; 2018,Nov,11; 2018,Jan,8; 2017,Jan,8; 2016,Jan,13; 2015,Jan,16; 2014,Jan,11

36557 **Insertion of tunneled centrally inserted central venous catheter, without subcutaneous port or pump; younger than 5 years of age** A

(76937, 77001)
9.21   29.0   **FUD** 010   T A2 80 50
AMA: 2018,Jan,8; 2017,Jan,8; 2016,Jan,13; 2015,Jan,16; 2014,Jan,11

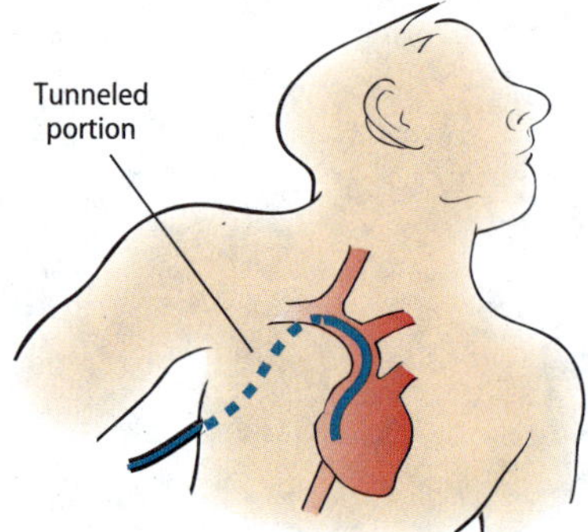

A tunneled centrally inserted CVC is inserted

36558 **age 5 years or older** A

EXCLUDES *Peripheral insertion (36571)*
(76937, 77001)
7.54   21.7   **FUD** 010   T A2 80 50
AMA: 2018,Jan,8; 2017,Jan,8; 2016,Jan,13; 2015,Jan,16; 2015,Jan,13; 2014,Jan,11

36560 **Insertion of tunneled centrally inserted central venous access device, with subcutaneous port; younger than 5 years of age** A

EXCLUDES *Peripheral insertion (36570)*
(76937, 77001)
11.0   37.1   **FUD** 010   T G2 80 50
AMA: 2018,Jan,8; 2017,Jan,8; 2016,Jan,13; 2015,Jan,16; 2014,Jan,11

36561 **age 5 years or older** A

EXCLUDES *Peripheral insertion (36571)*
(76937, 77001)
9.74   30.6   **FUD** 010   T A2 80 50
AMA: 2018,Jan,8; 2017,Jan,8; 2016,Jan,13; 2015,Jan,16; 2014,Jan,11

36563 **Insertion of tunneled centrally inserted central venous access device with subcutaneous pump**

(76937, 77001)
10.6   34.4   **FUD** 010   T A2 80
AMA: 2018,Jan,8; 2017,Jan,8; 2016,Jan,13; 2015,Jan,16; 2014,Jan,11

36565 **Insertion of tunneled centrally inserted central venous access device, requiring 2 catheters via 2 separate venous access sites; without subcutaneous port or pump (eg, Tesio type catheter)**

(76937, 77001)
9.63   24.8   **FUD** 010   T A2 80 50
AMA: 2018,Jan,8; 2017,Jan,8; 2016,Jan,13; 2015,Jan,16; 2014,Jan,11

36566 **with subcutaneous port(s)**

(76937, 77001)
10.4   135.   **FUD** 010   T A2 80 50
AMA: 2018,Jan,8; 2017,Jan,8; 2016,Jan,13; 2015,Jan,16; 2014,Jan,11

36568 **Insertion of peripherally inserted central venous catheter (PICC), without subcutaneous port or pump, without imaging guidance; younger than 5 years of age** A

EXCLUDES *Centrally inserted placement (36555)*
Imaging guidance (76937, 77001)
Peripherally inserted ([36572])
PICC line removal with codes for removal of tunneled central venous catheters; report appropriate E&M code
2.65   2.65   **FUD** 000   T A2
AMA: 2019,May,3; 2018,Jan,8; 2017,Jan,8; 2016,Jan,13; 2015,Jan,16; 2014,Jan,11

36569 **age 5 years or older** A

EXCLUDES *Centrally inserted placement (36556)*
Imaging guidance (76937, 77001)
Peripherally inserted ([36573])
PICC line removal with codes for removal of tunneled central venous catheters; report appropriate E&M code
2.72   2.72   **FUD** 000   T A2
AMA: 2019,May,3; 2018,Jan,8; 2017,Jan,8; 2016,Jan,13; 2015,Jan,16; 2014,Sep,13; 2014,Jan,11

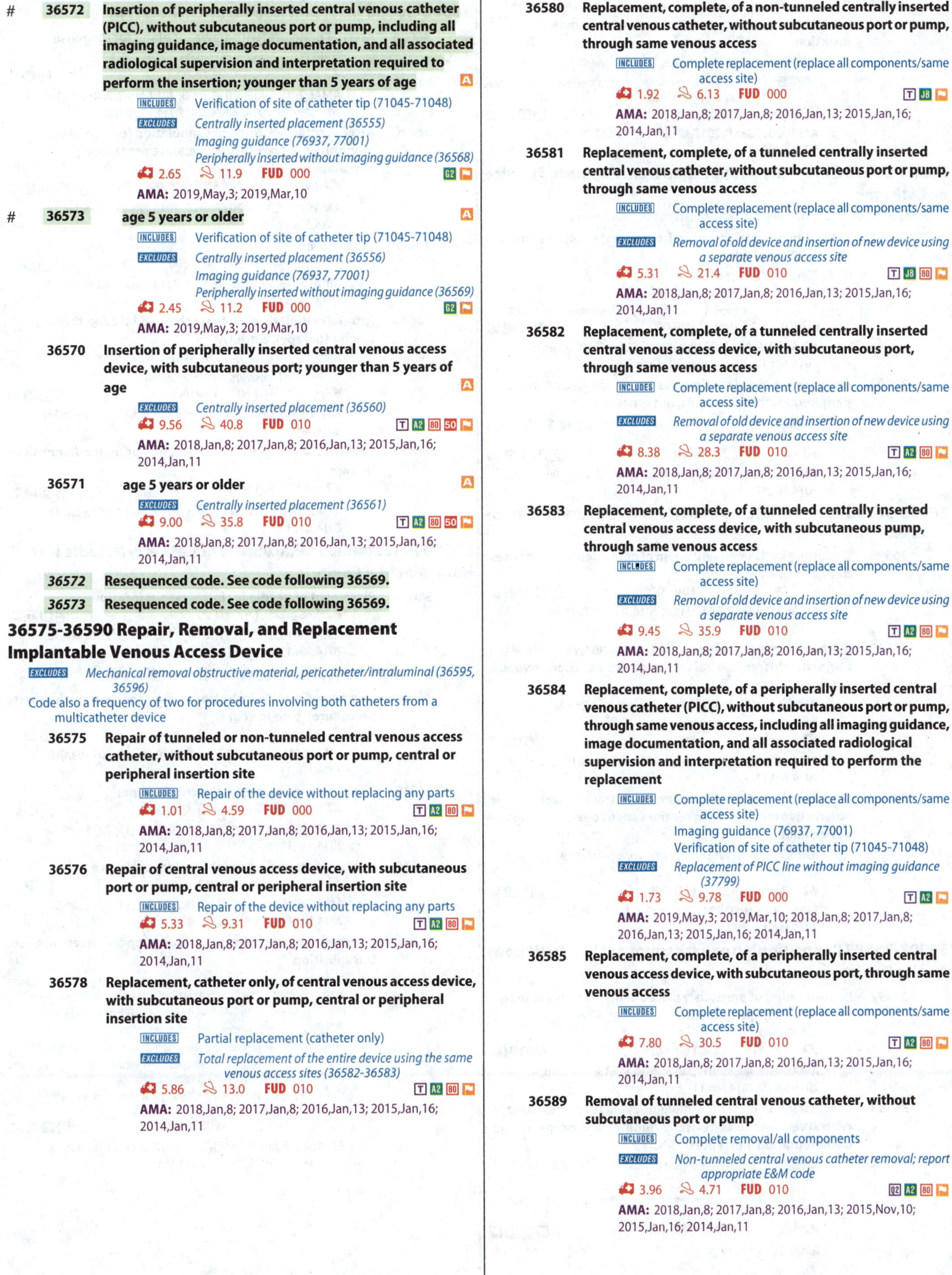

36572 **Insertion of peripherally inserted central venous catheter (PICC), without subcutaneous port or pump, including all imaging guidance, image documentation, and all associated radiological supervision and interpretation required to perform the insertion; younger than 5 years of age**

INCLUDES Verification of site of catheter tip (71045-71048)

EXCLUDES *Centrally inserted placement (36555)*
Imaging guidance (76937, 77001)
Peripherally inserted without imaging guidance (36568)

2.65 11.9 FUD 000 G2

AMA: 2019,May,3; 2019,Mar,10

36573 **age 5 years or older**

INCLUDES Verification of site of catheter tip (71045-71048)

EXCLUDES *Centrally inserted placement (36556)*
Imaging guidance (76937, 77001)
Peripherally inserted without imaging guidance (36569)

2.45 11.2 FUD 000 G2

AMA: 2019,May,3; 2019,Mar,10

36570 **Insertion of peripherally inserted central venous access device, with subcutaneous port; younger than 5 years of age**

EXCLUDES *Centrally inserted placement (36560)*

9.56 40.8 FUD 010 T A2 80 50

AMA: 2018,Jan,8; 2017,Jan,8; 2016,Jan,13; 2015,Jan,16; 2014,Jan,11

36571 **age 5 years or older**

EXCLUDES *Centrally inserted placement (36561)*

9.00 35.8 FUD 010 T A2 80 50

AMA: 2018,Jan,8; 2017,Jan,8; 2016,Jan,13; 2015,Jan,16; 2014,Jan,11

36572 **Resequenced code. See code following 36569.**

36573 **Resequenced code. See code following 36569.**

36575-36590 Repair, Removal, and Replacement Implantable Venous Access Device

EXCLUDES *Mechanical removal obstructive material, pericatheter/intraluminal (36595, 36596)*

Code also a frequency of two for procedures involving both catheters from a multicatheter device

36575 **Repair of tunneled or non-tunneled central venous access catheter, without subcutaneous port or pump, central or peripheral insertion site**

INCLUDES Repair of the device without replacing any parts

1.01 4.59 FUD 000 T A2 80

AMA: 2018,Jan,8; 2017,Jan,8; 2016,Jan,13; 2015,Jan,16; 2014,Jan,11

36576 **Repair of central venous access device, with subcutaneous port or pump, central or peripheral insertion site**

INCLUDES Repair of the device without replacing any parts

5.33 9.31 FUD 010 T A2 80

AMA: 2018,Jan,8; 2017,Jan,8; 2016,Jan,13; 2015,Jan,16; 2014,Jan,11

36578 **Replacement, catheter only, of central venous access device, with subcutaneous port or pump, central or peripheral insertion site**

INCLUDES Partial replacement (catheter only)

EXCLUDES *Total replacement of the entire device using the same venous access sites (36582-36583)*

5.86 13.0 FUD 010 T A2 80

AMA: 2018,Jan,8; 2017,Jan,8; 2016,Jan,13; 2015,Jan,16; 2014,Jan,11

36580 **Replacement, complete, of a non-tunneled centrally inserted central venous catheter, without subcutaneous port or pump, through same venous access**

INCLUDES Complete replacement (replace all components/same access site)

1.92 6.13 FUD 000 T J8

AMA: 2018,Jan,8; 2017,Jan,8; 2016,Jan,13; 2015,Jan,16; 2014,Jan,11

36581 **Replacement, complete, of a tunneled centrally inserted central venous catheter, without subcutaneous port or pump, through same venous access**

INCLUDES Complete replacement (replace all components/same access site)

EXCLUDES *Removal of old device and insertion of new device using a separate venous access site*

5.31 21.4 FUD 010 T J8 80

AMA: 2018,Jan,8; 2017,Jan,8; 2016,Jan,13; 2015,Jan,16; 2014,Jan,11

36582 **Replacement, complete, of a tunneled centrally inserted central venous access device, with subcutaneous port, through same venous access**

INCLUDES Complete replacement (replace all components/same access site)

EXCLUDES *Removal of old device and insertion of new device using a separate venous access site*

8.38 28.3 FUD 010 T A2 80

AMA: 2018,Jan,8; 2017,Jan,8; 2016,Jan,13; 2015,Jan,16; 2014,Jan,11

36583 **Replacement, complete, of a tunneled centrally inserted central venous access device, with subcutaneous pump, through same venous access**

INCLUDES Complete replacement (replace all components/same access site)

EXCLUDES *Removal of old device and insertion of new device using a separate venous access site*

9.45 35.9 FUD 010 T A2 80

AMA: 2018,Jan,8; 2017,Jan,8; 2016,Jan,13; 2015,Jan,16; 2014,Jan,11

36584 **Replacement, complete, of a peripherally inserted central venous catheter (PICC), without subcutaneous port or pump, through same venous access, including all imaging guidance, image documentation, and all associated radiological supervision and interpretation required to perform the replacement**

INCLUDES Complete replacement (replace all components/same access site)
Imaging guidance (76937, 77001)
Verification of site of catheter tip (71045-71048)

EXCLUDES *Replacement of PICC line without imaging guidance (37799)*

1.73 9.78 FUD 000 T A2

AMA: 2019,May,3; 2019,Mar,10; 2018,Jan,8; 2017,Jan,8; 2016,Jan,13; 2015,Jan,16; 2014,Jan,11

36585 **Replacement, complete, of a peripherally inserted central venous access device, with subcutaneous port, through same venous access**

INCLUDES Complete replacement (replace all components/same access site)

7.80 30.5 FUD 010 T A2 80

AMA: 2018,Jan,8; 2017,Jan,8; 2016,Jan,13; 2015,Jan,16; 2014,Jan,11

36589 **Removal of tunneled central venous catheter, without subcutaneous port or pump**

INCLUDES Complete removal/all components

EXCLUDES *Non-tunneled central venous catheter removal; report appropriate E&M code*

3.96 4.71 FUD 010 Q2 A2 80

AMA: 2018,Jan,8; 2017,Jan,8; 2016,Jan,13; 2015,Nov,10; 2015,Jan,16; 2014,Jan,11

36590 **Removal of tunneled central venous access device, with subcutaneous port or pump, central or peripheral insertion**

INCLUDES Complete removal/all components

EXCLUDES *Non-tunneled central venous catheter removal; report appropriate E&M code*

5.49 6.34 FUD 010 Q2 A2 80

AMA: 2018,Jan,8; 2017,Jan,8; 2016,Jan,13; 2015,Jan,16; 2014,Jan,11

36591-36592 Obtain Blood Specimen from Implanted Device or Catheter

EXCLUDES *Use of code with any other service except laboratory services*

36591 **Collection of blood specimen from a completely implantable venous access device**

EXCLUDES *Collection of:*
Capillary blood specimen (36416)
Venous blood specimen by venipuncture (36415)

0.69 0.69 FUD XXX Q1 N1 80 TC

AMA: 2019,Aug,8; 2018,Jan,8; 2017,Jan,8; 2016,Jan,13; 2015,Jan,16; 2014,May,4; 2014,Jan,11

36592 **Collection of blood specimen using established central or peripheral catheter, venous, not otherwise specified**

EXCLUDES *Collection of blood from an established arterial catheter (37799)*

0.77 0.77 FUD XXX Q1 N1 80 TC

AMA: 2018,Jan,8; 2017,Jan,8; 2016,Jan,13; 2015,Jan,16; 2014,Jan,11

36593-36596 Restore Patency of Occluded Catheter or Device

EXCLUDES *Venous catheterization (36010-36012)*

36593 **Declotting by thrombolytic agent of implanted vascular access device or catheter**

0.89 0.89 FUD XXX T P3 80 TC

AMA: 2018,Jan,8; 2017,Jan,8; 2016,Jan,13; 2015,Jan,16; 2014,Jan,11

36595 **Mechanical removal of pericatheter obstructive material (eg, fibrin sheath) from central venous device via separate venous access**

EXCLUDES *Declotting by thrombolytic agent (36593)*

(75901)

5.30 17.3 FUD 000 T J8

AMA: 2018,Jan,8; 2017,Jan,8; 2016,Jan,13; 2015,Jan,16; 2014,Jan,11

36596 **Mechanical removal of intraluminal (intracatheter) obstructive material from central venous device through device lumen**

EXCLUDES *Declotting by thrombolytic agent (36593)*

(75902)

1.28 3.57 FUD 000 T G2

AMA: 2018,Jan,8; 2017,Jan,8; 2016,Jan,13; 2015,Jan,16; 2014,Jan,11

36597-36598 Repositioning or Assessment of In Situ Venous Access Device

36597 **Repositioning of previously placed central venous catheter under fluoroscopic guidance**

(76000)

1.77 3.69 FUD 000 T G2

AMA: 2018,Jan,8; 2017,Jan,8; 2016,Jan,13; 2015,Jan,16; 2014,Sep,5; 2014,Jan,11

36598 **Contrast injection(s) for radiologic evaluation of existing central venous access device, including fluoroscopy, image documentation and report**

EXCLUDES *Complete venography studies (75820, 75825, 75827)*
Fluoroscopy (76000)
Mechanical removal of pericatheter obstructive material (36595-36596)

1.06 3.30 FUD 000 T P3 80 50

AMA: 2014,Jan,11

36600-36660 Insertion Needle or Catheter: Artery

36600 **Arterial puncture, withdrawal of blood for diagnosis**

EXCLUDES *Critical care services*

0.45 0.87 FUD XXX Q1 N1

AMA: 2019,Aug,8; 2018,Jan,8; 2017,Jan,8; 2016,Jan,13; 2015,Jan,16; 2014,May,4; 2014,Jan,11

36620 **Arterial catheterization or cannulation for sampling, monitoring or transfusion (separate procedure); percutaneous**

1.28 1.28 FUD 000 N N1

AMA: 2018,Jan,8; 2017,Jan,8; 2016,Jan,13; 2015,Jan,16; 2014,Jan,11

36625 **cutdown**

3.05 3.05 FUD 000 N N1

AMA: 2018,Jan,8; 2017,Jan,8; 2016,Jan,13; 2015,Jan,16; 2014,Jan,11

36640 **Arterial catheterization for prolonged infusion therapy (chemotherapy), cutdown**

EXCLUDES *Intra-arterial chemotherapy (96420-96425)*
Transcatheter embolization (75894)

3.30 3.30 FUD 000 T A2

AMA: 2018,Jan,8; 2017,Jan,8; 2016,Jan,13; 2015,Jan,16; 2014,Jan,11

36660 **Catheterization, umbilical artery, newborn, for diagnosis or therapy** A

1.98 1.98 FUD 000 63 C 80

AMA: 2018,Jan,8; 2017,Jan,8; 2016,Jan,13; 2015,Jan,16; 2014,Jan,11

36680 Percutaneous Placement of Catheter/Needle into Bone Marrow Cavity

36680 **Placement of needle for intraosseous infusion**

1.69 1.69 FUD 000 Q1 N1 80

AMA: 2018,Jan,8; 2017,Jan,8; 2016,Jan,13; 2015,Jan,16; 2014,Jan,11

36800-36821 Vascular Access for Hemodialysis

36800 **Insertion of cannula for hemodialysis, other purpose (separate procedure); vein to vein**

3.53 3.53 FUD 000 T G2

AMA: 2018,Jan,8; 2017,Jan,8; 2016,Jan,13; 2015,Jan,16; 2014,Jan,11

36810 **arteriovenous, external (Scribner type)**

6.05 6.05 FUD 000 T A2

AMA: 2018,Jan,8; 2017,Jan,8; 2016,Jan,13; 2015,Jan,16; 2014,Jan,11

36815 **arteriovenous, external revision, or closure**

3.91 3.91 FUD 000 T A2

AMA: 2018,Jan,8; 2017,Jan,8; 2016,Jan,13; 2015,Jan,16; 2014,Jan,11

36818 **Arteriovenous anastomosis, open; by upper arm cephalic vein transposition**

INCLUDES Two incisions in the upper arm; a medial incision over the brachial artery and a lateral incision for exposure of a portion of the cephalic vein

EXCLUDES *When performed unilaterally with:*
Arteriovenous anastomosis, open (36819-36820)
Creation of arteriovenous fistula by other than direct arteriovenous anastomosis (36830)

Code also modifier 50 or 59, as appropriate, for a bilateral procedure

20.1 20.1 FUD 090 T A2 80

AMA: 2018,Jan,8; 2017,Mar,3; 2017,Jan,8; 2016,Mar,10; 2016,Jan,13; 2015,Jan,16; 2014,Jan,11

36819 **by upper arm basilic vein transposition**

EXCLUDES *When performed unilaterally with:*
Arteriovenous anastomosis, open (36818, 36820-36821)
Creation of arteriovenous fistula by other than direct arteriovenous anastomosis (36830)

Code also modifier 50 or 59, as appropriate, for bilateral procedure

21.1 21.1 FUD 090 T A2 80

AMA: 2018,Jan,8; 2017,Mar,3; 2017,Jan,8; 2016,Jan,13; 2015,Jan,16; 2014,Jan,11

36820 **by forearm vein transposition**

21.2 21.2 FUD 090 T A2 80 50

AMA: 2018,Jan,8; 2017,Mar,3; 2017,Jan,8; 2016,Jan,13; 2015,Jan,16; 2014,Jan,11

36821 **direct, any site (eg, Cimino type) (separate procedure)**

19.2 19.2 FUD 090 T A2 80

AMA: 2018,Jan,8; 2017,Mar,3; 2017,Jan,8; 2016,Jan,13; 2015,Aug,8; 2015,Jan,16; 2014,Jan,11

36823 Vascular Access for Extracorporeal Circulation

INCLUDES Chemotherapy perfusion

EXCLUDES *Chemotherapy administration (96409-96425)*
Maintenance for extracorporeal circulation (33946-33949)

36823 **Insertion of arterial and venous cannula(s) for isolated extracorporeal circulation including regional chemotherapy perfusion to an extremity, with or without hyperthermia, with removal of cannula(s) and repair of arteriotomy and venotomy sites**

40.5 40.5 FUD 090 C

AMA: 2018,Jan,8; 2017,Mar,3; 2014,Jan,11

36825-36835 Permanent Vascular Access Procedures

36825 **Creation of arteriovenous fistula by other than direct arteriovenous anastomosis (separate procedure); autogenous graft**

EXCLUDES *Direct arteriovenous (AV) anastomosis (36821)*

23.0 23.0 FUD 090 T A2 80

AMA: 2018,Jan,8; 2017,Mar,3; 2017,Jan,8; 2016,Jan,13; 2015,Jan,16; 2014,Jan,11

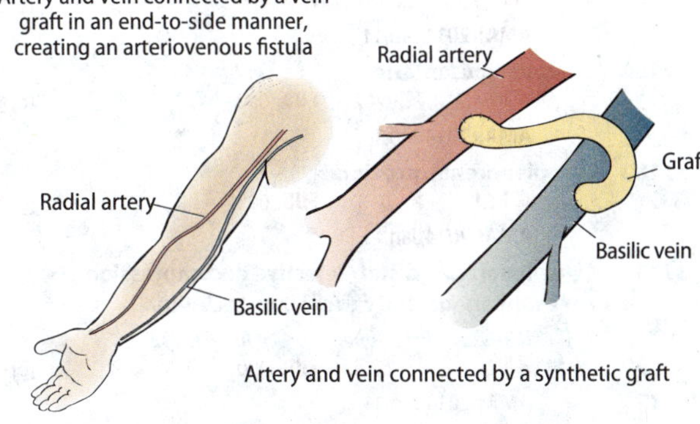

36830 **nonautogenous graft (eg, biological collagen, thermoplastic graft)**

EXCLUDES *Direct arteriovenous (AV) anastomosis (36821)*

19.3 19.3 FUD 090 T A2 80

AMA: 2018,Jan,8; 2017,Mar,3; 2017,Jan,8; 2016,Jan,13; 2015,Jan,16; 2015,Jan,13; 2014,Jan,11

36831 **Thrombectomy, open, arteriovenous fistula without revision, autogenous or nonautogenous dialysis graft (separate procedure)**

17.8 17.8 FUD 090 T A2 80

AMA: 2018,Jan,8; 2017,Mar,3; 2017,Jan,8; 2016,Jan,13; 2015,Jan,16; 2014,Jan,11

36832 **Revision, open, arteriovenous fistula; without thrombectomy, autogenous or nonautogenous dialysis graft (separate procedure)**

INCLUDES Revision of an arteriovenous access fistula or graft

21.9 21.9 FUD 090 T A2 80

AMA: 2018,Jan,8; 2017,Mar,3; 2017,Jan,8; 2016,Jan,13; 2015,Jan,16; 2014,Jan,11

36833 **with thrombectomy, autogenous or nonautogenous dialysis graft (separate procedure)**

EXCLUDES *Hemodialysis circuit procedures (36901-36906)*

23.5 23.5 FUD 090 T A2 80

AMA: 2018,Jan,8; 2017,Mar,3; 2017,Jan,8; 2016,Jan,13; 2015,Jan,16; 2014,Jan,11

36835 **Insertion of Thomas shunt (separate procedure)**

13.8 13.8 FUD 090 T A2

AMA: 2014,Jan,11

36838 DRIL Procedure for Ischemic Steal Syndrome

EXCLUDES *Bypass graft, with vein (35512, 35522-35523)*
Ligation (37607, 37618)
Revision, open, arteriovenous fistula (36832)

36838 **Distal revascularization and interval ligation (DRIL), upper extremity hemodialysis access (steal syndrome)**

33.1 33.1 FUD 090 T 80 50

AMA: 2014,Jan,11

36860-36861 Restore Patency of Occluded Cannula or Arteriovenous Fistula

36860 **External cannula declotting (separate procedure); without balloon catheter**

(76000)

3.20 7.17 FUD 000 T A2

AMA: 2018,Jan,8; 2017,Jan,8; 2016,Jan,13; 2015,Jan,16; 2014,Jan,11

36861 **with balloon catheter**

(76000)

4.02 4.02 FUD 000 T A2

AMA: 2018,Jan,8; 2017,Jan,8; 2016,Jan,13; 2015,Jan,16; 2014,Jan,11

36901-36909 Hemodialysis Circuit Procedures

EXCLUDES *Arteriography to assess inflow to hemodialysis circuit when performed (76937)*

36901 **Introduction of needle(s) and/or catheter(s), dialysis circuit, with diagnostic angiography of the dialysis circuit, including all direct puncture(s) and catheter placement(s), injection(s) of contrast, all necessary imaging from the arterial anastomosis and adjacent artery through entire venous outflow including the inferior or superior vena cava, fluoroscopic guidance, radiological supervision and interpretation and image documentation and report;**

INCLUDES Access
Catheter advancement (e.g., imaging of accessory veins, assess all sections of circuit)
Contrast injection

EXCLUDES *Balloon angioplasty of peripheral segment (36902)*
Open revision with thrombectomy of arteriovenous fistula (36833)
Percutaneous transluminal procedures of peripheral segment (36904-36906)
Stent placement in peripheral segment (36903)
Use of code more than one time per procedure

4.90 16.9 FUD 000 T P3

AMA: 2018,Jan,8; 2017,Mar,3

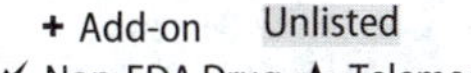
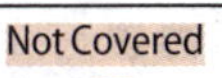

36902 **with transluminal balloon angioplasty, peripheral dialysis segment, including all imaging and radiological supervision and interpretation necessary to perform the angioplasty**

EXCLUDES *Open revision with thrombectomy of arteriovenous fistula (36833)*
Percutaneous transluminal procedures of peripheral segment (36904-36906)
Stent placement in peripheral segment (36903)
Use of code more than one time per procedure

6.98 36.0 FUD 000 J G2

AMA: 2018,Jan,8; 2017,Jul,3; 2017,Mar,3

36903 **with transcatheter placement of intravascular stent(s), peripheral dialysis segment, including all imaging and radiological supervision and interpretation necessary to perform the stenting, and all angioplasty within the peripheral dialysis segment**

INCLUDES Balloon angioplasty of peripheral segment (36902)

EXCLUDES *Central hemodialysis circuit procedures (36907-36908)*
Open revision with thrombectomy of arteriovenous fistula (36833)
Percutaneous transluminal procedures of peripheral segment (36904-36906)
Use of code more than one time per procedure

9.23 152. FUD 000 J J8

AMA: 2018,Jan,8; 2017,Jul,3; 2017,Mar,3

36904 **Percutaneous transluminal mechanical thrombectomy and/or infusion for thrombolysis, dialysis circuit, any method, including all imaging and radiological supervision and interpretation, diagnostic angiography, fluoroscopic guidance, catheter placement(s), and intraprocedural pharmacological thrombolytic injection(s);**

EXCLUDES *Open thrombectomy of arteriovenous fistula with/without revision (36831, 36833)*
Use of code more than one time per procedure

10.7 53.1 FUD 000 J G2

AMA: 2018,Jan,8; 2017,Jul,3; 2017,Mar,3

36905 **with transluminal balloon angioplasty, peripheral dialysis segment, including all imaging and radiological supervision and interpretation necessary to perform the angioplasty**

INCLUDES Percutaneous mechanical thrombectomy (36904)

EXCLUDES *Use of code more than one time per procedure*

12.9 66.8 FUD 000 J G2

AMA: 2018,Jan,8; 2017,Jul,3; 2017,Mar,3

36906 **with transcatheter placement of intravascular stent(s), peripheral dialysis segment, including all imaging and radiological supervision and interpretation necessary to perform the stenting, and all angioplasty within the peripheral dialysis circuit**

INCLUDES Percutaneous transluminal balloon angioplasty (36905)
Percutaneous transluminal thrombectomy (36904)

EXCLUDES *Hemodialysis circuit procedures provided by catheter or needle access (36901-36903)*
Use of code more than one time per procedure

Code also balloon angioplasty of central veins, when performed (36907)

Code also stent placement in central veins, when performed (36908)

14.9 193. FUD 000 J J8

AMA: 2018,Jan,8; 2017,Jul,3; 2017,Mar,3

\+ 36907 **Transluminal balloon angioplasty, central dialysis segment, performed through dialysis circuit, including all imaging and radiological supervision and interpretation required to perform the angioplasty (List separately in addition to code for primary procedure)**

INCLUDES All central hemodialysis segment angiography

EXCLUDES *Angiography with stent placement (36908)*

Code first (36818-36833, 36901-36906)

4.26 20.4 FUD ZZZ N N1

AMA: 2018,Jan,8; 2017,Jul,3; 2017,Mar,3

\+ 36908 **Transcatheter placement of intravascular stent(s), central dialysis segment, performed through dialysis circuit, including all imaging and radiological supervision and interpretation required to perform the stenting, and all angioplasty in the central dialysis segment (List separately in addition to code for primary procedure)**

INCLUDES All central hemodialysis segment stent(s) placed
Balloon angioplasty central dialysis segment (36907)

Code first when performed (36818-36833, 36901-36906)

6.03 68.0 FUD ZZZ N N1

AMA: 2018,Jan,8; 2017,Jul,3; 2017,Mar,3

\+ 36909 **Dialysis circuit permanent vascular embolization or occlusion (including main circuit or any accessory veins), endovascular, including all imaging and radiological supervision and interpretation necessary to complete the intervention (List separately in addition to code for primary procedure)**

INCLUDES All embolization/occlusion procedures performed in the hemodialysis circuit

EXCLUDES *Banding/ligation of arteriovenous fistula (37607)*
Use of code more than one time per day

Code first (36901-36906)

5.84 54.9 FUD ZZZ N N1

AMA: 2018,Jan,8; 2017,Mar,3

37140-37181 Open Decompression of Portal Circulation

EXCLUDES *Peritoneal-venous shunt (49425)*

37140 **Venous anastomosis, open; portocaval**

67.4 67.4 FUD 090 C

AMA: 2014,Jan,11

37145 **renoportal**

62.5 62.5 FUD 090 C 80

AMA: 2014,Jan,11

37160 **caval-mesenteric**

64.2 64.2 FUD 090 C 80

AMA: 2014,Jan,11

37180 **splenorenal, proximal**

61.7 61.7 FUD 090 C 80

AMA: 2014,Jan,11

37181 **splenorenal, distal (selective decompression of esophagogastric varices, any technique)**

EXCLUDES *Percutaneous procedure (37182)*

67.4 67.4 FUD 090 C 80

AMA: 2014,Jan,11

37182-37183 Transvenous Decompression of Portal Circulation

INCLUDES Percutaneous transhepatic portography (75885, 75887)

37182 **Insertion of transvenous intrahepatic portosystemic shunt(s) (TIPS) (includes venous access, hepatic and portal vein catheterization, portography with hemodynamic evaluation, intrahepatic tract formation/dilatation, stent placement and all associated imaging guidance and documentation)**

EXCLUDES *Open procedure (37140)*

23.7 23.7 FUD 000 C 80

AMA: 2018,Jan,8; 2017,Jan,8; 2016,Jan,13; 2015,Jan,16; 2014,Jan,11

37183 Revision of transvenous intrahepatic portosystemic shunt(s) (TIPS) (includes venous access, hepatic and portal vein catheterization, portography with hemodynamic evaluation, intrahepatic tract recanulization/dilatation, stent placement and all associated imaging guidance and documentation)

EXCLUDES *Arteriovenous (AV) aneurysm repair (36832)*

10.8 170. FUD 000 J 80

AMA: 2018,Jan,8; 2017,Jan,8; 2016,Jan,13; 2015,Jan,16; 2014,Jan,11

37184-37188 Removal of Thrombus from Vessel: Percutaneous

INCLUDES Fluoroscopic guidance (76000)
Injection(s) of thrombolytics during the procedure
Postprocedure evaluation
Pretreatment planning

EXCLUDES *Continuous infusion of thrombolytics prior to and after the procedure (37211-37214)*
Diagnostic studies
Intracranial arterial mechanical thrombectomy or infusion (61645)
Mechanical thrombectomy, coronary (92973)
Other interventions performed percutaneously (e.g., balloon angioplasty)
Placement of catheters
Radiological supervision/interpretation

37184 Primary percutaneous transluminal mechanical thrombectomy, noncoronary, non-intracranial, arterial or arterial bypass graft, including fluoroscopic guidance and intraprocedural pharmacological thrombolytic injection(s); initial vessel

EXCLUDES *Intracranial arterial mechanical thrombectomy (61645)*
Mechanical thrombectomy for embolus/thrombus complicating another percutaneous interventional procedure (37186)
Mechanical thrombectomy of another vascular family/separate access site, append modifier 59 to the primary service
Therapeutic, prophylactic, or diagnostic injection (96374)

12.9 60.2 FUD 000 J J8 50

AMA: 2019,Sep,5; 2018,Jan,8; 2017,Jan,8; 2016,Jul,6; 2016,Mar,3; 2016,Jan,13; 2015,Nov,3; 2015,Apr,10; 2015,Jan,16; 2014,Jan,11

\+ **37185 second and all subsequent vessel(s) within the same vascular family (List separately in addition to code for primary mechanical thrombectomy procedure)**

INCLUDES Treatment of second and all succeeding vessel(s) in same vascular family

EXCLUDES *Intravenous drug injections administered subsequent to an initial service*
Mechanical thrombectomy for treating of embolus/thrombus complicating another percutaneous interventional procedure (37186)
Therapeutic, prophylactic, or diagnostic injection (96375)

Code first (37184)

4.85 18.5 FUD ZZZ N N1

AMA: 2019,Sep,5; 2018,Jan,8; 2017,Jan,8; 2016,Jul,6; 2016,Jan,13; 2015,Nov,3; 2015,Apr,10; 2015,Jan,16; 2014,Jan,11

\+ **37186 Secondary percutaneous transluminal thrombectomy (eg, nonprimary mechanical, snare basket, suction technique), noncoronary, non-intracranial, arterial or arterial bypass graft, including fluoroscopic guidance and intraprocedural pharmacological thrombolytic injections, provided in conjunction with another percutaneous intervention other than primary mechanical thrombectomy (List separately in addition to code for primary procedure)**

INCLUDES Removal of small emboli/thrombi prior to or after another percutaneous procedure

EXCLUDES *Primary percutaneous transluminal mechanical thrombectomy, noncoronary, non-intracranial (37184-37185)*
Therapeutic, prophylactic, or diagnostic injection (96375)

Code first primary procedure

7.10 37.4 FUD ZZZ N N1

AMA: 2019,Sep,5; 2018,Jan,8; 2017,Jan,8; 2016,Jul,6; 2016,Jan,13; 2015,Nov,3; 2015,Jan,16; 2014,Jan,11

37187 Percutaneous transluminal mechanical thrombectomy, vein(s), including intraprocedural pharmacological thrombolytic injections and fluoroscopic guidance

INCLUDES Secondary or subsequent intravenous injection after another initial service

EXCLUDES *Therapeutic, prophylactic, or diagnostic injection (96375)*

11.4 55.5 FUD 000 J J8 50

AMA: 2018,Jan,8; 2017,Jan,8; 2016,Jul,6; 2016,Mar,3; 2016,Jan,13; 2015,Nov,3; 2015,Jan,16; 2014,Jan,11

37188 Percutaneous transluminal mechanical thrombectomy, vein(s), including intraprocedural pharmacological thrombolytic injections and fluoroscopic guidance, repeat treatment on subsequent day during course of thrombolytic therapy

EXCLUDES *Therapeutic, prophylactic, or diagnostic injection (96375)*

8.03 46.7 FUD 000 T G2 50

AMA: 2018,Jan,8; 2017,Jan,8; 2016,Jul,6; 2016,Mar,3; 2016,Jan,13; 2015,Nov,3; 2015,Jan,16; 2014,Jan,11

37191-37193 Vena Cava Filters

37191 Insertion of intravascular vena cava filter, endovascular approach including vascular access, vessel selection, and radiological supervision and interpretation, intraprocedural roadmapping, and imaging guidance (ultrasound and fluoroscopy), when performed

EXCLUDES *Open ligation of inferior vena cava via laparotomy or retroperitoneal approach (37619)*

6.49 69.9 FUD 000 T

AMA: 2018,Jan,8; 2017,Feb,14; 2017,Jan,8; 2016,May,11; 2016,Jan,13; 2015,Jan,16; 2014,Jan,11

37192 Repositioning of intravascular vena cava filter, endovascular approach including vascular access, vessel selection, and radiological supervision and interpretation, intraprocedural roadmapping, and imaging guidance (ultrasound and fluoroscopy), when performed

EXCLUDES *Insertion of intravascular vena cava filter (37191)*

9.98 37.4 FUD 000 T

AMA: 2018,Jan,8; 2017,Jan,8; 2016,May,11; 2016,Jan,13; 2015,Jan,16; 2014,Jan,11

37193 Retrieval (removal) of intravascular vena cava filter, endovascular approach including vascular access, vessel selection, and radiological supervision and interpretation, intraprocedural roadmapping, and imaging guidance (ultrasound and fluoroscopy), when performed

EXCLUDES *Transcatheter retrieval, percutaneous, of intravascular foreign body (37197)*

10.1 44.0 FUD 000 T

AMA: 2018,Jan,8; 2017,Jan,8; 2016,May,11; 2016,Jan,13; 2015,Jan,16; 2014,Jan,11

37195 Intravenous Cerebral Thrombolysis

37195 Thrombolysis, cerebral, by intravenous infusion

0.00 0.00 FUD XXX T 80

AMA: 2014,Jan,11

37197-37214 Transcatheter Procedures: Infusions, Biopsy, Foreign Body Removal

37197 Transcatheter retrieval, percutaneous, of intravascular foreign body (eg, fractured venous or arterial catheter), includes radiological supervision and interpretation, and imaging guidance (ultrasound or fluoroscopy), when performed

EXCLUDES *Percutaneous vena cava filter retrieval (37193)*
Removal leadless pacemaker system ([33275])

8.78 43.4 FUD 000 T G2

AMA: 2018,Jan,8; 2017,Feb,14; 2017,Jan,8; 2016,May,11; 2016,Jan,13; 2015,Jan,16; 2014,Jan,11

37200 Transcatheter biopsy

(75970)

6.30 6.30 FUD 000 T G2

AMA: 2014,Jan,11

37211 Transcatheter therapy, arterial infusion for thrombolysis other than coronary or intracranial, any method, including radiological supervision and interpretation, initial treatment day

INCLUDES Catheter change or position change
E&M services on the day of and related to thrombolysis
First day of transcatheter thrombolytic infusion
Fluoroscopic guidance
Follow-up arteriography or venography
Radiologic supervision and interpretation

EXCLUDES *Angiography through existing catheter for follow-up study for transcatheter therapy, embolization, or infusion, other than for thrombolysis (75898)*
Catheter placement
Declotting of implanted catheter or vascular access device by thrombolytic agent (36593)
Diagnostic studies
Intracranial arterial mechanical thrombectomy or infusion (61645)
Percutaneous interventions
Procedure performed more than one time per date of service
Ultrasound guidance (76937)

Code also significant, separately identifiable E&M service on the day of thrombolysis using modifier 25

11.2 11.2 FUD 000 T G2 50

AMA: 2019,Sep,6; 2018,Jan,8; 2017,Jan,8; 2016,Jul,6; 2016,Mar,3; 2016,Jan,13; 2015,Nov,3; 2015,Jan,16; 2014,Jan,11

37212 Transcatheter therapy, venous infusion for thrombolysis, any method, including radiological supervision and interpretation, initial treatment day

INCLUDES Catheter change or position change
E&M services on the day of and related to thrombolysis

EXCLUDES *Angiography through existing catheter for follow-up study for transcatheter therapy, embolization, or infusion, other than for thrombolysis (75898)*
Catheter placement
First day of transcatheter thrombolytic infusion
Declotting of implanted catheter or vascular access device by thrombolytic agent (36593)
Fluoroscopic guidance
Follow-up arteriography or venography
Diagnostic studies
Initiation and completion of thrombolysis on same date of service
Percutaneous interventions
Radiologic supervision and interpretation
Procedure performed more than one time per date of service
Ultrasound guidance (76937)

Code also significant, separately identifiable E&M service on the day of thrombolysis using modifier 25

9.81 9.81 FUD 000 T G2 50

AMA: 2019,Sep,6; 2018,Jan,8; 2017,Jan,8; 2016,Jul,6; 2016,Mar,3; 2016,Jan,13; 2015,Nov,3; 2015,Jan,16; 2014,Jan,11

37213 Transcatheter therapy, arterial or venous infusion for thrombolysis other than coronary, any method, including radiological supervision and interpretation, continued treatment on subsequent day during course of thrombolytic therapy, including follow-up catheter contrast injection, position change, or exchange, when performed;

INCLUDES Continued thrombolytic infusions on subsequent days besides the initial and last days of treatment
E&M services on the day of and related to thrombolysis
Fluoroscopic guidance
Radiologic supervision and interpretation

EXCLUDES *Angiography through existing catheter for follow-up study for transcatheter therapy, embolization, or infusion, other than for thrombolysis (75898)*
Catheter placement
Declotting of implanted catheter or vascular access device by thrombolytic agent (36593)
Diagnostic studies
Percutaneous interventions
Procedure performed more than one time per date of service
Ultrasound guidance (76937)

Code also significant, separately identifiable E&M service on the day of thrombolysis using modifier 25

6.76 6.76 FUD 000 T

AMA: 2019,Sep,6; 2018,Jan,8; 2017,Jan,8; 2016,Jul,6; 2016,Mar,3; 2016,Jan,13; 2015,Nov,3; 2015,Jan,16; 2014,Jan,11

37214 **cessation of thrombolysis including removal of catheter and vessel closure by any method**

INCLUDES E&M services on the day of and related to thrombolysis
Fluoroscopic guidance
Last day of transcatheter thrombolytic infusions
Radiologic supervision and interpretation

EXCLUDES *Angiography through existing catheter for follow-up study for transcatheter therapy, embolization, or infusion, other than for thrombolysis (75898)*
Catheter placement
Declotting of implanted catheter or vascular access device by thrombolytic agent (36593)
Diagnostic studies
Percutaneous interventions
Procedure performed more than one time per date of service
Ultrasound guidance (76937)

Code also significant, separately identifiable E&M service on the day of thrombolysis using modifier 25

3.57 3.57 **FUD** 000 T

AMA: 2019,Sep,6; 2018,Jan,8; 2017,Jan,8; 2016,Jul,6; 2016,Mar,3; 2016,Jan,13; 2015,Nov,3; 2015,Jan,16; 2014,Jan,11

37215-37216 Stenting of Cervical Carotid Artery with/without Insertion Distal Embolic Protection Device

INCLUDES Carotid stenting, if required
Ipsilateral cerebral and cervical carotid diagnostic imaging/supervision and interpretation
Ipsilateral selective carotid catheterization

EXCLUDES *Carotid catheterization and imaging, if carotid stenting not required*
Selective catheter placement, common carotid or innominate artery (36222-36224)
Transcatheter placement extracranial vertebral artery stents, open or percutaneous (0075T, 0076T)

37215 **Transcatheter placement of intravascular stent(s), cervical carotid artery, open or percutaneous, including angioplasty, when performed, and radiological supervision and interpretation; with distal embolic protection**

29.2 29.2 **FUD** 090 C 80 50

AMA: 2018,Jan,8; 2017,Jul,3; 2017,Jan,8; 2016,Jan,13; 2015,Jan,16; 2014,Mar,8; 2014,Jan,11

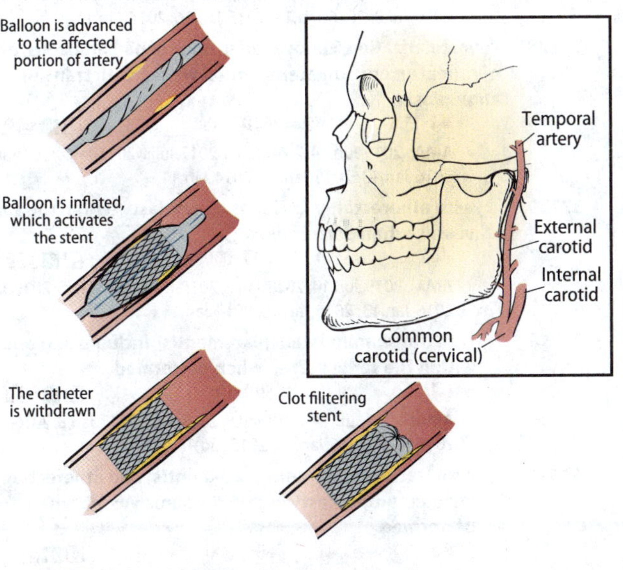

37216 **without distal embolic protection**

29.2 29.2 **FUD** 090 E

AMA: 2018,Jan,8; 2017,Jul,3; 2017,Jan,8; 2016,Jan,13; 2015,Jan,16; 2014,Mar,8; 2014,Jan,11

37217-37218 Stenting of Intrathoracic Carotid Artery/Innominate Artery

INCLUDES Access to vessel (open)
Arteriotomy closure by suture
Catheterization of the vessel (selective)
Imaging during and after the procedure
Radiological supervision and interpretation

EXCLUDES *Transcatheter insertion extracranial vertebral artery stents, open or percutaneous (0075T-0076T)*
Transcatheter insertion intracranial stents (61635)
Transcatheter insertion intravascular cervical carotid artery stents, open or percutaneous (37215-37216)

37217 **Transcatheter placement of intravascular stent(s), intrathoracic common carotid artery or innominate artery by retrograde treatment, open ipsilateral cervical carotid artery exposure, including angioplasty, when performed, and radiological supervision and interpretation**

31.3 31.3 **FUD** 090 C 80 50

AMA: 2018,Jan,8; 2017,Jul,3; 2017,Jan,8; 2016,Jan,13; 2015,May,7; 2015,Jan,16; 2014,Mar,8; 2014,Jan,11

37218 **Transcatheter placement of intravascular stent(s), intrathoracic common carotid artery or innominate artery, open or percutaneous antegrade approach, including angioplasty, when performed, and radiological supervision and interpretation**

EXCLUDES *Selective catheter placement, common carotid or innominate artery (36222-36224)*

23.7 23.7 **FUD** 090 C 80 50

AMA: 2018,Jan,8; 2017,Jul,3; 2017,Jan,8; 2016,Jan,13; 2015,May,7

37220-37235 Endovascular Revascularization Lower Extremities

INCLUDES Percutaneous and open interventional and associated procedures for lower extremity occlusive disease; unilateral
Accessing the vessel
Arteriotomy closure by suturing of puncture or pressure with application of arterial closure device
Atherectomy (e.g., directional, laser, rotational)
Balloon angioplasty (e.g., cryoplasty, cutting balloon, low-profile)
Catheterization of the vessel (selective)
Embolic protection
Imaging once procedure is complete
Radiological supervision and interpretation of intervention(s)
Stenting (e.g., bare metal, balloon-expandable, covered, drug-eluting, self-expanding)
Traversing the lesion
Reporting the most comprehensive treatment in a given vessel according to the following hierarchy:
1. Stent and atherectomy
2. Atherectomy
3. Stent
4. PTA
Revascularization procedures for three arterial vascular territories:
Femoral/popliteal vascular territory including the common, deep, and superficial femoral arteries, and the popliteal artery (one extremity = a single vessel) (37224-37227)
Iliac vascular territory: common iliac, external iliac, internal iliac (37220-37223)
Tibial/peroneal territory: includes anterior tibial, peroneal artery, posterior tibial (37228-37235)

EXCLUDES *Assignment of more than one code from this family for each lower extremity vessel treated*
Assignment of more than one code when multiple vessels are treated in the femoral/popliteal territory (report the most complex service for more than one lesion in the territory); when a contiguous lesion that spans from one territory to another can be opened with a single procedure; or when more than one stent is deployed in the same vessel
Extensive repair or replacement of artery (35226, 35286)
Mechanical thrombectomy and/or thrombolysis

Code also add-on codes for different vessels, but not different lesions in the same vessel; and for multiple territories in the same leg
Code also modifier 59 if same territory(ies) of both legs are treated during the same surgical session
Code first one primary code for the initial service in each leg

37220 Revascularization, endovascular, open or percutaneous, iliac artery, unilateral, initial vessel; with transluminal angioplasty
Code also only when transluminal angioplasty is performed outside the treatment target zone of (34701-34708, 34709, [34718], 34710-34711, 34845-34848)
11.6 | 83.7 | FUD 000 | J G2 50
AMA: 2019,Jun,14; 2018,Jan,8; 2017,Jul,3; 2017,Jan,8; 2016,Jul,8; 2016,Jan,13; 2015,Jan,16; 2014,Jan,11

37221 with transluminal stent placement(s), includes angioplasty within the same vessel, when performed
Code also only when transluminal angioplasty is performed outside the treatment target zone of (34701-34708, 34709, [34718], 34710-34711, 34845-34848)
14.4 | 118. | FUD 000 | J J8 80 50
AMA: 2019,Jun,14; 2018,Jan,8; 2017,Dec,3; 2017,Jul,3; 2017,Jan,8; 2016,Jul,6; 2016,Jul,8; 2016,Jan,13; 2015,Jan,13; 2015,Jan,16; 2014,Jan,11

\+ **37222 Revascularization, endovascular, open or percutaneous, iliac artery, each additional ipsilateral iliac vessel; with transluminal angioplasty (List separately in addition to code for primary procedure)**
Code also only when transluminal angioplasty is performed outside the treatment target zone of (34701-34708, 34709, [34718], 34710-34711, 34845-34848)
Code first (37220-37221)
5.42 | 22.6 | FUD ZZZ | N N1 80 50
AMA: 2019,Jun,14; 2018,Jan,8; 2017,Jul,3; 2017,Jan,8; 2016,Jul,8; 2016,Jan,13; 2015,Jan,16; 2014,Jan,11

\+ **37223 with transluminal stent placement(s), includes angioplasty within the same vessel, when performed (List separately in addition to code for primary procedure)**
Code also only when transluminal angioplasty is performed outside the treatment target zone of (34701-34708, 34709, [34718], 34710-34711, 34845-34848)
Code first (37221)
6.20 | 62.6 | FUD ZZZ | N N1 80 50
AMA: 2019,Jun,14; 2018,Jan,8; 2017,Dec,3; 2017,Jul,3; 2017,Jan,8; 2016,Jul,8; 2016,Jul,6; 2016,Jan,13; 2015,Jan,16; 2014,Jan,11

37224 Revascularization, endovascular, open or percutaneous, femoral, popliteal artery(s), unilateral; with transluminal angioplasty
EXCLUDES *Revascularization with intravascular stent grafts in femoral-popliteal segment (0505T)*
12.9 | 100. | FUD 000 | J J8 80 50
AMA: 2019,Jun,14; 2018,Jan,8; 2017,Jul,3; 2017,Jan,8; 2016,Jul,8; 2016,Jan,13; 2015,Jan,16; 2014,Jan,11

37225 with atherectomy, includes angioplasty within the same vessel, when performed
EXCLUDES *Revascularization with intravascular stent grafts in femoral-popliteal segment (0505T)*
17.6 | 345. | FUD 000 | J J8 80 50
AMA: 2019,Jun,14; 2018,Jan,8; 2017,Jul,3; 2017,Jan,8; 2016,Jul,8; 2016,Jan,13; 2015,Jan,16; 2014,Jan,11

37226 with transluminal stent placement(s), includes angioplasty within the same vessel, when performed
EXCLUDES *Revascularization with intravascular stent grafts in femoral-popliteal segment (0505T)*
15.1 | 299. | FUD 000 | J J8 80 50
AMA: 2019,Jun,14; 2018,Jan,8; 2017,Jul,3; 2017,Jan,8; 2016,Jul,6; 2016,Jul,8; 2016,Jan,13; 2015,Jan,16; 2014,Jan,11

37227 with transluminal stent placement(s) and atherectomy, includes angioplasty within the same vessel, when performed
EXCLUDES *Revascularization with intravascular stent grafts in femoral-popliteal segment (0505T)*
21.1 | 444. | FUD 000 | J J8 80 50
AMA: 2019,Jun,14; 2018,Jan,8; 2017,Jul,3; 2017,Jan,8; 2016,Jul,6; 2016,Jul,8; 2016,Jan,13; 2015,Jan,16; 2014,Jan,11

37228 Revascularization, endovascular, open or percutaneous, tibial, peroneal artery, unilateral, initial vessel; with transluminal angioplasty
15.8 | 145. | FUD 000 | J J8 80 50
AMA: 2019,Jun,14; 2018,Jan,8; 2017,Jul,3; 2017,Jan,8; 2016,Jul,8; 2016,Jan,13; 2015,Jan,16; 2014,Jan,11

37229 with atherectomy, includes angioplasty within the same vessel, when performed
20.5 | 345. | FUD 000 | J J8 80 50
AMA: 2019,Jun,14; 2018,Jan,8; 2017,Jul,3; 2017,Jan,8; 2016,Jul,8; 2016,Jan,13; 2015,Jan,16; 2014,Jan,11

37230 with transluminal stent placement(s), includes angioplasty within the same vessel, when performed
20.3 | 294. | FUD 000 | J J8 80 50
AMA: 2019,Jun,14; 2018,Jan,8; 2017,Jul,3; 2017,Jan,8; 2016,Jul,8; 2016,Jul,6; 2016,Jan,13; 2015,Jan,16; 2014,Jan,11

37231 with transluminal stent placement(s) and atherectomy, includes angioplasty within the same vessel, when performed
22.1 | 422. | FUD 000 | J J8 80 50
AMA: 2019,Jun,14; 2018,Jan,8; 2017,Jul,3; 2017,Jan,8; 2016,Jul,8; 2016,Jul,6; 2016,Jan,13; 2015,Jan,16; 2014,Jan,11

+ **37232** **Revascularization, endovascular, open or percutaneous, tibial/peroneal artery, unilateral, each additional vessel; with transluminal angioplasty (List separately in addition to code for primary procedure)**

Code first (37228-37231)

5.85 31.1 FUD ZZZ N N1 80 50

AMA: 2019,Jun,14; 2018,Jan,8; 2017,Jul,3; 2017,Jan,8; 2016,Jul,8; 2016,Jan,13; 2015,Jan,16; 2014,Jan,11

+ **37233** **with atherectomy, includes angioplasty within the same vessel, when performed (List separately in addition to code for primary procedure)**

Code first (37229, 37231)

9.53 37.9 FUD ZZZ N N1 80 50

AMA: 2019,Jun,14; 2018,Jan,8; 2017,Jul,3; 2017,Jan,8; 2016,Jul,8; 2016,Jan,13; 2015,Jan,16; 2014,Jan,11

+ **37234** **with transluminal stent placement(s), includes angioplasty within the same vessel, when performed (List separately in addition to code for primary procedure)**

Code first (37229-37231)

8.32 109. FUD ZZZ N N1 80 50

AMA: 2019,Jun,14; 2018,Jan,8; 2017,Jul,3; 2017,Jan,8; 2016,Jul,8; 2016,Jul,6; 2016,Jan,13; 2015,Jan,16; 2014,Jan,11

+ **37235** **with transluminal stent placement(s) and atherectomy, includes angioplasty within the same vessel, when performed (List separately in addition to code for primary procedure)**

Code first (37231)

11.6 119. FUD ZZZ N N1 80 50

AMA: 2019,Jun,14; 2018,Jan,8; 2017,Jul,3; 2017,Jan,8; 2016,Jul,6; 2016,Jul,8; 2016,Jan,13; 2015,Jan,16; 2014,Jan,11

37246-37249 [37246, 37247, 37248, 37249] Transluminal Balloon Angioplasty

INCLUDES Open and percutaneous balloon angioplasty
Radiological supervision and interpretation (37220-37235)

EXCLUDES *Angioplasty of other vessels:*
Aortic/visceral arteries (with endovascular repair) (34841-34848)
Coronary artery (92920-92944)
Intracranial artery (61630, 61635)
Performed in a hemodialysis circuit (36901-36909)
Percutaneous removal of thrombus/infusion of thrombolytics (37184-37188, 37211-37214)
Pulmonary artery (92997-92998)
Use of codes more than one time for all services performed in a single vessel or treatable with one angioplasty procedure

Code also angioplasty of different vessel, when performed ([37247], [37249])
Code also extensive repair or replacement of artery, when performed (35226, 35286)
Code also intravascular ultrasound, when performed (37252-37253)

37246 **Transluminal balloon angioplasty (except lower extremity artery(ies) for occlusive disease, intracranial, coronary, pulmonary, or dialysis circuit), open or percutaneous, including all imaging and radiological supervision and interpretation necessary to perform the angioplasty within the same artery; initial artery**

EXCLUDES *Intravascular stent placement except lower extremities (37236-37237)*
Revascularization lower extremities (37220-37235)
Stent placement:
Cervical carotid artery (37215-37216)
Intrathoracic carotid or innominate artery (37217-37218)

Code first (37239)

10.1 59.2 FUD 000 J G2 50

AMA: 2018,Jan,8; 2017,Aug,10; 2017,Jul,3

+ # **37247** **each additional artery (List separately in addition to code for primary procedure)**

EXCLUDES *Intravascular stent placement except lower extremities (37236-37237)*
Revascularization lower extremities (37220-37235)
Stent placement:
Cervical carotid artery (37215-37216)
Intrathoracic carotid or innominate artery (37217-37218)

Code first ([37246])

4.97 22.5 FUD ZZZ N N1 50

AMA: 2018,Jan,8; 2017,Aug,10; 2017,Jul,3

37248 **Transluminal balloon angioplasty (except dialysis circuit), open or percutaneous, including all imaging and radiological supervision and interpretation necessary to perform the angioplasty within the same vein; initial vein**

EXCLUDES *Placement of intravascular (venous) stent in same vein, same session as (37238-37239)*
Revascularization with intravascular stent grafts in femoral-popliteal segment (0505T)

8.66 42.3 FUD 000 J G2 50

AMA: 2018,Jan,8; 2017,Aug,10; 2017,Jul,3; 2017,Mar,3

+ # **37249** **each additional vein (List separately in addition to code for primary procedure)**

EXCLUDES *Placement of intravascular (venous) stent in same vein, same session as (37238-37239)*
Revascularization with intravascular stent grafts in femoral-popliteal segment (0505T)

Code first (37239)

4.22 16.7 FUD ZZZ N N1 50

AMA: 2018,Jan,8; 2017,Aug,10; 2017,Jul,3; 2017,Mar,3

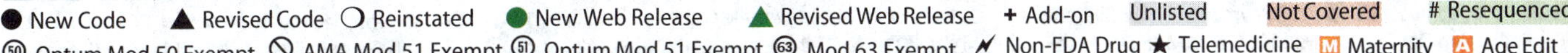

37236-37239 Endovascular Revascularization Excluding Lower Extremities

INCLUDES Arteriotomy closure by suturing of a puncture, pressure or application of arterial closure device
Balloon angioplasty
Post-dilation after stent deployment
Predilation performed as primary or secondary angioplasty
Treatment of lesion inside same vessel but outside of stented portion
Treatment using different-sized balloons to accomplish the procedure
Endovascular revascularization of arteries and veins other than carotid, coronary, extracranial, intracranial, lower extremities
Imaging once procedure is complete
Radiological supervision and interpretation
Stent placement provided as the only treatment

EXCLUDES *Angioplasty in an unrelated vessel*
Extensive repair or replacement of an artery (35226, 35286)
Insertion of multiple stents in a single vessel using more than one code
Intravascular ultrasound (37252-37253)
Mechanical thrombectomy (37184-37188)
Selective and nonselective catheterization (36005, 36010-36015, 36200, 36215-36218, 36245-36248)
Stent placement in:
Arteries of the lower extremities for occlusive disease (37221, 37223, 37226-37227, 37230-37231, 37234-37235)
Cervical carotid artery (37215-37216)
Extracranial vertebral (0075T-0076T)
Hemodialysis circuit (36903, 36905, 36908)
Intracoronary (92928-92929, 92933-92934, 92937-92938, 92941, 92943-92944)
Intracranial (61635)
Intrathoracic common carotid or innominate artery, retrograde or antegrade approach (37218)
Visceral arteries with fenestrated aortic repair (34841-34848)
Thrombolytic therapy (37211-37214)
Ultrasound guidance (76937)

Code also add-on codes for different vessels treated during the same operative session

37236 Transcatheter placement of an intravascular stent(s) (except lower extremity artery(s) for occlusive disease, cervical carotid, extracranial vertebral or intrathoracic carotid, intracranial, or coronary), open or percutaneous, including radiological supervision and interpretation and including all angioplasty within the same vessel, when performed; initial artery

EXCLUDES *Procedures in the same target treatment zone with (34841-34848)*

Facility RVU 12.9 Non-Facility RVU 101. FUD 000 J J8 80 50

AMA: 2018,Jan,8; 2017,Dec,3; 2017,Jul,3; 2017,Jan,8; 2016,Jul,3; 2016,Jul,6; 2016,Mar,5; 2016,Jan,13; 2015,May,7; 2015,Jan,16; 2014,Jan,11

+ **37237 each additional artery (List separately in addition to code for primary procedure)**

EXCLUDES *Procedures in the same target treatment zone with (34841-34848)*

Code first (37236)

Facility RVU 6.19 Non-Facility RVU 60.3 FUD ZZZ N N1 80 50

AMA: 2018,Jan,8; 2017,Dec,3; 2017,Jul,3; 2017,Jan,8; 2016,Jul,6; 2016,Mar,5; 2016,Jan,13; 2015,Jan,16; 2014,Jan,11

37238 Transcatheter placement of an intravascular stent(s), open or percutaneous, including radiological supervision and interpretation and including angioplasty within the same vessel, when performed; initial vein

EXCLUDES *Revascularization with intravascular stent grafts in femoral-popliteal segment (0505T)*

Facility RVU 8.82 Non-Facility RVU 102. FUD 000 J J8 80 50

AMA: 2018,Jan,8; 2017,Jul,3; 2017,Mar,3; 2017,Jan,8; 2016,Jul,6; 2016,Jun,8; 2014,Jan,11

+ **37239 each additional vein (List separately in addition to code for primary procedure)**

EXCLUDES *Revascularization with intravascular stent grafts in femoral-popliteal segment (0505T)*

Code first (37238)

Facility RVU 4.42 Non-Facility RVU 48.9 FUD ZZZ N N1 80 50

AMA: 2018,Jan,8; 2017,Jul,3; 2017,Mar,3; 2017,Jan,8; 2016,Jul,6; 2014,Jan,11

37241-37249 Therapeutic Vascular Embolization/ Occlusion

INCLUDES Embolization or occlusion of arteries, lymphatics, and veins except for head/neck and central nervous system
Imaging once procedure is complete
Intraprocedural guidance
Radiological supervision and interpretation
Roadmapping
Stent placement provided as support for embolization

EXCLUDES *Embolization code assigned more than once per operative field*
Head, neck, or central nervous system embolization (61624, 61626, 61710)
Multiple codes for indications that overlap, code only the indication needing the most immediate attention
Stent deployment as primary management of aneurysm, pseudoaneurysm, or vascular extravasation
Vein destruction with sclerosing solution (36468-36471)

Code also additional embolization procedure(s) and the appropriate modifiers (eg, modifier 59) when embolization procedures are performed in multiple operative fields

Code also diagnostic angiography and catheter placement using modifier 59 when appropriate

37241 Vascular embolization or occlusion, inclusive of all radiological supervision and interpretation, intraprocedural roadmapping, and imaging guidance necessary to complete the intervention; venous, other than hemorrhage (eg, congenital or acquired venous malformations, venous and capillary hemangiomas, varices, varicoceles)

EXCLUDES *Embolization of side branch(s) of an outflow vein from a hemodialysis access (36909)*
Procedure in same operative field with:
Endovenous ablation therapy of incompetent vein (36475-36479)
Injection of sclerosing solution; single vein (36470-36471)
Transcatheter embolization procedures (75894, 75898)
Vein destruction (36468-36479 [36465, 36466])

Facility RVU 12.8 Non-Facility RVU 137. FUD 000 J P2

AMA: 2019,Sep,6; 2018,Mar,3; 2018,Jan,8; 2017,Mar,3; 2017,Jan,8; 2016,Nov,3; 2016,Jan,13; 2015,Nov,3; 2015,Aug,8; 2015,Apr,10; 2015,Jan,16; 2014,Oct,6; 2014,Aug,14; 2014,Jan,11

37242 arterial, other than hemorrhage or tumor (eg, congenital or acquired arterial malformations, arteriovenous malformations, arteriovenous fistulas, aneurysms, pseudoaneurysms)

EXCLUDES *Percutaneous treatment of pseudoaneurysm of an extremity (36002)*

Facility RVU 13.8 Non-Facility RVU 211. FUD 000 J J8

AMA: 2019,Sep,6; 2018,Jul,14; 2018,Mar,3; 2018,Jan,8; 2017,Jan,8; 2016,Jan,13; 2015,Nov,3; 2015,Jan,16; 2014,Oct,6; 2014,Jan,11

37243 for tumors, organ ischemia, or infarction

INCLUDES Embolization of uterine fibroids (37244)

EXCLUDES *Procedure in same operative field:*
Angiography (75898)
Transcatheter embolization in same operative field (75894)

Code also chemotherapy when provided with embolization procedure (96420-96425)

Code also injection of radioisotopes when provided with embolization procedure (79445)

Facility RVU 16.3 Non-Facility RVU 273. FUD 000 J G2

AMA: 2019,Sep,6; 2018,Mar,3; 2018,Jan,8; 2017,Jan,8; 2016,Jan,13; 2015,Nov,3; 2015,Jan,16; 2014,Oct,6; 2014,Jan,11

37244 for arterial or venous hemorrhage or lymphatic extravasation

INCLUDES Embolization of uterine arteries for hemorrhage

Facility RVU 19.3 Non-Facility RVU 195. FUD 000 J

AMA: 2019,Sep,6; 2018,Jul,14; 2018,Mar,3; 2018,Jan,8; 2017,Oct,9; 2017,Jan,8; 2016,Jan,13; 2015,Nov,3; 2015,Jan,16; 2014,Oct,6; 2014,Aug,14; 2014,Jan,11

37246 **Resequenced code. See code following 37235.**

37247 **Resequenced code. See code following 37235.**

37248 **Resequenced code. See code following 37235.**

37249 **Resequenced code. See code following 37235.**

37252-37253 Intravascular Ultrasound: Noncoronary

INCLUDES Manipulation and repositioning of the transducer prior to and after therapeutic interventional procedures

EXCLUDES *Selective or non-selective catheter placement for access (36005-36248)*
Transcatheter procedures (37200, 37236-37239, 37241-37244, 61624, 61626)
Vena cava filter procedures (37191-37193, 37197)

Code first (33361-33369, 33477, 33880-33886, 34701-34708, 34709, [34718], 34710-34711, 34712, 34841-34848, 36010-36015, 36100-36218, 36221-36228, 36245-36248, 36251-36254, 36481, 36555-36571 [36572, 36573], 36578, 36580-36585, 36595, 36901-36909, 37184-37188, 37200, 37211-37218, 37220-37239 [37246, 37247, 37248, 37249], 37241-37244, 61623, 75600-75635, 75705-75774, 75805, 75807, 75810, 75820-75833, 75860-75872, 75885-75898, 75901-75902, 75956-75959, 75970, 76000, 77001, 0075T-0076T, 0234T-0238T, 0338T)

\+ **37252** **Intravascular ultrasound (noncoronary vessel) during diagnostic evaluation and/or therapeutic intervention, including radiological supervision and interpretation; initial noncoronary vessel (List separately in addition to code for primary procedure)**
Code first primary procedure
2.65 35.7 FUD ZZZ N N1 80
AMA: 2018,Jan,8; 2017,Dec,3; 2017,Aug,10; 2017,Mar,3; 2017,Jan,8; 2016,Jul,6; 2016,May,11

\+ **37253** **each additional noncoronary vessel (List separately in addition to code for primary procedure)**
Code first (37252)
2.13 5.60 FUD ZZZ N N1 80
AMA: 2018,Jan,8; 2017,Dec,3; 2017,Aug,10; 2017,Mar,3; 2017,Jan,8; 2016,Jul,6; 2016,May,11

37500-37501 Vascular Endoscopic Procedures

INCLUDES Diagnostic endoscopy

EXCLUDES *Open procedure (37760)*

37500 **Vascular endoscopy, surgical, with ligation of perforator veins, subfascial (SEPS)**
18.3 18.3 FUD 090 T A2 50
AMA: 2018,Jan,8; 2017,Jan,8; 2016,Jan,13; 2015,Jan,16; 2014,Jan,11

37501 **Unlisted vascular endoscopy procedure**
0.00 0.00 FUD YYY T 50
AMA: 2014,Jan,11

37565-37606 Ligation Procedures: Jugular Vein, Carotid Arteries

CMS: 100-03,160.8 Electroencephalographic Monitoring During Cerebral Vasculature Surgery

EXCLUDES *Arterial balloon occlusion, endovascular, temporary (61623)*
Suture of arteries and veins (35201-35286)
Transcatheter arterial embolization/occlusion, permanent (61624-61626)
Treatment of intracranial aneurysm (61703)

37565 **Ligation, internal jugular vein**
20.7 20.7 FUD 090 T 80 50
AMA: 2014,Jan,11

37600 **Ligation; external carotid artery**
21.0 21.0 FUD 090 T 80
AMA: 2014,Jan,11

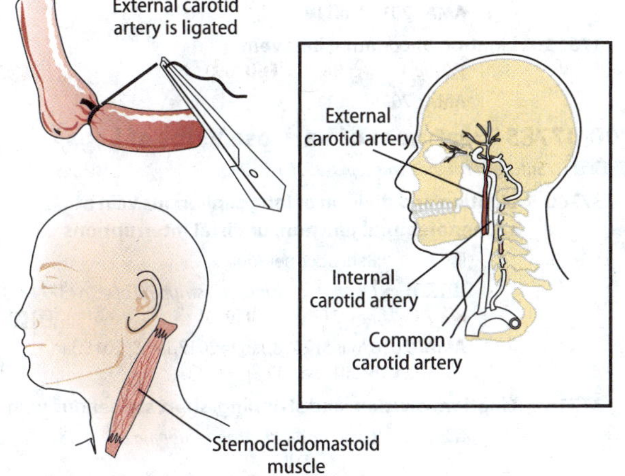

37605 **internal or common carotid artery**
21.3 21.3 FUD 090 T 80
AMA: 2014,Jan,11

37606 **internal or common carotid artery, with gradual occlusion, as with Selverstone or Crutchfield clamp**
20.9 20.9 FUD 090 T 80
AMA: 2014,Jan,11

37607-37609 Ligation Hemodialysis Angioaccess or Temporal Artery

EXCLUDES *Suture of arteries and veins (35201-35286)*

37607 **Ligation or banding of angioaccess arteriovenous fistula**
10.8 10.8 FUD 090 T A2
AMA: 2014,Jan,11

37609 **Ligation or biopsy, temporal artery**
5.94 8.87 FUD 010 J A2 50
AMA: 2014,Jan,11

37615-37618 Arterial Ligation, Major Vessel, for Injury/Rupture

EXCLUDES *Suture of arteries and veins (35201-35286)*

37615 **Ligation, major artery (eg, post-traumatic, rupture); neck**
INCLUDES Touroff ligation
15.2 15.2 FUD 090 T 80
AMA: 2014,Jan,11

37616 **chest**
INCLUDES Bardenheurer operation
32.0 32.0 FUD 090 C 80
AMA: 2014,Jan,11

37617 **abdomen**
38.8 38.8 FUD 090 C 80
AMA: 2018,Jan,8; 2017,Jan,8; 2016,Jan,13; 2015,Jan,16; 2014,Jan,11

37618 **extremity**
11.1 11.1 FUD 090 C 80
AMA: 2014,Jan,11

37619 Ligation Inferior Vena Cava

EXCLUDES *Suture of arteries and veins (35201-35286)*
Endovascular delivery of inferior vena cava filter (37191)

37619 **Ligation of inferior vena cava**
50.1 50.1 FUD 090 T 80
AMA: 2018,Jan,8; 2017,Jan,8; 2016,Jan,13; 2015,Jan,16; 2014,Jan,11

37650-37660 Venous Ligation, Femoral and Common Iliac

EXCLUDES *Suture of arteries and veins (35201-35286)*

37650 Ligation of femoral vein
13.2 13.2 FUD 090 T A2 50
AMA: 2014,Jan,11

37660 Ligation of common iliac vein
38.1 38.1 FUD 090 C 80 50
AMA: 2014,Jan,11

37700-37785 Treatment of Varicose Veins of Legs

EXCLUDES *Suture of arteries and veins (35201-35286)*

37700 Ligation and division of long saphenous vein at saphenofemoral junction, or distal interruptions
INCLUDES Babcock operation
EXCLUDES *Ligation, division, and stripping of vein (37718, 37722)*
7.07 7.07 FUD 090 T A2 50
AMA: 2018,Mar,3; 2018,Jan,8; 2017,Jan,8; 2016,Jan,13; 2015,Jan,16; 2014,Jan,11

37718 Ligation, division, and stripping, short saphenous vein
EXCLUDES *Ligation, division, and stripping of vein (37700, 37735, 37780)*
12.4 12.4 FUD 090 T A2 50
AMA: 2018,Mar,3; 2018,Jan,8; 2017,Jan,8; 2014,Jan,11

37722 Ligation, division, and stripping, long (greater) saphenous veins from saphenofemoral junction to knee or below
EXCLUDES *Ligation, division, and stripping of vein (37700, 37718, 37735)*
13.7 13.7 FUD 090 T A2 50
AMA: 2018,Mar,3; 2018,Jan,8; 2017,Jan,8; 2014,Jan,11

37735 Ligation and division and complete stripping of long or short saphenous veins with radical excision of ulcer and skin graft and/or interruption of communicating veins of lower leg, with excision of deep fascia
EXCLUDES *Ligation, division, and stripping of vein (37700, 37718, 37722, 37780)*
16.7 16.7 FUD 090 T A2 50
AMA: 2018,Mar,3; 2018,Jan,8; 2017,Jan,8; 2016,Jan,13; 2015,Jan,16; 2014,Jan,11

37760 Ligation of perforator veins, subfascial, radical (Linton type), including skin graft, when performed, open,1 leg
EXCLUDES *Duplex scan of extremity veins (93971)*
Ligation of subfascial perforator veins, endoscopic (37500)
Ultrasonic guidance (76937, 76942, 76998)
18.0 18.0 FUD 090 T A2 50
AMA: 2018,Mar,3; 2018,Jan,8; 2017,Jan,8; 2016,Jan,13; 2015,Jan,16; 2014,Jan,11

37761 Ligation of perforator vein(s), subfascial, open, including ultrasound guidance, when performed, 1 leg
EXCLUDES *Duplex scan of extremity veins (93971)*
Ligation of subfascial perforator veins, endoscopic (37500)
Ultrasonic guidance (76937, 76942, 76998)
15.6 15.6 FUD 090 T R2 80 50
AMA: 2018,Mar,3; 2018,Jan,8; 2017,Jan,8; 2016,Jan,13; 2015,Jan,16; 2014,Jan,11

37765 Stab phlebectomy of varicose veins, 1 extremity; 10-20 stab incisions
EXCLUDES *Fewer than 10 incisions (37799)*
More than 20 incisions (37766)
12.9 18.5 FUD 090 T P3 50
AMA: 2018,Mar,3; 2018,Jan,8; 2017,Jan,8; 2016,Nov,3; 2016,Jan,13; 2015,Jan,16; 2014,Oct,6; 2014,Jan,11

37766 more than 20 incisions
EXCLUDES *Fewer than 10 incisions (37799)*
10-20 incisions (37765)
15.8 22.0 FUD 090 T P3 50
AMA: 2018,Mar,3; 2018,Jan,8; 2017,Jan,8; 2016,Nov,3; 2016,Jan,13; 2015,Jan,16; 2014,Oct,6; 2014,Jan,11

37780 Ligation and division of short saphenous vein at saphenopopliteal junction (separate procedure)
6.75 6.75 FUD 090 T A2 50
AMA: 2018,Jan,8; 2017,Jan,8; 2016,Jan,13; 2015,Jan,16; 2014,Jan,11

37785 Ligation, division, and/or excision of varicose vein cluster(s), 1 leg
7.45 10.0 FUD 090 T A2 50
AMA: 2018,Jan,8; 2017,Jan,8; 2016,Jan,13; 2015,Jan,16; 2014,Jan,11

37788-37790 Treatment of Vascular Disease of the Penis

37788 Penile revascularization, artery, with or without vein graft ♂
36.5 36.5 FUD 090 C 80
AMA: 2014,Jan,11

37790 Penile venous occlusive procedure
14.0 14.0 FUD 090 J A2 80
AMA: 2014,Jan,11

37799 Unlisted Vascular Surgery Procedures

CMS: 100-04,32,161 Intracranial Percutaneous Transluminal Angioplasty (PTA) With Stenting; 100-04,4,180.3 Unlisted Service or Procedure

37799 Unlisted procedure, vascular surgery
0.00 0.00 FUD YYY T 80
AMA: 2018,Nov,11; 2018,Jan,8; 2017,Jan,8; 2016,Nov,3; 2016,Jan,13; 2015,Apr,10; 2015,Jan,16; 2014,Oct,6; 2014,Aug,14; 2014,Mar,8; 2014,Jan,11

38100-38200 Splenic Procedures

38100 Splenectomy; total (separate procedure)
33.4 33.4 FUD 090 C 80
AMA: 2018,Jan,8; 2017,Jan,8; 2016,Jan,13; 2015,Jan,16; 2014,Jan,11

38101 partial (separate procedure)
33.5 33.5 FUD 090 C 80
AMA: 2018,Jan,8; 2017,Jan,8; 2016,Jan,13; 2015,Jan,16; 2014,Jan,11

+ **38102 total, en bloc for extensive disease, in conjunction with other procedure (List in addition to code for primary procedure)**
Code first primary procedure
7.65 7.65 FUD ZZZ C 80
AMA: 2018,Jan,8; 2017,Jan,8; 2016,Jan,13; 2015,Jan,16; 2014,Jan,11

38115 **Repair of ruptured spleen (splenorrhaphy) with or without partial splenectomy**
37.0 37.0 FUD 090 C 80
AMA: 2018,Jan,8; 2017,Jan,8; 2016,Jan,13; 2015,Jan,16; 2014,Jan,11

38120 **Laparoscopy, surgical, splenectomy**
INCLUDES Diagnostic laparoscopy (49320)
30.5 30.5 FUD 090 J 80
AMA: 2018,Jan,8; 2017,Jan,8; 2016,Jan,13; 2015,Jan,16; 2014,Jan,11

38129 **Unlisted laparoscopy procedure, spleen**
0.00 0.00 FUD YYY J 80
AMA: 2018,Jan,8; 2017,Jan,8; 2016,Jan,13; 2015,Jan,16; 2014,Jan,11

38200 **Injection procedure for splenoportography**
(75810)
3.84 3.84 FUD 000 N N1 80
AMA: 2014,Jan,11

38204-38215 Hematopoietic Stem Cell Preparation

CMS: 100-03,110.23 Stem Cell Transplantation; 100-04,3,90.3 Stem Cell Transplantation; 100-04,3,90.3.1 Allogeneic Stem Cell Transplantation; 100-04,3,90.3.3 Billing for Allogeneic Stem Cell Transplants; 100-04,32,90 Billing for Stem Cell Transplantation; 100-04,32,90.2.1 Coding for Stem Cell Transplantation; 100-04,4,231.10 Billing for Autologous Stem Cell Transplants; 100-04,4,231.11 Billing for Allogeneic Stem Cell Transplants

INCLUDES Preservation, preparation, purification of stem cells before transplant or reinfusion

EXCLUDES *Procedure performed more than one time per day*

38204 **Management of recipient hematopoietic progenitor cell donor search and cell acquisition**
3.03 3.03 FUD XXX N N1
AMA: 2018,Jan,8; 2017,Jan,8; 2016,Jan,13; 2015,Jan,16; 2014,Jan,11

38205 **Blood-derived hematopoietic progenitor cell harvesting for transplantation, per collection; allogeneic**
2.38 2.38 FUD 000 B 80
AMA: 2018,May,3; 2018,Jan,8; 2017,Jan,8; 2016,Jan,13; 2015,Jan,16; 2014,Jan,11

38206 **autologous**
2.39 2.39 FUD 000 S G2 80
AMA: 2018,May,3; 2018,Jan,8; 2017,Jan,8; 2016,Jan,13; 2015,Jan,16; 2014,Jan,11

38207 **Transplant preparation of hematopoietic progenitor cells; cryopreservation and storage**
EXCLUDES *Flow cytometry (88182, 88184-88189)*
(88240)
1.35 1.35 FUD XXX S
AMA: 2018,Jan,8; 2017,Jan,8; 2016,Jan,13; 2015,Jan,16; 2014,Jan,11

38208 **thawing of previously frozen harvest, without washing, per donor**
EXCLUDES *Flow cytometry (88182, 88184-88189)*
(88241)
0.86 0.86 FUD XXX S
AMA: 2018,Jan,8; 2017,Jan,8; 2016,Jan,13; 2015,Jan,16; 2014,Jan,11

38209 **thawing of previously frozen harvest, with washing, per donor**
EXCLUDES *Flow cytometry (88182, 88184-88189)*
0.36 0.36 FUD XXX S
AMA: 2018,Jan,8; 2017,Jan,8; 2016,Jan,13; 2015,Jan,16; 2014,Jan,11

38210 **specific cell depletion within harvest, T-cell depletion**
EXCLUDES *Flow cytometry (88182, 88184-88189)*
2.40 2.40 FUD XXX S
AMA: 2018,Jan,8; 2017,Jan,8; 2016,Jan,13; 2015,Jan,16; 2014,Jan,11

38211 **tumor cell depletion**
EXCLUDES *Flow cytometry (88182, 88184-88189)*
2.16 2.16 FUD XXX S
AMA: 2018,Jan,8; 2017,Jan,8; 2016,Jan,13; 2015,Jan,16; 2014,Jan,11

38212 **red blood cell removal**
EXCLUDES *Flow cytometry (88182, 88184-88189)*
1.43 1.43 FUD XXX S
AMA: 2018,Jan,8; 2017,Jan,8; 2016,Jan,13; 2015,Jan,16; 2014,Jan,11

38213 **platelet depletion**
EXCLUDES *Flow cytometry (88182, 88184-88189)*
0.36 0.36 FUD XXX S
AMA: 2018,Jan,8; 2017,Jan,8; 2016,Jan,13; 2015,Jan,16; 2014,Jan,11

38214 **plasma (volume) depletion**
EXCLUDES *Flow cytometry (88182, 88184-88189)*
1.23 1.23 FUD XXX S
AMA: 2018,Jan,8; 2017,Jan,8; 2016,Jan,13; 2015,Jan,16; 2014,Jan,11

38215 **cell concentration in plasma, mononuclear, or buffy coat layer**
EXCLUDES *Flow cytometry (88182, 88184-88189)*
1.43 1.43 FUD XXX S
AMA: 2018,Jan,8; 2017,Jan,8; 2016,Jan,13; 2015,Jan,16; 2014,Jan,11

38220-38232 Bone Marrow Procedures

CMS: 100-03,110.23 Stem Cell Transplantation; 100-04,3,90.3 Stem Cell Transplantation; 100-04,32,90 Billing for Stem Cell Transplantation; 100-04,4,231.11 Billing for Allogeneic Stem Cell Transplants

38220 **Diagnostic bone marrow; aspiration(s)**
EXCLUDES *Aspiration of bone marrow for spinal graft (20939)*
Bone marrow biopsy (38221)
Bone marrow for platelet rich stem cell injection (0232T)
Code also biopsy bone marrow during same session (38222)
1.99 4.71 FUD XXX J P3 80 50
AMA: 2018,May,3; 2018,Jan,8; 2017,Jan,8; 2016,Jan,13; 2015,Mar,9; 2015,Jan,16; 2014,Jan,11

38221 **biopsy(ies)**
EXCLUDES *Aspiration and biopsy during same session (38222)*
Aspiration of bone marrow (38220)
(88305)
2.00 4.39 FUD XXX J P3 80 50
AMA: 2018,May,3; 2018,Jan,8; 2017,Jan,8; 2016,Jan,13; 2015,Mar,9; 2014,Jan,11

38222 **biopsy(ies) and aspiration(s)**
EXCLUDES *Aspiration of bone marrow only (38221)*
Biopsy of bone marrow only (38220)
(88305)
2.24 4.87 FUD XXX J P3 80 50
AMA: 2018,May,3

38230 **Bone marrow harvesting for transplantation; allogeneic**
EXCLUDES *Aspiration of bone marrow for platelet rich stem cell injection (0232T)*
Harvesting of blood-derived hematopoietic progenitor cells for transplant (allogeneic) (38205)
5.97 5.97 FUD 000 S G2 80
AMA: 2018,Jan,8; 2017,Jan,8; 2016,Jan,13; 2015,Jan,16; 2014,Jan,11

38232 **autologous**
EXCLUDES *Aspiration of bone marrow (38220, 38222)*
Aspiration of bone marrow for platelet rich stem cell injection (0232T)
Aspiration of bone marrow for spinal graft (20939)
Harvesting of blood-derived peripheral stem cells for transplant (allogenic/autologous) (38205-38206)
5.75 5.75 FUD 000 S G2 80
AMA: 2018,Jan,8; 2017,Jan,8; 2016,Jan,13; 2015,Jan,16; 2014,Jan,11

38240-38243 [38243] Hematopoietic Progenitor Cell Transplantation

CMS: 100-03,110.23 Stem Cell Transplantation; 100-04,3,90.3 Stem Cell Transplantation; 100-04,3,90.3.1 Allogeneic Stem Cell Transplantation; 100-04,3,90.3.2 Autologous Stem Cell Transplantation (AuSCT); 100-04,3,90.3.3 Billing for Allogeneic Stem Cell Transplants; 100-04,32,90 Billing for Stem Cell Transplantation; 100-04,32,90.2 Allogeneic Stem Cell Transplantation; 100-04,32,90.2.1 Coding for Stem Cell Transplantation; 100-04,32,90.3 Autologous Stem Cell Transplantation; 100-04,32,90.4 Edits Stem Cell Transplant; 100-04,32,90.6 Clinical Trials for Stem Cell Transplant for Myelodysplastic Syndrome (; 100-04,4,231.10 Billing for Autologous Stem Cell Transplants; 100-04,4,231.11 Billing for Allogeneic Stem Cell Transplants

INCLUDES Evaluation of patient prior to, during, and after the infusion
Management of uncomplicated adverse reactions such as hives or nausea
Monitoring of physiological parameters
Physician presence during the infusion
Supervision of clinical staff

EXCLUDES *Administration of fluids for the transplant or for incidental hydration separately*
Concurrent administration of medications with the infusion for the transplant
Cryopreservation, freezing, and storage of hematopoietic progenitor cells for transplant (38207)
Human leukocyte antigen (HLA) testing (81379-81383, 86812-86821)
Modification, treatment, processing of hematopoietic progenitor cell specimens for transplant (38210-38215)
Thawing and expansion of hematopoietic progenitor cells for transplant (38208-38209)

Code also administration of medications and/or fluids not related to the transplant with modifier 59

Code also E&M service for the treatment of more complicated adverse reactions after the infusion, as appropriate

Code also separately identifiable E&M service on the same date, using modifier 25 as appropriate (99211-99215, 99217-99220, [99224, 99225, 99226], 99221-99223, 99231-99239, 99471-99472, 99475-99476)

38240 **Hematopoietic progenitor cell (HPC); allogeneic transplantation per donor**

EXCLUDES *Allogeneic lymphocyte infusions on same date of service with (38242)*
Hematopoietic progenitor cell (HPC); HPC boost on same date of service with ([38243])

6.53 6.53 **FUD** XXX J 80

AMA: 2018,Jan,8; 2017,Jan,8; 2016,Jan,13; 2015,Jan,16; 2014,Jan,11

38241 **autologous transplantation**

4.88 4.88 **FUD** XXX S G2 80

AMA: 2018,Jan,8; 2017,Jan,8; 2016,Jan,13; 2015,Jan,16; 2014,Jan,11

\# **38243** **HPC boost**

EXCLUDES *Allogeneic lymphocyte infusions on same date of service with (38242)*
Hematopoietic progenitor cell (HPC); allogeneic transplantation per donor on same date of service with (38240)

3.47 3.47 **FUD** 000 S R2 80

AMA: 2018,Jan,8; 2017,Jan,8; 2016,Jan,13; 2015,Feb,10; 2015,Jan,16; 2014,Jan,11

38242 **Allogeneic lymphocyte infusions**

EXCLUDES *Aspiration of bone marrow (38220, 38222)*
Aspiration of bone marrow for platelet rich stem cell injection (0232T)
Aspiration of bone marrow for spinal graft (20939)
Hematopoietic progenitor cell (HPC); allogeneic transplantation per donor on same date of service with (38240)
Hematopoietic progenitor cell (HPC); HPC boost on same date of service with ([38243])

(81379-81383, 86812-86813, 86816-86817, 86821)

3.45 3.45 **FUD** 000 S R2 80

AMA: 2018,Jan,8; 2017,Jan,8; 2016,Jan,13; 2015,Jan,16; 2014,Jan,11

38243 **Resequenced code. See code following 38241.**

38300-38382 Incision Lymphatic Vessels

38300 **Drainage of lymph node abscess or lymphadenitis; simple**

5.86 9.20 **FUD** 010 J A2

AMA: 2014,Jan,11

38305 **extensive**

14.0 14.0 **FUD** 090 J A2

AMA: 2014,Jan,11

38308 **Lymphangiotomy or other operations on lymphatic channels**

13.0 13.0 **FUD** 090 J A2 80

AMA: 2014,Jan,11

38380 **Suture and/or ligation of thoracic duct; cervical approach**

16.3 16.3 **FUD** 090 C 80

AMA: 2014,Jan,11

38381 **thoracic approach**

23.2 23.2 **FUD** 090 C 80

AMA: 2014,Jan,11

38382 **abdominal approach**

19.4 19.4 **FUD** 090 C 80

AMA: 2014,Jan,11

38500-38555 Biopsy/Excision Lymphatic Vessels

EXCLUDES *Injection for sentinel node identification (38792)*
Percutaneous needle biopsy retroperitoneal mass (49180)

38500 **Biopsy or excision of lymph node(s); open, superficial**

EXCLUDES *Lymphadenectomy (38700-38780)*

7.36 9.58 **FUD** 010 J A2 50

AMA: 2019,Feb,8; 2018,Jan,8; 2017,Jan,8; 2016,Jan,13; 2015,Jan,16; 2014,Jan,11

38505 **by needle, superficial (eg, cervical, inguinal, axillary)**

EXCLUDES *Fine needle aspiration (10004-10012, 10021)*

(88172-88173)

(76942, 77002, 77012, 77021)

2.02 3.56 **FUD** 000 J A2 50

AMA: 2019,Feb,8; 2018,Jan,8; 2017,Jan,8; 2016,Jan,13; 2015,Jan,16; 2014,Jan,11

38510 **open, deep cervical node(s)**

12.0 14.9 **FUD** 010 J A2 50

AMA: 2019,Feb,8; 2018,Jan,8; 2017,Jan,8; 2016,Jan,13; 2015,Jan,16; 2014,Jan,11

38520 **open, deep cervical node(s) with excision scalene fat pad**

13.4 13.4 **FUD** 090 J A2 50

AMA: 2019,Feb,8; 2018,Jan,8; 2017,Jan,8; 2016,Jan,13; 2015,Jan,16; 2014,Jan,11

38525 **open, deep axillary node(s)**

12.6 12.6 **FUD** 090 J A2 50

AMA: 2019,Feb,8; 2018,Jan,8; 2017,Jan,8; 2016,Jan,13; 2015,Mar,5; 2015,Jan,16; 2014,Apr,10; 2014,Jan,11

38530 **open, internal mammary node(s)**

EXCLUDES *Fine needle aspiration (10005-10012)*
Lymphadenectomy (38720-38746)

16.1 16.1 **FUD** 090 J A2 80 50

AMA: 2019,Feb,8; 2018,Jan,8; 2017,Jan,8; 2016,Jan,13; 2015,Jan,16; 2014,Apr,10; 2014,Jan,11

38531 **open, inguinofemoral node(s)**

12.6 12.6 **FUD** 090 80 50

AMA: 2019,Feb,8

38542 **Dissection, deep jugular node(s)**

EXCLUDES *Complete cervical lymphadenectomy (38720)*

14.8 14.8 **FUD** 090 J A2 80 50

AMA: 2019,Feb,8; 2018,Jan,8; 2017,Jan,8; 2016,Jan,13; 2015,Jan,16; 2014,Jan,11

38550 **Excision of cystic hygroma, axillary or cervical; without deep neurovascular dissection**

14.7 14.7 **FUD** 090 J A2 80

AMA: 2014,Jan,11

38555 **with deep neurovascular dissection**

29.2 29.2 **FUD** 090 J A2 80

AMA: 2014,Jan,11

38562-38564 Limited Lymphadenectomy: Staging

38562 **Limited lymphadenectomy for staging (separate procedure); pelvic and para-aortic**

EXCLUDES *Prostatectomy (55812, 55842)*
Radioactive substance inserted into prostate (55862)

20.4 20.4 FUD 090 C 80

AMA: 2019,Feb,8; 2018,Jan,8; 2017,Jan,8; 2016,Jan,13; 2015,Jan,16; 2014,Jan,11

38564 **retroperitoneal (aortic and/or splenic)**

20.4 20.4 FUD 090 C 80

AMA: 2019,Feb,8; 2014,Jan,11

38570-38589 Laparoscopic Lymph Node Procedures

INCLUDES Diagnostic laparoscopy (49320)

EXCLUDES *Laparoscopy with draining of lymphocele to peritoneal cavity (49323)*
Limited lymphadenectomy:
Pelvic (38562)
Retroperitoneal (38564)

38570 **Laparoscopy, surgical; with retroperitoneal lymph node sampling (biopsy), single or multiple**

14.7 14.7 FUD 010 J A2 80

AMA: 2019,Feb,8; 2018,Jan,8; 2017,Jan,8; 2016,Jan,13; 2015,Jan,16; 2014,Jan,11

38571 **with bilateral total pelvic lymphadenectomy**

19.1 19.1 FUD 010 J A2 80

AMA: 2019,Feb,8; 2018,Jan,8; 2017,Jan,8; 2016,Jan,13; 2015,Jan,16; 2014,Jan,11

38572 **with bilateral total pelvic lymphadenectomy and peri-aortic lymph node sampling (biopsy), single or multiple**

EXCLUDES *Lymphocele drainage into peritoneal cavity (49323)*

26.7 26.7 FUD 010 J A2 80

AMA: 2019,Feb,8; 2018,Jan,8; 2017,Jan,8; 2016,Jan,13; 2015,Jan,13; 2015,Jan,16; 2014,Jan,11

38573 **with bilateral total pelvic lymphadenectomy and peri-aortic lymph node sampling, peritoneal washings, peritoneal biopsy(ies), omentectomy, and diaphragmatic washings, including diaphragmatic and other serosal biopsy(ies), when performed**

EXCLUDES *Laparoscopic hysterectomy procedures (58541-58554)*
Laparoscopic omentopexy (separate procedure) (49326)
Laparoscopy abdomen, diagnostic (separate procedure)(49320)
Laparoscopy unlisted (38589)
Laparoscopy without omentectomy (38570-38572)
Lymphadenectomy for staging (38562-38564)
Omentectomy (separate procedure) (49255)
Pelvic lymphadenectomy of external iliac, hypogastric, and obturator nodes (38770)
Retroperitoneal lymphadenectomy of aortic, pelvic, and renal nodes (separate procedure)(38780)

33.7 33.7 FUD 010 J G2 80

AMA: 2019,Mar,5; 2018,Apr,10

38589 **Unlisted laparoscopy procedure, lymphatic system**

0.00 0.00 FUD YYY J 80 50

AMA: 2018,Apr,10; 2018,Jan,8; 2017,Jan,8; 2016,Jan,13; 2015,Jan,16; 2014,Jan,11

38700-38780 Lymphadenectomy Procedures

INCLUDES Lymph node biopsy/excision (38500)

EXCLUDES *Excision of lymphedematous skin and subcutaneous tissue (15004-15005)*
Limited lymphadenectomy
Pelvic (38562)
Retroperitoneal (38564)
Repair of lymphedematous skin and tissue (15570-15650)

38700 **Suprahyoid lymphadenectomy**

23.1 23.1 FUD 090 J G2 80 50

AMA: 2019,Feb,8; 2018,Jan,8; 2017,Jan,8; 2016,Jan,13; 2015,Jan,16; 2014,Jan,11

38720 **Cervical lymphadenectomy (complete)**

38.6 38.6 FUD 090 J 80 50

AMA: 2019,Feb,8; 2018,Jan,8; 2017,Jan,8; 2016,Jan,13; 2015,Jan,16; 2014,Jan,11

38724 **Cervical lymphadenectomy (modified radical neck dissection)**

41.6 41.6 FUD 090 C 80 50

AMA: 2019,Mar,10; 2019,Feb,8; 2018,Jan,8; 2017,Jan,8; 2016,Jan,13; 2015,Jan,16; 2014,Jan,11

38740 **Axillary lymphadenectomy; superficial**

20.1 20.1 FUD 090 J A2 80 50

AMA: 2019,Feb,8; 2018,Jan,8; 2017,Jan,8; 2016,Jan,13; 2015,Jan,16; 2014,Apr,10; 2014,Jan,11

38745 **complete**

25.4 25.4 FUD 090 J A2 80 50

AMA: 2019,Feb,8; 2014,Jan,11

\+ **38746** **Thoracic lymphadenectomy by thoracotomy, mediastinal and regional lymphadenectomy (List separately in addition to code for primary procedure)**

INCLUDES Left side
Aortopulmonary window
Inferior pulmonary ligament
Paraesophageal
Subcarinal
Right side
Inferior pulmonary ligament
Paraesophageal
Paratracheal
Subcarinal

EXCLUDES *Thoracoscopic mediastinal and regional lymphadenectomy (32674)*

Code first (21601, 31760, 31766, 31786, 32096-32200, 32220-32320, 32440-32491, 32503-32505, 33025, 33030, 33050-33130, 39200-39220, 39560-39561, 43101, 43112, 43117-43118, 43122-43123, 43351, 60270, 60505)

6.23 6.23 FUD ZZZ C 80

AMA: 2019,Feb,8; 2018,Jan,8; 2017,Jan,8; 2016,Jan,13; 2015,Jan,16; 2014,May,3; 2014,Jan,11

Parasternal nodes
Central nodes

\+ **38747** **Abdominal lymphadenectomy, regional, including celiac, gastric, portal, peripancreatic, with or without para-aortic and vena caval nodes (List separately in addition to code for primary procedure)**

Code first primary procedure

7.77 7.77 FUD ZZZ C 80

AMA: 2019,Feb,8; 2014,Jan,11

38760 **Inguinofemoral lymphadenectomy, superficial, including Cloquet's node (separate procedure)**

24.3 24.3 FUD 090 J A2 80 50

AMA: 2019,Feb,8; 2018,Jan,8; 2017,Jan,8; 2016,Jan,13; 2015,Jan,16; 2014,Jan,11

38765 **Inguinofemoral lymphadenectomy, superficial, in continuity with pelvic lymphadenectomy, including external iliac, hypogastric, and obturator nodes (separate procedure)**
37.6 37.6 FUD 090 C 80 50
AMA: 2019,Feb,8; 2018,Jan,8; 2017,Jan,8; 2016,Jan,13; 2015,Jan,16; 2014,Jan,11

38770 **Pelvic lymphadenectomy, including external iliac, hypogastric, and obturator nodes (separate procedure)**
23.4 23.4 FUD 090 C 80 50
AMA: 2019,Feb,8; 2014,Jan,11

38780 **Retroperitoneal transabdominal lymphadenectomy, extensive, including pelvic, aortic, and renal nodes (separate procedure)**
29.7 29.7 FUD 090 C 80
AMA: 2019,Feb,8; 2014,Jan,11

38790-38999 Cannulation/Injection/Other Procedures

38790 **Injection procedure; lymphangiography**
(75801-75807)
2.39 2.39 FUD 000 N N1 50
AMA: 2014,Jan,11

38792 **radioactive tracer for identification of sentinel node**
EXCLUDES *Sentinel node excision (38500-38542)*
Sentinel node(s) identification (mapping) intraoperative with nonradioactive dye injection (38900)
(78195)
0.96 2.34 FUD 000 Q1 N1 50
AMA: 2019,Feb,8; 2018,Jan,8; 2017,Jan,8; 2016,Jan,13; 2015,Mar,5; 2015,Jan,16; 2014,Jan,11

38794 **Cannulation, thoracic duct**
8.57 8.57 FUD 090 N N1 80
AMA: 2014,Jan,11

\+ **38900** **Intraoperative identification (eg, mapping) of sentinel lymph node(s) includes injection of non-radioactive dye, when performed (List separately in addition to code for primary procedure)**
EXCLUDES *Injection of tracer for sentinel node identification (38792)*
Code first (19302, 19307, 38500, 38510, 38520, 38525, 38530-38531, 38542, 38562-38564, 38570-38572, 38740, 38745, 38760, 38765, 38770, 38780, 56630-56634, 56637, 56640)
4.00 4.00 FUD ZZZ N N1 80 50
AMA: 2019,Feb,8; 2018,Jan,8; 2017,Jan,8; 2016,Jan,13; 2015,Mar,5; 2014,Jan,11

38999 **Unlisted procedure, hemic or lymphatic system**
0.00 0.00 FUD YYY S 80
AMA: 2018,Jan,8; 2017,Jan,8; 2016,Jan,13; 2015,Jan,16; 2014,Jan,11

39000-39499 Surgical Procedures: Mediastinum

39000 **Mediastinotomy with exploration, drainage, removal of foreign body, or biopsy; cervical approach**
14.3 14.3 FUD 090 C 80
AMA: 2014,Jan,11

39010 **transthoracic approach, including either transthoracic or median sternotomy**
EXCLUDES *ECMO/ECLS insertion or reposition of cannula (33955-33956, [33963, 33964])*
Video-assisted thoracic surgery (VATS) pericardial biopsy (32604)
22.7 22.7 FUD 090 C 80
AMA: 2018,Jan,8; 2017,Jan,8; 2016,Jan,13; 2015,Jul,3; 2015,Jan,16; 2014,Jan,11; 2014,Jan,5

39200 **Resection of mediastinal cyst**
25.2 25.2 FUD 090 C 80
AMA: 2014,Jan,11

39220 **Resection of mediastinal tumor**
EXCLUDES *Thymectomy (60520)*
Thyroidectomy, substernal (60270)
Video-assisted thoracic surgery (VATS) resection cyst, mass, or tumor of mediastinum (32662)
32.7 32.7 FUD 090 C 80
AMA: 2014,Jan,11

39401 **Mediastinoscopy; includes biopsy(ies) of mediastinal mass (eg, lymphoma), when performed**
8.96 8.96 FUD 000 J
AMA: 2018,Jan,8; 2017,Jan,8; 2016,Jun,4

39402 **with lymph node biopsy(ies) (eg, lung cancer staging)**
11.7 11.7 FUD 000 J
AMA: 2018,Jan,8; 2017,Jan,8; 2016,Jun,4

39499 **Unlisted procedure, mediastinum**
0.00 0.00 FUD YYY C 80
AMA: 2014,Jan,11

39501-39599 Surgical Procedures: Diaphragm

EXCLUDES *Esophagogastric fundoplasty, with fundic patch (43325)*
Repair of diaphragmatic (esophageal) hernias:
Laparoscopic with fundoplication (43280-43282)
Laparotomy (43332-43333)
Thoracoabdominal (43336-43337)
Thoracotomy (43334-43335)

39501 **Repair, laceration of diaphragm, any approach**
24.6 24.6 FUD 090 C 80
AMA: 2018,Jan,8; 2017,Jan,8; 2016,Jan,13; 2015,Jan,16; 2014,Dec,16; 2014,Dec,16; 2014,Jan,11

39503 **Repair, neonatal diaphragmatic hernia, with or without chest tube insertion and with or without creation of ventral hernia** A
173. 173. FUD 090 63 C 80
AMA: 2018,Jan,8; 2017,Jan,8; 2016,Jan,13; 2015,Jan,16; 2014,Jan,11

Trachea
Lungs
Diaphragm

A defect of the diaphragm can allow abdominal contents to herniate into the thoracic cavity

39540 **Repair, diaphragmatic hernia (other than neonatal), traumatic; acute**
25.2 25.2 FUD 090 C 80
AMA: 2018,Jan,8; 2017,Jan,8; 2016,Jan,13; 2015,Jan,16; 2014,Jan,11

39541 **chronic**
27.2 27.2 FUD 090 C 80
AMA: 2018,Jan,8; 2017,Jan,8; 2016,Jan,13; 2015,Jan,16; 2014,Jan,11

39545 **Imbrication of diaphragm for eventration, transthoracic or transabdominal, paralytic or nonparalytic**
25.7 25.7 FUD 090 C 80
AMA: 2018,Jan,8; 2017,Jan,8; 2016,Jan,13; 2015,Jan,16; 2014,Jan,11

39560 **Resection, diaphragm; with simple repair (eg, primary suture)**
23.1 23.1 **FUD** 090 C 80
AMA: 2018,Jan,8; 2017,Jan,8; 2016,Jan,13; 2015,Jan,16; 2014,Jan,11

39561 **with complex repair (eg, prosthetic material, local muscle flap)**
35.9 35.9 **FUD** 090 C 80
AMA: 2018,Jan,8; 2017,Jan,8; 2016,Jan,13; 2015,Jan,16; 2014,Jan,11

39599 **Unlisted procedure, diaphragm**
0.00 0.00 **FUD** YYY C 80
AMA: 2014,Jan,11

40490-40799 Resection and Repair Procedures of the Lips

EXCLUDES *Procedures on the skin of lips-see integumentary section codes*

40490 Biopsy of lip
2.09 3.59 FUD 000 T P3
AMA: 2019,Jan,9; 2014,Jan,11

40500 Vermilionectomy (lip shave), with mucosal advancement
10.4 14.6 FUD 090 J A2
AMA: 2014,Jan,11

40510 Excision of lip; transverse wedge excision with primary closure
EXCLUDES *Excision of mucous lesions (40810-40816)*
10.1 13.9 FUD 090 J A2
AMA: 2014,Jan,11

40520 V-excision with primary direct linear closure
EXCLUDES *Excision of mucous lesions (40810-40816)*
10.2 14.1 FUD 090 J A2
AMA: 2014,Jan,11

40525 full thickness, reconstruction with local flap (eg, Estlander or fan)
15.8 15.8 FUD 090 J A2
AMA: 2014,Jan,11

40527 full thickness, reconstruction with cross lip flap (Abbe-Estlander)
INCLUDES *Cleft lip repair with cross lip pedicle flap (Abbe-Estlander type), without pedicle sectioning and insertion*
EXCLUDES *Cleft lip repair with cross lip pedicle flap (Abbe-Estlander type), with pedicle sectioning and insertion (40761)*
17.7 17.7 FUD 090 J A2 80
AMA: 2014,Jan,11

40530 Resection of lip, more than one-fourth, without reconstruction
EXCLUDES *Reconstruction (13131-13153)*
11.5 15.5 FUD 090 J A2
AMA: 2014,Jan,11

40650 Repair lip, full thickness; vermilion only
8.71 13.0 FUD 090 T A2 80
AMA: 2018,Jan,8; 2017,Jan,8; 2016,Nov,7; 2016,Jan,13; 2015,Jan,16; 2014,Jan,11

40652 up to half vertical height
10.1 14.2 FUD 090 T A2 80
AMA: 2018,Jan,8; 2017,Jan,8; 2016,Nov,7; 2016,Jan,13; 2015,Jan,16; 2014,Jan,11

40654 over one-half vertical height, or complex
12.2 16.4 FUD 090 T A2
AMA: 2018,Jan,8; 2017,Jan,8; 2016,Nov,7; 2014,Jan,11

40700 Plastic repair of cleft lip/nasal deformity; primary, partial or complete, unilateral
EXCLUDES *Cleft lip repair with cross lip pedicle flap (Abbe-Estlander type):*
With pedicle sectioning and insertion (40761)
Without pedicle sectioning and insertion (40527)
Rhinoplasty for nasal deformity secondary to congenital cleft lip (30460, 30462)
29.0 29.0 FUD 090 J A2 80
AMA: 2018,Jan,8; 2017,Jan,8; 2016,Jan,13; 2015,Jan,16; 2014,Dec,18; 2014,Jan,11

40701 primary bilateral, 1-stage procedure
EXCLUDES *Cleft lip repair with cross lip pedicle flap (Abbe-Estlander type):*
With pedicle sectioning and insertion (40761)
Without pedicle sectioning and insertion (40527)
Rhinoplasty for nasal deformity secondary to congenital cleft lip (30460, 30462)
34.4 34.4 FUD 090 J A2 80
AMA: 2018,Jan,8; 2017,Jan,8; 2016,Jan,13; 2015,Jan,16; 2014,Dec,18; 2014,Jan,11

40702 primary bilateral, 1 of 2 stages
EXCLUDES *Cleft lip repair with cross lip pedicle flap (Abbe-Estlander type):*
With pedicle sectioning and insertion (40761)
Without pedicle sectioning and insertion (40527)
Rhinoplasty for nasal deformity secondary to congenital cleft lip (30460, 30462)
28.9 28.9 FUD 090 J R2 80
AMA: 2018,Jan,8; 2017,Jan,8; 2016,Jan,13; 2015,Jan,16; 2014,Dec,18; 2014,Jan,11

40720 secondary, by recreation of defect and reclosure
EXCLUDES *Cleft lip repair with cross lip pedicle flap (Abbe-Estlander type):*
With pedicle sectioning and insertion (40761)
Without pedicle sectioning and insertion (40527)
Rhinoplasty for nasal deformity secondary to congenital cleft lip (30460, 30462)
29.7 29.7 FUD 090 J A2 80 50
AMA: 2018,Jan,8; 2017,Jan,8; 2016,Jan,13; 2015,Jan,16; 2014,Dec,18; 2014,Jan,11

40761 with cross lip pedicle flap (Abbe-Estlander type), including sectioning and inserting of pedicle
EXCLUDES *Cleft lip repair with cross lip pedicle flap (Abbe-Estlander type) without sectioning and insertion of pedicle (40527)*
Cleft palate repair (42200-42225)
Other reconstructive procedures (14060-14061, 15120-15261, 15574, 15576, 15630)
31.3 31.3 FUD 090 J A2
AMA: 2014,Jan,11

40799 Unlisted procedure, lips
0.00 0.00 FUD YYY T 80
AMA: 2014,Jan,11

40800-40819 Incision and Resection of Buccal Cavity

INCLUDES Mucosal/submucosal tissue of lips/cheeks
Oral cavity outside the dentoalveolar structures

40800 Drainage of abscess, cyst, hematoma, vestibule of mouth; simple
3.72 6.08 FUD 010 T P3
AMA: 2014,Jan,11

40801 complicated
6.26 8.86 FUD 010 T A2
AMA: 2014,Jan,11

Digestive System 40490 — 40801

40804 **Removal of embedded foreign body, vestibule of mouth; simple**
3.36 5.47 FUD 010 Q1 N1 80
AMA: 2014,Jan,11

40805 **complicated**
6.43 8.91 FUD 010 T P3 80
AMA: 2014,Jan,11

40806 **Incision of labial frenum (frenotomy)**
0.93 2.91 FUD 000 T P3 80
AMA: 2014,Jan,11

40808 **Biopsy, vestibule of mouth**
3.06 5.37 FUD 010 T P3
AMA: 2019,Jan,9; 2014,Jan,11

40810 **Excision of lesion of mucosa and submucosa, vestibule of mouth; without repair**
3.64 5.99 FUD 010 J P3
AMA: 2014,Jan,11

40812 **with simple repair**
5.63 8.30 FUD 010 J P3
AMA: 2014,Jan,11

40814 **with complex repair**
8.71 11.0 FUD 090 J A2
AMA: 2014,Jan,11

40816 **complex, with excision of underlying muscle**
9.02 11.5 FUD 090 J A2
AMA: 2014,Jan,11

40818 **Excision of mucosa of vestibule of mouth as donor graft**
7.91 10.5 FUD 090 T A2 80
AMA: 2014,Jan,11

40819 **Excision of frenum, labial or buccal (frenumectomy, frenulectomy, frenectomy)**
6.79 9.05 FUD 090 T A2 80
AMA: 2014,Jan,11

40820 Destruction of Lesion of Buccal Cavity

CMS: 100-03,140.5 Laser Procedures

INCLUDES Mucosal/submucosal tissue of lips/cheeks
Oral cavity outside the dentoalveolar structures

40820 **Destruction of lesion or scar of vestibule of mouth by physical methods (eg, laser, thermal, cryo, chemical)**
4.91 7.54 FUD 010 J P3
AMA: 2014,Jan,11

40830-40899 Repair Procedures of the Buccal Cavity

INCLUDES Mucosal/submucosal tissue of lips/cheeks
Oral cavity outside the dentoalveolar structures

EXCLUDES *Skin grafts (15002-15630)*

40830 **Closure of laceration, vestibule of mouth; 2.5 cm or less**
4.79 7.78 FUD 010 T G2 80
AMA: 2014,Jan,11

40831 **over 2.5 cm or complex**
6.55 9.95 FUD 010 T A2 80
AMA: 2014,Jan,11

40840 **Vestibuloplasty; anterior**
18.0 23.5 FUD 090 J A2 80
AMA: 2014,Jan,11

40842 **posterior, unilateral**
17.7 22.8 FUD 090 J A2 80
AMA: 2014,Jan,11

40843 **posterior, bilateral**
23.6 30.1 FUD 090 J A2 80
AMA: 2014,Jan,11

40844 **entire arch**
31.8 39.2 FUD 090 J A2 80
AMA: 2014,Jan,11

40845 **complex (including ridge extension, muscle repositioning)**
35.2 42.2 FUD 090 J A2 80
AMA: 2014,Jan,11

40899 **Unlisted procedure, vestibule of mouth**
0.00 0.00 FUD YYY T 80
AMA: 2014,Jan,11

41000-41018 Surgical Incision of Floor of Mouth or Tongue

EXCLUDES *Frenoplasty (41520)*

41000 **Intraoral incision and drainage of abscess, cyst, or hematoma of tongue or floor of mouth; lingual**
3.22 4.65 FUD 010 T P3
AMA: 2014,Jan,11

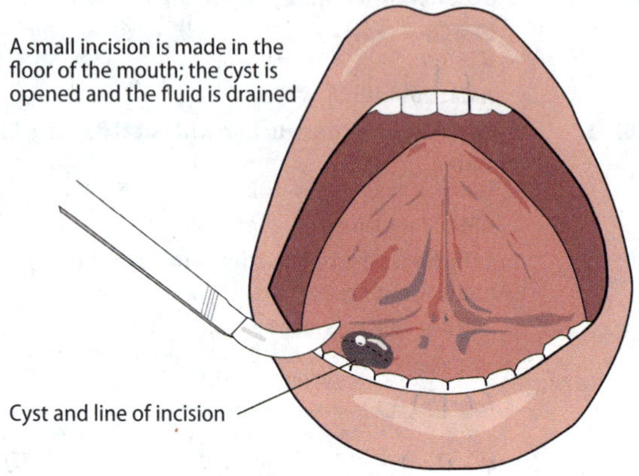

41005 **sublingual, superficial**
3.54 6.34 FUD 010 T A2 80
AMA: 2014,Jan,11

41006 **sublingual, deep, supramylohyoid**
7.36 10.2 FUD 090 T A2 80
AMA: 2014,Jan,11

41007 **submental space**
7.12 10.0 FUD 090 T A2 80
AMA: 2014,Jan,11

41008 **submandibular space**
7.74 11.0 FUD 090 J A2 80
AMA: 2014,Jan,11

41009 **masticator space**
8.46 11.8 FUD 090 T A2 80
AMA: 2014,Jan,11

41010 **Incision of lingual frenum (frenotomy)**
3.11 5.90 FUD 010 T A2 80
AMA: 2018,Jan,8; 2017,Nov,10; 2017,Sep,14; 2014,Jan,11

41015 **Extraoral incision and drainage of abscess, cyst, or hematoma of floor of mouth; sublingual**
9.53 12.0 FUD 090 T A2 80
AMA: 2014,Jan,11

41016 **submental**
10.0 12.8 FUD 090 J A2 80
AMA: 2014,Jan,11

41017 **submandibular**
10.1 13.0 FUD 090 J A2 80
AMA: 2014,Jan,11

41018 **masticator space**
11.8 14.7 FUD 090 T A2 80
AMA: 2014,Jan,11

41019 Placement of Devices for Brachytherapy

EXCLUDES *Application of interstitial radioelements (77770-77772, 77778)*
Intracranial brachytherapy radiation sources with stereotactic insertion (61770)

41019 **Placement of needles, catheters, or other device(s) into the head and/or neck region (percutaneous, transoral, or transnasal) for subsequent interstitial radioelement application**
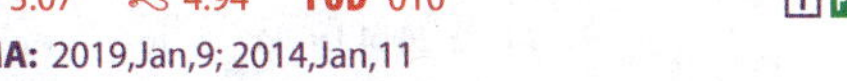
(76942, 77002, 77012, 77021)
13.7 13.7 FUD 000 J G2 80
AMA: 2018,Jan,8; 2017,Jan,8; 2016,Jan,13; 2015,Jan,16; 2014,Jan,11

41100-41599 Resection and Repair of the Tongue

41100 **Biopsy of tongue; anterior two-thirds**
3.07 4.94 FUD 010 T P3
AMA: 2019,Jan,9; 2014,Jan,11

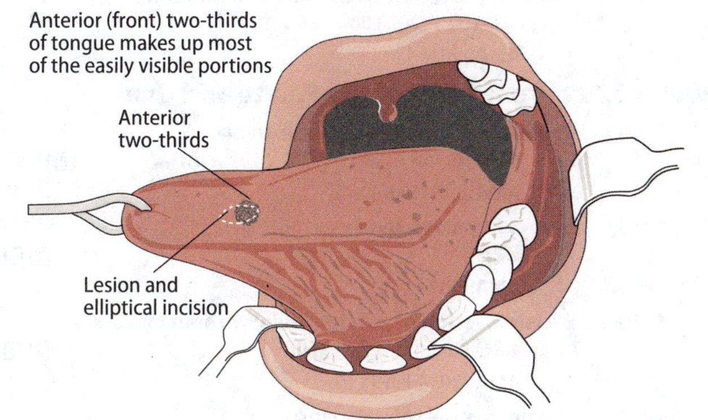

41105 **posterior one-third**
3.19 5.02 FUD 010 J P3
AMA: 2014,Jan,11

41108 **Biopsy of floor of mouth**
2.58 4.37 FUD 010 J P3
AMA: 2019,Jan,9; 2014,Jan,11

41110 **Excision of lesion of tongue without closure**
3.77 6.21 FUD 010 J P3
AMA: 2014,Jan,11

41112 **Excision of lesion of tongue with closure; anterior two-thirds**
7.22 9.65 FUD 090 J A2
AMA: 2014,Jan,11

41113 **posterior one-third**
7.98 10.5 FUD 090 J A2
AMA: 2014,Jan,11

41114 **with local tongue flap**
INCLUDES Excision lesion of tongue with closure anterior/posterior two-thirds (41112-41113)
18.1 18.1 FUD 090 J A2 80
AMA: 2014,Jan,11

41115 **Excision of lingual frenum (frenectomy)**
4.17 7.17 FUD 010 T P3 80
AMA: 2018,Jan,8; 2017,Nov,10; 2017,Sep,14; 2014,Jan,11

41116 **Excision, lesion of floor of mouth**
6.31 9.55 FUD 090 J A2
AMA: 2014,Jan,11

41120 **Glossectomy; less than one-half tongue**
30.8 30.8 FUD 090 J A2 80
AMA: 2018,Jan,8; 2017,Jan,8; 2016,Jan,13; 2015,Jan,16; 2014,Jan,11

41130 **hemiglossectomy**
38.0 38.0 FUD 090 C 80
AMA: 2018,Jan,8; 2017,Jan,8; 2016,Jan,13; 2015,Jan,16; 2014,Jan,11

41135 **partial, with unilateral radical neck dissection**
62.9 62.9 FUD 090 C 80
AMA: 2018,Jan,8; 2017,Jan,8; 2016,Jan,13; 2015,Jan,16; 2014,Jan,11

41140 **complete or total, with or without tracheostomy, without radical neck dissection**
INCLUDES Regnoli's excision
63.0 63.0 FUD 090 C 80
AMA: 2018,Jan,8; 2017,Jan,8; 2016,Jan,13; 2015,Jan,16; 2014,Jan,11

41145 **complete or total, with or without tracheostomy, with unilateral radical neck dissection**
79.8 79.8 FUD 090 C 80
AMA: 2018,Jan,8; 2017,Jan,8; 2016,Jan,13; 2015,Jan,16; 2014,Jan,11

41150 **composite procedure with resection floor of mouth and mandibular resection, without radical neck dissection**
63.5 63.5 FUD 090 C 80
AMA: 2018,Jan,8; 2017,Jan,8; 2016,Jan,13; 2015,Jan,16; 2014,Jan,11

41153 **composite procedure with resection floor of mouth, with suprahyoid neck dissection**
68.8 68.8 FUD 090 C 80
AMA: 2018,Jan,8; 2017,Jan,8; 2016,Jan,13; 2015,Jan,16; 2014,Jan,11

41155 **composite procedure with resection floor of mouth, mandibular resection, and radical neck dissection (Commando type)**
87.2 87.2 FUD 090 C 80
AMA: 2018,Jan,8; 2017,Jan,8; 2016,Jan,13; 2015,Jan,16; 2014,Jan,11

41250 **Repair of laceration 2.5 cm or less; floor of mouth and/or anterior two-thirds of tongue**
4.42 7.84 FUD 010 Q1 N1 80
AMA: 2014,Jan,11

41251 **posterior one-third of tongue**
5.33 8.79 FUD 010 T A2 80
AMA: 2014,Jan,11

41252 **Repair of laceration of tongue, floor of mouth, over 2.6 cm or complex**
6.01 9.13 FUD 010 T A2 80
AMA: 2014,Jan,11

41510 **Suture of tongue to lip for micrognathia (Douglas type procedure)**
13.0 13.0 FUD 090 J A2 80
AMA: 2018,Jan,8; 2017,Jan,8; 2016,Jan,13; 2015,Jan,16; 2014,Jan,11

41512 **Tongue base suspension, permanent suture technique**
EXCLUDES *Suture tongue to lip for micrognathia (41510)*
18.9 18.9 FUD 090 J G2 80
AMA: 2018,Jan,8; 2017,Jan,8; 2016,Jan,13; 2015,Jan,16; 2014,Jan,11

41520 **Frenoplasty (surgical revision of frenum, eg, with Z-plasty)**
EXCLUDES *Frenotomy (40806, 41010)*
7.11 10.1 FUD 090 J A2 80
AMA: 2018,Jan,8; 2017,Nov,10; 2017,Sep,14; 2014,Jan,11

41530 **Submucosal ablation of the tongue base, radiofrequency, 1 or more sites, per session**
10.7 27.4 FUD 000 J P3 80
AMA: 2018,Jan,8; 2017,Jan,8; 2016,Jan,13; 2015,Jan,16; 2014,Jan,11

41599 **Unlisted procedure, tongue, floor of mouth**
0.00 0.00 FUD YYY T 80
AMA: 2018,Jan,8; 2017,Jan,8; 2016,Jan,13; 2015,Jan,16; 2014,Jan,11

Digestive System

41019 — 41599

41800-41899 Procedures of the Teeth and Supporting Structures

41800 **Drainage of abscess, cyst, hematoma from dentoalveolar structures**
4.35 8.29 FUD 010 Q1 N1
AMA: 2014,Jan,11

41805 **Removal of embedded foreign body from dentoalveolar structures; soft tissues**
5.44 8.28 FUD 010 T P3 80
AMA: 2014,Jan,11

41806 **bone**
7.97 11.3 FUD 010 T P3 80
AMA: 2014,Jan,11

41820 **Gingivectomy, excision gingiva, each quadrant**
0.00 0.00 FUD 000 J R2 80
AMA: 2014,Jan,11

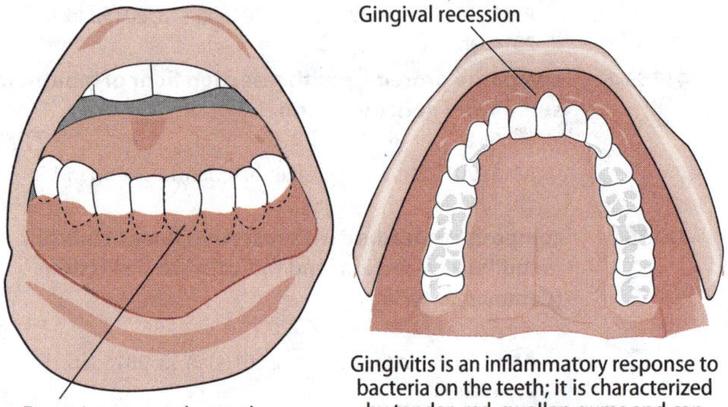

Gingival recession

Excessive mucosal growth

Gingivitis is an inflammatory response to bacteria on the teeth; it is characterized by tender, red, swollen gums and can lead to gingival recession

41821 **Operculectomy, excision pericoronal tissues**
0.00 0.00 FUD 000 T G2 80
AMA: 2014,Jan,11

41822 **Excision of fibrous tuberosities, dentoalveolar structures**
5.08 8.17 FUD 010 T P3 80
AMA: 2014,Jan,11

41823 **Excision of osseous tuberosities, dentoalveolar structures**
9.27 12.6 FUD 090 J P3 80
AMA: 2014,Jan,11

41825 **Excision of lesion or tumor (except listed above), dentoalveolar structures; without repair**
EXCLUDES *Lesion destruction nonexcisional (41850)*
3.53 6.19 FUD 010 J P3
AMA: 2014,Jan,11

41826 **with simple repair**
EXCLUDES *Lesion destruction nonexcisional (41850)*
6.10 9.09 FUD 010 J P3
AMA: 2014,Jan,11

41827 **with complex repair**
EXCLUDES *Lesion destruction nonexcisional (41850)*
8.85 12.8 FUD 090 J A2
AMA: 2014,Jan,11

41828 **Excision of hyperplastic alveolar mucosa, each quadrant (specify)**
6.05 9.02 FUD 010 J P3 80
AMA: 2014,Jan,11

41830 **Alveolectomy, including curettage of osteitis or sequestrectomy**
8.07 11.4 FUD 010 J P3 80
AMA: 2014,Jan,11

41850 **Destruction of lesion (except excision), dentoalveolar structures**
0.00 0.00 FUD 000 T R2 80
AMA: 2014,Jan,11

41870 **Periodontal mucosal grafting**
0.00 0.00 FUD 000 J G2 80
AMA: 2014,Jan,11

41872 **Gingivoplasty, each quadrant (specify)**
7.69 11.2 FUD 090 J P3 80
AMA: 2014,Jan,11

41874 **Alveoloplasty, each quadrant (specify)**
EXCLUDES *Fracture reduction (21421-21490)*
Laceration closure (40830-40831)
Maxilla osteotomy, segmental (21206)
7.41 11.1 FUD 090 J P3 80
AMA: 2014,Jan,11

41899 **Unlisted procedure, dentoalveolar structures**
0.00 0.00 FUD YYY T 80
AMA: 2014,Jan,11

42000-42299 Procedures of the Palate and Uvula

42000 **Drainage of abscess of palate, uvula**
2.98 4.45 FUD 010 T A2 80
AMA: 2014,Jan,11

42100 **Biopsy of palate, uvula**
3.14 4.28 FUD 010 T P3
AMA: 2014,Jan,11

42104 **Excision, lesion of palate, uvula; without closure**
3.98 6.20 FUD 010 J P3
AMA: 2014,Jan,11

42106 **with simple primary closure**
5.06 7.79 FUD 010 J P3
AMA: 2014,Jan,11

42107 **with local flap closure**
EXCLUDES *Mucosal graft (40818)*
Skin graft (14040-14302)
9.94 13.3 FUD 090 J A2
AMA: 2014,Jan,11

42120 **Resection of palate or extensive resection of lesion**
EXCLUDES *Palate reconstruction using extraoral tissue (14040-14302, 15050, 15120, 15240, 15576)*
29.1 29.1 FUD 090 J A2 80
AMA: 2014,Jan,11

42140 **Uvulectomy, excision of uvula**
4.46 7.67 FUD 090 J A2
AMA: 2014,Jan,11

42145 **Palatopharyngoplasty (eg, uvulopalatopharyngoplasty, uvulopharyngoplasty)**
EXCLUDES *Excision of maxillary torus palatinus (21032)*
Excision of torus mandibularis (21031)
19.9 19.9 FUD 090 J A2
AMA: 2018,Jan,8; 2017,Jan,8; 2016,Jan,13; 2015,Jan,16; 2014,Jan,11

42160 **Destruction of lesion, palate or uvula (thermal, cryo or chemical)**
4.21 6.69 FUD 010 J P3 80
AMA: 2018,Jan,8; 2017,Jan,8; 2016,Jan,13; 2015,Jan,16; 2014,Jan,11

42180 **Repair, laceration of palate; up to 2 cm**
5.28 7.08 FUD 010 T A2 80
AMA: 2014,Jan,11

42182 **over 2 cm or complex**
7.35 9.26 FUD 010 J A2 80
AMA: 2014,Jan,11

42200 Palatoplasty for cleft palate, soft and/or hard palate only
27.3 27.3 FUD 090 J A2 80
AMA: 2018,Jan,8; 2017,Jan,8; 2016,Jan,13; 2015,Mar,9; 2015,Jan,16; 2014,Jul,8; 2014,Jan,11

42205 Palatoplasty for cleft palate, with closure of alveolar ridge; soft tissue only
28.4 28.4 FUD 090 J A2 80
AMA: 2014,Jan,11

42210 with bone graft to alveolar ridge (includes obtaining graft)
31.7 31.7 FUD 090 J A2 80
AMA: 2014,Jan,11

42215 Palatoplasty for cleft palate; major revision
20.7 20.7 FUD 090 J A2 80
AMA: 2014,Jan,11

42220 secondary lengthening procedure
17.0 17.0 FUD 090 J A2 80
AMA: 2014,Jan,11

42225 attachment pharyngeal flap
28.4 28.4 FUD 090 J G2 80
AMA: 2018,Jan,8; 2017,Jan,8; 2016,Jan,13; 2015,Jan,16; 2014,Jan,11

42226 Lengthening of palate, and pharyngeal flap
25.3 25.3 FUD 090 J A2 80
AMA: 2014,Jan,11

42227 Lengthening of palate, with island flap
23.8 23.8 FUD 090 J G2 80
AMA: 2014,Jan,11

42235 Repair of anterior palate, including vomer flap
EXCLUDES *Oronasal fistula repair (30600)*
20.9 20.9 FUD 090 J A2 80
AMA: 2018,Jan,8; 2017,Jan,8; 2016,Jan,13; 2015,Mar,9; 2015,Jan,16; 2014,Jul,8; 2014,Jan,11

42260 Repair of nasolabial fistula
EXCLUDES *Cleft lip repair (40700-40761)*
18.9 23.5 FUD 090 J A2 80
AMA: 2014,Jan,11

42280 Maxillary impression for palatal prosthesis
3.21 5.10 FUD 010 T P3 80
AMA: 2014,Jan,11

42281 Insertion of pin-retained palatal prosthesis
4.75 6.56 FUD 010 J G2 80
AMA: 2014,Jan,11

42299 Unlisted procedure, palate, uvula
0.00 0.00 FUD YYY T 80
AMA: 2018,Jan,8; 2017,Jan,8; 2016,Jan,13; 2015,Jan,16; 2014,Jul,8; 2014,Jan,11

42300-42699 Procedures of the Salivary Ducts and Glands

42300 Drainage of abscess; parotid, simple
4.38 6.02 FUD 010 T A2
AMA: 2014,Jan,11

42305 parotid, complicated
12.3 12.3 FUD 090 J A2 80
AMA: 2014,Jan,11

42310 Drainage of abscess; submaxillary or sublingual, intraoral
3.92 5.08 FUD 010 T A2 80
AMA: 2014,Jan,11

42320 submaxillary, external
5.05 7.24 FUD 010 T A2 80
AMA: 2014,Jan,11

42330 Sialolithotomy; submandibular (submaxillary), sublingual or parotid, uncomplicated, intraoral
4.72 6.65 FUD 010 J P3
AMA: 2014,Jan,11

42335 submandibular (submaxillary), complicated, intraoral
7.38 11.1 FUD 090 J P3
AMA: 2014,Jan,11

42340 parotid, extraoral or complicated intraoral
9.73 13.8 FUD 090 J A2 80 50
AMA: 2014,Jan,11

42400 Biopsy of salivary gland; needle
EXCLUDES *Fine needle aspiration (10021, [10004, 10005, 10006, 10007, 10008, 10009, 10010, 10011, 10012])*
(76942, 77002, 77012, 77021)
(88172-88173)
1.55 2.95 FUD 000 T P3
AMA: 2019,Apr,4; 2014,Jan,11

42405 incisional
(76942, 77002, 77012, 77021)
6.50 8.59 FUD 010 J A2
AMA: 2014,Jan,11

42408 Excision of sublingual salivary cyst (ranula)
10.2 14.7 FUD 090 J A2 80
AMA: 2014,Jan,11

42409 Marsupialization of sublingual salivary cyst (ranula)
6.41 9.99 FUD 090 J A2 80
AMA: 2014,Jan,11

42410 Excision of parotid tumor or parotid gland; lateral lobe, without nerve dissection
EXCLUDES *Facial nerve suture or graft (64864, 64865, 69740, 69745)*
17.9 17.9 FUD 090 J A2 80 50
AMA: 2014,Jan,11

42415 lateral lobe, with dissection and preservation of facial nerve
EXCLUDES *Facial nerve suture or graft (64864, 64865, 69740, 69745)*
30.3 30.3 FUD 090 J A2 80 50
AMA: 2014,Jan,11

42420 total, with dissection and preservation of facial nerve
EXCLUDES *Facial nerve suture or graft (64864, 64865, 69740, 69745)*
34.0 34.0 FUD 090 J A2 80 50
AMA: 2014,Jan,11

42425 total, en bloc removal with sacrifice of facial nerve
EXCLUDES *Facial nerve suture or graft (64864, 64865, 69740, 69745)*
23.9 23.9 FUD 090 J A2 80 50
AMA: 2014,Jan,11

42426 total, with unilateral radical neck dissection
EXCLUDES *Facial nerve suture or graft (64864, 64865, 69740, 69745)*
38.8 38.8 FUD 090 C 80 50
AMA: 2018,Jan,8; 2017,Jan,8; 2016,Jan,13; 2015,Jan,16; 2014,Jan,11

42440 Excision of submandibular (submaxillary) gland
11.8 11.8 FUD 090 J A2 80 50
AMA: 2014,Jan,11

42450 Excision of sublingual gland
10.2 13.0 FUD 090 J A2 80
AMA: 2014,Jan,11

42500 Plastic repair of salivary duct, sialodochoplasty; primary or simple
9.80 12.4 FUD 090 J A2 80
AMA: 2014,Jan,11

42505 secondary or complicated
12.9 15.9 FUD 090 J A2
AMA: 2014,Jan,11

42507 Parotid duct diversion, bilateral (Wilke type procedure);
14.4 14.4 FUD 090 J A2 80
AMA: 2014,Jan,11

42509 with excision of both submandibular glands
23.9 23.9 FUD 090 J A2 80
AMA: 2014,Jan,11

42510 with ligation of both submandibular (Wharton's) ducts
17.7 17.7 FUD 090 J A2 80
AMA: 2014,Jan,11

42550 Injection procedure for sialography
(70390)
1.84 4.17 FUD 000 N N1
AMA: 2014,Jan,11

42600 Closure salivary fistula
10.0 14.1 FUD 090 J A2 80
AMA: 2014,Jan,11

42650 Dilation salivary duct
1.66 2.31 FUD 000 T P3
AMA: 2014,Jan,11

42660 Dilation and catheterization of salivary duct, with or without injection
2.57 3.61 FUD 000 T P3 80
AMA: 2014,Jan,11

42665 Ligation salivary duct, intraoral
5.96 9.42 FUD 090 J A2 80
AMA: 2014,Jan,11

42699 Unlisted procedure, salivary glands or ducts
0.00 0.00 FUD YYY T 80
AMA: 2014,Jan,11

42700-42999 Procedures of the Adenoids/Throat/Tonsils

42700 Incision and drainage abscess; peritonsillar
3.88 5.43 FUD 010 T A2
AMA: 2014,Jan,11

42720 retropharyngeal or parapharyngeal, intraoral approach
11.2 13.0 FUD 010 J A2 80
AMA: 2014,Jan,11

42725 retropharyngeal or parapharyngeal, external approach
23.5 23.5 FUD 090 J A2 80
AMA: 2014,Jan,11

42800 Biopsy; oropharynx
EXCLUDES *Laryngoscopy with biopsy (31510, 31535-31536, 31576)*
3.23 4.50 FUD 010 J P3
AMA: 2014,Jan,11

42804 nasopharynx, visible lesion, simple
EXCLUDES *Laryngoscopy with biopsy (31510, 31535-31536)*
3.28 5.65 FUD 010 J A2
AMA: 2014,Jan,11

42806 nasopharynx, survey for unknown primary lesion
EXCLUDES *Laryngoscopy with biopsy (31510, 31535-31536)*
3.81 6.32 FUD 010 J A2
AMA: 2014,Jan,11

42808 Excision or destruction of lesion of pharynx, any method
4.67 6.52 FUD 010 J A2
AMA: 2014,Jan,11

42809 Removal of foreign body from pharynx
3.53 5.75 FUD 010 Q1 N1
AMA: 2014,Jan,11

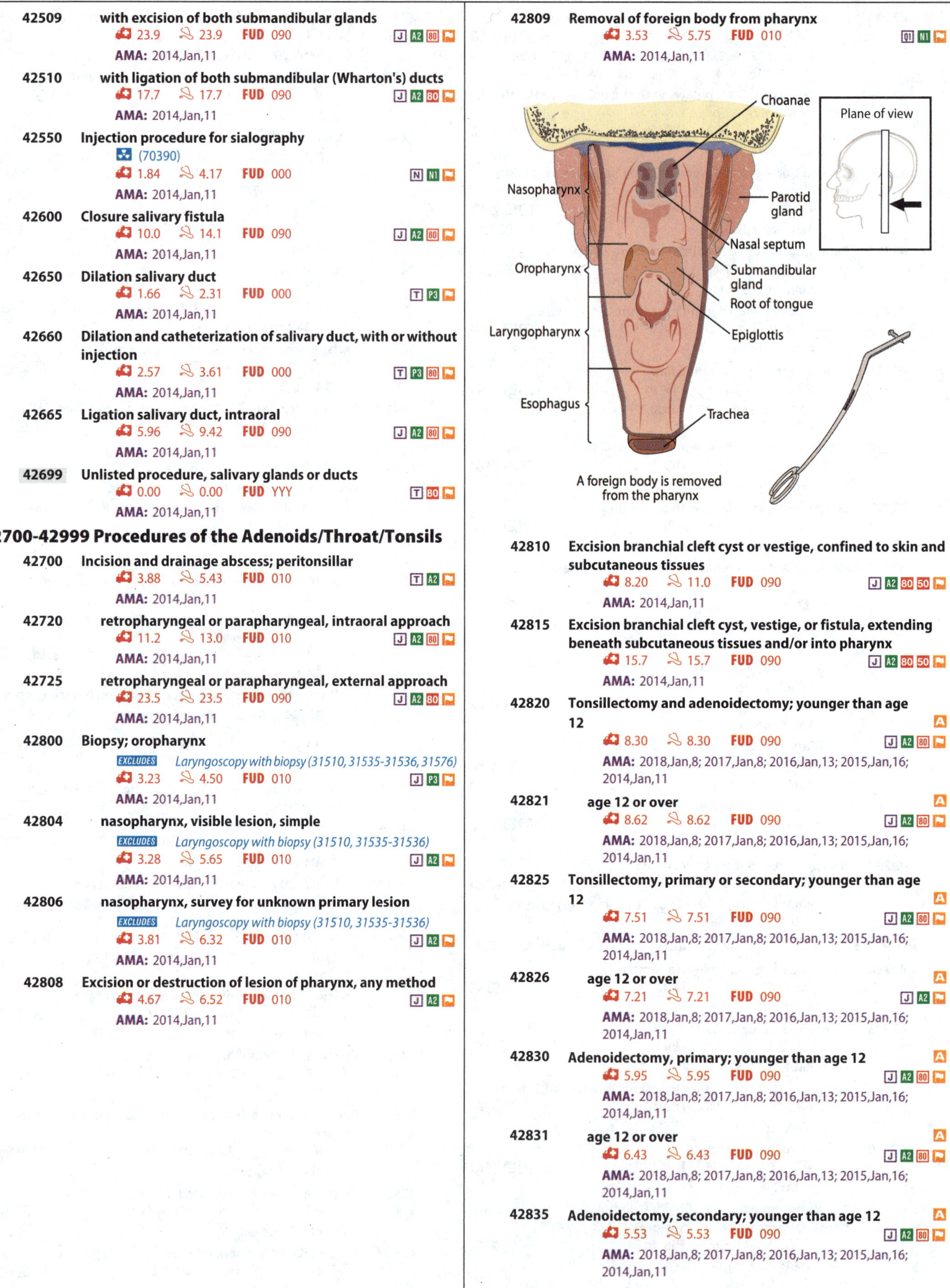

A foreign body is removed from the pharynx

42810 Excision branchial cleft cyst or vestige, confined to skin and subcutaneous tissues
8.20 11.0 FUD 090 J A2 80 50
AMA: 2014,Jan,11

42815 Excision branchial cleft cyst, vestige, or fistula, extending beneath subcutaneous tissues and/or into pharynx
15.7 15.7 FUD 090 J A2 80 50
AMA: 2014,Jan,11

42820 Tonsillectomy and adenoidectomy; younger than age 12 A
8.30 8.30 FUD 090 J A2 80
AMA: 2018,Jan,8; 2017,Jan,8; 2016,Jan,13; 2015,Jan,16; 2014,Jan,11

42821 age 12 or over A
8.62 8.62 FUD 090 J A2 80
AMA: 2018,Jan,8; 2017,Jan,8; 2016,Jan,13; 2015,Jan,16; 2014,Jan,11

42825 Tonsillectomy, primary or secondary; younger than age 12 A
7.51 7.51 FUD 090 J A2 80
AMA: 2018,Jan,8; 2017,Jan,8; 2016,Jan,13; 2015,Jan,16; 2014,Jan,11

42826 age 12 or over A
7.21 7.21 FUD 090 J A2
AMA: 2018,Jan,8; 2017,Jan,8; 2016,Jan,13; 2015,Jan,16; 2014,Jan,11

42830 Adenoidectomy, primary; younger than age 12 A
5.95 5.95 FUD 090 J A2 80
AMA: 2018,Jan,8; 2017,Jan,8; 2016,Jan,13; 2015,Jan,16; 2014,Jan,11

42831 age 12 or over A
6.43 6.43 FUD 090 J A2 80
AMA: 2018,Jan,8; 2017,Jan,8; 2016,Jan,13; 2015,Jan,16; 2014,Jan,11

42835 Adenoidectomy, secondary; younger than age 12 A
5.53 5.53 FUD 090 J A2 80
AMA: 2018,Jan,8; 2017,Jan,8; 2016,Jan,13; 2015,Jan,16; 2014,Jan,11

42836 age 12 or over
6.90 6.90 FUD 090
AMA: 2018,Jan,8; 2017,Jan,8; 2016,Jan,13; 2015,Jan,16; 2014,Jan,11

42842 Radical resection of tonsil, tonsillar pillars, and/or retromolar trigone; without closure
29.0 29.0 FUD 090
AMA: 2018,Jan,8; 2017,Jan,8; 2016,Jan,13; 2015,Jan,16; 2014,Jan,11

42844 closure with local flap (eg, tongue, buccal)
39.9 39.9 FUD 090
AMA: 2018,Jan,8; 2017,Jan,8; 2016,Jan,13; 2015,Jan,16; 2014,Jan,11

42845 closure with other flap
Code also closure with other flap(s)
Code also radical neck dissection when combined (38720)
64.3 64.3 FUD 090
AMA: 2018,Jan,8; 2017,Jan,8; 2016,Jan,13; 2015,Jan,16; 2014,Jan,11

42860 Excision of tonsil tags
5.39 5.39 FUD 090
AMA: 2014,Jan,11

Tonsillar tags or polyps are removed

42870 Excision or destruction lingual tonsil, any method (separate procedure)
EXCLUDES *Nasopharynx resection (juvenile angiofibroma) by transzygomatic/bicoronal approach (61586, 61600)*
17.0 17.0 FUD 090
AMA: 2014,Jan,11

42890 Limited pharyngectomy
Code also radical neck dissection when combined (38720)
41.2 41.2 FUD 090
AMA: 2014,Jan,11

42892 Resection of lateral pharyngeal wall or pyriform sinus, direct closure by advancement of lateral and posterior pharyngeal walls
Code also radical neck dissection when combined (38720)
54.2 54.2 FUD 090
AMA: 2018,Jan,8; 2017,Jan,8; 2016,Jan,13; 2015,Jan,16; 2014,Jan,11

42894 Resection of pharyngeal wall requiring closure with myocutaneous or fasciocutaneous flap or free muscle, skin, or fascial flap with microvascular anastomosis
EXCLUDES *Flap used for reconstruction (15730, 15733-15734, 15756-15758)*
Code also radical neck dissection when combined (38720)
68.5 68.5 FUD 090
AMA: 2018,Jan,8; 2017,Jan,8; 2016,Jan,13; 2015,Jan,16; 2014,Jan,11

42900 Suture pharynx for wound or injury
9.65 9.65 FUD 010
AMA: 2014,Jan,11

42950 Pharyngoplasty (plastic or reconstructive operation on pharynx)
EXCLUDES *Pharyngeal flap (42225)*
23.2 23.2 FUD 090
AMA: 2018,Jan,8; 2017,Jan,8; 2016,Apr,8; 2014,Jan,11

42953 Pharyngoesophageal repair
Code also closure using myocutaneous or other flap
27.9 27.9 FUD 090
AMA: 2014,Jan,11

42955 Pharyngostomy (fistulization of pharynx, external for feeding)
22.0 22.0 FUD 090
AMA: 2014,Jan,11

42960 Control oropharyngeal hemorrhage, primary or secondary (eg, post-tonsillectomy); simple
4.83 4.83 FUD 010
AMA: 2014,Jan,11

42961 complicated, requiring hospitalization
11.9 11.9 FUD 090
AMA: 2014,Jan,11

42962 with secondary surgical intervention
14.8 14.8 FUD 090
AMA: 2014,Jan,11

42970 Control of nasopharyngeal hemorrhage, primary or secondary (eg, postadenoidectomy); simple, with posterior nasal packs, with or without anterior packs and/or cautery
11.8 11.8 FUD 090
AMA: 2014,Jan,11

42971 complicated, requiring hospitalization
13.0 13.0 FUD 090
AMA: 2014,Jan,11

42972 with secondary surgical intervention
14.6 14.6 FUD 090
AMA: 2014,Jan,11

42999 Unlisted procedure, pharynx, adenoids, or tonsils
0.00 0.00 FUD YYY
AMA: 2018,Jan,8; 2017,Jan,8; 2016,Jan,13; 2015,Jan,16; 2014,Feb,11; 2014,Jan,11

43020-43135 Incision/Resection of Esophagus

EXCLUDES *Gastrointestinal reconstruction for previous esophagectomy (43360-43361)*
Gastrotomy with intraluminal tube insertion (43510)

43020 Esophagotomy, cervical approach, with removal of foreign body
EXCLUDES *Laparotomy with esophageal intubation (43510)*
16.1 16.1 FUD 090
AMA: 2014,Jan,11

43030 Cricopharyngeal myotomy
EXCLUDES *Laparotomy with esophageal intubation (43510)*
14.9 14.9 FUD 090
AMA: 2014,Jan,11

43045 **Esophagotomy, thoracic approach, with removal of foreign body**

EXCLUDES *Laparotomy with esophageal intubation (43510)*

37.6 37.6 FUD 090 C 80

AMA: 2014,Jan,11

43100 **Excision of lesion, esophagus, with primary repair; cervical approach**

EXCLUDES *Wide excision of malignant lesion of cervical esophagus, with total laryngectomy:*
With radical neck dissection (31365, 43107, 43116, 43124)
Without radical neck dissection (31360, 43107, 43116, 43124)

18.0 18.0 FUD 090 C 80

AMA: 2014,Jan,11

43101 **thoracic or abdominal approach**

EXCLUDES *Wide excision of malignant lesion of cervical esophagus with total laryngectomy:*
With radical neck dissection (31365, 43107, 43116, 43124)
Without radical neck dissection (31360, 43107, 43116, 43124)

29.1 29.1 FUD 090 C 80

AMA: 2018,Jan,8; 2017,Jan,8; 2016,Jan,13; 2015,Jan,16; 2014,Jan,11

43107 **Total or near total esophagectomy, without thoracotomy; with pharyngogastrostomy or cervical esophagogastrostomy, with or without pyloroplasty (transhiatal)**

86.5 86.5 FUD 090 C 80

AMA: 2014,Jan,11

43108 **with colon interposition or small intestine reconstruction, including intestine mobilization, preparation and anastomosis(es)**

129. 129. FUD 090 C 80

AMA: 2014,Jan,11

43112 **Total or near total esophagectomy, with thoracotomy; with pharyngogastrostomy or cervical esophagogastrostomy, with or without pyloroplasty (ie, McKeown esophagectomy or tri-incisional esophagectomy)**

101. 101. FUD 090 C 80

AMA: 2018,Jul,7; 2018,Jan,8; 2017,Jan,8; 2016,Jan,13; 2015,Jan,16; 2014,Jan,11

43113 **with colon interposition or small intestine reconstruction, including intestine mobilization, preparation, and anastomosis(es)**

126. 126. FUD 090 C 80

AMA: 2014,Jan,11

43116 **Partial esophagectomy, cervical, with free intestinal graft, including microvascular anastomosis, obtaining the graft and intestinal reconstruction**

INCLUDES Operating microscope (69990)

EXCLUDES *Free jejunal graft with microvascular anastomosis done by a different physician (43496)*

Code also modifier 52 if intestinal or free jejunal graft with microvascular anastomosis is done by another physician

145. 145. FUD 090 C 80

AMA: 2016,Feb,12; 2014,Jan,11

43117 **Partial esophagectomy, distal two-thirds, with thoracotomy and separate abdominal incision, with or without proximal gastrectomy; with thoracic esophagogastrostomy, with or without pyloroplasty (Ivor Lewis)**

EXCLUDES *Esophagogastrectomy (lower third) and vagotomy (43122)*
Total esophagectomy with gastropharyngostomy (43107, 43124)

94.3 94.3 FUD 090 C 80

AMA: 2014,Jan,11

43118 **with colon interposition or small intestine reconstruction, including intestine mobilization, preparation, and anastomosis(es)**

EXCLUDES *Esophagogastrectomy (lower third) and vagotomy (43122)*
Total esophagectomy with gastropharyngostomy (43107, 43124)

105. 105. FUD 090 C 80

AMA: 2014,Jan,11

43121 **Partial esophagectomy, distal two-thirds, with thoracotomy only, with or without proximal gastrectomy, with thoracic esophagogastrostomy, with or without pyloroplasty**

83.0 83.0 FUD 090 C 80

AMA: 2014,Jan,11

43122 **Partial esophagectomy, thoracoabdominal or abdominal approach, with or without proximal gastrectomy; with esophagogastrostomy, with or without pyloroplasty**

74.1 74.1 FUD 090 C 80

AMA: 2014,Jan,11

43123 **with colon interposition or small intestine reconstruction, including intestine mobilization, preparation, and anastomosis(es)**

131. 131. FUD 090 C 80

AMA: 2014,Jan,11

43124 **Total or partial esophagectomy, without reconstruction (any approach), with cervical esophagostomy**

110. 110. FUD 090 C 80

AMA: 2018,Jan,8; 2017,Jan,8; 2016,Jan,13; 2015,Jan,16; 2014,Jan,11

43130 **Diverticulectomy of hypopharynx or esophagus, with or without myotomy; cervical approach**

EXCLUDES *Diverticulectomy hypopharynx or cervical esophagus, endoscopic (43180)*

22.6 22.6 FUD 090 J G2 80

AMA: 2018,Jan,8; 2017,Jan,8; 2016,Jan,13; 2015,Jan,16; 2014,Jan,11

43135 **thoracic approach**

EXCLUDES *Diverticulectomy hypopharynx or cervical esophagus, endoscopic (43180)*

42.7 42.7 FUD 090 C 80

AMA: 2018,Jan,8; 2017,Jan,8; 2016,Jan,13; 2015,Jan,16; 2014,Jan,11

43180-43233 [43211, 43212, 43213, 43214] Endoscopic Procedures: Esophagus

INCLUDES Control of bleeding as a result of endoscopic procedure during same operative session
Diagnostic endoscopy with surgical endoscopy
Examination of upper esophageal sphincter (cricopharyngeus muscle) to/including the gastroesophageal junction
Retroflexion examination of proximal region of stomach

43180 **Esophagoscopy, rigid, transoral with diverticulectomy of hypopharynx or cervical esophagus (eg, Zenker's diverticulum), with cricopharyngeal myotomy, includes use of telescope or operating microscope and repair, when performed**

INCLUDES Operating microscope (69990)

EXCLUDES *Esophagogastroduodenoscopy, flexible, transoral; with esophagogastric fundoplasty (43210)*
Open diverticulectomy hypopharynx or esophagus (43130-43135)

15.7 15.7 FUD 090 J G2

AMA: 2018,Jan,8; 2017,Jan,8; 2016,Feb,12; 2016,Jan,13; 2015,Nov,8

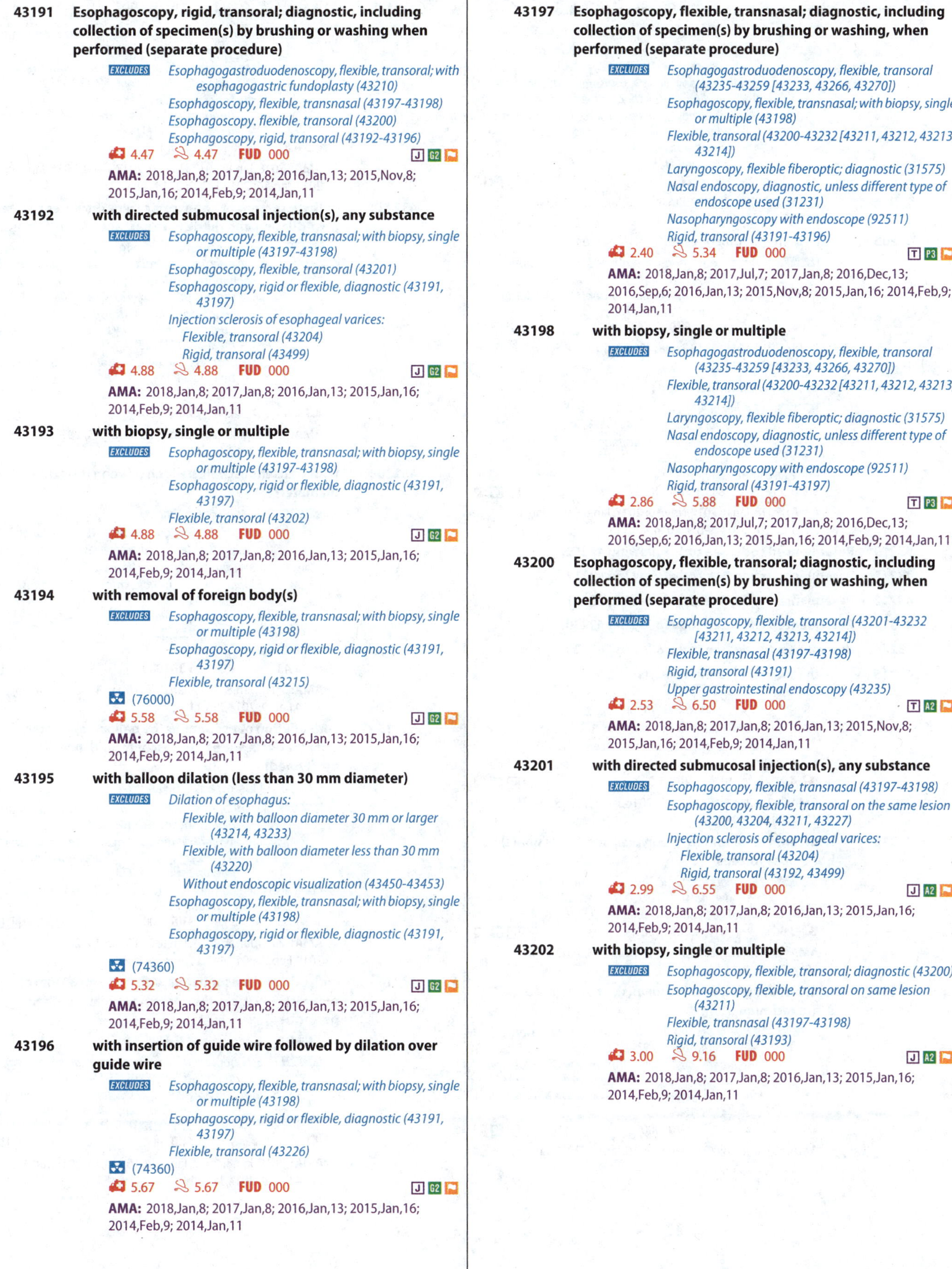

43191 Esophagoscopy, rigid, transoral; diagnostic, including collection of specimen(s) by brushing or washing when performed (separate procedure)

EXCLUDES *Esophagogastroduodenoscopy, flexible, transoral; with esophagogastric fundoplasty (43210)*
Esophagoscopy, flexible, transnasal (43197-43198)
Esophagoscopy. flexible, transoral (43200)
Esophagoscopy, rigid, transoral (43192-43196)

4.47 4.47 FUD 000 J G2

AMA: 2018,Jan,8; 2017,Jan,8; 2016,Jan,13; 2015,Nov,8; 2015,Jan,16; 2014,Feb,9; 2014,Jan,11

43192 with directed submucosal injection(s), any substance

EXCLUDES *Esophagoscopy, flexible, transnasal; with biopsy, single or multiple (43197-43198)*
Esophagoscopy, flexible, transoral (43201)
Esophagoscopy, rigid or flexible, diagnostic (43191, 43197)
Injection sclerosis of esophageal varices:
Flexible, transoral (43204)
Rigid, transoral (43499)

4.88 4.88 FUD 000 J G2

AMA: 2018,Jan,8; 2017,Jan,8; 2016,Jan,13; 2015,Jan,16; 2014,Feb,9; 2014,Jan,11

43193 with biopsy, single or multiple

EXCLUDES *Esophagoscopy, flexible, transnasal; with biopsy, single or multiple (43197-43198)*
Esophagoscopy, rigid or flexible, diagnostic (43191, 43197)
Flexible, transoral (43202)

4.88 4.88 FUD 000 J G2

AMA: 2018,Jan,8; 2017,Jan,8; 2016,Jan,13; 2015,Jan,16; 2014,Feb,9; 2014,Jan,11

43194 with removal of foreign body(s)

EXCLUDES *Esophagoscopy, flexible, transnasal; with biopsy, single or multiple (43198)*
Esophagoscopy, rigid or flexible, diagnostic (43191, 43197)
Flexible, transoral (43215)

(76000)

5.58 5.58 FUD 000 J G2

AMA: 2018,Jan,8; 2017,Jan,8; 2016,Jan,13; 2015,Jan,16; 2014,Feb,9; 2014,Jan,11

43195 with balloon dilation (less than 30 mm diameter)

EXCLUDES *Dilation of esophagus:*
Flexible, with balloon diameter 30 mm or larger (43214, 43233)
Flexible, with balloon diameter less than 30 mm (43220)
Without endoscopic visualization (43450-43453)
Esophagoscopy, flexible, transnasal; with biopsy, single or multiple (43198)
Esophagoscopy, rigid or flexible, diagnostic (43191, 43197)

(74360)

5.32 5.32 FUD 000 J G2

AMA: 2018,Jan,8; 2017,Jan,8; 2016,Jan,13; 2015,Jan,16; 2014,Feb,9; 2014,Jan,11

43196 with insertion of guide wire followed by dilation over guide wire

EXCLUDES *Esophagoscopy, flexible, transnasal; with biopsy, single or multiple (43198)*
Esophagoscopy, rigid or flexible, diagnostic (43191, 43197)
Flexible, transoral (43226)

(74360)

5.67 5.67 FUD 000 J G2

AMA: 2018,Jan,8; 2017,Jan,8; 2016,Jan,13; 2015,Jan,16; 2014,Feb,9; 2014,Jan,11

43197 Esophagoscopy, flexible, transnasal; diagnostic, including collection of specimen(s) by brushing or washing, when performed (separate procedure)

EXCLUDES *Esophagogastroduodenoscopy, flexible, transoral (43235-43259 [43233, 43266, 43270])*
Esophagoscopy, flexible, transnasal; with biopsy, single or multiple (43198)
Flexible, transoral (43200-43232 [43211, 43212, 43213, 43214])
Laryngoscopy, flexible fiberoptic; diagnostic (31575)
Nasal endoscopy, diagnostic, unless different type of endoscope used (31231)
Nasopharyngoscopy with endoscope (92511)
Rigid, transoral (43191-43196)

2.40 5.34 FUD 000 T P3

AMA: 2018,Jan,8; 2017,Jul,7; 2017,Jan,8; 2016,Dec,13; 2016,Sep,6; 2016,Jan,13; 2015,Nov,8; 2015,Jan,16; 2014,Feb,9; 2014,Jan,11

43198 with biopsy, single or multiple

EXCLUDES *Esophagogastroduodenoscopy, flexible, transoral (43235-43259 [43233, 43266, 43270])*
Flexible, transoral (43200-43232 [43211, 43212, 43213, 43214])
Laryngoscopy, flexible fiberoptic; diagnostic (31575)
Nasal endoscopy, diagnostic, unless different type of endoscope used (31231)
Nasopharyngoscopy with endoscope (92511)
Rigid, transoral (43191-43197)

2.86 5.88 FUD 000 T P3

AMA: 2018,Jan,8; 2017,Jul,7; 2017,Jan,8; 2016,Dec,13; 2016,Sep,6; 2016,Jan,13; 2015,Jan,16; 2014,Feb,9; 2014,Jan,11

43200 Esophagoscopy, flexible, transoral; diagnostic, including collection of specimen(s) by brushing or washing, when performed (separate procedure)

EXCLUDES *Esophagoscopy, flexible, transoral (43201-43232 [43211, 43212, 43213, 43214])*
Flexible, transnasal (43197-43198)
Rigid, transoral (43191)
Upper gastrointestinal endoscopy (43235)

2.53 6.50 FUD 000 T A2

AMA: 2018,Jan,8; 2017,Jan,8; 2016,Jan,13; 2015,Nov,8; 2015,Jan,16; 2014,Feb,9; 2014,Jan,11

43201 with directed submucosal injection(s), any substance

EXCLUDES *Esophagoscopy, flexible, transnasal (43197-43198)*
Esophagoscopy, flexible, transoral on the same lesion (43200, 43204, 43211, 43227)
Injection sclerosis of esophageal varices:
Flexible, transoral (43204)
Rigid, transoral (43192, 43499)

2.99 6.55 FUD 000 J A2

AMA: 2018,Jan,8; 2017,Jan,8; 2016,Jan,13; 2015,Jan,16; 2014,Feb,9; 2014,Jan,11

43202 with biopsy, single or multiple

EXCLUDES *Esophagoscopy, flexible, transoral; diagnostic (43200)*
Esophagoscopy, flexible, transoral on same lesion (43211)
Flexible, transnasal (43197-43198)
Rigid, transoral (43193)

3.00 9.16 FUD 000 J A2

AMA: 2018,Jan,8; 2017,Jan,8; 2016,Jan,13; 2015,Jan,16; 2014,Feb,9; 2014,Jan,11

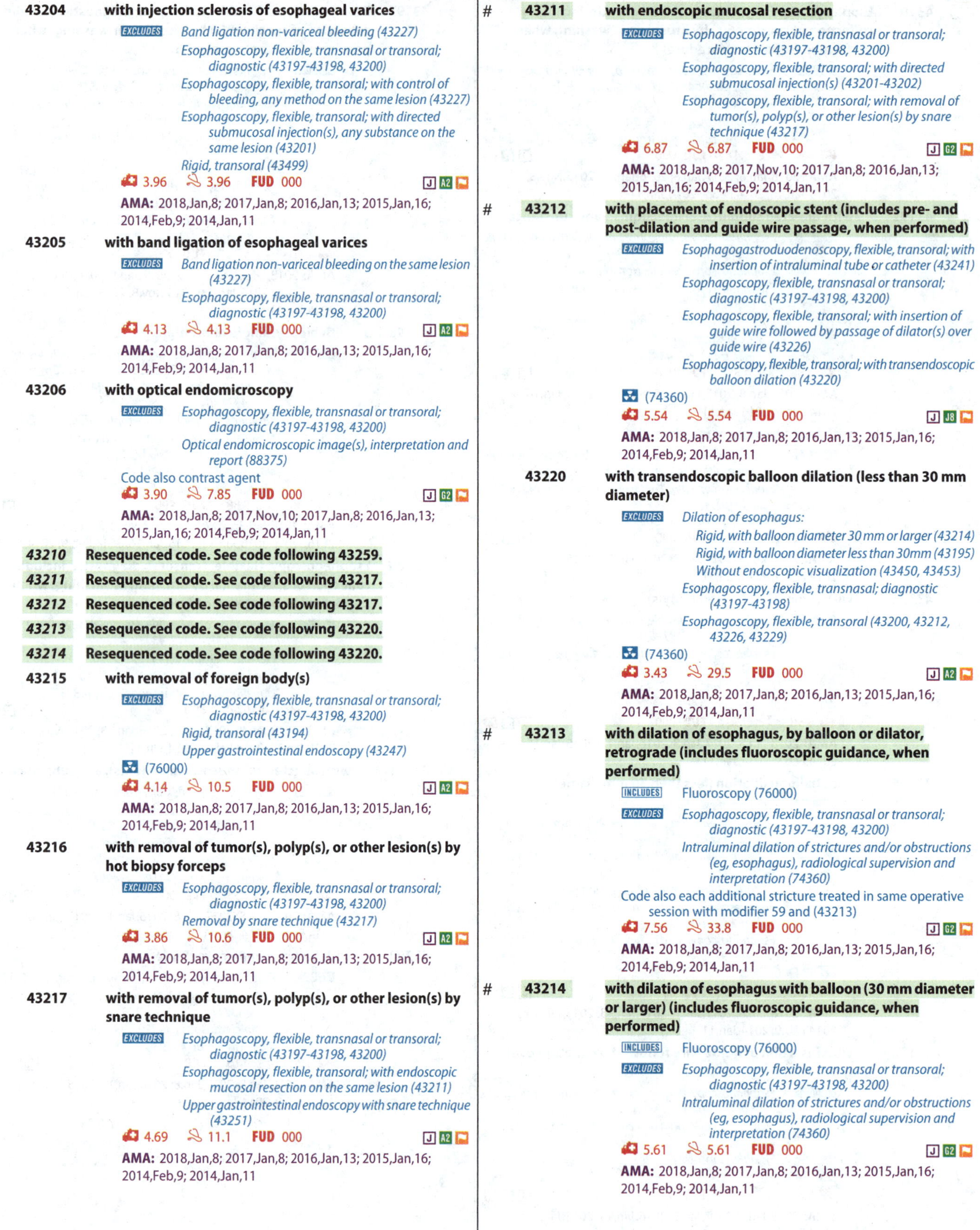

43204 **with injection sclerosis of esophageal varices**

EXCLUDES *Band ligation non-variceal bleeding (43227)*
Esophagoscopy, flexible, transnasal or transoral; diagnostic (43197-43198, 43200)
Esophagoscopy, flexible, transoral; with control of bleeding, any method on the same lesion (43227)
Esophagoscopy, flexible, transoral; with directed submucosal injection(s), any substance on the same lesion (43201)
Rigid, transoral (43499)

3.96 3.96 FUD 000 J A2

AMA: 2018,Jan,8; 2017,Jan,8; 2016,Jan,13; 2015,Jan,16; 2014,Feb,9; 2014,Jan,11

43205 **with band ligation of esophageal varices**

EXCLUDES *Band ligation non-variceal bleeding on the same lesion (43227)*
Esophagoscopy, flexible, transnasal or transoral; diagnostic (43197-43198, 43200)

4.13 4.13 FUD 000 J A2

AMA: 2018,Jan,8; 2017,Jan,8; 2016,Jan,13; 2015,Jan,16; 2014,Feb,9; 2014,Jan,11

43206 **with optical endomicroscopy**

EXCLUDES *Esophagoscopy, flexible, transnasal or transoral; diagnostic (43197-43198, 43200)*
Optical endomicroscopic image(s), interpretation and report (88375)

Code also contrast agent

3.90 7.85 FUD 000 J G2

AMA: 2018,Jan,8; 2017,Nov,10; 2017,Jan,8; 2016,Jan,13; 2015,Jan,16; 2014,Feb,9; 2014,Jan,11

43210 **Resequenced code. See code following 43259.**

43211 **Resequenced code. See code following 43217.**

43212 **Resequenced code. See code following 43217.**

43213 **Resequenced code. See code following 43220.**

43214 **Resequenced code. See code following 43220.**

43215 **with removal of foreign body(s)**

EXCLUDES *Esophagoscopy, flexible, transnasal or transoral; diagnostic (43197-43198, 43200)*
Rigid, transoral (43194)
Upper gastrointestinal endoscopy (43247)

(76000)

4.14 10.5 FUD 000 J A2

AMA: 2018,Jan,8; 2017,Jan,8; 2016,Jan,13; 2015,Jan,16; 2014,Feb,9; 2014,Jan,11

43216 **with removal of tumor(s), polyp(s), or other lesion(s) by hot biopsy forceps**

EXCLUDES *Esophagoscopy, flexible, transnasal or transoral; diagnostic (43197-43198, 43200)*
Removal by snare technique (43217)

3.86 10.6 FUD 000 J A2

AMA: 2018,Jan,8; 2017,Jan,8; 2016,Jan,13; 2015,Jan,16; 2014,Feb,9; 2014,Jan,11

43217 **with removal of tumor(s), polyp(s), or other lesion(s) by snare technique**

EXCLUDES *Esophagoscopy, flexible, transnasal or transoral; diagnostic (43197-43198, 43200)*
Esophagoscopy, flexible, transoral; with endoscopic mucosal resection on the same lesion (43211)
Upper gastrointestinal endoscopy with snare technique (43251)

4.69 11.1 FUD 000 J A2

AMA: 2018,Jan,8; 2017,Jan,8; 2016,Jan,13; 2015,Jan,16; 2014,Feb,9; 2014,Jan,11

\# **43211** **with endoscopic mucosal resection**

EXCLUDES *Esophagoscopy, flexible, transnasal or transoral; diagnostic (43197-43198, 43200)*
Esophagoscopy, flexible, transoral; with directed submucosal injection(s) (43201-43202)
Esophagoscopy, flexible, transoral; with removal of tumor(s), polyp(s), or other lesion(s) by snare technique (43217)

6.87 6.87 FUD 000 J G2

AMA: 2018,Jan,8; 2017,Nov,10; 2017,Jan,8; 2016,Jan,13; 2015,Jan,16; 2014,Feb,9; 2014,Jan,11

\# **43212** **with placement of endoscopic stent (includes pre- and post-dilation and guide wire passage, when performed)**

EXCLUDES *Esophagogastroduodenoscopy, flexible, transoral; with insertion of intraluminal tube or catheter (43241)*
Esophagoscopy, flexible, transnasal or transoral; diagnostic (43197-43198, 43200)
Esophagoscopy, flexible, transoral; with insertion of guide wire followed by passage of dilator(s) over guide wire (43226)
Esophagoscopy, flexible, transoral; with transendoscopic balloon dilation (43220)

(74360)

5.54 5.54 FUD 000 J J8

AMA: 2018,Jan,8; 2017,Jan,8; 2016,Jan,13; 2015,Jan,16; 2014,Feb,9; 2014,Jan,11

43220 **with transendoscopic balloon dilation (less than 30 mm diameter)**

EXCLUDES *Dilation of esophagus:*
Rigid, with balloon diameter 30 mm or larger (43214)
Rigid, with balloon diameter less than 30mm (43195)
Without endoscopic visualization (43450, 43453)
Esophagoscopy, flexible, transnasal; diagnostic (43197-43198)
Esophagoscopy, flexible, transoral (43200, 43212, 43226, 43229)

(74360)

3.43 29.5 FUD 000 J A2

AMA: 2018,Jan,8; 2017,Jan,8; 2016,Jan,13; 2015,Jan,16; 2014,Feb,9; 2014,Jan,11

\# **43213** **with dilation of esophagus, by balloon or dilator, retrograde (includes fluoroscopic guidance, when performed)**

INCLUDES Fluoroscopy (76000)

EXCLUDES *Esophagoscopy, flexible, transnasal or transoral; diagnostic (43197-43198, 43200)*
Intraluminal dilation of strictures and/or obstructions (eg, esophagus), radiological supervision and interpretation (74360)

Code also each additional stricture treated in same operative session with modifier 59 and (43213)

7.56 33.8 FUD 000 J G2

AMA: 2018,Jan,8; 2017,Jan,8; 2016,Jan,13; 2015,Jan,16; 2014,Feb,9; 2014,Jan,11

\# **43214** **with dilation of esophagus with balloon (30 mm diameter or larger) (includes fluoroscopic guidance, when performed)**

INCLUDES Fluoroscopy (76000)

EXCLUDES *Esophagoscopy, flexible, transnasal or transoral; diagnostic (43197-43198, 43200)*
Intraluminal dilation of strictures and/or obstructions (eg, esophagus), radiological supervision and interpretation (74360)

5.61 5.61 FUD 000 J G2

AMA: 2018,Jan,8; 2017,Jan,8; 2016,Jan,13; 2015,Jan,16; 2014,Feb,9; 2014,Jan,11

43226 **with insertion of guide wire followed by passage of dilator(s) over guide wire**

EXCLUDES *Esophagoscopy, flexible, transnasal or transoral; diagnostic (43197-43198, 43200)*
Esophagoscopy, flexible, transoral; with ablation of tumor(s), polyp(s), or other lesion(s) on the same lesion (43229)
Esophagoscopy, flexible, transoral; with placement of endoscopic stent (43212)
Esophagoscopy, flexible, transoral; with transendoscopic balloon dilation (43220)
Rigid, transoral (43196)

(74360)

3.80 9.59 FUD 000 J A2

AMA: 2018,Jan,8; 2017,Jan,8; 2016,Jan,13; 2015,Jan,16; 2014,Feb,9; 2014,Jan,11

43227 **with control of bleeding, any method**

EXCLUDES *Esophagoscopy, flexible, transnasal or transoral; diagnostic (43197-43198, 43200)*
Esophagoscopy, flexible, transoral; with directed submucosal injection(s) on the same lesion (43201)
Esophagoscopy, flexible, transoral; with injection sclerosis of esophageal varices on the same lesion (43204-43205)

4.84 17.7 FUD 000 J A2

AMA: 2018,Jan,8; 2017,Jan,8; 2016,Jan,13; 2015,Jan,16; 2014,Feb,9; 2014,Feb,11; 2014,Jan,11

43229 **with ablation of tumor(s), polyp(s), or other lesion(s) (includes pre- and post-dilation and guide wire passage, when performed)**

EXCLUDES *Esophagoscopy, flexible, transnasal or transoral; diagnostic (43197-43198, 43200)*
Esophagoscopy, flexible, transoral; with insertion of guide wire followed by passage of dilator(s) over guide wire on the same lesion (43226)
Esophagoscopy, flexible, transoral; with transendoscopic balloon dilation on the same lesion (43220)

Code also esophagoscopic photodynamic therapy, when performed (96570-96571)

5.77 19.0 FUD 000 J G2

AMA: 2018,Jan,8; 2017,Jan,8; 2016,Jan,13; 2015,Jan,16; 2014,Feb,9; 2014,Jan,11

43231 **with endoscopic ultrasound examination**

EXCLUDES *Esophagoscopy, flexible, transnasal or transoral; diagnostic (43197-43198, 43200)*
Esophagoscopy, flexible, transoral; with transendoscopic ultrasound-guided intramural or transmural fine needle aspiration/biopsy(s) (43232)
Gastrointestinal endoscopic ultrasound, supervision, and interpretation (76975)
Procedure performed more than one time per operative session

4.65 9.79 FUD 000 J A2

AMA: 2018,Jan,8; 2017,Jan,8; 2016,Jan,13; 2015,Jan,16; 2014,Feb,9; 2014,Jan,11

43232 **with transendoscopic ultrasound-guided intramural or transmural fine needle aspiration/biopsy(s)**

EXCLUDES *Esophagoscopy, flexible, transnasal or transoral; diagnostic (43197-43198, 43200)*
Esophagoscopy, flexible, transoral; with endoscopic ultrasound examination (43231)
Gastrointestinal endoscopic ultrasound, supervision and interpretation (76975)
Procedure performed more than one time per operative session
Ultrasonic guidance (76942)

5.82 11.8 FUD 000 J A2

AMA: 2018,Jan,8; 2017,Jan,8; 2016,Jan,13; 2015,Jan,16; 2014,Feb,9; 2014,Jan,11

43233 **Resequenced code. See code following 43249.**

43235-43210 [43210, 43233, 43266, 43270] Endoscopic Procedures: Esophagogastroduodenoscopy (EGD)

INCLUDES Control of bleeding as result of the endoscopic procedure during same operative session
Diagnostic endoscopy with surgical endoscopy

EXCLUDES *Exam of jejunum distal to the anastomosis in surgically altered stomach, including post-gastroenterostomy (Billroth II) and gastric bypass (43235-43259 [43233, 43266, 43270])*
Exam of upper esophageal sphincter (cricopharyngeus muscle) to/including gastroesophageal junction and/or retroflexion exam of proximal region of stomach (43197-43232 [43211, 43212, 43213, 43214])

Code also modifier 52 when duodenum is not examined either deliberately or due to significant issues and repeat procedure will not be performed

Code also modifier 53 when duodenum is not examined either deliberately or due to significant issues and repeat procedure is planned

43235 **Esophagogastroduodenoscopy, flexible, transoral; diagnostic, including collection of specimen(s) by brushing or washing, when performed (separate procedure)**

EXCLUDES *Endoscopy of small intestine (44360-44379)*
Esophagogastroduodenoscopy, flexible, transoral; with esophagogastric fundoplasty (43210)
Esophagoscopy, flexible, transnasal; diagnostic (43197-43198)
Procedure performed with surgical endoscopy (43236-43259 [43233, 43266, 43270])

3.58 7.61 FUD 000 T A2

AMA: 2018,Jul,14; 2018,Jan,8; 2017,Jul,10; 2017,Jan,8; 2016,Jan,13; 2015,Nov,8; 2015,Jan,16; 2014,Jan,11

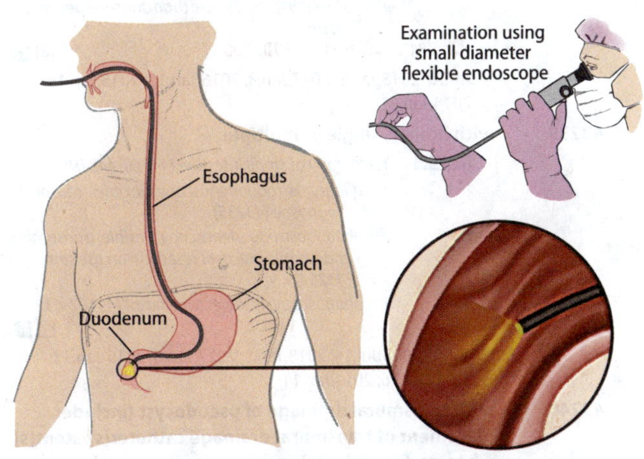

43236 **with directed submucosal injection(s), any substance**

EXCLUDES *Endoscopy of small intestine (44360-44379)*
Esophagogastroduodenoscopy, flexible, transoral; with control of bleeding, any method (43255)
Esophagogastroduodenoscopy, flexible, transoral; with endoscopic mucosal resection on the same lesion (43254)
Esophagogastroduodenoscopy, flexible, transoral; with injection sclerosis of esophageal/gastric varices on the same lesion (43243)
Esophagoscopy, flexible, transnasal or transoral; diagnostic (43197-43198, 43235)
Injection sclerosis of varices, esophageal/gastric (43243)

4.05 10.0 FUD 000 T A2

AMA: 2018,Jan,8; 2017,Jan,8; 2016,Jan,13; 2015,Jan,16; 2014,Jan,11

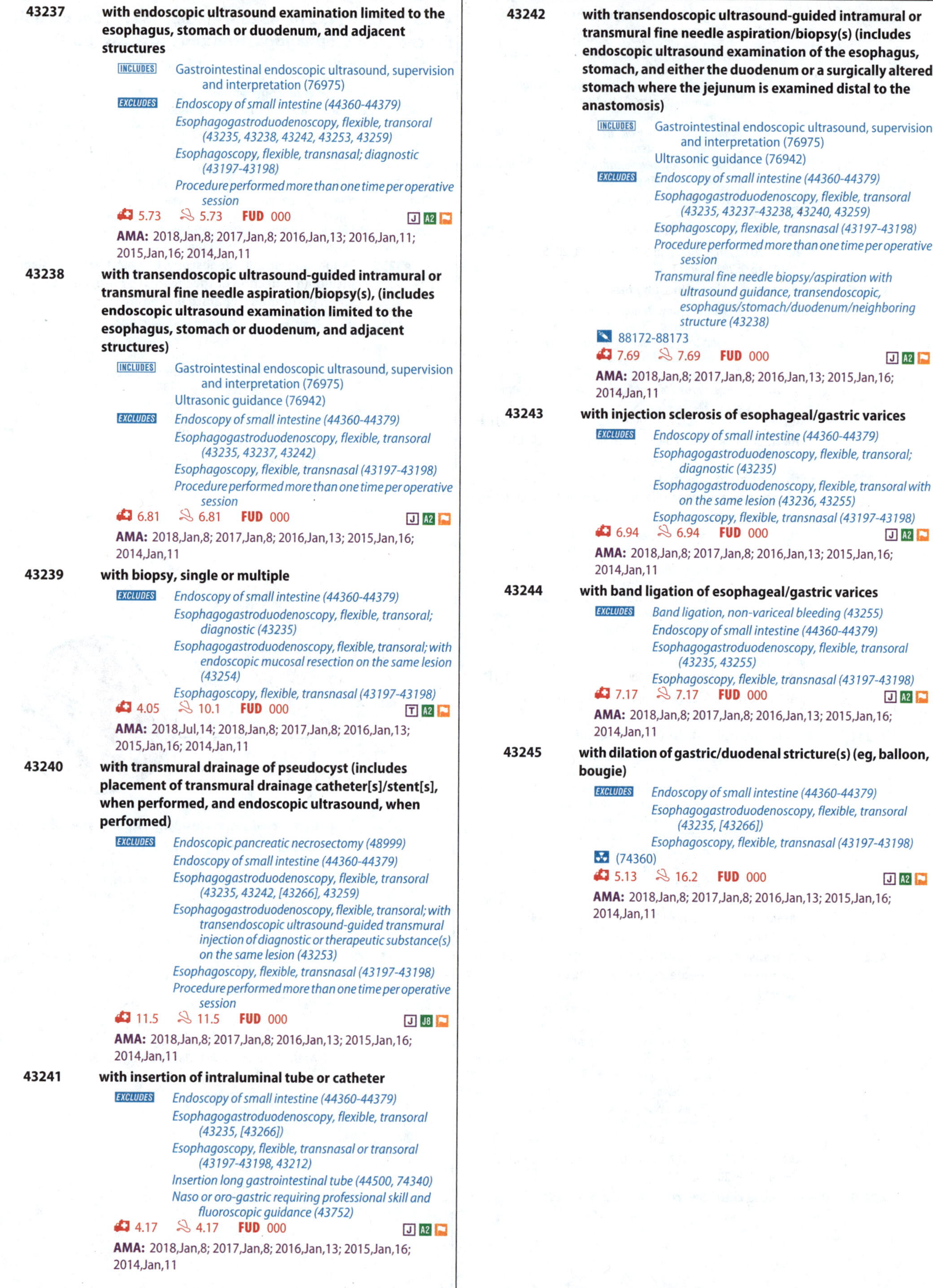

43237 **with endoscopic ultrasound examination limited to the esophagus, stomach or duodenum, and adjacent structures**

INCLUDES Gastrointestinal endoscopic ultrasound, supervision and interpretation (76975)

EXCLUDES *Endoscopy of small intestine (44360-44379)*
Esophagogastroduodenoscopy, flexible, transoral (43235, 43238, 43242, 43253, 43259)
Esophagoscopy, flexible, transnasal; diagnostic (43197-43198)
Procedure performed more than one time per operative session

5.73 5.73 FUD 000 J A2

AMA: 2018,Jan,8; 2017,Jan,8; 2016,Jan,13; 2016,Jan,11; 2015,Jan,16; 2014,Jan,11

43238 **with transendoscopic ultrasound-guided intramural or transmural fine needle aspiration/biopsy(s), (includes endoscopic ultrasound examination limited to the esophagus, stomach or duodenum, and adjacent structures)**

INCLUDES Gastrointestinal endoscopic ultrasound, supervision and interpretation (76975)
Ultrasonic guidance (76942)

EXCLUDES *Endoscopy of small intestine (44360-44379)*
Esophagogastroduodenoscopy, flexible, transoral (43235, 43237, 43242)
Esophagoscopy, flexible, transnasal (43197-43198)
Procedure performed more than one time per operative session

6.81 6.81 FUD 000 J A2

AMA: 2018,Jan,8; 2017,Jan,8; 2016,Jan,13; 2015,Jan,16; 2014,Jan,11

43239 **with biopsy, single or multiple**

EXCLUDES *Endoscopy of small intestine (44360-44379)*
Esophagogastroduodenoscopy, flexible, transoral; diagnostic (43235)
Esophagogastroduodenoscopy, flexible, transoral; with endoscopic mucosal resection on the same lesion (43254)
Esophagoscopy, flexible, transnasal (43197-43198)

4.05 10.1 FUD 000 T A2

AMA: 2018,Jul,14; 2018,Jan,8; 2017,Jan,8; 2016,Jan,13; 2015,Jan,16; 2014,Jan,11

43240 **with transmural drainage of pseudocyst (includes placement of transmural drainage catheter[s]/stent[s], when performed, and endoscopic ultrasound, when performed)**

EXCLUDES *Endoscopic pancreatic necrosectomy (48999)*
Endoscopy of small intestine (44360-44379)
Esophagogastroduodenoscopy, flexible, transoral (43235, 43242, [43266], 43259)
Esophagogastroduodenoscopy, flexible, transoral; with transendoscopic ultrasound-guided transmural injection of diagnostic or therapeutic substance(s) on the same lesion (43253)
Esophagoscopy, flexible, transnasal (43197-43198)
Procedure performed more than one time per operative session

11.5 11.5 FUD 000 J J8

AMA: 2018,Jan,8; 2017,Jan,8; 2016,Jan,13; 2015,Jan,16; 2014,Jan,11

43241 **with insertion of intraluminal tube or catheter**

EXCLUDES *Endoscopy of small intestine (44360-44379)*
Esophagogastroduodenoscopy, flexible, transoral (43235, [43266])
Esophagoscopy, flexible, transnasal or transoral (43197-43198, 43212)
Insertion long gastrointestinal tube (44500, 74340)
Naso or oro-gastric requiring professional skill and fluoroscopic guidance (43752)

4.17 4.17 FUD 000 J A2

AMA: 2018,Jan,8; 2017,Jan,8; 2016,Jan,13; 2015,Jan,16; 2014,Jan,11

43242 **with transendoscopic ultrasound-guided intramural or transmural fine needle aspiration/biopsy(s) (includes endoscopic ultrasound examination of the esophagus, stomach, and either the duodenum or a surgically altered stomach where the jejunum is examined distal to the anastomosis)**

INCLUDES Gastrointestinal endoscopic ultrasound, supervision and interpretation (76975)
Ultrasonic guidance (76942)

EXCLUDES *Endoscopy of small intestine (44360-44379)*
Esophagogastroduodenoscopy, flexible, transoral (43235, 43237-43238, 43240, 43259)
Esophagoscopy, flexible, transnasal (43197-43198)
Procedure performed more than one time per operative session
Transmural fine needle biopsy/aspiration with ultrasound guidance, transendoscopic, esophagus/stomach/duodenum/neighboring structure (43238)

88172-88173

7.69 7.69 FUD 000 J A2

AMA: 2018,Jan,8; 2017,Jan,8; 2016,Jan,13; 2015,Jan,16; 2014,Jan,11

43243 **with injection sclerosis of esophageal/gastric varices**

EXCLUDES *Endoscopy of small intestine (44360-44379)*
Esophagogastroduodenoscopy, flexible, transoral; diagnostic (43235)
Esophagogastroduodenoscopy, flexible, transoral with on the same lesion (43236, 43255)
Esophagoscopy, flexible, transnasal (43197-43198)

6.94 6.94 FUD 000 J A2

AMA: 2018,Jan,8; 2017,Jan,8; 2016,Jan,13; 2015,Jan,16; 2014,Jan,11

43244 **with band ligation of esophageal/gastric varices**

EXCLUDES *Band ligation, non-variceal bleeding (43255)*
Endoscopy of small intestine (44360-44379)
Esophagogastroduodenoscopy, flexible, transoral (43235, 43255)
Esophagoscopy, flexible, transnasal (43197-43198)

7.17 7.17 FUD 000 J A2

AMA: 2018,Jan,8; 2017,Jan,8; 2016,Jan,13; 2015,Jan,16; 2014,Jan,11

43245 **with dilation of gastric/duodenal stricture(s) (eg, balloon, bougie)**

EXCLUDES *Endoscopy of small intestine (44360-44379)*
Esophagogastroduodenoscopy, flexible, transoral (43235, [43266])
Esophagoscopy, flexible, transnasal (43197-43198)

(74360)

5.13 16.2 FUD 000 J A2

AMA: 2018,Jan,8; 2017,Jan,8; 2016,Jan,13; 2015,Jan,16; 2014,Jan,11

43246 **with directed placement of percutaneous gastrostomy tube**

EXCLUDES *Endoscopy of small intestine (44360-44372, 44376-44379)*
Esophagogastroduodenoscopy, flexible, transoral; diagnostic (43235)
Esophagoscopy, flexible, transnasal (43197-43198)
Gastrostomy tube replacement without endoscopy or imaging (43762-43763)
Percutaneous insertion of gastrostomy tube (49440)

5.86 5.86 FUD 000 J A2 80

AMA: 2019,Feb,5; 2018,Jan,8; 2017,Jan,8; 2016,Jan,13; 2015,Jan,16; 2014,Jan,11

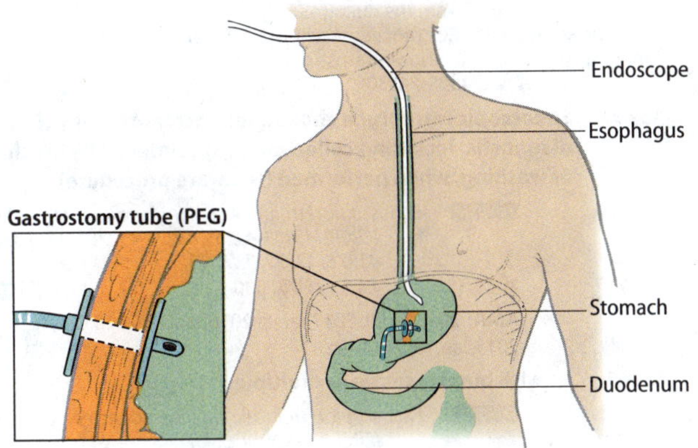

43247 **with removal of foreign body(s)**

EXCLUDES *Endoscopy of small intestine (44360-44379)*
Esophagogastroduodenoscopy, flexible, transoral; diagnostic (43235)
Esophagoscopy, flexible, transnasal (43197-43198)

(76000)

5.18 10.2 FUD 000 T A2

AMA: 2018,Jan,8; 2017,Jan,8; 2016,Jan,13; 2015,Jan,16; 2014,Jan,11

43248 **with insertion of guide wire followed by passage of dilator(s) through esophagus over guide wire**

EXCLUDES *Endoscopy of small intestine (44360-44379)*
Esophagogastroduodenoscopy, flexible, transoral (43235, [43266], [43270])
Esophagoscopy, flexible, transnasal (43197-43198)

(74360)

4.86 10.5 FUD 000 T A2

AMA: 2018,Jan,8; 2017,Jul,10; 2017,Jan,8; 2016,Jan,13; 2015,Jan,16; 2014,Jan,11

43249 **with transendoscopic balloon dilation of esophagus (less than 30 mm diameter)**

EXCLUDES *Endoscopy of small intestine (44360-44379)*
Esophagogastroduodenoscopy, flexible, transoral (43235, [43266], [43270])
Esophagoscopy, flexible, transnasal (43197-43198)

(74360)

4.49 29.9 FUD 000 J A2

AMA: 2018,Jul,14; 2018,Jan,8; 2017,Jan,8; 2016,Jan,13; 2015,Jan,16; 2014,Jan,11

\# **43233** **with dilation of esophagus with balloon (30 mm diameter or larger) (includes fluoroscopic guidance, when performed)**

INCLUDES Fluoroscopy (76000)

EXCLUDES *Endoscopy of small intestine (44360-44379)*
Esophagogastroduodenoscopy, flexible, transoral (43235, [43266], [43270])
Esophagoscopy, flexible, transnasal (43197-43198)
Intraluminal dilation of strictures and/or obstructions (e.g., esophagus), radiological supervision and interpretation (74360)

6.68 6.68 FUD 000 J G2

AMA: 2018,Jan,8; 2017,Jan,8; 2016,Jan,13; 2015,Jan,16; 2014,Jan,11

43250 **with removal of tumor(s), polyp(s), or other lesion(s) by hot biopsy forceps**

EXCLUDES *Endoscopy of small intestine (44360-44379)*
Esophagogastroduodenoscopy, flexible, transoral (43235)
Esophagoscopy, flexible, transnasal (43197-43198)

4.97 11.8 FUD 000 J A2

AMA: 2018,Jan,8; 2017,Jan,8; 2016,Jan,13; 2015,Jan,16; 2014,Jan,11

43251 **with removal of tumor(s), polyp(s), or other lesion(s) by snare technique**

EXCLUDES *Endoscopic mucosal resection when performed on same lesion (43254)*
Endoscopy of small intestine (44360-44379)
Esophagogastroduodenoscopy, flexible, transoral (43235)
Esophagoscopy, flexible, transnasal (43197-43198)

5.74 13.0 FUD 000 J A2

AMA: 2018,Jan,8; 2017,Jan,8; 2016,Jan,13; 2015,Jan,16; 2014,Jan,11

43252 **with optical endomicroscopy**

EXCLUDES *Endoscopy of small intestine (44360-44379)*
Esophagogastroduodenoscopy, flexible, transoral (43235)
Esophagoscopy, flexible, transnasal (43197-43198)
Optical endomicroscopic image(s), interpretation and report (88375)

Code also contrast agent

4.95 8.96 FUD 000 J G2

AMA: 2018,Jan,8; 2017,Jan,8; 2016,Jan,13; 2015,Jan,16; 2014,Jan,11

43253 **with transendoscopic ultrasound-guided transmural injection of diagnostic or therapeutic substance(s) (eg, anesthetic, neurolytic agent) or fiducial marker(s) (includes endoscopic ultrasound examination of the esophagus, stomach, and either the duodenum or a surgically altered stomach where the jejunum is examined distal to the anastomosis)**

INCLUDES Gastrointestinal endoscopic ultrasound, supervision and interpretation (76975)
Ultrasonic guidance (76942)

EXCLUDES *Endoscopy of small intestine (44360-44379)*
Esophagogastroduodenoscopy, flexible, transoral (43235, 43237, 43259)
Esophagogastroduodenoscopy, flexible, transoral; with transmural drainage of pseudocyst on the same lesion with (43240)
Esophagoscopy, flexible, transnasal (43197-43198)
Procedure performed more than one time per operative session
Transmural fine needle biopsy/aspiration with ultrasound guidance, transendoscopic, esophagus/stomach/duodenum/neighboring structures (43238, 43242)

7.70 7.70 FUD 000 J G2

AMA: 2018,Apr,10; 2018,Jan,8; 2017,Jan,8; 2016,Jan,13; 2015,Jan,16; 2014,Jan,11

43254 **with endoscopic mucosal resection**

EXCLUDES *Endoscopy of small intestine (44360-44379)*
Esophagogastroduodenoscopy, flexible, transoral; diagnostic (43235)
Esophagogastroduodenoscopy, flexible, transoral on the same lesion (43236, 43239, 43251)
Esophagoscopy, flexible, transnasal (43197-43198)

7.91 7.91 FUD 000 J G2

AMA: 2018,Jan,8; 2017,Jan,8; 2016,Jan,13; 2015,Jan,16; 2014,Jan,11

43255 **with control of bleeding, any method**

EXCLUDES *Endoscopy of small intestine (44360-44379)*
Esophagogastroduodenoscopy, flexible, transoral (43235)
Esophagogastroduodenoscopy, flexible, transoral on the same lesion (43236, 43243-43244)
Esophagoscopy, flexible, transnasal (43197-43198)

5.87 18.7 FUD 000 J A2

AMA: 2018,Jan,8; 2017,Jan,8; 2016,Jan,13; 2015,Jan,16; 2014,Jan,11

\# **43266** **with placement of endoscopic stent (includes pre- and post-dilation and guide wire passage, when performed)**

6.39 6.39 FUD 000 J J8

AMA: 2018,Jan,8; 2017,Jan,8; 2016,Jan,13; 2015,Jan,16; 2014,Jan,11

43257 **with delivery of thermal energy to the muscle of lower esophageal sphincter and/or gastric cardia, for treatment of gastroesophageal reflux disease**

EXCLUDES *Endoscopy small intestine (44360-44379)*
Esophageal lesion ablation (43229, [43270])
Esophagogastroduodenoscopy, flexible, transoral; diagnostic (43235)
Esophagoscopy, flexible, transnasal (43197-43198)

6.80 6.80 FUD 000 J A2

AMA: 2018,Jan,8; 2017,Jan,8; 2016,Jan,13; 2015,Jan,16; 2014,Jan,11

\# **43270** **with ablation of tumor(s), polyp(s), or other lesion(s) (includes pre- and post-dilation and guide wire passage, when performed)**

INCLUDES Endoscopic dilation performed on same lesion (43248-43249)

EXCLUDES *Endoscopy small intestine (44360-44379)*
Esophagogastroduodenoscopy, flexible, transoral (43235)
Esophagoscopy, flexible, transnasal (43197-43198)

Code also photodynamic therapy, if performed (96570-96571)

6.57 19.6 FUD 000 J G2

AMA: 2018,Jan,8; 2017,Jan,8; 2016,Jan,13; 2015,Jan,16; 2014,Jan,11

43259 **with endoscopic ultrasound examination, including the esophagus, stomach, and either the duodenum or a surgically altered stomach where the jejunum is examined distal to the anastomosis**

INCLUDES Gastrointestinal endoscopic ultrasound, supervision and interpretation (76975)

EXCLUDES *Endoscopy of small intestine (44360-44379)*
Esophagogastroduodenoscopy, flexible, transoral (43235, 43237, 43240, 43242, 43253)
Esophagoscopy, flexible, transnasal (43197-43198)
Procedure performed more than one time per operative session

6.62 6.62 FUD 000 J A2

AMA: 2018,Jan,8; 2017,Jan,8; 2016,Jan,13; 2016,Jan,11; 2015,Jan,16; 2014,Jan,11

\# **43210** **with esophagogastric fundoplasty, partial or complete, includes duodenoscopy when performed**

EXCLUDES *Esophagoscopy, flexible, transnasal (43197)*
Esophagoscopy, flexible, transoral (43200, 43235)
Esophagoscopy, rigid, transoral (43180, 43191)

12.5 12.5 FUD 000 J G2

AMA: 2018,Jan,8; 2017,Jan,8; 2016,Jan,13; 2015,Nov,8

43260-43278 [43274, 43275, 43276, 43278] Endoscopic Procedures: ERCP

INCLUDES Diagnostic endoscopy with surgical endoscopy
Pancreaticobiliary system:
Biliary tree (right and left hepatic ducts, cystic duct/gallbladder, and common bile ducts)
Pancreas (major and minor ducts)

EXCLUDES *ERCP via Roux-en-Y anatomy (for instance post-gastric or bariatric bypass or post total gastrectomy) or via gastrostomy (open or laparoscopic) (47999, 48999)*
Optical endomicroscopy of biliary tract and pancreas, report one time per session (0397T)
Percutaneous biliary catheter procedures (47490-47544)

Code also appropriate endoscopy of each anatomic site examined
Code also sphincteroplasty or ductal stricture dilation, when performed prior to the debris/stone removal from the duct ([43277])
Code also the appropriate ERCP procedure when performed on altered postoperative anatomy (i.e. Billroth II gastroenterostomy)

(74328-74330)

43260 **Endoscopic retrograde cholangiopancreatography (ERCP); diagnostic, including collection of specimen(s) by brushing or washing, when performed (separate procedure)**

EXCLUDES *Endoscopic retrograde cholangiopancreatography (ERCP) (43261-43265, 43274-43278 [43274, 43275, 43276, 43277, 43278])*

9.45 9.45 FUD 000 J A2

AMA: 2018,Jan,8; 2017,Jan,8; 2016,Jan,13; 2015,Dec,3; 2015,Jan,16; 2014,Jan,11

43261 **with biopsy, single or multiple**

EXCLUDES *Endoscopic retrograde cholangiopancreatography (ERCP); diagnostic (43260)*
Percutaneous endoluminal biopsy of biliary tree (47543)

9.92 9.92 FUD 000 J A2

AMA: 2018,Jan,8; 2017,Jan,8; 2016,Jan,13; 2015,Dec,3; 2015,Jan,16; 2014,Jan,11

43262 **with sphincterotomy/papillotomy**

EXCLUDES *Endoscopic retrograde cholangiopancreatography (ERCP) (43260, [43277])*
Endoscopic retrograde cholangiopancreatography (ERCP) with placement or exchange of stent in the same location ([43274])
Endoscopic retrograde cholangiopancreatography (ERCP) with removal foreign body in the same location ([43276])
Esophagogastroduodenoscopy, flexible, transoral with ablation of tumor(s), polyp(s), or other lesion(s) in the same location ([43270])
Percutaneous balloon dilation biliary duct or ampulla (47542)

Code also procedure performed with sphincterotomy (43261, 43263-43265, [43275], [43278])

10.4 10.4 FUD 000 J A2

AMA: 2018,Jan,8; 2017,Jan,8; 2016,Jan,13; 2015,Dec,3; 2015,Jan,16; 2014,Jan,11

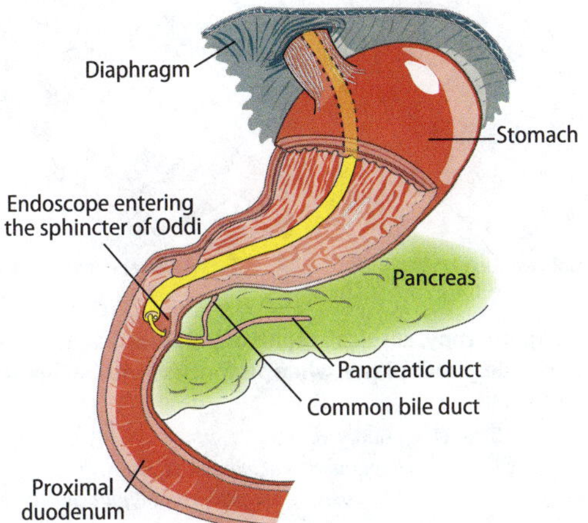

An endoscope is fed through the stomach and into the duodenum Usually a smaller sub-scope is fed up the sphincter of Oddi and into the ducts that drain the pancreas and the gallbladder (common bile)

43263 **with pressure measurement of sphincter of Oddi**

EXCLUDES *Endoscopic retrograde cholangiopancreatography (ERCP); diagnostic (43260)*
Procedure performed more than one time per session

10.4 10.4 FUD 000 J A2

AMA: 2018,Jan,8; 2017,Jan,8; 2016,Jan,13; 2015,Jan,16; 2014,Jan,11

43264 **with removal of calculi/debris from biliary/pancreatic duct(s)**

INCLUDES Incidental dilation due to passage of instrument

EXCLUDES *Endoscopic retrograde cholangiopancreatography (ERCP) (43260, 43265)*
Findings without debris or calculi, even if balloon was used
Percutaneous calculus/debris removal (47544)

Code also sphincteroplasty when dilation is necessary in order to access the area of debris/stones ([43277])

10.6 10.6 FUD 000 J A2

AMA: 2018,Jan,8; 2017,Jan,8; 2016,Jan,13; 2015,Dec,3; 2015,Jan,16; 2014,Jan,11

43265 **with destruction of calculi, any method (eg, mechanical, electrohydraulic, lithotripsy)**

INCLUDES Incidental dilation due to passage of instrument
Stone removal when in the same ductal system

EXCLUDES *Endoscopic retrograde cholangiopancreatography (ERCP) (43260, 43264)*
Findings without debris or calculi, even if balloon was used
Percutaneous calculus/debris removal (47544)

Code also sphincteroplasty when dilation is necessary in order to access the area of debris/stones ([43277])

12.6 12.6 FUD 000 J A2

AMA: 2018,Jan,8; 2017,Jan,8; 2016,Jan,13; 2015,Dec,3; 2015,Jan,16; 2014,Jan,11

43266 **Resequenced code. See code following 43255.**

43270 **Resequenced code. See code following 43257.**

43274 **with placement of endoscopic stent into biliary or pancreatic duct, including pre- and post-dilation and guide wire passage, when performed, including sphincterotomy, when performed, each stent**

INCLUDES Balloon dilation when in the same duct
Tube placement for naso-pancreatic or naso-biliary drainage

EXCLUDES *Percutaneous placement biliary stent (47538-47540)*
Procedures for stent placement or exchange in the same duct (43262, [43275], [43276], [43277])

Code also for each additional stent placement in different ducts or side by side in same duct in same session/day, using modifier 59 with ([43274])

13.5 13.5 FUD 000 J G2

AMA: 2018,Jan,8; 2017,Jan,8; 2016,Jan,13; 2015,Jan,16; 2014,Jan,11

43275 **with removal of foreign body(s) or stent(s) from biliary/pancreatic duct(s)**

EXCLUDES *Endoscopic retrograde cholangiopancreatography (ERCP) (43260, [43274], [43276])*
Pancreatic or biliary duct stent removal without ERCP (43247)
Percutaneous calculus/debris removal (47544)
Procedure performed more than one time per session

11.0 11.0 FUD 000 J G2

AMA: 2018,Jan,8; 2017,Jan,8; 2016,Jan,13; 2015,Jan,16; 2014,Jan,11

43276 **with removal and exchange of stent(s), biliary or pancreatic duct, including pre- and post-dilation and guide wire passage, when performed, including sphincterotomy, when performed, each stent exchanged**

INCLUDES Balloon dilation when in the same duct
Stent placement or exchange of one stent

EXCLUDES *Endoscopic retrograde cholangiopancreatography (ERCP) (43260, [43275])*
Procedures for stent insertion or exchange of stent in same duct (43262, [43274])

Code also each additional stent exchanged in same session/day, using modifier 59 with ([43276])

14.1 14.1 FUD 000 J G2

AMA: 2018,Jan,8; 2017,Jan,8; 2016,Jan,13; 2015,Jan,16; 2014,Jan,11

\# **43277** **with trans-endoscopic balloon dilation of biliary/pancreatic duct(s) or of ampulla (sphincteroplasty), including sphincterotomy, when performed, each duct**

EXCLUDES *Endoscopic retrograde cholangiopancreatography (ERCP) (43260, 43262, [43274], [43276])*
Endoscopic retrograde cholangiopancreatography (ERCP); with ablation of tumor(s), polyp(s), or other lesion(s) for the same lesion ([43278])
Percutaneous dilation biliary duct/ampulla (47542)
Removal of stone/debris, dilation incidental to instrument passage (43264-43265)

Code also both right and left hepatic duct (bilateral) balloon dilation, using ([43277]) and append modifier 59 to second procedure

Code also each additional balloon dilation in different ducts or side by side in same duct in same session/day, using modifier 59 with ([43277])

Code also same session sphincterotomy without sphincteroplasty in different duct, using modifier 59 with (43262)

11.0 11.0 **FUD** 000 J G2

AMA: 2018,Jan,8; 2017,Jan,8; 2016,Jan,13; 2015,Dec,3; 2015,Jan,16; 2014,Jan,11

\# **43278** **with ablation of tumor(s), polyp(s), or other lesion(s), including pre- and post-dilation and guide wire passage, when performed**

EXCLUDES *Ampullectomy (43254)*
Endoscopic retrograde cholangiopancreatography (ERCP); diagnostic (43260)
Endoscopic retrograde cholangiopancreatography (ERCP); with trans-endoscopic balloon dilation of biliary/pancreatic duct(s) or of ampulla (sphincteroplasty) on the same lesion with ([43277])

12.6 12.6 **FUD** 000 J G2

AMA: 2018,Jan,8; 2017,Jan,8; 2016,Jan,13; 2015,Jan,16; 2014,Jan,11

\+ **43273** **Endoscopic cannulation of papilla with direct visualization of pancreatic/common bile duct(s) (List separately in addition to code(s) for primary procedure)**

3.49 3.49 **FUD** ZZZ N N1 80

AMA: 2018,Jan,8; 2017,Jan,8; 2016,Jan,13; 2015,Jan,16; 2014,Jan,11

43274 **Resequenced code. See code following numeric code 43270.**

43275 **Resequenced code. See code following numeric code 43270.**

43276 **Resequenced code. See code following numeric code 43270.**

43277 **Resequenced code. See code following numeric code 43270.**

43278 **Resequenced code. See code following numeric code 43270.**

43279-43289 Laparoscopic Procedures of Esophagus

INCLUDES Diagnostic laparoscopy with surgical laparoscopy (49320)

43279 **Laparoscopy, surgical, esophagomyotomy (Heller type), with fundoplasty, when performed**

EXCLUDES *Esophagomyotomy, open method (43330-43331)*
Laparoscopy, surgical, esophagogastric fundoplasty (43280)

37.3 37.3 **FUD** 090 C 80

AMA: 2018,Jan,8; 2017,Aug,6; 2017,Jan,8; 2016,Jan,13; 2015,Jan,16; 2014,Jan,11

43280 **Laparoscopy, surgical, esophagogastric fundoplasty (eg, Nissen, Toupet procedures)**

EXCLUDES *Esophagogastric fundoplasty, open method (43327-43328)*
Esophagogastroduodenoscopy fundoplasty, transoral (43210)
Laparoscopy, surgical, esophageal sphincter augmentation (43284-43285)
Laparoscopy, surgical, esophagomyotomy (43279)
Laparoscopy, surgical, fundoplasty (43281-43282)

31.3 31.3 **FUD** 090 J 80

AMA: 2018,Jan,8; 2017,Aug,6; 2017,Jan,8; 2016,Jan,13; 2015,Nov,8; 2015,Jan,16; 2014,Dec,16; 2014,Dec,16; 2014,Jan,11

Esophagus
Diaphragm
Fundus of stomach

Normal stomach After surgery

43281 **Laparoscopy, surgical, repair of paraesophageal hernia, includes fundoplasty, when performed; without implantation of mesh**

EXCLUDES *Dilation of esophagus (43450, 43453)*
Implantation of mesh or other prosthesis (49568)
Laparoscopy, surgical, esophagogastric fundoplasty (43280)
Transabdominal repair of paraesophageal hiatal hernia (43332-43333)
Transthoracic repair of diaphragmatic hernia (43334-43335)

44.7 44.7 **FUD** 090 J 80

AMA: 2018,Nov,11; 2018,Sep,14; 2018,Jan,8; 2017,Aug,6; 2017,Jan,8; 2016,Jan,13; 2015,Jan,16; 2014,Dec,16; 2014,Dec,16; 2014,Jan,11

43282 **with implantation of mesh**

EXCLUDES *Dilation of esophagus (43450, 43453)*
Laparoscopy, surgical, esophagogastric fundoplasty (43280)
Transabdominal paraesophageal hernia repair (43332-43333)
Transthoracic paraesophageal hernia repair (43334-43335)

50.3 50.3 **FUD** 090 J 80

AMA: 2018,Jan,8; 2017,Aug,6; 2017,Jan,8; 2016,Aug,9; 2016,Jan,13; 2015,Jan,16; 2014,Dec,16; 2014,Dec,16; 2014,Jan,11

\+ **43283** **Laparoscopy, surgical, esophageal lengthening procedure (eg, Collis gastroplasty or wedge gastroplasty) (List separately in addition to code for primary procedure)**

Code first (43280-43282)

4.60 4.60 **FUD** ZZZ C 80

AMA: 2018,Jan,8; 2017,Jan,8; 2016,Jan,13; 2015,Jan,16; 2014,Jan,11

43284 **Laparoscopy, surgical, esophageal sphincter augmentation procedure, placement of sphincter augmentation device (ie, magnetic band), including cruroplasty when performed**

EXCLUDES *Performed during the same session (43279-43282)*

18.6 18.6 **FUD** 090 J J8 80

AMA: 2019,Apr,10; 2018,Sep,14; 2018,Jan,8; 2017,Aug,6

43285 **Removal of esophageal sphincter augmentation device**

19.0 19.0 **FUD** 090 02 G2 80

AMA: 2018,Jan,8; 2017,Aug,6

43286 **Esophagectomy, total or near total, with laparoscopic mobilization of the abdominal and mediastinal esophagus and proximal gastrectomy, with laparoscopic pyloric drainage procedure if performed, with open cervical pharyngogastrostomy or esophagogastrostomy (ie, laparoscopic transhiatal esophagectomy)**
90.9 90.9 FUD 090 C 80
AMA: 2018,Jul,7

43287 **Esophagectomy, distal two-thirds, with laparoscopic mobilization of the abdominal and lower mediastinal esophagus and proximal gastrectomy, with laparoscopic pyloric drainage procedure if performed, with separate thoracoscopic mobilization of the middle and upper mediastinal esophagus and thoracic esophagogastrostomy (ie, laparoscopic thoracoscopic esophagectomy, Ivor Lewis esophagectomy)**
EXCLUDES *Right tube thoracostomy (32551)*
104. 104. FUD 090 C 80
AMA: 2018,Jul,7

43288 **Esophagectomy, total or near total, with thoracoscopic mobilization of the upper, middle, and lower mediastinal esophagus, with separate laparoscopic proximal gastrectomy, with laparoscopic pyloric drainage procedure if performed, with open cervical pharyngogastrostomy or esophagogastrostomy (ie, thoracoscopic, laparoscopic and cervical incision esophagectomy, McKeown esophagectomy, tri-incisional esophagectomy)**
EXCLUDES *Right tube thoracostomy (32551)*
108. 108. FUD 090 C 80
AMA: 2018,Jul,7

43289 **Unlisted laparoscopy procedure, esophagus**
0.00 0.00 FUD YYY J 80 50
AMA: 2018,Jul,7; 2018,Jan,8; 2017,Jan,8; 2016,Jan,13; 2015,Jan,16; 2014,Dec,16; 2014,Dec,16; 2014,Jan,11

43300-43425 Open Esophageal Repair Procedures

43300 **Esophagoplasty (plastic repair or reconstruction), cervical approach; without repair of tracheoesophageal fistula**
17.6 17.6 FUD 090 C 80
AMA: 2014,Jan,11

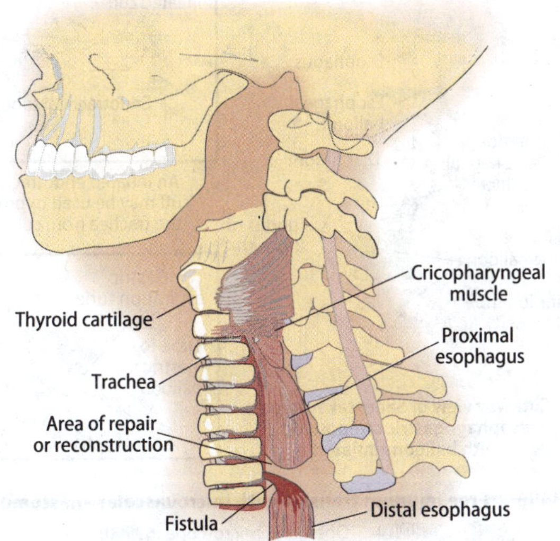

Example of esophageal atresia where the proximal esophagus fails to communicate with the lower portion; note that a fistula has developed from the trachea

43305 **with repair of tracheoesophageal fistula**
31.3 31.3 FUD 090 C 80
AMA: 2014,Jan,11

43310 **Esophagoplasty (plastic repair or reconstruction), thoracic approach; without repair of tracheoesophageal fistula**
43.0 43.0 FUD 090 C 80
AMA: 2014,Jan,11

43312 **with repair of tracheoesophageal fistula**
46.3 46.3 FUD 090 C 80
AMA: 2014,Jan,11

43313 **Esophagoplasty for congenital defect (plastic repair or reconstruction), thoracic approach; without repair of congenital tracheoesophageal fistula**
79.3 79.3 FUD 090 63 C 80
AMA: 2014,Jan,11

43314 **with repair of congenital tracheoesophageal fistula**
85.4 85.4 FUD 090 63 C 80
AMA: 2014,Jan,11

43320 **Esophagogastrostomy (cardioplasty), with or without vagotomy and pyloroplasty, transabdominal or transthoracic approach**
EXCLUDES *Laparoscopic approach (43280)*
40.5 40.5 FUD 090 C 80
AMA: 2014,Jan,11

43325 **Esophagogastric fundoplasty, with fundic patch (Thal-Nissen procedure)**
EXCLUDES *Myotomy, cricopharyngeal (43030)*
39.4 39.4 FUD 090 C 80
AMA: 2014,Jan,11

43327 **Esophagogastric fundoplasty partial or complete; laparotomy**
23.7 23.7 FUD 090 C 80
AMA: 2018,Jan,8; 2017,Jan,8; 2016,Jan,13; 2015,Nov,8; 2015,Jan,16; 2014,Jan,11

43328 **thoracotomy**
EXCLUDES *Esophagogastroduodenoscopy fundoplasty, transoral (43210)*
32.6 32.6 FUD 090 C 80
AMA: 2018,Jan,8; 2017,Jan,8; 2016,Jan,13; 2015,Nov,8; 2015,Jan,16; 2014,Jan,11

43330 **Esophagomyotomy (Heller type); abdominal approach**
EXCLUDES *Esophagomyotomy, laparoscopic method (43279)*
38.7 38.7 FUD 090 C 80
AMA: 2018,Jan,8; 2017,Jan,8; 2016,Jan,13; 2015,Jan,16; 2014,Jan,11

43331 **thoracic approach**
EXCLUDES *Thoracoscopy with esophagomyotomy (32665)*
38.7 38.7 FUD 090 C 80
AMA: 2018,Jan,8; 2017,Jan,8; 2016,Jan,13; 2015,Jan,16; 2014,Jan,11

43332 **Repair, paraesophageal hiatal hernia (including fundoplication), via laparotomy, except neonatal; without implantation of mesh or other prosthesis**
EXCLUDES *Neonatal diaphragmatic hernia repair (39503)*
33.6 33.6 FUD 090 C 80
AMA: 2018,Jan,8; 2017,Jan,8; 2016,Jan,13; 2015,Jan,16; 2014,Jan,11

43333 **with implantation of mesh or other prosthesis**
EXCLUDES *Neonatal diaphragmatic hernia repair (39503)*
36.5 36.5 FUD 090 C 80
AMA: 2018,Jan,8; 2017,Jan,8; 2016,Jan,13; 2015,Jan,16; 2014,Jan,11

43334 **Repair, paraesophageal hiatal hernia (including fundoplication), via thoracotomy, except neonatal; without implantation of mesh or other prosthesis**
EXCLUDES *Neonatal diaphragmatic hernia repair (39503)*
36.2 36.2 FUD 090 C 80
AMA: 2018,Jan,8; 2017,Jan,8; 2016,Jan,13; 2015,Jan,16; 2014,Jan,11

43335 with implantation of mesh or other prosthesis

EXCLUDES *Neonatal diaphragmatic hernia repair (39503)*

38.8 38.8 FUD 090 C 80

AMA: 2018,Jan,8; 2017,Jan,8; 2016,Jan,13; 2015,Jan,16; 2014,Jan,11

43336 **Repair, paraesophageal hiatal hernia, (including fundoplication), via thoracoabdominal incision, except neonatal; without implantation of mesh or other prosthesis**

EXCLUDES *Neonatal diaphragmatic hernia repair (39503)*

43.8 43.8 FUD 090 C 80

AMA: 2018,Jan,8; 2017,Jan,8; 2016,Jan,13; 2015,Jan,16; 2014,Jan,11

43337 with implantation of mesh or other prosthesis

EXCLUDES *Neonatal diaphragmatic hernia repair (39503)*

44.9 44.9 FUD 090 C 80

AMA: 2018,Jan,8; 2017,Jan,8; 2016,Jan,13; 2015,Jan,16; 2014,Jan,11

+ **43338** **Esophageal lengthening procedure (eg, Collis gastroplasty or wedge gastroplasty) (List separately in addition to code for primary procedure)**

Code first (43280, 43327-43337)

3.37 3.37 FUD ZZZ C 80

AMA: 2018,Jan,8; 2017,Jan,8; 2016,Jan,13; 2015,Jan,16; 2014,Jan,11

43340 **Esophagojejunostomy (without total gastrectomy); abdominal approach**

40.0 40.0 FUD 090 C 80

AMA: 2014,Jan,11

43341 thoracic approach

40.6 40.6 FUD 090 C 80

AMA: 2014,Jan,11

43351 **Esophagostomy, fistulization of esophagus, external; thoracic approach**

38.1 38.1 FUD 090 C 80

AMA: 2014,Jan,11

43352 cervical approach

30.8 30.8 FUD 090 C 80

AMA: 2014,Jan,11

43360 **Gastrointestinal reconstruction for previous esophagectomy, for obstructing esophageal lesion or fistula, or for previous esophageal exclusion; with stomach, with or without pyloroplasty**

65.3 65.3 FUD 090 C 80

AMA: 2014,Jan,11

43361 with colon interposition or small intestine reconstruction, including intestine mobilization, preparation, and anastomosis(es)

78.3 78.3 FUD 090 C 80

AMA: 2014,Jan,11

43400 **Ligation, direct, esophageal varices**

44.2 44.2 FUD 090 C 80

AMA: 2014,Jan,11

~~**43401** **Transection of esophagus with repair, for esophageal varices**~~

43405 **Ligation or stapling at gastroesophageal junction for pre-existing esophageal perforation**

42.1 42.1 FUD 090 C 80

AMA: 2014,Jan,11

43410 **Suture of esophageal wound or injury; cervical approach**

29.4 29.4 FUD 090 C 80

AMA: 2018,Jan,8; 2017,Jan,8; 2016,Jan,13; 2015,Jan,16; 2014,Jan,11

43415 transthoracic or transabdominal approach

74.6 74.6 FUD 090 C 80

AMA: 2014,Jan,11

43420 **Closure of esophagostomy or fistula; cervical approach**

EXCLUDES *Paraesophageal hiatal hernia repair:*
Transabdominal (43332-43333)
Transthoracic (43334-43335)

29.1 29.1 FUD 090 J 80

AMA: 2014,Jan,11

43425 transthoracic or transabdominal approach

EXCLUDES *Paraesophageal hiatal hernia repair:*
Transabdominal (43332-43333)
Transthoracic (43334-43335)

41.8 41.8 FUD 090 C 80

AMA: 2014,Jan,11

43450-43453 Esophageal Dilation

43450 **Dilation of esophagus, by unguided sound or bougie, single or multiple passes**

(74220, 74360)

2.31 4.70 FUD 000 T A2

AMA: 2018,Jan,8; 2017,Jul,10; 2017,Jan,8; 2016,Jan,13; 2015,Jan,16; 2014,Jan,11

43453 **Dilation of esophagus, over guide wire**

EXCLUDES *Dilation performed with direct visualization (43195, 43226)*
Endoscopic dilation by dilator or balloon:
Balloon diameter 30 mm or larger (43214, 43233)
Balloon diameter less than 30 mm (43195, 43220, 43249)

(74220, 74360)

2.50 25.4 FUD 000 J A2

AMA: 2018,Jan,8; 2017,Jan,8; 2016,Jan,13; 2015,Jan,16; 2014,Jan,11

43460-43499 Other/Unlisted Esophageal Procedures

43460 **Esophagogastric tamponade, with balloon (Sengstaken type)**

EXCLUDES *Removal of foreign body of the esophagus with balloon catheter (43499, 74235)*

(74220)

6.22 6.22 FUD 000 C

AMA: 2014,Jan,11

Inflated cuff
Endotracheal tube
An inflated endotracheal cuff may be used to protect the trachea from collapse
Esophagus
Esophageal balloon
Inferior esophageal sphincter
Diaphragm
Fundus of stomach
Gastric balloon and aspiration tube
Gastric aspiration tube
Tube to gastric balloon
Tube to esophageal balloon

Cutaway view of Sengstaken-type esophagogastric tamponade with balloons inflated

43496 **Free jejunum transfer with microvascular anastomosis**

INCLUDES Operating microscope (69990)

0.00 0.00 FUD 090 C 80

AMA: 2018,Jan,8; 2017,Jan,8; 2016,Feb,12; 2016,Jan,13; 2015,Jan,16; 2014,Jan,11

43499 **Unlisted procedure, esophagus**

0.00 0.00 FUD YYY T

AMA: 2018,Jul,7; 2018,Jan,8; 2017,Jan,8; 2016,Jan,13; 2015,Nov,10; 2015,Nov,8; 2015,Jan,16; 2014,Jan,11

43500-43641 Open Gastric Incisional and Resection Procedures

43500 **Gastrotomy; with exploration or foreign body removal**
22.7 22.7 **FUD** 090 C 80
AMA: 2014,Jan,11

43501 **with suture repair of bleeding ulcer**
39.0 39.0 **FUD** 090 C 80
AMA: 2014,Jan,11

43502 **with suture repair of pre-existing esophagogastric laceration (eg, Mallory-Weiss)**
44.3 44.3 **FUD** 090 C 80
AMA: 2014,Jan,11

43510 **with esophageal dilation and insertion of permanent intraluminal tube (eg, Celestin or Mousseaux-Barbin)**
27.4 27.4 **FUD** 090 T 80
AMA: 2014,Jan,11

43520 **Pyloromyotomy, cutting of pyloric muscle (Fredet-Ramstedt type operation)**
19.9 19.9 **FUD** 090 63 C 80
AMA: 2014,Jan,11

43605 **Biopsy of stomach, by laparotomy**
24.3 24.3 **FUD** 090 C 80
AMA: 2014,Jan,11

43610 **Excision, local; ulcer or benign tumor of stomach**
28.5 28.5 **FUD** 090 C 80
AMA: 2014,Jan,11

43611 **malignant tumor of stomach**
35.5 35.5 **FUD** 090 C 80
AMA: 2014,Jan,11

43620 **Gastrectomy, total; with esophagoenterostomy**
57.0 57.0 **FUD** 090 C 80
AMA: 2014,Jan,11

43621 **with Roux-en-Y reconstruction**
65.9 65.9 **FUD** 090 C 80
AMA: 2014,Jan,11

43622 **with formation of intestinal pouch, any type**
67.2 67.2 **FUD** 090 C 80
AMA: 2014,Jan,11

43631 **Gastrectomy, partial, distal; with gastroduodenostomy**
INCLUDES Billroth operation
42.0 42.0 **FUD** 090 C 80
AMA: 2014,Jan,11

43632 **with gastrojejunostomy**
INCLUDES Polya anastomosis
59.0 59.0 **FUD** 090 C 80
AMA: 2014,Jan,11

43633 **with Roux-en-Y reconstruction**
55.8 55.8 **FUD** 090 C 80
AMA: 2014,Jan,11

43634 **with formation of intestinal pouch**
61.8 61.8 **FUD** 090 C 80
AMA: 2014,Jan,11

\+ **43635** **Vagotomy when performed with partial distal gastrectomy (List separately in addition to code[s] for primary procedure)**
Code first as appropriate (43631-43634)
3.26 3.26 **FUD** ZZZ C 80
AMA: 2014,Jan,11

43640 **Vagotomy including pyloroplasty, with or without gastrostomy; truncal or selective**
EXCLUDES *Pyloroplasty (43800)*
Vagotomy (64755, 64760)
34.1 34.1 **FUD** 090 C 80
AMA: 2014,Jan,11

43641 **parietal cell (highly selective)**
EXCLUDES *Upper gastrointestinal endoscopy (43235-43259 [43233, 43266, 43270])*
34.9 34.9 **FUD** 090 C 80
AMA: 2014,Jan,11

43644-43645 Laparoscopic Gastric Bypass with Small Bowel Resection

CMS: 100-03,100.1 Bariatric Surgery for Treatment Co-morbid Conditions Due to Morbid Obesity; 100-04,32,150.1 Bariatric Surgery: Treatment of Co-Morbid Conditions Due to Morbid Obesity; 100-04,32,150.2 HCPCS Procedure Codes for Bariatric Surgery; 100-04,32,150.5 ICD Diagnosis Codes for BMI ≥35; 100-04,32,150.6 Bariatric Surgery Claims Guidance

INCLUDES Diagnostic laparoscopy (49320)
EXCLUDES *Endoscopy, upper gastrointestinal, (esophagus/stomach/duodenum/jejunum) (43235-43259 [43233, 43266, 43270])*

43644 **Laparoscopy, surgical, gastric restrictive procedure; with gastric bypass and Roux-en-Y gastroenterostomy (roux limb 150 cm or less)**
EXCLUDES *Roux limb less than 150 cm (43846)*
Roux limb greater than 150 cm (43645)
50.2 50.2 **FUD** 090 C 80
AMA: 2014,Jan,11

43645 **with gastric bypass and small intestine reconstruction to limit absorption**
EXCLUDES *Roux limb less than 150 cm (43847)*
53.7 53.7 **FUD** 090 C 80
AMA: 2018,Jan,8; 2017,Jan,8; 2016,Jan,13; 2015,Jan,16; 2014,Jan,11

43647-43659 Other and Unlisted Laparoscopic Gastric Procedures

INCLUDES Diagnostic laparoscopy (49320)
EXCLUDES *Endoscopy, upper gastrointestinal, (esophagus/stomach/duodenum/jejunum) (43235-43259 [43233, 43266, 43270])*

43647 **Laparoscopy, surgical; implantation or replacement of gastric neurostimulator electrodes, antrum**
EXCLUDES *Electronic analysis/programming gastric neurostimulator (95980-95982)*
Insertion gastric neurostimulator pulse generator (64590)
Laparoscopy with implantation, removal, or revision of gastric neurostimulator electrodes on the lesser curvature of the stomach (43659)
Open method (43881)
Vagus nerve blocking pulse generator and/or neurostimulator electrode array implantation, reprogramming, replacement, revision, or removal at the esophagogastric junction performed laparoscopically (0312T-0317T)
0.00 0.00 **FUD** YYY J 80
AMA: 2019,Feb,6; 2018,Jan,8; 2017,Jan,8; 2016,Jan,13; 2015,Jan,16; 2014,Jan,11

43648 **revision or removal of gastric neurostimulator electrodes, antrum**
EXCLUDES *Electronic analysis/programming gastric neurostimulator (95980-95982)*
Laparoscopy with implantation, removal, or revision of gastric neurostimulator electrodes on the lesser curvature of the stomach (43659)
Open method (43882)
Revision/removal gastric neurostimulator pulse generator (64595)
Vagus nerve blocking pulse generator and/or neurostimulator electrode array implantation, reprogramming, replacement, revision, or removal at the esophagogastric junction performed laparoscopically (0312T-0317T)
0.00 0.00 **FUD** YYY J 80
AMA: 2019,Feb,6; 2018,Jan,8; 2017,Jan,8; 2016,Jan,13; 2015,Jan,16; 2014,Jan,11

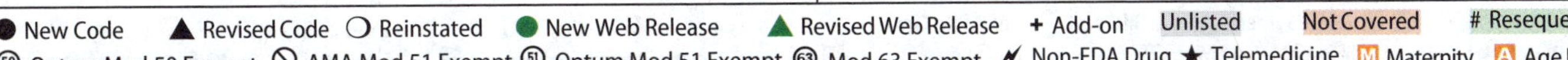

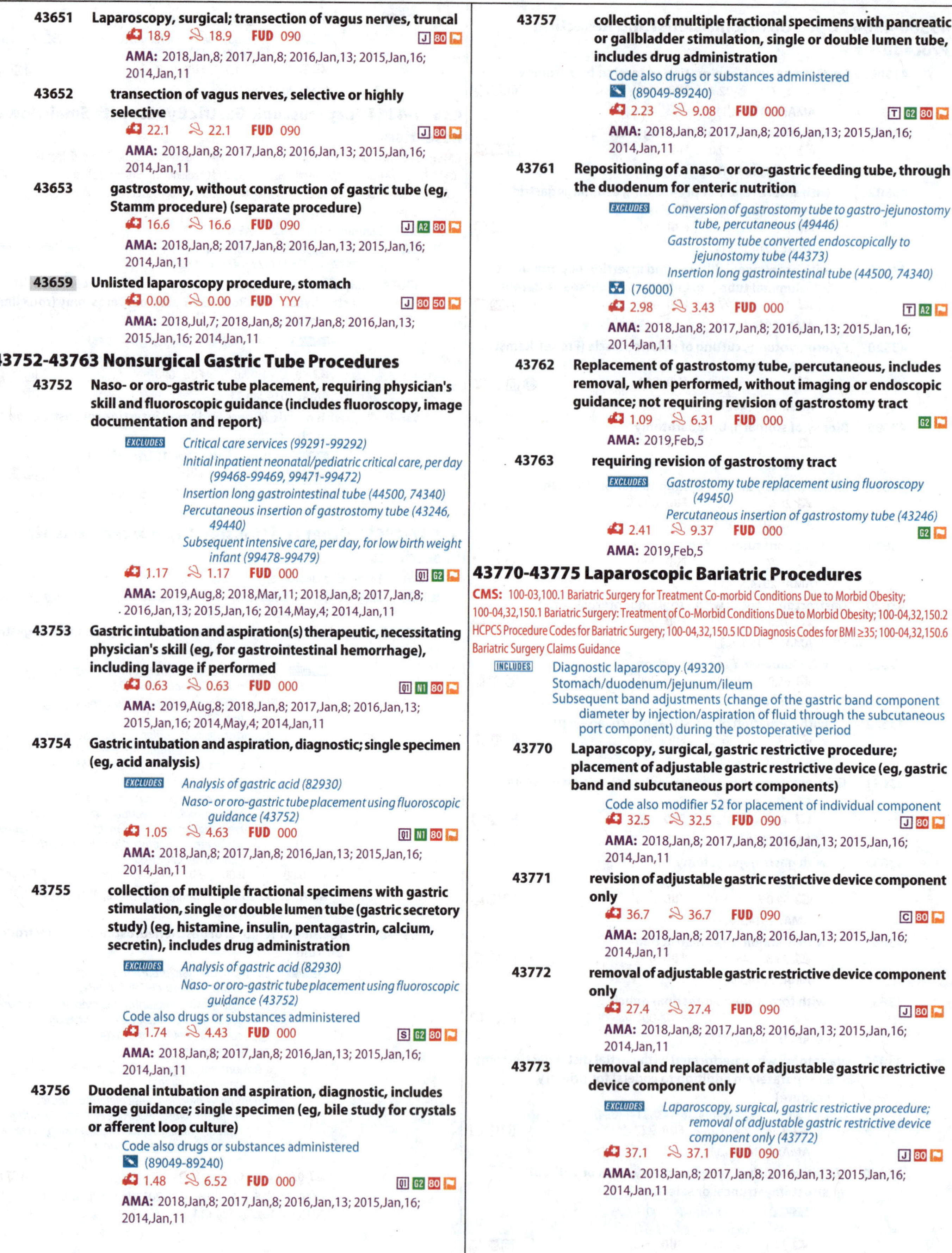

43651 **Laparoscopy, surgical; transection of vagus nerves, truncal**
18.9 18.9 FUD 090 J 80
AMA: 2018,Jan,8; 2017,Jan,8; 2016,Jan,13; 2015,Jan,16; 2014,Jan,11

43652 **transection of vagus nerves, selective or highly selective**
22.1 22.1 FUD 090 J 80
AMA: 2018,Jan,8; 2017,Jan,8; 2016,Jan,13; 2015,Jan,16; 2014,Jan,11

43653 **gastrostomy, without construction of gastric tube (eg, Stamm procedure) (separate procedure)**
16.6 16.6 FUD 090 J A2 80
AMA: 2018,Jan,8; 2017,Jan,8; 2016,Jan,13; 2015,Jan,16; 2014,Jan,11

43659 **Unlisted laparoscopy procedure, stomach**
0.00 0.00 FUD YYY J 80 50
AMA: 2018,Jul,7; 2018,Jan,8; 2017,Jan,8; 2016,Jan,13; 2015,Jan,16; 2014,Jan,11

43752-43763 Nonsurgical Gastric Tube Procedures

43752 **Naso- or oro-gastric tube placement, requiring physician's skill and fluoroscopic guidance (includes fluoroscopy, image documentation and report)**
EXCLUDES *Critical care services (99291-99292)*
Initial inpatient neonatal/pediatric critical care, per day (99468-99469, 99471-99472)
Insertion long gastrointestinal tube (44500, 74340)
Percutaneous insertion of gastrostomy tube (43246, 49440)
Subsequent intensive care, per day, for low birth weight infant (99478-99479)
1.17 1.17 FUD 000 Q1 G2
AMA: 2019,Aug,8; 2018,Mar,11; 2018,Jan,8; 2017,Jan,8; 2016,Jan,13; 2015,Jan,16; 2014,May,4; 2014,Jan,11

43753 **Gastric intubation and aspiration(s) therapeutic, necessitating physician's skill (eg, for gastrointestinal hemorrhage), including lavage if performed**
0.63 0.63 FUD 000 Q1 N1 80
AMA: 2019,Aug,8; 2018,Jan,8; 2017,Jan,8; 2016,Jan,13; 2015,Jan,16; 2014,May,4; 2014,Jan,11

43754 **Gastric intubation and aspiration, diagnostic; single specimen (eg, acid analysis)**
EXCLUDES *Analysis of gastric acid (82930)*
Naso- or oro-gastric tube placement using fluoroscopic guidance (43752)
1.05 4.63 FUD 000 Q1 N1 80
AMA: 2018,Jan,8; 2017,Jan,8; 2016,Jan,13; 2015,Jan,16; 2014,Jan,11

43755 **collection of multiple fractional specimens with gastric stimulation, single or double lumen tube (gastric secretory study) (eg, histamine, insulin, pentagastrin, calcium, secretin), includes drug administration**
EXCLUDES *Analysis of gastric acid (82930)*
Naso- or oro-gastric tube placement using fluoroscopic guidance (43752)
Code also drugs or substances administered
1.74 4.43 FUD 000 S G2 80
AMA: 2018,Jan,8; 2017,Jan,8; 2016,Jan,13; 2015,Jan,16; 2014,Jan,11

43756 **Duodenal intubation and aspiration, diagnostic, includes image guidance; single specimen (eg, bile study for crystals or afferent loop culture)**
Code also drugs or substances administered
(89049-89240)
1.48 6.52 FUD 000 Q1 G2 80
AMA: 2018,Jan,8; 2017,Jan,8; 2016,Jan,13; 2015,Jan,16; 2014,Jan,11

43757 **collection of multiple fractional specimens with pancreatic or gallbladder stimulation, single or double lumen tube, includes drug administration**
Code also drugs or substances administered
(89049-89240)
2.23 9.08 FUD 000 T G2 80
AMA: 2018,Jan,8; 2017,Jan,8; 2016,Jan,13; 2015,Jan,16; 2014,Jan,11

43761 **Repositioning of a naso- or oro-gastric feeding tube, through the duodenum for enteric nutrition**
EXCLUDES *Conversion of gastrostomy tube to gastro-jejunostomy tube, percutaneous (49446)*
Gastrostomy tube converted endoscopically to jejunostomy tube (44373)
Insertion long gastrointestinal tube (44500, 74340)
(76000)
2.98 3.43 FUD 000 T A2
AMA: 2018,Jan,8; 2017,Jan,8; 2016,Jan,13; 2015,Jan,16; 2014,Jan,11

43762 **Replacement of gastrostomy tube, percutaneous, includes removal, when performed, without imaging or endoscopic guidance; not requiring revision of gastrostomy tract**
1.09 6.31 FUD 000 G2
AMA: 2019,Feb,5

43763 **requiring revision of gastrostomy tract**
EXCLUDES *Gastrostomy tube replacement using fluoroscopy (49450)*
Percutaneous insertion of gastrostomy tube (43246)
2.41 9.37 FUD 000 G2
AMA: 2019,Feb,5

43770-43775 Laparoscopic Bariatric Procedures

CMS: 100-03,100.1 Bariatric Surgery for Treatment Co-morbid Conditions Due to Morbid Obesity; 100-04,32,150.1 Bariatric Surgery: Treatment of Co-Morbid Conditions Due to Morbid Obesity; 100-04,32,150.2 HCPCS Procedure Codes for Bariatric Surgery; 100-04,32,150.5 ICD Diagnosis Codes for BMI ≥35; 100-04,32,150.6 Bariatric Surgery Claims Guidance

INCLUDES Diagnostic laparoscopy (49320)
Stomach/duodenum/jejunum/ileum
Subsequent band adjustments (change of the gastric band component diameter by injection/aspiration of fluid through the subcutaneous port component) during the postoperative period

43770 **Laparoscopy, surgical, gastric restrictive procedure; placement of adjustable gastric restrictive device (eg, gastric band and subcutaneous port components)**
Code also modifier 52 for placement of individual component
32.5 32.5 FUD 090 J 80
AMA: 2018,Jan,8; 2017,Jan,8; 2016,Jan,13; 2015,Jan,16; 2014,Jan,11

43771 **revision of adjustable gastric restrictive device component only**
36.7 36.7 FUD 090 C 80
AMA: 2018,Jan,8; 2017,Jan,8; 2016,Jan,13; 2015,Jan,16; 2014,Jan,11

43772 **removal of adjustable gastric restrictive device component only**
27.4 27.4 FUD 090 J 80
AMA: 2018,Jan,8; 2017,Jan,8; 2016,Jan,13; 2015,Jan,16; 2014,Jan,11

43773 **removal and replacement of adjustable gastric restrictive device component only**
EXCLUDES *Laparoscopy, surgical, gastric restrictive procedure; removal of adjustable gastric restrictive device component only (43772)*
37.1 37.1 FUD 090 J 80
AMA: 2018,Jan,8; 2017,Jan,8; 2016,Jan,13; 2015,Jan,16; 2014,Jan,11

43774 **removal of adjustable gastric restrictive device and subcutaneous port components**

EXCLUDES *Removal/replacement of subcutaneous port components and gastric band (43659)*

27.8 27.8 FUD 090 J 80

AMA: 2018,Jan,8; 2017,Jan,8; 2016,Jan,13; 2015,Jan,16; 2014,Jan,11

43775 **longitudinal gastrectomy (ie, sleeve gastrectomy)**

EXCLUDES *Open gastric restrictive procedure for morbid obesity, without gastric bypass, other than vertical-banded gastroplasty (43843)*

Vagus nerve blocking pulse generator and/or neurostimulator electrode array implantation, reprogramming, replacement, revision, or removal at the esophagogastric junction performed laparoscopically (0312T-0317T)

32.3 32.3 FUD 090 C 80

AMA: 2014,Jan,11

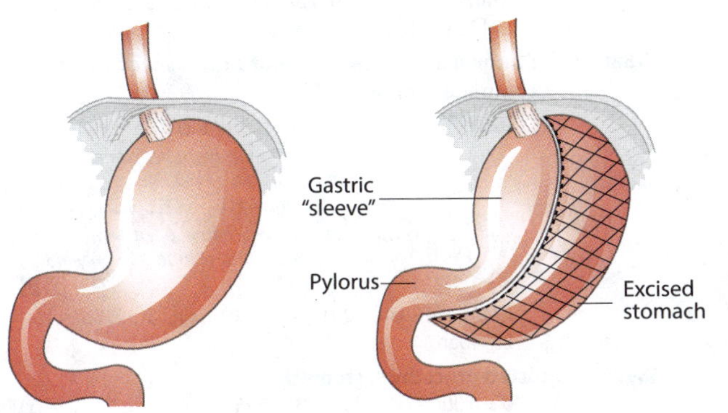

43800-43840 Open Gastric Incisional/Repair/Resection Procedures

43800 **Pyloroplasty**

EXCLUDES *Vagotomy with pyloroplasty (43640)*

26.9 26.9 FUD 090 C 80

AMA: 2014,Jan,11

43810 **Gastroduodenostomy**

29.5 29.5 FUD 090 C 80

AMA: 2014,Jan,11

43820 **Gastrojejunostomy; without vagotomy**

38.9 38.9 FUD 090 C 80

AMA: 2014,Jan,11

43825 **with vagotomy, any type**

38.0 38.0 FUD 090 C 80

AMA: 2014,Jan,11

43830 **Gastrostomy, open; without construction of gastric tube (eg, Stamm procedure) (separate procedure)**

20.3 20.3 FUD 090 J 80

AMA: 2019,Feb,5; 2018,Jan,8; 2017,Jan,8; 2016,Jan,13; 2015,Jan,16; 2014,Jan,11

43831 **neonatal, for feeding** A

EXCLUDES *Change of gastrostomy tube (43762-43763)*

Gastrostomy tube replacement using fluoroscopy (49450)

17.3 17.3 FUD 090 63 T 80

AMA: 2019,Feb,5; 2018,Jan,8; 2017,Jan,8; 2016,Jan,13; 2015,Jan,16; 2014,Jan,11

43832 **with construction of gastric tube (eg, Janeway procedure)**

EXCLUDES *Endoscopic placement of percutaneous gastrostomy tube (43246)*

30.0 30.0 FUD 090 C 80

AMA: 2018,Jan,8; 2017,Jan,8; 2016,Jan,13; 2015,Jan,16; 2014,Jan,11

43840 **Gastrorrhaphy, suture of perforated duodenal or gastric ulcer, wound, or injury**

39.4 39.4 FUD 090 C 80

AMA: 2014,Jan,11

43842-43848 Open Bariatric Procedures for Morbid Obesity

CMS: 100-03,100.1 Bariatric Surgery for Treatment Co-morbid Conditions Due to Morbid Obesity; 100-04,32,150.1 Bariatric Surgery: Treatment of Co-Morbid Conditions Due to Morbid Obesity; 100-04,32,150.2 HCPCS Procedure Codes for Bariatric Surgery; 100-04,32,150.5 ICD Diagnosis Codes for BMI ≥35; 100-04,32,150.6 Bariatric Surgery Claims Guidance

43842 **Gastric restrictive procedure, without gastric bypass, for morbid obesity; vertical-banded gastroplasty**

34.5 34.5 FUD 090 E

AMA: 2018,Jan,8; 2017,Jan,8; 2016,Jan,13; 2015,Jan,16; 2014,Jan,11

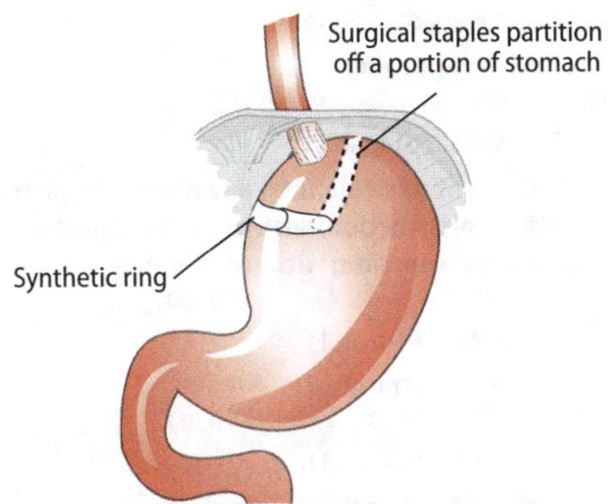

The stomach is surgically restricted to treat morbid obesity; a vertical-banded partitioning technique gives the patient a sensation of fullness, thus decreasing daily caloric intake

43843 **other than vertical-banded gastroplasty**

EXCLUDES *Laparoscopic longitudinal gastrectomy (e.g., sleeve gastrectomy) (43775)*

37.2 37.2 FUD 090 C 80

AMA: 2018,Jan,8; 2017,Jan,8; 2016,Jan,13; 2015,Jan,16; 2014,Jan,11

43845 **Gastric restrictive procedure with partial gastrectomy, pylorus-preserving duodenoileostomy and ileoileostomy (50 to 100 cm common channel) to limit absorption (biliopancreatic diversion with duodenal switch)**

EXCLUDES *Enteroenterostomy, anastomosis of intestine (44130)*

Exploratory laparotomy, exploratory celiotomy (49000)

Gastrectomy, partial, distal; with Roux-en-Y reconstruction (43633)

Gastric restrictive procedure, with gastric bypass for morbid obesity; with small intestine reconstruction (43847)

56.5 56.5 FUD 090 C 80

AMA: 2018,Jan,8; 2017,Jan,8; 2016,Jan,13; 2015,Jan,16; 2014,Jan,11

43846 **Gastric restrictive procedure, with gastric bypass for morbid obesity; with short limb (150 cm or less) Roux-en-Y gastroenterostomy**

EXCLUDES *Performed laparoscopically (43644)*

Roux limb more than 150 cm (43847)

47.0 47.0 FUD 090 C 80

AMA: 2018,Jan,8; 2017,Jan,8; 2016,Jan,13; 2015,Jan,16; 2014,Jan,11

43847 **with small intestine reconstruction to limit absorption**

EXCLUDES *Performed laparoscopically (43645)*

52.4 52.4 FUD 090 C 80

AMA: 2018,Jan,8; 2017,Jan,8; 2016,Jan,13; 2015,Jan,16; 2014,Jan,11

43848 **Revision, open, of gastric restrictive procedure for morbid obesity, other than adjustable gastric restrictive device (separate procedure)**

EXCLUDES *Gastric restrictive port procedures (43886-43888)*
Procedures for adjustable gastric restrictive devices (43770-43774)

55.9 55.9 FUD 090 C 80

AMA: 2018,Jan,8; 2017,Jan,8; 2016,Jan,13; 2015,Jan,16; 2014,Jan,11

43850-43882 Open Gastric Procedures: Closure/Implantation/Replacement/Revision

43850 **Revision of gastroduodenal anastomosis (gastroduodenostomy) with reconstruction; without vagotomy**

47.3 47.3 FUD 090 C 80

AMA: 2014,Jan,11

43855 **with vagotomy**

49.1 49.1 FUD 090 C 80

AMA: 2014,Jan,11

43860 **Revision of gastrojejunal anastomosis (gastrojejunostomy) with reconstruction, with or without partial gastrectomy or intestine resection; without vagotomy**

47.4 47.4 FUD 090 C 80

AMA: 2014,Jan,11

43865 **with vagotomy**

49.7 49.7 FUD 090 C 80

AMA: 2014,Jan,11

43870 **Closure of gastrostomy, surgical**

20.6 20.6 FUD 090 J A2 80

AMA: 2018,Jul,14; 2014,Jan,11

43880 **Closure of gastrocolic fistula**

46.1 46.1 FUD 090 C 80

AMA: 2014,Jan,11

43881 **Implantation or replacement of gastric neurostimulator electrodes, antrum, open**

EXCLUDES *Electronic analysis and programming (95980-95982)*
Implantation/removal/revision gastric neurostimulator electrodes, lesser curvature or vagal trunk (EGJ):
Laparoscopically (43659)
Open, lesser curvature (43999)
Implantation/replacement performed laparoscopically (43647)
Insertion of gastric neurostimulator pulse generator (64590)
Vagus nerve blocking pulse generator and/or neurostimulator electrode array implantation, reprogramming, replacement, revision, or removal at the esophagogastric junction performed laparoscopically (0312T-0317T)

0.00 0.00 FUD YYY C 80

AMA: 2019,Feb,6; 2018,Jan,8; 2017,Jan,8; 2016,Jan,13; 2015,Jan,16; 2014,Jan,11

43882 **Revision or removal of gastric neurostimulator electrodes, antrum, open**

EXCLUDES *Electronic analysis and programming (95980-95982)*
Implantation/removal/revision gastric neurostimulator electrodes, lesser curvature or vagal trunk (EGJ):
Laparoscopic (43659)
Open, lesser curvature (43999)
Revision/removal gastric neurostimulator electrodes, antrum, performed laparoscopically (43648)
Revision/removal gastric neurostimulator pulse generator (64595)
Vagus nerve blocking pulse generator and/or neurostimulator electrode array implantation, reprogramming, replacement, revision, or removal at the esophagogastric junction performed laparoscopically (0312T-0317T)

0.00 0.00 FUD YYY C 80

AMA: 2019,Feb,6; 2018,Jan,8; 2017,Jan,8; 2016,Jan,13; 2015,Jan,16; 2014,Jan,11

43886-43999 Bariatric Procedures: Removal/Replacement/Revision Port Components

CMS: 100-04,32,150.1 Bariatric Surgery: Treatment of Co-Morbid Conditions Due to Morbid Obesity; 100-04,32,150.2 HCPCS Procedure Codes for Bariatric Surgery; 100-04,32,150.5 ICD Diagnosis Codes for BMI ≥35; 100-04,32,150.6 Bariatric Surgery Claims Guidance

43886 **Gastric restrictive procedure, open; revision of subcutaneous port component only**

10.5 10.5 FUD 090 T G2 80

AMA: 2018,Jan,8; 2017,Jan,8; 2016,Jan,13; 2015,Jan,16; 2014,Jan,11

43887 **removal of subcutaneous port component only**

EXCLUDES *Gastric band and subcutaneous port components:*
Removal and replacement performed laparoscopically (43659)
Removal performed laparoscopically (43774)

9.48 9.48 FUD 090 Q2 G2 80

AMA: 2018,Jan,8; 2017,Jan,8; 2016,Jan,13; 2015,Jan,16; 2014,Jan,11

43888 **removal and replacement of subcutaneous port component only**

EXCLUDES *Gastric band and subcutaneous port components:*
Removal and replacement performed laparoscopically (43659)
Removal performed laparoscopically (43774)
Gastric restrictive procedure, open; removal of subcutaneous port component only (43887)

13.3 13.3 FUD 090 T G2 80

AMA: 2018,Jan,8; 2017,Jan,8; 2016,Jan,13; 2015,Jan,16; 2014,Jan,11

43999 **Unlisted procedure, stomach**

0.00 0.00 FUD YYY T 80

AMA: 2018,Dec,10; 2018,Dec,10; 2018,Jul,14; 2018,Jan,8; 2017,Jan,8; 2016,Jan,13; 2015,Jan,16; 2014,Jan,11

44005-44130 Incisional and Resection Procedures of Bowel

44005 **Enterolysis (freeing of intestinal adhesion) (separate procedure)**

EXCLUDES *Enterolysis performed laparoscopically (44180)*
Excision of ileoanal reservoir with ileostomy (45136)

31.7 31.7 FUD 090 C 80

AMA: 2018,Feb,11; 2018,Jan,8; 2017,Jan,8; 2016,Jan,13; 2015,Jan,16; 2014,Jan,11

44010 **Duodenotomy, for exploration, biopsy(s), or foreign body removal**

24.9 24.9 FUD 090 C 80

AMA: 2014,Jan,11

The duodenum is surgically accessed and explored A foreign body may be removed and/or a biopsy specimen taken

+ **44015** **Tube or needle catheter jejunostomy for enteral alimentation, intraoperative, any method (List separately in addition to primary procedure)**
Code first the primary procedure
4.13 4.13 FUD ZZZ C 80
AMA: 2018,Jan,8; 2017,Jan,8; 2016,Jan,13; 2015,Jan,16; 2014,Jan,11

44020 **Enterotomy, small intestine, other than duodenum; for exploration, biopsy(s), or foreign body removal**
28.2 28.2 FUD 090 C 80
AMA: 2014,Jan,11

44021 **for decompression (eg, Baker tube)**
28.3 28.3 FUD 090 C 80
AMA: 2014,Jan,11

44025 **Colotomy, for exploration, biopsy(s), or foreign body removal**
INCLUDES Amussat's operation
EXCLUDES *Intestine exteriorization (Mikulicz resection with crushing of spur) (44602-44605)*
28.5 28.5 FUD 090 C 80
AMA: 2014,Jan,11

44050 **Reduction of volvulus, intussusception, internal hernia, by laparotomy**
27.1 27.1 FUD 090 C 80
AMA: 2014,Jan,11

44055 **Correction of malrotation by lysis of duodenal bands and/or reduction of midgut volvulus (eg, Ladd procedure)**
43.4 43.4 FUD 090 63 C 80
AMA: 2014,Jan,11

44100 **Biopsy of intestine by capsule, tube, peroral (1 or more specimens)**
3.14 3.14 FUD 000 T A2
AMA: 2014,Jan,11

44110 **Excision of 1 or more lesions of small or large intestine not requiring anastomosis, exteriorization, or fistulization; single enterotomy**
24.6 24.6 FUD 090 C 80
AMA: 2014,Jan,11

44111 **multiple enterotomies**
28.5 28.5 FUD 090 C 80
AMA: 2014,Jan,11

44120 **Enterectomy, resection of small intestine; single resection and anastomosis**
EXCLUDES *Excision of ileoanal reservoir with ileostomy (45136)*
35.4 35.4 FUD 090 C 80
AMA: 2018,Nov,11; 2018,Jan,8; 2017,Jan,8; 2016,Jan,13; 2015,Jan,16; 2014,Jan,11

+ **44121** **each additional resection and anastomosis (List separately in addition to code for primary procedure)**
Code first (44120)
7.04 7.04 FUD ZZZ C 80
AMA: 2014,Jan,11

44125 **with enterostomy**
34.2 34.2 FUD 090 C 80
AMA: 2014,Jan,11

44126 **Enterectomy, resection of small intestine for congenital atresia, single resection and anastomosis of proximal segment of intestine; without tapering**
71.7 71.7 FUD 090 63 C 80
AMA: 2014,Jan,11

44127 **with tapering**
82.9 82.9 FUD 090 63 C 80
AMA: 2014,Jan,11

+ **44128** **each additional resection and anastomosis (List separately in addition to code for primary procedure)**
Code first single resection of small intestine (44126, 44127)
7.10 7.10 FUD ZZZ 63 C 80
AMA: 2014,Jan,11

44130 **Enteroenterostomy, anastomosis of intestine, with or without cutaneous enterostomy (separate procedure)**
38.1 38.1 FUD 090 C 80
AMA: 2014,Jan,11

44132-44137 Intestine Transplant Procedures

CMS: 100-03,260.5 Intestinal and Multi-Visceral Transplantation; 100-04,3,90.6 Intestinal and Multi-Visceral Transplants

44132 **Donor enterectomy (including cold preservation), open; from cadaver donor**
INCLUDES Graft:
Cold preservation
Harvest
EXCLUDES *Preparation/reconstruction of backbench intestinal graft (44715, 44720-44721)*
0.00 0.00 FUD XXX C 80
AMA: 2014,Jan,11

44133 **partial, from living donor**
INCLUDES Donor care
Graft:
Cold preservation
Harvest
EXCLUDES *Preparation/reconstruction of backbench intestinal graft (44715, 44720-44721)*
0.00 0.00 FUD XXX C 80
AMA: 2014,Jan,11

44135 **Intestinal allotransplantation; from cadaver donor**
INCLUDES Allograft transplantation
Recipient care
0.00 0.00 FUD XXX C 80
AMA: 2014,Jan,11

44136 **from living donor**
INCLUDES Allograft transplantation
Recipient care
0.00 0.00 FUD XXX C 80
AMA: 2014,Jan,11

44137 **Removal of transplanted intestinal allograft, complete**
EXCLUDES *Partial removal of transplant allograft (44120-44121, 44140)*
0.00 0.00 FUD XXX C 80
AMA: 2014,Jan,11

44139-44160 Colon Resection Procedures

+ **44139** **Mobilization (take-down) of splenic flexure performed in conjunction with partial colectomy (List separately in addition to primary procedure)**
Code first partial colectomy (44140-44147)
3.51 3.51 FUD ZZZ C 80
AMA: 2014,Jan,11

44140 **Colectomy, partial; with anastomosis**
EXCLUDES *Laparoscopic method (44204)*
38.9 38.9 FUD 090 C 80
AMA: 2018,Jan,8; 2017,Jan,8; 2016,Jan,13; 2015,Jan,16; 2014,Jan,11

44141 **with skin level cecostomy or colostomy**
52.9 52.9 FUD 090 C 80
AMA: 2018,Jan,8; 2017,Jan,8; 2016,Jan,13; 2015,Jan,16; 2014,Jan,11

44143 **with end colostomy and closure of distal segment (Hartmann type procedure)**
EXCLUDES *Laparoscopic method (44206)*
48.2 48.2 FUD 090 C 80
AMA: 2018,Jan,8; 2017,Jan,8; 2016,Jan,13; 2015,Jan,16; 2014,Jan,11

44144 **with resection, with colostomy or ileostomy and creation of mucofistula**
51.3 51.3 **FUD** 090 C 80
AMA: 2018,Jan,8; 2017,Jan,8; 2016,Jan,13; 2015,Jan,16; 2014,Jan,11

44145 **with coloproctostomy (low pelvic anastomosis)**
EXCLUDES *Laparoscopic method (44207)*
48.0 48.0 **FUD** 090 C 80
AMA: 2014,Jan,11

44146 **with coloproctostomy (low pelvic anastomosis), with colostomy**
EXCLUDES *Laparoscopic method (44208)*
61.3 61.3 **FUD** 090 C 80
AMA: 2018,Jun,11; 2018,Jan,8; 2017,Jan,8; 2016,Jan,13; 2015,Jan,16; 2014,Jan,11

44147 **abdominal and transanal approach**
56.3 56.3 **FUD** 090 C 80
AMA: 2018,Jan,8; 2017,Jan,8; 2016,Jan,13; 2015,Jan,16; 2014,Jan,11

44150 **Colectomy, total, abdominal, without proctectomy; with ileostomy or ileoproctostomy**
INCLUDES Lane's operation
EXCLUDES *Laparoscopic method (44210)*
54.0 54.0 **FUD** 090 C 80
AMA: 2014,Jan,11

44151 **with continent ileostomy**
62.7 62.7 **FUD** 090 C 80
AMA: 2014,Jan,11

44155 **Colectomy, total, abdominal, with proctectomy; with ileostomy**
INCLUDES Miles' colectomy
EXCLUDES *Laparoscopic method (44212)*
60.1 60.1 **FUD** 090 C 80
AMA: 2014,Jan,11

44156 **with continent ileostomy**
67.1 67.1 **FUD** 090 C 80
AMA: 2014,Jan,11

44157 **with ileoanal anastomosis, includes loop ileostomy, and rectal mucosectomy, when performed**
63.6 63.6 **FUD** 090 C 80
AMA: 2014,Jan,11

44158 **with ileoanal anastomosis, creation of ileal reservoir (S or J), includes loop ileostomy, and rectal mucosectomy, when performed**
EXCLUDES *Laparoscopic method (44211)*
65.2 65.2 **FUD** 090 C 80
AMA: 2014,Jan,11

44160 **Colectomy, partial, with removal of terminal ileum with ileocolostomy**
EXCLUDES *Laparoscopic method (44205)*
36.0 36.0 **FUD** 090 C 80
AMA: 2018,Jan,8; 2017,Jan,8; 2016,Jan,13; 2015,Jan,16; 2014,Jan,11

44180 Laparoscopic Enterolysis

INCLUDES Diagnostic laparoscopy (49320)
EXCLUDES *Laparoscopic salpingolysis/ovariolysis (58660)*

44180 **Laparoscopy, surgical, enterolysis (freeing of intestinal adhesion) (separate procedure)**
26.6 26.6 **FUD** 090 J 80
AMA: 2018,Feb,11; 2018,Jan,8; 2017,Jan,8; 2016,Jan,13; 2015,Jan,16; 2014,Jan,11

44186-44238 Laparoscopic Enterostomy Procedures

INCLUDES Diagnostic laparoscopy (49320)

44186 **Laparoscopy, surgical; jejunostomy (eg, for decompression or feeding)**
18.8 18.8 **FUD** 090 J 80
AMA: 2018,Jan,8; 2017,Jan,8; 2016,Jan,13; 2015,Jan,16; 2014,Jan,11

44187 **ileostomy or jejunostomy, non-tube**
EXCLUDES *Open method (44310)*
31.8 31.8 **FUD** 090 C 80
AMA: 2019,Sep,10; 2018,Jan,8; 2017,Jan,8; 2016,Jan,13; 2015,Jan,16; 2014,Jan,11

44188 **Laparoscopy, surgical, colostomy or skin level cecostomy**
EXCLUDES *Laparoscopy, surgical, appendectomy (44970)*
Open method (44320)
35.4 35.4 **FUD** 090 C 80
AMA: 2018,Jan,8; 2017,Jan,8; 2016,Jan,13; 2015,Jan,16; 2014,Jan,11

44202 **Laparoscopy, surgical; enterectomy, resection of small intestine, single resection and anastomosis**
EXCLUDES *Open method (44120)*
40.1 40.1 **FUD** 090 C 80
AMA: 2018,Jan,8; 2017,Jan,8; 2016,Jan,13; 2015,Jan,16; 2014,Jan,11

+ 44203 **each additional small intestine resection and anastomosis (List separately in addition to code for primary procedure)**
EXCLUDES *Open method (44121)*
Code first single resection of small intestine (44202)
6.96 6.96 **FUD** ZZZ C 80
AMA: 2018,Jan,8; 2017,Jan,8; 2016,Jan,13; 2015,Jan,16; 2014,Jan,11

44204 **colectomy, partial, with anastomosis**
EXCLUDES *Open method (44140)*
44.6 44.6 **FUD** 090 C 80
AMA: 2018,Jan,8; 2017,Dec,14; 2017,Jan,8; 2016,Jan,13; 2015,Jan,16; 2014,Jan,11

44205 **colectomy, partial, with removal of terminal ileum with ileocolostomy**
EXCLUDES *Open method (44160)*
38.7 38.7 **FUD** 090 C 80
AMA: 2018,Jan,8; 2017,Jan,8; 2016,Jan,13; 2015,Jan,16; 2014,Jan,11

44206 **colectomy, partial, with end colostomy and closure of distal segment (Hartmann type procedure)**
EXCLUDES *Open method (44143)*
50.6 50.6 **FUD** 090 C 80
AMA: 2018,Jan,8; 2017,Jan,8; 2016,Jan,13; 2015,Jan,16; 2014,Jan,11

44207 **colectomy, partial, with anastomosis, with coloproctostomy (low pelvic anastomosis)**
EXCLUDES *Open method (44145)*
52.6 52.6 **FUD** 090 C 80
AMA: 2018,Jan,8; 2017,Jan,8; 2016,Jan,13; 2015,Jan,16; 2014,Jan,11

44208 **colectomy, partial, with anastomosis, with coloproctostomy (low pelvic anastomosis) with colostomy**
EXCLUDES *Open method (44146)*
57.4 57.4 **FUD** 090 C 80
AMA: 2018,Jan,8; 2017,Jan,8; 2016,Jan,13; 2015,Jan,16; 2014,Jan,11

44210 **colectomy, total, abdominal, without proctectomy, with ileostomy or ileoproctostomy**

EXCLUDES *Open method (44150)*

51.5 51.5 FUD 090 C 80

AMA: 2018,Jan,8; 2017,Jan,8; 2016,Jan,13; 2015,Jan,16; 2014,Jan,11

44211 **colectomy, total, abdominal, with proctectomy, with ileoanal anastomosis, creation of ileal reservoir (S or J), with loop ileostomy, includes rectal mucosectomy, when performed**

EXCLUDES *Open method (44157-44158)*

62.9 62.9 FUD 090 C 80

AMA: 2018,Jan,8; 2017,Jan,8; 2016,Jan,13; 2015,Jan,16; 2014,Jan,11

44212 **colectomy, total, abdominal, with proctectomy, with ileostomy**

EXCLUDES *Open method (44155)*

59.1 59.1 FUD 090 C 80

AMA: 2018,Jan,8; 2017,Jan,8; 2016,Jan,13; 2015,Jan,16; 2014,Jan,11

+ **44213** **Laparoscopy, surgical, mobilization (take-down) of splenic flexure performed in conjunction with partial colectomy (List separately in addition to primary procedure)**

EXCLUDES *Open method (44139)*

Code first partial colectomy (44204-44208)

5.45 5.45 FUD ZZZ C 80

AMA: 2018,Jan,8; 2017,Jan,8; 2016,Jan,13; 2015,Jan,16; 2014,Jan,11

44227 **Laparoscopy, surgical, closure of enterostomy, large or small intestine, with resection and anastomosis**

EXCLUDES *Open method (44625-44626)*

48.2 48.2 FUD 090 C 80

AMA: 2018,Jan,8; 2017,Jan,8; 2016,Jan,13; 2015,Jan,16; 2014,Jan,11

44238 **Unlisted laparoscopy procedure, intestine (except rectum)**

0.00 0.00 FUD YYY J 80 50

AMA: 2018,Jan,8; 2017,Jul,10; 2017,Jan,8; 2016,Jan,13; 2015,Jan,16; 2014,Jan,11

44300-44346 Open Enterostomy Procedures

44300 **Placement, enterostomy or cecostomy, tube open (eg, for feeding or decompression) (separate procedure)**

EXCLUDES *Intraoperative lavage, colon (44701)*
Other gastrointestinal tube(s) placed percutaneously with fluoroscopic imaging guidance (49441-49442)

24.4 24.4 FUD 090 C 80

AMA: 2018,Jan,8; 2017,Jan,8; 2016,Jan,13; 2015,Jan,16; 2014,Jan,11

44310 **Ileostomy or jejunostomy, non-tube**

EXCLUDES *Colectomy, partial; with resection, with colostomy or ileostomy and creation of mucofistula (44144)*
Colectomy, total, abdominal (44150-44151, 44155-44156)
Excision of ileoanal reservoir with ileostomy (45136)
Laparoscopic method (44187)
Proctectomy (45113, 45119)

30.2 30.2 FUD 090 C 80

AMA: 2018,Jan,8; 2017,Jan,8; 2016,Jan,13; 2015,Jan,16; 2014,Jan,11

44312 **Revision of ileostomy; simple (release of superficial scar) (separate procedure)**

17.1 17.1 FUD 090 T A2 80

AMA: 2014,Jan,11

44314 **complicated (reconstruction in-depth) (separate procedure)**

29.1 29.1 FUD 090 C 80

AMA: 2014,Jan,11

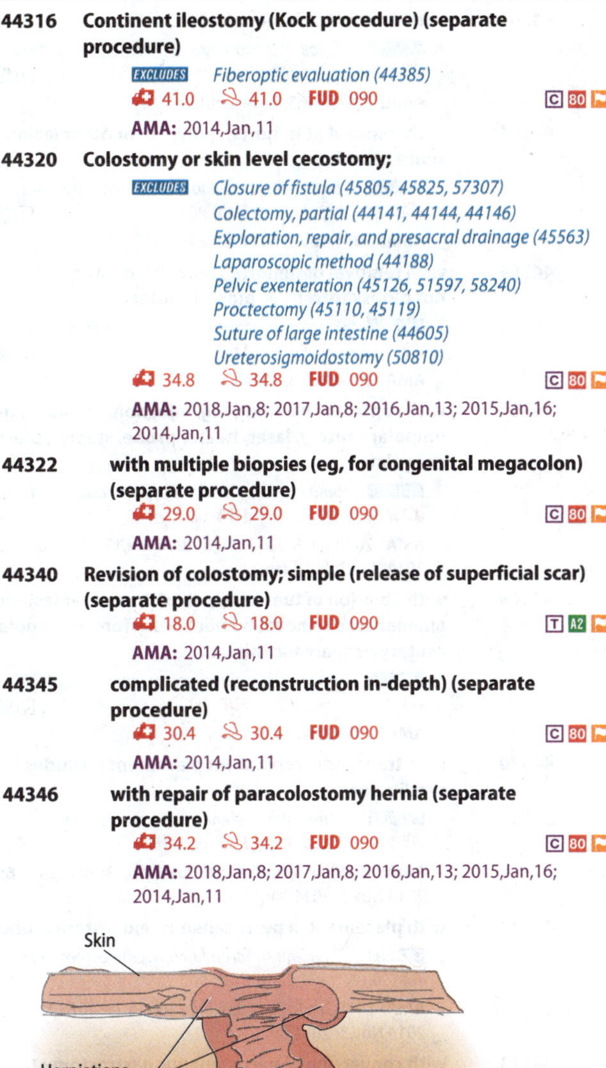

44316 **Continent ileostomy (Kock procedure) (separate procedure)**

EXCLUDES *Fiberoptic evaluation (44385)*

41.0 41.0 FUD 090 C 80

AMA: 2014,Jan,11

44320 **Colostomy or skin level cecostomy;**

EXCLUDES *Closure of fistula (45805, 45825, 57307)*
Colectomy, partial (44141, 44144, 44146)
Exploration, repair, and presacral drainage (45563)
Laparoscopic method (44188)
Pelvic exenteration (45126, 51597, 58240)
Proctectomy (45110, 45119)
Suture of large intestine (44605)
Ureterosigmoidostomy (50810)

34.8 34.8 FUD 090 C 80

AMA: 2018,Jan,8; 2017,Jan,8; 2016,Jan,13; 2015,Jan,16; 2014,Jan,11

44322 **with multiple biopsies (eg, for congenital megacolon) (separate procedure)**

29.0 29.0 FUD 090 C 80

AMA: 2014,Jan,11

44340 **Revision of colostomy; simple (release of superficial scar) (separate procedure)**

18.0 18.0 FUD 090 T A2

AMA: 2014,Jan,11

44345 **complicated (reconstruction in-depth) (separate procedure)**

30.4 30.4 FUD 090 C 80

AMA: 2014,Jan,11

44346 **with repair of paracolostomy hernia (separate procedure)**

34.2 34.2 FUD 090 C 80

AMA: 2018,Jan,8; 2017,Jan,8; 2016,Jan,13; 2015,Jan,16; 2014,Jan,11

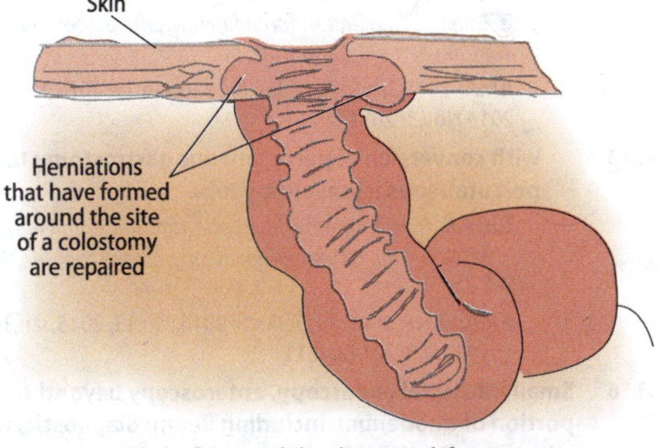

The colon is mobilized, trimmed if necessary, and a new stoma is often created

44360-44379 Endoscopy of Small Intestine

INCLUDES Control of bleeding as a result of endoscopic procedure during same operative session

EXCLUDES *Esophagogastroduodenoscopy, flexible, transoral (43235-43259 [43233, 43266, 43270])*
Retrograde exam through anus/colon stoma (44799)

44360 **Small intestinal endoscopy, enteroscopy beyond second portion of duodenum, not including ileum; diagnostic, including collection of specimen(s) by brushing or washing, when performed (separate procedure)**

EXCLUDES *Small intestinal endoscopy, enteroscopy (44376-44379)*

4.20 4.20 FUD 000 J A2

AMA: 2018,Jan,8; 2017,Jan,8; 2016,Jan,13; 2015,Jan,16; 2014,Nov,3; 2014,Jan,11

44361 **with biopsy, single or multiple**

EXCLUDES *Small intestinal endoscopy, enteroscopy (44376-44379)*

4.65 4.65 FUD 000 J A2

AMA: 2014,Nov,3; 2014,Jan,11

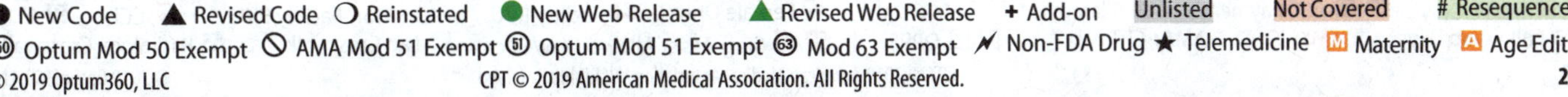

44363 **with removal of foreign body(s)**
EXCLUDES *Small intestinal endoscopy, enteroscopy (44376-44379)*
5.62 5.62 FUD 000 J A2 80
AMA: 2014,Nov,3; 2014,Jan,11

44364 **with removal of tumor(s), polyp(s), or other lesion(s) by snare technique**
EXCLUDES *Small intestinal endoscopy, enteroscopy (44376-44379)*
5.99 5.99 FUD 000 J A2 80
AMA: 2014,Nov,3; 2014,Jan,11

44365 **with removal of tumor(s), polyp(s), or other lesion(s) by hot biopsy forceps or bipolar cautery**
EXCLUDES *Small intestinal endoscopy, enteroscopy (44376-44379)*
5.32 5.32 FUD 000 J A2 80
AMA: 2014,Nov,3; 2014,Jan,11

44366 **with control of bleeding (eg, injection, bipolar cautery, unipolar cautery, laser, heater probe, stapler, plasma coagulator)**
EXCLUDES *Small intestinal endoscopy, enteroscopy (44376-44379)*
7.02 7.02 FUD 000 J A2
AMA: 2018,Jan,8; 2017,Jan,8; 2016,Jan,13; 2015,Jan,16; 2014,Nov,3; 2014,Jan,11

44369 **with ablation of tumor(s), polyp(s), or other lesion(s) not amenable to removal by hot biopsy forceps, bipolar cautery or snare technique**
EXCLUDES *Small intestinal endoscopy, enteroscopy (44376-44379)*
7.19 7.19 FUD 000 J A2 80
AMA: 2014,Nov,3; 2014,Jan,11

44370 **with transendoscopic stent placement (includes predilation)**
EXCLUDES *Small intestinal endoscopy, enteroscopy (44376-44379)*
7.80 7.80 FUD 000 J J8 80
AMA: 2018,Jan,8; 2017,Jan,8; 2016,Jan,13; 2015,Jan,16; 2014,Nov,3; 2014,Jan,11

44372 **with placement of percutaneous jejunostomy tube**
EXCLUDES *Small intestinal endoscopy, enteroscopy (44376-44379)*
7.02 7.02 FUD 000 J A2
AMA: 2018,Jan,8; 2017,Jan,8; 2016,Jan,13; 2015,Jan,16; 2014,Nov,3; 2014,Jan,11

44373 **with conversion of percutaneous gastrostomy tube to percutaneous jejunostomy tube**
EXCLUDES *Jejunostomy, fiberoptic, through stoma (43235)*
Small intestinal endoscopy, enteroscopy (44376-44379)
5.62 5.62 FUD 000 J A2
AMA: 2018,Jan,8; 2017,Jan,8; 2016,Jan,13; 2015,Jan,16; 2014,Nov,3; 2014,Jan,11

44376 **Small intestinal endoscopy, enteroscopy beyond second portion of duodenum, including ileum; diagnostic, with or without collection of specimen(s) by brushing or washing (separate procedure)**
EXCLUDES *Small intestinal endoscopy, enteroscopy (44360-44373)*
8.33 8.33 FUD 000 J A2 80
AMA: 2018,Jan,8; 2017,Jan,8; 2016,Jan,13; 2015,Jan,16; 2014,Nov,3; 2014,Jan,11

44377 **with biopsy, single or multiple**
EXCLUDES *Small intestinal endoscopy, enteroscopy (44360-44373)*
8.77 8.77 FUD 000 J A2 80
AMA: 2018,Jan,8; 2017,Jan,8; 2016,Jan,13; 2015,Jan,16; 2014,Nov,3; 2014,Jan,11

44378 **with control of bleeding (eg, injection, bipolar cautery, unipolar cautery, laser, heater probe, stapler, plasma coagulator)**
EXCLUDES *Small intestinal endoscopy, enteroscopy (44360-44373)*
11.2 11.2 FUD 000 J A2 80
AMA: 2018,Jan,8; 2017,Jan,8; 2016,Jan,13; 2015,Jan,16; 2014,Nov,3; 2014,Jan,11

44379 **with transendoscopic stent placement (includes predilation)**
EXCLUDES *Small intestinal endoscopy, enteroscopy (44360-44373)*
11.9 11.9 FUD 000 J A2 80
AMA: 2018,Jan,8; 2017,Jan,8; 2016,Jan,13; 2015,Jan,16; 2014,Nov,3; 2014,Jan,11

44380-44384 [44381] Ileoscopy Via Stoma

INCLUDES Control of bleeding as result of endoscopic procedure during same operative session
EXCLUDES *Computed tomographic colonography (74261-74263)*
Code also exam of nonfunctional distal colon/rectum, when performed, with:
Anoscopy (46600, 46604-46606, 46608-46615)
Proctosigmoidoscopy (45300-45327)
Sigmoidoscopy (45330-45347 [45346])

44380 **Ileoscopy, through stoma; diagnostic, including collection of specimen(s) by brushing or washing, when performed (separate procedure)**
EXCLUDES *Ileoscopy, through stoma (44382-44384 [44381])*
1.64 4.97 FUD 000 T A2
AMA: 2018,Jan,8; 2017,Jan,8; 2016,Jan,13; 2015,Jan,16; 2014,Dec,3; 2014,Nov,3; 2014,Jan,11

44381 **Resequenced code. See code following 44382.**

44382 **with biopsy, single or multiple**
EXCLUDES *Ileoscopy, through stoma; diagnostic (44380)*
2.14 7.80 FUD 000 T A2
AMA: 2018,Jan,8; 2017,Jan,8; 2016,Jan,13; 2015,Jan,16; 2014,Dec,3; 2014,Nov,3; 2014,Jan,11

44381 **with transendoscopic balloon dilation**
EXCLUDES *Ileoscopy, through stoma (44380, 44384)*
Code also each additional stricture dilated in same session, using modifier 59 with (44381)
(74360)
2.44 27.0 FUD 000 J G2
AMA: 2018,Jan,8; 2017,Jan,8; 2016,Jan,13; 2015,Jan,16; 2014,Dec,3; 2014,Nov,3

44384 **with placement of endoscopic stent (includes pre- and post-dilation and guide wire passage, when performed)**
EXCLUDES *Ileoscopy, through stoma (44380-44381)*
(74360)
4.47 4.47 FUD 000 J G2
AMA: 2018,Jan,8; 2017,Jan,8; 2016,Jan,13; 2015,Jan,16; 2014,Dec,3; 2014,Nov,3

44385-44386 Endoscopy of Small Intestinal Pouch

INCLUDES Control of bleeding as result of the endoscopic procedure during same operative session
EXCLUDES *Computed tomographic colonography (74261-74263)*

44385 **Endoscopic evaluation of small intestinal pouch (eg, Kock pouch, ileal reservoir [S or J]); diagnostic, including collection of specimen(s) by brushing or washing, when performed (separate procedure)**
EXCLUDES *Endoscopic evaluation of small intestinal pouch (44386)*
2.09 5.60 FUD 000 T A2
AMA: 2018,Jan,8; 2017,Jan,8; 2016,Jan,13; 2015,Jan,16; 2014,Dec,3; 2014,Nov,3; 2014,Jan,11

44386 **with biopsy, single or multiple**
EXCLUDES *Endoscopic evaluation of small intestinal pouch (44385)*
2.60 8.36 FUD 000 T A2
AMA: 2018,Jan,8; 2017,Jan,8; 2016,Jan,13; 2015,Jan,16; 2014,Dec,3; 2014,Nov,3; 2014,Jan,11

44388-44408 [44401] Colonoscopy Via Stoma

INCLUDES Control of bleeding as result of endoscopic procedure during same operative session

EXCLUDES *Colonoscopy via rectum (45378, 45392-45393 [45390, 45398])*
Computed tomographic colonography (74261-74263)

Code also exam of nonfunctional distal colon/rectum, when performed, with:
Anoscopy (46600, 46604-46606, 46608-46615)
Proctosigmoidoscopy (45300-45327)
Sigmoidoscopy (45330-45347 [45346])

44388 **Colonoscopy through stoma; diagnostic, including collection of specimen(s) by brushing or washing, when performed (separate procedure)**

EXCLUDES *Colonoscopy through stoma (44389-44408 [44401])*
Code also modifier 53 when planned total colonoscopy cannot be completed
4.56 8.42 FUD 000 T A2
AMA: 2018,Jan,8; 2017,Jan,8; 2016,Jan,13; 2015,Jan,16; 2014,Dec,3; 2014,Nov,3; 2014,Jan,11

44389 **with biopsy, single or multiple**

EXCLUDES *Colonoscopy through stoma; diagnostic (44388)*
Colonoscopy through stoma; with endoscopic mucosal resection on the same lesion (44403)
Code also modifier 52 when colonoscope fails to reach the junction of the small intestine
5.02 11.0 FUD 000 T A2
AMA: 2018,Jan,8; 2017,Jan,8; 2016,Jan,13; 2015,Jan,16; 2014,Dec,3; 2014,Nov,3; 2014,Jan,11

44390 **with removal of foreign body(s)**

EXCLUDES *Colonoscopy through stoma; diagnostic (44388)*
Code also modifier 52 when colonoscope fails to reach the junction of the small intestine
(76000)
6.17 10.9 FUD 000 T A2
AMA: 2018,Jan,8; 2017,Jan,8; 2016,Jan,13; 2015,Jan,16; 2014,Dec,3; 2014,Nov,3; 2014,Jan,11

44391 **with control of bleeding, any method**

EXCLUDES *Colonoscopy through stoma; diagnostic (44388)*
Colonoscopy through stoma; with directed submucosal injection(s) on the same lesion (44404)
Code also modifier 52 when colonoscope fails to reach the junction of the small intestine
6.72 19.3 FUD 000 T A2
AMA: 2018,Jan,8; 2017,Jan,8; 2016,Jan,13; 2015,Jan,16; 2014,Dec,3; 2014,Nov,3; 2014,Jan,11

44392 **with removal of tumor(s), polyp(s), or other lesion(s) by hot biopsy forceps**

EXCLUDES *Colonoscopy through stoma; diagnostic (44388)*
Code also modifier 52 when colonoscope fails to reach the junction of the small intestine
5.82 10.2 FUD 000 T A2
AMA: 2018,Jan,8; 2017,Jan,8; 2016,Jan,13; 2015,Jan,16; 2014,Dec,3; 2014,Nov,3; 2014,Jan,11

44401 **with ablation of tumor(s), polyp(s), or other lesion(s) (includes pre-and post-dilation and guide wire passage, when performed)**

EXCLUDES *Colonoscopy through stoma; diagnostic (44388)*
Colonoscopy through stoma; with transendoscopic balloon dilation on the same lesion (44405)
Code also modifier 52 when colonoscope fails to reach the junction of the small intestine
7.09 86.2 FUD 000 T G2
AMA: 2018,Jan,8; 2017,Jan,8; 2016,Jan,13; 2015,Jan,16; 2014,Dec,3; 2014,Nov,3

44394 **with removal of tumor(s), polyp(s), or other lesion(s) by snare technique**

EXCLUDES *Colonoscopy through stoma; diagnostic (44388)*
Colonoscopy through stoma; with endoscopic mucosal resection on the same lesion (44403)
Code also modifier 52 when colonoscope fails to reach the junction of the small intestine
6.60 11.7 FUD 000 T A2
AMA: 2018,Jan,8; 2017,Jan,8; 2016,Jan,13; 2015,Jan,16; 2014,Dec,3; 2014,Nov,3; 2014,Jan,11

44401 **Resequenced code. See code following 44392.**

44402 **with endoscopic stent placement (including pre- and post-dilation and guide wire passage, when performed)**

EXCLUDES *Colonoscopy through stoma (44388, 44405)*
Code also modifier 52 when colonoscope fails to reach the junction of the small intestine
(74360)
7.66 7.66 FUD 000 J J8
AMA: 2018,Jan,8; 2017,Jan,8; 2016,Jan,13; 2015,Jan,16; 2014,Dec,3; 2014,Nov,3

44403 **with endoscopic mucosal resection**

EXCLUDES *Colonoscopy through stoma; diagnostic (44388)*
Colonoscopy through stoma on the same lesion (44389, 44394, 44404)
Code also modifier 52 when colonoscope fails to reach the junction of the small intestine
8.89 8.89 FUD 000 T G2
AMA: 2018,Jan,8; 2017,Jan,8; 2016,Jan,13; 2015,Jan,16; 2014,Dec,3; 2014,Nov,3

44404 **with directed submucosal injection(s), any substance**

EXCLUDES *Colonoscopy through stoma; diagnostic (44388)*
Colonoscopy through stoma on the same lesion (44391, 44403)
Code also modifier 52 when colonoscope fails to reach the junction of the small intestine
5.03 10.8 FUD 000 T G2
AMA: 2018,Jan,8; 2017,Jan,8; 2016,Jan,13; 2015,Jan,16; 2014,Dec,3; 2014,Nov,3

44405 **with transendoscopic balloon dilation**

EXCLUDES *Colonoscopy through stoma (44388, [44401], 44402)*
Code also each additional stricture dilated in same session, using modifier 59 with (44405)
Code also modifier 52 when colonoscope fails to reach the junction of the small intestine
(74360)
5.37 15.5 FUD 000 T G2
AMA: 2018,Jan,8; 2017,Jan,8; 2016,Jan,13; 2015,Jan,16; 2014,Dec,3; 2014,Nov,3

44406 **with endoscopic ultrasound examination, limited to the sigmoid, descending, transverse, or ascending colon and cecum and adjacent structures**

INCLUDES Gastrointestinal endoscopic ultrasound, supervision and interpretation (76975)

EXCLUDES *Colonoscopy through stoma (44388, 44407)*
Procedure performed more than one time per operative session
Code also modifier 52 when colonoscope fails to reach the junction of the small intestine
6.73 6.73 FUD 000 T G2
AMA: 2018,Jan,8; 2017,Jan,8; 2016,Jan,13; 2015,Jan,16; 2014,Dec,3; 2014,Nov,3

Digestive System

44388 — 44406

44407 with transendoscopic ultrasound guided intramural or transmural fine needle aspiration/biopsy(s), includes endoscopic ultrasound examination limited to the sigmoid, descending, transverse, or ascending colon and cecum and adjacent structures

INCLUDES Gastrointestinal endoscopic ultrasound, supervision and interpretation (76975)
Ultrasonic guidance (76942)

EXCLUDES *Colonoscopy through stoma (44388, 44406)*
Procedure performed more than one time per operative session

Code also modifier 52 when colonoscope fails to reach the junction of the small intestine

8.08 8.08 FUD 000 T G2

AMA: 2018,Jan,8; 2017,Jan,8; 2016,Jan,13; 2015,Jan,16; 2014,Dec,3; 2014,Nov,3

44408 with decompression (for pathologic distention) (eg, volvulus, megacolon), including placement of decompression tube, when performed

EXCLUDES *Colonoscopy through stoma; diagnostic (44388)*
Procedure performed more than one time per operative session

6.79 6.79 FUD 000 T G2

AMA: 2018,Jan,8; 2017,Jan,8; 2016,Jan,13; 2015,Jan,16; 2014,Dec,3; 2014,Nov,3

44500 Gastrointestinal Intubation

44500 Introduction of long gastrointestinal tube (eg, Miller-Abbott) (separate procedure)

EXCLUDES *Placement of oro- or naso-gastric tube (43752)*

(74340)

0.56 0.56 FUD 000 T G2 80

AMA: 2018,Jan,8; 2017,Jan,8; 2016,Sep,9; 2016,Jan,13; 2015,Jan,16; 2014,Jan,11

44602-44680 Open Repair Procedures of Intestines

44602 Suture of small intestine (enterorrhaphy) for perforated ulcer, diverticulum, wound, injury or rupture; single perforation

40.9 40.9 FUD 090 C 80

AMA: 2014,Jan,11

44603 multiple perforations

47.0 47.0 FUD 090 C 80

AMA: 2014,Jan,11

44604 Suture of large intestine (colorrhaphy) for perforated ulcer, diverticulum, wound, injury or rupture (single or multiple perforations); without colostomy

30.7 30.7 FUD 090 C 80

AMA: 2014,Jan,11

44605 with colostomy

37.7 37.7 FUD 090 C 80

AMA: 2014,Jan,11

44615 Intestinal stricturoplasty (enterotomy and enterorrhaphy) with or without dilation, for intestinal obstruction

31.1 31.1 FUD 090 C 80

AMA: 2014,Jan,11

44620 Closure of enterostomy, large or small intestine;

EXCLUDES *Laparoscopic method (44227)*

25.1 25.1 FUD 090 C 80

AMA: 2014,Jan,11

44625 with resection and anastomosis other than colorectal

EXCLUDES *Laparoscopic method (44227)*

29.4 29.4 FUD 090 C 80

AMA: 2014,Jan,11

44626 with resection and colorectal anastomosis (eg, closure of Hartmann type procedure)

EXCLUDES *Laparoscopic method (44227)*

46.4 46.4 FUD 090 C 80

AMA: 2014,Jan,11

44640 Closure of intestinal cutaneous fistula

40.6 40.6 FUD 090 C 80

AMA: 2014,Jan,11

44650 Closure of enteroenteric or enterocolic fistula

41.8 41.8 FUD 090 C 80

AMA: 2014,Jan,11

44660 Closure of enterovesical fistula; without intestinal or bladder resection

EXCLUDES *Closure of fistula:*
Gastrocolic (43880)
Rectovesical (45800, 45805)
Renocolic (50525-50526)

38.7 38.7 FUD 090 C 80

AMA: 2014,Jan,11

44661 with intestine and/or bladder resection

EXCLUDES *Closure of fistula:*
Gastrocolic (43880)
Rectovesical (45800, 45805)
Renocolic (50525-50526)

44.9 44.9 FUD 090 C 80

AMA: 2014,Jan,11

44680 Intestinal plication (separate procedure)

INCLUDES Noble intestinal plication

31.0 31.0 FUD 090 C 80

AMA: 2014,Jan,11

44700-44705 Other Intestinal Procedures

44700 Exclusion of small intestine from pelvis by mesh or other prosthesis, or native tissue (eg, bladder or omentum)

EXCLUDES *Therapeutic radiation clinical treatment (77261-77799 [77295, 77385, 77386, 77387, 77424, 77425])*

29.1 29.1 FUD 090 C 80

AMA: 2014,Jan,11

\+ **44701** Intraoperative colonic lavage (List separately in addition to code for primary procedure)

EXCLUDES *Appendectomy (44950-44960)*

Code first as appropriate (44140, 44145, 44150, 44604)

4.95 4.95 FUD ZZZ N N1 80

AMA: 2014,Jan,11

44705 Preparation of fecal microbiota for instillation, including assessment of donor specimen

EXCLUDES *Fecal instillation by enema or oro-nasogastric tube (44799)*
Therapeutic enema (74283)

2.16 3.25 FUD XXX B

AMA: 2018,Jan,8; 2017,Jan,8; 2016,Jan,13; 2015,Jan,16; 2014,Jan,11

44715-44799 Backbench Transplant Procedures

CMS: 100-04,3,90.6 Intestinal and Multi-Visceral Transplants

44715 Backbench standard preparation of cadaver or living donor intestine allograft prior to transplantation, including mobilization and fashioning of the superior mesenteric artery and vein

INCLUDES Mobilization/fashioning of superior mesenteric vein/artery

0.00 0.00 FUD XXX C 80

AMA: 2014,Jan,11

44720 Backbench reconstruction of cadaver or living donor intestine allograft prior to transplantation; venous anastomosis, each

7.99 7.99 FUD XXX C 80

AMA: 2014,Jan,11

44721 arterial anastomosis, each

11.1 11.1 FUD XXX C 80

AMA: 2018,Jan,8; 2017,Jan,8; 2016,Jan,13; 2015,Jan,16; 2014,Jan,11

44799 **Unlisted procedure, small intestine**

EXCLUDES *Unlisted colon procedure (45399)*

Unlisted intestinal procedure performed laparoscopically (44238)

Unlisted rectal procedure (45499, 45999)

0.00 0.00 FUD YYY T

AMA: 2018,Jan,8; 2017,Jan,8; 2016,Jan,13; 2015,Jan,16; 2014,Nov,3; 2014,Jan,11

44800-44899 Meckel's Diverticulum and Mesentery Procedures

44800 **Excision of Meckel's diverticulum (diverticulectomy) or omphalomesenteric duct**

22.2 22.2 FUD 090 C 80

AMA: 2014,Jan,11

44820 **Excision of lesion of mesentery (separate procedure)**

EXCLUDES *Resection of intestine (44120-44128, 44140-44160)*

24.2 24.2 FUD 090 C 80

AMA: 2014,Jan,11

44850 **Suture of mesentery (separate procedure)**

EXCLUDES *Internal hernia repair/reduction (44050)*

21.7 21.7 FUD 090 C 80

AMA: 2014,Jan,11

44899 **Unlisted procedure, Meckel's diverticulum and the mesentery**

0.00 0.00 FUD YYY C 80

AMA: 2014,Jan,11

44900-44979 Open and Endoscopic Appendix Procedures

44900 **Incision and drainage of appendiceal abscess, open**

EXCLUDES *Image guided percutaneous catheter drainage (49406)*

22.4 22.4 FUD 090 C 80

AMA: 2014,Jan,11

44950 **Appendectomy;**

INCLUDES Battle's operation

EXCLUDES *Procedure performed with other intra-abdominal procedure(s) when appendectomy is incidental*

18.6 18.6 FUD 090 J 80

AMA: 2018,Jan,8; 2017,Jan,8; 2016,Jan,13; 2015,Jan,16; 2014,Jan,11

Cecum

Swollen and inflamed appendix

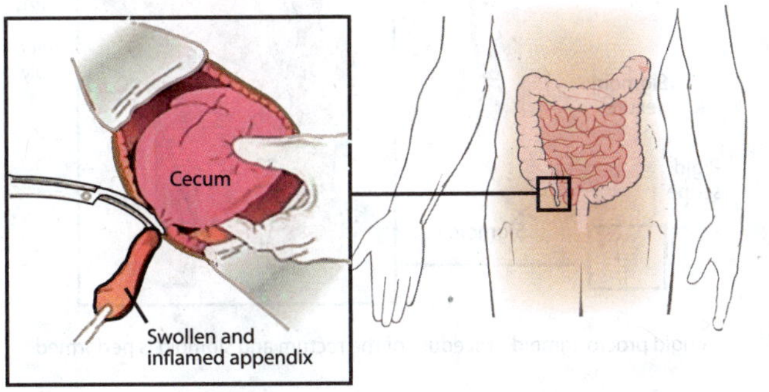

\+ **44955** **when done for indicated purpose at time of other major procedure (not as separate procedure) (List separately in addition to code for primary procedure)**

Code first primary procedure

2.45 2.45 FUD ZZZ N 80

AMA: 2018,Jan,8; 2017,Jan,8; 2016,Jan,13; 2015,Jan,16; 2014,Jan,11

44960 **for ruptured appendix with abscess or generalized peritonitis**

INCLUDES Battle's operation

25.4 25.4 FUD 090 C 80

AMA: 2018,Jan,8; 2017,Jan,8; 2016,Jan,13; 2015,Jan,16; 2014,Jan,11

44970 **Laparoscopy, surgical, appendectomy**

INCLUDES Diagnostic laparoscopy

17.4 17.4 FUD 090 J 80

AMA: 2018,Jan,8; 2017,Jan,8; 2016,Jan,13; 2015,Mar,3; 2015,Jan,16; 2014,Jan,11

44979 **Unlisted laparoscopy procedure, appendix**

0.00 0.00 FUD YYY J 80 50

AMA: 2018,Jan,8; 2017,Jan,8; 2016,Jan,13; 2015,Jan,16; 2014,Jan,11

45000-45190 Open and Transrectal Procedures of Rectum

45000 **Transrectal drainage of pelvic abscess**

EXCLUDES *Image guided transrectal catheter drainage (49407)*

12.2 12.2 FUD 090 T A2

AMA: 2014,Jan,11

45005 **Incision and drainage of submucosal abscess, rectum**

4.66 8.14 FUD 010 T A2

AMA: 2014,Jan,11

45020 **Incision and drainage of deep supralevator, pelvirectal, or retrorectal abscess**

EXCLUDES *Incision and drainage of perianal, ischiorectal, intramural abscess (46050, 46060)*

16.5 16.5 FUD 090 J A2

AMA: 2014,Jan,11

45100 **Biopsy of anorectal wall, anal approach (eg, congenital megacolon)**

EXCLUDES *Biopsy performed endoscopically (45305)*

8.64 8.64 FUD 090 J A2

AMA: 2014,Jan,11

45108 **Anorectal myomectomy**

10.7 10.7 FUD 090 J A2

AMA: 2014,Jan,11

45110 **Proctectomy; complete, combined abdominoperineal, with colostomy**

EXCLUDES *Laparoscopic method (45395)*

53.3 53.3 FUD 090 C 80

AMA: 2014,Jan,11

45111 **partial resection of rectum, transabdominal approach**

INCLUDES Luschka proctectomy

31.4 31.4 FUD 090 C 80

AMA: 2014,Jan,11

45112 **Proctectomy, combined abdominoperineal, pull-through procedure (eg, colo-anal anastomosis)**

EXCLUDES *Proctectomy for colo-anal anastomosis with creation of colonic pouch or reservoir (45119)*

54.0 54.0 FUD 090 C 80

AMA: 2014,Jan,11

45113 **Proctectomy, partial, with rectal mucosectomy, ileoanal anastomosis, creation of ileal reservoir (S or J), with or without loop ileostomy**

54.7 54.7 FUD 090 C 80

AMA: 2014,Jan,11

45114 **Proctectomy, partial, with anastomosis; abdominal and transsacral approach**

52.8 52.8 FUD 090 C 80

AMA: 2014,Jan,11

45116 **transsacral approach only (Kraske type)**

45.1 45.1 FUD 090 C 80

AMA: 2014,Jan,11

45119 **Proctectomy, combined abdominoperineal pull-through procedure (eg, colo-anal anastomosis), with creation of colonic reservoir (eg, J-pouch), with diverting enterostomy when performed**

EXCLUDES *Laparoscopic method (45397)*

55.9 55.9 FUD 090 C 80

AMA: 2018,Jan,8; 2017,Jan,8; 2016,Jan,13; 2015,Jan,16; 2014,Jan,11

45120 **Proctectomy, complete (for congenital megacolon), abdominal and perineal approach; with pull-through procedure and anastomosis (eg, Swenson, Duhamel, or Soave type operation)**
Facility RVU 46.2 Non-Facility RVU 46.2 **FUD** 090 C 80
AMA: 2014,Jan,11

45121 **with subtotal or total colectomy, with multiple biopsies**
Facility RVU 50.5 Non-Facility RVU 50.5 **FUD** 090 C 80
AMA: 2014,Jan,11

45123 **Proctectomy, partial, without anastomosis, perineal approach**
Facility RVU 32.4 Non-Facility RVU 32.4 **FUD** 090 C 80
AMA: 2014,Jan,11

45126 **Pelvic exenteration for colorectal malignancy, with proctectomy (with or without colostomy), with removal of bladder and ureteral transplantations, and/or hysterectomy, or cervicectomy, with or without removal of tube(s), with or without removal of ovary(s), or any combination thereof**
Facility RVU 80.5 Non-Facility RVU 80.5 **FUD** 090 C 80
AMA: 2014,Jan,11

45130 **Excision of rectal procidentia, with anastomosis; perineal approach**
INCLUDES Altemeier procedure
Facility RVU 31.4 Non-Facility RVU 31.4 **FUD** 090 C 80
AMA: 2014,Jan,11

45135 **abdominal and perineal approach**
INCLUDES Altemeier procedure
Facility RVU 37.6 Non-Facility RVU 37.6 **FUD** 090 C 80
AMA: 2014,Jan,11

45136 **Excision of ileoanal reservoir with ileostomy**
EXCLUDES *Enterolysis (44005)*
Ileostomy or jejunostomy, non-tube (44310)
Facility RVU 53.3 Non-Facility RVU 53.3 **FUD** 090 C 80
AMA: 2014,Jan,11

45150 **Division of stricture of rectum**
Facility RVU 12.0 Non-Facility RVU 12.0 **FUD** 090 T A2 80
AMA: 2014,Jan,11

45160 **Excision of rectal tumor by proctotomy, transsacral or transcoccygeal approach**
Facility RVU 29.7 Non-Facility RVU 29.7 **FUD** 090 J A2 80
AMA: 2014,Jan,11

45171 **Excision of rectal tumor, transanal approach; not including muscularis propria (ie, partial thickness)**
EXCLUDES *Transanal destruction of rectal tumor (45190)*
Transanal endoscopic microsurgical tumor excision (TEMS) (0184T)
Facility RVU 17.4 Non-Facility RVU 17.4 **FUD** 090 J G2 80
AMA: 2018,Jan,8; 2017,Jan,8; 2016,Jan,13; 2015,Jan,16; 2014,Jan,11

45172 **including muscularis propria (ie, full thickness)**
EXCLUDES *Transanal destruction of rectal tumor (45190)*
Transanal endoscopic microsurgical tumor excision (TEMS) (0184T)
Facility RVU 23.5 Non-Facility RVU 23.5 **FUD** 090 J G2 80
AMA: 2018,Feb,11; 2018,Jan,8; 2017,Jan,8; 2016,Jan,13; 2015,Jan,16; 2014,Jan,11

45190 **Destruction of rectal tumor (eg, electrodesiccation, electrosurgery, laser ablation, laser resection, cryosurgery) transanal approach**
EXCLUDES *Transanal endoscopic microsurgical tumor excision (TEMS) (0184T)*
Transanal excision of rectal tumor (45171-45172)
Facility RVU 20.1 Non-Facility RVU 20.1 **FUD** 090 J A2
AMA: 2018,Jan,8; 2017,Jan,8; 2016,Jan,13; 2015,Jan,16; 2014,Jan,11

45300-45327 Rigid Proctosigmoidoscopy Procedures

INCLUDES Control of bleeding as result of the endoscopic procedure during same operative session
Exam of:
Entire rectum
Portion of sigmoid colon

EXCLUDES *Computed tomographic colonography (74261-74263)*

Code also examination of colon through stoma:
Colonoscopy via stoma (44388-44408 [44401])
Ileoscopy via stoma (44380-44384 [44381])

45300 **Proctosigmoidoscopy, rigid; diagnostic, with or without collection of specimen(s) by brushing or washing (separate procedure)**
(74360)
Facility RVU 1.41 Non-Facility RVU 3.47 **FUD** 000 T P3
AMA: 2018,Jan,8; 2017,Jan,8; 2016,Jan,13; 2015,Jan,16; 2014,Jan,11

45303 **with dilation (eg, balloon, guide wire, bougie)**
(74360)
Facility RVU 2.47 Non-Facility RVU 26.3 **FUD** 000 T P2
AMA: 2018,Jan,8; 2017,Jan,8; 2016,Jan,13; 2015,Jan,16; 2014,Jan,11

45305 **with biopsy, single or multiple**
Facility RVU 2.11 Non-Facility RVU 4.38 **FUD** 000 T A2
AMA: 2018,Jan,8; 2017,Jan,8; 2016,Jan,13; 2015,Jan,16; 2014,Jan,11

45307 **with removal of foreign body**
Facility RVU 2.79 Non-Facility RVU 5.03 **FUD** 000 J A2 80
AMA: 2018,Jan,8; 2017,Jan,8; 2016,Jan,13; 2015,Jan,16; 2014,Jan,11

45308 **with removal of single tumor, polyp, or other lesion by hot biopsy forceps or bipolar cautery**
Facility RVU 2.43 Non-Facility RVU 4.93 **FUD** 000 J A2
AMA: 2018,Jan,8; 2017,Jan,8; 2016,Jan,13; 2015,Jan,16; 2014,Jan,11

A rigid proctosigmoid procedure of the rectum and sigmoid is performed

45309 **with removal of single tumor, polyp, or other lesion by snare technique**
Facility RVU 2.59 Non-Facility RVU 5.11 **FUD** 000 T A2
AMA: 2018,Jan,8; 2017,Jan,8; 2016,Jan,13; 2015,Jan,16; 2014,Jan,11

45315 **with removal of multiple tumors, polyps, or other lesions by hot biopsy forceps, bipolar cautery or snare technique**
Facility RVU 3.07 Non-Facility RVU 5.61 **FUD** 000 T A2
AMA: 2018,Jan,8; 2017,Jan,8; 2016,Jan,13; 2015,Jan,16; 2014,Jan,11

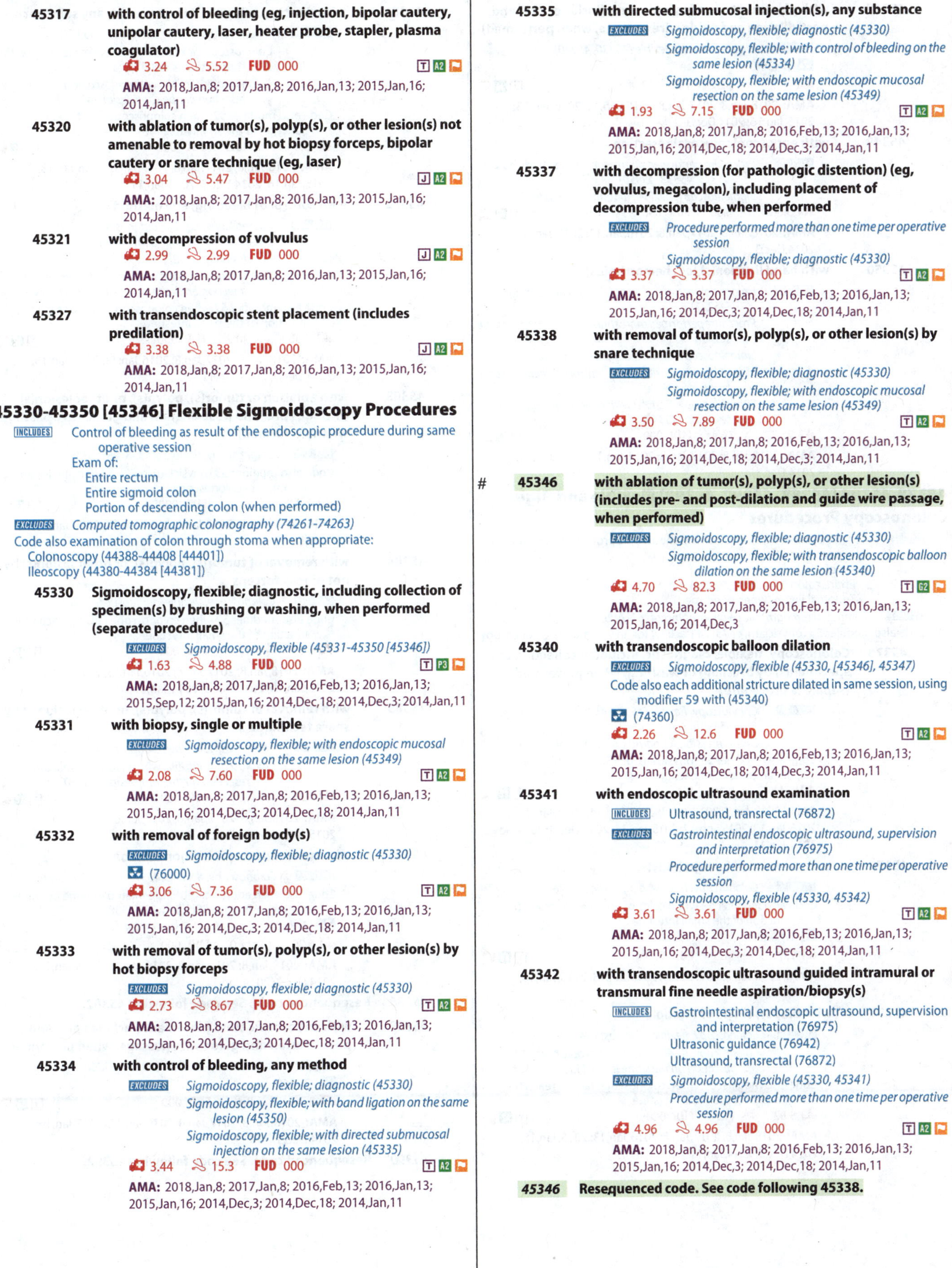

45317 **with control of bleeding (eg, injection, bipolar cautery, unipolar cautery, laser, heater probe, stapler, plasma coagulator)**
3.24 5.52 FUD 000 T A2
AMA: 2018,Jan,8; 2017,Jan,8; 2016,Jan,13; 2015,Jan,16; 2014,Jan,11

45320 **with ablation of tumor(s), polyp(s), or other lesion(s) not amenable to removal by hot biopsy forceps, bipolar cautery or snare technique (eg, laser)**
3.04 5.47 FUD 000 J A2
AMA: 2018,Jan,8; 2017,Jan,8; 2016,Jan,13; 2015,Jan,16; 2014,Jan,11

45321 **with decompression of volvulus**
2.99 2.99 FUD 000 J A2
AMA: 2018,Jan,8; 2017,Jan,8; 2016,Jan,13; 2015,Jan,16; 2014,Jan,11

45327 **with transendoscopic stent placement (includes predilation)**
3.38 3.38 FUD 000 J A2
AMA: 2018,Jan,8; 2017,Jan,8; 2016,Jan,13; 2015,Jan,16; 2014,Jan,11

45330-45350 [45346] Flexible Sigmoidoscopy Procedures

INCLUDES Control of bleeding as result of the endoscopic procedure during same operative session
Exam of:
Entire rectum
Entire sigmoid colon
Portion of descending colon (when performed)

EXCLUDES *Computed tomographic colonography (74261-74263)*

Code also examination of colon through stoma when appropriate:
Colonoscopy (44388-44408 [44401])
Ileoscopy (44380-44384 [44381])

45330 **Sigmoidoscopy, flexible; diagnostic, including collection of specimen(s) by brushing or washing, when performed (separate procedure)**
EXCLUDES *Sigmoidoscopy, flexible (45331-45350 [45346])*
1.63 4.88 FUD 000 T P3
AMA: 2018,Jan,8; 2017,Jan,8; 2016,Feb,13; 2016,Jan,13; 2015,Sep,12; 2015,Jan,16; 2014,Dec,18; 2014,Dec,3; 2014,Jan,11

45331 **with biopsy, single or multiple**
EXCLUDES *Sigmoidoscopy, flexible; with endoscopic mucosal resection on the same lesion (45349)*
2.08 7.60 FUD 000 T A2
AMA: 2018,Jan,8; 2017,Jan,8; 2016,Feb,13; 2016,Jan,13; 2015,Jan,16; 2014,Dec,3; 2014,Dec,18; 2014,Jan,11

45332 **with removal of foreign body(s)**
EXCLUDES *Sigmoidoscopy, flexible; diagnostic (45330)*
(76000)
3.06 7.36 FUD 000 T A2
AMA: 2018,Jan,8; 2017,Jan,8; 2016,Feb,13; 2016,Jan,13; 2015,Jan,16; 2014,Dec,3; 2014,Dec,18; 2014,Jan,11

45333 **with removal of tumor(s), polyp(s), or other lesion(s) by hot biopsy forceps**
EXCLUDES *Sigmoidoscopy, flexible; diagnostic (45330)*
2.73 8.67 FUD 000 T A2
AMA: 2018,Jan,8; 2017,Jan,8; 2016,Feb,13; 2016,Jan,13; 2015,Jan,16; 2014,Dec,3; 2014,Dec,18; 2014,Jan,11

45334 **with control of bleeding, any method**
EXCLUDES *Sigmoidoscopy, flexible; diagnostic (45330)*
Sigmoidoscopy, flexible; with band ligation on the same lesion (45350)
Sigmoidoscopy, flexible; with directed submucosal injection on the same lesion (45335)
3.44 15.3 FUD 000 T A2
AMA: 2018,Jan,8; 2017,Jan,8; 2016,Feb,13; 2016,Jan,13; 2015,Jan,16; 2014,Dec,3; 2014,Dec,18; 2014,Jan,11

45335 **with directed submucosal injection(s), any substance**
EXCLUDES *Sigmoidoscopy, flexible; diagnostic (45330)*
Sigmoidoscopy, flexible; with control of bleeding on the same lesion (45334)
Sigmoidoscopy, flexible; with endoscopic mucosal resection on the same lesion (45349)
1.93 7.15 FUD 000 T A2
AMA: 2018,Jan,8; 2017,Jan,8; 2016,Feb,13; 2016,Jan,13; 2015,Jan,16; 2014,Dec,18; 2014,Dec,3; 2014,Jan,11

45337 **with decompression (for pathologic distention) (eg, volvulus, megacolon), including placement of decompression tube, when performed**
EXCLUDES *Procedure performed more than one time per operative session*
Sigmoidoscopy, flexible; diagnostic (45330)
3.37 3.37 FUD 000 T A2
AMA: 2018,Jan,8; 2017,Jan,8; 2016,Feb,13; 2016,Jan,13; 2015,Jan,16; 2014,Dec,3; 2014,Dec,18; 2014,Jan,11

45338 **with removal of tumor(s), polyp(s), or other lesion(s) by snare technique**
EXCLUDES *Sigmoidoscopy, flexible; diagnostic (45330)*
Sigmoidoscopy, flexible; with endoscopic mucosal resection on the same lesion (45349)
3.50 7.89 FUD 000 T A2
AMA: 2018,Jan,8; 2017,Jan,8; 2016,Feb,13; 2016,Jan,13; 2015,Jan,16; 2014,Dec,18; 2014,Dec,3; 2014,Jan,11

45346 **with ablation of tumor(s), polyp(s), or other lesion(s) (includes pre- and post-dilation and guide wire passage, when performed)**
EXCLUDES *Sigmoidoscopy, flexible; diagnostic (45330)*
Sigmoidoscopy, flexible; with transendoscopic balloon dilation on the same lesion (45340)
4.70 82.3 FUD 000 T G2
AMA: 2018,Jan,8; 2017,Jan,8; 2016,Feb,13; 2016,Jan,13; 2015,Jan,16; 2014,Dec,3

45340 **with transendoscopic balloon dilation**
EXCLUDES *Sigmoidoscopy, flexible (45330, [45346], 45347)*
Code also each additional stricture dilated in same session, using modifier 59 with (45340)
(74360)
2.26 12.6 FUD 000 T A2
AMA: 2018,Jan,8; 2017,Jan,8; 2016,Feb,13; 2016,Jan,13; 2015,Jan,16; 2014,Dec,18; 2014,Dec,3; 2014,Jan,11

45341 **with endoscopic ultrasound examination**
INCLUDES Ultrasound, transrectal (76872)
EXCLUDES *Gastrointestinal endoscopic ultrasound, supervision and interpretation (76975)*
Procedure performed more than one time per operative session
Sigmoidoscopy, flexible (45330, 45342)
3.61 3.61 FUD 000 T A2
AMA: 2018,Jan,8; 2017,Jan,8; 2016,Feb,13; 2016,Jan,13; 2015,Jan,16; 2014,Dec,3; 2014,Dec,18; 2014,Jan,11

45342 **with transendoscopic ultrasound guided intramural or transmural fine needle aspiration/biopsy(s)**
INCLUDES Gastrointestinal endoscopic ultrasound, supervision and interpretation (76975)
Ultrasonic guidance (76942)
Ultrasound, transrectal (76872)
EXCLUDES *Sigmoidoscopy, flexible (45330, 45341)*
Procedure performed more than one time per operative session
4.96 4.96 FUD 000 T A2
AMA: 2018,Jan,8; 2017,Jan,8; 2016,Feb,13; 2016,Jan,13; 2015,Jan,16; 2014,Dec,3; 2014,Dec,18; 2014,Jan,11

45346 **Resequenced code. See code following 45338.**

Digestive System 45317 — 45346

45347 **with placement of endoscopic stent (includes pre- and post-dilation and guide wire passage, when performed)**

EXCLUDES *Sigmoidoscopy, flexible (45330, 45340)*

(74360)

4.52 4.52 FUD 000 J J8

AMA: 2018,Jan,8; 2017,Jan,8; 2016,Feb,13; 2016,Jan,13; 2015,Jan,16; 2014,Dec,3

45349 **with endoscopic mucosal resection**

EXCLUDES *Procedure performed on the same lesion with (45331, 45335, 45338, 45350)*
Sigmoidoscopy, flexible; diagnostic (45330)

5.80 5.80 FUD 000 T G2

AMA: 2018,Jan,8; 2017,Jan,8; 2016,Jan,13; 2015,Jan,16; 2014,Dec,3

45350 **with band ligation(s) (eg, hemorrhoids)**

EXCLUDES *Hemorrhoidectomy, internal, by rubber band ligation (46221)*
Procedure performed more than one time per operative session
Sigmoidoscopy, flexible; diagnostic (45330)
Sigmoidoscopy, flexible; with control of bleeding, same lesion (45334)
Sigmoidoscopy, flexible; with endoscopic mucosal resection (45349)

2.94 16.4 FUD 000 T G2

AMA: 2018,Jan,8; 2017,Jan,8; 2016,Jan,13; 2015,Jan,16; 2014,Dec,3

45378-45398 [45388, 45390, 45398] Flexible and Rigid Colonoscopy Procedures

INCLUDES Control of bleeding as result of the endoscopic procedure during same operative session
Exam of:
Entire colon (rectum to cecum)
Terminal ileum (when performed)

EXCLUDES *Computed tomographic colonography (74261-74263)*

Code also modifier 53 (physician), or 73, 74 (facility) for an incomplete colonoscopy

45378 **Colonoscopy, flexible; diagnostic, including collection of specimen(s) by brushing or washing, when performed (separate procedure)**

EXCLUDES *Colonoscopy, flexible (45379-45393 [45388, 45390, 45398])*
Decompression for pathological distention (45393)

Code also modifier 53 (physician), or 73, 74 (facility) for an incomplete colonoscopy

5.41 9.18 FUD 000 T A2

AMA: 2018,Jan,7; 2018,Jan,8; 2017,Sep,14; 2017,Jan,8; 2016,Jan,13; 2015,Sep,12; 2015,Jan,16; 2014,Dec,3; 2014,Nov,3; 2014,Jan,11

45379 **with removal of foreign body(s)**

EXCLUDES *Colonoscopy, flexible; diagnostic (45378)*

Code also modifier 52 when colonoscope fails to reach the junction of the small intestine

(76000)

7.00 11.8 FUD 000 T A2

AMA: 2018,Jan,8; 2017,Jan,8; 2016,Jan,13; 2015,Jan,16; 2014,Dec,3; 2014,Jan,11

45380 **with biopsy, single or multiple**

EXCLUDES *Colonoscopy, flexible; diagnostic (45378)*
Colonoscopy, flexible; with endoscopic mucosal resection on the same lesion (45390)

Code also modifier 52 when colonoscope fails to reach the junction of the small intestine

5.87 11.7 FUD 000 T A2

AMA: 2018,Jan,8; 2017,Jan,8; 2016,Jan,13; 2015,Jan,16; 2014,Dec,3; 2014,Jan,11

45381 **with directed submucosal injection(s), any substance**

EXCLUDES *Colonoscopy, flexible; diagnostic (45378)*
Colonoscopy, flexible; with control of bleeding on the same lesion (45382)
Colonoscopy, flexible; with endoscopic mucosal resection on the same lesion (45390)

Code also modifier 52 when colonoscope fails to reach the junction of the small intestine

5.87 11.5 FUD 000 T A2

AMA: 2018,Jan,8; 2017,Jan,8; 2017,Jan,6; 2016,Jan,13; 2015,Jan,16; 2014,Dec,3; 2014,Jan,11

45382 **with control of bleeding, any method**

EXCLUDES *Colonoscopy, flexible; diagnostic (45378)*
Colonoscopy, flexible; with band ligation on the same lesion ([45398])
Colonoscopy, flexible; with directed submucosal injection on the same lesion (45381)

Code also modifier 52 when colonoscope fails to reach the junction of the small intestine

7.58 20.2 FUD 000 T A2

AMA: 2018,Jan,8; 2017,Jan,8; 2016,Jan,13; 2015,Jan,16; 2014,Dec,3; 2014,Jan,11

\# **45388** **with ablation of tumor(s), polyp(s), or other lesion(s) (includes pre- and post-dilation and guide wire passage, when performed)**

EXCLUDES *Colonoscopy, flexible (45378, 45386)*

Code also modifier 53 (physician), or 73, 74 (facility) for an incomplete colonoscopy

7.92 86.8 FUD 000 T G2

AMA: 2018,Jan,8; 2017,Jan,8; 2016,Jan,13; 2015,Jan,16; 2014,Dec,3

45384 **with removal of tumor(s), polyp(s), or other lesion(s) by hot biopsy forceps**

EXCLUDES *Colonoscopy, flexible; diagnostic (45378)*

Code also modifier 52 when colonoscope fails to reach the junction of the small intestine

6.68 13.1 FUD 000 T A2

AMA: 2018,Jan,8; 2017,Jan,8; 2016,Jan,13; 2015,Jun,10; 2015,Jan,16; 2014,Dec,3; 2014,Jan,11

45385 **with removal of tumor(s), polyp(s), or other lesion(s) by snare technique**

EXCLUDES *Colonoscopy, flexible; diagnostic (45378)*
Colonoscopy, flexible; with endoscopic mucosal resection on the same lesion (45390)

7.45 12.3 FUD 000 T A2

AMA: 2018,Jan,8; 2017,Jan,8; 2017,Jan,6; 2016,Jan,13; 2015,Jan,16; 2014,Dec,3; 2014,Jan,11

45386 **with transendoscopic balloon dilation**

EXCLUDES *Colonoscopy, flexible (45378, [45388], 45389)*

Code also each additional stricture dilated in same operative session, using modifier 59 with (45386)

(74360)

6.20 17.0 FUD 000 T A2

AMA: 2018,Jan,8; 2017,Jan,8; 2016,Jan,13; 2015,Jan,16; 2014,Dec,3; 2014,Jan,11

45388 **Resequenced code. See code following 45382.**

45389 **with endoscopic stent placement (includes pre- and post-dilation and guide wire passage, when performed)**

EXCLUDES *Colonoscopy, flexible (45378, 45386)*

(74360)

8.49 8.49 FUD 000 J J8

AMA: 2018,Jan,8; 2017,Jan,8; 2016,Jan,13; 2015,Jan,16; 2014,Dec,3

45390 **Resequenced code. See code following 45392.**

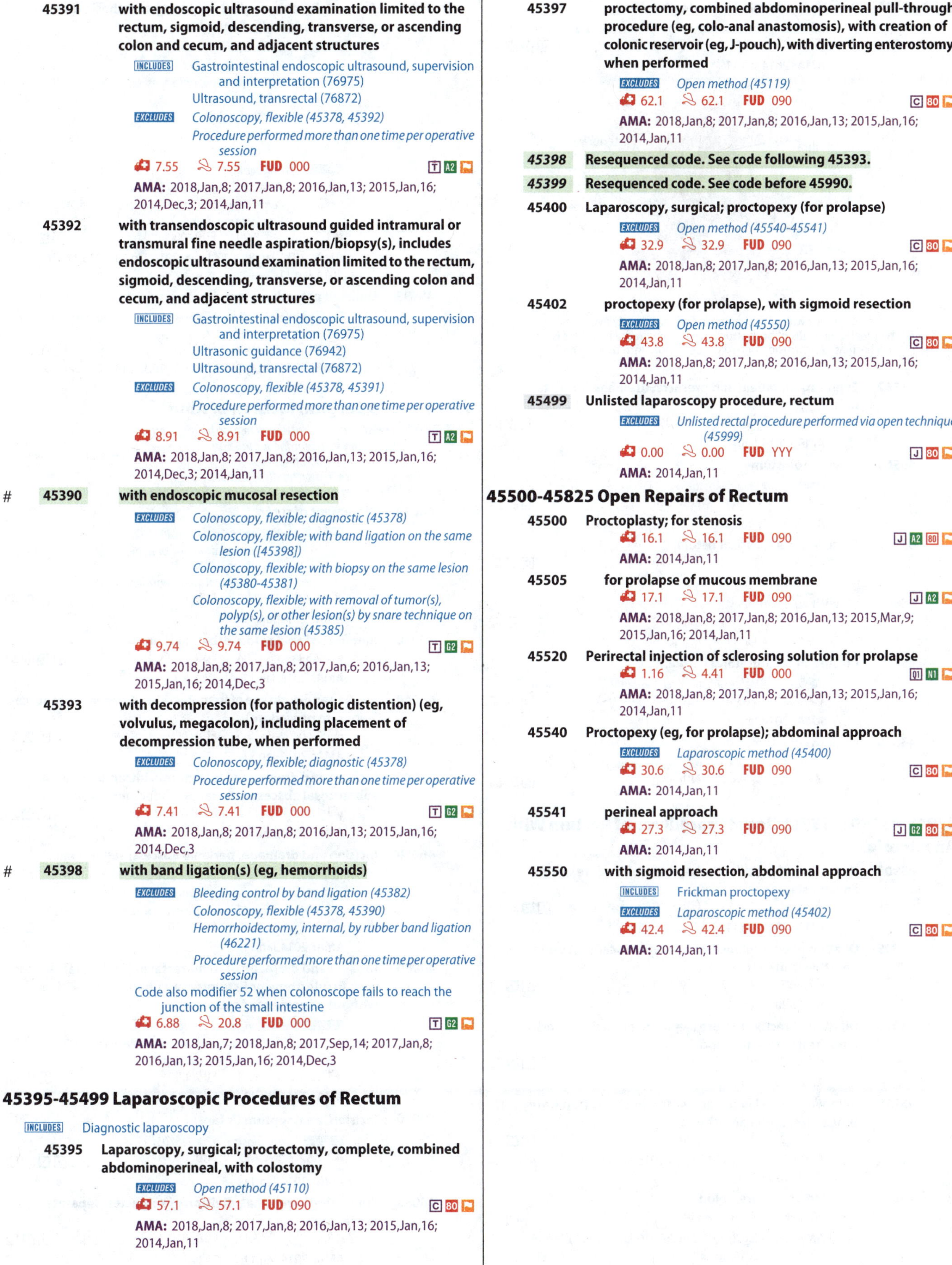

45391 with endoscopic ultrasound examination limited to the rectum, sigmoid, descending, transverse, or ascending colon and cecum, and adjacent structures

INCLUDES Gastrointestinal endoscopic ultrasound, supervision and interpretation (76975)
Ultrasound, transrectal (76872)

EXCLUDES *Colonoscopy, flexible (45378, 45392)*
Procedure performed more than one time per operative session

7.55 7.55 FUD 000 T A2

AMA: 2018,Jan,8; 2017,Jan,8; 2016,Jan,13; 2015,Jan,16; 2014,Dec,3; 2014,Jan,11

45392 with transendoscopic ultrasound guided intramural or transmural fine needle aspiration/biopsy(s), includes endoscopic ultrasound examination limited to the rectum, sigmoid, descending, transverse, or ascending colon and cecum, and adjacent structures

INCLUDES Gastrointestinal endoscopic ultrasound, supervision and interpretation (76975)
Ultrasonic guidance (76942)
Ultrasound, transrectal (76872)

EXCLUDES *Colonoscopy, flexible (45378, 45391)*
Procedure performed more than one time per operative session

8.91 8.91 FUD 000 T A2

AMA: 2018,Jan,8; 2017,Jan,8; 2016,Jan,13; 2015,Jan,16; 2014,Dec,3; 2014,Jan,11

45390 with endoscopic mucosal resection

EXCLUDES *Colonoscopy, flexible; diagnostic (45378)*
Colonoscopy, flexible; with band ligation on the same lesion ([45398])
Colonoscopy, flexible; with biopsy on the same lesion (45380-45381)
Colonoscopy, flexible; with removal of tumor(s), polyp(s), or other lesion(s) by snare technique on the same lesion (45385)

9.74 9.74 FUD 000 T G2

AMA: 2018,Jan,8; 2017,Jan,8; 2017,Jan,6; 2016,Jan,13; 2015,Jan,16; 2014,Dec,3

45393 with decompression (for pathologic distention) (eg, volvulus, megacolon), including placement of decompression tube, when performed

EXCLUDES *Colonoscopy, flexible; diagnostic (45378)*
Procedure performed more than one time per operative session

7.41 7.41 FUD 000 T G2

AMA: 2018,Jan,8; 2017,Jan,8; 2016,Jan,13; 2015,Jan,16; 2014,Dec,3

45398 with band ligation(s) (eg, hemorrhoids)

EXCLUDES *Bleeding control by band ligation (45382)*
Colonoscopy, flexible (45378, 45390)
Hemorrhoidectomy, internal, by rubber band ligation (46221)
Procedure performed more than one time per operative session

Code also modifier 52 when colonoscope fails to reach the junction of the small intestine

6.88 20.8 FUD 000 T G2

AMA: 2018,Jan,7; 2018,Jan,8; 2017,Sep,14; 2017,Jan,8; 2016,Jan,13; 2015,Jan,16; 2014,Dec,3

45395-45499 Laparoscopic Procedures of Rectum

INCLUDES Diagnostic laparoscopy

45395 Laparoscopy, surgical; proctectomy, complete, combined abdominoperineal, with colostomy

EXCLUDES *Open method (45110)*

57.1 57.1 FUD 090 C 80

AMA: 2018,Jan,8; 2017,Jan,8; 2016,Jan,13; 2015,Jan,16; 2014,Jan,11

45397 proctectomy, combined abdominoperineal pull-through procedure (eg, colo-anal anastomosis), with creation of colonic reservoir (eg, J-pouch), with diverting enterostomy, when performed

EXCLUDES *Open method (45119)*

62.1 62.1 FUD 090 C 80

AMA: 2018,Jan,8; 2017,Jan,8; 2016,Jan,13; 2015,Jan,16; 2014,Jan,11

45398 Resequenced code. See code following 45393.

45399 Resequenced code. See code before 45990.

45400 Laparoscopy, surgical; proctopexy (for prolapse)

EXCLUDES *Open method (45540-45541)*

32.9 32.9 FUD 090 C 80

AMA: 2018,Jan,8; 2017,Jan,8; 2016,Jan,13; 2015,Jan,16; 2014,Jan,11

45402 proctopexy (for prolapse), with sigmoid resection

EXCLUDES *Open method (45550)*

43.8 43.8 FUD 090 C 80

AMA: 2018,Jan,8; 2017,Jan,8; 2016,Jan,13; 2015,Jan,16; 2014,Jan,11

45499 Unlisted laparoscopy procedure, rectum

EXCLUDES *Unlisted rectal procedure performed via open technique (45999)*

0.00 0.00 FUD YYY J 80

AMA: 2014,Jan,11

45500-45825 Open Repairs of Rectum

45500 Proctoplasty; for stenosis

16.1 16.1 FUD 090 J A2 80

AMA: 2014,Jan,11

45505 for prolapse of mucous membrane

17.1 17.1 FUD 090 J A2

AMA: 2018,Jan,8; 2017,Jan,8; 2016,Jan,13; 2015,Mar,9; 2015,Jan,16; 2014,Jan,11

45520 Perirectal injection of sclerosing solution for prolapse

1.16 4.41 FUD 000 Q1 N1

AMA: 2018,Jan,8; 2017,Jan,8; 2016,Jan,13; 2015,Jan,16; 2014,Jan,11

45540 Proctopexy (eg, for prolapse); abdominal approach

EXCLUDES *Laparoscopic method (45400)*

30.6 30.6 FUD 090 C 80

AMA: 2014,Jan,11

45541 perineal approach

27.3 27.3 FUD 090 J G2 80

AMA: 2014,Jan,11

45550 with sigmoid resection, abdominal approach

INCLUDES Frickman proctopexy

EXCLUDES *Laparoscopic method (45402)*

42.4 42.4 FUD 090 C 80

AMA: 2014,Jan,11

45560 **Repair of rectocele (separate procedure)**

EXCLUDES *Posterior colporrhaphy with rectocele repair (57250)*

19.7 19.7 FUD 090 J A2 80

AMA: 2014,Jan,11

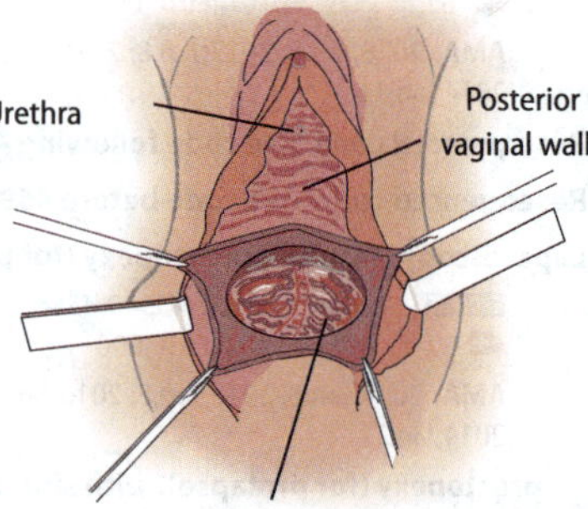

Urethra

Posterior vaginal wall

The posterior wall of the vagina is opened directly over the rectocele; the walls of both structures are repaired; a rectocele is a herniated protrusion of part of the rectum into the vagina

45562 **Exploration, repair, and presacral drainage for rectal injury;**

32.4 32.4 FUD 090 C 80

AMA: 2014,Jan,11

45563 **with colostomy**

INCLUDES Maydl colostomy

47.9 47.9 FUD 090 C 80

AMA: 2014,Jan,11

45800 **Closure of rectovesical fistula;**

36.4 36.4 FUD 090 C 80

AMA: 2014,Jan,11

45805 **with colostomy**

42.5 42.5 FUD 090 C 80

AMA: 2014,Jan,11

45820 **Closure of rectourethral fistula;**

EXCLUDES *Closure of fistula, rectovaginal (57300-57308)*

36.7 36.7 FUD 090 C 80

AMA: 2014,Jan,11

45825 **with colostomy**

EXCLUDES *Closure of fistula, rectovaginal (57300-57308)*

44.4 44.4 FUD 090 C 80

AMA: 2014,Jan,11

45900-45999 [45399] Closed Procedures of Rectum With Anesthesia

45900 **Reduction of procidentia (separate procedure) under anesthesia**

5.83 5.83 FUD 010 T A2 80

AMA: 2014,Jan,11

45905 **Dilation of anal sphincter (separate procedure) under anesthesia other than local**

4.87 4.87 FUD 010 T A2

AMA: 2014,Jan,11

45910 **Dilation of rectal stricture (separate procedure) under anesthesia other than local**

5.53 5.53 FUD 010 T A2

AMA: 2014,Jan,11

45915 **Removal of fecal impaction or foreign body (separate procedure) under anesthesia**

6.59 9.70 FUD 010 T A2

AMA: 2018,Jan,8; 2017,Jan,8; 2016,Jan,13; 2015,Jan,16; 2014,Jan,11

45399 **Unlisted procedure, colon**

0.00 0.00 FUD YYY T

AMA: 2018,Jan,8; 2017,Jan,8; 2016,Jan,13; 2015,Jan,16; 2014,Dec,3; 2014,Nov,3

45990 **Anorectal exam, surgical, requiring anesthesia (general, spinal, or epidural), diagnostic**

INCLUDES Diagnostic:
- Anoscopy
- Proctoscopy, rigid

Exam:
- Pelvic (when performed)
- Perineal, external
- Rectal, digital

EXCLUDES *Anogenital examination (99170)*
Anoscopy; diagnostic (46600)
Pelvic examination under anesthesia (57410)
Proctosigmoidoscopy, rigid (45300-45327)

3.09 3.09 FUD 000 J A2 80

AMA: 2018,Jan,8; 2017,Jan,8; 2016,Jan,13; 2015,Jan,16; 2014,Jan,11

45999 **Unlisted procedure, rectum**

EXCLUDES *Unlisted rectal procedure performed laparoscopically (45499)*

0.00 0.00 FUD YYY T 80

AMA: 2018,Jan,8; 2017,Jan,8; 2016,Jan,13; 2015,Jan,16; 2014,Jan,11

46020-46083 Surgical Incision of Anus

EXCLUDES *Cryosurgical destruction of hemorrhoid(s) (46999)*
Fistulotomy, subcutaneous (46270)
Hemorrhoidopexy ([46947])
Injection of hemorrhoid(s) (46500)
Thermal energy destruction of internal hemorrhoid(s) (46930)

46020 **Placement of seton**

EXCLUDES *Anoscopy; diagnostic (46600)*
Incision and drainage of ischiorectal or intramural abscess (46060)
Surgical anal fistula treatment (46280)

6.79 8.00 FUD 010 J A2

AMA: 2014,Jan,11

46030 **Removal of anal seton, other marker**

2.59 4.04 FUD 010 T A2 80

AMA: 2014,Jan,11

46040 **Incision and drainage of ischiorectal and/or perirectal abscess (separate procedure)**

12.0 15.5 FUD 090 T A2

AMA: 2014,Jan,11

46045 **Incision and drainage of intramural, intramuscular, or submucosal abscess, transanal, under anesthesia**

12.5 12.5 FUD 090 J A2

AMA: 2014,Jan,11

46050 **Incision and drainage, perianal abscess, superficial**

EXCLUDES *Incision and drainage abscess:*
Ischiorectal/intramural (46060)
Supralevator/pelvirectal/retrorectal (45020)

2.82 5.98 FUD 010 T A2

AMA: 2014,Jan,11

46060 **Incision and drainage of ischiorectal or intramural abscess, with fistulectomy or fistulotomy, submuscular, with or without placement of seton**

EXCLUDES *Incision and drainage abscess:*
Supralevator/pelvirectal/retrorectal (45020)
Placement of seton (46020)

13.8 13.8 FUD 090 J A2

AMA: 2014,Jan,11

46070 **Incision, anal septum (infant)** A

EXCLUDES *Anoplasty (46700-46705)*

7.52 7.52 FUD 090 63 J G2 80

AMA: 2014,Jan,11

46080 **Sphincterotomy, anal, division of sphincter (separate procedure)**

4.59 7.41 FUD 010 J A2

AMA: 2014,Jan,11

46083 **Incision of thrombosed hemorrhoid, external**
3.08 5.24 FUD 010 T P2
AMA: 2018,Jan,8; 2017,Jan,8; 2016,Jan,13; 2015,Jan,16; 2014,Jan,11

46200-46262 [46220, 46320, 46945, 46946, 46948] Anal Resection and Hemorrhoidectomies

EXCLUDES *Cryosurgical destruction of hemorrhoid(s) (46999)*
Hemorrhoidopexy ([46947])
Injection of hemorrhoid(s) (46500)
Thermal energy destruction of internal hemorrhoid(s) (46930)

46200 **Fissurectomy, including sphincterotomy, when performed**
9.45 13.0 FUD 090 J A2
AMA: 2014,Jan,11

46220 **Resequenced code. See code before 46230.**

46221 **Hemorrhoidectomy, internal, by rubber band ligation(s)**
EXCLUDES *Colonoscopy or sigmoidoscopy, flexible; with band ligation (45350, [45398])*
Transanal hemorrhoidal dearterialization, two or more columns/groups ([46948])
5.51 7.77 FUD 010 T P3
AMA: 2018,Jan,7; 2018,Jan,8; 2017,Sep,14; 2017,Jan,8; 2016,Jan,13; 2015,Apr,10; 2015,Jan,16; 2014,Dec,3; 2014,Jan,11

▲ # 46945 **Hemorrhoidectomy, internal, by ligation other than rubber band; single hemorrhoid column/group, without imaging guidance**
EXCLUDES *Transanal hemorrhoidal dearterialization, two or more columns/groups ([46948])*
Ultrasonic guidance (76942)
Ultrasonic guidance, intraoperative (76998)
Ultrasound, transrectal (76872)
6.54 9.08 FUD 090 J P3
AMA: 2018,Jan,8; 2017,Jan,8; 2016,Jan,13; 2015,Apr,10; 2014,Jan,11

▲ # 46946 **2 or more hemorrhoid columns/groups, without imaging guidance**
EXCLUDES *Transanal hemorrhoidal dearterialization, two or more columns/groups ([46948])*
Ultrasonic guidance (76942)
Ultrasonic guidance, intraoperative (76998)
Ultrasound, transrectal (76872)
6.50 9.17 FUD 090 J A2
AMA: 2018,Jan,8; 2017,Jan,8; 2016,Jan,13; 2015,Apr,10; 2014,Jan,11

● # 46948 **Hemorrhoidectomy, internal, by transanal hemorrhoidal dearterialization, 2 or more hemorrhoid columns/groups, including ultrasound guidance, with mucopexy, when performed**
0.00 0.00 FUD 000
EXCLUDES *Transanal hemorrhoidal dearterialization, single column/group (46999)*
Ultrasonic guidance (76942)
Ultrasonic guidance, intraoperative (76998)
Ultrasound, transrectal (76872)

46220 **Excision of single external papilla or tag, anus**
3.44 6.22 FUD 010 T A2
AMA: 2014,Jan,11

46230 **Excision of multiple external papillae or tags, anus**
4.99 8.11 FUD 010 J A2
AMA: 2014,Jan,11

46320 **Excision of thrombosed hemorrhoid, external**
3.22 5.43 FUD 010 T P3
AMA: 2014,Jan,11

46250 **Hemorrhoidectomy, external, 2 or more columns/groups**
EXCLUDES *Hemorrhoidectomy, external, single column/group (46999)*
Transanal hemorrhoidal dearterialization, two or more columns/groups ([46948])
9.13 13.4 FUD 090 J A2
AMA: 2014,Jan,11

46255 **Hemorrhoidectomy, internal and external, single column/group;**
EXCLUDES *Transanal hemorrhoidal dearterialization, two or more columns/groups ([46948])*
10.2 14.7 FUD 090 J A2
AMA: 2018,Jan,8; 2017,Jan,8; 2016,Jan,13; 2015,Jan,16; 2014,Oct,14; 2014,Jan,11

46257 **with fissurectomy**
EXCLUDES *Transanal hemorrhoidal dearterialization, two or more columns/groups ([46948])*
12.2 12.2 FUD 090 J A2
AMA: 2014,Jan,11

46258 **with fistulectomy, including fissurectomy, when performed**
EXCLUDES *Transanal hemorrhoidal dearterialization, two or more columns/groups ([46948])*
13.5 13.5 FUD 090 J A2 80
AMA: 2014,Jan,11

46260 **Hemorrhoidectomy, internal and external, 2 or more columns/groups;**
INCLUDES Whitehead hemorrhoidectomy
EXCLUDES *Transanal hemorrhoidal dearterialization, two or more columns/groups ([46948])*
13.7 13.7 FUD 090 J A2
AMA: 2014,Jan,11

46261 **with fissurectomy**
EXCLUDES *Transanal hemorrhoidal dearterialization, two or more columns/groups ([46948])*
15.0 15.0 FUD 090 J A2
AMA: 2014,Jan,11

46262 **with fistulectomy, including fissurectomy, when performed**
EXCLUDES *Transanal hemorrhoidal dearterialization, two or more columns/groups ([46948])*
16.0 16.0 FUD 090 J A2
AMA: 2018,Jan,8; 2017,Jan,8; 2016,Jan,13; 2015,Jan,16; 2014,Jan,11

46270-46320 Resection of Anal Fistula

46270 **Surgical treatment of anal fistula (fistulectomy/fistulotomy); subcutaneous**
11.3 14.8 FUD 090 J A2
AMA: 2014,Jan,11

46275 **intersphincteric**
11.9 15.6 FUD 090 J A2
AMA: 2014,Jan,11

46280 **transsphincteric, suprasphincteric, extrasphincteric or multiple, including placement of seton, when performed**
EXCLUDES *Placement of seton (46020)*
13.6 13.6 FUD 090 J A2
AMA: 2014,Jan,11

46285 **second stage**
11.9 15.5 FUD 090 J A2
AMA: 2014,Jan,11

46288 **Closure of anal fistula with rectal advancement flap**
15.8 15.8 FUD 090 J A2
AMA: 2014,Jan,11

46320 **Resequenced code. See code following 46230.**

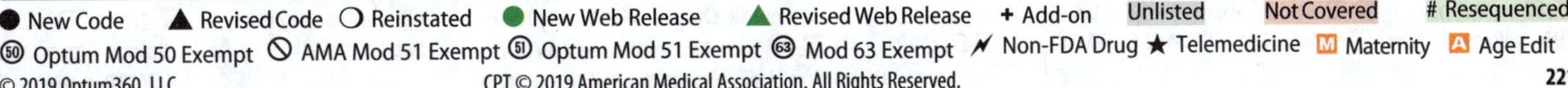

46500 Other Hemorrhoid Procedures

EXCLUDES *Anoscopic injection of bulking agent, submucosal, for fecal incontinence (46999)*

46500 **Injection of sclerosing solution, hemorrhoids**
5.12 8.23 FUD 010 T P3
AMA: 2018,Jan,8; 2017,Jan,8; 2016,Jan,13; 2015,Jan,16; 2014,Jan,11

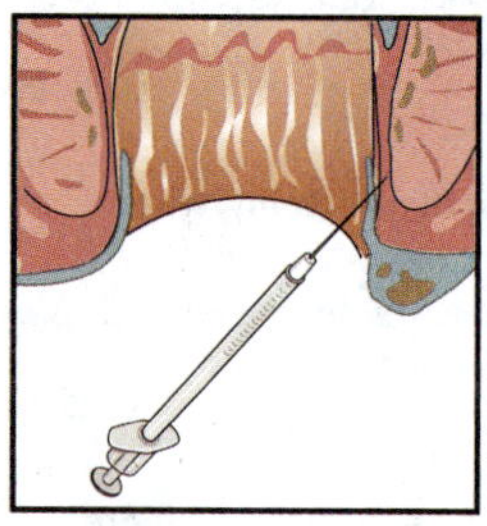

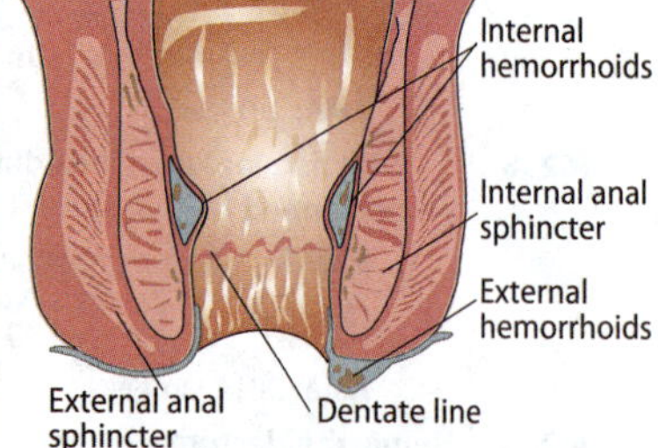

A sclerosing agent is injected into the tissues underlying hemorrhoids

46505 Chemodenervation Anal Sphincter

EXCLUDES *Chemodenervation of:*
Extremity muscles (64642-64645)
Muscles/facial nerve (64612)
Neck muscles (64616)
Other peripheral nerve/branch (64640)
Pudendal nerve (64630)
Trunk muscles (64646-64647)

Code also drug(s)/substance(s) given

46505 **Chemodenervation of internal anal sphincter**
6.93 8.35 FUD 010 T G2 50
AMA: 2019,Apr,9; 2018,Jan,8; 2017,Jan,8; 2016,Jan,13; 2015,Jan,16; 2014,Jan,11

46600-46615 Anoscopic Procedures

EXCLUDES *Delivery of thermal energy via anoscope to the muscle of the anal canal (46999)*
Injection of bulking agent, submucosal, for fecal incontinence (46999)

46600 **Anoscopy; diagnostic, including collection of specimen(s) by brushing or washing, when performed (separate procedure)**
EXCLUDES *Excision of rectal tumor, transanal endoscopic microsurgical approach (ie, TEMS) (0184T)*
High-resolution anoscopy (HRA), diagnostic (46601)
Surgical incision of anus (46020-46761 [46220, 46320, 46320, 46945, 46946, 46947, 46948])
1.18 2.72 FUD 000 Q1 N1
AMA: 2018,Jan,7; 2018,Jan,8; 2017,Jan,8; 2016,Jan,13; 2015,Jan,16; 2014,Jan,11

46601 **diagnostic, with high-resolution magnification (HRA) (eg, colposcope, operating microscope) and chemical agent enhancement, including collection of specimen(s) by brushing or washing, when performed**
INCLUDES Operating microscope (69990)
2.70 3.97 FUD 000 Q1 N1
AMA: 2018,Oct,11; 2016,Feb,12

46604 **with dilation (eg, balloon, guide wire, bougie)**
1.90 18.3 FUD 000 T P2
AMA: 2018,Jan,8; 2017,Jan,8; 2016,Jan,13; 2015,Jan,16; 2014,Jan,11

46606 **with biopsy, single or multiple**
EXCLUDES *High resolution anoscopy (HRA) with biopsy (46607)*
2.17 6.89 FUD 000 T P3
AMA: 2019,Sep,10; 2018,Jan,8; 2017,Jan,8; 2016,Jan,13; 2015,Jan,16; 2014,Jan,11

46607 **with high-resolution magnification (HRA) (eg, colposcope, operating microscope) and chemical agent enhancement, with biopsy, single or multiple**
INCLUDES Operating microscope (69990)
3.64 5.59 FUD 000 T G2
AMA: 2018,Oct,11; 2016,Feb,12

46608 **with removal of foreign body**
2.43 7.26 FUD 000 T A2
AMA: 2018,Jan,8; 2017,Jan,8; 2016,Jan,13; 2015,Jan,16; 2014,Jan,11

46610 **with removal of single tumor, polyp, or other lesion by hot biopsy forceps or bipolar cautery**
2.32 6.89 FUD 000 J A2
AMA: 2018,Jan,8; 2017,Jan,8; 2016,Jan,13; 2015,Jan,16; 2014,Jan,11

46611 **with removal of single tumor, polyp, or other lesion by snare technique**
2.33 5.43 FUD 000 T A2
AMA: 2018,Jan,8; 2017,Jan,8; 2016,Jan,13; 2015,Jan,16; 2014,Jan,11

46612 **with removal of multiple tumors, polyps, or other lesions by hot biopsy forceps, bipolar cautery or snare technique**
2.75 8.39 FUD 000 J A2
AMA: 2018,Jan,8; 2017,Jan,8; 2016,Jan,13; 2015,Jan,16; 2014,Jan,11

46614 **with control of bleeding (eg, injection, bipolar cautery, unipolar cautery, laser, heater probe, stapler, plasma coagulator)**
1.87 3.97 FUD 000 T P3
AMA: 2018,Jan,8; 2017,Jan,8; 2016,Jan,13; 2015,Jan,16; 2014,Jan,11

46615 **with ablation of tumor(s), polyp(s), or other lesion(s) not amenable to removal by hot biopsy forceps, bipolar cautery or snare technique**
2.64 4.34 FUD 000 J A2
AMA: 2018,Jan,8; 2017,Jan,8; 2016,Jan,13; 2015,Jan,16; 2014,Jan,11

46700-46947 [46947] Anal Repairs and Stapled Hemorrhoidopexy

46700 **Anoplasty, plastic operation for stricture; adult**
18.9 18.9 FUD 090 J A2
AMA: 2014,Jan,11

46705 **infant** A
EXCLUDES *Anal septum incision (46070)*
16.1 16.1 FUD 090 63 C 80
AMA: 2014,Jan,11

46706 **Repair of anal fistula with fibrin glue**
5.10 5.10 FUD 010 J A2
AMA: 2014,Jan,11

46707 **Repair of anorectal fistula with plug (eg, porcine small intestine submucosa [SIS])**
14.2 14.2 FUD 090 J G2 80
AMA: 2018,Jan,8; 2017,Jan,8; 2016,Jan,13; 2015,Jan,16; 2014,Jan,11

46710 **Repair of ileoanal pouch fistula/sinus (eg, perineal or vaginal), pouch advancement; transperineal approach**
32.1 32.1 FUD 090 C 80
AMA: 2018,Jan,8; 2017,Jan,8; 2016,Jan,13; 2015,Jan,16; 2014,Jan,11

46712 **combined transperineal and transabdominal approach**
64.7 64.7 FUD 090 C 80
AMA: 2018,Jan,8; 2017,Jan,8; 2016,Jan,13; 2015,Jan,16; 2014,Jan,11

46715 Repair of low imperforate anus; with anoperineal fistula (cut-back procedure)
15.7 15.7 FUD 090
AMA: 2014,Jan,11

46716 with transposition of anoperineal or anovestibular fistula
35.1 35.1 FUD 090
AMA: 2014,Jan,11

46730 Repair of high imperforate anus without fistula; perineal or sacroperineal approach
57.0 57.0 FUD 090
AMA: 2014,Jan,11

46735 combined transabdominal and sacroperineal approaches
65.8 65.8 FUD 090
AMA: 2014,Jan,11

46740 Repair of high imperforate anus with rectourethral or rectovaginal fistula; perineal or sacroperineal approach
62.3 62.3 FUD 090
AMA: 2014,Jan,11

46742 combined transabdominal and sacroperineal approaches
72.2 72.2 FUD 090
AMA: 2014,Jan,11

46744 Repair of cloacal anomaly by anorectovaginoplasty and urethroplasty, sacroperineal approach ♀
102. 102. FUD 090
AMA: 2014,Jan,11

46746 Repair of cloacal anomaly by anorectovaginoplasty and urethroplasty, combined abdominal and sacroperineal approach; ♀
113. 113. FUD 090
AMA: 2014,Jan,11

46748 with vaginal lengthening by intestinal graft or pedicle flaps ♀
122. 122. FUD 090
AMA: 2014,Jan,11

46750 Sphincteroplasty, anal, for incontinence or prolapse; adult
21.6 21.6 FUD 090
AMA: 2014,Jan,11

46751 child
19.0 19.0 FUD 090
AMA: 2014,Jan,11

46753 Graft (Thiersch operation) for rectal incontinence and/or prolapse
17.7 17.7 FUD 090
AMA: 2014,Jan,11

46754 Removal of Thiersch wire or suture, anal canal
6.75 9.03 FUD 010
AMA: 2014,Jan,11

46760 Sphincteroplasty, anal, for incontinence, adult; muscle transplant
31.7 31.7 FUD 090
AMA: 2014,Jan,11

46761 levator muscle imbrication (Park posterior anal repair)
26.4 26.4 FUD 090
AMA: 2014,Jan,11

46947 Hemorrhoidopexy (eg, for prolapsing internal hemorrhoids) by stapling
11.0 11.0 FUD 090
AMA: 2018,Jan,8; 2017,Jan,8; 2016,Jan,13; 2015,Jan,16; 2014,Jan,11

46900-46999 Destruction Procedures: Anus

46900 Destruction of lesion(s), anus (eg, condyloma, papilloma, molluscum contagiosum, herpetic vesicle), simple; chemical
3.92 6.76 FUD 010
AMA: 2014,Jan,11

46910 electrodesiccation
3.86 7.39 FUD 010
AMA: 2014,Jan,11

46916 cryosurgery
4.14 6.83 FUD 010
AMA: 2014,Jan,11

46917 laser surgery
3.73 12.2 FUD 010
AMA: 2014,Jan,11

46922 surgical excision
3.92 8.00 FUD 010
AMA: 2014,Jan,11

46924 Destruction of lesion(s), anus (eg, condyloma, papilloma, molluscum contagiosum, herpetic vesicle), extensive (eg, laser surgery, electrosurgery, cryosurgery, chemosurgery)
5.21 15.1 FUD 010
AMA: 2014,Jan,11

46930 Destruction of internal hemorrhoid(s) by thermal energy (eg, infrared coagulation, cautery, radiofrequency)

EXCLUDES *Other hemorrhoid procedures:*
Cryosurgery destruction (46999)
Excision ([46320], 46250-46262)
Hemorrhoidopexy ([46947])
Incision (46083)
Injection sclerosing solution (46500)
Ligation (46221, [46945, 46946])

4.28 6.02 FUD 090
AMA: 2018,Jan,8; 2017,Jan,8; 2016,Jul,8; 2016,Jan,13; 2015,Apr,10; 2014,Jan,11

46940 Curettage or cautery of anal fissure, including dilation of anal sphincter (separate procedure); initial
4.20 6.79 FUD 010
AMA: 2014,Jan,11

46942 subsequent
3.78 6.48 FUD 010
AMA: 2014,Jan,11

46945 **Resequenced code. See code following 46221.**

46946 **Resequenced code. See code following resequenced code 46945.**

46947 **Resequenced code. See code following 46761.**

46948 **Resequenced code. See code before resequenced code 46220.**

46999 Unlisted procedure, anus
0.00 0.00 FUD YYY
AMA: 2018,Oct,11; 2018,Jan,8; 2017,Jan,8; 2016,Jan,13; 2015,Apr,10; 2015,Jan,16; 2014,Jan,11

47000-47001 Needle Biopsy of Liver

EXCLUDES *Fine needle aspiration (10021, [10004, 10005, 10006, 10007, 10008, 10009, 10010, 10011, 10012])*

47000 Biopsy of liver, needle; percutaneous
(76942, 77002, 77012, 77021)
(88172-88173)
2.58 8.72 FUD 000
AMA: 2019,Apr,4; 2018,Jan,8; 2017,Jan,8; 2016,Jan,13; 2015,Jan,16; 2014,Jan,11

Digestive System

46715 — 47000

● New Code ▲ Revised Code ○ Reinstated ● New Web Release ▲ Revised Web Release + Add-on Unlisted Not Covered # Resequenced
Optum Mod 50 Exempt AMA Mod 51 Exempt Optum Mod 51 Exempt Mod 63 Exempt Non-FDA Drug ★ Telemedicine Maternity Age Edit

+ **47001** **when done for indicated purpose at time of other major procedure (List separately in addition to code for primary procedure)**

Code first primary procedure

(76942, 77002)

(88172-88173)

3.02 3.02 FUD ZZZ N NI

AMA: 2018,Jan,8; 2017,Jan,8; 2016,Jan,13; 2015,Jan,16; 2014,Jan,11

47010-47130 Open Incisional and Resection Procedures of Liver

47010 **Hepatotomy, for open drainage of abscess or cyst, 1 or 2 stages**

EXCLUDES *Image guided percutaneous catheter drainage (49505)*

35.1 35.1 FUD 090 C 80

AMA: 2014,Jan,11

47015 **Laparotomy, with aspiration and/or injection of hepatic parasitic (eg, amoebic or echinococcal) cyst(s) or abscess(es)**

33.7 33.7 FUD 090 C 80

AMA: 2014,Jan,11

47100 **Biopsy of liver, wedge**

24.5 24.5 FUD 090 C 80

AMA: 2014,Jan,11

47120 **Hepatectomy, resection of liver; partial lobectomy**

67.7 67.7 FUD 090 C 80

AMA: 2018,Jan,8; 2017,Jan,8; 2016,Oct,11; 2016,Jan,13; 2015,Jan,16; 2014,Sep,13; 2014,Jan,11

47122 **trisegmentectomy**

99.6 99.6 FUD 090 C 80

AMA: 2014,Jan,11

47125 **total left lobectomy**

89.5 89.5 FUD 090 C 80

AMA: 2014,Jan,11

47130 **total right lobectomy**

96.2 96.2 FUD 090 C 80

AMA: 2014,Jan,11

47133-47147 Liver Transplant Procedures

CMS: 100-03,260.1 Adult Liver Transplantation; 100-03,260.2 Pediatric Liver Transplantation; 100-04,3,90.4 Liver Transplants; 100-04,3,90.4.1 Standard Liver Acquisition Charge; 100-04,3,90.4.2 Billing for Liver Transplant and Acquisition Services; 100-04,3,90.6 Intestinal and Multi-Visceral Transplants

47133 **Donor hepatectomy (including cold preservation), from cadaver donor**

INCLUDES Graft:
- Cold preservation
- Harvest

0.00 0.00 FUD XXX C

AMA: 2014,Jan,11

47135 **Liver allotransplantation, orthotopic, partial or whole, from cadaver or living donor, any age**

INCLUDES Partial/whole recipient hepatectomy
Partial/whole transplant of allograft
Recipient care

156. 156. FUD 090 C 80

AMA: 2018,Jan,8; 2017,Jan,8; 2016,Jan,13; 2015,Jan,16; 2014,Jan,11

47140 **Donor hepatectomy (including cold preservation), from living donor; left lateral segment only (segments II and III)**

INCLUDES Donor care
Graft:
- Cold preservation
- Harvest

103. 103. FUD 090 C 80

AMA: 2018,Jan,8; 2017,Jan,8; 2016,Jan,13; 2015,Jan,16; 2014,Jan,11

47141 **total left lobectomy (segments II, III and IV)**

INCLUDES Donor care
Graft:
- Cold preservation
- Harvest

124. 124. FUD 090 C 80

AMA: 2014,Jan,11

47142 **total right lobectomy (segments V, VI, VII and VIII)**

INCLUDES Donor care
Graft:
- Cold preservation
- Harvest

136. 136. FUD 090 C 80

AMA: 2014,Jan,11

47143 **Backbench standard preparation of cadaver donor whole liver graft prior to allotransplantation, including cholecystectomy, if necessary, and dissection and removal of surrounding soft tissues to prepare the vena cava, portal vein, hepatic artery, and common bile duct for implantation; without trisegment or lobe split**

EXCLUDES *Cholecystectomy (47600, 47610)*
Hepatectomy (47120-47125)

0.00 0.00 FUD XXX C 80

AMA: 2018,Jan,8; 2017,Jan,8; 2016,Jan,13; 2015,Jan,16; 2014,Jan,11

47144 **with trisegment split of whole liver graft into 2 partial liver grafts (ie, left lateral segment [segments II and III] and right trisegment [segments I and IV through VIII])**

EXCLUDES *Cholecystectomy (47600, 47610)*
Hepatectomy (47120-47125)

0.00 0.00 FUD 090 C 80

AMA: 2014,Jan,11

47145 **with lobe split of whole liver graft into 2 partial liver grafts (ie, left lobe [segments II, III, and IV] and right lobe [segments I and V through VIII])**

EXCLUDES *Cholecystectomy (47600, 47610)*
Hepatectomy (47120-47125)

0.00 0.00 FUD XXX C 80

AMA: 2014,Jan,11

47146 **Backbench reconstruction of cadaver or living donor liver graft prior to allotransplantation; venous anastomosis, each**

EXCLUDES *Cholecystectomy (47600, 47610)*
Hepatectomy (47120-47125)

9.43 9.43 FUD XXX C 80

AMA: 2014,Jan,11

47147 **arterial anastomosis, each**

EXCLUDES *Cholecystectomy (47600, 47610)*
Hepatectomy (47120-47125)

11.1 11.1 FUD XXX C 80

AMA: 2014,Jan,11

47300-47362 Open Repair of Liver

47300 **Marsupialization of cyst or abscess of liver**
32.8 32.8 FUD 090 C 80
AMA: 2014,Jan,11

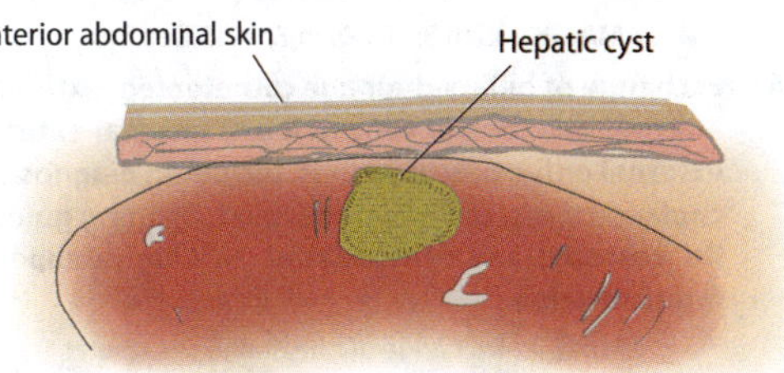

Cutaway view of liver

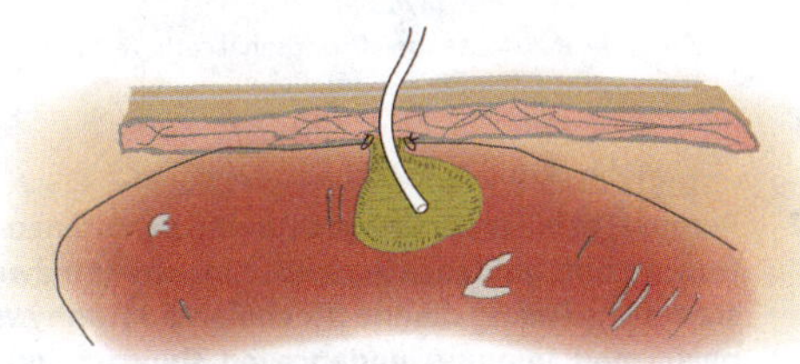
Marsupialization of cyst

A liver cyst or abscess is marsupialized; this method involves surgical access to the cyst and making an incision into it; the edges of the cyst are sutured to the abdominal wall and drainage, open or closed, is placed into the cyst

47350 **Management of liver hemorrhage; simple suture of liver wound or injury**
39.7 39.7 FUD 090 C 80
AMA: 2014,Jan,11

47360 **complex suture of liver wound or injury, with or without hepatic artery ligation**
54.5 54.5 FUD 090 C 80
AMA: 2014,Jan,11

47361 **exploration of hepatic wound, extensive debridement, coagulation and/or suture, with or without packing of liver**
88.0 88.0 FUD 090 C 80
AMA: 2014,Jan,11

47362 **re-exploration of hepatic wound for removal of packing**
42.1 42.1 FUD 090 C 80
AMA: 2014,Jan,11

47370-47379 Laparoscopic Ablation Liver Tumors

INCLUDES Diagnostic laparoscopy (49320)

47370 **Laparoscopy, surgical, ablation of 1 or more liver tumor(s); radiofrequency**
(76940)
36.2 36.2 FUD 090 J 80
AMA: 2018,Jan,8; 2017,Jan,8; 2016,Jan,13; 2015,Jan,16; 2014,Jan,11

47371 **cryosurgical**
(76940)
36.5 36.5 FUD 090 J 80
AMA: 2014,Jan,11

47379 **Unlisted laparoscopic procedure, liver**
0.00 0.00 FUD YYY J 80
AMA: 2018,Aug,10; 2018,Jan,8; 2017,Jan,8; 2016,Jan,13; 2015,Jan,16; 2014,Dec,18; 2014,Jan,11

47380-47399 Open/Percutaneous Ablation Liver Tumors

47380 **Ablation, open, of 1 or more liver tumor(s); radiofrequency**
(76940)
41.8 41.8 FUD 090 C 80
AMA: 2018,Jan,8; 2017,Jan,8; 2016,Jan,13; 2015,Jan,16; 2014,Jan,11

47381 **cryosurgical**
(76940)
43.0 43.0 FUD 090 C 80
AMA: 2014,Jan,11

47382 **Ablation, 1 or more liver tumor(s), percutaneous, radiofrequency**
(76940, 77013, 77022)
21.5 130. FUD 010 J G2
AMA: 2018,Jan,8; 2017,Jan,8; 2016,Jan,13; 2015,Jan,16; 2014,Jan,11

47383 **Ablation, 1 or more liver tumor(s), percutaneous, cryoablation**
(76940, 77013, 77022)
13.2 196. FUD 010 J J8
AMA: 2018,Jan,8; 2017,Jan,8; 2016,Jan,13; 2015,Jan,16; 2014,Dec,18

47399 **Unlisted procedure, liver**
0.00 0.00 FUD YYY T
AMA: 2018,Jan,8; 2017,Mar,10; 2017,Jan,8; 2016,Jan,13; 2015,Jan,16; 2014,Dec,18; 2014,Jan,11

47400-47490 Biliary Tract Procedures

47400 **Hepaticotomy or hepaticostomy with exploration, drainage, or removal of calculus**
62.6 62.6 FUD 090 C 80
AMA: 2014,Jan,11

47420 **Choledochotomy or choledochostomy with exploration, drainage, or removal of calculus, with or without cholecystotomy; without transduodenal sphincterotomy or sphincteroplasty**
38.9 38.9 FUD 090 C 80
AMA: 2014,Jan,11

47425 **with transduodenal sphincterotomy or sphincteroplasty**
39.7 39.7 FUD 090 C 80
AMA: 2014,Jan,11

47460 **Transduodenal sphincterotomy or sphincteroplasty, with or without transduodenal extraction of calculus (separate procedure)**
36.8 36.8 FUD 090 C 80
AMA: 2014,Jan,11

47480 **Cholecystotomy or cholecystostomy, open, with exploration, drainage, or removal of calculus (separate procedure)**
EXCLUDES *Percutaneous cholecystostomy (47490)*
25.4 25.4 FUD 090 C 80
AMA: 2018,Jan,8; 2017,Jan,8; 2016,Jan,13; 2015,Jan,16; 2014,Jan,11

47490 **Cholecystostomy, percutaneous, complete procedure, including imaging guidance, catheter placement, cholecystogram when performed, and radiological supervision and interpretation**

INCLUDES Radiological guidance (75989, 76942, 77002, 77012, 77021)

EXCLUDES *Injection procedure for cholangiography (47531-47532)*
Open cholecystostomy (47480)

9.56 9.56 FUD 010 J

AMA: 2018,Jan,8; 2017,Jan,8; 2016,Jan,13; 2015,Dec,3; 2015,Jan,16; 2014,Jan,11

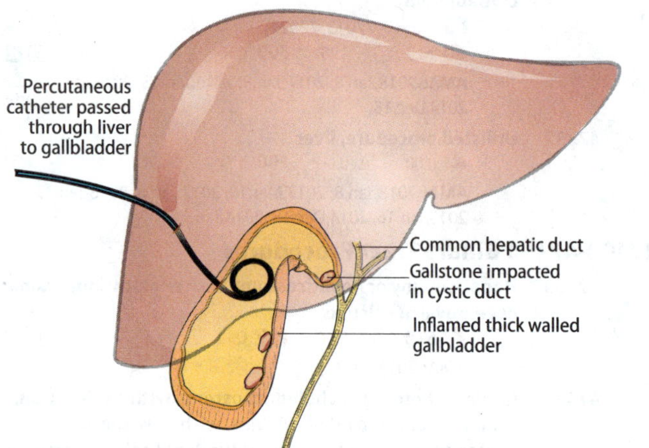

47531-47532 Injection/Insertion Procedures of Biliary Tract

INCLUDES Contrast material injection
Radiologic supervision and interpretation

EXCLUDES *Intraoperative cholangiography (74300-74301)*
Procedures performed via the same access (47490, 47533-47541)

47531 **Injection procedure for cholangiography, percutaneous, complete diagnostic procedure including imaging guidance (eg, ultrasound and/or fluoroscopy) and all associated radiological supervision and interpretation; existing access**

2.06 9.89 FUD 000 Q2 N1

AMA: 2018,Jan,8; 2017,Jan,8; 2015,Dec,3

47532 **new access (eg, percutaneous transhepatic cholangiogram)**

6.18 23.2 FUD 000 Q2 N1

AMA: 2018,Jan,8; 2017,Jan,8; 2015,Dec,3

47533-47544 Percutaneous Procedures of the Biliary Tract

47533 **Placement of biliary drainage catheter, percutaneous, including diagnostic cholangiography when performed, imaging guidance (eg, ultrasound and/or fluoroscopy), and all associated radiological supervision and interpretation; external**

EXCLUDES *Conversion to internal-external drainage catheter (47535)*
Percutaneous placement stent in bile duct (47538)
Placement stent into bile duct, new access (47540)
Replacement existing internal drainage catheter (47536)

7.74 35.2 FUD 000 J G2

AMA: 2018,Jan,8; 2017,Jan,8; 2015,Dec,3

47534 **internal-external**

EXCLUDES *Conversion to external only drainage catheter (47536)*
Percutaneous placement stent in bile duct (47538)
Placement stent into bile duct, new access (47540)

10.8 41.0 FUD 000 J G2

AMA: 2018,Jan,8; 2017,Jan,8; 2015,Dec,3

47535 **Conversion of external biliary drainage catheter to internal-external biliary drainage catheter, percutaneous, including diagnostic cholangiography when performed, imaging guidance (eg, fluoroscopy), and all associated radiological supervision and interpretation**

5.75 28.4 FUD 000 J G2

AMA: 2018,Jan,8; 2017,Jan,8; 2015,Dec,3

47536 **Exchange of biliary drainage catheter (eg, external, internal-external, or conversion of internal-external to external only), percutaneous, including diagnostic cholangiography when performed, imaging guidance (eg, fluoroscopy), and all associated radiological supervision and interpretation**

INCLUDES Exchange of one drainage catheter

EXCLUDES *Placement of stent(s) into a bile duct, percutaneous (47538)*

Code also exchange of additional catheters in same session with modifier 59 (47536)

3.84 19.5 FUD 000 J G2

AMA: 2018,Jan,8; 2017,Jan,8; 2015,Dec,3

47537 **Removal of biliary drainage catheter, percutaneous, requiring fluoroscopic guidance (eg, with concurrent indwelling biliary stents), including diagnostic cholangiography when performed, imaging guidance (eg, fluoroscopy), and all associated radiological supervision and interpretation**

EXCLUDES *Placement of stent(s) into a bile duct via the same access (47538)*
Removal without use of fluoroscopic guidance; report with appropriate E&M service code

2.79 11.5 FUD 000 Q2 G2

AMA: 2018,Jan,8; 2017,Jan,8; 2015,Dec,3

47538 **Placement of stent(s) into a bile duct, percutaneous, including diagnostic cholangiography, imaging guidance (eg, fluoroscopy and/or ultrasound), balloon dilation, catheter exchange(s) and catheter removal(s) when performed, and all associated radiological supervision and interpretation; existing access**

EXCLUDES *Drainage catheter inserted following stent placement (47536)*
Procedures performed via the same access (47536-47537)
Treatment of same lesion in same operative session ([43277], 47542, 47555-47556)

Code also multiple stents placed during same session when: (47538-47540)
Serial stents placed within the same bile duct;
Stent placement via two or more percutaneous access sites or the space between two other stents
Two or more stents inserted through the same percutaneous access

6.88 121. FUD 000 J J8

AMA: 2018,Jan,8; 2017,Jan,8; 2016,Mar,10; 2015,Dec,3

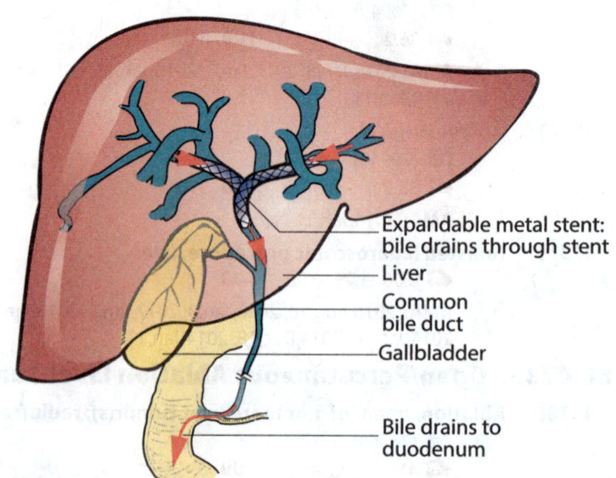

47539 **new access, without placement of separate biliary drainage catheter**

EXCLUDES *Treatment of same lesion in same session ([43277], 47542, 47555-47556)*

Code also multiple stents placed during same session when: (47538-47540)

Serial stents placed within the same bile duct

Stent placement via two or more percutaneous access sites or the space between two other stents

Two or more stents inserted through the same percutaneous access

12.4 135. FUD 000 J J8

AMA: 2018,Jan,8; 2017,Jan,8; 2016,Mar,10; 2015,Dec,3

47540 **new access, with placement of separate biliary drainage catheter (eg, external or internal-external)**

EXCLUDES *Procedure performed via the same access (47533-47534)*

Treatment of same lesion in same session ([43277], 47542, 47555-47556)

Code also multiple stents placed during same session when: (47538-47540)

Serial stents placed within the same bile duct;

Stent placement via two or more percutaneous access sites or the space between two other stents;

Two or more stents inserted through the same percutaneous access

12.8 137. FUD 000 J J8

AMA: 2018,Jan,8; 2017,Jan,8; 2016,Mar,10; 2015,Dec,3

47541 **Placement of access through the biliary tree and into small bowel to assist with an endoscopic biliary procedure (eg, rendezvous procedure), percutaneous, including diagnostic cholangiography when performed, imaging guidance (eg, ultrasound and/or fluoroscopy), and all associated radiological supervision and interpretation, new access**

EXCLUDES *Access through biliary tree into small bowel for endoscopic biliary procedure (47535-47537)*

Conversion, exchange, or removal of external biliary drainage catheter (47535-47537)

Injection procedure for cholangiography (47531-47532)

Placement of biliary drainage catheter (47533-47534)

Placement of stent(s) into a bile duct (47538-47540)

Procedure performed when previous catheter access exists

9.64 33.8 FUD 000 J G2

AMA: 2018,Jan,8; 2017,Jan,8; 2015,Dec,3

\+ **47542** **Balloon dilation of biliary duct(s) or of ampulla (sphincteroplasty), percutaneous, including imaging guidance (eg, fluoroscopy), and all associated radiological supervision and interpretation, each duct (List separately in addition to code for primary procedure)**

EXCLUDES *Biliary endoscopy, with dilation of biliary duct stricture (47555-47556)*

Endoscopic balloon dilation ([43277], 47555-47556)

Endoscopic retrograde cholangiopancreatography (ERCP) (43262, [43277])

Placement of stent(s) into a bile duct (47538-47540)

Procedure performed with balloon used to remove calculi, debris, sludge without dilation (47544)

Code also one additional dilation code when more than one dilation performed in same session, using modifier 59 with (47542)

Code first (47531-47537, 47541)

3.94 13.9 FUD ZZZ N N1

AMA: 2018,Jan,8; 2017,Jan,8; 2015,Dec,3

\+ **47543** **Endoluminal biopsy(ies) of biliary tree, percutaneous, any method(s) (eg, brush, forceps, and/or needle), including imaging guidance (eg, fluoroscopy), and all associated radiological supervision and interpretation, single or multiple (List separately in addition to code for primary procedure)**

EXCLUDES *Endoscopic biopsy (46261, 47553)*

Endoscopic brushings (43260, 47552)

Procedure performed more than one time per session

Code first (47531-47540)

4.20 13.3 FUD ZZZ N N1

AMA: 2018,Jan,8; 2017,Jan,8; 2015,Dec,3

\+ **47544** **Removal of calculi/debris from biliary duct(s) and/or gallbladder, percutaneous, including destruction of calculi by any method (eg, mechanical, electrohydraulic, lithotripsy) when performed, imaging guidance (eg, fluoroscopy), and all associated radiological supervision and interpretation (List separately in addition to code for primary procedure)**

EXCLUDES *Device deployment without findings of calculi/debris*

Endoscopic calculi removal/destruction (43264-43265, 47554)

Endoscopic retrograde cholangiopancreatography (ERCP); with removal of calculi/debris from biliary/pancreatic duct(s) (43264)

Procedures with removal of incidental debris (47531-47543)

Code first when debris removal not incidental, as appropriate (47531-47540)

4.61 29.2 FUD ZZZ N N1

AMA: 2018,Jan,8; 2017,Jan,8; 2015,Dec,3

47550-47556 Endoscopic Procedures of the Biliary Tract

INCLUDES Diagnostic endoscopy (49320)

EXCLUDES *Endoscopic retrograde cholangiopancreatography (ERCP) (43260-43265, [43274], [43275], [43276], [43277], [43278], 74328-74330, 74363)*

\+ **47550** **Biliary endoscopy, intraoperative (choledochoscopy) (List separately in addition to code for primary procedure)**

Code first primary procedure

4.80 4.80 FUD ZZZ C 80

AMA: 2014,Jan,11

47552 **Biliary endoscopy, percutaneous via T-tube or other tract; diagnostic, with collection of specimen(s) by brushing and/or washing, when performed (separate procedure)**

9.01 9.01 FUD 000 J A2

AMA: 2018,Jan,8; 2017,Jan,8; 2016,Jan,13; 2015,Dec,3; 2015,Jan,16; 2014,Jan,11

47553 **with biopsy, single or multiple**

8.91 8.91 FUD 000 J A2

AMA: 2018,Jan,8; 2017,Jan,8; 2016,Jan,13; 2015,Dec,3; 2015,Jan,16; 2014,Jan,11

47554 **with removal of calculus/calculi**

14.9 14.9 FUD 000 J A2

AMA: 2018,Jan,8; 2017,Jan,8; 2016,Jan,13; 2015,Dec,3; 2015,Jan,16; 2014,Jan,11

47555 **with dilation of biliary duct stricture(s) without stent**

(74363)

9.46 9.46 FUD 000 J A2

AMA: 2018,Jan,8; 2017,Jan,8; 2016,Jan,13; 2015,Dec,3; 2015,Jan,16; 2014,Jan,11

47556 **with dilation of biliary duct stricture(s) with stent**

(74363)

10.7 10.7 FUD 000 J J8

AMA: 2018,Jan,8; 2017,Jan,8; 2016,Jan,13; 2015,Dec,3; 2015,Jan,16; 2014,Jan,11

47562-47579 Laparoscopic Gallbladder Procedures

INCLUDES Diagnostic laparoscopy (49320)

47562 **Laparoscopy, surgical; cholecystectomy**

19.0 19.0 FUD 090 J G2 80

AMA: 2018,Jan,8; 2017,Jan,8; 2016,Jan,13; 2015,Jan,16; 2014,Jan,11

47563 **cholecystectomy with cholangiography**
EXCLUDES *Percutaneous cholangiography (47531-47532)*
Code also intraoperative radiology supervision and interpretation (74300-74301)
20.7 20.7 FUD 090 J G2 80
AMA: 2019,Mar,10; 2018,Jan,8; 2017,Jan,8; 2016,Jan,13; 2015,Jan,16; 2014,Jan,11

47564 **cholecystectomy with exploration of common duct**
32.2 32.2 FUD 090 J G2 80
AMA: 2018,Jan,8; 2017,Jan,8; 2016,Jan,13; 2015,Jan,16; 2014,Jan,11

47570 **cholecystoenterostomy**
22.5 22.5 FUD 090 C 80
AMA: 2018,Jan,8; 2017,Jan,8; 2016,Jan,13; 2015,Jan,16; 2014,Jan,11

47579 **Unlisted laparoscopy procedure, biliary tract**
0.00 0.00 FUD YYY J 80 50
AMA: 2018,Jan,8; 2017,Jan,8; 2016,Jan,13; 2015,Jan,16; 2014,Jan,11

47600-47620 Open Gallbladder Procedures

47600 **Cholecystectomy;**
EXCLUDES *Laparoscopic method (47562-47564)*
30.9 30.9 FUD 090 C 80
AMA: 2018,Jan,8; 2017,Jan,8; 2016,Jan,13; 2015,Jan,16; 2014,Jan,11

47605 **with cholangiography**
EXCLUDES *Laparoscopic method (47563-47564)*
32.6 32.6 FUD 090 C 80
AMA: 2018,Jan,8; 2017,Jan,8; 2016,Jan,13; 2015,Jan,16; 2014,Jan,11

47610 **Cholecystectomy with exploration of common duct;**
EXCLUDES *Laparoscopic method (47564)*
Code also biliary endoscopy when performed in conjunction with cholecystectomy with exploration of common duct (47550)
36.3 36.3 FUD 090 C 80
AMA: 2018,Jan,8; 2017,Jan,8; 2016,Jan,13; 2015,Jan,16; 2014,Jan,11

47612 **with choledochoenterostomy**
36.6 36.6 FUD 090 C 80
AMA: 2014,Jan,11

47620 **with transduodenal sphincterotomy or sphincteroplasty, with or without cholangiography**
40.0 40.0 FUD 090 C 80
AMA: 2014,Jan,11

47700-47999 Open Resection and Repair of Biliary Tract

47700 **Exploration for congenital atresia of bile ducts, without repair, with or without liver biopsy, with or without cholangiography**
30.6 30.6 FUD 090 63 C 80
AMA: 2014,Jan,11

47701 **Portoenterostomy (eg, Kasai procedure)**
49.5 49.5 FUD 090 63 C 80
AMA: 2014,Jan,11

47711 **Excision of bile duct tumor, with or without primary repair of bile duct; extrahepatic**
EXCLUDES *Anastomosis (47760-47800)*
45.1 45.1 FUD 090 C 80
AMA: 2014,Jan,11

47712 **intrahepatic**
EXCLUDES *Anastomosis (47760-47800)*
58.1 58.1 FUD 090 C 80
AMA: 2014,Jan,11

47715 **Excision of choledochal cyst**
38.6 38.6 FUD 090 C 80
AMA: 2018,Jan,8; 2017,Jan,8; 2016,Jan,13; 2015,Jan,16; 2014,Jan,11

47720 **Cholecystoenterostomy; direct**
EXCLUDES *Laparoscopic method (47570)*
33.4 33.4 FUD 090 C 80
AMA: 2018,Jan,8; 2017,Jan,8; 2016,Jan,13; 2015,Jan,16; 2014,Jan,11

47721 **with gastroenterostomy**
39.3 39.3 FUD 090 C 80
AMA: 2014,Jan,11

47740 **Roux-en-Y**
37.7 37.7 FUD 090 C 80
AMA: 2014,Jan,11

47741 **Roux-en-Y with gastroenterostomy**
42.8 42.8 FUD 090 C 80
AMA: 2014,Jan,11

47760 **Anastomosis, of extrahepatic biliary ducts and gastrointestinal tract**
65.4 65.4 FUD 090 C 80
AMA: 2014,Jan,11

47765 **Anastomosis, of intrahepatic ducts and gastrointestinal tract**
INCLUDES Longmire anastomosis
88.4 88.4 FUD 090 C 80
AMA: 2014,Jan,11

47780 **Anastomosis, Roux-en-Y, of extrahepatic biliary ducts and gastrointestinal tract**
71.8 71.8 FUD 090 C 80
AMA: 2014,Jan,11

47785 **Anastomosis, Roux-en-Y, of intrahepatic biliary ducts and gastrointestinal tract**
94.4 94.4 FUD 090 C 80
AMA: 2014,Jan,11

47800 **Reconstruction, plastic, of extrahepatic biliary ducts with end-to-end anastomosis**
45.5 45.5 FUD 090 C 80
AMA: 2014,Jan,11

47801 **Placement of choledochal stent**
32.3 32.3 FUD 090 C 80
AMA: 2018,Jan,8; 2017,Jan,8; 2016,Jan,13; 2015,Jan,16; 2014,Jan,11

47802 **U-tube hepaticoenterostomy**
44.3 44.3 FUD 090 C 80
AMA: 2014,Jan,11

47900 **Suture of extrahepatic biliary duct for pre-existing injury (separate procedure)**
39.7 39.7 FUD 090 C 80
AMA: 2014,Jan,11

47999 **Unlisted procedure, biliary tract**
0.00 0.00 FUD YYY T
AMA: 2018,Jan,8; 2017,Jan,8; 2016,Jan,13; 2015,Jan,16; 2014,Jan,11

48000-48548 Open Procedures of the Pancreas

EXCLUDES *Peroral pancreatic procedures performed endoscopically (43260-43265, [43274], [43275], [43276], [43277], [43278])*

48000 Placement of drains, peripancreatic, for acute pancreatitis;
54.6 54.6 FUD 090 C 80
AMA: 2014,Jan,11

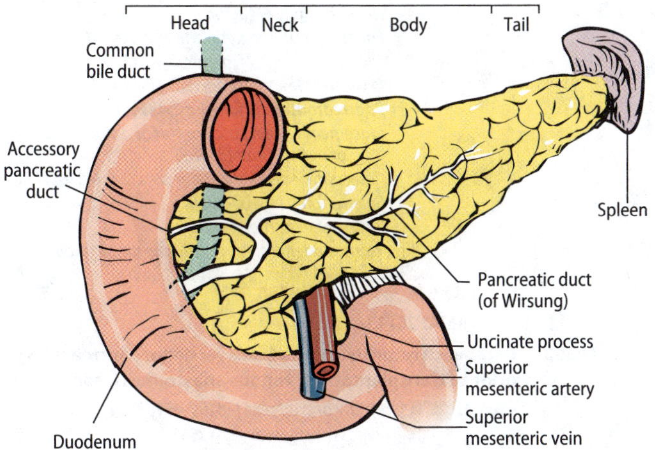

48001 with cholecystostomy, gastrostomy, and jejunostomy
66.6 66.6 FUD 090 C 80
AMA: 2014,Jan,11

48020 Removal of pancreatic calculus
34.1 34.1 FUD 090 C 80
AMA: 2014,Jan,11

48100 Biopsy of pancreas, open (eg, fine needle aspiration, needle core biopsy, wedge biopsy)
25.8 25.8 FUD 090 C 80
AMA: 2014,Jan,11

Pancreas tissue may be defined by placing surgical staples

Example of wedge biopsy

Pancreas tissue is collected in an open surgical session for biopsy purposes

Biopsy needle for fine needle aspiration or percutaneous removal

48102 Biopsy of pancreas, percutaneous needle
EXCLUDES *Fine needle aspiration ([10005, 10006, 10007, 10008, 10009, 10010, 10011, 10012])*
(76942, 77002, 77012, 77021)
(88172-88173)
6.95 15.2 FUD 010 J A2
AMA: 2019,Apr,4; 2014,Jan,11

48105 Resection or debridement of pancreas and peripancreatic tissue for acute necrotizing pancreatitis
82.4 82.4 FUD 090 C 80
AMA: 2014,Jan,11

48120 Excision of lesion of pancreas (eg, cyst, adenoma)
32.0 32.0 FUD 090 C 80
AMA: 2014,Jan,11

48140 Pancreatectomy, distal subtotal, with or without splenectomy; without pancreaticojejunostomy
45.4 45.4 FUD 090 C 80
AMA: 2018,Jan,8; 2017,Jul,10; 2014,Jan,11

48145 with pancreaticojejunostomy
47.4 47.4 FUD 090 C 80
AMA: 2014,Jan,11

48146 Pancreatectomy, distal, near-total with preservation of duodenum (Child-type procedure)
54.5 54.5 FUD 090 C 80
AMA: 2014,Jan,11

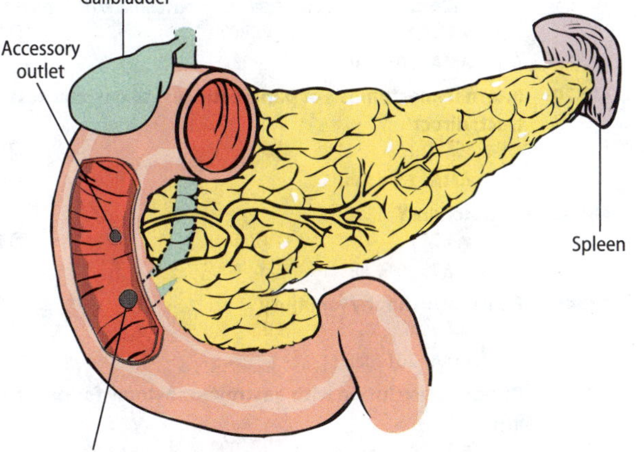

48148 Excision of ampulla of Vater
36.2 36.2 FUD 090 C 80
AMA: 2014,Jan,11

48150 Pancreatectomy, proximal subtotal with total duodenectomy, partial gastrectomy, choledochoenterostomy and gastrojejunostomy (Whipple-type procedure); with pancreatojejunostomy
90.6 90.6 FUD 090 C 80
AMA: 2018,Jan,8; 2017,Jan,8; 2016,Jan,13; 2015,Dec,16; 2014,Jan,11

48152 without pancreatojejunostomy
84.0 84.0 FUD 090 C 80
AMA: 2014,Jan,11

48153 Pancreatectomy, proximal subtotal with near-total duodenectomy, choledochoenterostomy and duodenojejunostomy (pylorus-sparing, Whipple-type procedure); with pancreatojejunostomy
90.1 90.1 FUD 090 C 80
AMA: 2014,Jan,11

48154 without pancreatojejunostomy
84.3 84.3 FUD 090 C 80
AMA: 2014,Jan,11

48155 Pancreatectomy, total
52.6 52.6 FUD 090 C 80
AMA: 2014,Jan,11

48160 **Pancreatectomy, total or subtotal, with autologous transplantation of pancreas or pancreatic islet cells**

EXCLUDES *Laparoscopic pancreatic islet cell transplantation (0585T)*
Open pancreatic islet cell transplantation (0586T)
Percutaneous pancreatic islet cell transplantation (0584T)

0.00 0.00 FUD XXX E

AMA: 2014,Jan,11

\+ **48400** **Injection procedure for intraoperative pancreatography (List separately in addition to code for primary procedure)**

Code first primary procedure
(74300-74301)

3.07 3.07 FUD ZZZ C 80

AMA: 2018,Jan,8; 2017,Jan,8; 2016,Jan,13; 2015,Jan,16; 2014,Jan,11

48500 **Marsupialization of pancreatic cyst**

33.4 33.4 FUD 090 C 80

AMA: 2014,Jan,11

48510 **External drainage, pseudocyst of pancreas, open**

EXCLUDES *Image guided percutaneous catheter drainage (49405)*

31.8 31.8 FUD 090 C 80

AMA: 2014,Jan,11

48520 **Internal anastomosis of pancreatic cyst to gastrointestinal tract; direct**

31.5 31.5 FUD 090 C 80

AMA: 2014,Jan,11

48540 **Roux-en-Y**

37.8 37.8 FUD 090 C 80

AMA: 2014,Jan,11

48545 **Pancreatorrhaphy for injury**

39.0 39.0 FUD 090 C 80

AMA: 2014,Jan,11

48547 **Duodenal exclusion with gastrojejunostomy for pancreatic injury**

51.9 51.9 FUD 090 C 80

AMA: 2014,Jan,11

48548 **Pancreaticojejunostomy, side-to-side anastomosis (Puestow-type operation)**

48.2 48.2 FUD 090 C 80

AMA: 2014,Jan,11

48550-48999 Pancreas Transplant Procedures

CMS: 100-03,260.3 Pancreas Transplants; 100-04,3,90.5 Pancreas Transplants with Kidney Transplants; 100-04,3,90.5.1 Pancreas Transplants Alone

48550 **Donor pancreatectomy (including cold preservation), with or without duodenal segment for transplantation**

INCLUDES Graft:
Cold preservation
Harvest (with or without duodenal segment)

0.00 0.00 FUD XXX E

AMA: 2018,Jan,8; 2017,Jan,8; 2016,Jan,13; 2015,Jan,16; 2014,Jan,11

48551 **Backbench standard preparation of cadaver donor pancreas allograft prior to transplantation, including dissection of allograft from surrounding soft tissues, splenectomy, duodenotomy, ligation of bile duct, ligation of mesenteric vessels, and Y-graft arterial anastomoses from iliac artery to superior mesenteric artery and to splenic artery**

EXCLUDES *Biopsy of pancreas (48100-48102)*
Bypass graft, with vein (35531, 35563)
Duodenotomy (44010)
Endoscopic procedures of the biliary tract (47550-47556)
Excision of lesion of mesentery (44820)
Excision of lesion of pancreas (48120)
Pancreatorrhaphy for injury (48545)
Placement of vein patch or cuff at distal anastomosis of bypass graft (35685)
Resection or debridement of pancreas (48105)
Splenectomy (38100-38102)
Suture of mesentery (44850)
Transduodenal sphincterotomy, sphincteroplasty (47460)

0.00 0.00 FUD XXX C 80

AMA: 2014,Jan,11

48552 **Backbench reconstruction of cadaver donor pancreas allograft prior to transplantation, venous anastomosis, each**

EXCLUDES *Biopsy of pancreas (48100-48102)*
Bypass graft, with vein (35531, 35563)
Duodenotomy (44010)
Endoscopic procedures of the biliary tract (47550-47556)
Excision of lesion of mesentery (44820)
Excision of lesion of pancreas (48120)
Pancreatorrhaphy for injury (48545)
Placement of vein patch or cuff at distal anastomosis of bypass graft (35685)
Resection or debridement of pancreas (48105)
Splenectomy (38100-38102)
Suture of mesentery (44850)
Transduodenal sphincterotomy, sphincteroplasty (47460)

6.87 6.87 FUD XXX C 80

AMA: 2014,Jan,11

48554 **Transplantation of pancreatic allograft**

INCLUDES Allograft transplant
Recipient care

73.9 73.9 FUD 090 C 80

AMA: 2014,Jan,11

48556 **Removal of transplanted pancreatic allograft**

36.9 36.9 FUD 090 C 80

AMA: 2014,Jan,11

48999 **Unlisted procedure, pancreas**

0.00 0.00 FUD YYY T 80

AMA: 2018,Jan,8; 2017,Jan,8; 2016,Jan,13; 2015,Jan,16; 2014,Jan,11

49000-49084 Exploratory and Drainage Procedures: Abdomen/Peritoneum

49000 **Exploratory laparotomy, exploratory celiotomy with or without biopsy(s) (separate procedure)**

EXCLUDES *Exploration of penetrating wound without laparotomy (20102)*

22.3 22.3 FUD 090 C 80

AMA: 2018,Jan,8; 2017,Dec,3; 2017,Jan,8; 2016,Jan,13; 2015,Jan,16; 2014,Jan,11

49002 **Reopening of recent laparotomy**

EXCLUDES *Hepatic wound re-exploration for packing removal (47362)*
Pelvic wound re-exploration for packing removal/repacking (49014)

30.3 30.3 FUD 090 C 80

AMA: 2018,Jan,8; 2017,Jan,8; 2016,Jan,13; 2015,Jan,16; 2014,Jan,11

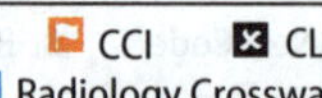

49010 **Exploration, retroperitoneal area with or without biopsy(s) (separate procedure)**

EXCLUDES *Exploration of penetrating wound without laparotomy (20102)*

26.9 26.9 FUD 090 C 80

AMA: 2014,Jan,11

● **49013** **Preperitoneal pelvic packing for hemorrhage associated with pelvic trauma, including local exploration**

● **49014** **Re-exploration of pelvic wound with removal of preperitoneal pelvic packing, including repacking, when performed**

49020 **Drainage of peritoneal abscess or localized peritonitis, exclusive of appendiceal abscess, open**

EXCLUDES *Appendiceal abscess (44900)*
Image guided percutaneous catheter drainage of abscess/peritonitis via catheter (49406)
Image-guided transrectal/transvaginal drainage of peritoneal abscess via catheter (49407)

46.1 46.1 FUD 090 C 80

AMA: 2014,Jan,11

49040 **Drainage of subdiaphragmatic or subphrenic abscess, open**

EXCLUDES *Image-guided percutaneous drainage of subdiaphragmatic/subphrenic abscess via catheter (49406)*

28.9 28.9 FUD 090 C 80

AMA: 2014,Jan,11

49060 **Drainage of retroperitoneal abscess, open**

EXCLUDES *Image-guided percutaneous drainage of retroperitoneal abscess via catheter (49406)*
Transrectal/transvaginal image-guided drainage of retroperitoneal abscess via catheter (49407)

31.8 31.8 FUD 090 C

AMA: 2018,Jan,8; 2017,Jan,8; 2016,Jan,13; 2015,Jan,16; 2014,Jan,11

49062 **Drainage of extraperitoneal lymphocele to peritoneal cavity, open**

EXCLUDES *Drainage of lymphocele to peritoneal cavity, laparoscopic (49323)*
Image-guided percutaneous drainage of retroperitoneal lymphocele via catheter (49406)

21.3 21.3 FUD 090 C 80

AMA: 2018,Jan,8; 2017,Jan,8; 2016,Jan,13; 2015,Jan,16; 2014,Jan,11

49082 **Abdominal paracentesis (diagnostic or therapeutic); without imaging guidance**

2.12 5.67 FUD 000 T G2

AMA: 2018,Jan,8; 2017,Jan,8; 2016,Jan,13; 2015,Jan,16; 2014,Jan,11

49083 **with imaging guidance**

INCLUDES Radiological guidance (76942, 77002, 77012, 77021)

EXCLUDES *Image-guided percutaneous drainage of retroperitoneal abscess via catheter (49406)*

3.11 8.44 FUD 000 T G2

AMA: 2018,Jan,8; 2017,Jan,8; 2016,Jan,13; 2015,Jan,16; 2014,Mar,13; 2014,Jan,11

49084 **Peritoneal lavage, including imaging guidance, when performed**

INCLUDES Radiological guidance (76942, 77002, 77012, 77021)

EXCLUDES *Image-guided percutaneous drainage of retroperitoneal abscess via catheter (49406)*

3.13 3.13 FUD 000 T G2

AMA: 2018,Jan,8; 2017,Jan,8; 2016,Jan,13; 2015,Jan,16; 2014,Jan,11

49180 Biopsy of Mass: Abdomen/Retroperitoneum

EXCLUDES *Fine needle aspiration (10021, [10004, 10005, 10006, 10007, 10008, 10009, 10010, 10011, 10012])*
Lysis of intestinal adhesions (44005)

49180 **Biopsy, abdominal or retroperitoneal mass, percutaneous needle**

(76942, 77002, 77012, 77021)

(88172-88173)

2.46 4.71 FUD 000 J A2

AMA: 2019,Feb,8; 2019,Apr,4; 2018,Jan,8; 2017,Jan,8; 2016,Jan,13; 2015,Jan,16; 2014,Jan,11

49185 Sclerotherapy of a Fluid Collection

49185 **Sclerotherapy of a fluid collection (eg, lymphocele, cyst, or seroma), percutaneous, including contrast injection(s), sclerosant injection(s), diagnostic study, imaging guidance (eg, ultrasound, fluoroscopy) and radiological supervision and interpretation when performed**

INCLUDES Multiple lesions treated via same access

EXCLUDES *Contrast injection for assessment of abscess or cyst (49424)*
Pleurodesis (32560)
Radiologic examination, abscess, fistula or sinus tract stud (76080)
Sclerosis of veins/endovenous ablation of incompetent veins of extremity (36468, 36470-36471, 36475-36476, 36478-36479)
Sclerotherapy of lymphatic/vascular malformation (37241)

Code also access or drainage via needle or catheter (10030, 10160, 49405-49407, 50390)

Code also existing catheter exchange pre- or post-sclerosant injection (49423, 75984)

Code also modifier 59 for treatment of multiple lesions in same session via separate access

3.48 30.2 FUD 000 T

AMA: 2018,Jan,8; 2017,Jan,8; 2016,Mar,10

49203-49205 Open Destruction or Excision: Abdominal Tumors

EXCLUDES *Ablation, open, 1 or more renal mass lesion(s), cryosurgical*
Biopsy of kidney or ovary (50205, 58900)
Cryoablation of renal tumor (50250, 50593)
Excision of perinephric cyst (50290)
Excision of presacral or sacrococcygeal tumor (49215)
Exploration, renal or retroperitoneal area (49010, 50010)
Exploratory laparotomy (49000)
Laparotomy, for staging or restaging of ovarian, tubal, or primary peritoneal malignancy (58960)
Nephrectomy (50225, 50236)
Oophorectomy (58940-58958)
Ovarian cystectomy (58925)
Pelvic or retroperitoneal lymphadenectomy (38770, 38780)
Primary, recurrent ovarian, uterine, or tubal resection (58957-58958)
Wedge resection or bisection of ovary (58920)

Code also colectomy (44140)
Code also nephrectomy (50220, 50240)
Code also small bowel resection (44120)
Code also vena caval resection with reconstruction (37799)

49203 **Excision or destruction, open, intra-abdominal tumors, cysts or endometriomas, 1 or more peritoneal, mesenteric, or retroperitoneal primary or secondary tumors; largest tumor 5 cm diameter or less**

34.7 34.7 FUD 090 C 80

AMA: 2018,Jan,8; 2017,Jan,8; 2016,Jan,13; 2015,Jan,16; 2014,Jan,11

49204 **largest tumor 5.1-10.0 cm diameter**

44.3 44.3 FUD 090 C 80

AMA: 2018,Jan,8; 2017,Jan,8; 2016,Jan,13; 2015,Jan,16; 2014,Jan,11

49205 **largest tumor greater than 10.0 cm diameter**

51.0 51.0 FUD 090 C 80

AMA: 2018,Jan,8; 2017,Jan,8; 2016,Jan,13; 2015,Jan,16; 2014,Jan,11

49215 Resection Presacral/Sacrococcygeal Tumor

49215 **Excision of presacral or sacrococcygeal tumor**
64.2 64.2 FUD 090 63 C 80
AMA: 2014,Jan,11

49220-49255 Other Open Abdominal Procedures

EXCLUDES *Lysis of intestinal adhesions (44005)*

49220 **Staging laparotomy for Hodgkins disease or lymphoma (includes splenectomy, needle or open biopsies of both liver lobes, possibly also removal of abdominal nodes, abdominal node and/or bone marrow biopsies, ovarian repositioning)**
28.2 28.2 FUD 090 C 80
AMA: 2014,Jan,11

49250 **Umbilectomy, omphalectomy, excision of umbilicus (separate procedure)**
17.0 17.0 FUD 090 J A2
AMA: 2014,Jan,11

49255 **Omentectomy, epiploectomy, resection of omentum (separate procedure)**
22.9 22.9 FUD 090 C 80
AMA: 2018,Mar,11; 2018,Jan,8; 2017,Jan,8; 2016,Jan,13; 2015,Jan,16; 2014,Jan,11

49320-49329 Laparoscopic Procedures of the Abdomen/Peritoneum/Omentum

INCLUDES Diagnostic laparoscopy (49320)
EXCLUDES *Fulguration/excision of lesions of ovary/pelvic viscera/peritoneal surface, performed laparoscopically (58662)*

49320 **Laparoscopy, abdomen, peritoneum, and omentum, diagnostic, with or without collection of specimen(s) by brushing or washing (separate procedure)**
9.43 9.43 FUD 010 J A2 80
AMA: 2018,Jan,8; 2017,Apr,7; 2017,Jan,8; 2016,Jan,13; 2015,Dec,16; 2015,Jan,16; 2014,Jan,11

49321 **Laparoscopy, surgical; with biopsy (single or multiple)**
9.97 9.97 FUD 010 J A2 80
AMA: 2018,Aug,10; 2018,Jan,8; 2017,Jan,8; 2016,Jan,13; 2015,Jan,16; 2014,Jan,11

49322 **with aspiration of cavity or cyst (eg, ovarian cyst) (single or multiple)**
10.7 10.7 FUD 010 J A2 80
AMA: 2018,Jan,8; 2017,Jan,8; 2016,Jan,13; 2015,Jan,16; 2014,Jan,11

49323 **with drainage of lymphocele to peritoneal cavity**
EXCLUDES *Open drainage of lymphocele to peritoneal cavity (49062)*
18.3 18.3 FUD 090 J 80
AMA: 2018,Jan,8; 2017,Jan,8; 2016,Jan,13; 2015,Jan,16; 2014,Jan,11

49324 **with insertion of tunneled intraperitoneal catheter**
EXCLUDES *Open approach (49421)*
Code also insertion of subcutaneous extension to intraperitoneal cannula with remote chest exit site, when appropriate (49435)
11.2 11.2 FUD 010 J G2 80
AMA: 2014,Jan,11

49325 **with revision of previously placed intraperitoneal cannula or catheter, with removal of intraluminal obstructive material if performed**
11.9 11.9 FUD 010 J G2 80
AMA: 2014,Jan,11

\+ **49326** **with omentopexy (omental tacking procedure) (List separately in addition to code for primary procedure)**
Code first laparoscopy with permanent intraperitoneal cannula or catheter insertion or revision of previously placed catheter/cannula (49324, 49325)
5.47 5.47 FUD ZZZ N N1 80
AMA: 2014,Jan,11

\+ **49327** **with placement of interstitial device(s) for radiation therapy guidance (eg, fiducial markers, dosimeter), intra-abdominal, intrapelvic, and/or retroperitoneum, including imaging guidance, if performed, single or multiple (List separately in addition to code for primary procedure)**
EXCLUDES *Open approach (49412)*
Percutaneous approach (49411)
Code first laparoscopic abdominal, pelvic or retroperitoneal procedures
3.79 3.79 FUD ZZZ N N1 80
AMA: 2014,Jan,11

49329 **Unlisted laparoscopy procedure, abdomen, peritoneum and omentum**
0.00 0.00 FUD YYY J 80 50
AMA: 2019,Mar,10; 2018,Jan,8; 2017,Jan,8; 2016,Jan,13; 2015,Jan,16; 2014,Jan,11

49400-49436 Peritoneal and Visceral Procedures: Drainage/Insertion/Modifications/Removal

49400 **Injection of air or contrast into peritoneal cavity (separate procedure)**
(74190)
2.68 3.93 FUD 000 N N1
AMA: 2018,Jan,8; 2017,Jan,8; 2016,Jan,13; 2015,Jan,16; 2014,Jan,11

49402 **Removal of peritoneal foreign body from peritoneal cavity**
EXCLUDES *Enterolysis (44005)*
Percutaneous or open drainage or lavage (49020, 49040, 49082-49084, 49406)
Percutaneous tunneled intraperitoneal catheter insertion without subcutaneous port (49418)
24.8 24.8 FUD 090 J A2
AMA: 2014,Jan,11

49405 **Image-guided fluid collection drainage by catheter (eg, abscess, hematoma, seroma, lymphocele, cyst); visceral (eg, kidney, liver, spleen, lung/mediastinum), percutaneous**
INCLUDES Radiological guidance (75989, 76942, 77002-77003, 77012, 77021)
EXCLUDES *Open drainage (47010, 48510, 50020)*
Percutaneous cholecystostomy (47490)
Percutaneous pleural drainage (32556-32557)
Pneumonostomy (32200)
Thoracentesis (32554-32555)
Code also each individual collection drained per separate catheter
5.72 23.9 FUD 000 J
AMA: 2018,Jan,8; 2017,Jan,8; 2016,Jan,13; 2015,Jan,16; 2014,May,9; 2014,Jan,11

49406 **peritoneal or retroperitoneal, percutaneous**
INCLUDES Radiological guidance (75989, 76942, 77002-77003, 77012, 77021)
EXCLUDES *Diagnostic or therapeutic percutaneous abdominal paracentesis (49082-49083)*
Open peritoneal/retroperitoneal drainage (44900, 49020-49062, 49084, 50020, 58805, 58822)
Open transrectal drainage pelvic abscess (45000)
Percutaneous tunneled intraperitoneal catheter insertion without subcutaneous port (49418)
Transrectal/transvaginal image-guided peritoneal/retroperitoneal drainage via catheter (49407)
Code also each individual collection drained per separate catheter
5.72 23.9 FUD 000 J G2
AMA: 2018,Jan,8; 2017,Jan,8; 2016,Jan,13; 2015,Jan,16; 2014,May,9; 2014,Jan,11

49407 **peritoneal or retroperitoneal, transvaginal or transrectal**

INCLUDES Radiological guidance (75989, 76942, 77002-77003, 77012, 77021)

EXCLUDES *Image guided percutaneous catheter drainage of soft tissue (eg, abdominal wall, neck, extremity) (10030)*

Open transrectal/transvaginal drainage (45000, 58800, 58820)

Percutaneous pleural drainage (32556-32557)

Peritoneal drainage or lavage, open or percutaneous (49020, 49040, 49060)

Thoracentesis (32554-32555)

Code also each individual collection drained per separate catheter

6.06 19.4 FUD 000 J G2

AMA: 2018,Jan,8; 2017,Jan,8; 2016,Jan,13; 2015,Jan,16; 2014,May,9; 2014,Jan,11

49411 **Placement of interstitial device(s) for radiation therapy guidance (eg, fiducial markers, dosimeter), percutaneous, intra-abdominal, intra-pelvic (except prostate), and/or retroperitoneum, single or multiple**

EXCLUDES *Placement (percutaneous) of interstitial device(s) for intrathoracic radiation therapy guidance (32553)*

Code also supply of device

(76942, 77002, 77012, 77021)

5.34 13.7 FUD 000 S P3 80

AMA: 2018,Jan,8; 2017,Jan,8; 2016,Jun,3; 2016,Jan,13; 2015,Jan,16; 2014,Jan,11

\+ **49412** **Placement of interstitial device(s) for radiation therapy guidance (eg, fiducial markers, dosimeter), open, intra-abdominal, intrapelvic, and/or retroperitoneum, including image guidance, if performed, single or multiple (List separately in addition to code for primary procedure)**

EXCLUDES *Laparoscopic approach (49327)*

Percutaneous approach (49411)

Code first open abdominal, pelvic or retroperitoneal procedure(s)

2.41 2.41 FUD ZZZ C 80

AMA: 2014,Jan,11

49418 **Insertion of tunneled intraperitoneal catheter (eg, dialysis, intraperitoneal chemotherapy instillation, management of ascites), complete procedure, including imaging guidance, catheter placement, contrast injection when performed, and radiological supervision and interpretation, percutaneous**

5.89 36.1 FUD 000 J G2 80

AMA: 2014,Jan,11

49419 **Insertion of tunneled intraperitoneal catheter, with subcutaneous port (ie, totally implantable)**

EXCLUDES *Removal of catheter/cannula (49422)*

12.7 12.7 FUD 090 T A2

AMA: 2014,Jan,11

49421 **Insertion of tunneled intraperitoneal catheter for dialysis, open**

EXCLUDES *Laparoscopic approach (49324)*

Code also insertion of subcutaneous extension to intraperitoneal cannula with remote chest exit site, when appropriate (49435)

6.64 6.64 FUD 000 J G2

AMA: 2018,Jan,8; 2017,Jan,8; 2016,Jan,13; 2015,Jan,16; 2014,Jan,11

49422 **Removal of tunneled intraperitoneal catheter**

EXCLUDES *Removal temporary catheter or cannula (Use appropriate E&M code)*

6.46 6.46 FUD 000 Q2 A2

AMA: 2014,Jan,11

49423 **Exchange of previously placed abscess or cyst drainage catheter under radiological guidance (separate procedure)**

(75984)

2.07 16.1 FUD 000 J G2 80

AMA: 2018,Jan,8; 2017,Jan,8; 2016,Jan,13; 2015,Jan,16; 2014,Jan,11

49424 **Contrast injection for assessment of abscess or cyst via previously placed drainage catheter or tube (separate procedure)**

(76080)

1.10 4.35 FUD 000 N N1 80

AMA: 2018,Jan,8; 2017,Jan,8; 2016,Jan,13; 2015,Jan,16; 2014,Jan,11

49425 **Insertion of peritoneal-venous shunt**

20.8 20.8 FUD 090 C 80

AMA: 2014,Jan,11

49426 **Revision of peritoneal-venous shunt**

EXCLUDES *Shunt patency test (78291)*

17.8 17.8 FUD 090 J A2

AMA: 2014,Jan,11

49427 **Injection procedure (eg, contrast media) for evaluation of previously placed peritoneal-venous shunt**

(75809, 78291)

1.32 1.32 FUD 000 N N1 80

AMA: 2014,Jan,11

49428 **Ligation of peritoneal-venous shunt**

12.5 12.5 FUD 010 C

AMA: 2014,Jan,11

49429 **Removal of peritoneal-venous shunt**

13.3 13.3 FUD 010 Q2 G2

AMA: 2014,Jan,11

\+ **49435** **Insertion of subcutaneous extension to intraperitoneal cannula or catheter with remote chest exit site (List separately in addition to code for primary procedure)**

Code first permanent insertion of intraperitoneal catheter/cannula (49324, 49421)

3.45 3.45 FUD ZZZ N N1 80

AMA: 2014,Jan,11

49436 **Delayed creation of exit site from embedded subcutaneous segment of intraperitoneal cannula or catheter**

5.36 5.36 FUD 010 J G2 80

AMA: 2014,Jan,11

49440-49442 Insertion of Percutaneous Gastrointestinal Tube

EXCLUDES *Naso- or oro-gastric tube placement (43752)*

49440 **Insertion of gastrostomy tube, percutaneous, under fluoroscopic guidance including contrast injection(s), image documentation and report**

INCLUDES Needle placement with fluoroscopic guidance (77002)

Code also gastrostomy to gastro-jejunostomy tube conversion with initial gastrostomy tube insertion, when performed (49446)

5.96 26.9 FUD 010 J G2 80

AMA: 2018,Jan,8; 2017,Jan,8; 2016,Jan,13; 2015,Jan,16; 2014,Dec,18; 2014,Sep,5; 2014,Jan,11

49441 **Insertion of duodenostomy or jejunostomy tube, percutaneous, under fluoroscopic guidance including contrast injection(s), image documentation and report**

EXCLUDES *Gastrostomy tube to gastrojejunostomy tube conversion (49446)*

7.00 30.6 FUD 010 J G2 80

AMA: 2018,Jan,8; 2017,Jan,8; 2016,Jan,13; 2015,Jan,16; 2014,Dec,18; 2014,Sep,5; 2014,Jan,11

49442 **Insertion of cecostomy or other colonic tube, percutaneous, under fluoroscopic guidance including contrast injection(s), image documentation and report**
6.04 25.4 FUD 010 T G2 80
AMA: 2018,Jan,8; 2017,Jan,8; 2016,Jan,13; 2015,Jan,16; 2014,Dec,18; 2014,Sep,5; 2014,Jan,11

49446 Percutaneous Conversion: Gastrostomy to Gastro-jejunostomy Tube

EXCLUDES *Code also initial gastrostomy tube insertion (49440) when conversion is performed at the same time*

49446 **Conversion of gastrostomy tube to gastro-jejunostomy tube, percutaneous, under fluoroscopic guidance including contrast injection(s), image documentation and report**
4.30 25.9 FUD 000 J G2 80
AMA: 2018,Jan,8; 2017,Jan,8; 2016,Jan,13; 2015,Jan,16; 2014,Sep,5; 2014,Jan,11

49450-49452 Replacement Gastrointestinal Tube

EXCLUDES *Placement of new tube whether gastrostomy, jejunostomy, duodenostomy, gastro-jejunostomy, or cecostomy at different percutaneous site (49440-49442)*

49450 **Replacement of gastrostomy or cecostomy (or other colonic) tube, percutaneous, under fluoroscopic guidance including contrast injection(s), image documentation and report**
EXCLUDES *Change of gastrostomy tube, percutaneous, without imaging or endoscopic guidance (43762-43763)*
1.92 18.8 FUD 000 T G2 80
AMA: 2019,Feb,5; 2018,Jan,8; 2017,Jan,8; 2016,Jan,13; 2015,Jan,16; 2014,Sep,5; 2014,Jan,11

49451 **Replacement of duodenostomy or jejunostomy tube, percutaneous, under fluoroscopic guidance including contrast injection(s), image documentation and report**
2.62 20.4 FUD 000 T G2 80
AMA: 2018,Jan,8; 2017,Jan,8; 2016,Jan,13; 2015,Jan,16; 2014,Dec,18; 2014,Sep,5; 2014,Jan,11

49452 **Replacement of gastro-jejunostomy tube, percutaneous, under fluoroscopic guidance including contrast injection(s), image documentation and report**
4.01 25.1 FUD 000 T G2 80
AMA: 2018,Jan,8; 2017,Jan,8; 2016,Jan,13; 2015,Jan,16; 2014,Sep,5; 2014,Jan,11

49460-49465 Removal of Obstruction/Injection for Contrast Through Gastrointestinal Tube

49460 **Mechanical removal of obstructive material from gastrostomy, duodenostomy, jejunostomy, gastro-jejunostomy, or cecostomy (or other colonic) tube, any method, under fluoroscopic guidance including contrast injection(s), if performed, image documentation and report**
INCLUDES Contrast injection (49465)
EXCLUDES *Replacement of gastrointestinal tube (49450-49452)*
1.39 20.4 FUD 000 T G2 80
AMA: 2018,Jan,8; 2017,Jan,8; 2016,Jan,13; 2015,Jan,16; 2014,Sep,5; 2014,Jan,11

49465 **Contrast injection(s) for radiological evaluation of existing gastrostomy, duodenostomy, jejunostomy, gastro-jejunostomy, or cecostomy (or other colonic) tube, from a percutaneous approach including image documentation and report**
EXCLUDES *Mechanical removal of obstructive material from gastrointestinal tube (49460)*
Replacement of gastrointestinal tube (49450-49452)
0.89 4.48 FUD 000 Q1 G2 80
AMA: 2018,Jan,8; 2017,Jan,8; 2016,Jan,13; 2015,Jan,16; 2014,Sep,5; 2014,Jan,11

49491-49492 Inguinal Hernia Repair on Premature Infant

INCLUDES Hernia repairs done on preterm infants younger than or equal to 50 weeks postconception age but younger than 6 months of age since birth
Initial repair: no previous repair required
Mesh or other prosthesis
EXCLUDES *Abdominal wall debridement (11042, 11043)*
Intra-abdominal hernia repair/reduction (44050)
Code also repair or excision of testicle(s), intestine, ovaries if performed (44120, 54520, 58940)

49491 **Repair, initial inguinal hernia, preterm infant (younger than 37 weeks gestation at birth), performed from birth up to 50 weeks postconception age, with or without hydrocelectomy; reducible** A
23.0 23.0 FUD 090 63 J 80 50
AMA: 2018,Jan,8; 2017,Jan,8; 2016,Jan,13; 2015,Jan,16; 2014,Jan,11

49492 **incarcerated or strangulated** A
27.7 27.7 FUD 090 63 J 80 50
AMA: 2018,Jan,8; 2017,Jan,8; 2016,Jan,13; 2015,Jan,16; 2014,Jan,11

49495-49557 Hernia Repair: Femoral/Inguinal /Lumbar

INCLUDES Initial repair: no previous repair required
Mesh or other prosthesis
Recurrent repair: required previous repair(s)
EXCLUDES *Abdominal wall debridement (11042, 11043)*
Intra-abdominal hernia repair/reduction (44050)
Code also repair or excision of testicle(s), intestine, ovaries if performed (44120, 54520, 58940)

49495 **Repair, initial inguinal hernia, full term infant younger than age 6 months, or preterm infant older than 50 weeks postconception age and younger than age 6 months at the time of surgery, with or without hydrocelectomy; reducible** A
INCLUDES Hernia repairs done on preterm infants older than 50 weeks postconception age and younger than 6 months
11.8 11.8 FUD 090 63 J A2 80 50
AMA: 2018,Jan,8; 2017,Jan,8; 2016,Jan,13; 2015,Jan,16; 2014,Jan,11

49496 **incarcerated or strangulated** A
INCLUDES Hernia repairs done on preterm infants older than 50 weeks postconception age and younger than 6 months
17.7 17.7 FUD 090 63 J A2 80 50
AMA: 2018,Jan,8; 2017,Jan,8; 2016,Jan,13; 2015,Jan,16; 2014,Jan,11

49500 **Repair initial inguinal hernia, age 6 months to younger than 5 years, with or without hydrocelectomy; reducible** A
INCLUDES Repairs performed on patients 6 months to younger than 5 years old
11.9 11.9 FUD 090 J A2 80 50
AMA: 2018,Jan,8; 2017,Jan,8; 2016,Jan,13; 2015,Jan,16; 2014,Nov,14; 2014,Jan,11

49501 **incarcerated or strangulated** A
INCLUDES Repairs performed on patients 6 months to younger than 5 years old
17.5 17.5 FUD 090 J A2 80 50
AMA: 2018,Jan,8; 2017,Jan,8; 2016,Jan,13; 2015,Jan,16; 2014,Jan,11

49505 **Repair initial inguinal hernia, age 5 years or older; reducible** A
INCLUDES MacEwen hernia repair
Code also when performed:
Excision of hydrocele (55040)
Excision of spermatocele (54840)
Simple orchiectomy (54520)
15.0 15.0 FUD 090 J A2 80 50
AMA: 2018,Jan,8; 2017,Jan,8; 2016,Jan,13; 2015,Jan,16; 2014,Jan,11

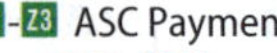 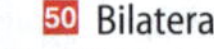  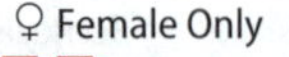 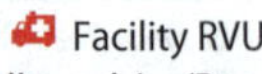 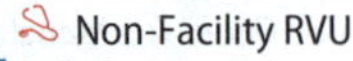 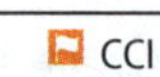

26/TC PC/TC Only A2-Z3 ASC Payment 50 Bilateral ♂ Male Only ♀ Female Only Facility RVU Non-Facility RVU CCI CLIA
FUD Follow-up Days CMS: IOM AMA: CPT Asst A-Y OPPSI 80/80 Surg Assist Allowed / w/Doc Lab Crosswalk Radiology Crosswalk

49507 **incarcerated or strangulated** [A]

Code also when performed:

Excision of hydrocele (55040)

Excision of spermatocele (54840)

Simple orchiectomy (54520)

16.9 16.9 FUD 090 J A2 80 50

AMA: 2018,Jan,8; 2017,Jan,8; 2016,Jan,13; 2015,Jan,16; 2014,Jan,11

49520 **Repair recurrent inguinal hernia, any age; reducible**

18.3 18.3 FUD 090 J A2 80 50

AMA: 2018,Jan,8; 2017,Jan,8; 2016,Jan,13; 2015,Jan,16; 2014,Jan,11

49521 **incarcerated or strangulated**

20.7 20.7 FUD 090 J A2 80 50

AMA: 2018,Jan,8; 2017,Jan,8; 2016,Jan,13; 2015,Jan,16; 2014,Jan,11

49525 **Repair inguinal hernia, sliding, any age**

EXCLUDES *Inguinal hernia repair, incarcerated/strangulated (49496, 49501, 49507, 49521)*

16.6 16.6 FUD 090 J A2 80 50

AMA: 2018,Jan,8; 2017,Jan,8; 2016,Jan,13; 2015,Jan,16; 2014,Jan,11

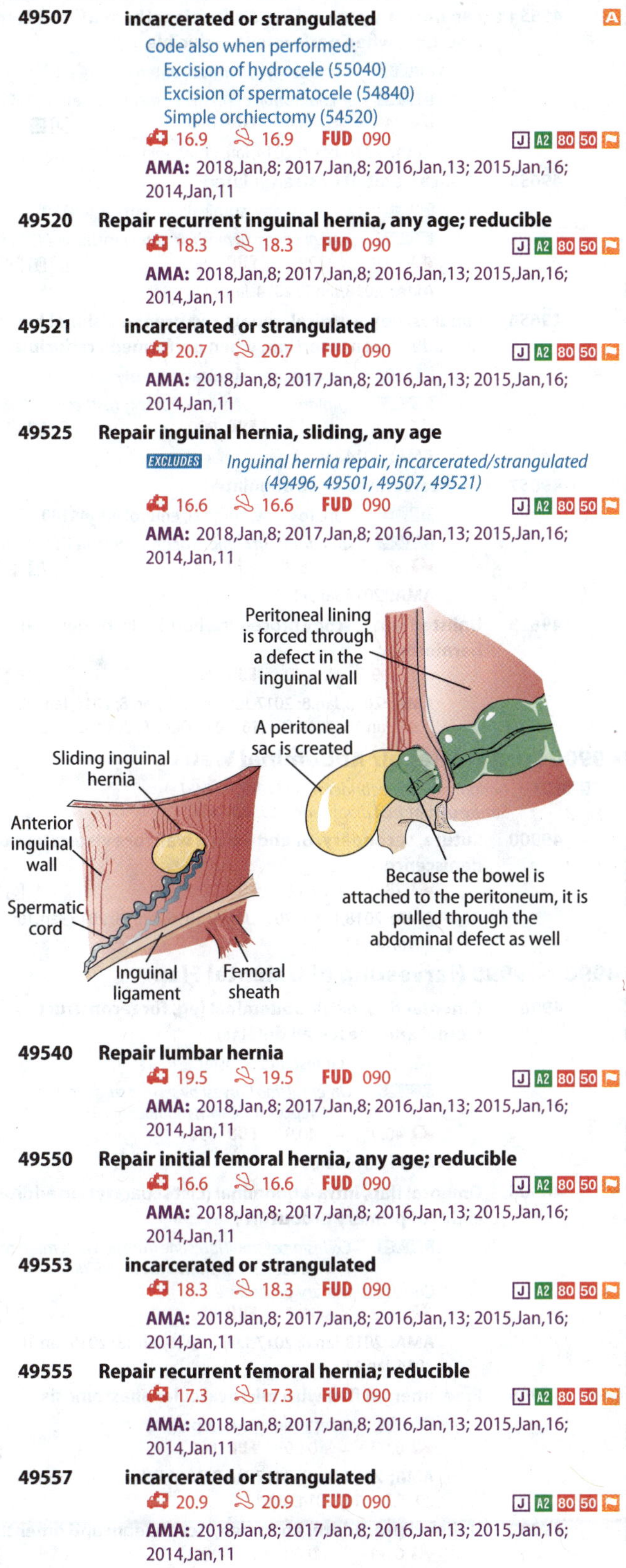

49540 **Repair lumbar hernia**

19.5 19.5 FUD 090 J A2 80 50

AMA: 2018,Jan,8; 2017,Jan,8; 2016,Jan,13; 2015,Jan,16; 2014,Jan,11

49550 **Repair initial femoral hernia, any age; reducible**

16.6 16.6 FUD 090 J A2 80 50

AMA: 2018,Jan,8; 2017,Jan,8; 2016,Jan,13; 2015,Jan,16; 2014,Jan,11

49553 **incarcerated or strangulated**

18.3 18.3 FUD 090 J A2 80 50

AMA: 2018,Jan,8; 2017,Jan,8; 2016,Jan,13; 2015,Jan,16; 2014,Jan,11

49555 **Repair recurrent femoral hernia; reducible**

17.3 17.3 FUD 090 J A2 80 50

AMA: 2018,Jan,8; 2017,Jan,8; 2016,Jan,13; 2015,Jan,16; 2014,Jan,11

49557 **incarcerated or strangulated**

20.9 20.9 FUD 090 J A2 80 50

AMA: 2018,Jan,8; 2017,Jan,8; 2016,Jan,13; 2015,Jan,16; 2014,Jan,11

49560-49568 Hernia Repair: Incisional/Ventral

INCLUDES Initial repair: no previous repair required

Recurrent repair: required previous repair(s)

EXCLUDES *Abdominal wall debridement (11042, 11043)*

Intra-abdominal hernia repair/reduction (44050)

Code also repair or excision of testicle(s), intestine, ovaries if performed (44120, 54520, 58940)

49560 **Repair initial incisional or ventral hernia; reducible**

Code also implantation of mesh or other prosthesis if performed (49568)

21.3 21.3 FUD 090 J A2 80 50

AMA: 2018,Jan,8; 2017,Jan,8; 2016,Jan,13; 2015,Jan,16; 2014,Jan,11

49561 **incarcerated or strangulated**

Code also implantation of mesh or other prosthesis if performed (49568)

26.9 26.9 FUD 090 J A2 80 50

AMA: 2018,Jul,14; 2018,Mar,11; 2018,Jan,8; 2017,Jan,8; 2016,Jan,13; 2015,Jan,16; 2014,Jan,11

49565 **Repair recurrent incisional or ventral hernia; reducible**

Code also implantation of mesh or other prosthesis if performed (49568)

22.2 22.2 FUD 090 J A2 80 50

AMA: 2018,Jan,8; 2017,Jan,8; 2016,Jan,13; 2015,Jan,16; 2014,Jan,11

49566 **incarcerated or strangulated**

Code also implantation of mesh or other prosthesis if performed (49568)

27.1 27.1 FUD 090 J A2 80 50

AMA: 2018,Jan,8; 2017,Jan,8; 2016,Jan,13; 2015,Jan,16; 2014,Jan,11

\+ **49568** **Implantation of mesh or other prosthesis for open incisional or ventral hernia repair or mesh for closure of debridement for necrotizing soft tissue infection (List separately in addition to code for the incisional or ventral hernia repair)**

EXCLUDES *Reporting with modifier 50. Report once for each side when performed bilaterally*

Code first (11004-11006, 49560-49566)

7.77 7.77 FUD ZZZ 50 N N1 80

AMA: 2018,Jan,8; 2017,Jan,8; 2016,Jan,13; 2015,Jan,16; 2014,Jan,11

49570-49590 Hernia Repair: Epigastric/Lateral Ventral/Umbilical

INCLUDES Mesh or other prosthesis

EXCLUDES *Abdominal wall debridement (11042, 11043)*

Intra-abdominal hernia repair/reduction (44050)

Code also repair or excision of testicle(s), intestine, ovaries if performed (44120, 54520, 58940)

49570 **Repair epigastric hernia (eg, preperitoneal fat); reducible (separate procedure)**

12.0 12.0 FUD 090 J A2 80 50

AMA: 2018,Jan,8; 2017,Jan,8; 2016,Jan,13; 2015,Jan,16; 2014,Jan,11

49572 **incarcerated or strangulated**

14.9 14.9 FUD 090 J A2 80 50

AMA: 2018,Jan,8; 2017,Jan,8; 2016,Jan,13; 2015,Jan,16; 2014,Jan,11

49580 **Repair umbilical hernia, younger than age 5 years; reducible** [A]

9.63 9.63 FUD 090 J A2 80

AMA: 2018,Jan,8; 2017,Jan,8; 2016,Jan,13; 2015,Jan,16; 2014,Jan,11

49582 **incarcerated or strangulated** [A]

13.9 13.9 FUD 090 J A2 80

AMA: 2018,Jan,8; 2017,Jan,8; 2016,Jan,13; 2015,Jan,16; 2014,Jan,11

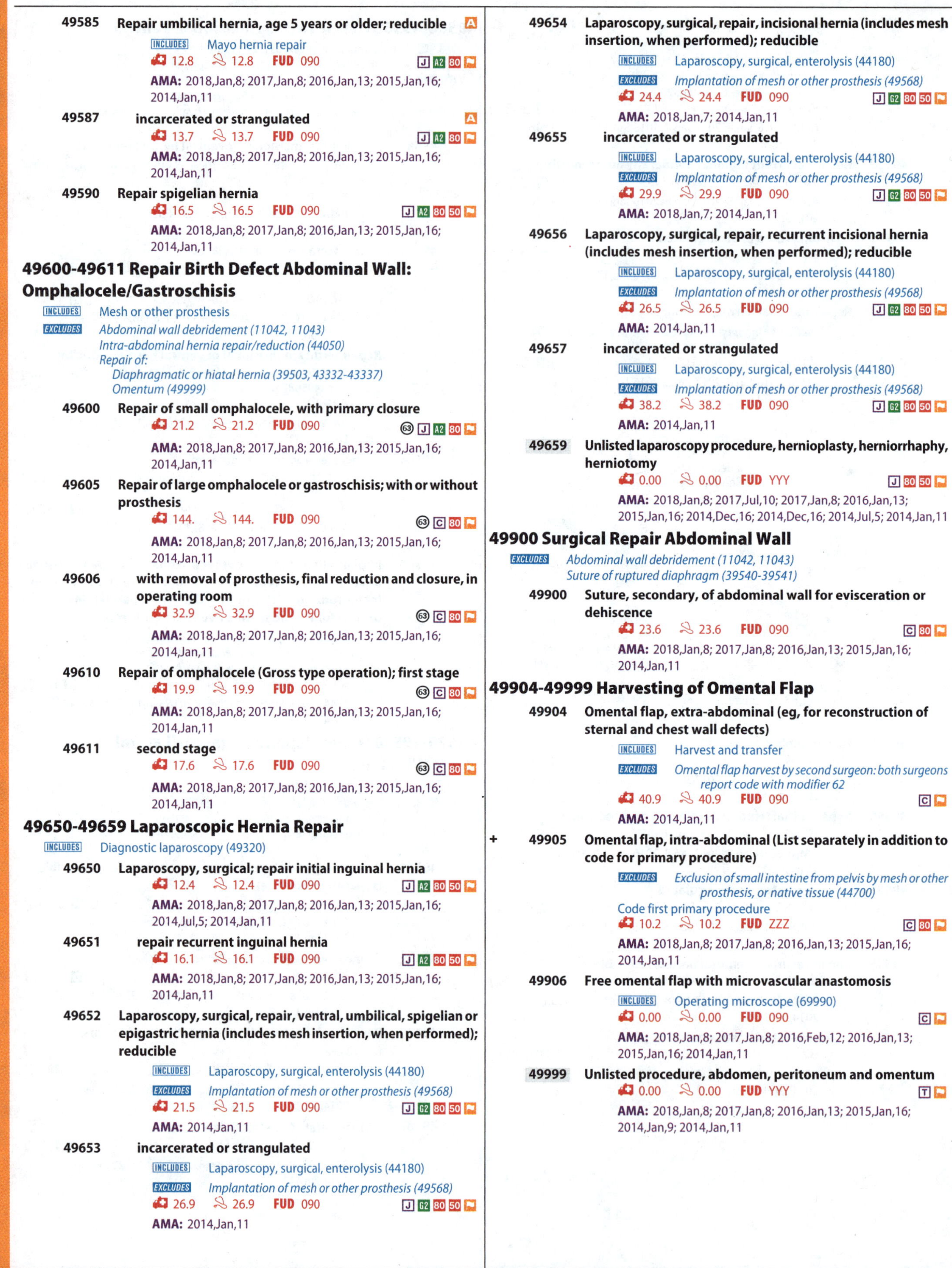

49585 **Repair umbilical hernia, age 5 years or older; reducible** A

INCLUDES Mayo hernia repair

12.8 12.8 FUD 090 J A2 80

AMA: 2018,Jan,8; 2017,Jan,8; 2016,Jan,13; 2015,Jan,16; 2014,Jan,11

49587 **incarcerated or strangulated** A

13.7 13.7 FUD 090 J A2 80

AMA: 2018,Jan,8; 2017,Jan,8; 2016,Jan,13; 2015,Jan,16; 2014,Jan,11

49590 **Repair spigelian hernia**

16.5 16.5 FUD 090 J A2 80 50

AMA: 2018,Jan,8; 2017,Jan,8; 2016,Jan,13; 2015,Jan,16; 2014,Jan,11

49600-49611 Repair Birth Defect Abdominal Wall: Omphalocele/Gastroschisis

INCLUDES Mesh or other prosthesis

EXCLUDES *Abdominal wall debridement (11042, 11043)*
Intra-abdominal hernia repair/reduction (44050)
Repair of:
Diaphragmatic or hiatal hernia (39503, 43332-43337)
Omentum (49999)

49600 **Repair of small omphalocele, with primary closure**

21.2 21.2 FUD 090 63 J A2 80

AMA: 2018,Jan,8; 2017,Jan,8; 2016,Jan,13; 2015,Jan,16; 2014,Jan,11

49605 **Repair of large omphalocele or gastroschisis; with or without prosthesis**

144. 144. FUD 090 63 C 80

AMA: 2018,Jan,8; 2017,Jan,8; 2016,Jan,13; 2015,Jan,16; 2014,Jan,11

49606 **with removal of prosthesis, final reduction and closure, in operating room**

32.9 32.9 FUD 090 63 C 80

AMA: 2018,Jan,8; 2017,Jan,8; 2016,Jan,13; 2015,Jan,16; 2014,Jan,11

49610 **Repair of omphalocele (Gross type operation); first stage**

19.9 19.9 FUD 090 63 C 80

AMA: 2018,Jan,8; 2017,Jan,8; 2016,Jan,13; 2015,Jan,16; 2014,Jan,11

49611 **second stage**

17.6 17.6 FUD 090 63 C 80

AMA: 2018,Jan,8; 2017,Jan,8; 2016,Jan,13; 2015,Jan,16; 2014,Jan,11

49650-49659 Laparoscopic Hernia Repair

INCLUDES Diagnostic laparoscopy (49320)

49650 **Laparoscopy, surgical; repair initial inguinal hernia**

12.4 12.4 FUD 090 J A2 80 50

AMA: 2018,Jan,8; 2017,Jan,8; 2016,Jan,13; 2015,Jan,16; 2014,Jul,5; 2014,Jan,11

49651 **repair recurrent inguinal hernia**

16.1 16.1 FUD 090 J A2 80 50

AMA: 2018,Jan,8; 2017,Jan,8; 2016,Jan,13; 2015,Jan,16; 2014,Jan,11

49652 **Laparoscopy, surgical, repair, ventral, umbilical, spigelian or epigastric hernia (includes mesh insertion, when performed); reducible**

INCLUDES Laparoscopy, surgical, enterolysis (44180)

EXCLUDES *Implantation of mesh or other prosthesis (49568)*

21.5 21.5 FUD 090 J G2 80 50

AMA: 2014,Jan,11

49653 **incarcerated or strangulated**

INCLUDES Laparoscopy, surgical, enterolysis (44180)

EXCLUDES *Implantation of mesh or other prosthesis (49568)*

26.9 26.9 FUD 090 J G2 80 50

AMA: 2014,Jan,11

49654 **Laparoscopy, surgical, repair, incisional hernia (includes mesh insertion, when performed); reducible**

INCLUDES Laparoscopy, surgical, enterolysis (44180)

EXCLUDES *Implantation of mesh or other prosthesis (49568)*

24.4 24.4 FUD 090 J G2 80 50

AMA: 2018,Jan,7; 2014,Jan,11

49655 **incarcerated or strangulated**

INCLUDES Laparoscopy, surgical, enterolysis (44180)

EXCLUDES *Implantation of mesh or other prosthesis (49568)*

29.9 29.9 FUD 090 J G2 80 50

AMA: 2018,Jan,7; 2014,Jan,11

49656 **Laparoscopy, surgical, repair, recurrent incisional hernia (includes mesh insertion, when performed); reducible**

INCLUDES Laparoscopy, surgical, enterolysis (44180)

EXCLUDES *Implantation of mesh or other prosthesis (49568)*

26.5 26.5 FUD 090 J G2 80 50

AMA: 2014,Jan,11

49657 **incarcerated or strangulated**

INCLUDES Laparoscopy, surgical, enterolysis (44180)

EXCLUDES *Implantation of mesh or other prosthesis (49568)*

38.2 38.2 FUD 090 J G2 80 50

AMA: 2014,Jan,11

49659 **Unlisted laparoscopy procedure, hernioplasty, herniorrhaphy, herniotomy**

0.00 0.00 FUD YYY J 80 50

AMA: 2018,Jan,8; 2017,Jul,10; 2017,Jan,8; 2016,Jan,13; 2015,Jan,16; 2014,Dec,16; 2014,Dec,16; 2014,Jul,5; 2014,Jan,11

49900 Surgical Repair Abdominal Wall

EXCLUDES *Abdominal wall debridement (11042, 11043)*
Suture of ruptured diaphragm (39540-39541)

49900 **Suture, secondary, of abdominal wall for evisceration or dehiscence**

23.6 23.6 FUD 090 C 80

AMA: 2018,Jan,8; 2017,Jan,8; 2016,Jan,13; 2015,Jan,16; 2014,Jan,11

49904-49999 Harvesting of Omental Flap

49904 **Omental flap, extra-abdominal (eg, for reconstruction of sternal and chest wall defects)**

INCLUDES Harvest and transfer

EXCLUDES *Omental flap harvest by second surgeon: both surgeons report code with modifier 62*

40.9 40.9 FUD 090 C

AMA: 2014,Jan,11

\+ **49905** **Omental flap, intra-abdominal (List separately in addition to code for primary procedure)**

EXCLUDES *Exclusion of small intestine from pelvis by mesh or other prosthesis, or native tissue (44700)*

Code first primary procedure

10.2 10.2 FUD ZZZ C 80

AMA: 2018,Jan,8; 2017,Jan,8; 2016,Jan,13; 2015,Jan,16; 2014,Jan,11

49906 **Free omental flap with microvascular anastomosis**

INCLUDES Operating microscope (69990)

0.00 0.00 FUD 090 C

AMA: 2018,Jan,8; 2017,Jan,8; 2016,Feb,12; 2016,Jan,13; 2015,Jan,16; 2014,Jan,11

49999 **Unlisted procedure, abdomen, peritoneum and omentum**

0.00 0.00 FUD YYY T

AMA: 2018,Jan,8; 2017,Jan,8; 2016,Jan,13; 2015,Jan,16; 2014,Jan,9; 2014,Jan,11

50010-50045 Kidney Procedures for Exploration or Drainage

EXCLUDES *Donor nephrectomy performed laparoscopically (50547)*
Retroperitoneal
Abscess drainage (49060)
Exploration (49010)
Tumor/cyst excision (49203-49205)

50010 Renal exploration, not necessitating other specific procedures

EXCLUDES *Laparoscopic ablation of mass lesions of kidney (50542)*
21.2 21.2 FUD 090 C 80 50
AMA: 2014,Jan,11

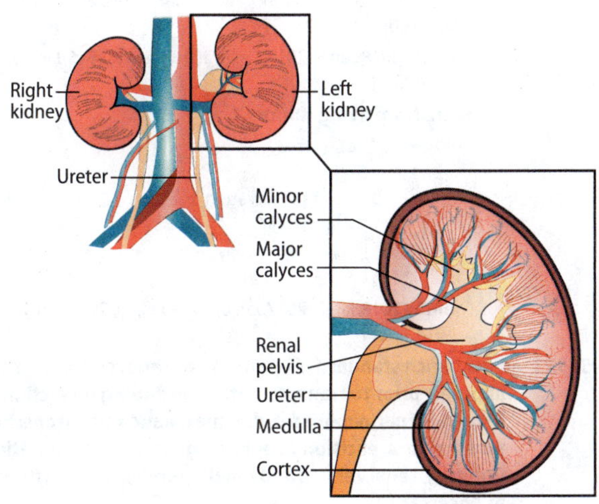

50020 Drainage of perirenal or renal abscess, open

EXCLUDES *Image-guided percutaneous drainage of perirenal or renal abscess (49405)*
29.3 29.3 FUD 090 J
AMA: 2018,Jan,8; 2017,Jan,8; 2016,Jan,13; 2015,Jan,16; 2014,May,9; 2014,Jan,11

50040 Nephrostomy, nephrotomy with drainage

26.8 26.8 FUD 090 C 50
AMA: 2018,Jan,8; 2017,Jan,8; 2016,Jan,13; 2015,Jan,16; 2014,Jan,11

50045 Nephrotomy, with exploration

EXCLUDES *Renal endoscopy through nephrotomy (50570-50580)*
26.9 26.9 FUD 090 C 80 50
AMA: 2018,Jan,8; 2017,Jan,8; 2016,Jan,13; 2015,Jan,16; 2014,Jan,11

50060-50081 Treatment of Kidney Stones

CMS: 100-03,230.1 NCD for Treatment of Kidney Stones

EXCLUDES *Retroperitoneal:*
Abscess drainage (49060)
Exploration (49010)
Tumor/cyst excision (49203-49205)

50060 Nephrolithotomy; removal of calculus

33.0 33.0 FUD 090 C 80 50
AMA: 2018,Jan,8; 2017,Jan,8; 2016,Jan,13; 2015,Jan,16; 2014,Jan,11

50065 secondary surgical operation for calculus

34.9 34.9 FUD 090 C 80 50
AMA: 2018,Jan,8; 2017,Jan,8; 2016,Jan,13; 2015,Jan,16; 2014,Jan,11

50070 complicated by congenital kidney abnormality

34.3 34.3 FUD 090 C 80 50
AMA: 2018,Jan,8; 2017,Jan,8; 2016,Jan,13; 2015,Jan,16; 2014,Jan,11

50075 removal of large staghorn calculus filling renal pelvis and calyces (including anatrophic pyelolithotomy)

42.1 42.1 FUD 090 C 80 50
AMA: 2018,Jan,8; 2017,Jan,8; 2016,Jan,13; 2015,Jan,16; 2014,Jan,11

50080 Percutaneous nephrostolithotomy or pyelostolithotomy, with or without dilation, endoscopy, lithotripsy, stenting, or basket extraction; up to 2 cm

EXCLUDES *Dilation of existing tract by same provider ([50436, 50437])*
Nephrostomy without nephrostolithotomy (50040, [50432, 50433], 52334)
(76000)
25.1 25.1 FUD 090 J G2 50
AMA: 2018,Jan,8; 2017,Jan,8; 2016,Jan,13; 2015,Jan,16; 2014,Jan,11

50081 over 2 cm

EXCLUDES *Dilation of existing tract by same provider ([50436, 50437])*
Nephrostomy without nephrostolithotomy (50040, [50432, 50433], 52334)
(76000)
36.9 36.9 FUD 090 J G2 80 50
AMA: 2018,Jan,8; 2017,Jan,8; 2016,Jan,13; 2015,Jan,16; 2014,Jan,11

50100 Repair of Anomalous Vessels of the Kidney

EXCLUDES *Retroperitoneal:*
Abscess drainage (49060)
Exploration (49010)
Tumor/cyst excision (49203-49205)

50100 Transection or repositioning of aberrant renal vessels (separate procedure)

31.3 31.3 FUD 090 C 80 50
AMA: 2018,Jan,8; 2017,Jan,8; 2016,Jan,13; 2015,Jan,16; 2014,Jan,11

50120-50135 Procedures of Renal Pelvis

EXCLUDES *Retroperitoneal:*
Abscess drainage (49060)
Exploration (49010)
Tumor/cyst excision (49203-49205)

50120 Pyelotomy; with exploration

INCLUDES Gol-Vernet pyelotomy
EXCLUDES *Renal endoscopy through pyelotomy (50570-50580)*
27.4 27.4 FUD 090 C 80 50
AMA: 2018,Jan,8; 2017,Jan,8; 2016,Jan,13; 2015,Jan,16; 2014,Jan,11

50125 with drainage, pyelostomy

28.4 28.4 FUD 090 C 80 50
AMA: 2018,Jan,8; 2017,Jan,8; 2016,Jan,13; 2015,Jan,16; 2014,Jan,11

50130 with removal of calculus (pyelolithotomy, pelviolithotomy, including coagulum pyelolithotomy)

29.9 29.9 FUD 090 C 80 50
AMA: 2018,Jan,8; 2017,Jan,8; 2016,Jan,13; 2015,Jan,16; 2014,Jan,11

50135 complicated (eg, secondary operation, congenital kidney abnormality)

32.4 32.4 FUD 090 C 80 50
AMA: 2018,Jan,8; 2017,Jan,8; 2016,Jan,13; 2015,Jan,16; 2014,Jan,11

50200-50205 Biopsy of Kidney

EXCLUDES *Laparoscopic renal mass lesion ablation (50542)*
Retroperitoneal tumor/cyst excision (49203-49205)

50200 Renal biopsy; percutaneous, by trocar or needle

EXCLUDES *Fine needle aspiration ([10005, 10006, 10007, 10008, 10009, 10010, 10011, 10012])*
(76942, 77002, 77012, 77021)
(88172-88173)
3.71 15.2 FUD 000 J A2 50
AMA: 2019,Apr,4; 2018,Jan,8; 2017,Jan,8; 2016,Jan,13; 2015,Jan,16; 2014,Jan,11

Urinary System

50010 — 50200

50205 by surgical exposure of kidney
21.8 21.8 FUD 090 C 80 50
AMA: 2018,Jan,8; 2017,Jan,8; 2016,Jan,13; 2015,Jan,16; 2014,Jan,11

50220-50240 Nephrectomy Procedures

EXCLUDES *Laparoscopic renal mass lesion ablation (50542)*
Retroperitoneal tumor/cyst excision (49203-49205)

50220 **Nephrectomy, including partial ureterectomy, any open approach including rib resection;**
30.3 30.3 FUD 090 C 80 50
AMA: 2018,Jan,8; 2017,Jan,8; 2016,Jan,13; 2015,Jan,16; 2014,Jan,11

50225 **complicated because of previous surgery on same kidney**
34.8 34.8 FUD 090 C 80 50
AMA: 2018,Jan,8; 2017,Jan,8; 2016,Jan,13; 2015,Jan,16; 2014,Jan,11

50230 **radical, with regional lymphadenectomy and/or vena caval thrombectomy**
EXCLUDES *Vena caval resection with reconstruction (37799)*
37.1 37.1 FUD 090 C 80 50
AMA: 2018,Jan,8; 2017,Jan,8; 2016,Jan,13; 2015,Jan,16; 2014,Jan,11

50234 **Nephrectomy with total ureterectomy and bladder cuff; through same incision**
37.7 37.7 FUD 090 C 80 50
AMA: 2018,Jan,8; 2017,Jan,8; 2016,Jan,13; 2015,Jan,16; 2014,Jan,11

50236 **through separate incision**
42.4 42.4 FUD 090 C 80 50
AMA: 2018,Jan,8; 2017,Jan,8; 2016,Jan,13; 2015,Jan,16; 2014,Jan,11

50240 **Nephrectomy, partial**
EXCLUDES *Laparoscopic partial nephrectomy (50543)*
38.3 38.3 FUD 090 C 80 50
AMA: 2018,Jan,8; 2017,Jan,8; 2016,Jan,13; 2015,Jan,16; 2014,Jan,11

50250-50290 Open Removal Kidney Lesions

EXCLUDES *Open destruction or excision intra-abdominal tumors (49203-49205)*

50250 **Ablation, open, 1 or more renal mass lesion(s), cryosurgical, including intraoperative ultrasound guidance and monitoring, if performed**
EXCLUDES *Laparoscopic renal mass lesion ablation (50542)*
Percutaneous renal tumor ablation (50592-50593)
35.1 35.1 FUD 090 C 80
AMA: 2018,Jan,8; 2017,Jan,8; 2016,Jan,13; 2015,Jan,16; 2014,Jan,11

50280 **Excision or unroofing of cyst(s) of kidney**
EXCLUDES *Renal cyst laparoscopic ablation (50541)*
27.6 27.6 FUD 090 C 80 50
AMA: 2018,Jan,8; 2017,Jan,8; 2016,Jan,13; 2015,Jan,16; 2014,Jan,11

50290 **Excision of perinephric cyst**
25.9 25.9 FUD 090 C 80
AMA: 2018,Jan,8; 2017,Jan,8; 2016,Jan,13; 2015,Jan,16; 2014,Jan,11

50300-50380 Kidney Transplant Procedures

CMS: 100-04,3,90.1 Kidney Transplant - General; 100-04,3,90.1.1 Standard Kidney Acquisition Charge; 100-04,3,90.1.2 Billing for Kidney Transplant and Acquisition Services; 100-04,3,90.5 Pancreas Transplants with Kidney Transplants

EXCLUDES *Dialysis procedures (90935-90999)*
Lymphocele drainage to peritoneal cavity performed laparoscopically (49323)

50300 **Donor nephrectomy (including cold preservation); from cadaver donor, unilateral or bilateral**
INCLUDES Graft:
Cold preservation
Harvesting
EXCLUDES *Donor nephrectomy performed laparoscopically (50547)*
0.00 0.00 FUD XXX C
AMA: 2018,Jan,8; 2017,Jan,8; 2016,Jan,13; 2015,Jan,16; 2014,Jan,11

50320 **open, from living donor**
INCLUDES Donor care
Graft:
Cold preservation
Harvesting
EXCLUDES *Donor nephrectomy performed laparoscopically (50547)*
43.5 43.5 FUD 090 C 80 50
AMA: 2018,Jan,8; 2017,Jan,8; 2016,Jan,13; 2015,Jan,16; 2014,Jan,11

50323 **Backbench standard preparation of cadaver donor renal allograft prior to transplantation, including dissection and removal of perinephric fat, diaphragmatic and retroperitoneal attachments, excision of adrenal gland, and preparation of ureter(s), renal vein(s), and renal artery(s), ligating branches, as necessary**
EXCLUDES *Adrenalectomy (60540, 60545)*
0.00 0.00 FUD XXX C 80
AMA: 2018,Jan,8; 2017,Jan,8; 2016,Jan,13; 2015,Jan,16; 2014,Jan,11

50325 **Backbench standard preparation of living donor renal allograft (open or laparoscopic) prior to transplantation, including dissection and removal of perinephric fat and preparation of ureter(s), renal vein(s), and renal artery(s), ligating branches, as necessary**
0.00 0.00 FUD XXX C 80
AMA: 2014,Jan,11

50327 **Backbench reconstruction of cadaver or living donor renal allograft prior to transplantation; venous anastomosis, each**
6.29 6.29 FUD XXX C 80
AMA: 2014,Jan,11

50328 **arterial anastomosis, each**
5.51 5.51 FUD XXX C 80
AMA: 2014,Jan,11

50329 **ureteral anastomosis, each**
5.24 5.24 FUD XXX C 80
AMA: 2014,Jan,11

50340 **Recipient nephrectomy (separate procedure)**
27.4 27.4 FUD 090 C 80 50
AMA: 2014,Jan,11

50360 **Renal allotransplantation, implantation of graft; without recipient nephrectomy**
INCLUDES Allograft transplantation
Recipient care
Code also backbench work (50323, 50325, 50327-50329)
Code also donor nephrectomy (cadaver or living donor) (50300, 50320, 50547)
70.0 70.0 FUD 090 C 80
AMA: 2014,Jan,11

50365 **with recipient nephrectomy**
INCLUDES Allograft transplantation
Recipient care
83.0 83.0 FUD 090 C 80 50
AMA: 2018,Jan,8; 2017,Jan,8; 2016,Jan,13; 2015,Jan,16; 2014,Jan,11

50370 **Removal of transplanted renal allograft**
34.8 34.8 FUD 090 C 80
AMA: 2014,Jan,11

50380 **Renal autotransplantation, reimplantation of kidney**
INCLUDES Reimplantation of autograft
EXCLUDES *Secondary procedures:*
Nephrolithotomy (50060-50075)
Partial nephrectomy (50240, 50543)
58.1 58.1 FUD 090 C 80
AMA: 2019,Sep,10; 2018,Jan,8; 2017,Jan,8; 2016,Jan,13; 2015,Jan,16; 2014,Jan,11

50382-50386 Removal With/Without Replacement Internal Ureteral Stent

INCLUDES Radiological supervision and interpretation

50382 **Removal (via snare/capture) and replacement of internally dwelling ureteral stent via percutaneous approach, including radiological supervision and interpretation**
EXCLUDES *Dilation existing tract, percutaneous for endourologic procedure ([50436, 50437])*
Removal and replacement of an internally dwelling ureteral stent using a transurethral approach (50385)
7.46 31.3 FUD 000 J G2 50
AMA: 2018,Jan,8; 2017,Jan,8; 2016,Jan,13; 2016,Jan,3; 2015,Jan,16; 2014,Jan,11

50384 **Removal (via snare/capture) of internally dwelling ureteral stent via percutaneous approach, including radiological supervision and interpretation**
EXCLUDES *Dilation existing tract, percutaneous for endourologic procedure ([50436, 50437])*
Removal of an internally dwelling ureteral stent using a transurethral approach (50386)
6.68 25.0 FUD 000 Q2 G2 50
AMA: 2018,Jan,8; 2017,Jan,8; 2016,Jan,13; 2016,Jan,3; 2015,Jan,16; 2014,Jan,11

50385 **Removal (via snare/capture) and replacement of internally dwelling ureteral stent via transurethral approach, without use of cystoscopy, including radiological supervision and interpretation**
6.34 30.7 FUD 000 J G2 80 50
AMA: 2018,Jan,8; 2017,Jan,8; 2016,Jan,13; 2016,Jan,3; 2015,Jan,16; 2014,Jan,11

50386 **Removal (via snare/capture) of internally dwelling ureteral stent via transurethral approach, without use of cystoscopy, including radiological supervision and interpretation**
4.70 20.3 FUD 000 Q2 P3 80 50
AMA: 2018,Jan,8; 2017,Jan,8; 2016,Jan,3; 2016,Jan,13; 2015,Jan,16; 2014,Jan,11

50387 Remove/Replace Accessible Ureteral Stent

EXCLUDES *Removal and replacement of ureteral stent through ureterostomy tube or ileal conduit (50688)*
Removal without replacement of externally accessible ureteral stent without fluoroscopic guidance, report with appropriate E&M code

50387 **Removal and replacement of externally accessible nephroureteral catheter (eg, external/internal stent) requiring fluoroscopic guidance, including radiological supervision and interpretation**
2.43 14.6 FUD 000 J G2 80 50
AMA: 2018,Jan,8; 2017,Jan,8; 2016,Mar,10; 2016,Jan,13; 2016,Jan,3; 2015,Oct,5; 2015,Jan,16; 2014,Jan,11

50389-50435 [50430, 50431, 50432, 50433, 50434, 50435, 50436, 50437] Percutaneous and Injection Procedures With/Without Indwelling Tube/Catheter Access

50389 **Removal of nephrostomy tube, requiring fluoroscopic guidance (eg, with concurrent indwelling ureteral stent)**
EXCLUDES *Nephrostomy tube removal without fluoroscopic guidance, report with appropriate E&M code*
1.56 9.49 FUD 000 Q2 G2 50
AMA: 2018,Jan,8; 2017,Jan,8; 2016,Jan,13; 2016,Jan,3; 2015,Oct,5; 2015,Jan,16; 2014,Jan,11

50390 **Aspiration and/or injection of renal cyst or pelvis by needle, percutaneous**
EXCLUDES *Antegrade nephrostogram/pyelogram ([50430, 50431])*
(74425, 74470, 76942, 77002, 77012, 77021)
2.78 2.78 FUD 000 T A2 50
AMA: 2018,Jan,8; 2017,Jan,8; 2016,Jan,13; 2015,Oct,5; 2015,Jan,16; 2014,Jan,11

50391 **Instillation(s) of therapeutic agent into renal pelvis and/or ureter through established nephrostomy, pyelostomy or ureterostomy tube (eg, anticarcinogenic or antifungal agent)**
Code also therapeutic agent
2.84 3.52 FUD 000 T P3 50
AMA: 2018,Jan,8; 2017,Jan,8; 2016,Jan,13; 2015,Oct,5; 2015,Jan,16; 2014,Jan,11

50436 **Dilation of existing tract, percutaneous, for an endourologic procedure including imaging guidance (eg, ultrasound and/or fluoroscopy) and all associated radiological supervision and interpretation, with postprocedure tube placement, when performed**
4.37 4.37 FUD 000 G2 50
EXCLUDES *Percutaneous nephrostolithotomy (50080-50081)*
Procedure performed for same renal collecting system/ureter ([50430, 50431, 50432, 50433], 52334, 74485)
Removal, replacement internally dwelling ureteral stent (50382, 50384)

50437 **including new access into the renal collecting system**
7.29 7.29 FUD 000 G2 50
EXCLUDES *Percutaneous nephrostolithotomy (50080-50081)*
Procedure performed for same renal collecting system/ureter ([50430, 50431, 50432, 50433], 52334, 74485)
Removal, replacement internally dwelling ureteral stent (50382, 50384)

50396 **Manometric studies through nephrostomy or pyelostomy tube, or indwelling ureteral catheter**
(74425)
3.38 3.38 FUD 000 J A2 80 50
AMA: 2018,Jan,8; 2017,Jan,8; 2016,Jan,13; 2015,Jan,16; 2014,Jan,11

\# **50430** **Injection procedure for antegrade nephrostogram and/or ureterogram, complete diagnostic procedure including imaging guidance (eg, ultrasound and fluoroscopy) and all associated radiological supervision and interpretation; new access**

INCLUDES Renal pelvis and associated ureter as a single element

EXCLUDES *Procedure performed for same renal collecting system/ureter ([50432, 50433, 50434, 50435], 50693-50695, 74425)*

4.46 14.5 FUD 000

AMA: 2018,Jan,8; 2017,Jan,8; 2016,Jan,3; 2016,Jan,13; 2015,Oct,5

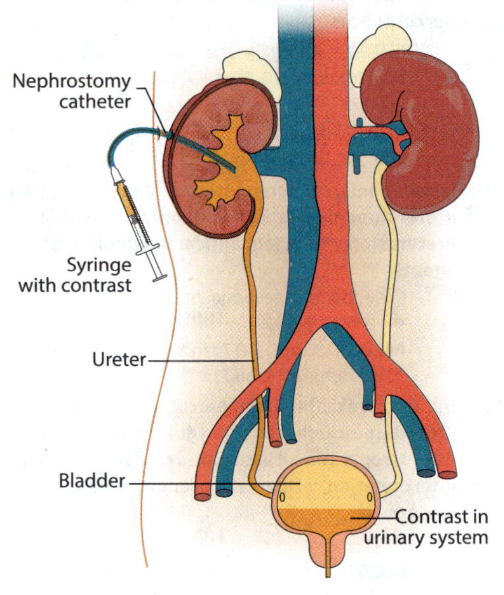

\# **50431** **existing access**

INCLUDES Renal pelvis and associated ureter as a single element

EXCLUDES *Procedure performed for same renal collecting system/ureter ([50432, 50433, 50434, 50435], 50693-50695, 74425)*

1.90 6.03 FUD 000

AMA: 2018,Jan,8; 2017,Jan,8; 2016,Jan,3; 2016,Jan,13; 2015,Oct,5

\# **50432** **Placement of nephrostomy catheter, percutaneous, including diagnostic nephrostogram and/or ureterogram when performed, imaging guidance (eg, ultrasound and/or fluoroscopy) and all associated radiological supervision and interpretation**

INCLUDES Renal pelvis and associated ureter as a single element

EXCLUDES *Dilation of nephroureteral catheter tract ([50436, 50437])*

Procedure performed for same renal collecting system/ureter ([50430, 50431], [50433], 50694-50695, 74425)

5.98 23.5 FUD 000

AMA: 2018,Mar,11; 2018,Jan,8; 2017,Jan,8; 2016,Jan,3; 2016,Jan,13; 2015,Oct,5

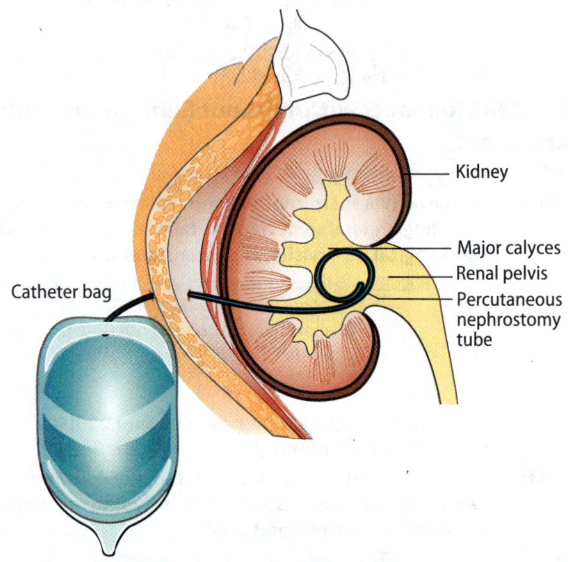

\# **50433** **Placement of nephroureteral catheter, percutaneous, including diagnostic nephrostogram and/or ureterogram when performed, imaging guidance (eg, ultrasound and/or fluoroscopy) and all associated radiological supervision and interpretation, new access**

INCLUDES Renal pelvis and associated ureter as a single element

EXCLUDES *Dilation of nephroureteral catheter tract ([50436, 50437])*

Nephroureteral catheter removal/replacement (50387)

Procedures performed for same renal collecting system/ureter ([50430, 50431, 50432], 50693-50695, 74425)

7.44 31.2 FUD 000

AMA: 2018,Mar,11; 2018,Jan,8; 2017,Jan,8; 2016,Jan,3; 2016,Jan,13; 2015,Oct,5

\# **50434** **Convert nephrostomy catheter to nephroureteral catheter, percutaneous, including diagnostic nephrostogram and/or ureterogram when performed, imaging guidance (eg, ultrasound and/or fluoroscopy) and all associated radiological supervision and interpretation, via pre-existing nephrostomy tract**

INCLUDES Renal pelvis and associated ureter as a single element

EXCLUDES *Procedure performed for same renal collecting system/ureter ([50430, 50431], [50435], 50684, 50693, 74425)*

5.60 24.6 FUD 000

AMA: 2018,Jan,8; 2017,Jan,8; 2016,Jan,3; 2016,Jan,13; 2015,Oct,5

\# **50435** **Exchange nephrostomy catheter, percutaneous, including diagnostic nephrostogram and/or ureterogram when performed, imaging guidance (eg, ultrasound and/or fluoroscopy) and all associated radiological supervision and interpretation**

INCLUDES Renal pelvis and associated ureter as a single element

EXCLUDES *Procedure performed for same renal collecting system/ureter ([50430, 50431], [50434], 50693, 74425)*

Removal nephrostomy catheter that requires fluoroscopic guidance (50389)

2.90 14.6 FUD 000 J G2 50

AMA: 2018,Mar,11; 2018,Jan,8; 2017,Jan,8; 2016,Jan,3; 2016,Jan,13; 2015,Oct,5

50400-50540 Open Surgical Procedures of Kidney

50400 **Pyeloplasty (Foley Y-pyeloplasty), plastic operation on renal pelvis, with or without plastic operation on ureter, nephropexy, nephrostomy, pyelostomy, or ureteral splinting; simple**

EXCLUDES *Laparoscopic pyeloplasty (50544)*

33.5 33.5 FUD 090 C 80 50

AMA: 2018,Jan,8; 2017,Jan,8; 2016,Jan,13; 2015,Jan,16; 2014,Jan,11

50405 **complicated (congenital kidney abnormality, secondary pyeloplasty, solitary kidney, calycoplasty)**

EXCLUDES *Laparoscopic pyeloplasty (50544)*

40.4 40.4 FUD 090 C 80 50

AMA: 2018,Jan,8; 2017,Jan,8; 2016,Jan,13; 2015,Jan,16; 2014,Jan,11

50430 **Resequenced code. See code following 50396.**

50431 **Resequenced code. See code following 50396.**

50432 **Resequenced code. See code following 50396.**

50433 **Resequenced code. See code following 50396.**

50434 **Resequenced code. See code following 50396.**

50435 **Resequenced code. See code following 50396.**

50436 **Resequenced code. See code following 50391.**

50437 **Resequenced code. See code following 50391.**

50500 **Nephrorrhaphy, suture of kidney wound or injury**

37.3 37.3 FUD 090 C 80

AMA: 2014,Jan,11

Schematic of nephron

50520 **Closure of nephrocutaneous or pyelocutaneous fistula**

33.6 33.6 FUD 090 C 80

AMA: 2014,Jan,11

50525 **Closure of nephrovisceral fistula (eg, renocolic), including visceral repair; abdominal approach**

42.6 42.6 FUD 090 C 80

AMA: 2014,Jan,11

50526 **thoracic approach**

45.7 45.7 FUD 090 C 80

AMA: 2014,Jan,11

50540 **Symphysiotomy for horseshoe kidney with or without pyeloplasty and/or other plastic procedure, unilateral or bilateral (1 operation)**

33.2 33.2 FUD 090 C 80

AMA: 2014,Jan,11

50541-50549 Laparoscopic Surgical Procedures of the Kidney

INCLUDES Diagnostic laparoscopy (49320)

EXCLUDES *Laparoscopic drainage of lymphocele to peritoneal cavity (49323)*

50541 **Laparoscopy, surgical; ablation of renal cysts**

26.5 26.5 FUD 090 J 80 50

AMA: 2018,Jan,8; 2017,Jan,8; 2016,Jan,13; 2015,Jan,16; 2014,Jan,11

50542 **ablation of renal mass lesion(s), including intraoperative ultrasound guidance and monitoring, when performed**

EXCLUDES *Open ablation of renal mass lesions (50250)*

Percutaneous ablation of renal tumors (50592-50593)

33.7 33.7 FUD 090 J 80 50

AMA: 2018,Jan,8; 2017,Jan,8; 2016,Jan,13; 2015,Jan,16; 2014,Jan,11

50543 **partial nephrectomy**

EXCLUDES *Partial nephrectomy, open approach (50240)*

43.0 43.0 FUD 090 J 80 50

AMA: 2018,Jan,8; 2017,Jan,8; 2016,Jan,13; 2015,Jan,16; 2014,Jan,11

50544 **pyeloplasty**

36.0 36.0 FUD 090 J 80 50

AMA: 2018,Jan,8; 2017,Jan,8; 2016,Jan,13; 2015,Jan,16; 2014,Jan,11

50545 **radical nephrectomy (includes removal of Gerota's fascia and surrounding fatty tissue, removal of regional lymph nodes, and adrenalectomy)**

EXCLUDES *Radical nephrectomy, open approach (50230)*

38.7 38.7 FUD 090 C 80 50

AMA: 2018,Jan,8; 2017,Jan,8; 2016,Jan,13; 2015,Jan,16; 2014,Jan,11

50546 **nephrectomy, including partial ureterectomy**

34.8 34.8 FUD 090 C 80 50

AMA: 2018,Jan,8; 2017,Jan,8; 2016,Jan,13; 2015,Jan,16; 2014,Jan,11

50547 **donor nephrectomy (including cold preservation), from living donor**

INCLUDES Donor care

Graft:

Cold preservation

Harvesting

EXCLUDES *Backbench reconstruction renal allograft prior to transplantation (50327-50329)*

Backbench standard preparation of living donor renal allograft prior to transplantation (50325)

Donor nephrectomy, open approach (50320)

46.4 46.4 FUD 090 C 80 50

AMA: 2018,Jan,8; 2017,Jan,8; 2016,Jan,13; 2015,Jan,16; 2014,Jan,11

50548 **nephrectomy with total ureterectomy**

EXCLUDES *Nephrectomy, open approach (50234, 50236)*

38.9 38.9 FUD 090 C 80 50

AMA: 2018,Jan,8; 2017,Jan,8; 2016,Jan,13; 2015,Jan,16; 2014,Jan,11

50549 **Unlisted laparoscopy procedure, renal**
0.00 0.00 FUD YYY J 80 50
AMA: 2018,Jan,8; 2017,Jan,8; 2016,Jan,13; 2015,Jan,16; 2014,Jan,11

50551-50562 Endoscopic Procedures of Kidney via Established Nephrostomy/Pyelostomy Access

50551 **Renal endoscopy through established nephrostomy or pyelostomy, with or without irrigation, instillation, or ureteropyelography, exclusive of radiologic service;**
8.54 10.4 FUD 000 J A2 80 50
AMA: 2018,Jan,8; 2017,Jan,8; 2016,Jan,13; 2015,Jan,16; 2014,Jan,11

50553 **with ureteral catheterization, with or without dilation of ureter**
EXCLUDES *Image-guided ureter dilation without endoscopic guidance (50706)*
9.09 11.1 FUD 000 J A2 50
AMA: 2018,Jan,8; 2017,Jan,8; 2016,Jan,3; 2016,Jan,13; 2015,Jan,16; 2014,Jan,11

50555 **with biopsy**
EXCLUDES *Image-guided biopsy ureter/renal pelvis without endoscopic guidance (50606)*
9.88 11.9 FUD 000 J A2 80 50
AMA: 2018,Jan,8; 2017,Jan,8; 2016,Jan,3; 2016,Jan,13; 2015,Jan,16; 2014,Jan,11

50557 **with fulguration and/or incision, with or without biopsy**
10.0 12.1 FUD 000 J A2 80 50
AMA: 2018,Jan,8; 2017,Jan,8; 2016,Jan,13; 2015,Jan,16; 2014,Jan,11

50561 **with removal of foreign body or calculus**
11.4 13.7 FUD 000 J A2 80 50
AMA: 2018,Jan,8; 2017,Jan,8; 2016,Jan,13; 2015,Jan,16; 2014,Jan,11

50562 **with resection of tumor**
16.8 16.8 FUD 090 J G2 80
AMA: 2018,Jan,8; 2017,Jan,8; 2016,Jan,13; 2015,Jan,16; 2014,Jan,11

50570-50580 Endoscopic Procedures of Kidney via Nephrotomy/Pyelotomy Access

Code also if provided service is significant and identifiable (50045, 50120)

50570 **Renal endoscopy through nephrotomy or pyelotomy, with or without irrigation, instillation, or ureteropyelography, exclusive of radiologic service;**
14.2 14.2 FUD 000 J G2 80 50
AMA: 2018,Jan,8; 2017,Jan,8; 2016,Jan,13; 2015,Jan,16; 2014,Jan,11

50572 **with ureteral catheterization, with or without dilation of ureter**
EXCLUDES *Image-guided ureter dilation without endoscopic guidance (50706)*
15.4 15.4 FUD 000 T G2 80 50
AMA: 2018,Jan,8; 2017,Jan,8; 2016,Jan,3; 2016,Jan,13; 2015,Jan,16; 2014,Jan,11

50574 **with biopsy**
EXCLUDES *Image-guide ureter/renal pelvis biopsy without endoscopic guidance (50606)*
16.3 16.3 FUD 000 J G2 80 50
AMA: 2018,Jan,8; 2017,Jan,8; 2016,Jan,3; 2016,Jan,13; 2015,Jan,16; 2014,Jan,11

50575 **with endopyelotomy (includes cystoscopy, ureteroscopy, dilation of ureter and ureteral pelvic junction, incision of ureteral pelvic junction and insertion of endopyelotomy stent)**
20.6 20.6 FUD 000 J G2 50
AMA: 2018,Jan,8; 2017,Jan,8; 2016,Jan,13; 2015,Jan,16; 2014,Jan,11

50576 **with fulguration and/or incision, with or without biopsy**
16.3 16.3 FUD 000 J G2 80 50
AMA: 2018,Jan,8; 2017,Jan,8; 2016,Jan,13; 2015,Jan,16; 2014,Jan,11

50580 **with removal of foreign body or calculus**
17.5 17.5 FUD 000 J G2 80 50
AMA: 2018,Jan,8; 2017,Jan,8; 2016,Jan,13; 2015,Jan,16; 2014,Jan,11

50590-50593 Noninvasive and Minimally Invasive Procedures of the Kidney

50590 **Lithotripsy, extracorporeal shock wave**
16.4 21.0 FUD 090 J G2 50
AMA: 2018,Jan,8; 2017,Jan,8; 2016,Jan,13; 2015,Jan,16; 2014,Jan,11

50592 **Ablation, 1 or more renal tumor(s), percutaneous, unilateral, radiofrequency**
(76940, 77013, 77022)
9.93 92.3 FUD 010 J G2 50
AMA: 2014,Jan,11

50593 **Ablation, renal tumor(s), unilateral, percutaneous, cryotherapy**
(76940, 77013, 77022)
13.3 125. FUD 010 J J8 80 50
AMA: 2018,Jan,8; 2014,Jan,11

50600-50940 Open and Injection Procedures of Ureter

50600 **Ureterotomy with exploration or drainage (separate procedure)**
Code also ureteral endoscopy through ureterotomy when procedures constitute a significant identifiable service (50970-50980)
27.1 27.1 FUD 090 C 80 50
AMA: 2014,Jan,11

50605 **Ureterotomy for insertion of indwelling stent, all types**
28.6 28.6 FUD 090 C 80 50
AMA: 2018,Jan,8; 2017,Jan,8; 2016,Jan,13; 2015,Jan,16; 2014,Jan,11

+ **50606 Endoluminal biopsy of ureter and/or renal pelvis, non-endoscopic, including imaging guidance (eg, ultrasound and/or fluoroscopy) and all associated radiological supervision and interpretation (List separately in addition to code for primary procedure)**

INCLUDES Renal pelvis and associated ureter as a single element

EXCLUDES *Procedure performed for same renal collecting system/associated ureter with (50555, 50574, 50955, 50974, 52007, 74425)*

Code first (50382-50389, [50430, 50431, 50432, 50433, 50434, 50435], 50684, 50688, 50690, 50693-50695, 51610)

4.43 18.8 FUD ZZZ N N1 50

AMA: 2018,Jan,8; 2017,Jan,8; 2016,Jan,3

50610 Ureterolithotomy; upper one-third of ureter

EXCLUDES *Cystotomy with calculus basket extraction of ureteral calculus (51065)*
Transvesical ureterolithotomy (51060)
Ureteral calculus manipulation/extraction performed endoscopically (50080-50081, 50561, 50961, 50980, 52320-52330, 52352-52353, [52356])
Ureterolithotomy performed laparoscopically (50945)

27.3 27.3 FUD 090 C 80 50

AMA: 2018,Jan,8; 2017,Jan,8; 2016,Jan,13; 2015,Jan,16; 2014,Jan,11

50620 middle one-third of ureter

EXCLUDES *Cystotomy with calculus basket extraction of ureteral calculus (51065)*
Transvesical ureterolithotomy (51060)
Ureteral calculus manipulation/extraction performed endoscopically (50080-50081, 50561, 50961, 50980, 52320-52330, 52352-52353, [52356])
Ureterolithotomy performed laparoscopically (50945)

26.1 26.1 FUD 090 C 80 50

AMA: 2018,Jan,8; 2017,Jan,8; 2016,Jan,13; 2015,Jan,16; 2014,Jan,11

50630 lower one-third of ureter

EXCLUDES *Cystotomy with calculus basket extraction of ureteral calculus (51065)*
Transvesical ureterolithotomy (51060)
Ureteral calculus manipulation/extraction performed endoscopically (50080-50081, 50561, 50961, 50980, 52320-52330, 52352-52353, [52356])
Ureterolithotomy performed laparoscopically (50945)

25.8 25.8 FUD 090 C 80 50

AMA: 2018,Jan,8; 2017,Jan,8; 2016,Jan,13; 2015,Jan,16; 2014,May,3; 2014,Jan,11

50650 Ureterectomy, with bladder cuff (separate procedure)

EXCLUDES *Ureterocele (51535, 52300)*

30.0 30.0 FUD 090 C 80 50

AMA: 2014,Jan,11

50660 Ureterectomy, total, ectopic ureter, combination abdominal, vaginal and/or perineal approach

EXCLUDES *Ureterocele (51535, 52300)*

33.1 33.1 FUD 090 C 80

AMA: 2014,Jan,11

50684 Injection procedure for ureterography or ureteropyelography through ureterostomy or indwelling ureteral catheter

EXCLUDES *Placement of nephroureteral catheter ([50433, 50434])*
Placement of ureteral stent (50693-50695)

(74425)

1.45 3.10 FUD 000 N N1 50

AMA: 2018,Jan,8; 2017,Jan,8; 2016,Jan,3; 2015,Oct,5; 2014,Jan,11

50686 Manometric studies through ureterostomy or indwelling ureteral catheter

2.55 3.99 FUD 000 S P2 80

AMA: 2014,Jan,11

50688 Change of ureterostomy tube or externally accessible ureteral stent via ileal conduit

(75984)

2.25 2.25 FUD 010 J A2

AMA: 2018,Jan,8; 2017,Jan,8; 2016,Jan,3; 2014,Jan,11

50690 Injection procedure for visualization of ileal conduit and/or ureteropyelography, exclusive of radiologic service

(74425)

2.02 2.87 FUD 000 N N1

AMA: 2018,Jan,8; 2017,Jan,8; 2016,Jan,3; 2014,Jan,11

50693 Placement of ureteral stent, percutaneous, including diagnostic nephrostogram and/or ureterogram when performed, imaging guidance (eg, ultrasound and/or fluoroscopy), and all associated radiological supervision and interpretation; pre-existing nephrostomy tract

INCLUDES Renal pelvis and associated ureter as a single element

EXCLUDES *Procedure performed for the same renal collecting system/ureter ([50430, 50431, 50432, 50433, 50434, 50435], 50684, 74425)*

5.94 28.7 FUD 000 J G2 50

AMA: 2018,Jan,8; 2017,Jan,8; 2016,Jan,3; 2016,Jan,13; 2015,Oct,5

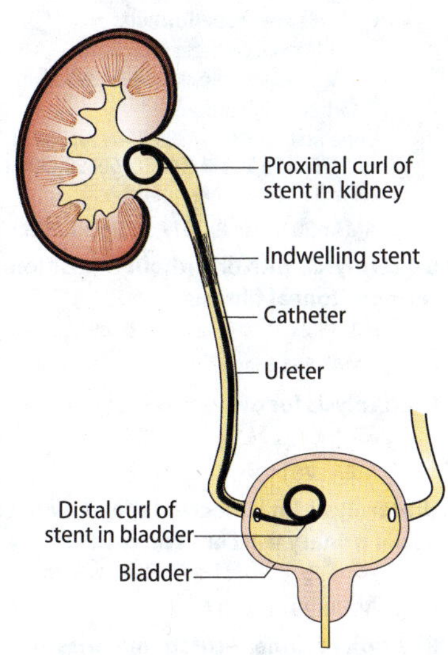

50694 new access, without separate nephrostomy catheter

INCLUDES Renal pelvis and associated ureter as a single element

EXCLUDES *Procedure performed for the same renal collecting system/ureter ([50430, 50431, 50432, 50433, 50434, 50435], 50684, 74425)*

7.77 31.7 FUD 000 J G2 50

AMA: 2018,Jan,8; 2017,Jan,8; 2016,Jan,3; 2016,Jan,13; 2015,Oct,5

50695 new access, with separate nephrostomy catheter

INCLUDES Placement of separate ureteral stent and nephrostomy catheter into a ureter/associated renal pelvis through a new access
Renal pelvis and associated ureter as a single element

EXCLUDES *Procedure performed for the same renal collecting system/ureter ([50430, 50431, 50432, 50433, 50434, 50435], 50684, 74425)*

9.95 38.7 FUD 000 J G2 50

AMA: 2018,Jan,8; 2017,Jan,8; 2016,Jan,3; 2016,Jan,13; 2015,Oct,5

50700 Ureteroplasty, plastic operation on ureter (eg, stricture)

26.7 26.7 FUD 090 C 80 50

AMA: 2014,Jan,11

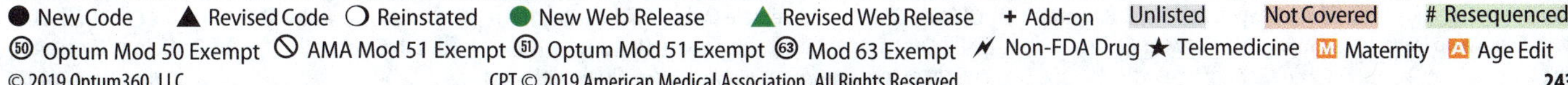

\+ **50705 Ureteral embolization or occlusion, including imaging guidance (eg, ultrasound and/or fluoroscopy) and all associated radiological supervision and interpretation (List separately in addition to code for primary procedure)**

INCLUDES Renal pelvis and associated ureter as a single element

Code also when performed:
- Additional catheter insertions
- Diagnostic pyelography/ureterography
- Other interventions

Code first (50382-50389, [50430, 50431, 50432, 50433, 50434, 50435], 50684, 50688, 50690, 50693-50695, 51610)

5.69 | 56.8 | FUD ZZZ | N N1 50

AMA: 2018,Jan,8; 2017,Jan,8; 2016,Jan,3

\+ **50706 Balloon dilation, ureteral stricture, including imaging guidance (eg, ultrasound and/or fluoroscopy) and all associated radiological supervision and interpretation (List separately in addition to code for primary procedure)**

INCLUDES Dilation of nephrostomy, ureters, or urethra (74485)
Renal pelvis and associated ureter as a single element

EXCLUDES *Cystourethroscopy (52341, 52344-52345)*
Renal endoscopy (50553, 50572)
Ureteral endoscopy (50953, 50972)

Code also when performed:
- Additional catheter insertions
- Diagnostic pyelography/ureterography
- Other interventions

Code first (50382-50389, [50430, 50431, 50432, 50433, 50434, 50435], 50684, 50688, 50690, 50693-50695, 51610)

5.31 | 27.4 | FUD ZZZ | N N1 50

AMA: 2018,Jan,8; 2017,Jan,8; 2016,Jan,3

50715 Ureterolysis, with or without repositioning of ureter for retroperitoneal fibrosis

35.2 | 35.2 | FUD 090 | C 80 50

AMA: 2014,Jan,11

50722 Ureterolysis for ovarian vein syndrome ♀

29.1 | 29.1 | FUD 090 | C 80

AMA: 2014,Jan,11

50725 Ureterolysis for retrocaval ureter, with reanastomosis of upper urinary tract or vena cava

31.9 | 31.9 | FUD 090 | C 80

AMA: 2014,Jan,11

50727 Revision of urinary-cutaneous anastomosis (any type urostomy);

14.7 | 14.7 | FUD 090 | J G2 80

AMA: 2014,Jan,11

50728 with repair of fascial defect and hernia

21.2 | 21.2 | FUD 090 | C 80

AMA: 2014,Jan,11

50740 Ureteropyelostomy, anastomosis of ureter and renal pelvis

35.4 | 35.4 | FUD 090 | C 80 50

AMA: 2018,Jan,8; 2017,Jan,8; 2016,Jan,13; 2015,Jan,16; 2014,Jan,11

50750 Ureterocalycostomy, anastomosis of ureter to renal calyx

33.3 | 33.3 | FUD 090 | C 80 50

AMA: 2018,Jan,8; 2017,Jan,8; 2016,Jan,13; 2015,Jan,16; 2014,Jan,11

50760 Ureteroureterostomy

32.6 | 32.6 | FUD 090 | C 80 50

AMA: 2018,Jan,8; 2017,Jan,8; 2016,Jan,13; 2015,Jan,16; 2014,Jan,11

50770 Transureteroureterostomy, anastomosis of ureter to contralateral ureter

33.3 | 33.3 | FUD 090 | C 80

AMA: 2014,Jan,11

50780 Ureteroneocystostomy; anastomosis of single ureter to bladder

INCLUDES Minor procedures to prevent vesicoureteral reflux

EXCLUDES *Cystourethroplasty with ureteroneocystostomy (51820)*

31.9 | 31.9 | FUD 090 | C 80 50

AMA: 2018,Feb,11; 2018,Jan,8; 2017,Jan,8; 2016,Jan,13; 2015,Jan,16; 2014,Jan,11

50782 anastomosis of duplicated ureter to bladder

INCLUDES Minor procedures to prevent vesicoureteral reflux

31.1 | 31.1 | FUD 090 | C 80 50

AMA: 2018,Jan,8; 2017,Jan,8; 2016,Jan,13; 2015,Jan,16; 2014,Jan,11

50783 with extensive ureteral tailoring

INCLUDES Minor procedures to prevent vesicoureteral reflux

32.6 | 32.6 | FUD 090 | C 80 50

AMA: 2018,Jan,8; 2017,Jan,8; 2016,Jan,13; 2015,Jan,16; 2014,Jan,11

50785 with vesico-psoas hitch or bladder flap

INCLUDES Minor procedures to prevent vesicoureteral reflux

35.1 | 35.1 | FUD 090 | C 80 50

AMA: 2018,Jan,8; 2017,Jan,8; 2016,Jan,13; 2015,Jan,16; 2014,Jan,11

50800 Ureteroenterostomy, direct anastomosis of ureter to intestine

EXCLUDES *Cystectomy with ureterosigmoidostomy/ureteroileal conduit (51580-51595)*

26.8 | 26.8 | FUD 090 | C 80 50

AMA: 2018,Jan,8; 2017,Jan,8; 2016,Jan,13; 2015,Jan,16; 2014,Jan,11

50810 Ureterosigmoidostomy, with creation of sigmoid bladder and establishment of abdominal or perineal colostomy, including intestine anastomosis

EXCLUDES *Cystectomy with ureterosigmoidostomy/ureteroileal conduit (51580-51595)*

40.5 | 40.5 | FUD 090 | C 80

AMA: 2018,Jan,8; 2017,Jan,8; 2016,Jan,13; 2015,Jan,16; 2014,Jan,11

50815 Ureterocolon conduit, including intestine anastomosis

EXCLUDES *Cystectomy with ureterosigmoidostomy/ureteroileal conduit (51580-51595)*

35.3 | 35.3 | FUD 090 | C 80 50

AMA: 2018,Jan,8; 2017,Jan,8; 2016,Jan,13; 2015,Jan,16; 2014,Jan,11

50820 Ureteroileal conduit (ileal bladder), including intestine anastomosis (Bricker operation)

EXCLUDES *Cystectomy with ureterosigmoidostomy/ureteroileal conduit (51580-51595)*

38.0 | 38.0 | FUD 090 | C 80 50

AMA: 2018,Jan,8; 2017,Jan,8; 2016,Jan,13; 2015,Jan,16; 2014,Jan,11

50825 Continent diversion, including intestine anastomosis using any segment of small and/or large intestine (Kock pouch or Camey enterocystoplasty)

48.0 | 48.0 | FUD 090 | C 80

AMA: 2018,Jan,8; 2017,Jan,8; 2016,Jan,13; 2015,Jan,16; 2014,Jan,11

50830 Urinary undiversion (eg, taking down of ureteroileal conduit, ureterosigmoidostomy or ureteroenterostomy with ureteroureterostomy or ureteroneocystostomy)

52.1 | 52.1 | FUD 090 | C 80

AMA: 2018,Jan,8; 2017,Jan,8; 2016,Jan,13; 2015,Jan,16; 2014,Jan,11

50840 Replacement of all or part of ureter by intestine segment, including intestine anastomosis

35.5 | 35.5 | FUD 090 | C 80 50

AMA: 2018,Jan,8; 2017,Jan,8; 2016,Jan,13; 2015,Jan,16; 2014,Jan,11

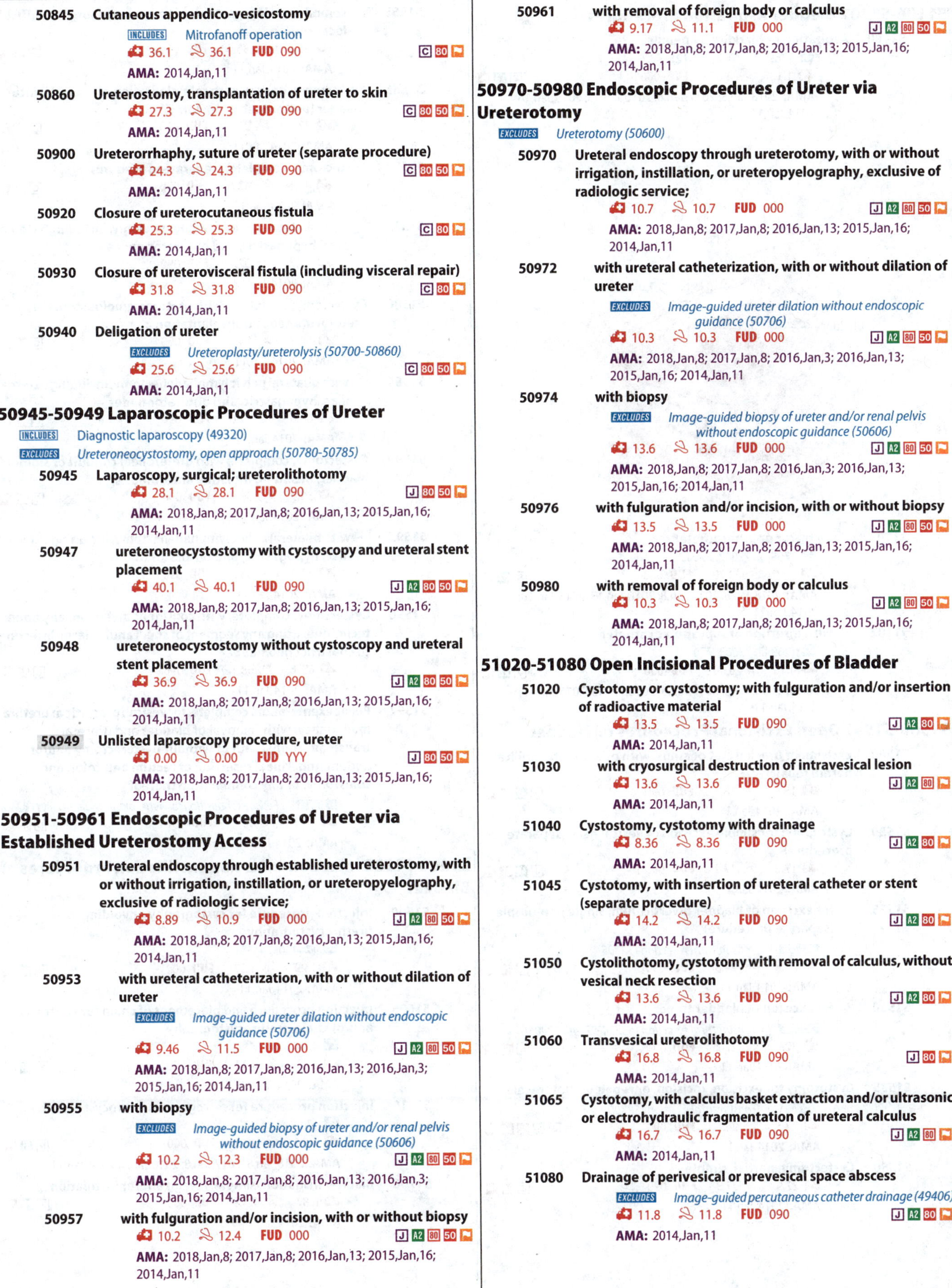

50845 **Cutaneous appendico-vesicostomy**
INCLUDES Mitrofanoff operation
36.1 36.1 FUD 090 C 80
AMA: 2014,Jan,11

50860 **Ureterostomy, transplantation of ureter to skin**
27.3 27.3 FUD 090 C 80 50
AMA: 2014,Jan,11

50900 **Ureterorrhaphy, suture of ureter (separate procedure)**
24.3 24.3 FUD 090 C 80 50
AMA: 2014,Jan,11

50920 **Closure of ureterocutaneous fistula**
25.3 25.3 FUD 090 C 80
AMA: 2014,Jan,11

50930 **Closure of ureterovisceral fistula (including visceral repair)**
31.8 31.8 FUD 090 C 80
AMA: 2014,Jan,11

50940 **Deligation of ureter**
EXCLUDES *Ureteroplasty/ureterolysis (50700-50860)*
25.6 25.6 FUD 090 C 80 50
AMA: 2014,Jan,11

50945-50949 Laparoscopic Procedures of Ureter

INCLUDES Diagnostic laparoscopy (49320)
EXCLUDES *Ureteroneocystostomy, open approach (50780-50785)*

50945 **Laparoscopy, surgical; ureterolithotomy**
28.1 28.1 FUD 090 J 80 50
AMA: 2018,Jan,8; 2017,Jan,8; 2016,Jan,13; 2015,Jan,16; 2014,Jan,11

50947 **ureteroneocystostomy with cystoscopy and ureteral stent placement**
40.1 40.1 FUD 090 J A2 80 50
AMA: 2018,Jan,8; 2017,Jan,8; 2016,Jan,13; 2015,Jan,16; 2014,Jan,11

50948 **ureteroneocystostomy without cystoscopy and ureteral stent placement**
36.9 36.9 FUD 090 J A2 80 50
AMA: 2018,Jan,8; 2017,Jan,8; 2016,Jan,13; 2015,Jan,16; 2014,Jan,11

50949 **Unlisted laparoscopy procedure, ureter**
0.00 0.00 FUD YYY J 80 50
AMA: 2018,Jan,8; 2017,Jan,8; 2016,Jan,13; 2015,Jan,16; 2014,Jan,11

50951-50961 Endoscopic Procedures of Ureter via Established Ureterostomy Access

50951 **Ureteral endoscopy through established ureterostomy, with or without irrigation, instillation, or ureteropyelography, exclusive of radiologic service;**
8.89 10.9 FUD 000 J A2 80 50
AMA: 2018,Jan,8; 2017,Jan,8; 2016,Jan,13; 2015,Jan,16; 2014,Jan,11

50953 **with ureteral catheterization, with or without dilation of ureter**
EXCLUDES *Image-guided ureter dilation without endoscopic guidance (50706)*
9.46 11.5 FUD 000 J A2 80 50
AMA: 2018,Jan,8; 2017,Jan,8; 2016,Jan,13; 2016,Jan,3; 2015,Jan,16; 2014,Jan,11

50955 **with biopsy**
EXCLUDES *Image-guided biopsy of ureter and/or renal pelvis without endoscopic guidance (50606)*
10.2 12.3 FUD 000 J A2 80 50
AMA: 2018,Jan,8; 2017,Jan,8; 2016,Jan,13; 2016,Jan,3; 2015,Jan,16; 2014,Jan,11

50957 **with fulguration and/or incision, with or without biopsy**
10.2 12.4 FUD 000 J A2 80 50
AMA: 2018,Jan,8; 2017,Jan,8; 2016,Jan,13; 2015,Jan,16; 2014,Jan,11

50961 **with removal of foreign body or calculus**
9.17 11.1 FUD 000 J A2 80 50
AMA: 2018,Jan,8; 2017,Jan,8; 2016,Jan,13; 2015,Jan,16; 2014,Jan,11

50970-50980 Endoscopic Procedures of Ureter via Ureterotomy

EXCLUDES *Ureterotomy (50600)*

50970 **Ureteral endoscopy through ureterotomy, with or without irrigation, instillation, or ureteropyelography, exclusive of radiologic service;**
10.7 10.7 FUD 000 J A2 80 50
AMA: 2018,Jan,8; 2017,Jan,8; 2016,Jan,13; 2015,Jan,16; 2014,Jan,11

50972 **with ureteral catheterization, with or without dilation of ureter**
EXCLUDES *Image-guided ureter dilation without endoscopic guidance (50706)*
10.3 10.3 FUD 000 J A2 80 50
AMA: 2018,Jan,8; 2017,Jan,8; 2016,Jan,3; 2016,Jan,13; 2015,Jan,16; 2014,Jan,11

50974 **with biopsy**
EXCLUDES *Image-guided biopsy of ureter and/or renal pelvis without endoscopic guidance (50606)*
13.6 13.6 FUD 000 J A2 80 50
AMA: 2018,Jan,8; 2017,Jan,8; 2016,Jan,3; 2016,Jan,13; 2015,Jan,16; 2014,Jan,11

50976 **with fulguration and/or incision, with or without biopsy**
13.5 13.5 FUD 000 J A2 80 50
AMA: 2018,Jan,8; 2017,Jan,8; 2016,Jan,13; 2015,Jan,16; 2014,Jan,11

50980 **with removal of foreign body or calculus**
10.3 10.3 FUD 000 J A2 80 50
AMA: 2018,Jan,8; 2017,Jan,8; 2016,Jan,13; 2015,Jan,16; 2014,Jan,11

51020-51080 Open Incisional Procedures of Bladder

51020 **Cystotomy or cystostomy; with fulguration and/or insertion of radioactive material**
13.5 13.5 FUD 090 J A2 80
AMA: 2014,Jan,11

51030 **with cryosurgical destruction of intravesical lesion**
13.6 13.6 FUD 090 J A2 80
AMA: 2014,Jan,11

51040 **Cystostomy, cystotomy with drainage**
8.36 8.36 FUD 090 J A2 80
AMA: 2014,Jan,11

51045 **Cystotomy, with insertion of ureteral catheter or stent (separate procedure)**
14.2 14.2 FUD 090 J A2 80
AMA: 2014,Jan,11

51050 **Cystolithotomy, cystotomy with removal of calculus, without vesical neck resection**
13.6 13.6 FUD 090 J A2 80
AMA: 2014,Jan,11

51060 **Transvesical ureterolithotomy**
16.8 16.8 FUD 090 J 80
AMA: 2014,Jan,11

51065 **Cystotomy, with calculus basket extraction and/or ultrasonic or electrohydraulic fragmentation of ureteral calculus**
16.7 16.7 FUD 090 J A2 80
AMA: 2014,Jan,11

51080 **Drainage of perivesical or prevesical space abscess**
EXCLUDES *Image-guided percutaneous catheter drainage (49406)*
11.8 11.8 FUD 090 J A2 80
AMA: 2014,Jan,11

51100-51102 Bladder Aspiration Procedures

51100 Aspiration of bladder; by needle
(76942, 77002, 77012)
1.13 1.84 FUD 000 T P3
AMA: 2018,Jan,8; 2017,Jan,8; 2016,Jan,13; 2015,Jan,16; 2014,Jan,11

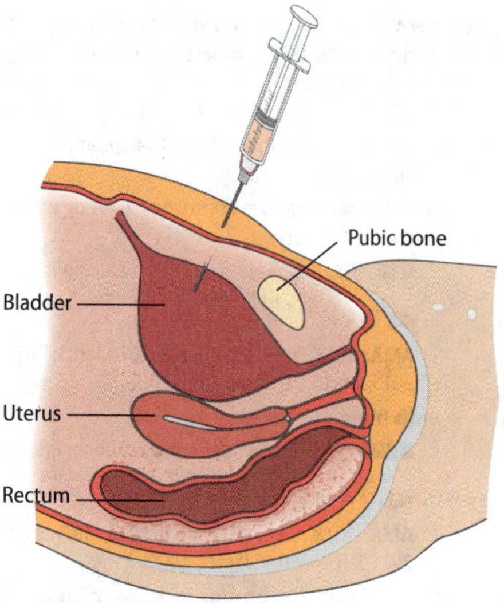

51101 by trocar or intracatheter
(76942, 77002, 77012)
1.50 3.79 FUD 000 S P3
AMA: 2018,Jan,8; 2017,Jan,8; 2016,Jan,13; 2015,Jan,16; 2014,Jan,11

51102 with insertion of suprapubic catheter
(76942, 77002, 77012)
4.18 6.60 FUD 000 J A2
AMA: 2018,Jan,8; 2017,Jan,8; 2016,Jan,13; 2015,Jan,16; 2014,Jan,11

51500-51597 Open Excisional Procedures of Bladder

51500 Excision of urachal cyst or sinus, with or without umbilical hernia repair
18.4 18.4 FUD 090 J A2 80
AMA: 2014,Jan,11

51520 Cystotomy; for simple excision of vesical neck (separate procedure)
17.2 17.2 FUD 090 J A2 80
AMA: 2014,Jan,11

51525 for excision of bladder diverticulum, single or multiple (separate procedure)
EXCLUDES *Transurethral resection (52305)*
24.8 24.8 FUD 090 C 80
AMA: 2014,Jan,11

51530 for excision of bladder tumor
EXCLUDES *Transurethral resection (52234-52240, 52305)*
22.2 22.2 FUD 090 C 80
AMA: 2014,Jan,11

51535 Cystotomy for excision, incision, or repair of ureterocele
EXCLUDES *Transurethral excision (52300)*
22.5 22.5 FUD 090 J G2 80 50
AMA: 2014,Jan,11

51550 Cystectomy, partial; simple
27.9 27.9 FUD 090 C 80
AMA: 2014,Jan,11

51555 complicated (eg, postradiation, previous surgery, difficult location)
36.6 36.6 FUD 090 C 80
AMA: 2014,Jan,11

51565 Cystectomy, partial, with reimplantation of ureter(s) into bladder (ureteroneocystostomy)
37.5 37.5 FUD 090 C 80
AMA: 2014,Jan,11

51570 Cystectomy, complete; (separate procedure)
42.6 42.6 FUD 090 C 80
AMA: 2014,Jan,11

51575 with bilateral pelvic lymphadenectomy, including external iliac, hypogastric, and obturator nodes
52.7 52.7 FUD 090 C 80
AMA: 2014,Jan,11

51580 Cystectomy, complete, with ureterosigmoidostomy or ureterocutaneous transplantations;
54.7 54.7 FUD 090 C 80
AMA: 2014,Jan,11

51585 with bilateral pelvic lymphadenectomy, including external iliac, hypogastric, and obturator nodes
61.0 61.0 FUD 090 C 80
AMA: 2014,Jan,11

51590 Cystectomy, complete, with ureteroileal conduit or sigmoid bladder, including intestine anastomosis;
55.9 55.9 FUD 090 C 80
AMA: 2014,Jan,11

51595 with bilateral pelvic lymphadenectomy, including external iliac, hypogastric, and obturator nodes
63.3 63.3 FUD 090 C 80
AMA: 2014,Jan,11

51596 Cystectomy, complete, with continent diversion, any open technique, using any segment of small and/or large intestine to construct neobladder
68.1 68.1 FUD 090 C 80
AMA: 2014,Jan,11

51597 Pelvic exenteration, complete, for vesical, prostatic or urethral malignancy, with removal of bladder and ureteral transplantations, with or without hysterectomy and/or abdominoperineal resection of rectum and colon and colostomy, or any combination thereof
EXCLUDES *Pelvic exenteration for gynecologic malignancy (58240)*
66.3 66.3 FUD 090 C 80
AMA: 2014,Jan,11

51600-51720 Injection/Insertion/Instillation Procedures of Bladder

51600 Injection procedure for cystography or voiding urethrocystography
(74430, 74455)
1.29 5.57 FUD 000 N N1
AMA: 2014,Jan,11

51605 Injection procedure and placement of chain for contrast and/or chain urethrocystography
(74430)
1.11 1.11 FUD 000 N N1
AMA: 2014,Jan,11

51610 Injection procedure for retrograde urethrocystography
(74450)
1.85 3.21 FUD 000 N N1
AMA: 2018,Jan,8; 2017,Jan,8; 2016,Jan,3; 2014,Jan,11

51700 Bladder irrigation, simple, lavage and/or instillation
0.87 2.12 FUD 000 T P3
AMA: 2014,Jan,11

51701 **Insertion of non-indwelling bladder catheter (eg, straight catheterization for residual urine)**
EXCLUDES *Catheterization for specimen collection (P9612)*
Insertion of catheter as an inclusive component of another procedure
0.73 1.27 FUD 000 Q1 N1
AMA: 2018,Jan,8; 2017,Jan,8; 2016,Jan,13; 2015,Jan,16; 2014,Jan,11

51702 **Insertion of temporary indwelling bladder catheter; simple (eg, Foley)**
EXCLUDES *Focused ultrasound ablation of uterine leiomyomata (0071T-0072T)*
Insertion of catheter as an inclusive component of another procedure
0.73 1.76 FUD 000 Q1 N1
AMA: 2018,Jan,8; 2017,Jan,8; 2016,Jan,13; 2015,Jan,16; 2014,May,3; 2014,Jan,11

51703 **complicated (eg, altered anatomy, fractured catheter/balloon)**
2.23 3.78 FUD 000 S P2
AMA: 2018,Jan,8; 2017,Jan,8; 2016,Jan,13; 2015,Jan,16; 2014,Jan,11

51705 **Change of cystostomy tube; simple**
1.50 2.67 FUD 000 T P3
AMA: 2018,Jan,8; 2017,Jan,8; 2016,Jan,13; 2015,Jan,16; 2014,Jan,11

51710 **complicated**
(75984)
2.30 3.69 FUD 000 T A2
AMA: 2018,Jan,8; 2017,Jan,8; 2016,Jan,13; 2015,Jan,16; 2014,Jan,11

51715 **Endoscopic injection of implant material into the submucosal tissues of the urethra and/or bladder neck**
EXCLUDES *Injection of bulking agent (submucosal) for fecal incontinence, via anoscope (46999)*
5.76 9.07 FUD 000 J J8 80
AMA: 2014,Jan,11

51720 **Bladder instillation of anticarcinogenic agent (including retention time)**
Code also bacillus Calmette-Guerin vaccine (BCG) (90586)
1.27 2.40 FUD 000 T P3
AMA: 2018,Jan,8; 2017,Jan,8; 2016,Jan,13; 2015,Jan,16; 2014,Jan,11

51725-51798 [51797] Uroflowmetric Evaluations

INCLUDES Equipment
Fees for services of technician
Medications
Supplies

Code also modifier 26 if physician/other qualified health care professional provides only interpretation of results and/or operates the equipment

51725 **Simple cystometrogram (CMG) (eg, spinal manometer)**
5.69 5.69 FUD 000 T P2 80
AMA: 2018,Jan,8; 2017,Jan,8; 2016,Jan,13; 2015,Jan,16; 2014,Jan,11

51726 **Complex cystometrogram (ie, calibrated electronic equipment);**
7.94 7.94 FUD 000 T A2
AMA: 2018,Jan,8; 2017,Jan,8; 2016,Jan,13; 2015,Jan,16; 2014,Jan,11

51727 **with urethral pressure profile studies (ie, urethral closure pressure profile), any technique**
9.39 9.39 FUD 000 T P3 80
AMA: 2018,Jan,8; 2017,Jan,8; 2016,Jan,13; 2015,Jan,16; 2014,Jan,11

51728 **with voiding pressure studies (ie, bladder voiding pressure), any technique**
9.55 9.55 FUD 000 T P3 80
AMA: 2018,Jan,8; 2017,Jan,8; 2016,Jan,13; 2015,Jan,16; 2014,Jan,11

51729 **with voiding pressure studies (ie, bladder voiding pressure) and urethral pressure profile studies (ie, urethral closure pressure profile), any technique**
10.2 10.2 FUD 000 T P3 80
AMA: 2018,Jan,8; 2017,Jan,8; 2016,Jan,13; 2015,Jan,16; 2014,Jan,11

+ # **51797** **Voiding pressure studies, intra-abdominal (ie, rectal, gastric, intraperitoneal) (List separately in addition to code for primary procedure)**
Code first (51728-51729)
3.95 3.95 FUD ZZZ N N1 80
AMA: 2018,Jan,8; 2017,Jan,8; 2016,Jan,13; 2015,Jan,16; 2014,Jan,11

51736 **Simple uroflowmetry (UFR) (eg, stop-watch flow rate, mechanical uroflowmeter)**
0.40 0.40 FUD XXX Q1 N1 80
AMA: 2018,Jan,8; 2017,Jan,8; 2016,Jan,13; 2015,Jan,16; 2014,Jan,11

51741 **Complex uroflowmetry (eg, calibrated electronic equipment)**
0.41 0.41 FUD XXX Q1 N1
AMA: 2018,Jan,8; 2017,Jan,8; 2016,Jan,13; 2015,Jan,16; 2014,Sep,13; 2014,Jan,11

51784 **Electromyography studies (EMG) of anal or urethral sphincter, other than needle, any technique**
EXCLUDES *Stimulus evoked response (51792)*
1.93 1.93 FUD XXX S P3
AMA: 2018,Jan,8; 2017,Jan,8; 2016,Jan,13; 2015,Jan,16; 2014,Sep,13; 2014,Feb,11; 2014,Jan,11

51785 **Needle electromyography studies (EMG) of anal or urethral sphincter, any technique**
9.17 9.17 FUD XXX T A2 80
AMA: 2018,Jan,8; 2017,Jan,8; 2016,Jan,13; 2015,Jan,16; 2014,Jan,11

51792 **Stimulus evoked response (eg, measurement of bulbocavernosus reflex latency time)**
EXCLUDES *Electromyography studies (EMG) of anal or urethral sphincter (51784)*
6.57 6.57 FUD 000 Q1 N1 80
AMA: 2018,Jan,8; 2017,Jan,8; 2016,Jan,13; 2015,Jan,16; 2014,Feb,11; 2014,Jan,11

51797 **Resequenced code. See code following 51729.**

51798 **Measurement of post-voiding residual urine and/or bladder capacity by ultrasound, non-imaging**
0.36 0.36 FUD XXX Q1 N1 80 TC
AMA: 2018,Jun,11; 2018,Jan,8; 2017,Jan,8; 2016,Jan,13; 2015,Jan,16; 2014,Jan,11

51800-51980 Open Repairs Urinary System

51800 **Cystoplasty or cystourethroplasty, plastic operation on bladder and/or vesical neck (anterior Y-plasty, vesical fundus resection), any procedure, with or without wedge resection of posterior vesical neck**
30.3 30.3 FUD 090 C 80
AMA: 2014,Jan,11

51820 **Cystourethroplasty with unilateral or bilateral ureteroneocystostomy**
31.3 31.3 FUD 090 C 80
AMA: 2014,Jan,11

51840 **Anterior vesicourethropexy, or urethropexy (eg, Marshall-Marchetti-Krantz, Burch); simple**
EXCLUDES *Pereyra type urethropexy (57289)*
19.3 19.3 FUD 090 C 80
AMA: 2018,Jan,8; 2017,Jan,8; 2016,Jan,13; 2015,Jan,16; 2014,Jan,11

51841 **complicated (eg, secondary repair)**

EXCLUDES *Pereyra type urethropexy (57289)*

22.4 22.4 FUD 090 C 80

AMA: 2018,Jan,8; 2017,Jan,8; 2016,Jan,13; 2015,Jan,16; 2014,Jan,11

51845 **Abdomino-vaginal vesical neck suspension, with or without endoscopic control (eg, Stamey, Raz, modified Pereyra)** ♀

16.8 16.8 FUD 090 J 80

AMA: 2018,Jan,8; 2017,Jan,8; 2016,Jan,13; 2015,Jan,16; 2014,Jan,11

51860 **Cystorrhaphy, suture of bladder wound, injury or rupture; simple**

21.5 21.5 FUD 090 J 80

AMA: 2014,Jan,11

51865 **complicated**

25.9 25.9 FUD 090 C 80

AMA: 2014,Jan,11

51880 **Closure of cystostomy (separate procedure)**

13.5 13.5 FUD 090 J A2 80

AMA: 2014,Jan,11

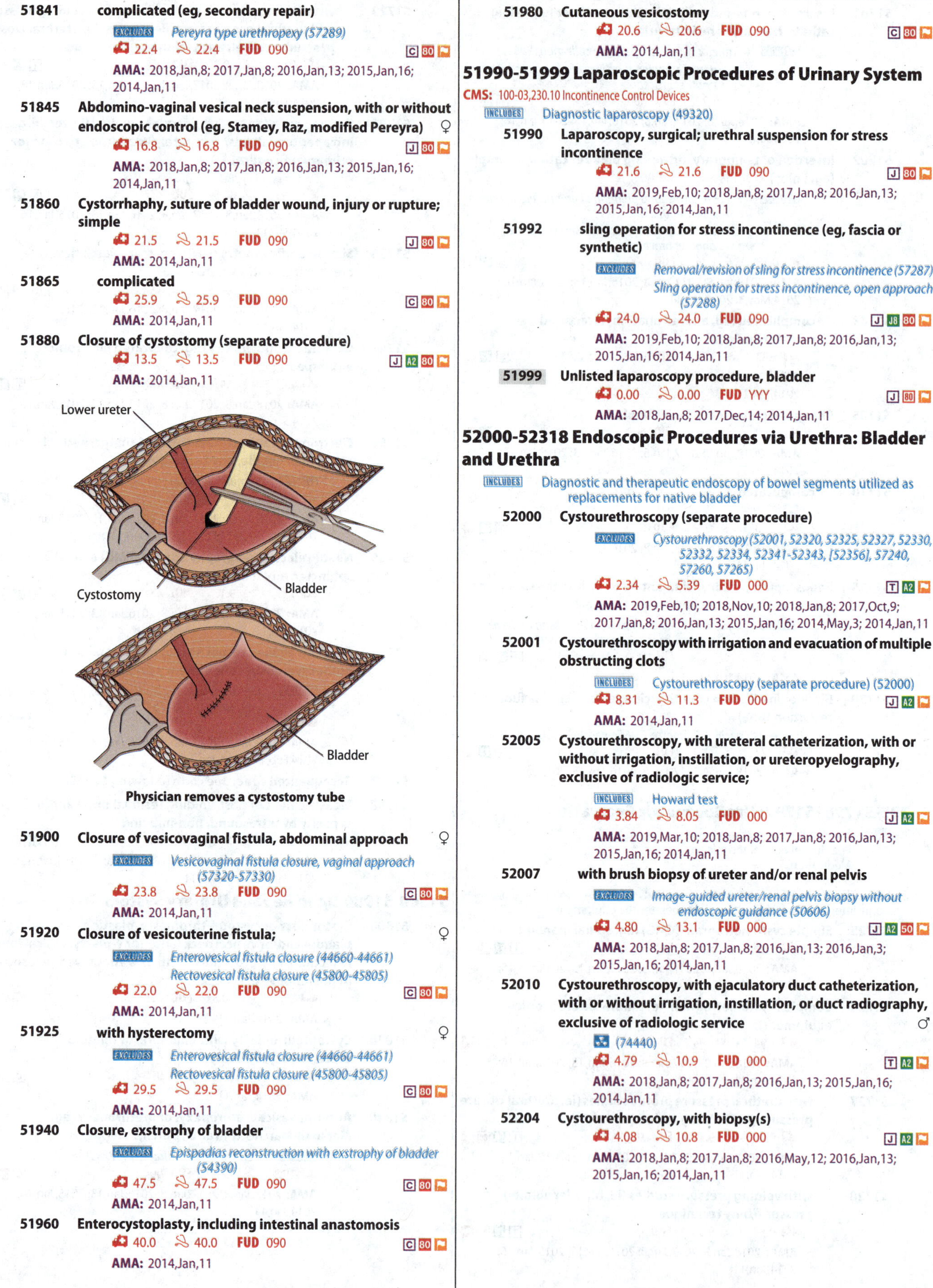

Physician removes a cystostomy tube

51900 **Closure of vesicovaginal fistula, abdominal approach** ♀

EXCLUDES *Vesicovaginal fistula closure, vaginal approach (57320-57330)*

23.8 23.8 FUD 090 C 80

AMA: 2014,Jan,11

51920 **Closure of vesicouterine fistula;** ♀

EXCLUDES *Enterovesical fistula closure (44660-44661)*
Rectovesical fistula closure (45800-45805)

22.0 22.0 FUD 090 C 80

AMA: 2014,Jan,11

51925 **with hysterectomy** ♀

EXCLUDES *Enterovesical fistula closure (44660-44661)*
Rectovesical fistula closure (45800-45805)

29.5 29.5 FUD 090 C 80

AMA: 2014,Jan,11

51940 **Closure, exstrophy of bladder**

EXCLUDES *Epispadias reconstruction with exstrophy of bladder (54390)*

47.5 47.5 FUD 090 C 80

AMA: 2014,Jan,11

51960 **Enterocystoplasty, including intestinal anastomosis**

40.0 40.0 FUD 090 C 80

AMA: 2014,Jan,11

51980 **Cutaneous vesicostomy**

20.6 20.6 FUD 090 C 80

AMA: 2014,Jan,11

51990-51999 Laparoscopic Procedures of Urinary System

CMS: 100-03,230.10 Incontinence Control Devices

INCLUDES Diagnostic laparoscopy (49320)

51990 **Laparoscopy, surgical; urethral suspension for stress incontinence**

21.6 21.6 FUD 090 J 80

AMA: 2019,Feb,10; 2018,Jan,8; 2017,Jan,8; 2016,Jan,13; 2015,Jan,16; 2014,Jan,11

51992 **sling operation for stress incontinence (eg, fascia or synthetic)**

EXCLUDES *Removal/revision of sling for stress incontinence (57287)*
Sling operation for stress incontinence, open approach (57288)

24.0 24.0 FUD 090 J J8 80

AMA: 2019,Feb,10; 2018,Jan,8; 2017,Jan,8; 2016,Jan,13; 2015,Jan,16; 2014,Jan,11

51999 **Unlisted laparoscopy procedure, bladder**

0.00 0.00 FUD YYY J 80

AMA: 2018,Jan,8; 2017,Dec,14; 2014,Jan,11

52000-52318 Endoscopic Procedures via Urethra: Bladder and Urethra

INCLUDES Diagnostic and therapeutic endoscopy of bowel segments utilized as replacements for native bladder

52000 **Cystourethroscopy (separate procedure)**

EXCLUDES *Cystourethroscopy (52001, 52320, 52325, 52327, 52330, 52332, 52334, 52341-52343, [52356], 57240, 57260, 57265)*

2.34 5.39 FUD 000 T A2

AMA: 2019,Feb,10; 2018,Nov,10; 2018,Jan,8; 2017,Oct,9; 2017,Jan,8; 2016,Jan,13; 2015,Jan,16; 2014,May,3; 2014,Jan,11

52001 **Cystourethroscopy with irrigation and evacuation of multiple obstructing clots**

INCLUDES Cystourethroscopy (separate procedure) (52000)

8.31 11.3 FUD 000 J A2

AMA: 2014,Jan,11

52005 **Cystourethroscopy, with ureteral catheterization, with or without irrigation, instillation, or ureteropyelography, exclusive of radiologic service;**

INCLUDES Howard test

3.84 8.05 FUD 000 J A2

AMA: 2019,Mar,10; 2018,Jan,8; 2017,Jan,8; 2016,Jan,13; 2015,Jan,16; 2014,Jan,11

52007 **with brush biopsy of ureter and/or renal pelvis**

EXCLUDES *Image-guided ureter/renal pelvis biopsy without endoscopic guidance (50606)*

4.80 13.1 FUD 000 J A2 50

AMA: 2018,Jan,8; 2017,Jan,8; 2016,Jan,13; 2016,Jan,3; 2015,Jan,16; 2014,Jan,11

52010 **Cystourethroscopy, with ejaculatory duct catheterization, with or without irrigation, instillation, or duct radiography, exclusive of radiologic service** ♂

(74440)

4.79 10.9 FUD 000 T A2

AMA: 2018,Jan,8; 2017,Jan,8; 2016,Jan,13; 2015,Jan,16; 2014,Jan,11

52204 **Cystourethroscopy, with biopsy(s)**

4.08 10.8 FUD 000 J A2

AMA: 2018,Jan,8; 2017,Jan,8; 2016,May,12; 2016,Jan,13; 2015,Jan,16; 2014,Jan,11

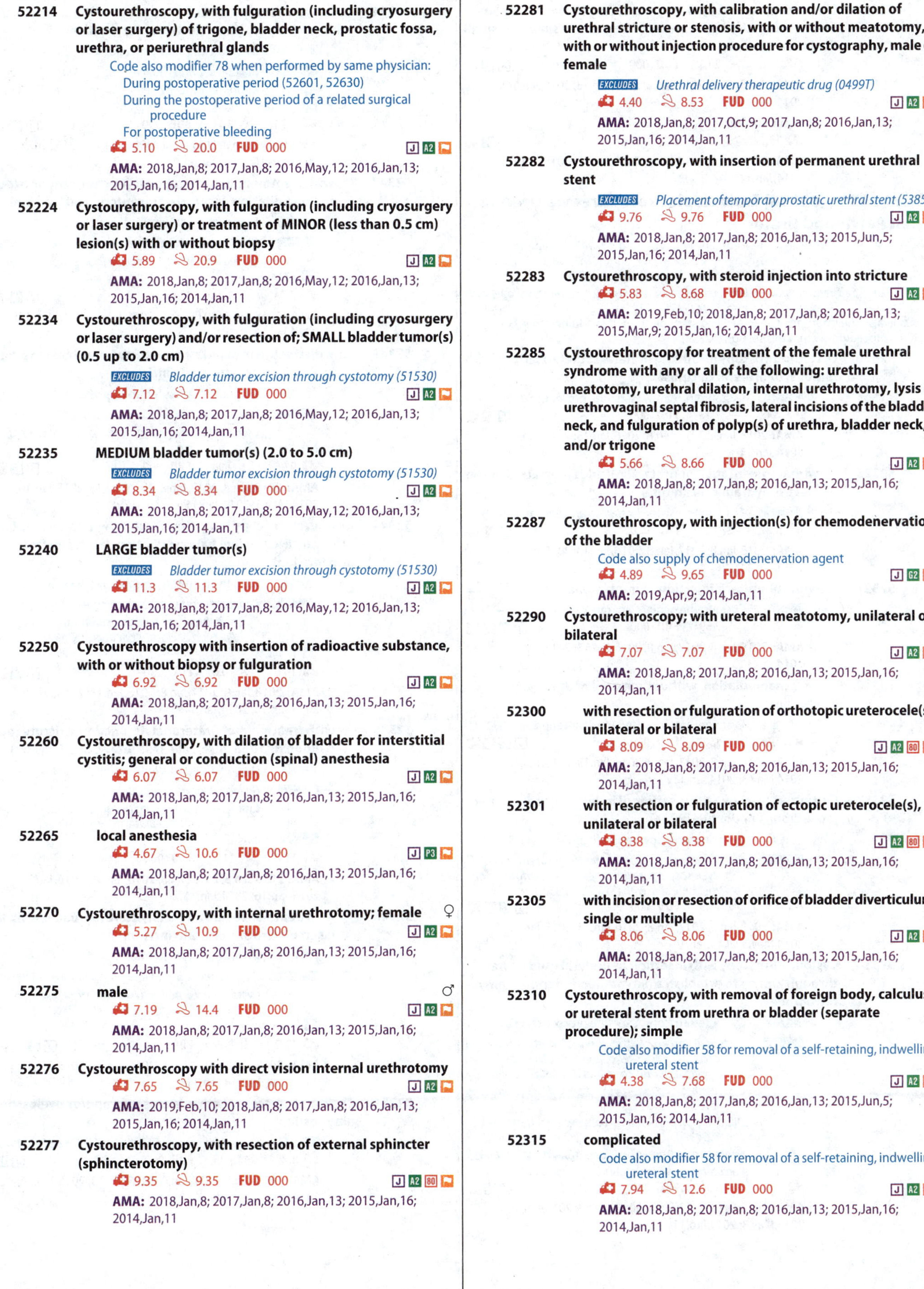

52214 **Cystourethroscopy, with fulguration (including cryosurgery or laser surgery) of trigone, bladder neck, prostatic fossa, urethra, or periurethral glands**

Code also modifier 78 when performed by same physician:
- During postoperative period (52601, 52630)
- During the postoperative period of a related surgical procedure
- For postoperative bleeding

5.10 20.0 FUD 000 J A2

AMA: 2018,Jan,8; 2017,Jan,8; 2016,May,12; 2016,Jan,13; 2015,Jan,16; 2014,Jan,11

52224 **Cystourethroscopy, with fulguration (including cryosurgery or laser surgery) or treatment of MINOR (less than 0.5 cm) lesion(s) with or without biopsy**

5.89 20.9 FUD 000 J A2

AMA: 2018,Jan,8; 2017,Jan,8; 2016,May,12; 2016,Jan,13; 2015,Jan,16; 2014,Jan,11

52234 **Cystourethroscopy, with fulguration (including cryosurgery or laser surgery) and/or resection of; SMALL bladder tumor(s) (0.5 up to 2.0 cm)**

EXCLUDES *Bladder tumor excision through cystotomy (51530)*

7.12 7.12 FUD 000 J A2

AMA: 2018,Jan,8; 2017,Jan,8; 2016,May,12; 2016,Jan,13; 2015,Jan,16; 2014,Jan,11

52235 **MEDIUM bladder tumor(s) (2.0 to 5.0 cm)**

EXCLUDES *Bladder tumor excision through cystotomy (51530)*

8.34 8.34 FUD 000 J A2

AMA: 2018,Jan,8; 2017,Jan,8; 2016,May,12; 2016,Jan,13; 2015,Jan,16; 2014,Jan,11

52240 **LARGE bladder tumor(s)**

EXCLUDES *Bladder tumor excision through cystotomy (51530)*

11.3 11.3 FUD 000 J A2

AMA: 2018,Jan,8; 2017,Jan,8; 2016,May,12; 2016,Jan,13; 2015,Jan,16; 2014,Jan,11

52250 **Cystourethroscopy with insertion of radioactive substance, with or without biopsy or fulguration**

6.92 6.92 FUD 000 J A2

AMA: 2018,Jan,8; 2017,Jan,8; 2016,Jan,13; 2015,Jan,16; 2014,Jan,11

52260 **Cystourethroscopy, with dilation of bladder for interstitial cystitis; general or conduction (spinal) anesthesia**

6.07 6.07 FUD 000 J A2

AMA: 2018,Jan,8; 2017,Jan,8; 2016,Jan,13; 2015,Jan,16; 2014,Jan,11

52265 **local anesthesia**

4.67 10.6 FUD 000 J P3

AMA: 2018,Jan,8; 2017,Jan,8; 2016,Jan,13; 2015,Jan,16; 2014,Jan,11

52270 **Cystourethroscopy, with internal urethrotomy; female** ♀

5.27 10.9 FUD 000 J A2

AMA: 2018,Jan,8; 2017,Jan,8; 2016,Jan,13; 2015,Jan,16; 2014,Jan,11

52275 **male** ♂

7.19 14.4 FUD 000 J A2

AMA: 2018,Jan,8; 2017,Jan,8; 2016,Jan,13; 2015,Jan,16; 2014,Jan,11

52276 **Cystourethroscopy with direct vision internal urethrotomy**

7.65 7.65 FUD 000 J A2

AMA: 2019,Feb,10; 2018,Jan,8; 2017,Jan,8; 2016,Jan,13; 2015,Jan,16; 2014,Jan,11

52277 **Cystourethroscopy, with resection of external sphincter (sphincterotomy)**

9.35 9.35 FUD 000 J A2 80

AMA: 2018,Jan,8; 2017,Jan,8; 2016,Jan,13; 2015,Jan,16; 2014,Jan,11

52281 **Cystourethroscopy, with calibration and/or dilation of urethral stricture or stenosis, with or without meatotomy, with or without injection procedure for cystography, male or female**

EXCLUDES *Urethral delivery therapeutic drug (0499T)*

4.40 8.53 FUD 000 J A2

AMA: 2018,Jan,8; 2017,Oct,9; 2017,Jan,8; 2016,Jan,13; 2015,Jan,16; 2014,Jan,11

52282 **Cystourethroscopy, with insertion of permanent urethral stent**

EXCLUDES *Placement of temporary prostatic urethral stent (53855)*

9.76 9.76 FUD 000 J A2

AMA: 2018,Jan,8; 2017,Jan,8; 2016,Jan,13; 2015,Jun,5; 2015,Jan,16; 2014,Jan,11

52283 **Cystourethroscopy, with steroid injection into stricture**

5.83 8.68 FUD 000 J A2

AMA: 2019,Feb,10; 2018,Jan,8; 2017,Jan,8; 2016,Jan,13; 2015,Mar,9; 2015,Jan,16; 2014,Jan,11

52285 **Cystourethroscopy for treatment of the female urethral syndrome with any or all of the following: urethral meatotomy, urethral dilation, internal urethrotomy, lysis of urethrovaginal septal fibrosis, lateral incisions of the bladder neck, and fulguration of polyp(s) of urethra, bladder neck, and/or trigone** ♀

5.66 8.66 FUD 000 J A2

AMA: 2018,Jan,8; 2017,Jan,8; 2016,Jan,13; 2015,Jan,16; 2014,Jan,11

52287 **Cystourethroscopy, with injection(s) for chemodenervation of the bladder**

Code also supply of chemodenervation agent

4.89 9.65 FUD 000 J G2

AMA: 2019,Apr,9; 2014,Jan,11

52290 **Cystourethroscopy; with ureteral meatotomy, unilateral or bilateral**

7.07 7.07 FUD 000 J A2

AMA: 2018,Jan,8; 2017,Jan,8; 2016,Jan,13; 2015,Jan,16; 2014,Jan,11

52300 **with resection or fulguration of orthotopic ureterocele(s), unilateral or bilateral**

8.09 8.09 FUD 000 J A2 80

AMA: 2018,Jan,8; 2017,Jan,8; 2016,Jan,13; 2015,Jan,16; 2014,Jan,11

52301 **with resection or fulguration of ectopic ureterocele(s), unilateral or bilateral**

8.38 8.38 FUD 000 J A2 80

AMA: 2018,Jan,8; 2017,Jan,8; 2016,Jan,13; 2015,Jan,16; 2014,Jan,11

52305 **with incision or resection of orifice of bladder diverticulum, single or multiple**

8.06 8.06 FUD 000 J A2

AMA: 2018,Jan,8; 2017,Jan,8; 2016,Jan,13; 2015,Jan,16; 2014,Jan,11

52310 **Cystourethroscopy, with removal of foreign body, calculus, or ureteral stent from urethra or bladder (separate procedure); simple**

Code also modifier 58 for removal of a self-retaining, indwelling ureteral stent

4.38 7.68 FUD 000 J A2

AMA: 2018,Jan,8; 2017,Jan,8; 2016,Jan,13; 2015,Jun,5; 2015,Jan,16; 2014,Jan,11

52315 **complicated**

Code also modifier 58 for removal of a self-retaining, indwelling ureteral stent

7.94 12.6 FUD 000 J A2

AMA: 2018,Jan,8; 2017,Jan,8; 2016,Jan,13; 2015,Jan,16; 2014,Jan,11

52317 **Litholapaxy: crushing or fragmentation of calculus by any means in bladder and removal of fragments; simple or small (less than 2.5 cm)**

10.0 24.1 FUD 000 J A2

AMA: 2018,Jan,8; 2017,Jan,8; 2016,Jan,13; 2015,Jan,16; 2014,Jan,11

52318 **complicated or large (over 2.5 cm)**

13.7 13.7 FUD 000 J A2

AMA: 2018,Jan,8; 2017,Jan,8; 2016,Jan,13; 2015,Jan,16; 2014,Jan,11

52320-52356 [52356] Endoscopic Procedures via Urethra: Renal Pelvis and Ureter

INCLUDES Diagnostic cystourethroscopy when performed with therapeutic cystourethroscopy

Insertion/removal of temporary ureteral catheter (52005)

EXCLUDES *Self-retaining/indwelling ureteral stent removal by cystourethroscope, with modifier 58 if appropriate (52310, 52315)*

Code also the insertion of an indwelling stent performed in addition to other procedures within this section (52332)

52320 **Cystourethroscopy (including ureteral catheterization); with removal of ureteral calculus**

INCLUDES Cystourethroscopy (separate procedure) (52000)

7.13 7.13 FUD 000 J A2 50

AMA: 2018,Jan,8; 2017,Jan,8; 2016,Jan,13; 2015,Jan,16; 2014,Jan,11

52325 **with fragmentation of ureteral calculus (eg, ultrasonic or electro-hydraulic technique)**

INCLUDES Cystourethroscopy (separate procedure) (52000)

9.27 9.27 FUD 000 J A2 50

AMA: 2018,Jan,8; 2017,Jan,8; 2016,Jan,13; 2015,Jan,16; 2014,Jan,11

52327 **with subureteric injection of implant material**

INCLUDES Cystourethroscopy (separate procedure) (52000)

7.59 7.59 FUD 000 J J8 50

AMA: 2018,Jan,8; 2017,Jan,8; 2016,Jan,13; 2015,Jan,16; 2014,Jan,11

52330 **with manipulation, without removal of ureteral calculus**

INCLUDES Cystourethroscopy (separate procedure) (52000)

7.63 15.4 FUD 000 J A2 50

AMA: 2018,Jan,8; 2017,Jan,8; 2016,Jan,13; 2015,Jan,16; 2014,May,3; 2014,Jan,11

52332 **Cystourethroscopy, with insertion of indwelling ureteral stent (eg, Gibbons or double-J type)**

INCLUDES Cystourethroscopy (separate procedure) (52000)

EXCLUDES *Cystourethroscopy, with ureteroscopy and/or pyeloscopy; with lithotripsy when performed on the same side with (52353, [52356])*

4.50 13.5 FUD 000 J A2 50

AMA: 2018,Jan,8; 2017,Jan,8; 2016,Jan,13; 2015,Jan,16; 2014,May,3; 2014,Jan,11

52334 **Cystourethroscopy with insertion of ureteral guide wire through kidney to establish a percutaneous nephrostomy, retrograde**

INCLUDES Cystourethroscopy (separate procedure) (52000)

EXCLUDES *Cystourethroscopy with incision/fulguration/resection of congenital posterior urethral valves/obstructive hypertrophic mucosal folds (52400)*

Cystourethroscopy with pyeloscopy and/or ureteroscopy (52351-52353 [52356])

Dilation of nephroureteral catheter tract ([50436], [50437])

Nephrostomy tract establishment only ([50432, 50433])

Percutaneous nephrostolithotomy (50080, 50081)

5.30 5.30 FUD 000 J A2

AMA: 2018,Jan,8; 2017,Jan,8; 2016,Jan,13; 2015,Jan,16; 2014,May,3; 2014,Jan,11

52341 **Cystourethroscopy; with treatment of ureteral stricture (eg, balloon dilation, laser, electrocautery, and incision)**

INCLUDES Diagnostic cystourethroscopy (52351)

EXCLUDES *Balloon dilation with imaging guidance (50706)*

Cystourethroscopy, separate procedure (52000)

(74485)

8.21 8.21 FUD 000 J A2 50

AMA: 2018,Jan,8; 2017,Jan,8; 2016,Jan,13; 2016,Jan,3; 2015,Jan,16; 2014,Jan,11

52342 **with treatment of ureteropelvic junction stricture (eg, balloon dilation, laser, electrocautery, and incision)**

INCLUDES Diagnostic cystourethroscopy (52351)

EXCLUDES *Balloon dilation with imaging guidance (50706)*

Cystourethroscopy (separate procedure) (52000)

(74485)

8.93 8.93 FUD 000 J A2 50

AMA: 2018,Jan,8; 2017,Jan,8; 2016,Jan,13; 2015,Jan,16; 2014,Jan,11

52343 **with treatment of intra-renal stricture (eg, balloon dilation, laser, electrocautery, and incision)**

INCLUDES Diagnostic cystourethroscopy (52351)

EXCLUDES *Balloon dilation with imaging guidance (50706)*

Cystourethroscopy (separate procedure) (52000)

(74485)

9.96 9.96 FUD 000 J A2 50

AMA: 2018,Jan,8; 2017,Jan,8; 2016,Jan,13; 2015,Jan,16; 2014,May,3; 2014,Jan,11

52344 **Cystourethroscopy with ureteroscopy; with treatment of ureteral stricture (eg, balloon dilation, laser, electrocautery, and incision)**

INCLUDES Diagnostic cystourethroscopy (52351)

EXCLUDES *Balloon dilation, ureteral stricture (50706)*

Cystourethroscopy with transurethral resection or incision of ejaculatory ducts (52402)

(74485)

10.6 10.6 FUD 000 J A2 50

AMA: 2018,Jan,8; 2017,Jan,8; 2016,Jan,13; 2016,Jan,3; 2015,Jan,16; 2014,Jan,11

52345 **with treatment of ureteropelvic junction stricture (eg, balloon dilation, laser, electrocautery, and incision)**

INCLUDES Diagnostic cystourethroscopy (52351)

EXCLUDES *Balloon dilation, ureteral stricture (50706)*

Cystourethroscopy with transurethral resection or incision of ejaculatory ducts (52402)

(74485)

11.4 11.4 FUD 000 J A2 80 50

AMA: 2018,Jan,8; 2017,Jan,8; 2016,Jan,13; 2016,Jan,3; 2015,Jan,16; 2014,Jan,11

52346 **with treatment of intra-renal stricture (eg, balloon dilation, laser, electrocautery, and incision)**

INCLUDES Diagnostic cystourethroscopy (52351)

EXCLUDES *Balloon dilation with imaging guidance (50706)*

Cystourethroscopy with transurethral resection or incision of ejaculatory ducts (52402)

(74485)

12.9 12.9 FUD 000 J A2 80 50

AMA: 2018,Jan,8; 2017,Jan,8; 2016,Jan,13; 2015,Jan,16; 2014,May,3; 2014,Jan,11

52351 **Cystourethroscopy, with ureteroscopy and/or pyeloscopy; diagnostic**

EXCLUDES *Cystourethroscopy (52341-52346, 52352-52353 [52356])*

8.75 8.75 FUD 000 J A2

AMA: 2018,Jan,8; 2017,Jan,8; 2016,Jan,13; 2015,Jan,16; 2014,May,3; 2014,Jan,11

52352 **with removal or manipulation of calculus (ureteral catheterization is included)**

INCLUDES Diagnostic cystourethroscopy (52351)

10.2 10.2 FUD 000 J A2 50

AMA: 2018,Jan,8; 2017,Jan,8; 2016,Jan,13; 2015,Jan,16; 2014,Jan,11

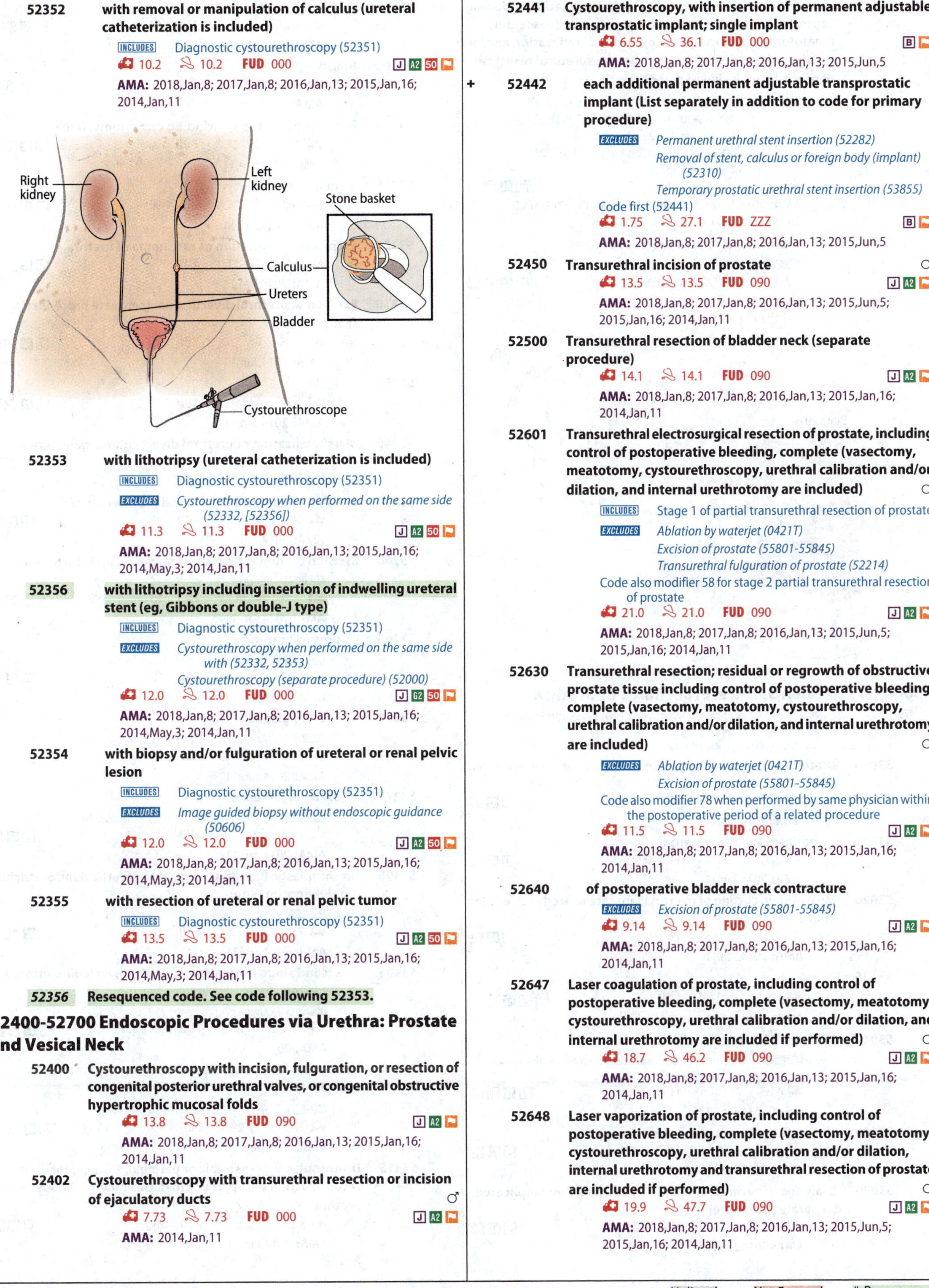

52353 **with lithotripsy (ureteral catheterization is included)**

INCLUDES Diagnostic cystourethroscopy (52351)

EXCLUDES *Cystourethroscopy when performed on the same side (52332, [52356])*

11.3 11.3 FUD 000 J A2 50

AMA: 2018,Jan,8; 2017,Jan,8; 2016,Jan,13; 2015,Jan,16; 2014,May,3; 2014,Jan,11

52356 **with lithotripsy including insertion of indwelling ureteral stent (eg, Gibbons or double-J type)**

INCLUDES Diagnostic cystourethroscopy (52351)

EXCLUDES *Cystourethroscopy when performed on the same side with (52332, 52353)*

Cystourethroscopy (separate procedure) (52000)

12.0 12.0 FUD 000 J G2 50

AMA: 2018,Jan,8; 2017,Jan,8; 2016,Jan,13; 2015,Jan,16; 2014,May,3; 2014,Jan,11

52354 **with biopsy and/or fulguration of ureteral or renal pelvic lesion**

INCLUDES Diagnostic cystourethroscopy (52351)

EXCLUDES *Image guided biopsy without endoscopic guidance (50606)*

12.0 12.0 FUD 000 J A2 50

AMA: 2018,Jan,8; 2017,Jan,8; 2016,Jan,13; 2015,Jan,16; 2014,May,3; 2014,Jan,11

52355 **with resection of ureteral or renal pelvic tumor**

INCLUDES Diagnostic cystourethroscopy (52351)

13.5 13.5 FUD 000 J A2 50

AMA: 2018,Jan,8; 2017,Jan,8; 2016,Jan,13; 2015,Jan,16; 2014,May,3; 2014,Jan,11

52356 **Resequenced code. See code following 52353.**

52400-52700 Endoscopic Procedures via Urethra: Prostate and Vesical Neck

52400 **Cystourethroscopy with incision, fulguration, or resection of congenital posterior urethral valves, or congenital obstructive hypertrophic mucosal folds**

13.8 13.8 FUD 090 J A2

AMA: 2018,Jan,8; 2017,Jan,8; 2016,Jan,13; 2015,Jan,16; 2014,Jan,11

52402 **Cystourethroscopy with transurethral resection or incision of ejaculatory ducts** ♂

7.73 7.73 FUD 000 J A2

AMA: 2014,Jan,11

52441 **Cystourethroscopy, with insertion of permanent adjustable transprostatic implant; single implant**

6.55 36.1 FUD 000 B

AMA: 2018,Jan,8; 2017,Jan,8; 2016,Jan,13; 2015,Jun,5

\+ 52442 **each additional permanent adjustable transprostatic implant (List separately in addition to code for primary procedure)**

EXCLUDES *Permanent urethral stent insertion (52282)*

Removal of stent, calculus or foreign body (implant) (52310)

Temporary prostatic urethral stent insertion (53855)

Code first (52441)

1.75 27.1 FUD ZZZ B

AMA: 2018,Jan,8; 2017,Jan,8; 2016,Jan,13; 2015,Jun,5

52450 **Transurethral incision of prostate** ♂

13.5 13.5 FUD 090 J A2

AMA: 2018,Jan,8; 2017,Jan,8; 2016,Jan,13; 2015,Jun,5; 2015,Jan,16; 2014,Jan,11

52500 **Transurethral resection of bladder neck (separate procedure)**

14.1 14.1 FUD 090 J A2

AMA: 2018,Jan,8; 2017,Jan,8; 2016,Jan,13; 2015,Jan,16; 2014,Jan,11

52601 **Transurethral electrosurgical resection of prostate, including control of postoperative bleeding, complete (vasectomy, meatotomy, cystourethroscopy, urethral calibration and/or dilation, and internal urethrotomy are included)** ♂

INCLUDES Stage 1 of partial transurethral resection of prostate

EXCLUDES *Ablation by waterjet (0421T)*

Excision of prostate (55801-55845)

Transurethral fulguration of prostate (52214)

Code also modifier 58 for stage 2 partial transurethral resection of prostate

21.0 21.0 FUD 090 J A2

AMA: 2018,Jan,8; 2017,Jan,8; 2016,Jan,13; 2015,Jun,5; 2015,Jan,16; 2014,Jan,11

52630 **Transurethral resection; residual or regrowth of obstructive prostate tissue including control of postoperative bleeding, complete (vasectomy, meatotomy, cystourethroscopy, urethral calibration and/or dilation, and internal urethrotomy are included)** ♂

EXCLUDES *Ablation by waterjet (0421T)*

Excision of prostate (55801-55845)

Code also modifier 78 when performed by same physician within the postoperative period of a related procedure

11.5 11.5 FUD 090 J A2

AMA: 2018,Jan,8; 2017,Jan,8; 2016,Jan,13; 2015,Jan,16; 2014,Jan,11

52640 **of postoperative bladder neck contracture**

EXCLUDES *Excision of prostate (55801-55845)*

9.14 9.14 FUD 090 J A2

AMA: 2018,Jan,8; 2017,Jan,8; 2016,Jan,13; 2015,Jan,16; 2014,Jan,11

52647 **Laser coagulation of prostate, including control of postoperative bleeding, complete (vasectomy, meatotomy, cystourethroscopy, urethral calibration and/or dilation, and internal urethrotomy are included if performed)** ♂

18.7 46.2 FUD 090 J A2

AMA: 2018,Jan,8; 2017,Jan,8; 2016,Jan,13; 2015,Jan,16; 2014,Jan,11

52648 **Laser vaporization of prostate, including control of postoperative bleeding, complete (vasectomy, meatotomy, cystourethroscopy, urethral calibration and/or dilation, internal urethrotomy and transurethral resection of prostate are included if performed)** ♂

19.9 47.7 FUD 090 J A2

AMA: 2018,Jan,8; 2017,Jan,8; 2016,Jan,13; 2015,Jun,5; 2015,Jan,16; 2014,Jan,11

52649 **Laser enucleation of the prostate with morcellation, including control of postoperative bleeding, complete (vasectomy, meatotomy, cystourethroscopy, urethral calibration and/or dilation, internal urethrotomy and transurethral resection of prostate are included if performed)** ♂

INCLUDES Cystourethroscopy (52000, 52276, 52281)
Laser coagulation of prostate (52647-52648)
Meatotomy (53020)
Transurethral resection of prostate (52601)
Vasectomy (55250)

23.8 23.8 FUD 090 J G2 80

AMA: 2018,Jan,8; 2017,Jan,8; 2016,Jan,13; 2015,Jun,5; 2014,Jan,11

52700 **Transurethral drainage of prostatic abscess** ♂

EXCLUDES *Litholapaxy (52317, 52318)*

12.7 12.7 FUD 090 J A2 80

AMA: 2018,Jan,8; 2017,Jan,8; 2016,Jan,13; 2015,Jan,16; 2014,Jan,11

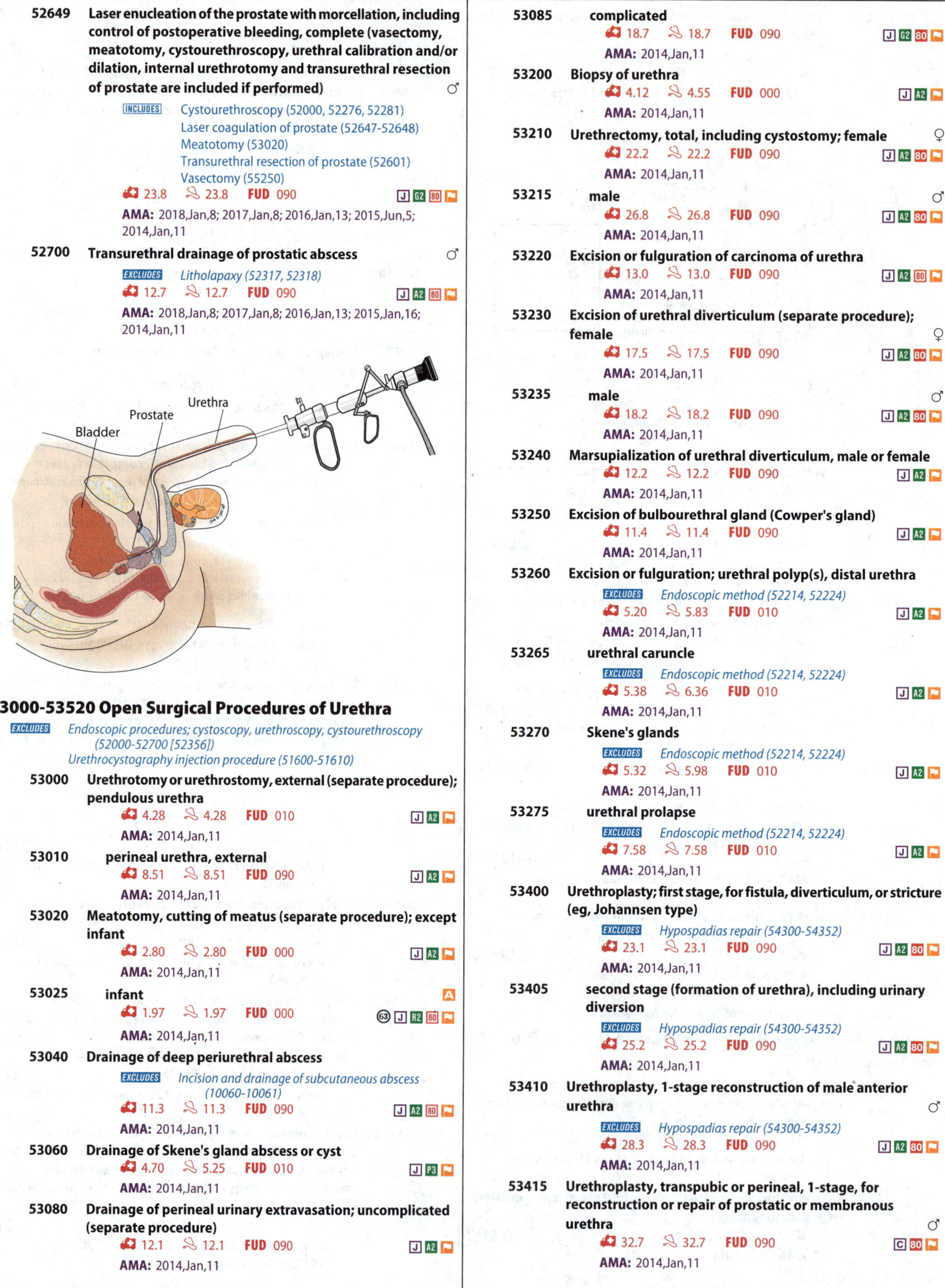

53000-53520 Open Surgical Procedures of Urethra

EXCLUDES *Endoscopic procedures; cystoscopy, urethroscopy, cystourethroscopy (52000-52700 [52356])*
Urethrocystography injection procedure (51600-51610)

53000 **Urethrotomy or urethrostomy, external (separate procedure); pendulous urethra**

4.28 4.28 FUD 010 J A2

AMA: 2014,Jan,11

53010 **perineal urethra, external**

8.51 8.51 FUD 090 J A2

AMA: 2014,Jan,11

53020 **Meatotomy, cutting of meatus (separate procedure); except infant**

2.80 2.80 FUD 000 J A2

AMA: 2014,Jan,11

53025 **infant** A

1.97 1.97 FUD 000 63 J R2 80

AMA: 2014,Jan,11

53040 **Drainage of deep periurethral abscess**

EXCLUDES *Incision and drainage of subcutaneous abscess (10060-10061)*

11.3 11.3 FUD 090 J A2 80

AMA: 2014,Jan,11

53060 **Drainage of Skene's gland abscess or cyst**

4.70 5.25 FUD 010 J P3

AMA: 2014,Jan,11

53080 **Drainage of perineal urinary extravasation; uncomplicated (separate procedure)**

12.1 12.1 FUD 090 J A2

AMA: 2014,Jan,11

53085 **complicated**

18.7 18.7 FUD 090 J G2 80

AMA: 2014,Jan,11

53200 **Biopsy of urethra**

4.12 4.55 FUD 000 J A2

AMA: 2014,Jan,11

53210 **Urethrectomy, total, including cystostomy; female** ♀

22.2 22.2 FUD 090 J A2 80

AMA: 2014,Jan,11

53215 **male** ♂

26.8 26.8 FUD 090 J A2 80

AMA: 2014,Jan,11

53220 **Excision or fulguration of carcinoma of urethra**

13.0 13.0 FUD 090 J A2 80

AMA: 2014,Jan,11

53230 **Excision of urethral diverticulum (separate procedure); female** ♀

17.5 17.5 FUD 090 J A2 80

AMA: 2014,Jan,11

53235 **male** ♂

18.2 18.2 FUD 090 J A2 80

AMA: 2014,Jan,11

53240 **Marsupialization of urethral diverticulum, male or female**

12.2 12.2 FUD 090 J A2

AMA: 2014,Jan,11

53250 **Excision of bulbourethral gland (Cowper's gland)**

11.4 11.4 FUD 090 J A2

AMA: 2014,Jan,11

53260 **Excision or fulguration; urethral polyp(s), distal urethra**

EXCLUDES *Endoscopic method (52214, 52224)*

5.20 5.83 FUD 010 J A2

AMA: 2014,Jan,11

53265 **urethral caruncle**

EXCLUDES *Endoscopic method (52214, 52224)*

5.38 6.36 FUD 010 J A2

AMA: 2014,Jan,11

53270 **Skene's glands**

EXCLUDES *Endoscopic method (52214, 52224)*

5.32 5.98 FUD 010 J A2

AMA: 2014,Jan,11

53275 **urethral prolapse**

EXCLUDES *Endoscopic method (52214, 52224)*

7.58 7.58 FUD 010 J A2

AMA: 2014,Jan,11

53400 **Urethroplasty; first stage, for fistula, diverticulum, or stricture (eg, Johannsen type)**

EXCLUDES *Hypospadias repair (54300-54352)*

23.1 23.1 FUD 090 J A2 80

AMA: 2014,Jan,11

53405 **second stage (formation of urethra), including urinary diversion**

EXCLUDES *Hypospadias repair (54300-54352)*

25.2 25.2 FUD 090 J A2 80

AMA: 2014,Jan,11

53410 **Urethroplasty, 1-stage reconstruction of male anterior urethra** ♂

EXCLUDES *Hypospadias repair (54300-54352)*

28.3 28.3 FUD 090 J A2 80

AMA: 2014,Jan,11

53415 **Urethroplasty, transpubic or perineal, 1-stage, for reconstruction or repair of prostatic or membranous urethra** ♂

32.7 32.7 FUD 090 C 80

AMA: 2014,Jan,11

53420 **Urethroplasty, 2-stage reconstruction or repair of prostatic or membranous urethra; first stage** ♂
24.3 24.3 FUD 090 J A2
AMA: 2014,Jan,11

53425 **second stage** ♂
27.1 27.1 FUD 090 J A2 80
AMA: 2014,Jan,11

53430 **Urethroplasty, reconstruction of female urethra** ♀
27.9 27.9 FUD 090 J A2 80
AMA: 2014,Jan,11

53431 **Urethroplasty with tubularization of posterior urethra and/or lower bladder for incontinence (eg, Tenago, Leadbetter procedure)**
33.4 33.4 FUD 090 J A2 80
AMA: 2014,Jan,11

53440 **Sling operation for correction of male urinary incontinence (eg, fascia or synthetic)** ♂
21.7 21.7 FUD 090 J J8 80
AMA: 2014,Jan,11

53442 **Removal or revision of sling for male urinary incontinence (eg, fascia or synthetic)** ♂
22.6 22.6 FUD 090 J A2 80
AMA: 2014,Jan,11

53444 **Insertion of tandem cuff (dual cuff)**
22.9 22.9 FUD 090 J J8 80
AMA: 2014,Jan,11

53445 **Insertion of inflatable urethral/bladder neck sphincter, including placement of pump, reservoir, and cuff**
21.7 21.7 FUD 090 J J8 80
AMA: 2014,Jan,11

53446 **Removal of inflatable urethral/bladder neck sphincter, including pump, reservoir, and cuff**
18.5 18.5 FUD 090 Q2 A2 80
AMA: 2014,Jan,11

53447 **Removal and replacement of inflatable urethral/bladder neck sphincter including pump, reservoir, and cuff at the same operative session**
23.3 23.3 FUD 090 J J8 80
AMA: 2014,Jan,11

53448 **Removal and replacement of inflatable urethral/bladder neck sphincter including pump, reservoir, and cuff through an infected field at the same operative session including irrigation and debridement of infected tissue**
INCLUDES Debridement (11042, 11043)
37.0 37.0 FUD 090 C 80
AMA: 2014,Jan,11

53449 **Repair of inflatable urethral/bladder neck sphincter, including pump, reservoir, and cuff**
17.6 17.6 FUD 090 J A2 80
AMA: 2014,Jan,11

53450 **Urethromeatoplasty, with mucosal advancement**
EXCLUDES *Meatotomy (53020, 53025)*
11.8 11.8 FUD 090 J A2
AMA: 2018,Jan,8; 2017,Jan,8; 2016,Jan,13; 2015,Jan,16; 2014,Jan,11

53460 **Urethromeatoplasty, with partial excision of distal urethral segment (Richardson type procedure)**
13.2 13.2 FUD 090 J A2 80
AMA: 2014,Jan,11

53500 **Urethrolysis, transvaginal, secondary, open, including cystourethroscopy (eg, postsurgical obstruction, scarring)**
INCLUDES Cystourethroscopy (separate procedure) (52000)
EXCLUDES *Retropubic approach (53899)*
21.5 21.5 FUD 090 J 80
AMA: 2018,Jan,8; 2017,Jan,8; 2016,Jan,13; 2015,Jan,16; 2014,Jan,11

53502 **Urethrorrhaphy, suture of urethral wound or injury, female** ♀
14.0 14.0 FUD 090 J A2
AMA: 2014,Jan,11

53505 **Urethrorrhaphy, suture of urethral wound or injury; penile** ♂
14.0 14.0 FUD 090 J A2 80
AMA: 2014,Jan,11

53510 **perineal** ♂
18.2 18.2 FUD 090 J A2 80
AMA: 2014,Jan,11

53515 **prostatomembranous** ♂
23.0 23.0 FUD 090 J A2 80
AMA: 2014,Jan,11

53520 **Closure of urethrostomy or urethrocutaneous fistula, male (separate procedure)** ♂
EXCLUDES *Closure of fistula:*
Urethrorectal (45820, 45825)
Urethrovaginal (57310)
16.1 16.1 FUD 090 J A2
AMA: 2014,Jan,11

53600-53665 Urethral Dilation

EXCLUDES *Endoscopic procedures; cystoscopy, urethroscopy, cystourethroscopy (52000-52700 [52356])*
Urethral catheterization (51701-51703)
Urethrocystography injection procedure (51600-51610)
(74485)

53600 **Dilation of urethral stricture by passage of sound or urethral dilator, male; initial** ♂
1.84 2.39 FUD 000 T P3
AMA: 2014,Jan,11

53601 **subsequent** ♂
1.55 2.29 FUD 000 Q1 N1
AMA: 2014,Jan,11

53605 **Dilation of urethral stricture or vesical neck by passage of sound or urethral dilator, male, general or conduction (spinal) anesthesia** ♂
EXCLUDES *Procedure performed under local anesthesia (53600-53601, 53620-53621)*
1.87 1.87 FUD 000 J A2
AMA: 2014,Jan,11

53620 **Dilation of urethral stricture by passage of filiform and follower, male; initial** ♂
2.52 3.79 FUD 000 T P3
AMA: 2014,Jan,11

53621 **subsequent** ♂
2.09 3.56 FUD 000 T P3
AMA: 2014,Jan,11

53660 **Dilation of female urethra including suppository and/or instillation; initial** ♀

1.20 1.99 FUD 000 S P3

AMA: 2014,Jan,11

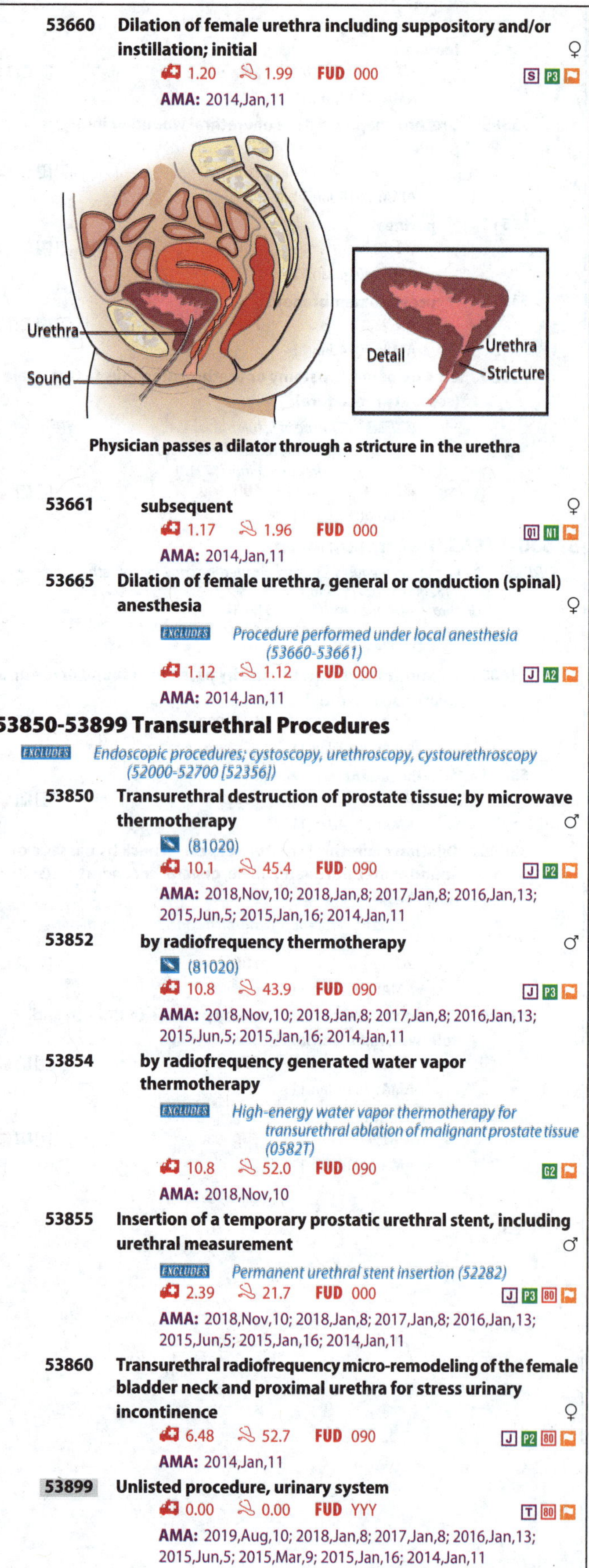

Physician passes a dilator through a stricture in the urethra

53661 **subsequent** ♀

1.17 1.96 FUD 000 Q1 N1

AMA: 2014,Jan,11

53665 **Dilation of female urethra, general or conduction (spinal) anesthesia** ♀

EXCLUDES *Procedure performed under local anesthesia (53660-53661)*

1.12 1.12 FUD 000 J A2

AMA: 2014,Jan,11

53850-53899 Transurethral Procedures

EXCLUDES *Endoscopic procedures; cystoscopy, urethroscopy, cystourethroscopy (52000-52700 [52356])*

53850 **Transurethral destruction of prostate tissue; by microwave thermotherapy** ♂

(81020)

10.1 45.4 FUD 090 J P2

AMA: 2018,Nov,10; 2018,Jan,8; 2017,Jan,8; 2016,Jan,13; 2015,Jun,5; 2015,Jan,16; 2014,Jan,11

53852 **by radiofrequency thermotherapy** ♂

(81020)

10.8 43.9 FUD 090 J P3

AMA: 2018,Nov,10; 2018,Jan,8; 2017,Jan,8; 2016,Jan,13; 2015,Jun,5; 2015,Jan,16; 2014,Jan,11

53854 **by radiofrequency generated water vapor thermotherapy**

EXCLUDES *High-energy water vapor thermotherapy for transurethral ablation of malignant prostate tissue (0582T)*

10.8 52.0 FUD 090 G2

AMA: 2018,Nov,10

53855 **Insertion of a temporary prostatic urethral stent, including urethral measurement** ♂

EXCLUDES *Permanent urethral stent insertion (52282)*

2.39 21.7 FUD 000 J P3 80

AMA: 2018,Nov,10; 2018,Jan,8; 2017,Jan,8; 2016,Jan,13; 2015,Jun,5; 2015,Jan,16; 2014,Jan,11

53860 **Transurethral radiofrequency micro-remodeling of the female bladder neck and proximal urethra for stress urinary incontinence** ♀

6.48 52.7 FUD 090 J P2 80

AMA: 2014,Jan,11

53899 **Unlisted procedure, urinary system**

0.00 0.00 FUD YYY T 80

AMA: 2019,Aug,10; 2018,Jan,8; 2017,Jan,8; 2016,Jan,13; 2015,Jun,5; 2015,Mar,9; 2015,Jan,16; 2014,Jan,11

54000-54015 Procedures of Penis: Incisional

EXCLUDES *Debridement of abdominal perineal gangrene (11004-11006)*

54000 **Slitting of prepuce, dorsal or lateral (separate procedure); newborn**
3.14 4.40 FUD 010
AMA: 2014,Jan,11

54001 **except newborn**
4.02 5.44 FUD 010
AMA: 2014,Jan,11

54015 **Incision and drainage of penis, deep**
EXCLUDES *Abscess, skin/subcutaneous (10060-10160)*
8.92 8.92 FUD 010
AMA: 2014,Jan,11

The physician incises the penis to drain an abscess or hematoma

54050-54065 Destruction of Penis Lesions: Multiple Methods

EXCLUDES *Excision/destruction other lesions (11420-11426, 11620-11626, 17000-17250, 17270-17276)*

54050 **Destruction of lesion(s), penis (eg, condyloma, papilloma, molluscum contagiosum, herpetic vesicle), simple; chemical**
3.05 3.80 FUD 010
AMA: 2014,Jan,11

54055 **electrodesiccation**
2.69 3.49 FUD 010
AMA: 2014,Jan,11

54056 **cryosurgery**
3.18 4.03 FUD 010
AMA: 2014,Jan,11

54057 **laser surgery**
2.76 3.97 FUD 010
AMA: 2014,Jan,11

54060 **surgical excision**
3.76 5.29 FUD 010
AMA: 2014,Jan,11

54065 **Destruction of lesion(s), penis (eg, condyloma, papilloma, molluscum contagiosum, herpetic vesicle), extensive (eg, laser surgery, electrosurgery, cryosurgery, chemosurgery)**
4.97 6.31 FUD 010
AMA: 2014,Jan,11

54100-54115 Procedures of Penis: Excisional

54100 **Biopsy of penis; (separate procedure)**
3.59 5.64 FUD 000
AMA: 2019,Jan,9; 2018,Jan,8; 2017,Jan,8; 2016,Jan,13; 2015,Jan,16; 2014,Jan,11

54105 **deep structures**
6.16 7.68 FUD 010
AMA: 2014,Jan,11

54110 **Excision of penile plaque (Peyronie disease);**
18.0 18.0 FUD 090
AMA: 2014,Jan,11

54111 **with graft to 5 cm in length**
23.1 23.1 FUD 090
AMA: 2018,Jan,8; 2017,Jan,8; 2016,Jan,13; 2015,Jan,16; 2014,Jan,11

54112 **with graft greater than 5 cm in length**
27.1 27.1 FUD 090
AMA: 2014,Jan,11

54115 **Removal foreign body from deep penile tissue (eg, plastic implant)**
12.2 13.0 FUD 090
AMA: 2014,Jan,11

54120-54135 Amputation of Penis

EXCLUDES *Lymphadenectomy (separate procedure) (38760-38770)*

54120 **Amputation of penis; partial**
18.2 18.2 FUD 090
AMA: 2014,Jan,11

54125 **complete**
23.5 23.5 FUD 090
AMA: 2014,Jan,11

54130 **Amputation of penis, radical; with bilateral inguinofemoral lymphadenectomy**
34.5 34.5 FUD 090
AMA: 2014,Jan,11

54135 **in continuity with bilateral pelvic lymphadenectomy, including external iliac, hypogastric and obturator nodes**
43.7 43.7 FUD 090
AMA: 2014,Jan,11

54150-54164 Circumcision Procedures

54150 **Circumcision, using clamp or other device with regional dorsal penile or ring block**
Code also modifier 52 when performed without dorsal penile or ring block
2.83 4.42 FUD 000
AMA: 2018,Jan,8; 2017,Jan,8; 2016,Jan,13; 2015,Jan,16; 2014,Jan,11

54160 **Circumcision, surgical excision other than clamp, device, or dorsal slit; neonate (28 days of age or less)**
4.17 6.32 FUD 010
AMA: 2018,Jan,8; 2017,Jan,8; 2016,Jan,13; 2015,Jan,16; 2014,Jan,11

54161 **older than 28 days of age**
5.70 5.70 FUD 010
AMA: 2018,Jan,8; 2017,Jan,8; 2016,Jan,13; 2015,Jan,16; 2014,Jan,11

54162 **Lysis or excision of penile post-circumcision adhesions**
5.77 7.42 FUD 010
AMA: 2014,Jan,11

54163 **Repair incomplete circumcision**
6.31 6.31 FUD 010
AMA: 2014,Jan,11

54164 **Frenulotomy of penis**
EXCLUDES *Circumcision (54150-54163)*
5.60 5.60 FUD 010
AMA: 2014,Jan,11

54200-54250 Evaluation and Treatment of Erectile Abnormalities

54200 Injection procedure for Peyronie disease; ♂
2.42 3.13 FUD 010 T P3
AMA: 2014,Jan,11

54205 with surgical exposure of plaque ♂
15.4 15.4 FUD 090 J A2 80
AMA: 2014,Jan,11

54220 Irrigation of corpora cavernosa for priapism ♂
3.87 5.97 FUD 000 T A2
AMA: 2014,Jan,11

54230 Injection procedure for corpora cavernosography ♂
(74445)
2.30 2.82 FUD 000 N N1
AMA: 2014,Jan,11

54231 Dynamic cavernosometry, including intracavernosal injection of vasoactive drugs (eg, papaverine, phentolamine) ♂
3.36 4.08 FUD 000 J P3
AMA: 2014,Jan,11

54235 Injection of corpora cavernosa with pharmacologic agent(s) (eg, papaverine, phentolamine) ♂
2.11 2.56 FUD 000 T P3
AMA: 2018,Jan,8; 2017,Jan,8; 2016,Jan,13; 2015,Jan,16; 2014,Jan,11

54240 Penile plethysmography ♂
2.97 2.97 FUD 000 S P3 80
AMA: 2014,Jan,11

54250 Nocturnal penile tumescence and/or rigidity test ♂
3.50 3.50 FUD 000 T P3 80
AMA: 2014,Jan,11

54300-54390 Hypospadias Repair and Related Procedures

EXCLUDES *Other urethroplasties (53400-53430)*
Revascularization of penis (37788)

54300 Plastic operation of penis for straightening of chordee (eg, hypospadias), with or without mobilization of urethra ♂
18.6 18.6 FUD 090 J A2 80
AMA: 2018,Jan,8; 2017,Jan,8; 2016,Jan,13; 2015,Jan,16; 2014,Dec,16; 2014,Dec,16; 2014,Jan,11

54304 Plastic operation on penis for correction of chordee or for first stage hypospadias repair with or without transplantation of prepuce and/or skin flaps ♂
21.6 21.6 FUD 090 J A2 80
AMA: 2014,Jan,11

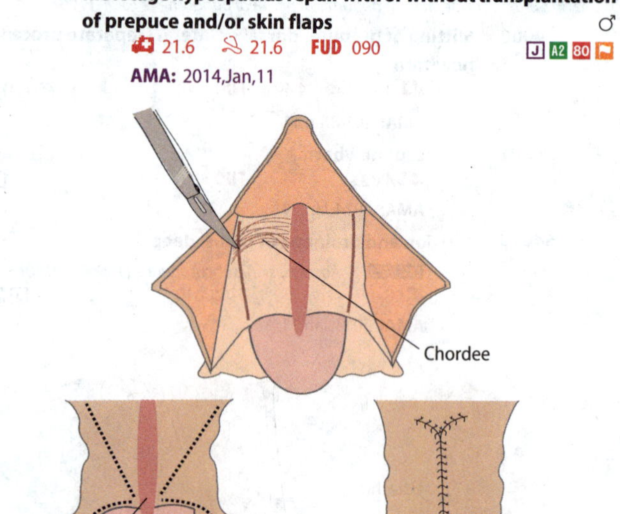

The foreskin is used in either a free graft or a flap graft to cover the ventral skin defects created to correct the chordee

54308 Urethroplasty for second stage hypospadias repair (including urinary diversion); less than 3 cm ♂
20.6 20.6 FUD 090 J A2 80
AMA: 2014,Jan,11

54312 greater than 3 cm ♂
23.6 23.6 FUD 090 J A2 80
AMA: 2014,Jan,11

54316 Urethroplasty for second stage hypospadias repair (including urinary diversion) with free skin graft obtained from site other than genitalia ♂
28.8 28.8 FUD 090 J A2 80
AMA: 2014,Jan,11

54318 Urethroplasty for third stage hypospadias repair to release penis from scrotum (eg, third stage Cecil repair) ♂
20.5 20.5 FUD 090 J A2 80
AMA: 2014,Jan,11

54322 1-stage distal hypospadias repair (with or without chordee or circumcision); with simple meatal advancement (eg, Magpi, V-flap) ♂
22.6 22.6 FUD 090 J A2 80
AMA: 2014,Jan,11

54324 with urethroplasty by local skin flaps (eg, flip-flap, prepucial flap) ♂
INCLUDES Browne's operation
28.0 28.0 FUD 090 J A2 80
AMA: 2014,Jan,11

54326 with urethroplasty by local skin flaps and mobilization of urethra ♂
27.3 27.3 FUD 090 J A2 80
AMA: 2014,Jan,11

54328 with extensive dissection to correct chordee and urethroplasty with local skin flaps, skin graft patch, and/or island flap ♂
EXCLUDES *Urethroplasty/straightening of chordee (54308)*
27.1 27.1 FUD 090 J A2 80
AMA: 2018,Jan,8; 2017,Jan,8; 2016,Jan,13; 2015,Jan,16; 2014,Jan,11

54332 **1-stage proximal penile or penoscrotal hypospadias repair requiring extensive dissection to correct chordee and urethroplasty by use of skin graft tube and/or island flap** ♂
29.3 29.3 FUD 090 J 80
AMA: 2018,Jan,8; 2017,Jan,8; 2016,Jan,13; 2015,Jan,16; 2014,Jan,11

54336 **1-stage perineal hypospadias repair requiring extensive dissection to correct chordee and urethroplasty by use of skin graft tube and/or island flap** ♂
34.4 34.4 FUD 090 J 80
AMA: 2018,Jan,8; 2017,Jan,8; 2016,Jan,13; 2015,Jan,16; 2014,Jan,11

54340 **Repair of hypospadias complications (ie, fistula, stricture, diverticula); by closure, incision, or excision, simple** ♂
16.4 16.4 FUD 090 J A2 80
AMA: 2014,Jan,11

54344 **requiring mobilization of skin flaps and urethroplasty with flap or patch graft** ♂
27.4 27.4 FUD 090 J A2 80
AMA: 2014,Jan,11

54348 **requiring extensive dissection and urethroplasty with flap, patch or tubed graft (includes urinary diversion)** ♂
29.3 29.3 FUD 090 J A2 80
AMA: 2014,Jan,11

54352 **Repair of hypospadias cripple requiring extensive dissection and excision of previously constructed structures including re-release of chordee and reconstruction of urethra and penis by use of local skin as grafts and island flaps and skin brought in as flaps or grafts** ♂
41.0 41.0 FUD 090 J A2 80
AMA: 2014,Jan,11

54360 **Plastic operation on penis to correct angulation** ♂
20.8 20.8 FUD 090 J A2 80
AMA: 2014,Jan,11

54380 **Plastic operation on penis for epispadias distal to external sphincter;** ♂
INCLUDES Lowsley's operation
23.1 23.1 FUD 090 J A2 80
AMA: 2014,Jan,11

54385 **with incontinence** ♂
26.8 26.8 FUD 090 J A2 80
AMA: 2014,Jan,11

54390 **with exstrophy of bladder** ♂
35.9 35.9 FUD 090 C 80
AMA: 2014,Jan,11

54400-54417 Procedures to Treat Impotence

CMS: 100-03,230.4 Diagnosis and Treatment of Impotence

EXCLUDES *Other urethroplasties (53400-53430)*
Revascularization of penis (37788)

54400 **Insertion of penile prosthesis; non-inflatable (semi-rigid)** ♂
EXCLUDES *Replacement/removal penile prosthesis (54415, 54416)*
15.3 15.3 FUD 090 J J8
AMA: 2014,Jan,11

54401 **inflatable (self-contained)** ♂
EXCLUDES *Replacement/removal penile prosthesis (54415, 54416)*
18.9 18.9 FUD 090 J J8
AMA: 2014,Jan,11

54405 **Insertion of multi-component, inflatable penile prosthesis, including placement of pump, cylinders, and reservoir** ♂
Code also modifier 52 for reduced services
23.4 23.4 FUD 090 J J8 80
AMA: 2014,Jan,11

54406 **Removal of all components of a multi-component, inflatable penile prosthesis without replacement of prosthesis** ♂
Code also modifier 52 for reduced services
21.1 21.1 FUD 090 Q2 A2 80
AMA: 2014,Jan,11

54408 **Repair of component(s) of a multi-component, inflatable penile prosthesis** ♂
22.8 22.8 FUD 090 J A2 80
AMA: 2014,Jan,11

54410 **Removal and replacement of all component(s) of a multi-component, inflatable penile prosthesis at the same operative session** ♂
24.8 24.8 FUD 090 J J8 80
AMA: 2014,Jan,11

54411 **Removal and replacement of all components of a multi-component inflatable penile prosthesis through an infected field at the same operative session, including irrigation and debridement of infected tissue** ♂
INCLUDES Debridement (11042, 11043)
Code also modifier 52 for reduced services
29.7 29.7 FUD 090 J 80
AMA: 2014,Jan,11

54415 **Removal of non-inflatable (semi-rigid) or inflatable (self-contained) penile prosthesis, without replacement of prosthesis** ♂
15.3 15.3 FUD 090 Q2 A2 80
AMA: 2014,Jan,11

54416 **Removal and replacement of non-inflatable (semi-rigid) or inflatable (self-contained) penile prosthesis at the same operative session** ♂
20.5 20.5 FUD 090 J J8 80
AMA: 2014,Jan,11

54417 **Removal and replacement of non-inflatable (semi-rigid) or inflatable (self-contained) penile prosthesis through an infected field at the same operative session, including irrigation and debridement of infected tissue** ♂
INCLUDES Debridement (11042, 11043)
25.9 25.9 FUD 090 J 80
AMA: 2014,Jan,11

54420-54450 Other Procedures of the Penis

EXCLUDES *Other urethroplasties (53400-53430)*
Revascularization of penis (37788)

54420 **Corpora cavernosa-saphenous vein shunt (priapism operation), unilateral or bilateral** ♂
20.3 20.3 FUD 090 J A2 80
AMA: 2014,Jan,11

54430 **Corpora cavernosa-corpus spongiosum shunt (priapism operation), unilateral or bilateral** ♂
18.5 | 18.5 | FUD 090 | C 80
AMA: 2014,Jan,11

Cross section of penis

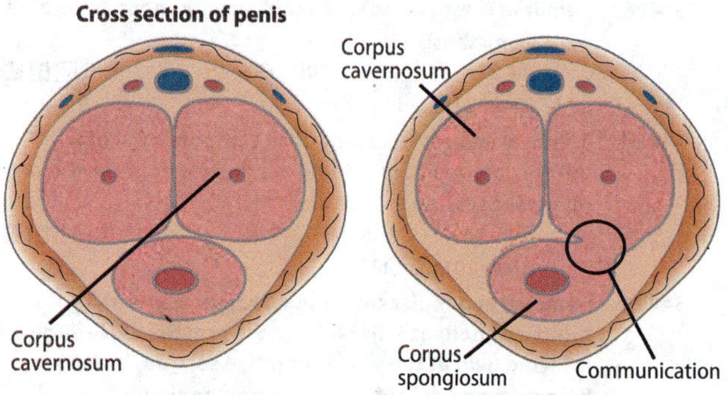

Corpus cavernosum

Corpus cavernosum

Corpus spongiosum

Communication

The physician creates a communication between the corpus cavernosum and the corpus spongiosum

54435 **Corpora cavernosa-glans penis fistulization (eg, biopsy needle, Winter procedure, rongeur, or punch) for priapism** ♂
12.0 | 12.0 | FUD 090 | J A2
AMA: 2014,Jan,11

54437 **Repair of traumatic corporeal tear(s)** ♂
19.4 | 19.4 | FUD 090 | J G2 80
EXCLUDES *Urethral repair (53410, 53415)*

54438 **Replantation, penis, complete amputation including urethral repair** ♂
38.7 | 38.7 | FUD 090 | C 80
EXCLUDES *Replantation/repair of corporeal tear in incomplete amputation penis (54437)*
Replantation/urethral repair in incomplete amputation penis (53410-53415)

54440 **Plastic operation of penis for injury** ♂
0.00 | 0.00 | FUD 090 | J A2 80
AMA: 2014,Jan,11

54450 **Foreskin manipulation including lysis of preputial adhesions and stretching** ♂
1.67 | 1.99 | FUD 000 | T A2
AMA: 2014,Jan,11

54500-54560 Testicular Procedures: Incisional

EXCLUDES *Debridement of abdominal perineal gangrene (11004-11006)*

54500 **Biopsy of testis, needle (separate procedure)** ♂
EXCLUDES *Fine needle aspiration (10021, [10004, 10005, 10006, 10007, 10008, 10009, 10010, 10011, 10012])*
(88172-88173)
2.15 | 2.15 | FUD 000 | J A2 80 50
AMA: 2019,Apr,4; 2014,Jan,11

54505 **Biopsy of testis, incisional (separate procedure)** ♂
Code also when combined with epididymogram, seminal vesiculogram or vasogram (55300)
6.07 | 6.07 | FUD 010 | J A2 80 50
AMA: 2018,Jan,8; 2017,Jan,8; 2016,Jan,13; 2015,Jan,16; 2014,Jan,11

54512 **Excision of extraparenchymal lesion of testis** ♂
15.6 | 15.6 | FUD 090 | J A2 50
AMA: 2018,Jan,8; 2017,Jan,8; 2016,Jan,13; 2015,Jan,16; 2014,Jan,11

54520 **Orchiectomy, simple (including subcapsular), with or without testicular prosthesis, scrotal or inguinal approach** ♂
INCLUDES Huggins' orchiectomy
EXCLUDES *Lymphadenectomy, radical retroperitoneal (38780)*
Code also hernia repair if performed (49505, 49507)
9.45 | 9.45 | FUD 090 | J A2 50
AMA: 2018,Jan,8; 2017,Jan,8; 2016,Jan,13; 2015,Jan,16; 2014,Jan,11

54522 **Orchiectomy, partial** ♂
EXCLUDES *Lymphadenectomy, radical retroperitoneal (38780)*
17.0 | 17.0 | FUD 090 | J A2 80 50
AMA: 2018,Jan,8; 2017,Jan,8; 2016,Jan,13; 2015,Jan,16; 2014,Jan,11

54530 **Orchiectomy, radical, for tumor; inguinal approach** ♂
EXCLUDES *Lymphadenectomy, radical retroperitoneal (38780)*
14.6 | 14.6 | FUD 090 | J A2 80 50
AMA: 2018,Jan,8; 2017,Jan,8; 2016,Jan,13; 2015,Jan,16; 2014,Jan,11

54535 **with abdominal exploration** ♂
EXCLUDES *Lymphadenectomy, radical retroperitoneal (38780)*
21.5 | 21.5 | FUD 090 | J 80 50
AMA: 2018,Jan,8; 2017,Jan,8; 2016,Jan,13; 2015,Jan,16; 2014,Jan,11

54550 **Exploration for undescended testis (inguinal or scrotal area)** ♂
14.2 | 14.2 | FUD 090 | J A2 80 50
AMA: 2018,Jan,8; 2017,Mar,10; 2017,Jan,8; 2016,Jan,13; 2015,Jan,16; 2014,Jan,11

54560 **Exploration for undescended testis with abdominal exploration** ♂
19.8 | 19.8 | FUD 090 | J G2 80 50
AMA: 2018,Jan,8; 2017,Jan,8; 2016,Jan,13; 2015,Jan,16; 2014,Jan,11

54600-54699 Open and Laparoscopic Testicular Procedures

54600 **Reduction of torsion of testis, surgical, with or without fixation of contralateral testis** ♂
13.1 | 13.1 | FUD 090 | J A2 50
AMA: 2018,Jan,8; 2017,Jan,8; 2016,Jan,13; 2015,Jan,16; 2014,Jan,11

Normal testes

Torsion of testis

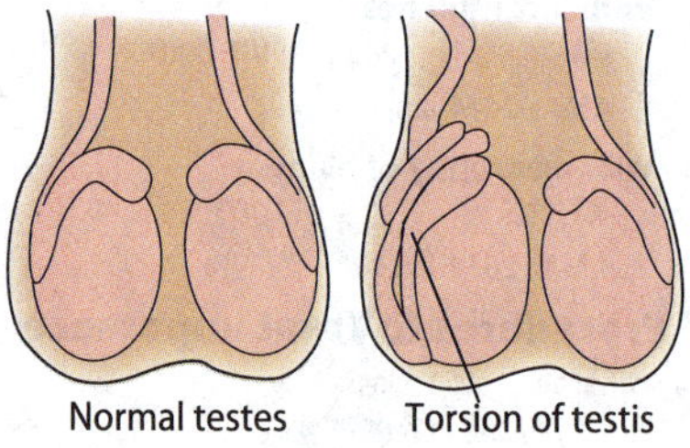

54620 **Fixation of contralateral testis (separate procedure)** ♂
8.66 | 8.66 | FUD 010 | J A2 50
AMA: 2014,Jan,11

▲ **54640** **Orchiopexy, inguinal or scrotal approach** ♂
INCLUDES Bevan's operation
Koop inguinal orchiopexy
Prentice orchiopexy
EXCLUDES *Repair inguinal hernia with inguinal orchiopexy (49495-49525)*
13.8 | 13.8 | FUD 090 | J A2 80 50
AMA: 2018,Jan,8; 2017,Mar,10; 2017,Jan,8; 2016,Jan,13; 2015,Jan,16; 2014,Jan,11

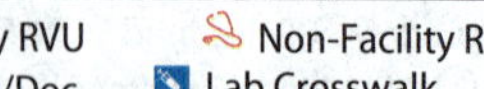

54650 **Orchiopexy, abdominal approach, for intra-abdominal testis (eg, Fowler-Stephens)** ♂
EXCLUDES *Laparoscopic orchiopexy (54692)*
20.5 20.5 FUD 090 J 80 50
AMA: 2018,Jan,8; 2017,Jan,8; 2016,Jan,13; 2015,Jan,16; 2014,Jan,11

54660 **Insertion of testicular prosthesis (separate procedure)** ♂
10.3 10.3 FUD 090 J J8 80 50
AMA: 2018,Jan,8; 2017,Jan,8; 2016,Jan,13; 2015,Jan,16; 2014,Jan,11

54670 **Suture or repair of testicular injury** ♂
11.7 11.7 FUD 090 J A2 80 50
AMA: 2018,Jan,8; 2017,Jan,8; 2016,Jan,13; 2015,Jan,16; 2014,Jan,11

54680 **Transplantation of testis(es) to thigh (because of scrotal destruction)** ♂
22.7 22.7 FUD 090 J A2 80 50
AMA: 2018,Jan,8; 2017,Jan,8; 2016,Jan,13; 2015,Jan,16; 2014,Jan,11

54690 **Laparoscopy, surgical; orchiectomy** ♂
INCLUDES Diagnostic laparoscopy (49320)
18.9 18.9 FUD 090 J A2 80 50
AMA: 2019,Feb,10; 2018,Jan,8; 2017,Jan,8; 2016,Jan,13; 2015,Jan,16; 2014,Jan,11

54692 **orchiopexy for intra-abdominal testis** ♂
INCLUDES Diagnostic laparoscopy (49320)
21.9 21.9 FUD 090 J G2 50
AMA: 2018,Jan,8; 2017,Jan,8; 2016,Jan,13; 2015,Jan,16; 2014,Jan,11

54699 **Unlisted laparoscopy procedure, testis** ♂
0.00 0.00 FUD YYY J 80 50
AMA: 2018,Jan,8; 2017,Jan,8; 2016,Jan,13; 2015,Jan,16; 2014,Jan,11

54700-54901 Open Procedures of the Epididymis

54700 **Incision and drainage of epididymis, testis and/or scrotal space (eg, abscess or hematoma)** ♂
EXCLUDES *Debridement of genitalia for necrotizing soft tissue infection (11004-11006)*
6.16 6.16 FUD 010 J A2 50
AMA: 2018,Jan,8; 2017,Jan,8; 2016,Jan,13; 2015,Jan,16; 2014,Jan,11

54800 **Biopsy of epididymis, needle** ♂
EXCLUDES *Fine needle aspiration (10021, [10004, 10005, 10006, 10007, 10008, 10009, 10010, 10011, 10012])*
88172-88173
3.64 3.64 FUD 000 J A2 80 50
AMA: 2019,Apr,4; 2018,Jan,8; 2017,Jan,8; 2016,Jan,13; 2015,Jan,16; 2014,Jan,11

54830 **Excision of local lesion of epididymis** ♂
10.7 10.7 FUD 090 J A2 80 50
AMA: 2018,Jan,8; 2017,Jan,8; 2016,Jan,13; 2015,Jan,16; 2014,Jan,11

54840 **Excision of spermatocele, with or without epididymectomy** ♂
9.29 9.29 FUD 090 J A2 50
AMA: 2018,Jan,8; 2017,Jan,8; 2016,Jan,13; 2015,Jan,16; 2014,Jan,11

54860 **Epididymectomy; unilateral** ♂
12.1 12.1 FUD 090 J A2
AMA: 2014,Jan,11

54861 **bilateral** ♂
16.3 16.3 FUD 090 J A2 80
AMA: 2014,Jan,11

54865 **Exploration of epididymis, with or without biopsy** ♂
10.3 10.3 FUD 090 J A2 80
AMA: 2014,Jan,11

54900 **Epididymovasostomy, anastomosis of epididymis to vas deferens; unilateral** ♂
EXCLUDES *Operating microscope (69990)*
23.1 23.1 FUD 090 J A2 80
AMA: 2018,Jan,8; 2017,Jan,8; 2016,Jan,13; 2015,Jan,16; 2014,Jan,11

54901 **bilateral** ♂
EXCLUDES *Operating microscope (69990)*
30.5 30.5 FUD 090 J A2 80
AMA: 2018,Jan,8; 2017,Jan,8; 2016,Jan,13; 2015,Jan,16; 2014,Jan,11

55000-55180 Procedures of the Tunica Vaginalis and Scrotum

55000 **Puncture aspiration of hydrocele, tunica vaginalis, with or without injection of medication** ♂
2.45 3.34 FUD 000 T P3 50
AMA: 2014,Jan,11

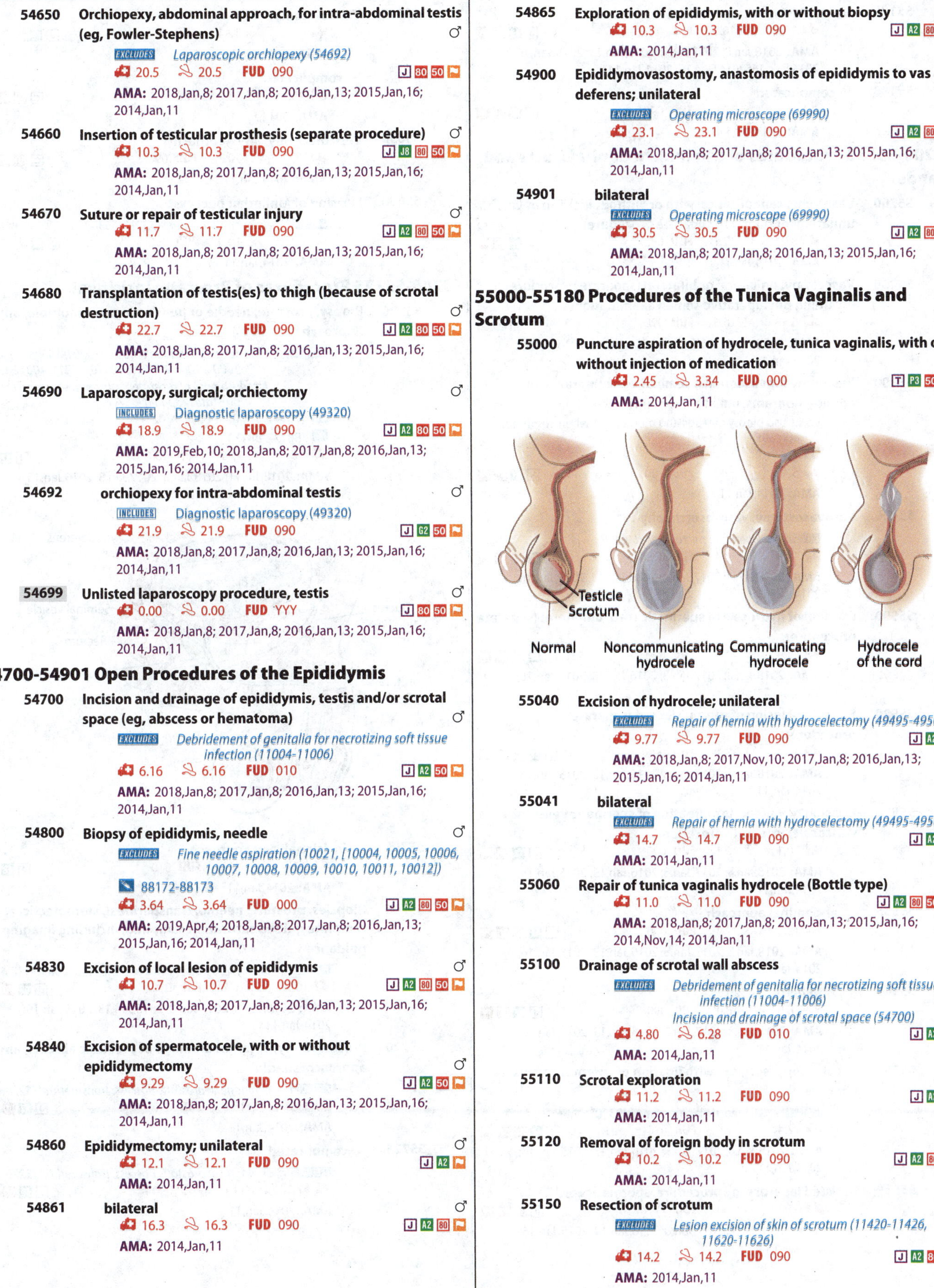

55040 **Excision of hydrocele; unilateral** ♂
EXCLUDES *Repair of hernia with hydrocelectomy (49495-49501)*
9.77 9.77 FUD 090 J A2
AMA: 2018,Jan,8; 2017,Nov,10; 2017,Jan,8; 2016,Jan,13; 2015,Jan,16; 2014,Jan,11

55041 **bilateral** ♂
EXCLUDES *Repair of hernia with hydrocelectomy (49495-49501)*
14.7 14.7 FUD 090 J A2
AMA: 2014,Jan,11

55060 **Repair of tunica vaginalis hydrocele (Bottle type)** ♂
11.0 11.0 FUD 090 J A2 80 50
AMA: 2018,Jan,8; 2017,Jan,8; 2016,Jan,13; 2015,Jan,16; 2014,Nov,14; 2014,Jan,11

55100 **Drainage of scrotal wall abscess** ♂
EXCLUDES *Debridement of genitalia for necrotizing soft tissue infection (11004-11006)*
Incision and drainage of scrotal space (54700)
4.80 6.28 FUD 010 J A2
AMA: 2014,Jan,11

55110 **Scrotal exploration** ♂
11.2 11.2 FUD 090 J A2
AMA: 2014,Jan,11

55120 **Removal of foreign body in scrotum** ♂
10.2 10.2 FUD 090 J A2 80
AMA: 2014,Jan,11

55150 **Resection of scrotum** ♂
EXCLUDES *Lesion excision of skin of scrotum (11420-11426, 11620-11626)*
14.2 14.2 FUD 090 J A2 80
AMA: 2014,Jan,11

55175 **Scrotoplasty; simple** ♂
Facility RVU 10.5 Non-Facility RVU 10.5 **FUD** 090 J A2 80 CCI
AMA: 2018,Jan,8; 2017,Jan,8; 2016,Jan,13; 2015,Jan,16; 2014,Dec,16; 2014,Dec,16; 2014,Jan,11

55180 **complicated** ♂
Facility RVU 19.9 Non-Facility RVU 19.9 **FUD** 090 J A2 80 CCI
AMA: 2014,Jan,11

55200-55680 Procedures of Other Male Genital Ducts and Glands

55200 **Vasotomy, cannulization with or without incision of vas, unilateral or bilateral (separate procedure)** ♂
Facility RVU 8.04 Non-Facility RVU 12.1 **FUD** 090 J A2 80 CCI
AMA: 2014,Jan,11

55250 **Vasectomy, unilateral or bilateral (separate procedure), including postoperative semen examination(s)** ♂
Facility RVU 6.58 Non-Facility RVU 10.6 **FUD** 090 J A2 CCI
AMA: 2018,Jan,8; 2017,Jan,8; 2016,Jan,13; 2015,Jan,16; 2014,Jan,11

55300 **Vasotomy for vasograms, seminal vesiculograms, or epididymograms, unilateral or bilateral** ♂
Code also biopsy of testis and modifier 51 when combined (54505)
Radiology Crosswalk (74440)
Facility RVU 5.42 Non-Facility RVU 5.42 **FUD** 000 N N1 80 CCI
AMA: 2014,Jan,11

55400 **Vasovasostomy, vasovasorrhaphy** ♂
EXCLUDES *Operating microscope (69990)*
Facility RVU 14.4 Non-Facility RVU 14.4 **FUD** 090 J A2 80 50 CCI
AMA: 2018,Jan,8; 2017,Jan,8; 2016,Jan,13; 2015,Jan,16; 2014,Jan,11

55500 **Excision of hydrocele of spermatic cord, unilateral (separate procedure)** ♂
Facility RVU 11.4 Non-Facility RVU 11.4 **FUD** 090 J A2 80 50 CCI
AMA: 2018,Jan,8; 2017,Jan,8; 2016,Jan,13; 2015,Jan,16; 2014,Jan,11

55520 **Excision of lesion of spermatic cord (separate procedure)** ♂
Facility RVU 13.1 Non-Facility RVU 13.1 **FUD** 090 J A2 80 50 CCI
AMA: 2018,Jan,8; 2017,Jan,8; 2016,Jan,13; 2015,Jan,16; 2014,Jan,11

55530 **Excision of varicocele or ligation of spermatic veins for varicocele; (separate procedure)** ♂
Facility RVU 10.1 Non-Facility RVU 10.1 **FUD** 090 J A2 50 CCI
AMA: 2018,Jan,8; 2017,Jan,8; 2016,Jan,13; 2015,Jan,16; 2014,Jan,11

55535 **abdominal approach** ♂
Facility RVU 12.4 Non-Facility RVU 12.4 **FUD** 090 J A2 80 50 CCI
AMA: 2018,Jan,8; 2017,Jan,8; 2016,Jan,13; 2015,Jan,16; 2014,Jan,11

55540 **with hernia repair** ♂
Facility RVU 16.0 Non-Facility RVU 16.0 **FUD** 090 J A2 50 CCI
AMA: 2018,Jan,8; 2017,Jan,8; 2016,Jan,13; 2015,Jan,16; 2014,Jan,11

55550 **Laparoscopy, surgical, with ligation of spermatic veins for varicocele** ♂
INCLUDES Diagnostic laparoscopy (49320)
Facility RVU 12.4 Non-Facility RVU 12.4 **FUD** 090 J A2 80 50 CCI
AMA: 2018,Jan,8; 2017,Jan,8; 2016,Jan,13; 2015,Jan,16; 2014,Jan,11

55559 **Unlisted laparoscopy procedure, spermatic cord** ♂
Facility RVU 0.00 Non-Facility RVU 0.00 **FUD** YYY J 80 50 CCI
AMA: 2018,Jan,8; 2017,Jan,8; 2016,Jan,13; 2015,Jan,16; 2014,Jan,11

55600 **Vesiculotomy;** ♂
Facility RVU 12.1 Non-Facility RVU 12.1 **FUD** 090 J R2 80 50 CCI
AMA: 2014,Jan,11

55605 **complicated** ♂
Facility RVU 15.1 Non-Facility RVU 15.1 **FUD** 090 C 80 50 CCI
AMA: 2014,Jan,11

55650 **Vesiculectomy, any approach** ♂
Facility RVU 20.7 Non-Facility RVU 20.7 **FUD** 090 C 80 50 CCI
AMA: 2014,Jan,11

55680 **Excision of Mullerian duct cyst** ♂
EXCLUDES *Injection procedure (52010, 55300)*
Facility RVU 10.0 Non-Facility RVU 10.0 **FUD** 090 J A2 80 50 CCI
AMA: 2014,Jan,11

55700-55725 Procedures of Prostate: Incisional

55700 **Biopsy, prostate; needle or punch, single or multiple, any approach** ♂
EXCLUDES *Fine needle aspiration (10021, [10004, 10005, 10006, 10007, 10008, 10009, 10010, 10011, 10012])*
Needle biopsy of prostate, saturation sampling for prostate mapping (55706)
Radiology Crosswalk (76942, 77002, 77012, 77021)
Lab Crosswalk (88172-88173)
Facility RVU 3.77 Non-Facility RVU 7.12 **FUD** 000 J A2 CCI
AMA: 2018,Jul,11; 2018,Jan,8; 2017,Jan,8; 2016,Jan,13; 2015,Jan,16; 2014,Jan,11

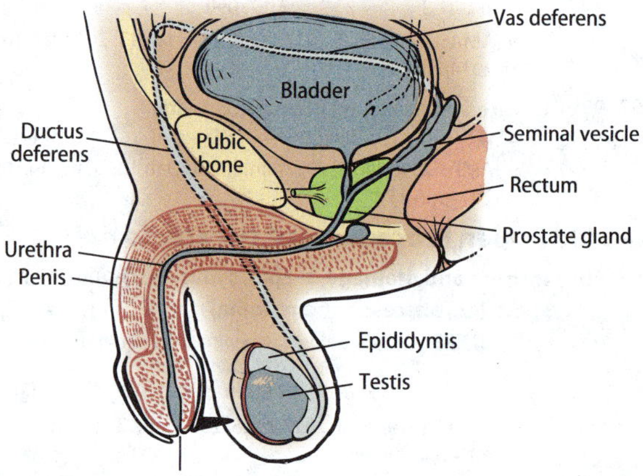

55705 **incisional, any approach** ♂
Facility RVU 7.68 Non-Facility RVU 7.68 **FUD** 010 J A2 CCI
AMA: 2014,Jan,11

55706 **Biopsies, prostate, needle, transperineal, stereotactic template guided saturation sampling, including imaging guidance** ♂
EXCLUDES *Biopsy, prostate; needle or punch (55700)*
Facility RVU 10.7 Non-Facility RVU 10.7 **FUD** 010 J G2 80 CCI
AMA: 2018,Jan,8; 2017,Jan,8; 2016,Jan,13; 2015,Jan,16; 2014,Jan,11

55720 **Prostatotomy, external drainage of prostatic abscess, any approach; simple** ♂
EXCLUDES *Drainage of prostatic abscess, transurethral (52700)*
Facility RVU 13.0 Non-Facility RVU 13.0 **FUD** 090 J A2 80 CCI
AMA: 2014,Jan,11

55725 **complicated** ♂
EXCLUDES *Drainage of prostatic abscess, transurethral (52700)*
Facility RVU 17.1 Non-Facility RVU 17.1 **FUD** 090 J A2 80 CCI
AMA: 2014,Jan,11

55801-55845 Open Prostatectomy

EXCLUDES *Limited pelvic lymphadenectomy for staging (separate procedure) (38562)*
Node dissection, independent (38770-38780)
Transurethral prostate
Destruction (53850-53852)
Resection (52601-52640)

55801 **Prostatectomy, perineal, subtotal (including control of postoperative bleeding, vasectomy, meatotomy, urethral calibration and/or dilation, and internal urethrotomy)** ♂
31.6 31.6 FUD 090 C 80
AMA: 2014,Jan,11

55810 **Prostatectomy, perineal radical;** ♂
INCLUDES Walsh modified radical prostatectomy
38.0 38.0 FUD 090 C 80
AMA: 2014,Jan,11

55812 **with lymph node biopsy(s) (limited pelvic lymphadenectomy)** ♂
46.5 46.5 FUD 090 C 80
AMA: 2014,Jan,11

55815 **with bilateral pelvic lymphadenectomy, including external iliac, hypogastric and obturator nodes** ♂
EXCLUDES *When performed on separate days, report: (38770, 55810)*
Pelvic lymphadenectomy, bilateral, and append modifier 50 (38770)
Perineal radical prostatectomy (55810)
51.0 51.0 FUD 090 C 80
AMA: 2014,Jan,11

55821 **Prostatectomy (including control of postoperative bleeding, vasectomy, meatotomy, urethral calibration and/or dilation, and internal urethrotomy); suprapubic, subtotal, 1 or 2 stages** ♂
25.2 25.2 FUD 090 C 80
AMA: 2014,Jan,11

55831 **retropubic, subtotal** ♂
27.3 27.3 FUD 090 C 80
AMA: 2014,Jan,11

55840 **Prostatectomy, retropubic radical, with or without nerve sparing;** ♂
EXCLUDES *Prostatectomy, radical retropubic, performed laparoscopically (55866)*
33.9 33.9 FUD 090 C 80
AMA: 2014,Jan,11

55842 **with lymph node biopsy(s) (limited pelvic lymphadenectomy)** ♂
EXCLUDES *Prostatectomy, retropubic radical, performed laparoscopically (55866)*
33.9 33.9 FUD 090 C 80
AMA: 2014,Jan,11

55845 **with bilateral pelvic lymphadenectomy, including external iliac, hypogastric, and obturator nodes** ♂
EXCLUDES *Prostatectomy, retropubic radical, performed laparoscopically (55866)*
When performed on separate days, report: (38770, 55840)
Pelvic lymphadenectomy, bilateral, and append modifier 50 (38770)
Radical prostatectomy, retropubic, with or without nerve sparing (55840)
39.4 39.4 FUD 090 C 80
AMA: 2014,Jan,11

55860-55865 Prostate Exposure for Radiation Source Application

55860 **Exposure of prostate, any approach, for insertion of radioactive substance;** ♂
EXCLUDES *Interstitial radioelement application (77770-77772, 77778)*
25.3 25.3 FUD 090 J G2
AMA: 2014,Jan,11

55862 **with lymph node biopsy(s) (limited pelvic lymphadenectomy)** ♂
31.7 31.7 FUD 090 C 80
AMA: 2014,Jan,11

55865 **with bilateral pelvic lymphadenectomy, including external iliac, hypogastric and obturator nodes** ♂
38.6 38.6 FUD 090 C 80
AMA: 2014,Jan,11

55866 Laparoscopic Prostatectomy

55866 **Laparoscopy, surgical prostatectomy, retropubic radical, including nerve sparing, includes robotic assistance, when performed** ♂
INCLUDES Diagnostic laparoscopy (49320)
EXCLUDES *Open method (55840)*
41.7 41.7 FUD 090 J 80
AMA: 2018,Jan,8; 2017,Jan,8; 2016,Jan,13; 2015,Jan,16; 2014,Jan,11

55870-55899 Miscellaneous Prostate Procedures

55870 **Electroejaculation** ♂
EXCLUDES *Artificial insemination (58321-58322)*
4.10 5.04 FUD 000 T P3
AMA: 2014,Jan,11

55873 **Cryosurgical ablation of the prostate (includes ultrasonic guidance and monitoring)** ♂
22.1 176. FUD 090 J J8
AMA: 2019,Sep,10; 2018,Jan,8; 2017,Jan,8; 2016,Jan,13; 2015,Sep,12; 2015,Jan,16; 2014,Jan,11

55874 **Transperineal placement of biodegradable material, peri-prostatic, single or multiple injection(s), including image guidance, when performed** ♂
4.80 98.6 FUD 000 T G2
INCLUDES Ultrasound guidance (76942)

55875 **Transperineal placement of needles or catheters into prostate for interstitial radioelement application, with or without cystoscopy** ♂
Code also interstitial radioelement application (77770-77772, 77778)
(76965)
22.1 22.1 FUD 090 J A2 80
AMA: 2018,Jan,8; 2017,Jan,8; 2016,Jan,13; 2015,Jan,16; 2014,Jan,11

55876 **Placement of interstitial device(s) for radiation therapy guidance (eg, fiducial markers, dosimeter), prostate (via needle, any approach), single or multiple** ♂
Code also supply of device
(76942, 77002, 77012, 77021)
2.91 4.05 FUD 000 S P3
AMA: 2018,Jan,8; 2017,Jan,8; 2016,Jun,3; 2016,Jan,13; 2015,Jan,16; 2014,Jan,11

55899 **Unlisted procedure, male genital system** ♂
0.00 0.00 FUD YYY T 80
AMA: 2019,Jun,14; 2018,Jan,8; 2017,Jan,8; 2017,Jan,6; 2016,Jan,13; 2015,Jun,5; 2015,Jan,16; 2014,Jan,11

55920 Insertion Brachytherapy Catheters/Needles Pelvis/Genitalia, Male/Female

55920 **Placement of needles or catheters into pelvic organs and/or genitalia (except prostate) for subsequent interstitial radioelement application**

EXCLUDES *Insertion of Heyman capsules for purposes of brachytherapy (58346)*
Insertion of vaginal ovoids and/or uterine tandems for purposes of brachytherapy (57155)
Placement of catheters or needles, prostate (55875)

13.0 13.0 FUD 000 J G2 80

AMA: 2018,Jan,8; 2017,Jan,8; 2016,Jan,13; 2015,Jan,16; 2014,Jan,11

55970-55980 Transsexual Surgery

CMS: 100-02,16,10 Exclusions from Coverage; 100-02,16,180 Services Related to Noncovered Procedures

55970 **Intersex surgery; male to female** ♂

0.00 0.00 FUD YYY J

AMA: 2014,Jan,11

55980 **female to male** ♀

0.00 0.00 FUD YYY J

AMA: 2014,Jan,11

56405-56420 Incision and Drainage of Abscess

EXCLUDES *Incision and drainage Skene's gland cyst/abscess (53060)*
Incision and drainage subcutaneous abscess/cyst/furuncle (10040, 10060, 10061)

56405 **Incision and drainage of vulva or perineal abscess** ♀

3.22 3.25 FUD 010 T P3

AMA: 2019,Jul,6; 2014,Jan,11

56420 **Incision and drainage of Bartholin's gland abscess** ♀

2.75 3.86 FUD 010 T P3

AMA: 2019,Jul,6; 2014,Jan,11

56440-56442 Other Female Genital Incisional Procedures

EXCLUDES *Incision and drainage subcutaneous abscess/cyst/furuncle (10040, 10060, 10061)*

56440 **Marsupialization of Bartholin's gland cyst** ♀

5.15 5.15 FUD 010 J A2

AMA: 2019,Jul,6; 2014,Jan,11

56441 **Lysis of labial adhesions** ♀

4.09 4.33 FUD 010 J A2 80

AMA: 2019,Jul,6; 2014,Jan,11

56442 **Hymenotomy, simple incision** ♀

1.34 1.34 FUD 000 J A2 80

AMA: 2019,Jul,6; 2014,Jan,11

56501-56515 Destruction of Vulvar Lesions, Any Method

EXCLUDES *Excision/fulguration/destruction*
Skene's glands (53270)
Urethral caruncle (53265)

56501 **Destruction of lesion(s), vulva; simple (eg, laser surgery, electrosurgery, cryosurgery, chemosurgery)** ♀

3.41 4.10 FUD 010 T P3

AMA: 2019,Aug,10; 2019,Jul,6; 2014,Jan,11

56515 **extensive (eg, laser surgery, electrosurgery, cryosurgery, chemosurgery)** ♀

5.80 6.72 FUD 010 T A2

AMA: 2019,Aug,10; 2019,Jul,6; 2014,Jan,11

56605-56606 Vulvar and Perineal Biopsies

EXCLUDES *Excision local lesion (11420-11426, 11620-11626)*

56605 **Biopsy of vulva or perineum (separate procedure); 1 lesion** ♀

1.71 2.43 FUD 000 T P3

AMA: 2019,Jul,6; 2019,Jan,9; 2018,Jan,8; 2017,Jan,8; 2016,Jan,13; 2015,Jan,16; 2014,Jan,11

\+ **56606** **each separate additional lesion (List separately in addition to code for primary procedure)** ♀

Code first (56605)

0.85 1.09 FUD ZZZ N N1

AMA: 2019,Jul,6; 2019,Jan,9; 2014,Jan,11

56620-56640 Vulvectomy Procedures

INCLUDES Removal of:
Greater than 80% of the vulvar area - complete procedure
Less than 80% of the vulvar area - partial procedure
Skin and deep subcutaneous tissue - radical procedure
Skin and superficial subcutaneous tissues - simple procedure

EXCLUDES *Skin graft (15004-15005, 15120-15121, 15240-15241)*

56620 **Vulvectomy simple; partial** ♀

15.5 15.5 FUD 090 J A2 80

AMA: 2019,Jul,6; 2019,Jan,14; 2018,Jan,8; 2017,Jan,8; 2016,Jan,13; 2015,Jan,16; 2014,Jan,11

56625 **complete** ♀

18.5 18.5 FUD 090 J A2 80

AMA: 2019,Jul,6; 2014,Jan,11

56630 **Vulvectomy, radical, partial;** ♀

Code also lymph node biopsy/excision when partial radical vulvectomy with inguinofemoral lymph node biopsy without inguinofemoral lymphadenectomy is performed (38531)

27.2 27.2 FUD 090 C 80

AMA: 2019,Jul,6; 2019,Feb,8; 2014,Jan,11

56631 **with unilateral inguinofemoral lymphadenectomy** ♀

INCLUDES Bassett's operation

34.4 34.4 FUD 090 C 80

AMA: 2019,Jul,6; 2019,Feb,8; 2014,Jan,11

56632 **with bilateral inguinofemoral lymphadenectomy** ♀

INCLUDES Bassett's operation

40.6 40.6 FUD 090 C 80

AMA: 2019,Jul,6; 2019,Feb,8; 2014,Jan,11

56633 **Vulvectomy, radical, complete;** ♀

INCLUDES Bassett's operation

35.3 35.3 FUD 090 C 80

AMA: 2019,Jul,6; 2019,Feb,8; 2014,Jan,11

56634 **with unilateral inguinofemoral lymphadenectomy** ♀

INCLUDES Bassett's operation

38.1 38.1 FUD 090 C 80

AMA: 2019,Jul,6; 2019,Feb,8; 2014,Jan,11

56637 **with bilateral inguinofemoral lymphadenectomy** ♀

INCLUDES Bassett's operation

Code also lymph node biopsy/excision when complete radical vulvectomy with inguinofemoral lymph node biopsy without inguinofemoral lymphadenectomy is performed (38531)

43.9 43.9 **FUD** 090 C 80

AMA: 2019,Jul,6; 2019,Feb,8; 2014,Jan,11

56640 **Vulvectomy, radical, complete, with inguinofemoral, iliac, and pelvic lymphadenectomy** ♀

INCLUDES Bassett's operation

EXCLUDES *Lymphadenectomy (38760-38780)*

44.8 44.8 **FUD** 090 C 80 50

AMA: 2019,Jul,6; 2019,Feb,8; 2014,Jan,11

56700-56740 Other Excisional Procedures: External Female Genitalia

56700 **Partial hymenectomy or revision of hymenal ring** ♀

5.38 5.38 **FUD** 010 J A2 80

AMA: 2019,Jul,6; 2014,Jan,11

56740 **Excision of Bartholin's gland or cyst** ♀

EXCLUDES *Excision/fulguration/marsupialization:*
Skene's glands (53270)
Urethral carcinoma (53220)
Urethral caruncle (53265)
Urethral diverticulum (53230, 53240)

8.66 8.66 **FUD** 010 J A2 50

AMA: 2019,Jul,6; 2014,Jan,11

56800-56810 Repair/Reconstruction External Female Genitalia

EXCLUDES *Repair of urethra for mucosal prolapse (53275)*

56800 **Plastic repair of introitus** ♀

INCLUDES Emmet's operation

6.92 6.92 **FUD** 010 J A2 80

AMA: 2019,Jul,6; 2014,Jan,11

56805 **Clitoroplasty for intersex state** ♀

32.5 32.5 **FUD** 090 J G2 80

AMA: 2019,Jul,6; 2014,Jan,11

56810 **Perineoplasty, repair of perineum, nonobstetrical (separate procedure)** ♀

INCLUDES Emmet's operation

EXCLUDES *Genitalia wound repair (12001-12007, 12041-12047, 13131-13133)*
Introitus plastic repair (56800)
Sphincteroplasty, anal (46750-46751)
Vaginal/perineum recent injury repair, nonobstetrical (57210)

7.49 7.49 **FUD** 010 J A2 80

AMA: 2019,Jul,6; 2014,Jan,11

56820-56821 Vulvar Colposcopy with/without Biopsy

EXCLUDES *Colposcopic procedures and/or examinations:*
Cervix (57452-57461)
Vagina (57420-57421)

56820 **Colposcopy of the vulva;** ♀

2.46 3.28 **FUD** 000 T P3

AMA: 2019,Jul,6; 2018,Jan,8; 2017,Jan,8; 2016,Jan,13; 2015,Jan,16; 2014,Jan,11

56821 **with biopsy(s)** ♀

3.28 4.36 **FUD** 000 T P3

AMA: 2019,Jul,6; 2018,Jan,8; 2017,Jan,8; 2016,Jan,13; 2015,Jan,16; 2014,Jan,11

57000-57023 Incisional Procedures: Vagina

57000 **Colpotomy; with exploration** ♀

5.44 5.44 **FUD** 010 J A2 80

AMA: 2019,Jul,6; 2018,Jan,8; 2017,Jan,8; 2016,Jan,13; 2015,Jan,16; 2014,Jan,11

57010 **with drainage of pelvic abscess** ♀

INCLUDES Laroyenne operation

12.4 12.4 **FUD** 090 J A2 80

AMA: 2019,Jul,6; 2014,Jan,11

57020 **Colpocentesis (separate procedure)** ♀

2.29 2.77 **FUD** 000 J A2 80

AMA: 2019,Jul,6; 2014,Jan,11

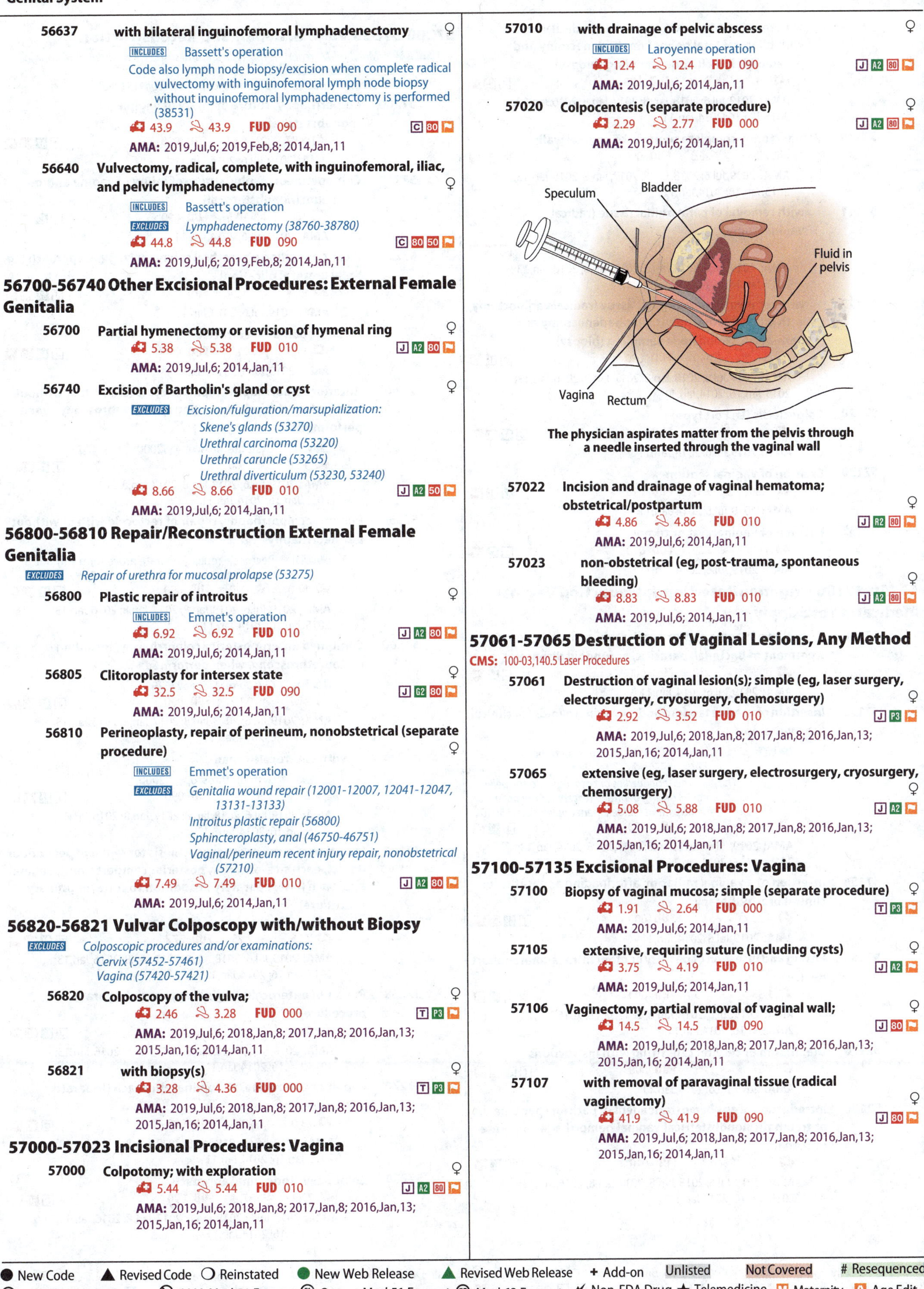

The physician aspirates matter from the pelvis through a needle inserted through the vaginal wall

57022 **Incision and drainage of vaginal hematoma; obstetrical/postpartum** ♀

4.86 4.86 **FUD** 010 J R2 80

AMA: 2019,Jul,6; 2014,Jan,11

57023 **non-obstetrical (eg, post-trauma, spontaneous bleeding)** ♀

8.83 8.83 **FUD** 010 J A2 80

AMA: 2019,Jul,6; 2014,Jan,11

57061-57065 Destruction of Vaginal Lesions, Any Method

CMS: 100-03,140.5 Laser Procedures

57061 **Destruction of vaginal lesion(s); simple (eg, laser surgery, electrosurgery, cryosurgery, chemosurgery)** ♀

2.92 3.52 **FUD** 010 J P3

AMA: 2019,Jul,6; 2018,Jan,8; 2017,Jan,8; 2016,Jan,13; 2015,Jan,16; 2014,Jan,11

57065 **extensive (eg, laser surgery, electrosurgery, cryosurgery, chemosurgery)** ♀

5.08 5.88 **FUD** 010 J A2

AMA: 2019,Jul,6; 2018,Jan,8; 2017,Jan,8; 2016,Jan,13; 2015,Jan,16; 2014,Jan,11

57100-57135 Excisional Procedures: Vagina

57100 **Biopsy of vaginal mucosa; simple (separate procedure)** ♀

1.91 2.64 **FUD** 000 T P3

AMA: 2019,Jul,6; 2014,Jan,11

57105 **extensive, requiring suture (including cysts)** ♀

3.75 4.19 **FUD** 010 J A2

AMA: 2019,Jul,6; 2014,Jan,11

57106 **Vaginectomy, partial removal of vaginal wall;** ♀

14.5 14.5 **FUD** 090 J 80

AMA: 2019,Jul,6; 2018,Jan,8; 2017,Jan,8; 2016,Jan,13; 2015,Jan,16; 2014,Jan,11

57107 **with removal of paravaginal tissue (radical vaginectomy)** ♀

41.9 41.9 **FUD** 090 J 80

AMA: 2019,Jul,6; 2018,Jan,8; 2017,Jan,8; 2016,Jan,13; 2015,Jan,16; 2014,Jan,11

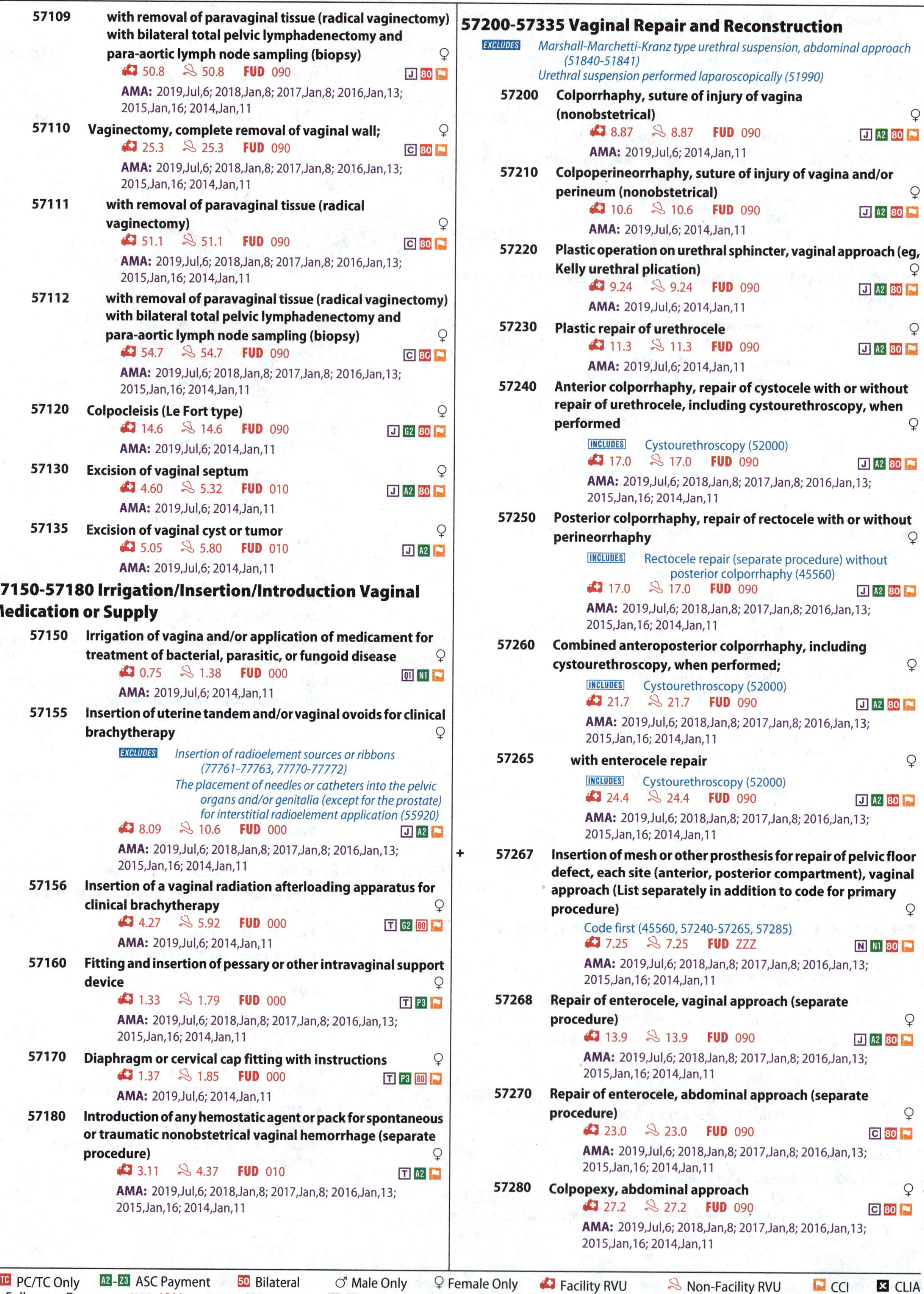

57109 with removal of paravaginal tissue (radical vaginectomy) with bilateral total pelvic lymphadenectomy and para-aortic lymph node sampling (biopsy) ♀
50.8 50.8 FUD 090 C 80
AMA: 2019,Jul,6; 2018,Jan,8; 2017,Jan,8; 2016,Jan,13; 2015,Jan,16; 2014,Jan,11

57110 Vaginectomy, complete removal of vaginal wall; ♀
25.3 25.3 FUD 090 C 80
AMA: 2019,Jul,6; 2018,Jan,8; 2017,Jan,8; 2016,Jan,13; 2015,Jan,16; 2014,Jan,11

57111 with removal of paravaginal tissue (radical vaginectomy) ♀
51.1 51.1 FUD 090 C 80
AMA: 2019,Jul,6; 2018,Jan,8; 2017,Jan,8; 2016,Jan,13; 2015,Jan,16; 2014,Jan,11

57112 with removal of paravaginal tissue (radical vaginectomy) with bilateral total pelvic lymphadenectomy and para-aortic lymph node sampling (biopsy) ♀
54.7 54.7 FUD 090 C 80
AMA: 2019,Jul,6; 2018,Jan,8; 2017,Jan,8; 2016,Jan,13; 2015,Jan,16; 2014,Jan,11

57120 Colpocleisis (Le Fort type) ♀
14.6 14.6 FUD 090 J G2 80
AMA: 2019,Jul,6; 2014,Jan,11

57130 Excision of vaginal septum ♀
4.60 5.32 FUD 010 J A2 80
AMA: 2019,Jul,6; 2014,Jan,11

57135 Excision of vaginal cyst or tumor ♀
5.05 5.80 FUD 010 J A2
AMA: 2019,Jul,6; 2014,Jan,11

57150-57180 Irrigation/Insertion/Introduction Vaginal Medication or Supply

57150 Irrigation of vagina and/or application of medicament for treatment of bacterial, parasitic, or fungoid disease ♀
0.75 1.38 FUD 000 Q1 N1
AMA: 2019,Jul,6; 2014,Jan,11

57155 Insertion of uterine tandem and/or vaginal ovoids for clinical brachytherapy ♀
EXCLUDES *Insertion of radioelement sources or ribbons (77761-77763, 77770-77772)*
The placement of needles or catheters into the pelvic organs and/or genitalia (except for the prostate) for interstitial radioelement application (55920)
8.09 10.6 FUD 000 J A2
AMA: 2019,Jul,6; 2018,Jan,8; 2017,Jan,8; 2016,Jan,13; 2015,Jan,16; 2014,Jan,11

57156 Insertion of a vaginal radiation afterloading apparatus for clinical brachytherapy ♀
4.27 5.92 FUD 000 T G2 80
AMA: 2019,Jul,6; 2014,Jan,11

57160 Fitting and insertion of pessary or other intravaginal support device ♀
1.33 1.79 FUD 000 T P3
AMA: 2019,Jul,6; 2018,Jan,8; 2017,Jan,8; 2016,Jan,13; 2015,Jan,16; 2014,Jan,11

57170 Diaphragm or cervical cap fitting with instructions ♀
1.37 1.85 FUD 000 T P3 80
AMA: 2019,Jul,6; 2014,Jan,11

57180 Introduction of any hemostatic agent or pack for spontaneous or traumatic nonobstetrical vaginal hemorrhage (separate procedure) ♀
3.11 4.37 FUD 010 T A2
AMA: 2019,Jul,6; 2018,Jan,8; 2017,Jan,8; 2016,Jan,13; 2015,Jan,16; 2014,Jan,11

57200-57335 Vaginal Repair and Reconstruction

EXCLUDES *Marshall-Marchetti-Kranz type urethral suspension, abdominal approach (51840-51841)*
Urethral suspension performed laparoscopically (51990)

57200 Colporrhaphy, suture of injury of vagina (nonobstetrical) ♀
8.87 8.87 FUD 090 J A2 80
AMA: 2019,Jul,6; 2014,Jan,11

57210 Colpoperineorrhaphy, suture of injury of vagina and/or perineum (nonobstetrical) ♀
10.6 10.6 FUD 090 J A2 80
AMA: 2019,Jul,6; 2014,Jan,11

57220 Plastic operation on urethral sphincter, vaginal approach (eg, Kelly urethral plication) ♀
9.24 9.24 FUD 090 J A2 80
AMA: 2019,Jul,6; 2014,Jan,11

57230 Plastic repair of urethrocele ♀
11.3 11.3 FUD 090 J A2 80
AMA: 2019,Jul,6; 2014,Jan,11

57240 Anterior colporrhaphy, repair of cystocele with or without repair of urethrocele, including cystourethroscopy, when performed ♀
INCLUDES Cystourethroscopy (52000)
17.0 17.0 FUD 090 J A2 80
AMA: 2019,Jul,6; 2018,Jan,8; 2017,Jan,8; 2016,Jan,13; 2015,Jan,16; 2014,Jan,11

57250 Posterior colporrhaphy, repair of rectocele with or without perineorrhaphy ♀
INCLUDES Rectocele repair (separate procedure) without posterior colporrhaphy (45560)
17.0 17.0 FUD 090 J A2 80
AMA: 2019,Jul,6; 2018,Jan,8; 2017,Jan,8; 2016,Jan,13; 2015,Jan,16; 2014,Jan,11

57260 Combined anteroposterior colporrhaphy, including cystourethroscopy, when performed; ♀
INCLUDES Cystourethroscopy (52000)
21.7 21.7 FUD 090 J A2 80
AMA: 2019,Jul,6; 2018,Jan,8; 2017,Jan,8; 2016,Jan,13; 2015,Jan,16; 2014,Jan,11

57265 with enterocele repair ♀
INCLUDES Cystourethroscopy (52000)
24.4 24.4 FUD 090 J A2 80
AMA: 2019,Jul,6; 2018,Jan,8; 2017,Jan,8; 2016,Jan,13; 2015,Jan,16; 2014,Jan,11

+ **57267** Insertion of mesh or other prosthesis for repair of pelvic floor defect, each site (anterior, posterior compartment), vaginal approach (List separately in addition to code for primary procedure) ♀
Code first (45560, 57240-57265, 57285)
7.25 7.25 FUD ZZZ N N1 80
AMA: 2019,Jul,6; 2018,Jan,8; 2017,Jan,8; 2016,Jan,13; 2015,Jan,16; 2014,Jan,11

57268 Repair of enterocele, vaginal approach (separate procedure) ♀
13.9 13.9 FUD 090 J A2 80
AMA: 2019,Jul,6; 2018,Jan,8; 2017,Jan,8; 2016,Jan,13; 2015,Jan,16; 2014,Jan,11

57270 Repair of enterocele, abdominal approach (separate procedure) ♀
23.0 23.0 FUD 090 C 80
AMA: 2019,Jul,6; 2018,Jan,8; 2017,Jan,8; 2016,Jan,13; 2015,Jan,16; 2014,Jan,11

57280 Colpopexy, abdominal approach ♀
27.2 27.2 FUD 090 C 80
AMA: 2019,Jul,6; 2018,Jan,8; 2017,Jan,8; 2016,Jan,13; 2015,Jan,16; 2014,Jan,11

57282 **Colpopexy, vaginal; extra-peritoneal approach (sacrospinous, iliococcygeus)** ♀
14.5 14.5 FUD 090 J 80
AMA: 2019,Jul,6; 2018,Jan,8; 2017,Jan,8; 2016,Jan,13; 2015,Jan,16; 2014,Jan,11

57283 **intra-peritoneal approach (uterosacral, levator myorrhaphy)** ♀
EXCLUDES *Excision of cervical stump (57556)*
Vaginal hysterectomy (58263, 58270, 58280, 58292, 58294)
19.6 19.6 FUD 090 J 80
AMA: 2019,Jul,6; 2018,Jan,8; 2017,Jan,8; 2016,Jan,13; 2015,Jan,16; 2014,Jan,11

57284 **Paravaginal defect repair (including repair of cystocele, if performed); open abdominal approach** ♀
EXCLUDES *Anterior colporrhaphy (57240)*
Anterior vesicourethropexy (51840-51841)
Combined anteroposterior colporrhaphy (57260-57265)
Hysterectomy (58152, 58267)
Laparoscopy, surgical; urethral suspension for stress incontinence (51990)
23.3 23.3 FUD 090 J 80
AMA: 2019,Jul,6; 2018,Jan,8; 2017,Jan,8; 2016,Jan,13; 2015,Jan,16; 2014,Jan,11

57285 **vaginal approach** ♀
EXCLUDES *Anterior colporrhaphy (57240)*
Combined anteroposterior colporrhaphy (57260-57265)
Laparoscopy, surgical; urethral suspension for stress incontinence (51990)
Vaginal hysterectomy (58267)
19.2 19.2 FUD 090 J 80
AMA: 2019,Jul,6; 2018,Jan,8; 2017,Jan,8; 2016,Jan,13; 2015,Jan,16; 2014,Jan,11

57287 **Removal or revision of sling for stress incontinence (eg, fascia or synthetic)** ♀
19.9 19.9 FUD 090 Q2 G2 80
AMA: 2019,Jul,6; 2018,Jan,8; 2017,Jan,8; 2016,Jan,13; 2015,Jan,16; 2014,Jan,11

57288 **Sling operation for stress incontinence (eg, fascia or synthetic)** ♀
INCLUDES Millin-Read operation
EXCLUDES *Sling operation for stress incontinence performed laparoscopically (51992)*
20.6 20.6 FUD 090 J J8 80
AMA: 2019,Jul,6; 2019,Feb,10; 2018,Jan,8; 2017,Jan,8; 2016,Jan,13; 2015,Jan,16; 2014,Jan,11

57289 **Pereyra procedure, including anterior colporrhaphy** ♀
21.7 21.7 FUD 090 J A2 80
AMA: 2019,Jul,6; 2018,Jan,8; 2017,Jan,8; 2016,Jan,13; 2015,Jan,16; 2014,Jan,11

57291 **Construction of artificial vagina; without graft** ♀
INCLUDES McIndoe vaginal construction
15.1 15.1 FUD 090 J A2 80
AMA: 2019,Jul,6; 2014,Jan,11

57292 **with graft** ♀
23.1 23.1 FUD 090 J 80
AMA: 2019,Jul,6; 2014,Jan,11

57295 **Revision (including removal) of prosthetic vaginal graft; vaginal approach** ♀
EXCLUDES *Laparoscopic approach (57426)*
13.7 13.7 FUD 090 J G2 80
AMA: 2019,Jul,6; 2014,Jan,11

57296 **open abdominal approach** ♀
EXCLUDES *Laparoscopic approach (57426)*
26.9 26.9 FUD 090 C 80
AMA: 2019,Jul,6; 2014,Jan,11

57300 **Closure of rectovaginal fistula; vaginal or transanal approach** ♀
16.4 16.4 FUD 090 J A2 80
AMA: 2019,Jul,6; 2014,Jan,11

57305 **abdominal approach** ♀
27.3 27.3 FUD 090 C 80
AMA: 2019,Jul,6; 2014,Jan,11

57307 **abdominal approach, with concomitant colostomy** ♀
29.9 29.9 FUD 090 C 80
AMA: 2019,Jul,6; 2014,Jan,11

57308 **transperineal approach, with perineal body reconstruction, with or without levator plication** ♀
19.0 19.0 FUD 090 C 80
AMA: 2019,Jul,6; 2014,Jan,11

57310 **Closure of urethrovaginal fistula;** ♀
13.5 13.5 FUD 090 J G2 80
AMA: 2019,Jul,6; 2014,Jan,11

57311 **with bulbocavernosus transplant** ♀
15.4 15.4 FUD 090 C 80
AMA: 2019,Jul,6; 2014,Jan,11

57320 **Closure of vesicovaginal fistula; vaginal approach** ♀
EXCLUDES *Cystostomy, concomitant (51020-51040, 51101-51102)*
15.5 15.5 FUD 090 J G2 80
AMA: 2019,Jul,6; 2014,Jan,11

57330 **transvesical and vaginal approach** ♀
EXCLUDES *Vesicovaginal fistula closure, abdominal approach (51900)*
21.6 21.6 FUD 090 J 80
AMA: 2019,Jul,6; 2014,Jan,11

57335 **Vaginoplasty for intersex state** ♀
32.8 32.8 FUD 090 J 80
AMA: 2019,Jul,6; 2014,Jan,11

57400-57415 Treatment of Vaginal Disorders Under Anesthesia

57400 **Dilation of vagina under anesthesia (other than local)** ♀
3.81 3.81 FUD 000 J A2 80
AMA: 2019,Jul,6; 2014,Jan,11

57410 **Pelvic examination under anesthesia (other than local)** ♀
3.05 3.05 FUD 000 J A2
AMA: 2019,Jul,6; 2018,Jan,8; 2017,Jan,8; 2016,Jan,13; 2015,Jan,16; 2014,Jan,11

57415 **Removal of impacted vaginal foreign body (separate procedure) under anesthesia (other than local)** ♀
EXCLUDES *Removal of impacted vaginal foreign body without anesthesia, report with appropriate E&M code*
4.70 4.70 FUD 010 J A2 80
AMA: 2019,Jul,6; 2014,Jan,11

57420-57426 Endoscopic Vaginal Procedures

57420 **Colposcopy of the entire vagina, with cervix if present;** ♀
EXCLUDES *Colposcopic procedures and/or examinations:*
Cervix (57452-57461)
Vulva (56820-56821)
Code also endometrial sampling (biopsy) performed at the same time as colposcopy (58110)
Code also modifier 51 for colposcopic procedures of different sites, as appropriate
2.62 3.45 FUD 000 T P3
AMA: 2019,Jul,6; 2018,Jan,8; 2017,Jan,8; 2016,Jan,13; 2015,Jan,16; 2014,Jan,11

57421 **with biopsy(s) of vagina/cervix** ♀

EXCLUDES *Colposcopic procedures and/or examinations:*
Cervix (57452-57461)
Vulva (56820-56821)
Code also endometrial sampling (biopsy) performed at the same time as colposcopy (58110)
Code also modifier 51 for colposcopic procedures of multiple sites, as appropriate

3.52 4.62 FUD 000 T P3

AMA: 2019,Jul,6; 2018,Jan,8; 2017,Jan,8; 2016,Jan,13; 2015,Jan,16; 2014,Jan,11

57423 **Paravaginal defect repair (including repair of cystocele, if performed), laparoscopic approach** ♀

EXCLUDES *Anterior colporrhaphy (57240)*
Anterior vesicourethropexy (51840-51841)
Combined anteroposterior colporrhaphy (57260)
Diagnostic laparoscopy (49320)
Hysterectomy (58152, 58267)
Laparoscopy, surgical; urethral suspension for stress incontinence (51990)

26.1 26.1 FUD 090 J 80

AMA: 2019,Jul,6; 2018,Jan,8; 2017,Jan,8; 2016,Jan,13; 2015,Jan,16; 2014,Jan,11

57425 **Laparoscopy, surgical, colpopexy (suspension of vaginal apex)** ♀

27.6 27.6 FUD 090 J 80

AMA: 2019,Jul,6; 2014,Jan,11

57426 **Revision (including removal) of prosthetic vaginal graft, laparoscopic approach** ♀

EXCLUDES *Open abdominal approach (57296)*
Vaginal approach (57295)

24.2 24.2 FUD 090 J G2 80

AMA: 2019,Jul,6; 2014,Jan,11

57452-57461 Endoscopic Cervical Procedures

EXCLUDES *Colposcopic procedures and/or examinations:*
Vagina (57420-57421)
Vulva (56820-56821)
Code also endometrial sampling (biopsy) performed at the same time as colposcopy (58110)

57452 **Colposcopy of the cervix including upper/adjacent vagina;** ♀

2.62 3.25 FUD 000 T P3

AMA: 2019,Jul,6; 2018,Jan,8; 2017,Jan,8; 2016,Jan,13; 2015,Jan,16; 2014,Jan,11

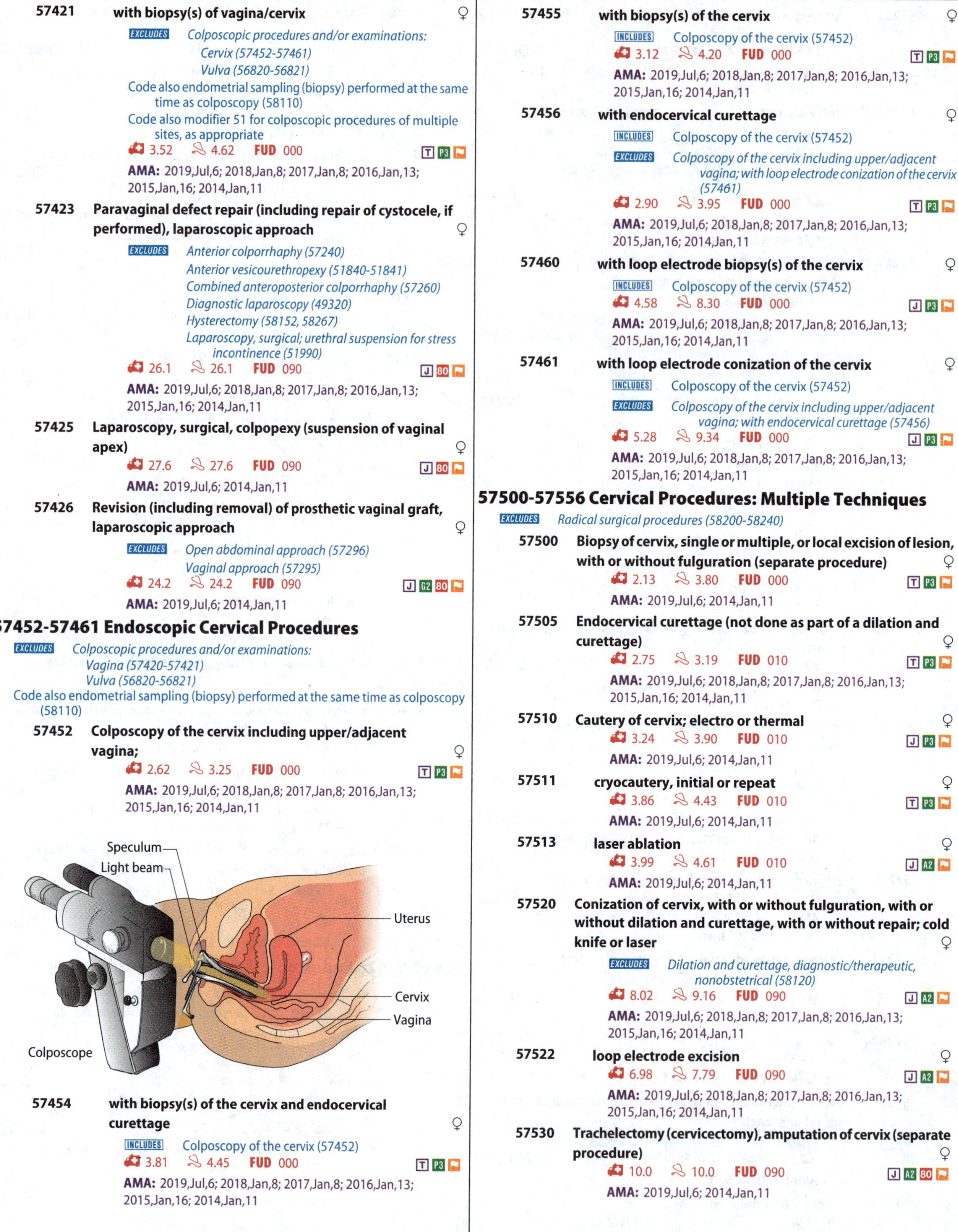

57454 **with biopsy(s) of the cervix and endocervical curettage** ♀

INCLUDES Colposcopy of the cervix (57452)

3.81 4.45 FUD 000 T P3

AMA: 2019,Jul,6; 2018,Jan,8; 2017,Jan,8; 2016,Jan,13; 2015,Jan,16; 2014,Jan,11

57455 **with biopsy(s) of the cervix** ♀

INCLUDES Colposcopy of the cervix (57452)

3.12 4.20 FUD 000 T P3

AMA: 2019,Jul,6; 2018,Jan,8; 2017,Jan,8; 2016,Jan,13; 2015,Jan,16; 2014,Jan,11

57456 **with endocervical curettage** ♀

INCLUDES Colposcopy of the cervix (57452)
EXCLUDES *Colposcopy of the cervix including upper/adjacent vagina; with loop electrode conization of the cervix (57461)*

2.90 3.95 FUD 000 T P3

AMA: 2019,Jul,6; 2018,Jan,8; 2017,Jan,8; 2016,Jan,13; 2015,Jan,16; 2014,Jan,11

57460 **with loop electrode biopsy(s) of the cervix** ♀

INCLUDES Colposcopy of the cervix (57452)

4.58 8.30 FUD 000 J P3

AMA: 2019,Jul,6; 2018,Jan,8; 2017,Jan,8; 2016,Jan,13; 2015,Jan,16; 2014,Jan,11

57461 **with loop electrode conization of the cervix** ♀

INCLUDES Colposcopy of the cervix (57452)
EXCLUDES *Colposcopy of the cervix including upper/adjacent vagina; with endocervical curettage (57456)*

5.28 9.34 FUD 000 J P3

AMA: 2019,Jul,6; 2018,Jan,8; 2017,Jan,8; 2016,Jan,13; 2015,Jan,16; 2014,Jan,11

57500-57556 Cervical Procedures: Multiple Techniques

EXCLUDES *Radical surgical procedures (58200-58240)*

57500 **Biopsy of cervix, single or multiple, or local excision of lesion, with or without fulguration (separate procedure)** ♀

2.13 3.80 FUD 000 T P3

AMA: 2019,Jul,6; 2014,Jan,11

57505 **Endocervical curettage (not done as part of a dilation and curettage)** ♀

2.75 3.19 FUD 010 T P3

AMA: 2019,Jul,6; 2018,Jan,8; 2017,Jan,8; 2016,Jan,13; 2015,Jan,16; 2014,Jan,11

57510 **Cautery of cervix; electro or thermal** ♀

3.24 3.90 FUD 010 J P3

AMA: 2019,Jul,6; 2014,Jan,11

57511 **cryocautery, initial or repeat** ♀

3.86 4.43 FUD 010 T P3

AMA: 2019,Jul,6; 2014,Jan,11

57513 **laser ablation** ♀

3.99 4.61 FUD 010 J A2

AMA: 2019,Jul,6; 2014,Jan,11

57520 **Conization of cervix, with or without fulguration, with or without dilation and curettage, with or without repair; cold knife or laser** ♀

EXCLUDES *Dilation and curettage, diagnostic/therapeutic, nonobstetrical (58120)*

8.02 9.16 FUD 090 J A2

AMA: 2019,Jul,6; 2018,Jan,8; 2017,Jan,8; 2016,Jan,13; 2015,Jan,16; 2014,Jan,11

57522 **loop electrode excision** ♀

6.98 7.79 FUD 090 J A2

AMA: 2019,Jul,6; 2018,Jan,8; 2017,Jan,8; 2016,Jan,13; 2015,Jan,16; 2014,Jan,11

57530 **Trachelectomy (cervicectomy), amputation of cervix (separate procedure)** ♀

10.0 10.0 FUD 090 J A2 80

AMA: 2019,Jul,6; 2014,Jan,11

57531 **Radical trachelectomy, with bilateral total pelvic lymphadenectomy and para-aortic lymph node sampling biopsy, with or without removal of tube(s), with or without removal of ovary(s)** ♀

EXCLUDES *Radical hysterectomy (58210)*

47.8 47.8 FUD 090 C 80

AMA: 2019,Jul,6; 2014,Jan,11

57540 **Excision of cervical stump, abdominal approach;** ♀

22.0 22.0 FUD 090 C 80

AMA: 2019,Jul,6; 2014,Jan,11

57545 **with pelvic floor repair** ♀

23.3 23.3 FUD 090 C 80

AMA: 2019,Jul,6; 2014,Jan,11

57550 **Excision of cervical stump, vaginal approach;** ♀

11.6 11.6 FUD 090 J A2 80

AMA: 2019,Jul,6; 2014,Jan,11

57555 **with anterior and/or posterior repair** ♀

17.1 17.1 FUD 090 J 80

AMA: 2019,Jul,6; 2014,Jan,11

57556 **with repair of enterocele** ♀

EXCLUDES *Insertion of hemostatic agent/pack for spontaneous/traumatic nonobstetrical vaginal hemorrhage (57180)*
Intrauterine device insertion (58300)

16.2 16.2 FUD 090 J A2 80

AMA: 2019,Jul,6; 2014,Jan,11

57558-57800 Cervical Procedures: Dilation, Suturing, or Instrumentation

57558 **Dilation and curettage of cervical stump** ♀

EXCLUDES *Radical surgical procedures (58200-58240)*

3.33 3.80 FUD 010 J A2

AMA: 2019,Jul,6; 2014,Jan,11

57700 **Cerclage of uterine cervix, nonobstetrical** ♀

INCLUDES McDonald cerclage
Shirodker operation

9.13 9.13 FUD 090 J A2 80

AMA: 2019,Jul,6; 2014,Jan,11

57720 **Trachelorrhaphy, plastic repair of uterine cervix, vaginal approach** ♀

INCLUDES Emmet operation

8.89 8.89 FUD 090 J A2 80

AMA: 2019,Jul,6; 2014,Jan,11

57800 **Dilation of cervical canal, instrumental (separate procedure)** ♀

1.37 1.85 FUD 000 J P3

AMA: 2019,Jul,6; 2014,Jan,11

58100-58120 Procedures Involving the Endometrium

58100 **Endometrial sampling (biopsy) with or without endocervical sampling (biopsy), without cervical dilation, any method (separate procedure)** ♀

EXCLUDES *Endocervical curettage only (57505)*
Endometrial sampling (biopsy) performed in conjunction with colposcopy (58110)

2.01 2.64 FUD 000 T P3

AMA: 2019,Jul,6; 2014,Jan,11

\+ **58110** **Endometrial sampling (biopsy) performed in conjunction with colposcopy (List separately in addition to code for primary procedure)** ♀

Code first colposcopy (57420-57421, 57452-57461)

1.17 1.44 FUD ZZZ N N1 80

AMA: 2019,Jul,6; 2018,Jan,8; 2017,Jan,8; 2016,Jan,13; 2015,Jan,16; 2014,Jan,11

58120 **Dilation and curettage, diagnostic and/or therapeutic (nonobstetrical)** ♀

EXCLUDES *Postpartum hemorrhage (59160)*

6.35 7.66 FUD 010 J A2

AMA: 2019,Jul,6; 2018,Jan,8; 2017,Jan,8; 2016,Jan,13; 2015,Jan,16; 2014,Jan,11

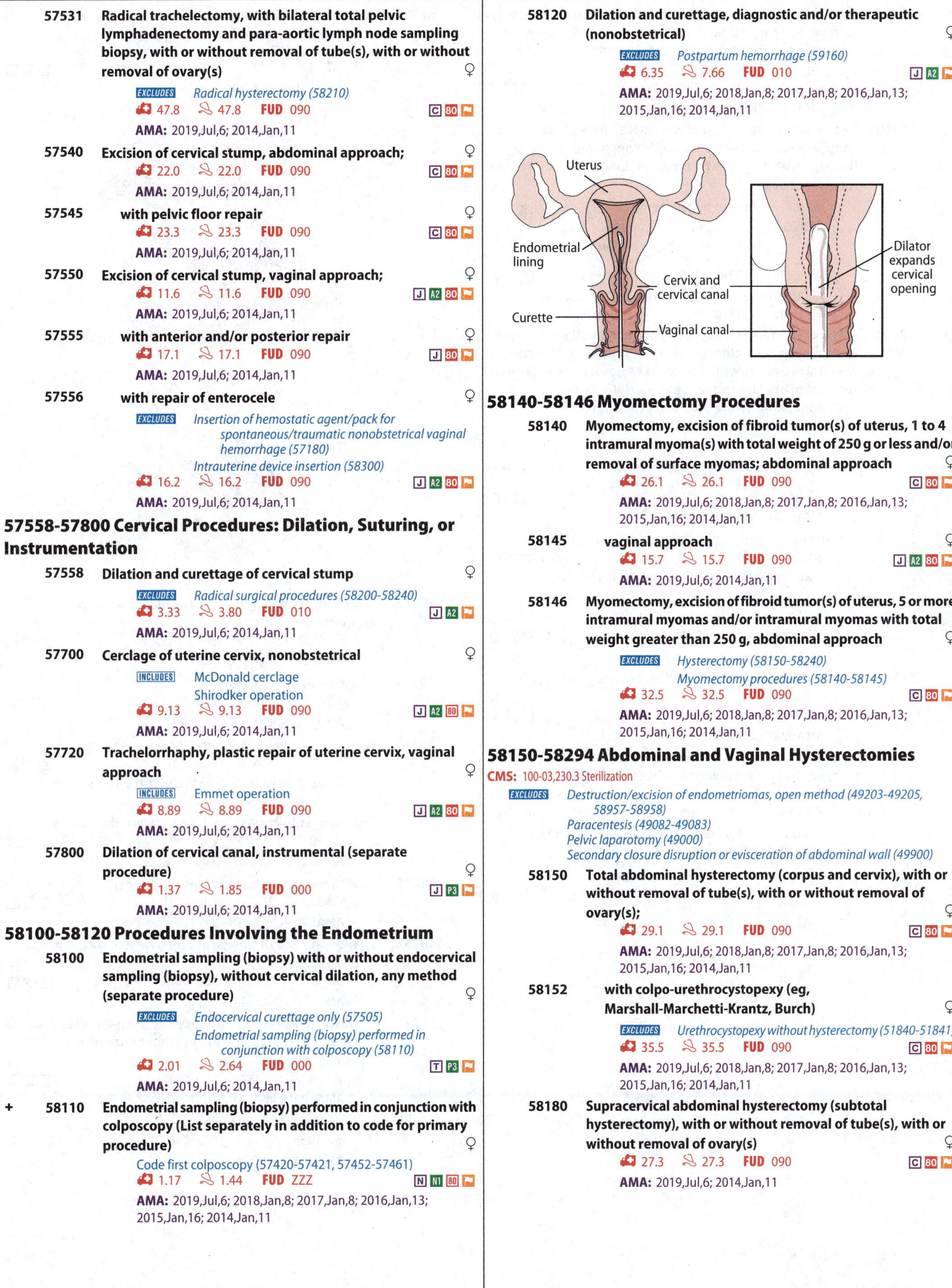

58140-58146 Myomectomy Procedures

58140 **Myomectomy, excision of fibroid tumor(s) of uterus, 1 to 4 intramural myoma(s) with total weight of 250 g or less and/or removal of surface myomas; abdominal approach** ♀

26.1 26.1 FUD 090 C 80

AMA: 2019,Jul,6; 2018,Jan,8; 2017,Jan,8; 2016,Jan,13; 2015,Jan,16; 2014,Jan,11

58145 **vaginal approach** ♀

15.7 15.7 FUD 090 J A2 80

AMA: 2019,Jul,6; 2014,Jan,11

58146 **Myomectomy, excision of fibroid tumor(s) of uterus, 5 or more intramural myomas and/or intramural myomas with total weight greater than 250 g, abdominal approach** ♀

EXCLUDES *Hysterectomy (58150-58240)*
Myomectomy procedures (58140-58145)

32.5 32.5 FUD 090 C 80

AMA: 2019,Jul,6; 2018,Jan,8; 2017,Jan,8; 2016,Jan,13; 2015,Jan,16; 2014,Jan,11

58150-58294 Abdominal and Vaginal Hysterectomies

CMS: 100-03,230.3 Sterilization

EXCLUDES *Destruction/excision of endometriomas, open method (49203-49205, 58957-58958)*
Paracentesis (49082-49083)
Pelvic laparotomy (49000)
Secondary closure disruption or evisceration of abdominal wall (49900)

58150 **Total abdominal hysterectomy (corpus and cervix), with or without removal of tube(s), with or without removal of ovary(s);** ♀

29.1 29.1 FUD 090 C 80

AMA: 2019,Jul,6; 2018,Jan,8; 2017,Jan,8; 2016,Jan,13; 2015,Jan,16; 2014,Jan,11

58152 **with colpo-urethrocystopexy (eg, Marshall-Marchetti-Krantz, Burch)** ♀

EXCLUDES *Urethrocystopexy without hysterectomy (51840-51841)*

35.5 35.5 FUD 090 C 80

AMA: 2019,Jul,6; 2018,Jan,8; 2017,Jan,8; 2016,Jan,13; 2015,Jan,16; 2014,Jan,11

58180 **Supracervical abdominal hysterectomy (subtotal hysterectomy), with or without removal of tube(s), with or without removal of ovary(s)** ♀

27.3 27.3 FUD 090 C 80

AMA: 2019,Jul,6; 2014,Jan,11

58200 **Total abdominal hysterectomy, including partial vaginectomy, with para-aortic and pelvic lymph node sampling, with or without removal of tube(s), with or without removal of ovary(s)** ♀
39.7 39.7 FUD 090 C 80
AMA: 2019,Jul,6; 2014,Jan,11

58210 **Radical abdominal hysterectomy, with bilateral total pelvic lymphadenectomy and para-aortic lymph node sampling (biopsy), with or without removal of tube(s), with or without removal of ovary(s)** ♀
INCLUDES Wertheim hysterectomy
EXCLUDES *Chemotherapy (96401-96549)*
Hysterectomy, radical, with transposition of ovary(s) (58825)
53.4 53.4 FUD 090 C 80
AMA: 2019,Jul,6; 2018,Jan,8; 2017,Jan,8; 2016,Jan,13; 2015,Jan,16; 2014,Jan,11

58240 **Pelvic exenteration for gynecologic malignancy, with total abdominal hysterectomy or cervicectomy, with or without removal of tube(s), with or without removal of ovary(s), with removal of bladder and ureteral transplantations, and/or abdominoperineal resection of rectum and colon and colostomy, or any combination thereof** ♀
EXCLUDES *Chemotherapy (96401-96549)*
Pelvic exenteration for male genital malignancy or lower urinary tract (51597)
84.8 84.8 FUD 090 C 80
AMA: 2019,Jul,6; 2014,Jan,11

58260 **Vaginal hysterectomy, for uterus 250 g or less;** ♀
23.4 23.4 FUD 090 J G2 80
AMA: 2019,Jul,6; 2018,Jan,8; 2017,Jan,8; 2016,Jan,13; 2015,Jan,16; 2014,Jan,11

58262 **with removal of tube(s), and/or ovary(s)** ♀
26.1 26.1 FUD 090 J G2 80
AMA: 2019,Jul,6; 2014,Jan,11

58263 **with removal of tube(s), and/or ovary(s), with repair of enterocele** ♀
28.0 28.0 FUD 090 J 80
AMA: 2019,Jul,6; 2014,Jan,11

58267 **with colpo-urethrocystopexy (Marshall-Marchetti-Krantz type, Pereyra type) with or without endoscopic control** ♀
29.8 29.8 FUD 090 C 80
AMA: 2019,Jul,6; 2018,Jan,8; 2017,Jan,8; 2016,Jan,13; 2015,Jan,16; 2014,Jan,11

58270 **with repair of enterocele** ♀
EXCLUDES *Vaginal hysterectomy with repair of enterocele and removal of tubes and/or ovaries (58263)*
25.0 25.0 FUD 090 J 80
AMA: 2019,Jul,6; 2014,Jan,11

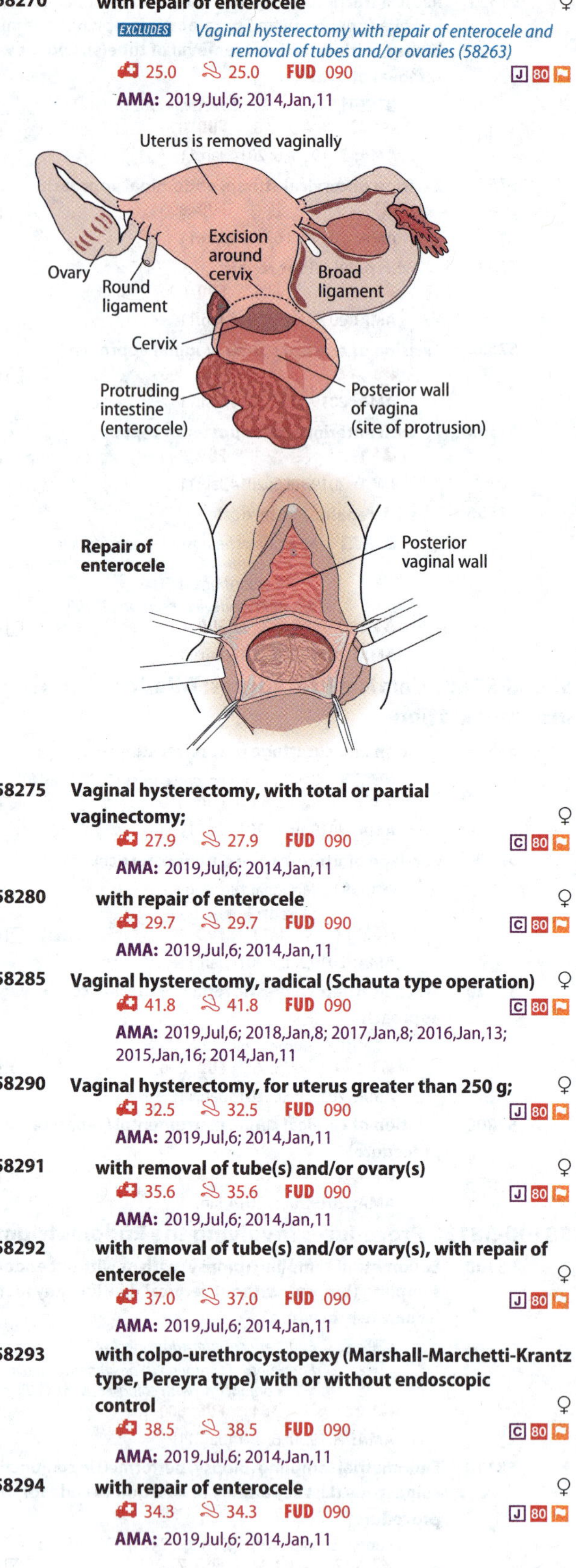

58275 **Vaginal hysterectomy, with total or partial vaginectomy;** ♀
27.9 27.9 FUD 090 C 80
AMA: 2019,Jul,6; 2014,Jan,11

58280 **with repair of enterocele** ♀
29.7 29.7 FUD 090 C 80
AMA: 2019,Jul,6; 2014,Jan,11

58285 **Vaginal hysterectomy, radical (Schauta type operation)** ♀
41.8 41.8 FUD 090 C 80
AMA: 2019,Jul,6; 2018,Jan,8; 2017,Jan,8; 2016,Jan,13; 2015,Jan,16; 2014,Jan,11

58290 **Vaginal hysterectomy, for uterus greater than 250 g;** ♀
32.5 32.5 FUD 090 J 80
AMA: 2019,Jul,6; 2014,Jan,11

58291 **with removal of tube(s) and/or ovary(s)** ♀
35.6 35.6 FUD 090 J 80
AMA: 2019,Jul,6; 2014,Jan,11

58292 **with removal of tube(s) and/or ovary(s), with repair of enterocele** ♀
37.0 37.0 FUD 090 J 80
AMA: 2019,Jul,6; 2014,Jan,11

58293 **with colpo-urethrocystopexy (Marshall-Marchetti-Krantz type, Pereyra type) with or without endoscopic control** ♀
38.5 38.5 FUD 090 C 80
AMA: 2019,Jul,6; 2014,Jan,11

58294 **with repair of enterocele** ♀
34.3 34.3 FUD 090 J 80
AMA: 2019,Jul,6; 2014,Jan,11

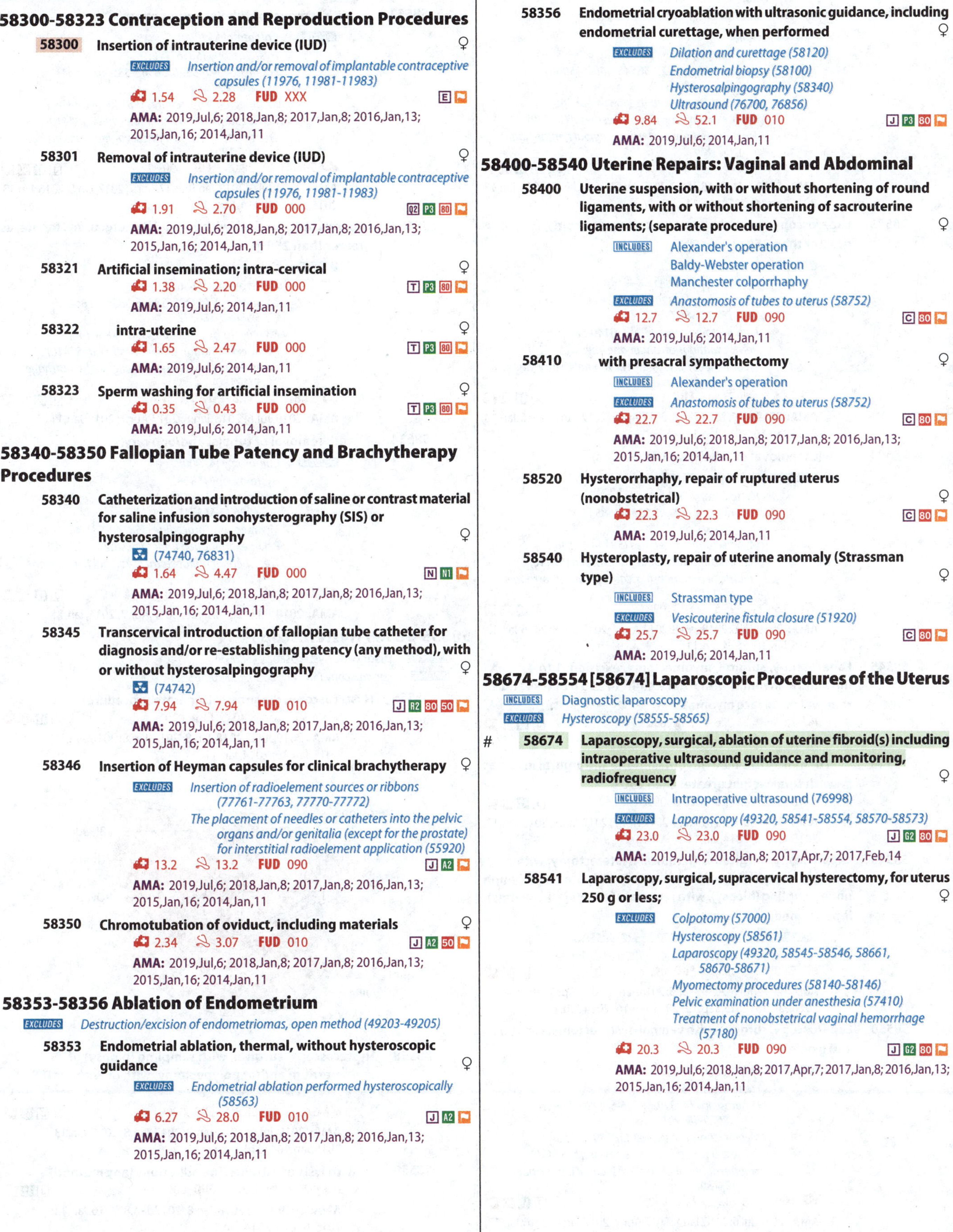

58300-58323 Contraception and Reproduction Procedures

58300 **Insertion of intrauterine device (IUD)** ♀

EXCLUDES *Insertion and/or removal of implantable contraceptive capsules (11976, 11981-11983)*

1.54 | 2.28 | FUD XXX | E

AMA: 2019,Jul,6; 2018,Jan,8; 2017,Jan,8; 2016,Jan,13; 2015,Jan,16; 2014,Jan,11

58301 **Removal of intrauterine device (IUD)** ♀

EXCLUDES *Insertion and/or removal of implantable contraceptive capsules (11976, 11981-11983)*

1.91 | 2.70 | FUD 000 | Q2 P3 80

AMA: 2019,Jul,6; 2018,Jan,8; 2017,Jan,8; 2016,Jan,13; 2015,Jan,16; 2014,Jan,11

58321 **Artificial insemination; intra-cervical** ♀

1.38 | 2.20 | FUD 000 | T P3 80

AMA: 2019,Jul,6; 2014,Jan,11

58322 **intra-uterine** ♀

1.65 | 2.47 | FUD 000 | T P3 80

AMA: 2019,Jul,6; 2014,Jan,11

58323 **Sperm washing for artificial insemination** ♀

0.35 | 0.43 | FUD 000 | T P3 80

AMA: 2019,Jul,6; 2014,Jan,11

58340-58350 Fallopian Tube Patency and Brachytherapy Procedures

58340 **Catheterization and introduction of saline or contrast material for saline infusion sonohysterography (SIS) or hysterosalpingography** ♀

(74740, 76831)

1.64 | 4.47 | FUD 000 | N N1

AMA: 2019,Jul,6; 2018,Jan,8; 2017,Jan,8; 2016,Jan,13; 2015,Jan,16; 2014,Jan,11

58345 **Transcervical introduction of fallopian tube catheter for diagnosis and/or re-establishing patency (any method), with or without hysterosalpingography** ♀

(74742)

7.94 | 7.94 | FUD 010 | J R2 80 50

AMA: 2019,Jul,6; 2018,Jan,8; 2017,Jan,8; 2016,Jan,13; 2015,Jan,16; 2014,Jan,11

58346 **Insertion of Heyman capsules for clinical brachytherapy** ♀

EXCLUDES *Insertion of radioelement sources or ribbons (77761-77763, 77770-77772)*
The placement of needles or catheters into the pelvic organs and/or genitalia (except for the prostate) for interstitial radioelement application (55920)

13.2 | 13.2 | FUD 090 | J A2

AMA: 2019,Jul,6; 2018,Jan,8; 2017,Jan,8; 2016,Jan,13; 2015,Jan,16; 2014,Jan,11

58350 **Chromotubation of oviduct, including materials** ♀

2.34 | 3.07 | FUD 010 | J A2 50

AMA: 2019,Jul,6; 2018,Jan,8; 2017,Jan,8; 2016,Jan,13; 2015,Jan,16; 2014,Jan,11

58353-58356 Ablation of Endometrium

EXCLUDES *Destruction/excision of endometriomas, open method (49203-49205)*

58353 **Endometrial ablation, thermal, without hysteroscopic guidance** ♀

EXCLUDES *Endometrial ablation performed hysteroscopically (58563)*

6.27 | 28.0 | FUD 010 | J A2

AMA: 2019,Jul,6; 2018,Jan,8; 2017,Jan,8; 2016,Jan,13; 2015,Jan,16; 2014,Jan,11

58356 **Endometrial cryoablation with ultrasonic guidance, including endometrial curettage, when performed** ♀

EXCLUDES *Dilation and curettage (58120)*
Endometrial biopsy (58100)
Hysterosalpingography (58340)
Ultrasound (76700, 76856)

9.84 | 52.1 | FUD 010 | J P3 80

AMA: 2019,Jul,6; 2014,Jan,11

58400-58540 Uterine Repairs: Vaginal and Abdominal

58400 **Uterine suspension, with or without shortening of round ligaments, with or without shortening of sacrouterine ligaments; (separate procedure)** ♀

INCLUDES Alexander's operation
Baldy-Webster operation
Manchester colporrhaphy

EXCLUDES *Anastomosis of tubes to uterus (58752)*

12.7 | 12.7 | FUD 090 | C 80

AMA: 2019,Jul,6; 2014,Jan,11

58410 **with presacral sympathectomy** ♀

INCLUDES Alexander's operation

EXCLUDES *Anastomosis of tubes to uterus (58752)*

22.7 | 22.7 | FUD 090 | C 80

AMA: 2019,Jul,6; 2018,Jan,8; 2017,Jan,8; 2016,Jan,13; 2015,Jan,16; 2014,Jan,11

58520 **Hysterorrhaphy, repair of ruptured uterus (nonobstetrical)** ♀

22.3 | 22.3 | FUD 090 | C 80

AMA: 2019,Jul,6; 2014,Jan,11

58540 **Hysteroplasty, repair of uterine anomaly (Strassman type)** ♀

INCLUDES Strassman type

EXCLUDES *Vesicouterine fistula closure (51920)*

25.7 | 25.7 | FUD 090 | C 80

AMA: 2019,Jul,6; 2014,Jan,11

58674-58554 [58674] Laparoscopic Procedures of the Uterus

INCLUDES Diagnostic laparoscopy

EXCLUDES *Hysteroscopy (58555-58565)*

\# **58674** **Laparoscopy, surgical, ablation of uterine fibroid(s) including intraoperative ultrasound guidance and monitoring, radiofrequency** ♀

INCLUDES Intraoperative ultrasound (76998)

EXCLUDES *Laparoscopy (49320, 58541-58554, 58570-58573)*

23.0 | 23.0 | FUD 090 | J G2 80

AMA: 2019,Jul,6; 2018,Jan,8; 2017,Apr,7; 2017,Feb,14

58541 **Laparoscopy, surgical, supracervical hysterectomy, for uterus 250 g or less;** ♀

EXCLUDES *Colpotomy (57000)*
Hysteroscopy (58561)
Laparoscopy (49320, 58545-58546, 58661, 58670-58671)
Myomectomy procedures (58140-58146)
Pelvic examination under anesthesia (57410)
Treatment of nonobstetrical vaginal hemorrhage (57180)

20.3 | 20.3 | FUD 090 | J G2 80

AMA: 2019,Jul,6; 2018,Jan,8; 2017,Apr,7; 2017,Jan,8; 2016,Jan,13; 2015,Jan,16; 2014,Jan,11

58542 **with removal of tube(s) and/or ovary(s)** ♀

EXCLUDES *Colpotomy (57000)*
Hysteroscopy (58561)
Laparoscopy (49320, 58545-58546, 58661, 58670-58671)
Myomectomy procedures (58140-58146)
Pelvic examination under anesthesia (57410)
Treatment of nonobstetrical vaginal hemorrhage (57180)

23.2 23.2 FUD 090 J G2 80

AMA: 2019,Jul,6; 2018,Jan,8; 2017,Apr,7; 2017,Jan,8; 2016,Jan,13; 2015,Jan,16; 2014,Jan,11

58543 **Laparoscopy, surgical, supracervical hysterectomy, for uterus greater than 250 g;** ♀

EXCLUDES *Colpotomy (57000)*
Hysteroscopy (58561)
Laparoscopy (49320, 58545-58546, 58661, 58670-58671)
Myomectomy procedures (58140-58146)
Pelvic examination under anesthesia (57410)
Treatment of nonobstetrical vaginal hemorrhage (57180)

23.5 23.5 FUD 090 J G2 80

AMA: 2019,Jul,6; 2018,Jan,8; 2017,Apr,7; 2017,Jan,8; 2016,Jan,13; 2015,Jan,16; 2014,Jan,11

58544 **with removal of tube(s) and/or ovary(s)** ♀

EXCLUDES *Colpotomy (57000)*
Hysteroscopy (58561)
Laparoscopy (49320, 58545-58546, 58661, 58670-58671)
Myomectomy procedures (58140-58146)
Pelvic examination under anesthesia (57410)
Treatment of nonobstetrical vaginal hemorrhage (57180)

25.5 25.5 FUD 090 J G2 80

AMA: 2019,Jul,6; 2018,Jan,8; 2017,Apr,7; 2017,Jan,8; 2016,Jan,13; 2015,Jan,16; 2014,Jan,11

58545 **Laparoscopy, surgical, myomectomy, excision; 1 to 4 intramural myomas with total weight of 250 g or less and/or removal of surface myomas** ♀

25.6 25.6 FUD 090 J A2 80

AMA: 2019,Jul,6; 2017,Apr,7; 2014,Jan,11

58546 **5 or more intramural myomas and/or intramural myomas with total weight greater than 250 g** ♀

31.6 31.6 FUD 090 J A2 80

AMA: 2019,Jul,6; 2018,Jan,8; 2017,Apr,7; 2017,Jan,8; 2016,Jan,13; 2015,Jan,16; 2014,Jan,11

58548 **Laparoscopy, surgical, with radical hysterectomy, with bilateral total pelvic lymphadenectomy and para-aortic lymph node sampling (biopsy), with removal of tube(s) and ovary(s), if performed** ♀

EXCLUDES *Laparoscopy (38570-38572, 58550-58554)*
Radical hysterectomy (58210, 58285)

55.0 55.0 FUD 090 C 80

AMA: 2019,Jul,6; 2019,Mar,5; 2018,Jan,8; 2017,Apr,7; 2017,Jan,8; 2016,Jan,13; 2015,Sep,12; 2015,Jan,16; 2014,Jan,11

58550 **Laparoscopy, surgical, with vaginal hysterectomy, for uterus 250 g or less;** ♀

EXCLUDES *Colpotomy (57000)*
Hysteroscopy (58561)
Laparoscopy (49320, 58545-58546, 58661, 58670-58671)
Myomectomy procedures (58140-58146)
Pelvic examination under anesthesia (57410)
Treatment of nonobstetrical vaginal hemorrhage (57180)

24.9 24.9 FUD 090 J A2 80

AMA: 2019,Jul,6; 2018,Jan,8; 2017,Apr,7; 2017,Jan,8; 2016,Jan,13; 2015,Jan,16; 2014,Jan,11

58552 **with removal of tube(s) and/or ovary(s)** ♀

EXCLUDES *Colpotomy (57000)*
Hysteroscopy (58561)
Laparoscopy (49320, 58545-58546, 58661, 58670-58671)
Myomectomy procedures (58140-58146)
Pelvic examination under anesthesia (57410)
Treatment of nonobstetrical vaginal hemorrhage (57180)

28.0 28.0 FUD 090 J G2 80

AMA: 2019,Jul,6; 2018,Jan,8; 2017,Apr,7; 2017,Jan,8; 2016,Jan,13; 2015,Jan,16; 2014,Jan,11

58553 **Laparoscopy, surgical, with vaginal hysterectomy, for uterus greater than 250 g;** ♀

EXCLUDES *Colpotomy (57000)*
Hysteroscopy (58561)
Laparoscopy (49320, 58545-58546, 58661, 58670-58671)
Myomectomy procedures (58140-58146)
Pelvic examination under anesthesia (57410)
Treatment of nonobstetrical vaginal hemorrhage (57180)

31.8 31.8 FUD 090 J G2 80

AMA: 2019,Jul,6; 2018,Jan,8; 2017,Apr,7; 2014,Jan,11

58554 **with removal of tube(s) and/or ovary(s)** ♀

EXCLUDES *Colpotomy (57000)*
Hysteroscopy (58561)
Laparoscopy (49320, 58545-58546, 58661, 58670-58671)
Myomectomy procedures (58140-58146)
Pelvic examination under anesthesia (57410)
Treatment of nonobstetrical vaginal hemorrhage (57180)

37.6 37.6 FUD 090 J G2 80

AMA: 2019,Jul,6; 2018,Jan,8; 2017,Apr,7; 2014,Jan,11

58555-58565 Hysteroscopy

INCLUDES Diagnostic hysteroscopy (58555)
EXCLUDES *Laparoscopy (58541-58554, 58570-58578)*

58555 **Hysteroscopy, diagnostic (separate procedure)** ♀

4.35 8.40 FUD 000 J A2 80

AMA: 2019,Jul,6; 2018,Jan,8; 2017,Jan,8; 2016,Jan,13; 2015,Jan,16; 2014,Jan,11

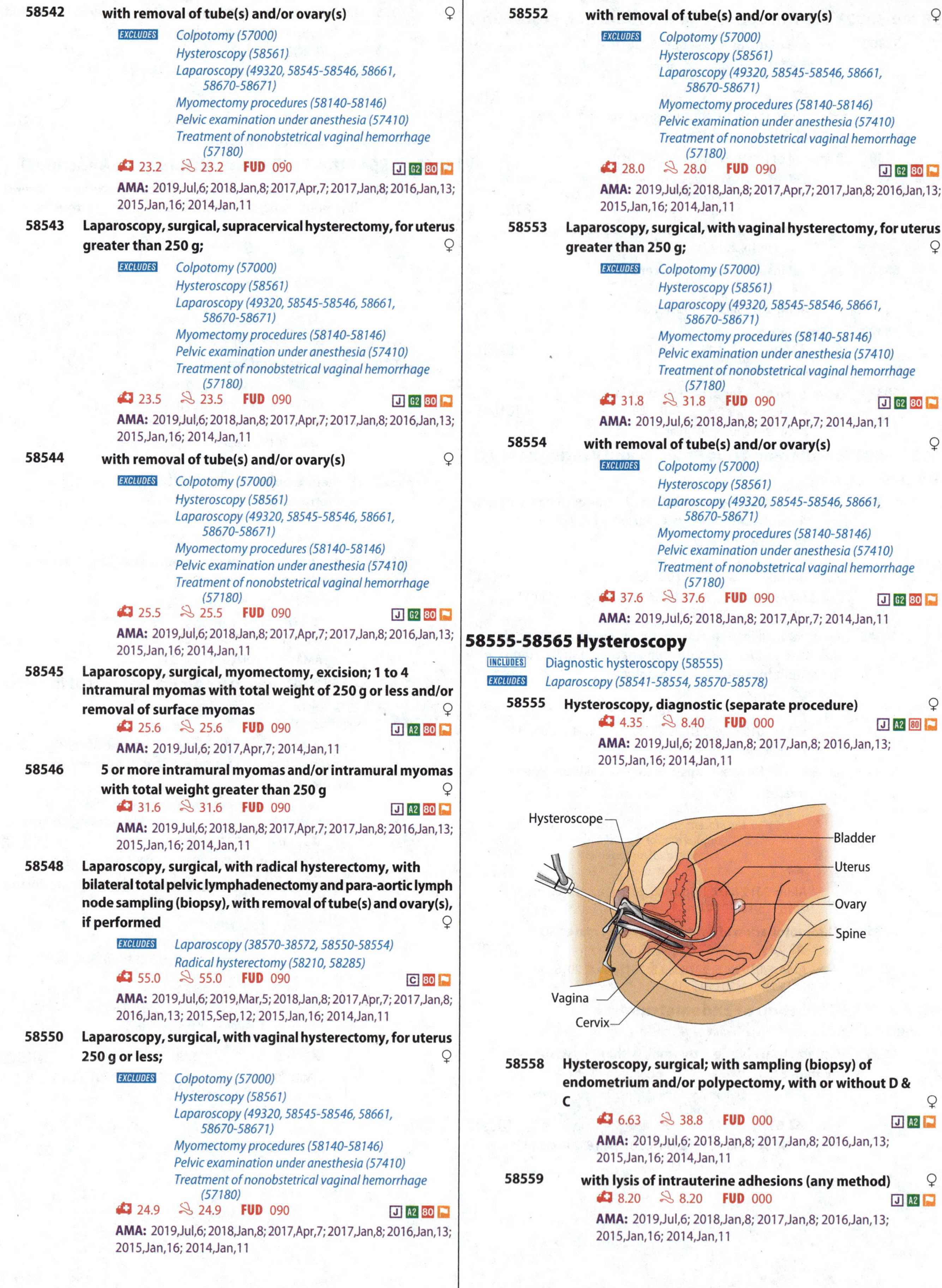

58558 **Hysteroscopy, surgical; with sampling (biopsy) of endometrium and/or polypectomy, with or without D & C** ♀

6.63 38.8 FUD 000 J A2

AMA: 2019,Jul,6; 2018,Jan,8; 2017,Jan,8; 2016,Jan,13; 2015,Jan,16; 2014,Jan,11

58559 **with lysis of intrauterine adhesions (any method)** ♀

8.20 8.20 FUD 000 J A2

AMA: 2019,Jul,6; 2018,Jan,8; 2017,Jan,8; 2016,Jan,13; 2015,Jan,16; 2014,Jan,11

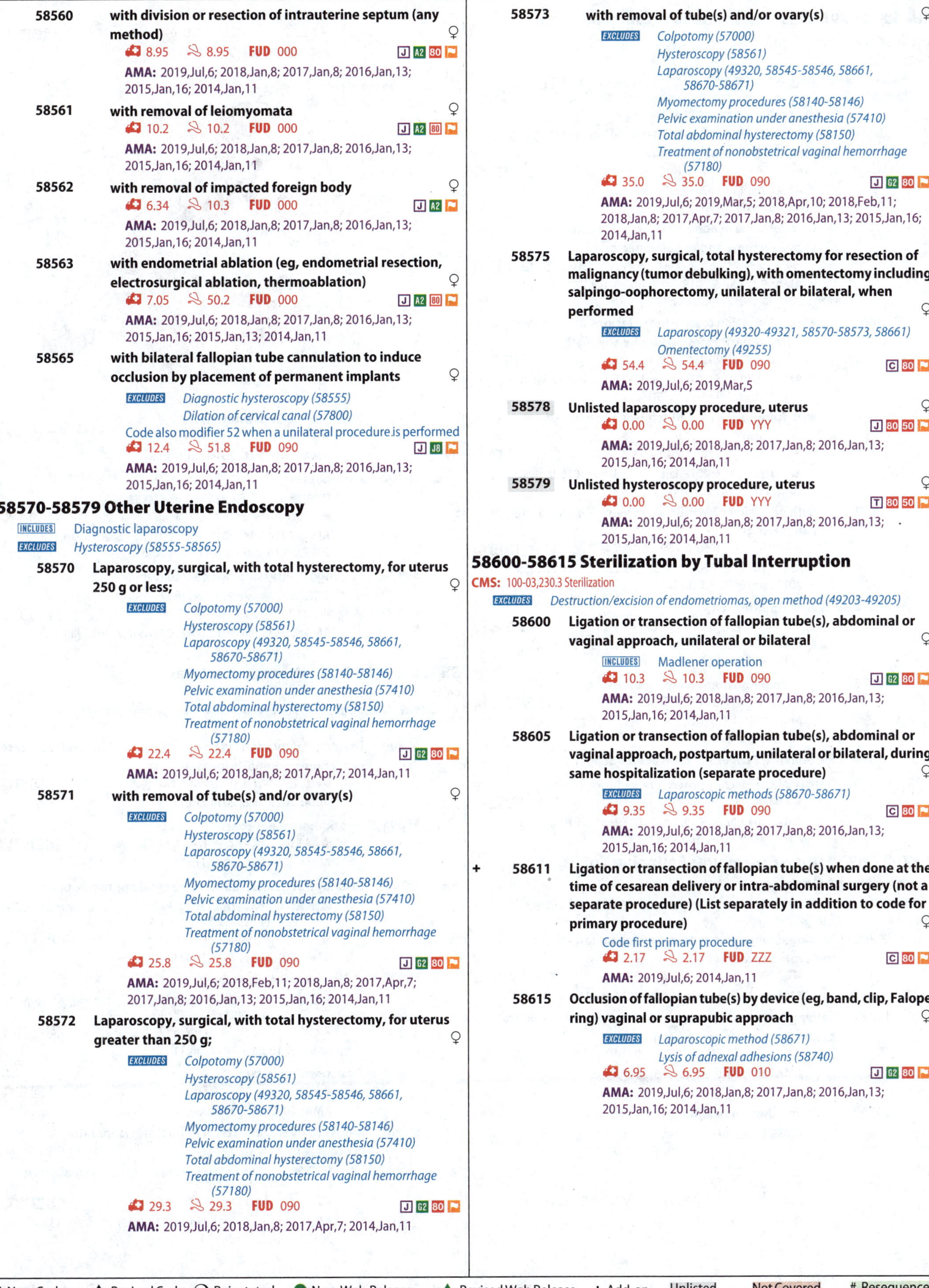

58560 **with division or resection of intrauterine septum (any method)** ♀
8.95 | 8.95 | FUD 000 | J A2 80
AMA: 2019,Jul,6; 2018,Jan,8; 2017,Jan,8; 2016,Jan,13; 2015,Jan,16; 2014,Jan,11

58561 **with removal of leiomyomata** ♀
10.2 | 10.2 | FUD 000 | J A2 80
AMA: 2019,Jul,6; 2018,Jan,8; 2017,Jan,8; 2016,Jan,13; 2015,Jan,16; 2014,Jan,11

58562 **with removal of impacted foreign body** ♀
6.34 | 10.3 | FUD 000 | J A2
AMA: 2019,Jul,6; 2018,Jan,8; 2017,Jan,8; 2016,Jan,13; 2015,Jan,16; 2014,Jan,11

58563 **with endometrial ablation (eg, endometrial resection, electrosurgical ablation, thermoablation)** ♀
7.05 | 50.2 | FUD 000 | J A2 80
AMA: 2019,Jul,6; 2018,Jan,8; 2017,Jan,8; 2016,Jan,13; 2015,Jan,16; 2015,Jan,13; 2014,Jan,11

58565 **with bilateral fallopian tube cannulation to induce occlusion by placement of permanent implants** ♀
EXCLUDES *Diagnostic hysteroscopy (58555)*
Dilation of cervical canal (57800)
Code also modifier 52 when a unilateral procedure is performed
12.4 | 51.8 | FUD 090 | J J8
AMA: 2019,Jul,6; 2018,Jan,8; 2017,Jan,8; 2016,Jan,13; 2015,Jan,16; 2014,Jan,11

58570-58579 Other Uterine Endoscopy

INCLUDES Diagnostic laparoscopy
EXCLUDES *Hysteroscopy (58555-58565)*

58570 **Laparoscopy, surgical, with total hysterectomy, for uterus 250 g or less;** ♀
EXCLUDES *Colpotomy (57000)*
Hysteroscopy (58561)
Laparoscopy (49320, 58545-58546, 58661, 58670-58671)
Myomectomy procedures (58140-58146)
Pelvic examination under anesthesia (57410)
Total abdominal hysterectomy (58150)
Treatment of nonobstetrical vaginal hemorrhage (57180)
22.4 | 22.4 | FUD 090 | J G2 80
AMA: 2019,Jul,6; 2018,Jan,8; 2017,Apr,7; 2014,Jan,11

58571 **with removal of tube(s) and/or ovary(s)** ♀
EXCLUDES *Colpotomy (57000)*
Hysteroscopy (58561)
Laparoscopy (49320, 58545-58546, 58661, 58670-58671)
Myomectomy procedures (58140-58146)
Pelvic examination under anesthesia (57410)
Total abdominal hysterectomy (58150)
Treatment of nonobstetrical vaginal hemorrhage (57180)
25.8 | 25.8 | FUD 090 | J G2 80
AMA: 2019,Jul,6; 2018,Feb,11; 2018,Jan,8; 2017,Apr,7; 2017,Jan,8; 2016,Jan,13; 2015,Jan,16; 2014,Jan,11

58572 **Laparoscopy, surgical, with total hysterectomy, for uterus greater than 250 g;** ♀
EXCLUDES *Colpotomy (57000)*
Hysteroscopy (58561)
Laparoscopy (49320, 58545-58546, 58661, 58670-58671)
Myomectomy procedures (58140-58146)
Pelvic examination under anesthesia (57410)
Total abdominal hysterectomy (58150)
Treatment of nonobstetrical vaginal hemorrhage (57180)
29.3 | 29.3 | FUD 090 | J G2 80
AMA: 2019,Jul,6; 2018,Jan,8; 2017,Apr,7; 2014,Jan,11

58573 **with removal of tube(s) and/or ovary(s)** ♀
EXCLUDES *Colpotomy (57000)*
Hysteroscopy (58561)
Laparoscopy (49320, 58545-58546, 58661, 58670-58671)
Myomectomy procedures (58140-58146)
Pelvic examination under anesthesia (57410)
Total abdominal hysterectomy (58150)
Treatment of nonobstetrical vaginal hemorrhage (57180)
35.0 | 35.0 | FUD 090 | J G2 80
AMA: 2019,Jul,6; 2019,Mar,5; 2018,Apr,10; 2018,Feb,11; 2018,Jan,8; 2017,Apr,7; 2017,Jan,8; 2016,Jan,13; 2015,Jan,16; 2014,Jan,11

58575 **Laparoscopy, surgical, total hysterectomy for resection of malignancy (tumor debulking), with omentectomy including salpingo-oophorectomy, unilateral or bilateral, when performed** ♀
EXCLUDES *Laparoscopy (49320-49321, 58570-58573, 58661)*
Omentectomy (49255)
54.4 | 54.4 | FUD 090 | C 80
AMA: 2019,Jul,6; 2019,Mar,5

58578 **Unlisted laparoscopy procedure, uterus** ♀
0.00 | 0.00 | FUD YYY | J 80 50
AMA: 2019,Jul,6; 2018,Jan,8; 2017,Jan,8; 2016,Jan,13; 2015,Jan,16; 2014,Jan,11

58579 **Unlisted hysteroscopy procedure, uterus** ♀
0.00 | 0.00 | FUD YYY | T 80 50
AMA: 2019,Jul,6; 2018,Jan,8; 2017,Jan,8; 2016,Jan,13; 2015,Jan,16; 2014,Jan,11

58600-58615 Sterilization by Tubal Interruption

CMS: 100-03,230.3 Sterilization
EXCLUDES *Destruction/excision of endometriomas, open method (49203-49205)*

58600 **Ligation or transection of fallopian tube(s), abdominal or vaginal approach, unilateral or bilateral** ♀
INCLUDES Madlener operation
10.3 | 10.3 | FUD 090 | J G2 80
AMA: 2019,Jul,6; 2018,Jan,8; 2017,Jan,8; 2016,Jan,13; 2015,Jan,16; 2014,Jan,11

58605 **Ligation or transection of fallopian tube(s), abdominal or vaginal approach, postpartum, unilateral or bilateral, during same hospitalization (separate procedure)** ♀
EXCLUDES *Laparoscopic methods (58670-58671)*
9.35 | 9.35 | FUD 090 | C 80
AMA: 2019,Jul,6; 2018,Jan,8; 2017,Jan,8; 2016,Jan,13; 2015,Jan,16; 2014,Jan,11

\+ **58611** **Ligation or transection of fallopian tube(s) when done at the time of cesarean delivery or intra-abdominal surgery (not a separate procedure) (List separately in addition to code for primary procedure)** ♀
Code first primary procedure
2.17 | 2.17 | FUD ZZZ | C 80
AMA: 2019,Jul,6; 2014,Jan,11

58615 **Occlusion of fallopian tube(s) by device (eg, band, clip, Falope ring) vaginal or suprapubic approach** ♀
EXCLUDES *Laparoscopic method (58671)*
Lysis of adnexal adhesions (58740)
6.95 | 6.95 | FUD 010 | J G2 80
AMA: 2019,Jul,6; 2018,Jan,8; 2017,Jan,8; 2016,Jan,13; 2015,Jan,16; 2014,Jan,11

● New Code ▲ Revised Code ○ Reinstated ● New Web Release ▲ Revised Web Release + Add-on Unlisted Not Covered # Resequenced
Ⓢ Optum Mod 50 Exempt ⊘ AMA Mod 51 Exempt Ⓢ Optum Mod 51 Exempt Ⓢ Mod 63 Exempt Non-FDA Drug ★ Telemedicine M Maternity A Age Edit

58660-58679 Endoscopic Procedures Fallopian Tubes and/or Ovaries

CMS: 100-03,230.3 Sterilization

INCLUDES Diagnostic laparoscopy (49320)

EXCLUDES *Laparoscopy with biopsy of fallopian tube or ovary (49321)*
Laparoscopy with ovarian cyst aspiration (49322)

58660 **Laparoscopy, surgical; with lysis of adhesions (salpingolysis, ovariolysis) (separate procedure)** ♀
19.2 19.2 FUD 090 J A2 80
AMA: 2019,Jul,6; 2018,Jan,8; 2017,Jan,8; 2016,Jan,13; 2015,Jan,16; 2014,Jan,11

58661 **with removal of adnexal structures (partial or total oophorectomy and/or salpingectomy)** ♀
18.5 18.5 FUD 010 J A2 80 50
AMA: 2019,Jul,6; 2018,Jan,8; 2017,Jan,8; 2016,Jan,13; 2015,Jan,16; 2014,Jan,11

58662 **with fulguration or excision of lesions of the ovary, pelvic viscera, or peritoneal surface by any method** ♀
20.2 20.2 FUD 090 J A2 80
AMA: 2019,Jul,6; 2018,Jan,8; 2017,Dec,14; 2017,Jan,8; 2016,Jan,13; 2015,Jan,16; 2014,Jan,11

58670 **with fulguration of oviducts (with or without transection)** ♀
10.3 10.3 FUD 090 J A2
AMA: 2019,Jul,6; 2018,Jan,8; 2017,Jan,8; 2016,Jan,13; 2015,Jan,16; 2014,Jan,11

58671 **with occlusion of oviducts by device (eg, band, clip, or Falope ring)** ♀
10.3 10.3 FUD 090 J A2
AMA: 2019,Jul,6; 2018,Jan,8; 2017,Jan,8; 2016,Jan,13; 2015,Jan,16; 2014,Jan,11

58672 **with fimbrioplasty** ♀
20.7 20.7 FUD 090 J A2 80 50
AMA: 2019,Jul,6; 2018,Jan,8; 2017,Jan,8; 2016,Jan,13; 2015,Jan,16; 2014,Jan,11

58673 **with salpingostomy (salpingoneostomy)** ♀
22.5 22.5 FUD 090 J A2 80 50
AMA: 2019,Jul,6; 2018,Jan,8; 2017,Jan,8; 2016,Jan,13; 2015,Jan,16; 2014,Jan,11

58674 **Resequenced code. See code before 58541.**

58679 **Unlisted laparoscopy procedure, oviduct, ovary** ♀
0.00 0.00 FUD YYY J 80 50
AMA: 2019,Jul,6; 2018,Jan,8; 2017,Jan,8; 2016,Jan,13; 2015,Jan,16; 2014,Jan,11

58700-58770 Open Procedures Fallopian Tubes, with/without Ovaries

EXCLUDES *Destruction/excision of endometriomas, open method (49203-49205, 58957-58958)*

58700 **Salpingectomy, complete or partial, unilateral or bilateral (separate procedure)** ♀
22.3 22.3 FUD 090 C 80
AMA: 2019,Jul,6; 2018,Sep,14; 2014,Jan,11

58720 **Salpingo-oophorectomy, complete or partial, unilateral or bilateral (separate procedure)** ♀
21.3 21.3 FUD 090 C 80
AMA: 2019,Jul,6; 2018,Jan,8; 2017,Jan,8; 2016,Jan,13; 2015,Jan,16; 2014,Jan,11

58740 **Lysis of adhesions (salpingolysis, ovariolysis)** ♀
EXCLUDES *Excision/fulguration of lesions performed laparoscopically (58662)*
Laparoscopic method (58660)
25.5 25.5 FUD 090 C 80
AMA: 2019,Jul,6; 2018,Jan,8; 2017,Jan,8; 2016,Jan,13; 2015,Jan,16; 2014,Jan,11

58750 **Tubotubal anastomosis** ♀
25.5 25.5 FUD 090 C 80 50
AMA: 2019,Jul,6; 2014,Jan,11

58752 **Tubouterine implantation** ♀
25.4 25.4 FUD 090 C 80 50
AMA: 2019,Jul,6; 2014,Jan,11

58760 **Fimbrioplasty** ♀
EXCLUDES *Laparoscopic method (58672)*
22.9 22.9 FUD 090 C 80 50
AMA: 2019,Jul,6; 2018,Jan,8; 2017,Jan,8; 2016,Jan,13; 2015,Jan,16; 2014,Jan,11

58770 **Salpingostomy (salpingoneostomy)** ♀
EXCLUDES *Laparoscopic method (58673)*
24.1 24.1 FUD 090 J 80 50
AMA: 2019,Jul,6; 2018,Jan,8; 2017,Jan,8; 2016,Jan,13; 2015,Jan,16; 2014,Jan,11

58800-58925 Open Procedures: Ovary

CMS: 100-03,230.3 Sterilization

EXCLUDES *Destruction/excision of endometriomas, open method (49203-49205, 58957-58958)*

58800 **Drainage of ovarian cyst(s), unilateral or bilateral (separate procedure); vaginal approach** ♀
8.55 9.35 FUD 090 J A2
AMA: 2019,Jul,6; 2014,Jan,11

58805 **abdominal approach** ♀
11.6 11.6 FUD 090 J G2 80
AMA: 2019,Jul,6; 2014,Jan,11

58820 **Drainage of ovarian abscess; vaginal approach, open** ♀
EXCLUDES *Transrectal fluid drainage using catheter, image guided (49407)*
9.02 9.02 FUD 090 J A2 80 50
AMA: 2019,Jul,6; 2014,Jan,11

58822 **abdominal approach** ♀
EXCLUDES *Transrectal fluid drainage using catheter, image guided (49407)*
19.8 19.8 FUD 090 C 80 50
AMA: 2019,Jul,6; 2014,Jan,11

58825 **Transposition, ovary(s)** ♀
19.7 19.7 FUD 090 C 80
AMA: 2019,Jul,6; 2014,Jan,11

58900 **Biopsy of ovary, unilateral or bilateral (separate procedure)** ♀
EXCLUDES *Laparoscopy with biopsy of fallopian tube or ovary (49321)*
11.8 11.8 FUD 090 J A2 80
AMA: 2019,Jul,6; 2018,Jan,8; 2017,Jan,8; 2016,Jan,13; 2015,Jan,16; 2014,Jan,11

26/TC PC/TC Only A2-Z3 ASC Payment 50 Bilateral ♂ Male Only ♀ Female Only Facility RVU Non-Facility RVU CCI CLIA
FUD Follow-up Days CMS: IOM AMA: CPT Asst A-Y OPPSI 80/80 Surg Assist Allowed / w/Doc Lab Crosswalk Radiology Crosswalk

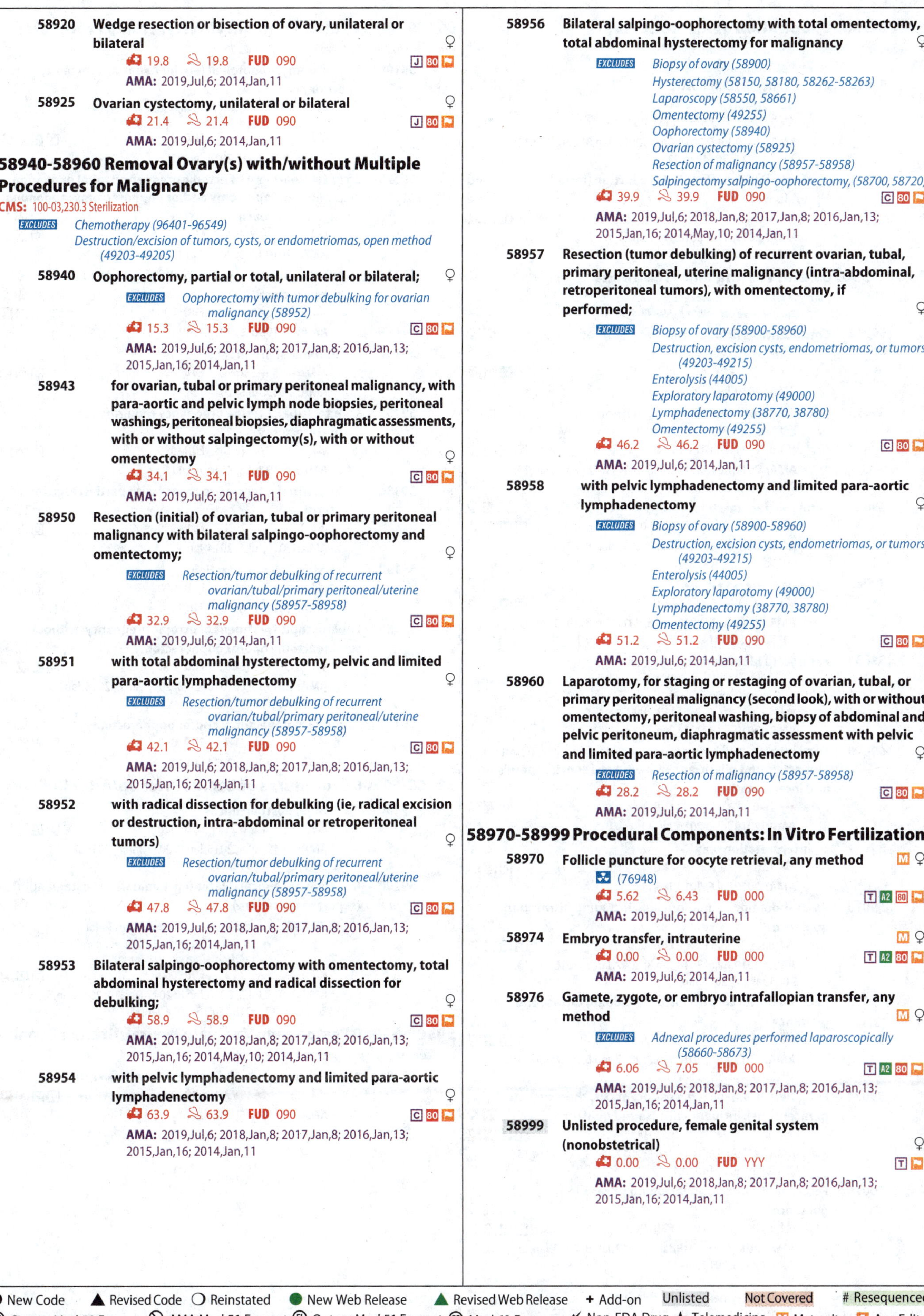

58920 **Wedge resection or bisection of ovary, unilateral or bilateral** ♀
19.8 19.8 FUD 090 J 80
AMA: 2019,Jul,6; 2014,Jan,11

58925 **Ovarian cystectomy, unilateral or bilateral** ♀
21.4 21.4 FUD 090 J 80
AMA: 2019,Jul,6; 2014,Jan,11

58940-58960 Removal Ovary(s) with/without Multiple Procedures for Malignancy

CMS: 100-03,230.3 Sterilization

EXCLUDES *Chemotherapy (96401-96549)*
Destruction/excision of tumors, cysts, or endometriomas, open method (49203-49205)

58940 **Oophorectomy, partial or total, unilateral or bilateral;** ♀
EXCLUDES *Oophorectomy with tumor debulking for ovarian malignancy (58952)*
15.3 15.3 FUD 090 C 80
AMA: 2019,Jul,6; 2018,Jan,8; 2017,Jan,8; 2016,Jan,13; 2015,Jan,16; 2014,Jan,11

58943 **for ovarian, tubal or primary peritoneal malignancy, with para-aortic and pelvic lymph node biopsies, peritoneal washings, peritoneal biopsies, diaphragmatic assessments, with or without salpingectomy(s), with or without omentectomy** ♀
34.1 34.1 FUD 090 C 80
AMA: 2019,Jul,6; 2014,Jan,11

58950 **Resection (initial) of ovarian, tubal or primary peritoneal malignancy with bilateral salpingo-oophorectomy and omentectomy;** ♀
EXCLUDES *Resection/tumor debulking of recurrent ovarian/tubal/primary peritoneal/uterine malignancy (58957-58958)*
32.9 32.9 FUD 090 C 80
AMA: 2019,Jul,6; 2014,Jan,11

58951 **with total abdominal hysterectomy, pelvic and limited para-aortic lymphadenectomy** ♀
EXCLUDES *Resection/tumor debulking of recurrent ovarian/tubal/primary peritoneal/uterine malignancy (58957-58958)*
42.1 42.1 FUD 090 C 80
AMA: 2019,Jul,6; 2018,Jan,8; 2017,Jan,8; 2016,Jan,13; 2015,Jan,16; 2014,Jan,11

58952 **with radical dissection for debulking (ie, radical excision or destruction, intra-abdominal or retroperitoneal tumors)** ♀
EXCLUDES *Resection/tumor debulking of recurrent ovarian/tubal/primary peritoneal/uterine malignancy (58957-58958)*
47.8 47.8 FUD 090 C 80
AMA: 2019,Jul,6; 2018,Jan,8; 2017,Jan,8; 2016,Jan,13; 2015,Jan,16; 2014,Jan,11

58953 **Bilateral salpingo-oophorectomy with omentectomy, total abdominal hysterectomy and radical dissection for debulking;** ♀
58.9 58.9 FUD 090 C 80
AMA: 2019,Jul,6; 2018,Jan,8; 2017,Jan,8; 2016,Jan,13; 2015,Jan,16; 2014,May,10; 2014,Jan,11

58954 **with pelvic lymphadenectomy and limited para-aortic lymphadenectomy** ♀
63.9 63.9 FUD 090 C 80
AMA: 2019,Jul,6; 2018,Jan,8; 2017,Jan,8; 2016,Jan,13; 2015,Jan,16; 2014,Jan,11

58956 **Bilateral salpingo-oophorectomy with total omentectomy, total abdominal hysterectomy for malignancy** ♀
EXCLUDES *Biopsy of ovary (58900)*
Hysterectomy (58150, 58180, 58262-58263)
Laparoscopy (58550, 58661)
Omentectomy (49255)
Oophorectomy (58940)
Ovarian cystectomy (58925)
Resection of malignancy (58957-58958)
Salpingectomy salpingo-oophorectomy, (58700, 58720)
39.9 39.9 FUD 090 C 80
AMA: 2019,Jul,6; 2018,Jan,8; 2017,Jan,8; 2016,Jan,13; 2015,Jan,16; 2014,May,10; 2014,Jan,11

58957 **Resection (tumor debulking) of recurrent ovarian, tubal, primary peritoneal, uterine malignancy (intra-abdominal, retroperitoneal tumors), with omentectomy, if performed;** ♀
EXCLUDES *Biopsy of ovary (58900-58960)*
Destruction, excision cysts, endometriomas, or tumors (49203-49215)
Enterolysis (44005)
Exploratory laparotomy (49000)
Lymphadenectomy (38770, 38780)
Omentectomy (49255)
46.2 46.2 FUD 090 C 80
AMA: 2019,Jul,6; 2014,Jan,11

58958 **with pelvic lymphadenectomy and limited para-aortic lymphadenectomy** ♀
EXCLUDES *Biopsy of ovary (58900-58960)*
Destruction, excision cysts, endometriomas, or tumors (49203-49215)
Enterolysis (44005)
Exploratory laparotomy (49000)
Lymphadenectomy (38770, 38780)
Omentectomy (49255)
51.2 51.2 FUD 090 C 80
AMA: 2019,Jul,6; 2014,Jan,11

58960 **Laparotomy, for staging or restaging of ovarian, tubal, or primary peritoneal malignancy (second look), with or without omentectomy, peritoneal washing, biopsy of abdominal and pelvic peritoneum, diaphragmatic assessment with pelvic and limited para-aortic lymphadenectomy** ♀
EXCLUDES *Resection of malignancy (58957-58958)*
28.2 28.2 FUD 090 C 80
AMA: 2019,Jul,6; 2014,Jan,11

58970-58999 Procedural Components: In Vitro Fertilization

58970 **Follicle puncture for oocyte retrieval, any method** M ♀
(76948)
5.62 6.43 FUD 000 T A2 80
AMA: 2019,Jul,6; 2014,Jan,11

58974 **Embryo transfer, intrauterine** M ♀
0.00 0.00 FUD 000 T A2 80
AMA: 2019,Jul,6; 2014,Jan,11

58976 **Gamete, zygote, or embryo intrafallopian transfer, any method** M ♀
EXCLUDES *Adnexal procedures performed laparoscopically (58660-58673)*
6.06 7.05 FUD 000 T A2 80
AMA: 2019,Jul,6; 2018,Jan,8; 2017,Jan,8; 2016,Jan,13; 2015,Jan,16; 2014,Jan,11

58999 **Unlisted procedure, female genital system (nonobstetrical)** ♀
0.00 0.00 FUD YYY T
AMA: 2019,Jul,6; 2018,Jan,8; 2017,Jan,8; 2016,Jan,13; 2015,Jan,16; 2014,Jan,11

● New Code ▲ Revised Code ○ Reinstated ● New Web Release ▲ Revised Web Release + Add-on Unlisted Not Covered # Resequenced
Optum Mod 50 Exempt AMA Mod 51 Exempt Optum Mod 51 Exempt Mod 63 Exempt Non-FDA Drug ★ Telemedicine M Maternity A Age Edit

59000-59001 Aspiration of Amniotic Fluid

EXCLUDES *Intrauterine fetal transfusion (36460)*
Unlisted fetal invasive procedure (59897)

59000 Amniocentesis; diagnostic M ♀
(76946)
2.33 3.53 FUD 000 T P3
AMA: 2019,Jul,6; 2018,Jan,8; 2017,Jan,8; 2016,Jan,13; 2015,Jan,16; 2014,Jan,11

59001 therapeutic amniotic fluid reduction (includes ultrasound guidance) M ♀
5.15 5.15 FUD 000 T R2
AMA: 2019,Jul,6; 2018,Jan,8; 2017,Jan,8; 2016,Jan,13; 2015,Jan,16; 2014,Jan,11

59012-59076 Fetal Testing and Treatment

EXCLUDES *Intrauterine fetal transfusion (36460)*
Unlisted fetal invasive procedures (59897)

59012 Cordocentesis (intrauterine), any method M ♀
(76941)
5.82 5.82 FUD 000 T G2 80
AMA: 2019,Jul,6; 2014,Jan,11

59015 Chorionic villus sampling, any method M ♀
(76945)
3.78 4.47 FUD 000 T P3 80
AMA: 2019,Jul,6; 2018,Jan,8; 2017,Jan,8; 2016,Jan,13; 2015,Jan,16; 2014,Jan,11

59020 Fetal contraction stress test M ♀
1.99 1.99 FUD 000 T P3 80
AMA: 2019,Jul,6; 2018,Jan,8; 2017,Jan,8; 2016,Jan,13; 2015,Jan,16; 2014,Jan,11

59025 Fetal non-stress test M ♀
1.37 1.37 FUD 000 T P3 80
AMA: 2019,Jul,6; 2018,Jan,8; 2017,Jan,8; 2016,Jan,13; 2015,Jan,16; 2014,Jan,11

59030 Fetal scalp blood sampling M ♀
Code also modifier 76 or 77, as appropriate, for repeat fetal scalp blood sampling
3.25 3.25 FUD 000 T 80
AMA: 2019,Jul,6; 2014,Jan,11

59050 Fetal monitoring during labor by consulting physician (ie, non-attending physician) with written report; supervision and interpretation M ♀
1.46 1.46 FUD XXX M 80
AMA: 2019,Jul,6; 2014,Jan,11

59051 interpretation only M ♀
1.21 1.21 FUD XXX B 80
AMA: 2019,Jul,6; 2014,Jan,11

59070 Transabdominal amnioinfusion, including ultrasound guidance M ♀
8.92 11.5 FUD 000 T G2 80
AMA: 2019,Jul,6; 2018,Jan,8; 2017,Jan,8; 2016,Jan,13; 2015,Jan,16; 2014,Jan,11

59072 Fetal umbilical cord occlusion, including ultrasound guidance M ♀
15.0 15.0 FUD 000 T G2
AMA: 2019,Jul,6; 2018,Jan,8; 2017,Jan,8; 2016,Jan,13; 2015,Jan,16; 2014,Jan,11

59074 Fetal fluid drainage (eg, vesicocentesis, thoracocentesis, paracentesis), including ultrasound guidance M ♀
8.92 11.1 FUD 000 T G2 80
AMA: 2019,Jul,6; 2018,Jan,8; 2017,Jan,8; 2016,Jan,13; 2015,Jan,16; 2014,Jan,11

59076 Fetal shunt placement, including ultrasound guidance M ♀
15.0 15.0 FUD 000 T G2 80
AMA: 2019,Jul,6; 2018,Jan,8; 2017,Jan,8; 2016,Jan,13; 2015,Jan,16; 2014,Jan,11

59100-59151 Tubal Pregnancy/Hysterotomy Procedures

CMS: 100-03,230.3 Sterilization

59100 Hysterotomy, abdominal (eg, for hydatidiform mole, abortion) M ♀
Code also ligation of fallopian tubes when performed at the same time as hysterotomy (58611)
24.1 24.1 FUD 090 J R2 80
AMA: 2019,Jul,6; 2014,Jan,11

59120 Surgical treatment of ectopic pregnancy; tubal or ovarian, requiring salpingectomy and/or oophorectomy, abdominal or vaginal approach M ♀
23.0 23.0 FUD 090 C 80
AMA: 2019,Jul,6; 2014,Jan,11

59121 tubal or ovarian, without salpingectomy and/or oophorectomy M ♀
23.0 23.0 FUD 090 C 80
AMA: 2019,Jul,6; 2014,Jan,11

59130 abdominal pregnancy M ♀
26.8 26.8 FUD 090 C 80
AMA: 2019,Jul,6; 2014,Jan,11

59135 interstitial, uterine pregnancy requiring total hysterectomy M ♀
26.5 26.5 FUD 090 C 80
AMA: 2019,Jul,6; 2014,Jan,11

59136 interstitial, uterine pregnancy with partial resection of uterus M ♀
25.4 25.4 FUD 090 C 80
AMA: 2019,Jul,6; 2014,Jan,11

59140 cervical, with evacuation M ♀
11.6 11.6 FUD 090 C 80
AMA: 2019,Jul,6; 2014,Jan,11

59150 Laparoscopic treatment of ectopic pregnancy; without salpingectomy and/or oophorectomy M ♀
22.3 22.3 FUD 090 J G2 80
AMA: 2019,Jul,6; 2018,Jan,8; 2017,Jan,8; 2016,Jan,13; 2015,Jan,16; 2014,Jan,11

59151 with salpingectomy and/or oophorectomy M ♀
21.7 21.7 FUD 090 J G2 80
AMA: 2019,Jul,6; 2014,Jan,11

59160-59200 Procedures of Uterus Prior To/After Delivery

59160 Curettage, postpartum M ♀
5.11 6.21 FUD 010 J A2 80
AMA: 2019,Jul,6; 2018,Jan,8; 2017,Jan,8; 2016,Jan,13; 2015,Jan,16; 2014,Jan,11

59200 Insertion of cervical dilator (eg, laminaria, prostaglandin) (separate procedure) M ♀
EXCLUDES *Fetal transfusion, intrauterine (36460)*
Hypertonic solution/prostaglandin introduction for labor initiation (59850-59857)
1.29 2.23 FUD 000 T P3
AMA: 2019,Jul,6; 2018,Jan,8; 2017,Dec,14; 2017,Jan,8; 2016,Jan,13; 2015,Jan,16; 2014,Jan,11

59300-59350 Postpartum Vaginal/Cervical/Uterine Repairs

EXCLUDES *Nonpregnancy-related cerclage (57700)*

59300 Episiotomy or vaginal repair, by other than attending M ♀
4.26 5.77 FUD 000 J P3 80
AMA: 2019,Jul,6; 2014,Jan,11

59320 **Cerclage of cervix, during pregnancy; vaginal** M ♀

4.37 4.37 FUD 000 J A2 80

AMA: 2019,Jul,6; 2018,Jan,8; 2017,Jan,8; 2016,Jan,13; 2015,Jan,16; 2014,Jan,11

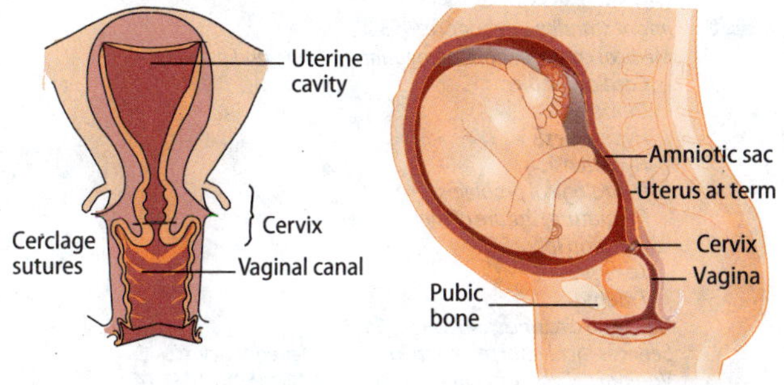

59325 **abdominal** M ♀

6.96 6.96 FUD 000 C 80

AMA: 2019,Jul,6; 2018,Jan,8; 2017,Jan,8; 2016,Jan,13; 2015,Jan,16; 2014,Jan,11

59350 **Hysterorrhaphy of ruptured uterus** M ♀

8.08 8.08 FUD 000 C 80

AMA: 2019,Jul,6; 2014,Jan,11

59400-59410 Vaginal Delivery: Comprehensive and Component Services

CMS: 100-02,15,180 Nurse-Midwife (CNM) Services; 100-02,15,20.1 Physician Expense for Surgery, Childbirth, and Treatment for Infertility

INCLUDES Care provided for an uncomplicated pregnancy including delivery as well as antepartum and postpartum care:
- Admission history
- Admission to hospital
- Artificial rupture of membranes
- Management of uncomplicated labor
- Physical exam
- Vaginal delivery with or without episiotomy or forceps

EXCLUDES *Medical complications of pregnancy, labor, and delivery:*
- *Cardiac problems*
- *Diabetes*
- *Hyperemesis*
- *Hypertension*
- *Neurological problems*
- *Premature rupture of membranes*
- *Pre-term labor*
- *Toxemia*
- *Trauma*

Newborn circumcision (54150, 54160)

Services incidental to or unrelated to the pregnancy

59400 **Routine obstetric care including antepartum care, vaginal delivery (with or without episiotomy, and/or forceps) and postpartum care** M ♀

INCLUDES Fetal heart tones
- Hospital/office visits following cesarean section or vaginal delivery
- Initial/subsequent history
- Physical exams
- Recording of weight/blood pressures
- Routine chemical urinalysis
- Routine prenatal visits:
  - Each month up to 28 weeks gestation
  - Every other week from 29 to 36 weeks gestation
  - Weekly from 36 weeks until delivery

60.4 60.4 FUD MMM B

AMA: 2019,Jul,6; 2018,Jan,8; 2017,Jan,8; 2016,Jan,13; 2015,Jan,16; 2014,Jan,11

59409 **Vaginal delivery only (with or without episiotomy and/or forceps);** M ♀

Code also inpatient management after delivery/discharge services (99217-99239 [99224, 99225, 99226])

23.3 23.3 FUD MMM J 80

AMA: 2019,Jul,6; 2018,Jan,8; 2017,Jan,8; 2016,Jan,13; 2015,Jan,16; 2014,Jan,11

59410 **including postpartum care** M ♀

INCLUDES Hospital/office visits following cesarean section or vaginal delivery

29.9 29.9 FUD MMM B

AMA: 2019,Jul,6; 2014,Jan,11

59412-59414 Other Maternity Services

CMS: 100-02,15,180 Nurse-Midwife (CNM) Services; 100-02,15,20.1 Physician Expense for Surgery, Childbirth, and Treatment for Infertility

59412 **External cephalic version, with or without tocolysis** M ♀

Code also delivery code(s)

2.95 2.95 FUD MMM J G2 80

AMA: 2019,Jul,6; 2014,Jan,11

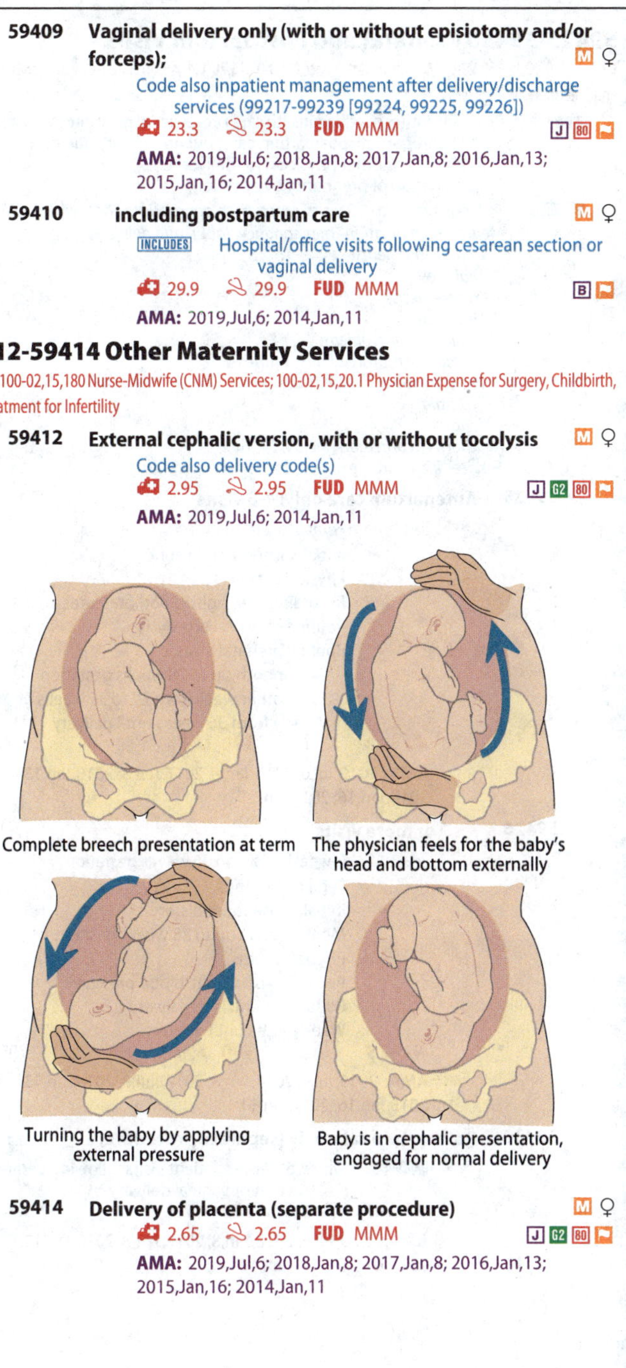

Complete breech presentation at term

The physician feels for the baby's head and bottom externally

Turning the baby by applying external pressure

Baby is in cephalic presentation, engaged for normal delivery

59414 **Delivery of placenta (separate procedure)** M ♀

2.65 2.65 FUD MMM J G2 80

AMA: 2019,Jul,6; 2018,Jan,8; 2017,Jan,8; 2016,Jan,13; 2015,Jan,16; 2014,Jan,11

59425-59430 Prenatal and Postpartum Visits

CMS: 100-02,15,180 Nurse-Midwife (CNM) Services; 100-02,15,20.1 Physician Expense for Surgery, Childbirth, and Treatment for Infertility

INCLUDES Physician/other qualified health care professional providing all or a portion of antepartum/postpartum care, but no delivery due to:
- Referral to another physician for delivery
- Termination of pregnancy by abortion

EXCLUDES *Antepartum care, 1-3 visits, report with appropriate E&M service code*
Medical complications of pregnancy, labor, and delivery:
- *Cardiac problems*
- *Diabetes*
- *Hyperemesis*
- *Hypertension*
- *Neurological problems*
- *Premature rupture of membranes*
- *Pre-term labor*
- *Toxemia*
- *Trauma*

Newborn circumcision (54150, 54160)
Services incidental to or unrelated to the pregnancy

59425 Antepartum care only; 4-6 visits M ♀

INCLUDES Fetal heart tones
Initial/subsequent history
Physical exams
Recording of weight/blood pressures
Routine chemical urinalysis
Routine prenatal visits:
- Each month up to 28 weeks gestation
- Every other week from 29 to 36 weeks gestation
- Weekly from 36 weeks until delivery

10.2 13.1 FUD MMM B 80

AMA: 2019,Jul,6; 2018,Jan,8; 2017,Jan,8; 2016,Jan,13; 2015,Jan,16; 2014,Jan,11

59426 7 or more visits M ♀

INCLUDES Biweekly visits to 36 weeks gestation
Fetal heart tones
Initial/subsequent history
Monthly visits up to 28 weeks gestation
Physical exams
Recording of weight/blood pressures
Routine chemical urinalysis
Weekly visits until delivery

17.9 23.5 FUD MMM B 80

AMA: 2019,Jul,6; 2018,Jan,8; 2017,Jan,8; 2016,Jan,13; 2015,Jan,16; 2014,Jan,11

59430 Postpartum care only (separate procedure) M ♀

INCLUDES Office/other outpatient visits following cesarean section or vaginal delivery

3.97 5.57 FUD MMM B

AMA: 2019,Jul,6; 2018,Jan,8; 2017,Jan,8; 2016,Jan,13; 2015,Jan,16; 2014,Jan,11

59510-59525 Cesarean Section Delivery: Comprehensive and Components of Care

CMS: 100-02,15,20.1 Physician Expense for Surgery, Childbirth, and Treatment for Infertility

INCLUDES Classic cesarean section
Low cervical cesarean section

EXCLUDES *Infant standby attendance (99360)*
Medical complications of pregnancy, labor, and delivery:
- *Cardiac problems*
- *Diabetes*
- *Hyperemesis*
- *Hypertension*
- *Neurological problems*
- *Premature rupture of membranes*
- *Pre-term labor*
- *Toxemia*
- *Trauma*

Newborn circumcision (54150, 54160)
Services incidental to or unrelated to the pregnancy
Vaginal delivery after prior cesarean section (59610-59614)

59510 Routine obstetric care including antepartum care, cesarean delivery, and postpartum care M ♀

INCLUDES Admission history
Admission to hospital
Cesarean delivery
Fetal heart tones
Hospital/office visits following cesarean section
Initial/subsequent history
Management of uncomplicated labor
Physical exam
Recording of weight/blood pressures
Routine chemical urinalysis
Routine prenatal visits:
- Each month up to 28 weeks gestation
- Every other week 29 to 36 weeks gestation
- Weekly from 36 weeks until delivery

EXCLUDES *Medical problems complicating labor and delivery*

67.0 67.0 FUD MMM B

AMA: 2019,Jul,6; 2018,Jan,8; 2017,Jan,8; 2016,Jan,13; 2015,Jan,16; 2014,Jan,11

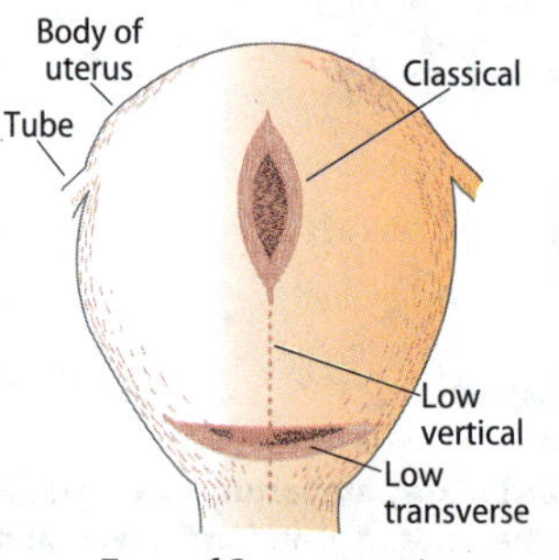

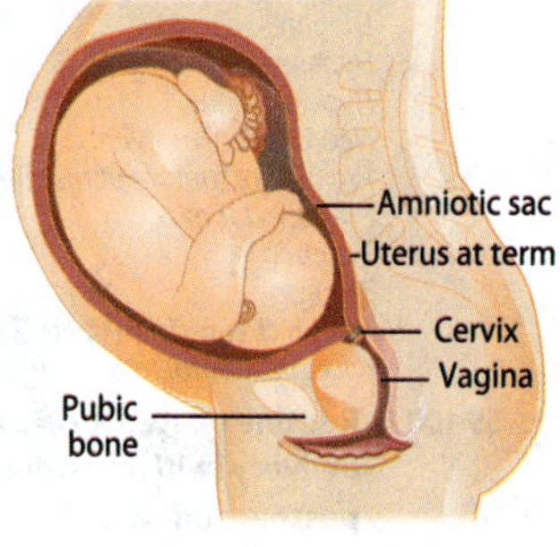

Types of Cesarean section are classified by uterine incision

59514 Cesarean delivery only; M ♀

INCLUDES Admission history
Admission to hospital
Cesarean delivery
Management of uncomplicated labor
Physical exam

EXCLUDES *Medical problems complicating labor and delivery*

Code also inpatient management after delivery/discharge services (99217-99239 [99224, 99225, 99226])

26.3 26.3 FUD MMM C 80

AMA: 2019,Jul,6; 2018,Jan,8; 2017,Jan,8; 2016,Jan,13; 2015,Jan,16; 2014,Jan,11

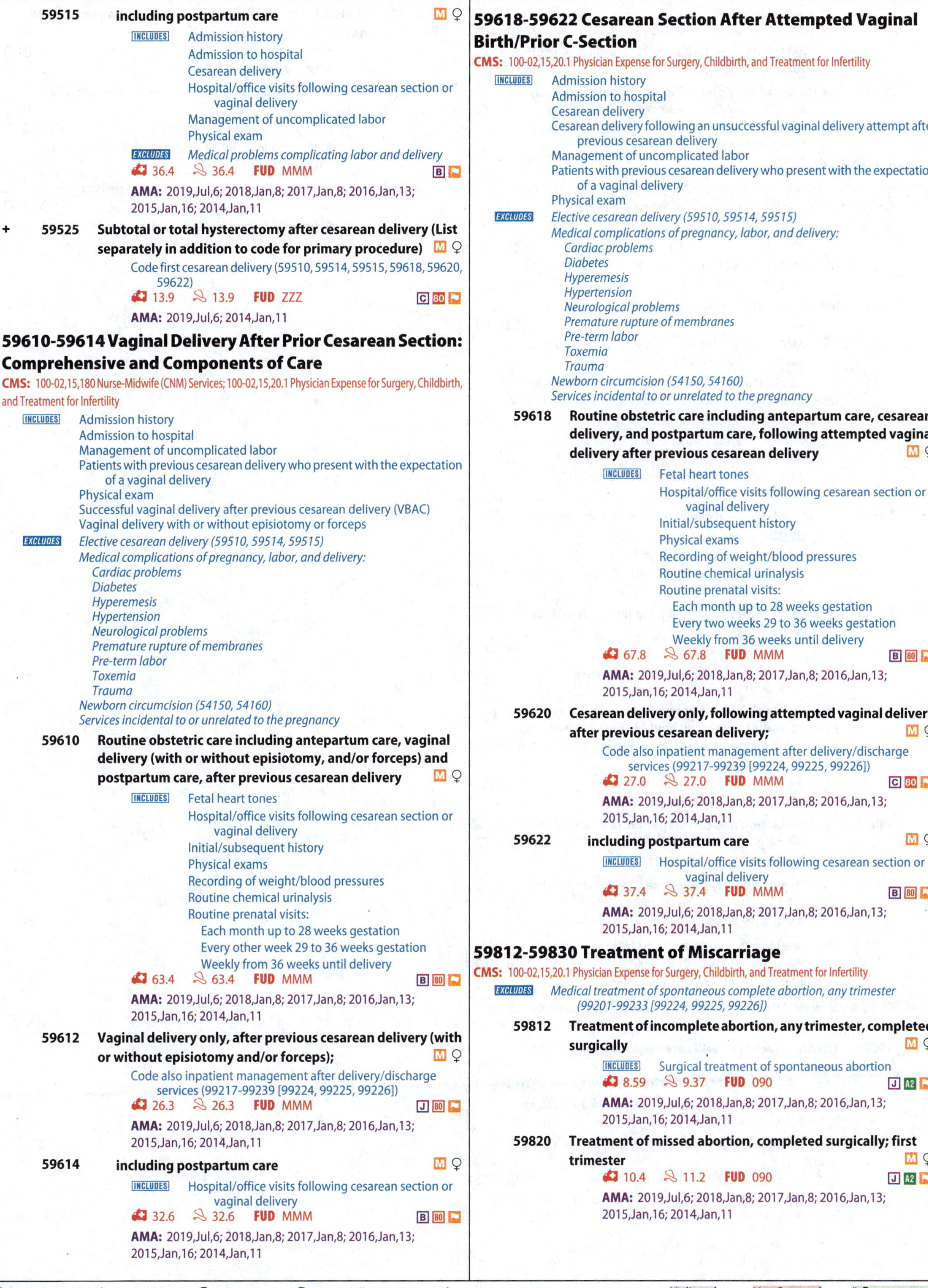

59515 including postpartum care M ♀

INCLUDES Admission history
Admission to hospital
Cesarean delivery
Hospital/office visits following cesarean section or vaginal delivery
Management of uncomplicated labor
Physical exam

EXCLUDES *Medical problems complicating labor and delivery*

36.4 36.4 FUD MMM B

AMA: 2019,Jul,6; 2018,Jan,8; 2017,Jan,8; 2016,Jan,13; 2015,Jan,16; 2014,Jan,11

\+ 59525 **Subtotal or total hysterectomy after cesarean delivery (List separately in addition to code for primary procedure)** M ♀

Code first cesarean delivery (59510, 59514, 59515, 59618, 59620, 59622)

13.9 13.9 FUD ZZZ C 80

AMA: 2019,Jul,6; 2014,Jan,11

59610-59614 Vaginal Delivery After Prior Cesarean Section: Comprehensive and Components of Care

CMS: 100-02,15,180 Nurse-Midwife (CNM) Services; 100-02,15,20.1 Physician Expense for Surgery, Childbirth, and Treatment for Infertility

INCLUDES Admission history
Admission to hospital
Management of uncomplicated labor
Patients with previous cesarean delivery who present with the expectation of a vaginal delivery
Physical exam
Successful vaginal delivery after previous cesarean delivery (VBAC)
Vaginal delivery with or without episiotomy or forceps

EXCLUDES *Elective cesarean delivery (59510, 59514, 59515)*
Medical complications of pregnancy, labor, and delivery:
Cardiac problems
Diabetes
Hyperemesis
Hypertension
Neurological problems
Premature rupture of membranes
Pre-term labor
Toxemia
Trauma
Newborn circumcision (54150, 54160)
Services incidental to or unrelated to the pregnancy

59610 **Routine obstetric care including antepartum care, vaginal delivery (with or without episiotomy, and/or forceps) and postpartum care, after previous cesarean delivery** M ♀

INCLUDES Fetal heart tones
Hospital/office visits following cesarean section or vaginal delivery
Initial/subsequent history
Physical exams
Recording of weight/blood pressures
Routine chemical urinalysis
Routine prenatal visits:
Each month up to 28 weeks gestation
Every other week 29 to 36 weeks gestation
Weekly from 36 weeks until delivery

63.4 63.4 FUD MMM B 80

AMA: 2019,Jul,6; 2018,Jan,8; 2017,Jan,8; 2016,Jan,13; 2015,Jan,16; 2014,Jan,11

59612 **Vaginal delivery only, after previous cesarean delivery (with or without episiotomy and/or forceps);** M ♀

Code also inpatient management after delivery/discharge services (99217-99239 [99224, 99225, 99226])

26.3 26.3 FUD MMM J 80

AMA: 2019,Jul,6; 2018,Jan,8; 2017,Jan,8; 2016,Jan,13; 2015,Jan,16; 2014,Jan,11

59614 including postpartum care M ♀

INCLUDES Hospital/office visits following cesarean section or vaginal delivery

32.6 32.6 FUD MMM B 80

AMA: 2019,Jul,6; 2018,Jan,8; 2017,Jan,8; 2016,Jan,13; 2015,Jan,16; 2014,Jan,11

59618-59622 Cesarean Section After Attempted Vaginal Birth/Prior C-Section

CMS: 100-02,15,20.1 Physician Expense for Surgery, Childbirth, and Treatment for Infertility

INCLUDES Admission history
Admission to hospital
Cesarean delivery
Cesarean delivery following an unsuccessful vaginal delivery attempt after previous cesarean delivery
Management of uncomplicated labor
Patients with previous cesarean delivery who present with the expectation of a vaginal delivery
Physical exam

EXCLUDES *Elective cesarean delivery (59510, 59514, 59515)*
Medical complications of pregnancy, labor, and delivery:
Cardiac problems
Diabetes
Hyperemesis
Hypertension
Neurological problems
Premature rupture of membranes
Pre-term labor
Toxemia
Trauma
Newborn circumcision (54150, 54160)
Services incidental to or unrelated to the pregnancy

59618 **Routine obstetric care including antepartum care, cesarean delivery, and postpartum care, following attempted vaginal delivery after previous cesarean delivery** M ♀

INCLUDES Fetal heart tones
Hospital/office visits following cesarean section or vaginal delivery
Initial/subsequent history
Physical exams
Recording of weight/blood pressures
Routine chemical urinalysis
Routine prenatal visits:
Each month up to 28 weeks gestation
Every two weeks 29 to 36 weeks gestation
Weekly from 36 weeks until delivery

67.8 67.8 FUD MMM B 80

AMA: 2019,Jul,6; 2018,Jan,8; 2017,Jan,8; 2016,Jan,13; 2015,Jan,16; 2014,Jan,11

59620 **Cesarean delivery only, following attempted vaginal delivery after previous cesarean delivery;** M ♀

Code also inpatient management after delivery/discharge services (99217-99239 [99224, 99225, 99226])

27.0 27.0 FUD MMM C 80

AMA: 2019,Jul,6; 2018,Jan,8; 2017,Jan,8; 2016,Jan,13; 2015,Jan,16; 2014,Jan,11

59622 including postpartum care M ♀

INCLUDES Hospital/office visits following cesarean section or vaginal delivery

37.4 37.4 FUD MMM B 80

AMA: 2019,Jul,6; 2018,Jan,8; 2017,Jan,8; 2016,Jan,13; 2015,Jan,16; 2014,Jan,11

59812-59830 Treatment of Miscarriage

CMS: 100-02,15,20.1 Physician Expense for Surgery, Childbirth, and Treatment for Infertility

EXCLUDES *Medical treatment of spontaneous complete abortion, any trimester (99201-99233 [99224, 99225, 99226])*

59812 **Treatment of incomplete abortion, any trimester, completed surgically** M ♀

INCLUDES Surgical treatment of spontaneous abortion

8.59 9.37 FUD 090 J A2

AMA: 2019,Jul,6; 2018,Jan,8; 2017,Jan,8; 2016,Jan,13; 2015,Jan,16; 2014,Jan,11

59820 **Treatment of missed abortion, completed surgically; first trimester** M ♀

10.4 11.2 FUD 090 J A2

AMA: 2019,Jul,6; 2018,Jan,8; 2017,Jan,8; 2016,Jan,13; 2015,Jan,16; 2014,Jan,11

59821 **second trimester**
10.3 11.2 FUD 090
AMA: 2019,Jul,6; 2018,Jan,8; 2017,Jan,8; 2016,Jan,13; 2015,Jan,16; 2014,Jan,11

59830 **Treatment of septic abortion, completed surgically**
12.7 12.7 FUD 090
AMA: 2019,Jul,6; 2018,Jan,8; 2017,Jan,8; 2016,Jan,13; 2015,Jan,16; 2014,Jan,11

59840-59866 Elective Abortions

CMS: 100-02,1,90 Termination of Pregnancy; 100-02,15,20.1 Physician Expense for Surgery, Childbirth, and Treatment for Infertility; 100-03,140.1 Abortion; 100-04,3,100.1 Billing for Abortion Services

59840 **Induced abortion, by dilation and curettage**
6.08 6.50 FUD 010
AMA: 2019,Jul,6; 2018,Jan,8; 2017,Jan,8; 2016,Jan,13; 2015,Jan,16; 2014,Jan,11

59841 **Induced abortion, by dilation and evacuation**
10.4 11.2 FUD 010
AMA: 2019,Jul,6; 2018,Jan,8; 2017,Jan,8; 2016,Jan,13; 2015,Jan,16; 2014,Jan,11

59850 **Induced abortion, by 1 or more intra-amniotic injections (amniocentesis-injections), including hospital admission and visits, delivery of fetus and secundines;**
EXCLUDES *Cervical dilator insertion (59200)*
10.1 10.1 FUD 090
AMA: 2019,Jul,6; 2018,Jan,8; 2017,Jan,8; 2016,Jan,13; 2015,Jan,16; 2014,Jan,11

59851 **with dilation and curettage and/or evacuation**
EXCLUDES *Cervical dilator insertion (59200)*
10.9 10.9 FUD 090
AMA: 2019,Jul,6; 2018,Jan,8; 2017,Jan,8; 2016,Jan,13; 2015,Jan,16; 2014,Jan,11

59852 **with hysterotomy (failed intra-amniotic injection)**
EXCLUDES *Cervical dilator insertion (59200)*
15.0 15.0 FUD 090
AMA: 2019,Jul,6; 2018,Jan,8; 2017,Jan,8; 2016,Jan,13; 2015,Jan,16; 2014,Jan,11

59855 **Induced abortion, by 1 or more vaginal suppositories (eg, prostaglandin) with or without cervical dilation (eg, laminaria), including hospital admission and visits, delivery of fetus and secundines;**
12.0 12.0 FUD 090
AMA: 2019,Jul,6; 2014,Jan,11

59856 **with dilation and curettage and/or evacuation**
14.1 14.1 FUD 090
AMA: 2019,Jul,6; 2014,Jan,11

59857 **with hysterotomy (failed medical evacuation)**
15.0 15.0 FUD 090
AMA: 2019,Jul,6; 2014,Jan,11

59866 **Multifetal pregnancy reduction(s) (MPR)**
6.22 6.22 FUD 000
AMA: 2019,Jul,6; 2014,Jan,11

59870-59899 Miscellaneous Obstetrical Procedures

CMS: 100-02,15,20.1 Physician Expense for Surgery, Childbirth, and Treatment for Infertility

59870 **Uterine evacuation and curettage for hydatidiform mole**
14.0 14.0 FUD 090
AMA: 2019,Jul,6; 2018,Jan,8; 2017,Jan,8; 2016,Jan,13; 2015,Jan,16; 2014,Jan,11

59871 **Removal of cerclage suture under anesthesia (other than local)**
3.83 3.83 FUD 000
AMA: 2019,Jul,6; 2018,Jan,8; 2017,Jan,8; 2016,Jan,13; 2015,Jan,16; 2014,Jan,11

59897 **Unlisted fetal invasive procedure, including ultrasound guidance, when performed**
0.00 0.00 FUD YYY
AMA: 2019,Jul,6; 2014,Jan,11

59898 **Unlisted laparoscopy procedure, maternity care and delivery**
0.00 0.00 FUD YYY
AMA: 2019,Jul,6; 2018,Jan,8; 2017,Jan,8; 2016,Jan,13; 2015,Jan,16; 2014,Jan,11

59899 **Unlisted procedure, maternity care and delivery**
0.00 0.00 FUD YYY
AMA: 2019,Jul,6; 2018,Jan,8; 2017,Jan,8; 2016,Jan,13; 2015,Jan,16; 2014,Jan,11

60000 I&D of Infected Thyroglossal Cyst

60000 **Incision and drainage of thyroglossal duct cyst, infected**
4.36 4.88 FUD 010 T A2 80
AMA: 2014,Jan,11

60100 Core Needle Biopsy: Thyroid

EXCLUDES *Fine needle aspiration (10021, [10004, 10005, 10006, 10007, 10008, 10009, 10010, 10011, 10012])*

60100 **Biopsy thyroid, percutaneous core needle**
(76942, 77002, 77012, 77021)
(88172-88173)
2.27 3.20 FUD 000 T P3
AMA: 2019,Apr,4; 2018,Jan,8; 2017,Jan,8; 2016,Jan,13; 2015,Jan,16; 2014,Jan,11

60200 Surgical Removal Thyroid Cyst or Mass; Division of Isthmus

60200 **Excision of cyst or adenoma of thyroid, or transection of isthmus**
19.0 19.0 FUD 090 J A2 80
AMA: 2018,Jan,8; 2017,Jan,8; 2016,Jan,13; 2015,Jan,16; 2014,Jan,11

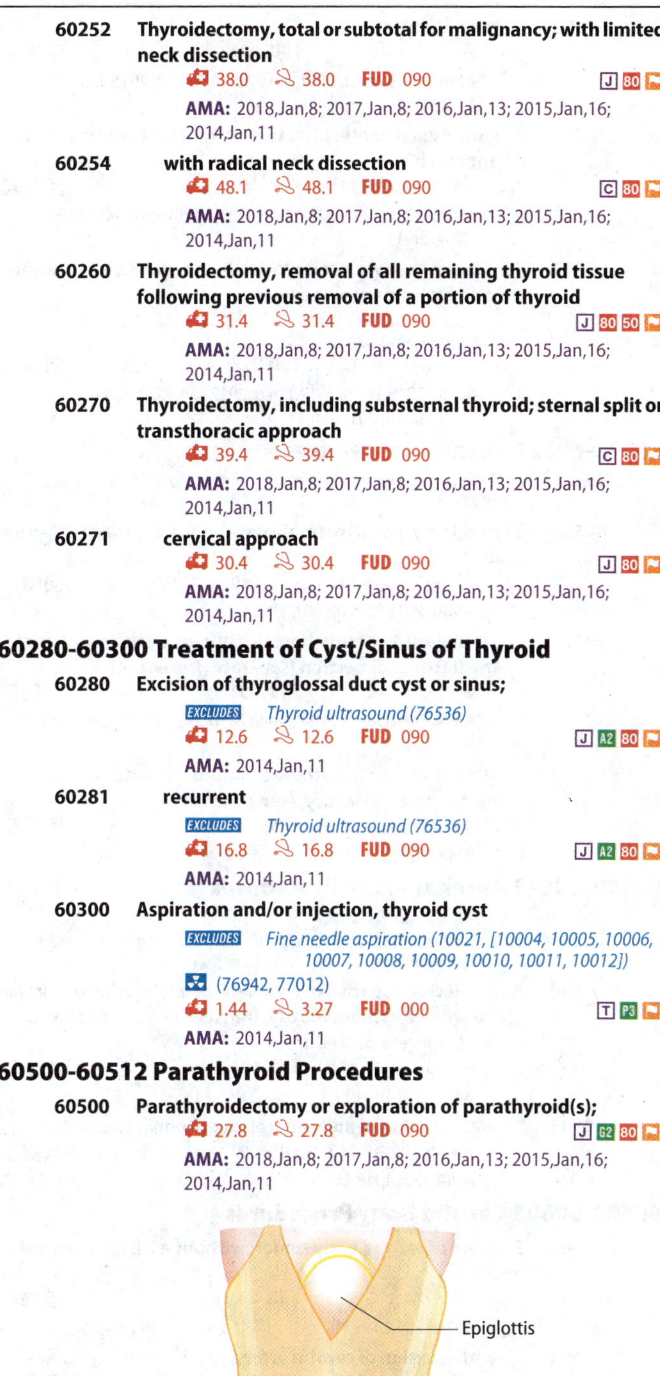

60210-60225 Subtotal Thyroidectomy

60210 **Partial thyroid lobectomy, unilateral; with or without isthmusectomy**
20.3 20.3 FUD 090 J G2 80
AMA: 2018,Jan,8; 2017,Jan,8; 2016,Jan,13; 2015,Jan,16; 2014,Jan,11

60212 **with contralateral subtotal lobectomy, including isthmusectomy**
29.0 29.0 FUD 090 J G2 80
AMA: 2018,Jan,8; 2017,Jan,8; 2016,Jan,13; 2015,Jan,16; 2014,Jan,11

60220 **Total thyroid lobectomy, unilateral; with or without isthmusectomy**
20.3 20.3 FUD 090 J G2 80
AMA: 2018,Jan,8; 2017,Jan,8; 2016,Jan,13; 2015,Jan,16; 2014,Jan,11

60225 **with contralateral subtotal lobectomy, including isthmusectomy**
26.7 26.7 FUD 090 J G2 80
AMA: 2018,Jan,8; 2017,Jan,8; 2016,Jan,13; 2015,Jan,16; 2014,Jan,11

60240-60271 Complete Thyroidectomy Procedures

60240 **Thyroidectomy, total or complete**
EXCLUDES *Subtotal or partial thyroidectomy (60271)*
26.4 26.4 FUD 090 J G2 80
AMA: 2018,Jan,8; 2017,Jan,8; 2016,Jan,13; 2015,Jan,16; 2014,Jan,11

60252 **Thyroidectomy, total or subtotal for malignancy; with limited neck dissection**
38.0 38.0 FUD 090 J 80
AMA: 2018,Jan,8; 2017,Jan,8; 2016,Jan,13; 2015,Jan,16; 2014,Jan,11

60254 **with radical neck dissection**
48.1 48.1 FUD 090 C 80
AMA: 2018,Jan,8; 2017,Jan,8; 2016,Jan,13; 2015,Jan,16; 2014,Jan,11

60260 **Thyroidectomy, removal of all remaining thyroid tissue following previous removal of a portion of thyroid**
31.4 31.4 FUD 090 J 80 50
AMA: 2018,Jan,8; 2017,Jan,8; 2016,Jan,13; 2015,Jan,16; 2014,Jan,11

60270 **Thyroidectomy, including substernal thyroid; sternal split or transthoracic approach**
39.4 39.4 FUD 090 C 80
AMA: 2018,Jan,8; 2017,Jan,8; 2016,Jan,13; 2015,Jan,16; 2014,Jan,11

60271 **cervical approach**
30.4 30.4 FUD 090 J 80
AMA: 2018,Jan,8; 2017,Jan,8; 2016,Jan,13; 2015,Jan,16; 2014,Jan,11

60280-60300 Treatment of Cyst/Sinus of Thyroid

60280 **Excision of thyroglossal duct cyst or sinus;**
EXCLUDES *Thyroid ultrasound (76536)*
12.6 12.6 FUD 090 J A2 80
AMA: 2014,Jan,11

60281 **recurrent**
EXCLUDES *Thyroid ultrasound (76536)*
16.8 16.8 FUD 090 J A2 80
AMA: 2014,Jan,11

60300 **Aspiration and/or injection, thyroid cyst**
EXCLUDES *Fine needle aspiration (10021, [10004, 10005, 10006, 10007, 10008, 10009, 10010, 10011, 10012])*
(76942, 77012)
1.44 3.27 FUD 000 T P3
AMA: 2014,Jan,11

60500-60512 Parathyroid Procedures

60500 **Parathyroidectomy or exploration of parathyroid(s);**
27.8 27.8 FUD 090 J G2 80
AMA: 2018,Jan,8; 2017,Jan,8; 2016,Jan,13; 2015,Jan,16; 2014,Jan,11

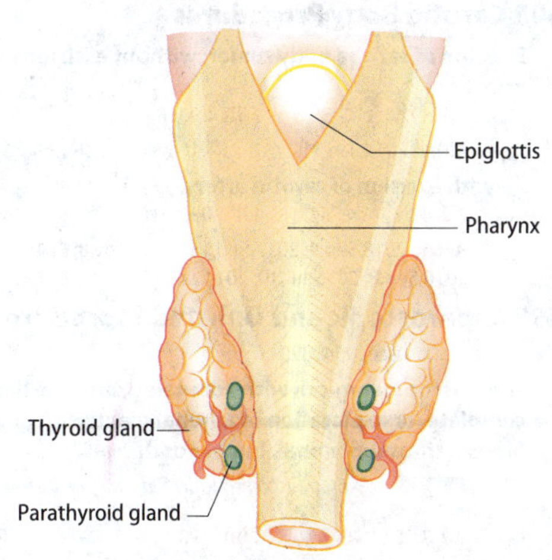

Posterior view of pharynx, thyroid glands, and parathyroid glands

60502 **re-exploration**
37.2 37.2 FUD 090 J 80
AMA: 2018,Jan,8; 2017,Jan,8; 2016,Jan,13; 2015,Jan,16; 2014,Jan,11

60505 **with mediastinal exploration, sternal split or transthoracic approach**
40.1 40.1 FUD 090 C 80
AMA: 2018,Jan,8; 2017,Jan,8; 2016,Jan,13; 2015,Jan,16; 2014,Jan,11

+ 60512 **Parathyroid autotransplantation (List separately in addition to code for primary procedure)**
Code first (60212, 60225, 60240, 60252, 60254, 60260, 60270-60271, 60500, 60502, 60505)
7.03 7.03 FUD ZZZ N 80
AMA: 2018,Jan,8; 2017,Jan,8; 2017,Jan,6; 2016,Jan,13; 2015,Jan,16; 2014,Jan,11

60520-60522 Thymus Procedures

EXCLUDES *Surgical thoracoscopy (video-assisted thoracic surgery (VATS) thymectomy (32673)*

60520 **Thymectomy, partial or total; transcervical approach (separate procedure)**
30.2 30.2 FUD 090 J 80
AMA: 2019,Mar,10; 2014,Jan,11

60521 **sternal split or transthoracic approach, without radical mediastinal dissection (separate procedure)**
32.4 32.4 FUD 090 C 80
AMA: 2018,Jan,8; 2017,Jan,8; 2016,Jan,13; 2015,Jan,16; 2014,Jan,11

60522 **sternal split or transthoracic approach, with radical mediastinal dissection (separate procedure)**
39.5 39.5 FUD 090 C 80
AMA: 2014,Jan,11

60540-60545 Adrenal Gland Procedures

EXCLUDES *Laparoscopic approach (60650)*
Removal of remote or disseminated pheochromocytoma (49203-49205)
Standard backbench preparation of cadaver donor (50323)

60540 **Adrenalectomy, partial or complete, or exploration of adrenal gland with or without biopsy, transabdominal, lumbar or dorsal (separate procedure);**
30.8 30.8 FUD 090 C 80 50
AMA: 2014,Jan,11

60545 **with excision of adjacent retroperitoneal tumor**
35.3 35.3 FUD 090 C 80 50
AMA: 2014,Jan,11

60600-60605 Carotid Body Procedures

60600 **Excision of carotid body tumor; without excision of carotid artery**
39.6 39.6 FUD 090 C 80
AMA: 2014,Jan,11

60605 **with excision of carotid artery**
47.9 47.9 FUD 090 C 80
AMA: 2018,Sep,9; 2017,Sep,13; 2016,Nov,8; 2016,Oct,10; 2016,Sep,8; 2016,Jul,10; 2014,Jan,11

60650-60699 Laparoscopic and Unlisted Procedures

INCLUDES Diagnostic laparoscopy (49320)

60650 **Laparoscopy, surgical, with adrenalectomy, partial or complete, or exploration of adrenal gland with or without biopsy, transabdominal, lumbar or dorsal**
EXCLUDES *Peritoneoscopy performed as separate procedure (49320)*
34.5 34.5 FUD 090 C 80 50
AMA: 2018,Jan,8; 2017,Jan,8; 2016,Jan,13; 2015,Jan,16; 2014,Jan,11

60659 **Unlisted laparoscopy procedure, endocrine system**
0.00 0.00 FUD YYY J 80 50
AMA: 2018,Jan,8; 2017,Jan,8; 2016,Jan,13; 2015,Jan,16; 2014,Jan,11

60699 **Unlisted procedure, endocrine system**
0.00 0.00 FUD YYY J 80
AMA: 2018,Jan,8; 2017,Jan,8; 2016,Jan,13; 2015,Jan,16; 2014,Jan,11

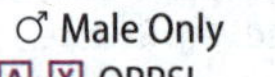
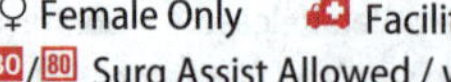
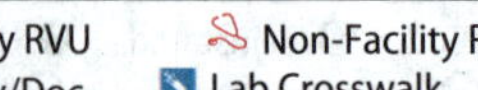
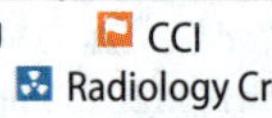

61000-61253 Transcranial Access via Puncture, Burr Hole, Twist Hole, or Trephine

EXCLUDES *Injection for:*
Cerebral angiography (36100-36218)

61000 **Subdural tap through fontanelle, or suture, infant, unilateral or bilateral; initial**

EXCLUDES *Injection for:*
Pneumoencephalography (61055)
Ventriculography (61026, 61120)

3.19 3.19 FUD 000 T R2

AMA: 2014,Jan,11

Overhead view of newborn skull

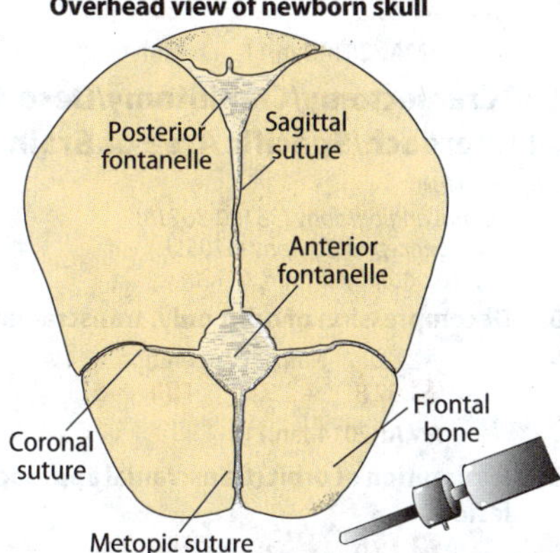

An initial tap through to the subdural level is performed on an infant via a fontanelle or suture, either unilateral or bilateral

61001 **subsequent taps**

3.16 3.16 FUD 000 T R2

AMA: 2014,Jan,11

61020 **Ventricular puncture through previous burr hole, fontanelle, suture, or implanted ventricular catheter/reservoir; without injection**

2.87 2.87 FUD 000 T A2

AMA: 2014,Jan,11

61026 **with injection of medication or other substance for diagnosis or treatment**

INCLUDES Injection for ventriculography

3.05 3.05 FUD 000 T A2

AMA: 2014,Jan,11

61050 **Cisternal or lateral cervical (C1-C2) puncture; without injection (separate procedure)**

2.45 2.45 FUD 000 T A2 80

AMA: 2014,Jan,11

61055 **with injection of medication or other substance for diagnosis or treatment**

INCLUDES Injection for pneumoencephalography

EXCLUDES *Myelography via lumbar injection (62302-62305)*
Radiology procedures except when furnished by a different provider

3.62 3.62 FUD 000 T A2

AMA: 2014,Sep,3; 2014,Jan,11

61070 **Puncture of shunt tubing or reservoir for aspiration or injection procedure**

(75809)

1.64 1.64 FUD 000 T A2

AMA: 2018,Jan,8; 2017,Jan,8; 2016,Jan,13; 2015,Jan,16; 2014,Jan,11

61105 **Twist drill hole for subdural or ventricular puncture**

13.5 13.5 FUD 090 C 80

AMA: 2014,Jan,11

61107 **Twist drill hole(s) for subdural, intracerebral, or ventricular puncture; for implanting ventricular catheter, pressure recording device, or other intracerebral monitoring device**

Code also intracranial neuroendoscopic ventricular catheter insertion or reinsertion, when performed (62160)

9.20 9.20 FUD 000 ⊘ C

AMA: 2014,Jan,11

61108 **for evacuation and/or drainage of subdural hematoma**

26.0 26.0 FUD 090 C

AMA: 2014,Jan,11

61120 **Burr hole(s) for ventricular puncture (including injection of gas, contrast media, dye, or radioactive material)**

INCLUDES Includes: Injection for ventriculography

21.8 21.8 FUD 090 C 80

AMA: 2014,Jan,11

61140 **Burr hole(s) or trephine; with biopsy of brain or intracranial lesion**

36.9 36.9 FUD 090 C 80

AMA: 2014,Jan,11

61150 **with drainage of brain abscess or cyst**

39.8 39.8 FUD 090 C

AMA: 2014,Jan,11

61151 **with subsequent tapping (aspiration) of intracranial abscess or cyst**

29.1 29.1 FUD 090 C

AMA: 2014,Jan,11

61154 **Burr hole(s) with evacuation and/or drainage of hematoma, extradural or subdural**

37.1 37.1 FUD 090 C 80 50

AMA: 2014,Jan,11

61156 **Burr hole(s); with aspiration of hematoma or cyst, intracerebral**

36.5 36.5 FUD 090 C 80

AMA: 2014,Jan,11

61210 **for implanting ventricular catheter, reservoir, EEG electrode(s), pressure recording device, or other cerebral monitoring device (separate procedure)**

Code also intracranial neuroendoscopic ventricular catheter insertion or reinsertion, when performed (62160)

10.8 10.8 FUD 000 C

AMA: 2018,Jan,8; 2017,Jan,8; 2016,Jan,13; 2015,Jan,16; 2014,Jan,11

61215 **Insertion of subcutaneous reservoir, pump or continuous infusion system for connection to ventricular catheter**

EXCLUDES *Chemotherapy (96450)*
Refilling and maintenance of implantable infusion pump (95990)

14.8 14.8 FUD 090 J A2

AMA: 2018,Jan,8; 2017,Jan,8; 2016,Jan,13; 2015,Jan,16; 2014,Jan,11

61250 **Burr hole(s) or trephine, supratentorial, exploratory, not followed by other surgery**

EXCLUDES *Burr hole or trephine followed by craniotomy at same operative session (61304-61321)*

25.4 25.4 FUD 090 C 80 50

AMA: 2014,Jan,11

61253 **Burr hole(s) or trephine, infratentorial, unilateral or bilateral**

EXCLUDES *Burr hole or trephine followed by craniotomy at same operative session (61304-61321)*

29.1 29.1 FUD 090 C 80

AMA: 2018,Jan,8; 2017,Jan,8; 2016,Jan,13; 2015,Jan,16; 2014,Jan,11

61304-61323 Craniectomy/Craniotomy: By Indication/Specific Area of Brain

EXCLUDES *Injection for:*
Cerebral angiography (36100-36218)
Pneumoencephalography (61055)
Ventriculography (61026, 61120)

61304 Craniectomy or craniotomy, exploratory; supratentorial

EXCLUDES *Other craniectomy/craniotomy procedures when performed at the same anatomical site and during the same surgical encounter*

48.1 48.1 FUD 090 C 80

AMA: 2014,Jan,11

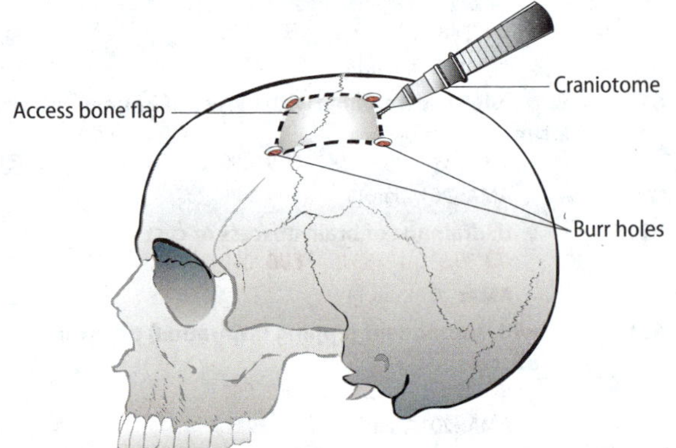

61305 infratentorial (posterior fossa)

EXCLUDES *Other craniectomy/craniotomy procedures when performed at the same anatomical site and during the same surgical encounter*

58.6 58.6 FUD 090 C 80

AMA: 2014,Jan,11

61312 Craniectomy or craniotomy for evacuation of hematoma, supratentorial; extradural or subdural

60.8 60.8 FUD 090 C 80

AMA: 2018,Jan,8; 2017,Jan,8; 2016,Jan,13; 2015,Jan,16; 2014,Jan,11

61313 intracerebral

58.0 58.0 FUD 090 C 80

AMA: 2014,Jan,11

61314 Craniectomy or craniotomy for evacuation of hematoma, infratentorial; extradural or subdural

53.2 53.2 FUD 090 C 80

AMA: 2014,Jan,11

61315 intracerebellar

60.4 60.4 FUD 090 C 80

AMA: 2014,Jan,11

+ **61316 Incision and subcutaneous placement of cranial bone graft (List separately in addition to code for primary procedure)**

Code first (61304, 61312-61313, 61322-61323, 61340, 61570-61571, 61680-61705)

2.60 2.60 FUD ZZZ C

AMA: 2014,Jan,11

61320 Craniectomy or craniotomy, drainage of intracranial abscess; supratentorial

55.5 55.5 FUD 090 C 80

AMA: 2014,Jan,11

61321 infratentorial

62.7 62.7 FUD 090 C 80

AMA: 2014,Jan,11

61322 Craniectomy or craniotomy, decompressive, with or without duraplasty, for treatment of intracranial hypertension, without evacuation of associated intraparenchymal hematoma; without lobectomy

EXCLUDES *Craniectomy or craniotomy for evacuation of hematoma (61313)*
Subtemporal decompression (61340)

69.7 69.7 FUD 090 C 80

AMA: 2018,Aug,10; 2014,Jan,11

61323 with lobectomy

EXCLUDES *Craniectomy or craniotomy for evacuation of hematoma (61313)*
Subtemporal decompression (61340)

69.8 69.8 FUD 090 C 80

AMA: 2014,Jan,11

61330-61530 Craniectomy/Craniotomy/Decompression Brain By Surgical Approach/Specific Area of Brain

EXCLUDES *Injection for:*
Cerebral angiography (36100-36218)
Pneumoencephalography (61055)
Ventriculography (61026, 61120)

61330 Decompression of orbit only, transcranial approach

INCLUDES Naffziger operation

52.8 52.8 FUD 090 J G2 80 50

AMA: 2014,Jan,11

61333 Exploration of orbit (transcranial approach); with removal of lesion

59.6 59.6 FUD 090 C 80 50

AMA: 2014,Jan,11

61340 Subtemporal cranial decompression (pseudotumor cerebri, slit ventricle syndrome)

EXCLUDES *Decompression craniotomy or craniectomy for intracranial hypertension, without hematoma removal (61322-61323)*

42.4 42.4 FUD 090 C 80 50

AMA: 2014,Jan,11

61343 Craniectomy, suboccipital with cervical laminectomy for decompression of medulla and spinal cord, with or without dural graft (eg, Arnold-Chiari malformation)

64.0 64.0 FUD 090 C 80

AMA: 2014,Jan,11

61345 Other cranial decompression, posterior fossa

EXCLUDES *Kroenlein procedure (67445)*
Orbital decompression using a lateral wall approach (67445)

60.1 60.1 FUD 090 C 80

AMA: 2014,Jan,11

61450 Craniectomy, subtemporal, for section, compression, or decompression of sensory root of gasserian ganglion

INCLUDES Frazier-Spiller procedure
Hartley-Krause
Krause decompression
Taarnhoj procedure

56.6 56.6 FUD 090 C 80

AMA: 2014,Jan,11

61458 Craniectomy, suboccipital; for exploration or decompression of cranial nerves

INCLUDES Jannetta decompression

58.8 58.8 FUD 090 C 80

AMA: 2014,Jan,11

61460 **for section of 1 or more cranial nerves**
61.7 61.7 FUD 090 C 80
AMA: 2014,Jan,11

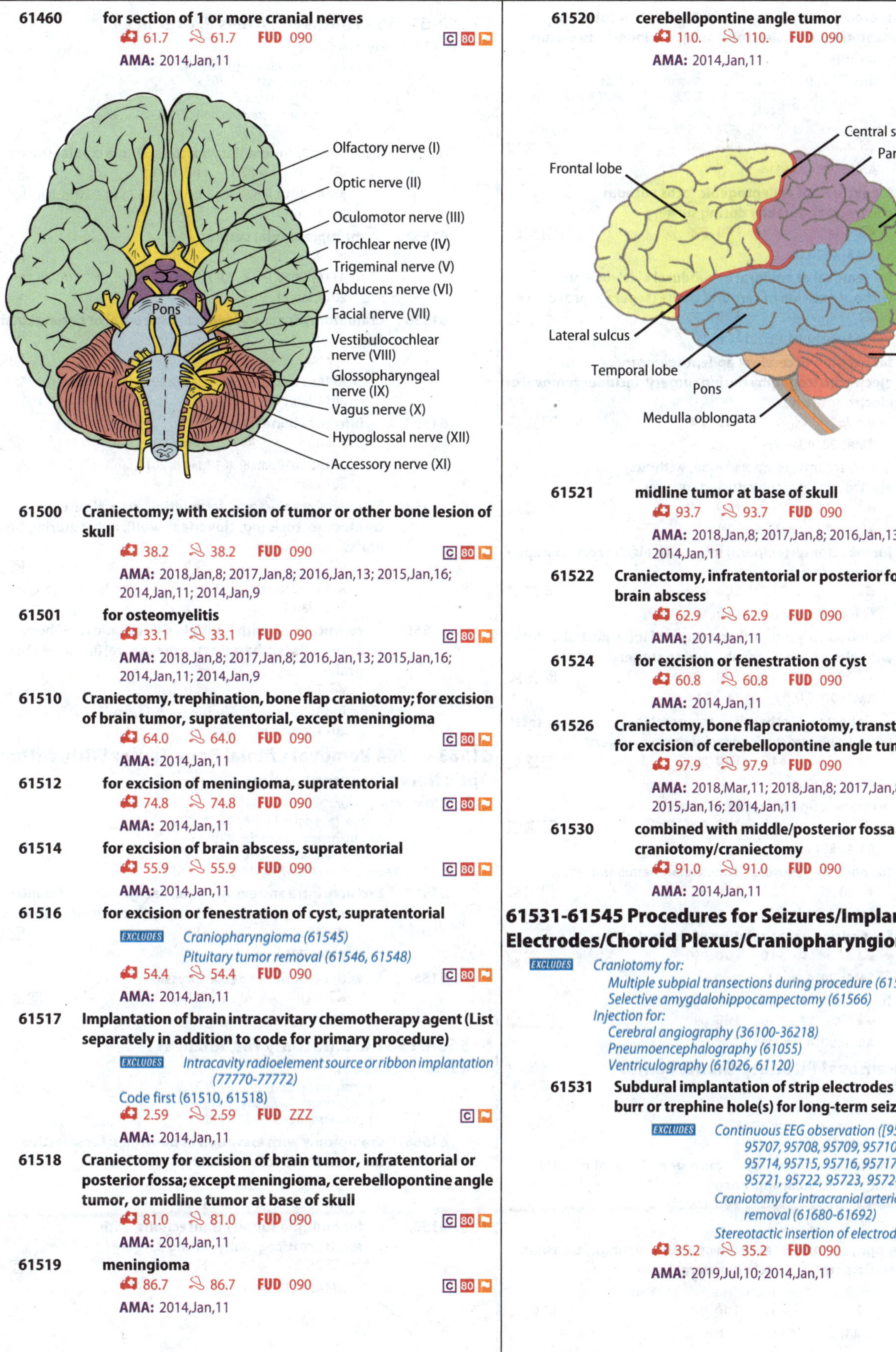

61500 **Craniectomy; with excision of tumor or other bone lesion of skull**
38.2 38.2 FUD 090 C 80
AMA: 2018,Jan,8; 2017,Jan,8; 2016,Jan,13; 2015,Jan,16; 2014,Jan,11; 2014,Jan,9

61501 **for osteomyelitis**
33.1 33.1 FUD 090 C 80
AMA: 2018,Jan,8; 2017,Jan,8; 2016,Jan,13; 2015,Jan,16; 2014,Jan,11; 2014,Jan,9

61510 **Craniectomy, trephination, bone flap craniotomy; for excision of brain tumor, supratentorial, except meningioma**
64.0 64.0 FUD 090 C 80
AMA: 2014,Jan,11

61512 **for excision of meningioma, supratentorial**
74.8 74.8 FUD 090 C 80
AMA: 2014,Jan,11

61514 **for excision of brain abscess, supratentorial**
55.9 55.9 FUD 090 C 80
AMA: 2014,Jan,11

61516 **for excision or fenestration of cyst, supratentorial**
EXCLUDES *Craniopharyngioma (61545)*
Pituitary tumor removal (61546, 61548)
54.4 54.4 FUD 090 C 80
AMA: 2014,Jan,11

\+ **61517** **Implantation of brain intracavitary chemotherapy agent (List separately in addition to code for primary procedure)**
EXCLUDES *Intracavity radioelement source or ribbon implantation (77770-77772)*
Code first (61510, 61518)
2.59 2.59 FUD ZZZ C
AMA: 2014,Jan,11

61518 **Craniectomy for excision of brain tumor, infratentorial or posterior fossa; except meningioma, cerebellopontine angle tumor, or midline tumor at base of skull**
81.0 81.0 FUD 090 C 80
AMA: 2014,Jan,11

61519 **meningioma**
86.7 86.7 FUD 090 C 80
AMA: 2014,Jan,11

61520 **cerebellopontine angle tumor**
110. 110. FUD 090 C 80
AMA: 2014,Jan,11

61521 **midline tumor at base of skull**
93.7 93.7 FUD 090 C 80
AMA: 2018,Jan,8; 2017,Jan,8; 2016,Jan,13; 2015,Jan,16; 2014,Jan,11

61522 **Craniectomy, infratentorial or posterior fossa; for excision of brain abscess**
62.9 62.9 FUD 090 C 80
AMA: 2014,Jan,11

61524 **for excision or fenestration of cyst**
60.8 60.8 FUD 090 C 80
AMA: 2014,Jan,11

61526 **Craniectomy, bone flap craniotomy, transtemporal (mastoid) for excision of cerebellopontine angle tumor;**
97.9 97.9 FUD 090 C
AMA: 2018,Mar,11; 2018,Jan,8; 2017,Jan,8; 2016,Jan,13; 2015,Jan,16; 2014,Jan,11

61530 **combined with middle/posterior fossa craniotomy/craniectomy**
91.0 91.0 FUD 090 C
AMA: 2014,Jan,11

61531-61545 Procedures for Seizures/Implanted Electrodes/Choroid Plexus/Craniopharyngioma

EXCLUDES *Craniotomy for:*
Multiple subpial transections during procedure (61567)
Selective amygdalohippocampectomy (61566)
Injection for:
Cerebral angiography (36100-36218)
Pneumoencephalography (61055)
Ventriculography (61026, 61120)

61531 **Subdural implantation of strip electrodes through 1 or more burr or trephine hole(s) for long-term seizure monitoring**
EXCLUDES *Continuous EEG observation ([95700, 95705, 95706, 95707, 95708, 95709, 95710, 95711, 95712, 95713, 95714, 95715, 95716, 95717, 95718, 95719, 95720, 95721, 95722, 95723, 95724, 95725, 95726])*
Craniotomy for intracranial arteriovenous malformation removal (61680-61692)
Stereotactic insertion of electrodes (61760)
35.2 35.2 FUD 090 C 80
AMA: 2019,Jul,10; 2014,Jan,11

61533 **Craniotomy with elevation of bone flap; for subdural implantation of an electrode array, for long-term seizure monitoring**

EXCLUDES *Continuous EEG monitoring ([95700, 95705, 95706, 95707, 95708, 95709, 95710, 95711, 95712, 95713, 95714, 95715, 95716, 95717, 95718, 95719, 95720, 95721, 95722, 95723, 95724, 95725, 95726])*

44.4 44.4 FUD 090 C 80

AMA: 2014,Jan,11

61534 **for excision of epileptogenic focus without electrocorticography during surgery**

47.4 47.4 FUD 090 C 80

AMA: 2014,Jan,11

61535 **for removal of epidural or subdural electrode array, without excision of cerebral tissue (separate procedure)**

29.1 29.1 FUD 090 C 80

AMA: 2019,Jul,10; 2014,Jan,11

61536 **for excision of cerebral epileptogenic focus, with electrocorticography during surgery (includes removal of electrode array)**

76.1 76.1 FUD 090 C 80

AMA: 2014,Jan,11

61537 **for lobectomy, temporal lobe, without electrocorticography during surgery**

72.4 72.4 FUD 090 C 80

AMA: 2014,Jan,11

61538 **for lobectomy, temporal lobe, with electrocorticography during surgery**

78.2 78.2 FUD 090 C 80

AMA: 2019,Mar,6; 2014,Jan,11

61539 **for lobectomy, other than temporal lobe, partial or total, with electrocorticography during surgery**

69.6 69.6 FUD 090 C 80

AMA: 2019,Mar,6; 2014,Jan,11

61540 **for lobectomy, other than temporal lobe, partial or total, without electrocorticography during surgery**

64.2 64.2 FUD 090 C 80

AMA: 2014,Jan,11

61541 **for transection of corpus callosum**

63.3 63.3 FUD 090 C 80

AMA: 2014,Jan,11

61543 **for partial or subtotal (functional) hemispherectomy**

61.7 61.7 FUD 090 C 80

AMA: 2014,Jan,11

61544 **for excision or coagulation of choroid plexus**

56.0 56.0 FUD 090 C 80

AMA: 2014,Jan,11

61545 **for excision of craniopharyngioma**

93.0 93.0 FUD 090 C 80

AMA: 2014,Jan,11

61546-61548 Removal Pituitary Gland/Tumor

EXCLUDES *Injection for:*
Cerebral angiography (36100-36218)
Pneumoencephalography (61055)
Ventriculography (61026, 61120)

61546 **Craniotomy for hypophysectomy or excision of pituitary tumor, intracranial approach**

68.0 68.0 FUD 090 C 80

AMA: 2014,Jan,11

61548 **Hypophysectomy or excision of pituitary tumor, transnasal or transseptal approach, nonstereotactic**

INCLUDES Operating microscope (69990)

45.8 45.8 FUD 090 C 80

AMA: 2016,Feb,12; 2014,Jan,11

61550-61559 Craniosynostosis Procedures

EXCLUDES *Injection for:*
Cerebral angiography (36100-36218)
Pneumoencephalography (61055)
Ventriculography (61026, 61120)
Orbital hypertelorism reconstruction (21260-21263)
Reconstruction (21172-21180)

61550 **Craniectomy for craniosynostosis; single cranial suture**

32.1 32.1 FUD 090 C 80

AMA: 2018,Jan,8; 2017,Jan,8; 2016,Jan,13; 2015,Jan,16; 2014,Jan,11

61552 **multiple cranial sutures**

43.5 43.5 FUD 090 C 80

AMA: 2018,Jan,8; 2017,Jan,8; 2016,Jan,13; 2015,Jan,16; 2014,Jan,11

61556 **Craniotomy for craniosynostosis; frontal or parietal bone flap**

50.1 50.1 FUD 090 C 80

AMA: 2018,Jan,8; 2017,Jan,8; 2016,Jan,13; 2015,Jan,16; 2014,Jan,11

61557 **bifrontal bone flap**

49.4 49.4 FUD 090 C 80

AMA: 2018,Jan,8; 2017,Jan,8; 2016,Jan,13; 2015,Jan,16; 2014,Jan,11

61558 **Extensive craniectomy for multiple cranial suture craniosynostosis (eg, cloverleaf skull); not requiring bone grafts**

55.2 55.2 FUD 090 C 80

AMA: 2018,Jan,8; 2017,Jan,8; 2016,Jan,13; 2015,Jan,16; 2014,Jan,11

61559 **recontouring with multiple osteotomies and bone autografts (eg, barrel-stave procedure) (includes obtaining grafts)**

70.5 70.5 FUD 090 C 80

AMA: 2018,Jan,8; 2017,Jan,8; 2016,Jan,13; 2015,Jan,16; 2014,Jan,11

61563-61564 Removal Cranial Bone Tumor With/Without Optic Nerve Decompression

EXCLUDES *Injection for:*
Cerebral angiography (36100-36218)
Pneumoencephalography (61055)
Ventriculography (61026, 61120)
Reconstruction (21181-21183)

61563 **Excision, intra and extracranial, benign tumor of cranial bone (eg, fibrous dysplasia); without optic nerve decompression**

57.5 57.5 FUD 090 C 80

AMA: 2014,Jan,11

61564 **with optic nerve decompression**

70.9 70.9 FUD 090 C 80 50

AMA: 2014,Jan,11

61566-61567 Craniotomy for Seizures

EXCLUDES *Injection for:*
Cerebral angiography (36100-36218)
Pneumoencephalography (61055)
Ventriculography (61026, 61120)

61566 **Craniotomy with elevation of bone flap; for selective amygdalohippocampectomy**

66.1 66.1 FUD 090 C 80

AMA: 2018,Nov,7; 2014,Jan,11

61567 **for multiple subpial transections, with electrocorticography during surgery**

75.5 75.5 FUD 090 C 80

AMA: 2014,Jan,11

61570-61571 Removal of Foreign Body from Brain

EXCLUDES *Injection for:*
Cerebral angiography (36100-36218)
Pneumoencephalography (61055)
Ventriculography (61026, 61120)
Sequestrectomy for osteomyelitis (61501)

61570 **Craniectomy or craniotomy; with excision of foreign body from brain**
54.5 54.5 FUD 090 C 80
AMA: 2014,Jan,11

61571 **with treatment of penetrating wound of brain**
57.3 57.3 FUD 090 C 80
AMA: 2014,Jan,11

61575-61576 Transoral Approach Posterior Cranial Fossa/Upper Cervical Cord

EXCLUDES *Arthrodesis (22548)*
Injection for:
Cerebral angiography (36100-36218)
Pneumoencephalography (61055)
Ventriculography (61026, 61120)

61575 **Transoral approach to skull base, brain stem or upper spinal cord for biopsy, decompression or excision of lesion;**
73.6 73.6 FUD 090 C 80
AMA: 2014,Jan,11

61576 **requiring splitting of tongue and/or mandible (including tracheostomy)**
121. 121. FUD 090 C 80
AMA: 2014,Jan,11

61580-61598 Surgical Approach: Cranial Fossae

EXCLUDES *Definitive surgery (61600-61616)*
Dural repair and/or reconstruction (61618-61619)
Injection for:
Cerebral angiography (36100-36218)
Pneumoencephalography (61055)
Ventriculography (61026, 61120)
Primary closure (15730, 15733, 15756-15758)

61580 **Craniofacial approach to anterior cranial fossa; extradural, including lateral rhinotomy, ethmoidectomy, sphenoidectomy, without maxillectomy or orbital exenteration**
70.3 70.3 FUD 090 C 50
AMA: 2018,Jan,8; 2017,Jan,8; 2016,Jan,13; 2015,Jan,16; 2014,Jan,11

61581 **extradural, including lateral rhinotomy, orbital exenteration, ethmoidectomy, sphenoidectomy and/or maxillectomy**
76.1 76.1 FUD 090 C 50
AMA: 2018,Jan,8; 2017,Jan,8; 2016,Jan,13; 2015,Jan,16; 2014,Jan,11

61582 **extradural, including unilateral or bifrontal craniotomy, elevation of frontal lobe(s), osteotomy of base of anterior cranial fossa**
88.5 88.5 FUD 090 C 80
AMA: 2018,Jan,8; 2017,Jan,8; 2016,Jan,13; 2015,Jan,16; 2014,Jan,11

61583 **intradural, including unilateral or bifrontal craniotomy, elevation or resection of frontal lobe, osteotomy of base of anterior cranial fossa**
84.2 84.2 FUD 090 C 80
AMA: 2018,Jan,8; 2017,Dec,13; 2017,Jan,8; 2016,Jan,13; 2015,Jan,16; 2014,Jan,11

61584 **Orbitocranial approach to anterior cranial fossa, extradural, including supraorbital ridge osteotomy and elevation of frontal and/or temporal lobe(s); without orbital exenteration**
83.7 83.7 FUD 090 C 80 50
AMA: 2018,Jan,8; 2017,Jan,8; 2016,Jan,13; 2015,Jan,16; 2014,Jan,11

61585 **with orbital exenteration**
95.1 95.1 FUD 090 C 80 50
AMA: 2018,Jan,8; 2017,Jan,8; 2016,Jan,13; 2015,Jan,16; 2014,Jan,11

61586 **Bicoronal, transzygomatic and/or LeFort I osteotomy approach to anterior cranial fossa with or without internal fixation, without bone graft**
70.5 70.5 FUD 090 C 80
AMA: 2014,Jan,11

61590 **Infratemporal pre-auricular approach to middle cranial fossa (parapharyngeal space, infratemporal and midline skull base, nasopharynx), with or without disarticulation of the mandible, including parotidectomy, craniotomy, decompression and/or mobilization of the facial nerve and/or petrous carotid artery**
88.1 88.1 FUD 090 C 80 50
AMA: 2018,Jan,8; 2017,Jan,8; 2016,Jan,13; 2015,Jan,16; 2014,Jan,11

61591 **Infratemporal post-auricular approach to middle cranial fossa (internal auditory meatus, petrous apex, tentorium, cavernous sinus, parasellar area, infratemporal fossa) including mastoidectomy, resection of sigmoid sinus, with or without decompression and/or mobilization of contents of auditory canal or petrous carotid artery**
89.1 89.1 FUD 090 C 80 50
AMA: 2018,Jan,8; 2017,Jan,8; 2016,Jan,13; 2015,Jan,16; 2014,Jan,11

61592 **Orbitocranial zygomatic approach to middle cranial fossa (cavernous sinus and carotid artery, clivus, basilar artery or petrous apex) including osteotomy of zygoma, craniotomy, extra- or intradural elevation of temporal lobe**
92.5 92.5 FUD 090 C 80 50
AMA: 2018,Jan,8; 2017,Jan,8; 2016,Jan,13; 2015,Jan,16; 2014,Jan,11

61595 **Transtemporal approach to posterior cranial fossa, jugular foramen or midline skull base, including mastoidectomy, decompression of sigmoid sinus and/or facial nerve, with or without mobilization**
68.1 68.1 FUD 090 C 50
AMA: 2018,Mar,11; 2018,Jan,8; 2017,Jan,8; 2016,Jan,13; 2015,Jan,16; 2014,Jan,11

61596 **Transcochlear approach to posterior cranial fossa, jugular foramen or midline skull base, including labyrinthectomy, decompression, with or without mobilization of facial nerve and/or petrous carotid artery**
70.1 70.1 FUD 090 C 80 50
AMA: 2018,Jan,8; 2017,Jan,8; 2016,Jan,13; 2015,Jan,16; 2014,Jan,11

61597 **Transcondylar (far lateral) approach to posterior cranial fossa, jugular foramen or midline skull base, including occipital condylectomy, mastoidectomy, resection of C1-C3 vertebral body(s), decompression of vertebral artery, with or without mobilization**
85.5 85.5 FUD 090 C 80 50
AMA: 2018,Jan,8; 2017,Jan,8; 2016,Jan,13; 2015,Jan,16; 2014,Jan,11

61598 **Transpetrosal approach to posterior cranial fossa, clivus or foramen magnum, including ligation of superior petrosal sinus and/or sigmoid sinus**
82.9 82.9 FUD 090 C 80
AMA: 2018,Jan,8; 2017,Jan,8; 2016,Jan,13; 2015,Jan,16; 2014,Jan,11

61600-61616 Definitive Procedures: Cranial Fossae

EXCLUDES *Dural repair and/or reconstruction (61618-61619)*
Injection for:
Cerebral angiography (36100-36218)
Pneumoencephalography (61055)
Ventriculography (61026, 61120)
Primary closure (15730, 15733, 15756-15758)
Surgical approach (61580-61598)

61600 Resection or excision of neoplastic, vascular or infectious lesion of base of anterior cranial fossa; extradural
61.5 61.5 FUD 090 C 80
AMA: 2018,Jan,8; 2017,Jan,8; 2016,Jan,13; 2015,Jan,16; 2014,Jan,11

61601 intradural, including dural repair, with or without graft
70.1 70.1 FUD 090 C 80
AMA: 2018,Jan,8; 2017,Jan,8; 2016,Jan,13; 2015,Jan,16; 2014,Jan,11

61605 Resection or excision of neoplastic, vascular or infectious lesion of infratemporal fossa, parapharyngeal space, petrous apex; extradural
62.1 62.1 FUD 090 C 80
AMA: 2018,Jan,8; 2017,Jan,8; 2016,Jan,13; 2015,Jan,16; 2014,Jan,11

61606 intradural, including dural repair, with or without graft
85.7 85.7 FUD 090 C 80
AMA: 2018,Jan,8; 2017,Jan,8; 2016,Jan,13; 2015,Jan,16; 2014,Jan,11

61607 Resection or excision of neoplastic, vascular or infectious lesion of parasellar area, cavernous sinus, clivus or midline skull base; extradural
77.8 77.8 FUD 090 C 80
AMA: 2018,Jan,8; 2017,Jan,8; 2016,Jan,13; 2015,Jan,16; 2014,Jan,11

61608 intradural, including dural repair, with or without graft
95.7 95.7 FUD 090 C 80
AMA: 2018,Jan,8; 2017,Jan,8; 2016,Jan,13; 2015,Jan,16; 2014,Jan,11

\+ **61611 Transection or ligation, carotid artery in petrous canal; without repair (List separately in addition to code for primary procedure)**
Code first (61605-61608)
13.8 13.8 FUD ZZZ C 80
AMA: 2018,Jan,8; 2017,Jan,8; 2016,Jan,13; 2015,Jan,16; 2014,Jan,11

61613 Obliteration of carotid aneurysm, arteriovenous malformation, or carotid-cavernous fistula by dissection within cavernous sinus
96.9 96.9 FUD 090 C 80 50
AMA: 2018,Jan,8; 2017,Jan,8; 2016,Jan,13; 2015,Jan,16; 2014,Jan,11

61615 Resection or excision of neoplastic, vascular or infectious lesion of base of posterior cranial fossa, jugular foramen, foramen magnum, or C1-C3 vertebral bodies; extradural
81.9 81.9 FUD 090 C 80
AMA: 2018,Jan,8; 2017,Jan,8; 2016,Jan,13; 2015,Jan,16; 2014,Jan,11

61616 intradural, including dural repair, with or without graft
97.3 97.3 FUD 090 C 80
AMA: 2018,Mar,11; 2018,Jan,8; 2017,Jan,8; 2016,Jan,13; 2015,Jan,16; 2014,Jan,11

61618-61619 Reconstruction Post-Surgical Cranial Fossae Defects

EXCLUDES *Definitive surgery (61600-61616)*
Injection for:
Cerebral angiography (36100-36218)
Pneumoencephalography (61055)
Ventriculography (61026, 61120)
Primary closure (15730, 15733, 15756-15758)
Surgical approach (61580-61598)

61618 Secondary repair of dura for cerebrospinal fluid leak, anterior, middle or posterior cranial fossa following surgery of the skull base; by free tissue graft (eg, pericranium, fascia, tensor fascia lata, adipose tissue, homologous or synthetic grafts)
37.5 37.5 FUD 090 C 80
AMA: 2018,Jan,8; 2017,Jan,8; 2016,Jan,13; 2015,Jan,16; 2014,Jan,11

61619 by local or regionalized vascularized pedicle flap or myocutaneous flap (including galea, temporalis, frontalis or occipitalis muscle)
41.3 41.3 FUD 090 C 80
AMA: 2018,Jan,8; 2017,Jan,8; 2016,Jan,13; 2015,Jan,16; 2014,Jan,11

61623-61651 Neurovascular Interventional Procedures

61623 Endovascular temporary balloon arterial occlusion, head or neck (extracranial/intracranial) including selective catheterization of vessel to be occluded, positioning and inflation of occlusion balloon, concomitant neurological monitoring, and radiologic supervision and interpretation of all angiography required for balloon occlusion and to exclude vascular injury post occlusion

EXCLUDES *Diagnostic angiography of target artery just before temporary occlusion; report only radiological supervision and interpretation*
Selective catheterization and angiography of artery besides the target artery; report catheterization and radiological supervision and interpretation codes as appropriate

16.6 16.6 FUD 000 J
AMA: 2018,Jan,8; 2017,Jan,8; 2016,Jan,13; 2015,Jan,16; 2014,Jan,11

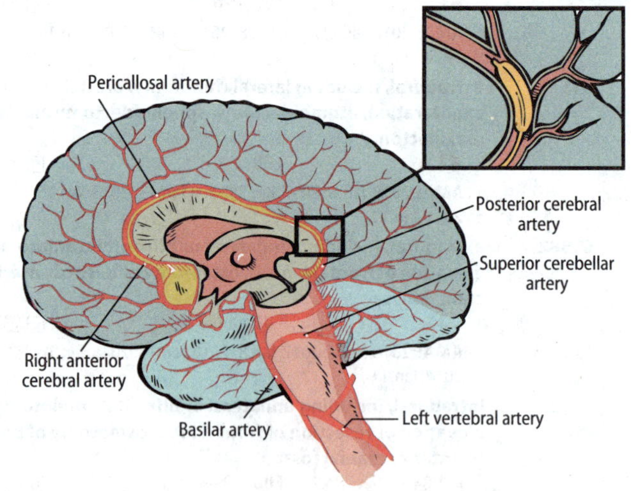

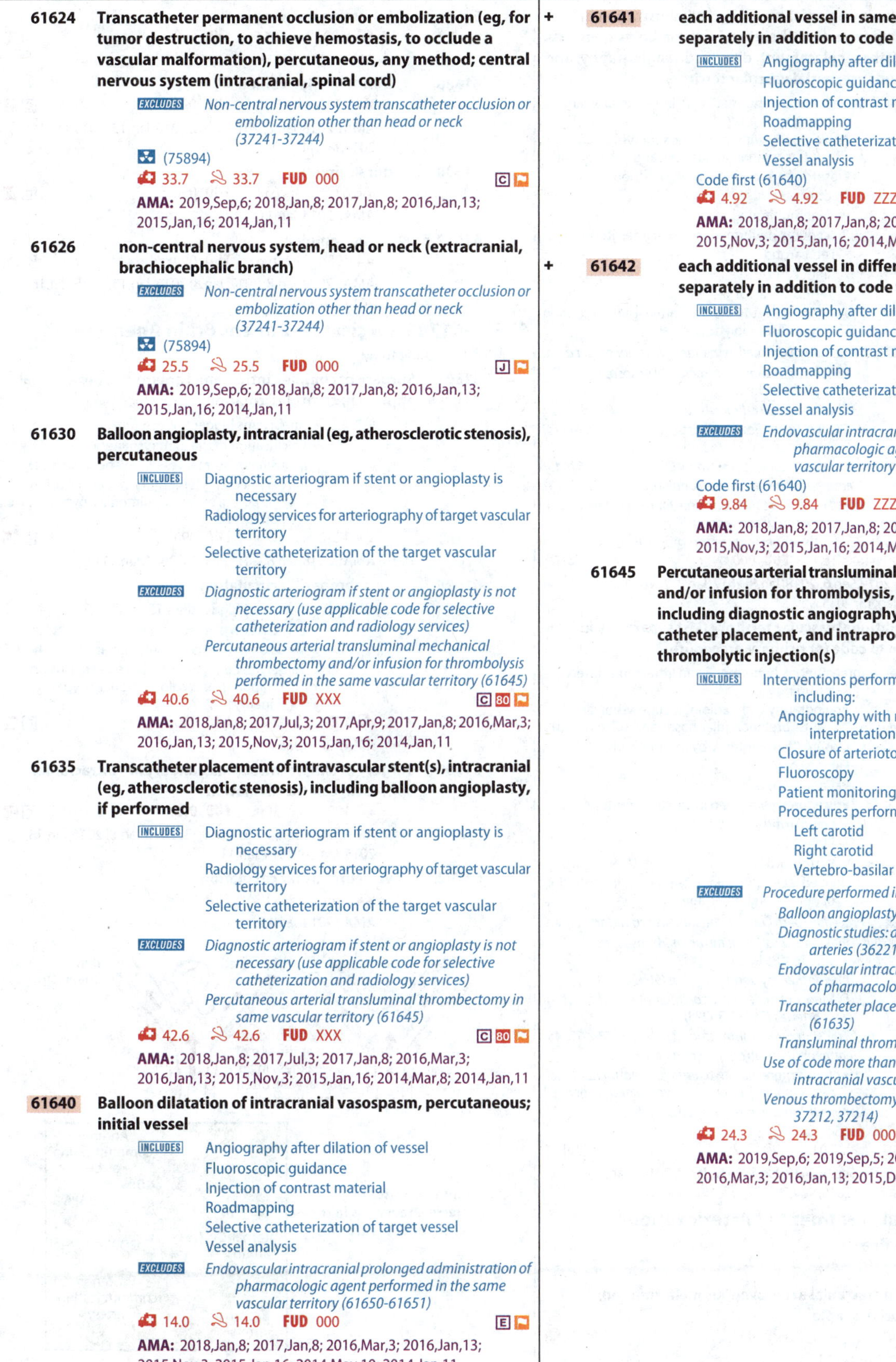

61624 Transcatheter permanent occlusion or embolization (eg, for tumor destruction, to achieve hemostasis, to occlude a vascular malformation), percutaneous, any method; central nervous system (intracranial, spinal cord)

EXCLUDES *Non-central nervous system transcatheter occlusion or embolization other than head or neck (37241-37244)*

(75894)

33.7 33.7 FUD 000 C

AMA: 2019,Sep,6; 2018,Jan,8; 2017,Jan,8; 2016,Jan,13; 2015,Jan,16; 2014,Jan,11

61626 non-central nervous system, head or neck (extracranial, brachiocephalic branch)

EXCLUDES *Non-central nervous system transcatheter occlusion or embolization other than head or neck (37241-37244)*

(75894)

25.5 25.5 FUD 000 J

AMA: 2019,Sep,6; 2018,Jan,8; 2017,Jan,8; 2016,Jan,13; 2015,Jan,16; 2014,Jan,11

61630 Balloon angioplasty, intracranial (eg, atherosclerotic stenosis), percutaneous

INCLUDES Diagnostic arteriogram if stent or angioplasty is necessary
Radiology services for arteriography of target vascular territory
Selective catheterization of the target vascular territory

EXCLUDES *Diagnostic arteriogram if stent or angioplasty is not necessary (use applicable code for selective catheterization and radiology services)*
Percutaneous arterial transluminal mechanical thrombectomy and/or infusion for thrombolysis performed in the same vascular territory (61645)

40.6 40.6 FUD XXX C 80

AMA: 2018,Jan,8; 2017,Jul,3; 2017,Apr,9; 2017,Jan,8; 2016,Mar,3; 2016,Jan,13; 2015,Nov,3; 2015,Jan,16; 2014,Jan,11

61635 Transcatheter placement of intravascular stent(s), intracranial (eg, atherosclerotic stenosis), including balloon angioplasty, if performed

INCLUDES Diagnostic arteriogram if stent or angioplasty is necessary
Radiology services for arteriography of target vascular territory
Selective catheterization of the target vascular territory

EXCLUDES *Diagnostic arteriogram if stent or angioplasty is not necessary (use applicable code for selective catheterization and radiology services)*
Percutaneous arterial transluminal thrombectomy in same vascular territory (61645)

42.6 42.6 FUD XXX C 80

AMA: 2018,Jan,8; 2017,Jul,3; 2017,Jan,8; 2016,Mar,3; 2016,Jan,13; 2015,Nov,3; 2015,Jan,16; 2014,Mar,8; 2014,Jan,11

61640 Balloon dilatation of intracranial vasospasm, percutaneous; initial vessel

INCLUDES Angiography after dilation of vessel
Fluoroscopic guidance
Injection of contrast material
Roadmapping
Selective catheterization of target vessel
Vessel analysis

EXCLUDES *Endovascular intracranial prolonged administration of pharmacologic agent performed in the same vascular territory (61650-61651)*

14.0 14.0 FUD 000 E

AMA: 2018,Jan,8; 2017,Jan,8; 2016,Mar,3; 2016,Jan,13; 2015,Nov,3; 2015,Jan,16; 2014,May,10; 2014,Jan,11

+ **61641 each additional vessel in same vascular territory (List separately in addition to code for primary procedure)**

INCLUDES Angiography after dilation of vessel
Fluoroscopic guidance
Injection of contrast material
Roadmapping
Selective catheterization of target vessel
Vessel analysis

Code first (61640)

4.92 4.92 FUD ZZZ E

AMA: 2018,Jan,8; 2017,Jan,8; 2016,Mar,3; 2016,Jan,13; 2015,Nov,3; 2015,Jan,16; 2014,May,10; 2014,Jan,11

+ **61642 each additional vessel in different vascular territory (List separately in addition to code for primary procedure))**

INCLUDES Angiography after dilation of vessel
Fluoroscopic guidance
Injection of contrast material
Roadmapping
Selective catheterization of target vessel
Vessel analysis

EXCLUDES *Endovascular intracranial prolonged administration of pharmacologic agent performed in the same vascular territory (61650-61651)*

Code first (61640)

9.84 9.84 FUD ZZZ E

AMA: 2018,Jan,8; 2017,Jan,8; 2016,Mar,3; 2016,Jan,13; 2015,Nov,3; 2015,Jan,16; 2014,May,10; 2014,Jan,11

61645 Percutaneous arterial transluminal mechanical thrombectomy and/or infusion for thrombolysis, intracranial, any method, including diagnostic angiography, fluoroscopic guidance, catheter placement, and intraprocedural pharmacological thrombolytic injection(s)

INCLUDES Interventions performed in an intracranial artery including:
- Angiography with radiologic supervision and interpretation (diagnostic and subsequent)
- Closure of arteriotomy by any method
- Fluoroscopy
- Patient monitoring
- Procedures performed in vascular territories:
  - Left carotid
  - Right carotid
  - Vertebro-basilar

EXCLUDES *Procedure performed in the same vascular target area:*
- *Balloon angioplasty, intracranial (61630)*
- *Diagnostic studies: aortic arch, carotid, and vertebral arteries (36221-36228)*
- *Endovascular intracranial prolonged administration of pharmacologic agent (61650-61651)*
- *Transcatheter placement of intravascular stent (61635)*
- *Transluminal thrombectomy (37184, 37186)*

Use of code more than one time for treatment of each intracranial vascular territory
Venous thrombectomy or thrombolysis (37187-37188, 37212, 37214)

24.3 24.3 FUD 000 C 80 50

AMA: 2019,Sep,6; 2019,Sep,5; 2018,Jan,8; 2017,Jan,8; 2016,Mar,3; 2016,Jan,13; 2015,Dec,18; 2015,Nov,3

Nervous System

61624 — 61645

61650 **Endovascular intracranial prolonged administration of pharmacologic agent(s) other than for thrombolysis, arterial, including catheter placement, diagnostic angiography, and imaging guidance; initial vascular territory**

INCLUDES Interventions performed in an intracranial artery, including:
- Angiography with radiologic supervision and interpretation (diagnostic and subsequent)
- Closure of arteriotomy by any method
- Fluoroscopy
- Patient monitoring
- Procedures performed in vascular territories:
  - Left carotid
  - Right carotid
  - Vertebro-basilar

Prolonged (at least 10 minutes) arterial administration of non-thrombolytic agents

EXCLUDES *Procedure performed in the same vascular target area:*
- *Balloon dilatation of intracranial vasospasm (61640-61642)*
- *Chemotherapy administration (96420-96425)*
- *Diagnostic studies: aortic arch, carotid, and vertebral arteries (36221-36228)*
- *Transluminal thrombectomy (37184, 37186, 61645)*

Treatment of an iatrogenic condition

Use of code more than one time for treatment of each intracranial vascular territory

Venous thrombectomy or thrombolysis

16.1 16.1 **FUD** 000 C

AMA: 2019,Sep,6; 2018,Jan,8; 2017,Jan,8; 2016,Mar,3; 2016,Jan,13; 2015,Nov,3

\+ **61651** **each additional vascular territory (List separately in addition to code for primary procedure)**

INCLUDES Interventions performed in an intracranial artery including:
- Angiography with radiologic supervision and interpretation (diagnostic and subsequent)
- Closure of arteriotomy by any method
- Fluoroscopy
- Patient monitoring
- Procedures performed in vascular territories:
  - Left carotid
  - Right carotid
  - Vertebro-basilar

Prolonged (at least 10 minutes) arterial administration of non-thrombolytic agents

EXCLUDES *Procedure performed in the same vascular target area:*
- *Balloon dilatation of intracranial vasospasm (61640-61642)*
- *Chemotherapy administration (96420-96425)*
- *Diagnostic studies: aortic arch, carotid, and vertebral arteries (36221-36228)*
- *Transluminal thrombectomy (37184, 37186, 61645)*

Treatment of an iatrogenic condition

Use of code more than two times for treatment of the two remaining intracranial vascular territory(ies)

Venous thrombectomy or thrombolysis

Code first (61650)

7.01 7.01 **FUD** ZZZ C

AMA: 2019,Sep,6; 2018,Jan,8; 2017,Jan,8; 2016,Mar,3; 2016,Jan,13; 2015,Nov,3

61680-61692 Surgical Treatment of Arteriovenous Malformation of the Brain

INCLUDES Craniotomy

61680 **Surgery of intracranial arteriovenous malformation; supratentorial, simple**

66.1 66.1 **FUD** 090 C 80

AMA: 2014,Jan,11

61682 **supratentorial, complex**

123. 123. **FUD** 090 C 80

AMA: 2018,Jan,8; 2017,Jan,8; 2016,Jan,13; 2015,Jan,16; 2014,Jan,11

61684 **infratentorial, simple**

84.0 84.0 **FUD** 090 C 80

AMA: 2014,Jan,11

61686 **infratentorial, complex**

136. 136. **FUD** 090 C 80

AMA: 2018,Jan,8; 2017,Jan,8; 2016,Jan,13; 2015,Jan,16; 2014,Jan,11

61690 **dural, simple**

63.6 63.6 **FUD** 090 C 80

AMA: 2014,Jan,11

61692 **dural, complex**

108. 108. **FUD** 090 C 80

AMA: 2018,Jan,8; 2017,Jan,8; 2016,Jan,13; 2015,Jan,16; 2014,Jan,11

61697-61703 Surgical Treatment Brain Aneurysm

INCLUDES Craniotomy

61697 **Surgery of complex intracranial aneurysm, intracranial approach; carotid circulation**

INCLUDES Aneurysms bigger than 15 mm
- Calcification of the aneurysm neck
- Inclusion of normal vessels in aneurysm neck
- Surgery needing temporary vessel occlusion, trapping, or cardiopulmonary bypass to treat aneurysm

125. 125. **FUD** 090 C 80

AMA: 2018,Jan,8; 2017,Dec,13; 2014,Jan,11

61698 **vertebrobasilar circulation**

INCLUDES Aneurysm bigger than 15 mm
- Calcification of aneurysm neck
- Inclusion of normal vessels into aneurysm neck
- Surgery needing temporary vessel occlusion, trapping, or cardiopulmonary bypass to treat aneurysm

140. 140. **FUD** 090 C 80

AMA: 2014,Jan,11

61700 **Surgery of simple intracranial aneurysm, intracranial approach; carotid circulation**

100. 100. **FUD** 090 C 80

AMA: 2018,Jan,8; 2017,Dec,13; 2017,Jan,8; 2016,Jan,13; 2015,Jan,16; 2014,Jan,11

61702 **vertebrobasilar circulation**

118. 118. **FUD** 090 C 80

AMA: 2014,Jan,11

Berry aneurysm

Berry aneurysms form at the site of a weakness in an arterial wall, often at a junction

Common sites of berry aneurysms in the circle of Willis arteries

Anterior communicating artery
40%
34%
Internal carotid
4%
20%
Posterior communicating artery
Basilar artery

61703 **Surgery of intracranial aneurysm, cervical approach by application of occluding clamp to cervical carotid artery (Selverstone-Crutchfield type)**

EXCLUDES *Cervical approach for direct ligation of carotid artery (37600-37606)*

39.9 39.9 **FUD** 090 C 80

AMA: 2014,Jan,11

61705-61710 Other Procedures for Aneurysm, Arteriovenous Malformation, and Carotid-Cavernous Fistula

INCLUDES Craniotomy

61705 **Surgery of aneurysm, vascular malformation or carotid-cavernous fistula; by intracranial and cervical occlusion of carotid artery**

73.6 73.6 **FUD** 090 C 80

AMA: 2014,Jan,11

61708 **by intracranial electrothrombosis**

EXCLUDES *Ligation or gradual occlusion of internal or common carotid artery (37605-37606)*

75.1 75.1 **FUD** 090 C 80

AMA: 2014,Jan,11

61710 **by intra-arterial embolization, injection procedure, or balloon catheter**

63.3 63.3 **FUD** 090 C 80

AMA: 2018,Jan,8; 2017,Jan,8; 2016,Jan,13; 2015,Jan,16; 2014,Jan,11

61711 Extracranial-Intracranial Bypass

CMS: 100-02,16,10 Exclusions from Coverage; 100-03,20.2 Extracranial-intracranial (EC-IC) Arterial Bypass Surgery

INCLUDES Craniotomy

EXCLUDES *Carotid or vertebral thromboendarterectomy (35301)*

Code also operating microscope when appropriate (69990)

61711 **Anastomosis, arterial, extracranial-intracranial (eg, middle cerebral/cortical) arteries**

75.8 75.8 **FUD** 090 C 80

AMA: 2014,Jan,11

61720-61791 Stereotactic Procedures of the Brain

61720 **Creation of lesion by stereotactic method, including burr hole(s) and localizing and recording techniques, single or multiple stages; globus pallidus or thalamus**

37.3 37.3 **FUD** 090 J

AMA: 2018,Jan,8; 2017,Jan,8; 2016,Jan,13; 2015,Jan,16; 2014,Jul,8; 2014,Jan,11

61735 **subcortical structure(s) other than globus pallidus or thalamus**

46.8 46.8 **FUD** 090 C

AMA: 2014,Jul,8; 2014,Jan,11

61750 **Stereotactic biopsy, aspiration, or excision, including burr hole(s), for intracranial lesion;**

41.4 41.4 **FUD** 090 C

AMA: 2018,Jan,8; 2017,Jan,8; 2016,Jan,13; 2015,Jan,16; 2014,Jul,8; 2014,Jan,11

61751 **with computed tomography and/or magnetic resonance guidance**

(70450, 70460, 70470, 70551-70553)

40.4 40.4 **FUD** 090 C

AMA: 2018,Jan,8; 2017,Jan,8; 2016,Jan,13; 2015,Jan,16; 2014,Jul,8; 2014,Jan,11

61760 **Stereotactic implantation of depth electrodes into the cerebrum for long-term seizure monitoring**

46.0 46.0 **FUD** 090 C

AMA: 2014,Jul,8; 2014,Jan,11

61770 **Stereotactic localization, including burr hole(s), with insertion of catheter(s) or probe(s) for placement of radiation source**

47.7 47.7 **FUD** 090 J G2

AMA: 2018,Jan,8; 2017,Jan,8; 2016,Jan,13; 2015,Jan,16; 2014,Jul,8; 2014,Jan,11

+ **61781** **Stereotactic computer-assisted (navigational) procedure; cranial, intradural (List separately in addition to code for primary procedure)**

EXCLUDES *Creation of lesion by stereotactic method (61720-61791)*
Extradural stereotactic computer-assisted procedure for same surgical session by same individual (61782)
Radiation treatment delivery, stereotactic radiosurgery (SRS) (77371-77373)
Stereotactic implantation of neurostimulator electrode array (61863-61868)
Stereotactic radiation treatment management (77432)
Stereotactic radiosurgery (61796-61799)
Ventriculocisternostomy (62201)

Code first primary procedure

6.94 6.94 **FUD** ZZZ N N1 80

AMA: 2018,Jan,8; 2017,Jan,8; 2016,Jan,13; 2015,Jan,16; 2014,Sep,13; 2014,Jul,8; 2014,Jan,11

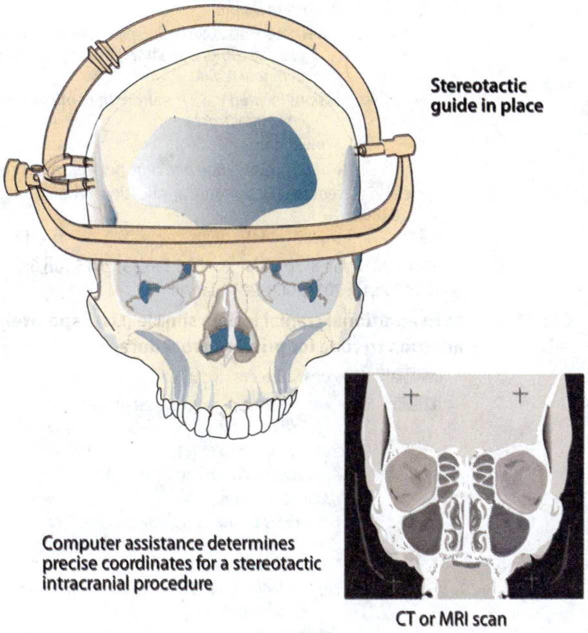

Stereotactic guide in place

Computer assistance determines precise coordinates for a stereotactic intracranial procedure

CT or MRI scan

+ **61782** **cranial, extradural (List separately in addition to code for primary procedure)**

EXCLUDES *Intradural stereotactic computer-assisted procedure for same surgical session by same individual (61781)*
Stereotactic radiosurgery (61796-61799)

Code first primary procedure

5.02 5.02 **FUD** ZZZ N N1 80

AMA: 2018,Apr,3; 2018,Jan,8; 2017,Jan,8; 2016,Jan,13; 2015,Jan,16; 2014,Jul,8; 2014,Jan,11

+ **61783** **spinal (List separately in addition to code for primary procedure)**

EXCLUDES *Stereotactic radiosurgery (61796-61799, 63620-63621)*

Code first primary procedure

6.80 6.80 **FUD** ZZZ N N1 80

AMA: 2018,Jan,8; 2017,Jan,8; 2016,Jan,13; 2015,Jan,16; 2014,Jul,8; 2014,Jan,11

61790 **Creation of lesion by stereotactic method, percutaneous, by neurolytic agent (eg, alcohol, thermal, electrical, radiofrequency); gasserian ganglion**

25.7 25.7 **FUD** 090 J A2 50

AMA: 2014,Jul,8; 2014,Jan,11

61791 **trigeminal medullary tract**

33.0 33.0 **FUD** 090 J A2 80 50

AMA: 2018,Jan,8; 2017,Jan,8; 2016,Jan,13; 2015,Jan,16; 2014,Jul,8; 2014,Jan,11

61796-61800 Stereotactic Radiosurgery (SRS): Brain

INCLUDES Planning, dosimetry, targeting, positioning or blocking performed by the neurosurgeon

EXCLUDES *Application of cranial tongs, caliper, or stereotactic frame (20660)*
Intensity modulated beam delivery plan and treatment (77301, 77385-77386)
Radiation treatment management and radiosurgery by the same provider (77427-77435)
Stereotactic body radiation therapy (77373, 77435)
Stereotactic radiosurgery more than once per lesion per treatment course
Treatment planning, physics and dosimetry, and treatment delivery performed by the radiation oncologist

61796 Stereotactic radiosurgery (particle beam, gamma ray, or linear accelerator); 1 simple cranial lesion

INCLUDES Lesions < 3.5 cm

EXCLUDES *Stereotactic computer-assisted procedures (61781-61783)*
Stereotactic radiosurgery (61798)
Treatment of complex lesions: (61798-61799)
Arteriovenous malformations (AVM)
Brainstem lesions
Cavernous sinus/parasellar/petroclival tumors, glomus tumors, pituitary tumors, and tumors of pineal region
Lesions located <= 5 mm from the optic nerve, chasm, or tract
Schwannomas
Use of code more than one time per treatment course

Code also stereotactic headframe application, when performed (61800)

29.7 29.7 FUD 090 B 80

AMA: 2018,Jan,8; 2017,Jan,8; 2016,Jan,13; 2015,Jun,6; 2015,Jan,16; 2014,Jul,8; 2014,Jan,11

\+ **61797 each additional cranial lesion, simple (List separately in addition to code for primary procedure)**

INCLUDES Lesions < 3.5 cm

EXCLUDES *Stereotactic computer-assisted procedures (61781-61783)*
Treatment of complex lesions: (61798-61799)
Arteriovenous malformations (AVM)
Brainstem lesion
Cavernous sinus/parasellar/petroclival tumors, glomus tumors, pituitary tumor, tumors of pineal region
Lesions located <= 5 mm from the optic nerve, chasm, or tract
Schwannomas
Use of code for additional stereotactic radiosurgery more than four times in total per treatment course when used alone or in combination with (61799)

Code first (61796, 61798)

6.48 6.48 FUD ZZZ B 80

AMA: 2018,Jan,8; 2017,Jan,8; 2016,Jan,13; 2015,Jun,6; 2015,Jan,16; 2014,Jul,8; 2014,Jan,11

61798 1 complex cranial lesion

INCLUDES All therapeutic lesion creation procedures
Treatment of complex lesions:
Arteriovenous malformations (AVM)
Brainstem lesions
Cavernous sinus, parasellar, petroclival, glomus, pineal region, and pituitary tumors
Lesions located <= 5 mm from the optic nerve, chasm, or tract
Lesions >= 3.5 cm
Schwannomas
Treatment of multiple lesions as long as one is complex

EXCLUDES *Stereotactic computer-assisted procedures (61781-61783)*
Stereotactic radiosurgery (61796)
Use of code more than one time per treatment course

Code also stereotactic headframe application, when performed (61800)

40.5 40.5 FUD 090 B 80

AMA: 2018,Jan,8; 2017,Jan,8; 2016,Jan,13; 2015,Jun,6; 2015,Jan,16; 2014,Jul,8; 2014,Jan,11

\+ **61799 each additional cranial lesion, complex (List separately in addition to code for primary procedure)**

INCLUDES All therapeutic lesion creation procedures
Treatment of complex lesions:
Arteriovenous malformations (AVM)
Brainstem lesions
Cavernous sinus, parasellar, petroclival, glomus, pineal region, and pituitary tumors
Lesions located <= 5 mm from the optic nerve, chasm, or tract
Lesions >= 3.5 cm
Schwannomas

EXCLUDES *Stereotactic computer-assisted procedures (61781-61783)*
Use of code for additional stereotactic radiosurgery more than four times in total per treatment course when used alone or in combination with (61797)

Code first (61798)

8.98 8.98 FUD ZZZ B 80

AMA: 2018,Jan,8; 2017,Jan,8; 2016,Jan,13; 2015,Jun,6; 2015,Jan,16; 2014,Jul,8; 2014,Jan,11

\+ **61800 Application of stereotactic headframe for stereotactic radiosurgery (List separately in addition to code for primary procedure)**

Code first (61796, 61798)

4.52 4.52 FUD ZZZ B 80

AMA: 2018,Jan,8; 2017,Jan,8; 2016,Jan,13; 2015,Jun,6; 2015,Jan,16; 2014,Jan,11

61850-61888 Intracranial Neurostimulation

INCLUDES Analysis of system at time of implantation (95970)
Microelectrode recording by operating surgeon

EXCLUDES *Electronic analysis and reprogramming of neurostimulator pulse generator (95970, 95976-95977, [95983, 95984])*
Neurophysiological mapping by another physician/qualified health care professional (95961-95962)

61850 Twist drill or burr hole(s) for implantation of neurostimulator electrodes, cortical

28.1 28.1 FUD 090 C 80

AMA: 2019,Feb,6; 2018,Jan,8; 2017,Jan,8; 2016,Jan,13; 2015,Jan,16; 2014,Jan,11

61860 Craniectomy or craniotomy for implantation of neurostimulator electrodes, cerebral, cortical

46.0 46.0 FUD 090 C 80

AMA: 2019,Feb,6; 2018,Jan,8; 2017,Jan,8; 2016,Jan,13; 2015,Jan,16; 2014,Jan,11

61863 Twist drill, burr hole, craniotomy, or craniectomy with stereotactic implantation of neurostimulator electrode array in subcortical site (eg, thalamus, globus pallidus, subthalamic nucleus, periventricular, periaqueductal gray), without use of intraoperative microelectrode recording; first array

43.9 43.9 FUD 090 C 80 50

AMA: 2019,Feb,6; 2018,Jan,8; 2017,Jan,8; 2016,Jan,13; 2015,Jan,16; 2014,Jul,8; 2014,Jan,11

\+ **61864 each additional array (List separately in addition to primary procedure)**

Code first (61863)

8.36 8.36 FUD ZZZ C 80

AMA: 2019,Feb,6; 2014,Jul,8; 2014,Jan,11

61867 Twist drill, burr hole, craniotomy, or craniectomy with stereotactic implantation of neurostimulator electrode array in subcortical site (eg, thalamus, globus pallidus, subthalamic nucleus, periventricular, periaqueductal gray), with use of intraoperative microelectrode recording; first array

66.8 66.8 FUD 090 C 80 50

AMA: 2019,Feb,6; 2014,Jul,8; 2014,Jan,11

\+ **61868 each additional array (List separately in addition to primary procedure)**

Code first (61867)

14.7 14.7 FUD ZZZ C 80

AMA: 2019,Feb,6; 2018,Jan,8; 2017,Jan,8; 2016,Jan,13; 2015,Jan,16; 2014,Jul,8; 2014,Jan,11

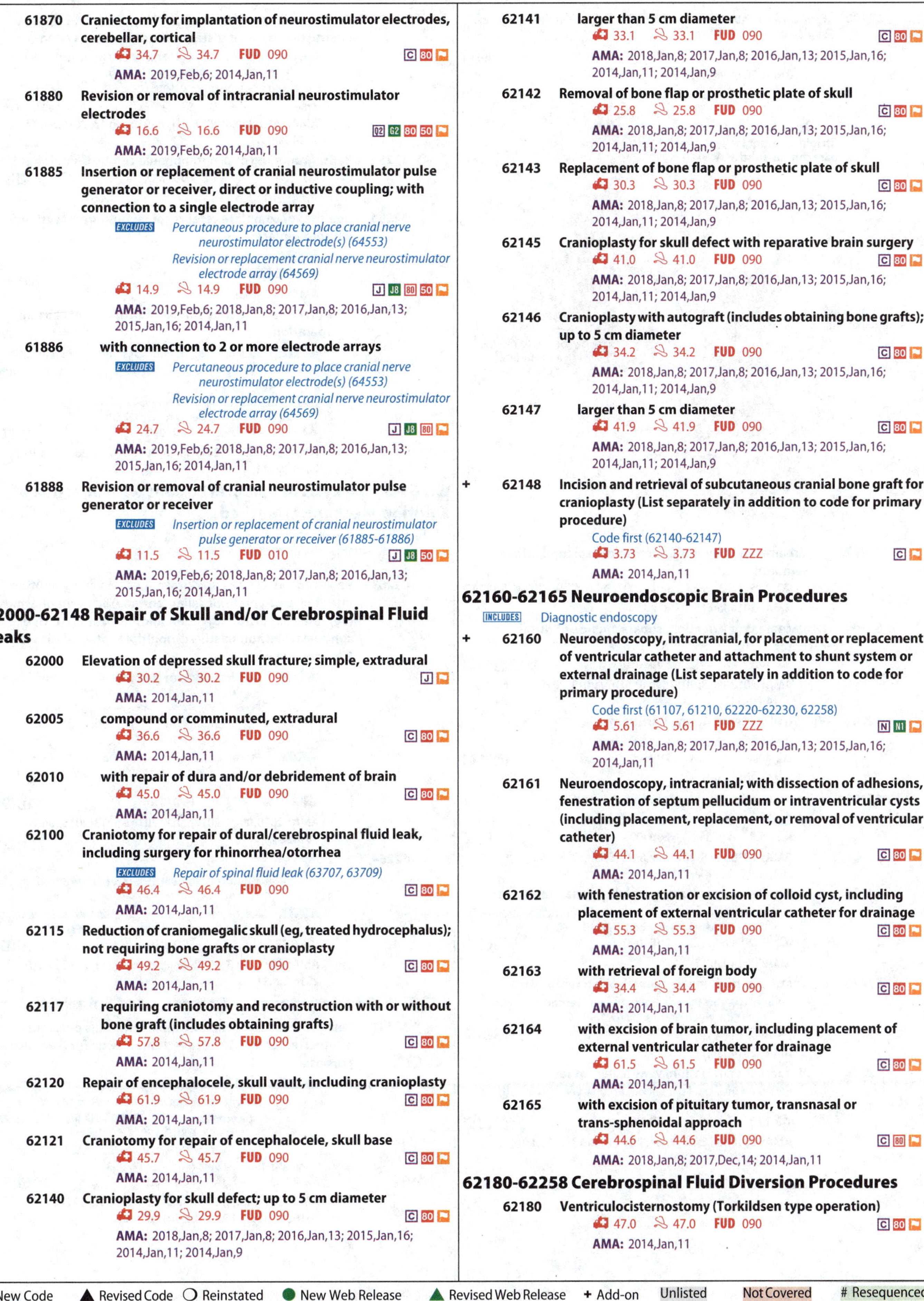

61870 **Craniectomy for implantation of neurostimulator electrodes, cerebellar, cortical**
34.7 34.7 FUD 090 C 80
AMA: 2019,Feb,6; 2014,Jan,11

61880 **Revision or removal of intracranial neurostimulator electrodes**
16.6 16.6 FUD 090 Q2 G2 80 50
AMA: 2019,Feb,6; 2014,Jan,11

61885 **Insertion or replacement of cranial neurostimulator pulse generator or receiver, direct or inductive coupling; with connection to a single electrode array**
EXCLUDES *Percutaneous procedure to place cranial nerve neurostimulator electrode(s) (64553)*
Revision or replacement cranial nerve neurostimulator electrode array (64569)
14.9 14.9 FUD 090 J J8 80 50
AMA: 2019,Feb,6; 2018,Jan,8; 2017,Jan,8; 2016,Jan,13; 2015,Jan,16; 2014,Jan,11

61886 **with connection to 2 or more electrode arrays**
EXCLUDES *Percutaneous procedure to place cranial nerve neurostimulator electrode(s) (64553)*
Revision or replacement cranial nerve neurostimulator electrode array (64569)
24.7 24.7 FUD 090 J J8 80
AMA: 2019,Feb,6; 2018,Jan,8; 2017,Jan,8; 2016,Jan,13; 2015,Jan,16; 2014,Jan,11

61888 **Revision or removal of cranial neurostimulator pulse generator or receiver**
EXCLUDES *Insertion or replacement of cranial neurostimulator pulse generator or receiver (61885-61886)*
11.5 11.5 FUD 010 J J8 50
AMA: 2019,Feb,6; 2018,Jan,8; 2017,Jan,8; 2016,Jan,13; 2015,Jan,16; 2014,Jan,11

62000-62148 Repair of Skull and/or Cerebrospinal Fluid Leaks

62000 **Elevation of depressed skull fracture; simple, extradural**
30.2 30.2 FUD 090 J
AMA: 2014,Jan,11

62005 **compound or comminuted, extradural**
36.6 36.6 FUD 090 C 80
AMA: 2014,Jan,11

62010 **with repair of dura and/or debridement of brain**
45.0 45.0 FUD 090 C 80
AMA: 2014,Jan,11

62100 **Craniotomy for repair of dural/cerebrospinal fluid leak, including surgery for rhinorrhea/otorrhea**
EXCLUDES *Repair of spinal fluid leak (63707, 63709)*
46.4 46.4 FUD 090 C 80
AMA: 2014,Jan,11

62115 **Reduction of craniomegalic skull (eg, treated hydrocephalus); not requiring bone grafts or cranioplasty**
49.2 49.2 FUD 090 C 80
AMA: 2014,Jan,11

62117 **requiring craniotomy and reconstruction with or without bone graft (includes obtaining grafts)**
57.8 57.8 FUD 090 C 80
AMA: 2014,Jan,11

62120 **Repair of encephalocele, skull vault, including cranioplasty**
61.9 61.9 FUD 090 C 80
AMA: 2014,Jan,11

62121 **Craniotomy for repair of encephalocele, skull base**
45.7 45.7 FUD 090 C 80
AMA: 2014,Jan,11

62140 **Cranioplasty for skull defect; up to 5 cm diameter**
29.9 29.9 FUD 090 C 80
AMA: 2018,Jan,8; 2017,Jan,8; 2016,Jan,13; 2015,Jan,16; 2014,Jan,11; 2014,Jan,9

62141 **larger than 5 cm diameter**
33.1 33.1 FUD 090 C 80
AMA: 2018,Jan,8; 2017,Jan,8; 2016,Jan,13; 2015,Jan,16; 2014,Jan,11; 2014,Jan,9

62142 **Removal of bone flap or prosthetic plate of skull**
25.8 25.8 FUD 090 C 80
AMA: 2018,Jan,8; 2017,Jan,8; 2016,Jan,13; 2015,Jan,16; 2014,Jan,11; 2014,Jan,9

62143 **Replacement of bone flap or prosthetic plate of skull**
30.3 30.3 FUD 090 C 80
AMA: 2018,Jan,8; 2017,Jan,8; 2016,Jan,13; 2015,Jan,16; 2014,Jan,11; 2014,Jan,9

62145 **Cranioplasty for skull defect with reparative brain surgery**
41.0 41.0 FUD 090 C 80
AMA: 2018,Jan,8; 2017,Jan,8; 2016,Jan,13; 2015,Jan,16; 2014,Jan,11; 2014,Jan,9

62146 **Cranioplasty with autograft (includes obtaining bone grafts); up to 5 cm diameter**
34.2 34.2 FUD 090 C 80
AMA: 2018,Jan,8; 2017,Jan,8; 2016,Jan,13; 2015,Jan,16; 2014,Jan,11; 2014,Jan,9

62147 **larger than 5 cm diameter**
41.9 41.9 FUD 090 C 80
AMA: 2018,Jan,8; 2017,Jan,8; 2016,Jan,13; 2015,Jan,16; 2014,Jan,11; 2014,Jan,9

\+ **62148** **Incision and retrieval of subcutaneous cranial bone graft for cranioplasty (List separately in addition to code for primary procedure)**
Code first (62140-62147)
3.73 3.73 FUD ZZZ C
AMA: 2014,Jan,11

62160-62165 Neuroendoscopic Brain Procedures

INCLUDES Diagnostic endoscopy

\+ **62160** **Neuroendoscopy, intracranial, for placement or replacement of ventricular catheter and attachment to shunt system or external drainage (List separately in addition to code for primary procedure)**
Code first (61107, 61210, 62220-62230, 62258)
5.61 5.61 FUD ZZZ N N1
AMA: 2018,Jan,8; 2017,Jan,8; 2016,Jan,13; 2015,Jan,16; 2014,Jan,11

62161 **Neuroendoscopy, intracranial; with dissection of adhesions, fenestration of septum pellucidum or intraventricular cysts (including placement, replacement, or removal of ventricular catheter)**
44.1 44.1 FUD 090 C 80
AMA: 2014,Jan,11

62162 **with fenestration or excision of colloid cyst, including placement of external ventricular catheter for drainage**
55.3 55.3 FUD 090 C 80
AMA: 2014,Jan,11

62163 **with retrieval of foreign body**
34.4 34.4 FUD 090 C 80
AMA: 2014,Jan,11

62164 **with excision of brain tumor, including placement of external ventricular catheter for drainage**
61.5 61.5 FUD 090 C 80
AMA: 2014,Jan,11

62165 **with excision of pituitary tumor, transnasal or trans-sphenoidal approach**
44.6 44.6 FUD 090 C 80
AMA: 2018,Jan,8; 2017,Dec,14; 2014,Jan,11

62180-62258 Cerebrospinal Fluid Diversion Procedures

62180 **Ventriculocisternostomy (Torkildsen type operation)**
47.0 47.0 FUD 090 C 80
AMA: 2014,Jan,11

62190 **Creation of shunt; subarachnoid/subdural-atrial, -jugular, -auricular**
27.1 27.1 FUD 090 C
AMA: 2014,Jan,11

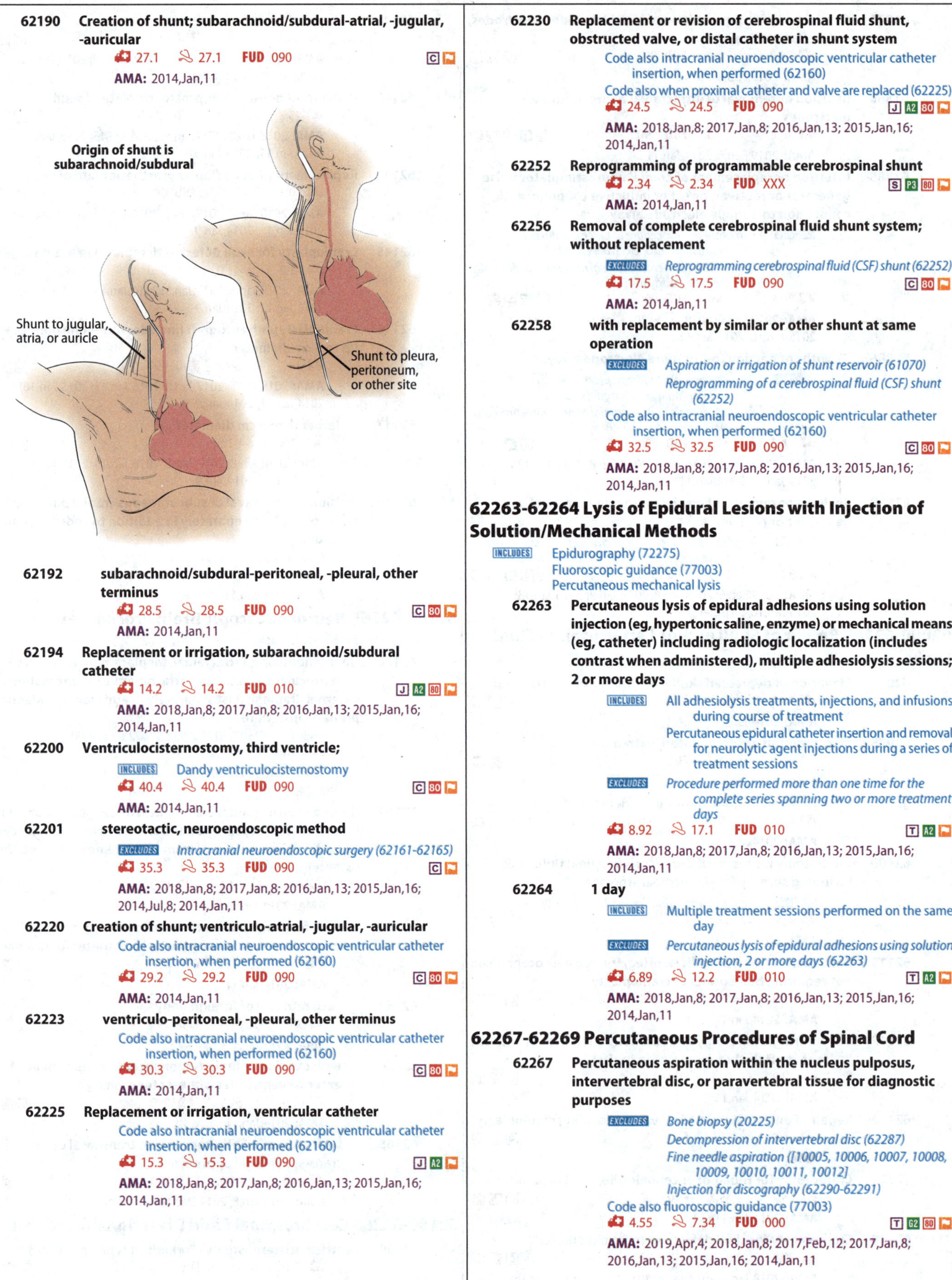

62192 **subarachnoid/subdural-peritoneal, -pleural, other terminus**
28.5 28.5 FUD 090 C 80
AMA: 2014,Jan,11

62194 **Replacement or irrigation, subarachnoid/subdural catheter**
14.2 14.2 FUD 010 J A2 80
AMA: 2018,Jan,8; 2017,Jan,8; 2016,Jan,13; 2015,Jan,16; 2014,Jan,11

62200 **Ventriculocisternostomy, third ventricle;**
INCLUDES Dandy ventriculocisternostomy
40.4 40.4 FUD 090 C 80
AMA: 2014,Jan,11

62201 **stereotactic, neuroendoscopic method**
EXCLUDES *Intracranial neuroendoscopic surgery (62161-62165)*
35.3 35.3 FUD 090 C
AMA: 2018,Jan,8; 2017,Jan,8; 2016,Jan,13; 2015,Jan,16; 2014,Jul,8; 2014,Jan,11

62220 **Creation of shunt; ventriculo-atrial, -jugular, -auricular**
Code also intracranial neuroendoscopic ventricular catheter insertion, when performed (62160)
29.2 29.2 FUD 090 C 80
AMA: 2014,Jan,11

62223 **ventriculo-peritoneal, -pleural, other terminus**
Code also intracranial neuroendoscopic ventricular catheter insertion, when performed (62160)
30.3 30.3 FUD 090 C 80
AMA: 2014,Jan,11

62225 **Replacement or irrigation, ventricular catheter**
Code also intracranial neuroendoscopic ventricular catheter insertion, when performed (62160)
15.3 15.3 FUD 090 J A2
AMA: 2018,Jan,8; 2017,Jan,8; 2016,Jan,13; 2015,Jan,16; 2014,Jan,11

62230 **Replacement or revision of cerebrospinal fluid shunt, obstructed valve, or distal catheter in shunt system**
Code also intracranial neuroendoscopic ventricular catheter insertion, when performed (62160)
Code also when proximal catheter and valve are replaced (62225)
24.5 24.5 FUD 090 J A2 80
AMA: 2018,Jan,8; 2017,Jan,8; 2016,Jan,13; 2015,Jan,16; 2014,Jan,11

62252 **Reprogramming of programmable cerebrospinal shunt**
2.34 2.34 FUD XXX S P3 80
AMA: 2014,Jan,11

62256 **Removal of complete cerebrospinal fluid shunt system; without replacement**
EXCLUDES *Reprogramming cerebrospinal fluid (CSF) shunt (62252)*
17.5 17.5 FUD 090 C 80
AMA: 2014,Jan,11

62258 **with replacement by similar or other shunt at same operation**
EXCLUDES *Aspiration or irrigation of shunt reservoir (61070)*
Reprogramming of a cerebrospinal fluid (CSF) shunt (62252)
Code also intracranial neuroendoscopic ventricular catheter insertion, when performed (62160)
32.5 32.5 FUD 090 C 80
AMA: 2018,Jan,8; 2017,Jan,8; 2016,Jan,13; 2015,Jan,16; 2014,Jan,11

62263-62264 Lysis of Epidural Lesions with Injection of Solution/Mechanical Methods

INCLUDES Epidurography (72275)
Fluoroscopic guidance (77003)
Percutaneous mechanical lysis

62263 **Percutaneous lysis of epidural adhesions using solution injection (eg, hypertonic saline, enzyme) or mechanical means (eg, catheter) including radiologic localization (includes contrast when administered), multiple adhesiolysis sessions; 2 or more days**
INCLUDES All adhesiolysis treatments, injections, and infusions during course of treatment
Percutaneous epidural catheter insertion and removal for neurolytic agent injections during a series of treatment sessions
EXCLUDES *Procedure performed more than one time for the complete series spanning two or more treatment days*
8.92 17.1 FUD 010 T A2
AMA: 2018,Jan,8; 2017,Jan,8; 2016,Jan,13; 2015,Jan,16; 2014,Jan,11

62264 **1 day**
INCLUDES Multiple treatment sessions performed on the same day
EXCLUDES *Percutaneous lysis of epidural adhesions using solution injection, 2 or more days (62263)*
6.89 12.2 FUD 010 T A2
AMA: 2018,Jan,8; 2017,Jan,8; 2016,Jan,13; 2015,Jan,16; 2014,Jan,11

62267-62269 Percutaneous Procedures of Spinal Cord

62267 **Percutaneous aspiration within the nucleus pulposus, intervertebral disc, or paravertebral tissue for diagnostic purposes**
EXCLUDES *Bone biopsy (20225)*
Decompression of intervertebral disc (62287)
Fine needle aspiration ([10005, 10006, 10007, 10008, 10009, 10010, 10011, 10012])
Injection for discography (62290-62291)
Code also fluoroscopic guidance (77003)
4.55 7.34 FUD 000 T G2 80
AMA: 2019,Apr,4; 2018,Jan,8; 2017,Feb,12; 2017,Jan,8; 2016,Jan,13; 2015,Jan,16; 2014,Jan,11

62268 **Percutaneous aspiration, spinal cord cyst or syrinx**

(76942, 77002, 77012)

7.40 7.40 FUD 000 T A2

AMA: 2018,Jan,8; 2017,Dec,13; 2014,Jan,11

62269 **Biopsy of spinal cord, percutaneous needle**

EXCLUDES *Fine needle aspiration [(10005, 1006, 1007, 1008, 1009, 10010, 10011, 10012)]*

(76942, 77002, 77012)

(88172-88173)

7.66 7.66 FUD 000 J A2 80

AMA: 2019,Apr,4; 2014,Jan,11

62270-62329 [62328, 62329] Spinal Puncture, Subarachnoid Space, Diagnostic/Therapeutic

Code also fluoroscopic guidance (77003)

▲ 62270 **Spinal puncture, lumbar, diagnostic;**

EXCLUDES *Radiological guidance (77003, 77012)*
Ultrasound or MRI guidance (76942, 77021)

2.23 4.22 FUD 000 T A2

AMA: 2018,Jan,8; 2017,Jan,8; 2016,Jan,13; 2015,Jan,16; 2014,Sep,3; 2014,Jan,11

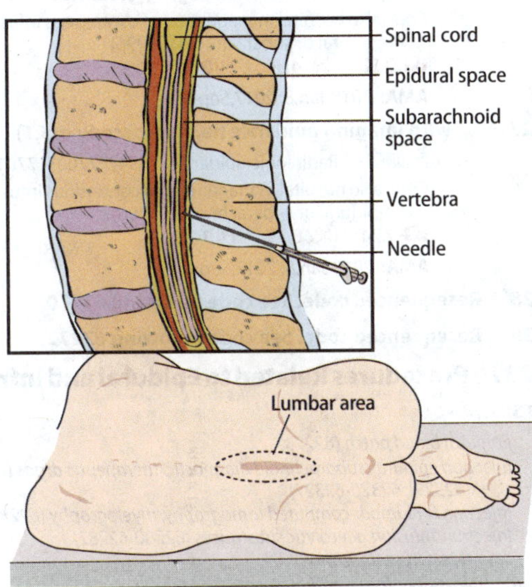

Common position to access vertebral interspace

● # 62328 **with fluoroscopic or CT guidance**

0.00 0.00 FUD 000

EXCLUDES *Radiological guidance (77003, 77012)*
Ultrasound or MRI guidance (76942, 77021)

▲ 62272 **Spinal puncture, therapeutic, for drainage of cerebrospinal fluid (by needle or catheter);**

EXCLUDES *Radiological guidance (77003, 77012)*
Ultrasound or MRI guidance (76942, 77021)

2.41 5.57 FUD 000 T A2

AMA: 2018,Jan,8; 2017,Jan,8; 2016,Jan,13; 2015,Jan,16; 2014,Jan,11

● # 62329 **with fluoroscopic or CT guidance**

0.00 0.00 FUD 000

EXCLUDES *Radiological guidance (77003, 77012)*
Ultrasound or MRI guidance (76942, 77021)

62273 Epidural Blood Patch

CMS: 100-03,10.5 NCD for Autogenous Epidural Blood Graft (10.5)

EXCLUDES *Injection of diagnostic or therapeutic material (62320-62327)*

Code also fluoroscopic guidance (77003)

62273 **Injection, epidural, of blood or clot patch**

3.26 4.93 FUD 000 T A2

AMA: 2018,Jan,8; 2017,Jan,8; 2016,Jan,13; 2015,Jan,16; 2014,Jan,11

62280-62282 Neurolysis

INCLUDES Contrast injection during fluoroscopic guidance/localization

EXCLUDES *Injection of diagnostic or therapeutic material only (62320-62327)*

Code also fluoroscopic guidance and localization unless a formal contrast study is performed (77003)

62280 **Injection/infusion of neurolytic substance (eg, alcohol, phenol, iced saline solutions), with or without other therapeutic substance; subarachnoid**

4.76 9.45 FUD 010 T A2

AMA: 2018,Jan,8; 2017,Jan,8; 2016,Jan,13; 2015,Jan,16; 2014,Jan,11

62281 **epidural, cervical or thoracic**

4.58 6.94 FUD 010 T A2

AMA: 2018,Jan,8; 2017,Jan,8; 2016,Jan,13; 2015,Jan,16; 2014,Jan,11

62282 **epidural, lumbar, sacral (caudal)**

4.16 8.63 FUD 010 T A2

AMA: 2018,Jan,8; 2017,Jan,8; 2016,Jan,13; 2015,Jan,16; 2014,Jan,11

62284-62294 Injection/Aspiration of Spine, Diagnostic/Therapeutic

62284 **Injection procedure for myelography and/or computed tomography, lumbar**

EXCLUDES *Injection at C1-C2 (61055)*
Myelography (62302-62305, 72240, 72255, 72265, 72270)

Code also fluoroscopic guidance (77003)

2.54 5.61 FUD 000 N N1

AMA: 2018,Jan,8; 2017,Jan,8; 2016,Jan,13; 2015,Jan,16; 2014,Sep,3; 2014,Jan,11

62287 **Decompression procedure, percutaneous, of nucleus pulposus of intervertebral disc, any method utilizing needle based technique to remove disc material under fluoroscopic imaging or other form of indirect visualization, with discography and/or epidural injection(s) at the treated level(s), when performed, single or multiple levels, lumbar**

INCLUDES Endoscopic approach

EXCLUDES *Injection for discography (62290)*
Injection of diagnostic or therapeutic substance(s) (62322)
Lumbar discography (72295)
Percutaneous aspiration, diagnostic (62267)
Percutaneous decompression of nucleus pulposus of an intervertebral disc, non-needle based technique (0274T-0275T)
Radiological guidance (77003, 77012)

16.7 16.7 FUD 090 J A2

AMA: 2018,Jan,8; 2017,Feb,12; 2017,Jan,8; 2016,Jan,13; 2015,Mar,9; 2015,Jan,16; 2014,Apr,10; 2014,Jan,11

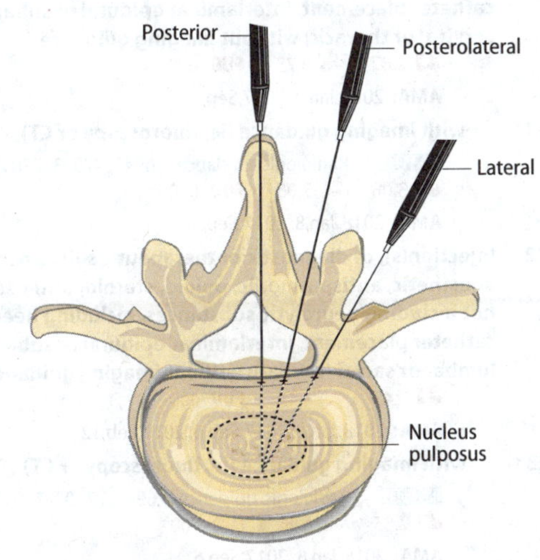

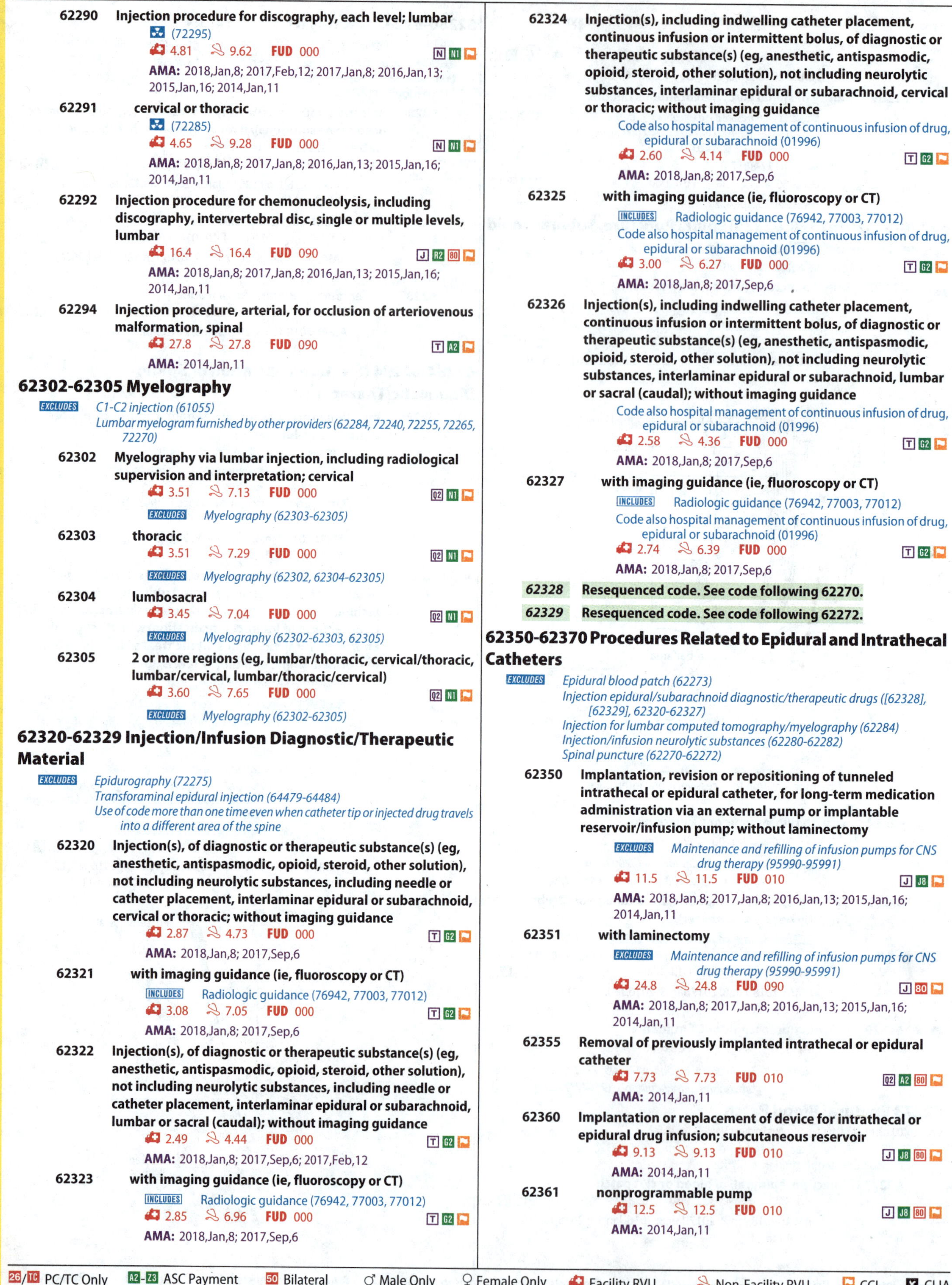

62290 **Injection procedure for discography, each level; lumbar**
(72295)
4.81 9.62 **FUD** 000 N N1
AMA: 2018,Jan,8; 2017,Feb,12; 2017,Jan,8; 2016,Jan,13; 2015,Jan,16; 2014,Jan,11

62291 **cervical or thoracic**
(72285)
4.65 9.28 **FUD** 000 N N1
AMA: 2018,Jan,8; 2017,Jan,8; 2016,Jan,13; 2015,Jan,16; 2014,Jan,11

62292 **Injection procedure for chemonucleolysis, including discography, intervertebral disc, single or multiple levels, lumbar**
16.4 16.4 **FUD** 090 J R2 80
AMA: 2018,Jan,8; 2017,Jan,8; 2016,Jan,13; 2015,Jan,16; 2014,Jan,11

62294 **Injection procedure, arterial, for occlusion of arteriovenous malformation, spinal**
27.8 27.8 **FUD** 090 T A2
AMA: 2014,Jan,11

62302-62305 Myelography

EXCLUDES *C1-C2 injection (61055)*
Lumbar myelogram furnished by other providers (62284, 72240, 72255, 72265, 72270)

62302 **Myelography via lumbar injection, including radiological supervision and interpretation; cervical**
3.51 7.13 **FUD** 000 Q2 N1
EXCLUDES *Myelography (62303-62305)*

62303 **thoracic**
3.51 7.29 **FUD** 000 Q2 N1
EXCLUDES *Myelography (62302, 62304-62305)*

62304 **lumbosacral**
3.45 7.04 **FUD** 000 Q2 N1
EXCLUDES *Myelography (62302-62303, 62305)*

62305 **2 or more regions (eg, lumbar/thoracic, cervical/thoracic, lumbar/cervical, lumbar/thoracic/cervical)**
3.60 7.65 **FUD** 000 Q2 N1
EXCLUDES *Myelography (62302-62305)*

62320-62329 Injection/Infusion Diagnostic/Therapeutic Material

EXCLUDES *Epidurography (72275)*
Transforaminal epidural injection (64479-64484)
Use of code more than one time even when catheter tip or injected drug travels into a different area of the spine

62320 **Injection(s), of diagnostic or therapeutic substance(s) (eg, anesthetic, antispasmodic, opioid, steroid, other solution), not including neurolytic substances, including needle or catheter placement, interlaminar epidural or subarachnoid, cervical or thoracic; without imaging guidance**
2.87 4.73 **FUD** 000 T G2
AMA: 2018,Jan,8; 2017,Sep,6

62321 **with imaging guidance (ie, fluoroscopy or CT)**
INCLUDES Radiologic guidance (76942, 77003, 77012)
3.08 7.05 **FUD** 000 T G2
AMA: 2018,Jan,8; 2017,Sep,6

62322 **Injection(s), of diagnostic or therapeutic substance(s) (eg, anesthetic, antispasmodic, opioid, steroid, other solution), not including neurolytic substances, including needle or catheter placement, interlaminar epidural or subarachnoid, lumbar or sacral (caudal); without imaging guidance**
2.49 4.44 **FUD** 000 T G2
AMA: 2018,Jan,8; 2017,Sep,6; 2017,Feb,12

62323 **with imaging guidance (ie, fluoroscopy or CT)**
INCLUDES Radiologic guidance (76942, 77003, 77012)
2.85 6.96 **FUD** 000 T G2
AMA: 2018,Jan,8; 2017,Sep,6

62324 **Injection(s), including indwelling catheter placement, continuous infusion or intermittent bolus, of diagnostic or therapeutic substance(s) (eg, anesthetic, antispasmodic, opioid, steroid, other solution), not including neurolytic substances, interlaminar epidural or subarachnoid, cervical or thoracic; without imaging guidance**
Code also hospital management of continuous infusion of drug, epidural or subarachnoid (01996)
2.60 4.14 **FUD** 000 T G2
AMA: 2018,Jan,8; 2017,Sep,6

62325 **with imaging guidance (ie, fluoroscopy or CT)**
INCLUDES Radiologic guidance (76942, 77003, 77012)
Code also hospital management of continuous infusion of drug, epidural or subarachnoid (01996)
3.00 6.27 **FUD** 000 T G2
AMA: 2018,Jan,8; 2017,Sep,6

62326 **Injection(s), including indwelling catheter placement, continuous infusion or intermittent bolus, of diagnostic or therapeutic substance(s) (eg, anesthetic, antispasmodic, opioid, steroid, other solution), not including neurolytic substances, interlaminar epidural or subarachnoid, lumbar or sacral (caudal); without imaging guidance**
Code also hospital management of continuous infusion of drug, epidural or subarachnoid (01996)
2.58 4.36 **FUD** 000 T G2
AMA: 2018,Jan,8; 2017,Sep,6

62327 **with imaging guidance (ie, fluoroscopy or CT)**
INCLUDES Radiologic guidance (76942, 77003, 77012)
Code also hospital management of continuous infusion of drug, epidural or subarachnoid (01996)
2.74 6.39 **FUD** 000 T G2
AMA: 2018,Jan,8; 2017,Sep,6

62328 **Resequenced code. See code following 62270.**

62329 **Resequenced code. See code following 62272.**

62350-62370 Procedures Related to Epidural and Intrathecal Catheters

EXCLUDES *Epidural blood patch (62273)*
Injection epidural/subarachnoid diagnostic/therapeutic drugs ([62328], [62329], 62320-62327)
Injection for lumbar computed tomography/myelography (62284)
Injection/infusion neurolytic substances (62280-62282)
Spinal puncture (62270-62272)

62350 **Implantation, revision or repositioning of tunneled intrathecal or epidural catheter, for long-term medication administration via an external pump or implantable reservoir/infusion pump; without laminectomy**
EXCLUDES *Maintenance and refilling of infusion pumps for CNS drug therapy (95990-95991)*
11.5 11.5 **FUD** 010 J J8
AMA: 2018,Jan,8; 2017,Jan,8; 2016,Jan,13; 2015,Jan,16; 2014,Jan,11

62351 **with laminectomy**
EXCLUDES *Maintenance and refilling of infusion pumps for CNS drug therapy (95990-95991)*
24.8 24.8 **FUD** 090 J 80
AMA: 2018,Jan,8; 2017,Jan,8; 2016,Jan,13; 2015,Jan,16; 2014,Jan,11

62355 **Removal of previously implanted intrathecal or epidural catheter**
7.73 7.73 **FUD** 010 Q2 A2 80
AMA: 2014,Jan,11

62360 **Implantation or replacement of device for intrathecal or epidural drug infusion; subcutaneous reservoir**
9.13 9.13 **FUD** 010 J J8 80
AMA: 2014,Jan,11

62361 **nonprogrammable pump**
12.5 12.5 **FUD** 010 J J8 80
AMA: 2014,Jan,11

62362 **programmable pump, including preparation of pump, with or without programming**
11.0 11.0 FUD 010 J J8 80
AMA: 2018,Jan,8; 2017,Jan,8; 2016,Jan,13; 2015,Jan,16; 2014,Jan,11

62365 **Removal of subcutaneous reservoir or pump, previously implanted for intrathecal or epidural infusion**
8.52 8.52 FUD 010 Q2 A2 80
AMA: 2014,Jan,11

62367 **Electronic analysis of programmable, implanted pump for intrathecal or epidural drug infusion (includes evaluation of reservoir status, alarm status, drug prescription status); without reprogramming or refill**
EXCLUDES *Maintenance and refilling of infusion pumps for CNS drug therapy (95990-95991)*
0.72 1.14 FUD XXX S P3
AMA: 2018,Jan,8; 2017,Jan,8; 2016,Jan,13; 2015,Jan,16; 2014,Jan,11

62368 **with reprogramming**
EXCLUDES *Maintenance and refilling of infusion pumps for CNS drug therapy (95990-95991)*
1.01 1.57 FUD XXX S P3
AMA: 2018,Jan,8; 2017,Jan,8; 2016,Jan,13; 2015,Jan,16; 2014,Jan,11

62369 **with reprogramming and refill**
EXCLUDES *Maintenance and refilling of infusion pumps for CNS drug therapy (95990-95991)*
1.01 3.34 FUD XXX S P3
AMA: 2018,Jan,8; 2017,Jan,8; 2016,Jan,13; 2015,Jan,16; 2014,Jan,11

62370 **with reprogramming and refill (requiring skill of a physician or other qualified health care professional)**
EXCLUDES *Maintenance and refilling of infusion pumps for CNS drug therapy (95990-95991)*
1.33 3.47 FUD XXX S P3
AMA: 2018,Jan,8; 2017,Jan,8; 2016,Jan,13; 2015,Jan,16; 2014,Jan,11

62380 Endoscopic Decompression/Laminectomy/Laminotomy

EXCLUDES *Open decompression (63030, 63056)*
Percutaneous decompression (62267, 0274T-0275T)
Code also operating microscope, when applicable (69990)

62380 **Endoscopic decompression of spinal cord, nerve root(s), including laminotomy, partial facetectomy, foraminotomy, discectomy and/or excision of herniated intervertebral disc, 1 interspace, lumbar**
0.00 0.00 FUD 090 J G2 80 50
AMA: 2018,Jan,8; 2017,Feb,12

63001-63048 Posterior Midline Approach: Laminectomy/Laminotomy/Decompression

INCLUDES Endoscopic assistance through open and direct visualization
EXCLUDES *Arthrodesis (22590-22614)*
Percutaneous decompression (62287, 0274T, 0275T)
Code also operating microscope, when applicable (69990)

63001 **Laminectomy with exploration and/or decompression of spinal cord and/or cauda equina, without facetectomy, foraminotomy or discectomy (eg, spinal stenosis), 1 or 2 vertebral segments; cervical**
36.0 36.0 FUD 090 J G2 80
AMA: 2018,Jan,8; 2017,Mar,7; 2017,Jan,8; 2016,Jan,13; 2015,Jan,16; 2014,Jan,11

63003 **thoracic**
36.0 36.0 FUD 090 J G2 80
AMA: 2018,Jan,8; 2017,Mar,7; 2017,Jan,8; 2016,Jan,13; 2015,Jan,16; 2014,Jan,11

63005 **lumbar, except for spondylolisthesis**
34.4 34.4 FUD 090 J G2 80
AMA: 2018,Jan,8; 2017,Mar,7; 2017,Feb,9; 2017,Jan,8; 2016,Jan,13; 2015,Jan,16; 2014,Jan,11

63011 **sacral**
31.6 31.6 FUD 090 J 80
AMA: 2018,Jan,8; 2017,Mar,7; 2017,Jan,8; 2016,Jan,13; 2015,Jan,16; 2014,Jan,11

63012 **Laminectomy with removal of abnormal facets and/or pars inter-articularis with decompression of cauda equina and nerve roots for spondylolisthesis, lumbar (Gill type procedure)**
34.6 34.6 FUD 090 J 80
AMA: 2018,Jan,8; 2017,Mar,7; 2017,Feb,9; 2017,Jan,8; 2016,Jan,13; 2015,Jan,16; 2014,Jan,11

63015 **Laminectomy with exploration and/or decompression of spinal cord and/or cauda equina, without facetectomy, foraminotomy or discectomy (eg, spinal stenosis), more than 2 vertebral segments; cervical**
43.2 43.2 FUD 090 J 80
AMA: 2018,Jan,8; 2017,Mar,7; 2017,Jan,8; 2016,Jan,13; 2015,Jan,16; 2014,Jan,11

63016 **thoracic**
44.3 44.3 FUD 090 J 80
AMA: 2018,Jan,8; 2017,Mar,7; 2017,Jan,8; 2016,Jan,13; 2015,Jan,16; 2014,Jan,11

63017 **lumbar**
36.7 36.7 FUD 090 J 80
AMA: 2018,Jan,8; 2017,Mar,7; 2017,Feb,9; 2017,Jan,8; 2016,Jan,13; 2015,Jan,16; 2014,Jan,11

Nerve root problems in C5 through C7 cause paralysis of the upper limb

C1 to C4

C5 to C7

Atlas (C1)

Axis (C2)

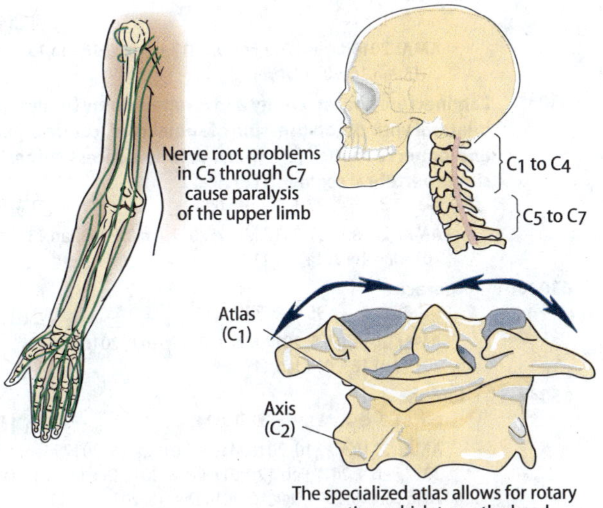

The specialized atlas allows for rotary motion, which turns the head

63020 **Laminotomy (hemilaminectomy), with decompression of nerve root(s), including partial facetectomy, foraminotomy and/or excision of herniated intervertebral disc; 1 interspace, cervical**
33.6 33.6 FUD 090 J G2 80 50
AMA: 2018,Jan,8; 2017,Mar,7; 2017,Jan,8; 2016,Jan,13; 2015,Jan,16; 2014,Jan,11

63030 **1 interspace, lumbar**
28.2 28.2 FUD 090 J G2 80 50
AMA: 2018,Jan,8; 2017,Mar,7; 2017,Feb,9; 2017,Feb,12; 2017,Jan,8; 2016,May,13; 2016,Jan,13; 2015,Jan,16; 2014,Jan,11

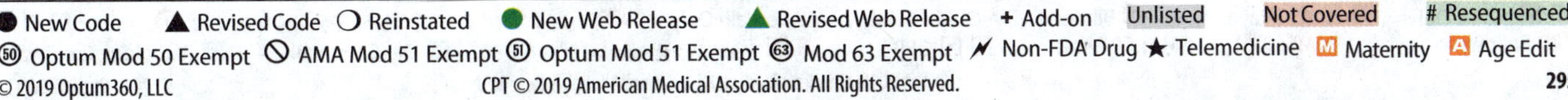

+ 63035 **each additional interspace, cervical or lumbar (List separately in addition to code for primary procedure)**

EXCLUDES *Reporting with modifier 50. Report once for each side when performed bilaterally*

Code first (63020-63030)

5.58 5.58 FUD ZZZ 50 N 80

AMA: 2018,Jan,8; 2017,Feb,9; 2017,Jan,8; 2016,Jan,13; 2015,Jan,16; 2014,Jan,11

63040 **Laminotomy (hemilaminectomy), with decompression of nerve root(s), including partial facetectomy, foraminotomy and/or excision of herniated intervertebral disc, reexploration, single interspace; cervical**

40.4 40.4 FUD 090 J 80 50

AMA: 2018,Jan,8; 2017,Mar,7; 2017,Jan,8; 2016,Jan,13; 2015,Jan,16; 2014,Jan,11

63042 **lumbar**

37.6 37.6 FUD 090 J G2 80 50

AMA: 2018,Jan,8; 2017,Mar,7; 2017,Feb,9; 2017,Jan,8; 2016,Jan,13; 2015,Jan,16; 2014,Jan,11

+ 63043 **each additional cervical interspace (List separately in addition to code for primary procedure)**

EXCLUDES *Reporting with modifier 50. Report once for each side when performed bilaterally*

Code first (63040)

0.00 0.00 FUD ZZZ 50 N 80

AMA: 2018,Jan,8; 2017,Jan,8; 2016,Jan,13; 2015,Jan,16; 2014,Jan,11

+ 63044 **each additional lumbar interspace (List separately in addition to code for primary procedure)**

EXCLUDES *Reporting with modifier 50. Report once for each side when performed bilaterally*

Code first (63042)

0.00 0.00 FUD ZZZ 50 N N1 80

AMA: 2018,Jan,8; 2017,Feb,9; 2017,Jan,8; 2016,Jan,13; 2015,Jan,16; 2014,Jan,11

63045 **Laminectomy, facetectomy and foraminotomy (unilateral or bilateral with decompression of spinal cord, cauda equina and/or nerve root[s], [eg, spinal or lateral recess stenosis]), single vertebral segment; cervical**

37.3 37.3 FUD 090 J G2 80

AMA: 2018,Jan,8; 2017,Mar,7; 2017,Jan,8; 2016,Jan,13; 2015,Jan,16; 2014,Jan,11

63046 **thoracic**

35.6 35.6 FUD 090 J G2 80

AMA: 2018,Jan,8; 2017,Mar,7; 2017,Jan,8; 2016,Jan,13; 2015,Jan,16; 2014,Jan,11

63047 **lumbar**

31.9 31.9 FUD 090 J G2 80

AMA: 2018,May,10; 2018,May,9; 2018,Jan,8; 2017,Mar,7; 2017,Feb,9; 2017,Feb,12; 2017,Jan,8; 2016,Oct,11; 2016,Jan,13; 2015,Jan,16; 2014,Dec,16; 2014,Dec,16; 2014,Jan,11

+ 63048 **each additional segment, cervical, thoracic, or lumbar (List separately in addition to code for primary procedure)**

Code first (63045-63047)

6.17 6.17 FUD ZZZ N 80

AMA: 2018,Jan,8; 2017,Feb,9; 2017,Jan,8; 2016,Jan,13; 2015,Jan,16; 2014,Jan,11

63050-63051 Cervical Laminoplasty: Posterior Midline Approach

EXCLUDES *Procedure performed on the same vertebral segment(s) (22600, 22614, 22840-22842, 63001, 63015, 63045, 63048, 63295)*

63050 **Laminoplasty, cervical, with decompression of the spinal cord, 2 or more vertebral segments;**

43.5 43.5 FUD 090 C 80

AMA: 2018,Jan,8; 2017,Mar,7; 2017,Jan,8; 2016,Jan,13; 2015,Jan,16; 2014,Jan,11

63051 **with reconstruction of the posterior bony elements (including the application of bridging bone graft and non-segmental fixation devices [eg, wire, suture, mini-plates], when performed)**

49.7 49.7 FUD 090 C 80

AMA: 2018,Jan,8; 2017,Mar,7; 2017,Jan,8; 2016,Jan,13; 2015,Jan,16; 2014,Jan,11

63055-63066 Spinal Cord/Nerve Root Decompression: Costovertebral or Transpedicular Approach

63055 **Transpedicular approach with decompression of spinal cord, equina and/or nerve root(s) (eg, herniated intervertebral disc), single segment; thoracic**

47.4 47.4 FUD 090 J G2 80

AMA: 2018,Jan,8; 2017,Mar,7; 2017,Jan,8; 2016,Jan,13; 2015,Jan,16; 2014,Jan,11

63056 **lumbar (including transfacet, or lateral extraforaminal approach) (eg, far lateral herniated intervertebral disc)**

43.2 43.2 FUD 090 J G2 80

AMA: 2018,Jan,8; 2017,Mar,7; 2017,Feb,12; 2017,Jan,8; 2016,Jan,13; 2015,Jan,16; 2014,Jan,11; 2014,Jan,9

+ 63057 **each additional segment, thoracic or lumbar (List separately in addition to code for primary procedure)**

Code first (63055-63056)

9.32 9.32 FUD ZZZ N 80

AMA: 2018,Jan,8; 2017,Jan,8; 2016,Jan,13; 2015,Jan,16; 2014,Jan,11

63064 **Costovertebral approach with decompression of spinal cord or nerve root(s) (eg, herniated intervertebral disc), thoracic; single segment**

EXCLUDES *Laminectomy with intraspinal thoracic lesion removal (63266, 63271, 63276, 63281, 63286)*

51.9 51.9 FUD 090 J 80

AMA: 2018,Jan,8; 2017,Mar,7; 2017,Jan,8; 2016,Jan,13; 2015,Jan,16; 2014,Jan,11

+ 63066 **each additional segment (List separately in addition to code for primary procedure)**

EXCLUDES *Laminectomy with intraspinal thoracic lesion removal (63266, 63271, 63276, 63281, 63286)*

Code first (63064)

6.09 6.09 FUD ZZZ N 80

AMA: 2014,Jan,11

63075-63078 Discectomy: Anterior or Anterolateral Approach

INCLUDES Operating microscope (69990)

63075 **Discectomy, anterior, with decompression of spinal cord and/or nerve root(s), including osteophytectomy; cervical, single interspace**

EXCLUDES *Anterior cervical discectomy and anterior interbody fusion at same level during same operative session (22551)*

Anterior interbody arthrodesis (even by another provider) (22554)

39.2 39.2 FUD 090 J 80

AMA: 2018,Jan,8; 2017,Mar,7; 2017,Jan,8; 2016,Feb,12; 2016,Jan,13; 2015,Apr,7; 2015,Jan,16; 2014,Jan,11

+ 63076 **cervical, each additional interspace (List separately in addition to code for primary procedure)**

EXCLUDES *Anterior cervical discectomy and anterior interbody fusion at same level during same operative session (22552)*

Anterior interbody arthrodesis (even by another provider) (22554)

Code first (63075)

7.20 7.20 FUD ZZZ N 80

AMA: 2018,Jan,8; 2017,Jan,8; 2016,Feb,12; 2016,Jan,13; 2015,Jan,16; 2014,Jan,11

63077 thoracic, single interspace
44.2 44.2 FUD 090 C 80
AMA: 2018,Jan,8; 2017,Mar,7; 2017,Jan,8; 2016,Feb,12; 2016,Jan,13; 2015,Jan,16; 2014,Jan,11

+ 63078 thoracic, each additional interspace (List separately in addition to code for primary procedure)
Code first (63077)
6.13 6.13 FUD ZZZ C 80
AMA: 2018,Jan,8; 2017,Jan,8; 2016,Feb,12; 2016,Jan,13; 2015,Jan,16; 2014,Jan,11

63081-63091 Vertebral Corpectomy, All Levels, Anterior Approach

INCLUDES Disc removal at the level below and/or above vertebral segment
Partial removal:
Cervical: Removal of ≥ 1/2 of vertebral body
Lumbar: Removal of ≥ 1/3 of vertebral body
Thoracic: Removal of ≥ 1/3 of vertebral body

EXCLUDES *Arthrodesis (22548-22812)*

Code also reconstruction (20930-20938, 22548-22812, 22840-22855 [22859])

63081 **Vertebral corpectomy (vertebral body resection), partial or complete, anterior approach with decompression of spinal cord and/or nerve root(s); cervical, single segment**
EXCLUDES *Transoral approach (61575-61576)*
51.1 51.1 FUD 090 C 80
AMA: 2018,Jan,8; 2017,Mar,7; 2017,Jan,8; 2016,Apr,8; 2016,Jan,13; 2015,Jun,10; 2015,Jan,16; 2014,Jan,11

+ 63082 cervical, each additional segment (List separately in addition to code for primary procedure)
EXCLUDES *Transoral approach (61575-61576)*
Code first (63081)
7.77 7.77 FUD ZZZ C 80
AMA: 2018,Jan,8; 2017,Jan,8; 2016,Apr,8; 2016,Jan,13; 2015,Jan,16; 2014,Jan,11

63085 **Vertebral corpectomy (vertebral body resection), partial or complete, transthoracic approach with decompression of spinal cord and/or nerve root(s); thoracic, single segment**
55.9 55.9 FUD 090 C 80
AMA: 2018,Jan,8; 2017,Mar,7; 2017,Jan,8; 2016,Apr,8; 2016,Jan,13; 2015,Jan,16; 2014,Jan,11

+ 63086 thoracic, each additional segment (List separately in addition to code for primary procedure)
Code first (63085)
5.58 5.58 FUD ZZZ C 80
AMA: 2018,Jan,8; 2017,Jan,8; 2016,Apr,8; 2016,Jan,13; 2015,Jan,16; 2014,Jan,11

63087 **Vertebral corpectomy (vertebral body resection), partial or complete, combined thoracolumbar approach with decompression of spinal cord, cauda equina or nerve root(s), lower thoracic or lumbar; single segment**
70.3 70.3 FUD 090 C 80
AMA: 2018,Jan,8; 2017,Mar,7; 2017,Jan,8; 2016,Apr,8; 2016,Jan,13; 2015,Jan,16; 2014,Jan,11

+ 63088 each additional segment (List separately in addition to code for primary procedure)
Code first (63087)
7.53 7.53 FUD ZZZ C 80
AMA: 2018,Jan,8; 2017,Jan,8; 2016,Apr,8; 2016,Jan,13; 2015,Jan,16; 2014,Jan,11

63090 **Vertebral corpectomy (vertebral body resection), partial or complete, transperitoneal or retroperitoneal approach with decompression of spinal cord, cauda equina or nerve root(s), lower thoracic, lumbar, or sacral; single segment**
56.9 56.9 FUD 090 C 80
AMA: 2018,Jan,8; 2017,Mar,7; 2017,Jan,8; 2016,Apr,8; 2016,Jan,13; 2015,Jan,16; 2014,Jan,11

+ 63091 each additional segment (List separately in addition to code for primary procedure)
Code first (63090)
5.18 5.18 FUD ZZZ C 80
AMA: 2018,Jan,8; 2017,Jan,8; 2016,Apr,8; 2016,Jan,13; 2015,Jan,16; 2014,Jan,11

63101-63103 Corpectomy: Lateral Extracavitary Approach

INCLUDES Partial removal:
Cervical: Removal of ≥ 1/2 of vertebral body
Lumbar: Removal of ≥ 1/3 of vertebral body
Thoracic: Removal of ≥ 1/3 of vertebral body

63101 **Vertebral corpectomy (vertebral body resection), partial or complete, lateral extracavitary approach with decompression of spinal cord and/or nerve root(s) (eg, for tumor or retropulsed bone fragments); thoracic, single segment**
67.8 67.8 FUD 090 C 80
AMA: 2018,Jan,8; 2017,Mar,7; 2017,Jan,8; 2016,Jan,13; 2015,Jan,16; 2014,Jan,11

63102 lumbar, single segment
66.0 66.0 FUD 090 C 80
AMA: 2018,Jan,8; 2017,Mar,7; 2017,Jan,8; 2016,Jan,13; 2015,Jan,16; 2014,Jan,11

+ 63103 thoracic or lumbar, each additional segment (List separately in addition to code for primary procedure)
Code first (63101-63102)
8.60 8.60 FUD ZZZ C 80
AMA: 2014,Jan,11

63170-63295 Laminectomies

63170 **Laminectomy with myelotomy (eg, Bischof or DREZ type), cervical, thoracic, or thoracolumbar**
46.8 46.8 FUD 090 C 80
AMA: 2018,Jan,8; 2017,Mar,7; 2017,Jan,8; 2016,Jan,13; 2015,Jan,16; 2014,Jan,11

63172 **Laminectomy with drainage of intramedullary cyst/syrinx; to subarachnoid space**
40.4 40.4 FUD 090 C 80
AMA: 2018,Jan,8; 2017,Mar,7; 2017,Jan,8; 2016,Jan,13; 2015,Jan,16; 2014,Jan,11

63173 to peritoneal or pleural space
50.7 50.7 FUD 090 C 80
AMA: 2018,Jan,8; 2017,Mar,7; 2017,Jan,8; 2016,Jan,13; 2015,Jan,16; 2014,Jan,11

63180 **Laminectomy and section of dentate ligaments, with or without dural graft, cervical; 1 or 2 segments**
43.6 43.6 FUD 090 C 80
AMA: 2018,Jan,8; 2017,Mar,7; 2017,Jan,8; 2016,Jan,13; 2015,Jan,16; 2014,Jan,11

63182 more than 2 segments
47.9 47.9 FUD 090 C 80
AMA: 2018,Jan,8; 2017,Mar,7; 2017,Jan,8; 2016,Jan,13; 2015,Jan,16; 2014,Jan,11

63185 **Laminectomy with rhizotomy; 1 or 2 segments**
INCLUDES Dana rhizotomy
Stoffel rhizotomy
33.2 33.2 FUD 090 C 80
AMA: 2018,Jan,8; 2017,Mar,7; 2017,Jan,8; 2016,Jan,13; 2015,Jan,16; 2014,Jan,11

63190 more than 2 segments
36.1 36.1 FUD 090 C 80
AMA: 2018,Jan,8; 2017,Mar,7; 2017,Jan,8; 2016,Jan,13; 2015,Jan,16; 2014,Jan,11

63191 **Laminectomy with section of spinal accessory nerve**
EXCLUDES *Division of sternocleidomastoid muscle for torticollis (21720)*
40.5 40.5 FUD 090 C 80 50
AMA: 2018,Jan,8; 2017,Mar,7; 2017,Jan,8; 2016,Jan,13; 2015,Jan,16; 2014,Jan,11

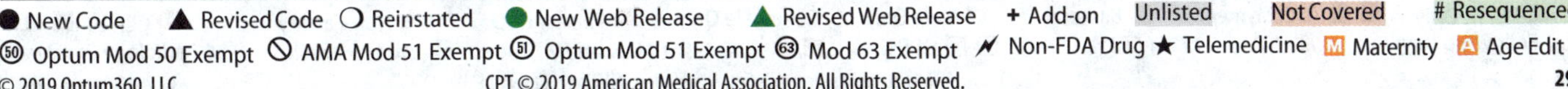

63194 **Laminectomy with cordotomy, with section of 1 spinothalamic tract, 1 stage; cervical**
46.9 46.9 FUD 090
AMA: 2018,Jan,8; 2017,Mar,7; 2017,Jan,8; 2016,Jan,13; 2015,Jan,16; 2014,Jan,11

63195 **thoracic**
45.1 45.1 FUD 090
AMA: 2018,Jan,8; 2017,Mar,7; 2017,Jan,8; 2016,Jan,13; 2015,Jan,16; 2014,Jan,11

63196 **Laminectomy with cordotomy, with section of both spinothalamic tracts, 1 stage; cervical**
52.4 52.4 FUD 090
AMA: 2018,Jan,8; 2017,Mar,7; 2017,Jan,8; 2016,Jan,13; 2015,Jan,16; 2014,Jan,11

63197 **thoracic**
50.3 50.3 FUD 090
AMA: 2018,Jan,8; 2017,Mar,7; 2017,Jan,8; 2016,Jan,13; 2015,Jan,16; 2014,Jan,11

63198 **Laminectomy with cordotomy with section of both spinothalamic tracts, 2 stages within 14 days; cervical**
INCLUDES Keen laminectomy
61.5 61.5 FUD 090
AMA: 2018,Jan,8; 2017,Mar,7; 2017,Jan,8; 2016,Jan,13; 2015,Jan,16; 2014,Jan,11

63199 **thoracic**
64.5 64.5 FUD 090
AMA: 2018,Jan,8; 2017,Mar,7; 2017,Jan,8; 2016,Jan,13; 2015,Jan,16; 2014,Jan,11

63200 **Laminectomy, with release of tethered spinal cord, lumbar**
44.7 44.7 FUD 090
AMA: 2018,Jan,8; 2017,Mar,7; 2017,Jan,8; 2016,Jan,13; 2015,Jan,16; 2014,Jan,11

63250 **Laminectomy for excision or occlusion of arteriovenous malformation of spinal cord; cervical**
87.8 87.8 FUD 090
AMA: 2018,Jan,8; 2017,Mar,7; 2017,Jan,8; 2016,Jan,13; 2015,Jan,16; 2014,Jan,11

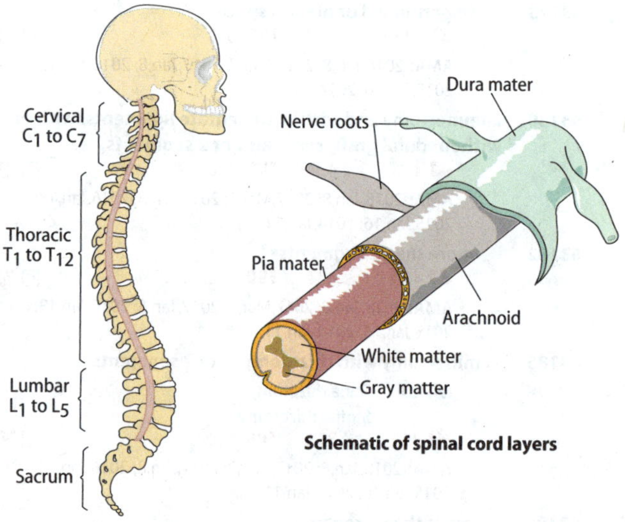

Schematic of spinal cord layers

63251 **thoracic**
89.7 89.7 FUD 090
AMA: 2018,Jan,8; 2017,Mar,7; 2017,Jan,8; 2016,Jan,13; 2015,Jan,16; 2014,Jan,11

63252 **thoracolumbar**
89.7 89.7 FUD 090
AMA: 2018,Jan,8; 2017,Mar,7; 2017,Jan,8; 2016,Jan,13; 2015,Jan,16; 2014,Jan,11

63265 **Laminectomy for excision or evacuation of intraspinal lesion other than neoplasm, extradural; cervical**
48.6 48.6 FUD 090
AMA: 2018,Jan,8; 2017,Mar,7; 2017,Jan,8; 2016,Jan,13; 2015,Jan,16; 2014,Jan,11

63266 **thoracic**
50.2 50.2 FUD 090
AMA: 2017,Mar,7; 2014,Jan,11

63267 **lumbar**
39.8 39.8 FUD 090
AMA: 2018,Jan,8; 2017,Mar,7; 2017,Jan,8; 2016,Jan,13; 2015,Jan,16; 2014,Jan,11

63268 **sacral**
41.2 41.2 FUD 090
AMA: 2018,Jan,8; 2017,Mar,7; 2017,Jan,8; 2016,Jan,13; 2015,Jan,16; 2014,Jan,11

63270 **Laminectomy for excision of intraspinal lesion other than neoplasm, intradural; cervical**
61.1 61.1 FUD 090
AMA: 2018,Jan,8; 2017,Mar,7; 2017,Jan,8; 2016,Jan,13; 2015,Jan,16; 2014,Jan,11

63271 **thoracic**
60.4 60.4 FUD 090
AMA: 2018,Jan,8; 2017,Mar,7; 2017,Jan,8; 2016,Jan,13; 2015,Jan,16; 2014,Jan,11

63272 **lumbar**
55.1 55.1 FUD 090
AMA: 2018,Jan,8; 2017,Mar,7; 2017,Jan,8; 2016,Jan,13; 2015,Jan,16; 2014,Jan,11

63273 **sacral**
54.9 54.9 FUD 090
AMA: 2018,Jan,8; 2017,Mar,7; 2017,Jan,8; 2016,Jan,13; 2015,Jan,16; 2014,Jan,11

63275 **Laminectomy for biopsy/excision of intraspinal neoplasm; extradural, cervical**
52.6 52.6 FUD 090
AMA: 2018,Jan,8; 2017,Mar,7; 2017,Jan,8; 2016,Jan,13; 2015,Jan,16; 2014,Jan,11

63276 **extradural, thoracic**
52.2 52.2 FUD 090
AMA: 2018,Jan,8; 2017,Mar,7; 2017,Jan,8; 2016,Jan,13; 2015,Jan,16; 2014,Jan,11

63277 **extradural, lumbar**
45.3 45.3 FUD 090
AMA: 2018,Jan,8; 2017,Mar,7; 2017,Jan,8; 2016,Jan,13; 2015,Jan,16; 2014,Jan,11

63278 **extradural, sacral**
46.7 46.7 FUD 090
AMA: 2018,Jan,8; 2017,Mar,7; 2017,Jan,8; 2016,Jan,13; 2015,Jan,16; 2014,Jan,11

63280 **intradural, extramedullary, cervical**
61.9 61.9 FUD 090
AMA: 2018,Jan,8; 2017,Mar,7; 2017,Jan,8; 2016,Jan,13; 2015,Jan,16; 2014,Jan,11

63281 **intradural, extramedullary, thoracic**
61.2 61.2 FUD 090
AMA: 2018,Jan,8; 2017,Mar,7; 2017,Jan,8; 2016,Jan,13; 2015,Jan,16; 2014,Jan,11

63282 **intradural, extramedullary, lumbar**
57.7 57.7 FUD 090
AMA: 2018,Jan,8; 2017,Mar,7; 2017,Jan,8; 2016,Jan,13; 2015,Jan,16; 2014,Jan,11

63283 **intradural, sacral**
55.3 55.3 FUD 090
AMA: 2018,Jan,8; 2017,Mar,7; 2017,Jan,8; 2016,Jan,13; 2015,Jan,16; 2014,Jan,11

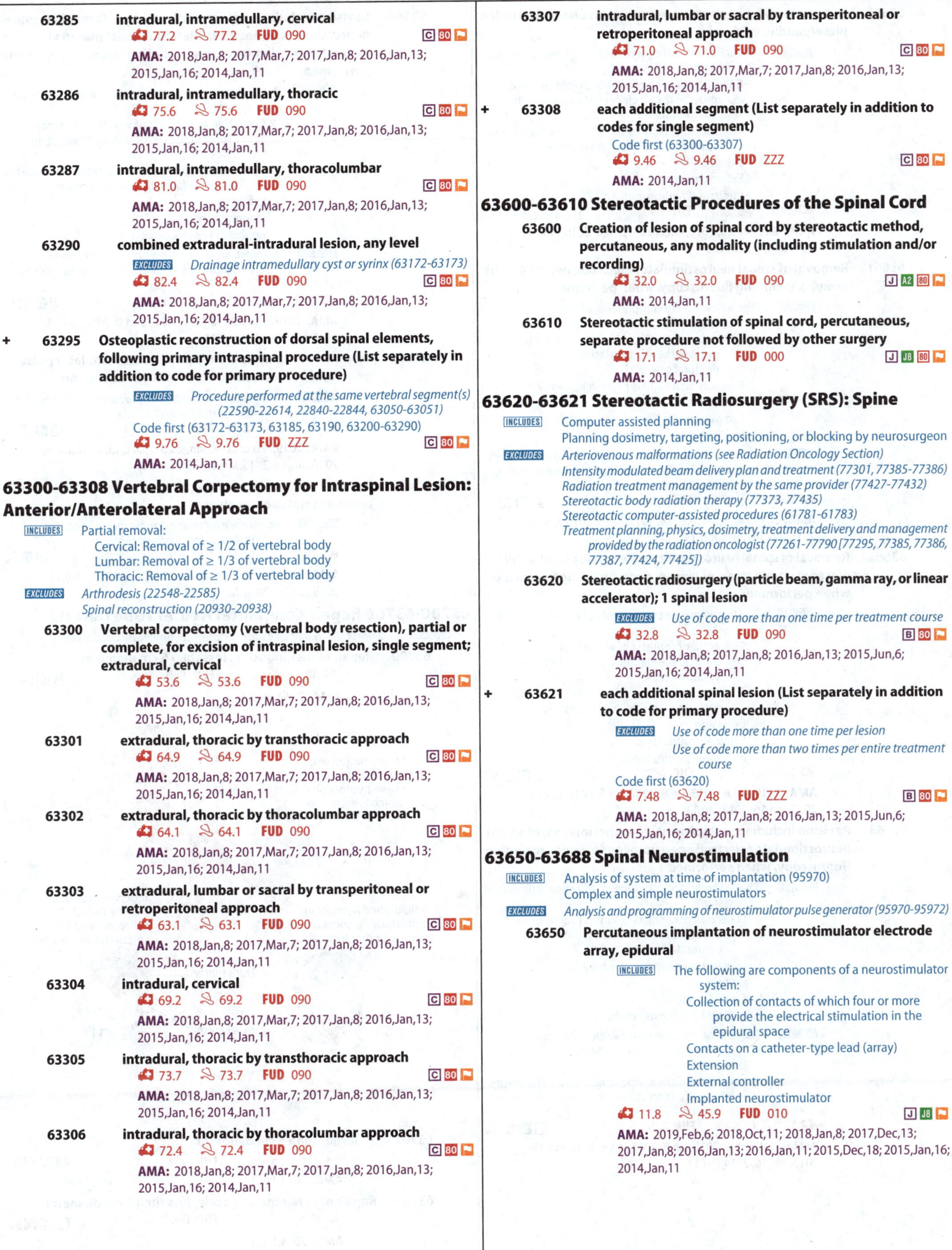

63285 **intradural, intramedullary, cervical**
77.2 77.2 FUD 090 C 80
AMA: 2018,Jan,8; 2017,Mar,7; 2017,Jan,8; 2016,Jan,13; 2015,Jan,16; 2014,Jan,11

63286 **intradural, intramedullary, thoracic**
75.6 75.6 FUD 090 C 80
AMA: 2018,Jan,8; 2017,Mar,7; 2017,Jan,8; 2016,Jan,13; 2015,Jan,16; 2014,Jan,11

63287 **intradural, intramedullary, thoracolumbar**
81.0 81.0 FUD 090 C 80
AMA: 2018,Jan,8; 2017,Mar,7; 2017,Jan,8; 2016,Jan,13; 2015,Jan,16; 2014,Jan,11

63290 **combined extradural-intradural lesion, any level**
EXCLUDES *Drainage intramedullary cyst or syrinx (63172-63173)*
82.4 82.4 FUD 090 C 80
AMA: 2018,Jan,8; 2017,Mar,7; 2017,Jan,8; 2016,Jan,13; 2015,Jan,16; 2014,Jan,11

+ **63295** **Osteoplastic reconstruction of dorsal spinal elements, following primary intraspinal procedure (List separately in addition to code for primary procedure)**
EXCLUDES *Procedure performed at the same vertebral segment(s) (22590-22614, 22840-22844, 63050-63051)*
Code first (63172-63173, 63185, 63190, 63200-63290)
9.76 9.76 FUD ZZZ C 80
AMA: 2014,Jan,11

63300-63308 Vertebral Corpectomy for Intraspinal Lesion: Anterior/Anterolateral Approach

INCLUDES Partial removal:
Cervical: Removal of ≥ 1/2 of vertebral body
Lumbar: Removal of ≥ 1/3 of vertebral body
Thoracic: Removal of ≥ 1/3 of vertebral body

EXCLUDES *Arthrodesis (22548-22585)*
Spinal reconstruction (20930-20938)

63300 **Vertebral corpectomy (vertebral body resection), partial or complete, for excision of intraspinal lesion, single segment; extradural, cervical**
53.6 53.6 FUD 090 C 80
AMA: 2018,Jan,8; 2017,Mar,7; 2017,Jan,8; 2016,Jan,13; 2015,Jan,16; 2014,Jan,11

63301 **extradural, thoracic by transthoracic approach**
64.9 64.9 FUD 090 C 80
AMA: 2018,Jan,8; 2017,Mar,7; 2017,Jan,8; 2016,Jan,13; 2015,Jan,16; 2014,Jan,11

63302 **extradural, thoracic by thoracolumbar approach**
64.1 64.1 FUD 090 C 80
AMA: 2018,Jan,8; 2017,Mar,7; 2017,Jan,8; 2016,Jan,13; 2015,Jan,16; 2014,Jan,11

63303 **extradural, lumbar or sacral by transperitoneal or retroperitoneal approach**
63.1 63.1 FUD 090 C 80
AMA: 2018,Jan,8; 2017,Mar,7; 2017,Jan,8; 2016,Jan,13; 2015,Jan,16; 2014,Jan,11

63304 **intradural, cervical**
69.2 69.2 FUD 090 C 80
AMA: 2018,Jan,8; 2017,Mar,7; 2017,Jan,8; 2016,Jan,13; 2015,Jan,16; 2014,Jan,11

63305 **intradural, thoracic by transthoracic approach**
73.7 73.7 FUD 090 C 80
AMA: 2018,Jan,8; 2017,Mar,7; 2017,Jan,8; 2016,Jan,13; 2015,Jan,16; 2014,Jan,11

63306 **intradural, thoracic by thoracolumbar approach**
72.4 72.4 FUD 090 C 80
AMA: 2018,Jan,8; 2017,Mar,7; 2017,Jan,8; 2016,Jan,13; 2015,Jan,16; 2014,Jan,11

63307 **intradural, lumbar or sacral by transperitoneal or retroperitoneal approach**
71.0 71.0 FUD 090 C 80
AMA: 2018,Jan,8; 2017,Mar,7; 2017,Jan,8; 2016,Jan,13; 2015,Jan,16; 2014,Jan,11

+ **63308** **each additional segment (List separately in addition to codes for single segment)**
Code first (63300-63307)
9.46 9.46 FUD ZZZ C 80
AMA: 2014,Jan,11

63600-63610 Stereotactic Procedures of the Spinal Cord

63600 **Creation of lesion of spinal cord by stereotactic method, percutaneous, any modality (including stimulation and/or recording)**
32.0 32.0 FUD 090 J A2 80
AMA: 2014,Jan,11

63610 **Stereotactic stimulation of spinal cord, percutaneous, separate procedure not followed by other surgery**
17.1 17.1 FUD 000 J J8 80
AMA: 2014,Jan,11

63620-63621 Stereotactic Radiosurgery (SRS): Spine

INCLUDES Computer assisted planning
Planning dosimetry, targeting, positioning, or blocking by neurosurgeon

EXCLUDES *Arteriovenous malformations (see Radiation Oncology Section)*
Intensity modulated beam delivery plan and treatment (77301, 77385-77386)
Radiation treatment management by the same provider (77427-77432)
Stereotactic body radiation therapy (77373, 77435)
Stereotactic computer-assisted procedures (61781-61783)
Treatment planning, physics, dosimetry, treatment delivery and management provided by the radiation oncologist (77261-77790 [77295, 77385, 77386, 77387, 77424, 77425])

63620 **Stereotactic radiosurgery (particle beam, gamma ray, or linear accelerator); 1 spinal lesion**
EXCLUDES *Use of code more than one time per treatment course*
32.8 32.8 FUD 090 B 80
AMA: 2018,Jan,8; 2017,Jan,8; 2016,Jan,13; 2015,Jun,6; 2015,Jan,16; 2014,Jan,11

+ **63621** **each additional spinal lesion (List separately in addition to code for primary procedure)**
EXCLUDES *Use of code more than one time per lesion*
Use of code more than two times per entire treatment course
Code first (63620)
7.48 7.48 FUD ZZZ B 80
AMA: 2018,Jan,8; 2017,Jan,8; 2016,Jan,13; 2015,Jun,6; 2015,Jan,16; 2014,Jan,11

63650-63688 Spinal Neurostimulation

INCLUDES Analysis of system at time of implantation (95970)
Complex and simple neurostimulators

EXCLUDES *Analysis and programming of neurostimulator pulse generator (95970-95972)*

63650 **Percutaneous implantation of neurostimulator electrode array, epidural**
INCLUDES The following are components of a neurostimulator system:
Collection of contacts of which four or more provide the electrical stimulation in the epidural space
Contacts on a catheter-type lead (array)
Extension
External controller
Implanted neurostimulator
11.8 45.9 FUD 010 J J8
AMA: 2019,Feb,6; 2018,Oct,11; 2018,Jan,8; 2017,Dec,13; 2017,Jan,8; 2016,Jan,13; 2016,Jan,11; 2015,Dec,18; 2015,Jan,16; 2014,Jan,11

63655 **Laminectomy for implantation of neurostimulator electrodes, plate/paddle, epidural**

INCLUDES The following are components of a neurostimulator system:
- Collection of contacts of which four or more provide the electrical stimulation in the epidural space
- Contacts on a plate or paddle-shaped surface for systems placed by open exposure
- Extension
- External controller
- Implanted neurostimulator

24.1 24.1 **FUD** 090 J J8 80

AMA: 2019,Feb,6; 2018,Jan,8; 2017,Jan,8; 2016,Jan,13; 2015,Jan,16; 2014,Jan,11

63661 **Removal of spinal neurostimulator electrode percutaneous array(s), including fluoroscopy, when performed**

INCLUDES The following are components of a neurostimulator system:
- Collection of contacts of which four or more provide the electrical stimulation in the epidural space
- Contacts on a catheter-type lead (array)
- Extension
- External controller
- Implanted neurostimulator

EXCLUDES *Use of code when removing or replacing a temporary array placed percutaneously for an external generator*

9.32 17.5 **FUD** 010 Q2 G2 80

AMA: 2019,Feb,6; 2018,Jan,8; 2017,Jan,8; 2016,Jan,13; 2015,Jan,16; 2014,Jan,11

63662 **Removal of spinal neurostimulator electrode plate/paddle(s) placed via laminotomy or laminectomy, including fluoroscopy, when performed**

INCLUDES The following are components of a neurostimulator system:
- Collection of contacts of which four or more provide the electrical stimulation in the epidural space
- Contacts on a plate or paddle-shaped surface for systems placed by open exposure
- Extension
- External controller
- Implanted neurostimulator

24.4 24.4 **FUD** 090 Q2 G2 80

AMA: 2019,Feb,6; 2018,Jan,8; 2017,Jan,8; 2016,Jan,13; 2015,Jan,16; 2014,Jan,11

63663 **Revision including replacement, when performed, of spinal neurostimulator electrode percutaneous array(s), including fluoroscopy, when performed**

INCLUDES The following are components of a neurostimulator system:
- Collection of contacts of which four or more provide the electrical stimulation in the epidural space
- Contacts on a catheter-type lead (array)
- Extension
- External controller
- Implanted neurostimulator

EXCLUDES *Removal of spinal neurostimulator electrode percutaneous array(s), plate/paddle(s) at same level (63661-63662)*

Use of code when removing or replacing a temporary array placed percutaneously for an external generator

12.9 23.4 **FUD** 010 J J8 80

AMA: 2019,Feb,6; 2018,Jan,8; 2017,Jan,8; 2016,Jan,13; 2015,Jan,16; 2014,Jan,11

63664 **Revision including replacement, when performed, of spinal neurostimulator electrode plate/paddle(s) placed via laminotomy or laminectomy, including fluoroscopy, when performed**

INCLUDES The following are components of a neurostimulator system:
- Collection of contacts of which four or more provide the electrical stimulation in the epidural space
- Contacts on a plate or paddle-shaped surface for systems placed by open exposure
- Extension
- External controller
- Implanted neurostimulator

EXCLUDES *Removal of spinal neurostimulator electrode percutaneous array(s), plate/paddle(s) at same level (63661-63662)*

25.2 25.2 **FUD** 090 J J8 80

AMA: 2019,Feb,6; 2018,Jan,8; 2017,Jan,8; 2016,Jan,13; 2015,Jan,16; 2014,Jan,11

63685 **Insertion or replacement of spinal neurostimulator pulse generator or receiver, direct or inductive coupling**

EXCLUDES *Use of code for insertion/replacement with code for revision/removal (63688)*

10.4 10.4 **FUD** 010 J J8 80

AMA: 2019,Feb,6; 2018,Jan,8; 2017,Dec,13; 2017,Jan,8; 2016,Jan,13; 2015,Jan,16; 2014,Jan,11

63688 **Revision or removal of implanted spinal neurostimulator pulse generator or receiver**

EXCLUDES *Use of code for revision/removal with code for insertion/replacement (63685)*

10.7 10.7 **FUD** 010 Q2 A2

AMA: 2019,Feb,6; 2018,Jan,8; 2017,Jan,8; 2016,Jan,13; 2015,Jan,16; 2014,Jan,11

63700-63706 Repair Congenital Neural Tube Defects

EXCLUDES *Complex skin repair (see appropriate integumentary closure code)*

63700 **Repair of meningocele; less than 5 cm diameter**

38.2 38.2 **FUD** 090 63 C 80

AMA: 2014,Jan,11

Most children with severe spina bifida also have hydrocephalus, which is excessive fluid in the skull

Cervical

Thoracic

Lumbar

A fluid-filled herniation that protrudes is spina bifida cystica, or meningocele

If nerves protrude into the defect, it is called rachischisis, or meningomyelocele

Dura mater

Spinal cord

Vertebra

63702 **larger than 5 cm diameter**

41.8 41.8 **FUD** 090 63 C 80

AMA: 2014,Jan,11

63704 **Repair of myelomeningocele; less than 5 cm diameter**

48.5 48.5 **FUD** 090 63 C 80

AMA: 2014,Jan,11

63706 **larger than 5 cm diameter**
54.0 54.0 FUD 090 ⑥③ C 80
AMA: 2014,Jan,11

63707-63710 Repair Dural Cerebrospinal Fluid Leak

63707 **Repair of dural/cerebrospinal fluid leak, not requiring laminectomy**
26.9 26.9 FUD 090 C 80
AMA: 2014,Jan,11

63709 **Repair of dural/cerebrospinal fluid leak or pseudomeningocele, with laminectomy**
32.0 32.0 FUD 090 C 80
AMA: 2014,Jan,11

63710 **Dural graft, spinal**
EXCLUDES *Laminectomy and section of dentate ligament (63180, 63182)*
31.6 31.6 FUD 090 C 80
AMA: 2014,Jan,11

63740-63746 Cerebrospinal Fluid (CSF) Shunt: Lumbar

EXCLUDES *Placement of subarachnoid catheter with reservoir and/or pump:*
Not requiring laminectomy (62350, 62360-62362)
With laminectomy (62351, 62360-62362)

63740 **Creation of shunt, lumbar, subarachnoid-peritoneal, -pleural, or other; including laminectomy**
28.5 28.5 FUD 090 C 80
AMA: 2014,Jan,11

63741 **percutaneous, not requiring laminectomy**
19.7 19.7 FUD 090 J 80
AMA: 2014,Jan,11

63744 **Replacement, irrigation or revision of lumbosubarachnoid shunt**
19.5 19.5 FUD 090 J J8 80
AMA: 2014,Jan,11

63746 **Removal of entire lumbosubarachnoid shunt system without replacement**
17.6 17.6 FUD 090 02 A2 80
AMA: 2014,Jan,11

64400-64463 Nerve Blocks

EXCLUDES *Epidural or subarachnoid injection (62320-62327)*
Nerve destruction (62280-62282, 64600-64681 [64633, 64634, 64635, 64636])

▲ 64400 **Injection(s), anesthetic agent(s) and/or steroid; trigeminal nerve, each branch (ie, ophthalmic, maxillary, mandibular)**
EXCLUDES *Destruction of genicular nerve branches ([64624])*
Imaging guidance and localization
Injection of genicular nerve branches (64454)
Use of code more than one time per encounter when multiple injections are required to block nerve and branches
2.08 3.88 FUD 000 T P3 50
AMA: 2018,Jan,8; 2017,Jan,8; 2016,Jan,13; 2015,Jan,16; 2014,Jan,11

~~64402~~ ~~**facial nerve**~~
To report, see (64999)

▲ 64405 **greater occipital nerve**
EXCLUDES *Destruction of genicular nerve branches ([64624])*
Imaging guidance and localization
Injection of genicular nerve branches (64454)
Use of code more than one time per encounter when multiple injections are required to block nerve and branches
1.54 2.37 FUD 000 T P3 50
AMA: 2018,Jan,8; 2017,Jan,8; 2016,Oct,11; 2016,Jan,13; 2015,Jan,16; 2014,Jan,11

▲ 64408 **vagus nerve**
EXCLUDES *Destruction of genicular nerve branches ([64624])*
Imaging guidance and localization
Injection of genicular nerve branches (64454)
Use of code more than one time per encounter when multiple injections are required to block nerve and branches
2.44 3.35 FUD 000 T P3 80 50
AMA: 2018,Jan,8; 2017,Jan,8; 2016,Jan,13; 2015,Jan,16; 2014,Jan,11

~~64410~~ ~~**phrenic nerve**~~
To report, see (64999)

~~64413~~ ~~**cervical plexus**~~
To report, see (64999)

▲ 64415 **brachial plexus**
EXCLUDES *Destruction of genicular nerve branches ([64624])*
Imaging guidance and localization
Injection of genicular nerve branches (64454)
Use of code more than one time per encounter when multiple injections are required to block nerve and branches
1.87 3.38 FUD 000 T A2 50
AMA: 2018,Jan,8; 2017,Jan,8; 2016,Jan,13; 2015,Jan,16; 2014,Jan,11

▲ 64416 **brachial plexus, continuous infusion by catheter (including catheter placement)**
EXCLUDES *Destruction of genicular nerve branches ([64624])*
Imaging guidance and localization
Injection of genicular nerve branches (64454)
Management of epidural or subarachnoid continuous drug administration (01996)
Use of code more than one time per encounter when multiple injections are required to block nerve and branches
2.28 2.28 FUD 000 T G2 50
AMA: 2018,Jan,8; 2017,Jan,8; 2016,Jan,13; 2015,Jan,16; 2014,Jan,11

▲ 64417 **axillary nerve**
EXCLUDES *Destruction of genicular nerve branches ([64624])*
Imaging guidance and localization
Injection of genicular nerve branches (64454)
Use of code more than one time per encounter when multiple injections are required to block nerve and branches
2.02 3.76 FUD 000 T A2 50
AMA: 2018,Jan,8; 2017,Jan,8; 2016,Jan,13; 2015,Jan,16; 2014,Jan,11

▲ 64418 **suprascapular nerve**
EXCLUDES *Destruction of genicular nerve branches ([64624])*
Imaging guidance and localization
Injection of genicular nerve branches (64454)
Use of code more than one time per encounter when multiple injections are required to block nerve and branches
1.64 2.71 FUD 000 T P3 50
AMA: 2018,Jan,8; 2017,Jan,8; 2016,Jan,13; 2015,Jan,16; 2014,Jan,11

▲ 64420 **intercostal nerve, single level**
EXCLUDES *Destruction of genicular nerve branches ([64624])*
Imaging guidance and localization
Injection of genicular nerve branches (64454)
Use of code more than one time per encounter when multiple injections are required to block nerve and branches
1.92 3.15 FUD 000 T A2
AMA: 2018,Jan,8; 2017,Jan,8; 2016,Jan,9; 2016,Jan,13; 2015,Jun,3; 2015,Jan,16; 2014,Jan,11

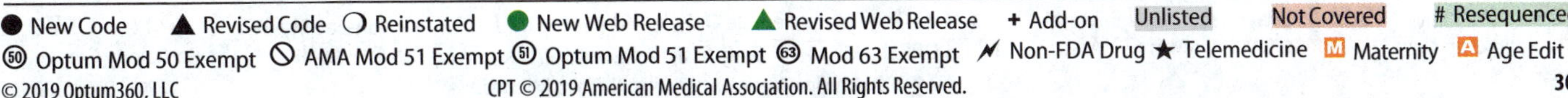

▲ + **64421** **intercostal nerve, each additional level (List separately in addition to code for primary procedure)**

EXCLUDES *Destruction of genicular nerve branches ([64624])*
Imaging guidance and localization
Injection of genicular nerve branches (64454)
Reporting with modifier 50. Report once for each side when performed bilaterally
Use of code more than one time per encounter when multiple injections are required to block nerve and branches

2.64 | 4.46 | **FUD** 000 | (50) T A2

AMA: 2018,Jan,8; 2017,Jan,8; 2016,Jan,9; 2016,Jan,13; 2015,Jun,3; 2015,Jan,16; 2014,Jan,11

▲ **64425** **ilioinguinal, iliohypogastric nerves**

EXCLUDES *Destruction of genicular nerve branches ([64624])*
Imaging guidance and localization
Injection of genicular nerve branches (64454)
Use of code more than one time per encounter when multiple injections are required to block nerve and branches

2.72 | 3.93 | **FUD** 000 | T P3 50

AMA: 2018,Jan,8; 2017,Jan,8; 2016,Jan,13; 2015,Jun,3; 2015,Jan,16; 2014,Jan,11

▲ **64430** **pudendal nerve**

EXCLUDES *Destruction of genicular nerve branches ([64624])*
Imaging guidance and localization
Injection of genicular nerve branches (64454)
Use of code more than one time per encounter when multiple injections are required to block nerve and branches

2.30 | 4.14 | **FUD** 000 | T A2 50

AMA: 2018,Jan,8; 2017,Jan,8; 2016,Jan,13; 2015,Jan,16; 2014,Jan,11

▲ **64435** **paracervical (uterine) nerve** ♀

EXCLUDES *Destruction of genicular nerve branches ([64624])*
Imaging guidance and localization
Injection of genicular nerve branches (64454)
Use of code more than one time per encounter when multiple injections are required to block nerve and branches

2.35 | 4.00 | **FUD** 000 | T P3 50

AMA: 2018,Jan,8; 2017,Jan,8; 2016,Jan,13; 2015,Jan,16; 2014,Jan,11

▲ **64445** **sciatic nerve**

EXCLUDES *Destruction of genicular nerve branches ([64624])*
Imaging guidance and localization
Injection of genicular nerve branches (64454)
Use of code more than one time per encounter when multiple injections are required to block nerve and branches

2.09 | 3.89 | **FUD** 000 | T P3 50

AMA: 2018,Jan,8; 2017,Jan,8; 2016,Jan,13; 2015,Jan,16; 2014,Jan,11

▲ **64446** **sciatic nerve, continuous infusion by catheter (including catheter placement)**

EXCLUDES *Destruction of genicular nerve branches ([64624])*
Imaging guidance and localization
Injection of genicular nerve branches (64454)
Management of epidural or subarachnoid continuous drug administration (01996)
Use of code more than one time per encounter when multiple injections are required to block nerve and branches

2.28 | 2.28 | **FUD** 000 | T G2 50

AMA: 2018,Jan,8; 2017,Jan,8; 2016,Jan,13; 2015,Jan,16; 2014,Jan,11

▲ **64447** **femoral nerve**

EXCLUDES *Destruction of genicular nerve branches ([64624])*
Imaging guidance and localization
Injection of genicular nerve branches (64454)
Management of epidural or subarachnoid continuous drug administration (01996)
Use of code more than one time per encounter when multiple injections are required to block nerve and branches

1.91 | 3.46 | **FUD** 000 | T P3 50

AMA: 2018,Jan,8; 2017,Jan,8; 2016,Jan,13; 2015,Sep,12; 2015,Jan,16; 2014,Dec,16; 2014,Dec,16; 2014,Nov,14; 2014,Jan,11

▲ **64448** **femoral nerve, continuous infusion by catheter (including catheter placement)**

EXCLUDES *Destruction of genicular nerve branches ([64624])*
Imaging guidance and localization
Injection of genicular nerve branches (64454)
Management of epidural or subarachnoid continuous drug administration (01996)
Use of code more than one time per encounter when multiple injections are required to block nerve and branches

2.05 | 2.05 | **FUD** 000 | T G2 50

AMA: 2018,Jan,8; 2017,Jan,8; 2016,Jan,13; 2015,Sep,12; 2015,Jan,16; 2014,Dec,16; 2014,Dec,16; 2014,Nov,14; 2014,Jan,11

▲ **64449** **lumbar plexus, posterior approach, continuous infusion by catheter (including catheter placement)**

EXCLUDES *Destruction of genicular nerve branches ([64624])*
Imaging guidance and localization
Injection of genicular nerve branches (64454)
Management of epidural or subarachnoid continuous drug administration (01996)
Use of code more than one time per encounter when multiple injections are required to block nerve and branches

2.44 | 2.44 | **FUD** 000 | T G2 50

AMA: 2018,Jan,8; 2017,Jan,8; 2016,Jan,13; 2015,Jan,16; 2014,Jan,11

▲ **64450** **other peripheral nerve or branch**

EXCLUDES *Destruction of genicular nerve branches ([64624])*
Imaging guidance and localization
Injection of genicular nerve branches (64454)
Injection of nerves innervating the sacroiliac joint (64451)
Use of code more than one time per encounter when multiple injections are required to block nerve and branches

1.28 | 2.19 | **FUD** 000 | T P3 50

AMA: 2018,Nov,10; 2018,Jan,8; 2017,Jan,8; 2016,Oct,11; 2016,Jan,13; 2015,Nov,10; 2015,Sep,12; 2015,Jun,3; 2015,Jan,16; 2014,Jan,11

● **64451** **nerves innervating the sacroiliac joint, with image guidance (ie, fluoroscopy or computed tomography)**

INCLUDES Imaging guidance and any contrast injection

EXCLUDES *Destruction of genicular nerve branches ([64624])*
Injection of genicular nerve branches (64454)
Use of code more than one time per encounter when multiple injections are required to block nerve and branches

● **64454** **genicular nerve branches, including imaging guidance, when performed**

INCLUDES Imaging guidance and any contrast injection

EXCLUDES *Destruction of genicular nerve branches ([64624])*
Injection of genicular nerve branches (64454)
Use of code more than one time per encounter when multiple injections are required to block nerve and branches

Modifier 52 for injection of fewer than all of the following genicular nerve branches: superolateral, superomedial, and inferomedial

64455 **Injection(s), anesthetic agent and/or steroid, plantar common digital nerve(s) (eg, Morton's neuroma)**

INCLUDES Single or multiple injections on the same site

EXCLUDES *Destruction by neurolytic agent; plantar common digital nerve (64632)*
Destruction of genicular nerve branches ([64624])
Imaging guidance and localization
Injection of genicular nerve branches (64454)
Use of code more than one time per encounter when multiple injections are required to block nerve and branches

1.00 1.36 FUD 000 T P3 80 50

AMA: 2018,Jan,8; 2017,Jan,8; 2016,Jan,13; 2015,Jan,16; 2014,Jan,11

64461 **Resequenced code. See code following 64484.**

64462 **Resequenced code. See code following 64484.**

64463 **Resequenced code. See code following 64484.**

64479-64484 Transforaminal Injection

INCLUDES Imaging guidance (fluoroscopy or CT) and contrast injection

EXCLUDES *Epidural or subarachnoid injection (62320-62327)*
Nerve destruction (62280-62282, 64600-64681 [64633, 64634, 64635, 64636])

64479 **Injection(s), anesthetic agent and/or steroid, transforaminal epidural, with imaging guidance (fluoroscopy or CT); cervical or thoracic, single level**

INCLUDES Imaging guidance and any contrast injection
Single or multiple injections on the same site
Transforaminal epidural injection at T12-L1 level

EXCLUDES *Transforaminal epidural injection using ultrasonic guidance (0228T)*

3.76 6.95 FUD 000 T A2 50

AMA: 2018,Jan,8; 2017,Jan,8; 2016,Jan,13; 2016,Jan,9; 2015,Jan,16; 2014,Jan,11

Thoracic vertebra (superior view)

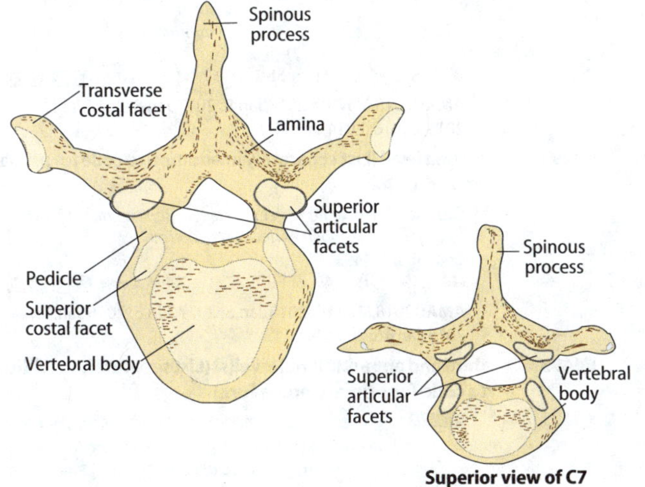

Superior view of C7

\+ **64480** **cervical or thoracic, each additional level (List separately in addition to code for primary procedure)**

INCLUDES Imaging guidance and any contrast injection
Single or multiple injections on the same site

EXCLUDES *Destruction of genicular nerve branches ([64624])*
Injection of genicular nerve branches (64454)
Reporting with modifier 50. Report once for each side when performed bilaterally
Transforaminal epidural injection at T12-L1 level
Transforaminal epidural injection using ultrasonic guidance (0229T)
Use of code more than one time per encounter when multiple injections are required to block nerve and branches

Code first (64479)

1.80 3.42 FUD ZZZ 50 N N1

AMA: 2018,Jan,8; 2017,Jan,8; 2016,Jan,9; 2016,Jan,13; 2015,Jan,16; 2014,Jan,11

64483 **lumbar or sacral, single level**

INCLUDES Imaging guidance and any contrast injection
Single or multiple injections on the same site

EXCLUDES *Destruction of genicular nerve branches ([64624])*
Injection of genicular nerve branches (64454)
Transforaminal epidural injection using ultrasonic guidance (0230T)
Use of code more than one time per encounter when multiple injections are required to block nerve and branches

3.19 6.44 FUD 000 T A2 50

AMA: 2018,Jan,8; 2017,Jan,8; 2016,Oct,11; 2016,Jan,13; 2016,Jan,9; 2015,Jan,16; 2014,Jan,11

\+ **64484** **lumbar or sacral, each additional level (List separately in addition to code for primary procedure)**

INCLUDES Imaging guidance and any contrast injection
Single or multiple injections on the same site

EXCLUDES *Destruction of genicular nerve branches ([64624])*
Injection of genicular nerve branches (64454)
Reporting with modifier 50. Report once for each side when performed bilaterally
Transforaminal epidural injection using ultrasonic guidance (0231T)
Use of code more than one time per encounter when multiple injections are required to block nerve and branches

Code first (64483)

1.49 2.79 FUD ZZZ 50 N N1

AMA: 2018,Jan,8; 2017,Jan,8; 2016,Jan,9; 2016,Jan,13; 2015,Jan,16; 2014,Jan,11

64461-64463 [64461, 64462, 64463] Paravertebral Blocks

INCLUDES Radiological guidance (76942, 77002-77003)

EXCLUDES *Injection of:*
Anesthetic agent (64420-64421, 64479-64480)
Diagnostic or therapeutic substance (62320, 62324, 64490-64492)

\# **64461** **Paravertebral block (PVB) (paraspinous block), thoracic; single injection site (includes imaging guidance, when performed)**

INCLUDES Imaging guidance and any contrast injection

EXCLUDES *Destruction of genicular nerve branches ([64624])*
Injection of genicular nerve branches (64454)
Use of code more than one time per encounter when multiple injections are required to block nerve and branches

2.33 3.96 FUD 000 T G2 50

AMA: 2018,Dec,8; 2018,Dec,8; 2018,Jan,8; 2017,Jan,8; 2016,Jan,9

+ # 64462 **second and any additional injection site(s) (includes imaging guidance, when performed) (List separately in addition to code for primary procedure)**

INCLUDES Imaging guidance and any contrast injection

EXCLUDES *Destruction of genicular nerve branches ([64624])*
Injection of genicular nerve branches (64454)
Procedure performed more than one time per day
Reporting with modifier 50. Report once for each side when performed bilaterally

Code first (64461)

1.47 2.20 FUD ZZZ (50) N N1 80

AMA: 2018,Dec,8; 2018,Dec,8; 2018,Jan,8; 2017,Jan,8; 2016,Jan,9

 # 64463 **continuous infusion by catheter (includes imaging guidance, when performed)**

INCLUDES Imaging guidance and any contrast injection

EXCLUDES *Destruction of genicular nerve branches ([64624])*
Injection of genicular nerve branches (64454)
Use of code more than one time per encounter when multiple injections are required to block nerve and branches

2.42 5.13 FUD 000 T G2 50

AMA: 2018,Dec,8; 2018,Dec,8; 2018,Jan,8; 2017,Jan,8; 2016,Jan,9

64486-64489 Transversus Abdominis Plane (TAP) Block

64486 **Transversus abdominis plane (TAP) block (abdominal plane block, rectus sheath block) unilateral; by injection(s) (includes imaging guidance, when performed)**

INCLUDES Imaging guidance and any contrast injection

EXCLUDES *Destruction of genicular nerve branches ([64624])*
Injection of genicular nerve branches (64454)
Use of code more than one time per encounter when multiple injections are required to block nerve and branches

1.61 3.12 FUD 000 N N1 50

AMA: 2018,Jan,8; 2017,Jan,8; 2016,Jan,13; 2015,Jun,3

64487 **by continuous infusion(s) (includes imaging guidance, when performed)**

INCLUDES Imaging guidance and any contrast injection

EXCLUDES *Destruction of genicular nerve branches ([64624])*
Injection of genicular nerve branches (64454)
Use of code more than one time per encounter when multiple injections are required to block nerve and branches

1.87 4.49 FUD 000 N N1 50

AMA: 2018,Jan,8; 2017,Jan,8; 2016,Jan,13; 2015,Jun,3

64488 **Transversus abdominis plane (TAP) block (abdominal plane block, rectus sheath block) bilateral; by injections (includes imaging guidance, when performed)**

INCLUDES Imaging guidance and any contrast injection

EXCLUDES *Destruction of genicular nerve branches ([64624])*
Injection of genicular nerve branches (64454)
Use of code more than one time per encounter when multiple injections are required to block nerve and branches

2.02 3.83 FUD 000 N N1

AMA: 2018,Jan,8; 2017,Jan,8; 2016,Jan,13; 2015,Jun,3

64489 **by continuous infusions (includes imaging guidance, when performed)**

INCLUDES Imaging guidance and any contrast injection

EXCLUDES *Destruction of genicular nerve branches ([64624])*
Injection of genicular nerve branches (64454)
Use of code more than one time per encounter when multiple injections are required to block nerve and branches

2.27 6.65 FUD 000 N N1

AMA: 2018,Jan,8; 2017,Jan,8; 2016,Jan,13; 2015,Jun,3

64490-64495 Paraspinal Nerve Injections

INCLUDES Image guidance (CT or fluoroscopy) and any contrast injection

EXCLUDES *Injection without imaging (20552-20553)*
Ultrasonic guidance (0213T-0218T)

64490 **Injection(s), diagnostic or therapeutic agent, paravertebral facet (zygapophyseal) joint (or nerves innervating that joint) with image guidance (fluoroscopy or CT), cervical or thoracic; single level**

INCLUDES Injection of T12-L1 joint and nerves that innervate that joint

3.03 5.39 FUD 000 T G2 80 50

AMA: 2018,Jan,8; 2017,Jan,8; 2016,Jan,9; 2016,Jan,13; 2015,Jan,16; 2014,Jan,11

+ 64491 **second level (List separately in addition to code for primary procedure)**

EXCLUDES *Reporting with modifier 50. Report once for each side when performed bilaterally*

Code first (64490)

1.72 2.68 FUD ZZZ (50) N N1 80

AMA: 2018,Jan,8; 2017,Jan,8; 2016,Jan,9; 2016,Jan,13; 2015,Jan,16; 2014,Jan,11

+ 64492 **third and any additional level(s) (List separately in addition to code for primary procedure)**

EXCLUDES *Procedure performed more than one time per day*
Reporting with modifier 50. Report once for each side when performed bilaterally

Code also when appropriate (64491)

Code first (64490)

1.74 2.70 FUD ZZZ (50) N N1 80

AMA: 2018,Jan,8; 2017,Jan,8; 2016,Jan,9; 2016,Jan,13; 2015,Jan,16; 2014,Jan,11

64493 **Injection(s), diagnostic or therapeutic agent, paravertebral facet (zygapophyseal) joint (or nerves innervating that joint) with image guidance (fluoroscopy or CT), lumbar or sacral; single level**

EXCLUDES *Injection of nerves innervating the sacroiliac joint (64451)*

2.58 4.91 FUD 000 T G2 80 50

AMA: 2018,May,10; 2018,Jan,8; 2017,Jan,8; 2016,Jan,13; 2015,Jan,16; 2014,Jan,11

+ 64494 **second level (List separately in addition to code for primary procedure)**

EXCLUDES *Reporting with modifier 50. Report once for each side when performed bilaterally*

Code first (64493)

1.49 2.49 FUD ZZZ (50) N N1 80

AMA: 2018,May,10; 2018,Jan,8; 2017,Jan,8; 2016,Jan,13; 2015,Jan,16; 2014,Jan,11

+ 64495 **third and any additional level(s) (List separately in addition to code for primary procedure)**

EXCLUDES *Procedure performed more than one time per day*
Reporting with modifier 50. Report once for each side when performed bilaterally

Code also when appropriate (64494)

Code first (64493)

1.51 2.49 FUD ZZZ (50) N N1 80

AMA: 2018,May,10; 2018,Jan,8; 2017,Jan,8; 2016,Jan,13; 2015,Jan,16; 2014,Jan,11

64505-64530 Sympathetic Nerve Blocks

64505 **Injection, anesthetic agent; sphenopalatine ganglion**

2.69 3.36 FUD 000 T P3 50

AMA: 2018,Jan,8; 2017,Jan,8; 2016,Jan,13; 2015,Jan,16; 2014,Jul,8; 2014,Jan,11

64510 **stellate ganglion (cervical sympathetic)**

2.13 3.78 FUD 000 T A2 50

AMA: 2018,Jan,8; 2017,Jan,8; 2016,Jan,13; 2015,Jan,16; 2014,Jan,11

64517 **superior hypogastric plexus**
3.60 | 5.43 | FUD 000 | T A2
AMA: 2018,Jan,8; 2017,Jan,8; 2016,Jan,13; 2015,Jan,16; 2014,Jan,11

64520 **lumbar or thoracic (paravertebral sympathetic)**
2.34 | 5.75 | FUD 000 | T A2 50
AMA: 2018,Jan,8; 2017,Jan,8; 2016,Jan,13; 2015,Jan,16; 2014,Jan,11

64530 **celiac plexus, with or without radiologic monitoring**
EXCLUDES *Transmural anesthetic injection with transendoscopic ultrasound-guidance (43253)*
2.63 | 5.73 | FUD 000 | T A2
AMA: 2018,Jan,8; 2017,Jan,8; 2016,Jan,13; 2015,Jan,16; 2014,Jan,11

64553-64570 Electrical Nerve Stimulation: Insertion/Replacement/Removal/Revision

INCLUDES Analysis of system at time of implantation (95970)
Simple and complex neurostimulators
EXCLUDES *Analysis and programming of neurostimulator pulse generator (95970-95972)*
TENS therapy (97014, 97032)

64553 **Percutaneous implantation of neurostimulator electrode array; cranial nerve**
INCLUDES Temporary and permanent percutaneous array placement
EXCLUDES *Open procedure (61885-61886)*
Percutaneous electrical stimulation of peripheral nerve with needle or needle electrodes (64999)
10.1 | 48.8 | FUD 010 | J J8 80
AMA: 2019,Feb,6; 2018,Oct,8; 2018,Jan,8; 2017,Jan,8; 2016,Jan,13; 2015,Jan,16; 2014,Jan,11

64555 **peripheral nerve (excludes sacral nerve)**
INCLUDES Temporary and permanent percutaneous array placement
EXCLUDES *Percutaneous electrical stimulation of a cranial nerve with needle or needle electrodes (64999)*
Posterior tibial neurostimulation (64566)
9.85 | 44.3 | FUD 010 | J J8
AMA: 2019,Feb,6; 2018,Oct,8; 2018,Aug,10; 2018,Jan,8; 2017,Dec,13; 2017,Jan,8; 2016,Feb,13; 2016,Jan,13; 2015,Jan,16; 2015,Jan,13; 2014,Jan,11

64561 **sacral nerve (transforaminal placement) including image guidance, if performed**
INCLUDES Temporary and permanent percutaneous array placement
EXCLUDES *Percutaneous electrical stimulation or neuromodulation with needle or needle electrodes (64999)*
8.75 | 20.9 | FUD 010 | J J8 50
AMA: 2019,Feb,6; 2018,Oct,8; 2018,Jan,8; 2017,Jan,8; 2016,Jan,13; 2015,Jan,16; 2014,Sep,5; 2014,Jan,11

64566 **Posterior tibial neurostimulation, percutaneous needle electrode, single treatment, includes programming**
EXCLUDES *Electronic analysis of implanted neurostimulator pulse generator system (95970-95972)*
Percutaneous implantation of neurostimulator electrode array; peripheral nerve (64555)
0.87 | 3.62 | FUD 000 | T P3 80
AMA: 2019,Feb,6; 2018,Oct,8; 2018,Jan,8; 2017,Jan,8; 2016,Jan,13; 2015,Jan,16; 2014,Jan,11

64568 **Incision for implantation of cranial nerve (eg, vagus nerve) neurostimulator electrode array and pulse generator**
EXCLUDES *Insertion chest wall respiratory sensor electrode or array with pulse generator connection (0466T)*
Insertion, replacement of cranial neurostimulator pulse generator or receiver (61885-61886)
Removal of neurostimulator electrode array and pulse generator (64570)
18.4 | 18.4 | FUD 090 | J J8 80 50
AMA: 2019,Feb,6; 2018,Mar,9; 2018,Jan,8; 2017,Jan,8; 2016,Nov,6; 2016,Jan,13; 2015,Jan,16; 2014,Jan,11

64569 **Revision or replacement of cranial nerve (eg, vagus nerve) neurostimulator electrode array, including connection to existing pulse generator**
EXCLUDES *Removal of neurostimulator electrode array and pulse generator (64570)*
Replacement of pulse generator (61885)
Revision or replacement chest wall respiratory sensor electrode with pulse generator connection (0467T)
Revision, removal pulse generator (61888)
22.1 | 22.1 | FUD 090 | J J8 80 50
AMA: 2019,Feb,6; 2018,Mar,9; 2018,Jan,8; 2017,Jan,8; 2016,Nov,6; 2016,Jan,13; 2015,Jan,16; 2014,Jan,11

64570 **Removal of cranial nerve (eg, vagus nerve) neurostimulator electrode array and pulse generator**
EXCLUDES *Laparoscopic revision, replacement, removal, or implantation of vagus nerve blocking neurostimulator pulse generator and/or electrode array at the esophagogastric junction (0312T-0317T)*
Removal of chest wall respiratory sensor electrode or array (0468T)
Revision, removal pulse generator (61888)
21.4 | 21.4 | FUD 090 | Q2 G2 80 50
AMA: 2019,Feb,6; 2018,Mar,9; 2018,Jan,8; 2017,Jan,8; 2016,Nov,6; 2016,Jan,13; 2015,Jan,16; 2014,Jan,11

64575-64595 Implantation/Revision/Removal Neurostimulators: Incisional

INCLUDES Simple and complex neurostimulators
EXCLUDES *Analysis and programming of neurostimulator pulse generator (95970-95972)*

64575 **Incision for implantation of neurostimulator electrode array; peripheral nerve (excludes sacral nerve)**
9.60 | 9.60 | FUD 090 | J J8
AMA: 2019,Feb,6; 2014,Jan,11

64580 **neuromuscular**
8.88 | 8.88 | FUD 090 | J G2 80
AMA: 2019,Feb,6; 2014,Jan,11

64581 **sacral nerve (transforaminal placement)**
19.0 | 19.0 | FUD 090 | J J8
AMA: 2019,Feb,6; 2018,Jan,8; 2017,Jan,8; 2016,Jan,13; 2015,Jan,16; 2014,Sep,5; 2014,Jan,11

64585 **Revision or removal of peripheral neurostimulator electrode array**
4.14 | 7.03 | FUD 010 | Q2 A2
AMA: 2019,Feb,6; 2014,Jan,11

64590 **Insertion or replacement of peripheral or gastric neurostimulator pulse generator or receiver, direct or inductive coupling**
EXCLUDES *Revision, removal of neurostimulator pulse generator (64595)*
4.64 | 7.60 | FUD 010 | J J8
AMA: 2019,Feb,6; 2018,Aug,10; 2018,Jan,8; 2017,Dec,13; 2017,Jan,8; 2016,Jan,13; 2015,Jan,13; 2015,Jan,16; 2014,Jan,11

64595 **Revision or removal of peripheral or gastric neurostimulator pulse generator or receiver**
EXCLUDES *Insertion, replacement of neurostimulator pulse generator (64590)*
3.63 | 6.89 | FUD 010 | Q2 J8
AMA: 2019,Feb,6; 2018,Jan,8; 2017,Jan,8; 2016,Jan,13; 2015,Jan,16; 2014,Jan,11

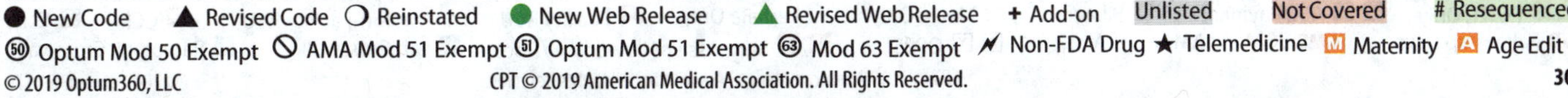

64600-64610 Chemical Denervation Trigeminal Nerve

INCLUDES Injection of therapeutic medication

EXCLUDES *Electromyography or muscle electric stimulation guidance (95873-95874)*
Nerve destruction of:
Anal sphincter (46505)
Bladder (52287)
Strabismus that involves the extraocular muscles (67345)
Treatments that do not destroy the target nerve (64999)

Code also chemodenervation agent

64600 Destruction by neurolytic agent, trigeminal nerve; supraorbital, infraorbital, mental, or inferior alveolar branch
6.66 12.3 FUD 010 T A2
AMA: 2019,Apr,9; 2018,Jan,8; 2017,Jan,8; 2016,Jan,13; 2015,Jan,16; 2014,Jan,11

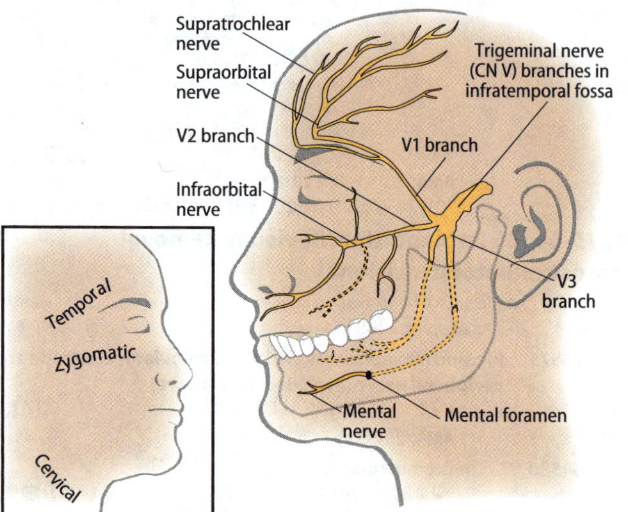

64605 second and third division branches at foramen ovale
10.0 16.8 FUD 010 J A2 80 50
AMA: 2019,Apr,9; 2018,Jan,8; 2017,Jan,8; 2016,Jan,13; 2015,Jan,16; 2014,Jan,11

64610 second and third division branches at foramen ovale under radiologic monitoring
14.2 22.0 FUD 010 J A2 50
AMA: 2019,Apr,9; 2018,Jan,8; 2017,Apr,9; 2017,Jan,8; 2016,Jan,13; 2015,Jan,16; 2014,Jan,11

64624 [64624] Chemical Denervation Genicular Nerve Branches

● # **64624 Destruction by neurolytic agent, genicular nerve branches including imaging guidance, when performed**
0.00 0.00 FUD 000

EXCLUDES *Injection of genicular nerve branches (64454)*

Code also modifier 52 for destruction of fewer than all of the following genicular nerve branches: superolateral, superomedial, and inferomedial

64625 [64625] Radiofrequency Ablation Sacroiliac Joint Nerves

● # **64625 Radiofrequency ablation, nerves innervating the sacroiliac joint, with image guidance (ie, fluoroscopy or computed tomography)**
0.00 0.00 FUD 000

INCLUDES CT needle guidance (77012)
Electrical stimulation or needle electromyelograph for guidance (95873-95874)
Fluoroscopic needle guidance or localization (77002-77003)

EXCLUDES *Destruction by neurolytic agent, paravertebral facet joint nerve ([64624])*
Radiofrequency ablation with ultrasound (76999)

64611-64617 Chemical Denervation Procedures Head and Neck

INCLUDES Injection of therapeutic medication

EXCLUDES *Electromyography or muscle electric stimulation guidance (95873-95874)*
Nerve destruction of:
Anal sphincter (46505)
Bladder (52287)
Extraocular muscles to treat strabismus (67345)
Treatments that do not destroy the target nerve (64999)

64611 Chemodenervation of parotid and submandibular salivary glands, bilateral
Code also modifier 52 for injection of fewer than four salivary glands
3.03 3.45 FUD 010 T P3 80
AMA: 2019,Apr,9; 2018,Jan,8; 2017,Jan,8; 2016,Jan,13; 2015,Jan,16; 2014,Jan,11

64612 Chemodenervation of muscle(s); muscle(s) innervated by facial nerve, unilateral (eg, for blepharospasm, hemifacial spasm)
3.39 3.83 FUD 010 T P3 50
AMA: 2019,Apr,9; 2018,Jan,8; 2017,Jan,8; 2016,Jan,13; 2015,Jan,16; 2014,May,5; 2014,Jan,11; 2014,Jan,6

64615 muscle(s) innervated by facial, trigeminal, cervical spinal and accessory nerves, bilateral (eg, for chronic migraine)
EXCLUDES *Chemodenervation (64612, 64616-64617, 64642-64647)*
Procedure performed more than one time per session
Code also any guidance by muscle electrical stimulation or needle electromyography but report only once (95873-95874)
3.58 4.27 FUD 010 T P3
AMA: 2019,Apr,9; 2018,Jan,8; 2017,Jan,8; 2016,Jan,13; 2015,Jan,16; 2014,Jan,11; 2014,Jan,6

64616 neck muscle(s), excluding muscles of the larynx, unilateral (eg, for cervical dystonia, spasmodic torticollis)
Code also guidance by muscle electrical stimulation or needle electromyography, but report only once (95873-95874)
3.18 3.80 FUD 010 T P3 50
AMA: 2019,Apr,9; 2018,Jan,8; 2017,Jan,8; 2016,Jan,13; 2015,Jan,16; 2014,May,5; 2014,Jan,6; 2014,Jan,11

64617 larynx, unilateral, percutaneous (eg, for spasmodic dysphonia), includes guidance by needle electromyography, when performed
EXCLUDES *Chemodenervation of larynx via direct laryngoscopy (31570-31571)*
Diagnostic needle electromyography of larynx (95865)
Electrical stimulation guidance for chemodenervation (95873-95874)
3.14 4.62 FUD 010 T P3 50
AMA: 2019,Apr,9; 2018,Jan,8; 2017,Jan,8; 2016,Jan,13; 2015,Jan,16; 2014,Jan,6; 2014,Jan,11

64620-64640 [64633, 64634, 64635, 64636] Chemical Denervation Intercostal, Facet Joint, Plantar, and Pudendal Nerve(s)

INCLUDES Injection of therapeutic medication

64620 Destruction by neurolytic agent, intercostal nerve
5.00 5.91 FUD 010 T A2
AMA: 2019,Apr,9; 2018,Jan,8; 2017,Jan,8; 2016,Jan,13; 2015,Jan,16; 2014,Jan,6; 2014,Jan,11

64624 **Resequenced code. See code following 64610.**

64625 **Resequenced code. See code before 64611.**

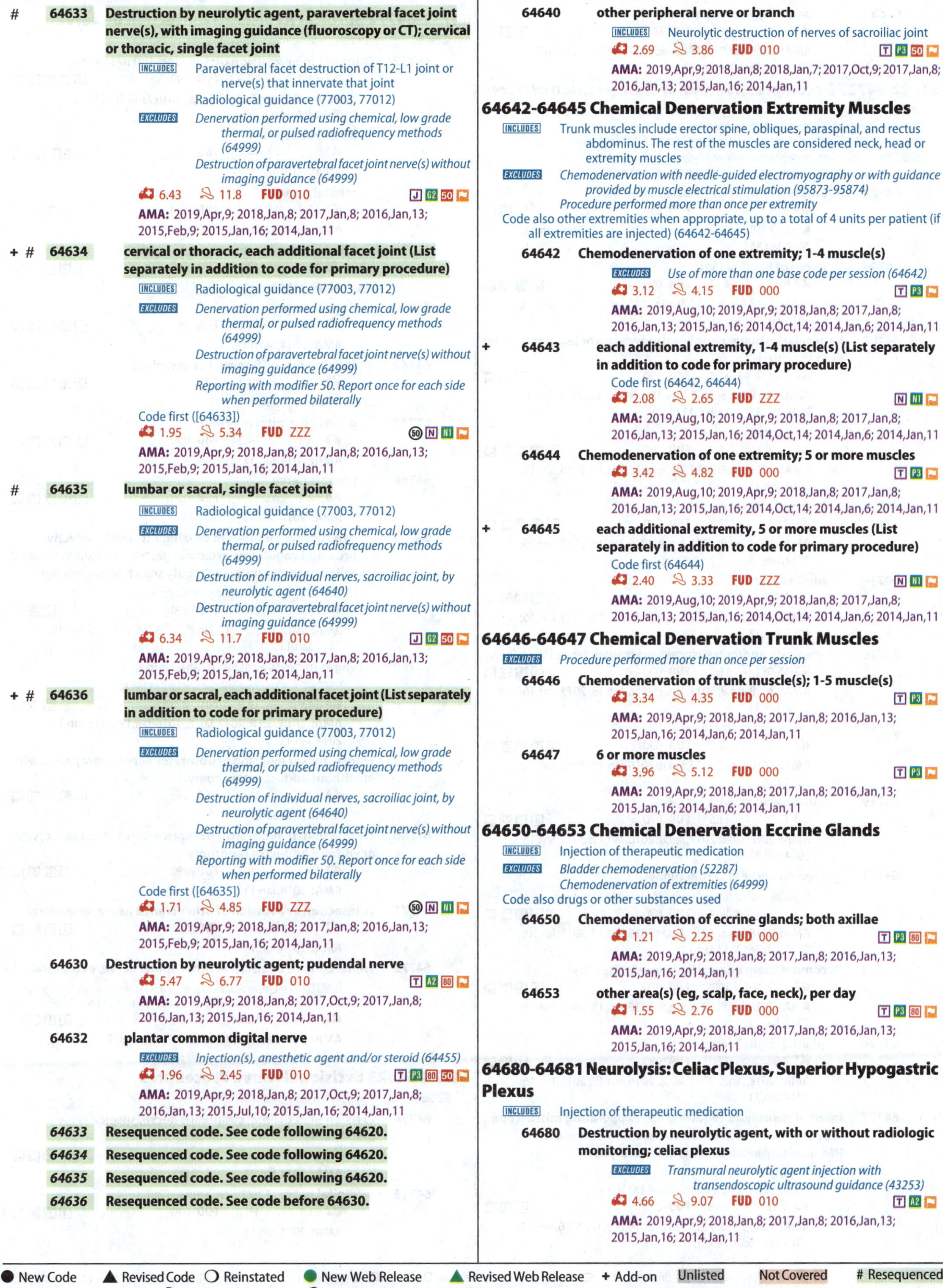

\# **64633** **Destruction by neurolytic agent, paravertebral facet joint nerve(s), with imaging guidance (fluoroscopy or CT); cervical or thoracic, single facet joint**

INCLUDES Paravertebral facet destruction of T12-L1 joint or nerve(s) that innervate that joint

Radiological guidance (77003, 77012)

EXCLUDES *Denervation performed using chemical, low grade thermal, or pulsed radiofrequency methods (64999)*

Destruction of paravertebral facet joint nerve(s) without imaging guidance (64999)

6.43 11.8 FUD 010 J G2 50

AMA: 2019,Apr,9; 2018,Jan,8; 2017,Jan,8; 2016,Jan,13; 2015,Feb,9; 2015,Jan,16; 2014,Jan,11

\+ # **64634** **cervical or thoracic, each additional facet joint (List separately in addition to code for primary procedure)**

INCLUDES Radiological guidance (77003, 77012)

EXCLUDES *Denervation performed using chemical, low grade thermal, or pulsed radiofrequency methods (64999)*

Destruction of paravertebral facet joint nerve(s) without imaging guidance (64999)

Reporting with modifier 50. Report once for each side when performed bilaterally

Code first ([64633])

1.95 5.34 FUD ZZZ 50 N N1

AMA: 2019,Apr,9; 2018,Jan,8; 2017,Jan,8; 2016,Jan,13; 2015,Feb,9; 2015,Jan,16; 2014,Jan,11

\# **64635** **lumbar or sacral, single facet joint**

INCLUDES Radiological guidance (77003, 77012)

EXCLUDES *Denervation performed using chemical, low grade thermal, or pulsed radiofrequency methods (64999)*

Destruction of individual nerves, sacroiliac joint, by neurolytic agent (64640)

Destruction of paravertebral facet joint nerve(s) without imaging guidance (64999)

6.34 11.7 FUD 010 J G2 50

AMA: 2019,Apr,9; 2018,Jan,8; 2017,Jan,8; 2016,Jan,13; 2015,Feb,9; 2015,Jan,16; 2014,Jan,11

\+ # **64636** **lumbar or sacral, each additional facet joint (List separately in addition to code for primary procedure)**

INCLUDES Radiological guidance (77003, 77012)

EXCLUDES *Denervation performed using chemical, low grade thermal, or pulsed radiofrequency methods (64999)*

Destruction of individual nerves, sacroiliac joint, by neurolytic agent (64640)

Destruction of paravertebral facet joint nerve(s) without imaging guidance (64999)

Reporting with modifier 50. Report once for each side when performed bilaterally

Code first ([64635])

1.71 4.85 FUD ZZZ 50 N N1

AMA: 2019,Apr,9; 2018,Jan,8; 2017,Jan,8; 2016,Jan,13; 2015,Feb,9; 2015,Jan,16; 2014,Jan,11

64630 **Destruction by neurolytic agent; pudendal nerve**

5.47 6.77 FUD 010 T A2 80

AMA: 2019,Apr,9; 2018,Jan,8; 2017,Oct,9; 2017,Jan,8; 2016,Jan,13; 2015,Jan,16; 2014,Jan,11

64632 **plantar common digital nerve**

EXCLUDES *Injection(s), anesthetic agent and/or steroid (64455)*

1.96 2.45 FUD 010 T P3 80 50

AMA: 2019,Apr,9; 2018,Jan,8; 2017,Oct,9; 2017,Jan,8; 2016,Jan,13; 2015,Jul,10; 2015,Jan,16; 2014,Jan,11

64633 **Resequenced code. See code following 64620.**

64634 **Resequenced code. See code following 64620.**

64635 **Resequenced code. See code following 64620.**

64636 **Resequenced code. See code before 64630.**

64640 **other peripheral nerve or branch**

INCLUDES Neurolytic destruction of nerves of sacroiliac joint

2.69 3.86 FUD 010 T P3 50

AMA: 2019,Apr,9; 2018,Jan,8; 2018,Jan,7; 2017,Oct,9; 2017,Jan,8; 2016,Jan,13; 2015,Jan,16; 2014,Jan,11

64642-64645 Chemical Denervation Extremity Muscles

INCLUDES Trunk muscles include erector spine, obliques, paraspinal, and rectus abdominus. The rest of the muscles are considered neck, head or extremity muscles

EXCLUDES *Chemodenervation with needle-guided electromyography or with guidance provided by muscle electrical stimulation (95873-95874)*

Procedure performed more than once per extremity

Code also other extremities when appropriate, up to a total of 4 units per patient (if all extremities are injected) (64642-64645)

64642 **Chemodenervation of one extremity; 1-4 muscle(s)**

EXCLUDES *Use of more than one base code per session (64642)*

3.12 4.15 FUD 000 T P3

AMA: 2019,Aug,10; 2019,Apr,9; 2018,Jan,8; 2017,Jan,8; 2016,Jan,13; 2015,Jan,16; 2014,Oct,14; 2014,Jan,6; 2014,Jan,11

\+ **64643** **each additional extremity, 1-4 muscle(s) (List separately in addition to code for primary procedure)**

Code first (64642, 64644)

2.08 2.65 FUD ZZZ N N1

AMA: 2019,Aug,10; 2019,Apr,9; 2018,Jan,8; 2017,Jan,8; 2016,Jan,13; 2015,Jan,16; 2014,Oct,14; 2014,Jan,6; 2014,Jan,11

64644 **Chemodenervation of one extremity; 5 or more muscles**

3.42 4.82 FUD 000 T P3

AMA: 2019,Aug,10; 2019,Apr,9; 2018,Jan,8; 2017,Jan,8; 2016,Jan,13; 2015,Jan,16; 2014,Oct,14; 2014,Jan,6; 2014,Jan,11

\+ **64645** **each additional extremity, 5 or more muscles (List separately in addition to code for primary procedure)**

Code first (64644)

2.40 3.33 FUD ZZZ N N1

AMA: 2019,Aug,10; 2019,Apr,9; 2018,Jan,8; 2017,Jan,8; 2016,Jan,13; 2015,Jan,16; 2014,Oct,14; 2014,Jan,6; 2014,Jan,11

64646-64647 Chemical Denervation Trunk Muscles

EXCLUDES *Procedure performed more than once per session*

64646 **Chemodenervation of trunk muscle(s); 1-5 muscle(s)**

3.34 4.35 FUD 000 T P3

AMA: 2019,Apr,9; 2018,Jan,8; 2017,Jan,8; 2016,Jan,13; 2015,Jan,16; 2014,Jan,6; 2014,Jan,11

64647 **6 or more muscles**

3.96 5.12 FUD 000 T P3

AMA: 2019,Apr,9; 2018,Jan,8; 2017,Jan,8; 2016,Jan,13; 2015,Jan,16; 2014,Jan,6; 2014,Jan,11

64650-64653 Chemical Denervation Eccrine Glands

INCLUDES Injection of therapeutic medication

EXCLUDES *Bladder chemodenervation (52287)*

Chemodenervation of extremities (64999)

Code also drugs or other substances used

64650 **Chemodenervation of eccrine glands; both axillae**

1.21 2.25 FUD 000 T P3 80

AMA: 2019,Apr,9; 2018,Jan,8; 2017,Jan,8; 2016,Jan,13; 2015,Jan,16; 2014,Jan,11

64653 **other area(s) (eg, scalp, face, neck), per day**

1.55 2.76 FUD 000 T P3 80

AMA: 2019,Apr,9; 2018,Jan,8; 2017,Jan,8; 2016,Jan,13; 2015,Jan,16; 2014,Jan,11

64680-64681 Neurolysis: Celiac Plexus, Superior Hypogastric Plexus

INCLUDES Injection of therapeutic medication

64680 **Destruction by neurolytic agent, with or without radiologic monitoring; celiac plexus**

EXCLUDES *Transmural neurolytic agent injection with transendoscopic ultrasound guidance (43253)*

4.66 9.07 FUD 010 T A2

AMA: 2019,Apr,9; 2018,Jan,8; 2017,Jan,8; 2016,Jan,13; 2015,Jan,16; 2014,Jan,11

64681 superior hypogastric plexus
7.87 16.4 **FUD** 010 T A2
AMA: 2019,Apr,9; 2018,Jan,8; 2017,Jan,8; 2016,Jan,13; 2015,Jan,16; 2014,Jan,11

64702-64727 Decompression and/or Transposition of Nerve

INCLUDES External neurolysis and/or transposition to repair or restore a nerve
Neuroplasty with nerve wrapping
Surgical decompression/freeing of nerve from scar tissue

EXCLUDES *Facial nerve decompression (69720)*
Percutaneous neurolysis (62263-62264, 62280-62282)

64702 Neuroplasty; digital, 1 or both, same digit
14.4 14.4 **FUD** 090 J A2
AMA: 2018,Jan,8; 2017,Jan,8; 2016,Jan,13; 2015,Jan,16; 2014,Jan,11

64704 nerve of hand or foot
9.23 9.23 **FUD** 090 J A2 80
AMA: 2018,Jan,8; 2017,Jan,8; 2016,Jan,13; 2015,Jan,16; 2014,Jan,11

64708 Neuroplasty, major peripheral nerve, arm or leg, open; other than specified
14.4 14.4 **FUD** 090 J G2 80
AMA: 2018,Jan,8; 2017,Nov,10; 2017,Jan,8; 2016,Jan,13; 2015,Jan,16; 2014,Jan,11

64712 sciatic nerve
16.7 16.7 **FUD** 090 J G2 80 50
AMA: 2018,Jan,8; 2017,Jan,8; 2016,Jan,13; 2015,Jan,16; 2014,Jan,11

64713 brachial plexus
22.4 22.4 **FUD** 090 J G2 80 50
AMA: 2018,Jan,8; 2017,Jan,8; 2016,Jan,13; 2015,Jan,16; 2014,Jan,11

64714 lumbar plexus
20.8 20.8 **FUD** 090 J G2 80 50
AMA: 2018,Jan,8; 2017,Jan,8; 2016,Jan,13; 2015,Jan,16; 2014,Jan,11

64716 Neuroplasty and/or transposition; cranial nerve (specify)
15.0 15.0 **FUD** 090 J A2 80
AMA: 2018,Jan,8; 2017,Jan,8; 2016,Jan,13; 2015,Jan,16; 2014,Jan,11

64718 ulnar nerve at elbow
17.0 17.0 **FUD** 090 J A2 80 50
AMA: 2018,Jan,8; 2017,Jan,8; 2016,Jan,13; 2015,Jan,16; 2014,Jan,11

64719 ulnar nerve at wrist
11.5 11.5 **FUD** 090 J A2 50
AMA: 2018,Jan,8; 2017,Jan,8; 2016,Jan,13; 2015,Jan,16; 2014,Jan,11

64721 median nerve at carpal tunnel
EXCLUDES *Arthroscopic procedure (29848)*
12.3 12.4 **FUD** 090 J A2 50
AMA: 2018,Jan,8; 2017,Jan,8; 2016,Jan,13; 2015,Jul,10; 2015,Jan,16; 2014,Jan,11

64722 Decompression; unspecified nerve(s) (specify)
10.2 10.2 **FUD** 090 J A2 80
AMA: 2018,Jan,8; 2017,Jan,8; 2016,Jan,13; 2015,Jan,16; 2014,Jan,11

64726 plantar digital nerve
7.80 7.80 **FUD** 090 J A2
AMA: 2018,Jan,8; 2017,Jan,8; 2016,Jan,13; 2015,Jan,16; 2014,Jan,11

\+ **64727 Internal neurolysis, requiring use of operating microscope (List separately in addition to code for neuroplasty) (Neuroplasty includes external neurolysis)**
INCLUDES Operating microscope (69990)
Code first neuroplasty (64702-64721)
5.31 5.31 **FUD** ZZZ N N1
AMA: 2018,Jan,8; 2017,Jan,8; 2016,Feb,12; 2016,Jan,13; 2015,Jan,16; 2014,Jan,11

64732-64772 Surgical Avulsion/Transection of Nerve

EXCLUDES *Stereotactic lesion of gasserian ganglion (61790)*

64732 Transection or avulsion of; supraorbital nerve
12.8 12.8 **FUD** 090 J A2 80 50
AMA: 2018,Jan,8; 2017,Jan,8; 2016,Jan,13; 2015,Jan,16; 2014,Jan,11

64734 infraorbital nerve
14.5 14.5 **FUD** 090 J A2 80 50
AMA: 2014,Jan,11

64736 mental nerve
10.7 10.7 **FUD** 090 J A2 80 50
AMA: 2014,Jan,11

64738 inferior alveolar nerve by osteotomy
13.3 13.3 **FUD** 090 J A2 80 50
AMA: 2014,Jan,11

64740 lingual nerve
14.0 14.0 **FUD** 090 J A2 80 50
AMA: 2014,Jan,11

64742 facial nerve, differential or complete
14.1 14.1 **FUD** 090 J A2 80 50
AMA: 2014,Jan,11

64744 greater occipital nerve
14.2 14.2 **FUD** 090 J A2 80 50
AMA: 2014,Jan,11

64746 phrenic nerve
12.4 12.4 **FUD** 090 J A2 80 50
AMA: 2014,Jan,11

64755 vagus nerves limited to proximal stomach (selective proximal vagotomy, proximal gastric vagotomy, parietal cell vagotomy, supra- or highly selective vagotomy)
EXCLUDES *Laparoscopic procedure (43652)*
26.6 26.6 **FUD** 090 C 80
AMA: 2018,Jan,8; 2017,Jan,8; 2016,Jan,13; 2015,Jan,16; 2014,Jan,11

64760 vagus nerve (vagotomy), abdominal
EXCLUDES *Laparoscopic procedure (43651)*
14.9 14.9 **FUD** 090 C 80
AMA: 2018,Jan,8; 2017,Jan,8; 2016,Jan,13; 2015,Jan,16; 2014,Jan,11

64763 Transection or avulsion of obturator nerve, extrapelvic, with or without adductor tenotomy
14.7 14.7 **FUD** 090 J G2 80 50
AMA: 2014,Jan,11

64766 Transection or avulsion of obturator nerve, intrapelvic, with or without adductor tenotomy
18.2 18.2 **FUD** 090 J G2 80 50
AMA: 2014,Jan,11

64771 Transection or avulsion of other cranial nerve, extradural
17.0 17.0 **FUD** 090 J A2 80
AMA: 2014,Jan,11

64772 Transection or avulsion of other spinal nerve, extradural
EXCLUDES *Removal of tender scar and soft tissue including neuroma if necessary (11400-11446, 13100-13153)*
16.2 16.2 **FUD** 090 J A2 80
AMA: 2018,Jan,8; 2017,Jan,8; 2016,Jan,13; 2015,Apr,10; 2014,Jan,11

64774-64823 Excisional Nerve Procedures

EXCLUDES *Morton neuroma excision (28080)*

64774 Excision of neuroma; cutaneous nerve, surgically identifiable
11.7 11.7 **FUD** 090 J A2
AMA: 2014,Jan,11

64776 digital nerve, 1 or both, same digit
11.1 11.1 **FUD** 090 J A2 80
AMA: 2014,Jan,11

+ **64778** **digital nerve, each additional digit (List separately in addition to code for primary procedure)**
Code first (64776)
5.30 5.30 FUD ZZZ N N1
AMA: 2014,Jan,11

64782 **hand or foot, except digital nerve**
13.2 13.2 FUD 090 J A2
AMA: 2014,Jan,11

+ **64783** **hand or foot, each additional nerve, except same digit (List separately in addition to code for primary procedure)**
Code first (64782)
6.33 6.33 FUD ZZZ N N1
AMA: 2014,Jan,11

64784 **major peripheral nerve, except sciatic**
20.9 20.9 FUD 090 J A2 80
AMA: 2014,Jan,11

64786 **sciatic nerve**
29.0 29.0 FUD 090 J A2 80 50
AMA: 2014,Jan,11

+ **64787** **Implantation of nerve end into bone or muscle (List separately in addition to neuroma excision)**
Code also, when appropriate (64774-64786)
6.96 6.96 FUD ZZZ N N1 80
AMA: 2014,Jan,11

64788 **Excision of neurofibroma or neurolemmoma; cutaneous nerve**
11.5 11.5 FUD 090 J A2
AMA: 2018,Jan,8; 2017,Jan,8; 2016,Apr,3; 2014,Jan,11

64790 **major peripheral nerve**
24.1 24.1 FUD 090 J A2 80
AMA: 2018,Jan,8; 2017,Jan,8; 2016,Apr,3; 2014,Jan,11

64792 **extensive (including malignant type)**
EXCLUDES *Destruction neurofibroma of skin (0419T-0420T)*
31.4 31.4 FUD 090 J A2 80
AMA: 2018,Jan,8; 2017,Jan,8; 2016,Apr,3; 2014,Jan,11

64795 **Biopsy of nerve**
5.64 5.64 FUD 000 J A2
AMA: 2014,Jan,11

64802 **Sympathectomy, cervical**
24.3 24.3 FUD 090 J A2 80 50
AMA: 2014,Jan,11

64804 **Sympathectomy, cervicothoracic**
34.7 34.7 FUD 090 J 80 50
AMA: 2014,Jan,11

64809 **Sympathectomy, thoracolumbar**
INCLUDES Leriche sympathectomy
31.8 31.8 FUD 090 C 80 50
AMA: 2014,Jan,11

64818 **Sympathectomy, lumbar**
22.5 22.5 FUD 090 C 80 50
AMA: 2014,Jan,11

64820 **Sympathectomy; digital arteries, each digit**
INCLUDES Operating microscope (69990)
20.5 20.5 FUD 090 J G2
AMA: 2018,Jan,8; 2017,Jan,8; 2016,Feb,12; 2016,Jan,13; 2015,Jan,16; 2014,Jan,11

64821 **radial artery**
INCLUDES Operating microscope (69990)
20.0 20.0 FUD 090 J A2 50
AMA: 2016,Feb,12; 2014,Jan,11

64822 **ulnar artery**
INCLUDES Operating microscope (69990)
20.0 20.0 FUD 090 J G2 50
AMA: 2016,Feb,12; 2014,Jan,11

64823 **superficial palmar arch**
INCLUDES Operating microscope (69990)
22.7 22.7 FUD 090 J G2 50
AMA: 2016,Feb,12; 2014,Jan,11

64831-64907 Nerve Repair: Suture and Nerve Grafts

64831 **Suture of digital nerve, hand or foot; 1 nerve**
19.7 19.7 FUD 090 J A2 50
AMA: 2018,Jan,8; 2017,Jan,8; 2016,Jan,13; 2015,Jan,16; 2014,Sep,13; 2014,Jan,11

+ **64832** **each additional digital nerve (List separately in addition to code for primary procedure)**
Code first (64831)
9.73 9.73 FUD ZZZ N N1 80
AMA: 2018,Jan,8; 2017,Jan,8; 2016,Jan,13; 2015,Jan,16; 2014,Jan,11

64834 **Suture of 1 nerve; hand or foot, common sensory nerve**
21.3 21.3 FUD 090 J A2 80 50
AMA: 2014,Jan,11

64835 **median motor thenar**
23.4 23.4 FUD 090 J A2 80 50
AMA: 2014,Jan,11

64836 **ulnar motor**
23.5 23.5 FUD 090 J A2 80 50
AMA: 2014,Jan,11

+ **64837** **Suture of each additional nerve, hand or foot (List separately in addition to code for primary procedure)**
Code first (64834-64836)
10.6 10.6 FUD ZZZ N N1 80
AMA: 2014,Jan,11

64840 **Suture of posterior tibial nerve**
27.8 27.8 FUD 090 J A2 80 50
AMA: 2014,Jan,11

64856 **Suture of major peripheral nerve, arm or leg, except sciatic; including transposition**
29.2 29.2 FUD 090 J A2
AMA: 2014,Jan,11

64857 **without transposition**
30.4 30.4 FUD 090 J A2 80
AMA: 2014,Jan,11

64858 **Suture of sciatic nerve**
34.0 34.0 FUD 090 J A2 80 50
AMA: 2014,Jan,11

+ **64859** **Suture of each additional major peripheral nerve (List separately in addition to code for primary procedure)**
Code first (64856-64857)
7.24 7.24 FUD ZZZ N N1 80
AMA: 2014,Jan,11

64861 **Suture of; brachial plexus**
44.5 44.5 FUD 090 J A2 80 50
AMA: 2014,Jan,11

64862 **lumbar plexus**
39.3 39.3 FUD 090 J A2 80 50
AMA: 2014,Jan,11

64864 **Suture of facial nerve; extracranial**
24.9 24.9 FUD 090 J A2 80
AMA: 2014,Jan,11

64865 **infratemporal, with or without grafting**
31.4 31.4 FUD 090 J A2 80
AMA: 2014,Jan,11

64866 **Anastomosis; facial-spinal accessory**
36.7 36.7 FUD 090 C 80
AMA: 2014,Jan,11

64868 **facial-hypoglossal**
INCLUDES Korte-Ballance anastomosis
28.8 28.8 FUD 090 C 80
AMA: 2014,Jan,11

+ **64872** **Suture of nerve; requiring secondary or delayed suture (List separately in addition to code for primary neurorrhaphy)**
Code first (64831-64865)
3.39 3.39 FUD ZZZ N N1 80
AMA: 2014,Jan,11

+ **64874** **requiring extensive mobilization, or transposition of nerve (List separately in addition to code for nerve suture)**
Code first (64831-64865)
5.06 5.06 FUD ZZZ N N1 80
AMA: 2014,Jan,11

+ **64876** **requiring shortening of bone of extremity (List separately in addition to code for nerve suture)**
Code first (64831-64865)
5.75 5.75 FUD ZZZ N N1 80
AMA: 2014,Jan,11

64885 **Nerve graft (includes obtaining graft), head or neck; up to 4 cm in length**
32.1 32.1 FUD 090 J J8 80
AMA: 2018,Jan,8; 2017,Dec,12; 2017,Jan,8; 2016,Jan,13; 2015,Jan,16; 2014,Jan,11

64886 **more than 4 cm length**
37.2 37.2 FUD 090 J J8 80
AMA: 2018,Jan,8; 2017,Dec,12; 2017,Jan,8; 2016,Jan,13; 2015,Jan,16; 2014,Jan,11

64890 **Nerve graft (includes obtaining graft), single strand, hand or foot; up to 4 cm length**
31.2 31.2 FUD 090 J J8 80
AMA: 2018,Jan,8; 2017,Dec,12; 2017,Jan,8; 2016,Jan,13; 2015,Aug,8; 2015,Apr,10; 2014,Jan,11

64891 **more than 4 cm length**
33.2 33.2 FUD 090 J G2 80
AMA: 2018,Jan,8; 2017,Dec,12; 2014,Jan,11

64892 **Nerve graft (includes obtaining graft), single strand, arm or leg; up to 4 cm length**
30.1 30.1 FUD 090 J A2 80
AMA: 2018,Jan,8; 2017,Dec,12; 2014,Jan,11

64893 **more than 4 cm length**
32.4 32.4 FUD 090 J G2 80
AMA: 2018,Jan,8; 2017,Dec,12; 2014,Jan,11

64895 **Nerve graft (includes obtaining graft), multiple strands (cable), hand or foot; up to 4 cm length**
38.4 38.4 FUD 090 J A2 80
AMA: 2018,Jan,8; 2017,Dec,12; 2017,Jan,8; 2016,Jan,13; 2015,Jan,16; 2014,Jan,11

64896 **more than 4 cm length**
41.4 41.4 FUD 090 J A2 80
AMA: 2018,Jan,8; 2017,Dec,12; 2017,Jan,8; 2016,Jan,13; 2015,Jan,16; 2014,Jan,11

64897 **Nerve graft (includes obtaining graft), multiple strands (cable), arm or leg; up to 4 cm length**
36.4 36.4 FUD 090 J G2 80
AMA: 2018,Jan,8; 2017,Dec,12; 2017,Jan,8; 2016,Jan,13; 2015,Jan,16; 2014,Jan,11

64898 **more than 4 cm length**
39.7 39.7 FUD 090 J A2 80
AMA: 2018,Jan,8; 2017,Dec,12; 2017,Jan,8; 2016,Jan,13; 2015,Jan,16; 2014,Jan,11

+ **64901** **Nerve graft, each additional nerve; single strand (List separately in addition to code for primary procedure)**
Code first (64885-64893)
17.4 17.4 FUD ZZZ N N1 80
AMA: 2018,Jan,8; 2017,Dec,12; 2017,Jan,8; 2016,Jan,13; 2015,Jan,16; 2014,Jan,11

+ **64902** **multiple strands (cable) (List separately in addition to code for primary procedure)**
Code first (64885-64886, 64895-64898)
20.1 20.1 FUD ZZZ N N1 80
AMA: 2018,Jan,8; 2017,Dec,12; 2017,Jan,8; 2016,Jan,13; 2015,Jan,16; 2014,Jan,11

64905 **Nerve pedicle transfer; first stage**
29.4 29.4 FUD 090 J A2 80
AMA: 2018,Jan,8; 2017,Dec,12; 2014,Jan,11

64907 **second stage**
37.7 37.7 FUD 090 J A2 80
AMA: 2018,Jan,8; 2017,Dec,12; 2014,Jan,11

64910-64999 Nerve Repair: Synthetic and Vein Grafts

64910 **Nerve repair; with synthetic conduit or vein allograft (eg, nerve tube), each nerve**
INCLUDES Operating microscope (69990)
22.8 22.8 FUD 090 J J8 80
AMA: 2018,Jan,8; 2017,Dec,12; 2017,Jan,8; 2016,Jan,13; 2015,Aug,8; 2015,Apr,10; 2015,Jan,16; 2014,Jan,11

Damaged nerve
Healthy nerve
Artificial nerve conduit

A synthetic "bridge" is affixed to each end of a severed nerve with sutures
The procedure is performed using an operating microscope

64911 **with autogenous vein graft (includes harvest of vein graft), each nerve**
INCLUDES Operating microscope (69990)
29.6 29.6 FUD 090 J 80
AMA: 2018,Jan,8; 2017,Dec,12; 2017,Jan,8; 2016,Jan,13; 2015,Jan,16; 2014,Jan,11

64912 **with nerve allograft, each nerve, first strand (cable)**
INCLUDES Operating microscope (69990)
22.3 22.3 FUD 090 J G2 80
AMA: 2018,Jan,8; 2017,Dec,12

+ **64913** **with nerve allograft, each additional strand (List separately in addition to code for primary procedure)**
INCLUDES Operating microscope (69990)
Code first (64912)
4.50 4.50 FUD ZZZ N N1 80
AMA: 2018,Jan,8; 2017,Dec,12

64999 **Unlisted procedure, nervous system**

0.00 0.00 **FUD** YYY T 80

AMA: 2019,Jul,10; 2019,May,10; 2019,Apr,9; 2018,Dec,8; 2018,Dec,8; 2018,Oct,8; 2018,Oct,11; 2018,Aug,10; 2018,Mar,9; 2018,Jan,7; 2018,Jan,8; 2017,Dec,13; 2017,Dec,14; 2017,Dec,12; 2017,Jan,8; 2016,Nov,6; 2016,Oct,11; 2016,Feb,13; 2016,Jan,13; 2015,Oct,9; 2015,Aug,8; 2015,Jul,10; 2015,Apr,10; 2015,Feb,9; 2015,Jan,16; 2014,Jul,8; 2014,Feb,11; 2014,Jan,11; 2014,Jan,9; 2014,Jan,8

65091-65093 Surgical Removal of Eyeball Contents

INCLUDES Operating microscope (69990)

65091 **Evisceration of ocular contents; without implant**
18.4 18.4 FUD 090 J A2 80 50
AMA: 2016,Feb,12; 2014,Jan,11

Conjunctiva

Sclera

Muscles are severed at their attachment to the eyeball

Evisceration involves removal of the contents of the eyeball: the vitreous; retina; choroid; lens; iris; and ciliary muscle. Only the scleral shell remains. A temporary or permanent implant is usually inserted

Enucleation involves severing the extraorbital muscles and optic nerve with removal of the eyeball. An implant is usually inserted and, if permanent, may involve attachment to the severed extraorbital muscles

65093 **with implant**
18.2 18.2 FUD 090 J A2 50
AMA: 2016,Feb,12; 2014,Jan,11

65101-65105 Surgical Removal of Eyeball

INCLUDES Operating microscope (69990)

EXCLUDES *Conjunctivoplasty following enucleation (68320-68328)*

65101 **Enucleation of eye; without implant**
21.3 21.3 FUD 090 J A2 50
AMA: 2016,Feb,12; 2014,Jan,11

65103 **with implant, muscles not attached to implant**
22.2 22.2 FUD 090 J A2 50
AMA: 2016,Feb,12; 2014,Jan,11

65105 **with implant, muscles attached to implant**
24.4 24.4 FUD 090 J A2 80 50
AMA: 2016,Feb,12; 2014,Jan,11

65110-65114 Surgical Removal of Orbital Contents

INCLUDES Operating microscope (69990)

EXCLUDES *Free full thickness graft (15260-15261)*
Repair more extensive than skin (67930-67975)
Skin graft (15120-15121)

65110 **Exenteration of orbit (does not include skin graft), removal of orbital contents; only**
35.0 35.0 FUD 090 J A2 80 50
AMA: 2016,Feb,12; 2014,Jan,11

65112 **with therapeutic removal of bone**
40.5 40.5 FUD 090 J A2 80 50
AMA: 2016,Feb,12; 2014,Jan,11

65114 **with muscle or myocutaneous flap**
42.5 42.5 FUD 090 J A2 80 50
AMA: 2016,Feb,12; 2014,Jan,11

65125-65175 Implant Procedures: Insertion, Removal, and Revision

INCLUDES Operating microscope (69990)

EXCLUDES *Orbital implant insertion outside muscle cone (67550)*
Orbital implant removal or revision outside muscle cone (67560)

65125 **Modification of ocular implant with placement or replacement of pegs (eg, drilling receptacle for prosthesis appendage) (separate procedure)**
8.32 13.0 FUD 090 J G2 50
AMA: 2016,Feb,12; 2014,Jan,11

65130 **Insertion of ocular implant secondary; after evisceration, in scleral shell**
21.1 21.1 FUD 090 J A2 50
AMA: 2016,Feb,12; 2014,Jan,11

65135 **after enucleation, muscles not attached to implant**
21.4 21.4 FUD 090 J A2 50
AMA: 2016,Feb,12; 2014,Jan,11

65140 **after enucleation, muscles attached to implant**
23.3 23.3 FUD 090 J A2 50
AMA: 2016,Feb,12; 2014,Jan,11

65150 **Reinsertion of ocular implant; with or without conjunctival graft**
16.8 16.8 FUD 090 J A2 80 50
AMA: 2016,Feb,12; 2014,Jan,11

65155 **with use of foreign material for reinforcement and/or attachment of muscles to implant**
24.4 24.4 FUD 090 J A2 50
AMA: 2016,Feb,12; 2014,Jan,11

65175 **Removal of ocular implant**
19.0 19.0 FUD 090 J A2 50
AMA: 2016,Feb,12; 2014,Jan,11

65205-65265 Foreign Body Removal By Area of Eye

INCLUDES Operating microscope (69990)

EXCLUDES *Removal:*
Anterior segment implant (65920)
Ocular implant (65175)
Orbital implant outside muscle cone (67560)
Posterior segment implant (67120)
Removal of foreign body:
Eyelid (67938)
Lacrimal system (68530)
Orbit:
Frontal approach (67413)
Lateral approach (67430)

65205 **Removal of foreign body, external eye; conjunctival superficial**
(70030, 76529)
1.02 1.31 FUD 000 Q1 N1 50
AMA: 2018,Jan,8; 2017,Jan,8; 2016,Feb,12; 2016,Jan,13; 2015,Jan,16; 2014,Jan,11

65210 **conjunctival embedded (includes concretions), subconjunctival, or scleral nonperforating**
(70030, 76529)
1.22 1.60 FUD 000 Q1 N1 50
AMA: 2016,Feb,12; 2014,Jan,11

65220 **corneal, without slit lamp**
EXCLUDES *Repair of corneal wound with foreign body (65275)*
(70030, 76529)
1.19 1.68 FUD 000 Q1 N1 50
AMA: 2018,Jan,8; 2017,Jan,8; 2016,Feb,12; 2016,Jan,13; 2015,Jan,16; 2014,Jan,11

65222 **corneal, with slit lamp**
EXCLUDES *Repair of corneal wound with foreign body (65275)*
(70030, 76529)
1.48 1.93 FUD 000 Q1 N1 50
AMA: 2018,Jan,8; 2017,Jan,8; 2016,Feb,12; 2016,Jan,13; 2015,Jan,16; 2014,Jan,11

65235 **Removal of foreign body, intraocular; from anterior chamber of eye or lens**
(70030, 76529)
20.2 20.2 FUD 090 J A2 80 50
AMA: 2018,Jan,8; 2017,Jan,8; 2016,Feb,12; 2016,Jan,13; 2015,Jan,16; 2014,Jan,11

65260 **from posterior segment, magnetic extraction, anterior or posterior route**
(70030, 76529)
27.4 27.4 FUD 090 J A2 80 50
AMA: 2016,Feb,12; 2014,Jan,11

65265 **from posterior segment, nonmagnetic extraction**

(70030, 76529)

30.7 30.7 FUD 090 [J] [A2] [80] [50]

AMA: 2016,Feb,12; 2014,Jan,11

65270-65290 Laceration Repair External Eye

INCLUDES Conjunctival flap
Operating microscope (69990)
Restoration of anterior chamber with air or saline injection

EXCLUDES *Repair:*
Ciliary body or iris (66680)
Eyelid laceration (12011-12018, 12051-12057, 13151-13160, 67930, 67935)
Lacrimal system injury (68700)
Surgical wound (66250)
Treatment of orbit fracture (21385-21408)

65270 **Repair of laceration; conjunctiva, with or without nonperforating laceration sclera, direct closure**

4.01 7.79 FUD 010 [J] [A2] [80] [50]

AMA: 2018,Jan,8; 2017,Jan,8; 2016,Feb,12; 2016,Jan,13; 2015,Jan,16; 2014,Jan,11

65272 **conjunctiva, by mobilization and rearrangement, without hospitalization**

10.0 14.5 FUD 090 [J] [A2] [50]

AMA: 2016,Feb,12; 2014,Jan,11

65273 **conjunctiva, by mobilization and rearrangement, with hospitalization**

10.8 10.8 FUD 090 [C] [50]

AMA: 2016,Feb,12; 2014,Jan,11

65275 **cornea, nonperforating, with or without removal foreign body**

13.1 16.5 FUD 090 [J] [A2] [80] [50]

AMA: 2016,Feb,12; 2014,Jan,11

65280 **cornea and/or sclera, perforating, not involving uveal tissue**

EXCLUDES *Procedure performed for surgical wound repair*

19.1 19.1 FUD 090 [J] [A2] [80] [50]

AMA: 2018,Jan,8; 2017,Jan,8; 2016,Feb,12; 2016,Jan,13; 2015,Jan,16; 2014,Jan,11

65285 **cornea and/or sclera, perforating, with reposition or resection of uveal tissue**

EXCLUDES *Procedure performed for surgical wound repair*

31.5 31.5 FUD 090 [J] [A2] [50]

AMA: 2018,Jan,8; 2017,Jan,8; 2016,Feb,12; 2016,Jan,13; 2015,Jan,16; 2014,Jan,11

65286 **application of tissue glue, wounds of cornea and/or sclera**

14.1 20.0 FUD 090 [J] [P3] [50]

AMA: 2018,Jan,8; 2017,Jan,8; 2016,Feb,12; 2016,Jan,13; 2015,Jan,16; 2014,Jan,11

65290 **Repair of wound, extraocular muscle, tendon and/or Tenon's capsule**

13.9 13.9 FUD 090 [J] [A2] [50]

AMA: 2016,Feb,12; 2014,Jan,11

65400-65600 Removal Corneal Lesions

INCLUDES Operating microscope (69990)

65400 **Excision of lesion, cornea (keratectomy, lamellar, partial), except pterygium**

17.1 19.4 FUD 090 [T] [A2] [50]

AMA: 2018,Jan,8; 2017,Jan,8; 2016,Feb,12; 2016,Jan,13; 2015,Jan,16; 2014,Jan,11

65410 **Biopsy of cornea**

2.96 4.11 FUD 000 [J] [A2] [80] [50]

AMA: 2018,Jan,8; 2017,Jan,8; 2016,Feb,12; 2016,Jan,13; 2015,Jan,16; 2014,Jan,11

65420 **Excision or transposition of pterygium; without graft**

10.7 14.9 FUD 090 [J] [A2] [50]

AMA: 2018,Jan,8; 2017,Jan,8; 2016,Feb,12; 2016,Jan,13; 2015,Jan,16; 2014,Jan,11

65426 **with graft**

13.6 18.7 FUD 090 [J] [A2] [50]

AMA: 2018,May,10; 2018,Jan,8; 2017,Jan,8; 2016,Feb,12; 2016,Jan,13; 2015,Jan,16; 2014,Jan,11

65430 **Scraping of cornea, diagnostic, for smear and/or culture**

2.94 3.31 FUD 000 [Q1] [N1] [50]

AMA: 2016,Feb,12; 2014,Jan,11

65435 **Removal of corneal epithelium; with or without chemocauterization (abrasion, curettage)**

EXCLUDES *Collagen cross-linking of cornea (0402T)*

1.98 2.32 FUD 000 [T] [P3] [50]

AMA: 2018,Jan,8; 2017,Jan,8; 2016,Feb,12; 2016,Jan,13; 2015,Jan,16; 2014,Jan,11

65436 **with application of chelating agent (eg, EDTA)**

10.5 11.0 FUD 090 [J] [P3] [50]

AMA: 2016,Feb,12; 2014,Jan,11

65450 **Destruction of lesion of cornea by cryotherapy, photocoagulation or thermocauterization**

9.15 9.30 FUD 090 [T] [G2] [50]

AMA: 2016,Feb,12; 2014,Jan,11

65600 **Multiple punctures of anterior cornea (eg, for corneal erosion, tattoo)**

9.74 11.3 FUD 090 [J] [P3] [50]

AMA: 2016,Feb,12; 2014,Jan,11

65710-65757 Corneal Transplants

CMS: 100-03,80.7 Refractive Keratoplasty

INCLUDES Operating microscope (69990)

EXCLUDES *Computerized corneal topography (92025)*
Processing, preserving, and transporting corneal tissue (V2785)

65710 **Keratoplasty (corneal transplant); anterior lamellar**

INCLUDES Use and preparation of fresh or preserved graft

EXCLUDES *Refractive keratoplasty surgery (65760-65767)*

31.7 31.7 FUD 090 [J] [A2] [80] [50]

AMA: 2018,Jan,8; 2017,Jan,8; 2016,Feb,12; 2016,Jan,13; 2015,Jan,16; 2014,Jan,11

65730 **penetrating (except in aphakia or pseudophakia)**

INCLUDES Use and preparation of fresh or preserved graft

EXCLUDES *Refractive keratoplasty surgery (65760-65767)*

35.1 35.1 FUD 090 [J] [A2] [80] [50]

AMA: 2018,Jan,8; 2017,Jan,8; 2016,Feb,12; 2016,Jan,13; 2015,Jan,16; 2014,Jan,11

65750 **penetrating (in aphakia)**

INCLUDES Use and preparation of fresh or preserved graft

EXCLUDES *Refractive keratoplasty surgery (65760-65767)*

35.3 35.3 FUD 090 [J] [A2] [80] [50]

AMA: 2018,Jan,8; 2017,Jan,8; 2016,Feb,12; 2016,Jan,13; 2015,Jan,16; 2014,Jan,11

65755 **penetrating (in pseudophakia)**
INCLUDES Use and preparation of fresh or preserved graft
EXCLUDES *Refractive keratoplasty surgery (65760-65767)*
35.1 35.1 FUD 090 J A2 80 50
AMA: 2018,Jan,8; 2017,Jan,8; 2016,Feb,12; 2016,Jan,13; 2015,Jan,16; 2014,Jan,11

65756 **endothelial**
EXCLUDES *Refractive keratoplasty surgery (65760-65767)*
Code also donor material
Code also if appropriate (65757)
33.6 33.6 FUD 090 J G2 80 50
AMA: 2018,Jan,8; 2017,Jan,8; 2016,Feb,12; 2016,Jan,13; 2015,Jan,16; 2014,Jan,11

+ 65757 **Backbench preparation of corneal endothelial allograft prior to transplantation (List separately in addition to code for primary procedure)**
Code first (65756)
0.00 0.00 FUD ZZZ N N1 80
AMA: 2018,Jan,8; 2017,Jan,8; 2016,Feb,12; 2016,Jan,13; 2015,Jan,16; 2014,Aug,14; 2014,Jan,11

65760-65785 Corneal Refractive Procedures

CMS: 100-03,80.7 Refractive Keratoplasty
INCLUDES Operating microscope (69990)
EXCLUDES *Unlisted corneal procedures (66999)*

65760 **Keratomileusis**
EXCLUDES *Computerized corneal topography (92025)*
0.00 0.00 FUD XXX E
AMA: 2016,Feb,12; 2014,Jan,11

65765 **Keratophakia**
EXCLUDES *Computerized corneal topography (92025)*
0.00 0.00 FUD XXX E
AMA: 2016,Feb,12; 2014,Jan,11

65767 **Epikeratoplasty**
EXCLUDES *Computerized corneal topography (92025)*
0.00 0.00 FUD XXX E
AMA: 2016,Feb,12; 2014,Jan,11

65770 **Keratoprosthesis**
EXCLUDES *Computerized corneal topography (92025)*
39.6 39.6 FUD 090 J J8 80 50
AMA: 2016,Feb,12; 2014,Jan,11

65771 **Radial keratotomy**
EXCLUDES *Computerized corneal topography (92025)*
0.00 0.00 FUD XXX E
AMA: 2016,Feb,12; 2014,Jan,11

65772 **Corneal relaxing incision for correction of surgically induced astigmatism**
11.5 12.8 FUD 090 T A2 50
AMA: 2016,Feb,12; 2014,Jan,11

65775 **Corneal wedge resection for correction of surgically induced astigmatism**
EXCLUDES *Fitting of contact lens to treat disease (92071-92072)*
15.8 15.8 FUD 090 J A2 50
AMA: 2018,Jan,8; 2017,Jan,8; 2016,Feb,12; 2016,Jan,13; 2015,Jan,16; 2014,Jan,11

65778 **Placement of amniotic membrane on the ocular surface; without sutures**
EXCLUDES *Ocular surface reconstruction (65780)*
Removal of corneal epithelium (65435)
Scraping of cornea, diagnostic (65430)
Use of tissue glue to place amniotic membrane (66999)
1.58 40.0 FUD 000 Q2 N1 80 50
AMA: 2018,Feb,11; 2018,Jan,8; 2017,Jan,8; 2016,Feb,12; 2016,Jan,13; 2015,Jan,16; 2014,May,5; 2014,Jan,11

65779 **single layer, sutured**
EXCLUDES *Ocular surface reconstruction (65780)*
Removal of corneal epithelium (65435)
Scraping of cornea, diagnostic (65430)
Use of tissue glue to place amniotic membrane (66999)
4.32 34.5 FUD 000 Q2 N1 80 50
AMA: 2018,Feb,11; 2018,Jan,8; 2017,Jan,8; 2016,Feb,12; 2016,Jan,13; 2015,Jan,16; 2014,May,5; 2014,Jan,11

65780 **Ocular surface reconstruction; amniotic membrane transplantation, multiple layers**
EXCLUDES *Placement amniotic membrane without reconstruction without sutures or single layer sutures (65778-65779)*
18.9 18.9 FUD 090 J A2 50
AMA: 2018,Feb,11; 2018,Jan,8; 2017,Jan,8; 2016,Feb,12; 2016,Jan,13; 2015,Jan,16; 2014,May,5; 2014,Jan,11

65781 **limbal stem cell allograft (eg, cadaveric or living donor)**
37.9 37.9 FUD 090 J A2 80 50
AMA: 2018,Jan,8; 2017,Jan,8; 2016,Feb,12; 2016,Jan,13; 2015,Jan,16; 2014,Jan,11

65782 **limbal conjunctival autograft (includes obtaining graft)**
EXCLUDES *Conjunctival allograft harvest from a living donor (68371)*
32.6 32.6 FUD 090 J A2 50
AMA: 2018,Jan,8; 2017,Jan,8; 2016,Feb,12; 2016,Jan,13; 2015,Jan,16; 2014,Jan,11

65785 **Implantation of intrastromal corneal ring segments**
12.5 69.5 FUD 090 J P2 50
AMA: 2016,Feb,12

65800-66030 Anterior Segment Procedures

INCLUDES Operating microscope (69990)
EXCLUDES *Unlisted procedures of anterior segment (66999)*

65800 **Paracentesis of anterior chamber of eye (separate procedure); with removal of aqueous**
EXCLUDES *Insertion of ocular telescope prosthesis (0308T)*
2.59 3.42 FUD 000 J A2 50
AMA: 2018,Jan,8; 2017,Jan,8; 2016,Feb,12; 2016,Jan,13; 2015,Jan,16; 2014,Jan,11

65810 **with removal of vitreous and/or discission of anterior hyaloid membrane, with or without air injection**
EXCLUDES *Insertion of ocular telescope prosthesis (0308T)*
13.2 13.2 FUD 090 J A2 50
AMA: 2018,Jan,8; 2017,Jan,8; 2016,Feb,12; 2016,Jan,13; 2015,Jan,16; 2014,Jan,11

65815 **with removal of blood, with or without irrigation and/or air injection**
EXCLUDES *Injection only (66020-66030)*
Insertion of ocular telescope prosthesis (0308T)
Removal of blood clot only (65930)
13.5 18.2 FUD 090 J A2 50
AMA: 2018,Jan,8; 2017,Jan,8; 2016,Feb,12; 2016,Jan,13; 2015,Jan,16; 2014,Jan,11

65820 **Goniotomy**
INCLUDES Barkan's operation
Code also ophthalmic endoscope if used (69990)
21.5 21.5 FUD 090 63 J A2 80 50
AMA: 2019,Sep,10; 2018,Dec,8; 2018,Dec,8; 2018,Jul,3; 2018,Jan,8; 2017,Jan,8; 2016,Feb,12; 2016,Jan,13; 2015,Jan,16; 2014,Jan,11

65850 **Trabeculotomy ab externo**
23.8 23.8 FUD 090 J A2 50
AMA: 2016,Feb,12; 2014,Jan,11

65855 **Trabeculoplasty by laser surgery**
EXCLUDES *Severing adhesions of anterior segment (65860-65880)*
Trabeculectomy ab externo (66170)
5.91 7.01 FUD 010 T P3 50
AMA: 2018,Jan,8; 2017,Jan,8; 2016,Feb,12; 2016,Jan,13; 2015,Jan,16; 2014,Jan,11

65860 **Severing adhesions of anterior segment, laser technique (separate procedure)**
7.18 8.81 FUD 090 T P3 80 50
AMA: 2016,Feb,12; 2014,Jan,11

65865 **Severing adhesions of anterior segment of eye, incisional technique (with or without injection of air or liquid) (separate procedure); goniosynechiae**
EXCLUDES *Laser trabeculectomy (65855)*
13.4 13.4 FUD 090 J A2 50
AMA: 2016,Feb,12; 2014,Jan,11

65870 **anterior synechiae, except goniosynechiae**
16.7 16.7 FUD 090 J A2 50
AMA: 2016,Feb,12; 2014,Jan,11

65875 **posterior synechiae**
Code also ophthalmic endoscope if used (66990)
17.9 17.9 FUD 090 J A2 50
AMA: 2018,Jan,8; 2017,Jan,8; 2016,Feb,12; 2016,Jan,13; 2015,Jan,16; 2014,Jan,11

65880 **corneovitreal adhesions**
EXCLUDES *Laser procedure (66821)*
18.8 18.8 FUD 090 J A2 50
AMA: 2016,Feb,12; 2014,Jan,11

65900 **Removal of epithelial downgrowth, anterior chamber of eye**
27.6 27.6 FUD 090 J A2 80 50
AMA: 2016,Feb,12; 2014,Jan,11

65920 **Removal of implanted material, anterior segment of eye**
Code also ophthalmic endoscope if used (66990)
22.4 22.4 FUD 090 J A2 50
AMA: 2018,Jan,8; 2017,Jan,8; 2016,Feb,12; 2016,Jan,13; 2015,Jan,16; 2014,Jan,11

65930 **Removal of blood clot, anterior segment of eye**
18.0 18.0 FUD 090 J A2 50
AMA: 2016,Feb,12; 2014,Jan,11

66020 **Injection, anterior chamber of eye (separate procedure); air or liquid**
EXCLUDES *Insertion of ocular telescope prosthesis (0308T)*
3.74 5.43 FUD 010 J A2 50
AMA: 2018,Jan,8; 2017,Jan,8; 2016,Feb,12; 2016,Jan,13; 2015,Jan,16; 2014,Jan,11

66030 **medication**
EXCLUDES *Insertion of ocular telescope prosthesis (0308T)*
3.16 4.87 FUD 010 J A2 50
AMA: 2016,Feb,12; 2014,Jan,11

66130 Excision Scleral Lesion

INCLUDES Operating microscope (69990)
EXCLUDES *Intraocular foreign body removal (65235)*
Surgery on posterior sclera (67250, 67255)

66130 **Excision of lesion, sclera**
16.1 19.9 FUD 090 J A2 80 50
AMA: 2016,Feb,12; 2014,Jan,11

66150-66185 Procedures for Glaucoma

INCLUDES Operating microscope (69990)
EXCLUDES *Intraocular foreign body removal (65235)*
Surgery on posterior sclera (67250, 67255)

66150 **Fistulization of sclera for glaucoma; trephination with iridectomy**
24.9 24.9 FUD 090 J A2 50
AMA: 2018,Jul,3; 2016,Feb,12; 2014,Jan,11

66155 **thermocauterization with iridectomy**
24.9 24.9 FUD 090 J A2 50
AMA: 2018,Jul,3; 2016,Feb,12; 2014,Jan,11

66160 **sclerectomy with punch or scissors, with iridectomy**
INCLUDES Knapp's operation
28.1 28.1 FUD 090 J A2 50
AMA: 2018,Jul,3; 2016,Feb,12; 2014,Jan,11

66170 **trabeculectomy ab externo in absence of previous surgery**
EXCLUDES *Repair of surgical wound (66250)*
Trabeculectomy ab externo (65850)
31.1 31.1 FUD 090 J A2 80 50
AMA: 2018,Dec,8; 2018,Dec,10; 2018,Dec,8; 2018,Dec,10; 2018,Jul,3; 2018,Jan,8; 2017,Jan,8; 2016,Feb,12; 2016,Jan,13; 2015,Jan,16; 2014,Jan,11

66172 **trabeculectomy ab externo with scarring from previous ocular surgery or trauma (includes injection of antifibrotic agents)**
33.9 33.9 FUD 090 J A2 80 50
AMA: 2019,Apr,7; 2018,Dec,10; 2018,Dec,10; 2018,Jul,3; 2018,Jan,8; 2017,Jan,8; 2016,Feb,12; 2016,Jan,13; 2015,Jan,16; 2014,Jan,11

66174 **Transluminal dilation of aqueous outflow canal; without retention of device or stent**
26.9 26.9 FUD 090 J A2 80 50
AMA: 2019,Sep,10; 2018,Dec,8; 2018,Dec,8; 2016,Feb,12; 2014,Jan,11

66175 **with retention of device or stent**
28.2 28.2 FUD 090 J A2 80 50
AMA: 2016,Feb,12; 2014,Jan,11

66179 **Aqueous shunt to extraocular equatorial plate reservoir, external approach; without graft**
30.6 30.6 FUD 090 J G2 80 50
AMA: 2018,Jul,3; 2018,Jan,8; 2017,Jan,8; 2016,Feb,12; 2016,Jan,13; 2015,Jan,10

66180 **with graft**
EXCLUDES *Scleral reinforcement (67255)*
32.3 32.3 FUD 090 J J8 80 50
AMA: 2018,Jul,3; 2018,Jan,8; 2017,Jan,8; 2016,Feb,12; 2016,Jan,13; 2015,Jan,16; 2015,Jan,10; 2014,Jan,11

66183 **Insertion of anterior segment aqueous drainage device, without extraocular reservoir, external approach**
29.2 29.2 FUD 090 J J8 80 50
AMA: 2018,Jul,3; 2018,Jan,8; 2017,Jan,8; 2016,Feb,12; 2016,Jan,13; 2015,Jan,16; 2014,May,5; 2014,Jan,11

66184 **Revision of aqueous shunt to extraocular equatorial plate reservoir; without graft**
22.3 22.3 FUD 090 J G2 80 50
AMA: 2018,Jan,8; 2017,Jan,8; 2016,Feb,12; 2016,Jan,13; 2015,Jan,10

66185 **with graft**
EXCLUDES *Implanted shunt removal (67120)*
Scleral reinforcement (67255)
24.0 24.0 FUD 090 J A2 80 50
AMA: 2018,Jan,8; 2017,Jan,8; 2016,Feb,12; 2016,Jan,13; 2015,Jan,10; 2014,Jan,11

66225 Staphyloma Repair

INCLUDES Operating microscope (69990)
EXCLUDES *Scleral procedures with retinal procedures (67101-67228)*
Scleral reinforcement (67250, 67255)

66225 **Repair of scleral staphyloma; with graft**
26.4 26.4 FUD 090 J A2 50
AMA: 2016,Feb,12; 2014,Jan,11

66250 Anterior Segment Operative Wound Revision or Repair

INCLUDES Operating microscope (69990)
EXCLUDES *Unlisted procedures of anterior sclera (66999)*

66250 **Revision or repair of operative wound of anterior segment, any type, early or late, major or minor procedure**
15.8 21.4 FUD 090 J A2 50
AMA: 2018,Dec,8; 2018,Dec,8; 2018,Jan,8; 2017,Jan,8; 2016,Feb,12; 2016,Jan,13; 2015,Jan,16; 2014,Jan,11

66500-66505 Iridotomy With/Without Transfixion

INCLUDES Operating microscope (69990)

EXCLUDES *Photocoagulation iridotomy (66761)*

66500 Iridotomy by stab incision (separate procedure); except transfixion

10.2 10.2 FUD 090 J A2 50

AMA: 2016,Feb,12; 2014,Jan,11

66505 with transfixion as for iris bombe

11.1 11.1 FUD 090 J A2 50

AMA: 2016,Feb,12; 2014,Jan,11

66600-66635 Iridectomy Procedures

INCLUDES Operating microscope (69990)

EXCLUDES *Insertion of ocular telescope prosthesis (0308T)*
Photocoagulation coreoplasty (66762)

66600 Iridectomy, with corneoscleral or corneal section; for removal of lesion

23.9 23.9 FUD 090 J A2 50

AMA: 2016,Feb,12; 2014,Jan,11

66605 with cyclectomy

30.3 30.3 FUD 090 J A2 50

AMA: 2016,Feb,12; 2014,Jan,11

66625 peripheral for glaucoma (separate procedure)

12.2 12.2 FUD 090 J A2 50

AMA: 2016,Feb,12; 2014,Jan,11

66630 sector for glaucoma (separate procedure)

16.1 16.1 FUD 090 J A2 50

AMA: 2016,Feb,12; 2014,Jan,11

66635 optical (separate procedure)

16.3 16.3 FUD 090 J A2 50

AMA: 2016,Feb,12; 2014,Jan,11

66680-66770 Other Procedures of the Uveal Tract

INCLUDES Operating microscope (69990)

EXCLUDES *Unlisted procedures of ciliary body or iris (66999)*

66680 Repair of iris, ciliary body (as for iridodialysis)

EXCLUDES *Resection or repositioning of uveal tissue for perforating laceration of cornea and/or sclera (65285)*

14.7 14.7 FUD 090 J A2 50

AMA: 2016,Feb,12; 2014,Jan,11

66682 Suture of iris, ciliary body (separate procedure) with retrieval of suture through small incision (eg, McCannel suture)

18.3 18.3 FUD 090 J A2 50

AMA: 2016,Feb,12; 2014,Jan,11

66700 Ciliary body destruction; diathermy

INCLUDES Heine's operation

11.1 12.8 FUD 090 J A2 80 50

AMA: 2016,Feb,12; 2014,Jan,11

66710 cyclophotocoagulation, transscleral

11.1 12.6 FUD 090 J A2 50

AMA: 2018,Jan,8; 2017,Jan,8; 2016,Feb,12; 2016,Jan,13; 2015,Jan,16; 2014,Jan,11

▲ **66711 cyclophotocoagulation, endoscopic, without concomitant removal of crystalline lens**

EXCLUDES *Endoscopic cyclophotocoagulation performed in conjunction with extracapsular cataract removal with insertion of lens ([66987], [66988])*

18.2 18.2 FUD 090 J A2 50

AMA: 2018,Jan,8; 2017,Jan,8; 2016,Feb,12; 2016,Jan,13; 2015,Jan,16; 2014,Jan,11

66720 cryotherapy

11.6 13.1 FUD 090 J A2 50

AMA: 2016,Feb,12; 2014,Jan,11

66740 cyclodialysis

11.1 12.5 FUD 090 J A2 50

AMA: 2016,Feb,12; 2014,Jan,11

66761 Iridotomy/iridectomy by laser surgery (eg, for glaucoma) (per session)

EXCLUDES *Insertion of ocular telescope prosthesis (0308T)*

6.71 8.50 FUD 010 T P3 50

AMA: 2018,Jan,8; 2017,Jan,8; 2016,Feb,12; 2016,Jan,13; 2015,Jan,16; 2014,Jan,11

66762 Iridoplasty by photocoagulation (1 or more sessions) (eg, for improvement of vision, for widening of anterior chamber angle)

12.0 13.5 FUD 090 T P2 50

AMA: 2018,Jan,8; 2017,Jan,8; 2016,Feb,12; 2016,Jan,13; 2015,Jan,16; 2014,Jan,11

66770 Destruction of cyst or lesion iris or ciliary body (nonexcisional procedure)

EXCLUDES *Excision:*
Epithelial downgrowth (65900)
Iris, ciliary body lesion (66600-66605)

13.7 15.0 FUD 090 T P2 50

AMA: 2016,Feb,12; 2014,Jan,11

66820-66825 Post-Cataract Surgery Procedures

INCLUDES Operating microscope (69990)

66820 Discission of secondary membranous cataract (opacified posterior lens capsule and/or anterior hyaloid); stab incision technique (Ziegler or Wheeler knife)

11.4 11.4 FUD 090 J G2 50

AMA: 2016,Feb,12; 2014,Jan,11

Cataract
Iris
Lens

Artificial lens
Cornea
Opaque lens capsule
Iris

An after-cataract is a cataract that develops in a lens tissue that remains after most of the lens has already been removed

66821 laser surgery (eg, YAG laser) (1 or more stages)

8.85 9.42 FUD 090 T A2 50

AMA: 2016,Feb,12; 2014,Jan,11

66825 Repositioning of intraocular lens prosthesis, requiring an incision (separate procedure)

EXCLUDES *Insertion of ocular telescope prosthesis (0308T)*

21.8 21.8 FUD 090 J A2 80 50

AMA: 2016,Feb,12; 2014,Jan,11

66830-66940 Cataract Extraction; Without Insertion Intraocular Lens

CMS: 100-03,80.10 Phacoemulsification Procedure--Cataract Extraction

INCLUDES Anterior and/or posterior capsulotomy
Enzymatic zonulysis
Iridectomy/iridotomy
Lateral canthotomy
Medications
Operating microscope (69990)
Subconjunctival injection
Subtenon injection
Use of viscoelastic material

EXCLUDES *Removal of intralenticular foreign body without lens excision (65235)*
Repair of surgical laceration (66250)

66830 **Removal of secondary membranous cataract (opacified posterior lens capsule and/or anterior hyaloid) with corneo-scleral section, with or without iridectomy (iridocapsulotomy, iridocapsulectomy)**

INCLUDES Graefe's operation

20.1 20.1 FUD 090 J A2 50

AMA: 2016,Feb,12; 2014,Jan,11

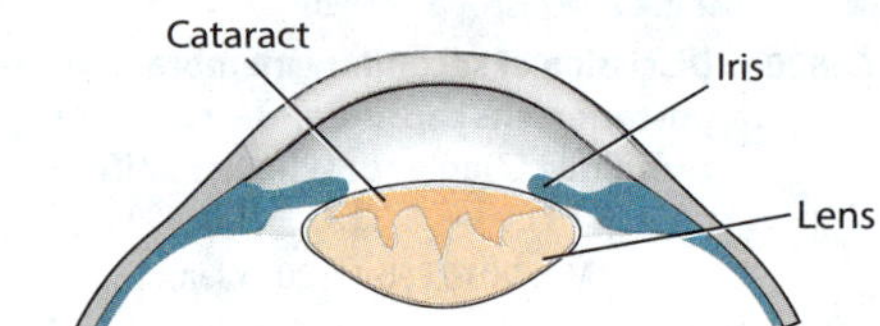

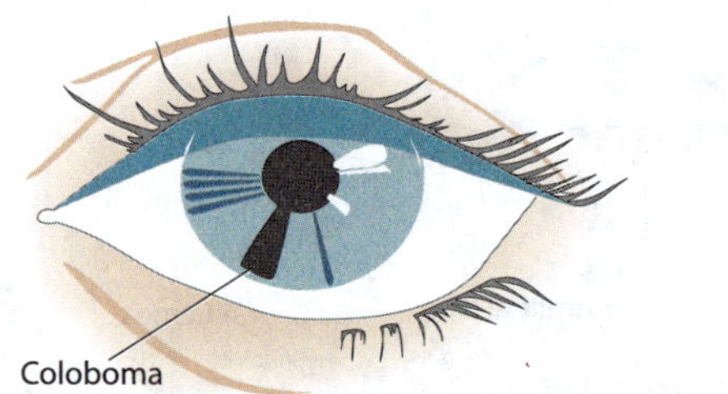

A congenital keyhole pupil is also called a coloboma of the iris

66840 **Removal of lens material; aspiration technique, 1 or more stages**

INCLUDES Fukala's operation

19.7 19.7 FUD 090 J A2 50

AMA: 2018,Jan,8; 2017,Jan,8; 2016,Sep,9; 2016,Jun,6; 2016,Apr,8; 2016,Feb,12; 2016,Jan,13; 2015,Jan,16; 2014,Jan,11

66850 **phacofragmentation technique (mechanical or ultrasonic) (eg, phacoemulsification), with aspiration**

22.5 22.5 FUD 090 J A2 50

AMA: 2018,Jan,8; 2017,Jan,8; 2016,Jun,6; 2016,Feb,12; 2016,Jan,13; 2015,Jan,16; 2014,Jan,11

66852 **pars plana approach, with or without vitrectomy**

23.9 23.9 FUD 090 J A2 80 50

AMA: 2018,Jan,8; 2017,Jan,8; 2016,Jun,6; 2016,Feb,12; 2016,Jan,13; 2015,Jan,16; 2014,Jan,11

66920 **intracapsular**

21.4 21.4 FUD 090 J A2 80 50

AMA: 2018,Jan,8; 2017,Jan,8; 2016,Feb,12; 2016,Jan,13; 2015,Jan,16; 2014,Jan,11

66930 **intracapsular, for dislocated lens**

24.3 24.3 FUD 090 J A2 80 50

AMA: 2018,Jan,8; 2017,Jan,8; 2016,Feb,12; 2016,Jan,13; 2015,Jan,16; 2014,Jan,11

66940 **extracapsular (other than 66840, 66850, 66852)**

22.2 22.2 FUD 090 J A2 80 50

AMA: 2018,Jan,8; 2017,Jan,8; 2016,Jun,6; 2016,Feb,12; 2016,Jan,13; 2015,Jan,16; 2014,Jan,11

66982-66988 [66987, 66988] Cataract Extraction: With Insertion Intraocular Lens

INCLUDES Anterior or posterior capsulotomy
Enzymatic zonulysis
Iridectomy/iridotomy
Lateral canthotomy
Medications
Operating microscope (69990)
Subconjunctival injection
Subtenon injection
Use of viscoelastic material

EXCLUDES *Implanted material removal from the anterior segment (65920)*
Insertion of ocular telescope prosthesis (0308T)
Secondary fixation (66682)
Supply of intraocular lens

▲ **66982** **Extracapsular cataract removal with insertion of intraocular lens prosthesis (1-stage procedure), manual or mechanical technique (eg, irrigation and aspiration or phacoemulsification), complex, requiring devices or techniques not generally used in routine cataract surgery (eg, iris expansion device, suture support for intraocular lens, or primary posterior capsulorrhexis) or performed on patients in the amblyogenic developmental stage; without endoscopic cyclophotocoagulation**

EXCLUDES *Complex extracapsular cataract removal in conjunction with endoscopic cyclophotocoagulation ([66987])*
Insertion of ocular telescope prosthesis (0308T)

(76519)

22.5 22.5 FUD 090 J A2 50

AMA: 2018,Dec,6; 2018,Dec,6; 2018,Jan,8; 2017,Dec,14; 2017,Jan,8; 2016,Mar,10; 2016,Feb,12; 2016,Jan,13; 2015,Jan,16; 2014,Jan,11

● # **66987** **with endoscopic cyclophotocoagulation**

0.00 0.00 FUD 000

EXCLUDES *Complex extracapsular cataract removal without endoscopic cyclophotocoagulation (66982)*
Insertion of ocular telescope prosthesis (0308T)

66983 **Intracapsular cataract extraction with insertion of intraocular lens prosthesis (1 stage procedure)**

(76519)

21.0 21.0 FUD 090 J A2 50

AMA: 2018,Jan,8; 2017,Jan,8; 2016,Feb,12; 2016,Jan,13; 2015,Jan,16; 2014,Jan,11

▲ **66984** **Extracapsular cataract removal with insertion of intraocular lens prosthesis (1 stage procedure), manual or mechanical technique (eg, irrigation and aspiration or phacoemulsification); without endoscopic cyclophotocoagulation**

EXCLUDES *Complex extracapsular cataract removal (66982)*
Extracapsular cataract removal in conjunction with endoscopic cyclophotocoagulation ([66988])
Insertion of ocular telescope prosthesis (0308T)

(76519)

18.1 18.1 FUD 090 J A2 50

AMA: 2018,Dec,6; 2018,Dec,6; 2018,Jan,8; 2017,Jan,8; 2016,Feb,12; 2016,Jan,13; 2015,Jan,16; 2014,Jan,11

● # **66988** **with endoscopic cyclophotocoagulation**

0.00 0.00 FUD 000

EXCLUDES *Complex extracapsular cataract removal in conjunction with endoscopic cyclophotocoagulation ([66987])*
Extracapsular cataract removal without endoscopic cyclophotocoagulation (66984)
Insertion of ocular telescope prosthesis (0308T)

66985-66988 Secondary Insertion or Replacement of Intraocular Lens

INCLUDES Operating microscope (69990)

EXCLUDES *Implanted material removal from the anterior segment (65920)*
Insertion of ocular telescope prosthesis (0308T)
Secondary fixation (66682)
Supply of intraocular lens

Code also ophthalmic endoscope if used (66990)

66985 Insertion of intraocular lens prosthesis (secondary implant), not associated with concurrent cataract removal

EXCLUDES *Insertion of lens at the time of cataract procedure (66982-66984)*

(76519)

21.8 21.8 FUD 090 J A2 50

AMA: 2018,Jan,8; 2017,Jan,8; 2016,Feb,12; 2016,Jan,13; 2015,Jan,16; 2014,Jan,11

66986 Exchange of intraocular lens

(76519)

25.8 25.8 FUD 090 J A2 50

AMA: 2018,Jan,8; 2017,Jan,8; 2016,Feb,12; 2016,Jan,13; 2015,Jan,16; 2014,Jan,11

66987 **Resequenced code. See code following 66982.**

66988 **Resequenced code. See code following 66984.**

66990-66999 Ophthalmic Endoscopy

INCLUDES Operating microscope (69990)

\+ **66990 Use of ophthalmic endoscope (List separately in addition to code for primary procedure)**

Code first (65820, 65875, 65920, 66985-66986, 67036, 67039-67043, 67113)

2.56 2.56 FUD ZZZ N N1

AMA: 2018,Jul,3; 2018,Jan,8; 2017,Jan,8; 2016,Sep,5; 2016,Feb,12; 2016,Jan,13; 2015,Jan,16; 2014,Jan,11

66999 Unlisted procedure, anterior segment of eye

0.00 0.00 FUD YYY J 80 50

AMA: 2018,Jan,8; 2017,Jan,8; 2016,Apr,8; 2016,Feb,12; 2016,Jan,13; 2015,Jan,16; 2014,Jan,11

67005-67015 Vitrectomy: Partial and Subtotal

INCLUDES Operating microscope (69990)

67005 Removal of vitreous, anterior approach (open sky technique or limbal incision); partial removal

EXCLUDES *Anterior chamber vitrectomy by paracentesis (65810)*
Severing of corneovitreal adhesions (65880)

13.4 13.4 FUD 090 J A2 50

AMA: 2018,Jan,8; 2017,Jan,8; 2016,Feb,12; 2016,Jan,13; 2015,Jan,16; 2014,Jan,11

67010 subtotal removal with mechanical vitrectomy

EXCLUDES *Anterior chamber vitrectomy by paracentesis (65810)*
Severing of corneovitreal adhesions (65880)

15.4 15.4 FUD 090 J A2 50

AMA: 2018,Jan,8; 2017,Jan,8; 2016,Feb,12; 2016,Jan,13; 2015,Jan,16; 2014,Jan,11

67015 Aspiration or release of vitreous, subretinal or choroidal fluid, pars plana approach (posterior sclerotomy)

16.5 16.5 FUD 090 J A2 50

AMA: 2018,Jan,8; 2017,Jan,8; 2016,Sep,5; 2016,Jun,6; 2016,Feb,12; 2014,Jan,11

67025-67028 Intravitreal Injection/Implantation

INCLUDES Operating microscope (69990)

67025 Injection of vitreous substitute, pars plana or limbal approach (fluid-gas exchange), with or without aspiration (separate procedure)

17.9 20.8 FUD 090 J A2 50

AMA: 2019,Aug,10; 2018,Feb,3; 2016,Feb,12; 2014,Jan,11

67027 Implantation of intravitreal drug delivery system (eg, ganciclovir implant), includes concomitant removal of vitreous

EXCLUDES *Removal of drug delivery system (67121)*

24.2 24.2 FUD 090 J A2 80 50

AMA: 2018,Feb,3; 2018,Jan,8; 2017,Jan,8; 2016,Feb,12; 2016,Jan,13; 2015,Jan,16; 2014,Jan,11

67028 Intravitreal injection of a pharmacologic agent (separate procedure)

2.83 2.89 FUD 000 S P3 50

AMA: 2018,Feb,3; 2018,Jan,8; 2017,Jan,8; 2016,Feb,12; 2016,Jan,13; 2015,Jan,16; 2014,Jan,11

67030-67031 Incision of Vitreous Strands/Membranes

INCLUDES Operating microscope (69990)

67030 Discission of vitreous strands (without removal), pars plana approach

15.2 15.2 FUD 090 J A2 50

AMA: 2016,Feb,12; 2014,Jan,11

67031 Severing of vitreous strands, vitreous face adhesions, sheets, membranes or opacities, laser surgery (1 or more stages)

10.1 11.1 FUD 090 T A2 50

AMA: 2016,Feb,12; 2014,Jan,11

67036-67043 Pars Plana Mechanical Vitrectomy

INCLUDES Operating microscope (69990)

EXCLUDES *Foreign body removal (65260, 65265)*
Lens removal (66850)
Unlisted vitreal procedures (67299)
Vitrectomy in retinal detachment (67108, 67113)

Code also ophthalmic endoscope if used (66990)

67036 Vitrectomy, mechanical, pars plana approach;

25.6 25.6 FUD 090 J A2 80 50

AMA: 2018,Jan,8; 2017,Jan,8; 2016,Sep,5; 2016,Feb,12; 2016,Jan,13; 2015,Jan,16; 2014,Jan,11

67039 with focal endolaser photocoagulation

27.4 27.4 FUD 090 J A2 80 50

AMA: 2018,Jan,8; 2017,Jan,8; 2016,Sep,5; 2016,Feb,12; 2016,Jan,13; 2015,Jan,16; 2014,Jan,11

67040 with endolaser panretinal photocoagulation

29.6 29.6 FUD 090 J A2 80 50

AMA: 2018,Jan,8; 2017,Jan,8; 2016,Sep,5; 2016,Feb,12; 2016,Jan,13; 2015,Jan,16; 2014,Jan,11

67041 with removal of preretinal cellular membrane (eg, macular pucker)

32.7 32.7 FUD 090 J G2 80 50

AMA: 2018,Jan,8; 2017,Jan,8; 2016,Sep,5; 2016,Feb,12; 2016,Jan,13; 2015,Jan,16; 2014,Jan,11

67042 with removal of internal limiting membrane of retina (eg, for repair of macular hole, diabetic macular edema), includes, if performed, intraocular tamponade (ie, air, gas or silicone oil)

32.7 32.7 FUD 090 J G2 80 50

AMA: 2018,Jan,8; 2017,Jan,8; 2016,Sep,5; 2016,Feb,12; 2016,Jan,13; 2015,Jan,16; 2014,Jan,11

67043 with removal of subretinal membrane (eg, choroidal neovascularization), includes, if performed, intraocular tamponade (ie, air, gas or silicone oil) and laser photocoagulation

34.5 34.5 FUD 090 J G2 80 50

AMA: 2018,Jan,8; 2017,Jan,8; 2016,Sep,5; 2016,Feb,12; 2016,Jan,13; 2015,Jan,16; 2014,Jan,11

67101-67115 Detached Retina Repair

INCLUDES Operating microscope (69990)
Primary technique when cryotherapy and/or diathermy and/or photocoagulation are used in combination

67101 Repair of retinal detachment, including drainage of subretinal fluid when performed; cryotherapy
8.10 9.40 FUD 010 J P3 50
AMA: 2018,Jan,8; 2017,Feb,14; 2017,Jan,8; 2016,Sep,5; 2016,Jun,6; 2016,Feb,12; 2016,Jan,13; 2015,Jan,16; 2014,Jan,11

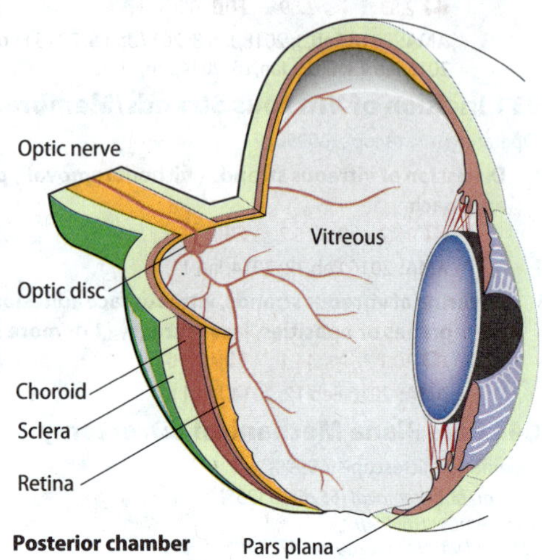

67105 photocoagulation
7.82 8.45 FUD 010 T P3 50
AMA: 2018,Jan,8; 2017,Feb,14; 2017,Jan,8; 2016,Sep,5; 2016,Jun,6; 2016,Feb,12; 2016,Jan,13; 2015,Jan,16; 2014,Jan,11

67107 Repair of retinal detachment; scleral buckling (such as lamellar scleral dissection, imbrication or encircling procedure), including, when performed, implant, cryotherapy, photocoagulation, and drainage of subretinal fluid
INCLUDES Gonin's operation
32.1 32.1 FUD 090 J G2 80 50
AMA: 2019,Aug,10; 2018,Jan,8; 2017,Jan,8; 2016,Sep,5; 2016,Jun,6; 2016,Feb,12; 2014,Jan,11

67108 with vitrectomy, any method, including, when performed, air or gas tamponade, focal endolaser photocoagulation, cryotherapy, drainage of subretinal fluid, scleral buckling, and/or removal of lens by same technique
34.1 34.1 FUD 090 J G2 80 50
AMA: 2018,Jan,8; 2017,Jan,8; 2016,Sep,5; 2016,Jun,6; 2016,Feb,12; 2016,Jan,13; 2015,Jan,16; 2014,Jan,11

67110 by injection of air or other gas (eg, pneumatic retinopexy)
23.1 25.0 FUD 090 J P3 50
AMA: 2018,Jan,8; 2017,Jan,8; 2016,Sep,5; 2016,Jun,6; 2016,Feb,12; 2014,Jan,11

67113 Repair of complex retinal detachment (eg, proliferative vitreoretinopathy, stage C-1 or greater, diabetic traction retinal detachment, retinopathy of prematurity, retinal tear of greater than 90 degrees), with vitrectomy and membrane peeling, including, when performed, air, gas, or silicone oil tamponade, cryotherapy, endolaser photocoagulation, drainage of subretinal fluid, scleral buckling, and/or removal of lens
EXCLUDES *Vitrectomy for other than retinal detachment, pars plana approach (67036-67043)*
Code also ophthalmic endoscope if used (66990)
38.0 38.0 FUD 090 J G2 80 50
AMA: 2018,Jan,8; 2017,Jan,8; 2016,Sep,5; 2016,Jun,6; 2016,Feb,12; 2016,Jan,13; 2015,Jan,16; 2014,Jan,11

67115 Release of encircling material (posterior segment)
14.1 14.1 FUD 090 J A2 50
AMA: 2016,Feb,12; 2014,Jan,11

67120-67121 Removal of Previously Implanted Prosthetic Device

INCLUDES Operating microscope (69990)
EXCLUDES *Foreign body removal (65260, 65265)*
Removal of implanted material anterior segment (65920)

67120 Removal of implanted material, posterior segment; extraocular
15.8 18.8 FUD 090 J A2 50
AMA: 2016,Feb,12; 2014,Jan,11

67121 intraocular
25.8 25.8 FUD 090 J A2 80 50
AMA: 2016,Feb,12; 2014,Jan,11

67141-67145 Retinal Detachment: Preventative Procedures

INCLUDES Operating microscope (69990)
Treatment at one or more sessions that may occur at different encounters
EXCLUDES *Procedure performed more than one time during a defined period of treatment*

67141 Prophylaxis of retinal detachment (eg, retinal break, lattice degeneration) without drainage, 1 or more sessions; cryotherapy, diathermy
13.8 14.9 FUD 090 T A2 50
AMA: 2018,Jan,8; 2017,Jan,8; 2016,Sep,5; 2016,Feb,12; 2016,Jan,13; 2015,Jan,16; 2014,Jan,11

67145 photocoagulation (laser or xenon arc)
14.1 15.0 FUD 090 T P2 50
AMA: 2018,Jan,8; 2017,Jan,8; 2016,Sep,5; 2016,Feb,12; 2016,Jan,13; 2015,Jan,16; 2014,Jan,11

67208-67218 Destruction of Retinal Lesions

INCLUDES Operating microscope (69990)
Treatment at one or more sessions that may occur at different encounters
EXCLUDES *Procedure performed more than one time during a defined period of treatment*
Unlisted retinal procedures (67299)

67208 Destruction of localized lesion of retina (eg, macular edema, tumors), 1 or more sessions; cryotherapy, diathermy
16.4 17.0 FUD 090 T P2 50
AMA: 2018,Jan,8; 2017,Jan,8; 2016,Feb,12; 2016,Jan,13; 2015,Jan,16; 2014,Jan,11

67210 photocoagulation
14.2 14.7 FUD 090 T P2 50
AMA: 2018,Jan,8; 2017,Jan,8; 2016,Feb,12; 2016,Jan,13; 2015,Jan,16; 2014,Jan,11

67218 radiation by implantation of source (includes removal of source)
39.3 39.3 FUD 090 J A2 50
AMA: 2018,Jan,8; 2017,Jan,8; 2016,Feb,12; 2016,Jan,13; 2015,Jan,16; 2014,Jan,11

67220-67225 Destruction of Choroidal Lesions

INCLUDES Operating microscope (69990)

67220 Destruction of localized lesion of choroid (eg, choroidal neovascularization); photocoagulation (eg, laser), 1 or more sessions
INCLUDES Treatment at one or more sessions that may occur at different encounters
EXCLUDES *Procedure performed more than one time during a defined period of treatment*
14.2 15.1 FUD 090 T P2 50
AMA: 2018,Jan,8; 2017,Jan,8; 2016,Feb,12; 2016,Jan,13; 2015,Jan,16; 2014,Jan,11

67221 photodynamic therapy (includes intravenous infusion)
6.05 8.07 FUD 000 T P3
AMA: 2018,Feb,10; 2018,Jan,8; 2017,Jan,8; 2016,Feb,12; 2016,Jan,13; 2015,Jan,16; 2014,Jan,11

+ 67225 **photodynamic therapy, second eye, at single session (List separately in addition to code for primary eye treatment)**
Code first (67221)
0.80 0.84 FUD ZZZ N N1
AMA: 2018,Jan,8; 2017,Jan,8; 2016,Feb,12; 2016,Jan,13; 2015,Jan,16; 2014,Jan,11

67227-67229 Destruction Retinopathy

INCLUDES Operating microscope (69990)
EXCLUDES *Unlisted retinal procedures (67299)*

67227 **Destruction of extensive or progressive retinopathy (eg, diabetic retinopathy), cryotherapy, diathermy**
7.30 8.34 FUD 010 J P3 50
AMA: 2018,Jan,8; 2017,Jan,8; 2016,Feb,12; 2016,Jan,13; 2015,Jan,16; 2014,Jan,11

67228 **Treatment of extensive or progressive retinopathy (eg, diabetic retinopathy), photocoagulation**
8.72 9.73 FUD 010 T P3 50
AMA: 2018,Jan,8; 2017,Jan,8; 2016,Feb,12; 2016,Jan,13; 2015,Jan,16; 2014,Jan,11

67229 **Treatment of extensive or progressive retinopathy, 1 or more sessions, preterm infant (less than 37 weeks gestation at birth), performed from birth up to 1 year of age (eg, retinopathy of prematurity), photocoagulation or cryotherapy**
INCLUDES Treatment at one or more sessions that may occur at different encounters
EXCLUDES *Procedure performed more than one time during a defined period of treatment*
33.1 33.1 FUD 090 T R2 50
AMA: 2018,Jan,8; 2017,Jan,8; 2016,Feb,12; 2016,Jan,13; 2015,Jan,16; 2014,Jan,11

67250-67255 Reinforcement of Posterior Sclera

INCLUDES Operating microscope (69990)
EXCLUDES *Removal of lesion of sclera (66130)*
Repair scleral staphyloma (66225)

67250 **Scleral reinforcement (separate procedure); without graft**
22.6 22.6 FUD 090 J A2 50
AMA: 2016,Feb,12; 2014,Jan,11

67255 **with graft**
EXCLUDES *Aqueous shunt to extraocular equatorial plate reservoir (66180)*
Revision of aqueous shunt to extraocular equatorial plate reservoir; with graft (66185)
19.4 19.4 FUD 090 J A2 80 50
AMA: 2018,Jan,8; 2017,Jan,8; 2016,Feb,12; 2016,Jan,13; 2015,Jan,16; 2015,Jan,10; 2014,Jan,11

67299 Unlisted Posterior Segment Procedure

CMS: 100-04,4,180.3 Unlisted Service or Procedure
INCLUDES Operating microscope (69990)

67299 **Unlisted procedure, posterior segment**
0.00 0.00 FUD YYY J 80 50
AMA: 2018,Jan,8; 2017,Jan,8; 2016,Feb,12; 2016,Jan,13; 2015,Jan,16; 2014,Jan,11

67311-67334 Strabismus Procedures on Extraocular Muscles

INCLUDES Operating microscope (69990)
Code also adjustable sutures (67335)

67311 **Strabismus surgery, recession or resection procedure; 1 horizontal muscle**
16.9 16.9 FUD 090 J A2 50
AMA: 2018,Jan,8; 2017,Jan,8; 2017,Jan,6; 2016,Feb,12; 2016,Jan,13; 2015,Jan,16; 2014,Jan,11

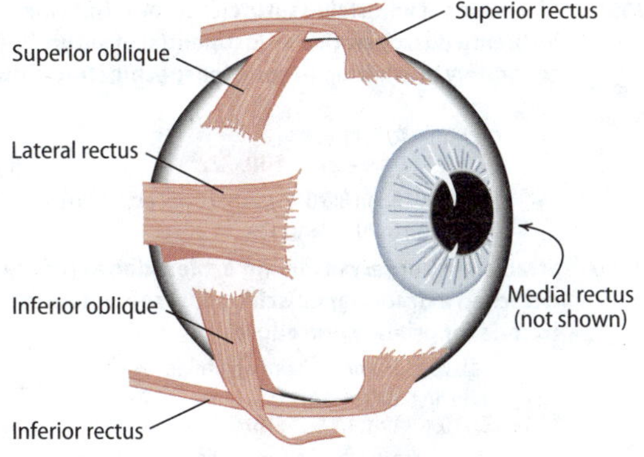

Muscles of the eyeball (right eye shown)

67312 **2 horizontal muscles**
20.2 20.2 FUD 090 J A2 50
AMA: 2018,Jan,8; 2017,Jan,8; 2016,Feb,12; 2016,Jan,13; 2015,Jan,16; 2014,Jan,11

67314 **1 vertical muscle (excluding superior oblique)**
19.1 19.1 FUD 090 J A2 50
AMA: 2018,Jan,8; 2017,Jan,8; 2016,Feb,12; 2016,Jan,13; 2015,Jan,16; 2014,Jan,11

67316 **2 or more vertical muscles (excluding superior oblique)**
22.7 22.7 FUD 090 J A2 80 50
AMA: 2018,Jan,8; 2017,Jan,8; 2016,Feb,12; 2016,Jan,13; 2015,Jan,16; 2014,Jan,11

67318 **Strabismus surgery, any procedure, superior oblique muscle**
19.9 19.9 FUD 090 J A2 50
AMA: 2018,Jan,8; 2017,Jan,8; 2016,Feb,12; 2016,Jan,13; 2015,Jan,16; 2014,Jan,11

+ 67320 **Transposition procedure (eg, for paretic extraocular muscle), any extraocular muscle (specify) (List separately in addition to code for primary procedure)**
Code first (67311-67318)
9.17 9.17 FUD ZZZ N N1
AMA: 2018,Jan,8; 2017,Jan,8; 2016,Feb,12; 2016,Jan,13; 2015,Jan,16; 2014,Jan,11

+ 67331 **Strabismus surgery on patient with previous eye surgery or injury that did not involve the extraocular muscles (List separately in addition to code for primary procedure)**
Code first (67311-67318)
8.70 8.70 FUD ZZZ N N1 50
AMA: 2018,Jan,8; 2017,Jan,8; 2016,Feb,12; 2016,Jan,13; 2015,Jan,16; 2014,Jan,11

+ 67332 **Strabismus surgery on patient with scarring of extraocular muscles (eg, prior ocular injury, strabismus or retinal detachment surgery) or restrictive myopathy (eg, dysthyroid ophthalmopathy) (List separately in addition to code for primary procedure)**
Code first (67311-67318)
9.44 9.44 FUD ZZZ N N1 50
AMA: 2018,Jan,8; 2017,Jan,8; 2016,Feb,12; 2016,Jan,13; 2015,Jan,16; 2014,Jan,11

+ **67334 Strabismus surgery by posterior fixation suture technique, with or without muscle recession (List separately in addition to code for primary procedure)**

Code first (67311-67318)

8.59 8.59 FUD ZZZ N N1 50

AMA: 2018,Jan,8; 2017,Jan,8; 2016,Feb,12; 2016,Jan,13; 2015,Jan,16; 2014,Jan,11

67335-67399 Other Procedures of Extraocular Muscles

INCLUDES Operating microscope (69990)

+ **67335 Placement of adjustable suture(s) during strabismus surgery, including postoperative adjustment(s) of suture(s) (List separately in addition to code for specific strabismus surgery)**

Code first (67311-67334)

4.21 4.21 FUD ZZZ N N1 50

AMA: 2018,Jan,8; 2017,Jan,8; 2016,Feb,12; 2016,Jan,13; 2015,Jan,16; 2014,Jan,11

+ **67340 Strabismus surgery involving exploration and/or repair of detached extraocular muscle(s) (List separately in addition to code for primary procedure)**

INCLUDES Hummelsheim operation

Code first (67311-67334)

10.1 10.1 FUD ZZZ N N1 80

AMA: 2018,Jan,8; 2017,Jan,8; 2016,Feb,12; 2016,Jan,13; 2015,Jan,16; 2014,Jan,11

67343 Release of extensive scar tissue without detaching extraocular muscle (separate procedure)

Code also if these procedures are performed on other than the affected muscle (67311-67340)

18.5 18.5 FUD 090 J A2 50

AMA: 2018,Jan,8; 2017,Jan,8; 2016,Feb,12; 2016,Jan,13; 2015,Jan,16; 2014,Jan,11

67345 Chemodenervation of extraocular muscle

EXCLUDES *Nerve destruction for blepharospasm and other neurological disorders (64612, 64616)*

6.22 6.96 FUD 010 T P3 50

AMA: 2019,Apr,9; 2018,Jan,8; 2017,Jan,8; 2016,Feb,12; 2016,Jan,13; 2015,Jan,16; 2014,May,5; 2014,Jan,11

67346 Biopsy of extraocular muscle

EXCLUDES *Repair laceration extraocular muscle, tendon, or Tenon's capsule (65290)*

5.50 5.50 FUD 000 J A2 80 50

AMA: 2016,Feb,12; 2014,Jan,11

67399 Unlisted procedure, extraocular muscle

0.00 0.00 FUD YYY T 80 50

AMA: 2018,Jan,8; 2017,Jul,10; 2016,Feb,12; 2014,Jan,11

67400-67415 Frontal Orbitotomy

INCLUDES Operating microscope (69990)

67400 Orbitotomy without bone flap (frontal or transconjunctival approach); for exploration, with or without biopsy

26.7 26.7 FUD 090 J A2 50

AMA: 2016,Feb,12; 2014,Jan,11

67405 with drainage only

22.8 22.8 FUD 090 J A2 50

AMA: 2018,Jan,8; 2017,Jan,8; 2016,Feb,12; 2016,Jan,13; 2015,Jan,16; 2014,Jan,11

67412 with removal of lesion

24.6 24.6 FUD 090 J A2 50

AMA: 2016,Feb,12; 2014,Jan,11

67413 with removal of foreign body

24.7 24.7 FUD 090 J A2 80 50

AMA: 2016,Feb,12; 2014,Jan,11

67414 with removal of bone for decompression

38.1 38.1 FUD 090 J G2 80 50

AMA: 2018,Jan,8; 2017,Jan,8; 2016,Feb,12; 2016,Jan,13; 2015,Jan,16; 2014,Jan,11

67415 Fine needle aspiration of orbital contents

EXCLUDES *Decompression optic nerve (67570)*
Exenteration, enucleation, and repair (65101-65175)

2.97 2.97 FUD 000 J A2 80 50

AMA: 2016,Feb,12; 2014,Jan,11

67420-67450 Lateral Orbitotomy

INCLUDES Operating microscope (69990)

EXCLUDES *Orbital implant (67550, 67560)*
Surgical removal of all or some of the orbital contents or repair after removal (65091-65175)
Transcranial approach orbitotomy (61330, 61333)

67420 Orbitotomy with bone flap or window, lateral approach (eg, Kroenlein); with removal of lesion

46.2 46.2 FUD 090 J A2 80 50

AMA: 2016,Feb,12; 2014,Jan,11

67430 with removal of foreign body

35.9 35.9 FUD 090 J A2 80 50

AMA: 2016,Feb,12; 2014,Jan,11

67440 with drainage

34.7 34.7 FUD 090 J A2 80 50

AMA: 2016,Feb,12; 2014,Jan,11

67445 with removal of bone for decompression

EXCLUDES *Decompression optic nerve sheath (67570)*

40.3 40.3 FUD 090 J A2 80 50

AMA: 2016,Feb,12; 2014,Jan,11

67450 for exploration, with or without biopsy

36.1 36.1 FUD 090 J A2 80 50

AMA: 2016,Feb,12; 2014,Jan,11

67500-67515 Eye Injections

INCLUDES Operating microscope (69990)

67500 Retrobulbar injection; medication (separate procedure, does not include supply of medication)

1.73 2.02 FUD 000 T G2 50

AMA: 2018,Jan,8; 2017,Jan,8; 2016,Feb,12; 2016,Jan,13; 2015,Jan,16; 2014,Jan,11

67505 alcohol

2.03 2.38 FUD 000 T P3 50

AMA: 2016,Feb,12; 2014,Jan,11

67515 Injection of medication or other substance into Tenon's capsule

EXCLUDES *Subconjunctival injection (68200)*

2.06 2.24 FUD 000 T P3 50

AMA: 2018,Jan,8; 2017,Jan,8; 2016,Feb,12; 2016,Jan,13; 2015,Jan,16; 2014,Jan,11

67550-67560 Orbital Implant

INCLUDES Operating microscope (69990)

EXCLUDES *Fracture repair malar area, orbit (21355-21408)*
Ocular implant inside muscle cone (65093-65105, 65130-65175)

67550 Orbital implant (implant outside muscle cone); insertion

27.8 27.8 FUD 090 J A2 50

AMA: 2016,Feb,12; 2014,Jan,11

67560 removal or revision

28.5 28.5 FUD 090 J A2 80 50

AMA: 2016,Feb,12; 2014,Jan,11

67570-67599 Other and Unlisted Orbital Procedures

INCLUDES Operating microscope (69990)

67570 Optic nerve decompression (eg, incision or fenestration of optic nerve sheath)

33.9 33.9 FUD 090 J A2 80 50

AMA: 2016,Feb,12; 2014,Jan,11

67599 Unlisted procedure, orbit

0.00 0.00 FUD YYY T 80 50

AMA: 2016,Feb,12; 2014,Jan,11

67700-67810 [67810] Incisional Procedures of Eyelids

INCLUDES Operating microscope (69990)

67700 Blepharotomy, drainage of abscess, eyelid
3.31 7.82 FUD 010 T P2 50
AMA: 2018,Jan,8; 2017,Jan,8; 2016,Feb,12; 2016,Jan,13; 2015,Jan,16; 2014,Jan,11

67710 Severing of tarsorrhaphy
2.77 6.56 FUD 010 T P3 50
AMA: 2018,Jan,8; 2017,Jan,8; 2016,Feb,12; 2016,Jan,13; 2015,Jan,16; 2014,Jan,11

67715 Canthotomy (separate procedure)
EXCLUDES *Canthoplasty (67950)*
Symblepharon division (68340)
3.08 7.07 FUD 010 J A2 50
AMA: 2018,Jan,8; 2017,Jan,8; 2016,Feb,12; 2016,Jan,13; 2015,Jan,16; 2014,Jan,11

\# **67810 Incisional biopsy of eyelid skin including lid margin**
EXCLUDES *Biopsy of eyelid skin (11102-11107)*
2.03 4.99 FUD 000 T P3 50
AMA: 2019,Jan,9; 2018,Jan,8; 2017,Jan,8; 2016,Feb,12; 2016,Jan,13; 2015,Jan,16; 2014,Jan,11

67800-67808 Excision of Chalazion (Meibomian Cyst)

INCLUDES Lesion removal requiring more than skin:
- Lid margin
- Palpebral conjunctiva
- Tarsus

Operating microscope (69990)

EXCLUDES *Blepharoplasty, graft, or reconstructive procedures (67930-67975)*
Excision/destruction skin lesion of eyelid (11310-11313, 11440-11446, 11640-11646, 17000-17004)

67800 Excision of chalazion; single
2.93 3.64 FUD 010 T P3
AMA: 2018,Jan,8; 2017,Jan,8; 2016,Feb,12; 2016,Jan,13; 2015,Jan,16; 2014,Jan,11

67801 multiple, same lid
3.79 4.64 FUD 010 T P3
AMA: 2016,Feb,12; 2014,Jan,11

67805 multiple, different lids
4.67 5.76 FUD 010 T P3
AMA: 2018,Jan,8; 2017,Jan,8; 2016,Feb,12; 2016,Jan,13; 2015,Jan,16; 2014,Jan,11

67808 under general anesthesia and/or requiring hospitalization, single or multiple
10.4 10.4 FUD 090 J A2
AMA: 2016,Feb,12; 2014,Jan,11

67810-67850 Other Eyelid Procedures

INCLUDES Operating microscope (69990)

67810 **Resequenced code. See code following 67715.**

67820 Correction of trichiasis; epilation, by forceps only
0.99 0.93 FUD 000 Q1 N1 50
AMA: 2018,Jan,8; 2017,Jan,8; 2016,Feb,12; 2016,Jan,13; 2015,Jan,16; 2014,Jan,11

67825 epilation by other than forceps (eg, by electrosurgery, cryotherapy, laser surgery)
3.46 3.71 FUD 010 T P3 50
AMA: 2018,Jan,8; 2017,Jan,8; 2016,Feb,12; 2016,Jan,13; 2015,Jan,16; 2014,Jan,11

67830 incision of lid margin
3.92 7.64 FUD 010 T A2 50
AMA: 2016,Feb,12; 2014,Jan,11

67835 incision of lid margin, with free mucous membrane graft
12.4 12.4 FUD 090 J A2 80 50
AMA: 2016,Feb,12; 2014,Jan,11

67840 Excision of lesion of eyelid (except chalazion) without closure or with simple direct closure
EXCLUDES *Eyelid resection and reconstruction (67961, 67966)*
4.49 7.91 FUD 010 T P3 50
AMA: 2019,Jan,14; 2016,Feb,12; 2014,Jan,11

67850 Destruction of lesion of lid margin (up to 1 cm)
EXCLUDES *Mohs micro procedures (17311-17315)*
Topical chemotherapy (99201-99215)
3.84 6.13 FUD 010 T P3 50
AMA: 2016,Feb,12; 2014,Jan,11

67875-67882 Suturing of the Eyelids

INCLUDES Operating microscope (69990)

EXCLUDES *Canthoplasty (67950)*
Canthotomy (67715)
Severing of tarsorrhaphy (67710)

67875 Temporary closure of eyelids by suture (eg, Frost suture)
2.75 4.96 FUD 000 T G2 50
AMA: 2016,Feb,12; 2014,Jan,11

67880 Construction of intermarginal adhesions, median tarsorrhaphy, or canthorrhaphy;
10.4 13.1 FUD 090 J A2 50
AMA: 2016,Feb,12; 2014,Jan,11

67882 with transposition of tarsal plate
13.4 16.1 FUD 090 J A2 50
AMA: 2016,Feb,12; 2014,Jan,11

67900-67912 Repair of Ptosis/Retraction Eyelids, Eyebrows

INCLUDES Operating microscope (69990)

67900 Repair of brow ptosis (supraciliary, mid-forehead or coronal approach)
EXCLUDES *Forehead rhytidectomy (15824)*
14.4 18.2 FUD 090 J A2 50
AMA: 2018,Jan,8; 2017,Jan,8; 2016,Feb,12; 2016,Jan,13; 2015,Jan,16; 2014,Jan,11

67901 Repair of blepharoptosis; frontalis muscle technique with suture or other material (eg, banked fascia)
16.5 21.9 FUD 090 J A2 50
AMA: 2018,Jan,8; 2017,Jul,10; 2017,Jan,8; 2016,Feb,12; 2016,Jan,13; 2015,Jan,16; 2014,Jan,11

67902 frontalis muscle technique with autologous fascial sling (includes obtaining fascia)
20.5 20.5 FUD 090 J A2 50
AMA: 2018,Jan,8; 2017,Jan,8; 2016,Feb,12; 2016,Jan,13; 2015,Jan,16; 2014,Jan,11

67903 (tarso) levator resection or advancement, internal approach
13.7 16.9 FUD 090 J A2 50
AMA: 2018,Jan,8; 2017,Jan,8; 2016,Feb,12; 2016,Jan,13; 2015,Jan,16; 2014,Jan,11

67904 (tarso) levator resection or advancement, external approach

INCLUDES Everbusch's operation

16.9 | 20.9 | FUD 090 | J A2 50

AMA: 2018,Jan,8; 2017,Jan,8; 2016,Feb,12; 2016,Jan,13; 2015,Jan,16; 2014,Jan,11

67906 superior rectus technique with fascial sling (includes obtaining fascia)

14.4 | 14.4 | FUD 090 | J A2 50

AMA: 2018,Jan,8; 2017,Jan,8; 2016,Feb,12; 2016,Jan,13; 2015,Jan,16; 2014,Jan,11

67908 conjunctivo-tarso-Muller's muscle-levator resection (eg, Fasanella-Servat type)

12.1 | 14.1 | FUD 090 | J A2 50

AMA: 2018,Jan,8; 2017,Jan,8; 2016,Feb,12; 2016,Jan,13; 2015,Jan,16; 2014,Jan,11

67909 Reduction of overcorrection of ptosis

12.4 | 15.3 | FUD 090 | J A2 50

AMA: 2018,Jan,8; 2017,Jan,8; 2016,Feb,12; 2016,Jan,13; 2015,Jan,16; 2014,Jan,11

67911 Correction of lid retraction

EXCLUDES *Autologous graft harvest ([15769], 20920, 20922)*
Lid defect correction using fat obtained via liposuction (15773-15774)
Mucous membrane graft repair of trichiasis (67835)

15.9 | 15.9 | FUD 090 | J A2 50

AMA: 2018,Jan,8; 2017,Jan,8; 2016,Feb,12; 2016,Jan,13; 2015,Jan,16; 2014,Jan,11

67912 Correction of lagophthalmos, with implantation of upper eyelid lid load (eg, gold weight)

13.8 | 25.4 | FUD 090 | J A2 50

AMA: 2018,Jan,8; 2017,Jan,8; 2016,Feb,12; 2016,Jan,13; 2015,Jan,16; 2014,Jan,11

67914-67924 Repair Ectropion/Entropion

INCLUDES Operating microscope (69990)

EXCLUDES *Cicatricial ectropion or entropion with scar excision or graft (67961-67966)*

67914 Repair of ectropion; suture

INCLUDES Canthoplasty (67950)

9.29 | 13.5 | FUD 090 | J A2 50

AMA: 2018,Jan,8; 2017,Jan,8; 2016,Feb,12; 2016,Jan,13; 2015,Jan,16; 2014,Jan,11

67915 thermocauterization

5.62 | 8.52 | FUD 090 | J P3 50

AMA: 2018,Jan,8; 2017,Jan,8; 2016,Feb,12; 2016,Jan,13; 2015,Jan,16; 2014,Jan,11

67916 excision tarsal wedge

12.2 | 17.0 | FUD 090 | J A2 50

AMA: 2018,Jan,8; 2017,Jan,8; 2016,Feb,12; 2016,Jan,13; 2015,Jan,16; 2014,Jan,11

67917 extensive (eg, tarsal strip operations)

EXCLUDES *Repair of everted punctum (68705)*

13.0 | 17.3 | FUD 090 | J A2 50

AMA: 2018,Jan,8; 2017,Jan,8; 2016,Feb,12; 2016,Jan,13; 2015,Jan,16; 2014,Jan,11

67921 Repair of entropion; suture

8.82 | 13.2 | FUD 090 | J A2 50

AMA: 2018,Jan,8; 2017,Jan,8; 2016,Feb,12; 2016,Jan,13; 2015,Jan,16; 2014,Jan,11

67922 thermocauterization

5.60 | 8.37 | FUD 090 | J P3 50

AMA: 2018,Jan,8; 2017,Jan,8; 2016,Feb,12; 2016,Jan,13; 2015,Jan,16; 2014,Jan,11

67923 excision tarsal wedge

12.2 | 17.0 | FUD 090 | J A2 50

AMA: 2018,Jan,8; 2017,Jan,8; 2016,Feb,12; 2016,Jan,13; 2015,Jan,16; 2014,Jan,11

67924 extensive (eg, tarsal strip or capsulopalpebral fascia repairs operation)

INCLUDES Canthoplasty (67950)

13.0 | 18.1 | FUD 090 | J A2 50

AMA: 2018,Jan,8; 2017,Jan,8; 2016,Feb,12; 2016,Jan,13; 2015,Jan,16; 2014,Jan,11

67930-67935 Repair Eyelid Wound

INCLUDES Operating microscope (69990)
Repairs involving more than skin:
Lid margin
Palpebral conjunctiva
Tarsus

EXCLUDES *Blepharoplasty for entropion or ectropion (67916-67917, 67923-67924)*
Correction of lid retraction and blepharoptosis (67901-67911)
Free graft (15120-15121, 15260-15261)
Graft preparation (15004)
Plastic repair of lacrimal canaliculi (68700)
Removal of eyelid lesion (67800 [67810], 67840-67850)
Repair involving skin of eyelid (12011-12018, 12051-12057, 13151-13153)
Repair of blepharochalasis (15820-15823)
Skin adjacent tissue transfer (14060-14061)
Tarsorrhaphy, canthorrhaphy (67880, 67882)

67930 Suture of recent wound, eyelid, involving lid margin, tarsus, and/or palpebral conjunctiva direct closure; partial thickness

6.82 | 10.4 | FUD 010 | J P3 50

AMA: 2016,Feb,12; 2014,Jan,11

67935 full thickness

12.6 | 16.9 | FUD 090 | J A2 50

AMA: 2016,Feb,12; 2014,Jan,11

67938-67999 Eyelid Reconstruction/Repair/Removal Deep Foreign Body

INCLUDES Operating microscope (69990)

EXCLUDES *Blepharoplasty for entropion or ectropion (67916-67917, 67923-67924)*
Correction of lid retraction and blepharoptosis (67901-67911)
Free graft (15120-15121, 15260-15261)
Graft preparation (15004)
Plastic repair of lacrimal canaliculi (68700)
Removal of eyelid lesion (67800-67808, 67840-67850)
Repair involving skin of eyelid (12011-12018, 12051-12057, 13151-13153)
Repair of blepharochalasis (15820-15823)
Skin adjacent tissue transfer (14060-14061)
Tarsorrhaphy, canthorrhaphy (67880, 67882)

67938 Removal of embedded foreign body, eyelid

3.31 | 7.19 | FUD 010 | T P2 50

AMA: 2018,Jan,8; 2017,Jan,8; 2016,Feb,12; 2016,Jan,13; 2015,Jan,16; 2014,May,5; 2014,Jan,11

67950 Canthoplasty (reconstruction of canthus)

13.1 | 16.3 | FUD 090 | J A2 50

AMA: 2016,Feb,12; 2014,Jan,11

67961 Excision and repair of eyelid, involving lid margin, tarsus, conjunctiva, canthus, or full thickness, may include preparation for skin graft or pedicle flap with adjacent tissue transfer or rearrangement; up to one-fourth of lid margin

INCLUDES Canthoplasty (67950)

EXCLUDES *Delay flap (15630)*
Flap attachment (15650)
Free skin grafts (15120-15121, 15260-15261)
Tubed pedicle flap preparation (15576)

12.9 | 16.4 | FUD 090 | J A2 80 50

AMA: 2018,Jan,8; 2017,Jan,8; 2016,Feb,12; 2016,Jan,13; 2015,Jan,16; 2014,Jan,11

67966 over one-fourth of lid margin

INCLUDES Canthoplasty (67950)

EXCLUDES *Delay flap (15630)*
Flap attachment (15650)
Free skin grafts (15120-15121, 15260-15261)
Tubed pedicle flap preparation (15576)

18.7 | 21.9 | FUD 090 | J A2 50

AMA: 2018,Jan,8; 2017,Jan,8; 2016,Feb,12; 2016,Jan,13; 2015,Jan,16; 2014,Jan,11

67971 **Reconstruction of eyelid, full thickness by transfer of tarsoconjunctival flap from opposing eyelid; up to two-thirds of eyelid, 1 stage or first stage**

INCLUDES Dupuy-Dutemp reconstruction
Landboldt's operation

20.5 20.5 FUD 090 J A2 50

AMA: 2016,Feb,12; 2014,Jan,11

67973 **total eyelid, lower, 1 stage or first stage**

INCLUDES Landboldt's operation

26.4 26.4 FUD 090 J A2 80 50

AMA: 2016,Feb,12; 2014,Jan,11

67974 **total eyelid, upper, 1 stage or first stage**

INCLUDES Landboldt's operation

26.4 26.4 FUD 090 J A2 80 50

AMA: 2016,Feb,12; 2014,Jan,11

67975 **second stage**

INCLUDES Landboldt's operation

19.4 19.4 FUD 090 J A2 50

AMA: 2016,Feb,12; 2014,Jan,11

67999 **Unlisted procedure, eyelids**

0.00 0.00 FUD YYY T 80 50

AMA: 2018,Jan,8; 2017,Jul,10; 2017,Jan,8; 2016,Feb,12; 2016,Jan,13; 2015,Jan,16; 2014,Jan,11

68020-68200 Conjunctival Biopsy/Injection/Treatment of Lesions

INCLUDES Operating microscope (69990)

EXCLUDES *Foreign body removal (65205-65265)*

68020 **Incision of conjunctiva, drainage of cyst**

3.15 3.44 FUD 010 T P3 50

AMA: 2016,Feb,12; 2014,Jan,11

68040 **Expression of conjunctival follicles (eg, for trachoma)**

EXCLUDES *Automated evacuation meibomian glands with heat/pressure (0207T)*
Manual evacuation of meibomian glands ([0563T])

1.41 1.78 FUD 000 T P3 50

AMA: 2018,Jan,8; 2017,Jan,8; 2016,Feb,12; 2016,Jan,13; 2015,Jan,16; 2014,May,5; 2014,Jan,11

68100 **Biopsy of conjunctiva**

2.75 4.97 FUD 000 J P3 50

AMA: 2019,Jan,9; 2016,Feb,12; 2014,Jan,11

68110 **Excision of lesion, conjunctiva; up to 1 cm**

4.22 6.56 FUD 010 J P3 50

AMA: 2018,Feb,11; 2018,Jan,8; 2017,Jan,6; 2016,Feb,12; 2014,Jan,11

68115 **over 1 cm**

5.23 9.07 FUD 010 J A2 50

AMA: 2018,Feb,11; 2016,Feb,12; 2014,Jan,11

68130 **with adjacent sclera**

11.7 15.4 FUD 090 J A2 50

AMA: 2016,Feb,12; 2014,Jan,11

68135 **Destruction of lesion, conjunctiva**

4.28 4.49 FUD 010 J P3 50

AMA: 2016,Feb,12; 2014,Jan,11

68200 **Subconjunctival injection**

EXCLUDES *Retrobulbar or Tenon's capsule injection (67500-67515)*

0.99 1.18 FUD 000 Q1 N1 50

AMA: 2018,Jan,8; 2017,Jan,8; 2016,Feb,12; 2016,Jan,13; 2015,Jan,16; 2014,Jan,11

68320-68340 Conjunctivoplasty Procedures

INCLUDES Operating microscope (69990)

EXCLUDES *Conjunctival foreign body removal (65205, 65210)*
Laceration repair (65270-65273)

68320 **Conjunctivoplasty; with conjunctival graft or extensive rearrangement**

15.3 20.8 FUD 090 J A2 50

AMA: 2018,Jan,8; 2017,Jan,8; 2016,Feb,12; 2016,Jan,13; 2015,Jan,16; 2014,Jan,11

68325 **with buccal mucous membrane graft (includes obtaining graft)**

18.6 18.6 FUD 090 J A2 50

AMA: 2016,Feb,12; 2014,Jan,11

68326 **Conjunctivoplasty, reconstruction cul-de-sac; with conjunctival graft or extensive rearrangement**

18.3 18.3 FUD 090 J A2 50

AMA: 2016,Feb,12; 2014,Jan,11

68328 **with buccal mucous membrane graft (includes obtaining graft)**

20.1 20.1 FUD 090 J A2 80 50

AMA: 2016,Feb,12; 2014,Jan,11

68330 **Repair of symblepharon; conjunctivoplasty, without graft**

13.1 17.3 FUD 090 J A2 80 50

AMA: 2016,Feb,12; 2014,Jan,11

68335 **with free graft conjunctiva or buccal mucous membrane (includes obtaining graft)**

18.4 18.4 FUD 090 J A2 50

AMA: 2016,Feb,12; 2014,Jan,11

68340 **division of symblepharon, with or without insertion of conformer or contact lens**

11.3 16.0 FUD 090 J A2 80 50

AMA: 2016,Feb,12; 2014,Jan,11

68360-68399 Conjunctival Flaps and Unlisted Procedures

INCLUDES Operating microscope (69990)

68360 **Conjunctival flap; bridge or partial (separate procedure)**

EXCLUDES *Conjunctival flap for injury (65280, 65285)*
Conjunctival foreign body removal (65205, 65210)
Surgical wound repair (66250)

11.7 15.3 FUD 090 J A2 50

AMA: 2016,Feb,12; 2014,Jan,11

68362 **total (such as Gunderson thin flap or purse string flap)**

EXCLUDES *Conjunctival flap for injury (65280, 65285)*
Conjunctival foreign body removal (65205, 65210)
Surgical wound repair (66250)

18.6 18.6 FUD 090 J A2 50

AMA: 2018,Jan,8; 2017,Jan,8; 2016,Feb,12; 2016,Jan,13; 2015,Jan,16; 2014,Jan,11

68371 **Harvesting conjunctival allograft, living donor**

11.7 11.7 FUD 010 J A2 50

AMA: 2018,Jan,8; 2017,Jan,8; 2016,Feb,12; 2016,Jan,13; 2015,Jan,16; 2014,Jan,11

68399 **Unlisted procedure, conjunctiva**

0.00 0.00 FUD YYY T 80 50

AMA: 2018,Jan,8; 2017,Jan,8; 2016,Feb,12; 2016,Jan,13; 2015,Jan,16; 2014,Jan,11

68400-68899 Nasolacrimal System Procedures

INCLUDES Operating microscope (69990)

68400 Incision, drainage of lacrimal gland
3.76 | 8.24 | FUD 010 | T P3 50
AMA: 2016,Feb,12; 2014,Jan,11

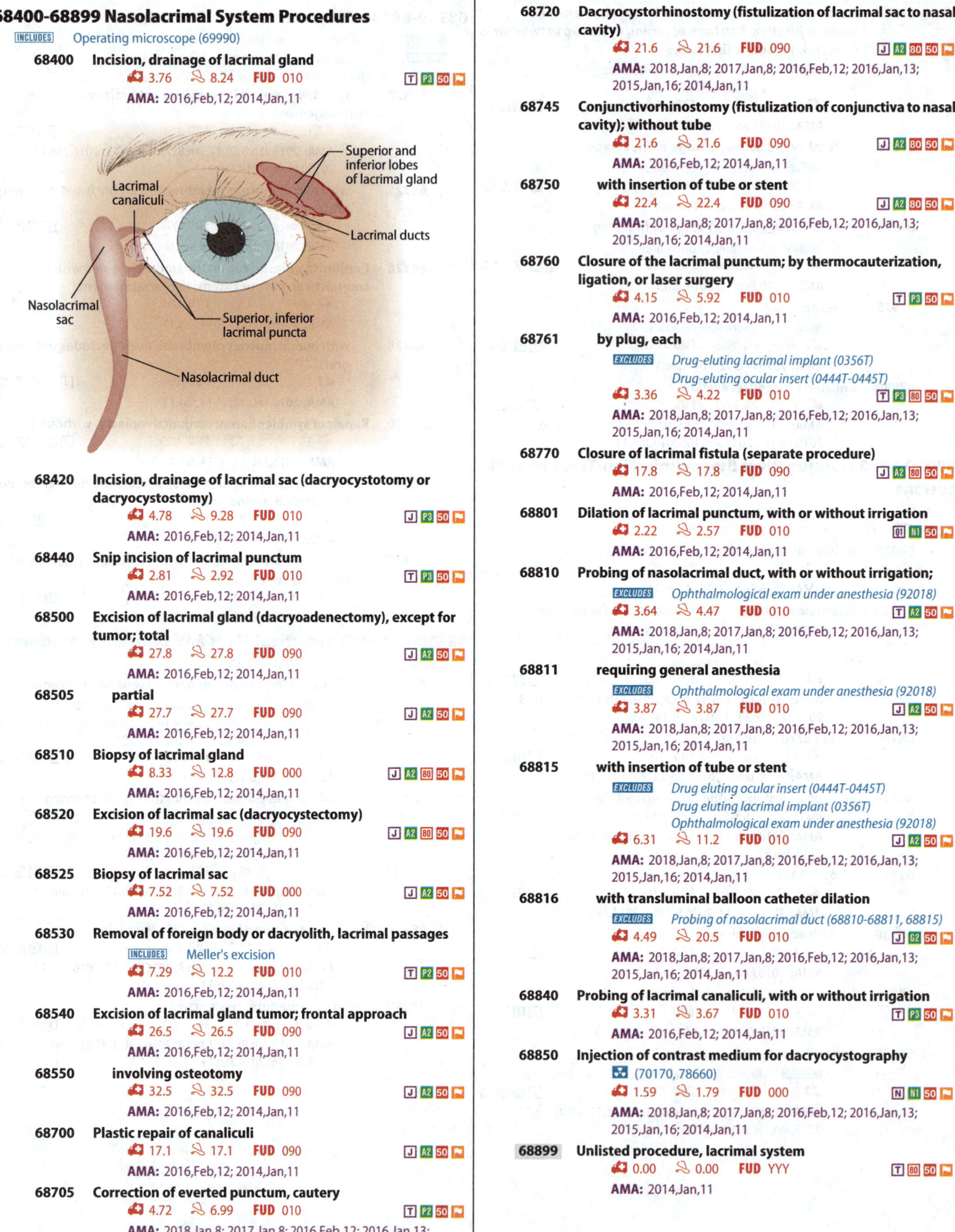

68420 Incision, drainage of lacrimal sac (dacryocystotomy or dacryocystostomy)
4.78 | 9.28 | FUD 010 | J P3 50
AMA: 2016,Feb,12; 2014,Jan,11

68440 Snip incision of lacrimal punctum
2.81 | 2.92 | FUD 010 | T P3 50
AMA: 2016,Feb,12; 2014,Jan,11

68500 Excision of lacrimal gland (dacryoadenectomy), except for tumor; total
27.8 | 27.8 | FUD 090 | J A2 50
AMA: 2016,Feb,12; 2014,Jan,11

68505 partial
27.7 | 27.7 | FUD 090 | J A2 50
AMA: 2016,Feb,12; 2014,Jan,11

68510 Biopsy of lacrimal gland
8.33 | 12.8 | FUD 000 | J A2 80 50
AMA: 2016,Feb,12; 2014,Jan,11

68520 Excision of lacrimal sac (dacryocystectomy)
19.6 | 19.6 | FUD 090 | J A2 80 50
AMA: 2016,Feb,12; 2014,Jan,11

68525 Biopsy of lacrimal sac
7.52 | 7.52 | FUD 000 | J A2 50
AMA: 2016,Feb,12; 2014,Jan,11

68530 Removal of foreign body or dacryolith, lacrimal passages
INCLUDES Meller's excision
7.29 | 12.2 | FUD 010 | T P2 50
AMA: 2016,Feb,12; 2014,Jan,11

68540 Excision of lacrimal gland tumor; frontal approach
26.5 | 26.5 | FUD 090 | J A2 50
AMA: 2016,Feb,12; 2014,Jan,11

68550 involving osteotomy
32.5 | 32.5 | FUD 090 | J A2 50
AMA: 2016,Feb,12; 2014,Jan,11

68700 Plastic repair of canaliculi
17.1 | 17.1 | FUD 090 | J A2 50
AMA: 2016,Feb,12; 2014,Jan,11

68705 Correction of everted punctum, cautery
4.72 | 6.99 | FUD 010 | T P2 50
AMA: 2018,Jan,8; 2017,Jan,8; 2016,Feb,12; 2016,Jan,13; 2015,Jan,16; 2014,Jan,11

68720 Dacryocystorhinostomy (fistulization of lacrimal sac to nasal cavity)
21.6 | 21.6 | FUD 090 | J A2 80 50
AMA: 2018,Jan,8; 2017,Jan,8; 2016,Feb,12; 2016,Jan,13; 2015,Jan,16; 2014,Jan,11

68745 Conjunctivorhinostomy (fistulization of conjunctiva to nasal cavity); without tube
21.6 | 21.6 | FUD 090 | J A2 80 50
AMA: 2016,Feb,12; 2014,Jan,11

68750 with insertion of tube or stent
22.4 | 22.4 | FUD 090 | J A2 80 50
AMA: 2018,Jan,8; 2017,Jan,8; 2016,Feb,12; 2016,Jan,13; 2015,Jan,16; 2014,Jan,11

68760 Closure of the lacrimal punctum; by thermocauterization, ligation, or laser surgery
4.15 | 5.92 | FUD 010 | T P3 50
AMA: 2016,Feb,12; 2014,Jan,11

68761 by plug, each
EXCLUDES *Drug-eluting lacrimal implant (0356T)*
Drug-eluting ocular insert (0444T-0445T)
3.36 | 4.22 | FUD 010 | T P3 80 50
AMA: 2018,Jan,8; 2017,Jan,8; 2016,Feb,12; 2016,Jan,13; 2015,Jan,16; 2014,Jan,11

68770 Closure of lacrimal fistula (separate procedure)
17.8 | 17.8 | FUD 090 | J A2 80 50
AMA: 2016,Feb,12; 2014,Jan,11

68801 Dilation of lacrimal punctum, with or without irrigation
2.22 | 2.57 | FUD 010 | Q1 N1 50
AMA: 2016,Feb,12; 2014,Jan,11

68810 Probing of nasolacrimal duct, with or without irrigation;
EXCLUDES *Ophthalmological exam under anesthesia (92018)*
3.64 | 4.47 | FUD 010 | T A2 50
AMA: 2018,Jan,8; 2017,Jan,8; 2016,Feb,12; 2016,Jan,13; 2015,Jan,16; 2014,Jan,11

68811 requiring general anesthesia
EXCLUDES *Ophthalmological exam under anesthesia (92018)*
3.87 | 3.87 | FUD 010 | J A2 50
AMA: 2018,Jan,8; 2017,Jan,8; 2016,Feb,12; 2016,Jan,13; 2015,Jan,16; 2014,Jan,11

68815 with insertion of tube or stent
EXCLUDES *Drug eluting ocular insert (0444T-0445T)*
Drug eluting lacrimal implant (0356T)
Ophthalmological exam under anesthesia (92018)
6.31 | 11.2 | FUD 010 | J A2 50
AMA: 2018,Jan,8; 2017,Jan,8; 2016,Feb,12; 2016,Jan,13; 2015,Jan,16; 2014,Jan,11

68816 with transluminal balloon catheter dilation
EXCLUDES *Probing of nasolacrimal duct (68810-68811, 68815)*
4.49 | 20.5 | FUD 010 | J G2 50
AMA: 2018,Jan,8; 2017,Jan,8; 2016,Feb,12; 2016,Jan,13; 2015,Jan,16; 2014,Jan,11

68840 Probing of lacrimal canaliculi, with or without irrigation
3.31 | 3.67 | FUD 010 | T P3 50
AMA: 2016,Feb,12; 2014,Jan,11

68850 Injection of contrast medium for dacryocystography
(70170, 78660)
1.59 | 1.79 | FUD 000 | N N1 50
AMA: 2018,Jan,8; 2017,Jan,8; 2016,Feb,12; 2016,Jan,13; 2015,Jan,16; 2014,Jan,11

68899 Unlisted procedure, lacrimal system
0.00 | 0.00 | FUD YYY | T 80 50
AMA: 2014,Jan,11

69000-69020 Treatment External Abscess/Hematoma

69000 **Drainage external ear, abscess or hematoma; simple**
3.42 5.29 FUD 010 T P3 50
AMA: 2018,Jan,8; 2017,Jan,8; 2016,Jan,13; 2015,Jan,16; 2014,Jan,11

An incision is made to drain the contents of an abscess or hematoma

69005 **complicated**
4.50 6.13 FUD 010 J P3 50
AMA: 2014,Jan,11

69020 **Drainage external auditory canal, abscess**
4.03 6.57 FUD 010 T P3 50
AMA: 2018,Jan,8; 2017,Jan,8; 2016,Jan,13; 2015,Jan,16; 2014,Jan,11

69090 Cosmetic Ear Piercing

CMS: 100-02,16,10 Exclusions from Coverage; 100-02,16,120 Cosmetic Procedures

69090 **Ear piercing**
0.00 0.00 FUD XXX E
AMA: 2014,Jan,11

69100-69222 External Ear/Auditory Canal Procedures

EXCLUDES *Reconstruction of ear (see integumentary section codes)*

69100 **Biopsy external ear**
1.40 2.79 FUD 000 T P3
AMA: 2019,Jan,9; 2014,Jan,11

69105 **Biopsy external auditory canal**
1.79 3.99 FUD 000 T P3 50
AMA: 2014,Jan,11

69110 **Excision external ear; partial, simple repair**
9.21 13.0 FUD 090 J A2 50
AMA: 2014,Jan,11

69120 **complete amputation**
11.3 11.3 FUD 090 J A2
AMA: 2014,Jan,11

69140 **Excision exostosis(es), external auditory canal**
25.0 25.0 FUD 090 J A2 80 50
AMA: 2014,Jan,11

69145 **Excision soft tissue lesion, external auditory canal**
7.04 11.1 FUD 090 J A2 50
AMA: 2014,Jan,11

69150 **Radical excision external auditory canal lesion; without neck dissection**
EXCLUDES *Skin graft (15004-15261)*
Temporal bone resection (69535)
29.5 29.5 FUD 090 J A2
AMA: 2014,Jan,11

69155 **with neck dissection**
EXCLUDES *Skin graft (15004-15261)*
Temporal bone resection (69535)
47.0 47.0 FUD 090 C 80
AMA: 2014,Jan,11

69200 **Removal foreign body from external auditory canal; without general anesthesia**
1.35 2.32 FUD 000 Q1 N1 50
AMA: 2014,Jan,11

69205 **with general anesthesia**
2.82 2.82 FUD 010 J A2 50
AMA: 2018,Jan,8; 2017,Jan,8; 2016,Jan,13; 2015,Jan,16; 2014,Jan,11

69209 **Removal impacted cerumen using irrigation/lavage, unilateral**
EXCLUDES *Removal impacted cerumen using instrumentation (69210)*
Removal of nonimpacted cerumen (see appropriate E&M code(s)) (99201-99233 [99224, 99225, 99226], 99241-99255, 99281-99285, 99304-99318, 99324-99337, 99341-99350)
0.40 0.40 FUD 000 Q1 N1 50
AMA: 2018,Jan,8; 2017,Jan,8; 2016,Mar,10; 2016,Feb,13; 2016,Jan,7

69210 **Removal impacted cerumen requiring instrumentation, unilateral**
EXCLUDES *Removal of impacted cerumen using irrigation or lavage (69209)*
Removal of nonimpacted cerumen (see appropriate E&M code(s)) (99201-99233 [99224, 99225, 99226], 99241-99255, 99281-99285, 99304-99318, 99324-99337, 99341-99350)
0.94 1.34 FUD 000 Q1 N1
AMA: 2018,Jan,8; 2017,Jan,8; 2016,Mar,10; 2016,Feb,13; 2016,Jan,13; 2016,Jan,7; 2015,Jan,16; 2014,Nov,14; 2014,Jan,11

69220 **Debridement, mastoidectomy cavity, simple (eg, routine cleaning)**
1.47 2.29 FUD 000 Q1 N1 50
AMA: 2014,Jan,11

69222 **Debridement, mastoidectomy cavity, complex (eg, with anesthesia or more than routine cleaning)**
3.84 6.12 FUD 010 T P3 50
AMA: 2014,Jan,11

69300 Plastic Surgery for Prominent Ears

CMS: 100-02,16,120 Cosmetic Procedures; 100-02,16,180 Services Related to Noncovered Procedures

EXCLUDES *Suture of laceration of external ear (12011-14302)*

69300 **Otoplasty, protruding ear, with or without size reduction**
13.8 18.1 FUD YYY J A2 80 50
AMA: 2014,Jan,11

69310-69399 Reconstruction Auditory Canal: Postaural Approach

EXCLUDES *Suture of laceration of external ear (12011-14302)*

69310 **Reconstruction of external auditory canal (meatoplasty) (eg, for stenosis due to injury, infection) (separate procedure)**
31.0 31.0 FUD 090 J A2 50
AMA: 2018,Jan,8; 2017,Jan,8; 2016,Jan,13; 2015,Jan,16; 2014,Jul,8; 2014,Jan,11; 2014,Jan,9

69320 **Reconstruction external auditory canal for congenital atresia, single stage**
EXCLUDES *Other reconstruction surgery with graft (13151-15760, 21230-21235)*
Tympanoplasty (69631, 69641)
43.5 43.5 FUD 090 J A2 80 50
AMA: 2014,Jan,11

69399 **Unlisted procedure, external ear**
EXCLUDES *Otoscopy under general anesthesia (92502)*
0.00 0.00 FUD YYY T 80
AMA: 2014,Jan,11

69420-69450 Ear Drum Procedures

69420 **Myringotomy including aspiration and/or eustachian tube inflation**

3.41 5.36 **FUD** 010 T P2 50

AMA: 2018,Jan,8; 2017,Jan,8; 2016,Jan,13; 2015,Jan,16; 2014,Jan,11

69421 **Myringotomy including aspiration and/or eustachian tube inflation requiring general anesthesia**

4.22 4.22 **FUD** 010 J A2 50

AMA: 2018,Jan,8; 2017,Jan,8; 2016,Jan,13; 2015,Jan,16; 2014,Jan,11

69424 **Ventilating tube removal requiring general anesthesia**

EXCLUDES *Cochlear device implantation (69930)*
Eardrum repair (69610-69646)
Foreign body removal (69205)
Implantation, replacement of electromagnetic bone conduction hearing device in temporal bone (69710-69745)
Labyrinth procedures (69801-69915)
Mastoid obliteration (69670)
Myringotomy (69420-69421)
Polyp, glomus tumor removal (69535-69554)
Removal impacted cerumen requiring instrumentation (69210)
Repair of window (69666-69667)
Revised mastoidectomy (69601-69605)
Stapes procedures (69650-69662)
Transmastoid excision (69501-69530)
Tympanic neurectomy (69676)
Tympanostomy, tympanolysis (69433-69450)

1.75 3.63 **FUD** 000 Q2 P3 50

AMA: 2018,Jan,8; 2017,Jan,8; 2016,Jan,13; 2015,Jan,16; 2014,Jan,11

69433 **Tympanostomy (requiring insertion of ventilating tube), local or topical anesthesia**

EXCLUDES *Tympanostomy with tube insertion using iontophoresis and automated tube delivery system (0583T)*

3.75 5.67 **FUD** 010 T P3 50

AMA: 2018,Feb,11; 2018,Jan,8; 2017,Jan,8; 2016,Jan,13; 2015,Jan,16; 2014,Jan,11

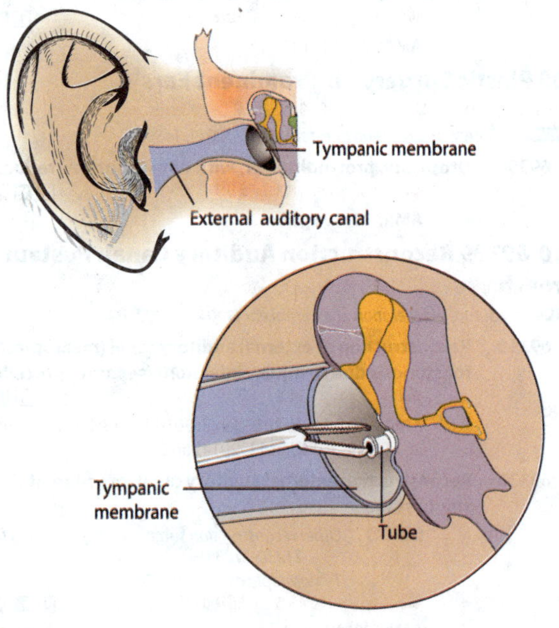

69436 **Tympanostomy (requiring insertion of ventilating tube), general anesthesia**

4.51 4.51 **FUD** 010 T A2 50

AMA: 2018,Feb,11; 2018,Jan,8; 2017,Jan,8; 2016,Jan,13; 2015,Jan,16; 2014,Jan,11

69440 **Middle ear exploration through postauricular or ear canal incision**

EXCLUDES *Atticotomy (69601-69605)*

19.5 19.5 **FUD** 090 J A2 50

AMA: 2014,Jan,11

69450 **Tympanolysis, transcanal**

15.4 15.4 **FUD** 090 J A2 80 50

AMA: 2014,Jan,11

69501-69530 Transmastoid Excision

EXCLUDES *Mastoidectomy cavity debridement (69220, 69222)*
Skin graft (15004-15770)

69501 **Transmastoid antrotomy (simple mastoidectomy)**

20.6 20.6 **FUD** 090 J A2 50

AMA: 2018,Jan,8; 2017,Jan,8; 2016,Jan,13; 2015,Jan,16; 2014,Jan,11

69502 **Mastoidectomy; complete**

27.3 27.3 **FUD** 090 J A2 80 50

AMA: 2018,Jan,8; 2017,Jan,8; 2016,Jan,13; 2015,Jan,16; 2014,Jan,11

69505 **modified radical**

34.2 34.2 **FUD** 090 J A2 80 50

AMA: 2018,Jan,8; 2017,Jan,8; 2016,Jan,13; 2015,Jan,16; 2014,Jan,11

69511 **radical**

35.1 35.1 **FUD** 090 J A2 80 50

AMA: 2018,Jan,8; 2017,Jan,8; 2016,Jan,13; 2015,Jan,16; 2014,Jan,11

69530 **Petrous apicectomy including radical mastoidectomy**

47.1 47.1 **FUD** 090 J A2 80 50

AMA: 2014,Jan,11

69535-69554 Polyp and Glomus Tumor Removal

69535 **Resection temporal bone, external approach**

EXCLUDES *Middle fossa approach (69950-69970)*

76.7 76.7 **FUD** 090 C 50

AMA: 2014,Jan,11

69540 **Excision aural polyp**

3.59 5.87 **FUD** 010 T P3 50

AMA: 2014,Jan,11

69550 **Excision aural glomus tumor; transcanal**

29.6 29.6 **FUD** 090 J A2 80 50

AMA: 2014,Jan,11

69552 **transmastoid**

44.7 44.7 **FUD** 090 J A2 80 50

AMA: 2014,Jan,11

69554 **extended (extratemporal)**

71.8 71.8 **FUD** 090 C 80 50

AMA: 2014,Jan,11

69601-69605 Revised Mastoidectomy

EXCLUDES *Skin graft (15120-15121, 15260-15261)*

69601 **Revision mastoidectomy; resulting in complete mastoidectomy**

29.5 29.5 **FUD** 090 J A2 80 50

AMA: 2018,Jan,8; 2017,Jan,8; 2016,Jan,13; 2015,Jan,16; 2014,Jan,11

69602 **resulting in modified radical mastoidectomy**

30.9 30.9 **FUD** 090 J A2 80 50

AMA: 2018,Jan,8; 2017,Jan,8; 2016,Jan,13; 2015,Jan,16; 2014,Jan,11

69603 resulting in radical mastoidectomy
35.9 35.9 FUD 090 J A2 80 50
AMA: 2018,Jan,8; 2017,Jan,8; 2016,Jan,13; 2015,Jan,16; 2014,Jan,11

69604 resulting in tympanoplasty
EXCLUDES *Secondary tympanoplasty following mastoidectomy (69631-69632)*
31.6 31.6 FUD 090 J A2 50
AMA: 2018,Jan,8; 2017,Jan,8; 2016,Jan,13; 2015,Jan,16; 2014,Jan,11

69605 with apicectomy
44.4 44.4 FUD 090 J A2 80 50
AMA: 2014,Jan,11

69610-69646 Eardrum Repair with/without Other Procedures

69610 **Tympanic membrane repair, with or without site preparation of perforation for closure, with or without patch**
8.27 10.8 FUD 010 J P3 50
AMA: 2018,Jan,8; 2017,Jan,8; 2016,Jan,13; 2015,May,10; 2015,Apr,10; 2015,Jan,16; 2014,Jan,11

69620 **Myringoplasty (surgery confined to drumhead and donor area)**
13.8 19.8 FUD 090 J A2 50
AMA: 2018,Jan,8; 2017,Jan,8; 2016,Jan,13; 2015,May,10; 2015,Apr,10; 2015,Jan,16; 2014,Jan,11

69631 **Tympanoplasty without mastoidectomy (including canalplasty, atticotomy and/or middle ear surgery), initial or revision; without ossicular chain reconstruction**
25.1 25.1 FUD 090 J A2 50
AMA: 2018,Jan,8; 2017,Jan,8; 2016,Jan,13; 2015,Jan,16; 2014,Jan,11

69632 with ossicular chain reconstruction (eg, postfenestration)
30.6 30.6 FUD 090 J A2 50
AMA: 2018,Jan,8; 2017,Jan,8; 2016,Jan,13; 2015,Jan,16; 2014,Jan,11

69633 with ossicular chain reconstruction and synthetic prosthesis (eg, partial ossicular replacement prosthesis [PORP], total ossicular replacement prosthesis [TORP])
29.7 29.7 FUD 090 J A2 50
AMA: 2018,Jan,8; 2017,Jan,8; 2016,Jan,13; 2015,Jan,16; 2014,Jan,11

69635 **Tympanoplasty with antrotomy or mastoidotomy (including canalplasty, atticotomy, middle ear surgery, and/or tympanic membrane repair); without ossicular chain reconstruction**
35.3 35.3 FUD 090 J A2 50
AMA: 2018,Jan,8; 2017,Jan,8; 2016,Jan,13; 2015,Jan,16; 2014,Jan,11

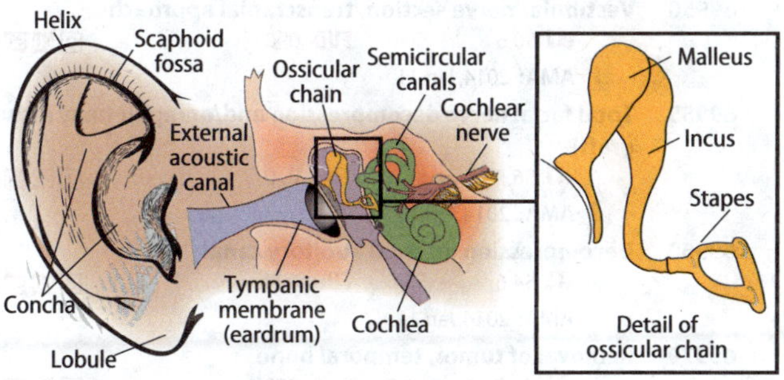

69636 with ossicular chain reconstruction
39.3 39.3 FUD 090 J A2 80 50
AMA: 2018,Jan,8; 2017,Jan,8; 2016,Jan,13; 2015,Jan,16; 2014,Jan,11

69637 with ossicular chain reconstruction and synthetic prosthesis (eg, partial ossicular replacement prosthesis [PORP], total ossicular replacement prosthesis [TORP])
39.9 39.9 FUD 090 J A2 80 50
AMA: 2018,Jan,8; 2017,Jan,8; 2016,Jan,13; 2015,Jan,16; 2014,Jan,11

69641 **Tympanoplasty with mastoidectomy (including canalplasty, middle ear surgery, tympanic membrane repair); without ossicular chain reconstruction**
29.6 29.6 FUD 090 J A2 50
AMA: 2018,Jan,8; 2017,Jan,8; 2016,Jan,13; 2015,Jan,16; 2014,Jan,11

69642 with ossicular chain reconstruction
38.0 38.0 FUD 090 J A2 50
AMA: 2018,Jan,8; 2017,Jan,8; 2016,Jan,13; 2015,Jan,16; 2014,Jan,11

69643 with intact or reconstructed wall, without ossicular chain reconstruction
34.7 34.7 FUD 090 J A2 50
AMA: 2018,Jan,8; 2017,Jan,8; 2016,Jan,13; 2015,Jan,16; 2014,Jan,11

69644 with intact or reconstructed canal wall, with ossicular chain reconstruction
42.1 42.1 FUD 090 J A2 50
AMA: 2018,Jan,8; 2017,Jan,8; 2016,Jan,13; 2015,Jan,16; 2014,Jan,11

69645 radical or complete, without ossicular chain reconstruction
41.4 41.4 FUD 090 J A2 50
AMA: 2018,Jan,8; 2017,Jan,8; 2016,Jan,13; 2015,Jan,16; 2014,Jan,11

69646 radical or complete, with ossicular chain reconstruction
44.1 44.1 FUD 090 J A2 80 50
AMA: 2018,Jan,8; 2017,Jan,8; 2016,Jan,13; 2015,Jan,16; 2014,Jan,11

69650-69662 Stapes Procedures

69650 **Stapes mobilization**
22.8 22.8 FUD 090 J A2 50
AMA: 2014,Jan,11

69660 **Stapedectomy or stapedotomy with reestablishment of ossicular continuity, with or without use of foreign material;**
26.3 26.3 FUD 090 J A2 50
AMA: 2014,Jan,11

69661 with footplate drill out
34.3 34.3 FUD 090 J A2 80 50
AMA: 2014,Jan,11

69662 **Revision of stapedectomy or stapedotomy**
32.9 32.9 FUD 090 J A2 50
AMA: 2014,Jan,11

69666-69700 Other Inner Ear Procedures

69666 **Repair oval window fistula**
22.9 22.9 FUD 090 J A2 80 50
AMA: 2014,Jan,11

69667 **Repair round window fistula**
23.0 23.0 FUD 090 J A2 80 50
AMA: 2014,Jan,11

69670 **Mastoid obliteration (separate procedure)**
26.8 26.8 FUD 090 J A2 80 50
AMA: 2014,Jan,11

69676 **Tympanic neurectomy**
23.6 23.6 FUD 090 J A2 50
AMA: 2014,Jan,11

69700 **Closure postauricular fistula, mastoid (separate procedure)**
19.3 19.3 **FUD** 090 T A2 50
AMA: 2014,Jan,11

69710-69718 Procedures Related to Hearing Aids/Auditory Implants

CMS: 100-02,16,100 Hearing Devices

69710 **Implantation or replacement of electromagnetic bone conduction hearing device in temporal bone**
INCLUDES Removal of existing device when performing replacement procedure
0.00 0.00 **FUD** XXX E
AMA: 2014,Jan,11

69711 **Removal or repair of electromagnetic bone conduction hearing device in temporal bone**
24.2 24.2 **FUD** 090 J A2 80 50
AMA: 2014,Jan,11

69714 **Implantation, osseointegrated implant, temporal bone, with percutaneous attachment to external speech processor/cochlear stimulator; without mastoidectomy**
30.4 30.4 **FUD** 090 J J8 50
AMA: 2018,Jan,8; 2017,Jan,8; 2016,Jan,13; 2015,Jan,16; 2014,Jan,11

69715 **with mastoidectomy**
37.6 37.6 **FUD** 090 J J8 50
AMA: 2014,Jan,11

69717 **Replacement (including removal of existing device), osseointegrated implant, temporal bone, with percutaneous attachment to external speech processor/cochlear stimulator; without mastoidectomy**
31.9 31.9 **FUD** 090 J J8 50
AMA: 2014,Jan,11

69718 **with mastoidectomy**
38.0 38.0 **FUD** 090 J G2 50
AMA: 2014,Jan,11

69720-69799 Procedures of the Facial Nerve

EXCLUDES *Extracranial suture of facial nerve (64864)*

69720 **Decompression facial nerve, intratemporal; lateral to geniculate ganglion**
34.1 34.1 **FUD** 090 J A2 80 50
AMA: 2014,Jan,11

69725 **including medial to geniculate ganglion**
53.5 53.5 **FUD** 090 J 80 50
AMA: 2014,Jan,11

69740 **Suture facial nerve, intratemporal, with or without graft or decompression; lateral to geniculate ganglion**
33.2 33.2 **FUD** 090 J A2 80 50
AMA: 2014,Jan,11

69745 **including medial to geniculate ganglion**
35.3 35.3 **FUD** 090 J A2 80 50
AMA: 2014,Jan,11

69799 **Unlisted procedure, middle ear**
0.00 0.00 **FUD** YYY T 80 50
AMA: 2019,Jan,14; 2018,Jan,8; 2017,Jan,8; 2016,Jan,13; 2015,Jan,16; 2014,Jan,11

69801-69915 Procedures of the Labyrinth

69801 **Labyrinthotomy, with perfusion of vestibuloactive drug(s), transcanal**
EXCLUDES *Myringotomy, tympanostomy on the same ear (69420-69421, 69433, 69436)*
Procedure performed more than one time per day
3.58 5.83 **FUD** 000 T P3 80 50
AMA: 2018,Jan,8; 2017,Jan,8; 2016,Jan,13; 2015,Jan,16; 2014,Jan,11

69805 **Endolymphatic sac operation; without shunt**
29.8 29.8 **FUD** 090 J A2 80 50
AMA: 2014,Jan,11

69806 **with shunt**
26.6 26.6 **FUD** 090 J A2 50
AMA: 2014,Jan,11

69905 **Labyrinthectomy; transcanal**
26.0 26.0 **FUD** 090 J A2 50
AMA: 2014,Jan,11

69910 **with mastoidectomy**
28.7 28.7 **FUD** 090 J A2 80 50
AMA: 2014,Jan,11

69915 **Vestibular nerve section, translabyrinthine approach**
EXCLUDES *Transcranial approach (69950)*
43.6 43.6 **FUD** 090 J A2 80 50
AMA: 2014,Jan,11

69930-69949 Cochlear Implantation

CMS: 100-02,16,100 Hearing Devices

69930 **Cochlear device implantation, with or without mastoidectomy**
34.8 34.8 **FUD** 090 J J8 80 50
AMA: 2014,Jan,11

The internal coil is secured to the temporal bone and an electrode is fed through the round window into the cochlea

69949 **Unlisted procedure, inner ear**
0.00 0.00 **FUD** YYY T 80 50
AMA: 2014,Jan,11

69950-69979 Inner Ear Procedures via Craniotomy

EXCLUDES *External approach (69535)*

69950 **Vestibular nerve section, transcranial approach**
50.6 50.6 **FUD** 090 C 80 50
AMA: 2014,Jan,11

69955 **Total facial nerve decompression and/or repair (may include graft)**
56.2 56.2 **FUD** 090 J 80 50
AMA: 2014,Jan,11

69960 **Decompression internal auditory canal**
54.6 54.6 **FUD** 090 J 80 50
AMA: 2014,Jan,11

69970 **Removal of tumor, temporal bone**
61.0 61.0 **FUD** 090 J 80 50
AMA: 2014,Jan,11

69979 **Unlisted procedure, temporal bone, middle fossa approach**
0.00 0.00 **FUD** YYY T 80 50
AMA: 2018,Jan,8; 2017,Jan,8; 2016,Jan,13; 2015,Jan,16; 2014,Sep,13; 2014,Jan,11

69990 Operating Microscope

EXCLUDES *Magnifying loupes*
Use of code with (15756-15758, 15842, 19364, 19368, 20955-20962, 20969-20973, 22551-22552, 22856-22857 [22858], 22861, 26551-26554, 26556, 31526, 31531, 31536, 31541-31546, 31561, 31571, 43116, 43180, 43496, 46601, 46607, 49906, 61548, 63075-63078, 64727, 64820-64823, 64912-64913, 65091-68850 [66987, 66988, 67810], 0184T, 0308T, 0402T, 0583T)

\+ **69990 Microsurgical techniques, requiring use of operating microscope (List separately in addition to code for primary procedure)**

Code first primary procedure

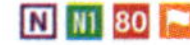

6.40 6.40 **FUD** ZZZ N N1 80

AMA: 2018,Feb,11; 2018,Jan,8; 2017,Dec,12; 2017,Dec,13; 2017,Dec,14; 2017,Jan,8; 2016,Feb,12; 2016,Jan,13; 2015,Jan,16; 2014,Sep,13; 2014,Apr,10; 2014,Jan,11; 2014,Jan,8

70010-70015 Radiography: Neurodiagnostic

70010 Myelography, posterior fossa, radiological supervision and interpretation
1.73 1.73 FUD XXX Q2 N1 80
AMA: 2018,Jan,8; 2017,Jan,8; 2016,Jan,13; 2015,Jan,16; 2014,Jan,11

70015 Cisternography, positive contrast, radiological supervision and interpretation
4.35 4.35 FUD XXX Q2 N1 80
AMA: 2014,Jan,11

70030-70390 Radiography: Head, Neck, Orofacial Structures

INCLUDES Minimum number of views or more views when needed to adequately complete the study
Radiographs that have to be repeated during the encounter due to substandard quality; only one unit of service is reported

EXCLUDES *Obtaining more films after review of initial films, based on the discretion of the radiologist, an order for the test, and a change in the patient's condition*

70030 Radiologic examination, eye, for detection of foreign body
0.83 0.83 FUD XXX Q1 N1 80
AMA: 2014,Jan,11

70100 Radiologic examination, mandible; partial, less than 4 views
0.97 0.97 FUD XXX Q1 N1 80
AMA: 2014,Jan,11

70110 complete, minimum of 4 views
1.13 1.13 FUD XXX Q1 N1 80
AMA: 2014,Jan,11

70120 Radiologic examination, mastoids; less than 3 views per side
0.97 0.97 FUD XXX Q1 N1 80
AMA: 2014,Jan,11

70130 complete, minimum of 3 views per side
1.61 1.61 FUD XXX Q1 N1 80
AMA: 2014,Jan,11

70134 Radiologic examination, internal auditory meati, complete
1.51 1.51 FUD XXX Q1 N1 80
AMA: 2014,Jan,11

70140 Radiologic examination, facial bones; less than 3 views
0.86 0.86 FUD XXX Q1 N1 80
AMA: 2014,Jan,11

70150 complete, minimum of 3 views
1.23 1.23 FUD XXX Q1 N1 80
AMA: 2014,Jan,11

70160 Radiologic examination, nasal bones, complete, minimum of 3 views
0.97 0.97 FUD XXX Q1 N1 80
AMA: 2014,Jan,11

70170 Dacryocystography, nasolacrimal duct, radiological supervision and interpretation
EXCLUDES *Injection of contrast (68850)*
0.00 0.00 FUD XXX Q2 N1 80
AMA: 2014,Jan,11

70190 Radiologic examination; optic foramina
1.03 1.03 FUD XXX Q1 N1 80
AMA: 2014,Jan,11

70200 orbits, complete, minimum of 4 views
1.24 1.24 FUD XXX Q1 N1 80
AMA: 2014,Jan,11

70210 Radiologic examination, sinuses, paranasal, less than 3 views
0.89 0.89 FUD XXX Q1 N1 80
AMA: 2014,Jan,11

70220 Radiologic examination, sinuses, paranasal, complete, minimum of 3 views
1.10 1.10 FUD XXX Q1 N1 80
AMA: 2014,Jan,11

70240 Radiologic examination, sella turcica
0.89 0.89 FUD XXX Q1 N1 80
AMA: 2014,Jan,11

70250 Radiologic examination, skull; less than 4 views
1.07 1.07 FUD XXX Q1 N1 80
AMA: 2014,Jan,11

70260 complete, minimum of 4 views
1.34 1.34 FUD XXX Q1 N1 80
AMA: 2014,Jan,11

70300 Radiologic examination, teeth; single view
0.40 0.40 FUD XXX Q1 N1 80
AMA: 2014,Jan,11

70310 partial examination, less than full mouth
1.06 1.06 FUD XXX Q1 N1 80
AMA: 2014,Jan,11

70320 **complete, full mouth**
1.53 | 1.53 | FUD XXX | Q1 N1 80
AMA: 2014,Jan,11

70328 **Radiologic examination, temporomandibular joint, open and closed mouth; unilateral**
0.89 | 0.89 | FUD XXX | Q1 N1 80
AMA: 2014,Jan,11

70330 **bilateral**
1.39 | 1.39 | FUD XXX | Q1 N1 80
AMA: 2018,Jan,8; 2017,Jan,8; 2016,Jan,13; 2015,Jan,16; 2014,Jan,11

70332 **Temporomandibular joint arthrography, radiological supervision and interpretation**
INCLUDES Fluoroscopic guidance (77002)
2.15 | 2.15 | FUD XXX | Q2 N1 80
AMA: 2018,Jan,8; 2017,Jan,8; 2016,Jan,13; 2015,Jan,16; 2014,Jan,11

70336 **Magnetic resonance (eg, proton) imaging, temporomandibular joint(s)**
8.86 | 8.86 | FUD XXX | Q3 Z2 80
AMA: 2018,Jan,8; 2017,Jan,8; 2016,Jan,13; 2015,Aug,6; 2015,Jan,16; 2014,Jan,11

70350 **Cephalogram, orthodontic**
0.53 | 0.53 | FUD XXX | Q1 N1 80
AMA: 2018,Jan,8; 2017,Jan,8; 2016,Jan,13; 2015,Jan,16; 2014,Jan,11

70355 **Orthopantogram (eg, panoramic x-ray)**
0.56 | 0.56 | FUD XXX | Q1 N1 80
AMA: 2014,Jan,11

70360 **Radiologic examination; neck, soft tissue**
0.85 | 0.85 | FUD XXX | Q1 N1 80
AMA: 2014,Jan,11

70370 **pharynx or larynx, including fluoroscopy and/or magnification technique**
2.27 | 2.27 | FUD XXX | Q1 N1 80
AMA: 2014,Jan,11

70371 **Complex dynamic pharyngeal and speech evaluation by cine or video recording**
EXCLUDES *Laryngeal computed tomography (70490-70492)*
2.77 | 2.77 | FUD XXX | Q1 N1 80
AMA: 2018,Jan,8; 2017,Jan,8; 2016,Jan,13; 2015,Jan,16; 2014,Jul,5; 2014,Jan,11

70380 **Radiologic examination, salivary gland for calculus**
0.95 | 0.95 | FUD XXX | Q1 N1 80
AMA: 2014,Jan,11

70390 **Sialography, radiological supervision and interpretation**
2.90 | 2.90 | FUD XXX | Q2 N1 80
AMA: 2014,Jan,11

70450-70492 Computerized Tomography: Head, Neck, Face

CMS: 100-04,4,250.16 Multiple Procedure Payment Reduction: Certain Diagnostic Imaging Procedures Rendered by Physicians

INCLUDES Imaging using tomographic technique enhanced by computer imaging to create a cross-sectional plane of the body
EXCLUDES *3D rendering (76376-76377)*

70450 **Computed tomography, head or brain; without contrast material**
3.26 | 3.26 | FUD XXX | Q3 Z2 80
AMA: 2018,Jan,8; 2017,Jan,8; 2016,Jan,13; 2015,Jan,16; 2014,Jan,11

70460 **with contrast material(s)**
4.61 | 4.61 | FUD XXX | Q3 Z2 80
AMA: 2018,Jan,8; 2017,Jan,8; 2016,Jan,13; 2015,Jan,16; 2014,Jan,11

70470 **without contrast material, followed by contrast material(s) and further sections**
5.39 | 5.39 | FUD XXX | Q3 Z2 80
AMA: 2018,Jan,8; 2017,Jan,8; 2016,Jan,13; 2015,Jan,16; 2014,Jan,11

70480 **Computed tomography, orbit, sella, or posterior fossa or outer, middle, or inner ear; without contrast material**
6.55 | 6.55 | FUD XXX | Q3 Z2 80
AMA: 2018,Jan,8; 2017,Jan,8; 2016,Jan,13; 2015,Jan,16; 2014,Jan,11

70481 **with contrast material(s)**
7.76 | 7.76 | FUD XXX | Q3 Z2 80
AMA: 2018,Jan,8; 2017,Jan,8; 2016,Jan,13; 2015,Jan,16; 2014,Jan,11

70482 **without contrast material, followed by contrast material(s) and further sections**
8.45 | 8.45 | FUD XXX | Q3 Z2 80
AMA: 2014,Jan,11

70486 **Computed tomography, maxillofacial area; without contrast material**
3.92 | 3.92 | FUD XXX | Q3 Z2 80
AMA: 2018,Jan,8; 2017,Jan,8; 2016,Jan,13; 2015,Jan,16; 2014,Jan,11

70487 **with contrast material(s)**
4.71 | 4.71 | FUD XXX | Q3 Z2 80
AMA: 2014,Jan,11

70488 **without contrast material, followed by contrast material(s) and further sections**
5.74 | 5.74 | FUD XXX | Q3 Z2 80
AMA: 2014,Jan,11

70490 **Computed tomography, soft tissue neck; without contrast material**
EXCLUDES *CT of the cervical spine (72125)*
4.63 | 4.63 | FUD XXX | Q3 Z2 80
AMA: 2014,Jan,11

70491 **with contrast material(s)**
EXCLUDES *CT of the cervical spine (72126)*
5.71 | 5.71 | FUD XXX | Q3 Z2 80
AMA: 2014,Jan,11

70492 **without contrast material followed by contrast material(s) and further sections**
EXCLUDES *CT of the cervical spine (72125-72127)*
6.88 | 6.88 | FUD XXX | Q3 Z2 80
AMA: 2014,Jan,11

70496-70498 Computerized Tomographic Angiography: Head and Neck

CMS: 100-04,4,250.16 Multiple Procedure Payment Reduction: Certain Diagnostic Imaging Procedures Rendered by Physicians

INCLUDES Use of computed tomography to visualize arterial and venous vessels of the body

70496 **Computed tomographic angiography, head, with contrast material(s), including noncontrast images, if performed, and image postprocessing**
8.31 | 8.31 | FUD XXX | Q3 Z2 80
AMA: 2018,Jan,8; 2017,Jan,8; 2016,Jan,13; 2015,Jan,16; 2014,Jan,11

70498 **Computed tomographic angiography, neck, with contrast material(s), including noncontrast images, if performed, and image postprocessing**
8.29 | 8.29 | FUD XXX | Q3 Z2 80
AMA: 2018,Jan,8; 2017,Jan,8; 2016,Jan,13; 2015,Jan,16; 2014,Jan,11

70540-70543 Magnetic Resonance Imaging: Face, Neck, Orbits

CMS: 100-04,4,250.16 Multiple Procedure Payment Reduction: Certain Diagnostic Imaging Procedures Rendered by Physicians

INCLUDES Application of an external magnetic field that forces alignment of hydrogen atom nuclei in soft tissues which converts to sets of tomographic images that can be displayed as three-dimensional images

EXCLUDES *Magnetic resonance angiography head/neck (70544-70549)*
Procedure performed more than one time per session

70540 Magnetic resonance (eg, proton) imaging, orbit, face, and/or neck; without contrast material(s)
7.48 7.48 FUD XXX Q3 Z2 80
AMA: 2018,Jan,8; 2017,Jan,8; 2016,Jan,13; 2015,Jan,16; 2014,Jan,11

70542 with contrast material(s)
8.89 8.89 FUD XXX Q3 Z2 80
AMA: 2018,Jan,8; 2017,Jan,8; 2016,Jan,13; 2015,Jan,16; 2014,Jan,11

70543 without contrast material(s), followed by contrast material(s) and further sequences
11.1 11.1 FUD XXX Q3 Z2 80
AMA: 2018,Jan,8; 2017,Jan,8; 2016,Jan,13; 2015,Jan,16; 2014,Jan,11

70544-70549 Magnetic Resonance Angiography: Head and Neck

CMS: 100-04,13,40.1.1 Magnetic Resonance Angiography; 100-04,13,40.1.2 HCPCS Coding Requirements; 100-04,4,250.16 Multiple Procedure Payment Reduction: Certain Diagnostic Imaging Procedures Rendered by Physicians

INCLUDES Use of magnetic fields and radio waves to produce detailed cross-sectional images of internal body structures

EXCLUDES *Use of code with the following unless a separate diagnostic MRI is performed (70551-70553)*

70544 Magnetic resonance angiography, head; without contrast material(s)
7.84 7.84 FUD XXX Q3 Z2 80
AMA: 2018,Jan,8; 2017,Jan,8; 2016,Jan,13; 2015,Jan,16; 2014,Jan,11

70545 with contrast material(s)
7.78 7.78 FUD XXX Q3 Z2 80
AMA: 2018,Jan,8; 2017,Jan,8; 2016,Jan,13; 2015,Jan,16; 2014,Jan,11

70546 without contrast material(s), followed by contrast material(s) and further sequences
11.5 11.5 FUD XXX Q3 Z2 80
AMA: 2018,Jan,8; 2017,Jan,8; 2016,Jan,13; 2015,Jan,16; 2014,Jan,11

70547 Magnetic resonance angiography, neck; without contrast material(s)
7.87 7.87 FUD XXX Q3 Z2 80
AMA: 2018,Jan,8; 2017,Jan,8; 2016,Jan,13; 2015,Jan,16; 2014,Jan,11

70548 with contrast material(s)
8.66 8.66 FUD XXX Q3 Z2 80
AMA: 2018,Jan,8; 2017,Jan,8; 2016,Jan,13; 2015,Jan,16; 2014,Jan,11

70549 without contrast material(s), followed by contrast material(s) and further sequences
12.0 12.0 FUD XXX Q3 Z2 80
AMA: 2018,Jan,8; 2017,Jan,8; 2016,Jan,13; 2015,Jan,16; 2014,Jan,11

70551-70553 Magnetic Resonance Imaging: Brain and Brain Stem

CMS: 100-04,4,200.3.2 Multi-Source Photon Stereotactic RadiosurgeryPlanning and Delivery; 100-04,4,250.16 Multiple Procedure Payment Reduction: Certain Diagnostic Imaging Procedures Rendered by Physicians

INCLUDES Application of an external magnetic field that forces alignment of hydrogen atom nuclei in soft tissues which converts to sets of tomographic images that can be displayed as three-dimensional images

EXCLUDES *Magnetic spectroscopy (76390)*

70551 Magnetic resonance (eg, proton) imaging, brain (including brain stem); without contrast material
6.38 6.38 FUD XXX Q3 Z2 80
AMA: 2018,Jan,8; 2017,Jan,8; 2016,Jan,13; 2015,Jan,16; 2014,Jan,11

70552 with contrast material(s)
8.86 8.86 FUD XXX Q3 Z2 80
AMA: 2018,Jan,8; 2017,Jan,8; 2016,Jan,13; 2015,Jan,16; 2014,Jan,11

70553 without contrast material, followed by contrast material(s) and further sequences
10.4 10.4 FUD XXX Q3 Z2 80
AMA: 2018,Jan,8; 2017,Jan,8; 2016,Jan,13; 2015,Jan,16; 2014,Jan,11

70554-70555 Magnetic Resonance Imaging: Brain Mapping

INCLUDES Neuroimaging technique using MRI to identify and map signals related to brain activity

EXCLUDES *Use of code with the following unless a separate diagnostic MRI is performed (70551-70553)*

70554 Magnetic resonance imaging, brain, functional MRI; including test selection and administration of repetitive body part movement and/or visual stimulation, not requiring physician or psychologist administration

EXCLUDES *Functional brain mapping (96020)*
Testing performed by a physician or psychologist (70555)

12.4 12.4 FUD XXX Q3 Z2 80
AMA: 2018,Jan,8; 2017,Jan,8; 2016,Jan,13; 2015,Jan,16; 2014,Jan,11

70555 requiring physician or psychologist administration of entire neurofunctional testing

EXCLUDES *Testing performed by a technologist, nonphysician, or nonpsychologist (70554)*

Code also (96020)
0.00 0.00 FUD XXX S Z2 80
AMA: 2018,Jan,8; 2017,Jan,8; 2016,Jan,13; 2015,Jan,16; 2014,Jan,11

70557-70559 Magnetic Resonance Imaging: Intraoperative

EXCLUDES *Intracranial lesion stereotaxic biopsy with magnetic resonance guidance (61751, 77021-77022)*
Procedures performed more than one time per surgical encounter
Use of codes unless a separate report is generated

Code also stereotactic biopsy, aspiration, or excision, when performed with magnetic resonance imaging (61751)

70557 Magnetic resonance (eg, proton) imaging, brain (including brain stem and skull base), during open intracranial procedure (eg, to assess for residual tumor or residual vascular malformation); without contrast material
0.00 0.00 FUD XXX S Z2 80
AMA: 2014,Jan,11

70558 with contrast material(s)
0.00 0.00 FUD XXX S Z2 80
AMA: 2014,Jan,11

70559 without contrast material(s), followed by contrast material(s) and further sequences
0.00 0.00 FUD XXX S Z2 80
AMA: 2014,Jan,11

71045-71130 Radiography: Thorax

71045 Radiologic examination, chest; single view

EXCLUDES *Acute abdomen series, complete (2 or more views) including a view of the chest (74022)*
Remotely performed CAD (0175T)

Code also concurrent computer-aided detection (CAD) (0174T)

0.70 0.70 FUD XXX Q3 Z3 80

AMA: 2019,Aug,8; 2019,May,10; 2019,Mar,10; 2018,Apr,7

71046 2 views

EXCLUDES *Acute abdomen series, complete (2 or more views) including a view of the chest (74022)*
Remotely performed CAD (0175T)

Code also concurrent computer-aided detection (CAD) (0174T)

0.89 0.89 FUD XXX Q3 Z3 80

AMA: 2019,Aug,8; 2019,Mar,10; 2018,Apr,7

71047 3 views

EXCLUDES *Complete acute abdomen series (2 or more views) that includes a view of the chest (74022)*
Remotely performed CAD (0175T)

Code also concurrent computer-aided detection (CAD) (0174T)

1.12 1.12 FUD XXX Q1 N1 80

AMA: 2019,Mar,10; 2018,Apr,7

71048 4 or more views

EXCLUDES *Acute abdomen series, complete (2 or more views) including a view of the chest (74022)*
Remotely performed CAD (0175T)

Code also concurrent computer-aided detection (CAD) (0174T)

1.21 1.21 FUD XXX Q1 N1 80

AMA: 2019,Mar,10; 2018,Apr,7

71100 Radiologic examination, ribs, unilateral; 2 views

0.97 0.97 FUD XXX Q1 N1 80

AMA: 2014,Jan,11

71101 including posteroanterior chest, minimum of 3 views

1.11 1.11 FUD XXX Q1 N1 80

AMA: 2014,Jan,11

71110 Radiologic examination, ribs, bilateral; 3 views

1.16 1.16 FUD XXX Q1 N1 80

AMA: 2014,Jan,11

71111 including posteroanterior chest, minimum of 4 views

1.38 1.38 FUD XXX Q1 N1 80

AMA: 2014,Jan,11

71120 Radiologic examination; sternum, minimum of 2 views

0.88 0.88 FUD XXX Q1 N1 80

AMA: 2014,Jan,11

71130 sternoclavicular joint or joints, minimum of 3 views

1.05 1.05 FUD XXX Q1 N1 80

AMA: 2014,Jan,11

71250-71270 Computerized Tomography: Thorax

CMS: 100-04,4,250.16 Multiple Procedure Payment Reduction: Certain Diagnostic Imaging Procedures Rendered by Physicians

INCLUDES Imaging using tomographic technique enhanced by computer imaging to create a cross-sectional plane of the body

EXCLUDES *3D rendering (76376-76377)*
CT of the heart (75571-75574)

71250 Computed tomography, thorax; without contrast material

4.47 4.47 FUD XXX Q3 Z2 80

AMA: 2018,Jan,8; 2017,Jan,8; 2016,Jan,13; 2015,Jan,16; 2014,Jan,11

71260 with contrast material(s)

5.53 5.53 FUD XXX Q3 Z2 80

AMA: 2018,Jan,8; 2017,Jan,8; 2016,Jan,13; 2015,Jan,16; 2014,Jan,11

71270 without contrast material, followed by contrast material(s) and further sections

6.56 6.56 FUD XXX Q3 Z2 80

AMA: 2018,Jan,8; 2017,Jan,8; 2016,Jan,13; 2015,Jan,16; 2014,Jan,11

71275 Computerized Tomographic Angiography: Thorax

CMS: 100-04,4,250.16 Multiple Procedure Payment Reduction: Certain Diagnostic Imaging Procedures Rendered by Physicians

INCLUDES Multiple rapid thin section CT scans to create cross-sectional images of bones, organs and tissues

EXCLUDES *CT angiography of coronary arteries that includes calcification score and/or cardiac morphology (75574)*

71275 Computed tomographic angiography, chest (noncoronary), with contrast material(s), including noncontrast images, if performed, and image postprocessing

8.50 8.50 FUD XXX Q3 Z2 80

AMA: 2018,Jan,8; 2017,Jan,8; 2016,Jan,13; 2015,Jan,16; 2014,Jan,11

71550-71552 Magnetic Resonance Imaging: Thorax

CMS: 100-04,4,250.16 Multiple Procedure Payment Reduction: Certain Diagnostic Imaging Procedures Rendered by Physicians

INCLUDES Application of an external magnetic field that forces alignment of hydrogen atom nuclei in soft tissues which converts to sets of tomographic images that can be displayed as three-dimensional images

EXCLUDES *MRI of the breast (77046-77049)*

71550 Magnetic resonance (eg, proton) imaging, chest (eg, for evaluation of hilar and mediastinal lymphadenopathy); without contrast material(s)

11.4 11.4 FUD XXX Q3 Z2 80

AMA: 2018,Jan,8; 2017,Jan,8; 2016,Jan,13; 2015,Jan,16; 2014,Jan,11

71551 with contrast material(s)

12.6 12.6 FUD XXX Q3 Z2 80

AMA: 2018,Jan,8; 2017,Jan,8; 2016,Jan,13; 2015,Jan,16; 2014,Jan,11

71552 without contrast material(s), followed by contrast material(s) and further sequences

15.9 15.9 FUD XXX Q3 Z2 80

AMA: 2018,Jan,8; 2017,Jan,8; 2016,Jan,13; 2015,Jan,16; 2014,Jan,11

71555 Magnetic Resonance Angiography: Thorax

CMS: 100-04,13,40.1.1 Magnetic Resonance Angiography; 100-04,13,40.1.2 HCPCS Coding Requirements; 100-04,4,250.16 Multiple Procedure Payment Reduction: Certain Diagnostic Imaging Procedures Rendered by Physicians

71555 Magnetic resonance angiography, chest (excluding myocardium), with or without contrast material(s)

11.0 11.0 FUD XXX B 80

AMA: 2018,Jan,8; 2017,Jan,8; 2016,Jan,13; 2015,Jan,16; 2014,Jan,11

72020-72120 Radiography: Spine

INCLUDES Minimum number of views or more views when needed to adequately complete the study
Radiographs that have to be repeated during the encounter due to substandard quality; only one unit of service is reported

EXCLUDES *Obtaining more films after review of initial films, based on the discretion of the radiologist, an order for the test, and a change in the patient's condition*

72020 **Radiologic examination, spine, single view, specify level**
EXCLUDES *Single view of entire thoracic and lumbar spine (72081)*
0.65 0.65 FUD XXX Q1 N1 80
AMA: 2018,Jan,8; 2017,Jan,8; 2016,Sep,4; 2016,Jan,13; 2015,Oct,9; 2015,Jan,16; 2014,Jan,11

72040 **Radiologic examination, spine, cervical; 2 or 3 views**
1.03 1.03 FUD XXX Q1 N1 80
AMA: 2018,Aug,10; 2018,Jan,8; 2017,Jan,8; 2016,Jan,13; 2015,Jan,16; 2014,Jan,11

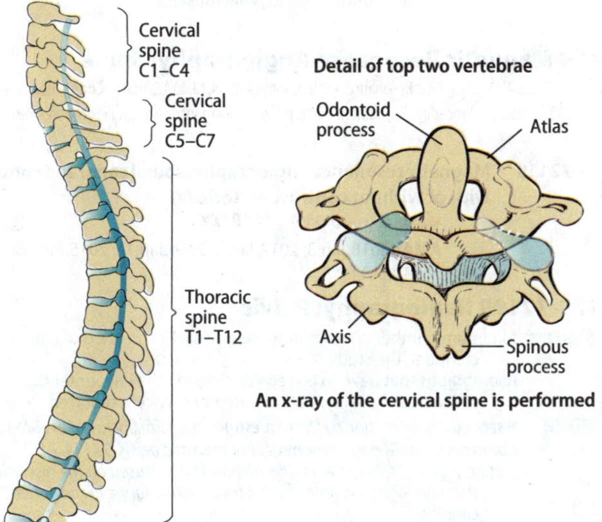

An x-ray of the cervical spine is performed

72050 **4 or 5 views**
1.42 1.42 FUD XXX Q1 N1 80
AMA: 2014,Jan,11

72052 **6 or more views**
1.69 1.69 FUD XXX Q1 N1 80
AMA: 2014,Jan,11

72070 **Radiologic examination, spine; thoracic, 2 views**
0.96 0.96 FUD XXX Q1 N1 80
AMA: 2018,Jan,8; 2017,Jan,8; 2016,Jan,13; 2015,Jan,16; 2014,Jan,11

72072 **thoracic, 3 views**
1.02 1.02 FUD XXX Q1 N1 80
AMA: 2018,Jan,8; 2017,Jan,8; 2016,Jan,13; 2015,Jan,16; 2014,Jan,11

72074 **thoracic, minimum of 4 views**
1.12 1.12 FUD XXX Q1 N1 80
AMA: 2018,Jan,8; 2017,Jan,8; 2016,Jan,13; 2015,Jan,16; 2014,Jan,11

72080 **thoracolumbar junction, minimum of 2 views**
EXCLUDES *Single view of thoracolumbar junction (72020)*
0.95 0.95 FUD XXX Q1 N1 80
AMA: 2018,Jan,8; 2017,Jan,8; 2016,Sep,4; 2016,Jan,13; 2015,Oct,9; 2015,Jan,16; 2014,Jan,11

72081 **Radiologic examination, spine, entire thoracic and lumbar, including skull, cervical and sacral spine if performed (eg, scoliosis evaluation); one view**
1.14 1.14 FUD XXX Q1 N1 80
AMA: 2018,Jan,8; 2017,Jan,8; 2016,Sep,4

72082 **2 or 3 views**
1.83 1.83 FUD XXX Q1 N1 80
AMA: 2018,Jan,8; 2017,Jan,8; 2016,Sep,4

72083 **4 or 5 views**
2.16 2.16 FUD XXX S Z2 80
AMA: 2018,Jan,8; 2017,Jan,8; 2016,Sep,4

72084 **minimum of 6 views**
2.52 2.52 FUD XXX S Z2 80
AMA: 2018,Jan,8; 2017,Jan,8; 2016,Sep,4

72100 **Radiologic examination, spine, lumbosacral; 2 or 3 views**
1.03 1.03 FUD XXX Q1 N1 80
AMA: 2018,Jan,8; 2017,Jan,8; 2016,Jan,13; 2015,Jan,16; 2014,Jan,11

72110 **minimum of 4 views**
1.44 1.44 FUD XXX Q1 N1 80
AMA: 2018,Jan,8; 2017,Jan,8; 2016,Jan,13; 2015,Jan,16; 2014,Jan,11

72114 **complete, including bending views, minimum of 6 views**
1.64 1.64 FUD XXX Q1 N1 80
AMA: 2014,Jan,11

72120 **bending views only, 2 or 3 views**
1.21 1.21 FUD XXX Q1 N1 80
AMA: 2018,Jan,8; 2017,Jan,8; 2016,Aug,7; 2014,Jan,11

72125-72133 Computerized Tomography: Spine

CMS: 100-04,12,20.4.7 Services Not Meeting National Electrical Manufacturers Association (NEMA) Standard; 100-04,4,20.6.12 Use of HCPCS Modifier – CT; 100-04,4,250.16 Multiple Procedure Payment Reduction: Certain Diagnostic Imaging Procedures Rendered by Physicians

INCLUDES Imaging using tomographic technique enhanced by computer imaging to create a cross-sectional plane of the body

EXCLUDES *3D rendering (76376-76377)*

Code also intrathecal injection procedure when performed (61055, 62284)

72125 **Computed tomography, cervical spine; without contrast material**
5.18 5.18 FUD XXX Q3 Z2 80
AMA: 2014,Jan,11

72126 **with contrast material**
6.40 6.40 FUD XXX Q3 Z3 80
AMA: 2018,Jan,8; 2017,Jan,8; 2016,Jan,13; 2015,Jan,16; 2014,Jan,11

72127 **without contrast material, followed by contrast material(s) and further sections**
7.58 7.58 FUD XXX Q3 Z2 80
AMA: 2014,Jan,11

72128 **Computed tomography, thoracic spine; without contrast material**
5.08 5.08 FUD XXX Q3 Z2 80
AMA: 2014,Jan,11

72129 **with contrast material**
6.44 6.44 FUD XXX Q3 Z2 80
AMA: 2019,Jan,14; 2018,Jan,8; 2017,Jan,8; 2016,Jan,13; 2015,Jan,16; 2014,Jan,11

72130 **without contrast material, followed by contrast material(s) and further sections**
7.59 7.59 FUD XXX Q3 Z2 80
AMA: 2014,Jan,11

72131 **Computed tomography, lumbar spine; without contrast material**
5.06 5.06 FUD XXX Q3 Z2 80
AMA: 2014,Jan,11

72132 **with contrast material**
6.41 6.41 FUD XXX Q3 Z3 80
AMA: 2019,Jan,14; 2018,Jan,8; 2017,Jan,8; 2016,Jan,13; 2015,Jan,16; 2014,Jan,11

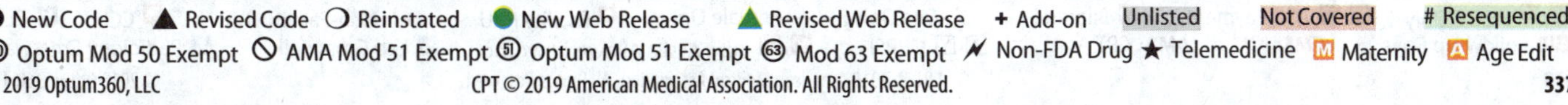

72133 **without contrast material, followed by contrast material(s) and further sections**
7.56 7.56 FUD XXX
AMA: 2014,Jan,11

72141-72158 Magnetic Resonance Imaging: Spine

CMS: 100-04,4,250.16 Multiple Procedure Payment Reduction: Certain Diagnostic Imaging Procedures Rendered by Physicians

INCLUDES Application of an external magnetic field that forces alignment of hydrogen atom nuclei in soft tissues which converts to sets of tomographic images that can be displayed as three-dimensional images

Code also intrathecal injection procedure when performed (61055, 62284)

72141 **Magnetic resonance (eg, proton) imaging, spinal canal and contents, cervical; without contrast material**
6.22 6.22 FUD XXX
AMA: 2018,Jan,8; 2017,Jan,8; 2016,Jan,13; 2015,Jan,16; 2014,Jun,14; 2014,Jan,11

72142 **with contrast material(s)**
EXCLUDES *MRI of cervical spinal canal performed without contrast followed by repeating the study with contrast (72156)*
9.03 9.03 FUD XXX
AMA: 2018,Jan,8; 2017,Jan,8; 2016,Jan,13; 2015,Jan,16; 2014,Jan,11

72146 **Magnetic resonance (eg, proton) imaging, spinal canal and contents, thoracic; without contrast material**
6.23 6.23 FUD XXX
AMA: 2018,Jan,8; 2017,Jan,8; 2016,Jan,13; 2015,Jan,16; 2014,Jun,14; 2014,Jan,11

72147 **with contrast material(s)**
EXCLUDES *MRI of thoracic spinal canal performed without contrast followed by repeating the study with contrast (72157)*
8.98 8.98 FUD XXX
AMA: 2018,Jan,8; 2017,Jan,8; 2016,Jan,13; 2015,Jan,16; 2014,Jan,11

72148 **Magnetic resonance (eg, proton) imaging, spinal canal and contents, lumbar; without contrast material**
6.23 6.23 FUD XXX
AMA: 2018,Jan,8; 2017,Jan,8; 2016,Jan,13; 2015,Jan,16; 2014,Jun,14; 2014,Jan,11

72149 **with contrast material(s)**
EXCLUDES *MRI of lumbar spinal canal performed without contrast followed by repeating the study with contrast (72158)*
8.92 8.92 FUD XXX
AMA: 2014,Jan,11

72156 **Magnetic resonance (eg, proton) imaging, spinal canal and contents, without contrast material, followed by contrast material(s) and further sequences; cervical**
10.5 10.5 FUD XXX
AMA: 2014,Jan,11

72157 **thoracic**
10.5 10.5 FUD XXX
AMA: 2014,Jan,11

72158 **lumbar**
10.5 10.5 FUD XXX
AMA: 2014,Jan,11

Superior view of thoracic spine and surrounding paraspinal muscles

72159 Magnetic Resonance Angiography: Spine

CMS: 100-04,13,40.1.1 Magnetic Resonance Angiography; 100-04,13,40.1.2 HCPCS Coding Requirements; 100-04,4,250.16 Multiple Procedure Payment Reduction: Certain Diagnostic Imaging Procedures Rendered by Physicians

72159 **Magnetic resonance angiography, spinal canal and contents, with or without contrast material(s)**
11.4 11.4 FUD XXX
AMA: 2018,Jan,8; 2017,Jan,8; 2016,Jan,13; 2015,Jan,16; 2014,Jan,11

72170-72190 Radiography: Pelvis

INCLUDES Minimum number of views or more views when needed to adequately complete the study
Radiographs that have to be repeated during the encounter due to substandard quality; only one unit of service is reported

EXCLUDES *A second interpretation by the requesting physician (included in E&M service)*
Combined CT or CT angiography of abdomen and pelvis (74174, 74176-74178)
Obtaining more films after review of initial films, based on the discretion of the radiologist, an order for the test, and a change in the patient's condition
Pelvimetry (74710)

72170 **Radiologic examination, pelvis; 1 or 2 views**
0.93 0.93 FUD XXX
AMA: 2018,Jan,8; 2017,Jan,8; 2016,Aug,7; 2016,Jun,5; 2016,Jan,13; 2015,Jan,16; 2014,Jan,11

72190 **complete, minimum of 3 views**
1.12 1.12 FUD XXX
AMA: 2016,Jun,5; 2014,Jan,11

72191 Computerized Tomographic Angiography: Pelvis

CMS: 100-04,4,250.16 Multiple Procedure Payment Reduction: Certain Diagnostic Imaging Procedures Rendered by Physicians

EXCLUDES *Computed tomographic angiography (73706, 74174-74175, 75635)*

72191 **Computed tomographic angiography, pelvis, with contrast material(s), including noncontrast images, if performed, and image postprocessing**
8.85 8.85 FUD XXX
AMA: 2018,Jan,8; 2017,Jan,8; 2016,Jan,13; 2015,Jan,16; 2014,Jan,11

72192-72194 Computerized Tomography: Pelvis

CMS: 100-04,4,250.16 Multiple Procedure Payment Reduction: Certain Diagnostic Imaging Procedures Rendered by Physicians

EXCLUDES *3D rendering (76376-76377)*
Combined CT of abdomen and pelvis (74176-74178)
CT colonography, diagnostic (74261-74262)
CT colonography, screening (74263)

72192 **Computed tomography, pelvis; without contrast material**
4.10 4.10 FUD XXX
AMA: 2018,Jan,8; 2017,Jan,8; 2016,Jan,13; 2015,Jan,16; 2014,Jan,11

72193 with contrast material(s)
6.59 6.59 FUD XXX 03 Z2 80
AMA: 2018,Jan,8; 2017,Jan,8; 2016,Jan,13; 2015,Jan,16; 2014,Jan,11

72194 without contrast material, followed by contrast material(s) and further sections
7.48 7.48 FUD XXX 03 Z2 80
AMA: 2018,Jan,8; 2017,Jan,8; 2016,Jan,13; 2015,Jan,16; 2014,Jan,11

72195-72197 Magnetic Resonance Imaging: Pelvis

CMS: 100-04,4,250.16 Multiple Procedure Payment Reduction: Certain Diagnostic Imaging Procedures Rendered by Physicians

INCLUDES Application of an external magnetic field that forces alignment of hydrogen atom nuclei in soft tissues which converts to sets of tomographic images that can be displayed as three-dimensional images

EXCLUDES *Magnetic resonance imaging of fetus(es) (74712-74713)*

72195 Magnetic resonance (eg, proton) imaging, pelvis; without contrast material(s)
7.62 7.62 FUD XXX 03 Z2 80
AMA: 2018,Jul,11; 2018,Jan,8; 2017,Jan,8; 2016,Jun,5; 2016,Jan,13; 2015,Jan,16; 2014,Jun,14; 2014,Jan,11

72196 with contrast material(s)
8.90 8.90 FUD XXX 03 Z2 80
AMA: 2018,Jul,11; 2018,Jan,8; 2017,Jan,8; 2016,Jun,5; 2016,Jan,13; 2015,Jan,16; 2014,Jan,11

72197 without contrast material(s), followed by contrast material(s) and further sequences
11.2 11.2 FUD XXX 03 Z2 80
AMA: 2018,Jul,11; 2018,Jan,8; 2017,Jan,8; 2016,Jun,5; 2016,Jan,13; 2015,Jan,16; 2014,Jan,11

72198 Magnetic Resonance Angiography: Pelvis

CMS: 100-04,13,40.1.1 Magnetic Resonance Angiography; 100-04,13,40.1.2 HCPCS Coding Requirements; 100-04,4,250.16 Multiple Procedure Payment Reduction: Certain Diagnostic Imaging Procedures Rendered by Physicians

INCLUDES Use of magnetic fields and radio waves to produce detailed cross-sectional images of the arteries and veins

72198 Magnetic resonance angiography, pelvis, with or without contrast material(s)
11.0 11.0 FUD XXX B 80
AMA: 2018,Jan,8; 2017,Jan,8; 2016,Jan,13; 2015,Jan,16; 2014,Jan,11

72200-72220 Radiography: Pelvisacral

INCLUDES Minimum number of views or more views when needed to adequately complete the study
Radiographs that have to be repeated during the encounter due to substandard quality; only one unit of service is reported

EXCLUDES *Obtaining more films after review of initial films, based on the discretion of the radiologist, an order for the test, and a change in the patient's condition*
Second interpretation by the requesting physician (included in E&M service)

72200 Radiologic examination, sacroiliac joints; less than 3 views
0.87 0.87 FUD XXX 01 N1 80
AMA: 2014,Jan,11

72202 3 or more views
0.98 0.98 FUD XXX 01 N1 80
AMA: 2014,Jan,11

72220 Radiologic examination, sacrum and coccyx, minimum of 2 views
0.86 0.86 FUD XXX 01 N1 80
AMA: 2014,Jan,11

72240-72270 Myelography with Contrast: Spinal Cord

CMS: 100-04,13,30.1.3.1 Payment for Low Osmolar Contrast Material

EXCLUDES *Injection procedure for myelography (62284)*
Myelography (62302-62305)

Code also injection at C1-C2 for complete myelography (61055)

72240 Myelography, cervical, radiological supervision and interpretation
2.94 2.94 FUD XXX 02 N1 80
AMA: 2018,Jan,8; 2017,Jan,8; 2016,Jan,13; 2015,Jan,16; 2014,Sep,3; 2014,Jan,11

72255 Myelography, thoracic, radiological supervision and interpretation
2.99 2.99 FUD XXX 02 N1 80
AMA: 2018,Jan,8; 2017,Jan,8; 2016,Jan,13; 2015,Jan,16; 2014,Sep,3; 2014,Jan,11

72265 Myelography, lumbosacral, radiological supervision and interpretation
2.75 2.75 FUD XXX 02 N1 80
AMA: 2018,Jan,8; 2017,Jan,8; 2016,Jan,13; 2015,Jan,16; 2014,Sep,3; 2014,Jan,11

72270 Myelography, 2 or more regions (eg, lumbar/thoracic, cervical/thoracic, lumbar/cervical, lumbar/thoracic/cervical), radiological supervision and interpretation
3.82 3.82 FUD XXX 02 N1 80
AMA: 2018,Jan,8; 2017,Jan,8; 2016,Jan,13; 2015,Jan,16; 2014,Sep,3; 2014,Jan,11

72275 Radiography: Epidural Space

INCLUDES Epidurogram, documentation of images, formal written report
Fluoroscopic guidance (77003)

EXCLUDES *Arthrodesis (22586)*
Second interpretation by the requesting physician (included in E&M service)

Code also injection procedure as appropriate (62280-62282, 62320-62327, 64479-64480, 64483-64484)

72275 Epidurography, radiological supervision and interpretation
3.48 3.48 FUD XXX N N1 80
AMA: 2018,Jan,8; 2017,Jan,8; 2016,Jan,13; 2015,Jan,16; 2014,Jan,11

72285 Radiography: Intervertebral Disc (Cervical/Thoracic)

CMS: 100-04,13,30.1.3.1 Payment for Low Osmolar Contrast Material

Code also discography injection procedure (62291)

72285 Discography, cervical or thoracic, radiological supervision and interpretation
3.32 3.32 FUD XXX 02 N1 80
AMA: 2018,Jan,8; 2017,Jan,8; 2016,Jan,13; 2015,Jan,16; 2014,Jan,11

72295 Radiography: Intervertebral Disc (Lumbar)

CMS: 100-04,13,30.1.3.1 Payment for Low Osmolar Contrast Material

Code also discography injection procedure (62290)

72295 Discography, lumbar, radiological supervision and interpretation
2.90 2.90 FUD XXX 02 N1 80
AMA: 2018,Jan,8; 2017,Feb,12; 2017,Jan,8; 2016,Jan,13; 2015,Jan,16; 2014,Jan,11

73000-73085 Radiography: Shoulder and Upper Arm

INCLUDES Minimum number of views or more views when needed to adequately complete the study
Radiographs that have to be repeated during the encounter due to substandard quality; only one unit of service is reported

EXCLUDES *Obtaining more films after review of initial films, based on the discretion of the radiologist, an order for the test, and a change in the patient's condition*
Second interpretation by the requesting physician (included in E&M service)
Stress views of upper body joint(s), when performed (77071)

73000 Radiologic examination; clavicle, complete
0.82 0.82 FUD XXX Q1 N1 80
AMA: 2014,Jan,11

Radiograph

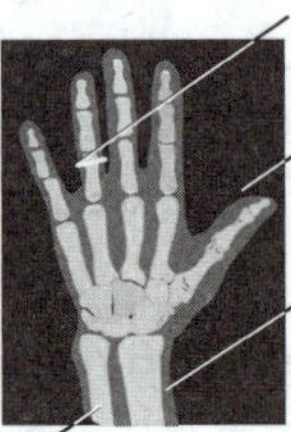

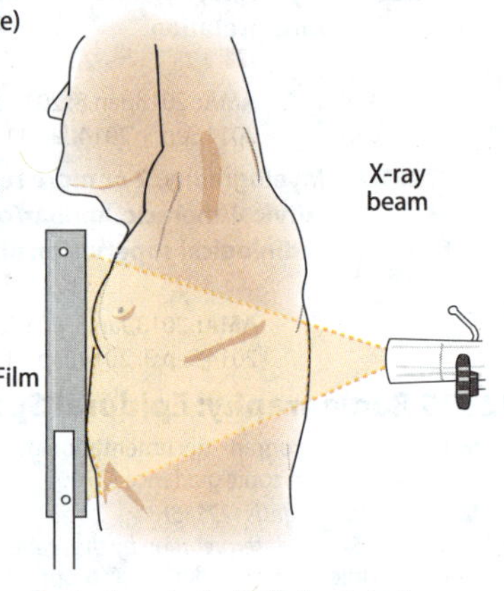

Posterioranterior (PA) chest study; lateral views also common

73010 scapula, complete
0.90 0.90 FUD XXX Q1 N1 80
AMA: 2014,Jan,11

73020 Radiologic examination, shoulder; 1 view
0.67 0.67 FUD XXX Q1 N1 80
AMA: 2014,Jan,11

73030 complete, minimum of 2 views
0.85 0.85 FUD XXX Q1 N1 80
AMA: 2014,Jan,11

73040 Radiologic examination, shoulder, arthrography, radiological supervision and interpretation
INCLUDES Fluoroscopic guidance (77002)
Code also arthrography injection procedure (23350)
3.12 3.12 FUD XXX Q2 N1 80
AMA: 2018,Jan,8; 2017,Jan,8; 2016,Jan,13; 2015,Jan,16; 2014,Jan,11

73050 Radiologic examination; acromioclavicular joints, bilateral, with or without weighted distraction
1.05 1.05 FUD XXX Q1 N1 80
AMA: 2014,Jan,11

73060 humerus, minimum of 2 views
0.85 0.85 FUD XXX Q1 N1 80
AMA: 2014,Jan,11

73070 Radiologic examination, elbow; 2 views
0.76 0.76 FUD XXX Q1 N1 80
AMA: 2018,Jan,8; 2017,Jan,8; 2016,Jan,13; 2015,Jan,16; 2014,Jan,11

73080 complete, minimum of 3 views
0.84 0.84 FUD XXX Q1 N1 80
AMA: 2014,Jan,11

73085 Radiologic examination, elbow, arthrography, radiological supervision and interpretation
INCLUDES Fluoroscopic guidance (77002)
Code also arthrography injection procedure (24220)
2.99 2.99 FUD XXX Q2 N1 80
AMA: 2018,Jan,8; 2017,Jan,8; 2016,Jan,13; 2015,Jan,16; 2014,Jan,11

73090-73140 Radiography: Forearm and Hand

INCLUDES Minimum number of views or more views when needed to adequately complete the study
Radiographs that have to be repeated during the encounter due to substandard quality; only one unit of service is reported

EXCLUDES *Obtaining more films after review of initial films, based on the discretion of the radiologist, an order for the test, and a change in the patient's condition*
Second interpretation by the requesting physician (included in E&M service)
Stress views of upper body joint(s), when performed (77071)

73090 Radiologic examination; forearm, 2 views
0.79 0.79 FUD XXX Q1 N1 80
AMA: 2018,Jan,8; 2017,Jan,8; 2016,Jan,13; 2015,Jan,16; 2014,Jan,11

73092 upper extremity, infant, minimum of 2 views A
0.81 0.81 FUD XXX Q1 N1 80
AMA: 2014,Jan,11

73100 Radiologic examination, wrist; 2 views
0.90 0.90 FUD XXX Q1 N1 80
AMA: 2018,Oct,11; 2018,Jan,8; 2017,Jan,8; 2016,Jan,13; 2015,Jan,16; 2014,Jan,11

73110 complete, minimum of 3 views
1.03 1.03 FUD XXX Q1 N1 80
AMA: 2018,Oct,11; 2018,Jan,8; 2017,Jan,8; 2016,Jan,13; 2015,Jan,16; 2014,Jan,11

73115 Radiologic examination, wrist, arthrography, radiological supervision and interpretation
INCLUDES Fluoroscopic guidance (77002)
Code also arthrography injection procedure (25246)
3.33 3.33 FUD XXX Q2 N1 80
AMA: 2018,Jan,8; 2017,Jan,8; 2016,Jan,13; 2015,Jan,16; 2014,Jan,11

73120 Radiologic examination, hand; 2 views
0.82 0.82 FUD XXX Q1 N1 80
AMA: 2018,Oct,11; 2014,Jan,11

73130 minimum of 3 views
0.94 0.94 FUD XXX Q1 N1 80
AMA: 2014,Jan,11

73140 Radiologic examination, finger(s), minimum of 2 views
0.95 0.95 FUD XXX Q1 N1 80
AMA: 2018,Jan,8; 2017,Jan,8; 2016,Jan,13; 2015,Jan,16; 2014,Jan,11

73200-73202 Computerized Tomography: Shoulder, Arm, Hand

CMS: 100-04,4,250.16 Multiple Procedure Payment Reduction: Certain Diagnostic Imaging Procedures Rendered by Physicians

INCLUDES Imaging using tomographic technique enhanced by computer imaging to create a cross-sectional plane of the body
Intravascular, intrathecal, or intra-articular contrast materials when noted in code descriptor

EXCLUDES *3D rendering (76376-76377)*

73200 Computed tomography, upper extremity; without contrast material
5.05 5.05 FUD XXX Q3 Z2 80
AMA: 2018,Jan,8; 2017,Jan,8; 2016,Jan,13; 2015,Jan,16; 2014,Jan,11

73201 with contrast material(s)
6.28 6.28 FUD XXX Q3 Z3 80
AMA: 2018,Jan,8; 2017,Jan,8; 2016,Jan,13; 2015,Aug,6; 2015,Jan,16; 2014,Jan,11

73000 — 73201

73202 **without contrast material, followed by contrast material(s) and further sections**
7.82 7.82 FUD XXX Q3 Z2 80
AMA: 2014,Jan,11

73206 Computerized Tomographic Angiography: Shoulder, Arm, and Hand

CMS: 100-04,4,250.16 Multiple Procedure Payment Reduction: Certain Diagnostic Imaging Procedures Rendered by Physicians

INCLUDES Intravascular, intrathecal, or intra-articular contrast materials when noted in code descriptor
Multiple rapid thin section CT scans to create cross-sectional images of the arteries and veins

73206 **Computed tomographic angiography, upper extremity, with contrast material(s), including noncontrast images, if performed, and image postprocessing**
9.24 9.24 FUD XXX Q3 Z2 80
AMA: 2018,Jan,8; 2017,Jan,8; 2016,Jan,13; 2015,Jan,16; 2014,Jan,11

73218-73223 Magnetic Resonance Imaging: Shoulder, Arm, Hand

CMS: 100-04,4,250.16 Multiple Procedure Payment Reduction: Certain Diagnostic Imaging Procedures Rendered by Physicians

INCLUDES Application of an external magnetic field that forces alignment of hydrogen atom nuclei in soft tissues which converts to sets of tomographic images that can be displayed as three-dimensional images
Intravascular, intrathecal, or intra-articular contrast materials when noted in code descriptor

73218 **Magnetic resonance (eg, proton) imaging, upper extremity, other than joint; without contrast material(s)**
10.1 10.1 FUD XXX Q3 Z2 80
AMA: 2018,Jan,8; 2017,Jan,8; 2016,Jan,13; 2015,Jan,16; 2014,Jan,11

73219 **with contrast material(s)**
11.1 11.1 FUD XXX Q3 Z2 80
AMA: 2018,Jan,8; 2017,Jan,8; 2016,Jan,13; 2015,Jan,16; 2014,Jan,11

73220 **without contrast material(s), followed by contrast material(s) and further sequences**
13.7 13.7 FUD XXX Q3 Z2 80
AMA: 2018,Jan,8; 2017,Jan,8; 2016,Jan,13; 2015,Jan,16; 2014,Jan,11

73221 **Magnetic resonance (eg, proton) imaging, any joint of upper extremity; without contrast material(s)**
6.57 6.57 FUD XXX Q3 Z2 80
AMA: 2018,Jan,8; 2017,Jan,8; 2016,Jan,13; 2015,Jan,16; 2014,Jan,11

73222 **with contrast material(s)**
10.4 10.4 FUD XXX Q3 Z3 80
AMA: 2018,Jan,8; 2017,Jan,8; 2016,Jan,13; 2015,Aug,6; 2015,Jan,16; 2014,Jan,11

73223 **without contrast material(s), followed by contrast material(s) and further sequences**
12.9 12.9 FUD XXX Q3 Z2 80
AMA: 2018,Jan,8; 2017,Jan,8; 2016,Jan,13; 2015,Jan,16; 2014,Jan,11

73225 Magnetic Resonance Angiography: Shoulder, Arm, Hand

CMS: 100-04,13,40.1.1 Magnetic Resonance Angiography; 100-04,4,250.16 Multiple Procedure Payment Reduction: Certain Diagnostic Imaging Procedures Rendered by Physicians

INCLUDES Intravascular, intrathecal, or intra-articular contrast materials when noted in code descriptor
Use of magnetic fields and radio waves to produce detailed cross-sectional images of the arteries and veins

73225 **Magnetic resonance angiography, upper extremity, with or without contrast material(s)**
10.9 10.9 FUD XXX B 80
AMA: 2018,Jan,8; 2017,Jan,8; 2016,Jan,13; 2015,Jan,16; 2014,Jan,11

73501-73552 Radiography: Pelvic Region and Thigh

EXCLUDES *Stress views of lower body joint(s), when performed (77071)*

73501 **Radiologic examination, hip, unilateral, with pelvis when performed; 1 view**
0.87 0.87 FUD XXX Q1 N1 80
AMA: 2018,Jan,8; 2017,Jan,8; 2016,Aug,7; 2016,Jun,8; 2016,Jan,13; 2015,Oct,9

73502 **2-3 views**
1.21 1.21 FUD XXX Q1 N1 80
AMA: 2018,Jan,8; 2017,Jan,8; 2016,Aug,7; 2016,Jun,8; 2016,Jan,13; 2015,Oct,9

73503 **minimum of 4 views**
1.51 1.51 FUD XXX Q1 N1 80
AMA: 2018,Jan,8; 2017,Jan,8; 2016,Aug,7; 2016,Jun,8; 2016,Jan,13; 2015,Oct,9

73521 **Radiologic examination, hips, bilateral, with pelvis when performed; 2 views**
1.08 1.08 FUD XXX Q1 N1 80
AMA: 2018,Jan,8; 2017,Jan,8; 2016,Aug,7; 2016,Jun,8; 2016,Jan,13; 2015,Oct,9

73522 **3-4 views**
1.41 1.41 FUD XXX Q1 N1 80
AMA: 2018,Jan,8; 2017,Jan,8; 2016,Aug,7; 2016,Jun,8; 2016,Jan,13; 2015,Oct,9

73523 **minimum of 5 views**
1.65 1.65 FUD XXX S N1 80
AMA: 2018,Jan,8; 2017,Jan,8; 2016,Aug,7; 2016,Jun,8; 2016,Jan,13; 2015,Oct,9

73525 **Radiologic examination, hip, arthrography, radiological supervision and interpretation**
INCLUDES Fluoroscopic guidance (77002)
3.18 3.18 FUD XXX Q2 N1 80
AMA: 2018,Jan,8; 2017,Jan,8; 2016,Nov,10; 2016,Aug,7; 2016,Jan,13; 2015,Jan,16; 2014,Jan,11

73551 **Radiologic examination, femur; 1 view**
0.80 0.80 FUD XXX Q1 N1 80
AMA: 2018,Jan,8; 2017,Jan,8; 2016,Aug,7

73552 **minimum 2 views**
0.94 0.94 FUD XXX Q1 N1 80
AMA: 2018,Jan,8; 2017,Nov,10; 2017,Jan,8; 2016,Aug,7

73560-73660 Radiography: Lower Leg, Ankle, and Foot

EXCLUDES *Stress views of lower body joint(s), when performed (77071)*

73560 **Radiologic examination, knee; 1 or 2 views**
0.91 0.91 FUD XXX Q1 N1 80
AMA: 2018,Jan,8; 2017,Jan,8; 2016,Jan,13; 2015,May,10; 2015,Feb,10; 2014,Jan,11

73562 **3 views**
1.05 1.05 FUD XXX Q1 N1 80
AMA: 2014,Jan,11

73564 **complete, 4 or more views**
1.17 1.17 FUD XXX Q1 N1 80
AMA: 2018,Jan,8; 2017,Jan,8; 2016,Jan,13; 2015,May,10; 2015,Feb,10; 2015,Jan,16; 2014,Jan,11

73565 **both knees, standing, anteroposterior**
1.05 1.05 FUD XXX Q1 N1 80
AMA: 2018,Jan,8; 2017,Jan,8; 2016,Jan,13; 2015,May,10; 2015,Feb,10; 2014,Jan,11

73580 **Radiologic examination, knee, arthrography, radiological supervision and interpretation**
INCLUDES Fluoroscopic guidance (77002)
3.59 3.59 FUD XXX Q2 N1 80
AMA: 2019,Aug,7; 2018,Jan,8; 2017,Jan,8; 2016,Jan,13; 2015,Aug,6; 2015,Jan,16; 2014,Jan,11

73590 Radiologic examination; tibia and fibula, 2 views
0.83 0.83 FUD XXX Q1 N1 80
AMA: 2018,Jan,8; 2017,Nov,10; 2017,Jan,8; 2016,Jan,13; 2015,Jan,16; 2014,Jan,11

73592 lower extremity, infant, minimum of 2 views A
0.81 0.81 FUD XXX Q1 N1 80
AMA: 2018,Jan,8; 2017,Nov,10; 2014,Jan,11

73600 Radiologic examination, ankle; 2 views
0.87 0.87 FUD XXX Q1 N1 80
AMA: 2018,Jan,8; 2017,Jan,8; 2016,Jan,13; 2015,Jan,16; 2014,Jan,11

73610 complete, minimum of 3 views
0.94 0.94 FUD XXX Q1 N1 80
AMA: 2018,Jan,8; 2017,Jan,8; 2016,Jan,13; 2015,Jan,16; 2014,Jan,11

73615 Radiologic examination, ankle, arthrography, radiological supervision and interpretation
INCLUDES Fluoroscopic guidance (77002)
3.34 3.34 FUD XXX Q2 N1 80
AMA: 2018,Jan,8; 2017,Jan,8; 2016,Jan,13; 2015,Jan,16; 2014,Jan,11

73620 Radiologic examination, foot; 2 views
0.76 0.76 FUD XXX Q1 N1 80
AMA: 2018,Jan,8; 2017,Jan,8; 2016,Jan,13; 2015,Jan,16; 2014,Jan,11

73630 complete, minimum of 3 views
0.88 0.88 FUD XXX Q1 N1 80
AMA: 2014,Jan,11

73650 Radiologic examination; calcaneus, minimum of 2 views
0.76 0.76 FUD XXX Q1 N1 80
AMA: 2014,Jan,11

73660 toe(s), minimum of 2 views
0.81 0.81 FUD XXX Q1 N1 80
AMA: 2014,Jan,11

73700-73702 Computerized Tomography: Leg, Ankle, and Foot

CMS: 100-04,4,250.16 Multiple Procedure Payment Reduction: Certain Diagnostic Imaging Procedures Rendered by Physicians

EXCLUDES *3D rendering (76376-76377)*

73700 Computed tomography, lower extremity; without contrast material
5.06 5.06 FUD XXX Q3 Z2 80
AMA: 2018,Jan,8; 2017,Jan,8; 2016,Jan,13; 2015,Jan,16; 2014,Jan,11

73701 with contrast material(s)
6.36 6.36 FUD XXX Q3 Z2 80
AMA: 2019,Aug,7; 2018,Jan,8; 2017,Jan,8; 2016,Jan,13; 2015,Jan,16; 2014,Jan,11

73702 without contrast material, followed by contrast material(s) and further sections
7.70 7.70 FUD XXX Q3 Z2 80
AMA: 2019,Aug,7; 2018,Jan,8; 2017,Jan,8; 2016,Jan,13; 2015,Jan,16; 2014,Jan,11

73706 Computerized Tomographic Angiography: Leg, Ankle, and Foot

CMS: 100-04,4,250.16 Multiple Procedure Payment Reduction: Certain Diagnostic Imaging Procedures Rendered by Physicians

EXCLUDES *CT angiography for aorto-iliofemoral runoff (75635)*

73706 Computed tomographic angiography, lower extremity, with contrast material(s), including noncontrast images, if performed, and image postprocessing
10.0 10.0 FUD XXX Q3 Z2 80
AMA: 2018,Jan,8; 2017,Jan,8; 2016,Jan,13; 2015,Jan,16; 2014,Jan,11

73718-73723 Magnetic Resonance Imaging: Leg, Ankle, and Foot

CMS: 100-04,4,250.16 Multiple Procedure Payment Reduction: Certain Diagnostic Imaging Procedures Rendered by Physicians

73718 Magnetic resonance (eg, proton) imaging, lower extremity other than joint; without contrast material(s)
7.39 7.39 FUD XXX Q3 Z2 80
AMA: 2018,Jan,8; 2017,Jan,8; 2016,Jan,13; 2015,Jan,16; 2014,Jan,11

73719 with contrast material(s)
8.74 8.74 FUD XXX Q3 Z2 80
AMA: 2019,Aug,7; 2018,Jan,8; 2017,Jan,8; 2016,Jan,13; 2015,Jan,16; 2014,Jan,11

73720 without contrast material(s), followed by contrast material(s) and further sequences
11.2 11.2 FUD XXX Q3 Z2 80
AMA: 2019,Aug,7; 2018,Jan,8; 2017,Jan,8; 2016,Jan,13; 2015,Jan,16; 2014,Jan,11

73721 Magnetic resonance (eg, proton) imaging, any joint of lower extremity; without contrast material
6.57 6.57 FUD XXX Q3 Z2 80
AMA: 2018,Jan,8; 2017,Jan,8; 2016,Jan,13; 2015,Jan,16; 2014,Jan,11

73722 with contrast material(s)
10.5 10.5 FUD XXX Q3 Z3 80
AMA: 2019,Aug,7; 2018,Jan,8; 2017,Jan,8; 2016,Jan,13; 2015,Aug,6; 2015,Jan,16; 2014,Jan,11

73723 without contrast material(s), followed by contrast material(s) and further sequences
12.9 12.9 FUD XXX Q3 Z2 80
AMA: 2019,Aug,7; 2018,Jan,8; 2017,Jan,8; 2016,Jan,13; 2015,Jan,16; 2014,Jan,11

73725 Magnetic Resonance Angiography: Leg, Ankle, and Foot

CMS: 100-04,13,40.1.2 HCPCS Coding Requirements; 100-04,4,250.16 Multiple Procedure Payment Reduction: Certain Diagnostic Imaging Procedures Rendered by Physicians

73725 Magnetic resonance angiography, lower extremity, with or without contrast material(s)
11.1 11.1 FUD XXX B 80
AMA: 2018,Jan,8; 2017,Jan,8; 2016,Jan,13; 2015,Jan,16; 2014,Jan,11

74018-74022 Radiography: Abdomen--General

74018 Radiologic examination, abdomen; 1 view
0.80 0.80 FUD XXX Q1 N1 80
AMA: 2019,May,10; 2018,Apr,7

74019 2 views
0.98 0.98 FUD XXX Q1 N1 80
AMA: 2018,Apr,7

74021 3 or more views
1.13 1.13 FUD XXX Q1 N1 80
AMA: 2018,Apr,7

26/TC PC/TC Only 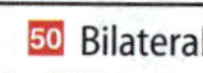 A2-Z3 ASC Payment 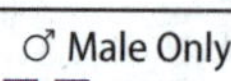 50 Bilateral 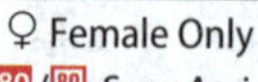 ♂ Male Only ♀ Female Only 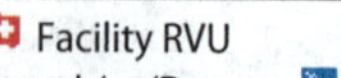 Facility RVU 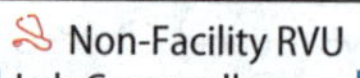 Non-Facility RVU CCI 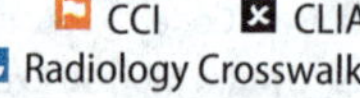 CLIA
FUD Follow-up Days CMS: IOM AMA: CPT Asst A-Y OPPSI 80/80 Surg Assist Allowed / w/Doc Lab Crosswalk Radiology Crosswalk

▲ **74022** **Radiologic examination, complete acute abdomen series, including 2 or more views of the abdomen (eg, supine, erect, decubitus), and a single view chest**
1.31 1.31 FUD XXX Q1 N1 80
AMA: 2019,May,10; 2018,Apr,7; 2016,Jun,5; 2014,Jan,11

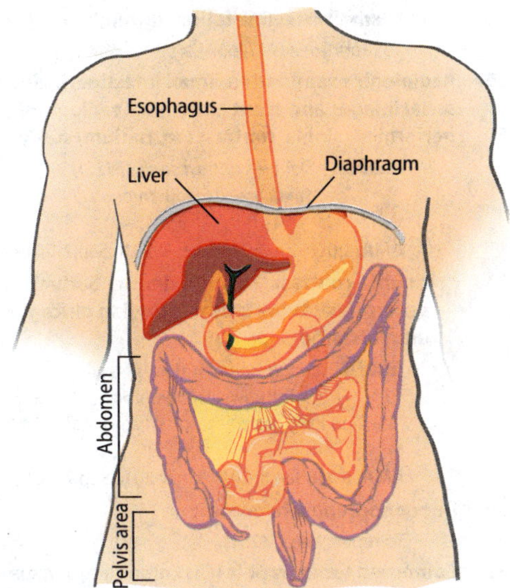

74150-74170 Computerized Tomography: Abdomen–General

CMS: 100-04,4,250.16 Multiple Procedure Payment Reduction: Certain Diagnostic Imaging Procedures Rendered by Physicians

EXCLUDES *3D rendering (76376-76377)*
Combined CT of abdomen and pelvis (74176-74178)
CT colonography, diagnostic (74261-74262)
CT colonography, screening (74263)

74150 **Computed tomography, abdomen; without contrast material**
4.22 4.22 FUD XXX Q3 Z2 80
AMA: 2018,Jan,8; 2017,Jan,8; 2016,Jun,5; 2016,Jan,13; 2015,Jan,16; 2014,Jan,11

74160 **with contrast material(s)**
6.72 6.72 FUD XXX Q3 Z2 80
AMA: 2018,Jan,8; 2017,Jan,8; 2016,Jun,5; 2016,Jan,13; 2015,Jan,16; 2014,Jan,11

74170 **without contrast material, followed by contrast material(s) and further sections**
7.62 7.62 FUD XXX Q3 Z2 80
AMA: 2018,Jan,8; 2017,Jan,8; 2016,Jun,5; 2016,Jan,13; 2015,Jan,16; 2014,Jan,11

74174-74175 Computerized Tomographic Angiography: Abdomen and Pelvis

CMS: 100-04,4,250.16 Multiple Procedure Payment Reduction: Certain Diagnostic Imaging Procedures Rendered by Physicians

EXCLUDES *CT angiography for aorto-iliofemoral runoff (75635)*
CT angiography, lower extremity (73706)
CT angiography, pelvis (72191)

74174 **Computed tomographic angiography, abdomen and pelvis, with contrast material(s), including noncontrast images, if performed, and image postprocessing**
EXCLUDES *3D rendering (76376-76377)*
Computed tomographic angiography abdomen (74175)
11.1 11.1 FUD XXX S Z2 80
AMA: 2014,Jan,11

74175 **Computed tomographic angiography, abdomen, with contrast material(s), including noncontrast images, if performed, and image postprocessing**
8.87 8.87 FUD XXX Q3 Z2 80
AMA: 2018,Jan,8; 2017,Jan,8; 2016,Jan,13; 2015,Jan,16; 2014,Jan,11

74176-74178 Computerized Tomography: Abdomen and Pelvis

CMS: 100-04,4,250.16 Multiple Procedure Payment Reduction: Certain Diagnostic Imaging Procedures Rendered by Physicians

EXCLUDES *Computed tomography of abdomen or pelvis alone (72192-72194, 74150-74170)*
Procedure performed more than one time for each combined examination of the abdomen and pelvis

74176 **Computed tomography, abdomen and pelvis; without contrast material**
5.65 5.65 FUD XXX Q3 Z3
AMA: 2018,Jan,8; 2017,Jan,8; 2016,Jan,13; 2015,Jan,16; 2014,Jan,11

74177 **with contrast material(s)**
8.99 8.99 FUD XXX Q3 Z2
AMA: 2018,Jan,8; 2017,Jan,8; 2016,Jan,13; 2015,Jan,16; 2014,Jan,11

74178 **without contrast material in one or both body regions, followed by contrast material(s) and further sections in one or both body regions**
10.1 10.1 FUD XXX Q3 Z2
AMA: 2018,Jan,8; 2017,Jan,8; 2016,Jan,13; 2015,Jan,16; 2014,Jan,11

74181-74183 Magnetic Resonance Imaging: Abdomen–General

CMS: 100-04,4,250.16 Multiple Procedure Payment Reduction: Certain Diagnostic Imaging Procedures Rendered by Physicians

74181 **Magnetic resonance (eg, proton) imaging, abdomen; without contrast material(s)**
6.88 6.88 FUD XXX Q3 Z2 80
AMA: 2018,Mar,11; 2018,Jan,8; 2017,Jan,8; 2016,Jan,13; 2015,Jan,16; 2014,Jan,11

74182 **with contrast material(s)**
10.1 10.1 FUD XXX Q3 Z2 80
AMA: 2018,Mar,11; 2018,Jan,8; 2017,Jan,8; 2016,Jan,13; 2015,Jan,16; 2014,Jan,11

74183 **without contrast material(s), followed by with contrast material(s) and further sequences**
11.2 11.2 FUD XXX Q3 Z2 80
AMA: 2018,Mar,11; 2018,Jan,8; 2017,Jan,8; 2016,Jan,13; 2015,Jan,16; 2014,Jan,11

74185 Magnetic Resonance Angiography: Abdomen–General

CMS: 100-04,13,40.1.1 Magnetic Resonance Angiography; 100-04,13,40.1.2 HCPCS Coding Requirements; 100-04,4,250.16 Multiple Procedure Payment Reduction: Certain Diagnostic Imaging Procedures Rendered by Physicians

74185 **Magnetic resonance angiography, abdomen, with or without contrast material(s)**
11.1 11.1 FUD XXX B 80
AMA: 2018,Jan,8; 2017,Jan,8; 2016,Jan,13; 2015,Jan,16; 2014,Jan,11

74190 Peritoneography

74190 **Peritoneogram (eg, after injection of air or contrast), radiological supervision and interpretation**
EXCLUDES *Computed tomography, pelvis or abdomen (72192, 74150)*
Code also injection procedure (49400)
0.00 0.00 FUD XXX Q2 N1 80
AMA: 2018,Jan,8; 2017,Jan,8; 2016,Jan,13; 2015,Jan,16; 2014,Jan,11

74210-74235 Radiography: Throat and Esophagus

EXCLUDES *Percutaneous placement of gastrostomy tube, endoscopic (43246)*
Percutaneous placement of gastrostomy tube, fluoroscopic guidance (49440)

▲ **74210 Radiologic examination, pharynx and/or cervical esophagus, including scout neck radiograph(s) and delayed image(s), when performed, contrast (eg, barium) study**
2.49 2.49 FUD XXX Q1 N1 80
AMA: 2014,Jan,11

▲ **74220 Radiologic examination, esophagus, including scout chest radiograph(s) and delayed image(s), when performed; single-contrast (eg, barium) study**
EXCLUDES *Double-contrast study (74221)*
Small bowel follow-through (74248)
Upper GI tract studies (74240-74246)
2.73 2.73 FUD XXX Q1 N1 80
AMA: 2014,Jan,11

● **74221 double-contrast (eg, high-density barium and effervescent agent) study**
EXCLUDES *Single-contrast study (74220)*
Small bowel follow-through (74248)
Upper GI tract studies (74240-74246)

▲ **74230 Radiologic examination, swallowing function, with cineradiography/videoradiography, including scout neck radiograph(s) and delayed image(s), when performed, contrast (eg, barium) study**
EXCLUDES *Swallowing function motion fluoroscopic examination (92611)*
3.59 3.59 FUD XXX Q1 N1 80
AMA: 2018,Jan,8; 2017,Jan,8; 2016,Jan,13; 2015,Jan,16; 2014,Jul,5; 2014,Jan,11

74235 Removal of foreign body(s), esophageal, with use of balloon catheter, radiological supervision and interpretation
Code also procedure (43499)
0.00 0.00 FUD XXX N N1 80
AMA: 2014,Jan,11

74240-74283 Radiography: Intestines

EXCLUDES *Percutaneous placement of gastrostomy tube, endoscopic (43246)*
Percutaneous placement of gastrostomy tube, fluoroscopic guidance (49440)

▲ **74240 Radiologic examination, upper gastrointestinal tract, including scout abdominal radiograph(s) and delayed image(s), when performed; single-contrast (eg, barium) study**
INCLUDES Upper GI with KUB
EXCLUDES *Double-contrast study (74246)*
Esophagus studies (74220-74221)
Small bowel follow-through when performed (74248)
3.45 3.45 FUD XXX Q1 Z3 80
AMA: 2018,Jan,8; 2017,Jan,8; 2016,Sep,7; 2014,Jan,11

~~74241 with or without delayed images, with KUB~~
To report, see (74240)

~~74245 with small intestine, includes multiple serial images~~
To report, see (74240, 74248)

▲ **74246 double-contrast (eg, high-density barium and effervescent agent) study, including glucagon, when administered**
INCLUDES Upper GI with KUB
EXCLUDES *Esophagus studies (74220-74221)*
Single-contrast study (74240)
3.84 3.84 FUD XXX Q1 Z2 80
AMA: 2018,Jan,8; 2017,Jan,8; 2016,Sep,7; 2014,Jan,11

~~74247 with or without delayed images, with KUB~~
To report, see (74246)

● + **74248 Radiologic small intestine follow-through study, including multiple serial images (List separately in addition to code for primary procedure for upper GI radiologic examination)**
0.00 0.00 FUD 000
EXCLUDES *Single- or double-contrast small intestine studies (74250-74251)*
Code first (74240, 74246)

~~74249 with small intestine follow-through~~
To report, see (74246, 74248)

▲ **74250 Radiologic examination, small intestine, including multiple serial images and scout abdominal radiograph(s), when performed; single-contrast (eg, barium) study**
EXCLUDES *Double-contrast study (74251)*
Small bowel follow-through (74248)
3.18 3.18 FUD XXX Q1 Z2 80
AMA: 2018,Jan,8; 2017,Jan,8; 2016,Sep,7; 2014,Jan,11

▲ **74251 double-contrast (eg, high-density barium and air via enteroclysis tube) study, including glucagon, when administered**
EXCLUDES *Single-contrast study (74250)*
Small bowel follow-through (74248)
Insertion long gastrointestinal tube (44500, 74340)
12.1 12.1 FUD XXX S Z2 80
AMA: 2018,Jan,8; 2017,Jan,8; 2016,Sep,7; 2014,Jan,11

~~74260 Duodenography, hypotonic~~
To report, see (74251)

74261 Computed tomographic (CT) colonography, diagnostic, including image postprocessing; without contrast material
EXCLUDES *3D rendering (76376-76377)*
Computed tomography of abdomen or pelvis alone (72192-72194, 74150-74170)
Screening computed tomographic (CT) colonography (74263)
13.5 13.5 FUD XXX Q3 Z2 80
AMA: 2018,Jan,8; 2017,Jan,8; 2016,Jan,13; 2015,Jan,16; 2014,Jan,11

74262 with contrast material(s) including non-contrast images, if performed
EXCLUDES *3D rendering (76376-76377)*
Computed tomography of abdomen or pelvis alone (72192-72194, 74150-74170)
Screening computed tomographic (CT) colonography (74263)
15.2 15.2 FUD XXX Q3 Z2 80
AMA: 2018,Jan,8; 2017,Jan,8; 2016,Jan,13; 2015,Jan,16; 2014,Jan,11

74263 Computed tomographic (CT) colonography, screening, including image postprocessing
EXCLUDES *3D rendering (76376-76377)*
Computed tomographic (CT) colonography (74261-74262)
Computed tomography of abdomen or pelvis alone (72192-72194, 74150-74170)
21.3 21.3 FUD XXX E
AMA: 2018,Jan,8; 2017,Jan,8; 2016,Jan,13; 2015,Jan,16; 2014,Jan,11

▲ **74270 Radiologic examination, colon, including scout abdominal radiograph(s) and delayed image(s), when performed; single-contrast (eg, barium) study**
EXCLUDES *Double-contrast study (74280)*
4.54 4.54 FUD XXX Q1 N1 80
AMA: 2018,Jan,8; 2017,Jan,8; 2016,Jan,13; 2015,Jan,16; 2014,Jan,11

▲ **74280 double-contrast (eg, high density barium and air) study, including glucagon, when administered**
EXCLUDES *Single-contrast study (74270)*
6.41 6.41 FUD XXX S Z2 80
AMA: 2014,Jan,11

74283 **Therapeutic enema, contrast or air, for reduction of intussusception or other intraluminal obstruction (eg, meconium ileus)**
6.61 6.61 FUD XXX S Z2 80
AMA: 2014,Jan,11

74290-74330 Radiography: Biliary Tract

74290 **Cholecystography, oral contrast**
2.15 2.15 FUD XXX Q1 N1 80
AMA: 2014,Jan,11

74300 **Cholangiography and/or pancreatography; intraoperative, radiological supervision and interpretation**
0.00 0.00 FUD XXX N N1 80
AMA: 2018,Jan,8; 2017,Jan,8; 2016,Jan,13; 2015,Dec,3; 2015,Jan,16; 2014,Jan,11

+ 74301 **additional set intraoperative, radiological supervision and interpretation (List separately in addition to code for primary procedure)**
Code first (74300)
0.00 0.00 FUD ZZZ N N1 80
AMA: 2015,Dec,3; 2014,Jan,11

74328 **Endoscopic catheterization of the biliary ductal system, radiological supervision and interpretation**
Code also ERCP(~43261-43265, 43274-43278 [43274, 43275, 43276, 43277,43278])
0.00 0.00 FUD XXX N N1 80
AMA: 2018,Jan,8; 2017,Jan,8; 2016,Jan,13; 2015,Jan,16; 2014,Jan,11

74329 **Endoscopic catheterization of the pancreatic ductal system, radiological supervision and interpretation**
Code also ERCP (~43261-43265, 43274-43278 [43274, 43275, 43276, 43277, 43278])
0.00 0.00 FUD XXX N N1 80
AMA: 2014,Jan,11

74330 **Combined endoscopic catheterization of the biliary and pancreatic ductal systems, radiological supervision and interpretation**
Code also ERCP (~43261-43265, 43274-43278 [43274, 43275, 43276, 43277, 43278])
0.00 0.00 FUD XXX N N1 80
AMA: 2014,Jan,11

74340-74363 Radiography: Bilidigestive Intubation

EXCLUDES *Percutaneous insertion of gastrostomy tube, endoscopic (43246)*
Percutaneous placement of gastrotomy tube, fluoroscopic guidance (49440)

74340 **Introduction of long gastrointestinal tube (eg, Miller-Abbott), including multiple fluoroscopies and images, radiological supervision and interpretation**
Code also placement of tube (44500)
0.00 0.00 FUD XXX N N1 80
AMA: 2018,Jan,8; 2017,Jan,8; 2016,Sep,9; 2014,Jan,11

74355 **Percutaneous placement of enteroclysis tube, radiological supervision and interpretation**
INCLUDES Fluoroscopic guidance (77002)
0.00 0.00 FUD XXX N N1 80
AMA: 2018,Jan,8; 2017,Jan,8; 2016,Jan,13; 2015,Jan,16; 2014,Jan,11

74360 **Intraluminal dilation of strictures and/or obstructions (eg, esophagus), radiological supervision and interpretation**
EXCLUDES *Esophagogastroduodenoscopy, flexible, transoral; with dilation of esophagus (43233)*
Esophagoscopy, flexible, transoral; with dilation of esophagus (43213-43214)
0.00 0.00 FUD XXX N N1 80
AMA: 2018,Jan,8; 2017,Jan,8; 2016,Jan,13; 2015,Jan,16; 2014,Jan,11

74363 **Percutaneous transhepatic dilation of biliary duct stricture with or without placement of stent, radiological supervision and interpretation**
EXCLUDES *Surgical procedure (47555-47556)*
0.00 0.00 FUD XXX N N1 80
AMA: 2014,Jan,11

74400-74775 Radiography: Urogenital

74400 **Urography (pyelography), intravenous, with or without KUB, with or without tomography**
3.36 3.36 FUD XXX S Z2 80
AMA: 2014,Jan,11

74410 **Urography, infusion, drip technique and/or bolus technique;**
3.41 3.41 FUD XXX S Z2 80
AMA: 2014,Jan,11

74415 **with nephrotomography**
4.07 4.07 FUD XXX S Z2 80
AMA: 2014,Jan,11

74420 **Urography, retrograde, with or without KUB**
2.02 2.02 FUD XXX S Z2 80
AMA: 2018,Jan,8; 2017,Jan,8; 2016,Jan,13; 2015,Jan,16; 2014,Jan,11

74425 **Urography, antegrade (pyelostogram, nephrostogram, loopogram), radiological supervision and interpretation**
EXCLUDES *Injection for antegrade nephrostogram and/or ureterogram ([50430, 50431, 50432, 50433, 50434, 50435])*
Ureteral stent placement (50693-50695)
0.00 0.00 FUD XXX Q2 N1 80
AMA: 2018,Jan,8; 2017,Jan,8; 2016,Jan,13; 2016,Jan,3; 2015,Oct,5; 2015,Jan,16; 2014,Jan,11

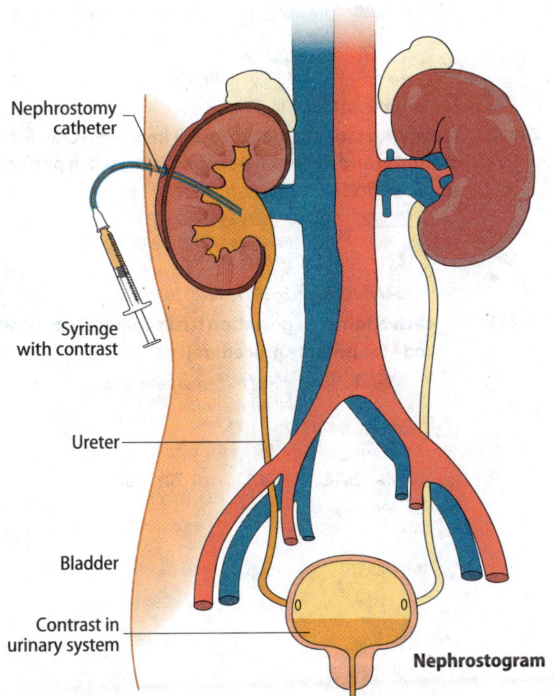

74430 **Cystography, minimum of 3 views, radiological supervision and interpretation**
1.11 1.11 FUD XXX Q2 N1 80
AMA: 2014,Jan,11

74440 **Vasography, vesiculography, or epididymography, radiological supervision and interpretation** ♂
2.44 2.44 FUD XXX Q2 N1 80
AMA: 2014,Jan,11

74445 **Corpora cavernosography, radiological supervision and interpretation** ♂

INCLUDES Needle placement with fluoroscopic guidance (77002)

0.00 0.00 FUD XXX Q2 N1 80

AMA: 2018,Jan,8; 2017,Jan,8; 2016,Jan,13; 2015,Jan,16; 2014,Jan,11

74450 **Urethrocystography, retrograde, radiological supervision and interpretation**

0.00 0.00 FUD XXX Q2 N1 80

AMA: 2014,Jan,11

74455 **Urethrocystography, voiding, radiological supervision and interpretation**

2.55 2.55 FUD XXX Q2 N1 80

AMA: 2014,Jan,11

74470 **Radiologic examination, renal cyst study, translumbar, contrast visualization, radiological supervision and interpretation**

INCLUDES Needle placement with fluoroscopic guidance (77002)

0.00 0.00 FUD XXX Q2 N1 80

AMA: 2018,Jan,8; 2017,Jan,8; 2016,Jan,13; 2015,Jan,16; 2014,Jan,11

74485 **Dilation of ureter(s) or urethra, radiological supervision and interpretation**

EXCLUDES *Change of pyelostomy/nephrostomy tube ([50435])*
Nephrostomy tract dilation for procedure ([50436, 50437])
Ureter dilation without radiologic guidance (52341, 52344)

3.02 3.02 FUD XXX Q2 N1 80

AMA: 2018,Jan,8; 2017,Jan,8; 2016,Jan,13; 2016,Jan,3; 2015,Oct,5; 2015,Jan,16; 2014,Jan,11

74710 **Pelvimetry, with or without placental localization** ♀

EXCLUDES *Imaging procedures on abdomen and pelvis (72170-72190, 74018-74019, 74021-74022, 74150-74170)*

1.08 1.08 FUD XXX Q1 N1 80

AMA: 2014,Jan,11

74712 **Magnetic resonance (eg, proton) imaging, fetal, including placental and maternal pelvic imaging when performed; single or first gestation** ♀

EXCLUDES *Imaging of maternal pelvis or placenta without fetal imaging (72195-72197)*

13.5 13.5 FUD XXX S Z2 80

AMA: 2018,Jan,8; 2017,Jan,8; 2016,Jun,5

\+ **74713** **each additional gestation (List separately in addition to code for primary procedure)** ♀

EXCLUDES *Imaging of maternal pelvis or placenta without fetal imaging (72195-72197)*

Code first (74712)

6.60 6.60 FUD ZZZ N N1 80

AMA: 2018,Jan,8; 2017,Jan,8; 2016,Jun,5

74740 **Hysterosalpingography, radiological supervision and interpretation** ♀

EXCLUDES *Imaging procedures on abdomen and pelvis (72170-72190, 74018-74019, 74021-74022, 74150-74170)*

Code also injection of saline/contrast (58340)

2.32 2.32 FUD XXX Q2 N1 80

AMA: 2018,Jan,8; 2017,Jan,8; 2016,Jan,13; 2015,Jan,16; 2014,Jan,11

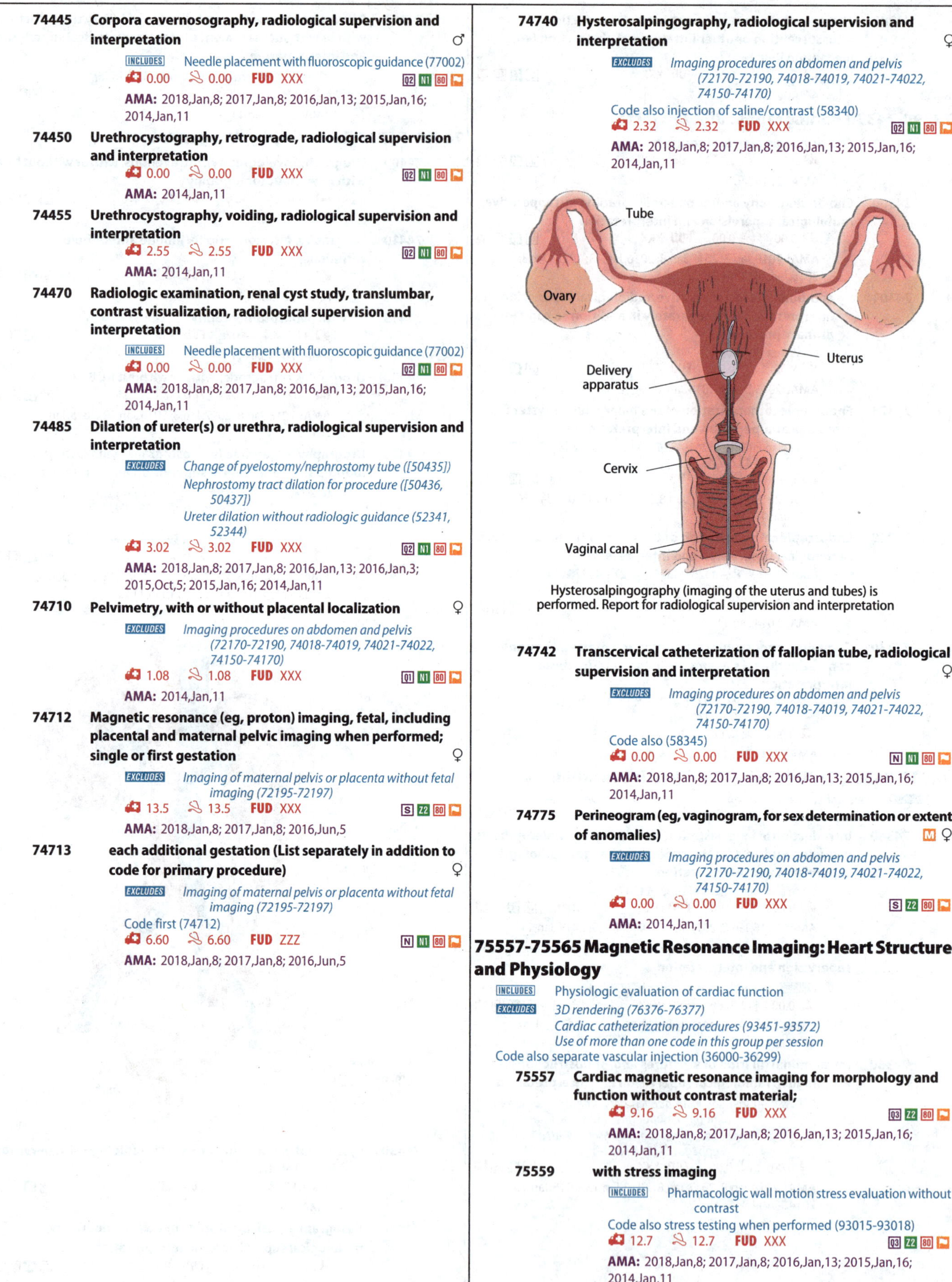

Hysterosalpingography (imaging of the uterus and tubes) is performed. Report for radiological supervision and interpretation

74742 **Transcervical catheterization of fallopian tube, radiological supervision and interpretation** ♀

EXCLUDES *Imaging procedures on abdomen and pelvis (72170-72190, 74018-74019, 74021-74022, 74150-74170)*

Code also (58345)

0.00 0.00 FUD XXX N N1 80

AMA: 2018,Jan,8; 2017,Jan,8; 2016,Jan,13; 2015,Jan,16; 2014,Jan,11

74775 **Perineogram (eg, vaginogram, for sex determination or extent of anomalies)** M ♀

EXCLUDES *Imaging procedures on abdomen and pelvis (72170-72190, 74018-74019, 74021-74022, 74150-74170)*

0.00 0.00 FUD XXX S Z2 80

AMA: 2014,Jan,11

75557-75565 Magnetic Resonance Imaging: Heart Structure and Physiology

INCLUDES Physiologic evaluation of cardiac function

EXCLUDES *3D rendering (76376-76377)*
Cardiac catheterization procedures (93451-93572)
Use of more than one code in this group per session

Code also separate vascular injection (36000-36299)

75557 **Cardiac magnetic resonance imaging for morphology and function without contrast material;**

9.16 9.16 FUD XXX Q3 Z2 80

AMA: 2018,Jan,8; 2017,Jan,8; 2016,Jan,13; 2015,Jan,16; 2014,Jan,11

75559 **with stress imaging**

INCLUDES Pharmacologic wall motion stress evaluation without contrast

Code also stress testing when performed (93015-93018)

12.7 12.7 FUD XXX Q3 Z2 80

AMA: 2018,Jan,8; 2017,Jan,8; 2016,Jan,13; 2015,Jan,16; 2014,Jan,11

75561 **Cardiac magnetic resonance imaging for morphology and function without contrast material(s), followed by contrast material(s) and further sequences;**

12.0 12.0 FUD XXX 03 Z2 80

AMA: 2018,Jan,8; 2017,Jan,8; 2016,Jan,13; 2015,Jan,16; 2014,Jan,11

75563 **with stress imaging**

INCLUDES Pharmacologic perfusion stress evaluation with contrast

Code also stress testing when performed (93015-93018)

14.2 14.2 FUD XXX 03 Z2 80

AMA: 2018,Jan,8; 2017,Jan,8; 2016,Jan,13; 2015,Jan,16; 2014,Jan,11

\+ **75565** **Cardiac magnetic resonance imaging for velocity flow mapping (List separately in addition to code for primary procedure)**

Code first (75557, 75559, 75561, 75563)

1.51 1.51 FUD ZZZ N N1 80

AMA: 2018,Jan,8; 2017,Jan,8; 2016,Jan,13; 2015,Jan,16; 2014,Jan,11

75571-75574 Computed Tomographic Imaging: Heart

CMS: 100-04,12,20.4.7 Services Not Meeting National Electrical Manufacturers Association (NEMA) Standard; 100-04,4,20.6.12 Use of HCPCS Modifier – CT; 100-04,4,250.16 Multiple Procedure Payment Reduction: Certain Diagnostic Imaging Procedures Rendered by Physicians

EXCLUDES *3D rendering (76376-76377)*
Use of more than one code in this group per session

75571 **Computed tomography, heart, without contrast material, with quantitative evaluation of coronary calcium**

2.92 2.92 FUD XXX 01 N1 80

AMA: 2018,Jan,8; 2017,Jan,8; 2016,Jan,13; 2015,Jan,16; 2014,Jan,11

75572 **Computed tomography, heart, with contrast material, for evaluation of cardiac structure and morphology (including 3D image postprocessing, assessment of cardiac function, and evaluation of venous structures, if performed)**

7.52 7.52 FUD XXX S Z2 80

AMA: 2018,Jan,8; 2017,Jan,8; 2016,Jan,13; 2015,Jan,16; 2014,Jan,11

75573 **Computed tomography, heart, with contrast material, for evaluation of cardiac structure and morphology in the setting of congenital heart disease (including 3D image postprocessing, assessment of LV cardiac function, RV structure and function and evaluation of venous structures, if performed)**

10.1 10.1 FUD XXX S Z2 80

AMA: 2018,Jan,8; 2017,Jan,8; 2016,Jan,13; 2015,Jan,16; 2014,Jan,11

75574 **Computed tomographic angiography, heart, coronary arteries and bypass grafts (when present), with contrast material, including 3D image postprocessing (including evaluation of cardiac structure and morphology, assessment of cardiac function, and evaluation of venous structures, if performed)**

11.0 11.0 FUD XXX S Z2 80

AMA: 2018,Jan,8; 2017,Jan,8; 2016,Jan,13; 2015,Jan,16; 2014,Jan,11

75600-75774 Radiography: Arterial

INCLUDES Diagnostic angiography specifically included in the interventional code description
The following diagnostic procedures with interventional supervision and interpretation:
- Angiography
- Contrast injection
- Fluoroscopic guidance for intervention
- Post-angioplasty/atherectomy/stent angiography
- Roadmapping
- Vessel measurement

EXCLUDES *Catheterization codes for diagnostic angiography of lower extremity when an access site other than the site used for the therapy is required*
Diagnostic angiogram during a separate encounter from the interventional procedure
Diagnostic angiography with interventional procedure if:
1. No previous catheter-based angiogram is accessible and a complete diagnostic procedure is performed and the decision to proceed with an interventional procedure is based on the diagnostic service, OR
2. The previous diagnostic angiogram is accessible but the documentation in the medical record specifies that:
A. the patient's condition has changed
B. there is insufficient imaging of the patient's anatomy and/or disease, OR
C. there is a clinical change during the procedure that necessitates a new examination away from the site of the intervention
3. Modifier 59 is appended to the code(s) for the diagnostic radiological supervision and interpretation service to indicate the guidelines were met
Intra-arterial procedures (36100-36248)
Intravenous procedures (36000, 36005-36015)

75600 **Aortography, thoracic, without serialography, radiological supervision and interpretation**

EXCLUDES *Supravalvular aortography (93567)*

5.63 5.63 FUD XXX 02 N1 80

AMA: 2014,Jan,11

75605 **Aortography, thoracic, by serialography, radiological supervision and interpretation**

EXCLUDES *Supravalvular aortography (93567)*

3.78 3.78 FUD XXX 02 N1 80

AMA: 2018,Jan,8; 2017,Jan,8; 2016,Jan,13; 2015,Jan,16; 2014,Jan,11

75625 **Aortography, abdominal, by serialography, radiological supervision and interpretation**

EXCLUDES *Supravalvular aortography (93567)*

3.73 3.73 FUD XXX 02 N1 80

AMA: 2018,Jan,8; 2017,Jan,8; 2016,Jan,13; 2015,Jan,16; 2014,Jan,11

75630 **Aortography, abdominal plus bilateral iliofemoral lower extremity, catheter, by serialography, radiological supervision and interpretation**

EXCLUDES *Supravalvular aortography (93567)*

4.68 4.68 FUD XXX 02 N1 80

AMA: 2018,Jan,8; 2017,Jan,8; 2016,Jan,13; 2015,Jan,16; 2014,Jan,11

75635 **Computed tomographic angiography, abdominal aorta and bilateral iliofemoral lower extremity runoff, with contrast material(s), including noncontrast images, if performed, and image postprocessing**

EXCLUDES *3D rendering (76376-76377)*
Computed tomographic angiography, abdomen, lower extremity, pelvis (72191, 73706, 74174-74175)

12.4 12.4 FUD XXX 02 N1 80

AMA: 2018,Jan,8; 2017,Jan,8; 2016,Jan,13; 2015,Jan,16; 2014,Jan,11

75705 **Angiography, spinal, selective, radiological supervision and interpretation**

7.13 7.13 FUD XXX 02 N1 80

AMA: 2014,Jan,11

75710 **Angiography, extremity, unilateral, radiological supervision and interpretation**
4.73 4.73 FUD XXX Q2 N1 80
AMA: 2018,Jan,8; 2017,Mar,3; 2017,Jan,8; 2016,Jan,13; 2015,Jan,16; 2014,Jan,11

75716 **Angiography, extremity, bilateral, radiological supervision and interpretation**
5.04 5.04 FUD XXX Q2 N1 80
AMA: 2018,Jan,8; 2017,Jan,8; 2016,Jan,13; 2015,Jan,16; 2014,Jan,11

75726 **Angiography, visceral, selective or supraselective (with or without flush aortogram), radiological supervision and interpretation**
EXCLUDES *Selective angiography, each additional visceral vessel examined after basic examination (75774)*
4.08 4.08 FUD XXX Q2 N1 80
AMA: 2014,Jan,11

75731 **Angiography, adrenal, unilateral, selective, radiological supervision and interpretation**
4.73 4.73 FUD XXX Q2 N1 80
AMA: 2014,Jan,11

75733 **Angiography, adrenal, bilateral, selective, radiological supervision and interpretation**
5.09 5.09 FUD XXX Q2 N1 80
AMA: 2014,Jan,11

75736 **Angiography, pelvic, selective or supraselective, radiological supervision and interpretation**
4.38 4.38 FUD XXX Q2 N1 80
AMA: 2014,Jan,11

75741 **Angiography, pulmonary, unilateral, selective, radiological supervision and interpretation**
4.13 4.13 FUD XXX Q2 N1 80
AMA: 2019,Jun,3; 2018,Jan,8; 2017,Jan,8; 2016,Jan,13; 2015,Jan,16; 2014,Jan,11

75743 **Angiography, pulmonary, bilateral, selective, radiological supervision and interpretation**
4.64 4.64 FUD XXX Q2 N1 80
AMA: 2019,Jun,3; 2018,Jan,8; 2017,Jan,8; 2016,Jan,13; 2015,Jan,16; 2014,Jan,11

75746 **Angiography, pulmonary, by nonselective catheter or venous injection, radiological supervision and interpretation**
EXCLUDES *Nonselective injection procedure or catheter introduction with cardiac cath (93568)*
4.16 4.16 FUD XXX Q2 N1 80
AMA: 2019,Jun,3; 2014,Jan,11

75756 **Angiography, internal mammary, radiological supervision and interpretation**
EXCLUDES *Internal mammary angiography with cardiac cath (93455, 93457, 93459, 93461, 93564)*
4.79 4.79 FUD XXX Q2 N1 80
AMA: 2018,Jan,8; 2017,Jan,8; 2016,Jan,13; 2015,Jan,16; 2014,Jan,11

+ **75774** **Angiography, selective, each additional vessel studied after basic examination, radiological supervision and interpretation (List separately in addition to code for primary procedure)**
EXCLUDES *Angiography (75600-75756)*
Cardiac cath procedures (93452-93462, 93531-93533, 93563-93568)
Catheterizations (36215-36248)
Dialysis circuit angiography (current access), use modifier 52 with (36901)
Nonselective catheter placement, thoracic aorta (36221-36228)
Code also diagnostic angiography of upper extremities and other vascular beds (except cervicocerebral vessels), when appropriate
Code first initial vessel
2.33 2.33 FUD ZZZ N N1 80
AMA: 2018,Jan,8; 2017,Jan,8; 2016,Jan,13; 2015,Jan,16; 2014,Jan,11

75801-75893 Radiography: Lymphatic and Venous

INCLUDES Diagnostic venography specifically included in the interventional code description
The following diagnostic procedures with interventional supervision and interpretation:
Contrast injection
Fluoroscopic guidance for intervention
Post-angioplasty/venography
Roadmapping
Venography
Vessel measurement

EXCLUDES *Diagnostic venogram during a separate encounter from the interventional procedure*
Diagnostic venography with interventional procedure if:
1. No previous catheter-based venogram is accessible and a complete diagnostic procedure is performed and the decision to proceed with an interventional procedure is based on the diagnostic service, OR
2. The previous diagnostic venogram is accessible but the documentation in the medical record specifies that:
A. The patient's condition has changed
B. There is insufficient imaging of the patient's anatomy and/or disease, OR
C. There is a clinical change during the procedure that necessitates a new examination away from the site of the intervention
Intravenous procedures (36000-36015, 36400-36510 [36465, 36466, 36482, 36483])
Lymphatic injection procedures (38790)

75801 **Lymphangiography, extremity only, unilateral, radiological supervision and interpretation**
0.00 0.00 FUD XXX Q2 N1 80
AMA: 2014,Jan,11

75803 **Lymphangiography, extremity only, bilateral, radiological supervision and interpretation**
0.00 0.00 FUD XXX Q2 N1 80
AMA: 2014,Jan,11

75805 **Lymphangiography, pelvic/abdominal, unilateral, radiological supervision and interpretation**
0.00 0.00 FUD XXX Q2 N1 80
AMA: 2014,Jan,11

75807 **Lymphangiography, pelvic/abdominal, bilateral, radiological supervision and interpretation**
0.00 0.00 FUD XXX Q2 N1 80
AMA: 2014,Jan,11

75809 **Shuntogram for investigation of previously placed indwelling nonvascular shunt (eg, LeVeen shunt, ventriculoperitoneal shunt, indwelling infusion pump), radiological supervision and interpretation**
Code also surgical procedure (49427, 61070)
2.69 2.69 FUD XXX Q2 N1 80
AMA: 2018,Jan,8; 2017,Jan,8; 2016,Jan,13; 2015,Jan,16; 2014,Jan,11

75810 **Splenoportography, radiological supervision and interpretation**
0.00 0.00 FUD XXX Q2 N1 80
AMA: 2018,Jan,8; 2017,Jan,8; 2016,Jan,13; 2015,Jan,16; 2014,Jan,11

75820 **Venography, extremity, unilateral, radiological supervision and interpretation**
3.15 3.15 FUD XXX Q2 N1 80
AMA: 2019,Mar,6; 2018,Jan,8; 2017,Jan,8; 2016,May,5; 2016,Jan,13; 2015,May,3; 2015,Jan,16; 2014,Jan,11

75822 **Venography, extremity, bilateral, radiological supervision and interpretation**
3.68 3.68 FUD XXX Q2 N1 80
AMA: 2014,Jan,11

75825 **Venography, caval, inferior, with serialography, radiological supervision and interpretation**
3.68 3.68 FUD XXX Q2 N1 80
AMA: 2018,Jan,8; 2017,Feb,14; 2017,Jan,8; 2016,Jan,13; 2015,Jan,16; 2014,Jan,11

75827 **Venography, caval, superior, with serialography, radiological supervision and interpretation**
3.82 3.82 FUD XXX 02 N1 80
AMA: 2018,Jan,8; 2017,Jan,8; 2016,Jan,13; 2015,Jan,16; 2014,Jan,11

75831 **Venography, renal, unilateral, selective, radiological supervision and interpretation**
3.84 3.84 FUD XXX 02 N1 80
AMA: 2014,Jan,11

75833 **Venography, renal, bilateral, selective, radiological supervision and interpretation**
4.55 4.55 FUD XXX 02 N1 80
AMA: 2014,Jan,11

75840 **Venography, adrenal, unilateral, selective, radiological supervision and interpretation**
4.08 4.08 FUD XXX 02 N1 80
AMA: 2014,Jan,11

75842 **Venography, adrenal, bilateral, selective, radiological supervision and interpretation**
4.95 4.95 FUD XXX 02 N1 80
AMA: 2014,Jan,11

75860 **Venography, venous sinus (eg, petrosal and inferior sagittal) or jugular, catheter, radiological supervision and interpretation**
3.99 3.99 FUD XXX 02 N1 80
AMA: 2014,Jan,11

75870 **Venography, superior sagittal sinus, radiological supervision and interpretation**
5.30 5.30 FUD XXX 02 N1 80
AMA: 2014,Jan,11

75872 **Venography, epidural, radiological supervision and interpretation**
4.08 4.08 FUD XXX 02 N1 80
AMA: 2014,Jan,11

75880 **Venography, orbital, radiological supervision and interpretation**
3.44 3.44 FUD XXX 02 N1 80
AMA: 2014,Jan,11

75885 **Percutaneous transhepatic portography with hemodynamic evaluation, radiological supervision and interpretation**
4.29 4.29 FUD XXX 02 N1 80
AMA: 2018,Jan,8; 2017,Jan,8; 2016,Jan,13; 2015,Jan,16; 2014,Jan,11

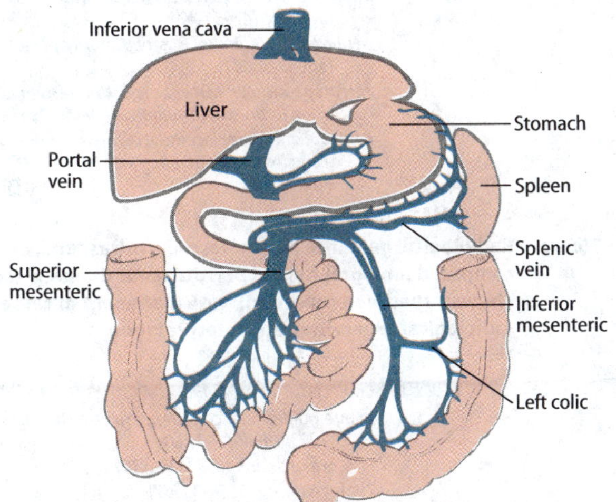

Schematic showing the portal vein

75887 **Percutaneous transhepatic portography without hemodynamic evaluation, radiological supervision and interpretation**
4.31 4.31 FUD XXX 02 N1 80
AMA: 2018,Jan,8; 2017,Jan,8; 2016,Jan,13; 2015,Jan,16; 2014,Jan,11

75889 **Hepatic venography, wedged or free, with hemodynamic evaluation, radiological supervision and interpretation**
3.93 3.93 FUD XXX 02 N1 80
AMA: 2014,Jan,11

75891 **Hepatic venography, wedged or free, without hemodynamic evaluation, radiological supervision and interpretation**
3.98 3.98 FUD XXX 02 N1 80
AMA: 2014,Jan,11

75893 **Venous sampling through catheter, with or without angiography (eg, for parathyroid hormone, renin), radiological supervision and interpretation**
Code also surgical procedure (36500)
3.32 3.32 FUD XXX 02 N1 80
AMA: 2014,Jan,11

75894-75902 Transcatheter Procedures

INCLUDES The following diagnostic procedures with interventional supervision and interpretation:
- Angiography/venography
- Completion angiography/venography except for those services allowed by (75898)
- Contrast injection
- Fluoroscopic guidance for intervention
- Roadmapping
- Vessel measurement

EXCLUDES *Diagnostic angiography/venography performed at the same session as transcatheter therapy unless it is specifically included in the code descriptor or is excluded in the venography/angiography notes (75600-75893)*

75894 **Transcatheter therapy, embolization, any method, radiological supervision and interpretation**
EXCLUDES *Endovenous ablation therapy of incompetent vein (36478-36479)*
Transluminal balloon angioplasty (36475-36476)
Vascular embolization or occlusion (37241-37244)
0.00 0.00 FUD XXX N N1 80
AMA: 2018,Mar,3; 2018,Jan,8; 2017,Jan,8; 2016,Nov,3; 2016,Jan,13; 2015,Jan,16; 2014,Oct,6; 2014,Jan,11

75898 **Angiography through existing catheter for follow-up study for transcatheter therapy, embolization or infusion, other than for thrombolysis**
EXCLUDES *Percutaneous arterial transluminal mechanical thrombectomy (61645)*
Prolonged endovascular intracranial administration of pharmacologic agent(s) (61650-61651)
Transcatheter therapy, arterial infusion for thrombolysis (37211-37214)
Vascular embolization or occlusion (37241-37244)
0.00 0.00 FUD XXX 02 N1 80
AMA: 2019,Sep,6; 2018,Jan,8; 2017,Jan,8; 2016,Jan,13; 2015,Nov,3; 2015,Jan,16; 2014,Oct,6; 2014,Jan,11

75901 **Mechanical removal of pericatheter obstructive material (eg, fibrin sheath) from central venous device via separate venous access, radiologic supervision and interpretation**
EXCLUDES *Venous catheterization (36010-36012)*
Code also surgical procedure (36595)
5.62 5.62 FUD XXX N N1 80
AMA: 2018,Jan,8; 2017,Jan,8; 2016,Jan,13; 2015,Jan,16; 2014,Jan,11

75902 **Mechanical removal of intraluminal (intracatheter) obstructive material from central venous device through device lumen, radiologic supervision and interpretation**

EXCLUDES *Venous catheterization (36010-36012)*

Code also surgical procedure (36596)

Facility RVU 2.22 Non-Facility RVU 2.22 FUD XXX N N1 80

AMA: 2018,Jan,8; 2017,Jan,8; 2016,Jan,13; 2015,Jan,16; 2014,Jan,11

75956-75959 Endovascular Aneurysm Repair

INCLUDES The following diagnostic procedures with interventional supervision and interpretation:
- Angiography/venography
- Completion angiography/venography except for those services allowed by (75898)
- Contrast injection
- Fluoroscopic guidance for intervention
- Injection procedure only for transcatheter therapy or biopsy (36100-36299)
- Percutaneous needle biopsy
  - Pancreas (48102)
  - Retroperitoneal lymph node/mass (49180)
- Roadmapping
- Vessel measurement

EXCLUDES *Diagnostic angiography/venography performed at the same session as transcatheter therapy unless it is specifically included in the code descriptor (75600-75893)*

Radiological supervision and interpretation for transluminal angioplasty in:
- *Femoral/popliteal arteries (37224-37227)*
- *Iliac artery (37220-37223)*
- *Tibial/peroneal artery (37228-37235)*

75956 **Endovascular repair of descending thoracic aorta (eg, aneurysm, pseudoaneurysm, dissection, penetrating ulcer, intramural hematoma, or traumatic disruption); involving coverage of left subclavian artery origin, initial endoprosthesis plus descending thoracic aortic extension(s), if required, to level of celiac artery origin, radiological supervision and interpretation**

Code also endovascular graft implantation (33880)

Facility RVU 0.00 Non-Facility RVU 0.00 FUD XXX C 80

AMA: 2018,Jan,8; 2017,Jan,8; 2016,Jan,13; 2015,Jan,16; 2014,Jan,11

75957 **not involving coverage of left subclavian artery origin, initial endoprosthesis plus descending thoracic aortic extension(s), if required, to level of celiac artery origin, radiological supervision and interpretation**

Code also endovascular graft implantation (33881)

Facility RVU 0.00 Non-Facility RVU 0.00 FUD XXX C 80

AMA: 2018,Jan,8; 2017,Jan,8; 2016,Jan,13; 2015,Jan,16; 2014,Jan,11

75958 **Placement of proximal extension prosthesis for endovascular repair of descending thoracic aorta (eg, aneurysm, pseudoaneurysm, dissection, penetrating ulcer, intramural hematoma, or traumatic disruption), radiological supervision and interpretation**

Code also placement of each additional proximal extension(s) (75958)

Code also proximal endovascular extension implantation (33883-33884)

Facility RVU 0.00 Non-Facility RVU 0.00 FUD XXX C 80

AMA: 2018,Jan,8; 2017,Jan,8; 2016,Jan,13; 2015,Jan,16; 2014,Jan,11

75959 **Placement of distal extension prosthesis(s) (delayed) after endovascular repair of descending thoracic aorta, as needed, to level of celiac origin, radiological supervision and interpretation**

INCLUDES Corresponding services for placement of distal thoracic endovascular extension(s) placed during procedure following the principal procedure

EXCLUDES *Endovascular repair of descending thoracic aorta (75956-75957)*

Use of code more than one time no matter how many modules are deployed

Code also placement of distal endovascular extension (33886)

Facility RVU 0.00 Non-Facility RVU 0.00 FUD XXX C 80

AMA: 2018,Jan,8; 2017,Jan,8; 2016,Jan,13; 2015,Jan,16; 2014,Jan,11

75970 Percutaneous Transluminal Angioplasty

INCLUDES The following diagnostic procedures with interventional supervision and interpretation:
- Angiography/venography
- Completion angiography/venography except for those services allowed by (75898)
- Contrast injection
- Fluoroscopic guidance for intervention
- Roadmapping
- Vessel measurement

EXCLUDES *Diagnostic angiography/venography performed at the same session as transcatheter therapy unless it is specifically included in the code descriptor (75600-75893)*

Injection procedure only for transcatheter therapy or biopsy (36100-36299)
- *Percutaneous needle biopsy (48102)*
- *Pancreas (48102)*
- *Retroperitoneal lymph node/mass (49180)*
- *Radiological supervision and interpretation for transluminal balloon angioplasty in:*
- *Femoral/popliteal arteries (37224-37227)*
- *Iliac artery (37220-37223)*
- *Tibial/peroneal artery (37228-37235)*

Transcatheter renal/ureteral biopsy (52007)

75970 **Transcatheter biopsy, radiological supervision and interpretation**

Facility RVU 0.00 Non-Facility RVU 0.00 FUD XXX N N1 80

AMA: 2018,Jan,8; 2014,Jan,11

75984-75989 Percutaneous Drainage

75984 **Change of percutaneous tube or drainage catheter with contrast monitoring (eg, genitourinary system, abscess), radiological supervision and interpretation**

EXCLUDES *Change only of nephrostomy/pyelostomy tube ([50435])*

Cholecystostomy, percutaneous (47490)

Introduction procedure only for percutaneous biliary drainage (47531-47544)

Nephrostolithotomy/pyelostolithotomy, percutaneous (50080-50081)

Percutaneous replacement of gastrointestinal tube using fluoroscopic guidance (49450-49452)

Removal and/or replacement of internal ureteral stent using transurethral approach (50385-50386)

Facility RVU 2.89 Non-Facility RVU 2.89 FUD XXX N N1 80

AMA: 2014,Jan,11

75989 **Radiological guidance (ie, fluoroscopy, ultrasound, or computed tomography), for percutaneous drainage (eg, abscess, specimen collection), with placement of catheter, radiological supervision and interpretation**

INCLUDES Imaging guidance

EXCLUDES *Cholecystostomy (47490)*

Image-guided fluid collection drainage by catheter (10030, 49405-49407)

Pericardial drainage (33017-33019)

Thoracentesis (32554-32557)

Facility RVU 3.42 Non-Facility RVU 3.42 FUD XXX N N1 80

AMA: 2018,Jan,8; 2017,Jan,8; 2016,Jan,13; 2015,Dec,3; 2015,Jan,16; 2014,May,9; 2014,Jan,11

76000-76140 Miscellaneous Techniques

EXCLUDES *Arthrography:*
Ankle (73615)
Elbow (73085)
Hip (73525)
Knee (73580)
Shoulder (73040)
Wrist (73115)
CT cerebral perfusion test (0042T)

76000 Fluoroscopy (separate procedure), up to 1 hour physician or other qualified health care professional time

EXCLUDES *Extracorporeal membrane oxygenation (ECMO)/extracorporeal life support (ECLS) (33957-33959, [33962, 33963, 33964])*
Insertion/removal/replacement wireless cardiac stimulator (0515T-0520T)
Insertion/replacement/removal leadless pacemaker ([33274, 33275])

1.33 1.33 FUD XXX S Z3 80

AMA: 2019,Sep,10; 2019,Sep,5; 2019,Jun,3; 2019,Mar,6; 2018,Apr,7; 2018,Mar,3; 2018,Jan,8; 2017,Jan,8; 2016,Nov,3; 2016,Aug,5; 2016,May,5; 2016,May,13; 2016,Mar,5; 2016,Jan,11; 2016,Jan,13; 2015,Nov,3; 2015,Sep,3; 2015,May,3; 2015,Jan,16; 2014,Dec,3; 2014,Nov,5; 2014,Oct,6; 2014,Sep,5; 2014,Jan,11

76010 Radiologic examination from nose to rectum for foreign body, single view, child A

0.77 0.77 FUD XXX Q1 N1 80

AMA: 2018,Jan,8; 2017,Jan,8; 2016,Jan,13; 2015,Jan,16; 2014,Jan,11

76080 Radiologic examination, abscess, fistula or sinus tract study, radiological supervision and interpretation

EXCLUDES *Contrast injections, radiology evaluation, and guidance via fluoroscopy of gastrostomy, duodenostomy, jejunostomy, gastro-jejunostomy, or cecostomy tube (49465)*

1.61 1.61 FUD XXX Q2 N1 80

AMA: 2018,Jan,8; 2017,Jan,8; 2016,Jan,13; 2015,Jan,16; 2014,Jan,11

76098 Radiological examination, surgical specimen

EXCLUDES *Breast biopsy with placement of breast localization device(s) (19081-19086)*

0.47 0.47 FUD XXX Q2 N1 80

AMA: 2012,Feb,9-10; 1997,Nov,1

76100 Radiologic examination, single plane body section (eg, tomography), other than with urography

2.67 2.67 FUD XXX Q1 N1 80

AMA: 2012,Feb,9-10; 1997,Nov,1

76101 Radiologic examination, complex motion (ie, hypercycloidal) body section (eg, mastoid polytomography), other than with urography; unilateral

EXCLUDES *Nephrotomography (74415)*
Panoramic x-ray (70355)
Procedure performed more than one time per day

2.65 2.65 FUD XXX Q1 Z2 80

AMA: 2012,Feb,9-10; 1997,Nov,1

76102 bilateral

EXCLUDES *Nephrotomography (74415)*
Panoramic x-ray (70355)
Procedure performed more than one time per day

4.88 4.88 FUD XXX S Z2 80

AMA: 2012,Feb,9-10; 1997,Nov,1

76120 Cineradiography/videoradiography, except where specifically included

2.87 2.87 FUD XXX Q1 N1 80

AMA: 2018,Jan,8; 2017,Jan,8; 2016,Jan,13; 2015,Jan,16; 2014,Jan,11

\+ **76125 Cineradiography/videoradiography to complement routine examination (List separately in addition to code for primary procedure)**

Code first primary procedure

0.00 0.00 FUD ZZZ N N1 80

AMA: 2018,Jan,8; 2017,Jan,8; 2016,Jan,13; 2015,Jan,16; 2014,Jan,11

76140 Consultation on X-ray examination made elsewhere, written report

0.00 0.00 FUD XXX E

AMA: 2018,Jan,8; 2017,Jan,8; 2016,Jan,13; 2015,Jan,16; 2014,Jan,11

76376-76377 Three-dimensional Manipulation

INCLUDES Concurrent physician supervision of image postprocessing
3D manipulation of volumetric data set
Rendering of image

EXCLUDES *Anatomic guide 3D-printed and designed from image data set (0561T-0562T)*
Anatomic model 3D-printed from image data set (0559T-0560T)
Arthrography:
Ankle (73615)
Elbow (73085)
Hip (73525)
Knee (73580)
Shoulder (73040)
Wrist (73115)
Cardiac magnetic resonance imaging (75557, 75559, 75561, 75563, 75565)
Computed tomographic angiography (70496, 70498, 71275, 72191, 73206, 73706, 74174-74175, 74261-74263, 75571-75574, 75635)
Computer-aided detection of MRI data for lesion, breast MRI (77046-77049)
CT cerebral perfusion test (0042T)
Digital breast tomosynthesis (77061-77063)
Echocardiography, transesophageal (TEE) for guidance (93355)
Magnetic resonance angiography (70544-70549, 71555, 72198, 73225, 73725, 74185)
Nuclear radiology procedures (78012-78999)
Physician planning of a patient-specific fenestrated visceral aortic endograft (34839)

Code also base imaging procedure(s)

76376 3D rendering with interpretation and reporting of computed tomography, magnetic resonance imaging, ultrasound, or other tomographic modality with image postprocessing under concurrent supervision; not requiring image postprocessing on an independent workstation

EXCLUDES *3D rendering (76377)*
Bronchoscopy, with computer-assisted, image-guided navigation (31627)

0.65 0.65 FUD XXX N N1 80

AMA: 2019,Aug,5; 2019,Sep,10; 2018,Jul,11; 2018,Jan,8; 2017,Jan,8; 2016,Apr,8; 2016,Jan,13; 2015,Jan,16; 2014,Jan,11

76377 requiring image postprocessing on an independent workstation

EXCLUDES *3D rendering (76376)*

2.01 2.01 FUD XXX N N1 80

AMA: 2019,Aug,5; 2019,Sep,10; 2018,Jul,11; 2018,Jan,8; 2017,Jan,8; 2016,Apr,8; 2016,Jan,13; 2015,Jan,16; 2014,Jan,11

76380 Computerized Tomography: Delimited

EXCLUDES *Arthrography:*
Ankle (73615)
Elbow (73085)
Hip (73525)
Knee (73580)
Shoulder (73040)
Wrist (73115)
CT cerebral perfusion test (0042T)

76380 Computed tomography, limited or localized follow-up study

4.07 4.07 FUD XXX Q1 N1 80

AMA: 2019,Mar,10; 2018,Jan,8; 2017,Jan,8; 2016,Jan,13; 2015,Jan,16; 2014,Jan,11

76390-76391 Magnetic Resonance Spectroscopy

EXCLUDES *Arthrography:*
Ankle (73615)
Elbow (73085)
Hip (73525)
Knee (73580)
Shoulder (73040)
Wrist (73115)
CT cerebral perfusion test (0042T)

76390 **Magnetic resonance spectroscopy**
EXCLUDES *MRI*
12.3 12.3 **FUD** XXX E
AMA: 2012,Feb,9-10; 1997,Nov,1

76391 **Magnetic resonance (eg, vibration) elastography**
6.66 6.66 **FUD** XXX Z2 80
AMA: 2019,Aug,3

76496-76499 Unlisted Radiology Procedures

76496 **Unlisted fluoroscopic procedure (eg, diagnostic, interventional)**
0.00 0.00 **FUD** XXX Q1 N1 80
AMA: 2012,Feb,9-10; 1997,Nov,1

76497 **Unlisted computed tomography procedure (eg, diagnostic, interventional)**
0.00 0.00 **FUD** XXX Q1 N1 80
AMA: 2018,Sep,10; 2018,Jan,8; 2017,Jan,8; 2016,Jan,13; 2015,Jan,16; 2014,Jan,11

76498 **Unlisted magnetic resonance procedure (eg, diagnostic, interventional)**
0.00 0.00 **FUD** XXX S Z2 80
AMA: 2019,Aug,5; 2018,Jul,11; 2018,Jan,8; 2017,Jan,8; 2016,Jan,13; 2015,Jan,16; 2014,Jan,11

76499 **Unlisted diagnostic radiographic procedure**
0.00 0.00 **FUD** XXX Q1 N1 80
AMA: 2018,Jan,8; 2017,Jan,8; 2016,Dec,15; 2016,Jul,8; 2016,Jan,13; 2015,Jan,16; 2014,Jan,11

76506 Ultrasound: Brain

INCLUDES Required permanent documentation of ultrasound images except when diagnostic purpose is biometric measurement
Written documentation
EXCLUDES *Noninvasive vascular studies, diagnostic (93880-93990)*
Ultrasound exam that does not include thorough assessment of organ or site, recorded image, and written report

76506 **Echoencephalography, real time with image documentation (gray scale) (for determination of ventricular size, delineation of cerebral contents, and detection of fluid masses or other intracranial abnormalities), including A-mode encephalography as secondary component where indicated**
3.26 3.26 **FUD** XXX Q1 N1 80
AMA: 2018,Jan,8; 2017,Jan,8; 2016,Jan,13; 2015,Jan,16; 2014,Jan,11

76510-76529 Ultrasound: Eyes

INCLUDES Required permanent documentation of ultrasound images except when diagnostic purpose is biometric measurement
Written documentation

76510 **Ophthalmic ultrasound, diagnostic; B-scan and quantitative A-scan performed during the same patient encounter**
3.15 3.15 **FUD** XXX Q1 N1 80
AMA: 2018,Jan,8; 2017,Jan,8; 2016,Jan,13; 2015,Jan,16; 2014,Jan,11

76511 **quantitative A-scan only**
1.93 1.93 **FUD** XXX Q1 N1 80
AMA: 2019,Jan,12; 2018,Jan,8; 2017,Jan,8; 2016,Jan,13; 2015,Jan,16; 2014,Jan,11

76512 **B-scan (with or without superimposed non-quantitative A-scan)**
1.73 1.73 **FUD** XXX Q1 N1 80
AMA: 2019,Jan,12; 2018,Jan,8; 2017,Jan,8; 2016,Jan,13; 2015,Jan,16; 2014,Jan,11

76513 **anterior segment ultrasound, immersion (water bath) B-scan or high resolution biomicroscopy**
EXCLUDES *Computerized ophthalmic testing other than by ultrasound (92132-92134)*
2.78 2.78 **FUD** XXX Q1 N1 80
AMA: 2019,Jan,12; 2018,Jan,8; 2017,Jan,8; 2016,Jan,13; 2015,Jan,16; 2014,Jan,11

76514 **corneal pachymetry, unilateral or bilateral (determination of corneal thickness)**
INCLUDES Biometric measurement for which permanent documentation of images is not required
EXCLUDES *Collagen cross-linking of cornea (0402T)*
0.36 0.36 **FUD** XXX Q1 N1 80
AMA: 2019,Jan,12; 2018,Jan,8; 2017,Jan,8; 2016,Feb,12; 2016,Jan,13; 2015,Jan,16; 2014,Jan,11

76516 **Ophthalmic biometry by ultrasound echography, A-scan;**
INCLUDES Biometric measurement for which permanent documentation of images is not required
1.53 1.53 **FUD** XXX Q1 N1 80
AMA: 2019,Jan,12; 2018,Jan,8; 2017,Jan,8; 2016,Jan,13; 2015,Jan,16; 2014,Jan,11

76519 **with intraocular lens power calculation**
INCLUDES Biometric measurement for which permanent documentation of images is not required
Written prescription that satisfies requirement for written report
EXCLUDES *Partial coherence interferometry (92136)*
1.87 1.87 **FUD** XXX Q1 N1 80
AMA: 2019,Jan,12; 2018,Jan,8; 2017,Jan,8; 2016,Jan,13; 2015,Jan,16; 2014,Jan,11

76529 **Ophthalmic ultrasonic foreign body localization**
2.33 2.33 **FUD** XXX Q1 N1 80
AMA: 2019,Jan,12; 2018,Jan,8; 2017,Jan,8; 2016,Jan,13; 2015,Jan,16; 2014,Jan,11

76536-76800 Ultrasound: Neck, Thorax, Abdomen, and Spine

INCLUDES Required permanent documentation of ultrasound images except when diagnostic purpose is biometric measurement
Written documentation
EXCLUDES *Focused ultrasound ablation of uterine leiomyomata (0071T-0072T)*
Ultrasound exam that does not include thorough assessment of organ or site, recorded image, and written report

76536 **Ultrasound, soft tissues of head and neck (eg, thyroid, parathyroid, parotid), real time with image documentation**
3.25 3.25 **FUD** XXX Q1 N1 80
AMA: 2018,Jan,8; 2017,Oct,9; 2017,Jan,8; 2016,Jan,13; 2015,Jan,16; 2014,Jan,11

76604 **Ultrasound, chest (includes mediastinum), real time with image documentation**
2.51 2.51 **FUD** XXX Q1 N1 80
AMA: 2018,Jan,8; 2017,Oct,9; 2017,Jan,8; 2016,Jan,13; 2015,Jan,16; 2014,Jan,11

76641 **Ultrasound, breast, unilateral, real time with image documentation, including axilla when performed; complete**
INCLUDES Complete examination of all four quadrants, retroareolar region, and axilla when performed
EXCLUDES *Procedure performed more than one time per breast per session*
3.02 3.02 **FUD** XXX Q1 N1 80 50
AMA: 2018,Jan,8; 2017,Oct,9; 2017,Jan,8; 2016,Jan,13; 2015,Aug,8

76642 **limited**
INCLUDES Examination not including all of the elements in complete examination
EXCLUDES *Procedure performed more than one time per breast per session*
2.47 2.47 **FUD** XXX Q1 N1 80 50
AMA: 2018,Jan,8; 2017,Oct,9

76700 Ultrasound, abdominal, real time with image documentation; complete

INCLUDES Real time scans of:
- Common bile duct
- Gall bladder
- Inferior vena cava
- Kidneys
- Liver
- Pancreas
- Spleen
- Upper abdominal aorta

3.43 3.43 FUD XXX Q3 Z2 80

AMA: 2018,Jan,8; 2017,Oct,9; 2017,Jan,8; 2016,Jan,13; 2015,Jan,16; 2014,Jan,11

76705 limited (eg, single organ, quadrant, follow-up)

2.56 2.56 FUD XXX Q3 Z2 80

AMA: 2018,Jan,8; 2017,Oct,9; 2017,Jan,8; 2016,Jan,13; 2015,Jan,16; 2014,Jan,11

76706 Ultrasound, abdominal aorta, real time with image documentation, screening study for abdominal aortic aneurysm (AAA)

EXCLUDES *Diagnostic ultrasound of aorta (76770-76775)*
Duplex scan of aorta (93978-93979)

3.20 3.20 FUD XXX S 80

AMA: 2018,Jan,8; 2017,Sep,11

76770 Ultrasound, retroperitoneal (eg, renal, aorta, nodes), real time with image documentation; complete

INCLUDES Complete assessment of kidneys and bladder if history indicates urinary pathology
Real time scans of:
- Abdominal aorta
- Common iliac artery origins
- Inferior vena cava
- Kidneys

3.18 3.18 FUD XXX Q3 Z2 80

AMA: 2018,Jan,8; 2017,Oct,9; 2017,Jan,8; 2016,Jan,13; 2015,Jan,16; 2014,Jan,11

76775 limited

1.65 1.65 FUD XXX Q1 N1 80

AMA: 2018,Jan,8; 2017,Oct,9; 2017,Jan,8; 2016,Jan,13; 2015,Jan,16; 2014,Jan,11

76776 Ultrasound, transplanted kidney, real time and duplex Doppler with image documentation

EXCLUDES *Abdominal/pelvic/scrotal contents/retroperitoneal duplex scan (93975-93976)*
Transplanted kidney ultrasound without duplex doppler (76775)

4.38 4.38 FUD XXX Q3 Z2 80

AMA: 2018,Jan,8; 2017,Jan,8; 2016,Jan,13; 2015,Jan,16; 2014,Jan,11

76800 Ultrasound, spinal canal and contents

4.04 4.04 FUD XXX Q1 N1 80

AMA: 2018,Jan,8; 2017,Jan,8; 2016,Jan,13; 2015,Jan,16; 2014,Jan,11

76801-76802 Ultrasound: Pregnancy Less Than 14 Weeks

INCLUDES Determination of the number of gestational sacs and fetuses
Gestational sac/fetal measurement appropriate for gestational age (younger than 14 weeks 0 days)
Inspection of the maternal uterus and adnexa
Quality analysis of amniotic fluid volume/gestational sac shape
Visualization of fetal and placental anatomic formation
Written documentation of each component of exam

EXCLUDES *Focused ultrasound ablation of uterine leiomyomata (0071T-0072T)*
Ultrasound exam that does not include thorough assessment of organ or site, recorded image, and written report

76801 Ultrasound, pregnant uterus, real time with image documentation, fetal and maternal evaluation, first trimester (< 14 weeks 0 days), transabdominal approach; single or first gestation M ♀

EXCLUDES *Fetal nuchal translucency measurement, first trimester (76813)*

3.46 3.46 FUD XXX S Z2 80

AMA: 2018,Jan,8; 2017,Jan,8; 2016,Jan,13; 2015,Jan,16; 2014,Jan,11

\+ **76802 each additional gestation (List separately in addition to code for primary procedure)** M ♀

EXCLUDES *Fetal nuchal translucency measurement, first trimester (76814)*

Code first (76801)

1.81 1.81 FUD ZZZ N N1 80

AMA: 2018,Jan,8; 2017,Jan,8; 2016,Jan,13; 2015,Jan,16; 2014,Jan,11

76805-76810 Ultrasound: Pregnancy of 14 Weeks or More

INCLUDES Determination of the number of gestational/chorionic sacs and fetuses
Evaluation of:
- Amniotic fluid
- Four chambered heart
- Intracranial, spinal, abdominal anatomy
- Placenta location
- Umbilical cord insertion site

Examination of maternal adnexa if visible
Gestational sac/fetal measurement appropriate for gestational age (older than or equal to 14 weeks 0 days)
Written documentation of each component of exam

EXCLUDES *Focused ultrasound ablation of uterine leiomyomata (0071T-0072T)*
Ultrasound exam that does not include thorough assessment of organ or site, recorded image, and written report

76805 Ultrasound, pregnant uterus, real time with image documentation, fetal and maternal evaluation, after first trimester (> or = 14 weeks 0 days), transabdominal approach; single or first gestation M ♀

3.97 3.97 FUD XXX S Z2 80

AMA: 2018,Jan,8; 2017,Jan,8; 2016,Jan,13; 2015,Jan,16; 2014,Jan,11

\+ **76810 each additional gestation (List separately in addition to code for primary procedure)** M ♀

Code first (76805)

2.63 2.63 FUD ZZZ N N1 80

AMA: 2018,Jan,8; 2017,Jan,8; 2016,Jan,13; 2015,Jan,16; 2014,Jan,11

76811-76812 Ultrasound: Pregnancy, with Additional Studies of Fetus

INCLUDES Determination of the number of gestational/chorionic sacs and fetuses
Evaluation of:
- Abdominal organ specific anatomy
- Amniotic fluid
- Chest anatomy
- Face
- Fetal brain/ventricles
- Four chambered heart
- Heart/outflow tracts and chest anatomy
- Intracranial, spinal, abdominal anatomy
- Limbs including number, length, and architecture
- Other fetal anatomy as indicated
- Placenta location
- Umbilical cord insertion site

Examination of maternal adnexa if visible
Gestational sac/fetal measurement appropriate for gestational age (older than or equal to 14 weeks 0 days)
Written documentation of each component of exam, including reason for nonvisualization, when applicable

EXCLUDES *Focused ultrasound ablation of uterine leiomyomata (0071T-0072T)*
Ultrasound exam that does not include thorough assessment organ or site, recorded image, and written report

76811 Ultrasound, pregnant uterus, real time with image documentation, fetal and maternal evaluation plus detailed fetal anatomic examination, transabdominal approach; single or first gestation M ♀
5.12 5.12 FUD XXX S Z3 80
AMA: 2018,Jan,8; 2017,Jan,8; 2016,Jan,13; 2015,Jan,16; 2014,Jan,11

\+ **76812 each additional gestation (List separately in addition to code for primary procedure)** M ♀
Code first (76811)
5.72 5.72 FUD ZZZ N N1 80
AMA: 2018,Jan,8; 2017,Jan,8; 2016,Jan,13; 2015,Jan,16; 2014,Jan,11

76813-76828 Ultrasound: Other Fetal Evaluations

INCLUDES Required permanent documentation of ultrasound images except when diagnostic purpose is biometric measurement
Written documentation

EXCLUDES *Focused ultrasound ablation of uterine leiomyomata (0071T-0072T)*
Ultrasound exam that does not include thorough assessment of organ or site, recorded image, and written report

76813 Ultrasound, pregnant uterus, real time with image documentation, first trimester fetal nuchal translucency measurement, transabdominal or transvaginal approach; single or first gestation M ♀
3.45 3.45 FUD XXX Q1 N1 80
AMA: 2018,Jan,8; 2017,Jan,8; 2016,Jan,13; 2015,Jan,16; 2014,Jan,11

\+ **76814 each additional gestation (List separately in addition to code for primary procedure)** M ♀
Code first (76813)
2.27 2.27 FUD XXX N N1 80
AMA: 2018,Jan,8; 2017,Jan,8; 2016,Jan,13; 2015,Jan,16; 2014,Jan,11

76815 Ultrasound, pregnant uterus, real time with image documentation, limited (eg, fetal heart beat, placental location, fetal position and/or qualitative amniotic fluid volume), 1 or more fetuses M ♀
INCLUDES Exam concentrating on one or more elements
Reporting only one time per exam, instead of per element
EXCLUDES *Fetal nuchal translucency measurement, first trimester (76813-76814)*
2.38 2.38 FUD XXX Q1 N1 80
AMA: 2018,Jan,8; 2017,Jan,8; 2016,Jan,13; 2015,Jan,16; 2014,Jan,11

76816 Ultrasound, pregnant uterus, real time with image documentation, follow-up (eg, re-evaluation of fetal size by measuring standard growth parameters and amniotic fluid volume, re-evaluation of organ system(s) suspected or confirmed to be abnormal on a previous scan), transabdominal approach, per fetus M ♀
INCLUDES Re-evaluation of fetal size, interval growth, or aberrancies noted on a prior ultrasound
Code also modifier 59 for examination of each additional fetus in a multiple pregnancy
3.23 3.23 FUD XXX Q1 N1 80
AMA: 2018,Jan,8; 2017,Jan,8; 2016,Jan,13; 2015,Jan,16; 2014,Jan,11

76817 Ultrasound, pregnant uterus, real time with image documentation, transvaginal M ♀
EXCLUDES *Transvaginal ultrasound, non-obstetrical (76830)*
Code also transabdominal obstetrical ultrasound, if performed
2.73 2.73 FUD XXX Q1 N1 80
AMA: 2018,Jan,8; 2017,Jan,8; 2016,Jan,13; 2015,Jan,16; 2014,Jan,11

76818 Fetal biophysical profile; with non-stress testing M ♀
Code also modifier 59 for each additional fetus
3.44 3.44 FUD XXX S Z2 80
AMA: 2018,Jan,8; 2017,Jan,8; 2016,Jan,13; 2015,Jan,16; 2014,Jan,11

76819 without non-stress testing M ♀
EXCLUDES *Amniotic fluid index without non-stress test (76815)*
Code also modifier 59 for each additional fetus
2.52 2.52 FUD XXX S Z3 80
AMA: 2018,Jan,8; 2017,Jan,8; 2016,Jan,13; 2015,Jan,16; 2014,Jan,11

76820 Doppler velocimetry, fetal; umbilical artery M
1.35 1.35 FUD XXX Q1 N1 80
AMA: 2018,Jan,8; 2017,Jan,8; 2016,Jul,8; 2016,Jan,13; 2015,Jan,16; 2014,Jan,11

76821 middle cerebral artery M
2.61 2.61 FUD XXX Q1 N1 80
AMA: 2018,Jan,8; 2017,Jan,8; 2016,Jan,13; 2015,Jan,16; 2014,Jan,11

76825 Echocardiography, fetal, cardiovascular system, real time with image documentation (2D), with or without M-mode recording; M ♀
7.79 7.79 FUD XXX S Z3 80
AMA: 2018,Jan,8; 2017,Sep,14; 2017,Jan,8; 2016,Jan,13; 2015,Jan,16; 2014,Jan,11

76826 follow-up or repeat study M ♀
4.62 4.62 FUD XXX S Z2 80
AMA: 2018,Jan,8; 2017,Sep,14

76827 Doppler echocardiography, fetal, pulsed wave and/or continuous wave with spectral display; complete M ♀
2.11 2.11 FUD XXX Q1 N1 80
AMA: 2018,Jan,8; 2017,Jan,8; 2016,Jan,13; 2015,Jan,16; 2014,Jan,11

76828 follow-up or repeat study M ♀
EXCLUDES *Color mapping (93325)*
1.51 1.51 FUD XXX Q1 N1 80
AMA: 2018,Jan,8; 2017,Jan,8; 2016,Jan,13; 2015,Jan,16; 2014,Jan,11

76830-76873 Ultrasound: Male and Female Genitalia

INCLUDES Required permanent documentation of ultrasound images except when diagnostic purpose is biometric measurement
Written documentation

EXCLUDES *Focused ultrasound ablation of uterine leiomyomata (0071T-0072T)*
Ultrasound exam that does not include thorough assessment of organ or site, recorded image, and written report

76830 Ultrasound, transvaginal ♀

EXCLUDES *Transvaginal ultrasound, obstetric (76817)*

Code also transabdominal non-obstetrical ultrasound, if performed

3.44 3.44 FUD XXX S Z2 80

AMA: 2018,Jan,8; 2017,Oct,9; 2017,Jan,8; 2016,Jan,13; 2015,Jan,16; 2014,Jan,11

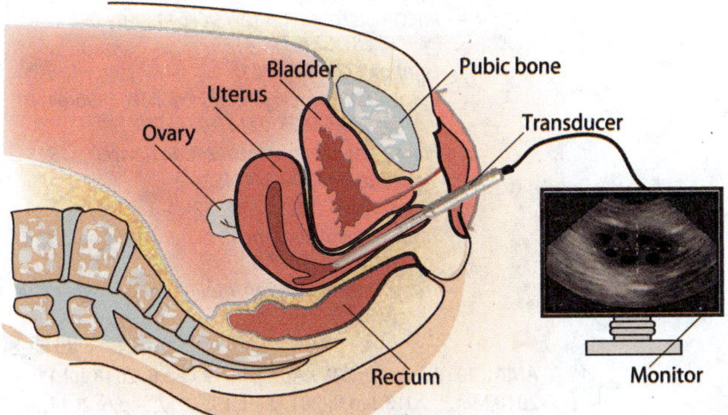

Ultrasound is performed in real time with image documentation by a transvaginal approach

76831 Saline infusion sonohysterography (SIS), including color flow Doppler, when performed ♀

Code also saline introduction for saline infusion sonohysterography (58340)

3.35 3.35 FUD XXX Q3 Z3 80

AMA: 2018,Jan,8; 2017,Jan,8; 2016,Jan,13; 2015,Jan,16; 2014,Jan,11

76856 Ultrasound, pelvic (nonobstetric), real time with image documentation; complete

INCLUDES Total examination of the female pelvic anatomy which includes:
- Bladder measurement
- Description and measurement of the uterus and adnexa
- Description of any pelvic pathology
- Measurement of the endometrium

Total examination of the male pelvis which includes:
- Bladder measurement
- Description of any pelvic pathology
- Evaluation of prostate and seminal vesicles

3.09 3.09 FUD XXX Q3 Z2 80

AMA: 2018,Jan,8; 2017,Oct,9; 2017,Jan,8; 2016,Aug,9; 2016,Jan,13; 2015,Jan,16; 2014,Jan,11

76857 limited or follow-up (eg, for follicles)

INCLUDES Focused evaluation limited to:
- Evaluation of one or more elements listed in 76856 and/or
- Reevaluation of one or more pelvic aberrancies noted on a prior ultrasound

Urinary bladder alone

EXCLUDES *Bladder volume or post-voided residual measurement without imaging the bladder (51798)*
Urinary bladder and kidneys (76770)

1.38 1.38 FUD XXX Q3 Z3 80

AMA: 2018,Jan,8; 2017,Oct,9; 2017,Jan,8; 2016,Jan,13; 2015,Jan,16; 2014,Jan,11

76870 Ultrasound, scrotum and contents ♂

2.97 2.97 FUD XXX Q1 N1 80

AMA: 2018,Jan,8; 2017,Oct,9

76872 Ultrasound, transrectal;

EXCLUDES *Colonoscopy (45391-45392)*
Hemorrhoidectomy by transanal hemorrhoidal dearterialization ([46948])
Sigmoidoscopy (45341-45342)
Transurethral prostate ablation (0421T)

3.62 3.62 FUD XXX S Z2 80

AMA: 2018,Nov,10; 2018,Jul,11; 2018,Jan,8; 2017,Oct,9; 2017,Jan,8; 2016,Jan,13; 2015,Jan,16; 2014,Jan,11

76873 prostate volume study for brachytherapy treatment planning (separate procedure) ♂

4.91 4.91 FUD XXX S Z2 80

AMA: 2018,Jan,8; 2017,Jan,8; 2016,Jan,13; 2015,Jan,16; 2014,Jan,11

76881-76886 Ultrasound: Extremities

EXCLUDES *Doppler studies of the extremities (93925-93926, 93930-93931, 93970-93971)*

76881 Ultrasound, complete joint (ie, joint space and peri-articular soft tissue structures) real-time with image documentation

INCLUDES Real time scans of a specific joint including assessment of:
- Joint space
- Muscles
- Other soft tissue
- Tendons

Required permanent documentation of images
Stress manipulations and dynamic imaging when performed
Written documentation including an explanation of any components of the joint that cannot be visualized

2.51 2.51 FUD XXX S Z3 80

AMA: 2018,Jan,8; 2017,Oct,9; 2017,Jan,8; 2016,Sep,9

76882 Ultrasound, limited, joint or other nonvascular extremity structure(s) (eg, joint space, peri-articular tendon[s], muscle[s], nerve[s], other soft tissue structure[s], or soft tissue mass[es]), real-time with image documentation

INCLUDES Limited examination of a joint or for evaluation of an extremity for a mass or other abnormality not requiring all of the components of a complete joint evaluation (76881)
Real time scans of a specific joint including assessment of:
- Joint space
- Muscles
- Other soft tissue
- Tendons

Required permanent documentation of images
Written documentation containing a description of all of the components of the joint visualized

1.62 1.62 FUD XXX Q1 N1 80

AMA: 2018,Jan,8; 2017,Oct,9; 2017,Jan,8; 2016,Sep,9

76885 Ultrasound, infant hips, real time with imaging documentation; dynamic (requiring physician or other qualified health care professional manipulation) A

4.05 4.05 FUD XXX Q1 N1 80

AMA: 2012,Feb,9-10; 2002,May,7

76886 limited, static (not requiring physician or other qualified health care professional manipulation) A

2.97 2.97 FUD XXX Q1 N1 80

AMA: 2012,Feb,9-10; 2002,May,7

76930-76970 Imaging Guidance: Ultrasound

INCLUDES Required permanent documentation of ultrasound images except when diagnostic purpose is biometric measurement
Written documentation

EXCLUDES *Focused ultrasound ablation of uterine leiomyomata (0071T-0072T)*
Ultrasound exam that does not include thorough assessment of organ or site, recorded image, and written report

~~**76930 Ultrasonic guidance for pericardiocentesis, imaging supervision and interpretation**~~

To report, see (33016-33018)

76932 Ultrasonic guidance for endomyocardial biopsy, imaging supervision and interpretation

0.00 0.00 FUD YYY N N1 80

AMA: 2012,Feb,9-10; 2001,Sep,4

76936 Ultrasound guided compression repair of arterial pseudoaneurysm or arteriovenous fistulae (includes diagnostic ultrasound evaluation, compression of lesion and imaging)

7.60 7.60 FUD XXX S Z2 80

AMA: 2012,Feb,9-10; 2002,May,7

+ **76937 Ultrasound guidance for vascular access requiring ultrasound evaluation of potential access sites, documentation of selected vessel patency, concurrent realtime ultrasound visualization of vascular needle entry, with permanent recording and reporting (List separately in addition to code for primary procedure)**

INCLUDES Ultrasonic guidance (76942)

EXCLUDES *Extremity venous noninvasive vascular diagnostic study performed separately from venous access guidance (93970-93971)*
Insertion of intravascular vena cava filter (37191-37193)
Insertion/replacement leadless pacemaker ([33274])
Ligation perforator veins (37760-37761)
Removal leadless pacemaker ([33275])
Revascularization with intravascular stent grafts in femoral-popliteal segment (0505T)

Code first primary procedure

0.96 0.96 FUD ZZZ N N1 80

AMA: 2019,May,3; 2019,Mar,6; 2018,Mar,3; 2018,Jan,8; 2017,Dec,3; 2017,Aug,10; 2017,Jul,3; 2017,Mar,3; 2017,Jan,8; 2016,Nov,3; 2016,Jul,6; 2016,Jan,13; 2015,Jul,10; 2015,Jan,16; 2014,Oct,6; 2014,Jan,11

76940 Ultrasound guidance for, and monitoring of, parenchymal tissue ablation

EXCLUDES *Ablation (20982-20983, [32994], 32998, 47370-47383, 50250, 50542, 50592-50593, 0582T)*
Ultrasound guidance:
Intraoperative (76998)
Needle placement (76942)

0.00 0.00 FUD YYY N N1 80

AMA: 2018,Jan,8; 2017,Nov,8; 2017,Jan,8; 2016,Jan,13; 2015,Jul,8; 2015,Jan,16; 2014,Jan,11

76941 Ultrasonic guidance for intrauterine fetal transfusion or cordocentesis, imaging supervision and interpretation M ♀

Code also surgical procedure (36460, 59012)

0.00 0.00 FUD XXX N N1 80

AMA: 2012,Feb,9-10; 2001,Sep,4

76942 Ultrasonic guidance for needle placement (eg, biopsy, aspiration, injection, localization device), imaging supervision and interpretation

EXCLUDES *Arthrocentesis (20604, 20606, 20611)*
Autologous WBC injection (0481T)
Breast biopsy with placement of localization device(s) (19083)
Esophagogastroduodenoscopy (43237, 43242)
Esophagoscopy (43232)
Fine needle aspiration biopsy ([10004], [10005], [10006], 10021)
Gastrointestinal endoscopic ultrasound (76975)
Hemorrhoidectomy by transanal hemorrhoidal dearterialization ([46948])
Image-guided fluid collection drainage by catheter (10030)
Injection procedures (27096, 64479-64484, 0228T-0232T)
Ligation (37760-37761)
Paravertebral facet joint injections (64490-64491, 64493-64495, 0213T-0218T)
Placement of breast localization device(s) (19285)
Sigmoidoscopy (45341-45342)
Thoracentesis (32554-32557)
Transperineal placement, periprostatic biodegradable material (55874)
Transurethral ablation, malignant prostate tissue (0582T)

1.61 1.61 FUD XXX N N1 80

AMA: 2019,Aug,10; 2019,Apr,4; 2019,Feb,8; 2018,Jul,11; 2018,Mar,3; 2018,Jan,8; 2017,Dec,13; 2017,Sep,6; 2017,Jun,10; 2017,Jan,8; 2016,Nov,3; 2016,Jun,3; 2016,Jan,9; 2016,Jan,13; 2015,Dec,3; 2015,Nov,10; 2015,Aug,8; 2015,Feb,6; 2015,Jan,16; 2014,Oct,6; 2014,Jan,11

76945 Ultrasonic guidance for chorionic villus sampling, imaging supervision and interpretation M ♀

Code also surgical procedure (59015)

0.00 0.00 FUD XXX N N1 80

AMA: 2012,Feb,9-10; 2001,Sep,4

76946 Ultrasonic guidance for amniocentesis, imaging supervision and interpretation M ♀

0.92 0.92 FUD XXX N N1 80

AMA: 2012,Feb,9-10; 2001,Sep,4

76948 Ultrasonic guidance for aspiration of ova, imaging supervision and interpretation M ♀

2.12 2.12 FUD XXX N N1 80

AMA: 2012,Feb,9-10; 2001,Sep,4

76965 Ultrasonic guidance for interstitial radioelement application

2.62 2.62 FUD XXX N N1 80

AMA: 2012,Feb,9-10; 1997,Nov,1

76970 Ultrasound study follow-up (specify)

2.54 2.54 FUD XXX Q1 N1 80

AMA: 2012,Feb,9-10; 1997,Nov,1

76975 Endoscopic Ultrasound

INCLUDES Required permanent documentation of ultrasound images except when diagnostic purpose is biometric measurement
Written documentation

EXCLUDES *Focused ultrasound ablation of uterine leiomyomata (0071T-0072T)*
Ultrasound exam that does not include thorough assessment of organ or site, recorded image, and written report

76975 Gastrointestinal endoscopic ultrasound, supervision and interpretation

INCLUDES Ultrasonic guidance (76942)

EXCLUDES *Colonoscopy (44406-44407, 45391-45392)*
Esophagogastroduodenoscopy (43237-43238, 43240, 43242, 43259)
Esophagoscopy (43231-43232)
Sigmoidoscopy (45341-45342)

0.00 0.00 FUD XXX Q2 N1 80

AMA: 2018,Jan,8; 2017,Jan,8; 2016,Jan,13; 2015,Jan,16; 2014,Jan,11

76977 Bone Density Measurements: Ultrasound

CMS: 100-02,15,80.5.5 Frequency Standards

INCLUDES Required permanent documentation of ultrasound images except when diagnostic purpose is biometric measurement
Written documentation

EXCLUDES *Ultrasound exam that does not include thorough assessment of organ or site, recorded image, and written report*

76977 **Ultrasound bone density measurement and interpretation, peripheral site(s), any method**
0.21 0.21 FUD XXX S Z3 80
AMA: 2012,Feb,9-10; 1998,Nov,1

76978-76979 Targeted Dynamic Microbubble Sonographic Contrast Characterization: Ultrasound

INCLUDES Intravenous injection (96374)

76978 **Ultrasound, targeted dynamic microbubble sonographic contrast characterization (non-cardiac); initial lesion**
9.18 9.18 FUD XXX Z2 80
AMA: 2019,Jun,9

\+ **76979** **each additional lesion with separate injection (List separately in addition to code for primary procedure)**
Code first (76978)
6.23 6.23 FUD ZZZ N1 80
AMA: 2019,Jun,9

76981-76983 Elastography: Ultrasound

EXCLUDES *Shear wave liver elastography (91200)*

76981 **Ultrasound, elastography; parenchyma (eg, organ)**
EXCLUDES *Use of code more than one time in each session for the same parenchymal organ and/or parenchymal organ and lesion*
3.04 3.04 FUD XXX Z2 80
AMA: 2019,Aug,3

76982 **first target lesion**
2.72 2.72 FUD XXX Z2 80
AMA: 2019,Aug,3

\+ **76983** **each additional target lesion (List separately in addition to code for primary procedure)**
EXCLUDES *Use of code more than two times for each organ*
Code first (76982)
1.67 1.67 FUD ZZZ N1 80
AMA: 2019,Aug,3

76998-76999 Imaging Guidance During Surgery: Ultrasound

INCLUDES Required permanent documentation of ultrasound images except when diagnostic purpose is biometric measurement
Written documentation

EXCLUDES *Focused ultrasound ablation of uterine leiomyomata (0071T-0072T)*
Ultrasound exam that does not include thorough assessment of organ or site, recorded image, and written report

76998 **Ultrasonic guidance, intraoperative**
EXCLUDES *Ablation (47370-47371, 47380-47382)*
Endovenous ablation therapy of incompetent vein (36475, 36479)
Hemorrhoidectomy by transanal hemorrhoidal dearterialization ([46948])
Ligation (37760-37761)
Wireless cardiac stimulator (0515T-0520T)
0.00 0.00 FUD XXX N N1 80
AMA: 2018,Mar,3; 2018,Jan,8; 2017,Apr,7; 2017,Jan,8; 2016,Nov,3; 2016,Jan,13; 2015,Aug,8; 2015,Jan,16; 2014,Oct,6; 2014,Jan,5; 2014,Jan,11

76999 **Unlisted ultrasound procedure (eg, diagnostic, interventional)**
0.00 0.00 FUD XXX Q1 N1 80
AMA: 2018,Jul,11; 2018,Jan,8; 2017,Jan,8; 2016,Jan,13; 2015,Jan,16; 2014,Jan,11

77001-77022 Imaging Guidance Techniques

\+ **77001** **Fluoroscopic guidance for central venous access device placement, replacement (catheter only or complete), or removal (includes fluoroscopic guidance for vascular access and catheter manipulation, any necessary contrast injections through access site or catheter with related venography radiologic supervision and interpretation, and radiographic documentation of final catheter position) (List separately in addition to code for primary procedure)**
INCLUDES Fluoroscopic guidance for needle placement (77002)
EXCLUDES *Any procedure codes that include fluoroscopic guidance in the code descriptor*
Extracorporeal membrane oxygenation (ECMO)/extracorporeal life support (ECLS) (33957-33959, [33962, 33963, 33964])
Formal extremity venography performed separately from venous access and interpreted separately (36005, 75820, 75822, 75825, 75827)
Insertion peripherally inserted central venous catheter (PICC) (36568-36569, [36572, 36573])
Replacement of peripherally inserted central venous catheter (PICC) (36584)
Code first primary procedure
2.55 2.55 FUD ZZZ N N1 80
AMA: 2019,May,3; 2018,Jan,8; 2017,Jan,8; 2016,Jan,13; 2015,Jan,16; 2014,Jan,11

\+ **77002** **Fluoroscopic guidance for needle placement (eg, biopsy, aspiration, injection, localization device) (List separately in addition to code for primary procedure)**
EXCLUDES *Ablation therapy (20982-20983)*
Any procedure codes that include fluoroscopic guidance in the code descriptor:
Radiological guidance for percutaneous drainage by catheter (75989)
Transhepatic portography (75885, 75887)
Arthrography procedure(s) (70332, 73040, 73085, 73115, 73525, 73580, 73615)
Biopsy, breast, with placement of breast localization device(s) (19081-19086)
Image-guided fluid collection drainage by catheter (10030)
Placement of breast localization device(s) (19281-19288)
Platelet rich plasma injection(s) (0232T)
Thoracentesis (32554-32557)
Code first surgical procedure (10160, 20206, 20220, 20225, 20520, 20525-20526, 20550-20555, 20600, 20605, 20610, 20612, 20615, 21116, 21550, 23350, 24220, 25246, 27093-27095, 27369, 27648, 32400-32405, 32553, 36002, 38220-38222, 38505, 38794, 41019, 42400-42405, 47000-47001, 48102, 49180, 49411, 50200, 50390, 51100-51102, 55700, 55876, 60100, 62268-62269, 64505, 64600-64605)
2.86 2.86 FUD ZZZ N N1 80
AMA: 2019,Aug,7; 2019,Mar,6; 2019,Apr,4; 2019,Feb,8; 2018,Dec,10; 2018,Dec,10; 2018,Jan,8; 2017,Jun,10; 2017,Jan,8; 2016,Sep,9; 2016,Aug,7; 2016,Jun,3; 2016,Jan,13; 2016,Jan,9; 2015,Dec,3; 2015,Aug,6; 2015,Jul,8; 2015,Feb,10; 2015,Feb,6; 2015,Jan,16; 2014,Jan,11

+ **77003** **Fluoroscopic guidance and localization of needle or catheter tip for spine or paraspinous diagnostic or therapeutic injection procedures (epidural or subarachnoid) (List separately in addition to code for primary procedure)**

EXCLUDES *Any procedure codes that include fluoroscopic guidance in the code descriptor*
Arthrodesis (22586)
Image-guided fluid collection drainage by catheter (10030)
Injection of medication (subarachnoid/interlaminar epidural) (62320, 62321, 62322, 62323, 62324, 62325, 62326, 62327)
Spinal puncture (62270, [62328], 62272, [62329])

Code first (61050-61055, 62267, 62273, 62280-62284, 64510, 64517, 64520, 64610, 96450)

2.77 2.77 FUD ZZZ N N1 80

AMA: 2018,Jan,8; 2017,Dec,13; 2017,Sep,6; 2017,Feb,9; 2017,Feb,12; 2017,Jan,8; 2016,Jan,9; 2016,Jan,13; 2016,Jan,11; 2015,Jan,16; 2014,Jan,11

77011 **Computed tomography guidance for stereotactic localization**

EXCLUDES *Arthrodesis (22586)*

6.47 6.47 FUD XXX N N1

AMA: 2018,Jan,8; 2017,Jan,8; 2016,Jan,13; 2015,Jan,16; 2014,Jan,11

77012 **Computed tomography guidance for needle placement (eg, biopsy, aspiration, injection, localization device), radiological supervision and interpretation**

EXCLUDES *Arthrodesis (22586)*
Autologous white blood cell concentrate (0481T)
Destruction of paravertebral facet joint nerve by neurolysis ([64633, 64634, 64635, 64636])
Fine needle aspiration biopsy using CT guidance ([10009, 10010])
Image-guided fluid collection drainage by catheter (10030)
Injection, paravertebral facet joint (64490-64495)
Platelet rich plasma injection(s) (0232T)
Sacroiliac joint arthrography (27096)
Spinal puncture (62270, [62328], 62272, [62329])
Thoracentesis (32554-32557)
Transforaminal epidural needle placement/injection (64479-64480, 64483-64484)

4.27 4.27 FUD XXX N N1

AMA: 2019,Feb,8; 2019,Apr,4; 2018,Jan,8; 2017,Sep,6; 2017,Feb,12; 2017,Jan,8; 2016,Jun,3; 2016,Jan,13; 2015,Dec,3; 2015,Feb,6; 2015,Jan,16; 2014,Jan,11

77013 **Computed tomography guidance for, and monitoring of, parenchymal tissue ablation**

EXCLUDES *Ablation therapy (20982-20983, 32994, 32998, 47382-47383, 50592-50593)*

0.00 0.00 FUD XXX N N1 80

AMA: 2018,Jan,8; 2017,Nov,8; 2017,Jan,8; 2016,Jan,13; 2015,Jul,8; 2015,Jan,16; 2014,Jan,11

77014 **Computed tomography guidance for placement of radiation therapy fields**

Code also placement of interstitial device(s) for radiation therapy guidance (31627, 32553, 49411, 55876)

3.41 3.41 FUD XXX N N1

AMA: 2018,Jan,8; 2017,Jan,8; 2016,Feb,3; 2016,Jan,13; 2015,Apr,10; 2015,Jan,16; 2014,Jan,11

77021 **Magnetic resonance imaging guidance for needle placement (eg, for biopsy, needle aspiration, injection, or placement of localization device) radiological supervision and interpretation**

EXCLUDES *Autologous white blood cell concentrate (0481T)*
Biopsy, breast, with placement of breast localization device(s) (19085)
Fine needle aspiration biopsy using MR guidance ([10011, 10012])
Image-guided fluid collection drainage by catheter (10030)
Placement of breast localization device(s) (19287)
Platelet rich plasma injection(s) (0232T)
Surgical procedure
Thoracentesis (32554-32557)

13.4 13.4 FUD XXX N N1

AMA: 2019,Feb,8; 2019,Apr,4; 2018,Jul,11; 2018,Jan,8; 2017,Jun,10; 2017,Jan,8; 2016,Jun,3; 2016,Jan,13; 2015,Dec,3; 2015,Feb,6; 2015,Jan,16; 2014,Jan,11

77022 **Magnetic resonance imaging guidance for, and monitoring of, parenchymal tissue ablation**

EXCLUDES *Ablation:*
Percutaneous radiofrequency (32994, 32998, 47382-47383, 50592-50593)
Reduction or eradication of 1 or more bone tumors (20982-20983)
Uterine leiomyomata by focused ablation (0071T-0072T)

0.00 0.00 FUD XXX N N1 80

AMA: 2019,Sep,10; 2018,Mar,3; 2018,Jan,8; 2017,Nov,8; 2017,Jan,8; 2016,Nov,3; 2016,Jan,13; 2015,Jul,8; 2015,Jan,16; 2014,Oct,6; 2014,Jan,11

77046-77067 Radiography: Breast

77046 **Magnetic resonance imaging, breast, without contrast material; unilateral**

7.02 7.02 FUD XXX Z2 80

AMA: 2019,Aug,5

77047 **bilateral**

7.21 7.21 FUD XXX Z2 80

AMA: 2019,Aug,5

77048 **Magnetic resonance imaging, breast, without and with contrast material(s), including computer-aided detection (CAD real-time lesion detection, characterization and pharmacokinetic analysis), when performed; unilateral**

11.1 11.1 FUD XXX 80

AMA: 2019,Aug,5

77049 **bilateral**

11.3 11.3 FUD XXX 80

AMA: 2019,Aug,5

77053 **Mammary ductogram or galactogram, single duct, radiological supervision and interpretation**

Code also injection procedure (19030)

1.62 1.62 FUD XXX Q2 N1

AMA: 2018,Jan,8; 2017,Jan,8; 2016,Jan,13; 2015,Jan,16; 2014,Jan,11

77054 **Mammary ductogram or galactogram, multiple ducts, radiological supervision and interpretation**

2.12 2.12 FUD XXX Q2 N1

AMA: 2018,Jan,8; 2017,Jan,8; 2016,Jan,13; 2015,Jan,16; 2014,Jan,11

77061 **Diagnostic digital breast tomosynthesis; unilateral**

EXCLUDES *3D rendering (76376-76377)*
Screening mammography (77067)

0.00 0.00 FUD XXX E

AMA: 2018,Jan,8

77062 **bilateral**

EXCLUDES *3D rendering (76376-76377)*

Screening mammography (77067)

0.00 0.00 FUD XXX E

AMA: 2018,Jan,8; 2017,Jan,8; 2016,Dec,15

+ 77063 **Screening digital breast tomosynthesis, bilateral (List separately in addition to code for primary procedure)**

EXCLUDES *3D rendering (76376-76377)*

Diagnostic mammography (77065-77066)

Code first (77067)

1.55 1.55 FUD ZZZ A

AMA: 2018,Jan,8; 2017,Jan,8; 2016,Dec,15

77065 **Diagnostic mammography, including computer-aided detection (CAD) when performed; unilateral**

3.77 3.77 FUD XXX A 80

AMA: 2019,Aug,5; 2018,Jan,8; 2017,Jan,8; 2016,Dec,15

77066 **bilateral**

4.77 4.77 FUD XXX A 80

AMA: 2019,Aug,5; 2018,Jan,8; 2017,Jan,8; 2016,Dec,15

77067 **Screening mammography, bilateral (2-view study of each breast), including computer-aided detection (CAD) when performed**

EXCLUDES *Breast scan, electrical impedance (76499)*

3.84 3.84 FUD XXX A 80

AMA: 2019,Aug,5; 2018,Jan,8; 2017,Jan,8; 2016,Dec,15

77071-77086 [77085, 77086] Additional Evaluations of Bones and Joints

77071 **Manual application of stress performed by physician or other qualified health care professional for joint radiography, including contralateral joint if indicated**

Code also interpretation of stressed images according to anatomical site and number of views

1.43 1.43 FUD XXX Q1 N1 80 26

AMA: 2018,Jan,8; 2017,Jan,8; 2016,Jan,13; 2015,Jan,16; 2014,Jan,11

77072 **Bone age studies**

0.68 0.68 FUD XXX Q1 N1 80

AMA: 2018,Jan,8; 2017,Jan,8; 2016,Jan,13; 2015,Jan,16; 2014,Jan,11

77073 **Bone length studies (orthoroentgenogram, scanogram)**

1.06 1.06 FUD XXX Q1 N1 80

AMA: 2018,Jan,8; 2017,Jan,8; 2016,Jan,13; 2015,Jan,16; 2014,Jan,11

77074 **Radiologic examination, osseous survey; limited (eg, for metastases)**

1.91 1.91 FUD XXX Q1 N1 80

AMA: 2018,Jan,8; 2017,Jan,8; 2016,Jan,13; 2015,Jan,16; 2014,Jan,11

77075 **complete (axial and appendicular skeleton)**

2.60 2.60 FUD XXX Q1 N1 80

AMA: 2018,Jan,8; 2017,Jan,8; 2016,Jan,13; 2015,Jan,16; 2014,Jan,11

77076 **Radiologic examination, osseous survey, infant**

2.85 2.85 FUD XXX Q1 N1 80

AMA: 2018,Jan,8; 2017,Jan,8; 2016,Jan,13; 2015,Jan,16; 2014,Jan,11

77077 **Joint survey, single view, 2 or more joints (specify)**

1.09 1.09 FUD XXX Q1 N1 80

AMA: 2018,Jan,8; 2017,Jan,8; 2016,Jan,13; 2015,Jan,16; 2014,Jan,11

77078 **Computed tomography, bone mineral density study, 1 or more sites, axial skeleton (eg, hips, pelvis, spine)**

3.24 3.24 FUD XXX S Z2 80

AMA: 2018,Jan,8; 2017,Jan,8; 2016,Jan,13; 2015,Jan,16; 2014,Jan,11

77080 **Dual-energy X-ray absorptiometry (DXA), bone density study, 1 or more sites; axial skeleton (eg, hips, pelvis, spine)**

EXCLUDES *Dual-energy x-ray absorptiometry (DXA), bone density study ([77085])*

Vertebral fracture assessment via dual-energy x-ray absorptiometry (DXA) ([77086])

1.13 1.13 FUD XXX S Z3 80

AMA: 2018,Jan,8; 2017,Jan,8; 2016,Jan,13; 2015,Jan,16; 2014,Jan,11

77081 **appendicular skeleton (peripheral) (eg, radius, wrist, heel)**

0.94 0.94 FUD XXX S Z3 80

AMA: 2018,Jan,8; 2017,Jan,8; 2016,Jan,13; 2015,Jan,16; 2014,Jan,11

77085 **axial skeleton (eg, hips, pelvis, spine), including vertebral fracture assessment**

1.54 1.54 FUD XXX Q1 N1 80

EXCLUDES *Dual-energy x-ray absorptiometry (DXA), bone density study (77080)*

Vertebral fracture assessment via dual-energy x-ray absorptiometry (DXA) ([77086])

77086 **Vertebral fracture assessment via dual-energy X-ray absorptiometry (DXA)**

0.99 0.99 FUD XXX Q1 N1 80

EXCLUDES *Dual-energy x-ray absorptiometry (DXA), bone density study (77080)*

Therapy performed more than one time for treatment to a specific area

Vertebral fracture assessment via dual-energy X-ray absorptiometry (DXA) ([77085])

77084 **Magnetic resonance (eg, proton) imaging, bone marrow blood supply**

10.7 10.7 FUD XXX S Z2 80

AMA: 2018,Jan,8; 2017,Jan,8; 2016,Jan,13; 2015,Jan,16; 2014,Jan,11

77085 **Resequenced code. See code following 77081.**

77086 **Resequenced code. See code before 77084.**

77261-77263 Therapeutic Radiology: Treatment Planning

INCLUDES Determination of:

- Appropriate treatment devices
- Number and size of treatment ports
- Treatment method
- Treatment time/dosage
- Treatment volume

Interpretation of special testing

Tumor localization

EXCLUDES *Brachytherapy (0394T-0395T)*

Radiation treatment delivery, superficial (77401)

77261 **Therapeutic radiology treatment planning; simple**

INCLUDES Planning for single treatment area included in a single port or simple parallel opposed ports with simple or no blocking

2.03 2.03 FUD XXX B 80 26

AMA: 2018,Jan,8; 2017,Jan,8; 2016,Feb,3; 2016,Jan,13; 2015,Jan,16; 2014,Jan,11

77262 **intermediate**

INCLUDES Planning for three or more converging ports, two separate treatment sites, multiple blocks, or special time dose constraints

3.06 3.06 FUD XXX B 80 26

AMA: 2018,Jan,8; 2017,Jan,8; 2016,Feb,3; 2016,Jan,13; 2015,Jan,16; 2014,Jan,11

77263 **complex**

INCLUDES Planning for very complex blocking, custom shielding blocks, tangential ports, special wedges or compensators, three or more separate treatment areas, rotational or special beam considerations, combination of treatment modalities

4.78 4.78 FUD XXX B 80 26

AMA: 2018,Jan,8; 2017,Jan,8; 2016,Feb,3; 2016,Jan,13; 2015,Jan,16; 2014,Jan,11

77280-77299 Radiation Therapy Simulation

77280 Therapeutic radiology simulation-aided field setting; simple

INCLUDES Simulation of a single treatment site

7.84 7.84 FUD XXX S Z2 80

AMA: 2018,Jan,8; 2017,Jan,8; 2016,Jan,13; 2015,Apr,10; 2015,Jan,16; 2014,Jan,11

77285 intermediate

INCLUDES Two different treatment sites

12.9 12.9 FUD XXX S Z2 80

AMA: 2018,Jan,8; 2017,Jan,8; 2016,Jan,13; 2015,Apr,10; 2015,Jan,16; 2014,Jan,11

77290 complex

INCLUDES Brachytherapy
Complex blocking
Contrast material
Custom shielding blocks
Hyperthermia probe verification
Rotation, arc or particle therapy
Simulation to ≥ 3 treatment sites

14.4 14.4 FUD XXX S Z2 80

AMA: 2018,Jan,8; 2017,Jan,8; 2016,Sep,9; 2016,Jan,13; 2015,Apr,10; 2015,Jan,16; 2014,Jan,11

+ **77293 Respiratory motion management simulation (List separately in addition to code for primary procedure)**

Code first (77295, 77301)

13.0 13.0 FUD ZZZ N N1 80

AMA: 2018,Jan,8; 2017,Jan,8; 2016,Jan,13; 2015,Dec,16

77295 **Resequenced code. See code before 77300.**

77299 Unlisted procedure, therapeutic radiology clinical treatment planning

0.00 0.00 FUD XXX S Z2 80

AMA: 2018,Jan,8; 2017,Jan,8; 2016,Jan,13; 2015,Jan,16; 2014,Jan,11

77295-77370 [77295] Radiation Physics Services

\# **77295 3-dimensional radiotherapy plan, including dose-volume histograms**

13.9 13.9 FUD XXX S Z3 80

AMA: 2018,Jan,8; 2017,Jan,8; 2016,Jan,13; 2015,Dec,16; 2015,Jun,6; 2015,Jan,16; 2014,Jan,11

77300 Basic radiation dosimetry calculation, central axis depth dose calculation, TDF, NSD, gap calculation, off axis factor, tissue inhomogeneity factors, calculation of non-ionizing radiation surface and depth dose, as required during course of treatment, only when prescribed by the treating physician

EXCLUDES *Brachytherapy (77316-77318, 77767-77772, 0394T-0395T)*
Teletherapy plan (77306-77307, 77321)

1.89 1.89 FUD XXX S Z3 80

AMA: 2018,Jan,8; 2017,Jan,8; 2016,Jan,13; 2015,Jan,16; 2014,Jan,11

77301 Intensity modulated radiotherapy plan, including dose-volume histograms for target and critical structure partial tolerance specifications

55.0 55.0 FUD XXX S Z2 80

AMA: 2018,Jan,8; 2017,Jan,8; 2016,Jan,13; 2015,Jan,16; 2014,Jan,11

77306 Teletherapy isodose plan; simple (1 or 2 unmodified ports directed to a single area of interest), includes basic dosimetry calculation(s)

EXCLUDES *Brachytherapy (0394T-0395T)*
Radiation dosimetry calculation (77300)
Radiation treatment delivery (77401)
Therapy performed more than one time for treatment to a specific area

4.25 4.25 FUD XXX S Z3 80

AMA: 2018,Jan,8; 2017,Jan,8; 2016,Feb,3

77307 complex (multiple treatment areas, tangential ports, the use of wedges, blocking, rotational beam, or special beam considerations), includes basic dosimetry calculation(s)

EXCLUDES *Brachytherapy (0394T-0395T)*
Radiation dosimetry calculation (77300)
Radiation treatment delivery (77401)
Therapy performed more than one time for treatment to a specific area

8.22 8.22 FUD XXX S Z3 80

AMA: 2018,Jan,8; 2017,Jan,8; 2016,Feb,3

77316 Brachytherapy isodose plan; simple (calculation[s] made from 1 to 4 sources, or remote afterloading brachytherapy, 1 channel), includes basic dosimetry calculation(s)

EXCLUDES *Brachytherapy (0394T-0395T)*
Radiation dosimetry calculation (77300)
Radiation treatment delivery (77401)

5.78 5.78 FUD XXX S Z3 80

AMA: 2018,Jan,8; 2017,Jan,8; 2016,Feb,3

77317 intermediate (calculation[s] made from 5 to 10 sources, or remote afterloading brachytherapy, 2-12 channels), includes basic dosimetry calculation(s)

EXCLUDES *Brachytherapy (0394T-0395T)*
Radiation dosimetry calculation (77300)
Radiation treatment delivery (77401)

7.57 7.57 FUD XXX S Z2 80

AMA: 2018,Jan,8; 2017,Jan,8

77318 complex (calculation[s] made from over 10 sources, or remote afterloading brachytherapy, over 12 channels), includes basic dosimetry calculation(s)

EXCLUDES *Brachytherapy (0394T-0395T)*
Radiation dosimetry calculation (77300)
Radiation treatment delivery (77401)

10.8 10.8 FUD XXX S Z2 80

AMA: 2018,Jan,8; 2017,Jan,8; 2016,Feb,3

77321 Special teletherapy port plan, particles, hemibody, total body

2.66 2.66 FUD XXX S Z3 80

AMA: 2018,Jan,8; 2017,Jan,8; 2016,Jan,13; 2015,Jan,16; 2014,Jan,11

77331 Special dosimetry (eg, TLD, microdosimetry) (specify), only when prescribed by the treating physician

1.84 1.84 FUD XXX S Z3 80

AMA: 2018,Jan,8; 2017,Jan,8; 2016,Jan,13; 2015,Jun,6; 2015,Jan,16; 2014,Jan,11

77332 Treatment devices, design and construction; simple (simple block, simple bolus)

EXCLUDES *Brachytherapy (0394T-0395T)*
Radiation treatment delivery (77401)

1.49 1.49 FUD XXX S Z3 80

AMA: 2018,Jan,8; 2017,Jan,8; 2016,Feb,3; 2016,Jan,13; 2015,Jan,16; 2014,Jan,11

77333 intermediate (multiple blocks, stents, bite blocks, special bolus)

EXCLUDES *Brachytherapy (0394T-0395T)*
Radiation treatment delivery (77401)

3.10 3.10 FUD XXX S Z2 80

AMA: 2018,Jan,8; 2017,Jan,8; 2016,Feb,3; 2016,Jan,13; 2015,Jan,16; 2014,Jan,11

77334 complex (irregular blocks, special shields, compensators, wedges, molds or casts)

EXCLUDES *Brachytherapy (0394T-0395T)*
Radiation treatment delivery (77401)

3.64 3.64 FUD XXX S Z3 80

AMA: 2018,Jan,8; 2017,Jan,8; 2016,Sep,9; 2016,Feb,3; 2016,Jan,13; 2015,Dec,16; 2015,Jan,16; 2014,Jan,11

77336 **Continuing medical physics consultation, including assessment of treatment parameters, quality assurance of dose delivery, and review of patient treatment documentation in support of the radiation oncologist, reported per week of therapy**

EXCLUDES *Brachytherapy (0394T-0395T)*
Radiation treatment delivery (77401)

2.26 2.26 FUD XXX S Z2 80 TC

AMA: 2018,Jan,8; 2017,Jan,8; 2016,Feb,3; 2016,Jan,13; 2015,Jan,16; 2014,Jan,11

77338 **Multi-leaf collimator (MLC) device(s) for intensity modulated radiation therapy (IMRT), design and construction per IMRT plan**

EXCLUDES *Immobilization in IMRT treatment (77332-77334)*
Intensity modulated radiation treatment delivery (IMRT) (77385)
Use of code more than one time per IMRT plan

14.1 14.1 FUD XXX S Z2 80

AMA: 2018,Jan,8; 2017,Jan,8; 2016,Jan,13; 2015,Jan,16; 2014,Jan,11

77370 **Special medical radiation physics consultation**

3.52 3.52 FUD XXX S Z2 80 TC

AMA: 2018,Jan,8; 2017,Jan,8; 2016,Feb,3; 2016,Jan,13; 2015,Jun,6; 2015,Jan,16; 2014,Jan,11

77371-77399 Stereotactic Radiosurgery (SRS) Planning and Delivery

77371 **Radiation treatment delivery, stereotactic radiosurgery (SRS), complete course of treatment of cranial lesion(s) consisting of 1 session; multi-source Cobalt 60 based**

EXCLUDES *Guidance with computed tomography for radiation therapy field placement (77014)*

0.00 0.00 FUD XXX J 80 TC

AMA: 2018,Jan,8; 2017,Jan,8; 2016,Jan,13; 2015,Jan,16; 2014,Jul,8; 2014,Jan,11

77372 **linear accelerator based**

EXCLUDES *Guidance with computed tomography for radiation therapy field placement (77014)*
Radiation treatment supervision (77432)

30.2 30.2 FUD XXX J 80 TC

AMA: 2018,Jan,8; 2017,Jan,8; 2016,Jan,13; 2015,Jan,16; 2014,Jul,8; 2014,Jan,11

77373 **Stereotactic body radiation therapy, treatment delivery, per fraction to 1 or more lesions, including image guidance, entire course not to exceed 5 fractions**

EXCLUDES *Guidance with computed tomography for radiation therapy field placement (77014)*
Intensity modulated radiation treatment delivery (IMRT) (77385-77386)
Radiation treatment delivery (77401-77402, 77407, 77412)
Single fraction cranial lesion(s) (77371-77372)

36.6 36.6 FUD XXX S 80 TC

AMA: 2018,Jan,8; 2017,Jan,8; 2016,Jan,13; 2015,Jun,6; 2015,Jan,16; 2014,Jul,8; 2014,Jan,11

77385 **Resequenced code. See code following 77417.**

77386 **Resequenced code. See code following 77417.**

77387 **Resequenced code. See code following 77417.**

77399 **Unlisted procedure, medical radiation physics, dosimetry and treatment devices, and special services**

0.00 0.00 FUD XXX S Z2 80

AMA: 2018,Jan,8; 2017,Jan,8; 2016,Jan,13; 2015,Jan,16; 2014,Jan,11

77401-77425 [77385, 77386, 77387, 77424, 77425] Radiation Treatment

INCLUDES Technical component and assorted energy levels

77401 **Radiation treatment delivery, superficial and/or ortho voltage, per day**

EXCLUDES *Continuing medical physics consultation (77336)*
Isodose plan:
Brachytherapy (77316-77318)
Teletherapy (77306-77307)
Management of:
Intraoperative radiation treatment (77469-77470)
Radiation therapy (77431-77432)
Radiation treatment (77427)
Stereotactic body radiation therapy (77435)
Stereotactic body radiation therapy, treatment delivery (77373)
Unlisted procedure, therapeutic radiology treatment management (77499)
Therapeutic radiology treatment planning (77261-77263)
Treatment devices, design and construction (77332-77334)

Code also E&M services when performed alone, as appropriate

0.70 0.70 FUD XXX S Z3 80 TC

AMA: 2018,Jan,8; 2017,Jan,8; 2016,Feb,3; 2016,Jan,13; 2015,Dec,14; 2015,Jan,16; 2014,Jan,11

77402 **Radiation treatment delivery, ≥1 MeV; simple**

EXCLUDES *Stereotactic body radiation therapy, treatment delivery (77373)*

0.00 0.00 FUD XXX S Z2 80 TC

AMA: 2018,Jan,8; 2017,Jan,8; 2016,Jun,9; 2016,Mar,7; 2016,Feb,3; 2016,Jan,13; 2015,Dec,14; 2015,Jan,16; 2014,Jan,11

77407 **intermediate**

EXCLUDES *Stereotactic body radiation therapy, treatment delivery (77373)*

0.00 0.00 FUD XXX S Z2 80 TC

AMA: 2018,Jan,8; 2017,Jan,8; 2016,Jun,9; 2016,Mar,7; 2016,Feb,3; 2016,Jan,13; 2015,Dec,14; 2015,Jan,16; 2014,Jan,11

77412 **complex**

0.00 0.00 FUD XXX S Z2 80 TC

AMA: 2018,Jan,8; 2017,Jan,8; 2016,Jun,9; 2016,Mar,7; 2016,Feb,3; 2016,Jan,13; 2015,Dec,14; 2015,Jan,16; 2014,Jan,11

77417 **Therapeutic radiology port image(s)**

0.32 0.32 FUD XXX N N1 80 TC

AMA: 2018,Jan,8; 2017,Dec,14; 2017,Jan,8; 2016,Jan,13; 2015,Dec,14; 2015,Jan,16; 2014,Jan,11

77385 **Intensity modulated radiation treatment delivery (IMRT), includes guidance and tracking, when performed; simple**

0.00 0.00 FUD XXX S Z2 80 TC

AMA: 2018,Jan,8; 2017,Jan,8; 2016,Feb,3

77386 **complex**

0.00 0.00 FUD XXX S Z2 80 TC

AMA: 2018,Jan,8; 2017,Jan,8; 2016,Feb,3

77387 **Guidance for localization of target volume for delivery of radiation treatment, includes intrafraction tracking, when performed**

0.00 0.00 FUD XXX N N1 80

AMA: 2018,Jan,8; 2017,Jan,8; 2016,Feb,3; 2016,Jan,13; 2015,Dec,16; 2015,Dec,14

77424 **Intraoperative radiation treatment delivery, x-ray, single treatment session**

0.00 0.00 FUD XXX J Z2

AMA: 2018,Jan,8; 2017,Jan,8; 2016,Jan,13; 2015,Dec,14

77425 **Intraoperative radiation treatment delivery, electrons, single treatment session**

0.00 0.00 FUD XXX J Z2

AMA: 2018,Jan,8; 2017,Jan,8; 2016,Jan,13; 2015,Dec,14; 2015,Jan,16; 2014,Jan,11

77423-77425 Neutron Therapy

77423 **High energy neutron radiation treatment delivery, 1 or more isocenter(s) with coplanar or non-coplanar geometry with blocking and/or wedge, and/or compensator(s)**
0.00 0.00 FUD XXX S Z3 80 TC
AMA: 2018,Jan,8; 2017,Jan,8; 2016,Jan,13; 2015,Dec,14; 2015,Jan,16; 2014,Jan,11

77424 **Resequenced code. See code following 77417.**

77425 **Resequenced code. See code following 77417.**

77427-77499 Radiation Therapy Management

INCLUDES Assessment of patient for medical evaluation and management (at least one per treatment management service) that includes:
Coordination of care/treatment
Evaluation of patient's response to treatment
Review of:
Dose delivery
Dosimetry
Lab tests
Patient treatment set-up
Port film
Treatment parameters
X-rays
Units of five fractions or treatment sessions regardless of time. Two or more fractions performed on the same day can be counted separately provided there is a distinct break in service between sessions and the fractions are of the character usually furnished on different days.

EXCLUDES *High dose rate electronic brachytherapy (0394T-0395T)*
Radiation treatment delivery (77401)

77427 **Radiation treatment management, 5 treatments**
5.37 5.37 FUD XXX B 26
AMA: 2018,Jan,8; 2017,Jan,8; 2016,Feb,3; 2016,Jan,13; 2015,Jun,6; 2015,Jan,16; 2014,Jan,11

77431 **Radiation therapy management with complete course of therapy consisting of 1 or 2 fractions only**
2.96 2.96 FUD XXX B 80 26
AMA: 2018,Jan,8; 2017,Jan,8; 2016,Feb,3; 2016,Jan,13; 2015,Jun,6; 2015,Jan,16; 2014,Jan,11

77432 **Stereotactic radiation treatment management of cranial lesion(s) (complete course of treatment consisting of 1 session)**
12.0 12.0 FUD XXX B 80 26
AMA: 2018,Jan,8; 2017,Jan,8; 2016,Feb,3; 2016,Jan,13; 2015,Dec,14; 2015,Dec,16; 2015,Jun,6; 2015,Jan,16; 2014,Jul,8; 2014,Jan,11

77435 **Stereotactic body radiation therapy, treatment management, per treatment course, to 1 or more lesions, including image guidance, entire course not to exceed 5 fractions**
18.1 18.1 FUD XXX N N1 80 26
AMA: 2018,Jan,8; 2017,Jan,8; 2016,Feb,3; 2016,Jan,13; 2015,Dec,14; 2015,Jun,6; 2015,Jan,16; 2014,Jan,11

77469 **Intraoperative radiation treatment management**
9.00 9.00 FUD XXX B 80
AMA: 2018,Jan,8; 2017,Jan,8; 2016,Feb,3; 2015,Jun,6

77470 **Special treatment procedure (eg, total body irradiation, hemibody radiation, per oral or endocavitary irradiation)**
3.75 3.75 FUD XXX S Z3 80
AMA: 2018,Jan,8; 2017,Jan,8; 2016,Feb,3; 2016,Jan,13; 2015,Jun,6; 2015,Jan,16; 2014,Jan,11

77499 **Unlisted procedure, therapeutic radiology treatment management**
0.00 0.00 FUD XXX B 80
AMA: 2018,Jan,8; 2017,Jan,8; 2016,Feb,3; 2016,Jan,13; 2015,Jun,6; 2015,Jan,16; 2014,Jan,11

77520-77525 Proton Therapy

EXCLUDES *High dose rate electronic brachytherapy, per fraction (0394T-0395T)*

77520 **Proton treatment delivery; simple, without compensation**
0.00 0.00 FUD XXX S Z2 80 TC
AMA: 2018,Jan,8; 2017,Jan,8; 2016,Jan,13; 2015,Jan,16; 2014,Jan,11

77522 **simple, with compensation**
0.00 0.00 FUD XXX S Z2 80 TC
AMA: 2012,Feb,9-10; 2010,Oct,3-4

77523 **intermediate**
0.00 0.00 FUD XXX S Z2 80 TC
AMA: 2018,Jan,8; 2017,Jan,8; 2016,Jan,13; 2015,Jan,16; 2014,Jan,11

77525 **complex**
0.00 0.00 FUD XXX S Z2 80 TC
AMA: 2012,Feb,9-10; 2010,Oct,3-4

77600-77620 Hyperthermia Treatment

CMS: 100-03,110.1 Hyperthermia for Treatment of Cancer

INCLUDES Interstitial insertion of temperature sensors
Management during the course of therapy
Normal follow-up care for three months after completion
Physics planning
Use of heat generating devices

EXCLUDES *Initial E&M service*
Radiation therapy treatment (77371-77373, 77401-77412, 77423)

77600 **Hyperthermia, externally generated; superficial (ie, heating to a depth of 4 cm or less)**
12.7 12.7 FUD XXX S Z2 80
AMA: 2018,Jan,8; 2017,Jan,8; 2016,Jan,13; 2015,Jan,16; 2014,Jan,11

77605 **deep (ie, heating to depths greater than 4 cm)**
22.0 22.0 FUD XXX S Z2 80
AMA: 2018,Jan,8; 2017,Jan,8; 2016,Jan,13; 2015,Jan,16; 2014,Jan,11

77610 **Hyperthermia generated by interstitial probe(s); 5 or fewer interstitial applicators**
19.6 19.6 FUD XXX S Z2 80
AMA: 2018,Jan,8; 2017,Jan,8; 2016,Jan,13; 2015,Jan,16; 2014,Jan,11

77615 **more than 5 interstitial applicators**
30.0 30.0 FUD XXX S Z2 80
AMA: 2018,Jan,8; 2017,Jan,8; 2016,Jan,13; 2015,Jan,16; 2014,Jan,11

77620 **Hyperthermia generated by intracavitary probe(s)**
14.6 14.6 FUD XXX S Z2 80
AMA: 2018,Jan,8; 2017,Jan,8; 2016,Jan,13; 2015,Jan,16; 2014,Jan,11

77750-77799 Brachytherapy

CMS: 100-04,13,70.4 Clinical Brachytherapy; 100-04,13,70.5 Radiation Physics Services; 100-04,4,61.4.4 Billing for Brachytherapy Source Supervision, Handling and Loading Costs

INCLUDES Hospital admission and daily visits

EXCLUDES *Placement of:*
Heyman capsules (58346)
Ovoids and tandems (57155)

77750 **Infusion or instillation of radioelement solution (includes 3-month follow-up care)**
10.7 10.7 FUD 090 S Z2 80
AMA: 2018,Jan,8; 2017,Jan,8; 2016,Jan,13; 2015,Jan,16; 2014,Jan,11

77761 **Intracavitary radiation source application; simple**
11.3 11.3 FUD 090 S Z3 80
AMA: 2018,Jan,8; 2017,Jan,8; 2016,Jan,13; 2015,Jan,16; 2014,Jan,11

77762 **intermediate**
15.0 15.0 FUD 090 S Z3 80
AMA: 2018,Jan,8; 2017,Jan,8; 2016,Jan,13; 2015,Jan,16; 2014,Jan,11

77763 **complex**
21.3 21.3 FUD 090 S Z3 80
AMA: 2018,Jan,8; 2017,Jan,8; 2016,Jan,13; 2015,Jan,16; 2014,Jan,11

77767 **Remote afterloading high dose rate radionuclide skin surface brachytherapy, includes basic dosimetry, when performed; lesion diameter up to 2.0 cm or 1 channel**
6.60 6.60 FUD XXX S Z2 80

77768 **lesion diameter over 2.0 cm and 2 or more channels, or multiple lesions**
10.1 10.1 FUD XXX S Z2 80

77770 **Remote afterloading high dose rate radionuclide interstitial or intracavitary brachytherapy, includes basic dosimetry, when performed; 1 channel**
9.36 9.36 FUD XXX S Z3 80

77771 **2-12 channels**
17.0 17.0 FUD XXX S Z2 80

77772 **over 12 channels**
25.8 25.8 FUD XXX S Z2 80

77778 **Interstitial radiation source application, complex, includes supervision, handling, loading of radiation source, when performed**
24.0 24.0 FUD 000 S Z2 80
AMA: 2018,Jan,8; 2017,Jan,8; 2016,Jan,13; 2015,Jan,16; 2014,Jan,11

77789 **Surface application of low dose rate radionuclide source**
3.49 3.49 FUD 000 S Z2 80
AMA: 2018,Jan,8; 2017,Jan,8; 2016,Jan,13; 2015,Jan,16; 2014,Jan,11

77790 **Supervision, handling, loading of radiation source**
0.43 0.43 FUD XXX N N1 80 TC
AMA: 2018,Jan,8; 2017,Jan,8; 2016,Jan,13; 2015,Jan,16; 2014,Jan,11

77799 **Unlisted procedure, clinical brachytherapy**
0.00 0.00 FUD XXX S Z2 80
AMA: 2018,Jan,8; 2017,Jan,8; 2016,Jan,13; 2015,Jan,16; 2014,Jan,11

78012-78099 Nuclear Radiology: Thyroid, Parathyroid, Adrenal

EXCLUDES *Diagnostic services (see appropriate sections)*
Follow-up care (see appropriate section)
Code also radiopharmaceutical(s) and/or drug(s) supplied

78012 **Thyroid uptake, single or multiple quantitative measurement(s) (including stimulation, suppression, or discharge, when performed)**
2.34 2.34 FUD XXX S Z2 80
AMA: 2018,Jan,8; 2017,Jan,8; 2016,Jan,13; 2015,Jan,16

78013 **Thyroid imaging (including vascular flow, when performed);**
5.54 5.54 FUD XXX S Z2 80
AMA: 2018,Jan,8; 2017,Jan,8; 2016,Jan,13; 2015,Jan,16

78014 **with single or multiple uptake(s) quantitative measurement(s) (including stimulation, suppression, or discharge, when performed)**
6.95 6.95 FUD XXX S Z2 80
AMA: 2018,Jan,8; 2017,Jan,8; 2016,Jan,13; 2015,Jan,16

78015 **Thyroid carcinoma metastases imaging; limited area (eg, neck and chest only)**
6.47 6.47 FUD XXX S Z2 80
AMA: 2018,Jan,8; 2017,Jan,8; 2016,Jan,13; 2015,Jan,16; 2014,Jan,11

78016 **with additional studies (eg, urinary recovery)**
8.12 8.12 FUD XXX S Z2 80
AMA: 2018,Jan,8; 2017,Jan,8; 2016,Jan,13; 2015,Jan,16; 2014,Jan,11

78018 **whole body**
9.03 9.03 FUD XXX S Z2 80
AMA: 2018,Jan,8; 2017,Jan,8; 2016,Jan,13; 2015,Jan,16; 2014,Jan,11

\+ **78020** **Thyroid carcinoma metastases uptake (List separately in addition to code for primary procedure)**
2.41 2.41 FUD ZZZ N N1 80
AMA: 2018,Jan,8; 2017,Jan,8; 2016,Jan,13; 2015,Jan,16; 2014,Jan,11

78070 **Parathyroid planar imaging (including subtraction, when performed);**
EXCLUDES *Distribution of radiopharmaceutical agents or tumor localization (78800-78802, [78804], 78803)*
Radiopharmaceutical quantification measurements ([78835])
SPECT with concurrently acquired CT transmission scan ([78830, 78831, 78832])
8.61 8.61 FUD XXX S Z2 80
AMA: 2018,Jan,8; 2017,Jan,8; 2016,Dec,9; 2016,Dec,16; 2016,Jan,13; 2015,Jan,16; 2014,Jan,11

78071 **with tomographic (SPECT)**
EXCLUDES *Distribution of radiopharmaceutical agents or tumor localization (78800-78802, [78804], 78803)*
Radiopharmaceutical quantification measurements ([78835])
SPECT with concurrently acquired CT transmission scan ([78830, 78831, 78832])
10.2 10.2 FUD XXX S Z2 80
AMA: 2018,Jan,8; 2017,Jan,8; 2016,Dec,16; 2016,Dec,9

78072 **with tomographic (SPECT), and concurrently acquired computed tomography (CT) for anatomical localization**
EXCLUDES *Distribution of radiopharmaceutical agents or tumor localization (78800-78802, [78804], 78803)*
Radiopharmaceutical quantification measurements ([78835])
SPECT with concurrently acquired CT transmission scan ([78830, 78831, 78832])
11.2 11.2 FUD XXX S Z2 80
AMA: 2018,Jan,8; 2017,Jan,8; 2016,Dec,16; 2016,Dec,9

78075 **Adrenal imaging, cortex and/or medulla**
13.0 13.0 FUD XXX S Z2 80
AMA: 2018,Jan,8; 2017,Jan,8; 2016,Jan,13; 2015,Jan,16; 2014,Jan,11

78099 **Unlisted endocrine procedure, diagnostic nuclear medicine**
0.00 0.00 FUD XXX S Z2 80
AMA: 2018,Jan,8; 2017,Jan,8; 2016,Dec,9; 2016,Jan,13; 2015,Jan,16; 2014,Jan,11

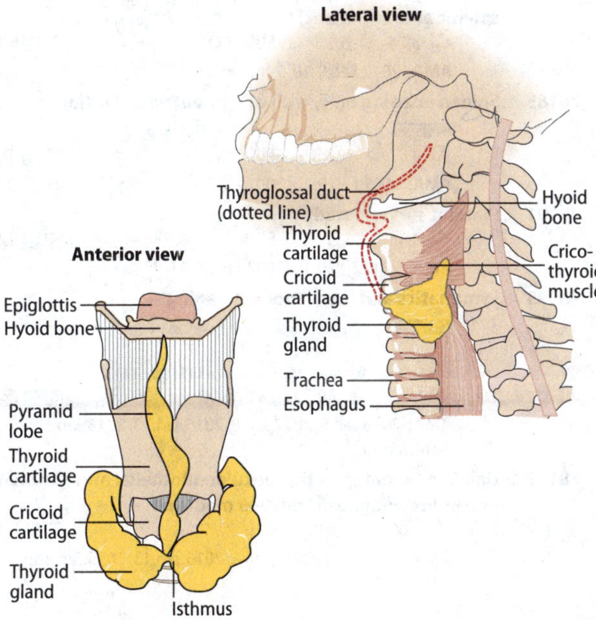

Lateral view
Thyroglossal duct (dotted line)
Hyoid bone
Thyroid cartilage
Crico-thyroid muscle
Cricoid cartilage
Thyroid gland
Trachea
Esophagus

Anterior view
Epiglottis
Hyoid bone
Pyramid lobe
Thyroid cartilage
Cricoid cartilage
Thyroid gland
Isthmus

Radiology
77767 — 78099

78102-78199 Nuclear Radiology: Blood Forming Organs

EXCLUDES *Diagnostic services (see appropriate sections)*
Follow-up care (see appropriate section)
Radioimmunoassays (82009-84999 [82042, 82652])

Code also radiopharmaceutical(s) and/or drug(s) supplied

78102 Bone marrow imaging; limited area
4.89 4.89 FUD XXX S Z2 80
AMA: 2018,Jan,8; 2017,Jan,8; 2016,Jan,13; 2015,Jan,16; 2014,Jan,11

78103 multiple areas
6.27 6.27 FUD XXX S Z2 80
AMA: 2012,Feb,9-10; 2007,Jan,28-31

78104 whole body
7.15 7.15 FUD XXX S Z2 80
AMA: 2012,Feb,9-10; 2007,Jan,28-31

78110 Plasma volume, radiopharmaceutical volume-dilution technique (separate procedure); single sampling
1.99 1.99 FUD XXX S Z2 80
AMA: 2012,Feb,9-10; 2007,Jan,28-31

78111 multiple samplings
2.11 2.11 FUD XXX S Z2 80
AMA: 2012,Feb,9-10; 2007,Jan,28-31

78120 Red cell volume determination (separate procedure); single sampling
2.04 2.04 FUD XXX S Z2 80
AMA: 2012,Feb,9-10; 2007,Jan,28-31

78121 multiple samplings
2.23 2.23 FUD XXX S Z2 80
AMA: 2012,Feb,9-10; 2007,Jan,28-31

78122 Whole blood volume determination, including separate measurement of plasma volume and red cell volume (radiopharmaceutical volume-dilution technique)
2.73 2.73 FUD XXX S Z2 80
AMA: 2012,Feb,9-10; 2007,Jan,28-31

78130 Red cell survival study;
3.56 3.56 FUD XXX S Z2 80
AMA: 2012,Feb,9-10; 2007,Jan,28-31

78135 differential organ/tissue kinetics (eg, splenic and/or hepatic sequestration)
8.02 8.02 FUD XXX S Z2 80
AMA: 2012,Feb,9-10; 2007,Jan,28-31

78140 Labeled red cell sequestration, differential organ/tissue (eg, splenic and/or hepatic)
3.14 3.14 FUD XXX S Z2 80
AMA: 2012,Feb,9-10; 2007,Jan,28-31

78185 Spleen imaging only, with or without vascular flow
EXCLUDES *Liver imaging (78215-78216)*
4.87 4.87 FUD XXX S Z2 80
AMA: 2012,Feb,9-10; 2007,Jan,28-31

78191 Platelet survival study
3.56 3.56 FUD XXX S Z2 80
AMA: 2012,Feb,9-10; 2007,Jan,28-31

78195 Lymphatics and lymph nodes imaging
EXCLUDES *Sentinel node identification without scintigraphy (38792)*
Sentinel node removal (38500-38542)
10.2 10.2 FUD XXX S Z2 80
AMA: 2018,Jan,8; 2017,Jan,8; 2016,Jan,13; 2015,Jan,16; 2014,Jan,11

78199 Unlisted hematopoietic, reticuloendothelial and lymphatic procedure, diagnostic nuclear medicine
0.00 0.00 FUD XXX S Z2 80
AMA: 2018,Jan,8; 2017,Jan,8; 2016,Jan,13; 2015,Jan,16; 2014,Jan,11

78201-78299 Nuclear Radiology: Digestive System

EXCLUDES *Diagnostic services (see appropriate sections)*
Follow-up care (see appropriate section)

Code also radiopharmaceutical(s) and/or drug(s) supplied

78201 Liver imaging; static only
EXCLUDES *Spleen imaging only (78185)*
5.49 5.49 FUD XXX S Z2 80
AMA: 2018,Jan,8; 2017,Jan,8; 2016,Jan,13; 2015,Jan,16; 2014,Jan,11

78202 with vascular flow
EXCLUDES *Spleen imaging only (78185)*
5.82 5.82 FUD XXX S Z2 80
AMA: 2012,Feb,9-10; 2007,Jan,28-31

~~78205 Liver imaging (SPECT);~~
To report, see (78803)

~~78206 with vascular flow~~
To report, see (78803)

78215 Liver and spleen imaging; static only
5.61 5.61 FUD XXX S Z2 80
AMA: 2012,Feb,9-10; 2007,Jan,28-31

78216 with vascular flow
3.68 3.68 FUD XXX S Z2 80
AMA: 2012,Feb,9-10; 2007,Jan,28-31

78226 Hepatobiliary system imaging, including gallbladder when present;
9.52 9.52 FUD XXX S Z2 80
AMA: 2012,Feb,9-10

78227 with pharmacologic intervention, including quantitative measurement(s) when performed
12.8 12.8 FUD XXX S Z2 80
AMA: 2012,Feb,9-10

78230 Salivary gland imaging;
5.03 5.03 FUD XXX S Z2 80
AMA: 2012,Feb,9-10; 2007,Jan,28-31

78231 with serial images
2.98 2.98 FUD XXX S Z2 80
AMA: 2012,Feb,9-10; 2007,Jan,28-31

78232 Salivary gland function study
2.92 2.92 FUD XXX S Z2 80
AMA: 2012,Feb,9-10; 2007,Jan,28-31

78258 Esophageal motility
6.31 6.31 FUD XXX S Z2 80
AMA: 2012,Feb,9-10; 2007,Jan,28-31

78261 Gastric mucosa imaging
5.83 5.83 FUD XXX S Z2 80
AMA: 2012,Feb,9-10; 2007,Jan,28-31

78262 Gastroesophageal reflux study
6.95 6.95 FUD XXX S Z2 80
AMA: 2018,Jan,8; 2017,Jan,8; 2016,Jan,13; 2015,Dec,11

78264 Gastric emptying imaging study (eg, solid, liquid, or both);
EXCLUDES *Procedure performed more than one time per study*
9.65 9.65 FUD XXX S Z2 80
AMA: 2018,Jan,8; 2017,Jan,8; 2016,Jan,13; 2015,Dec,11

78265 with small bowel transit
EXCLUDES *Procedure performed more than one time per study*
11.4 11.4 FUD XXX S Z2 80
AMA: 2018,Jan,8; 2017,Jan,8; 2015,Dec,11

78266 with small bowel and colon transit, multiple days
EXCLUDES *Procedure performed more than one time per study*
13.5 13.5 FUD XXX S Z2 80
AMA: 2018,Jan,8; 2017,Jan,8; 2015,Dec,11

78267 Urea breath test, C-14 (isotopic); acquisition for analysis
EXCLUDES *Breath hydrogen/methane test (91065)*
0.00 0.00 FUD XXX A
AMA: 2018,Jan,8; 2017,Jan,8; 2016,Jan,13; 2015,Jan,16; 2014,Jan,11

78268 analysis

EXCLUDES *Breath hydrogen/methane test (91065)*

0.00 0.00 FUD XXX A

AMA: 2018,Jan,8; 2017,Jan,8; 2016,Jan,13; 2015,Jan,16; 2014,Jan,11

78278 **Acute gastrointestinal blood loss imaging**

10.0 10.0 FUD XXX S Z2 80

AMA: 2012,Feb,9-10; 2007,Jan,28-31

78282 **Gastrointestinal protein loss**

0.00 0.00 FUD XXX S Z2 80

AMA: 2018,Jul,14

78290 **Intestine imaging (eg, ectopic gastric mucosa, Meckel's localization, volvulus)**

9.53 9.53 FUD XXX S Z2 80

AMA: 2012,Feb,9-10; 2007,Jan,28-31

78291 **Peritoneal-venous shunt patency test (eg, for LeVeen, Denver shunt)**

Code also (49427)

7.39 7.39 FUD XXX S Z2 80

AMA: 2012,Feb,9-10; 2007,Jan,28-31

78299 **Unlisted gastrointestinal procedure, diagnostic nuclear medicine**

0.00 0.00 FUD XXX S Z2 80

AMA: 2018,Jan,8; 2017,Jan,8; 2016,Jan,13; 2015,Jan,16; 2014,Jan,11

78300-78399 Nuclear Radiology: Bones and Joints

EXCLUDES *Diagnostic services (see appropriate sections)*
Follow-up care (see appropriate section)

Code also radiopharmaceutical(s) and/or drug(s) supplied

78300 **Bone and/or joint imaging; limited area**

6.63 6.63 FUD XXX S Z2 80

AMA: 2018,Jan,8; 2017,Jan,8; 2016,Jan,13; 2015,Jan,16; 2014,Jan,11

78305 **multiple areas**

8.08 8.08 FUD XXX S Z2 80

AMA: 2018,Jan,8; 2017,Jan,8; 2016,Jan,13; 2015,Jan,16; 2014,Jan,11

78306 **whole body**

8.71 8.71 FUD XXX S Z2 80

AMA: 2018,Jan,8; 2017,Jan,8; 2016,Jan,13; 2015,Jan,16; 2014,Jan,11

78315 **3 phase study**

9.98 9.98 FUD XXX S Z2 80

AMA: 2018,Jan,8; 2017,Jan,8; 2016,Jan,13; 2015,Jan,16; 2014,Jan,11

~~**78320** **tomographic (SPECT)**~~

To report, see (78803)

78350 **Bone density (bone mineral content) study, 1 or more sites; single photon absorptiometry**

0.93 0.93 FUD XXX E

AMA: 2012,Feb,9-10; 2007,Jan,28-31

78351 **dual photon absorptiometry, 1 or more sites**

0.44 0.44 FUD XXX E

AMA: 2012,Feb,9-10; 2007,Jan,28-31

78399 **Unlisted musculoskeletal procedure, diagnostic nuclear medicine**

0.00 0.00 FUD XXX S Z2 80

AMA: 2018,Jan,8; 2017,Jan,8; 2016,Jan,13; 2015,Jan,16; 2014,Jan,11

78414-78499 [78429, 78430, 78431, 78432, 78433, 78434] Nuclear Radiology: Heart and Vascular

EXCLUDES *Diagnostic services (see appropriate sections)*
Follow-up care (see appropriate section)

Code also radiopharmaceutical(s) and/or drug(s) supplied

78414 **Determination of central c-v hemodynamics (non-imaging) (eg, ejection fraction with probe technique) with or without pharmacologic intervention or exercise, single or multiple determinations**

0.00 0.00 FUD XXX S Z2 80

AMA: 2018,Jan,8; 2017,Jan,8; 2016,Jan,13; 2015,Jan,16; 2014,Jan,11

78428 **Cardiac shunt detection**

5.29 5.29 FUD XXX S Z2 80

AMA: 2018,Jan,8; 2017,Jan,8; 2016,Jan,13; 2015,Jan,16; 2014,Jan,11

78429 **Resequenced code. See code following 78459.**

78430 **Resequenced code. See code following 78491.**

78431 **Resequenced code. See code following 78492.**

78432 **Resequenced code. See code following 78492.**

78433 **Resequenced code. See code following 78492.**

78434 **Resequenced code. See code following 78492.**

78445 **Non-cardiac vascular flow imaging (ie, angiography, venography)**

5.38 5.38 FUD XXX S Z2 80

AMA: 2018,Jan,8; 2017,Jan,8; 2016,Jan,13; 2015,Jan,16; 2014,Jan,11

78451 **Myocardial perfusion imaging, tomographic (SPECT) (including attenuation correction, qualitative or quantitative wall motion, ejection fraction by first pass or gated technique, additional quantification, when performed); single study, at rest or stress (exercise or pharmacologic)**

EXCLUDES *Distribution of radiopharmaceutical agents or tumor localization (78800-78802, [78804], 78803)*
Radiopharmaceutical quantification measurements ([78835])
SPECT with concurrently acquired CT transmission scan ([78830, 78831, 78832])

Code also stress testing when performed (93015-93018)

9.77 9.77 FUD XXX S Z2 80

AMA: 2018,Jan,8; 2017,Jan,8; 2016,Jan,13; 2015,Jan,16; 2014,Jan,11

78452 **multiple studies, at rest and/or stress (exercise or pharmacologic) and/or redistribution and/or rest reinjection**

EXCLUDES *Distribution of radiopharmaceutical agents or tumor localization (78800-78802, [78804], 78803)*
Radiopharmaceutical quantification measurements ([78835])
SPECT with concurrently acquired CT transmission scan ([78830, 78831, 78832])

Code also stress testing when performed (93015-93018)

13.6 13.6 FUD XXX S Z2 80

AMA: 2018,Jan,8; 2017,Jan,8; 2016,Jan,13; 2015,Jan,16; 2014,Jan,11

78453 **Myocardial perfusion imaging, planar (including qualitative or quantitative wall motion, ejection fraction by first pass or gated technique, additional quantification, when performed); single study, at rest or stress (exercise or pharmacologic)**

Code also stress testing when performed (93015-93018)

8.78 8.78 FUD XXX S Z2 80

AMA: 2018,Jan,8; 2017,Jan,8; 2016,Jan,13; 2015,Jan,16; 2014,Jan,11

Radiology

78268 — 78453

78454 multiple studies, at rest and/or stress (exercise or pharmacologic) and/or redistribution and/or rest reinjection

Code also stress testing when performed (93015-93018)

12.5 12.5 FUD XXX S Z2 80

AMA: 2018,Jan,8; 2017,Jan,8; 2016,Jan,13; 2015,Jan,16; 2014,Jan,11

78456 Acute venous thrombosis imaging, peptide

8.93 8.93 FUD XXX S Z2

AMA: 2018,Jan,8; 2017,Jan,8; 2016,Jan,13; 2015,Jan,16; 2014,Jan,11

78457 Venous thrombosis imaging, venogram; unilateral

5.52 5.52 FUD XXX S Z2 80

AMA: 2018,Jan,8; 2017,Jan,8; 2016,Jan,13; 2015,Jan,16; 2014,Jan,11

78458 bilateral

5.92 5.92 FUD XXX S Z2 80

AMA: 2018,Jan,8; 2017,Jan,8; 2016,Jan,13; 2015,Jan,16; 2014,Jan,11

▲ **78459** Myocardial imaging, positron emission tomography (PET), metabolic evaluation study (including ventricular wall motion[s] and/or ejection fraction[s], when performed), single study;

INCLUDES Examination of CT transmission images for field of view anatomy review

EXCLUDES *CT coronary calcium scoring (75571)*
CT for other than attenuation correction/anatomical localization; use site-specific CT code with modifier 59
Myocardial perfusion studies (78491-78492)

0.00 0.00 FUD XXX S Z2 80

AMA: 2018,Jan,8; 2017,Jan,8; 2016,Jan,13; 2015,Jan,16; 2014,Jan,11

● # **78429** with concurrently acquired computed tomography transmission scan

0.00 0.00 FUD 000

INCLUDES Examination of CT transmission images for field of view anatomy review

EXCLUDES *CT coronary calcium scoring (75571)*
CT for other than attenuation correction/anatomical localization; use site-specific CT code with modifier 59

78466 Myocardial imaging, infarct avid, planar; qualitative or quantitative

5.67 5.67 FUD XXX S Z2 80

AMA: 2012,Feb,9-10; 2010,May,5-6

78468 with ejection fraction by first pass technique

5.88 5.88 FUD XXX S Z2 80

AMA: 2018,Jan,8; 2017,Jan,8; 2016,Jan,13; 2015,Jan,16; 2014,Jan,11

78469 tomographic SPECT with or without quantification

EXCLUDES *Distribution of radiopharmaceutical agents or tumor localization (78800-78802, [78804], 78803)*
Myocardial sympathetic innervation imaging (0331T-0332T)
Radiopharmaceutical quantification measurements ([78835])
SPECT with concurrently acquired CT transmission scan ([78830, 78831, 78832])

6.50 6.50 FUD XXX S Z2 80

AMA: 2018,Nov,11; 2018,Jan,8; 2017,Jan,8; 2016,Jan,13; 2015,Jan,16; 2014,Jan,11

78472 Cardiac blood pool imaging, gated equilibrium; planar, single study at rest or stress (exercise and/or pharmacologic), wall motion study plus ejection fraction, with or without additional quantitative processing

EXCLUDES *Cardiac blood pool imaging (78481, 78483, 78494)*
Myocardial perfusion imaging (78451-78454)
Right ventricular ejection fraction by first pass technique (78496)

Code also stress testing when performed (93015-93018)

6.59 6.59 FUD XXX S Z2 80

AMA: 2018,Jan,8; 2017,Jan,8; 2016,Jan,13; 2015,Jan,16; 2014,Jan,11

78473 multiple studies, wall motion study plus ejection fraction, at rest and stress (exercise and/or pharmacologic), with or without additional quantification

EXCLUDES *Cardiac blood pool imaging (78481, 78483, 78494)*
Myocardial perfusion imaging (78451-78454)

Code also stress testing when performed (93015-93018)

8.32 8.32 FUD XXX S Z2 80

AMA: 2018,Jan,8; 2017,Jan,8; 2016,Jan,13; 2015,Jan,16; 2014,Jan,11

78481 Cardiac blood pool imaging (planar), first pass technique; single study, at rest or with stress (exercise and/or pharmacologic), wall motion study plus ejection fraction, with or without quantification

EXCLUDES *Myocardial perfusion imaging (78451-78454)*

Code also stress testing when performed (93015-93018)

5.06 5.06 FUD XXX S Z2 80

AMA: 2018,Jan,8; 2017,Jan,8; 2016,Jan,13; 2015,Jan,16; 2014,Jan,11

78483 multiple studies, at rest and with stress (exercise and/or pharmacologic), wall motion study plus ejection fraction, with or without quantification

EXCLUDES *Blood flow studies of the brain (78610)*
Myocardial perfusion imaging (78451-78454)

Code also stress testing when performed (93015-93018)

6.83 6.83 FUD XXX S Z2 80

AMA: 2018,Jan,8; 2017,Jan,8; 2016,Jan,13; 2015,Jan,16; 2014,Jan,11

▲ **78491** Myocardial imaging, positron emission tomography (PET), perfusion study (including ventricular wall motion[s] and/or ejection fraction[s], when performed); single study, at rest or stress (exercise or pharmacologic)

Code also stress testing when performed (93015-93018)

0.00 0.00 FUD XXX S Z2 80

AMA: 2018,Jan,8; 2017,Jan,8; 2016,Jan,13; 2015,Jan,16; 2014,Jan,11

● # **78430** single study, at rest or stress (exercise or pharmacologic), with concurrently acquired computed tomography transmission scan

0.00 0.00 FUD 000

INCLUDES Examination of CT transmission images for field of view anatomy review

Code also stress testing when performed (93015-93018)

▲ **78492** multiple studies at rest and stress (exercise or pharmacologic)

Code also stress testing when performed (93015-93018)

0.00 0.00 FUD XXX S Z2 80

AMA: 2018,Jan,8; 2017,Jan,8; 2016,Jan,13; 2015,Jan,16; 2014,Jan,11

● # **78431** multiple studies at rest and stress (exercise or pharmacologic), with concurrently acquired computed tomography transmission scan

0.00 0.00 FUD 000

INCLUDES Examination of CT transmission images for field of view anatomy review

Code also stress testing when performed (93015-93018)

● # **78432** **Myocardial imaging, positron emission tomography (PET), combined perfusion with metabolic evaluation study (including ventricular wall motion[s] and/or ejection fraction[s], when performed), dual radiotracer (eg, myocardial viability);**

0.00 0.00 FUD 000

Code also stress testing when performed (93015-93018)

● # **78433** **with concurrently acquired computed tomography transmission scan**

0.00 0.00 FUD 000

INCLUDES Examination of CT transmission images for field of view anatomy review

EXCLUDES *CT for other than attenuation correction/anatomical localization; use site-specific CT code with modifier 59*

Code also stress testing when performed (93015-93018)

● + # **78434** **Absolute quantitation of myocardial blood flow (AQMBF), positron emission tomography (PET), rest and pharmacologic stress (List separately in addition to code for primary procedure)**

0.00 0.00 FUD 000

EXCLUDES *CT coronary calcium scoring (75571)*
Myocardial imaging by planar or SPECT (78451-78454)

Code first ([78431], 78492)

78494 **Cardiac blood pool imaging, gated equilibrium, SPECT, at rest, wall motion study plus ejection fraction, with or without quantitative processing**

EXCLUDES *Distribution of radiopharmaceutical agents or tumor localization (78800-78802, [78804], 78803)*
Radiopharmaceutical quantification measurements ([78835])
SPECT with concurrently acquired CT transmission scan ([78830, 78831, 78832])

6.51 6.51 FUD XXX S Z2 80

AMA: 2018,Jan,8; 2017,Jan,8; 2016,Jan,13; 2015,Jan,16; 2014,Jan,11

\+ **78496** **Cardiac blood pool imaging, gated equilibrium, single study, at rest, with right ventricular ejection fraction by first pass technique (List separately in addition to code for primary procedure)**

Code first (78472)

1.25 1.25 FUD ZZZ N N1 80

AMA: 2018,Jan,8; 2017,Jan,8; 2016,Jan,13; 2015,Jan,16; 2014,Jan,11

78499 **Unlisted cardiovascular procedure, diagnostic nuclear medicine**

0.00 0.00 FUD XXX S Z2 80

AMA: 2018,Jan,8; 2017,Jan,8; 2016,Jan,13; 2015,Jan,16; 2014,Jan,11

78579-78599 Nuclear Radiology: Lungs

EXCLUDES *Diagnostic services (see appropriate sections)*
Follow-up care (see appropriate sections)

Code also radiopharmaceutical(s) and/or drug(s) supplied

78579 **Pulmonary ventilation imaging (eg, aerosol or gas)**

EXCLUDES *Procedure performed more than one time per imaging session*

5.36 5.36 FUD XXX S Z2 80

AMA: 2012,Feb,9-10

78580 **Pulmonary perfusion imaging (eg, particulate)**

EXCLUDES *Myocardial perfusion imaging (78451-78454)*
Procedure performed more than one time per imaging session

6.87 6.87 FUD XXX S Z2 80

AMA: 2018,Jan,8; 2017,Jan,8; 2016,Jan,13; 2015,Jan,16; 2014,Jan,11

78582 **Pulmonary ventilation (eg, aerosol or gas) and perfusion imaging**

EXCLUDES *Myocardial perfusion imaging (78451-78454)*
Procedure performed more than one time per imaging session

9.64 9.64 FUD XXX S Z2 80

AMA: 2012,Feb,9-10

78597 **Quantitative differential pulmonary perfusion, including imaging when performed**

EXCLUDES *Myocardial perfusion imaging (78451-78454)*
Procedure performed more than one time per imaging session

5.79 5.79 FUD XXX S Z2 80

AMA: 2012,Feb,9-10

78598 **Quantitative differential pulmonary perfusion and ventilation (eg, aerosol or gas), including imaging when performed**

EXCLUDES *Myocardial perfusion imaging (78451-78454)*
Procedure performed more than one time per imaging session

8.80 8.80 FUD XXX S Z2 80

AMA: 2012,Feb,9-10

78599 **Unlisted respiratory procedure, diagnostic nuclear medicine**

0.00 0.00 FUD XXX S Z2 80

AMA: 2018,Jan,8; 2017,Jan,8; 2016,Jan,13; 2015,Jan,16; 2014,Jan,11

78600-78650 Nuclear Radiology: Brain/Cerebrospinal Fluid

EXCLUDES *Diagnostic services (see appropriate sections)*
Follow-up care (see appropriate section)

Code also radiopharmaceutical(s) and/or drug(s) supplied

78600 **Brain imaging, less than 4 static views;**

5.32 5.32 FUD XXX S Z2 80

AMA: 2018,Jan,8; 2017,Jan,8; 2016,Jan,13; 2015,Jan,16; 2014,Jan,11

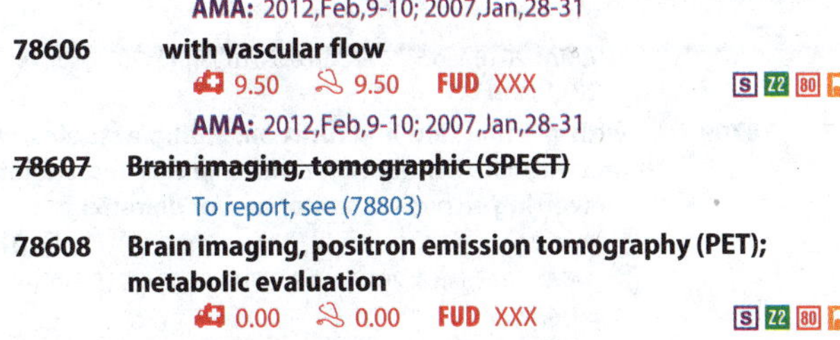

Schematic of frontal coronal CT section of skull

78601 **with vascular flow**

6.25 6.25 FUD XXX S Z2 80

AMA: 2012,Feb,9-10; 2007,Jan,28-31

78605 **Brain imaging, minimum 4 static views;**

5.74 5.74 FUD XXX S Z2 80

AMA: 2012,Feb,9-10; 2007,Jan,28-31

78606 **with vascular flow**

9.50 9.50 FUD XXX S Z2 80

AMA: 2012,Feb,9-10; 2007,Jan,28-31

~~**78607** **Brain imaging, tomographic (SPECT)**~~

To report, see (78803)

78608 **Brain imaging, positron emission tomography (PET); metabolic evaluation**

0.00 0.00 FUD XXX S Z2 80

AMA: 2012,Feb,9-10; 2007,Jan,28-31

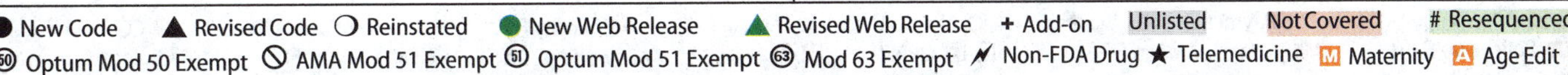
● New Code ▲ Revised Code ○ Reinstated ● New Web Release ▲ Revised Web Release + Add-on Unlisted Not Covered # Resequenced
Optum Mod 50 Exempt AMA Mod 51 Exempt Optum Mod 51 Exempt Mod 63 Exempt Non-FDA Drug ★ Telemedicine Maternity Age Edit

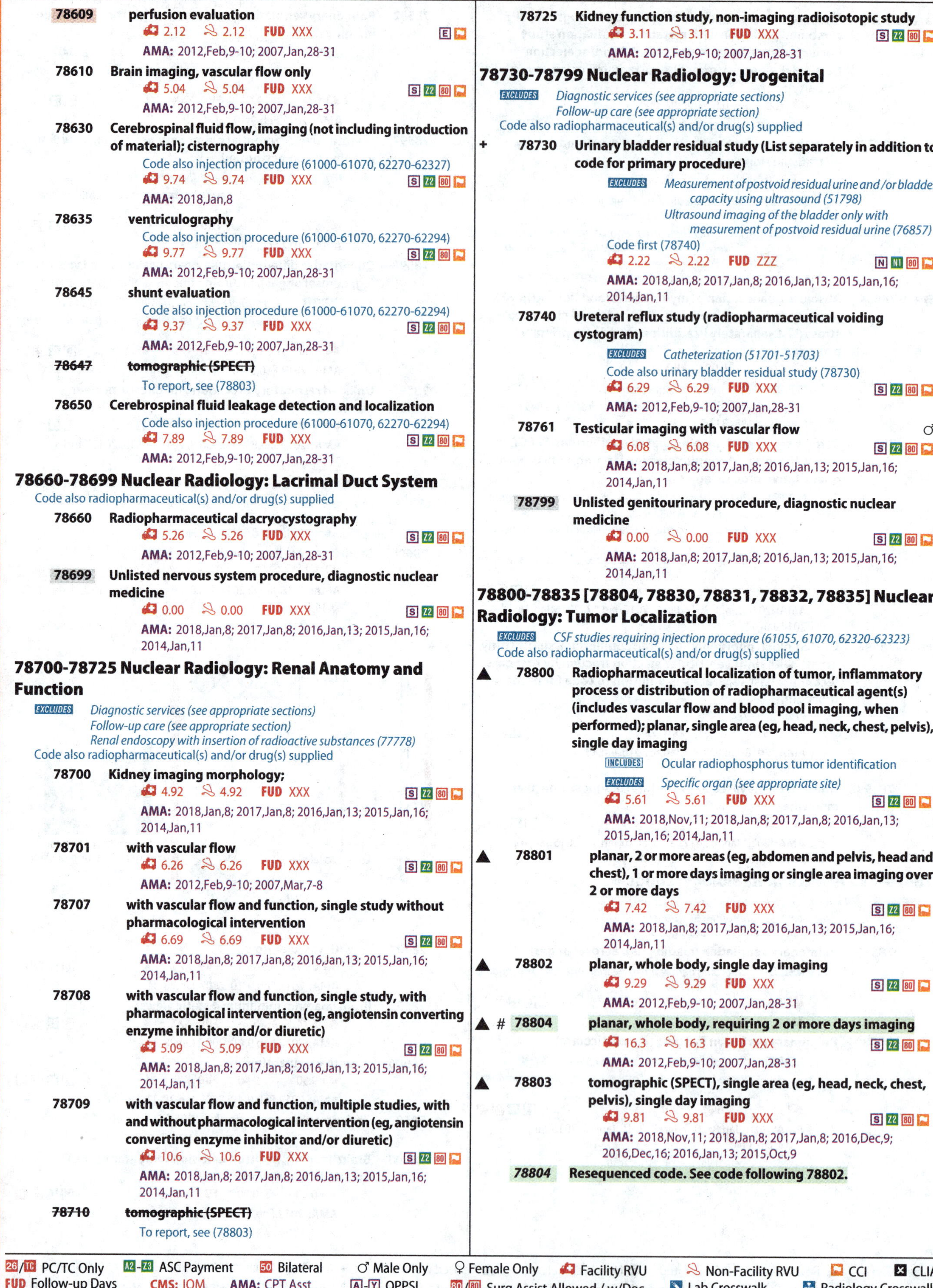

78609 perfusion evaluation
2.12 2.12 FUD XXX E
AMA: 2012,Feb,9-10; 2007,Jan,28-31

78610 **Brain imaging, vascular flow only**
5.04 5.04 FUD XXX S Z2 80
AMA: 2012,Feb,9-10; 2007,Jan,28-31

78630 **Cerebrospinal fluid flow, imaging (not including introduction of material); cisternography**
Code also injection procedure (61000-61070, 62270-62327)
9.74 9.74 FUD XXX S Z2 80
AMA: 2018,Jan,8

78635 ventriculography
Code also injection procedure (61000-61070, 62270-62294)
9.77 9.77 FUD XXX S Z2 80
AMA: 2012,Feb,9-10; 2007,Jan,28-31

78645 shunt evaluation
Code also injection procedure (61000-61070, 62270-62294)
9.37 9.37 FUD XXX S Z2 80
AMA: 2012,Feb,9-10; 2007,Jan,28-31

~~78647~~ ~~tomographic (SPECT)~~
To report, see (78803)

78650 **Cerebrospinal fluid leakage detection and localization**
Code also injection procedure (61000-61070, 62270-62294)
7.89 7.89 FUD XXX S Z2 80
AMA: 2012,Feb,9-10; 2007,Jan,28-31

78660-78699 Nuclear Radiology: Lacrimal Duct System

Code also radiopharmaceutical(s) and/or drug(s) supplied

78660 **Radiopharmaceutical dacryocystography**
5.26 5.26 FUD XXX S Z2 80
AMA: 2012,Feb,9-10; 2007,Jan,28-31

78699 **Unlisted nervous system procedure, diagnostic nuclear medicine**
0.00 0.00 FUD XXX S Z2 80
AMA: 2018,Jan,8; 2017,Jan,8; 2016,Jan,13; 2015,Jan,16; 2014,Jan,11

78700-78725 Nuclear Radiology: Renal Anatomy and Function

EXCLUDES *Diagnostic services (see appropriate sections)*
Follow-up care (see appropriate section)
Renal endoscopy with insertion of radioactive substances (77778)
Code also radiopharmaceutical(s) and/or drug(s) supplied

78700 **Kidney imaging morphology;**
4.92 4.92 FUD XXX S Z2 80
AMA: 2018,Jan,8; 2017,Jan,8; 2016,Jan,13; 2015,Jan,16; 2014,Jan,11

78701 with vascular flow
6.26 6.26 FUD XXX S Z2 80
AMA: 2012,Feb,9-10; 2007,Mar,7-8

78707 with vascular flow and function, single study without pharmacological intervention
6.69 6.69 FUD XXX S Z2 80
AMA: 2018,Jan,8; 2017,Jan,8; 2016,Jan,13; 2015,Jan,16; 2014,Jan,11

78708 with vascular flow and function, single study, with pharmacological intervention (eg, angiotensin converting enzyme inhibitor and/or diuretic)
5.09 5.09 FUD XXX S Z2 80
AMA: 2018,Jan,8; 2017,Jan,8; 2016,Jan,13; 2015,Jan,16; 2014,Jan,11

78709 with vascular flow and function, multiple studies, with and without pharmacological intervention (eg, angiotensin converting enzyme inhibitor and/or diuretic)
10.6 10.6 FUD XXX S Z2 80
AMA: 2018,Jan,8; 2017,Jan,8; 2016,Jan,13; 2015,Jan,16; 2014,Jan,11

~~78710~~ ~~tomographic (SPECT)~~
To report, see (78803)

78725 **Kidney function study, non-imaging radioisotopic study**
3.11 3.11 FUD XXX S Z2 80
AMA: 2012,Feb,9-10; 2007,Jan,28-31

78730-78799 Nuclear Radiology: Urogenital

EXCLUDES *Diagnostic services (see appropriate sections)*
Follow-up care (see appropriate section)
Code also radiopharmaceutical(s) and/or drug(s) supplied

+ **78730** **Urinary bladder residual study (List separately in addition to code for primary procedure)**
EXCLUDES *Measurement of postvoid residual urine and/or bladder capacity using ultrasound (51798)*
Ultrasound imaging of the bladder only with measurement of postvoid residual urine (76857)
Code first (78740)
2.22 2.22 FUD ZZZ N N1 80
AMA: 2018,Jan,8; 2017,Jan,8; 2016,Jan,13; 2015,Jan,16; 2014,Jan,11

78740 **Ureteral reflux study (radiopharmaceutical voiding cystogram)**
EXCLUDES *Catheterization (51701-51703)*
Code also urinary bladder residual study (78730)
6.29 6.29 FUD XXX S Z2 80
AMA: 2012,Feb,9-10; 2007,Jan,28-31

78761 **Testicular imaging with vascular flow** ♂
6.08 6.08 FUD XXX S Z2 80
AMA: 2018,Jan,8; 2017,Jan,8; 2016,Jan,13; 2015,Jan,16; 2014,Jan,11

78799 **Unlisted genitourinary procedure, diagnostic nuclear medicine**
0.00 0.00 FUD XXX S Z2 80
AMA: 2018,Jan,8; 2017,Jan,8; 2016,Jan,13; 2015,Jan,16; 2014,Jan,11

78800-78835 [78804, 78830, 78831, 78832, 78835] Nuclear Radiology: Tumor Localization

EXCLUDES *CSF studies requiring injection procedure (61055, 61070, 62320-62323)*
Code also radiopharmaceutical(s) and/or drug(s) supplied

▲ **78800** **Radiopharmaceutical localization of tumor, inflammatory process or distribution of radiopharmaceutical agent(s) (includes vascular flow and blood pool imaging, when performed); planar, single area (eg, head, neck, chest, pelvis), single day imaging**
INCLUDES Ocular radiophosphorus tumor identification
EXCLUDES *Specific organ (see appropriate site)*
5.61 5.61 FUD XXX S Z2 80
AMA: 2018,Nov,11; 2018,Jan,8; 2017,Jan,8; 2016,Jan,13; 2015,Jan,16; 2014,Jan,11

▲ **78801** planar, 2 or more areas (eg, abdomen and pelvis, head and chest), 1 or more days imaging or single area imaging over 2 or more days
7.42 7.42 FUD XXX S Z2 80
AMA: 2018,Jan,8; 2017,Jan,8; 2016,Jan,13; 2015,Jan,16; 2014,Jan,11

▲ **78802** planar, whole body, single day imaging
9.29 9.29 FUD XXX S Z2 80
AMA: 2012,Feb,9-10; 2007,Jan,28-31

▲ # **78804** planar, whole body, requiring 2 or more days imaging
16.3 16.3 FUD XXX S Z2 80
AMA: 2012,Feb,9-10; 2007,Jan,28-31

▲ **78803** tomographic (SPECT), single area (eg, head, neck, chest, pelvis), single day imaging
9.81 9.81 FUD XXX S Z2 80
AMA: 2018,Nov,11; 2018,Jan,8; 2017,Jan,8; 2016,Dec,9; 2016,Dec,16; 2016,Jan,13; 2015,Oct,9

78804 **Resequenced code. See code following 78802.**

~~78805 Radiopharmaceutical localization of inflammatory process; limited area~~

To report, see (78300, 78305-78306, 78315, 78800-78803, 78830-78832)

~~78806 whole body~~

To report, see (78300, 78305-78306, 78315, 78800-78803, 78830-78832)

~~78807 tomographic (SPECT)~~

To report, see (78300, 78305-78306, 78315, 78800-78803, 78830-78832)

● # **78830** **tomographic (SPECT) with concurrently acquired computed tomography (CT) transmission scan for anatomical review, localization and determination/detection of pathology, single area (eg, head, neck, chest, pelvis), single day imaging**

0.00 0.00 FUD 000

● # **78831** **tomographic (SPECT), minimum 2 areas (eg, pelvis and knees, abdomen and pelvis), single day imaging, or single area imaging over 2 or more days**

0.00 0.00 FUD 000

● # **78832** **tomographic (SPECT) with concurrently acquired computed tomography (CT) transmission scan for anatomical review, localization and determination/detection of pathology, minimum 2 areas (eg, pelvis and knees, abdomen and pelvis), single day imaging, or single area imaging over 2 or more days**

0.00 0.00 FUD 000

● + # **78835** **Radiopharmaceutical quantification measurement(s) single area (List separately in addition to code for primary procedure)**

0.00 0.00 FUD 000

78808 Intravenous Injection for Radiopharmaceutical Localization

Code also radiopharmaceutical(s) and/or drug(s) supplied

78808 **Injection procedure for radiopharmaceutical localization by non-imaging probe study, intravenous (eg, parathyroid adenoma)**

1.12 1.12 FUD XXX Q1 N1 80

AMA: 2018,Jan,8; 2017,Jan,8; 2016,Dec,9

78811-78999 Nuclear Radiology: Diagnosis, Staging, Restaging or Monitoring Cancer

CMS: 100-03,220.6.17 Positron Emission Tomography (FDG) for Oncologic Conditions; 100-03,220.6.19 NaF-18 PET to Identify Bone Metastasis of Cancer; 100-03,220.6.9 FDG PET for Refractory Seizures; 100-04,13,60 Positron Emission Tomography (PET) Scans - General Information; 100-04,13,60.13 Billing for PET Scans for Specific Indications of Cervical Cancer; 100-04,13,60.15 Billing for CMS-Approved Clinical Trials for PET Scans; 100-04,13,60.16 Billing and Coverage for PET Scans; 100-04,13,60.17 Billing and Coverage Changes for PET Scans for Cervical Cancer; 100-04,13,60.18 Billing and Coverage for PET (NaF-18) Scans to Identify Bone Metastasis; 100-04,13,60.2 Use of Gamma Cameras, Full and Partial Ring PET Scanners; 100-04,13,60.3 PET Scan Qualifying Conditions; 100-04,13,60.3.1 Appropriate Codes for PET Scans; 100-04,13,60.3.2 Tracer Codes Required for Positron Emission Tomography (PET) Scans

EXCLUDES *CT scan performed for other than attenuation correction and anatomical localization (report with the appropriate site-specific CT code and modifier 59)*
Ocular radiophosphorus tumor identification (78800)
PET brain scan (78608-78609)
PET myocardial imaging (78459, 78491-78492)
Procedure performed more than one time per imaging session

Code also radiopharmaceutical(s) and/or drug(s) supplied

78811 **Positron emission tomography (PET) imaging; limited area (eg, chest, head/neck)**

0.00 0.00 FUD XXX S Z2 80

AMA: 2018,Jan,8; 2017,Jan,8; 2016,Jan,13; 2015,Jan,16; 2014,Jan,11

78812 **skull base to mid-thigh**

0.00 0.00 FUD XXX S Z2 80

AMA: 2018,Jan,8; 2017,Jan,8; 2016,Jan,13; 2015,Jan,16; 2014,Jan,11

78813 **whole body**

0.00 0.00 FUD XXX S Z2 80

AMA: 2018,Jan,8; 2017,Jan,8; 2016,Jan,13; 2015,Jan,16; 2014,Jan,11

78814 **Positron emission tomography (PET) with concurrently acquired computed tomography (CT) for attenuation correction and anatomical localization imaging; limited area (eg, chest, head/neck)**

0.00 0.00 FUD XXX S Z2 80

AMA: 2018,Jan,8; 2017,Jan,8; 2016,Jan,13; 2015,Jan,16; 2014,Jan,11

78815 **skull base to mid-thigh**

0.00 0.00 FUD XXX S Z2 80

AMA: 2018,Jan,8; 2017,Jan,8; 2016,Jan,13; 2015,Jan,16; 2014,Jan,11

78816 **whole body**

0.00 0.00 FUD XXX S Z2 80

AMA: 2018,Jan,8; 2017,Jan,8; 2016,Jan,13; 2015,Jan,16; 2014,Jan,11

78830 **Resequenced code. See code following resequenced numeric code 78804.**

78831 **Resequenced code. See code following resequenced numeric code 78804.**

78832 **Resequenced code. See code following resequenced numeric code 78804.**

78835 **Resequenced code. See code following resequenced numeric code 78804.**

78999 **Unlisted miscellaneous procedure, diagnostic nuclear medicine**

0.00 0.00 FUD XXX S Z2 80

AMA: 2018,Jan,8; 2017,Jan,8; 2016,Dec,9; 2016,Dec,16; 2016,Jan,13; 2015,Oct,9; 2015,Jan,16; 2014,Jan,11

79005-79999 Systemic Radiopharmaceutical Therapy

EXCLUDES *Imaging guidance*
Injection into artery, body cavity, or joint (see appropriate injection codes)
Radiological supervision and interpretation

79005 **Radiopharmaceutical therapy, by oral administration**

EXCLUDES *Monoclonal antibody treatment (79403)*

3.91 3.91 FUD XXX S Z3 80

AMA: 2018,Jan,8; 2017,Jan,8; 2016,Jan,13; 2015,Jan,16; 2014,Jan,11

79101 **Radiopharmaceutical therapy, by intravenous administration**

EXCLUDES *Administration of nonantibody radioelement solution including follow-up care (77750)*
Hydration infusion (96360)
Intravenous injection, IV push (96374-96375, 96409)
Radiolabeled monoclonal antibody IV infusion (79403)
Venipuncture (36400, 36410)

4.18 4.18 FUD XXX S Z3 80

AMA: 2018,Jan,8; 2017,Jan,8; 2016,Jan,13; 2015,Jan,16; 2014,Jan,11

79200 **Radiopharmaceutical therapy, by intracavitary administration**

3.83 3.83 FUD XXX S Z3 80

AMA: 2018,Jan,8; 2017,Jan,8; 2016,Jan,13; 2015,Jan,16; 2014,Jan,11

79300 **Radiopharmaceutical therapy, by interstitial radioactive colloid administration**

0.00 0.00 FUD XXX S Z2 80

AMA: 2018,Jan,8; 2017,Jan,8; 2016,Jan,13; 2015,Jan,16; 2014,Jan,11

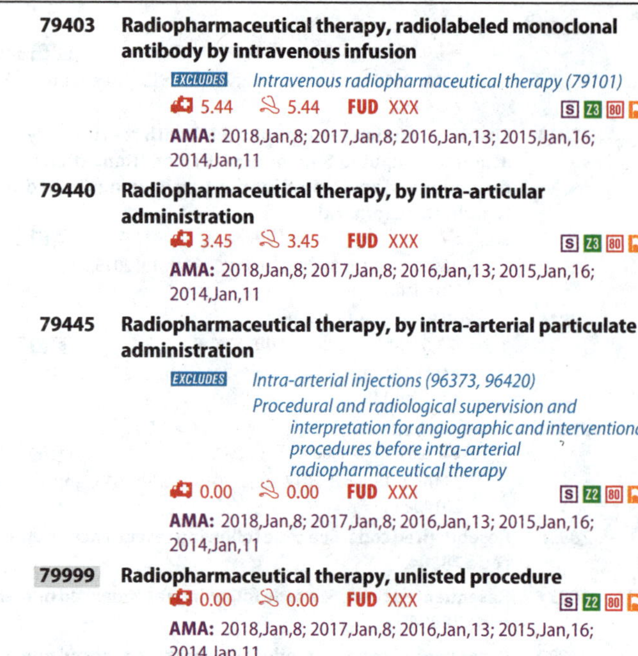

79403 **Radiopharmaceutical therapy, radiolabeled monoclonal antibody by intravenous infusion**

EXCLUDES *Intravenous radiopharmaceutical therapy (79101)*

5.44 5.44 FUD XXX S Z3 80

AMA: 2018,Jan,8; 2017,Jan,8; 2016,Jan,13; 2015,Jan,16; 2014,Jan,11

79440 **Radiopharmaceutical therapy, by intra-articular administration**

3.45 3.45 FUD XXX S Z3 80

AMA: 2018,Jan,8; 2017,Jan,8; 2016,Jan,13; 2015,Jan,16; 2014,Jan,11

79445 **Radiopharmaceutical therapy, by intra-arterial particulate administration**

EXCLUDES *Intra-arterial injections (96373, 96420)*

Procedural and radiological supervision and interpretation for angiographic and interventional procedures before intra-arterial radiopharmaceutical therapy

0.00 0.00 FUD XXX S Z2 80

AMA: 2018,Jan,8; 2017,Jan,8; 2016,Jan,13; 2015,Jan,16; 2014,Jan,11

79999 **Radiopharmaceutical therapy, unlisted procedure**

0.00 0.00 FUD XXX S Z2 80

AMA: 2018,Jan,8; 2017,Jan,8; 2016,Jan,13; 2015,Jan,16; 2014,Jan,11

80047-80081 [80081] Multi-test Laboratory Panels

INCLUDES Groups of specified tests that may be reported as a panel

EXCLUDES *Reporting two or more panel codes that include the same tests; report the panel with the highest number of tests in common to meet the definition of the panel code*

Code also individual tests that are not part of the panel, when appropriate

80047 Basic metabolic panel (Calcium, ionized)

INCLUDES Calcium, ionized (82330)
Carbon dioxide (bicarbonate) (82374)
Chloride (82435)
Creatinine (82565)
Glucose (82947)
Potassium (84132)
Sodium (84295)
Urea nitrogen (BUN) (84520)

0.00 0.00 FUD XXX

AMA: 2018,Jan,8; 2017,Jan,8; 2016,Jan,13; 2015,Jan,16; 2014,Jan,11

80048 Basic metabolic panel (Calcium, total)

INCLUDES Calcium, total (82310)
Carbon dioxide (bicarbonate) (82374)
Chloride (82435)
Creatinine (82565)
Glucose (82947)
Potassium (84132)
Sodium (84295)
Urea nitrogen (BUN) (84520)

0.00 0.00 FUD XXX

AMA: 2018,Jan,8; 2017,Jan,8; 2016,Jan,13; 2015,Jan,16; 2014,Jan,11

80050 General health panel

INCLUDES Complete blood count (CBC), automated, with:
Manual differential WBC count
Blood smear with manual differential AND complete (CBC), automated (85007, 85027)
Manual differential WBC count, buffy coat AND complete (CBC), automated (85009, 85027)
OR
Automated differential WBC count
Automated differential WBC count AND complete (CBC), automated/automated differential WBC count (85004, 85025)
Automated differential WBC count AND complete (CBC), automated (85004, 85027)
Comprehensive metabolic profile (80053)
Thyroid stimulating hormone (84443)

0.00 0.00 FUD XXX

AMA: 2018,Jan,8; 2017,Jan,8; 2016,Jan,13; 2015,Jan,16; 2014,Jan,11

80051 Electrolyte panel

INCLUDES Carbon dioxide (bicarbonate) (82374)
Chloride (82435)
Potassium (84132)
Sodium (84295)

0.00 0.00 FUD XXX

AMA: 2018,Jan,8; 2017,Jan,8; 2016,Jan,13; 2015,Jan,16; 2014,Jan,11

80053 Comprehensive metabolic panel

INCLUDES Albumin (82040)
Bilirubin, total (82247)
Calcium, total (82310)
Carbon dioxide (bicarbonate) (82374)
Chloride (82435)
Creatinine (82565)
Glucose (82947)
Phosphatase, alkaline (84075)
Potassium (84132)
Protein, total (84155)
Sodium (84295)
Transferase, alanine amino (ALT) (SGPT) (84460)
Transferase, aspartate amino (AST) (SGOT) (84450)
Urea nitrogen (BUN) (84520)

0.00 0.00 FUD XXX

AMA: 2018,Jan,8; 2017,Jan,8; 2016,Jan,13; 2015,Jan,16; 2014,Jan,11

80055 Obstetric panel M ♀

INCLUDES Complete blood count (CBC), automated, with:
Manual differential WBC count
Blood smear with manual differential AND complete (CBC), automated (85007, 85027)
Manual differential WBC count, buffy coat AND complete (CBC), automated (85009, 85027)
OR
Automated differential WBC count
Automated differential WBC count AND complete (CBC), automated/automated differential WBC count (85004, 85025)
Automated differential WBC count AND complete (CBC), automated (85004, 85027)
Blood typing, ABO and Rh (86900-86901)
Hepatitis B surface antigen (HBsAg) (87340)
RBC antibody screen, each serum technique (86850)
Rubella antibody (86762)
Syphilis test, non-treponemal antibody qualitative (86592)

EXCLUDES *Use of code when syphilis screening is provided using a treponemal antibody approach. Instead, assign individual codes for tests performed in the OB panel (86780)*

0.00 0.00 FUD XXX

AMA: 2018,Jan,8; 2017,Jan,8; 2016,Jan,13; 2015,Jan,16; 2014,Jan,11

80081 Obstetric panel (includes HIV testing) M ♀

INCLUDES Complete blood count (CBC), automated, with:
Manual differential WBC count
Blood smear with manual differential AND complete (CBC), automated (85007, 85027)
Manual differential WBC count, buffy count AND complete (CBC), automated (85009, 85027)
OR
Automated differential WBC count
Automated differential WBC count AND complete (CBC), automated/automated differential WBC count (85004, 85025)
Automated differential WBC count AND complete (CBC), automated (85004, 85027)
Blood typing, ABO and Rh (86900-86901)
Hepatitis B surface antigen (HBsAg) (87340)
HIV-1 antigens, with HIV-1 and HIV-2 antibodies, single result (87389)
RBC antibody screen, each serum technique (86850)
Rubella antibody (86762)
Syphilis test, non-treponemal antibody qualitative (86592)

EXCLUDES *Use of code when syphilis screening is provided using a treponemal antibody approach. Instead, assign individual codes for tests performed in the OB panel (86780)*

0.00 0.00 FUD XXX

AMA: 2018,Jan,8; 2017,Jan,8; 2016,Jan,13

80061 Lipid panel

INCLUDES Cholesterol, serum, total (82465)
Lipoprotein, direct measurement, high density cholesterol (HDL cholesterol) (83718)
Triglycerides (84478)

0.00 0.00 FUD XXX

AMA: 2018,Jan,8; 2017,Sep,11; 2017,Jan,8; 2016,Jan,13; 2015,Jan,16; 2014,Jan,11

80069 Renal function panel

INCLUDES Albumin (82040)
Calcium, total (82310)
Carbon dioxide (bicarbonate) (82374)
Chloride (82435)
Creatinine (82565)
Glucose (82947)
Phosphorus inorganic (phosphate) (84100)
Potassium (84132)
Sodium (84295)
Urea nitrogen (BUN) (84520)

0.00 0.00 FUD XXX

AMA: 2018,Jan,8; 2017,Jan,8; 2016,Jan,13; 2015,Jan,16; 2014,Jan,11

80074 Acute hepatitis panel

INCLUDES Hepatitis A antibody (HAAb) IgM (86709)
Hepatitis B core antibody (HBcAb), IgM (86705)
Hepatitis B surface antigen (HBsAg) (87340)
Hepatitis C antibody (86803)

0.00 0.00 FUD XXX

AMA: 2018,Jan,8; 2017,Jan,8; 2016,Jan,13; 2015,Jan,16; 2014,Jan,11

80076 Hepatic function panel

INCLUDES Albumin (82040)
Bilirubin, direct (82248)
Bilirubin, total (82247)
Phosphatase, alkaline (84075)
Protein, total (84155)
Transferase, alanine amino (ALT) (SGPT) (84460)
Transferase, aspartate amino (AST) (SGOT) (84450)

0.00 0.00 FUD XXX

AMA: 2018,Jan,8; 2017,Jan,8; 2016,Jan,13; 2015,Jan,16; 2014,Jan,11

80081 **Resequenced code. See code following 80055.**

80305-80307 [80305, 80306, 80307] Nonspecific Drug Screening

INCLUDES All testing procedures provided despite the number of tests performed per modality

EXCLUDES *Confirmatory drug testing ([80320, 80321, 80322, 80323, 80324, 80325, 80326, 80327, 80328, 80329, 80330, 80331, 80332, 80333, 80334, 80335, 80336, 80337, 80338, 80339, 80340, 80341, 80342, 80343, 80344, 80345, 80346, 80347, 80348, 80349, 80350, 80351, 80352, 80353, 80354, 80355, 80356, 80357, 80358, 80359, 80360, 80361, 80362, 80363, 80364, 80365, 80366, 80367, 80368, 80369, 80370, 80371, 80372, 80373, 80374, 80375, 80376, 80377, 83992], [83992])*
Validation testing

80305 Drug test(s), presumptive, any number of drug classes, any number of devices or procedures; capable of being read by direct optical observation only (eg, utilizing immunoassay [eg, dipsticks, cups, cards, or cartridges]), includes sample validation when performed, per date of service

0.00 0.00 FUD XXX

AMA: 2018,Jul,14; 2018,Jan,8; 2017,Mar,6

80306 read by instrument assisted direct optical observation (eg, utilizing immunoassay [eg, dipsticks, cups, cards, or cartridges]), includes sample validation when performed, per date of service

0.00 0.00 FUD XXX

AMA: 2018,Jan,8; 2017,Mar,6

80307 by instrument chemistry analyzers (eg, utilizing immunoassay [eg, EIA, ELISA, EMIT, FPIA, IA, KIMS, RIA]), chromatography (eg, GC, HPLC), and mass spectrometry either with or without chromatography, (eg, DART, DESI, GC-MS, GC-MS/MS, LC-MS, LC-MS/MS, LDTD, MALDI, TOF) includes sample validation when performed, per date of service

0.00 0.00 FUD XXX

AMA: 2018,Jan,8; 2017,Mar,6

80320-80377 [80320, 80321, 80322, 80323, 80324, 80325, 80326, 80327, 80328, 80329, 80330, 80331, 80332, 80333, 80334, 80335, 80336, 80337, 80338, 80339, 80340, 80341, 80342, 80343, 80344, 80345, 80346, 80347, 80348, 80349, 80350, 80351, 80352, 80353, 80354, 80355, 80356, 80357, 80358, 80359, 80360, 80361, 80362, 80363, 80364, 80365, 80366, 80367, 80368, 80369, 80370, 80371, 80372, 80373, 80374, 80375, 80376, 80377, 83992] Confirmatory Drug Testing

INCLUDES Antihistamine drug tests ([80375, 80376, 80377])
Detection of specific drugs using methods other than immunoassay or enzymatic technique

EXCLUDES *Metabolites separate from the code for the drug except when a distinct code is available*

80320 Alcohols

0.00 0.00 FUD XXX

AMA: 2018,Jan,8; 2017,Jan,8; 2016,Jan,13; 2015,Apr,3

80321 Alcohol biomarkers; 1 or 2

0.00 0.00 FUD XXX

AMA: 2015,Apr,3

80322 3 or more

0.00 0.00 FUD XXX

AMA: 2015,Apr,3

80323 Alkaloids, not otherwise specified

0.00 0.00 FUD XXX

AMA: 2015,Apr,3

80324 Amphetamines; 1 or 2

0.00 0.00 FUD XXX

AMA: 2015,Apr,3

80325 3 or 4

0.00 0.00 FUD XXX

AMA: 2015,Apr,3

80326 5 or more

0.00 0.00 FUD XXX

AMA: 2015,Apr,3

80327 Anabolic steroids; 1 or 2

0.00 0.00 FUD XXX

AMA: 2015,Apr,3

80328 3 or more

EXCLUDES *Analysis dihydrotestosterone for monitoring, endogenous levels of hormone (82642)*

0.00 0.00 FUD XXX

AMA: 2015,Apr,3

80329 Analgesics, non-opioid; 1 or 2

0.00 0.00 FUD XXX

AMA: 2015,Apr,3

80330 3-5

0.00 0.00 FUD XXX

AMA: 2015,Apr,3

80331 6 or more

0.00 0.00 FUD XXX

AMA: 2015,Apr,3

80332 Antidepressants, serotonergic class; 1 or 2

0.00 0.00 FUD XXX

AMA: 2015,Apr,3

80333 3-5
0.00 0.00 FUD XXX B
AMA: 2015,Apr,3

80334 6 or more
0.00 0.00 FUD XXX B
AMA: 2015,Apr,3

80335 **Antidepressants, tricyclic and other cyclicals; 1 or 2**
0.00 0.00 FUD XXX B
AMA: 2015,Apr,3

80336 3-5
0.00 0.00 FUD XXX B
AMA: 2015,Apr,3

80337 6 or more
0.00 0.00 FUD XXX B
AMA: 2015,Apr,3

80338 **Antidepressants, not otherwise specified**
0.00 0.00 FUD XXX B
AMA: 2015,Apr,3

80339 **Antiepileptics, not otherwise specified; 1-3**
0.00 0.00 FUD XXX B
AMA: 2015,Apr,3

80340 4-6
0.00 0.00 FUD XXX B
AMA: 2015,Apr,3

80341 7 or more
EXCLUDES *Definitive drug testing for antihistamines ([80375, 80376, 80377])*
0.00 0.00 FUD XXX B
AMA: 2015,Apr,3

80342 **Antipsychotics, not otherwise specified; 1-3**
0.00 0.00 FUD XXX B
AMA: 2015,Apr,3

80343 4-6
0.00 0.00 FUD XXX B
AMA: 2015,Apr,3

80344 7 or more
0.00 0.00 FUD XXX B
AMA: 2015,Apr,3

80345 **Barbiturates**
0.00 0.00 FUD XXX B
AMA: 2015,Apr,3

80346 **Benzodiazepines; 1-12**
0.00 0.00 FUD XXX B
AMA: 2015,Apr,3

80347 13 or more
0.00 0.00 FUD XXX B
AMA: 2015,Apr,3

80348 **Buprenorphine**
0.00 0.00 FUD XXX B
AMA: 2015,Apr,3

80349 **Cannabinoids, natural**
0.00 0.00 FUD XXX B
AMA: 2015,Apr,3

80350 **Cannabinoids, synthetic; 1-3**
0.00 0.00 FUD XXX B
AMA: 2015,Apr,3

80351 4-6
0.00 0.00 FUD XXX B
AMA: 2015,Apr,3

80352 7 or more
0.00 0.00 FUD XXX B
AMA: 2015,Apr,3

80353 **Cocaine**
0.00 0.00 FUD XXX B
AMA: 2015,Apr,3

80354 **Fentanyl**
0.00 0.00 FUD XXX B
AMA: 2015,Apr,3

80355 **Gabapentin, non-blood**
EXCLUDES *Therapeutic drug assay ([80171])*
0.00 0.00 FUD XXX B
AMA: 2018,Jan,8; 2017,Jan,8; 2016,Jan,13; 2015,Apr,3

80356 **Heroin metabolite**
0.00 0.00 FUD XXX B
AMA: 2015,Apr,3

80357 **Ketamine and norketamine**
0.00 0.00 FUD XXX B
AMA: 2015,Apr,3

80358 **Methadone**
0.00 0.00 FUD XXX B
AMA: 2015,Apr,3

80359 **Methylenedioxyamphetamines (MDA, MDEA, MDMA)**
0.00 0.00 FUD XXX B
AMA: 2015,Apr,3

80360 **Methylphenidate**
0.00 0.00 FUD XXX B
AMA: 2015,Apr,3

80361 **Opiates, 1 or more**
0.00 0.00 FUD XXX B
AMA: 2015,Apr,3

80362 **Opioids and opiate analogs; 1 or 2**
0.00 0.00 FUD XXX B
AMA: 2015,Apr,3

80363 3 or 4
0.00 0.00 FUD XXX B
AMA: 2015,Apr,3

80364 5 or more
0.00 0.00 FUD XXX B
AMA: 2015,Apr,3

80365 **Oxycodone**
0.00 0.00 FUD XXX B
AMA: 2015,Apr,3

83992 **Phencyclidine (PCP)**
0.00 0.00 FUD XXX E
AMA: 2018,Jan,8; 2017,Jan,8; 2016,Jan,13; 2015,Jun,10; 2015,Apr,3

80366 **Pregabalin**
0.00 0.00 FUD XXX B
AMA: 2015,Apr,3

80367 **Propoxyphene**
0.00 0.00 FUD XXX B
AMA: 2015,Apr,3

80368 **Sedative hypnotics (non-benzodiazepines)**
0.00 0.00 FUD XXX B
AMA: 2015,Apr,3

80369 **Skeletal muscle relaxants; 1 or 2**
0.00 0.00 FUD XXX B
AMA: 2015,Apr,3

80370 3 or more
0.00 0.00 FUD XXX B
AMA: 2015,Apr,3

80371 **Stimulants, synthetic**
0.00 0.00 FUD XXX B
AMA: 2015,Apr,3

80372 **Tapentadol**
0.00 0.00 FUD XXX
AMA: 2015,Apr,3

80373 **Tramadol**
0.00 0.00 FUD XXX
AMA: 2015,Apr,3

80374 **Stereoisomer (enantiomer) analysis, single drug class**
Code also index drug analysis if appropriate
0.00 0.00 FUD XXX
AMA: 2015,Apr,3

80375 **Drug(s) or substance(s), definitive, qualitative or quantitative, not otherwise specified; 1-3**
0.00 0.00 FUD XXX
AMA: 2018,Jan,8; 2017,Jan,8; 2016,Jan,13; 2015,Apr,3

80376 **4-6**
0.00 0.00 FUD XXX
AMA: 2018,Jan,8; 2017,Jan,8; 2016,Jan,13; 2015,Apr,3

80377 **7 or more**
EXCLUDES *Definitive drug testing for antihistamines ([80375, 80376, 80377])*
0.00 0.00 FUD XXX
AMA: 2018,Jan,8; 2017,Jan,8; 2016,Jan,13; 2015,Apr,3

80145-80377 [80164, 80165, 80171, 80230, 80235, 80280, 80285] Therapeutic Drug Levels

INCLUDES Testing of drug and metabolite(s) in primary code
Tests on specimens from blood and blood components, and spinal fluid

● **80145** **Adalimumab**

80150 **Amikacin**
0.00 0.00 FUD XXX
AMA: 2018,Jan,8; 2017,Jan,8; 2016,Jan,13; 2015,Apr,3; 2015,Jan,16; 2014,Jan,11

80155 **Caffeine**
0.00 0.00 FUD XXX
AMA: 2015,Apr,3; 2014,Jan,11

80156 **Carbamazepine; total**
0.00 0.00 FUD XXX
AMA: 2018,Jan,8; 2017,Jan,8; 2016,Jan,13; 2015,Apr,3; 2015,Jan,16; 2014,Jan,11

80157 **free**
0.00 0.00 FUD XXX
AMA: 2018,Jan,8; 2017,Jan,8; 2016,Jan,13; 2015,Apr,3; 2015,Jan,16; 2014,Jan,11

80158 **Cyclosporine**
0.00 0.00 FUD XXX
AMA: 2018,Jan,8; 2017,Jan,8; 2016,Jan,13; 2015,Apr,3; 2015,Jan,16; 2014,Jan,11

80159 **Clozapine**
0.00 0.00 FUD XXX
AMA: 2015,Apr,3; 2014,Jan,11

80162 **Digoxin; total**
0.00 0.00 FUD XXX
AMA: 2018,Jan,8; 2017,Jan,8; 2016,Jan,13; 2015,Apr,3; 2015,Jan,16; 2014,Jan,11

80163 **free**
0.00 0.00 FUD XXX
AMA: 2018,Jan,8; 2017,Jan,8; 2016,Jan,13; 2015,Apr,3

80164 **Resequenced code. See code following 80201.**

80165 **Resequenced code. See code following 80201.**

80168 **Ethosuximide**
0.00 0.00 FUD XXX
AMA: 2018,Jan,8; 2017,Jan,8; 2016,Jan,13; 2015,Apr,3; 2015,Jan,16; 2014,Jan,11

80169 **Everolimus**
0.00 0.00 FUD XXX
AMA: 2015,Apr,3; 2014,Jan,11

80171 **Gabapentin, whole blood, serum, or plasma**
0.00 0.00 FUD XXX
AMA: 2018,Jan,8; 2017,Jan,8; 2016,Jan,13; 2015,Apr,3; 2014,Jan,11

80170 **Gentamicin**
0.00 0.00 FUD XXX
AMA: 2018,Jan,8; 2017,Jan,8; 2016,Jan,13; 2015,Apr,3; 2015,Jan,16; 2014,Jan,11

80171 **Resequenced code. See code following 80169.**

80173 **Haloperidol**
0.00 0.00 FUD XXX
AMA: 2018,Jan,8; 2017,Jan,8; 2016,Jan,13; 2015,Apr,3; 2015,Jan,16; 2014,Jan,11

● # **80230** **Infliximab**
0.00 0.00 FUD 000

● # **80235** **Lacosamide**
0.00 0.00 FUD 000

80175 **Lamotrigine**
0.00 0.00 FUD XXX
AMA: 2015,Apr,3; 2014,Jan,11

80176 **Lidocaine**
0.00 0.00 FUD XXX
AMA: 2018,Jan,8; 2017,Jan,8; 2016,Jan,13; 2015,Apr,3; 2015,Jan,16; 2014,Jan,11

80177 **Levetiracetam**
0.00 0.00 FUD XXX
AMA: 2015,Apr,3; 2014,Jan,11

80178 **Lithium**
0.00 0.00 FUD XXX
AMA: 2018,Jan,8; 2017,Jan,8; 2016,Jan,13; 2015,Apr,3; 2015,Jan,16; 2014,Jan,11

80180 **Mycophenolate (mycophenolic acid)**
0.00 0.00 FUD XXX
AMA: 2015,Apr,3; 2014,Jan,11

80183 **Oxcarbazepine**
0.00 0.00 FUD XXX
AMA: 2015,Apr,3; 2014,Jan,11

80184 **Phenobarbital**
0.00 0.00 FUD XXX
AMA: 2018,Jan,8; 2017,Jan,8; 2016,Jan,13; 2015,Apr,3; 2015,Jan,16; 2014,Jan,11

80185 **Phenytoin; total**
0.00 0.00 FUD XXX
AMA: 2018,Jan,8; 2017,Jan,8; 2016,Jan,13; 2015,Apr,3; 2015,Jan,16; 2014,Jan,11

80186 **free**
0.00 0.00 FUD XXX
AMA: 2018,Jan,8; 2017,Jan,8; 2016,Jan,13; 2015,Apr,3; 2015,Jan,16; 2014,Jan,11

● **80187** **Posaconazole**

80188 **Primidone**
0.00 0.00 FUD XXX
AMA: 2018,Jan,8; 2017,Jan,8; 2016,Jan,13; 2015,Apr,3; 2015,Jan,16; 2014,Jan,11

80190 **Procainamide;**
0.00 0.00 FUD XXX
AMA: 2018,Jan,8; 2017,Jan,8; 2016,Jan,13; 2015,Apr,3; 2015,Jan,16; 2014,Jan,11

80192 **with metabolites (eg, n-acetyl procainamide)**
0.00 0.00 FUD XXX
AMA: 2018,Jan,8; 2017,Jan,8; 2016,Jan,13; 2015,Apr,3; 2015,Jan,16; 2014,Jan,11

80194 **Quinidine**
0.00 0.00 FUD XXX
AMA: 2018,Jan,8; 2017,Jan,8; 2016,Jan,13; 2015,Apr,3; 2015,Jan,16; 2014,Jan,11

80195 **Sirolimus**
0.00 0.00 FUD XXX
AMA: 2018,Jan,8; 2017,Jan,8; 2016,Jan,13; 2015,Apr,3; 2015,Jan,16; 2014,Jan,11

80197 **Tacrolimus**
0.00 0.00 FUD XXX
AMA: 2018,Jan,8; 2017,Jan,8; 2016,Jan,13; 2015,Apr,3; 2015,Jan,16; 2014,Jan,11

80198 **Theophylline**
0.00 0.00 FUD XXX
AMA: 2018,Jan,8; 2017,Jan,8; 2016,Jan,13; 2015,Apr,3; 2015,Jan,16; 2014,Jan,11

80199 **Tiagabine**
0.00 0.00 FUD XXX
AMA: 2015,Apr,3; 2014,Jan,11

80200 **Tobramycin**
0.00 0.00 FUD XXX
AMA: 2018,Jan,8; 2017,Jan,8; 2016,Jan,13; 2015,Apr,3; 2015,Jan,16; 2014,Jan,11

80201 **Topiramate**
0.00 0.00 FUD XXX
AMA: 2018,Jan,8; 2017,Jan,8; 2016,Jan,13; 2015,Apr,3; 2015,Jan,16; 2014,Jan,11

80164 **Valproic acid (dipropylacetic acid); total**
0.00 0.00 FUD XXX
AMA: 2018,Jan,8; 2017,Jan,8; 2016,Jan,13; 2015,Apr,3; 2015,Jan,16; 2014,Jan,11

80165 **free**
0.00 0.00 FUD XXX
AMA: 2018,Jan,8; 2017,Jan,8; 2016,Jan,13; 2015,Apr,3

80202 **Vancomycin**
0.00 0.00 FUD XXX
AMA: 2018,Jan,8; 2017,Jan,8; 2016,Jan,13; 2015,Apr,3; 2015,Jan,16; 2014,Jan,11

● # 80280 **Vedolizumab**
0.00 0.00 FUD 000

● # 80285 **Voriconazole**
0.00 0.00 FUD 000

80203 **Zonisamide**
0.00 0.00 FUD XXX
AMA: 2015,Apr,3; 2014,Jan,11

80230 **Resequenced code. See code following 80173.**

80235 **Resequenced code. See code before 80175.**

80280 **Resequenced code. See code following 80202.**

80285 **Resequenced code. See code before 80203.**

80299 **Quantitation of therapeutic drug, not elsewhere specified**
0.00 0.00 FUD XXX
AMA: 2018,Jan,8; 2017,Jan,8; 2016,Jan,13; 2015,Apr,3; 2015,Jan,16; 2014,Jan,11

80305 **Resequenced code. See code before 80145.**

80306 **Resequenced code. See code before 80145.**

80307 **Resequenced code. See code before 80145.**

80320 **Resequenced code. See code before 80145.**

80321 **Resequenced code. See code before 80145.**

80322 **Resequenced code. See code before 80145.**

80323 **Resequenced code. See code before 80145.**

80324 **Resequenced code. See code before 80145.**

80325 **Resequenced code. See code before 80145.**

80326 **Resequenced code. See code before 80145.**

80327 **Resequenced code. See code before 80145.**

80328 **Resequenced code. See code before 80145.**

80329 **Resequenced code. See code before 80145.**

80330 **Resequenced code. See code before 80145.**

80331 **Resequenced code. See code before 80145.**

80332 **Resequenced code. See code before 80145.**

80333 **Resequenced code. See code before 80145.**

80334 **Resequenced code. See code before 80145.**

80335 **Resequenced code. See code before 80145.**

80336 **Resequenced code. See code before 80145.**

80337 **Resequenced code. See code before 80145.**

80338 **Resequenced code. See code before 80145.**

80339 **Resequenced code. See code before 80145.**

80340 **Resequenced code. See code before 80145.**

80341 **Resequenced code. See code before 80145.**

80342 **Resequenced code. See code before 80145.**

80343 **Resequenced code. See code before 80145.**

80344 **Resequenced code. See code before 80145.**

80345 **Resequenced code. See code before 80145.**

80346 **Resequenced code. See code before 80145.**

80347 **Resequenced code. See code before 80145.**

80348 **Resequenced code. See code before 80145.**

80349 **Resequenced code. See code before 80145.**

80350 **Resequenced code. See code before 80145.**

80351 **Resequenced code. See code before 80145.**

80352 **Resequenced code. See code before 80145.**

80353 **Resequenced code. See code before 80145.**

80354 **Resequenced code. See code before 80145.**

80355 **Resequenced code. See code before 80145.**

80356 **Resequenced code. See code before 80145.**

80357 **Resequenced code. See code before 80145.**

80358 **Resequenced code. See code before 80145.**

80359 **Resequenced code. See code before 80145.**

80360 **Resequenced code. See code before 80145.**

80361 **Resequenced code. See code before 80145.**

80362 **Resequenced code. See code before 80145.**

80363 **Resequenced code. See code before 80145.**

80364 **Resequenced code. See code before 80145.**

80365 **Resequenced code. See code before 80145.**

80366 **Resequenced code. See code before 80145.**

80367 **Resequenced code. See code before 80145.**

80368 **Resequenced code. See code before 80145.**

80369 **Resequenced code. See code before 80145.**

80370 **Resequenced code. See code before 80145.**

80371 **Resequenced code. See code before 80145.**

80372 **Resequenced code. See code before 80145.**

80373 **Resequenced code. See code before 80145.**

80374 **Resequenced code. See code before 80145.**

80375 **Resequenced code. See code before 80145.**

80376 **Resequenced code. See code before 80145.**

80377 **Resequenced code. See code before 80145.**

80400-80439 Stimulation and Suppression Test Panels

EXCLUDES *Administration of evocative or suppressive material (96365-96368, 96372, 96374-96376, C8957)*
Evocative or suppression test substances, as applicable
Physician monitoring and attendance during test (see E&M services)

80400 ACTH stimulation panel; for adrenal insufficiency
INCLUDES Cortisol x 2 (82533)
0.00 0.00 FUD XXX
AMA: 2018,Jan,8; 2017,Jan,8; 2016,Jan,13; 2015,Jan,16; 2014,Jan,11

80402 for 21 hydroxylase deficiency
INCLUDES 17 hydroxyprogesterone X 2 (83498)
Cortisol x 2 (82533)
0.00 0.00 FUD XXX
AMA: 2014,Jan,11

80406 for 3 beta-hydroxydehydrogenase deficiency
INCLUDES 17 hydroxypregnenolone x 2 (84143)
Cortisol x 2 (82533)
0.00 0.00 FUD XXX
AMA: 2014,Jan,11

80408 Aldosterone suppression evaluation panel (eg, saline infusion)
INCLUDES Aldosterone x 2 (82088)
Renin x 2 (84244)
0.00 0.00 FUD XXX
AMA: 2014,Jan,11

80410 Calcitonin stimulation panel (eg, calcium, pentagastrin)
INCLUDES Calcitonin x 3 (82308)
0.00 0.00 FUD XXX
AMA: 2014,Jan,11

80412 Corticotropic releasing hormone (CRH) stimulation panel
INCLUDES Adrenocorticotropic hormone (ACTH) x 6 (82024)
Cortisol x 6 (82533)
0.00 0.00 FUD XXX
AMA: 2014,Jan,11

80414 Chorionic gonadotropin stimulation panel; testosterone response
INCLUDES Testosterone x 2 on three pooled blood samples (84403)
0.00 0.00 FUD XXX
AMA: 2014,Jan,11

80415 estradiol response
INCLUDES Estradiol x 2 on three pooled blood samples (82670)
0.00 0.00 FUD XXX
AMA: 2014,Jan,11

80416 Renal vein renin stimulation panel (eg, captopril)
INCLUDES Renin x 6 (84244)
0.00 0.00 FUD XXX
AMA: 2014,Jan,11

80417 Peripheral vein renin stimulation panel (eg, captopril)
INCLUDES Renin x 2 (84244)
0.00 0.00 FUD XXX
AMA: 2014,Jan,11

80418 Combined rapid anterior pituitary evaluation panel
INCLUDES Adrenocorticotropic hormone (ACTH) x 4 (82024)
Cortisol x 4 (82533)
Follicle stimulating hormone (FSH) x 4 (83001)
Human growth hormone x 4 (83003)
Luteinizing hormone (LH) x 4 (83002)
Prolactin x 4 (84146)
Thyroid stimulating hormone (TSH) x 4 (84443)
0.00 0.00 FUD XXX
AMA: 2014,Jan,11

80420 Dexamethasone suppression panel, 48 hour
INCLUDES Cortisol x 2 (82533)
Free cortisol, urine x 2 (82530)
Volume measurement for timed collection x 2 (81050)
EXCLUDES *Single dose dexamethasone (82533)*
0.00 0.00 FUD XXX
AMA: 2014,Jan,11

80422 Glucagon tolerance panel; for insulinoma
INCLUDES Glucose x 3 (82947)
Insulin x 3 (83525)
0.00 0.00 FUD XXX
AMA: 2014,Jan,11

80424 for pheochromocytoma
INCLUDES Catecholamines, fractionated x 2 (82384)
0.00 0.00 FUD XXX
AMA: 2014,Jan,11

80426 Gonadotropin releasing hormone stimulation panel
INCLUDES Follicle stimulating hormone (FSH) x 4 (83001)
Luteinizing hormone (LH) x 4 (83002)
0.00 0.00 FUD XXX
AMA: 2014,Jan,11

80428 Growth hormone stimulation panel (eg, arginine infusion, l-dopa administration)
INCLUDES Human growth hormone (HGH) x 4 (83003)
0.00 0.00 FUD XXX
AMA: 2014,Jan,11

80430 Growth hormone suppression panel (glucose administration)
INCLUDES Glucose x 3 (82947)
Human growth hormone (HGH) x 4 (83003)
0.00 0.00 FUD XXX
AMA: 2014,Jan,11

80432 Insulin-induced C-peptide suppression panel
INCLUDES C-peptide x 5 (84681)
Glucose x 5 (82947)
Insulin (83525)
0.00 0.00 FUD XXX
AMA: 2014,Jan,11

80434 Insulin tolerance panel; for ACTH insufficiency
INCLUDES Cortisol x 5 (82533)
Glucose x 5 (82947)
0.00 0.00 FUD XXX
AMA: 2014,Jan,11

80435 for growth hormone deficiency
INCLUDES Glucose x 5 (82947)
Human growth hormone (HGH) x 5 (83003)
0.00 0.00 FUD XXX
AMA: 2014,Jan,11

80436 Metyrapone panel
INCLUDES 11 deoxycortisol x 2 (82634)
Cortisol x 2 (82533)
0.00 0.00 FUD XXX
AMA: 2014,Jan,11

80438 Thyrotropin releasing hormone (TRH) stimulation panel; 1 hour

INCLUDES Thyroid stimulating hormone (TSH) x 3 (84443)

0.00 0.00 FUD XXX

AMA: 2014,Jan,11

80439 2 hour

INCLUDES Thyroid stimulating hormone (TSH) x 4 (84443)

0.00 0.00 FUD XXX

AMA: 2014,Jan,11

80500-80502 Consultation By Clinical Pathologist

INCLUDES Pharmacokinetic consultations
Written report by pathologist for tests requiring additional medical judgment and requested by a physician or other qualified health care professional

EXCLUDES *Consultations that include patient examination*
Use of code when a medical interpretive assessment is not provided

80500 Clinical pathology consultation; limited, without review of patient's history and medical records

0.56 0.65 FUD XXX

AMA: 2018,Jan,8; 2017,Jan,8; 2016,Jan,13; 2015,Jan,16; 2014,Jan,11

80502 comprehensive, for a complex diagnostic problem, with review of patient's history and medical records

2.01 2.10 FUD XXX

AMA: 2018,Jan,8; 2017,Jan,8; 2016,Jan,13; 2015,Jan,16; 2014,Jan,11

81000-81099 Urine Tests

81000 Urinalysis, by dip stick or tablet reagent for bilirubin, glucose, hemoglobin, ketones, leukocytes, nitrite, pH, protein, specific gravity, urobilinogen, any number of these constituents; non-automated, with microscopy

0.00 0.00 FUD XXX

AMA: 2018,Jul,14; 2018,Jan,8; 2017,Jan,8; 2016,Jan,13; 2015,Jan,16; 2014,Jan,11

81001 automated, with microscopy

0.00 0.00 FUD XXX

AMA: 2014,Jan,11

81002 non-automated, without microscopy

INCLUDES Mosenthal test

0.00 0.00 FUD XXX

AMA: 2018,Jan,8; 2017,Jan,8; 2016,Jan,13; 2015,Jan,16; 2014,Jan,11

81003 automated, without microscopy

0.00 0.00 FUD XXX

AMA: 2018,Jan,8; 2017,Jan,8; 2016,Jan,13; 2015,Jan,16; 2014,Jan,11

81005 Urinalysis; qualitative or semiquantitative, except immunoassays

INCLUDES Benedict test for dextrose

EXCLUDES *Immunoassay, qualitative or semiquantitative (83518)*
Microalbumin (82043-82044)
Nonimmunoassay reagent strip analysis (81000, 81002)

0.00 0.00 FUD XXX

AMA: 2018,Jan,8; 2017,Jan,8; 2016,Jan,13; 2015,Jan,16; 2014,Jan,11

81007 bacteriuria screen, except by culture or dipstick

EXCLUDES *Culture (87086-87088)*
Dipstick (81000, 81002)

0.00 0.00 FUD XXX

AMA: 2014,Jan,11

81015 microscopic only

EXCLUDES *Sperm evaluation for retrograde ejaculation (89331)*

0.00 0.00 FUD XXX

AMA: 2018,Jan,8; 2017,Nov,10; 2014,Jan,11

81020 2 or 3 glass test

INCLUDES Valentine's test

0.00 0.00 FUD XXX

AMA: 2014,Jan,11

81025 Urine pregnancy test, by visual color comparison methods

0.00 0.00 FUD XXX

AMA: 2018,Jan,8; 2017,Jan,8; 2016,Jan,13; 2015,Jan,16; 2014,Jan,11

81050 Volume measurement for timed collection, each

0.00 0.00 FUD XXX

AMA: 2014,Jan,11

81099 Unlisted urinalysis procedure

0.00 0.00 FUD XXX

AMA: 2018,Jan,8; 2017,Jan,8; 2016,Jan,13; 2015,Jan,16; 2014,Jan,11

81105-81364 [81105, 81106, 81107, 81108, 81109, 81110, 81111, 81112, 81120, 81121, 81161, 81162, 81163, 81164, 81165, 81166, 81167, 81173, 81174, 81184, 81185, 81186, 81187, 81188, 81189, 81190, 81200, 81201, 81202, 81203, 81204, 81205, 81206, 81207, 81208, 81209, 81210, 81219, 81227, 81230, 81231, 81233, 81234, 81238, 81239, 81245, 81246, 81250, 81257, 81258, 81259, 81261, 81262, 81263, 81264, 81265, 81266, 81267, 81268, 81269, 81271, 81274, 81277, 81283, 81284, 81285, 81286, 81287, 81288, 81289, 81291, 81292, 81293, 81294, 81295, 81301, 81302, 81303, 81304, 81306, 81307, 81308, 81309, 81312, 81320, 81324, 81325, 81326, 81332, 81334, 81336, 81337, 81343, 81344, 81345, 81361, 81362, 81363, 81364] Gene Analysis: Tier 1 Procedures

INCLUDES All analytical procedures in the evaluation such as:
- Amplification
- Cell lysis
- Detection
- Digestion
- Extraction
- Nucleic acid stabilization

Code selection based on specific gene being reviewed
Evaluation of constitutional or somatic gene variations
Evaluation of the presence of gene variants using the common gene variant name
Examples of proteins or diseases in the code description that are not all inclusive
Gene specific and genomic testing
Generally all the listed gene variants in the code description would be tested but lists are not all inclusive
Genes described using Human Genome Organization (HUGO) approved names
Qualitative results unless otherwise stated
Tier 1 molecular pathology codes (81105-81254 [81161, 81162, 81163, 81164, 81165, 81166, 81167, 81173, 81174, 81184, 81185, 81186, 81187, 81188, 81189, 81190, 81200, 81201, 81202, 81203, 81204, 81205, 81206, 81207, 81208, 81209, 81210, 81219, 81227, 81230, 81231, 81233, 81234, 81238, 81239, 81245, 81246, 81250, 81257, 81258, 81259, 81265, 81266, 81267, 81268, 81269, 81284, 81285, 81286, 81289, 81361, 81362, 81363, 81364])

EXCLUDES *Full gene sequencing using separate gene variant assessment codes unless it is specifically stated in the code description*
In situ hybridization analyses (88271-88275, 88365-88368 [88364, 88373, 88374])
Microbial identification (87149-87153, 87471-87801 [87623, 87624, 87625], 87900-87904 [87906, 87910, 87912])
Other related gene variants not listed in code
Tier 1 molecular pathology codes (81370-81383)
Tier 2 codes (81400-81408)
Unlisted molecular pathology procedures ([81479])

Code also modifier 26 when only interpretation and report are performed
Code also services required before cell lysis

81105 **Resequenced code. See code before 81260.**

81106 **Resequenced code. See code before 81260.**

81107 **Resequenced code. See code before 81260.**

81108 Resequenced code. See code before 81260.

81109 Resequenced code. See code before 81260.

81110 Resequenced code. See code before 81260.

81111 Resequenced code. See code before 81260.

81112 Resequenced code. See code before 81260.

81120 Resequenced code. See code before 81260.

81121 Resequenced code. See code before 81260.

81161 Resequenced code. See code following numeric code 81231.

81162 Resequenced code. See code following resequenced code 81210.

81163 Resequenced code. See code following resequenced code 81210.

81164 Resequenced code. See code following resequenced code 81210.

81165 Resequenced code. See code following 81212.

81166 Resequenced code. See code following 81212.

81167 Resequenced code. See code following 81216.

81170 *ABL1 (ABL proto-oncogene 1, non-receptor tyrosine kinase)* (eg, acquired imatinib tyrosine kinase inhibitor resistance), gene analysis, variants in the kinase domain
0.00 0.00 FUD XXX A
AMA: 2018,Jan,8; 2017,Jan,8; 2016,Aug,9

81171 *AFF2 (AF4/FMR2 family, member 2 [FMR2])* (eg, fragile X mental retardation 2 [FRAXE]) gene analysis; evaluation to detect abnormal (eg, expanded) alleles
0.00 0.00 FUD XXX

81172 characterization of alleles (eg, expanded size and methylation status)
0.00 0.00 FUD XXX

81173 Resequenced code. See code following resequenced code 81204.

81174 Resequenced code. See code following resequenced code 81204.

\# 81201 *APC (adenomatous polyposis coli)* (eg, familial adenomatosis polyposis [FAP], attenuated FAP) gene analysis; full gene sequence
0.00 0.00 FUD XXX A
AMA: 2018,Nov,9; 2018,Jan,8; 2017,Jan,8; 2016,Aug,9; 2016,Jan,13; 2015,Jan,16; 2014,Jan,11

\# 81202 known familial variants
0.00 0.00 FUD XXX A
AMA: 2018,Nov,9; 2018,Jan,8; 2017,Jan,8; 2016,Aug,9; 2016,Jan,13; 2015,Jan,16; 2014,Jan,11

\# 81203 duplication/deletion variants
0.00 0.00 FUD XXX A
AMA: 2018,Nov,9; 2018,Jan,8; 2017,Jan,8; 2016,Aug,9; 2016,Jan,13; 2015,Jan,16; 2014,Jan,11

\# 81204 *AR (androgen receptor)* (eg, spinal and bulbar muscular atrophy, Kennedy disease, X chromosome inactivation) gene analysis; characterization of alleles (eg, expanded size or methylation status)
0.00 0.00 FUD XXX
AMA: 2018,Nov,9

\# 81173 full gene sequence
0.00 0.00 FUD XXX

\# 81174 known familial variant
0.00 0.00 FUD XXX

\# 81200 *ASPA (aspartoacylase)* (eg, Canavan disease) gene analysis, common variants (eg, E285A, Y231X)
0.00 0.00 FUD XXX A
AMA: 2018,Nov,9; 2018,Jan,8; 2017,Jan,8; 2016,Aug,9; 2016,Jan,13; 2015,Jan,16; 2014,Jan,11

81175 *ASXL1 (additional sex combs like 1, transcriptional regulator)* (eg, myelodysplastic syndrome, myeloproliferative neoplasms, chronic myelomonocytic leukemia), gene analysis; full gene sequence
0.00 0.00 FUD XXX A

81176 targeted sequence analysis (eg, exon 12)
0.00 0.00 FUD XXX A

81177 *ATN1 (atrophin 1)* (eg, dentatorubral-pallidoluysian atrophy) gene analysis, evaluation to detect abnormal (eg, expanded) alleles
0.00 0.00 FUD XXX

81178 *ATXN1 (ataxin 1)* (eg, spinocerebellar ataxia) gene analysis, evaluation to detect abnormal (eg, expanded) alleles
0.00 0.00 FUD XXX
AMA: 2019,Sep,7

81179 *ATXN2 (ataxin 2)* (eg, spinocerebellar ataxia) gene analysis, evaluation to detect abnormal (eg, expanded) alleles
0.00 0.00 FUD XXX
AMA: 2019,Sep,7

81180 *ATXN3 (ataxin 3)* (eg, spinocerebellar ataxia, Machado-Joseph disease) gene analysis, evaluation to detect abnormal (eg, expanded) alleles
0.00 0.00 FUD XXX
AMA: 2019,Sep,7

81181 *ATXN7 (ataxin 7)* (eg, spinocerebellar ataxia) gene analysis, evaluation to detect abnormal (eg, expanded) alleles
0.00 0.00 FUD XXX
AMA: 2019,Sep,7

81182 *ATXN8OS (ATXN8 opposite strand [non-protein coding])* (eg, spinocerebellar ataxia) gene analysis, evaluation to detect abnormal (eg, expanded) alleles
0.00 0.00 FUD XXX
AMA: 2019,Sep,7

81183 *ATXN10 (ataxin 10)* (eg, spinocerebellar ataxia) gene analysis, evaluation to detect abnormal (eg, expanded) alleles
0.00 0.00 FUD XXX
AMA: 2019,Sep,7

81184 Resequenced code. See code following resequenced code 81233.

81185 Resequenced code. See code following resequenced code 81233.

81186 Resequenced code. See code following resequenced code 81233.

81187 Resequenced code. See code following resequenced code 81268.

81188 Resequenced code. See code following resequenced code 81266.

81189 Resequenced code. See code following resequenced code 81266.

81190 Resequenced code. See code following resequenced code 81266.

81200 Resequenced code. See code before 81175.

81201 Resequenced code. See code following numeric code 81174.

81202 Resequenced code. See code following numeric code 81174.

81203 Resequenced code. See code following numeric code 81174.

81204 Resequenced code. See code following numeric code 81174.

81205 Resequenced code. See code following numeric code 81210.

81206 Resequenced code. See code following numeric code 81210.

81207 **Resequenced code. See code following numeric code 81210.**

81208 **Resequenced code. See code following numeric code 81210.**

81209 **Resequenced code. See code following numeric code 81210.**

81210 **Resequenced code. See code following resequenced code 81209.**

\# **81205** ***BCKDHB (branched-chain keto acid dehydrogenase E1, beta polypeptide)*** **(eg, maple syrup urine disease) gene analysis, common variants (eg, R183P, G278S, E422X)**

0.00 0.00 FUD XXX

AMA: 2018,Nov,9; 2018,Jan,8; 2017,Jan,8; 2016,Aug,9; 2016,Jan,13; 2015,Jan,16; 2014,Jan,11

\# **81206** ***BCR/ABL1 (t(9;22))*** **(eg, chronic myelogenous leukemia) translocation analysis; major breakpoint, qualitative or quantitative**

0.00 0.00 FUD XXX

AMA: 2018,Nov,9; 2018,Jan,8; 2017,Jan,8; 2016,Aug,9; 2016,Jan,13; 2015,Jan,16; 2014,Jan,11

\# **81207** **minor breakpoint, qualitative or quantitative**

0.00 0.00 FUD XXX

AMA: 2018,Nov,9; 2018,Jan,8; 2017,Jan,8; 2016,Aug,9; 2016,Jan,13; 2015,Jan,16; 2014,Jan,11

\# **81208** **other breakpoint, qualitative or quantitative**

0.00 0.00 FUD XXX

AMA: 2018,Nov,9; 2018,Jan,8; 2017,Jan,8; 2016,Aug,9; 2016,Jan,13; 2015,Jan,16; 2014,Jan,11

\# **81209** ***BLM (Bloom syndrome, RecQ helicase-like)*** **(eg, Bloom syndrome) gene analysis, 2281del6ins7 variant**

0.00 0.00 FUD XXX

AMA: 2018,Nov,9; 2018,Jan,8; 2017,Jan,8; 2016,Aug,9; 2016,Jan,13; 2015,Jan,16; 2014,Jan,11

\# **81210** ***BRAF (B-Raf proto-oncogene, serine/threonine kinase)*** **(eg, colon cancer, melanoma), gene analysis, V600 variant(s)**

0.00 0.00 FUD XXX

AMA: 2018,Nov,9; 2018,Jan,8; 2017,Jan,8; 2016,Aug,9; 2016,Jan,13; 2015,Jan,16; 2014,Jan,11

\# **81162** ***BRCA1 (BRCA1, DNA repair associated), BRCA2 (BRCA2, DNA repair associated)*** **(eg, hereditary breast and ovarian cancer) gene analysis; full sequence analysis and full duplication/deletion analysis (ie, detection of large gene rearrangements)**

EXCLUDES *BRCA1 common duplication/deletion variant ([81479])*
BRCA1, BRCA2 full duplication/deletion analysis only (81164, 81166-81167, 81216)
BRCA1, BRCA2 full sequence analysis only (81163, 81165)
BRCA1, BRCA2 known familial variant only (81217)
Hereditary breast cancer genomic sequence analysis panel (81432)

0.00 0.00 FUD XXX

AMA: 2019,May,5; 2018,Jan,8; 2017,Jan,8; 2016,Aug,9

\# **81163** **full sequence analysis**

EXCLUDES *BRCA1 common duplication/deletion variant ([81479])*
BRCA1, BRCA2 full duplication/deletion analysis only (81164, 81216)
BRCA1, BRCA2 full sequence analysis and full duplication/deletion analysis (81162)
BRCA1, BRCA2 full sequence analysis only (81165)
Hereditary breast cancer genomic sequence analysis panel (81432)

0.00 0.00 FUD XXX

AMA: 2019,May,5

\# **81164** **full duplication/deletion analysis (ie, detection of large gene rearrangements)**

EXCLUDES *BRCA1 common duplication/deletion variant ([81479])*
BRCA1, BRCA2 full sequence analysis and full duplication/deletion analysis (81162)
BRCA1, BRCA2 full sequence analysis only (81163)
BRCA1, BRCA2 full duplication/deletion analysis only (81166-81167)
BRCA1, BRCA2 known familial variant only (81217)

0.00 0.00 FUD XXX

AMA: 2019,May,5

81212 **185delAG, 5385insC, 6174delT variants**

0.00 0.00 FUD XXX

AMA: 2019,May,5; 2018,Nov,9; 2018,Jan,8; 2017,Jan,8; 2016,Aug,9; 2016,Jan,13; 2015,Jan,16; 2014,Jan,11

\# **81165** ***BRCA1 (BRCA1, DNA repair associated)*** **(eg, hereditary breast and ovarian cancer) gene analysis; full sequence analysis**

EXCLUDES *BRCA1 common duplication/deletion variant ([81479])*
BRCA1, BRCA2 full sequence analysis and full duplication/deletion analysis (81162)
BRCA1, BRCA2 full sequence analysis only (81163)
Hereditary breast cancer genomic sequence analysis panel (81432)

0.00 0.00 FUD XXX

AMA: 2019,May,5

\# **81166** **full duplication/deletion analysis (ie, detection of large gene rearrangements)**

EXCLUDES *BRCA1 common duplication/deletion variant ([81479])*
BRCA1, BRCA2 full duplication/deletion analysis only (81164)
BRCA1, BRCA2 full sequence analysis and full duplication/deletion analysis (81162)

0.00 0.00 FUD XXX

AMA: 2019,May,5

81215 **known familial variant**

EXCLUDES *BRCA1 common duplication/deletion variant ([81479])*

0.00 0.00 FUD XXX

AMA: 2019,May,5; 2018,Nov,9; 2018,Jan,8; 2017,Jan,8; 2016,Aug,9; 2016,Jan,13; 2015,Jan,16; 2014,Jan,11

81216 ***BRCA2 (BRCA2, DNA repair associated)*** **(eg, hereditary breast and ovarian cancer) gene analysis; full sequence analysis**

EXCLUDES *BRCA1, BRCA2 full sequence analysis only (81163)*
BRCA1, BRCA2 full sequence analysis and full duplication/deletion analysis (81162)
Hereditary breast cancer genomic sequence analysis panel (81432)

0.00 0.00 FUD XXX

AMA: 2019,May,5; 2018,Nov,9; 2018,Jan,8; 2017,Jan,8; 2016,Aug,9; 2016,Jan,13; 2015,Jan,16; 2014,Jan,11

\# **81167** **full duplication/deletion analysis (ie, detection of large gene rearrangements)**

EXCLUDES *BRCA1, BRCA2 full duplication/deletion analysis only (81164, 81167)*
BRCA1, BRCA2 full sequence analysis and full duplication/deletion analysis (81162)

0.00 0.00 FUD XXX

AMA: 2019,May,5

81217 **known familial variant**

EXCLUDES *BRCA1, BRCA2 full duplication/deletion analysis only (81164, 81167)*
BRCA1, BRCA2 full sequence analysis and full duplication/deletion analysis (81162)

0.00 0.00 FUD XXX

AMA: 2019,May,5; 2018,Nov,9; 2018,Jan,8; 2017,Jan,8; 2016,Aug,9; 2016,Jan,13; 2015,Jan,16; 2014,Jan,11

\# **81233** ***BTK (Bruton's tyrosine kinase)*** **(eg, chronic lymphocytic leukemia) gene analysis, common variants (eg, C481S, C481R, C481F)**

0.00 0.00 FUD XXX

AMA: 2018,Nov,9

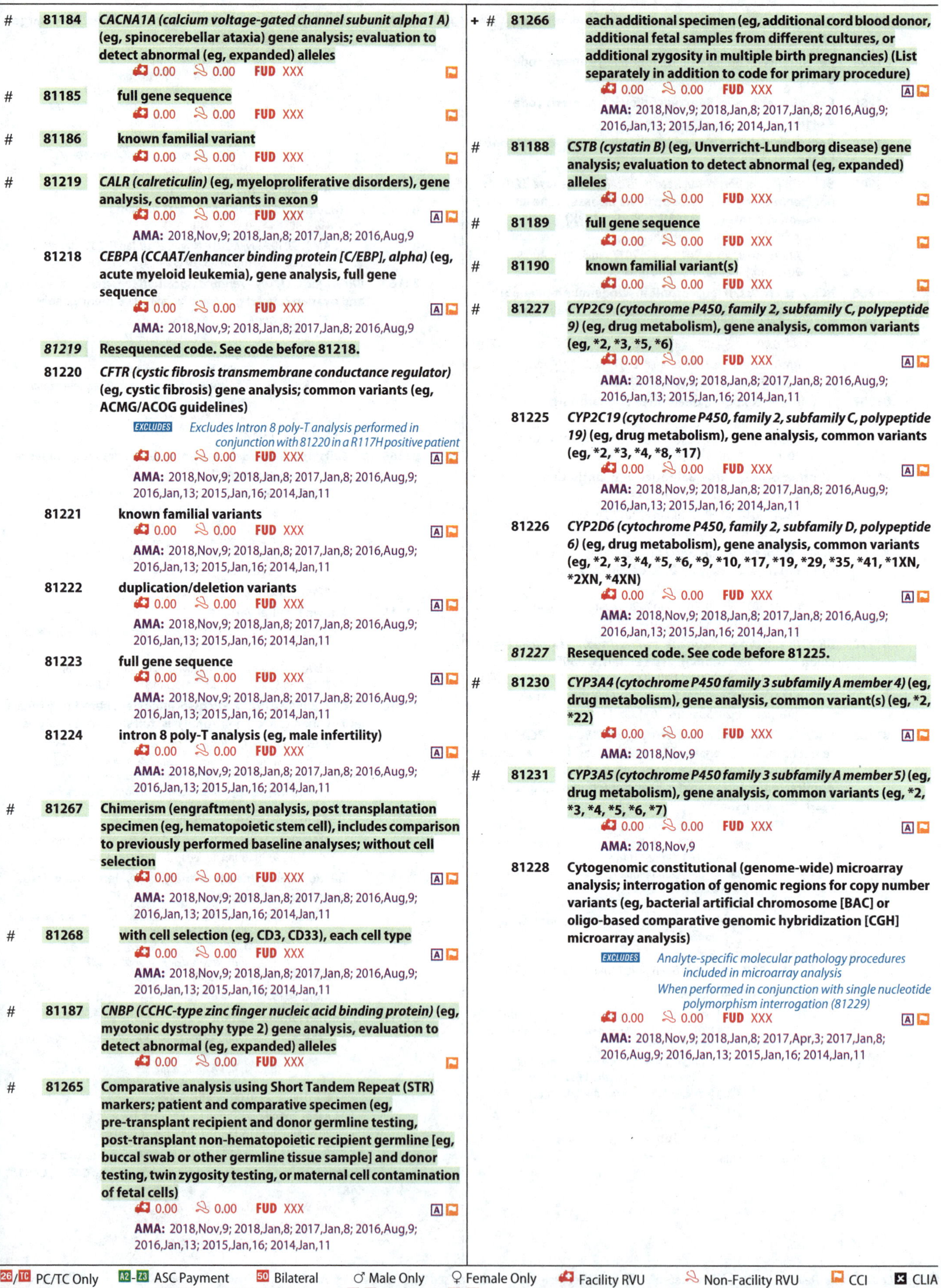

\# **81184** ***CACNA1A (calcium voltage-gated channel subunit alpha1 A)*** **(eg, spinocerebellar ataxia) gene analysis; evaluation to detect abnormal (eg, expanded) alleles**
0.00 0.00 FUD XXX

\# **81185** **full gene sequence**
0.00 0.00 FUD XXX

\# **81186** **known familial variant**
0.00 0.00 FUD XXX

\# **81219** ***CALR (calreticulin)*** **(eg, myeloproliferative disorders), gene analysis, common variants in exon 9**
0.00 0.00 FUD XXX
AMA: 2018,Nov,9; 2018,Jan,8; 2017,Jan,8; 2016,Aug,9

81218 ***CEBPA (CCAAT/enhancer binding protein [C/EBP], alpha)*** **(eg, acute myeloid leukemia), gene analysis, full gene sequence**
0.00 0.00 FUD XXX
AMA: 2018,Nov,9; 2018,Jan,8; 2017,Jan,8; 2016,Aug,9

81219 **Resequenced code. See code before 81218.**

81220 ***CFTR (cystic fibrosis transmembrane conductance regulator)*** **(eg, cystic fibrosis) gene analysis; common variants (eg, ACMG/ACOG guidelines)**
EXCLUDES *Excludes Intron 8 poly-T analysis performed in conjunction with 81220 in a R117H positive patient*
0.00 0.00 FUD XXX
AMA: 2018,Nov,9; 2018,Jan,8; 2017,Jan,8; 2016,Aug,9; 2016,Jan,13; 2015,Jan,16; 2014,Jan,11

81221 **known familial variants**
0.00 0.00 FUD XXX
AMA: 2018,Nov,9; 2018,Jan,8; 2017,Jan,8; 2016,Aug,9; 2016,Jan,13; 2015,Jan,16; 2014,Jan,11

81222 **duplication/deletion variants**
0.00 0.00 FUD XXX
AMA: 2018,Nov,9; 2018,Jan,8; 2017,Jan,8; 2016,Aug,9; 2016,Jan,13; 2015,Jan,16; 2014,Jan,11

81223 **full gene sequence**
0.00 0.00 FUD XXX
AMA: 2018,Nov,9; 2018,Jan,8; 2017,Jan,8; 2016,Aug,9; 2016,Jan,13; 2015,Jan,16; 2014,Jan,11

81224 **intron 8 poly-T analysis (eg, male infertility)**
0.00 0.00 FUD XXX
AMA: 2018,Nov,9; 2018,Jan,8; 2017,Jan,8; 2016,Aug,9; 2016,Jan,13; 2015,Jan,16; 2014,Jan,11

\# **81267** **Chimerism (engraftment) analysis, post transplantation specimen (eg, hematopoietic stem cell), includes comparison to previously performed baseline analyses; without cell selection**
0.00 0.00 FUD XXX
AMA: 2018,Nov,9; 2018,Jan,8; 2017,Jan,8; 2016,Aug,9; 2016,Jan,13; 2015,Jan,16; 2014,Jan,11

\# **81268** **with cell selection (eg, CD3, CD33), each cell type**
0.00 0.00 FUD XXX
AMA: 2018,Nov,9; 2018,Jan,8; 2017,Jan,8; 2016,Aug,9; 2016,Jan,13; 2015,Jan,16; 2014,Jan,11

\# **81187** ***CNBP (CCHC-type zinc finger nucleic acid binding protein)*** **(eg, myotonic dystrophy type 2) gene analysis, evaluation to detect abnormal (eg, expanded) alleles**
0.00 0.00 FUD XXX

\# **81265** **Comparative analysis using Short Tandem Repeat (STR) markers; patient and comparative specimen (eg, pre-transplant recipient and donor germline testing, post-transplant non-hematopoietic recipient germline [eg, buccal swab or other germline tissue sample] and donor testing, twin zygosity testing, or maternal cell contamination of fetal cells)**
0.00 0.00 FUD XXX
AMA: 2018,Nov,9; 2018,Jan,8; 2017,Jan,8; 2016,Aug,9; 2016,Jan,13; 2015,Jan,16; 2014,Jan,11

\+ # **81266** **each additional specimen (eg, additional cord blood donor, additional fetal samples from different cultures, or additional zygosity in multiple birth pregnancies) (List separately in addition to code for primary procedure)**
0.00 0.00 FUD XXX
AMA: 2018,Nov,9; 2018,Jan,8; 2017,Jan,8; 2016,Aug,9; 2016,Jan,13; 2015,Jan,16; 2014,Jan,11

\# **81188** ***CSTB (cystatin B)*** **(eg, Unverricht-Lundborg disease) gene analysis; evaluation to detect abnormal (eg, expanded) alleles**
0.00 0.00 FUD XXX

\# **81189** **full gene sequence**
0.00 0.00 FUD XXX

\# **81190** **known familial variant(s)**
0.00 0.00 FUD XXX

\# **81227** ***CYP2C9 (cytochrome P450, family 2, subfamily C, polypeptide 9)*** **(eg, drug metabolism), gene analysis, common variants (eg, *2, *3, *5, *6)**
0.00 0.00 FUD XXX
AMA: 2018,Nov,9; 2018,Jan,8; 2017,Jan,8; 2016,Aug,9; 2016,Jan,13; 2015,Jan,16; 2014,Jan,11

81225 ***CYP2C19 (cytochrome P450, family 2, subfamily C, polypeptide 19)*** **(eg, drug metabolism), gene analysis, common variants (eg, *2, *3, *4, *8, *17)**
0.00 0.00 FUD XXX
AMA: 2018,Nov,9; 2018,Jan,8; 2017,Jan,8; 2016,Aug,9; 2016,Jan,13; 2015,Jan,16; 2014,Jan,11

81226 ***CYP2D6 (cytochrome P450, family 2, subfamily D, polypeptide 6)*** **(eg, drug metabolism), gene analysis, common variants (eg, *2, *3, *4, *5, *6, *9, *10, *17, *19, *29, *35, *41, *1XN, *2XN, *4XN)**
0.00 0.00 FUD XXX
AMA: 2018,Nov,9; 2018,Jan,8; 2017,Jan,8; 2016,Aug,9; 2016,Jan,13; 2015,Jan,16; 2014,Jan,11

81227 **Resequenced code. See code before 81225.**

\# **81230** ***CYP3A4 (cytochrome P450 family 3 subfamily A member 4)*** **(eg, drug metabolism), gene analysis, common variant(s) (eg, *2, *22)**
0.00 0.00 FUD XXX
AMA: 2018,Nov,9

\# **81231** ***CYP3A5 (cytochrome P450 family 3 subfamily A member 5)*** **(eg, drug metabolism), gene analysis, common variants (eg, *2, *3, *4, *5, *6, *7)**
0.00 0.00 FUD XXX
AMA: 2018,Nov,9

81228 **Cytogenomic constitutional (genome-wide) microarray analysis; interrogation of genomic regions for copy number variants (eg, bacterial artificial chromosome [BAC] or oligo-based comparative genomic hybridization [CGH] microarray analysis)**
EXCLUDES *Analyte-specific molecular pathology procedures included in microarray analysis*
When performed in conjunction with single nucleotide polymorphism interrogation (81229)
0.00 0.00 FUD XXX
AMA: 2018,Nov,9; 2018,Jan,8; 2017,Apr,3; 2017,Jan,8; 2016,Aug,9; 2016,Jan,13; 2015,Jan,16; 2014,Jan,11

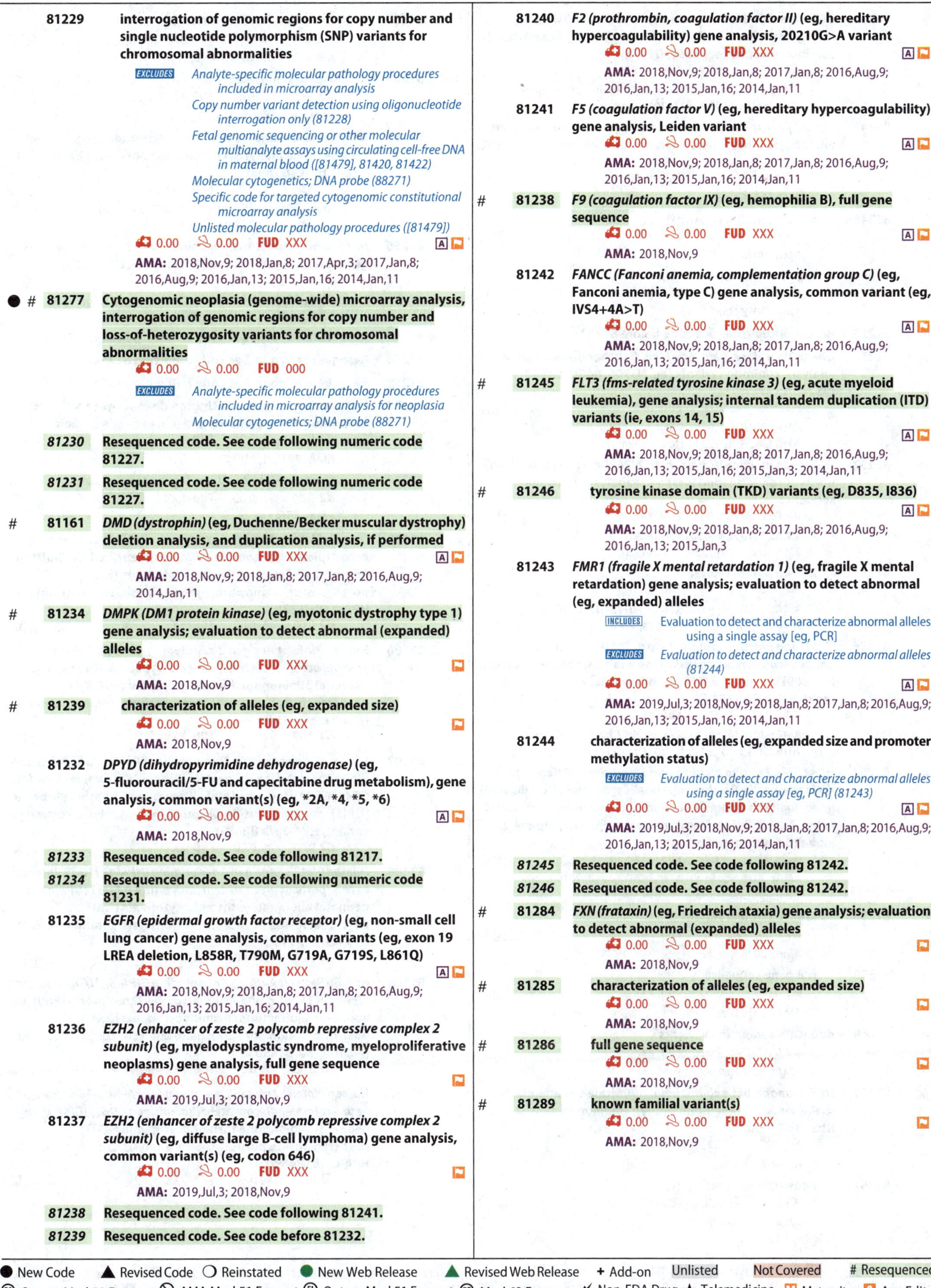

81229 **interrogation of genomic regions for copy number and single nucleotide polymorphism (SNP) variants for chromosomal abnormalities**

EXCLUDES *Analyte-specific molecular pathology procedures included in microarray analysis*
Copy number variant detection using oligonucleotide interrogation only (81228)
Fetal genomic sequencing or other molecular multianalyte assays using circulating cell-free DNA in maternal blood ([81479], 81420, 81422)
Molecular cytogenetics; DNA probe (88271)
Specific code for targeted cytogenomic constitutional microarray analysis
Unlisted molecular pathology procedures ([81479])

0.00 0.00 FUD XXX A

AMA: 2018,Nov,9; 2018,Jan,8; 2017,Apr,3; 2017,Jan,8; 2016,Aug,9; 2016,Jan,13; 2015,Jan,16; 2014,Jan,11

● # **81277** **Cytogenomic neoplasia (genome-wide) microarray analysis, interrogation of genomic regions for copy number and loss-of-heterozygosity variants for chromosomal abnormalities**

0.00 0.00 FUD 000

EXCLUDES *Analyte-specific molecular pathology procedures included in microarray analysis for neoplasia*
Molecular cytogenetics; DNA probe (88271)

81230 **Resequenced code. See code following numeric code 81227.**

81231 **Resequenced code. See code following numeric code 81227.**

\# **81161** ***DMD (dystrophin)*** **(eg, Duchenne/Becker muscular dystrophy) deletion analysis, and duplication analysis, if performed**

0.00 0.00 FUD XXX A

AMA: 2018,Nov,9; 2018,Jan,8; 2017,Jan,8; 2016,Aug,9; 2014,Jan,11

\# **81234** ***DMPK (DM1 protein kinase)*** **(eg, myotonic dystrophy type 1) gene analysis; evaluation to detect abnormal (expanded) alleles**

0.00 0.00 FUD XXX

AMA: 2018,Nov,9

\# **81239** **characterization of alleles (eg, expanded size)**

0.00 0.00 FUD XXX

AMA: 2018,Nov,9

81232 ***DPYD (dihydropyrimidine dehydrogenase)*** **(eg, 5-fluorouracil/5-FU and capecitabine drug metabolism), gene analysis, common variant(s) (eg, *2A, *4, *5, *6)**

0.00 0.00 FUD XXX A

AMA: 2018,Nov,9

81233 **Resequenced code. See code following 81217.**

81234 **Resequenced code. See code following numeric code 81231.**

81235 ***EGFR (epidermal growth factor receptor)*** **(eg, non-small cell lung cancer) gene analysis, common variants (eg, exon 19 LREA deletion, L858R, T790M, G719A, G719S, L861Q)**

0.00 0.00 FUD XXX A

AMA: 2018,Nov,9; 2018,Jan,8; 2017,Jan,8; 2016,Aug,9; 2016,Jan,13; 2015,Jan,16; 2014,Jan,11

81236 ***EZH2 (enhancer of zeste 2 polycomb repressive complex 2 subunit)*** **(eg, myelodysplastic syndrome, myeloproliferative neoplasms) gene analysis, full gene sequence**

0.00 0.00 FUD XXX

AMA: 2019,Jul,3; 2018,Nov,9

81237 ***EZH2 (enhancer of zeste 2 polycomb repressive complex 2 subunit)*** **(eg, diffuse large B-cell lymphoma) gene analysis, common variant(s) (eg, codon 646)**

0.00 0.00 FUD XXX

AMA: 2019,Jul,3; 2018,Nov,9

81238 **Resequenced code. See code following 81241.**

81239 **Resequenced code. See code before 81232.**

81240 ***F2 (prothrombin, coagulation factor II)*** **(eg, hereditary hypercoagulability) gene analysis, 20210G>A variant**

0.00 0.00 FUD XXX A

AMA: 2018,Nov,9; 2018,Jan,8; 2017,Jan,8; 2016,Aug,9; 2016,Jan,13; 2015,Jan,16; 2014,Jan,11

81241 ***F5 (coagulation factor V)*** **(eg, hereditary hypercoagulability) gene analysis, Leiden variant**

0.00 0.00 FUD XXX A

AMA: 2018,Nov,9; 2018,Jan,8; 2017,Jan,8; 2016,Aug,9; 2016,Jan,13; 2015,Jan,16; 2014,Jan,11

\# **81238** ***F9 (coagulation factor IX)*** **(eg, hemophilia B), full gene sequence**

0.00 0.00 FUD XXX A

AMA: 2018,Nov,9

81242 ***FANCC (Fanconi anemia, complementation group C)*** **(eg, Fanconi anemia, type C) gene analysis, common variant (eg, IVS4+4A>T)**

0.00 0.00 FUD XXX A

AMA: 2018,Nov,9; 2018,Jan,8; 2017,Jan,8; 2016,Aug,9; 2016,Jan,13; 2015,Jan,16; 2014,Jan,11

\# **81245** ***FLT3 (fms-related tyrosine kinase 3)*** **(eg, acute myeloid leukemia), gene analysis; internal tandem duplication (ITD) variants (ie, exons 14, 15)**

0.00 0.00 FUD XXX A

AMA: 2018,Nov,9; 2018,Jan,8; 2017,Jan,8; 2016,Aug,9; 2016,Jan,13; 2015,Jan,16; 2015,Jan,3; 2014,Jan,11

\# **81246** **tyrosine kinase domain (TKD) variants (eg, D835, I836)**

0.00 0.00 FUD XXX A

AMA: 2018,Nov,9; 2018,Jan,8; 2017,Jan,8; 2016,Aug,9; 2016,Jan,13; 2015,Jan,3

81243 ***FMR1 (fragile X mental retardation 1)*** **(eg, fragile X mental retardation) gene analysis; evaluation to detect abnormal (eg, expanded) alleles**

INCLUDES Evaluation to detect and characterize abnormal alleles using a single assay [eg, PCR]

EXCLUDES *Evaluation to detect and characterize abnormal alleles (81244)*

0.00 0.00 FUD XXX A

AMA: 2019,Jul,3; 2018,Nov,9; 2018,Jan,8; 2017,Jan,8; 2016,Aug,9; 2016,Jan,13; 2015,Jan,16; 2014,Jan,11

81244 **characterization of alleles (eg, expanded size and promoter methylation status)**

EXCLUDES *Evaluation to detect and characterize abnormal alleles using a single assay [eg, PCR] (81243)*

0.00 0.00 FUD XXX A

AMA: 2019,Jul,3; 2018,Nov,9; 2018,Jan,8; 2017,Jan,8; 2016,Aug,9; 2016,Jan,13; 2015,Jan,16; 2014,Jan,11

81245 **Resequenced code. See code following 81242.**

81246 **Resequenced code. See code following 81242.**

\# **81284** ***FXN (frataxin)*** **(eg, Friedreich ataxia) gene analysis; evaluation to detect abnormal (expanded) alleles**

0.00 0.00 FUD XXX

AMA: 2018,Nov,9

\# **81285** **characterization of alleles (eg, expanded size)**

0.00 0.00 FUD XXX

AMA: 2018,Nov,9

\# **81286** **full gene sequence**

0.00 0.00 FUD XXX

AMA: 2018,Nov,9

\# **81289** **known familial variant(s)**

0.00 0.00 FUD XXX

AMA: 2018,Nov,9

\# **81250** ***G6PC (glucose-6-phosphatase, catalytic subunit)*** **(eg, Glycogen storage disease, type 1a, von Gierke disease) gene analysis, common variants (eg, R83C, Q347X)**
0.00 0.00 FUD XXX
AMA: 2018,Nov,9; 2018,Jan,8; 2017,Jan,8; 2016,Aug,9; 2016,Jan,13; 2015,Jan,16; 2014,Jan,11

81247 ***G6PD (glucose-6-phosphate dehydrogenase)*** **(eg, hemolytic anemia, jaundice), gene analysis; common variant(s) (eg, A, A-)**
0.00 0.00 FUD XXX
AMA: 2018,Nov,9

81248 **known familial variant(s)**
0.00 0.00 FUD XXX
AMA: 2018,Nov,9

81249 **full gene sequence**
0.00 0.00 FUD XXX
AMA: 2018,Nov,9

81250 **Resequenced code. See code before 81247.**

81251 ***GBA (glucosidase, beta, acid)*** **(eg, Gaucher disease) gene analysis, common variants (eg, N370S, 84GG, L444P, IVS2+1G>A)**
0.00 0.00 FUD XXX
AMA: 2018,Nov,9; 2018,Jan,8; 2017,Jan,8; 2016,Aug,9; 2016,Jan,13; 2015,Jan,16; 2014,Jan,11

81252 ***GJB2 (gap junction protein, beta 2, 26kDa, connexin 26)*** **(eg, nonsyndromic hearing loss) gene analysis; full gene sequence**
0.00 0.00 FUD XXX
AMA: 2018,Nov,9; 2018,Jan,8; 2017,Jan,8; 2016,Aug,9; 2016,Jan,13; 2015,Jan,16; 2014,Jan,11

81253 **known familial variants**
0.00 0.00 FUD XXX
AMA: 2018,Nov,9; 2018,Jan,8; 2017,Jan,8; 2016,Aug,9; 2016,Jan,13; 2015,Jan,16; 2014,Jan,11

81254 ***GJB6 (gap junction protein, beta 6, 30kDa, connexin 30)*** **(eg, nonsyndromic hearing loss) gene analysis, common variants (eg, 309kb [del(GJB6-D13S1830)] and 232kb [del(GJB6-D13S1854)])**
0.00 0.00 FUD XXX
AMA: 2018,Nov,9; 2018,Jan,8; 2017,Jan,8; 2016,Aug,9; 2016,Jan,13; 2015,Jan,16; 2014,Jan,11

\# **81257** ***HBA1/HBA2 (alpha globin 1 and alpha globin 2)*** **(eg, alpha thalassemia, Hb Bart hydrops fetalis syndrome, HbH disease), gene analysis; common deletions or variant (eg, Southeast Asian, Thai, Filipino, Mediterranean, alpha3.7, alpha4.2, alpha20.5, Constant Spring)**
0.00 0.00 FUD XXX
AMA: 2018,Nov,9; 2018,Jan,8; 2017,Jan,8; 2016,Aug,9; 2016,Jan,13; 2015,Jan,16; 2014,Jan,11

\# **81258** **known familial variant**
0.00 0.00 FUD XXX
AMA: 2018,Nov,9

\# **81259** **full gene sequence**
0.00 0.00 FUD XXX
AMA: 2018,Nov,9

\# **81269** **duplication/deletion variants**
0.00 0.00 FUD XXX
AMA: 2018,Nov,9

\# **81361** ***HBB (hemoglobin, subunit beta)*** **(eg, sickle cell anemia, beta thalassemia, hemoglobinopathy); common variant(s) (eg, HbS, HbC, HbE)**
0.00 0.00 FUD XXX
AMA: 2018,Nov,9

\# **81362** **known familial variant(s)**
0.00 0.00 FUD XXX
AMA: 2018,Nov,9

\# **81363** **duplication/deletion variant(s)**
0.00 0.00 FUD XXX
AMA: 2018,Nov,9; 2018,Sep,14

\# **81364** **full gene sequence**
0.00 0.00 FUD XXX
AMA: 2018,Nov,9; 2018,Sep,14

81255 ***HEXA (hexosaminidase A [alpha polypeptide])*** **(eg, Tay-Sachs disease) gene analysis, common variants (eg, 1278insTATC, 1421+1G>C, G269S)**
0.00 0.00 FUD XXX
AMA: 2018,Nov,9; 2018,Jan,8; 2017,Jan,8; 2016,Aug,9; 2016,Jan,13; 2015,Jan,16; 2014,Jan,11

81256 ***HFE (hemochromatosis)*** **(eg, hereditary hemochromatosis) gene analysis, common variants (eg, C282Y, H63D)**
0.00 0.00 FUD XXX
AMA: 2018,Nov,9; 2018,Jan,8; 2017,Jan,8; 2016,Aug,9; 2016,Jan,13; 2015,Jan,16; 2014,Jan,11

81257 **Resequenced code. See code following 81254.**

81258 **Resequenced code. See code following 81254.**

81259 **Resequenced code. See code following 81254.**

\# **81271** ***HTT (huntingtin)*** **(eg, Huntington disease) gene analysis; evaluation to detect abnormal (eg, expanded) alleles**
0.00 0.00 FUD XXX
AMA: 2018,Nov,9

\# **81274** **characterization of alleles (eg, expanded size)**
0.00 0.00 FUD XXX
AMA: 2018,Nov,9

\# **81105** ***Human Platelet Antigen 1 genotyping (HPA-1), ITGB3 (integrin, beta 3 [platelet glycoprotein IIIa], antigen CD61 [GPIIIa])*** **(eg, neonatal alloimmune thrombocytopenia [NAIT], post-transfusion purpura), gene analysis, common variant, HPA-1a/b (L33P)**
0.00 0.00 FUD XXX

\# **81106** ***Human Platelet Antigen 2 genotyping (HPA-2), GP1BA (glycoprotein Ib [platelet], alpha polypeptide [GPIba])*** **(eg, neonatal alloimmune thrombocytopenia [NAIT], post-transfusion purpura), gene analysis, common variant, HPA-2a/b (T145M)**
0.00 0.00 FUD XXX

\# **81107** ***Human Platelet Antigen 3 genotyping (HPA-3), ITGA2B (integrin, alpha 2b [platelet glycoprotein IIb of IIb/IIIa complex], antigen CD41 [GPIIb])*** **(eg, neonatal alloimmune thrombocytopenia [NAIT], post-transfusion purpura), gene analysis, common variant, HPA-3a/b (I843S)**
0.00 0.00 FUD XXX

\# **81108** ***Human Platelet Antigen 4 genotyping (HPA-4), ITGB3 (integrin, beta 3 [platelet glycoprotein IIIa], antigen CD61 [GPIIIa])*** **(eg, neonatal alloimmune thrombocytopenia [NAIT], post-transfusion purpura), gene analysis, common variant, HPA-4a/b (R143Q)**
0.00 0.00 FUD XXX

\# **81109** ***Human Platelet Antigen 5 genotyping (HPA-5), ITGA2 (integrin, alpha 2 [CD49B, alpha 2 subunit of VLA-2 receptor] [GPIa])*** **(eg, neonatal alloimmune thrombocytopenia [NAIT], post-transfusion purpura), gene analysis, common variant (eg, HPA-5a/b (K505E))**
0.00 0.00 FUD XXX

\# **81110** ***Human Platelet Antigen 6 genotyping (HPA-6w), ITGB3 (integrin, beta 3 [platelet glycoprotein IIIa, antigen CD61] [GPIIIa])*** **(eg, neonatal alloimmune thrombocytopenia [NAIT], post-transfusion purpura), gene analysis, common variant, HPA-6a/b (R489Q)**
0.00 0.00 FUD XXX

\# **81111** ***Human Platelet Antigen 9 genotyping (HPA-9w), ITGA2B (integrin, alpha 2b [platelet glycoprotein IIb of IIb/IIIa complex, antigen CD41] [GPIIb])*** **(eg, neonatal alloimmune thrombocytopenia [NAIT], post-transfusion purpura), gene analysis, common variant, HPA-9a/b (V837M)**
0.00 0.00 FUD XXX A

\# **81112** ***Human Platelet Antigen 15 genotyping (HPA-15), CD109 (CD109 molecule)*** **(eg, neonatal alloimmune thrombocytopenia [NAIT], post-transfusion purpura), gene analysis, common variant, HPA-15a/b (S682Y)**
0.00 0.00 FUD XXX A

\# **81120** ***IDH1 (isocitrate dehydrogenase 1 [NADP+], soluble)*** **(eg, glioma), common variants (eg, R132H, R132C)**
0.00 0.00 FUD XXX A

\# **81121** ***IDH2 (isocitrate dehydrogenase 2 [NADP+], mitochondrial)*** **(eg, glioma), common variants (eg, R140W, R172M)**
0.00 0.00 FUD XXX A

\# **81283** ***IFNL3 (interferon, lambda 3)*** **(eg, drug response), gene analysis, rs12979860 variant**
0.00 0.00 FUD XXX A
AMA: 2018,Nov,9

\# **81261** ***IGH@ (Immunoglobulin heavy chain locus)*** **(eg, leukemias and lymphomas, B-cell), gene rearrangement analysis to detect abnormal clonal population(s); amplified methodology (eg, polymerase chain reaction)**
0.00 0.00 FUD XXX A
AMA: 2018,Nov,9; 2018,Jan,8; 2017,Jan,8; 2016,Aug,9; 2016,Jan,13; 2015,Jan,16; 2014,Jan,11

\# **81262** **direct probe methodology (eg, Southern blot)**
0.00 0.00 FUD XXX A
AMA: 2018,Nov,9; 2018,Jan,8; 2017,Jan,8; 2016,Aug,9; 2016,Jan,13; 2015,Jan,16; 2014,Jan,11

\# **81263** ***IGH@ (Immunoglobulin heavy chain locus)*** **(eg, leukemia and lymphoma, B-cell), variable region somatic mutation analysis**
0.00 0.00 FUD XXX A
AMA: 2018,Nov,9; 2018,Jan,8; 2017,Jan,8; 2016,Aug,9; 2016,Jan,13; 2015,Jan,16; 2014,Jan,11

\# **81264** ***IGK@ (Immunoglobulin kappa light chain locus)*** **(eg, leukemia and lymphoma, B-cell), gene rearrangement analysis, evaluation to detect abnormal clonal population(s)**
0.00 0.00 FUD XXX A
AMA: 2018,Nov,9; 2018,Jan,8; 2017,Jan,8; 2016,Aug,9; 2016,Jan,13; 2015,Jan,16; 2014,Jan,11

81260 ***IKBKAP (inhibitor of kappa light polypeptide gene enhancer in B-cells, kinase complex-associated protein)*** **(eg, familial dysautonomia) gene analysis, common variants (eg, 2507+6T>C, R696P)**
0.00 0.00 FUD XXX A
AMA: 2018,Nov,9; 2018,Jan,8; 2017,Jan,8; 2016,Aug,9; 2016,Jan,13; 2015,Jan,16; 2014,Jan,11

81261 **Resequenced code. See code before 81260.**

81262 **Resequenced code. See code before 81260.**

81263 **Resequenced code. See code following resequenced code 81262.**

81264 **Resequenced code. See code before 81260.**

81265 **Resequenced code. See code following resequenced code 81187.**

81266 **Resequenced code. See code following resequenced code 81265.**

81267 **Resequenced code. See code following 81224.**

81268 **Resequenced code. See code following 81224.**

81269 **Resequenced code. See code following resequenced code 81259.**

81270 ***JAK2 (Janus kinase 2)*** **(eg, myeloproliferative disorder) gene analysis, p.Val617Phe (V617F) variant**
0.00 0.00 FUD XXX A
AMA: 2018,Nov,9; 2018,Jan,8; 2017,Jan,8; 2016,Aug,9; 2016,Jan,13; 2015,Jan,16; 2014,Jan,11

81271 **Resequenced code. See code following numeric code 81259.**

81272 ***KIT (v-kit Hardy-Zuckerman 4 feline sarcoma viral oncogene homolog)*** **(eg, gastrointestinal stromal tumor [GIST], acute myeloid leukemia, melanoma), gene analysis, targeted sequence analysis (eg, exons 8, 11, 13, 17, 18)**
0.00 0.00 FUD XXX A
AMA: 2018,Nov,9; 2018,Jan,8; 2017,Jan,8; 2016,Aug,9

81273 ***KIT (v-kit Hardy-Zuckerman 4 feline sarcoma viral oncogene homolog)*** **(eg, mastocytosis), gene analysis, D816 variant**
0.00 0.00 FUD XXX A
AMA: 2018,Nov,9; 2018,Jan,8; 2017,Jan,8; 2016,Aug,9

81274 **Resequenced code. See code following resequenced code 81271.**

81275 ***KRAS (Kirsten rat sarcoma viral oncogene homolog)*** **(eg, carcinoma) gene analysis; variants in exon 2 (eg, codons 12 and 13)**
0.00 0.00 FUD XXX A
AMA: 2018,Nov,9; 2018,Jan,8; 2017,Jan,8; 2016,Aug,9; 2016,Jan,13; 2015,Jan,16; 2014,Jan,11

81276 **additional variant(s) (eg, codon 61, codon 146)**
0.00 0.00 FUD XXX A
AMA: 2018,Nov,9; 2018,Jan,8; 2017,Jan,8; 2016,Aug,9

81277 **Resequenced code. See code following 81229.**

81283 **Resequenced code. See code following resequenced code 81121.**

81284 **Resequenced code. See code following numeric code 81246.**

81285 **Resequenced code. See code following numeric code 81246.**

81286 **Resequenced code. See code following numeric code 81246.**

81287 **Resequenced code. See code following resequenced code 81304.**

81288 **Resequenced code. See code following resequenced code 81292.**

81289 **Resequenced code. See code following numeric code 81246.**

81290 ***MCOLN1 (mucolipin 1)*** **(eg, Mucolipidosis, type IV) gene analysis, common variants (eg, IVS3-2A>G, del6.4kb)**
0.00 0.00 FUD XXX A
AMA: 2018,Nov,9; 2018,Jan,8; 2017,Jan,8; 2016,Aug,9; 2016,Jan,13; 2015,Jan,16; 2014,Jan,11

\# **81302** ***MECP2 (methyl CpG binding protein 2)*** **(eg, Rett syndrome) gene analysis; full sequence analysis**
0.00 0.00 FUD XXX A
AMA: 2018,Nov,9; 2018,Jan,8; 2017,Jan,8; 2016,Aug,9; 2016,Jan,13; 2015,Jan,16; 2014,Jan,11

\# **81303** **known familial variant**
0.00 0.00 FUD XXX A
AMA: 2018,Nov,9; 2018,Jan,8; 2017,Jan,8; 2016,Aug,9; 2016,Jan,13; 2015,Jan,16; 2014,Jan,11

\# **81304** **duplication/deletion variants**
0.00 0.00 FUD XXX A
AMA: 2018,Nov,9; 2018,Jan,8; 2017,Jan,8; 2016,Aug,9; 2016,Jan,13; 2015,Jan,16; 2014,Jan,11

\# **81287** ***MGMT (O-6-methylguanine-DNA methyltransferase)*** **(eg, glioblastoma multiforme), promoter methylation analysis**
0.00 0.00 FUD XXX
AMA: 2019,Jul,3; 2018,Dec,10; 2018,Dec,10; 2018,Nov,9; 2018,Jan,8; 2017,Jan,8; 2016,Aug,9; 2014,Jan,11

\# **81301** **Microsatellite instability analysis (eg, hereditary non-polyposis colorectal cancer, Lynch syndrome) of markers for mismatch repair deficiency (eg, BAT25, BAT26), includes comparison of neoplastic and normal tissue, if performed**
0.00 0.00 FUD XXX
AMA: 2018,Nov,9; 2018,Jan,8; 2017,Jan,8; 2016,Aug,9; 2016,Jan,13; 2015,Jan,16; 2014,Jan,11

\# **81292** ***MLH1 (mutL homolog 1, colon cancer, nonpolyposis type 2)*** **(eg, hereditary non-polyposis colorectal cancer, Lynch syndrome) gene analysis; full sequence analysis**
0.00 0.00 FUD XXX
AMA: 2018,Nov,9; 2018,Jan,8; 2017,Jan,8; 2016,Aug,9; 2016,Jan,13; 2015,Jan,16; 2015,Jan,3; 2014,Jan,11

\# **81288** **promoter methylation analysis**
0.00 0.00 FUD XXX
AMA: 2018,Nov,9; 2018,Jan,8; 2017,Jan,8; 2016,Aug,9; 2016,Jan,13; 2015,Jan,3

\# **81293** **known familial variants**
0.00 0.00 FUD XXX
AMA: 2018,Nov,9; 2018,Jan,8; 2017,Jan,8; 2016,Aug,9; 2016,Jan,13; 2015,Jan,16; 2014,Jan,11

\# **81294** **duplication/deletion variants**
0.00 0.00 FUD XXX
AMA: 2018,Nov,9; 2018,Jan,8; 2017,Jan,8; 2016,Aug,9; 2016,Jan,13; 2015,Jan,16; 2014,Jan,11

\# **81295** ***MSH2 (mutS homolog 2, colon cancer, nonpolyposis type 1)*** **(eg, hereditary non-polyposis colorectal cancer, Lynch syndrome) gene analysis; full sequence analysis**
0.00 0.00 FUD XXX
AMA: 2018,Nov,9; 2018,Jan,8; 2017,Jan,8; 2016,Aug,9; 2016,Jan,13; 2015,Jan,16; 2014,Jan,11

81291 **Resequenced code. See code before 81305.**

81292 **Resequenced code. See code before numeric code 81291.**

81293 **Resequenced code. See code before numeric code 81291.**

81294 **Resequenced code. See code before numeric code 81291.**

81295 **Resequenced code. See code before numeric code 81291.**

81296 **known familial variants**
0.00 0.00 FUD XXX
AMA: 2018,Nov,9; 2018,Jan,8; 2017,Jan,8; 2016,Aug,9; 2016,Jan,13; 2015,Jan,16; 2014,Jan,11

81297 **duplication/deletion variants**
0.00 0.00 FUD XXX
AMA: 2018,Nov,9; 2018,Jan,8; 2017,Jan,8; 2016,Aug,9; 2016,Jan,13; 2015,Jan,16; 2014,Jan,11

81298 ***MSH6 (mutS homolog 6 [E. coli])*** **(eg, hereditary non-polyposis colorectal cancer, Lynch syndrome) gene analysis; full sequence analysis**
0.00 0.00 FUD XXX
AMA: 2018,Nov,9; 2018,Jan,8; 2017,Jan,8; 2016,Aug,9; 2016,Jan,13; 2015,Jan,16; 2014,Jan,11

81299 **known familial variants**
0.00 0.00 FUD XXX
AMA: 2018,Nov,9; 2018,Jan,8; 2017,Jan,8; 2016,Aug,9; 2016,Jan,13; 2015,Jan,16; 2014,Jan,11

81300 **duplication/deletion variants**
0.00 0.00 FUD XXX
AMA: 2018,Nov,9; 2018,Jan,8; 2017,Jan,8; 2016,Aug,9; 2016,Jan,13; 2015,Jan,16; 2014,Jan,11

81301 **Resequenced code. See code following resequenced code 81287.**

81302 **Resequenced code. See code following 81290.**

81303 **Resequenced code. See code following 81290.**

81304 **Resequenced code. See code following 81290.**

\# **81291** ***MTHFR (5,10-methylenetetrahydrofolate reductase)*** **(eg, hereditary hypercoagulability) gene analysis, common variants (eg, 677T, 1298C)**
0.00 0.00 FUD XXX
AMA: 2018,Nov,9; 2018,Jan,8; 2017,Jan,8; 2016,Aug,9; 2016,Jan,13; 2015,Jan,16; 2014,Jan,11

81305 ***MYD88 (myeloid differentiation primary response 88)*** **(eg, Waldenstrom's macroglobulinemia, lymphoplasmacytic leukemia) gene analysis, p.Leu265Pro (L265P) variant**
0.00 0.00 FUD XXX
AMA: 2019,Jul,3; 2018,Nov,9

81306 **Resequenced code. See code following numeric code 81312.**

81307 **Resequenced code. See code before 81313.**

81308 **Resequenced code. See code before 81313.**

81309 **Resequenced code. See code following 81314.**

81310 ***NPM1 (nucleophosmin)*** **(eg, acute myeloid leukemia) gene analysis, exon 12 variants**
0.00 0.00 FUD XXX
AMA: 2018,Nov,9; 2018,Jan,8; 2017,Jan,8; 2016,Aug,9; 2016,Jan,13; 2015,Jan,16; 2014,Jan,11

81311 ***NRAS (neuroblastoma RAS viral [v-ras] oncogene homolog)*** **(eg, colorectal carcinoma), gene analysis, variants in exon 2 (eg, codons 12 and 13) and exon 3 (eg, codon 61)**
0.00 0.00 FUD XXX
AMA: 2018,Nov,9; 2018,Jan,8; 2017,Jan,8; 2016,Aug,9

81312 **Resequenced code. See code following resequenced code 81306.**

\# **81306** ***NUDT15 (nudix hydrolase 15)*** **(eg, drug metabolism) gene analysis, common variant(s) (eg, *2, *3, *4, *5, *6)**
0.00 0.00 FUD XXX
AMA: 2019,Jul,3; 2018,Nov,9

\# **81312** ***PABPN1 (poly[A] binding protein nuclear 1)*** **(eg, oculopharyngeal muscular dystrophy) gene analysis, evaluation to detect abnormal (eg, expanded) alleles**
0.00 0.00 FUD XXX
AMA: 2018,Nov,9

● # **81307** ***PALB2 (partner and localizer of BRCA2)*** **(eg, breast and pancreatic cancer) gene analysis; full gene sequence**
0.00 0.00 FUD 000

● # **81308** **known familial variant**
0.00 0.00 FUD 000

81313 ***PCA3/KLK3 (prostate cancer antigen 3 [non-protein coding]/kallikrein-related peptidase 3 [prostate specific antigen])*** **ratio (eg, prostate cancer)**
0.00 0.00 FUD XXX
AMA: 2018,Nov,9; 2018,Jan,8; 2017,Jan,8; 2016,Aug,9; 2016,Jan,13; 2015,Jan,3

81314 ***PDGFRA (platelet-derived growth factor receptor, alpha polypeptide)*** **(eg, gastrointestinal stromal tumor [GIST]), gene analysis, targeted sequence analysis (eg, exons 12, 18)**
0.00 0.00 FUD XXX
AMA: 2018,Nov,9; 2018,Jan,8; 2017,Jan,8; 2016,Aug,9

● # **81309** ***PIK3CA (phosphatidylinositol-4, 5-biphosphate 3-kinase, catalytic subunit alpha)*** **(eg, colorectal and breast cancer) gene analysis, targeted sequence analysis (eg, exons 7, 9, 20)**
0.00 0.00 FUD 000

\# **81320** ***PLCG2 (phospholipase C gamma 2)*** **(eg, chronic lymphocytic leukemia) gene analysis, common variants (eg, R665W, S707F, L845F)**
0.00 0.00 FUD XXX
AMA: 2019,Jul,3; 2018,Nov,9

81315 ***PML/RARalpha, (t(15;17)), (promyelocytic leukemia/retinoic acid receptor alpha)*** **(eg, promyelocytic leukemia) translocation analysis; common breakpoints (eg, intron 3 and intron 6), qualitative or quantitative**
0.00 0.00 FUD XXX A
AMA: 2018,Nov,9; 2018,Jan,8; 2017,Jan,8; 2016,Aug,9; 2016,Jan,13; 2015,Jan,16; 2014,Jan,11

81316 **single breakpoint (eg, intron 3, intron 6 or exon 6), qualitative or quantitative**
0.00 0.00 FUD XXX A
AMA: 2018,Nov,9; 2018,Jan,8; 2017,Jan,8; 2016,Aug,9; 2016,Jan,13; 2015,Jan,16; 2014,Jan,11

81324 ***PMP22 (peripheral myelin protein 22)*** **(eg, Charcot-Marie-Tooth, hereditary neuropathy with liability to pressure palsies) gene analysis; duplication/deletion analysis**
0.00 0.00 FUD XXX A
AMA: 2018,Nov,9; 2018,Jan,8; 2017,Jan,8; 2016,Aug,9; 2016,Jan,13; 2015,Jan,16; 2014,Jan,11

81325 **full sequence analysis**
0.00 0.00 FUD XXX A
AMA: 2018,Nov,9; 2018,May,6; 2018,Jan,8; 2017,Jan,8; 2016,Aug,9; 2016,Jan,13; 2015,Jan,16; 2014,Jan,11

81326 **known familial variant**
0.00 0.00 FUD XXX A
AMA: 2018,Nov,9; 2018,Jan,8; 2017,Jan,8; 2016,Aug,9; 2016,Jan,13; 2015,Jan,16; 2014,Jan,11

81317 ***PMS2 (postmeiotic segregation increased 2 [S. cerevisiae])*** **(eg, hereditary non-polyposis colorectal cancer, Lynch syndrome) gene analysis; full sequence analysis**
0.00 0.00 FUD XXX A
AMA: 2018,Nov,9; 2018,Jan,8; 2017,Jan,8; 2016,Aug,9; 2016,Jan,13; 2015,Jan,16; 2014,Jan,11

81318 **known familial variants**
0.00 0.00 FUD XXX A
AMA: 2018,Nov,9; 2018,Jan,8; 2017,Jan,8; 2016,Aug,9; 2016,Jan,13; 2015,Jan,16; 2014,Jan,11

81319 **duplication/deletion variants**
0.00 0.00 FUD XXX A
AMA: 2018,Nov,9; 2018,Jan,8; 2017,Jan,8; 2016,Aug,9; 2016,Jan,13; 2015,Jan,16; 2014,Jan,11

81320 **Resequenced code. See code before 81315.**

81343 ***PPP2R2B (protein phosphatase 2 regulatory subunit Bbeta)*** **(eg, spinocerebellar ataxia) gene analysis, evaluation to detect abnormal (eg, expanded) alleles**
0.00 0.00 FUD XXX
AMA: 2018,Nov,9

81321 ***PTEN (phosphatase and tensin homolog)*** **(eg, Cowden syndrome, PTEN hamartoma tumor syndrome) gene analysis; full sequence analysis**
0.00 0.00 FUD XXX A
AMA: 2018,Nov,9; 2018,Jan,8; 2017,Jan,8; 2016,Aug,9; 2016,Jan,13; 2015,Jan,16; 2014,Jan,11

81322 **known familial variant**
0.00 0.00 FUD XXX A
AMA: 2018,Nov,9; 2018,Jan,8; 2017,Jan,8; 2016,Aug,9; 2016,Jan,13; 2015,Jan,16; 2014,Jan,11

81323 **duplication/deletion variant**
0.00 0.00 FUD XXX A
AMA: 2018,Nov,9; 2018,Jan,8; 2017,Jan,8; 2016,Aug,9; 2016,Jan,13; 2015,Jan,16; 2014,Jan,11

81324 **Resequenced code. See code following 81316.**

81325 **Resequenced code. See code following 81316.**

81326 **Resequenced code. See code following 81316.**

81334 ***RUNX1 (runt related transcription factor 1)*** **(eg, acute myeloid leukemia, familial platelet disorder with associated myeloid malignancy), gene analysis, targeted sequence analysis (eg, exons 3-8)**
0.00 0.00 FUD XXX A
AMA: 2018,Nov,9

81327 ***SEPT9 (Septin9)*** **(eg, colorectal cancer) promoter methylation analysis**
0.00 0.00 FUD XXX A
AMA: 2019,Jul,3; 2018,Nov,9

81332 ***SERPINA1 (serpin peptidase inhibitor, clade A, alpha-1 antiproteinase, antitrypsin, member 1)*** **(eg, alpha-1-antitrypsin deficiency), gene analysis, common variants (eg, *S and *Z)**
0.00 0.00 FUD XXX A
AMA: 2018,Nov,9; 2018,Jan,8; 2017,Jan,8; 2016,Aug,9; 2016,Jan,13; 2015,Jan,16; 2014,Jan,11

81328 ***SLCO1B1 (solute carrier organic anion transporter family, member 1B1)*** **(eg, adverse drug reaction), gene analysis, common variant(s) (eg, *5)**
0.00 0.00 FUD XXX A
AMA: 2018,Nov,9

81329 ***SMN1 (survival of motor neuron 1, telomeric)*** **(eg, spinal muscular atrophy) gene analysis; dosage/deletion analysis (eg, carrier testing), includes SMN2 (survival of motor neuron 2, centromeric) analysis, if performed**
0.00 0.00 FUD XXX
AMA: 2019,Jul,3; 2018,Nov,9

81336 **full gene sequence**
0.00 0.00 FUD XXX
AMA: 2019,Jul,3; 2018,Nov,9

81337 **known familial sequence variant(s)**
0.00 0.00 FUD XXX
AMA: 2019,Jul,3; 2018,Nov,9

81330 ***SMPD1(sphingomyelin phosphodiesterase 1, acid lysosomal)*** **(eg, Niemann-Pick disease, Type A) gene analysis, common variants (eg, R496L, L302P, fsP330)**
0.00 0.00 FUD XXX A
AMA: 2018,Nov,9; 2018,Jan,8; 2017,Jan,8; 2016,Aug,9; 2016,Jan,13; 2015,Jan,16; 2014,Jan,11

81331 ***SNRPN/UBE3A (small nuclear ribonucleoprotein polypeptide N and ubiquitin protein ligase E3A)*** **(eg, Prader-Willi syndrome and/or Angelman syndrome), methylation analysis**
0.00 0.00 FUD XXX A
AMA: 2018,Nov,9; 2018,Jan,8; 2017,Jan,8; 2016,Aug,9; 2016,Jan,13; 2015,Jan,16; 2014,Jan,11

81332 **Resequenced code. See code following 81327.**

81344 ***TBP (TATA box binding protein)*** **(eg, spinocerebellar ataxia) gene analysis, evaluation to detect abnormal (eg, expanded) alleles**
0.00 0.00 FUD XXX
AMA: 2018,Nov,9

81345 ***TERT (telomerase reverse transcriptase)*** **(eg, thyroid carcinoma, glioblastoma multiforme) gene analysis, targeted sequence analysis (eg, promoter region)**
0.00 0.00 FUD XXX
AMA: 2019,Jul,3; 2018,Nov,9

81333 ***TGFBI (transforming growth factor beta-induced)*** **(eg, corneal dystrophy) gene analysis, common variants (eg, R124H, R124C, R124L, R555W, R555Q)**
0.00 0.00 FUD XXX
AMA: 2019,Jul,3; 2018,Nov,9

81334 **Resequenced code. See code following numeric code 81326.**

81335 ***TPMT (thiopurine S-methyltransferase)*** **(eg, drug metabolism), gene analysis, common variants (eg, *2, *3)**
0.00 0.00 FUD XXX A
AMA: 2018,Nov,9

81336 **Resequenced code. See code following 81329.**

81337 **Resequenced code. See code following 81329.**

81340 ***TRB@ (T cell antigen receptor, beta)* (eg, leukemia and lymphoma), gene rearrangement analysis to detect abnormal clonal population(s); using amplification methodology (eg, polymerase chain reaction)**
0.00 0.00 FUD XXX
AMA: 2018,Nov,9; 2018,Jan,8; 2017,Jan,8; 2016,Aug,9; 2016,Jan,13; 2015,Jan,16; 2014,Jan,11

81341 **using direct probe methodology (eg, Southern blot)**
0.00 0.00 FUD XXX
AMA: 2018,Nov,9; 2018,Jan,8; 2017,Jan,8; 2016,Aug,9; 2016,Jan,13; 2015,Jan,16; 2014,Jan,11

81342 ***TRG@ (T cell antigen receptor, gamma)* (eg, leukemia and lymphoma), gene rearrangement analysis, evaluation to detect abnormal clonal population(s)**
0.00 0.00 FUD XXX
AMA: 2018,Nov,9; 2018,Jan,8; 2017,Jan,8; 2016,Aug,9; 2016,Jan,13; 2015,Jan,16; 2014,Jan,11

81343 **Resequenced code. See code following numeric code 81320.**

81344 **Resequenced code. See code following numeric code 81332.**

81345 **Resequenced code. See code following numeric code 81332.**

81346 ***TYMS (thymidylate synthetase)* (eg, 5-fluorouracil/5-FU drug metabolism), gene analysis, common variant(s) (eg, tandem repeat variant)**
0.00 0.00 FUD XXX
AMA: 2018,Nov,9

▲ 81350 ***UGT1A1 (UDP glucuronosyltransferase 1 family, polypeptide A1)* (eg, drug metabolism, hereditary unconjugated hyperbilirubinemia [Gilbert syndrome]) gene analysis, common variants (eg, *28, *36, *37)**
0.00 0.00 FUD XXX
AMA: 2018,Nov,9; 2018,Jan,8; 2017,Jan,8; 2016,Aug,9; 2016,Jan,13; 2015,Jan,16; 2014,Jan,11

81355 ***VKORC1 (vitamin K epoxide reductase complex, subunit 1)* (eg, warfarin metabolism), gene analysis, common variant(s) (eg, -1639G>A, c.173+1000C>T)**
0.00 0.00 FUD XXX
AMA: 2018,Nov,9; 2018,Jan,8; 2017,Jan,8; 2016,Aug,9; 2016,Jan,13; 2015,Jan,16; 2014,Jan,11

81361 **Resequenced code. See code following 81254.**

81362 **Resequenced code. See code following 81254.**

81363 **Resequenced code. See code following 81254.**

81364 **Resequenced code. See code following 81254.**

81370-81383 Human Leukocyte Antigen (HLA) Testing

INCLUDES Additional testing that must be performed to resolve ambiguous allele combinations for high-resolution typing
All analytical procedures in the evaluation such as:
- Amplification
- Cell lysis
- Detection
- Digestion
- Extraction
- Nucleic acid stabilization

Analysis to identify human leukocyte antigen (HLA) alleles and allele groups connected to specific diseases and individual response to drug therapy in addition to other clinical uses
Code selection based on specific gene being reviewed
Evaluation of the presence of gene variants using the common gene variant name
Examples of proteins or diseases in the code description that are not all inclusive
Generally all the listed gene variants in the code description would be tested but lists are not all inclusive
Genes described using Human Genome Organization (HUGO) approved names
High-resolution typing resolves the common well-defined (CWD) alleles and is usually identified by at least four-digits. There are some instances when high-resolution typing may include some ambiguities for rare alleles, and those may be reported as a string of alleles or an NMDP code
Histocompatibility antigen testing
Intermediate resolution HLA testing is identified by a string of alleles or a National Marrow Donor Program (NMDP) code
Low and intermediate resolution are considered low resolution for code assignment
Low-resolution HLA type reporting is identified by two-digit HLA name
Multiple variant alleles or allele groups that can be identified by typing
One or more HLA genes in specific clinical circumstances
Qualitative results unless otherwise stated
Typing performed to determine the compatibility of recipients and potential donors undergoing solid organ or hematopoietic stem cell pretransplantation testing

EXCLUDES *Full gene sequencing using separate gene variant assessment codes unless it is specifically stated in the code description*
HLA antigen typing by nonmolecular pathology methods (86812-86821)
In situ hybridization analyses (88271-88275, 88368-88375 [88377])
Microbial identification (87149-87153, 87471-87801 [87623, 87624, 87625], 87900-87904 [87906, 87910, 87912])
Other related gene variants not listed in code
Tier 1 molecular pathology codes (81105-81254 [81161, 81162, 81163, 81164, 81165, 81166, 81167, 81173, 81174, 81184, 81185, 81186, 81187, 81188, 81189, 81190, 81200, 81201, 81202, 81203, 81204, 81205, 81206, 81207, 81208, 81209, 81210, 81219, 81227, 81230, 81231, 81233, 81234, 81238, 81239, 81245, 81246, 81250, 81257, 81258, 81259, 81265, 81266, 81267, 81268, 81269, 81284, 81285, 81286, 81289, 81361, 81362, 81363, 81364])
Tier 2 and unlisted molecular pathology procedures (81400-81408, [81479])

Code also modifier 26 when only interpretation and report are performed
Code also services required before cell lysis

81370 **HLA Class I and II typing, low resolution (eg, antigen equivalents); *HLA-A, -B, -C, -DRB1/3/4/5, and -DQB1***
0.00 0.00 FUD XXX
AMA: 2018,Nov,9; 2018,Jan,8; 2017,Jan,8; 2016,Aug,9; 2016,Jan,13; 2015,Jan,16; 2014,Jan,11

81371 ***HLA-A, -B, and -DRB1* (eg, verification typing)**
0.00 0.00 FUD XXX
AMA: 2018,Nov,9; 2018,Jan,8; 2017,Jan,8; 2016,Aug,9; 2016,Jan,13; 2015,Jan,16; 2014,Jan,11

81372 **HLA Class I typing, low resolution (eg, antigen equivalents); complete *(ie, HLA-A, -B, and -C)***
EXCLUDES *Class I and II low-resolution HLA typing for HLA-A, -B, -C, -DRB1/3/4/5, and -DQB1 (81370)*
0.00 0.00 FUD XXX
AMA: 2018,Nov,9; 2018,Jan,8; 2017,Jan,8; 2016,Aug,9; 2016,Jan,13; 2015,Jan,16; 2014,Jan,11

81373 **one locus *(eg, HLA-A, -B, or -C)*, each**

EXCLUDES *A complete Class 1 (HLA-A, -B, and -C) low-resolution typing (81372)*

Reporting the presence or absence of a single antigen equivalent using low-resolution methodology (81374)

0.00 0.00 FUD XXX A

AMA: 2018,Nov,9; 2018,Jan,8; 2017,Jan,8; 2016,Aug,9; 2016,Jan,13; 2015,Jan,16; 2014,Jan,11

81374 **one antigen equivalent *(eg, B*27)*, each**

EXCLUDES *Testing for the presence or absence of more than 2 antigen equivalents at a locus, use the following code for each locus test (81373)*

0.00 0.00 FUD XXX A

AMA: 2018,Nov,9; 2018,Jan,8; 2017,Jan,8; 2016,Aug,9; 2016,Jan,13; 2015,Jan,16; 2014,Jan,11

81375 **HLA Class II typing, low resolution (eg, antigen equivalents); *HLA-DRB1/3/4/5 and -DQB1***

EXCLUDES *Class I and II low-resolution HLA typing for HLA-A, -B, -C, -DRB 1/3/4/5, and DQB1 (81370)*

0.00 0.00 FUD XXX A

AMA: 2018,Nov,9; 2018,Jan,8; 2017,Jan,8; 2016,Aug,9; 2016,Jan,13; 2015,Jan,16; 2014,Jan,11

81376 **one locus *(eg, HLA-DRB1, -DRB3/4/5, -DQB1, -DQA1, -DPB1, or -DPA1)*, each**

INCLUDES Low-resolution typing, HLA-DRB1/3/4/5 reported as a single locus

EXCLUDES *Low-resolution typing for HLA-DRB1/3/4/5 and -DQB1 (81375)*

0.00 0.00 FUD XXX A

AMA: 2018,Nov,9; 2018,Jan,8; 2017,Jan,8; 2016,Aug,9; 2016,Jan,13; 2015,Jan,16; 2014,Jan,11

81377 **one antigen equivalent, each**

EXCLUDES *Testing for presence or absence of more than two antigen equivalents at a locus (81376)*

0.00 0.00 FUD XXX A

AMA: 2018,Nov,9; 2018,Jan,8; 2017,Jan,8; 2016,Aug,9; 2016,Jan,13; 2015,Jan,16; 2014,Jan,11

81378 **HLA Class I and II typing, high resolution (ie, alleles or allele groups), *HLA-A, -B, -C, and -DRB1***

0.00 0.00 FUD XXX A

AMA: 2018,Nov,9; 2018,Jan,8; 2017,Jan,8; 2016,Aug,9; 2016,Jan,13; 2015,Jan,16; 2014,Jan,11

81379 **HLA Class I typing, high resolution (ie, alleles or allele groups); complete (ie, *HLA-A, -B, and -C*)**

0.00 0.00 FUD XXX A

AMA: 2018,Nov,9; 2018,Jan,8; 2017,Jan,8; 2016,Aug,9; 2016,Jan,13; 2015,Jan,16; 2014,Jan,11

81380 **one locus (eg, *HLA-A, -B, or -C*), each**

EXCLUDES *Complete Class I high-resolution typing for HLA-A, -B, and -C (81379)*

Testing for presence or absence of a single allele or allele group using high-resolution methodology (81381)

0.00 0.00 FUD XXX A

AMA: 2018,Nov,9; 2018,Jan,8; 2017,Jan,8; 2016,Aug,9; 2016,Jan,13; 2015,Jan,16; 2014,Jan,11

81381 **one allele or allele group (eg, *B*57:01P*), each**

EXCLUDES *Testing for the presence or absence of more than two alleles or allele groups of locus, report the following code for each locus (81380)*

0.00 0.00 FUD XXX A

AMA: 2018,Nov,9; 2018,Jan,8; 2017,Jan,8; 2016,Aug,9; 2016,Jan,13; 2015,Jan,16; 2014,Jan,11

81382 **HLA Class II typing, high resolution (ie, alleles or allele groups); one locus (eg, *HLA-DRB1, -DRB3/4/5, -DQB1, -DQA1, -DPB1, or -DPA1*), each**

INCLUDES Typing of one or all of the DRB3/4/5 genes is regarded as one locus

EXCLUDES *Testing for just the presence or absence of a single allele or allele group using high-resolution methodology (81383)*

0.00 0.00 FUD XXX A

AMA: 2018,Nov,9; 2018,Jan,8; 2017,Jan,8; 2016,Jan,13; 2015,Jan,16; 2014,Jan,11

81383 **one allele or allele group (eg, *HLA-DQB1*06:02P*), each**

EXCLUDES *For testing for the presence or absence of more than two alleles or allele groups at a locus, report the following code for each locus (81382)*

0.00 0.00 FUD XXX A

AMA: 2018,Nov,9; 2018,Jan,8; 2017,Jan,8; 2016,Jan,13; 2015,Jan,16; 2014,Jan,11

81400-81479 [81479] Molecular Pathology Tier 2 Procedures

INCLUDES All analytical procedures in the evaluation such as:

- Amplification
- Cell lysis
- Detection
- Digestion
- Extraction
- Nucleic acid stabilization

Code selection based on specific gene being reviewed

Codes that are arranged by level of technical resources and work involved

Evaluation of the presence of a gene variant using the common gene variant name

Examples of proteins or diseases in the code description (not all inclusive)

Generally all the listed gene variants in the code description would be tested but lists are not all inclusive

Genes described using the Human Genome Organization (HUGO) approved names

Histocompatibility testing

Qualitative results unless otherwise stated

Specific analytes listed after the code description to use for selecting the appropriate molecular pathology procedure

Targeted genomic testing (81410-81471 [81448])

Testing for diseases that are more rare

EXCLUDES *Full gene sequencing using separate gene variant assessment codes unless it is specifically stated in the code description*

In situ hybridization analyses (88271-88275, 88365-88368 [88364, 88373, 88374])

Microbial identification (87149-87153, 87471-87801 [87623, 87624, 87625], 87900-87904 [87906, 87910, 87912])

Other related gene variants not listed in code

Tier 1 molecular pathology (81105-81254 [81161, 81162, 81163, 81164, 81165, 81166, 81167, 81173, 81174, 81184, 81185, 81186, 81187, 81188, 81189, 81190, 81200, 81201, 81202, 81203, 81204, 81205, 81206, 81207, 81208, 81209, 81210, 81219, 81227, 81230, 81231, 81233, 81234, 81238, 81239, 81245, 81246, 81250, 81257, 81258, 81259, 81265, 81266, 81267, 81268, 81269, 81284, 81285, 81286, 81289, 81361, 81362, 81363, 81364])

Unlisted molecular pathology procedures ([81479])

Code also modifier 26 when only interpretation and report are performed

Code also services required before cell lysis

81400 **Molecular pathology procedure, Level 1 (eg, identification of single germline variant [eg, SNP] by techniques such as restriction enzyme digestion or melt curve analysis)**

ACADM (acyl-CoA dehydrogenase, C-4 to C-12 straight chain, MCAD) (eg, medium chain acyl dehydrogenase deficiency), K304E variant

ACE (angiotensin converting enzyme) (eg, hereditary blood pressure regulation), insertion/deletion variant

AGTR1 (angiotensin II receptor, type 1) (eg, essential hypertension), 1166A>C variant

BCKDHA (branched chain keto acid dehydrogenase E1, alpha polypeptide) (eg, maple syrup urine disease, type 1A), Y438N variant

CCR5 (chemokine C-C motif receptor 5) (eg, HIV resistance), 32-bp deletion mutation/794 825del32 deletion

CLRN1 (clarin 1) (eg, Usher syndrome, type 3), N48K variant

F2 (coagulation factor 2) (eg, hereditary hypercoagulability), 1199G>A variant

F5 (coagulation factor V) (eg, hereditary hypercoagulability), HR2 variant

F7 (coagulation factor VII [serum prothrombin conversion accelerator]) (eg, hereditary hypercoagulability), R353Q variant

F13B (coagulation factor XIII, B polypeptide) (eg, hereditary hypercoagulability), V34L variant

FGB (fibrinogen beta chain) (eg, hereditary ischemic heart disease), -455G>A variant

FGFR1 (fibroblast growth factor receptor 1) (eg, Pfeiffer syndrome type 1, craniosynostosis), P252R variant

FGFR3 (fibroblast growth factor receptor 3) (eg, Muenke syndrome), P250R variant

FKTN (fukutin) (eg, Fukuyama congenital muscular dystrophy), retrotransposon insertion variant

GNE (glucosamine [UDP-N-acetyl]-2 -epimerase/N-acetylmannosamine kinase) (eg, inclusion body myopathy 2 [IBM2], Nonaka myopathy), M712T variant

IVD (isovaleryl-CoA dehydrogenase) (eg, isovaleric acidemia), A282V variant

LCT (lactase-phlorizin hydrolase) (eg, lactose intolerance), 13910 C>T variant

NEB (nebulin) (eg, nemaline myopathy 2), exon 55 deletion variant

PCDH15 (protocadherin-related 15) (eg, Usher syndrome type 1F), R245X variant

SERPINE1 (serpine peptidase inhibitor clade E, member 1, plasminogen activator inhibitor -1, PAI-1) (eg, thrombophilia), 4G variant

SHOC2 (soc-2 suppressor of clear homolog) (eg, Noonan-like syndrome with loose anagen hair), S2G variant

SRY (sex determining region Y) (eg, 46,XX testicular disorder of sex development, gonadal dysgenesis), gene analysis

TOR1A (torsin family 1, member A [torsin A]) (eg, early-onset primary dystonia [DYT1]), 907_909delGAG (904_906delGAG) variant

0.00 0.00 **FUD** XXX A

AMA: 2019,Jul,3; 2018,Nov,9; 2018,Jan,8; 2017,Jan,8; 2016,Aug,9; 2016,Jan,13; 2015,Jan,16; 2015,Jan,3; 2014,Jan,11

81401 **Molecular pathology procedure, Level 2 (eg, 2-10 SNPs, 1 methylated variant, or 1 somatic variant [typically using nonsequencing target variant analysis], or detection of a dynamic mutation disorder/triplet repeat)**

ABCC8 (ATP-binding cassette, sub-family C [CFTR/MRP], member 8) (eg, familial hyperinsulinism), common variants (eg, c.3898-9G>A [c.3992-9G>A], F1388del)

ABL1 (ABL proto oncogene 1, non-receptor tyrosine kinase) (eg, acquired imatinib resistance), T315I variant

ACADM (acyl-CoA dehydrogenase, C-4 to C-12 straight chain, MCAD) (eg, medium chain acyl dehydrogenase deficiency), common variants (eg, K304E, Y42H)

ADRB2 (adrenergic beta-2 receptor surface) (eg, drug metabolism), common variants (eg, G16R, Q27E)

APOB (apolipoprotein B) (eg, familial hypercholesterolemia type B), common variants (eg, R3500Q, R3500W)

*APOE (apolipoprotein E) (eg, hyperlipoproteinemia type III, cardiovascular disease, Alzheimer disease), common variants (eg, *2, *3, *4)*

CBFB/MYH11 (inv(16)) (eg, acute myeloid leukemia), qualitative, and quantitative, if performed

CBS (cystathionine-beta-synthase) (eg, homocystinuria, cystathionine beta-synthase deficiency), common variants (eg, I278T, G307S)

CCND1/IGH (BCL1/IgH, t(11;14)) (eg, mantle cell lymphoma) translocation analysis, major breakpoint, qualitative and quantitative, if performed

CFH/ARMS2 (complement factor H/age-related maculopathy susceptibility 2) (eg, macular degeneration), common variants (eg, Y402H [CFH], A69S [ARMS2])

DEK/NUP214 (t(6;9))(eg, acute myeloid leukemia), translocation analysis, qualitative, and quantitative, if performed

E2A/PBX1 (t(1;19)) (eg, acute lymphocytic leukemia), translocation analysis, qualitative, and quantitative, if performed

EML4/ALK (inv(2)) (eg, non-small cell lung cancer), translocation or inversion analysis

ETV6/NTRK3 (t(12;15)) (eg, congenital/infantile fibrosarcoma), translocation analysis, qualitative, and quantitative, if performed

ETV6/RUNX1 (t(12;21)) (eg, acute lymphocytic leukemia), translocation analysis, qualitative and quantitative, if performed

EWSR1/ATF1 (t(12;22)) (eg, clear cell sarcoma), translocation analysis, qualitative, and quantitative, if performed

EWSR1/ERG (t(21;22)) (eg, Ewing sarcoma/peripheral neuroectodermal tumor), translocation analysis, qualitative and quantitative, if performed

EWSR1/FLI1 (t(11;22)) (eg, Ewing sarcoma/peripheral neuroectodermal tumor), translocation analysis, qualitative and quantitative, if performed

EWSR1/WT1 (t(11;22)) (eg, desmoplastic small round cell tumor), translocation analysis, qualitative and quantitative, if performed

F11 (coagulation factor XI) (eg, coagulation disorder), common variants (eg, E117X [Type II], F283L [Type III], IVS14del14, and IVS14+1G>A [Type I])

FGFR3 (fibroblast growth factor receptor 3) (eg, achondroplasia, hypochondroplasia), common variants (eg, 1138G>A, 1138G>C, 1620C>A, 1620C>G)

FIP1L1/PDGFRA (del[4q12]) (eg, imatinib-sensitive chronic eosinophilic leukemia), qualitative and quantitative, if performed

FLG (filaggrin) (eg, ichthyosis vulgaris), common variants (eg, R501X, 2282del4, R2447X, S3247X, 3702delG)

FOXO1/PAX3 (t(2;13)) (eg, alveolar rhabdomyosarcoma), translocation analysis, qualitative and quantitative, if performed

FOXO1/PAX7 (t(1;13)) (eg, alveolar rhabdomyosarcoma), translocation analysis, qualitative and quantitative, if performed

FUS/DDIT3 (t(12;16)) (eg, myxoid liposarcoma), translocation analysis, qualitative, and quantitative, if performed

GALC (galactosylceramidase) (eg, Krabbe disease), common variants (eg, c.857G>A, 30-kb deletion)

GALT (galactose-1-phosphate uridylyltransferase) (eg, galactosemia), common variants (eg, Q188R, S135L, K285N, T138M, L195P, Y209C, IVS2-2A>G, P171S, del5kb, N314D, L218L/N314D)

H19 (imprinted maternally expressed transcript [non-protein coding]) (eg, Beckwith-Wiedemann syndrome), methylation analysis

IGH@/BCL2 (t(14;18)) (eg, follicular lymphoma), translocation and analysis; single breakpoint (eg) major breakpoint region [MBR] or minor cluster region [mcr]), qualitative or quantitative(When both MBR and mcr breakpoints are performed, use 81402)

KCNQ10T1 (KCNQ1 overlapping transcript 1 [non-protein coding]) (e.g, Beckwith-Wiedemann syndrome), methylation analysis

LINC00518 (long intergenic non-protein coding RNA 518) (eg, melanoma), expression analysis

LRRK2 (leucine-rich repeat kinase 2) (eg, Parkinson disease), common variants (eg, R1441G, G2019S, I2020T)

MED12 (mediator complex subunit 12) (eg, FG syndrome type 1, Lujan syndrome), common variants (eg, R961W, N1007S)

MEG3/DLK1 (maternally expressed 3 [non-protein coding]/delta-like 1 homolog [Drosophila]) (eg, intrauterine growth retardation), methylation analysis

MLL/AFF1 (t(4;11)) (eg acute lymphoblastic leukemia), translocation analysis, qualitative and quantitative, if performed

MLL/MLLT3 (t(9;11)) (eg, acute myeloid leukemia) translocation analysis, qualitative and quantitative, if performed

MT-RNR1 (mitochondrially encoded 12S RNA) (eg, nonsyndromic hearing loss), common variants (eg, m.1555>G, m1494C>T)

MUTYH (mutY homolog [E.coli]) (eg, MYH-associated polyposis), common variants (eg, Y165C, G382D)

MT-ATP6 (mitochondrially encoded ATP synthase 6) (eg, neuropathy with ataxia and retinitis pigmentosa [NARP], Leigh syndrome), common variants (eg, m.8993T>G, m.8993T>C)

MT-ND4, MT-ND6 (mitochondrially encoded NADH dehydrogenase 4, mitochondrially encoded NADH dehydrogenase 6) (eg, Leber hereditary optic neuropathy [LHON]), common variants (eg m.11778G>A, m3460G>A, m14484T>C)

MT-ND5 (mitochondrially encoded tRNA leucine 1 [UUA/G], mitochondrially encoded NADH dehydrogenase 5) (eg, mitochondrial encephalopathy with lactic acidosis and stroke-like episodes [MELAS]), common variants (eg, m.3243A>G, m.3271T>C, m.3252A>G, m.13513G>A)

MT-TK (mitochondrially encoded tRNA lysine) (eg, myoclonic epilepsy with ragged-red fibers [MERRF]), common variants (eg, m8344A>G, m.8356T>C)

MT-TL1 (mitochondrially encoded tRNA leucine 1[UUA/G]) (eg, diabetes and hearing loss), common variants (eg, m.3243A>G, m.14709 T>C) MT-TL1

MT-TS1, MT-RNR1 (mitochondrially encoded tRNA serine 1 [UCN], mitochondrially encoded 12S RNA) (eg, nonsyndromic sensorineural deafness [including aminoglycoside-induced nonsyndromic deafness]) common variants (eg, m.7445A>G, m.1555A>G)

NOD2 (nucleotide-binding oligomerization domain containing 2) (eg, Crohn's disease, Blau syndrome), common variants (eg, SNP 8, SNP 12, SNP 13)

NPM/ALK (t(2;5)) (eg, anaplastic large cell lymphoma), translocation analysis

PAX8/PPARG (t(2;3) (q13;p25)) (eg, follicular thyroid carcinoma), translocation analysis

PRAME (preferentially expressed antigen in melanoma)(eg, melanoma), expression analysis

PRSS1 (protease, serine, 1 [trypsin 1]) (eg, hereditary pancreatitis), common variants (eg, N29I, A16V, R122H)

PYGM (phosphorylase, glycogen, muscle) (eg, glycogen storage disease type V, McArdle disease), common variants (eg, R50X, G205S)

RUNX1/RUNX1T1 (t(8;21)) (eg, acute myeloid leukemia) translocation analysis, qualitative and quantitative, if performed

SS18/SSX1 (t(X;18)) (eg, synovial sarcoma), translocation analysis, qualitative and quantitative, if performed

SS18/SSX2 (t(X;18)) (eg, synovial sarcoma), translocation analysis, qualitative and quantitative, if performed

VWF (von Willebrand factor) (eg, von Willebrand disease type 2N), common variants (eg, T791M, R816W, R854Q)

0.00 0.00 FUD XXX A

AMA: 2019,Sep,7; 2019,Jul,3; 2018,Nov,9; 2018,Jan,8; 2017,Jan,8; 2016,Aug,9; 2016,Jan,13; 2015,Jan,16; 2015,Jan,3; 2014,Jan,11

81402 Molecular pathology procedure, Level 3 (eg, >10 SNPs, 2-10 methylated variants, or 2-10 somatic variants [typically using non-sequencing target variant analysis], immunoglobulin and T-cell receptor gene rearrangements, duplication/deletion variants of 1 exon, loss of heterozygosity [LOH], uniparental disomy [UPD])

Chromosome 1p-/19q- (eg, glial tumors), deletion analysis

Chromosome 18q- (eg, D18S55, D18S58, D18S61, D18S64, and D18S69) (eg, colon cancer), allelic imbalance assessment (ie, loss of heterozygosity)

COL1A1/PDGFB (t(17;22)) (eg, dermatofibrosarcoma protuberans), translocation analysis, multiple breakpoints, qualitative, and quantitative, if performed

CYP21A2 (cytochrome P450, family 21, subfamily A, polypeptide 2) (eg, congenital adrenal hyperplasia, 21-hydroxylase deficiency), common variants (eg, IVS2-13G, P30L, I172N, exon 6 mutation cluster [I235N, V236E, M238K], V281L, L307FfsX6, Q318X, R356W, P453S, G110VfsX21, 30-kb deletion variant)

ESR1/PGR (receptor 1/progesterone receptor) ratio (eg, breast cancer)

IGH@/BCL2 (t(14;18)) (eg, follicular lymphoma), translocation analysis; major breakpoint region (MBR) and minor cluster region (mcr) breakpoints, qualitative or quantitative

MEFV (Mediterranean fever) (eg, familial Mediterranean fever), common variants (eg, E148Q, P369S, F479L, M680I, I692del, M694V, M694I, K695R, V726A, A744S, R761H)

MPL (myeloproliferative leukemia virus oncogene, thrombopoietin receptor, TPOR) (eg, myeloproliferative disorder), common variants (eg, W515A, W515K, W515L, W515R)

TRD@ (T cell antigen receptor, delta) (eg, leukemia and lymphoma), gene rearrangement analysis, evaluation to detect abnormal clonal population

Uniparental disomy (UPD) (eg, Russell-Silver syndrome, Prader-Willi/Angelman syndrome), short tandem repeat (STR) analysis

0.00 0.00 FUD XXX A

AMA: 2018,Nov,9; 2018,Jan,8; 2017,Jan,8; 2016,Aug,9; 2016,Jan,13; 2015,Jan,16; 2015,Jan,3; 2014,Jan,11

81403 Molecular pathology procedure, Level 4 (eg, analysis of single exon by DNA sequence analysis, analysis of >10 amplicons using multiplex PCR in 2 or more independent reactions, mutation scanning or duplication/deletion variants of 2-5 exons)

ANG (angiogenin, ribonuclease, RNase A family, 5) (eg, amyotrophic lateral sclerosis), full gene sequence

ARX (aristaless-related homeobox) (eg, X-linked lissencephaly with ambiguous genitalia, X-linked mental retardation), duplication/deletion analysis

CEL (carboxyl ester lipase [bile salt-stimulated lipase]) (eg, maturity-onset diabetes of the young [MODY]), targeted sequence analysis of exon 11 (eg, c.1785delC, c.1686delT)

CTNNB1 (catenin [cadherin-associated protein], beta 1, 88kDa) (eg, desmoid tumors), targeted sequence analysis (eg, exon 3)

DAZ/SRY (deleted in azoospermia and sex determining region Y) (eg, male infertility), common deletions (eg, AZFa, AZFb, AZFc, AZFd)

DNMT3A (DNA [cytosine-5-]-methyltransferase 3 alpha) (eg, acute myeloid leukemia), targeted sequence analysis (eg, exon 23)

EPCAM (epithelial cell adhesion molecule) (eg, Lynch syndrome), duplication/deletion analysis

F8 (coagulation factor VIII) (eg, hemophilia A), inversion analysis, intron 1 and intron 22A

F12 (coagulation factor XII [Hageman factor]) (eg, angioedema, hereditary, type III; factor XII deficiency), targeted sequence analysis of exon 9

FGFR3 (fibroblast growth factor receptor 3) (eg, isolated craniosynostosis), targeted sequence analysis (eg, exon 7)

(For targeted sequence analysis of multiple FGFR3 exons, use 81404) (81404)

GJB1 (gap junction protein, beta 1) (eg, Charcot-Marie-Tooth X-linked), full gene sequence

GNAQ (guanine nucleotide-binding protein G[q] subunit alpha) (eg, uveal melanoma), common variants (eg, R183, Q209)

HRAS (v-Ha-ras Harvey rat sarcoma viral oncogene homolog) (eg, Costello syndrome), exon 2 sequence

Human erythrocyte antigen gene analyses (eg, SLC14A1 [Kidd blood group], BCAM [Lutheran blood group], ICAM4 [Landsteiner-Wiener blood group], SLC4A1 [Diego blood group], AQP1 [Colton blood group], ERMAP [Scianna blood group], RHCE [Rh blood group, CcEe antigens], KEL [Kell blood group], DARC [Duffy blood group], GYPA, GYPB, GYPE [MNS blood group], ART4 [Dombrock blood group]) (eg, sickle-cell disease, thalassemia, hemolytic transfusion reactions, hemolytic disease of the fetus or newborn), common variants

JAK2 (Janus kinase 2) (eg, myeloproliferative disorder), exon 12 sequence and exon 13 sequence, if performed

KCNC3 (potassium voltage-gated channel, Shaw-related subfamily, member 3) (eg, spinocerebellar ataxia), targeted sequence analysis (eg, exon 2)

KCNJ2 (potassium inwardly-rectifying channel, subfamily J, member 2) (eg, Andersen-Tawil syndrome), full gene sequence

KCNJ11 (potassium inwardly-rectifying channel, subfamily J, member 11) (eg, familial hyperinsulinism), full gene sequence

Killer cell immunoglobulin-like receptor (KIR) gene family (eg, hematopoietic stem cell transplantation), genotyping of KIR family genes

Known familial variant, not otherwise specified, for gene listed in Tier 1 or Tier 2, or identified during a genomic sequencing procedure, DNA sequence analysis, each variant exon

(For a known familial variant that is considered a common variant, use specific common variant Tier 1 or Tier 2 code)

MC4R (melanocortin 4 receptor) (eg, obesity), full gene sequence

*MICA (MHC class I polypeptide-related sequence A) (eg, solid organ transplantation), common variants (eg, *001, *002)*

MPL (myeloproliferative leukemia virus oncogene, thrombopoietin receptor, TPOR) (eg, myeloproliferative disorder), exon 10 sequence

MT-RNR1 (mitochondrially encoded 12S RNA) (eg, nonsyndromic hearing loss), full gene sequence

MT-TS1 (mitochondrially encoded tRNA serine 1) (eg, nonsyndromic hearing loss), full gene sequence

NDP (Norrie disease [pseudoglioma]) (eg, Norrie disease), duplication/deletion analysis

NHLRC1 (NHL repeat containing 1) (eg, progressive myoclonus epilepsy), full gene sequence

PHOX2B (paired-like homeobox 2b) (eg, congenital central hypoventilation syndrome), duplication/deletion analysis

PLN (phospholamban) (eg, dilated cardiomyopathy, hypertrophic cardiomyopathy), full gene sequence

RHD (Rh blood group, D antigen) (eg, hemolytic disease of the fetus and newborn, Rh maternal/fetal compatibility), deletion analysis (eg, exons 4, 5, and 7, pseudogene)

RHD (Rh blood group, D antigen) (eg, hemolytic disease of the fetus and newborn, Rh maternal/fetal compatibility), deletion analysis (eg, exons 4, 5, and 7, pseudogene), performed on cell-free fetal DNA in maternal blood

(For human erythrocyte gene analysis of RHD, use a separate unit of 81403)

SH2D1A (SH2 domain containing 1A) (eg, X-linked lymphoproliferative syndrome), duplication/deletion analysis

TWIST1 (twist homolog 1 [Drosophila]) (eg, Saethre-Chotzen syndrome), duplication/deletion analysis

UBA1 (ubiquitin-like modifier activating enzyme 1) (eg, spinal muscular atrophy, X-linked), targeted sequence analysis (eg, exon 15)

VHL (von Hippel-Lindau tumor suppressor) (eg, von Hippel-Lindau familial cancer syndrome), deletion/duplication analysis

VWF (von Willebrand factor) (eg, von Willebrand disease types 2A, 2B, 2M), targeted sequence analysis (eg, exon 28)

0.00 0.00 **FUD** XXX A

AMA: 2019,Jul,3; 2018,Nov,9; 2018,May,6; 2018,Jan,8; 2017,Jan,8; 2016,Aug,9; 2016,Jan,13; 2015,Jan,16; 2015,Jan,3; 2014,Jan,11

▲ **81404 Molecular pathology procedure, Level 5 (eg, analysis of 2-5 exons by DNA sequence analysis, mutation scanning or duplication/deletion variants of 6-10 exons, or characterization of a dynamic mutation disorder/triplet repeat by Southern blot analysis)**

ACADS (acyl-CoA dehydrogenase, C-2 to C-3 short chain) (eg, short chain acyl-CoA dehydrogenase deficiency), targeted sequence analysis (eg, exons 5 and 6)

AQP2 (aquaporin 2 [collecting duct]) (eg, nephrogenic diabetes insipidus), full gene sequence

ARX (aristaless related homeobox) (eg, X-linked lissencephaly with ambiguous genitalia, X-linked mental retardation), full gene sequence

AVPR2 (arginine vasopressin receptor 2) (eg, nephrogenic diabetes insipidus), full gene sequence

BBS10 (Bardet-Biedl syndrome 10) (eg, Bardet-Biedl syndrome), full gene sequence

BTD (biotinidase) (eg, biotinidase deficiency), full gene sequence

C10orf2 (chromosome 10 open reading frame 2) (eg, mitochondrial DNA depletion syndrome), full gene sequence

CAV3 (caveolin 3) (eg, CAV3-related distal myopathy, limb-girdle muscular dystrophy type 1C), full gene sequence

CD40LG (CD40 ligand) (eg, X-linked hyper IgM syndrome), full gene sequence

CDKN2A (cyclin-dependent kinase inhibitor 2A) (eg, CDKN2A-related cutaneous malignant melanoma, familial atypical mole-malignant melanoma syndrome), full gene sequence

CLRN1 (clarin 1) (eg, Usher syndrome, type 3), full gene sequence

COX6B1 (cytochrome c oxidase subunit VIb polypeptide 1) (eg, mitochondrial respiratory chain complex IV deficiency), full gene sequence

CPT2 (carnitine palmitoyltransferase 2) (eg, carnitine palmitoyltransferase II deficiency), full gene sequence

CRX (cone-rod homeobox) (eg, cone-rod dystrophy 2, Leber congenital amaurosis), full gene sequence

CYP1B1 (cytochrome P450, family 1, subfamily B, polypeptide 1) (eg, primary congenital glaucoma), full gene sequence

EGR2 (early growth response 2) (eg, Charcot-Marie-Tooth), full gene sequence

EMD (emerin) (eg, Emery-Dreifuss muscular dystrophy), duplication/deletion analysis

EPM2A (epilepsy, progressive myoclonus type 2A, Lafora disease [laforin]) (eg, progressive myoclonus epilepsy), full gene sequence

FGF23 (fibroblast growth factor 23) (eg, hypophosphatemic rickets), full gene sequence

FGFR2 (fibroblast growth factor receptor 2) (eg, craniosynostosis, Apert syndrome, Crouzon syndrome), targeted sequence analysis (eg, exons 8, 10)

FGFR3 (fibroblast growth factor receptor 3) (eg, achondroplasia, hypochondroplasia), targeted sequence analysis (eg, exons 8, 11, 12, 13)

FHL1 (four and a half LIM domains 1) (eg, Emery-Dreifuss muscular dystrophy), full gene sequence

FKRP (Fukutin related protein) (eg, congenital muscular dystrophy type 1C [MDC1C], limb-girdle muscular dystrophy [LGMD] type 2I), full gene sequence

FOXG1 (forkhead box G1) (eg, Rett syndrome), full gene sequence

FSHMD1A (facioscapulohumeral muscular dystrophy 1A) (eg, facioscapulohumeral muscular dystrophy), evaluation to detect abnormal (eg, deleted) alleles

FSHMD1A (facioscapulohumeral muscular dystrophy 1A) (eg, facioscapulohumeral muscular dystrophy), characterization of haplotype(s) (ie, chromosome 4A and 4B haplotypes)

26/TC PC/TC Only 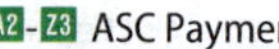 ASC Payment 50 Bilateral ♂ Male Only ♀ Female Only Facility RVU Non-Facility RVU CCI CLIA
FUD Follow-up Days **CMS:** IOM **AMA:** CPT Asst A-Y OPPSI 80/80 Surg Assist Allowed / w/Doc Lab Crosswalk Radiology Crosswalk

GH1 (growth hormone 1) (eg, growth hormone deficiency), full gene sequence

GP1BB (glycoprotein Ib [platelet], beta polypeptide) (eg, Bernard-Soulier syndrome type B), full gene sequence

(For common deletion variants of alpha globin 1 and alpha globin 2 genes, use 81257)

HNF1B (HNF1 homeobox B) (eg, maturity-onset diabetes of the young [MODY]), duplication/deletion analysis

HRAS (v-Ha-ras Harvey rat sarcoma viral oncogene homolog) (eg, Costello syndrome), full gene sequence

HSD3B2 (hydroxy-delta-5-steroid dehydrogenase, 3 beta- and steroid delta-isomerase 2) (eg, 3-beta-hydroxysteroid dehydrogenase type II deficiency), full gene sequence

HSD11B2 (hydroxysteroid [11-beta] dehydrogenase 2) (eg, mineralocorticoid excess syndrome), full gene sequence

HSPB1 (heat shock 27kDa protein 1) (eg, Charcot-Marie-Tooth disease), full gene sequence

INS (insulin) (eg, diabetes mellitus), full gene sequence

KCNJ1 (potassium inwardly-rectifying channel, subfamily J, member 1) (eg, Bartter syndrome), full gene sequence

KCNJ10 (potassium inwardly-rectifying channel, subfamily J, member 10) (eg, SeSAME syndrome, EAST syndrome, sensorineural hearing loss), full gene sequence

LITAF (lipopolysaccharide-induced TNF factor) (eg, Charcot-Marie-Tooth), full gene sequence

MEFV (Mediterranean fever) (eg, familial Mediterranean fever), full gene sequence

MEN1 (multiple endocrine neoplasia I) (eg, multiple endocrine neoplasia type 1, Wermer syndrome), duplication/deletion analysis

MMACHC (methylmalonic aciduria [cobalamin deficiency] cblC type, with homocystinuria) (eg, methylmalonic acidemia and homocystinuria), full gene sequence

MPV17 (MpV17 mitochondrial inner membrane protein) (eg, mitochondrial DNA depletion syndrome), duplication/deletion analysis

NDP (Norrie disease [pseudoglioma]) (eg, Norrie disease), full gene sequence

NDUFA1 (NADH dehydrogenase [ubiquinone] 1 alpha subcomplex, 1, 7.5kDa) (eg, Leigh syndrome, mitochondrial complex I deficiency), full gene sequence

NDUFAF2 (NADH dehydrogenase [ubiquinone] 1 alpha subcomplex, assembly factor 2) (eg, Leigh syndrome, mitochondrial complex I deficiency), full gene sequence

NDUFS4 (NADH dehydrogenase [ubiquinone] Fe-S protein 4, 18kDa [NADH-coenzyme Q reductase]) (eg, Leigh syndrome, mitochondrial complex I deficiency), full gene sequence

NIPA1 (non-imprinted in Prader-Willi/Angelman syndrome 1) (eg, spastic paraplegia), full gene sequence

NLGN4X (neuroligin 4, X-linked) (eg, autism spectrum disorders), duplication/deletion analysis

NPC2 (Niemann-Pick disease, type C2 [epididymal secretory protein E1]) (eg, Niemann-Pick disease type C2), full gene sequence

NR0B1 (nuclear receptor subfamily 0, group B, member 1) (eg, congenital adrenal hypoplasia), full gene sequence

PDX1 (pancreatic and duodenal homeobox 1) (eg, maturity-onset diabetes of the young [MODY]), full gene sequence

PHOX2B (paired-like homeobox 2b) (eg, congenital central hypoventilation syndrome), full gene sequence

PIK3CA (phosphatidylinositol-4,5-bisphosphate 3-kinase, catalytic subunit alpha) (eg, colorectal cancer), targeted sequence analysis (eg, exons 9 and 20)

PLP1 (proteolipid protein 1) (eg, Pelizaeus-Merzbacher disease, spastic paraplegia), duplication/deletion analysis

PQBP1 (polyglutamine binding protein 1) (eg, Renpenning syndrome), duplication/deletion analysis

PRNP (prion protein) (eg, genetic prion disease), full gene sequence

PROP1 (PROP paired-like homeobox 1) (eg, combined pituitary hormone deficiency), full gene sequence

PRPH2 (peripherin 2 [retinal degeneration, slow]) (eg, retinitis pigmentosa), full gene sequence

PRSS1 (protease, serine, 1 [trypsin 1]) (eg, hereditary pancreatitis), full gene sequence

RAF1 (v-raf-1 murine leukemia viral oncogene homolog 1) (eg, LEOPARD syndrome), targeted sequence analysis (eg, exons 7, 12, 14, 17)

RET (ret proto-oncogene) (eg, multiple endocrine neoplasia, type 2B and familial medullary thyroid carcinoma), common variants (eg, M918T, 2647_2648delinsTT, A883F)

RHO (rhodopsin) (eg, retinitis pigmentosa), full gene sequence

RP1 (retinitis pigmentosa 1) (eg, retinitis pigmentosa), full gene sequence

SCN1B (sodium channel, voltage-gated, type I, beta) (eg, Brugada syndrome), full gene sequence

SCO2 (SCO cytochrome oxidase deficient homolog 2 [SCO1L]) (eg, mitochondrial respiratory chain complex IV deficiency), full gene sequence

SDHC (succinate dehydrogenase complex, subunit C, integral membrane protein, 15kDa) (eg, hereditary paraganglioma-pheochromocytoma syndrome), duplication/deletion analysis

SDHD (succinate dehydrogenase complex, subunit D, integral membrane protein) (eg, hereditary paraganglioma), full gene sequence

SGCG (sarcoglycan, gamma [35kDa dystrophin-associated glycoprotein]) (eg, limb-girdle muscular dystrophy), duplication/deletion analysis

SH2D1A (SH2 domain containing 1A) (eg, X-linked lymphoproliferative syndrome), full gene sequence

SLC16A2 (solute carrier family 16, member 2 [thyroid hormone transporter]) (eg, specific thyroid hormone cell transporter deficiency, Allan-Herndon-Dudley syndrome), duplication/deletion analysis

SLC25A20 (solute carrier family 25 [carnitine/acylcarnitine translocase], member 20) (eg, carnitine-acylcarnitine translocase deficiency), duplication/deletion analysis

SLC25A4 (solute carrier family 25 [mitochondrial carrier; adenine nucleotide translocation], member 4) (eg, progressive external ophthalmoplegia), full gene sequence

SOD1 (superoxide dismutase 1, soluble) (eg, amyotrophic lateral sclerosis), full gene sequence

SPINK1 (serine peptidase inhibitor, Kazal type 1) (eg, hereditary pancreatitis), full gene sequence

STK11 (serine/threonine kinase 11) (eg, Peutz-Jeghers syndrome), duplication/deletion analysis

TACO1 (translational activator of mitochondrial encoded cytochrome c oxidase I) (eg, mitochondrial respiratory chain complex IV deficiency), full gene sequence

THAP1 (THAP domain containing, apoptosis associated protein 1) (eg, torsion dystonia), full gene sequence

TOR1A (torsin family 1, member A [torsin A]) (eg, torsion dystonia), full gene sequence

TP53 (tumor protein 53) (eg, tumor samples), targeted sequence analysis of 2-5 exons

TTPA (tocopherol [alpha] transfer protein) (eg, ataxia), full gene sequence

TTR (transthyretin) (eg, familial transthyretin amyloidosis), full gene sequence

TWIST1 (twist homolog 1 [Drosophila]) (eg, Saethre-Chotzen syndrome), full gene sequence

TYR (tyrosinase [oculocutaneous albinism IA]) (eg, oculocutaneous albinism IA), full gene sequence

USH1G (Usher syndrome 1G [autosomal recessive]) (eg, Usher syndrome, type 1), full gene sequence

VWF (von Willebrand factor) (eg, von Willebrand disease type 1C), targeted sequence analysis (eg, exons 26, 27, 37)

VHL (von Hippel-Lindau tumor suppressor) (eg, von Hippel-Lindau familial cancer syndrome), full gene sequence

ZEB2 (zinc finger E-box binding homeobox 2) (eg, Mowat-Wilson syndrome), duplication/deletion analysis

ZNF41 (zinc finger protein 41) (eg, X-linked mental retardation 89), full gene sequence

0.00 0.00 **FUD** XXX

AMA: 2019,Jul,3; 2018,Nov,9; 2018,May,6; 2018,Jan,8; 2017,Jan,8; 2016,Aug,9; 2016,Jan,13; 2015,Jan,16; 2015,Jan,3; 2014,Jan,11

81405 Molecular pathology procedure, Level 6 (eg, analysis of 6-10 exons by DNA sequence analysis, mutation scanning or duplication/deletion variants of 11-25 exons, regionally targeted cytogenomic array analysis)

ABCD1 (ATP-binding cassette, sub-family D [ALD], member 1) (eg, adrenoleukodystrophy), full gene sequence

ACADS (acyl-CoA dehydrogenase, C-2 to C-3 short chain) (eg, short chain acyl-CoA dehydrogenase deficiency), full gene sequence

ACTA2 (actin, alpha 2, smooth muscle, aorta) (eg, thoracic aortic aneurysms and aortic dissections), full gene sequence

ACTC1 (actin, alpha, cardiac muscle 1) (eg, familial hypertrophic cardiomyopathy), full gene sequence

ANKRD1 (ankyrin repeat domain 1) (eg, dilated cardiomyopathy), full gene sequence

APTX (aprataxin) (eg, ataxia with oculomotor apraxia 1), full gene sequence

ARSA (arylsulfatase A) (eg, arylsulfatase A deficiency), full gene sequence

BCKDHA (branched chain keto acid dehydrogenase E1, alpha polypeptide) (eg, maple syrup urine disease, type 1A), full gene sequence

BCS1L (BCS1-like [S. cerevisiae]) (eg, Leigh syndrome, mitochondrial complex III deficiency, GRACILE syndrome), full gene sequence

BMPR2 (bone morphogenetic protein receptor, type II [serine/threonine kinase]) (eg, heritable pulmonary arterial hypertension), duplication/deletion analysis

CASQ2 (calsequestrin 2 [cardiac muscle]) (eg, catecholaminergic polymorphic ventricular tachycardia), full gene sequence

CASR (calcium-sensing receptor) (eg, hypocalcemia), full gene sequence

CDKL5 (cyclin-dependent kinase-like 5) (eg, early infantile epileptic encephalopathy), duplication/deletion analysis

CHRNA4 (cholinergic receptor, nicotinic, alpha 4) (eg, nocturnal frontal lobe epilepsy), full gene sequence

CHRNB2 (cholinergic receptor, nicotinic, beta 2 [neuronal]) (eg, nocturnal frontal lobe epilepsy), full gene sequence

COX10 (COX10 homolog, cytochrome c oxidase assembly protein) (eg, mitochondrial respiratory chain complex IV deficiency), full gene sequence

COX15 (COX15 homolog, cytochrome c oxidase assembly protein) (eg, mitochondrial respiratory chain complex IV deficiency), full gene sequence

CPOX (coproporphyrinogen oxidase) (eg, hereditary coproporphyria), full gene sequence

CTRC (chymotrypsin C) (eg, hereditary pancreatitis), full gene sequence

CYP11B1 (cytochrome P450, family 11, subfamily B, polypeptide 1) (eg, congenital adrenal hyperplasia), full gene sequence

CYP17A1 (cytochrome P450, family 17, subfamily A, polypeptide 1) (eg, congenital adrenal hyperplasia), full gene sequence

CYP21A2 (cytochrome P450, family 21, subfamily A, polypeptide2) (eg, steroid 21-hydroxylase isoform, congenital adrenal hyperplasia), full gene sequence

Cytogenomic constitutional targeted microarray analysis of chromosome 22q13 by interrogation of genomic regions for copy number and single nucleotide polymorphism (SNP) variants for chromosomal abnormalities

(When performing genome-wide cytogenomic constitutional microarray analysis, see 81228, 81229) (81228-81229)

(Do not report analyte-specific molecular pathology procedures separately when the specific analytes are included as part of the microarray analysis of chromosome 22q13)

(Do not report 88271 when performing cytogenomic microarray analysis)

DBT (dihydrolipoamide branched chain transacylase E2) (eg, maple syrup urine disease, type 2), duplication/deletion analysis

DCX (doublecortin) (eg, X-linked lissencephaly), full gene sequence

DES (desmin) (eg, myofibrillar myopathy), full gene sequence

DFNB59 (deafness, autosomal recessive 59) (eg, autosomal recessive nonsyndromic hearing impairment), full gene sequence

DGUOK (deoxyguanosine kinase) (eg, hepatocerebral mitochondrial DNA depletion syndrome), full gene sequence

DHCR7 (7-dehydrocholesterol reductase) (eg, Smith-Lemli-Opitz syndrome), full gene sequence

EIF2B2 (eukaryotic translation initiation factor 2B, subunit 2 beta, 39kDa) (eg, leukoencephalopathy with vanishing white matter), full gene sequence

EMD (emerin) (eg, Emery-Dreifuss muscular dystrophy), full gene sequence

ENG (endoglin) (eg, hereditary hemorrhagic telangiectasia, type 1), duplication/deletion analysis

EYA1 (eyes absent homolog 1 [Drosophila]) (eg, branchio-oto-renal [BOR] spectrum disorders), duplication/deletion analysis

FGFR1 (fibroblast growth factor receptor 1) (eg, Kallmann syndrome 2), full gene sequence

FH (fumarate hydratase) (eg, fumarate hydratase deficiency, hereditary leiomyomatosis with renal cell cancer), full gene sequence

FKTN (fukutin) (eg, limb-girdle muscular dystrophy [LGMD] type 2M or 2L), full gene sequence

FTSJ1 (FtsJ RNA methyltransferase homolog 1 [E. coli]) (eg, X-linked mental retardation 9), duplication/deletion analysis

GABRG2 (gamma-aminobutyric acid [GABA] A receptor, gamma 2) (eg, generalized epilepsy with febrile seizures), full gene sequence

GCH1 (GTP cyclohydrolase 1) (eg, autosomal dominant dopa-responsive dystonia), full gene sequence

GDAP1 (ganglioside-induced differentiation-associated protein 1) (eg, Charcot-Marie-Tooth disease), full gene sequence

GFAP (glial fibrillary acidic protein) (eg, Alexander disease), full gene sequence

GHR (growth hormone receptor) (eg, Laron syndrome), full gene sequence

GHRHR (growth hormone releasing hormone receptor) (eg, growth hormone deficiency), full gene sequence

GLA (galactosidase, alpha) (eg, Fabry disease), full gene sequence

HNF1A (HNF1 homeobox A) (eg, maturity-onset diabetes of the young [MODY]), full gene sequence

HNF1B (HNF1 homeobox B) (eg, maturity-onset diabetes of the young [MODY]), full gene sequence

HTRA1 (HtrA serine peptidase 1) (eg, macular degeneration), full gene sequence

IDS (iduronate 2-sulfatase) (eg, mucopolysaccharidosis, type II), full gene sequence

IL2RG (interleukin 2 receptor, gamma) (eg, X-linked severe combined immunodeficiency), full gene sequence

ISPD (isoprenoid synthase domain containing) (eg, muscle-eye-brain disease, Walker-Warburg syndrome), full gene sequence

KRAS (Kirsten rat sarcoma viral oncogene homolog) (eg, Noonan syndrome), full gene sequence

LAMP2 (lysosomal-associated membrane protein 2) (eg, Danon disease), full gene sequence

LDLR (low density lipoprotein receptor) (eg, familial hypercholesterolemia), duplication/deletion analysis

MEN1 (multiple endocrine neoplasia I) (eg, multiple endocrine neoplasia type 1, Wermer syndrome), full gene sequence

MMAA (methylmalonic aciduria [cobalamine deficiency] type A) (eg, MMAA-related methylmalonic acidemia), full gene sequence

MMAB (methylmalonic aciduria [cobalamine deficiency] type B) (eg, MMAA-related methylmalonic acidemia), full gene sequence

MPI (mannose phosphate isomerase) (eg, congenital disorder of glycosylation 1b), full gene sequence

MPV17 (MpV17 mitochondrial inner membrane protein) (eg, mitochondrial DNA depletion syndrome), full gene sequence

MPZ (myelin protein zero) (eg, Charcot-Marie-Tooth), full gene sequence

MTM1 (myotubularin 1) (eg, X-linked centronuclear myopathy), duplication/deletion analysis

MYL2 (myosin, light chain 2, regulatory, cardiac, slow) (eg, familial hypertrophic cardiomyopathy), full gene sequence

MYL3 (myosin, light chain 3, alkali, ventricular, skeletal, slow) (eg, familial hypertrophic cardiomyopathy), full gene sequence

MYOT (myotilin) (eg, limb-girdle muscular dystrophy), full gene sequence

NDUFS7 (NADH dehydrogenase [ubiquinone] Fe-S protein 7, 20kDa [NADH-coenzyme Q reductase]) (eg, Leigh syndrome, mitochondrial complex I deficiency), full gene sequence

NDUFS8 (NADH dehydrogenase [ubiquinone] Fe-S protein 8, 23kDa [NADH-coenzyme Q reductase]) (eg, Leigh syndrome, mitochondrial complex I deficiency), full gene sequence

NDUFV1 (NADH dehydrogenase [ubiquinone] flavoprotein 1, 51kDa) (eg, Leigh syndrome, mitochondrial complex I deficiency), full gene sequence

NEFL (neurofilament, light polypeptide) (eg, Charcot-Marie-Tooth), full gene sequence

NF2 (neurofibromin 2 [merlin]) (eg, neurofibromatosis, type 2), duplication/deletion analysis

NLGN3 (neuroligin 3) (eg, autism spectrum disorders), full gene sequence

NLGN4X (neuroligin 4, X-linked) (eg, autism spectrum disorders), full gene sequence

NPHP1 (nephronophthisis 1 [juvenile]) (eg, Joubert syndrome), deletion analysis, and duplication analysis, if performed

NPHS2 (nephrosis 2, idiopathic, steroid-resistant [podocin]) (eg, steroid-resistant nephrotic syndrome), full gene sequence

NSD1 (nuclear receptor binding SET domain protein 1) (eg, Sotos syndrome), duplication/deletion analysis

OTC (ornithine carbamoyltransferase) (eg, ornithine transcarbamylase deficiency), full gene sequence

PAFAH1B1 (platelet-activating factor acetylhydrolase 1b, regulatory subunit 1 [45kDa]) (eg, lissencephaly, Miller-Dieker syndrome), duplication/deletion analysis

PARK2 (Parkinson protein 2, E3 ubiquitin protein ligase [parkin]) (eg, Parkinson disease), duplication/deletion analysis

PCCA (propionyl CoA carboxylase, alpha polypeptide) (eg, propionic acidemia, type 1), duplication/deletion analysis

PCDH19 (protocadherin 19) (eg, epileptic encephalopathy), full gene sequence

PDHA1 (pyruvate dehydrogenase [lipoamide] alpha 1) (eg, lactic acidosis), duplication/deletion analysis

PDHB (pyruvate dehydrogenase [lipoamide] beta) (eg, lactic acidosis), full gene sequence

PINK1 (PTEN induced putative kinase 1) (eg, Parkinson disease), full gene sequence

PKLR (pyruvate kinase, liver and RBC) (eg, pyruvate kinase deficiency), full gene sequence

PLP1 (proteolipid protein 1) (eg, Pelizaeus-Merzbacher disease, spastic paraplegia), full gene sequence

POU1F1 (POU class 1 homeobox 1) (eg, combined pituitary hormone deficiency), full gene sequence

PQBP1 (polyglutamine binding protein 1) (eg, Renpenning syndrome), full gene sequence

PRX (periaxin) (eg, Charcot-Marie-Tooth disease), full gene sequence

PSEN1 (presenilin 1) (eg, Alzheimer's disease), full gene sequence

RAB7A (RAB7A, member RAS oncogene family) (eg, Charcot-Marie-Tooth disease), full gene sequence

RAI1 (retinoic acid induced 1) (eg, Smith-Magenis syndrome), full gene sequence

REEP1 (receptor accessory protein 1) (eg, spastic paraplegia), full gene sequence

RET (ret proto-oncogene) (eg, multiple endocrine neoplasia, type 2A and familial medullary thyroid carcinoma), targeted sequence analysis (eg, exons 10, 11, 13-16)

RPS19 (ribosomal protein S19) (eg, Diamond-Blackfan anemia), full gene sequence

RRM2B (ribonucleotide reductase M2 B [TP53 inducible]) (eg, mitochondrial DNA depletion), full gene sequence

SCO1 (SCO cytochrome oxidase deficient homolog 1) (eg, mitochondrial respiratory chain complex IV deficiency), full gene sequence

SDHB (succinate dehydrogenase complex, subunit B, iron sulfur) (eg, hereditary paraganglioma), full gene sequence

SDHC (succinate dehydrogenase complex, subunit C, integral membrane protein, 15kDa) (eg, hereditary paraganglioma-pheochromocytoma syndrome), full gene sequence

SGCA (sarcoglycan, alpha [50kDa dystrophin-associated glycoprotein]) (eg, limb-girdle muscular dystrophy), full gene sequence

SGCB (sarcoglycan, beta [43kDa dystrophin-associated glycoprotein]) (eg, limb-girdle muscular dystrophy), full gene sequence

SGCD (sarcoglycan, delta [35kDa dystrophin-associated glycoprotein]) (eg, limb-girdle muscular dystrophy), full gene sequence

SGCE (sarcoglycan, epsilon) (eg, myoclonic dystonia), duplication/deletion analysis

SGCG (sarcoglycan, gamma [35kDa dystrophin-associated glycoprotein]) (eg, limb-girdle muscular dystrophy), full gene sequence

SHOC2 (soc-2 suppressor of clear homolog) (eg, Noonan-like syndrome with loose anagen hair), full gene sequence

SHOX (short stature homeobox) (eg, Langer mesomelic dysplasia), full gene sequence

SIL1 (SIL1 homolog, endoplasmic reticulum chaperone [S. cerevisiae]) (eg, ataxia), full gene sequence

SLC2A1 (solute carrier family 2 [facilitated glucose transporter], member 1) (eg, glucose transporter type 1 [GLUT 1] deficiency syndrome), full gene sequence

SLC16A2 (solute carrier family 16, member 2 [thyroid hormone transporter]) (eg, specific thyroid hormone cell transporter deficiency, Allan-Herndon-Dudley syndrome), full gene sequence

SLC22A5 (solute carrier family 22 [organic cation/carnitine transporter], member 5) (eg, systemic primary carnitine deficiency), full gene sequence

SLC25A20 (solute carrier family 25 [carnitine/acylcarnitine translocase], member 20) (eg, carnitine-acylcarnitine translocase deficiency), full gene sequence

SMAD4 (SMAD family member 4) (eg, hemorrhagic telangiectasia syndrome, juvenile polyposis), duplication/deletion analysis

SPAST (spastin) (eg, spastic paraplegia), duplication/deletion analysis

SPG7 (spastic paraplegia 7 [pure and complicated autosomal recessive]) (eg, spastic paraplegia), duplication/deletion analysis

SPRED1 (sprouty-related, EVH1 domain containing 1) (eg, Legius syndrome), full gene sequence

STAT3 (signal transducer and activator of transcription 3 [acute-phase response factor]) (eg, autosomal dominant hyper-IgE syndrome), targeted sequence analysis (eg, exons 12, 13, 14, 16, 17, 20, 21)

STK11 (serine/threonine kinase 11) (eg, Peutz-Jeghers syndrome), full gene sequence

SURF1 (surfeit 1) (eg, mitochondrial respiratory chain complex IV deficiency), full gene sequence

TARDBP (TAR DNA binding protein) (eg, amyotrophic lateral sclerosis), full gene sequence

TBX5 (T-box 5) (eg, Holt-Oram syndrome), full gene sequence

TCF4 (transcription factor 4) (eg, Pitt-Hopkins syndrome), duplication/deletion analysis

TGFBR1 (transforming growth factor, beta receptor 1) (eg, Marfan syndrome), full gene sequence

TGFBR2 (transforming growth factor, beta receptor 2) (eg, Marfan syndrome), full gene sequence

THRB (thyroid hormone receptor, beta) (eg, thyroid hormone resistance, thyroid hormone beta receptor deficiency), full gene sequence or targeted sequence analysis of >5 exons

TK2 (thymidine kinase 2, mitochondrial) (eg, mitochondrial DNA depletion syndrome), full gene sequence

TNNC1 (troponin C type 1 [slow]) (eg, hypertrophic cardiomyopathy or dilated cardiomyopathy), full gene sequence

TNNI3 (troponin 1, type 3 [cardiac]) (eg, familial hypertrophic cardiomyopathy), full gene sequence

TP53 (tumor protein 53) (eg, Li-Fraumeni syndrome, tumor samples), full gene sequence or targeted sequence analysis of >5 exons

TPM1 (tropomyosin 1 [alpha]) (eg, familial hypertrophic cardiomyopathy), full gene sequence

TSC1 (tuberous sclerosis 1) (eg, tuberous sclerosis), duplication/deletion analysis

TYMP (thymidine phosphorylase) (eg, mitochondrial DNA depletion syndrome), full gene sequence

VWF (von Willebrand factor) (eg, von Willebrand disease type 2N), targeted sequence analysis (eg, exons 18-20, 23-25)

WT1 (Wilms tumor 1) (eg, Denys-Drash syndrome, familial Wilms tumor), full gene sequence

ZEB2 (zinc finger E-box binding homeobox 2) (eg, Mowat-Wilson syndrome), full gene sequence

0.00 0.00 **FUD** XXX A

AMA: 2019,Jul,3; 2018,Nov,9; 2018,Sep,14; 2018,May,6; 2018,Jan,8; 2017,Jan,8; 2016,Aug,9; 2016,Jan,13; 2015,Jan,16; 2015,Jan,3; 2014,Jan,11

▲ **81406 Molecular pathology procedure, Level 7 (eg, analysis of 11-25 exons by DNA sequence analysis, mutation scanning or duplication/deletion variants of 26-50 exons)**

ACADVL (acyl-CoA dehydrogenase, very long chain) (eg, very long chain acyl-coenzyme A dehydrogenase deficiency), full gene sequence

ACTN4 (actinin, alpha 4) (eg, focal segmental glomerulosclerosis), full gene sequence

AFG3L2 (AFG3 ATPase family gene 3-like 2 [S. cerevisiae]) (eg, spinocerebellar ataxia), full gene sequence

AIRE (autoimmune regulator) (eg, autoimmune polyendocrinopathy syndrome type 1), full gene sequence

ALDH7A1 (aldehyde dehydrogenase 7 family, member A1) (eg, pyridoxine-dependent epilepsy), full gene sequence

ANO5 (anoctamin 5) (eg, limb-girdle muscular dystrophy), full gene sequence

ANOS1 (anosim-1) (eg, Kallmann syndrome 1), full gene sequence

APP (amyloid beta [A4] precursor protein) (eg, Alzheimer's disease), full gene sequence

ASS1 (argininosuccinate synthase 1) (eg, citrullinemia type I), full gene sequence

ATL1 (atlastin GTPase 1) (eg, spastic paraplegia), full gene sequence

ATP1A2 (ATPase, Na+/K+ transporting, alpha 2 polypeptide) (eg, familial hemiplegic migraine), full gene sequence

ATP7B (ATPase, Cu++ transporting, beta polypeptide) (eg, Wilson disease), full gene sequence

BBS1 (Bardet-Biedl syndrome 1) (eg, Bardet-Biedl syndrome), full gene sequence

BBS2 (Bardet-Biedl syndrome 2) (eg, Bardet-Biedl syndrome), full gene sequence

BCKDHB (branched-chain keto acid dehydrogenase E1, beta polypeptide) (eg, maple syrup urine disease, type 1B), full gene sequence

BEST1 (bestrophin 1) (eg, vitelliform macular dystrophy), full gene sequence

BMPR2 (bone morphogenetic protein receptor, type II [serine/threonine kinase]) (eg, heritable pulmonary arterial hypertension), full gene sequence

BRAF (B-Raf proto-oncogene, serine/threonine kinase) (eg, Noonan syndrome), full gene sequence

BSCL2 (Berardinelli-Seip congenital lipodystrophy 2 [seipin]) (eg, Berardinelli-Seip congenital lipodystrophy), full gene sequence

BTK (Bruton agammaglobulinemia tyrosine kinase) (eg, X-linked agammaglobulinemia), full gene sequence

CACNB2 (calcium channel, voltage-dependent, beta 2 subunit) (eg, Brugada syndrome), full gene sequence

CAPN3 (calpain 3) (eg, limb-girdle muscular dystrophy [LGMD] type 2A, calpainopathy), full gene sequence

CBS (cystathionine-beta-synthase) (eg, homocystinuria, cystathionine beta-synthase deficiency), full gene sequence

CDH1 (cadherin 1, type 1, E-cadherin [epithelial]) (eg, hereditary diffuse gastric cancer), full gene sequence

CDKL5 (cyclin-dependent kinase-like 5) (eg, early infantile epileptic encephalopathy), full gene sequence

CLCN1 (chloride channel 1, skeletal muscle) (eg, myotonia congenita), full gene sequence

CLCNKB (chloride channel, voltage-sensitive Kb) (eg, Bartter syndrome 3 and 4b), full gene sequence

CNTNAP2 (contactin-associated protein-like 2) (eg, Pitt-Hopkins-like syndrome 1), full gene sequence

COL6A2 (collagen, type VI, alpha 2) (eg, collagen type VI-related disorders), duplication/deletion analysis

CPT1A (carnitine palmitoyltransferase 1A [liver]) (eg, carnitine palmitoyltransferase 1A [CPT1A] deficiency), full gene sequence

CRB1 (crumbs homolog 1 [Drosophila]) (eg, Leber congenital amaurosis), full gene sequence

CREBBP (CREB binding protein) (eg, Rubinstein-Taybi syndrome), duplication/deletion analysis

DBT (dihydrolipoamide branched chain transacylase E2) (eg, maple syrup urine disease, type 2), full gene sequence

DLAT (dihydrolipoamide S-acetyltransferase) (eg, pyruvate dehydrogenase E2 deficiency), full gene sequence

DLD (dihydrolipoamide dehydrogenase) (eg, maple syrup urine disease, type III), full gene sequence

DSC2 (desmocollin) (eg, arrhythmogenic right ventricular dysplasia/cardiomyopathy 11), full gene sequence

DSG2 (desmoglein 2) (eg, arrhythmogenic right ventricular dysplasia/cardiomyopathy 10), full gene sequence

DSP (desmoplakin) (eg, arrhythmogenic right ventricular dysplasia/cardiomyopathy 8), full gene sequence

EFHC1 (EF-hand domain [C-terminal] containing 1) (eg, juvenile myoclonic epilepsy), full gene sequence

EIF2B3 (eukaryotic translation initiation factor 2B, subunit 3 gamma, 58kDa) (eg, leukoencephalopathy with vanishing white matter), full gene sequence

EIF2B4 (eukaryotic translation initiation factor 2B, subunit 4 delta, 67kDa) (eg, leukoencephalopathy with vanishing white matter), full gene sequence

EIF2B5 (eukaryotic translation initiation factor 2B, subunit 5 epsilon, 82kDa) (eg, childhood ataxia with central nervous system hypomyelination/vanishing white matter), full gene sequence

ENG (endoglin) (eg, hereditary hemorrhagic telangiectasia, type 1), full gene sequence

EYA1 (eyes absent homolog 1 [Drosophila]) (eg, branchio-oto-renal [BOR] spectrum disorders), full gene sequence

F8 (coagulation factor VIII) (eg, hemophilia A), duplication/deletion analysis

FAH (fumarylacetoacetate hydrolase [fumarylacetoacetase]) (eg, tyrosinemia, type 1), full gene sequence

FASTKD2 (FAST kinase domains 2) (eg, mitochondrial respiratory chain complex IV deficiency), full gene sequence

FIG4 (FIG4 homolog, SAC1 lipid phosphatase domain containing [S. cerevisiae]) (eg, Charcot-Marie-Tooth disease), full gene sequence

FTSJ1 (FtsJ RNA methyltransferase homolog 1 [E. coli]) (eg, X-linked mental retardation 9), full gene sequence

FUS (fused in sarcoma) (eg, amyotrophic lateral sclerosis), full gene sequence

GAA (glucosidase, alpha; acid) (eg, glycogen storage disease type II [Pompe disease]), full gene sequence

GALC (galactosylceramidase) (eg, Krabbe disease), full gene sequence

GALT (galactose-1-phosphate uridylyltransferase) (eg, galactosemia), full gene sequence

GARS (glycyl-tRNA synthetase) (eg, Charcot-Marie-Tooth disease), full gene sequence

GCDH (glutaryl-CoA dehydrogenase) (eg, glutaricacidemia type 1), full gene sequence

GCK (glucokinase [hexokinase 4]) (eg, maturity-onset diabetes of the young [MODY]), full gene sequence

GLUD1 (glutamate dehydrogenase 1) (eg, familial hyperinsulinism), full gene sequence

GNE (glucosamine [UDP-N-acetyl]-2-epimerase/N-acetylmannosamine kinase) (eg, inclusion body myopathy 2 [IBM2], Nonaka myopathy), full gene sequence

GRN (granulin) (eg, frontotemporal dementia), full gene sequence

HADHA (hydroxyacyl-CoA dehydrogenase/3-ketoacyl-CoA thiolase/enoyl-CoA hydratase [trifunctional protein] alpha subunit) (eg, long chain acyl-coenzyme A dehydrogenase deficiency), full gene sequence

HADHB (hydroxyacyl-CoA dehydrogenase/3-ketoacyl-CoA thiolase/enoyl-CoA hydratase [trifunctional protein], beta subunit) (eg, trifunctional protein deficiency), full gene sequence

HEXA (hexosaminidase A, alpha polypeptide) (eg, Tay-Sachs disease), full gene sequence

HLCS (HLCS holocarboxylase synthetase) (eg, holocarboxylase synthetase deficiency), full gene sequence

HMBS (hydroxymethylbilane synthase) (eg, acute intermittent porphyria), full gene sequence

HNF4A (hepatocyte nuclear factor 4, alpha) (eg, maturity-onset diabetes of the young [MODY]), full gene sequence

IDUA (iduronidase, alpha-L-) (eg, mucopolysaccharidosis type I), full gene sequence

INF2 (inverted formin, FH2 and WH2 domain containing) (eg, focal segmental glomerulosclerosis), full gene sequence

IVD (isovaleryl-CoA dehydrogenase) (eg, isovaleric acidemia), full gene sequence

JAG1 (jagged 1) (eg, Alagille syndrome), duplication/deletion analysis

JUP (junction plakoglobin) (eg, arrhythmogenic right ventricular dysplasia/cardiomyopathy 11), full gene sequence

KCNH2 (potassium voltage-gated channel, subfamily H [eag-related], member 2) (eg, short QT syndrome, long QT syndrome), full gene sequence

KCNQ1 (potassium voltage-gated channel, KQT-like subfamily, member 1) (eg, short QT syndrome, long QT syndrome), full gene sequence

KCNQ2 (potassium voltage-gated channel, KQT-like subfamily, member 2) (eg, epileptic encephalopathy), full gene sequence

LDB3 (LIM domain binding 3) (eg, familial dilated cardiomyopathy, myofibrillar myopathy), full gene sequence

LDLR (low density lipoprotein receptor) (eg, familial hypercholesterolemia), full gene sequence

LEPR (leptin receptor(eg, obesity with hypogonadism), full gene sequence

LHCGR (luteinizing hormone/choriogonadotropin receptor) (eg, precocious male puberty), full gene sequence

LMNA (lamin A/C) (eg, Emery-Dreifuss muscular dystrophy [EDMD1, 2 and 3] limb-girdle muscular dystrophy [LGMD] type 1B, dilated cardiomyopathy [CMD1A], familial partial lipodystrophy [FPLD2]), full gene sequence

LRP5 (low density lipoprotein receptor-related protein 5) (eg, osteopetrosis), full gene sequence

MAP2K1 (mitogen-activated protein kinase 1) (eg, cardiofaciocutaneous syndrome), full gene sequence

MAP2K2 (mitogen-activated protein kinase 2) (eg, cardiofaciocutaneous syndrome), full gene sequence

MAPT (microtubule-associated protein tau) (eg, frontotemporal dementia), full gene sequence

MCCC1 (methylcrotonoyl-CoA carboxylase 1 [alpha]) (eg, 3-methylcrotonyl-CoA carboxylase deficiency), full gene sequence

MCCC2 (methylcrotonoyl-CoA carboxylase 2 [beta]) (eg, 3-methylcrotonyl carboxylase deficiency), full gene sequence

MFN2 (mitofusin 2) (eg, Charcot-Marie-Tooth disease), full gene sequence

MTM1 (myotubularin 1) (eg, X-linked centronuclear myopathy), full gene sequence

MUT (methylmalonyl CoA mutase) (eg, methylmalonic acidemia), full gene sequence

MUTYH (mutY homolog [E. coli]) (eg, MYH-associated polyposis), full gene sequence

NDUFS1 (NADH dehydrogenase [ubiquinone] Fe-S protein 1, 75kDa [NADH-coenzyme Q reductase]) (eg, Leigh syndrome, mitochondrial complex I deficiency), full gene sequence

NF2 (neurofibromin 2 [merlin]) (eg, neurofibromatosis, type 2), full gene sequence

NOTCH3 (notch 3) (eg, cerebral autosomal dominant arteriopathy with subcortical infarcts and leukoencephalopathy [CADASIL]), targeted sequence analysis (eg, exons 1-23)

NPC1 (Niemann-Pick disease, type C1) (eg, Niemann-Pick disease), full gene sequence

NPHP1 (nephronophthisis 1 [juvenile]) (eg, Joubert syndrome), full gene sequence

NSD1 (nuclear receptor binding SET domain protein 1) (eg, Sotos syndrome), full gene sequence

OPA1 (optic atrophy 1) (eg, optic atrophy), duplication/deletion analysis

OPTN (optineurin) (eg, amyotrophic lateral sclerosis), full gene sequence

PAFAH1B1 (platelet-activating factor acetylhydrolase 1b, regulatory subunit 1 [45kDa]) (eg, lissencephaly, Miller-Dieker syndrome), full gene sequence

PAH (phenylalanine hydroxylase) (eg, phenylketonuria), full gene sequence

PALB2 (partner and localizer of BRCA2) (eg, breast and pancreatic cancer), full gene sequence

PARK2 (Parkinson protein 2, E3 ubiquitin protein ligase [parkin]) (eg, Parkinson disease), full gene sequence

PAX2 (paired box 2) (eg, renal coloboma syndrome), full gene sequence

PC (pyruvate carboxylase) (eg, pyruvate carboxylase deficiency), full gene sequence

PCCA (propionyl CoA carboxylase, alpha polypeptide) (eg, propionic acidemia, type 1), full gene sequence

PCCB (propionyl CoA carboxylase, beta polypeptide) (eg, propionic acidemia), full gene sequence

PCDH15 (protocadherin-related 15) (eg, Usher syndrome type 1F), duplication/deletion analysis

PCSK9 (proprotein convertase subtilisin/kexin type 9) (eg familial hypercholesterolemia), full gene sequence

PDHA1 (pyruvate dehydrogenase [lipoamide] alpha 1) (eg, lactic acidosis), full gene sequence

PDHX (pyruvate dehydrogenase complex, component X) (eg, lactic acidosis), full gene sequence

PHEX (phosphate-regulating endopeptidase homolog, X-linked) (eg, hypophosphatemic rickets), full gene sequence

PKD2 (polycystic kidney disease 2 [autosomal dominant]) (eg, polycystic kidney disease), full gene sequence

PKP2 (plakophilin 2) (eg, arrhythmogenic right ventricular dysplasia/cardiomyopathy 9), full gene sequence

PNKD (eg, paroxysmal nonkinesigenic dyskinesia), full gene sequence

POLG (polymerase [DNA directed], gamma) (eg, Alpers-Huttenlocher syndrome, autosomal dominant progressive external ophthalmoplegia), full gene sequence

POMGNT1 (protein O-linked mannose beta1, 2-N acetylglucosaminyltransferase) (eg, muscle-eye-brain disease, Walker-Warburg syndrome), full gene sequence

POMT1 (protein-O-mannosyltransferase 1) (eg, limb-girdle muscular dystrophy [LGMD] type 2K, Walker-Warburg syndrome), full gene sequence

POMT2 (protein-O-mannosyltransferase 2) (eg, limb-girdle muscular dystrophy [LGMD] type 2N, Walker-Warburg syndrome), full gene sequence

PPOX (protoporphyrinogen oxidase) (eg, variegate porphyria), full gene sequence

PRKAG2 (protein kinase, AMP-activated, gamma 2 non-catalytic subunit) (eg, familial hypertrophic cardiomyopathy with Wolff-Parkinson-White syndrome, lethal congenital glycogen storage disease of heart), full gene sequence

PRKCG (protein kinase C, gamma) (eg, spinocerebellar ataxia), full gene sequence

PSEN2 (presenilin 2[Alzheimer's disease 4]) (eg, Alzheimer's disease), full gene sequence

PTPN11 (protein tyrosine phosphatase, non-receptor type 11) (eg, Noonan syndrome, LEOPARD syndrome), full gene sequence

PYGM (phosphorylase, glycogen, muscle) (eg, glycogen storage disease type V, McArdle disease), full gene sequence

RAF1 (v-raf-1 murine leukemia viral oncogene homolog 1) (eg, LEOPARD syndrome), full gene sequence

RET (ret proto-oncogene) (eg, Hirschsprung disease), full gene sequence

RPE65 (retinal pigment epithelium-specific protein 65kDa) (eg, retinitis pigmentosa, Leber congenital amaurosis), full gene sequence

RYR1 (ryanodine receptor 1, skeletal) (eg, malignant hyperthermia), targeted sequence analysis of exons with functionally-confirmed mutations

SCN4A (sodium channel, voltage-gated, type IV, alpha subunit) (eg, hyperkalemic periodic paralysis), full gene sequence

SCNN1A (sodium channel, nonvoltage-gated 1 alpha) (eg, pseudohypoaldosteronism), full gene sequence

SCNN1B (sodium channel, nonvoltage-gated 1, beta) (eg, Liddle syndrome, pseudohypoaldosteronism), full gene sequence

SCNN1G (sodium channel, nonvoltage-gated 1, gamma) (eg, Liddle syndrome, pseudohypoaldosteronism), full gene sequence

SDHA (succinate dehydrogenase complex, subunit A, flavoprotein [Fp]) (eg, Leigh syndrome, mitochondrial complex II deficiency), full gene sequence

SETX (senataxin) (eg, ataxia), full gene sequence

SGCE (sarcoglycan, epsilon) (eg, myoclonic dystonia), full gene sequence

SH3TC2 (SH3 domain and tetratricopeptide repeats 2) (eg, Charcot-Marie-Tooth disease), full gene sequence

SLC9A6 (solute carrier family 9 [sodium/hydrogen exchanger], member 6) (eg, Christianson syndrome), full gene sequence

SLC26A4 (solute carrier family 26, member 4) (eg, Pendred syndrome), full gene sequence

SLC37A4 (solute carrier family 37 [glucose-6-phosphate transporter], member 4) (eg, glycogen storage disease type Ib), full gene sequence

SMAD4 (SMAD family member 4) (eg, hemorrhagic telangiectasia syndrome, juvenile polyposis), full gene sequence

SOS1 (son of sevenless homolog 1) (eg, Noonan syndrome, gingival fibromatosis), full gene sequence

SPAST (spastin) (eg, spastic paraplegia), full gene sequence

SPG7 (spastic paraplegia 7 [pure and complicated autosomal recessive]) (eg, spastic paraplegia), full gene sequence

STXBP1 (syntaxin-binding protein 1) (eg, epileptic encephalopathy), full gene sequence

TAZ (tafazzin) (eg, methylglutaconic aciduria type 2, Barth syndrome), full gene sequence

TCF4 (transcription factor 4) (eg, Pitt-Hopkins syndrome), full gene sequence

TH (tyrosine hydroxylase) (eg, Segawa syndrome), full gene sequence

TMEM43 (transmembrane protein 43) (eg, arrhythmogenic right ventricular cardiomyopathy), full gene sequence

TNNT2 (troponin T, type 2 [cardiac]) (eg, familial hypertrophic cardiomyopathy), full gene sequence

TRPC6 (transient receptor potential cation channel, subfamily C, member 6) (eg, focal segmental glomerulosclerosis), full gene sequence

TSC1 (tuberous sclerosis 1) (eg, tuberous sclerosis), full gene sequence

TSC2 (tuberous sclerosis 2) (eg, tuberous sclerosis), duplication/deletion analysis

UBE3A (ubiquitin protein ligase E3A) (eg, Angelman syndrome) full gene sequence

UMOD (uromodulin) (eg, glomerulocystic kidney disease with hyperuricemia and isosthenuria), full gene sequence

VWF (von Willebrand factor) (von Willebrand disease type 2A), extended targeted sequence analysis (eg, exons 11-16, 24-26, 51, 52)

WAS (Wiskott-Aldrich syndrome [eczema-thrombocytopenia]) (eg, Wiskott-Aldrich syndrome), full gene sequence

0.00 0.00 **FUD** XXX A

AMA: 2018,Nov,9; 2018,May,6; 2018,Jan,8; 2017,Apr,9; 2017,Jan,8; 2016,Aug,9; 2016,Jan,13; 2015,Jan,16; 2015,Jan,3; 2014,Jan,11

▲ **81407** **Molecular pathology procedure, Level 8 (eg, analysis of 26-50 exons by DNA sequence analysis, mutation scanning or duplication/deletion variants of >50 exons, sequence analysis of multiple genes on one platform)**

ABCC8 (ATP-binding cassette, sub-family C [CFTR/MRP], member 8) (eg, familial hyperinsulinism), full gene sequence

AGL (amylo-alpha-1, 6-glucosidase, 4-alpha-glucanotransferase) (eg, glycogen storage disease type III), full gene sequence

AHI1 (Abelson helper integration site 1) (eg, Joubert syndrome), full gene sequence

APOB (apolipoprotein B) (eg, familial hypercholesterolemia type B) full gene sequence

ASPM (asp [abnormal spindle] homolog, microcephaly associated [Drosophila]) (eg, primary microcephaly), full gene sequence

CHD7 (chromodomain helicase DNA binding protein 7) (eg, CHARGE syndrome), full gene sequence

COL4A4 (collagen, type IV, alpha 4) (eg, Alport syndrome), full gene sequence

COL4A5 (collagen, type IV, alpha 5) (eg, Alport syndrome), duplication/deletion analysis

COL6A1 (collagen, type VI, alpha 1) (eg, collagen type VI-related disorders), full gene sequence

COL6A2 (collagen, type VI, alpha 2) (eg, collagen type VI-related disorders), full gene sequence

COL6A3 (collagen, type VI, alpha 3) (eg, collagen type VI-related disorders), full gene sequence

CREBBP (CREB binding protein) (eg, Rubinstein-Taybi syndrome), full gene sequence

F8 (coagulation factor VIII) (eg, hemophilia A), full gene sequence

JAG1 (jagged 1) (eg, Alagille syndrome), full gene sequence

KDM5C (lysine [K]-specific demethylase 5C) (eg, X-linked mental retardation), full gene sequence

KIAA0196 (KIAA0196) (eg, spastic paraplegia), full gene sequence

L1CAM (L1 cell adhesion molecule) (eg, MASA syndrome, X-linked hydrocephaly), full gene sequence

LAMB2 (laminin, beta 2 [laminin S]) (eg, Pierson syndrome), full gene sequence

MYBPC3 (myosin binding protein C, cardiac) (eg, familial hypertrophic cardiomyopathy), full gene sequence

MYH6 (myosin, heavy chain 6, cardiac muscle, alpha) (eg, familial dilated cardiomyopathy), full gene sequence

MYH7 (myosin, heavy chain 7, cardiac muscle, beta) (eg, familial hypertrophic cardiomyopathy, Liang distal myopathy), full gene sequence

MYO7A (myosin VIIA) (eg, Usher syndrome, type 1), full gene sequence

NOTCH1 (notch 1) (eg, aortic valve disease), full gene sequence

NPHS1 (nephrosis 1, congenital, Finnish type [nephrin]) (eg, congenital Finnish nephrosis), full gene sequence

OPA1 (optic atrophy 1) (eg, optic atrophy), full gene sequence

PCDH15 (protocadherin-related 15) (eg, Usher syndrome, type 1), full gene sequence

PKD1 (polycystic kidney disease 1 [autosomal dominant]) (eg, polycystic kidney disease), full gene sequence

PLCE1 (phospholipase C, epsilon 1) (eg, nephrotic syndrome type 3), full gene sequence

SCN1A (sodium channel, voltage-gated, type 1, alpha subunit) (eg, generalized epilepsy with febrile seizures), full gene sequence

SCN5A (sodium channel, voltage-gated, type V, alpha subunit) (eg, familial dilated cardiomyopathy), full gene sequence

SLC12A1 (solute carrier family 12 [sodium/potassium/chloride transporters], member 1) (eg, Bartter syndrome), full gene sequence

SLC12A3 (solute carrier family 12 [sodium/chloride transporters], member 3) (eg, Gitelman syndrome), full gene sequence

SPG11 (spastic paraplegia 11 [autosomal recessive]) (eg, spastic paraplegia), full gene sequence

SPTBN2 (spectrin, beta, non-erythrocytic 2) (eg, spinocerebellar ataxia), full gene sequence

TMEM67 (transmembrane protein 67) (eg, Joubert syndrome), full gene sequence

TSC2 (tuberous sclerosis 2) (eg, tuberous sclerosis), full gene sequence

USH1C (Usher syndrome 1C [autosomal recessive, severe]) (eg, Usher syndrome, type 1), full gene sequence

VPS13B (vacuolar protein sorting 13 homolog B [yeast]) (eg, Cohen syndrome), duplication/deletion analysis

WDR62 (WD repeat domain 62) (eg, primary autosomal recessive microcephaly), full gene sequence

0.00 0.00 **FUD** XXX A

AMA: 2019,Jul,3; 2018,Nov,9; 2018,May,6; 2018,Jan,8; 2017,Jan,8; 2016,Aug,9; 2016,Jan,13; 2015,Jan,16; 2015,Jan,3; 2014,Jan,11

81408 **Molecular pathology procedure, Level 9 (eg, analysis of >50 exons in a single gene by DNA sequence analysis)**

ABCA4 (ATP-binding cassette, sub-family A [ABC1], member 4) (eg, Stargardt disease, age-related macular degeneration), full gene sequence

ATM (ataxia telangiectasia mutated) (eg, ataxia telangiectasia), full gene sequence

CDH23 (cadherin-related 23) (eg, Usher syndrome, type 1), full gene sequence

CEP290 (centrosomal protein 290kDa) (eg, Joubert syndrome), full gene sequence

COL1A1 (collagen, type I, alpha 1) (eg, osteogenesis imperfecta, type I), full gene sequence

COL1A2 (collagen, type I, alpha 2) (eg, osteogenesis imperfecta, type I), full gene sequence

COL4A1 (collagen, type IV, alpha 1) (eg, brain small-vessel disease with hemorrhage), full gene sequence

COL4A3 (collagen, type IV, alpha 3 [Goodpasture antigen]) (eg, Alport syndrome), full gene sequence

COL4A5 (collagen, type IV, alpha 5) (eg, Alport syndrome), full gene sequence

DMD (dystrophin) (eg, Duchenne/Becker muscular dystrophy), full gene sequence

DYSF (dysferlin, limb girdle muscular dystrophy 2B [autosomal recessive]) (eg, limb-girdle muscular dystrophy), full gene sequence

FBN1 (fibrillin 1) (eg, Marfan syndrome), full gene sequence

ITPR1 (inositol 1,4,5-trisphosphate receptor, type 1) (eg, spinocerebellar ataxia), full gene sequence

LAMA2 (laminin, alpha 2) (eg, congenital muscular dystrophy), full gene sequence

LRRK2 (leucine-rich repeat kinase 2) (eg, Parkinson disease), full gene sequence

MYH11 (myosin, heavy chain 11, smooth muscle) (eg, thoracic aortic aneurysms and aortic dissections), full gene sequence

NEB (nebulin) (eg, nemaline myopathy 2), full gene sequence

NF1 (neurofibromin 1) (eg, neurofibromatosis, type 1), full gene sequence

PKHD1 (polycystic kidney and hepatic disease 1) (eg, autosomal recessive polycystic kidney disease), full gene sequence

RYR1 (ryanodine receptor 1, skeletal) (eg, malignant hyperthermia), full gene sequence

RYR2 (ryanodine receptor 2 [cardiac]) (eg, catecholaminergic polymorphic ventricular tachycardia, arrhythmogenic right ventricular dysplasia), full gene sequence or targeted sequence analysis of > 50 exons

USH2A (Usher syndrome 2A [autosomal recessive, mild]) (eg, Usher syndrome, type 2), full gene sequence

VPS13B (vacuolar protein sorting 13 homolog B [yeast]) (eg, Cohen syndrome), full gene sequence

VWF (von Willebrand factor) (eg, von Willebrand disease types 1 and 3), full gene sequence

0.00 0.00 **FUD** XXX A

AMA: 2018,Nov,9; 2018,May,6; 2018,Jan,8; 2017,Jan,8; 2016,Aug,9; 2016,Jan,13; 2015,Jan,16; 2015,Jan,3; 2014,Jan,11

\# **81479** **Unlisted molecular pathology procedure**

0.00 0.00 **FUD** XXX A

AMA: 2019,Jun,11; 2019,May,5; 2018,Dec,10; 2018,Dec,10; 2018,Nov,9; 2018,Sep,14; 2018,Jun,8; 2018,May,6; 2018,Jan,8; 2017,Apr,9; 2017,Jan,8; 2016,Sep,9; 2016,Aug,9; 2016,Apr,4; 2016,Jan,13; 2015,Jan,3; 2015,Jan,16; 2014,Jan,11

81410-81479 [81443, 81448] Genomic Sequencing

EXCLUDES *In situ hybridization analyses (88271-88275, 88365-88368 [88364, 88373, 88374])*

Microbial identification (87149-87153, 87471-87801 [87623, 87624, 87625], 87900-87904 [87906, 87910, 87912])

81410 **Aortic dysfunction or dilation (eg, Marfan syndrome, Loeys Dietz syndrome, Ehler Danlos syndrome type IV, arterial tortuosity syndrome); genomic sequence analysis panel, must include sequencing of at least 9 genes, including *FBN1, TGFBR1, TGFBR2, COL3A1, MYH11, ACTA2, SLC2A10, SMAD3,* and *MYLK***

0.00 0.00 **FUD** XXX A

AMA: 2018,Jan,8; 2017,Jan,8; 2016,Jan,13; 2015,Jan,3

81411 **duplication/deletion analysis panel, must include analyses for *TGFBR1, TGFBR2, MYH11, and COL3A1***

0.00 0.00 **FUD** XXX A

AMA: 2018,Jan,8; 2017,Jan,8; 2016,Jan,13; 2015,Jan,3

81412 **Ashkenazi Jewish associated disorders (eg, Bloom syndrome, Canavan disease, cystic fibrosis, familial dysautonomia, Fanconi anemia group C, Gaucher disease, Tay-Sachs disease), genomic sequence analysis panel, must include sequencing of at least 9 genes, including *ASPA, BLM, CFTR, FANCC, GBA, HEXA, IKBKAP, MCOLN1,* and *SMPD1***

0.00 0.00 **FUD** XXX A

AMA: 2018,Nov,9; 2018,Jan,8; 2017,Jan,8; 2016,Apr,4

81413 **Cardiac ion channelopathies (eg, Brugada syndrome, long QT syndrome, short QT syndrome, catecholaminergic polymorphic ventricular tachycardia); genomic sequence analysis panel, must include sequencing of at least 10 genes, including ANK2, CASQ2, CAV3, KCNE1, KCNE2, KCNH2, KCNJ2, KCNQ1, RYR2, and SCN5A**

EXCLUDES *Evaluation of cardiomyopathy (81439)*

0.00 0.00 **FUD** XXX A

AMA: 2018,Jan,8; 2017,Apr,3

81414 **duplication/deletion gene analysis panel, must include analysis of at least 2 genes, including KCNH2 and KCNQ1**

EXCLUDES *Evaluation of cardiomyopathy (81439)*

0.00 0.00 **FUD** XXX A

AMA: 2018,Jan,8; 2017,Apr,3

81415 **Exome (eg, unexplained constitutional or heritable disorder or syndrome); sequence analysis**

0.00 0.00 **FUD** XXX A

AMA: 2018,Jan,8; 2017,Jan,8; 2016,Jan,13; 2015,Jan,3

\+ **81416** **sequence analysis, each comparator exome (eg, parents, siblings) (List separately in addition to code for primary procedure)**

Code first (81415)

0.00 0.00 **FUD** XXX A

AMA: 2018,Jan,8; 2017,Jan,8; 2016,Jan,13; 2015,Jan,3

81417 **re-evaluation of previously obtained exome sequence (eg, updated knowledge or unrelated condition/syndrome)**

EXCLUDES *Microarray assessment (81228-81229)*

Results that are incidental

0.00 0.00 **FUD** XXX A

AMA: 2018,Jan,8; 2017,Jan,8; 2016,Jan,13; 2015,Jan,3

81420 **Fetal chromosomal aneuploidy (eg, trisomy 21, monosomy X) genomic sequence analysis panel, circulating cell-free fetal DNA in maternal blood, must include analysis of chromosomes 13, 18, and 21** M

EXCLUDES *Genome-wide microarray analysis (81228-81229)*

Molecular cytogenetics (88271)

0.00 0.00 **FUD** XXX A

AMA: 2018,Apr,10; 2018,Jan,8; 2017,Jan,8; 2016,Jan,13; 2015,Dec,18; 2015,Jan,3

81422 **Fetal chromosomal microdeletion(s) genomic sequence analysis (eg, DiGeorge syndrome, Cri-du-chat syndrome), circulating cell-free fetal DNA in maternal blood**

EXCLUDES *Genome-wide microarray analysis (81228-81229)*

Molecular cytogenetics (88271)

0.00 0.00 **FUD** XXX A

AMA: 2018,Jan,8; 2017,Apr,3

\# **81443** **Genetic testing for severe inherited conditions (eg, cystic fibrosis, Ashkenazi Jewish-associated disorders [eg, Bloom syndrome, Canavan disease, Fanconi anemia type C, mucolipidosis type VI, Gaucher disease, Tay-Sachs disease], beta hemoglobinopathies, phenylketonuria, galactosemia), genomic sequence analysis panel, must include sequencing of at least 15 genes (eg, *ACADM, ARSA, ASPA, ATP7B, BCKDHA, BCKDHB, BLM, CFTR, DHCR7, FANCC, G6PC, GAA, GALT, GBA, GBE1, HBB, HEXA, IKBKAP, MCOLN1, PAH*)**

0.00 0.00 **FUD** XXX

AMA: 2019,Jul,3; 2018,Nov,9

81425 **Genome (eg, unexplained constitutional or heritable disorder or syndrome); sequence analysis**
0.00 0.00 FUD XXX A
AMA: 2018,Jan,8; 2017,Jan,8; 2016,Jan,13; 2015,Jan,3

\+ 81426 **sequence analysis, each comparator genome (eg, parents, siblings) (List separately in addition to code for primary procedure)**
Code first (81425)
0.00 0.00 FUD XXX A
AMA: 2018,Jan,8; 2017,Jan,8; 2016,Jan,13; 2015,Jan,3

81427 **re-evaluation of previously obtained genome sequence (eg, updated knowledge or unrelated condition/syndrome)**
EXCLUDES *Genome-wide microarray analysis (81228-81229)*
Results that are incidental
0.00 0.00 FUD XXX A
AMA: 2018,Jan,8; 2017,Jan,8; 2016,Jan,13; 2015,Jan,3

81430 **Hearing loss (eg, nonsyndromic hearing loss, Usher syndrome, Pendred syndrome); genomic sequence analysis panel, must include sequencing of at least 60 genes, including *CDH23, CLRN1, GJB2, GPR98, MTRNR1, MYO7A, MYO15A, PCDH15, OTOF, SLC26A4, TMC1, TMPRSS3, USH1C, USH1G, USH2A*, and *WFS1***
0.00 0.00 FUD XXX A
AMA: 2018,Jan,8; 2017,Jan,8; 2016,Jan,13; 2015,Jan,3

81431 **duplication/deletion analysis panel, must include copy number analyses for *STRC* and *DFNB1* deletions in *GJB2* and *GJB6* genes**
0.00 0.00 FUD XXX A
AMA: 2018,Jan,8; 2017,Jan,8; 2016,Jan,13; 2015,Jan,3

81432 **Hereditary breast cancer-related disorders (eg, hereditary breast cancer, hereditary ovarian cancer, hereditary endometrial cancer); genomic sequence analysis panel, must include sequencing of at least 10 genes, always including *BRCA1, BRCA2, CDH1, MLH1, MSH2, MSH6, PALB2, PTEN, STK11, and TP53***
0.00 0.00 FUD XXX A
AMA: 2019,May,5; 2018,Jan,8; 2017,Jan,8; 2016,Apr,4

81433 **duplication/deletion analysis panel, must include analyses for *BRCA1, BRCA2, MLH1, MSH2*, and *STK11***
0.00 0.00 FUD XXX A
AMA: 2018,Jan,8; 2017,Jan,8; 2016,Apr,4

81434 **Hereditary retinal disorders (eg, retinitis pigmentosa, Leber congenital amaurosis, cone-rod dystrophy), genomic sequence analysis panel, must include sequencing of at least 15 genes, including *ABCA4, CNGA1, CRB1, EYS, PDE6A, PDE6B, PRPF31, PRPH2, RDH12, RHO, RP1, RP2, RPE65, RPGR*, and *USH2A***
0.00 0.00 FUD XXX A
AMA: 2018,Jan,8; 2017,Jan,8; 2016,Apr,4

81435 **Hereditary colon cancer disorders (eg, Lynch syndrome, PTEN hamartoma syndrome, Cowden syndrome, familial adenomatosis polyposis); genomic sequence analysis panel, must include sequencing of at least 10 genes, including *APC, BMPR1A, CDH1, MLH1, MSH2, MSH6, MUTYH, PTEN, SMAD4*, and *STK11***
0.00 0.00 FUD XXX A
AMA: 2018,Jan,8; 2017,Jan,8; 2016,Apr,4; 2016,Jan,13; 2015,Jan,3

81436 **duplication/deletion analysis panel, must include analysis of at least 5 genes, including *MLH1, MSH2, EPCAM, SMAD4*, and *STK11***
0.00 0.00 FUD XXX A
AMA: 2018,Jan,8; 2017,Jan,8; 2016,Apr,4; 2016,Jan,13; 2015,Jan,3

81437 **Hereditary neuroendocrine tumor disorders (eg, medullary thyroid carcinoma, parathyroid carcinoma, malignant pheochromocytoma or paraganglioma); genomic sequence analysis panel, must include sequencing of at least 6 genes, including *MAX, SDHB, SDHC, SDHD, TMEM127*, and *VHL***
0.00 0.00 FUD XXX A
AMA: 2018,Jan,8; 2017,Jan,8; 2016,Apr,4

81438 **duplication/deletion analysis panel, must include analyses for *SDHB, SDHC, SDHD*, and *VHL***
0.00 0.00 FUD XXX A
AMA: 2018,Jan,8; 2017,Jan,8; 2016,Apr,4

\# 81448 **Hereditary peripheral neuropathies (eg, Charcot-Marie-Tooth, spastic paraplegia), genomic sequence analysis panel, must include sequencing of at least 5 peripheral neuropathy-related genes (eg, *BSCL2, GJB1, MFN2, MPZ, REEP1, SPAST, SPG11, SPTLC1*)**
0.00 0.00 FUD XXX A
AMA: 2018,May,6

81439 **Hereditary cardiomyopathy (eg, hypertrophic cardiomyopathy, dilated cardiomyopathy, arrhythmogenic right ventricular cardiomyopathy), genomic sequence analysis panel, must include sequencing of at least 5 cardiomyopathy-related genes (eg, *DSG2, MYBPC3, MYH7, PKP2, TTN*)**
EXCLUDES *Genetic tests of cardiac ion channelopathies (81413-81414)*
0.00 0.00 FUD XXX A
AMA: 2018,Sep,14; 2018,Jan,8; 2017,Apr,3

81440 **Nuclear encoded mitochondrial genes (eg, neurologic or myopathic phenotypes), genomic sequence panel, must include analysis of at least 100 genes, including *BCS1L, C10orf2, COQ2, COX10, DGUOK, MPV17, OPA1, PDSS2, POLG, POLG2, RRM2B, SCO1, SCO2, SLC25A4, SUCLA2, SUCLG1, TAZ, TK2*, and *TYMP***
0.00 0.00 FUD XXX A
AMA: 2018,Jan,8; 2017,Jan,8; 2016,Jan,13; 2015,Jan,3

81442 **Noonan spectrum disorders (eg, Noonan syndrome, cardio-facio-cutaneous syndrome, Costello syndrome, LEOPARD syndrome, Noonan-like syndrome), genomic sequence analysis panel, must include sequencing of at least 12 genes, including *BRAF, CBL, HRAS, KRAS, MAP2K1, MAP2K2, NRAS, PTPN11, RAF1, RIT1, SHOC2*, and *SOS1***
0.00 0.00 FUD XXX A
AMA: 2018,Jan,8; 2017,Jan,8; 2016,Apr,4

81443 **Resequenced code. See code following 81422.**

81445 **Targeted genomic sequence analysis panel, solid organ neoplasm, DNA analysis, and RNA analysis when performed, 5-50 genes (eg, *ALK, BRAF, CDKN2A, EGFR, ERBB2, KIT, KRAS, NRAS, MET, PDGFRA, PDGFRB, PGR, PIK3CA, PTEN, RET*), interrogation for sequence variants and copy number variants or rearrangements, if performed**
EXCLUDES *Microarray copy number assessment (81406)*
0.00 0.00 FUD XXX A
AMA: 2018,Jan,8; 2017,Jan,8; 2016,Apr,4; 2016,Jan,13; 2015,Jan,3

81448 **Resequenced code. See code following 81438.**

81450 **Targeted genomic sequence analysis panel, hematolymphoid neoplasm or disorder, DNA analysis, and RNA analysis when performed, 5-50 genes (eg, *BRAF, CEBPA, DNMT3A, EZH2, FLT3, IDH1, IDH2, JAK2, KRAS, KIT, MLL, NRAS, NPM1, NOTCH1*), interrogation for sequence variants, and copy number variants or rearrangements, or isoform expression or mRNA expression levels, if performed**
EXCLUDES *Microarray copy number assessment (81406)*
0.00 0.00 FUD XXX A
AMA: 2018,Jan,8; 2017,Jan,8; 2016,Apr,4; 2016,Jan,13; 2015,Jan,3

81455 Targeted genomic sequence analysis panel, solid organ or hematolymphoid neoplasm, DNA analysis, and RNA analysis when performed, 51 or greater genes (eg, *ALK, BRAF, CDKN2A, CEBPA, DNMT3A, EGFR, ERBB2, EZH2, FLT3, IDH1, IDH2, JAK2, KIT, KRAS, MLL, NPM1, NRAS, MET, NOTCH1, PDGFRA, PDGFRB, PGR, PIK3CA, PTEN, RET*), interrogation for sequence variants and copy number variants or rearrangements, if performed

EXCLUDES *Microarray copy number assessment (81406)*

0.00 0.00 FUD XXX A

AMA: 2018,Jan,8; 2017,Jan,8; 2016,Apr,4; 2016,Jan,13; 2015,Jan,3

81460 Whole mitochondrial genome (eg, Leigh syndrome, mitochondrial encephalomyopathy, lactic acidosis, and stroke-like episodes [MELAS], myoclonic epilepsy with ragged-red fibers [MERFF], neuropathy, ataxia, and retinitis pigmentosa [NARP], Leber hereditary optic neuropathy [LHON]), genomic sequence, must include sequence analysis of entire mitochondrial genome with heteroplasmy detection

0.00 0.00 FUD XXX A

AMA: 2018,Jan,8; 2017,Jan,8; 2016,Jan,13; 2015,Jan,3

81465 Whole mitochondrial genome large deletion analysis panel (eg, Kearns-Sayre syndrome, chronic progressive external ophthalmoplegia), including heteroplasmy detection, if performed

0.00 0.00 FUD XXX A

AMA: 2018,Jan,8; 2017,Jan,8; 2016,Jan,13; 2015,Jan,3

81470 X-linked intellectual disability (XLID) (eg, syndromic and non-syndromic XLID); genomic sequence analysis panel, must include sequencing of at least 60 genes, including *ARX, ATRX, CDKL5, FGD1, FMR1, HUWE1, IL1RAPL, KDM5C, L1CAM, MECP2, MED12, MID1, OCRL, RPS6KA3,* and *SLC16A2*

0.00 0.00 FUD XXX A

AMA: 2018,Jan,8; 2017,Jan,8; 2016,Jan,13; 2015,Jan,3

81471 duplication/deletion gene analysis, must include analysis of at least 60 genes, including *ARX, ATRX, CDKL5, FGD1, FMR1, HUWE1, IL1RAPL, KDM5C, L1CAM, MECP2, MED12, MID1, OCRL, RPS6KA3,* and *SLC16A2*

0.00 0.00 FUD XXX A

AMA: 2018,Jan,8; 2017,Jan,8; 2016,Jan,13; 2015,Jan,3

81479 **Resequenced code. See code following 81408.**

81490-81599 [81522] Multianalyte Assays

INCLUDES Procedures using results of multiple assay panels (eg, molecular pathology, fluorescent in situ hybridization, non-nucleic acid-based) and other patient information to perform algorithmic analysis
Required analytical services (eg, amplification, cell lysis, detection, digestion, extraction, hybridization, nucleic acid stabilization) and algorithmic analysis

EXCLUDES *Genomic resequencing tests (81410-81471 [81448])*
In situ hybridization analyses (88271-88275, 88365-88368 [88364, 88373, 88374])
Microbial identification (87149-87153, 87471-87801 [87623, 87624, 87625], 87900-87904 [87906, 87910, 87912])
Multianalyte assays with algorithmic analyses without a Category I code (0002M-0007M, 0011M-0013M)

Code also procedures performed prior to cell lysis (eg, microdissection) (88380-88381)

81490 Autoimmune (rheumatoid arthritis), analysis of 12 biomarkers using immunoassays, utilizing serum, prognostic algorithm reported as a disease activity score

0.00 0.00 FUD XXX Q

EXCLUDES *C-reactive protein (86140)*

81493 Coronary artery disease, mRNA, gene expression profiling by real-time RT-PCR of 23 genes, utilizing whole peripheral blood, algorithm reported as a risk score

0.00 0.00 FUD XXX A

81500 Oncology (ovarian), biochemical assays of two proteins (CA-125 and HE4), utilizing serum, with menopausal status, algorithm reported as a risk score ♀

EXCLUDES *Human epididymis protein 4 (HE4) (86305)*
Immunoassay for tumor antigen, quantitative; CA 125 (86304)

0.00 0.00 FUD XXX E

AMA: 2019,Jun,11; 2015,Jan,3; 2014,Jan,11

81503 Oncology (ovarian), biochemical assays of five proteins (CA-125, apolipoprotein A1, beta-2 microglobulin, transferrin, and pre-albumin), utilizing serum, algorithm reported as a risk score ♀

EXCLUDES *Apolipoprotein (82172)*
Beta-2 microglobulin (82232)
Immunoassay for tumor antigen, quantitative; CA 125 (86304)
Prealbumin (84134)
Transferrin (84466)

0.00 0.00 FUD XXX Q

AMA: 2019,Jun,11; 2015,Jan,3; 2014,Jan,11

81504 Oncology (tissue of origin), microarray gene expression profiling of > 2000 genes, utilizing formalin-fixed paraffin-embedded tissue, algorithm reported as tissue similarity scores

0.00 0.00 FUD XXX A

AMA: 2019,Jun,11; 2015,Jan,3; 2014,Jan,11

81506 Endocrinology (type 2 diabetes), biochemical assays of seven analytes (glucose, HbA1c, insulin, hs-CRP, adiponectin, ferritin, interleukin 2-receptor alpha), utilizing serum or plasma, algorithm reporting a risk score

EXCLUDES *C-reactive protein; high sensitivity (hsCRP) (86141)*
Ferritin (82728)
Glucose (82947)
Hemoglobin; glycosylated (A1C) (83036)
Immunoassay for analyte other than infectious agent antibody or infectious agent antigen (83520)
Insulin; total (83525)
Unlisted chemistry procedure (84999)

0.00 0.00 FUD XXX E

AMA: 2019,Jun,11; 2015,Jan,3; 2014,Jan,11

81507 Fetal aneuploidy (trisomy 21, 18, and 13) DNA sequence analysis of selected regions using maternal plasma, algorithm reported as a risk score for each trisomy ♀

EXCLUDES *Genome-wide microarray analysis (81228-81229)*
Molecular cytogenetics (88271)

0.00 0.00 FUD XXX A

AMA: 2019,Jun,11; 2018,Apr,10; 2015,Jan,3; 2014,Jan,11

81508 Fetal congenital abnormalities, biochemical assays of two proteins (PAPP-A, hCG [any form]), utilizing maternal serum, algorithm reported as a risk score ♀

EXCLUDES *Gonadotropin, chorionic (hCG) (84702)*
Pregnancy-associated plasma protein-A (PAPP-A) (84163)

0.00 0.00 FUD XXX E

AMA: 2019,Jun,11; 2015,Jan,3; 2014,Jan,11

81509 Fetal congenital abnormalities, biochemical assays of three proteins (PAPP-A, hCG [any form], DIA), utilizing maternal serum, algorithm reported as a risk score ♀

EXCLUDES *Gonadotropin, chorionic (hCG) (84702)*
Inhibin A (86336)
Pregnancy-associated plasma protein-A (PAPP-A) (84163)

0.00 0.00 FUD XXX E

AMA: 2019,Jun,11; 2015,Jan,3; 2014,Jan,11

81510 **Fetal congenital abnormalities, biochemical assays of three analytes (AFP, uE3, hCG [any form]), utilizing maternal serum, algorithm reported as a risk score** ♀

EXCLUDES *Alpha-fetoprotein (AFP) (82105)*
Estriol (82677)
Gonadotropin, chorionic (hCG) (84702)

0.00 0.00 FUD XXX E

AMA: 2019,Jun,11; 2015,Jan,3; 2014,Jan,11

81511 **Fetal congenital abnormalities, biochemical assays of four analytes (AFP, uE3, hCG [any form], DIA) utilizing maternal serum, algorithm reported as a risk score (may include additional results from previous biochemical testing)** ♀

EXCLUDES *Alpha-fetoprotein (AFP) (82105)*
Estriol (82677)
Gonadotropin, chorionic (hCG) (84702)
Inhibin A (86336)

0.00 0.00 FUD XXX E

AMA: 2019,Jun,11; 2015,Jan,3; 2014,Jan,11

81512 **Fetal congenital abnormalities, biochemical assays of five analytes (AFP, uE3, total hCG, hyperglycosylated hCG, DIA) utilizing maternal serum, algorithm reported as a risk score** ♀

EXCLUDES *Alpha-fetoprotein (AFP) (82105)*
Estriol (82677)
Gonadotropin, chorionic (hCG) (84702)
Inhibin A (86336)

0.00 0.00 FUD XXX E

AMA: 2019,Jun,11; 2015,Jan,3; 2014,Jan,11

81518 **Oncology (breast), mRNA, gene expression profiling by real-time RT-PCR of 11 genes (7 content and 4 housekeeping), utilizing formalin-fixed paraffin-embedded tissue, algorithms reported as percentage risk for metastatic recurrence and likelihood of benefit from extended endocrine therapy**

0.00 0.00 FUD XXX

AMA: 2019,Jun,11; 2019,Jul,3

● # **81522** **Oncology (breast), mRNA, gene expression profiling by RT-PCR of 12 genes (8 content and 4 housekeeping), utilizing formalin-fixed paraffin-embedded tissue, algorithm reported as recurrence risk score**

0.00 0.00 FUD 000

81519 **Oncology (breast), mRNA, gene expression profiling by real-time RT-PCR of 21 genes, utilizing formalin-fixed paraffin embedded tissue, algorithm reported as recurrence score**

0.00 0.00 FUD XXX A

AMA: 2019,Jun,11; 2018,Jan,8; 2017,Jan,8; 2016,Jan,13; 2015,Jan,3

81520 **Oncology (breast), mRNA gene expression profiling by hybrid capture of 58 genes (50 content and 8 housekeeping), utilizing formalin-fixed paraffin-embedded tissue, algorithm reported as a recurrence risk score**

0.00 0.00 FUD XXX A

AMA: 2019,Jun,11; 2018,Jun,8

81521 **Oncology (breast), mRNA, microarray gene expression profiling of 70 content genes and 465 housekeeping genes, utilizing fresh frozen or formalin-fixed paraffin-embedded tissue, algorithm reported as index related to risk of distant metastasis**

0.00 0.00 FUD XXX A

AMA: 2019,Jun,11; 2018,Jun,8

81522 **Resequenced code. See code following 81518.**

81525 **Oncology (colon), mRNA, gene expression profiling by real-time RT-PCR of 12 genes (7 content and 5 housekeeping), utilizing formalin-fixed paraffin-embedded tissue, algorithm reported as a recurrence score**

0.00 0.00 FUD XXX A

AMA: 2019,Jun,11

81528 **Oncology (colorectal) screening, quantitative real-time target and signal amplification of 10 DNA markers (*KRAS* mutations, promoter methylation of *NDRG4* and *BMP3*) and fecal hemoglobin, utilizing stool, algorithm reported as a positive or negative result**

EXCLUDES *Blood, occult, by fecal hemoglobin (82274)*
KRAS (Kirsten rat sarcoma viral oncogene homolog) (81275)

0.00 0.00 FUD XXX A

AMA: 2019,Jun,11

81535 **Oncology (gynecologic), live tumor cell culture and chemotherapeutic response by DAPI stain and morphology, predictive algorithm reported as a drug response score; first single drug or drug combination**

0.00 0.00 FUD XXX Q

AMA: 2019,Jun,11

\+ **81536** **each additional single drug or drug combination (List separately in addition to code for primary procedure)**

Code first (81535)

0.00 0.00 FUD XXX Q

AMA: 2019,Jun,11

81538 **Oncology (lung), mass spectrometric 8-protein signature, including amyloid A, utilizing serum, prognostic and predictive algorithm reported as good versus poor overall survival**

0.00 0.00 FUD XXX Q

AMA: 2019,Jun,11

81539 **Oncology (high-grade prostate cancer), biochemical assay of four proteins (Total PSA, Free PSA, Intact PSA, and human kallikrein-2 [hK2]), utilizing plasma or serum, prognostic algorithm reported as a probability score** ♂

0.00 0.00 FUD XXX Q

AMA: 2019,Jun,11; 2018,Jan,8; 2017,Apr,3

81540 **Oncology (tumor of unknown origin), mRNA, gene expression profiling by real-time RT-PCR of 92 genes (87 content and 5 housekeeping) to classify tumor into main cancer type and subtype, utilizing formalin-fixed paraffin-embedded tissue, algorithm reported as a probability of a predicted main cancer type and subtype**

0.00 0.00 FUD XXX A

AMA: 2019,Jun,11

81541 **Oncology (prostate), mRNA gene expression profiling by real-time RT-PCR of 46 genes (31 content and 15 housekeeping), utilizing formalin-fixed paraffin-embedded tissue, algorithm reported as a disease-specific mortality risk score**

0.00 0.00 FUD XXX A

AMA: 2019,Jun,11; 2018,Aug,8

● **81542** **Oncology (prostate), mRNA, microarray gene expression profiling of 22 content genes, utilizing formalin-fixed paraffin-embedded tissue, algorithm reported as metastasis risk score**

81545 **Oncology (thyroid), gene expression analysis of 142 genes, utilizing fine needle aspirate, algorithm reported as a categorical result (eg, benign or suspicious)**

0.00 0.00 FUD XXX A

AMA: 2019,Jun,11

81551 **Oncology (prostate), promoter methylation profiling by real-time PCR of 3 genes (*GSTP1, APC, RASSF1*), utilizing formalin-fixed paraffin-embedded tissue, algorithm reported as a likelihood of prostate cancer detection on repeat biopsy**

0.00 0.00 FUD XXX A

AMA: 2019,Jun,11; 2018,Aug,8

Pathology and Laboratory

81510 — 81551

● New Code ▲ Revised Code ○ Reinstated ● New Web Release ▲ Revised Web Release + Add-on Unlisted Not Covered # Resequenced
⑩ Optum Mod 50 Exempt ⊘ AMA Mod 51 Exempt ⑤ Optum Mod 51 Exempt ⑥ Mod 63 Exempt ✗ Non-FDA Drug ★ Telemedicine M Maternity A Age Edit

● **81552** **Oncology (uveal melanoma), mRNA, gene expression profiling by real-time RT-PCR of 15 genes (12 content and 3 housekeeping), utilizing fine needle aspirate or formalin-fixed paraffin-embedded tissue, algorithm reported as risk of metastasis**

81595 **Cardiology (heart transplant), mRNA, gene expression profiling by real-time quantitative PCR of 20 genes (11 content and 9 housekeeping), utilizing subfraction of peripheral blood, algorithm reported as a rejection risk score**
0.00 0.00 FUD XXX
AMA: 2019,Jun,11

81596 **Infectious disease, chronic hepatitis C virus (HCV) infection, six biochemical assays (ALT, A2-macroglobulin, apolipoprotein A-1, total bilirubin, GGT, and haptoglobin) utilizing serum, prognostic algorithm reported as scores for fibrosis and necroinflammatory activity in liver**
0.00 0.00 FUD XXX
AMA: 2019,Jun,11; 2019,Jul,3

81599 **Unlisted multianalyte assay with algorithmic analysis**
0.00 0.00 FUD XXX
AMA: 2019,Jun,11; 2018,Jun,8; 2018,Apr,10; 2015,Jan,3; 2014,Jan,11

82009-82030 Chemistry: Acetaldehyde—Adenosine

INCLUDES Clinical information not requested by the ordering physician
Mathematically calculated results
Quantitative analysis unless otherwise specified
Specimens from any source unless otherwise specified

EXCLUDES *Analytes from nonrequested laboratory analysis*
Calculated results that represent a score or probability that was derived by algorithm
Drug testing ([80305, 80306, 80307], [80324, 80325, 80326, 80327, 80328, 80329, 80330, 80331, 80332, 80333, 80334, 80335, 80336, 80337, 80338, 80339, 80340, 80341, 80342, 80343, 80344, 80345, 80346, 80347, 80348, 80349, 80350, 80351, 80352, 80353, 80354, 80355, 80356, 80357, 80358, 80359, 80360, 80361, 80362, 80363, 80364, 80365, 80366, 80367, 80368, 80369, 80370, 80371, 80372, 80373, 80374, 80375, 80376, 80377, 83992])
Organ or disease panels (80048-80076 [80081])
Therapeutic drug assays (80150-80299 [80164, 80165, 80171])

82009 **Ketone body(s) (eg, acetone, acetoacetic acid, beta-hydroxybutyrate); qualitative**
0.00 0.00 FUD XXX
AMA: 2018,Jan,8; 2017,Jan,8; 2016,Jan,13; 2015,Jun,10; 2015,Apr,3; 2015,Jan,16; 2014,Jan,11

82010 **quantitative**
0.00 0.00 FUD XXX
AMA: 2018,Jan,8; 2017,Jan,8; 2016,Jan,13; 2015,Jun,10; 2015,Apr,3; 2015,Jan,16; 2014,Jan,11

82013 **Acetylcholinesterase**
EXCLUDES *Acid phosphatase (84060-84066)*
Gastric acid analysis (82930)
0.00 0.00 FUD XXX
AMA: 2015,Jun,10; 2015,Apr,3; 2014,Jan,11

82016 **Acylcarnitines; qualitative, each specimen**
0.00 0.00 FUD XXX
AMA: 2015,Jun,10; 2015,Apr,3; 2014,Jan,11

82017 **quantitative, each specimen**
EXCLUDES *Carnitine (82379)*
0.00 0.00 FUD XXX
AMA: 2015,Jun,10; 2015,Apr,3; 2014,Jan,11

82024 **Adrenocorticotropic hormone (ACTH)**
0.00 0.00 FUD XXX
AMA: 2015,Jun,10; 2015,Apr,3; 2014,Jan,11

82030 **Adenosine, 5-monophosphate, cyclic (cyclic AMP)**
0.00 0.00 FUD XXX
AMA: 2015,Jun,10; 2015,Apr,3; 2014,Jan,11

82040-82045 [82042] Chemistry: Albumin

INCLUDES Clinical information not requested by the ordering physician
Mathematically calculated results
Quantitative analysis unless otherwise specified
Specimens from any other sources unless otherwise specified

EXCLUDES *Analytes from nonrequested laboratory analysis*
Calculated results that represent a score or probability that was derived by algorithm
Drug testing ([80305, 80306, 80307], [80324, 80325, 80326, 80327, 80328, 80329, 80330, 80331, 80332, 80333, 80334, 80335, 80336, 80337, 80338, 80339, 80340, 80341, 80342, 80343, 80344, 80345, 80346, 80347, 80348, 80349, 80350, 80351, 80352, 80353, 80354, 80355, 80356, 80357, 80358, 80359, 80360, 80361, 80362, 80363, 80364, 80365, 80366, 80367, 80368, 80369, 80370, 80371, 80372, 80373, 80374, 80375, 80376, 80377, 83992])
Organ or disease panels (80048-80076 [80081])
Therapeutic drug assays (80150-80299 [80164, 80165, 80171])

82040 **Albumin; serum, plasma or whole blood**
0.00 0.00 FUD XXX
AMA: 2018,Jan,8; 2017,Jan,8; 2016,Jan,13; 2015,Jun,10; 2015,Apr,3; 2015,Jan,16; 2014,Jan,11

82042 **Resequenced code. See code following 82045.**

82043 **urine (eg, microalbumin), quantitative**
0.00 0.00 FUD XXX
AMA: 2018,Jan,8; 2017,Jan,8; 2016,Jan,13; 2015,Jun,10; 2015,Apr,3; 2015,Jan,16; 2014,Jan,11

82044 **urine (eg, microalbumin), semiquantitative (eg, reagent strip assay)**
EXCLUDES *Prealbumin (84134)*
0.00 0.00 FUD XXX
AMA: 2018,Jan,8; 2017,Jan,8; 2016,Jan,13; 2015,Jun,10; 2015,Apr,3; 2015,Jan,16; 2014,Jan,11

82045 **ischemia modified**
0.00 0.00 FUD XXX
AMA: 2015,Jun,10; 2015,Apr,3

\# **82042** **other source, quantitative, each specimen**
EXCLUDES *Total protein (84155-84157, 84160)*
0.00 0.00 FUD XXX
AMA: 2015,Jun,10; 2015,Apr,3; 2014,Jan,11

82075-82107 Chemistry: Alcohol—Alpha-fetoprotein (AFP)

INCLUDES Clinical information not requested by the ordering physician
Mathematically calculated results
Quantitative analysis unless otherwise specified
Specimens from any source unless otherwise specified

EXCLUDES *Analytes from nonrequested laboratory analysis*
Calculated results that represent a score or probability that was derived by algorithm
Drug testing ([80305, 80306, 80307], [80324, 80325, 80326, 80327, 80328, 80329, 80330, 80331, 80332, 80333, 80334, 80335, 80336, 80337, 80338, 80339, 80340, 80341, 80342, 80343, 80344, 80345, 80346, 80347, 80348, 80349, 80350, 80351, 80352, 80353, 80354, 80355, 80356, 80357, 80358, 80359, 80360, 80361, 80362, 80363, 80364, 80365, 80366, 80367, 80368, 80369, 80370, 80371, 80372, 80373, 80374, 80375, 80376, 80377, 83992])
Organ or disease panels (80048-80076 [80081])
Therapeutic drug assays (80150-80299 [80164, 80165, 80171])

82075 **Alcohol (ethanol), breath**
0.00 0.00 FUD XXX
AMA: 2015,Jun,10; 2015,Apr,3

82085 **Aldolase**
0.00 0.00 FUD XXX
AMA: 2015,Jun,10; 2015,Apr,3

82088 **Aldosterone**
EXCLUDES *Alkaline phosphatase (84075, 84080)*
Alphaketoglutarate (82009-82010)
Alphatocopherol (VitaminE) (84446)
0.00 0.00 FUD XXX
AMA: 2015,Jun,10; 2015,Apr,3

82103 **Alpha-1-antitrypsin; total**
0.00 0.00 FUD XXX
AMA: 2015,Jun,10; 2015,Apr,3

82104 **phenotype**
0.00 0.00 FUD XXX
AMA: 2015,Jun,10; 2015,Apr,3

82105 **Alpha-fetoprotein (AFP); serum**
0.00 0.00 FUD XXX
AMA: 2015,Jun,10; 2015,Apr,3

82106 **amniotic fluid**
0.00 0.00 FUD XXX
AMA: 2015,Jun,10; 2015,Apr,3

82107 **AFP-L3 fraction isoform and total AFP (including ratio)**
0.00 0.00 FUD XXX
AMA: 2015,Jun,10; 2015,Apr,3

82108 Chemistry: Aluminum

CMS: 100-02,11,20.2 ESRD Laboratory Services

INCLUDES Clinical information not requested by the ordering physician
Mathematically calculated results
Quantitative analysis unless otherwise specified
Specimens from any source unless otherwise specified

EXCLUDES *Analytes from nonrequested laboratory analysis*
Calculated results that represent a score or probability that was derived by algorithm
Drug testing ([80305, 80306, 80307], [80324, 80325, 80326, 80327, 80328, 80329, 80330, 80331, 80332, 80333, 80334, 80335, 80336, 80337, 80338, 80339, 80340, 80341, 80342, 80343, 80344, 80345, 80346, 80347, 80348, 80349, 80350, 80351, 80352, 80353, 80354, 80355, 80356, 80357, 80358, 80359, 80360, 80361, 80362, 80363, 80364, 80365, 80366, 80367, 80368, 80369, 80370, 80371, 80372, 80373, 80374, 80375, 80376, 80377, 83992])
Organ or disease panels (80048-80076 [80081])
Therapeutic drug assays (80150-80299 [80164, 80165, 80171])

82108 **Aluminum**
0.00 0.00 FUD XXX
AMA: 2015,Jun,10; 2015,Apr,3

82120-82261 Chemistry: Amines—Biotinidase

INCLUDES Clinical information not requested by the ordering physician
Mathematically calculated results
Quantitative analysis unless otherwise specified
Specimens from any source unless otherwise specified

EXCLUDES *Analytes from nonrequested laboratory analysis*
Calculated results that represent a score or probability that was derived by algorithm
Drug testing ([80305, 80306, 80307], [80324, 80325, 80326, 80327, 80328, 80329, 80330, 80331, 80332, 80333, 80334, 80335, 80336, 80337, 80338, 80339, 80340, 80341, 80342, 80343, 80344, 80345, 80346, 80347, 80348, 80349, 80350, 80351, 80352, 80353, 80354, 80355, 80356, 80357, 80358, 80359, 80360, 80361, 80362, 80363, 80364, 80365, 80366, 80367, 80368, 80369, 80370, 80371, 80372, 80373, 80374, 80375, 80376, 80377, 83992])
Organ or disease panels (80048-80076 [80081])
Therapeutic drug assays (80150-80299 [80164, 80165, 80171])

82120 **Amines, vaginal fluid, qualitative** ♀
EXCLUDES *Combined pH and amines test for vaginitis (82120, 83986)*
0.00 0.00 FUD XXX
AMA: 2018,Jan,8; 2017,Jan,8; 2016,Jan,13; 2015,Jun,10; 2015,Apr,3; 2015,Jan,16; 2014,Jan,11

82127 **Amino acids; single, qualitative, each specimen**
0.00 0.00 FUD XXX
AMA: 2015,Jun,10; 2015,Apr,3

82128 **multiple, qualitative, each specimen**
0.00 0.00 FUD XXX
AMA: 2015,Jun,10; 2015,Apr,3

82131 **single, quantitative, each specimen**
INCLUDES Van Slyke method
0.00 0.00 FUD XXX
AMA: 2018,Jan,8; 2017,Jan,8; 2016,Jan,13; 2015,Jun,10; 2015,Apr,3; 2015,Jan,16; 2014,Jan,11

82135 **Aminolevulinic acid, delta (ALA)**
0.00 0.00 FUD XXX
AMA: 2015,Jun,10; 2015,Apr,3

82136 **Amino acids, 2 to 5 amino acids, quantitative, each specimen**
0.00 0.00 FUD XXX
AMA: 2015,Jun,10; 2015,Apr,3

82139 **Amino acids, 6 or more amino acids, quantitative, each specimen**
0.00 0.00 FUD XXX
AMA: 2015,Jun,10; 2015,Apr,3

82140 **Ammonia**
0.00 0.00 FUD XXX
AMA: 2015,Jun,10; 2015,Apr,3

82143 **Amniotic fluid scan (spectrophotometric)** M ♀
EXCLUDES *Amobarbital ([80345])*
L/S ratio (83661)
0.00 0.00 FUD XXX
AMA: 2015,Jun,10; 2015,Apr,3

82150 **Amylase**
0.00 0.00 FUD XXX
AMA: 2015,Jun,10; 2015,Apr,3

82154 **Androstanediol glucuronide**
0.00 0.00 FUD XXX
AMA: 2018,Jan,8; 2017,Jan,8; 2016,Jan,13; 2015,Jun,10; 2015,Apr,3; 2015,Jan,16; 2014,Jan,11

82157 **Androstenedione**
0.00 0.00 FUD XXX
AMA: 2015,Jun,10; 2015,Apr,3

82160 **Androsterone**
0.00 0.00 FUD XXX
AMA: 2015,Jun,10; 2015,Apr,3

82163 **Angiotensin II**
0.00 0.00 FUD XXX
AMA: 2015,Jun,10; 2015,Apr,3

82164 **Angiotensin I - converting enzyme (ACE)**
EXCLUDES *Antidiuretic hormone (ADH) (84588)*
Antimony (83015)
Antitrypsin, alpha-1- (82103-82104)
0.00 0.00 FUD XXX
AMA: 2015,Jun,10; 2015,Apr,3

82172 **Apolipoprotein, each**
0.00 0.00 FUD XXX
AMA: 2015,Jun,10; 2015,Apr,3

82175 **Arsenic**
EXCLUDES *Heavy metal screening (83015)*
0.00 0.00 FUD XXX
AMA: 2015,Jun,10; 2015,Apr,3

82180 **Ascorbic acid (Vitamin C), blood**
EXCLUDES *Aspirin (acetylsalicylic acid) ([80329, 80330, 80331])*
Atherogenic index, blood, ultracentrifugation, quantitative (83701)
0.00 0.00 FUD XXX
AMA: 2015,Jun,10; 2015,Apr,3

82190 **Atomic absorption spectroscopy, each analyte**
0.00 0.00 FUD XXX
AMA: 2015,Jun,10; 2015,Apr,3

82232 **Beta-2 microglobulin**
0.00 0.00 FUD XXX
AMA: 2015,Jun,10; 2015,Apr,3

82239 **Bile acids; total**
0.00 0.00 FUD XXX
AMA: 2015,Jun,10; 2015,Apr,3

82240 **cholylglycine**
EXCLUDES *Bile pigments, urine (81000-81005)*
0.00 0.00 FUD XXX
AMA: 2015,Jun,10; 2015,Apr,3

Pathology and Laboratory

82104 — 82240

● New Code ▲ Revised Code ○ Reinstated ● New Web Release ▲ Revised Web Release + Add-on Unlisted Not Covered # Resequenced
⊛ Optum Mod 50 Exempt ⊘ AMA Mod 51 Exempt ⊛ Optum Mod 51 Exempt ⊛ Mod 63 Exempt ⁄ Non-FDA Drug ★ Telemedicine M Maternity A Age Edit

82247 **Bilirubin; total**

INCLUDES Van Den Bergh test

0.00 0.00 FUD XXX

AMA: 2018,Jan,8; 2017,Jan,8; 2016,Jan,13; 2015,Jun,10; 2015,Apr,3; 2015,Jan,16; 2014,Jan,11

82248 **direct**

0.00 0.00 FUD XXX

AMA: 2018,Jan,8; 2017,Jan,8; 2016,Jan,13; 2015,Jun,10; 2015,Apr,3; 2015,Jan,16; 2014,Jan,11

82252 **feces, qualitative**

0.00 0.00 FUD XXX

AMA: 2015,Jun,10; 2015,Apr,3

82261 **Biotinidase, each specimen**

0.00 0.00 FUD XXX

AMA: 2015,Jun,10; 2015,Apr,3

82270-82274 Chemistry: Occult Blood

CMS: 100-04,16,70.8 CLIA Waived Tests; 100-04,18,60 Colorectal Cancer Screening

INCLUDES Clinical information not requested by the ordering physician
Mathematically calculated results
Quantitative analysis unless otherwise specified
Specimens from any source unless otherwise specified

EXCLUDES *Analytes from nonrequested laboratory analysis*
Calculated results that represent a score or probability that was derived by algorithm
Drug testing ([80305, 80306, 80307], [80324, 80325, 80326, 80327, 80328, 80329, 80330, 80331, 80332, 80333, 80334, 80335, 80336, 80337, 80338, 80339, 80340, 80341, 80342, 80343, 80344, 80345, 80346, 80347, 80348, 80349, 80350, 80351, 80352, 80353, 80354, 80355, 80356, 80357, 80358, 80359, 80360, 80361, 80362, 80363, 80364, 80365, 80366, 80367, 80368, 80369, 80370, 80371, 80372, 80373, 80374, 80375, 80376, 80377, 83992])
Organ or disease panels (80048-80076 [80081])
Therapeutic drug assays (80150-80299 [80164, 80165, 80171])

82270 **Blood, occult, by peroxidase activity (eg, guaiac), qualitative; feces, consecutive collected specimens with single determination, for colorectal neoplasm screening (ie, patient was provided 3 cards or single triple card for consecutive collection)**

INCLUDES Day test

0.00 0.00 FUD XXX

AMA: 2018,Jan,8; 2017,Jan,8; 2016,Jan,13; 2015,Jun,10; 2015,Apr,3; 2015,Jan,16; 2014,Jan,11

82271 **other sources**

0.00 0.00 FUD XXX

AMA: 2015,Jun,10; 2015,Apr,3

82272 **Blood, occult, by peroxidase activity (eg, guaiac), qualitative, feces, 1-3 simultaneous determinations, performed for other than colorectal neoplasm screening**

0.00 0.00 FUD XXX

AMA: 2018,Jan,8; 2017,Jan,8; 2016,Jan,13; 2015,Jun,10; 2015,Apr,3; 2015,Jan,16; 2014,Jan,11

82274 **Blood, occult, by fecal hemoglobin determination by immunoassay, qualitative, feces, 1-3 simultaneous determinations**

0.00 0.00 FUD XXX

AMA: 2015,Jun,10; 2015,Apr,3

82286-82308 [82652] Chemistry: Bradykinin—Calcitonin

INCLUDES Clinical information not requested by the ordering physician
Mathematically calculated results
Quantitative analysis unless otherwise specified
Specimens from any source unless otherwise specified

EXCLUDES *Analytes from nonrequested laboratory analysis*
Calculated results that represent a score or probability that was derived by algorithm
Drug testing ([80305, 80306, 80307], [80324, 80325, 80326, 80327, 80328, 80329, 80330, 80331, 80332, 80333, 80334, 80335, 80336, 80337, 80338, 80339, 80340, 80341, 80342, 80343, 80344, 80345, 80346, 80347, 80348, 80349, 80350, 80351, 80352, 80353, 80354, 80355, 80356, 80357, 80358, 80359, 80360, 80361, 80362, 80363, 80364, 80365, 80366, 80367, 80368, 80369, 80370, 80371, 80372, 80373, 80374, 80375, 80376, 80377, 83992])
Organ or disease panels (80048-80076 [80081])
Therapeutic drug assays (80150-80299 [80164, 80165, 80171])

82286 **Bradykinin**

0.00 0.00 FUD XXX

AMA: 2015,Jun,10; 2015,Apr,3

82300 **Cadmium**

0.00 0.00 FUD XXX

AMA: 2015,Jun,10; 2015,Apr,3

82306 **Vitamin D; 25 hydroxy, includes fraction(s), if performed**

0.00 0.00 FUD XXX

AMA: 2015,Jun,10; 2015,Apr,3

82652 **1, 25 dihydroxy, includes fraction(s), if performed**

0.00 0.00 FUD XXX

AMA: 2015,Jun,10; 2015,Apr,3

82308 **Calcitonin**

0.00 0.00 FUD XXX

AMA: 2015,Jun,10; 2015,Apr,3

82310-82373 Chemistry: Calcium, total; Carbohydrate Deficient Transferrin

INCLUDES Clinical information not requested by the ordering physician
Mathematically calculated results
Quantitative analysis unless otherwise specified
Specimens from any source unless otherwise specified

EXCLUDES *Analytes from nonrequested laboratory analysis*
Calculated results that represent a score or probability that was derived by algorithm
Drug testing ([80305, 80306, 80307], [80324, 80325, 80326, 80327, 80328, 80329, 80330, 80331, 80332, 80333, 80334, 80335, 80336, 80337, 80338, 80339, 80340, 80341, 80342, 80343, 80344, 80345, 80346, 80347, 80348, 80349, 80350, 80351, 80352, 80353, 80354, 80355, 80356, 80357, 80358, 80359, 80360, 80361, 80362, 80363, 80364, 80365, 80366, 80367, 80368, 80369, 80370, 80371, 80372, 80373, 80374, 80375, 80376, 80377, 83992])
Organ or disease panels (80048-80076 [80081])
Therapeutic drug assays (80150-80299 [80164, 80165, 80171])

82310 **Calcium; total**

0.00 0.00 FUD XXX

AMA: 2018,Jan,8; 2017,Jan,8; 2016,Jan,13; 2015,Jun,10; 2015,Apr,3; 2015,Jan,16; 2014,Jan,11

82330 **ionized**

0.00 0.00 FUD XXX

AMA: 2018,Jan,8; 2017,Jan,8; 2016,Jan,13; 2015,Jun,10; 2015,Apr,3; 2015,Jan,16; 2014,Jan,11

82331 **after calcium infusion test**

0.00 0.00 FUD XXX

AMA: 2015,Jun,10; 2015,Apr,3

82340 **urine quantitative, timed specimen**

0.00 0.00 FUD XXX

AMA: 2015,Jun,10; 2015,Apr,3

82355 **Calculus; qualitative analysis**

0.00 0.00 FUD XXX

AMA: 2015,Jun,10; 2015,Apr,3

82360 **quantitative analysis, chemical**

0.00 0.00 FUD XXX

AMA: 2015,Jun,10; 2015,Apr,3

82365 infrared spectroscopy
0.00 0.00 FUD XXX
AMA: 2015,Jun,10; 2015,Apr,3

82370 X-ray diffraction
0.00 0.00 FUD XXX
AMA: 2015,Jun,10; 2015,Apr,3

82373 Carbohydrate deficient transferrin
0.00 0.00 FUD XXX
AMA: 2015,Jun,10; 2015,Apr,3

82374 Chemistry: Carbon Dioxide

CMS: 100-02,11,20.2 ESRD Laboratory Services; 100-02,11,30.2.2 Automated Multi-Channel Chemistry (AMCC) Tests; 100-04,16,40.6.1 Automated Multi-Channel Chemistry (AMCC) Tests for ESRD Beneficiaries; 100-04,16,70.8 CLIA Waived Tests; 100-04,16,90.2 Organ or Disease Oriented Panels

INCLUDES Clinical information not requested by the ordering physician
Mathematically calculated results
Quantitative analysis unless otherwise specified
Specimens from any source unless otherwise specified

EXCLUDES *Analytes from nonrequested laboratory analysis*
Calculated results that represent a score or probability that was derived by algorithm
Drug testing ([80305, 80306, 80307], [80324, 80325, 80326, 80327, 80328, 80329, 80330, 80331, 80332, 80333, 80334, 80335, 80336, 80337, 80338, 80339, 80340, 80341, 80342, 80343, 80344, 80345, 80346, 80347, 80348, 80349, 80350, 80351, 80352, 80353, 80354, 80355, 80356, 80357, 80358, 80359, 80360, 80361, 80362, 80363, 80364, 80365, 80366, 80367, 80368, 80369, 80370, 80371, 80372, 80373, 80374, 80375, 80376, 80377, 83992])
Organ or disease panels (80048-80076 [80081])
Therapeutic drug assays (80150-80299 [80164, 80165, 80171])

82374 Carbon dioxide (bicarbonate)
EXCLUDES *Blood gases (82803)*
0.00 0.00 FUD XXX
AMA: 2018,Jan,8; 2017,Jan,8; 2016,Jan,13; 2015,Jun,10; 2015,Apr,3; 2015,Jan,16; 2014,Jan,11

82375-82376 Chemistry: Carboxyhemoglobin (Carbon Monoxide)

INCLUDES Clinical information not requested by the ordering physician
Mathematically calculated results
Specimens from any source unless otherwise specified

EXCLUDES *Analytes from nonrequested laboratory analysis*
Calculated results that represent a score or probability that was derived by algorithm
Drug testing ([80305, 80306, 80307], [80324, 80325, 80326, 80327, 80328, 80329, 80330, 80331, 80332, 80333, 80334, 80335, 80336, 80337, 80338, 80339, 80340, 80341, 80342, 80343, 80344, 80345, 80346, 80347, 80348, 80349, 80350, 80351, 80352, 80353, 80354, 80355, 80356, 80357, 80358, 80359, 80360, 80361, 80362, 80363, 80364, 80365, 80366, 80367, 80368, 80369, 80370, 80371, 80372, 80373, 80374, 80375, 80376, 80377, 83992])
Organ or disease panels (80048-80076 [80081])
Transcutaneous measurement of carboxyhemoglobin (88740)

82375 Carboxyhemoglobin; quantitative
0.00 0.00 FUD XXX
AMA: 2018,Jan,8; 2017,Jan,8; 2016,Jan,13; 2015,Jun,10; 2015,Apr,3; 2015,Jan,16; 2014,Jan,11

82376 qualitative
0.00 0.00 FUD XXX
AMA: 2015,Jun,10; 2015,Apr,3

82378 Chemistry: Carcinoembryonic Antigen (CEA)

CMS: 100-03,190.26 Carcinoembryonic Antigen (CEA)

INCLUDES Clinical information not requested by the ordering physician

EXCLUDES *Analytes from nonrequested laboratory analysis*
Calculated results that represent a score or probability that was derived by algorithm

82378 Carcinoembryonic antigen (CEA)
0.00 0.00 FUD XXX
AMA: 2018,Jan,8; 2017,Jan,8; 2016,Jan,13; 2015,Jun,10; 2015,Apr,3; 2015,Jan,16; 2014,Jan,11

82379-82415 Chemistry: Carnitine—Chloramphenicol

INCLUDES Clinical information not requested by the ordering physician
Mathematically calculated results
Quantitative analysis unless otherwise specified
Specimens from any source unless otherwise specified

EXCLUDES *Analytes from nonrequested laboratory analysis*
Calculated results that represent a score or probability that was derived by algorithm
Drug testing ([80305, 80306, 80307], [80324, 80325, 80326, 80327, 80328, 80329, 80330, 80331, 80332, 80333, 80334, 80335, 80336, 80337, 80338, 80339, 80340, 80341, 80342, 80343, 80344, 80345, 80346, 80347, 80348, 80349, 80350, 80351, 80352, 80353, 80354, 80355, 80356, 80357, 80358, 80359, 80360, 80361, 80362, 80363, 80364, 80365, 80366, 80367, 80368, 80369, 80370, 80371, 80372, 80373, 80374, 80375, 80376, 80377, 83992])
Organ or disease panels (80048-80076 [80081])
Therapeutic drug assays (80150-80299 [80164, 80165, 80171])

82379 Carnitine (total and free), quantitative, each specimen
EXCLUDES *Acylcarnitine (82016-82017)*
0.00 0.00 FUD XXX
AMA: 2015,Jun,10; 2015,Apr,3

82380 Carotene
0.00 0.00 FUD XXX
AMA: 2015,Jun,10; 2015,Apr,3

82382 Catecholamines; total urine
0.00 0.00 FUD XXX
AMA: 2015,Jun,10; 2015,Apr,3

82383 blood
0.00 0.00 FUD XXX
AMA: 2015,Jun,10; 2015,Apr,3

82384 fractionated
EXCLUDES *Urine metabolites (83835, 84585)*
0.00 0.00 FUD XXX
AMA: 2015,Jun,10; 2015,Apr,3

82387 Cathepsin-D
0.00 0.00 FUD XXX
AMA: 2015,Jun,10; 2015,Apr,3

82390 Ceruloplasmin
0.00 0.00 FUD XXX
AMA: 2015,Jun,10; 2015,Apr,3

82397 Chemiluminescent assay
0.00 0.00 FUD XXX
AMA: 2018,Jan,8; 2017,Jan,8; 2016,Jan,13; 2015,Jun,10; 2015,Apr,3; 2015,Jan,16; 2014,Jan,11

82415 Chloramphenicol
0.00 0.00 FUD XXX
AMA: 2015,Jun,10; 2015,Apr,3

82435-82438 Chemistry: Chloride

INCLUDES Clinical information not requested by the ordering physician
Mathematically calculated results
Quantitative analysis unless otherwise specified
Specimens from any source unless otherwise specified

EXCLUDES *Analytes from nonrequested laboratory analysis*
Calculated results that represent a score or probability that was derived by algorithm
Organ or disease panels (80048-80076 [80081])
Therapeutic drug assays (80150-80299 [80164, 80165, 80171])

82435 Chloride; blood
0.00 0.00 FUD XXX
AMA: 2018,Jan,8; 2017,Jan,8; 2016,Jan,13; 2015,Jun,10; 2015,Apr,3; 2015,Jan,16; 2014,Jan,11

82436 urine
0.00 0.00 FUD XXX
AMA: 2015,Jun,10; 2015,Apr,3

82438 other source
EXCLUDES *Sweat collections by iontophoresis (89230)*
0.00 0.00 FUD XXX
AMA: 2018,Jan,8; 2017,Jan,8; 2016,Jan,13; 2015,Jun,10; 2015,Apr,3; 2015,Jan,16; 2014,Jan,11

82441 Chemistry: Chlorinated Hydrocarbons

INCLUDES Clinical information not requested by the ordering physician
Mathematically calculated results
Quantitative analysis unless otherwise specified
Specimens from any source unless otherwise specified

EXCLUDES *Analytes from nonrequested laboratory analysis*
Calculated results that represent a score or probability that was derived by algorithm

82441 Chlorinated hydrocarbons, screen

EXCLUDES *Cholecalciferol (Vitamin D) (82306)*
0.00 0.00 FUD XXX
AMA: 2015,Jun,10; 2015,Apr,3

82465 Chemistry: Cholesterol, Total

CMS: 100-03,190.23 Lipid Testing; 100-04,16,40.6.1 Automated Multi-Channel Chemistry (AMCC) Tests for ESRD Beneficiaries; 100-04,16,70.8 CLIA Waived Tests; 100-04,16,90.2 Organ or Disease Oriented Panels

INCLUDES Clinical information not requested by the ordering physician
Mathematically calculated results
Quantitative analysis unless otherwise specified

EXCLUDES *Analytes from nonrequested laboratory analysis*
Calculated results that represent a score or probability that was derived by algorithm
Organ or disease panels (80048-80076 [80081])

82465 Cholesterol, serum or whole blood, total

EXCLUDES *High density lipoprotein (HDL) (83718)*
0.00 0.00 FUD XXX
AMA: 2018,Jan,8; 2017,Jan,8; 2016,Jan,13; 2015,Jun,10; 2015,Apr,3; 2015,Jan,16; 2014,Jan,11

82480-82507 Chemistry: Cholinesterase—Citrate

INCLUDES Clinical information not requested by the ordering physician
Mathematically calculated results
Quantitative analysis unless otherwise specified
Specimens from any source unless otherwise specified

EXCLUDES *Analytes from nonrequested laboratory analysis*
Calculated results that represent a score or probability that was derived by algorithm
Drug testing ([80305, 80306, 80307], [80324, 80325, 80326, 80327, 80328, 80329, 80330, 80331, 80332, 80333, 80334, 80335, 80336, 80337, 80338, 80339, 80340, 80341, 80342, 80343, 80344, 80345, 80346, 80347, 80348, 80349, 80350, 80351, 80352, 80353, 80354, 80355, 80356, 80357, 80358, 80359, 80360, 80361, 80362, 80363, 80364, 80365, 80366, 80367, 80368, 80369, 80370, 80371, 80372, 80373, 80374, 80375, 80376, 80377, 83992])
Organ or disease panels (80048-80076 [80081])
Therapeutic drug assays (80150-80299 [80164, 80165, 80171])

82480 Cholinesterase; serum
0.00 0.00 FUD XXX
AMA: 2015,Jun,10; 2015,Apr,3

82482 RBC
0.00 0.00 FUD XXX
AMA: 2015,Jun,10; 2015,Apr,3

82485 Chondroitin B sulfate, quantitative

EXCLUDES *Chorionic gonadotropin (84702-84703)*
0.00 0.00 FUD XXX
AMA: 2015,Jun,10; 2015,Apr,3

82495 Chromium
0.00 0.00 FUD XXX
AMA: 2015,Jun,10; 2015,Apr,3

82507 Citrate

EXCLUDES *Cocaine, qualitative analysis ([80353])*
Codeine, qualitative analysis ([80361])
Complement (86160-86162)
0.00 0.00 FUD XXX
AMA: 2015,Jun,10; 2015,Apr,3

82523 Chemistry: Collagen Crosslinks, Any Method

CMS: 100-03,190.19 NCD for Collagen Crosslinks, Any Method; 100-04,16,70.8 CLIA Waived Tests

INCLUDES Clinical information not requested by the ordering physician
Mathematically calculated results
Quantitative analysis unless otherwise specified
Specimens from any source unless otherwise specified

EXCLUDES *Analytes from nonrequested laboratory analysis*
Calculated results that represent a score or probability that was derived by algorithm
Organ or disease panels (80048-80076 [80081])
Therapeutic drug assays (80150-80299 [80164, 80165, 80171])

82523 Collagen cross links, any method
0.00 0.00 FUD XXX
AMA: 2015,Jun,10; 2015,Apr,3

82525-82735 Chemistry: Copper—Fluoride

INCLUDES Clinical information not requested by the ordering physician
Mathematically calculated results
Quantitative analysis unless otherwise specified
Specimens from any source unless otherwise specified

EXCLUDES *Analytes from nonrequested laboratory analysis*
Calculated results that represent a score or probability that was derived by algorithm
Drug testing ([80305, 80306, 80307], [80324, 80325, 80326, 80327, 80328, 80329, 80330, 80331, 80332, 80333, 80334, 80335, 80336, 80337, 80338, 80339, 80340, 80341, 80342, 80343, 80344, 80345, 80346, 80347, 80348, 80349, 80350, 80351, 80352, 80353, 80354, 80355, 80356, 80357, 80358, 80359, 80360, 80361, 80362, 80363, 80364, 80365, 80366, 80367, 80368, 80369, 80370, 80371, 80372, 80373, 80374, 80375, 80376, 80377, 83992])
Organ or disease panels (80048-80076 [80081])
Therapeutic drug assays (80150-80299 [80164, 80165, 80171])

82525 Copper

EXCLUDES *Coproporphyrin (84119-84120)*
Corticosteroids (83491)
0.00 0.00 FUD XXX
AMA: 2015,Jun,10; 2015,Apr,3

82528 Corticosterone

INCLUDES Porter-Silber test
0.00 0.00 FUD XXX
AMA: 2015,Jun,10; 2015,Apr,3

82530 Cortisol; free
0.00 0.00 FUD XXX
AMA: 2018,Jan,8; 2017,Jan,8; 2016,Jan,13; 2015,Jun,10; 2015,Apr,3; 2015,Jan,16; 2014,Jan,11

82533 total
0.00 0.00 FUD XXX
AMA: 2018,Jan,8; 2017,Jan,8; 2016,Jan,13; 2015,Jun,10; 2015,Apr,3; 2015,Jan,16; 2014,Jan,11

82540 Creatine
0.00 0.00 FUD XXX
AMA: 2015,Jun,10; 2015,Apr,3

82542 Column chromatography, includes mass spectrometry, if performed (eg, HPLC, LC, LC/MS, LC/MS-MS, GC, GC/MS-MS, GC/MS, HPLC/MS), non-drug analyte(s) not elsewhere specified, qualitative or quantitative, each specimen

EXCLUDES *Column chromatography/mass spectrometry of drugs/substances ([80305, 80306, 80307], [80320, 80321, 80322, 80323, 80324, 80325, 80326, 80327, 80328, 80329, 80330, 80331, 80332, 80333, 80334, 80335, 80336, 80337, 80338, 80339, 80340, 80341, 80342, 80343, 80344, 80345, 80346, 80347, 80348, 80349, 80350, 80351, 80352, 80353, 80354, 80355, 80356, 80357, 80358, 80359, 80360, 80361, 80362, 80363, 80364, 80365, 80366, 80367, 80368, 80369, 80370, 80371, 80372, 80373, 80374, 80375, 80376, 80377, 83992])*
Procedure performed more than one time per specimen
0.00 0.00 FUD XXX
AMA: 2018,Jan,8; 2017,Jan,8; 2016,Jan,13; 2015,Jun,10; 2015,Apr,3

82550 Creatine kinase (CK), (CPK); total
0.00 0.00 FUD XXX
AMA: 2018,Jan,8; 2017,Jan,8; 2016,Jan,13; 2015,Jun,10; 2015,Apr,3; 2015,Jan,16; 2014,Jan,11

82552 isoenzymes
0.00 0.00 FUD XXX
AMA: 2018,Jan,8; 2017,Jan,8; 2016,Jan,13; 2015,Jun,10; 2015,Apr,3; 2015,Jan,16; 2014,Jan,11

82553 MB fraction only
0.00 0.00 FUD XXX
AMA: 2018,Jan,8; 2017,Jan,8; 2016,Jan,13; 2015,Jun,10; 2015,Apr,3; 2015,Jan,16; 2014,Jan,11

82554 isoforms
0.00 0.00 FUD XXX
AMA: 2018,Jan,8; 2017,Jan,8; 2016,Jan,13; 2015,Jun,10; 2015,Apr,3; 2015,Jan,16; 2014,Jan,11

82565 **Creatinine; blood**
0.00 0.00 FUD XXX
AMA: 2018,Jan,8; 2017,Jan,8; 2016,Jan,13; 2015,Jun,10; 2015,Apr,3; 2015,Jan,16; 2014,Jan,11

82570 other source
0.00 0.00 FUD XXX
AMA: 2015,Jun,10; 2015,Apr,3

82575 clearance
INCLUDES Holten test
0.00 0.00 FUD XXX
AMA: 2015,Jun,10; 2015,Apr,3

82585 **Cryofibrinogen**
0.00 0.00 FUD XXX
AMA: 2015,Jun,10; 2015,Apr,3

82595 **Cryoglobulin, qualitative or semi-quantitative (eg, cryocrit)**
EXCLUDES *Crystals, pyrophosphate vs urate (89060)*
Quantitative, cryoglobulin (82784-82785)
0.00 0.00 FUD XXX
AMA: 2015,Jun,10; 2015,Apr,3

82600 **Cyanide**
0.00 0.00 FUD XXX
AMA: 2015,Jun,10; 2015,Apr,3

82607 **Cyanocobalamin (Vitamin B-12);**
EXCLUDES *Cyclic AMP (82030)*
Cyclosporine (80158)
0.00 0.00 FUD XXX
AMA: 2015,Jun,10; 2015,Apr,3

82608 unsaturated binding capacity
EXCLUDES *Cyclic AMP (82030)*
Cyclosporine (80158)
0.00 0.00 FUD XXX
AMA: 2015,Jun,10; 2015,Apr,3

82610 **Cystatin C**
0.00 0.00 FUD XXX
AMA: 2018,Jan,8; 2017,Jan,8; 2016,Jan,13; 2015,Jun,10; 2015,Apr,3; 2015,Jan,16; 2014,Jan,11

82615 **Cystine and homocystine, urine, qualitative**
0.00 0.00 FUD XXX
AMA: 2015,Jun,10; 2015,Apr,3

82626 **Dehydroepiandrosterone (DHEA)**
EXCLUDES *Anabolic steroids ([80327, 80328])*
0.00 0.00 FUD XXX
AMA: 2018,Jan,8; 2017,Jan,8; 2016,Jan,13; 2015,Jun,10; 2015,Apr,3; 2015,Jan,16; 2014,Jan,11

82627 **Dehydroepiandrosterone-sulfate (DHEA-S)**
EXCLUDES *Delta-aminolevulinicacid (ALA) (82135)*
0.00 0.00 FUD XXX
AMA: 2018,Jan,8; 2017,Jan,8; 2016,Jan,13; 2015,Jun,10; 2015,Apr,3; 2015,Jan,16; 2014,Jan,11

82633 **Desoxycorticosterone, 11-**
0.00 0.00 FUD XXX
AMA: 2015,Jun,10; 2015,Apr,3

82634 **Deoxycortisol, 11-**
EXCLUDES *Dexamethasone suppression test (80420)*
Diastase, urine (82150)
0.00 0.00 FUD XXX
AMA: 2015,Jun,10; 2015,Apr,3

82638 **Dibucaine number**
EXCLUDES *Dichloroethane (82441)*
Dichloromethane (82441)
Diethylether (84600)
0.00 0.00 FUD XXX
AMA: 2015,Jun,10; 2015,Apr,3

82642 **Dihydrotestosterone (DHT)**
0.00 0.00 FUD XXX
EXCLUDES *Anabolic drug testing analysis of dihydrotestosterone ([80327, 80328])*
Dipropylaceticacid ([80164])
Dopamine (82382)
Duodenal contents, individual enzymes for intubation and collection (43756-43757)

82652 **Resequenced code. See code following 82306.**

82656 **Elastase, pancreatic (EL-1), fecal, qualitative or semi-quantitative**
0.00 0.00 FUD XXX
AMA: 2018,Jan,8; 2017,Jan,8; 2016,Jan,13; 2015,Jun,10; 2015,Apr,3; 2015,Jan,16; 2014,Jan,11

82657 **Enzyme activity in blood cells, cultured cells, or tissue, not elsewhere specified; nonradioactive substrate, each specimen**
0.00 0.00 FUD XXX
AMA: 2015,Jun,10; 2015,Apr,3

82658 radioactive substrate, each specimen
0.00 0.00 FUD XXX
AMA: 2015,Jun,10; 2015,Apr,3

82664 **Electrophoretic technique, not elsewhere specified**
EXCLUDES *Endocrine receptor assays (84233-84235)*
0.00 0.00 FUD XXX
AMA: 2015,Jun,10; 2015,Apr,3

82668 **Erythropoietin**
0.00 0.00 FUD XXX
AMA: 2015,Jun,10; 2015,Apr,3

82670 **Estradiol**
0.00 0.00 FUD XXX
AMA: 2015,Jun,10; 2015,Apr,3

82671 **Estrogens; fractionated**
EXCLUDES *Estrogen receptor assay (84233)*
0.00 0.00 FUD XXX
AMA: 2015,Jun,10; 2015,Apr,3

82672 total
EXCLUDES *Estrogen receptor assay (84233)*
0.00 0.00 FUD XXX
AMA: 2015,Jun,10; 2015,Apr,3

82677 **Estriol**
0.00 0.00 FUD XXX
AMA: 2015,Jun,10; 2015,Apr,3

82679 **Estrone**
EXCLUDES *Ethanol ([80320])*
0.00 0.00 FUD XXX
AMA: 2015,Jun,10; 2015,Apr,3

82693 **Ethylene glycol**
0.00 0.00 FUD XXX
AMA: 2015,Jun,10; 2015,Apr,3

82696 **Etiocholanolone**
EXCLUDES *Fractionation of ketosteroids (83593)*
0.00 0.00 FUD XXX
AMA: 2015,Jun,10; 2015,Apr,3

Pathology and Laboratory

82552 — 82696

82705 **Fat or lipids, feces; qualitative**
0.00 0.00 FUD XXX
AMA: 2015,Jun,10; 2015,Apr,3

82710 **quantitative**
0.00 0.00 FUD XXX
AMA: 2015,Jun,10; 2015,Apr,3

82715 **Fat differential, feces, quantitative**
0.00 0.00 FUD XXX
AMA: 2015,Jun,10; 2015,Apr,3

82725 **Fatty acids, nonesterified**
0.00 0.00 FUD XXX
AMA: 2015,Jun,10; 2015,Apr,3

82726 **Very long chain fatty acids**
EXCLUDES *Long-chain (C20-22) omega-3 fatty acids in red blood cell (RBC) membranes (0111T)*
0.00 0.00 FUD XXX
AMA: 2015,Jun,10; 2015,Apr,3

82728 **Ferritin**
EXCLUDES *Fetal hemoglobin (83030, 83033, 85460)*
Fetoprotein, alpha-1 (82105-82106)
0.00 0.00 FUD XXX
AMA: 2015,Jun,10; 2015,Apr,3

82731 **Fetal fibronectin, cervicovaginal secretions, semi-quantitative** M ♀
0.00 0.00 FUD XXX
AMA: 2015,Jun,10; 2015,Apr,3

82735 **Fluoride**
EXCLUDES *Foam stability test (83662)*
0.00 0.00 FUD XXX
AMA: 2015,Jun,10; 2015,Apr,3

82746-82941 Chemistry: Folic Acid—Gastrin

INCLUDES Clinical information not requested by the ordering physician
Mathematically calculated results
Quantitative analysis unless otherwise specified
Specimens from any source unless otherwise specified

EXCLUDES *Analytes from nonrequested laboratory analysis*
Calculated results that represent a score or probability that was derived by algorithm
Drug testing ([80305, 80306, 80307], [80324, 80325, 80326, 80327, 80328, 80329, 80330, 80331, 80332, 80333, 80334, 80335, 80336, 80337, 80338, 80339, 80340, 80341, 80342, 80343, 80344, 80345, 80346, 80347, 80348, 80349, 80350, 80351, 80352, 80353, 80354, 80355, 80356, 80357, 80358, 80359, 80360, 80361, 80362, 80363, 80364, 80365, 80366, 80367, 80368, 80369, 80370, 80371, 80372, 80373, 80374, 80375, 80376, 80377, 83992])
Organ or disease panels (80048-80076 [80081])
Therapeutic drug assays (80150-80299 [80164, 80165, 80171])

82746 **Folic acid; serum**
0.00 0.00 FUD XXX
AMA: 2015,Jun,10; 2015,Apr,3

82747 **RBC**
EXCLUDES *Follicle stimulating hormone (FSH) (83001)*
0.00 0.00 FUD XXX
AMA: 2015,Jun,10; 2015,Apr,3

82757 **Fructose, semen**
EXCLUDES *Fructosamine (82985)*
Fructose, TLC screen (84375)
0.00 0.00 FUD XXX
AMA: 2015,Jun,10; 2015,Apr,3

82759 **Galactokinase, RBC**
0.00 0.00 FUD XXX
AMA: 2015,Jun,10; 2015,Apr,3

82760 **Galactose**
0.00 0.00 FUD XXX
AMA: 2015,Jun,10; 2015,Apr,3

82775 **Galactose-1-phosphate uridyl transferase; quantitative**
0.00 0.00 FUD XXX
AMA: 2015,Jun,10; 2015,Apr,3

82776 **screen**
0.00 0.00 FUD XXX
AMA: 2015,Jun,10; 2015,Apr,3

82777 **Galectin-3**
0.00 0.00 FUD XXX
AMA: 2015,Jun,10; 2015,Apr,3

82784 **Gammaglobulin (immunoglobulin); IgA, IgD, IgG, IgM, each**
INCLUDES Farr test
0.00 0.00 FUD XXX
AMA: 2018,Jan,8; 2017,Jan,8; 2016,Jan,13; 2015,Jun,10; 2015,Apr,3; 2015,Jan,16; 2014,Jan,11

82785 **IgE**
INCLUDES Farr test
EXCLUDES *Allergen specific, IgE (86003, 86005)*
0.00 0.00 FUD XXX
AMA: 2018,Jan,8; 2017,Jan,8; 2016,Jan,13; 2015,Jun,10; 2015,Apr,3; 2015,Jan,16; 2014,Jan,11

82787 **immunoglobulin subclasses (eg, IgG1, 2, 3, or 4), each**
EXCLUDES *Gamma-glutamyltransferase (GGT) (82977)*
0.00 0.00 FUD XXX
AMA: 2015,Jun,10; 2015,Apr,3

82800 **Gases, blood, pH only**
0.00 0.00 FUD XXX
AMA: 2015,Jun,10; 2015,Apr,3

82803 **Gases, blood, any combination of pH, pCO2, pO2, CO2, HCO3 (including calculated O2 saturation);**
INCLUDES Two or more of the listed analytes
0.00 0.00 FUD XXX
AMA: 2015,Jun,10; 2015,Apr,3

82805 **with O2 saturation, by direct measurement, except pulse oximetry**
0.00 0.00 FUD XXX
AMA: 2015,Jun,10; 2015,Apr,3

82810 **Gases, blood, O2 saturation only, by direct measurement, except pulse oximetry**
EXCLUDES *Pulse oximetry (94760)*
0.00 0.00 FUD XXX
AMA: 2015,Jun,10; 2015,Apr,3

82820 **Hemoglobin-oxygen affinity (pO2 for 50% hemoglobin saturation with oxygen)**
EXCLUDES *Gastric acid analysis (82930)*
0.00 0.00 FUD XXX
AMA: 2015,Jun,10; 2015,Apr,3

82930 **Gastric acid analysis, includes pH if performed, each specimen**
0.00 0.00 FUD XXX
AMA: 2018,Jan,8; 2017,Jan,8; 2016,Jan,13; 2015,Jun,10; 2015,Apr,3; 2015,Jan,16; 2014,Jan,11

82938 **Gastrin after secretin stimulation**
0.00 0.00 FUD XXX
AMA: 2015,Jun,10; 2015,Apr,3

82941 **Gastrin**
EXCLUDES *Gentamicin (80170)*
GGT (82977)
Qualitative column chromatography report specific analyte or (82542)
0.00 0.00 FUD XXX
AMA: 2015,Jun,10; 2015,Apr,3

82943-82962 Chemistry: Glucagon—Glucose Testing

CMS: 100-03,190.20 Blood Glucose Testing

INCLUDES Clinical information not requested by the ordering physician
Mathematically calculated results
Quantitative analysis unless otherwise specified
Specimens from any source unless otherwise specified

EXCLUDES *Analytes from nonrequested laboratory analysis*
Calculated results that represent a score or probability that was derived by algorithm
Organ or disease panels (80048-80076 [80081])
Therapeutic drug assays (80150-80299 [80164, 80165, 80171])

Code also glucose administration injection (96374)

82943 Glucagon
0.00 0.00 FUD XXX
AMA: 2015,Jun,10; 2015,Apr,3

82945 Glucose, body fluid, other than blood
0.00 0.00 FUD XXX
AMA: 2015,Jun,10; 2015,Apr,3

82946 Glucagon tolerance test
0.00 0.00 FUD XXX
AMA: 2015,Jun,10; 2015,Apr,3

82947 Glucose; quantitative, blood (except reagent strip)
0.00 0.00 FUD XXX
AMA: 2018,Jan,8; 2017,Jan,8; 2016,Jan,13; 2015,Jun,10; 2015,Apr,3; 2015,Jan,16; 2014,Jan,11

82948 blood, reagent strip
0.00 0.00 FUD XXX
AMA: 2018,Jan,8; 2017,Jan,8; 2016,Jan,13; 2015,Jun,10; 2015,Apr,3; 2015,Jan,16; 2014,Jan,11

82950 post glucose dose (includes glucose)
0.00 0.00 FUD XXX
AMA: 2018,Jan,8; 2017,Jan,8; 2016,Jan,13; 2015,Jun,10; 2015,Apr,3; 2015,Jan,16; 2014,Jan,11

82951 tolerance test (GTT), 3 specimens (includes glucose)
0.00 0.00 FUD XXX
AMA: 2018,Jan,8; 2017,Jan,8; 2016,Jan,13; 2015,Jun,10; 2015,Apr,3; 2015,Jan,16; 2014,Jan,11

+ **82952 tolerance test, each additional beyond 3 specimens (List separately in addition to code for primary procedure)**
EXCLUDES *Insulin tolerance test (80434-80435)*
Leucine tolerance test (80428)
Semiquantitative urine glucose (81000, 81002, 81005, 81099)
Code first (82951)
0.00 0.00 FUD XXX
AMA: 2018,Jan,8; 2017,Jan,8; 2016,Jan,13; 2015,Jun,10; 2015,Apr,3; 2015,Jan,16; 2014,Jan,11

82955 Glucose-6-phosphate dehydrogenase (G6PD); quantitative
Code also glucose tolerance test with medication, when performed (96374)
0.00 0.00 FUD XXX
AMA: 2015,Jun,10; 2015,Apr,3

82960 screen
Code also glucose tolerance test with medication, when performed (96374)
0.00 0.00 FUD XXX
AMA: 2015,Jun,10; 2015,Apr,3

82962 Glucose, blood by glucose monitoring device(s) cleared by the FDA specifically for home use
0.00 0.00 FUD XXX
AMA: 2018,Jan,8; 2017,Jan,8; 2016,Jan,13; 2015,Jun,10; 2015,Apr,3; 2015,Jan,16; 2014,Jan,11

82963-83690 Chemistry: Glucosidase—Lipase

INCLUDES Clinical information not requested by the ordering physician
Mathematically calculated results
Quantitative analysis unless otherwise specified
Specimens from any source unless otherwise specified

EXCLUDES *Analytes from nonrequested laboratory analysis*
Calculated results that represent a score or probability that was derived by algorithm
Drug testing ([80305, 80306, 80307], [80324, 80325, 80326, 80327, 80328, 80329, 80330, 80331, 80332, 80333, 80334, 80335, 80336, 80337, 80338, 80339, 80340, 80341, 80342, 80343, 80344, 80345, 80346, 80347, 80348, 80349, 80350, 80351, 80352, 80353, 80354, 80355, 80356, 80357, 80358, 80359, 80360, 80361, 80362, 80363, 80364, 80365, 80366, 80367, 80368, 80369, 80370, 80371, 80372, 80373, 80374, 80375, 80376, 80377, 83992])
Organ or disease panels (80048-80076 [80081])
Therapeutic drug assays (80150-80299 [80164, 80165, 80171])

82963 Glucosidase, beta
0.00 0.00 FUD XXX
AMA: 2015,Jun,10; 2015,Apr,3

82965 Glutamate dehydrogenase
0.00 0.00 FUD XXX
AMA: 2015,Jun,10; 2015,Apr,3

82977 Glutamyltransferase, gamma (GGT)
0.00 0.00 FUD XXX
AMA: 2018,Jan,8; 2017,Jan,8; 2016,Jan,13; 2015,Jun,10; 2015,Apr,3; 2015,Jan,16; 2014,Jan,11

82978 Glutathione
0.00 0.00 FUD XXX
AMA: 2015,Jun,10; 2015,Apr,3

82979 Glutathione reductase, RBC
EXCLUDES *Glycohemoglobin (83036)*
0.00 0.00 FUD XXX
AMA: 2015,Jun,10; 2015,Apr,3

82985 Glycated protein
EXCLUDES *Gonadotropin chorionic (hCG) (84702-84703)*
0.00 0.00 FUD XXX
AMA: 2018,Jan,8; 2017,Jan,8; 2016,Jan,13; 2015,Jun,10; 2015,Apr,3; 2015,Jan,16; 2014,Jan,11

83001 Gonadotropin; follicle stimulating hormone (FSH)
0.00 0.00 FUD XXX
AMA: 2015,Jun,10; 2015,Apr,3

83002 luteinizing hormone (LH)
EXCLUDES *Luteinizing releasing factor (LRH) (83727)*
0.00 0.00 FUD XXX
AMA: 2015,Jun,10; 2015,Apr,3

83003 Growth hormone, human (HGH) (somatotropin)
EXCLUDES *Antibody to human growth hormone (86277)*
0.00 0.00 FUD XXX
AMA: 2015,Jun,10; 2015,Apr,3

83006 Growth stimulation expressed gene 2 (ST2, Interleukin 1 receptor like-1)
0.00 0.00 FUD XXX
AMA: 2015,Jun,10; 2015,Apr,3

83009 Helicobacter pylori, blood test analysis for urease activity, non-radioactive isotope (eg, C-13)
EXCLUDES *H. pylori, breath test analysis for urease activity (83013-83014)*
0.00 0.00 FUD XXX
AMA: 2015,Jun,10; 2015,Apr,3

83010 Haptoglobin; quantitative
0.00 0.00 FUD XXX
AMA: 2015,Jun,10; 2015,Apr,3

83012 phenotypes
0.00 0.00 FUD XXX
AMA: 2015,Jun,10; 2015,Apr,3

Pathology and Laboratory
82943 — 83012

83013 **Helicobacter pylori; breath test analysis for urease activity, non-radioactive isotope (eg, C-13)**
0.00 0.00 FUD XXX
AMA: 2018,Jan,8; 2017,Jan,8; 2016,Jan,13; 2015,Jun,10; 2015,Apr,3; 2015,Jan,16; 2014,Jan,11

83014 **drug administration**
EXCLUDES *H. pylori:*
Blood test analysis for urease activity (83009)
Enzyme immunoassay (87339)
Liquid scintillation counter (78267-78268)
Stool (87338)
0.00 0.00 FUD XXX
AMA: 2018,Jan,8; 2017,Jan,8; 2016,Jan,13; 2015,Jun,10; 2015,Apr,3; 2015,Jan,16; 2014,Jan,11

83015 **Heavy metal (eg, arsenic, barium, beryllium, bismuth, antimony, mercury); qualitative, any number of analytes**
INCLUDES Reinsch test
0.00 0.00 FUD XXX
AMA: 2015,Jun,10; 2015,Apr,3

83018 **quantitative, each, not elsewhere specified**
EXCLUDES *Evaluation of a known heavy metal with a specific code*
0.00 0.00 FUD XXX
AMA: 2015,Jun,10; 2015,Apr,3

83020 **Hemoglobin fractionation and quantitation; electrophoresis (eg, A2, S, C, and/or F)**
0.00 0.00 FUD XXX
AMA: 2015,Jun,10; 2015,Apr,3

83021 **chromatography (eg, A2, S, C, and/or F)**
EXCLUDES *Analysis of glycosylated (A1c) hemoglobin by chromatography or electrophoresis without an identified hemoglobin variant (83036)*
0.00 0.00 FUD XXX
AMA: 2018,Jan,8; 2017,Jan,8; 2016,Jan,13; 2015,Jun,10; 2015,Apr,3; 2015,Jan,16; 2014,Jan,11

83026 **Hemoglobin; by copper sulfate method, non-automated**
0.00 0.00 FUD XXX
AMA: 2015,Jun,10; 2015,Apr,3

83030 **F (fetal), chemical**
0.00 0.00 FUD XXX
AMA: 2015,Jun,10; 2015,Apr,3

83033 **F (fetal), qualitative**
0.00 0.00 FUD XXX
AMA: 2015,Jun,10; 2015,Apr,3

83036 **glycosylated (A1C)**
EXCLUDES *Analysis of glycosylated (A1c) hemoglobin by chromatography or electrophoresis without an identified hemoglobin variant (83020-83021)*
Detection of hemoglobin, fecal, by immunoassay (82274)
0.00 0.00 FUD XXX
AMA: 2018,Jan,8; 2017,Jan,8; 2016,Jan,13; 2015,Jun,10; 2015,Apr,3; 2015,Jan,16; 2014,Jan,11

83037 **glycosylated (A1C) by device cleared by FDA for home use**
0.00 0.00 FUD XXX
AMA: 2018,Jan,8; 2017,Jan,8; 2016,Jan,13; 2015,Jun,10; 2015,Apr,3; 2015,Jan,16; 2014,Jan,11

83045 **methemoglobin, qualitative**
0.00 0.00 FUD XXX
AMA: 2015,Jun,10; 2015,Apr,3

83050 **methemoglobin, quantitative**
EXCLUDES *Transcutaneous methemoglobin test (88741)*
0.00 0.00 FUD XXX
AMA: 2018,Jan,8; 2017,Jan,8; 2016,Jan,13; 2015,Jun,10; 2015,Apr,3; 2015,Jan,16; 2014,Jan,11

83051 **plasma**
0.00 0.00 FUD XXX
AMA: 2015,Jun,10; 2015,Apr,3

83060 **sulfhemoglobin, quantitative**
0.00 0.00 FUD XXX
AMA: 2015,Jun,10; 2015,Apr,3

83065 **thermolabile**
0.00 0.00 FUD XXX
AMA: 2015,Jun,10; 2015,Apr,3

83068 **unstable, screen**
0.00 0.00 FUD XXX
AMA: 2015,Jun,10; 2015,Apr,3

83069 **urine**
0.00 0.00 FUD XXX
AMA: 2015,Jun,10; 2015,Apr,3

83070 **Hemosiderin, qualitative**
EXCLUDES *HIAA (83497)*
Qualitative column chromatography report specific analyte or (82542)
0.00 0.00 FUD XXX
AMA: 2015,Jun,10; 2015,Apr,3

83080 **b-Hexosaminidase, each assay**
0.00 0.00 FUD XXX
AMA: 2015,Jun,10; 2015,Apr,3

83088 **Histamine**
EXCLUDES *Hollander test (43754-43755)*
0.00 0.00 FUD XXX
AMA: 2015,Jun,10; 2015,Apr,3

83090 **Homocysteine**
0.00 0.00 FUD XXX
AMA: 2018,Jan,8; 2017,Jan,8; 2016,Jan,13; 2015,Jun,10; 2015,Apr,3; 2015,Jan,16; 2014,Jan,11

83150 **Homovanillic acid (HVA)**
EXCLUDES *Hormone testing report from alphabetic list in Chemistry section*
Hydrogen/methane breath test (91065)
0.00 0.00 FUD XXX
AMA: 2015,Jun,10; 2015,Apr,3

83491 **Hydroxycorticosteroids, 17- (17-OHCS)**
EXCLUDES *Cortisol (82530, 82533)*
Deoxycortisol (82634)
0.00 0.00 FUD XXX
AMA: 2015,Jun,10; 2015,Apr,3

83497 **Hydroxyindolacetic acid, 5-(HIAA)**
EXCLUDES *5-Hydroxytryptamine (84260)*
Urine qualitative test (81005)
0.00 0.00 FUD XXX
AMA: 2015,Jun,10; 2015,Apr,3

83498 **Hydroxyprogesterone, 17-d**
0.00 0.00 FUD XXX
AMA: 2015,Jun,10; 2015,Apr,3

83500 **Hydroxyproline; free**
0.00 0.00 FUD XXX
AMA: 2015,Jun,10; 2015,Apr,3

83505 **total**
0.00 0.00 FUD XXX
AMA: 2015,Jun,10; 2015,Apr,3

83516 **Immunoassay for analyte other than infectious agent antibody or infectious agent antigen; qualitative or semiquantitative, multiple step method**
0.00 0.00 FUD XXX
AMA: 2015,Jun,10; 2015,Apr,3

83518 **qualitative or semiquantitative, single step method (eg, reagent strip)**
0.00 0.00 FUD XXX
AMA: 2015,Jun,10; 2015,Apr,3

83519 quantitative, by radioimmunoassay (eg, RIA)
0.00 0.00 FUD XXX
AMA: 2018,Jan,8; 2017,Jan,8; 2016,Jan,13; 2015,Jun,10; 2015,Apr,3; 2015,Jan,16; 2014,Jan,11

83520 quantitative, not otherwise specified
EXCLUDES *Immunoassays for antibodies to infectious agent antigen report specific analyte/method from Immunology*
Immunoassay of tumor antigens not elsewhere specified (86316)
Immunoglobulins (82784, 82785)
0.00 0.00 FUD XXX
AMA: 2015,Jun,10; 2015,Apr,3

83525 Insulin; total
EXCLUDES *Proinsulin (84206)*
0.00 0.00 FUD XXX
AMA: 2015,Jun,10; 2015,Apr,3

83527 free
0.00 0.00 FUD XXX
AMA: 2018,Jan,8; 2017,Jan,8; 2016,Jan,13; 2015,Jun,10; 2015,Apr,3; 2015,Jan,16; 2014,Jan,11

83528 Intrinsic factor
EXCLUDES *Intrinsic factor antibodies (86340)*
0.00 0.00 FUD XXX
AMA: 2015,Jun,10; 2015,Apr,3

83540 Iron
0.00 0.00 FUD XXX
AMA: 2018,Jan,8; 2017,Jan,8; 2016,Jan,13; 2015,Jun,10; 2015,Apr,3; 2015,Jan,16; 2014,Jan,11

83550 Iron binding capacity
0.00 0.00 FUD XXX
AMA: 2015,Jun,10; 2015,Apr,3

83570 Isocitric dehydrogenase (IDH)
EXCLUDES *Isonicotinic acid hydrazide, INH, report specific method*
Isopropyl alcohol ([80320])
0.00 0.00 FUD XXX
AMA: 2015,Jun,10; 2015,Apr,3

83582 Ketogenic steroids, fractionation
EXCLUDES *Ketone bodies:*
Serum (82009, 82010)
Urine (81000-81003)
0.00 0.00 FUD XXX
AMA: 2015,Jun,10; 2015,Apr,3

83586 Ketosteroids, 17- (17-KS); total
0.00 0.00 FUD XXX
AMA: 2015,Jun,10; 2015,Apr,3

83593 fractionation
0.00 0.00 FUD XXX
AMA: 2015,Jun,10; 2015,Apr,3

83605 Lactate (lactic acid)
0.00 0.00 FUD XXX
AMA: 2015,Jun,10; 2015,Apr,3

83615 Lactate dehydrogenase (LD), (LDH);
0.00 0.00 FUD XXX
AMA: 2018,Jan,8; 2017,Jan,8; 2016,Jan,13; 2015,Jun,10; 2015,Apr,3; 2015,Jan,16; 2014,Jan,11

83625 isoenzymes, separation and quantitation
0.00 0.00 FUD XXX
AMA: 2018,Jan,8; 2017,Jan,8; 2016,Jan,13; 2015,Jun,10; 2015,Apr,3; 2015,Jan,16; 2014,Jan,11

83630 Lactoferrin, fecal; qualitative
0.00 0.00 FUD XXX
AMA: 2018,Jan,8; 2017,Jan,8; 2016,Jan,13; 2015,Jun,10; 2015,Apr,3; 2015,Jan,16; 2014,Jan,11

83631 quantitative
0.00 0.00 FUD XXX
AMA: 2018,Jan,8; 2017,Jan,8; 2016,Jan,13; 2015,Jun,10; 2015,Apr,3; 2015,Jan,16; 2014,Jan,11

83632 Lactogen, human placental (HPL) human chorionic somatomammotropin M
0.00 0.00 FUD XXX
AMA: 2015,Jun,10; 2015,Apr,3

83633 Lactose, urine, qualitative
EXCLUDES *Lactase deficiency breath hydrogen/methane test (91065)*
Lactose tolerance test (82951, 82952)
0.00 0.00 FUD XXX
AMA: 2015,Jun,10; 2015,Apr,3

83655 Lead
0.00 0.00 FUD XXX
AMA: 2015,Jun,10; 2015,Apr,3

83661 Fetal lung maturity assessment; lecithin sphingomyelin (L/S) ratio M
0.00 0.00 FUD XXX
AMA: 2018,Jan,8; 2017,Jan,8; 2016,Jan,13; 2015,Jun,10; 2015,Apr,3; 2015,Jan,16; 2014,Jan,11

83662 foam stability test M
0.00 0.00 FUD XXX
AMA: 2015,Jun,10; 2015,Apr,3

83663 fluorescence polarization M
0.00 0.00 FUD XXX
AMA: 2015,Jun,10; 2015,Apr,3

83664 lamellar body density M
EXCLUDES *Phosphatidylglycerol (84081)*
0.00 0.00 FUD XXX
AMA: 2015,Jun,10; 2015,Apr,3

83670 Leucine aminopeptidase (LAP)
0.00 0.00 FUD XXX
AMA: 2015,Jun,10; 2015,Apr,3

83690 Lipase
0.00 0.00 FUD XXX
AMA: 2015,Jun,10; 2015,Apr,3

83695-83727 Chemistry: Lipoprotein—Luteinizing Releasing Factor

INCLUDES Clinical information not requested by the ordering physician
Mathematically calculated results
Quantitative analysis unless otherwise specified
Specimens from any source unless otherwise specified

EXCLUDES *Analytes from nonrequested laboratory analysis*
Calculated results that represent a score or probability that was derived by algorithm
Organ or disease panels (80048-80076 [80081])
Therapeutic drug assays (80150-80299 [80164, 80165, 80171])

83695 Lipoprotein (a)
0.00 0.00 FUD XXX
AMA: 2018,Jan,8; 2017,Jan,8; 2016,Jan,13; 2015,Jun,10; 2015,Apr,3; 2015,Jan,16; 2014,Jan,11

83698 Lipoprotein-associated phospholipase A2 (Lp-PLA2)
EXCLUDES *Secretory type II phospholipase A2 (sPLA2-IIA) (0423T)*
0.00 0.00 FUD XXX
AMA: 2015,Jun,10; 2015,Apr,3

83700 Lipoprotein, blood; electrophoretic separation and quantitation
0.00 0.00 FUD XXX
AMA: 2018,Jan,8; 2017,Jan,8; 2016,Jan,13; 2015,Jun,10; 2015,Apr,3; 2015,Jan,16; 2014,Jan,11

83701 **high resolution fractionation and quantitation of lipoproteins including lipoprotein subclasses when performed (eg, electrophoresis, ultracentrifugation)**
0.00 0.00 FUD XXX
AMA: 2018,Jan,8; 2017,Jan,8; 2016,Jan,13; 2015,Jun,10; 2015,Apr,3; 2015,Jan,16; 2014,Jan,11

83704 **quantitation of lipoprotein particle number(s) (eg, by nuclear magnetic resonance spectroscopy), includes lipoprotein particle subclass(es), when performed**
0.00 0.00 FUD XXX
AMA: 2018,Jan,8; 2017,Jan,8; 2016,Jan,13; 2015,Jun,10; 2015,Apr,3; 2015,Jan,16; 2014,Jan,11

83718 **Lipoprotein, direct measurement; high density cholesterol (HDL cholesterol)**
0.00 0.00 FUD XXX
AMA: 2018,Jan,8; 2017,Jan,8; 2016,Jan,13; 2015,Jun,10; 2015,Apr,3; 2015,Jan,16; 2014,Jan,11

83719 **VLDL cholesterol**
0.00 0.00 FUD XXX
AMA: 2018,Jan,8; 2017,Jan,8; 2016,Jan,13; 2015,Jun,10; 2015,Apr,3; 2015,Jan,16; 2014,Jan,11

83721 **LDL cholesterol**
EXCLUDES *Fractionation by high resolution electrophoresis or ultracentrifugation (83701)*
Lipoprotein particle numbers and subclasses analysis by nuclear magnetic resonance spectroscopy (83704)
0.00 0.00 FUD XXX
AMA: 2018,Jan,8; 2017,Jan,8; 2016,Jan,13; 2015,Jun,10; 2015,Apr,3; 2015,Jan,16; 2014,Jan,11

83722 **small dense LDL cholesterol**
0.00 0.00 FUD XXX
EXCLUDES *Fractionation by high resolution electrophoresis or ultracentrifugation (83701)*
Lipoprotein particle numbers/subclass analysis by nuclear magnetic resonance spectroscopy (83704)

83727 **Luteinizing releasing factor (LRH)**
EXCLUDES *alpha-2-Macroglobulin (86329)*
Luteinizing hormone (LH) (83002)
0.00 0.00 FUD XXX
AMA: 2015,Jun,10; 2015,Apr,3

83735-83885 Chemistry: Magnesium—Nickel

INCLUDES Clinical information not requested by the ordering physician
Mathematically calculated results
Quantitative analysis unless otherwise specified
Specimens from any source unless otherwise specified

EXCLUDES *Analytes from nonrequested laboratory analysis*
Calculated results that represent a score or probability that was derived by algorithm
Organ or disease panels (80048-80076 [80081])
Therapeutic drug assays (80150-80299 [80164, 80165, 80171])

83735 **Magnesium**
0.00 0.00 FUD XXX
AMA: 2015,Jun,10; 2015,Apr,3

83775 **Malate dehydrogenase**
EXCLUDES *Maltose tolerance (82951, 82952)*
Mammotropin (84146)
0.00 0.00 FUD XXX
AMA: 2015,Jun,10; 2015,Apr,3

83785 **Manganese**
0.00 0.00 FUD XXX
AMA: 2015,Jun,10; 2015,Apr,3

83789 **Mass spectrometry and tandem mass spectrometry (eg, MS, MS/MS, MALDI, MS-TOF, QTOF), non-drug analyte(s) not elsewhere specified, qualitative or quantitative, each specimen**
EXCLUDES *Column chromatography/mass spectrometry of drugs or substances ([80305], [80306], [80307], [80320, 80321, 80322, 80323, 80324, 80325, 80326, 80327, 80328, 80329, 80330, 80331, 80332, 80333, 80334, 80335, 80336, 80337, 80338, 80339, 80340, 80341, 80342, 80343, 80344, 80345, 80346, 80347, 80348, 80349, 80350, 80351, 80352, 80353, 80354, 80355, 80356, 80357, 80358, 80359, 80360, 80361, 80362, 80363, 80364, 80365, 80366, 80367, 80368, 80369, 80370, 80371, 80372, 80373, 80374, 80375, 80376, 80377, 83992])*
Procedure performed more than one time per specimen
Report specific analyte testing with code(s) from Chemistry section
0.00 0.00 FUD XXX
AMA: 2015,Jun,10; 2015,Apr,3

83825 **Mercury, quantitative**
EXCLUDES *Mercury screen (83015)*
0.00 0.00 FUD XXX
AMA: 2015,Jun,10; 2015,Apr,3

83835 **Metanephrines**
EXCLUDES *Catecholamines (82382-82384)*
Methamphetamine ([80324], [80325], [80326])
Methane breath test (91065)
0.00 0.00 FUD XXX
AMA: 2015,Jun,10; 2015,Apr,3

83857 **Methemalbumin**
EXCLUDES *Methemoglobin (83045, 83050)*
Methyl alcohol ([80320])
Microalbumin
Quantitative (82043)
Semiquantitative (82044)
0.00 0.00 FUD XXX
AMA: 2015,Jun,10; 2015,Apr,3

83861 **Microfluidic analysis utilizing an integrated collection and analysis device, tear osmolarity**
EXCLUDES *beta-2 Microglobulin (82232)*
Code also when performed on both eyes 83861 X 2
0.00 0.00 FUD XXX
AMA: 2015,Jun,10; 2015,Apr,3

83864 **Mucopolysaccharides, acid, quantitative**
0.00 0.00 FUD XXX
AMA: 2015,Jun,10; 2015,Apr,3

83872 **Mucin, synovial fluid (Ropes test)**
0.00 0.00 FUD XXX
AMA: 2015,Jun,10; 2015,Apr,3

83873 **Myelin basic protein, cerebrospinal fluid**
EXCLUDES *Oligoclonal bands (83916)*
0.00 0.00 FUD XXX
AMA: 2015,Jun,10; 2015,Apr,3

83874 **Myoglobin**
0.00 0.00 FUD XXX
AMA: 2018,Jan,8; 2017,Jan,8; 2016,Jan,13; 2015,Jun,10; 2015,Apr,3; 2015,Jan,16; 2014,Jan,11

83876 **Myeloperoxidase (MPO)**
0.00 0.00 FUD XXX
AMA: 2015,Jun,10; 2015,Apr,3

83880 **Natriuretic peptide**
0.00 0.00 FUD XXX
AMA: 2018,Jan,8; 2017,Jan,8; 2016,Jan,13; 2015,Jun,10; 2015,Apr,3; 2015,Jan,16; 2014,Jan,11

83883 **Nephelometry, each analyte not elsewhere specified**
0.00 0.00 FUD XXX
AMA: 2015,Jun,10; 2015,Apr,3

83885 **Nickel**
0.00 0.00 FUD XXX
AMA: 2015,Jun,10; 2015,Apr,3

83915-84066 Chemistry: Nucleotidase 5'-—Phosphatase (Acid)

INCLUDES Clinical information not requested by the ordering physician
Mathematically calculated results
Quantitative analysis unless otherwise specified
Specimens from any source unless otherwise specified

EXCLUDES *Analytes from nonrequested laboratory analysis*
Calculated results that represent a score or probability that was derived by algorithm
Drug testing ([80305, 80306, 80307], [80324, 80325, 80326, 80327, 80328, 80329, 80330, 80331, 80332, 80333, 80334, 80335, 80336, 80337, 80338, 80339, 80340, 80341, 80342, 80343, 80344, 80345, 80346, 80347, 80348, 80349, 80350, 80351, 80352, 80353, 80354, 80355, 80356, 80357, 80358, 80359, 80360, 80361, 80362, 80363, 80364, 80365, 80366, 80367, 80368, 80369, 80370, 80371, 80372, 80373, 80374, 80375, 80376, 80377, 83992])
Organ or disease panels (80048-80076 [80081])
Therapeutic drug assays (80150-80299 [80164, 80165, 80171])

83915 **Nucleotidase 5'-**
0.00 0.00 FUD XXX
AMA: 2015,Jun,10; 2015,Apr,3

83916 **Oligoclonal immune (oligoclonal bands)**
0.00 0.00 FUD XXX
AMA: 2015,Jun,10; 2015,Apr,3

83918 **Organic acids; total, quantitative, each specimen**
0.00 0.00 FUD XXX
AMA: 2018,Jan,8; 2017,Jan,8; 2016,Jan,13; 2015,Jun,10; 2015,Apr,3; 2015,Jan,16; 2014,Jan,11

83919 **qualitative, each specimen**
0.00 0.00 FUD XXX
AMA: 2015,Jun,10; 2015,Apr,3

83921 **Organic acid, single, quantitative**
0.00 0.00 FUD XXX
AMA: 2015,Jun,10; 2015,Apr,3

83930 **Osmolality; blood**
EXCLUDES *Tear osmolarity (83861)*
0.00 0.00 FUD XXX
AMA: 2015,Jun,10; 2015,Apr,3

83935 **urine**
EXCLUDES *Tear osmolarity (83861)*
0.00 0.00 FUD XXX
AMA: 2015,Jun,10; 2015,Apr,3

83937 **Osteocalcin (bone g1a protein)**
0.00 0.00 FUD XXX
AMA: 2018,Jan,8; 2017,Jan,8; 2016,Jan,13; 2015,Jun,10; 2015,Apr,3; 2015,Jan,16; 2014,Jan,11

83945 **Oxalate**
0.00 0.00 FUD XXX
AMA: 2015,Jun,10; 2015,Apr,3

83950 **Oncoprotein; HER-2/neu**
EXCLUDES *Tissue (88342, 88365)*
0.00 0.00 FUD XXX
AMA: 2015,Jun,10; 2015,Apr,3

83951 **des-gamma-carboxy-prothrombin (DCP)**
0.00 0.00 FUD XXX
AMA: 2015,Jun,10; 2015,Apr,3

83970 **Parathormone (parathyroid hormone)**
EXCLUDES *Chlorinated hydrocarbon screen (82441)*
Quantitative pesticide report code for specific method
0.00 0.00 FUD XXX
AMA: 2015,Jun,10; 2015,Apr,3

83986 **pH; body fluid, not otherwise specified**
EXCLUDES *Blood pH (82800, 82803)*
0.00 0.00 FUD XXX
AMA: 2018,Jan,8; 2017,Jan,8; 2016,May,13; 2016,Jan,13; 2015,Jun,10; 2015,Apr,3; 2015,Jan,16

83987 **exhaled breath condensate**
EXCLUDES *Blood pH (82800, 82803)*
Phenobarbital ([80345])
0.00 0.00 FUD XXX
AMA: 2015,Jun,10; 2015,Apr,3

83992 **Resequenced code. See code following resequenced code 80365.**

83993 **Calprotectin, fecal**
0.00 0.00 FUD XXX
AMA: 2018,Jan,8; 2017,Jan,8; 2016,Jan,13; 2015,Jun,10; 2015,Apr,3; 2015,Jan,16; 2014,Jan,11

84030 **Phenylalanine (PKU), blood**
INCLUDES Guthrie test
EXCLUDES *Phenylalanine-tyrosine ratio (84030, 84510)*
0.00 0.00 FUD XXX
AMA: 2015,Jun,10; 2015,Apr,3

84035 **Phenylketones, qualitative**
0.00 0.00 FUD XXX
AMA: 2015,Jun,10; 2015,Apr,3

84060 **Phosphatase, acid; total**
0.00 0.00 FUD XXX
AMA: 2015,Jun,10; 2015,Apr,3

84066 **prostatic**
0.00 0.00 FUD XXX
AMA: 2015,Jun,10; 2015,Apr,3

84075-84080 Chemistry: Phosphatase (Alkaline)

CMS: 100-03,160.17 Payment for L-Dopa /Associated Inpatient Hospital Services

INCLUDES Clinical information not requested by the ordering physician
Mathematically calculated results
Quantitative analysis unless otherwise specified
Specimens from any source unless otherwise specified

EXCLUDES *Analytes from nonrequested laboratory analysis*
Calculated results that represent a score or probability that was derived by algorithm
Organ or disease panels (80048-80076 [80081])

84075 **Phosphatase, alkaline;**
0.00 0.00 FUD XXX
AMA: 2018,Jan,8; 2017,Jan,8; 2016,Jan,13; 2015,Jun,10; 2015,Apr,3; 2015,Jan,16; 2014,Jan,11

84078 **heat stable (total not included)**
0.00 0.00 FUD XXX
AMA: 2015,Jun,10; 2015,Apr,3

84080 **isoenzymes**
0.00 0.00 FUD XXX
AMA: 2015,Jun,10; 2015,Apr,3

84081-84150 Chemistry: Phosphatidylglycerol—Prostaglandin

INCLUDES Clinical information not requested by the ordering physician
Mathematically calculated results
Quantitative analysis unless otherwise specified
Specimens from any source unless otherwise specified

EXCLUDES *Analytes from nonrequested laboratory analysis*
Calculated results that represent a score or probability that was derived by algorithm
Organ or disease panels (80048-80076 [80081])
Therapeutic drug assays (80150-80299 [80164, 80165, 80171])

84081 **Phosphatidylglycerol**
EXCLUDES *Cholinesterase (82480, 82482)*
Inorganic phosphates (84100)
Organic phosphates, report code for specific method
0.00 0.00 FUD XXX
AMA: 2015,Jun,10; 2015,Apr,3

84085 **Phosphogluconate, 6-, dehydrogenase, RBC**
0.00 0.00 FUD XXX
AMA: 2015,Jun,10; 2015,Apr,3

84087 **Phosphohexose isomerase**
0.00 0.00 FUD XXX
AMA: 2015,Jun,10; 2015,Apr,3

84100 **Phosphorus inorganic (phosphate);**
0.00 0.00 FUD XXX
AMA: 2018,Jan,8; 2017,Jan,8; 2016,Jan,13; 2015,Jun,10; 2015,Apr,3; 2015,Jan,16; 2014,Jan,11

84105 **urine**
EXCLUDES *Pituitary gonadotropins (83001-83002)*
PKU (84030, 84035)
0.00 0.00 FUD XXX
AMA: 2015,Jun,10; 2015,Apr,3

84106 **Porphobilinogen, urine; qualitative**
0.00 0.00 FUD XXX
AMA: 2015,Jun,10; 2015,Apr,3

84110 **quantitative**
0.00 0.00 FUD XXX
AMA: 2015,Jun,10; 2015,Apr,3

84112 **Evaluation of cervicovaginal fluid for specific amniotic fluid protein(s) (eg, placental alpha microglobulin-1 [PAMG-1], placental protein 12 [PP12], alpha-fetoprotein), qualitative, each specimen** ♀
0.00 0.00 FUD XXX
AMA: 2015,Jun,10; 2015,Apr,3

84119 **Porphyrins, urine; qualitative**
0.00 0.00 FUD XXX
AMA: 2015,Jun,10; 2015,Apr,3

84120 **quantitation and fractionation**
0.00 0.00 FUD XXX
AMA: 2015,Jun,10; 2015,Apr,3

84126 **Porphyrins, feces, quantitative**
EXCLUDES *Porphyrin precursors (82135, 84106, 84110)*
Protoporphyrin, RBC (84202, 84203)
0.00 0.00 FUD XXX
AMA: 2015,Jun,10; 2015,Apr,3

84132 **Potassium; serum, plasma or whole blood**
0.00 0.00 FUD XXX
AMA: 2018,Jan,8; 2017,Jan,8; 2016,Jan,13; 2015,Jun,10; 2015,Apr,3; 2015,Jan,16; 2014,Jan,11

84133 **urine**
0.00 0.00 FUD XXX
AMA: 2015,Jun,10; 2015,Apr,3

84134 **Prealbumin**
EXCLUDES *Microalbumin (82043-82044)*
0.00 0.00 FUD XXX
AMA: 2015,Jun,10; 2015,Apr,3

84135 **Pregnanediol** ♀
0.00 0.00 FUD XXX
AMA: 2015,Jun,10; 2015,Apr,3

84138 **Pregnanetriol** ♀
0.00 0.00 FUD XXX
AMA: 2015,Jun,10; 2015,Apr,3

84140 **Pregnenolone**
0.00 0.00 FUD XXX
AMA: 2018,Jan,8; 2017,Jan,8; 2016,Jan,13; 2015,Jun,10; 2015,Apr,3; 2015,Jan,16; 2014,Jan,11

84143 **17-hydroxypregnenolone**
0.00 0.00 FUD XXX
AMA: 2018,Jan,8; 2017,Jan,8; 2016,Jan,13; 2015,Jun,10; 2015,Apr,3; 2015,Jan,16; 2014,Jan,11

84144 **Progesterone**
EXCLUDES *Progesterone receptor assay (84234)*
Proinsulin (84206)
0.00 0.00 FUD XXX
AMA: 2015,Jun,10; 2015,Apr,3

84145 **Procalcitonin (PCT)**
0.00 0.00 FUD XXX
AMA: 2015,Jun,10; 2015,Apr,3

84146 **Prolactin**
0.00 0.00 FUD XXX
AMA: 2015,Jun,10; 2015,Apr,3

84150 **Prostaglandin, each**
0.00 0.00 FUD XXX
AMA: 2015,Jun,10; 2015,Apr,3

84152-84154 Chemistry: Prostate Specific Antigen

CMS: 100-03,190.31 Prostate Specific Antigen (PSA); 100-03,210.1 Prostate Cancer Screening Tests

INCLUDES Clinical information not requested by the ordering physician
Mathematically calculated results
Quantitative analysis unless otherwise specified

EXCLUDES *Analytes from nonrequested laboratory analysis*
Calculated results that represent a score or probability that was derived by algorithm

84152 **Prostate specific antigen (PSA); complexed (direct measurement)** ♂
0.00 0.00 FUD XXX
AMA: 2015,Jun,10; 2015,Apr,3

84153 **total** ♂
0.00 0.00 FUD XXX
AMA: 2018,Jan,8; 2017,Jan,8; 2016,Jan,13; 2015,Jun,10; 2015,Apr,3; 2015,Jan,16; 2014,Jan,11

84154 **free** ♂
0.00 0.00 FUD XXX
AMA: 2018,Jan,8; 2017,Jan,8; 2016,Jan,13; 2015,Jun,10; 2015,Apr,3; 2015,Jan,16; 2014,Jan,11

84155-84157 Chemistry: Protein, Total (Not by Refractometry)

INCLUDES Clinical information not requested by the ordering physician
Mathematically calculated results

EXCLUDES *Analytes from nonrequested laboratory analysis*
Calculated results that represent a score or probability that was derived by algorithm
Organ or disease panels (80048-80076 [80081])

84155 **Protein, total, except by refractometry; serum, plasma or whole blood**
0.00 0.00 FUD XXX
AMA: 2018,Jan,8; 2017,Jan,8; 2016,Jan,13; 2015,Jun,10; 2015,Apr,3; 2015,Jan,16; 2014,Jan,11

84156 **urine**
0.00 0.00 FUD XXX
AMA: 2015,Jun,10; 2015,Apr,3

84157 **other source (eg, synovial fluid, cerebrospinal fluid)**
0.00 0.00 FUD XXX
AMA: 2015,Jun,10; 2015,Apr,3

84160-84432 Chemistry: Protein, Total (Refractometry)—Thyroglobulin

INCLUDES Clinical information not requested by the ordering physician
Mathematically calculated results
Quantitative analysis unless otherwise specified
Specimens from any source unless otherwise specified

EXCLUDES *Analytes from nonrequested laboratory analysis*
Calculated results that represent a score or probability that was derived by algorithm
Drug testing ([80305, 80306, 80307], [80324, 80325, 80326, 80327, 80328, 80329, 80330, 80331, 80332, 80333, 80334, 80335, 80336, 80337, 80338, 80339, 80340, 80341, 80342, 80343, 80344, 80345, 80346, 80347, 80348, 80349, 80350, 80351, 80352, 80353, 80354, 80355, 80356, 80357, 80358, 80359, 80360, 80361, 80362, 80363, 80364, 80365, 80366, 80367, 80368, 80369, 80370, 80371, 80372, 80373, 80374, 80375, 80376, 80377, 83992])
Organ or disease panels (80048-80076 [80081])
Therapeutic drug assays (80150-80299 [80164, 80165, 80171])

84160 **Protein, total, by refractometry, any source**
EXCLUDES *Urine total protein, dipstick method (81000-81003)*
0.00 0.00 FUD XXX
AMA: 2015,Jun,10; 2015,Apr,3

84163 **Pregnancy-associated plasma protein-A (PAPP-A)** ♀
0.00 0.00 FUD XXX
AMA: 2015,Jun,10; 2015,Apr,3

84165 Protein; electrophoretic fractionation and quantitation, serum
0.00 0.00 FUD XXX
AMA: 2015,Jun,10; 2015,Apr,3

84166 electrophoretic fractionation and quantitation, other fluids with concentration (eg, urine, CSF)
0.00 0.00 FUD XXX
AMA: 2015,Jun,10; 2015,Apr,3

84181 Western Blot, with interpretation and report, blood or other body fluid
0.00 0.00 FUD XXX
AMA: 2015,Jun,10; 2015,Apr,3

84182 Western Blot, with interpretation and report, blood or other body fluid, immunological probe for band identification, each
EXCLUDES *Western Blot tissue analysis (88371)*
0.00 0.00 FUD XXX
AMA: 2015,Jun,10; 2015,Apr,3

84202 Protoporphyrin, RBC; quantitative
0.00 0.00 FUD XXX
AMA: 2015,Jun,10; 2015,Apr,3

84203 screen
0.00 0.00 FUD XXX
AMA: 2015,Jun,10; 2015,Apr,3

84206 Proinsulin
EXCLUDES *Pseudocholinesterase (82480)*
0.00 0.00 FUD XXX
AMA: 2015,Jun,10; 2015,Apr,3

84207 Pyridoxal phosphate (Vitamin B-6)
0.00 0.00 FUD XXX
AMA: 2015,Jun,10; 2015,Apr,3

84210 Pyruvate
0.00 0.00 FUD XXX
AMA: 2015,Jun,10; 2015,Apr,3

84220 Pyruvate kinase
0.00 0.00 FUD XXX
AMA: 2015,Jun,10; 2015,Apr,3

84228 Quinine
0.00 0.00 FUD XXX
AMA: 2018,Jan,8; 2017,Jan,8; 2016,Jan,13; 2015,Jun,10; 2015,Apr,3

84233 Receptor assay; estrogen
0.00 0.00 FUD XXX
AMA: 2015,Jun,10; 2015,Apr,3

84234 progesterone
0.00 0.00 FUD XXX
AMA: 2015,Jun,10; 2015,Apr,3

84235 endocrine, other than estrogen or progesterone (specify hormone)
0.00 0.00 FUD XXX
AMA: 2015,Jun,10; 2015,Apr,3

84238 non-endocrine (specify receptor)
0.00 0.00 FUD XXX
AMA: 2018,Jan,8; 2017,Jan,8; 2016,Jan,13; 2015,Jun,10; 2015,Apr,3; 2015,Jan,16; 2014,Jan,11

84244 Renin
0.00 0.00 FUD XXX
AMA: 2015,Jun,10; 2015,Apr,3

84252 Riboflavin (Vitamin B-2)
EXCLUDES *Salicylates ([80329], [80330], [80331])*
Secretin test reported with appropriate analyses (43756, 43757, 99070)
0.00 0.00 FUD XXX
AMA: 2015,Jun,10; 2015,Apr,3

84255 Selenium
0.00 0.00 FUD XXX
AMA: 2015,Jun,10; 2015,Apr,3

84260 Serotonin
EXCLUDES *Urine metabolites (HIAA) (83497)*
0.00 0.00 FUD XXX
AMA: 2015,Jun,10; 2015,Apr,3

84270 Sex hormone binding globulin (SHBG)
0.00 0.00 FUD XXX
AMA: 2018,Jan,8; 2017,Jan,8; 2016,Jan,13; 2015,Jun,10; 2015,Apr,3; 2015,Jan,16; 2014,Jan,11

84275 Sialic acid
EXCLUDES *Sickle hemoglobin (85660)*
0.00 0.00 FUD XXX
AMA: 2015,Jun,10; 2015,Apr,3

84285 Silica
0.00 0.00 FUD XXX
AMA: 2015,Jun,10; 2015,Apr,3

84295 Sodium; serum, plasma or whole blood
0.00 0.00 FUD XXX
AMA: 2018,Jan,8; 2017,Jan,8; 2016,Jan,13; 2015,Jun,10; 2015,Apr,3; 2015,Jan,16; 2014,Jan,11

84300 urine
0.00 0.00 FUD XXX
AMA: 2015,Jun,10; 2015,Apr,3

84302 other source
EXCLUDES *Somatomammotropin (83632)*
Somatotropin (83003)
0.00 0.00 FUD XXX
AMA: 2018,Jan,8; 2017,Jan,8; 2016,Jan,13; 2015,Jun,10; 2015,Apr,3; 2015,Jan,16; 2014,Jan,11

84305 Somatomedin
0.00 0.00 FUD XXX
AMA: 2018,Jan,8; 2017,Jan,8; 2016,Jan,13; 2015,Jun,10; 2015,Apr,3; 2015,Jan,16; 2014,Jan,11

84307 Somatostatin
0.00 0.00 FUD XXX
AMA: 2018,Jan,8; 2017,Jan,8; 2016,Jan,13; 2015,Jun,10; 2015,Apr,3; 2015,Jan,16; 2014,Jan,11

84311 Spectrophotometry, analyte not elsewhere specified
0.00 0.00 FUD XXX
AMA: 2015,Jun,10; 2015,Apr,3

84315 Specific gravity (except urine)
EXCLUDES *Stone analysis (82355-82370)*
Suppression of growth stimulation expressed gene 2 [ST2] testing (83006)
Urine specific gravity (81000-81003)
0.00 0.00 FUD XXX
AMA: 2015,Jun,10; 2015,Apr,3

84375 Sugars, chromatographic, TLC or paper chromatography
0.00 0.00 FUD XXX
AMA: 2015,Jun,10; 2015,Apr,3

84376 Sugars (mono-, di-, and oligosaccharides); single qualitative, each specimen
0.00 0.00 FUD XXX
AMA: 2018,Jan,8; 2017,Jan,8; 2016,Jan,13; 2015,Jun,10; 2015,Apr,3; 2015,Jan,16; 2014,Jan,11

84377 multiple qualitative, each specimen
0.00 0.00 FUD XXX
AMA: 2018,Jan,8; 2017,Jan,8; 2016,Jan,13; 2015,Jun,10; 2015,Apr,3; 2015,Jan,16; 2014,Jan,11

84378 single quantitative, each specimen
0.00 0.00 FUD XXX
AMA: 2015,Jun,10; 2015,Apr,3

84379 multiple quantitative, each specimen
0.00 0.00 FUD XXX
AMA: 2018,Jan,8; 2017,Jan,8; 2016,Jan,13; 2015,Jun,10; 2015,Apr,3; 2015,Jan,16; 2014,Jan,11

84392 Sulfate, urine
EXCLUDES *Sulfhemoglobin (83060)*
T-3 (84479-84481)
T-4 (84436-84439)
0.00 0.00 FUD XXX
AMA: 2015,Jun,10; 2015,Apr,3

84402 Testosterone; free
EXCLUDES *Anabolic steroids ([80327, 80328])*
0.00 0.00 FUD XXX
AMA: 2015,Jun,10; 2015,Apr,3

84403 total
EXCLUDES *Anabolic steroids ([80327, 80328])*
0.00 0.00 FUD XXX
AMA: 2015,Jun,10; 2015,Apr,3

84410 bioavailable, direct measurement (eg, differential precipitation)
0.00 0.00 FUD XXX

84425 Thiamine (Vitamin B-1)
0.00 0.00 FUD XXX
AMA: 2015,Jun,10; 2015,Apr,3

84430 Thiocyanate
0.00 0.00 FUD XXX
AMA: 2015,Jun,10; 2015,Apr,3

84431 Thromboxane metabolite(s), including thromboxane if performed, urine
Code also for determination of concurrent urine creatinine (82570)
0.00 0.00 FUD XXX
AMA: 2015,Jun,10; 2015,Apr,3

84432 Thyroglobulin
EXCLUDES *Thyroglobulin antibody (86800)*
Thyrotropin releasing hormone (TRH) (80438, 80439)
0.00 0.00 FUD XXX
AMA: 2018,Jan,8; 2017,Jan,8; 2016,Jan,13; 2015,Jun,10; 2015,Apr,3; 2015,Jan,16; 2014,Jan,11

84436-84445 Chemistry: Thyroid Tests

CMS: 100-03,190.22 Thyroid Testing

INCLUDES Clinical information not requested by the ordering physician
Mathematically calculated results
Quantitative analysis unless otherwise specified
Specimens from any source unless otherwise specified

EXCLUDES *Analytes from nonrequested laboratory analysis*
Calculated results that represent a score or probability that was derived by algorithm
Organ or disease panels (80048-80076 [80081])
Therapeutic drug assays (80150-80299 [80164, 80165, 80171])

84436 Thyroxine; total
0.00 0.00 FUD XXX
AMA: 2018,Jan,8; 2017,Jan,8; 2016,Jan,13; 2015,Jun,10; 2015,Apr,3; 2015,Jan,16; 2014,Jan,11

84437 requiring elution (eg, neonatal)
0.00 0.00 FUD XXX
AMA: 2015,Jun,10; 2015,Apr,3

84439 free
0.00 0.00 FUD XXX
AMA: 2015,Jun,10; 2015,Apr,3

84442 Thyroxine binding globulin (TBG)
0.00 0.00 FUD XXX
AMA: 2015,Jun,10; 2015,Apr,3

84443 Thyroid stimulating hormone (TSH)
0.00 0.00 FUD XXX
AMA: 2015,Jun,10; 2015,Apr,3

84445 Thyroid stimulating immune globulins (TSI)
EXCLUDES *Tobramycin (80200)*
0.00 0.00 FUD XXX
AMA: 2018,Jan,8; 2017,Jan,8; 2016,Jan,13; 2015,Jun,10; 2015,Apr,3; 2015,Jan,16; 2014,Jan,11

84446-84449 Chemistry: Tocopherol Alpha—Transcortin

INCLUDES Clinical information not requested by the ordering physician
Mathematically calculated results
Quantitative analysis unless otherwise specified
Specimens from any source unless otherwise specified

EXCLUDES *Analytes from nonrequested laboratory analysis*
Calculated results that represent a score or probability that was derived by algorithm
Organ or disease panels (80048-80076 [80081])
Therapeutic drug assays (80150-80299 [80164, 80165, 80171])

84446 Tocopherol alpha (Vitamin E)
0.00 0.00 FUD XXX
AMA: 2015,Jun,10; 2015,Apr,3

84449 Transcortin (cortisol binding globulin)
0.00 0.00 FUD XXX
AMA: 2018,Jan,8; 2017,Jan,8; 2016,Jan,13; 2015,Jun,10; 2015,Apr,3; 2015,Jan,16; 2014,Jan,11

84450-84460 Chemistry: Transferase

CMS: 100-02,11,30.2.2 Automated Multi-Channel Chemistry (AMCC) Tests; 100-03,160.17 Payment for L-Dopa /Associated Inpatient Hospital Services; 100-04,16,40.6.1 Automated Multi-Channel Chemistry (AMCC) Tests for ESRD Beneficiaries; 100-04,16,70.8 CLIA Waived Tests

INCLUDES Clinical information not requested by the ordering physician
Mathematically calculated results
Quantitative analysis unless otherwise specified

EXCLUDES *Analytes from nonrequested laboratory analysis*
Calculated results that represent a score or probability that was derived by algorithm

84450 Transferase; aspartate amino (AST) (SGOT)
0.00 0.00 FUD XXX
AMA: 2018,Jan,8; 2017,Jan,8; 2016,Jan,13; 2015,Jun,10; 2015,Apr,3; 2015,Jan,16; 2014,Jan,11

84460 alanine amino (ALT) (SGPT)
0.00 0.00 FUD XXX
AMA: 2018,Jan,8; 2017,Jan,8; 2016,Jan,13; 2015,Jun,10; 2015,Apr,3; 2015,Jan,16; 2014,Jan,11

84466 Chemistry: Transferrin

CMS: 100-02,11,20.2 ESRD Laboratory Services; 100-03,190.18 Serum Iron Studies

INCLUDES Clinical information not requested by the ordering physician
Mathematically calculated results
Quantitative analysis unless otherwise specified

EXCLUDES *Analytes from nonrequested laboratory analysis*
Calculated results that represent a score or probability that was derived by algorithm

84466 Transferrin
EXCLUDES *Iron binding capacity (83550)*
0.00 0.00 FUD XXX
AMA: 2018,Jan,8; 2017,Jan,8; 2016,Jan,13; 2015,Jun,10; 2015,Apr,3; 2015,Jan,16; 2014,Jan,11

84478 Chemistry: Triglycerides

CMS: 100-02,11,30.2.2 Automated Multi-Channel Chemistry (AMCC) Tests; 100-03,190.23 Lipid Testing; 100-04,16,70.8 CLIA Waived Tests; 100-04,16,90.2 Organ or Disease Oriented Panels

INCLUDES Clinical information not requested by the ordering physician
Mathematically calculated results

EXCLUDES *Analytes from nonrequested laboratory analysis*
Calculated results that represent a score or probability that was derived by algorithm
Organ or disease panels (80048-80076 [80081])

84478 Triglycerides
0.00 0.00 FUD XXX
AMA: 2018,Jan,8; 2017,Jan,8; 2016,Jan,13; 2015,Jun,10; 2015,Apr,3; 2015,Jan,16; 2014,Jan,11

84479-84482 Chemistry: Thyroid Hormone—Triiodothyronine

CMS: 100-03,190.22 Thyroid Testing

INCLUDES Clinical information not requested by the ordering physician
Mathematically calculated results
Quantitative analysis unless otherwise specified
Specimens from any source unless otherwise specified

EXCLUDES *Analytes from nonrequested laboratory analysis*
Calculated results that represent a score or probability that was derived by algorithm
Organ or disease panels (80048-80076 [80081])

84479 Thyroid hormone (T3 or T4) uptake or thyroid hormone binding ratio (THBR)
0.00 0.00 FUD XXX
AMA: 2018,Jan,8; 2017,Jan,8; 2016,Jan,13; 2015,Jun,10; 2015,Apr,3; 2015,Jan,16; 2014,Jan,11

84480 Triiodothyronine T3; total (TT-3)
0.00 0.00 FUD XXX
AMA: 2015,Jun,10; 2015,Apr,3

84481 free
0.00 0.00 FUD XXX
AMA: 2015,Jun,10; 2015,Apr,3

84482 reverse
0.00 0.00 FUD XXX
AMA: 2018,Jan,8; 2017,Jan,8; 2016,Jan,13; 2015,Jun,10; 2015,Apr,3; 2015,Jan,16; 2014,Jan,11

84484-84512 Chemistry: Troponin (Quantitative)—Troponin (Qualitative)

INCLUDES Clinical information not requested by the ordering physician
Mathematically calculated results
Specimens from any source unless otherwise specified

EXCLUDES *Analytes from nonrequested laboratory analysis*
Calculated results that represent a score or probability that was derived by algorithm
Organ or disease panels

84484 Troponin, quantitative
EXCLUDES *Qualitative troponin assay (84512)*
0.00 0.00 FUD XXX
AMA: 2018,Jan,8; 2017,Jan,8; 2016,Jan,13; 2015,Jun,10; 2015,Apr,3; 2015,Jan,16; 2014,Jan,11

84485 Trypsin; duodenal fluid
0.00 0.00 FUD XXX
AMA: 2015,Jun,10; 2015,Apr,3

84488 feces, qualitative
0.00 0.00 FUD XXX
AMA: 2015,Jun,10; 2015,Apr,3

84490 feces, quantitative, 24-hour collection
0.00 0.00 FUD XXX
AMA: 2015,Jun,10; 2015,Apr,3

84510 Tyrosine
EXCLUDES *Urate crystal identification (89060)*
0.00 0.00 FUD XXX
AMA: 2015,Jun,10; 2015,Apr,3

84512 Troponin, qualitative
EXCLUDES *Quantitative troponin assay (84484)*
0.00 0.00 FUD XXX
AMA: 2018,Jan,8; 2017,Jan,8; 2016,Jan,13; 2015,Jun,10; 2015,Apr,3; 2015,Jan,16; 2014,Jan,11

84520-84525 Chemistry: Urea Nitrogen (Blood)

CMS: 100-03,160.17 Payment for L-Dopa /Associated Inpatient Hospital Services

INCLUDES Clinical information not requested by the ordering physician
Mathematically calculated results

EXCLUDES *Analytes from nonrequested laboratory analysis*
Calculated results that represent a score or probability that was derived by algorithm
Organ or disease panels (80048-80076 [80081])

84520 Urea nitrogen; quantitative
0.00 0.00 FUD XXX
AMA: 2018,Jan,8; 2017,Jan,8; 2016,Jan,13; 2015,Jun,10; 2015,Apr,3; 2015,Jan,16; 2014,Jan,11

84525 semiquantitative (eg, reagent strip test)
INCLUDES Patterson's test
0.00 0.00 FUD XXX
AMA: 2018,Jan,8; 2017,Jan,8; 2016,Jan,13; 2015,Jun,10; 2015,Apr,3; 2015,Jan,16; 2014,Jan,11

84540-84630 Chemistry: Urea Nitrogen (Urine)—Zinc

INCLUDES Clinical information not requested by the ordering physician
Mathematically calculated results
Quantitative analysis unless otherwise specified
Specimens from any source unless otherwise specified

EXCLUDES *Analytes from nonrequested laboratory analysis*
Calculated results that represent a score or probability that was derived by algorithm
Organ or disease panels (80048-80076 [80081])
Therapeutic drug assays (80150-80299 [80164, 80165, 80171])

84540 Urea nitrogen, urine
0.00 0.00 FUD XXX
AMA: 2015,Jun,10; 2015,Apr,3

84545 Urea nitrogen, clearance
0.00 0.00 FUD XXX
AMA: 2015,Jun,10; 2015,Apr,3

84550 Uric acid; blood
0.00 0.00 FUD XXX
AMA: 2018,Jan,8; 2017,Jan,8; 2016,Jan,13; 2015,Jun,10; 2015,Apr,3; 2015,Jan,16; 2014,Jan,11

84560 other source
0.00 0.00 FUD XXX
AMA: 2015,Jun,10; 2015,Apr,3

84577 Urobilinogen, feces, quantitative
0.00 0.00 FUD XXX
AMA: 2015,Jun,10; 2015,Apr,3

84578 Urobilinogen, urine; qualitative
0.00 0.00 FUD XXX
AMA: 2015,Jun,10; 2015,Apr,3

84580 quantitative, timed specimen
0.00 0.00 FUD XXX
AMA: 2015,Jun,10; 2015,Apr,3

84583 semiquantitative
EXCLUDES *Uroporphyrins (84120)*
Valproic acid (dipropylacetic acid) ([80164])
0.00 0.00 FUD XXX
AMA: 2015,Jun,10; 2015,Apr,3

84585 Vanillylmandelic acid (VMA), urine
0.00 0.00 FUD XXX
AMA: 2015,Jun,10; 2015,Apr,3

84586 Vasoactive intestinal peptide (VIP)
0.00 0.00 FUD XXX
AMA: 2018,Jan,8; 2017,Jan,8; 2016,Jan,13; 2015,Jun,10; 2015,Apr,3; 2015,Jan,16; 2014,Jan,11

84588 Vasopressin (antidiuretic hormone, ADH)
0.00 0.00 FUD XXX
AMA: 2018,Jan,7; 2015,Jun,10; 2015,Apr,3

84590 **Vitamin A**

EXCLUDES *Vitamin B-1 (84425)*
Vitamin B-2 (84252)
Vitamin B-6 (84207)
Vitamin B-12 (82607)
Vitamin C (82180)
Vitamin D (82306, [82652])
Vitamin E (84446)

0.00 0.00 FUD XXX

AMA: 2015,Jun,10; 2015,Apr,3

84591 **Vitamin, not otherwise specified**

0.00 0.00 FUD XXX

AMA: 2015,Jun,10; 2015,Apr,3

84597 **Vitamin K**

EXCLUDES *Vanillylmandelic acid (VMA) (84585)*

0.00 0.00 FUD XXX

AMA: 2015,Jun,10; 2015,Apr,3

84600 **Volatiles (eg, acetic anhydride, diethylether)**

EXCLUDES *Carbon tetrachloride, dichloroethane, dichloromethane (82441)*
Isopropyl alcohol and methanol ([80320])
Volume, blood, RISA, or Cr-51 (78110, 78111)

0.00 0.00 FUD XXX

AMA: 2015,Jun,10; 2015,Apr,3

84620 **Xylose absorption test, blood and/or urine**

EXCLUDES *Administration (99070)*

0.00 0.00 FUD XXX

AMA: 2015,Jun,10; 2015,Apr,3

84630 **Zinc**

0.00 0.00 FUD XXX

AMA: 2015,Jun,10; 2015,Apr,3

84681-84999 Other and Unlisted Chemistry Tests

INCLUDES Clinical information not requested by the ordering physician
Mathematically calculated results
Quantitative analysis unless otherwise specified
Specimens from any source unless otherwise specified

EXCLUDES *Analytes from nonrequested laboratory analysis*
Calculated results that represent a score or probability that was derived by algorithm
Confirmational testing of a not otherwise specified drug ([80375, 80376, 80377], 80299)
Organ or disease panels (80048-80076 [80081])

84681 **C-peptide**

0.00 0.00 FUD XXX

AMA: 2015,Jun,10; 2015,Apr,3

84702 **Gonadotropin, chorionic (hCG); quantitative**

0.00 0.00 FUD XXX

AMA: 2015,Jun,10; 2015,Apr,3

84703 **qualitative**

EXCLUDES *Urine pregnancy test by visual color comparison (81025)*

0.00 0.00 FUD XXX

AMA: 2015,Jun,10; 2015,Apr,3

84704 **free beta chain**

0.00 0.00 FUD XXX

AMA: 2018,Jan,8; 2017,Jan,8; 2016,Jan,13; 2015,Jun,10; 2015,Apr,3; 2015,Jan,16; 2014,Jan,11

84830 **Ovulation tests, by visual color comparison methods for human luteinizing hormone** ♀

0.00 0.00 FUD XXX

AMA: 2018,Jan,8; 2017,Jan,8; 2016,Jan,13; 2015,Jun,10; 2015,Apr,3

84999 **Unlisted chemistry procedure**

EXCLUDES *Definitive drug testing, not otherwise specified ([80375], [80376], [80377], 80299)*

0.00 0.00 FUD XXX

AMA: 2018,Jan,8; 2017,Jan,8; 2016,Jan,13; 2015,Apr,3; 2015,Jan,16; 2014,Jan,11

85002 Bleeding Time Test

EXCLUDES *Agglutinins (86000, 86156, 86157)*
Antiplasmin (85410)
Antithrombin III (85300, 85301)
Blood banking procedures (86077-86079)

85002 **Bleeding time**

0.00 0.00 FUD XXX

AMA: 2018,Jan,8; 2017,Jan,8; 2016,Jan,13; 2015,Jan,16; 2014,Jan,11

85004-85049 Blood Counts

CMS: 100-03,190.15 Blood Counts

EXCLUDES *Agglutinins (86000, 86156-86157)*
Antiplasmin (85410)
Antithrombin III (85300-85301)
Blood banking procedures (86850-86999)

85004 **Blood count; automated differential WBC count**

0.00 0.00 FUD XXX

AMA: 2018,Jan,8; 2017,Jan,8; 2016,Jan,13; 2015,Jan,16; 2014,Jan,11

85007 **blood smear, microscopic examination with manual differential WBC count**

0.00 0.00 FUD XXX

AMA: 2018,Jan,8; 2017,Jan,8; 2016,Jan,13; 2015,Jan,16; 2014,Jan,11

85008 **blood smear, microscopic examination without manual differential WBC count**

EXCLUDES *Cell count other fluids (eg, CSF) (89050-89051)*

0.00 0.00 FUD XXX

AMA: 2018,Jan,8; 2017,Jan,8; 2016,Jan,13; 2015,Jan,16; 2014,Jan,11

85009 **manual differential WBC count, buffy coat**

EXCLUDES *Eosinophils, nasal smear (89190)*

0.00 0.00 FUD XXX

AMA: 2018,Jan,8; 2017,Jan,8; 2016,Jan,13; 2015,Jan,16; 2014,Jan,11

85013 **spun microhematocrit**

0.00 0.00 FUD XXX

AMA: 2005,Aug,7-8; 2005,Jul,11-12

85014 **hematocrit (Hct)**

0.00 0.00 FUD XXX

AMA: 2018,Jan,8; 2017,Jan,8; 2016,Jan,13; 2015,Jan,16; 2014,Jan,11

85018 **hemoglobin (Hgb)**

EXCLUDES *Immunoassay, hemoglobin, fecal (82274)*
Other hemoglobin determination (83020-83069)
Transcutaneous hemoglobin measurement (88738)

0.00 0.00 FUD XXX

AMA: 2018,Jan,8; 2017,Jan,8; 2016,Jan,13; 2015,Jan,16; 2014,Jan,11

85025 **complete (CBC), automated (Hgb, Hct, RBC, WBC and platelet count) and automated differential WBC count**

0.00 0.00 FUD XXX

AMA: 2018,Jan,8; 2017,Jan,8; 2016,Jan,13; 2015,Jan,16; 2014,Jan,11

85027 **complete (CBC), automated (Hgb, Hct, RBC, WBC and platelet count)**

0.00 0.00 FUD XXX

AMA: 2018,Jan,8; 2017,Jan,8; 2016,Jan,13; 2015,Jan,16; 2014,Jan,11

85032 **manual cell count (erythrocyte, leukocyte, or platelet) each**

0.00 0.00 FUD XXX

AMA: 2018,Jan,8; 2017,Jan,8; 2016,Jan,13; 2015,Jan,16; 2014,Jan,11

85041 **red blood cell (RBC), automated**
EXCLUDES *Complete blood count (85025, 85027)*
0.00 0.00 FUD XXX
AMA: 2018,Jan,8; 2017,Jan,8; 2016,Jan,13; 2015,Jan,16; 2014,Jan,11

85044 **reticulocyte, manual**
0.00 0.00 FUD XXX
AMA: 2018,Jan,8; 2017,Jan,8; 2016,Jan,13; 2015,Jan,16; 2014,Jan,11

85045 **reticulocyte, automated**
0.00 0.00 FUD XXX
AMA: 2018,Jan,8; 2017,Jan,8; 2016,Jan,13; 2015,Jan,16; 2014,Jan,11

85046 **reticulocytes, automated, including 1 or more cellular parameters (eg, reticulocyte hemoglobin content [CHr], immature reticulocyte fraction [IRF], reticulocyte volume [MRV], RNA content), direct measurement**
0.00 0.00 FUD XXX
AMA: 2005,Aug,7-8; 2005,Jul,11-12

85048 **leukocyte (WBC), automated**
0.00 0.00 FUD XXX
AMA: 2018,Jan,8; 2017,Jan,8; 2016,Jan,13; 2015,Jan,16; 2014,Jan,11

85049 **platelet, automated**
0.00 0.00 FUD XXX
AMA: 2005,Aug,7-8; 2005,Jul,11-12

85055-85705 Coagulopathy Testing

EXCLUDES *Agglutinins (86000, 86156-86157)*
Antiplasmin (85410)
Antithrombin III (85300-85301)
Blood banking procedures (86850-86999)

85055 **Reticulated platelet assay**
0.00 0.00 FUD XXX
AMA: 2005,Aug,7-8; 2005,Jul,11-12

85060 **Blood smear, peripheral, interpretation by physician with written report**
0.70 0.70 FUD XXX B 80
AMA: 2005,Aug,7-8; 2005,Jul,11-12

85097 **Bone marrow, smear interpretation**
EXCLUDES *Bone biopsy (20220, 20225, 20240, 20245, 20250-20251)*
Special stains (88312-88313)
1.42 2.11 FUD XXX Q2 80
AMA: 2018,Jan,8; 2017,Jan,8; 2016,Jan,13; 2015,Jan,16; 2014,Jan,11

85130 **Chromogenic substrate assay**
EXCLUDES *Circulating anticoagulant screen (mixing studies) (85611, 85732)*
0.00 0.00 FUD XXX
AMA: 2005,Aug,7-8; 2005,Jul,11-12

85170 **Clot retraction**
0.00 0.00 FUD XXX
AMA: 2005,Aug,7-8; 2005,Jul,11-12

85175 **Clot lysis time, whole blood dilution**
EXCLUDES *Clotting factor I (fibrinogen) (85384, 85385)*
0.00 0.00 FUD XXX
AMA: 2005,Aug,7-8; 2005,Jul,11-12

85210 **Clotting; factor II, prothrombin, specific**
EXCLUDES *Prothrombin time (85610-85611)*
Russell viper venom time (85612-85613)
0.00 0.00 FUD XXX
AMA: 2005,Aug,7-8; 2005,Jul,11-12

85220 **factor V (AcG or proaccelerin), labile factor**
0.00 0.00 FUD XXX
AMA: 2005,Aug,7-8; 2005,Jul,11-12

85230 **factor VII (proconvertin, stable factor)**
0.00 0.00 FUD XXX
AMA: 2005,Aug,7-8; 2005,Jul,11-12

85240 **factor VIII (AHG), 1-stage**
0.00 0.00 FUD XXX
AMA: 2005,Aug,7-8; 2005,Jul,11-12

85244 **factor VIII related antigen**
0.00 0.00 FUD XXX
AMA: 2005,Aug,7-8; 2005,Jul,11-12

85245 **factor VIII, VW factor, ristocetin cofactor**
0.00 0.00 FUD XXX
AMA: 2005,Aug,7-8; 2005,Jul,11-12

85246 **factor VIII, VW factor antigen**
0.00 0.00 FUD XXX
AMA: 2005,Aug,7-8; 2005,Jul,11-12

85247 **factor VIII, von Willebrand factor, multimetric analysis**
0.00 0.00 FUD XXX
AMA: 2005,Aug,7-8; 2005,Jul,11-12

85250 **factor IX (PTC or Christmas)**
0.00 0.00 FUD XXX
AMA: 2005,Aug,7-8; 2005,Jul,11-12

85260 **factor X (Stuart-Prower)**
0.00 0.00 FUD XXX
AMA: 2005,Aug,7-8; 2005,Jul,11-12

85270 **factor XI (PTA)**
0.00 0.00 FUD XXX
AMA: 2005,Aug,7-8; 2005,Jul,11-12

85280 **factor XII (Hageman)**
0.00 0.00 FUD XXX
AMA: 2005,Aug,7-8; 2005,Jul,11-12

85290 **factor XIII (fibrin stabilizing)**
0.00 0.00 FUD XXX
AMA: 2005,Aug,7-8; 2005,Jul,11-12

85291 **factor XIII (fibrin stabilizing), screen solubility**
0.00 0.00 FUD XXX
AMA: 2005,Aug,7-8; 2005,Jul,11-12

85292 **prekallikrein assay (Fletcher factor assay)**
0.00 0.00 FUD XXX
AMA: 2005,Aug,7-8; 2005,Jul,11-12

85293 **high molecular weight kininogen assay (Fitzgerald factor assay)**
0.00 0.00 FUD XXX
AMA: 2005,Aug,7-8; 2005,Jul,11-12

85300 **Clotting inhibitors or anticoagulants; antithrombin III, activity**
0.00 0.00 FUD XXX
AMA: 2005,Aug,7-8; 2005,Jul,11-12

85301 **antithrombin III, antigen assay**
0.00 0.00 FUD XXX
AMA: 2005,Aug,7-8; 2005,Jul,11-12

85302 **protein C, antigen**
0.00 0.00 FUD XXX
AMA: 2005,Aug,7-8; 2005,Jul,11-12

85303 **protein C, activity**
0.00 0.00 FUD XXX
AMA: 2005,Aug,7-8; 2005,Jul,11-12

85305 **protein S, total**
0.00 0.00 FUD XXX
AMA: 2005,Jul,11-12; 2005,Aug,7-8

85306 **protein S, free**
0.00 0.00 FUD XXX
AMA: 2005,Aug,7-8; 2005,Jul,11-12

85307 **Activated Protein C (APC) resistance assay**
0.00 0.00 FUD XXX
AMA: 2005,Aug,7-8; 2005,Jul,11-12

85335 **Factor inhibitor test**
0.00 0.00 FUD XXX
AMA: 2005,Aug,7-8; 2005,Jul,11-12

85337 Thrombomodulin
EXCLUDES *Mixing studies for inhibitors (85732)*
0.00 0.00 FUD XXX
AMA: 2005,Aug,7-8; 2005,Jul,11-12

85345 Coagulation time; Lee and White
0.00 0.00 FUD XXX
AMA: 2005,Aug,7-8; 2005,Jul,11-12

85347 activated
0.00 0.00 FUD XXX
AMA: 2019,Apr,10

85348 other methods
EXCLUDES *Differential count (85007-85009, 85025)*
Duke bleeding time (85002)
Eosinophils, nasal smear (89190)
0.00 0.00 FUD XXX
AMA: 2005,Aug,7-8; 2005,Jul,11-12

85360 Euglobulin lysis
EXCLUDES *Fetal hemoglobin (83030, 83033, 85460)*
0.00 0.00 FUD XXX
AMA: 2005,Aug,7-8; 2005,Jul,11-12

85362 Fibrin(ogen) degradation (split) products (FDP) (FSP); agglutination slide, semiquantitative
EXCLUDES *Immunoelectrophoresis (86320)*
0.00 0.00 FUD XXX
AMA: 2005,Aug,7-8; 2005,Jul,11-12

85366 paracoagulation
0.00 0.00 FUD XXX
AMA: 2005,Aug,7-8; 2005,Jul,11-12

85370 quantitative
0.00 0.00 FUD XXX
AMA: 2005,Aug,7-8; 2005,Jul,11-12

85378 Fibrin degradation products, D-dimer; qualitative or semiquantitative
0.00 0.00 FUD XXX
AMA: 2018,Jan,8; 2017,Jan,8; 2016,Jan,13; 2015,Jan,16; 2014,Jan,11

85379 quantitative
INCLUDES Ultrasensitive and standard sensitivity quantitative D-dimer (85379)
0.00 0.00 FUD XXX
AMA: 2005,Aug,7-8; 2005,Jul,11-12

85380 ultrasensitive (eg, for evaluation for venous thromboembolism), qualitative or semiquantitative
0.00 0.00 FUD XXX
AMA: 2018,Jan,8; 2017,Jan,8; 2016,Jan,13; 2015,Jan,16; 2014,Jan,11

85384 Fibrinogen; activity
0.00 0.00 FUD XXX
AMA: 2019,Apr,10

85385 antigen
0.00 0.00 FUD XXX
AMA: 2005,Jul,11-12; 2005,Aug,7-8

85390 Fibrinolysins or coagulopathy screen, interpretation and report
0.00 0.00 FUD XXX
AMA: 2019,Apr,10

85396 Coagulation/fibrinolysis assay, whole blood (eg, viscoelastic clot assessment), including use of any pharmacologic additive(s), as indicated, including interpretation and written report, per day
0.58 0.58 FUD XXX
AMA: 2019,Apr,10

85397 Coagulation and fibrinolysis, functional activity, not otherwise specified (eg, ADAMTS-13), each analyte
0.00 0.00 FUD XXX

85400 Fibrinolytic factors and inhibitors; plasmin
0.00 0.00 FUD XXX
AMA: 2005,Aug,7-8; 2005,Jul,11-12

85410 alpha-2 antiplasmin
0.00 0.00 FUD XXX
AMA: 2005,Aug,7-8; 2005,Jul,11-12

85415 plasminogen activator
0.00 0.00 FUD XXX
AMA: 2005,Aug,7-8; 2005,Jul,11-12

85420 plasminogen, except antigenic assay
0.00 0.00 FUD XXX
AMA: 2005,Aug,7-8; 2005,Jul,11-12

85421 plasminogen, antigenic assay
EXCLUDES *Fragility, red blood cell (85547, 85555-85557)*
0.00 0.00 FUD XXX
AMA: 2005,Aug,7-8; 2005,Jul,11-12

85441 Heinz bodies; direct
0.00 0.00 FUD XXX
AMA: 2005,Aug,7-8; 2005,Jul,11-12

85445 induced, acetyl phenylhydrazine
EXCLUDES *Hematocrit (PCV) (85014, 85025, 85027)*
Hemoglobin (83020-83068, 85018, 85025, 85027)
0.00 0.00 FUD XXX
AMA: 2005,Aug,7-8; 2005,Jul,11-12

85460 Hemoglobin or RBCs, fetal, for fetomaternal hemorrhage; differential lysis (Kleihauer-Betke) M ♀
EXCLUDES *Hemoglobin F (83030, 83033)*
Hemolysins (86940-86941)
0.00 0.00 FUD XXX
AMA: 2018,Jan,8; 2017,Jan,8; 2016,Jan,13; 2015,Jan,16; 2014,Jan,11

85461 rosette M ♀
0.00 0.00 FUD XXX
AMA: 2005,Jul,11-12; 2005,Aug,7-8

85475 Hemolysin, acid
INCLUDES Ham test
EXCLUDES *Hemolysins and agglutinins (86940-86941)*
0.00 0.00 FUD XXX
AMA: 2005,Aug,7-8; 2005,Jul,11-12

85520 Heparin assay
0.00 0.00 FUD XXX
AMA: 2005,Aug,7-8; 2005,Jul,11-12

85525 Heparin neutralization
0.00 0.00 FUD XXX
AMA: 2018,Jan,8; 2017,Aug,9

85530 Heparin-protamine tolerance test
0.00 0.00 FUD XXX
AMA: 2005,Aug,7-8; 2005,Jul,11-12

85536 Iron stain, peripheral blood
EXCLUDES *Iron stains on bone marrow or other tissues with physician evaluation (88313)*
0.00 0.00 FUD XXX
AMA: 2005,Aug,7-8; 2005,Jul,11-12

85540 Leukocyte alkaline phosphatase with count
0.00 0.00 FUD XXX
AMA: 2005,Aug,7-8; 2005,Jul,11-12

85547 Mechanical fragility, RBC
0.00 0.00 FUD XXX
AMA: 2005,Aug,7-8; 2005,Jul,11-12

85549 Muramidase
EXCLUDES *Nitroblue tetrazolium dye test (86384)*
0.00 0.00 FUD XXX
AMA: 2005,Aug,7-8; 2005,Jul,11-12

85555 **Osmotic fragility, RBC; unincubated**
0.00 0.00 FUD XXX
AMA: 2005,Aug,7-8; 2005,Jul,11-12

85557 **incubated**
EXCLUDES *Packed cell volume (85013)*
Parasites, blood (eg, malaria smears) (87207)
Partial thromboplastin time (85730, 85732)
Plasmin (85400)
Plasminogen (85420)
Plasminogen activator (85415)
0.00 0.00 FUD XXX
AMA: 2005,Aug,7-8; 2005,Jul,11-12

85576 **Platelet, aggregation (in vitro), each agent**
EXCLUDES *Thromboxane metabolite(s), including thromboxane, when performed, in urine (84431)*
0.00 0.00 FUD XXX
AMA: 2019,Apr,10; 2018,Jan,8; 2017,Jan,8; 2016,Jan,13; 2015,Jan,16; 2014,Jan,11

85597 **Phospholipid neutralization; platelet**
0.00 0.00 FUD XXX
AMA: 2018,Jan,8; 2017,Jan,8; 2016,Jan,13; 2015,Jan,16; 2014,Jan,11

85598 **hexagonal phospholipid**
0.00 0.00 FUD XXX
AMA: 2018,Jan,8; 2017,Jan,8; 2016,Jan,13; 2015,Jan,16; 2014,Jan,11

85610 **Prothrombin time;**
0.00 0.00 FUD XXX
AMA: 2005,Aug,7-8; 2005,Jul,11-12

85611 **substitution, plasma fractions, each**
0.00 0.00 FUD XXX
AMA: 2005,Aug,7-8; 2005,Jul,11-12

85612 **Russell viper venom time (includes venom); undiluted**
0.00 0.00 FUD XXX
AMA: 2005,Aug,7-8; 2005,Jul,11-12

85613 **diluted**
EXCLUDES *Red blood cell count (85025, 85027, 85041)*
0.00 0.00 FUD XXX
AMA: 2005,Aug,7-8; 2005,Jul,11-12

85635 **Reptilase test**
EXCLUDES *Reticulocyte count (85044-85045)*
0.00 0.00 FUD XXX
AMA: 2005,Aug,7-8; 2005,Jul,11-12

85651 **Sedimentation rate, erythrocyte; non-automated**
0.00 0.00 FUD XXX
AMA: 2005,Aug,7-8; 2005,Jul,11-12

85652 **automated**
INCLUDES Westergren test
0.00 0.00 FUD XXX
AMA: 2005,Aug,7-8; 2005,Jul,11-12

85660 **Sickling of RBC, reduction**
EXCLUDES *Hemoglobin electrophoresis (83020)*
Smears (87207)
0.00 0.00 FUD XXX
AMA: 2005,Aug,7-8; 2005,Jul,11-12

85670 **Thrombin time; plasma**
0.00 0.00 FUD XXX
AMA: 2005,Jul,11-12; 2005,Aug,7-8

85675 **titer**
0.00 0.00 FUD XXX
AMA: 2005,Jul,11-12; 2005,Aug,7-8

85705 **Thromboplastin inhibition, tissue**
EXCLUDES *Individual clotting factors (85245-85247)*
0.00 0.00 FUD XXX
AMA: 2005,Aug,7-8; 2005,Jul,11-12

85730-85732 Partial Thromboplastin Time (PTT)

EXCLUDES *Agglutinins (86000, 86156-86157)*
Antiplasmin (85410)
Antithrombin III (85300-85301)
Blood banking procedures (86850-86999)

85730 **Thromboplastin time, partial (PTT); plasma or whole blood**
INCLUDES Hicks-Pitney test
0.00 0.00 FUD XXX
AMA: 2005,Aug,7-8; 2005,Jul,11-12

85732 **substitution, plasma fractions, each**
0.00 0.00 FUD XXX
AMA: 2018,Jan,8; 2017,Jan,8; 2016,Jan,13; 2015,Jan,16; 2014,Jan,11

85810-85999 Blood Viscosity and Unlisted Hematology Procedures

85810 **Viscosity**
EXCLUDES *von Willebrand factor assay (85245-85247)*
WBC count (85025, 85027, 85048, 89050)
0.00 0.00 FUD XXX
AMA: 2018,Jan,8; 2017,Jan,8; 2016,Jan,13; 2015,Jan,16; 2014,Jan,11

85999 **Unlisted hematology and coagulation procedure**
0.00 0.00 FUD XXX
AMA: 2018,Jan,8; 2017,Aug,9; 2017,Jan,8; 2016,Jan,13; 2015,Jan,16; 2014,Jan,11

86000-86063 Antibody Testing

86000 **Agglutinins, febrile (eg, Brucella, Francisella, Murine typhus, Q fever, Rocky Mountain spotted fever, scrub typhus), each antigen**
EXCLUDES *Infectious agent antibodies (86602-86804)*
0.00 0.00 FUD XXX
AMA: 2018,Jan,8; 2017,Jan,8; 2016,Jan,13; 2015,Jan,16; 2014,Jan,11

86001 **Allergen specific IgG quantitative or semiquantitative, each allergen**
EXCLUDES *Agglutinins and autohemolysins (86940-86941)*
0.00 0.00 FUD XXX
AMA: 2005,Aug,7-8; 2005,Jul,11-12

86003 **Allergen specific IgE; quantitative or semiquantitative, crude allergen extract, each**
EXCLUDES *Total quantitative IgE (82785)*
0.00 0.00 FUD XXX
AMA: 2018,Jan,8; 2017,Jan,8; 2016,Jan,13; 2015,Jan,16; 2014,Jan,11

86005 **qualitative, multiallergen screen (eg, disk, sponge, card)**
EXCLUDES *Total qualitative IgE (83518)*
0.00 0.00 FUD XXX
AMA: 2018,Jan,8; 2017,Jan,8; 2016,Jan,13; 2015,Jan,16; 2014,Jan,11

86008 **quantitative or semiquantitative, recombinant or purified component, each**
0.00 0.00 FUD XXX
EXCLUDES *Alpha-1 antitrypsin (82103, 82104)*
Alpha-1 feto-protein (82105, 82106)
Anti-AChR (acetylcholine receptor) antibody titer (86255, 86256)
Anticardiolipin antibody (86147)
Anti-deoxyribonuclease titer (86215)
Anti-DNA (86225)

86021 **Antibody identification; leukocyte antibodies**
0.00 0.00 FUD XXX
AMA: 2005,Jul,11-12; 2005,Aug,7-8

86022 **platelet antibodies**
0.00 0.00 FUD XXX
AMA: 2005,Jul,11-12; 2005,Aug,7-8

Pathology and Laboratory
85555 — 86022

● New Code ▲ Revised Code ○ Reinstated ● New Web Release ▲ Revised Web Release + Add-on Unlisted Not Covered # Resequenced
⑩ Optum Mod 50 Exempt ⊘ AMA Mod 51 Exempt ⑤ Optum Mod 51 Exempt ⑥ Mod 63 Exempt ✓ Non-FDA Drug ★ Telemedicine M Maternity A Age Edit

86023 **platelet associated immunoglobulin assay**
0.00 0.00 FUD XXX
AMA: 2005,Jul,11-12; 2005,Aug,7-8

86038 **Antinuclear antibodies (ANA);**
0.00 0.00 FUD XXX
AMA: 2005,Aug,7-8; 2005,Jul,11-12

86039 **titer**
EXCLUDES *Antistreptococcal antibody, ie, anti-DNAse (86215)*
Antistreptokinase titer (86590)
0.00 0.00 FUD XXX
AMA: 2005,Aug,7-8; 2005,Jul,11-12

86060 **Antistreptolysin 0; titer**
EXCLUDES *Antibodies, infectious agents (86602-86804)*
0.00 0.00 FUD XXX
AMA: 2005,Jul,11-12; 2005,Aug,7-8

86063 **screen**
EXCLUDES *Antibodies to blastomyces (86612)*
Antibodies, infectious agents (86602-86804)
0.00 0.00 FUD XXX
AMA: 2005,Jul,11-12; 2005,Aug,7-8

86077-86079 Blood Bank Services

86077 **Blood bank physician services; difficult cross match and/or evaluation of irregular antibody(s), interpretation and written report**
1.46 1.57 FUD XXX
AMA: 2005,Aug,7-8; 2005,Jul,11-12

86078 **investigation of transfusion reaction including suspicion of transmissible disease, interpretation and written report**
1.46 1.57 FUD XXX
AMA: 2005,Aug,7-8; 2005,Jul,11-12

86079 **authorization for deviation from standard blood banking procedures (eg, use of outdated blood, transfusion of Rh incompatible units), with written report**
EXCLUDES *Brucella antibodies (86622)*
Candida antibodies (86628)
Candida skin test (86485)
1.46 1.56 FUD XXX
AMA: 2005,Aug,7-8; 2005,Jul,11-12

86140-86344 [86152, 86153] Diagnostic Immunology Testing

86140 **C-reactive protein;**
EXCLUDES *Candidiasis (86628)*
0.00 0.00 FUD XXX
AMA: 2005,Aug,7-8; 2005,Jul,11-12

86141 **high sensitivity (hsCRP)**
0.00 0.00 FUD XXX
AMA: 2005,Aug,7-8; 2005,Jul,11-12

86146 **Beta 2 Glycoprotein I antibody, each**
0.00 0.00 FUD XXX
AMA: 2005,Aug,7-8; 2005,Jul,11-12

86147 **Cardiolipin (phospholipid) antibody, each Ig class**
0.00 0.00 FUD XXX
AMA: 2005,Aug,7-8; 2005,Jul,11-12

86152 **Cell enumeration using immunologic selection and identification in fluid specimen (eg, circulating tumor cells in blood);**
0.00 0.00 FUD XXX
EXCLUDES *Flow cytometric immunophenotyping (88184-88189)*
Flow cytometric quantitation (86355-86357, 86359-86361, 86367)
Code also physician interpretation/report when performed ([86153])

86153 **physician interpretation and report, when required**
0.00 0.00 FUD 000
EXCLUDES *Flow cytometric immunophenotyping (88184-88189)*
Flow cytometric quantitation (86355-86357, 86359-86361, 86367)
Code first cell enumeration, when performed ([86152])

86148 **Anti-phosphatidylserine (phospholipid) antibody**
EXCLUDES *Antiprothrombin (phospholipid cofactor) antibody (86849)*
0.00 0.00 FUD XXX
AMA: 2018,Jan,8; 2017,Jan,8; 2016,Jan,13; 2015,Jan,16; 2014,Jan,11

86152 **Resequenced code. See code following 86147.**

86153 **Resequenced code. See code before 86148.**

86155 **Chemotaxis assay, specify method**
EXCLUDES *Antibodies, coccidioides (86635)*
Clostridium difficile toxin (87230)
Skin test, coccidioides (86490)
0.00 0.00 FUD XXX
AMA: 2005,Aug,7-8; 2005,Jul,11-12

86156 **Cold agglutinin; screen**
0.00 0.00 FUD XXX
AMA: 2005,Aug,7-8; 2005,Jul,11-12

86157 **titer**
0.00 0.00 FUD XXX
AMA: 2005,Aug,7-8; 2005,Jul,11-12

86160 **Complement; antigen, each component**
0.00 0.00 FUD XXX
AMA: 2005,Aug,7-8; 2005,Jul,11-12

86161 **functional activity, each component**
0.00 0.00 FUD XXX
AMA: 2005,Aug,7-8; 2005,Jul,11-12

86162 **total hemolytic (CH50)**
0.00 0.00 FUD XXX
AMA: 2005,Aug,7-8; 2005,Jul,11-12

86171 **Complement fixation tests, each antigen**
EXCLUDES *Coombs test*
0.00 0.00 FUD XXX
AMA: 2005,Aug,7-8; 2005,Jul,11-12

86200 **Cyclic citrullinated peptide (CCP), antibody**
0.00 0.00 FUD XXX
AMA: 2018,Jan,8; 2017,Jan,8; 2016,Jan,13; 2015,Jan,16; 2014,Jan,11

86215 **Deoxyribonuclease, antibody**
0.00 0.00 FUD XXX
AMA: 2005,Aug,7-8; 2005,Jul,11-12

86225 **Deoxyribonucleic acid (DNA) antibody; native or double stranded**
EXCLUDES *Echinococcus antibodies, report code for specific method*
HIV antibody tests (86701-86703)
0.00 0.00 FUD XXX
AMA: 2005,Aug,7-8; 2005,Jul,11-12

86226 **single stranded**
EXCLUDES *Anti D.S, DNA, IFA, eg, using C. Lucilae (86255-86256)*
0.00 0.00 FUD XXX
AMA: 2005,Aug,7-8; 2005,Jul,11-12

86235 **Extractable nuclear antigen, antibody to, any method (eg, nRNP, SS-A, SS-B, Sm, RNP, Sc170, J01), each antibody**
0.00 0.00 FUD XXX
AMA: 2005,Aug,7-8; 2005,Jul,11-12

86255 **Fluorescent noninfectious agent antibody; screen, each antibody**
0.00 0.00 FUD XXX
AMA: 2005,Aug,9-10; 2005,Aug,7-8

86256 **titer, each antibody**

EXCLUDES *Fluorescent technique for antigen identification in tissue (88346, [88350])*
FTA (86780)
Gel (agar) diffusion tests (86331)
Indirect fluorescence (88346, [88350])

0.00 0.00 FUD XXX

AMA: 2005,Aug,9-10; 2005,Aug,7-8

86277 **Growth hormone, human (HGH), antibody**

0.00 0.00 FUD XXX

AMA: 2005,Aug,7-8; 2005,Jul,11-12

86280 **Hemagglutination inhibition test (HAI)**

EXCLUDES *Antibodies to infectious agents (86602-86804)*
Rubella (86762)

0.00 0.00 FUD XXX

AMA: 2005,Aug,7-8; 2005,Jul,11-12

86294 **Immunoassay for tumor antigen, qualitative or semiquantitative (eg, bladder tumor antigen)**

EXCLUDES *Qualitative NMP22 protein (86386)*

0.00 0.00 FUD XXX

AMA: 2005,Aug,7-8; 2005,Jul,11-12

86300 **Immunoassay for tumor antigen, quantitative; CA 15-3 (27.29)**

0.00 0.00 FUD XXX

AMA: 2005,Aug,7-8; 2005,Jul,11-12

86301 **CA 19-9**

0.00 0.00 FUD XXX

AMA: 2005,Aug,7-8; 2005,Jul,11-12

86304 **CA 125**

EXCLUDES *Antibody, hepatitis delta agent (86692)*
Measurement of serum HER-2/neu oncoprotein (83950)

0.00 0.00 FUD XXX

AMA: 2005,Aug,7-8; 2005,Jul,11-12

86305 **Human epididymis protein 4 (HE4)**

0.00 0.00 FUD XXX

86308 **Heterophile antibodies; screening**

EXCLUDES *Antibodies to infectious agents (86602-86804)*

0.00 0.00 FUD XXX

AMA: 2005,Jul,11-12; 2005,Aug,7-8

86309 **titer**

EXCLUDES *Antibodies to infectious agents (86602-86804)*

0.00 0.00 FUD XXX

AMA: 2005,Jul,11-12; 2005,Aug,7-8

86310 **titers after absorption with beef cells and guinea pig kidney**

EXCLUDES *Antibodies, infectious agents (86602-86804)*
Histoplasma antibodies (86698)
Histoplasmosis skin test (86510)
Human growth hormone antibody (86277)

0.00 0.00 FUD XXX

AMA: 2005,Jul,11-12; 2005,Aug,7-8

86316 **Immunoassay for tumor antigen, other antigen, quantitative (eg, CA 50, 72-4, 549), each**

0.00 0.00 FUD XXX

AMA: 2018,Jan,8; 2017,Jan,8; 2016,Jan,13; 2015,Jan,16; 2014,Jan,11

86317 **Immunoassay for infectious agent antibody, quantitative, not otherwise specified**

EXCLUDES *Immunoassay techniques for antigens (83516, 83518-83520, 87301-87450, 87810-87899)*
Particle agglutination test (86403)

0.00 0.00 FUD XXX

AMA: 2005,Jul,11-12; 2005,Aug,7-8

86318 **Immunoassay for infectious agent antibody, qualitative or semiquantitative, single step method (eg, reagent strip)**

0.00 0.00 FUD XXX

AMA: 2018,Jan,8; 2017,Jan,8; 2016,Jan,13; 2015,Jan,16; 2014,Jan,11

86320 **Immunoelectrophoresis; serum**

0.00 0.00 FUD XXX

AMA: 2005,Jul,11-12; 2005,Aug,7-8

86325 **other fluids (eg, urine, cerebrospinal fluid) with concentration**

0.00 0.00 FUD XXX

AMA: 2005,Jul,11-12; 2005,Aug,7-8

86327 **crossed (2-dimensional assay)**

0.00 0.00 FUD XXX

AMA: 2005,Jul,11-12; 2005,Aug,7-8

86329 **Immunodiffusion; not elsewhere specified**

0.00 0.00 FUD XXX

AMA: 2018,Jan,8; 2017,Jan,8; 2016,Jan,13; 2015,Jan,16; 2014,Jan,11

86331 **gel diffusion, qualitative (Ouchterlony), each antigen or antibody**

0.00 0.00 FUD XXX

AMA: 2005,Aug,7-8; 2005,Jul,11-12

86332 **Immune complex assay**

0.00 0.00 FUD XXX

AMA: 2005,Aug,7-8; 2005,Jul,11-12

86334 **Immunofixation electrophoresis; serum**

0.00 0.00 FUD XXX

AMA: 2005,Jul,11-12; 2005,Aug,7-8

86335 **other fluids with concentration (eg, urine, CSF)**

0.00 0.00 FUD XXX

AMA: 2005,Aug,7-8; 2005,Jul,11-12

86336 **Inhibin A**

0.00 0.00 FUD XXX

AMA: 2005,Aug,7-8; 2005,Jul,11-12

86337 **Insulin antibodies**

0.00 0.00 FUD XXX

AMA: 2005,Aug,7-8; 2005,Jul,11-12

86340 **Intrinsic factor antibodies**

EXCLUDES *Antibodies, leptospira (86720)*
Leukoagglutinins (86021)

0.00 0.00 FUD XXX

AMA: 2005,Jul,11-12; 2005,Aug,7-8

86341 **Islet cell antibody**

0.00 0.00 FUD XXX

AMA: 2018,Jan,8; 2017,Jan,8; 2016,Jan,13; 2015,Jan,16; 2014,Jan,11

86343 **Leukocyte histamine release test (LHR)**

0.00 0.00 FUD XXX

AMA: 2005,Aug,7-8; 2005,Jul,11-12

86344 **Leukocyte phagocytosis**

0.00 0.00 FUD XXX

AMA: 2005,Aug,7-8; 2005,Jul,11-12

86352 Assay Cellular Function

86352 **Cellular function assay involving stimulation (eg, mitogen or antigen) and detection of biomarker (eg, ATP)**

0.00 0.00 FUD XXX

86353 Lymphocyte Mitogen Response Assay

CMS: 100-03,190.8 Lymphocyte Mitogen Response Assays

86353 **Lymphocyte transformation, mitogen (phytomitogen) or antigen induced blastogenesis**

EXCLUDES *Cellular function assay with stimulation and detection of biomarker (86352)*
Malaria antibodies (86750)

0.00 0.00 FUD XXX

AMA: 2005,Aug,7-8; 2005,Jul,11-12

86355-86593 Additional Diagnostic Immunology Testing

86355 **B cells, total count**
EXCLUDES *Flow cytometry interpretation (88187-88189)*
0.00 0.00 FUD XXX
AMA: 2018,Jan,8; 2017,Jan,8; 2016,Jan,13; 2015,Jan,16; 2014,Jan,11

86356 **Mononuclear cell antigen, quantitative (eg, flow cytometry), not otherwise specified, each antigen**
EXCLUDES *Flow cytometry interpretation (88187-88189)*
0.00 0.00 FUD XXX
AMA: 2018,Jan,8; 2017,Jan,8; 2016,Jan,13; 2015,Jan,16; 2014,Jan,11

86357 **Natural killer (NK) cells, total count**
EXCLUDES *Flow cytometry interpretation (88187-88189)*
0.00 0.00 FUD XXX
AMA: 2018,Jan,8; 2017,Jan,8; 2016,Jan,13; 2015,Jan,16; 2014,Jan,11

86359 **T cells; total count**
EXCLUDES *Flow cytometry interpretation (88187-88189)*
0.00 0.00 FUD XXX
AMA: 2018,Jan,8; 2017,Jan,8; 2016,Jan,13; 2015,Jan,16; 2014,Jan,11

86360 **absolute CD4 and CD8 count, including ratio**
EXCLUDES *Flow cytometry interpretation (88187-88189)*
0.00 0.00 FUD XXX
AMA: 2018,Jan,8; 2017,Jan,8; 2016,Jan,13; 2015,Jan,16; 2014,Jan,11

86361 **absolute CD4 count**
EXCLUDES *Flow cytometry interpretation (88187-88189)*
0.00 0.00 FUD XXX
AMA: 2018,Jan,8; 2017,Jan,8; 2016,Jan,13; 2015,Jan,16; 2014,Jan,11

86367 **Stem cells (ie, CD34), total count**
EXCLUDES *Flow cytometric immunophenotyping, potential hematolymphoid neoplasia assessment (88184-88189)*
Flow cytometry interpretation (88187-88189)
0.00 0.00 FUD XXX
AMA: 2018,Jan,8; 2017,Jan,8; 2016,Jan,13; 2015,Jan,16; 2014,Jan,11

86376 **Microsomal antibodies (eg, thyroid or liver-kidney), each**
0.00 0.00 FUD XXX
AMA: 2005,Jul,11-12; 2005,Aug,7-8

86382 **Neutralization test, viral**
0.00 0.00 FUD XXX
AMA: 2005,Aug,7-8; 2005,Jul,11-12

86384 **Nitroblue tetrazolium dye test (NTD)**
0.00 0.00 FUD XXX
AMA: 2005,Aug,7-8; 2005,Jul,11-12

86386 **Nuclear Matrix Protein 22 (NMP22), qualitative**
0.00 0.00 FUD XXX
EXCLUDES *Ouchterlony diffusion (86331)*
Platelet antibodies (86022, 86023)

86403 **Particle agglutination; screen, each antibody**
0.00 0.00 FUD XXX
AMA: 2005,Jul,11-12; 2005,Aug,7-8

86406 **titer, each antibody**
EXCLUDES *Pregnancy test (84702, 84703)*
Rapid plasma reagin test (RPR) (86592, 86593)
0.00 0.00 FUD XXX
AMA: 2005,Jul,11-12; 2005,Aug,7-8

86430 **Rheumatoid factor; qualitative**
0.00 0.00 FUD XXX
AMA: 2005,Aug,7-8; 2005,Jul,11-12

86431 **quantitative**
EXCLUDES *Serologic syphilis testing (86592, 86593)*
0.00 0.00 FUD XXX
AMA: 2005,Aug,7-8; 2005,Jul,11-12

86480 **Tuberculosis test, cell mediated immunity antigen response measurement; gamma interferon**
0.00 0.00 FUD XXX
AMA: 2018,Jan,8; 2017,Jan,8; 2016,Jan,13; 2015,Jan,16; 2014,Jan,11

86481 **enumeration of gamma interferon-producing T-cells in cell suspension**
0.00 0.00 FUD XXX
AMA: 2010,Dec,7-10

86485 **Skin test; candida**
EXCLUDES *Candida antibody (86628)*
0.00 0.00 FUD XXX
AMA: 2005,Jul,11-12; 2005,Aug,7-8

86486 **unlisted antigen, each**
0.15 0.15 FUD XXX
AMA: 2008,Apr,5-7

86490 **coccidioidomycosis**
2.49 2.49 FUD XXX
AMA: 2005,Aug,7-8; 2005,Jul,11-12

86510 **histoplasmosis**
EXCLUDES *Histoplasma antibody (86698)*
0.19 0.19 FUD XXX
AMA: 2005,Aug,7-8; 2005,Jul,11-12

86580 **tuberculosis, intradermal**
INCLUDES Heaf test
Intradermal Mantoux test
EXCLUDES *Antibodies to sporothrix, report code for specific method*
Skin test for allergy (95012-95199)
Smooth muscle antibody (86255-86256)
Tuberculosis test, cell mediated immunity measurement of gamma interferon antigen response (86480)
0.24 0.24 FUD XXX
AMA: 2005,Aug,7-8; 2005,Jul,11-12

86590 **Streptokinase, antibody**
EXCLUDES *Antibodies, infectious agents (86602-86804)*
Streptolysin O antibody, antistreptolysin O (86060, 86063)
0.00 0.00 FUD XXX
AMA: 2005,Jul,11-12; 2005,Aug,7-8

86592 **Syphilis test, non-treponemal antibody; qualitative (eg, VDRL, RPR, ART)**
INCLUDES Wasserman test
EXCLUDES *Antibodies to infectious agents (86602-86804)*
0.00 0.00 FUD XXX
AMA: 2005,Jul,11-12; 2005,Aug,7-8

86593 **quantitative**
EXCLUDES *Antibodies, infectious agents (86602-86804)*
Tetanus antibody (86774)
Thyroglobulin (84432)
Thyroglobulin antibody (86800)
Thyroid microsomal antibody (86376)
Toxoplasma antibody (86777-86778)
0.00 0.00 FUD XXX
AMA: 2005,Jul,11-12; 2005,Aug,7-8

86602-86698 Testing for Antibodies to Infectious Agents: Actinomyces- Histoplasma

INCLUDES Qualitative or semiquantitative immunoassays performed by multiple-step methods for the detection of antibodies to infectious agents

EXCLUDES *Detection of:*
Antibodies other than those to infectious agents, see specific antibody or method
Infectious agent/antigen (87260-87899 [87623, 87624, 87625, 87806])
Immunoassays by single-step method (86318)

86602 Antibody; actinomyces
0.00 0.00 FUD XXX
AMA: 2018,Jan,8; 2017,Jan,8; 2016,Jan,13; 2015,Jan,16; 2014,Jan,11

86603 adenovirus
0.00 0.00 FUD XXX
AMA: 2005,Jul,11-12; 2005,Aug,7-8

86606 Aspergillus
0.00 0.00 FUD XXX
AMA: 2005,Jul,11-12; 2005,Aug,7-8

86609 bacterium, not elsewhere specified
0.00 0.00 FUD XXX
AMA: 2005,Jul,11-12; 2005,Aug,7-8

86611 Bartonella
0.00 0.00 FUD XXX
AMA: 2005,Jul,11-12; 2005,Aug,7-8

86612 Blastomyces
0.00 0.00 FUD XXX
AMA: 2005,Jul,11-12; 2005,Aug,7-8

86615 Bordetella
0.00 0.00 FUD XXX
AMA: 2005,Jul,11-12; 2005,Aug,7-8

86617 Borrelia burgdorferi (Lyme disease) confirmatory test (eg, Western Blot or immunoblot)
0.00 0.00 FUD XXX
AMA: 2005,Jul,11-12; 2005,Aug,7-8

86618 Borrelia burgdorferi (Lyme disease)
0.00 0.00 FUD XXX
AMA: 2005,Jul,11-12; 2005,Aug,7-8

86619 Borrelia (relapsing fever)
0.00 0.00 FUD XXX
AMA: 2005,Jul,11-12; 2005,Aug,7-8

86622 Brucella
0.00 0.00 FUD XXX
AMA: 2005,Jul,11-12; 2005,Aug,7-8

86625 Campylobacter
0.00 0.00 FUD XXX
AMA: 2005,Jul,11-12; 2005,Aug,7-8

86628 Candida
EXCLUDES *Candida skin test (86485)*
0.00 0.00 FUD XXX
AMA: 2005,Jul,11-12; 2005,Aug,7-8

86631 Chlamydia
0.00 0.00 FUD XXX
AMA: 2005,Jul,11-12; 2005,Aug,7-8

86632 Chlamydia, IgM
EXCLUDES *Chlamydia antigen (87270, 87320)*
Fluorescent antibody technique (86255-86256)
0.00 0.00 FUD XXX
AMA: 2005,Jul,11-12; 2005,Aug,7-8

86635 Coccidioides
0.00 0.00 FUD XXX
AMA: 2005,Jul,11-12; 2005,Aug,7-8

86638 Coxiella burnetii (Q fever)
0.00 0.00 FUD XXX
AMA: 2005,Jul,11-12; 2005,Aug,7-8

86641 Cryptococcus
0.00 0.00 FUD XXX
AMA: 2005,Jul,11-12; 2005,Aug,7-8

86644 cytomegalovirus (CMV)
0.00 0.00 FUD XXX
AMA: 2005,Jul,11-12; 2005,Aug,7-8

86645 cytomegalovirus (CMV), IgM
0.00 0.00 FUD XXX
AMA: 2018,Jan,8; 2017,Jan,8; 2016,Jan,13; 2015,Jan,16; 2014,Jan,11

86648 Diphtheria
0.00 0.00 FUD XXX
AMA: 2005,Jul,11-12; 2005,Aug,7-8

86651 encephalitis, California (La Crosse)
0.00 0.00 FUD XXX
AMA: 2005,Jul,11-12; 2005,Aug,7-8

86652 encephalitis, Eastern equine
0.00 0.00 FUD XXX
AMA: 2005,Jul,11-12; 2005,Aug,7-8

86653 encephalitis, St. Louis
0.00 0.00 FUD XXX
AMA: 2005,Jul,11-12; 2005,Aug,7-8

86654 encephalitis, Western equine
0.00 0.00 FUD XXX
AMA: 2005,Jul,11-12; 2005,Aug,7-8

86658 enterovirus (eg, coxsackie, echo, polio)
EXCLUDES *Antibodies to:*
Trichinella (86784)
Trypanosoma—see code for specific methodology
Tuberculosis (86580)
Viral—see code for specific methodology
0.00 0.00 FUD XXX
AMA: 2005,Jul,11-12; 2005,Aug,7-8

86663 Epstein-Barr (EB) virus, early antigen (EA)
0.00 0.00 FUD XXX
AMA: 2005,Jul,11-12; 2005,Aug,7-8

86664 Epstein-Barr (EB) virus, nuclear antigen (EBNA)
0.00 0.00 FUD XXX
AMA: 2005,Jul,11-12; 2005,Aug,7-8

86665 Epstein-Barr (EB) virus, viral capsid (VCA)
0.00 0.00 FUD XXX
AMA: 2005,Jul,11-12; 2005,Aug,7-8

86666 Ehrlichia
0.00 0.00 FUD XXX
AMA: 2005,Jul,11-12; 2005,Aug,7-8

86668 Francisella tularensis
0.00 0.00 FUD XXX
AMA: 2005,Jul,11-12; 2005,Aug,7-8

86671 fungus, not elsewhere specified
0.00 0.00 FUD XXX
AMA: 2005,Jul,11-12; 2005,Aug,7-8

86674 Giardia lamblia
0.00 0.00 FUD XXX
AMA: 2005,Jul,11-12; 2005,Aug,7-8

86677 Helicobacter pylori
0.00 0.00 FUD XXX
AMA: 2018,Jan,8; 2017,Jan,8; 2016,Jan,13; 2015,Jan,16; 2014,Jan,11

86682 helminth, not elsewhere specified
0.00 0.00 FUD XXX
AMA: 2005,Jul,11-12; 2005,Aug,7-8

86684 Haemophilus influenza
0.00 0.00 FUD XXX
AMA: 2005,Jul,11-12; 2005,Aug,7-8

86687 HTLV-I
0.00 0.00 FUD XXX
AMA: 2005,Jul,11-12; 2005,Aug,7-8

86688 HTLV-II
0.00 0.00 FUD XXX
AMA: 2005,Jul,11-12; 2005,Aug,7-8

86689 HTLV or HIV antibody, confirmatory test (eg, Western Blot)
0.00 0.00 FUD XXX
AMA: 2018,Jan,8; 2017,Jan,8; 2016,Jan,13; 2015,Jan,16; 2014,Jan,11

86692 hepatitis, delta agent
EXCLUDES *Hepatitis delta agent, antigen (87380)*
0.00 0.00 FUD XXX
AMA: 2005,Jul,11-12; 2005,Aug,7-8

86694 herpes simplex, non-specific type test
0.00 0.00 FUD XXX
AMA: 2005,Jul,11-12; 2005,Aug,7-8

86695 herpes simplex, type 1
0.00 0.00 FUD XXX
AMA: 2018,Jan,8; 2017,Jan,8; 2016,Jan,13; 2015,Jan,16; 2014,Jan,11

86696 herpes simplex, type 2
0.00 0.00 FUD XXX
AMA: 2005,Jul,11-12; 2005,Aug,7-8

86698 histoplasma
0.00 0.00 FUD XXX
AMA: 2005,Jul,11-12; 2005,Aug,7-8

86701-86703 Testing for HIV Antibodies

CMS: 100-03,190.14 Human Immunodeficiency Virus Testing (Diagnosis); 100-03,190.9 Serologic Testing for Acquired Immunodeficiency Syndrome (AIDS)

INCLUDES Qualitative or semiquantitative immunoassays performed by multiple-step methods for the detection of antibodies to infectious agents

EXCLUDES *Confirmatory test for HIV antibody (86689)*
HIV-1 antigen (87390)
HIV-1 antigen(s) with HIV 1 and 2 antibodies, single result (87389)
HIV-2 antigen (87391)
Immunoassays by single-step method (86318)

Code also modifier 92 for test performed using a kit or transportable instrument comprising all or part of a single-use, disposable analytical chamber

86701 Antibody; HIV-1
0.00 0.00 FUD XXX
AMA: 2018,Jan,8; 2017,Jan,8; 2016,Jan,13; 2015,Jan,16; 2014,Jan,11

86702 HIV-2
0.00 0.00 FUD XXX
AMA: 2018,Jan,8; 2017,Jan,8; 2016,Jan,13; 2015,Jan,16; 2014,Jan,11

86703 HIV-1 and HIV-2, single result
0.00 0.00 FUD XXX
AMA: 2018,Jan,8; 2017,Jan,8; 2016,Jan,13; 2015,Jan,16; 2014,Jan,11

86704-86804 Testing for Infectious Disease Antibodies: Hepatitis—Yersinia

INCLUDES Qualitative or semiquantitative immunoassays performed by multiple-step methods for the detection of antibodies to infectious agents

EXCLUDES *Detection of:*
Antibodies other than those to infectious agents, see specific antibody or method
Infectious agent/antigen (87260-87899 [87623, 87624, 87625, 87806])
Immunoassays by single-step method (86318)

86704 Hepatitis B core antibody (HBcAb); total
0.00 0.00 FUD XXX
AMA: 2018,Jan,8; 2017,Jan,8; 2016,Jan,13; 2015,Jan,16; 2014,Jan,11

86705 IgM antibody
0.00 0.00 FUD XXX
AMA: 2018,Jan,8; 2017,Jan,8; 2016,Jan,13; 2015,Jan,16; 2014,Jan,11

86706 Hepatitis B surface antibody (HBsAb)
0.00 0.00 FUD XXX
AMA: 2005,Jul,11-12; 2005,Aug,7-8

86707 Hepatitis Be antibody (HBeAb)
0.00 0.00 FUD XXX
AMA: 2005,Jul,11-12; 2005,Aug,7-8

86708 Hepatitis A antibody (HAAb)
0.00 0.00 FUD XXX
AMA: 2018,Jan,8; 2017,Jan,8; 2016,Jan,13; 2015,Jan,16; 2014,Jan,11

86709 Hepatitis A antibody (HAAb), IgM antibody
0.00 0.00 FUD XXX
AMA: 2018,Jan,8; 2017,Jan,8; 2016,Jan,13; 2015,Jan,16; 2014,Jan,11

86710 Antibody; influenza virus
0.00 0.00 FUD XXX
AMA: 2018,Jan,8; 2017,Jan,8; 2016,Jan,13; 2015,Jan,16; 2014,Jan,11

86711 JC (John Cunningham) virus
0.00 0.00 FUD XXX

86713 Legionella
0.00 0.00 FUD XXX
AMA: 2005,Jul,11-12; 2005,Aug,7-8

86717 Leishmania
0.00 0.00 FUD XXX
AMA: 2005,Jul,11-12; 2005,Aug,7-8

86720 Leptospira
0.00 0.00 FUD XXX
AMA: 2005,Jul,11-12; 2005,Aug,7-8

86723 Listeria monocytogenes
0.00 0.00 FUD XXX
AMA: 2005,Jul,11-12; 2005,Aug,7-8

86727 lymphocytic choriomeningitis
0.00 0.00 FUD XXX
AMA: 2005,Jul,11-12; 2005,Aug,7-8

86732 mucormycosis
0.00 0.00 FUD XXX
AMA: 2005,Jul,11-12; 2005,Aug,7-8

86735 mumps
0.00 0.00 FUD XXX
AMA: 2018,Jan,8; 2017,Jan,8; 2016,Jan,13; 2015,Jan,16; 2014,Jan,11

86738 mycoplasma
0.00 0.00 FUD XXX
AMA: 2005,Jul,11-12; 2005,Aug,7-8

86741 Neisseria meningitidis
0.00 0.00 FUD XXX
AMA: 2005,Jul,11-12; 2005,Aug,7-8

86744 Nocardia
0.00 0.00 FUD XXX
AMA: 2005,Jul,11-12; 2005,Aug,7-8

86747 parvovirus
0.00 0.00 FUD XXX
AMA: 2005,Jul,11-12; 2005,Aug,7-8

86750 Plasmodium (malaria)
0.00 0.00 FUD XXX
AMA: 2005,Jul,11-12; 2005,Aug,7-8

86753 protozoa, not elsewhere specified
0.00 0.00 FUD XXX
AMA: 2005,Jul,11-12; 2005,Aug,7-8

86756 respiratory syncytial virus
0.00 0.00 FUD XXX
AMA: 2005,Jul,11-12; 2005,Aug,7-8

86757 **Rickettsia**
0.00 0.00 FUD XXX
AMA: 2005,Jul,11-12; 2005,Aug,7-8

86759 **rotavirus**
0.00 0.00 FUD XXX
AMA: 2005,Jul,11-12; 2005,Aug,7-8

86762 **rubella**
0.00 0.00 FUD XXX
AMA: 2005,Jul,11-12; 2005,Aug,7-8

86765 **rubeola**
0.00 0.00 FUD XXX
AMA: 2005,Jul,11-12; 2005,Aug,7-8

86768 **Salmonella**
0.00 0.00 FUD XXX
AMA: 2005,Jul,11-12; 2005,Aug,7-8

86771 **Shigella**
0.00 0.00 FUD XXX
AMA: 2005,Jul,11-12; 2005,Aug,7-8

86774 **tetanus**
0.00 0.00 FUD XXX
AMA: 2005,Jul,11-12; 2005,Aug,7-8

86777 **Toxoplasma**
0.00 0.00 FUD XXX
AMA: 2005,Jul,11-12; 2005,Aug,7-8

86778 **Toxoplasma, IgM**
0.00 0.00 FUD XXX
AMA: 2005,Jul,11-12; 2005,Aug,7-8

86780 **Treponema pallidum**
0.00 0.00 FUD XXX
EXCLUDES *Nontreponemal antibody analysis syphilis testing (86592-86593)*

86784 **Trichinella**
0.00 0.00 FUD XXX
AMA: 2005,Jul,11-12; 2005,Aug,7-8

86787 **varicella-zoster**
0.00 0.00 FUD XXX
AMA: 2005,Jul,11-12; 2005,Aug,7-8

86788 **West Nile virus, IgM**
0.00 0.00 FUD XXX

86789 **West Nile virus**
0.00 0.00 FUD XXX

86790 **virus, not elsewhere specified**
0.00 0.00 FUD XXX
AMA: 2005,Jul,11-12; 2005,Aug,7-8

86793 **Yersinia**
0.00 0.00 FUD XXX
AMA: 2005,Jul,11-12; 2005,Aug,7-8

86794 **Zika virus, IgM**
0.00 0.00 FUD XXX

86800 **Thyroglobulin antibody**
EXCLUDES *Thyroglobulin (84432)*
0.00 0.00 FUD XXX
AMA: 2005,Jul,11-12; 2005,Aug,7-8

86803 **Hepatitis C antibody;**
0.00 0.00 FUD XXX
AMA: 2005,Jul,11-12; 2005,Aug,7-8

86804 **confirmatory test (eg, immunoblot)**
0.00 0.00 FUD XXX
AMA: 2018,Jan,8; 2017,Jan,8; 2016,Jan,13; 2015,Jan,16; 2014,Jan,11

86805-86808 Pre-Transplant Antibody Cross Matching

86805 **Lymphocytotoxicity assay, visual crossmatch; with titration**
0.00 0.00 FUD XXX
AMA: 2018,Jan,8; 2017,Jan,8; 2016,Jan,13; 2015,Jan,16; 2014,Jan,11

86806 **without titration**
0.00 0.00 FUD XXX
AMA: 2005,Aug,7-8; 2005,Jul,11-12

86807 **Serum screening for cytotoxic percent reactive antibody (PRA); standard method**
0.00 0.00 FUD XXX
AMA: 2018,Jan,8; 2017,Jan,8; 2016,Jan,13; 2015,Jan,16; 2014,Jan,11

86808 **quick method**
0.00 0.00 FUD XXX
AMA: 2018,Jan,8; 2017,Jan,8; 2016,Jan,13; 2015,Jan,16; 2014,Jan,11

86812-86826 Histocompatibility Testing

CMS: 100-03,110.23 Stem Cell Transplantation; 100-03,190.1 Histocompatibility Testing; 100-04,3,90.3 Stem Cell Transplantation; 100-04,3,90.3.1 Allogeneic Stem Cell Transplantation; 100-04,3,90.3.3 Billing for Allogeneic Stem Cell Transplants; 100-04,32,90 Billing for Stem Cell Transplantation; 100-04,4,231.11 Billing for Allogeneic Stem Cell Transplants

EXCLUDES *HLA typing by molecular pathology techniques (81370-81383)*

86812 **HLA typing; A, B, or C (eg, A10, B7, B27), single antigen**
0.00 0.00 FUD XXX
AMA: 2018,Jan,8; 2017,Jan,8; 2016,Jan,13; 2015,Jan,16; 2014,Jan,11

86813 **A, B, or C, multiple antigens**
0.00 0.00 FUD XXX
AMA: 2018,Jan,8; 2017,Jan,8; 2016,Jan,13; 2015,Jan,16; 2014,Jan,11

86816 **DR/DQ, single antigen**
0.00 0.00 FUD XXX
AMA: 2018,Jan,8; 2017,Jan,8; 2016,Jan,13; 2015,Jan,16; 2014,Jan,11

86817 **DR/DQ, multiple antigens**
0.00 0.00 FUD XXX
AMA: 2018,Jan,8; 2017,Jan,8; 2016,Jan,13; 2015,Jan,16; 2014,Jan,11

86821 **lymphocyte culture, mixed (MLC)**
0.00 0.00 FUD XXX
AMA: 2018,Jan,8; 2017,Jan,8; 2016,Jan,13; 2015,Jan,16; 2014,Jan,11

86825 **Human leukocyte antigen (HLA) crossmatch, non-cytotoxic (eg, using flow cytometry); first serum sample or dilution**
0.00 0.00 FUD XXX
INCLUDES Autologous HLA crossmatch
EXCLUDES *B cells (86355)*
Flow cytometry (88184-88189)
Lymphocytotoxicity visual crossmatch (86805-86806)
T cells (86359)

+ 86826 **each additional serum sample or sample dilution (List separately in addition to primary procedure)**
0.00 0.00 FUD XXX
INCLUDES Autologous HLA crossmatch
EXCLUDES *B cells (86355)*
Flow cytometry (88184-88189)
Lymphocytotoxicity visual crossmatch (86805-86806)
T cells (86359)
Code first (86825)

86828-86849 HLA Antibodies

86828 **Antibody to human leukocyte antigens (HLA), solid phase assays (eg, microspheres or beads, ELISA, flow cytometry); qualitative assessment of the presence or absence of antibody(ies) to HLA Class I and Class II HLA antigens**
0.00 0.00 FUD XXX Q
Code also solid phase testing of untreated and treated specimens of either class of HLA after treatment (86828-86833)

86829 **qualitative assessment of the presence or absence of antibody(ies) to HLA Class I or Class II HLA antigens**
0.00 0.00 FUD XXX Q
Code also solid phase testing of untreated and treated specimens of either class of HLA after treatment (86828-86833)

86830 **antibody identification by qualitative panel using complete HLA phenotypes, HLA Class I**
0.00 0.00 FUD XXX Q
Code also solid phase testing of untreated and treated specimens of either class of HLA after treatment (86828-86833)

86831 **antibody identification by qualitative panel using complete HLA phenotypes, HLA Class II**
0.00 0.00 FUD XXX Q
Code also solid phase testing of untreated and treated specimens of either class of HLA after treatment (86828-86833)

86832 **high definition qualitative panel for identification of antibody specificities (eg, individual antigen per bead methodology), HLA Class I**
0.00 0.00 FUD XXX Q
Code also solid phase testing of untreated and treated specimens of either class of HLA after treatment (86828-86833)

86833 **high definition qualitative panel for identification of antibody specificities (eg, individual antigen per bead methodology), HLA Class II**
0.00 0.00 FUD XXX Q
Code also solid phase testing of untreated and treated specimens of either class of HLA after treatment (86828-86833)

86834 **semi-quantitative panel (eg, titer), HLA Class I**
0.00 0.00 FUD XXX Q

86835 **semi-quantitative panel (eg, titer), HLA Class II**
0.00 0.00 FUD XXX Q

86849 **Unlisted immunology procedure**
0.00 0.00 FUD XXX N
AMA: 2018,Jan,8; 2017,Jan,8; 2016,Jan,13; 2015,Jan,16; 2014,Jan,11

86850-86999 Transfusion Services

EXCLUDES *Apheresis (36511-36512)*
Therapeutic phlebotomy (99195)

86850 **Antibody screen, RBC, each serum technique**
0.00 0.00 FUD XXX Q1
AMA: 2018,Jan,8; 2017,Jan,8; 2016,Jan,13; 2015,Jan,16; 2014,Jan,11

86860 **Antibody elution (RBC), each elution**
0.00 0.00 FUD XXX Q1
AMA: 2005,Jul,11-12; 2005,Aug,7-8

86870 **Antibody identification, RBC antibodies, each panel for each serum technique**
0.00 0.00 FUD XXX Q2
AMA: 2018,Jan,8; 2017,Jan,8; 2016,Jan,13; 2015,Jan,16; 2014,Jan,11

86880 **Antihuman globulin test (Coombs test); direct, each antiserum**
0.00 0.00 FUD XXX Q1
AMA: 2005,Aug,7-8; 2005,Jul,11-12

86885 **indirect, qualitative, each reagent red cell**
0.00 0.00 FUD XXX Q1
AMA: 2018,Jan,8; 2017,Jan,8; 2016,Jan,13; 2015,Jan,16; 2014,Jan,11

86886 **indirect, each antibody titer**
EXCLUDES *Indirect antihuman globulin (Coombs) test for RBC antibody identification using reagent red cell panels (86870)*
Indirect antihuman globulin (Coombs) test for RBC antibody screening (86850)
0.00 0.00 FUD XXX Q1
AMA: 2018,Jan,8; 2017,Jan,8; 2016,Jan,13; 2015,Jan,16; 2014,Jan,11

86890 **Autologous blood or component, collection processing and storage; predeposited**
0.00 0.00 FUD XXX Q1
AMA: 2018,Jan,8; 2017,Jan,8; 2016,Jan,13; 2015,Jan,16; 2014,Jan,11

86891 **intra- or postoperative salvage**
0.00 0.00 FUD XXX Q1
AMA: 2005,Aug,7-8; 2005,Jul,11-12

86900 **Blood typing, serologic; ABO**
0.00 0.00 FUD XXX Q1
AMA: 2005,Jul,11-12; 2005,Aug,7-8

86901 **Rh (D)**
0.00 0.00 FUD XXX Q1
AMA: 2018,Jan,8; 2017,Jan,8; 2016,Jan,13; 2015,Jan,16; 2014,Jan,11

86902 **antigen testing of donor blood using reagent serum, each antigen test**
Code also one time for each antigen for each unit of blood when multiple units are tested for the same antigen
0.00 0.00 FUD XXX Q1
AMA: 2010,Dec,7-10

86904 **antigen screening for compatible unit using patient serum, per unit screened**
0.00 0.00 FUD XXX Q1
AMA: 2005,Aug,7-8; 2005,Jul,11-12

86905 **RBC antigens, other than ABO or Rh (D), each**
0.00 0.00 FUD XXX Q1
AMA: 2005,Jul,11-12; 2005,Aug,7-8

86906 **Rh phenotyping, complete**
EXCLUDES *Use of molecular pathology procedures for human erythrocyte antigen typing (81403)*
0.00 0.00 FUD XXX Q1
AMA: 2005,Jul,11-12; 2005,Aug,7-8

86910 **Blood typing, for paternity testing, per individual; ABO, Rh and MN**
0.00 0.00 FUD XXX E
AMA: 2005,Jul,11-12; 2005,Aug,7-8

86911 **each additional antigen system**
0.00 0.00 FUD XXX E
AMA: 2005,Jul,11-12; 2005,Aug,7-8

86920 **Compatibility test each unit; immediate spin technique**
0.00 0.00 FUD XXX Q1
AMA: 2018,Jan,8; 2017,Jan,8; 2016,Jan,13; 2015,Jan,16; 2014,Jan,11

86921 **incubation technique**
0.00 0.00 FUD XXX Q1
AMA: 2018,Jan,8; 2017,Jan,8; 2016,Jan,13; 2015,Jan,16; 2014,Jan,11

86922 **antiglobulin technique**
0.00 0.00 FUD XXX Q1
AMA: 2018,Jan,8; 2017,Jan,8; 2016,Jan,13; 2015,Jan,16; 2014,Jan,11

86923 **electronic**
EXCLUDES *Other compatibility test techniques (86920-86922)*
0.00 0.00 FUD XXX Q1
AMA: 2018,Jan,8; 2017,Jan,8; 2016,Jan,13; 2015,Jan,16; 2014,Jan,11

86927 **Fresh frozen plasma, thawing, each unit**
0.00 0.00 FUD XXX
AMA: 2005,Aug,7-8; 2005,Jul,11-12

86930 **Frozen blood, each unit; freezing (includes preparation)**
0.00 0.00 FUD XXX
AMA: 2018,Jan,8; 2017,Jan,8; 2016,Jan,13; 2015,Jan,16; 2014,Jan,11

86931 **thawing**
0.00 0.00 FUD XXX
AMA: 2018,Jan,8; 2017,Jan,8; 2016,Jan,13; 2015,Jan,16; 2014,Jan,11

86932 **freezing (includes preparation) and thawing**
0.00 0.00 FUD XXX
AMA: 2018,Jan,8; 2017,Jan,8; 2016,Jan,13; 2015,Jan,16; 2014,Jan,11

86940 **Hemolysins and agglutinins; auto, screen, each**
0.00 0.00 FUD XXX
AMA: 2005,Aug,7-8; 2005,Jul,11-12

86941 **incubated**
0.00 0.00 FUD XXX
AMA: 2005,Jul,11-12; 2005,Aug,7-8

86945 **Irradiation of blood product, each unit**
0.00 0.00 FUD XXX
AMA: 2018,Jan,8; 2017,Jan,8; 2016,Jan,13; 2015,Jan,16; 2014,Jan,11

86950 **Leukocyte transfusion**
EXCLUDES *Infusion allogeneic lymphocytes (38242)*
Leukapheresis (36511)
0.00 0.00 FUD XXX
AMA: 2018,Jan,8; 2017,Jan,8; 2016,Jan,13; 2015,Jan,16

86960 **Volume reduction of blood or blood product (eg, red blood cells or platelets), each unit**
0.00 0.00 FUD XXX
AMA: 2018,Jan,8; 2017,Jan,8; 2016,Jan,13; 2015,Jan,16; 2014,Jan,11

86965 **Pooling of platelets or other blood products**
EXCLUDES *Autologous WBC injection (0481T)*
Injection of platelet rich plasma (0232T)
0.00 0.00 FUD XXX
AMA: 2018,Jan,8; 2017,Jan,8; 2016,Jan,13; 2015,Jan,16; 2014,Jan,11

86970 **Pretreatment of RBCs for use in RBC antibody detection, identification, and/or compatibility testing; incubation with chemical agents or drugs, each**
0.00 0.00 FUD XXX
AMA: 2005,Jul,11-12; 2005,Aug,7-8

86971 **incubation with enzymes, each**
0.00 0.00 FUD XXX
AMA: 2005,Jul,11-12; 2005,Aug,7-8

86972 **by density gradient separation**
0.00 0.00 FUD XXX
AMA: 2005,Jul,11-12; 2005,Aug,7-8

86975 **Pretreatment of serum for use in RBC antibody identification; incubation with drugs, each**
0.00 0.00 FUD XXX
AMA: 2005,Jul,11-12; 2005,Aug,7-8

86976 **by dilution**
0.00 0.00 FUD XXX
AMA: 2005,Jul,11-12; 2005,Aug,7-8

86977 **incubation with inhibitors, each**
0.00 0.00 FUD XXX
AMA: 2005,Jul,11-12; 2005,Aug,7-8

86978 **by differential red cell absorption using patient RBCs or RBCs of known phenotype, each absorption**
0.00 0.00 FUD XXX
AMA: 2005,Jul,11-12; 2005,Aug,7-8

86985 **Splitting of blood or blood products, each unit**
0.00 0.00 FUD XXX
AMA: 2018,Jan,8; 2017,Jan,8; 2016,Jan,13; 2015,Jan,16; 2014,Jan,11

86999 **Unlisted transfusion medicine procedure**
0.00 0.00 FUD XXX
AMA: 2018,Jan,8; 2017,Jan,8; 2016,Jan,13; 2015,Jan,16; 2014,Jan,11

87003-87118 Identification of Microorganisms

INCLUDES Bacteriology, mycology, parasitology, and virology
EXCLUDES *Additional tests using molecular probes, chromatography, nucleic acid resequencing, or immunologic techniques (87140-87158)*
Code also modifier 59 for multiple specimens or sites
Code also modifier 91 for repeat procedures performed on the same day

87003 **Animal inoculation, small animal, with observation and dissection**
0.00 0.00 FUD XXX
AMA: 2005,Aug,7-8; 2005,Jul,11-12

87015 **Concentration (any type), for infectious agents**
EXCLUDES *Direct smear for ova and parasites (87177)*
0.00 0.00 FUD XXX
AMA: 2005,Aug,7-8; 2005,Jul,11-12

87040 **Culture, bacterial; blood, aerobic, with isolation and presumptive identification of isolates (includes anaerobic culture, if appropriate)**
0.00 0.00 FUD XXX
AMA: 2018,Jan,8; 2017,Jan,8; 2016,Jan,13; 2015,Jan,16; 2014,Jan,11

87045 **stool, aerobic, with isolation and preliminary examination (eg, KIA, LIA), Salmonella and Shigella species**
0.00 0.00 FUD XXX
AMA: 2005,Aug,7-8; 2005,Jul,11-12

87046 **stool, aerobic, additional pathogens, isolation and presumptive identification of isolates, each plate**
0.00 0.00 FUD XXX
AMA: 2018,Jan,8; 2017,Jan,8; 2016,Jan,13; 2015,Jan,16; 2014,Jan,11

87070 **any other source except urine, blood or stool, aerobic, with isolation and presumptive identification of isolates**
EXCLUDES *Urine (87088)*
0.00 0.00 FUD XXX
AMA: 2018,Jan,8; 2017,Jan,8; 2016,Jan,13; 2015,Jan,16; 2014,Jan,11

87071 **quantitative, aerobic with isolation and presumptive identification of isolates, any source except urine, blood or stool**
EXCLUDES *Urine (87088)*
0.00 0.00 FUD XXX
AMA: 2018,Jan,8; 2017,Jan,8; 2016,Jan,13; 2015,Jan,16; 2014,Jan,11

87073 **quantitative, anaerobic with isolation and presumptive identification of isolates, any source except urine, blood or stool**
EXCLUDES *Definitive identification of isolates (87076, 87077)*
Typing of isolates (87140-87158)
0.00 0.00 FUD XXX
AMA: 2018,Jan,8; 2017,Jan,8; 2016,Jan,13; 2015,Jan,16; 2014,Jan,11

87075 **any source, except blood, anaerobic with isolation and presumptive identification of isolates**
0.00 0.00 FUD XXX
AMA: 2005,Aug,7-8; 2005,Jul,11-12

87076 **anaerobic isolate, additional methods required for definitive identification, each isolate**
0.00 0.00 FUD XXX
AMA: 2018,Jan,8; 2017,Jan,8; 2016,Jan,13; 2015,Jan,16; 2014,Jan,11

87077 **aerobic isolate, additional methods required for definitive identification, each isolate**
0.00 0.00 FUD XXX
AMA: 2018,Jan,8; 2017,Jan,8; 2016,Jan,13; 2015,Jan,16; 2014,Jan,11

87081 **Culture, presumptive, pathogenic organisms, screening only;**
0.00 0.00 FUD XXX
AMA: 2018,Jan,8; 2017,Jan,8; 2016,Jan,13; 2015,Jan,16; 2014,Jan,11

87084 **with colony estimation from density chart**
0.00 0.00 FUD XXX
AMA: 2005,Aug,7-8; 2005,Jul,11-12

87086 **Culture, bacterial; quantitative colony count, urine**
0.00 0.00 FUD XXX
AMA: 2018,Jan,8; 2017,Jan,8; 2016,Jan,13; 2015,Jan,16; 2014,Jan,11

87088 **with isolation and presumptive identification of each isolate, urine**
0.00 0.00 FUD XXX
AMA: 2018,Jan,8; 2017,Jan,8; 2016,Jan,13; 2015,Jan,16; 2014,Jan,11

87101 **Culture, fungi (mold or yeast) isolation, with presumptive identification of isolates; skin, hair, or nail**
0.00 0.00 FUD XXX
AMA: 2018,Jan,8; 2017,Jan,8; 2016,Jan,13; 2015,Jan,16; 2014,Jan,11

87102 **other source (except blood)**
0.00 0.00 FUD XXX
AMA: 2005,Aug,7-8; 2005,Jul,11-12

87103 **blood**
0.00 0.00 FUD XXX
AMA: 2005,Aug,7-8; 2005,Jul,11-12

87106 **Culture, fungi, definitive identification, each organism; yeast**
0.00 0.00 FUD XXX
AMA: 2005,Aug,7-8; 2005,Jul,11-12

87107 **mold**
0.00 0.00 FUD XXX
AMA: 2005,Aug,7-8; 2005,Jul,11-12

87109 **Culture, mycoplasma, any source**
0.00 0.00 FUD XXX
AMA: 2005,Aug,7-8; 2005,Jul,11-12

87110 **Culture, chlamydia, any source**
EXCLUDES *Immunofluorescence staining of shell vials (87140)*
0.00 0.00 FUD XXX
AMA: 2005,Aug,7-8; 2005,Jul,11-12

87116 **Culture, tubercle or other acid-fast bacilli (eg, TB, AFB, mycobacteria) any source, with isolation and presumptive identification of isolates**
EXCLUDES *Concentration (87015)*
0.00 0.00 FUD XXX
AMA: 2005,Aug,7-8; 2005,Jul,11-12

87118 **Culture, mycobacterial, definitive identification, each isolate**
0.00 0.00 FUD XXX
AMA: 2005,Aug,7-8; 2005,Jul,11-12

87140-87158 Additional Culture Typing Techniques

INCLUDES Bacteriology, mycology, parasitology, and virology
EXCLUDES *Use of molecular procedure codes as a substitute for codes in this range (81105-81183 [81173, 81174, 81200, 81201, 81202, 81203, 81204], 81400-81408, [81479])*
Code also definitive identification
Code also modifier 59 for multiple specimens or sites
Code also modifier 91 for repeat procedures performed on the same day

87140 **Culture, typing; immunofluorescent method, each antiserum**
0.00 0.00 FUD XXX
AMA: 2018,Jan,8; 2017,Jan,8; 2016,Jan,13; 2015,Jan,16; 2014,Jan,11

87143 **gas liquid chromatography (GLC) or high pressure liquid chromatography (HPLC) method**
0.00 0.00 FUD XXX
AMA: 2005,Aug,7-8; 2005,Jul,11-12

87147 **immunologic method, other than immunofluorescence (eg, agglutination grouping), per antiserum**
0.00 0.00 FUD XXX
AMA: 2018,Jan,8; 2017,Jan,8; 2016,Jan,13; 2015,Jan,16; 2014,Jan,11

87149 **identification by nucleic acid (DNA or RNA) probe, direct probe technique, per culture or isolate, each organism probed**
0.00 0.00 FUD XXX
AMA: 2018,Jan,8; 2017,Jan,8; 2016,Jan,13; 2015,Jan,16; 2014,Jan,11

87150 **identification by nucleic acid (DNA or RNA) probe, amplified probe technique, per culture or isolate, each organism probed**
0.00 0.00 FUD XXX
AMA: 2018,Jan,8; 2017,Jan,8; 2016,Jan,13; 2015,Jan,16; 2014,Jan,11

87152 **identification by pulse field gel typing**
0.00 0.00 FUD XXX
AMA: 2018,Jan,8; 2017,Jan,8; 2016,Jan,13; 2015,Jan,16; 2014,Jan,11

87153 **identification by nucleic acid sequencing method, each isolate (eg, sequencing of the 16S rRNA gene)**
0.00 0.00 FUD XXX
AMA: 2018,Jan,8; 2017,Jan,8; 2016,Jan,13; 2015,Jan,16

87158 **other methods**
0.00 0.00 FUD XXX
AMA: 2018,Jan,8; 2017,Jan,8; 2016,Jan,13; 2015,Jan,16; 2014,Jan,11

87164-87255 Identification of Organism from Primary Source and Sensitivity Studies

INCLUDES Bacteriology, mycology, parasitology, and virology
EXCLUDES *Additional tests using molecular probes, chromatography, or immunologic techniques (87140-87158)*
Code also modifier 59 for multiple specimens or sites
Code also modifier 91 for repeat procedures performed on the same day

87164 **Dark field examination, any source (eg, penile, vaginal, oral, skin); includes specimen collection**
0.00 0.00 FUD XXX
AMA: 2005,Jul,11-12; 2005,Aug,7-8

87166 **without collection**
0.00 0.00 FUD XXX
AMA: 2005,Aug,7-8; 2005,Jul,11-12

87168 **Macroscopic examination; arthropod**
0.00 0.00 FUD XXX
AMA: 2005,Aug,7-8; 2005,Jul,11-12

87169 **parasite**
0.00 0.00 FUD XXX
AMA: 2005,Aug,7-8; 2005,Jul,11-12

87172 **Pinworm exam (eg, cellophane tape prep)**
0.00 0.00 FUD XXX
AMA: 2005,Aug,7-8; 2005,Jul,11-12

87176 **Homogenization, tissue, for culture**
0.00 0.00 FUD XXX
AMA: 2005,Aug,7-8; 2005,Jul,11-12

87177 **Ova and parasites, direct smears, concentration and identification**
EXCLUDES *Coccidia or microsporidia exam (87207)*
Complex special stain (trichrome, iron hematoxylin) (87209)
Concentration for infectious agents (87015)
Direct smears from primary source (87207)
Nucleic acid probes in cytologic material (88365)
0.00 0.00 FUD XXX
AMA: 2018,Jan,8; 2017,Jan,8; 2016,Jan,13; 2015,Jan,16; 2014,Jan,11

87181 **Susceptibility studies, antimicrobial agent; agar dilution method, per agent (eg, antibiotic gradient strip)**
0.00 0.00 FUD XXX
AMA: 2018,Jan,8; 2017,Jan,8; 2016,Jan,13; 2015,Jan,16; 2014,Jan,11

87184 **disk method, per plate (12 or fewer agents)**
0.00 0.00 FUD XXX
AMA: 2018,Jan,8; 2017,Jan,8; 2016,Jan,13; 2015,Jan,16; 2014,Jan,11

87185 **enzyme detection (eg, beta lactamase), per enzyme**
0.00 0.00 FUD XXX
AMA: 2018,Jan,8; 2017,Jan,8; 2016,Jan,13; 2015,Jan,16; 2014,Jan,11

87186 **microdilution or agar dilution (minimum inhibitory concentration [MIC] or breakpoint), each multi-antimicrobial, per plate**
0.00 0.00 FUD XXX
AMA: 2018,Jan,8; 2017,Jan,8; 2016,Jan,13; 2015,Jan,16; 2014,Jan,11

+ 87187 **microdilution or agar dilution, minimum lethal concentration (MLC), each plate (List separately in addition to code for primary procedure)**
Code first (87186, 87188)
0.00 0.00 FUD XXX
AMA: 2018,Jan,8; 2017,Jan,8; 2016,Jan,13; 2015,Jan,16; 2014,Jan,11

87188 **macrobroth dilution method, each agent**
0.00 0.00 FUD XXX
AMA: 2018,Jan,8; 2017,Jan,8; 2016,Jan,13; 2015,Jan,16; 2014,Jan,11

87190 **mycobacteria, proportion method, each agent**
EXCLUDES *Other mycobacterial susceptibility studies (87181, 87184, 87186, 87188)*
0.00 0.00 FUD XXX
AMA: 2005,Aug,7-8; 2005,Jul,11-12

87197 **Serum bactericidal titer (Schlichter test)**
0.00 0.00 FUD XXX
AMA: 2005,Aug,7-8; 2005,Jul,11-12

87205 **Smear, primary source with interpretation; Gram or Giemsa stain for bacteria, fungi, or cell types**
0.00 0.00 FUD XXX
AMA: 2018,Jan,8; 2017,Jan,8; 2016,Jan,13; 2015,Jan,16; 2014,Jan,11

87206 **fluorescent and/or acid fast stain for bacteria, fungi, parasites, viruses or cell types**
0.00 0.00 FUD XXX
AMA: 2005,Aug,7-8; 2005,Jul,11-12

87207 **special stain for inclusion bodies or parasites (eg, malaria, coccidia, microsporidia, trypanosomes, herpes viruses)**
EXCLUDES *Direct smears with concentration and identification (87177)*
Fat, fibers, meat, nasal eosinophils, starch (89049-89240)
Thick smear preparation (87015)
0.00 0.00 FUD XXX
AMA: 2018,Jan,8; 2017,Jan,8; 2016,Jan,13; 2015,Jan,16; 2014,Jan,11

87209 **complex special stain (eg, trichrome, iron hemotoxylin) for ova and parasites**
0.00 0.00 FUD XXX
AMA: 2018,Jan,8; 2017,Jan,8; 2016,Jan,13; 2015,Jan,16; 2014,Jan,11

87210 **wet mount for infectious agents (eg, saline, India ink, KOH preps)**
EXCLUDES *KOH evaluation of skin, hair, or nails (87220)*
0.00 0.00 FUD XXX
AMA: 2018,Jan,8; 2017,Jan,8; 2016,May,13

87220 **Tissue examination by KOH slide of samples from skin, hair, or nails for fungi or ectoparasite ova or mites (eg, scabies)**
0.00 0.00 FUD XXX
AMA: 2005,Aug,7-8; 2005,Jul,11-12

87230 **Toxin or antitoxin assay, tissue culture (eg, Clostridium difficile toxin)**
0.00 0.00 FUD XXX
AMA: 2005,Aug,7-8; 2005,Jul,11-12

87250 **Virus isolation; inoculation of embryonated eggs, or small animal, includes observation and dissection**
0.00 0.00 FUD XXX
AMA: 2005,Aug,7-8; 2005,Jul,11-12

87252 **tissue culture inoculation, observation, and presumptive identification by cytopathic effect**
0.00 0.00 FUD XXX
AMA: 2005,Aug,7-8; 2005,Jul,11-12

87253 **tissue culture, additional studies or definitive identification (eg, hemabsorption, neutralization, immunofluorescence stain), each isolate**
EXCLUDES *Electron microscopy (88348)*
Inclusion bodies in:
Fluids (88106)
Smears (87207-87210)
Tissue sections (88304-88309)
0.00 0.00 FUD XXX
AMA: 2005,Aug,7-8; 2005,Jul,11-12

87254 **centrifuge enhanced (shell vial) technique, includes identification with immunofluorescence stain, each virus**
Code also (87252)
0.00 0.00 FUD XXX
AMA: 2018,Jan,8; 2017,Jan,8; 2016,Jan,13; 2015,Jan,16; 2014,Jan,11

87255 **including identification by non-immunologic method, other than by cytopathic effect (eg, virus specific enzymatic activity)**
0.00 0.00 FUD XXX
AMA: 2018,Jan,8; 2017,Jan,8; 2016,Jan,13; 2015,Jan,16; 2014,Jan,11

87260-87300 Fluorescence Microscopy by Organism

INCLUDES Primary source only

EXCLUDES *Comparable tests on culture material (87140-87158)*
Identification of antibodies (86602-86804)
Nonspecific agent detection (87299, 87449-87450, 87797-87799, 87899)

Code also modifier 59 for different species or strains reported by the same code

87260 Infectious agent antigen detection by immunofluorescent technique; adenovirus
0.00 0.00 FUD XXX
AMA: 2005,Jul,11-12; 2005,Aug,7-8

87265 Bordetella pertussis/parapertussis
0.00 0.00 FUD XXX
AMA: 2005,Jul,11-12; 2005,Aug,7-8

87267 Enterovirus, direct fluorescent antibody (DFA)
0.00 0.00 FUD XXX
AMA: 2018,Jan,8; 2017,Jan,8; 2016,Jan,13; 2015,Jan,16; 2014,Jan,11

87269 giardia
0.00 0.00 FUD XXX
AMA: 2005,Jul,11-12; 2005,Aug,7-8

87270 Chlamydia trachomatis
0.00 0.00 FUD XXX
AMA: 2005,Jul,11-12; 2005,Aug,7-8

87271 Cytomegalovirus, direct fluorescent antibody (DFA)
0.00 0.00 FUD XXX
AMA: 2018,Jan,8; 2017,Jan,8; 2016,Jan,13; 2015,Jan,16; 2014,Jan,11

87272 cryptosporidium
0.00 0.00 FUD XXX
AMA: 2005,Jul,11-12; 2005,Aug,7-8

87273 Herpes simplex virus type 2
0.00 0.00 FUD XXX
AMA: 2005,Jul,11-12; 2005,Aug,7-8

87274 Herpes simplex virus type 1
0.00 0.00 FUD XXX
AMA: 2005,Jul,11-12; 2005,Aug,7-8

87275 influenza B virus
0.00 0.00 FUD XXX
AMA: 2018,Jan,8; 2017,Jan,8; 2016,Jan,13; 2015,Jan,16; 2014,Jan,11

87276 influenza A virus
0.00 0.00 FUD XXX
AMA: 2018,Jan,8; 2017,Jan,8; 2016,Jan,13; 2015,Jan,16; 2014,Jan,11

87278 Legionella pneumophila
0.00 0.00 FUD XXX
AMA: 2005,Jul,11-12; 2005,Aug,7-8

87279 Parainfluenza virus, each type
0.00 0.00 FUD XXX
AMA: 2005,Jul,11-12; 2005,Aug,7-8

87280 respiratory syncytial virus
0.00 0.00 FUD XXX
AMA: 2005,Jul,11-12; 2005,Aug,7-8

87281 Pneumocystis carinii
0.00 0.00 FUD XXX
AMA: 2005,Jul,11-12; 2005,Aug,7-8

87283 Rubeola
0.00 0.00 FUD XXX
AMA: 2005,Jul,11-12; 2005,Aug,7-8

87285 Treponema pallidum
0.00 0.00 FUD XXX
AMA: 2005,Jul,11-12; 2005,Aug,7-8

87290 Varicella zoster virus
0.00 0.00 FUD XXX
AMA: 2005,Jul,11-12; 2005,Aug,7-8

87299 not otherwise specified, each organism
0.00 0.00 FUD XXX
AMA: 2018,Jan,8; 2017,Jan,8; 2016,Jan,13; 2015,Jan,16; 2014,Jan,11

87300 Infectious agent antigen detection by immunofluorescent technique, polyvalent for multiple organisms, each polyvalent antiserum
EXCLUDES *Physician evaluation of infectious disease agents by immunofluorescence (88346)*
0.00 0.00 FUD XXX
AMA: 2005,Jul,11-12; 2005,Aug,7-8

87301-87451 Enzyme Immunoassay Technique by Organism

INCLUDES Primary source only

EXCLUDES *Comparable tests on culture material (87140-87158)*
Identification of antibodies (86602-86804)
Nonspecific agent detection (87449-87450, 87797-87799, 87899)

Code also modifier 59 for different species or strains reported by the same code

87301 Infectious agent antigen detection by immunoassay technique, (eg, enzyme immunoassay [EIA], enzyme-linked immunosorbent assay [ELISA], immunochemiluminometric assay [IMCA]) qualitative or semiquantitative, multiple-step method; adenovirus enteric types 40/41
0.00 0.00 FUD XXX
AMA: 2018,Jan,8; 2017,Jan,8; 2016,Jan,13; 2015,Jan,16; 2014,Jan,11

87305 Aspergillus
0.00 0.00 FUD XXX

87320 Chlamydia trachomatis
0.00 0.00 FUD XXX
AMA: 2005,Jul,11-12; 2005,Aug,7-8

87324 Clostridium difficile toxin(s)
0.00 0.00 FUD XXX
AMA: 2005,Jul,11-12; 2005,Aug,7-8

87327 Cryptococcus neoformans
EXCLUDES *Cryptococcus latex agglutination (86403)*
0.00 0.00 FUD XXX
AMA: 2005,Jul,11-12; 2005,Aug,7-8

87328 cryptosporidium
0.00 0.00 FUD XXX
AMA: 2005,Jul,11-12; 2005,Aug,7-8

87329 giardia
0.00 0.00 FUD XXX
AMA: 2005,Jul,11-12; 2005,Aug,7-8

87332 cytomegalovirus
0.00 0.00 FUD XXX
AMA: 2005,Jul,11-12; 2005,Aug,7-8

87335 Escherichia coli 0157
EXCLUDES *Giardia antigen (87329)*
0.00 0.00 FUD XXX
AMA: 2005,Jul,11-12; 2005,Aug,7-8

87336 Entamoeba histolytica dispar group
0.00 0.00 FUD XXX
AMA: 2005,Jul,11-12; 2005,Aug,7-8

87337 Entamoeba histolytica group
0.00 0.00 FUD XXX
AMA: 2005,Jul,11-12; 2005,Aug,7-8

87338 Helicobacter pylori, stool
0.00 0.00 FUD XXX
AMA: 2018,Jan,8; 2017,Jan,8; 2016,Jan,13; 2015,Jan,16; 2014,Jan,11

87339 **Helicobacter pylori**

EXCLUDES *H. pylori:*

Breath and blood by mass spectrometry (83013-83014)

Liquid scintillation counter (78267-78268)

Stool (87338)

0.00 0.00 FUD XXX

AMA: 2005,Jul,11-12; 2005,Aug,7-8

87340 **hepatitis B surface antigen (HBsAg)**

0.00 0.00 FUD XXX

AMA: 2018,Jan,8; 2017,Jan,8; 2016,Jan,13; 2015,Jan,16; 2014,Jan,11

87341 **hepatitis B surface antigen (HBsAg) neutralization**

0.00 0.00 FUD XXX

AMA: 2005,Jul,11-12; 2005,Aug,7-8

87350 **hepatitis Be antigen (HBeAg)**

0.00 0.00 FUD XXX

AMA: 2005,Jul,11-12; 2005,Aug,7-8

87380 **hepatitis, delta agent**

0.00 0.00 FUD XXX

AMA: 2005,Jul,11-12; 2005,Aug,7-8

87385 **Histoplasma capsulatum**

0.00 0.00 FUD XXX

AMA: 2005,Jul,11-12; 2005,Aug,7-8

87389 **HIV-1 antigen(s), with HIV-1 and HIV-2 antibodies, single result**

0.00 0.00 FUD XXX

Code also modifier 92 for test performed using a kit or transportable instrument that is all or in part consists of a single-use, disposable analytical chamber

87390 **HIV-1**

0.00 0.00 FUD XXX

AMA: 2005,Jul,11-12; 2005,Aug,7-8

87391 **HIV-2**

0.00 0.00 FUD XXX

AMA: 2005,Jul,11-12; 2005,Aug,7-8

87400 **Influenza, A or B, each**

0.00 0.00 FUD XXX

AMA: 2018,Jan,8; 2017,Jan,8; 2016,Jan,13; 2015,Jan,16; 2014,Jan,11

87420 **respiratory syncytial virus**

0.00 0.00 FUD XXX

AMA: 2005,Jul,11-12; 2005,Aug,7-8

87425 **rotavirus**

0.00 0.00 FUD XXX

AMA: 2005,Jul,11-12; 2005,Aug,7-8

87427 **Shiga-like toxin**

0.00 0.00 FUD XXX

AMA: 2005,Jul,11-12; 2005,Aug,7-8

87430 **Streptococcus, group A**

0.00 0.00 FUD XXX

AMA: 2018,Jan,8; 2017,Jan,8; 2016,Jan,13; 2015,Jan,16

87449 **Infectious agent antigen detection by immunoassay technique, (eg, enzyme immunoassay [EIA], enzyme-linked immunosorbent assay [ELISA], immunochemiluminometric assay [IMCA]), qualitative or semiquantitative; multiple-step method, not otherwise specified, each organism**

0.00 0.00 FUD XXX

AMA: 2018,Jan,8; 2017,Jan,8; 2016,Jan,13; 2015,Jan,16; 2014,Jan,11

87450 **single step method, not otherwise specified, each organism**

0.00 0.00 FUD XXX

AMA: 2005,Jul,11-12; 2005,Aug,7-8

87451 **multiple step method, polyvalent for multiple organisms, each polyvalent antiserum**

0.00 0.00 FUD XXX

AMA: 2005,Jul,11-12; 2005,Aug,7-8

87471-87801 [87623, 87624, 87625] Detection Infectious Agent by Probe Techniques

INCLUDES Primary source only

EXCLUDES *Comparable tests on culture material (87140-87158)*

Identification of antibodies (86602-86804)

Nonspecific agent detection (87299, 87449-87450, 87797-87799, 87899)

Use of molecular procedure codes as a substitute for codes in this range (81161-81408 [81105, 81106, 81107, 81108, 81109, 81110, 81111, 81112, 81120, 81121, 81161, 81162, 81230, 81231, 81238, 81269, 81283, 81287, 81288, 81334])

Code also modifier 59 for different species or strains reported by the same code

87471 **Infectious agent detection by nucleic acid (DNA or RNA); Bartonella henselae and Bartonella quintana, amplified probe technique**

0.00 0.00 FUD XXX

AMA: 2018,Jan,8; 2017,Jan,8; 2016,Jan,13; 2015,Jan,16

87472 **Bartonella henselae and Bartonella quintana, quantification**

0.00 0.00 FUD XXX

AMA: 2018,Jan,8; 2017,Jan,8; 2016,Jan,13; 2015,Jan,16

87475 **Borrelia burgdorferi, direct probe technique**

0.00 0.00 FUD XXX

AMA: 2018,Jan,8; 2017,Jan,8; 2016,Jan,13; 2015,Jan,16

87476 **Borrelia burgdorferi, amplified probe technique**

0.00 0.00 FUD XXX

AMA: 2018,Jan,8; 2017,Jan,8; 2016,Jan,13; 2015,Jan,16

87480 **Candida species, direct probe technique**

0.00 0.00 FUD XXX

AMA: 2018,Jan,8; 2017,Jan,8; 2016,Jan,13; 2015,Jan,16

87481 **Candida species, amplified probe technique**

0.00 0.00 FUD XXX

AMA: 2018,Jan,8; 2017,Jan,8; 2016,Jan,13; 2015,Jan,16

87482 **Candida species, quantification**

0.00 0.00 FUD XXX

AMA: 2018,Jan,8; 2017,Jan,8; 2016,Jan,13; 2015,Jan,16

87483 **central nervous system pathogen (eg, Neisseria meningitidis, Streptococcus pneumoniae, Listeria, Haemophilus influenzae, E. coli, Streptococcus agalactiae, enterovirus, human parechovirus, herpes simplex virus type 1 and 2, human herpesvirus 6, cytomegalovirus, varicella zoster virus, Cryptococcus), includes multiplex reverse transcription, when performed, and multiplex amplified probe technique, multiple types or subtypes, 12-25 targets**

0.00 0.00 FUD XXX

87485 **Chlamydia pneumoniae, direct probe technique**

0.00 0.00 FUD XXX

AMA: 2018,Jan,8; 2017,Jan,8; 2016,Jan,13; 2015,Jan,16

87486 **Chlamydia pneumoniae, amplified probe technique**

0.00 0.00 FUD XXX

AMA: 2018,Jan,8; 2017,Jan,8; 2016,Jan,13; 2015,Jan,16

87487 **Chlamydia pneumoniae, quantification**

0.00 0.00 FUD XXX

AMA: 2018,Jan,8; 2017,Jan,8; 2016,Jan,13; 2015,Jan,16

87490 **Chlamydia trachomatis, direct probe technique**

0.00 0.00 FUD XXX

AMA: 2018,Jan,8; 2017,Jan,8; 2016,Jan,13; 2015,Jan,16

87491 **Chlamydia trachomatis, amplified probe technique**

0.00 0.00 FUD XXX

AMA: 2018,Jan,8; 2017,Jan,8; 2016,Jan,13; 2015,Jan,16

87492 **Chlamydia trachomatis, quantification**

0.00 0.00 FUD XXX

AMA: 2018,Jan,8; 2017,Jan,8; 2016,Jan,13; 2015,Jan,16

87493 **Clostridium difficile, toxin gene(s), amplified probe technique**
0.00 0.00 FUD XXX
AMA: 2018,Jan,8; 2017,Jan,8; 2016,Jan,13; 2015,Jan,16; 2014,Jan,11

87495 **cytomegalovirus, direct probe technique**
0.00 0.00 FUD XXX
AMA: 2018,Jan,8; 2017,Jan,8; 2016,Jan,13; 2015,Jan,16

87496 **cytomegalovirus, amplified probe technique**
0.00 0.00 FUD XXX
AMA: 2018,Jan,8; 2017,Jan,8; 2016,Jan,13; 2015,Jan,16

87497 **cytomegalovirus, quantification**
0.00 0.00 FUD XXX
AMA: 2018,Jan,8; 2017,Jan,8; 2016,Jan,13; 2015,Jan,16

87498 **enterovirus, amplified probe technique, includes reverse transcription when performed**
0.00 0.00 FUD XXX
AMA: 2018,Jan,8; 2017,Jan,8; 2016,Jan,13; 2015,Jan,16

87500 **vancomycin resistance (eg, enterococcus species van A, van B), amplified probe technique**
0.00 0.00 FUD XXX
AMA: 2018,Jan,8; 2017,Jan,8; 2016,Jan,13; 2015,Jan,16; 2014,Jan,11

87501 **influenza virus, includes reverse transcription, when performed, and amplified probe technique, each type or subtype**
0.00 0.00 FUD XXX
AMA: 2018,Jan,8; 2017,Jan,8; 2016,Jan,13; 2015,Jan,16

87502 **influenza virus, for multiple types or sub-types, includes multiplex reverse transcription, when performed, and multiplex amplified probe technique, first 2 types or sub-types**
0.00 0.00 FUD XXX
AMA: 2018,Jan,8; 2017,Jan,8; 2016,Jan,13; 2015,Jan,16

\+ 87503 **influenza virus, for multiple types or sub-types, includes multiplex reverse transcription, when performed, and multiplex amplified probe technique, each additional influenza virus type or sub-type beyond 2 (List separately in addition to code for primary procedure)**
Code first (87502)
0.00 0.00 FUD XXX
AMA: 2018,Jan,8; 2017,Jan,8; 2016,Jan,13; 2015,Jan,16

87505 **gastrointestinal pathogen (eg, Clostridium difficile, E. coli, Salmonella, Shigella, norovirus, Giardia), includes multiplex reverse transcription, when performed, and multiplex amplified probe technique, multiple types or subtypes, 3-5 targets**
0.00 0.00 FUD XXX

87506 **gastrointestinal pathogen (eg, Clostridium difficile, E. coli, Salmonella, Shigella, norovirus, Giardia), includes multiplex reverse transcription, when performed, and multiplex amplified probe technique, multiple types or subtypes, 6-11 targets**
0.00 0.00 FUD XXX

87507 **gastrointestinal pathogen (eg, Clostridium difficile, E. coli, Salmonella, Shigella, norovirus, Giardia), includes multiplex reverse transcription, when performed, and multiplex amplified probe technique, multiple types or subtypes, 12-25 targets**
0.00 0.00 FUD XXX

87510 **Gardnerella vaginalis, direct probe technique**
0.00 0.00 FUD XXX
AMA: 2018,Jan,8; 2017,Jan,8; 2016,Jan,13; 2015,Jan,16

87511 **Gardnerella vaginalis, amplified probe technique**
0.00 0.00 FUD XXX
AMA: 2018,Jan,8; 2017,Jan,8; 2016,Jan,13; 2015,Jan,16

87512 **Gardnerella vaginalis, quantification**
0.00 0.00 FUD XXX
AMA: 2018,Jan,8; 2017,Jan,8; 2016,Jan,13; 2015,Jan,16

87516 **hepatitis B virus, amplified probe technique**
0.00 0.00 FUD XXX
AMA: 2018,Jan,8; 2017,Jan,8; 2016,Jan,13; 2015,Jan,16

87517 **hepatitis B virus, quantification**
0.00 0.00 FUD XXX
AMA: 2018,Jan,8; 2017,Jan,8; 2016,Jan,13; 2015,Jan,16

87520 **hepatitis C, direct probe technique**
0.00 0.00 FUD XXX
AMA: 2018,Jan,8; 2017,Jan,8; 2016,Jan,13; 2015,Jan,16

87521 **hepatitis C, amplified probe technique, includes reverse transcription when performed**
0.00 0.00 FUD XXX
AMA: 2018,Jan,8; 2017,Jan,8; 2016,Jan,13; 2015,Jan,16

87522 **hepatitis C, quantification, includes reverse transcription when performed**
0.00 0.00 FUD XXX
AMA: 2018,Jan,8; 2017,Jan,8; 2016,Jan,13; 2015,Jan,16

87525 **hepatitis G, direct probe technique**
0.00 0.00 FUD XXX
AMA: 2018,Jan,8; 2017,Jan,8; 2016,Jan,13; 2015,Jan,16

87526 **hepatitis G, amplified probe technique**
0.00 0.00 FUD XXX
AMA: 2018,Jan,8; 2017,Jan,8; 2016,Jan,13; 2015,Jan,16

87527 **hepatitis G, quantification**
0.00 0.00 FUD XXX
AMA: 2018,Jan,8; 2017,Jan,8; 2016,Jan,13; 2015,Jan,16

87528 **Herpes simplex virus, direct probe technique**
0.00 0.00 FUD XXX
AMA: 2018,Jan,8; 2017,Jan,8; 2016,Jan,13; 2015,Jan,16

87529 **Herpes simplex virus, amplified probe technique**
0.00 0.00 FUD XXX
AMA: 2018,Jan,8; 2017,Jan,8; 2016,Jan,13; 2015,Jan,16

87530 **Herpes simplex virus, quantification**
0.00 0.00 FUD XXX
AMA: 2018,Jan,8; 2017,Jan,8; 2016,Jan,13; 2015,Jan,16

87531 **Herpes virus-6, direct probe technique**
0.00 0.00 FUD XXX
AMA: 2018,Jan,8; 2017,Jan,8; 2016,Jan,13; 2015,Jan,16

87532 **Herpes virus-6, amplified probe technique**
0.00 0.00 FUD XXX
AMA: 2018,Jan,8; 2017,Jan,8; 2016,Jan,13; 2015,Jan,16

87533 **Herpes virus-6, quantification**
0.00 0.00 FUD XXX
AMA: 2018,Jan,8; 2017,Jan,8; 2016,Jan,13; 2015,Jan,16

87534 **HIV-1, direct probe technique**
0.00 0.00 FUD XXX
AMA: 2018,Jan,8; 2017,Jan,8; 2016,Jan,13; 2015,Jan,16

87535 **HIV-1, amplified probe technique, includes reverse transcription when performed**
0.00 0.00 FUD XXX
AMA: 2018,Jan,8; 2017,Jan,8; 2016,Jan,13; 2015,Jan,16; 2014,Jan,11

87536 **HIV-1, quantification, includes reverse transcription when performed**
0.00 0.00 FUD XXX
AMA: 2018,Jan,8; 2017,Jan,8; 2016,Jan,13; 2015,Jan,16; 2014,Jan,11

87537 **HIV-2, direct probe technique**
0.00 0.00 FUD XXX
AMA: 2018,Jan,8; 2017,Jan,8; 2016,Jan,13; 2015,Jan,16

87538 HIV-2, amplified probe technique, includes reverse transcription when performed
0.00 0.00 FUD XXX
AMA: 2018,Jan,8; 2017,Jan,8; 2016,Jan,13; 2015,Jan,16

87539 HIV-2, quantification, includes reverse transcription when performed
0.00 0.00 FUD XXX
AMA: 2018,Jan,8; 2017,Jan,8; 2016,Jan,13; 2015,Jan,16

87623 Human Papillomavirus (HPV), low-risk types (eg, 6, 11, 42, 43, 44)
0.00 0.00 FUD XXX

87624 Human Papillomavirus (HPV), high-risk types (eg, 16, 18, 31, 33, 35, 39, 45, 51, 52, 56, 58, 59, 68)
INCLUDES Low- and high-risk types in one assay
0.00 0.00 FUD XXX
AMA: 2018,Jan,8; 2017,Jan,8; 2016,Jan,13; 2015,Oct,9

87625 Human Papillomavirus (HPV), types 16 and 18 only, includes type 45, if performed
EXCLUDES *HPV detection (genotyping) (0500T)*
0.00 0.00 FUD XXX
AMA: 2018,Jan,8; 2017,Jan,8; 2016,Jan,13; 2015,Oct,9; 2015,Jun,10

87540 Legionella pneumophila, direct probe technique
0.00 0.00 FUD XXX
AMA: 2018,Jan,8; 2017,Jan,8; 2016,Jan,13; 2015,Jan,16

87541 Legionella pneumophila, amplified probe technique
0.00 0.00 FUD XXX
AMA: 2018,Jan,8; 2017,Jan,8; 2016,Jan,13; 2015,Jan,16

87542 Legionella pneumophila, quantification
0.00 0.00 FUD XXX
AMA: 2018,Jan,8; 2017,Jan,8; 2016,Jan,13; 2015,Jan,16

87550 Mycobacteria species, direct probe technique
0.00 0.00 FUD XXX
AMA: 2018,Jan,8; 2017,Jan,8; 2016,Jan,13; 2015,Jan,16

87551 Mycobacteria species, amplified probe technique
0.00 0.00 FUD XXX
AMA: 2018,Jan,8; 2017,Jan,8; 2016,Jan,13; 2015,Jan,16

87552 Mycobacteria species, quantification
0.00 0.00 FUD XXX
AMA: 2018,Jan,8; 2017,Jan,8; 2016,Jan,13; 2015,Jan,16

87555 Mycobacteria tuberculosis, direct probe technique
0.00 0.00 FUD XXX
AMA: 2018,Jan,8; 2017,Jan,8; 2016,Jan,13; 2015,Jan,16

87556 Mycobacteria tuberculosis, amplified probe technique
0.00 0.00 FUD XXX
AMA: 2018,Jan,8; 2017,Jan,8; 2016,Jan,13; 2015,Jan,16

87557 Mycobacteria tuberculosis, quantification
0.00 0.00 FUD XXX
AMA: 2018,Jan,8; 2017,Jan,8; 2016,Jan,13; 2015,Jan,16

87560 Mycobacteria avium-intracellulare, direct probe technique
0.00 0.00 FUD XXX
AMA: 2018,Jan,8; 2017,Jan,8; 2016,Jan,13; 2015,Jan,16

87561 Mycobacteria avium-intracellulare, amplified probe technique
0.00 0.00 FUD XXX
AMA: 2018,Jan,8; 2017,Jan,8; 2016,Jan,13; 2015,Jan,16

87562 Mycobacteria avium-intracellulare, quantification
0.00 0.00 FUD XXX
AMA: 2018,Jan,8; 2017,Jan,8; 2016,Jan,13; 2015,Jan,16

● 87563 Mycoplasma genitalium, amplified probe technique

87580 Mycoplasma pneumoniae, direct probe technique
0.00 0.00 FUD XXX
AMA: 2018,Jan,8; 2017,Jan,8; 2016,Jan,13; 2015,Jan,16

87581 Mycoplasma pneumoniae, amplified probe technique
0.00 0.00 FUD XXX
AMA: 2018,Jan,8; 2017,Jan,8; 2016,Jan,13; 2015,Jan,16

87582 Mycoplasma pneumoniae, quantification
0.00 0.00 FUD XXX
AMA: 2018,Jan,8; 2017,Jan,8; 2016,Jan,13; 2015,Jan,16

87590 Neisseria gonorrhoeae, direct probe technique
0.00 0.00 FUD XXX
AMA: 2018,Jan,8; 2017,Jan,8; 2016,Jan,13; 2015,Jan,16

87591 Neisseria gonorrhoeae, amplified probe technique
0.00 0.00 FUD XXX
AMA: 2018,Jan,8; 2017,Jan,8; 2016,Jan,13; 2015,Jan,16

87592 Neisseria gonorrhoeae, quantification
0.00 0.00 FUD XXX
AMA: 2018,Jan,8; 2017,Jan,8; 2016,Jan,13; 2015,Jan,16

87623 Resequenced code. See code following 87539.

87624 Resequenced code. See code following 87539.

87625 Resequenced code. See code before 87540.

87631 respiratory virus (eg, adenovirus, influenza virus, coronavirus, metapneumovirus, parainfluenza virus, respiratory syncytial virus, rhinovirus), includes multiplex reverse transcription, when performed, and multiplex amplified probe technique, multiple types or subtypes, 3-5 targets
INCLUDES Detection of multiple respiratory viruses with one test
EXCLUDES *Assays for typing or subtyping influenza viruses only (87501-87503)*
Single test for detection of multiple infectious organisms (87800-87801)
0.00 0.00 FUD XXX
AMA: 2018,Jan,8; 2017,Jan,8; 2016,Jan,13; 2015,Jan,16

87632 respiratory virus (eg, adenovirus, influenza virus, coronavirus, metapneumovirus, parainfluenza virus, respiratory syncytial virus, rhinovirus), includes multiplex reverse transcription, when performed, and multiplex amplified probe technique, multiple types or subtypes, 6-11 targets
INCLUDES Detection of multiple respiratory viruses with one test
EXCLUDES *Assays for typing or subtyping influenza viruses only (87501-87503)*
Single test to detect multiple infectious organisms (87800-87801)
0.00 0.00 FUD XXX
AMA: 2018,Jan,8; 2017,Jan,8; 2016,Jan,13; 2015,Jan,16

87633 respiratory virus (eg, adenovirus, influenza virus, coronavirus, metapneumovirus, parainfluenza virus, respiratory syncytial virus, rhinovirus), includes multiplex reverse transcription, when performed, and multiplex amplified probe technique, multiple types or subtypes, 12-25 targets
INCLUDES Detection of multiple respiratory viruses with one test
EXCLUDES *Assays for typing or subtyping influenza viruses only (87501-87503)*
Single test to detect multiple infectious organisms (87800-87801)
0.00 0.00 FUD XXX
AMA: 2018,Jan,8; 2017,Jan,8; 2016,Jan,13; 2015,Jan,16

87634 respiratory syncytial virus, amplified probe technique
0.00 0.00 FUD XXX
EXCLUDES *Assays for RSV with other respiratory viruses (87631-87633)*

87640 Staphylococcus aureus, amplified probe technique
0.00 0.00 FUD XXX
AMA: 2018,Jan,8; 2017,Jan,8; 2016,Jan,13; 2015,Jan,16; 2014,Jan,11

87641 **Staphylococcus aureus, methicillin resistant, amplified probe technique**

EXCLUDES *Assays that detect methicillin resistance and identify Staphylococcus aureus using a single nucleic acid sequence (87641)*

0.00 0.00 FUD XXX

AMA: 2018,Jan,8; 2017,Jan,8; 2016,Jan,13; 2015,Jan,16; 2014,Jan,11

87650 **Streptococcus, group A, direct probe technique**

0.00 0.00 FUD XXX

AMA: 2018,Jan,8; 2017,Jan,8; 2016,Jan,13; 2015,Jan,16

87651 **Streptococcus, group A, amplified probe technique**

0.00 0.00 FUD XXX

AMA: 2018,Jan,8; 2017,Jan,8; 2016,Jan,13; 2015,Jan,16

87652 **Streptococcus, group A, quantification**

0.00 0.00 FUD XXX

AMA: 2018,Jan,8; 2017,Jan,8; 2016,Jan,13; 2015,Jan,16

87653 **Streptococcus, group B, amplified probe technique**

0.00 0.00 FUD XXX

AMA: 2018,Jan,8; 2017,Jan,8; 2016,Jan,13; 2015,Jan,16; 2014,Jan,11

87660 **Trichomonas vaginalis, direct probe technique**

0.00 0.00 FUD XXX

AMA: 2018,Jan,8; 2017,Jan,8; 2016,Jan,13; 2015,Jan,16

87661 **Trichomonas vaginalis, amplified probe technique**

0.00 0.00 FUD XXX

87662 **Zika virus, amplified probe technique**

0.00 0.00 FUD XXX

87797 **Infectious agent detection by nucleic acid (DNA or RNA), not otherwise specified; direct probe technique, each organism**

0.00 0.00 FUD XXX

AMA: 2018,Jan,8; 2017,Jan,8; 2016,Aug,9; 2016,Jan,13; 2015,Jan,16; 2014,Jan,11

87798 **amplified probe technique, each organism**

0.00 0.00 FUD XXX

AMA: 2018,Jan,8; 2017,Jan,8; 2016,Jan,13; 2015,Jan,16; 2014,Jan,11

87799 **quantification, each organism**

0.00 0.00 FUD XXX

AMA: 2018,Jan,8; 2017,Jan,8; 2016,Jan,13; 2015,Jan,16

87800 **Infectious agent detection by nucleic acid (DNA or RNA), multiple organisms; direct probe(s) technique**

INCLUDES Single test to detect multiple infectious organisms

EXCLUDES *Detection of specific infectious agents not otherwise specified (87797-87799)*

Each specific organism nucleic acid detection from a primary source (87471-87660 [87623, 87624, 87625])

0.00 0.00 FUD XXX

AMA: 2018,Jan,8; 2017,Jan,8; 2016,Aug,9; 2016,Jan,13; 2015,Jan,16

87801 **amplified probe(s) technique**

INCLUDES Single test to detect multiple infectious organisms

EXCLUDES *Detection of multiple respiratory viruses with one test (87631-87633)*

Detection of specific infectious agents not otherwise specified (87797-87799)

Each specific organism nucleic acid detection from a primary source (87471-87660 [87623, 87624, 87625])

0.00 0.00 FUD XXX

AMA: 2018,Jan,8; 2017,Jan,8; 2016,Jan,13; 2015,Jan,16; 2014,Jan,11

87802-87899 [87806] Detection Infectious Agent by Immunoassay with Direct Optical Observation

87802 **Infectious agent antigen detection by immunoassay with direct optical observation; Streptococcus, group B**

0.00 0.00 FUD XXX

AMA: 2005,Aug,7-8; 2005,Jul,11-12

87803 **Clostridium difficile toxin A**

0.00 0.00 FUD XXX

AMA: 2005,Aug,7-8; 2005,Jul,11-12

87806 **HIV-1 antigen(s), with HIV-1 and HIV-2 antibodies**

0.00 0.00 FUD XXX

87804 **Influenza**

0.00 0.00 FUD XXX

AMA: 2018,Jan,8; 2017,Jan,8; 2016,Jan,13; 2015,Jan,16; 2014,Jan,11

87806 **Resequenced code. See code following 87803.**

87807 **respiratory syncytial virus**

0.00 0.00 FUD XXX

AMA: 2005,Jul,11-12; 2005,Aug,7-8

87808 **Trichomonas vaginalis**

0.00 0.00 FUD XXX

87809 **adenovirus**

0.00 0.00 FUD XXX

AMA: 2018,Jan,8; 2017,Jan,8; 2016,Jan,13; 2015,Jan,16; 2014,Jan,11

87810 **Chlamydia trachomatis**

0.00 0.00 FUD XXX

AMA: 2018,Jan,8; 2017,Jan,8; 2016,Jan,13; 2015,Jan,16; 2014,Jan,11

87850 **Neisseria gonorrhoeae**

0.00 0.00 FUD XXX

AMA: 2018,Jan,8; 2017,Jan,8; 2016,Jan,13; 2015,Jan,16; 2014,Jan,11

87880 **Streptococcus, group A**

0.00 0.00 FUD XXX

AMA: 2018,Jan,8; 2017,Jan,8; 2016,Jan,13; 2015,Jan,16; 2014,Jan,11

87899 **not otherwise specified**

0.00 0.00 FUD XXX

AMA: 2018,Jan,8; 2017,Jan,8; 2016,Jan,13; 2015,Jan,16; 2014,Jan,11

87900-87999 [87906, 87910, 87912] Drug Sensitivity Genotype/Phenotype

87900 **Infectious agent drug susceptibility phenotype prediction using regularly updated genotypic bioinformatics**

0.00 0.00 FUD XXX

AMA: 2018,Jan,8; 2017,Jan,8; 2016,Jan,13; 2015,Dec,18; 2015,Jan,16; 2014,Jan,11

87910 **Infectious agent genotype analysis by nucleic acid (DNA or RNA); cytomegalovirus**

EXCLUDES *HPV detection (genotyping) (0500T)*

HIV-1 infectious agent phenotype prediction (87900)

0.00 0.00 FUD XXX

AMA: 2018,Jan,8; 2017,Jan,8; 2016,Jan,13; 2015,Jan,16

87901 **HIV-1, reverse transcriptase and protease regions**

EXCLUDES *Infectious agent drug susceptibility phenotype prediction for HIV-1 (87900)*

0.00 0.00 FUD XXX

AMA: 2018,Jan,8; 2017,Jan,8; 2016,Jan,13; 2015,Jan,16; 2014,Jan,11

87906 **HIV-1, other region (eg, integrase, fusion)**

EXCLUDES *HIV-1 infectious agent phenotype prediction (87900)*

0.00 0.00 FUD XXX

AMA: 2018,Jan,8; 2017,Jan,8; 2016,Jan,13; 2015,Jan,16

\# **87912** **Hepatitis B virus**
0.00 0.00 FUD XXX
AMA: 2018,Jan,8; 2017,Jan,8; 2016,Jan,13; 2015,Jan,16

87902 **Hepatitis C virus**
0.00 0.00 FUD XXX
AMA: 2018,Jan,8; 2017,Jan,8; 2016,Jan,13; 2015,Dec,18; 2015,Nov,10; 2015,Jan,16; 2014,Jan,11

87903 **Infectious agent phenotype analysis by nucleic acid (DNA or RNA) with drug resistance tissue culture analysis, HIV 1; first through 10 drugs tested**
0.00 0.00 FUD XXX
AMA: 2018,Jan,8; 2017,Jan,8; 2016,Jan,13; 2015,Jan,16; 2014,Jan,11

\+ **87904** **each additional drug tested (List separately in addition to code for primary procedure)**
Code first (87903)
0.00 0.00 FUD XXX
AMA: 2018,Jan,8; 2017,Jan,8; 2016,Jan,13; 2015,Jan,16; 2014,Jan,11

87905 **Infectious agent enzymatic activity other than virus (eg, sialidase activity in vaginal fluid)**
0.00 0.00 FUD XXX
EXCLUDES *Isolation of a virus identified by a nonimmunologic method, and by noncytopathic effect (87255)*

87906 **Resequenced code. See code following 87901.**

87910 **Resequenced code. See code following 87900.**

87912 **Resequenced code. See code before 87902.**

87999 **Unlisted microbiology procedure**
0.00 0.00 FUD XXX
AMA: 2018,Jan,8; 2017,Jan,8; 2016,Jan,13; 2015,Jan,16; 2014,Jan,11

88000-88099 Autopsy Services

CMS: 100-02,15,80.1 Payment for Clinical Laboratory Services

INCLUDES Services for physicians only

88000 **Necropsy (autopsy), gross examination only; without CNS**
0.00 0.00 FUD XXX
AMA: 2018,Jan,8; 2017,Jan,8; 2016,Jan,13; 2015,Jan,16; 2014,Jan,11

88005 **with brain**
0.00 0.00 FUD XXX
AMA: 2005,Jul,11-12; 2005,Aug,7-8

88007 **with brain and spinal cord**
0.00 0.00 FUD XXX
AMA: 2005,Jul,11-12; 2005,Aug,7-8

88012 **infant with brain**
0.00 0.00 FUD XXX
AMA: 2005,Jul,11-12; 2005,Aug,7-8

88014 **stillborn or newborn with brain**
0.00 0.00 FUD XXX
AMA: 2005,Jul,11-12; 2005,Aug,7-8

88016 **macerated stillborn**
0.00 0.00 FUD XXX
AMA: 2005,Jul,11-12; 2005,Aug,7-8

88020 **Necropsy (autopsy), gross and microscopic; without CNS**
0.00 0.00 FUD XXX
AMA: 2005,Jul,11-12; 2005,Aug,7-8

88025 **with brain**
0.00 0.00 FUD XXX
AMA: 2005,Jul,11-12; 2005,Aug,7-8

88027 **with brain and spinal cord**
0.00 0.00 FUD XXX
AMA: 2005,Jul,11-12; 2005,Aug,7-8

88028 **infant with brain**
0.00 0.00 FUD XXX
AMA: 2005,Jul,11-12; 2005,Aug,7-8

88029 **stillborn or newborn with brain**
0.00 0.00 FUD XXX
AMA: 2005,Jul,11-12; 2005,Aug,7-8

88036 **Necropsy (autopsy), limited, gross and/or microscopic; regional**
0.00 0.00 FUD XXX
AMA: 2005,Jul,11-12; 2005,Aug,7-8

88037 **single organ**
0.00 0.00 FUD XXX
AMA: 2005,Jul,11-12; 2005,Aug,7-8

88040 **Necropsy (autopsy); forensic examination**
0.00 0.00 FUD XXX
AMA: 2005,Jul,11-12; 2005,Aug,7-8

88045 **coroner's call**
0.00 0.00 FUD XXX
AMA: 2005,Jul,11-12; 2005,Aug,7-8

88099 **Unlisted necropsy (autopsy) procedure**
0.00 0.00 FUD XXX
AMA: 2018,Jan,8; 2017,Jan,8; 2016,Jan,13; 2015,Jan,16; 2014,Jan,11

88104-88140 Cytopathology: Other Than Cervical/Vaginal

88104 **Cytopathology, fluids, washings or brushings, except cervical or vaginal; smears with interpretation**
1.98 1.98 FUD XXX
AMA: 2018,Jan,8; 2017,Jan,8; 2016,Jan,13; 2015,Jan,16; 2014,Jan,11

88106 **simple filter method with interpretation**
EXCLUDES *Cytopathology smears with interpretation (88104)*
Selective cellular enhancement (nongynecological) including filter transfer techniques (88112)
1.81 1.81 FUD XXX
AMA: 2018,Jan,8; 2017,Jan,8; 2016,Jan,13; 2015,Jan,16; 2014,Jan,11

88108 **Cytopathology, concentration technique, smears and interpretation (eg, Saccomanno technique)**
EXCLUDES *Cervical or vaginal smears (88150-88155)*
Gastric intubation with lavage (43754-43755)
(74340)
1.71 1.71 FUD XXX
AMA: 2018,Jan,8; 2017,Jan,8; 2016,Jan,13; 2015,Jan,16; 2014,Jan,11

88112 **Cytopathology, selective cellular enhancement technique with interpretation (eg, liquid based slide preparation method), except cervical or vaginal**
EXCLUDES *Cytopathology cellular enhancement technique (88108)*
1.90 1.90 FUD XXX
AMA: 2005,Aug,7-8; 2005,Jul,11-12

88120 **Cytopathology, in situ hybridization (eg, FISH), urinary tract specimen with morphometric analysis, 3-5 molecular probes, each specimen; manual**
EXCLUDES *More than five probes (88399)*
Morphometric in situ hybridization on specimens other than urinary tract (88367-88368 [88373, 88374])
16.8 16.8 FUD XXX
AMA: 2010,Dec,7-10

88121 **using computer-assisted technology**
EXCLUDES *More than five probes (88399)*
Morphometric in situ hybridization on specimens other than urinary tract (88367-88368 [88373, 88374])
13.5 13.5 FUD XXX
AMA: 2010,Dec,7-10

88125 **Cytopathology, forensic (eg, sperm)**
0.75 0.75 FUD XXX
AMA: 2005,Aug,7-8; 2005,Jul,11-12

88130 **Sex chromatin identification; Barr bodies**
0.00 0.00 FUD XXX
AMA: 2005,Aug,7-8; 2005,Jul,11-12

88140 peripheral blood smear, polymorphonuclear drumsticks

EXCLUDES *Guard stain (88313)*

0.00 0.00 FUD XXX

AMA: 2018,Jan,8; 2017,Jan,8; 2016,Jan,13; 2015,Jan,16; 2014,Jan,11

88141-88155 Pap Smears

CMS: 100-03,210.2 Screening Pap Smears/Pelvic Examinations for Early Cancer Detection

EXCLUDES *Non-Bethesda method (88150-88153)*

88141 Cytopathology, cervical or vaginal (any reporting system), requiring interpretation by physician ♀

Code also (88142-88153, 88164-88167, 88174-88175)

0.90 0.90 FUD XXX

AMA: 2018,Jan,8; 2017,Jan,8; 2016,Jan,13; 2015,Jan,16; 2014,Jan,11

88142 Cytopathology, cervical or vaginal (any reporting system), collected in preservative fluid, automated thin layer preparation; manual screening under physician supervision ♀

INCLUDES Bethesda or non-Bethesda method

0.00 0.00 FUD XXX

AMA: 2018,Jan,8; 2017,Jan,8; 2016,Jan,13; 2015,Jan,16; 2014,Jan,11

88143 with manual screening and rescreening under physician supervision ♀

INCLUDES Bethesda or non-Bethesda method

EXCLUDES *Automated screening of automated thin layer preparation (88174-88175)*

0.00 0.00 FUD XXX

AMA: 2018,Jan,8; 2017,Jan,8; 2016,Jan,13; 2015,Jan,16; 2014,Jan,11

88147 Cytopathology smears, cervical or vaginal; screening by automated system under physician supervision ♀

0.00 0.00 FUD XXX

AMA: 2018,Jan,8; 2017,Jan,8; 2016,Jan,13; 2015,Jan,16; 2014,Jan,11

88148 screening by automated system with manual rescreening under physician supervision ♀

0.00 0.00 FUD XXX

AMA: 2018,Jan,8; 2017,Jan,8; 2016,Jan,13; 2015,Jan,16; 2014,Jan,11

88150 Cytopathology, slides, cervical or vaginal; manual screening under physician supervision ♀

EXCLUDES *Bethesda method Pap smears (88164-88167)*

0.00 0.00 FUD XXX

AMA: 2018,Jan,8; 2017,Jan,8; 2016,Jan,13; 2015,Jan,16; 2014,Jan,11

88152 with manual screening and computer-assisted rescreening under physician supervision

EXCLUDES *Bethesda method Pap smears (88164-88167)*

0.00 0.00 FUD XXX

AMA: 2018,Jan,8; 2017,Jan,8; 2016,Jan,13; 2015,Jan,16; 2014,Jan,11

88153 with manual screening and rescreening under physician supervision ♀

EXCLUDES *Bethesda method Pap smears (88164-88167)*

0.00 0.00 FUD XXX

AMA: 2018,Jan,8; 2017,Jan,8; 2016,Jan,13; 2015,Jan,16; 2014,Jan,11

+ **88155** Cytopathology, slides, cervical or vaginal, definitive hormonal evaluation (eg, maturation index, karyopyknotic index, estrogenic index) (List separately in addition to code[s] for other technical and interpretation services) ♀

Code first (88142-88153, 88164-88167, 88174-88175)

0.00 0.00 FUD XXX

AMA: 2018,Jan,8; 2017,Jan,8; 2016,Jan,13; 2015,Jan,16; 2014,Jan,11

88160-88162 Cytopathology Smears (Other Than Pap)

88160 Cytopathology, smears, any other source; screening and interpretation

2.01 2.01 FUD XXX

AMA: 2006,Dec,10-12; 2005,Jul,11-12

88161 preparation, screening and interpretation

1.87 1.87 FUD XXX

AMA: 2018,Jan,8; 2017,Jan,8; 2016,Jan,13; 2015,Jan,16; 2014,Jan,11

88162 extended study involving over 5 slides and/or multiple stains

EXCLUDES *Aerosol collection of sputum (89220)*
Special stains (88312-88314)

2.70 2.70 FUD XXX

AMA: 2005,Aug,7-8; 2005,Jul,11-12

88164-88167 Pap Smears: Bethesda System

CMS: 100-03,210.2 Screening Pap Smears/Pelvic Examinations for Early Cancer Detection

EXCLUDES *Non-Bethesda method (88150-88153)*

88164 Cytopathology, slides, cervical or vaginal (the Bethesda System); manual screening under physician supervision ♀

0.00 0.00 FUD XXX

AMA: 2018,Jan,8; 2017,Jan,8; 2016,Jan,13; 2015,Jan,16; 2014,Jan,11

88165 with manual screening and rescreening under physician supervision ♀

0.00 0.00 FUD XXX

AMA: 2018,Jan,8; 2017,Jan,8; 2016,Jan,13; 2015,Jan,16; 2014,Jan,11

88166 with manual screening and computer-assisted rescreening under physician supervision ♀

0.00 0.00 FUD XXX

AMA: 2018,Jan,8; 2017,Jan,8; 2016,Jan,13; 2015,Jan,16; 2014,Jan,11

88167 with manual screening and computer-assisted rescreening using cell selection and review under physician supervision ♀

EXCLUDES *Fine needle aspiration ([10004, 10005, 10006, 10007, 10008, 10009, 10010, 10011, 10012])*

0.00 0.00 FUD XXX

AMA: 2018,Jan,8; 2017,Jan,8; 2016,Jan,13; 2015,Jan,16; 2014,Jan,11

88172-88177 [88177] Cytopathology of Needle Biopsy

EXCLUDES *Fine needle aspiration (10021, [10004, 10005, 10006, 10007, 10008, 10009, 10010, 10011, 10012])*

88172 Cytopathology, evaluation of fine needle aspirate; immediate cytohistologic study to determine adequacy for diagnosis, first evaluation episode, each site

INCLUDES The submission of a complete set of cytologic material for evaluation regardless of the number of needle passes performed or slides prepared from each site

EXCLUDES *Cytologic examination during intraoperative pathology consultation (88333-88334)*

1.60 1.60 FUD XXX

AMA: 2019,Feb,8; 2019,Apr,4; 2018,Jan,8; 2017,Jan,8; 2016,Jan,13; 2016,Jan,11; 2015,Jan,16; 2014,Jan,11

88173 interpretation and report

INCLUDES The interpretation and report from each anatomical site no matter how many passes or evaluation episodes are performed during the aspiration

EXCLUDES *Cytologic examination during intraoperative pathology consultation (88333-88334)*

4.32 4.32 FUD XXX

AMA: 2019,Feb,8; 2019,Apr,4; 2018,Jan,8; 2017,Jan,8; 2016,Jan,13; 2015,Jan,16; 2014,Jan,11

+ # **88177** **immediate cytohistologic study to determine adequacy for diagnosis, each separate additional evaluation episode, same site (List separately in addition to code for primary procedure)**

Code also each additional immediate repeat evaluation episode(s) required from the same site (e.g., previous sample is inadequate)

Code first (88172)

0.84 0.84 FUD ZZZ N 80

AMA: 2019,Apr,4; 2018,Jan,8; 2017,Jan,8; 2016,Jan,11

88174-88177 Pap Smears: Automated Screening

EXCLUDES *Non-Bethesda method (88150-88153)*

88174 **Cytopathology, cervical or vaginal (any reporting system), collected in preservative fluid, automated thin layer preparation; screening by automated system, under physician supervision** ♀

INCLUDES Bethesda or non-Bethesda method

0.00 0.00 FUD XXX Q

AMA: 2018,Jan,8; 2017,Jan,8; 2016,Jan,13; 2015,Jan,16; 2014,Jan,11

88175 **with screening by automated system and manual rescreening or review, under physician supervision** ♀

INCLUDES Bethesda or non-Bethesda method

EXCLUDES *Manual screening (88142-88143)*

0.00 0.00 FUD XXX Q

AMA: 2018,Jan,8; 2017,Jan,8; 2016,Jan,13; 2015,Jan,16; 2014,Jan,11

88177 **Resequenced code. See code following 88173.**

88182-88199 Cytopathology Using the Fluorescence-Activated Cell Sorter

88182 **Flow cytometry, cell cycle or DNA analysis**

EXCLUDES *DNA ploidy analysis by morphometric technique (88358)*

3.79 3.79 FUD XXX Q2 80

AMA: 2018,Jan,8; 2017,Jan,8; 2016,Jan,13; 2015,Jan,16

88184 **Flow cytometry, cell surface, cytoplasmic, or nuclear marker, technical component only; first marker**

1.88 1.88 FUD XXX Q2 80 TC

AMA: 2018,Jan,8; 2017,Jan,8; 2016,Jan,13; 2015,Jan,16; 2014,Jan,11

+ **88185** **each additional marker (List separately in addition to code for first marker)**

Code first (88184)

0.69 0.69 FUD ZZZ N 80 TC

AMA: 2018,Jan,8; 2017,Jan,8; 2016,Jan,13; 2015,Jan,16; 2014,Jan,11

88187 **Flow cytometry, interpretation; 2 to 8 markers**

EXCLUDES *Antibody assessment by flow cytometry (83516-83520, 86000-86849 [86152, 86153])*
Cell enumeration by immunologic selection and identification ([86152, 86153])
Interpretation (86355-86357, 86359-86361, 86367)

1.08 1.08 FUD XXX B 80 26

AMA: 2018,Jan,8; 2017,Jan,8; 2016,Jan,13; 2015,Jan,16; 2014,Jan,11

88188 **9 to 15 markers**

EXCLUDES *Antibody assessment by flow cytometry (83516-83520, 86000-86849 [86152, 86153])*
Cell enumeration by immunologic selection and identification ([86152, 86153])
Interpretation (86355-86357, 86359-86361, 86367)

1.83 1.83 FUD XXX B 80 26

AMA: 2018,Jan,8; 2017,Jan,8; 2016,Jan,13; 2015,Jan,16; 2014,Jan,11

88189 **16 or more markers**

EXCLUDES *Antibody assessment by flow cytometry (83516-83520, 86000-86849 [86152, 86153])*
Cell enumeration using immunologic selection and identification in fluid sample ([86152, 86153])
Interpretation (86355-86357, 86359-86361, 86367)

2.45 2.45 FUD XXX B 80 26

AMA: 2018,Jan,8; 2017,Jan,8; 2016,Jan,13; 2015,Jan,16; 2014,Jan,11

88199 **Unlisted cytopathology procedure**

EXCLUDES *Electron microscopy (88348)*

0.00 0.00 FUD XXX Q1 80

AMA: 2018,Jan,8; 2017,Jan,8; 2016,Jan,13; 2015,Jan,16; 2014,Jan,11

88230-88299 Cytogenic Studies

CMS: 100-03,190.3 Cytogenic Studies

EXCLUDES *Acetylcholinesterase (82013)*
Alpha-fetoprotein (amniotic fluid or serum) (82105-82106)
Microdissection (88380)
Molecular pathology codes (81105-81383 [81105, 81106, 81107, 81108, 81109, 81110, 81111, 81112, 81120, 81121, 81161, 81162, 81163, 81164, 81165, 81166, 81167, 81173, 81174, 81184, 81185, 81186, 81187, 81188, 81189, 81190, 81200, 81201, 81202, 81203, 81204, 81205, 81206, 81207, 81208, 81209, 81210, 81219, 81227, 81230, 81231, 81233, 81234, 81238, 81239, 81245, 81246, 81250, 81257, 81258, 81259, 81261, 81262, 81263, 81264, 81265, 81266, 81267, 81268, 81269, 81271, 81274, 81283, 81284, 81285, 81286, 81287, 81288, 81289, 81291, 81292, 81293, 81294, 81295, 81301, 81302, 81303, 81304, 81306, 81312, 81320, 81324, 81325, 81326, 81332, 81334, 81336, 81337, 81343, 81344, 81345, 81361, 81362, 81363, 81364], 81400-81408, [81479], 81410-81471 [81448], 81500-81512, 81599)

88230 **Tissue culture for non-neoplastic disorders; lymphocyte**

0.00 0.00 FUD XXX Q

AMA: 2018,Jan,8; 2017,Jan,8; 2016,Jan,13; 2015,Jan,16; 2014,Jan,11

88233 **skin or other solid tissue biopsy**

0.00 0.00 FUD XXX Q

AMA: 2018,Jan,8; 2017,Jan,8; 2016,Jan,13; 2015,Jan,16; 2014,Jan,11

88235 **amniotic fluid or chorionic villus cells** M

0.00 0.00 FUD XXX Q

AMA: 2018,Jan,8; 2017,Jan,8; 2016,Jan,13; 2015,Jan,16; 2014,Jan,11

88237 **Tissue culture for neoplastic disorders; bone marrow, blood cells**

0.00 0.00 FUD XXX Q

AMA: 2018,Jan,8; 2017,Jan,8; 2016,Jan,13; 2015,Jan,16; 2014,Jan,11

88239 **solid tumor**

0.00 0.00 FUD XXX Q

AMA: 2018,Jan,8; 2017,Jan,8; 2016,Jan,13; 2015,Jan,16; 2014,Jan,11

88240 **Cryopreservation, freezing and storage of cells, each cell line**

EXCLUDES *Therapeutic cryopreservation and storage (38207)*

0.00 0.00 FUD XXX Q

AMA: 2018,Jan,8; 2017,Jan,8; 2016,Jan,13; 2015,Jan,16; 2014,Jan,11

88241 **Thawing and expansion of frozen cells, each aliquot**

EXCLUDES *Therapeutic thawing of prior harvest (38208)*

0.00 0.00 FUD XXX Q

AMA: 2018,Jan,8; 2017,Jan,8; 2016,Jan,13; 2015,Jan,16; 2014,Jan,11

88245 **Chromosome analysis for breakage syndromes; baseline Sister Chromatid Exchange (SCE), 20-25 cells**

0.00 0.00 FUD XXX Q

AMA: 2018,Jan,8; 2017,Jan,8; 2016,Jan,13; 2015,Jan,16; 2014,Jan,11

88248 baseline breakage, score 50-100 cells, count 20 cells, 2 karyotypes (eg, for ataxia telangiectasia, Fanconi anemia, fragile X)
0.00 0.00 FUD XXX
AMA: 2018,Jan,8; 2017,Jan,8; 2016,Jan,13; 2015,Jan,16; 2014,Jan,11

88249 score 100 cells, clastogen stress (eg, diepoxybutane, mitomycin C, ionizing radiation, UV radiation)
0.00 0.00 FUD XXX
AMA: 2018,Jan,8; 2017,Jan,8; 2016,Jan,13; 2015,Jan,16; 2014,Jan,11

88261 Chromosome analysis; count 5 cells, 1 karyotype, with banding
0.00 0.00 FUD XXX
AMA: 2018,Jan,8; 2017,Jan,8; 2016,Jan,13; 2015,Jan,16; 2014,Jan,11

88262 count 15-20 cells, 2 karyotypes, with banding
0.00 0.00 FUD XXX
AMA: 2019,Aug,10; 2018,Jan,8; 2017,Jan,8; 2016,Jan,13; 2015,Jan,16; 2014,Jan,11

88263 count 45 cells for mosaicism, 2 karyotypes, with banding
0.00 0.00 FUD XXX
AMA: 2018,Jan,8; 2017,Jan,8; 2016,Jan,13; 2015,Jan,16; 2014,Jan,11

88264 analyze 20-25 cells
0.00 0.00 FUD XXX
AMA: 2019,Aug,10; 2018,Jan,8; 2017,Jan,8; 2016,Jan,13; 2015,Jan,16; 2014,Jan,11

88267 Chromosome analysis, amniotic fluid or chorionic villus, count 15 cells, 1 karyotype, with banding M ♀
0.00 0.00 FUD XXX
AMA: 2018,Jan,8; 2017,Jan,8; 2016,Jan,13; 2015,Jan,16; 2014,Jan,11

88269 Chromosome analysis, in situ for amniotic fluid cells, count cells from 6-12 colonies, 1 karyotype, with banding M ♀
0.00 0.00 FUD XXX
AMA: 2018,Jan,8; 2017,Jan,8; 2016,Jan,13; 2015,Jan,16; 2014,Jan,11

88271 Molecular cytogenetics; DNA probe, each (eg, FISH)
EXCLUDES *Cytogenomic microarray analysis (81228-81229, 81405-81406, [81479])*
Fetal chromosome analysis using maternal blood (81420-81422)
0.00 0.00 FUD XXX
AMA: 2018,Jan,8; 2017,Apr,3; 2017,Jan,8; 2016,Jan,13; 2015,Jan,16; 2014,Jan,11

88272 chromosomal in situ hybridization, analyze 3-5 cells (eg, for derivatives and markers)
0.00 0.00 FUD XXX
AMA: 2018,Jan,8; 2017,Jan,8; 2016,Jan,13; 2015,Jan,16; 2014,Jan,11

88273 chromosomal in situ hybridization, analyze 10-30 cells (eg, for microdeletions)
0.00 0.00 FUD XXX
AMA: 2018,Jan,8; 2017,Jan,8; 2016,Jan,13; 2015,Jan,16; 2014,Jan,11

88274 interphase in situ hybridization, analyze 25-99 cells
0.00 0.00 FUD XXX
AMA: 2018,Jan,8; 2017,Jan,8; 2016,Jan,13; 2015,Jan,16; 2014,Jan,11

88275 interphase in situ hybridization, analyze 100-300 cells
0.00 0.00 FUD XXX
AMA: 2018,Jan,8; 2017,Jan,8; 2016,Jan,13; 2015,Jan,16; 2014,Jan,11

88280 Chromosome analysis; additional karyotypes, each study
0.00 0.00 FUD XXX
AMA: 2018,Jan,8; 2017,Jan,8; 2016,Jan,13; 2015,Jan,16; 2014,Jan,11

88283 additional specialized banding technique (eg, NOR, C-banding)
0.00 0.00 FUD XXX
AMA: 2018,Jan,8; 2017,Jan,8; 2016,Jan,13; 2015,Jan,16; 2014,Jan,11

88285 additional cells counted, each study
0.00 0.00 FUD XXX
AMA: 2018,Jan,8; 2017,Jan,8; 2016,Jan,13; 2015,Jan,16; 2014,Jan,11

88289 additional high resolution study
0.00 0.00 FUD XXX
AMA: 2018,Jan,8; 2017,Jan,8; 2016,Jan,13; 2015,Jan,16; 2014,Jan,11

88291 Cytogenetics and molecular cytogenetics, interpretation and report
0.94 0.94 FUD XXX M 80 26
AMA: 2018,Jan,8; 2017,Jan,8; 2016,Jan,13; 2015,Jan,16; 2014,Jan,11

88299 Unlisted cytogenetic study
0.00 0.00 FUD XXX Q1 80
AMA: 2018,Jan,8; 2017,Jan,8; 2016,Jan,13; 2015,Jan,16; 2014,Jan,11

88300 Evaluation of Surgical Specimen: Gross Anatomy

CMS: 100-02,15,80.1 Payment for Clinical Laboratory Services

INCLUDES Attainment, examination, and reporting
Unit of service is the specimen

EXCLUDES *Additional procedures (88311-88365 [88341, 88350], 88399)*
Microscopic exam (88302-88309)

88300 Level I - Surgical pathology, gross examination only
0.45 0.45 FUD XXX Q1 80
AMA: 2018,Jan,8; 2017,Jan,8; 2016,Jan,13; 2015,Jan,16; 2014,Jan,11

88302-88309 Evaluation of Surgical Specimens: Gross and Microscopic Anatomy

CMS: 100-02,15,80.1 Payment for Clinical Laboratory Services

INCLUDES Attainment, examination, and reporting
Unit of service is the specimen

EXCLUDES *Additional procedures (88311-88365 [88341, 88350], 88399)*
Mohs surgery (17311-17315)

88302 Level II - Surgical pathology, gross and microscopic examination

INCLUDES Confirming identification and absence of disease:
- Appendix, incidental
- Fallopian tube, sterilization
- Fingers or toes traumatic amputation
- Foreskin, newborn
- Hernia sac, any site
- Hydrocele sac
- Nerve
- Skin, plastic repair
- Sympathetic ganglion
- Testis, castration
- Vaginal mucosa, incidental
- Vas deferens, sterilization

0.87 0.87 FUD XXX Q1 80
AMA: 2018,Jan,8; 2017,Jan,8; 2016,Jan,13; 2015,Jan,16; 2014,Feb,10; 2014,Jan,11

88304 Level III - Surgical pathology, gross and microscopic examination

INCLUDES
- Abortion, induced
- Abscess
- Anal tag
- Aneurysm-atrial/ventricular
- Appendix, other than incidental
- Artery, atheromatous plaque
- Bartholin's gland cyst
- Bone fragment(s), other than pathologic fracture
- Bursa/ synovial cyst
- Carpal tunnel tissue
- Cartilage, shavings
- Cholesteatoma
- Colon, colostomy stoma
- Conjunctiva-biopsy/pterygium
- Cornea
- Diverticulum-esophagus/small intestine
- Dupuytren's contracture tissue
- Femoral head, other than fracture
- Fissure/fistula
- Foreskin, other than newborn
- Gallbladder
- Ganglion cyst
- Hematoma
- Hemorrhoids
- Hydatid of Morgagni
- Intervertebral disc
- Joint, loose body
- Meniscus
- Mucocele, salivary
- Neuroma-Morton's/traumatic
- Pilonidal cyst/sinus
- Polyps, inflammatory-nasal/sinusoidal
- Skin-cyst/tag/debridement
- Soft tissue, debridement
- Soft tissue, lipoma
- Spermatocele
- Tendon/tendon sheath
- Testicular appendage
- Thrombus or embolus
- Tonsil and/or adenoids
- Varicocele
- Vas deferens, other than sterilization
- Vein, varicosity

1.14 1.14 FUD XXX Q1 80

AMA: 2018,Jan,8; 2017,Jan,8; 2016,Jan,13; 2015,Jan,16; 2014,Feb,10; 2014,Jan,11

88305 Level IV - Surgical pathology, gross and microscopic examination

INCLUDES
- Abortion, spontaneous/missed
- Artery, biopsy
- Bone exostosis
- Bone marrow, biopsy
- Brain/meninges, other than for tumor resection
- Breast biopsy without microscopic assessment of surgical margin
- Breast reduction mammoplasty
- Bronchus, biopsy
- Cell block, any source
- Cervix, biopsy
- Colon, biopsy
- Duodenum, biopsy
- Endocervix, curettings/biopsy
- Endometrium, curettings/biopsy
- Esophagus, biopsy
- Extremity, amputation, traumatic
- Fallopian tube, biopsy
- Fallopian tube, ectopic pregnancy
- Femoral head, fracture
- Finger/toes, amputation, nontraumatic
- Gingiva/oral mucosa, biopsy
- Heart valve
- Joint resection
- Kidney biopsy
- Larynx biopsy
- Leiomyoma(s), uterine myomectomy-without uterus
- Lip, biopsy/wedge resection
- Lung, transbronchial biopsy
- Lymph node, biopsy
- Muscle, biopsy
- Nasal mucosa, biopsy
- Nasopharynx/oropharynx, biopsy
- Nerve biopsy
- Odontogenic/dental cyst
- Omentum, biopsy
- Ovary, biopsy/wedge resection
- Ovary with or without tube, nonneoplastic
- Parathyroid gland
- Peritoneum, biopsy
- Pituitary tumor
- Placenta, other than third trimester
- Pleura/pericardium-biopsy/tissue
- Polyp:
  - Cervical/endometrial
  - Colorectal
  - Stomach/small intestine
- Prostate:
  - Needle biopsy
  - TUR
- Salivary gland, biopsy
- Sinus, paranasal biopsy
- Skin, other than cyst/tag/debridement/plastic repair
- Small intestine, biopsy
- Soft tissue, other than tumor/mas/lipoma/debridement
- Spleen
- Stomach biopsy
- Synovium
- Testis, other than tumor/biopsy, castration
- Thyroglossal duct/brachial cleft cyst
- Tongue, biopsy
- Tonsil, biopsy
- Trachea biopsy
- Ureter, biopsy
- Urethra, biopsy
- Urinary bladder, biopsy
- Uterus, with or without tubes and ovaries, for prolapse
- Vagina biopsy
- Vulva/labial biopsy

1.95 1.95 FUD XXX Q1 80

AMA: 2018,May,3; 2018,Jan,8; 2017,Jan,8; 2016,Jan,13; 2015,Jan,16; 2014,Feb,10; 2014,Jan,11

88307 **Level V - Surgical pathology, gross and microscopic examination**

INCLUDES Adrenal resection
Bone, biopsy/curettings
Bone fragment(s), pathologic fractures
Brain, biopsy
Brain meninges, tumor resection
Breast, excision of lesion, requiring microscopic evaluation of surgical margins
Breast, mastectomy-partial/simple
Cervix, conization
Colon, segmental resection, other than for tumor
Extremity, amputation, nontraumatic
Eye, enucleation
Kidney, partial/total nephrectomy
Larynx, partial/total resection
Liver
  Biopsy, needle/wedge
  Partial resection
Lung, wedge biopsy
Lymph nodes, regional resection
Mediastinum, mass
Myocardium, biopsy
Odontogenic tumor
Ovary with or without tube, neoplastic
Pancreas, biopsy
Placenta, third trimester
Prostate, except radical resection
Salivary gland
Sentinel lymph node
Small intestine, resection, other than for tumor
Soft tissue mass (except lipoma)-biopsy/simple excision
Stomach-subtotal/total resection, other than for tumor
Testis, biopsy
Thymus, tumor
Thyroid, total/lobe
Ureter, resection
Urinary bladder, TUR
Uterus, with or without tubes and ovaries, other than neoplastic/prolapse

7.59 7.59 FUD XXX Q2 80

AMA: 2018,Jan,8; 2017,Jan,8; 2016,Jan,13; 2015,Jan,16; 2014,Feb,10; 2014,Jan,11

88309 **Level VI - Surgical pathology, gross and microscopic examination**

INCLUDES Bone resection
Breast, mastectomy-with regional lymph nodes
Colon:
  Segmental resection for tumor
  Total resection
Esophagus, partial/total resection
Extremity, disarticulation
Fetus, with dissection
Larynx, partial/total resection-with regional lymph nodes
Lung-total/lobe/segment resection
Pancreas, total/subtotal resection
Prostate, radical resection
Small intestine, resection for tumor
Soft tissue tumor, extensive resection
Stomach, subtotal/total resection for tumor
Testis, tumor
Tongue/tonsil, resection for tumor
Urinary bladder, partial/total resection
Uterus, with or without tubes and ovaries, neoplastic
Vulva, total/subtotal resection

EXCLUDES *Evaluation of fine needle aspirate (88172-88173)*
Fine needle aspiration (10021, [10004, 10005, 10006, 10007, 10008, 10009, 10010, 10011, 10012])

11.5 11.5 FUD XXX Q2 80

AMA: 2018,Jan,8; 2017,Jan,8; 2016,Jan,13; 2015,Jan,16; 2014,Feb,10; 2014,Jan,11

88311-88399 [88341, 88350, 88364, 88373, 88374, 88377] Additional Surgical Pathology Services

CMS: 100-02,15,80.1 Payment for Clinical Laboratory Services

\+ **88311** **Decalcification procedure (List separately in addition to code for surgical pathology examination)**

Code first surgical pathology exam (88302-88309)

0.61 0.61 FUD XXX N 80

AMA: 2018,Jan,8; 2017,Jan,8; 2016,Jan,13; 2015,Jan,16; 2014,Jan,11

88312 **Special stain including interpretation and report; Group I for microorganisms (eg, acid fast, methenamine silver)**

INCLUDES Reporting one unit for each special stain performed on a surgical pathology block, cytologic sample, or hematologic smear

2.83 2.83 FUD XXX Q1 80

AMA: 2018,Jan,8; 2017,Jan,8; 2016,Jan,13; 2015,Jan,16; 2014,Jan,11

88313 **Group II, all other (eg, iron, trichrome), except stain for microorganisms, stains for enzyme constituents, or immunocytochemistry and immunohistochemistry**

INCLUDES Reporting one unit for each special stain performed on a surgical pathology block, cytologic sample, or hematologic smear

EXCLUDES *Immunocytochemistry and immunohistochemistry (88342)*

2.05 2.05 FUD XXX Q1 80

AMA: 2018,Jan,8; 2017,Jan,8; 2016,Jan,13; 2015,Jan,16; 2014,Jan,11

\+ **88314** **histochemical stain on frozen tissue block (List separately in addition to code for primary procedure)**

INCLUDES Reporting one unit for each special stain on each frozen surgical pathology block

EXCLUDES *Routine frozen section stain during Mohs surgery (17311-17315)*
Special stain performed on frozen tissue section specimen to identify enzyme constituents (88319)

Code also modifier 59 for nonroutine histochemical stain on frozen section during Mohs surgery

Code first (17311-17315, 88302-88309, 88331-88332)

2.60 2.60 FUD XXX N 80

AMA: 2018,Jan,8; 2017,Jan,8; 2016,Jan,13; 2015,Jan,16; 2014,Jan,11

88319 **Group III, for enzyme constituents**

INCLUDES Reporting one unit for each special stain on each frozen surgical pathology block

EXCLUDES *Detection of enzyme constituents by immunohistochemical or immunocytochemical methodology (88342)*

2.74 2.74 FUD XXX Q2 80

AMA: 2018,Jan,8; 2017,Jan,8; 2016,Jan,13; 2015,Jan,16; 2014,Jan,11

88321 **Consultation and report on referred slides prepared elsewhere**

2.42 2.85 FUD XXX Q1 80

AMA: 2018,Jan,8; 2017,Jan,8; 2016,Jan,13; 2015,Jan,16; 2014,Jan,11

88323 **Consultation and report on referred material requiring preparation of slides**

3.28 3.28 FUD XXX Q1 80

AMA: 2018,Jan,8; 2017,Jan,8; 2016,Jan,13; 2015,Jan,16; 2014,Jan,11

88325 **Consultation, comprehensive, with review of records and specimens, with report on referred material**

4.29 5.12 FUD XXX Q1 80

AMA: 2018,Jan,8; 2017,Jan,8; 2016,Jan,13; 2015,Jan,16; 2014,Jan,11

88329 **Pathology consultation during surgery;**

1.04 1.47 FUD XXX Q1 80

AMA: 2018,Jan,8; 2017,Jan,8; 2016,Jan,13; 2015,Jan,16; 2014,Feb,10; 2014,Jan,11

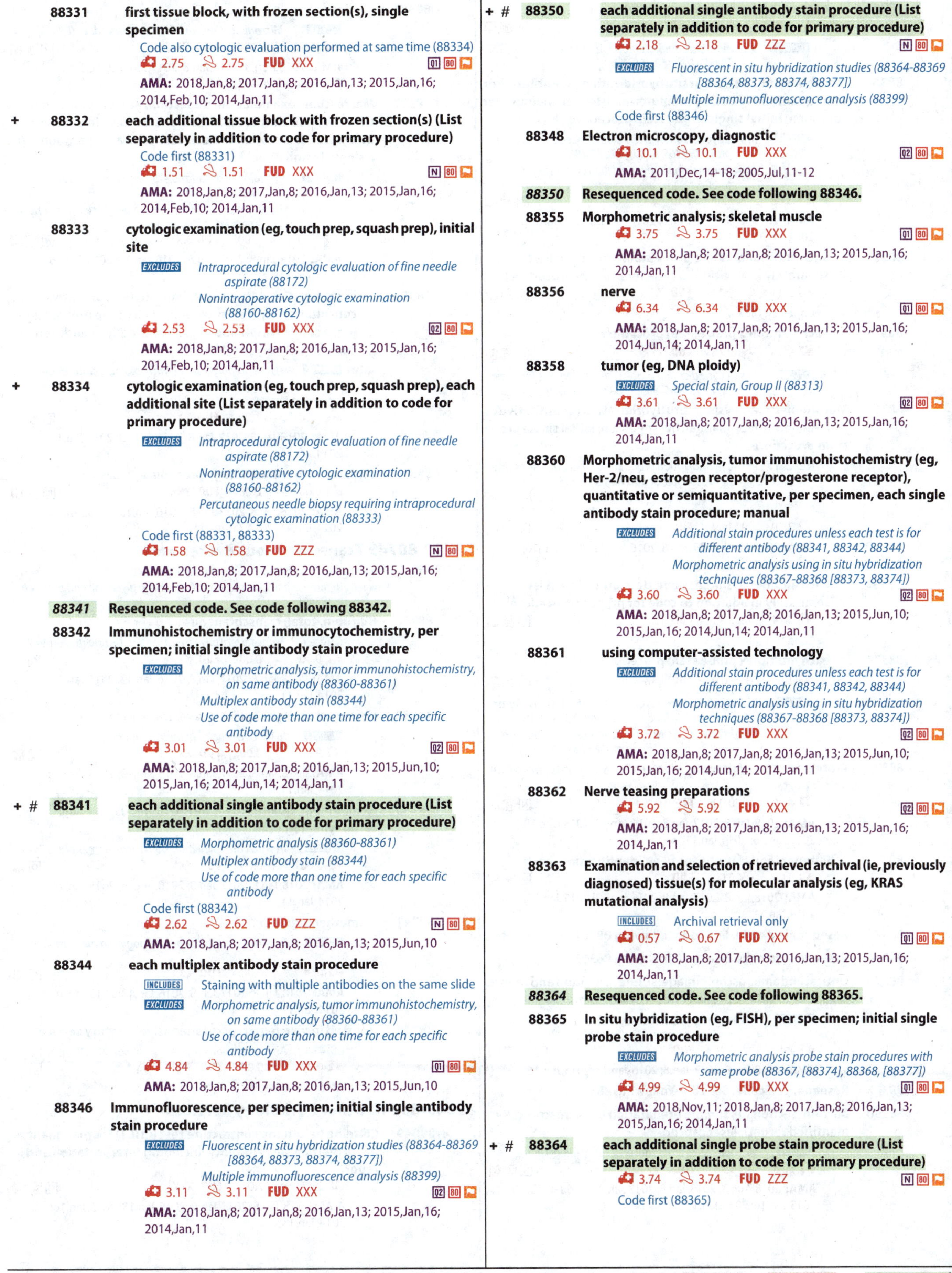

88331 **first tissue block, with frozen section(s), single specimen**

Code also cytologic evaluation performed at same time (88334)

2.75 2.75 FUD XXX 01 80

AMA: 2018,Jan,8; 2017,Jan,8; 2016,Jan,13; 2015,Jan,16; 2014,Feb,10; 2014,Jan,11

\+ 88332 **each additional tissue block with frozen section(s) (List separately in addition to code for primary procedure)**

Code first (88331)

1.51 1.51 FUD XXX N 80

AMA: 2018,Jan,8; 2017,Jan,8; 2016,Jan,13; 2015,Jan,16; 2014,Feb,10; 2014,Jan,11

88333 **cytologic examination (eg, touch prep, squash prep), initial site**

EXCLUDES *Intraprocedural cytologic evaluation of fine needle aspirate (88172)*

Nonintraoperative cytologic examination (88160-88162)

2.53 2.53 FUD XXX 02 80

AMA: 2018,Jan,8; 2017,Jan,8; 2016,Jan,13; 2015,Jan,16; 2014,Feb,10; 2014,Jan,11

\+ 88334 **cytologic examination (eg, touch prep, squash prep), each additional site (List separately in addition to code for primary procedure)**

EXCLUDES *Intraprocedural cytologic evaluation of fine needle aspirate (88172)*

Nonintraoperative cytologic examination (88160-88162)

Percutaneous needle biopsy requiring intraprocedural cytologic examination (88333)

Code first (88331, 88333)

1.58 1.58 FUD ZZZ N 80

AMA: 2018,Jan,8; 2017,Jan,8; 2016,Jan,13; 2015,Jan,16; 2014,Feb,10; 2014,Jan,11

88341 **Resequenced code. See code following 88342.**

88342 **Immunohistochemistry or immunocytochemistry, per specimen; initial single antibody stain procedure**

EXCLUDES *Morphometric analysis, tumor immunohistochemistry, on same antibody (88360-88361)*

Multiplex antibody stain (88344)

Use of code more than one time for each specific antibody

3.01 3.01 FUD XXX 02 80

AMA: 2018,Jan,8; 2017,Jan,8; 2016,Jan,13; 2015,Jun,10; 2015,Jan,16; 2014,Jun,14; 2014,Jan,11

\+ # 88341 **each additional single antibody stain procedure (List separately in addition to code for primary procedure)**

EXCLUDES *Morphometric analysis (88360-88361)*

Multiplex antibody stain (88344)

Use of code more than one time for each specific antibody

Code first (88342)

2.62 2.62 FUD ZZZ N 80

AMA: 2018,Jan,8; 2017,Jan,8; 2016,Jan,13; 2015,Jun,10

88344 **each multiplex antibody stain procedure**

INCLUDES Staining with multiple antibodies on the same slide

EXCLUDES *Morphometric analysis, tumor immunohistochemistry, on same antibody (88360-88361)*

Use of code more than one time for each specific antibody

4.84 4.84 FUD XXX 01 80

AMA: 2018,Jan,8; 2017,Jan,8; 2016,Jan,13; 2015,Jun,10

88346 **Immunofluorescence, per specimen; initial single antibody stain procedure**

EXCLUDES *Fluorescent in situ hybridization studies (88364-88369 [88364, 88373, 88374, 88377])*

Multiple immunofluorescence analysis (88399)

3.11 3.11 FUD XXX 02 80

AMA: 2018,Jan,8; 2017,Jan,8; 2016,Jan,13; 2015,Jan,16; 2014,Jan,11

\+ # 88350 **each additional single antibody stain procedure (List separately in addition to code for primary procedure)**

2.18 2.18 FUD ZZZ N 80

EXCLUDES *Fluorescent in situ hybridization studies (88364-88369 [88364, 88373, 88374, 88377])*

Multiple immunofluorescence analysis (88399)

Code first (88346)

88348 **Electron microscopy, diagnostic**

10.1 10.1 FUD XXX 02 80

AMA: 2011,Dec,14-18; 2005,Jul,11-12

88350 **Resequenced code. See code following 88346.**

88355 **Morphometric analysis; skeletal muscle**

3.75 3.75 FUD XXX 01 80

AMA: 2018,Jan,8; 2017,Jan,8; 2016,Jan,13; 2015,Jan,16; 2014,Jan,11

88356 **nerve**

6.34 6.34 FUD XXX 01 80

AMA: 2018,Jan,8; 2017,Jan,8; 2016,Jan,13; 2015,Jan,16; 2014,Jun,14; 2014,Jan,11

88358 **tumor (eg, DNA ploidy)**

EXCLUDES *Special stain, Group II (88313)*

3.61 3.61 FUD XXX 02 80

AMA: 2018,Jan,8; 2017,Jan,8; 2016,Jan,13; 2015,Jan,16; 2014,Jan,11

88360 **Morphometric analysis, tumor immunohistochemistry (eg, Her-2/neu, estrogen receptor/progesterone receptor), quantitative or semiquantitative, per specimen, each single antibody stain procedure; manual**

EXCLUDES *Additional stain procedures unless each test is for different antibody (88341, 88342, 88344)*

Morphometric analysis using in situ hybridization techniques (88367-88368 [88373, 88374])

3.60 3.60 FUD XXX 02 80

AMA: 2018,Jan,8; 2017,Jan,8; 2016,Jan,13; 2015,Jun,10; 2015,Jan,16; 2014,Jun,14; 2014,Jan,11

88361 **using computer-assisted technology**

EXCLUDES *Additional stain procedures unless each test is for different antibody (88341, 88342, 88344)*

Morphometric analysis using in situ hybridization techniques (88367-88368 [88373, 88374])

3.72 3.72 FUD XXX 02 80

AMA: 2018,Jan,8; 2017,Jan,8; 2016,Jan,13; 2015,Jun,10; 2015,Jan,16; 2014,Jun,14; 2014,Jan,11

88362 **Nerve teasing preparations**

5.92 5.92 FUD XXX 02 80

AMA: 2018,Jan,8; 2017,Jan,8; 2016,Jan,13; 2015,Jan,16; 2014,Jan,11

88363 **Examination and selection of retrieved archival (ie, previously diagnosed) tissue(s) for molecular analysis (eg, KRAS mutational analysis)**

INCLUDES Archival retrieval only

0.57 0.67 FUD XXX 01 80

AMA: 2018,Jan,8; 2017,Jan,8; 2016,Jan,13; 2015,Jan,16; 2014,Jan,11

88364 **Resequenced code. See code following 88365.**

88365 **In situ hybridization (eg, FISH), per specimen; initial single probe stain procedure**

EXCLUDES *Morphometric analysis probe stain procedures with same probe (88367, [88374], 88368, [88377])*

4.99 4.99 FUD XXX 01 80

AMA: 2018,Nov,11; 2018,Jan,8; 2017,Jan,8; 2016,Jan,13; 2015,Jan,16; 2014,Jan,11

\+ # 88364 **each additional single probe stain procedure (List separately in addition to code for primary procedure)**

3.74 3.74 FUD ZZZ N 80

Code first (88365)

88366 **each multiplex probe stain procedure**
7.44 7.44 FUD XXX Q1 80

EXCLUDES *Morphometric analysis probe stain procedures (88367, [88374], 88368, [88377])*

88367 **Morphometric analysis, in situ hybridization (quantitative or semi-quantitative), using computer-assisted technology, per specimen; initial single probe stain procedure**

EXCLUDES *In situ hybridization probe stain procedures for same probe (88365, 88366, 88368, [88377])*
Morphometric in situ hybridization evaluation of urinary tract cytologic specimens (88120-88121)

3.08 3.08 FUD XXX Q2 80

AMA: 2018,Jan,8; 2017,Jan,8; 2016,Jan,13; 2015,Jan,16; 2014,Jan,11

\+ # 88373 **each additional single probe stain procedure (List separately in addition to code for primary procedure)**
2.11 2.11 FUD ZZZ N 80

Code first (88367)

\# 88374 **each multiplex probe stain procedure**
9.18 9.18 FUD XXX Q1 80

EXCLUDES *In situ hybridization probe stain procedures for same probe (88365, 88366, 88368, [88377])*

88368 **Morphometric analysis, in situ hybridization (quantitative or semi-quantitative), manual, per specimen; initial single probe stain procedure**

EXCLUDES *In situ hybridization probe stain procedures for same probe (88365, 88366-88367, [88374])*
Morphometric in situ hybridization evaluation of urinary tract cytologic specimens (88120-88121)

3.59 3.59 FUD XXX Q2 80

AMA: 2018,Jan,8; 2017,Jan,8; 2016,Jan,13; 2015,Jan,16; 2014,Jan,11

\+ 88369 **each additional single probe stain procedure (List separately in addition to code for primary procedure)**
3.14 3.14 FUD ZZZ N 80

Code first (88368)

\# 88377 **each multiplex probe stain procedure**
10.9 10.9 FUD XXX Q1 80

EXCLUDES *In situ hybridization probe stain procedures for same probe (88365, 88366-88367, [88374])*
Morphometric in situ hybridization evaluation, urinary tract cytologic specimens (88120-88121)

88371 **Protein analysis of tissue by Western Blot, with interpretation and report;**
0.00 0.00 FUD XXX N 80

AMA: 2018,Jan,8; 2017,Jan,8; 2016,Jan,13; 2015,Dec,18; 2015,Jan,16; 2014,Jan,11

88372 **immunological probe for band identification, each**
0.00 0.00 FUD XXX N 80

AMA: 2018,Jan,8; 2017,Jan,8; 2016,Jan,13; 2015,Jan,16; 2014,Jan,11

88373 **Resequenced code. See code following 88367.**

88374 **Resequenced code. See code following 88367.**

88375 **Optical endomicroscopic image(s), interpretation and report, real-time or referred, each endoscopic session**

EXCLUDES *Endoscopic procedures that include optical endomicroscopy (43206, 43252, 0397T)*

1.42 1.42 FUD XXX B 80 26

AMA: 2018,Jan,8; 2017,Jan,8; 2016,Jan,13; 2015,Jan,16

88377 **Resequenced code. See code following 88369.**

88380 **Microdissection (ie, sample preparation of microscopically identified target); laser capture**

EXCLUDES *Microdissection, manual procedure (88381)*

3.78 3.78 FUD XXX N 80

AMA: 2018,Aug,3; 2018,Jan,8; 2017,Jan,8; 2016,Jan,13; 2015,Jan,16; 2014,Jan,11

88381 **manual**

EXCLUDES *Microdissection, laser capture procedure (88380)*

4.34 4.34 FUD XXX N 80

AMA: 2018,Aug,3; 2018,Jan,8; 2017,Jan,8; 2016,Jan,13; 2015,Jan,16; 2014,Jan,11

88387 **Macroscopic examination, dissection, and preparation of tissue for non-microscopic analytical studies (eg, nucleic acid-based molecular studies); each tissue preparation (eg, a single lymph node)**

EXCLUDES *Pathology consultation during surgery (88329-88334, 88388)*
Tissue preparation for microbiologic cultures or flow cytometric studies

1.00 1.00 FUD XXX N 80

AMA: 2018,Jan,8; 2017,Jan,8; 2016,Jan,13; 2015,Jan,16; 2014,Jan,11

\+ 88388 **in conjunction with a touch imprint, intraoperative consultation, or frozen section, each tissue preparation (eg, a single lymph node) (List separately in addition to code for primary procedure)**

EXCLUDES *Tissue preparation for microbiologic cultures or flow cytometric studies*

Code first (88329-88334)

1.00 1.00 FUD XXX N 80

AMA: 2018,Jan,8; 2017,Jan,8; 2016,Jan,13; 2015,Jan,16; 2014,Jan,11

88399 **Unlisted surgical pathology procedure**
0.00 0.00 FUD XXX Q1 80

AMA: 2018,Jan,8; 2017,Jan,8; 2016,Jan,13; 2015,Jan,16; 2014,Jun,14; 2014,Jan,11

88720-88749 Transcutaneous Procedures

EXCLUDES *Transcutaneous oxyhemoglobin measurement (0493T)*
Wavelength fluorescent spectroscopy of advanced glycation end products (skin) (88749)

88720 **Bilirubin, total, transcutaneous**

EXCLUDES *Transdermal oxygen saturation testing (94760-94762)*

0.00 0.00 FUD XXX Q

AMA: 2018,Jan,8; 2017,Jan,8; 2016,Jan,13; 2015,Jan,16; 2014,Jan,11

88738 **Hemoglobin (Hgb), quantitative, transcutaneous**

EXCLUDES *In vitro hemoglobin measurement (85018)*

0.00 0.00 FUD XXX Q

AMA: 2018,Jan,8; 2017,Jan,8; 2016,Jan,13; 2015,Jan,16; 2014,Jan,11

88740 **Hemoglobin, quantitative, transcutaneous, per day; carboxyhemoglobin**

EXCLUDES *In vitro carboxyhemoglobin measurement (82375)*

0.00 0.00 FUD XXX Q

AMA: 2018,Jan,8; 2017,Jan,8; 2016,Jan,13; 2015,Jan,16; 2014,Jan,11

88741 **methemoglobin**

EXCLUDES *In vitro quantitative methemoglobin measurement (83050)*

0.00 0.00 FUD XXX Q

AMA: 2018,Jan,8; 2017,Jan,8; 2016,Jan,13; 2015,Jan,16; 2014,Jan,11

88749 **Unlisted in vivo (eg, transcutaneous) laboratory service**

INCLUDES All in vivo measurements not specifically listed

0.00 0.00 FUD XXX Q

AMA: 2010,Dec,7-10

89049-89240 Other Pathology Services

89049 **Caffeine halothane contracture test (CHCT) for malignant hyperthermia susceptibility, including interpretation and report**
1.77 7.06 FUD XXX Q1 80

AMA: 2018,Jan,8; 2017,Jan,8; 2016,Jan,13; 2015,Jan,16; 2014,Jan,11

89050 **Cell count, miscellaneous body fluids (eg, cerebrospinal fluid, joint fluid), except blood;**
0.00 0.00 FUD XXX
AMA: 2018,Jan,8; 2017,Jan,8; 2016,Jan,13; 2015,Jan,16; 2014,Jan,11

89051 **with differential count**
0.00 0.00 FUD XXX
AMA: 2018,Jan,8; 2017,Jan,8; 2016,Jan,13; 2015,Jan,16; 2014,Jan,11

89055 **Leukocyte assessment, fecal, qualitative or semiquantitative**
0.00 0.00 FUD XXX
AMA: 2018,Jan,8; 2017,Jan,8; 2016,Jan,13; 2015,Jan,16; 2014,Jan,11

89060 **Crystal identification by light microscopy with or without polarizing lens analysis, tissue or any body fluid (except urine)**
EXCLUDES *Crystal identification on paraffin embedded tissue*
0.00 0.00 FUD XXX
AMA: 2018,Jan,8; 2017,Jan,8; 2016,Jan,13; 2015,Jan,16; 2014,Jan,11

89125 **Fat stain, feces, urine, or respiratory secretions**
0.00 0.00 FUD XXX
AMA: 2018,Jan,8; 2017,Jan,8; 2016,Jan,13; 2015,Jan,16; 2014,Jan,11

89160 **Meat fibers, feces**
0.00 0.00 FUD XXX
AMA: 2018,Jan,8; 2017,Jan,8; 2016,Jan,13; 2015,Jan,16; 2014,Jan,11

89190 **Nasal smear for eosinophils**
EXCLUDES *Occult blood feces (82270)*
Paternity tests (86910)
0.00 0.00 FUD XXX
AMA: 2018,Jan,8; 2017,Jan,8; 2016,Jan,13; 2015,Jan,16; 2014,Jan,11

89220 **Sputum, obtaining specimen, aerosol induced technique (separate procedure)**
0.46 0.46 FUD XXX
AMA: 2018,Jan,8; 2017,Jan,8; 2016,Jan,13; 2015,Jan,16; 2014,Jan,11

89230 **Sweat collection by iontophoresis**
0.08 0.08 FUD XXX
AMA: 2018,Jan,8; 2017,Jan,8; 2016,Jan,13; 2015,Jan,16; 2014,Jan,11

89240 **Unlisted miscellaneous pathology test**
0.00 0.00 FUD XXX
AMA: 2018,Jan,8; 2017,Jan,8; 2016,Jan,13; 2015,Jan,16; 2014,Jan,11

89250-89398 Infertility Treatment Services

CMS: 100-02,1,100 Treatment for Infertility

89250 **Culture of oocyte(s)/embryo(s), less than 4 days;**
0.00 0.00 FUD XXX
AMA: 2018,Jan,8; 2017,Jan,8; 2016,Jan,13; 2015,Jan,16; 2014,Jan,11

89251 **with co-culture of oocyte(s)/embryos**
EXCLUDES *Extended culture of oocyte(s)/embryo(s) (89272)*
0.00 0.00 FUD XXX
AMA: 2018,Jan,8; 2017,Jan,8; 2016,Jan,13; 2015,Jan,16; 2014,Jan,11

89253 **Assisted embryo hatching, microtechniques (any method)**
0.00 0.00 FUD XXX
AMA: 2018,Jan,8; 2017,Jan,8; 2016,Jan,13; 2015,Jan,16; 2014,Jan,11

89254 **Oocyte identification from follicular fluid**
0.00 0.00 FUD XXX
AMA: 2018,Jan,8; 2017,Jan,8; 2016,Jan,13; 2015,Jan,16; 2014,Jan,11

89255 **Preparation of embryo for transfer (any method)**
0.00 0.00 FUD XXX
AMA: 2018,Jan,8; 2017,Jan,8; 2016,Jan,13; 2015,Jan,16; 2014,Jan,11

89257 **Sperm identification from aspiration (other than seminal fluid)**
EXCLUDES *Semen analysis (89300-89320)*
Sperm identification from testis tissue (89264)
0.00 0.00 FUD XXX
AMA: 2018,Jan,8; 2017,Jan,8; 2016,Jan,13; 2015,Jan,16; 2014,Jan,11

89258 **Cryopreservation; embryo(s)**
0.00 0.00 FUD XXX
AMA: 2018,Jan,8; 2017,Jan,8; 2016,Jan,13; 2015,Jan,16; 2014,Jan,11

89259 **sperm**
EXCLUDES *Cryopreservation of testicular reproductive tissue (89335)*
0.00 0.00 FUD XXX
AMA: 2018,Jan,8; 2017,Jan,8; 2016,Jan,13; 2015,Jan,16; 2014,Jan,11

89260 **Sperm isolation; simple prep (eg, sperm wash and swim-up) for insemination or diagnosis with semen analysis**
0.00 0.00 FUD XXX
AMA: 2018,Jan,8; 2017,Jan,8; 2016,Jan,13; 2015,Jan,16; 2014,Jan,11

89261 **complex prep (eg, Percoll gradient, albumin gradient) for insemination or diagnosis with semen analysis**
EXCLUDES *Semen analysis without sperm wash or swim-up (89320)*
0.00 0.00 FUD XXX
AMA: 2018,Jan,8; 2017,Jan,8; 2016,Jan,13; 2015,Jan,16; 2014,Jan,11

89264 **Sperm identification from testis tissue, fresh or cryopreserved** ♂
EXCLUDES *Biopsy of testis (54500, 54505)*
Semen analysis (89300-89320)
Sperm identification from aspiration (89257)
0.00 0.00 FUD XXX
AMA: 2018,Jan,8; 2017,Jan,8; 2016,Jan,13; 2015,Jan,16; 2014,Jan,11

89268 **Insemination of oocytes**
0.00 0.00 FUD XXX
AMA: 2018,Jan,8; 2017,Jan,8; 2016,Jan,13; 2015,Jan,16; 2014,Jan,11

89272 **Extended culture of oocyte(s)/embryo(s), 4-7 days**
0.00 0.00 FUD XXX
AMA: 2018,Jan,8; 2017,Jan,8; 2016,Jan,13; 2015,Jan,16; 2014,Jan,11

89280 **Assisted oocyte fertilization, microtechnique; less than or equal to 10 oocytes**
0.00 0.00 FUD XXX
AMA: 2018,Jan,8; 2017,Jan,8; 2016,Jan,13; 2015,Jan,16; 2014,Jan,11

89281 **greater than 10 oocytes**
0.00 0.00 FUD XXX
AMA: 2018,Jan,8; 2017,Jan,8; 2016,Jan,13; 2015,Jan,16; 2014,Jan,11

89290 **Biopsy, oocyte polar body or embryo blastomere, microtechnique (for pre-implantation genetic diagnosis); less than or equal to 5 embryos**
0.00 0.00 FUD XXX
AMA: 2018,Jan,8; 2017,Jan,8; 2016,Jan,13; 2015,Jan,16; 2014,Jan,11

89291 **greater than 5 embryos**
0.00 0.00 FUD XXX
AMA: 2018,Jan,8; 2017,Jan,8; 2016,Jan,13; 2015,Jan,16; 2014,Jan,11

89300 **Semen analysis; presence and/or motility of sperm including Huhner test (post coital)** ♀
0.00 0.00 FUD XXX
AMA: 2018,Jan,8; 2017,Jan,8; 2016,Jan,13; 2015,Jan,16; 2014,Jan,11

89310 **motility and count (not including Huhner test)** ♂
0.00 0.00 FUD XXX
AMA: 2018,Jan,8; 2017,Jan,8; 2016,Jan,13; 2015,Jan,16; 2014,Jan,11

89320 **volume, count, motility, and differential** ♂
EXCLUDES *Skin testing (86485-86580, 95012-95199)*
0.00 0.00 FUD XXX
AMA: 2018,Jan,8; 2017,Jan,8; 2016,Jan,13; 2015,Jan,16; 2014,Jan,11

89321 **sperm presence and motility of sperm, if performed** ♂
EXCLUDES *Hyaluronan binding assay (HBA) (89398)*
0.00 0.00 FUD XXX
AMA: 2018,Jan,8; 2017,Jan,8; 2016,Jan,13; 2015,Jan,16; 2014,Jan,11

89322 **volume, count, motility, and differential using strict morphologic criteria (eg, Kruger)** ♂
0.00 0.00 FUD XXX
AMA: 2018,Jan,8; 2017,Jan,8; 2016,Jan,13; 2015,Jan,16; 2014,Jan,11

89325 **Sperm antibodies** ♂
EXCLUDES *Medicolegal identification of sperm (88125)*
0.00 0.00 FUD XXX
AMA: 2018,Jan,8; 2017,Jan,8; 2016,Jan,13; 2015,Jan,16; 2014,Jan,11

89329 **Sperm evaluation; hamster penetration test** ♂
0.00 0.00 FUD XXX
AMA: 2018,Jan,8; 2017,Jan,8; 2016,Jan,13; 2015,Jan,16; 2014,Jan,11

89330 **cervical mucus penetration test, with or without spinnbarkeit test** ♂
0.00 0.00 FUD XXX
AMA: 2018,Jan,8; 2017,Jan,8; 2016,Jan,13; 2015,Jan,16; 2014,Jan,11

89331 **Sperm evaluation, for retrograde ejaculation, urine (sperm concentration, motility, and morphology, as indicated)** ♂
EXCLUDES *Detection of sperm in urine (81015)*
Code also semen analysis on concurrent sperm specimen (89300-89322)
0.00 0.00 FUD XXX
AMA: 2018,Jan,8; 2017,Jan,8; 2016,Jan,13; 2015,Jan,16; 2014,Jan,11

89335 **Cryopreservation, reproductive tissue, testicular**
EXCLUDES *Cryopreservation of:*
Embryo(s) (89258)
Mature oocytes (89337)
Ovarian tissue, oocytes (0058T)
Sperm (89259)
0.00 0.00 FUD XXX
AMA: 2018,Jan,8; 2017,Jan,8; 2016,Jan,13; 2015,Jan,16; 2014,Jan,11

89337 **Cryopreservation, mature oocyte(s)** ♀
EXCLUDES *Cryopreservation of immature oocyte[s] (89398)*
0.00 0.00 FUD XXX
AMA: 2018,Jan,8; 2017,Jan,8; 2016,Jan,13; 2015,Jan,16

89342 **Storage (per year); embryo(s)**
0.00 0.00 FUD XXX
AMA: 2018,Jan,8; 2017,Jan,8; 2016,Jan,13; 2015,Jan,16; 2014,Jan,11

89343 **sperm/semen**
0.00 0.00 FUD XXX
AMA: 2018,Jan,8; 2017,Jan,8; 2016,Jan,13; 2015,Jan,16; 2014,Jan,11

89344 **reproductive tissue, testicular/ovarian**
0.00 0.00 FUD XXX
AMA: 2018,Jan,8; 2017,Jan,8; 2016,Jan,13; 2015,Jan,16; 2014,Jan,11

89346 **oocyte(s)**
0.00 0.00 FUD XXX
AMA: 2018,Jan,8; 2017,Jan,8; 2016,Jan,13; 2015,Jan,16; 2014,Jan,11

89352 **Thawing of cryopreserved; embryo(s)**
0.00 0.00 FUD XXX
AMA: 2018,Jan,8; 2017,Jan,8; 2016,Jan,13; 2015,Jan,16; 2014,Jan,11

89353 **sperm/semen, each aliquot**
0.00 0.00 FUD XXX
AMA: 2018,Jan,8; 2017,Jan,8; 2016,Jan,13; 2015,Jan,16; 2014,Jan,11

89354 **reproductive tissue, testicular/ovarian**
0.00 0.00 FUD XXX
AMA: 2018,Jan,8; 2017,Jan,8; 2016,Jan,13; 2015,Jan,16; 2014,Jan,11

89356 **oocytes, each aliquot**
0.00 0.00 FUD XXX
AMA: 2018,Jan,8; 2017,Jan,8; 2016,Jan,13; 2015,Jan,16; 2014,Jan,11

89398 **Unlisted reproductive medicine laboratory procedure**
0.00 0.00 FUD XXX
INCLUDES Hyaluronan binding assay (HBA)

0001U-0162U Proprietary Laboratory Analysis (PLA)

INCLUDES All necessary investigative services
PLA codes take priority over other CPT codes
EXCLUDES *Additional procedures necessary before cell lysis (88380-88381)*

0001U **Red blood cell antigen typing, DNA, human erythrocyte antigen gene analysis of 35 antigens from 11 blood groups, utilizing whole blood, common RBC alleles reported**
INCLUDES PreciseType® HEA Test, Immucor, Inc
0.00 0.00 FUD 000
AMA: 2019,Jun,11

0002U **Oncology (colorectal), quantitative assessment of three urine metabolites (ascorbic acid, succinic acid and carnitine) by liquid chromatography with tandem mass spectrometry (LC-MS/MS) using multiple reaction monitoring acquisition, algorithm reported as likelihood of adenomatous polyps**
INCLUDES PolypDX™, Atlantic Diagnostic Laboratories, LLC, Metabolomic Technologies Inc
0.00 0.00 FUD 000
AMA: 2018,Aug,3

0003U **Oncology (ovarian) biochemical assays of five proteins (apolipoprotein A-1, CA 125 II, follicle stimulating hormone, human epididymis protein 4, transferrin), utilizing serum, algorithm reported as a likelihood score**
0.00 0.00 FUD 000
INCLUDES Overa (OVA1 Next Generation), Aspira Labs, Inc, Vermillion, Inc

0005U **Oncology (prostate) gene expression profile by real-time RT-PCR of 3 genes (ERG, PCA3, and SPDEF), urine, algorithm reported as risk score**
0.00 0.00 FUD 000
INCLUDES ExosomeDx® Prostate (IntelliScore), Exosome Diagnostics, Inc, Exosome Diagnostics, Inc

0006U **Detection of interacting medications, substances, supplements and foods, 120 or more analytes, definitive chromatography with mass spectrometry, urine, description and severity of each interaction identified, per date of service**
0.00 0.00 FUD 000
INCLUDES Drug-substance Identification and Interaction, Aegis Sciences Corporation

0007U **Drug test(s), presumptive, with definitive confirmation of positive results, any number of drug classes, urine, includes specimen verification including DNA authentication in comparison to buccal DNA, per date of service**

INCLUDES ToxProtect, Genotox Laboratories Ltd

0.00 0.00 FUD 000 Q

AMA: 2018,Jan,6

▲ **0008U** **Helicobacter pylori detection and antibiotic resistance, DNA, 16S and 23S rRNA, gyrA, pbp1, rdxA and rpoB, next-generation sequencing, formalin-fixed paraffin-embedded or fresh tissue or fecal sample, predictive, reported as positive or negative for resistance to clarithromycin, fluoroquinolones, metronidazole, amoxicillin, tetracycline, and rifabutin**

0.00 0.00 FUD 000 A

INCLUDES AmHPR® H. pylori Antibiotic Resistance Panel, American Molecular Laboratories, Inc

0009U **Oncology (breast cancer), ERBB2 (HER2) copy number by FISH, tumor cells from formalin fixed paraffin embedded tissue isolated using image-based dielectrophoresis (DEP) sorting, reported as ERBB2 gene amplified or non-amplified**

0.00 0.00 FUD 000 Q

INCLUDES DEPArray™ HER2, PacificDx

0010U **Infectious disease (bacterial), strain typing by whole genome sequencing, phylogenetic-based report of strain relatedness, per submitted isolate**

0.00 0.00 FUD 000 A

INCLUDES Bacterial Typing by Whole Genome Sequencing, Mayo Clinic

0011U **Prescription drug monitoring, evaluation of drugs present by LC-MS/MS, using oral fluid, reported as a comparison to an estimated steady-state range, per date of service including all drug compounds and metabolites**

0.00 0.00 FUD 000 Q

INCLUDES Cordant CORE™, Cordant Health Solutions

0012U **Germline disorders, gene rearrangement detection by whole genome next-generation sequencing, DNA, whole blood, report of specific gene rearrangement(s)**

0.00 0.00 FUD 000 A

INCLUDES MatePair Targeted Rearrangements, Congenital, Mayo Clinic

0013U **Oncology (solid organ neoplasia), gene rearrangement detection by whole genome next-generation sequencing, DNA, fresh or frozen tissue or cells, report of specific gene rearrangement(s)**

0.00 0.00 FUD 000 A

INCLUDES MatePair Targeted Rearrangements, Oncology, Mayo Clinic

0014U **Hematology (hematolymphoid neoplasia), gene rearrangement detection by whole genome next-generation sequencing, DNA, whole blood or bone marrow, report of specific gene rearrangement(s)**

0.00 0.00 FUD 000 A

INCLUDES MatePair Targeted Rearrangements, Hematologic, Mayo Clinic

0016U **Oncology (hematolymphoid neoplasia), RNA, BCR/ABL1 major and minor breakpoint fusion transcripts, quantitative PCR amplification, blood or bone marrow, report of fusion not detected or detected with quantitation**

0.00 0.00 FUD 000 A

INCLUDES BCR-ABL1 major and minor breakpoint fusion transcripts, University of Iowa, Department of Pathology, Asuragen

0017U **Oncology (hematolymphoid neoplasia), JAK2 mutation, DNA, PCR amplification of exons 12-14 and sequence analysis, blood or bone marrow, report of JAK2 mutation not detected or detected**

0.00 0.00 FUD 000 A

INCLUDES *JAK2* Mutation, University of Iowa, Department of Pathology

0018U **Oncology (thyroid), microRNA profiling by RT-PCR of 10 microRNA sequences, utilizing fine needle aspirate, algorithm reported as a positive or negative result for moderate to high risk of malignancy**

0.00 0.00 FUD 000 A

INCLUDES ThyraMIR™, Interpace Diagnostics

0019U **Oncology, RNA, gene expression by whole transcriptome sequencing, formalin-fixed paraffin embedded tissue or fresh frozen tissue, predictive algorithm reported as potential targets for therapeutic agents**

0.00 0.00 FUD 000 A

INCLUDES OncoTarget/OncoTreat, Columbia University Department of Pathology and Cell Biology, Darwin Health

0021U **Oncology (prostate), detection of 8 autoantibodies (ARF 6, NKX3-1, 5'-UTR-BMI1, CEP 164, 3'-UTR-Ropporin, Desmocollin, AURKAIP-1, CSNK2A2), multiplexed immunoassay and flow cytometry serum, algorithm reported as risk score**

0.00 0.00 FUD 000 Q

INCLUDES Apifiny®, Armune BioScience, Inc

0022U **Targeted genomic sequence analysis panel, non-small cell lung neoplasia, DNA and RNA analysis, 23 genes, interrogation for sequence variants and rearrangements, reported as presence/absence of variants and associated therapy(ies) to consider**

0.00 0.00 FUD 000 A

INCLUDES Oncomine™ Dx Target Test, Thermo Fisher Scientific

0023U **Oncology (acute myelogenous leukemia), DNA, genotyping of internal tandem duplication, p.D835, p.I836, using mononuclear cells, reported as detection or non-detection of FLT3 mutation and indication for or against the use of midostaurin**

0.00 0.00 FUD 000 A

INCLUDES LeukoStrat® CDx *FLT3* Mutation Assay, LabPMM LLC, an Invivoscribe Technologies, Inc Company, Invivoscribe Technologies, Inc

0024U **Glycosylated acute phase proteins (GlycA), nuclear magnetic resonance spectroscopy, quantitative**

0.00 0.00 FUD 000 Q

INCLUDES GlycA, Laboratory Corporation of America, Laboratory Corporation of America

0025U **Tenofovir, by liquid chromatography with tandem mass spectrometry (LC-MS/MS), urine, quantitative**

0.00 0.00 FUD 000 Q

INCLUDES UrSure Tenofovir Quantification Test, Synergy Medical Laboratories, UrSure Inc

0026U **Oncology (thyroid), DNA and mRNA of 112 genes, next-generation sequencing, fine needle aspirate of thyroid nodule, algorithmic analysis reported as a categorical result ("Positive, high probability of malignancy" or "Negative, low probability of malignancy")**

0.00 0.00 FUD 000 A

INCLUDES Thyroseq Genomic Classifier, CBLPath, Inc, University of Pittsburgh Medical Center

0027U ***JAK2 (Janus kinase 2)* (eg, myeloproliferative disorder) gene analysis, targeted sequence analysis exons 12-15**

0.00 0.00 FUD 000 A

INCLUDES *JAK2* Exons 12 to 15 Sequencing, Mayo Clinic, Mayo Clinic

0029U **Drug metabolism (adverse drug reactions and drug response), targeted sequence analysis (ie, *CYP1A2, CYP2C19, CYP2C9, CYP2D6, CYP3A4, CYP3A5, CYP4F2, SLCO1B1, VKORC1* and rs12777823)**
0.00 0.00 FUD 000 A

INCLUDES Focused Pharmacogenomics Panel, Mayo Clinic, Mayo Clinic

0030U **Drug metabolism (warfarin drug response), targeted sequence analysis (ie, *CYP2C9, CYP4F2, VKORC1*, rs12777823)**
0.00 0.00 FUD 000 A

INCLUDES Warfarin Response Genotype, Mayo Clinic, Mayo Clinic

0031U ***CYP1A2 (cytochrome P450 family 1, subfamily A, member 2)*(eg, drug metabolism) gene analysis, common variants (ie, *1F, *1K, *6, *7)**
0.00 0.00 FUD 000 A

INCLUDES Cytochrome P450 1A2 Genotype, Mayo Clinic, Mayo Clinic

0032U ***COMT (catechol-O-methyltransferase)(drug metabolism)* gene analysis, c.472G>A (rs4680) variant**
0.00 0.00 FUD 000 A

INCLUDES Catechol-O-Methyltransferase (*COMT*) Genotype, Mayo Clinic, Mayo Clinic

0033U ***HTR2A (5-hydroxytryptamine receptor 2A), HTR2C (5-hydroxytryptamine receptor 2C)* (eg, citalopram metabolism) gene analysis, common variants (ie, *HTR2A* rs7997012 [c.614-2211T>C], *HTR2C* rs3813929 [c.-759C>T] and rs1414334 [c.551-3008C>G])**
0.00 0.00 FUD 000 A

INCLUDES Serotonin Receptor Genotype (*HTR2A* and *HTR2C*), Mayo Clinic, Mayo Clinic

0034U ***TPMT (thiopurine S-methyltransferase), NUDT15 (nudix hydroxylase 15)(eg, thiopurine metabolism)*, gene analysis, common variants (ie, *TPMT* *2, *3A, *3B, *3C, *4, *5, *6, *8, *12; *NUDT15* *3, *4, *5)**
0.00 0.00 FUD 000 A

INCLUDES Thiopurine Methyltransferase (*TPMT*) and Nudix Hydrolase (*NUDT15*) Genotyping, Mayo Clinic, Mayo Clinic

0035U **Neurology (prion disease), cerebrospinal fluid, detection of prion protein by quaking-induced conformational conversion, qualitative**
0.00 0.00 FUD 000

INCLUDES Real-time quaking-induced conversion for prion detection (RT-QuIC), National Prion Disease Pathology Surveillance Center

0036U **Exome (ie, somatic mutations), paired formalin-fixed paraffin-embedded tumor tissue and normal specimen, sequence analyses**
0.00 0.00 FUD 000

INCLUDES EXaCT-1 Whole Exome Testing, Lab of Oncology-Molecular Detection, Weill Cornell Medicine- Clinical Genomics Laboratory

0037U **Targeted genomic sequence analysis, solid organ neoplasm, DNA analysis of 324 genes, interrogation for sequence variants, gene copy number amplifications, gene rearrangements, microsatellite instability and tumor mutational burden**
0.00 0.00 FUD 000

INCLUDES FoundationOne CDx™ (F1CDx), Foundation Medicine, Inc, Foundation Medicine, Inc

0038U **Vitamin D, 25 hydroxy D2 and D3, by LC-MS/MS, serum microsample, quantitative**
0.00 0.00 FUD 000

INCLUDES Sensieva™ Droplet 25OH Vitamin D2/D3 Microvolume LC/MS Assay, InSource Diagnostics, InSource Diagnostics

0039U **Deoxyribonucleic acid (DNA) antibody, double stranded, high avidity**
0.00 0.00 FUD 000

INCLUDES Anti-dsDNA, High Salt/Avidity, University of Washington, Department of Laboratory Medicine, Bio-Rad

0040U ***BCR/ABL1 (t(9;22))* (eg, chronic myelogenous leukemia) translocation analysis, major breakpoint, quantitative**
0.00 0.00 FUD 000

INCLUDES MRDx BCR-ABL Test, MolecularMD, MolecularMD

0041U **Borrelia burgdorferi, antibody detection of 5 recombinant protein groups, by immunoblot, IgM**
0.00 0.00 FUD 000

INCLUDES Lyme ImmunoBlot IgM, IGeneX Inc, ID-FISH Technology Inc. (ASR) (Lyme ImmunoBlot IgM Strips Only)

0042U **Borrelia burgdorferi, antibody detection of 12 recombinant protein groups, by immunoblot, IgG**
0.00 0.00 FUD 000

INCLUDES Lyme ImmunoBlot IgG, IGeneX Inc, ID-FISH Technology Inc (ASR) (Lyme ImmunoBlot IgG Strips Only)

0043U **Tick-borne relapsing fever Borrelia group, antibody detection to 4 recombinant protein groups, by immunoblot, IgM**
0.00 0.00 FUD 000

INCLUDES Tick-Borne Relapsing Fever (TBRF) Borrelia ImmunoBlots IgM Test, IGeneX Inc, ID-FISH Technology Inc (Provides TBRF ImmunoBlot IgM Strips)

0044U **Tick-borne relapsing fever Borrelia group, antibody detection to 4 recombinant protein groups, by immunoblot, IgG**
0.00 0.00 FUD 000

INCLUDES Tick-Borne Relapsing Fever (TBRF) Borrelia ImmunoBlots IgG Test, IGeneX Inc., ID-FISH Technology Inc (Provides TBRF ImmunoBlot IgG Strips)

0045U **Oncology (breast ductal carcinoma in situ), mRNA, gene expression profiling by real-time RT-PCR of 12 genes (7 content and 5 housekeeping), utilizing formalin-fixed paraffin-embedded tissue, algorithm reported as recurrence score**
0.00 0.00 FUD 000

INCLUDES The Oncotype DX® Breast DCIS Score™ Test, Genomic Health, Inc, Genomic Health, Inc

0046U ***FLT3* (fms-related tyrosine kinase 3) (eg, acute myeloid leukemia) internal tandem duplication (ITD) variants, quantitative**
0.00 0.00 FUD 000

INCLUDES FLT3 ITD MRD by NGS, LabPMM LLC, an Invivoscribe Technologies, Inc Company

0047U **Oncology (prostate), mRNA, gene expression profiling by real-time RT-PCR of 17 genes (12 content and 5 housekeeping), utilizing formalin-fixed paraffin-embedded tissue, algorithm reported as a risk score**
0.00 0.00 FUD 000

INCLUDES Oncotype DX Genomic Prostate Score, Genomic Health, Inc, Genomic Health, Inc

0048U **Oncology (solid organ neoplasia), DNA, targeted sequencing of protein-coding exons of 468 cancer-associated genes, including interrogation for somatic mutations and microsatellite instability, matched with normal specimens, utilizing formalin-fixed paraffin-embedded tumor tissue, report of clinically significant mutation(s)**
0.00 0.00 FUD 000

INCLUDES MSK-IMPACT (Integrated Mutation Profiling of Actionable Cancer Targets), Memorial Sloan Kettering Cancer Center

0049U NPM1 (nucleophosmin) (eg, acute myeloid leukemia) gene analysis, quantitative
0.00 0.00 FUD 000
INCLUDES *NPM1* MRD by NGS, LabPMM LLC, an Invivoscribe Technologies, Inc Company

0050U Targeted genomic sequence analysis panel, acute myelogenous leukemia, DNA analysis, 194 genes, interrogation for sequence variants, copy number variants or rearrangements
0.00 0.00 FUD 000
INCLUDES MyAML NGS Panel, LabPMM LLC, an Invivoscribe Technologies, Inc Company

0051U Prescription drug monitoring, evaluation of drugs present by LC-MS/MS, urine, 31 drug panel, reported as quantitative results, detected or not detected, per date of service
0.00 0.00 FUD 000
INCLUDES UCompliDx, Elite Medical Laboratory Solutions, LLC, Elite Medical Laboratory Solutions, LLC (LDT)

0052U Lipoprotein, blood, high resolution fractionation and quantitation of lipoproteins, including all five major lipoprotein classes and subclasses of HDL, LDL, and VLDL by vertical auto profile ultracentrifugation
0.00 0.00 FUD 000
INCLUDES VAP Cholesterol Test, VAP Diagnostics Laboratory, Inc, VAP Diagnostics Laboratory, Inc

0053U Oncology (prostate cancer), FISH analysis of 4 genes (*ASAP1, HDAC9, CHD1* and *PTEN*, needle biopsy specimen, algorithm reported as probability of higher tumor grade
0.00 0.00 FUD 000
INCLUDES Prostate Cancer Risk Panel, Mayo Clinic, Laboratory Developed Test

0054U Prescription drug monitoring, 14 or more classes of drugs and substances, definitive tandem mass spectrometry with chromatography, capillary blood, quantitative report with therapeutic and toxic ranges, including steady-state range for the prescribed dose when detected, per date of service
0.00 0.00 FUD 000
INCLUDES AssuranceRx Micro Serum, Firstox Laboratories, LLC, Firstox Laboratories, LLC

0055U Cardiology (heart transplant), cell-free DNA, PCR assay of 96 DNA target sequences (94 single nucleotide polymorphism targets and two control targets), plasma
0.00 0.00 FUD 000
INCLUDES myTAIHEART, TAI Diagnostics, Inc, TAI Diagnostics, Inc

0056U Hematology (acute myelogenous leukemia), DNA, whole genome next-generation sequencing to detect gene rearrangement(s), blood or bone marrow, report of specific gene rearrangement(s)
0.00 0.00 FUD 000
INCLUDES MatePair Acute Myeloid Leukemia Panel, Mayo Clinic, Laboratory Developed Test

~~**0057U Oncology (solid organ neoplasia), mRNA, gene expression profiling by massively parallel sequencing for analysis of 51 genes, utilizing formalin-fixed paraffin-embedded tissue, algorithm reported as a normalized percentile rank**~~

0058U Oncology (Merkel cell carcinoma), detection of antibodies to the Merkel cell polyoma virus oncoprotein (small T antigen), serum, quantitative
0.00 0.00 FUD 000
INCLUDES Merkel SmT Oncoprotein Antibody Titer, University of Washington, Department of Laboratory Medicine

0059U Oncology (Merkel cell carcinoma), detection of antibodies to the Merkel cell polyoma virus capsid protein (VP1), serum, reported as positive or negative
0.00 0.00 FUD 000
INCLUDES Merkel Virus VP1 Capsid Antibody, University of Washington, Department of Laboratory Medicine

0060U Twin zygosity, genomic targeted sequence analysis of chromosome 2, using circulating cell-free fetal DNA in maternal blood
0.00 0.00 FUD 000
INCLUDES Twins Zygosity PLA, Natera, Inc, Natera, Inc

0061U Transcutaneous measurement of five biomarkers (tissue oxygenation [StO2], oxyhemoglobin [ctHbO2], deoxyhemoglobin [ctHbR], papillary and reticular dermal hemoglobin concentrations [ctHb1 and ctHb2]), using spatial frequency domain imaging (SFDI) and multi-spectral analysis
0.00 0.00 FUD 000
INCLUDES Transcutaneous multispectral measurement of tissue oxygenation and hemoglobin using spatial frequency domain imaging (SFDI), Modulated Imaging, Inc, Modulated Imaging, Inc

● **0062U Autoimmune (systemic lupus erythematosus), IgG and IgM analysis of 80 biomarkers, utilizing serum, algorithm reported with a risk score**
0.00 0.00 FUD 000
INCLUDES SLE-key® Rule Out, Veracis Inc, Veracis Inc

● **0063U Neurology (autism), 32 amines by LC-MS/MS, using plasma, algorithm reported as metabolic signature associated with autism spectrum disorder**
0.00 0.00 FUD 000
INCLUDES NPDX ASD ADM Panel I, Stemina Biomarker Discovery, Inc, Stemina Biomarker Discovery, Inc d/b/a NeuroPointDX

● **0064U Antibody, Treponema pallidum, total and rapid plasma reagin (RPR), immunoassay, qualitative**
0.00 0.00 FUD 000
INCLUDES BioPlex 2200 Syphilis Total & RPR Assay, Bio-Rad Laboratories, Bio-Rad Laboratories

● **0065U Syphilis test, non-treponemal antibody, immunoassay, qualitative (RPR)**
0.00 0.00 FUD 000
INCLUDES BioPlex 2200 RPR Assay, Bio-Rad Laboratories, Bio-Rad Laboratories

● **0066U Placental alpha-micro globulin-1 (PAMG-1), immunoassay with direct optical observation, cervico-vaginal fluid, each specimen**
0.00 0.00 FUD 000
INCLUDES PartoSure™ Test, Parsagen Diagnostics, Inc, Parsagen Diagnostics, Inc, a QIAGEN Company

● **0067U Oncology (breast), immunohistochemistry, protein expression profiling of 4 biomarkers (matrix metalloproteinase-1 [MMP-1], carcinoembryonic antigen-related cell adhesion molecule 6 [CEACAM6], hyaluronoglucosaminidase [HYAL1], highly expressed in cancer protein [HEC1]), formalin-fixed paraffin-embedded precancerous breast tissue, algorithm reported as carcinoma risk score**
0.00 0.00 FUD 000
INCLUDES BBDRisk Dx™, Silbiotech, Inc, Silbiotech, Inc

● **0068U Candida species panel (*C. albicans, C. glabrata, C. parapsilosis, C. kruseii, C tropicalis, and C. auris*), amplified probe technique with qualitative report of the presence or absence of each species**
0.00 0.00 FUD 000
INCLUDES MYCODART Dual Amplification Real Time PCR Panel for 6 Candida species, RealTime Laboratories, Inc, RealTime Laboratories, Inc

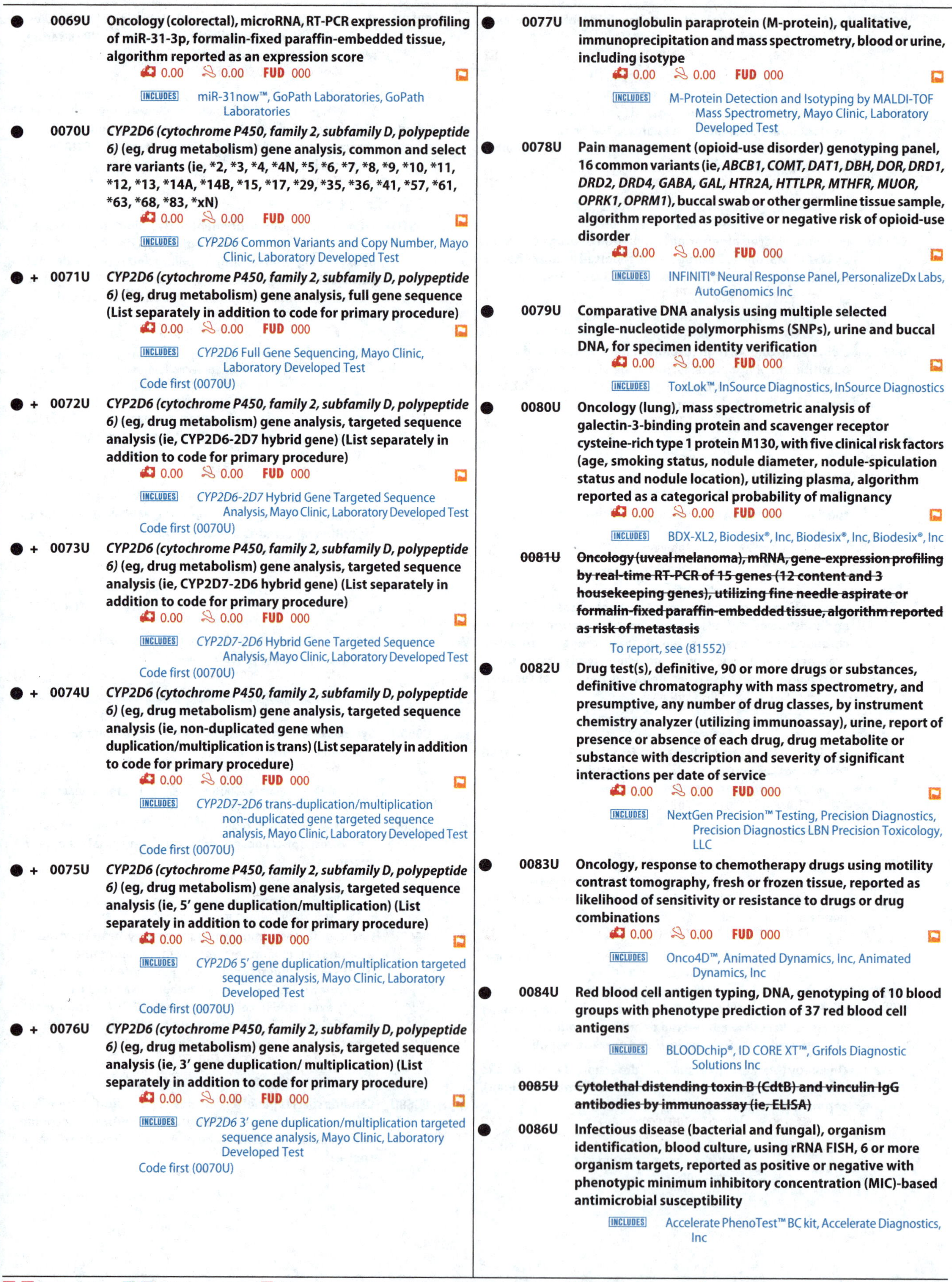

● **0069U** **Oncology (colorectal), microRNA, RT-PCR expression profiling of miR-31-3p, formalin-fixed paraffin-embedded tissue, algorithm reported as an expression score**

0.00 0.00 FUD 000

INCLUDES miR-31now™, GoPath Laboratories, GoPath Laboratories

● **0070U** ***CYP2D6 (cytochrome P450, family 2, subfamily D, polypeptide 6)* (eg, drug metabolism) gene analysis, common and select rare variants (ie, *2, *3, *4, *4N, *5, *6, *7, *8, *9, *10, *11, *12, *13, *14A, *14B, *15, *17, *29, *35, *36, *41, *57, *61, *63, *68, *83, *xN)**

0.00 0.00 FUD 000

INCLUDES *CYP2D6* Common Variants and Copy Number, Mayo Clinic, Laboratory Developed Test

● + **0071U** ***CYP2D6 (cytochrome P450, family 2, subfamily D, polypeptide 6)* (eg, drug metabolism) gene analysis, full gene sequence (List separately in addition to code for primary procedure)**

0.00 0.00 FUD 000

INCLUDES *CYP2D6* Full Gene Sequencing, Mayo Clinic, Laboratory Developed Test

Code first (0070U)

● + **0072U** ***CYP2D6 (cytochrome P450, family 2, subfamily D, polypeptide 6)* (eg, drug metabolism) gene analysis, targeted sequence analysis (ie, CYP2D6-2D7 hybrid gene) (List separately in addition to code for primary procedure)**

0.00 0.00 FUD 000

INCLUDES *CYP2D6-2D7* Hybrid Gene Targeted Sequence Analysis, Mayo Clinic, Laboratory Developed Test

Code first (0070U)

● + **0073U** ***CYP2D6 (cytochrome P450, family 2, subfamily D, polypeptide 6)* (eg, drug metabolism) gene analysis, targeted sequence analysis (ie, CYP2D7-2D6 hybrid gene) (List separately in addition to code for primary procedure)**

0.00 0.00 FUD 000

INCLUDES *CYP2D7-2D6* Hybrid Gene Targeted Sequence Analysis, Mayo Clinic, Laboratory Developed Test

Code first (0070U)

● + **0074U** ***CYP2D6 (cytochrome P450, family 2, subfamily D, polypeptide 6)* (eg, drug metabolism) gene analysis, targeted sequence analysis (ie, non-duplicated gene when duplication/multiplication is trans) (List separately in addition to code for primary procedure)**

0.00 0.00 FUD 000

INCLUDES *CYP2D7-2D6* trans-duplication/multiplication non-duplicated gene targeted sequence analysis, Mayo Clinic, Laboratory Developed Test

Code first (0070U)

● + **0075U** ***CYP2D6 (cytochrome P450, family 2, subfamily D, polypeptide 6)* (eg, drug metabolism) gene analysis, targeted sequence analysis (ie, 5' gene duplication/multiplication) (List separately in addition to code for primary procedure)**

0.00 0.00 FUD 000

INCLUDES *CYP2D6* 5' gene duplication/multiplication targeted sequence analysis, Mayo Clinic, Laboratory Developed Test

Code first (0070U)

● + **0076U** ***CYP2D6 (cytochrome P450, family 2, subfamily D, polypeptide 6)* (eg, drug metabolism) gene analysis, targeted sequence analysis (ie, 3' gene duplication/ multiplication) (List separately in addition to code for primary procedure)**

0.00 0.00 FUD 000

INCLUDES *CYP2D6* 3' gene duplication/multiplication targeted sequence analysis, Mayo Clinic, Laboratory Developed Test

Code first (0070U)

● **0077U** **Immunoglobulin paraprotein (M-protein), qualitative, immunoprecipitation and mass spectrometry, blood or urine, including isotype**

0.00 0.00 FUD 000

INCLUDES M-Protein Detection and Isotyping by MALDI-TOF Mass Spectrometry, Mayo Clinic, Laboratory Developed Test

● **0078U** **Pain management (opioid-use disorder) genotyping panel, 16 common variants (ie, *ABCB1, COMT, DAT1, DBH, DOR, DRD1, DRD2, DRD4, GABA, GAL, HTR2A, HTTLPR, MTHFR, MUOR, OPRK1, OPRM1*), buccal swab or other germline tissue sample, algorithm reported as positive or negative risk of opioid-use disorder**

0.00 0.00 FUD 000

INCLUDES INFINITI® Neural Response Panel, PersonalizeDx Labs, AutoGenomics Inc

● **0079U** **Comparative DNA analysis using multiple selected single-nucleotide polymorphisms (SNPs), urine and buccal DNA, for specimen identity verification**

0.00 0.00 FUD 000

INCLUDES ToxLok™, InSource Diagnostics, InSource Diagnostics

● **0080U** **Oncology (lung), mass spectrometric analysis of galectin-3-binding protein and scavenger receptor cysteine-rich type 1 protein M130, with five clinical risk factors (age, smoking status, nodule diameter, nodule-spiculation status and nodule location), utilizing plasma, algorithm reported as a categorical probability of malignancy**

0.00 0.00 FUD 000

INCLUDES BDX-XL2, Biodesix®, Inc, Biodesix®, Inc, Biodesix®, Inc

~~**0081U**~~ ~~**Oncology (uveal melanoma), mRNA, gene-expression profiling by real-time RT-PCR of 15 genes (12 content and 3 housekeeping genes), utilizing fine needle aspirate or formalin-fixed paraffin-embedded tissue, algorithm reported as risk of metastasis**~~

To report, see (81552)

● **0082U** **Drug test(s), definitive, 90 or more drugs or substances, definitive chromatography with mass spectrometry, and presumptive, any number of drug classes, by instrument chemistry analyzer (utilizing immunoassay), urine, report of presence or absence of each drug, drug metabolite or substance with description and severity of significant interactions per date of service**

0.00 0.00 FUD 000

INCLUDES NextGen Precision™ Testing, Precision Diagnostics, Precision Diagnostics LBN Precision Toxicology, LLC

● **0083U** **Oncology, response to chemotherapy drugs using motility contrast tomography, fresh or frozen tissue, reported as likelihood of sensitivity or resistance to drugs or drug combinations**

0.00 0.00 FUD 000

INCLUDES Onco4D™, Animated Dynamics, Inc, Animated Dynamics, Inc

● **0084U** **Red blood cell antigen typing, DNA, genotyping of 10 blood groups with phenotype prediction of 37 red blood cell antigens**

INCLUDES BLOODchip®, ID CORE XT™, Grifols Diagnostic Solutions Inc

~~**0085U**~~ ~~**Cytolethal distending toxin B (CdtB) and vinculin IgG antibodies by immunoassay (ie, ELISA)**~~

● **0086U** **Infectious disease (bacterial and fungal), organism identification, blood culture, using rRNA FISH, 6 or more organism targets, reported as positive or negative with phenotypic minimum inhibitory concentration (MIC)-based antimicrobial susceptibility**

INCLUDES Accelerate PhenoTest™ BC kit, Accelerate Diagnostics, Inc

● **0087U** **Cardiology (heart transplant), mRNA gene expression profiling by microarray of 1283 genes, transplant biopsy tissue, allograft rejection and injury algorithm reported as a probability score**

INCLUDES Molecular Microscope® MMDx—Heart, Kashi Clinical Laboratories

● **0088U** **Transplantation medicine (kidney allograft rejection), microarray gene expression profiling of 1494 genes, utilizing transplant biopsy tissue, algorithm reported as a probability score for rejection**

INCLUDES Molecular Microscope® MMDx—Kidney, Kashi Clinical Laboratories

● **0089U** **Oncology (melanoma), gene expression profiling by RTqPCR, *PRAME* and *LINC00518*, superficial collection using adhesive patch(es)**

INCLUDES Pigmented Lesion Assay (PLA), DermTech

● **0090U** **Oncology (cutaneous melanoma), mRNA gene expression profiling by RT-PCR of 23 genes (14 content and 9 housekeeping), utilizing formalin-fixed paraffin-embedded tissue, algorithm reported as a categorical result (ie, benign, indeterminate, malignant)**

INCLUDES myPath® Melanoma, Myriad Genetic Laboratories

● **0091U** **Oncology (colorectal) screening, cell enumeration of circulating tumor cells, utilizing whole blood, algorithm, for the presence of adenoma or cancer, reported as a positive or negative result**

INCLUDES FirstSight^{CRC}, CellMax Life

● **0092U** **Oncology (lung), three protein biomarkers, immunoassay using magnetic nanosensor technology, plasma, algorithm reported as risk score for likelihood of malignancy**

INCLUDES REVEAL Lung Nodule Characterization, MagArray, Inc

● **0093U** **Prescription drug monitoring, evaluation of 65 common drugs by LC-MS/MS, urine, each drug reported detected or not detected**

INCLUDES ComplyRX, Claro Labs

● **0094U** **Genome (eg, unexplained constitutional or heritable disorder or syndrome), rapid sequence analysis**

INCLUDES RCIGM Rapid Whole Genome Sequencing, Rady Children's Institute for Genomic Medicine (RCIGM)

● **0095U** **Inflammation (eosinophilic esophagitis), ELISA analysis of eotaxin-3 *(CCL26 [C-C motif chemokine ligand 26])* and major basic protein *(PRG2 [proteoglycan 2, pro eosinophil major basic protein])*, specimen obtained by swallowed nylon string, algorithm reported as predictive probability index for active eosinophilic esophagitis**

INCLUDES Esophageal String Test™ (EST), Cambridge Biomedical, Inc

● **0096U** **Human papillomavirus (HPV), high-risk types (ie, 16, 18, 31, 33, 35, 39, 45, 51, 52, 56, 58, 59, 66, 68), male urine**

INCLUDES HPV, High-Risk, Male Urine, Molecular Testing Labs

● **0097U** **Gastrointestinal pathogen, multiplex reverse transcription and multiplex amplified probe technique, multiple types or subtypes, 22 targets (Campylobacter [C. jejuni/C. coli/C. upsaliensis], Clostridium difficile [C. difficile] toxin A/B, Plesiomonas shigelloides, Salmonella, Vibrio [V. parahaemolyticus/V. vulnificus/V. cholerae], including specific identification of Vibrio cholerae, Yersinia enterocolitica, Enteroaggregative Escherichia coli [EAEC], Enteropathogenic Escherichia coli [EPEC], Enterotoxigenic Escherichia coli [ETEC] lt/st, Shiga-like toxin-producing Escherichia coli [STEC] stx1/stx2 [including specific identification of the E. coli O157 serogroup within STEC], Shigella/Enteroinvasive Escherichia coli [EIEC], Cryptosporidium, Cyclospora cayetanensis, Entamoeba histolytica, Giardia lamblia [also known as G. intestinalis and G. duodenalis], adenovirus F 40/41, astrovirus, norovirus GI/GII, rotavirus A, sapovirus [Genogroups I, II, IV, and V])**

INCLUDES BioFire® FilmArray® Gastrointestinal (GI) Panel, BioFire® Diagnostics

● **0098U** **Respiratory pathogen, multiplex reverse transcription and multiplex amplified probe technique, multiple types or subtypes, 14 targets (adenovirus, coronavirus, human metapneumovirus, influenza A, influenza A subtype H1, influenza A subtype H3, influenza A subtype H1-2009, influenza B, parainfluenza virus, human rhinovirus/enterovirus, respiratory syncytial virus, Bordetella pertussis, Chlamydophila pneumoniae, Mycoplasma pneumoniae)**

INCLUDES BioFire® FilmArray® Respiratory Panel (RP) EZ, BioFire® Diagnostics

● **0099U** **Respiratory pathogen, multiplex reverse transcription and multiplex amplified probe technique, multiple types or subtypes, 20 targets (adenovirus, coronavirus 229E, coronavirus HKU1, coronavirus, coronavirus OC43, human metapneumovirus, influenza A, influenza A subtype, influenza A subtype H3, influenza A subtype H1-2009, influenza, parainfluenza virus, parainfluenza virus 2, parainfluenza virus 3, parainfluenza virus 4, human rhinovirus/enterovirus, respiratory syncytial virus, Bordetella pertussis, Chlamydophila pneumonia, Mycoplasma pneumoniae)**

INCLUDES BioFire® FilmArray® Respiratory Panel (RP), BioFire® Diagnostics

● **0100U** **Respiratory pathogen, multiplex reverse transcription and multiplex amplified probe technique, multiple types or subtypes, 21 targets (adenovirus, coronavirus 229E, coronavirus HKU1, coronavirus NL63, coronavirus OC43, human metapneumovirus, human rhinovirus/enterovirus, influenza A, including subtypes H1, H1-2009, and H3, influenza B, parainfluenza virus 1, parainfluenza virus 2, parainfluenza virus 3, parainfluenza virus 4, respiratory syncytial virus, Bordetella parapertussis [IS1001], Bordetella pertussis [ptxP], Chlamydia pneumoniae, Mycoplasma pneumoniae)**

INCLUDES BioFire® FilmArray® Respiratory Panel 2 (RP2), BioFire® Diagnostics

● **0101U** **Hereditary colon cancer disorders (eg, Lynch syndrome, *PTEN* hamartoma syndrome, Cowden syndrome, familial adenomatosis polyposis), genomic sequence analysis panel utilizing a combination of NGS, Sanger, MLPA, and array CGH, with MRNA analytics to resolve variants of unknown significance when indicated (15 genes [sequencing and deletion/duplication], *EPCAM* and *GREM1* [deletion/duplication only])**

INCLUDES ColoNext®, Ambry Genetics®, Ambry Genetics®

● **0102U** **Hereditary breast cancer-related disorders (eg, hereditary breast cancer, hereditary ovarian cancer, hereditary endometrial cancer), genomic sequence analysis panel utilizing a combination of NGS, Sanger, MLPA, and array CGH, with MRNA analytics to resolve variants of unknown significance when indicated (17 genes [sequencing and deletion/duplication])**

INCLUDES BreastNext®, Ambry Genetics®, Ambry Genetics®

● **0103U** **Hereditary ovarian cancer (eg, hereditary ovarian cancer, hereditary endometrial cancer), genomic sequence analysis panel utilizing a combination of NGS, Sanger, MLPA, and array CGH, with MRNA analytics to resolve variants of unknown significance when indicated (24 genes [sequencing and deletion/duplication], *EPCAM* [deletion/duplication only])**

INCLUDES OvaNext®, Ambry Genetics®, Ambry Genetics®

~~**0104U** **Hereditary pan cancer (eg, hereditary breast and ovarian cancer, hereditary endometrial cancer, hereditary colorectal cancer), genomic sequence analysis panel utilizing a combination of NGS, Sanger, MLPA, and array CGH, with MRNA analytics to resolve variants of unknown significance when indicated (32 genes [sequencing and deletion/duplication], *EPCAM* and *GREM1* [deletion/duplication only])**~~

● **0105U** **Nephrology (chronic kidney disease), multiplex electrochemiluminescent immunoassay (ECLIA) of tumor necrosis factor receptor 1A, receptor superfamily 2 *(TNFR1, TNFR2)*, and kidney injury molecule-1 (KIM-1) combined with longitudinal clinical data, including *APOL1* genotype if available, and plasma (isolated fresh or frozen), algorithm reported as probability score for rapid kidney function decline (RKFD)**

INCLUDES KidneyIntelX™, RenalytixAI, RenalytixAI

● **0106U** **Gastric emptying, serial collection of 7 timed breath specimens, non-radioisotope carbon-13 (^{13}C) spirulina substrate, analysis of each specimen by gas isotope ratio mass spectrometry, reported as rate of $^{13}CO_2$ excretion**

INCLUDES 13C-Spirulina Gastric Emptying Breath Test (GEBT), Cairn Diagnostics d/b/a Advanced Breath Diagnostics, LLC, Cairn Diagnostics d/b/a Advanced Breath Diagnostics, LLC

● **0107U** **Clostridium difficile toxin(s) antigen detection by immunoassay technique, stool, qualitative, multiple-step method**

INCLUDES Singulex Clarity C.diff toxins A/B assay, Singulex

● **0108U** **Gastroenterology (Barrett's esophagus), whole slide-digital imaging, including morphometric analysis, computer-assisted quantitative immunolabeling of 9 protein biomarkers (p16, AMACR, p53, CD68, COX-2, CD45RO, HIF1a, HER-2, K20) and morphology, formalin-fixed paraffin-embedded tissue, algorithm reported as risk of progression to high-grade dysplasia or cancer**

INCLUDES TissueCypher® Barrett's Esophagus Assay, Cernostics, Cernostics

● **0109U** **Infectious disease (Aspergillus species), real-time PCR for detection of DNA from 4 species *(A. fumigatus, A. terreus, A. niger,* and *A. flavus)*, blood, lavage fluid, or tissue, qualitative reporting of presence or absence of each species**

INCLUDES MYCODART Dual Amplification Real Time PCR Panel for 4 Aspergillus species, RealTime Laboratories, Inc/MycoDART, Inc

● **0110U** **Prescription drug monitoring, one or more oral oncology drug(s) and substances, definitive tandem mass spectrometry with chromatography, serum or plasma from capillary blood or venous blood, quantitative report with steady-state range for the prescribed drug(s) when detected**

INCLUDES Oral OncolyticAssuranceRX, Firstox Laboratories, LLC, Firstox Laboratories, LLC

● **0111U** **Oncology (colon cancer), targeted *KRAS* (codons 12, 13, and 61) and *NRAS* (codons 12, 13, and 61) gene analysis utilizing formalin-fixed paraffin-embedded tissue**

INCLUDES Praxis(™) Extended RAS Panel, Illumina, Illumina

● **0112U** **Infectious agent detection and identification, targeted sequence analysis (16S and 18S rRNA genes) with drug-resistance gene**

INCLUDES MicroGenDX qPCR & NGS For Infection, MicroGenDX, MicroGenDX

● **0113U** **Oncology (prostate), measurement of *PCA3* and *TMPRSS2-ERG* in urine and PSA in serum following prostatic massage, by RNA amplification and fluorescence-based detection, algorithm reported as risk score**

INCLUDES MiPS (Mi-Prostate Score), MLabs, MLabs

● **0114U** **Gastroenterology (Barrett's esophagus), *VIM* and *CCNA1* methylation analysis, esophageal cells, algorithm reported as likelihood for Barrett's esophagus**

INCLUDES EsoGuard™, Lucid Diagnostics, Lucid Diagnostics

● **0115U** **Respiratory infectious agent detection by nucleic acid (DNA and RNA), 18 viral types and subtypes and 2 bacterial targets, amplified probe technique, including multiplex reverse transcription for RNA targets, each analyte reported as detected or not detected**

INCLUDES ePlex Respiratory Pathogen (RP) Panel, GenMark Diagnostics, Inc, GenMark Diagnostics, Inc

● **0116U** **Prescription drug monitoring, enzyme immunoassay of 35 or more drugs confirmed with LC-MS/MS, oral fluid, algorithm results reported as a patient-compliance measurement with risk of drug to drug interactions for prescribed medications**

INCLUDES Snapshot Oral Fluid Compliance, Ethos Laboratories

● **0117U** **Pain management, analysis of 11 endogenous analytes (methylmalonic acid, xanthurenic acid, homocysteine, pyroglutamic acid, vanilmandelate, 5-hydroxyindoleacetic acid, hydroxymethylglutarate, ethylmalonate, 3-hydroxypropyl mercapturic acid (3-HPMA), quinolinic acid, kynurenic acid), LC-MS/MS, urine, algorithm reported as a pain-index score with likelihood of atypical biochemical function associated with pain**

INCLUDES Foundation PI☒, Ethos Laboratories

● **0118U** **Transplantation medicine, quantification of donor-derived cell-free DNA using whole genome next-generation sequencing, plasma, reported as percentage of donor-derived cell-free DNA in the total cell-free DNA**

INCLUDES Viracor TRAC™ dd-cfDNA, Viracor Eurofins, Viracor Eurofins

● **0119U** **Cardiology, ceramides by liquid chromatography-tandem mass spectrometry, plasma, quantitative report with risk score for major cardiovascular events**

INCLUDES MI-HEART Ceramides, Plasma, Mayo Clinic, Laboratory Developed Test

● **0120U** **Oncology (B-cell lymphoma classification), mRNA, gene expression profiling by fluorescent probe hybridization of 58 genes (45 content and 13 housekeeping genes), formalin-fixed paraffin-embedded tissue, algorithm reported as likelihood for primary mediastinal B-cell lymphoma (PMBCL) and diffuse large B-cell lymphoma (DLBCL) with cell of origin subtyping in the latter**

INCLUDES Lymph3Cx Lymphoma Molecular Subtyping Assay, Mayo Clinic, Laboratory Developed Test

● **0121U** **Sickle cell disease, microfluidic flow adhesion (VCAM-1), whole blood**

INCLUDES Flow Adhesion of Whole Blood on VCAM-1 (FAB-V), Functional Fluidics, Functional Fluidics

● **0122U** **Sickle cell disease, microfluidic flow adhesion (P-Selectin), whole blood**

INCLUDES Flow Adhesion of Whole Blood to P-SELECTIN (WB-PSEL), Functional Fluidics, Functional Fluidics

● **0123U** **Mechanical fragility, RBC, shear stress and spectral analysis profiling**

INCLUDES Mechanical Fragility, RBC by shear stress profiling and spectral analysis, Functional Fluidics, Functional Fluidics

● **0124U** **Fetal congenital abnormalities, biochemical assays of 3 analytes (free beta-hCG, PAPP-A, AFP), time-resolved fluorescence immunoassay, maternal dried-blood spot, algorithm reported as risk scores for fetal trisomies 13/18 and 21**

INCLUDES First Trimester Screen | FB⊠, Eurofins NTD, LLC, Eurofins NTD, LLC

● **0125U** **Fetal congenital abnormalities and perinatal complications, biochemical assays of 5 analytes (free beta-hCG, PAPP-A, AFP, placental growth factor, and inhibin-A), time-resolved fluorescence immunoassay, maternal serum, algorithm reported as risk scores for fetal trisomies 13/18, 21, and preeclampsia**

INCLUDES Maternal Fetal Screen | T1⊠, Eurofins NTD, LLC, Eurofins NTD, LLC

● **0126U** **Fetal congenital abnormalities and perinatal complications, biochemical assays of 5 analytes (free beta-hCG, PAPP-A, AFP, placental growth factor, and inhibin-A), time-resolved fluorescence immunoassay, includes qualitative assessment of Y chromosome in cell-free fetal DNA, maternal serum and plasma, predictive algorithm reported as a risk scores for fetal trisomies 13/18, 21, and preeclampsia**

INCLUDES Maternal Fetal Screen | T1 + Y Chromosome ⊠, Eurofins NTD, LLC, Eurofins NTD, LLC

● **0127U** **Obstetrics (preeclampsia), biochemical assays of 3 analytes (PAPP-A, AFP, and placental growth factor), time-resolved fluorescence immunoassay, maternal serum, predictive algorithm reported as a risk score for preeclampsia**

INCLUDES Preeclampsia Screen | T1⊠, Eurofins NTD, LLC, Eurofins NTD, LLC

● **0128U** **Obstetrics (preeclampsia), biochemical assays of 3 analytes (PAPP-A, AFP, and placental growth factor), time-resolved fluorescence immunoassay, includes qualitative assessment of Y chromosome in cell-free fetal DNA, maternal serum and plasma, predictive algorithm reported as a risk score for preeclampsia**

INCLUDES Preeclampsia Screen | T1 + Y Chromosome⊠, Eurofins NTD, LLC, Eurofins NTD, LLC

● **0129U** **Hereditary breast cancer-related disorders (eg, hereditary breast cancer, hereditary ovarian cancer, hereditary endometrial cancer), genomic sequence analysis and deletion/duplication analysis panel *(ATM, BRCA1, BRCA2, CDH1, CHEK2, PALB2, PTEN,* and *TP53)***

INCLUDES BRCAplus, Ambry Genetics

● + **0130U** **Hereditary colon cancer disorders (eg, Lynch syndrome, PTEN hamartoma syndrome, Cowden syndrome, familial adenomatosis polyposis), targeted mRNA sequence analysis panel *(APC, CDH1, CHEK2, MLH1, MSH2, MSH6, MUTYH, PMS2, PTEN,* and *TP53)* (List separately in addition to code for primary procedure)**

0.00 0.00 FUD 000

INCLUDES +RNAinsight™ for ColoNext®, Ambry Genetics

Code first (81435, 0101U)

● + **0131U** **Hereditary breast cancer-related disorders (eg, hereditary breast cancer, hereditary ovarian cancer, hereditary endometrial cancer), targeted mRNA sequence analysis panel (13 genes) (List separately in addition to code for primary procedure)**

0.00 0.00 FUD 000

INCLUDES +RNAinsight™ for BreastNext®, Ambry Genetics

Code first ([81162], 81432, 0102U)

● + **0132U** **Hereditary ovarian cancer-related disorders (eg, hereditary breast cancer, hereditary ovarian cancer, hereditary endometrial cancer), targeted mRNA sequence analysis panel (17 genes) (List separately in addition to code for primary procedure)**

0.00 0.00 FUD 000

INCLUDES +RNAinsight™ for OvaNext®, Ambry Genetics

Code first ([81162], 81432, 0103U)

● + **0133U** **Hereditary prostate cancer-related disorders, targeted mRNA sequence analysis panel (11 genes) (List separately in addition to code for primary procedure)**

0.00 0.00 FUD 000

INCLUDES +RNAinsight™ for ProstateNext®, Ambry Genetics

Code first ([81162])

● + **0134U** **Hereditary pan cancer (eg, hereditary breast and ovarian cancer, hereditary endometrial cancer, hereditary colorectal cancer), targeted mRNA sequence analysis panel (18 genes) (List separately in addition to code for primary procedure)**

0.00 0.00 FUD 000

INCLUDES +RNAinsight™ for CancerNext®, Ambry Genetics

Code first ([81162], 81432, 81435)

● + **0135U** **Hereditary gynecological cancer (eg, hereditary breast and ovarian cancer, hereditary endometrial cancer, hereditary colorectal cancer), targeted mRNA sequence analysis panel (12 genes) (List separately in addition to code for primary procedure)**

0.00 0.00 FUD 000

INCLUDES +RNAinsight™ for GYNPlus®, Ambry Genetics

Code first ([81162])

● + **0136U** ***ATM (ataxia telangiectasia mutated)* (eg, ataxia telangiectasia) mRNA sequence analysis (List separately in addition to code for primary procedure)**

0.00 0.00 FUD 000

INCLUDES +RNAinsight™ for *ATM*, Ambry Genetics

Code first (81408)

● + **0137U** ***PALB2 (partner and localizer of BRCA2)* (eg, breast and pancreatic cancer) mRNA sequence analysis (List separately in addition to code for ...**

0.00 0.00 FUD 000

INCLUDES +RNAinsight™ for *PALB2*, Ambry Genetics

Code first (81406)

● + **0138U** ***BRCA1 (BRCA1, DNA repair associated), BRCA2 (BRCA2, DNA repair associated)* (eg, hereditary breast and ovarian cancer) mRNA sequence analysis (List separately in addition to code for primary procedure)**

0.00 0.00 FUD 000

INCLUDES +RNAinsight™ for *BRCA1/2*, Ambry Genetics

Code first ([81162])

● **0139U** **Neurology (autism spectrum disorder [ASD]), quantitative measurements of 6 central carbon metabolites (ie, α-ketoglutarate, alanine, lactate, phenylalanine, pyruvate, and succinate), LC-MS/MS, plasma, algorithmic analysis with result reported as negative or positive (with metabolic subtypes of ASD)**

NPDX ASD Energy Metabolism, Stemina Biomarker Discovery, Inc, Stemina Biomarker Discovery, Inc.

● **0140U** **Infectious disease (fungi), fungal pathogen identification, DNA (15 fungal targets), blood culture, amplified probe technique, each target reported as detected or not detected**

INCLUDES ePlex® BCID Fungal Pathogens Panel, GenMark Diagnostics, Inc, GenMark Diagnostics, Inc

● **0141U** **Infectious disease (bacteria and fungi), gram-positive organism identification and drug resistance element detection, DNA (20 gram-positive bacterial targets, 4 resistance genes, 1 pan gram-negative bacterial target, 1 pan Candida target), blood culture, amplified probe technique, each target reported as detected or not detected**

INCLUDES ePlex® BCID Gram-Positive Panel, GenMark Diagnostics, Inc, GenMark Diagnostics, Inc

● **0142U** **Infectious disease (bacteria and fungi), gram-negative bacterial identification and drug resistance element detection, DNA (21 gram-negative bacterial targets, 6 resistance genes, 1 pan gram-positive bacterial target, 1 pan Candida target), amplified probe technique, each target reported as detected or not detected**

INCLUDES ePlex® BCID Gram-Negative Panel, GenMark Diagnostics, Inc, GenMark Diagnostics, Inc

● **0143U** **Drug assay, definitive, 120 or more drugs or metabolites, urine, quantitative liquid chromatography with tandem mass spectrometry (LC-MS/MS) using multiple reaction monitoring (MRM), with drug or metabolite description, comments including sample validation, per date of service**

INCLUDES CareViewRx, Newstar Medical Laboratories, LLC, Newstar Medical Laboratories, LLC

EXCLUDES *PsychViewRx Plus analysis by Newstar Medical Laboratories, LLC. To report, see (0150U)*

● **0144U** **Drug assay, definitive, 160 or more drugs or metabolites, urine, quantitative liquid chromatography with tandem mass spectrometry (LC-MS/MS) using multiple reaction monitoring (MRM), with drug or metabolite description, comments including sample validation, per date of service**

EXCLUDES *CareViewRx Plus, Newstar Medical Laboratories, LLC, Newstar Medical Laboratories, LLC*

● **0145U** **Drug assay, definitive, 65 or more drugs or metabolites, urine, quantitative liquid chromatography with tandem mass spectrometry (LC-MS/MS) using multiple reaction monitoring (MRM), with drug or metabolite description, comments including sample validation, per date of service**

EXCLUDES *PainViewRx, Newstar Medical Laboratories, LLC, Newstar Medical Laboratories, LLC*

● **0146U** **Drug assay, definitive, 80 or more drugs or metabolites, urine, by quantitative liquid chromatography with tandem mass spectrometry (LC-MS/MS) using multiple reaction monitoring (MRM), with drug or metabolite description, comments including sample validation, per date of service**

INCLUDES PainViewRx Plus, Newstar Medical Laboratories, LLC, Newstar Medical Laboratories, LLC

● **0147U** **Drug assay, definitive, 85 or more drugs or metabolites, urine, quantitative liquid chromatography with tandem mass spectrometry (LC-MS/MS) using multiple reaction monitoring (MRM), with drug or metabolite description, comments including sample validation, per date of service**

INCLUDES RiskViewRx, Newstar Medical Laboratories, LLC, Newstar Medical Laboratories, LLC

● **0148U** **Drug assay, definitive, 100 or more drugs or metabolites, urine, quantitative liquid chromatography with tandem mass spectrometry (LC-MS/MS) using multiple reaction monitoring (MRM), with drug or metabolite description, comments including sample validation, per date of service**

INCLUDES RiskViewRx Plus, Newstar Medical Laboratories, LLC, Newstar Medical Laboratories, LLC

● **0149U** **Drug assay, definitive, 60 or more drugs or metabolites, urine, quantitative liquid chromatography with tandem mass spectrometry (LC-MS/MS) using multiple reaction monitoring (MRM), with drug or metabolite description, comments including sample validation, per date of service**

INCLUDES PsychViewRx, Newstar Medical Laboratories, LLC, Newstar Medical Laboratories, LLC

● **0150U** **Drug assay, definitive, 120 or more drugs or metabolites, urine, quantitative liquid chromatography with tandem mass spectrometry (LC-MS/MS) using multiple reaction monitoring (MRM), with drug or metabolite description, comments including sample validation, per date of service**

INCLUDES PsychViewRx Plus, Newstar Medical Laboratories, LLC, Newstar Medical Laboratories, LLC

EXCLUDES *CareViewRx analysis by Newstar Medical Laboratories, LLC. To report, see (0143U)*

● **0151U** **Infectious disease (bacterial or viral respiratory tract infection), pathogen specific nucleic acid (DNA or RNA), 33 targets, real-time semi-quantitative PCR, bronchoalveolar lavage, sputum, or endotracheal aspirate, detection of 33 organismal and antibiotic resistance genes with limited semi-quantitative results**

INCLUDES BioFire® FilmArray® Pneumonia Panel, BioFire® Diagnostics, BioFire® Diagnostics

● **0152U** **Infectious disease (bacteria, fungi, parasites, and DNA viruses), DNA, PCR and next-generation sequencing, plasma, detection of >1,000 potential microbial organisms for significant positive pathogens**

INCLUDES Karius® Test, Karius Inc, Karius Inc

● **0153U** **Oncology (breast), mRNA, gene expression profiling by next-generation sequencing of 101 genes, utilizing formalin-fixed paraffin-embedded tissue, algorithm reported as a triple negative breast cancer clinical subtype(s) with information on immune cell involvement**

INCLUDES Insight TNBCtype™, Insight Molecular Labs

● **0154U** ***FGFR3 (fibroblast growth factor receptor 3)*** **gene analysis (ie, p.R248C [c.742C>T], p.S249C [c.746C>G], p.G370C [c.1108G>T], p.Y373C [c.1118A>G], FGFR3-TACC3v1, and FGFR3-TACC3v3)**

INCLUDES therascreen® *FGFR* RGQ RT-PCR Kit, QIAGEN, QIAGEN GmbH

● **0155U** ***PIK3CA (phosphatidylinositol-4,5-bisphosphate 3-kinase, catalytic subunit alpha)*** **(eg, breast cancer) gene analysis (ie, p.C420R, p.E542K, p.E545A, p.E545D [g.1635G>T only], p.E545G, p.E545K, p.Q546E, p.Q546R, p.H1047L, p.H1047R, p.H1047Y)**

INCLUDES therascreen *PIK3CA* RGQ PCR Kit, QIAGEN, QIAGEN GmbH

● **0156U** **Copy number (eg, intellectual disability, dysmorphology), sequence analysis**

INCLUDES SMASH™, New York Genome Center, Marvel Genomics™

● + **0157U** ***APC (APC regulator of WNT signaling pathway)*** **(eg, familial adenomatosis polyposis [FAP]) mRNA sequence analysis (List separately in addition to code for primary procedure)**

0.00 0.00 FUD 000

INCLUDES CustomNext + RNA: *APC*, Ambry Genetics®, Ambry Genetics®

● + **0158U** ***MLH1 (mutL homolog 1)*** **(eg, hereditary non-polyposis colorectal cancer, Lynch syndrome) mRNA sequence analysis (List separately in addition to code for primary procedure)**

0.00 0.00 FUD 000

INCLUDES CustomNext + RNA: *MLH1*, Ambry Genetics®, Ambry Genetics®

● + 0159U ***MSH2 (mutS homolog 2)*** **(eg, hereditary colon cancer, Lynch syndrome) mRNA sequence analysis (List separately in addition to code for primary procedure)**
0.00 0.00 FUD 000

INCLUDES CustomNext + RNA: *MSH2*, Ambry Genetics®, Ambry Genetics®

● + 0160U ***MSH6 (mutS homolog 6)*** **(eg, hereditary colon cancer, Lynch syndrome) mRNA sequence analysis (List separately in addition to code for primary procedure)**
0.00 0.00 FUD 000

INCLUDES CustomNext + RNA: *MSH6*, Ambry Genetics®, Ambry Genetics®

● + 0161U ***PMS2 (PMS1 homolog 2, mismatch repair system component)*** **(eg, hereditary non-polyposis colorectal cancer, Lynch syndrome) mRNA sequence analysis (List separately in addition to code for primary procedure)**
0.00 0.00 FUD 000

INCLUDES CustomNext + RNA: *PMS2*, Ambry Genetics®, Ambry Genetics®

● + 0162U **Hereditary colon cancer (Lynch syndrome), targeted mRNA sequence analysis panel *(MLH1, MSH2, MSH6, PMS2)* (List separately in addition to code for primary procedure)**
0.00 0.00 FUD 000

INCLUDES CustomNext + RNA: Lynch *(MLH1, MSH2, MSH6, PMS2)*, Ambry Genetics®, Ambry Genetics®

90281-90399 Immunoglobulin Products

INCLUDES Immune globulin product only
Anti-infectives
Antitoxins
Isoantibodies
Monoclonal antibodies
Code also (96365-96372, 96374-96375)

90281 Immune globulin (Ig), human, for intramuscular use
INCLUDES Gamastan
0.00 0.00 FUD XXX
AMA: 2018,Jan,8; 2017,Jan,8; 2016,Jan,13; 2015,Jan,16; 2014,Jan,11

90283 Immune globulin (IgIV), human, for intravenous use
0.00 0.00 FUD XXX
AMA: 2018,Jan,8; 2017,Jan,8; 2016,Jan,13; 2015,Jan,16; 2014,Jan,11

90284 Immune globulin (SCIg), human, for use in subcutaneous infusions, 100 mg, each
0.00 0.00 FUD XXX
AMA: 2018,Jan,8; 2017,Jan,8; 2016,Jan,13; 2015,Jan,16

90287 Botulinum antitoxin, equine, any route
0.00 0.00 FUD XXX
AMA: 2018,Jan,8; 2017,Jan,8; 2016,Jan,13; 2015,Jan,16; 2014,Jan,11

90288 Botulism immune globulin, human, for intravenous use
0.00 0.00 FUD XXX
AMA: 2018,Jan,8; 2017,Jan,8; 2016,Jan,13; 2015,Jan,16; 2014,Jan,11

90291 Cytomegalovirus immune globulin (CMV-IgIV), human, for intravenous use
INCLUDES Cytogram
0.00 0.00 FUD XXX
AMA: 2018,Jan,8; 2017,Jan,8; 2016,Jan,13; 2015,Jan,16; 2014,Jan,11

90296 Diphtheria antitoxin, equine, any route
0.00 0.00 FUD XXX
AMA: 2018,Jan,8; 2017,Jan,8; 2016,Jan,13; 2015,Jan,16; 2014,Jan,11

90371 Hepatitis B immune globulin (HBIg), human, for intramuscular use
INCLUDES HBIG
0.00 0.00 FUD XXX
AMA: 2018,Jan,8; 2017,Jan,8; 2016,Jan,13; 2015,Jan,16; 2014,Jan,11

90375 Rabies immune globulin (RIg), human, for intramuscular and/or subcutaneous use
INCLUDES HyperRAB
0.00 0.00 FUD XXX
AMA: 2018,Jan,8; 2017,Jan,8; 2016,Jan,13; 2015,Jan,16

90376 Rabies immune globulin, heat-treated (RIg-HT), human, for intramuscular and/or subcutaneous use
0.00 0.00 FUD XXX
AMA: 2018,Jan,8; 2017,Jan,8; 2016,Jan,13; 2015,Jan,16

90378 Respiratory syncytial virus, monoclonal antibody, recombinant, for intramuscular use, 50 mg, each
INCLUDES Synagis
0.00 0.00 FUD XXX
AMA: 2018,Jan,8; 2017,Jan,8; 2016,Jan,13; 2015,Jan,16; 2014,Jan,11

90384 Rho(D) immune globulin (RhIg), human, full-dose, for intramuscular use
0.00 0.00 FUD XXX
AMA: 2018,Jan,8; 2017,Jan,8; 2016,Jan,13; 2015,Jan,16; 2014,Jan,11

90385 Rho(D) immune globulin (RhIg), human, mini-dose, for intramuscular use
0.00 0.00 FUD XXX
AMA: 2018,Jan,8; 2017,Jan,8; 2016,Jan,13; 2015,Jan,16; 2014,Jan,11

90386 Rho(D) immune globulin (RhIgIV), human, for intravenous use
0.00 0.00 FUD XXX
AMA: 2018,Jan,8; 2017,Jan,8; 2016,Jan,13; 2015,Jan,16; 2014,Jan,11

90389 Tetanus immune globulin (TIg), human, for intramuscular use
INCLUDES HyperTET S/D (Tetanus Immune Globulin)
0.00 0.00 FUD XXX
AMA: 2018,Jan,8; 2017,Jan,8; 2016,Jan,13; 2015,Jan,16; 2014,Jan,11

90393 Vaccinia immune globulin, human, for intramuscular use
0.00 0.00 FUD XXX
AMA: 2018,Jan,8; 2017,Jan,8; 2016,Jan,13; 2015,Jan,16; 2014,Jan,11

90396 Varicella-zoster immune globulin, human, for intramuscular use
INCLUDES VariZIG
0.00 0.00 FUD XXX
AMA: 2018,Jan,8; 2017,Jan,8; 2016,Jan,13; 2015,Jan,16; 2014,Jan,11

90399 Unlisted immune globulin
0.00 0.00 FUD XXX
AMA: 2018,Jan,8; 2017,Jan,8; 2016,Jan,13; 2015,Jan,16; 2014,Jan,11

90460-90461 Injections Provided with Counseling

INCLUDES All components of influenza vaccine, report X 1 only
Combination vaccines which comprise multiple vaccine components
Components (all antigens) in vaccines to prevent disease due to specific organisms
Counseling by physician or other qualified health care professional
Multi-valent antigens or multiple antigen serotypes against single organisms are considered one component
Patient/family face-to-face counseling by doctor or qualified health care professional for patients 18 years of age and younger

EXCLUDES *Administration of influenza and pneumococcal vaccine for Medicare patients (G0008-G0009)*
Allergy testing (95004-95028)
Bacterial/viral/fungal skin tests (86485-86580)
Diagnostic or therapeutic injections (96365-96372, 96374-96375)
Vaccines provided without face-to-face counseling from a physician or qualified health care professional or to patients over the age of 18 (90471-90474)

Code also significant, separately identifiable E&M service when appropriate
Code also toxoid/vaccine (90476-90749 [90620, 90621, 90625, 90630, 90644, 90672, 90673, 90674, 90750, 90756])

90460 Immunization administration through 18 years of age via any route of administration, with counseling by physician or other qualified health care professional; first or only component of each vaccine or toxoid administered
Code also each additional component in a vaccine (e.g., A 5-year-old receives DtaP-IPV IM administration, and MMR/Varicella vaccines SQ administration. Report initial component X 2, and additional components X 6)
0.47 0.47 FUD XXX
AMA: 2018,Nov,7; 2018,Jan,8; 2017,Jan,8; 2016,Oct,6; 2016,Jan,13; 2015,May,6; 2015,Apr,9; 2015,Apr,10; 2015,Jan,16; 2014,Mar,10; 2014,Jan,11

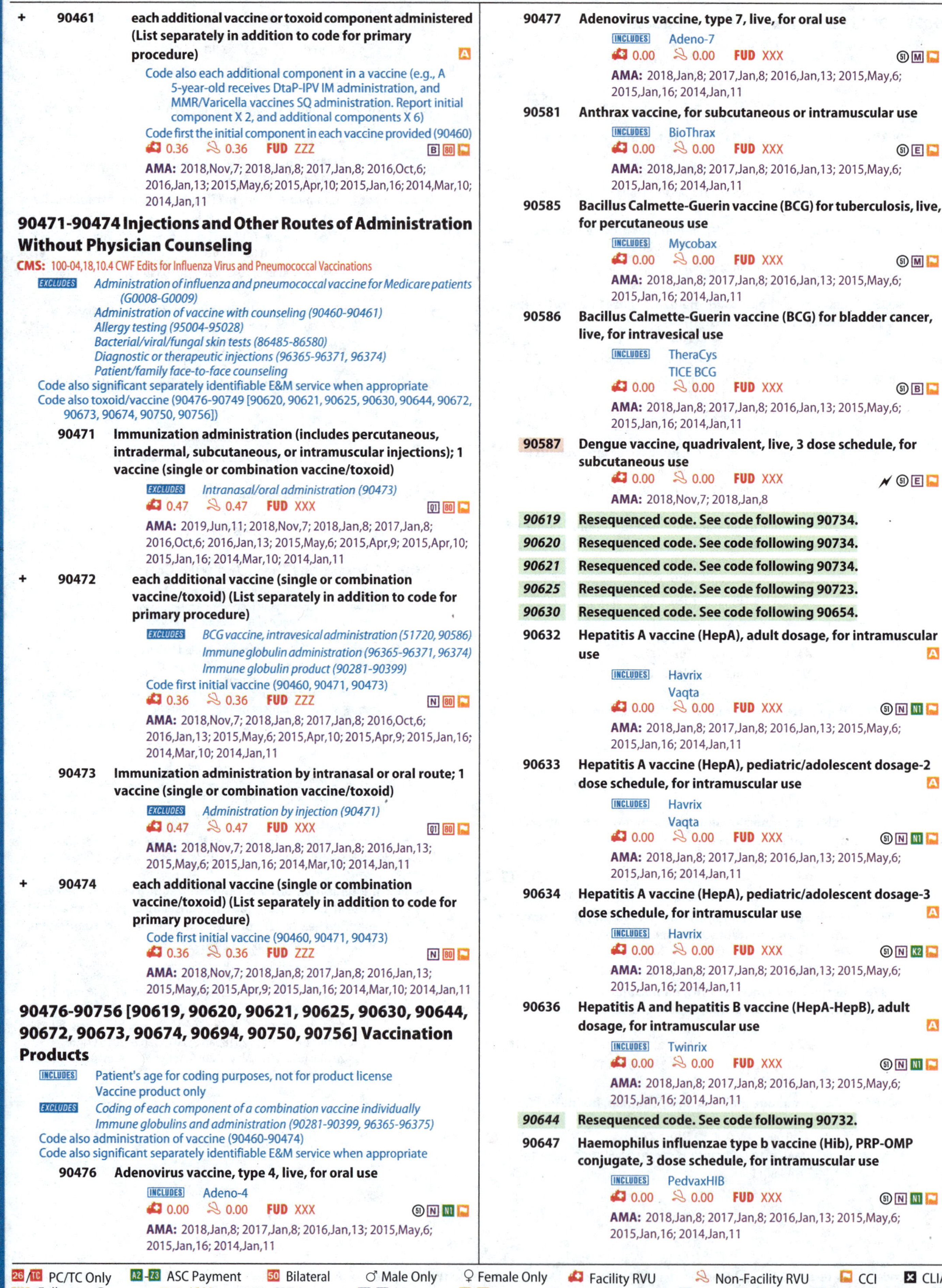

+ **90461** **each additional vaccine or toxoid component administered (List separately in addition to code for primary procedure)**

Code also each additional component in a vaccine (e.g., A 5-year-old receives DtaP-IPV IM administration, and MMR/Varicella vaccines SQ administration. Report initial component X 2, and additional components X 6)

Code first the initial component in each vaccine provided (90460)

0.36 0.36 FUD ZZZ

AMA: 2018,Nov,7; 2018,Jan,8; 2017,Jan,8; 2016,Oct,6; 2016,Jan,13; 2015,May,6; 2015,Apr,10; 2015,Jan,16; 2014,Mar,10; 2014,Jan,11

90471-90474 Injections and Other Routes of Administration Without Physician Counseling

CMS: 100-04,18,10.4 CWF Edits for Influenza Virus and Pneumococcal Vaccinations

EXCLUDES *Administration of influenza and pneumococcal vaccine for Medicare patients (G0008-G0009)*
Administration of vaccine with counseling (90460-90461)
Allergy testing (95004-95028)
Bacterial/viral/fungal skin tests (86485-86580)
Diagnostic or therapeutic injections (96365-96371, 96374)
Patient/family face-to-face counseling

Code also significant separately identifiable E&M service when appropriate

Code also toxoid/vaccine (90476-90749 [90620, 90621, 90625, 90630, 90644, 90672, 90673, 90674, 90750, 90756])

90471 **Immunization administration (includes percutaneous, intradermal, subcutaneous, or intramuscular injections); 1 vaccine (single or combination vaccine/toxoid)**

EXCLUDES *Intranasal/oral administration (90473)*

0.47 0.47 FUD XXX

AMA: 2019,Jun,11; 2018,Nov,7; 2018,Jan,8; 2017,Jan,8; 2016,Oct,6; 2016,Jan,13; 2015,May,6; 2015,Apr,9; 2015,Apr,10; 2015,Jan,16; 2014,Mar,10; 2014,Jan,11

+ **90472** **each additional vaccine (single or combination vaccine/toxoid) (List separately in addition to code for primary procedure)**

EXCLUDES *BCG vaccine, intravesical administration (51720, 90586)*
Immune globulin administration (96365-96371, 96374)
Immune globulin product (90281-90399)

Code first initial vaccine (90460, 90471, 90473)

0.36 0.36 FUD ZZZ

AMA: 2018,Nov,7; 2018,Jan,8; 2017,Jan,8; 2016,Oct,6; 2016,Jan,13; 2015,May,6; 2015,Apr,10; 2015,Apr,9; 2015,Jan,16; 2014,Mar,10; 2014,Jan,11

90473 **Immunization administration by intranasal or oral route; 1 vaccine (single or combination vaccine/toxoid)**

EXCLUDES *Administration by injection (90471)*

0.47 0.47 FUD XXX

AMA: 2018,Nov,7; 2018,Jan,8; 2017,Jan,8; 2016,Jan,13; 2015,May,6; 2015,Jan,16; 2014,Mar,10; 2014,Jan,11

+ **90474** **each additional vaccine (single or combination vaccine/toxoid) (List separately in addition to code for primary procedure)**

Code first initial vaccine (90460, 90471, 90473)

0.36 0.36 FUD ZZZ

AMA: 2018,Nov,7; 2018,Jan,8; 2017,Jan,8; 2016,Jan,13; 2015,May,6; 2015,Apr,9; 2015,Jan,16; 2014,Mar,10; 2014,Jan,11

90476-90756 [90619, 90620, 90621, 90625, 90630, 90644, 90672, 90673, 90674, 90694, 90750, 90756] Vaccination Products

INCLUDES Patient's age for coding purposes, not for product license
Vaccine product only

EXCLUDES *Coding of each component of a combination vaccine individually*
Immune globulins and administration (90281-90399, 96365-96375)

Code also administration of vaccine (90460-90474)

Code also significant separately identifiable E&M service when appropriate

90476 **Adenovirus vaccine, type 4, live, for oral use**

INCLUDES Adeno-4

0.00 0.00 FUD XXX

AMA: 2018,Jan,8; 2017,Jan,8; 2016,Jan,13; 2015,May,6; 2015,Jan,16; 2014,Jan,11

90477 **Adenovirus vaccine, type 7, live, for oral use**

INCLUDES Adeno-7

0.00 0.00 FUD XXX

AMA: 2018,Jan,8; 2017,Jan,8; 2016,Jan,13; 2015,May,6; 2015,Jan,16; 2014,Jan,11

90581 **Anthrax vaccine, for subcutaneous or intramuscular use**

INCLUDES BioThrax

0.00 0.00 FUD XXX

AMA: 2018,Jan,8; 2017,Jan,8; 2016,Jan,13; 2015,May,6; 2015,Jan,16; 2014,Jan,11

90585 **Bacillus Calmette-Guerin vaccine (BCG) for tuberculosis, live, for percutaneous use**

INCLUDES Mycobax

0.00 0.00 FUD XXX

AMA: 2018,Jan,8; 2017,Jan,8; 2016,Jan,13; 2015,May,6; 2015,Jan,16; 2014,Jan,11

90586 **Bacillus Calmette-Guerin vaccine (BCG) for bladder cancer, live, for intravesical use**

INCLUDES TheraCys
TICE BCG

0.00 0.00 FUD XXX

AMA: 2018,Jan,8; 2017,Jan,8; 2016,Jan,13; 2015,May,6; 2015,Jan,16; 2014,Jan,11

90587 **Dengue vaccine, quadrivalent, live, 3 dose schedule, for subcutaneous use**

0.00 0.00 FUD XXX

AMA: 2018,Nov,7; 2018,Jan,8

90619 **Resequenced code. See code following 90734.**

90620 **Resequenced code. See code following 90734.**

90621 **Resequenced code. See code following 90734.**

90625 **Resequenced code. See code following 90723.**

90630 **Resequenced code. See code following 90654.**

90632 **Hepatitis A vaccine (HepA), adult dosage, for intramuscular use**

INCLUDES Havrix
Vaqta

0.00 0.00 FUD XXX

AMA: 2018,Jan,8; 2017,Jan,8; 2016,Jan,13; 2015,May,6; 2015,Jan,16; 2014,Jan,11

90633 **Hepatitis A vaccine (HepA), pediatric/adolescent dosage-2 dose schedule, for intramuscular use**

INCLUDES Havrix
Vaqta

0.00 0.00 FUD XXX

AMA: 2018,Jan,8; 2017,Jan,8; 2016,Jan,13; 2015,May,6; 2015,Jan,16; 2014,Jan,11

90634 **Hepatitis A vaccine (HepA), pediatric/adolescent dosage-3 dose schedule, for intramuscular use**

INCLUDES Havrix

0.00 0.00 FUD XXX

AMA: 2018,Jan,8; 2017,Jan,8; 2016,Jan,13; 2015,May,6; 2015,Jan,16; 2014,Jan,11

90636 **Hepatitis A and hepatitis B vaccine (HepA-HepB), adult dosage, for intramuscular use**

INCLUDES Twinrix

0.00 0.00 FUD XXX

AMA: 2018,Jan,8; 2017,Jan,8; 2016,Jan,13; 2015,May,6; 2015,Jan,16; 2014,Jan,11

90644 **Resequenced code. See code following 90732.**

90647 **Haemophilus influenzae type b vaccine (Hib), PRP-OMP conjugate, 3 dose schedule, for intramuscular use**

INCLUDES PedvaxHIB

0.00 0.00 FUD XXX

AMA: 2018,Jan,8; 2017,Jan,8; 2016,Jan,13; 2015,May,6; 2015,Jan,16; 2014,Jan,11

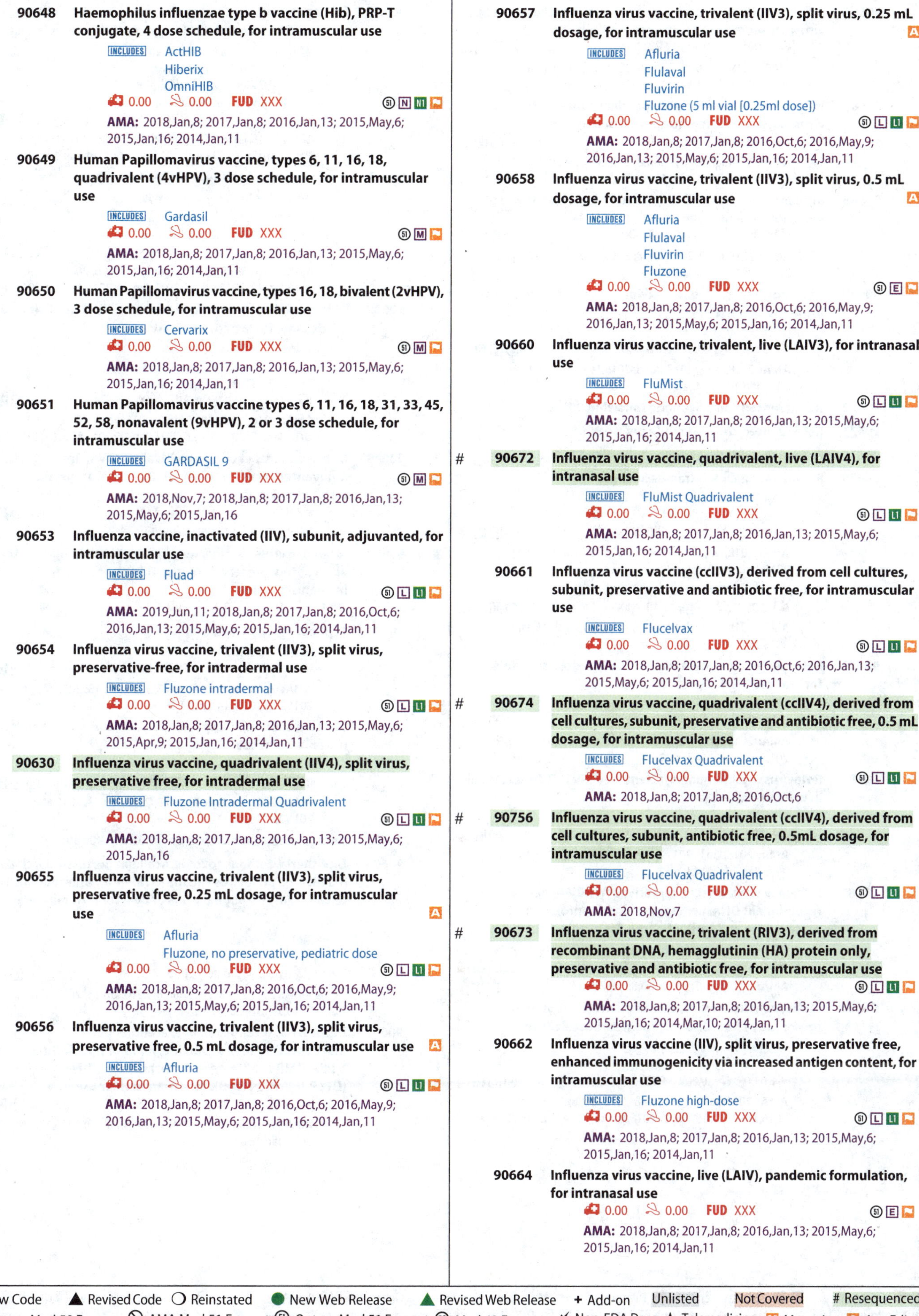

90648 **Haemophilus influenzae type b vaccine (Hib), PRP-T conjugate, 4 dose schedule, for intramuscular use**

INCLUDES ActHIB
Hiberix
OmniHIB

0.00 0.00 FUD XXX

AMA: 2018,Jan,8; 2017,Jan,8; 2016,Jan,13; 2015,May,6; 2015,Jan,16; 2014,Jan,11

90649 **Human Papillomavirus vaccine, types 6, 11, 16, 18, quadrivalent (4vHPV), 3 dose schedule, for intramuscular use**

INCLUDES Gardasil

0.00 0.00 FUD XXX

AMA: 2018,Jan,8; 2017,Jan,8; 2016,Jan,13; 2015,May,6; 2015,Jan,16; 2014,Jan,11

90650 **Human Papillomavirus vaccine, types 16, 18, bivalent (2vHPV), 3 dose schedule, for intramuscular use**

INCLUDES Cervarix

0.00 0.00 FUD XXX

AMA: 2018,Jan,8; 2017,Jan,8; 2016,Jan,13; 2015,May,6; 2015,Jan,16; 2014,Jan,11

90651 **Human Papillomavirus vaccine types 6, 11, 16, 18, 31, 33, 45, 52, 58, nonavalent (9vHPV), 2 or 3 dose schedule, for intramuscular use**

INCLUDES GARDASIL 9

0.00 0.00 FUD XXX

AMA: 2018,Nov,7; 2018,Jan,8; 2017,Jan,8; 2016,Jan,13; 2015,May,6; 2015,Jan,16

90653 **Influenza vaccine, inactivated (IIV), subunit, adjuvanted, for intramuscular use**

INCLUDES Fluad

0.00 0.00 FUD XXX

AMA: 2019,Jun,11; 2018,Jan,8; 2017,Jan,8; 2016,Oct,6; 2016,Jan,13; 2015,May,6; 2015,Jan,16; 2014,Jan,11

90654 **Influenza virus vaccine, trivalent (IIV3), split virus, preservative-free, for intradermal use**

INCLUDES Fluzone intradermal

0.00 0.00 FUD XXX

AMA: 2018,Jan,8; 2017,Jan,8; 2016,Jan,13; 2015,May,6; 2015,Apr,9; 2015,Jan,16; 2014,Jan,11

90630 **Influenza virus vaccine, quadrivalent (IIV4), split virus, preservative free, for intradermal use**

INCLUDES Fluzone Intradermal Quadrivalent

0.00 0.00 FUD XXX

AMA: 2018,Jan,8; 2017,Jan,8; 2016,Jan,13; 2015,May,6; 2015,Jan,16

90655 **Influenza virus vaccine, trivalent (IIV3), split virus, preservative free, 0.25 mL dosage, for intramuscular use** A

INCLUDES Afluria
Fluzone, no preservative, pediatric dose

0.00 0.00 FUD XXX

AMA: 2018,Jan,8; 2017,Jan,8; 2016,Oct,6; 2016,May,9; 2016,Jan,13; 2015,May,6; 2015,Jan,16; 2014,Jan,11

90656 **Influenza virus vaccine, trivalent (IIV3), split virus, preservative free, 0.5 mL dosage, for intramuscular use** A

INCLUDES Afluria

0.00 0.00 FUD XXX

AMA: 2018,Jan,8; 2017,Jan,8; 2016,Oct,6; 2016,May,9; 2016,Jan,13; 2015,May,6; 2015,Jan,16; 2014,Jan,11

90657 **Influenza virus vaccine, trivalent (IIV3), split virus, 0.25 mL dosage, for intramuscular use** A

INCLUDES Afluria
Flulaval
Fluvirin
Fluzone (5 ml vial [0.25ml dose])

0.00 0.00 FUD XXX

AMA: 2018,Jan,8; 2017,Jan,8; 2016,Oct,6; 2016,May,9; 2016,Jan,13; 2015,May,6; 2015,Jan,16; 2014,Jan,11

90658 **Influenza virus vaccine, trivalent (IIV3), split virus, 0.5 mL dosage, for intramuscular use** A

INCLUDES Afluria
Flulaval
Fluvirin
Fluzone

0.00 0.00 FUD XXX

AMA: 2018,Jan,8; 2017,Jan,8; 2016,Oct,6; 2016,May,9; 2016,Jan,13; 2015,May,6; 2015,Jan,16; 2014,Jan,11

90660 **Influenza virus vaccine, trivalent, live (LAIV3), for intranasal use**

INCLUDES FluMist

0.00 0.00 FUD XXX

AMA: 2018,Jan,8; 2017,Jan,8; 2016,Jan,13; 2015,May,6; 2015,Jan,16; 2014,Jan,11

90672 **Influenza virus vaccine, quadrivalent, live (LAIV4), for intranasal use**

INCLUDES FluMist Quadrivalent

0.00 0.00 FUD XXX

AMA: 2018,Jan,8; 2017,Jan,8; 2016,Jan,13; 2015,May,6; 2015,Jan,16; 2014,Jan,11

90661 **Influenza virus vaccine (ccIIV3), derived from cell cultures, subunit, preservative and antibiotic free, for intramuscular use**

INCLUDES Flucelvax

0.00 0.00 FUD XXX

AMA: 2018,Jan,8; 2017,Jan,8; 2016,Oct,6; 2016,Jan,13; 2015,May,6; 2015,Jan,16; 2014,Jan,11

90674 **Influenza virus vaccine, quadrivalent (ccIIV4), derived from cell cultures, subunit, preservative and antibiotic free, 0.5 mL dosage, for intramuscular use**

INCLUDES Flucelvax Quadrivalent

0.00 0.00 FUD XXX

AMA: 2018,Jan,8; 2017,Jan,8; 2016,Oct,6

90756 **Influenza virus vaccine, quadrivalent (ccIIV4), derived from cell cultures, subunit, antibiotic free, 0.5mL dosage, for intramuscular use**

INCLUDES Flucelvax Quadrivalent

0.00 0.00 FUD XXX

AMA: 2018,Nov,7

90673 **Influenza virus vaccine, trivalent (RIV3), derived from recombinant DNA, hemagglutinin (HA) protein only, preservative and antibiotic free, for intramuscular use**

0.00 0.00 FUD XXX

AMA: 2018,Jan,8; 2017,Jan,8; 2016,Jan,13; 2015,May,6; 2015,Jan,16; 2014,Mar,10; 2014,Jan,11

90662 **Influenza virus vaccine (IIV), split virus, preservative free, enhanced immunogenicity via increased antigen content, for intramuscular use**

INCLUDES Fluzone high-dose

0.00 0.00 FUD XXX

AMA: 2018,Jan,8; 2017,Jan,8; 2016,Jan,13; 2015,May,6; 2015,Jan,16; 2014,Jan,11

90664 **Influenza virus vaccine, live (LAIV), pandemic formulation, for intranasal use**

0.00 0.00 FUD XXX

AMA: 2018,Jan,8; 2017,Jan,8; 2016,Jan,13; 2015,May,6; 2015,Jan,16; 2014,Jan,11

90666 **Influenza virus vaccine (IIV), pandemic formulation, split virus, preservative free, for intramuscular use**

0.00 0.00 FUD XXX

AMA: 2018,Jan,8; 2017,Jan,8; 2016,Jan,13; 2015,May,6; 2015,Jan,16; 2014,Jan,11

90667 **Influenza virus vaccine (IIV), pandemic formulation, split virus, adjuvanted, for intramuscular use**

0.00 0.00 FUD XXX

AMA: 2018,Jan,8; 2017,Jan,8; 2016,Jan,13; 2015,May,6; 2015,Jan,16; 2014,Jan,11

90668 **Influenza virus vaccine (IIV), pandemic formulation, split virus, for intramuscular use**

0.00 0.00 FUD XXX

AMA: 2018,Jan,8; 2017,Jan,8; 2016,Jan,13; 2015,May,6; 2015,Jan,16; 2014,Jan,11

90670 **Pneumococcal conjugate vaccine, 13 valent (PCV13), for intramuscular use**

INCLUDES Prevnar 13

0.00 0.00 FUD XXX

AMA: 2018,Jan,8; 2017,Jan,8; 2016,Jan,13; 2015,May,6; 2015,Jan,16; 2014,Jan,11

90672 **Resequenced code. See code following 90660.**

90673 **Resequenced code. See code before 90662.**

90674 **Resequenced code. See code following 90661.**

90675 **Rabies vaccine, for intramuscular use**

INCLUDES Imovax
RabAvert

0.00 0.00 FUD XXX

AMA: 2018,Jan,8; 2017,Jan,8; 2016,Jan,13; 2015,May,6; 2015,Jan,16; 2014,Jan,11

90676 **Rabies vaccine, for intradermal use**

0.00 0.00 FUD XXX

AMA: 2018,Jan,8; 2017,Jan,8; 2016,Jan,13; 2015,May,6; 2015,Jan,16; 2014,Jan,11

90680 **Rotavirus vaccine, pentavalent (RV5), 3 dose schedule, live, for oral use**

INCLUDES RotaTeq

0.00 0.00 FUD XXX

AMA: 2018,Jan,8; 2017,Jan,8; 2016,Jan,13; 2015,May,6; 2015,Jan,16; 2014,Jan,11

90681 **Rotavirus vaccine, human, attenuated (RV1), 2 dose schedule, live, for oral use**

INCLUDES Rotarix

0.00 0.00 FUD XXX

AMA: 2018,Jan,8; 2017,Jan,8; 2016,Jan,13; 2015,May,6; 2015,Jan,16; 2014,Jan,11

90682 **Influenza virus vaccine, quadrivalent (RIV4), derived from recombinant DNA, hemagglutinin (HA) protein only, preservative and antibiotic free, for intramuscular use**

INCLUDES Flublok Quadrivalent

0.00 0.00 FUD XXX

AMA: 2018,Nov,7; 2018,Jan,8; 2017,Jan,8

90685 **Influenza virus vaccine, quadrivalent (IIV4), split virus, preservative free, 0.25 mL, for intramuscular use** A

INCLUDES Afluria Quadrivalent
Fluzone Quadrivalent

0.00 0.00 FUD XXX

AMA: 2018,Jan,8; 2017,Jan,8; 2016,Oct,6; 2016,May,9; 2016,Jan,13; 2015,May,6; 2015,Jan,16; 2014,Mar,10; 2014,Jan,11

90686 **Influenza virus vaccine, quadrivalent (IIV4), split virus, preservative free, 0.5 mL dosage, for intramuscular use** A

INCLUDES Afluria Quadrivalent
Fluarix Quadrivalent
FluLaval Quadrivalent
Fluzone Quadrivalent

0.00 0.00 FUD XXX

AMA: 2018,Jan,8; 2017,Jan,8; 2016,Oct,6; 2016,May,9; 2016,Jan,13; 2015,May,6; 2015,Jan,16; 2014,Mar,10; 2014,Jan,11

90687 **Influenza virus vaccine, quadrivalent (IIV4), split virus, 0.25 mL dosage, for intramuscular use** A

INCLUDES Afluria Quadrivalent
Fluzone Quadrivalent

0.00 0.00 FUD XXX

AMA: 2018,Jan,8; 2017,Jan,8; 2016,Oct,6; 2016,May,9; 2016,Jan,13; 2015,May,6; 2015,Jan,16; 2014,Mar,10; 2014,Jan,11

90688 **Influenza virus vaccine, quadrivalent (IIV4), split virus, 0.5 mL dosage, for intramuscular use** A

INCLUDES Afluria Quadrivalent
Flulaval Quadrivalent
Fluzone Quadrivalent

0.00 0.00 FUD XXX

AMA: 2018,Jan,8; 2017,Jan,8; 2016,Oct,6; 2016,May,9; 2016,Jan,13; 2015,May,6; 2015,Jan,16; 2014,Mar,10; 2014,Jan,11

90689 **Influenza virus vaccine quadrivalent (IIV4), inactivated, adjuvanted, preservative free, 0.25 mL dosage, for intramuscular use**

0.00 0.00 FUD XXX

AMA: 2019,Jul,10; 2018,Nov,7

● # **90694** **Influenza virus vaccine, quadrivalent (aIIV4), inactivated, adjuvanted, preservative free, 0.5 mL dosage, for intramuscular use**

0.00 0.00 FUD 000

90690 **Typhoid vaccine, live, oral**

INCLUDES Vivotif

0.00 0.00 FUD XXX

AMA: 2018,Jan,8; 2017,Jan,8; 2016,Jan,13; 2015,May,6; 2015,Jan,16; 2014,Jan,11

90691 **Typhoid vaccine, Vi capsular polysaccharide (ViCPs), for intramuscular use**

INCLUDES Typhim Vi

0.00 0.00 FUD XXX

AMA: 2018,Jan,8; 2017,Jan,8; 2016,Jan,13; 2015,May,6; 2015,Jan,16; 2014,Jan,11

90694 **Resequenced code. See code following 90689.**

90696 **Diphtheria, tetanus toxoids, acellular pertussis vaccine and inactivated poliovirus vaccine (DTaP-IPV), when administered to children 4 through 6 years of age, for intramuscular use** A

INCLUDES KINRIX
Quadracel

0.00 0.00 FUD XXX

AMA: 2018,Jan,8; 2017,Jan,8; 2016,Jan,13; 2015,May,6; 2015,Jan,16; 2014,Jan,11

90697 **Diphtheria, tetanus toxoids, acellular pertussis vaccine, inactivated poliovirus vaccine, Haemophilus influenzae type b PRP-OMP conjugate vaccine, and hepatitis B vaccine (DTaP-IPV-Hib-HepB), for intramuscular use**

0.00 0.00 FUD XXX

AMA: 2018,Jan,8; 2017,Jan,8; 2016,Jan,13; 2015,May,6; 2015,Jan,16

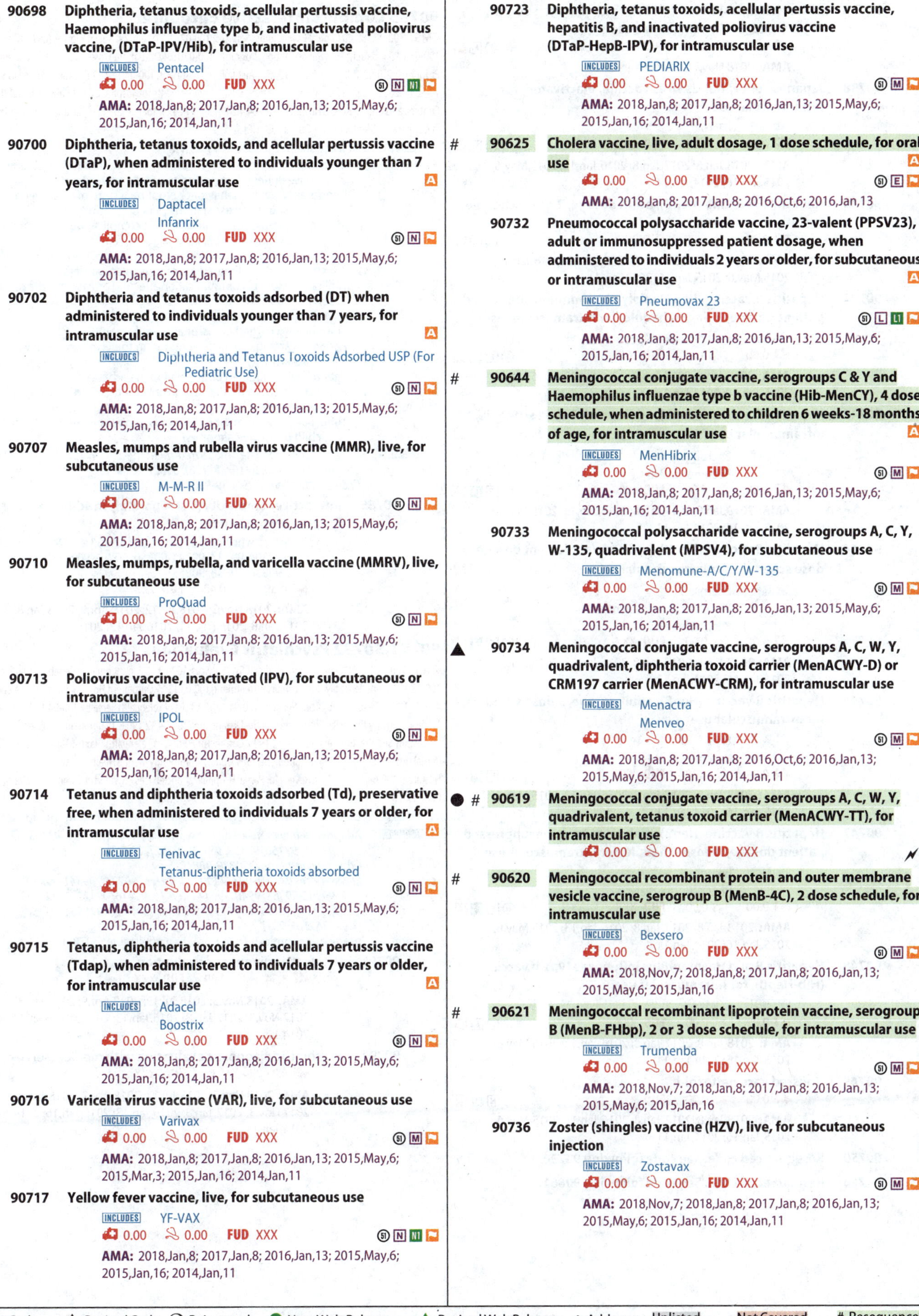

90698 **Diphtheria, tetanus toxoids, acellular pertussis vaccine, Haemophilus influenzae type b, and inactivated poliovirus vaccine, (DTaP-IPV/Hib), for intramuscular use**
INCLUDES Pentacel
0.00 0.00 FUD XXX
AMA: 2018,Jan,8; 2017,Jan,8; 2016,Jan,13; 2015,May,6; 2015,Jan,16; 2014,Jan,11

90700 **Diphtheria, tetanus toxoids, and acellular pertussis vaccine (DTaP), when administered to individuals younger than 7 years, for intramuscular use**
INCLUDES Daptacel
Infanrix
0.00 0.00 FUD XXX
AMA: 2018,Jan,8; 2017,Jan,8; 2016,Jan,13; 2015,May,6; 2015,Jan,16; 2014,Jan,11

90702 **Diphtheria and tetanus toxoids adsorbed (DT) when administered to individuals younger than 7 years, for intramuscular use**
INCLUDES Diphtheria and Tetanus Toxoids Adsorbed USP (For Pediatric Use)
0.00 0.00 FUD XXX
AMA: 2018,Jan,8; 2017,Jan,8; 2016,Jan,13; 2015,May,6; 2015,Jan,16; 2014,Jan,11

90707 **Measles, mumps and rubella virus vaccine (MMR), live, for subcutaneous use**
INCLUDES M-M-R II
0.00 0.00 FUD XXX
AMA: 2018,Jan,8; 2017,Jan,8; 2016,Jan,13; 2015,May,6; 2015,Jan,16; 2014,Jan,11

90710 **Measles, mumps, rubella, and varicella vaccine (MMRV), live, for subcutaneous use**
INCLUDES ProQuad
0.00 0.00 FUD XXX
AMA: 2018,Jan,8; 2017,Jan,8; 2016,Jan,13; 2015,May,6; 2015,Jan,16; 2014,Jan,11

90713 **Poliovirus vaccine, inactivated (IPV), for subcutaneous or intramuscular use**
INCLUDES IPOL
0.00 0.00 FUD XXX
AMA: 2018,Jan,8; 2017,Jan,8; 2016,Jan,13; 2015,May,6; 2015,Jan,16; 2014,Jan,11

90714 **Tetanus and diphtheria toxoids adsorbed (Td), preservative free, when administered to individuals 7 years or older, for intramuscular use**
INCLUDES Tenivac
Tetanus-diphtheria toxoids absorbed
0.00 0.00 FUD XXX
AMA: 2018,Jan,8; 2017,Jan,8; 2016,Jan,13; 2015,May,6; 2015,Jan,16; 2014,Jan,11

90715 **Tetanus, diphtheria toxoids and acellular pertussis vaccine (Tdap), when administered to individuals 7 years or older, for intramuscular use**
INCLUDES Adacel
Boostrix
0.00 0.00 FUD XXX
AMA: 2018,Jan,8; 2017,Jan,8; 2016,Jan,13; 2015,May,6; 2015,Jan,16; 2014,Jan,11

90716 **Varicella virus vaccine (VAR), live, for subcutaneous use**
INCLUDES Varivax
0.00 0.00 FUD XXX
AMA: 2018,Jan,8; 2017,Jan,8; 2016,Jan,13; 2015,May,6; 2015,Mar,3; 2015,Jan,16; 2014,Jan,11

90717 **Yellow fever vaccine, live, for subcutaneous use**
INCLUDES YF-VAX
0.00 0.00 FUD XXX
AMA: 2018,Jan,8; 2017,Jan,8; 2016,Jan,13; 2015,May,6; 2015,Jan,16; 2014,Jan,11

90723 **Diphtheria, tetanus toxoids, acellular pertussis vaccine, hepatitis B, and inactivated poliovirus vaccine (DTaP-HepB-IPV), for intramuscular use**
INCLUDES PEDIARIX
0.00 0.00 FUD XXX
AMA: 2018,Jan,8; 2017,Jan,8; 2016,Jan,13; 2015,May,6; 2015,Jan,16; 2014,Jan,11

90625 **Cholera vaccine, live, adult dosage, 1 dose schedule, for oral use**
0.00 0.00 FUD XXX
AMA: 2018,Jan,8; 2017,Jan,8; 2016,Oct,6; 2016,Jan,13

90732 **Pneumococcal polysaccharide vaccine, 23-valent (PPSV23), adult or immunosuppressed patient dosage, when administered to individuals 2 years or older, for subcutaneous or intramuscular use**
INCLUDES Pneumovax 23
0.00 0.00 FUD XXX
AMA: 2018,Jan,8; 2017,Jan,8; 2016,Jan,13; 2015,May,6; 2015,Jan,16; 2014,Jan,11

90644 **Meningococcal conjugate vaccine, serogroups C & Y and Haemophilus influenzae type b vaccine (Hib-MenCY), 4 dose schedule, when administered to children 6 weeks-18 months of age, for intramuscular use**
INCLUDES MenHibrix
0.00 0.00 FUD XXX
AMA: 2018,Jan,8; 2017,Jan,8; 2016,Jan,13; 2015,May,6; 2015,Jan,16; 2014,Jan,11

90733 **Meningococcal polysaccharide vaccine, serogroups A, C, Y, W-135, quadrivalent (MPSV4), for subcutaneous use**
INCLUDES Menomune-A/C/Y/W-135
0.00 0.00 FUD XXX
AMA: 2018,Jan,8; 2017,Jan,8; 2016,Jan,13; 2015,May,6; 2015,Jan,16; 2014,Jan,11

▲ **90734** **Meningococcal conjugate vaccine, serogroups A, C, W, Y, quadrivalent, diphtheria toxoid carrier (MenACWY-D) or CRM197 carrier (MenACWY-CRM), for intramuscular use**
INCLUDES Menactra
Menveo
0.00 0.00 FUD XXX
AMA: 2018,Jan,8; 2017,Jan,8; 2016,Oct,6; 2016,Jan,13; 2015,May,6; 2015,Jan,16; 2014,Jan,11

● # **90619** **Meningococcal conjugate vaccine, serogroups A, C, W, Y, quadrivalent, tetanus toxoid carrier (MenACWY-TT), for intramuscular use**
0.00 0.00 FUD XXX

90620 **Meningococcal recombinant protein and outer membrane vesicle vaccine, serogroup B (MenB-4C), 2 dose schedule, for intramuscular use**
INCLUDES Bexsero
0.00 0.00 FUD XXX
AMA: 2018,Nov,7; 2018,Jan,8; 2017,Jan,8; 2016,Jan,13; 2015,May,6; 2015,Jan,16

90621 **Meningococcal recombinant lipoprotein vaccine, serogroup B (MenB-FHbp), 2 or 3 dose schedule, for intramuscular use**
INCLUDES Trumenba
0.00 0.00 FUD XXX
AMA: 2018,Nov,7; 2018,Jan,8; 2017,Jan,8; 2016,Jan,13; 2015,May,6; 2015,Jan,16

90736 **Zoster (shingles) vaccine (HZV), live, for subcutaneous injection**
INCLUDES Zostavax
0.00 0.00 FUD XXX
AMA: 2018,Nov,7; 2018,Jan,8; 2017,Jan,8; 2016,Jan,13; 2015,May,6; 2015,Jan,16; 2014,Jan,11

● New Code ▲ Revised Code ○ Reinstated ● New Web Release ▲ Revised Web Release + Add-on Unlisted Not Covered # Resequenced
Optum Mod 50 Exempt AMA Mod 51 Exempt Optum Mod 51 Exempt Mod 63 Exempt Non-FDA Drug ★ Telemedicine Maternity Age Edit

90750 **Zoster (shingles) vaccine (HZV), recombinant, subunit, adjuvanted, for intramuscular use**

0.00 0.00 FUD XXX

AMA: 2018,Nov,7

90738 **Japanese encephalitis virus vaccine, inactivated, for intramuscular use**

INCLUDES Ixiaro

0.00 0.00 FUD XXX

AMA: 2018,Jan,8; 2017,Jan,8; 2016,Jan,13; 2015,May,6; 2015,Jan,16; 2014,Jan,11

90739 **Hepatitis B vaccine (HepB), adult dosage, 2 dose schedule, for intramuscular use**

0.00 0.00 FUD XXX

AMA: 2018,Nov,7; 2018,Jan,8; 2017,Jan,8; 2016,Jan,13; 2015,May,6; 2015,Jan,16; 2014,Jan,11

90740 **Hepatitis B vaccine (HepB), dialysis or immunosuppressed patient dosage, 3 dose schedule, for intramuscular use**

INCLUDES Recombivax HB

0.00 0.00 FUD XXX

AMA: 2018,Jan,8; 2017,Jan,8; 2016,Jan,13; 2015,May,6; 2015,Jan,16; 2014,Jan,11

90743 **Hepatitis B vaccine (HepB), adolescent, 2 dose schedule, for intramuscular use**

INCLUDES Energix-B
Recombivax HB

0.00 0.00 FUD XXX

AMA: 2018,Jan,8; 2017,Jan,8; 2016,Jan,13; 2015,May,6; 2015,Jan,16; 2014,Jan,11

90744 **Hepatitis B vaccine (HepB), pediatric/adolescent dosage, 3 dose schedule, for intramuscular use**

INCLUDES Energix-B
Flucelvax Quadrivalent
Recombivax HB

0.00 0.00 FUD XXX

AMA: 2018,Jan,8; 2017,Jan,8; 2016,Jan,13; 2015,May,6; 2015,Jan,16; 2014,Jan,11

90746 **Hepatitis B vaccine (HepB), adult dosage, 3 dose schedule, for intramuscular use**

INCLUDES Energix-B
Recombivax HB

0.00 0.00 FUD XXX

AMA: 2018,Jan,8; 2017,Jan,8; 2016,Jan,13; 2015,May,6; 2015,Jan,16; 2014,Jan,11

90747 **Hepatitis B vaccine (HepB), dialysis or immunosuppressed patient dosage, 4 dose schedule, for intramuscular use**

INCLUDES Energix-B
RECOMBIVAX dialysis

0.00 0.00 FUD XXX

AMA: 2018,Jan,8; 2017,Jan,8; 2016,Jan,13; 2015,May,6; 2015,Jan,16; 2014,Jan,11

90748 **Hepatitis B and Haemophilus influenzae type b vaccine (Hib-HepB), for intramuscular use**

INCLUDES COMVAX

0.00 0.00 FUD XXX

AMA: 2018,Jan,8; 2017,Jan,8; 2016,Jan,13; 2015,May,6; 2015,Jan,16; 2014,Jan,11

90749 **Unlisted vaccine/toxoid**

0.00 0.00 FUD XXX

AMA: 2018,Jan,8; 2017,Jan,8; 2016,Jan,13; 2015,May,6; 2015,Jan,16; 2014,Jan,11

90750 **Resequenced code. See code following 90736.**

90756 **Resequenced code. See code following 90661.**

90785 Complex Interactive Encounter

CMS: 100-02,15,160 Clinical Psychologist Services; 100-02,15,170 Clinical Social Worker (CSW) Services; 100-03,10.3 Inpatient Pain Rehabilitation Programs; 100-03,10.4 Outpatient Hospital Pain Rehabilitation Programs; 100-03,130.1 Inpatient Stays for Alcoholism Treatment; 100-04,12,100 Teaching Physician Services; 100-04,4,260.1 Special Partial Hospitalization Billing Requirements forHospitals, Community Mental Health Centers, and Critical Access Hospitals; 100-04,4,260.1.1 Bill Review for Partial Hospitalization Services Provided in Community Mental Health Centers (CMHC)

INCLUDES At least one of the following activities:
- Discussion of a sentinel event demanding third-party involvement (eg, abuse or neglect reported to a state agency)
- Interference by the behavior or emotional state of caregiver to understand and assist in the plan of treatment
- Managing discordant communication complicating care among participating members (eg, arguing, reactivity)
- Use of nonverbal communication methods (eg, toys, other devices, or translator) to eliminate communication barriers

Complicated issues of communication affecting provision of the psychiatric service

Involved communication with:
- Emotionally charged or dissonant family members
- Patients wanting others present during the visit (e.g., family member, translator)
- Patients with impaired or undeveloped verbal skills
- Patients with third parties responsible for their care (eg, parents, guardians)
- Third-party involvement (eg, schools, probation and parole officers, child protective agencies)

EXCLUDES *Adaptive behavior assessment/treatment ([97151, 97152, 97153, 97154, 97155, 97156, 97157, 97158], 0362T, 0373T)*
Crisis psychotherapy (90839-90840)

\+ **90785** **Interactive complexity (List separately in addition to the code for primary procedure)**

Code first, when performed (99201-99255 [99224, 99225, 99226], 99304-99337, 99341-99350, 90791-90792, 90832-90834, 90836-90838, 90853)

0.39 0.42 FUD ZZZ

AMA: 2018,Nov,3; 2018,Jul,12; 2018,Apr,9; 2018,Jan,8; 2017,Jan,8; 2016,Dec,11; 2016,Jan,13; 2015,Jan,16

90791-90792 Psychiatric Evaluations

CMS: 100-02,15,170 Clinical Social Worker (CSW) Services; 100-03,10.3 Inpatient Pain Rehabilitation Programs; 100-03,130.1 Inpatient Stays for Alcoholism Treatment; 100-03,130.2 Outpatient Hospital Services for Alcoholism; 100-04,12,100 Teaching Physician Services; 100-04,12,190.3 List of Telehealth Services; 100-04,12,190.6 Payment Methodology for Physician/Practitioner at the Distant Site ; 100-04,12,190.6.1 Submission of Telehealth Claims for Distant Site Practitioners; 100-04,12,190.7 Contractor Editing of Telehealth Claims; 100-04,4,260.1 Special Partial Hospitalization Billing Requirements forHospitals, Community Mental Health Centers, and Critical Access Hospitals; 100-04,4,260.1.1 Bill Review for Partial Hospitalization Services Provided in Community Mental Health Centers (CMHC)

INCLUDES Diagnostic assessment or reassessment without psychotherapy services

EXCLUDES *Adaptive behavior assessment/treatment ([97151, 97152, 97153, 97154, 97155, 97156, 97157, 97158], 0362T, 0373T)*
Crisis psychotherapy (90839-90840)
E&M services (99201-99337 [99224, 99225, 99226], 99341-99350, 99366-99368, 99401-99443 [99415, 99416, 99421, 99422, 99423], [97151], [97152], [97153], [97154], [97155], [97156], [97157], [97158], 0362T, 0373T)

Code also interactive complexity services when applicable (90785)

90791 **Psychiatric diagnostic evaluation**

3.54 3.89 FUD XXX ★

AMA: 2018,Nov,3; 2018,Jul,12; 2018,Apr,9; 2018,Jan,8; 2017,Nov,3; 2017,Jan,8; 2016,Jan,13; 2015,Jan,16; 2014,Jun,3; 2014,Jan,11

90792 **Psychiatric diagnostic evaluation with medical services**

4.01 4.37 FUD XXX ★

AMA: 2018,Nov,3; 2018,Jul,12; 2018,Apr,9; 2018,Jan,8; 2017,Nov,3; 2017,Jan,8; 2016,Jan,13; 2015,Jan,16; 2014,Jun,3; 2014,Jan,11

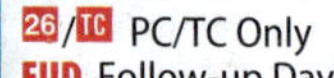 PC/TC Only 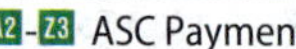 ASC Payment 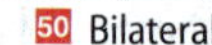 Bilateral 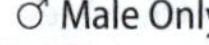 Male Only 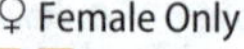 Female Only Facility RVU Non-Facility RVU CCI CLIA
FUD Follow-up Days CMS: IOM AMA: CPT Asst A-Y OPPSI 80/80 Surg Assist Allowed / w/Doc Lab Crosswalk Radiology Crosswalk

90832-90838 Psychotherapy Services

CMS: 100-02,15,160 Clinical Psychologist Services; 100-02,15,170 Clinical Social Worker (CSW) Services; 100-03,130.1 Inpatient Stays for Alcoholism Treatment; 100-03,130.2 Outpatient Hospital Services for Alcoholism; 100-03,130.3 Chemical Aversion Therapy for Treatment of Alcoholism; 100-04,12,100 Teaching Physician Services; 100-04,12,160 Independent Psychologist Services; 100-04,12,170 Clinical Psychologist Services; 100-04,12,190.3 List of Telehealth Services; 100-04,12,190.6 Payment Methodology for Physician/Practitioner at the Distant Site ; 100-04,12,190.6.1 Submission of Telehealth Claims for Distant Site Practitioners; 100-04,12,190.7 Contractor Editing of Telehealth Claims

INCLUDES Face-to-face time with patient (family, other informers may also be present)
Pharmacologic management in time allocated to psychotherapy service codes
Psychotherapy only (90832, 90834, 90837)
Psychotherapy with separately identifiable medical E&M services includes add-on codes (90833, 90836, 90838)
Service times of no less than 16 minutes
Services provided in all settings
Therapeutic communication to:
Ameliorate the patient's mental and behavioral symptoms
Modify behavior
Support and encourage personality growth and development
Treatment for:
Behavior disturbances
Mental illness

EXCLUDES *Adaptive behavior assessment/treatment ([97151, 97152, 97153, 97154, 97155, 97156, 97157, 97158], 0362T, 0373T)*
Crisis psychotherapy (90839-90840)
Family psychotherapy (90846-90847)

Code also interactive complexity services with the time the provider spends performing the service reflected in the time for the appropriate psychotherapy code (90785)

90832 Psychotherapy, 30 minutes with patient
1.76 1.90 FUD XXX ★ 03
AMA: 2018,Nov,3; 2018,Jul,12; 2018,Jan,8; 2017,Nov,3; 2017,Sep,11; 2017,Jan,8; 2016,Dec,11; 2016,Jan,13; 2015,Oct,9; 2015,Jan,16; 2014,Aug,5; 2014,Feb,3

\+ **90833 Psychotherapy, 30 minutes with patient when performed with an evaluation and management service (List separately in addition to the code for primary procedure)**
Code first (99201-99255 [99224, 99225, 99226], 99304-99337, 99341-99350)
1.84 1.97 FUD ZZZ 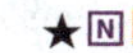
AMA: 2018,Nov,3; 2018,Jul,12; 2018,Jan,8; 2017,Nov,3; 2017,Jan,8; 2016,Dec,11; 2016,Jan,13; 2015,Oct,9; 2015,Jan,16; 2014,Aug,5; 2014,Feb,3

90834 Psychotherapy, 45 minutes with patient
2.35 2.53 FUD XXX 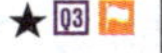
AMA: 2018,Nov,3; 2018,Jul,12; 2018,Jan,8; 2017,Nov,3; 2017,Jan,8; 2016,Dec,11; 2016,Jan,13; 2015,Oct,9; 2015,Jan,16; 2014,Jun,3; 2014,Feb,3

\+ **90836 Psychotherapy, 45 minutes with patient when performed with an evaluation and management service (List separately in addition to the code for primary procedure)**
Code first (99201-99255 [99224, 99225, 99226], 99304-99337, 99341-99350)
2.33 2.49 FUD ZZZ 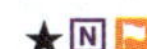
AMA: 2018,Nov,3; 2018,Jul,12; 2018,Jan,8; 2017,Nov,3; 2017,Jan,8; 2016,Dec,11; 2016,Jan,13; 2015,Oct,9; 2015,Jan,16; 2014,Feb,3

90837 Psychotherapy, 60 minutes with patient
Code also prolonged service for psychotherapy performed without E&M service face-to-face with the patient lasting 90 minutes or longer (99354-99357)
3.53 3.80 FUD XXX ★ 03
AMA: 2018,Nov,3; 2018,Jul,12; 2018,Jan,8; 2017,Nov,3; 2017,Jan,8; 2016,Dec,11; 2016,Jan,13; 2015,Oct,3; 2015,Oct,9; 2015,Jan,16; 2014,Apr,6; 2014,Feb,3

\+ **90838 Psychotherapy, 60 minutes with patient when performed with an evaluation and management service (List separately in addition to the code for primary procedure)**
Code first (99201-99255 [99224, 99225, 99226], 99304-99337, 99341-99350)
3.08 3.29 FUD ZZZ ★ N
AMA: 2018,Nov,3; 2018,Jul,12; 2018,Jan,8; 2017,Nov,3; 2017,Jan,8; 2016,Dec,11; 2016,Jan,13; 2015,Oct,9; 2015,Jan,16; 2014,Apr,6; 2014,Feb,3

90839-90840 Services for Patients in Crisis

CMS: 100-02,15,170 Clinical Social Worker (CSW) Services; 100-03,130.1 Inpatient Stays for Alcoholism Treatment; 100-03,130.3 Chemical Aversion Therapy for Treatment of Alcoholism; 100-04,12,100 Teaching Physician Services; 100-04,12,160 Independent Psychologist Services; 100-04,12,160.1 Payment of Independent Psychologist Services; 100-04,12,170 Clinical Psychologist Services

INCLUDES 30 minutes or more of face-to-face time with the patient (for all or part of the service) and/or family providing crisis psychotherapy
All time spent exclusively with patient (for all or part of the service) and/or family, even if time is not continuous
Emergent care to a patient in severe distress (eg, life threatening or complex)
Institute interventions to minimize psychological trauma
Measures to ease the crisis and reestablish safety
Psychotherapy

EXCLUDES *Adaptive behavior assessment/treatment ([97151, 97152, 97153, 97154, 97155, 97156, 97157, 97158], 0362T, 0373T)*
Other psychiatric services (90785-90899)

90839 Psychotherapy for crisis; first 60 minutes
INCLUDES First 30-74 minutes of crisis psychotherapy per day
EXCLUDES *Use of code more than one time per day, even when service is not continuous on that date.*
3.69 3.96 FUD XXX 03 80
AMA: 2018,Nov,3; 2018,Jul,12; 2018,Jan,8; 2017,Nov,3; 2017,Jan,8; 2016,Jan,13; 2015,Oct,9; 2015,Jan,16; 2014,Aug,5

\+ **90840 each additional 30 minutes (List separately in addition to code for primary service)**
INCLUDES Up to 30 minutes of time beyond the initial 74 minutes
Code first (90839)
1.76 1.90 FUD ZZZ N 80
AMA: 2018,Nov,3; 2018,Jul,12; 2018,Jan,8; 2017,Nov,3; 2017,Jan,8; 2016,Jan,13; 2015,Oct,9; 2015,Jan,16; 2014,Aug,5

90845-90863 Additional Psychotherapy Services

CMS: 100-02,15,170 Clinical Social Worker (CSW) Services; 100-03,10.3 Inpatient Pain Rehabilitation Programs; 100-03,10.4 Outpatient Hospital Pain Rehabilitation Programs

EXCLUDES *Adaptive behavior assessment/treatment ([97151, 97152, 97153, 97154, 97155, 97156, 97157, 97158], 0362T, 0373T)*
Analysis/programming of neurostimulators for vagus nerve stimulation therapy (95970, 95976-95977)
Crisis psychotherapy (90839-90840)

90845 Psychoanalysis
2.52 2.70 FUD XXX ★ 03 80
AMA: 2018,Nov,3; 2018,Jul,12; 2018,Jan,8; 2017,Jan,8; 2016,Jan,13; 2015,Oct,9; 2015,Jan,16; 2014,Jan,11

90846 Family psychotherapy (without the patient present), 50 minutes
EXCLUDES *Service times of less than 26 minutes*
2.85 3.06 FUD XXX ★ 03 80
AMA: 2018,Nov,3; 2018,Jul,12; 2018,Jan,8; 2017,Nov,3; 2017,Mar,10; 2017,Jan,8; 2016,Dec,11; 2016,Jan,13; 2015,Oct,9; 2015,Jan,16; 2014,Jan,11

90847 Family psychotherapy (conjoint psychotherapy) (with patient present), 50 minutes
EXCLUDES *Service times of less than 26 minutes*
Service times of more than 80 minutes, see prolonged services (99354-99357)
2.96 3.18 FUD XXX ★ 03 80
AMA: 2018,Nov,3; 2018,Jul,12; 2018,Jan,8; 2017,Nov,3; 2017,Jan,8; 2016,Dec,11; 2016,Jan,13; 2015,Oct,9; 2015,Jan,16; 2014,Jan,11

90849 Multiple-family group psychotherapy
0.87 1.17 FUD XXX
AMA: 2018,Nov,3; 2018,Jul,12; 2018,Jan,8; 2017,Nov,3; 2017,Jan,8; 2016,Jan,13; 2015,Oct,9; 2015,Jan,16; 2014,Aug,14; 2014,Jan,11

90853 Group psychotherapy (other than of a multiple-family group)
Code also group psychotherapy with interactive complexity (90785)
0.70 0.76 FUD XXX
AMA: 2018,Nov,3; 2018,Jul,12; 2018,Jan,8; 2017,Nov,3; 2017,Mar,10; 2017,Jan,8; 2016,Jan,13; 2015,Oct,9; 2015,Jan,16; 2014,Aug,14; 2014,Jun,3; 2014,Jan,11

\+ **90863 Pharmacologic management, including prescription and review of medication, when performed with psychotherapy services (List separately in addition to the code for primary procedure)**
INCLUDES Pharmacologic management in time allocated to psychotherapy service codes
Code first (90832, 90834, 90837)
0.70 0.74 FUD XXX ★
AMA: 2018,Nov,3; 2018,Jul,12; 2018,Jan,8; 2017,Jan,8; 2016,Jan,13; 2015,Jan,16

90865-90870 Other Psychiatric Treatment

EXCLUDES *Adaptive behavior assessment/treatment ([97151, 97152, 97153, 97154, 97155, 97156, 97157, 97158], 0362T, 0373T)*
Analysis/programming of neurostimulators for vagus nerve stimulation therapy (95970, 95976-95977)
Crisis psychotherapy (90839-90840)

90865 Narcosynthesis for psychiatric diagnostic and therapeutic purposes (eg, sodium amobarbital (Amytal) interview)
3.59 4.79 FUD XXX
AMA: 2018,Nov,3; 2018,Jul,12; 2018,Jan,8; 2017,Jan,8; 2016,Jan,13; 2015,Jan,16; 2014,Jan,11

90867 Therapeutic repetitive transcranial magnetic stimulation (TMS) treatment; initial, including cortical mapping, motor threshold determination, delivery and management
INCLUDES Evaluation E&M services related directly to:
Cortical mapping
Delivery and management of TMS services
Motor threshold determination
EXCLUDES *Electromyography (95860, 95870)*
Evoked potential studies (95928-95929)
Medication management
Navigated transcranial magnetic stimulation (nTMS) motor function mapping for treatment planning, upper and lower extremity (90868-90869)
Significant, separately identifiable E&M service
Significant, separately identifiable psychotherapy service
Use of code more than one time for each course of treatment
0.00 0.00 FUD 000
AMA: 2018,Nov,3; 2018,Jul,12

90868 subsequent delivery and management, per session
INCLUDES E&M services related directly to:
Cortical mapping
Delivery and management of TMS services
Motor threshold determination
EXCLUDES *Medication management*
Navigated transcranial magnetic stimulation (nTMS) motor function mapping for treatment planning, upper and lower extremity (64999)
Significant, separately identifiable E&M service
Significant, separately identifiable psychotherapy service
0.00 0.00 FUD 000
AMA: 2018,Nov,3; 2018,Jul,12

90869 subsequent motor threshold re-determination with delivery and management
INCLUDES E&M services related directly to:
Cortical mapping
Delivery and management of TMS services
Motor threshold determination
EXCLUDES *Electromyography (95860, 95870)*
Evoked potential studies (95928-95929)
Medication management
Navigated transcranial magnetic stimulation (nTMS) motor function mapping for treatment planning, upper and lower extremity (64999)
Significant, separately identifiable E&M service
Significant, separately identifiable psychotherapy service
0.00 0.00 FUD 000
AMA: 2018,Nov,3; 2018,Jul,12

90870 Electroconvulsive therapy (includes necessary monitoring)
3.12 4.96 FUD 000
AMA: 2018,Nov,3; 2018,Jul,12; 2018,Jan,8; 2017,Jan,8; 2016,Jan,13; 2015,Jan,16; 2014,Jan,11

90875-90880 Psychiatric Therapy with Biofeedback or Hypnosis

CMS: 100-02,15,170 Clinical Social Worker (CSW) Services; 100-04,12,160 Independent Psychologist Services; 100-04,12,160.1 Payment of Independent Psychologist Services; 100-04,12,170 Clinical Psychologist Services
EXCLUDES *Adaptive behavior assessment/treatment ([97151, 97152, 97153, 97154, 97155, 97156, 97157, 97158], 0362T, 0373T)*
Analysis/programming of neurostimulators for vagus nerve stimulation therapy (95970, 95976-95977)
Crisis psychotherapy (90839-90840)

90875 Individual psychophysiological therapy incorporating biofeedback training by any modality (face-to-face with the patient), with psychotherapy (eg, insight oriented, behavior modifying or supportive psychotherapy); 30 minutes
1.73 1.80 FUD XXX
AMA: 2018,Nov,3; 2018,Jul,12; 2018,Jan,8; 2017,Jan,8; 2016,Jan,13; 2015,Jan,16; 2014,Jan,11

90876 45 minutes
2.74 3.05 FUD XXX
AMA: 2018,Nov,3; 2018,Jul,12; 2018,Jan,8; 2017,Jan,8; 2016,Jan,13; 2015,Jan,16; 2014,Jan,11

90880 Hypnotherapy
2.58 2.98 FUD XXX
AMA: 2018,Nov,3; 2018,Jul,12; 2018,Jan,8; 2017,Jan,8; 2016,Jan,13; 2015,Jan,16; 2014,Jan,11

90882-90899 Psychiatric Services without Patient Face-to-Face Contact

CMS: 100-04,12,160 Independent Psychologist Services; 100-04,12,160.1 Payment of Independent Psychologist Services
EXCLUDES *Analysis/programming of neurostimulators for vagus nerve stimulation therapy (95970, 95976-95977)*
Crisis psychotherapy (90839-90840)

90882 Environmental intervention for medical management purposes on a psychiatric patient's behalf with agencies, employers, or institutions
0.00 0.00 FUD XXX
AMA: 2018,Nov,3; 2018,Jul,12; 2018,Jan,8; 2017,Jan,8; 2016,Jan,13; 2015,Jan,16; 2014,Jan,11

90885 Psychiatric evaluation of hospital records, other psychiatric reports, psychometric and/or projective tests, and other accumulated data for medical diagnostic purposes
1.41 1.41 FUD XXX
AMA: 2018,Nov,3; 2018,Jul,12; 2018,Jan,8; 2017,Jan,8; 2016,Jan,13; 2015,Jan,16; 2014,Jan,11

90887 **Interpretation or explanation of results of psychiatric, other medical examinations and procedures, or other accumulated data to family or other responsible persons, or advising them how to assist patient**

EXCLUDES *Adaptive behavior assessment/treatment ([97151, 97152, 97153, 97154, 97155, 97156, 97157, 97158], 0362T, 0373T)*

2.14 2.48 FUD XXX N

AMA: 2018,Nov,3; 2018,Jul,12; 2018,Jan,8; 2017,Jan,8; 2016,Jan,13; 2015,Jan,16; 2014,Jan,11

90889 **Preparation of report of patient's psychiatric status, history, treatment, or progress (other than for legal or consultative purposes) for other individuals, agencies, or insurance carriers**

0.00 0.00 FUD XXX N

AMA: 2018,Nov,3; 2018,Jul,12; 2018,Jan,8; 2017,Jan,8; 2016,Jan,13; 2015,Jan,16; 2014,Jan,11

90899 **Unlisted psychiatric service or procedure**

0.00 0.00 FUD XXX Q3 80

AMA: 2018,Nov,3; 2018,Jul,12; 2018,Jan,8; 2017,Jan,8; 2016,Jan,13; 2015,Jan,16; 2014,Jan,11

90901-90913 Biofeedback Therapy

EXCLUDES *Psychophysiological therapy utilizing biofeedback training (90875-90876)*

90901 **Biofeedback training by any modality**

0.57 1.13 FUD 000 A 80

AMA: 2018,Jan,8; 2017,Jan,8; 2016,Jan,13; 2015,Jan,16; 2014,Jan,11

90911 ~~**Biofeedback training, perineal muscles, anorectal or urethral sphincter, including EMG and/or manometry**~~

To report, see (90912-90913)

● **90912** **Biofeedback training, perineal muscles, anorectal or urethral sphincter, including EMG and/or manometry, when performed; initial 15 minutes of one-on-one physician or other qualified health care professional contact with the patient**

EXCLUDES *Incontinence treatment using pulsed magnetic neuromodulation (53899)*
Testing of rectal sensation, tone, and compliance (91120)

● + **90913** **each additional 15 minutes of one-on-one physician or other qualified health care professional contact with the patient (List separately in addition to code for primary procedure)**

0.00 0.00 FUD 000

EXCLUDES *Incontinence treatment using pulsed magnetic neuromodulation (53899)*
Testing of rectal sensation, tone, and compliance (91120)

Code first (90912)

90935-90940 Hemodialysis Services: Inpatient ESRD and Outpatient Non-ESRD

CMS: 100-02,11,20 Renal Dialysis Items and Services; 100-04,3,100.6 Inpatient Renal Services

EXCLUDES *Attendance by physician or other qualified health care provider for a prolonged period of time (99354-99360 [99415, 99416])*
Blood specimen collection from partial/complete implantable venous access device (36591)
Declotting of cannula (36831, 36833, 36860-36861)
Hemodialysis home visit by non-physician health care professional (99512)
Therapeutic apheresis procedures (36511-36516)
Thrombolytic agent declotting of implanted vascular access device/catheter (36593)

Code also significant separately identifiable E&M service not related to dialysis procedure or renal failure with modifier 25 (99201-99215, 99217-99223 [99224, 99225, 99226], 99231-99239, 99241-99245, 99281-99285, 99291-99292, 99304-99318, 99324-99337, 99341-99350, 99466-99467, 99468-99476, 99477-99480)

90935 **Hemodialysis procedure with single evaluation by a physician or other qualified health care professional**

INCLUDES All E&M services related to the patient's renal disease rendered on a day dialysis is performed
Inpatient ESRD and non-ESRD procedures
Only one evaluation of the patient related to hemodialysis procedure
Outpatient non-ESRD dialysis

2.07 2.07 FUD 000 S 80

AMA: 2018,Jan,8; 2017,Jan,8; 2016,Jan,13; 2015,Jan,16; 2014,Jan,11

90937 **Hemodialysis procedure requiring repeated evaluation(s) with or without substantial revision of dialysis prescription**

INCLUDES All E&M services related to the patient's renal disease rendered on a day dialysis is performed
Inpatient ESRD and non-ESRD procedures
Outpatient non-ESRD dialysis
Re-evaluation of the patient during hemodialysis procedure

2.95 2.95 FUD 000 B 80

AMA: 2018,Jan,8; 2017,Jan,8; 2016,Jan,13; 2015,Jan,16; 2014,Jan,11

90940 **Hemodialysis access flow study to determine blood flow in grafts and arteriovenous fistulae by an indicator method**

EXCLUDES *Hemodialysis access duplex scan (93990)*

0.00 0.00 FUD XXX N

AMA: 2018,Jan,8; 2017,Jan,8; 2016,Jan,13; 2015,Jan,16; 2014,Jan,11

90945-90947 Dialysis Techniques Other Than Hemodialysis

CMS: 100-04,12,40.3 Global Surgery Review; 100-04,3,100.6 Inpatient Renal Services

INCLUDES All E&M services related to the patient's renal disease rendered on the day dialysis is performed
Procedures other than hemodialysis:
Continuous renal replacement therapies
Hemofiltration
Peritoneal dialysis

EXCLUDES *Attendance by physician or other qualified health care provider for a prolonged period of time (99354-99360 [99415, 99416])*
Hemodialysis
Tunneled intraperitoneal catheter insertion
Open (49421)
Percutaneous (49418)

Code also significant, separately identifiable E&M service not related to dialysis procedure or renal failure with modifier 25 (99201-99215, 99217-99223 [99224, 99225, 99226], 99231-99239, 99241-99245, 99281-99285, 99291-99292, 99304-99318, 99324-99337, 99341-99350, 99466-99480 [99485, 99486])

90945 **Dialysis procedure other than hemodialysis (eg, peritoneal dialysis, hemofiltration, or other continuous renal replacement therapies), with single evaluation by a physician or other qualified health care professional**

INCLUDES Only one evaluation of the patient related to the procedure

EXCLUDES *Peritoneal dialysis home infusion (99601, 99602)*

2.42 2.42 FUD 000 V 80

AMA: 2018,Jan,8; 2017,Jan,8; 2016,Jan,13; 2015,Jan,16; 2014,Jan,11

90947 **Dialysis procedure other than hemodialysis (eg, peritoneal dialysis, hemofiltration, or other continuous renal replacement therapies) requiring repeated evaluations by a physician or other qualified health care professional, with or without substantial revision of dialysis prescription**

EXCLUDES *Re-evaluation during a procedure*

3.51 3.51 **FUD** 000 B 80

AMA: 2018,Jan,8; 2017,Jan,8; 2016,Jan,13; 2015,Jan,16; 2014,Jan,11

90951-90962 End-stage Renal Disease Monthly Outpatient Services

CMS: 100-02,11,20 Renal Dialysis Items and Services; 100-04,12,190.3 List of Telehealth Services; 100-04,12,190.3.4 ESRD-Related Services as a Telehealth Service; 100-04,8,140.1 ESRD-Related Services Under the Monthly Capitation Payment

INCLUDES Establishing dialyzing cycle
Management of dialysis visits
Outpatient E&M of dialysis visits
Patient management during dialysis for a month
Telephone calls

EXCLUDES *ESRD/non-ESRD dialysis services performed in an inpatient setting (90935-90937, 90945-90947)*
Non-ESRD dialysis services performed in an outpatient setting (90935-90937, 90945-90947)
Non-ESRD related E&M services that cannot be performed during the dialysis session
Services provided during the time transitional care management services are being provided (99495-99496)
Services provided in the same month with chronic care management (99487-99489)

90951 **End-stage renal disease (ESRD) related services monthly, for patients younger than 2 years of age to include monitoring for the adequacy of nutrition, assessment of growth and development, and counseling of parents; with 4 or more face-to-face visits by a physician or other qualified health care professional per month** A

26.6 26.6 **FUD** XXX ★ M 80

AMA: 2018,Feb,11; 2018,Jan,8; 2017,Jan,8; 2016,Jan,13; 2015,Jan,16; 2014,Oct,3; 2014,Jan,11

90952 **with 2-3 face-to-face visits by a physician or other qualified health care professional per month** A

0.00 0.00 **FUD** XXX ★ M 80

AMA: 2018,Feb,11; 2018,Jan,8; 2017,Jan,8; 2016,Jan,13; 2015,Jan,16; 2014,Oct,3; 2014,Jan,11

90953 **with 1 face-to-face visit by a physician or other qualified health care professional per month** A

0.00 0.00 **FUD** XXX M 80

AMA: 2018,Feb,11; 2018,Jan,8; 2017,Jan,8; 2016,Jan,13; 2015,Jan,16; 2014,Oct,3; 2014,Jan,11

90954 **End-stage renal disease (ESRD) related services monthly, for patients 2-11 years of age to include monitoring for the adequacy of nutrition, assessment of growth and development, and counseling of parents; with 4 or more face-to-face visits by a physician or other qualified health care professional per month** A

22.9 22.9 **FUD** XXX ★ M 80

AMA: 2018,Feb,11; 2018,Jan,8; 2017,Jan,8; 2016,Jan,13; 2015,Jan,16; 2014,Oct,3; 2014,Jan,11

90955 **with 2-3 face-to-face visits by a physician or other qualified health care professional per month** A

12.9 12.9 **FUD** XXX ★ M 80

AMA: 2018,Feb,11; 2018,Jan,8; 2017,Jan,8; 2016,Jan,13; 2015,Jan,16; 2014,Oct,3; 2014,Jan,11

90956 **with 1 face-to-face visit by a physician or other qualified health care professional per month** A

9.00 9.00 **FUD** XXX M 80

AMA: 2018,Feb,11; 2018,Jan,8; 2017,Jan,8; 2016,Jan,13; 2015,Jan,16; 2014,Oct,3; 2014,Jan,11

90957 **End-stage renal disease (ESRD) related services monthly, for patients 12-19 years of age to include monitoring for the adequacy of nutrition, assessment of growth and development, and counseling of parents; with 4 or more face-to-face visits by a physician or other qualified health care professional per month** A

18.1 18.1 **FUD** XXX ★ M 80

AMA: 2018,Feb,11; 2018,Jan,8; 2017,Jan,8; 2016,Jan,13; 2015,Jan,16; 2014,Oct,3; 2014,Jan,11

90958 **with 2-3 face-to-face visits by a physician or other qualified health care professional per month** A

12.3 12.3 **FUD** XXX ★ M 80

AMA: 2018,Feb,11; 2018,Jan,8; 2017,Jan,8; 2016,Jan,13; 2015,Jan,16; 2014,Oct,3; 2014,Jan,11

90959 **with 1 face-to-face visit by a physician or other qualified health care professional per month** A

8.40 8.40 **FUD** XXX M 80

AMA: 2018,Feb,11; 2018,Jan,8; 2017,Jan,8; 2016,Jan,13; 2015,Jan,16; 2014,Oct,3; 2014,Jan,11

90960 **End-stage renal disease (ESRD) related services monthly, for patients 20 years of age and older; with 4 or more face-to-face visits by a physician or other qualified health care professional per month** A

8.02 8.02 **FUD** XXX ★ M 80

AMA: 2018,Feb,11; 2018,Jan,8; 2017,Jan,8; 2016,Jan,13; 2015,Jan,16; 2014,Oct,3; 2014,Jan,11

90961 **with 2-3 face-to-face visits by a physician or other qualified health care professional per month** A

6.74 6.74 **FUD** XXX ★ M 80

AMA: 2018,Feb,11; 2018,Jan,8; 2017,Jan,8; 2016,Jan,13; 2015,Jan,16; 2014,Oct,3; 2014,Jan,11

90962 **with 1 face-to-face visit by a physician or other qualified health care professional per month** A

5.21 5.21 **FUD** XXX M 80

AMA: 2018,Feb,11; 2018,Jan,8; 2017,Jan,8; 2016,Jan,13; 2015,Jan,16; 2014,Oct,3; 2014,Jan,11

90963-90966 End-stage Renal Disease Monthly Home Dialysis Services

CMS: 100-02,11,20 Renal Dialysis Items and Services; 100-04,12,190.3.4 ESRD-Related Services as a Telehealth Service; 100-04,8,140.1 ESRD-Related Services Under the Monthly Capitation Payment; 100-04,8,140.1.1 Payment for Managing Patients on Home Dialysis

INCLUDES ESRD services for home dialysis patients
Services provided for a full month

EXCLUDES *Services provided during the time transitional care management services are being provided (99495-99496)*
Services provided in the same month with chronic care management (99487-99489)

90963 **End-stage renal disease (ESRD) related services for home dialysis per full month, for patients younger than 2 years of age to include monitoring for the adequacy of nutrition, assessment of growth and development, and counseling of parents** A

15.4 15.4 **FUD** XXX M 80

AMA: 2018,Feb,11; 2018,Jan,8; 2017,Jan,8; 2016,Jan,13; 2015,Jan,16; 2014,Oct,3; 2014,Jan,11

90964 **End-stage renal disease (ESRD) related services for home dialysis per full month, for patients 2-11 years of age to include monitoring for the adequacy of nutrition, assessment of growth and development, and counseling of parents** A

13.4 13.4 **FUD** XXX M 80

AMA: 2018,Feb,11; 2018,Jan,8; 2017,Jan,8; 2016,Jan,13; 2015,Jan,16; 2014,Oct,3; 2014,Jan,11

90965 **End-stage renal disease (ESRD) related services for home dialysis per full month, for patients 12-19 years of age to include monitoring for the adequacy of nutrition, assessment of growth and development, and counseling of parents** A
12.8 12.8 FUD XXX M 80
AMA: 2018,Feb,11; 2018,Jan,8; 2017,Jan,8; 2016,Jan,13; 2015,Jan,16; 2014,Oct,3; 2014,Jan,11

90966 **End-stage renal disease (ESRD) related services for home dialysis per full month, for patients 20 years of age and older** A
6.72 6.72 FUD XXX M 80
AMA: 2018,Feb,11; 2018,Jan,8; 2017,Jan,8; 2016,Jan,13; 2015,Jan,16; 2014,Oct,3; 2014,Jan,11

90967-90970 End-stage Renal Disease Services: Partial Month

CMS: 100-02,11,20 Renal Dialysis Items and Services

INCLUDES ESRD services for less than a full month, such as:
A patient who is transient, dies, recovers, or undergoes kidney transplant
Outpatient ESRD-related services initiated prior to completion of assessment
Patient spending part of the month as a hospital inpatient
Services reported on a daily basis, less the days of hospitalization

EXCLUDES *Services provided during the time transitional care management services are being provided (99495-99496)*
Services provided in the same month with chronic care management (99487-99489)

90967 **End-stage renal disease (ESRD) related services for dialysis less than a full month of service, per day; for patients younger than 2 years of age** A
0.51 0.51 FUD XXX M 80
AMA: 2018,Feb,11; 2018,Jan,8; 2017,Jan,8; 2016,Jan,13; 2015,Jan,16; 2014,Oct,3; 2014,Jan,11

90968 **for patients 2-11 years of age** A
0.45 0.45 FUD XXX M 80
AMA: 2018,Feb,11; 2018,Jan,8; 2017,Jan,8; 2016,Jan,13; 2015,Jan,16; 2014,Oct,3; 2014,Jan,11

90969 **for patients 12-19 years of age** A
0.43 0.43 FUD XXX M 80
AMA: 2018,Feb,11; 2018,Jan,8; 2017,Jan,8; 2016,Jan,13; 2015,Jan,16; 2014,Oct,3; 2014,Jan,11

90970 **for patients 20 years of age and older** A
0.22 0.22 FUD XXX M 80
AMA: 2018,Feb,11; 2018,Jan,8; 2017,Jan,8; 2016,Jan,13; 2015,Jan,16; 2014,Oct,3; 2014,Jan,11

90989-90993 Dialysis Training Services

CMS: 100-04,3,100.6 Inpatient Renal Services

90989 **Dialysis training, patient, including helper where applicable, any mode, completed course**
0.00 0.00 FUD XXX B
AMA: 2018,Feb,11; 2018,Jan,8; 2017,Jan,8; 2016,Jan,13; 2015,Jan,16; 2014,Jan,11

90993 **Dialysis training, patient, including helper where applicable, any mode, course not completed, per training session**
0.00 0.00 FUD XXX B
AMA: 2018,Feb,11; 2018,Jan,8; 2017,Jan,8; 2016,Jan,13; 2015,Jan,16; 2014,Jan,11

90997-90999 Hemoperfusion and Unlisted Dialysis Procedures

CMS: 100-04,3,100.6 Inpatient Renal Services

90997 **Hemoperfusion (eg, with activated charcoal or resin)**
2.53 2.53 FUD 000 B 80
AMA: 2018,Feb,11

90999 **Unlisted dialysis procedure, inpatient or outpatient**
0.00 0.00 FUD XXX B 80
AMA: 2018,Feb,11

91010-91022 Esophageal Manometry

91010 **Esophageal motility (manometric study of the esophagus and/or gastroesophageal junction) study with interpretation and report;**
EXCLUDES *Esophageal motility studies with high-resolution esophageal pressure topography (91299)*
Code also for esophageal motility studies with stimulant or perfusion (91013)
5.38 5.38 FUD 000 S 80
AMA: 2018,Feb,11

\+ **91013** **with stimulation or perfusion (eg, stimulant, acid or alkali perfusion) (List separately in addition to code for primary procedure)**
EXCLUDES *Esophageal motility studies with high-resolution esophageal pressure topography (91299)*
Use of code more than one time for each session
Code first (91010)
0.73 0.73 FUD ZZZ N 80
AMA: 2018,Feb,11

91020 **Gastric motility (manometric) studies**
EXCLUDES *Gastrointestinal imaging by wireless capsule (91112)*
7.01 7.01 FUD 000 S 80
AMA: 2018,Feb,11; 2018,Jan,8; 2017,Jan,8; 2016,Jan,13; 2015,Jan,16

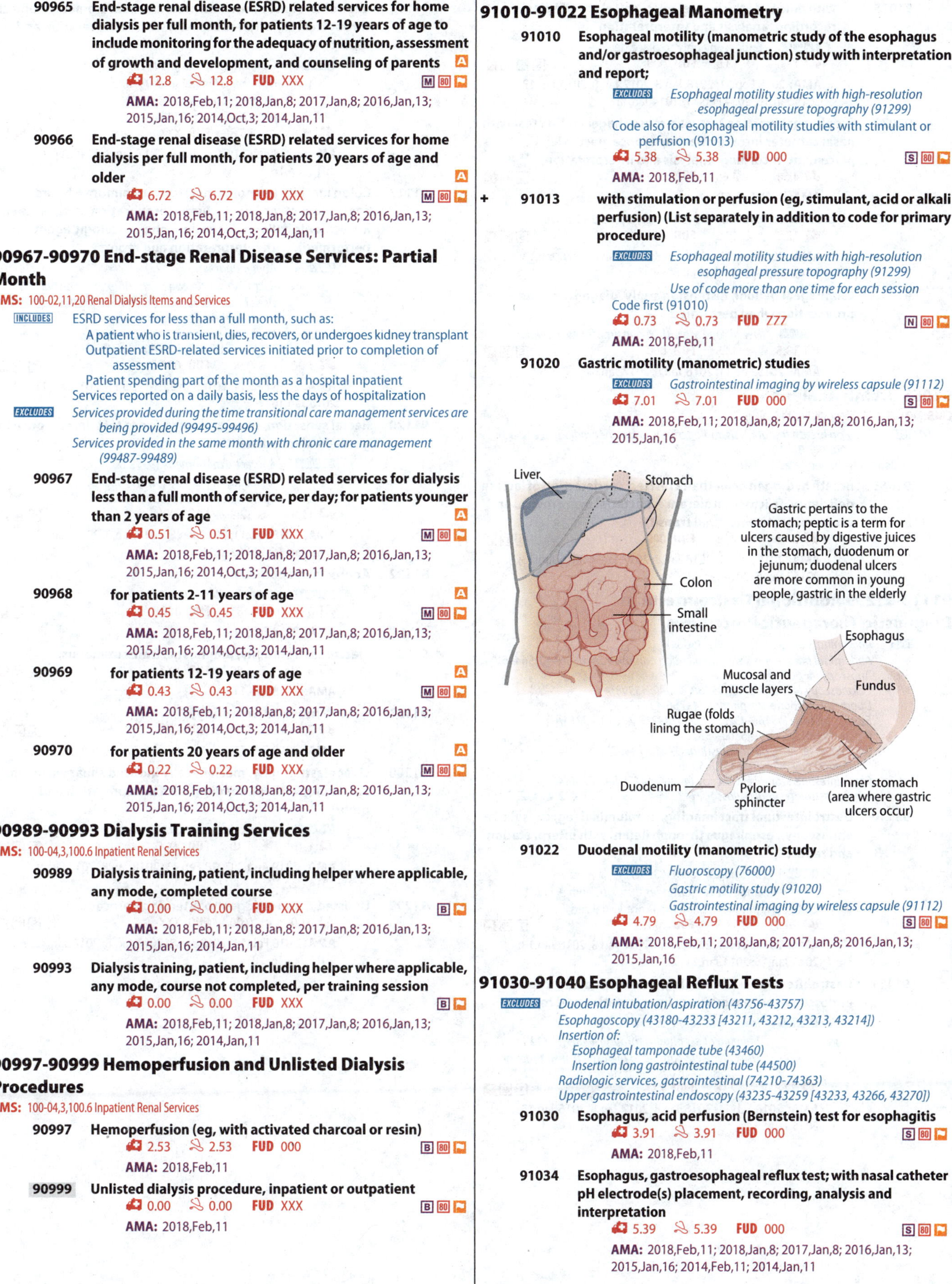

Gastric pertains to the stomach; peptic is a term for ulcers caused by digestive juices in the stomach, duodenum or jejunum; duodenal ulcers are more common in young people, gastric in the elderly

91022 **Duodenal motility (manometric) study**
EXCLUDES *Fluoroscopy (76000)*
Gastric motility study (91020)
Gastrointestinal imaging by wireless capsule (91112)
4.79 4.79 FUD 000 S 80
AMA: 2018,Feb,11; 2018,Jan,8; 2017,Jan,8; 2016,Jan,13; 2015,Jan,16

91030-91040 Esophageal Reflux Tests

EXCLUDES *Duodenal intubation/aspiration (43756-43757)*
Esophagoscopy (43180-43233 [43211, 43212, 43213, 43214])
Insertion of:
Esophageal tamponade tube (43460)
Insertion long gastrointestinal tube (44500)
Radiologic services, gastrointestinal (74210-74363)
Upper gastrointestinal endoscopy (43235-43259 [43233, 43266, 43270])

91030 **Esophagus, acid perfusion (Bernstein) test for esophagitis**
3.91 3.91 FUD 000 S 80
AMA: 2018,Feb,11

91034 **Esophagus, gastroesophageal reflux test; with nasal catheter pH electrode(s) placement, recording, analysis and interpretation**
5.39 5.39 FUD 000 S 80
AMA: 2018,Feb,11; 2018,Jan,8; 2017,Jan,8; 2016,Jan,13; 2015,Jan,16; 2014,Feb,11; 2014,Jan,11

91035 **with mucosal attached telemetry pH electrode placement, recording, analysis and interpretation**

INCLUDES Endoscopy only to place device

13.6 13.6 **FUD** 000 S Z2 80

AMA: 2018,Feb,11; 2018,Jan,8; 2017,Jan,8; 2016,Jan,13; 2015,Jan,16; 2014,Feb,11; 2014,Jan,11

91037 **Esophageal function test, gastroesophageal reflux test with nasal catheter intraluminal impedance electrode(s) placement, recording, analysis and interpretation;**

4.66 4.66 **FUD** 000 S 80

AMA: 2018,Feb,11

91038 **prolonged (greater than 1 hour, up to 24 hours)**

12.5 12.5 **FUD** 000 S 80

AMA: 2018,Feb,11; 2018,Jan,8; 2017,Jan,8; 2016,Jan,13; 2015,Jan,16; 2014,Feb,11

91040 **Esophageal balloon distension study, diagnostic, with provocation when performed**

EXCLUDES *Use of code more than one time for each session*

13.5 13.5 **FUD** 000 S 80

AMA: 2018,Feb,11; 2018,Jan,8; 2017,Jan,6

91065 Breath Analysis

CMS: 100-03,100.5 Diagnostic Breath Analysis

EXCLUDES *H. pylori breath test analysis, radioactive (C-14) or nonradioactive (C-13) (78268, 83013)*

Code also each challenge administered

91065 **Breath hydrogen or methane test (eg, for detection of lactase deficiency, fructose intolerance, bacterial overgrowth, or oro-cecal gastrointestinal transit)**

2.13 2.13 **FUD** 000 S 80

AMA: 2018,Feb,11; 2018,Jan,8; 2017,Jan,8; 2016,Jan,13; 2015,Jan,16; 2014,Jan,11

91110-91299 Additional Gastrointestinal Diagnostic/Therapeutic Procedures

EXCLUDES *Abdominal paracentesis (49082-49084)*
Abdominal paracentesis with medication administration (96440, 96446)
Anoscopy (46600-46615)
Colonoscopy (45378-45393 [45388, 45390, 45398])
Duodenal intubation/aspiration (43756-43757)
Esophagoscopy (43180-43233 [43211, 43212, 43213, 43214])
Proctosigmoidoscopy (45300-45327)
Radiologic services, gastrointestinal (74210-74363)
Sigmoidoscopy (45330-45350 [45346])
Small intestine/stomal endoscopy (44360-44408 [44381, 44401])
Upper gastrointestinal endoscopy (43235-43259 [43233, 43266, 43270])

91110 **Gastrointestinal tract imaging, intraluminal (eg, capsule endoscopy), esophagus through ileum, with interpretation and report**

EXCLUDES *Imaging of colon (0355T)*
Imaging of esophagus through ileum (91111)

Code also modifier 52 if ileum is not visualized

24.9 24.9 **FUD** XXX T 80

AMA: 2018,Feb,11; 2018,Jan,8; 2017,Jan,8; 2016,Jan,13; 2015,Jan,16; 2014,Jan,11

91111 **Gastrointestinal tract imaging, intraluminal (eg, capsule endoscopy), esophagus with interpretation and report**

EXCLUDES *Imaging of colon (0355T)*
Imaging of esophagus through ileum (91111)
Use of wireless capsule to measure transit times or pressure in gastrointestinal tract (91112)

22.8 22.8 **FUD** XXX T 80

AMA: 2018,Feb,11; 2018,Jan,8; 2017,Jan,8; 2016,Jan,13; 2015,Jan,16

91112 **Gastrointestinal transit and pressure measurement, stomach through colon, wireless capsule, with interpretation and report**

EXCLUDES *Colon motility study (91117)*
Duodenal motility study (91022)
Gastric motility studies (91020)
pH of body fluid (83986)

35.8 35.8 **FUD** XXX T 80

AMA: 2018,Feb,11; 2018,Jan,8; 2017,Jan,8; 2016,Jan,13; 2015,Jan,16

91117 **Colon motility (manometric) study, minimum 6 hours continuous recording (including provocation tests, eg, meal, intracolonic balloon distension, pharmacologic agents, if performed), with interpretation and report**

EXCLUDES *Anal manometry (91122)*
Rectal sensation, tone and compliance testing (91120)
Use of code more than one time regardless of the number of provocations
Use of wireless capsule to measure transit times or pressure in gastrointestinal tract (91112)

3.96 3.96 **FUD** 000 T 80

AMA: 2018,Feb,11; 2018,Jan,8; 2017,Jan,8; 2016,Jan,13; 2015,Jan,16

91120 **Rectal sensation, tone, and compliance test (ie, response to graded balloon distention)**

EXCLUDES *Anorectal manometry (91122)*
Biofeedback training (90912, 90913)
Colon motility study (91117)

12.9 12.9 **FUD** XXX S 80

AMA: 2018,Feb,11; 2018,Jan,8; 2017,Jan,8; 2016,Jan,13; 2015,Jan,16; 2014,Jan,11

91122 **Anorectal manometry**

EXCLUDES *Colon motility study (91117)*

6.85 6.85 **FUD** 000 T 80

AMA: 2018,Feb,11

91132 **Electrogastrography, diagnostic, transcutaneous;**

6.80 6.80 **FUD** XXX S 80

AMA: 2018,Feb,11

91133 **with provocative testing**

7.44 7.44 **FUD** XXX Q1 80

AMA: 2018,Feb,11

91200 **Liver elastography, mechanically induced shear wave (eg, vibration), without imaging, with interpretation and report**

EXCLUDES *Ultrasound elastography parenchyma (76981-76983)*

1.10 1.10 **FUD** XXX Q1 80

AMA: 2019,Aug,3; 2018,Feb,11; 2018,Jan,8; 2017,Oct,9; 2014,Dec,13

91299 **Unlisted diagnostic gastroenterology procedure**

0.00 0.00 **FUD** XXX S 80

AMA: 2018,Feb,11; 2018,Jan,8; 2017,Jan,8; 2016,Jan,13; 2015,Jan,16; 2014,Jan,11

92002-92014 Ophthalmic Medical Services

CMS: 100-02,15,30.4 Optometrist's Services

INCLUDES Routine ophthalmoscopy
Services provided to established patients who have received professional services from the physician or other qualified health care provider or another physician or other qualified health care professional within the same group practice of the exact same specialty and subspecialty within the past three years
Services provided to new patients who have received no professional services from the physician or other qualified health care provider or another physician or other qualified health care professional within the same group practice of the exact same specialty and subspecialty within the past three years

EXCLUDES *Retinal polarization scan (0469T)*
Surgical procedures on the eye/ocular adnexa (65091-68899 [67810])
Visual screening tests (99173-99174 [99177])

92002 Ophthalmological services: medical examination and evaluation with initiation of diagnostic and treatment program; intermediate, new patient

INCLUDES Evaluation of new/existing condition complicated by new diagnostic or management problem
Integrated services where medical decision making cannot be separated from examination methods
Other diagnostic procedures
- Biomicroscopy
- Mydriasis
- Ophthalmoscopy
- Tonometry

Problems not related to primary diagnosis
The following for intermediate services:
- External ocular/adnexal examination
- General medical observation
- History

1.36 2.37 FUD XXX V 80

AMA: 2018,Feb,11; 2018,Feb,3; 2018,Jan,8; 2017,Sep,14; 2017,Jan,8; 2016,Jan,13; 2015,Jan,16; 2014,Jan,11

92004 comprehensive, new patient, 1 or more visits

INCLUDES General evaluation of complete visual system
Integrated services where medical decision making cannot be separated from examination methods
Single service that need not be performed at one session
The following for comprehensive services:
- Basic sensorimotor examination
- Biomicroscopy
- Dilation (cycloplegia)
- External examinations
- General medical observation
- Gross visual fields
- History
- Initiation of diagnostic/treatment programs
- Mydriasis
- Ophthalmoscopic examinations
- Other diagnostic procedures
- Prescription of medication
- Special diagnostic/treatment services
- Tonometry

2.81 4.26 FUD XXX V 80

AMA: 2018,Feb,11; 2018,Feb,3; 2018,Jan,8; 2017,Sep,14; 2017,Jan,8; 2016,Nov,9; 2016,Jan,13; 2015,Jan,16; 2014,Jan,11

92012 Ophthalmological services: medical examination and evaluation, with initiation or continuation of diagnostic and treatment program; intermediate, established patient

INCLUDES Evaluation of new/existing condition complicated by new diagnostic or management problem
Integrated services where medical decision making cannot be separated from examination methods
Problems not related to primary diagnosis
The following for intermediate services:
- External ocular/adnexal examination
- General medical observation
- History
- Other diagnostic procedures:
  - Biomicroscopy
  - Mydriasis
  - Ophthalmoscopy
  - Tonometry

1.49 2.49 FUD XXX V 80

AMA: 2018,Feb,11; 2018,Feb,3; 2018,Jan,8; 2017,Sep,14; 2017,Jan,8; 2016,Jan,13; 2015,Jan,16; 2014,Jan,11

92014 comprehensive, established patient, 1 or more visits

INCLUDES General evaluation of complete visual system
Integrated services where medical decision making cannot be separated from examination methods
Single service that need not be performed at one session
The following for comprehensive services:
- Basic sensorimotor examination
- Biomicroscopy
- Dilation (cycloplegia)
- External examinations
- General medical observation
- Gross visual fields
- History
- Initiation of diagnostic/treatment programs
- Mydriasis
- Ophthalmoscopic examinations
- Other diagnostic procedures
- Prescription of medication
- Special diagnostic/treatment services
- Tonometry

2.25 3.57 FUD XXX V 80

AMA: 2018,Feb,11; 2018,Feb,3; 2018,Jan,8; 2017,Sep,14; 2017,Jan,8; 2016,Nov,9; 2016,Jan,13; 2015,Jan,16; 2014,Jan,11

92015-92145 Ophthalmic Special Services

INCLUDES Routine ophthalmoscopy
Surgical procedures on the eye/ocular adnexa (65091-68899 [67810])

Code also E&M services, when performed
Code also general ophthalmological services, when performed (92002-92014)

92015 Determination of refractive state

INCLUDES Lens prescription
- Absorptive factor
- Axis
- Impact resistance
- Lens power
- Prism
- Specification of lens type:
  - Bifocal
  - Monofocal

EXCLUDES *Ocular screening, instrument based (99173-99174 [99177])*

0.55 0.56 FUD XXX E

AMA: 2018,Feb,11; 2018,Jan,8; 2017,Jan,8; 2016,Mar,10; 2016,Jan,13; 2015,Jan,16; 2014,Jan,11

92018 Ophthalmological examination and evaluation, under general anesthesia, with or without manipulation of globe for passive range of motion or other manipulation to facilitate diagnostic examination; complete

4.13 4.13 FUD XXX J 80

AMA: 2018,Feb,11; 2018,Jan,8; 2017,Jan,8; 2016,Jan,13; 2015,Jan,16; 2014,Jan,11

92019 **limited**
2.05 2.05 FUD XXX J 80
AMA: 2018,Feb,11; 2018,Jan,8; 2017,Jan,8; 2016,Jan,13; 2015,Jan,16; 2014,Jan,11

92020 **Gonioscopy (separate procedure)**
EXCLUDES *Gonioscopy under general anesthesia (92018)*
0.60 0.78 FUD XXX Q1 80
AMA: 2018,Feb,11; 2018,Jan,8; 2017,Jan,8; 2016,Jan,13; 2015,Jan,16; 2014,Jan,11

92025 **Computerized corneal topography, unilateral or bilateral, with interpretation and report**
EXCLUDES *Corneal transplant procedures (65710-65771)*
Manual keratoscopy
1.07 1.07 FUD XXX Q1 80
AMA: 2018,Feb,11; 2018,Jan,8; 2017,Jan,8; 2016,Jan,13; 2015,Jan,16; 2014,Jan,11

92060 **Sensorimotor examination with multiple measurements of ocular deviation (eg, restrictive or paretic muscle with diplopia) with interpretation and report (separate procedure)**
1.82 1.82 FUD XXX Q1 80
AMA: 2018,Feb,11; 2018,Jan,8; 2017,Jan,8; 2016,Jan,13; 2015,Jan,16; 2014,Jan,11

92065 **Orthoptic and/or pleoptic training, with continuing medical direction and evaluation**
1.51 1.51 FUD XXX Q1 80
AMA: 2018,Feb,11; 2018,Jan,8; 2017,Jan,8; 2016,Jan,13; 2015,Jan,16; 2014,Jan,11

92071 **Fitting of contact lens for treatment of ocular surface disease**
EXCLUDES *Contact lens service for keratoconus (92072)*
Code also supply of lens with appropriate supply code or (99070)
0.95 1.07 FUD XXX N 80 50
AMA: 2018,Feb,11

92072 **Fitting of contact lens for management of keratoconus, initial fitting**
EXCLUDES *Contact lens service for disease of ocular surface (92071)*
Subsequent fittings (99211-99215, 92012-92014)
Code also supply of lens with appropriate supply code or (99070)
2.84 3.72 FUD XXX N 80
AMA: 2018,Feb,11; 2018,Jan,8; 2017,Sep,14; 2017,Jan,8; 2016,Jan,13; 2015,Jan,16; 2014,Jan,11

92081 **Visual field examination, unilateral or bilateral, with interpretation and report; limited examination (eg, tangent screen, Autoplot, arc perimeter, or single stimulus level automated test, such as Octopus 3 or 7 equivalent)**
INCLUDES Gross visual testing/confrontation testing
0.96 0.96 FUD XXX Q1 80
AMA: 2018,Feb,11; 2018,Jan,8; 2017,Jan,8; 2016,Jan,13; 2015,Jan,16; 2014,Jan,11

92082 **intermediate examination (eg, at least 2 isopters on Goldmann perimeter, or semiquantitative, automated suprathreshold screening program, Humphrey suprathreshold automatic diagnostic test, Octopus program 33)**
INCLUDES Gross visual testing/confrontation testing
1.35 1.35 FUD XXX Q1 80
AMA: 2018,Feb,11; 2018,Jan,8; 2017,Jan,8; 2016,Jan,13; 2015,Jan,16; 2014,Jan,11

92083 **extended examination (eg, Goldmann visual fields with at least 3 isopters plotted and static determination within the central 30°, or quantitative, automated threshold perimetry, Octopus program G-1, 32 or 42, Humphrey visual field analyzer full threshold programs 30-2, 24-2, or 30/60-2)**
INCLUDES Gross visual field testing/confrontation testing
EXCLUDES *Assessment of visual field by transmission of data by patient to a surveillance center (0378T-0379T)*
1.81 1.81 FUD XXX Q1 80
AMA: 2018,Feb,11; 2018,Jan,8; 2017,Jan,8; 2016,Jan,13; 2015,Jan,16; 2014,Jan,11

92100 **Serial tonometry (separate procedure) with multiple measurements of intraocular pressure over an extended time period with interpretation and report, same day (eg, diurnal curve or medical treatment of acute elevation of intraocular pressure)**
EXCLUDES *Intraocular pressure monitoring for 24 hours or more (0329T)*
Ocular blood flow measurements (0198T)
Single-episode tonometry (99201-99215, 92002-92004)
0.96 2.32 FUD XXX N 80
AMA: 2018,Feb,11; 2018,Jan,8; 2017,Jan,8; 2016,Jan,13; 2015,Jan,16; 2014,May,5; 2014,Jan,11

92132 **Scanning computerized ophthalmic diagnostic imaging, anterior segment, with interpretation and report, unilateral or bilateral**
EXCLUDES *Imaging of anterior segment with specular microscopy and endothelial cell analysis (92286)*
Scanning computerized ophthalmic diagnostic imaging of optic nerve and retina (92133-92134)
Tear film imaging (0330T)
0.89 0.89 FUD XXX Q1 80
AMA: 2018,Feb,11; 2018,Jan,8; 2017,Jan,8; 2016,Jan,13; 2015,Jan,16; 2014,May,5; 2014,Jan,11

92133 **Scanning computerized ophthalmic diagnostic imaging, posterior segment, with interpretation and report, unilateral or bilateral; optic nerve**
EXCLUDES *Remote imaging for retinal disease (92227-92228)*
Scanning computerized ophthalmic imaging of retina at same visit (92134)
1.05 1.05 FUD XXX Q1 80
AMA: 2018,Feb,11; 2018,Jan,8; 2017,Jan,8; 2016,Jan,13; 2015,Jan,16; 2014,Nov,10; 2014,Jan,11

92134 **retina**
EXCLUDES *Remote imaging for retinal disease (92227-92228)*
Scanning computerized ophthalmic imaging of optic nerve at same visit (92133)
1.16 1.16 FUD XXX Q1 80
AMA: 2018,Feb,11; 2018,Jan,8; 2017,Jan,8; 2016,Jan,13; 2015,Jan,16; 2014,Nov,10; 2014,Jan,11

92136 **Ophthalmic biometry by partial coherence interferometry with intraocular lens power calculation**
EXCLUDES *Tear film imaging (0330T)*
1.98 1.98 FUD XXX Q1 80
AMA: 2018,Feb,11; 2018,Jan,8; 2017,Jan,8; 2016,Jan,13; 2015,Jan,16; 2014,May,5; 2014,Jan,11

92145 **Corneal hysteresis determination, by air impulse stimulation, unilateral or bilateral, with interpretation and report**
0.49 0.49 FUD XXX Q1 80
AMA: 2018,Feb,11

92201-92287 Other Ophthalmology Services

EXCLUDES *Prescription, fitting, and/or medical supervision of ocular prosthesis adaptation by physician (99201-99215, 99241-99245, 92002-92014)*

● **92201** **Ophthalmoscopy, extended; with retinal drawing and scleral depression of peripheral retinal disease (eg, for retinal tear, retinal detachment, retinal tumor) with interpretation and report, unilateral or bilateral**
EXCLUDES *Fundus photography with interpretation and report (92250)*

● **92202** **with drawing of optic nerve or macula (eg, for glaucoma, macular pathology, tumor) with interpretation and report, unilateral or bilateral**

EXCLUDES *Fundus photography with interpretation and report (92250)*

~~92225~~ **~~Ophthalmoscopy, extended, with retinal drawing (eg, for retinal detachment, melanoma), with interpretation and report; initial~~**

To report, see (92201-92202)

~~92226~~ **~~subsequent~~**

To report, see (92201-92202)

92227 **Remote imaging for detection of retinal disease (eg, retinopathy in a patient with diabetes) with analysis and report under physician supervision, unilateral or bilateral**

EXCLUDES *When services provided with E&M services as part of a single organ system or (92002-92014, 92133-92134, 92228, 92250)*

0.40 0.40 FUD XXX ★ Q1 80 TC

AMA: 2019,Aug,10; 2018,Feb,11; 2018,Jan,8; 2017,Jan,8; 2016,Jul,8; 2016,Jan,13; 2015,Jan,16; 2014,Jan,11

92228 **Remote imaging for monitoring and management of active retinal disease (eg, diabetic retinopathy) with physician review, interpretation and report, unilateral or bilateral**

EXCLUDES *When services provided with E&M services as part of a single organ system or (92002-92014, 92133-92134, 92227, 92250)*

0.97 0.97 FUD XXX ★ Q1 80

AMA: 2018,Feb,11; 2018,Jan,8; 2017,Jan,8; 2016,Jan,13; 2015,Jan,16; 2014,Jan,11

92230 **Fluorescein angioscopy with interpretation and report**

0.95 1.83 FUD XXX Q1 80

AMA: 2018,Feb,11; 2018,Jan,8; 2017,Jan,8; 2016,Jan,13; 2015,Jan,16; 2014,Jan,11

92235 **Fluorescein angiography (includes multiframe imaging) with interpretation and report, unilateral or bilateral**

EXCLUDES *Fluorescein and indocyanine-green angiography (92242)*

2.59 2.59 FUD XXX S 80

AMA: 2018,Feb,11; 2018,Jan,8; 2017,Jun,8; 2017,Jan,8; 2016,Jan,13; 2015,Jan,16; 2014,Jan,11

92240 **Indocyanine-green angiography (includes multiframe imaging) with interpretation and report, unilateral or bilateral**

EXCLUDES *Fluorescein and indocyanine-green angiography (92242)*

5.83 5.83 FUD XXX S 80

AMA: 2018,Feb,11; 2018,Jan,8; 2017,Jun,8; 2017,Jan,8; 2016,Jan,13; 2015,Jan,16; 2014,Jan,11

92242 **Fluorescein angiography and indocyanine-green angiography (includes multiframe imaging) performed at the same patient encounter with interpretation and report, unilateral or bilateral**

6.48 6.48 FUD XXX S 80

AMA: 2018,Feb,11; 2018,Jan,8; 2017,Jun,8

92250 **Fundus photography with interpretation and report**

1.43 1.43 FUD XXX Q1 80

AMA: 2018,Feb,11; 2018,Jan,8; 2017,Jan,8; 2016,Jul,8; 2016,Jan,13; 2015,May,9; 2015,Jan,16; 2014,Dec,16; 2014,Dec,16; 2014,Nov,10; 2014,Jan,11

92260 **Ophthalmodynamometry**

0.31 0.55 FUD XXX Q1 80

AMA: 2018,Feb,11; 2018,Jan,8; 2017,Jan,8; 2016,Jan,13; 2015,Jan,16; 2014,Jan,11

92265 **Needle oculoelectromyography, 1 or more extraocular muscles, 1 or both eyes, with interpretation and report**

2.48 2.48 FUD XXX Q1 80

AMA: 2018,Feb,11; 2018,Jan,8; 2017,Jan,8; 2016,Jan,13; 2015,Jan,16; 2014,Jan,11

92270 **Electro-oculography with interpretation and report**

EXCLUDES *Recording saccadic eye movement (92700)*
Vestibular function testing (92537-92538, 92540-92542, 92544-92549)

2.70 2.70 FUD XXX Q1 80

AMA: 2018,Feb,11; 2018,Jan,8; 2017,Jan,8; 2016,Jan,13; 2015,Sep,7; 2015,Jan,16; 2014,Jan,11

92273 **Electroretinography (ERG), with interpretation and report; full field (ie, ffERG, flash ERG, Ganzfeld ERG)**

3.78 3.78 FUD XXX 80

AMA: 2019,Jan,12

92274 **multifocal (mfERG)**

2.56 2.56 FUD XXX 80

AMA: 2019,Jan,12

92283 **Color vision examination, extended, eg, anomaloscope or equivalent**

1.52 1.52 FUD XXX Q1 80

AMA: 2018,Feb,11; 2018,Jan,8; 2017,Jan,8; 2016,Jan,13; 2015,Jan,16; 2014,Jan,11

92284 **Dark adaptation examination with interpretation and report**

1.74 1.74 FUD XXX Q1 80

AMA: 2018,Feb,11; 2018,Jan,8; 2017,Jan,8; 2016,Jan,13; 2015,Jan,16; 2014,Jan,11

92285 **External ocular photography with interpretation and report for documentation of medical progress (eg, close-up photography, slit lamp photography, goniophotography, stereo-photography)**

0.61 0.61 FUD XXX Q1 80

AMA: 2018,Feb,11; 2018,Jan,8; 2017,Jan,8; 2016,Jan,13; 2015,Jan,16; 2014,May,5; 2014,Jan,11

92286 **Anterior segment imaging with interpretation and report; with specular microscopy and endothelial cell analysis**

1.10 1.10 FUD XXX Q1 80

AMA: 2018,Feb,11; 2018,Jan,8; 2017,Jan,8; 2016,Jan,13; 2015,Jan,16; 2014,Jan,11

92287 **with fluorescein angiography**

4.13 4.13 FUD XXX Q1 80

AMA: 2018,Feb,11; 2018,Jan,8; 2017,Jan,8; 2016,Jan,13; 2015,Jan,16; 2014,Jan,11

92310-92326 Services Related to Contact Lenses

CMS: 100-02,15,30.4 Optometrist's Services

INCLUDES Incidental revision of lens during training period
Patient training/instruction
Specification of optical/physical characteristics:
- Curvature
- Flexibility
- Gas-permeability
- Power
- Size

EXCLUDES *Extended wear lenses follow up (92012-92014)*
General ophthalmological services
Therapeutic/surgical use of contact lens (68340, 92071-92072)

92310 **Prescription of optical and physical characteristics of and fitting of contact lens, with medical supervision of adaptation; corneal lens, both eyes, except for aphakia**

1.69 2.80 FUD XXX E

AMA: 2018,Feb,11; 2018,Jan,8; 2017,Jan,8; 2016,Jan,13; 2015,Jan,16; 2014,Jan,11

92311 **corneal lens for aphakia, 1 eye**

1.57 2.94 FUD XXX Q1 80

AMA: 2018,Feb,11; 2018,Jan,8; 2017,Jan,8; 2016,Jan,13; 2015,Jan,16; 2014,Jan,11

92312 **corneal lens for aphakia, both eyes**

1.81 3.40 FUD XXX Q1 80

AMA: 2018,Feb,11; 2018,Jan,8; 2017,Jan,8; 2016,Jan,13; 2015,Jan,16; 2014,Jan,11

92313 **corneoscleral lens**
1.31 2.78 **FUD** XXX
AMA: 2018,Feb,11; 2018,Jan,8; 2017,Jan,8; 2016,Jan,13; 2015,Jan,16; 2014,Jan,11

92314 **Prescription of optical and physical characteristics of contact lens, with medical supervision of adaptation and direction of fitting by independent technician; corneal lens, both eyes except for aphakia**
1.00 2.36 **FUD** XXX
AMA: 2018,Feb,11; 2018,Jan,8; 2017,Jan,8; 2016,Jan,13; 2015,Jan,16; 2014,Jan,11

92315 **corneal lens for aphakia, 1 eye**
0.62 2.19 **FUD** XXX
AMA: 2018,Feb,11; 2018,Jan,8; 2017,Jan,8; 2016,Jan,13; 2015,Jan,16; 2014,Jan,11

92316 **corneal lens for aphakia, both eyes**
0.93 2.72 **FUD** XXX
AMA: 2018,Feb,11; 2018,Jan,8; 2017,Jan,8; 2016,Jan,13; 2015,Jan,16; 2014,Jan,11

92317 **corneoscleral lens**
0.62 2.29 **FUD** XXX
AMA: 2018,Feb,11; 2018,Jan,8; 2017,Jan,8; 2016,Jan,13; 2015,Jan,16; 2014,Jan,11

92325 **Modification of contact lens (separate procedure), with medical supervision of adaptation**
1.24 1.24 **FUD** XXX
AMA: 2018,Feb,11; 2018,Jan,8; 2017,Jan,8; 2016,Jan,13; 2015,Jan,16; 2014,Jan,11

92326 **Replacement of contact lens**
1.05 1.05 **FUD** XXX
AMA: 2018,Feb,11; 2018,Jan,8; 2017,Jan,8; 2016,Jan,13; 2015,Jan,16; 2014,Jan,11

92340-92499 Services Related to Eyeglasses

CMS: 100-02,15,30.4 Optometrist's Services

INCLUDES Anatomical facial characteristics measurement
Final adjustment of spectacles to visual axes/anatomical topography
Written laboratory specifications

EXCLUDES *Supply of materials*

92340 **Fitting of spectacles, except for aphakia; monofocal**
0.53 0.99 **FUD** XXX
AMA: 2018,Feb,11; 2018,Jan,8; 2017,Jan,8; 2016,Jan,13; 2015,Jan,16; 2014,Jan,11

92341 **bifocal**
0.68 1.14 **FUD** XXX
AMA: 2018,Feb,11; 2018,Jan,8; 2017,Jan,8; 2016,Jan,13; 2015,Jan,16; 2014,Jan,11

92342 **multifocal, other than bifocal**
0.77 1.23 **FUD** XXX
AMA: 2018,Feb,11; 2018,Jan,8; 2017,Jan,8; 2016,Jan,13; 2015,Jan,16; 2014,Jan,11

92352 **Fitting of spectacle prosthesis for aphakia; monofocal**
0.53 1.17 **FUD** XXX
AMA: 2018,Feb,11; 2018,Jan,8; 2017,Jan,8; 2016,Jan,13; 2015,Jan,16; 2014,Jan,11

92353 **multifocal**
0.72 1.36 **FUD** XXX
AMA: 2018,Feb,11; 2018,Jan,8; 2017,Jan,8; 2016,Jan,13; 2015,Jan,16; 2014,Jan,11

92354 **Fitting of spectacle mounted low vision aid; single element system**
0.38 0.38 **FUD** XXX
AMA: 2018,Feb,11; 2018,Jan,8; 2017,Jan,8; 2016,Jan,13; 2015,Jan,16; 2014,Jan,11

92355 **telescopic or other compound lens system**
0.59 0.59 **FUD** XXX
AMA: 2018,Feb,11; 2018,Jan,8; 2017,Jan,8; 2016,Jan,13; 2015,Jan,16; 2014,Jan,11

92358 **Prosthesis service for aphakia, temporary (disposable or loan, including materials)**
0.32 0.32 **FUD** XXX
AMA: 2018,Feb,11; 2018,Jan,8; 2017,Jan,8; 2016,Jan,13; 2015,Jan,16; 2014,Jan,11

92370 **Repair and refitting spectacles; except for aphakia**
0.46 0.88 **FUD** XXX
AMA: 2018,Feb,11; 2018,Jan,8; 2017,Jan,8; 2016,Jan,13; 2015,Jan,16; 2014,Jan,11

92371 **spectacle prosthesis for aphakia**
0.33 0.33 **FUD** XXX
AMA: 2018,Feb,11; 2018,Jan,8; 2017,Jan,8; 2016,Jan,13; 2015,Jan,16; 2014,Jan,11

92499 **Unlisted ophthalmological service or procedure**
0.00 0.00 **FUD** XXX
AMA: 2019,Jan,12; 2018,Jul,3; 2018,Feb,11; 2018,Jan,8; 2017,Jan,8; 2016,Jan,13; 2015,Jan,16; 2014,Jan,11

92502-92526 Special Procedures of the Ears/Nose/Throat

INCLUDES Anterior rhinoscopy, tuning fork testing, otoscopy, or removal non-impacted cerumen
Diagnostic/treatment services not generally included in an E&M service

EXCLUDES *Laryngoscopy with stroboscopy (31579)*

92502 **Otolaryngologic examination under general anesthesia**
2.73 2.73 **FUD** 000
AMA: 2018,Feb,11; 2018,Jan,8; 2017,Jan,8; 2016,Sep,6

92504 **Binocular microscopy (separate diagnostic procedure)**
0.27 0.83 **FUD** XXX
AMA: 2018,Feb,11; 2018,Jan,8; 2017,Jan,8; 2016,Sep,6; 2016,Jan,13; 2015,Jan,16; 2014,Jan,11

92507 **Treatment of speech, language, voice, communication, and/or auditory processing disorder; individual**

EXCLUDES *Adaptive behavior treatment ([97153], [97155])*
Auditory rehabilitation:
Postlingual hearing loss (92633)
Prelingual hearing loss (92630)
Programming of cochlear implant (92601-92604)

2.23 2.23 **FUD** XXX
AMA: 2018,Dec,7; 2018,Dec,7; 2018,Nov,3; 2018,Feb,11; 2018,Jan,8; 2017,Jan,8; 2016,Sep,6; 2016,Jan,13; 2015,Jan,16; 2014,Jan,11

92508 **group, 2 or more individuals**

EXCLUDES *Adaptive behavior treatment ([97154], [97158])*
Auditory rehabilitation:
Postlingual hearing loss (92633)
Prelingual hearing loss (92630)
Programming of cochlear implant (92601-92604)

0.67 0.67 **FUD** XXX
AMA: 2018,Nov,3; 2018,Feb,11; 2018,Jan,8; 2017,Jan,8; 2016,Sep,6; 2016,Jan,13; 2015,Jan,16; 2014,Jun,3; 2014,Jan,11

92511 **Nasopharyngoscopy with endoscope (separate procedure)**

EXCLUDES *Diagnostic flexible laryngoscopy (31575)*
Transnasal esophagoscopy (43197-43198)

1.08 3.15 **FUD** 000
AMA: 2018,Feb,11; 2018,Jan,8; 2017,Jul,7; 2017,Jan,8; 2016,Dec,13; 2016,Sep,6

92512 **Nasal function studies (eg, rhinomanometry)**
0.80 1.68 **FUD** XXX
AMA: 2018,Feb,11; 2018,Jan,8; 2017,Jan,8; 2016,Sep,6

92516 **Facial nerve function studies (eg, electroneuronography)**
0.65 1.94 **FUD** XXX
AMA: 2018,Feb,11; 2018,Jan,8; 2017,Jan,8; 2016,Sep,6

92520 **Laryngeal function studies (ie, aerodynamic testing and acoustic testing)**

EXCLUDES *Other laryngeal function testing (92700)*
Swallowing/laryngeal sensory testing with flexible fiberoptic endoscope (92611-92617)

Code also modifier 52 for single test

1.15 2.23 FUD XXX

AMA: 2018,Feb,11; 2018,Jan,8; 2017,Jan,8; 2016,Sep,6; 2016,Jan,13; 2015,Jan,16; 2014,Jan,11

92521 **Evaluation of speech fluency (eg, stuttering, cluttering)**

INCLUDES Ability to execute motor movements needed for speech
Comprehension of written and verbal expression
Determination of patient's ability to create and communicate expressive thought
Evaluation of the ability to produce speech sound

3.21 3.21 FUD XXX

AMA: 2018,Feb,11; 2018,Jan,8; 2017,Jan,8; 2016,Sep,6; 2016,Jan,13; 2015,Jan,16; 2014,Jun,3

92522 **Evaluation of speech sound production (eg, articulation, phonological process, apraxia, dysarthria);**

INCLUDES Ability to execute motor movements needed for speech
Comprehension of written and verbal expression
Determination of patient's ability to create and communicate expressive thought
Evaluation of the ability to produce speech sound

2.60 2.60 FUD XXX

AMA: 2018,Feb,11; 2018,Jan,8; 2017,Jan,8; 2016,Sep,6; 2016,Jan,13; 2015,Jan,16; 2014,Jun,3

92523 **with evaluation of language comprehension and expression (eg, receptive and expressive language)**

INCLUDES Ability to execute motor movements needed for speech
Comprehension of written and verbal expression
Determination of patient's ability to create and communicate expressive thought
Evaluation of the ability to produce speech sound

5.54 5.54 FUD XXX

AMA: 2018,Feb,11; 2018,Jan,8; 2017,Jan,8; 2016,Sep,6; 2016,Jan,13; 2015,Jan,16; 2014,Jun,3

92524 **Behavioral and qualitative analysis of voice and resonance**

INCLUDES Ability to execute motor movements needed for speech
Comprehension of written and verbal expression
Determination of patient's ability to create and communicate expressive thought
Evaluation of the ability to produce speech sound

2.51 2.51 FUD XXX

AMA: 2018,Feb,11; 2018,Jan,8; 2017,Jan,8; 2016,Sep,6; 2016,Jan,13; 2015,Jan,16; 2014,Jun,3

92526 **Treatment of swallowing dysfunction and/or oral function for feeding**

2.44 2.44 FUD XXX

AMA: 2018,Feb,11; 2018,Jan,8; 2017,Jan,8; 2016,Sep,6

92531-92549 Vestibular Function Tests

92531 **Spontaneous nystagmus, including gaze**

EXCLUDES *When performed with E&M services (99201-99215, 99218-99223 [99224, 99225, 99226], 99231-99236, 99241-99245, 99304-99318, 99324-99337)*

0.00 0.00 FUD XXX

AMA: 2018,Feb,11

92532 **Positional nystagmus test**

EXCLUDES *When performed with E&M services (99201-99215, 99218-99223 [99224, 99225, 99226], 99231-99236, 99241-99245, 99304-99318, 99324-99337)*

0.00 0.00 FUD XXX

AMA: 2018,Feb,11

92533 **Caloric vestibular test, each irrigation (binaural, bithermal stimulation constitutes 4 tests)**

INCLUDES Barany caloric test

0.00 0.00 FUD XXX

AMA: 2018,Feb,11; 2018,Jan,8; 2017,Jan,8; 2016,Jan,13; 2015,Jan,16; 2014,Jan,11

92534 **Optokinetic nystagmus test**

0.00 0.00 FUD XXX

AMA: 2018,Feb,11

92537 **Caloric vestibular test with recording, bilateral; bithermal (ie, one warm and one cool irrigation in each ear for a total of four irrigations)**

EXCLUDES *Electro-oculography (92270)*
Monothermal caloric vestibular test (92538)

Code also modifier 52 when only three irrigations are performed

1.16 1.16 FUD XXX

AMA: 2018,Feb,11; 2015,Sep,7

92538 **monothermal (ie, one irrigation in each ear for a total of two irrigations)**

EXCLUDES *Electro-oculography (92270)*
Monothermal caloric vestibular test (92538)

Code also modifier 52 if only one irrigation is performed

0.60 0.60 FUD XXX

AMA: 2018,Feb,11; 2015,Sep,7

92540 **Basic vestibular evaluation, includes spontaneous nystagmus test with eccentric gaze fixation nystagmus, with recording, positional nystagmus test, minimum of 4 positions, with recording, optokinetic nystagmus test, bidirectional foveal and peripheral stimulation, with recording, and oscillating tracking test, with recording**

EXCLUDES *Vestibular function tests (92270, 92541-92542, 92544-92545)*

2.95 2.95 FUD XXX

AMA: 2018,Feb,11; 2018,Jan,8; 2017,Jan,8; 2016,Jan,13; 2015,Sep,7

92541 **Spontaneous nystagmus test, including gaze and fixation nystagmus, with recording**

EXCLUDES *Vestibular function tests (92270, 92540, 92542, 92544-92545)*

0.71 0.71 FUD XXX

AMA: 2019,Jan,12; 2018,Feb,11; 2018,Jan,8; 2017,Jan,8; 2016,Jan,13; 2015,Sep,7; 2015,Jan,16; 2014,Jan,11

92542 **Positional nystagmus test, minimum of 4 positions, with recording**

EXCLUDES *Vestibular function tests (92270, 92540-92541, 92544-92545)*

0.82 0.82 FUD XXX

AMA: 2018,Feb,11; 2018,Jan,8; 2017,Jan,8; 2016,Jan,13; 2015,Sep,7; 2015,Jan,16; 2014,Jan,11

92544 **Optokinetic nystagmus test, bidirectional, foveal or peripheral stimulation, with recording**

EXCLUDES *Vestibular function tests (92270, 92540-92542, 92545)*

0.49 0.49 FUD XXX

AMA: 2018,Feb,11; 2018,Jan,8; 2017,Jan,8; 2016,Jan,13; 2015,Sep,7; 2015,Jan,16; 2014,Jan,11

92545 **Oscillating tracking test, with recording**

EXCLUDES *Vestibular function tests (92270, 92540-92542, 92544)*

0.46 0.46 FUD XXX

AMA: 2018,Feb,11; 2018,Jan,8; 2017,Jan,8; 2016,Jan,13; 2015,Sep,7; 2015,Jan,16; 2014,Jan,11

92546 **Sinusoidal vertical axis rotational testing**

EXCLUDES *Electro-oculography (92270)*

2.95 2.95 FUD XXX

AMA: 2018,Feb,11; 2018,Jan,8; 2017,Jan,8; 2016,Jan,13; 2015,Sep,7; 2015,Jan,16; 2014,Jan,11

\+ **92547** **Use of vertical electrodes (List separately in addition to code for primary procedure)**

EXCLUDES *Electro-oculography (92700)*

Code first (92540-92546)

0.21 0.21 FUD ZZZ N 80 TC

AMA: 2018,Feb,11; 2018,Jan,8; 2017,Jan,8; 2016,Jan,13; 2015,Sep,7; 2015,Jan,16; 2014,Jan,11

▲ **92548** **Computerized dynamic posturography sensory organization test (CDP-SOT), 6 conditions (ie, eyes open, eyes closed, visual sway, platform sway, eyes closed platform sway, platform and visual sway), including interpretation and report;**

EXCLUDES *Electro-oculography (92270)*

2.72 2.72 FUD XXX Q1 80

AMA: 2018,Feb,11; 2018,Jan,8; 2017,Jan,8; 2016,Jan,13; 2015,Sep,7; 2015,Jan,16; 2014,Jan,11

● **92549** **with motor control test (MCT) and adaptation test (ADT)**

EXCLUDES *Electro-oculography (92270)*

92550-92597 [92558] Hearing and Speech Tests

INCLUDES Diagnostic/treatment services not generally included in a comprehensive otorhinolaryngologic evaluation or office visit

Testing of both ears

Tuning fork and whisper tests

Use of calibrated electronic equipment, recording of results, and a report with interpretation

EXCLUDES *Evaluation of speech/language/hearing problems using observation/assessment of performance (92521-92524)*

Code also modifier 52 for unilateral testing

92550 **Tympanometry and reflex threshold measurements**

INCLUDES Tympanometry, acoustic reflex testing individual codes (92567-92568)

0.62 0.62 FUD XXX Q1 80

AMA: 2018,Feb,11; 2018,Jan,8; 2017,Jan,8; 2016,Jan,13; 2015,Jan,16; 2014,Aug,3

92551 **Screening test, pure tone, air only**

0.33 0.33 FUD XXX E

AMA: 2018,Feb,11; 2018,Jan,8; 2017,Jan,8; 2016,Jan,13; 2015,Jan,16; 2014,Aug,3

92552 **Pure tone audiometry (threshold); air only**

EXCLUDES *Automated test (0208T)*

0.89 0.89 FUD XXX Q1 80 TC

AMA: 2018,Feb,11; 2018,Jan,8; 2017,Jan,8; 2016,Jan,13; 2015,Jan,16; 2014,Aug,3

92553 **air and bone**

EXCLUDES *Automated test (0209T)*

1.08 1.08 FUD XXX Q1 80 TC

AMA: 2018,Feb,11; 2018,Jan,8; 2017,Jan,8; 2016,Jan,13; 2015,Jan,16; 2014,Aug,3; 2014,Jan,11

92555 **Speech audiometry threshold;**

EXCLUDES *Automated test (0210T)*

0.68 0.68 FUD XXX Q1 80 TC

AMA: 2018,Feb,11; 2018,Jan,8; 2017,Jan,8; 2016,Jan,13; 2015,Jan,16; 2014,Aug,3

92556 **with speech recognition**

EXCLUDES *Automated test (0211T)*

1.07 1.07 FUD XXX Q1 80 TC

AMA: 2018,Feb,11; 2018,Jan,8; 2017,Jan,8; 2016,Jan,13; 2015,Jan,16; 2014,Aug,3; 2014,Jan,11

92557 **Comprehensive audiometry threshold evaluation and speech recognition (92553 and 92556 combined)**

EXCLUDES *Automated test (0208T-0212T)*

Evaluation/selection of hearing aid (92590-92595)

0.93 1.08 FUD XXX Q1 80

AMA: 2018,Feb,11; 2018,Jan,8; 2017,Jan,8; 2016,Jan,13; 2015,Jan,16; 2014,Aug,3; 2014,Jan,11

92558 **Resequenced code. See code following 92586.**

92559 **Audiometric testing of groups**

INCLUDES For group testing, indicate tests performed

0.00 0.00 FUD XXX E

AMA: 2018,Feb,11; 2018,Jan,8; 2017,Jan,8; 2016,Jan,13; 2015,Jan,16; 2014,Aug,3

92560 **Bekesy audiometry; screening**

0.00 0.00 FUD XXX E

AMA: 2018,Feb,11; 2018,Jan,8; 2017,Jan,8; 2016,Jan,13; 2015,Jan,16; 2014,Aug,3

92561 **diagnostic**

1.10 1.10 FUD XXX Q1 80 TC

AMA: 2018,Feb,11; 2018,Jan,8; 2017,Jan,8; 2016,Jan,13; 2015,Jan,16; 2014,Aug,3

92562 **Loudness balance test, alternate binaural or monaural**

INCLUDES ABLB test

1.28 1.28 FUD XXX Q1 80 TC

AMA: 2018,Feb,11; 2018,Jan,8; 2017,Jan,8; 2016,Jan,13; 2015,Jan,16; 2014,Aug,3

92563 **Tone decay test**

0.87 0.87 FUD XXX Q1 80 TC

AMA: 2018,Feb,11; 2018,Jan,8; 2017,Jan,8; 2016,Jan,13; 2015,Jan,16; 2014,Aug,3

92564 **Short increment sensitivity index (SISI)**

0.71 0.71 FUD XXX Q1 80 TC

AMA: 2018,Feb,11; 2018,Jan,8; 2017,Jan,8; 2016,Jan,13; 2015,Jan,16; 2014,Aug,3; 2014,Jan,11

92565 **Stenger test, pure tone**

0.43 0.43 FUD XXX Q1 80 TC

AMA: 2018,Feb,11; 2018,Jan,8; 2017,Jan,8; 2016,Jan,13; 2015,Jan,16; 2014,Aug,3

92567 **Tympanometry (impedance testing)**

0.31 0.43 FUD XXX Q1 80

AMA: 2018,Feb,11; 2018,Jan,8; 2017,Jan,8; 2016,Jan,13; 2015,Jan,16; 2014,Aug,3; 2014,Jan,11

92568 **Acoustic reflex testing, threshold**

0.44 0.45 FUD XXX Q1 80

AMA: 2018,Feb,11; 2018,Jan,8; 2017,Jan,8; 2016,Jan,13; 2015,Jan,16; 2014,Aug,3; 2014,Jan,11

92570 **Acoustic immittance testing, includes tympanometry (impedance testing), acoustic reflex threshold testing, and acoustic reflex decay testing**

INCLUDES Tympanometry, acoustic reflex testing individual codes (92567-92568)

0.85 0.92 FUD XXX Q1 80

AMA: 2018,Feb,11; 2018,Jan,8; 2017,Jan,8; 2016,Jan,13; 2015,Jan,16; 2014,Aug,3

92571 **Filtered speech test**

0.76 0.76 FUD XXX Q1 80 TC

AMA: 2018,Feb,11; 2018,Jan,8; 2017,Jan,8; 2016,Jan,13; 2015,Jan,16; 2014,Aug,3; 2014,Jan,11

92572 **Staggered spondaic word test**

1.21 1.21 FUD XXX Q1 80 TC

AMA: 2018,Feb,11; 2018,Jan,8; 2017,Jan,8; 2016,Jan,13; 2015,Jan,16; 2014,Aug,3; 2014,Jan,11

92575 **Sensorineural acuity level test**

1.79 1.79 FUD XXX Q1 80 TC

AMA: 2018,Feb,11; 2018,Jan,8; 2017,Jan,8; 2016,Jan,13; 2015,Jan,16; 2014,Aug,3

92576 **Synthetic sentence identification test**

1.03 1.03 FUD XXX Q1 80 TC

AMA: 2018,Feb,11; 2018,Jan,8; 2017,Jan,8; 2016,Jan,13; 2015,Jan,16; 2014,Aug,3; 2014,Jan,11

92577 **Stenger test, speech**

0.39 0.39 FUD XXX Q1 80 TC

AMA: 2018,Feb,11; 2018,Jan,8; 2017,Jan,8; 2016,Jan,13; 2015,Jan,16; 2014,Aug,3

92579 **Visual reinforcement audiometry (VRA)**
1.09 1.31 FUD XXX Q1 80
AMA: 2018,Feb,11; 2018,Jan,8; 2017,Jan,8; 2016,Jan,13; 2015,Jan,16; 2014,Aug,3

92582 **Conditioning play audiometry**
2.06 2.06 FUD XXX Q1 80 TC
AMA: 2018,Feb,11; 2018,Jan,8; 2017,Jan,8; 2016,Jan,13; 2015,Jan,16; 2014,Aug,3

92583 **Select picture audiometry**
1.35 1.35 FUD XXX Q1 80 TC
AMA: 2018,Feb,11; 2018,Jan,8; 2017,Jan,8; 2016,Jan,13; 2015,Jan,16; 2014,Aug,3

92584 **Electrocochleography**
2.09 2.09 FUD XXX S 80 TC
AMA: 2018,Feb,11; 2018,Jan,8; 2017,Jan,8; 2016,Jan,13; 2015,Jan,16; 2014,Aug,3; 2014,Jan,11

92585 **Auditory evoked potentials for evoked response audiometry and/or testing of the central nervous system; comprehensive**
3.81 3.81 FUD XXX S 80
AMA: 2018,Feb,11; 2018,Jan,8; 2017,Jan,8; 2016,Jan,13; 2015,Jan,16; 2014,Aug,3

92586 **limited**
2.61 2.61 FUD XXX S 80 TC
AMA: 2018,Feb,11; 2018,Jan,8; 2017,Jan,8; 2016,Jan,13; 2015,Jan,16; 2014,Aug,3

\# **92558** **Evoked otoacoustic emissions, screening (qualitative measurement of distortion product or transient evoked otoacoustic emissions), automated analysis**
0.25 0.28 FUD XXX E
AMA: 2018,Feb,11; 2018,Jan,8; 2017,Jan,8; 2016,Jan,13; 2015,Jan,16; 2014,Aug,3

92587 **Distortion product evoked otoacoustic emissions; limited evaluation (to confirm the presence or absence of hearing disorder, 3-6 frequencies) or transient evoked otoacoustic emissions, with interpretation and report**
0.62 0.62 FUD XXX S 80
AMA: 2018,Feb,11; 2018,Jan,8; 2017,Jan,8; 2016,Jan,13; 2015,Jan,16; 2014,Aug,3; 2014,Jan,11

92588 **comprehensive diagnostic evaluation (quantitative analysis of outer hair cell function by cochlear mapping, minimum of 12 frequencies), with interpretation and report**
EXCLUDES *Evaluation of central auditory function (92620-92621)*
0.94 0.94 FUD XXX S 80
AMA: 2018,Feb,11; 2018,Jan,8; 2017,Jan,8; 2016,Jan,13; 2015,Jan,16; 2014,Aug,3

92590 **Hearing aid examination and selection; monaural**
0.00 0.00 FUD XXX E
AMA: 2018,Feb,11; 2018,Jan,8; 2017,Jan,8; 2016,Jan,13; 2015,Jan,16; 2014,Aug,3; 2014,Jul,4

92591 **binaural**
0.00 0.00 FUD XXX E
AMA: 2018,Feb,11; 2018,Jan,8; 2017,Jan,8; 2016,Jan,13; 2015,Jan,16; 2014,Aug,3

92592 **Hearing aid check; monaural**
0.00 0.00 FUD XXX E
AMA: 2018,Feb,11; 2018,Jan,8; 2017,Jan,8; 2016,Jan,13; 2015,Jan,16; 2014,Aug,3

92593 **binaural**
0.00 0.00 FUD XXX E
AMA: 2018,Feb,11; 2018,Jan,8; 2017,Jan,8; 2016,Jan,13; 2015,Jan,16; 2014,Aug,3

92594 **Electroacoustic evaluation for hearing aid; monaural**
0.00 0.00 FUD XXX E
AMA: 2018,Feb,11; 2018,Jan,8; 2017,Jan,8; 2016,Jan,13; 2015,Jan,16; 2014,Aug,3

92595 **binaural**
0.00 0.00 FUD XXX E
AMA: 2018,Feb,11; 2018,Jan,8; 2017,Jan,8; 2016,Jan,13; 2015,Jan,16; 2014,Aug,3

92596 **Ear protector attenuation measurements**
1.89 1.89 FUD XXX Q1 80 TC
AMA: 2018,Feb,11; 2018,Jan,8; 2017,Jan,8; 2016,Jan,13; 2015,Jan,16; 2014,Aug,3

92597 **Resequenced code. See code following 92604.**

92601-92609 [92597, 92618] Services Related to Hearing and Speech Devices

INCLUDES Diagnostic/treatment services not generally included in a comprehensive otorhinolaryngologic evaluation or office visit

92601 **Diagnostic analysis of cochlear implant, patient younger than 7 years of age; with programming** A
INCLUDES Connection to cochlear implant
Postoperative analysis/fitting of previously placed external devices
Stimulator programming
EXCLUDES *Cochlear implant placement (69930)*
3.57 4.68 FUD XXX S 80
AMA: 2018,Feb,11; 2018,Jan,8; 2017,Jan,8; 2016,Sep,6; 2016,Jan,13; 2015,Jan,16; 2014,Jul,4; 2014,Jan,11

92602 **subsequent reprogramming** A
INCLUDES Internal stimulator re-programming
Subsequent sessions for external transmitter measurements/adjustment
EXCLUDES *Analysis with programming (92601)*
Aural rehabilitation services after a cochlear implant (92626-92627, 92630-92633)
Cochlear implant placement (69930)
2.02 2.92 FUD XXX S 80
AMA: 2018,Feb,11; 2018,Jan,8; 2017,Jan,8; 2016,Sep,6; 2016,Jan,13; 2015,Jan,16; 2014,Jul,4; 2014,Jan,11

92603 **Diagnostic analysis of cochlear implant, age 7 years or older; with programming** A
INCLUDES Connection to cochlear implant
Post-operative analysis/fitting of previously placed external devices
Stimulator programming
EXCLUDES *Cochlear implant placement (69930)*
3.47 4.37 FUD XXX S 80
AMA: 2018,Feb,11; 2018,Jan,8; 2017,Jan,8; 2016,Sep,6; 2016,Jan,13; 2015,Jan,16; 2014,Jul,4; 2014,Jan,11

92604 **subsequent reprogramming** A
INCLUDES Internal stimulator re-programming
Subsequent sessions for external transmitter measurements/adjustment
EXCLUDES *Analysis with programming (92603)*
Cochlear implant placement (69930)
1.94 2.60 FUD XXX S 80
AMA: 2018,Feb,11; 2018,Jan,8; 2017,Jan,8; 2016,Sep,6; 2016,Jan,13; 2015,Jan,16; 2014,Jul,4; 2014,Jan,11

\# **92597** **Evaluation for use and/or fitting of voice prosthetic device to supplement oral speech**
EXCLUDES *Augmentative or alternative communication device services (92605, [92618], 92607-92608)*
2.06 2.06 FUD XXX A 80
AMA: 2018,Feb,11; 2018,Jan,8; 2017,Jan,8; 2016,Jan,13; 2015,Jan,16; 2014,Jan,11

92605 **Evaluation for prescription of non-speech-generating augmentative and alternative communication device, face-to-face with the patient; first hour**
EXCLUDES *Prosthetic voice device fitting or use evaluation (92597)*
2.53 2.65 FUD XXX A
AMA: 2018,Feb,11; 2018,Jan,8; 2017,Jan,8; 2016,Jan,13; 2015,Jan,16; 2014,Jan,11

+ # **92618** **each additional 30 minutes (List separately in addition to code for primary procedure)**

Code first (92605)

0.94 0.96 FUD ZZZ A

AMA: 2018,Feb,11

92606 **Therapeutic service(s) for the use of non-speech-generating device, including programming and modification**

2.02 2.35 FUD XXX A

AMA: 2018,Feb,11; 2018,Jan,8; 2017,Jan,8; 2016,Jan,13; 2015,Jan,16; 2014,Jan,11

92607 **Evaluation for prescription for speech-generating augmentative and alternative communication device, face-to-face with the patient; first hour**

EXCLUDES *Evaluation for prescription of non-speech generating device (92605)*

Evaluation for use/fitting of voice prosthetic (92597)

3.69 3.69 FUD XXX A 80

AMA: 2018,Feb,11; 2018,Jan,8; 2017,Jan,8; 2016,Jan,13; 2015,Jan,16; 2014,Jan,11

+ **92608** **each additional 30 minutes (List separately in addition to code for primary procedure)**

Code first initial hour (92607)

1.47 1.47 FUD ZZZ A 80

AMA: 2018,Feb,11; 2018,Jan,8; 2017,Jan,8; 2016,Jan,13; 2015,Jan,16; 2014,Jan,11

92609 **Therapeutic services for the use of speech-generating device, including programming and modification**

EXCLUDES *Therapeutic services for use of non-speech generating device (92606)*

3.08 3.08 FUD XXX A 80

AMA: 2018,Feb,11; 2018,Jan,8; 2017,Jan,8; 2016,Jan,13; 2015,Jan,16; 2014,Jan,11

92610-92618 Swallowing Evaluations

92610 **Evaluation of oral and pharyngeal swallowing function**

EXCLUDES *Evaluation with flexible endoscope (92612-92617)*

Motion fluoroscopic evaluation of swallowing function (92611)

2.06 2.45 FUD XXX A 80

AMA: 2018,Feb,11; 2018,Jan,8; 2017,Apr,8; 2017,Jan,8; 2016,Jan,13; 2015,Jan,16; 2014,Jan,11

92611 **Motion fluoroscopic evaluation of swallowing function by cine or video recording**

EXCLUDES *Diagnostic flexible laryngoscopy (31575)*

Evaluation of oral/pharyngeal swallowing function (92610)

(74230)

2.55 2.55 FUD XXX A 80

AMA: 2018,Feb,11; 2018,Jan,8; 2017,Apr,8; 2017,Jan,8; 2016,Sep,6; 2016,Jan,13; 2015,Jan,16; 2014,Jul,5; 2014,Jan,11

92612 **Flexible endoscopic evaluation of swallowing by cine or video recording;**

EXCLUDES *Diagnostic flexible fiberoptic laryngoscopy (31575)*

Flexible endoscopic examination/testing without cine or video recording (92700)

1.94 5.42 FUD XXX A 80

AMA: 2018,Feb,11; 2018,Jan,8; 2017,Jul,7; 2017,Apr,8; 2017,Jan,8; 2016,Dec,13; 2016,Sep,6; 2016,Jan,13; 2015,Jan,16; 2014,Jan,11

92613 **interpretation and report only**

EXCLUDES *Diagnostic flexible laryngoscopy (31575)*

Oral/pharyngeal swallowing function examination (92610)

Swallowing function motion fluoroscopic examination (92611)

1.07 1.07 FUD XXX B 80

AMA: 2018,Feb,11; 2018,Jan,8; 2017,Jul,7; 2017,Apr,8; 2017,Jan,8; 2016,Dec,13; 2016,Sep,6; 2016,Jan,13; 2015,Jan,16; 2014,Jan,11

92614 **Flexible endoscopic evaluation, laryngeal sensory testing by cine or video recording;**

EXCLUDES *Diagnostic flexible laryngoscopy (31575)*

Flexible endoscopic examination/testing without cine or video recording (92700)

1.90 4.03 FUD XXX A 80

AMA: 2018,Feb,11; 2018,Jan,8; 2017,Jul,7; 2017,Apr,8; 2017,Jan,8; 2016,Dec,13; 2016,Sep,6; 2016,Jan,13; 2015,Jan,16; 2014,Jan,11

92615 **interpretation and report only**

EXCLUDES *Diagnostic flexible laryngoscopy (31575)*

0.94 0.94 FUD XXX E 80

AMA: 2018,Feb,11; 2018,Jan,8; 2017,Jul,7; 2017,Apr,8; 2017,Jan,8; 2016,Dec,13; 2016,Sep,6; 2016,Jan,13; 2015,Jan,16; 2014,Jan,11

92616 **Flexible endoscopic evaluation of swallowing and laryngeal sensory testing by cine or video recording;**

EXCLUDES *Diagnostic flexible fiberoptic laryngoscopy (31575)*

Flexible endoscopic examination/testing without cine or video recording (92700)

2.84 5.85 FUD XXX A 80

AMA: 2018,Feb,11; 2018,Jan,8; 2017,Jul,7; 2017,Apr,8; 2017,Jan,8; 2016,Dec,13; 2016,Sep,6; 2016,Jan,13; 2015,Jan,16; 2014,Jan,11

92617 **interpretation and report only**

EXCLUDES *Diagnostic flexible laryngoscopy (31575)*

1.18 1.18 FUD XXX E 80

AMA: 2018,Feb,11; 2018,Jan,8; 2017,Jul,7; 2017,Apr,8; 2017,Jan,8; 2016,Dec,13; 2016,Sep,6; 2016,Jan,13; 2015,Jan,16; 2014,Jan,11

92618 **Resequenced code. See code following 92605.**

92620-92700 Diagnostic Hearing Evaluations and Rehabilitation

INCLUDES Diagnostic/treatment services not generally included in a comprehensive otorhinolaryngologic evaluation or office visit

92620 **Evaluation of central auditory function, with report; initial 60 minutes**

EXCLUDES *Voice analysis (92521-92524)*

2.32 2.67 FUD XXX Q1 80

AMA: 2018,Feb,11; 2018,Jan,8; 2017,Jan,8; 2016,Jan,13; 2015,Jan,16; 2014,Aug,3

+ **92621** **each additional 15 minutes (List separately in addition to code for primary procedure)**

EXCLUDES *Voice analysis (92521-92524)*

Code first (92620)

0.54 0.64 FUD ZZZ N 80

AMA: 2018,Feb,11; 2018,Jan,8; 2017,Jan,8; 2016,Jan,13; 2015,Jan,16; 2014,Aug,3

92625 **Assessment of tinnitus (includes pitch, loudness matching, and masking)**

EXCLUDES *Loudness test (92562)*

Code also modifier 52 for unilateral procedure

1.78 1.99 FUD XXX Q1 80

AMA: 2018,Feb,11; 2018,Jan,8; 2017,Jan,8; 2016,Jan,13; 2015,Jan,16; 2014,Aug,3

▲ **92626** **Evaluation of auditory function for surgically implanted device(s) candidacy or postoperative status of a surgically implanted device(s); first hour**

INCLUDES Assessment to determine patient's proficiency in the use of remaining hearing to identify speech

Face-to-face time spent with the patient or family

EXCLUDES *Hearing aid evaluation, fitting, follow-up, or selection (92590-92591, 92592-92593, 92594-92595)*

2.16 2.55 FUD XXX Q1 80

AMA: 2018,Feb,11; 2018,Jan,8; 2017,Jan,8; 2016,Sep,6; 2016,Jan,13; 2015,Jan,16; 2014,Jul,4; 2014,May,10; 2014,Jan,11

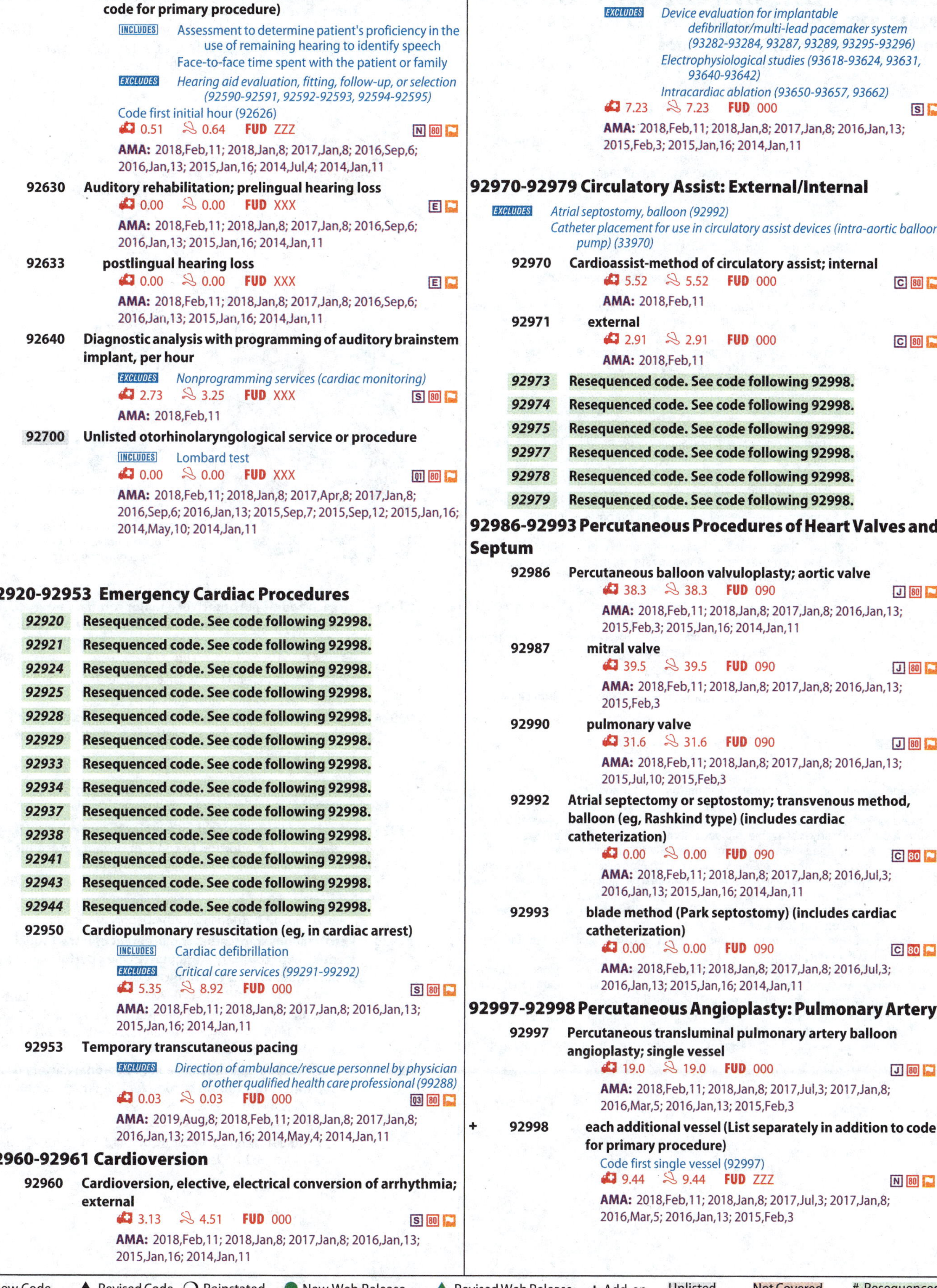

▲ + 92627 **each additional 15 minutes (List separately in addition to code for primary procedure)**

INCLUDES Assessment to determine patient's proficiency in the use of remaining hearing to identify speech
Face-to-face time spent with the patient or family

EXCLUDES *Hearing aid evaluation, fitting, follow-up, or selection (92590-92591, 92592-92593, 92594-92595)*

Code first initial hour (92626)

0.51 0.64 FUD ZZZ N 80

AMA: 2018,Feb,11; 2018,Jan,8; 2017,Jan,8; 2016,Sep,6; 2016,Jan,13; 2015,Jan,16; 2014,Jul,4; 2014,Jan,11

92630 **Auditory rehabilitation; prelingual hearing loss**

0.00 0.00 FUD XXX E

AMA: 2018,Feb,11; 2018,Jan,8; 2017,Jan,8; 2016,Sep,6; 2016,Jan,13; 2015,Jan,16; 2014,Jan,11

92633 **postlingual hearing loss**

0.00 0.00 FUD XXX E

AMA: 2018,Feb,11; 2018,Jan,8; 2017,Jan,8; 2016,Sep,6; 2016,Jan,13; 2015,Jan,16; 2014,Jan,11

92640 **Diagnostic analysis with programming of auditory brainstem implant, per hour**

EXCLUDES *Nonprogramming services (cardiac monitoring)*

2.73 3.25 FUD XXX S 80

AMA: 2018,Feb,11

92700 **Unlisted otorhinolaryngological service or procedure**

INCLUDES Lombard test

0.00 0.00 FUD XXX Q1 80

AMA: 2018,Feb,11; 2018,Jan,8; 2017,Apr,8; 2017,Jan,8; 2016,Sep,6; 2016,Jan,13; 2015,Sep,7; 2015,Sep,12; 2015,Jan,16; 2014,May,10; 2014,Jan,11

92920-92953 Emergency Cardiac Procedures

92920 **Resequenced code. See code following 92998.**

92921 **Resequenced code. See code following 92998.**

92924 **Resequenced code. See code following 92998.**

92925 **Resequenced code. See code following 92998.**

92928 **Resequenced code. See code following 92998.**

92929 **Resequenced code. See code following 92998.**

92933 **Resequenced code. See code following 92998.**

92934 **Resequenced code. See code following 92998.**

92937 **Resequenced code. See code following 92998.**

92938 **Resequenced code. See code following 92998.**

92941 **Resequenced code. See code following 92998.**

92943 **Resequenced code. See code following 92998.**

92944 **Resequenced code. See code following 92998.**

92950 **Cardiopulmonary resuscitation (eg, in cardiac arrest)**

INCLUDES Cardiac defibrillation

EXCLUDES *Critical care services (99291-99292)*

5.35 8.92 FUD 000 S 80

AMA: 2018,Feb,11; 2018,Jan,8; 2017,Jan,8; 2016,Jan,13; 2015,Jan,16; 2014,Jan,11

92953 **Temporary transcutaneous pacing**

EXCLUDES *Direction of ambulance/rescue personnel by physician or other qualified health care professional (99288)*

0.03 0.03 FUD 000 Q3 80

AMA: 2019,Aug,8; 2018,Feb,11; 2018,Jan,8; 2017,Jan,8; 2016,Jan,13; 2015,Jan,16; 2014,May,4; 2014,Jan,11

92960-92961 Cardioversion

92960 **Cardioversion, elective, electrical conversion of arrhythmia; external**

3.13 4.51 FUD 000 S 80

AMA: 2018,Feb,11; 2018,Jan,8; 2017,Jan,8; 2016,Jan,13; 2015,Jan,16; 2014,Jan,11

92961 **internal (separate procedure)**

EXCLUDES *Device evaluation for implantable defibrillator/multi-lead pacemaker system (93282-93284, 93287, 93289, 93295-93296)*
Electrophysiological studies (93618-93624, 93631, 93640-93642)
Intracardiac ablation (93650-93657, 93662)

7.23 7.23 FUD 000 S

AMA: 2018,Feb,11; 2018,Jan,8; 2017,Jan,8; 2016,Jan,13; 2015,Feb,3; 2015,Jan,16; 2014,Jan,11

92970-92979 Circulatory Assist: External/Internal

EXCLUDES *Atrial septostomy, balloon (92992)*
Catheter placement for use in circulatory assist devices (intra-aortic balloon pump) (33970)

92970 **Cardioassist-method of circulatory assist; internal**

5.52 5.52 FUD 000 C 80

AMA: 2018,Feb,11

92971 **external**

2.91 2.91 FUD 000 C 80

AMA: 2018,Feb,11

92973 **Resequenced code. See code following 92998.**

92974 **Resequenced code. See code following 92998.**

92975 **Resequenced code. See code following 92998.**

92977 **Resequenced code. See code following 92998.**

92978 **Resequenced code. See code following 92998.**

92979 **Resequenced code. See code following 92998.**

92986-92993 Percutaneous Procedures of Heart Valves and Septum

92986 **Percutaneous balloon valvuloplasty; aortic valve**

38.3 38.3 FUD 090 J 80

AMA: 2018,Feb,11; 2018,Jan,8; 2017,Jan,8; 2016,Jan,13; 2015,Feb,3; 2015,Jan,16; 2014,Jan,11

92987 **mitral valve**

39.5 39.5 FUD 090 J 80

AMA: 2018,Feb,11; 2018,Jan,8; 2017,Jan,8; 2016,Jan,13; 2015,Feb,3

92990 **pulmonary valve**

31.6 31.6 FUD 090 J 80

AMA: 2018,Feb,11; 2018,Jan,8; 2017,Jan,8; 2016,Jan,13; 2015,Jul,10; 2015,Feb,3

92992 **Atrial septectomy or septostomy; transvenous method, balloon (eg, Rashkind type) (includes cardiac catheterization)**

0.00 0.00 FUD 090 C 80

AMA: 2018,Feb,11; 2018,Jan,8; 2017,Jan,8; 2016,Jul,3; 2016,Jan,13; 2015,Jan,16; 2014,Jan,11

92993 **blade method (Park septostomy) (includes cardiac catheterization)**

0.00 0.00 FUD 090 C 80

AMA: 2018,Feb,11; 2018,Jan,8; 2017,Jan,8; 2016,Jul,3; 2016,Jan,13; 2015,Jan,16; 2014,Jan,11

92997-92998 Percutaneous Angioplasty: Pulmonary Artery

92997 **Percutaneous transluminal pulmonary artery balloon angioplasty; single vessel**

19.0 19.0 FUD 000 J 80

AMA: 2018,Feb,11; 2018,Jan,8; 2017,Jul,3; 2017,Jan,8; 2016,Mar,5; 2016,Jan,13; 2015,Feb,3

\+ 92998 **each additional vessel (List separately in addition to code for primary procedure)**

Code first single vessel (92997)

9.44 9.44 FUD ZZZ N 80

AMA: 2018,Feb,11; 2018,Jan,8; 2017,Jul,3; 2017,Jan,8; 2016,Mar,5; 2016,Jan,13; 2015,Feb,3

92920-92944 [92920, 92921, 92924, 92925, 92928, 92929, 92933, 92934, 92937, 92938, 92941, 92943, 92944]

Intravascular Coronary Procedures

Additional procedures performed in a third branch of a major coronary artery

INCLUDES Accessing the vessel
All procedures performed in all segments of branches of coronary arteries
Branches of left anterior descending (diagonals), left circumflex (marginals), and right (posterior descending, posterolaterals)
Distal, proximal, and mid segments
All procedures performed in all segments of major coronary arteries through the native vessels:
Distal, proximal, and mid segments
Left main, left anterior descending, left circumflex, right, and ramus intermedius arteries
All procedures performed in major coronary arteries or recognized coronary artery branches through a coronary artery bypass graft
A sequential bypass graft with more than a single distal anastomosis as one graft
Branching bypass grafts (eg, "Y" grafts) include a coronary vessel for the primary graft, with each branch off the primary graft making up an additional coronary vessel
Each coronary artery bypass graft denotes a single coronary vessel
Embolic protection devices when used
Arteriotomy closure through the access sheath
Atherectomy (eg, directional, laser, rotational)
Balloon angioplasty (eg, cryoplasty, cutting balloon, wired balloons)
Cardiac catheterization and related procedures when included in the coronary revascularization service (93454-93461, 93563-93564)
Imaging once procedure is complete
Percutaneous coronary interventions (PCI) for disease of coronary vessels, native and bypass grafts
Procedures in branches of the left main and ramus intermedius coronary arteries as they are unrecognized for purposes of individual code assignment
Radiological supervision and interpretation of intervention(s)
Reporting the most comprehensive treatment in a given vessel according to a hierarchy of intensity for the base and add-on codes:
Add-on codes: 92944 = 92938 > 92934 > 92925 > 92929 > 92921
Base codes (report only one): 92943 = 92941 = 92933 > 92924 > 92937 = 92928 > 92920
Revascularization achieved with a single procedure when a single lesion continues from one target vessel (major artery, branch, or bypass graft) to ...
Selective vessel catheterization
Stenting (eg, balloon expandable, bare metal, covered, drug eluting, self-expanding)
Traversing of the lesion

EXCLUDES *Application of intravascular radioelements (77770-77772)*
Insertion of device for coronary intravascular brachytherapy (92974)
Reduction of septum (eg, alcohol ablation) (93799)

Code also add-on codes for procedures performed during the same session in additional recognized branches of the target vessel
Code also diagnostic angiography at the time of the interventional procedure when:
A previous study is available, but documentation states the patient's condition has changed since the previous study or visualization of the anatomy/pathology is inadequate, or a change occurs during the procedure warranting additional evaluation of an area outside the current target area
No previous catheter-based coronary angiography study is available, and a full diagnostic study is performed, with the decision to perform the intervention based on that study, or
Code also diagnostic angiography performed at a session separate from the interventional procedure
Code also individual base codes for treatment of a segment of a major native coronary artery and another segment of the same artery that requires treatment through a bypass graft when performed at the same time
Code also procedures for both vessels for a bifurcation lesion
Code also procedures performed in second branch of a major coronary artery
Code also treatment of arterial segment requiring access through a bypass graft

\# **92920** **Percutaneous transluminal coronary angioplasty; single major coronary artery or branch**
15.4 15.4 FUD 000 J 80
AMA: 2018,Feb,11; 2018,Jan,8; 2017,Jul,3; 2017,Jan,8; 2016,Jan,13; 2015,Jan,16; 2014,Dec,6

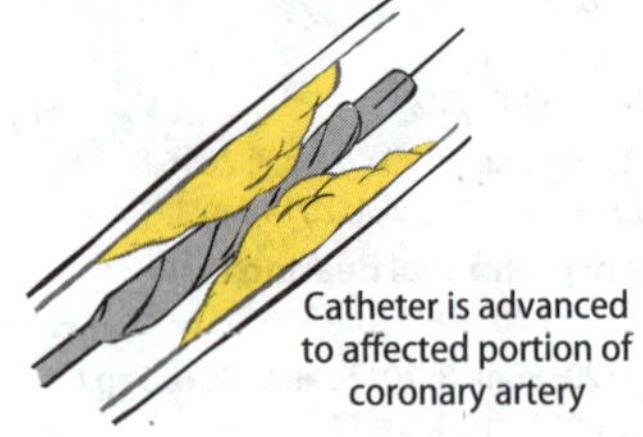

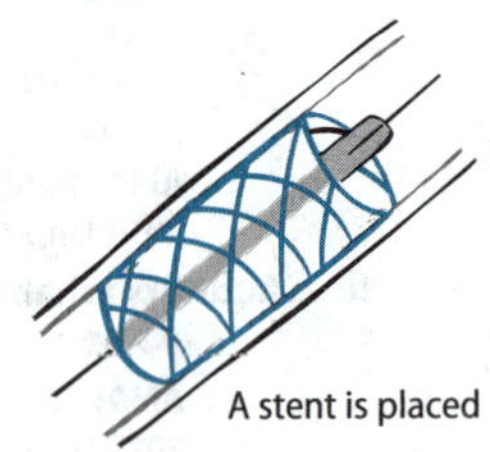

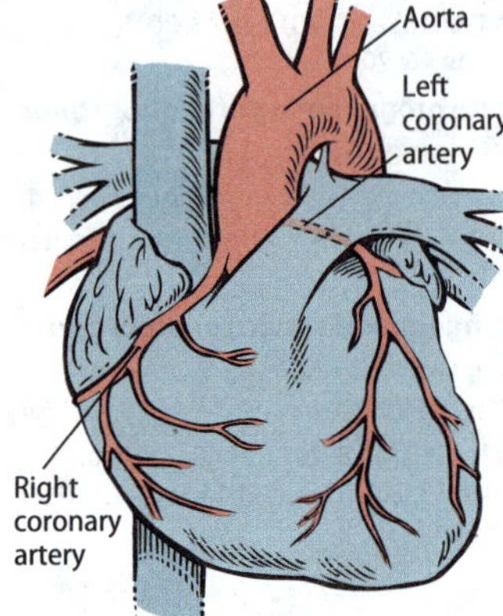

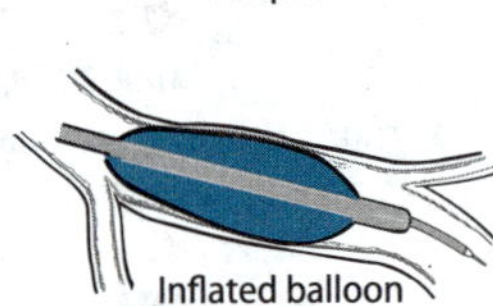

A balloon may be inflated or other intravascular therapy may accompany the procedure

\+ # **92921** **each additional branch of a major coronary artery (List separately in addition to code for primary procedure)**
Code first (92920, 92924, 92928, 92933, 92937, 92941, 92943)
0.00 0.00 FUD ZZZ N
AMA: 2018,Feb,11; 2018,Jan,8; 2017,Jul,3; 2017,Jan,8; 2016,Jan,13; 2015,Jan,16; 2014,Dec,6; 2014,Sep,13

\# **92924** **Percutaneous transluminal coronary atherectomy, with coronary angioplasty when performed; single major coronary artery or branch**
18.4 18.4 FUD 000 J 80
AMA: 2018,Feb,11; 2018,Jan,8; 2017,Jul,3; 2017,Jan,8; 2016,Jan,13; 2015,Jan,16; 2014,Dec,6

\+ # **92925** **each additional branch of a major coronary artery (List separately in addition to code for primary procedure)**
Code first (92924, 92928, 92933, 92937, 92941, 92943)
0.00 0.00 FUD ZZZ N
AMA: 2018,Feb,11; 2018,Jan,8; 2017,Jul,3; 2017,Jan,8; 2016,Jan,13; 2015,Jan,16; 2014,Dec,6; 2014,Sep,13

\# **92928** **Percutaneous transcatheter placement of intracoronary stent(s), with coronary angioplasty when performed; single major coronary artery or branch**
17.2 17.2 FUD 000 J 80
AMA: 2018,Feb,11; 2018,Jan,8; 2017,Jul,3; 2017,Feb,14; 2017,Jan,8; 2017,Jan,6; 2016,Jan,13; 2015,Jan,16; 2014,Dec,6; 2014,Sep,13; 2014,Mar,13; 2014,Jan,3

\+ # **92929** **each additional branch of a major coronary artery (List separately in addition to code for primary procedure)**
Code first (92928, 92933, 92937, 92941, 92943)
0.00 0.00 FUD ZZZ N
AMA: 2018,Feb,11; 2018,Jan,8; 2017,Jul,3; 2017,Jan,8; 2017,Jan,6; 2016,Jan,13; 2015,Jan,16; 2014,Dec,6; 2014,Sep,13

92933 **Percutaneous transluminal coronary atherectomy, with intracoronary stent, with coronary angioplasty when performed; single major coronary artery or branch**
19.3 19.3 FUD 000 J 80
AMA: 2018,Feb,11; 2018,Jan,8; 2017,Jul,3; 2017,Jan,8; 2016,Jan,13; 2015,Jan,16; 2014,Dec,6

+ # 92934 **each additional branch of a major coronary artery (List separately in addition to code for primary procedure)**
Code first (92933, 92937, 92941, 92943)
0.00 0.00 FUD ZZZ N
AMA: 2018,Feb,11; 2018,Jan,8; 2017,Jul,3; 2017,Jan,8; 2016,Jan,13; 2015,Jan,16; 2014,Dec,6; 2014,Sep,13

92937 **Percutaneous transluminal revascularization of or through coronary artery bypass graft (internal mammary, free arterial, venous), any combination of intracoronary stent, atherectomy and angioplasty, including distal protection when performed; single vessel**
17.2 17.2 FUD 000 J 80
AMA: 2018,Feb,11; 2018,Jan,8; 2017,Jul,3; 2017,Feb,14; 2017,Jan,8; 2016,Jan,13; 2015,Jan,16; 2014,Dec,6; 2014,Mar,13

+ # 92938 **each additional branch subtended by the bypass graft (List separately in addition to code for primary procedure)**
Code first (92937)
0.00 0.00 FUD ZZZ N
AMA: 2018,Feb,11; 2018,Jan,8; 2017,Jul,3; 2017,Jan,8; 2016,Jan,13; 2015,Jan,16; 2014,Dec,6; 2014,Sep,13; 2014,Mar,13

92941 **Percutaneous transluminal revascularization of acute total/subtotal occlusion during acute myocardial infarction, coronary artery or coronary artery bypass graft, any combination of intracoronary stent, atherectomy and angioplasty, including aspiration thrombectomy when performed, single vessel**
INCLUDES Aspiration thrombectomy, when performed
Embolic protection
Rheolytic thrombectomy
Code also treatment of additional vessels, when appropriate (92920-92938, 92943-92944)
19.3 19.3 FUD 000 C 80
AMA: 2018,Feb,11; 2018,Jan,8; 2017,Jul,3; 2017,Feb,14; 2017,Jan,8; 2016,Jan,13; 2015,Jan,16; 2014,Dec,6; 2014,Mar,13; 2014,Jan,3

92943 **Percutaneous transluminal revascularization of chronic total occlusion, coronary artery, coronary artery branch, or coronary artery bypass graft, any combination of intracoronary stent, atherectomy and angioplasty; single vessel**
INCLUDES Lack of antegrade flow with angiography and clinical criteria indicative of chronic total occlusion
19.3 19.3 FUD 000 J 80
AMA: 2018,Feb,11; 2018,Jan,8; 2017,Jul,3; 2017,Jan,8; 2016,Jan,13; 2015,Jan,16; 2014,Dec,6

+ # 92944 **each additional coronary artery, coronary artery branch, or bypass graft (List separately in addition to code for primary procedure)**
EXCLUDES *Application of intravascular radioelements (77770-77772)*
Code first (92924, 92928, 92933, 92937, 92941, 92943)
0.00 0.00 FUD ZZZ N
AMA: 2018,Feb,11; 2018,Jan,8; 2017,Jul,3; 2017,Jan,8; 2016,Jan,13; 2015,Jan,16; 2014,Dec,6; 2014,Sep,13

92973-92979 [92973, 92974, 92975, 92977, 92978, 92979] Additional Coronary Artery Procedures

+ # 92973 **Percutaneous transluminal coronary thrombectomy mechanical (List separately in addition to code for primary procedure)**
EXCLUDES *Aspiration thrombectomy*
Code first (92920, 92924, 92928, 92933, 92937, 92941, 92943, 92975, 93454-93461, 93563-93564)
5.15 5.15 FUD ZZZ N 80
AMA: 2018,Feb,11; 2018,Jan,8; 2017,Feb,14; 2017,Jan,8; 2016,Jan,13; 2015,Jan,16; 2014,Dec,6; 2014,Jan,11

+ # 92974 **Transcatheter placement of radiation delivery device for subsequent coronary intravascular brachytherapy (List separately in addition to code for primary procedure)**
EXCLUDES *Application of intravascular radioelements (77770-77772)*
Code first (92920, 92924, 92928, 92933, 92937, 92941, 92943, 93454-93461)
4.72 4.72 FUD ZZZ N 80
AMA: 2018,Feb,11; 2018,Jan,8; 2017,Feb,14; 2017,Jan,8; 2016,Jan,13; 2015,Jan,16; 2014,Dec,6; 2014,Jan,11

92975 **Thrombolysis, coronary; by intracoronary infusion, including selective coronary angiography**
EXCLUDES *Thrombolysis, cerebral (37195)*
Thrombolysis other than coronary ([37211, 37212, 37213, 37214])
10.9 10.9 FUD 000 C 80
AMA: 2018,Feb,11

92977 **by intravenous infusion**
EXCLUDES *Thrombolysis, cerebral (37195)*
Thrombolysis other than coronary ([37211, 37212, 37213, 37214])
1.56 1.56 FUD XXX T 80
AMA: 2018,Feb,11

+ # 92978 **Endoluminal imaging of coronary vessel or graft using intravascular ultrasound (IVUS) or optical coherence tomography (OCT) during diagnostic evaluation and/or therapeutic intervention including imaging supervision, interpretation and report; initial vessel (List separately in addition to code for primary procedure)**
Code first primary procedure (92920, 92924, 92928, 92933, 92937, 92941, 92943, 92975, 93454-93461, 93563-93564)
0.00 0.00 FUD ZZZ N 80
AMA: 2018,Feb,11; 2018,Jan,8; 2017,Jan,8; 2016,Jan,13; 2015,Jan,16; 2014,Dec,6; 2014,Jan,11

+ # 92979 **each additional vessel (List separately in addition to code for primary procedure)**
INCLUDES Transducer manipulations/repositioning in the vessel examined, before and after therapeutic intervention
EXCLUDES *Intravascular spectroscopy (93799)*
Code first initial vessel (92978)
0.00 0.00 FUD ZZZ N 80
AMA: 2018,Feb,11; 2018,Jan,8; 2017,Jan,8; 2016,Jan,13; 2015,Jan,16; 2014,Dec,6; 2014,Jan,11

93000-93010 Electrocardiographic Services

INCLUDES Specific order for the service, a separate written and signed report, and documentation of medical necessity
EXCLUDES *Acoustic cardiography (93799)*
Echocardiography (93303-93350)
Intracardiac ischemia monitoring system (0525T-0532T)
Use of these codes for the review of telemetry monitoring strips

93000 **Electrocardiogram, routine ECG with at least 12 leads; with interpretation and report**
0.48 0.48 FUD XXX M 80
AMA: 2018,Feb,11; 2018,Jan,8; 2017,Oct,3; 2017,Jan,8; 2016,Jan,13; 2015,Jan,16; 2014,Jan,11

93005 tracing only, without interpretation and report
0.24 0.24 **FUD** XXX Q1 80 TC
AMA: 2018,Feb,11; 2018,Jan,8; 2017,Oct,3; 2017,Jan,8; 2016,Apr,8; 2016,Jan,13; 2015,Jan,16; 2014,Jan,11

93010 interpretation and report only
0.24 0.24 **FUD** XXX B 80 26
AMA: 2018,Feb,11; 2018,Jan,8; 2017,Oct,3; 2017,Jan,8; 2016,Apr,8; 2016,Jan,13; 2015,Jan,16; 2014,Jan,11

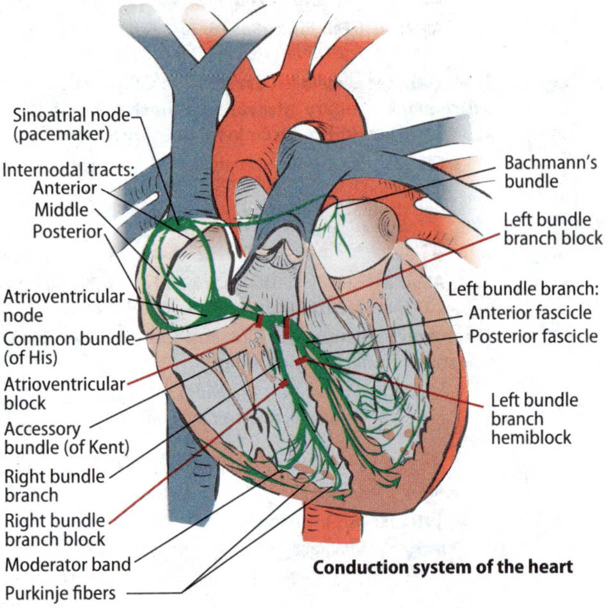

Conduction system of the heart

93015-93018 Stress Test

93015 Cardiovascular stress test using maximal or submaximal treadmill or bicycle exercise, continuous electrocardiographic monitoring, and/or pharmacological stress; with supervision, interpretation and report
2.01 2.01 **FUD** XXX B 80
AMA: 2018,Feb,11; 2018,Jan,8; 2017,Oct,3; 2017,Jan,8; 2016,Jan,13; 2015,Jan,16; 2014,Jan,11

93016 supervision only, without interpretation and report
0.63 0.63 **FUD** XXX B 80 26
AMA: 2018,Feb,11; 2018,Jan,8; 2017,Oct,3; 2017,Jan,8; 2016,Jan,13; 2015,Jan,16; 2014,Jan,11

93017 tracing only, without interpretation and report
0.96 0.96 **FUD** XXX Q1 80 TC
AMA: 2018,Feb,11; 2018,Jan,8; 2017,Oct,3; 2017,Jan,8; 2016,Jan,13; 2015,Jan,16; 2014,Jan,11

93018 interpretation and report only
0.42 0.42 **FUD** XXX B 80 26
AMA: 2018,Feb,11; 2018,Jan,8; 2017,Oct,3; 2017,Jan,8; 2016,Jan,13; 2015,Jan,16; 2014,Jan,11

93024 Provocation Test for Coronary Vasospasm

93024 Ergonovine provocation test
3.12 3.12 **FUD** XXX Q1 80
AMA: 2018,Feb,11

93025 Microvolt T-Wave Alternans

CMS: 100-03,20.30 Microvolt T-Wave Alternans (MTWA); 100-04,32,370 Microvolt T-wave Alternans; 100-04,32,370.1 Coding and Claims Processing for MTWA; 100-04,32,370.2 Messaging for MTWA

INCLUDES Specific order for the service, a separate written and signed report, and documentation of medical necessity

EXCLUDES *Echocardiography (93303-93350)*
Use of these codes for the review of telemetry monitoring strips

93025 Microvolt T-wave alternans for assessment of ventricular arrhythmias
4.23 4.23 **FUD** XXX S 80
AMA: 2018,Feb,11; 2018,Jan,8; 2017,Jan,8; 2016,Jan,13; 2015,Jan,16; 2014,Jan,11

93040-93042 Rhythm Strips

INCLUDES Specific order for the service, a separate written and signed report, and documentation of medical necessity

EXCLUDES *Device evaluation ([93261], 93279-93289 [93260], 93291-93296, 93298)*
Echocardiography (93303-93350)
Use of these codes for the review of telemetry monitoring strips

93040 Rhythm ECG, 1-3 leads; with interpretation and report
0.36 0.36 **FUD** XXX B 80
AMA: 2018,Feb,11; 2018,Jan,8; 2017,Oct,3; 2017,Jan,8; 2016,Jan,13; 2015,Jan,16; 2014,Jan,11

93041 tracing only without interpretation and report
0.16 0.16 **FUD** XXX Q1 80 TC
AMA: 2018,Feb,11; 2018,Jan,8; 2017,Oct,3; 2017,Jan,8; 2016,Jan,13; 2015,Jan,16; 2014,Jan,11

93042 interpretation and report only
0.20 0.20 **FUD** XXX B 80 26
AMA: 2018,Feb,11; 2018,Jan,8; 2017,Oct,3; 2017,Jan,8; 2016,Jan,13; 2015,Jan,16; 2014,Jan,11

93050 Arterial Waveform Analysis

EXCLUDES *Use of code with any intra-arterial diagnostic or interventional procedure*

93050 Arterial pressure waveform analysis for assessment of central arterial pressures, includes obtaining waveform(s), digitization and application of nonlinear mathematical transformations to determine central arterial pressures and augmentation index, with interpretation and report, upper extremity artery, non-invasive
0.46 0.46 **FUD** XXX Q1 80
AMA: 2018,Feb,11

93224-93227 Holter Monitor

INCLUDES Cardiac monitoring using in-person as well as remote technology for the assessment of electrocardiographic data
Up to 48 hours of recording on a continuous basis

EXCLUDES *Echocardiography (93303-93355)*
Implantable patient activated cardiac event recorders (93285, 93291, 93297-93298)
More than 48 hours of monitoring (0295T-0298T)

Code also modifier 52 when less than 12 hours of continuous recording is provided

93224 External electrocardiographic recording up to 48 hours by continuous rhythm recording and storage; includes recording, scanning analysis with report, review and interpretation by a physician or other qualified health care professional
2.51 2.51 **FUD** XXX M 80
AMA: 2018,Feb,11; 2018,Jan,8; 2017,Jan,8; 2016,Jan,13; 2015,Jan,16; 2014,Jan,11

93225 recording (includes connection, recording, and disconnection)
0.73 0.73 **FUD** XXX Q1 80 TC
AMA: 2018,Feb,11; 2018,Jan,8; 2017,Jan,8; 2016,Jan,13; 2015,Jan,16; 2014,Jan,11

93226 scanning analysis with report
1.03 1.03 **FUD** XXX Q1 80 TC
AMA: 2018,Feb,11; 2018,Jan,8; 2017,Jan,8; 2016,Jan,13; 2015,Jan,16; 2014,Jan,11

Medicine

93227 **review and interpretation by a physician or other qualified health care professional**

0.75 0.75 FUD XXX M 80 26

AMA: 2018,Mar,5; 2018,Feb,11; 2018,Jan,8; 2017,Jan,8; 2016,Jan,13; 2015,Jan,16; 2014,Jan,11

93228-93229 Remote Cardiovascular Telemetry

INCLUDES Cardiac monitoring using in-person as well as remote technology for the assessment of electrocardiographic data
Mobile telemetry monitors with the capacity to:
Detect arrhythmias
Real-time data analysis for the evaluation quality of the signal
Records ECG rhythm on a continuous basis using external electrodes on the patient
Transmit a tracing at any time
Transmit data to an attended surveillance center where a technician is available to respond to device or rhythm alerts and contact the physician or qualified health care professional if needed

EXCLUDES *Use of code more than one time in a 30-day period*

93228 **External mobile cardiovascular telemetry with electrocardiographic recording, concurrent computerized real time data analysis and greater than 24 hours of accessible ECG data storage (retrievable with query) with ECG triggered and patient selected events transmitted to a remote attended surveillance center for up to 30 days; review and interpretation with report by a physician or other qualified health care professional**

EXCLUDES *Cardiovascular monitors that do not perform automatic ECG triggered transmissions to an attended surveillance center (93224-93227, 93268-93272)*

0.74 0.74 FUD XXX ★ M 80 26

AMA: 2018,Feb,11; 2018,Jan,8; 2017,Jan,8; 2016,Jan,13; 2015,Jan,16; 2014,Jan,11

93229 **technical support for connection and patient instructions for use, attended surveillance, analysis and transmission of daily and emergent data reports as prescribed by a physician or other qualified health care professional**

19.9 19.9 FUD XXX ★ S 80 TC

AMA: 2018,Feb,11; 2018,Jan,8; 2017,Jan,8; 2016,Jan,13; 2015,Jan,16; 2014,Jan,11

93260-93272 Event Monitors

INCLUDES ECG rhythm derived elements, which differ from physiologic data and include rhythm of the heart, rate, ST analysis, heart rate variability, T-wave alternans, among others
Event monitors that:
Record parts of ECGs in response to patient activation or an automatic detection algorithm (or both)
Require attended surveillance
Transmit data upon request (although not immediately when activated)

EXCLUDES *Monitoring of cardiovascular devices (93279-93289 [93260], 93291-93296, 93298)*

93260 **Resequenced code. See code following 93284.**

93261 **Resequenced code. See code following 93289.**

93264 **Resequenced code. See code before 93279.**

93268 **External patient and, when performed, auto activated electrocardiographic rhythm derived event recording with symptom-related memory loop with remote download capability up to 30 days, 24-hour attended monitoring; includes transmission, review and interpretation by a physician or other qualified health care professional**

EXCLUDES *Implantable patient activated cardiac event recorders (93285, 93291, 93298)*
Subcutaneous cardiac rhythm monitor (33285)

5.70 5.70 FUD XXX ★ M 80

AMA: 2018,Feb,11; 2018,Jan,8; 2017,Jan,8; 2016,Jan,13; 2015,Jan,16; 2014,Jan,11

93270 **recording (includes connection, recording, and disconnection)**

0.26 0.26 FUD XXX ★ Q1 80 TC

AMA: 2018,Feb,11; 2018,Jan,8; 2017,Jan,8; 2016,Jan,13; 2015,Jan,16; 2014,Jan,11

93271 **transmission and analysis**

4.72 4.72 FUD XXX ★ S 80 TC

AMA: 2018,Feb,11; 2018,Jan,8; 2017,Jan,8; 2016,Jan,13; 2015,Jan,16; 2014,Jan,11

93272 **review and interpretation by a physician or other qualified health care professional**

EXCLUDES *Implantable patient activated cardiac event recorders (93285, 93291, 93298)*
Subcutaneous cardiac rhythm monitor (33285)

0.72 0.72 FUD XXX ★ M 80 26

AMA: 2018,Mar,5; 2018,Feb,11; 2018,Jan,8; 2017,Jan,8; 2016,Jan,13; 2015,Jan,16; 2014,Jan,11

93278 Signal-averaged Electrocardiography

EXCLUDES *Echocardiography (93303-93355)*
Code also modifier 26 for the interpretation and report only

93278 **Signal-averaged electrocardiography (SAECG), with or without ECG**

0.87 0.87 FUD XXX Q1 80

AMA: 2018,Feb,11; 2018,Jan,8; 2017,Jan,8; 2016,Jan,13; 2015,Jan,16; 2014,Jan,11

93264 [93264] Wireless Pulmonary Artery Pressure Sensor Monitoring

INCLUDES Collection of data from an internal sensor in pulmonary artery
Downloads, interpretation, analysis, and report that must occur at least one time per week
Transmission and storage of data

EXCLUDES *Use of code if monitoring is for less than a 30-day period*
Use of code more than one time in 30 days

\# 93264 **Remote monitoring of a wireless pulmonary artery pressure sensor for up to 30 days, including at least weekly downloads of pulmonary artery pressure recordings, interpretation(s), trend analysis, and report(s) by a physician or other qualified health care professional**

1.02 1.44 FUD XXX 80

AMA: 2019,Jun,3

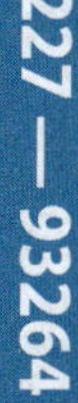

93279-93299 [93260, 93261] Monitoring of Cardiovascular Devices

INCLUDES Implantable cardiovascular monitor (ICM) interrogation:
- Analysis of at least one recorded physiologic cardiovascular data element from either internal or external sensors
- Programmed parameters

Implantable defibrillator interrogation:
- Battery
- Capture and sensing functions
- Leads
- Presence or absence of therapy for ventricular tachyarrhythmias
- Programmed parameters
- Underlying heart rhythm

Implantable loop recorder (ILR) interrogation:
- Heart rate and rhythm during recorded episodes from both patient-initiated and device detected events
- Programmed parameters

In-person interrogation/device evaluation (93288)

In-person peri-procedural device evaluation/programming of device system parameters (93286)

Interrogation evaluation of device

Pacemaker interrogation:
- Battery
- Capture and sensing functions
- Heart rhythm
- Leads
- Programmed parameters

Time period established by the initiation of remote monitoring or the 91st day of implantable defibrillator or pacemaker monitoring or the 31st day of ILR monitoring and extending for the succeeding 30- or 90-day period

EXCLUDES *Wearable device monitoring (93224-93272)*

93279 **Programming device evaluation (in person) with iterative adjustment of the implantable device to test the function of the device and select optimal permanent programmed values with analysis, review and report by a physician or other qualified health care professional; single lead pacemaker system or leadless pacemaker system in one cardiac chamber**

EXCLUDES *External ECG event recording up to 30 days (93268-93272)*
Peri-procedural and interrogation device evaluation (93286, 93288)
Rhythm strips (93040-93042)

1.56 1.56 **FUD** XXX Q1 80

AMA: 2019,Mar,6; 2018,Feb,11; 2018,Jan,8; 2017,Jan,8; 2016,Aug,5; 2016,May,5; 2016,Jan,13; 2015,Jan,16; 2014,Nov,5; 2014,Jul,3; 2014,Jan,11

93280 **dual lead pacemaker system**

EXCLUDES *External ECG event recording up to 30 days (93268-93272)*
Peri-procedural and interrogation device evaluation (93286, 93288)
Rhythm strips (93040-93042)

1.83 1.83 **FUD** XXX Q1 80

AMA: 2018,Feb,11; 2018,Jan,8; 2017,Jan,8; 2016,Aug,5; 2016,May,5; 2016,Jan,13; 2015,Jan,16; 2014,Nov,5; 2014,Jul,3; 2014,Jan,11

93281 **multiple lead pacemaker system**

EXCLUDES *External ECG event recording up to 30 days (93268-93272)*
Peri-procedural and interrogation device evaluation (93286, 93288)
Rhythm strips (93040-93042)

1.97 1.97 **FUD** XXX Q1 80

AMA: 2018,Feb,11; 2018,Jan,8; 2017,Jan,8; 2016,Aug,5; 2016,May,5; 2016,Jan,13; 2015,Jan,16; 2014,Nov,5; 2014,Jul,3; 2014,Jan,11

93282 **single lead transvenous implantable defibrillator system**

EXCLUDES *Device evaluation subcutaneous lead defibrillator system (93260)*
External ECG event recording up to 30 days (93268-93272)
Peri-procedural and interrogation device evaluation (93287, 93289)
Rhythm strips (93040-93042)
Wearable cardio-defibrillator system services (93745)

1.90 1.90 **FUD** XXX Q1 80

AMA: 2018,Feb,11; 2018,Jan,8; 2017,Jan,8; 2016,Aug,5; 2016,Jan,13; 2015,Jan,16; 2014,Nov,5; 2014,Jul,3; 2014,Jan,11

93283 **dual lead transvenous implantable defibrillator system**

EXCLUDES *External ECG event recording up to 30 days (93268-93272)*
Peri-procedural and interrogation device evaluation (93287, 93289)
Rhythm strips (93040-93042)

2.39 2.39 **FUD** XXX Q1 80

AMA: 2018,Feb,11; 2018,Jan,8; 2017,Jan,8; 2016,Aug,5; 2016,Jan,13; 2015,Jan,16; 2014,Nov,5; 2014,Jul,3; 2014,Jan,11

93284 **multiple lead transvenous implantable defibrillator system**

EXCLUDES *External ECG event recording up to 30 days (93268-93272)*
Peri-procedural and interrogation device evaluation (93287, 93289)
Rhythm strips (93040-93042)

2.59 2.59 **FUD** XXX Q1 80

AMA: 2018,Feb,11; 2018,Jan,8; 2017,Jan,8; 2016,Aug,5; 2016,Jan,13; 2015,Jan,16; 2014,Nov,5; 2014,Jul,3; 2014,Jan,11

93260 **implantable subcutaneous lead defibrillator system**

EXCLUDES *Device evaluation (93261, 93282, 93287)*
External ECG event recording up to 30 days (93268-93272)
Insertion/removal/replacement implantable defibrillator (33240, 33241, [33262], [33270, 33271, 33272, 33273])
Rhythm strips (93040-93042)

1.93 1.93 **FUD** XXX Q1 80

AMA: 2018,Feb,11; 2018,Jan,8; 2017,Jan,8; 2016,Aug,5; 2016,Jan,13; 2015,Jan,16; 2014,Nov,5

93285 **subcutaneous cardiac rhythm monitor system**

EXCLUDES *Device evaluation (93279-93284, 93291)*
External ECG event recording up to 30 days (93268-93272)
Insertion subcutaneous cardiac rhythm monitor (33285)
Rhythm strips (93040-93042)

1.37 1.37 **FUD** XXX Q1 80

AMA: 2019,Apr,3; 2018,Feb,11; 2018,Jan,8; 2017,Jan,8; 2016,Aug,5; 2016,Jan,13; 2015,Jan,16; 2014,Nov,5; 2014,Jul,3; 2014,Jan,11

93286 **Peri-procedural device evaluation (in person) and programming of device system parameters before or after a surgery, procedure, or test with analysis, review and report by a physician or other qualified health care professional; single, dual, or multiple lead pacemaker system, or leadless pacemaker system**

INCLUDES One evaluation and programming (if performed once before and once after, report as two units)

EXCLUDES *Device evaluation (93279-93281, 93288)*
External ECG event recording up to 30 days (93268-93272)
Rhythm strips (93040-93042)
Services related to cardiac contractility modulation systems (0408T-0411T, 0414T-0415T)
Subcutaneous implantable defibrillator peri-procedural device evaluation and programming (93260, 93261)

0.99 0.99 FUD XXX N 80

AMA: 2019,Mar,6; 2018,Feb,11; 2018,Jan,8; 2017,Jan,8; 2016,Aug,5; 2016,May,5; 2016,Jan,13; 2015,Jan,16; 2014,Nov,5; 2014,Jul,3; 2014,Jan,11

93287 **single, dual, or multiple lead implantable defibrillator system**

INCLUDES One evaluation and programming (if performed once before and once after, report as two units)

EXCLUDES *Device evaluation (93282-93284, 93289)*
External ECG event recording up to 30 days (93268-93272)
Rhythm strips (93040-93042)
Services related to cardiac contractility modulation systems (0408T-0411T, 0414T-0415T)
Subcutaneous implantable defibrillator peri-procedural device evaluation and programming (93260, 93261)

1.22 1.22 FUD XXX N 80

AMA: 2018,Feb,11; 2018,Jan,8; 2017,Jan,8; 2016,Aug,5; 2016,May,5; 2016,Jan,13; 2015,Jan,16; 2014,Nov,5; 2014,Jul,3; 2014,Jan,11

93288 **Interrogation device evaluation (in person) with analysis, review and report by a physician or other qualified health care professional, includes connection, recording and disconnection per patient encounter; single, dual, or multiple lead pacemaker system, or leadless pacemaker system**

EXCLUDES *Device evaluation (93279-93281, 93286, 93294-93295)*
External ECG event recording up to 30 days (93268-93272)
Rhythm strips (93040-93042)

1.25 1.25 FUD XXX Q1 80

AMA: 2019,Mar,6; 2018,Feb,11; 2018,Jan,8; 2017,Jan,8; 2016,Aug,5; 2016,May,5; 2016,Jan,13; 2015,Jan,16; 2014,Nov,5; 2014,Jul,3; 2014,Jan,11

93289 **single, dual, or multiple lead transvenous implantable defibrillator system, including analysis of heart rhythm derived data elements**

EXCLUDES *Monitoring physiologic cardiovascular data elements derived from an implantable defibrillator (93290)*

EXCLUDES *Device evaluation (93261, 93282-93284, 93287, 93295-93296)*
External ECG event recording up to 30 days (93268-93272)
Rhythm strips (93040-93042)

1.70 1.70 FUD XXX Q1 80

AMA: 2018,Feb,11; 2018,Jan,8; 2017,Jan,8; 2016,Aug,5; 2016,May,5; 2016,Jan,13; 2015,Jan,16; 2014,Nov,5; 2014,Jul,3; 2014,Jan,11

\# **93261** **implantable subcutaneous lead defibrillator system**

EXCLUDES *Device evaluation (93260, 93287, 93289)*
External ECG event recording up to 30 days (93268-93272)
Insertion/removal/replacement implantable defibrillator (33240, 33241, [33262], [33270, 33271, 33272, 33273])
Rhythm strips (93040-93042)

1.77 1.77 FUD XXX Q1 80

AMA: 2018,Feb,11; 2018,Jan,8; 2017,Jan,8; 2016,Aug,5; 2016,Jan,13; 2015,Jan,16; 2014,Nov,5

93290 **implantable cardiovascular physiologic monitor system, including analysis of 1 or more recorded physiologic cardiovascular data elements from all internal and external sensors**

EXCLUDES *Device evaluation (93297)*
Heart rhythm derived data (93289)

1.19 1.19 FUD XXX Q1 80

AMA: 2018,Feb,11; 2018,Jan,8; 2017,Jan,8; 2016,Aug,5; 2016,Jan,13; 2015,Jan,16; 2014,Nov,5; 2014,Jul,3; 2014,Jan,11

93291 **subcutaneous cardiac rhythm monitor system, including heart rhythm derived data analysis**

EXCLUDES *Device evaluation (93288-93290 [93261], 93298)*
External ECG event recording up to 30 days (93268-93272)
Insertion subcutaneous cardiac rhythm monitor (33285)
Rhythm strips (93040-93042)

1.07 1.07 FUD XXX Q1 80

AMA: 2019,Apr,3; 2018,Feb,11; 2018,Jan,8; 2017,Jan,8; 2016,Aug,5; 2016,Jan,13; 2015,Jan,16; 2014,Nov,5; 2014,Jul,3; 2014,Jan,11

93292 **wearable defibrillator system**

EXCLUDES *External ECG event recording up to 30 days (93268-93272)*
Rhythm strips (93040-93042)
Wearable cardioverter-defibrillator system (93745)

1.14 1.14 FUD XXX Q1 80

AMA: 2018,Feb,11; 2018,Jan,8; 2017,Jan,8; 2016,Aug,5; 2016,Jan,13; 2015,Jan,16; 2014,Nov,5; 2014,Jul,3; 2014,Jan,11

93293 **Transtelephonic rhythm strip pacemaker evaluation(s) single, dual, or multiple lead pacemaker system, includes recording with and without magnet application with analysis, review and report(s) by a physician or other qualified health care professional, up to 90 days**

EXCLUDES *Device evaluation (93294)*
External ECG event recording up to 30 days (93268-93272)
Rhythm strips (93040-93042)
Use of code more than one time in a 90-day period
Use of code when monitoring period is less than 30 days

1.48 1.48 FUD XXX Q1 80

AMA: 2018,Feb,11; 2018,Jan,8; 2017,Jan,8; 2016,Aug,5; 2016,Jan,13; 2015,Jan,16; 2014,Nov,5; 2014,Jul,3; 2014,Jan,11

93294 **Interrogation device evaluation(s) (remote), up to 90 days; single, dual, or multiple lead pacemaker system, or leadless pacemaker system with interim analysis, review(s) and report(s) by a physician or other qualified health care professional**

EXCLUDES *Device evaluation (93288, 93293)*
External ECG event recording up to 30 days (93268-93272)
Rhythm strips (93040-93042)
Use of code more than one time in a 90-day period
Use of code when monitoring period is less than 30 days

0.87 0.87 FUD XXX M 80 26

AMA: 2019,Mar,6; 2018,Feb,11; 2018,Jan,8; 2017,Jan,8; 2016,Aug,5; 2016,Jan,13; 2015,Jan,16; 2014,Nov,5; 2014,Jul,3; 2014,Jan,11

93295 **single, dual, or multiple lead implantable defibrillator system with interim analysis, review(s) and report(s) by a physician or other qualified health care professional**

EXCLUDES *Device evaluation (93289)*
External ECG event recording up to 30 days (93268-93272)
Remote interrogation device evaluation implantable cardioverter-defibrillator with substernal lead (0578T, 0579T)
Remote monitoring of physiological cardiovascular data (93297)
Rhythm strips (93040-93042)
Use of code more than one time in a 90-day period
Use of code when monitoring period is less than 30 days

1.26 1.26 FUD XXX M 80 26

AMA: 2018,Feb,11; 2018,Jan,8; 2017,Jan,8; 2016,Aug,5; 2016,Jan,13; 2015,Jan,16; 2014,Nov,5; 2014,Jul,3; 2014,Jan,11

93296 **single, dual, or multiple lead pacemaker system, leadless pacemaker system, or implantable defibrillator system, remote data acquisition(s), receipt of transmissions and technician review, technical support and distribution of results**

EXCLUDES *Device evaluation (93288-93289)*
External ECG event recording up to 30 days (93268-93272)
Remote interrogation device evaluation implantable cardioverter-defibrillator with substernal lead (0578T, 0579T)
Rhythm strips (93040-93042)
Use of code more than one time in a 90-day period
Use of code when monitoring period is less than 30 days

0.72 0.72 FUD XXX 01 80 TC

AMA: 2019,Mar,6; 2019,Jan,6; 2018,Feb,11; 2018,Jan,8; 2017,Jan,8; 2016,Aug,5; 2016,Jan,13; 2015,Jan,16; 2014,Nov,5; 2014,Jul,3; 2014,Jan,11

93297 **Interrogation device evaluation(s), (remote) up to 30 days; implantable cardiovascular physiologic monitor system, including analysis of 1 or more recorded physiologic cardiovascular data elements from all internal and external sensors, analysis, review(s) and report(s) by a physician or other qualified health care professional**

EXCLUDES *Collection and interpretation of physiologic data digitally stored and/or transmitted ([99091])*
Device evaluation (93290, 93298)
Heart rhythm derived data (93295)
Remote monitoring of a wireless pulmonary artery pressure sensor (93264)
Remote monitoring of physiologic parameter(s) with daily recording(s) or programmed alert(s) ([99454])
Use of code more than one time in a 30-day period
Use of code when monitoring period is less than 10 days

0.75 0.75 FUD XXX M 80 26

AMA: 2018,Feb,11; 2018,Jan,8; 2017,Jan,8; 2016,Aug,5; 2016,Jan,13; 2015,Jan,16; 2014,Nov,5; 2014,Jul,3; 2014,Jan,11

93298 **subcutaneous cardiac rhythm monitor system, including analysis of recorded heart rhythm data, analysis, review(s) and report(s) by a physician or other qualified health care professional**

EXCLUDES *Collection and interpretation of physiologic data digitally stored and/or transmitted ([99091])*
Device evaluation (93291, 93297)
External ECG event recording up to 30 days (93268-93272)
Implantation of patient-activated cardiac event recorder (33285)
Remote monitoring of physiologic parameter(s) with daily recording(s) or programmed alert(s) ([99454])
Rhythm strips (93040-93042)
Use of code more than one time in a 30-day period
Use of code when monitoring period is less than 10 days

0.75 0.75 FUD XXX M 80 26

AMA: 2019,Apr,3; 2018,Feb,11; 2018,Jan,8; 2017,Jan,8; 2016,Aug,5; 2016,Jan,13; 2015,Jan,16; 2014,Nov,5; 2014,Jul,3; 2014,Jan,11

93299 **~~implantable cardiovascular physiologic monitor system or subcutaneous cardiac rhythm monitor system, remote data acquisition(s), receipt of transmissions and technician review, technical support and distribution of results~~**

To report, see (93297-93298)

93303-93356 [93356] Echocardiography

INCLUDES Interpretation and report
Obtaining ultrasonic signals from heart/great arteries
Report of study which includes:
Description of recognized abnormalities
Documentation of all clinically relevant findings which includes obtained quantitative measurements
Interpretation of all information obtained
Two-dimensional image/doppler ultrasonic signal documentation
Ultrasound exam of:
Adjacent great vessels
Cardiac chambers/valves
Pericardium

EXCLUDES *Contrast agents and/or drugs used for pharmacological stress*
Echocardiography, fetal (76825-76828)
Ultrasound with thorough examination of the organ(s) or anatomic region/documentation of the image/final written report

93303 **Transthoracic echocardiography for congenital cardiac anomalies; complete**

6.65 6.65 FUD XXX S 80

AMA: 2018,Feb,11; 2018,Jan,8; 2017,Jan,8; 2016,Jan,13; 2015,May,10; 2015,Jan,16; 2014,Jan,11

93304 **follow-up or limited study**

4.53 4.53 FUD XXX S 80

AMA: 2018,Feb,11; 2018,Jan,8; 2017,Jan,8; 2016,Jan,13; 2015,May,10; 2015,Jan,16; 2014,Jan,11

93306 **Echocardiography, transthoracic, real-time with image documentation (2D), includes M-mode recording, when performed, complete, with spectral Doppler echocardiography, and with color flow Doppler echocardiography**

INCLUDES Doppler and color flow
Two-dimensional and M-mode

EXCLUDES *Transthoracic without spectral and color doppler (93307)*

5.84 5.84 FUD XXX S 80

AMA: 2018,Dec,10; 2018,Dec,10; 2018,Feb,11; 2018,Jan,8; 2017,Jan,8; 2016,Apr,8; 2016,Jan,13; 2015,May,10; 2015,Jan,16

93307 **Echocardiography, transthoracic, real-time with image documentation (2D), includes M-mode recording, when performed, complete, without spectral or color Doppler echocardiography**

INCLUDES Additional structures that may be viewed such as pulmonary vein or artery, pulmonic valve, inferior vena cava
Obtaining/recording appropriate measurements
Two-dimensional/selected M-mode exam of:
Adjacent portions of the aorta
Aortic/mitral/tricuspid valves
Left/right atria
Left/right ventricles
Pericardium
Using multiple views as required to obtain a complete functional/anatomic evaluation

EXCLUDES *Doppler echocardiography (93320-93321, 93325)*

3.97 3.97 FUD XXX S 80

AMA: 2018,Feb,11; 2018,Jan,8; 2017,Jan,8; 2016,Apr,8; 2016,Jan,13; 2015,May,10; 2015,Jan,16; 2014,Jan,11

93308 **Echocardiography, transthoracic, real-time with image documentation (2D), includes M-mode recording, when performed, follow-up or limited study**

INCLUDES An exam that does not evaluate/document the attempt to evaluate all the structures that comprise the complete echocardiographic exam

2.78 2.78 FUD XXX S 80

AMA: 2018,Dec,10; 2018,Dec,10; 2018,Feb,11; 2018,Jan,8; 2017,Jan,8; 2016,Apr,8; 2016,Jan,13; 2015,May,10; 2015,Jan,16; 2014,Jan,11

93312 Echocardiography, transesophageal, real-time with image documentation (2D) (with or without M-mode recording); including probe placement, image acquisition, interpretation and report

EXCLUDES *Transesophageal echocardiography (93355)*

6.97 6.97 FUD XXX S 80

AMA: 2018,Feb,11; 2018,Jan,8; 2017,Jan,8; 2016,Jan,13; 2015,Jan,16; 2014,Jul,8; 2014,Jan,11

93313 placement of transesophageal probe only

EXCLUDES *Excludes procedure if performed by same person performing transesophageal echocardiography (93355)*

0.33 0.33 FUD XXX S 80

AMA: 2018,Feb,11; 2018,Jan,8; 2017,Jan,8; 2016,Jan,13; 2015,Jan,16; 2014,Jul,8; 2014,Jan,11

93314 image acquisition, interpretation and report only

EXCLUDES *Transesophageal echocardiography (93355)*

6.73 6.73 FUD XXX N 80

AMA: 2018,Feb,11; 2018,Jan,8; 2017,Jan,8; 2016,Jan,13; 2015,Jan,16; 2014,Jul,8; 2014,Jan,11

93315 Transesophageal echocardiography for congenital cardiac anomalies; including probe placement, image acquisition, interpretation and report

EXCLUDES *Transesophageal echocardiography (93355)*

0.00 0.00 FUD XXX S 80

AMA: 2018,Feb,11; 2018,Jan,8; 2017,Jan,8; 2016,Jan,13; 2015,Jan,16; 2014,Jul,8; 2014,Jan,11

93316 placement of transesophageal probe only

EXCLUDES *Transesophageal echocardiography (93355)*

0.79 0.79 FUD XXX S 80

AMA: 2018,Feb,11; 2018,Jan,8; 2017,Jan,8; 2016,Jan,13; 2015,Jan,16; 2014,Jan,11

93317 image acquisition, interpretation and report only

EXCLUDES *Transesophageal echocardiography (93355)*

0.00 0.00 FUD XXX N 80

AMA: 2018,Feb,11; 2018,Jan,8; 2017,Jan,8; 2016,Jan,13; 2015,Jan,16; 2014,Jan,11

93318 Echocardiography, transesophageal (TEE) for monitoring purposes, including probe placement, real time 2-dimensional image acquisition and interpretation leading to ongoing (continuous) assessment of (dynamically changing) cardiac pumping function and to therapeutic measures on an immediate time basis

EXCLUDES *Transesophageal echocardiography (93355)*

0.00 0.00 FUD XXX S 80

AMA: 2018,Feb,11; 2018,Jan,8; 2017,Jan,8; 2016,Jan,13; 2015,Jan,16; 2014,Jan,11

\+ **93320 Doppler echocardiography, pulsed wave and/or continuous wave with spectral display (List separately in addition to codes for echocardiographic imaging); complete**

EXCLUDES *Transesophageal echocardiography (93355)*

Code first (93303-93304, 93312, 93314-93315, 93317, 93350-93351)

1.51 1.51 FUD ZZZ N 80

AMA: 2018,Feb,11; 2018,Jan,8; 2017,Jan,8; 2016,Jan,13; 2015,Jan,16; 2014,Jan,11

\+ **93321 follow-up or limited study (List separately in addition to codes for echocardiographic imaging)**

EXCLUDES *Transesophageal echocardiography (93355)*

Code first (93303-93304, 93308, 93312, 93314-93315, 93317, 93350-93351)

0.76 0.76 FUD ZZZ N 80

AMA: 2018,Feb,11; 2018,Jan,8; 2017,Jan,8; 2016,Jan,13; 2015,Jan,16; 2014,Jan,11

\+ **93325 Doppler echocardiography color flow velocity mapping (List separately in addition to codes for echocardiography)**

EXCLUDES *Transesophageal echocardiography (93355)*

Code first (76825-76828, 93303-93304, 93308, 93312, 93314-93315, 93317, 93350-93351)

0.71 0.71 FUD ZZZ N 80

AMA: 2018,Feb,11; 2018,Jan,8; 2017,Jan,8; 2016,Jul,8; 2016,Jan,13; 2015,Jan,16; 2014,Jan,11

93350 Echocardiography, transthoracic, real-time with image documentation (2D), includes M-mode recording, when performed, during rest and cardiovascular stress test using treadmill, bicycle exercise and/or pharmacologically induced stress, with interpretation and report;

EXCLUDES *Cardiovascular stress test, complete procedure (93015)*

Code also exercise stress testing (93016-93018)

5.31 5.31 FUD XXX S 80

AMA: 2018,Feb,11; 2018,Jan,8; 2017,Jan,8; 2016,Apr,8; 2016,Jan,13; 2015,Jan,16; 2014,Jul,8; 2014,Jan,11

93351 including performance of continuous electrocardiographic monitoring, with supervision by a physician or other qualified health care professional

INCLUDES Stress echocardiogram performed with a complete cardiovascular stress test

EXCLUDES *Cardiovascular stress test (93015-93018)*
Echocardiography (93350)
Professional only components of complete stress test and stress echocardiogram performed in a facility by same physician, report with modifier 26
Use of code for professional component (modifier 26 appended) with (93016, 93018, 93350)

Code also components of cardiovascular stress test when professional services not performed by same physician performing stress echocardiogram (93016-93018)

6.57 6.57 FUD XXX S

AMA: 2018,Feb,11; 2018,Jan,8; 2017,Jan,8; 2016,Apr,8; 2016,Jan,13; 2015,Jan,16; 2014,Jul,8; 2014,Jan,11

● + # **93356 Myocardial strain imaging using speckle tracking-derived assessment of myocardial mechanics (List separately in addition to codes for echocardiography imaging)**

0.00 0.00 FUD 000

EXCLUDES *Use of code more than one time for each session*

Code first (93303-93304, 93306, 93307, 93308, 93350-93351)

\+ **93352 Use of echocardiographic contrast agent during stress echocardiography (List separately in addition to code for primary procedure)**

EXCLUDES *Use of code more than one time for each stress echocardiogram*

Code first (93350, 93351)

0.95 0.95 FUD ZZZ M 80

AMA: 2018,Feb,11; 2018,Jan,8; 2017,Jan,8; 2016,Jan,13; 2015,Jan,16; 2014,Jan,11

93355 Echocardiography, transesophageal (TEE) for guidance of a transcatheter intracardiac or great vessel(s) structural intervention(s) (eg,TAVR, transcatheter pulmonary valve replacement, mitral valve repair, paravalvular regurgitation repair, left atrial appendage occlusion/closure, ventricular septal defect closure) (peri-and intra-procedural), real-time image acquisition and documentation, guidance with quantitative measurements, probe manipulation, interpretation, and report, including diagnostic transesophageal echocardiography and, when performed, administration of ultrasound contrast, Doppler, color flow, and 3D

EXCLUDES *3D rendering (76376-76377)*
Doppler echocardiography (93320-93321, 93325)
Transesophageal echocardiography (93312-93318)
Transesophageal probe positioning by different provider (93313)

6.57 6.57 FUD XXX N 80

AMA: 2018,Feb,11

93356 **Resequenced code. See code following 93351.**

93451-93505 Heart Catheterization

INCLUDES Access site imaging and placement of closure device
Catheter insertion and positioning
Contrast injection (except as listed below)
Imaging and insertion of closure device
Radiology supervision and interpretation
Roadmapping angiography

EXCLUDES *Congenital cardiac cath procedures (93530-93533)*

Code also separately identifiable:
- Aortography (93567)
- Noncardiac angiography (see radiology and vascular codes)
- Pulmonary angiography (93568)
- Right ventricular or atrial injection (93566)

93451 Right heart catheterization including measurement(s) of oxygen saturation and cardiac output, when performed

INCLUDES Cardiac output review
Insertion catheter into 1+ right cardiac chambers or areas
Obtaining samples for blood gas

EXCLUDES *Catheterization procedures that include right side of heart (93453, 93456-93457, 93460-93461)*
Implantation wireless pulmonary artery pressure sensor (33289)
Indicator dilution studies (93561-93562)
Percutaneous repair congenital interatrial defect (93580)
Swan-Ganz catheter insertion (93503)
Valve repair or annulus reconstruction (33418, 0345T, 0483T, 0484T, 0544T, 0545T)

Code also administration of medication or exercise to repeat assessment of hemodynamic measurement (93463-93464)

22.1 22.1 FUD 000 J G2 80

AMA: 2019,Jun,3; 2019,Mar,6; 2018,Dec,10; 2018,Dec,10; 2018,Feb,11; 2018,Jan,8; 2017,Dec,13; 2017,Jul,3; 2017,Jan,8; 2016,Mar,5; 2016,Jan,13; 2015,Sep,3; 2015,Jan,16; 2014,Jul,3; 2014,Jan,11

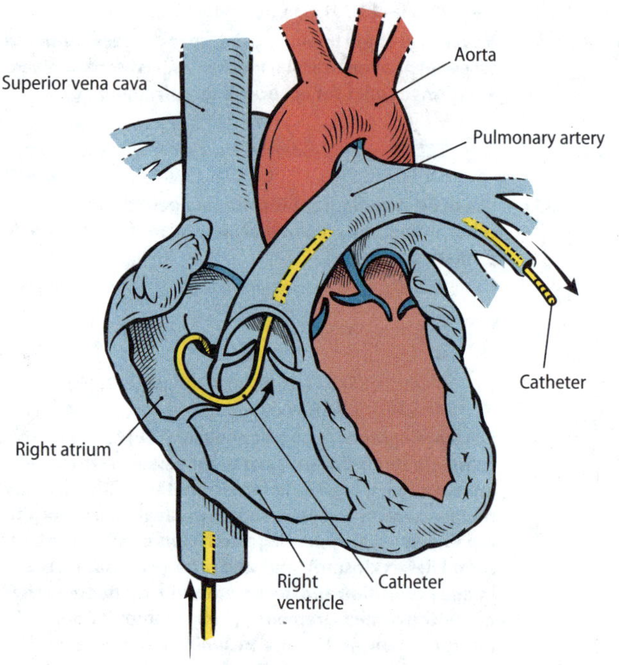

93452 Left heart catheterization including intraprocedural injection(s) for left ventriculography, imaging supervision and interpretation, when performed

INCLUDES Insertion of catheter into left cardiac chambers

EXCLUDES *Catheterization procedures that include injections for left ventriculography (93453, 93458-93461)*
Injection procedures (93561-93565)
Percutaneous repair congenital interatrial defect (93580)
Services related to cardiac contractility modulation systems (0408T-0411T, 0414T-0415T)
Swan-Ganz catheter insertion (93503)
Valve repair or annulus reconstruction (33418, 0345T, 0483T, 0484T, 0544T, 0545T)

Code also administration of medication or exercise to repeat assessment of hemodynamic measurement (93463-93464)

Code also transapical or transseptal puncture (93462)

24.6 24.6 FUD 000 J G2 80

AMA: 2018,Feb,11; 2018,Jan,8; 2017,Jul,3; 2017,Jan,8; 2016,Jan,13; 2015,Jan,16; 2014,Jul,3; 2014,Jan,11

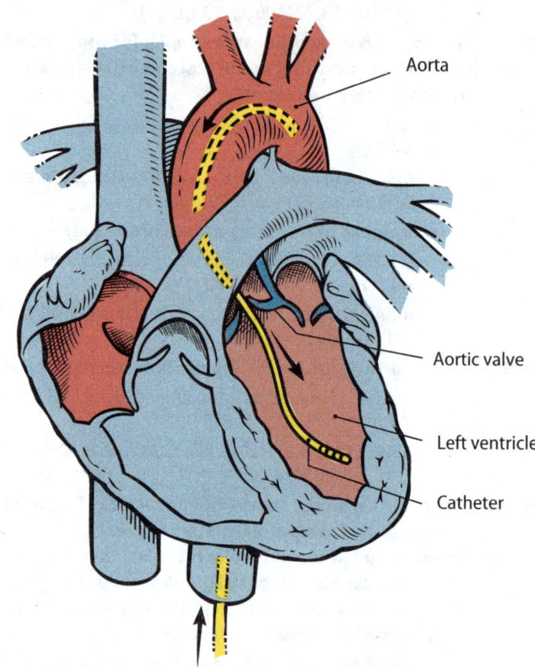

93453 Combined right and left heart catheterization including intraprocedural injection(s) for left ventriculography, imaging supervision and interpretation, when performed

INCLUDES Cardiac output review
Insertion catheter into 1+ right cardiac chambers or areas
Insertion of catheter into left cardiac chambers
Obtaining samples for blood gas

EXCLUDES *Catheterization procedures (93451-93452, 93456-93461)*
Injection procedures (93561-93565)
Percutaneous repair congenital interatrial defect (93580)
Services related to cardiac contractility modulation systems (0408T-0411T, 0414T-0415T)
Swan-Ganz catheter insertion (93503)
Valve repair or annulus reconstruction (33418, 0345T, 0483T, 0484T, 0544T, 0545T)

Code also administration of medication or exercise to repeat assessment of hemodynamic measurement (93463-93464)

Code also transapical or transseptal puncture (93462)

31.9 31.9 FUD 000 J G2 80

AMA: 2019,Jun,3; 2019,Mar,6; 2018,Feb,11; 2018,Jan,8; 2017,Jul,3; 2017,Jan,8; 2016,Mar,5; 2016,Jan,13; 2015,Sep,3; 2015,Jan,16; 2014,Jul,3; 2014,Jan,11

93454 Catheter placement in coronary artery(s) for coronary angiography, including intraprocedural injection(s) for coronary angiography, imaging supervision and interpretation;

EXCLUDES *Injection procedures (93561-93565)*
Swan-Ganz catheter insertion (93503)
Valve repair or annulus reconstruction (33418, 0345T, 0483T, 0484T, 0544T, 0545T)

24.8 24.8 FUD 000 J G2 80

AMA: 2018,Feb,11; 2018,Jan,8; 2017,Feb,14; 2017,Jan,8; 2016,Mar,5; 2016,Jan,13; 2015,Jan,16; 2014,Dec,6; 2014,Jul,3; 2014,Jan,11

93455 with catheter placement(s) in bypass graft(s) (internal mammary, free arterial, venous grafts) including intraprocedural injection(s) for bypass graft angiography

EXCLUDES *Injection procedures (93561-93565)*
Percutaneous repair congenital interatrial defect (93580)
Swan-Ganz catheter insertion (93503)
Valve repair or annulus reconstruction (33418, 0345T, 0483T, 0484T, 0544T, 0545T)

28.6 28.6 FUD 000 J G2 80

AMA: 2018,Feb,11; 2018,Jan,8; 2017,Jan,8; 2016,Mar,5; 2016,Jan,13; 2015,Jan,16; 2014,Dec,6; 2014,Jul,3; 2014,Jan,11

93456 with right heart catheterization

INCLUDES Cardiac output review
Insertion catheter into 1+ right cardiac chambers or areas
Obtaining samples for blood gas

EXCLUDES *Injection procedures (93561-93565)*
Percutaneous repair congenital interatrial defect (93580)
Swan-Ganz catheter insertion (93503)
Valve repair or annulus reconstruction (33418, 0345T, 0483T, 0484T, 0544T, 0545T)

Code also administration of medication or exercise to repeat assessment of hemodynamic measurement (93463-93464)

31.4 31.4 FUD 000 ⊘ J G2 80

AMA: 2019,Jun,3; 2019,Mar,6; 2018,Feb,11; 2018,Jan,8; 2017,Jul,3; 2017,Jan,8; 2016,Mar,5; 2016,Jan,13; 2015,Sep,3; 2015,Jan,16; 2014,Dec,6; 2014,Jul,3; 2014,Jan,11

93457 with catheter placement(s) in bypass graft(s) (internal mammary, free arterial, venous grafts) including intraprocedural injection(s) for bypass graft angiography and right heart catheterization

INCLUDES Cardiac output review
Insertion catheter into 1+ right cardiac chambers or areas
Obtaining samples for blood gas

EXCLUDES *Injection procedures (93561-93565)*
Percutaneous repair congenital interatrial defect (93580)
Swan-Ganz catheter insertion (93503)
Valve repair or annulus reconstruction (33418, 0345T, 0483T, 0484T, 0544T, 0545T)

Code also administration of medication or exercise to repeat assessment of hemodynamic measurement (93463-93464)

35.1 35.1 FUD 000 J G2 80

AMA: 2019,Jun,3; 2019,Mar,6; 2018,Feb,11; 2018,Jan,8; 2017,Jan,8; 2016,Mar,5; 2016,Jan,13; 2015,Sep,3; 2015,Jan,16; 2014,Dec,6; 2014,Jul,3; 2014,Jan,11

93458 with left heart catheterization including intraprocedural injection(s) for left ventriculography, when performed

INCLUDES Insertion of catheter into left cardiac chambers

EXCLUDES *Injection procedures (93561-93565)*
Percutaneous repair congenital interatrial defect (93580)
Services related to cardiac contractility modulation systems (0408T-0411T, 0414T-0415T)
Swan-Ganz catheter insertion (93503)
Valve repair or annulus reconstruction (33418, 0345T, 0483T, 0484T, 0544T, 0545T)

Code also administration of medication or exercise to repeat assessment of hemodynamic measurement (93463-93464)
Code also transapical or transseptal puncture (93462)

29.5 29.5 FUD 000 J G2 80

AMA: 2018,Feb,11; 2018,Jan,8; 2017,Jul,3; 2017,Jan,8; 2016,Mar,5; 2016,Jan,13; 2015,Sep,3; 2015,Jan,16; 2014,Dec,6; 2014,Jul,3; 2014,Jan,11

93459 with left heart catheterization including intraprocedural injection(s) for left ventriculography, when performed, catheter placement(s) in bypass graft(s) (internal mammary, free arterial, venous grafts) with bypass graft angiography

INCLUDES Insertion of catheter into left cardiac chambers

EXCLUDES *Injection procedures (93561-93565)*
Percutaneous repair congenital interatrial defect (93580)
Services related to cardiac contractility modulation systems (0408T-0411T, 0414T-0415T)
Swan-Ganz catheter insertion (93503)
Valve repair or annulus reconstruction (33418, 0345T, 0483T, 0484T, 0544T, 0545T)

Code also administration of medication or exercise to repeat assessment of hemodynamic measurement (93463-93464)
Code also transapical or transseptal puncture (93462)

32.4 32.4 FUD 000 J G2 80

AMA: 2018,Feb,11; 2018,Jan,8; 2017,Jul,3; 2017,Jan,8; 2016,Mar,5; 2016,Jan,13; 2015,Sep,3; 2015,Jan,16; 2014,Dec,6; 2014,Jul,3; 2014,Jan,11

93460 with right and left heart catheterization including intraprocedural injection(s) for left ventriculography, when performed

INCLUDES Cardiac output review
Insertion catheter into 1+ right cardiac chambers or areas
Insertion of catheter into left cardiac chambers
Obtaining samples for blood gas

EXCLUDES *Injection procedures (93561-93565)*
Percutaneous repair congenital interatrial defect (93580)
Services related to cardiac contractility modulation systems (0408T-0411T, 0414T-0415T)
Swan-Ganz catheter insertion (93503)
Valve repair or annulus reconstruction (33418, 0345T, 0483T, 0484T, 0544T, 0545T)

Code also administration of medication or exercise to repeat assessment of hemodynamic measurement (93463-93464)
Code also transapical or transseptal puncture (93462)

35.4 35.4 FUD 000 J G2 80

AMA: 2019,Jun,3; 2019,Mar,6; 2018,Feb,11; 2018,Jan,8; 2017,Jul,3; 2017,Jan,8; 2016,Mar,5; 2016,Jan,13; 2015,Sep,3; 2015,Jan,16; 2014,Dec,6; 2014,Jul,3; 2014,Jan,11

93461 **with right and left heart catheterization including intraprocedural injection(s) for left ventriculography, when performed, catheter placement(s) in bypass graft(s) (internal mammary, free arterial, venous grafts) with bypass graft angiography**

INCLUDES Cardiac output review
Insertion catheter into 1+ right cardiac chambers or areas
Insertion of catheter into left cardiac chambers
Obtaining samples for blood gas

EXCLUDES *Injection procedures (93561-93565)*
Percutaneous repair congenital interatrial defect (93580)
Services related to cardiac contractility modulation systems (0408T-0411T, 0414T-0415T)
Swan-Ganz catheter insertion (93503)
Valve repair or annulus reconstruction (33418, 0345T, 0483T, 0484T, 0544T, 0545T)

Code also administration of medication or exercise to repeat assessment of hemodynamic measurement (93463-93464)
Code also transapical or transseptal puncture (93462)

40.0 40.0 FUD 000 J G2 80

AMA: 2019,Jun,3; 2019,Mar,6; 2018,Feb,11; 2018,Jan,8; 2017,Jul,3; 2017,Jan,8; 2016,Mar,5; 2016,Jan,13; 2015,Sep,3; 2015,Jan,16; 2014,Dec,6; 2014,Jul,3; 2014,Jan,11

+ **93462** **Left heart catheterization by transseptal puncture through intact septum or by transapical puncture (List separately in addition to code for primary procedure)**

INCLUDES Insertion of catheter into left cardiac chambers

EXCLUDES *Comprehensive electrophysiologic evaluation (93656)*
Transseptal approach for percutaneous closure paravalvular leak (93590)
Valve repair or annulus reconstruction unless performed with transapical puncture (0345T, 0544T)

Code also percutaneous closure paravalvular leak when a transapical puncture is performed (93590-93591)
Code first (33477, 93452-93453, 93458-93461, 93582, 93653-93654)

6.11 6.11 FUD ZZZ N N1 80

AMA: 2018,Feb,11; 2018,Jan,8; 2017,Sep,3; 2017,Jul,3; 2017,Jan,8; 2016,Jan,13; 2015,Sep,3; 2015,Jan,16; 2014,Jul,3; 2014,Jan,11

+ **93463** **Pharmacologic agent administration (eg, inhaled nitric oxide, intravenous infusion of nitroprusside, dobutamine, milrinone, or other agent) including assessing hemodynamic measurements before, during, after and repeat pharmacologic agent administration, when performed (List separately in addition to code for primary procedure)**

EXCLUDES *Coronary interventional procedures (92920-92944, 92975, 92977)*
Use of code more than one time per catheterization

Code first (33477, 93451-93453, 93456-93461, 93530-93533, 93580-93581)

2.82 2.82 FUD ZZZ N 80

AMA: 2018,Feb,11; 2018,Jan,8; 2017,Jan,8; 2016,Jan,13; 2015,Jan,16; 2014,Dec,6; 2014,Jul,3; 2014,Jan,11

+ **93464** **Physiologic exercise study (eg, bicycle or arm ergometry) including assessing hemodynamic measurements before and after (List separately in addition to code for primary procedure)**

EXCLUDES *Administration of pharmacologic agent (93463)*
Bundle of His recording (93600)
Use of code more than one time per catheterization

Code first (33477, 93451-93453, 93456-93461, 93530-93533)

7.04 7.04 FUD ZZZ N 80

AMA: 2018,Feb,11; 2018,Jan,8; 2017,Jan,8; 2016,Jan,13; 2015,Jan,16; 2014,Jul,3; 2014,Jan,11

93503 **Insertion and placement of flow directed catheter (eg, Swan-Ganz) for monitoring purposes**

EXCLUDES *Diagnostic cardiac catheterization (93451-93461, 93530-93533)*
Subsequent monitoring (99356-99357)

2.55 2.55 FUD 000 T 80

AMA: 2018,Feb,11; 2018,Jan,8; 2017,Jan,8; 2016,Jan,13; 2015,Jan,16; 2014,Jan,11

93505 **Endomyocardial biopsy**

EXCLUDES *Intravascular brachytherapy radionuclide insertion (77770-77772)*
Transcatheter insertion of brachytherapy delivery device (92974)

19.9 19.9 FUD 000 T 80

AMA: 2018,Feb,11; 2018,Jan,8; 2017,Dec,13; 2017,Jan,8; 2016,Jan,13; 2015,Jan,16; 2014,Jan,11

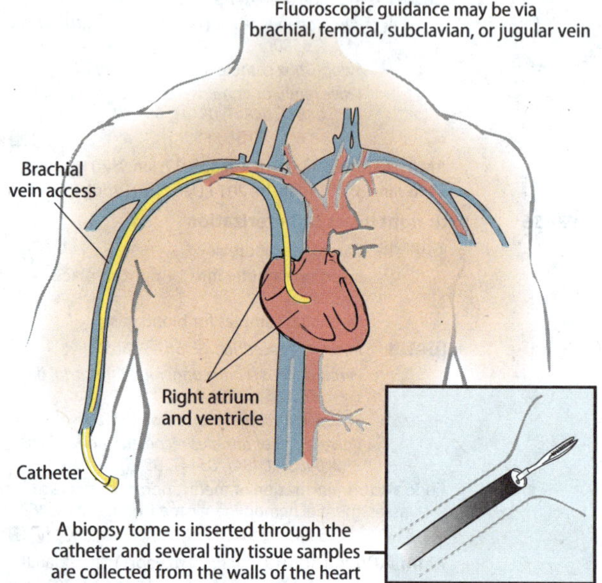

93530-93533 Congenital Heart Defect Catheterization

INCLUDES Access site imaging and placement of closure device
Cardiac output review
Insertion catheter into 1+ right cardiac chambers or areas
Obtaining samples for blood gas
Radiology supervision and interpretation
Roadmapping angiography

EXCLUDES *Cardiac cath on noncongenital heart (93451-93453, 93456-93461)*
Percutaneous repair congenital interatrial defect (93580)
Swan-Ganz catheter insertion (93503)

Code also (93563-93568)

93530 **Right heart catheterization, for congenital cardiac anomalies**

0.00 0.00 FUD 000 J 80

AMA: 2019,Jun,3; 2019,Mar,6; 2018,Feb,11; 2018,Jan,8; 2017,Jul,3; 2017,Jan,8; 2016,Mar,5; 2016,Jan,13; 2015,Sep,3; 2015,Jan,16; 2014,Jul,3; 2014,Jan,11

93531 **Combined right heart catheterization and retrograde left heart catheterization, for congenital cardiac anomalies**

0.00 0.00 FUD 000 J 80

AMA: 2019,Jun,3; 2019,Mar,6; 2018,Feb,11; 2018,Jan,8; 2017,Jul,3; 2017,Jan,8; 2016,Mar,5; 2016,Jan,13; 2015,Sep,3; 2015,Jan,16; 2014,Jul,3; 2014,Jan,11

93532 **Combined right heart catheterization and transseptal left heart catheterization through intact septum with or without retrograde left heart catheterization, for congenital cardiac anomalies**

0.00 0.00 FUD 000

AMA: 2019,Jun,3; 2019,Mar,6; 2018,Feb,11; 2018,Jan,8; 2017,Jul,3; 2017,Jan,8; 2016,Mar,5; 2016,Jan,13; 2015,Sep,3; 2015,Jan,16; 2014,Jul,3; 2014,Jan,11

93533 **Combined right heart catheterization and transseptal left heart catheterization through existing septal opening, with or without retrograde left heart catheterization, for congenital cardiac anomalies**

0.00 0.00 FUD 000

AMA: 2019,Jun,3; 2019,Mar,6; 2018,Feb,11; 2018,Jan,8; 2017,Jul,3; 2017,Jan,8; 2016,Mar,5; 2016,Jan,13; 2015,Sep,3; 2015,Jan,16; 2014,Jul,3; 2014,Jan,11

93561-93568 Injection Procedures

INCLUDES Catheter repositioning
Radiology supervision and interpretation
Using automatic power injector

93561 **Indicator dilution studies such as dye or thermodilution, including arterial and/or venous catheterization; with cardiac output measurement (separate procedure)**

EXCLUDES *Cardiac output, radioisotope method (78472-78473, 78481)*
Catheterization procedures (93451-93462)
Percutaneous closure patent ductus arteriosus (93582)

0.00 0.00 FUD ZZZ

AMA: 2019,Aug,8; 2018,Feb,11; 2018,Jan,8; 2017,Jan,8; 2016,Jan,13; 2015,Jan,16; 2014,Jul,3; 2014,Jan,11

93562 **subsequent measurement of cardiac output**

EXCLUDES *Cardiac output, radioisotope method (78472-78473, 78481)*
Catheterization procedures (93451-93462)
Percutaneous closure patent ductus arteriosus (93582)

0.00 0.00 FUD ZZZ

AMA: 2019,Aug,8; 2018,Feb,11; 2018,Jan,8; 2017,Jan,8; 2016,Jan,13; 2015,Jan,16; 2014,Jul,3; 2014,May,4; 2014,Jan,11

\+ **93563** **Injection procedure during cardiac catheterization including imaging supervision, interpretation, and report; for selective coronary angiography during congenital heart catheterization (List separately in addition to code for primary procedure)**

EXCLUDES *Catheterization procedures (93452-93461)*
Valve repair or annulus reconstruction (33418, 0345T, 0483T, 0484T, 0544T, 0545T)

Code first (93530-93533)

1.69 1.69 FUD ZZZ

AMA: 2018,Feb,11; 2018,Jan,8; 2017,Jan,8; 2016,Mar,5; 2016,Jan,13; 2015,Jan,16; 2014,Dec,6; 2014,Jan,11

\+ **93564** **for selective opacification of aortocoronary venous or arterial bypass graft(s) (eg, aortocoronary saphenous vein, free radial artery, or free mammary artery graft) to one or more coronary arteries and in situ arterial conduits (eg, internal mammary), whether native or used for bypass to one or more coronary arteries during congenital heart catheterization, when performed (List separately in addition to code for primary procedure)**

Percutaneous repair congenital interatrial defect (93580)
Valve repair or annulus reconstruction (33418, 0345T, 0483T, 0484T, 0544T, 0545T)

Code first (93530-93533)

EXCLUDES *Catheterization procedures (93452-93461)*

1.79 1.79 FUD ZZZ

AMA: 2018,Feb,11; 2018,Jan,8; 2017,Jan,8; 2016,Mar,5; 2016,Jan,13; 2015,Jan,16; 2014,Dec,6; 2014,Jan,11

\+ **93565** **for selective left ventricular or left atrial angiography (List separately in addition to code for primary procedure)**

EXCLUDES *Catheterization procedures (93452-93461)*
Percutaneous repair congenital interatrial defect (93580)

Code first (93530-93533)

1.31 1.31 FUD ZZZ

AMA: 2018,Feb,11; 2018,Jan,8; 2017,Jan,8; 2016,Jan,13; 2015,Jan,16; 2014,Jan,11

\+ **93566** **for selective right ventricular or right atrial angiography (List separately in addition to code for primary procedure)**

EXCLUDES *Annulus reconstruction (0545T)*
Percutaneous repair congenital interatrial defect (93580)
Use for right ventriculography when performed during insertion leadless pacemaker ([33274])

Code first (93451, 93453, 93456-93457, 93460-93461, 93530-93533)

1.35 4.38 FUD ZZZ

AMA: 2019,Mar,6; 2018,Feb,11; 2018,Jan,8; 2017,Jan,8; 2016,Aug,5; 2016,May,5; 2016,Mar,5; 2016,Jan,13; 2015,May,3; 2015,Jan,16; 2014,Jan,11

\+ **93567** **for supravalvular aortography (List separately in addition to code for primary procedure)**

EXCLUDES *Abdominal aortography or non-supravalvular thoracic aortography at same time as cardiac catheterization (36221, 75600-75630)*

Code first (93451-93461, 93530-93533)

1.53 3.71 FUD ZZZ

AMA: 2018,Feb,11; 2018,Jan,8; 2017,Jan,8; 2016,Mar,5; 2016,Jan,13; 2015,Jan,16; 2014,Jan,11

\+ **93568** **for pulmonary angiography (List separately in addition to code for primary procedure)**

Code first (93451, 93453, 93456-93457, 93460-93461, 93530-93533)

1.38 3.97 FUD ZZZ

AMA: 2019,Jun,3; 2019,Apr,10; 2018,Feb,11; 2018,Jan,8; 2017,Jan,8; 2016,Mar,5; 2016,Jan,13; 2015,Jan,16; 2014,Jan,11

93571-93572 Coronary Artery Doppler Studies

INCLUDES Doppler transducer manipulations/repositioning within the vessel examined, during coronary angiography/therapeutic intervention (angioplasty)

EXCLUDES *Intraprocedural coronary fractional flow reserve (FFR) ([0523T])*

\+ **93571** **Intravascular Doppler velocity and/or pressure derived coronary flow reserve measurement (coronary vessel or graft) during coronary angiography including pharmacologically induced stress; initial vessel (List separately in addition to code for primary procedure)**

Code first (92920, 92924, 92928, 92933, 92937, 92941, 92943, 92975, 93454-93461, 93563-93564)

0.00 0.00 FUD ZZZ

AMA: 2018,Feb,11; 2018,Jan,8; 2017,Jan,8; 2016,Jan,13; 2015,Dec,18; 2015,May,10; 2015,Jan,16; 2014,Dec,6; 2014,Jan,11

\+ **93572** **each additional vessel (List separately in addition to code for primary procedure)**

Code first initial vessel (93571)

0.00 0.00 FUD ZZZ

AMA: 2018,Feb,11; 2018,Jan,8; 2017,Jan,8; 2016,Jan,13; 2015,Dec,18; 2015,May,10; 2015,Jan,16; 2014,Dec,6; 2014,Jan,11

Medicine

93532 — 93572

93580-93583 Percutaneous Repair of Congenital Heart Defects

93580 Percutaneous transcatheter closure of congenital interatrial communication (ie, Fontan fenestration, atrial septal defect) with implant

INCLUDES Injection of contrast for right heart atrial/ventricular angiograms (93564-93566)
Right heart catheterization (93451, 93453, 93456-93457, 93460-93461, 93530-93533)

EXCLUDES *Bypass graft angiography (93455)*
Injection of contrast for left heart atrial/ventricular angiograms (93458-93459)
Left heart catheterization (93452, 93458-93459)

Code also echocardiography, when performed (93303-93317, 93662)

28.4 28.4 FUD 000 J 80

AMA: 2018,Feb,11; 2018,Jan,8; 2017,Jan,8; 2016,Jan,13; 2015,Jan,16; 2014,Jan,11

93581 Percutaneous transcatheter closure of a congenital ventricular septal defect with implant

INCLUDES Injection of contrast for right heart atrial/ventricular angiograms (93564-93566)
Right heart catheterization (93451, 93453, 93456-93457, 93460-93461, 93530-93533)

EXCLUDES *Bypass graft angiography (93455)*
Injection of contrast for left heart atrial/ventricular angiograms (93458-93459)
Left heart catheterization (93452, 93458-93459)

Code also echocardiography, when performed (93303-93317, 93662)

38.7 38.7 FUD 000 J 80

AMA: 2018,Feb,11; 2018,Jan,8; 2017,Jan,8; 2016,Jan,13; 2015,Jan,16; 2014,Jan,11

93582 Percutaneous transcatheter closure of patent ductus arteriosus

INCLUDES Aorta catheter placement (36200)
Aortography (75600-75605, 93567)
Heart catheterization (93451-93461, 93530-93533)

EXCLUDES *Catheterization pulmonary artery (36013-36014)*
Intracardiac echocardiographic services (93662)
Left heart catheterization performed via transapical puncture or transseptal puncture through intact septum (93462)
Ligation repair (33820, 33822, 33824)
Other cardiac angiographic procedures (93563-93566, 93568)
Other echocardiographic services by different provider (93315-93317)

19.4 19.4 FUD 000 J 80

AMA: 2019,Apr,10; 2018,Feb,11; 2018,Jan,8; 2017,Jan,8; 2016,Jan,13; 2015,Jan,16; 2014,Jul,3

93583 Percutaneous transcatheter septal reduction therapy (eg, alcohol septal ablation) including temporary pacemaker insertion when performed

INCLUDES Alcohol injection (93463)
Coronary angiography during the procedure to roadmap, guide the intervention, measure the vessel, and complete the angiography (93454-93461, 93531-93533, 93563, 93563, 93565)
Left heart catheterization (93452-93453, 93458-93461, 93531-93533)
Temporary pacemaker insertion (33210)

EXCLUDES *Intracardiac echocardiographic services when performed (93662)*
Myectomy (surgical ventriculomyotomy) to treat idiopathic hypertrophic subaortic stenosis (33416)
Other echocardiographic services rendered by different provider (93312-93317)

Code also diagnostic cardiac catheterization procedures if the patient's condition (clinical indication) has changed since the intervention or prior study, there is no available prior catheter-based diagnostic study of the treatment zone, or the prior study is not adequate (93451, 93454-93457, 93530, 93563-93564, 93566-93568)

21.6 21.6 FUD 000 C 80

AMA: 2018,Feb,11

93590-93592 Percutaneous Repair Paravalvular Leak

INCLUDES Access with insertion and positioning of device
Angiography
Fluoroscopy (76000)
Imaging guidance
Left heart catheterization (93452-93453, 93459-93461, 93531-93533)

Code also diagnostic right heart catheterization and angiography performed:
If a previous study is available but documentation states the patient's condition has changed since the previous study; visualization is insufficient; or a change necessitates reevaluation; append modifier 59
When there is no previous study and a complete diagnostic study is performed; append modifier 59

93590 Percutaneous transcatheter closure of paravalvular leak; initial occlusion device, mitral valve

INCLUDES Transseptal puncture (93462)

Code also for transapical puncture (93462)

31.2 31.2 FUD 000 J 80

AMA: 2018,Feb,11; 2018,Jan,8; 2017,Sep,3

93591 initial occlusion device, aortic valve

EXCLUDES *Transapical or transseptal puncture (93462)*

25.7 25.7 FUD 000 J 80

AMA: 2018,Feb,11; 2018,Jan,8; 2017,Sep,3

+ **93592 each additional occlusion device (List separately in addition to code for primary procedure)**

Code first (93590-93591)

11.3 11.3 FUD ZZZ N 80

AMA: 2018,Feb,11; 2018,Jan,8; 2017,Sep,3

93600-93603 Recording of Intracardiac Electrograms

INCLUDES Unusual situations where there may be recording/pacing/attempt at arrhythmia induction from only one side of the heart

EXCLUDES *Comprehensive electrophysiological studies (93619-93620, 93653-93654, 93656)*

93600 Bundle of His recording

0.00 0.00 FUD 000 J 80

AMA: 2018,Feb,11; 2018,Jan,8; 2017,Jan,8; 2016,Jan,13; 2015,Jan,16; 2014,Apr,3; 2014,Jan,11

93602 Intra-atrial recording

0.00 0.00 FUD 000 J 80

AMA: 2018,Feb,11; 2018,Jan,8; 2017,Jan,8; 2016,Jan,13; 2015,Jan,16; 2014,Apr,3; 2014,Jan,11

93603 Right ventricular recording

0.00 0.00 FUD 000 J 80

AMA: 2018,Feb,11; 2018,Jan,8; 2017,Jan,8; 2016,Jan,13; 2015,Jan,16; 2014,Apr,3; 2014,Jan,11

93609-93613 Intracardiac Mapping and Pacing

\+ **93609** **Intraventricular and/or intra-atrial mapping of tachycardia site(s) with catheter manipulation to record from multiple sites to identify origin of tachycardia (List separately in addition to code for primary procedure)**

EXCLUDES *Intracardiac 3D mapping (93613)*
Intracardiac ablation with 3D mapping (93654)

Code first (93620, 93653, 93656)
0.00 0.00 FUD ZZZ N 80
AMA: 2018,Feb,11; 2018,Jan,8; 2017,Jan,8; 2016,Jan,13; 2015,Jan,16; 2014,Apr,3; 2014,Jan,11

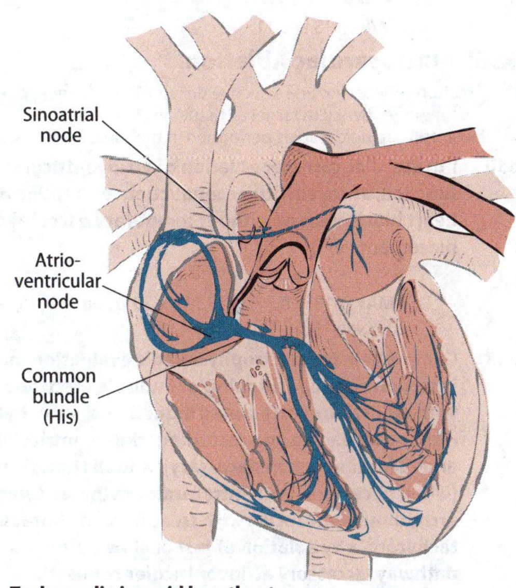

Tachycardia is rapid heartbeat

93610 **Intra-atrial pacing**

INCLUDES Unusual situations where there may be recording/pacing/attempt at arrhythmia induction from only one side of the heart

EXCLUDES *Comprehensive electrophysiological studies (93619-93620)*
Intracardiac ablation (93653-93654, 93656)

0.00 0.00 FUD 000 J 80
AMA: 2018,Feb,11; 2018,Jan,8; 2017,Jan,8; 2016,Jan,13; 2015,Jan,16; 2014,Apr,3; 2014,Jan,11

93612 **Intraventricular pacing**

INCLUDES Unusual situations where there may be recording/pacing/attempt at arrhythmia induction from only one side of the heart

EXCLUDES *Comprehensive electrophysiological studies (93619-93622)*
Intracardiac ablation (93653-93654, 93656)

0.00 0.00 FUD 000 J 80
AMA: 2018,Feb,11; 2018,Jan,8; 2017,Jan,8; 2016,Jan,13; 2015,Jan,16; 2014,Apr,3; 2014,Jan,11

\+ **93613** **Intracardiac electrophysiologic 3-dimensional mapping (List separately in addition to code for primary procedure)**

EXCLUDES *Intracardiac ablation with 3D mapping (93654)*
Mapping of tachycardia site (93609)

Code first (93620, 93653, 93656)
8.63 8.63 FUD ZZZ N 80
AMA: 2018,Feb,11; 2018,Jan,8; 2017,Jan,8; 2016,Jan,13; 2015,Jan,16; 2014,Apr,3; 2014,Jan,11

93615-93616 Recording and Pacing via Esophagus

93615 **Esophageal recording of atrial electrogram with or without ventricular electrogram(s);**

0.00 0.00 FUD 000 J 80
AMA: 2018,Feb,11; 2018,Jan,8; 2017,Jan,8; 2016,Jan,13; 2015,Jan,16; 2014,Jan,11

93616 **with pacing**

0.00 0.00 FUD 000 J 80
AMA: 2018,Feb,11; 2018,Jan,8; 2017,Jan,8; 2016,Jan,13; 2015,Jan,16; 2014,Jan,11

93618 Pacing to Produce an Arrhythmia

CMS: 100-03,20.12 Diagnostic Endocardial Electrical Stimulation (Pacing)

INCLUDES Unusual situations where there may be recording/pacing/attempt at arrhythmia induction from only one side of the heart

EXCLUDES *Comprehensive electrophysiological studies (93619-93622)*
Intracardiac ablation (93653-93654, 93656)
Intracardiac phonocardiogram (93799)

93618 **Induction of arrhythmia by electrical pacing**

0.00 0.00 FUD 000 J 80
AMA: 2018,Feb,11; 2018,Jan,8; 2017,Jan,8; 2016,Jan,13; 2015,Jan,16; 2014,Apr,3; 2014,Jan,11

93619-93623 Comprehensive Electrophysiological Studies

CMS: 100-03,20.12 Diagnostic Endocardial Electrical Stimulation (Pacing)

93619 **Comprehensive electrophysiologic evaluation with right atrial pacing and recording, right ventricular pacing and recording, His bundle recording, including insertion and repositioning of multiple electrode catheters, without induction or attempted induction of arrhythmia**

INCLUDES Evaluation of sinus node/atrioventricular node/His-Purkinje conduction system without arrhythmia induction

EXCLUDES *Comprehensive electrophysiological studies (93620-93622)*
Intracardiac ablation (93653-93657)
Intracardiac pacing (93610, 93612, 93618)
Recording of intracardiac electrograms (93600-93603)

0.00 0.00 FUD 000 J 80
AMA: 2018,Feb,11; 2018,Jan,8; 2017,Jan,8; 2016,Jan,13; 2015,Jan,16; 2014,Apr,3; 2014,Jan,11

93620 **Comprehensive electrophysiologic evaluation including insertion and repositioning of multiple electrode catheters with induction or attempted induction of arrhythmia; with right atrial pacing and recording, right ventricular pacing and recording, His bundle recording**

INCLUDES Recording/pacing/attempted arrhythmia induction from one or more site(s) in the heart

EXCLUDES *Comprehensive electrophysiological study without induction/attempted induction arrhythmia (93619)*
Intracardiac ablation (93653-93657)
Intracardiac pacing (93610, 93612, 93618)
Recording of intracardiac electrograms (93600-93603)

0.00 0.00 FUD 000 J 80
AMA: 2018,Feb,11; 2018,Jan,8; 2017,Jan,8; 2016,Jan,13; 2015,Jan,16; 2014,Apr,3; 2014,Jan,11

\+ **93621** **with left atrial pacing and recording from coronary sinus or left atrium (List separately in addition to code for primary procedure)**

INCLUDES Recording/pacing/attempted arrhythmia induction from one or more site(s) in the heart

EXCLUDES *Intracardiac ablation (93656)*

Code first (93620, 93653-93654)
0.00 0.00 FUD ZZZ N 80
AMA: 2018,Feb,11; 2018,Jan,8; 2017,Jan,8; 2016,Jan,13; 2015,Jan,16; 2014,Apr,3; 2014,Jan,11

+ 93622 **with left ventricular pacing and recording (List separately in addition to code for primary procedure)**

EXCLUDES *Intracardiac ablation (93654)*

Code first (93620, 93653, 93656)

0.00 0.00 FUD ZZZ N 80

AMA: 2018,Feb,11; 2018,Jan,8; 2017,Jan,8; 2016,Jan,13; 2015,Jan,16; 2014,Apr,3; 2014,Jan,11

+ 93623 **Programmed stimulation and pacing after intravenous drug infusion (List separately in addition to code for primary procedure)**

INCLUDES Recording/pacing/attempted arrhythmia induction from one or more site(s) in the heart

EXCLUDES *Use of code more than one time per day*

Code first comprehensive electrophysiologic evaluation (93610, 93612, 93619-93620, 93653-93654, 93656)

0.00 0.00 FUD ZZZ N 80

AMA: 2018,Feb,11; 2018,Jan,8; 2017,Jan,8; 2016,Jan,13; 2015,Jan,16; 2014,Apr,3; 2014,Jan,11

93624-93631 Followup and Intraoperative Electrophysiologic Studies

CMS: 100-03,20.12 Diagnostic Endocardial Electrical Stimulation (Pacing)

93624 **Electrophysiologic follow-up study with pacing and recording to test effectiveness of therapy, including induction or attempted induction of arrhythmia**

INCLUDES Recording/pacing/attempted arrhythmia induction from one or more site(s) in the heart

0.00 0.00 FUD 000 J 80

AMA: 2018,Feb,11; 2018,Jan,8; 2017,Jan,8; 2016,Jan,13; 2015,Jan,16; 2014,Jan,11

93631 **Intra-operative epicardial and endocardial pacing and mapping to localize the site of tachycardia or zone of slow conduction for surgical correction**

EXCLUDES *Operative ablation of an arrhythmogenic focus or pathway by a separate provider (33250-33261)*

0.00 0.00 FUD 000 N 80

AMA: 2018,Feb,11; 2018,Jan,8; 2017,Jan,8; 2016,Jan,13; 2015,Jan,16; 2014,Jan,11

93640-93644 Electrophysiologic Studies of Cardioverter-Defibrillators

INCLUDES Recording/pacing/attempted arrhythmia induction from one or more site(s) in the heart

93640 **Electrophysiologic evaluation of single or dual chamber pacing cardioverter-defibrillator leads including defibrillation threshold evaluation (induction of arrhythmia, evaluation of sensing and pacing for arrhythmia termination) at time of initial implantation or replacement;**

0.00 0.00 FUD 000 N 80

AMA: 2018,Feb,11; 2018,Jan,8; 2017,Jan,8; 2016,Jan,13; 2015,Jan,16; 2014,Jan,11

93641 **with testing of single or dual chamber pacing cardioverter-defibrillator pulse generator**

EXCLUDES *Single/dual chamber pacing cardioverter-defibrillators reprogramming/electronic analysis, subsequent/periodic (93282-93283, 93289, 93292, 93295, 93642)*

0.00 0.00 FUD 000 N 80

AMA: 2018,Feb,11; 2018,Jan,8; 2017,Jan,8; 2016,Jan,13; 2015,Jan,16; 2014,Apr,3; 2014,Jan,11

93642 **Electrophysiologic evaluation of single or dual chamber transvenous pacing cardioverter-defibrillator (includes defibrillation threshold evaluation, induction of arrhythmia, evaluation of sensing and pacing for arrhythmia termination, and programming or reprogramming of sensing or therapeutic parameters)**

9.78 9.78 FUD 000 J 80

AMA: 2018,Feb,11; 2018,Jan,8; 2017,Jan,8; 2016,Jan,13; 2015,Jan,16; 2014,Apr,3; 2014,Jan,11

93644 **Electrophysiologic evaluation of subcutaneous implantable defibrillator (includes defibrillation threshold evaluation, induction of arrhythmia, evaluation of sensing for arrhythmia termination, and programming or reprogramming of sensing or therapeutic parameters)**

EXCLUDES *Electrophysiological evaluation subcutaneous implantable defibrillator system with substernal electrode (0577T)*

Insertion/replacement subcutaneous implantable defibrillator ([33270])

Subcutaneous cardioverter-defibrillator electrophysiologic evaluation, subsequent/periodic (93260-93261)

5.65 5.65 FUD 000 N 80

AMA: 2018,Feb,11

93650-93657 Intracardiac Ablation

INCLUDES Ablation services include selective delivery of cryo-energy or radiofrequency to targeted tissue

Electrophysiologic studies performed in the same session with ablation

93650 **Intracardiac catheter ablation of atrioventricular node function, atrioventricular conduction for creation of complete heart block, with or without temporary pacemaker placement**

17.2 17.2 FUD 000 J 80

AMA: 2018,Feb,11; 2018,Jan,8; 2017,Jan,8; 2016,Jan,13; 2015,Jan,16; 2014,Jan,11

93653 **Comprehensive electrophysiologic evaluation including insertion and repositioning of multiple electrode catheters with induction or attempted induction of an arrhythmia with right atrial pacing and recording, right ventricular pacing and recording (when necessary), and His bundle recording (when necessary) with intracardiac catheter ablation of arrhythmogenic focus; with treatment of supraventricular tachycardia by ablation of fast or slow atrioventricular pathway, accessory atrioventricular connection, cavo-tricuspid isthmus or other single atrial focus or source of atrial re-entry**

EXCLUDES *Comprehensive electrophysiological studies (93619-93620)*

Electrophysiologic evaluation pacing cardioverter defibrillator (93642)

Intracardiac ablation with transseptal catheterization (93656)

Intracardiac ablation with treatment ventricular arrhythmia (93654)

Intracardiac pacing (93610, 93612, 93618)

Recording of intracardiac electrograms (93600-93603)

24.3 24.3 FUD 000 J 80

AMA: 2018,Feb,11; 2018,Jan,8; 2017,Jan,8; 2016,Jan,13; 2015,Jan,16; 2014,Apr,3

93654 **with treatment of ventricular tachycardia or focus of ventricular ectopy including intracardiac electrophysiologic 3D mapping, when performed, and left ventricular pacing and recording, when performed**

EXCLUDES *Comprehensive electrophysiological studies (93619-93620, 93622)*

Device evaluation (93279-93284, 93286-93289)

Electrophysiologic evaluation pacing cardioverter defibrillator (93642)

Intracardiac ablation with transseptal catheterization (93656)

Intracardiac ablation with treatment supraventricular tachycardia (93653)

Intracardiac pacing (93609-93613, 93618)

Recording of intracardiac electrograms (93600-93603)

32.6 32.6 FUD 000 J 80

AMA: 2018,Feb,11; 2018,Jan,8; 2017,Jan,8; 2016,Jan,13; 2015,Jan,16; 2014,Apr,3

+ **93655** **Intracardiac catheter ablation of a discrete mechanism of arrhythmia which is distinct from the primary ablated mechanism, including repeat diagnostic maneuvers, to treat a spontaneous or induced arrhythmia (List separately in addition to code for primary procedure)**

Code first (93653-93654, 93656)

12.4 12.4 FUD ZZZ N 80

AMA: 2018,Feb,11; 2018,Jan,8; 2017,Jan,8; 2016,Jan,13; 2015,Jan,16; 2014,Apr,3

93656 **Comprehensive electrophysiologic evaluation including transseptal catheterizations, insertion and repositioning of multiple electrode catheters with induction or attempted induction of an arrhythmia including left or right atrial pacing/recording when necessary, right ventricular pacing/recording when necessary, and His bundle recording when necessary with intracardiac catheter ablation of atrial fibrillation by pulmonary vein isolation**

INCLUDES His bundle recording when indicated
Left atrial pacing/recording
Right ventricular pacing/recording

EXCLUDES *Comprehensive electrophysiological studies (93619-93621)*
Device evaluation (93279-93284, 93286-93289)
Electrophysiologic evaluation with treatment ventricular tachycardia (93654)
Intracardiac ablation with treatment supraventricular tachycardia (93653)
Intracardiac pacing (93610, 93612, 93618)
Left heart catheterization by transseptal puncture (93462)
Recording of intracardiac electrograms (93600-93603)

32.7 32.7 FUD 000 J 80

AMA: 2019,Sep,10; 2018,Feb,11; 2018,Jan,8; 2017,Jan,8; 2016,Jan,13; 2015,Jan,16; 2014,Apr,3

+ **93657** **Additional linear or focal intracardiac catheter ablation of the left or right atrium for treatment of atrial fibrillation remaining after completion of pulmonary vein isolation (List separately in addition to code for primary procedure)**

Code first (93656)

12.3 12.3 FUD ZZZ N 80

AMA: 2019,Sep,10; 2018,Feb,11; 2018,Jan,8; 2017,Jan,8; 2016,Jan,13; 2015,Jan,16; 2014,Apr,3

93660-93662 Other Tests for Cardiac Function

93660 **Evaluation of cardiovascular function with tilt table evaluation, with continuous ECG monitoring and intermittent blood pressure monitoring, with or without pharmacological intervention**

EXCLUDES *Autonomic nervous system function testing (95921, 95924, [95943])*

4.51 4.51 FUD 000 S 80

AMA: 2018,Feb,11; 2018,Jan,8; 2017,Jan,8; 2016,Jan,13; 2015,Jan,16; 2014,Jan,11

+ **93662** **Intracardiac echocardiography during therapeutic/diagnostic intervention, including imaging supervision and interpretation (List separately in addition to code for primary procedure)**

EXCLUDES *Internal cardioversion (92961)*
Transcatheter tricuspid valve repair with prosthesis, percutaneous approach (0569T-0570T)

Code first (as appropriate) (92987, 93453, 93460-93462, 93532, 93580-93581, 93620-93622, 93653-93654, 93656)

0.00 0.00 FUD ZZZ N 80

AMA: 2018,Feb,11; 2018,Jan,8; 2017,Jan,8; 2016,Jan,13; 2015,Jan,16; 2014,Jan,11

93668 Rehabilitation Services: Peripheral Arterial Disease

CMS: 100-03,1,20.35 Supervised Exercise Therapy (SET) for Symptomatic Peripheral Artery Disease (PAD)(Effective May 25, 2017; 100-04,32,390 Supervised exercise therapy (SET) Symptomatic Peripheral Artery Disease; 100-04,32,390.1 General Billing Requirements for Supervised exercise therapy (SET) for PAD; 100-04,32,390.2 Coding Requirements for SET for PAD; 100-04,32,390.3 Special Billing Requirements for Professional Claims; 100-04,32,390.4 Special Billing Requirements for Institutional Claims; 100-04,32,390.5 Common Working File (CWF) Requirements; 100-04,32,390.6 Applicable Medicare Summary Notice (MSN), Remittance Advice Remark Codes (RARCs), and Claim Adjustment Reason Code (CARC) Messaging

INCLUDES Monitoring:
Other cardiovascular limitations for adjustment of workload
Patient's claudication threshold
Motorized treadmill or track
Sessions lasting 45-60 minutes
Supervision by exercise physiologist/nurse

Code also appropriate E&M service, when performed

93668 **Peripheral arterial disease (PAD) rehabilitation, per session**

0.50 0.50 FUD XXX S 80 TC

AMA: 2018,Feb,11

93701-93702 Thoracic Electrical Bioimpedance

EXCLUDES *Bioelectrical impedance analysis whole body (0358T)*
Indirect measurement of left ventricular filling pressure by computerized calibration of the arterial waveform response to Valsalva (93799)

93701 **Bioimpedance-derived physiologic cardiovascular analysis**

0.71 0.71 FUD XXX Q1 80 TC

AMA: 2018,Feb,11; 2018,Jan,8; 2017,Jan,8; 2016,Jan,13; 2015,Jan,16; 2014,Jan,11

93702 **Bioimpedance spectroscopy (BIS), extracellular fluid analysis for lymphedema assessment(s)**

3.57 3.57 FUD XXX S 80 TC

AMA: 2018,Feb,11

93724 Electronic Analysis of Pacemaker Function

93724 **Electronic analysis of antitachycardia pacemaker system (includes electrocardiographic recording, programming of device, induction and termination of tachycardia via implanted pacemaker, and interpretation of recordings)**

7.89 7.89 FUD 000 S 80

AMA: 2018,Feb,11; 2018,Jan,8; 2017,Jan,8; 2016,Jan,13; 2015,Jan,16; 2014,Jan,11

93740 Temperature Gradient Assessment

93740 **Temperature gradient studies**

0.23 0.23 FUD XXX Q1

AMA: 2018,Feb,11

93745 Wearable Cardioverter-Defibrillator System Services

EXCLUDES *Device evaluation (93282, 93292)*

93745 **Initial set-up and programming by a physician or other qualified health care professional of wearable cardioverter-defibrillator includes initial programming of system, establishing baseline electronic ECG, transmission of data to data repository, patient instruction in wearing system and patient reporting of problems or events**

0.00 0.00 FUD XXX S 80

AMA: 2018,Feb,11

Medicine

93655 — 93745

93750 Ventricular Assist Device (VAD) Interrogation

CMS: 100-03,20.9 Artificial Hearts and Related Devices; 100-03,20.9.1 Ventricular Assist Devices; 100-04,32,320.1 Artificial Hearts Prior to May 1, 2008; 100-04,32,320.2 Coding for Artificial Hearts After May 1, 2008; 100-04,32,320.3 Ventricular Assist Devices; 100-04,32,320.3.1 Post-cardiotomy; 100-04,32,320.3.2 Bridge- to -Transplantation

EXCLUDES *Insertion of ventricular assist device (33975-33976, 33979)*
Removal/replacement ventricular assist device (33981-33983)

93750 **Interrogation of ventricular assist device (VAD), in person, with physician or other qualified health care professional analysis of device parameters (eg, drivelines, alarms, power surges), review of device function (eg, flow and volume status, septum status, recovery), with programming, if performed, and report**

1.32 1.58 FUD XXX S 80

AMA: 2018,Dec,10; 2018,Dec,10; 2018,Feb,11; 2018,Jan,8; 2017,Jan,8; 2016,Jan,13; 2015,Jan,16; 2014,Jan,11

93770 Peripheral Venous Blood Pressure Assessment

CMS: 100-03,20.19 Ambulatory Blood Pressure Monitoring (20.19)

EXCLUDES *Cannulization, central venous (36500, 36555-36556)*

93770 **Determination of venous pressure**

0.23 0.23 FUD XXX N

AMA: 2018,Feb,11

93784-93790 Ambulatory Blood Pressure Monitoring

CMS: 100-03,20.19 Ambulatory Blood Pressure Monitoring (20.19); 100-04,32,10.1 Ambulatory Blood Pressure Monitoring Billing Requirements

EXCLUDES *Self-measured blood pressure monitoring ([99473, 99474])*

▲ **93784** **Ambulatory blood pressure monitoring, utilizing report-generating software, automated, worn continuously for 24 hours or longer; including recording, scanning analysis, interpretation and report**

1.51 1.51 FUD XXX B 80

AMA: 2018,Feb,11

▲ **93786** **recording only**

0.83 0.83 FUD XXX Q1 80 TC

AMA: 2018,Feb,11

▲ **93788** **scanning analysis with report**

0.15 0.15 FUD XXX Q1 80 TC

AMA: 2018,Feb,11

▲ **93790** **review with interpretation and report**

0.53 0.53 FUD XXX M 80 26

AMA: 2018,Feb,11

93792-93793 INR Monitoring

CMS: 100-03,190.11 Home PT/INR Monitoring for Anticoagulation Management; 100-04,32,60.4.1 Anticoagulation Management: Covered Diagnosis Codes

EXCLUDES *Chronic care management ([99490], 99487, 99489)*
Online digital evaluation and management services by a physician or other qualified health care professional ([99421, 99422, 99423])
Telephone assessment and management service by nonphysician healthcare professional (98966-98968)
Telephone evaluation and management service by physician or other qualified healthcare professional (99441-99443)
Transitional care management (99495-99496)

93792 **Patient/caregiver training for initiation of home international normalized ratio (INR) monitoring under the direction of a physician or other qualified health care professional, face-to-face, including use and care of the INR monitor, obtaining blood sample, instructions for reporting home INR test results, and documentation of patient's/caregiver's ability to perform testing and report results**

Code also INR home monitoring equipment with appropriate supply code or (99070)

Code also significantly separately identifiable E&M service on same date of service using modifier 25

1.48 1.48 FUD XXX B 80 TC

AMA: 2018,Mar,7; 2018,Feb,11

93793 **Anticoagulant management for a patient taking warfarin, must include review and interpretation of a new home, office, or lab international normalized ratio (INR) test result, patient instructions, dosage adjustment (as needed), and scheduling of additional test(s), when performed**

EXCLUDES *E&M services on same date of service (99201-99215, 99241-99245)*
Use of code more than one time per day

0.34 0.34 FUD XXX B 80 26

AMA: 2018,Mar,7; 2018,Feb,11; 2018,Jan,8; 2017,Nov,10

93797-93799 Cardiac Rehabilitation

CMS: 100-02,15,232 Cardiac Rehabilitation (CR) and Intensive Cardiac Rehabilitation (ICR) Services Furnished On or After January 1, 2010; 100-04,32,140.2 Cardiac Rehabilitation On or After January 1, 2010; 100-04,32,140.2.1 Coding Cardiac Rehabilitation Services On or After January 1, 2010; 100-04,32,140.2.2.2 Institutional Claims for CR and ICR Services; 100-04,32,140.2.2.4 CR Services Exceeding 36 Sessions; 100-04,32,140.3 Intensive Cardiac Rehabilitation Program Services Furnished On or After January 1, 2010; 100-08,15,4.2.8 Cardiac Rehabilitation (CR) and Intensive Cardiac Rehabilitation (ICR)

93797 **Physician or other qualified health care professional services for outpatient cardiac rehabilitation; without continuous ECG monitoring (per session)**

0.25 0.46 FUD 000 S 80

AMA: 2018,Feb,11

93798 **with continuous ECG monitoring (per session)**

0.40 0.72 FUD 000 S 80

AMA: 2018,Feb,11

93799 **Unlisted cardiovascular service or procedure**

0.00 0.00 FUD XXX S 80

AMA: 2018,Dec,10; 2018,Dec,10; 2018,Sep,10; 2018,Aug,10; 2018,Feb,11; 2018,Jan,8; 2017,Jan,8; 2016,May,5; 2016,Jan,13; 2015,Jan,16; 2014,Jan,11

93880-93895 Noninvasive Tests Extracranial/Intracranial Arteries

INCLUDES Patient care required to perform/supervise studies and interpret results

EXCLUDES *Hand-held dopplers that do not provide a hard copy or vascular flow bidirectional analysis (See E&M codes)*

93880 **Duplex scan of extracranial arteries; complete bilateral study**

EXCLUDES *Common carotid intima-media thickness (IMT) studies (93895, 0126T)*

5.70 5.70 FUD XXX S 80

AMA: 2018,Feb,11; 2018,Jan,8; 2017,Jan,8; 2016,Jan,13; 2015,Jan,16; 2014,Jan,11

93882 **unilateral or limited study**

EXCLUDES *Common carotid intima-media thickness (IMT) studies (93895, 0126T)*

3.64 3.64 FUD XXX S 80

AMA: 2018,Feb,11; 2018,Jan,8; 2017,Jan,8; 2016,Jan,13; 2015,Jan,16; 2014,Jan,11

93886 **Transcranial Doppler study of the intracranial arteries; complete study**

INCLUDES Complete transcranial doppler (TCD) study
Ultrasound evaluation of right/left anterior circulation territories and posterior circulation territory

7.67 7.67 FUD XXX S 80

AMA: 2018,Feb,11; 2018,Jan,8; 2017,Jan,8; 2016,Jan,13; 2015,Jan,16; 2014,Jan,11

93888 **limited study**

INCLUDES Limited TCD study
Ultrasound examination of two or fewer of these territories (right/left anterior circulation, posterior circulation)

4.47 4.47 FUD XXX S 80

AMA: 2018,Feb,11; 2018,Jan,8; 2017,Jan,8; 2016,Jan,13; 2015,Jan,16; 2014,Jan,11

93890 **vasoreactivity study**

EXCLUDES *Limited TCD study (93888)*

7.82 7.82 FUD XXX Q1 80

AMA: 2018,Feb,11; 2018,Jan,8; 2017,Jan,8; 2016,Jan,13; 2015,Jan,16; 2014,Jan,11

93892 **emboli detection without intravenous microbubble injection**

EXCLUDES *Limited TCD study (93888)*

8.81 8.81 FUD XXX 01 80

AMA: 2018,Feb,11; 2018,Jan,8; 2017,Jan,8; 2016,Jan,13; 2015,Jan,16; 2014,Jan,11

93893 **emboli detection with intravenous microbubble injection**

EXCLUDES *Limited TCD study (93888)*

9.81 9.81 FUD XXX 01 80

AMA: 2018,Feb,11; 2018,Jan,8; 2017,Jan,8; 2016,Jan,13; 2015,Jan,16; 2014,Jan,11

93895 **Quantitative carotid intima media thickness and carotid atheroma evaluation, bilateral**

EXCLUDES *Common carotid intima-media thickness (IMT) study (0126T)*

Complete and limited duplex studies (93880, 93882)

0.00 0.00 FUD XXX E 80

AMA: 2018,Feb,11

93922-93971 Noninvasive Vascular Studies: Extremities

CMS: 100-04,8,180 Noninvasive Studies for ESRD Patients

INCLUDES Patient care required to perform/supervise studies and interpret results

EXCLUDES *Hand-held dopplers that do not provide a hard copy or provided vascular flow bidirectional analysis (see E&M codes)*

93922 **Limited bilateral noninvasive physiologic studies of upper or lower extremity arteries, (eg, for lower extremity: ankle/brachial indices at distal posterior tibial and anterior tibial/dorsalis pedis arteries plus bidirectional, Doppler waveform recording and analysis at 1-2 levels, or ankle/brachial indices at distal posterior tibial and anterior tibial/dorsalis pedis arteries plus volume plethysmography at 1-2 levels, or ankle/brachial indices at distal posterior tibial and anterior tibial/dorsalis pedis arteries with, transcutaneous oxygen tension measurement at 1-2 levels)**

INCLUDES Evaluation of:

- Doppler analysis of bidirectional blood flow
- Nonimaging physiologic recordings of pressure
- Oxygen tension measurements and/or plethysmography

Lower extremity (potential levels include high thigh, low thigh, calf, ankle, metatarsal and toes) limited study includes either:

- Ankle/brachial indices at distal posterior tibial and anterior tibial/dorsalis pedis arteries plus bidirectional Doppler waveform recording and analysis as 1-2 levels; OR
- Ankle/brachial indices at distal posterior tibial and anterior tibial/dorsalis pedis arteries plus volume plethysmography at 1-2 levels; OR
- Ankle/brachial indices at distal posterior tibial and anterior tibial/dorsalis pedis arteries with transcutaneous oxygen tension measurements at 1-2 levels

Unilateral provocative functional measurement

Unilateral study of 3 or move levels

Upper extremity (potential levels include arm, forearm, wrist, and digits) limited study includes:

- Doppler-determined systolic pressures and bidirectional waveform recording with analysis at 1-2 levels; OR
- Doppler-determined systolic pressures and transcutaneous oxygen tension measurements at 1-2 levels; OR
- Doppler-determined systolic pressures and volume plethysmography at 1-2 levels

EXCLUDES *Transcutaneous oxyhemoglobin measurement (0493T)*

Use of code more than one time for the lower extremity(s)

Use of code more than one time for the upper extremity(s)

Code also modifier 52 for unilateral study of 1-2 levels

Code also twice with modifier 59 for upper and lower extremity study

2.44 2.44 FUD XXX 01 80

AMA: 2018,Feb,11; 2018,Jan,8; 2017,Jan,8; 2016,Jan,13; 2015,Jan,16; 2014,Jan,9; 2014,Jan,11

93923 **Complete bilateral noninvasive physiologic studies of upper or lower extremity arteries, 3 or more levels (eg, for lower extremity: ankle/brachial indices at distal posterior tibial and anterior tibial/dorsalis pedis arteries plus segmental blood pressure measurements with bidirectional Doppler waveform recording and analysis, at 3 or more levels, or ankle/brachial indices at distal posterior tibial and anterior tibial/dorsalis pedis arteries plus segmental volume plethysmography at 3 or more levels, or ankle/brachial indices at distal posterior tibial and anterior tibial/dorsalis pedis arteries plus segmental transcutaneous oxygen tension measurements at 3 or more levels), or single level study with provocative functional maneuvers (eg, measurements with postural provocative tests, or measurements with reactive hyperemia)**

INCLUDES Evaluation of:
- Doppler analysis of bidirectional blood flow
- Nonimaging physiologic recordings of pressures
- Oxygen tension measurements

Lower extremity:
- Ankle/brachial indices at distal posterior tibial and anterior tibial/dorsalis pedis arteries plus bidirectional Doppler waveform recording and analysis at 3 or more levels; OR
- Ankle/brachial indices at distal posterior tibial and anterior tibial/dorsalis pedis arteries with transcutaneous oxygen tension measurements at 3 or more levels; OR
- Ankle/brachial indices at distal posterior tibial and anterior tibial/dorsalis pedis arteries plus volume plethysmography at 3 or more levels; OR

Provocative functional maneuvers and measurement at a single level

Upper extremity complete study:
- Doppler-determined systolic pressures and bidirectional waveform recording with analysis at 3 or more levels; OR
- Doppler-determined systolic pressures and transcutaneous oxygen tension measurements at 3 or more levels; OR
- Doppler-determined systolic pressures and volume plethysmography at 3 or more levels; OR
- Provocative functional maneuvers and measurement at a single level

EXCLUDES *Unilateral study at 3 or more levels (93922)*
Use of code more than one time for the lower extremity(s)
Use of code more than one time for the upper extremity(s)

Code also twice with modifier 59 for upper and lower extremity study

3.78 3.78 FUD XXX S 80

AMA: 2018,Feb,11; 2018,Jan,8; 2017,Jan,8; 2016,Jan,13; 2015,Jan,16; 2014,Jan,11; 2014,Jan,9

93924 **Noninvasive physiologic studies of lower extremity arteries, at rest and following treadmill stress testing, (ie, bidirectional Doppler waveform or volume plethysmography recording and analysis at rest with ankle/brachial indices immediately after and at timed intervals following performance of a standardized protocol on a motorized treadmill plus recording of time of onset of claudication or other symptoms, maximal walking time, and time to recovery) complete bilateral study**

INCLUDES Evaluation of:
- Doppler analysis of bidirectional blood flow
- Non-imaging physiologic recordings of pressures
- Oxygen tension measurements
- Plethysmography

EXCLUDES *Noninvasive vascular studies of extremities (93922-93923)*
Other types of exercise

4.67 4.67 FUD XXX S 80

AMA: 2018,Feb,11; 2018,Jan,8; 2017,Jan,8; 2016,Jan,13; 2015,Jan,16; 2014,Jan,9; 2014,Jan,11

93925 **Duplex scan of lower extremity arteries or arterial bypass grafts; complete bilateral study**

EXCLUDES *Preoperative arterial inflow and venous outflow duplex scan for creation of hemodialysis access, same extremities (93985)*

7.25 7.25 FUD XXX S 80

AMA: 2018,Feb,11; 2018,Jan,8; 2017,Jan,8; 2016,Sep,9; 2016,Jan,13; 2015,Jan,16; 2014,Jan,11

93926 **unilateral or limited study**

EXCLUDES *Preoperative arterial inflow and venous outflow duplex scan for creation of hemodialysis access, same extremity (93986)*

4.26 4.26 FUD XXX S 80

AMA: 2018,Feb,11; 2018,Jan,8; 2017,Jan,8; 2016,Sep,9; 2016,Jan,13; 2015,Jan,16; 2014,Jan,11

93930 **Duplex scan of upper extremity arteries or arterial bypass grafts; complete bilateral study**

EXCLUDES *Preoperative arterial inflow and venous outflow duplex scan for creation of hemodialysis access, same extremity(ies) (93985-93986)*

5.82 5.82 FUD XXX S 80

AMA: 2018,Feb,11; 2018,Jan,8; 2017,Jan,8; 2016,Sep,9; 2016,Jan,13; 2015,Jan,16; 2014,Jan,11

93931 **unilateral or limited study**

EXCLUDES *Preoperative arterial inflow and venous outflow duplex scan for creation of hemodialysis access, same extremity (93985-93986)*

3.63 3.63 FUD XXX S 80

AMA: 2018,Feb,11; 2018,Jan,8; 2017,Jan,8; 2016,Sep,9; 2016,Jan,13; 2015,Jan,16; 2014,Jan,11

93970 **Duplex scan of extremity veins including responses to compression and other maneuvers; complete bilateral study**

EXCLUDES *Endovenous ablation (36475-36476, 36478-36479)*
Preoperative arterial inflow and venous outflow duplex scan for creation of hemodialysis access, same extremity(ies) (93985-93986)

5.52 5.52 FUD XXX S 80

AMA: 2018,Mar,3; 2018,Feb,11; 2018,Jan,8; 2017,Jan,8; 2016,Nov,3; 2016,Sep,9; 2016,Jan,13; 2015,Jan,16; 2014,Oct,6; 2014,Jan,11

93971 **unilateral or limited study**

EXCLUDES *Endovenous ablation (36475-36476, 36478-36479)*
Preoperative arterial inflow and venous outflow duplex scan for creation of hemodialysis access, same extremity (93985-93986)

3.42 3.42 FUD XXX S 80

AMA: 2018,Mar,3; 2018,Feb,11; 2018,Jan,8; 2017,Jan,8; 2016,Nov,3; 2016,Sep,9; 2016,Jan,13; 2015,Aug,8; 2015,Jan,16; 2014,Oct,6; 2014,Jan,11

93975-93981 Noninvasive Vascular Studies: Abdomen/Chest/Pelvis

93975 **Duplex scan of arterial inflow and venous outflow of abdominal, pelvic, scrotal contents and/or retroperitoneal organs; complete study**

7.88 7.88 FUD XXX S 80

AMA: 2018,Feb,11; 2018,Jan,8; 2017,Jan,8; 2016,Aug,9; 2016,Jan,13; 2015,Mar,9; 2015,Jan,16; 2014,Jun,14; 2014,Jan,11

93976 **limited study**

4.64 4.64 FUD XXX S 80

AMA: 2018,Feb,11; 2018,Jan,8; 2017,Jan,8; 2016,Aug,9; 2016,Jan,13; 2015,Mar,9; 2015,Jan,16; 2014,Jan,11

93978 **Duplex scan of aorta, inferior vena cava, iliac vasculature, or bypass grafts; complete study**

EXCLUDES *Ultrasound screening for abdominal aortic aneurysm (76706)*

5.34 5.34 FUD XXX S 80

AMA: 2018,Feb,11; 2018,Jan,8; 2017,Jan,8; 2016,Jan,13; 2015,Jan,16; 2014,Jan,11

93979 **unilateral or limited study**

EXCLUDES *Ultrasound screening for abdominal aortic aneurysm (76706)*

3.40 3.40 FUD XXX

AMA: 2018,Feb,11; 2018,Jan,8; 2017,Jan,8; 2016,Jan,13; 2015,Jan,16; 2014,Jun,14; 2014,Jan,11

93980 **Duplex scan of arterial inflow and venous outflow of penile vessels; complete study**

3.53 3.53 FUD XXX

AMA: 2018,Feb,11; 2018,Jan,8; 2017,Jan,8; 2016,Jan,13; 2015,Jan,16; 2014,Jan,11

93981 **follow-up or limited study**

2.15 2.15 FUD XXX

AMA: 2018,Feb,11; 2018,Jan,8; 2017,Jan,8; 2016,Jan,13; 2015,Jan,16; 2014,Jan,11

93985-93998 Noninvasive Vascular Studies: Hemodialysis Access

● 93985 **Duplex scan of arterial inflow and venous outflow for preoperative vessel assessment prior to creation of hemodialysis access; complete bilateral study**

EXCLUDES *Duplex scan of body of hemodialysis access, arterial inflow and venous outflow, same extremity(ies) (93990)*

Duplex scan of extremity arteries only, same extremity(ies) (93925, 93930)

Duplex scan of extremity veins only, same extremity(ies) (93970)

Physiologic arterial evaluation of extremities (93922-93924)

● 93986 **complete unilateral study**

EXCLUDES *Duplex scan of body of hemodialysis access, arterial inflow and venous outflow, same extremity (93990)*

Duplex scan of extremity arteries only, same extremity (93926, 93931)

Duplex scan of extremity veins only, same extremity (93971)

Physiologic arterial evaluation of extremities (93922-93924)

93990 **Duplex scan of hemodialysis access (including arterial inflow, body of access and venous outflow)**

EXCLUDES *Hemodialysis access flow measurement by indicator method (90940)*

4.42 4.42 FUD XXX

AMA: 2018,Feb,11; 2018,Jan,8; 2017,Jan,8; 2016,Jan,13; 2015,Jan,16; 2014,Jan,11

93998 **Unlisted noninvasive vascular diagnostic study**

0.00 0.00 FUD XXX

AMA: 2018,Feb,11; 2018,Jan,8; 2017,Jan,8; 2016,Jan,13; 2015,Jan,16; 2014,Jan,9

94002-94005 Ventilator Management Services

94002 **Ventilation assist and management, initiation of pressure or volume preset ventilators for assisted or controlled breathing; hospital inpatient/observation, initial day**

EXCLUDES *E&M services*

2.64 2.64 FUD XXX

AMA: 2019,Aug,8; 2018,Feb,11; 2018,Jan,8; 2017,Jan,8; 2016,Jan,13; 2015,Jan,16; 2014,Oct,8; 2014,May,4; 2014,Jan,11

94003 **hospital inpatient/observation, each subsequent day**

EXCLUDES *E&M services*

1.89 1.89 FUD XXX

AMA: 2019,Aug,8; 2018,Feb,11; 2018,Jan,8; 2017,Jan,8; 2016,Jan,13; 2015,Jan,16; 2014,Oct,8; 2014,May,4; 2014,Jan,11

94004 **nursing facility, per day**

EXCLUDES *E&M services*

1.40 1.40 FUD XXX

AMA: 2019,Aug,8; 2018,Feb,11; 2018,Jan,8; 2017,Jan,8; 2016,Jan,13; 2015,Jan,16; 2014,Oct,8; 2014,Jan,11

94005 **Home ventilator management care plan oversight of a patient (patient not present) in home, domiciliary or rest home (eg, assisted living) requiring review of status, review of laboratories and other studies and revision of orders and respiratory care plan (as appropriate), within a calendar month, 30 minutes or more**

Code also when a different provider reports care plan oversight in the same 30 days (99339-99340, 99374-99378)

2.61 2.61 FUD XXX

AMA: 2018,Feb,11; 2018,Jan,8; 2017,Jan,8; 2016,Jan,13; 2015,Jan,16; 2014,Oct,8; 2014,Jan,11

94010-94799 Respiratory Services: Diagnostic and Therapeutic

INCLUDES Laboratory procedure(s)

Test results interpretation

EXCLUDES *Separately identifiable E&M service*

94010 **Spirometry, including graphic record, total and timed vital capacity, expiratory flow rate measurement(s), with or without maximal voluntary ventilation**

INCLUDES Measurement of expiratory airflow and volumes

EXCLUDES *Diffusing capacity (94729)*

Other respiratory function services (94150, 94200, 94375, 94728)

1.00 1.00 FUD XXX

AMA: 2019,May,10; 2019,Mar,10; 2019,Apr,10; 2018,Feb,11; 2018,Jan,8; 2017,Jan,8; 2016,Jan,13; 2015,Sep,9; 2015,Jan,16; 2014,Mar,11; 2014,Jan,11

94011 **Measurement of spirometric forced expiratory flows in an infant or child through 2 years of age**

2.48 2.48 FUD XXX

AMA: 2019,Mar,10; 2018,Feb,11; 2018,Jan,8; 2017,Jan,8; 2016,Jan,13; 2015,Jan,16; 2014,Jan,11

94012 **Measurement of spirometric forced expiratory flows, before and after bronchodilator, in an infant or child through 2 years of age**

4.02 4.02 FUD XXX

AMA: 2019,Mar,10; 2018,Feb,11; 2018,Jan,8; 2017,Jan,8; 2016,Jan,13; 2015,Jan,16; 2014,Jan,11

94013 **Measurement of lung volumes (ie, functional residual capacity [FRC], forced vital capacity [FVC], and expiratory reserve volume [ERV]) in an infant or child through 2 years of age**

0.55 0.55 FUD XXX

AMA: 2019,Mar,10; 2018,Feb,11; 2018,Jan,8; 2017,Jan,8; 2016,Jan,13; 2015,Jan,16; 2014,Jan,11

94014 **Patient-initiated spirometric recording per 30-day period of time; includes reinforced education, transmission of spirometric tracing, data capture, analysis of transmitted data, periodic recalibration and review and interpretation by a physician or other qualified health care professional**

1.58 1.58 FUD XXX

AMA: 2019,Mar,10; 2018,Feb,11; 2018,Jan,8; 2017,Jan,8; 2016,Jan,13; 2015,Jan,16; 2014,Jan,11

94015 **recording (includes hook-up, reinforced education, data transmission, data capture, trend analysis, and periodic recalibration)**

0.86 0.86 FUD XXX

AMA: 2019,Mar,10; 2018,Feb,11; 2018,Jan,8; 2017,Jan,8; 2016,Jan,13; 2015,Jan,16; 2014,Jan,11

94016 **review and interpretation only by a physician or other qualified health care professional**

0.72 0.72 FUD XXX

AMA: 2019,Mar,10; 2018,Feb,11; 2018,Jan,8; 2017,Jan,8; 2016,Jan,13; 2015,Jan,16; 2014,Jan,11

● New Code ▲ Revised Code ○ Reinstated ● New Web Release ▲ Revised Web Release + Add-on Unlisted Not Covered # Resequenced
Optum Mod 50 Exempt AMA Mod 51 Exempt Optum Mod 51 Exempt Mod 63 Exempt Non-FDA Drug ★ Telemedicine Maternity Age Edit

94060 Bronchodilation responsiveness, spirometry as in 94010, pre- and post-bronchodilator administration

INCLUDES Spirometry performed prior to and after a bronchodilator has been administered

EXCLUDES *Bronchospasm prolonged exercise test with pre- and post-spirometry (94617)*
Diffusing capacity (94729)
Other respiratory function services (94150, 94200, 94375, 94640, 94728)

Code also bronchodilator supply with appropriate supply code or (99070)

1.68 1.68 FUD XXX S 80

AMA: 2019,Mar,10; 2019,Apr,10; 2018,Feb,11; 2018,Jan,8; 2017,Jan,8; 2016,Jan,13; 2015,Sep,9; 2015,Jan,16; 2014,Mar,11; 2014,Jan,11

94070 Bronchospasm provocation evaluation, multiple spirometric determinations as in 94010, with administered agents (eg, antigen[s], cold air, methacholine)

EXCLUDES *Diffusing capacity (94729)*
Inhalation treatment (diagnostic or therapeutic) (94640)

Code also antigen(s) administration with appropriate supply code or (99070)

1.69 1.69 FUD XXX S 80

AMA: 2019,Mar,10; 2018,Feb,11; 2018,Jan,8; 2017,Jan,8; 2016,Jan,13; 2015,Sep,9; 2015,Jan,16; 2014,Jan,11

94150 Vital capacity, total (separate procedure)

EXCLUDES *Other respiratory function services (94010, 94060, 94728)*
Thoracic gas volumes (94726-94727)

0.72 0.72 FUD XXX Q1

AMA: 2019,Mar,10; 2018,Sep,14; 2018,Feb,11; 2018,Jan,8; 2017,Jan,8; 2016,Jan,13; 2015,Jan,16; 2014,Mar,11; 2014,Jan,11

94200 Maximum breathing capacity, maximal voluntary ventilation

EXCLUDES *Other respiratory function services (94010, 94060)*

0.78 0.78 FUD XXX Q1 80

AMA: 2019,Mar,10; 2018,Feb,11; 2018,Jan,8; 2017,Jan,8; 2016,Jan,13; 2015,Jan,16; 2014,Mar,11; 2014,Jan,11

94250 Expired gas collection, quantitative, single procedure (separate procedure)

EXCLUDES *Complex pulmonary stress test (94621)*

0.78 0.78 FUD XXX Q1 80

AMA: 2019,Mar,10; 2018,Feb,11; 2018,Jan,8; 2017,Oct,3; 2017,Jan,8; 2016,Jan,13; 2015,Dec,16; 2015,Jan,16; 2014,Jan,11

94375 Respiratory flow volume loop

INCLUDES Identification of obstruction patterns in central or peripheral airways (inspiratory and/or expiratory)

EXCLUDES *Diffusing capacity (94729)*
Other respiratory function services (94010, 94060, 94728)

1.12 1.12 FUD XXX Q1 80

AMA: 2019,Mar,10; 2018,Feb,11; 2018,Jan,8; 2017,Jan,8; 2016,Jan,13; 2015,Jan,16; 2014,Mar,11; 2014,Jan,11

94400 Breathing response to CO2 (CO2 response curve)

EXCLUDES *Inhalation treatment (diagnostic or therapeutic) (94640)*

1.61 1.61 FUD XXX Q1 80

AMA: 2019,Mar,10; 2018,Feb,11; 2018,Jan,8; 2017,Jan,8; 2016,Jan,13; 2015,Sep,9; 2015,Jan,16; 2014,Mar,11; 2014,Jan,11

94450 Breathing response to hypoxia (hypoxia response curve)

EXCLUDES *HAST - high altitude simulation test (94452, 94453)*

2.06 2.06 FUD XXX Q1 80

AMA: 2019,Mar,10; 2018,Feb,11; 2018,Jan,8; 2017,Jan,8; 2016,Jan,13; 2015,Jan,16; 2014,Jan,11

94452 High altitude simulation test (HAST), with interpretation and report by a physician or other qualified health care professional;

EXCLUDES *HAST test with supplemental oxygen titration (94453)*
Noninvasive pulse oximetry (94760-94761)
Obtaining arterial blood gases (36600)

1.55 1.55 FUD XXX Q1 80

AMA: 2019,Mar,10; 2018,Feb,11; 2018,Jan,8; 2017,Jan,8; 2016,Jan,13; 2015,Jan,16; 2014,Jan,11

94453 with supplemental oxygen titration

EXCLUDES *HAST test without supplemental oxygen titration (94452)*
Noninvasive pulse oximetry (94760-94761)
Obtaining arterial blood gases (36600)

2.14 2.14 FUD XXX Q1 80

AMA: 2019,Mar,10; 2018,Feb,11; 2018,Jan,8; 2017,Jan,8; 2016,Jan,13; 2015,Jan,16; 2014,Jan,11

94610 Intrapulmonary surfactant administration by a physician or other qualified health care professional through endotracheal tube

INCLUDES Reporting once per dosing episode

EXCLUDES *Intubation, endotracheal (31500)*
Neonatal critical care (99468-99472)

1.59 1.59 FUD XXX ⊘ Q1 80

AMA: 2019,Mar,10; 2018,Feb,11; 2018,Jan,8; 2017,Jan,8; 2016,Jan,13; 2015,Jan,16; 2014,Jan,11

94617 Exercise test for bronchospasm, including pre- and post-spirometry, electrocardiographic recording(s), and pulse oximetry

EXCLUDES *Cardiovascular stress test (93015-93018)*
ECG monitoring (93000-93010, 93040-93042)
Pulse oximetry (94760-94761)

2.66 2.66 FUD XXX Q1 80

AMA: 2019,May,10; 2019,Mar,10; 2018,Feb,11; 2018,Jan,8; 2017,Oct,3

94618 Pulmonary stress testing (eg, 6-minute walk test), including measurement of heart rate, oximetry, and oxygen titration, when performed

EXCLUDES *Pulse oximetry (94760-94761)*

0.96 0.96 FUD XXX Q1 80

AMA: 2019,May,10; 2019,Mar,10; 2018,Feb,11; 2018,Jan,8; 2017,Oct,3

94621 Cardiopulmonary exercise testing, including measurements of minute ventilation, CO2 production, O2 uptake, and electrocardiographic recordings

EXCLUDES *Cardiovascular stress test (93015-93018)*
ECG monitoring (93000-93010, 93040-93042)
Expired gas collection (94250)
Oxygen uptake expired gas analysis (94680-94690)
Pulse oximetry (94760-94761)

4.54 4.54 FUD XXX S 80

AMA: 2019,May,10; 2019,Mar,10; 2018,Feb,11; 2018,Jan,8; 2017,Oct,3; 2017,Jan,8; 2016,Jan,13; 2015,Jan,16; 2014,Jan,11

94640 Pressurized or nonpressurized inhalation treatment for acute airway obstruction for therapeutic purposes and/or for diagnostic purposes such as sputum induction with an aerosol generator, nebulizer, metered dose inhaler or intermittent positive pressure breathing (IPPB) device

EXCLUDES *1 hour or more of continuous inhalation treatment (94644, 94645)*
Other respiratory function services (94060, 94070, 94400)

Code also modifier 76 when more than 1 inhalation treatment is performed on the same date

0.51 0.51 FUD XXX Q1 80

AMA: 2019,Mar,10; 2018,Feb,11; 2018,Jan,8; 2017,Jan,8; 2016,Jan,13; 2015,Sep,9; 2015,Jan,16; 2014,Mar,11; 2014,Jan,11

94642 **Aerosol inhalation of pentamidine for pneumocystis carinii pneumonia treatment or prophylaxis**
0.00 0.00 FUD XXX
AMA: 2019,Mar,10; 2018,Feb,11; 2018,Jan,8; 2017,Jan,8; 2016,Jan,13; 2015,Jan,16; 2014,Jan,11

94644 **Continuous inhalation treatment with aerosol medication for acute airway obstruction; first hour**
EXCLUDES *Services that are less than 1 hour (94640)*
1.40 1.40 FUD XXX
AMA: 2019,Mar,10; 2018,Feb,11; 2018,Jan,8; 2017,Jan,8; 2016,Jan,13; 2015,Sep,9; 2015,Jan,16; 2014,Mar,11; 2014,Jan,11

+ **94645** **each additional hour (List separately in addition to code for primary procedure)**
Code first initial hour (94644)
0.47 0.47 FUD XXX
AMA: 2019,Mar,10; 2018,Feb,11; 2018,Jan,8; 2017,Jan,8; 2016,Jan,13; 2015,Sep,9; 2015,Jan,16; 2014,Mar,11; 2014,Jan,11

94660 **Continuous positive airway pressure ventilation (CPAP), initiation and management**
1.09 1.81 FUD XXX
AMA: 2019,Aug,8; 2019,Mar,10; 2018,Feb,11; 2018,Jan,8; 2017,Jan,8; 2016,Jan,13; 2015,Jan,16; 2014,Oct,8; 2014,May,4; 2014,Jan,11

94662 **Continuous negative pressure ventilation (CNP), initiation and management**
1.03 1.03 FUD XXX
AMA: 2019,Aug,8; 2019,Mar,10; 2018,Feb,11; 2018,Jan,8; 2017,Jan,8; 2016,Jan,13; 2015,Jan,16; 2014,May,4; 2014,Jan,11

94664 **Demonstration and/or evaluation of patient utilization of an aerosol generator, nebulizer, metered dose inhaler or IPPB device**
INCLUDES Reporting only one time per day of service
0.48 0.48 FUD XXX
AMA: 2019,Mar,10; 2018,Feb,11; 2018,Jan,8; 2017,Jan,8; 2016,Jan,13; 2015,Jan,16; 2014,Jan,11

94667 **Manipulation chest wall, such as cupping, percussing, and vibration to facilitate lung function; initial demonstration and/or evaluation**
0.71 0.71 FUD XXX
AMA: 2019,Mar,10; 2018,Feb,11; 2018,Jan,8; 2017,Jan,8; 2016,Jan,13; 2015,Sep,9; 2015,Jan,16; 2014,Mar,11; 2014,Jan,11

94668 **subsequent**
0.92 0.92 FUD XXX
AMA: 2019,Mar,10; 2018,Feb,11; 2018,Jan,8; 2017,Jan,8; 2016,Jan,13; 2015,Sep,9; 2015,Jan,16; 2014,Mar,11; 2014,Jan,11

94669 **Mechanical chest wall oscillation to facilitate lung function, per session**
INCLUDES Application of an external wrap or vest to provide mechanical oscillation
0.90 0.90 FUD XXX
AMA: 2019,Mar,10; 2018,Feb,11; 2018,Jan,8; 2017,Jan,8; 2016,Jan,13; 2015,Jan,16; 2014,Jan,11

94680 **Oxygen uptake, expired gas analysis; rest and exercise, direct, simple**
EXCLUDES *Cardiopulmonary stress testing (94621)*
1.57 1.57 FUD XXX
AMA: 2019,Mar,10; 2018,Feb,11; 2018,Jan,8; 2017,Oct,3; 2017,Jan,8; 2016,Jan,13; 2015,Jan,16; 2014,Jan,11

94681 **including CO2 output, percentage oxygen extracted**
EXCLUDES *Cardiopulmonary stress testing (94621)*
1.55 1.55 FUD XXX
AMA: 2019,Mar,10; 2018,Feb,11; 2018,Jan,8; 2017,Oct,3; 2017,Jan,8; 2016,Jan,13; 2015,Jan,16; 2014,Jan,11

94690 **rest, indirect (separate procedure)**
EXCLUDES *Arterial puncture (36600)*
Cardiopulmonary stress testing (94621)
1.49 1.49 FUD XXX
AMA: 2019,Mar,10; 2018,Feb,11; 2018,Jan,8; 2017,Oct,3; 2017,Jan,8; 2016,Jan,13; 2015,Jan,16; 2014,Jan,11

94726 **Plethysmography for determination of lung volumes and, when performed, airway resistance**
INCLUDES Airway resistance
Determination of:
Functional residual capacity
Residual volume
Total lung capacity
EXCLUDES *Airway resistance (94728)*
Bronchial provocation (94070)
Diffusing capacity (94729)
Gas dilution or washout (94727)
Spirometry (94010, 94060)
1.52 1.52 FUD XXX
AMA: 2019,Mar,10; 2018,Feb,11; 2018,Jan,8; 2017,Jan,8; 2016,Jan,13; 2015,Jan,16; 2014,Jan,11

94727 **Gas dilution or washout for determination of lung volumes and, when performed, distribution of ventilation and closing volumes**
INCLUDES Closing volume
Distribution of ventilation
Lung volume measurement
EXCLUDES *Bronchial provocation (94070)*
Diffusing capacity (94729)
Plethysmography for lung volume/airway resistance (94726)
Spirometry (94010, 94060)
1.23 1.23 FUD XXX
AMA: 2019,Mar,10; 2018,Feb,11; 2018,Jan,8; 2017,Jan,8; 2016,Jan,13; 2015,Jan,16; 2014,Jan,11

▲ **94728** **Airway resistance by oscillometry**
EXCLUDES *Diffusing capacity (94729)*
Gas dilution techniques
Other respiratory function services (94010, 94060, 94070, 94375, 94726)
1.15 1.15 FUD XXX
AMA: 2019,Mar,10; 2018,Feb,11; 2018,Jan,8; 2017,Jan,8; 2016,Jan,13; 2015,Jan,16; 2014,Mar,11; 2014,Jan,11

+ **94729** **Diffusing capacity (eg, carbon monoxide, membrane) (List separately in addition to code for primary procedure)**
Code first (94010, 94060, 94070, 94375, 94726-94728)
1.56 1.56 FUD ZZZ
AMA: 2019,Mar,10; 2018,Feb,11; 2018,Jan,8; 2017,Jan,8; 2016,Jan,13; 2015,Jan,16; 2014,Jan,11

94750 **Pulmonary compliance study (eg, plethysmography, volume and pressure measurements)**
2.40 2.40 FUD XXX
AMA: 2019,Mar,10; 2018,Feb,11; 2018,Jan,8; 2017,Jan,8; 2016,Jan,13; 2015,Jan,16; 2014,Jan,11

94760 **Noninvasive ear or pulse oximetry for oxygen saturation; single determination**
EXCLUDES *Blood gases (82803-82810)*
Cardiopulmonary stress testing (94621)
Exercise test for bronchospasm (94617)
Pulmonary stress testing (94618)
0.07 0.07 FUD XXX
AMA: 2019,Aug,8; 2019,Mar,10; 2019,Jan,6; 2018,Feb,11; 2018,Jan,8; 2017,Oct,3; 2017,Jan,8; 2016,Jan,13; 2015,Jan,16; 2014,May,4; 2014,Jan,11

94761 **multiple determinations (eg, during exercise)**

EXCLUDES *Cardiopulmonary stress testing (94621)*
Exercise test for bronchospasm (94617)
Pulmonary stress testing (94618)

0.12 0.12 FUD XXX N 80 TC

AMA: 2019,Aug,8; 2019,Mar,10; 2018,Feb,11; 2018,Jan,8; 2017,Oct,3; 2017,Jan,8; 2016,Jan,13; 2015,Jan,16; 2014,May,4; 2014,Jan,11

94762 **by continuous overnight monitoring (separate procedure)**

0.71 0.71 FUD XXX Q3 80 TC

AMA: 2019,Aug,8; 2019,Mar,10; 2018,Feb,11; 2018,Jan,8; 2017,Jan,8; 2016,Jan,13; 2015,Jan,16; 2014,May,4; 2014,Jan,11

94770 **Carbon dioxide, expired gas determination by infrared analyzer**

EXCLUDES *Arterial catheterization/cannulation (36620)*
Arterial puncture (36600)
Bronchoscopy (31622-31654 [31651])
Flow directed catheter placement (93503)
Needle biopsy of the lung (32405)
Orotracheal/nasotracheal intubation (31500)
Placement of central venous catheter (36555-36556)
Therapeutic phlebotomy (99195)
Thoracentesis (32554-32555)
Venipuncture (36410)

0.21 0.21 FUD XXX S 80

AMA: 2019,Mar,10; 2018,Feb,11; 2018,Jan,8; 2017,Jan,8; 2016,Jan,13; 2015,Jan,16; 2014,Mar,11; 2014,Jan,11

94772 **Circadian respiratory pattern recording (pediatric pneumogram), 12-24 hour continuous recording, infant** A

EXCLUDES *Electromyograms/EEG/ECG/respiration recordings*

0.00 0.00 FUD XXX S 80

AMA: 2019,Mar,10; 2018,Feb,11; 2018,Jan,8; 2017,Jan,8; 2016,Jan,13; 2015,Jan,16; 2014,Jan,11

94774 **Pediatric home apnea monitoring event recording including respiratory rate, pattern and heart rate per 30-day period of time; includes monitor attachment, download of data, review, interpretation, and preparation of a report by a physician or other qualified health care professional** A

INCLUDES Oxygen saturation monitoring

EXCLUDES *Event monitors (93268-93272)*
Holter monitor (93224-93227)
Pediatric home apnea services (94775-94777)
Remote cardiovascular telemetry (93228-93229)
Sleep testing (95805-95811 [95800, 95801])

0.00 0.00 FUD YYY B 80

AMA: 2019,Mar,10; 2018,Feb,11; 2018,Jan,8; 2017,Jan,8; 2016,Jan,13; 2015,Jan,16; 2014,Jan,11

94775 **monitor attachment only (includes hook-up, initiation of recording and disconnection)** A

INCLUDES Oxygen saturation monitoring

EXCLUDES *Event monitors (93268-93272)*
Holter monitor (93224-93227)
Remote cardiovascular telemetry (93228-93229)
Sleep testing (95805-95811 [95800, 95801])

0.00 0.00 FUD YYY S 80 TC

AMA: 2019,Mar,10; 2018,Feb,11; 2018,Jan,8; 2017,Jan,8; 2016,Jan,13; 2015,Jan,16; 2014,Jan,11

94776 **monitoring, download of information, receipt of transmission(s) and analyses by computer only** A

INCLUDES Oxygen saturation monitoring

EXCLUDES *Event monitors (93268-93272)*
Holter monitor (93224-93227)
Remote cardiovascular telemetry (93228-93229)
Sleep testing (95805-95811 [95800, 95801])

0.00 0.00 FUD YYY S 80 TC

AMA: 2019,Mar,10; 2018,Feb,11; 2018,Jan,8; 2017,Jan,8; 2016,Jan,13; 2015,Jan,16; 2014,Jan,11

94777 **review, interpretation and preparation of report only by a physician or other qualified health care professional** A

INCLUDES Oxygen saturation monitoring

EXCLUDES *Event monitors (93268-93272)*
Holter monitor (93224-93227)
Remote cardiovascular telemetry (93228-93229)
Sleep testing (95805-95811 [95800, 95801])

0.00 0.00 FUD YYY B 80 26

AMA: 2019,Mar,10; 2018,Feb,11; 2018,Jan,8; 2017,Jan,8; 2016,Jan,13; 2015,Jan,16; 2014,Jan,11

94780 **Car seat/bed testing for airway integrity, for infants through 12 months of age, with continual clinical staff observation and continuous recording of pulse oximetry, heart rate and respiratory rate, with interpretation and report; 60 minutes** A

EXCLUDES *Pediatric and neonatal critical care services (99468-99476, 99477-99480)*
Pulse oximetry (94760-94761)
Rhythm strips (93040-93042)
Use of code for less than 60 minutes of service

0.68 1.45 FUD XXX Q1

AMA: 2019,Mar,10; 2018,Feb,11; 2018,Jan,8; 2017,Jan,8; 2016,Jan,13; 2015,May,10; 2015,Jan,16; 2014,Jan,11

\+ **94781** **each additional full 30 minutes (List separately in addition to code for primary procedure)** A

Code first (94780)

0.24 0.57 FUD ZZZ N

AMA: 2019,Mar,10; 2018,Feb,11; 2018,Jan,8; 2017,Jan,8; 2016,Jan,13; 2015,May,10; 2015,Jan,16; 2014,Jan,11

94799 **Unlisted pulmonary service or procedure**

0.00 0.00 FUD XXX Q1 80

AMA: 2019,Mar,10; 2018,Sep,14; 2018,Feb,11; 2018,Jan,8; 2017,Jan,8; 2016,Jan,13; 2015,Dec,16; 2015,May,10; 2015,Jan,16; 2014,Jan,11

95004-95071 Allergy Tests

EXCLUDES *Drugs administered for intractable/severe allergic reaction (eg, antihistamines, epinephrine, steroids) (96372)*
E&M services when reporting test interpretation/report
Laboratory tests for allergies (86000-86999 [86152, 86153])

Code also medical conferences regarding use of equipment (eg, air filters, humidifiers, dehumidifiers), climate therapy, physical, occupational, and recreation therapy using appropriate E&M codes

Code also significant, separately identifiable E&M services using modifier 25, when performed (99201-99215, 99217-99223 [99224, 99225, 99226], 99231-99233, 99241-99255, 99281-99285, 99304-99318, 99324-99337, 99341-99350, 99381-99429)

95004 **Percutaneous tests (scratch, puncture, prick) with allergenic extracts, immediate type reaction, including test interpretation and report, specify number of tests**

0.12 0.12 FUD XXX Q1 80

AMA: 2018,Feb,11; 2018,Jan,8; 2017,Jan,8; 2016,Jan,13; 2015,Jan,16; 2014,Jan,11

95012 **Nitric oxide expired gas determination**

0.57 0.57 FUD XXX Q1 80

AMA: 2018,Feb,11; 2018,Jan,8; 2017,Jan,8; 2016,Jan,13; 2015,Jan,16; 2014,Mar,11; 2014,Jan,11

95017 **Allergy testing, any combination of percutaneous (scratch, puncture, prick) and intracutaneous (intradermal), sequential and incremental, with venoms, immediate type reaction, including test interpretation and report, specify number of tests**

0.11 0.23 FUD XXX Q1 80

AMA: 2018,Feb,11; 2018,Jan,8; 2017,Jan,8; 2016,Jan,13; 2015,Jul,9; 2015,Jan,16

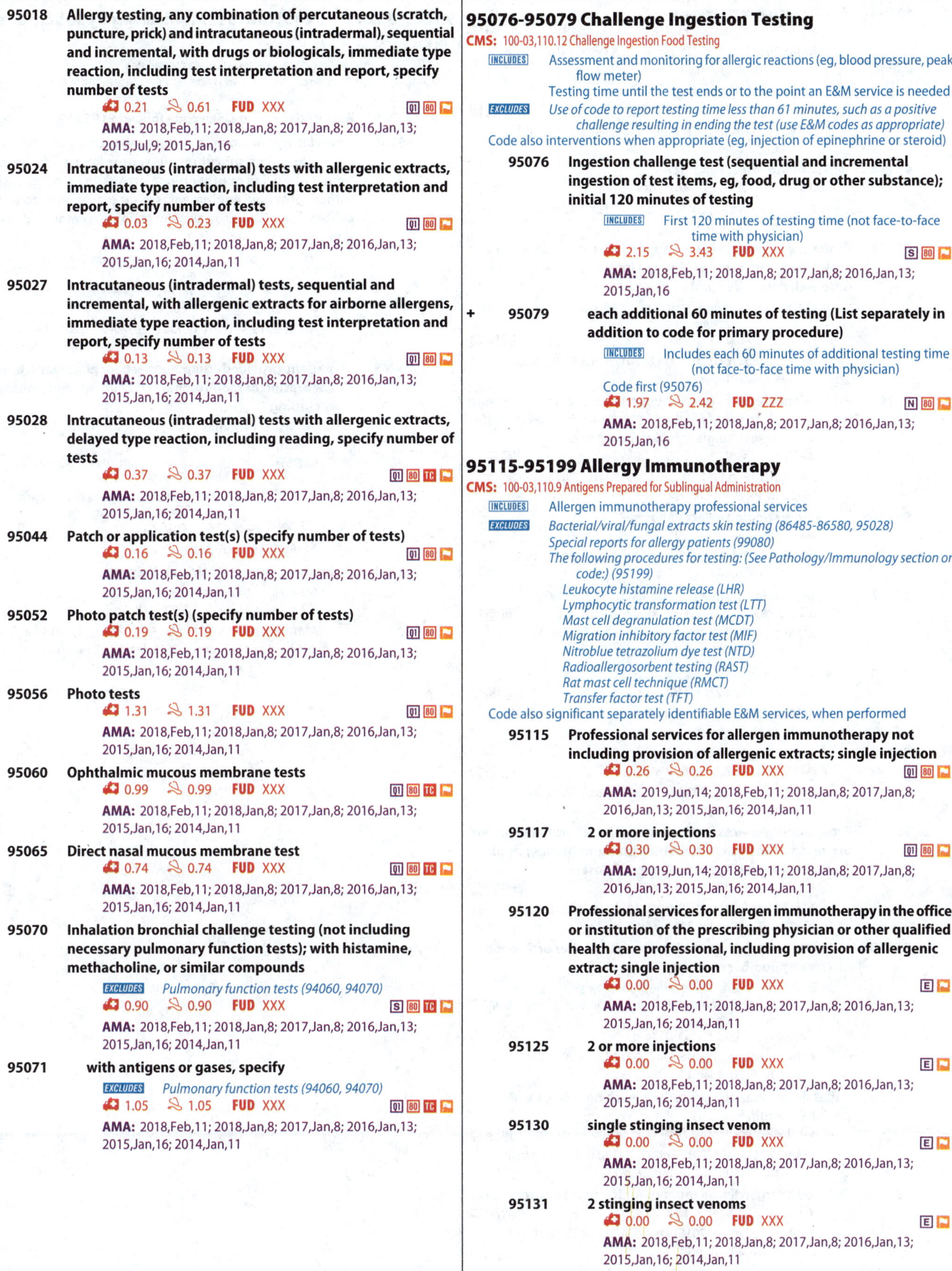

95018 **Allergy testing, any combination of percutaneous (scratch, puncture, prick) and intracutaneous (intradermal), sequential and incremental, with drugs or biologicals, immediate type reaction, including test interpretation and report, specify number of tests**
0.21 0.61 FUD XXX Q1 80
AMA: 2018,Feb,11; 2018,Jan,8; 2017,Jan,8; 2016,Jan,13; 2015,Jul,9; 2015,Jan,16

95024 **Intracutaneous (intradermal) tests with allergenic extracts, immediate type reaction, including test interpretation and report, specify number of tests**
0.03 0.23 FUD XXX Q1 80
AMA: 2018,Feb,11; 2018,Jan,8; 2017,Jan,8; 2016,Jan,13; 2015,Jan,16; 2014,Jan,11

95027 **Intracutaneous (intradermal) tests, sequential and incremental, with allergenic extracts for airborne allergens, immediate type reaction, including test interpretation and report, specify number of tests**
0.13 0.13 FUD XXX Q1 80
AMA: 2018,Feb,11; 2018,Jan,8; 2017,Jan,8; 2016,Jan,13; 2015,Jan,16; 2014,Jan,11

95028 **Intracutaneous (intradermal) tests with allergenic extracts, delayed type reaction, including reading, specify number of tests**
0.37 0.37 FUD XXX Q1 80 TC
AMA: 2018,Feb,11; 2018,Jan,8; 2017,Jan,8; 2016,Jan,13; 2015,Jan,16; 2014,Jan,11

95044 **Patch or application test(s) (specify number of tests)**
0.16 0.16 FUD XXX Q1 80
AMA: 2018,Feb,11; 2018,Jan,8; 2017,Jan,8; 2016,Jan,13; 2015,Jan,16; 2014,Jan,11

95052 **Photo patch test(s) (specify number of tests)**
0.19 0.19 FUD XXX Q1 80
AMA: 2018,Feb,11; 2018,Jan,8; 2017,Jan,8; 2016,Jan,13; 2015,Jan,16; 2014,Jan,11

95056 **Photo tests**
1.31 1.31 FUD XXX Q1 80
AMA: 2018,Feb,11; 2018,Jan,8; 2017,Jan,8; 2016,Jan,13; 2015,Jan,16; 2014,Jan,11

95060 **Ophthalmic mucous membrane tests**
0.99 0.99 FUD XXX Q1 80 TC
AMA: 2018,Feb,11; 2018,Jan,8; 2017,Jan,8; 2016,Jan,13; 2015,Jan,16; 2014,Jan,11

95065 **Direct nasal mucous membrane test**
0.74 0.74 FUD XXX Q1 80 TC
AMA: 2018,Feb,11; 2018,Jan,8; 2017,Jan,8; 2016,Jan,13; 2015,Jan,16; 2014,Jan,11

95070 **Inhalation bronchial challenge testing (not including necessary pulmonary function tests); with histamine, methacholine, or similar compounds**
EXCLUDES *Pulmonary function tests (94060, 94070)*
0.90 0.90 FUD XXX S 80 TC
AMA: 2018,Feb,11; 2018,Jan,8; 2017,Jan,8; 2016,Jan,13; 2015,Jan,16; 2014,Jan,11

95071 **with antigens or gases, specify**
EXCLUDES *Pulmonary function tests (94060, 94070)*
1.05 1.05 FUD XXX Q1 80 TC
AMA: 2018,Feb,11; 2018,Jan,8; 2017,Jan,8; 2016,Jan,13; 2015,Jan,16; 2014,Jan,11

95076-95079 Challenge Ingestion Testing

CMS: 100-03,110.12 Challenge Ingestion Food Testing
INCLUDES Assessment and monitoring for allergic reactions (eg, blood pressure, peak flow meter)
Testing time until the test ends or to the point an E&M service is needed
EXCLUDES *Use of code to report testing time less than 61 minutes, such as a positive challenge resulting in ending the test (use E&M codes as appropriate)*
Code also interventions when appropriate (eg, injection of epinephrine or steroid)

95076 **Ingestion challenge test (sequential and incremental ingestion of test items, eg, food, drug or other substance); initial 120 minutes of testing**
INCLUDES First 120 minutes of testing time (not face-to-face time with physician)
2.15 3.43 FUD XXX S 80
AMA: 2018,Feb,11; 2018,Jan,8; 2017,Jan,8; 2016,Jan,13; 2015,Jan,16

+ **95079** **each additional 60 minutes of testing (List separately in addition to code for primary procedure)**
INCLUDES Includes each 60 minutes of additional testing time (not face-to-face time with physician)
Code first (95076)
1.97 2.42 FUD ZZZ N 80
AMA: 2018,Feb,11; 2018,Jan,8; 2017,Jan,8; 2016,Jan,13; 2015,Jan,16

95115-95199 Allergy Immunotherapy

CMS: 100-03,110.9 Antigens Prepared for Sublingual Administration
INCLUDES Allergen immunotherapy professional services
EXCLUDES *Bacterial/viral/fungal extracts skin testing (86485-86580, 95028)*
Special reports for allergy patients (99080)
The following procedures for testing: (See Pathology/Immunology section or code:) (95199)
Leukocyte histamine release (LHR)
Lymphocytic transformation test (LTT)
Mast cell degranulation test (MCDT)
Migration inhibitory factor test (MIF)
Nitroblue tetrazolium dye test (NTD)
Radioallergosorbent testing (RAST)
Rat mast cell technique (RMCT)
Transfer factor test (TFT)
Code also significant separately identifiable E&M services, when performed

95115 **Professional services for allergen immunotherapy not including provision of allergenic extracts; single injection**
0.26 0.26 FUD XXX Q1 80
AMA: 2019,Jun,14; 2018,Feb,11; 2018,Jan,8; 2017,Jan,8; 2016,Jan,13; 2015,Jan,16; 2014,Jan,11

95117 **2 or more injections**
0.30 0.30 FUD XXX Q1 80
AMA: 2019,Jun,14; 2018,Feb,11; 2018,Jan,8; 2017,Jan,8; 2016,Jan,13; 2015,Jan,16; 2014,Jan,11

95120 **Professional services for allergen immunotherapy in the office or institution of the prescribing physician or other qualified health care professional, including provision of allergenic extract; single injection**
0.00 0.00 FUD XXX E
AMA: 2018,Feb,11; 2018,Jan,8; 2017,Jan,8; 2016,Jan,13; 2015,Jan,16; 2014,Jan,11

95125 **2 or more injections**
0.00 0.00 FUD XXX E
AMA: 2018,Feb,11; 2018,Jan,8; 2017,Jan,8; 2016,Jan,13; 2015,Jan,16; 2014,Jan,11

95130 **single stinging insect venom**
0.00 0.00 FUD XXX E
AMA: 2018,Feb,11; 2018,Jan,8; 2017,Jan,8; 2016,Jan,13; 2015,Jan,16; 2014,Jan,11

95131 **2 stinging insect venoms**
0.00 0.00 FUD XXX E
AMA: 2018,Feb,11; 2018,Jan,8; 2017,Jan,8; 2016,Jan,13; 2015,Jan,16; 2014,Jan,11

Medicine

95018 — 95131

● New Code ▲ Revised Code ○ Reinstated ● New Web Release ▲ Revised Web Release + Add-on Unlisted Not Covered # Resequenced
Optum Mod 50 Exempt ⊘ AMA Mod 51 Exempt Optum Mod 51 Exempt Mod 63 Exempt Non-FDA Drug ★ Telemedicine Maternity Age Edit

95132 **3 stinging insect venoms**
0.00 0.00 FUD XXX E
AMA: 2018,Feb,11; 2018,Jan,8; 2017,Jan,8; 2016,Jan,13; 2015,Jan,16; 2014,Jan,11

95133 **4 stinging insect venoms**
0.00 0.00 FUD XXX E
AMA: 2018,Feb,11; 2018,Jan,8; 2017,Jan,8; 2016,Jan,13; 2015,Jan,16; 2014,Jan,11

95134 **5 stinging insect venoms**
0.00 0.00 FUD XXX E
AMA: 2018,Feb,11; 2018,Jan,8; 2017,Jan,8; 2016,Jan,13; 2015,Jan,16; 2014,Jan,11

95144 **Professional services for the supervision of preparation and provision of antigens for allergen immunotherapy, single dose vial(s) (specify number of vials)**
INCLUDES Single dose vial/single dose of antigen administered in one injection
0.09 0.41 FUD XXX Q1 80
AMA: 2018,Feb,11; 2018,Jan,8; 2017,Jan,8; 2016,Jan,13; 2015,Jan,16; 2014,Jan,11

95145 **Professional services for the supervision of preparation and provision of antigens for allergen immunotherapy (specify number of doses); single stinging insect venom**
0.09 0.81 FUD XXX Q1 80
AMA: 2018,Feb,11; 2018,Jan,8; 2017,Jan,8; 2016,Jan,13; 2015,Jan,16; 2014,Jan,11

95146 **2 single stinging insect venoms**
0.09 1.50 FUD XXX Q1 80
AMA: 2018,Feb,11; 2018,Jan,8; 2017,Jan,8; 2016,Jan,13; 2015,Jan,16; 2014,Jan,11

95147 **3 single stinging insect venoms**
0.09 1.55 FUD XXX Q1 80
AMA: 2018,Feb,11; 2018,Jan,8; 2017,Jan,8; 2016,Jan,13; 2015,Jan,16; 2014,Jan,11

95148 **4 single stinging insect venoms**
0.09 2.23 FUD XXX Q1 80
AMA: 2018,Feb,11; 2018,Jan,8; 2017,Jan,8; 2016,Jan,13; 2015,Jan,16; 2014,Jan,11

95149 **5 single stinging insect venoms**
0.09 2.97 FUD XXX Q1 80
AMA: 2018,Feb,11; 2018,Jan,8; 2017,Jan,8; 2016,Jan,13; 2015,Jan,16; 2014,Jan,11

95165 **Professional services for the supervision of preparation and provision of antigens for allergen immunotherapy; single or multiple antigens (specify number of doses)**
0.09 0.40 FUD XXX Q1 80
AMA: 2018,Feb,11; 2018,Jan,8; 2017,Jan,8; 2016,Jan,13; 2015,Jan,16; 2014,Jan,11

95170 **whole body extract of biting insect or other arthropod (specify number of doses)**
INCLUDES A dose which is the amount of antigen(s) administered in a single injection from a multiple dose vial
0.09 0.30 FUD XXX Q1 80
AMA: 2018,Feb,11; 2018,Jan,8; 2017,Jan,8; 2016,Jan,13; 2015,Jan,16; 2014,Jan,11

95180 **Rapid desensitization procedure, each hour (eg, insulin, penicillin, equine serum)**
2.96 3.92 FUD XXX Q1 80
AMA: 2019,Jun,14; 2018,Feb,11; 2018,Jan,8; 2017,Jan,8; 2016,Jan,13; 2015,Jan,16; 2014,Jan,11

95199 **Unlisted allergy/clinical immunologic service or procedure**
0.00 0.00 FUD XXX Q1 80
AMA: 2018,Feb,11; 2018,Jan,8; 2017,Jan,8; 2016,Jan,13; 2015,Jan,16; 2014,Jan,11

95249-95251 [95249] Glucose Monitoring By Subcutaneous Device

EXCLUDES *Physiologic data collection/interpretation (99091)*
Code also when data receiver owned by patient for placement of sensor, hook-up, monitor calibration, training, and printout (95999)

95249 **Resequenced code. See code following 95250.**

95250 **Ambulatory continuous glucose monitoring of interstitial tissue fluid via a subcutaneous sensor for a minimum of 72 hours; physician or other qualified health care professional (office) provided equipment, sensor placement, hook-up, calibration of monitor, patient training, removal of sensor, and printout of recording**
EXCLUDES *Subcutaneous pocket with insertion interstitial glucose monitor (0446T)*
Use of code more than one time per month
4.26 4.26 FUD XXX V 80 TC
AMA: 2019,Jan,6; 2018,Jun,6; 2018,Mar,5; 2018,Feb,11; 2018,Jan,8; 2017,Jan,8; 2016,Jan,13; 2015,Jan,16; 2014,Jan,11

\# **95249** **patient-provided equipment, sensor placement, hook-up, calibration of monitor, patient training, and printout of recording**
INCLUDES Performing complete collection of initial data in the provider's office
EXCLUDES *Subcutaneous pocket with insertion interstitial glucose monitor (0446T)*
Use of code more than one time during the period the patient owns the data receiver
1.56 1.56 FUD XXX S 80 TC
AMA: 2018,Jun,6; 2018,Feb,11

95251 **analysis, interpretation and report**
EXCLUDES *Use of code more than one time per month*
1.01 1.01 FUD XXX B 80 26
AMA: 2018,Jun,6; 2018,Mar,5; 2018,Feb,11; 2018,Jan,8; 2017,Jan,8; 2016,Jan,13; 2015,Jan,16; 2014,Jan,11

95700-95783 Sleep Studies

INCLUDES Assessment of sleep disorders in adults and children
Continuous and simultaneous monitoring and recording of physiological sleep parameters of 6 hours or more
Evaluation of patient's response to therapies
Physician:
- Interpretation
- Recording
- Report

Recording sessions may be:
- Attended studies that include the presence of a technologist or qualified health care professional to respond to the needs of the patient or technical issues at the bedside
- Remote without the presence of a technologist or a qualified health professional
- Unattended without the presence of a technologist or qualified health care professional

Testing parameters include:
- Actigraphy: Use of a noninvasive portable device to record gross motor movements to approximate periods of sleep and wakefulness
- Electrooculogram (EOG): Records electrical activity associated with eye movements
- Maintenance of wakefulness test (MWT): An attended study used to determine the patient's ability to stay awake
- Multiple sleep latency test (MSLT): Attended study to determine the tendency of the patient to fall asleep
- Peripheral arterial tonometry (PAT): Pulsatile volume changes in a digit are measured to determine activity in the sympathetic nervous system for respiratory analysis
- Polysomnography: An attended continuous, simultaneous recording of physiological parameters of sleep for at least 6 hours in a sleep laboratory setting that also includes four or more of the following:
  1. Airflow-oral and/or nasal
  2. Bilateral anterior tibialis EMG
  3. Electrocardiogram (ECG)
  4. Oxyhemoglobin saturation, SpO2
  5. Respiratory effort
- Positive airway pressure (PAP): Noninvasive devices used to treat sleep-related disorders
- Respiratory airflow (ventilation): Assessment of air movement during inhalation and exhalation as measured by nasal pressure sensors and thermistor
- Respiratory analysis: Assessment of components of respiration obtained by other methods such as airflow or peripheral arterial tone
- Respiratory effort: Use of the diaphragm and/or intercostal muscle for airflow is measured using transducers to estimate thoracic and abdominal motion
- Respiratory movement: Measures the movement of the chest and abdomen during respiration
- Sleep latency: Pertains to the time it takes to get to sleep
- Sleep staging: Determination of the separate levels of sleep according to physiological measurements
- Total sleep time: Determined by the use of actigraphy and other methods

Use of portable and in-laboratory technology

EXCLUDES *E&M services*

95700 **Resequenced code. See code following 95967.**
95705 **Resequenced code. See code following 95967.**
95706 **Resequenced code. See code following 95967.**
95707 **Resequenced code. See code following 95967.**
95708 **Resequenced code. See code following 95967.**
95709 **Resequenced code. See code following 95967.**
95710 **Resequenced code. See code following 95967.**
95711 **Resequenced code. See code following 95967.**
95712 **Resequenced code. See code following 95967.**
95713 **Resequenced code. See code following 95967.**
95714 **Resequenced code. See code following 95967.**
95715 **Resequenced code. See code following 95967.**
95716 **Resequenced code. See code following 95967.**
95717 **Resequenced code. See code following 95967.**
95718 **Resequenced code. See code following 95967.**
95719 **Resequenced code. See code following 95967.**
95720 **Resequenced code. See code following 95967.**
95721 **Resequenced code, See code following 95967.**
95722 **Resequenced code. See code following 95967.**
95723 **Resequenced code. See code following 95967.**
95724 **Resequenced code. See code following 95967.**
95725 **Resequenced code. See code following 95967.**
95726 **Resequenced code. See code following 95967.**
95782 **Resequenced code. See code following 95811.**
95783 **Resequenced code. See code following 95811.**
95800 **Resequenced code. See code following 95806.**
95801 **Resequenced code. See code following 95806.**

95803 **Actigraphy testing, recording, analysis, interpretation, and report (minimum of 72 hours to 14 consecutive days of recording)**

EXCLUDES *Sleep studies (95806-95811 [95800, 95801])*
Use of code more than one time in a 14-day period

4.06 4.06 FUD XXX 01 80

AMA: 2018,Feb,11; 2018,Jan,8; 2017,Jan,8; 2016,Jan,13; 2015,Jan,16; 2014,Jan,11

95805 **Multiple sleep latency or maintenance of wakefulness testing, recording, analysis and interpretation of physiological measurements of sleep during multiple trials to assess sleepiness**

INCLUDES Physiological sleep parameters as measured by:
- Frontal, central, and occipital EEG leads (3 leads)
- Left and right EOG
- Submental EMG lead

EXCLUDES *Polysomnography (95808-95811)*
Sleep study, not attended (95806)

Code also modifier 52 when less than four nap opportunities are recorded

11.8 11.8 FUD XXX S 80

AMA: 2018,Feb,11; 2018,Jan,8; 2017,Jan,8; 2016,Jan,13; 2015,Jan,16; 2014,Jan,11

95806 **Sleep study, unattended, simultaneous recording of, heart rate, oxygen saturation, respiratory airflow, and respiratory effort (eg, thoracoabdominal movement)**

EXCLUDES *Arterial waveform analysis (93050)*
Event monitors (93268-93272)
Holter monitor (93224-93227)
Remote cardiovascular telemetry (93228-93229)
Rhythm strips (93041-93042)
Unattended sleep study with measurement of a minimum heart rate, oxygen saturation, and respiratory analysis (95801)
Unattended sleep study with measurement of heart rate, oxygen saturation, respiratory analysis, and sleep time (95800)

Code also modifier 52 for fewer than 6 hours of recording

3.90 3.90 FUD XXX S 80

AMA: 2018,Feb,11; 2018,Jan,8; 2017,Jan,8; 2016,Jan,13; 2015,Jan,16; 2014,Jan,11

\# **95800** **Sleep study, unattended, simultaneous recording; heart rate, oxygen saturation, respiratory analysis (eg, by airflow or peripheral arterial tone), and sleep time**

4.79 4.79 FUD XXX S 80

AMA: 2018,Feb,11; 2018,Jan,8; 2017,Jan,8; 2016,Jan,13; 2015,Jan,16; 2014,Jan,11

\# **95801** **minimum of heart rate, oxygen saturation, and respiratory analysis (eg, by airflow or peripheral arterial tone)**

2.57 2.57 FUD XXX 01 80

AMA: 2018,Feb,11; 2018,Jan,8; 2017,Jan,8; 2016,Jan,13; 2015,Jan,16; 2014,Jan,11

95807 **Sleep study, simultaneous recording of ventilation, respiratory effort, ECG or heart rate, and oxygen saturation, attended by a technologist**

EXCLUDES *Polysomnography (95808-95811)*
Sleep study, not attended (95806)

Code also modifier 52 for fewer than 6 hours of recording

12.1 12.1 FUD XXX S 80

AMA: 2018,Feb,11; 2018,Jan,8; 2017,Jan,8; 2016,Jan,13; 2015,Jan,16; 2014,Jan,11

95808 **Polysomnography; any age, sleep staging with 1-3 additional parameters of sleep, attended by a technologist**

EXCLUDES *Sleep study, not attended (95806)*

18.9 18.9 FUD XXX S 80

AMA: 2018,Feb,11; 2018,Jan,8; 2017,Jan,8; 2016,Jan,13; 2015,Jan,16; 2014,Jan,11

95810 **age 6 years or older, sleep staging with 4 or more additional parameters of sleep, attended by a technologist** A

EXCLUDES *Sleep study, not attended (95806)*

Code also modifier 52 for fewer than 6 hours of recording

17.3 17.3 FUD XXX S 80

AMA: 2018,Feb,11; 2018,Jan,8; 2017,Jan,8; 2016,Jan,13; 2015,Jan,16; 2014,Jan,11

95811 **age 6 years or older, sleep staging with 4 or more additional parameters of sleep, with initiation of continuous positive airway pressure therapy or bilevel ventilation, attended by a technologist** A

EXCLUDES *Sleep study, not attended (95806)*

Code also modifier 52 for fewer than 6 hours of recording

18.1 18.1 FUD XXX S 80

AMA: 2018,Feb,11; 2018,Jan,8; 2017,Jan,8; 2016,Jan,13; 2015,Jan,16; 2014,Oct,8; 2014,Jan,11

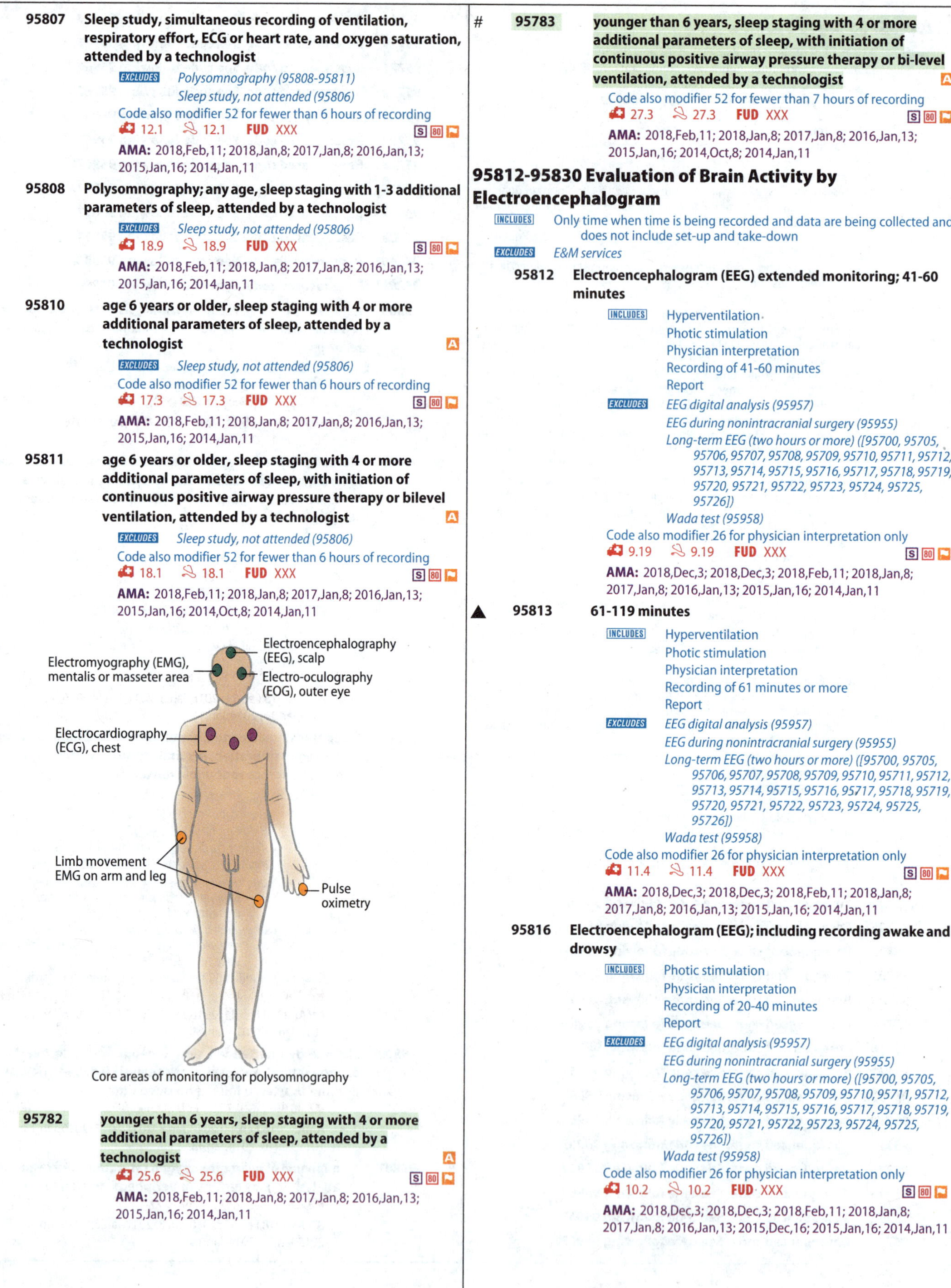

Core areas of monitoring for polysomnography

\# **95782** **younger than 6 years, sleep staging with 4 or more additional parameters of sleep, attended by a technologist** A

25.6 25.6 FUD XXX S 80

AMA: 2018,Feb,11; 2018,Jan,8; 2017,Jan,8; 2016,Jan,13; 2015,Jan,16; 2014,Jan,11

\# **95783** **younger than 6 years, sleep staging with 4 or more additional parameters of sleep, with initiation of continuous positive airway pressure therapy or bi-level ventilation, attended by a technologist** A

Code also modifier 52 for fewer than 7 hours of recording

27.3 27.3 FUD XXX S 80

AMA: 2018,Feb,11; 2018,Jan,8; 2017,Jan,8; 2016,Jan,13; 2015,Jan,16; 2014,Oct,8; 2014,Jan,11

95812-95830 Evaluation of Brain Activity by Electroencephalogram

INCLUDES Only time when time is being recorded and data are being collected and does not include set-up and take-down

EXCLUDES *E&M services*

95812 **Electroencephalogram (EEG) extended monitoring; 41-60 minutes**

INCLUDES Hyperventilation
Photic stimulation
Physician interpretation
Recording of 41-60 minutes
Report

EXCLUDES *EEG digital analysis (95957)*
EEG during nonintracranial surgery (95955)
Long-term EEG (two hours or more) ([95700, 95705, 95706, 95707, 95708, 95709, 95710, 95711, 95712, 95713, 95714, 95715, 95716, 95717, 95718, 95719, 95720, 95721, 95722, 95723, 95724, 95725, 95726])
Wada test (95958)

Code also modifier 26 for physician interpretation only

9.19 9.19 FUD XXX S 80

AMA: 2018,Dec,3; 2018,Dec,3; 2018,Feb,11; 2018,Jan,8; 2017,Jan,8; 2016,Jan,13; 2015,Jan,16; 2014,Jan,11

▲ **95813** **61-119 minutes**

INCLUDES Hyperventilation
Photic stimulation
Physician interpretation
Recording of 61 minutes or more
Report

EXCLUDES *EEG digital analysis (95957)*
EEG during nonintracranial surgery (95955)
Long-term EEG (two hours or more) ([95700, 95705, 95706, 95707, 95708, 95709, 95710, 95711, 95712, 95713, 95714, 95715, 95716, 95717, 95718, 95719, 95720, 95721, 95722, 95723, 95724, 95725, 95726])
Wada test (95958)

Code also modifier 26 for physician interpretation only

11.4 11.4 FUD XXX S 80

AMA: 2018,Dec,3; 2018,Dec,3; 2018,Feb,11; 2018,Jan,8; 2017,Jan,8; 2016,Jan,13; 2015,Jan,16; 2014,Jan,11

95816 **Electroencephalogram (EEG); including recording awake and drowsy**

INCLUDES Photic stimulation
Physician interpretation
Recording of 20-40 minutes
Report

EXCLUDES *EEG digital analysis (95957)*
EEG during nonintracranial surgery (95955)
Long-term EEG (two hours or more) ([95700, 95705, 95706, 95707, 95708, 95709, 95710, 95711, 95712, 95713, 95714, 95715, 95716, 95717, 95718, 95719, 95720, 95721, 95722, 95723, 95724, 95725, 95726])
Wada test (95958)

Code also modifier 26 for physician interpretation only

10.2 10.2 FUD XXX S 80

AMA: 2018,Dec,3; 2018,Dec,3; 2018,Feb,11; 2018,Jan,8; 2017,Jan,8; 2016,Jan,13; 2015,Dec,16; 2015,Jan,16; 2014,Jan,11

95819 **including recording awake and asleep**

INCLUDES Hyperventilation
Photic stimulation
Physician interpretation
Recording of 20-40 minutes
Report

EXCLUDES *EEG digital analysis (95957)*
EEG during nonintracranial surgery (95955)
Long-term EEG (two hours or more) ([95700, 95705, 95706, 95707, 95708, 95709, 95710, 95711, 95712, 95713, 95714, 95715, 95716, 95717, 95718, 95719, 95720, 95721, 95722, 95723, 95724, 95725, 95726])
Wada test (95958)

Code also modifier 26 for interpretation only

12.0 12.0 FUD XXX S 80

AMA: 2018,Dec,3; 2018,Dec,3; 2018,Feb,11; 2018,Jan,8; 2017,Jan,8; 2016,Jan,13; 2015,Dec,16; 2015,Jan,16; 2014,Jan,11

95822 **recording in coma or sleep only**

INCLUDES Hyperventilation
Photic stimulation
Physician interpretation
Recording of 20-40 minutes
Report

EXCLUDES *EEG digital analysis (95957)*
EEG during nonintracranial surgery (95955)
Long-term EEG (two hours or more) ([95700, 95705, 95706, 95707, 95708, 95709, 95710, 95711, 95712, 95713, 95714, 95715, 95716, 95717, 95718, 95719, 95720, 95721, 95722, 95723, 95724, 95725, 95726])
Wada test (95958)

Code also modifier 26 for interpretation only

10.9 10.9 FUD XXX S 80

AMA: 2018,Dec,3; 2018,Dec,3; 2018,Feb,11; 2018,Jan,8; 2017,Jan,8; 2016,Jan,13; 2015,Jan,16; 2014,Dec,18; 2014,Jan,11

95824 **cerebral death evaluation only**

INCLUDES Physician interpretation
Recording
Report

EXCLUDES *EEG digital analysis (95957)*
EEG during nonintracranial surgery (95955)
Long-term EEG (two hours or more) ([95700, 95705, 95706, 95707, 95708, 95709, 95710, 95711, 95712, 95713, 95714, 95715, 95716, 95717, 95718, 95719, 95720, 95721, 95722, 95723, 95724, 95725, 95726])
Wada test (95958)

Code also modifier 26 for physician interpretation only

0.00 0.00 FUD XXX S 80

AMA: 2018,Feb,11

95827 ~~**all night recording**~~

To report, see ([97505-95707], [95711], [95713], [95717-95718])

95829 **Resequenced code. See code following 95830.**

95830 **Insertion by physician or other qualified health care professional of sphenoidal electrodes for electroencephalographic (EEG) recording**

2.64 10.9 FUD XXX B 80

AMA: 2018,Feb,11

[95829, 95836] Evaluation of Brain Activity by Electrocorticography

\# 95829 **Electrocorticogram at surgery (separate procedure)**

INCLUDES EEG recording from electrodes placed in or on the brain
Interpretation and review during the surgical procedure

Code also modifier 26 for interpretation only

53.6 53.6 FUD XXX N 80

AMA: 2018,Dec,3; 2018,Dec,3; 2018,Feb,11

\# 95836 **Electrocorticogram from an implanted brain neurostimulator pulse generator/transmitter, including recording, with interpretation and written report, up to 30 days**

INCLUDES Intracranial recordings for up to 30 days (unattended) with storage for review at a later time

EXCLUDES *Programming of neurostimulator during the 30-day period ([95983, 95984])*
Use of code more than one time for the documented 30-day period

3.14 3.14 FUD XXX 80

AMA: 2018,Dec,3; 2018,Dec,3

95831-95857 Evaluation of Muscles and Range of Motion

CMS: 100-02,15,230.4 Services By a Physical/Occupational Therapist in Private Practice

EXCLUDES *E&M services*

95831 ~~**Muscle testing, manual (separate procedure) with report; extremity (excluding hand) or trunk**~~

To report, see ([97161], [97162], [97163], [97164], [97165], [97166], [97167], [97168], [97169], [97170], [97171], [97172])

95832 ~~**hand, with or without comparison with normal side**~~

To report, see ([97161], [97162], [97163], [97164], [97165], [97166], [97167], [97168], [97169], [97170], [97171], [97172])

95833 ~~**total evaluation of body, excluding hands**~~

To report, see ([97161], [97162], [97163], [97164], [97165], [97166], [97167], [97168], [97169], [97170], [97171], [97172])

95834 ~~**total evaluation of body, including hands**~~

To report, see ([97161], [97162], [97163], [97164], [97165], [97166], [97167], [97168], [97169], [97170], [97171], [97172])

95836 **Resequenced code. See code following 95830.**

95851 **Range of motion measurements and report (separate procedure); each extremity (excluding hand) or each trunk section (spine)**

0.22 0.59 FUD XXX A 80

AMA: 2018,Feb,11; 2018,Jan,8; 2017,Jan,8; 2016,Dec,16; 2016,Jan,13; 2015,Jan,16; 2014,Jan,11

95852 **hand, with or without comparison with normal side**

0.17 0.53 FUD XXX A 80

AMA: 2018,Feb,11; 2018,Jan,8; 2017,Jan,8; 2016,Jan,13; 2015,Jan,16; 2014,Jan,11

95857 **Cholinesterase inhibitor challenge test for myasthenia gravis**

0.85 1.54 FUD XXX S 80

AMA: 2018,Feb,11; 2018,Jan,8; 2017,Jan,8; 2016,Jan,13; 2015,Jan,16; 2014,Jan,11

95860-95887 [95885, 95886, 95887] Evaluation of Nerve and Muscle Function: EMGs with/without Nerve Conduction Studies

INCLUDES Physician interpretation
Recording
Report

EXCLUDES *E&M services*

95860 **Needle electromyography; 1 extremity with or without related paraspinal areas**

INCLUDES Testing of five or more muscles per extremity

EXCLUDES *Dynamic electromyography during motion analysis studies (96002-96003)*
Guidance for chemodenervation (95873-95874)

Code also modifier 26 for interpretation only

3.43 3.43 FUD XXX Q1 80

AMA: 2018,Feb,11; 2018,Jan,8; 2017,Jan,8; 2016,Jan,13; 2015,Mar,6; 2015,Jan,16; 2014,Jan,11

95861 **2 extremities with or without related paraspinal areas**

INCLUDES Testing of five or more muscles per extremity

EXCLUDES *Dynamic electromyography during motion analysis studies (96002-96003)*

Guidance for chemodenervation (95873-95874)

Code also modifier 26 for interpretation only

4.90 4.90 FUD XXX Q1 80

AMA: 2018,Feb,11; 2018,Jan,8; 2017,Jan,8; 2016,Jan,13; 2015,Mar,6; 2015,Jan,16; 2014,Jan,11

95863 **3 extremities with or without related paraspinal areas**

INCLUDES Testing of five or more muscles per extremity

EXCLUDES *Dynamic electromyography during motion analysis studies (96002-96003)*

Guidance for chemodenervation (95873-95874)

Code also modifier 26 for interpretation only

6.15 6.15 FUD XXX S 80

AMA: 2018,Feb,11; 2018,Jan,8; 2017,Jan,8; 2016,Jan,13; 2015,Mar,6; 2015,Jan,16; 2014,Jan,11

95864 **4 extremities with or without related paraspinal areas**

INCLUDES Testing of five or more muscles per extremity

EXCLUDES *Dynamic electromyography during motion analysis studies (96002-96003)*

Guidance for chemodenervation (95873-95874)

Code also modifier 26 for interpretation only

7.07 7.07 FUD XXX S 80

AMA: 2018,Feb,11; 2018,Jan,8; 2017,Jan,8; 2016,Jan,13; 2015,Mar,6; 2015,Jan,16; 2014,Jan,11

95865 **larynx**

EXCLUDES *Dynamic electromyography during motion analysis studies (96002-96003)*

Guidance for chemodenervation (95873-95874)

Code also modifier 26 for interpretation only

Code also modifier 52 for unilateral procedure

4.25 4.25 FUD XXX Q1 80

AMA: 2018,Feb,11; 2018,Jan,8; 2017,Jan,8; 2016,Jan,13; 2015,Mar,6; 2015,Jan,16; 2014,Jan,6; 2014,Jan,11

95866 **hemidiaphragm**

EXCLUDES *Dynamic electromyography during motion analysis studies (96002-96003)*

Guidance for chemodenervation (95873-95874)

Code also modifier 26 for interpretation only

3.90 3.90 FUD XXX Q1 80

AMA: 2018,Feb,11; 2018,Jan,8; 2017,Jan,8; 2016,Jan,13; 2015,Mar,6; 2015,Jan,16; 2014,Jan,11

95867 **cranial nerve supplied muscle(s), unilateral**

EXCLUDES *Guidance for chemodenervation (95873-95874)*

Code also modifier 26 for interpretation only

3.00 3.00 FUD XXX S 80

AMA: 2018,Feb,11; 2018,Jan,8; 2017,Jan,8; 2016,Jan,13; 2015,Mar,6; 2015,Jan,16; 2014,Jan,11

95868 **cranial nerve supplied muscles, bilateral**

EXCLUDES *Guidance for chemodenervation (95873-95874)*

3.93 3.93 FUD XXX S 80

AMA: 2018,Feb,11; 2018,Jan,8; 2017,Jan,8; 2016,Jan,13; 2015,Mar,6; 2015,Jan,16; 2014,Jan,11

95869 **thoracic paraspinal muscles (excluding T1 or T12)**

EXCLUDES *Dynamic electromyography during motion analysis studies (96002-96003)*

Guidance for chemodenervation (95873-95874)

2.67 2.67 FUD XXX Q1 80

AMA: 2018,Feb,11; 2018,Jan,8; 2017,Jan,8; 2016,Jan,13; 2015,Mar,6; 2015,Jan,16; 2014,Jan,11

95870 **limited study of muscles in 1 extremity or non-limb (axial) muscles (unilateral or bilateral), other than thoracic paraspinal, cranial nerve supplied muscles, or sphincters**

INCLUDES Adson test

Testing of four or less muscles per extremity

EXCLUDES *Anal/urethral sphincter/detrusor/urethra/perineum musculature (51785-51792)*

Complete study of extremities (95860-95864)

Dynamic electromyography during motion analysis studies (96002-96003)

Eye muscles (92265)

Guidance for chemodenervation (95873-95874)

2.58 2.58 FUD XXX Q1 80

AMA: 2018,Feb,11; 2018,Jan,8; 2017,Jan,8; 2016,Jan,13; 2015,Mar,6; 2015,Jan,16; 2014,Jan,11

95872 **Needle electromyography using single fiber electrode, with quantitative measurement of jitter, blocking and/or fiber density, any/all sites of each muscle studied**

EXCLUDES *Dynamic electromyography during motion analysis studies (96002-96003)*

5.64 5.64 FUD XXX S 80

AMA: 2018,Feb,11; 2018,Jan,8; 2017,Jan,8; 2016,Jan,13; 2015,Mar,6; 2015,Jan,16; 2014,Jan,11

+ # **95885** **Needle electromyography, each extremity, with related paraspinal areas, when performed, done with nerve conduction, amplitude and latency/velocity study; limited (List separately in addition to code for primary procedure)**

1.73 1.73 FUD ZZZ N 80

AMA: 2018,Feb,11; 2018,Jan,8; 2017,Jul,10; 2017,Jan,8; 2016,Jan,13; 2015,Mar,6; 2015,Jan,16; 2014,Jan,11

+ # **95886** **complete, five or more muscles studied, innervated by three or more nerves or four or more spinal levels (List separately in addition to code for primary procedure)**

2.68 2.68 FUD ZZZ N 80

AMA: 2018,Feb,11; 2018,Jan,8; 2017,Jul,10; 2017,Jan,8; 2016,Jan,13; 2015,Mar,6; 2015,Jan,16; 2014,Jan,11

+ # **95887** **Needle electromyography, non-extremity (cranial nerve supplied or axial) muscle(s) done with nerve conduction, amplitude and latency/velocity study (List separately in addition to code for primary procedure)**

2.33 2.33 FUD ZZZ N 80

AMA: 2018,Feb,11; 2018,Jan,8; 2017,Jul,10; 2017,Jan,8; 2016,Jan,13; 2015,Mar,6; 2015,Jan,16; 2014,Jan,11; 2014,Jan,8

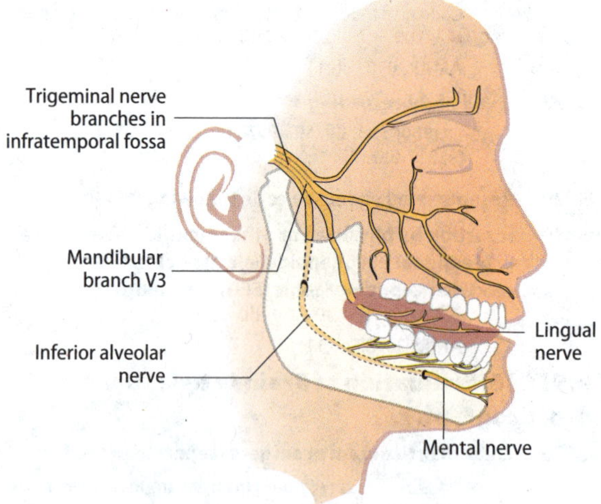

Trigeminal nerve branches in infratemporal fossa

Mandibular branch V3

Inferior alveolar nerve

Lingual nerve

Mental nerve

Cranial nerves: trigeminal branches of lower face and select facial nerves

Needle EMG is performed to determine conduction, amplitude, and latency/velocity

+ **95873 Electrical stimulation for guidance in conjunction with chemodenervation (List separately in addition to code for primary procedure)**

EXCLUDES *Chemodenervation larynx (64617)*
Injection of anesthetic or steroid, sacroiliac joint (64451)
Needle electromyography (95860-95870)
Needle electromyography guidance for chemodenervation (95874)
Radiofrequency ablation, sacroiliac joint ([64625])
Use of more than one guidance code for each code for chemodenervation

Code first chemodenervation (64612, 64615-64616, 64642-64647)

2.13 2.13 FUD ZZZ N 80

AMA: 2019,Apr,9; 2018,Feb,11; 2018,Jan,8; 2017,Jan,8; 2016,Jan,13; 2015,Mar,6; 2015,Jan,16; 2014,Jan,6; 2014,Jan,11

+ **95874 Needle electromyography for guidance in conjunction with chemodenervation (List separately in addition to code for primary procedure)**

EXCLUDES *Chemodenervation larynx (64617)*
Injection of anesthetic or steroid, sacroiliac joint (64451)
Needle electromyography (95860-95870)
Needle electromyography guidance for chemodenervation (95873)
Radiofrequency ablation, sacroiliac joint ([64625])
Use of more than one guidance code for each code for chemodenervation

Code first chemodenervation (64612, 64615-64616, 64642-64647)

2.18 2.18 FUD ZZZ N 80

AMA: 2019,Apr,9; 2018,Feb,11; 2018,Jan,8; 2017,Jan,8; 2016,Jan,13; 2015,Mar,6; 2015,Jan,16; 2014,Oct,14; 2014,Jan,6; 2014,Jan,11

95875 Ischemic limb exercise test with serial specimen(s) acquisition for muscle(s) metabolite(s)

3.75 3.75 FUD XXX S 80

AMA: 2018,Feb,11; 2018,Jan,8; 2017,Jan,8; 2016,Jan,13; 2015,Mar,6; 2015,Jan,16; 2014,Jan,11

95885 **Resequenced code. See code following 95872.**

95886 **Resequenced code. See code following 95872.**

95887 **Resequenced code. See code before 95873.**

95905-95913 Evaluation of Nerve Function: Nerve Conduction Studies

INCLUDES Conduction studies of motor and sensory nerves
Reports from on-site examiner including the work product of the interpretation of results using established methodologies, calculations, comparisons to normal studies, and interpretation by physician or other qualified health care professional
Single conduction study comprising a sensory and motor conduction test with/without F or H wave testing, and all orthodromic and antidromic impulses
Total number of tests performed indicate which code is appropriate

EXCLUDES *Use of code for more than one study when multiple sites on the same nerve are tested*

Code also electromyography performed with nerve conduction studies, as appropriate ([95885, 95886, 95887])

95905 Motor and/or sensory nerve conduction, using preconfigured electrode array(s), amplitude and latency/velocity study, each limb, includes F-wave study when performed, with interpretation and report

INCLUDES Study with preconfigured electrodes that are customized to a specific body location

EXCLUDES *Needle electromyography ([95885, 95886])*
Nerve conduction studies (95907-95913)
Use of this code more than one time for each limb studied

1.80 1.80 FUD XXX ⊘ Q1 80

AMA: 2018,Feb,11; 2018,Jan,8; 2017,Jan,8; 2016,Jan,13; 2015,Jan,16; 2014,Jan,11

95907 Nerve conduction studies; 1-2 studies

2.72 2.72 FUD XXX S 80

AMA: 2018,Aug,10; 2018,Feb,11; 2018,Jan,8; 2017,Dec,14; 2017,Jan,8; 2016,Jan,13; 2015,Jan,16; 2014,Jan,11

95908 3-4 studies

3.52 3.52 FUD XXX S 80

AMA: 2018,Aug,10; 2018,Feb,11; 2018,Jan,8; 2017,Jan,8; 2016,Jan,13; 2015,Mar,6; 2015,Jan,16; 2014,Jan,11

95909 5-6 studies

4.20 4.20 FUD XXX S 80

AMA: 2018,Aug,10; 2018,Feb,11; 2018,Jan,8; 2017,Jan,8; 2016,Jan,13; 2015,Jan,16; 2014,Jan,11

95910 7-8 studies

5.51 5.51 FUD XXX S 80

AMA: 2018,Aug,10; 2018,Feb,11; 2018,Jan,8; 2017,Jan,8; 2016,Jan,13; 2015,Jan,16; 2014,Jan,11

95911 9-10 studies

6.62 6.62 FUD XXX S 80

AMA: 2018,Aug,10; 2018,Feb,11; 2018,Jan,8; 2017,Jan,8; 2016,Jan,13; 2015,Jan,16; 2014,Jan,11

95912 11-12 studies

7.44 7.44 FUD XXX S 80

AMA: 2018,Aug,10; 2018,Feb,11; 2018,Jan,8; 2017,Jan,8; 2016,Jan,13; 2015,Jan,16; 2014,Jan,11

95913 13 or more studies

8.59 8.59 FUD XXX S 80

AMA: 2018,Aug,10; 2018,Feb,11; 2018,Jan,8; 2017,Jan,8; 2016,Jan,13; 2015,Jan,16; 2014,Jan,11

95940-95941 [95940, 95941] Intraoperative Neurophysiological Monitoring

INCLUDES Monitoring, testing, and data evaluation during surgical procedures by a monitoring professional dedicated only to performing the necessary testing and monitoring
Monitoring services provided by the anesthesiologist or surgeon separately

EXCLUDES *Baseline neurophysiologic monitoring*
EEG during nonintracranial surgery (95955)
Electrocorticography (95829)
Intraoperative cortical and subcortical mapping (95961-95962)
Neurostimulator programming/analysis (95971-95972, 95976-95977, [95983, 95984])
Time required for set-up, recording, interpretation, and removal of electrodes

Code also baseline studies (eg, EMGs, NCVs), no more than one time per operative session
Code also services provided after midnight using the date when monitoring started and the total monitoring time
Code also standby time prior to procedure (99360)
Code first (92585, 95822, 95860-95870, 95907-95913, 95925-95937 [95938, 95939])

+ # **95940 Continuous intraoperative neurophysiology monitoring in the operating room, one on one monitoring requiring personal attendance, each 15 minutes (List separately in addition to code for primary procedure)**

INCLUDES 15 minute increments of monitoring service
A total of all monitoring time for procedures overlapping midnight
Based on time spent monitoring, regardless of number of tests or parameters monitored
Continuous intraoperative neurophysiologic monitoring by a dedicated monitoring professional in the operating room providing one-on-one patient care
Monitoring time may begin prior to the incision
Monitoring time that is distinct from baseline neurophysiologic study/s time or other services (eg, mapping)

EXCLUDES *Time spent in executing or interpreting the baseline neurophysiologic study or studies*

Code also monitoring from outside of the operative room, when applicable ([95941])

0.93 0.93 FUD XXX N 80

AMA: 2018,Feb,11; 2018,Jan,8; 2017,Aug,8; 2017,Jan,8; 2016,Jan,13; 2015,Jan,16; 2014,Apr,5; 2014,Apr,10

+ # **95941** **Continuous intraoperative neurophysiology monitoring, from outside the operating room (remote or nearby) or for monitoring of more than one case while in the operating room, per hour (List separately in addition to code for primary procedure)**

INCLUDES Based on time spent monitoring, regardless of number of tests or parameters monitored
Monitoring time that is distinct from baseline neurophysiologic study/s time or other services (eg, mapping)
One hour increments of monitoring service

0.00 0.00 FUD XXX N

AMA: 2018,Feb,11; 2018,Jan,8; 2017,Aug,8; 2017,Jan,8; 2016,Jan,13; 2015,Jan,16; 2014,Dec,18; 2014,Apr,10; 2014,Apr,5; 2014,Jan,11

95921-95943 [95943] Evaluation of Autonomic Nervous System

INCLUDES Physician interpretation
Recording
Report
Testing for autonomic dysfunction including site and autonomic subsystems

95921 **Testing of autonomic nervous system function; cardiovagal innervation (parasympathetic function), including 2 or more of the following: heart rate response to deep breathing with recorded R-R interval, Valsalva ratio, and 30:15 ratio**

INCLUDES Display on a monitor
Minimum of two of the following elements are performed:
Cardiovascular function as indicated by a 30:15 ration (R/R interval at beat 30)/(R-R interval at beat 15)
Heart rate response to deep breathing obtained by visual quantitative analysis of recordings with patient taking 5-6 breaths per minute
Valsalva ratio (at least 2) obtained by dividing the highest heart rate by the lowest
Monitoring of heart rate by electrocardiography of rate obtained from time between two successive R waves (R-R interval)
Storage of data for waveform analysis
Testing most usually in prone position
Tilt table testing, when performed

EXCLUDES *Autonomic nervous system testing with sympathetic adrenergic function testing (95922, 95924)*
Simultaneous measures of parasympathetic and sympathetic function ([95943])

2.36 2.36 FUD XXX S 80

AMA: 2018,Feb,11; 2018,Jan,8; 2017,Jan,8; 2016,Jan,13; 2015,Jan,16; 2014,Jan,11

95922 **vasomotor adrenergic innervation (sympathetic adrenergic function), including beat-to-beat blood pressure and R-R interval changes during Valsalva maneuver and at least 5 minutes of passive tilt**

EXCLUDES *Autonomic nervous system testing with parasympathetic function (95921, 95924)*
Simultaneous measures of parasympathetic and sympathetic function ([95943])

2.70 2.70 FUD XXX Q1 80

AMA: 2018,Feb,11; 2018,Jan,8; 2017,Jan,8; 2016,Jan,13; 2015,Jan,16; 2014,Jan,11

95923 **sudomotor, including 1 or more of the following: quantitative sudomotor axon reflex test (QSART), silastic sweat imprint, thermoregulatory sweat test, and changes in sympathetic skin potential**

3.64 3.64 FUD XXX Q1 80

AMA: 2018,Feb,11; 2018,Jan,8; 2017,Jan,8; 2016,Jan,13; 2015,Jan,16; 2014,Jan,11

95924 **combined parasympathetic and sympathetic adrenergic function testing with at least 5 minutes of passive tilt**

INCLUDES Tilt table testing of adrenergic and parasympathetic function

EXCLUDES *Autonomic nervous system testing with parasympathetic function (95921-95922)*
Simultaneous measures of parasympathetic and sympathetic function ([95943])

4.25 4.25 FUD XXX S 80

AMA: 2018,Feb,11; 2018,Jan,8; 2017,Jan,8; 2016,Jan,13; 2015,Jan,16

95943 **Simultaneous, independent, quantitative measures of both parasympathetic function and sympathetic function, based on time-frequency analysis of heart rate variability concurrent with time-frequency analysis of continuous respiratory activity, with mean heart rate and blood pressure measures, during rest, paced (deep) breathing, Valsalva maneuvers, and head-up postural change**

EXCLUDES *Autonomic nervous system testing (95921-95922, 95924)*
Rhythm ECG (93040)

0.00 0.00 FUD XXX S 80

AMA: 2018,Feb,11; 2018,Jan,8; 2017,Jan,8; 2016,Jan,13; 2015,Jan,16

95925-95943 [95938, 95939] Neurotransmission Studies

95925 **Short-latency somatosensory evoked potential study, stimulation of any/all peripheral nerves or skin sites, recording from the central nervous system; in upper limbs**

EXCLUDES *Auditory evoked potentials (92585)*
Evoked potential study in both upper and lower limbs ([95938])
Evoked potential study in lower limbs (95926)

3.73 3.73 FUD XXX S 80

AMA: 2018,Feb,11; 2018,Jan,8; 2017,Jan,8; 2016,Jan,13; 2015,Jan,16; 2014,Jan,11

95926 **in lower limbs**

EXCLUDES *Auditory evoked potentials (92585)*
Evoked potential study in both upper and lower limbs ([95938])
Evoked potential study in upper limbs (95925)

3.61 3.61 FUD XXX S 80

AMA: 2018,Feb,11; 2018,Jan,8; 2017,Jan,8; 2016,Jan,13; 2015,Jan,16; 2014,Jan,11

95938 **in upper and lower limbs**

9.79 9.79 FUD XXX S 80

AMA: 2018,Feb,11; 2018,Jan,8; 2017,Jan,8; 2016,Jan,13; 2015,Jan,16; 2014,Jan,11

95927 **in the trunk or head**

EXCLUDES *Auditory evoked potentials (92585)*
Code also modifier 52 for unilateral test

3.74 3.74 FUD XXX S 80

AMA: 2018,Feb,11; 2018,Jan,8; 2017,Jan,8; 2016,Jan,13; 2015,Jan,16; 2014,Jan,11

95928 **Central motor evoked potential study (transcranial motor stimulation); upper limbs**

EXCLUDES *Central motor evoked potential study lower limbs (95929)*

6.20 6.20 FUD XXX S 80

AMA: 2018,Feb,11; 2018,Jan,8; 2017,Jan,8; 2016,Jan,13; 2015,Jan,16

95929 **lower limbs**

EXCLUDES *Central motor evoked potential study upper limbs (95928)*

6.35 6.35 FUD XXX S 80

AMA: 2018,Feb,11; 2018,Jan,8; 2017,Jan,8; 2016,Jan,13; 2015,Jan,16; 2014,Dec,6

95939 **in upper and lower limbs**

EXCLUDES *Central motor evoked potential study of either lower or upper limbs (95928-95929)*

14.5 14.5 FUD XXX S 80

AMA: 2018,Feb,11; 2018,Jan,8; 2017,Jan,8; 2016,Jan,13; 2015,Jan,16; 2014,Jan,11

95930 **Visual evoked potential (VEP) checkerboard or flash testing, central nervous system except glaucoma, with interpretation and report**

EXCLUDES *Visual acuity screening using automated visual evoked potential devices (0333T)*
Visual evoked glaucoma testing ([0464T])

1.94 1.94 FUD XXX S 80

AMA: 2018,Feb,11; 2018,Feb,3; 2018,Jan,8; 2017,Jan,8; 2016,Jan,13; 2015,Jan,16; 2014,Aug,8

95933 **Orbicularis oculi (blink) reflex, by electrodiagnostic testing**

2.30 2.30 FUD XXX Q1 80

AMA: 2018,Feb,11; 2018,Jan,8; 2017,Jul,10; 2017,Jan,8; 2016,Jan,13; 2015,Jan,16

95937 **Neuromuscular junction testing (repetitive stimulation, paired stimuli), each nerve, any 1 method**

2.48 2.48 FUD XXX S 80

AMA: 2018,Feb,11; 2018,Jan,8; 2017,Jan,8; 2016,Feb,13; 2016,Jan,13; 2015,Jan,16; 2014,Jan,11

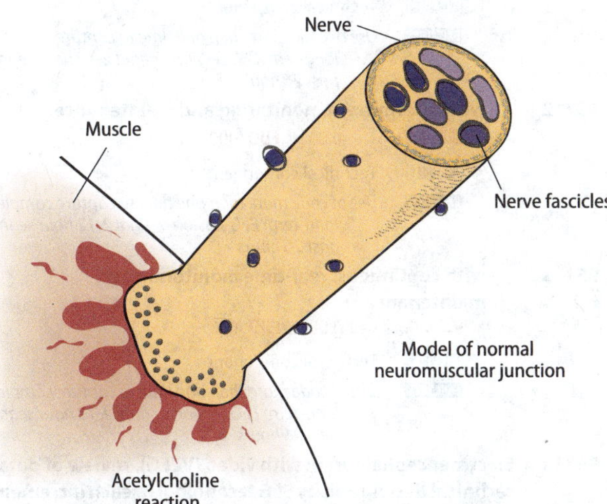

A selected neuromusular junction is repeatedly stimulated. The test is useful to demonstrate reduced muscle action potential from fatigue

95938 **Resequenced code. See code following 95926.**

95939 **Resequenced code. See code following 95929.**

95940 **Resequenced code. See code following 95913.**

95941 **Resequenced code. See code following 95913.**

95943 **Resequenced code. See code following 95924.**

95950-95962 Electroencephalography For Seizure Monitoring/Intraoperative Use

EXCLUDES *E&M services*

95950 ~~**Monitoring for identification and lateralization of cerebral seizure focus, electroencephalographic (eg, 8 channel EEG) recording and interpretation, each 24 hours**~~

To report, see ([95700-95726])

95951 ~~**Monitoring for localization of cerebral seizure focus by cable or radio, 16 or more channel telemetry, combined electroencephalographic (EEG) and video recording and interpretation (eg, for presurgical localization), each 24 hours**~~

To report, see ([95700-95726])

95953 ~~**Monitoring for localization of cerebral seizure focus by computerized portable 16 or more channel EEG, electroencephalographic (EEG) recording and interpretation, each 24 hours, unattended**~~

To report, see ([95700-95726])

95954 **Pharmacological or physical activation requiring physician or other qualified health care professional attendance during EEG recording of activation phase (eg, thiopental activation test)**

11.3 11.3 FUD XXX S 80

AMA: 2018,Feb,11; 2018,Jan,8; 2017,Jan,8; 2016,Jan,13; 2015,Jan,16; 2014,Jan,11

95955 **Electroencephalogram (EEG) during nonintracranial surgery (eg, carotid surgery)**

5.95 5.95 FUD XXX N 80

AMA: 2018,Feb,11; 2018,Jan,8; 2017,Jan,8; 2016,Jan,13; 2015,Jan,16; 2014,Dec,18

95956 ~~**Monitoring for localization of cerebral seizure focus by cable or radio, 16 or more channel telemetry, electroencephalographic (EEG) recording and interpretation, each 24 hours, attended by a technologist or nurse**~~

To report, see ([95700-95726])

95957 **Digital analysis of electroencephalogram (EEG) (eg, for epileptic spike analysis)**

EXCLUDES *Use of automated spike and seizure detection/trending software, when performed ([95700, 95705, 95706, 95707, 95708, 95709, 95710, 95711, 95712, 95713, 95714, 95715, 95716, 95717, 95718, 95719, 95720, 95721, 95722, 95723, 95724, 95725, 95726])*

7.62 7.62 FUD XXX N 80

AMA: 2018,Dec,3; 2018,Dec,3; 2018,Feb,11; 2018,Jan,8; 2017,Jan,8; 2016,Jan,13; 2015,Jan,16; 2014,Jan,11

95958 **Wada activation test for hemispheric function, including electroencephalographic (EEG) monitoring**

16.3 16.3 FUD XXX S 80

AMA: 2018,Feb,11

95961 **Functional cortical and subcortical mapping by stimulation and/or recording of electrodes on brain surface, or of depth electrodes, to provoke seizures or identify vital brain structures; initial hour of attendance by a physician or other qualified health care professional**

INCLUDES One hour of attendance by physician or other qualified health care professional

Code also each additional hour of attendance by physician or other qualified health care professional, when appropriate (95962)

Code also long-term EEG (two hours or more), when performed ([95700, 95705, 95706, 95707, 95708, 95709, 95710, 95711, 95712, 95713, 95714, 95715, 95716, 95717, 95718, 95719, 95720, 95721, 95722, 95723, 95724, 95725, 95726])

Code also modifier 52 for 30 minutes or less of attendance by physician or other qualified health care professional

8.69 8.69 FUD XXX S 80

AMA: 2018,Dec,3; 2018,Dec,3; 2018,Feb,11; 2018,Jan,8; 2017,Jan,8; 2016,Jan,13; 2015,Jan,16; 2014,Jan,11

\+ 95962 **each additional hour of attendance by a physician or other qualified health care professional (List separately in addition to code for primary procedure)**

INCLUDES One hour of attendance by physician or other qualified health care professional

Code also long-term EEG (two hours or more), when performed ([95700, 95705, 95706, 95707, 95708, 95709, 95710, 95711, 95712, 95713, 95714, 95715, 95716, 95717, 95718, 95719, 95720, 95721, 95722, 95723, 95724, 95725, 95726])

Code first initial hour (95961)

7.46 7.46 FUD ZZZ N 80

AMA: 2018,Feb,11; 2018,Jan,8; 2017,Jan,8; 2016,Jan,13; 2015,Jan,16; 2014,Jan,11

95965-95967 Magnetoencephalography

INCLUDES Physician interpretation
Recording
Report

EXCLUDES *CT provided along with magnetoencephalography (70450-70470, 70496)*
Electroencephalography provided along with magnetoencephalography (95812-95824)
E&M services
MRI provided along with magnetoencephalography (70551-70553)
Somatosensory evoked potentials/auditory evoked potentials/visual evoked potentials provided along with magnetic evoked field responses (92585, 95925, 95926, 95930)

95965 Magnetoencephalography (MEG), recording and analysis; for spontaneous brain magnetic activity (eg, epileptic cerebral cortex localization)
0.00 0.00 FUD XXX S 80
AMA: 2018,Feb,11

95966 for evoked magnetic fields, single modality (eg, sensory, motor, language, or visual cortex localization)
0.00 0.00 FUD XXX S 80
AMA: 2018,Feb,11

+ **95967 for evoked magnetic fields, each additional modality (eg, sensory, motor, language, or visual cortex localization) (List separately in addition to code for primary procedure)**
Code first single modality (95966)
0.00 0.00 FUD ZZZ N 80
AMA: 2018,Feb,11

95700-95726 [95700, 95705, 95706, 95707, 95708, 95709, 95710, 95711, 95712, 95713, 95714, 95715, 95716, 95717, 95718, 95719, 95720, 95721, 95722, 95723, 95724, 95725, 95726] Electronencephalogram (EEG)

INCLUDES Determination of:
Eligibility for epilepsy surgery
Location and type of seizures
Differentiation of seizures from other conditions
Monitoring of:
Seizure treatment
Status epilepticus
Use of automated spike and seizure detection/trending software, when performed

EXCLUDES *Diagnostic EEG recording time less than two hours*
Routine EEG (95812-95813, 95816, 95819, 95822)

Code also cortical or subcortical mapping, when performed (95961-95962)

● # **95700 Electroencephalogram (EEG) continuous recording, with video when performed, setup, patient education, and takedown when performed, administered in person by EEG technologist, minimum of 8 channels**
0.00 0.00 FUD 000
INCLUDES Technical component
EXCLUDES *EEG performed using patient-placed electrodes, performed by non-EEG technologist, or remote supervision by an EEG technologist (95999)*
Use of code more than one time for each session

● # **95705 Electroencephalogram (EEG), without video, review of data, technical description by EEG technologist, 2-12 hours; unmonitored**
0.00 0.00 FUD 000
INCLUDES Technical component
EXCLUDES *Use of code more than one time to capture complete long-term EEG session or final 2-12 hour segment past 26 hours*

● # **95706 with intermittent monitoring and maintenance**
0.00 0.00 FUD 000
INCLUDES Technical component
EXCLUDES *Use of code more than one time to capture complete long-term EEG session or final 2-12 hour segment past 26 hours*

● # **95707 with continuous, real-time monitoring and maintenance**
0.00 0.00 FUD 000
INCLUDES Technical component
EXCLUDES *Use of code more than one time to capture complete long-term EEG session or final 2-12 hour segment past 26 hours*

● # **95708 Electroencephalogram (EEG), without video, review of data, technical description by EEG technologist, each increment of 12-26 hours; unmonitored**
0.00 0.00 FUD 000
INCLUDES Technical component

● # **95709 with intermittent monitoring and maintenance**
0.00 0.00 FUD 000
INCLUDES Technical component

● # **95710 with continuous, real-time monitoring and maintenance**
0.00 0.00 FUD 000
INCLUDES Technical component

● # **95711 Electroencephalogram with video (VEEG), review of data, technical description by EEG technologist, 2-12 hours; unmonitored**
0.00 0.00 FUD 000
INCLUDES Technical component
EXCLUDES *Use of code more than one time to capture complete long-term EEG session or final 2-12 hour segment past 26 hours*

● # **95712 with intermittent monitoring and maintenance**
0.00 0.00 FUD 000
INCLUDES Technical component
EXCLUDES *Use of code more than one time to capture complete long-term EEG session or final 2-12 hour segment past 26 hours*

● # **95713 with continuous, real-time monitoring and maintenance**
0.00 0.00 FUD 000
INCLUDES Technical component
EXCLUDES *Use of code more than one time to capture complete long-term EEG session or final 2-12 hour segment past 26 hours*

● # **95714 Electroencephalogram with video (VEEG), review of data, technical description by EEG technologist, each increment of 12-26 hours; unmonitored**
0.00 0.00 FUD 000
INCLUDES Technical component

● # **95715 with intermittent monitoring and maintenance**
0.00 0.00 FUD 000
INCLUDES Technical component

● # **95716 with continuous, real-time monitoring and maintenance**
0.00 0.00 FUD 000
INCLUDES Technical component

● # **95717 Electroencephalogram (EEG), continuous recording, physician or other qualified health care professional review of recorded events, analysis of spike and seizure detection, interpretation and report, 2-12 hours of EEG recording; without video**
0.00 0.00 FUD 000
INCLUDES Professional component
EXCLUDES *Professional interpretation for recordings greater than 36 hours and for which the entire professional report is generated retroactively ([95721, 95722, 95723, 95724, 95725, 95726])*
Use of code more than one time to capture complete long-term EEG session or final 2-12 hour segment past 24 hours

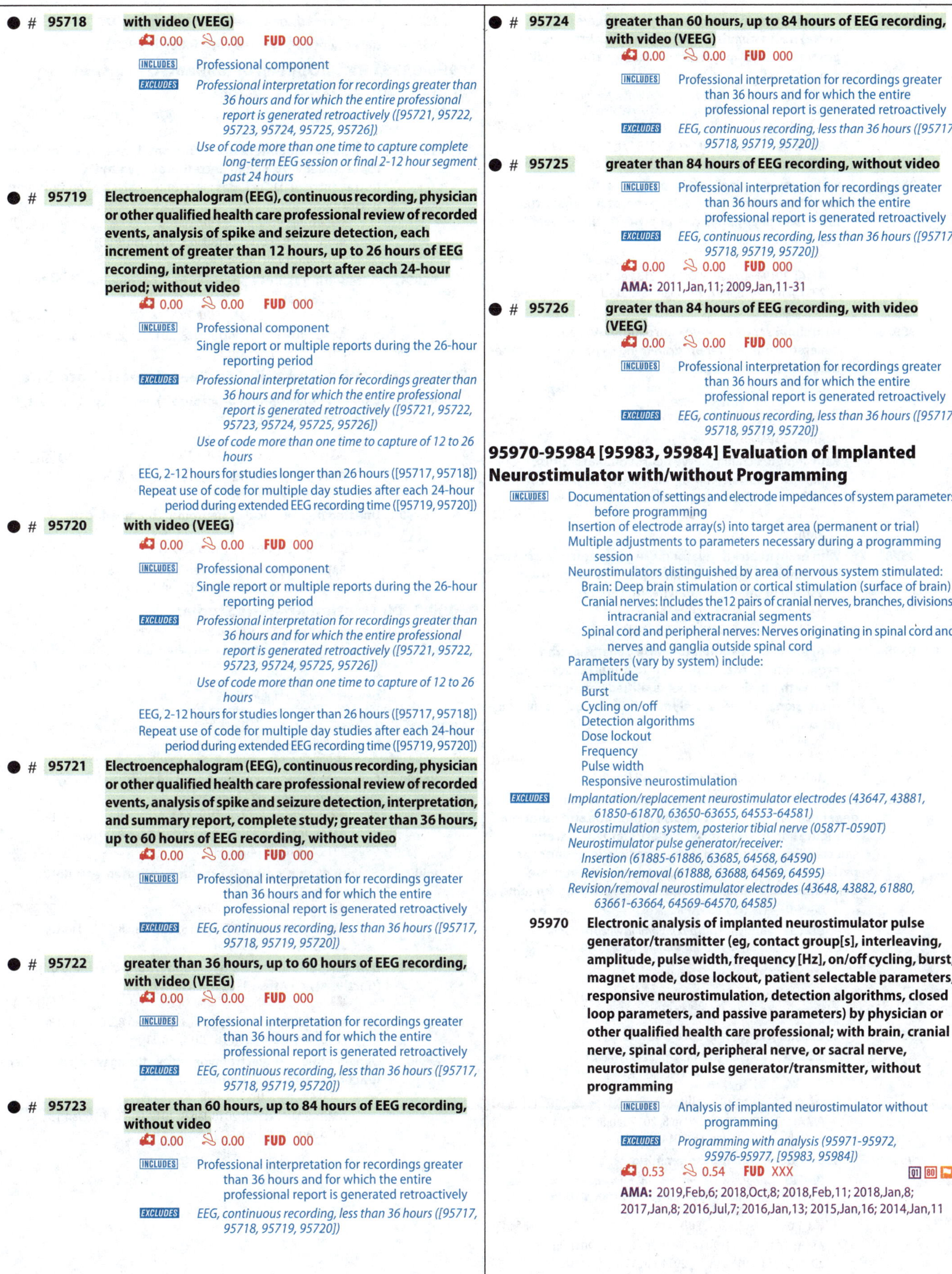

● # **95718** **with video (VEEG)**
0.00 0.00 FUD 000
INCLUDES Professional component
EXCLUDES *Professional interpretation for recordings greater than 36 hours and for which the entire professional report is generated retroactively ([95721, 95722, 95723, 95724, 95725, 95726])*
Use of code more than one time to capture complete long-term EEG session or final 2-12 hour segment past 24 hours

● # **95719** **Electroencephalogram (EEG), continuous recording, physician or other qualified health care professional review of recorded events, analysis of spike and seizure detection, each increment of greater than 12 hours, up to 26 hours of EEG recording, interpretation and report after each 24-hour period; without video**
0.00 0.00 FUD 000
INCLUDES Professional component
Single report or multiple reports during the 26-hour reporting period
EXCLUDES *Professional interpretation for recordings greater than 36 hours and for which the entire professional report is generated retroactively ([95721, 95722, 95723, 95724, 95725, 95726])*
Use of code more than one time to capture of 12 to 26 hours
EEG, 2-12 hours for studies longer than 26 hours ([95717, 95718])
Repeat use of code for multiple day studies after each 24-hour period during extended EEG recording time ([95719, 95720])

● # **95720** **with video (VEEG)**
0.00 0.00 FUD 000
INCLUDES Professional component
Single report or multiple reports during the 26-hour reporting period
EXCLUDES *Professional interpretation for recordings greater than 36 hours and for which the entire professional report is generated retroactively ([95721, 95722, 95723, 95724, 95725, 95726])*
Use of code more than one time to capture of 12 to 26 hours
EEG, 2-12 hours for studies longer than 26 hours ([95717, 95718])
Repeat use of code for multiple day studies after each 24-hour period during extended EEG recording time ([95719, 95720])

● # **95721** **Electroencephalogram (EEG), continuous recording, physician or other qualified health care professional review of recorded events, analysis of spike and seizure detection, interpretation, and summary report, complete study; greater than 36 hours, up to 60 hours of EEG recording, without video**
0.00 0.00 FUD 000
INCLUDES Professional interpretation for recordings greater than 36 hours and for which the entire professional report is generated retroactively
EXCLUDES *EEG, continuous recording, less than 36 hours ([95717, 95718, 95719, 95720])*

● # **95722** **greater than 36 hours, up to 60 hours of EEG recording, with video (VEEG)**
0.00 0.00 FUD 000
INCLUDES Professional interpretation for recordings greater than 36 hours and for which the entire professional report is generated retroactively
EXCLUDES *EEG, continuous recording, less than 36 hours ([95717, 95718, 95719, 95720])*

● # **95723** **greater than 60 hours, up to 84 hours of EEG recording, without video**
0.00 0.00 FUD 000
INCLUDES Professional interpretation for recordings greater than 36 hours and for which the entire professional report is generated retroactively
EXCLUDES *EEG, continuous recording, less than 36 hours ([95717, 95718, 95719, 95720])*

● # **95724** **greater than 60 hours, up to 84 hours of EEG recording, with video (VEEG)**
0.00 0.00 FUD 000
INCLUDES Professional interpretation for recordings greater than 36 hours and for which the entire professional report is generated retroactively
EXCLUDES *EEG, continuous recording, less than 36 hours ([95717, 95718, 95719, 95720])*

● # **95725** **greater than 84 hours of EEG recording, without video**
INCLUDES Professional interpretation for recordings greater than 36 hours and for which the entire professional report is generated retroactively
EXCLUDES *EEG, continuous recording, less than 36 hours ([95717, 95718, 95719, 95720])*
0.00 0.00 FUD 000
AMA: 2011,Jan,11; 2009,Jan,11-31

● # **95726** **greater than 84 hours of EEG recording, with video (VEEG)**
0.00 0.00 FUD 000
INCLUDES Professional interpretation for recordings greater than 36 hours and for which the entire professional report is generated retroactively
EXCLUDES *EEG, continuous recording, less than 36 hours ([95717, 95718, 95719, 95720])*

95970-95984 [95983, 95984] Evaluation of Implanted Neurostimulator with/without Programming

INCLUDES Documentation of settings and electrode impedances of system parameters before programming
Insertion of electrode array(s) into target area (permanent or trial)
Multiple adjustments to parameters necessary during a programming session
Neurostimulators distinguished by area of nervous system stimulated:
Brain: Deep brain stimulation or cortical stimulation (surface of brain)
Cranial nerves: Includes the12 pairs of cranial nerves, branches, divisions, intracranial and extracranial segments
Spinal cord and peripheral nerves: Nerves originating in spinal cord and nerves and ganglia outside spinal cord
Parameters (vary by system) include:
Amplitude
Burst
Cycling on/off
Detection algorithms
Dose lockout
Frequency
Pulse width
Responsive neurostimulation
EXCLUDES *Implantation/replacement neurostimulator electrodes (43647, 43881, 61850-61870, 63650-63655, 64553-64581)*
Neurostimulation system, posterior tibial nerve (0587T-0590T)
Neurostimulator pulse generator/receiver:
Insertion (61885-61886, 63685, 64568, 64590)
Revision/removal (61888, 63688, 64569, 64595)
Revision/removal neurostimulator electrodes (43648, 43882, 61880, 63661-63664, 64569-64570, 64585)

95970 **Electronic analysis of implanted neurostimulator pulse generator/transmitter (eg, contact group[s], interleaving, amplitude, pulse width, frequency [Hz], on/off cycling, burst, magnet mode, dose lockout, patient selectable parameters, responsive neurostimulation, detection algorithms, closed loop parameters, and passive parameters) by physician or other qualified health care professional; with brain, cranial nerve, spinal cord, peripheral nerve, or sacral nerve, neurostimulator pulse generator/transmitter, without programming**
INCLUDES Analysis of implanted neurostimulator without programming
EXCLUDES *Programming with analysis (95971-95972, 95976-95977, [95983, 95984])*
0.53 0.54 FUD XXX Q1 80
AMA: 2019,Feb,6; 2018,Oct,8; 2018,Feb,11; 2018,Jan,8; 2017,Jan,8; 2016,Jul,7; 2016,Jan,13; 2015,Jan,16; 2014,Jan,11

95971 **with simple spinal cord or peripheral nerve (eg, sacral nerve) neurostimulator pulse generator/transmitter programming by physician or other qualified health care professional**

EXCLUDES *Programming of neurostimulator for complex spinal cord or peripheral nerve (95972)*

1.17 1.44 FUD XXX S 80

AMA: 2019,Feb,6; 2018,Oct,8; 2018,Feb,11; 2018,Jan,8; 2017,Jan,8; 2016,Jul,7; 2016,Jan,13; 2015,Jan,16; 2014,Jan,11

95972 **with complex spinal cord or peripheral nerve (eg, sacral nerve) neurostimulator pulse generator/transmitter programming by physician or other qualified health care professional**

1.19 1.62 FUD XXX S 80

AMA: 2019,Feb,6; 2018,Oct,8; 2018,Feb,11; 2018,Jan,8; 2017,Jan,8; 2016,Jul,7; 2016,Jan,13; 2015,Jan,16; 2014,Aug,5; 2014,Jan,11

95976 **with simple cranial nerve neurostimulator pulse generator/transmitter programming by physician or other qualified health care professional**

EXCLUDES *Programming of neurostimulator for complex cranial nerve (95977)*

1.14 1.16 FUD XXX 80

AMA: 2019,Feb,6

95977 **with complex cranial nerve neurostimulator pulse generator/transmitter programming by physician or other qualified health care professional**

1.52 1.54 FUD XXX 80

AMA: 2019,Feb,6

\# **95983** **with brain neurostimulator pulse generator/transmitter programming, first 15 minutes face-to-face time with physician or other qualified health care professional**

1.44 1.46 FUD XXX 80

AMA: 2019,Feb,6; 2018,Dec,3; 2018,Dec,3

\+ # **95984** **with brain neurostimulator pulse generator/transmitter programming, each additional 15 minutes face-to-face time with physician or other qualified health care professional (List separately in addition to code for primary procedure)**

Code first ([95983])

1.26 1.27 FUD ZZZ 80

AMA: 2019,Feb,6; 2018,Dec,3; 2018,Dec,3

95980 **Electronic analysis of implanted neurostimulator pulse generator system (eg, rate, pulse amplitude and duration, configuration of wave form, battery status, electrode selectability, output modulation, cycling, impedance and patient measurements) gastric neurostimulator pulse generator/transmitter; intraoperative, with programming**

INCLUDES Gastric neurostimulator of lesser curvature

EXCLUDES *Analysis, with programming when performed, of vagus nerve trunk stimulator for morbid obesity (0312T, 0317T)*

1.32 1.32 FUD XXX N 80

AMA: 2018,Feb,11; 2018,Jan,8; 2017,Jan,8; 2016,Jul,7; 2016,Jan,13; 2015,Jan,16; 2014,Jan,11

95981 **subsequent, without reprogramming**

EXCLUDES *Analysis, with programming when performed, of vagus nerve trunk stimulator for morbid obesity (0312T, 0317T)*

0.51 0.97 FUD XXX Q1 80

AMA: 2018,Feb,11; 2018,Jan,8; 2017,Jan,8; 2016,Jul,7; 2016,Jan,13; 2015,Jan,16; 2014,Jan,11

95982 **subsequent, with reprogramming**

EXCLUDES *Analysis, with programming when performed, of vagus nerve trunk stimulator for morbid obesity (0312T, 0317T)*

1.04 1.55 FUD XXX Q1 80

AMA: 2018,Feb,11; 2018,Jan,8; 2017,Jan,8; 2016,Jul,7; 2016,Jan,13; 2015,Jan,16; 2014,Jan,11

95983 **Resequenced code. See code following 95977.**

95984 **Resequenced code. See code following 95977.**

95990-95991 Refill/Upkeep of Implanted Drug Delivery Pump to Central Nervous System

EXCLUDES *Analysis/reprogramming of implanted pump for infusion (62367-62370)*
E&M services

95990 **Refilling and maintenance of implantable pump or reservoir for drug delivery, spinal (intrathecal, epidural) or brain (intraventricular), includes electronic analysis of pump, when performed;**

2.62 2.62 FUD XXX S 80

AMA: 2018,Feb,11; 2018,Jan,8; 2017,Jan,8; 2016,Jan,13; 2015,Jan,16; 2014,Jan,11

95991 **requiring skill of a physician or other qualified health care professional**

1.14 3.30 FUD XXX T 80

AMA: 2018,Feb,11; 2018,Jan,8; 2017,Jan,8; 2016,Jan,13; 2015,Jan,16; 2014,Jan,11

95992-95999 Other and Unlisted Neurological Procedures

95992 **Canalith repositioning procedure(s) (eg, Epley maneuver, Semont maneuver), per day**

EXCLUDES *Nystagmus testing (92531-92532)*

1.07 1.25 FUD XXX A 80

AMA: 2018,Feb,11; 2018,Jan,8; 2017,Jan,8; 2016,Jan,13; 2015,Jan,16; 2014,Jan,11

95999 **Unlisted neurological or neuromuscular diagnostic procedure**

0.00 0.00 FUD XXX Q1 80

AMA: 2018,Aug,10; 2018,Feb,11; 2018,Jan,8; 2017,Jan,8; 2016,Jan,13; 2015,Aug,8; 2015,Jan,16; 2014,Jan,11

96000-96004 Motion Analysis Studies

CMS: 100-02,15,230.4 Services By a Physical/Occupational Therapist in Private Practice

INCLUDES Services provided as part of major therapeutic/diagnostic decision making
Services provided in a dedicated motion analysis department capable of:
3-D kinetics/dynamic electromyography
Computerized 3-D kinematics
Videotaping from the front/back/both sides

EXCLUDES *E&M services*
Gait training (97116)
Needle electromyography (95860-95872 [95885, 95886, 95887])

96000 **Comprehensive computer-based motion analysis by video-taping and 3D kinematics;**

2.72 2.72 FUD XXX S 80

AMA: 2018,Feb,11; 2018,Jan,8; 2017,Jan,8; 2016,Jan,13; 2015,Jan,16; 2014,Jan,11

96001 **with dynamic plantar pressure measurements during walking**

3.65 3.65 FUD XXX S 80

AMA: 2018,Feb,11; 2018,Jan,8; 2017,Jan,8; 2016,Jan,13; 2015,Jan,16; 2014,Jan,11

96002 **Dynamic surface electromyography, during walking or other functional activities, 1-12 muscles**

0.63 0.63 FUD XXX S 80

AMA: 2018,Feb,11; 2018,Jan,8; 2017,Jan,8; 2016,Jan,13; 2015,Aug,8; 2015,Jan,16; 2014,Jan,11

96003 **Dynamic fine wire electromyography, during walking or other functional activities, 1 muscle**

0.49 0.49 FUD XXX Q1 80

AMA: 2018,Feb,11; 2018,Jan,8; 2017,Jan,8; 2016,Jan,13; 2015,Jan,16; 2014,Jan,11

96004 **Review and interpretation by physician or other qualified health care professional of comprehensive computer-based motion analysis, dynamic plantar pressure measurements, dynamic surface electromyography during walking or other functional activities, and dynamic fine wire electromyography, with written report**

3.27 3.27 **FUD** XXX B 80 26

AMA: 2018,Feb,11; 2018,Jan,8; 2017,Jan,8; 2016,Jan,13; 2015,Aug,8; 2015,Jan,16; 2014,Jan,11

96020 Neurofunctional Brain Testing

INCLUDES Selection/administration of testing of:
- Cognition
- Determination of validity of neurofunctional testing relative to separately interpreted functional magnetic resonance images
- Functional neuroimaging
- Language
- Memory
- Monitoring performance of testing
- Movement
- Other neurological functions
- Sensation

EXCLUDES *Clinical depression treatment by repetitive transcranial magnetic stimulation (90867-90868)*
Developmental test administration (96112-96113)
E&M services on the same date
MRI of the brain (70554-70555)
Neurobehavioral status examination (96116, 96121)
Neuropsychological testing (96132-96133)
Psychological testing (96130-96131)

96020 **Neurofunctional testing selection and administration during noninvasive imaging functional brain mapping, with test administered entirely by a physician or other qualified health care professional (ie, psychologist), with review of test results and report**

0.00 0.00 **FUD** XXX N 80

AMA: 2018,Feb,11; 2018,Jan,8; 2017,Jan,8; 2016,Jan,13; 2015,Jan,16; 2014,Jan,11

96040 Genetic Counseling Services

INCLUDES Analysis for genetic risk assessment
Counseling of patient/family
Counseling services
Face-to-face interviews
Obtaining structured family genetic history
Pedigree construction
Review of medical data/family information
Services provided by trained genetic counselor
Services provided during one or more sessions
Thirty minutes of face-to-face time and is reported one time for each 16-30 minutes of the service

EXCLUDES *Education/genetic counseling by a physician or other qualified health care provider to a group (99078)*
Education/genetic counseling by a physician or other qualified health care provider to an individual; use appropriate E&M code
Education regarding genetic risks by a nonphysician to a group (98961, 98962)
Genetic counseling and/or risk factor reduction intervention from a physician or other qualified health care provider provided to patients without symptoms/diagnosis (99401-99412)
Use of code when 15 minutes or less of face-to-face time is provided

96040 **Medical genetics and genetic counseling services, each 30 minutes face-to-face with patient/family**

1.30 1.30 **FUD** XXX ★ B

AMA: 2018,Feb,11; 2018,Jan,8; 2017,Jan,8; 2016,Jan,13; 2015,Jan,16; 2014,Jan,11

97151-97158 [97151, 97152, 97153, 97154, 97155, 97156, 97157, 97158] Adaptive Behavior Assessments and Treatments

INCLUDES Adaptive behavior deficits (e.g., impairment in social, communication, self care skills)
Assessment and treatment that focuses on:
- Maladaptive behaviors (e.g., repetitive movements, risk of harm to self, others, property)
- Secondary functional impairment due to consequences of deficient adaptive and maladaptive behaviors (e.g. communication, play, leisure, social interactions)
- Treatment determined based on goals and targets identified in assessments

\# 97151 **Behavior identification assessment, administered by a physician or other qualified health care professional, each 15 minutes of the physician's or other qualified health care professional's time face-to-face with patient and/or guardian(s)/caregiver(s) administering assessments and discussing findings and recommendations, and non-face-to-face analyzing past data, scoring/interpreting the assessment, and preparing the report/treatment plan**

EXCLUDES *Health and behavior assessment and intervention (96156, 96158-96159, [96164, 96165], [96167, 96168], [96170, 96171])*
Medical team conference (99366-99368)
Neurobehavioral status examination (96116, 96121)
Neuropsychological testing (96132-96133, 96136-96139, 96146)
Psychiatric diagnostic evaluation (90791-90792)
Speech evaluations (92521-92524)

Code also more than one time on same or different days until assessment is complete
Code also supporting assessment depending on time patient spends face-to-face with one or more technicians (counting only the time spent by one of the technicians) ([97152], 0362T)

0.00 0.00 **FUD** XXX 80

AMA: 2018,Nov,3

\# 97152 **Behavior identification-supporting assessment, administered by one technician under the direction of a physician or other qualified health care professional, face-to-face with the patient, each 15 minutes**

EXCLUDES *Health and behavior assessment and intervention (96156, 96158-96159, [96164, 96165], [96167, 96168], [96170, 96171])*
Medical team conference (99366-99368)
Neurobehavioral status examination (96116, 96121)
Neuropsychological testing (96132-96133, 96136-96139, 96146)
Psychiatric diagnostic evaluation (90791-90792)
Speech evaluations (92521-92524)

Code also more than one time on same or different days until assessment is complete
Code also supporting assessment depending on time patient spends face-to-face with one or more technicians (counting only the time spent by one of the technicians) ([97151], 0362T)

0.00 0.00 **FUD** XXX 80

AMA: 2018,Nov,3

97153 **Adaptive behavior treatment by protocol, administered by technician under the direction of a physician or other qualified health care professional, face-to-face with one patient, each 15 minutes**

INCLUDES Face-to-face service with one patient only
Provided by technician under physician/other qualified healthcare professional direction

EXCLUDES *Aphasia and cognitive performance testing (96105, [96125])*
Behavioral/developmental screening/testing (96110-96113 [96127])
Health and behavior assessment and intervention (96156, 96158-96159, [96164, 96165], [96167, 96168], [96170, 96171])
Health risk assessment (96160-96161)
Neurobehavioral status examination (96116, 96121)
Psychiatric services (90785-90899)
Testing administration with scoring (96136-96139, 96146)
Testing evaluation (96130-96133)
Therapeutic procedure(s), individual patient (97129)
Treatment speech disorders (individual) (92507)

0.00 0.00 FUD XXX 80

AMA: 2018,Nov,3

97154 **Group adaptive behavior treatment by protocol, administered by technician under the direction of a physician or other qualified health care professional, face-to-face with two or more patients, each 15 minutes**

INCLUDES Face-to-face service with one patient only
Provided by technician under physician/other qualified healthcare professional direction

EXCLUDES *Aphasia and cognitive performance testing (96105, [96125])*
Behavioral/developmental screening/testing (96110-96113, [96127])
Health and behavior assessment and intervention (96156, 96158-96159, [96164, 96165], [96167, 96168], [96170, 96171])
Neurobehavioral status examination (96116, 96121)
Psychiatric services (90785-90899)
Testing administration with scoring (96136-96139, 96146)
Testing evaluation (96130-96133)
Therapeutic procedure(s) group of two or more patients (97150)
Treatment speech disorders (group) (92508)

0.00 0.00 FUD XXX 80

AMA: 2018,Nov,3

97155 **Adaptive behavior treatment with protocol modification, administered by physician or other qualified health care professional, which may include simultaneous direction of technician, face-to-face with one patient, each 15 minutes**

INCLUDES Face-to-face service with one patient only
Provided by technician under physician/other qualified healthcare professional direction

EXCLUDES *Aphasia and cognitive performance testing (96105, [96125])*
Behavioral/developmental screening/testing (96110-96113, [96127])
Health and behavior assessment and intervention (96156, 96158-96159, [96164, 96165], [96167, 96168], [96170, 96171])
Neurobehavioral status examination (96116, 96121)
Psychiatric services (90785-90899)
Testing administration with scoring (96136-96139, 96146)
Testing evaluation (96130-96133)
Therapeutic procedure(s), individual patient (97129)
Treatment speech disorders (individual) (92507)

0.00 0.00 FUD XXX 80

AMA: 2018,Nov,3

97156 **Family adaptive behavior treatment guidance, administered by physician or other qualified health care professional (with or without the patient present), face-to-face with guardian(s)/caregiver(s), each 15 minutes**

INCLUDES Provided by physician/other qualified healthcare professional
Without patient presence

EXCLUDES *Aphasia and cognitive performance testing (96105, [96125])*
Behavioral/developmental screening/testing (96110-96113 [96127])
Health and behavior assessment and intervention (96156, 96158-96159, [96164, 96165], [96167, 96168], [96170, 96171])
Neurobehavioral status examination (96116, 96121)
Psychiatric services (90785-90899)
Testing administration with scoring (96136-96139, 96146)
Testing evaluation (96130-96133)

0.00 0.00 FUD XXX 80

AMA: 2018,Nov,3

97157 **Multiple-family group adaptive behavior treatment guidance, administered by physician or other qualified health care professional (without the patient present), face-to-face with multiple sets of guardians/caregivers, each 15 minutes**

INCLUDES Provided by physician/other qualified healthcare professional
Without patient presence

EXCLUDES *Aphasia and cognitive performance testing (96105, [96125])*
Behavioral/developmental screening/testing (96110-96113 [96127])
Groups of more than 8 families
Health and behavior assessment and intervention (96156, 96158-96159, [96164, 96165], [96167, 96168], [96170, 96171])
Neurobehavioral status examination (96116, 96121)
Psychiatric services (90785-90899)
Testing administration with scoring (96136-96139, 96146)
Testing evaluation (96130-96133)

0.00 0.00 FUD XXX 80

AMA: 2018,Nov,3

97158 **Group adaptive behavior treatment with protocol modification, administered by physician or other qualified health care professional, face-to-face with multiple patients, each 15 minutes**

INCLUDES Face-to-face service with one patient only
Provided by technician under physician/other qualified healthcare professional direction

EXCLUDES *Aphasia and cognitive performance testing (96105, [96125])*
Behavioral/developmental screening/testing (96110-96113 [96127])
Groups of more than 8 patients
Health and behavior assessment and intervention (96156, 96158-96159, [96164, 96165], [96167, 96168], [96170, 96171])
Neurobehavioral status examination (96116, 96121)
Psychiatric services (90785-90899)
Testing administration with scoring (96136-96139, 96146)
Testing evaluation (96130-96133)
Therapeutic procedure(s) group of two or more patients (97150)
Treatment speech disorders (group) (92508)

0.00 0.00 FUD XXX 80

AMA: 2018,Nov,3

96105-96146 [96125, 96127] Testing Services

INCLUDES Interpretation and report when performed by qualified healthcare professional
Results when automatically generated

EXCLUDES *Adaptive behavior assessments and treatments ([97151, 97152, 97153, 97154, 97155, 97156, 97157, 97158], 0362T, 0373T)*
Cognitive skills development (97129, 97533)

96105 Assessment of aphasia (includes assessment of expressive and receptive speech and language function, language comprehension, speech production ability, reading, spelling, writing, eg, by Boston Diagnostic Aphasia Examination) with interpretation and report, per hour

EXCLUDES *Use of code for less than 31 minutes of time*
2.96 2.96 FUD XXX A 80
AMA: 2018,Nov,3; 2018,Oct,5; 2018,Feb,11; 2018,Jan,8; 2017,Jan,8; 2016,Jan,13; 2015,Aug,5; 2015,Jan,16; 2014,Jan,11

\# **96125 Standardized cognitive performance testing (eg, Ross Information Processing Assessment) per hour of a qualified health care professional's time, both face-to-face time administering tests to the patient and time interpreting these test results and preparing the report**

EXCLUDES *Neuropsychological testing (96132-96139, 96146)*
3.12 3.12 FUD XXX A 80
AMA: 2018,Nov,3; 2018,Oct,5; 2018,Feb,11; 2018,Jan,8; 2017,Jan,8; 2016,Jan,13; 2015,Aug,5; 2015,Jan,16; 2014,Jan,11

96110 Developmental screening (eg, developmental milestone survey, speech and language delay screen), with scoring and documentation, per standardized instrument

EXCLUDES *Emotional/behavioral assessment ([96127])*
0.28 0.28 FUD XXX E
AMA: 2018,Nov,3; 2018,Feb,11; 2018,Jan,8; 2017,Feb,14; 2017,Jan,8; 2016,Jan,13; 2015,Aug,5; 2015,Jan,16; 2014,Jun,3; 2014,Jan,11

96112 Developmental test administration (including assessment of fine and/or gross motor, language, cognitive level, social, memory and/or executive functions by standardized developmental instruments when performed), by physician or other qualified health care professional, with interpretation and report; first hour

EXCLUDES *Use of code for less than 31 minutes of time*
3.61 3.83 FUD XXX 80
AMA: 2018,Nov,3

\+ **96113 each additional 30 minutes (List separately in addition to code for primary procedure)**

EXCLUDES *Use of code for less than 16 minutes of time*
1.65 1.71 FUD ZZZ 80
AMA: 2018,Nov,3

\# **96127 Brief emotional/behavioral assessment (eg, depression inventory, attention-deficit/hyperactivity disorder [ADHD] scale), with scoring and documentation, per standardized instrument**

0.15 0.15 FUD XXX 01 80 TC
AMA: 2018,Nov,3; 2018,Oct,5; 2018,Apr,9; 2018,Feb,11; 2018,Jan,8; 2017,Feb,14; 2017,Jan,8; 2016,Jan,13; 2015,Aug,5

96116 Neurobehavioral status exam (clinical assessment of thinking, reasoning and judgment, [eg, acquired knowledge, attention, language, memory, planning and problem solving, and visual spatial abilities]), by physician or other qualified health care professional, both face-to-face time with the patient and time interpreting test results and preparing the report; first hour

EXCLUDES *Neuropsychological testing (96132-96139, 96146)*
Use of code for less than 31 minutes of time
2.41 2.70 FUD XXX ★ 03 80
AMA: 2018,Nov,3; 2018,Oct,5; 2018,Feb,11; 2018,Jan,8; 2017,Jan,8; 2016,Jan,13; 2015,Aug,5; 2015,Jan,16; 2014,Jun,3; 2014,Jan,11

\+ **96121 each additional hour (List separately in addition to code for primary procedure)**

EXCLUDES *Use of code for less than 31 minutes of time*
Code first (96116)
2.21 2.32 FUD ZZZ 80
AMA: 2018,Nov,3

96125 **Resequenced code. See code following 96105.**

96127 **Resequenced code. See code following 96113.**

96130 Psychological testing evaluation services by physician or other qualified health care professional, including integration of patient data, interpretation of standardized test results and clinical data, clinical decision making, treatment planning and report, and interactive feedback to the patient, family member(s) or caregiver(s), when performed; first hour

EXCLUDES *Use of code for less than 31 minutes of time*
3.10 3.30 FUD XXX 80
AMA: 2019,Sep,10; 2018,Nov,3

\+ **96131 each additional hour (List separately in addition to code for primary procedure)**

EXCLUDES *Use of code for less than 31 minutes of time*
2.36 2.51 FUD ZZZ 80
AMA: 2019,Sep,10; 2018,Nov,3

96132 Neuropsychological testing evaluation services by physician or other qualified health care professional, including integration of patient data, interpretation of standardized test results and clinical data, clinical decision making, treatment planning and report, and interactive feedback to the patient, family member(s) or caregiver(s), when performed; first hour

EXCLUDES *Use of code for less than 31 minutes of time*
3.04 3.71 FUD XXX 80
AMA: 2019,Sep,10; 2018,Nov,3

\+ **96133 each additional hour (List separately in addition to code for primary procedure)**

EXCLUDES *Use of code for less than 31 minutes of time*
2.33 2.83 FUD ZZZ 80
AMA: 2019,Sep,10; 2018,Nov,3

96136 Psychological or neuropsychological test administration and scoring by physician or other qualified health care professional, two or more tests, any method; first 30 minutes

EXCLUDES *Use of code for less than 16 minutes of time*
Code also testing evaluation on same or different days (96130-96133)
0.70 1.33 FUD XXX 80
AMA: 2019,Sep,10; 2018,Nov,3

\+ **96137 each additional 30 minutes (List separately in addition to code for primary procedure)**

EXCLUDES *Use of code for less than 16 minutes of time*
Code also testing evaluation on same or different days (96130-96133)
0.55 1.23 FUD ZZZ 80
AMA: 2019,Sep,10; 2018,Nov,3

96138 Psychological or neuropsychological test administration and scoring by technician, two or more tests, any method; first 30 minutes

EXCLUDES *Use of code for less than 16 minutes of time*
Code also testing evaluation on same or different days (96130-96133)
1.08 1.08 FUD XXX 80
AMA: 2018,Nov,3

\+ **96139 each additional 30 minutes (List separately in addition to code for primary procedure)**

EXCLUDES *Use of code for less than 16 minutes of time*
Code also testing evaluation on same or different days (96130-96133)
1.08 1.08 FUD ZZZ 80
AMA: 2018,Nov,3

96146 **Psychological or neuropsychological test administration, with single automated, standardized instrument via electronic platform, with automated result only**

EXCLUDES *Testing provided by physician, other qualified healthcare professional, or technician ([96127], 96136-96139)*

0.06 0.06 FUD XXX

AMA: 2018,Nov,3

96150-96171 [96164, 96165, 96167, 96168, 96170, 96171] Biopsychosocial Assessment/Intervention

INCLUDES Services for patients that have primary physical illnesses/diagnoses/symptoms who may benefit from assessments/interventions that focus on the biopsychosocial factors related to the patient's health status

Services used to identify the following factors which are important to the prevention/treatment/management of physical health problems:

- Behavioral
- Cognitive
- Emotional
- Psychological
- Social

EXCLUDES *Adaptive behavior services ([97151, 97152, 97153, 97154, 97155, 97156, 97157, 97158], 0362T, 0373T)*

E&M services on the same date

Health and behavior assessment and intervention (96156, 96158-96159)

Preventive medicine counseling services (99401-99412)

96150 ~~Health and behavior assessment (eg, health-focused clinical interview, behavioral observations, psychophysiological monitoring, health-oriented questionnaires), each 15 minutes face-to-face with the patient; initial assessment~~

To report, see (96156, 96158-96159)

96151 ~~re-assessment~~

To report, see (96156, 96158-96159)

96152 ~~Health and behavior intervention, each 15 minutes, face-to-face; individual~~

To report, see (96156, 96158-96159)

96153 ~~group (2 or more patients)~~

To report, see ([96164-96165])

96154 ~~family (with the patient present)~~

To report, see ([96167-96168])

96155 ~~family (without the patient present)~~

To report, see ([96170-96171])

● 96156 **Health behavior assessment, or re-assessment (ie, health-focused clinical interview, behavioral observations, clinical decision making)**

EXCLUDES *Psychotherapy services (90785-90899)*

● 96158 **Health behavior intervention, individual, face-to-face; initial 30 minutes**

EXCLUDES *Psychotherapy services (90785-90899)*

● + 96159 **each additional 15 minutes (List separately in addition to code for primary service)**

0.00 0.00 FUD 000

EXCLUDES *Psychotherapy services (90785-90899)*

Code first (96158)

● # 96164 **Health behavior intervention, group (2 or more patients), face-to-face; initial 30 minutes**

0.00 0.00 FUD 000

EXCLUDES *Psychotherapy services (90785-90899)*

● + # 96165 **each additional 15 minutes (List separately in addition to code for primary service)**

0.00 0.00 FUD 000

EXCLUDES *Psychotherapy services (90785-90899)*

Code first ([96164])

● # 96167 **Health behavior intervention, family (with the patient present), face-to-face; initial 30 minutes**

0.00 0.00 FUD 000

EXCLUDES *Psychotherapy services (90785-90899)*

● + # 96168 **each additional 15 minutes (List separately in addition to code for primary service)**

0.00 0.00 FUD 000

EXCLUDES *Psychotherapy services (90785-90899)*

Code first ([96167])

● # 96170 **Health behavior intervention, family (without the patient present), face-to-face; initial 30 minutes**

0.00 0.00 FUD 000

EXCLUDES *Psychotherapy services (90785-90899)*

● + # 96171 **each additional 15 minutes (List separately in addition to code for primary service)**

0.00 0.00 FUD 000

EXCLUDES *Psychotherapy services (90785-90899)*

Code first ([96170])

96160-96171 Health Risk Assessments

96160 **Administration of patient-focused health risk assessment instrument (eg, health hazard appraisal) with scoring and documentation, per standardized instrument**

0.11 0.11 FUD ZZZ

AMA: 2018,Feb,11; 2018,Jan,8; 2017,Feb,14; 2017,Jan,8; 2016,Nov,5

96161 **Administration of caregiver-focused health risk assessment instrument (eg, depression inventory) for the benefit of the patient, with scoring and documentation, per standardized instrument**

0.11 0.11 FUD ZZZ

AMA: 2018,Feb,11; 2018,Jan,8; 2017,Feb,14; 2017,Jan,8; 2016,Nov,5

96164 **Resequenced code. See code following 96159.**

96165 **Resequenced code. See code following 96159.**

96167 **Resequenced code. See code following 96159.**

96168 **Resequenced code. See code following 96159.**

96170 **Resequenced code. See code following 96159.**

96171 **Resequenced code. See code following 96159.**

96360-96361 Intravenous Fluid Infusion for Hydration (Nonchemotherapy)

CMS: 100-04,4,230.2 OPPS Drug Administration

INCLUDES Administration of prepackaged fluids and electrolytes
Coding hierarchy rules for facility reporting only:
Chemotherapy services are primary to diagnostic, prophylactic, and therapeutic services
Diagnostic, prophylactic, and therapeutic services are primary to hydration services
Infusions are primary to pushes
Pushes are primary to injections
Constant observation/attendance of person administering the drug or substance
Infusion of 15 minutes or less
Direct supervision by physician or other qualified health care provider:
Direction of personnel
Minimal supervision for:
Consent
Safety oversight
Supervision of personnel
Report the initial code for the primary reason for the visit regardless of the order in which the infusions or injections are given
The following if done to facilitate the injection/infusion:
Flush at the end of infusion
Indwelling IV, subcutaneous catheter/port access
Local anesthesia
Start of IV
Supplies/tubing/syringes
Treatment plan verification

EXCLUDES *Catheter/port declotting (36593)*
Drugs/other substances
Minimal infusion to keep the vein open or during other therapeutic infusions
Services provided by physicians or other qualified health care providers in facility settings
Significant separately identifiable E&M service if performed
Use of a code for a second initial service on the same date for accessing a multi-lumen catheter, restarting an IV, or when two IV lines are needed to meet an infusion rate
Use of code for infusion for hydration that is 31 minutes or less

96360 Intravenous infusion, hydration; initial, 31 minutes to 1 hour

EXCLUDES *Use of code if service is performed as a concurrent infusion*

1.07 1.07 FUD XXX S 80

AMA: 2019,Jun,5; 2018,Feb,11; 2018,Jan,8; 2017,Jan,8; 2016,Jan,13; 2015,Jan,16; 2014,May,10; 2014,Jan,11

+ 96361 each additional hour (List separately in addition to code for primary procedure)

INCLUDES Hydration infusion of more than 30 minutes beyond 1 hour
Hydration provided as a secondary or subsequent service after a different initial service via the same IV access site

Code first (96360)

0.38 0.38 FUD ZZZ S 80

AMA: 2019,Jun,5; 2018,Feb,11; 2018,Jan,8; 2017,Jan,8; 2016,Jan,13; 2015,Jan,16; 2014,May,10; 2014,Jan,11

96365-96371 Infusions: Diagnostic/Preventive/Therapeutic

CMS: 100-04,4,230.2 OPPS Drug Administration

INCLUDES Administration of fluid
Administration of substances/drugs
An infusion of 16 minutes or more
Coding hierarchy rules for facility reporting:
Chemotherapy services are primary to diagnostic, prophylactic, and therapeutic services
Diagnostic, prophylactic, and therapeutic services are primary to hydration services
Infusions are primary to pushes
Pushes are primary to injections
Constant presence of health care professional administering the substance/drug
Direct supervision of physician or other qualified health care provider:
Consent
Direction of personnel
Patient assessment
Safety oversight
Supervision of personnel
The following if done to facilitate the injection/infusion:
Flush at the end of infusion
Indwelling IV, subcutaneous catheter/port access
Local anesthesia
Start of IV
Supplies/tubing/syringes
Training to assess patient and monitor vital signs
Training to prepare/dose/dispose
Treatment plan verification

EXCLUDES *Catheter/port declotting (36593)*
Services provided by physicians or other qualified health care providers in facility settings
Significant separately identifiable E&M service, when performed
Use of a code for a second initial service on the same date for accessing a multi-lumen catheter, restarting an IV, or when two IV lines are needed to meet an infusion rate
Use of code with other procedures for which IV push or infusion is an integral part of the procedure

Code also drugs/materials

96365 Intravenous infusion, for therapy, prophylaxis, or diagnosis (specify substance or drug); initial, up to 1 hour

Code also second initial service with modifier 59 when patient's condition or drug protocol mandates the use of two IV lines

2.02 2.02 FUD XXX S 80

AMA: 2018,Dec,8; 2018,Dec,8; 2018,Sep,14; 2018,May,10; 2018,Feb,11; 2018,Jan,8; 2017,Jan,8; 2016,Jan,13; 2015,Jan,16; 2014,Jan,11

+ 96366 each additional hour (List separately in addition to code for primary procedure)

INCLUDES Additional hours of sequential infusion
Infusion intervals of more than 30 minutes beyond one hour
Second and subsequent infusions of the same drug or substance

Code also additional infusion, when appropriate (96367)
Code first (96365)

0.61 0.61 FUD ZZZ S 80

AMA: 2018,Sep,14; 2018,Feb,11; 2018,Jan,8; 2017,Jan,8; 2016,Jan,13; 2015,Jan,16; 2014,Jan,11

+ 96367 additional sequential infusion of a new drug/substance, up to 1 hour (List separately in addition to code for primary procedure)

INCLUDES A secondary or subsequent service with a new drug or substance after a different initial service via the same IV access

EXCLUDES *Use of code more than one time per sequential infusion of the same mix*

Code first (96365, 96374, 96409, 96413)

0.88 0.88 FUD ZZZ S 80

AMA: 2018,Feb,11; 2018,Jan,8; 2017,Jan,8; 2016,Jan,13; 2015,Jan,16; 2014,Jan,11

\+ **96368** **concurrent infusion (List separately in addition to code for primary procedure)**

EXCLUDES *Use of code more than one time per date of service*

Code first (96365, 96366, 96413, 96415, 96416)

0.59 0.59 FUD ZZZ N 80

AMA: 2018,Feb,11; 2018,Jan,8; 2017,Jan,8; 2016,Jan,13; 2015,Jan,16; 2014,Jan,11

96369 **Subcutaneous infusion for therapy or prophylaxis (specify substance or drug); initial, up to 1 hour, including pump set-up and establishment of subcutaneous infusion site(s)**

EXCLUDES *Infusions of 15 minutes or less (96372)*

Use of code more than one time per encounter

4.69 4.69 FUD XXX S 80

AMA: 2018,Feb,11; 2018,Jan,8; 2017,Jan,8; 2016,Jan,13; 2015,Jan,16; 2014,Jan,11

\+ **96370** **each additional hour (List separately in addition to code for primary procedure)**

INCLUDES Infusions of more than 30 minutes beyond one hour

Code first (96369)

0.44 0.44 FUD ZZZ S 80

AMA: 2018,Feb,11; 2018,Jan,8; 2017,Jan,8; 2016,Jan,13; 2015,Jan,16; 2014,Jan,11

\+ **96371** **additional pump set-up with establishment of new subcutaneous infusion site(s) (List separately in addition to code for primary procedure)**

EXCLUDES *Use of code more than one time per encounter*

Code first (96369)

1.84 1.84 FUD ZZZ Q1 80

AMA: 2018,Feb,11; 2018,Jan,8; 2017,Jan,8; 2016,Jan,13; 2015,Jan,16; 2014,Jan,11

96372-96379 Injections: Diagnostic/Preventive/Therapeutic

CMS: 100-04,4,230.2 OPPS Drug Administration

INCLUDES Administration of fluid
Administration of substances/drugs
Coding hierarchy rules for facility reporting:
- Chemotherapy services are primary to diagnostic, prophylactic, and therapeutic services
- Infusions are primary to pushes
- Pushes are primary to injections

Constant presence of health care professional administering the substance/drug
Direct supervision by physician or other qualified health care provider:
- Consent
- Direction of personnel
- Patient assessment
- Safety oversight
- Supervision of personnel

Infusion of 15 minutes or less
The following if done to facilitate the injection/infusion:
- Flush at the end of infusion
- Indwelling IV, subcutaneous catheter/port access
- Local anesthesia
- Start of IV
- Supplies/tubing/syringes

Training to assess patient and monitor vital signs
Training to prepare/dose/dispose
Treatment plan verification

EXCLUDES *Catheter/port declotting (36593)*
Services provided by physicians or other qualified health care providers in facility settings
Significant separately identifiable E&M service, when performed
Use of a code for a second initial service on the same date for accessing a multi-lumen catheter, restarting an IV, or when two IV lines are needed to meet an infusion rate
Use of code with other procedures for which IV push or infusion is an integral part of the procedure

Code also drugs/materials

96372 **Therapeutic, prophylactic, or diagnostic injection (specify substance or drug); subcutaneous or intramuscular**

INCLUDES Direct supervision by physician or other qualified health care provider when reported by the physician/other qualified health care provider. When reported by a hospital, physician/other qualified health care provider need not be present.
Hormonal therapy injections (non-antineoplastic) (96372)

EXCLUDES *Administration of vaccines/toxoids (90460-90474)*
Allergen immunotherapy injections (95115-95117)
Antineoplastic hormonal injections (96402)
Antineoplastic nonhormonal injections (96401)
Injections administered without direct supervision by physician or other qualified health care provider (99211)

0.47 0.47 FUD XXX Q1 80

AMA: 2018,Dec,10; 2018,Dec,10; 2018,Feb,11; 2018,Jan,8; 2017,Jan,8; 2016,Oct,9; 2016,Jan,13; 2015,Jan,16; 2014,Jan,11; 2014,Jan,9

96373 **intra-arterial**

0.53 0.53 FUD XXX S 80

AMA: 2018,Feb,11; 2018,Jan,8; 2017,Jan,8; 2016,Jan,13; 2015,Jan,16; 2014,Jan,11

96374 **intravenous push, single or initial substance/drug**

Code also second initial service with modifier 59 when patient's condition or drug protocol mandates the use of two IV lines

1.10 1.10 FUD XXX S 80

AMA: 2019,Sep,5; 2019,Jun,9; 2018,Feb,11; 2018,Jan,8; 2017,Jan,8; 2016,Jan,13; 2015,Nov,3; 2015,Jan,16; 2014,Jan,11

\+ **96375** **each additional sequential intravenous push of a new substance/drug (List separately in addition to code for primary procedure)**

INCLUDES IV push of a new substance/drug provided as a secondary or subsequent service after a different initial service via same IV access site

Code first (96365, 96374, 96409, 96413)

0.47 0.47 FUD ZZZ S 80

AMA: 2019,Sep,5; 2018,Feb,11; 2018,Jan,8; 2017,Jan,8; 2016,Jan,13; 2015,Nov,3; 2015,Jan,16; 2014,Jan,11

\+ **96376** **each additional sequential intravenous push of the same substance/drug provided in a facility (List separately in addition to code for primary procedure)**

INCLUDES Facilities only

EXCLUDES *IV push performed within 30 minutes of a reported push of the same substance or drug*

Services performed by any nonfacilty provider

Code first (96365, 96374, 96409, 96413)

0.00 0.00 FUD ZZZ N

AMA: 2018,Dec,8; 2018,Dec,8; 2018,Feb,11; 2018,Jan,8; 2017,Jan,8; 2016,Jan,13; 2015,Jan,16; 2014,Nov,14; 2014,Jan,11

96377 **Application of on-body injector (includes cannula insertion) for timed subcutaneous injection**

0.57 0.57 FUD XXX Q1 80

AMA: 2018,Feb,11; 2018,Jan,8; 2017,Jan,8; 2016,Oct,9

96379 **Unlisted therapeutic, prophylactic, or diagnostic intravenous or intra-arterial injection or infusion**

0.00 0.00 FUD XXX Q1 80

AMA: 2018,Feb,11; 2018,Jan,8; 2017,Jan,8; 2016,Jan,13; 2015,Jan,16; 2014,Jan,11

96401-96411 Chemotherapy and Other Complex Drugs, Biologicals: Injection and IV Push

CMS: 100-03,110.2 Certain Drugs Distributed by the National Cancer Institute; 100-03,110.6 Scalp Hypothermia During Chemotherapy, to Prevent Hair Loss; 100-04,4,230.2 OPPS Drug Administration

INCLUDES Highly complex services that require direct supervision for:
- Consent
- Patient assessment
- Safety oversight
- Supervision

More intense work and monitoring of clinical staff by physician or other qualified health care provider due to greater risk of severe patient reactions

Parenteral administration of:
- Anti-neoplastic agents for noncancer diagnoses
- Monoclonal antibody agents
- Nonradionuclide antineoplastic drugs
- Other biologic response modifiers

EXCLUDES *Use of a code for a second initial service on the same date for accessing a multi-lumen catheter, restarting an IV, or when two IV lines are needed to meet an infusion rate*

96401 **Chemotherapy administration, subcutaneous or intramuscular; non-hormonal anti-neoplastic**

EXCLUDES *Services performed by physicians or other qualified health care providers in facility settings*

2.24 2.24 FUD XXX Q1 80

AMA: 2018,Feb,11; 2018,Jan,8; 2017,Jan,8; 2016,Jan,13; 2015,Jan,16; 2014,Jan,11

96402 **hormonal anti-neoplastic**

EXCLUDES *Services performed by physicians or other qualified health care providers in facility settings*

0.87 0.87 FUD XXX Q1 80

AMA: 2018,Feb,11; 2018,Jan,8; 2017,Jan,8; 2016,Jan,13; 2015,Jan,16; 2014,Jan,11

96405 **Chemotherapy administration; intralesional, up to and including 7 lesions**

0.84 2.31 FUD 000 Q1

AMA: 2018,Feb,11; 2018,Jan,8; 2017,Jan,8; 2016,Jan,13; 2015,Jan,16; 2014,Jan,11

96406 **intralesional, more than 7 lesions**

1.31 3.46 FUD 000 S

AMA: 2018,Feb,11; 2018,Jan,8; 2017,Jan,8; 2016,Jan,13; 2015,Jan,16; 2014,Jan,11

96409 **intravenous, push technique, single or initial substance/drug**

INCLUDES Push technique includes:
- Administration of injection directly into vessel or access line by health care professional; or
- Infusion less than or equal to 15 minutes

EXCLUDES *Insertion of arterial and venous cannula(s) for extracorporeal circulation (36823)*

Services performed by physicians or other qualified health care providers in facility settings

Code also second initial service with modifier 59 when patient's condition or drug protocol mandates the use of two IV lines

3.05 3.05 FUD XXX S 80

AMA: 2018,Feb,11; 2018,Jan,8; 2017,Jan,8; 2016,Jan,13; 2015,Jan,16; 2014,Jan,11

\+ **96411** **intravenous, push technique, each additional substance/drug (List separately in addition to code for primary procedure)**

INCLUDES Push technique includes:
- Administration of injection directly into vessel or access line by health care professional; or
- Infusion less than or equal to 15 minutes

EXCLUDES *Insertion of arterial and venous cannula(s) for extracorporeal circulation (36823)*

Services performed by physicians or other qualified health care providers in facility settings

Code first initial substance/drug (96409, 96413)

1.65 1.65 FUD ZZZ S 80

AMA: 2018,Feb,11; 2018,Jan,8; 2017,Jan,8; 2016,Jan,13; 2015,Jan,16; 2014,Jan,11

96413-96417 Chemotherapy and Complex Drugs, Biologicals: Intravenous Infusion

CMS: 100-03,110.2 Certain Drugs Distributed by the National Cancer Institute; 100-03,110.6 Scalp Hypothermia During Chemotherapy, to Prevent Hair Loss; 100-04,4,230.2 OPPS Drug Administration

INCLUDES Highly complex services that require direct supervision for:
- Consent
- Patient assessment
- Safety oversight
- Supervision

More intense work and monitoring of clinical staff by physician or other qualified health care provider due to greater risk of severe patient reactions

Parenteral administration of:
- Anti-neoplastic agents for noncancer diagnoses
- Monoclonal antibody agents
- Nonradionuclide antineoplastic drugs
- Other biologic response modifiers

The following in the administration:
- Access to IV/catheter/port
- Drug preparation
- Flushing at the completion of the infusion
- Hydration fluid
- Routine tubing/syringe/supplies
- Starting the IV
- Use of local anesthesia

EXCLUDES *Administration of nonchemotherapy agents such as antibiotics/steroids/analgesics*
Declotting of catheter/port (36593)
Home infusion (99601-99602)
Insertion of arterial and venous cannula(s) for extracorpororeal circulation (36823)
Services provided by physicians or other qualified health care providers in facility settings
Use of a code for a second initial service on the same date for accessing a multi-lumen catheter, restarting an IV, or when two IV lines are needed to meet an infusion rate

Code also drug or substance
Code also significant separately identifiable E&M service, when performed

96413 Chemotherapy administration, intravenous infusion technique; up to 1 hour, single or initial substance/drug

INCLUDES Push technique includes:
- Administration of injection directly into vessel or access line by health care professional; or
- Infusion less than or equal to 15 minutes

EXCLUDES *Hydration administered as secondary or subsequent service via same IV access site (96361)*
Therapeutic/prophylactic/diagnostic drug infusion/injection through the same intravenous access (96366, 96367, 96375)

Code also second initial service with modifier 59 when patient's condition or drug protocol mandates the use of two IV lines

3.97 3.97 **FUD** XXX S 80

AMA: 2018,Feb,11; 2018,Jan,8; 2017,Jan,8; 2016,Jan,13; 2015,Jan,16; 2014,Jan,11

+ **96415 each additional hour (List separately in addition to code for primary procedure)**

INCLUDES Infusion intervals of more than 30 minutes past 1-hour increments

Code first initial hour (96413)

0.86 0.86 **FUD** ZZZ S 80

AMA: 2018,Feb,11; 2018,Jan,8; 2017,Jan,8; 2016,Jan,13; 2015,Jan,16; 2014,Jan,11

96416 initiation of prolonged chemotherapy infusion (more than 8 hours), requiring use of a portable or implantable pump

EXCLUDES *Portable or implantable infusion pump/reservoir refilling/maintenance for drug delivery (96521-96523)*

3.98 3.98 **FUD** XXX S 80

AMA: 2018,Feb,11; 2018,Jan,8; 2017,Jan,8; 2016,Jan,13; 2015,Jan,16; 2014,Jan,11

+ **96417 each additional sequential infusion (different substance/drug), up to 1 hour (List separately in addition to code for primary procedure)**

INCLUDES Push technique includes:
- Administration of injection directly into vessel or access line by health care professional; or
- Infusion less than or equal to 15 minutes

EXCLUDES *Additional hour(s) of sequential infusion (96415)*
Use of code more than one time per sequential infusion

Code first initial substance/drug (96413)

1.92 1.92 **FUD** ZZZ S 80

AMA: 2018,Feb,11; 2018,Jan,8; 2017,Jan,8; 2016,Jan,13; 2015,Jan,16; 2014,Jan,11

96420-96425 Chemotherapy and Complex Drugs, Biologicals: Intra-arterial

CMS: 100-03,110.2 Certain Drugs Distributed by the National Cancer Institute; 100-03,110.6 Scalp Hypothermia During Chemotherapy, to Prevent Hair Loss; 100-04,4,230.2 OPPS Drug Administration

INCLUDES Highly complex services that require direct supervision for:
- Consent
- Patient assessment
- Safety oversight
- Supervision

More intense work and monitoring of clinical staff by physician or other qualified health care provider due to greater risk of severe patient reactions

Parenteral administration of:
- Anti-neoplastic agents for noncancer diagnoses
- Monoclonal antibody agents
- Non-radionuclide antineoplastic drugs
- Other biologic response modifiers

The following in the administration:
- Access to IV/catheter/port
- Drug preparation
- Flushing at the completion of the infusion
- Hydration fluid
- Routine tubing/syringe/supplies
- Starting the IV
- Use of local anesthesia

EXCLUDES *Administration of non-chemotherapy agents such as antibiotics/steroids/analgesics*
Declotting of catheter/port (36593)
Home infusion (99601-99602)
Services provided by physicians or other qualified health care providers in facility settings
Use of a code for a second initial service on the same date for accessing a multi-lumen catheter, restarting an IV, or when two IV lines are needed

Code also drug or substance
Code also significant separately identifiable E&M service, when performed

96420 Chemotherapy administration, intra-arterial; push technique

INCLUDES Push technique includes:
- Administration of injection directly into vessel or access line by health care professional; or
- Infusion less than or equal to 15 minutes

Regional chemotherapy perfusion

EXCLUDES *Insertion of arterial and venous cannula(s) for extracorpororeal circulation (36823)*
Placement of intra-arterial catheter

2.95 2.95 **FUD** XXX S 80

AMA: 2018,Feb,11; 2018,Jan,8; 2017,Jan,8; 2016,Mar,3; 2016,Jan,13; 2015,Nov,3; 2015,Jan,16; 2014,Jan,11

96422 infusion technique, up to 1 hour

INCLUDES Push technique includes:
- Administration of injection directly into vessel or access line by health care professional; or
- Infusion less than or equal to 15 minutes

Regional chemotherapy perfusion

EXCLUDES *Insertion of arterial and venous cannula(s) for extracorpororeal circulation (36823)*
Placement of intra-arterial catheter

4.85 4.85 **FUD** XXX S 80

AMA: 2018,Feb,11; 2018,Jan,8; 2017,Jan,8; 2016,Mar,3; 2016,Jan,13; 2015,Nov,3; 2015,Jan,16; 2014,Jan,11

+ **96423** **infusion technique, each additional hour (List separately in addition to code for primary procedure)**

INCLUDES Infusion intervals of more than 30 minutes past 1-hour increments
Regional chemotherapy perfusion

EXCLUDES *Insertion of arterial and venous cannula(s) for extracorpororeal circulation (36823)*
Placement of intra-arterial catheter

Code first initial hour (96422)

2.24 2.24 FUD ZZZ S 80

AMA: 2018,Feb,11; 2018,Jan,8; 2017,Jan,8; 2016,Mar,3; 2016,Jan,13; 2015,Nov,3; 2015,Jan,16; 2014,Jan,11

96425 **infusion technique, initiation of prolonged infusion (more than 8 hours), requiring the use of a portable or implantable pump**

INCLUDES Regional chemotherapy perfusion

EXCLUDES *Insertion of arterial and venous cannula(s) for extracorpororeal circulation (36823)*
Placement of intra-arterial catheter
Portable or implantable infusion pump/reservoir refilling/maintenance for drug delivery (96521-96523)

5.14 5.14 FUD XXX S 80

AMA: 2018,Feb,11; 2018,Jan,8; 2017,Jan,8; 2016,Mar,3; 2016,Jan,13; 2015,Nov,3; 2015,Jan,16; 2014,Jan,11

96440-96450 Chemotherapy Administration: Intrathecal/Peritoneal Cavity/Pleural Cavity

CMS: 100-03,110.2 Certain Drugs Distributed by the National Cancer Institute; 100-04,4,230.2 OPPS Drug Administration

96440 **Chemotherapy administration into pleural cavity, requiring and including thoracentesis**

3.57 23.6 FUD 000 S 80

AMA: 2018,Feb,11; 2018,Jan,8; 2017,Jan,8; 2016,Jan,13; 2015,Jan,16; 2014,Jan,11

96446 **Chemotherapy administration into the peritoneal cavity via indwelling port or catheter**

0.79 5.78 FUD XXX S 80

AMA: 2018,Feb,11; 2018,Jan,8; 2017,Jan,8; 2016,Jan,13; 2015,Jan,16; 2014,Jan,11

96450 **Chemotherapy administration, into CNS (eg, intrathecal), requiring and including spinal puncture**

EXCLUDES *Chemotherapy administration, intravesical/bladder (51720)*
Fluoroscopy (77003)
Insertion of catheter/reservoir:
Intraventricular (61210, 61215)
Subarachnoid (62350-62351, 62360-62362)

2.27 5.13 FUD 000 S 80

AMA: 2018,Feb,11; 2018,Jan,8; 2017,Jan,8; 2016,Jan,13; 2015,Jan,16; 2014,Jan,11

96521-96523 Refill/Upkeep of Drug Delivery Device

CMS: 100-04,4,230.2 OPPS Drug Administration

INCLUDES Highly complex services that require direct supervision for:
Consent
Patient assessment
Safety oversight
Supervision
Parenteral administration of:
Anti-neoplastic agents for noncancer diagnoses
Monoclonal antibody agents
Non-radionuclide antineoplastic drugs
Other biologic response modifiers
The following in the administration:
Access to IV/catheter/port
Drug preparation
Flushing at the completion of the infusion
Hydration fluid
Routine tubing/syringe/supplies
Starting the IV
Use of local anesthesia
Therapeutic drugs other than chemotherapy

EXCLUDES *Administration of non-chemotherapy agents such as antibiotics/steroids/analgesics*
Blood specimen collection from completely implantable venous access device (36591)
Declotting of catheter/port (36593)
Home infusion (99601-99602)
Services provided by physicians or other qualified health care providers in facility settings

Code also drug or substance
Code also significant separately identifiable E&M service, when performed

96521 **Refilling and maintenance of portable pump**

4.13 4.13 FUD XXX S 80

AMA: 2018,Feb,11; 2018,Jan,8; 2017,Jan,8; 2016,Jan,13; 2015,Jan,16; 2014,Jan,11

96522 **Refilling and maintenance of implantable pump or reservoir for drug delivery, systemic (eg, intravenous, intra-arterial)**

EXCLUDES *Implantable infusion pump refilling/maintenance for spinal/brain drug delivery (95990-95991)*

3.39 3.39 FUD XXX S 80

AMA: 2018,Feb,11; 2018,Jan,8; 2017,Jan,8; 2016,Jan,13; 2015,Jan,16; 2014,Jan,11

96523 **Irrigation of implanted venous access device for drug delivery systems**

EXCLUDES *Direct supervision by physician or other qualified health care provider in facility settings*
Use of code with any other services on the same date of service

0.77 0.77 FUD XXX Q1 80

AMA: 2018,Feb,11; 2018,Jan,8; 2017,Jan,8; 2016,Jan,13; 2015,Jan,16; 2014,Jan,11

96542-96549 Chemotherapy Injection Into Brain

CMS: 100-04,4,230.2 OPPS Drug Administration

INCLUDES Highly complex services that require direct supervision for:
- Consent
- Patient assessment
- Safety oversight
- Supervision

Parenteral administration of:
- Anti-neoplastic agents for noncancer diagnoses
- Monoclonal antibody agents
- Non-radionuclide antineoplastic drugs
- Other biologic response modifiers

The following in the administration:
- Access to IV/catheter/port
- Drug preparation
- Flushing at the completion of the infusion
- Hydration fluid
- Routine tubing/syringe/supplies
- Starting the IV
- Use of local anesthesia

EXCLUDES *Administration of non-chemotherapy agents such as antibiotics/steroids/analgesics*
Blood specimen collection from completely implantable venous access device (36591)
Declotting of catheter/port (36593)
Home infusion (99601-99602)

Code also drug or substance
Code also significant separately identifiable E&M service, when performed

96542 Chemotherapy injection, subarachnoid or intraventricular via subcutaneous reservoir, single or multiple agents

EXCLUDES *Oral radioactive isotope therapy (79005)*

1.19 3.77 FUD XXX S 80

AMA: 2018,Feb,11; 2018,Jan,8; 2017,Jan,8; 2016,Jan,13; 2015,Jan,16; 2014,Jan,11

96549 Unlisted chemotherapy procedure

0.00 0.00 FUD XXX Q1 80

AMA: 2018,Feb,11; 2018,Jan,8; 2017,Jan,8; 2016,Jan,13; 2015,Jan,16; 2014,Jan,11

96567-96574 Destruction of Lesions: Photodynamic Therapy

EXCLUDES *Ocular photodynamic therapy (67221)*

96567 Photodynamic therapy by external application of light to destroy premalignant lesions of the skin and adjacent mucosa with application and illumination/activation of photosensitive drug(s), per day

INCLUDES Services provided without direct participation by physician or other qualified healthcare professional

3.50 3.50 FUD XXX Q1 80

AMA: 2018,Jul,14; 2018,Feb,10; 2018,Feb,11; 2018,Jan,8; 2017,Jan,8; 2016,Jan,13; 2015,Jan,16; 2014,Jan,11

\+ **96570 Photodynamic therapy by endoscopic application of light to ablate abnormal tissue via activation of photosensitive drug(s); first 30 minutes (List separately in addition to code for endoscopy or bronchoscopy procedures of lung and gastrointestinal tract)**

Code also for 38-52 minutes (96571)
Code also modifier 52 when services with report are less than 23 minutes
Code first (31641, 43229)

1.48 1.48 FUD ZZZ N

AMA: 2018,Feb,11; 2018,Jan,8; 2017,Jan,8; 2016,Jan,13; 2015,Jan,16; 2014,Jan,11

\+ **96571 each additional 15 minutes (List separately in addition to code for endoscopy or bronchoscopy procedures of lung and gastrointestinal tract)**

EXCLUDES *23-37 minutes of service (96570)*

Code first (96570)
Code first when appropriate (31641, 43229)

0.83 0.83 FUD ZZZ N

AMA: 2018,Feb,11; 2018,Jan,8; 2017,Jan,8; 2016,Jan,13; 2015,Jan,16; 2014,Jan,11

96573 Photodynamic therapy by external application of light to destroy premalignant lesions of the skin and adjacent mucosa with application and illumination/activation of photosensitizing drug(s) provided by a physician or other qualified health care professional, per day

INCLUDES Application of photosensitizer to lesions at an anatomical site
Debridement, when performed
Use of light to activate photosensitizer for destruction of premalignant lesions

EXCLUDES *Debridement lesion with photodynamic therapy provided by physician or other qualified healthcare professional (96574)*
Photodynamic therapy by external application of light to same anatomical site (96567)
Services provided to same area on same date of services as photodynamic therapy:
- *Biopsy (11102-11107)*
- *Debridement (11000-11001, 11004-11005)*
- *Excision of lesion (11400-11471)*
- *Shaving of lesion (11300-11313)*

5.70 5.70 FUD 000 Q1 80

AMA: 2018,Jul,14; 2018,Feb,11; 2018,Feb,10

96574 Debridement of premalignant hyperkeratotic lesion(s) (ie, targeted curettage, abrasion) followed with photodynamic therapy by external application of light to destroy premalignant lesions of the skin and adjacent mucosa with application and illumination/activation of photosensitizing drug(s) provided by a physician or other qualified health care professional, per day

INCLUDES Application of photosensitizer to lesions at an anatomical site
Debridement, when performed
Use of light to activate photosensitizer for destruction of premalignant lesions

EXCLUDES *Photodynamic therapy by external application of light for destruction of premalignant lesions (96573)*
Photodynamic therapy by external application of light to same anatomical site (96567)
Services provided to same area on same date of services as photodynamic therapy:
- *Biopsy (11102-11107)*
- *Debridement (11000-11001, 11004-11005)*
- *Excision of lesion (11400-11471)*
- *Shaving of lesion (11300-11313)*

7.25 7.25 FUD 000 Q1 80

AMA: 2018,Feb,10; 2018,Feb,11

96900-96999 Diagnostic/Therapeutic Skin Procedures

EXCLUDES *E&M services*
Injection, intralesional (11900-11901)

96900 Actinotherapy (ultraviolet light)

EXCLUDES *Rhinophototherapy (30999)*

(88160-88161)

0.61 0.61 FUD XXX Q1 80

AMA: 2018,Feb,11; 2018,Jan,8; 2017,Jan,8; 2016,Nov,9; 2016,Sep,3; 2016,Jan,13; 2015,Jan,16; 2014,Jan,11

96902 Microscopic examination of hairs plucked or clipped by the examiner (excluding hair collected by the patient) to determine telogen and anagen counts, or structural hair shaft abnormality

(88160-88161)

0.59 0.62 FUD XXX N

AMA: 2018,Feb,11

96904 Whole body integumentary photography, for monitoring of high risk patients with dysplastic nevus syndrome or a history of dysplastic nevi, or patients with a personal or familial history of melanoma

(88160-88161)

1.82 1.82 FUD XXX N 80

AMA: 2018,Feb,11

96910 Photochemotherapy; tar and ultraviolet B (Goeckerman treatment) or petrolatum and ultraviolet B

(88160-88161)

3.24 3.24 FUD XXX

AMA: 2018,Feb,11; 2018,Jan,8; 2017,Jan,8; 2016,Sep,3; 2016,Jan,13; 2015,Jan,16; 2014,Jan,11

96912 psoralens and ultraviolet A (PUVA)

(88160-88161)

2.75 2.75 FUD XXX

AMA: 2018,Feb,11; 2018,Jan,8; 2017,Jan,8; 2016,Sep,3; 2016,Jan,13; 2015,Jan,16; 2014,Jan,11

96913 Photochemotherapy (Goeckerman and/or PUVA) for severe photoresponsive dermatoses requiring at least 4-8 hours of care under direct supervision of the physician (includes application of medication and dressings)

(88160-88161)

3.91 3.91 FUD XXX

AMA: 2018,Feb,11; 2018,Jan,8; 2017,Jan,8; 2016,Sep,3

96920 Laser treatment for inflammatory skin disease (psoriasis); total area less than 250 sq cm

EXCLUDES *Destruction by laser of:*
- *Benign lesions (17110-17111)*
- *Cutaneous vascular proliferative lesions (17106-17108)*
- *Malignant lesions (17260-17286)*
- *Premalignant lesions (17000-17004)*

(88160-88161)

1.90 4.64 FUD 000

AMA: 2018,Feb,11; 2018,Jan,8; 2017,Jan,8; 2016,Sep,3; 2016,Jan,13; 2015,Jan,16; 2014,Jan,11

96921 250 sq cm to 500 sq cm

EXCLUDES *Destruction by laser of:*
- *Benign lesions (17110-17111)*
- *Cutaneous vascular proliferative lesions (17106-17108)*
- *Malignant lesions (17260-17286)*
- *Premalignant lesions (17000-17004)*

(88160-88161)

2.14 5.09 FUD 000

AMA: 2018,Feb,11; 2018,Jan,8; 2017,Jan,8; 2016,Sep,3; 2016,Jan,13; 2015,Jan,16; 2014,Jan,11

96922 over 500 sq cm

EXCLUDES *Destruction by laser of:*
- *Benign lesions (17110-17111)*
- *Cutaneous vascular proliferative lesions (17106-17108)*
- *Malignant lesions (17260-17286)*
- *Premalignant lesions (17000-17004)*

(88160-88161)

3.43 6.91 FUD 000

AMA: 2018,Feb,11; 2018,Jan,8; 2017,Jan,8; 2016,Sep,3; 2016,Jan,13; 2015,Jan,16; 2014,Jan,11

96931 Reflectance confocal microscopy (RCM) for cellular and sub-cellular imaging of skin; image acquisition and interpretation and report, first lesion

EXCLUDES *Optical coherence tomography for skin imaging (0470T-0471T)*
Reflectance confocal microscopy examination without generated mosaic images (96999)

4.83 4.83 FUD XXX

AMA: 2018,Feb,11; 2018,Jan,8; 2017,Sep,9

96932 image acquisition only, first lesion

EXCLUDES *Optical coherence tomography for skin imaging (0470T-0471T)*
Reflectance confocal microscopy examination without generated mosaic images (96999)

3.51 3.51 FUD XXX

AMA: 2018,Feb,11; 2018,Jan,8; 2017,Sep,9

96933 interpretation and report only, first lesion

EXCLUDES *Optical coherence tomography for skin imaging (0470T-0471T)*
Reflectance confocal microscopy examination without generated mosaic images (96999)

1.32 1.32 FUD XXX

AMA: 2018,Feb,11; 2018,Jan,8; 2017,Sep,9

+ 96934 image acquisition and interpretation and report, each additional lesion (List separately in addition to code for primary procedure)

EXCLUDES *Optical coherence tomography for skin imaging (0470T-0471T)*
Reflectance confocal microscopy examination without generated mosaic images (96999)

Code first (96931)

2.74 2.74 FUD ZZZ

AMA: 2018,Feb,11; 2018,Jan,8; 2017,Sep,9

+ 96935 image acquisition only, each additional lesion (List separately in addition to code for primary procedure)

EXCLUDES *Optical coherence tomography for skin imaging (0470T-0471T)*
Reflectance confocal microscopy examination without generated mosaic images (96999)

Code first (96932)

1.26 1.26 FUD ZZZ

AMA: 2018,Feb,11; 2018,Jan,8; 2017,Sep,9

+ 96936 interpretation and report only, each additional lesion (List separately in addition to code for primary procedure)

EXCLUDES *Optical coherence tomography for skin imaging (0470T-0471T)*
Reflectance confocal microscopy examination without generated mosaic images (96999)

Code first (96933)

1.26 1.26 FUD ZZZ

AMA: 2018,Feb,11; 2018,Jan,8; 2017,Sep,9

96999 Unlisted special dermatological service or procedure

0.00 0.00 FUD XXX

AMA: 2018,Feb,11; 2018,Jan,8; 2017,Sep,9; 2017,Jan,8; 2016,Sep,3; 2016,Jan,13; 2015,Jan,16; 2014,Jan,11

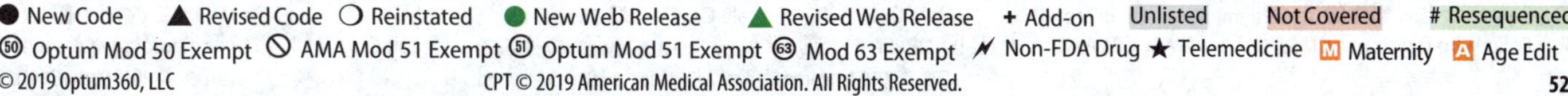

97161-97164 [97161, 97162, 97163, 97164] Assessment: Physical Therapy

CMS: 100-02,15,220 Coverage of Outpatient Rehabilitation Therapy Services; 100-02,15,220.4 Functional Reporting; 100-02,15,230 Practice of Physical Therapy, Occupational Therapy, and Speech-Language Pathology; 100-02,15,230.1 Practice of Physical Therapy; 100-02,15,230.4 Services By a Physical/Occupational Therapist in Private Practice; 100-04,5,10.3.2 Therapy Cap Exceptions; 100-04,5,10.3.3 Use of the KX Modifier; 100-04,5,10.6 Functional Reporting; 100-04,5,20.2 Reporting Units of Service

INCLUDES Creation of care plan
Evaluation of body systems as defined in the 1997 E&M documentation guidelines:
- Cardiovascular system: Vital signs, edema of extremities
- Integumentary system: Inspection for abnormalities of skin
- Mental status: Orientation, judgment, thought processes
- Musculoskeletal system: Evaluation of gait and station, range of motion, muscle strength, height and weight
- Neuromuscular evaluation: Balance, abnormal movements

EXCLUDES *Biofeedback traning via EMG (90901)*
Joint range of motion (95851-95852)
Transcutaneous nerve stimulation (TENS) (97014, 97032)

97161 **Physical therapy evaluation: low complexity, requiring these components: A history with no personal factors and/or comorbidities that impact the plan of care; An examination of body system(s) using standardized tests and measures addressing 1-2 elements from any of the following: body structures and functions, activity limitations, and/or participation restrictions; A clinical presentation with stable and/or uncomplicated characteristics; and Clinical decision making of low complexity using standardized patient assessment instrument and/or measurable assessment of functional outcome. Typically, 20 minutes are spent face-to-face with the patient and/or family.**

2.38 2.38 **FUD** XXX A 80

AMA: 2018,May,5; 2018,Feb,11; 2018,Jan,8; 2017,Aug,3; 2017,Jun,6; 2017,Jan,8

97162 **Physical therapy evaluation: moderate complexity, requiring these components: A history of present problem with 1-2 personal factors and/or comorbidities that impact the plan of care; An examination of body systems using standardized tests and measures in addressing a total of 3 or more elements from any of the following: body structures and functions, activity limitations, and/or participation restrictions; An evolving clinical presentation with changing characteristics; and Clinical decision making of moderate complexity using standardized patient assessment instrument and/or measurable assessment of functional outcome. Typically, 30 minutes are spent face-to-face with the patient and/or family.**

2.38 2.38 **FUD** XXX A 80

AMA: 2018,May,5; 2018,Feb,11; 2018,Jan,8; 2017,Aug,3; 2017,Jun,6; 2017,Jan,8

97163 **Physical therapy evaluation: high complexity, requiring these components: A history of present problem with 3 or more personal factors and/or comorbidities that impact the plan of care; An examination of body systems using standardized tests and measures addressing a total of 4 or more elements from any of the following: body structures and functions, activity limitations, and/or participation restrictions; A clinical presentation with unstable and unpredictable characteristics; and Clinical decision making of high complexity using standardized patient assessment instrument and/or measurable assessment of functional outcome. Typically, 45 minutes are spent face-to-face with the patient and/or family.**

2.38 2.38 **FUD** XXX A 80

AMA: 2018,May,5; 2018,Feb,11; 2018,Jan,8; 2017,Aug,3; 2017,Jun,6; 2017,Jan,8

97164 **Re-evaluation of physical therapy established plan of care, requiring these components: An examination including a review of history and use of standardized tests and measures is required; and Revised plan of care using a standardized patient assessment instrument and/or measurable assessment of functional outcome Typically, 20 minutes are spent face-to-face with the patient and/or family.**

1.61 1.61 **FUD** XXX A 80

AMA: 2018,May,5; 2018,Feb,11; 2018,Jan,8; 2017,Aug,3; 2017,Jun,6; 2017,Jan,8

97165-97168 [97165, 97166, 97167, 97168] Assessment: Occupational Therapy

CMS: 100-02,15,220 Coverage of Outpatient Rehabilitation Therapy Services; 100-02,15,220.4 Functional Reporting; 100-02,15,230 Practice of Physical Therapy, Occupational Therapy, and Speech-Language Pathology; 100-02,15,230.1 Practice of Physical Therapy; 100-02,15,230.2 Practice of Occupational Therapy; 100-02,15,230.4 Services By a Physical/Occupational Therapist in Private Practice; 100-04,5,10.3.2 Exceptions Process; 100-04,5,10.3.3 Use of the KX Modifier; 100-04,5,10.6 Functional Reporting; 100-04,5,20.2 Reporting Units of Service

INCLUDES Creation of care plan
Evaluations as appropriate
Medical history
Occupational status
Past history of therapy

97165 **Occupational therapy evaluation, low complexity, requiring these components: An occupational profile and medical and therapy history, which includes a brief history including review of medical and/or therapy records relating to the presenting problem; An assessment(s) that identifies 1-3 performance deficits (ie, relating to physical, cognitive, or psychosocial skills) that result in activity limitations and/or participation restrictions; and Clinical decision making of low complexity, which includes an analysis of the occupational profile, analysis of data from problem-focused assessment(s), and consideration of a limited number of treatment options. Patient presents with no comorbidities that affect occupational performance. Modification of tasks or assistance (eg, physical or verbal) with assessment(s) is not necessary to enable completion of evaluation component. Typically, 30 minutes are spent face-to-face with the patient and/or family.**

2.57 2.57 **FUD** XXX A 80

AMA: 2018,May,5; 2018,Feb,11; 2018,Jan,8; 2017,Jun,6; 2017,Feb,3; 2017,Jan,8

97166 **Occupational therapy evaluation, moderate complexity, requiring these components: An occupational profile and medical and therapy history, which includes an expanded review of medical and/or therapy records and additional review of physical, cognitive, or psychosocial history related to current functional performance; An assessment(s) that identifies 3-5 performance deficits (ie, relating to physical, cognitive, or psychosocial skills) that result in activity limitations and/or participation restrictions; and Clinical decision making of moderate analytic complexity, which includes an analysis of the occupational profile, analysis of data from detailed assessment(s), and consideration of several treatment options. Patient may present with comorbidities that affect occupational performance. Minimal to moderate modification of tasks or assistance (eg, physical or verbal) with assessment(s) is necessary to enable patient to complete evaluation component. Typically, 45 minutes are spent face-to-face with the patient and/or family.**

2.57 2.57 **FUD** XXX A 80

AMA: 2018,May,5; 2018,Feb,11; 2018,Jan,8; 2017,Jun,6; 2017,Feb,3; 2017,Jan,8

\# **97167** **Occupational therapy evaluation, high complexity, requiring these components: An occupational profile and medical and therapy history, which includes review of medical and/or therapy records and extensive additional review of physical, cognitive, or psychosocial history related to current functional performance; An assessment(s) that identifies 5 or more performance deficits (ie, relating to physical, cognitive, or psychosocial skills) that result in activity limitations and/or participation restrictions; and Clinical decision making of high analytic complexity, which includes an analysis of the patient profile, analysis of data from comprehensive assessment(s), and consideration of multiple treatment options. Patient presents with comorbidities that affect occupational performance. Significant modification of tasks or assistance (eg, physical or verbal) with assessment(s) is necessary to enable patient to complete evaluation component. Typically, 60 minutes are spent face-to-face with the patient and/or family.**

2.58 2.58 FUD XXX A 80

AMA: 2018,May,5; 2018,Feb,11; 2018,Jan,8; 2017,Jun,6; 2017,Feb,3; 2017,Jan,8

\# **97168** **Re-evaluation of occupational therapy established plan of care, requiring these components: An assessment of changes in patient functional or medical status with revised plan of care; An update to the initial occupational profile to reflect changes in condition or environment that affect future interventions and/or goals; and A revised plan of care. A formal reevaluation is performed when there is a documented change in functional status or a significant change to the plan of care is required. Typically, 30 minutes are spent face-to-face with the patient and/or family.**

1.75 1.75 FUD XXX A 80

AMA: 2018,May,5; 2018,Feb,11; 2018,Jan,8; 2017,Jun,6; 2017,Feb,3; 2017,Jan,8

97169-97172 [97169, 97170, 97171, 97172] Assessment: Athletic Training

CMS: 100-02,15,220 Coverage of Outpatient Rehabilitation Therapy Services; 100-02,15,230 Practice of Physical Therapy, Occupational Therapy, and Speech-Language Pathology; 100-02,15,230.1 Practice of Physical Therapy

INCLUDES Creation of care plan
Evaluation of body systems as defined in the 1997 E&M documentation guidelines:
- Cardiovascular system: Vital signs, edema of extremities
- Integumentary system: Inspection for abnormalities of skin
- Musculoskeletal system: Evaluation of gait and station, range of motion, muscle strength, height and weight
- Neuromuscular evaluation: Balance, abnormal movements

\# **97169** **Athletic training evaluation, low complexity, requiring these components: A history and physical activity profile with no comorbidities that affect physical activity; An examination of affected body area and other symptomatic or related systems addressing 1-2 elements from any of the following: body structures, physical activity, and/or participation deficiencies; and Clinical decision making of low complexity using standardized patient assessment instrument and/or measurable assessment of functional outcome. Typically, 15 minutes are spent face-to-face with the patient and/or family.**

0.00 0.00 FUD XXX E

AMA: 2018,May,5; 2018,Feb,11; 2018,Jan,8; 2017,Jun,6; 2017,Jan,8

\# **97170** **Athletic training evaluation, moderate complexity, requiring these components: A medical history and physical activity profile with 1-2 comorbidities that affect physical activity; An examination of affected body area and other symptomatic or related systems addressing a total of 3 or more elements from any of the following: body structures, physical activity, and/or participation deficiencies; and Clinical decision making of moderate complexity using standardized patient assessment instrument and/or measurable assessment of functional outcome. Typically, 30 minutes are spent face-to-face with the patient and/or family.**

0.00 0.00 FUD XXX E

AMA: 2018,May,5; 2018,Feb,11; 2018,Jan,8; 2017,Jun,6; 2017,Jan,8

\# **97171** **Athletic training evaluation, high complexity, requiring these components: A medical history and physical activity profile, with 3 or more comorbidities that affect physical activity; A comprehensive examination of body systems using standardized tests and measures addressing a total of 4 or more elements from any of the following: body structures, physical activity, and/or participation deficiencies; Clinical presentation with unstable and unpredictable characteristics; and Clinical decision making of high complexity using standardized patient assessment instrument and/or measurable assessment of functional outcome. Typically, 45 minutes are spent face-to-face with the patient and/or family.**

0.00 0.00 FUD XXX E

AMA: 2018,May,5; 2018,Feb,11; 2018,Jan,8; 2017,Jun,6; 2017,Jan,8

\# **97172** **Re-evaluation of athletic training established plan of care requiring these components: An assessment of patient's current functional status when there is a documented change; and A revised plan of care using a standardized patient assessment instrument and/or measurable assessment of functional outcome with an update in management options, goals, and interventions. Typically, 20 minutes are spent face-to-face with the patient and/or family.**

0.00 0.00 FUD XXX E

AMA: 2018,May,5; 2018,Feb,11; 2018,Jan,8; 2017,Jun,6; 2017,Jan,8

97010-97028 Physical Therapy Treatment Modalities: Supervised

CMS: 100-02,15,220 Coverage of Outpatient Rehabilitation Therapy Services; 100-02,15,220.4 Functional Reporting; 100-02,15,230 Practice of Physical Therapy, Occupational Therapy, and Speech-Language Pathology; 100-02,15,230.1 Practice of Physical Therapy; 100-02,15,230.2 Practice of Occupational Therapy; 100-02,15,230.4 Services By a Physical/Occupational Therapist in Private Practice; 100-03,10.3 Inpatient Pain Rehabilitation Programs; 100-03,10.4 Outpatient Hospital Pain Rehabilitation Programs; 100-03,160.17 Payment for L-Dopa /Associated Inpatient Hospital Services; 100-04,5,10 Part B Outpatient Rehabilitation and Comprehensive Outpatient Rehabilitation Facility (CORF) Services - General; 100-04,5,10.2 Financial Limitation for Outpatient Rehabilitation Services; 100-04,5,10.3.2 Therapy Cap Exceptions; 100-04,5,10.3.3 Use of the KX Modifier; 100-04,5,20.2 Reporting Units of Service

INCLUDES Adding incremental intervals of treatment time for the same visit to calculate the total service time

EXCLUDES *Direct patient contact by the provider*
Electromyography (95860-95872 [95885, 95886, 95887])
EMG biofeedback training (90901)
Muscle and range of motion tests ([97161, 97162, 97163, 97164, 97165, 97166, 97167, 97168, 97169, 97170, 97171, 97172])
Nerve conduction studies (95905-95913)

97010 **Application of a modality to 1 or more areas; hot or cold packs**

0.18 0.18 FUD XXX ⑤ A

AMA: 2018,May,5; 2018,Feb,11; 2018,Jan,8; 2017,Jan,8; 2016,Jun,8; 2016,Jan,13; 2015,Jan,16; 2014,Jan,11

97012 **traction, mechanical**

0.42 0.42 FUD XXX ⑤ A 80

AMA: 2018,May,5; 2018,Feb,11; 2018,Jan,8; 2017,Jan,8; 2016,Jun,8; 2016,Jan,13; 2015,Jan,16; 2014,Jan,11

97014 **electrical stimulation (unattended)**

EXCLUDES *Acupuncture with electrical stimulation (97813, 97814)*

0.42 0.42 FUD XXX

AMA: 2019,Jul,10; 2018,Oct,11; 2018,Oct,8; 2018,May,5; 2018,Feb,11; 2018,Jan,8; 2017,Jan,8; 2016,Jan,13; 2015,Jan,16; 2014,Jan,11

97016 **vasopneumatic devices**

0.36 0.36 FUD XXX

AMA: 2018,May,5; 2018,Feb,11; 2018,Jan,8; 2017,Jan,8; 2016,Jan,13; 2015,Jan,16; 2014,Jan,11

97018 **paraffin bath**

0.20 0.20 FUD XXX

AMA: 2018,May,5; 2018,Feb,11; 2018,Jan,8; 2017,Jan,8; 2016,Jan,13; 2015,Jan,16; 2014,Jan,11

97022 **whirlpool**

0.51 0.51 FUD XXX

AMA: 2018,May,5; 2018,Feb,11; 2018,Jan,8; 2017,Jan,8; 2016,Jan,13; 2015,Jan,16; 2014,Jan,11

97024 **diathermy (eg, microwave)**

0.20 0.20 FUD XXX

AMA: 2018,May,5; 2018,Feb,11; 2018,Jan,8; 2017,Jan,8; 2016,Jan,13; 2015,Jan,16; 2014,Jan,11

97026 **infrared**

0.18 0.18 FUD XXX

AMA: 2018,May,5; 2018,Feb,11; 2018,Jan,8; 2017,Jan,8; 2016,Jan,13; 2015,Jan,16; 2014,Jan,11

97028 **ultraviolet**

0.23 0.23 FUD XXX

AMA: 2018,May,5; 2018,Feb,11; 2018,Jan,8; 2017,Jan,8; 2016,Jan,13; 2015,Jan,16; 2014,Jan,11

97032-97039 Physical Therapy Treatment Modalities: Constant Attendance

CMS: 100-02,15,220 Coverage of Outpatient Rehabilitation Therapy Services; 100-02,15,220.4 Functional Reporting; 100-02,15,230 Practice of Physical Therapy, Occupational Therapy, and Speech-Language Pathology; 100-02,15,230.1 Practice of Physical Therapy; 100-02,15,230.2 Practice of Occupational Therapy; 100-02,15,230.4 Services By a Physical/Occupational Therapist in Private Practice; 100-03,10.3 Inpatient Pain Rehabilitation Programs; 100-03,10.4 Outpatient Hospital Pain Rehabilitation Programs; 100-03,160.17 Payment for L-Dopa /Associated Inpatient Hospital Services; 100-04,5,10 Part B Outpatient Rehabilitation and Comprehensive Outpatient Rehabilitation Facility (CORF) Services - General; 100-04,5,10.3.2 Exceptions Process; 100-04,5,10.3.3 Use of the KX Modifier; 100-04,5,20.2 Reporting Units of Service

INCLUDES Adding incremental intervals of treatment time for the same visit to calculate the total service time
Direct patient contact by the provider

EXCLUDES *Electromyography (95860-95872 [95885, 95886, 95887])*
EMG biofeedback training (90901)
Muscle and range of motion tests ([97161, 97162, 97163, 97164, 97165, 97166, 97167, 97168, 97169, 97170, 97171, 97172])
Nerve conduction studies (95905-95913)

97032 **Application of a modality to 1 or more areas; electrical stimulation (manual), each 15 minutes**

EXCLUDES *Transcutaneous electrical modulation pain reprocessing (TEMPR) (scrambler therapy) (0278T)*

0.42 0.42 FUD XXX

AMA: 2019,Jul,10; 2018,Oct,11; 2018,Oct,8; 2018,May,5; 2018,Feb,11; 2018,Jan,8; 2017,Jan,8; 2016,Jan,13; 2015,Jan,16; 2014,Jan,11

97033 **iontophoresis, each 15 minutes**

0.59 0.59 FUD XXX

AMA: 2018,May,5; 2018,Feb,11; 2018,Jan,8; 2017,Jan,8; 2016,Jan,13; 2015,Jan,16; 2014,Jan,11

97034 **contrast baths, each 15 minutes**

0.43 0.43 FUD XXX

AMA: 2018,May,5; 2018,Feb,11; 2018,Jan,8; 2017,Jan,8; 2016,Jan,13; 2015,Jan,16; 2014,Jan,11

97035 **ultrasound, each 15 minutes**

0.39 0.39 FUD XXX

AMA: 2018,May,5; 2018,Feb,11; 2018,Jan,8; 2017,Jan,8; 2016,Jan,13; 2015,Jan,16; 2014,Jan,11

97036 **Hubbard tank, each 15 minutes**

0.99 0.99 FUD XXX

AMA: 2018,May,5; 2018,Feb,11; 2018,Jan,8; 2017,Jan,8; 2016,Jan,13; 2015,Jan,16; 2014,Jan,11

97039 **Unlisted modality (specify type and time if constant attendance)**

0.00 0.00 FUD XXX

AMA: 2018,May,5; 2018,Feb,11; 2018,Jan,8; 2017,Jan,8; 2016,Nov,9; 2016,Jun,8; 2016,Jan,13; 2015,Jan,16; 2014,Jan,11

97110-97546 Other Therapeutic Techniques With Direct Patient Contact

CMS: 100-02,15,220 Coverage of Outpatient Rehabilitation Therapy Services; 100-02,15,230 Practice of Physical Therapy, Occupational Therapy, and Speech-Language Pathology; 100-02,15,230.1 Practice of Physical Therapy; 100-02,15,230.2 Practice of Occupational Therapy; 100-02,15,230.4 Services By a Physical/Occupational Therapist in Private Practice; 100-03,10.3 Inpatient Pain Rehabilitation Programs; 100-03,10.4 Outpatient Hospital Pain Rehabilitation Programs; 100-04,5,10 Part B Outpatient Rehabilitation and Comprehensive Outpatient Rehabilitation Facility (CORF) Services - General; 100-04,5,10.2 Financial Limitation for Outpatient Rehabilitation Services; 100-04,5,20.2 Reporting Units of Service

INCLUDES Application of clinical skills/services to improve function
Direct patient contact by the provider

EXCLUDES *Electromyography (95860-95872 [95885, 95886, 95887])*
EMG biofeedback training (90901)
Muscle and range of motion tests ([97161, 97162, 97163, 97164, 97165, 97166, 97167, 97168, 97169, 97170, 97171, 97172])
Nerve conduction studies (95905-95913)

97110 **Therapeutic procedure, 1 or more areas, each 15 minutes; therapeutic exercises to develop strength and endurance, range of motion and flexibility**

0.87 0.87 FUD XXX

AMA: 2019,Jun,14; 2018,Dec,7; 2018,Dec,7; 2018,May,5; 2018,Feb,11; 2018,Jan,8; 2017,Dec,14; 2017,Jan,8; 2016,Jun,8; 2016,Jan,13; 2015,Jan,16; 2014,Aug,5; 2014,Mar,13; 2014,Jan,11

97112 **neuromuscular reeducation of movement, balance, coordination, kinesthetic sense, posture, and/or proprioception for sitting and/or standing activities**

0.99 0.99 FUD XXX

AMA: 2018,May,5; 2018,Feb,11; 2018,Jan,8; 2017,Jan,8; 2016,Jan,13; 2015,Jan,16; 2014,Mar,13; 2014,Jan,11

97113 **aquatic therapy with therapeutic exercises**

1.10 1.10 FUD XXX

AMA: 2018,May,5; 2018,Feb,11; 2018,Jan,8; 2017,Jan,8; 2016,Jan,13; 2015,Jan,16; 2014,Mar,13; 2014,Jan,11

97116 **gait training (includes stair climbing)**

EXCLUDES *Comprehensive gait/motion analysis (96000-96003)*

0.86 0.86 FUD XXX

AMA: 2018,May,5; 2018,Feb,11; 2018,Jan,8; 2017,Jan,8; 2016,Jan,13; 2015,Jan,16; 2014,Mar,13; 2014,Jan,11

97124 **massage, including effleurage, petrissage and/or tapotement (stroking, compression, percussion)**

EXCLUDES *Myofascial release (97140)*

0.81 0.81 FUD XXX

AMA: 2019,Jun,14; 2018,May,5; 2018,Feb,11; 2018,Jan,8; 2017,Jan,8; 2016,Jun,8; 2016,Jan,13; 2015,Jan,16; 2014,Mar,13; 2014,Jan,11

97127 ~~**Therapeutic interventions that focus on cognitive function (eg, attention, memory, reasoning, executive function, problem solving, and/or pragmatic functioning) and compensatory strategies to manage the performance of an activity (eg, managing time or schedules, initiating, organizing and sequencing tasks), direct (one-on-one) patient contact**~~

To report, see (97129)

● **97129** **Therapeutic interventions that focus on cognitive function (eg, attention, memory, reasoning, executive function, problem solving, and/or pragmatic functioning) and compensatory strategies to manage the performance of an activity (eg, managing time or schedules, initiating, organizing, and sequencing tasks), direct (one-on-one) patient contact; initial 15 minutes**

0.00 0.00 FUD 000 (51)

EXCLUDES *Adaptive behavior treatment ([97153], [97155])*

Use of code more than one time per day

● + **97130** **each additional 15 minutes (List separately in addition to code for primary procedure)**

0.00 0.00 FUD 000 (51)

EXCLUDES *Adaptive behavior treatment ([97153], [97155])*

Code first (97129)

97139 **Unlisted therapeutic procedure (specify)**

0.00 0.00 FUD XXX A 80

AMA: 2018,May,5; 2018,Feb,11; 2018,Jan,8; 2017,Jan,8; 2016,Jan,13; 2015,Jan,16; 2014,Mar,13; 2014,Jan,11

97140 **Manual therapy techniques (eg, mobilization/ manipulation, manual lymphatic drainage, manual traction), 1 or more regions, each 15 minutes**

EXCLUDES *Insertion of needle without injection ([20560, 20561])*

0.79 0.79 FUD XXX (51) A 80

AMA: 2019,Jun,14; 2018,May,5; 2018,Feb,11; 2018,Jan,8; 2017,Jan,8; 2016,Nov,9; 2016,Sep,9; 2016,Aug,3; 2016,Jan,13; 2015,Mar,9; 2015,Jan,16; 2014,Mar,13; 2014,Jan,11

97150 **Therapeutic procedure(s), group (2 or more individuals)**

INCLUDES Constant attendance by the physician/therapist

Reporting this procedure for each member of group

EXCLUDES *Adaptive behavior services ([97154], [97158])*

Osteopathic manipulative treatment (98925-98929)

0.52 0.52 FUD XXX (51) A 80

AMA: 2018,Nov,3; 2018,May,5; 2018,Feb,11; 2018,Jan,8; 2017,Jan,8; 2016,Jan,13; 2015,Jan,16; 2014,Mar,13; 2014,Jan,11

97151 **Resequenced code. See code following 96040.**

97152 **Resequenced code. See code following 96040.**

97153 **Resequenced code. See code following 96040.**

97154 **Resequenced code. See code following 96040.**

97155 **Resequenced code. See code following 96040.**

97156 **Resequenced code. See code following 96040.**

97157 **Resequenced code. See code following 96040.**

97158 **Resequenced code. See code following 96040.**

97161 **Resequenced code. See code before 97010.**

97162 **Resequenced code. See code before 97010.**

97163 **Resequenced code. See code before 97010.**

97164 **Resequenced code. See code before 97010.**

97165 **Resequenced code. See code before 97010.**

97166 **Resequenced code. See code before 97010.**

97167 **Resequenced code. See code before 97010.**

97168 **Resequenced code. See code before 97010.**

97169 **Resequenced code. See code before 97010.**

97170 **Resequenced code. See code before 97010.**

97171 **Resequenced code. See code before 97010.**

97172 **Resequenced code. See code before 97010.**

97530 **Therapeutic activities, direct (one-on-one) patient contact (use of dynamic activities to improve functional performance), each 15 minutes**

1.13 1.13 FUD XXX (51) A 80

AMA: 2018,Dec,7; 2018,Dec,7; 2018,May,5; 2018,Feb,11; 2018,Jan,8; 2017,Jan,8; 2016,Jan,13; 2015,Jan,16; 2014,Mar,13; 2014,Jan,11

97533 **Sensory integrative techniques to enhance sensory processing and promote adaptive responses to environmental demands, direct (one-on-one) patient contact, each 15 minutes**

1.21 1.21 FUD XXX (51) A 80

AMA: 2018,May,5; 2018,Feb,11; 2018,Jan,8; 2017,Jan,8; 2016,Jan,13; 2015,Jan,16; 2014,Mar,13; 2014,Jan,11

97535 **Self-care/home management training (eg, activities of daily living (ADL) and compensatory training, meal preparation, safety procedures, and instructions in use of assistive technology devices/adaptive equipment) direct one-on-one contact, each 15 minutes**

0.97 0.97 FUD XXX (51) A 80

AMA: 2018,May,5; 2018,Feb,11; 2018,Jan,8; 2017,Jan,8; 2016,Aug,3; 2016,Jan,13; 2015,Jun,10; 2015,Mar,9; 2015,Jan,16; 2014,Mar,13; 2014,Jan,11

97537 **Community/work reintegration training (eg, shopping, transportation, money management, avocational activities and/or work environment/modification analysis, work task analysis, use of assistive technology device/adaptive equipment), direct one-on-one contact, each 15 minutes**

EXCLUDES *Wheelchair management/propulsion training (97542)*

0.93 0.93 FUD XXX (51) A 80

AMA: 2018,May,5; 2018,Feb,11; 2018,Jan,8; 2017,Jan,8; 2016,Jan,13; 2015,Jan,16; 2014,Mar,13; 2014,Jan,11

97542 **Wheelchair management (eg, assessment, fitting, training), each 15 minutes**

0.94 0.94 FUD XXX (51) A 80

AMA: 2018,May,5; 2018,Feb,11; 2018,Jan,8; 2017,Jan,8; 2016,Jan,13; 2015,Jun,10; 2015,Jan,16; 2014,Mar,13; 2014,Jan,11

97545 **Work hardening/conditioning; initial 2 hours**

0.00 0.00 FUD XXX (51) A 80

AMA: 2018,May,5; 2018,Feb,11; 2018,Jan,8; 2017,Jan,8; 2016,Jan,13; 2015,Jan,16; 2014,Mar,13; 2014,Jan,11

+ **97546** **each additional hour (List separately in addition to code for primary procedure)**

Code first initial 2 hours (97545)

0.00 0.00 FUD ZZZ (51) A 80

AMA: 2018,May,5; 2018,Feb,11; 2018,Jan,8; 2017,Jan,8; 2016,Jan,13; 2015,Jan,16; 2014,Mar,13; 2014,Jan,11

97597-97610 Treatment of Wounds

CMS: 100-02,15,220.4 Functional Reporting; 100-02,15,230.4 Services By a Physical/Occupational Therapist in Private Practice; 100-03,270.3 Blood-derived Products for Chronic Nonhealing Wounds; 100-04,4,200.9 Billing for "Sometimes Therapy" Services that May be Paid as Non-Therapy Services; 100-04,5,10 Part B Outpatient Rehabilitation and Comprehensive Outpatient Rehabilitation Facility (CORF) Services - General; 100-04,5,10.3.2 Exceptions Process; 100-04,5,10.3.3 Use of the KX Modifier

INCLUDES Direct patient contact
Removing devitalized/necrotic tissue and promoting healing

EXCLUDES *Burn wound debridement (16020-16030)*

97597 **Debridement (eg, high pressure waterjet with/without suction, sharp selective debridement with scissors, scalpel and forceps), open wound, (eg, fibrin, devitalized epidermis and/or dermis, exudate, debris, biofilm), including topical application(s), wound assessment, use of a whirlpool, when performed and instruction(s) for ongoing care, per session, total wound(s) surface area; first 20 sq cm or less**

INCLUDES Chemical cauterization (17250)

0.68 2.52 **FUD** 000 ⑤ T 80

AMA: 2018,May,5; 2018,Feb,11; 2018,Jan,8; 2017,Jan,8; 2016,Oct,3; 2016,Aug,9; 2016,Jan,13; 2015,Jan,16; 2014,Jun,11; 2014,Jan,11

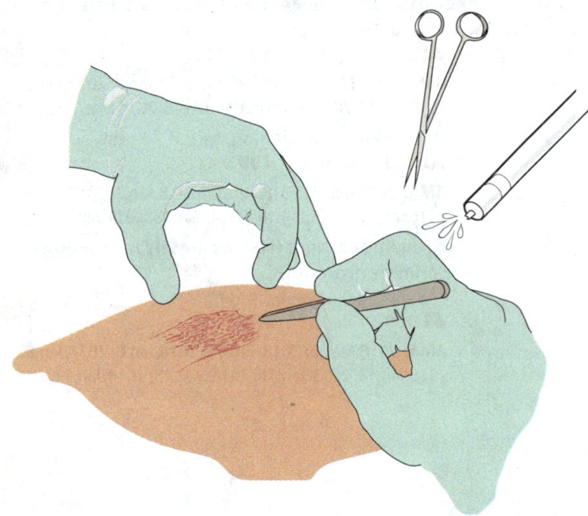

Wound may be washed, addressed with scissors, and/or tweezers and scalpel

\+ **97598** **each additional 20 sq cm, or part thereof (List separately in addition to code for primary procedure)**

INCLUDES Chemical cauterization (17250)

Code first (97597)

0.32 0.79 **FUD** ZZZ ⑤ N 80

AMA: 2018,May,5; 2018,Feb,11; 2018,Jan,8; 2017,Jan,8; 2016,Oct,3; 2016,Aug,9; 2016,Jan,13; 2015,Jan,16; 2014,Jun,11; 2014,Jan,11

97602 **Removal of devitalized tissue from wound(s), non-selective debridement, without anesthesia (eg, wet-to-moist dressings, enzymatic, abrasion, larval therapy), including topical application(s), wound assessment, and instruction(s) for ongoing care, per session**

INCLUDES Chemical cauterization (17250)

0.00 0.00 **FUD** XXX ⑤ Q1

AMA: 2018,May,5; 2018,Feb,11; 2018,Jan,8; 2017,Jan,8; 2016,Oct,3; 2016,Jan,13; 2015,Jan,16; 2014,Jun,11; 2014,Jan,11

97605 **Negative pressure wound therapy (eg, vacuum assisted drainage collection), utilizing durable medical equipment (DME), including topical application(s), wound assessment, and instruction(s) for ongoing care, per session; total wound(s) surface area less than or equal to 50 square centimeters**

EXCLUDES *Negative pressure wound therapy using disposable medical equipment (97607-97608)*

0.74 1.24 **FUD** XXX ⑤ Q1 80

AMA: 2018,May,5; 2018,Feb,11; 2018,Jan,8; 2017,Jan,8; 2016,Feb,13; 2016,Jan,13; 2015,Jan,16; 2014,Nov,8; 2014,Jan,11

97606 **total wound(s) surface area greater than 50 square centimeters**

EXCLUDES *Negative pressure wound therapy using disposable medical equipment (97607-97608)*

0.80 1.46 **FUD** XXX ⑤ Q1 80

AMA: 2018,May,5; 2018,Feb,11; 2018,Jan,8; 2017,Jan,8; 2016,Feb,13; 2016,Jan,13; 2015,Jan,16; 2014,Nov,8; 2014,Jan,11

97607 **Negative pressure wound therapy, (eg, vacuum assisted drainage collection), utilizing disposable, non-durable medical equipment including provision of exudate management collection system, topical application(s), wound assessment, and instructions for ongoing care, per session; total wound(s) surface area less than or equal to 50 square centimeters**

EXCLUDES *Negative pressure wound therapy using durable medical equipment (97605-97606)*

0.00 0.00 **FUD** XXX ⑤ T 80

AMA: 2018,May,5; 2018,Feb,11; 2018,Jan,8; 2017,Jan,8; 2016,Jan,13; 2015,Jan,16; 2014,Nov,8

97608 **total wound(s) surface area greater than 50 square centimeters**

EXCLUDES *Negative pressure wound therapy using durable medical equipment (97605-97606)*

0.00 0.00 **FUD** XXX ⑤ T 80

AMA: 2018,May,5; 2018,Feb,11; 2018,Jan,8; 2017,Jan,8; 2016,Jan,13; 2015,Jan,16; 2014,Nov,8

97610 **Low frequency, non-contact, non-thermal ultrasound, including topical application(s), when performed, wound assessment, and instruction(s) for ongoing care, per day**

0.48 6.39 **FUD** XXX ⑤ Q1 80

AMA: 2018,May,5; 2018,Feb,11; 2018,Jan,8; 2017,Jan,8; 2016,Jan,13; 2015,Jan,16; 2014,Jun,11

97750-97799 Assessments and Training

CMS: 100-02,15,220 Coverage of Outpatient Rehabilitation Therapy Services; 100-02,15,220.4 Functional Reporting; 100-02,15,230 Practice of Physical Therapy, Occupational Therapy, and Speech-Language Pathology; 100-02,15,230.1 Practice of Physical Therapy; 100-02,15,230.2 Practice of Occupational Therapy; 100-02,15,230.4 Services By a Physical/Occupational Therapist in Private Practice; 100-04,5,10 Part B Outpatient Rehabilitation and Comprehensive Outpatient Rehabilitation Facility (CORF) Services - General; 100-04,5,10.3.2 Therapy Cap Exceptions; 100-04,5,10.3.3 Use of the KX Modifier

97750 **Physical performance test or measurement (eg, musculoskeletal, functional capacity), with written report, each 15 minutes**

INCLUDES Direct patient contact

EXCLUDES *Electromyography (95860-95872, [95885, 95886, 95887])*
Joint range of motion (95851-95852)
Nerve velocity determination (95905, 95907-95913)

0.99 0.99 **FUD** XXX ⑤ A 80

AMA: 2018,May,5; 2018,Feb,11; 2018,Jan,8; 2017,Jan,8; 2016,Jan,13; 2015,Jan,16; 2014,Jan,11

97755 **Assistive technology assessment (eg, to restore, augment or compensate for existing function, optimize functional tasks and/or maximize environmental accessibility), direct one-on-one contact, with written report, each 15 minutes**

INCLUDES Direct patient contact

EXCLUDES *Augmentative/alternative communication device (92605, 92607)*
Electromyography (95860-95872, [95885, 95886, 95887])
Joint range of motion (95851-95852)
Nerve velocity determination (95905, 95907-95913)

1.08 1.08 FUD XXX

AMA: 2018,May,5; 2018,Feb,11

97760 **Orthotic(s) management and training (including assessment and fitting when not otherwise reported), upper extremity(ies), lower extremity(ies) and/or trunk, initial orthotic(s) encounter, each 15 minutes**

EXCLUDES *Gait training, if performed on the same extremity (97116)*

1.35 1.35 FUD XXX

AMA: 2018,May,5; 2018,Feb,11; 2018,Jan,8; 2017,Jan,8; 2016,Jan,13; 2015,Jan,16; 2014,Jan,11

97761 **Prosthetic(s) training, upper and/or lower extremity(ies), initial prosthetic(s) encounter, each 15 minutes**

1.16 1.16 FUD XXX

AMA: 2018,May,5; 2018,Feb,11; 2018,Jan,8; 2017,Jan,8; 2016,Jan,13; 2015,Jan,16; 2014,Jan,11

97763 **Orthotic(s)/prosthetic(s) management and/or training, upper extremity(ies), lower extremity(ies), and/or trunk, subsequent orthotic(s)/prosthetic(s) encounter, each 15 minutes**

EXCLUDES *Initial encounter for orthotics and prosthetics management and training (97760-97761)*

1.43 1.43 FUD XXX

AMA: 2018,May,5; 2018,Feb,11

97799 **Unlisted physical medicine/rehabilitation service or procedure**

0.00 0.00 FUD XXX

AMA: 2018,May,5; 2018,Feb,11; 2018,Jan,8; 2017,Jan,8; 2016,Nov,9; 2016,Jan,13; 2015,Jan,16; 2014,Jan,11

97802-97804 Medical Nutrition Therapy Services

CMS: 100-02,13,220 Preventive Health Services; 100-03,180.1 Medical Nutrition Therapy; 100-04,12,190.3 List of Telehealth Services; 100-04,12,190.6 Payment Methodology for Physician/Practitioner at the Distant Site ; 100-04,12,190.6.1 Submission of Telehealth Claims for Distant Site Practitioners; 100-04,12,190.7 Contractor Editing of Telehealth Claims; 100-04,4,300 Medical Nutrition Therapy Services; 100-04,4,300.6 CWF Edits for MNT/DSMT

EXCLUDES *Medical nutrition therapy assessment/intervention provided by physician or other qualified health care provider; use appropriate E&M codes*

97802 **Medical nutrition therapy; initial assessment and intervention, individual, face-to-face with the patient, each 15 minutes**

0.96 1.05 FUD XXX ★

AMA: 2018,Feb,11; 2018,Jan,8; 2017,Jan,8; 2016,Jan,13; 2015,Jan,16; 2014,Jan,11

97803 **re-assessment and intervention, individual, face-to-face with the patient, each 15 minutes**

0.82 0.91 FUD XXX ★

AMA: 2018,Feb,11; 2018,Jan,8; 2017,Jan,8; 2016,Jan,13; 2015,Jan,16; 2014,Jan,11

97804 **group (2 or more individual(s)), each 30 minutes**

0.45 0.48 FUD XXX ★

AMA: 2018,Feb,11; 2018,Jan,8; 2017,Jan,8; 2016,Jan,13; 2015,Jan,16; 2014,Jan,11

97810-97814 Acupuncture

CMS: 100-03,10.3 Inpatient Pain Rehabilitation Programs; 100-03,10.4 Outpatient Hospital Pain Rehabilitation Programs; 100-03,30.3 Acupuncture; 100-03,30.3.1 Acupuncture for Fibromyalgia; 100-03,30.3.2 Acupuncture for Osteoarthritis

INCLUDES 15 minute increments of face-to-face contact with the patient
Reporting only one code for each 15 minute increment

EXCLUDES *Insertion of needle without injection ([20560, 20561])*

Code also significant separately identifiable E&M service using modifier 25, when performed

97810 **Acupuncture, 1 or more needles; without electrical stimulation, initial 15 minutes of personal one-on-one contact with the patient**

EXCLUDES *Treatment with electrical stimulation (97813-97814)*

0.87 1.03 FUD XXX

AMA: 2018,Feb,11; 2018,Jan,8; 2017,Jan,8; 2016,Jan,13; 2015,Jan,16; 2014,Jan,11

\+ **97811** **without electrical stimulation, each additional 15 minutes of personal one-on-one contact with the patient, with re-insertion of needle(s) (List separately in addition to code for primary procedure)**

EXCLUDES *Treatment with electrical stimulation (97813-97814)*

Code first initial 15 minutes (97810)

0.72 0.78 FUD ZZZ

AMA: 2018,Feb,11; 2018,Jan,8; 2017,Jan,8; 2016,Jan,13; 2015,Jan,16; 2014,Jan,11

97813 **with electrical stimulation, initial 15 minutes of personal one-on-one contact with the patient**

EXCLUDES *Treatment without electrical stimulation (97813-97814)*

0.94 1.13 FUD XXX

AMA: 2018,Feb,11; 2018,Jan,8; 2017,Jan,8; 2016,Jan,13; 2015,Jan,16; 2014,Jan,11

\+ **97814** **with electrical stimulation, each additional 15 minutes of personal one-on-one contact with the patient, with re-insertion of needle(s) (List separately in addition to code for primary procedure)**

EXCLUDES *Treatment without electrical stimulation (97813-97814)*

Code first initial 15 minutes (97813)

0.79 0.91 FUD ZZZ

AMA: 2018,Feb,11; 2018,Jan,8; 2017,Jan,8; 2016,Jan,13; 2015,Jan,16; 2014,Jan,11

98925-98929 Osteopathic Manipulation

CMS: 100-03,150.1 Manipulation

INCLUDES Physician applied manual treatment done to eliminate/alleviate somatic dysfunction and related disorders using a variety of techniques
The following body regions:
- Abdomen/visceral region
- Cervical region
- Head region
- Lower extremities
- Lumbar region
- Pelvic region
- Rib cage region
- Sacral region
- Thoracic region
- Upper extremities

Code also significant separately identifiable E&M service using modifier 25, when performed

98925 **Osteopathic manipulative treatment (OMT); 1-2 body regions involved**

0.68 0.89 FUD 000

AMA: 2018,Aug,9; 2018,Feb,11; 2018,Jan,8; 2017,Dec,14; 2017,Jan,8; 2016,Jan,13; 2015,Jan,16; 2014,Jan,11

98926 **3-4 body regions involved**

1.02 1.28 FUD 000

AMA: 2018,Aug,9; 2018,Feb,11; 2018,Jan,8; 2017,Jan,8; 2016,Jan,13; 2015,Jan,16; 2014,Jan,11

98927 **5-6 body regions involved**

1.35 1.68 FUD 000

AMA: 2018,Aug,9; 2018,Feb,11; 2018,Jan,8; 2017,Jan,8; 2016,Jan,13; 2015,Jan,16; 2014,Jan,11

98928 **7-8 body regions involved**
1.69 2.04 FUD 000
AMA: 2018,Aug,9; 2018,Feb,11; 2018,Jan,8; 2017,Jan,8; 2016,Jan,13; 2015,Jan,16; 2014,Jan,11

98929 **9-10 body regions involved**
2.05 2.44 FUD 000
AMA: 2018,Aug,9; 2018,Feb,11; 2018,Jan,8; 2017,Jan,8; 2016,Jan,13; 2015,Jan,16; 2014,Jan,11

98940-98943 Chiropractic Manipulation

CMS: 100-01,5,70.6 Chiropractors; 100-02,15,240 Chiropractic Services - General; 100-02,15,240.1.3 Necessity for Treatment; 100-02,15,30.5 Chiropractor's Services; 100-03,150.1 Manipulation

INCLUDES Form of manual treatment performed to influence joint/neurophysical function
The following five extraspinal regions:
- Abdomen
- Head, including temporomandibular joint, excluding atlanto-occipital region
- Lower extremities
- Rib cage, not including costotransverse/costovertebral joints
- Upper extremities

The following five spinal regions:
- Cervical region (atlanto-occipital joint)
- Lumbar region
- Pelvic region (sacro-iliac joint)
- Sacral region
- Thoracic region (costovertebral/costotransverse joints)

Code also significant separately identifiable E&M service using modifier 25 when performed

98940 **Chiropractic manipulative treatment (CMT); spinal, 1-2 regions**
0.64 0.80 FUD 000
AMA: 2018,Nov,11; 2018,Feb,11; 2018,Jan,8; 2017,Jan,8; 2016,Jan,13; 2015,Jan,16; 2014,Jan,11

98941 **spinal, 3-4 regions**
0.98 1.16 FUD 000
AMA: 2018,Nov,11; 2018,Feb,11; 2018,Jan,8; 2017,Jan,8; 2016,Jan,13; 2015,Jan,16; 2014,Jan,11

98942 **spinal, 5 regions**
1.33 1.50 FUD 000
AMA: 2018,Nov,11; 2018,Feb,11; 2018,Jan,8; 2017,Jan,8; 2016,Jan,13; 2015,Jan,16; 2014,Jan,11

98943 **extraspinal, 1 or more regions**
0.67 0.77 FUD XXX
AMA: 2018,Nov,11; 2018,Feb,11; 2018,Jan,8; 2017,Jan,8; 2016,Jan,13; 2015,Jan,16; 2014,Jan,11

98960-98962 Self-Management Training

INCLUDES Education/training services:
- Prescribed by a physician or other qualified health care professional
- Provided by a qualified nonphysician health care provider

Standardized curriculum that may be modified as necessary for:
- Clinical needs
- Cultural norms
- Health literacy

Teaching the patient how to manage the illness/delay the comorbidity(s)

EXCLUDES *Genetic counseling education services (96040, 98961-98962)*
Health and behavior assessment and intervention (96156, 96158-96159, [96164, 96165], [96167, 96168], [96170, 96171])
Medical nutrition therapy (97802-97804)
The following services:
- *Counseling/education to a group (99078)*
- *Collection/interpretation of physiologic data ([99091])*
- *Complex chronic care management (99487, 99489)*
- *Counseling/risk factor reduction without symptoms/established disease (99401-99412)*
- *Physician supervision in home, domiciliary, or rest home (99339, 99340, 99374-99375, 99379-99380)*
- *Services provided with cumulative time of less than 5 minutes*
- *Services provided in which time would be reported with other services*
- *Supervision of hospice patient (99377-99378)*
- *Transitional care management (99495, 99496)*

98960 **Education and training for patient self-management by a qualified, nonphysician health care professional using a standardized curriculum, face-to-face with the patient (could include caregiver/family) each 30 minutes; individual patient**
0.77 0.77 FUD XXX ★
AMA: 2018,Aug,6; 2018,Feb,11; 2018,Jan,8; 2017,Jan,8; 2016,Jan,13; 2015,Jan,16; 2014,Oct,3; 2014,Jan,11

98961 **2-4 patients**
INCLUDES Group education regarding genetic risks
0.38 0.38 FUD XXX ★
AMA: 2018,Aug,6; 2018,Feb,11; 2018,Jan,8; 2017,Jan,8; 2016,Jan,13; 2015,Jan,16; 2014,Oct,3; 2014,Jan,11

98962 **5-8 patients**
INCLUDES Group education regarding genetic risks
0.28 0.28 FUD XXX ★
AMA: 2018,Aug,6; 2018,Feb,11; 2018,Jan,8; 2017,Jan,8; 2016,Jan,13; 2015,Jan,16; 2014,Oct,3; 2014,Jan,11

98966-98968 Nonphysician Telephone Services

INCLUDES Assessment and management services provided by telephone by a qualified health care professional
Episode of care initiated by an established patient or his/her guardian

EXCLUDES *Call initiated by the qualified health care professional*
Calls during the postoperative period of a procedure
Decision to see the patient at the next available urgent care appointment
Decision to see the patient within 24 hours of the call
Monitoring of INR (93792-93793)
Patient management services during same time frame as (99487-99489, 99495-99496)
Telephone services provided by a physician (99441-99443)
Telephone services that are considered a part of a previous or subsequent service
Use of codes if same codes billed within the past seven days

98966 **Telephone assessment and management service provided by a qualified nonphysician health care professional to an established patient, parent, or guardian not originating from a related assessment and management service provided within the previous 7 days nor leading to an assessment and management service or procedure within the next 24 hours or soonest available appointment; 5-10 minutes of medical discussion**
0.36 0.39 FUD XXX
AMA: 2018,Mar,7; 2018,Feb,11; 2018,Jan,8; 2017,Jan,8; 2016,Jan,13; 2015,Jan,16; 2014,Oct,3; 2014,Jan,11

98967 **11-20 minutes of medical discussion**
0.72 0.76 FUD XXX
AMA: 2018,Mar,7; 2018,Feb,11; 2018,Jan,8; 2017,Jan,8; 2016,Jan,13; 2015,Jan,16; 2014,Oct,3; 2014,Jan,11

98968 21-30 minutes of medical discussion
1.08 1.12 FUD XXX E
AMA: 2018,Mar,7; 2018,Feb,11; 2018,Jan,8; 2017,Jan,8; 2016,Jan,13; 2015,Jan,16; 2014,Oct,3; 2014,Jan,11

98969-98972 Nonphysician Online Service

Timely reply to the patient as well as:
- Ordering laboratory services
- Permanent record of the service; either hard copy or electronic
- Providing a prescription
- Related telephone calls

EXCLUDES *Monitoring of INR (93792-93793)*
Online digital assessment and management service provided by a qualified health care professional ([99421, 99422, 99423])
Online evaluation service:
- *Provided during the postoperative period of a procedure*
- *Provided more than once in a seven day period*
- *Related to a service provided in the previous seven days*
- *Provided with cumulative time of less than 5 minutes*
- *Where time would be reported as part of another service*

Patient management services during same time frame as:
- *Collection/interpretation of physiologic data ([99091])*
- *Complex chronic care management (99487-99489)*
- *Physician supervision in home, domiciliary, or rest home (99339-99340, 99374-99375, 99379-99380)*
- *Supervision of hospice patient (99377-99378)*
- *Transitional care management (99495-99496)*

98969 ~~Online assessment and management service provided by a qualified nonphysician health care professional to an established patient or guardian, not originating from a related assessment and management service provided within the previous 7 days, using the Internet or similar electronic communications network~~
To report, see (98970-98972)

● **98970** Qualified nonphysician health care professional online digital evaluation and management service, for an established patient, for up to 7 days, cumulative time during the 7 days; 5-10 minutes

● **98971** 11-20 minutes

● **98972** 21 or more minutes

99000-99091 Supplemental Services and Supplies

INCLUDES Supplemental reporting for services adjunct to the basic service provided

99000 Handling and/or conveyance of specimen for transfer from the office to a laboratory
0.00 0.00 FUD XXX E
AMA: 2018,Dec,10; 2018,Dec,10; 2018,Feb,11; 2018,Jan,8; 2017,Jan,8; 2016,Jan,13; 2015,Jan,16; 2014,Jan,11

99001 Handling and/or conveyance of specimen for transfer from the patient in other than an office to a laboratory (distance may be indicated)
0.00 0.00 FUD XXX E
AMA: 2018,Dec,10; 2018,Dec,10; 2018,Feb,11; 2018,Jan,8; 2017,Jan,8; 2016,Jan,13; 2015,Jan,16; 2014,Jan,11

99002 Handling, conveyance, and/or any other service in connection with the implementation of an order involving devices (eg, designing, fitting, packaging, handling, delivery or mailing) when devices such as orthotics, protectives, prosthetics are fabricated by an outside laboratory or shop but which items have been designed, and are to be fitted and adjusted by the attending physician or other qualified health care professional
EXCLUDES *Venous blood routine collection (36415)*
0.00 0.00 FUD XXX B
AMA: 2018,Dec,10; 2018,Dec,10; 2018,Feb,11; 2018,Jan,8; 2017,Jan,8; 2016,Jan,13; 2015,Jan,16; 2014,Jan,11

99024 Postoperative follow-up visit, normally included in the surgical package, to indicate that an evaluation and management service was performed during a postoperative period for a reason(s) related to the original procedure
0.00 0.00 FUD XXX B
AMA: 2018,Dec,10; 2018,Dec,10; 2018,Feb,11; 2018,Jan,8; 2017,Jul,9; 2017,Jan,3; 2017,Jan,8; 2016,Jan,13; 2015,Mar,3; 2015,Jan,16; 2014,Jan,11

99026 Hospital mandated on call service; in-hospital, each hour
EXCLUDES *Physician stand-by services with prolonged physician attendance (99360)*
Time spent providing procedures or services that may be separately reported
0.00 0.00 FUD XXX E
AMA: 2018,Dec,10; 2018,Dec,10; 2018,Feb,11; 2018,Jan,8; 2017,Jan,8; 2016,Jan,13; 2015,Jan,16; 2014,Jan,11

99027 out-of-hospital, each hour
EXCLUDES *Physician stand-by services with prolonged physician attendance (99360)*
Time spent providing procedures or services that may be separately reported
0.00 0.00 FUD XXX E
AMA: 2018,Dec,10; 2018,Dec,10; 2018,Feb,11; 2018,Jan,8; 2017,Jan,8; 2016,Jan,13; 2015,Jan,16; 2014,Jan,11

99050 Services provided in the office at times other than regularly scheduled office hours, or days when the office is normally closed (eg, holidays, Saturday or Sunday), in addition to basic service
Code also more than one adjunct code per encounter when appropriate
Code first basic service provided
0.00 0.00 FUD XXX Ⓢ B
AMA: 2018,Dec,10; 2018,Dec,10; 2018,Feb,11; 2018,Jan,8; 2017,Jan,8; 2016,Jan,13; 2015,Jan,16; 2014,Jan,11

99051 Service(s) provided in the office during regularly scheduled evening, weekend, or holiday office hours, in addition to basic service
Code also more than one adjunct code per encounter when appropriate
Code first basic service provided
0.00 0.00 FUD XXX Ⓢ B
AMA: 2018,Dec,10; 2018,Dec,10; 2018,Feb,11; 2018,Jan,8; 2017,Jan,8; 2016,Jan,13; 2015,Jan,16; 2014,Jan,11

99053 Service(s) provided between 10:00 PM and 8:00 AM at 24-hour facility, in addition to basic service
Code also more than one adjunct code per encounter when appropriate
Code first basic service provided
0.00 0.00 FUD XXX Ⓢ B
AMA: 2018,Dec,10; 2018,Dec,10; 2018,Feb,11; 2018,Jan,8; 2017,Jan,8; 2016,Jan,13; 2015,Jan,16; 2014,Jan,11

99056 Service(s) typically provided in the office, provided out of the office at request of patient, in addition to basic service
Code also more than one adjunct code per encounter when appropriate
Code first basic service provided
0.00 0.00 FUD XXX Ⓢ B
AMA: 2018,Dec,10; 2018,Dec,10; 2018,Feb,11; 2018,Jan,8; 2017,Jan,8; 2016,Jan,13; 2015,Jan,16; 2014,Jan,11

99058 Service(s) provided on an emergency basis in the office, which disrupts other scheduled office services, in addition to basic service
Code also more than one adjunct code per encounter when appropriate
Code first basic service provided
0.00 0.00 FUD XXX Ⓢ B
AMA: 2018,Dec,10; 2018,Dec,10; 2018,Feb,11; 2018,Jan,8; 2017,Jan,8; 2016,Jan,13; 2015,Jan,16; 2014,Jan,11

99060 **Service(s) provided on an emergency basis, out of the office, which disrupts other scheduled office services, in addition to basic service**

Code also more than one adjunct code per encounter when appropriate

Code first basic service provided

0.00 0.00 FUD XXX

AMA: 2018,Dec,10; 2018,Dec,10; 2018,Feb,11; 2018,Jan,8; 2017,Jan,8; 2016,Jan,13; 2015,Jan,16; 2014,Jan,11

99070 **Supplies and materials (except spectacles), provided by the physician or other qualified health care professional over and above those usually included with the office visit or other services rendered (list drugs, trays, supplies, or materials provided)**

EXCLUDES *Spectacles supply*

0.00 0.00 FUD XXX

AMA: 2019,Apr,10; 2019,Feb,10; 2018,Dec,10; 2018,Dec,10; 2018,Jun,11; 2018,Mar,7; 2018,Jan,8; 2018,Jan,3; 2017,Sep,14; 2017,Jan,6; 2017,Jan,8; 2016,Jan,13; 2015,Jan,16; 2014,Mar,11; 2014,Jan,11

99071 **Educational supplies, such as books, tapes, and pamphlets, for the patient's education at cost to physician or other qualified health care professional**

0.00 0.00 FUD XXX

AMA: 2018,Dec,10; 2018,Dec,10; 2018,Jan,8; 2017,Jan,8; 2016,Jan,13; 2015,Jan,16; 2014,Oct,3; 2014,Jan,11

99075 **Medical testimony**

0.00 0.00 FUD XXX

AMA: 2018,Dec,10; 2018,Dec,10; 2018,Jan,8; 2017,Jan,8; 2016,Jan,13; 2015,Jan,16; 2014,Jan,11

99078 **Physician or other qualified health care professional qualified by education, training, licensure/regulation (when applicable) educational services rendered to patients in a group setting (eg, prenatal, obesity, or diabetic instructions)**

0.00 0.00 FUD XXX

AMA: 2018,Dec,10; 2018,Dec,10; 2018,Jan,8; 2017,Jan,8; 2016,Jan,13; 2015,Jan,16; 2014,Oct,3; 2014,Jan,11

99080 **Special reports such as insurance forms, more than the information conveyed in the usual medical communications or standard reporting form**

EXCLUDES *Completion of workmen's compensation forms (99455-99456)*

0.00 0.00 FUD XXX

AMA: 2018,Dec,10; 2018,Dec,10; 2018,Jan,8; 2017,Jan,8; 2016,Jan,13; 2015,Jan,16; 2014,Oct,3; 2014,Jan,11

99082 **Unusual travel (eg, transportation and escort of patient)**

0.00 0.00 FUD XXX

AMA: 2018,Dec,10; 2018,Dec,10; 2018,Jan,8; 2017,Jan,8; 2016,Jan,13; 2015,Jan,16; 2014,Jan,11

99091 **Resequenced code. See code following resequenced code 99454.**

99100-99140 Modifying Factors for Anesthesia Services

CMS: 100-04,12,140.3 Payment for Qualified Nonphysician Anesthetists; 100-04,12,140.3.3 Billing Modifiers; 100-04,12,140.3.4 General Billing Instructions; 100-04,12,140.4.1 Anesthesiologist/Qualified Nonphysican Anesthetist; 100-04,12,140.4.2 Anesthetist and Anesthesiologist in a Single Procedure; 100-04,12,140.4.4 Conversion Factors for Anesthesia Services; 100-04,4,250.3.2 Anesthesia in a Hospital Outpatient Setting

Code first primary anesthesia procedure

\+ **99100** **Anesthesia for patient of extreme age, younger than 1 year and older than 70 (List separately in addition to code for primary anesthesia procedure)**

EXCLUDES *Anesthesia services for infants one year old or less at the time of surgery (00326, 00561, 00834, 00836)*

0.00 0.00 FUD ZZZ

AMA: 2018,Jan,8; 2017,Dec,8; 2017,Jan,8; 2016,Jan,13; 2015,Jan,16; 2014,Jan,11

\+ **99116** **Anesthesia complicated by utilization of total body hypothermia (List separately in addition to code for primary anesthesia procedure)**

EXCLUDES *Anesthesia for procedures on heart/pericardial sac/great vessels of chest with pump oxygenator (00561)*

0.00 0.00 FUD ZZZ

AMA: 2018,Jan,8; 2017,Dec,8; 2017,Jan,8; 2016,Jan,13; 2015,Jan,16; 2014,Jan,11

\+ **99135** **Anesthesia complicated by utilization of controlled hypotension (List separately in addition to code for primary anesthesia procedure)**

EXCLUDES *Anesthesia for procedures on heart/pericardial sac/great vessels of chest with pump oxygenator (00561)*

0.00 0.00 FUD ZZZ

AMA: 2018,Jan,8; 2017,Dec,8; 2017,Jan,8; 2016,Jan,13; 2015,Jan,16; 2014,Jan,11

\+ **99140** **Anesthesia complicated by emergency conditions (specify) (List separately in addition to code for primary anesthesia procedure)**

INCLUDES Conditions where postponement of treatment could be dangerous to life or health

0.00 0.00 FUD ZZZ

AMA: 2018,Jan,8; 2017,Dec,8; 2017,Jan,8; 2016,Jan,13; 2015,Jan,16; 2014,Jan,11

99151-99157 Moderate Sedation Services

INCLUDES Intraservice work that begins with administration of the sedation drugs and ends when the procedure is over
Monitoring of:
Patient response to the drugs
Vital signs
Ordering and providing the drug to the patient (first and subsequent)
Pre- and postservice procedures

99151 **Moderate sedation services provided by the same physician or other qualified health care professional performing the diagnostic or therapeutic service that the sedation supports, requiring the presence of an independent trained observer to assist in the monitoring of the patient's level of consciousness and physiological status; initial 15 minutes of intraservice time, patient younger than 5 years of age**

INCLUDES First 15 minutes of intraservice time for patients under age 5
Services provided to patients by same provider of the service for which moderate sedation is necessary with monitoring by a trained observer

0.70 2.20 FUD XXX

AMA: 2019,Feb,10; 2018,Jan,8; 2017,Sep,11; 2017,Jun,3; 2017,Jan,3

99152 **initial 15 minutes of intraservice time, patient age 5 years or older**

INCLUDES First 15 minutes of intraservice time for patients age 5 and over
Services provided to patients by same provider of the service for which moderate sedation is necessary with monitoring by a trained observer

0.36 1.46 FUD XXX

AMA: 2019,May,10; 2019,Feb,10; 2018,Jan,8; 2017,Sep,11; 2017,Jun,3; 2017,Jan,3

\+ **99153** **each additional 15 minutes intraservice time (List separately in addition to code for primary service)**

INCLUDES Services provided to patients by same provider of the service for which moderate sedation is necessary with monitoring by a trained observer (99155-99157)

EXCLUDES *Services provided to patients by a physician/other qualified health care professional other than the provider rendering the service*

Code first (99151-99152)

0.31 0.31 FUD ZZZ

AMA: 2019,May,10; 2019,Feb,10; 2018,Jan,8; 2017,Sep,11; 2017,Jun,3; 2017,Jan,3

99155 **Moderate sedation services provided by a physician or other qualified health care professional other than the physician or other qualified health care professional performing the diagnostic or therapeutic service that the sedation supports; initial 15 minutes of intraservice time, patient younger than 5 years of age**

INCLUDES First 15 minutes of intraservice time for patients under age 5
Services provided to patients by a physician/other qualified health care professional other than the provider rendering the service for which moderate sedation is necessary

2.74 2.74 FUD XXX N

AMA: 2019,Feb,10; 2018,Jan,8; 2017,Sep,11; 2017,Jun,3; 2017,Jan,3

99156 **initial 15 minutes of intraservice time, patient age 5 years or older**

INCLUDES First 15 minutes of intraservice time for patients age 5 and over
Services provided to patients by a physician/other qualified health care professional other than the provider rendering the service for which moderate sedation is necessary

2.15 2.15 FUD XXX N

AMA: 2019,Feb,10; 2018,Jan,8; 2017,Sep,11; 2017,Jun,3; 2017,Jan,3

\+ 99157 **each additional 15 minutes intraservice time (List separately in addition to code for primary service)**

INCLUDES Each subsequent 15 minutes of services
Services provided to patients by a physician/other qualified health care professional other than the provider rendering the service for which moderate sedation is necessary (99151-99152)

EXCLUDES *Services provided to patients by same provider of the service for which moderate sedation is necessary with monitoring by a trained observer (99151-99152)*

Code first (99155-99156)

1.64 1.64 FUD ZZZ N

AMA: 2019,Feb,10; 2018,Jan,8; 2017,Sep,11; 2017,Jun,3; 2017,Jan,3

99170 Specialized Examination of Child

EXCLUDES *Moderate sedation (99151-99157)*

99170 **Anogenital examination, magnified, in childhood for suspected trauma, including image recording when performed** A

2.47 4.48 FUD 000 T

AMA: 2018,Jan,8; 2017,Jan,8; 2016,Jan,13; 2015,Jan,16; 2014,Sep,7; 2014,Jan,11

99172-99173 Visual Acuity Screening Tests

INCLUDES Graduated visual acuity stimuli that allow a quantitative determination/estimation of visual acuity

EXCLUDES *General ophthalmological or E&M services*

99172 **Visual function screening, automated or semi-automated bilateral quantitative determination of visual acuity, ocular alignment, color vision by pseudoisochromatic plates, and field of vision (may include all or some screening of the determination[s] for contrast sensitivity, vision under glare)**

EXCLUDES *Screening for visual acuity, amblyogenic factors, retinal polarization scan (99173, 99174 [99177], 0469T)*

0.00 0.00 FUD XXX E

AMA: 2018,Jan,8; 2017,Jan,8; 2016,Jan,13; 2015,Jan,16; 2014,Jan,11

99173 **Screening test of visual acuity, quantitative, bilateral**

EXCLUDES *Screening for visual function, amblyogenic factors (99172, 99174, [99177])*

0.08 0.08 FUD XXX E

AMA: 2018,Jan,8; 2017,Jan,8; 2016,Jan,13; 2015,Jan,16; 2014,Jan,11

99174-99177 [99177] Screening For Amblyogenic Factors

EXCLUDES *General ophthalmological services (92002-92014)*
Screening for visual acuity (99172-99173, [99177])

99174 **Instrument-based ocular screening (eg, photoscreening, automated-refraction), bilateral; with remote analysis and report**

EXCLUDES *Ocular screening on-site analysis ([99177])*

0.16 0.16 FUD XXX E

AMA: 2018,Feb,3; 2018,Jan,8; 2017,Jan,8; 2016,Mar,10; 2016,Jan,13; 2015,Jan,16; 2014,Jan,11

\# 99177 **with on-site analysis**

EXCLUDES *Remote ocular screening (99174)*
Retinal polarization scan (0469T)

0.13 0.13 FUD XXX E

AMA: 2018,Feb,3; 2018,Jan,8; 2017,Jan,8; 2016,Mar,10

99175-99177 Drug Administration to Induce Vomiting

EXCLUDES *Diagnostic gastric lavage (43754-43755)*
Diagnostic gastric intubation (43754-43755)

99175 **Ipecac or similar administration for individual emesis and continued observation until stomach adequately emptied of poison**

0.73 0.73 FUD XXX N 80

AMA: 1997,Nov,1

99177 **Resequenced code. See code following 99174.**

99183-99184 Hyperbaric Oxygen Therapy

CMS: 100-03,20.29 Hyperbaric Oxygen Therapy; 100-04,32,30.1 HBO Therapy for Lower Extremity Diabetic Wounds

EXCLUDES *E&M services, when performed*
Other procedures such as wound debridement, when performed

99183 **Physician or other qualified health care professional attendance and supervision of hyperbaric oxygen therapy, per session**

3.12 3.12 FUD XXX B 80 26

AMA: 2018,Jan,8; 2017,Jan,8; 2016,Jan,13; 2015,Jan,16; 2014,Jan,11

99184 **Initiation of selective head or total body hypothermia in the critically ill neonate, includes appropriate patient selection by review of clinical, imaging and laboratory data, confirmation of esophageal temperature probe location, evaluation of amplitude EEG, supervision of controlled hypothermia, and assessment of patient tolerance of cooling** A

EXCLUDES *Use of code more than one time per hospitalization*

6.33 6.33 FUD XXX C 80

AMA: 2018,Jan,8; 2017,Jan,8; 2016,Jan,13; 2015,Oct,8

99188 Topical Fluoride Application

99188 **Application of topical fluoride varnish by a physician or other qualified health care professional**

0.29 0.35 FUD XXX E 80

99190-99192 Assemble and Manage Pump with Oxygenator/Heat Exchange

99190 **Assembly and operation of pump with oxygenator or heat exchanger (with or without ECG and/or pressure monitoring); each hour**

0.00 0.00 FUD XXX C

AMA: 1997,Nov,1

99191 **45 minutes**

0.00 0.00 FUD XXX C

AMA: 1997,Nov,1

99192 **30 minutes**

0.00 0.00 FUD XXX C

AMA: 1997,Nov,1

Medicine

99155 — 99192

99195-99199 Therapeutic Phlebotomy and Unlisted Procedures

99195 **Phlebotomy, therapeutic (separate procedure)**
2.86 2.86 FUD XXX Q1 80
AMA: 2018,Jan,8; 2017,Jan,8; 2016,Jan,13; 2015,Jan,16; 2014,Jan,11

99199 **Unlisted special service, procedure or report**
0.00 0.00 FUD XXX B 80
AMA: 2018,Jan,8; 2017,Jan,8; 2016,Jan,13; 2015,Jan,16; 2014,Jan,11

99500-99602 Home Visit By Non-Physician Professionals

INCLUDES Services performed by non-physician providers
Services provided in patient's:
- Assisted living apartment
- Custodial care facility
- Group home
- Non-traditional private home
- Residence
- School

EXCLUDES *Home visits performed by physicians (99341-99350)*
Other services/procedures provided by physicians to patients at home

Code also home visit E&M codes if health care provider is authorized to use (99341-99350)
Code also significant separately identifiable E&M service, when performed

99500 **Home visit for prenatal monitoring and assessment to include fetal heart rate, non-stress test, uterine monitoring, and gestational diabetes monitoring** M ♀
0.00 0.00 FUD XXX E
AMA: 2018,Jan,8; 2017,Jan,8; 2016,Jan,13; 2015,Jan,16; 2014,Jan,11

99501 **Home visit for postnatal assessment and follow-up care** M ♀
0.00 0.00 FUD XXX E
AMA: 2018,Jan,8; 2017,Jan,8; 2016,Jan,13; 2015,Jan,16; 2014,Jan,11

99502 **Home visit for newborn care and assessment** A
0.00 0.00 FUD XXX E
AMA: 2018,Jan,8; 2017,Jan,8; 2016,Jan,13; 2015,Jan,16; 2014,Jan,11

99503 **Home visit for respiratory therapy care (eg, bronchodilator, oxygen therapy, respiratory assessment, apnea evaluation)**
0.00 0.00 FUD XXX E
AMA: 2018,Jan,8; 2017,Jan,8; 2016,Jan,13; 2015,Jan,16; 2014,Jan,11

99504 **Home visit for mechanical ventilation care**
0.00 0.00 FUD XXX E
AMA: 2018,Jan,8; 2017,Jan,8; 2016,Jan,13; 2015,Jan,16; 2014,Jan,11

99505 **Home visit for stoma care and maintenance including colostomy and cystostomy**
0.00 0.00 FUD XXX E
AMA: 2018,Jan,8; 2017,Jan,8; 2016,Jan,13; 2015,Jan,16; 2014,Jan,11

99506 **Home visit for intramuscular injections**
0.00 0.00 FUD XXX E
AMA: 2018,Jan,8; 2017,Jan,8; 2016,Jan,13; 2015,Jan,16; 2014,Jan,11

99507 **Home visit for care and maintenance of catheter(s) (eg, urinary, drainage, and enteral)**
0.00 0.00 FUD XXX E
AMA: 2018,Jan,8; 2017,Jan,8; 2016,Jan,13; 2015,Jan,16; 2014,Jan,11

99509 **Home visit for assistance with activities of daily living and personal care**
EXCLUDES *Medical nutrition therapy/assessment home services (97802-97804)*
Self-care/home management training (97535)
Speech therapy home services (92507-92508)
0.00 0.00 FUD XXX E
AMA: 2018,Jan,8; 2017,Jan,8; 2016,Jan,13; 2015,Jan,16; 2014,Jan,11

99510 **Home visit for individual, family, or marriage counseling**
0.00 0.00 FUD XXX E
AMA: 2018,Jan,8; 2017,Jan,8; 2016,Jan,13; 2015,Jan,16; 2014,Jan,11

99511 **Home visit for fecal impaction management and enema administration**
0.00 0.00 FUD XXX E
AMA: 2018,Jan,8; 2017,Jan,8; 2016,Jan,13; 2015,Jan,16; 2014,Jan,11

99512 **Home visit for hemodialysis**
EXCLUDES *Peritoneal dialysis home infusion (99601-99602)*
0.00 0.00 FUD XXX E
AMA: 2018,Jan,8; 2017,Jan,8; 2016,Jan,13; 2015,Jan,16; 2014,Jan,11

99600 **Unlisted home visit service or procedure**
0.00 0.00 FUD XXX E
AMA: 2018,Jan,8; 2017,Jan,8; 2016,Jan,13; 2015,Jan,16; 2014,Jan,11

99601 **Home infusion/specialty drug administration, per visit (up to 2 hours);**
0.00 0.00 FUD XXX E
AMA: 2005,Nov,1-9; 2003,Oct,7

\+ **99602** **each additional hour (List separately in addition to code for primary procedure)**
Code first (99601)
0.00 0.00 FUD XXX E
AMA: 2005,Nov,1-9; 2003,Oct,7

99605-99607 Medication Management By Pharmacist

INCLUDES Direct (face-to-face) assessment and intervention by a pharmacist for the purpose of:
- Managing medication complications and/or interactions
- Maximizing the patient's response to drug therapy

Documenting the following required elements:
- Advice given regarding improvement of treatment compliance and outcomes
- Profile of medications (prescription and nonprescription)
- Review of applicable patient history

EXCLUDES *Routine tasks associated with dispensing and related activities (e.g., providing product information)*

99605 **Medication therapy management service(s) provided by a pharmacist, individual, face-to-face with patient, with assessment and intervention if provided; initial 15 minutes, new patient**
0.00 0.00 FUD XXX E
AMA: 2018,Apr,9; 2018,Jan,8; 2017,Jan,8; 2016,Jan,13; 2015,Jan,16; 2014,Oct,3; 2014,Jan,11

99606 **initial 15 minutes, established patient**
0.00 0.00 FUD XXX E
AMA: 2018,Apr,9; 2018,Jan,8; 2017,Jan,8; 2016,Jan,13; 2015,Jan,16; 2014,Oct,3; 2014,Jan,11

\+ **99607** **each additional 15 minutes (List separately in addition to code for primary service)**
Code first (99605, 99606)
0.00 0.00 FUD XXX E
AMA: 2018,Apr,9; 2018,Jan,8; 2017,Jan,8; 2016,Jan,13; 2015,Jan,16; 2014,Oct,3; 2014,Jan,11

Evaluation and Management (E/M) Services Guidelines

Information unique to this section is defined or identified below.

For additional information about evaluation and management services, see Appendix C: Evaluation and Management Extended Guidelines. This appendix includes comprehensive explanations and instructions for the correct selection of an E&M service code based on federal documentation standards.

Classification of Evaluation and Management (E/M) Services

The E/M section is divided into broad categories such as office visits, hospital visits, and consultations. Most of the categories are further divided into two or more subcategories of E/M services. For example, there are two subcategories of office visits (new patient and established patient) and there are two subcategories of hospital visits (initial and subsequent). The subcategories of E/M services are further classified into levels of E/M services that are identified by specific codes. This classification is important because the nature of work varies by type of service, place of service, and the patient's status.

The basic format of the levels of E/M services is the same for most categories. First, a unique code number is listed. Second, the place and/or type of service is specified, eg, office consultation. Third, the content of the service is defined, eg, comprehensive history and comprehensive examination. (See "Levels of E/M Services," for details on the content of E/M services.) Fourth, the nature of the presenting problem(s) usually associated with a given level is described. Fifth, the time typically required to provide the service is specified. (A detailed discussion of time is provided separately.)

Definitions of Commonly Used Terms

Certain key words and phrases are used throughout the E/M section. The following definitions are intended to reduce the potential for differing interpretations and to increase the consistency of reporting by physicians in differing specialties. E/M services may also be reported by other qualified health care professionals who are authorized to perform such services within the scope of their practice.

New and Established Patient

Solely for the purposes of distinguishing between new and established patients, professional services are those face-to-face services rendered by physicians and other qualified health care professionals who may report E/M services with a specific CPT® code or codes. A new patient is one who has not received any professional services from the physician/qualified health care professional or another physician/qualified health care professional of the exact same specialty and subspecialty who belongs to the same group practice, within the past three years.

An established patient is one who has received professional services from the physician/qualified health care professional or another physician/qualified health care professional of the exact same specialty and subspecialty who belongs to the same group practice, within the past three years. See the decision tree at right.

When a physician/qualified health care professional is on call or covering for another physician/qualified health care professional, the patient's encounter is classified as it would have been by the physician/qualified health care professional who is not available. When advanced practice nurses and physician assistants are working with physicians, they are considered as working in the exact same specialty and exact same subspecialties as the physician.

No distinction is made between new and established patients in the emergency department. E/M services in the emergency department category may be reported for any new or established patient who presents for treatment in the emergency department.

The decision tree in the next column is provided to aid in determining whether to report the E/M service provided as a new or an established patient encounter.

Chief Complaint

A chief complaint is a concise statement describing the symptom, problem, condition, diagnosis, or other factor that is the reason for the encounter, usually stated in the patient's words.

Concurrent Care and Transfer of Care

Concurrent care is the provision of similar services (e.g., hospital visits) to the same patient by more than one physician or other qualified health care professional on the same day. When concurrent care is provided, no special reporting is required. Transfer of care is the process whereby a physician or other qualified health care professional who is managing some or all of a patient's problems relinquishes this responsibility to another physician or other qualified health care professional who explicitly agrees to accept this responsibility and who, from the initial encounter, is not providing consultative services. The physician or other qualified health care professional transferring care is then no longer providing care for these problems though he or she may continue providing care for other conditions when appropriate. Consultation codes should not be reported by the physician or other qualified health care professional who has agreed to accept transfer of care before an initial evaluation, but they are appropriate to report if the decision to accept transfer of care cannot be made until after the initial consultation evaluation, regardless of site of service.

Decision Tree for New vs Established Patients

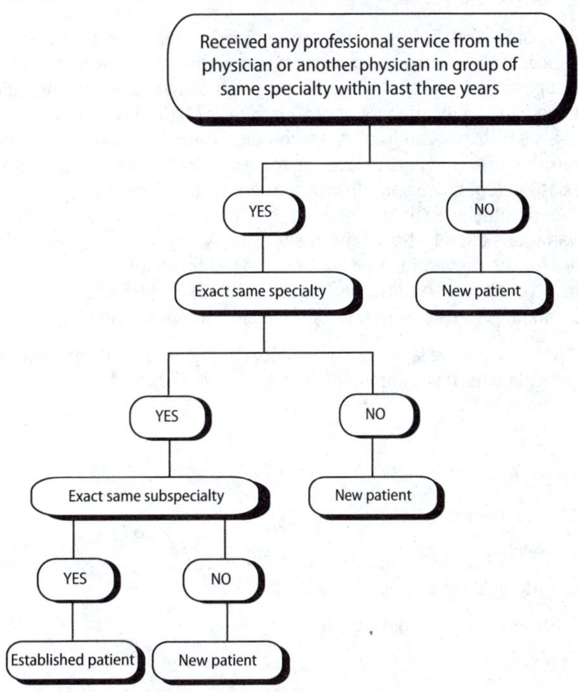

Counseling

Counseling is a discussion with a patient and/or family concerning one or more of the following areas:

- Diagnostic results, impressions, and/or recommended diagnostic studies
- Prognosis
- Risks and benefits of management (treatment) options
- Instructions for management (treatment) and/or follow-up
- Importance of compliance with chosen management (treatment) options
- Risk factor reduction
- Patient and family education (For psychotherapy, see 90832–90834, 90836–90840)

Family History

A review of medical events in the patient's family that includes significant information about:

- The health status or cause of death of parents, siblings, and children
- Specific diseases related to problems identified in the Chief Complaint or History of the Present Illness, and/or System Review
- Diseases of family members that may be hereditary or place the patient at risk

History of Present Illness

A chronological description of the development of the patient's present illness from the first sign and/or symptom to the present. This includes a description of location, quality, severity, timing, context, modifying factors, and associated signs and symptoms significantly related to the presenting problem(s).

Levels of E/M Services

Within each category or subcategory of E/M service, there are three to five levels of E/M services available for reporting purposes. Levels of E/M services are not interchangeable among the different categories or subcategories of service. For example, the first level of E/M services in the subcategory of office visit, new patient, does not have the same definition as the first level of E/M services in the subcategory of office visit, established patient.

The levels of E/M services include examinations, evaluations, treatments, conferences with or concerning patients, preventive pediatric and adult health supervision, and similar medical services, such as the determination of the need and/or location for appropriate care. Medical screening includes the history, examination, and medical decision-making required to determine the need and/or location for appropriate care and treatment of the patient (eg, office and other outpatient setting, emergency department, nursing facility). The levels of E/M services encompass the wide variations in skill, effort, time, responsibility, and medical knowledge required for the prevention or diagnosis and treatment of illness or injury and the promotion of optimal health. Each level of E/M services may be used by all physicians or other qualified health care professionals.

The descriptors for the levels of E/M services recognize seven components, six of which are used in defining the levels of E/M services. These components are:

- History
- Examination
- Medical decision making
- Counseling
- Coordination of care
- Nature of presenting problem
- Time

The first three of these components (history, examination, and medical decision making) are considered the key components in selecting a level of E/M services. (See "Determine the Extent of History Obtained.")

The next three components (counseling, coordination of care, and the nature of the presenting problem) are considered contributory factors in the majority of encounters. Although the first two of these contributory factors are important E/M services, it is not required that these services be provided at every patient encounter.

Coordination of care with other physicians, other qualified health care professionals, or agencies without a patient encounter on that day is reported using the case management codes.

The final component, time, is discussed in detail below.

Any specifically identifiable procedure (ie, identified with a specific CPT code) performed on or subsequent to the date of initial or subsequent E/M services should be reported separately.

The actual performance and/or interpretation of diagnostic tests/studies ordered during a patient encounter are not included in the levels of E/M services. Physician performance of diagnostic tests/studies for which specific CPT codes are available may be reported separately, in addition to the appropriate E/M code. The physician's interpretation of the results of diagnostic tests/studies (ie, professional component) with preparation of a separate distinctly identifiable signed written report may also be reported separately, using the appropriate CPT code with modifier 26 appended.

The physician or other health care professional may need to indicate that on the day a procedure or service identified by a CPT code was performed, the patient's condition required a significant separately identifiable E/M service above and beyond other services provided or beyond the usual preservice and postservice care associated with the procedure that was performed. The E/M service may be caused or prompted by the symptoms or condition for which the procedure and/or service was provided. This circumstance may be reported by adding modifier 25 to the appropriate level of E/M service. As such, different diagnoses are not required for reporting of the procedure and the E/M services on the same date.

Nature of Presenting Problem

A presenting problem is a disease, condition, illness, injury, symptom, sign, finding, complaint, or other reason for encounter, with or without a diagnosis being established at the time of the encounter. The E/M codes recognize five types of presenting problems that are defined as follows:

Minimal: A problem that may not require the presence of the physician or other qualified health care professional, but service is provided under the physician's or other qualified health care professional's supervision.

Self-limited or minor: A problem that runs a definite and prescribed course, is transient in nature, and is not likely to permanently alter health status OR has a good prognosis with management/compliance.

Low severity: A problem where the risk of morbidity without treatment is low; there is little to no risk of mortality without treatment; full recovery without functional impairment is expected.

Moderate severity: A problem where the risk of morbidity without treatment is moderate; there is moderate risk of mortality without treatment; uncertain prognosis OR increased probability of prolonged functional impairment.

High severity: A problem where the risk of morbidity without treatment is high to extreme; there is a moderate to high risk of mortality without treatment OR high probability of severe, prolonged functional impairment.

Past History

A review of the patient's past experiences with illnesses, injuries, and treatments that includes significant information about:

- Prior major illnesses and injuries
- Prior operations
- Prior hospitalizations
- Current medications
- Allergies (eg, drug, food)
- Age appropriate immunization status
- Age appropriate feeding/dietary status

Social History

An age appropriate review of past and current activities that includes significant information about:

- Marital status and/or living arrangements
- Current employment
- Occupational history
- Military history
- Use of drugs, alcohol, and tobacco
- Level of education
- Sexual history
- Other relevant social factors

System Review (Review of Systems)
An inventory of body systems obtained through a series of questions seeking to identify signs and/or symptoms that the patient may be experiencing or has experienced. For the purposes of the CPT codebook the following elements of a system review have been identified:

- Constitutional symptoms (fever, weight loss, etc)
- Eyes
- Ears, nose, mouth, throat
- Cardiovascular
- Respiratory
- Gastrointestinal
- Genitourinary
- Musculoskeletal
- Integumentary (skin and/or breast)
- Neurological
- Psychiatric
- Endocrine
- Hematologic/lymphatic
- Allergic/immunologic

The review of systems helps define the problem, clarify the differential diagnosis, identify needed testing, or serves as baseline data on other systems that might be affected by any possible management options.

Time
The inclusion of time in the definitions of levels of E/M services has been implicit in prior editions of the CPT codebook. The inclusion of time as an explicit factor beginning in *CPT 1992* is done to assist in selecting the most appropriate level of E/M services. It should be recognized that the specific times expressed in the visit code descriptors are averages and, therefore, represent a range of times that may be higher or lower depending on actual clinical circumstances.

Time is not a descriptive component for the emergency department levels of E/M services because emergency department services are typically provided on a variable intensity basis, often involving multiple encounters with several patients over an extended period of time. Therefore, it is often difficult to provide accurate estimates of the time spent face-to-face with the patient.

Studies to establish levels of E/M services employed surveys of practicing physicians to obtain data on the amount of time and work associated with typical E/M services. Since "work" is not easily quantifiable, the codes must rely on other objective, verifiable measures that correlate with physicians' estimates of their "work." It has been demonstrated that estimations of intraservice time, both within and across specialties, is a variable that is predictive of the "work" of E/M services. This same research has shown there is a strong relationship between intraservice time and total time for E/M services. Intraservice time, rather than total time, was chosen for inclusion with the codes because of its relative ease of measurement and because of its direct correlation with measurements of the total amount of time and work associated with typical E/M services.

Intraservice times are defined as face-to-face time for office and other outpatient visits and as unit/floor time for hospital and other inpatient visits. This distinction is necessary because most of the work of typical office visits takes place during the face-to-face time with the patient, while most of the work of typical hospital visits takes place during the time spent on the patient's floor or unit. When prolonged time occurs in either the office or the inpatient areas, the appropriate add-on code should be reported.

Face-to-face time (office and other outpatient visits and office consultations): For coding purposes, face-to-face time for these services is defined as only that time spent face-to-face with the patient and/or family. This includes the time spent performing such tasks as obtaining a history, performing an examination, and counseling the patient.

Time is also spent doing work before or after the face-to-face time with the patient, performing such tasks as reviewing records and tests, arranging for further services, and communicating further with other professionals and the patient through written reports and telephone contact.

This non-face-to-face time for office services—also called pre- and postencounter time—is not included in the time component described in the E/M codes. However, the pre- and post-non-face-to-face work associated with an encounter was included in calculating the total work of typical services in physician surveys.

Thus, the face-to-face time associated with the services described by any E/M code is a valid proxy for the total work done before, during, and after the visit.

Unit/floor time (hospital observation services, inpatient hospital care, initial inpatient hospital consultations, nursing facility): For reporting purposes, intraservice time for these services is defined as unit/floor time, which includes the time present on the patient's hospital unit and at the bedside rendering services for that patient. This includes the time to establish and/or review the patient's chart, examine the patient, write notes, and communicate with other professionals and the patient's family.

In the hospital, pre- and post-time includes time spent off the patient's floor performing such tasks as reviewing pathology and radiology findings in another part of the hospital.

This pre- and postvisit time is not included in the time component described in these codes. However, the pre- and postwork performed during the time spent off the floor or unit was included in calculating the total work of typical services in physician surveys.

Thus, the unit/floor time associated with the services described by any code is a valid proxy for the total work done before, during, and after the visit.

Unlisted Service
An E/M service may be provided that is not listed in this section of the CPT codebook. When reporting such a service, the appropriate unlisted code may be used to indicate the service, identifying it by "Special Report," as discussed in the following paragraph. The "Unlisted Services" and accompanying codes for the E/M section are as follows:

99429	**Unlisted preventive medicine service**
99499	**Unlisted evaluation and management service**

Special Report
An unlisted service or one that is unusual, variable, or new may require a special report demonstrating the medical appropriateness of the service. Pertinent information should include an adequate definition or description of the nature, extent, and need for the procedure and the time, effort, and equipment necessary to provide the service. Additional items that may be included are complexity of symptoms, final diagnosis, pertinent physical findings, diagnostic and therapeutic procedures, concurrent problems, and follow-up care.

Instructions for Selecting a Level of E/M Service

Review the Reporting Instructions for the Selected Category or Subcategory
Most of the categories and many of the subcategories of service have special guidelines or instructions unique to that category or subcategory. Where these are indicated, eg, "Inpatient Hospital Care," special instructions will be presented preceding the levels of E/M services.

Review the Level of E/M Service Descriptors and Examples in the Selected Category or Subcategory
The descriptors for the levels of E/M services recognize seven components, six of which are used in defining the levels of E/M services. These components are:

- History
- Examination
- Medical decision making

- Counseling
- Coordination of care
- Nature of presenting problem
- Time

The first three of these components (ie, history, examination, and medical decision making) should be considered the key components in selecting the level of E/M services. An exception to this rule is in the case of visits that consist predominantly of counseling or coordination of care.

The nature of the presenting problem and time are provided in some levels to assist the physician in determining the appropriate level of E/M service.

Determine the Extent of History Obtained

The extent of the history is dependent upon clinical judgment and on the nature of the presenting problem(s). The levels of E/M services recognize four types of history that are defined as follows:

Problem focused: Chief complaint; brief history of present illness or problem.

Expanded problem focused: Chief complaint; brief history of present illness; problem pertinent system review.

Detailed: Chief complaint; extended history of present illness; problem pertinent system review extended to include a review of a limited number of additional systems; pertinent past, family, and/or social history directly related to the patient's problems.

Comprehensive: Chief complaint; extended history of present illness; review of systems that is directly related to the problem(s) identified in the history of the present illness plus a review of all additional body systems; complete past, family, and social history.

The comprehensive history obtained as part of the preventive medicine E/M service is not problem-oriented and does not involve a chief complaint or present illness. It does, however, include a comprehensive system review and comprehensive or interval past, family, and social history as well as a comprehensive assessment/history of pertinent risk factors.

Determine the Extent of Examination Performed

The extent of the examination performed is dependent on clinical judgment and on the nature of the presenting problem(s). The levels of E/M services recognize four types of examination that are defined as follows:

Problem focused: A limited examination of the affected body area or organ system.

Expanded problem focused: A limited examination of the affected body area or organ system and other symptomatic or related organ system(s).

Detailed: An extended examination of the affected body area(s) and other symptomatic or related organ system(s).

Comprehensive: A general multisystem examination or a complete examination of a single organ system. Note: The comprehensive examination performed as part of the preventive medicine E/M service is multisystem, but its extent is based on age and risk factors identified.

For the purposes of these CPT definitions, the following body areas are recognized:

- Head, including the face
- Neck
- Chest, including breasts and axilla
- Abdomen
- Genitalia, groin, buttocks
- Back
- Each extremity

For the purposes of these CPT definitions, the following organ systems are recognized:

- Eyes
- Ears, nose, mouth, and throat
- Cardiovascular
- Respiratory
- Gastrointestinal
- Genitourinary
- Musculoskeletal
- Skin
- Neurologic
- Psychiatric
- Hematologic/lymphatic/immunologic

Determine the Complexity of Medical Decision Making

Medical decision making refers to the complexity of establishing a diagnosis and/or selecting a management option as measured by:

- The number of possible diagnoses and/or the number of management options that must be considered
- The amount and/or complexity of medical records, diagnostic tests, and/or other information that must be obtained, reviewed, and analyzed
- The risk of significant complications, morbidity, and/or mortality, as well as comorbidities associated with the patient's presenting problem(s), the diagnostic procedure(s), and/or the possible management options

Four types of medical decision making are recognized: straightforward, low complexity, moderate complexity, and high complexity. To qualify for a given type of decision making, two of the three elements in Table 1 must be met or exceeded.

Comorbidities and underlying diseases, in and of themselves, are not considered in selecting a level of E/M services unless their presence significantly increases the complexity of the medical decision making.

Select the Appropriate Level of E/M Services Based on the Following

For the following categories/subcategories, all of the key components, ie, history, examination, and medical decision making, must meet or exceed the stated requirements to qualify for a particular level of E/M service: office, new patient; hospital observation services; initial hospital care; office consultations; initial inpatient consultations; emergency department services; initial nursing facility care; domiciliary care, new patient; and home, new patient.

For the following categories/subcategories, two of the three key components (ie, history, examination, and medical decision making) must meet or exceed the stated requirements to qualify for a particular level of E/M services: office, established patient; subsequent hospital care; subsequent nursing facility care; domiciliary care, established patient; and home, established patient.

When counseling and/or coordination of care dominates (more than 50 percent) the encounter with the patient and/or family (face-to-face time in the office or other outpatient setting or floor/unit time in the hospital or nursing facility), then time shall be considered the key or controlling factor to qualify for a particular level of E/M services. This includes time spent with parties who have assumed responsibility for the care of the patient or decision making whether or not they are family members (e.g., foster parents, person acting in loco parentis, legal guardian). The extent of counseling and/or coordination of care must be documented in the medical record.

CONSULTATION CODES AND MEDICARE REIMBURSEMENT

The Centers for Medicare and Medicaid Services (CMS) no longer provides benefits for CPT consultation codes. CMS has, however, redistributed the value of the consultation codes across the other E/M codes for services which are covered by Medicare. CMS has retained codes 99241 - 99251 in the Medicare Physician Fee Schedule for those private payers that use this data for reimbursement. Note that private payers may choose to follow CMS or CPT guidelines, and the use of consultation codes should be verified with individual payers.

Table 1

Complexity of Medical Decision Making

Number of Diagnoses or Management Options	*Amount and/or Complexity of Data to Be Reviewed*	*Risk of Complications and/or Morbidity or Mortality*	*Type of Decision Making*
minimal	minimal or none	minimal	straightforward
limited	limited	low	low complexity
multiple	moderate	moderate	moderate complexity
extensive	extensive	high	high complexity

99201-99215 Outpatient and Other Visits

CMS: 100-04,11,40.1.3 Independent Attending Physician Services; 100-04,12,190.3 List of Telehealth Services; 100-04,12,190.6 Payment Methodology for Physician/Practitioner at the Distant Site ; 100-04,12,190.6.1 Submission of Telehealth Claims for Distant Site Practitioners; 100-04,12,190.7 Contractor Editing of Telehealth Claims; 100-04,12,230 Primary Care Incentive Payment Program; 100-04,12,230.1 Definition of Primary Care Practitioners and Services; 100-04,12,230.2 Coordination with Other Payments; 100-04,12,230.3 Claims Processing and Payment; 100-04,12,30.6.10 Consultation Services; 100-04,12,30.6.15.1 Prolonged Services With Direct Face-to-Face Patient Contact; 100-04,12,30.6.4 Services Furnished Incident to Physician's Service; 100-04,12,30.6.7 Payment for Office or Other Outpatient E&M Visits; 100-04,12,40.3 Global Surgery Review; 100-04,18,80.2 Contractor Billing Requirements; 100-04,32,12.1 Counseling to Prevent Tobacco Use HCPCS and Diagnosis Coding; 100-04,32,130.1 Billing and Payment of External counterpulsation (ECP)

INCLUDES Established patients: received prior professional services from the physician or qualified health care professional or another physician or qualified health care professional in the practice of the exact same specialty and subspecialty in the previous three years (99211-99215)
New patients: have not received professional services from the physician or qualified health care professional or any other physician or qualified health care professional in the same practice in the exact same specialty and subspecialty in the previous three years (99201-99205)
Office visits
Outpatient services (including services prior to a formal admission to a facility)

EXCLUDES *Services provided in:*
Emergency department (99281-99285)
Hospital observation (99217-99220 [99224, 99225, 99226])
Hospital observation or inpatient with same day admission and discharge (99234-99236)

99201 **Office or other outpatient visit for the evaluation and management of a new patient, which requires these 3 key components: A problem focused history; A problem focused examination; Straightforward medical decision making. Counseling and/or coordination of care with other physicians, other qualified health care professionals, or agencies are provided consistent with the nature of the problem(s) and the patient's and/or family's needs. Usually, the presenting problem(s) are self limited or minor. Typically, 10 minutes are spent face-to-face with the patient and/or family.**

0.76 1.29 FUD XXX ★ B 80

AMA: 2019,Feb,3; 2019,Jan,3; 2018,Sep,14; 2018,Apr,10; 2018,Apr,9; 2018,Mar,7; 2018,Jan,8; 2017,Aug,3; 2017,Jun,6; 2017,Jan,8; 2016,Dec,11; 2016,Sep,6; 2016,Mar,10; 2016,Jan,7; 2016,Jan,13; 2015,Dec,3; 2015,Oct,3; 2015,Jan,16; 2015,Jan,12; 2014,Nov,14; 2014,Oct,3; 2014,Oct,8; 2014,Aug,3; 2014,Jan,11

99202 **Office or other outpatient visit for the evaluation and management of a new patient, which requires these 3 key components: An expanded problem focused history; An expanded problem focused examination; Straightforward medical decision making. Counseling and/or coordination of care with other physicians, other qualified health care professionals, or agencies are provided consistent with the nature of the problem(s) and the patient's and/or family's needs. Usually, the presenting problem(s) are of low to moderate severity. Typically, 20 minutes are spent face-to-face with the patient and/or family.**

1.43 2.15 FUD XXX ★ B 80

AMA: 2019,Feb,3; 2019,Jan,3; 2018,Sep,14; 2018,Apr,10; 2018,Apr,9; 2018,Mar,7; 2018,Jan,8; 2017,Aug,3; 2017,Jun,6; 2017,Jan,8; 2016,Dec,11; 2016,Sep,6; 2016,Mar,10; 2016,Jan,7; 2016,Jan,13; 2015,Dec,3; 2015,Oct,3; 2015,Jan,16; 2015,Jan,12; 2014,Nov,14; 2014,Oct,3; 2014,Oct,8; 2014,Aug,3; 2014,Jan,11

99203 **Office or other outpatient visit for the evaluation and management of a new patient, which requires these 3 key components: A detailed history; A detailed examination; Medical decision making of low complexity. Counseling and/or coordination of care with other physicians, other qualified health care professionals, or agencies are provided consistent with the nature of the problem(s) and the patient's and/or family's needs. Usually, the presenting problem(s) are of moderate severity. Typically, 30 minutes are spent face-to-face with the patient and/or family.**

2.15 3.05 FUD XXX ★ B 80

AMA: 2019,Feb,3; 2019,Jan,3; 2018,Sep,14; 2018,Apr,9; 2018,Apr,10; 2018,Mar,7; 2018,Jan,8; 2017,Aug,3; 2017,Jun,6; 2017,Jan,8; 2016,Dec,11; 2016,Sep,6; 2016,Mar,10; 2016,Jan,7; 2016,Jan,13; 2015,Dec,3; 2015,Oct,3; 2015,Jan,12; 2015,Jan,16; 2014,Nov,14; 2014,Oct,3; 2014,Oct,8; 2014,Aug,3; 2014,Jan,11

99204 **Office or other outpatient visit for the evaluation and management of a new patient, which requires these 3 key components: A comprehensive history; A comprehensive examination; Medical decision making of moderate complexity. Counseling and/or coordination of care with other physicians, other qualified health care professionals, or agencies are provided consistent with the nature of the problem(s) and the patient's and/or family's needs. Usually, the presenting problem(s) are of moderate to high severity. Typically, 45 minutes are spent face-to-face with the patient and/or family.**

3.64 4.63 FUD XXX ★ B 80

AMA: 2019,Feb,3; 2019,Jan,3; 2018,Sep,14; 2018,Apr,9; 2018,Apr,10; 2018,Mar,7; 2018,Jan,8; 2017,Aug,3; 2017,Jun,6; 2017,Jan,8; 2016,Dec,11; 2016,Sep,6; 2016,Mar,10; 2016,Jan,7; 2016,Jan,13; 2015,Dec,3; 2015,Oct,3; 2015,Jan,12; 2015,Jan,16; 2014,Nov,14; 2014,Oct,3; 2014,Oct,8; 2014,Aug,3; 2014,Jan,11

99205 **Office or other outpatient visit for the evaluation and management of a new patient, which requires these 3 key components: A comprehensive history; A comprehensive examination; Medical decision making of high complexity. Counseling and/or coordination of care with other physicians, other qualified health care professionals, or agencies are provided consistent with the nature of the problem(s) and the patient's and/or family's needs. Usually, the presenting problem(s) are of moderate to high severity. Typically, 60 minutes are spent face-to-face with the patient and/or family.**

4.75 5.82 FUD XXX ★ B 80

AMA: 2019,Feb,3; 2019,Jan,3; 2018,Sep,14; 2018,Apr,9; 2018,Apr,10; 2018,Mar,7; 2018,Jan,8; 2017,Aug,3; 2017,Jun,6; 2017,Jan,8; 2016,Dec,11; 2016,Sep,6; 2016,Mar,10; 2016,Jan,7; 2016,Jan,13; 2015,Dec,3; 2015,Oct,3; 2015,Jan,12; 2015,Jan,16; 2014,Nov,14; 2014,Oct,3; 2014,Oct,8; 2014,Aug,3; 2014,Jan,11

99211 **Office or other outpatient visit for the evaluation and management of an established patient, that may not require the presence of a physician or other qualified health care professional. Usually, the presenting problem(s) are minimal. Typically, 5 minutes are spent performing or supervising these services.**

0.26 0.64 FUD XXX B 80

AMA: 2019,Feb,3; 2019,Jan,3; 2018,Sep,14; 2018,Apr,10; 2018,Apr,9; 2018,Mar,7; 2018,Jan,8; 2017,Aug,3; 2017,Jun,6; 2017,Mar,10; 2017,Jan,8; 2016,Dec,11; 2016,Sep,6; 2016,Mar,10; 2016,Jan,7; 2016,Jan,13; 2015,Dec,3; 2015,Oct,3; 2015,Jan,12; 2015,Jan,16; 2014,Nov,14; 2014,Oct,3; 2014,Oct,8; 2014,Aug,3; 2014,Mar,13; 2014,Jan,11

99212 **Office or other outpatient visit for the evaluation and management of an established patient, which requires at least 2 of these 3 key components: A problem focused history; A problem focused examination; Straightforward medical decision making. Counseling and/or coordination of care with other physicians, other qualified health care professionals, or agencies are provided consistent with the nature of the problem(s) and the patient's and/or family's needs. Usually, the presenting problem(s) are self limited or minor. Typically, 10 minutes are spent face-to-face with the patient and/or family.**

0.72 1.27 FUD XXX ★ B 80

AMA: 2019,Feb,3; 2019,Jan,3; 2018,Sep,14; 2018,Apr,9; 2018,Apr,10; 2018,Mar,7; 2018,Jan,8; 2017,Oct,5; 2017,Aug,3; 2017,Jun,6; 2017,Jan,8; 2016,Dec,11; 2016,Sep,6; 2016,Mar,10; 2016,Jan,7; 2016,Jan,13; 2015,Dec,3; 2015,Oct,3; 2015,Jan,12; 2015,Jan,16; 2014,Nov,14; 2014,Oct,3; 2014,Oct,8; 2014,Aug,3; 2014,Jan,11

99213 **Office or other outpatient visit for the evaluation and management of an established patient, which requires at least 2 of these 3 key components: An expanded problem focused history; An expanded problem focused examination; Medical decision making of low complexity. Counseling and coordination of care with other physicians, other qualified health care professionals, or agencies are provided consistent with the nature of the problem(s) and the patient's and/or family's needs. Usually, the presenting problem(s) are of low to moderate severity. Typically, 15 minutes are spent face-to-face with the patient and/or family.**

1.44 2.09 FUD XXX ★ B 80

AMA: 2019,Feb,3; 2019,Jan,3; 2018,Sep,14; 2018,Apr,9; 2018,Apr,10; 2018,Mar,7; 2018,Jan,8; 2017,Aug,3; 2017,Jun,6; 2017,Jan,8; 2016,Dec,11; 2016,Sep,6; 2016,Mar,10; 2016,Jan,7; 2016,Jan,13; 2015,Dec,3; 2015,Oct,3; 2015,Jan,12; 2015,Jan,16; 2014,Nov,14; 2014,Oct,8; 2014,Oct,3; 2014,Aug,3; 2014,Jan,11

99214 **Office or other outpatient visit for the evaluation and management of an established patient, which requires at least 2 of these 3 key components: A detailed history; A detailed examination; Medical decision making of moderate complexity. Counseling and/or coordination of care with other physicians, other qualified health care professionals, or agencies are provided consistent with the nature of the problem(s) and the patient's and/or family's needs. Usually, the presenting problem(s) are of moderate to high severity. Typically, 25 minutes are spent face-to-face with the patient and/or family.**

2.22 3.06 FUD XXX 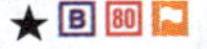

AMA: 2019,Feb,3; 2019,Jan,3; 2018,Sep,14; 2018,Apr,9; 2018,Apr,10; 2018,Mar,7; 2018,Jan,8; 2017,Aug,3; 2017,Jun,6; 2017,Jan,8; 2016,Dec,11; 2016,Sep,6; 2016,Mar,10; 2016,Jan,13; 2016,Jan,7; 2015,Dec,3; 2015,Oct,3; 2015,Jan,12; 2015,Jan,16; 2014,Nov,14; 2014,Oct,8; 2014,Oct,3; 2014,Aug,3; 2014,Jan,11

99215 **Office or other outpatient visit for the evaluation and management of an established patient, which requires at least 2 of these 3 key components: A comprehensive history; A comprehensive examination; Medical decision making of high complexity. Counseling and/or coordination of care with other physicians, other qualified health care professionals, or agencies are provided consistent with the nature of the problem(s) and the patient's and/or family's needs. Usually, the presenting problem(s) are of moderate to high severity. Typically, 40 minutes are spent face-to-face with the patient and/or family.**

3.13 4.10 FUD XXX ★ B 80

AMA: 2019,Feb,3; 2019,Jan,3; 2018,Sep,14; 2018,Apr,9; 2018,Apr,10; 2018,Mar,7; 2018,Jan,8; 2017,Aug,3; 2017,Jun,6; 2017,Jan,8; 2016,Dec,11; 2016,Sep,6; 2016,Mar,10; 2016,Jan,7; 2016,Jan,13; 2015,Dec,3; 2015,Oct,3; 2015,Jan,12; 2015,Jan,16; 2014,Nov,14; 2014,Oct,8; 2014,Oct,3; 2014,Aug,3; 2014,Jan,11

99217-99220 Facility Observation Visits: Initial and Discharge

CMS: 100-04,11,40.1.3 Independent Attending Physician Services; 100-04,12,30.6.4 Services Furnished Incident to Physician's Service; 100-04,12,30.6.8 Payment for Hospital Observation Services; 100-04,12,40.3 Global Surgery Review; 100-04,32,130.1 Billing and Payment of External counterpulsation (ECP)

INCLUDES Services provided on the same date in other settings or departments associated with the observation status admission (99201-99215, 99281-99285, 99304-99318, 99324-99337, 99341-99350, 99381-99429)

Services provided to new and established patients admitted to a hospital specifically for observation (not required to be a designated area of the hospital)

EXCLUDES *Services provided by physicians or another qualified health care professional other than the admitting physician ([99224, 99225, 99226], 99241-99245)*

Services provided to a patient admitted and discharged from observation status on the same date (99234-99236)

Services provided to a patient admitted to the hospital following observation status (99221-99223)

Services provided to a patient discharged from inpatient care (99238-99239)

99217 **Observation care discharge day management (This code is to be utilized to report all services provided to a patient on discharge from outpatient hospital "observation status" if the discharge is on other than the initial date of "observation status." To report services to a patient designated as "observation status" or "inpatient status" and discharged on the same date, use the codes for Observation or Inpatient Care Services [including Admission and Discharge Services, 99234-99236 as appropriate.])**

INCLUDES Discussing the observation admission with the patient

Final patient evaluation:

- Discharge instructions
- Sign off on discharge medical records

2.06 2.06 FUD XXX B 80

AMA: 2019,Jul,10; 2018,Jan,8; 2017,Aug,3; 2017,Jun,6; 2017,Jan,8; 2016,Dec,11; 2016,Jan,13; 2016,Jan,7; 2015,Dec,3; 2015,Jan,16; 2014,Nov,14; 2014,Oct,8; 2014,Jan,11

99218 **Initial observation care, per day, for the evaluation and management of a patient which requires these 3 key components: A detailed or comprehensive history; A detailed or comprehensive examination; and Medical decision making that is straightforward or of low complexity. Counseling and/or coordination of care with other physicians, other qualified health care professionals, or agencies are provided consistent with the nature of the problem(s) and the patient's and/or family's needs. Usually, the problem(s) requiring admission to outpatient hospital "observation status" are of low severity. Typically, 30 minutes are spent at the bedside and on the patient's hospital floor or unit.**

2.81 2.81 FUD XXX B 80

AMA: 2019,Jul,10; 2018,Dec,8; 2018,Dec,8; 2018,Jan,8; 2017,Aug,3; 2017,Jun,6; 2017,Jan,8; 2016,Dec,11; 2016,Jan,7; 2016,Jan,13; 2015,Dec,3; 2015,Jul,3; 2015,Mar,3; 2015,Jan,16; 2014,Nov,14; 2014,Oct,8; 2014,Jan,11

99219 **Initial observation care, per day, for the evaluation and management of a patient, which requires these 3 key components: A comprehensive history; A comprehensive examination; and Medical decision making of moderate complexity. Counseling and/or coordination of care with other physicians, other qualified health care professionals, or agencies are provided consistent with the nature of the problem(s) and the patient's and/or family's needs. Usually, the problem(s) requiring admission to outpatient hospital "observation status" are of moderate severity. Typically, 50 minutes are spent at the bedside and on the patient's hospital floor or unit.**

3.83 3.83 FUD XXX B 80

AMA: 2019,Jul,10; 2018,Dec,8; 2018,Dec,8; 2018,Jan,8; 2017,Aug,3; 2017,Jun,6; 2017,Jan,8; 2016,Dec,11; 2016,Jan,7; 2016,Jan,13; 2015,Dec,3; 2015,Jul,3; 2015,Jan,16; 2014,Nov,14; 2014,Oct,8; 2014,Jan,11

99220 **Initial observation care, per day, for the evaluation and management of a patient, which requires these 3 key components: A comprehensive history; A comprehensive examination; and Medical decision making of high complexity. Counseling and/or coordination of care with other physicians, other qualified health care professionals, or agencies are provided consistent with the nature of the problem(s) and the patient's and/or family's needs. Usually, the problem(s) requiring admission to outpatient hospital "observation status" are of high severity. Typically, 70 minutes are spent at the bedside and on the patient's hospital floor or unit.**

5.23 5.23 FUD XXX B 80

AMA: 2019,Jul,10; 2018,Dec,8; 2018,Dec,8; 2018,Jan,8; 2017,Aug,3; 2017,Jun,6; 2017,Jan,8; 2016,Dec,11; 2016,Jan,7; 2016,Jan,13; 2015,Dec,3; 2015,Jul,3; 2015,Jan,16; 2014,Nov,14; 2014,Oct,8; 2014,Jan,11

99224-99226 [99224, 99225, 99226] Facility Observation Visits: Subsequent

CMS: 100-04,11,40.1.3 Independent Attending Physician Services; 100-04,12,30.6.4 Services Furnished Incident to Physician's Service; 100-04,12,30.6.8 Payment for Hospital Observation Services; 100-04,12,30.6.9.1 Initial Hospital Care and Observation or Inpatient Care Services

INCLUDES Changes in patient's status (e.g., physical condition, history; response to medical management)
Medical record review
Review of diagnostic test results
Services provided on the same date in other settings or departments associated with the observation status admission (99201-99215, 99281-99285, 99304-99318, 99324-99337, 99341-99350, 99381-99429)

EXCLUDES *Observation admission and discharge on the same day (99234-99236)*

\# **99224** **Subsequent observation care, per day, for the evaluation and management of a patient, which requires at least 2 of these 3 key components: Problem focused interval history; Problem focused examination; Medical decision making that is straightforward or of low complexity. Counseling and/or coordination of care with other physicians, other qualified health care professionals, or agencies are provided consistent with the nature of the problem(s) and the patient's and/or family's needs. Usually, the patient is stable, recovering, or improving. Typically, 15 minutes are spent at the bedside and on the patient's hospital floor or unit.**

1.12 1.12 FUD XXX B 80

AMA: 2019,Jul,10; 2018,Jan,8; 2017,Aug,3; 2017,Jun,6; 2017,Jan,8; 2016,Dec,11; 2016,Jan,7; 2016,Jan,13; 2015,Dec,3; 2015,Jan,16; 2014,Nov,14; 2014,Oct,8; 2014,Jan,11

\# **99225** **Subsequent observation care, per day, for the evaluation and management of a patient, which requires at least 2 of these 3 key components: An expanded problem focused interval history; An expanded problem focused examination; Medical decision making of moderate complexity. Counseling and/or coordination of care with other physicians, other qualified health care professionals, or agencies are provided consistent with the nature of the problem(s) and the patient's and/or family's needs. Usually, the patient is responding inadequately to therapy or has developed a minor complication. Typically, 25 minutes are spent at the bedside and on the patient's hospital floor or unit.**

2.06 2.06 FUD XXX B 80

AMA: 2019,Jul,10; 2018,Jan,8; 2017,Aug,3; 2017,Jun,6; 2017,Jan,8; 2016,Dec,11; 2016,Jan,7; 2016,Jan,13; 2015,Dec,3; 2015,Jan,16; 2014,Nov,14; 2014,Oct,8; 2014,Jan,11

\# **99226** **Subsequent observation care, per day, for the evaluation and management of a patient, which requires at least 2 of these 3 key components: A detailed interval history; A detailed examination; Medical decision making of high complexity. Counseling and/or coordination of care with other physicians, other qualified health care professionals, or agencies are provided consistent with the nature of the problem(s) and the patient's and/or family's needs. Usually, the patient is unstable or has developed a significant complication or a significant new problem. Typically, 35 minutes are spent at the bedside and on the patient's hospital floor or unit.**

2.95 2.95 FUD XXX B 80

AMA: 2019,Jul,10; 2018,Jan,8; 2017,Aug,3; 2017,Jun,6; 2017,Jan,8; 2016,Dec,11; 2016,Jan,7; 2016,Jan,13; 2015,Dec,3; 2015,Jan,16; 2014,Nov,14; 2014,Oct,8; 2014,Jan,11

99221-99233 Inpatient Hospital Visits: Initial and Subsequent

CMS: 100-04,11,40.1.3 Independent Attending Physician Services; 100-04,12,30.6.10 Consultation Services; 100-04,12,30.6.15.1 Prolonged Services With Direct Face-to-Face Patient Contact; 100-04,12,30.6.4 Services Furnished Incident to Physician's Service; 100-04,12,30.6.9 Hospital Visit and Critical Care on Same Day

INCLUDES Initial physician services provided to the patient in the hospital or "partial" hospital settings (99221-99223)
Services provided on the date of admission in other settings or departments associated with an observation status admission (99201-99215, 99281-99285, 99304-99318, 99324-99337, 99341-99350, 99381-99397)
Services provided to a new or established patient

EXCLUDES *Inpatient admission and discharge on the same date (99234-99236)*
Inpatient E&M services provided by other than the admitting physician

99221 **Initial hospital care, per day, for the evaluation and management of a patient, which requires these 3 key components: A detailed or comprehensive history; A detailed or comprehensive examination; and Medical decision making that is straightforward or of low complexity. Counseling and/or coordination of care with other physicians, other qualified health care professionals, or agencies are provided consistent with the nature of the problem(s) and the patient's and/or family's needs. Usually, the problem(s) requiring admission are of low severity. Typically, 30 minutes are spent at the bedside and on the patient's hospital floor or unit.**

2.86 2.86 FUD XXX B 80

AMA: 2018,Dec,8; 2018,Dec,8; 2018,Jan,8; 2017,Aug,3; 2017,Jun,6; 2017,Jan,8; 2016,Dec,11; 2016,Mar,10; 2016,Jan,13; 2016,Jan,7; 2015,Dec,3; 2015,Dec,18; 2015,Jul,3; 2015,Jan,16; 2014,Nov,14; 2014,Oct,8; 2014,Jan,11

99222 **Initial hospital care, per day, for the evaluation and management of a patient, which requires these 3 key components: A comprehensive history; A comprehensive examination; and Medical decision making of moderate complexity. Counseling and/or coordination of care with other physicians, other qualified health care professionals, or agencies are provided consistent with the nature of the problem(s) and the patient's and/or family's needs. Usually, the problem(s) requiring admission are of moderate severity. Typically, 50 minutes are spent at the bedside and on the patient's hospital floor or unit.**

3.86 3.86 FUD XXX B 80

AMA: 2018,Dec,8; 2018,Dec,8; 2018,Jan,8; 2017,Aug,3; 2017,Jun,6; 2017,Jan,8; 2016,Dec,11; 2016,Mar,10; 2016,Jan,7; 2016,Jan,13; 2015,Dec,3; 2015,Dec,18; 2015,Jul,3; 2015,Mar,3; 2015,Jan,16; 2014,Nov,14; 2014,Oct,8; 2014,Jan,11

99223 **Initial hospital care, per day, for the evaluation and management of a patient, which requires these 3 key components: A comprehensive history; A comprehensive examination; and Medical decision making of high complexity. Counseling and/or coordination of care with other physicians, other qualified health care professionals, or agencies are provided consistent with the nature of the problem(s) and the patient's and/or family's needs. Usually, the problem(s) requiring admission are of high severity. Typically, 70 minutes are spent at the bedside and on the patient's hospital floor or unit.**

5.70 5.70 FUD XXX B 80

AMA: 2018,Dec,8; 2018,Dec,8; 2018,Jan,8; 2017,Aug,3; 2017,Jun,6; 2017,Jan,8; 2016,Dec,11; 2016,Mar,10; 2016,Jan,7; 2016,Jan,13; 2015,Dec,3; 2015,Dec,18; 2015,Jul,3; 2015,Jan,16; 2014,Nov,14; 2014,Oct,8; 2014,Jan,11

99224 **Resequenced code. See code following 99220.**

99225 **Resequenced code. See code following 99220.**

99226 **Resequenced code. See code following 99220.**

99231 **Subsequent hospital care, per day, for the evaluation and management of a patient, which requires at least 2 of these 3 key components: A problem focused interval history; A problem focused examination; Medical decision making that is straightforward or of low complexity. Counseling and/or coordination of care with other physicians, other qualified health care professionals, or agencies are provided consistent with the nature of the problem(s) and the patient's and/or family's needs. Usually, the patient is stable, recovering or improving. Typically, 15 minutes are spent at the bedside and on the patient's hospital floor or unit.**

1.11 1.11 FUD XXX 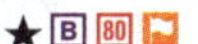

AMA: 2018,Dec,8; 2018,Dec,8; 2018,Jan,8; 2017,Aug,3; 2017,Jun,6; 2017,Jan,8; 2016,Dec,11; 2016,Jan,13; 2016,Jan,7; 2015,Dec,3; 2015,Jul,3; 2015,Jan,16; 2014,Nov,14; 2014,Oct,8; 2014,May,4; 2014,Jan,11

99232 **Subsequent hospital care, per day, for the evaluation and management of a patient, which requires at least 2 of these 3 key components: An expanded problem focused interval history; An expanded problem focused examination; Medical decision making of moderate complexity. Counseling and/or coordination of care with other physicians, other qualified health care professionals, or agencies are provided consistent with the nature of the problem(s) and the patient's and/or family's needs. Usually, the patient is responding inadequately to therapy or has developed a minor complication. Typically, 25 minutes are spent at the bedside and on the patient's hospital floor or unit.**

2.05 2.05 FUD XXX 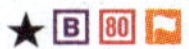

AMA: 2018,Dec,8; 2018,Dec,8; 2018,Jan,8; 2017,Aug,3; 2017,Jun,6; 2017,Jan,8; 2016,Dec,11; 2016,Oct,8; 2016,Jan,7; 2016,Jan,13; 2015,Dec,3; 2015,Jul,3; 2015,Jan,16; 2014,Nov,14; 2014,Oct,8; 2014,Jan,11

99233 **Subsequent hospital care, per day, for the evaluation and management of a patient, which requires at least 2 of these 3 key components: A detailed interval history; A detailed examination; Medical decision making of high complexity. Counseling and/or coordination of care with other physicians, other qualified health care professionals, or agencies are provided consistent with the nature of the problem(s) and the patient's and/or family's needs. Usually, the patient is unstable or has developed a significant complication or a significant new problem. Typically, 35 minutes are spent at the bedside and on the patient's hospital floor or unit.**

2.93 2.93 FUD XXX ★ B 80

AMA: 2018,Dec,8; 2018,Dec,8; 2018,Jan,8; 2017,Aug,3; 2017,Jun,6; 2017,Jan,8; 2016,Dec,11; 2016,Oct,8; 2016,Jan,13; 2016,Jan,7; 2015,Dec,3; 2015,Jul,3; 2015,Jan,16; 2014,Nov,14; 2014,Oct,8; 2014,May,4; 2014,Jan,11

99234-99236 Observation/Inpatient Visits: Admitted/Discharged on Same Date

CMS: 100-04,11,40.1.3 Independent Attending Physician Services; 100-04,12,30.6.4 Services Furnished Incident to Physician's Service; 100-04,12,30.6.8 Payment for Hospital Observation Services; 100-04,12,30.6.9 Payment for Inpatient Hospital Visits - General; 100-04,12,30.6.9.1 Initial Hospital Care and Observation or Inpatient Care Services; 100-04,12,30.6.9.2 Subsequent Hospital Visit and Discharge Management; 100-04,12,40.3 Global Surgery Review

INCLUDES Admission and discharge services on the same date in an observation or inpatient setting

All services provided by admitting physician or other qualified health care professional on same date of service, even when initiated in another setting (e.g., emergency department, nursing facility, office)

EXCLUDES *Services provided to patients admitted to observation and discharged on a different date (99217-99220, [99224, 99225, 99226])*

99234 **Observation or inpatient hospital care, for the evaluation and management of a patient including admission and discharge on the same date, which requires these 3 key components: A detailed or comprehensive history; A detailed or comprehensive examination; and Medical decision making that is straightforward or of low complexity. Counseling and/or coordination of care with other physicians, other qualified health care professionals, or agencies are provided consistent with the nature of the problem(s) and the patient's and/or family's needs. Usually the presenting problem(s) requiring admission are of low severity. Typically, 40 minutes are spent at the bedside and on the patient's hospital floor or unit.**

3.75 3.75 FUD XXX 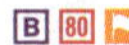

AMA: 2018,Dec,8; 2018,Dec,8; 2018,Apr,10; 2018,Jan,8; 2017,Aug,3; 2017,Jun,6; 2017,Jan,8; 2016,Dec,11; 2016,Jan,13; 2015,Jul,3; 2015,Jan,16; 2014,Oct,8; 2014,Jan,11

99235 **Observation or inpatient hospital care, for the evaluation and management of a patient including admission and discharge on the same date, which requires these 3 key components: A comprehensive history; A comprehensive examination; and Medical decision making of moderate complexity. Counseling and/or coordination of care with other physicians, other qualified health care professionals, or agencies are provided consistent with the nature of the problem(s) and the patient's and/or family's needs. Usually the presenting problem(s) requiring admission are of moderate severity. Typically, 50 minutes are spent at the bedside and on the patient's hospital floor or unit.**

4.77 4.77 FUD XXX B 80

AMA: 2018,Dec,8; 2018,Dec,8; 2018,Apr,10; 2018,Jan,8; 2017,Aug,3; 2017,Jun,6; 2017,Jan,8; 2016,Dec,11; 2016,Jan,13; 2015,Jul,3; 2015,Jan,16; 2014,Oct,8; 2014,Jan,11

99236 **Observation or inpatient hospital care, for the evaluation and management of a patient including admission and discharge on the same date, which requires these 3 key components: A comprehensive history; A comprehensive examination; and Medical decision making of high complexity. Counseling and/or coordination of care with other physicians, other qualified health care professionals, or agencies are provided consistent with the nature of the problem(s) and the patient's and/or family's needs. Usually the presenting problem(s) requiring admission are of high severity. Typically, 55 minutes are spent at the bedside and on the patient's hospital floor or unit.**

6.13 6.13 FUD XXX 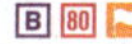

AMA: 2018,Dec,8; 2018,Dec,8; 2018,Apr,10; 2018,Jan,8; 2017,Aug,3; 2017,Jun,6; 2017,Jan,8; 2016,Dec,11; 2016,Jan,13; 2015,Jul,3; 2015,Jan,16; 2014,Oct,8; 2014,Jan,11

99238-99239 Inpatient Hospital Discharge Services

CMS: 100-04,11,40.1.3 Independent Attending Physician Services; 100-04,12,30.6.4 Services Furnished Incident to Physician's Service; 100-04,12,30.6.9 Swing Bed Visits; 100-04,12,30.6.9.1 Initial Hospital Care and Observation or Inpatient Care Services; 100-04,12,30.6.9.2 Subsequent Hospital Visit and Discharge Management; 100-04,12,40.3 Global Surgery Review

INCLUDES All services on discharge day when discharge and admission are not the same day
Discharge instructions
Final patient evaluation
Final preparation of the patient's medical records
Provision of prescriptions/referrals, as needed
Review of the inpatient admission

EXCLUDES *Admission/discharge on same date (99234-99236)*
Discharge from observation (99217)
Discharge from nursing facility (99315-99316)
Healthy newborn evaluated and discharged on same date (99463)
Services provided by other than attending physician or other qualified health care professional on date of discharge (99231-99233)

99238 **Hospital discharge day management; 30 minutes or less**
2.06 2.06 FUD XXX B 80
AMA: 2018,Dec,8; 2018,Dec,8; 2018,Jan,8; 2017,Aug,3; 2017,Jun,6; 2017,Jan,8; 2016,Dec,11; 2016,Jan,13; 2015,Jan,16; 2014,Oct,8; 2014,Jan,11

99239 **more than 30 minutes**
3.02 3.02 FUD XXX B 80
AMA: 2018,Dec,8; 2018,Dec,8; 2018,Jan,8; 2017,Aug,3; 2017,Jun,6; 2017,Jan,8; 2016,Dec,11; 2016,Jan,13; 2015,Jan,16; 2014,Oct,8; 2014,Jan,11

99241-99245 Consultations: Office and Outpatient

CMS: 100-04,11,40.1.3 Independent Attending Physician Services; 100-04,12,190.6 Payment Methodology for Physician/Practitioner at the Distant Site ; 100-04,12,190.6.1 Submission of Telehealth Claims for Distant Site Practitioners; 100-04,12,190.7 Contractor Editing of Telehealth Claims; 100-04,12,30.6.10 Consultation Services; 100-04,12,30.6.15.1 Prolonged Services With Direct Face-to-Face Patient Contact; 100-04,12,30.6.4 Services Furnished Incident to Physician's Service; 100-04,12,30.6.9.1 Initial Hospital Care and Observation or Inpatient Care Services; 100-04,12,40.3 Global Surgery Review; 100-04,32,130.1 Billing and Payment of External counterpulsation (ECP); 100-04,4,160 Clinic and Emergency Visits Under OPPS

INCLUDES A third-party mandated consultation; append modifier 32
All outpatient consultations provided in the office, outpatient or other ambulatory facility, domiciliary/rest home, emergency department, patient's home, and hospital observation
Documentation of a request for a consultation from an appropriate source
Documentation of the need for consultation in the patient's medical record
One consultation per consultant
Provision by a physician or qualified nonphysician practitioner whose advice, opinion, recommendation, suggestion, direction, or counsel, etc., is requested for evaluating/treating a patient since that individual's expertise in a specific medical area is beyond the scope of knowledge of the requesting physician
Provision of a written report of findings/recommendations from the consultant to the referring physician

EXCLUDES *Another appropriately requested and documented consultation pertaining to the same/new problem; repeat use of consultation codes*
Any distinctly recognizable procedure/service provided on or following the consultation
Assumption of care (all or partial); report subsequent codes as appropriate for the place of service (99211-99215, 99334-99337, 99347-99350)
Consultation prompted by the patient/family; report codes for office, domiciliary/rest home, or home visits instead (99201-99215, 99324-99337, 99341-99350)
Services provided to Medicare patients; E&M code as appropriate for the place of service or HCPCS code (99201-99215, 99221-99223, 99231-99233, G0406-G0408, G0425-G0427)

99241 **Office consultation for a new or established patient, which requires these 3 key components: A problem focused history; A problem focused examination; and Straightforward medical decision making. Counseling and/or coordination of care with other physicians, other qualified health care professionals, or agencies are provided consistent with the nature of the problem(s) and the patient's and/or family's needs. Usually, the presenting problem(s) are self limited or minor. Typically, 15 minutes are spent face-to-face with the patient and/or family.**
0.92 1.34 FUD XXX ★ E
AMA: 2018,Apr,9; 2018,Apr,10; 2018,Mar,7; 2018,Jan,8; 2017,Aug,3; 2017,Jun,6; 2017,Jan,8; 2016,Dec,11; 2016,Sep,6; 2016,Jan,13; 2016,Jan,7; 2015,Jan,12; 2015,Jan,16; 2014,Nov,14; 2014,Oct,8; 2014,Sep,13; 2014,Aug,3; 2014,Jan,11

99242 **Office consultation for a new or established patient, which requires these 3 key components: An expanded problem focused history; An expanded problem focused examination; and Straightforward medical decision making. Counseling and/or coordination of care with other physicians, other qualified health care professionals, or agencies are provided consistent with the nature of the problem(s) and the patient's and/or family's needs. Usually, the presenting problem(s) are of low severity. Typically, 30 minutes are spent face-to-face with the patient and/or family.**
1.93 2.52 FUD XXX ★ E
AMA: 2018,Apr,10; 2018,Apr,9; 2018,Mar,7; 2018,Jan,8; 2017,Aug,3; 2017,Jun,6; 2017,Jun,8; 2017,Jan,8; 2016,Dec,11; 2016,Sep,6; 2016,Jan,7; 2016,Jan,13; 2015,Jan,12; 2015,Jan,16; 2014,Nov,14; 2014,Oct,8; 2014,Sep,13; 2014,Aug,3; 2014,Jan,11

99243 **Office consultation for a new or established patient, which requires these 3 key components: A detailed history; A detailed examination; and Medical decision making of low complexity. Counseling and/or coordination of care with other physicians, other qualified health care professionals, or agencies are provided consistent with the nature of the problem(s) and the patient's and/or family's needs. Usually, the presenting problem(s) are of moderate severity. Typically, 40 minutes are spent face-to-face with the patient and/or family.**

2.70 3.45 FUD XXX ★ E

AMA: 2018,Apr,10; 2018,Apr,9; 2018,Mar,7; 2018,Jan,8; 2017,Aug,3; 2017,Jun,6; 2017,Jan,8; 2016,Dec,11; 2016,Sep,6; 2016,Jan,7; 2016,Jan,13; 2015,Jan,16; 2015,Jan,12; 2014,Nov,14; 2014,Oct,8; 2014,Sep,13; 2014,Aug,3; 2014,Jan,11

99244 **Office consultation for a new or established patient, which requires these 3 key components: A comprehensive history; A comprehensive examination; and Medical decision making of moderate complexity. Counseling and/or coordination of care with other physicians, other qualified health care professionals, or agencies are provided consistent with the nature of the problem(s) and the patient's and/or family's needs. Usually, the presenting problem(s) are of moderate to high severity. Typically, 60 minutes are spent face-to-face with the patient and/or family.**

4.34 5.16 FUD XXX ★ E

AMA: 2018,Apr,10; 2018,Apr,9; 2018,Mar,7; 2018,Jan,8; 2017,Aug,3; 2017,Jun,6; 2017,Jan,8; 2016,Dec,11; 2016,Sep,6; 2016,Jan,7; 2016,Jan,13; 2015,Jan,16; 2015,Jan,12; 2014,Nov,14; 2014,Oct,8; 2014,Sep,13; 2014,Aug,3; 2014,Jan,11

99245 **Office consultation for a new or established patient, which requires these 3 key components: A comprehensive history; A comprehensive examination; and Medical decision making of high complexity. Counseling and/or coordination of care with other physicians, other qualified health care professionals, or agencies are provided consistent with the nature of the problem(s) and the patient's and/or family's needs. Usually, the presenting problem(s) are of moderate to high severity. Typically, 80 minutes are spent face-to-face with the patient and/or family.**

5.37 6.29 FUD XXX ★ E

AMA: 2018,Apr,10; 2018,Apr,9; 2018,Mar,7; 2018,Jan,8; 2017,Aug,3; 2017,Jun,6; 2017,Jan,8; 2016,Dec,11; 2016,Sep,6; 2016,Jan,7; 2016,Jan,13; 2015,Jan,16; 2015,Jan,12; 2014,Nov,14; 2014,Oct,8; 2014,Sep,13; 2014,Aug,3; 2014,Jan,11

99251-99255 Consultations: Inpatient

CMS: 100-04,11,40.1.3 Independent Attending Physician Services; 100-04,12,190.6 Payment Methodology for Physician/Practitioner at the Distant Site ; 100-04,12,190.6.1 Submission of Telehealth Claims for Distant Site Practitioners; 100-04,12,190.7 Contractor Editing of Telehealth Claims; 100-04,12,30.6.10 Consultation Services; 100-04,12,30.6.15.1 Prolonged Services With Direct Face-to-Face Patient Contact; 100-04,12,30.6.4 Services Furnished Incident to Physician's Service; 100-04,12,30.6.9.1 Initial Hospital Care and Observation or Inpatient Care Services; 100-04,12,40.3 Global Surgery Review

INCLUDES
- A third-party mandated consultation; append modifier 32
- All inpatient consultations include services provided in the hospital inpatient or partial hospital settings and nursing facilities
- Consultation services provided outpatient for the same inpatient hospitalization (99241-99245)
- Documentation of a request for a consultation from an appropriate source
- Documentation of the need for consultation in the patient's medical record
- One consultation by consultant per admission
- Provision by a physician or qualified nonphysician practitioner whose advice, opinion, recommendation, suggestion, direction, or counsel, etc. is requested for evaluating/treating a patient since that individual's expertise in a specific medical area is beyond the scope of knowledge of the requesting physician
- Provision of a written report of findings/recommendations from the consultant to the referring physician

EXCLUDES
- *Another appropriately requested and documented consultation pertaining to the same/new problem: repeat use of consultation codes*
- *Any distinctly recognizable procedure/service provided on or following the consultation*
- *Assumption of care (all or partial): report subsequent codes as appropriate for the place of service (99231-99233, 99307-99310)*
- *Consultation prompted by the patient/family: report codes for office, domiciliary/rest home, or home visits instead (99201-99215, 99324-99337, 99341-99350)*
- *Services provided to Medicare patients; E&M code as appropriate for the place of service or HCPCS code (99201-99215, 99221-99223, 99231-99233, G0406-G0408, G0425-G0427)*

99251 **Inpatient consultation for a new or established patient, which requires these 3 key components: A problem focused history; A problem focused examination; and Straightforward medical decision making. Counseling and/or coordination of care with other physicians, other qualified health care professionals, or agencies are provided consistent with the nature of the problem(s) and the patient's and/or family's needs. Usually, the presenting problem(s) are self limited or minor. Typically, 20 minutes are spent at the bedside and on the patient's hospital floor or unit.**

1.38 1.38 FUD XXX ★ E

AMA: 2018,Jan,8; 2017,Aug,3; 2017,Jun,6; 2017,Jan,8; 2016,Dec,11; 2016,Jan,7; 2016,Jan,13; 2015,Jan,16; 2014,Nov,14; 2014,Oct,8; 2014,Jan,11

99252 **Inpatient consultation for a new or established patient, which requires these 3 key components: An expanded problem focused history; An expanded problem focused examination; and Straightforward medical decision making. Counseling and/or coordination of care with other physicians, other qualified health care professionals, or agencies are provided consistent with the nature of the problem(s) and the patient's and/or family's needs. Usually, the presenting problem(s) are of low severity. Typically, 40 minutes are spent at the bedside and on the patient's hospital floor or unit.**

2.11 2.11 FUD XXX ★ E

AMA: 2018,Jan,8; 2017,Aug,3; 2017,Jun,6; 2017,Jan,8; 2016,Dec,11; 2016,Jan,7; 2016,Jan,13; 2015,Jan,16; 2014,Nov,14; 2014,Oct,8; 2014,Jan,11

99253 **Inpatient consultation for a new or established patient, which requires these 3 key components: A detailed history; A detailed examination; and Medical decision making of low complexity. Counseling and/or coordination of care with other physicians, other qualified health care professionals, or agencies are provided consistent with the nature of the problem(s) and the patient's and/or family's needs. Usually, the presenting problem(s) are of moderate severity. Typically, 55 minutes are spent at the bedside and on the patient's hospital floor or unit.**

3.25 3.25 FUD XXX ★ E

AMA: 2018,Jan,8; 2017,Aug,3; 2017,Jun,6; 2017,Jan,8; 2016,Dec,11; 2016,Jan,7; 2016,Jan,13; 2015,Jan,16; 2014,Nov,14; 2014,Oct,8; 2014,Jan,11

99254 **Inpatient consultation for a new or established patient, which requires these 3 key components: A comprehensive history; A comprehensive examination; and Medical decision making of moderate complexity. Counseling and/or coordination of care with other physicians, other qualified health care professionals, or agencies are provided consistent with the nature of the problem(s) and the patient's and/or family's needs. Usually, the presenting problem(s) are of moderate to high severity. Typically, 80 minutes are spent at the bedside and on the patient's hospital floor or unit.**

4.72 4.72 FUD XXX ★ E

AMA: 2018,Jan,8; 2017,Aug,3; 2017,Jun,6; 2017,Jan,8; 2016,Dec,11; 2016,Jan,7; 2016,Jan,13; 2015,Jan,16; 2014,Nov,14; 2014,Oct,8; 2014,Jan,11

99255 **Inpatient consultation for a new or established patient, which requires these 3 key components: A comprehensive history; A comprehensive examination; and Medical decision making of high complexity. Counseling and/or coordination of care with other physicians, other qualified health care professionals, or agencies are provided consistent with the nature of the problem(s) and the patient's and/or family's needs. Usually, the presenting problem(s) are of moderate to high severity. Typically, 110 minutes are spent at the bedside and on the patient's hospital floor or unit.**

5.68 5.68 FUD XXX ★ E

AMA: 2018,Jan,8; 2017,Aug,3; 2017,Jun,6; 2017,Jan,8; 2016,Dec,11; 2016,Jan,7; 2016,Jan,13; 2015,Jan,16; 2014,Nov,14; 2014,Oct,8; 2014,Jan,11

99281-99288 Emergency Department Visits

CMS: 100-04,11,40.1.3 Independent Attending Physician Services; 100-04,12,30.6.11 Emergency Department Visits; 100-04,4,160 Clinic and Emergency Visits Under OPPS

INCLUDES Any amount of time spent with the patient, which usually involves a series of encounters while the patient is in the emergency department
Care provided to new and established patients

EXCLUDES *Critical care services (99291-99292)*
Observation services (99217-99220, 99234-99236)

99281 **Emergency department visit for the evaluation and management of a patient, which requires these 3 key components: A problem focused history; A problem focused examination; and Straightforward medical decision making. Counseling and/or coordination of care with other physicians, other qualified health care professionals, or agencies are provided consistent with the nature of the problem(s) and the patient's and/or family's needs. Usually, the presenting problem(s) are self limited or minor.**

0.60 0.60 FUD XXX J 80

AMA: 2019,Jul,10; 2018,Jan,8; 2017,Aug,3; 2017,Jun,6; 2017,Jan,8; 2016,Jan,7; 2016,Jan,13; 2015,Jan,16; 2015,Jan,12; 2014,Nov,14; 2014,Oct,8; 2014,Jan,11

99282 **Emergency department visit for the evaluation and management of a patient, which requires these 3 key components: An expanded problem focused history; An expanded problem focused examination; and Medical decision making of low complexity. Counseling and/or coordination of care with other physicians, other qualified health care professionals, or agencies are provided consistent with the nature of the problem(s) and the patient's and/or family's needs. Usually, the presenting problem(s) are of low to moderate severity.**

1.17 1.17 FUD XXX J 80

AMA: 2019,Jul,10; 2018,Jan,8; 2017,Aug,3; 2017,Jun,6; 2017,Jan,8; 2016,Jan,7; 2016,Jan,13; 2015,Jan,16; 2015,Jan,12; 2014,Nov,14; 2014,Oct,8; 2014,Jan,11

99283 **Emergency department visit for the evaluation and management of a patient, which requires these 3 key components: An expanded problem focused history; An expanded problem focused examination; and Medical decision making of moderate complexity. Counseling and/or coordination of care with other physicians, other qualified health care professionals, or agencies are provided consistent with the nature of the problem(s) and the patient's and/or family's needs. Usually, the presenting problem(s) are of moderate severity.**

1.75 1.75 FUD XXX J 80

AMA: 2019,Jul,10; 2018,Jan,8; 2017,Aug,3; 2017,Jun,6; 2017,Jan,8; 2016,Jan,13; 2016,Jan,7; 2015,Jan,16; 2015,Jan,12; 2014,Nov,14; 2014,Oct,8; 2014,Jan,11

99284 **Emergency department visit for the evaluation and management of a patient, which requires these 3 key components: A detailed history; A detailed examination; and Medical decision making of moderate complexity. Counseling and/or coordination of care with other physicians, other qualified health care professionals, or agencies are provided consistent with the nature of the problem(s) and the patient's and/or family's needs. Usually, the presenting problem(s) are of high severity, and require urgent evaluation by the physician, or other qualified health care professionals but do not pose an immediate significant threat to life or physiologic function.**

3.32 3.32 FUD XXX J 80

AMA: 2019,Jul,10; 2018,Jan,8; 2017,Aug,3; 2017,Jun,6; 2017,Jan,8; 2016,Jan,7; 2016,Jan,13; 2015,Jan,16; 2015,Jan,12; 2014,Nov,14; 2014,Oct,8; 2014,Jan,11

99285 **Emergency department visit for the evaluation and management of a patient, which requires these 3 key components within the constraints imposed by the urgency of the patient's clinical condition and/or mental status: A comprehensive history; A comprehensive examination; and Medical decision making of high complexity. Counseling and/or coordination of care with other physicians, other qualified health care professionals, or agencies are provided consistent with the nature of the problem(s) and the patient's and/or family's needs. Usually, the presenting problem(s) are of high severity and pose an immediate significant threat to life or physiologic function.**

4.89 4.89 FUD XXX J 80

AMA: 2019,Jul,10; 2018,Jan,8; 2017,Aug,3; 2017,Jun,6; 2017,Jan,8; 2016,Jan,7; 2016,Jan,13; 2015,Jan,16; 2015,Jan,12; 2014,Nov,14; 2014,Oct,8; 2014,Jan,11

99288 **Physician or other qualified health care professional direction of emergency medical systems (EMS) emergency care, advanced life support**

INCLUDES Management provided by an emergency/intensive care based physician or other qualified health care professional via voice contact to ambulance/rescue staff for services such as heart monitoring and drug administration

0.00 0.00 FUD XXX B

AMA: 2018,Jan,8; 2017,Aug,3; 2017,Jun,6; 2017,Jan,8; 2016,Jan,13; 2015,Jan,16; 2014,Oct,8; 2014,Jan,11

99291-99292 Critical Care Visits: Patients 72 Months of Age and Older

CMS: 100-04,11,40.1.3 Independent Attending Physician Services; 100-04,12,30.6.4 Services Furnished Incident to Physician's Service; 100-04,12,30.6.9 Swing Bed Visits; 100-04,12,40.3 Global Surgery Review; 100-04,4,160 Clinic and Emergency Visits Under OPPS; 100-04,4,160.1 Critical Care Services

INCLUDES 30 minutes or more of direct care provided by the physician or other qualified health care professional to a critically ill or injured patient, regardless of the location
All activities performed outside of the unit or off the floor
All time spent exclusively with patient/family/caregivers on the nursing unit or elsewhere
Outpatient critical care provided to neonates and pediatric patients up through 71 months of age
Physician or other qualified health care professional presence during interfacility transfer for critically ill/injured patients over 24 months of age
Professional services for interpretation of:
- Blood gases
- Chest films (71045-71046)
- Measurement of cardiac output (93561-93562)
- Other computer stored information
- Pulse oximetry (94760-94762)

Professional services for:
- Gastric intubation (43752-43753)
- Transcutaneous pacing, temporary (92953)
- Venous access, arterial puncture (36000, 36410, 36415, 36591, 36600)
- Ventilation assistance and management, includes CPAP, CNP (94002-94004, 94660, 94662)

EXCLUDES *All services that are less than 30 minutes; report appropriate E&M code*
Inpatient critical care services provided to child 2 through 5 years of age (99475-99476)
Inpatient critical care services provided to infants 29 days through 24 months of age (99471-99472)
Inpatient critical care services provided to neonates that are age 28 days or less (99468-99469)
Other procedures not listed as included performed by the physician or other qualified health care professional rendering critical care
Patients who are not critically ill but in the critical care department (report appropriate E&M code)
Physician or other qualified health care professional presence during interfacility transfer for critically ill/injured patients under 24 months of age (99466-99467)
Supervisory services of control physician during interfacility transfer for critically ill/injured patients under 24 months of age ([99485, 99486])

99291 **Critical care, evaluation and management of the critically ill or critically injured patient; first 30-74 minutes**

6.28 7.82 FUD XXX J 80

AMA: 2019,Aug,8; 2019,Jul,10; 2018,Dec,8; 2018,Dec,8; 2018,Jun,9; 2018,Jan,8; 2017,Aug,3; 2017,Jun,6; 2017,Jan,8; 2016,Oct,8; 2016,Aug,9; 2016,May,3; 2016,Jan,13; 2015,Jul,3; 2015,Feb,10; 2015,Jan,16; 2014,Oct,8; 2014,Oct,14; 2014,Aug,5; 2014,May,4; 2014,Jan,11

+ 99292 **each additional 30 minutes (List separately in addition to code for primary service)**

Code first (99291)

3.15 3.46 FUD ZZZ N 80

AMA: 2019,Aug,8; 2019,Jul,10; 2018,Dec,8; 2018,Dec,8; 2018,Jun,9; 2018,Jan,8; 2017,Aug,3; 2017,Jun,6; 2017,Jan,8; 2016,Aug,9; 2016,May,3; 2016,Jan,13; 2015,Jul,3; 2015,Feb,10; 2015,Jan,16; 2014,Oct,8; 2014,Oct,14; 2014,Aug,5; 2014,May,4; 2014,Jan,11

99304-99310 Nursing Facility Visits

CMS: 100-04,11,40.1.3 Independent Attending Physician Services; 100-04,12,230 Primary Care Incentive Payment Program; 100-04,12,230.1 Definition of Primary Care Practitioners and Services; 100-04,12,230.2 Coordination with Other Payments; 100-04,12,230.3 Claims Processing and Payment; 100-04,12,30.6.10 Consultation Services; 100-04,12,30.6.13 Nursing Facility Visits; 100-04,12,30.6.15.1 Prolonged Services With Direct Face-to-Face Patient Contact; 100-04,12,30.6.4 Services Furnished Incident to Physician's Service; 100-04,12,30.6.9 Swing Bed Visits

INCLUDES All E&M services provided by the admitting physician on the date of nursing facility admission in other locations (e.g., office, emergency department)
Initial care, subsequent care, discharge, and yearly assessments
Initial services include patient assessment and physician participation in developing a plan of care (99304-99306)
Services provided in a psychiatric residential treatment center
Services provided to new and established patients in a nursing facility (skilled, intermediate, and long-term care facilities)
Subsequent services include physician review of medical records, reassessment, and review of test results (99307-99310)

EXCLUDES *Care plan oversight services (99379-99380)*

Code also hospital discharge services on the same date of admission or readmission to the nursing home (99217, 99234-99236, 99238-99239)

99304 **Initial nursing facility care, per day, for the evaluation and management of a patient, which requires these 3 key components: A detailed or comprehensive history; A detailed or comprehensive examination; and Medical decision making that is straightforward or of low complexity. Counseling and/or coordination of care with other physicians, other qualified health care professionals, or agencies are provided consistent with the nature of the problem(s) and the patient's and/or family's needs. Usually, the problem(s) requiring admission are of low severity. Typically, 25 minutes are spent at the bedside and on the patient's facility floor or unit.**

2.54 2.54 FUD XXX B 80

AMA: 2018,Jan,8; 2017,Aug,3; 2017,Jun,6; 2017,Jan,8; 2016,Dec,11; 2016,Jan,13; 2016,Jan,7; 2015,Jan,16; 2014,Nov,14; 2014,Oct,8; 2014,Jan,11

99305 **Initial nursing facility care, per day, for the evaluation and management of a patient, which requires these 3 key components: A comprehensive history; A comprehensive examination; and Medical decision making of moderate complexity. Counseling and/or coordination of care with other physicians, other qualified health care professionals, or agencies are provided consistent with the nature of the problem(s) and the patient's and/or family's needs. Usually, the problem(s) requiring admission are of moderate severity. Typically, 35 minutes are spent at the bedside and on the patient's facility floor or unit.**

3.67 3.67 FUD XXX B 80

AMA: 2018,Jan,8; 2017,Aug,3; 2017,Jun,6; 2017,Jan,8; 2016,Dec,11; 2016,Jan,13; 2016,Jan,7; 2015,Jan,16; 2014,Nov,14; 2014,Oct,8; 2014,Jan,11

99306 **Initial nursing facility care, per day, for the evaluation and management of a patient, which requires these 3 key components: A comprehensive history; A comprehensive examination; and Medical decision making of high complexity. Counseling and/or coordination of care with other physicians, other qualified health care professionals, or agencies are provided consistent with the nature of the problem(s) and the patient's and/or family's needs. Usually, the problem(s) requiring admission are of high severity. Typically, 45 minutes are spent at the bedside and on the patient's facility floor or unit.**

4.70 4.70 FUD XXX B 80

AMA: 2018,Jan,8; 2017,Aug,3; 2017,Jun,6; 2017,Jan,8; 2016,Dec,11; 2016,Jan,13; 2016,Jan,7; 2015,Jan,16; 2014,Nov,14; 2014,Oct,8; 2014,Jan,11

99307 **Subsequent nursing facility care, per day, for the evaluation and management of a patient, which requires at least 2 of these 3 key components: A problem focused interval history; A problem focused examination; Straightforward medical decision making. Counseling and/or coordination of care with other physicians, other qualified health care professionals, or agencies are provided consistent with the nature of the problem(s) and the patient's and/or family's needs. Usually, the patient is stable, recovering, or improving. Typically, 10 minutes are spent at the bedside and on the patient's facility floor or unit.**

1.24 1.24 **FUD** XXX ★ B 80

AMA: 2018,Jan,8; 2017,Aug,3; 2017,Jun,6; 2017,Jan,8; 2016,Dec,11; 2016,Jan,13; 2016,Jan,7; 2015,Jan,16; 2014,Nov,14; 2014,Oct,8; 2014,Jan,11

99308 **Subsequent nursing facility care, per day, for the evaluation and management of a patient, which requires at least 2 of these 3 key components: An expanded problem focused interval history; An expanded problem focused examination; Medical decision making of low complexity. Counseling and/or coordination of care with other physicians, other qualified health care professionals, or agencies are provided consistent with the nature of the problem(s) and the patient's and/or family's needs. Usually, the patient is responding inadequately to therapy or has developed a minor complication. Typically, 15 minutes are spent at the bedside and on the patient's facility floor or unit.**

1.94 1.94 **FUD** XXX 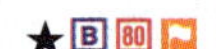

AMA: 2018,Jan,8; 2017,Aug,3; 2017,Jun,6; 2017,Jan,8; 2016,Dec,11; 2016,Jan,13; 2016,Jan,7; 2015,Jan,16; 2014,Nov,14; 2014,Oct,8; 2014,Jan,11

99309 **Subsequent nursing facility care, per day, for the evaluation and management of a patient, which requires at least 2 of these 3 key components: A detailed interval history; A detailed examination; Medical decision making of moderate complexity. Counseling and/or coordination of care with other physicians, other qualified health care professionals, or agencies are provided consistent with the nature of the problem(s) and the patient's and/or family's needs. Usually, the patient has developed a significant complication or a significant new problem. Typically, 25 minutes are spent at the bedside and on the patient's facility floor or unit.**

2.58 2.58 **FUD** XXX 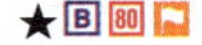

AMA: 2018,Jan,8; 2017,Aug,3; 2017,Jun,6; 2017,Jan,8; 2016,Dec,11; 2016,Jan,13; 2016,Jan,7; 2015,Jan,16; 2014,Nov,14; 2014,Oct,8; 2014,Jan,11

99310 **Subsequent nursing facility care, per day, for the evaluation and management of a patient, which requires at least 2 of these 3 key components: A comprehensive interval history; A comprehensive examination; Medical decision making of high complexity. Counseling and/or coordination of care with other physicians, other qualified health care professionals, or agencies are provided consistent with the nature of the problem(s) and the patient's and/or family's needs. The patient may be unstable or may have developed a significant new problem requiring immediate physician attention. Typically, 35 minutes are spent at the bedside and on the patient's facility floor or unit.**

3.82 3.82 **FUD** XXX ★ B 80

AMA: 2018,Jan,8; 2017,Aug,3; 2017,Jun,6; 2017,Jan,8; 2016,Dec,11; 2016,Jan,13; 2016,Jan,7; 2015,Jan,16; 2014,Nov,14; 2014,Oct,8; 2014,Jan,11

99315-99316 Nursing Home Discharge

CMS: 100-04,11,40.1.3 Independent Attending Physician Services; 100-04,12,230 Primary Care Incentive Payment Program; 100-04,12,230.1 Definition of Primary Care Practitioners and Services; 100-04,12,230.2 Coordination with Other Payments; 100-04,12,230.3 Claims Processing and Payment; 100-04,12,30.6.13 Nursing Facility Visits; 100-04,12,30.6.4 Services Furnished Incident to Physician's Service; 100-04,12,40.3 Global Surgery Review

INCLUDES Discharge services include all time spent by the physician or other qualified health care professional for:
- Completion of discharge records
- Discharge instructions for patient and caregivers
- Discussion regarding the stay in the facility
- Final patient examination
- Provide prescriptions and referrals as appropriate

99315 **Nursing facility discharge day management; 30 minutes or less**

2.07 2.07 **FUD** XXX B 80

AMA: 2018,Jan,8; 2017,Aug,3; 2017,Jun,6; 2017,Jan,8; 2016,Dec,11; 2016,Jan,13; 2016,Jan,7; 2015,Jan,16; 2014,Nov,14; 2014,Oct,8; 2014,Jan,11

99316 **more than 30 minutes**

2.98 2.98 **FUD** XXX B 80

AMA: 2018,Jan,8; 2017,Aug,3; 2017,Jun,6; 2017,Jan,8; 2016,Dec,11; 2016,Jan,13; 2016,Jan,7; 2015,Jan,16; 2014,Nov,14; 2014,Oct,8; 2014,Jan,11

99318 Annual Nursing Home Assessment

CMS: 100-04,11,40.1.3 Independent Attending Physician Services; 100-04,12,230 Primary Care Incentive Payment Program; 100-04,12,230.1 Definition of Primary Care Practitioners and Services; 100-04,12,230.2 Coordination with Other Payments; 100-04,12,230.3 Claims Processing and Payment; 100-04,12,30.6.13 Nursing Facility Visits; 100-04,12,30.6.15.1 Prolonged Services With Direct Face-to-Face Patient Contact; 100-04,12,30.6.4 Services Furnished Incident to Physician's Service; 100-04,12,30.6.9 Swing Bed Visits

INCLUDES Includes nursing facility visits on same date of service as (99304-99316)

99318 **Evaluation and management of a patient involving an annual nursing facility assessment, which requires these 3 key components: A detailed interval history; A comprehensive examination; and Medical decision making that is of low to moderate complexity. Counseling and/or coordination of care with other physicians, other qualified health care professionals, or agencies are provided consistent with the nature of the problem(s) and the patient's and/or family's needs. Usually, the patient is stable, recovering, or improving. Typically, 30 minutes are spent at the bedside and on the patient's facility floor or unit.**

2.70 2.70 **FUD** XXX B 80

AMA: 2018,Jan,8; 2017,Aug,3; 2017,Jun,6; 2017,Jan,8; 2016,Dec,11; 2016,Jan,7; 2016,Jan,13; 2015,Jan,16; 2014,Nov,14; 2014,Oct,8; 2014,Jan,11

99324-99337 Domiciliary Care, Rest Home, Assisted Living Visits

CMS: 100-04,12,230 Primary Care Incentive Payment Program; 100-04,12,230.1 Definition of Primary Care Practitioners and Services; 100-04,12,230.2 Coordination with Other Payments; 100-04,12,230.3 Claims Processing and Payment; 100-04,12,30.6.14 Domiciliary Care, Rest Home, Assisted Living Visits; 100-04,12,30.6.15.1 Prolonged Services With Direct Face-to-Face Patient Contact; 100-04,12,30.6.4 Services Furnished Incident to Physician's Service

INCLUDES E&M services for patients residing in assisted living, domiciliary care, and rest homes where medical care is not included

Services provided to new patients or established patients (99324-99328, 99334-99337)

EXCLUDES *Care plan oversight services provided to a patient in a rest home under the care of a home health agency (99374-99375)*

Care plan oversight services provided to a patient under the care of a hospice agency (99377-99378)

99324 **Domiciliary or rest home visit for the evaluation and management of a new patient, which requires these 3 key components: A problem focused history; A problem focused examination; and Straightforward medical decision making. Counseling and/or coordination of care with other physicians, other qualified health care professionals, or agencies are provided consistent with the nature of the problem(s) and the patient's and/or family's needs. Usually, the presenting problem(s) are of low severity. Typically, 20 minutes are spent with the patient and/or family or caregiver.**

1.56 1.56 FUD XXX B 80

AMA: 2018,Apr,9; 2018,Jan,8; 2017,Aug,3; 2017,Jun,6; 2017,Jan,8; 2016,Dec,11; 2016,Jan,13; 2016,Jan,7; 2015,Jan,16; 2014,Nov,14; 2014,Oct,8; 2014,Oct,3; 2014,Jan,11

99325 **Domiciliary or rest home visit for the evaluation and management of a new patient, which requires these 3 key components: An expanded problem focused history; An expanded problem focused examination; and Medical decision making of low complexity. Counseling and/or coordination of care with other physicians, other qualified health care professionals, or agencies are provided consistent with the nature of the problem(s) and the patient's and/or family's needs. Usually, the presenting problem(s) are of moderate severity. Typically, 30 minutes are spent with the patient and/or family or caregiver.**

2.26 2.26 FUD XXX B 80

AMA: 2018,Apr,9; 2018,Jan,8; 2017,Aug,3; 2017,Jun,6; 2017,Jan,8; 2016,Dec,11; 2016,Jan,13; 2016,Jan,7; 2015,Jan,16; 2014,Nov,14; 2014,Oct,8; 2014,Oct,3; 2014,Jan,11

99326 **Domiciliary or rest home visit for the evaluation and management of a new patient, which requires these 3 key components: A detailed history; A detailed examination; and Medical decision making of moderate complexity. Counseling and/or coordination of care with other physicians, other qualified health care professionals, or agencies are provided consistent with the nature of the problem(s) and the patient's and/or family's needs. Usually, the presenting problem(s) are of moderate to high severity. Typically, 45 minutes are spent with the patient and/or family or caregiver.**

3.92 3.92 FUD XXX B 80

AMA: 2018,Apr,9; 2018,Jan,8; 2017,Aug,3; 2017,Jun,6; 2017,Jan,8; 2016,Dec,11; 2016,Jan,13; 2016,Jan,7; 2015,Jan,16; 2014,Nov,14; 2014,Oct,8; 2014,Oct,3; 2014,Jan,11

99327 **Domiciliary or rest home visit for the evaluation and management of a new patient, which requires these 3 key components: A comprehensive history; A comprehensive examination; and Medical decision making of moderate complexity. Counseling and/or coordination of care with other physicians, other qualified health care professionals, or agencies are provided consistent with the nature of the problem(s) and the patient's and/or family's needs. Usually, the presenting problem(s) are of high severity. Typically, 60 minutes are spent with the patient and/or family or caregiver.**

5.26 5.26 FUD XXX B 80

AMA: 2018,Apr,9; 2018,Jan,8; 2017,Aug,3; 2017,Jun,6; 2017,Jan,8; 2016,Dec,11; 2016,Jan,13; 2016,Jan,7; 2015,Jan,16; 2014,Nov,14; 2014,Oct,8; 2014,Oct,3; 2014,Jan,11

99328 **Domiciliary or rest home visit for the evaluation and management of a new patient, which requires these 3 key components: A comprehensive history; A comprehensive examination; and Medical decision making of high complexity. Counseling and/or coordination of care with other physicians, other qualified health care professionals, or agencies are provided consistent with the nature of the problem(s) and the patient's and/or family's needs. Usually, the patient is unstable or has developed a significant new problem requiring immediate physician attention. Typically, 75 minutes are spent with the patient and/or family or caregiver.**

6.19 6.19 FUD XXX B 80

AMA: 2018,Apr,9; 2018,Jan,8; 2017,Aug,3; 2017,Jun,6; 2017,Jan,8; 2016,Dec,11; 2016,Jan,13; 2016,Jan,7; 2015,Jan,16; 2014,Nov,14; 2014,Oct,8; 2014,Oct,3; 2014,Jan,11

99334 **Domiciliary or rest home visit for the evaluation and management of an established patient, which requires at least 2 of these 3 key components: A problem focused interval history; A problem focused examination; Straightforward medical decision making. Counseling and/or coordination of care with other physicians, other qualified health care professionals, or agencies are provided consistent with the nature of the problem(s) and the patient's and/or family's needs. Usually, the presenting problem(s) are self-limited or minor. Typically, 15 minutes are spent with the patient and/or family or caregiver.**

1.70 1.70 FUD XXX B 80

AMA: 2018,Apr,9; 2018,Jan,8; 2017,Aug,3; 2017,Jun,6; 2017,Jan,8; 2016,Dec,11; 2016,Jan,13; 2016,Jan,7; 2015,Jan,16; 2014,Nov,14; 2014,Oct,8; 2014,Oct,3; 2014,Jan,11

99335 **Domiciliary or rest home visit for the evaluation and management of an established patient, which requires at least 2 of these 3 key components: An expanded problem focused interval history; An expanded problem focused examination; Medical decision making of low complexity. Counseling and/or coordination of care with other physicians, other qualified health care professionals, or agencies are provided consistent with the nature of the problem(s) and the patient's and/or family's needs. Usually, the presenting problem(s) are of low to moderate severity. Typically, 25 minutes are spent with the patient and/or family or caregiver.**

2.68 2.68 FUD XXX B 80

AMA: 2018,Apr,9; 2018,Jan,8; 2017,Aug,3; 2017,Jun,6; 2017,Jan,8; 2016,Dec,11; 2016,Jan,13; 2016,Jan,7; 2015,Jan,16; 2014,Nov,14; 2014,Oct,8; 2014,Oct,3; 2014,Jan,11

99336 **Domiciliary or rest home visit for the evaluation and management of an established patient, which requires at least 2 of these 3 key components: A detailed interval history; A detailed examination; Medical decision making of moderate complexity. Counseling and/or coordination of care with other physicians, other qualified health care professionals, or agencies are provided consistent with the nature of the problem(s) and the patient's and/or family's needs. Usually, the presenting problem(s) are of moderate to high severity. Typically, 40 minutes are spent with the patient and/or family or caregiver.**

3.82 3.82 FUD XXX B 80

AMA: 2018,Apr,9; 2018,Jan,8; 2017,Aug,3; 2017,Jun,6; 2017,Jan,8; 2016,Dec,11; 2016,Jan,13; 2016,Jan,7; 2015,Jan,16; 2014,Nov,14; 2014,Oct,8; 2014,Oct,3; 2014,Jan,11

99337 **Domiciliary or rest home visit for the evaluation and management of an established patient, which requires at least 2 of these 3 key components: A comprehensive interval history; A comprehensive examination; Medical decision making of moderate to high complexity. Counseling and/or coordination of care with other physicians, other qualified health care professionals, or agencies are provided consistent with the nature of the problem(s) and the patient's and/or family's needs. Usually, the presenting problem(s) are of moderate to high severity. The patient may be unstable or may have developed a significant new problem requiring immediate physician attention. Typically, 60 minutes are spent with the patient and/or family or caregiver.**

5.47 5.47 FUD XXX B 80

AMA: 2018,Apr,9; 2018,Jan,8; 2017,Aug,3; 2017,Jun,6; 2017,Jan,8; 2016,Dec,11; 2016,Jan,13; 2016,Jan,7; 2015,Jan,16; 2014,Nov,14; 2014,Oct,8; 2014,Oct,3; 2014,Jan,11

99339-99340 Care Plan Oversight: Rest Home, Domiciliary Care, Assisted Living, and Home

CMS: 100-04,12,180 Payment of Care Plan Oversight (CPO); 100-04,12,180.1 Billing for Care Plan Oversight (CPO); 100-04,12,230 Primary Care Incentive Payment Program; 100-04,12,230.1 Definition of Primary Care Practitioners and Services; 100-04,12,230.2 Coordination with Other Payments; 100-04,12,230.3 Claims Processing and Payment; 100-04,12,30.6.14 Domiciliary Care, Rest Home, Assisted Living Visits; 100-04,12,30.6.4 Services Furnished Incident to Physician's Service

INCLUDES Care plan oversight for patients residing in assisted living, domiciliary care, private residences, and rest homes

Patient management services during same time frame as ([99421, 99422, 99423], 99441-99443, 98966-98968)

EXCLUDES *Care plan oversight services furnished under a home health agency, nursing facility, or hospice (99374-99380)*

99339 **Individual physician supervision of a patient (patient not present) in home, domiciliary or rest home (eg, assisted living facility) requiring complex and multidisciplinary care modalities involving regular physician development and/or revision of care plans, review of subsequent reports of patient status, review of related laboratory and other studies, communication (including telephone calls) for purposes of assessment or care decisions with health care professional(s), family member(s), surrogate decision maker(s) (eg, legal guardian) and/or key caregiver(s) involved in patient's care, integration of new information into the medical treatment plan and/or adjustment of medical therapy, within a calendar month; 15-29 minutes**

2.17 2.17 FUD XXX B

AMA: 2019,Jan,6; 2018,Oct,9; 2018,Jan,8; 2017,Aug,3; 2017,Jun,6; 2017,Jan,8; 2016,Jan,13; 2015,Jan,16; 2014,Oct,3; 2014,Oct,8; 2014,Jan,11

99340 **30 minutes or more**

3.05 3.05 FUD XXX B

AMA: 2019,Jan,6; 2018,Oct,9; 2018,Jan,8; 2017,Aug,3; 2017,Jun,6; 2017,Jan,8; 2016,Jan,13; 2015,Jan,16; 2014,Oct,3; 2014,Oct,8; 2014,Jan,11

99341-99350 Home Visits

CMS: 100-04,11,40.1.3 Independent Attending Physician Services; 100-04,12,230 Primary Care Incentive Payment Program; 100-04,12,230.1 Definition of Primary Care Practitioners and Services; 100-04,12,230.2 Coordination with Other Payments; 100-04,12,230.3 Claims Processing and Payment; 100-04,12,30.6.14 Domiciliary Care, Rest Home, Assisted Living Visits; 100-04,12,30.6.14.1 Home Visits; 100-04,12,30.6.15.1 Prolonged Services With Direct Face-to-Face Patient Contact; 100-04,12,30.6.4 Services Furnished Incident to Physician's Service; 100-04,12,40.3 Global Surgery Review; 100-04,30.6.14.1 Home Services (Codes 99341 - 99350)

INCLUDES Services for a new patient or an established patient (99341-99345, 99347-99350)

Services provided to a patient in a private home (e.g., private residence, temporary or short-term housing such as campground, cruise ship, hostel or hotel)

EXCLUDES *Services provided to patients under home health agency or hospice care (99374-99378)*

99341 **Home visit for the evaluation and management of a new patient, which requires these 3 key components: A problem focused history; A problem focused examination; and Straightforward medical decision making. Counseling and/or coordination of care with other physicians, other qualified health care professionals, or agencies are provided consistent with the nature of the problem(s) and the patient's and/or family's needs. Usually, the presenting problem(s) are of low severity. Typically, 20 minutes are spent face-to-face with the patient and/or family.**

1.56 1.56 FUD XXX B 80

AMA: 2018,Apr,9; 2018,Jan,8; 2017,Aug,3; 2017,Jun,6; 2017,Jan,8; 2016,Dec,11; 2016,Jan,13; 2016,Jan,7; 2015,Jan,16; 2014,Nov,14; 2014,Oct,8; 2014,Oct,3; 2014,Jan,11

99342 **Home visit for the evaluation and management of a new patient, which requires these 3 key components: An expanded problem focused history; An expanded problem focused examination; and Medical decision making of low complexity. Counseling and/or coordination of care with other physicians, other qualified health care professionals, or agencies are provided consistent with the nature of the problem(s) and the patient's and/or family's needs. Usually, the presenting problem(s) are of moderate severity. Typically, 30 minutes are spent face-to-face with the patient and/or family.**

2.25 2.25 FUD XXX B 80

AMA: 2018,Apr,9; 2018,Jan,8; 2017,Aug,3; 2017,Jun,6; 2017,Jan,8; 2016,Dec,11; 2016,Jan,13; 2016,Jan,7; 2015,Jan,16; 2014,Nov,14; 2014,Oct,8; 2014,Oct,3; 2014,Jan,11

99343 **Home visit for the evaluation and management of a new patient, which requires these 3 key components: A detailed history; A detailed examination; and Medical decision making of moderate complexity. Counseling and/or coordination of care with other physicians, other qualified health care professionals, or agencies are provided consistent with the nature of the problem(s) and the patient's and/or family's needs. Usually, the presenting problem(s) are of moderate to high severity. Typically, 45 minutes are spent face-to-face with the patient and/or family.**

3.67 3.67 FUD XXX B 80

AMA: 2018,Apr,9; 2018,Jan,8; 2017,Aug,3; 2017,Jun,6; 2017,Jan,8; 2016,Dec,11; 2016,Jan,13; 2016,Jan,7; 2015,Jan,16; 2014,Nov,14; 2014,Oct,8; 2014,Oct,3; 2014,Jan,11

99344 **Home visit for the evaluation and management of a new patient, which requires these 3 key components: A comprehensive history; A comprehensive examination; and Medical decision making of moderate complexity. Counseling and/or coordination of care with other physicians, other qualified health care professionals, or agencies are provided consistent with the nature of the problem(s) and the patient's and/or family's needs. Usually, the presenting problem(s) are of high severity. Typically, 60 minutes are spent face-to-face with the patient and/or family.**

5.14 5.14 **FUD** XXX B 80

AMA: 2018,Apr,9; 2018,Jan,8; 2017,Aug,3; 2017,Jun,6; 2017,Jan,8; 2016,Dec,11; 2016,Jan,7; 2016,Jan,13; 2015,Jan,16; 2014,Nov,14; 2014,Oct,8; 2014,Oct,3; 2014,Jan,11

99345 **Home visit for the evaluation and management of a new patient, which requires these 3 key components: A comprehensive history; A comprehensive examination; and Medical decision making of high complexity. Counseling and/or coordination of care with other physicians, other qualified health care professionals, or agencies are provided consistent with the nature of the problem(s) and the patient's and/or family's needs. Usually, the patient is unstable or has developed a significant new problem requiring immediate physician attention. Typically, 75 minutes are spent face-to-face with the patient and/or family.**

6.25 6.25 **FUD** XXX B 80

AMA: 2018,Apr,9; 2018,Jan,8; 2017,Aug,3; 2017,Jun,6; 2017,Jan,8; 2016,Dec,11; 2016,Jan,7; 2016,Jan,13; 2015,Jan,16; 2014,Nov,14; 2014,Oct,8; 2014,Oct,3; 2014,Jan,11

99347 **Home visit for the evaluation and management of an established patient, which requires at least 2 of these 3 key components: A problem focused interval history; A problem focused examination; Straightforward medical decision making. Counseling and/or coordination of care with other physicians, other qualified health care professionals, or agencies are provided consistent with the nature of the problem(s) and the patient's and/or family's needs. Usually, the presenting problem(s) are self limited or minor. Typically, 15 minutes are spent face-to-face with the patient and/or family.**

1.56 1.56 **FUD** XXX B 80

AMA: 2018,Apr,9; 2018,Jan,8; 2017,Aug,3; 2017,Jun,6; 2017,Jan,8; 2016,Dec,11; 2016,Jan,7; 2016,Jan,13; 2015,Jan,16; 2014,Nov,14; 2014,Oct,8; 2014,Oct,3; 2014,Jan,11

99348 **Home visit for the evaluation and management of an established patient, which requires at least 2 of these 3 key components: An expanded problem focused interval history; An expanded problem focused examination; Medical decision making of low complexity. Counseling and/or coordination of care with other physicians, other qualified health care professionals, or agencies are provided consistent with the nature of the problem(s) and the patient's and/or family's needs. Usually, the presenting problem(s) are of low to moderate severity. Typically, 25 minutes are spent face-to-face with the patient and/or family.**

2.37 2.37 **FUD** XXX B 80

AMA: 2018,Apr,9; 2018,Jan,8; 2017,Aug,3; 2017,Jun,6; 2017,Jan,8; 2016,Dec,11; 2016,Jan,7; 2016,Jan,13; 2015,Jan,16; 2014,Nov,14; 2014,Oct,8; 2014,Oct,3; 2014,Jan,11

99349 **Home visit for the evaluation and management of an established patient, which requires at least 2 of these 3 key components: A detailed interval history; A detailed examination; Medical decision making of moderate complexity. Counseling and/or coordination of care with other physicians, other qualified health care professionals, or agencies are provided consistent with the nature of the problem(s) and the patient's and/or family's needs. Usually, the presenting problem(s) are moderate to high severity. Typically, 40 minutes are spent face-to-face with the patient and/or family.**

3.64 3.64 **FUD** XXX B 80

AMA: 2018,Apr,9; 2018,Jan,8; 2017,Aug,3; 2017,Jun,6; 2017,Jan,8; 2016,Dec,11; 2016,Jan,7; 2016,Jan,13; 2015,Jan,16; 2014,Nov,14; 2014,Oct,8; 2014,Oct,3; 2014,Jan,11

99350 **Home visit for the evaluation and management of an established patient, which requires at least 2 of these 3 key components: A comprehensive interval history; A comprehensive examination; Medical decision making of moderate to high complexity. Counseling and/or coordination of care with other physicians, other qualified health care professionals, or agencies are provided consistent with the nature of the problem(s) and the patient's and/or family's needs. Usually, the presenting problem(s) are of moderate to high severity. The patient may be unstable or may have developed a significant new problem requiring immediate physician attention. Typically, 60 minutes are spent face-to-face with the patient and/or family.**

5.05 5.05 **FUD** XXX B 80

AMA: 2018,Apr,9; 2018,Jan,8; 2017,Aug,3; 2017,Jun,6; 2017,Jan,8; 2016,Dec,11; 2016,Jan,7; 2016,Jan,13; 2015,Jan,16; 2014,Nov,14; 2014,Oct,8; 2014,Oct,3; 2014,Jan,11

99354-99357 Prolonged Services Direct Contact

CMS: 100-04,11,40.1.3 Independent Attending Physician Services; 100-04,12,30.6.15.1 Prolonged Services With Direct Face-to-Face Patient Contact; 100-04,12,30.6.4 Services Furnished Incident to Physician's Service

INCLUDES Personal contact with the patient by the physician or other qualified health professional
Services extending beyond the customary service provided in the inpatient or outpatient setting
Time spent providing additional indirect contact services on the floor or unit of the hospital or nursing facility during the same session as the direct contact
Time spent providing prolonged services on a date of service, even when the time is not continuous

EXCLUDES *Services less than 30 minutes, less than 15 minutes after the first hour, or after the final 30 minutes*
Services provided independent of the date of personal contact with the patient (99358-99359)

Code first E&M service code, as appropriate

+ **99354** **Prolonged evaluation and management or psychotherapy service(s) (beyond the typical service time of the primary procedure) in the office or other outpatient setting requiring direct patient contact beyond the usual service; first hour (List separately in addition to code for office or other outpatient Evaluation and Management or psychotherapy service)**

EXCLUDES *Prolonged service provided by clinical staff under supervision ([99415, 99416])*
Use of code more than one time per date of service

Code first (99201-99215, 99241-99245, 99324-99337, 99341-99350, 90837, 90847)

3.44 3.67 **FUD** ZZZ ★ N 80

AMA: 2019,Jun,7; 2018,Jan,8; 2017,Jan,8; 2016,Dec,11; 2016,Jan,13; 2015,Oct,9; 2015,Oct,3; 2015,Jan,16; 2014,Oct,8; 2014,Jun,14; 2014,Apr,6; 2014,Jan,11

\+ **99355** **each additional 30 minutes (List separately in addition to code for prolonged service)**

EXCLUDES *Prolonged service provided by clinical staff under supervision ([99415, 99416])*

Code first (99354)

2.60 2.80 FUD ZZZ ★ N 80

AMA: 2019,Jun,7; 2018,Jan,8; 2017,Jan,8; 2016,Dec,11; 2016,Jan,13; 2015,Oct,9; 2015,Oct,3; 2015,Jan,16; 2014,Oct,8; 2014,Jun,14; 2014,Apr,6; 2014,Jan,11

\+ **99356** **Prolonged service in the inpatient or observation setting, requiring unit/floor time beyond the usual service; first hour (List separately in addition to code for inpatient Evaluation and Management service)**

EXCLUDES *Use of code more than one time per date of service*

Code first (99218-99223 [99224, 99225, 99226], 99231-99236, 99251-99255, 99304-99310, 90837, 90847)

2.60 2.60 FUD ZZZ C 80

AMA: 2019,Jun,7; 2018,Jan,8; 2017,Jan,8; 2016,Dec,11; 2016,Jan,13; 2015,Oct,9; 2015,Oct,3; 2015,Jan,16; 2014,Oct,8; 2014,Jun,14; 2014,Apr,6; 2014,Jan,11

\+ **99357** **each additional 30 minutes (List separately in addition to code for prolonged service)**

Code first (99356)

2.61 2.61 FUD ZZZ C 80

AMA: 2019,Jun,7; 2018,Jan,8; 2017,Jan,8; 2016,Dec,11; 2016,Jan,13; 2015,Oct,9; 2015,Oct,3; 2015,Jan,16; 2014,Oct,8; 2014,Jun,14; 2014,Apr,6; 2014,Jan,11

99358-99359 Prolonged Services Indirect Contact

CMS: 100-04,11,40.1.3 Independent Attending Physician Services; 100-04,12,30.6.15.2 Prolonged Services Without Face to Face Service; 100-04,12,30.6.4 Services Furnished Incident to Physician's Service

INCLUDES Services extending beyond the customary service
Time spent providing indirect contact services by the physician or other qualified health care professional in relation to patient management where face-to-face services have or will occur on a different date
Time spent providing prolonged services performed on a date of service (which may be other than the date of the primary service) that are not continuous

EXCLUDES *Any additional unit or floor time in the hospital or nursing facility during the same evaluation and management session*
Behavioral health integration care management services (99484)
Care plan oversight (99339-99340, 99374-99380)
Chronic care management services provided during the same month ([99490], [99491])
INR monitoring services (93792-93793)
Online medical services ([99421, 99422, 99423])
Patient management services during same time frame as (99487-99489, 99495-99496)
Psychiatric collaborative care management services during the same month (99492-99494)
Services less than 30 minutes, less than 15 minutes after the first hour, or after the final 30 minutes
Time spent in medical team conference (99366-99368)
Use of code more than one time per date of service

Code also E&M or other services provided

99358 **Prolonged evaluation and management service before and/or after direct patient care; first hour**

EXCLUDES *Use of code more than one time per date of service*

3.15 3.15 FUD XXX N 80

AMA: 2019,Jun,7, 2019,Jan,13, 2018,Oct,9, 2018,Jan,8, 2017,Jan,8; 2016,Jan,13; 2015,Jan,16; 2014,Oct,8; 2014,Oct,3; 2014,Jan,11

\+ **99359** **each additional 30 minutes (List separately in addition to code for prolonged service)**

Code first (99358)

1.52 1.52 FUD ZZZ N 80

AMA: 2019,Jun,7; 2019,Jan,13; 2018,Oct,9; 2018,Jan,8; 2017,Jan,8; 2016,Jan,13; 2015,Jan,16; 2014,Oct,8; 2014,Oct,3; 2014,Jan,11

99415-99416 [99415, 99416] Prolonged Clinical Staff Services Under Supervision

CMS: 100-04,11,40.1.3 Independent Attending Physician Services

INCLUDES Time spent by clinical staff providing prolonged face-to-face services extending beyond the customary service under the supervision of a physician or other qualified health professional
Time spent by clinical staff providing prolonged services on a date of service, even when the time is not continuous

EXCLUDES *Prolonged service provided by physician or other qualified health care professional (99354-99357)*
Services less than 45 minutes
Services provided to more than two patients at the same time

Code also E&M or other services provided

\+ # **99415** **Prolonged clinical staff service (the service beyond the typical service time) during an evaluation and management service in the office or outpatient setting, direct patient contact with physician supervision; first hour (List separately in addition to code for outpatient Evaluation and Management service)**

EXCLUDES *Use of code more than one time per date of service*

Code first (99201-99215)

0.28 0.28 FUD ZZZ N 80 TC

AMA: 2018,Jan,8; 2017,Jan,8; 2016,Mar,8; 2016,Feb,13; 2016,Jan,13; 2015,Oct,3

\+ # **99416** **each additional 30 minutes (List separately in addition to code for prolonged service)**

EXCLUDES *Services less than 30 minutes, less than 15 minutes after the first hour, or after the final 30 minutes*

Code first ([99415])

0.12 0.12 FUD ZZZ N 80 TC

AMA: 2018,Jan,8; 2017,Jan,8; 2016,Mar,8; 2016,Feb,13; 2016,Jan,13; 2015,Oct,3

99360 Standby Services

CMS: 100-04,11,40.1.3 Independent Attending Physician Services; 100-04,12,30.6.15.3 Standby Services; 100-04,12,30.6.4 Services Furnished Incident to Physician's Service

INCLUDES Services requested by physician or qualified health care professional that involve no direct patient contact
Total standby time for the day

EXCLUDES *Delivery attendance (99464)*
Less than 30 minutes of standby time
On-call services mandated by the hospital (99026-99027)

Code also as appropriate (99460, 99465)

99360 **Standby service, requiring prolonged attendance, each 30 minutes (eg, operative standby, standby for frozen section, for cesarean/high risk delivery, for monitoring EEG)**

1.73 1.73 FUD XXX B

AMA: 2018,Jan,8; 2017,Jan,8; 2016,Jan,13; 2015,Jan,16; 2014,Oct,8; 2014,Apr,5; 2014,Jan,11

99366-99368 Interdisciplinary Conferences

CMS: 100-04,11,40.1.3 Independent Attending Physician Services

INCLUDES Documentation of participation, contribution, and recommendations of the conference
Face-to-face participation by minimum of three qualified people from different specialties or disciplines
Only participants who have performed face-to-face evaluations or direct treatment to the patient within the previous 60 days
Start of the review of an individual patient and ends at conclusion of review

EXCLUDES *Conferences of less than 30 minutes (not reportable)*
More than one individual from the same specialty at the same encounter
Patient management services during same time frame as (99487-99489, 99495-99496)
Time spent record keeping or writing a report

99366 Medical team conference with interdisciplinary team of health care professionals, face-to-face with patient and/or family, 30 minutes or more, participation by nonphysician qualified health care professional

INCLUDES Team conferences of 30 minutes or more

EXCLUDES *Team conferences by a physician with patient or family present, see appropriate evaluation and management service code*

1.19 1.21 FUD XXX N

AMA: 2018,Apr,9; 2018,Jan,8; 2017,Jan,8; 2016,Jan,13; 2015,Jan,16; 2014,Oct,8; 2014,Oct,3; 2014,Jun,3; 2014,Jan,11

99367 Medical team conference with interdisciplinary team of health care professionals, patient and/or family not present, 30 minutes or more; participation by physician

INCLUDES Team conferences of 30 minutes or more

1.60 1.60 FUD XXX N

AMA: 2018,Apr,9; 2018,Jan,8; 2017,Jan,8; 2016,Jan,13; 2015,Jan,16; 2014,Oct,8; 2014,Oct,3; 2014,Jun,3; 2014,Jan,11

99368 participation by nonphysician qualified health care professional

INCLUDES Team conferences of 30 minutes or more

1.04 1.04 FUD XXX N

AMA: 2018,Apr,9; 2018,Jan,8; 2017,Jan,8; 2016,Jan,13; 2015,Jan,16; 2014,Oct,8; 2014,Oct,3; 2014,Jun,3; 2014,Jan,11

99374-99380 Care Plan Oversight: Patient Under Care of HHA, Hospice, or Nursing Facility

CMS: 100-04,11,40.1.3 Independent Attending Physician Services; 100-04,12,180 Payment of Care Plan Oversight (CPO); 100-04,12,180.1 Billing for Care Plan Oversight (CPO); 100-04,12,30.6.4 Services Furnished Incident to Physician's Service

INCLUDES Analysis of reports, diagnostic tests, treatment plans
Discussions with other health care providers, outside of the practice, involved in the patient's care
Establishment of and revisions to care plans within a 30-day period
Payment to one physician per month for covered care plan oversight services (must be the same one who signed the plan of care)

EXCLUDES *Care plan oversight services provided in a hospice agency (99377-99378)*
Care plan oversight services provided in assisted living, domiciliary care, or private residence, not under care of a home health agency or hospice (99339-99340)
Patient management services during same time frame as ([99421, 99422, 99423], 99441-99443, 98966-98968)
Routine postoperative care provided during a global surgery period
Time discussing treatment with patient and/or caregivers

Code also office/outpatient visits, hospital, home, nursing facility, domiciliary, or non-face-to-face services

99374 Supervision of a patient under care of home health agency (patient not present) in home, domiciliary or equivalent environment (eg, Alzheimer's facility) requiring complex and multidisciplinary care modalities involving regular development and/or revision of care plans by that individual, review of subsequent reports of patient status, review of related laboratory and other studies, communication (including telephone calls) for purposes of assessment or care decisions with health care professional(s), family member(s), surrogate decision maker(s) (eg, legal guardian) and/or key caregiver(s) involved in patient's care, integration of new information into the medical treatment plan and/or adjustment of medical therapy, within a calendar month; 15-29 minutes

1.60 1.96 FUD XXX B

AMA: 2019,Jan,6; 2018,Jan,8; 2017,Jan,8; 2016,Jan,13; 2015,Jan,16; 2014,Oct,8; 2014,Oct,3; 2014,Jan,11

99375 30 minutes or more

2.50 2.94 FUD XXX E

AMA: 2019,Jan,6; 2018,Jan,8; 2017,Jan,8; 2016,Jan,13; 2015,Jan,16; 2014,Oct,8; 2014,Oct,3; 2014,Jan,11

99377 Supervision of a hospice patient (patient not present) requiring complex and multidisciplinary care modalities involving regular development and/or revision of care plans by that individual, review of subsequent reports of patient status, review of related laboratory and other studies, communication (including telephone calls) for purposes of assessment or care decisions with health care professional(s), family member(s), surrogate decision maker(s) (eg, legal guardian) and/or key caregiver(s) involved in patient's care, integration of new information into the medical treatment plan and/or adjustment of medical therapy, within a calendar month; 15-29 minutes

1.60 1.96 FUD XXX B

AMA: 2019,Jan,6; 2018,Jan,8; 2017,Jan,8; 2016,Jan,13; 2015,Jan,16; 2014,Oct,8; 2014,Oct,3; 2014,Jan,11

99378 30 minutes or more

2.50 2.94 FUD XXX E

AMA: 2019,Jan,6; 2018,Jan,8; 2017,Jan,8; 2016,Jan,13; 2015,Jan,16; 2014,Oct,8; 2014,Oct,3; 2014,Jan,11

99379 **Supervision of a nursing facility patient (patient not present) requiring complex and multidisciplinary care modalities involving regular development and/or revision of care plans by that individual, review of subsequent reports of patient status, review of related laboratory and other studies, communication (including telephone calls) for purposes of assessment or care decisions with health care professional(s), family member(s), surrogate decision maker(s) (eg, legal guardian) and/or key caregiver(s) involved in patient's care, integration of new information into the medical treatment plan and/or adjustment of medical therapy, within a calendar month; 15-29 minutes**

1.60 1.96 FUD XXX B

AMA: 2019,Jan,6; 2018,Jan,8; 2017,Jan,8; 2016,Jan,13; 2015,Jan,16; 2014,Oct,8; 2014,Oct,3; 2014,Jan,11

99380 **30 minutes or more**

2.50 2.94 FUD XXX B

AMA: 2019,Jan,6; 2018,Jan,8; 2017,Jan,8; 2016,Jan,13; 2015,Jan,16; 2014,Oct,8; 2014,Oct,3; 2014,Jan,11

99381-99397 Preventive Medicine Visits

CMS: 100-04,11,40.1.3 Independent Attending Physician Services; 100-04,12,30.6.2 Medically Necessary and Preventive Medicine Service on Same Date; 100-04,12,30.6.4 Services Furnished Incident to Physician's Service

INCLUDES Care of a small problem or preexisting condition that requires no extra work
New patients or established patients (99381-99387, 99391-99397)
Regular preventive care (e.g., well-child exams) for all age groups

EXCLUDES *Behavioral change interventions (99406-99409)*
Counseling/risk factor reduction interventions not provided with a preventive medical examination (99401-99412)
Diagnostic tests and other procedures

Code also immunization counseling, administration, and product (90460-90461, 90471-90474, 90476-90749 [90620, 90621, 90625, 90630, 90644, 90672, 90673, 90674, 90750, 90756])

Code also significant, separately identifiable E&M service on the same date for substantial problems requiring additional work using modifier 25 and (99201-99215)

99381 **Initial comprehensive preventive medicine evaluation and management of an individual including an age and gender appropriate history, examination, counseling/anticipatory guidance/risk factor reduction interventions, and the ordering of laboratory/diagnostic procedures, new patient; infant (age younger than 1 year)** A

2.17 3.13 FUD XXX E

AMA: 2018,Jan,8; 2017,Jan,8; 2016,Mar,8; 2016,Jan,13; 2015,Jan,16; 2014,Oct,8; 2014,Jan,11

99382 **early childhood (age 1 through 4 years)** A

2.32 3.28 FUD XXX E

AMA: 2018,Jan,8; 2017,Jan,8; 2016,Mar,8; 2016,Jan,13; 2015,Jan,16; 2014,Oct,8; 2014,Jan,11

99383 **late childhood (age 5 through 11 years)** A

2.46 3.41 FUD XXX E

AMA: 2018,Jan,8; 2017,Jan,8; 2016,Mar,8; 2016,Jan,13; 2015,Jan,16; 2014,Oct,8; 2014,Jan,11

99384 **adolescent (age 12 through 17 years)** A

2.88 3.85 FUD XXX E

AMA: 2018,Jan,8; 2017,Jan,8; 2016,Mar,8; 2016,Jan,13; 2015,Jan,12; 2015,Jan,16; 2014,Oct,8; 2014,Jan,11

99385 **18-39 years** A

2.76 3.72 FUD XXX E

AMA: 2018,Jan,8; 2017,Jan,8; 2016,Mar,8; 2016,Jan,13; 2015,Jan,12; 2015,Jan,16; 2014,Oct,8; 2014,Jan,11

99386 **40-64 years** A

3.36 4.32 FUD XXX E

AMA: 2018,Jan,8; 2017,Jan,8; 2016,Mar,8; 2016,Jan,13; 2015,Jan,12; 2015,Jan,16; 2014,Oct,8; 2014,Jan,11

99387 **65 years and older** A

3.61 4.68 FUD XXX E

AMA: 2018,Jan,8; 2017,Jan,8; 2016,Mar,8; 2016,Jan,13; 2015,Jan,16; 2014,Oct,8; 2014,Jan,11

99391 **Periodic comprehensive preventive medicine reevaluation and management of an individual including an age and gender appropriate history, examination, counseling/anticipatory guidance/risk factor reduction interventions, and the ordering of laboratory/diagnostic procedures, established patient; infant (age younger than 1 year)** A

1.98 2.82 FUD XXX E

AMA: 2018,Jan,8; 2017,Jan,8; 2016,Mar,8; 2016,Jan,13; 2015,Jan,16; 2014,Oct,8; 2014,Jan,11

99392 **early childhood (age 1 through 4 years)** A

2.17 3.01 FUD XXX E

AMA: 2018,Jan,8; 2017,Jan,8; 2016,Mar,8; 2016,Jan,13; 2015,Jan,16; 2014,Oct,8; 2014,Jan,11

99393 **late childhood (age 5 through 11 years)** A

2.17 3.00 FUD XXX E

AMA: 2018,Jan,8; 2017,Jan,8; 2016,Mar,8; 2016,Jan,13; 2015,Jan,16; 2014,Oct,8; 2014,Jan,11

99394 **adolescent (age 12 through 17 years)** A

2.46 3.29 FUD XXX E

AMA: 2018,Jan,8; 2017,Jan,8; 2016,Mar,8; 2016,Jan,13; 2015,Jan,12; 2015,Jan,16; 2014,Oct,8; 2014,Jan,11

99395 **18-39 years** A

2.53 3.36 FUD XXX E

AMA: 2018,Jan,8; 2017,Jan,8; 2016,Mar,8; 2016,Jan,13; 2015,Jan,16; 2015,Jan,12; 2014,Oct,8; 2014,Jan,11

99396 **40-64 years** A

2.74 3.58 FUD XXX E

AMA: 2018,Jan,8; 2017,Sep,11; 2017,Jan,8; 2016,Mar,8; 2016,Jan,13; 2015,Jan,12; 2015,Jan,16; 2014,Oct,8; 2014,Jan,11

99397 **65 years and older** A

2.88 3.85 FUD XXX E

AMA: 2018,Jan,8; 2017,Jan,8; 2016,Mar,8; 2016,Jan,13; 2015,Jan,16; 2014,Oct,8; 2014,Jan,11

99401-99423 Counseling Services: Risk Factor and Behavioral Change Modification

INCLUDES Face-to-face services for new and established patients based on time increments of 15 to 60 minutes
Health and behavioral services provided on the same day (96156-96159 [96164, 96165, 96167, 96168, 96170, 96171])
Issues such as a healthy diet, exercise, alcohol and drug abuse
Services provided by a physician or other qualified healthcare professional for the purpose of promoting health and reducing illness and injury

EXCLUDES *Counseling and risk factor reduction interventions included in preventive medicine services (99381-99397)*
Counseling services provided to patient groups with existing symptoms or illness (99078)

Code also significant, separately identifiable E&M services when performed and append modifier 25 to that service

99401 **Preventive medicine counseling and/or risk factor reduction intervention(s) provided to an individual (separate procedure); approximately 15 minutes**

0.70 1.10 FUD XXX E

AMA: 2018,Jan,8; 2017,Jan,8; 2016,Mar,8; 2016,Jan,13; 2015,Jan,16; 2014,Oct,8; 2014,Aug,5; 2014,Jan,11

99402 **approximately 30 minutes**

1.42 1.81 FUD XXX E

AMA: 2018,Jan,8; 2017,Jan,8; 2016,Mar,8; 2016,Jan,13; 2015,Jan,16; 2014,Oct,8; 2014,Aug,5; 2014,Jan,11

99403 **approximately 45 minutes**

2.12 2.51 FUD XXX E

AMA: 2018,Jan,8; 2017,Jan,8; 2016,Mar,8; 2016,Jan,13; 2015,Jan,16; 2014,Oct,8; 2014,Aug,5; 2014,Jan,11

99404 **approximately 60 minutes**

2.81 3.21 FUD XXX E

AMA: 2018,Jan,8; 2017,Jan,8; 2016,Mar,8; 2016,Jan,13; 2015,Jan,16; 2014,Oct,8; 2014,Aug,5; 2014,Jan,11

99406 **Smoking and tobacco use cessation counseling visit; intermediate, greater than 3 minutes up to 10 minutes**

0.35 0.42 FUD XXX ★ S 80

AMA: 2018,Jan,8; 2017,Nov,3; 2017,Jan,8; 2016,Mar,8; 2016,Jan,13; 2015,Jan,16; 2014,Oct,8; 2014,Jan,11

99407 **intensive, greater than 10 minutes**

INCLUDES Time duration of (99406)

0.73 0.80 FUD XXX ★ S 80

AMA: 2018,Jan,8; 2017,Nov,3; 2017,Jan,8; 2016,Mar,8; 2016,Jan,13; 2015,Jan,16; 2014,Oct,8; 2014,Jan,11

99408 **Alcohol and/or substance (other than tobacco) abuse structured screening (eg, AUDIT, DAST), and brief intervention (SBI) services; 15 to 30 minutes**

INCLUDES Health risk assessment (96160-96161)
Only initial screening and brief intervention
Services of 15 minutes or more

0.94 1.01 FUD XXX ★ E

AMA: 2018,Jan,8; 2017,Nov,3; 2017,Jan,8; 2016,Nov,5; 2016,Mar,8; 2016,Jan,13; 2015,Jan,16; 2014,Oct,8; 2014,Jan,11

99409 **greater than 30 minutes**

INCLUDES Health risk assessment (96160-96161)
Only initial screening and brief intervention
Time duration of (99408)

1.88 1.95 FUD XXX ★ E

AMA: 2018,Jan,8; 2017,Nov,3; 2017,Jan,8; 2016,Nov,5; 2016,Mar,8; 2016,Jan,13; 2015,Jan,16; 2014,Oct,8; 2014,Jan,11

99411 **Preventive medicine counseling and/or risk factor reduction intervention(s) provided to individuals in a group setting (separate procedure); approximately 30 minutes**

0.22 0.55 FUD XXX E

AMA: 2018,Jan,8; 2017,Jan,8; 2016,Mar,8; 2016,Jan,13; 2015,Jan,16; 2014,Oct,8; 2014,Jan,11

99412 **approximately 60 minutes**

0.36 0.69 FUD XXX E

AMA: 2018,Jan,8; 2017,Jan,8; 2016,Mar,8; 2016,Jan,13; 2015,Jan,16; 2014,Oct,8; 2014,Jan,11

99415 **Resequenced code. See code following 99359.**

99416 **Resequenced code. See code following 99359.**

99421 **Resequenced code. See code following 99443.**

99422 **Resequenced code. See code following 99443.**

99423 **Resequenced code. See code following 99443.**

99429 Other Preventive Medicine

99429 **Unlisted preventive medicine service**

0.00 0.00 FUD XXX E

AMA: 2018,Jan,8; 2017,Jan,8; 2016,Mar,8; 2016,Jan,13; 2015,Jan,16; 2014,Oct,8; 2014,Jan,11

99441-99443 Telephone Calls for Patient Management

CMS: 100-04,11,40.1.3 Independent Attending Physician Services

INCLUDES Episodes of care initiated by an established patient or the patient or guardian of an established patient
Non-face-to-face E&M services provided by a physician or other health care provider qualified to report E&M services
Related E&M services provided within:
Postoperative period of a completed procedure
Seven days prior to the service

EXCLUDES *Patient management services during same time frame as (99339-99340, 99374-99380, 99487-99489, 99495-99496, 93792-93793)*
Services provided by a qualified nonphysician health care professional unable to report E&M codes (98966-98968)
Use of codes more than one time for telephone and online services when reported within a seven day period of time by the same provider

99441 **Telephone evaluation and management service by a physician or other qualified health care professional who may report evaluation and management services provided to an established patient, parent, or guardian not originating from a related E/M service provided within the previous 7 days nor leading to an E/M service or procedure within the next 24 hours or soonest available appointment; 5-10 minutes of medical discussion**

0.36 0.39 FUD XXX E

AMA: 2019,Mar,8; 2018,Mar,7; 2018,Jan,8; 2017,Jan,8; 2016,Jan,13; 2015,Jan,16; 2014,Oct,3; 2014,Oct,8; 2014,Jan,11

99442 **11-20 minutes of medical discussion**

0.72 0.76 FUD XXX E

AMA: 2019,Mar,8; 2018,Mar,7; 2018,Jan,8; 2017,Jan,8; 2016,Jan,13; 2015,Jan,16; 2014,Oct,3; 2014,Oct,8; 2014,Jan,11

99443 **21-30 minutes of medical discussion**

1.08 1.12 FUD XXX E

AMA: 2019,Mar,8; 2018,Mar,7; 2018,Jan,8; 2017,Jan,8; 2016,Jan,13; 2015,Jan,16; 2014,Oct,3; 2014,Oct,8; 2014,Jan,11

99421-99423 [99421, 99422, 99423] Digital Evaluation and Management Services

CMS: 100-04,11,40.1.3 Independent Attending Physician Services

INCLUDES Cumulative service time within a 7 day time frame needed to evaluate, assess, and manage the patient:
Ordering of tests
Prescription generation
Separate digital inquiry for new and unrelated problem
Subsequent communication that is digitally supported (i.e., email, online, telephone)
Digital service initiated by an established patient

EXCLUDES *Clinical staff time*
Digital evaluation by a qualified nonphysician health care professional (98970-98972)
Digital evaluation peformed with separately reportable E&M services during same time frame for new or established patient:
Inquiries related to previously completed procedure and within the postoperative period
INR monitoring (93792-93793)
Office consultation (99241-99245)
Office or other outpatient visit (99201-99205, 99212-99215)
Patient management services (99339-99340, 99374-99380, [99091], 99487-99489, 99495-99496)
Digital service less than 5 minutes
Use of code more than one time in 7 days

● # **99421** **Online digital evaluation and management service, for an established patient, for up to 7 days, cumulative time during the 7 days; 5-10 minutes**

0.00 0.00 FUD 000

● # **99422** **11-20 minutes**

0.00 0.00 FUD 000

● # **99423** **21 or more minutes**

0.00 0.00 FUD 000

99444 Online Patient Management Services

99444 ~~**Online evaluation and management service provided by a physician or other qualified health care professional who may report evaluation and management services provided to an established patient or guardian, not originating from a related E/M service provided within the previous 7 days, using the Internet or similar electronic communications network**~~

To report, see (99421-99423)

99446-99452 [99451, 99452] Online and Telephone Consultative Services

INCLUDES Multiple telephone and/or internet contact needed to complete the consultation (e.g., test result(s) follow-up)
New or established patient with new problem or exacerbation of existing problem and not seen within the last 14 days
Review of pertinent lab, imaging and/or pathology studies, medical records, medications

EXCLUDES *Any service less than 5 minutes*
Communication with family with or without the patient present ([99421, 99422, 99423], 99441-99443, 98966-98967)
Transfer of care only

99446 **Interprofessional telephone/Internet/electronic health record assessment and management service provided by a consultative physician, including a verbal and written report to the patient's treating/requesting physician or other qualified health care professional; 5-10 minutes of medical consultative discussion and review**

INCLUDES Verbal and written reports from the consultant to the requesting provider

EXCLUDES *Prolonged services without direct patient contact (99358-99359)*
Use of code more than one time in 7 days

0.51 0.51 FUD XXX E 80

AMA: 2019,Jun,7; 2019,Jan,3; 2018,Jan,8; 2017,Jan,8; 2016,Jan,13; 2015,Jan,16; 2014,Oct,8; 2014,Jun,14

99447 **11-20 minutes of medical consultative discussion and review**

INCLUDES Verbal and written reports from the consultant to the requesting provider

EXCLUDES *Prolonged services without direct patient contact (99358-99359)*
Use of code more than one time in 7 days

1.01 1.01 FUD XXX E 80

AMA: 2019,Jun,7; 2019,Jan,3; 2018,Jan,8; 2017,Jan,8; 2016,Jan,13; 2015,Jan,16; 2014,Oct,8; 2014,Jun,14

99448 **21-30 minutes of medical consultative discussion and review**

INCLUDES Verbal and written reports from the consultant to the requesting provider

EXCLUDES *Prolonged services without direct patient contact (99358-99359)*
Use of code more than one time in 7 days

1.52 1.52 FUD XXX E 80

AMA: 2019,Jun,7; 2019,Jan,3; 2018,Jan,8; 2017,Jan,8; 2016,Jan,13; 2015,Jan,16; 2014,Oct,8; 2014,Jun,14

99449 **31 minutes or more of medical consultative discussion and review**

INCLUDES Verbal and written reports from the consultant to the requesting provider

EXCLUDES *Prolonged services without direct patient contact (99358-99359)*
Use of code more than one time in 7 days

2.02 2.02 FUD XXX E 80

AMA: 2019,Jun,7; 2019,Jan,3; 2018,Jan,8; 2017,Jan,8; 2016,Jan,13; 2015,Jan,16; 2014,Oct,8; 2014,Jun,14

\# **99451** **Interprofessional telephone/Internet/electronic health record assessment and management service provided by a consultative physician, including a written report to the patient's treating/requesting physician or other qualified health care professional, 5 minutes or more of medical consultative time**

INCLUDES Verbal and written reports from the consultant to the requesting provider

EXCLUDES *Prolonged services without direct patient contact (99358-99359)*
Use of code more than one time in 7 days

1.04 1.04 FUD XXX 80

AMA: 2019,Jun,7; 2019,Jan,3

\# **99452** **Interprofessional telephone/Internet/electronic health record referral service(s) provided by a treating/requesting physician or other qualified health care professional, 30 minutes**

INCLUDES Time preparing for referral of 16 to 30 minutes

EXCLUDES *Requesting physician's time 30 minutes over the typical E&M service, patient not on site (99358-99359)*
Requesting physician's time 30 minutes over the typical E&M service, patient on site (99354-99357)
Use of code more than one time every 14 days

1.04 1.04 FUD XXX 80

AMA: 2019,Jun,7; 2019,Jan,3

99453-99474 [99091, 99453, 99454, 99473, 99474] Remote Monitoring/Collection Biological Data

\# **99453** **Remote monitoring of physiologic parameter(s) (eg, weight, blood pressure, pulse oximetry, respiratory flow rate), initial; set-up and patient education on use of equipment**

INCLUDES 30 day period of physiologic monitoring of parameters such as weight, blood pressure, pulse oximetry
Services ordered by physician or other qualified healthcare professional
Services provided for each episode of care (starts when monitoring begins and ends when treatment goals achieved)
Set-up and instructions for use
Use of device approved by the FDA

EXCLUDES *Use for monitoring of less than 16 days*
Use of codes when services are included in other monitoring services (e.g., 93296, 94760, 95250)

0.54 0.54 FUD XXX 80

AMA: 2019,Mar,10; 2019,Jan,3; 2019,Jan,6

\# **99454** **device(s) supply with daily recording(s) or programmed alert(s) transmission, each 30 days**

INCLUDES 30 day period of physiologic monitoring of parameters such as weight, blood pressure, pulse oximetry
Service ordered by physician or other qualified healthcare professional
Supply of device
Use of device approved by the FDA

EXCLUDES *Remote monitoring treatment management*
Self-measured blood pressure monitoring ([99473, 99474])
Use for monitoring of less than 16 days
Use of codes when services are included in other monitoring services (e.g., 93296, 94760, 95250)

1.78 1.78 FUD XXX 80

AMA: 2019,Mar,10; 2019,Jan,3; 2019,Jan,6

99091 Collection and interpretation of physiologic data (eg, ECG, blood pressure, glucose monitoring) digitally stored and/or transmitted by the patient and/or caregiver to the physician or other qualified health care professional, qualified by education, training, licensure/regulation (when applicable) requiring a minimum of 30 minutes of time, each 30 days

INCLUDES E&M services provided on the same date of service

EXCLUDES *Care plan oversight services within 30 days (99339-99340, 99374-99375, 99378-99380)*
Remote physiologic monitoring treatment management within 30 days ([99457])
Use of code more than one time in 30 days
Use of codes when services are included in other monitoring services such as (93227, 93272, 95250)

1.62 1.62 FUD XXX N 80

AMA: 2019,Jun,3; 2019,Jan,6; 2018,Dec,10; 2018,Dec,10; 2018,Jun,6; 2018,Mar,5; 2018,Feb,7; 2018,Jan,8; 2017,Jan,8; 2016,Jan,13; 2015,Jan,16; 2014,Oct,3; 2014,Jan,11

● # **99473** Self-measured blood pressure using a device validated for clinical accuracy; patient education/training and device calibration

0.00 0.00 FUD 000

EXCLUDES *Use of codes when services are included in the same calendar month as:*
Ambulatory blood pressure monitoring (93784-93790)
Chronic care management service ([99490, 99491], 99487-99489)
Remote physiologic monitoring, collection and interpretation ([99453, 99454], [99091], [99457])
Use of code more than once per device

● # **99474** separate self-measurements of two readings one minute apart, twice daily over a 30-day period (minimum of 12 readings), collection of data reported by the patient and/or caregiver to the physician or other qualified health care professional, with report of average systolic and diastolic pressures and subsequent communication of a treatment plan to the patient

0.00 0.00 FUD 000

EXCLUDES *Use of codes when services are included in the same calendar month as:*
Ambulatory blood pressure monitoring (93784-93790)
Chronic care management services ([99490, 99491], 99487-99489)
Remote physiologic monitoring, collection and interpretation services ([99453, 99454], [99091], [99457])
Use of code more than once per calendar month

99457-99458 [99457, 99458] Remote Monitoring Management

CMS: 100-04,11,40.1.3 Independent Attending Physician Services

INCLUDES Interactive live communication with patient for at least 20 minutes per month
Results of remote monitoring used for patient management
Service ordered by physician or other qualified healthcare professional
Time managing care when more specific service codes are not available
Use of code each 30 days no matter the number of parameters monitored
Use of device approved by the FDA

EXCLUDES *Use of code for services lasting less than 20 mintues*
Use of code on same date of service as E&M services (99201-99215, 99221-99223, 99231-99233, 99251-99255, 99324-99328, 99334-99337, 99341-99350)

▲ # **99457** Remote physiologic monitoring treatment management services, clinical staff/physician/other qualified health care professional time in a calendar month requiring interactive communication with the patient/caregiver during the month; first 20 minutes

EXCLUDES *Collection and interpretation of physiologic data ([99091])*

0.90 1.43 FUD XXX 80

AMA: 2019,Jun,3; 2019,Jan,3; 2019,Jan,6

● + # **99458** each additional 20 minutes (List separately in addition to code for primary procedure)

0.00 0.00 FUD 000

EXCLUDES *Use of code if 20 minutes of additional treatment time is not obtained ([99457])*

Code first ([99457])

99450-99458 Life/Disability Insurance Eligibility Visits

INCLUDES Assessment services for insurance eligibility and work-related disability without medical management of the patient's illness/injury
Services provided to new/established patients at any site of service

EXCLUDES *Any additional E&M services or procedures performed on the same date of service: report with appropriate code*

99450 Basic life and/or disability examination that includes: Measurement of height, weight, and blood pressure; Completion of a medical history following a life insurance pro forma; Collection of blood sample and/or urinalysis complying with "chain of custody" protocols; and Completion of necessary documentation/certificates.

0.00 0.00 FUD XXX E

AMA: 2019,Jun,7; 2018,Jan,8; 2017,Jan,8; 2016,Jan,13; 2015,Jan,16; 2014,Oct,8; 2014,Jan,11

99451 Resequenced code. See code following 99449.

99452 Resequenced code. See code following 99449.

99453 Resequenced code. See code following 99449.

99454 Resequenced code. See code following 99449.

99455 Work related or medical disability examination by the treating physician that includes: Completion of a medical history commensurate with the patient's condition; Performance of an examination commensurate with the patient's condition; Formulation of a diagnosis, assessment of capabilities and stability, and calculation of impairment; Development of future medical treatment plan; and Completion of necessary documentation/certificates and report.

INCLUDES Special reports (99080)

0.00 0.00 FUD XXX B 80

AMA: 2018,Jan,8; 2017,Jan,8; 2016,Jan,13; 2015,Jan,16; 2014,Oct,8; 2014,Jan,11

99456 Work related or medical disability examination by other than the treating physician that includes: Completion of a medical history commensurate with the patient's condition; Performance of an examination commensurate with the patient's condition; Formulation of a diagnosis, assessment of capabilities and stability, and calculation of impairment; Development of future medical treatment plan; and Completion of necessary documentation/certificates and report.

INCLUDES Special reports (99080)

0.00 0.00 FUD XXX B 80

AMA: 2018,Jan,8; 2017,Jan,8; 2016,Jan,13; 2015,Jan,16; 2014,Oct,8; 2014,Jan,11

99457 Resequenced code. See code before resequenced code 99474.

99458 Resequenced code. See code before 99450.

99460-99463 Evaluation and Management Services for Age 28 Days or Less

CMS: 100-04,12,30.6.4 Services Furnished Incident to Physician's Service

INCLUDES Family consultation
Healthy newborn history and physical
Medical record documentation
Ordering of diagnostic test and treatments
Services provided to healthy newborns age 28 days or less

EXCLUDES *Neonatal intensive and critical care services (99466-99469 [99485, 99486], 99477-99480)*
Newborn follow up services in an office or outpatient setting (99201-99215, 99381, 99391)
Newborn hospital discharge services if provided on a date subsequent to the admission date (99238-99239)
Nonroutine neonatal inpatient evaluation and management services (99221-99233)

Code also attendance at delivery (99464)
Code also circumcision (54150)
Code also emergency resuscitation services (99465)

99460 **Initial hospital or birthing center care, per day, for evaluation and management of normal newborn infant** A
2.71 2.71 FUD XXX V 80
AMA: 2018,Jan,8; 2017,Jan,8; 2016,Jan,13; 2015,Jan,16; 2014,Oct,8; 2014,Jan,11

99461 **Initial care, per day, for evaluation and management of normal newborn infant seen in other than hospital or birthing center** A
1.78 2.58 FUD XXX M 80
AMA: 2018,Jan,8; 2017,Jan,8; 2016,Jan,13; 2015,Jan,16; 2014,Oct,8; 2014,Jan,11

99462 **Subsequent hospital care, per day, for evaluation and management of normal newborn** A
1.19 1.19 FUD XXX C 80
AMA: 2018,Jan,8; 2017,Jan,8; 2016,Jan,13; 2015,Jan,16; 2014,Oct,8; 2014,Jan,11

99463 **Initial hospital or birthing center care, per day, for evaluation and management of normal newborn infant admitted and discharged on the same date** A
3.13 3.13 FUD XXX V 80
AMA: 2018,Jan,8; 2017,Jan,8; 2016,Jan,13; 2015,Jan,16; 2014,Oct,8; 2014,Jan,11

99464-99465 Newborn Delivery Attendance/Resuscitation

CMS: 100-04,12,30.6.4 Services Furnished Incident to Physician's Service

99464 **Attendance at delivery (when requested by the delivering physician or other qualified health care professional) and initial stabilization of newborn** A
EXCLUDES *Resuscitation at delivery (99465)*
2.12 2.12 FUD XXX N 80
AMA: 2018,Jan,8; 2017,Jan,8; 2016,Jan,13; 2015,Jan,16; 2014,Oct,8; 2014,Jan,11

99465 **Delivery/birthing room resuscitation, provision of positive pressure ventilation and/or chest compressions in the presence of acute inadequate ventilation and/or cardiac output** A
EXCLUDES *Attendance at delivery (99464)*
Code also any necessary procedures performed as part of the resuscitation
4.13 4.13 FUD XXX S 80
AMA: 2018,Jan,8; 2017,Jan,8; 2016,Jan,13; 2015,Jan,16; 2014,Oct,8; 2014,Jan,11

99466-99467 Critical Care Transport Age 24 Months or Younger

CMS: 100-04,12,30.6.4 Services Furnished Incident to Physician's Service

INCLUDES Face-to-face care starting when the physician assumes responsibility of the patient at the referring facility until the receiving facility accepts the patient
Physician presence during interfacility transfer of critically ill/injured patient 24 months of age or less
Services provided by the physician during transport:
- Blood gases
- Chest x-rays (71045-71046)
- Data stored in computers (e.g., ECGs, blood pressures, hematologic data)
- Gastric intubation (43752-43753)
- Interpretation of cardiac output measurements (93562)
- Pulse oximetry (94760-94762)
- Routine monitoring:
  - Heart rate
  - Respiratory rate
- Temporary transcutaneous pacing (92953)
- Vascular access procedures (36000, 36400, 36405-36406, 36415, 36591, 36600)
- Ventilatory management (94002-94003, 94660, 94662)

EXCLUDES *Neonatal hypothermia (99184)*
Patient critical care transport services with personal contact with patient of less than 30 minutes
Physician directed emergency care via two-way voice communication with transporting staff (99288, [99485, 99486])
Services less than 30 minutes in duration (see E&M codes)
Services of the physician directing transport (control physician) ([99485, 99486])

Code also any services not designated as included in the critical care transport service

99466 **Critical care face-to-face services, during an interfacility transport of critically ill or critically injured pediatric patient, 24 months of age or younger; first 30-74 minutes of hands-on care during transport** A
6.75 6.75 FUD XXX N 80
AMA: 2018,Jun,9; 2018,Jan,8; 2017,Jan,8; 2016,Jan,13; 2015,Jan,16; 2014,Oct,8; 2014,Jan,11

\+ **99467** **each additional 30 minutes (List separately in addition to code for primary service)** A
Code first (99466)
3.37 3.37 FUD ZZZ N 80
AMA: 2018,Jun,9; 2018,Jan,8; 2017,Jan,8; 2016,Jan,13; 2015,Jan,16; 2014,Oct,8; 2014,Jan,11

99485-99486 [99485, 99486] Critical Care Transport Supervision Age 24 Months or Younger

INCLUDES Advice for treatment to the transport team from the control physician
Non face-to-face care starts with first contact by the control physician with the transport team and ends when patient responsibility is assumed by the receiving facility

EXCLUDES *Emergency systems physician direction for pediatric patient older than 24 months (99288)*
Services provided by transport team
Services less than 15 minutes
Services performed by control physician for the same time period
Services performed by same physician providing critical care transport (99466-99467)

\# **99485** **Supervision by a control physician of interfacility transport care of the critically ill or critically injured pediatric patient, 24 months of age or younger, includes two-way communication with transport team before transport, at the referring facility and during the transport, including data interpretation and report; first 30 minutes** A
2.17 2.17 FUD XXX B
AMA: 2018,Jun,9; 2018,Jan,8; 2017,Jan,8; 2016,Jan,13; 2015,Jan,16; 2014,Oct,8

\+ # **99486** **each additional 30 minutes (List separately in addition to code for primary procedure)** A
Code first ([99485])
1.88 1.88 FUD XXX B
AMA: 2018,Jun,9; 2018,Jan,8; 2017,Jan,8; 2016,Jan,13; 2015,Jan,16; 2014,Oct,8

99468-99476 Critical Care Age 5 Years or Younger

CMS: 100-04,12,30.6.4 Services Furnished Incident to Physician's Service

INCLUDES All services included in codes 99291-99292 as well as the following which may be reported by facilities only:
- Administration of blood/blood components (36430, 36440)
- Administration of intravenous fluids (96360-96361)
- Administration of surfactant (94610)
- Bladder aspiration, suprapubic (51100)
- Bladder catheterization (51701, 51702)
- Car seat evaluation (94780-94781)
- Catheterization umbilical artery (36660)
- Catheterization umbilical vein (36510)
- Central venous catheter, centrally inserted (36555)
- Endotracheal intubation (31500)
- Lumbar puncture (62270)
- Oral or nasogastric tube placement (43752)
- Pulmonary function testing, performed at the bedside (94375)
- Pulse or ear oximetry (94760-94762)
- Vascular access, arteries (36140, 36620)
- Vascular access, venous (36400-36406, 36420, 36600)
- Ventilatory management (94002-94004, 94660)

Initial and subsequent care provided to a critically ill infant or child

Other hospital care or intensive care services by same group or individual done on same day that patient was transferred to initial neonatal/pediatric critical care

Readmission to critical unit on same day or during the same stay (subsequent care)

EXCLUDES *Critical care services for patients 6 years of age or older (99291-99292)*

Critical care services provided by a second physician or physician of a different specialty (99291-99292)

Interfacility transport services by same or different individual of same or different specialty or group on same date of service (99466-99467, [99485, 99486])

Neonatal hypothermia (99184)

Services performed by individual in another group receiving a patient transferred to a lower level of care (99231-99233, 99478-99480)

Services performed by individual transferring a patient to a lower level of care (99231-99233, 99291-99292)

Services performed by same or different individual in same group on same day (99291-99292)

Services performed by transferring individual prior to transfer of patient to an individual in a different group (99221-99233, 99291-99292, 99460-99462, 99477-99480)

Code also normal newborn care if done on same day by same group or individual that provides critical care. Report modifier 25 with initial critical care code (99460-99462)

99468 Initial inpatient neonatal critical care, per day, for the evaluation and management of a critically ill neonate, 28 days of age or younger A

26.0 26.0 FUD XXX C 80

AMA: 2018,Dec,8; 2018,Dec,8; 2018,Jun,9; 2018,Jan,8; 2017,Jan,8; 2016,May,3; 2016,Jan,13; 2015,Oct,8; 2015,Jul,3; 2015,Feb,10; 2015,Jan,16; 2014,Oct,8; 2014,May,4; 2014,Jan,11

99469 Subsequent inpatient neonatal critical care, per day, for the evaluation and management of a critically ill neonate, 28 days of age or younger A

11.2 11.2 FUD XXX C 80

AMA: 2018,Dec,8; 2018,Dec,8; 2018,Jun,9; 2018,Jan,8; 2017,Jan,8; 2016,May,3; 2016,Jan,13; 2015,Oct,8; 2015,Jul,3; 2015,Feb,10; 2015,Jan,16; 2014,Oct,8; 2014,May,4; 2014,Jan,11

99471 Initial inpatient pediatric critical care, per day, for the evaluation and management of a critically ill infant or young child, 29 days through 24 months of age A

22.5 22.5 FUD XXX C 80

AMA: 2018,Dec,8; 2018,Dec,8; 2018,Jun,9; 2018,Jan,8; 2017,Jan,8; 2016,May,3; 2016,Jan,13; 2015,Jul,3; 2015,Feb,10; 2015,Jan,16; 2014,Oct,8; 2014,Jan,11

99472 Subsequent inpatient pediatric critical care, per day, for the evaluation and management of a critically ill infant or young child, 29 days through 24 months of age A

11.5 11.5 FUD XXX C 80

AMA: 2018,Dec,8; 2018,Dec,8; 2018,Jun,9; 2018,Jan,8; 2017,Jan,8; 2016,May,3; 2016,Jan,13; 2015,Jul,3; 2015,Feb,10; 2015,Jan,16; 2014,Oct,8; 2014,Jan,11

99473 **Resequenced code. See code before 99450.**

99474 **Resequenced code. See code before 99450.**

99475 Initial inpatient pediatric critical care, per day, for the evaluation and management of a critically ill infant or young child, 2 through 5 years of age A

15.8 15.8 FUD XXX C 80

AMA: 2018,Dec,8; 2018,Dec,8; 2018,Jun,9; 2018,Jan,8; 2017,Jan,8; 2016,May,3; 2016,Jan,13; 2015,Jul,3; 2015,Feb,10; 2015,Jan,16; 2014,Oct,8; 2014,Jan,11

99476 Subsequent inpatient pediatric critical care, per day, for the evaluation and management of a critically ill infant or young child, 2 through 5 years of age A

9.86 9.86 FUD XXX C 80

AMA: 2018,Dec,8; 2018,Dec,8; 2018,Jun,9; 2018,Jan,8; 2017,Jan,8; 2016,May,3; 2016,Jan,13; 2015,Jul,3; 2015,Feb,10; 2015,Jan,16; 2014,Oct,8; 2014,Jan,11

99477-99480 Initial Inpatient Neonatal Intensive Care and Other Services

CMS: 100-04,12,30.6.4 Services Furnished Incident to Physician's Service

INCLUDES All services included in codes 99291-99292 as well as the following that may be reported by facilities only:
- Adjustments to enteral and/or parenteral nutrition
- Airway and ventilator management (31500, 94002-94004, 94375, 94610, 94660)
- Bladder catheterization (51701-51702)
- Blood transfusion (36430, 36440)
- Car seat evaluation (94780-94781)
- Constant and/or frequent monitoring of vital signs
- Continuous observation by the healthcare team
- Heat maintenance
- Intensive cardiac or respiratory monitoring
- Oral or nasogastric tube insertion (43752)
- Oxygen saturation (94760-94762)
- Spinal puncture (62270)
- Suprapubic catheterization (51100)
- Vascular access procedures (36000, 36140, 36400, 36405-36406, 36420, 36510, 36555, 36600, 36620, 36660)

EXCLUDES *Critical care services for patient transferred after initial or subsequent intensive care is provided (99291-99292)*

Initial day intensive care provided by transferring individual same day neonate/infant transferred to a lower level of care (99477)

Inpatient neonatal/pediatric critical care services received on same day (99468-99476)

Necessary resuscitation services done as part of delivery care prior to admission

Neonatal hypothermia (99184)

Services provided by receiving individual when patient is transferred for critical care (99468-99476)

Services for receiving provider when patient improves after the initial day and is transferred to a lower level of care (99231-99233, 99478-99480)

Subsequent care of a sick neonate, under 28 days of age, more than 5000 grams, not requiring critical or intensive care services (99231-99233)

Code also care provided by receiving individual when patient is transferred to an individual in different group (99231-99233, 99462)

Code also initial neonatal intensive care service when physician or other qualified health care professional is present for delivery and/or neonate requires resuscitation (99464-99465); append modifier 25 to (99477)

99477 Initial hospital care, per day, for the evaluation and management of the neonate, 28 days of age or younger, who requires intensive observation, frequent interventions, and other intensive care services A

EXCLUDES *Initiation of care of a critically ill neonate (99468)*

Initiation of inpatient care of a normal newborn (99460)

9.85 9.85 FUD XXX C 80

AMA: 2018,Dec,8; 2018,Dec,8; 2018,Jan,8; 2017,Jan,8; 2016,Jan,13; 2015,Jul,3; 2015,Jan,16; 2014,Oct,8; 2014,Jan,11

99478 Subsequent intensive care, per day, for the evaluation and management of the recovering very low birth weight infant (present body weight less than 1500 grams) A

3.87 3.87 FUD XXX C 80

AMA: 2018,Dec,8; 2018,Dec,8; 2018,Jun,11; 2018,Jan,8; 2017,Jan,8; 2016,Jan,13; 2015,Jul,3; 2015,Jan,16; 2014,Oct,8; 2014,Jan,11

99479 **Subsequent intensive care, per day, for the evaluation and management of the recovering low birth weight infant (present body weight of 1500-2500 grams)**

3.52 3.52 FUD XXX

AMA: 2018,Dec,8; 2018,Dec,8; 2018,Jun,11; 2018,Jan,8; 2017,Jan,8; 2016,Jan,13; 2015,Jul,3; 2015,Jan,16; 2014,Oct,8; 2014,Jan,11

99480 **Subsequent intensive care, per day, for the evaluation and management of the recovering infant (present body weight of 2501-5000 grams)**

3.37 3.37 FUD XXX

AMA: 2018,Dec,8; 2018,Dec,8; 2018,Jun,11; 2018,Jan,8; 2017,Jan,8; 2016,Jan,13; 2015,Jul,3; 2015,Jan,16; 2014,Oct,8; 2014,Jan,11

99483-99486 Cognitive Impairment Services

INCLUDES Evaluation and care plans for new or existing patients with symptoms of cognitive impairment
- Assessment and care plan services during the same time frame as:
  - E&M services (99201-99215, 99241-99245, 99324-99337, 99341-99350, 99366-99368, 99497-99498)
  - Medication management (99605-99607)
  - Need for services evaluation (e.g., legal, financial, meals, personal care)
  - Patient and caregiver focused risk assessment (96160-96161)
  - Psychiatric and psychological services (90785, 90791-90792, [96127])
  - Psychological or neuropsychological tests (96146)
- Consideration of other conditions that may cause cognitive impairment (e.g., infection, hydrocephalus, stroke, medications)

EXCLUDES *Use of code more than one time per 180 day period*

99483 **Assessment of and care planning for a patient with cognitive impairment, requiring an independent historian, in the office or other outpatient, home or domiciliary or rest home, with all of the following required elements: Cognition-focused evaluation including a pertinent history and examination; Medical decision making of moderate or high complexity; Functional assessment (eg, basic and instrumental activities of daily living), including decision-making capacity; Use of standardized instruments for staging of dementia (eg, functional assessment staging test [FAST], clinical dementia rating [CDR]); Medication reconciliation and review for high-risk medications; Evaluation for neuropsychiatric and behavioral symptoms, including depression, including use of standardized screening instrument(s); Evaluation of safety (eg, home), including motor vehicle operation; Identification of caregiver(s), caregiver knowledge, caregiver needs, social supports, and the willingness of caregiver to take on caregiving tasks; Development, updating or revision, or review of an Advance Care Plan; Creation of a written care plan, including initial plans to address any neuropsychiatric symptoms, neuro-cognitive symptoms, functional limitations, and referral to community resources as needed (eg, rehabilitation services, adult day programs, support groups) shared with the patient and/or caregiver with initial education and support. Typically, 50 minutes are spent face-to-face with the patient and/or family or caregiver.**

5.09 7.32 FUD XXX

AMA: 2018,Jul,12; 2018,Apr,9; 2018,Jan,8

99484 **Resequenced code. See code following 99498.**

99485 **Resequenced code. See code following 99467.**

99486 **Resequenced code. See code following 99467.**

99490-99491 [99490, 99491] Coordination of Services for Chronic Care

CMS: 100-04,11,40.1.3 Independent Attending Physician Services

INCLUDES Case management services provided to patients that:
- Have two or more conditions anticipated to endure more than 12 months or until the patient's death
- Require at least 20 minutes of staff time monthly
- Risk is high that conditions will result in decompensation, deterioration, or death

Patient management services during same time frame as (99339-99340, 99487-99489)

EXCLUDES *Psychiatric collaborative care management (99484, 99492-99494)*
Use of code with ESRD services during the same month (90951-90970)

\# **99490** **Chronic care management services, at least 20 minutes of clinical staff time directed by a physician or other qualified health care professional, per calendar month, with the following required elements: multiple (two or more) chronic conditions expected to last at least 12 months, or until the death of the patient; chronic conditions place the patient at significant risk of death, acute exacerbation/decompensation, or functional decline; comprehensive care plan established, implemented, revised, or monitored.**

INCLUDES Patient management services during same time frame as (99358-99359, 99366-99368, 99374-99380, [99421, 99422, 99423], 99441-99443, [99091], 99495-99496, 93792-93793, 98960-98962, 99071, 99078, 99080, 99605-99607)

EXCLUDES *Chronic care management provided personally by physician or other qualified health care professional ([99491])*

0.90 1.17 FUD XXX

AMA: 2019,Jan,6; 2018,Oct,9; 2018,Jul,12; 2018,Apr,9; 2018,Mar,5; 2018,Mar,7; 2018,Feb,7; 2018,Jan,8; 2017,Jan,8; 2016,Jan,13; 2015,Feb,3; 2015,Jan,16; 2014,Oct,3

\# **99491** **Chronic care management services, provided personally by a physician or other qualified health care professional, at least 30 minutes of physician or other qualified health care professional time, per calendar month, with the following required elements: multiple (two or more) chronic conditions expected to last at least 12 months, or until the death of the patient; chronic conditions place the patient at significant risk of death, acute exacerbation/decompensation, or functional decline; comprehensive care plan established, implemented, revised, or monitored**

2.33 2.33 FUD XXX

EXCLUDES *Chronic care management provided by medically directed clinical staff only ([99490])*

99487-99491 [99490, 99491] Coordination of Complex Services for Chronic Care

INCLUDES All clinical non-face-to-face time with patient, family, and caregivers
Only services given by physician or other qualified health caregiver who has the role of care coordination for the patient for the month
Patient management services during same time frame as (99339-99340, 99358-99359, 99374-99380, 99441-99443, [99091], 99495-99496, 90951-90970, 93792-93793, 98960-98962, 98966-98968, 99071, 99078, 99080, 99605-99607)
Services provided to patients in a rest home, domiciliary, assisted living facility, or at home that include:
Caregiver education to family or patient, addressing independent living and self-management
Communication with patient and all caregivers and professionals regarding care
Determining which community and health resources would benefit the patient
Developing and maintaining a care plan
Facilitation of services and care
Health outcomes data and registry documentation
Providing communication with home health and other patient utilized services
Support for treatment and medication adherence
Services that address activities of daily living, psychosocial, and medical needs

EXCLUDES *E&M services by same/different individual during time frame of care management services*
Psychiatric collaborative care management (99484, 99492-99494)

99487 **Complex chronic care management services, with the following required elements: multiple (two or more) chronic conditions expected to last at least 12 months, or until the death of the patient, chronic conditions place the patient at significant risk of death, acute exacerbation/decompensation, or functional decline, establishment or substantial revision of a comprehensive care plan, moderate or high complexity medical decision making; 60 minutes of clinical staff time directed by a physician or other qualified health care professional, per calendar month**

INCLUDES Clinical services, 60 to 74 minutes, during a calendar month
1.47 2.58 FUD XXX S 80
AMA: 2019,Jan,6; 2018,Oct,9; 2018,Jul,12; 2018,Apr,9; 2018,Mar,5; 2018,Mar,7; 2018,Feb,7; 2018,Jan,8; 2017,Apr,9; 2017,Jan,8; 2016,Jan,13; 2015,Jan,16; 2014,Oct,8; 2014,Oct,3; 2014,Jun,3; 2014,Feb,3; 2014,Jan,11

\+ **99489** **each additional 30 minutes of clinical staff time directed by a physician or other qualified health care professional, per calendar month (List separately in addition to code for primary procedure)**

EXCLUDES *Clinical services less than 30 minutes beyond the initial 60 minutes of care, per calendar month*
Code first (99487)
0.74 1.29 FUD ZZZ N 80
AMA: 2019,Jan,6; 2018,Oct,9; 2018,Jul,12; 2018,Apr,9; 2018,Mar,5; 2018,Mar,7; 2018,Feb,7; 2018,Jan,8; 2017,Apr,9; 2017,Jan,8; 2016,Jan,13; 2015,Jan,16; 2014,Oct,8; 2014,Oct,3; 2014,Jun,3; 2014,Jan,11

99490 **Resequenced code. See code before 99487.**

99491 **Resequenced code. See code before 99487.**

99492-99494 Psychiatric Collaborative Care

INCLUDES Services provided during a calendar month by a physician or other qualified healthcare profession for patients with a psychiatric diagnosis
Assessment of behavioral health status
Creation of and updating a care plan
Treatment provided during an episode of care during which goals may be met, not achieved, or there is a lack of services during a period of six months

EXCLUDES *Additional services provided by a behavioral health care manager during the same calendar month period (do not count as time for 99492-99494):*
Psychiatric evaluation (90791-90792)
Psychotherapy (99406-99407, 99408-99409, 90832-90834, 90836-90838, 90839-90840, 90846-90847, 90849, 90853)
Services provided by a psychiatric consultant (do not count as time for 99492-99494): (E&M services) and psychiatric evaluation (90791-90792)

99492 **Initial psychiatric collaborative care management, first 70 minutes in the first calendar month of behavioral health care manager activities, in consultation with a psychiatric consultant, and directed by the treating physician or other qualified health care professional, with the following required elements: outreach to and engagement in treatment of a patient directed by the treating physician or other qualified health care professional; initial assessment of the patient, including administration of validated rating scales, with the development of an individualized treatment plan; review by the psychiatric consultant with modifications of the plan if recommended; entering patient in a registry and tracking patient follow-up and progress using the registry, with appropriate documentation, and participation in weekly caseload consultation with the psychiatric consultant; and provision of brief interventions using evidence-based techniques such as behavioral activation, motivational interviewing, and other focused treatment strategies.**

EXCLUDES *Services of less than 36 minutes*
Subsequent collaborative care managment in same calendar month (99493)
2.51 4.50 FUD XXX S 80
AMA: 2019,Jan,6; 2018,Jul,12; 2018,Mar,5; 2018,Feb,7; 2018,Jan,8; 2017,Nov,3

99493 **Subsequent psychiatric collaborative care management, first 60 minutes in a subsequent month of behavioral health care manager activities, in consultation with a psychiatric consultant, and directed by the treating physician or other qualified health care professional, with the following required elements: tracking patient follow-up and progress using the registry, with appropriate documentation; participation in weekly caseload consultation with the psychiatric consultant; ongoing collaboration with and coordination of the patient's mental health care with the treating physician or other qualified health care professional and any other treating mental health providers; additional review of progress and recommendations for changes in treatment, as indicated, including medications, based on recommendations provided by the psychiatric consultant; provision of brief interventions using evidence-based techniques such as behavioral activation, motivational interviewing, and other focused treatment strategies; monitoring of patient outcomes using validated rating scales; and relapse prevention planning with patients as they achieve remission of symptoms and/or other treatment goals and are prepared for discharge from active treatment.**

EXCLUDES *Initial collaborative care managment in same calendar month (99492)*
2.27 3.59 FUD XXX S 80
AMA: 2019,Jan,6; 2018,Jul,12; 2018,Mar,5; 2018,Feb,7; 2018,Jan,8; 2017,Nov,3

\+ **99494** **Initial or subsequent psychiatric collaborative care management, each additional 30 minutes in a calendar month of behavioral health care manager activities, in consultation with a psychiatric consultant, and directed by the treating physician or other qualified health care professional (List separately in addition to code for primary procedure)**

INCLUDES Coordination of care with emergency department staff

Code first (99492, 99493)

1.22 1.86 **FUD** ZZZ N 80

AMA: 2019,Jan,6; 2018,Jul,12; 2018,Mar,5; 2018,Feb,7; 2018,Jan,8; 2017,Nov,3

99495-99496 Management of Transitional Care Services

CMS: 100-02,13,230.1 Transitional Care Management Services; 100-04,11,40.1.3 Independent Attending Physician Services; 100-04,12,190.3 List of Telehealth Services

INCLUDES First interaction (face-to-face, by telephone, or electronic) with patient or his/her caregiver and must be done within 2 working days of discharge
Initial face-to-face; must be done within code time frame and include medication management
New or established patient with moderate to high complexity medical decision making needs during care transitions
Patient management services during same time frame as (99339-99340, 99358-99359, 99366-99368, 99374-99380, 99441-99443, [99091], 99487-99489, 90951-90970, 93792-93793, 98960-98962, 98966-98968, 99071, 99078, 99080, 99605-99607)
Services from discharge day up to 29 days post discharge
Subsequent discharge within 30 days
Without face-to-face patient care given by physician or other qualified health care professional includes:
Arrangement of follow-up and referrals with community resources and providers
Contacting qualified health care professionals for specific problems of patient
Discharge information review
Need for follow-up care review based on tests and treatments
Patient, family, and caregiver education
Without face-to-face patient care given by staff under the guidance of physician or other qualified health care professional includes:
Caregiver education to family or patient, addressing independent living and self-management
Communication with patient and all caregivers and professionals regarding care
Determining which community and health resources would benefit the patient
Providing communication with home health and other patient utilized services
Support for treatment and medication adherence
The facilitation of services and care

EXCLUDES *E&M services after the first face-to-face visit*

99495 **Transitional Care Management Services with the following required elements: Communication (direct contact, telephone, electronic) with the patient and/or caregiver within 2 business days of discharge Medical decision making of at least moderate complexity during the service period Face-to-face visit, within 14 calendar days of discharge**

3.11 4.62 **FUD** XXX ★ V 80

AMA: 2019,Jan,6; 2018,Jul,12; 2018,Apr,9; 2018,Mar,5; 2018,Mar,7; 2018,Feb,7; 2018,Jan,8; 2017,Jan,8; 2016,Jan,13; 2015,Jan,16; 2014,Oct,3; 2014,Oct,8; 2014,Mar,13; 2014,Jan,11

99496 **Transitional Care Management Services with the following required elements: Communication (direct contact, telephone, electronic) with the patient and/or caregiver within 2 business days of discharge Medical decision making of high complexity during the service period Face-to-face visit, within 7 calendar days of discharge**

4.51 6.52 **FUD** XXX ★ V 80

AMA: 2019,Jan,6; 2018,Jul,12; 2018,Apr,9; 2018,Mar,5; 2018,Mar,7; 2018,Feb,7; 2018,Jan,8; 2017,Jan,8; 2016,Jan,13; 2015,Jan,16; 2014,Oct,3; 2014,Oct,8; 2014,Mar,13; 2014,Jan,11

99497-99498 Advance Directive Guidance

CMS: 100-02,15,280.5.1 Advance Care Planning with an Annual Wellness Visit; 100-04,11,40.1.3 Independent Attending Physician Services; 100-04,18,140.8 Advance Care Planning with an Annual Wellness Visit (AWV); 100-04,4,200.11 Advance Care Planning as an Optional Element of an Annual Wellness Visit

EXCLUDES *Critical care services (99291-99292, 99468-99469, 99471-99472, 99475-99476, 99477-99480)*
Services for cognitive care (99483)
Treatment/management for an active problem (see appropriate E&M service)

99497 **Advance care planning including the explanation and discussion of advance directives such as standard forms (with completion of such forms, when performed), by the physician or other qualified health care professional; first 30 minutes, face-to-face with the patient, family member(s), and/or surrogate**

2.23 2.40 **FUD** XXX Q1 80

AMA: 2018,Apr,9; 2018,Jan,8; 2017,Jan,8; 2016,Feb,7; 2016,Jan,13; 2015,Jan,16; 2014,Dec,11

\+ **99498** **each additional 30 minutes (List separately in addition to code for primary procedure)**

Code first (99497)

2.10 2.11 **FUD** ZZZ N 80

AMA: 2018,Apr,9; 2018,Jan,8; 2017,Jan,8; 2016,Feb,7; 2016,Jan,13; 2015,Jan,16; 2014,Dec,11

99484 [99484] Behavioral Health Integration Care

CMS: 100-02,13,230.2 Chronic Care Management and General Behavioral Health Integration Services

INCLUDES Care management services requiring 20 minutes or more per calendar month
Coordination of care with emergency department staff
Face to face services when necessary
Provided as an outpatient service
Provision of services by clinical staff and reported by supervising physician or other qualified healthcare professional
Provision of services to patients with whom there is an ongoing relationship
Treatment plan and specific service components

EXCLUDES *Other services for which the time or activities associated with that service aren't used to meet requirements for 99484:*
Chronic care management ([99490], 99487-99489)
Psychiatric collaborative care in same calendar month (99492-99494)
Psychotherapy services (90785-90899)

\# **99484** **Care management services for behavioral health conditions, at least 20 minutes of clinical staff time, directed by a physician or other qualified health care professional, per calendar month, with the following required elements: initial assessment or follow-up monitoring, including the use of applicable validated rating scales; behavioral health care planning in relation to behavioral/psychiatric health problems, including revision for patients who are not progressing or whose status changes; facilitating and coordinating treatment such as psychotherapy, pharmacotherapy, counseling and/or psychiatric consultation; and continuity of care with a designated member of the care team.**

0.91 1.35 **FUD** XXX S 80

AMA: 2019,Jan,6; 2018,Jul,12; 2018,Mar,5; 2018,Feb,7; 2018,Jan,8

99499 Unlisted Evaluation and Management Services

CMS: 100-04,12,30.6.10 Consultation Services; 100-04,12,30.6.4 Services Furnished Incident to Physician's Service; 100-04,12,30.6.9.1 Initial Hospital Care and Observation or Inpatient Care Services

99499 **Unlisted evaluation and management service**

0.00 0.00 **FUD** XXX B 80

AMA: 2019,Aug,8; 2018,Jan,8; 2017,Jan,8; 2016,Jan,13; 2015,Jan,16; 2014,Oct,8; 2014,Jan,11

0001F-0015F Quality Measures with Multiple Components

INCLUDES Several measures grouped within a single code descriptor to make possible reporting for clinical conditions when all of the components have been met

0001F **Heart failure assessed (includes assessment of all the following components) (CAD): Blood pressure measured (2000F) Level of activity assessed (1003F) Clinical symptoms of volume overload (excess) assessed (1004F) Weight, recorded (2001F) Clinical signs of volume overload (excess) assessed (2002F)**

INCLUDES Blood pressure measured (2000F)
Clinical signs of volume overload (excess) assessed (2002F)
Clinical symptoms of volume overload (excess) assessed (1004F)
Level of activity assessed (1003F)
Weight recorded (2001F)

0.00 0.00 FUD XXX E

AMA: 2018,Jan,8; 2017,Jan,8; 2016,Jan,13; 2015,Jan,16; 2014,Jan,11

0005F **Osteoarthritis assessed (OA) Includes assessment of all the following components: Osteoarthritis symptoms and functional status assessed (1006F) Use of anti-inflammatory or over-the-counter (OTC) analgesic medications assessed (1007F) Initial examination of the involved joint(s) (includes visual inspection, palpation, range of motion) (2004F)**

INCLUDES Initial examination of the involved joint(s) (includes visual inspection/palpation/range of motion) (2004F)
Osteoarthritis symptoms and functional status assessed (1006F)
Use of anti-inflammatory or over-the-counter (OTC) analgesic medications assessed (1007F)

0.00 0.00 FUD XXX E

AMA: 2005,Oct,1-5

0012F **Community-acquired bacterial pneumonia assessment (includes all of the following components) (CAP): Co-morbid conditions assessed (1026F) Vital signs recorded (2010F) Mental status assessed (2014F) Hydration status assessed (2018F)**

0.00 0.00 FUD XXX E

INCLUDES Co-morbid conditions assessed (1026F)
Hydration status assessed (2018F)
Mental status assessed (2014F)
Vital signs recorded (2010F)

0014F **Comprehensive preoperative assessment performed for cataract surgery with intraocular lens (IOL) placement (includes assessment of all of the following components) (EC): Dilated fundus evaluation performed within 12 months prior to cataract surgery (2020F) Pre-surgical (cataract) axial length, corneal power measurement and method of intraocular lens power calculation documented (must be performed within 12 months prior to surgery) (3073F) Preoperative assessment of functional or medical indication(s) for surgery prior to the cataract surgery with intraocular lens placement (must be performed within 12 months prior to cataract surgery) (3325F)**

INCLUDES Evaluation of dilated fundus done within 12 months prior to surgery (2020F)
Preoperative assessment of functional or medical indications done within 12 months prior to surgery (3325F)
Presurgical measurement of axial length, corneal power, and IOL power calculation performed within 12 months prior to surgery (3073F)

0.00 0.00 FUD XXX E

AMA: 2008,Mar,8-12

0015F **Melanoma follow up completed (includes assessment of all of the following components) (ML): History obtained regarding new or changing moles (1050F) Complete physical skin exam performed (2029F) Patient counseled to perform a monthly self skin examination (5005F)**

INCLUDES Complete physical skin exam (2029F)
Counseling to perform monthly skin self-examination (5005F)
History obtained of new or changing moles (1050F)

0.00 0.00 FUD XXX E

AMA: 2008,Mar,8-12

0500F-0584F Care Provided According to Prevailing Guidelines

INCLUDES Measures of utilization or patient care provided for certain clinical purposes

0500F **Initial prenatal care visit (report at first prenatal encounter with health care professional providing obstetrical care. Report also date of visit and, in a separate field, the date of the last menstrual period [LMP]) (Prenatal)** M ♀

0.00 0.00 FUD XXX E

AMA: 2018,Jan,8; 2017,Jan,8; 2016,Jan,13; 2015,Jan,16; 2014,Jan,11

0501F **Prenatal flow sheet documented in medical record by first prenatal visit (documentation includes at minimum blood pressure, weight, urine protein, uterine size, fetal heart tones, and estimated date of delivery). Report also: date of visit and, in a separate field, the date of the last menstrual period [LMP] (Note: If reporting 0501F Prenatal flow sheet, it is not necessary to report 0500F Initial prenatal care visit) (Prenatal)** M ♀

0.00 0.00 FUD XXX E

AMA: 2004,Nov,1

0502F **Subsequent prenatal care visit (Prenatal) [Excludes: patients who are seen for a condition unrelated to pregnancy or prenatal care (eg, an upper respiratory infection; patients seen for consultation only, not for continuing care)]** M ♀

EXCLUDES *Patients seen for an unrelated pregnancy/prenatal care condition (e.g., upper respiratory infection; patients seen for consultation only, not for continuing care)*

0.00 0.00 FUD XXX E

AMA: 2004,Nov,1

0503F **Postpartum care visit (Prenatal)** M ♀

0.00 0.00 FUD XXX E

AMA: 2004,Nov,1

0505F **Hemodialysis plan of care documented (ESRD, P-ESRD)**

0.00 0.00 FUD XXX E

AMA: 2008,Mar,8-12

0507F **Peritoneal dialysis plan of care documented (ESRD)**

0.00 0.00 FUD XXX E

AMA: 2008,Mar,8-12

0509F **Urinary incontinence plan of care documented (GER)**

0.00 0.00 FUD XXX M

0513F **Elevated blood pressure plan of care documented (CKD)**

0.00 0.00 FUD XXX M

AMA: 2008,Mar,8-12

0514F **Plan of care for elevated hemoglobin level documented for patient receiving Erythropoiesis-Stimulating Agent therapy (ESA) (CKD)**

0.00 0.00 FUD XXX E

AMA: 2008,Mar,8-12

0516F **Anemia plan of care documented (ESRD)**

0.00 0.00 FUD XXX E

AMA: 2008,Mar,8-12

0517F **Glaucoma plan of care documented (EC)**

0.00 0.00 FUD XXX M

AMA: 2008,Mar,8-12

0518F Falls plan of care documented (GER)
0.00 0.00 FUD XXX M
AMA: 2008,Mar,8-12

0519F Planned chemotherapy regimen, including at a minimum: drug(s) prescribed, dose, and duration, documented prior to initiation of a new treatment regimen (ONC)
0.00 0.00 FUD XXX E
AMA: 2008,Mar,8-12

0520F Radiation dose limits to normal tissues established prior to the initiation of a course of 3D conformal radiation for a minimum of 2 tissue/organ (ONC)
0.00 0.00 FUD XXX M
AMA: 2008,Mar,8-12

0521F Plan of care to address pain documented (COA) (ONC)
0.00 0.00 FUD XXX M
AMA: 2008,Mar,8-12

0525F Initial visit for episode (BkP)
0.00 0.00 FUD XXX E
AMA: 2008,Mar,8-12

0526F Subsequent visit for episode (BkP)
0.00 0.00 FUD XXX M
AMA: 2008,Mar,8-12

0528F Recommended follow-up interval for repeat colonoscopy of at least 10 years documented in colonoscopy report (End/Polyp)
0.00 0.00 FUD XXX M

0529F Interval of 3 or more years since patient's last colonoscopy, documented (End/Polyp)
0.00 0.00 FUD XXX M

0535F Dyspnea management plan of care, documented (Pall Cr)
0.00 0.00 FUD XXX E

0540F Glucorticoid Management Plan Documented (RA)
0.00 0.00 FUD XXX M

0545F Plan for follow-up care for major depressive disorder, documented (MDD ADOL)
0.00 0.00 FUD XXX E

0550F Cytopathology report on routine nongynecologic specimen finalized within two working days of accession date (PATH)
0.00 0.00 FUD XXX E

0551F Cytopathology report on nongynecologic specimen with documentation that the specimen was non-routine (PATH)
0.00 0.00 FUD XXX E

0555F Symptom management plan of care documented (HF)
0.00 0.00 FUD XXX E

0556F Plan of care to achieve lipid control documented (CAD)
0.00 0.00 FUD XXX E

0557F Plan of care to manage anginal symptoms documented (CAD)
0.00 0.00 FUD XXX E

0575F HIV RNA control plan of care, documented (HIV)
0.00 0.00 FUD XXX E

0580F Multidisciplinary care plan developed or updated (ALS)
0.00 0.00 FUD XXX E

0581F Patient transferred directly from anesthetizing location to critical care unit (Peri2)
0.00 0.00 FUD XXX M

0582F Patient not transferred directly from anesthetizing location to critical care unit (Peri2)
0.00 0.00 FUD XXX E

0583F Transfer of care checklist used (Peri2)
0.00 0.00 FUD XXX M

0584F Transfer of care checklist not used (Peri2)
0.00 0.00 FUD XXX E

1000F-1505F Elements of History/Review of Systems

INCLUDES Measures for specific aspects of patient history or review of systems

1000F Tobacco use assessed (CAD, CAP, COPD, PV) (DM)
0.00 0.00 FUD XXX E
AMA: 2018,Jan,8; 2017,Jan,8; 2016,Jan,13; 2015,Jan,16; 2014,Jan,11

1002F Anginal symptoms and level of activity assessed (NMA-No Measure Associated)
0.00 0.00 FUD XXX E
AMA: 2004,Nov,1

1003F Level of activity assessed (NMA-No Measure Associated)
0.00 0.00 FUD XXX E
AMA: 2006,Dec,10-12

1004F Clinical symptoms of volume overload (excess) assessed (NMA-No Measure Associated)
0.00 0.00 FUD XXX E
AMA: 2006,Dec,10-12

1005F Asthma symptoms evaluated (includes documentation of numeric frequency of symptoms or patient completion of an asthma assessment tool/survey/questionnaire) (NMA-No Measure Associated)
0.00 0.00 FUD XXX E

1006F Osteoarthritis symptoms and functional status assessed (may include the use of a standardized scale or the completion of an assessment questionnaire, such as the SF-36, AAOS Hip & Knee Questionnaire) (OA) [Instructions: Report when osteoarthritis is addressed during the patient encounter]
0.00 0.00 FUD XXX M

INCLUDES Osteoarthritis when it is addressed during the patient encounter

1007F Use of anti-inflammatory or analgesic over-the-counter (OTC) medications for symptom relief assessed (OA)
0.00 0.00 FUD XXX E

1008F Gastrointestinal and renal risk factors assessed for patients on prescribed or OTC non-steroidal anti-inflammatory drug (NSAID) (OA)
0.00 0.00 FUD XXX E

1010F Severity of angina assessed by level of activity (CAD)
0.00 0.00 FUD XXX E

1011F Angina present (CAD)
0.00 0.00 FUD XXX E

1012F Angina absent (CAD)
0.00 0.00 FUD XXX E

1015F Chronic obstructive pulmonary disease (COPD) symptoms assessed (Includes assessment of at least 1 of the following: dyspnea, cough/sputum, wheezing), or respiratory symptom assessment tool completed (COPD)
0.00 0.00 FUD XXX E

1018F Dyspnea assessed, not present (COPD)
0.00 0.00 FUD XXX E

1019F Dyspnea assessed, present (COPD)
0.00 0.00 FUD XXX E

1022F Pneumococcus immunization status assessed (CAP, COPD)
0.00 0.00 FUD XXX E
AMA: 2010,Jul,3-5; 2008,Mar,8-12

1026F Co-morbid conditions assessed (eg, includes assessment for presence or absence of: malignancy, liver disease, congestive heart failure, cerebrovascular disease, renal disease, chronic obstructive pulmonary disease, asthma, diabetes, other co-morbid conditions) (CAP)
0.00 0.00 FUD XXX E

1030F Influenza immunization status assessed (CAP)
0.00 0.00 FUD XXX E
AMA: 2008,Mar,8-12

1031F Smoking status and exposure to second hand smoke in the home assessed (Asthma)
0.00 0.00 FUD XXX E

1032F Current tobacco smoker or currently exposed to secondhand smoke (Asthma)
0.00 0.00 FUD XXX E

1033F Current tobacco non-smoker and not currently exposed to secondhand smoke (Asthma)
0.00 0.00 FUD XXX E

1034F Current tobacco smoker (CAD, CAP, COPD, PV) (DM)
0.00 0.00 FUD XXX E
AMA: 2008,Mar,8-12

1035F Current smokeless tobacco user (eg, chew, snuff) (PV)
0.00 0.00 FUD XXX E
AMA: 2008,Mar,8-12

1036F Current tobacco non-user (CAD, CAP, COPD, PV) (DM) (IBD)
0.00 0.00 FUD XXX M
AMA: 2008,Mar,8-12

1038F Persistent asthma (mild, moderate or severe) (Asthma)
0.00 0.00 FUD XXX M
AMA: 2018,Jan,8; 2017,Jan,8; 2016,Jan,13; 2015,Jan,16; 2014,Jan,11

1039F Intermittent asthma (Asthma)
0.00 0.00 FUD XXX M
AMA: 2018,Jan,8; 2017,Jan,8; 2016,Jan,13; 2015,Jan,16; 2014,Jan,11

1040F DSM-5 criteria for major depressive disorder documented at the initial evaluation (MDD, MDD ADOL)
0.00 0.00 FUD XXX E
AMA: 2008,Mar,8-12

1050F History obtained regarding new or changing moles (ML)
0.00 0.00 FUD XXX E
AMA: 2008,Mar,8-12

1052F Type, anatomic location, and activity all assessed (IBD)
0.00 0.00 FUD XXX E

1055F Visual functional status assessed (EC)
0.00 0.00 FUD XXX E

1060F Documentation of permanent or persistent or paroxysmal atrial fibrillation (STR)
0.00 0.00 FUD XXX E

1061F Documentation of absence of permanent and persistent and paroxysmal atrial fibrillation (STR)
0.00 0.00 FUD XXX E

1065F Ischemic stroke symptom onset of less than 3 hours prior to arrival (STR)
0.00 0.00 FUD XXX E

1066F Ischemic stroke symptom onset greater than or equal to 3 hours prior to arrival (STR)
0.00 0.00 FUD XXX E

1070F Alarm symptoms (involuntary weight loss, dysphagia, or gastrointestinal bleeding) assessed; none present (GERD)
0.00 0.00 FUD XXX E

1071F 1 or more present (GERD)
0.00 0.00 FUD XXX E

1090F Presence or absence of urinary incontinence assessed (GER)
0.00 0.00 FUD XXX M

1091F Urinary incontinence characterized (eg, frequency, volume, timing, type of symptoms, how bothersome) (GER)
0.00 0.00 FUD XXX E

1100F Patient screened for future fall risk; documentation of 2 or more falls in the past year or any fall with injury in the past year (GER)
0.00 0.00 FUD XXX M
AMA: 2008,Mar,8-12

1101F documentation of no falls in the past year or only 1 fall without injury in the past year (GER)
0.00 0.00 FUD XXX M
AMA: 2008,Mar,8-12

1110F Patient discharged from an inpatient facility (eg, hospital, skilled nursing facility, or rehabilitation facility) within the last 60 days (GER)
0.00 0.00 FUD XXX E

1111F Discharge medications reconciled with the current medication list in outpatient medical record (COA) (GER)
0.00 0.00 FUD XXX M

1116F Auricular or periauricular pain assessed (AOE)
0.00 0.00 FUD XXX E
AMA: 2008,Mar,8-12

1118F GERD symptoms assessed after 12 months of therapy (GERD)
0.00 0.00 FUD XXX E
AMA: 2008,Mar,8-12

1119F Initial evaluation for condition (HEP C)(EPI, DSP)
0.00 0.00 FUD XXX E
AMA: 2008,Mar,8-12

1121F Subsequent evaluation for condition (HEP C)(EPI)
0.00 0.00 FUD XXX E
AMA: 2008,Mar,8-12

1123F Advance Care Planning discussed and documented advance care plan or surrogate decision maker documented in the medical record (DEM) (GER, Pall Cr)
0.00 0.00 FUD XXX M
AMA: 2008,Mar,8-12

1124F Advance Care Planning discussed and documented in the medical record, patient did not wish or was not able to name a surrogate decision maker or provide an advance care plan (DEM) (GER, Pall Cr)
0.00 0.00 FUD XXX M
AMA: 2008,Mar,8-12

1125F Pain severity quantified; pain present (COA) (ONC)
0.00 0.00 FUD XXX M
AMA: 2008,Mar,8-12

1126F no pain present (COA) (ONC)
0.00 0.00 FUD XXX M
AMA: 2008,Mar,8-12

1127F New episode for condition (NMA-No Measure Associated)
0.00 0.00 FUD XXX E
AMA: 2008,Mar,8-12

1128F Subsequent episode for condition (NMA-No Measure Associated)
0.00 0.00 FUD XXX E
AMA: 2008,Mar,8-12

1130F Back pain and function assessed, including all of the following: Pain assessment and functional status and patient history, including notation of presence or absence of "red flags" (warning signs) and assessment of prior treatment and response, and employment status (BkP)
0.00 0.00 FUD XXX E
AMA: 2008,Mar,8-12

1134F Episode of back pain lasting 6 weeks or less (BkP)
0.00 0.00 FUD XXX E
AMA: 2008,Mar,8-12

1135F Episode of back pain lasting longer than 6 weeks (BkP)
0.00 0.00 FUD XXX E
AMA: 2008,Mar,8-12

1136F Episode of back pain lasting 12 weeks or less (BkP)
0.00 0.00 FUD XXX E
AMA: 2008,Mar,8-12

1137F Episode of back pain lasting longer than 12 weeks (BkP)
0.00 0.00 FUD XXX E
AMA: 2008,Mar,8-12

1150F Documentation that a patient has a substantial risk of death within 1 year (Pall Cr)
0.00 0.00 FUD XXX E

1151F Documentation that a patient does not have a substantial risk of death within one year (Pall Cr)
0.00 0.00 FUD XXX E

1152F Documentation of advanced disease diagnosis, goals of care prioritize comfort (Pall Cr)
0.00 0.00 FUD XXX E

1153F Documentation of advanced disease diagnosis, goals of care do not prioritize comfort (Pall Cr)
0.00 0.00 FUD XXX E

1157F Advance care plan or similar legal document present in the medical record (COA)
0.00 0.00 FUD XXX E

1158F Advance care planning discussion documented in the medical record (COA)
0.00 0.00 FUD XXX M

1159F Medication list documented in medical record (COA)
0.00 0.00 FUD XXX E

1160F Review of all medications by a prescribing practitioner or clinical pharmacist (such as, prescriptions, OTCs, herbal therapies and supplements) documented in the medical record (COA)
0.00 0.00 FUD XXX E

1170F Functional status assessed (COA) (RA)
0.00 0.00 FUD XXX M

1175F Functional status for dementia assessed and results reviewed (DEM)
0.00 0.00 FUD XXX E

1180F All specified thromboembolic risk factors assessed (AFIB)
0.00 0.00 FUD XXX E

1181F Neuropsychiatric symptoms assessed and results reviewed (DEM)
0.00 0.00 FUD XXX E

1182F Neuropsychiatric symptoms, one or more present (DEM)
0.00 0.00 FUD XXX E

1183F Neuropsychiatric symptoms, absent (DEM)
0.00 0.00 FUD XXX E

1200F Seizure type(s) and current seizure frequency(ies) documented (EPI)
0.00 0.00 FUD XXX E

1205F Etiology of epilepsy or epilepsy syndrome(s) reviewed and documented (EPI)
0.00 0.00 FUD XXX E

1220F Patient screened for depression (SUD)
0.00 0.00 FUD XXX E

1400F Parkinson's disease diagnosis reviewed (Prkns)
0.00 0.00 FUD XXX E

1450F Symptoms improved or remained consistent with treatment goals since last assessment (HF)
0.00 0.00 FUD XXX E

1451F Symptoms demonstrated clinically important deterioration since last assessment (HF)
0.00 0.00 FUD XXX E

1460F Qualifying cardiac event/diagnosis in previous 12 months (CAD)
0.00 0.00 FUD XXX M

1461F No qualifying cardiac event/diagnosis in previous 12 months (CAD)
0.00 0.00 FUD XXX M

1490F Dementia severity classified, mild (DEM)
0.00 0.00 FUD XXX E

1491F Dementia severity classified, moderate (DEM)
0.00 0.00 FUD XXX E

1493F Dementia severity classified, severe (DEM)
0.00 0.00 FUD XXX E

1494F Cognition assessed and reviewed (DEM)
0.00 0.00 FUD XXX E

1500F Symptoms and signs of distal symmetric polyneuropathy reviewed and documented (DSP)
0.00 0.00 FUD XXX E

1501F Not initial evaluation for condition (DSP)
0.00 0.00 FUD XXX E

1502F Patient queried about pain and pain interference with function using a valid and reliable instrument (DSP)
0.00 0.00 FUD XXX E

1503F Patient queried about symptoms of respiratory insufficiency (ALS)
0.00 0.00 FUD XXX E

1504F Patient has respiratory insufficiency (ALS)
0.00 0.00 FUD XXX E

1505F Patient does not have respiratory insufficiency (ALS)
0.00 0.00 FUD XXX E

2000F-2060F [2033F] Elements of Examination

INCLUDES Components of clinical assessment or physical exam

2000F Blood pressure measured (CKD)(DM)
0.00 0.00 FUD XXX M
AMA: 2018,Jan,8; 2017,Jan,8; 2016,Jan,13; 2015,Jan,16; 2014,Jan,11

2001F Weight recorded (PAG)
0.00 0.00 FUD XXX E
AMA: 2006,Dec,10-12

2002F Clinical signs of volume overload (excess) assessed (NMA-No Measure Associated)
0.00 0.00 FUD XXX E
AMA: 2006,Dec,10-12

2004F Initial examination of the involved joint(s) (includes visual inspection, palpation, range of motion) (OA) [Instructions: Report only for initial osteoarthritis visit or for visits for new joint involvement]
INCLUDES Visits for initial osteoarthritis examination or new joint involvement
0.00 0.00 FUD XXX E
AMA: 2004,Feb,3; 2003,Aug,1

2010F Vital signs (temperature, pulse, respiratory rate, and blood pressure) documented and reviewed (CAP) (EM)
0.00 0.00 FUD XXX E

2014F Mental status assessed (CAP) (EM)
0.00 0.00 FUD XXX E

2015F Asthma impairment assessed (Asthma)
0.00 0.00 FUD XXX E

2016F Asthma risk assessed (Asthma)
0.00 0.00 FUD XXX E

2018F Hydration status assessed (normal/mildly dehydrated/severely dehydrated) (CAP)
0.00 0.00 FUD XXX E

2019F Dilated macular exam performed, including documentation of the presence or absence of macular thickening or hemorrhage and the level of macular degeneration severity (EC)
0.00 0.00 FUD XXX E

2020F Dilated fundus evaluation performed within 12 months prior to cataract surgery (EC)
0.00 0.00 FUD XXX E
AMA: 2008,Mar,8-12

2021F Dilated macular or fundus exam performed, including documentation of the presence or absence of macular edema and level of severity of retinopathy (EC)
0.00 0.00 FUD XXX E

▲ 2022F Dilated retinal eye exam with interpretation by an ophthalmologist or optometrist documented and reviewed; with evidence of retinopathy (DM)
0.00 0.00 FUD XXX M
AMA: 2008,Mar,8-12

2023F without evidence of retinopathy (DM)
0.00 0.00 FUD 000

▲ 2024F 7 standard field stereoscopic retinal photos with interpretation by an ophthalmologist or optometrist documented and reviewed; with evidence of retinopathy (DM)
0.00 0.00 FUD XXX M
AMA: 2008,Mar,8-12

2025F without evidence of retinopathy (DM)
0.00 0.00 FUD 000

▲ 2026F Eye imaging validated to match diagnosis from 7 standard field stereoscopic retinal photos results documented and reviewed; with evidence of retinopathy (DM)
0.00 0.00 FUD XXX M
AMA: 2008,Mar,8-12

● # 2033F without evidence of retinopathy (DM)
0.00 0.00 FUD 000

2027F Optic nerve head evaluation performed (EC)
0.00 0.00 FUD XXX M

2028F Foot examination performed (includes examination through visual inspection, sensory exam with monofilament, and pulse exam - report when any of the 3 components are completed) (DM)
0.00 0.00 FUD XXX E

2029F Complete physical skin exam performed (ML)
0.00 0.00 FUD XXX E
AMA: 2008,Mar,8-12

2030F Hydration status documented, normally hydrated (PAG)
0.00 0.00 FUD XXX E

2031F Hydration status documented, dehydrated (PAG)
0.00 0.00 FUD XXX E

2033F Resequenced code. See code following 2026F.

2035F Tympanic membrane mobility assessed with pneumatic otoscopy or tympanometry (OME)
0.00 0.00 FUD XXX E
AMA: 2008,Mar,8-12

2040F Physical examination on the date of the initial visit for low back pain performed, in accordance with specifications (BkP)
0.00 0.00 FUD XXX E
AMA: 2008,Mar,8-12

2044F Documentation of mental health assessment prior to intervention (back surgery or epidural steroid injection) or for back pain episode lasting longer than 6 weeks (BkP)
0.00 0.00 FUD XXX E
AMA: 2008,Mar,8-12

2050F Wound characteristics including size and nature of wound base tissue and amount of drainage prior to debridement documented (CWC)
0.00 0.00 FUD XXX E

2060F Patient interviewed directly on or before date of diagnosis of major depressive disorder (MDD ADOL)
0.00 0.00 FUD XXX E

3006F-3776F [3051F, 3052F] Findings from Diagnostic or Screening Tests

INCLUDES Results and medical decision making with regards to ordered tests:
- Clinical laboratory tests
- Other examination procedures
- Radiological examinations

3006F Chest X-ray results documented and reviewed (CAP)
0.00 0.00 FUD XXX E
AMA: 2018,Jan,8; 2017,Jan,8; 2016,Jan,13; 2015,Jan,16; 2014,Jan,11

3008F Body Mass Index (BMI), documented (PV)
0.00 0.00 FUD XXX E

3011F Lipid panel results documented and reviewed (must include total cholesterol, HDL-C, triglycerides and calculated LDL-C) (CAD)
0.00 0.00 FUD XXX E

3014F Screening mammography results documented and reviewed (PV)
0.00 0.00 FUD XXX E
AMA: 2008,Mar,8-12

3015F Cervical cancer screening results documented and reviewed (PV) ♀
0.00 0.00 FUD XXX E

3016F Patient screened for unhealthy alcohol use using a systematic screening method (PV) (DSP)
0.00 0.00 FUD XXX E

3017F Colorectal cancer screening results documented and reviewed (PV)
0.00 0.00 FUD XXX M
AMA: 2008,Mar,8-12

3018F Pre-procedure risk assessment and depth of insertion and quality of the bowel prep and complete description of polyp(s) found, including location of each polyp, size, number and gross morphology and recommendations for follow-up in final colonoscopy report documented (End/Polyp)
0.00 0.00 FUD XXX E

3019F Left ventricular ejection fraction (LVEF) assessment planned post discharge (HF)
0.00 0.00 FUD XXX E

3020F Left ventricular function (LVF) assessment (eg, echocardiography, nuclear test, or ventriculography) documented in the medical record (Includes quantitative or qualitative assessment results) (NMA-No Measure Associated)
0.00 0.00 FUD XXX E
AMA: 2006,Dec,10-12

3021F Left ventricular ejection fraction (LVEF) less than 40% or documentation of moderately or severely depressed left ventricular systolic function (CAD, HF)
0.00 0.00 FUD XXX M

3022F Left ventricular ejection fraction (LVEF) greater than or equal to 40% or documentation as normal or mildly depressed left ventricular systolic function (CAD, HF)
0.00 0.00 FUD XXX M

3023F Spirometry results documented and reviewed (COPD)
0.00 0.00 FUD XXX M

3025F Spirometry test results demonstrate FEV1/FVC less than 70% with COPD symptoms (eg, dyspnea, cough/sputum, wheezing) (CAP, COPD)
0.00 0.00 FUD XXX E

3027F Spirometry test results demonstrate FEV1/FVC greater than or equal to 70% or patient does not have COPD symptoms (COPD)
0.00 0.00 FUD XXX E

3028F Oxygen saturation results documented and reviewed (includes assessment through pulse oximetry or arterial blood gas measurement) (CAP, COPD) (EM)
0.00 0.00 FUD XXX E

3035F Oxygen saturation less than or equal to 88% or a PaO2 less than or equal to 55 mm Hg (COPD)
0.00 0.00 FUD XXX E

3037F Oxygen saturation greater than 88% or PaO2 greater than 55 mm Hg (COPD)
0.00 0.00 FUD XXX E

3038F Pulmonary function test performed within 12 months prior to surgery (Lung/Esop Cx)
0.00 0.00 FUD XXX E

3040F Functional expiratory volume (FEV1) less than 40% of predicted value (COPD)
0.00 0.00 FUD XXX E

3042F Functional expiratory volume (FEV1) greater than or equal to 40% of predicted value (COPD)
0.00 0.00 FUD XXX E

3044F Most recent hemoglobin A1c (HbA1c) level less than 7.0% (DM)
0.00 0.00 FUD XXX M

● # **3051F** Most recent hemoglobin A1c (HbA1c) level greater than or equal to 7.0% and less than 8.0% (DM)
0.00 0.00 FUD 000

3045F ~~Most recent hemoglobin A1c (HbA1c) level 7.0-9.0% (DM)~~
To report, see ([3051F], [3052F])

● # **3052F** Most recent hemoglobin A1c (HbA1c) level greater than or equal to 8.0% and less than or equal to 9.0% (DM)
0.00 0.00 FUD 000

▲ **3046F** Most recent hemoglobin A1c level greater than 9.0% (DM)
0.00 0.00 FUD XXX M

EXCLUDES *Levels of hemoglobin A1c less than or equal to 9.0% (3044F, [3051F], [3052F])*

3048F Most recent LDL-C less than 100 mg/dL (CAD) (DM)
0.00 0.00 FUD XXX E

3049F Most recent LDL-C 100-129 mg/dL (CAD) (DM)
0.00 0.00 FUD XXX E

3050F Most recent LDL-C greater than or equal to 130 mg/dL (CAD) (DM)
0.00 0.00 FUD XXX E

3051F Resequenced code. See code following 3044F.

3052F Resequenced code. See code before 3046F.

3055F Left ventricular ejection fraction (LVEF) less than or equal to 35% (HF)
0.00 0.00 FUD XXX E

3056F Left ventricular ejection fraction (LVEF) greater than 35% or no LVEF result available (HF)
0.00 0.00 FUD XXX E

3060F Positive microalbuminuria test result documented and reviewed (DM)
0.00 0.00 FUD XXX M

3061F Negative microalbuminuria test result documented and reviewed (DM)
0.00 0.00 FUD XXX M

3062F Positive macroalbuminuria test result documented and reviewed (DM)
0.00 0.00 FUD XXX M

3066F Documentation of treatment for nephropathy (eg, patient receiving dialysis, patient being treated for ESRD, CRF, ARF, or renal insufficiency, any visit to a nephrologist) (DM)
0.00 0.00 FUD XXX M

3072F Low risk for retinopathy (no evidence of retinopathy in the prior year) (DM)
0.00 0.00 FUD XXX M
AMA: 2008,Mar,8-12

3073F Pre-surgical (cataract) axial length, corneal power measurement and method of intraocular lens power calculation documented within 12 months prior to surgery (EC)
0.00 0.00 FUD XXX E
AMA: 2008,Mar,8-12

3074F Most recent systolic blood pressure less than 130 mm Hg (DM), (HTN, CKD, CAD)
0.00 0.00 FUD XXX E
AMA: 2008,Mar,8-12

3075F Most recent systolic blood pressure 130-139 mm Hg (DM) (HTN, CKD, CAD)
0.00 0.00 FUD XXX E
AMA: 2008,Mar,8-12

3077F Most recent systolic blood pressure greater than or equal to 140 mm Hg (HTN, CKD, CAD) (DM)
0.00 0.00 FUD XXX E
AMA: 2008,Mar,8-12

3078F Most recent diastolic blood pressure less than 80 mm Hg (HTN, CKD, CAD) (DM)
0.00 0.00 FUD XXX E
AMA: 2008,Mar,8-12

3079F Most recent diastolic blood pressure 80-89 mm Hg (HTN, CKD, CAD) (DM)
0.00 0.00 FUD XXX E
AMA: 2008,Mar,8-12

3080F Most recent diastolic blood pressure greater than or equal to 90 mm Hg (HTN, CKD, CAD) (DM)
0.00 0.00 FUD XXX E
AMA: 2008,Mar,8-12

3082F Kt/V less than 1.2 (Clearance of urea [Kt]/volume [V]) (ESRD, P-ESRD)
0.00 0.00 FUD XXX E
AMA: 2008,Mar,8-12

3083F Kt/V equal to or greater than 1.2 and less than 1.7 (Clearance of urea [Kt]/volume [V]) (ESRD, P-ESRD)
0.00 0.00 FUD XXX E
AMA: 2008,Mar,8-12

3084F Kt/V greater than or equal to 1.7 (Clearance of urea [Kt]/volume [V]) (ESRD, P-ESRD)
0.00 0.00 FUD XXX E
AMA: 2008,Mar,8-12

3085F Suicide risk assessed (MDD, MDD ADOL)
0.00 0.00 FUD XXX E

3088F Major depressive disorder, mild (MDD)
0.00 0.00 FUD XXX E

3089F Major depressive disorder, moderate (MDD)
0.00 0.00 FUD XXX E

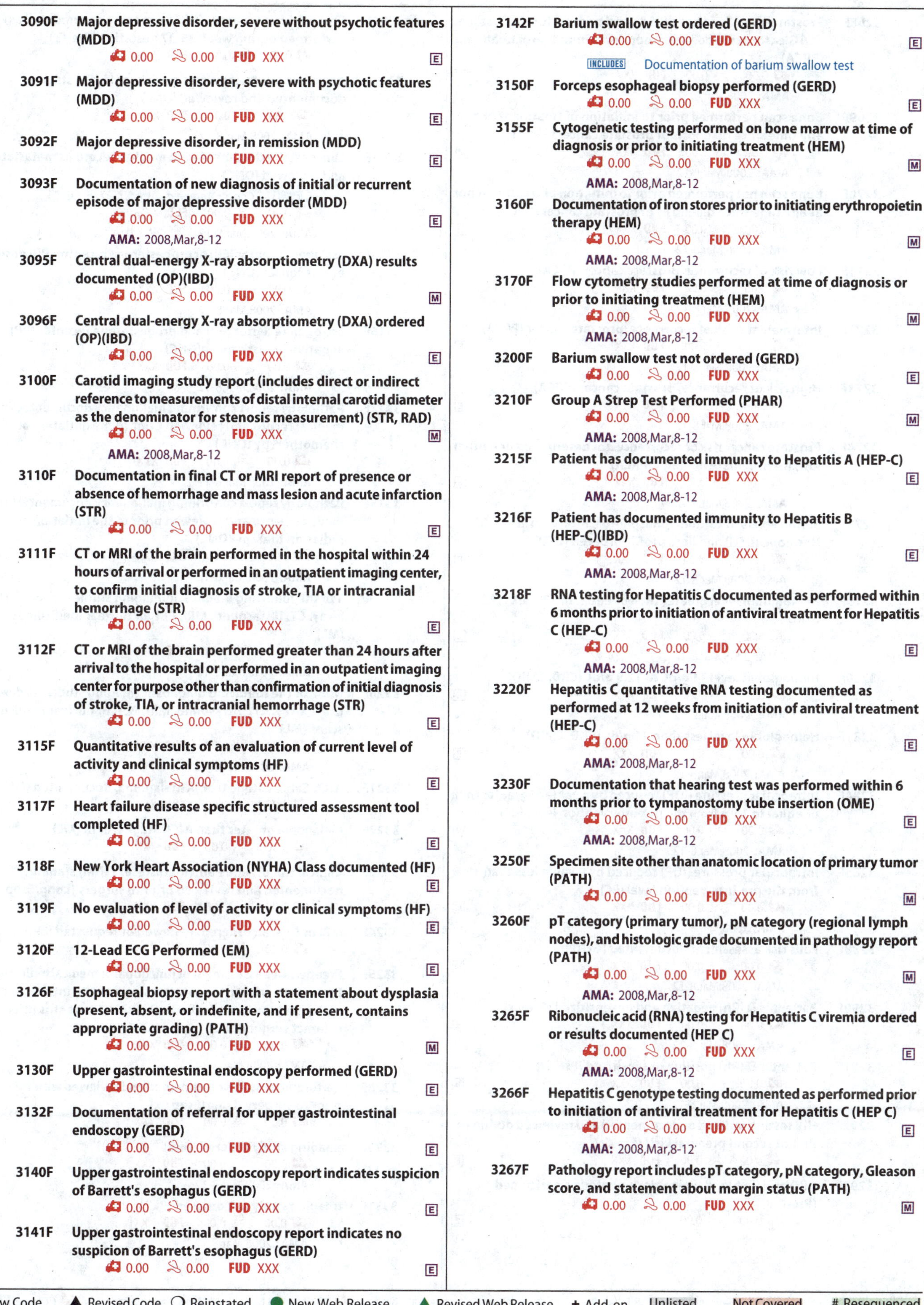

3090F Major depressive disorder, severe without psychotic features (MDD)
0.00 0.00 FUD XXX E

3091F Major depressive disorder, severe with psychotic features (MDD)
0.00 0.00 FUD XXX E

3092F Major depressive disorder, in remission (MDD)
0.00 0.00 FUD XXX E

3093F Documentation of new diagnosis of initial or recurrent episode of major depressive disorder (MDD)
0.00 0.00 FUD XXX E
AMA: 2008,Mar,8-12

3095F Central dual-energy X-ray absorptiometry (DXA) results documented (OP)(IBD)
0.00 0.00 FUD XXX M

3096F Central dual-energy X-ray absorptiometry (DXA) ordered (OP)(IBD)
0.00 0.00 FUD XXX E

3100F Carotid imaging study report (includes direct or indirect reference to measurements of distal internal carotid diameter as the denominator for stenosis measurement) (STR, RAD)
0.00 0.00 FUD XXX M
AMA: 2008,Mar,8-12

3110F Documentation in final CT or MRI report of presence or absence of hemorrhage and mass lesion and acute infarction (STR)
0.00 0.00 FUD XXX E

3111F CT or MRI of the brain performed in the hospital within 24 hours of arrival or performed in an outpatient imaging center, to confirm initial diagnosis of stroke, TIA or intracranial hemorrhage (STR)
0.00 0.00 FUD XXX E

3112F CT or MRI of the brain performed greater than 24 hours after arrival to the hospital or performed in an outpatient imaging center for purpose other than confirmation of initial diagnosis of stroke, TIA, or intracranial hemorrhage (STR)
0.00 0.00 FUD XXX E

3115F Quantitative results of an evaluation of current level of activity and clinical symptoms (HF)
0.00 0.00 FUD XXX E

3117F Heart failure disease specific structured assessment tool completed (HF)
0.00 0.00 FUD XXX E

3118F New York Heart Association (NYHA) Class documented (HF)
0.00 0.00 FUD XXX E

3119F No evaluation of level of activity or clinical symptoms (HF)
0.00 0.00 FUD XXX E

3120F 12-Lead ECG Performed (EM)
0.00 0.00 FUD XXX E

3126F Esophageal biopsy report with a statement about dysplasia (present, absent, or indefinite, and if present, contains appropriate grading) (PATH)
0.00 0.00 FUD XXX M

3130F Upper gastrointestinal endoscopy performed (GERD)
0.00 0.00 FUD XXX E

3132F Documentation of referral for upper gastrointestinal endoscopy (GERD)
0.00 0.00 FUD XXX E

3140F Upper gastrointestinal endoscopy report indicates suspicion of Barrett's esophagus (GERD)
0.00 0.00 FUD XXX E

3141F Upper gastrointestinal endoscopy report indicates no suspicion of Barrett's esophagus (GERD)
0.00 0.00 FUD XXX E

3142F Barium swallow test ordered (GERD)
0.00 0.00 FUD XXX E
INCLUDES Documentation of barium swallow test

3150F Forceps esophageal biopsy performed (GERD)
0.00 0.00 FUD XXX E

3155F Cytogenetic testing performed on bone marrow at time of diagnosis or prior to initiating treatment (HEM)
0.00 0.00 FUD XXX M
AMA: 2008,Mar,8-12

3160F Documentation of iron stores prior to initiating erythropoietin therapy (HEM)
0.00 0.00 FUD XXX M
AMA: 2008,Mar,8-12

3170F Flow cytometry studies performed at time of diagnosis or prior to initiating treatment (HEM)
0.00 0.00 FUD XXX M
AMA: 2008,Mar,8-12

3200F Barium swallow test not ordered (GERD)
0.00 0.00 FUD XXX E

3210F Group A Strep Test Performed (PHAR)
0.00 0.00 FUD XXX M
AMA: 2008,Mar,8-12

3215F Patient has documented immunity to Hepatitis A (HEP-C)
0.00 0.00 FUD XXX E
AMA: 2008,Mar,8-12

3216F Patient has documented immunity to Hepatitis B (HEP-C)(IBD)
0.00 0.00 FUD XXX E
AMA: 2008,Mar,8-12

3218F RNA testing for Hepatitis C documented as performed within 6 months prior to initiation of antiviral treatment for Hepatitis C (HEP-C)
0.00 0.00 FUD XXX E
AMA: 2008,Mar,8-12

3220F Hepatitis C quantitative RNA testing documented as performed at 12 weeks from initiation of antiviral treatment (HEP-C)
0.00 0.00 FUD XXX E
AMA: 2008,Mar,8-12

3230F Documentation that hearing test was performed within 6 months prior to tympanostomy tube insertion (OME)
0.00 0.00 FUD XXX E
AMA: 2008,Mar,8-12

3250F Specimen site other than anatomic location of primary tumor (PATH)
0.00 0.00 FUD XXX M

3260F pT category (primary tumor), pN category (regional lymph nodes), and histologic grade documented in pathology report (PATH)
0.00 0.00 FUD XXX M
AMA: 2008,Mar,8-12

3265F Ribonucleic acid (RNA) testing for Hepatitis C viremia ordered or results documented (HEP C)
0.00 0.00 FUD XXX E
AMA: 2008,Mar,8-12

3266F Hepatitis C genotype testing documented as performed prior to initiation of antiviral treatment for Hepatitis C (HEP C)
0.00 0.00 FUD XXX E
AMA: 2008,Mar,8-12

3267F Pathology report includes pT category, pN category, Gleason score, and statement about margin status (PATH)
0.00 0.00 FUD XXX M

3268F Prostate-specific antigen (PSA), and primary tumor (T) stage, and Gleason score documented prior to initiation of treatment (PRCA)
0.00 0.00 FUD XXX E
AMA: 2008,Mar,8-12

3269F Bone scan performed prior to initiation of treatment or at any time since diagnosis of prostate cancer (PRCA)
0.00 0.00 FUD XXX M
AMA: 2008,Mar,8-12

3270F Bone scan not performed prior to initiation of treatment nor at any time since diagnosis of prostate cancer (PRCA)
0.00 0.00 FUD XXX M
AMA: 2008,Mar,8-12

3271F Low risk of recurrence, prostate cancer (PRCA)
0.00 0.00 FUD XXX E
AMA: 2008,Mar,8-12

3272F Intermediate risk of recurrence, prostate cancer (PRCA)
0.00 0.00 FUD XXX E
AMA: 2008,Mar,8-12

3273F High risk of recurrence, prostate cancer (PRCA)
0.00 0.00 FUD XXX E
AMA: 2008,Mar,8-12

3274F Prostate cancer risk of recurrence not determined or neither low, intermediate nor high (PRCA)
0.00 0.00 FUD XXX E
AMA: 2008,Mar,8-12

3278F Serum levels of calcium, phosphorus, intact Parathyroid Hormone (PTH) and lipid profile ordered (CKD)
0.00 0.00 FUD XXX E
AMA: 2008,Mar,8-12

3279F Hemoglobin level greater than or equal to 13 g/dL (CKD, ESRD)
0.00 0.00 FUD XXX E
AMA: 2008,Mar,8-12

3280F Hemoglobin level 11 g/dL to 12.9 g/dL (CKD, ESRD)
0.00 0.00 FUD XXX E
AMA: 2008,Mar,8-12

3281F Hemoglobin level less than 11 g/dL (CKD, ESRD)
0.00 0.00 FUD XXX E
AMA: 2008,Mar,8-12

3284F Intraocular pressure (IOP) reduced by a value of greater than or equal to 15% from the pre-intervention level (EC)
0.00 0.00 FUD XXX M
AMA: 2008,Mar,8-12

3285F Intraocular pressure (IOP) reduced by a value less than 15% from the pre-intervention level (EC)
0.00 0.00 FUD XXX M
AMA: 2008,Mar,8-12

3288F Falls risk assessment documented (GER)
0.00 0.00 FUD XXX M
AMA: 2008,Mar,8-12

3290F Patient is D (Rh) negative and unsensitized (Pre-Cr)
0.00 0.00 FUD XXX E
AMA: 2008,Mar,8-12

3291F Patient is D (Rh) positive or sensitized (Pre-Cr)
0.00 0.00 FUD XXX E
AMA: 2008,Mar,8-12

3292F HIV testing ordered or documented and reviewed during the first or second prenatal visit (Pre-Cr)
0.00 0.00 FUD XXX E

3293F ABO and Rh blood typing documented as performed (Pre-Cr)
0.00 0.00 FUD XXX E

3294F Group B Streptococcus (GBS) screening documented as performed during week 35-37 gestation (Pre-Cr)
0.00 0.00 FUD XXX E

3300F American Joint Committee on Cancer (AJCC) stage documented and reviewed (ONC)
0.00 0.00 FUD XXX M
AMA: 2008,Mar,8-12

3301F Cancer stage documented in medical record as metastatic and reviewed (ONC)
EXCLUDES *Cancer staging measures (3321F-3390F)*
0.00 0.00 FUD XXX M
AMA: 2008,Mar,8-12

3315F Estrogen receptor (ER) or progesterone receptor (PR) positive breast cancer (ONC)
0.00 0.00 FUD XXX E
AMA: 2008,Mar,8-12

3316F Estrogen receptor (ER) and progesterone receptor (PR) negative breast cancer (ONC)
0.00 0.00 FUD XXX E
AMA: 2008,Mar,8-12

3317F Pathology report confirming malignancy documented in the medical record and reviewed prior to the initiation of chemotherapy (ONC)
0.00 0.00 FUD XXX E
AMA: 2008,Mar,8-12

3318F Pathology report confirming malignancy documented in the medical record and reviewed prior to the initiation of radiation therapy (ONC)
0.00 0.00 FUD XXX E
AMA: 2008,Mar,8-12

3319F 1 of the following diagnostic imaging studies ordered: chest x-ray, CT, Ultrasound, MRI, PET, or nuclear medicine scans (ML)
0.00 0.00 FUD XXX M
AMA: 2008,Mar,8-12

3320F None of the following diagnostic imaging studies ordered: chest X-ray, CT, Ultrasound, MRI, PET, or nuclear medicine scans (ML)
0.00 0.00 FUD XXX M
AMA: 2008,Mar,8-12

3321F AJCC Cancer Stage 0 or IA Melanoma, documented (ML)
0.00 0.00 FUD XXX M

3322F Melanoma greater than AJCC Stage 0 or IA (ML)
0.00 0.00 FUD XXX M

3323F Clinical tumor, node and metastases (TNM) staging documented and reviewed prior to surgery (Lung/Esop Cx)
0.00 0.00 FUD XXX E

3324F MRI or CT scan ordered, reviewed or requested (EPI)
0.00 0.00 FUD XXX E

3325F Preoperative assessment of functional or medical indication(s) for surgery prior to the cataract surgery with intraocular lens placement (must be performed within 12 months prior to cataract surgery) (EC)
0.00 0.00 FUD XXX E
AMA: 2008,Mar,8-12

3328F Performance status documented and reviewed within 2 weeks prior to surgery (Lung/Esop Cx)
0.00 0.00 FUD XXX E

3330F Imaging study ordered (BkP)
0.00 0.00 FUD XXX E
AMA: 2008,Mar,8-12

3331F Imaging study not ordered (BkP)
0.00 0.00 FUD XXX E
AMA: 2008,Mar,8-12

3340F Mammogram assessment category of "incomplete: need additional imaging evaluation" documented (RAD)
0.00 0.00 FUD XXX M
AMA: 2008,Mar,8-12

3341F Mammogram assessment category of "negative," documented (RAD)
0.00 0.00 FUD XXX M
AMA: 2008,Mar,8-12

3342F Mammogram assessment category of "benign," documented (RAD)
0.00 0.00 FUD XXX M
AMA: 2008,Mar,8-12

3343F Mammogram assessment category of "probably benign," documented (RAD)
0.00 0.00 FUD XXX M
AMA: 2008,Mar,8-12

3344F Mammogram assessment category of "suspicious," documented (RAD)
0.00 0.00 FUD XXX M
AMA: 2008,Mar,8-12

3345F Mammogram assessment category of "highly suggestive of malignancy," documented (RAD)
0.00 0.00 FUD XXX M
AMA: 2008,Mar,8-12

3350F Mammogram assessment category of "known biopsy proven malignancy," documented (RAD)
0.00 0.00 FUD XXX M
AMA: 2008,Mar,8-12

3351F Negative screen for depressive symptoms as categorized by using a standardized depression screening/assessment tool (MDD)
0.00 0.00 FUD XXX E

3352F No significant depressive symptoms as categorized by using a standardized depression assessment tool (MDD)
0.00 0.00 FUD XXX E

3353F Mild to moderate depressive symptoms as categorized by using a standardized depression screening/assessment tool (MDD)
0.00 0.00 FUD XXX E

3354F Clinically significant depressive symptoms as categorized by using a standardized depression screening/assessment tool (MDD)
0.00 0.00 FUD XXX E

3370F AJCC Breast Cancer Stage 0 documented (ONC)
0.00 0.00 FUD XXX E

3372F AJCC Breast Cancer Stage I: T1mic, T1a or T1b (tumor size ≤ 1 cm) documented (ONC)
0.00 0.00 FUD XXX E

3374F AJCC Breast Cancer Stage I: T1c (tumor size > 1 cm to 2 cm) documented (ONC)
0.00 0.00 FUD XXX E

3376F AJCC Breast Cancer Stage II documented (ONC)
0.00 0.00 FUD XXX E

3378F AJCC Breast Cancer Stage III documented (ONC)
0.00 0.00 FUD XXX E

3380F AJCC Breast Cancer Stage IV documented (ONC)
0.00 0.00 FUD XXX E

3382F AJCC colon cancer, Stage 0 documented (ONC)
0.00 0.00 FUD XXX E

3384F AJCC colon cancer, Stage I documented (ONC)
0.00 0.00 FUD XXX E

3386F AJCC colon cancer, Stage II documented (ONC)
0.00 0.00 FUD XXX E

3388F AJCC colon cancer, Stage III documented (ONC)
0.00 0.00 FUD XXX E

3390F AJCC colon cancer, Stage IV documented (ONC)
0.00 0.00 FUD XXX E

3394F Quantitative HER2 immunohistochemistry (IHC) evaluation of breast cancer consistent with the scoring system defined in the ASCO/CAP guidelines (PATH)
0.00 0.00 FUD XXX M

3395F Quantitative non-HER2 immunohistochemistry (IHC) evaluation of breast cancer (eg, testing for estrogen or progesterone receptors [ER/PR]) performed (PATH)
0.00 0.00 FUD XXX M

3450F Dyspnea screened, no dyspnea or mild dyspnea (Pall Cr)
0.00 0.00 FUD XXX E

3451F Dyspnea screened, moderate or severe dyspnea (Pall Cr)
0.00 0.00 FUD XXX E

3452F Dyspnea not screened (Pall Cr)
0.00 0.00 FUD XXX E

3455F TB screening performed and results interpreted within six months prior to initiation of first-time biologic disease modifying anti-rheumatic drug therapy for RA (RA)
0.00 0.00 FUD XXX M

3470F Rheumatoid arthritis (RA) disease activity, low (RA)
0.00 0.00 FUD XXX M

3471F Rheumatoid arthritis (RA) disease activity, moderate (RA)
0.00 0.00 FUD XXX M

3472F Rheumatoid arthritis (RA) disease activity, high (RA)
0.00 0.00 FUD XXX M

3475F Disease prognosis for rheumatoid arthritis assessed, poor prognosis documented (RA)
0.00 0.00 FUD XXX M

3476F Disease prognosis for rheumatoid arthritis assessed, good prognosis documented (RA)
0.00 0.00 FUD XXX M

3490F History of AIDS-defining condition (HIV)
0.00 0.00 FUD XXX E

3491F HIV indeterminate (infants of undetermined HIV status born of HIV-infected mothers) (HIV)
0.00 0.00 FUD XXX E

3492F History of nadir CD4+ cell count <350 cells/mm3 (HIV)
0.00 0.00 FUD XXX E

3493F No history of nadir CD4+ cell count <350 cells/mm3 and no history of AIDS-defining condition (HIV)
0.00 0.00 FUD XXX E

3494F CD4+ cell count <200 cells/mm3 (HIV)
0.00 0.00 FUD XXX E

3495F CD4+ cell count 200 - 499 cells/mm3 (HIV)
0.00 0.00 FUD XXX E

3496F CD4+ cell count ≥ 500 cells/mm3 (HIV)
0.00 0.00 FUD XXX E

3497F CD4+ cell percentage <15% (HIV)
0.00 0.00 FUD XXX E

3498F CD4+ cell percentage ≥ 15% (HIV)
0.00 0.00 FUD XXX E

3500F CD4+ cell count or CD4+ cell percentage documented as performed (HIV)
0.00 0.00 FUD XXX E

3502F HIV RNA viral load below limits of quantification (HIV)
0.00 0.00 FUD XXX E

3503F HIV RNA viral load not below limits of quantification (HIV)
0.00 0.00 FUD XXX E

3510F Documentation that tuberculosis (TB) screening test performed and results interpreted (HIV) (IBD)
0.00 0.00 FUD XXX E

3511F Chlamydia and gonorrhea screenings documented as performed (HIV)
0.00 0.00 FUD XXX E

3512F Syphilis screening documented as performed (HIV)
0.00 0.00 FUD XXX E

3513F Hepatitis B screening documented as performed (HIV)
0.00 0.00 FUD XXX E

3514F Hepatitis C screening documented as performed (HIV)
0.00 0.00 FUD XXX E

3515F Patient has documented immunity to Hepatitis C (HIV)
0.00 0.00 FUD XXX E

3517F Hepatitis B Virus (HBV) status assessed and results interpreted within one year prior to receiving a first course of anti-TNF (tumor necrosis factor) therapy (IBD)
0.00 0.00 FUD XXX E

3520F Clostridium difficile testing performed (IBD)
0.00 0.00 FUD XXX E

3550F Low risk for thromboembolism (AFIB)
0.00 0.00 FUD XXX E

3551F Intermediate risk for thromboembolism (AFIB)
0.00 0.00 FUD XXX E

3552F High risk for thromboembolism (AFIB)
0.00 0.00 FUD XXX E

3555F Patient had International Normalized Ratio (INR) measurement performed (AFIB)
0.00 0.00 FUD XXX E
AMA: 2010,Jul,3-5

3570F Final report for bone scintigraphy study includes correlation with existing relevant imaging studies (eg, X-ray, MRI, CT) corresponding to the same anatomical region in question (NUC_MED)
0.00 0.00 FUD XXX M

3572F Patient considered to be potentially at risk for fracture in a weight-bearing site (NUC_MED)
0.00 0.00 FUD XXX E

3573F Patient not considered to be potentially at risk for fracture in a weight-bearing site (NUC_MED)
0.00 0.00 FUD XXX E

3650F Electroencephalogram (EEG) ordered, reviewed or requested (EPI)
0.00 0.00 FUD XXX E

3700F Psychiatric disorders or disturbances assessed (Prkns)
0.00 0.00 FUD XXX E

3720F Cognitive impairment or dysfunction assessed (Prkns)
0.00 0.00 FUD XXX M

3725F Screening for depression performed (DEM)
0.00 0.00 FUD XXX M

3750F Patient not receiving dose of corticosteroids greater than or equal to 10mg/day for 60 or greater consecutive days (IBD)
0.00 0.00 FUD XXX E

3751F Electrodiagnostic studies for distal symmetric polyneuropathy conducted (or requested), documented, and reviewed within 6 months of initial evaluation for condition (DSP)
0.00 0.00 FUD XXX E

3752F Electrodiagnostic studies for distal symmetric polyneuropathy not conducted (or requested), documented, or reviewed within 6 months of initial evaluation for condition (DSP)
0.00 0.00 FUD XXX E

3753F Patient has clear clinical symptoms and signs that are highly suggestive of neuropathy AND cannot be attributed to another condition, AND has an obvious cause for the neuropathy (DSP)
0.00 0.00 FUD XXX E

3754F Screening tests for diabetes mellitus reviewed, requested, or ordered (DSP)
0.00 0.00 FUD XXX E

3755F Cognitive and behavioral impairment screening performed (ALS)
0.00 0.00 FUD XXX E

3756F Patient has pseudobulbar affect, sialorrhea, or ALS-related symptoms (ALS)
0.00 0.00 FUD XXX E

3757F Patient does not have pseudobulbar affect, sialorrhea, or ALS-related symptoms (ALS)
0.00 0.00 FUD XXX E

3758F Patient referred for pulmonary function testing or peak cough expiratory flow (ALS)
0.00 0.00 FUD XXX E

3759F Patient screened for dysphagia, weight loss, and impaired nutrition, and results documented (ALS)
0.00 0.00 FUD XXX E

3760F Patient exhibits dysphagia, weight loss, or impaired nutrition (ALS)
0.00 0.00 FUD XXX E

3761F Patient does not exhibit dysphagia, weight loss, or impaired nutrition (ALS)
0.00 0.00 FUD XXX E

3762F Patient is dysarthric (ALS)
0.00 0.00 FUD XXX E

3763F Patient is not dysarthric (ALS)
0.00 0.00 FUD XXX E

3775F Adenoma(s) or other neoplasm detected during screening colonoscopy (SCADR)
0.00 0.00 FUD XXX E

3776F Adenoma(s) or other neoplasm not detected during screening colonoscopy (SCADR)
0.00 0.00 FUD XXX E

4000F-4563F Therapies Provided (Includes Preventive Services)

INCLUDES Behavioral/pharmacologic/procedural therapies
Preventive services including patient education/counseling

4000F Tobacco use cessation intervention, counseling (COPD, CAP, CAD, Asthma) (DM) (PV)
0.00 0.00 FUD XXX E
AMA: 2018,Jan,8; 2017,Jan,8; 2016,Jan,13; 2015,Jan,16; 2014,Jan,11

4001F Tobacco use cessation intervention, pharmacologic therapy (COPD, CAD, CAP, PV, Asthma) (DM) (PV)
0.00 0.00 FUD XXX E
AMA: 2008,Mar,8-12; 2004,Nov,1

4003F Patient education, written/oral, appropriate for patients with heart failure, performed (NMA-No Measure Associated)
0.00 0.00 FUD XXX E
AMA: 2004,Nov,1

4004F Patient screened for tobacco use and received tobacco cessation intervention (counseling, pharmacotherapy, or both), if identified as a tobacco user (PV, CAD)
0.00 0.00 FUD XXX M

4005F Pharmacologic therapy (other than minerals/vitamins) for osteoporosis prescribed (OP) (IBD)
0.00 0.00 FUD XXX E

4008F Beta-blocker therapy prescribed or currently being taken (CAD,HF)
0.00 0.00 FUD XXX M

4010F Angiotensin Converting Enzyme (ACE) Inhibitor or Angiotensin Receptor Blocker (ARB) therapy prescribed or currently being taken (CAD, CKD, HF) (DM)
0.00 0.00 FUD XXX M

4011F Oral antiplatelet therapy prescribed (CAD)
0.00 0.00 FUD XXX E
AMA: 2004,Nov,1

4012F Warfarin therapy prescribed (NMA-No Measure Associated)
0.00 0.00 FUD XXX E

4013F Statin therapy prescribed or currently being taken (CAD)
0.00 0.00 FUD XXX E

4014F Written discharge instructions provided to heart failure patients discharged home (Instructions include all of the following components: activity level, diet, discharge medications, follow-up appointment, weight monitoring, what to do if symptoms worsen) (NMA-No Measure Associated)
0.00 0.00 FUD XXX E

4015F Persistent asthma, preferred long term control medication or an acceptable alternative treatment, prescribed (NMA-No Measure Associated)
0.00 0.00 FUD XXX E
EXCLUDES *Use of code with modifier 1P*
Code also modifier 2P for patient reasons for not prescribing

4016F Anti-inflammatory/analgesic agent prescribed (OA) (Use for prescribed or continued medication[s], including over-the-counter medication[s])
0.00 0.00 FUD XXX E
INCLUDES Over-the-counter medication(s)
Prescribed/continued medication(s)

4017F Gastrointestinal prophylaxis for NSAID use prescribed (OA)
0.00 0.00 FUD XXX E

4018F Therapeutic exercise for the involved joint(s) instructed or physical or occupational therapy prescribed (OA)
0.00 0.00 FUD XXX E

4019F Documentation of receipt of counseling on exercise and either both calcium and vitamin D use or counseling regarding both calcium and vitamin D use (OP)
0.00 0.00 FUD XXX E

4025F Inhaled bronchodilator prescribed (COPD)
0.00 0.00 FUD XXX E

4030F Long-term oxygen therapy prescribed (more than 15 hours per day) (COPD)
0.00 0.00 FUD XXX E

4033F Pulmonary rehabilitation exercise training recommended (COPD)
0.00 0.00 FUD XXX E
Code also dyspnea assessed, present (1019F)

4035F Influenza immunization recommended (COPD) (IBD)
0.00 0.00 FUD XXX E
AMA: 2008,Mar,8-12

4037F Influenza immunization ordered or administered (COPD, PV, CKD, ESRD)(IBD)
0.00 0.00 FUD XXX E
AMA: 2008,Mar,8-12

4040F Pneumococcal vaccine administered or previously received (COPD) (PV), (IBD)
0.00 0.00 FUD XXX M
AMA: 2008,Mar,8-12

4041F Documentation of order for cefazolin OR cefuroxime for antimicrobial prophylaxis (PERI 2)
0.00 0.00 FUD XXX E

4042F Documentation that prophylactic antibiotics were neither given within 4 hours prior to surgical incision nor given intraoperatively (PERI 2)
0.00 0.00 FUD XXX E

4043F Documentation that an order was given to discontinue prophylactic antibiotics within 48 hours of surgical end time, cardiac procedures (PERI 2)
0.00 0.00 FUD XXX E

4044F Documentation that an order was given for venous thromboembolism (VTE) prophylaxis to be given within 24 hours prior to incision time or 24 hours after surgery end time (PERI 2)
0.00 0.00 FUD XXX M

4045F Appropriate empiric antibiotic prescribed (CAP), (EM)
0.00 0.00 FUD XXX E

4046F Documentation that prophylactic antibiotics were given within 4 hours prior to surgical incision or given intraoperatively (PERI 2)
0.00 0.00 FUD XXX E

4047F Documentation of order for prophylactic parenteral antibiotics to be given within 1 hour (if fluoroquinolone or vancomycin, 2 hours) prior to surgical incision (or start of procedure when no incision is required) (PERI 2)
0.00 0.00 FUD XXX E

4048F Documentation that administration of prophylactic parenteral antibiotic was initiated within 1 hour (if fluoroquinolone or vancomycin, 2 hours) prior to surgical incision (or start of procedure when no incision is required) as ordered (PERI 2)
0.00 0.00 FUD XXX E

4049F Documentation that order was given to discontinue prophylactic antibiotics within 24 hours of surgical end time, non-cardiac procedure (PERI 2)
0.00 0.00 FUD XXX E

4050F Hypertension plan of care documented as appropriate (NMA-No Measure Associated)
0.00 0.00 FUD XXX E

4051F Referred for an arteriovenous (AV) fistula (ESRD, CKD)
0.00 0.00 FUD XXX E
AMA: 2008,Mar,8-12

4052F Hemodialysis via functioning arteriovenous (AV) fistula (ESRD)
0.00 0.00 FUD XXX E
AMA: 2008,Mar,8-12

4053F Hemodialysis via functioning arteriovenous (AV) graft (ESRD)
0.00 0.00 FUD XXX E
AMA: 2008,Mar,8-12

4054F Hemodialysis via catheter (ESRD)
0.00 0.00 FUD XXX E
AMA: 2008,Mar,8-12

4055F Patient receiving peritoneal dialysis (ESRD)
0.00 0.00 FUD XXX E
AMA: 2008,Mar,8-12

4056F Appropriate oral rehydration solution recommended (PAG)
0.00 0.00 FUD XXX E

4058F Pediatric gastroenteritis education provided to caregiver (PAG)
0.00 0.00 FUD XXX E

4060F Psychotherapy services provided (MDD, MDD ADOL)
0.00 0.00 FUD XXX E

4062F Patient referral for psychotherapy documented (MDD, MDD ADOL)
0.00 0.00 FUD XXX E

4063F Antidepressant pharmacotherapy considered and not prescribed (MDD ADOL)
0.00 0.00 FUD XXX E

4064F Antidepressant pharmacotherapy prescribed (MDD, MDD ADOL)
0.00 0.00 FUD XXX E

4065F Antipsychotic pharmacotherapy prescribed (MDD)
0.00 0.00 FUD XXX E

4066F Electroconvulsive therapy (ECT) provided (MDD)
0.00 0.00 FUD XXX E

4067F Patient referral for electroconvulsive therapy (ECT) documented (MDD)
0.00 0.00 FUD XXX E

4069F Venous thromboembolism (VTE) prophylaxis received (IBD)
0.00 0.00 FUD XXX E

4070F Deep vein thrombosis (DVT) prophylaxis received by end of hospital day 2 (STR)
0.00 0.00 FUD XXX E

4073F Oral antiplatelet therapy prescribed at discharge (STR)
0.00 0.00 FUD XXX E

4075F Anticoagulant therapy prescribed at discharge (STR)
0.00 0.00 FUD XXX E

4077F Documentation that tissue plasminogen activator (t-PA) administration was considered (STR)
0.00 0.00 FUD XXX E

4079F Documentation that rehabilitation services were considered (STR)
0.00 0.00 FUD XXX E

4084F Aspirin received within 24 hours before emergency department arrival or during emergency department stay (EM)
0.00 0.00 FUD XXX E

4086F Aspirin or clopidogrel prescribed or currently being taken (CAD)
0.00 0.00 FUD XXX M

4090F Patient receiving erythropoietin therapy (HEM)
0.00 0.00 FUD XXX M
AMA: 2008,Mar,8-12

4095F Patient not receiving erythropoietin therapy (HEM)
0.00 0.00 FUD XXX E
AMA: 2008,Mar,8-12

4100F Bisphosphonate therapy, intravenous, ordered or received (HEM)
0.00 0.00 FUD XXX M
AMA: 2008,Mar,8-12

4110F Internal mammary artery graft performed for primary, isolated coronary artery bypass graft procedure (CABG)
0.00 0.00 FUD XXX M

4115F Beta blocker administered within 24 hours prior to surgical incision (CABG)
0.00 0.00 FUD XXX M

4120F Antibiotic prescribed or dispensed (URI, PHAR), (A-BRONCH)
0.00 0.00 FUD XXX M
AMA: 2008,Mar,8-12

4124F Antibiotic neither prescribed nor dispensed (URI, PHAR), (A-BRONCH)
0.00 0.00 FUD XXX M
AMA: 2008,Mar,8-12

4130F Topical preparations (including OTC) prescribed for acute otitis externa (AOE)
0.00 0.00 FUD XXX M
AMA: 2010,Jan,6-7; 2008,Mar,8-12

4131F Systemic antimicrobial therapy prescribed (AOE)
0.00 0.00 FUD XXX M
AMA: 2008,Mar,8-12

4132F Systemic antimicrobial therapy not prescribed (AOE)
0.00 0.00 FUD XXX M
AMA: 2008,Mar,8-12

4133F Antihistamines or decongestants prescribed or recommended (OME)
0.00 0.00 FUD XXX E
AMA: 2008,Mar,8-12

4134F Antihistamines or decongestants neither prescribed nor recommended (OME)
0.00 0.00 FUD XXX E
AMA: 2008,Mar,8-12

4135F Systemic corticosteroids prescribed (OME)
0.00 0.00 FUD XXX E
AMA: 2008,Mar,8-12

4136F Systemic corticosteroids not prescribed (OME)
0.00 0.00 FUD XXX E
AMA: 2008,Mar,8-12

4140F Inhaled corticosteroids prescribed (Asthma)
0.00 0.00 FUD XXX E

4142F Corticosteroid sparing therapy prescribed (IBD)
0.00 0.00 FUD XXX E

4144F Alternative long-term control medication prescribed (Asthma)
0.00 0.00 FUD XXX E

4145F Two or more anti-hypertensive agents prescribed or currently being taken (CAD, HTN)
0.00 0.00 FUD XXX E

4148F Hepatitis A vaccine injection administered or previously received (HEP-C)
0.00 0.00 FUD XXX E

4149F Hepatitis B vaccine injection administered or previously received (HEP-C, HIV) (IBD)
0.00 0.00 FUD XXX E

4150F Patient receiving antiviral treatment for Hepatitis C (HEP-C)
0.00 0.00 FUD XXX E
AMA: 2008,Mar,8-12

4151F Patient did not start or is not receiving antiviral treatment for Hepatitis C during the measurement period (HEP-C)
0.00 0.00 FUD XXX E
AMA: 2008,Mar,8-12

4153F Combination peginterferon and ribavirin therapy prescribed (HEP-C)
0.00 0.00 FUD XXX E
AMA: 2008,Mar,8-12

4155F Hepatitis A vaccine series previously received (HEP-C)
0.00 0.00 FUD XXX E
AMA: 2008,Mar,8-12

4157F Hepatitis B vaccine series previously received (HEP-C)
0.00 0.00 FUD XXX E
AMA: 2008,Mar,8-12

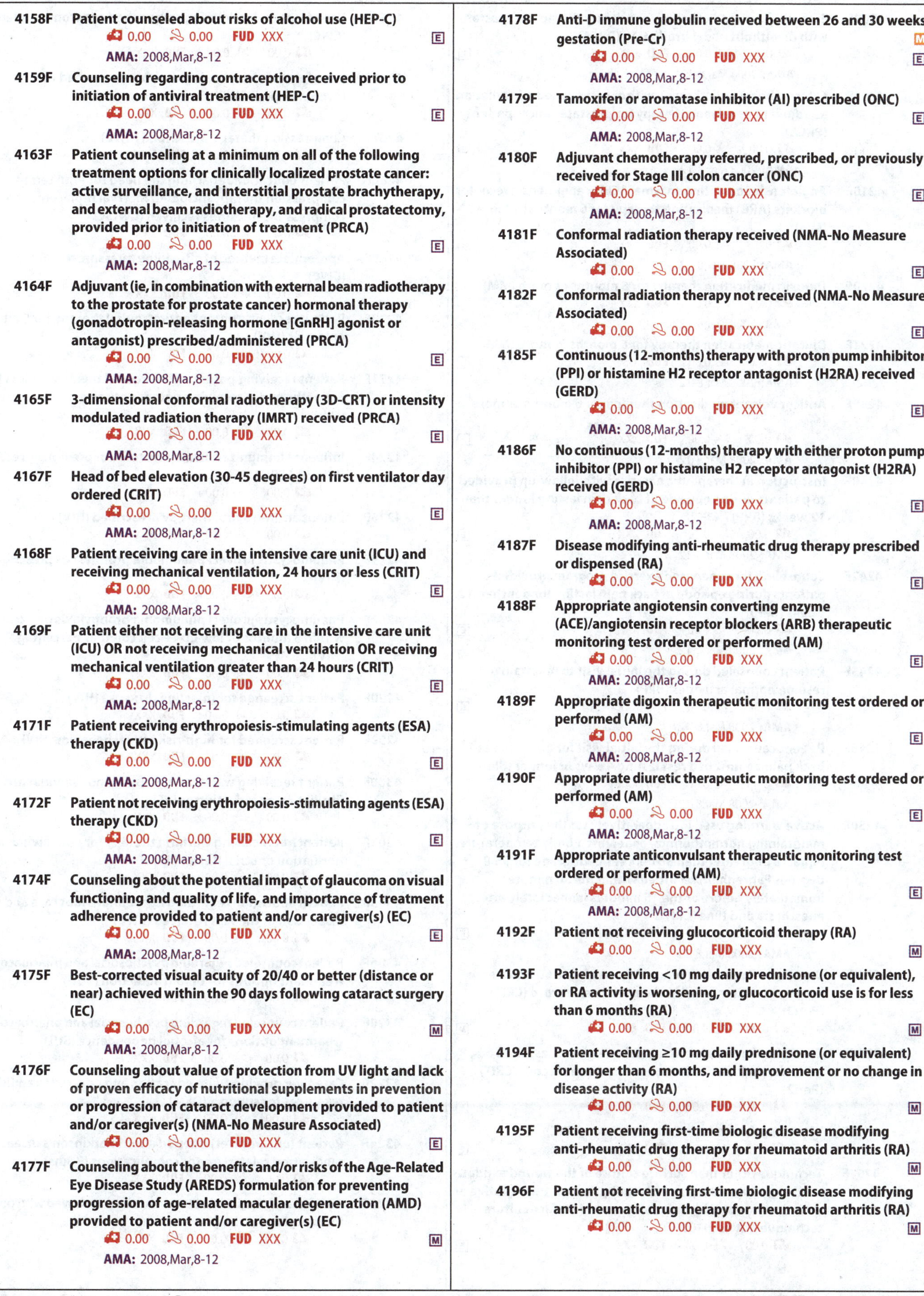

4158F Patient counseled about risks of alcohol use (HEP-C)
0.00 0.00 FUD XXX E
AMA: 2008,Mar,8-12

4159F Counseling regarding contraception received prior to initiation of antiviral treatment (HEP-C)
0.00 0.00 FUD XXX E
AMA: 2008,Mar,8-12

4163F Patient counseling at a minimum on all of the following treatment options for clinically localized prostate cancer: active surveillance, and interstitial prostate brachytherapy, and external beam radiotherapy, and radical prostatectomy, provided prior to initiation of treatment (PRCA)
0.00 0.00 FUD XXX E
AMA: 2008,Mar,8-12

4164F Adjuvant (ie, in combination with external beam radiotherapy to the prostate for prostate cancer) hormonal therapy (gonadotropin-releasing hormone [GnRH] agonist or antagonist) prescribed/administered (PRCA)
0.00 0.00 FUD XXX E
AMA: 2008,Mar,8-12

4165F 3-dimensional conformal radiotherapy (3D-CRT) or intensity modulated radiation therapy (IMRT) received (PRCA)
0.00 0.00 FUD XXX E
AMA: 2008,Mar,8-12

4167F Head of bed elevation (30-45 degrees) on first ventilator day ordered (CRIT)
0.00 0.00 FUD XXX E
AMA: 2008,Mar,8-12

4168F Patient receiving care in the intensive care unit (ICU) and receiving mechanical ventilation, 24 hours or less (CRIT)
0.00 0.00 FUD XXX E
AMA: 2008,Mar,8-12

4169F Patient either not receiving care in the intensive care unit (ICU) OR not receiving mechanical ventilation OR receiving mechanical ventilation greater than 24 hours (CRIT)
0.00 0.00 FUD XXX E
AMA: 2008,Mar,8-12

4171F Patient receiving erythropoiesis-stimulating agents (ESA) therapy (CKD)
0.00 0.00 FUD XXX E
AMA: 2008,Mar,8-12

4172F Patient not receiving erythropoiesis-stimulating agents (ESA) therapy (CKD)
0.00 0.00 FUD XXX E
AMA: 2008,Mar,8-12

4174F Counseling about the potential impact of glaucoma on visual functioning and quality of life, and importance of treatment adherence provided to patient and/or caregiver(s) (EC)
0.00 0.00 FUD XXX E
AMA: 2008,Mar,8-12

4175F Best-corrected visual acuity of 20/40 or better (distance or near) achieved within the 90 days following cataract surgery (EC)
0.00 0.00 FUD XXX M
AMA: 2008,Mar,8-12

4176F Counseling about value of protection from UV light and lack of proven efficacy of nutritional supplements in prevention or progression of cataract development provided to patient and/or caregiver(s) (NMA-No Measure Associated)
0.00 0.00 FUD XXX E

4177F Counseling about the benefits and/or risks of the Age-Related Eye Disease Study (AREDS) formulation for preventing progression of age-related macular degeneration (AMD) provided to patient and/or caregiver(s) (EC)
0.00 0.00 FUD XXX M
AMA: 2008,Mar,8-12

4178F Anti-D immune globulin received between 26 and 30 weeks gestation (Pre-Cr) M
0.00 0.00 FUD XXX E
AMA: 2008,Mar,8-12

4179F Tamoxifen or aromatase inhibitor (AI) prescribed (ONC)
0.00 0.00 FUD XXX E
AMA: 2008,Mar,8-12

4180F Adjuvant chemotherapy referred, prescribed, or previously received for Stage III colon cancer (ONC)
0.00 0.00 FUD XXX E
AMA: 2008,Mar,8-12

4181F Conformal radiation therapy received (NMA-No Measure Associated)
0.00 0.00 FUD XXX E

4182F Conformal radiation therapy not received (NMA-No Measure Associated)
0.00 0.00 FUD XXX E

4185F Continuous (12-months) therapy with proton pump inhibitor (PPI) or histamine H2 receptor antagonist (H2RA) received (GERD)
0.00 0.00 FUD XXX E
AMA: 2008,Mar,8-12

4186F No continuous (12-months) therapy with either proton pump inhibitor (PPI) or histamine H2 receptor antagonist (H2RA) received (GERD)
0.00 0.00 FUD XXX E
AMA: 2008,Mar,8-12

4187F Disease modifying anti-rheumatic drug therapy prescribed or dispensed (RA)
0.00 0.00 FUD XXX E

4188F Appropriate angiotensin converting enzyme (ACE)/angiotensin receptor blockers (ARB) therapeutic monitoring test ordered or performed (AM)
0.00 0.00 FUD XXX E
AMA: 2008,Mar,8-12

4189F Appropriate digoxin therapeutic monitoring test ordered or performed (AM)
0.00 0.00 FUD XXX E
AMA: 2008,Mar,8-12

4190F Appropriate diuretic therapeutic monitoring test ordered or performed (AM)
0.00 0.00 FUD XXX E
AMA: 2008,Mar,8-12

4191F Appropriate anticonvulsant therapeutic monitoring test ordered or performed (AM)
0.00 0.00 FUD XXX E
AMA: 2008,Mar,8-12

4192F Patient not receiving glucocorticoid therapy (RA)
0.00 0.00 FUD XXX M

4193F Patient receiving <10 mg daily prednisone (or equivalent), or RA activity is worsening, or glucocorticoid use is for less than 6 months (RA)
0.00 0.00 FUD XXX M

4194F Patient receiving ≥10 mg daily prednisone (or equivalent) for longer than 6 months, and improvement or no change in disease activity (RA)
0.00 0.00 FUD XXX M

4195F Patient receiving first-time biologic disease modifying anti-rheumatic drug therapy for rheumatoid arthritis (RA)
0.00 0.00 FUD XXX M

4196F Patient not receiving first-time biologic disease modifying anti-rheumatic drug therapy for rheumatoid arthritis (RA)
0.00 0.00 FUD XXX M

Category II Codes

4158F — 4196F

● New Code ▲ Revised Code ○ Reinstated ● New Web Release ▲ Revised Web Release + Add-on Unlisted Not Covered # Resequenced
⑤⓪ Optum Mod 50 Exempt ⃠ AMA Mod 51 Exempt ⑤① Optum Mod 51 Exempt ⑥③ Mod 63 Exempt Non-FDA Drug ★ Telemedicine M Maternity A Age Edit

4200F External beam radiotherapy as primary therapy to prostate with or without nodal irradiation (PRCA)
0.00 0.00 FUD XXX E
AMA: 2008,Mar,8-12

4201F External beam radiotherapy with or without nodal irradiation as adjuvant or salvage therapy for prostate cancer patient (PRCA)
0.00 0.00 FUD XXX E
AMA: 2008,Mar,8-12

4210F Angiotensin converting enzyme (ACE) or angiotensin receptor blockers (ARB) medication therapy for 6 months or more (MM)
0.00 0.00 FUD XXX E
AMA: 2008,Mar,8-12

4220F Digoxin medication therapy for 6 months or more (MM)
0.00 0.00 FUD XXX E
AMA: 2008,Mar,8-12

4221F Diuretic medication therapy for 6 months or more (MM)
0.00 0.00 FUD XXX E
AMA: 2008,Mar,8-12

4230F Anticonvulsant medication therapy for 6 months or more (MM)
0.00 0.00 FUD XXX E
AMA: 2008,Mar,8-12

4240F Instruction in therapeutic exercise with follow-up provided to patients during episode of back pain lasting longer than 12 weeks (BkP)
0.00 0.00 FUD XXX E
AMA: 2008,Mar,8-12

4242F Counseling for supervised exercise program provided to patients during episode of back pain lasting longer than 12 weeks (BkP)
0.00 0.00 FUD XXX E
AMA: 2008,Mar,8-12

4245F Patient counseled during the initial visit to maintain or resume normal activities (BkP)
0.00 0.00 FUD XXX E
AMA: 2008,Mar,8-12

4248F Patient counseled during the initial visit for an episode of back pain against bed rest lasting 4 days or longer (BkP)
0.00 0.00 FUD XXX E
AMA: 2008,Mar,8-12

4250F Active warming used intraoperatively for the purpose of maintaining normothermia, or at least 1 body temperature equal to or greater than 36 degrees Centigrade (or 96.8 degrees Fahrenheit) recorded within the 30 minutes immediately before or the 15 minutes immediately after anesthesia end time (CRIT)
0.00 0.00 FUD XXX E
AMA: 2008,Mar,8-12

4255F Duration of general or neuraxial anesthesia 60 minutes or longer, as documented in the anesthesia record (CRIT) (Peri2)
0.00 0.00 FUD XXX M

4256F Duration of general or neuraxial anesthesia less than 60 minutes, as documented in the anesthesia record (CRIT) (Peri2)
0.00 0.00 FUD XXX E

4260F Wound surface culture technique used (CWC)
0.00 0.00 FUD XXX E

4261F Technique other than surface culture of the wound exudate used (eg, Levine/deep swab technique, semi-quantitative or quantitative swab technique) or wound surface culture technique not used (CWC)
0.00 0.00 FUD XXX E

4265F Use of wet to dry dressings prescribed or recommended (CWC)
0.00 0.00 FUD XXX E

4266F Use of wet to dry dressings neither prescribed nor recommended (CWC)
0.00 0.00 FUD XXX E

4267F Compression therapy prescribed (CWC)
0.00 0.00 FUD XXX E

4268F Patient education regarding the need for long term compression therapy including interval replacement of compression stockings received (CWC)
0.00 0.00 FUD XXX E

4269F Appropriate method of offloading (pressure relief) prescribed (CWC)
0.00 0.00 FUD XXX E

4270F Patient receiving potent antiretroviral therapy for 6 months or longer (HIV)
0.00 0.00 FUD XXX E

4271F Patient receiving potent antiretroviral therapy for less than 6 months or not receiving potent antiretroviral therapy (HIV)
0.00 0.00 FUD XXX E

4274F Influenza immunization administered or previously received (HIV) (P-ESRD)
0.00 0.00 FUD XXX E

4276F Potent antiretroviral therapy prescribed (HIV)
0.00 0.00 FUD XXX E

4279F Pneumocystis jiroveci pneumonia prophylaxis prescribed (HIV)
0.00 0.00 FUD XXX E

4280F Pneumocystis jiroveci pneumonia prophylaxis prescribed within 3 months of low CD4+ cell count or percentage (HIV)
0.00 0.00 FUD XXX E

4290F Patient screened for injection drug use (HIV)
0.00 0.00 FUD XXX E

4293F Patient screened for high-risk sexual behavior (HIV)
0.00 0.00 FUD XXX E

4300F Patient receiving warfarin therapy for nonvalvular atrial fibrillation or atrial flutter (AFIB)
0.00 0.00 FUD XXX E

4301F Patient not receiving warfarin therapy for nonvalvular atrial fibrillation or atrial flutter (AFIB)
0.00 0.00 FUD XXX E

4305F Patient education regarding appropriate foot care and daily inspection of the feet received (CWC)
0.00 0.00 FUD XXX E

4306F Patient counseled regarding psychosocial and pharmacologic treatment options for opioid addiction (SUD)
0.00 0.00 FUD XXX E

4320F Patient counseled regarding psychosocial and pharmacologic treatment options for alcohol dependence (SUD)
0.00 0.00 FUD XXX E

4322F Caregiver provided with education and referred to additional resources for support (DEM)
0.00 0.00 FUD XXX M

4324F Patient (or caregiver) queried about Parkinson's disease medication related motor complications (Prkns)
0.00 0.00 FUD XXX E

4325F Medical and surgical treatment options reviewed with patient (or caregiver) (Prkns)
0.00 0.00 FUD XXX M

4326F Patient (or caregiver) queried about symptoms of autonomic dysfunction (Prkns)
0.00 0.00 FUD XXX E

4328F Patient (or caregiver) queried about sleep disturbances (Prkns)
0.00 0.00 FUD XXX E

4330F Counseling about epilepsy specific safety issues provided to patient (or caregiver(s)) (EPI)
0.00 0.00 FUD XXX E

4340F Counseling for women of childbearing potential with epilepsy (EPI)
0.00 0.00 FUD XXX M

4350F Counseling provided on symptom management, end of life decisions, and palliation (DEM)
0.00 0.00 FUD XXX E

4400F Rehabilitative therapy options discussed with patient (or caregiver) (Prkns)
0.00 0.00 FUD XXX M

4450F Self-care education provided to patient (HF)
0.00 0.00 FUD XXX E

4470F Implantable cardioverter-defibrillator (ICD) counseling provided (HF)
0.00 0.00 FUD XXX E

4480F Patient receiving ACE inhibitor/ARB therapy and beta-blocker therapy for 3 months or longer (HF)
0.00 0.00 FUD XXX E

4481F Patient receiving ACE inhibitor/ARB therapy and beta-blocker therapy for less than 3 months or patient not receiving ACE inhibitor/ARB therapy and beta-blocker therapy (HF)
0.00 0.00 FUD XXX E

4500F Referred to an outpatient cardiac rehabilitation program (CAD)
0.00 0.00 FUD XXX M

4510F Previous cardiac rehabilitation for qualifying cardiac event completed (CAD)
0.00 0.00 FUD XXX M

4525F Neuropsychiatric intervention ordered (DEM)
0.00 0.00 FUD XXX E

4526F Neuropsychiatric intervention received (DEM)
0.00 0.00 FUD XXX E

4540F Disease modifying pharmacotherapy discussed (ALS)
0.00 0.00 FUD XXX E

4541F Patient offered treatment for pseudobulbar affect, sialorrhea, or ALS-related symptoms (ALS)
0.00 0.00 FUD XXX E

4550F Options for noninvasive respiratory support discussed with patient (ALS)
0.00 0.00 FUD XXX E

4551F Nutritional support offered (ALS)
0.00 0.00 FUD XXX E

4552F Patient offered referral to a speech language pathologist (ALS)
0.00 0.00 FUD XXX E

4553F Patient offered assistance in planning for end of life issues (ALS)
0.00 0.00 FUD XXX E

4554F Patient received inhalational anesthetic agent (Peri2)
0.00 0.00 FUD XXX M

4555F Patient did not receive inhalational anesthetic agent (Peri2)
0.00 0.00 FUD XXX E

4556F Patient exhibits 3 or more risk factors for post-operative nausea and vomiting (Peri2)
0.00 0.00 FUD XXX M

4557F Patient does not exhibit 3 or more risk factors for post-operative nausea and vomiting (Peri2)
0.00 0.00 FUD XXX E

4558F Patient received at least 2 prophylactic pharmacologic anti-emetic agents of different classes preoperatively and intraoperatively (Peri2)
0.00 0.00 FUD XXX E

4559F At least 1 body temperature measurement equal to or greater than 35.5 degrees Celsius (or 95.9 degrees Fahrenheit) recorded within the 30 minutes immediately before or the 15 minutes immediately after anesthesia end time (Peri2)
0.00 0.00 FUD XXX E

4560F Anesthesia technique did not involve general or neuraxial anesthesia (Peri2)
0.00 0.00 FUD XXX E

4561F Patient has a coronary artery stent (Peri2)
0.00 0.00 FUD XXX E

4562F Patient does not have a coronary artery stent (Peri2)
0.00 0.00 FUD XXX E

4563F Patient received aspirin within 24 hours prior to anesthesia start time (Peri2)
0.00 0.00 FUD XXX E

5005F-5250F Results Conveyed and Documented

INCLUDES Patient's:
- Functional status
- Morbidity/mortality
- Satisfaction/experience with care

Review/communication of test results to patients

5005F Patient counseled on self-examination for new or changing moles (ML)
0.00 0.00 FUD XXX E
AMA: 2008,Mar,8-12

5010F Findings of dilated macular or fundus exam communicated to the physician or other qualified health care professional managing the diabetes care (EC)
0.00 0.00 FUD XXX M

5015F Documentation of communication that a fracture occurred and that the patient was or should be tested or treated for osteoporosis (OP)
0.00 0.00 FUD XXX M

5020F Treatment summary report communicated to physician(s) or other qualified health care professional(s) managing continuing care and to the patient within 1 month of completing treatment (ONC)
0.00 0.00 FUD XXX E
AMA: 2008,Mar,8-12

5050F Treatment plan communicated to provider(s) managing continuing care within 1 month of diagnosis (ML)
0.00 0.00 FUD XXX M
AMA: 2008,Mar,8-12

5060F Findings from diagnostic mammogram communicated to practice managing patient's on-going care within 3 business days of exam interpretation (RAD)
0.00 0.00 FUD XXX E
AMA: 2008,Mar,8-12

5062F Findings from diagnostic mammogram communicated to the patient within 5 days of exam interpretation (RAD)
0.00 0.00 FUD XXX E
AMA: 2008,Mar,8-12

5100F Potential risk for fracture communicated to the referring physician or other qualified health care professional within 24 hours of completion of the imaging study (NUC_MED)
0.00 0.00 FUD XXX E

5200F Consideration of referral for a neurological evaluation of appropriateness for surgical therapy for intractable epilepsy within the past 3 years (EPI)
0.00 0.00 FUD XXX E

5250F Asthma discharge plan provided to patient (Asthma)
0.00 0.00 FUD XXX E

6005F-6150F Elements Related to Patient Safety Processes

INCLUDES Patient safety practices

6005F Rationale (eg, severity of illness and safety) for level of care (eg, home, hospital) documented (CAP)
0.00 0.00 FUD XXX E
AMA: 2018,Jan,8; 2017,Jan,8; 2016,Jan,13; 2015,Jan,16; 2014,Jan,11

6010F Dysphagia screening conducted prior to order for or receipt of any foods, fluids, or medication by mouth (STR)
0.00 0.00 FUD XXX E

6015F Patient receiving or eligible to receive foods, fluids, or medication by mouth (STR)
0.00 0.00 FUD XXX E

6020F NPO (nothing by mouth) ordered (STR)
0.00 0.00 FUD XXX E

6030F All elements of maximal sterile barrier technique, hand hygiene, skin preparation and, if ultrasound is used, sterile ultrasound techniques followed (CRIT)
0.00 0.00 FUD XXX M
AMA: 2008,Mar,8-12

6040F Use of appropriate radiation dose reduction devices OR manual techniques for appropriate moderation of exposure, documented (RAD)
0.00 0.00 FUD XXX E

6045F Radiation exposure or exposure time in final report for procedure using fluoroscopy, documented (RAD)
0.00 0.00 FUD XXX E
AMA: 2008,Mar,8-12

6070F Patient queried and counseled about anti-epileptic drug (AED) side effects (EPI)
0.00 0.00 FUD XXX E

6080F Patient (or caregiver) queried about falls (Prkns, DSP)
0.00 0.00 FUD XXX E

6090F Patient (or caregiver) counseled about safety issues appropriate to patient's stage of disease (Prkns)
0.00 0.00 FUD XXX E

6100F Timeout to verify correct patient, correct site, and correct procedure, documented (PATH)
0.00 0.00 FUD XXX E

6101F Safety counseling for dementia provided (DEM)
0.00 0.00 FUD XXX E

6102F Safety counseling for dementia ordered (DEM)
0.00 0.00 FUD XXX E

6110F Counseling provided regarding risks of driving and the alternatives to driving (DEM)
0.00 0.00 FUD XXX E

6150F Patient not receiving a first course of anti-TNF (tumor necrosis factor) therapy (IBD)
0.00 0.00 FUD XXX E

7010F-7025F Recall/Reminder System in Place

INCLUDES Capabilities of the provider
Measures that address the setting or system of care provided

7010F Patient information entered into a recall system that includes: target date for the next exam specified and a process to follow up with patients regarding missed or unscheduled appointments (ML)
0.00 0.00 FUD XXX M
AMA: 2008,Mar,8-12

7020F Mammogram assessment category (eg, Mammography Quality Standards Act [MQSA], Breast Imaging Reporting and Data System [BI-RADS], or FDA approved equivalent categories) entered into an internal database to allow for analysis of abnormal interpretation (recall) rate (RAD)
0.00 0.00 FUD XXX E
AMA: 2008,Mar,8-12

7025F Patient information entered into a reminder system with a target due date for the next mammogram (RAD)
0.00 0.00 FUD XXX M
AMA: 2008,Mar,8-12

9001F-9007F No Measure Associated

INCLUDES Aspects of care not associated with measures at the current time

9001F Aortic aneurysm less than 5.0 cm maximum diameter on centerline formatted CT or minor diameter on axial formatted CT (NMA-No Measure Associated)
0.00 0.00 FUD XXX E

9002F Aortic aneurysm 5.0 - 5.4 cm maximum diameter on centerline formatted CT or minor diameter on axial formatted CT (NMA-No Measure Associated)
0.00 0.00 FUD XXX E

9003F Aortic aneurysm 5.5 - 5.9 cm maximum diameter on centerline formatted CT or minor diameter on axial formatted CT (NMA-No Measure Associated)
0.00 0.00 FUD XXX M

9004F Aortic aneurysm 6.0 cm or greater maximum diameter on centerline formatted CT or minor diameter on axial formatted CT (NMA-No Measure Associated)
0.00 0.00 FUD XXX M

9005F Asymptomatic carotid stenosis: No history of any transient ischemic attack or stroke in any carotid or vertebrobasilar territory (NMA-No Measure Associated)
0.00 0.00 FUD XXX E

9006F Symptomatic carotid stenosis: Ipsilateral carotid territory TIA or stroke less than 120 days prior to procedure (NMA-No Measure Associated)
0.00 0.00 FUD XXX M

9007F Other carotid stenosis: Ipsilateral TIA or stroke 120 days or greater prior to procedure or any prior contralateral carotid territory or vertebrobasilar TIA or stroke (NMA-No Measure Associated)
0.00 0.00 FUD XXX M

0042T

0042T Cerebral perfusion analysis using computed tomography with contrast administration, including post-processing of parametric maps with determination of cerebral blood flow, cerebral blood volume, and mean transit time

0.00 0.00 FUD XXX N 80

AMA: 2003,Nov,5

0054T-0055T

\+ **0054T Computer-assisted musculoskeletal surgical navigational orthopedic procedure, with image-guidance based on fluoroscopic images (List separately in addition to code for primary procedure)**

Code first primary procedure

0.00 0.00 FUD XXX N 80

AMA: 2018,Jan,8; 2017,Jan,8; 2016,Jan,13; 2015,Jan,16; 2014,Jan,11

\+ **0055T Computer-assisted musculoskeletal surgical navigational orthopedic procedure, with image-guidance based on CT/MRI images (List separately in addition to code for primary procedure)**

INCLUDES Performance of both CT and MRI in same session (1 unit)

Code first primary procedure

0.00 0.00 FUD XXX N 80

AMA: 2018,Jan,8; 2017,Jan,8; 2016,Jan,13; 2015,Jan,16; 2014,Jan,11

0058T

EXCLUDES *Cryopreservation of:*
- *Embryos (89258)*
- *Oocyte(s), immature (89398)*
- *Oocyte(s), mature (89337)*
- *Sperm (89259)*
- *Testicular reproductive tissue (89335)*

0058T Cryopreservation; reproductive tissue, ovarian

0.00 0.00 FUD XXX Q1 80

AMA: 2004,Apr,1; 2004,Jun,7

0071T-0072T

EXCLUDES *Insertion bladder catheter (51702)*
MRI guidance for parenchymal tissue ablation (77022)

0071T Focused ultrasound ablation of uterine leiomyomata, including MR guidance; total leiomyomata volume less than 200 cc of tissue ♀

0.00 0.00 FUD XXX J 80

AMA: 2005,Mar,1-6; 2005,Dec,3-6

0072T total leiomyomata volume greater or equal to 200 cc of tissue ♀

0.00 0.00 FUD XXX J 80

AMA: 2005,Mar,1-6; 2005,Dec,3-6

0075T-0076T

INCLUDES All diagnostic services for stenting
Ipsilateral extracranial vertebral selective catheterization when confirming the need for stenting

EXCLUDES *Selective catheterization and imaging when stenting is not required (report only selective catheterization codes)*

0075T Transcatheter placement of extracranial vertebral artery stent(s), including radiologic supervision and interpretation, open or percutaneous; initial vessel

0.00 0.00 FUD XXX C 80

AMA: 2018,Jan,8; 2017,Jan,8; 2016,Jan,13; 2015,Jan,16; 2014,Mar,8

\+ **0076T each additional vessel (List separately in addition to code for primary procedure)**

Code first (0075T)

0.00 0.00 FUD XXX C 80

AMA: 2018,Jan,8; 2017,Jan,8; 2016,Jan,13; 2015,Jan,16; 2014,Mar,8

0085T

0085T Breath test for heart transplant rejection

0.00 0.00 FUD XXX E

AMA: 2005,May,7-12

0095T-0098T

INCLUDES Fluoroscopy

\+ **0095T Removal of total disc arthroplasty (artificial disc), anterior approach, each additional interspace, cervical (List separately in addition to code for primary procedure)**

EXCLUDES *Lumbar disc (0164T)*
Revision of total disc arthroplasty, cervical (22861)
Revision of total disc arthroplasty, lumbar (22862)

Code first (22864)

0.00 0.00 FUD XXX C 80

AMA: 2006,Feb,1-6; 2005,Jun,6-8

\+ **0098T Revision including replacement of total disc arthroplasty (artificial disc), anterior approach, each additional interspace, cervical (List separately in addition to code for primary procedure)**

EXCLUDES *Application of intervertebral biomechanical device(s) at the same level (22853-22854, [22859])*
Removal of total disc arthroplasty (0095T)
Spinal cord decompression (63001-63048)

Code first (22861)

0.00 0.00 FUD XXX C 80

AMA: 2006,Feb,1-6; 2005,Jun,6-8

0100T

0100T Placement of a subconjunctival retinal prosthesis receiver and pulse generator, and implantation of intra-ocular retinal electrode array, with vitrectomy

EXCLUDES *Evaluation and initial programming of implantable retinal electrode array device (0472T)*

0.00 0.00 FUD XXX T J8 80

AMA: 2018,Feb,3; 2018,Jan,8; 2017,Jan,8; 2016,Jan,13; 2015,Jan,16; 2014,Jan,11

0101T-0513T [0512T, 0513T]

0101T Extracorporeal shock wave involving musculoskeletal system, not otherwise specified, high energy

EXCLUDES *Extracorporeal shock wave therapy of the integumentary system not otherwise specified ([0512T, 0513T])*

0.00 0.00 FUD XXX J G2 80

AMA: 2018,Dec,5; 2018,Dec,5; 2018,Jan,8; 2017,Jan,8; 2016,Jan,13; 2015,Jan,16; 2014,Jan,11

0102T Extracorporeal shock wave, high energy, performed by a physician, requiring anesthesia other than local, involving lateral humeral epicondyle

0.00 0.00 FUD XXX J G2 80

AMA: 2019,Jun,11; 2018,Dec,5; 2018,Dec,5; 2018,Jan,8; 2017,Jan,8; 2016,Jan,13; 2015,Jan,16; 2014,Jan,11

\# **0512T Extracorporeal shock wave for integumentary wound healing, high energy, including topical application and dressing care; initial wound**

0.00 0.00 FUD YYY R2 80

AMA: 2018,Dec,5; 2018,Dec,5

\+ # **0513T each additional wound (List separately in addition to code for primary procedure)**

Code first ([0512T])

0.00 0.00 FUD ZZZ N1 80

AMA: 2018,Dec,5; 2018,Dec,5

0106T-0110T

0106T Quantitative sensory testing (QST), testing and interpretation per extremity; using touch pressure stimuli to assess large diameter sensation

0.00 0.00 FUD XXX Q1 80

AMA: 2018,Jan,8; 2017,Jan,8; 2016,Jan,13; 2015,Jan,16; 2014,Jan,11

Category III Codes

0107T—0200T

0107T using vibration stimuli to assess large diameter fiber sensation

0.00 0.00 FUD XXX Q1 80

AMA: 2018,Jan,8; 2017,Jan,8; 2016,Jan,13; 2015,Jan,16; 2014,Jan,11

0108T using cooling stimuli to assess small nerve fiber sensation and hyperalgesia

0.00 0.00 FUD XXX Q1 80

AMA: 2018,Jan,8; 2017,Jan,8; 2016,Jan,13; 2015,Jan,16; 2014,Jan,11

0109T using heat-pain stimuli to assess small nerve fiber sensation and hyperalgesia

0.00 0.00 FUD XXX Q1 80

AMA: 2018,Jan,8; 2017,Jan,8; 2016,Jan,13; 2015,Jan,16; 2014,Jan,11

0110T using other stimuli to assess sensation

0.00 0.00 FUD XXX Q1 80

AMA: 2018,Jan,8; 2017,Jan,8; 2016,Jan,13; 2015,Jan,16; 2014,Jan,11

0111T-0126T

0111T **Long-chain (C20-22) omega-3 fatty acids in red blood cell (RBC) membranes**

EXCLUDES *Very long chain fatty acids (82726)*

0.00 0.00 FUD XXX A

AMA: 2018,Jan,8; 2017,Jan,8; 2016,Jan,13; 2015,Jan,16; 2014,Jan,11

0126T **Common carotid intima-media thickness (IMT) study for evaluation of atherosclerotic burden or coronary heart disease risk factor assessment**

EXCLUDES *Duplex scan extracranial arteries (93880-93882)*
Evaluation carotid intima media and atheroma (93895)

0.00 0.00 FUD XXX Q1 80

AMA: 2018,Jan,8; 2017,Jan,8; 2016,Jan,13; 2015,Jan,16; 2014,Jan,11

0163T-0165T

CMS: 100-03,150.10 Lumbar Artificial Disc Replacement (LADR)

INCLUDES Fluoroscopy

EXCLUDES *Application of intervertebral biomechanical device(s) at the same level (22853-22854, [22859])*
Cervical disc procedures (22856)
Decompression (63001-63048)
Exploration retroperitoneal area at same level (49010)

\+ 0163T **Total disc arthroplasty (artificial disc), anterior approach, including discectomy to prepare interspace (other than for decompression), each additional interspace, lumbar (List separately in addition to code for primary procedure)**

Code first (22857)

0.00 0.00 FUD YYY C 80

AMA: 2018,Jan,8; 2017,Jan,8; 2016,Jan,13; 2015,Jan,16; 2014,Jan,11

\+ 0164T **Removal of total disc arthroplasty, (artificial disc), anterior approach, each additional interspace, lumbar (List separately in addition to code for primary procedure)**

Code first (22865)

0.00 0.00 FUD YYY C 80

AMA: 2018,Jan,8; 2017,Jan,8; 2016,Jan,13; 2015,Jan,16; 2014,Jan,11

\+ 0165T **Revision including replacement of total disc arthroplasty (artificial disc), anterior approach, each additional interspace, lumbar (List separately in addition to code for primary procedure)**

Code first (22862)

0.00 0.00 FUD YYY C 80

AMA: 2018,Jan,8; 2017,Jan,8; 2016,Jan,13; 2015,Jan,16; 2014,Jan,11

0174T-0175T

\+ 0174T **Computer-aided detection (CAD) (computer algorithm analysis of digital image data for lesion detection) with further physician review for interpretation and report, with or without digitization of film radiographic images, chest radiograph(s), performed concurrent with primary interpretation (List separately in addition to code for primary procedure)**

Code first (71045-71048)

0.00 0.00 FUD XXX N 80

AMA: 2018,Apr,7

0175T **Computer-aided detection (CAD) (computer algorithm analysis of digital image data for lesion detection) with further physician review for interpretation and report, with or without digitization of film radiographic images, chest radiograph(s), performed remote from primary interpretation**

INCLUDES Chest x-rays (71045-71048)

0.00 0.00 FUD XXX N 80

AMA: 2018,Apr,7

0184T

0184T **Excision of rectal tumor, transanal endoscopic microsurgical approach (ie, TEMS), including muscularis propria (ie, full thickness)**

INCLUDES Operating microscope (66990)
Proctosigmoidoscopy (45300, 45308-45309, 45315, 45317, 45320)

EXCLUDES *Nonendoscopic excision of rectal tumor (45160, 45171-45172)*

0.00 0.00 FUD XXX J 80

AMA: 2018,Feb,11; 2018,Jan,8; 2017,Jan,8; 2016,Feb,12; 2016,Jan,13; 2015,Jan,16; 2014,Jan,11

0191T-0253T [0253T, 0376T]

0191T **Insertion of anterior segment aqueous drainage device, without extraocular reservoir, internal approach, into the trabecular meshwork; initial insertion**

0.00 0.00 FUD XXX J J8 80

AMA: 2018,Jul,3; 2018,Feb,3; 2018,Jan,8; 2017,Jan,8; 2016,Jan,13; 2015,Jan,16; 2014,Jan,11

\+ # 0376T **each additional device insertion (List separately in addition to code for primary procedure)**

Code first (0191T)

0.00 0.00 FUD XXX N N1 80

AMA: 2018,Jul,3; 2018,Feb,3

\# 0253T **Insertion of anterior segment aqueous drainage device, without extraocular reservoir, internal approach, into the suprachoroidal space**

EXCLUDES *Insertion aqueous drainage device, external approach (66183)*

0.00 0.00 FUD YYY J G2 80

AMA: 2018,Jul,3

0198T

0198T **Measurement of ocular blood flow by repetitive intraocular pressure sampling, with interpretation and report**

0.00 0.00 FUD XXX Q1 80

AMA: 2018,Jan,8; 2017,Jan,8; 2016,Jan,13; 2015,Jan,16; 2014,Jan,11

0200T-0201T

INCLUDES Deep bone biopsy (20225)

0200T **Percutaneous sacral augmentation (sacroplasty), unilateral injection(s), including the use of a balloon or mechanical device, when used, 1 or more needles, includes imaging guidance and bone biopsy, when performed**

0.00 0.00 FUD XXX J G2 80 50

AMA: 2018,Jan,8; 2017,Jan,8; 2016,Jan,13; 2015,Dec,18; 2015,Apr,8; 2015,Jan,8

0201T **Percutaneous sacral augmentation (sacroplasty), bilateral injections, including the use of a balloon or mechanical device, when used, 2 or more needles, includes imaging guidance and bone biopsy, when performed**
0.00 0.00 FUD XXX J G2 80
AMA: 2018,Jan,8; 2017,Jan,8; 2016,Jan,13; 2015,Dec,18; 2015,Apr,8; 2015,Jan,8

0202T-0563T [0563T]

0202T **Posterior vertebral joint(s) arthroplasty (eg, facet joint[s] replacement), including facetectomy, laminectomy, foraminotomy, and vertebral column fixation, injection of bone cement, when performed, including fluoroscopy, single level, lumbar spine**
0.00 0.00 FUD XXX C 80

INCLUDES Instrumentation (22840, 22853-22854, [22859])
Laminectomy (63005, 63012, 63017, 63047)
Laminotomy (63030, 63042)
Lumbar arthroplasty (22857)
Percutaneous lumbar vertebral augmentation (22514)
Percutaneous vertebroplasty (22511)
Spinal cord decompression (63056)

~~**0205T** **Intravascular catheter-based coronary vessel or graft spectroscopy (eg, infrared) during diagnostic evaluation and/or therapeutic intervention including imaging supervision, interpretation, and report, each vessel (List separately in addition to code for primary procedure)**~~

~~**0206T** **Computerized database analysis of multiple cycles of digitized cardiac electrical data from two or more ECG leads, including transmission to a remote center, application of multiple nonlinear mathematical transformations, with coronary artery obstruction severity assessment**~~

0207T **Evacuation of meibomian glands, automated, using heat and intermittent pressure, unilateral**

EXCLUDES *Evacuation using:*
Heat through wearable device ([0563T])
Manual expression only, report appropriate E&M code

0.00 0.00 FUD XXX Q1 80
AMA: 2018,Jan,8; 2017,Jan,8; 2016,Jan,13; 2015,Jan,16; 2014,May,5

● # **0563T** **Evacuation of meibomian glands, using heat delivered through wearable, open-eye eyelid treatment devices and manual gland expression, bilateral**
0.00 0.00 FUD 000

EXCLUDES *Evacuation using:*
Heat and intermittent pressure (0207T)
Manual expression only, report appropriate E&M code

0208T-0212T

EXCLUDES *Manual audiometric testing by a qualified health care professional, using audiometers (92551-92557)*

0208T **Pure tone audiometry (threshold), automated; air only**
0.00 0.00 FUD XXX Q1 80 TC
AMA: 2018,Jan,8; 2017,Jan,8; 2016,Jan,13; 2015,Jan,16; 2014,Aug,3

0209T **air and bone**
0.00 0.00 FUD XXX Q1 80 TC
AMA: 2018,Jan,8; 2017,Jan,8; 2016,Jan,13; 2015,Jan,16; 2014,Aug,3; 2014,Jan,11

0210T **Speech audiometry threshold, automated;**
0.00 0.00 FUD XXX Q1 80 TC
AMA: 2014,Aug,3

0211T **with speech recognition**
0.00 0.00 FUD XXX Q1 80 TC
AMA: 2018,Jan,8; 2017,Jan,8; 2016,Jan,13; 2015,Jan,16; 2014,Aug,3; 2014,Jan,11

0212T **Comprehensive audiometry threshold evaluation and speech recognition (0209T, 0211T combined), automated**
0.00 0.00 FUD XXX Q1 80 TC
AMA: 2018,Jan,8; 2017,Jan,8; 2016,Jan,13; 2015,Jan,16; 2014,Aug,3; 2014,Jan,11

0213T-0215T

0213T **Injection(s), diagnostic or therapeutic agent, paravertebral facet (zygapophyseal) joint (or nerves innervating that joint) with ultrasound guidance, cervical or thoracic; single level**
0.00 0.00 FUD XXX T R2 80 50
AMA: 2018,Jan,8; 2017,Jan,8; 2016,Jan,13; 2015,Jan,16; 2014,Jan,11

+ **0214T** **second level (List separately in addition to code for primary procedure)**

EXCLUDES *Reporting with modifier 50. Report once for each side when performed bilaterally*

Code first (0213T)
0.00 0.00 FUD ZZZ 50 N N1 80
AMA: 2018,Jan,8; 2017,Jan,8; 2016,Jan,13; 2015,Jan,16; 2014,Jan,11

+ **0215T** **third and any additional level(s) (List separately in addition to code for primary procedure)**

EXCLUDES *Reporting with modifier 50. Report once for each side when performed bilaterally*
Use of code more than one time per date of service

Code first (0213T-0214T)
0.00 0.00 FUD ZZZ 50 N N1 80
AMA: 2018,Jan,8; 2017,Jan,8; 2016,Jan,13; 2015,Jan,16; 2014,Jan,11

0216T-0218T

EXCLUDES *Injection with CT or fluoroscopic guidance (64490-64495)*

0216T **Injection(s), diagnostic or therapeutic agent, paravertebral facet (zygapophyseal) joint (or nerves innervating that joint) with ultrasound guidance, lumbar or sacral; single level**
0.00 0.00 FUD XXX T R2 80 50
AMA: 2018,Jan,8; 2017,Jan,8; 2016,Jan,13; 2015,Jan,16; 2014,Jan,11

+ **0217T** **second level (List separately in addition to code for primary procedure)**

EXCLUDES *Reporting with modifier 50. Report once for each side when performed bilaterally*

Code first (0216T)
0.00 0.00 FUD ZZZ 50 N N1 80
AMA: 2018,Jan,8; 2017,Jan,8; 2016,Jan,13; 2015,Jan,16; 2014,Jan,11

+ **0218T** **third and any additional level(s) (List separately in addition to code for primary procedure)**

EXCLUDES *Reporting with modifier 50. Report once for each side when performed bilaterally*
Use of code more than one time per date of service

Code first (0216T-0217T)
0.00 0.00 FUD ZZZ 50 N N1 80
AMA: 2018,Jan,8; 2017,Jan,8; 2016,Jan,13; 2015,Jan,16; 2014,Jan,11

0219T-0222T

INCLUDES Allografts at same level (20930-20931)
Application of intervertebral biomechanical device(s) at the same level (22853-22854, [22859])
Arthrodesis at same level (22600-22614)
Instrumentation at same level (22840)
Radiologic services

0219T **Placement of a posterior intrafacet implant(s), unilateral or bilateral, including imaging and placement of bone graft(s) or synthetic device(s), single level; cervical**
0.00 0.00 FUD XXX C 80
AMA: 2018,Jan,8; 2017,Jan,8; 2016,Jan,13; 2015,Jan,16; 2014,Jan,11

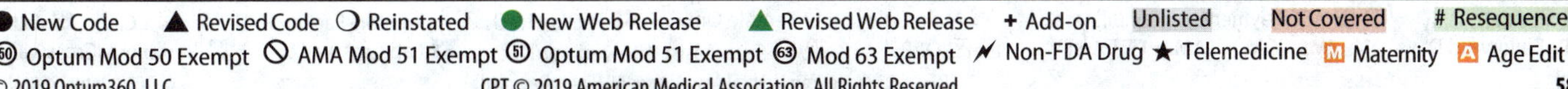

0220T **thoracic**
0.00 0.00 FUD XXX C 80
AMA: 2018,Jan,8; 2017,Jan,8; 2016,Jan,13; 2015,Jan,16; 2014,Jan,11

0221T **lumbar**
0.00 0.00 FUD XXX J 80
AMA: 2018,Jan,8; 2017,Jan,8; 2016,Jan,13; 2015,Jan,16; 2014,Jan,11

+ 0222T **each additional vertebral segment (List separately in addition to code for primary procedure)**
Code first (0219T-0221T)
0.00 0.00 FUD ZZZ N 80
AMA: 2018,Jan,8; 2017,Jan,8; 2016,Jan,13; 2015,Jan,16; 2014,Jan,11

0228T-0231T

INCLUDES Ultrasound guidance (76942, 76998-76999)

EXCLUDES *Injection performed with CT of fluoroscopic guidance (64479-64484)*

0228T **Injection(s), anesthetic agent and/or steroid, transforaminal epidural, with ultrasound guidance, cervical or thoracic; single level**
0.00 0.00 FUD XXX T G2 50
AMA: 2018,Jan,8; 2017,Jan,8; 2016,Jan,13; 2015,Jan,16; 2014,Jan,11

+ 0229T **each additional level (List separately in addition to code for primary procedure)**
Code first (0228T)
0.00 0.00 FUD XXX N N1 50
AMA: 2018,Jan,8; 2017,Jan,8; 2016,Jan,13; 2015,Jan,16; 2014,Jan,11

0230T **Injection(s), anesthetic agent and/or steroid, transforaminal epidural, with ultrasound guidance, lumbar or sacral; single level**
0.00 0.00 FUD XXX T G2 50
AMA: 2018,Jan,8; 2017,Jan,8; 2016,Jan,13; 2015,Jan,16; 2014,Jan,11

+ 0231T **each additional level (List separately in addition to code for primary procedure)**
Code first (0230T)
0.00 0.00 FUD XXX N N1 50
AMA: 2018,Jan,8; 2017,Jan,8; 2016,Jan,13; 2015,Jan,16; 2014,Jan,11

0232T

INCLUDES Arthrocentesis (20600-20611)
Blood collection (36415, 36592)
Fat and other soft tissue grafts ([15769], 15771-15774)
Imaging guidance (76942, 77002, 77012, 77021)
Injections (20550-20551)
Platelet/blood product pooling (86965)

EXCLUDES *Aspiration of bone marrow for grafting, biopsy, harvesting for transplant (38220-38221, 38230)*
Injections white cell concentrate (0481T)

0232T **Injection(s), platelet rich plasma, any site, including image guidance, harvesting and preparation when performed**
0.00 0.00 FUD XXX Q1 N1
AMA: 2019,Apr,10; 2018,May,3; 2018,Jan,8; 2017,Jan,8; 2016,Jan,13; 2015,Jan,16; 2014,Jan,11

0234T-0238T

INCLUDES Atherectomy by any technique in arteries above the inguinal ligaments
Radiology supervision and interpretation

EXCLUDES *Accessing and catheterization of the vessel*
Atherectomy performed below the inguinal ligaments (37225, 37227, 37229, 37231, 37233, 37235)
Closure of the arteriotomy by any technique
Negotiating the lesion
Other interventions to the same or different vessels
Protection from embolism

0234T **Transluminal peripheral atherectomy, open or percutaneous, including radiological supervision and interpretation; renal artery**
0.00 0.00 FUD YYY J 80
AMA: 2018,Jan,8; 2017,Jan,8; 2016,Jan,13; 2015,Jan,16; 2014,Jan,11

0235T **visceral artery (except renal), each vessel**
0.00 0.00 FUD YYY C 80
AMA: 2018,Jan,8; 2017,Jan,8; 2016,Jan,13; 2015,Jan,16; 2014,Jan,11

0236T **abdominal aorta**
0.00 0.00 FUD YYY J 80
AMA: 2018,Jan,8; 2017,Jan,8; 2016,Jan,13; 2015,Jan,16; 2014,Jan,11

0237T **brachiocephalic trunk and branches, each vessel**
0.00 0.00 FUD YYY J 80
AMA: 2018,Jan,8; 2017,Jan,8; 2016,Jan,13; 2015,Jan,16; 2014,Jan,11

0238T **iliac artery, each vessel**
0.00 0.00 FUD YYY J G2 80
AMA: 2018,Jan,8; 2017,Jan,8; 2016,Jan,13; 2015,Jan,16; 2014,Jan,11

0249T-0254T [0253T]

~~0249T~~ ~~**Ligation, hemorrhoidal vascular bundle(s), including ultrasound guidance**~~
To report, see (46948)

0253T **Resequenced code. See code before 0198T.**

~~0254T~~ ~~**Endovascular repair of iliac artery bifurcation (eg, aneurysm, pseudoaneurysm, arteriovenous malformation, trauma, dissection) using bifurcated endograft from the common iliac artery into both the external and internal iliac artery, including all selective and/or nonselective catheterization(s) required for device placement and all associated radiological supervision and interpretation, unilateral**~~
To report, see ([34717-34718])

0263T-0265T

EXCLUDES *Bone marrow and stem cell services (38204-38242 [38243])*

0263T **Intramuscular autologous bone marrow cell therapy, with preparation of harvested cells, multiple injections, one leg, including ultrasound guidance, if performed; complete procedure including unilateral or bilateral bone marrow harvest**
0.00 0.00 FUD XXX S G2 80
INCLUDES Duplex scan (93925-93926)
Ultrasound guidance (76942)

0264T **complete procedure excluding bone marrow harvest**
0.00 0.00 FUD XXX S G2 80
INCLUDES Bone marrow harvest only (0265T)
Duplex scan (93925-93926)
Ultrasound guidance (76942)

0265T **unilateral or bilateral bone marrow harvest only for intramuscular autologous bone marrow cell therapy**
0.00 0.00 FUD XXX S G2 80
EXCLUDES *Complete procedure (0263T-0264T)*

0266T-0273T

0266T Implantation or replacement of carotid sinus baroreflex activation device; total system (includes generator placement, unilateral or bilateral lead placement, intra-operative interrogation, programming, and repositioning, when performed)
0.00 0.00 FUD YYY C 80
INCLUDES Components of complete procedure (0267T-0268T)

0267T lead only, unilateral (includes intra-operative interrogation, programming, and repositioning, when performed)
0.00 0.00 FUD YYY T 80
EXCLUDES *Complete procedure (0266T)*
Device interrogation (0272T-0273T)
Removal/revision device or components (0269T-0271T)

0268T pulse generator only (includes intra-operative interrogation, programming, and repositioning, when performed)
0.00 0.00 FUD YYY J 80
EXCLUDES *Complete procedure (0266T)*
Device interrogation (0272T-0273T)
Removal/revision device or components (0269T-0271T)

0269T Revision or removal of carotid sinus baroreflex activation device; total system (includes generator placement, unilateral or bilateral lead placement, intra-operative interrogation, programming, and repositioning, when performed)
0.00 0.00 FUD XXX Q2 G2 80
EXCLUDES *Device interrogation (0272T-0273T)*
Implantation/replacement device and/or components (0266T-0268T)
Removal/revision device or components (0270T-0271T)

0270T lead only, unilateral (includes intra-operative interrogation, programming, and repositioning, when performed)
0.00 0.00 FUD XXX Q2 G2 80
EXCLUDES *Device interrogation (0272T-0273T)*
Implantation/replacement device and/or components (0266T-0269T)
Removal/revision device or components (0271T)

0271T pulse generator only (includes intra-operative interrogation, programming, and repositioning, when performed)
0.00 0.00 FUD XXX Q2 G2 80
EXCLUDES *Device interrogation (0272T-0273T)*
Implantation/replacement device and/or components (0266T-0268T)
Removal/revision device or components (0271T-0273T)

0272T Interrogation device evaluation (in person), carotid sinus baroreflex activation system, including telemetric iterative communication with the implantable device to monitor device diagnostics and programmed therapy values, with interpretation and report (eg, battery status, lead impedance, pulse amplitude, pulse width, therapy frequency, pathway mode, burst mode, therapy start/stop times each day);
0.00 0.00 FUD XXX S 80
EXCLUDES *Device interrogation (0273T)*
Implantation/replacement device and/or components (0266T-0268T)
Removal/revision device or components (0269T-0271T)

0273T with programming
0.00 0.00 FUD XXX S 80
EXCLUDES *Device interrogation (0272T)*
Implantation/replacement device and/or components (0266T-0268T)
Removal/revision device or components (0269T-0271T)

0274T-0275T

EXCLUDES *Laminotomy/hemilaminectomy by open and endoscopically assisted approach (63020-63035)*
Percutaneous decompression of nucleus pulposus of intervertebral disc by needle-based technique (62287)

0274T Percutaneous laminotomy/laminectomy (interlaminar approach) for decompression of neural elements, (with or without ligamentous resection, discectomy, facetectomy and/or foraminotomy), any method, under indirect image guidance (eg, fluoroscopic, CT), single or multiple levels, unilateral or bilateral; cervical or thoracic
0.00 0.00 FUD YYY J G2 80
AMA: 2018,Jan,8; 2017,Feb,12; 2017,Jan,8; 2016,Jan,13; 2015,Jan,16; 2014,Jan,11

0275T lumbar
0.00 0.00 FUD YYY J G2 80
AMA: 2018,Jan,8; 2017,Feb,12; 2017,Jan,8; 2016,Jan,13; 2015,Jan,16; 2014,Jan,11

0278T

0278T Transcutaneous electrical modulation pain reprocessing (eg, scrambler therapy), each treatment session (includes placement of electrodes)
0.00 0.00 FUD XXX Q1 N1 80

0290T

+ **0290T Corneal incisions in the recipient cornea created using a laser, in preparation for penetrating or lamellar keratoplasty (List separately in addition to code for primary procedure)**
Code first (65710, 65730, 65750, 65755)
0.00 0.00 FUD ZZZ N N1 80
AMA: 2018,Jan,8; 2017,Jan,8; 2016,Jan,13; 2015,Jan,16; 2014,Jan,11

0295T-0298T

EXCLUDES *External echocardiograph monitoring up to 48 hours (93224-93227)*
External electrocardiographic monitoring (93260-93272)
Mobile cardiovascular telemetry with echocardiograph recording (93228-93229)

0295T External electrocardiographic recording for more than 48 hours up to 21 days by continuous rhythm recording and storage; includes recording, scanning analysis with report, review and interpretation
0.00 0.00 FUD XXX M 80
AMA: 2018,Jan,8; 2017,Jan,8; 2016,Jan,13; 2015,Jan,16; 2014,Jan,11

0296T recording (includes connection and initial recording)
0.00 0.00 FUD XXX Q1 80
AMA: 2018,Jan,8; 2017,Jan,8; 2016,Jan,13; 2015,Jan,16; 2014,Jan,11

0297T scanning analysis with report
0.00 0.00 FUD XXX Q1 80
AMA: 2018,Jan,8; 2017,Jan,8; 2016,Jan,13; 2015,Jan,16; 2014,Jan,11

0298T review and interpretation
0.00 0.00 FUD XXX M 80
AMA: 2018,Jan,8; 2017,Jan,8; 2016,Jan,13; 2015,Jan,16; 2014,Jan,11

0308T

0308T Insertion of ocular telescope prosthesis including removal of crystalline lens or intraocular lens prosthesis
INCLUDES Injection procedures (66020, 66030)
Iridectomy when performed (66600-66635, 66761)
Operating microscope (69990)
Repositioning of intraocular lens (66825)
EXCLUDES *Cataract extraction (66982-66986)*
0.00 0.00 FUD YYY J J8 50
AMA: 2018,Jan,8; 2017,Jan,8; 2016,Jan,13; 2015,Jan,16; 2014,Jan,11

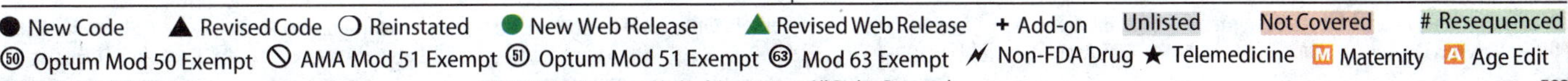

0312T-0317T

EXCLUDES *Analysis and/or programming (or reprogramming) of vagus nerve stimulator (95970, 95976-95977)*
Implantation, replacement, removal, and/or revision of vagus nerve neurostimulator (electrode array and/or pulse generator) for stimulation of vagus nerve other than at the esophagogastric junction (64568-64570)

0312T **Vagus nerve blocking therapy (morbid obesity); laparoscopic implantation of neurostimulator electrode array, anterior and posterior vagal trunks adjacent to esophagogastric junction (EGJ), with implantation of pulse generator, includes programming**
0.00 0.00 FUD XXX J 80
AMA: 2018,Jan,8; 2017,Jan,8; 2016,Jan,13; 2015,Jan,16

0313T **laparoscopic revision or replacement of vagal trunk neurostimulator electrode array, including connection to existing pulse generator**
0.00 0.00 FUD XXX T G2 80
AMA: 2018,Jan,8; 2017,Jan,8; 2016,Jan,13; 2015,Jan,16

0314T **laparoscopic removal of vagal trunk neurostimulator electrode array and pulse generator**
0.00 0.00 FUD XXX Q2 G2 80
AMA: 2018,Jan,8; 2017,Jan,8; 2016,Jan,13; 2015,Jan,16

0315T **removal of pulse generator**
EXCLUDES *Removal with replacement pulse generator (0316T)*
0.00 0.00 FUD XXX Q2 G2 80
AMA: 2018,Jan,8; 2017,Jan,8; 2016,Jan,13; 2015,Jan,16

0316T **replacement of pulse generator**
EXCLUDES *Removal without replacement pulse generator (0315T)*
0.00 0.00 FUD XXX J J8 80
AMA: 2018,Jan,8; 2017,Jan,8; 2016,Jan,13; 2015,Jan,16

0317T **neurostimulator pulse generator electronic analysis, includes reprogramming when performed**
EXCLUDES *Analysis and/or programming (or reprogramming) of vagus nerve stimulator (95970, 95976-95977)*
0.00 0.00 FUD XXX Q1 80
AMA: 2018,Jan,8; 2017,Jan,8; 2016,Jan,13; 2015,Jan,16

0329T-0330T

0329T **Monitoring of intraocular pressure for 24 hours or longer, unilateral or bilateral, with interpretation and report**
0.00 0.00 FUD YYY E
AMA: 2018,Jan,8; 2017,Jan,8; 2016,Jan,13; 2015,Jan,16; 2014,May,5

0330T **Tear film imaging, unilateral or bilateral, with interpretation and report**
0.00 0.00 FUD YYY Q1 N1
AMA: 2018,Jan,8; 2017,Jan,8; 2016,Jan,13; 2015,Jan,16; 2014,May,5

0331T-0332T

EXCLUDES *Myocardial infarction avid imaging (78466, 78468, 78469)*

0331T **Myocardial sympathetic innervation imaging, planar qualitative and quantitative assessment;**
0.00 0.00 FUD YYY S Z2
AMA: 2018,Jan,8; 2017,Jan,8; 2016,Jan,13; 2015,Jan,16; 2014,Jun,14

0332T **with tomographic SPECT**
0.00 0.00 FUD YYY S Z2
AMA: 2018,Jan,8; 2017,Jan,8; 2016,Jan,13; 2015,Jan,16; 2014,Jun,14

0333T-0464T [0464T]

0333T **Visual evoked potential, screening of visual acuity, automated, with report**
EXCLUDES *Visual evoked potential testing for glaucoma ([0464T])*
0.00 0.00 FUD YYY E
AMA: 2018,Feb,3; 2018,Jan,8; 2017,Jan,8; 2016,Jan,13; 2015,Jan,16; 2014,Aug,8

\# **0464T** **Visual evoked potential, testing for glaucoma, with interpretation and report**
EXCLUDES *Visual evoked potential for visual acuity (0333T)*
0.00 0.00 FUD YYY S
AMA: 2018,Feb,3

0335T-0511T [0510T, 0511T]

0335T **Insertion of sinus tarsi implant**
0.00 0.00 FUD YYY J J8
EXCLUDES *Arthroscopic subtalar arthrodesis (29907)*
Open talotarsal joint dislocation repair (28585)
Subtalar arthodesis (28725)

\# **0510T** **Removal of sinus tarsi implant**
0.00 0.00 FUD YYY G2 50

\# **0511T** **Removal and reinsertion of sinus tarsi implant**
0.00 0.00 FUD YYY J8 50

0338T-0339T

INCLUDES Selective catheter placement renal arteries (36251-36254)

0338T **Transcatheter renal sympathetic denervation, percutaneous approach including arterial puncture, selective catheter placement(s) renal artery(ies), fluoroscopy, contrast injection(s), intraprocedural roadmapping and radiological supervision and interpretation, including pressure gradient measurements, flush aortogram and diagnostic renal angiography when performed; unilateral**
0.00 0.00 FUD YYY J G2

0339T **bilateral**
0.00 0.00 FUD YYY J G2

0341T-0342T

~~0341T Quantitative pupillometry with interpretation and report, unilateral or bilateral~~

0342T **Therapeutic apheresis with selective HDL delipidation and plasma reinfusion**
0.00 0.00 FUD YYY S G2

0345T-0347T

0345T **Transcatheter mitral valve repair percutaneous approach via the coronary sinus**
INCLUDES Coronary angiography (93563-93564)
EXCLUDES *Diagnostic cardiac catheterization procedures integral to valve procedure (93451-93461, 93530-93533, 93563-93564)*
Repair of mitral valve including transseptal puncture (33418-33419)
Transcatheter implantation/replacement mitral valve (TMVI) (0483T-0484T)
Transcatheter mitral valve annulus reconstruction (0544T)
0.00 0.00 FUD YYY C
AMA: 2018,Jan,8; 2017,Jan,8; 2016,Jan,13; 2015,Sep,3

0347T **Placement of interstitial device(s) in bone for radiostereometric analysis (RSA)**
0.00 0.00 FUD YYY Q1 N1
AMA: 2018,Jan,8; 2017,Jan,8; 2016,Jan,13; 2015,Jun,8

0348T-0350T

0348T **Radiologic examination, radiostereometric analysis (RSA); spine, (includes cervical, thoracic and lumbosacral, when performed)**
0.00 0.00 FUD YYY Q1 N1
AMA: 2018,Jan,8; 2017,Jan,8; 2016,Jan,13; 2015,Jun,8

0349T **upper extremity(ies), (includes shoulder, elbow, and wrist, when performed)**
0.00 0.00 FUD YYY Q1 N1
AMA: 2018,Jan,8; 2017,Jan,8; 2016,Jan,13; 2015,Jun,8

0350T lower extremity(ies), (includes hip, proximal femur, knee, and ankle, when performed)
0.00 0.00 FUD YYY Q1 N1
AMA: 2018,Jan,8; 2017,Jan,8; 2016,Jan,13; 2015,Jun,8

0351T-0354T

0351T **Optical coherence tomography of breast or axillary lymph node, excised tissue, each specimen; real-time intraoperative**
INCLUDES Interpretation and report (0352T)
0.00 0.00 FUD YYY N N1
AMA: 2018,Jan,8; 2017,Jan,8; 2016,Jan,13; 2015,Apr,6

0352T **interpretation and report, real-time or referred**
INCLUDES Interpretation and report (0351T)
0.00 0.00 FUD YYY B
AMA: 2018,Jan,8; 2017,Jan,8; 2016,Jan,13; 2015,Apr,6

0353T **Optical coherence tomography of breast, surgical cavity; real-time intraoperative**
INCLUDES Interpretation and report (0354T)
EXCLUDES *Use of code more than one time per session*
0.00 0.00 FUD YYY N N1
AMA: 2018,Jan,8; 2017,Jan,8; 2016,Jan,13; 2015,Apr,6

0354T **interpretation and report, real time or referred**
0.00 0.00 FUD YYY B
AMA: 2018,Jan,8; 2017,Jan,8; 2016,Jan,13; 2015,Apr,6

0355T-0358T

0355T **Gastrointestinal tract imaging, intraluminal (eg, capsule endoscopy), colon, with interpretation and report**
0.00 0.00 FUD YYY J
INCLUDES Distal ileum imaging when performed
EXCLUDES *Capsule endoscopy esophagus only (91111)*
Capsule endoscopy esophagus through ileum (91110)

0356T **Insertion of drug-eluting implant (including punctal dilation and implant removal when performed) into lacrimal canaliculus, each**
EXCLUDES *Drug-eluting ocular insert (0444T-0445T)*
0.00 0.00 FUD YYY Q1 N1
AMA: 2018,Jan,8; 2017,Aug,7

~~0357T immature oocyte(s)~~

0358T **Bioelectrical impedance analysis whole body composition assessment, with interpretation and report**
0.00 0.00 FUD YYY Q1

0362T-0373T

INCLUDES Only the time of one technician when more than one is in attendance
Provided by physician/other qualified healthcare professional while on-site (immediately available during procedure), but does not need to be face-to-face
Provided in environment appropriate for patient
Provided to patients with destructive behaviors
EXCLUDES *Adaptive behavior services ([97153, 97154, 97155, 97156, 97157, 97158])*
Aphasia assessment (96105)
Behavioral/developmental screening/testing (96110-96113, [96127])
Behavior/health assessment (96156-96159 [96164, 96165, 96167, 96168, 96170, 96171])
Cognitive testing ([96125])
Neurobehavioral testing (96116-96121)
Psychiatric evaluations/psychotherapy/interactive complexity (90785-90899)
Psychological/neuropsychological evaluation/testing (96130-96146)

0362T **Behavior identification supporting assessment, each 15 minutes of technicians' time face-to-face with a patient, requiring the following components: administration by the physician or other qualified health care professional who is on site; with the assistance of two or more technicians; for a patient who exhibits destructive behavior; completion in an environment that is customized to the patient's behavior.**
INCLUDES Comprises:
Functional analysis and behavioral assessment
Procedures and instruments to assess functional impairment and levels of behavior
Structured observation with data collection not including direct patient involvement
EXCLUDES *Conferences by medical team (99366-99368)*
Occupational therapy evaluation ([97165, 97166, 97167, 97168])
Speech evaluation (92521-92524)
Code also when performed on different days until completion of behavioral and supporting assessments are complete
0.00 0.00 FUD YYY S
AMA: 2018,Nov,3; 2018,Jan,8; 2017,Jan,8; 2016,Jan,13; 2015,Jan,16; 2014,Jun,3

0373T **Adaptive behavior treatment with protocol modification, each 15 minutes of technicians' time face-to-face with a patient, requiring the following components: administration by the physician or other qualified health care professional who is on site; with the assistance of two or more technicians; for a patient who exhibits destructive behavior; completion in an environment that is customized to the patient's behavior.**
0.00 0.00 FUD YYY S
AMA: 2018,Nov,3; 2018,Jan,8; 2017,Jan,8; 2016,Jan,13; 2015,Jan,16; 2014,Jun,3

0375T

~~0375T Total disc arthroplasty (artificial disc), anterior approach, including discectomy with end plate preparation (includes osteophytectomy for nerve root or spinal cord decompression and microdissection), cervical, three or more levels~~

0376T-0377T [0376T]

0376T **Resequenced code. See code following 0191T.**

~~0377T Anoscopy with directed submucosal injection of bulking agent for fecal incontinence~~

0378T-0380T

0378T **Visual field assessment, with concurrent real time data analysis and accessible data storage with patient initiated data transmitted to a remote surveillance center for up to 30 days; review and interpretation with report by a physician or other qualified health care professional**
0.00 0.00 FUD XXX B 80
AMA: 2018,Jan,8; 2017,Jan,8; 2016,Jan,13; 2015,Jan,10

0379T technical support and patient instructions, surveillance, analysis and transmission of daily and emergent data reports as prescribed by a physician or other qualified health care professional
0.00 0.00 FUD XXX 01 N1 80
AMA: 2018,Jan,8; 2017,Jan,8; 2016,Jan,13; 2015,Jan,10

~~0380T Computer-aided animation and analysis of time series retinal images for the monitoring of disease progression, unilateral or bilateral, with interpretation and report~~

0381T-0386T

0381T External heart rate and 3-axis accelerometer data recording up to 14 days to assess changes in heart rate and to monitor motion analysis for the purposes of diagnosing nocturnal epilepsy seizure events; includes report, scanning analysis with report, review and interpretation by a physician or other qualified health care professional
0.00 0.00 FUD XXX M 80
EXCLUDES *External heart rate and data recording for 15 days or more (0383T-0386T)*

0382T review and interpretation only
0.00 0.00 FUD XXX M 80
EXCLUDES *External heart rate and data recording for 15 days or more (0383T-0386T)*

0383T External heart rate and 3-axis accelerometer data recording from 15 to 30 days to assess changes in heart rate and to monitor motion analysis for the purposes of diagnosing nocturnal epilepsy seizure events; includes report, scanning analysis with report, review and interpretation by a physician or other qualified health care professional
0.00 0.00 FUD XXX M 80
EXCLUDES *External heart rate and data recording for 14 days or less (0381T-0382T)*
External heart rate and data recording for 30 days or more (0385T-0386T)

0384T review and interpretation only
0.00 0.00 FUD XXX M 80
EXCLUDES *External heart rate and data recording for 14 days or less (0381T-0382T)*
External heart rate and data recording for 30 days or more (0385T-0386T)

0385T External heart rate and 3-axis accelerometer data recording more than 30 days to assess changes in heart rate and to monitor motion analysis for the purposes of diagnosing nocturnal epilepsy seizure events; includes report, scanning analysis with report, review and interpretation by a physician or other qualified health care professional
0.00 0.00 FUD XXX M 80
EXCLUDES *External heart rate and data recording for 30 days or less (0381T-0384T)*

0386T review and interpretation only
0.00 0.00 FUD XXX M 80
EXCLUDES *External heart rate and data recording for 30 days or less (0381T-0384T)*

0394T-0395T

EXCLUDES *Radiation oncology procedures (77261-77263, 77300, 77306-77307, 77316-77318, 77332-77334, 77336, 77427-77499, 77761-77772, 77778, 77789)*

0394T High dose rate electronic brachytherapy, skin surface application, per fraction, includes basic dosimetry, when performed
0.00 0.00 FUD XXX S Z2 80
EXCLUDES *Superficial non-brachytherapy radiation (77401)*

0395T High dose rate electronic brachytherapy, interstitial or intracavitary treatment, per fraction, includes basic dosimetry, when performed
0.00 0.00 FUD XXX S Z2 80
EXCLUDES *High dose rate skin surface application (0394T)*

0396T-0399T

+ 0396T Intra-operative use of kinetic balance sensor for implant stability during knee replacement arthroplasty (List separately in addition to code for primary procedure)
0.00 0.00 FUD XXX N N1 80
Code first (27445-27447, 27486-27488)

+ 0397T Endoscopic retrograde cholangiopancreatography (ERCP), with optical endomicroscopy (List separately in addition to code for primary procedure)
0.00 0.00 FUD XXX N N1 80
INCLUDES Optical endomicroscopic image(s) (88375)
EXCLUDES *Use of code more than one time per operative session*
Code first (43260-43265, [43274], [43275], [43276], [43277], [43278])

0398T Magnetic resonance image guided high intensity focused ultrasound (MRgFUS), stereotactic ablation lesion, intracranial for movement disorder including stereotactic navigation and frame placement when performed
0.00 0.00 FUD XXX S 80
INCLUDES Application stereotactic headframe (61800)
Stereotactic computer-assisted navigation (61781)

~~0399T Myocardial strain imaging (quantitative assessment of myocardial mechanics using image-based analysis of local myocardial dynamics) (List separately in addition to code for primary procedure)~~
To report, see (93356)

0400T-0401T

0400T Multi-spectral digital skin lesion analysis of clinically atypical cutaneous pigmented lesions for detection of melanomas and high risk melanocytic atypia; one to five lesions
0.00 0.00 FUD XXX N N1 80

0401T six or more lesions
0.00 0.00 FUD XXX N N1 80
INCLUDES Treatment of one to five lesions (0400T)

0402T

▲ 0402T Collagen cross-linking of cornea, including removal of the corneal epithelium and intraoperative pachymetry, when performed (Report medication separately)
INCLUDES Corneal epithelium removal (65435)
Corneal pachymetry (76514)
Operating microscope (69990)
0.00 0.00 FUD XXX J R2 80
AMA: 2018,Jun,11; 2018,Jan,8; 2017,Jan,8; 2016,Feb,12

0403T-0488T [0488T]

INCLUDES Intensive behavioral counseling by trained lifestyle coach
Standardized course with an emphasis on weight, exercise, stress management, and nutrition

0403T Preventive behavior change, intensive program of prevention of diabetes using a standardized diabetes prevention program curriculum, provided to individuals in a group setting, minimum 60 minutes, per day
EXCLUDES *Online/electronic diabetes prevention program ([0488T])*
Self-management training and education by nonphysician health care professional (98960-98962)
0.00 0.00 FUD XXX E 80
AMA: 2018,Aug,6; 2015,Aug,4

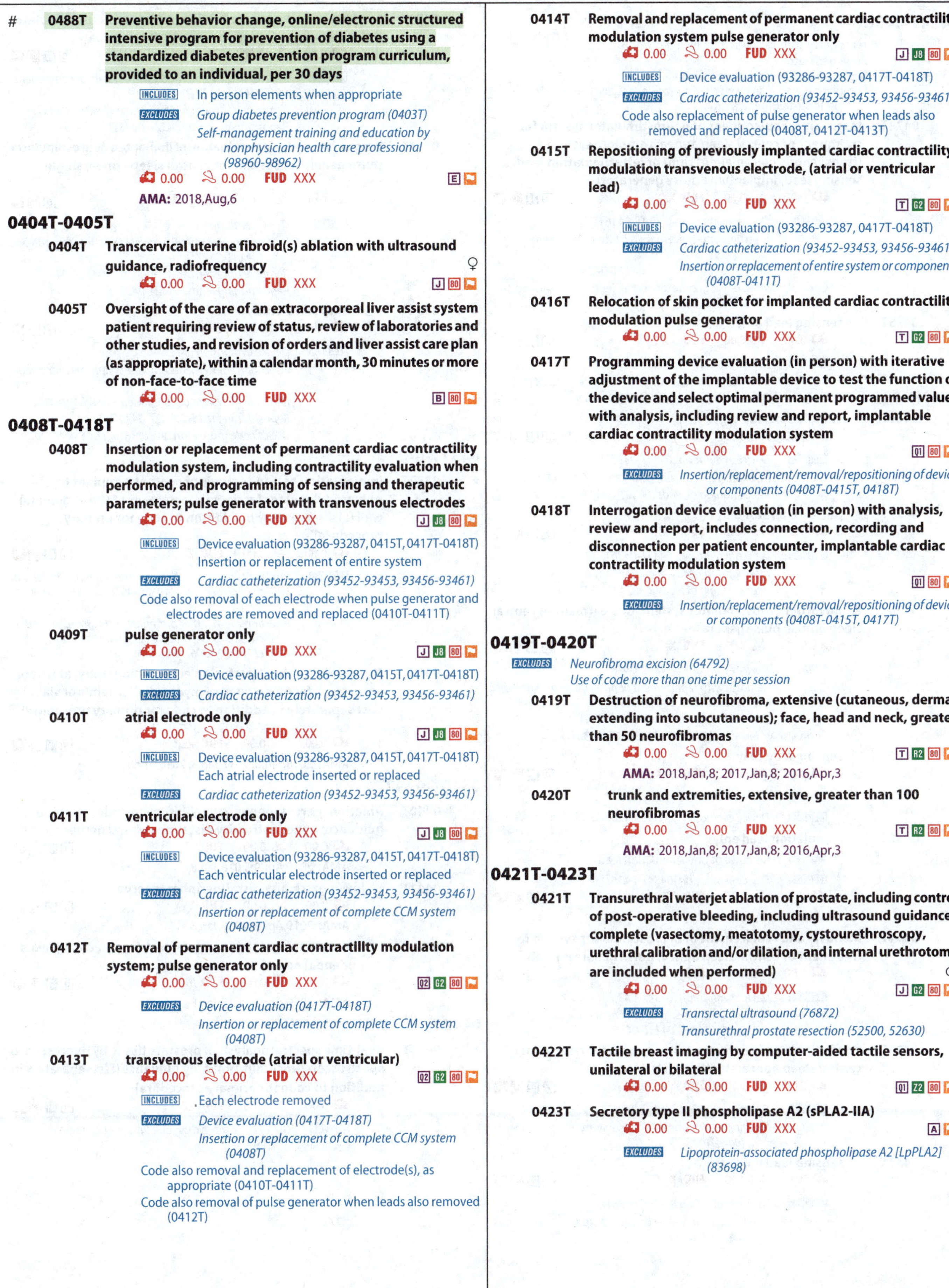

\# **0488T** **Preventive behavior change, online/electronic structured intensive program for prevention of diabetes using a standardized diabetes prevention program curriculum, provided to an individual, per 30 days**

INCLUDES In person elements when appropriate

EXCLUDES *Group diabetes prevention program (0403T)*
Self-management training and education by nonphysician health care professional (98960-98962)

0.00 0.00 FUD XXX E

AMA: 2018,Aug,6

0404T-0405T

0404T **Transcervical uterine fibroid(s) ablation with ultrasound guidance, radiofrequency** ♀

0.00 0.00 FUD XXX J 80

0405T **Oversight of the care of an extracorporeal liver assist system patient requiring review of status, review of laboratories and other studies, and revision of orders and liver assist care plan (as appropriate), within a calendar month, 30 minutes or more of non-face-to-face time**

0.00 0.00 FUD XXX B 80

0408T-0418T

0408T **Insertion or replacement of permanent cardiac contractility modulation system, including contractility evaluation when performed, and programming of sensing and therapeutic parameters; pulse generator with transvenous electrodes**

0.00 0.00 FUD XXX J J8 80

INCLUDES Device evaluation (93286-93287, 0415T, 0417T-0418T)
Insertion or replacement of entire system

EXCLUDES *Cardiac catheterization (93452-93453, 93456-93461)*

Code also removal of each electrode when pulse generator and electrodes are removed and replaced (0410T-0411T)

0409T **pulse generator only**

0.00 0.00 FUD XXX J J8 80

INCLUDES Device evaluation (93286-93287, 0415T, 0417T-0418T)

EXCLUDES *Cardiac catheterization (93452-93453, 93456-93461)*

0410T **atrial electrode only**

0.00 0.00 FUD XXX J J8 80

INCLUDES Device evaluation (93286-93287, 0415T, 0417T-0418T)
Each atrial electrode inserted or replaced

EXCLUDES *Cardiac catheterization (93452-93453, 93456-93461)*

0411T **ventricular electrode only**

0.00 0.00 FUD XXX J J8 80

INCLUDES Device evaluation (93286-93287, 0415T, 0417T-0418T)
Each ventricular electrode inserted or replaced

EXCLUDES *Cardiac catheterization (93452-93453, 93456-93461)*
Insertion or replacement of complete CCM system (0408T)

0412T **Removal of permanent cardiac contractility modulation system; pulse generator only**

0.00 0.00 FUD XXX Q2 G2 80

EXCLUDES *Device evaluation (0417T-0418T)*
Insertion or replacement of complete CCM system (0408T)

0413T **transvenous electrode (atrial or ventricular)**

0.00 0.00 FUD XXX Q2 G2 80

INCLUDES Each electrode removed

EXCLUDES *Device evaluation (0417T-0418T)*
Insertion or replacement of complete CCM system (0408T)

Code also removal and replacement of electrode(s), as appropriate (0410T-0411T)

Code also removal of pulse generator when leads also removed (0412T)

0414T **Removal and replacement of permanent cardiac contractility modulation system pulse generator only**

0.00 0.00 FUD XXX J J8 80

INCLUDES Device evaluation (93286-93287, 0417T-0418T)

EXCLUDES *Cardiac catheterization (93452-93453, 93456-93461)*

Code also replacement of pulse generator when leads also removed and replaced (0408T, 0412T-0413T)

0415T **Repositioning of previously implanted cardiac contractility modulation transvenous electrode, (atrial or ventricular lead)**

0.00 0.00 FUD XXX T G2 80

INCLUDES Device evaluation (93286-93287, 0417T-0418T)

EXCLUDES *Cardiac catheterization (93452-93453, 93456-93461)*
Insertion or replacement of entire system or components (0408T-0411T)

0416T **Relocation of skin pocket for implanted cardiac contractility modulation pulse generator**

0.00 0.00 FUD XXX T G2 80

0417T **Programming device evaluation (in person) with iterative adjustment of the implantable device to test the function of the device and select optimal permanent programmed values with analysis, including review and report, implantable cardiac contractility modulation system**

0.00 0.00 FUD XXX Q1 80

EXCLUDES *Insertion/replacement/removal/repositioning of device or components (0408T-0415T, 0418T)*

0418T **Interrogation device evaluation (in person) with analysis, review and report, includes connection, recording and disconnection per patient encounter, implantable cardiac contractility modulation system**

0.00 0.00 FUD XXX Q1 80

EXCLUDES *Insertion/replacement/removal/repositioning of device or components (0408T-0415T, 0417T)*

0419T-0420T

EXCLUDES *Neurofibroma excision (64792)*
Use of code more than one time per session

0419T **Destruction of neurofibroma, extensive (cutaneous, dermal extending into subcutaneous); face, head and neck, greater than 50 neurofibromas**

0.00 0.00 FUD XXX T R2 80

AMA: 2018,Jan,8; 2017,Jan,8; 2016,Apr,3

0420T **trunk and extremities, extensive, greater than 100 neurofibromas**

0.00 0.00 FUD XXX T R2 80

AMA: 2018,Jan,8; 2017,Jan,8; 2016,Apr,3

0421T-0423T

0421T **Transurethral waterjet ablation of prostate, including control of post-operative bleeding, including ultrasound guidance, complete (vasectomy, meatotomy, cystourethroscopy, urethral calibration and/or dilation, and internal urethrotomy are included when performed)** ♂

0.00 0.00 FUD XXX J G2 80

EXCLUDES *Transrectal ultrasound (76872)*
Transurethral prostate resection (52500, 52630)

0422T **Tactile breast imaging by computer-aided tactile sensors, unilateral or bilateral**

0.00 0.00 FUD XXX Q1 Z2 80

0423T **Secretory type II phospholipase A2 (sPLA2-IIA)**

0.00 0.00 FUD XXX A

EXCLUDES *Lipoprotein-associated phospholipase A2 [LpPLA2] (83698)*

0424T-0436T

INCLUDES Phrenic nerve stimulation system includes:
- Pulse generator
- Sensing lead (placed in azygos vein)
- Stimulation lead (placed into right brachiocephalic vein or left pericardiophrenic vein)

0424T **Insertion or replacement of neurostimulator system for treatment of central sleep apnea; complete system (transvenous placement of right or left stimulation lead, sensing lead, implantable pulse generator)**
0.00 0.00 FUD XXX J J8 80

INCLUDES Device evaluation (0434T-0436T)
Insertion or replacement system components (0425T-0427T)
Repositioning of leads (0432T-0433T)
Code also when pulse generator and all leads are removed and replaced (0428T-0430T)

0425T **sensing lead only**
0.00 0.00 FUD XXX J G2 80

EXCLUDES *Device evaluation (0434T-0436T)*
Insertion/replacement complete system (0424T)
Repositioning of leads (0432T-0433T)

0426T **stimulation lead only**
0.00 0.00 FUD XXX J G2 80

EXCLUDES *Device evaluation (0434T-0436T)*
Insertion/replacement complete system (0424T)
Repositioning of leads (0432T-0433T)

0427T **pulse generator only**
0.00 0.00 FUD XXX J G2 80

EXCLUDES *Device evaluation (0434T-0436T)*
Insertion/replacement complete system (0424T)
Repositioning of leads (0432T-0433T)

0428T **Removal of neurostimulator system for treatment of central sleep apnea; pulse generator only**
0.00 0.00 FUD XXX Q2 G2 80

EXCLUDES *Device evaluation (0434T-0436T)*
Removal with replacement of pulse generator and all leads (0424T, 0429T-0430T)
Repositioning of leads (0432T-0433T)
Code also when a lead is removed (0429T-0430T)

0429T **sensing lead only**
0.00 0.00 FUD XXX Q2 G2 80

INCLUDES Removal of one sensing lead
EXCLUDES *Device evaluation (0434T-0436T)*

0430T **stimulation lead only**

INCLUDES Removal of one stimulation lead
EXCLUDES *Device evaluation (0434T-0436T)*
0.00 0.00 FUD XXX Q2 G2 80
AMA: 2015,Aug,4

0431T **Removal and replacement of neurostimulator system for treatment of central sleep apnea, pulse generator only**
0.00 0.00 FUD XXX J G2 80

EXCLUDES *Device evaluation (0434T-0436T)*
Removal with replacement of generator and all three leads (0424T, 0428T-0430T)

0432T **Repositioning of neurostimulator system for treatment of central sleep apnea; stimulation lead only**
0.00 0.00 FUD XXX T G2 80

EXCLUDES *Device evaluation (0434T-0436T)*
Insertion/replacement complete system or components (0424T-0427T)

0433T **sensing lead only**
0.00 0.00 FUD XXX T G2 80

EXCLUDES *Device evaluation (0434T-0436T)*
Insertion/replacement complete system or components (0424T-0427T)

0434T **Interrogation device evaluation implanted neurostimulator pulse generator system for central sleep apnea**
0.00 0.00 FUD XXX S G2 80

EXCLUDES *Insertion/replacement complete system or components (0424T-0427T)*
Removal of system or components (0428T-0431T)
Repositioning leads (0432T-0433T)

0435T **Programming device evaluation of implanted neurostimulator pulse generator system for central sleep apnea; single session**
0.00 0.00 FUD XXX S 80

EXCLUDES *Device evaluation (0436T)*
Insertion/replacement complete system or components (0424T-0427T)
Removal of system or components (0428T-0431T)
Repositioning leads (0432T-0433T)

0436T **during sleep study**
0.00 0.00 FUD XXX S 80

EXCLUDES *Device evaluation (0435T)*
Insertion/replacement complete system or components (0424T-0427T)
Removal of system or components (0428T-0431T)
Repositioning leads (0432T-0433T)
Use of code more than one time for each sleep study

0437T-0439T

+ **0437T** **Implantation of non-biologic or synthetic implant (eg, polypropylene) for fascial reinforcement of the abdominal wall (List separately in addition to code for primary procedure)**
0.00 0.00 FUD ZZZ N N1 80

EXCLUDES *Implantation mesh, other material for repair incisional or ventral hernia (49560-49561, 49565-49566, 49568)*
Insertion mesh, other material for closure of wound caused by necrotizing soft tissue infection (11004-11006, 49568)

+ **0439T** **Myocardial contrast perfusion echocardiography, at rest or with stress, for assessment of myocardial ischemia or viability (List separately in addition to code for primary procedure)**
Code first (93306-93308, 93350-93351)
0.00 0.00 FUD ZZZ N N1 80
AMA: 2018,Jan,8; 2017,Jan,8; 2016,Apr,8

0440T-0442T

0440T **Ablation, percutaneous, cryoablation, includes imaging guidance; upper extremity distal/peripheral nerve**
0.00 0.00 FUD YYY J G2 80
AMA: 2019,Apr,9; 2018,Jan,8

0441T **lower extremity distal/peripheral nerve**
0.00 0.00 FUD YYY J G2 80
AMA: 2019,Apr,9; 2018,Jan,8

0442T **nerve plexus or other truncal nerve (eg, brachial plexus, pudendal nerve)**
0.00 0.00 FUD YYY J G2 80
AMA: 2019,Apr,9; 2018,Jan,8

0443T

+ **0443T** **Real-time spectral analysis of prostate tissue by fluorescence spectroscopy, including imaging guidance (List separately in addition to code for primary procedure)** ♂
0.00 0.00 FUD ZZZ N N1 80

EXCLUDES *Use of code more than one time for each session*
Code also (55700)

0444T-0445T

EXCLUDES *Insertion/removal drug-eluting stent into canaliculus (0356T)*

0444T Initial placement of a drug-eluting ocular insert under one or more eyelids, including fitting, training, and insertion, unilateral or bilateral

0.00 0.00 **FUD** YYY N N1 80

AMA: 2018,Jan,8; 2017,Aug,7

0445T Subsequent placement of a drug-eluting ocular insert under one or more eyelids, including re-training, and removal of existing insert, unilateral or bilateral

0.00 0.00 **FUD** YYY N N1 80

AMA: 2018,Jan,8; 2017,Aug,7

0446T-0448T

EXCLUDES *Placement non-implantable interstitial glucose sensor without pocket (95250)*

0446T Creation of subcutaneous pocket with insertion of implantable interstitial glucose sensor, including system activation and patient training

EXCLUDES *Interpretation/report of ambulatory glucose monitoring of interstitial tissue (95251)*
Removal interstitial glucose sensor (0447T-0448T)

0.00 0.00 **FUD** YYY T G2

AMA: 2018,Jun,6

0447T Removal of implantable interstitial glucose sensor from subcutaneous pocket via incision

0.00 0.00 **FUD** YYY Q2 G2

0448T Removal of implantable interstitial glucose sensor with creation of subcutaneous pocket at different anatomic site and insertion of new implantable sensor, including system activation

0.00 0.00 **FUD** YYY T G2

EXCLUDES *Initial insertion of sensor (0446T)*
Removal of sensor (0447T)

0449T-0450T

EXCLUDES *Removal by internal approach of aqueous drainage device without extraocular reservoir in subconjunctival space (92499)*

0449T Insertion of aqueous drainage device, without extraocular reservoir, internal approach, into the subconjunctival space; initial device

0.00 0.00 **FUD** YYY J J8

AMA: 2018,Sep,3; 2018,Jul,3

\+ **0450T each additional device (List separately in addition to code for primary procedure)**

Code first (0449T)

0.00 0.00 **FUD** YYY N N1

AMA: 2018,Jul,3

0451T-0463T

INCLUDES Access procedures (36000-36010)
Catheterization of vessel (36200-36228)
Diagnostic angiography (75600-75774)
Imaging guidance (76000, 76936-76937, 77001-77002, 77011-77012, 77021)
Injection procedures (93561-93572)
Radiological supervision and interpretation

EXCLUDES *Cardiac catheterization (93451-93533)*

0451T Insertion or replacement of a permanently implantable aortic counterpulsation ventricular assist system, endovascular approach, and programming of sensing and therapeutic parameters; complete system (counterpulsation device, vascular graft, implantable vascular hemostatic seal, mechano-electrical skin interface and subcutaneous electrodes)

EXCLUDES *Aortic counterpulsation ventricular assist system procedures (0452T-0458T)*
Insertion intra-aortic balloon assist device (33967, 33970, 33973)
Insertion/replacement extracorporeal ventricular assist device (33975-33976, 33981)
Insertion/replacement intracorporeal ventricular assist device (33979, 33982-33983)
Insertion ventricular assist device (33990-33991)

0.00 0.00 **FUD** YYY C

AMA: 2017,Dec,3

0452T aortic counterpulsation device and vascular hemostatic seal

EXCLUDES *Insertion intra-aortic balloon assist device (33973)*
Insertion intracorporeal ventricular assist device (33979, 33982-33983)
Insertion/replacement counterpulsation ventricular assist system procedures (0451T)
Insertion ventricular assist device (33990-33991)
Removal counterpulsation ventricular assist system (0455T-0456T)

0.00 0.00 **FUD** YYY C

AMA: 2017,Dec,3

0453T mechano-electrical skin interface

0.00 0.00 **FUD** YYY J

EXCLUDES *Insertion intra-aortic balloon assist device (33973)*
Insertion intracorporeal ventricular assist device (33979, 33982-33983)
Insertion/replacement counterpulsation ventricular assist system procedures (0451T)
Insertion ventricular assist device (33990-33991)
Removal counterpulsation ventricular assist system (0455T, 0457T)

0454T subcutaneous electrode

0.00 0.00 **FUD** YYY J

INCLUDES Each electrode inserted or replaced

EXCLUDES *Insertion intra-aortic balloon assist device (33973, 33982-33983)*
Insertion/replacement counterpulsation ventricular assist system (0451T)
Insertion/replacement intracorporeal ventricular assist device (33979, 33982-33983)
Insertion ventricular assist device (33990-33991)
Removal device or component (0455T, 0458T)

0455T **Removal of permanently implantable aortic counterpulsation ventricular assist system; complete system (aortic counterpulsation device, vascular hemostatic seal, mechano-electrical skin interface and electrodes)**

EXCLUDES *Insertion/replacement system or component (0451T-0454T)*
Removal:
Extracorporeal ventricular assist device (33977-33978)
Intra-aortic balloon assist device (33968, 33971, 33974)
Intracorporeal ventricular assist device (33980)
Percutaneous ventricular assist device (33992)
System or component (0456T-0458T)

0.00 0.00 FUD YYY C

AMA: 2017,Dec,3

0456T **aortic counterpulsation device and vascular hemostatic seal**

EXCLUDES *Insertion/replacement system or component (0451T-0452T)*
Removal:
Aortic counterpulsation ventricular assist system (0455T)
Intra-aortic balloon assist device (33974)
Intracorporeal ventricular assist device (33980)
Percutaneous ventricular assist device (33992)

0.00 0.00 FUD YYY C

AMA: 2017,Dec,3

0457T **mechano-electrical skin interface**

0.00 0.00 FUD YYY Q2

EXCLUDES *Insertion/replacement system or component (0451T, 0453T)*
Removal:
Aortic counterpulsation ventricular assist system (0455T)
Intra-aortic balloon assist device (33974)
Intracorporeal ventricular assist device (33980)
Percutaneous ventricular assist device (33992)

0458T **subcutaneous electrode**

0.00 0.00 FUD YYY Q2

INCLUDES Each electrode removed

EXCLUDES *Insertion/replacement system or component (0451T, 0454T)*
Removal:
Aortic counterpulsation ventricular assist system (0455T)
Intra-aortic balloon assist device (33974)
Intracorporeal ventricular assist device (33980)
Percutaneous ventricular assist device (33992)

0459T **Relocation of skin pocket with replacement of implanted aortic counterpulsation ventricular assist device, mechano-electrical skin interface and electrodes**

0.00 0.00 FUD YYY C

EXCLUDES *Repositioning percutaneous ventricular assist device (33993)*

0460T **Repositioning of previously implanted aortic counterpulsation ventricular assist device; subcutaneous electrode**

0.00 0.00 FUD YYY T

INCLUDES Reporting for repositioning of each electrode

EXCLUDES *Insertion/replacement system or component (0451T, 0454T)*
Repositioning of percutaneous ventricular assist device (33993)

0461T **aortic counterpulsation device**

0.00 0.00 FUD YYY C

EXCLUDES *Repositioning percutaneous ventricular assist device (33993)*

0462T **Programming device evaluation (in person) with iterative adjustment of the implantable mechano-electrical skin interface and/or external driver to test the function of the device and select optimal permanent programmed values with analysis, including review and report, implantable aortic counterpulsation ventricular assist system, per day**

0.00 0.00 FUD YYY S

EXCLUDES *Device evaluation (0463T)*
Insertion/replacement system or component (0451T-0454T)
Relocation of pocket (0459T)
Removal system or component (0455T-0458T)
Repositioning device (0460T-0461T)

0463T **Interrogation device evaluation (in person) with analysis, review and report, includes connection, recording and disconnection per patient encounter, implantable aortic counterpulsation ventricular assist system, per day**

0.00 0.00 FUD YYY S

EXCLUDES *Device evaluation (0462T)*
Insertion/replacement system or component (0451T-0454T)
Relocation of pocket (0459T)
Removal system or component (0455T-0458T)
Repositioning device (0460T-0461T)

0464T [0464T]

0464T **Resequenced code. See code following 0333T.**

0465T-0469T

EXCLUDES *Replacement/revision cranial nerve neurostimulator electrode array (64569)*

0465T **Suprachoroidal injection of a pharmacologic agent (does not include supply of medication)**

EXCLUDES *Intravitreal implantation or injection (67025-67028)*

0.00 0.00 FUD YYY T R2

AMA: 2018,Feb,3

\+ **0466T** **Insertion of chest wall respiratory sensor electrode or electrode array, including connection to pulse generator (List separately in addition to code for primary procedure)**

EXCLUDES *Revision/removal chest wall respiratory sensor electrode or array (0467T-0468T)*

Code first (64568)

0.00 0.00 FUD YYY N N1

AMA: 2018,Mar,9; 2018,Jan,8; 2017,Jan,8; 2016,Nov,6

0467T **Revision or replacement of chest wall respiratory sensor electrode or electrode array, including connection to existing pulse generator**

EXCLUDES *Insertion/removal chest wall respiratory sensor electrode or array (0466T, 0468T)*
Replacement/revision cranial nerve neurostimulator electrode array (64569)

0.00 0.00 FUD YYY Q2 N1

AMA: 2018,Mar,9; 2018,Jan,8; 2017,Jan,8; 2016,Nov,6

0468T **Removal of chest wall respiratory sensor electrode or electrode array**

EXCLUDES *Insertion/removal chest wall respiratory sensor electrode or array (0466T-0467T)*
Removal cranial neurostimulator electrode array (64570)

0.00 0.00 FUD YYY Q2 N1

AMA: 2018,Mar,9; 2018,Jan,8; 2017,Jan,8; 2016,Nov,6

0469T **Retinal polarization scan, ocular screening with on-site automated results, bilateral**

INCLUDES Ophthalmic medical services (92002-92014)

EXCLUDES *Ocular screening (99174, [99177])*

0.00 0.00 FUD XXX E

AMA: 2018,Feb,3

0470T-0471T

EXCLUDES *Optical coherence tomography of coronary vessel or graft (92978-92979)*
Reflectance confocal microscopy (RCM) for cellular and subcellular skin imaging (96931-96936)

0470T Optical coherence tomography (OCT) for microstructural and morphological imaging of skin, image acquisition, interpretation, and report; first lesion
0.00 0.00 FUD XXX M

\+ **0471T each additional lesion (List separately in addition to code for primary procedure)**
0.00 0.00 FUD XXX N N1
Code first (0470T)

0472T-0474T

0472T Device evaluation, interrogation, and initial programming of intraocular retinal electrode array (eg, retinal prosthesis), in person, with iterative adjustment of the implantable device to test functionality, select optimal permanent programmed values with analysis, including visual training, with review and report by a qualified health care professional
0.00 0.00 FUD XXX Q1
AMA: 2018,Feb,3

0473T Device evaluation and interrogation of intraocular retinal electrode array (eg, retinal prosthesis), in person, including reprogramming and visual training, when performed, with review and report by a qualified health care professional
INCLUDES Reprogramming of device (0473T)
EXCLUDES *Placement of intra-ocular retinal electrode display (0100T)*
0.00 0.00 FUD XXX Q1
AMA: 2018,Feb,3

0474T Insertion of anterior segment aqueous drainage device, with creation of intraocular reservoir, internal approach, into the supraciliary space
0.00 0.00 FUD XXX J
AMA: 2018,Dec,8; 2018,Dec,8; 2018,Jul,3; 2018,Feb,3

0475T-0478T

0475T Recording of fetal magnetic cardiac signal using at least 3 channels; patient recording and storage, data scanning with signal extraction, technical analysis and result, as well as supervision, review, and interpretation of report by a physician or other qualified health care professional
0.00 0.00 FUD XXX M

0476T patient recording, data scanning, with raw electronic signal transfer of data and storage
0.00 0.00 FUD XXX Q1

0477T signal extraction, technical analysis, and result
0.00 0.00 FUD XXX Q1

0478T review, interpretation, report by physician or other qualified health care professional
0.00 0.00 FUD XXX M

0479T-0480T

EXCLUDES *Ablative laser treatment for additional square cm for open wound (0492T)*
Cicatricial lesion excision (11400-11446)
Use of code more than one time per day

0479T Fractional ablative laser fenestration of burn and traumatic scars for functional improvement; first 100 cm2 or part thereof, or 1% of body surface area of infants and children
0.00 0.00 FUD 000 T G2
AMA: 2018,Jan,8; 2017,Dec,13

\+ **0480T each additional 100 cm2, or each additional 1% of body surface area of infants and children, or part thereof (List separately in addition to code for primary procedure)**
Code first (0479T)
0.00 0.00 FUD ZZZ N N1
AMA: 2018,Jan,8; 2017,Dec,13

0481T-0482T

0481T Injection(s), autologous white blood cell concentrate (autologous protein solution), any site, including image guidance, harvesting and preparation, when performed
0.00 0.00 FUD 000 Q1
EXCLUDES *Blood collection (36415, 36592)*
Bone marrow procedures (38220-38222, 38230)
Imaging guidance (76942, 77002, 77012, 77021)
Injection of platelet rich plasma (0232T)
Injections to tendon, ligament, or fascia (20550-20551)
Joint aspiration or injection (20600-20611)
Other tissue grafts ([15769], 15771-15774)
Pooling of platelets (86965)

~~**0482T Absolute quantitation of myocardial blood flow, positron emission tomography (PET), rest and stress (List separately in addition to code for primary procedure)**~~

0483T-0484T

INCLUDES Access and closure
Angiography
Balloon valvuloplasty
Contrast injections
Fluoroscopy
Radiological supervision and interpretation
Valve deployment and repositioning
Ventriculography
EXCLUDES *Diagnostic heart catheterization (93451-93453, 93456-93461, 93530-93533)*
Transcatheter mitral valve annulus reconstruction (0544T)
Transcatheter mitral valve repair through coronary sinus (0345T)
Transcatheter mitral valve repair with transseptal puncture, when performed (33418-33419)
Transcatheter tricuspid valve annulus reconstruction (0545T)
Code also cardiopulmonary bypass when provided (33367-33369)
Code also diagnostic cardiac catheterization procedures if there is no previous study available and append modifier 59 when:
The condition of the patient has changed
The previous study is inadequate

0483T Transcatheter mitral valve implantation/replacement (TMVI) with prosthetic valve; percutaneous approach, including transseptal puncture, when performed
0.00 0.00 FUD 000 C 80

0484T transthoracic exposure (eg, thoracotomy, transapical)
0.00 0.00 FUD 000 C 80

0485T-0486T

0485T Optical coherence tomography (OCT) of middle ear, with interpretation and report; unilateral
0.00 0.00 FUD XXX Q1 50

0486T bilateral
0.00 0.00 FUD XXX Q1

0487T-0488T [0488T]

0487T Biomechanical mapping, transvaginal, with report
0.00 0.00 FUD XXX Q1 N1

0488T **Resequenced code. See code following 0403T.**

0489T-0490T

EXCLUDES *Joint injection/aspiration (20600, 20604)*
Liposuction procedures (15876-15879)
Tissue grafts ([15769], 15771-15774)
Code also for complete procedure report both codes (0489T-0490T)

0489T Autologous adipose-derived regenerative cell therapy for scleroderma in the hands; adipose tissue harvesting, isolation and preparation of harvested cells including incubation with cell dissociation enzymes, removal of non-viable cells and debris, determination of concentration and dilution of regenerative cells
0.00 0.00 FUD 000 E
AMA: 2018,Sep,12

0490T multiple injections in one or both hands
EXCLUDES *Single injections*
0.00 0.00 FUD 000 E
AMA: 2018,Sep,12

0491T-0493T

0491T Ablative laser treatment, non-contact, full field and fractional ablation, open wound, per day, total treatment surface area; first 20 sq cm or less

0.00 0.00 FUD 000 T G2

+ **0492T each additional 20 sq cm, or part thereof (List separately in addition to code for primary procedure)**

0.00 0.00 FUD ZZZ N N1

EXCLUDES *Laser fenestration for scars (0479T-0480T)*

Code first (0491T)

0493T Near-infrared spectroscopy studies of lower extremity wounds (eg, for oxyhemoglobin measurement)

0.00 0.00 FUD XXX N N1

0494T-0496T

0494T Surgical preparation and cannulation of marginal (extended) cadaver donor lung(s) to ex vivo organ perfusion system, including decannulation, separation from the perfusion system, and cold preservation of the allograft prior to implantation, when performed

0.00 0.00 FUD XXX C 80

0495T Initiation and monitoring marginal (extended) cadaver donor lung(s) organ perfusion system by physician or qualified health care professional, including physiological and laboratory assessment (eg, pulmonary artery flow, pulmonary artery pressure, left atrial pressure, pulmonary vascular resistance, mean/peak and plateau airway pressure, dynamic compliance and perfusate gas analysis), including bronchoscopy and X ray when performed; first two hours in sterile field

0.00 0.00 FUD XXX C

+ **0496T each additional hour (List separately in addition to code for primary procedure)**

0.00 0.00 FUD ZZZ C

Code first (0495T)

0497T-0498T

EXCLUDES *ECG event monitoring (93268, 93271-93272)*
ECG rhythm strips (93040-93042)
External ECG monitoring for more than 48 hours and less than 21 days (0295T-0298T)
Remote telemetry (93228-93229)

0497T External patient-activated, physician- or other qualified health care professional-prescribed, electrocardiographic rhythm derived event recorder without 24 hour attended monitoring; in-office connection

0.00 0.00 FUD XXX Q1 TC

0498T review and interpretation by a physician or other qualified health care professional per 30 days with at least one patient-generated triggered event

0.00 0.00 FUD XXX M 26

0499T-0500T

0499T Cystourethroscopy, with mechanical dilation and urethral therapeutic drug delivery for urethral stricture or stenosis, including fluoroscopy, when performed

0.00 0.00 FUD 000 E

EXCLUDES *Cystourethroscopy for stricture (52281, 52283)*

0500T Infectious agent detection by nucleic acid (DNA or RNA), human papillomavirus (HPV) for five or more separately reported high-risk HPV types (eg, 16, 18, 31, 33, 35, 39, 45, 51, 52, 56, 58, 59, 68) (ie, genotyping)

0.00 0.00 FUD XXX A

EXCLUDES *Less than five high-risk HPV types ([87624, 87625])*

0501T-0523T [0523T]

EXCLUDES *Use of code more than one time for each CT angiogram*

0501T Noninvasive estimated coronary fractional flow reserve (FFR) derived from coronary computed tomography angiography data using computation fluid dynamics physiologic simulation software analysis of functional data to assess the severity of coronary artery disease; data preparation and transmission, analysis of fluid dynamics and simulated maximal coronary hyperemia, generation of estimated FFR model, with anatomical data review in comparison with estimated FFR model to reconcile discordant data, interpretation and report

INCLUDES All components of complete test (0501T-0504T)

0.00 0.00 FUD XXX M

AMA: 2018,Sep,10

0502T data preparation and transmission

0.00 0.00 FUD XXX N N1 TC

AMA: 2018,Sep,10

0503T analysis of fluid dynamics and simulated maximal coronary hyperemia, and generation of estimated FFR model

0.00 0.00 FUD XXX S N1 TC

AMA: 2018,Sep,10

0504T anatomical data review in comparison with estimated FFR model to reconcile discordant data, interpretation and report

0.00 0.00 FUD XXX M 26

AMA: 2018,Sep,10

+ # **0523T Intraprocedural coronary fractional flow reserve (FFR) with 3D functional mapping of color-coded FFR values for the coronary tree, derived from coronary angiogram data, for real-time review and interpretation of possible atherosclerotic stenosis(es) intervention (List separately in addition to code for primary procedure)**

0.00 0.00 FUD ZZZ N1 80

EXCLUDES *3-D rendering with interpretation (76376-76377)*
Coronary artery doppler studies (93571-93572)
Noninvasive estimated coronary fractional flow reserve (FFR) (0501T-0504T)
Procedure reported more than one time for each session

Code first (93454-93461)

0505T-0514T [0510T, 0511T, 0512T, 0513T]

0505T Endovenous femoral-popliteal arterial revascularization, with transcatheter placement of intravascular stent graft(s) and closure by any method, including percutaneous or open vascular access, ultrasound guidance for vascular access when performed, all catheterization(s) and intraprocedural roadmapping and imaging guidance necessary to complete the intervention, all associated radiological supervision and interpretation, when performed, with crossing of the occlusive lesion in an extraluminal fashion

0.00 0.00 FUD YYY 80

INCLUDES All procedures performed on the same side:
Catheterization (arterial and venous)
Diagnostic imaging for arteriography
Radiologic supervision and interpretation
Ultrasound guidance (76937)

EXCLUDES *Balloon angioplasty of arteries other than dialysis circuit ([37248, 37249])*
Revascularization femoral or popliteal artery (37224-37227)
Venous stenting (37238-37239)

0506T Macular pigment optical density measurement by heterochromatic flicker photometry, unilateral or bilateral, with interpretation and report

0.00 0.00 FUD XXX 80

AMA: 2018,Dec,6; 2018,Dec,6

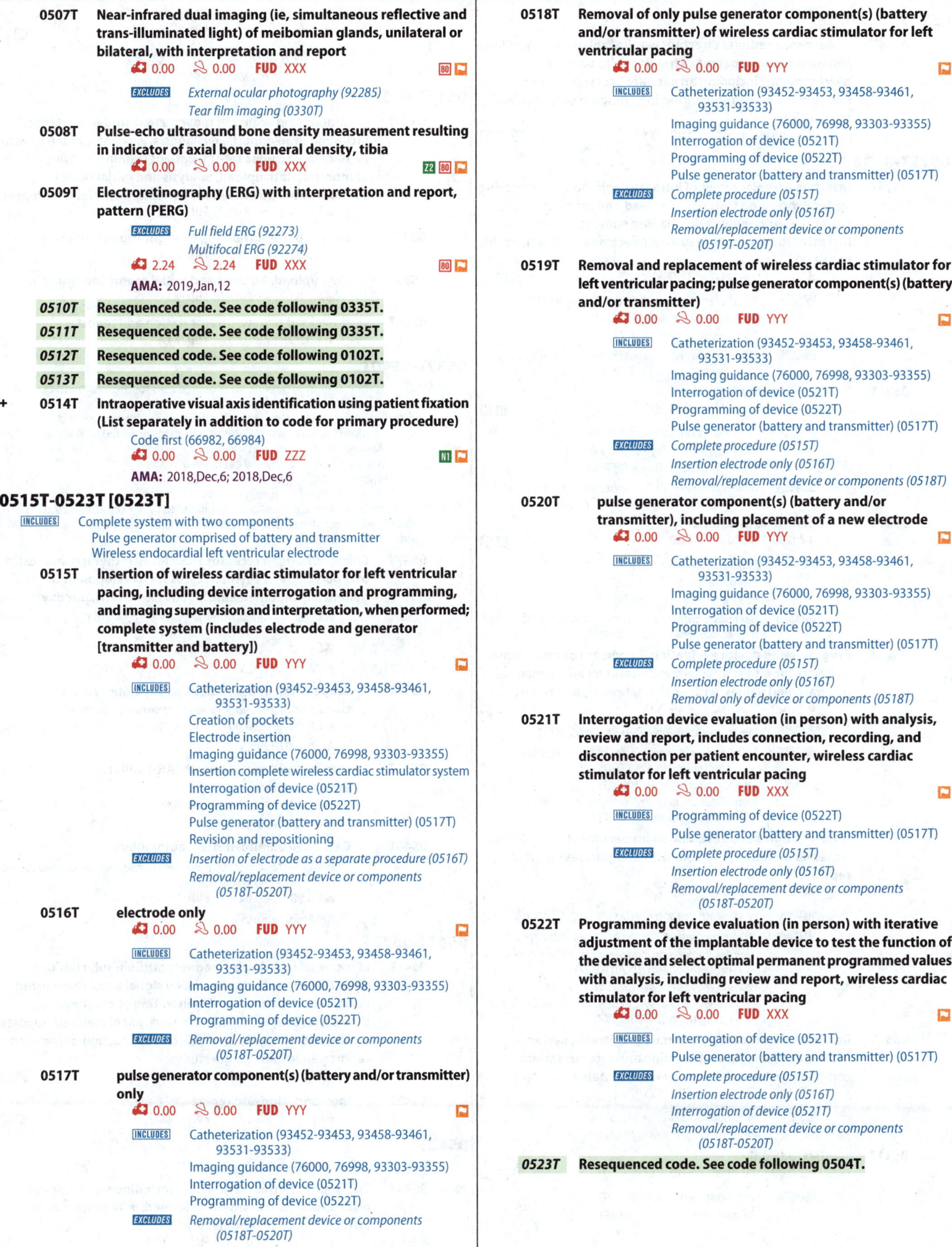

0507T **Near-infrared dual imaging (ie, simultaneous reflective and trans-illuminated light) of meibomian glands, unilateral or bilateral, with interpretation and report**
0.00 0.00 FUD XXX 80
EXCLUDES *External ocular photography (92285)*
Tear film imaging (0330T)

0508T **Pulse-echo ultrasound bone density measurement resulting in indicator of axial bone mineral density, tibia**
0.00 0.00 FUD XXX Z2 80

0509T **Electroretinography (ERG) with interpretation and report, pattern (PERG)**
EXCLUDES *Full field ERG (92273)*
Multifocal ERG (92274)
2.24 2.24 FUD XXX 80
AMA: 2019,Jan,12

0510T **Resequenced code. See code following 0335T.**

0511T **Resequenced code. See code following 0335T.**

0512T **Resequenced code. See code following 0102T.**

0513T **Resequenced code. See code following 0102T.**

\+ **0514T** **Intraoperative visual axis identification using patient fixation (List separately in addition to code for primary procedure)**
Code first (66982, 66984)
0.00 0.00 FUD ZZZ N1
AMA: 2018,Dec,6; 2018,Dec,6

0515T-0523T [0523T]

INCLUDES Complete system with two components
Pulse generator comprised of battery and transmitter
Wireless endocardial left ventricular electrode

0515T **Insertion of wireless cardiac stimulator for left ventricular pacing, including device interrogation and programming, and imaging supervision and interpretation, when performed; complete system (includes electrode and generator [transmitter and battery])**
0.00 0.00 FUD YYY
INCLUDES Catheterization (93452-93453, 93458-93461, 93531-93533)
Creation of pockets
Electrode insertion
Imaging guidance (76000, 76998, 93303-93355)
Insertion complete wireless cardiac stimulator system
Interrogation of device (0521T)
Programming of device (0522T)
Pulse generator (battery and transmitter) (0517T)
Revision and repositioning
EXCLUDES *Insertion of electrode as a separate procedure (0516T)*
Removal/replacement device or components (0518T-0520T)

0516T **electrode only**
0.00 0.00 FUD YYY
INCLUDES Catheterization (93452-93453, 93458-93461, 93531-93533)
Imaging guidance (76000, 76998, 93303-93355)
Interrogation of device (0521T)
Programming of device (0522T)
EXCLUDES *Removal/replacement device or components (0518T-0520T)*

0517T **pulse generator component(s) (battery and/or transmitter) only**
0.00 0.00 FUD YYY
INCLUDES Catheterization (93452-93453, 93458-93461, 93531-93533)
Imaging guidance (76000, 76998, 93303-93355)
Interrogation of device (0521T)
Programming of device (0522T)
EXCLUDES *Removal/replacement device or components (0518T-0520T)*

0518T **Removal of only pulse generator component(s) (battery and/or transmitter) of wireless cardiac stimulator for left ventricular pacing**
0.00 0.00 FUD YYY
INCLUDES Catheterization (93452-93453, 93458-93461, 93531-93533)
Imaging guidance (76000, 76998, 93303-93355)
Interrogation of device (0521T)
Programming of device (0522T)
Pulse generator (battery and transmitter) (0517T)
EXCLUDES *Complete procedure (0515T)*
Insertion electrode only (0516T)
Removal/replacement device or components (0519T-0520T)

0519T **Removal and replacement of wireless cardiac stimulator for left ventricular pacing; pulse generator component(s) (battery and/or transmitter)**
0.00 0.00 FUD YYY
INCLUDES Catheterization (93452-93453, 93458-93461, 93531-93533)
Imaging guidance (76000, 76998, 93303-93355)
Interrogation of device (0521T)
Programming of device (0522T)
Pulse generator (battery and transmitter) (0517T)
EXCLUDES *Complete procedure (0515T)*
Insertion electrode only (0516T)
Removal/replacement device or components (0518T)

0520T **pulse generator component(s) (battery and/or transmitter), including placement of a new electrode**
0.00 0.00 FUD YYY
INCLUDES Catheterization (93452-93453, 93458-93461, 93531-93533)
Imaging guidance (76000, 76998, 93303-93355)
Interrogation of device (0521T)
Programming of device (0522T)
Pulse generator (battery and transmitter) (0517T)
EXCLUDES *Complete procedure (0515T)*
Insertion electrode only (0516T)
Removal only of device or components (0518T)

0521T **Interrogation device evaluation (in person) with analysis, review and report, includes connection, recording, and disconnection per patient encounter, wireless cardiac stimulator for left ventricular pacing**
0.00 0.00 FUD XXX
INCLUDES Programming of device (0522T)
Pulse generator (battery and transmitter) (0517T)
EXCLUDES *Complete procedure (0515T)*
Insertion electrode only (0516T)
Removal/replacement device or components (0518T-0520T)

0522T **Programming device evaluation (in person) with iterative adjustment of the implantable device to test the function of the device and select optimal permanent programmed values with analysis, including review and report, wireless cardiac stimulator for left ventricular pacing**
0.00 0.00 FUD XXX
INCLUDES Interrogation of device (0521T)
Pulse generator (battery and transmitter) (0517T)
EXCLUDES *Complete procedure (0515T)*
Insertion electrode only (0516T)
Interrogation of device (0521T)
Removal/replacement device or components (0518T-0520T)

0523T **Resequenced code. See code following 0504T.**

0524T

0524T Endovenous catheter directed chemical ablation with balloon isolation of incompetent extremity vein, open or percutaneous, including all vascular access, catheter manipulation, diagnostic imaging, imaging guidance and monitoring
0.00 0.00 FUD YYY G2 50

0525T-0532T

0525T Insertion or replacement of intracardiac ischemia monitoring system, including testing of the lead and monitor, initial system programming, and imaging supervision and interpretation; complete system (electrode and implantable monitor)
0.00 0.00 FUD YYY J8

INCLUDES Electrocardiography (93000, 93005, 93010)
Interrogation of device (0529T)
Programming of device (0528T)

EXCLUDES *Removal of intracardiac ischemia monitor or components (0530T-0532T)*

0526T electrode only
0.00 0.00 FUD YYY J8

INCLUDES Electrocardiography (93000, 93005, 93010)
Interrogation of device (0529T)
Programming of device (0528T)

EXCLUDES *Removal of intracardiac ischemia monitor or components (0530T-0532T)*

0527T implantable monitor only
0.00 0.00 FUD YYY G2

INCLUDES Electrocardiography (93000, 93005, 93010)
Interrogation of device (0529T)
Programming of device (0528T)

EXCLUDES *Removal of intracardiac ischemia monitor or components (0530T-0532T)*

0528T Programming device evaluation (in person) of intracardiac ischemia monitoring system with iterative adjustment of programmed values, with analysis, review, and report
0.00 0.00 FUD XXX

INCLUDES Electrocardiography (93000, 93005, 93010)

EXCLUDES *Insertion/replacement intracardiac ischemia monitor or components (0525T-0527T)*
Interrogation of device (0529T)
Removal of intracardiac ischemia monitor or components (0530T-0532T)

0529T Interrogation device evaluation (in person) of intracardiac ischemia monitoring system with analysis, review, and report
0.00 0.00 FUD XXX

INCLUDES Electrocardiography (93000, 93005, 93010)

EXCLUDES *Insertion/replacement electrode only (0526T)*
Insertion/replacement intracardiac ischemia monitor or comoponents (0525T-0527T)
Programming of device (0528T)
Removal of intracardiac ischemia monitor or components (0530T-0532T)

0530T Removal of intracardiac ischemia monitoring system, including all imaging supervision and interpretation; complete system (electrode and implantable monitor)
0.00 0.00 FUD YYY G2

EXCLUDES *Interrogation of device (0529T)*
Programming of device (0528T)

0531T electrode only
0.00 0.00 FUD YYY G2

EXCLUDES *Interrogation of device (0529T)*
Programming of device (0528T)

0532T implantable monitor only
0.00 0.00 FUD YYY G2

EXCLUDES *Interrogation of device (0529T)*
Programming of device (0528T)

0533T-0536T

0533T Continuous recording of movement disorder symptoms, including bradykinesia, dyskinesia, and tremor for 6 days up to 10 days; includes set-up, patient training, configuration of monitor, data upload, analysis and initial report configuration, download review, interpretation and report
0.00 0.00 FUD XXX

0534T set-up, patient training, configuration of monitor
0.00 0.00 FUD XXX

0535T data upload, analysis and initial report configuration
0.00 0.00 FUD XXX

0536T download review, interpretation and report
0.00 0.00 FUD XXX

0537T-0540T

INCLUDES Administration of genetically modified cells for the treatment of serious diseases (e.g., cancer)
Evaluation prior to, during, and after CAR-T cell administration
Infusion of fluids and supportive medications provided with administration
Management of clinical staff
Management of untoward events (e.g, nausea)
Physician certification of processing of cells
Physician presence during cell administration

Code also care provided that is not directly related to CAR-T cell administration (e.g., other medical problems) may be reported separately using appropriate E&M code and modifier 25

0537T Chimeric antigen receptor T-cell (CAR-T) therapy; harvesting of blood-derived T lymphocytes for development of genetically modified autologous CAR-T cells, per day

EXCLUDES *Use more than one time per day despite number of times cells are collected*

0.00 0.00 FUD XXX

AMA: 2019,Jun,5

0538T preparation of blood-derived T lymphocytes for transportation (eg, cryopreservation, storage)
0.00 0.00 FUD XXX

AMA: 2019,Jun,5

0539T receipt and preparation of CAR-T cells for administration
0.00 0.00 FUD XXX

AMA: 2019,Jun,5

0540T CAR-T cell administration, autologous

EXCLUDES *Use more than one time per day despite number of units administered*

0.00 0.00 FUD YYY

AMA: 2019,Jun,5

0541T-0542T

0541T Myocardial imaging by magnetocardiography (MCG) for detection of cardiac ischemia, by signal acquisition using minimum 36 channel grid, generation of magnetic-field time-series images, quantitative analysis of magnetic dipoles, machine learning-derived clinical scoring, and automated report generation, single study;
0.00 0.00 FUD XXX TC

0542T interpretation and report
0.00 0.00 FUD XXX 26

0543T

EXCLUDES *Transesophageal echocardiography (93355)*

● **0543T Transapical mitral valve repair, including transthoracic echocardiography, when performed, with placement of artificial chordae tendineae**
0.00 0.00 FUD YYY 80

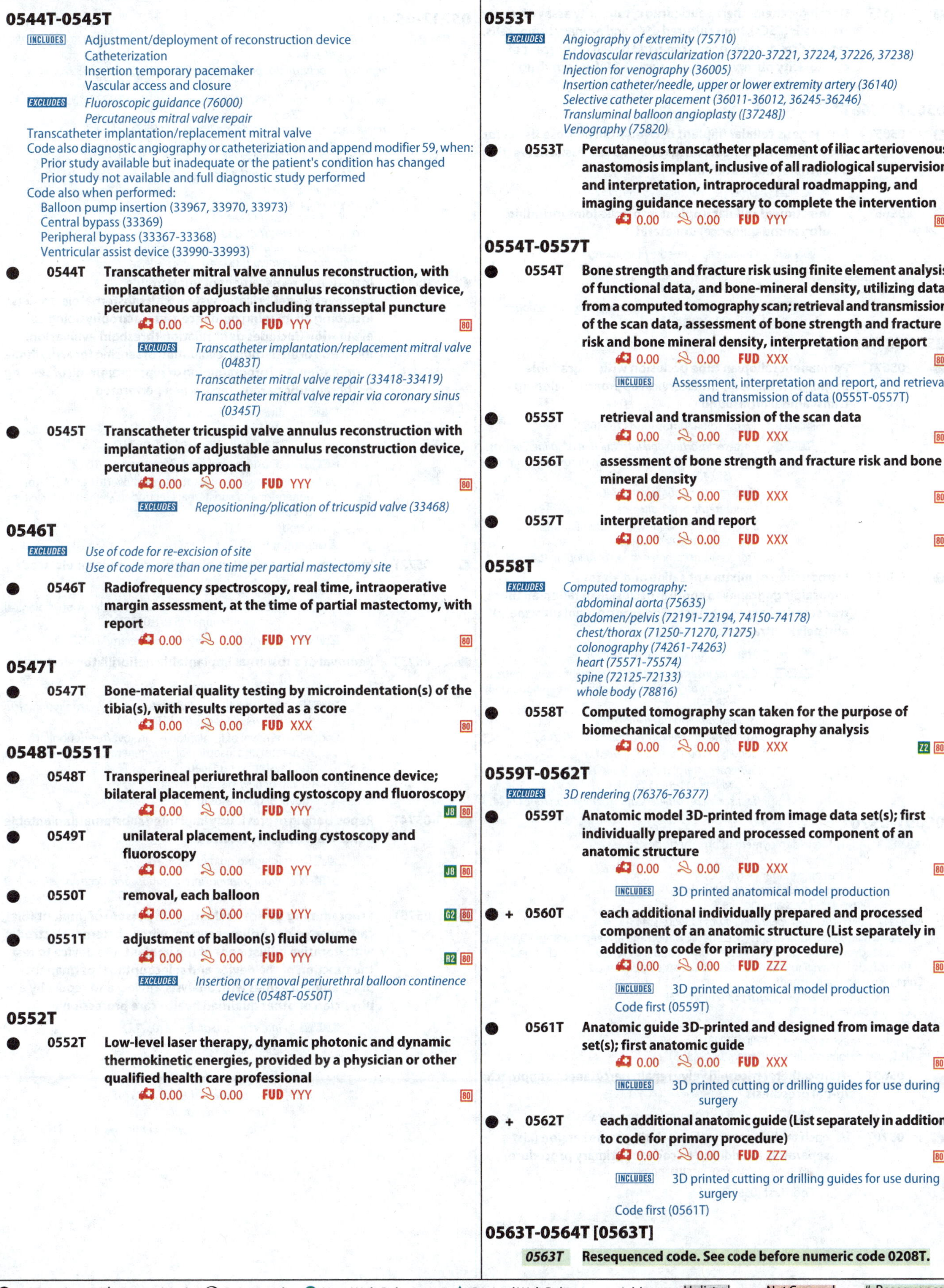

0544T-0545T

INCLUDES Adjustment/deployment of reconstruction device
Catheterization
Insertion temporary pacemaker
Vascular access and closure

EXCLUDES *Fluoroscopic guidance (76000)*
Percutaneous mitral valve repair

Transcatheter implantation/replacement mitral valve
Code also diagnostic angiography or catheteriziation and append modifier 59, when:
Prior study available but inadequate or the patient's condition has changed
Prior study not available and full diagnostic study performed
Code also when performed:
Balloon pump insertion (33967, 33970, 33973)
Central bypass (33369)
Peripheral bypass (33367-33368)
Ventricular assist device (33990-33993)

● 0544T **Transcatheter mitral valve annulus reconstruction, with implantation of adjustable annulus reconstruction device, percutaneous approach including transseptal puncture**
0.00 0.00 FUD YYY 80
EXCLUDES *Transcatheter implantation/replacement mitral valve (0483T)*
Transcatheter mitral valve repair (33418-33419)
Transcatheter mitral valve repair via coronary sinus (0345T)

● 0545T **Transcatheter tricuspid valve annulus reconstruction with implantation of adjustable annulus reconstruction device, percutaneous approach**
0.00 0.00 FUD YYY 80
EXCLUDES *Repositioning/plication of tricuspid valve (33468)*

0546T

EXCLUDES *Use of code for re-excision of site*
Use of code more than one time per partial mastectomy site

● 0546T **Radiofrequency spectroscopy, real time, intraoperative margin assessment, at the time of partial mastectomy, with report**
0.00 0.00 FUD YYY 80

0547T

● 0547T **Bone-material quality testing by microindentation(s) of the tibia(s), with results reported as a score**
0.00 0.00 FUD XXX 80

0548T-0551T

● 0548T **Transperineal periurethral balloon continence device; bilateral placement, including cystoscopy and fluoroscopy**
0.00 0.00 FUD YYY J8 80

● 0549T **unilateral placement, including cystoscopy and fluoroscopy**
0.00 0.00 FUD YYY J8 80

● 0550T **removal, each balloon**
0.00 0.00 FUD YYY G2 80

● 0551T **adjustment of balloon(s) fluid volume**
0.00 0.00 FUD YYY R2 80
EXCLUDES *Insertion or removal periurethral balloon continence device (0548T-0550T)*

0552T

● 0552T **Low-level laser therapy, dynamic photonic and dynamic thermokinetic energies, provided by a physician or other qualified health care professional**
0.00 0.00 FUD YYY 80

0553T

EXCLUDES *Angiography of extremity (75710)*
Endovascular revascularization (37220-37221, 37224, 37226, 37238)
Injection for venography (36005)
Insertion catheter/needle, upper or lower extremity artery (36140)
Selective catheter placement (36011-36012, 36245-36246)
Transluminal balloon angioplasty ([37248])
Venography (75820)

● 0553T **Percutaneous transcatheter placement of iliac arteriovenous anastomosis implant, inclusive of all radiological supervision and interpretation, intraprocedural roadmapping, and imaging guidance necessary to complete the intervention**
0.00 0.00 FUD YYY 80

0554T-0557T

● 0554T **Bone strength and fracture risk using finite element analysis of functional data, and bone-mineral density, utilizing data from a computed tomography scan; retrieval and transmission of the scan data, assessment of bone strength and fracture risk and bone mineral density, interpretation and report**
0.00 0.00 FUD XXX 80
INCLUDES Assessment, interpretation and report, and retrieval and transmission of data (0555T-0557T)

● 0555T **retrieval and transmission of the scan data**
0.00 0.00 FUD XXX 80

● 0556T **assessment of bone strength and fracture risk and bone mineral density**
0.00 0.00 FUD XXX 80

● 0557T **interpretation and report**
0.00 0.00 FUD XXX 80

0558T

EXCLUDES *Computed tomography:*
abdominal aorta (75635)
abdomen/pelvis (72191-72194, 74150-74178)
chest/thorax (71250-71270, 71275)
colonography (74261-74263)
heart (75571-75574)
spine (72125-72133)
whole body (78816)

● 0558T **Computed tomography scan taken for the purpose of biomechanical computed tomography analysis**
0.00 0.00 FUD XXX Z2 80

0559T-0562T

EXCLUDES *3D rendering (76376-76377)*

● 0559T **Anatomic model 3D-printed from image data set(s); first individually prepared and processed component of an anatomic structure**
0.00 0.00 FUD XXX 80
INCLUDES 3D printed anatomical model production

● + 0560T **each additional individually prepared and processed component of an anatomic structure (List separately in addition to code for primary procedure)**
0.00 0.00 FUD ZZZ 80
INCLUDES 3D printed anatomical model production
Code first (0559T)

● 0561T **Anatomic guide 3D-printed and designed from image data set(s); first anatomic guide**
0.00 0.00 FUD XXX 80
INCLUDES 3D printed cutting or drilling guides for use during surgery

● + 0562T **each additional anatomic guide (List separately in addition to code for primary procedure)**
0.00 0.00 FUD ZZZ 80
INCLUDES 3D printed cutting or drilling guides for use during surgery
Code first (0561T)

0563T-0564T [0563T]

0563T **Resequenced code. See code before numeric code 0208T.**

● **0564T** **Oncology, chemotherapeutic drug cytotoxicity assay of cancer stem cells (CSCs), from cultured CSCs and primary tumor cells, categorical drug response reported based on percent of cytotoxicity observed, a minimum of 14 drugs or drug combinations**

0565T-0566T

● **0565T** **Autologous cellular implant derived from adipose tissue for the treatment of osteoarthritis of the knees; tissue harvesting and cellular implant creation**

EXCLUDES *Other tissue grafts ([15769], 15771-15774)*

● **0566T** **injection of cellular implant into knee joint including ultrasound guidance, unilateral**

INCLUDES Guidance for needle placement:
- Fluoroscopy (77002)
- Ultrasound (76942)

EXCLUDES *Arthrocentesis, with or without imaging guidance (20610-20611)*

0567T-0568T

● **0567T** **Permanent fallopian tube occlusion with degradable biopolymer implant, transcervical approach, including transvaginal ultrasound**

INCLUDES Transvaginal ultrasound (76830)

EXCLUDES *Catheter insertion and introduction of saline/contrast for sonohysterography or hysterosalpingography (58340)*
Hysterosalpingography (74740)
Nonobstetric pelvic ultrasound (76856-76857)
Surgical hysteroscopy with bilateral occlusion of fallopian tube (58565)
Transcervical catheterization of fallopian tube (74742)

● **0568T** **Introduction of mixture of saline and air for sonosalpingography to confirm occlusion of fallopian tubes, transcervical approach, including transvaginal ultrasound and pelvic ultrasound**

INCLUDES Transvaginal ultrasound (76830)

EXCLUDES *Catheter insertion and introduction of saline/contrast for sonohysterography or hysterosalpingography (58340)*
Hysterosalpingography (74740)
Nonobstetric pelvic ultrasound (76856-76857)
Sonohysterography (SIS) (76831)
Surgical hysteroscopy with bilateral occlusion of fallopian tube (58565)
Transcervical catheterization of fallopian tube (74742)

0569T-0570T

INCLUDES Adjustment/deployment of prosthetic device
Catheterization
Fluoroscopic guidance (76000)
Intracardiac echocardiography (93662)
Vascular access and closure

EXCLUDES *Open tricuspid valve procedures (33460, 33463-33465, 33468)*

Code also diagnostic angiography or catheteriziation and append modifier 59, when:
- Prior study available but inadequate or the patient's condition has changed
- Prior study not available and full diagnostic study performed

Code also when performed:
- Balloon pump insertion (33967, 33970, 33973)
- Central bypass (33369)
- Peripheral bypass (33367-33368)
- Ventricular assist device (33990-33993)
- TEE, when done by different operator (93355)

● **0569T** **Transcatheter tricuspid valve repair, percutaneous approach; initial prosthesis**

EXCLUDES *Use of code more than once per session*

● + **0570T** **each additional prosthesis during same session (List separately in addition to code for primary procedure)**

0.00 0.00 FUD 000

Code first (0569T)

0571T-0580T

EXCLUDES *Defibrillator or pacemaker device evaluations (93279-93284, 93285-93289, 93290-93298)*
Implantable defibrillator procedures (33215-33220, 33223-33226, 33240-33249 [33230, 33231, 33262, 33263, 33264])
Pacemaker procedures (33202-33220 [33221], 33222-33226, 33233-33238 [33227, 33228, 33229])
Subcutaneous implantable defibrillator system procedures:
- *Electrophysiological evaluation (93644)*
- *Insertion of electrode ([33271])*
- *Insertion/replacement entire system ([33270])*
- *Interrogation ([93261])*
- *Programming ([93260])*
- *Removal of electrode ([33272])*
- *Repositioning of electrode ([33273])*

Transcatheter permanent leadless pacemaker procedures:
- *Insertion or replacement ([33274])*

● **0571T** **Insertion or replacement of implantable cardioverter-defibrillator system with substernal electrode(s), including all imaging guidance and electrophysiological evaluation (includes defibrillation threshold evaluation, induction of arrhythmia, evaluation of sensing for arrhythmia termination, and programming or reprogramming of sensing or therapeutic parameters), when performed**

INCLUDES Imaging guidance
Programming, interrogation, and electrophysiological evaluations (0575T-0577T)

EXCLUDES *Substernal electrode insertion only (0572T)*

Code also removal of implantable cardioverter-defibrillator generator and substernal electrode(s), when total system is replaced:
- Electrode(s) (0573T)
- Generator (0580T)

● **0572T** **Insertion of substernal implantable defibrillator electrode**

INCLUDES Imaging guidance
Programming, interrogation, and electrophysiological evaluations (0575T-0577T)

EXCLUDES *Insertion of generator and electrode (0571T)*

● **0573T** **Removal of substernal implantable defibrillator electrode**

INCLUDES Imaging guidance

EXCLUDES *Programming, interrogation, and electrophysiological evaluations (0575T-0577T)*

Code also removal of implantable cardioverter-defibrillator generator and insertion of new generator/electrode, when total system is replaced:
- Insertion of new system (0571T)
- Removal of generator (0580T)

● **0574T** **Repositioning of previously implanted substernal implantable defibrillator-pacing electrode**

INCLUDES Imaging guidance

EXCLUDES *Programming, interrogation, and electrophysiological evaluations (0575T-0577T)*

● **0575T** **Programming device evaluation (in person) of implantable cardioverter-defibrillator system with substernal electrode, with iterative adjustment of the implantable device to test the function of the device and select optimal permanent programmed values with analysis, review and report by a physician or other qualified health care professional**

EXCLUDES *Interrogation of device (0576T)*
Programming at time of:
- *Electrode insertion (0572T)*
- *Electrode removal (0573T)*
- *Electrode repositioning (0574T)*
- *Generator removal (0580T)*
- *Insertion/replacement entire system (0571T)*

● **0576T** **Interrogation device evaluation (in person) of implantable cardioverter-defibrillator system with substernal electrode, with analysis, review and report by a physician or other qualified health care professional, includes connection, recording and disconnection per patient encounter**

EXCLUDES *Interrogation at time of:*
Electrode insertion (0572T)
Electrode removal (0573T)
Electrode repositioning (0574T)
Insertion/replacement entire system (0571T)
Programming of device (0575T)

● **0577T** **Electrophysiological evaluation of implantable cardioverter-defibrillator system with substernal electrode (includes defibrillation threshold evaluation, induction of arrhythmia, evaluation of sensing for arrhythmia termination, and programming or reprogramming of sensing or therapeutic parameters)**

EXCLUDES *Electrophysiological evaluation at time of:*
Electrode insertion (0572T)
Electrode removal (0573T)
Electrode repositioning (0574T)
Generator removal (0580T)
Insertion/replacement entire system (0571T)

● **0578T** **Interrogation device evaluation(s) (remote), up to 90 days, substernal lead implantable cardioverter-defibrillator system with interim analysis, review(s) and report(s) by a physician or other qualified health care professional**

EXCLUDES *In person device interrogation (0576T)*
Use of code more than once per 90 days

● **0579T** **Interrogation device evaluation(s) (remote), up to 90 days, substernal lead implantable cardioverter-defibrillator system, remote data acquisition(s), receipt of transmissions and technician review, technical support and distribution of results**

EXCLUDES *In person device interrogation (0576T)*
Use of code more than once per 90 days

● **0580T** **Removal of substernal implantable defibrillator pulse generator only**

EXCLUDES *Programming, interrogation, and electrophysiological evaluations (0575T-0577T)*

Code also removal of substernal electrode and insertion of new generator/electrode, when total system is replaced:
Insertion of new system (0571T)
Removal of electrode (0573T)

0581T-0582T

● **0581T** **Ablation, malignant breast tumor(s), percutaneous, cryotherapy, including imaging guidance when performed, unilateral**

INCLUDES Ultrasound for:
Breast imaging (76641-76642)
Monitoring of tissue ablation (76940)
Needle placement (76942)

EXCLUDES *Cryoablation for breast fibroadenoma(s) (19105)*
Use of code more than once per treated breast

● **0582T** **Transurethral ablation of malignant prostate tissue by high-energy water vapor thermotherapy, including intraoperative imaging and needle guidance**

INCLUDES 3D rendering (76376-76377)
Cystourethroscopy (52000)
Imaging guidance for:
Needle placement (76942, 77021)
Tissue ablation monitoring (76940, 77022)
MRI of pelvis (72195-72197)
Transrectal ultrasound (76872)

EXCLUDES *Destruction by radiofrequency-generated water vapor thermotherapy for benign prostatic hypertrophy (BPH) (53854)*

0583T

● **0583T** **Tympanostomy (requiring insertion of ventilating tube), using an automated tube delivery system, iontophoresis local anesthesia**

INCLUDES Binocular microscopy (92504)
Iontophoresis (97033)
Operating microscope (69990)

EXCLUDES *Myringotomy (69420-69421)*
Removal of impacted cerumen (69209-69210)
Tympanostomy without the use of automated delivery system (69433, 69436)

0584T-0586T

● **0584T** **Islet cell transplant, includes portal vein catheterization and infusion, including all imaging, including guidance, and radiological supervision and interpretation, when performed; percutaneous**

● **0585T** **laparoscopic**

● **0586T** **open**

0587T-0590T

● **0587T** **Percutaneous implantation or replacement of integrated single device neurostimulation system including electrode array and receiver or pulse generator, including analysis, programming, and imaging guidance when performed, posterior tibial nerve**

INCLUDES Electronic analysis (95970-95972, 0589T-0590T)

EXCLUDES *Insertion of other neurostimulator devices (64555, 64566, 64575, 64590)*
Revision or removal of integrated neurostimulation system (0588T)

● **0588T** **Revision or removal of integrated single device neurostimulation system including electrode array and receiver or pulse generator, including analysis, programming, and imaging guidance when performed, posterior tibial nerve**

INCLUDES Electronic analysis (95970-95972, 0589T-0590T)

EXCLUDES *Initial insertion or replacement of integrated neurostimulation system (0587T)*
Insertion of other neurostimulator devices (64555, 64566, 64575, 64590)

● **0589T** **Electronic analysis with simple programming of implanted integrated neurostimulation system (eg, electrode array and receiver), including contact group(s), amplitude, pulse width, frequency (Hz), on/off cycling, burst, dose lockout, patient-selectable parameters, responsive neurostimulation, detection algorithms, closed-loop parameters, and passive parameters, when performed by physician or other qualified health care professional, posterior tibial nerve, 1-3 parameters**

EXCLUDES *Electronic analysis of other implanted neurostimulators (95970-95977, [95983, 95984])*
Electronic analysis with complex programming (0590T)
Use of code at time of insertion, replacement, revision, or removal of integrated neurostimulation system (0587T-0588T)
Use of code at time of insertion, replacement, revision, or removal of other neurostimulator device (generator and/or electrode) (43647-43648, 43881-43882, 61850-61888, 63650, 63655, 63661-63688, 64553-64595)

● **0590T** **Electronic analysis with complex programming of implanted integrated neurostimulation system (eg, electrode array and receiver), including contact group(s), amplitude, pulse width, frequency (Hz), on/off cycling, burst, dose lockout, patient-selectable parameters, responsive neurostimulation, detection algorithms, closed-loop parameters, and passive parameters, when performed by physician or other qualified health care professional, posterior tibial nerve, 4 or more parameters**

EXCLUDES *Electronic analysis of other implanted neurostimulators (95970-95977, [95983, 95984])*
Electronic analysis with simple programming (0589T)
Use of code at time of insertion, replacement, revision, or removal of integrated neurostimulation system (0587T-0588T)
Use of code at time of insertion, replacement, revision, or removal of other neurostimulator device (generator and/or electrode) (43647-43648, 43881-43882, 61850-61888, 63650, 63655, 63661-63688, 64553-64595)

0591T-0593T

INCLUDES Nonphysician health care professional coach trained to assist patients in obtaining improved health and well-being goals through the use of:
Accountability
Active learning processes
Self discovery

● **0591T** **Health and well-being coaching face-to-face; individual, initial assessment**

EXCLUDES *Health and well-being coaching, follow-up session (0592T)*
Health and well-being coaching, group session (0593T)

● **0592T** **individual, follow-up session, at least 30 minutes**

EXCLUDES *Diabetic preventative behavior change program ([0488T])*
Education/training for self-management (98960)
Health and well-being coaching, group session (0593T)
Health and well-being coaching, initial session (0591T)
Health behavior assessment/intervention (96156-96159)
Medical nutrition therapy (97802-97804)

● **0593T** **group (2 or more individuals), at least 30 minutes**

EXCLUDES *Diabetic preventative behavior change program (0403T)*
Education/training for self-management (98961-98962)
Group therapy procedure (97150)
Health and well-being coaching, individual (0591T-0592T)
Health behavior assessment/intervention ([96164, 96165])

Category III Codes 0590T — 0593T

Appendix A — Modifiers

CPT Modifiers

A modifier is a two-position alpha or numeric code appended to a CPT® code to clarify the services being billed. Modifiers provide a means by which a service can be altered without changing the procedure code. They add more information, such as the anatomical site, to the code. In addition, they help to eliminate the appearance of duplicate billing and unbundling. Modifiers are used to increase accuracy in reimbursement, coding consistency, editing, and to capture payment data.

22 **Increased Procedural Services:** When the work required to provide a service is substantially greater than typically required, it may be identified by adding modifier 22 to the usual procedure code. Documentation must support the substantial additional work and the reason for the additional work (ie, increased intensity, time, technical difficulty of procedure, severity of patient's condition, physical and mental effort required).
Note: This modifier should not be appended to an E/M service.

23 **Unusual Anesthesia:** Occasionally, a procedure, which usually requires either no anesthesia or local anesthesia, because of unusual circumstances must be done under general anesthesia. This circumstance may be reported by adding modifier 23 to the procedure code of the basic service.

24 **Unrelated Evaluation and Management Service by the Same Physician or Other Qualified Health Care Professional During a Postoperative Period:** The physician or other qualified health care professional may need to indicate that an evaluation and management service was performed during a postoperative period for a reason(s) unrelated to the original procedure. This circumstance may be reported by adding modifier 24 to the appropriate level of E/M service.

25 **Significant, Separately Identifiable Evaluation and Management Service by the Same Physician or Other Qualified Health Care Professional on the Same Day of the Procedure or Other Service:** It may be necessary to indicate that on the day a procedure or service identified by a CPT code was performed, the patient's condition required a significant, separately identifiable E/M service above and beyond the other service provided or beyond the usual preoperative and postoperative care associated with the procedure that was performed. A significant, separately identifiable E/M service is defined or substantiated by documentation that satisfies the relevant criteria for the respective E/M service to be reported (see Evaluation and Management Services Guidelines for instructions on determining level of E/M service). The E/M service may be prompted by the symptom or condition for which the procedure and/or service was provided. As such, different diagnoses are not required for reporting of the E/M services on the same date. This circumstance may be reported by adding modifier 25 to the appropriate level of E/M service.
Note: This modifier is not used to report an E/M service that resulted in a decision to perform surgery. See modifier 57. For significant, separately identifiable non-E/M services, see modifier 59.

26 **Professional Component:** Certain procedures are a combination of a physician or other qualified health care professional component and a technical component. When the physician or other qualified health care professional component is reported separately, the service may be identified by adding modifier 26 to the usual procedure number.

32 **Mandated Services:** Services related to mandated consultation and/or related services (eg, third party payer, governmental, legislative or regulatory requirement) may be identified by adding modifier 32 to the basic procedure.

33 **Preventive Services:** When the primary purpose of the service is the delivery of an evidence based service in accordance with a US Preventive Services Task Force A or B rating in effect and other preventive services identified in preventive services mandates (legislative or regulatory), the service may be identified by adding 33 to the procedure. For separately reported services specifically identified as preventive, the modifier should not be used.

47 **Anesthesia by Surgeon:** Regional or general anesthesia provided by the surgeon may be reported by adding modifier 47 to the basic service. (This does not include local anesthesia.)
Note: Modifier 47 would not be used as a modifier for the anesthesia procedures.

50 **Bilateral Procedure:** Unless otherwise identified in the listings, bilateral procedures that are performed at the same session should be identified by adding modifier 50 to the appropriate 5 digit code.
Note: This modifier should not be appended to designated "add-on" codes (see Appendix F).

51 **Multiple Procedures:** When multiple procedures, other than E/M services, Physical Medicine and Rehabilitation services or provision of supplies (eg, vaccines), are performed at the same session by the same individual, the primary procedure or service may be reported as listed. The additional procedure(s) or service(s) may be identified by appending modifier 51 to the additional procedure or service code(s).
Note: This modifier should not be appended to designated "add-on" codes (see Appendix F).

52 **Reduced Services:** Under certain circumstances a service or procedure is partially reduced or eliminated at the discretion of the physician or other qualified health care professional. Under these circumstances the service provided can be identified by its usual procedure number and the addition of modifier 52, signifying that the service is reduced. This provides a means of reporting reduced services without disturbing the identification of the basic service.
Note: For hospital outpatient reporting of a previously scheduled procedure/service that is partially reduced or cancelled as a result of extenuating circumstances or those that threaten the well-being of the patient prior to or after administration of anesthesia, see modifiers 73 and 74 (see modifiers approved for ASC hospital outpatient use).

53 **Discontinued Procedure:** Under certain circumstances, the physician or other qualified health care professional may elect to terminate a surgical or diagnostic procedure. Due to extenuating circumstances or those that threaten the well being of the patient, it may be necessary to indicate that a surgical or diagnostic procedure was started but discontinued. This circumstance may be reported by adding modifier 53 to the code reported by the physician for the discontinued procedure.
Note: This modifier is not used to report the elective cancellation of a procedure prior to the patient's anesthesia induction and/or surgical preparation in the operating suite. For outpatient hospital/ambulatory surgery center (ASC) reporting of a previously scheduled procedure/service that is partially reduced or cancelled as a result of extenuating circumstances or those that threaten the well being of the patient prior to or after administration of anesthesia, see modifiers 73 and 74 (see modifiers approved for ASC hospital outpatient use).

54 **Surgical Care Only:** When 1 physician or other qualified health care professional performs a surgical procedure and another provides preoperative and/or postoperative management, surgical services may be identified by adding modifier 54 to the usual procedure number.

55 **Postoperative Management Only:** When 1 physician or other qualified health care professional performed the postoperative management and another performed the surgical procedure, the postoperative component may be identified by adding modifier 55 to the usual procedure number.

56 **Preoperative Management Only:** When 1 physician or other qualified health care professional performed the preoperative care and evaluation and another performed the surgical procedure, the preoperative component may be identified by adding modifier 56 to the usual procedure number.

57 **Decision for Surgery:** An evaluation and management service that resulted in the initial decision to perform the surgery may be identified by adding modifier 57 to the appropriate level of E/M service.

58 Staged or Related Procedure or Service by the Same Physician or Other Qualified Health Care Professional During the Postoperative Period: It may be necessary to indicate that the performance of a procedure or service during the postoperative period was (a) planned or anticipated (staged); (b) more extensive than the original procedure; or (c) for therapy following a surgical procedure. This circumstance may be reported by adding modifier 58 to the staged or related procedure.
Note: For treatment of a problem that requires a return to the operating/procedure room (eg, unanticipated clinical condition), see modifier 78.

59 Distinct Procedural Service: Under certain circumstances, it may be necessary to indicate that a procedure or service was distinct or independent from other non-E/M services performed on the same day. Modifier 59 is used to identify procedures/services, other than E/M services, that are not normally reported together but are appropriate under the circumstances. Documentation must support a different session, different procedure or surgery, different site or organ system, separate incision/excision, separate lesion, or separate injury (or area of injury in extensive injuries) not ordinarily encountered or performed on the same day by the same individual. However, when another already established modifier is appropriate it should be used rather than modifier 59. Only if no more descriptive modifier is available, and the use of modifier 59 best explains the circumstances, should modifier 59 be used.
Note: Modifier 59 should not be appended to an E/M service. To report a separate and distinct E/M service with a non-E/M service performed on the same date, see modifier 25.

62 Two Surgeons: When 2 surgeons work together as primary surgeons performing distinct part(s) of a procedure, each surgeon should report his/her distinct operative work by adding modifier 62 to the procedure code and any associated add-on code(s) for that procedure as long as both surgeons continue to work together as primary surgeons. Each surgeon should report the co-surgery once using the same procedure code. If additional procedure(s) (including add-on procedure[s]) are performed during the same surgical session, separate code(s) may also be reported with modifier 62 added.
Note: If a co-surgeon acts as an assistant in the performance of additional procedure(s), other than those reported with the modifier 62, during the same surgical session, those services may be reported using separate procedure code(s) with modifier 80 or modifier 82 added, as appropriate.

63 Procedure Performed on Infants less than 4 kg: Procedures performed on neonates and infants up to a present body weight of 4 kg may involve significantly increased complexity and physician or other qualified health care professional work commonly associated with these patients. This circumstance may be reported by adding modifier 63 to the procedure number.
Note: Unless otherwise designated, this modifier may only be appended to procedures/services listed in the 20100-69990 code series and 92920, 92928, 92953, 92960, 92986, 92987, 92990, 92997, 92998, 93312, 93313, 93314, 93315, 93316, 93317, 93318, 93452, 93505, 93530, 93531, 93532, 93533, 93561, 93562, 93563, 93564, 93568, 93580, 93582, 93590, 93591, 93592, 93615, 93616 from the Medicine/Cardiovascular section.

Modifier 63 should not be appended to any CPT codes listed in the Evaluation and Management Services, Anesthesia, Radiology, Pathology/Laboratory, or Medicine sections (other than those identified above from the Medicine/Cardiovascular section).

66 Surgical Team: Under some circumstances, highly complex procedures (requiring the concomitant services of several physicians or other qualified health care professionals, often of different specialties, plus other highly skilled, specially trained personnel, various types of complex equipment) are carried out under the "surgical team" concept. Such circumstances may be identified by each participating individual with the addition of modifier 66 to the basic procedure number used for reporting services.

76 Repeat Procedure or Service by Same Physician or Other Qualified Health Care Professional: It may be necessary to indicate that a procedure or service was repeated by the same physician or other qualified health care professional subsequent to the original procedure or service. This circumstance may be reported by adding modifier 76 to the repeated procedure or service.
Note: This modifier should not be appended to an E/M service.

77 Repeat Procedure by Another Physician or Other Qualified Health Care Professional: It may be necessary to indicate that a basic procedure or service was repeated by another physician or other qualified health care professional subsequent to the original procedure or service. This circumstance may be reported by adding modifier 77 to the repeated procedure or service.
Note: This modifier should not be appended to an E/M service.

78 Unplanned Return to the Operating/Procedure Room by the Same Physician or Other Qualified Health Care Professional Following Initial Procedure for a Related Procedure During the Postoperative Period: It may be necessary to indicate that another procedure was performed during the postoperative period of the initial procedure (unplanned procedure following initial procedure). When this procedure is related to the first, and requires the use of an operating/procedure room, it may be reported by adding modifier 78 to the related procedure. (For repeat procedures, see modifier 76.)

79 Unrelated Procedure or Service by the Same Physician or Other Qualified Health Care Professional During the Postoperative Period: The individual may need to indicate that the performance of a procedure or service during the postoperative period was unrelated to the original procedure. This circumstance may be reported by using modifier 79. (For repeat procedures on the same day, see modifier 76.)

80 Assistant Surgeon: Surgical assistant services may be identified by adding modifier 80 to the usual procedure number(s).

81 Minimum Assistant Surgeon: Minimum surgical assistant services are identified by adding modifier 81 to the usual procedure number.

82 Assistant Surgeon (when qualified resident surgeon not available): The unavailability of a qualified resident surgeon is a prerequisite for use of modifier 82 appended to the usual procedure code number(s).

90 Reference (Outside) Laboratory: When laboratory procedures are performed by a party other than the treating or reporting physician or other qualified health care professional, the procedure may be identified by adding modifier 90 to the usual procedure number.

91 Repeat Clinical Diagnostic Laboratory Test: In the course of treatment of the patient, it may be necessary to repeat the same laboratory test on the same day to obtain subsequent (multiple) test results. Under these circumstances, the laboratory test performed can be identified by its usual procedure number and the addition of modifier 91.
Note: This modifier may not be used when tests are rerun to confirm initial results; due to testing problems with specimens or equipment; or for any other reason when a normal, one-time, reportable result is all that is required. This modifier may not be used when other code(s) describe a series of test results (eg, glucose tolerance tests, evocative/suppression testing). This modifier may only be used for laboratory test(s) performed more than once on the same day on the same patient.

92 Alternative Laboratory Platform Testing: When laboratory testing is being performed using a kit or transportable instrument that wholly or in part consists of a single use, disposable analytical chamber, the service may be identified by adding modifier 92 to the usual laboratory procedure code (HIV testing 86701-86703, and 87389). The test does not require permanent dedicated space, hence by its design may be hand carried or transported to the vicinity of the patient for immediate testing at that site, although location of the testing is not in itself determinative of the use of this modifier.

95 **Synchronous Telemedicine Service Rendered Via a Real-Time Interactive Audio and Video Telecommunications System:** Synchronous telemedicine service is defined as a **real-time** interaction between a physician or other qualified health care professional and a patient who is located at a distant site from the physician or other qualified health care professional. The totality of the communication of information exchanged between the physician or other qualified health care professional and patient during the course of the synchronous telemedicine service must be of an amount and nature that would be sufficient to meet the key components and/or requirements of the same service when rendered via a face-to-face interaction. Modifier 95 may only be appended to the services listed in Appendix F. Appendix F is the list of CPT codes for services that are typically performed face-to-face, but may be rendered via real-time (synchronous) interactive audio and video telecommunications system.

96 **Habilitative Services:** When a service or procedure that may be either habilitative or rehabilitative in nature is provided for habilitative purposes, the physician or other qualified health care professional may add modifier 96 to the service or procedure code to indicate that the service or procedure provided was a habilitative service. Habilitative services help an individual learn skills and functioning for daily living that the individual has not yet developed, and then keep and/or improve those learned skills. Habilitative services also help an individual keep, learn, or improve skills and functioning for daily living.

97 **Rehabilitative Services:** When a service or procedure that may be either habilitative or rehabilitative in nature is provided for rehabilitative purposes, the physician or other qualified health care professional may add modifier 97 to the service or procedure code to indicate that the service or procedure provided was a rehabilitative service. Rehabilitative services help an individual keep, get back, or improve skills and functioning for daily living that have been lost or impaired because the individual was sick, hurt, or disabled.

99 **Multiple Modifiers:** Under certain circumstances 2 or more modifiers may be necessary to completely delineate a service. In such situations modifier 99 should be added to the basic procedure, and other applicable modifiers may be listed as part of the description of the service.

Anesthesia Physical Status Modifiers

All anesthesia services are reported by use of the five-digit anesthesia procedure code with the appropriate physical status modifier appended.

Under certain circumstances, when other modifier(s) are appropriate, they should be reported in addition to the physical status modifier.

P1 A normal healthy patient

P2 A patient with mild systemic disease

P3 A patient with severe systemic disease

P4 A patient with severe systemic disease that is a constant threat to life

P5 A moribund patient who is not expected to survive without the operation

P6 A declared brain-dead patient whose organs are being removed for donor purposes

Modifiers Approved for Ambulatory Surgery Center (ASC) Hospital Outpatient Use

CPT Level I Modifiers

25 **Significant, Separately Identifiable Evaluation and Management Service by the Same Physician or Other Qualified Health Care Professional on the Same Day of the Procedure or Other Service:** It may be necessary to indicate that on the day a procedure or service identified by a CPT code was performed, the patient's condition required a significant, separately identifiable E/M service above and beyond the other service provided or beyond the usual preoperative and postoperative care associated with the procedure that was performed. A significant, separately identifiable E/M service is defined or substantiated by documentation that satisfies the relevant criteria for the respective E/M service to be reported (see Evaluation and Management Services Guidelines for instructions on determining level of E/M service). The E/M service may be prompted by the symptom or condition for which the procedure and/or service was provided. As such, different diagnoses are not required for reporting of the E/M services on the same date. This circumstance may be reported by adding modifier 25 to the appropriate level of E/M service.
Note: This modifier is not used to report an E/M service that resulted in a decision to perform surgery. See modifier 57. For significant, separately identifiable non-E/M services, see modifier 59.

27 **Multiple Outpatient Hospital E/M Encounters on the Same Date:** For hospital outpatient reporting purposes, utilization of hospital resources related to separate and distinct E/M encounters performed in multiple outpatient hospital settings on the same date may be reported by adding modifier 27 to each appropriate level outpatient and/or emergency department E/M code(s). This modifier provides a means of reporting circumstances involving evaluation and management services provided by a physician(s) in more than one (multiple) outpatient hospital setting(s) (eg, hospital emergency department, clinic).
Note: This modifier is not to be used for physician reporting of multiple E/M services performed by the same physician on the same date. For physician reporting of all outpatient evaluation and management services provided by the same physician on the same date and performed in multiple outpatient settings (eg, hospital emergency department, clinic), see Evaluation and Management, Emergency Department, or Preventive Medicine Services codes.

33 **Preventive Services:** When the primary purpose of the service is the delivery of an evidence based service in accordance with a US Preventive Services Task Force A or B rating in effect and other preventive services identified in preventive services mandates (legislative or regulatory), the service may be identified by adding 33 to the procedure. For separately reported services specifically identified as preventive, the modifier should not be used.

50 **Bilateral Procedure:** Unless otherwise identified in the listings, bilateral procedures that are performed at the same session should be identified by adding modifier 50 to the appropriate 5 digit code.

Note: This modifier should not be appended to designated "add-on" codes (see appendix F).

52 **Reduced Services:** Under certain circumstances a service or procedure is partially reduced or eliminated at the discretion of the physician or other qualified health care professional. Under these circumstances the service provided can be identified by its usual procedure number and the addition of modifier 52, signifying that the service is reduced. This provides a means of reporting reduced services without disturbing the identification of the basic service.
Note: For hospital outpatient reporting of a previously scheduled procedure/service that is partially reduced or cancelled as a result of extenuating circumstances or those that threaten the well-being of the patient prior to or after administration of anesthesia, see modifiers 73 and 74 (see modifiers approved for ASC hospital outpatient use).

58 **Staged or Related Procedure or Service by the Same Physician or Other Qualified Health Care Professional During the Postoperative Period:** It may be necessary to indicate that the performance of a procedure or service during the postoperative period was (a) planned or anticipated (staged); (b) more extensive than the original procedure; or (c) for therapy following a surgical procedure. This circumstance may be reported by adding modifier 58 to the staged or related procedure.
Note: For treatment of a problem that requires a return to the operating or procedure room (eg, unanticipated clinical condition), see modifier 78.

59 **Distinct Procedural Service:** Under certain circumstances, it may be necessary to indicate that a procedure or service was distinct or independent from other non-E/M services performed on the same day. Modifier 59 is used to identify procedures/services, other than E/M services, that are not normally reported together but are appropriate under the circumstances. Documentation must

support a different session, different procedure or surgery, different site or organ system, separate incision/excision, separate lesion, or separate injury (or area of injury in extensive injuries) not ordinarily encountered or performed on the same day by the same individual. However, when another already established modifier is appropriate it should be used rather than modifier 59. Only if no more descriptive modifier is available, and the use of modifier 59 best explains the circumstances, should modifier 59 be used.
Note: Modifier 59 should not be appended to an E/M service. To report a separate and distinct E/M service with a non-E/M service performed on the same date, see modifier 25.

73 **Discontinued Out-Patient Hospital/Ambulatory Surgery Center (ASC) Procedure Prior to the Administration of Anesthesia:** Due to extenuating circumstances or those that threaten the well being of the patient, the physician may cancel a surgical or diagnostic procedure subsequent to the patient's surgical preparation (including sedation when provided, and being taken to the room where the procedure is to be performed), but prior to the administration of anesthesia (local, regional block(s) or general). Under these circumstances, the intended service that is prepared for but cancelled can be reported by its usual procedure number and the addition of modifier 73.
Note: The elective cancellation of a service prior to the administration of anesthesia and/or surgical preparation of the patient should not be reported. For physician reporting of a discontinued procedure, see modifier 53.

74 **Discontinued Out-Patient Hospital/Ambulatory Surgery Center (ASC) Procedure After Administration of Anesthesia:** Due to extenuating circumstances or those that threaten the well being of the patient, the physician may terminate a surgical or diagnostic procedure after the administration of anesthesia (local, regional block(s), general) or after the procedure was started (incision made, intubation started, scope inserted, etc.). Under these circumstances, the procedure started but terminated can be reported by its usual procedure number and the addition of modifier 74.
Note: The elective cancellation of a service prior to the administration of anesthesia and/or surgical preparation of the patient should not be reported. For physician reporting of a discontinued procedure, see modifier 53.

76 **Repeat Procedure or Service by Same Physician or Other Qualified Health Care Professional:** It may be necessary to indicate that a procedure or service was repeated by the same physician or other qualified health care professional subsequent to the original procedure or service. This circumstance may be reported by adding modifier 76 to the repeated procedure or service.
Note: This modifier should not be appended to an E/M service.

77 **Repeat Procedure by Another Physician or Other Qualified Health Care Professional:** It may be necessary to indicate that a basic procedure or service was repeated by another physician or other qualified health care professional subsequent to the original procedure or service. This circumstance may be reported by adding modifier 77 to the repeated procedure or service.
Note: This modifier should not be appended to an E/M service.

78 **Unplanned Return to the Operating/Procedure Room by the Same Physician or Other Qualified Health Care Professional Following Initial Procedure for a Related Procedure During the Postoperative Period:** It may be necessary to indicate that another procedure was performed during the postoperative period of the initial procedure (unplanned procedure following initial procedure). When this procedure is related to the first, and requires the use of an operating/procedure room, it may be reported by adding modifier 78 to the related procedure. (For repeat procedures, see modifier 76.)

79 **Unrelated Procedure or Service by the Same Physician During the Postoperative Period:** The individual may need to indicate that the performance of a procedure or service during the postoperative period was unrelated to the original procedure. This circumstance may be reported by using modifier 79. (For repeat procedures on the same day, see modifier 76.)

91 **Repeat Clinical Diagnostic Laboratory Test:** In the course of treatment of the patient, it may be necessary to repeat the same laboratory test on the same day to obtain subsequent (multiple) test results. Under these circumstances, the laboratory test performed can be identified by its usual procedure number and the addition of modifier 91.
Note: This modifier may not be used when tests are rerun to confirm initial results; due to testing problems with specimens or equipment; or for any other reason when a normal, one-time, reportable result is all that is required. This modifier may not be used when other code(s) describe a series of test results (eg, glucose tolerance tests, evocative/suppression testing). This modifier may only be used for laboratory test(s) performed more than once on the same day on the same patient.

Level II (HCPCS/National) Modifiers

The HCPCS Level II modifiers included here are those most commonly used when coding procedures. See your 2020 HCPCS Level II book for a complete listing.

Anatomical Modifiers

E1 Upper left, eyelid
E2 Lower left, eyelid
E3 Upper right, eyelid
E4 Lower right, eyelid
F1 Left hand, second digit
F2 Left hand, third digit
F3 Left hand, fourth digit
F4 Left hand, fifth digit
F5 Right hand, thumb
F6 Right hand, second digit
F7 Right hand, third digit
F8 Right hand, fourth digit
F9 Right hand, fifth digit
FA Left hand, thumb
LT Left side (used to identify procedures performed on the left side of the body)
RT Right side (used to identify procedures performed on the right side of the body)
T1 Left foot, second digit
T2 Left foot, third digit
T3 Left foot, fourth digit
T4 Left foot, fifth digit
T5 Right foot, great toe
T6 Right foot, second digit
T7 Right foot, third digit
T8 Right foot, fourth digit
T9 Right foot, fifth digit
TA Left foot, great toe

Anesthesia Modifiers

AA Anesthesia services performed personally by anesthesiologist
AD Medical supervision by a physician: more than four concurrent anesthesia procedures
G8 Monitored anesthesia care (MAC) for deep complex, complicated, or markedly invasive surgical procedure
G9 Monitored anesthesia care for patient who has history of severe cardiopulmonary condition
QK Medical direction of two, three, or four concurrent anesthesia procedures involving qualified individuals
QS Monitored anesthesiology care service
QX CRNA service: with medical direction by a physician
QY Medical direction of one certified registered nurse anesthetist (CRNA) by an anesthesiologist
QZ CRNA service: without medical direction by a physician

Coronary Artery Modifiers

LC Left circumflex coronary artery

LD Left anterior descending coronary artery

LM Left main coronary artery

RC Right coronary artery

RI Ramus intermedius coronary artery

Other Modifiers

CT Computed tomography services furnished using equipment that does not meet each of the attributes of the national electrical manufacturers association (NEMA) XR-29-2013 standard

EA Erythropoetic stimulating agent (ESA) administered to treat anemia due to anticancer chemotherapy

EB Erythropoetic stimulating agent (ESA) administered to treat anemia due to anticancer radiotherapy

EC Erythropoetic stimulating agent (ESA) administered to treat anemia not due to anticancer radiotherapy or anticancer chemotherapy

FP Service provided as part of family planning program

FX X-ray taken using film

G7 Pregnancy resulted from rape or incest or pregnancy certified by physician as life threatening

GA Waiver of liability statement issued as required by payer policy, individual case

GG Performance and payment of a screening mammogram and diagnostic mammogram on the same patient, same day

GH Diagnostic mammogram converted from screening mammogram on same day

GQ Via asynchronous telecommunications system

GT Via interactive audio and video telecommunication systems

GU Waiver of liability statement issued as required by payer policy, routine notice

GX Notice of liability issued, voluntary under payer policy

GY Item or service statutorily excluded, does not meet the definition of any Medicare benefit or, for non-Medicare insurers, is not a contract benefit

GZ Item or service expected to be denied as not reasonable and necessary

PI Positron emission tomography (PET) or PET/computed tomography (CT) to inform the initial treatment strategy of tumors that are biopsy proven or strongly suspected of being cancerous based on other diagnostic testing

PS Positron emission tomography (PET) or PET/computed tomography (CT) to inform the subsequent treatment strategy of cancerous tumors when the beneficiary's treating physician determines that the PET study is needed to inform subsequent antitumor strategy

PT Colorectal cancer screening test; converted to diagnostic test or other procedure

Q7 One Class A finding

Q8 Two Class B findings

Q9 One Class B and two Class C findings

QC Single channel monitoring

QM Ambulance service provided under arrangement by a provider of services

QN Ambulance service furnished directly by a provider of services

QW CLIA waived test

TC Technical component; under certain circumstances, a charge may be made for the technical component alone; under those circumstances the technical component charge is identified by adding modifier TC to the usual procedure number; technical component charges are institutional charges and not billed separately by physicians; however, portable x-ray suppliers only bill for technical component and should utilize modifier TC; the charge data from portable x-ray suppliers will then be used to build customary and prevailing profiles

* **XE** Separate encounter, a service that is distinct because it occurred during a separate encounter

* **XP** Separate practitioner, a service that is distinct because it was performed by a different practitioner

* **XS** Separate structure, a service that is distinct because it was performed on a separate organ/structure

* **XU** Unusual nonoverlapping service, the use of a service that is distinct because it does not overlap usual components of the main service

* CMS instituted additional HCPCS modifiers to define explicit subsets of modifier 59 Distinct Procedural Service.

Category II Modifiers

1P Performance Measure Exclusion Modifier due to Medical Reasons

Reasons include:

- Not indicated (absence of organ/limb, already received/performed, other)
- Contraindicated (patient allergic history, potential adverse drug interaction, other)
- Other medical reasons

2P Performance Measure Exclusion Modifier due to Patient Reasons

Reasons include:

- Patient declined
- Economic, social, or religious reasons
- Other patient reasons

3P Performance Measure Exclusion Modifier due to System Reasons

Reasons include:

- Resources to perform the services not available
- Insurance coverage/payor-related limitations
- Other reasons attributable to health care delivery system

Modifier 8P is intended to be used as a "reporting modifier" to allow the reporting of circumstances when an action described in a measure's numerator is not performed and the reason is not otherwise specified.

8P Performance measure reporting modifier-action not performed, reason not otherwise specified

Appendix B — New, Revised, and Deleted Codes

New Codes

0563T Evacuation of meibomian glands, using heat delivered through wearable, open-eye eyelid treatment devices and manual gland expression, bilateral

0564T Oncology, chemotherapeutic drug cytotoxicity assay of cancer stem cells (CSCs), from cultured CSCs and primary tumor cells, categorical drug response reported based on percent of cytotoxicity observed, a minimum of 14 drugs or drug combinations

0565T Autologous cellular implant derived from adipose tissue for the treatment of osteoarthritis of the knees; tissue harvesting and cellular implant creation

0566T Autologous cellular implant derived from adipose tissue for the treatment of osteoarthritis of the knees; injection of cellular implant into knee joint including ultrasound guidance, unilateral

0567T Permanent fallopian tube occlusion with degradable biopolymer implant, transcervical approach, including transvaginal ultrasound

0568T Introduction of mixture of saline and air for sonosalpingography to confirm occlusion of fallopian tubes, transcervical approach, including transvaginal ultrasound and pelvic ultrasound

0569T Transcatheter tricuspid valve repair, percutaneous approach; initial prosthesis

0570T Transcatheter tricuspid valve repair, percutaneous approach; each additional prosthesis during same session (List separately in addition to code for primary procedure)

0571T Insertion or replacement of implantable cardioverter-defibrillator system with substernal electrode(s), including all imaging guidance and electrophysiological evaluation (includes defibrillation threshold evaluation, induction of arrhythmia, evaluation of sensing for arrhythmia termination, and programming or reprogramming of sensing or therapeutic parameters), when performed

0572T Insertion of substernal implantable defibrillator electrode

0573T Removal of substernal implantable defibrillator electrode

0574T Repositioning of previously implanted substernal implantable defibrillator-pacing electrode

0575T Programming device evaluation (in person) of implantable cardioverter-defibrillator system with substernal electrode, with iterative adjustment of the implantable device to test the function of the device and select optimal permanent programmed values with analysis, review and report by a physician or other qualified health care professional

0576T Interrogation device evaluation (in person) of implantable cardioverter-defibrillator system with substernal electrode, with analysis, review and report by a physician or other qualified health care professional, includes connection, recording and disconnection per patient encounter

0577T Electrophysiological evaluation of implantable cardioverter-defibrillator system with substernal electrode (includes defibrillation threshold evaluation, induction of arrhythmia, evaluation of sensing for arrhythmia termination, and programming or reprogramming of sensing or therapeutic parameters)

0578T Interrogation device evaluation(s) (remote), up to 90 days, substernal lead implantable cardioverter-defibrillator system with interim analysis, review(s) and report(s) by a physician or other qualified health care professional

0579T Interrogation device evaluation(s) (remote), up to 90 days, substernal lead implantable cardioverter-defibrillator system, remote data acquisition(s), receipt of transmissions and technician review, technical support and distribution of results

0580T Removal of substernal implantable defibrillator pulse generator only

0581T Ablation, malignant breast tumor(s), percutaneous, cryotherapy, including imaging guidance when performed, unilateral

0582T Transurethral ablation of malignant prostate tissue by high-energy water vapor thermotherapy, including intraoperative imaging and needle guidance

0583T Tympanostomy (requiring insertion of ventilating tube), using an automated tube delivery system, iontophoresis local anesthesia

0584T Islet cell transplant, includes portal vein catheterization and infusion, including all imaging, including guidance, and radiological supervision and interpretation, when performed; percutaneous

0585T Islet cell transplant, includes portal vein catheterization and infusion, including all imaging, including guidance, and radiological supervision and interpretation, when performed; laparoscopic

0586T Islet cell transplant, includes portal vein catheterization and infusion, including all imaging, including guidance, and radiological supervision and interpretation, when performed; open

0587T Percutaneous implantation or replacement of integrated single device neurostimulation system including electrode array and receiver or pulse generator, including analysis, programming, and imaging guidance when performed, posterior tibial nerve

0588T Revision or removal of integrated single device neurostimulation system including electrode array and receiver or pulse generator, including analysis, programming, and imaging guidance when performed, posterior tibial nerve

0589T Electronic analysis with simple programming of implanted integrated neurostimulation system (eg, electrode array and receiver), including contact group(s), amplitude, pulse width, frequency (Hz), on/off cycling, burst, dose lockout, patient-selectable parameters, responsive neurostimulation, detection algorithms, closed-loop parameters, and passive parameters, when performed by physician or other qualified health care professional, posterior tibial nerve, 1-3 parameters

0590T Electronic analysis with complex programming of implanted integrated neurostimulation system (eg, electrode array and receiver), including contact group(s), amplitude, pulse width, frequency (Hz), on/off cycling, burst, dose lockout, patient-selectable parameters, responsive neurostimulation, detection algorithms, closed-loop parameters, and passive parameters, when performed by physician or other qualified health care professional, posterior tibial nerve, 4 or more parameters

0591T Health and well-being coaching face-to-face; individual, initial assessment

0592T Health and well-being coaching face-to-face; individual, follow-up session, at least 30 minutes

0593T Health and well-being coaching face-to-face; group (2 or more individuals), at least 30 minutes

15769 Grafting of autologous soft tissue, other, harvested by direct excision (eg, fat, dermis, fascia)

15771 Grafting of autologous fat harvested by liposuction technique to trunk, breasts, scalp, arms, and/or legs; 50 cc or less injectate

15772 Grafting of autologous fat harvested by liposuction technique to trunk, breasts, scalp, arms, and/or legs; each additional 50 cc injectate, or part thereof (List separately in addition to code for primary procedure)

15773 Grafting of autologous fat harvested by liposuction technique to face, eyelids, mouth, neck, ears, orbits, genitalia, hands, and/or feet; 25 cc or less injectate

15774 Grafting of autologous fat harvested by liposuction technique to face, eyelids, mouth, neck, ears, orbits, genitalia, hands, and/or feet; each additional 25 cc injectate, or part thereof (List separately in addition to code for primary procedure)

20560 Needle insertion(s) without injection(s); 1 or 2 muscle(s)

20561 Needle insertion(s) without injection(s); 3 or more muscles

20700 Manual preparation and insertion of drug-delivery device(s), deep (eg, subfascial) (List separately in addition to code for primary procedure)

20701 Removal of drug-delivery device(s), deep (eg, subfascial) (List separately in addition to code for primary procedure)

20702 Manual preparation and insertion of drug-delivery device(s), intramedullary (List separately in addition to code for primary procedure)

20703 Removal of drug-delivery device(s), intramedullary (List separately in addition to code for primary procedure)

20704 Manual preparation and insertion of drug-delivery device(s), intra-articular (List separately in addition to code for primary procedure)

20705 Removal of drug-delivery device(s), intra-articular (List separately in addition to code for primary procedure)

21601 Excision of chest wall tumor including rib(s)

21602 Excision of chest wall tumor involving rib(s), with plastic reconstruction; without mediastinal lymphadenectomy

21603 Excision of chest wall tumor involving rib(s), with plastic reconstruction; with mediastinal lymphadenectomy

33016 Pericardiocentesis, including imaging guidance, when performed

33017 Pericardial drainage with insertion of indwelling catheter, percutaneous, including fluoroscopy and/or ultrasound guidance, when performed; 6 years and older without congenital cardiac anomaly

33018 Pericardial drainage with insertion of indwelling catheter, percutaneous, including fluoroscopy and/or ultrasound guidance, when performed; birth through 5 years of age or any age with congenital cardiac anomaly

33019 Pericardial drainage with insertion of indwelling catheter, percutaneous, including CT guidance

33858 Ascending aorta graft, with cardiopulmonary bypass, includes valve suspension, when performed; for aortic dissection

33859 Ascending aorta graft, with cardiopulmonary bypass, includes valve suspension, when performed; for aortic disease other than dissection (eg, aneurysm)

33871 Transverse aortic arch graft, with cardiopulmonary bypass, with profound hypothermia, total circulatory arrest and isolated cerebral perfusion with reimplantation of arch vessel(s) (eg, island pedicle or individual arch vessel reimplantation)

34717 Endovascular repair of iliac artery at the time of aorto-iliac artery endograft placement by deployment of an iliac branched endograft including pre-procedure sizing and device selection, all ipsilateral selective iliac artery catheterization(s), all associated radiological supervision and interpretation, and all endograft extension(s) proximally to the aortic bifurcation and distally in the internal iliac, external iliac, and common femoral artery(ies), and treatment zone angioplasty/stenting, when performed, for rupture or other than rupture (eg, for aneurysm, pseudoaneurysm, dissection, arteriovenous malformation, penetrating ulcer, traumatic disruption), unilateral (List separately in addition to code for primary procedure)

34718 Endovascular repair of iliac artery, not associated with placement of an aorto-iliac artery endograft at the same session, by deployment of an iliac branched endograft, including pre-procedure sizing and device selection, all ipsilateral selective iliac artery catheterization(s), all associated radiological supervision and interpretation, and all endograft extension(s) proximally to the aortic bifurcation and distally in the internal iliac, external iliac, and common femoral artery(ies), and treatment zone angioplasty/stenting, when performed, for other than rupture (eg, for aneurysm, pseudoaneurysm, dissection, arteriovenous malformation, penetrating ulcer), unilateral

35702 Exploration not followed by surgical repair, artery; upper extremity (eg, axillary, brachial, radial, ulnar)

35703 Exploration not followed by surgical repair, artery; lower extremity (eg, common femoral, deep femoral, superficial femoral, popliteal, tibial, peroneal)

46948 Hemorrhoidectomy, internal, by transanal hemorrhoidal dearterialization, 2 or more hemorrhoid columns/groups, including ultrasound guidance, with mucopexy, when performed

49013 Preperitoneal pelvic packing for hemorrhage associated with pelvic trauma, including local exploration

49014 Re-exploration of pelvic wound with removal of preperitoneal pelvic packing, including repacking, when performed

62328 Spinal puncture, lumbar, diagnostic; with fluoroscopic or CT guidance

62329 Spinal puncture, therapeutic, for drainage of cerebrospinal fluid (by needle or catheter); with fluoroscopic or CT guidance

64451 Injection(s), anesthetic agent(s) and/or steroid; nerves innervating the sacroiliac joint, with image guidance (ie, fluoroscopy or computed tomography)

64454 Injection(s), anesthetic agent(s) and/or steroid; genicular nerve branches, including imaging guidance, when performed

64624 Destruction by neurolytic agent, genicular nerve branches including imaging guidance, when performed

64625 Radiofrequency ablation, nerves innervating the sacroiliac joint, with image guidance (ie, fluoroscopy or computed tomography)

66987 Extracapsular cataract removal with insertion of intraocular lens prosthesis (1-stage procedure), manual or mechanical technique (eg, irrigation and aspiration or phacoemulsification), complex, requiring devices or techniques not generally used in routine cataract surgery (eg, iris expansion device, suture support for intraocular lens, or primary posterior capsulorrhexis) or performed on patients in the amblyogenic developmental stage; with endoscopic cyclophotocoagulation

66988 Extracapsular cataract removal with insertion of intraocular lens prosthesis (1 stage procedure), manual or mechanical technique (eg, irrigation and aspiration or phacoemulsification); with endoscopic cyclophotocoagulation

74221 Radiologic examination, esophagus, including scout chest radiograph(s) and delayed image(s), when performed; double-contrast (eg, high-density barium and effervescent agent) study

74248 Radiologic small intestine follow-through study, including multiple serial images (List separately in addition to code for primary procedure for upper GI radiologic examination)

78429 Myocardial imaging, positron emission tomography (PET), metabolic evaluation study (including ventricular wall motion[s] and/or ejection fraction[s], when performed), single study; with concurrently acquired computed tomography transmission scan

78430 Myocardial imaging, positron emission tomography (PET), perfusion study (including ventricular wall motion[s] and/or ejection fraction[s], when performed); single study, at rest or stress (exercise or pharmacologic), with concurrently acquired computed tomography transmission scan

78431 Myocardial imaging, positron emission tomography (PET), perfusion study (including ventricular wall motion[s] and/or ejection fraction[s], when performed); multiple studies at rest and stress (exercise or pharmacologic), with concurrently acquired computed tomography transmission scan

78432 Myocardial imaging, positron emission tomography (PET), combined perfusion with metabolic evaluation study (including ventricular wall motion[s] and/or ejection fraction[s], when performed), dual radiotracer (eg, myocardial viability);

78433 Myocardial imaging, positron emission tomography (PET), combined perfusion with metabolic evaluation study (including ventricular wall motion[s] and/or ejection fraction[s], when performed), dual radiotracer (eg, myocardial viability); with concurrently acquired computed tomography transmission scan

78434 Absolute quantitation of myocardial blood flow (AQMBF), positron emission tomography (PET), rest and pharmacologic stress (List separately in addition to code for primary procedure)

78830 Radiopharmaceutical localization of tumor, inflammatory process or distribution of radiopharmaceutical agent(s) (includes vascular flow and blood pool imaging, when performed); tomographic (SPECT) with concurrently acquired computed tomography (CT) transmission scan for anatomical review, localization and determination/detection of pathology, single area (eg, head, neck, chest, pelvis), single day imaging

78831 Radiopharmaceutical localization of tumor, inflammatory process or distribution of radiopharmaceutical agent(s) (includes vascular flow and blood pool imaging, when performed); tomographic (SPECT), minimum 2 areas (eg, pelvis and knees, abdomen and pelvis), single day imaging, or single area imaging over 2 or more days

78832 Radiopharmaceutical localization of tumor, inflammatory process or distribution of radiopharmaceutical agent(s) (includes vascular flow and blood pool imaging, when performed); tomographic (SPECT) with concurrently acquired computed tomography (CT) transmission scan for anatomical review, localization and determination/detection of pathology, minimum 2 areas (eg, pelvis and knees, abdomen and pelvis), single day imaging, or single area imaging over 2 or more days

78835 Radiopharmaceutical quantification measurement(s) single area (List separately in addition to code for primary procedure)

80145 Adalimumab

80187 Posaconazole

80230 Infliximab

80235 Lacosamide

80280 Vedolizumab

80285 Voriconazole

81277 Cytogenomic neoplasia (genome-wide) microarray analysis, interrogation of genomic regions for copy number and loss-of-heterozygosity variants for chromosomal abnormalities

81307 PALB2 (partner and localizer of BRCA2) (eg, breast and pancreatic cancer) gene analysis; full gene sequence

81308 PALB2 (partner and localizer of BRCA2) (eg, breast and pancreatic cancer) gene analysis; known familial variant

81309 PIK3CA (phosphatidylinositol-4, 5-biphosphate 3-kinase, catalytic subunit alpha) (eg, colorectal and breast cancer) gene analysis, targeted sequence analysis (eg, exons 7, 9, 20)

81522 Oncology (breast), mRNA, gene expression profiling by RT-PCR of 12 genes (8 content and 4 housekeeping), utilizing formalin-fixed paraffin-embedded tissue, algorithm reported as recurrence risk score

81542 Oncology (prostate), mRNA, microarray gene expression profiling of 22 content genes, utilizing formalin-fixed paraffin-embedded tissue, algorithm reported as metastasis risk score

81552 Oncology (uveal melanoma), mRNA, gene expression profiling by real-time RT-PCR of 15 genes (12 content and 3 housekeeping), utilizing fine needle aspirate or formalin-fixed paraffin-embedded tissue, algorithm reported as risk of metastasis

87563 Infectious agent detection by nucleic acid (DNA or RNA); Mycoplasma genitalium, amplified probe technique

90694 Influenza virus vaccine, quadrivalent (aIIV4), inactivated, adjuvanted, preservative free, 0.5 mL dosage, for intramuscular use

90912 Biofeedback training, perineal muscles, anorectal or urethral sphincter, including EMG and/or manometry, when performed; initial 15 minutes of one-on-one physician or other qualified health care professional contact with the patient

90913 Biofeedback training, perineal muscles, anorectal or urethral sphincter, including EMG and/or manometry, when performed; each additional 15 minutes of one-on-one physician or other qualified health care professional contact with the patient (List separately in addition to code for primary procedure)

92201 Ophthalmoscopy, extended; with retinal drawing and scleral depression of peripheral retinal disease (eg, for retinal tear, retinal detachment, retinal tumor) with interpretation and report, unilateral or bilateral

92202 Ophthalmoscopy, extended; with drawing of optic nerve or macula (eg, for glaucoma, macular pathology, tumor) with interpretation and report, unilateral or bilateral

92549 Computerized dynamic posturography sensory organization test (CDP-SOT), 6 conditions (ie, eyes open, eyes closed, visual sway, platform sway, eyes closed platform sway, platform and visual sway), including interpretation and report; with motor control test (MCT) and adaptation test (ADT)

93356 Myocardial strain imaging using speckle tracking-derived assessment of myocardial mechanics (List separately in addition to codes for echocardiography imaging)

93985 Duplex scan of arterial inflow and venous outflow for preoperative vessel assessment prior to creation of hemodialysis access; complete bilateral study

93986 Duplex scan of arterial inflow and venous outflow for preoperative vessel assessment prior to creation of hemodialysis access; complete unilateral study

95700 Electroencephalogram (EEG) continuous recording, with video when performed, setup, patient education, and takedown when performed, administered in person by EEG technologist, minimum of 8 channels

95705 Electroencephalogram (EEG), without video, review of data, technical description by EEG technologist, 2-12 hours; unmonitored

95706 Electroencephalogram (EEG), without video, review of data, technical description by EEG technologist, 2-12 hours; with intermittent monitoring and maintenance

95707 Electroencephalogram (EEG), without video, review of data, technical description by EEG technologist, 2-12 hours; with continuous, real-time monitoring and maintenance

95708 Electroencephalogram (EEG), without video, review of data, technical description by EEG technologist, each increment of 12-26 hours; unmonitored

95709 Electroencephalogram (EEG), without video, review of data, technical description by EEG technologist, each increment of 12-26 hours; with intermittent monitoring and maintenance

95710 Electroencephalogram (EEG), without video, review of data, technical description by EEG technologist, each increment of 12-26 hours; with continuous, real-time monitoring and maintenance

95711 Electroencephalogram with video (VEEG), review of data, technical description by EEG technologist, 2-12 hours; unmonitored

95712 Electroencephalogram with video (VEEG), review of data, technical description by EEG technologist, 2-12 hours; with intermittent monitoring and maintenance

95713 Electroencephalogram with video (VEEG), review of data, technical description by EEG technologist, 2-12 hours; with continuous, real-time monitoring and maintenance

95714 Electroencephalogram with video (VEEG), review of data, technical description by EEG technologist, each increment of 12-26 hours; unmonitored

95715 Electroencephalogram with video (VEEG), review of data, technical description by EEG technologist, each increment of 12-26 hours; with intermittent monitoring and maintenance

95716 Electroencephalogram with video (VEEG), review of data, technical description by EEG technologist, each increment of 12-26 hours; with continuous, real-time monitoring and maintenance

95717 Electroencephalogram (EEG), continuous recording, physician or other qualified health care professional review of recorded events, analysis of spike and seizure detection, interpretation and report, 2-12 hours of EEG recording; without video

95718 Electroencephalogram (EEG), continuous recording, physician or other qualified health care professional review of recorded events, analysis of spike and seizure detection, interpretation and report, 2-12 hours of EEG recording; with video (VEEG)

95719 Electroencephalogram (EEG), continuous recording, physician or other qualified health care professional review of recorded events, analysis of spike and seizure detection, each increment of greater than 12 hours, up to 26 hours of EEG recording, interpretation and report after each 24-hour period; without video

95720 Electroencephalogram (EEG), continuous recording, physician or other qualified health care professional review of recorded events, analysis of spike and seizure detection, each increment of greater than 12 hours, up to 26 hours of EEG recording, interpretation and report after each 24-hour period; with video (VEEG)

95721 Electroencephalogram (EEG), continuous recording, physician or other qualified health care professional review of recorded events, analysis of spike and seizure detection, interpretation, and summary report, complete study; greater than 36 hours, up to 60 hours of EEG recording, without video

95722 Electroencephalogram (EEG), continuous recording, physician or other qualified health care professional review of recorded events, analysis of spike and seizure detection, interpretation, and summary report, complete study; greater than 36 hours, up to 60 hours of EEG recording, with video (VEEG)

95723 Electroencephalogram (EEG), continuous recording, physician or other qualified health care professional review of recorded events, analysis of spike and seizure detection, interpretation, and summary report, complete study; greater than 60 hours, up to 84 hours of EEG recording, without video

95724 Electroencephalogram (EEG), continuous recording, physician or other qualified health care professional review of recorded events, analysis of spike and seizure detection, interpretation, and summary report, complete study; greater than 60 hours, up to 84 hours of EEG recording, with video (VEEG)

95725 Electroencephalogram (EEG), continuous recording, physician or other qualified health care professional review of recorded events, analysis of spike and seizure detection, interpretation, and summary report, complete study; greater than 84 hours of EEG recording, without video

95726 Electroencephalogram (EEG), continuous recording, physician or other qualified health care professional review of recorded events, analysis of spike and seizure detection, interpretation, and summary report, complete study; greater than 84 hours of EEG recording, with video (VEEG)

96156 Health behavior assessment, or re-assessment (ie, health-focused clinical interview, behavioral observations, clinical decision making)

96158 Health behavior intervention, individual, face-to-face; initial 30 minutes

96159 Health behavior intervention, individual, face-to-face; each additional 15 minutes (List separately in addition to code for primary service)

96164 Health behavior intervention, group (2 or more patients), face-to-face; initial 30 minutes

96165 Health behavior intervention, group (2 or more patients), face-to-face; each additional 15 minutes (List separately in addition to code for primary service)

96167 Health behavior intervention, family (with the patient present), face-to-face; initial 30 minutes

96168 Health behavior intervention, family (with the patient present), face-to-face; each additional 15 minutes (List separately in addition to code for primary service)

96170 Health behavior intervention, family (without the patient present), face-to-face; initial 30 minutes

96171 Health behavior intervention, family (without the patient present), face-to-face; each additional 15 minutes (List separately in addition to code for primary service)

97129 Therapeutic interventions that focus on cognitive function (eg, attention, memory, reasoning, executive function, problem solving, and/or pragmatic functioning) and compensatory strategies to manage the performance of an activity (eg, managing time or schedules, initiating, organizing, and sequencing tasks), direct (one-on-one) patient contact; initial 15 minutes

97130 Therapeutic interventions that focus on cognitive function (eg, attention, memory, reasoning, executive function, problem solving, and/or pragmatic functioning) and compensatory strategies to manage the performance of an activity (eg, managing time or schedules, initiating, organizing, and sequencing tasks), direct (one-on-one) patient contact; each additional 15 minutes (List separately in addition to code for primary procedure)

98970 Qualified nonphysician health care professional online digital evaluation and management service, for an established patient, for up to 7 days, cumulative time during the 7 days; 5-10 minutes

98971 Qualified nonphysician health care professional online digital evaluation and management service, for an established patient, for up to 7 days, cumulative time during the 7 days; 11-20 minutes

98972 Qualified nonphysician health care professional online digital evaluation and management service, for an established patient, for up to 7 days, cumulative time during the 7 days; 21 or more minutes

99421 Online digital evaluation and management service, for an established patient, for up to 7 days, cumulative time during the 7 days; 5-10 minutes

99422 Online digital evaluation and management service, for an established patient, for up to 7 days, cumulative time during the 7 days; 11-20 minutes

99423 Online digital evaluation and management service, for an established patient, for up to 7 days, cumulative time during the 7 days; 21 or more minutes

99458 Remote physiologic monitoring treatment management services, clinical staff/physician/other qualified health care professional time in a calendar month requiring interactive communication with the patient/caregiver during the month; each additional 20 minutes (List separately in addition to code for primary procedure)

99473 Self-measured blood pressure using a device validated for clinical accuracy; patient education/training and device calibration

99474 Self-measured blood pressure using a device validated for clinical accuracy; separate self-measurements of two readings one minute apart, twice daily over a 30-day period (minimum of 12 readings), collection of data reported by the patient and/or caregiver to the physician or other qualified health care professional, with report of average systolic and diastolic pressures and subsequent communication of a treatment plan to the patient

Revised Codes

31233 Nasal/sinus endoscopy, diagnostic ~~with maxillary sinusoscopy (via inferior meatus or canine fossa puncture)~~; with maxillary sinusoscopy (via inferior meatus or canine fossa puncture)

31235 with sphenoid sinusoscopy (via puncture of sphenoidal face or cannulation of ostium)

31292 Nasal/sinus endoscopy, surgical, with orbital decompression; ~~with~~ medial or inferior ~~orbital~~ wall ~~decompression~~

31293 ~~with~~ medial ~~orbital wall~~ and inferior ~~orbital wall decompression~~

31294 Nasal/sinus endoscopy, surgical, with optic nerve decompression~~; with optic nerve decompression~~

31295 Nasal/sinus endoscopy, surgical, with dilation (eg, balloon dilation); ~~with dilation of~~ maxillary sinus ostium ~~(eg, balloon dilation)~~, transnasal or via canine fossa

31296 ~~with dilation of~~ frontal sinus ostium ~~(eg, balloon dilation)~~

31297 ~~with dilation of~~ sphenoid sinus ostium ~~(eg, balloon dilation)~~

31298 ~~with dilation of~~ frontal and sphenoid sinus ostia ~~(eg, balloon dilation)~~

33275 Transcatheter removal of permanent leadless pacemaker, right ventricular, including imaging guidance (eg, fluoroscopy, venous ultrasound, ventriculography, femoral venography), when performed

35701 Exploration ~~(~~not followed by surgical repair,~~), with or without lysis of~~ artery; neck (eg, carotid ~~artery~~, subclavian)

46945 Hemorrhoidectomy, internal, by ligation other than rubber band; single hemorrhoid column/group, without imaging guidance

46946 2 or more hemorrhoid columns/groups, without imaging guidance

54640 Orchiopexy, inguinal ~~approach, with~~ or ~~without hernia repair~~ scrotal approach

62270 Spinal puncture, lumbar, diagnostic;

62272 Spinal puncture, therapeutic, for drainage of cerebrospinal fluid (by needle or catheter);

64400 Injection(s), anesthetic agent(s) and/or steroid; trigeminal nerve, ~~any division or branch~~each branch (ie, ophthalmic, maxillary, mandibular)

64405 greater occipital nerve

64408 vagus nerve

64415 brachial plexus~~, single~~

64416 brachial plexus, continuous infusion by catheter (including catheter placement)

64417 axillary nerve

64418 suprascapular nerve

64420 intercostal nerve, single level

64421 intercostal nerve, ~~multiple, regional block~~ each additional level (List separately in addition to code for primary procedure)

64425 ilioinguinal, iliohypogastric nerves

64430 pudendal nerve

64435 paracervical (uterine) nerve

64445 sciatic nerve~~, single~~

64446 sciatic nerve, continuous infusion by catheter (including catheter placement)

64447 femoral nerve~~, single~~

64448 femoral nerve, continuous infusion by catheter (including catheter placement)

64449 lumbar plexus, posterior approach, continuous infusion by catheter (including catheter placement)

64450 other peripheral nerve or branch

66711 Ciliary body destruction; cyclophotocoagulation, endoscopic, without concomitant removal of crystalline lens

66982 Extracapsular cataract removal with insertion of intraocular lens prosthesis (1-stage procedure), manual or mechanical technique (eg, irrigation and aspiration or phacoemulsification), complex, requiring devices or techniques not generally used in routine cataract surgery (eg, iris expansion device, suture support for intraocular lens, or primary posterior capsulorrhexis) or performed on patients in the amblyogenic developmental stage; without endoscopic cyclophotocoagulation

66984 Extracapsular cataract removal with insertion of intraocular lens prosthesis (1 stage procedure), manual or mechanical technique (eg, irrigation and aspiration or phacoemulsification); without endoscopic cyclophotocoagulation

74022 Radiologic examination, ~~abdomen;~~ complete acute abdomen series, including 2 or more views of the abdomen (eg, supine, erect, ~~and/or~~ decubitus ~~views~~), and a single view chest

74210 Radiologic examination, pharynx and/or cervical esophagus, including scout neck radiograph(s) and delayed image(s), when performed, contrast (eg, barium) study~~; pharynx and/or cervical esophagus~~

74220 Radiologic examination, esophagus, including scout chest radiograph(s) and delayed image(s), when performed; ~~esophagus~~single-contrast (eg, barium) study

74230 ~~Swallowing~~Radiologic examination, swallowing function, with cineradiography/videoradiography, including scout neck radiograph(s) and delayed image(s), when performed, contrast (eg, barium) study

74240 Radiologic examination, upper gastrointestinal tract, including scout abdominal radiograph(s) and delayed image(s), ~~upper~~ when performed; ~~with or without delayed images~~single-contrast (eg, ~~without KUB~~ barium) study

74246 with or without delayed images double-contrast (eg, high-density barium and effervescent agent) study, including glucagon, ~~without KUB~~ when administered

74250 Radiologic examination, small intestine, ~~includes~~including multiple serial images and scout abdominal radiograph(s), when performed; single-contrast (eg, barium) study

74251 double-contrast (eg, high-density barium and air via enteroclysis tube) study, including glucagon, when administered

74270 Radiologic examination, colon, including scout abdominal radiograph(s) and delayed image(s), when performed; single-contrast (eg, barium) ~~enema, with or without KUB~~study

74280 air double-contrast ~~with specific~~(eg, high density barium and air) study, ~~with or without glucagon~~including glucagon, when administered

78459 Myocardial imaging, positron emission tomography (PET), metabolic evaluation study (including ventricular wall motion[s] and/or ejection fraction[s], when performed), single study;

78491 Myocardial imaging, positron emission tomography (PET), perfusion study (including ventricular wall motion[s] and/or ejection fraction[s], when performed); single study, at rest or stress (exercise or pharmacologic)

78492 multiple studies at rest and~~/or~~ stress (exercise or pharmacologic)

78800 Radiopharmaceutical localization of tumor, inflammatory process or distribution of radiopharmaceutical agent(s) (includes vascular flow and blood pool imaging, when performed); ~~limited~~planar, single area (eg, head, neck, chest, pelvis), single day imaging

78801 multiple planar, 2 or more areas (eg, abdomen and pelvis, head and chest), 1 or more days imaging or single area imaging over 2 or more days

78802 planar, whole body, single day imaging

78803 tomographic (SPECT), single area (eg, head, neck, chest, pelvis), single day imaging

78804 planar, whole body, requiring 2 or more days imaging

81350 UGT1A1 (UDP glucuronosyltransferase 1 family, polypeptide A1) (eg, ~~irinotecan~~ drug metabolism, hereditary unconjugated hyperbilirubinemia [Gilbert syndrome])~~,~~ gene analysis, common variants (eg, *28, *36, *37)

81404 Molecular pathology procedure, Level 5 (eg, analysis of 2-5 exons by DNA sequence analysis, mutation scanning or duplication/deletion variants of 6-10 exons, or characterization of a dynamic mutation disorder/triplet repeat by Southern blot analysis) ~~PIK3CA (phosphatidylinositol-4,5-bisphosphate 3-kinase, catalytic subunit alpha) (eg, colorectal cancer), targeted sequence analysis (eg, exons 9 and 20)~~ UGT1A1 (UDP glucuronosyltransferase 1 family, polypeptide A1) (eg, hereditary unconjugated hyperbilirubinemia [Crigler-Najjar syndrome]) full gene sequence

81406 Molecular pathology procedure, Level 7 (eg, analysis of 11-25 exons by DNA sequence analysis, mutation scanning or duplication/deletion variants of 26-50 exons~~, cytogenomic array analysis for neoplasia) Cytogenomic microarray analysis, neoplasia (eg, interrogation of copy number, and loss-of-heterozygosity via single nucleotide polymorphism [SNP]-based comparative genomic hybridization [CGH] microarray analysis) PALB2 (partner and localizer of BRCA2) (eg, breast and pancreatic cancer), full gene sequence~~

81407 Molecular pathology procedure, Level 8 (eg, analysis of 26-50 exons by DNA sequence analysis, mutation scanning or duplication/deletion variants of >50 exons, sequence analysis of multiple genes on one platform) APOB (apolipoprotein B) (eg, familial hypercholesterolemia type B) full gene sequence

90734 Meningococcal conjugate vaccine, serogroups A, C, W, Y ~~and W-135, quadrivalent (MCV4~~, quadrivalent, diphtheria toxoid carrier (MenACWY-D) or ~~MenACWY)~~CRM197 carrier (MenACWY-CRM), for intramuscular use

92548 Computerized dynamic posturography sensory organization test (CDP-SOT), 6 conditions (ie, eyes open, eyes closed, visual sway, platform sway, eyes closed platform sway, platform and visual sway), including interpretation and report;

92626 Evaluation of auditory ~~rehabilitation~~function for surgically implanted device(s) candidacy or postoperative status of a surgically implanted device(s); first hour

92627 each additional 15 minutes (List separately in addition to code for primary procedure)

93784 Ambulatory blood pressure monitoring, utilizing ~~a system such as magnetic tape and/or computer disk,~~report-generating software, automated, worn continuously for 24 hours or longer; including recording, scanning analysis, interpretation and report

Appendix B — New, Revised, and Deleted Codes

93786 recording only

93788 scanning analysis with report

93790 review with interpretation and report

94728 Airway resistance by ~~impulse~~ oscillometry

95813 Electroencephalogram (EEG) extended monitoring; ~~greater than 1 hour~~61-119 minutes

99457 Remote physiologic monitoring treatment management services, ~~20 minutes or more of~~ clinical staff/physician/other qualified health care professional time in a calendar month requiring interactive communication with the patient/caregiver during the month; first 20 minutes

0008U Helicobacter pylori detection and antibiotic resistance, DNA, 16S and 23S rRNA, gyrA, pbp1, rdxA and rpoB, next generation sequencing, formalin-fixed paraffin-embedded or fresh tissue or fecal sample, predictive, reported as positive or negative for resistance to clarithromycin, fluoroquinolones, metronidazole, amoxicillin, tetracycline, and rifabutin

0402T Collagen cross-linking of cornea ~~(~~, including removal of the corneal epithelium and intraoperative pachymetry, when performed (Report medication separately)

2022F Dilated retinal eye exam with interpretation by an ophthalmologist or optometrist documented and reviewed; with evidence of retinopathy (DM)[2,4]

2024F 7 standard field stereoscopic retinal photos with interpretation by an ophthalmologist or optometrist documented and reviewed; with evidence of retinopathy (DM)[2,4]

2026F Eye imaging validated to match diagnosis from 7 standard field stereoscopic retinal photos results documented and reviewed; with evidence of retinopathy (DM)[2,4]

Deleted Codes

0009M	0081U	0104U	0205T	0206T	0249T	0254T
0341T	0357T	0375T	0377T	0380T	0399T	0482T
19260	19271	19272	19304	20926	33010	33011
33015	33860	33870	35721	35741	35761	43401
64402	64410	64413	74241	74245	74247	74249
74260	76930	78205	78206	78320	78607	78647
78710	78805	78806	78807	90911	92225	92226
93299	95827	95831	95832	95833	95834	95950
95951	95953	95956	96150	96151	96152	96153
96154	96155	97127	98969	99444		

Resequenced Icon Added

15769	20560	20561	46948	62328	62329	64624
64625	66987	66988	78429	78430	78431	78432
78433	78434	78804	78830	78831	78832	78835
80230	80235	80280	80285	81277	81307	81308
81309	81433	81522	90619	90694	93356	95700
95705	95706	95707	95708	95709	95710	95711
95712	95713	95714	95715	95716	95717	95718
95719	95720	95721	95722	95723	95724	95725
95726	96164	96165	96167	96168	96170	96171
2033F	3051F	3052F	99421	99422	99423	99458
99473	99474					

Web Release New and Revised Codes

Codes indicated as "Web Release" codes indicate CPT codes that are in *Current Procedural Coding Expert* for the current year, but will not be in the AMA CPT book until the following year. This can also include those codes designated by the AMA as new or revised for 2020 but that actually appeared in the 2019 Optum360 book. These codes will have the appropriate new or revised icon appended to match the CPT code book, however. See the complete list that follows:

New codes, deleted codes, and revisions to codes in the 2020 *Current Procedural Coding Expert* that will not appear in the CPT code book until 2021

These codes are indicated with the following icons: ● ▲ These icons will be green in the body of the book.

New Codes

0139U Neurology (autism spectrum disorder [ASD]), quantitative measurements of 6 central carbon metabolites (ie, α-ketoglutarate, alanine, lactate, phenylalanine, pyruvate, and succinate), LC-MS/MS, plasma, algorithmic analysis with result reported as negative or positive (with metabolic subtypes of ASD)

0140U Infectious disease (fungi), fungal pathogen identification, DNA (15 fungal targets), blood culture, amplified probe technique, each target reported as detected or not detected

0141U Infectious disease (bacteria and fungi), gram-positive organism identification and drug resistance element detection, DNA (20 gram-positive bacterial targets, 4 resistance genes, 1 pan gram-negative bacterial target, 1 pan Candida target), blood culture, amplified probe technique, each target reported as detected or not detected

0142U Infectious disease (bacteria and fungi), gram-negative bacterial identification and drug resistance element detection, DNA (21 gram-negative bacterial targets, 6 resistance genes, 1 pan gram-positive bacterial target, 1 pan Candida target), amplified probe technique, each target reported as detected or not detected

0143U Drug assay, definitive, 120 or more drugs or metabolites, urine, quantitative liquid chromatography with tandem mass spectrometry (LC-MS/MS) using multiple reaction monitoring (MRM), with drug or metabolite description, comments including sample validation, per date of service

0144U Drug assay, definitive, 160 or more drugs or metabolites, urine, quantitative liquid chromatography with tandem mass spectrometry (LC-MS/MS) using multiple reaction monitoring (MRM), with drug or metabolite description, comments including sample validation, per date of service

0145U Drug assay, definitive, 65 or more drugs or metabolites, urine, quantitative liquid chromatography with tandem mass spectrometry (LC-MS/MS) using multiple reaction monitoring (MRM), with drug or metabolite description, comments including sample validation, per date of service

0146U Drug assay, definitive, 80 or more drugs or metabolites, urine, by quantitative liquid chromatography with tandem mass spectrometry (LC-MS/MS) using multiple reaction monitoring (MRM), with drug or metabolite description, comments including sample validation, per date of service

0147U Drug assay, definitive, 85 or more drugs or metabolites, urine, quantitative liquid chromatography with tandem mass spectrometry (LC-MS/MS) using multiple reaction monitoring (MRM), with drug or metabolite description, comments including sample validation, per date of service

0148U Drug assay, definitive, 100 or more drugs or metabolites, urine, quantitative liquid chromatography with tandem mass spectrometry (LC-MS/MS) using multiple reaction monitoring (MRM), with drug or metabolite description, comments including sample validation, per date of service

0149U Drug assay, definitive, 60 or more drugs or metabolites, urine, quantitative liquid chromatography with tandem mass spectrometry (LC-MS/MS) using multiple reaction monitoring (MRM), with drug or metabolite description, comments including sample validation, per date of service

0150U Drug assay, definitive, 120 or more drugs or metabolites, urine, quantitative liquid chromatography with tandem mass spectrometry (LC-MS/MS) using multiple reaction monitoring (MRM), with drug or metabolite description, comments including sample validation, per date of service

0151U Infectious disease (bacterial or viral respiratory tract infection), pathogen specific nucleic acid (DNA or RNA), 33 targets, real-time semi-quantitative PCR, bronchoalveolar lavage, sputum, or endotracheal aspirate, detection of 33 organismal and antibiotic resistance genes with limited semi-quantitative results

0152U Infectious disease (bacteria, fungi, parasites, and DNA viruses), DNA, PCR and next-generation sequencing, plasma, detection of >1,000 potential microbial organisms for significant positive pathogens

0153U Oncology (breast), mRNA, gene expression profiling by next-generation sequencing of 101 genes, utilizing formalin-fixed paraffin-embedded tissue, algorithm reported as a triple negative breast cancer clinical subtype(s) with information on immune cell involvement

0154U *FGFR3 (fibroblast growth factor receptor 3)* gene analysis (ie, p.R248C [c.742C>T], p.S249C [c.746C>G], p.G370C [c.1108G>T], p.Y373C [c.1118A>G], FGFR3-TACC3v1, and FGFR3-TACC3v3)

0155U *PIK3CA (phosphatidylinositol-4,5-bisphosphate 3-kinase, catalytic subunit alpha)* (eg, breast cancer) gene analysis (ie, p.C420R, p.E542K, p.E545A, p.E545D [g.1635G>T only], p.E545G, p.E545K, p.Q546E, p.Q546R, p.H1047L, p.H1047R, p.H1047Y)

0156U Copy number (eg, intellectual disability, dysmorphology), sequence analysis

0157U *APC (APC regulator of WNT signaling pathway)* (eg, familial adenomatosis polyposis [FAP]) mRNA sequence analysis (List separately in addition to code for primary procedure)

0158U *MLH1 (mutL homolog 1)* (eg, hereditary non-polyposis colorectal cancer, Lynch syndrome) mRNA sequence analysis (List separately in addition to code for primary procedure)

0159U *MSH2 (mutS homolog 2)* (eg, hereditary colon cancer, Lynch syndrome) mRNA sequence analysis (List separately in addition to code for primary procedure)

0160U *MSH6 (mutS homolog 6)* (eg, hereditary colon cancer, Lynch syndrome) mRNA sequence analysis (List separately in addition to code for primary procedure)

0161U *PMS2 (PMS1 homolog 2, mismatch repair system component)* (eg, hereditary non-polyposis colorectal cancer, Lynch syndrome) mRNA sequence analysis (List separately in addition to code for primary procedure)

0162U Hereditary colon cancer (Lynch syndrome), targeted mRNA sequence analysis panel *(MLH1, MSH2, MSH6, PMS2)* (List separately in addition to code for primary procedure)

Deleted Codes

0011M Oncology, prostate cancer, mRNA expression assay of 12 genes (10 content and 2 housekeeping), RT-PCR test utilizing blood plasma and urine, algorithms to predict high-grade prostate cancer risk

0012M Oncology (urothelial), mRNA, gene expression profiling by real-time quantitative PCR of five genes (*MDK, HOXA13, CDC2 [CDK1], IGFBP5*, and *CXCR2*), utilizing urine, algorithm reported as a risk score for having urothelial carcinoma

0013M Oncology (urothelial), mRNA, gene expression profiling by real-time quantitative PCR of five genes (*MDK, HOXA13, CDC2 [CDK1], IGFBP5*, and *CXCR2*), utilizing urine, algorithm reported as a risk score for having recurrent urothelial carcinoma

81518 Oncology (breast), mRNA, gene expression profiling by real-time RT-PCR of 11 genes (7 content and 4 housekeeping), utilizing formalin-fixed paraffin-embedded tissue, algorithms reported as percentage risk for metastatic recurrence and likelihood of benefit from extended endocrine therapy

0062U Autoimmune (systemic lupus erythematosus), IgG and IgM analysis of 80 biomarkers, utilizing serum, algorithm reported with a risk score

0063U Neurology (autism), 32 amines by LC-MS/MS, using plasma, algorithm reported as metabolic signature associated with autism spectrum disorder

0064U Antibody, Treponema pallidum, total and rapid plasma reagin (RPR), immunoassay, qualitative

0065U Syphilis test, non-treponemal antibody, immunoassay, qualitative (RPR)

0066U Placental alpha-micro globulin-1 (PAMG-1), immunoassay with direct optical observation, cervico-vaginal fluid, each specimen

0067U Oncology (breast), immunohistochemistry, protein expression profiling of 4 biomarkers (matrix metalloproteinase-1 [MMP-1], carcinoembryonic antigen-related cell adhesion molecule 6 [CEACAM6], hyaluronoglucosaminidase [HYAL1], highly expressed in cancer protein [HEC1]), formalin-fixed paraffin-embedded precancerous breast tissue, algorithm reported as carcinoma risk score

0068U Candida species panel *(C. albicans, C. glabrata, C. parapsilosis, C. kruseii, C tropicalis, and C. auris)*, amplified probe technique with qualitative report of the presence or absence of each species

0069U Oncology (colorectal), microRNA, RT-PCR expression profiling of miR-31-3p, formalin-fixed paraffin-embedded tissue, algorithm reported as an expression score

0070U *CYP2D6 (cytochrome P450, family 2, subfamily D, polypeptide 6)* (eg, drug metabolism) gene analysis, common and select rare variants (ie, *2, *3, *4, *4N, *5, *6, *7, *8, *9, *10, *11, *12, *13, *14A, *14B, *15, *17, *29, *35, *36, *41, *57, *61, *63, *68, *83, *xN)

0071U *CYP2D6 (cytochrome P450, family 2, subfamily D, polypeptide 6)* (eg, drug metabolism) gene analysis, full gene sequence (List separately in addition to code for primary procedure)

0072U *CYP2D6 (cytochrome P450, family 2, subfamily D, polypeptide 6)* (eg, drug metabolism) gene analysis, targeted sequence analysis (ie, CYP2D6-2D7 hybrid gene) (List separately in addition to code for primary procedure)

0073U *CYP2D6 (cytochrome P450, family 2, subfamily D, polypeptide 6)* (eg, drug metabolism) gene analysis, targeted sequence analysis (ie, CYP2D7-2D6 hybrid gene) (List separately in addition to code for primary procedure)

0074U *CYP2D6 (cytochrome P450, family 2, subfamily D, polypeptide 6)* (eg, drug metabolism) gene analysis, targeted sequence analysis (ie, non-duplicated gene when duplication/multiplication is trans) (List separately in addition to code for primary procedure)

0075U *CYP2D6 (cytochrome P450, family 2, subfamily D, polypeptide 6)* (eg, drug metabolism) gene analysis, targeted sequence analysis (ie, 5' gene duplication/multiplication) (List separately in addition to code for primary procedure)

0076U *CYP2D6 (cytochrome P450, family 2, subfamily D, polypeptide 6)* (eg, drug metabolism) gene analysis, targeted sequence analysis (ie, 3' gene duplication/ multiplication) (List separately in addition to code for primary procedure)

0077U Immunoglobulin paraprotein (M-protein), qualitative, immunoprecipitation and mass spectrometry, blood or urine, including isotype

0078U Pain management (opioid-use disorder) genotyping panel, 16 common variants (ie, *ABCB1, COMT, DAT1, DBH, DOR, DRD1, DRD2, DRD4, GABA, GAL, HTR2A, HTTLPR, MTHFR, MUOR, OPRK1, OPRM1*), buccal swab or other germline tissue sample, algorithm reported as positive or negative risk of opioid-use disorder

0079U Comparative DNA analysis using multiple selected single-nucleotide polymorphisms (SNPs), urine and buccal DNA, for specimen identity verification

Appendix C — Evaluation and Management Extended Guidelines

This appendix provides an overview of evaluation and management (E/M) services, tables that identify the documentation elements associated with each code, and the federal documentation guidelines with emphasis on the 1997 exam guidelines. This set of guidelines represents the most complete discussion of the elements of the currently accepted versions. The 1997 version identifies both general multi-system physical examinations and single-system examinations, but providers may also use the original 1995 version of the E/M guidelines; both are currently supported by the Centers for Medicare and Medicaid Services (CMS) for audit purposes.

The levels of E/M services define the wide variations in skill, effort, and time and are required for preventing and/or diagnosing and treating illness or injury, and promoting optimal health. These codes are intended to represent physician work, and because much of this work involves the amount of training, experience, expertise, and knowledge that a provider may employ when treating a given patient, the true indications of the level of this work may be difficult to recognize without some explanation.

Providers

The AMA advises coders that while a particular service or procedure may be assigned to a specific section, the service or procedure itself is not limited to use only by that specialty group (see paragraphs 2 and 3 under "Instructions for Use of the CPT® Codebook" on page xii of the AMA CPT Book). Additionally, the procedures and services listed throughout the book are for use by any qualified physician or other qualified health care professional or entity (e.g., hospitals, laboratories, or home health agencies).

The use of the phrase "physician or other qualified health care professional" (OQHCP) was adopted to identify a health care provider other than a physician. This type of provider is further described in CPT as an individual "qualified by education, training, licensure/regulation (when applicable), and facility privileging (when applicable)." State licensure guidelines determine the scope of practice and an OQHCP must practice within these guidelines, even if more restrictive than the CPT guidelines. The OQHCP may report services independently or under incident-to guidelines. The professionals within this definition are separate from "clinical staff" and are able to practice independently. CPT defines clinical staff as "a person who works under the supervision of a physician or OQHCP and who is allowed, by law, regulation, and facility policy to perform or assist in the performance of a specified professional service, but who does not individually report that professional service." Keep in mind that there may be other policies or guidance that can affect who may report a specific service.

Types of E/M Services

When approaching E/M, the first choice that a provider must make is what type of code to use. The following tables outline the E/M codes for different levels of care for:

- Office or other outpatient services—new patient
- Office or other outpatient services—established patient
- Hospital observation services—initial care, subsequent, and discharge
- Hospital inpatient services—initial care, subsequent, and discharge
- Observation or inpatient care (including admission and discharge services)
- Consultations—office or other outpatient
- Consultations—inpatient
- Emergency department services
- Critical care
- Nursing facility—initial services
- Nursing facility—subsequent services
- Nursing facility—discharge and annual assessment
- Domiciliary, rest home, or custodial care—new patient
- Domiciliary, rest home, or custodial care—established patient
- Home services—new patient
- Home services—established patient
- Newborn care services
- Neonatal and pediatric interfacility transport
- Neonatal and pediatric critical care—inpatient
- Neonate and infant intensive care services—initial and continuing

The specifics of the code components that determine code selection are listed in the table and discussed in the next section. Before a level of service is decided upon, the correct type of service is identified.

A new patient is a patient who has not received any face-to-face professional services from the physician or OQHCP within the past three years. An established patient is a patient who has received face-to-face professional services from the physician or OQHCP within the past three years. In the case of group practices, if a physician or OQHCP of the exact same specialty or subspecialty has seen the patient within three years, the patient is considered established.

If a physician or OQHCP is on call or covering for another physician or OQHCP, the patient's encounter is classified as it would have been by the physician or OQHCP who is not available. Thus, a locum tenens physician or OQHCP who sees a patient on behalf of the patient's attending physician or OQHCP may not bill a new patient code unless the attending physician or OQHCP has not seen the patient for any problem within three years.

Office or other outpatient services are E/M services provided in the physician or OQHCP office, the outpatient area, or other ambulatory facility. Until the patient is admitted to a health care facility, he/she is considered to be an outpatient. Hospital observation services are E/M services provided to patients who are designated or admitted as "observation status" in a hospital.

Codes 99218-99220 are used to indicate initial observation care. These codes include the initiation of the observation status, supervision of patient care including writing orders, and the performance of periodic reassessments. These codes are used only by the provider "admitting" the patient for observation.

Codes 99234-99236 are used to indicate evaluation and management services to a patient who is admitted to and discharged from observation status or hospital inpatient on the same day. If the patient is admitted as an inpatient from observation on the same day, use the appropriate level of Initial Hospital Care (99221-99223).

Code 99217 indicates discharge from observation status. It includes the final physical examination of the patient, instructions, and preparation of the discharge records. It should not be used when admission and discharge are on the same date of service. As mentioned above, report codes 99234-99236 to appropriately describe same day observation services.

If a patient is in observation longer than one day, subsequent observation care codes 99224-99226 should be reported. If the patient is discharged on the second day, observation discharge code 99217 should be reported. If the patient status is changed to inpatient on a subsequent date, the appropriate inpatient code, 99221-99233, should be reported.

Initial hospital care is defined as E/M services provided during the first hospital inpatient encounter with the patient by the admitting provider. (If a physician other than the admitting physician performs the initial inpatient encounter, refer to consultations or subsequent hospital care in the CPT book.) Subsequent hospital care includes all follow-up encounters with the patient by all physicians or OQHCP. As there may only be one admitting physician, HCPCS Level II modifier AI Principal physician of record, should be appended to the initial hospital care code by the attending physician or OQHCP.

A consultation is the provision of a physician or OQHCP's opinion or advice about a patient for a specific problem at the request of another physician or other appropriate source. CPT also states that a consultation may be performed when a physician or OQHCP is determining whether to accept the transfer of patient care at the request of another physician or appropriate source. An office or other outpatient consultation is a consultation provided in the consultant's office, in the emergency department, or in an outpatient or other ambulatory facility including hospital observation services, home services, domiciliary, rest home, or custodial care. An inpatient consultation is a consultation provided in the hospital or partial hospital nursing facility setting. Report only one inpatient consultation by a consultant for each admission to the hospital or nursing facility.

If a consultant participates in the patient's management after the opinion or advice is provided, use codes for subsequent hospital or observation care or for office or other outpatient services (established patient), as appropriate.

Under CMS guidelines, the inpatient and office/outpatient consultation codes contained in the CPT manual are not covered services.

All outpatient consultation services will be reported for Medicare using the appropriate new or established evaluation and management (E/M) codes. Inpatient consultation services for the initial encounter should be reported by the physician providing the service using initial hospital care codes 99221–99223, and subsequent inpatient care codes 99231–99233.

Codes 99487, 99489, 99490, and 99491 are used to report evaluation and management services for chronic care management. These codes represent management and support services provided by clinical staff, under the direction of a physician or OQHCP, to patients residing at home or in a domiciliary, rest home, or assisted living facility. The qualified provider oversees the management and/or coordination of services for all medical conditions, psychosocial needs, and activities of daily living. These codes are reported only once per calendar month and have specific time-based thresholds.

Codes 99497-99498 are used to report the discussion and explanation of advanced directives by a physician or OQHCP. These codes represent a face-to-face service between the provider and a patient, family member, or surrogate. These codes are time-based codes and, since no active management of the problem(s) is undertaken during this time, may be reported on the same day as another E/M service.

Certain codes that CPT considers appropriate telehealth services are identified with the ★ icon and reported with modifier 95 Synchronous telemedicine service rendered via a real-time interactive audio and video telecommunications system. Medicare recognizes certain CPT and HCPCS Level II G codes as telehealth services reported with modifier GT. Check with individual payers for telehealth modifier guidance.

Office or Other Outpatient Services—New Patient

CMS PROPOSED CHANGES FOR E&M SERVICES, CODES 99201–99215

The Centers for Medicare and Medicaid Services (CMS) has announced the following changes that are scheduled to become effective January 1, 2021:

- Separate payment will be assigned for each level of office/outpatient E&M services codes, as revised by the CPT Editorial Panel effective January 1, 2021, and resurveyed by the AMA RUC, with minor refinement. This would include deletion of CPT code 99201 (Level 1 new patient office/outpatient E&M visit) and adoption of the revised CPT code descriptors for CPT codes 99202–99215.
- The use of history and/or physical exam to select among code levels will be eliminated.
- Either time or medical decision making can be used to decide the level of office/outpatient E&M visit (using the revised CPT interpretive guidelines for medical decision making), with the exception of 99211 and emergency department levels.
- Time is face-to-face and will include non-face-to-face time before and after the encounter.
- CMS will adopt updated E&M guidelines.
- CPT descriptions will be revised.
- A new CPT add-on code will be created for level 5 to capture prolonged/extended visits of at least 15 additional minutes.

E/M Code	History[1]	Exam[1]	Medical Decision Making[1]	Problem Severity	Coordination of Care; Counseling	Time Spent Face-to-Face (avg.)
99201	Problem-focused	Problem-focused	Straight-forward	Minor or self-limited	Consistent with problem(s) and patient's needs	10 min.
99202	Expanded problem-focused	Expanded problem-focused	Straight-forward	Low to moderate	Consistent with problem(s) and patient's needs	20 min.
99203	Detailed	Detailed	Low complexity	Moderate	Consistent with problem(s) and patient's needs	30 min.
99204	Comprehensive	Comprehensive	Moderate complexity	Moderate to high	Consistent with problem(s) and patient's needs	45 min.
99205	Comprehensive	Comprehensive	High complexity	Moderate to high	Consistent with problem(s) and patient's needs	60 min.

1 Key component. For new patients, all three components (history, exam, and medical decision making) are crucial for selecting the correct code.

Office or Other Outpatient Services—Established Patient[1]

E/M Code	History[2]	Exam[2]	Medical Decision Making[2]	Problem Severity	Coordination of Care; Counseling	Time Spent Face-to-Face (avg.)
99211	—	—	Physician supervision, but presence not required	Minimal	Consistent with problem(s) and patient's needs	5 min.
99212	Problem-focused	Problem-focused	Straight-forward	Minor or self-limited	Consistent with problem(s) and patient's needs	10 min.
99213	Expanded problem-focused	Expanded problem-focused	Low complexity	Low to moderate	Consistent with problem(s) and patient's needs	15 min.
99214	Detailed	Detailed	Moderate complexity	Moderate to high	Consistent with problem(s) and patient's needs	25 min.
99215	Comprehensive	Comprehensive	High complexity	Moderate to high	Consistent with problem(s) and patient's needs	40 min.

1 Includes follow-up, periodic reevaluation, and evaluation and management of new problems.

2 Key component. For established patients, at least two of the three components (history, exam, and medical decision making) are needed to select the correct code.

Hospital Observation Services

E/M Code	History[1]	Exam[1]	Medical Decision Making[1]	Problem Severity	Coordination of Care; Counseling	Time Spent Bedside and on Unit/Floor (avg.)
99217	Observation care discharge day management					
99218	Detailed or comprehensive	Detailed or comprehensive	Straight-forward or low complexity	Low	Consistent with problem(s) and patient's needs	30 min.
99219	Comprehensive	Comprehensive	Moderate complexity	Moderate	Consistent with problem(s) and patient's needs	50 min.
99220	Comprehensive	Comprehensive	High complexity	High	Consistent with problem(s) and patient's needs	70 min.

1 Key component. All three components (history, exam, and medical decision making) are crucial for selecting the correct code.

Subsequent Hospital Observation Services[1]

E/M Code[2]	History[3]	Exam[3]	Medical Decision Making[3]	Problem Severity	Coordination of Care; Counseling	Time Spent Bedside and on Unit/Floor (avg.)
99224	Problem-focused interval	Problem-focused	Straight-forward or low complexity	Stable, recovering, or improving	Consistent with problem(s) and patient's needs	15 min.
99225	Expanded problem-focused interval	Expanded problem-focused	Moderate complexity	Inadequate response to treatment; minor complications	Consistent with problem(s) and patient's needs	25 min.
99226	Detailed interval	Detailed	High complexity	Unstable; significant new problem or significant complication	Consistent with problem(s) and patient's needs	35 min.

1 All subsequent levels of service include reviewing the medical record, diagnostic studies, and changes in the patient's status, such as history, physical condition, and response to treatment since the last assessment.

2 These codes are resequenced in CPT and are printed following codes 99217-99220.

3 Key component. For subsequent care, at least two of the three components (history, exam, and medical decision making) are needed to select the correct code.

Hospital Inpatient Services—Initial Care[1]

E/M Code	History[2]	Exam[2]	Medical Decision Making[2]	Problem Severity	Coordination of Care; Counseling	Time Spent Bedside and on Unit/Floor (avg.)
99221	Detailed or comprehensive	Detailed or comprehensive	Straight-forward or low complexity	Low	Consistent with problem(s) and patient's needs	30 min.
99222	Comprehensive	Comprehensive	Moderate complexity	Moderate	Consistent with problem(s) and patient's needs	50 min.
99223	Comprehensive	Comprehensive	High complexity	High	Consistent with problem(s) and patient's needs	70 min.

1 The admitting physician should append modifier AI, Principal physician of record, for Medicare patients
2 Key component. For initial care, all three components (history, exam, and medical decision making) are crucial for selecting the correct code.

Hospital Inpatient Services—Subsequent Care[1]

E/M Code	History[2]	Exam[2]	Medical Decision Making[2]	Problem Severity	Coordination of Care; Counseling	Time Spent Bedside and on Unit/Floor (avg.)
99231	Problem-focused interval	Problem-focused	Straight-forward or low complexity	Stable, recovering or Improving	Consistent with problem(s) and patient's needs	15 min.
99232	Expanded problem-focused interval	Expanded problem-focused	Moderate complexity	Inadequate response to treatment; minor complications	Consistent with problem(s) and patient's needs	25 min.
99233	Detailed interval	Detailed	High complexity	Unstable; significant new problem or significant complication	Consistent with problem(s) and patient's needs	35 min.
99238	Hospital discharge day management					30 min. or less
99239	Hospital discharge day management					> 30 min.

1 All subsequent levels of service include reviewing the medical record, diagnostic studies, and changes in the patient's status, such as history, physical condition, and response to treatment since the last assessment.
2 Key component. For subsequent care, at least two of the three components (history, exam, and medical decision making) are needed to select the correct code.

Observation or Inpatient Care Services (Including Admission and Discharge Services)

E/M Code	History[1]	Exam[1]	Medical Decision Making[1]	Problem Severity	Coordination of Care; Counseling	Time
99234	Detailed or comprehensive	Detailed or comprehensive	Straight-forward or low complexity	Low	Consistent with problem(s) and patient's needs	40 min.
99235	Comprehensive	Comprehensive	Moderate	Moderate	Consistent with problem(s) and patient's needs	50 min.
99236	Comprehensive	Comprehensive	High	High	Consistent with problem(s) and patient's needs	55 min.

1 Key component. All three components (history, exam, and medical decision making) are crucial for selecting the correct code.

Consultations—Office or Other Outpatient

E/M Code	History[1]	Exam[1]	Medical Decision Making[1]	Problem Severity	Coordination of Care; Counseling	Time Spent Face-to-Face (avg.)
99241	Problem-focused	Problem-focused	Straight-forward	Minor or self-limited	Consistent with problem(s) and patient's needs	15 min.
99242	Expanded problem-focused	Expanded problem-focused	Straight-forward	Low	Consistent with problem(s) and patient's needs	30 min.
99243	Detailed	Detailed	Low complexity	Moderate	Consistent with problem(s) and patient's needs	40 min.
99244	Comprehensive	Comprehensive	Moderate complexity	Moderate to high	Consistent with problem(s) and patient's needs	60 min.
99245	Comprehensive	Comprehensive	High complexity	Moderate to high	Consistent with problem(s) and patient's needs	80 min.

1 Key component. For office or other outpatient consultations, all three components (history, exam, and medical decision making) are crucial for selecting the correct code.

Consultations—Inpatient[1]

E/M Code	History[2]	Exam[2]	Medical Decision Making[2]	Problem Severity	Coordination of Care; Counseling	Time Spent Bedside and on Unit/Floor (avg.)
99251	Problem-focused	Problem-focused	Straight-forward	Minor or self-limited	Consistent with problem(s) and patient's needs	20 min.
99252	Expanded problem-focused	Expanded problem-focused	Straight-forward	Low	Consistent with problem(s) and patient's needs	40 min.
99253	Detailed	Detailed	Low complexity	Moderate	Consistent with problem(s) and patient's needs	55 min.
99254	Comprehensive	Comprehensive	Moderate complexity	Moderate to high	Consistent with problem(s) and patient's needs	80 min.
99255	Comprehensive	Comprehensive	High complexity	Moderate to high	Consistent with problem(s) and patient's needs	110 min.

1 These codes are used for hospital inpatients, residents of nursing facilities or patients in a partial hospital setting.
2 Key component. For initial inpatient consultations, all three components (history, exam, and medical decision making) are crucial for selecting the correct code.

Emergency Department Services, New or Established Patient

E/M Code	History[1]	Exam[1]	Medical Decision Making[1]	Problem Severity[3]	Coordination of Care; Counseling	Time Spent[2] Face-to-Face (avg.)
99281	Problem-focused	Problem-focused	Straight-forward	Minor or self-limited	Consistent with problem(s) and patient's needs	N/A
99282	Expanded problem-focused	Expanded problem-focused	Low complexity	Low to moderate	Consistent with problem(s) and patient's needs	N/A
99283	Expanded problem-focused	Expanded problem-focused	Moderate complexity	Moderate	Consistent with problem(s) and patient's needs	N/A
99284	Detailed	Detailed	Moderate complexity	High; requires urgent evaluation	Consistent with problem(s) and patient's needs	N/A
99285	Comprehensive	Comprehensive	High complexity	High; poses immediate/significant threat to life or physiologic function	Consistent with problem(s) and patient's needs	N/A
99288[4]			High complexity			N/A

1 Key component. For emergency department services, all three components (history, exam, and medical decision making) are crucial for selecting the correct code and must be adequately documented in the medical record to substantiate the level of service reported.

2 Typical times have not been established for this category of services.

3 NOTE: The severity of the patient's problem, while taken into consideration when evaluating and treating the patient, does not automatically determine the level of E/M service unless the medical record documentation reflects the severity of the patient's illness, injury, or condition in the details of the history, physical examination, and medical decision making process. Federal auditors will "downcode" the level of E/M service despite the nature of the patient's problem when the documentation does not support the E/M code reported.

4 Code 99288 is used to report two-way communication with emergency medical services personnel in the field.

Critical Care

E/M Code	Patient Status	Physician Attendance	Time[1]
99291	Critically ill or critically injured	Constant	First 30–74 minutes
99292	Critically ill or critically injured	Constant	Each additional 30 minutes beyond the first 74 minutes

1 Per the guidelines for time in *CPT 2016 page xv*, "A unit of time is attained when the mid-point is passed. For example, an hour is attained when 31 minutes have elapsed (more than midway between zero and 60 minutes)."

Nursing Facility Services—Initial Nursing Facility Care[1]

E/M Code	History[1]	Exam[1]	Medical Decision Making[1]	Problem Severity	Coordination of Care; Counseling
99304	Detailed or comprehensive	Detailed or comprehensive	Straight-forward or low complexity	Low	25 min.
99305	Comprehensive	Comprehensive	Moderate complexity	Moderate	35 min.
99306	Comprehensive	Comprehensive	High complexity	High	45 min.

1 These services must be performed by the physician. See CPT Corrections Document – CPT 2013 page 3 or guidelines CPT 2016 page 26.

2 Key component. For new patients, all three components (history, exam, and medical decision making) are crucial for selecting the correct code.

Nursing Facility Services—Subsequent Nursing Facility Care

E/M Code	History[1]	Exam[1]	Medical Decision Making[2]	Problem Severity	Coordination of Care; Counseling
99307	Problem-focused interval	Problem-focused	Straight-forward	Stable, recovering or improving	10 min.
99308	Expanded problem-focused interval	Expanded problem-focused	Low complexity	Responding inadequately or has developed a minor complication	15 min.
99309	Detailed interval	Detailed	Moderate complexity	Significant complication or a significant new problem	25 min.
99310	Comprehensive interval	Comprehensive	High complexity	Developed a significant new problem requiring immediate attention	35 min.

1 Key component. For established patients, at least two of the three components (history, exam, and medical decision making) are needed for selecting the correct code.

Nursing Facility Discharge and Annual Assessment

E/M Code	History[1]	Exam[1]	Medical Decision Making[1]	Problem Severity	Time Spent Bedside and on Unit/Floor (avg.)
99315	Nursing facility discharge day management				30 min. or less
99316	Nursing facility discharge day management				more than 30 min.
99318	Detailed interval	Comprehensive	Low to moderate complexity	Stable, recovering or improving	30 min.

1 Key component. For annual nursing facility assessment, all three components (history, exam, and medical decision making) are crucial for selecting the correct code.

Domiciliary, Rest Home (e.g., Boarding Home) or Custodial Care Services—New Patient

E/M Code	History[1]	Exam[1]	Medical Decision Making[1]	Problem Severity	Coordination of Care; Counseling	Time Spent Face-to-Face (avg.)
99324	Problem-focused	Problem-focused	Straight-forward	Low	Consistent with problem(s) and patient's needs	20 min.
99325	Expanded problem-focused	Expanded problem-focused	Low complexity	Moderate	Consistent with problem(s) and patient's needs	30 min.
99326	Detailed	Detailed	Moderate complexity	Moderate to high	Consistent with problem(s) and patient's needs	45 min.
99327	Comprehensive	Comprehensive	Moderate complexity	High	Consistent with problem(s) and patient's needs	60 min.
99328	Comprehensive	Comprehensive	High complexity	Unstable or developed a new problem requiring immediate physician attention	Consistent with problem(s) and patient's needs	75 min.

1 Key component. For new patients, all three components (history, exam, and medical decision making) are crucial for selecting the correct code and must be adequately documented in the medical record to substantiate the level of service reported.

Domiciliary, Rest Home (e.g., Boarding Home) or Custodial Care Services— Established Patient

E/M Code	History[1]	Exam[1]	Medical Decision Making[1]	Problem Severity	Coordination of Care; Counseling	Time Spent Face-to-Face (avg.)
99334	Problem-focused interval	Problem-focused	Straight-forward	Minor or self-limited	Consistent with problem(s) and patient's needs	15 min.
99335	Expanded problem-focused interval	Expanded problem-focused	Low complexity	Low to moderate	Consistent with problem(s) and patient's needs	25 min.
99336	Detailed interval	Detailed	Moderate complexity	Moderate to high	Consistent with problem(s) and patient's needs	40 min.
99337	Comprehensive interval	Comprehensive	Moderate to high complexity	Moderate to high	Consistent with problem(s) and patient's needs	60 min.

1 Key component. For established patients, at least two of the three components (history, exam, and medical decision making) are needed for selecting the correct code.

Domiciliary, Rest Home (e.g., Assisted Living Facility), or Home Care Plan Oversight Services

E/M Code	Intent of Service	Presence of Patient	Time
99339	Individual physician supervision of a patient (patient not present) in home, domiciliary or rest home (e.g., assisted living facility) requiring complex and multidisciplinary care modalities involving regular physician development and/or revision of care plans, review of subsequent reports of patient status, review of related laboratory and other studies, communication (including telephone calls) for purposes of assessment or care decisions with health care professional(s), family member(s), surrogate decision maker(s) (e.g., legal guardian) and/or key caregiver(s) involved in patient's care, integration of new information into the medical treatment plan and/or adjustment of medical therapy, within a calendar month	Patient not present	15–29 min.
99340	Same as 99339	Patient not present	30 min. or more

Home Services—New Patient

E/M Code	History[1]	Exam[1]	Medical Decision Making[1]	Problem Severity	Coordination of Care; Counseling	Time Spent Face-to-Face (avg.)
99341	Problem-focused	Problem-focused	Straight-forward complexity	Low	Consistent with problem(s) and patient's needs	20 min.
99342	Expanded problem-focused	Expanded problem-focused	Low complexity	Moderate	Consistent with problem(s) and patient's needs	30 min.
99343	Detailed	Detailed	Moderate complexity	Moderate to high	Consistent with problem(s) and patient's needs	45 min.
99344	Comprehensive	Comprehensive	Moderate complexity	High	Consistent with problem(s) and patient's needs	60 min.
99345	Comprehensive	Comprehensive	High complexity	Usually the patient has developed a significant new problem requiring immediate physician attention	Consistent with problem(s) and patient's needs	75 min.

1 Key component. For new patients, all three components (history, exam, and medical decision making) are crucial for selecting the correct code and must be adequately documented in the medical record to substantiate the level of service reported.

Home Services—Established Patient

E/M Code	History[1]	Exam[1]	Medical Decision Making[1]	Problem Severity	Coordination of Care; Counseling	Time Spent Face-to-Face (avg.)
99347	Problem-focused interval	Problem-focused	Straight-forward	Minor or self-limited	Consistent with problem(s) and patient's needs	15 min.
99348	Expanded problem-focused interval	Expanded problem-focused	Low complexity	Low to moderate	Consistent with problem(s) and patient's needs	25 min.
99349	Detailed interval	Detailed	Moderate complexity	Moderate to high	Consistent with problem(s) and patient's needs	40 min.
99350	Comprehensive interval	Comprehensive	Moderate to high complexity	Moderate to high Usually the patient has developed a significant new problem requiring immediate physician attention	Consistent with problem(s) and patient's needs	60 min.

1 Key component. For established patients, at least two of the three components (history, exam, and medical decision making) are needed for selecting the correct code.

Newborn Care Services

E/M Code	Patient Status	Type of Visit
99460	Normal newborn	Inpatient initial inpatient hospital or birthing center per day
99461	Normal newborn	Inpatient initial treatment not in hospital or birthing center per day
99462	Normal newborn	Inpatient subsequent per day
99463	Normal newborn	Inpatient initial inpatient and discharge in hospital or birthing center per day
99464	Unstable newborn	Attendance at delivery
99465	High-risk newborn at delivery	Resuscitation, ventilation, and cardiac treatment

Neonatal and Pediatric Interfacility Transportation

E/M Code	Patient Status	Type of Visit
99466	Critically ill or injured infant or young child, to 24 months	Face-to-face transportation from one facility to another, initial 30-74 minutes
99467	Critically ill or injured infant or young child, to 24 months	Face-to-face transportation from one facility to another, each additional 30 minutes
99485[1]	Critically ill or injured infant or young child, to 24 months	Supervision of patient transport from one facility to another, initial 30 minutes
99486[1]	Critically ill or injured infant or young child, to 24 months	Supervision of patient transport from one facility to another, each additional 30 minutes

1 These codes are resequenced in CPT and are printed following codes 99466-99467.

Inpatient Neonatal and Pediatric Critical Care

E/M Code	Patient Status	Type of Visit
99468[1]	Critically ill neonate, aged 28 days or less	Inpatient initial per day
99469[2]	Critically ill neonate, aged 28 days or less	Inpatient subsequent per day
99471	Critically ill infant or young child, aged 29 days to 24 months	Inpatient initial per day
99472	Critically ill infant or young child, aged 29 days to 24 months	Inpatient subsequent per day
99475	Critically ill infant or young child, 2 to 5 years[3]	Inpatient initial per day
99476	Critically ill infant or young child, 2 to 5 years	Inpatient subsequent per day

1 Codes 99468, 99471, and 99475 may be reported only once per admission.

2 Codes 99469, 99472, and 99476 may be reported only once per day and by only one provider.

3 See 99291-99292 for patients 6 years of age and older.

Neonate and Infant Initial and Continuing Intensive Care Services

E/M Code	Patient Status	Type of Visit
99477	Neonate, aged 28 days or less	Inpatient initial per day
99478	Infant with present body weight of less than 1500 grams, no longer critically ill	Inpatient subsequent per day
99479	Infant with present body weight of 1500-2500 grams, no longer critically ill	Inpatient subsequent per day
99480	Infant with present body weight of 2501-5000 grams, no longer critically ill	Inpatient subsequent per day

Levels of E/M Services

Confusion may be experienced when first approaching E/M due to the way that each description of a code component or element seems to have another layer of description beneath. The three key components—history, exam, and decision making—are each comprised of elements that combine to create varying levels of that component.

For example, an expanded problem-focused history includes the chief complaint, a brief history of the present illness, and a system review focusing on the patient's problems. The level of exam is not made up of different elements but rather distinguished by the extent of exam across body areas or organ systems.

The single largest source of confusion are the "labels" or names applied to the varying degrees of history, exam, and decision-making. Terms such as expanded problem-focused, detailed, and comprehensive are somewhat meaningless unless they are defined. The lack of definition in CPT guidelines relative to these terms is precisely what caused the first set of federal guidelines to be developed in 1995 and again in 1997.

Documentation Guidelines for Evaluation and Management Services

Both versions of the federal guidelines go well beyond CPT guidelines in defining specific code requirements. The current version of the CPT guidelines does not explain the number of history of present illness (HPI) elements or the specific number of organ systems or body areas to be examined as they are in the federal guidelines. Adherence to some version of the guidelines is required when billing E/M to federal payers, but at this time, the CPT guidelines do not incorporate this level of detail into the code definitions. Although that could be interpreted to mean that non-governmental payers have a lesser documentation standard, it is best to adopt one set of the federal versions for all payer types for both consistency and ease of use.

The 1997 guidelines supply a great amount of detail relative to history and exam and will give the provider clear direction to follow when documenting elements. With that stated, the 1995 guidelines are equally valid and place a lesser documentation burden on the provider in regards to the physical exam.

The 1995 guidelines ask only for a notation of "normal" on systems with normal findings. The only narrative required is for abnormal findings. The 1997 version calls for much greater detail, or an "elemental" or "bullet-point" approach to organ systems, although a notation of normal is sufficient when addressing the elements within a system. The 1997 version works well in a template or electronic health record (EHR) format for recording E/M services.

The 1997 version did produce the single system specialty exam guidelines. When reviewing the complete guidelines listed below, note the differences between exam requirements in the 1995 and 1997 versions.

A Comparison of 1995 and 1997 Exam Guidelines

There are four types of exams indicated in the levels of E/M codes. Although the descriptors or labels are the same under 1995 and 1997 guidelines, the degree of detail required is different. The remaining content on this topic references the 1997 general multi-system specialty examination, at the end of this chapter.

The levels under each set of guidelines are:

1995 Exam Guidelines:

Problem focused:	One body area or system
Expanded problem focused:	Two to seven body areas or organ systems
Detailed:	Two to seven body areas or organ systems
Comprehensive:	Eight or more organ systems or a complete single-system examination

1997 Exam Guidelines:

Problem-focused:	Perform and document examination of one to five bullet point elements in one or more organ systems/body areas from the general multi-system examination
OR	
	Perform or document examination of one to five bullet point elements from one of the 10 single-organ-system examinations, shaded or unshaded boxes
Expanded problem-focused:	Perform and document examination of at least six bullet point elements in one or more organ systems from the general multi-system examination
OR	
	Perform and document examination of at least six bullet point elements from one of the 10 single-organ-system examinations, shaded or unshaded boxes
Detailed:	Perform and document examination of at least six organ systems or body areas, including at least two bullet point elements for each organ system or body area from the general multi-system examination
OR	
	Perform and document examination of at least 12 bullet point elements in two or more organ systems or body areas from the general multisystem examination
OR	
	Perform and document examination of at least 12 bullet elements from one of the single-organ-system examinations, shaded or unshaded boxes
Comprehensive:	Perform and document examination of at least nine organ systems or body areas, with all bullet elements for each organ system or body area (unless specific instructions are expected to limit examination content with at least two bullet elements for each organ system or body area) from the general multi-system examination
OR	
	Perform and document examination of all bullet point elements from one of the 10 single-organ system examinations with documentation of every element in shaded boxes and at least one element in each unshaded box from the single-organ-system examination.

The Documentation Guidelines

The following guidelines were developed jointly by the American Medical Association (AMA) and the Centers for Medicare and Medicaid Services (CMS). Their mutual goal was to provide physicians and claims reviewers with advice about preparing or reviewing documentation for Evaluation and Management (E/M) services.

I. Introduction

What is Documentation and Why Is It Important?

Medical record documentation is required to record pertinent facts, findings, and observations about an individual's health history, including past and present illnesses, examinations, tests, treatments, and outcomes. The medical record chronologically documents the care of the patient and is an important element contributing to high quality care. The medical record facilitates:

- The ability of the physician and other health care professionals to evaluate and plan the patient's immediate treatment and to monitor his/her health care over time
- Communication and continuity of care among physicians and other health care professionals involved in the patient's care
- Accurate and timely claims review and payment
- Appropriate utilization review and quality of care evaluations
- Collection of data that may be useful for research and education

An appropriately documented medical record can reduce many of the problems associated with claims processing and may serve as a legal document to verify the care provided, if necessary.

What Do Payers Want and Why?

Because payers have a contractual obligation to enrollees, they may require reasonable documentation that services are consistent with the insurance coverage provided. They may request information to validate:

- The site of service
- The medical necessity and appropriateness of the diagnostic and/or therapeutic services provided
- Services provided have been accurately reported

II. General Principles of Medical Record Documentation

The principles of documentation listed below are applicable to all types of medical and surgical services in all settings. For Evaluation and Management (E/M) services, the nature and amount of physician work and documentation varies by type of service, place of service, and the patient's status. The general principles listed below may be modified to account for these variable circumstances in providing E/M services.

- The medical record should be complete and legible
- The documentation of each patient encounter should include:
  - A reason for the encounter and relevant history, physical examination findings, and prior diagnostic test results
  - Assessment, clinical impression, or diagnosis
  - Plan for care
  - Date and legible identity of the practitioner
- If not documented, the rationale for ordering diagnostic and other ancillary services should be easily inferred
- Past and present diagnoses should be accessible to the treating and/or consulting physician
- Appropriate health risk factors should be identified
- The patient's progress, response to, and changes in treatment and revision of diagnosis should be documented
- The CPT and ICD-9-CM codes reported on the health insurance claim form or billing statement should be supported by the documentation in the medical record

III. *Documentation of E/M Services 1995 and 1997*

The following information provides definitions and documentation guidelines for the three key components of E/M services and for visits that consist predominately of counseling or coordination of care. The three key components—history, examination, and medical decision making—appear in the descriptors for office and other outpatient services, hospital observation services, hospital inpatient services, consultations, emergency department services, nursing facility services, domiciliary care services, and home services. While some of the text of the CPT guidelines has been repeated in this document, the reader should refer to CMS or CPT for the complete descriptors for E/M services and instructions for selecting a level of service. Documentation guidelines are identified by the symbol DG.

The descriptors for the levels of E/M services recognize seven components that are used in defining the levels of E/M services. These components are:

- History
- Examination
- Medical decision making
- Counseling
- Coordination of care
- Nature of presenting problem
- Time

The first three of these components (i.e., history, examination, and medical decision making) are the key components in selecting the level of E/M services. In the case of visits that consist predominately of counseling or coordination of care, time is the key or controlling factor to qualify for a particular level of E/M service.

Because the level of E/M service is dependent on two or three key components, performance and documentation of one component (e.g., examination) at the highest level does not necessarily mean that the encounter in its entirety qualifies for the highest level of E/M service.

These Documentation Guidelines for E/M services reflect the needs of the typical adult population. For certain groups of patients, the recorded information may vary slightly from that described here. Specifically, the medical records of infants, children, adolescents, and pregnant women may have additional or modified information, as appropriate, recorded in each history and examination area.

As an example, newborn records may include under history of the present illness (HPI) the details of the mother's pregnancy and the infant's status at birth; social history will focus on family structure; and family history will focus on congenital anomalies and hereditary disorders in the family. In addition, the content of a pediatric examination will vary with the age and development of the child. Although not specifically defined in these documentation guidelines, these patient group variations on history and examination are appropriate.

A. *Documentation of History*

The levels of E/M services are based on four types of history (Problem Focused, Expanded Problem Focused, Detailed, and Comprehensive). Each type of history includes some or all of the following elements:

- Chief complaint (CC)
- History of present illness (HPI)
- Review of systems (ROS)
- Past, family, and/or social history (PFSH)

The extent of history of present illness, review of systems, and past, family, and/or social history that is obtained and documented is dependent upon clinical judgment and the nature of the presenting problem.

The chart below shows the progression of the elements required for each type of history. To qualify for a given type of history all three elements in the table must be met. (A chief complaint is indicated at all levels.)

- DG: The CC, ROS, and PFSH may be listed as separate elements of history or they may be included in the description of the history of present illness

- DG: A ROS and/or a PFSH obtained during an earlier encounter does not need to be re-recorded if there is evidence that the physician reviewed and updated the previous information. This may occur when a physician updates his/her own record or in an institutional setting or group practice where many physicians use a common record. The review and update may be documented by:
  - Describing any new ROS and/or PFSH information or noting there has been no change in the information
  - Noting the date and location of the earlier ROS and/or PFSH

- DG: The ROS and/or PFSH may be recorded by ancillary staff or on a form completed by the patient. To document that the physician reviewed the information, there must be a notation supplementing or confirming the information recorded by others

- DG: If the physician is unable to obtain a history from the patient or other source, the record should describe the patient's condition or other circumstance that precludes obtaining a history

Definitions and specific documentation guidelines for each of the elements of history are listed below.

Chief Complaint (CC)

The CC is a concise statement describing the symptom, problem, condition, diagnosis, physician recommended return, or other factor that is the reason for the encounter, usually stated in the patient's words.

- DG: The medical record should clearly reflect the chief complaint

History of Present Illness (HPI)

The HPI is a chronological description of the development of the patient's present illness from the first sign and/or symptom or from the previous encounter to the present. It includes the following elements:

- Location
- Quality
- Severity
- Duration
- Timing
- Context
- Modifying factors
- Associated signs and symptoms

Brief and extended HPIs are distinguished by the amount of detail needed to accurately characterize the clinical problem.

A brief HPI consists of one to three elements of the HPI.

- DG: The medical record should describe one to three elements of the present illness (HPI)

An extended HPI consists of at least four elements of the HPI or the status of at least three chronic or inactive conditions.

- DG: The medical record should describe at least four elements of the present illness (HPI) or the status of at least three chronic or inactive conditions

Beginning with services performed on or after September 10, 2013, CMS has stated that physicians and OQHCP will be able to use the 1997 guidelines for an extended history of present illness (HPI) in combination with other elements from the 1995 documentation guidelines to document a particular level of evaluation and management service.

History of Present Illness	Review of systems (ROS)	PFSH	Type of History
Brief	N/A	N/A	Problem-focused
Brief	Problem Pertinent	N/A	Expanded Problem-Focused
Extended	Extended	Pertinent	Detailed
Extended	Complete	Complete	Comprehensive

Review of Systems (ROS)

A ROS is an inventory of body systems obtained through a series of questions seeking to identify signs and/or symptoms that the patient may be experiencing or has experienced. For purposes of ROS, the following systems are recognized:

- Constitutional symptoms (e.g., fever, weight loss)
- Eyes
- Ears, nose, mouth, throat
- Cardiovascular
- Respiratory
- Gastrointestinal
- Genitourinary
- Musculoskeletal
- Integumentary (skin and/or breast)
- Neurological
- Psychiatric
- Endocrine
- Hematologic/lymphatic
- Allergic/immunologic

A problem pertinent ROS inquires about the system directly related to the problem identified in the HPI.

- DG: The patient's positive responses and pertinent negatives for the system related to the problem should be documented

An extended ROS inquires about the system directly related to the problem identified in the HPI and a limited number of additional systems.

- DG: The patient's positive responses and pertinent negatives for two to nine systems should be documented

A complete ROS inquires about the system directly related to the problem identified in the HPI plus all additional body systems.

- DG: At least 10 organ systems must be reviewed. Those systems with positive or pertinent negative responses must be individually documented. For the remaining systems, a notation indicating all other systems are negative is permissible. In the absence of such a notation, at least 10 systems must be individually documented

Past, Family, and/or Social History (PFSH)

The PFSH consists of a review of three areas:

- Past history (the patient's past experiences with illnesses, operations, injuries, and treatment)
- Family history (a review of medical events in the patient's family, including diseases that may be hereditary or place the patient at risk)
- Social history (an age appropriate review of past and current activities)

For certain categories of E/M services that include only an interval history, it is not necessary to record information about the PFSH. Those categories are subsequent hospital care, follow-up inpatient consultations, and subsequent nursing facility care.

A pertinent PFSH is a review of the history area directly related to the problem identified in the HPI.

- DG: At least one specific item from any of the three history areas must be documented for a pertinent PFSH

A complete PFSH is a review of two or all three of the PFSH history areas, depending on the category of the E/M service. A review of all three history areas is required for services that by their nature include a comprehensive assessment or reassessment of the patient. A review of two of the three history areas is sufficient for other services.

- DG: A least one specific item from two of the three history areas must be documented for a complete PFSH for the following categories of E/M services: office or other outpatient services, established patient; emergency department; domiciliary care, established patient; and home care, established patient

- DG: At least one specific item from each of the three history areas must be documented for a complete PFSH for the following categories of E/M services: office or other outpatient services, new patient; hospital observation services; hospital inpatient services, initial care; consultations; comprehensive nursing facility assessments; domiciliary care, new patient; and home care, new patient

B. Documentation of Examination 1997 Guidelines

The levels of E/M services are based on four types of examination:

- Problem Focused: A limited examination of the affected body area or organ system
- Expanded Problem Focused: A limited examination of the affected body area or organ system and any other symptomatic or related body area or organ system
- Detailed: An extended examination of the affected body area or organ system and any other symptomatic or related body area or organ system
- Comprehensive: A general multi-system examination or complete examination of a single organ system and other symptomatic or related body area or organ system

These types of examinations have been defined for general multi-system and the following single organ systems:

- Cardiovascular
- Ears, nose, mouth, and throat
- Eyes
- Genitourinary (Female)
- Genitourinary (Male)
- Hematologic/lymphatic/immunologic
- Musculoskeletal
- Neurological
- Psychiatric
- Respiratory
- Skin

Any physician regardless of specialty may perform a general multi-system examination or any of the single organ system examinations. The type (general multi-system or single organ system) and content of examination are selected by the examining physician and are based upon clinical judgment, the patient's history, and the nature of the presenting problem.

The content and documentation requirements for each type and level of examination are summarized below and described in detail in a table found later on in this document. In the table, organ systems and body areas recognized by CPT for purposes of describing examinations are shown in the left column. The content, or individual elements, of the examination pertaining to that body area or organ system are identified by bullets (•) in the right column.

Parenthetical examples "(e.g., ...)," have been used for clarification and to provide guidance regarding documentation. Documentation for each element must satisfy any numeric requirements (such as "Measurement of any three of the following seven...") included in the description of the element. Elements with multiple components but with no specific numeric requirement (such as "Examination of liver and spleen") require documentation of at least one component. It is possible for a given examination to be expanded beyond what is defined here. When that occurs, findings related to the additional systems and/or areas should be documented.

- DG: Specific abnormal and relevant negative findings from the examination of the affected or symptomatic body area or organ system should be documented. A notation of "abnormal" without elaboration is insufficient

- DG: Abnormal or unexpected findings from the examination of any asymptomatic body area or organ system should be described

- DG: A brief statement or notation indicating "negative" or "normal" is sufficient to document normal findings related to an unaffected areas or asymptomatic organ system

General Multi-System Examinations

General multi-system examinations are described in detail later in this document. To qualify for a given level of multi-system examination, the following content and documentation requirements should be met:

- Problem Focused Examination: It should include performance and documentation of one to five elements identified by a bullet (•) in one or more organ systems or body areas
- Expanded Problem Focused Examination: It should include performance and documentation of at least six elements identified by a bullet (•) in one or more organ systems or body areas
- Detailed Examination: It should include at least six organ systems or body areas. For each system/area selected, performance and documentation of at least two elements identified by a bullet (•) is expected. Alternatively, a detailed examination may include performance and documentation of at least 12 elements identified by a bullet (•) in two or more organ systems or body areas
- Comprehensive Examination: It should include at least nine organ systems or body areas. For each system/area selected, all elements of the examination identified by a bullet (•) should be performed, unless specific directions limit the content of the examination. For each area/system, documentation of at least two elements identified by a bullet (•) is expected

Single Organ System Examinations

The single organ system examinations recognized by CMS include eyes; ears, nose, mouth, and throat; cardiovascular; respiratory; genitourinary (male and female); musculoskeletal; neurologic; hematologic, lymphatic, and immunologic; skin; and psychiatric. Note that for each specific single organ examination type, the performance and documentation of the stated number of elements, identified by a bullet (•) should be included, whether in a box with a shaded or unshaded border. The following content and documentation requirements must be met to qualify for a given level:

- Problem Focused Examination: one to five elements
- Expanded Problem Focused Examination: at least six elements
- Detailed Examination: at least 12 elements (other than eye and psychiatric examinations)
- Comprehensive Examination: all elements (Documentation of every element in a box with a shaded border and at least one element in a box with an unshaded border is expected)

Content and Documentation Requirements

General Multisystem Examination 1997

System/Body Area	Elements of Examination
Constitutional	• Measurement of any three of the following seven vital signs: 1) sitting or standing blood pressure, 2) supine blood pressure, 3) pulse rate and regularity, 4) respiration, 5) temperature, 6) height, 7) weight (May be measured and recorded by ancillary staff). • General appearance of patient (e.g., development, nutrition, body habitus, deformities attention to grooming)
Eyes	• Inspection of conjunctivae and lids • Examination of pupils and irises (e.g., reaction to light and accommodation, size and symmetry) • Ophthalmoscopic examination of optic discs (e.g., size, C/D ratio, appearance) and posterior segments (e.g., vessel changes, exudates, hemorrhages)
Ears, nose, mouth, and throat	• External inspection of ears and nose (e.g., overall appearance, scars, lesions, masses) • Otoscopic examination of external auditory canals and tympanic membranes • Assessment of hearing (e.g., whispered voice, finger rub, tuning fork) • Inspection of nasal mucosa, septum and turbinates • Inspection of lips, teeth and gums • Examination of oropharynx: oral mucosa, salivary glands, hard and soft palates, tongue, tonsils and posterior pharynx
Neck	• Examination of neck (e.g., masses, overall appearance, symmetry, tracheal position, crepitus) • Examination of thyroid (e.g., enlargement, tenderness, mass)
Respiratory	• Assessment of respiratory effort (e.g., intercostal retractions, use of accessory muscles, diaphragmatic movement) • Percussion of chest (e.g., dullness, flatness, hyperresonance) • Palpation of chest (e.g., tactile fremitus) • Auscultation of lungs (e.g., breath sounds, adventitious sounds, rubs)
Cardiovascular	• Palpation of heart (e.g., location, size, thrills) • Auscultation of heart with notation of abnormal sounds and murmurs • Examination of: — carotid arteries (e.g., pulse amplitude, bruits) — abdominal aorta (e.g., size, bruits) — femoral arteries (e.g., pulse amplitude, bruits) — pedal pulses (e.g., pulse amplitude) — extremities for edema and/or varicosities
Chest (Breasts)	• Inspection of breasts (e.g., symmetry, nipple discharge) • Palpation of breasts and axillae (e.g., masses or lumps, tenderness)
Gastrointestinal (Abdomen)	• Examination of abdomen with notation of presence of masses or tenderness • Examination of liver and spleen • Examination for presence or absence of hernia • Examination (when indicated) of anus, perineum and rectum, including sphincter tone, presence of hemorrhoids, rectal masses • Obtain stool sample for occult blood test when indicated

System/Body Area	Elements of Examination
Genitourinary	**Male:** • Examination of the scrotal contents (e.g., hydrocele, spermatocele, tenderness of cord, testicular mass) • Examination of the penis • Digital rectal examination of prostate gland (e.g., size, symmetry, nodularity tenderness) **Female**: • Pelvic examination (with or without specimen collection for smears and cultures), including: — examination of external genitalia (e.g., general appearance, hair distribution, lesions) and vagina (e.g., general appearance, estrogen effect, discharge, lesions, pelvic support, cystocele, rectocele) — examination of urethra (e.g., masses, tenderness, scarring) — examination of bladder (e.g., fullness, masses, tenderness) • Cervix (e.g., general appearance, lesions, discharge) • Uterus (e.g., size, contour, position, mobility, tenderness, consistency, descent or support) • Adnexa/parametria (e.g., masses, tenderness)
Lymphatic	Palpation of lymph nodes in **two or more** areas: • Neck • Groin • Axillae • Other
Musculoskeletal	• Examination of gait and station *(if circled, add to total at bottom of column to the left) • Inspection and/or palpation of digits and nails (e.g., clubbing, cyanosis, inflammatory conditions, petechiae, ischemia, infections, nodes) *(if circled, add to total at bottom of column to the left) Examination of joints, bones and muscles of **one or more of the following six** areas: 1) head and neck; 2) spine, ribs, and pelvis; 3) right upper extremity; 4) left upper extremity; 5) right lower extremity; and 6) left lower extremity. The examination of a given area includes: • Inspection and/or palpation with notation of presence of any misalignment, asymmetry, crepitation, defects, tenderness, masses, effusions • Assessment of range of motion with notation of any pain, crepitation or contracture • Assessment of stability with notation of any dislocation (luxation), subluxation, or laxity • Assessment of muscle strength and tone (e.g., flaccid, cog wheel, spastic) with notation of any atrophy or abnormal movements
Skin	• Inspection of skin and subcutaneous tissue (e.g., rashes, lesions, ulcers) • Palpation of skin and subcutaneous tissue (e.g., induration, subcutaneous nodules, tightening)
Neurologic	• Test cranial nerves with notation of any deficits • Examination of deep tendon reflexes with notation of pathological reflexes (e.g., Babinski) • Examination of sensation (e.g., by touch, pin, vibration, proprioception)
Psychiatric	• Description of patient's judgment and insight • Brief assessment of mental status including: — Orientation to time, place and person — Recent and remote memory — Mood and affect (e.g., depression, anxiety, agitation)

Content and Documentation Requirements

Level of exam	Perform and document
Problem focused	**One to five** elements identified by a bullet
Expanded problem focused	**At least six** elements identified by a bullet
Detailed	**At least 12** elements identified by a bullet, whether in a box with a shaded or unshaded border
Comprehensive	Performance of **all** elements identified by a bullet; whether in a box or with a shaded or unshaded box. Documentation of every element in each with a shaded border and at least one element in a box with un shaded border is expected

Number of Diagnoses or Management Options	Amount and/or Complexity of Data to be Reviewed	Risk of Complications and/or Morbidity or Mortality	Type of Decision Making
Minimal	Minimal or None	Minimal	Straightforward
Limited	Limited	Low	Low Complexity
Multiple	Moderate	Moderate	Moderate Complexity
Extensive	Extensive	High	High Complexity

C. *Documentation of the Complexity of Medical Decision Making 1995 and 1997*

The levels of E/M services recognize four types of medical decision-making (straightforward, low complexity, moderate complexity, and high complexity). Medical decision-making refers to the complexity of establishing a diagnosis and/or selecting a management option as measured by:

- The number of possible diagnoses and/or the number of management options that must be considered
- The amount and/or complexity of medical records, diagnostic tests, and/or other information that must be obtained, reviewed, and analyzed
- The risk of significant complications, morbidity, and/or mortality, as well as comorbidities, associated with the patient's presenting problem, the diagnostic procedure, and/or the possible management options

The following chart shows the progression of the elements required for each level of medical decision-making. To qualify for a given type of decision-making, two of the three elements in the table must be either met or exceeded.

Each of the elements of medical decision-making is described below.

Number of Diagnoses or Management Options

The number of possible diagnoses and/or the number of management options that must be considered is based on the number and types of problems addressed during the encounter, the complexity of establishing a diagnosis, and the management decisions that are made by the physician.

Generally, decision making with respect to a diagnosed problem is easier than that for an identified but undiagnosed problem. The number and type of diagnostic tests employed may be an indicator of the number of possible diagnoses. Problems that are improving or resolving are less complex than those that are worsening or failing to change as expected. The need to seek advice from others is another indicator of complexity of diagnostic or management problems.

- DG: For each encounter, an assessment, clinical impression, or diagnosis should be documented. It may be explicitly stated or implied in documented decisions regarding management plans and/or further evaluation
  - For a presenting problem with an established diagnosis, the record should reflect whether the problem is: a) improved, well controlled, resolving, or resolved; or b) inadequately controlled, worsening, or failing to change as expected
  - For a presenting problem without an established diagnosis, the assessment or clinical impression may be stated in the form of a differential diagnosis or as a "possible," "probable," or "rule-out" (R/O) diagnosis
- DG: The initiation of, or changes in, treatment should be documented. Treatment includes a wide range of management options including patient instructions, nursing instructions, therapies, and medications
- DG: If referrals are made, consultations requested, or advice sought, the record should indicate to whom or where the referral or consultation is made or from whom the advice is requested

Amount and/or Complexity of Data to be Reviewed

The amount and complexity of data to be reviewed is based on the types of diagnostic testing ordered or reviewed. A decision to obtain and review old medical records and/or obtain history from sources other than the patient increases the amount and complexity of data to be reviewed.

Discussion of contradictory or unexpected test results with the physician who performed or interpreted the test is an indication of the complexity of data being reviewed. On occasion, the physician who ordered a test may personally review the image, tracing, or specimen to supplement information from the physician who prepared the test report or interpretation; this is another indication of the complexity of data being reviewed.

- DG: If a diagnostic service (test or procedure) is ordered, planned, scheduled, or performed at the time of the E/M encounter, the type of service (e.g., lab or x-ray) should be documented
- DG: The review of lab, radiology, and/or other diagnostic tests should be documented. A simple notation such as WBC elevated" or "chest x-ray unremarkable" is acceptable. Alternatively, the review may be documented by initialing and dating the report containing the test results
- DG: A decision to obtain old records or a decision to obtain additional history from the family, caretaker, or other source to supplement that obtained from the patient should be documented
- DG: Relevant findings from the review of old records and/or the receipt of additional history from the family, caretaker, or other source to supplement that obtained from the patient should be documented. If there is no relevant information beyond that already obtained, that fact should be documented. A notation of "old records reviewed" or "additional history obtained from family" without elaboration is insufficient
- DG: The results of discussion of laboratory, radiology, or other diagnostic tests with the physician who performed or interpreted the study should be documented
- DG: The direct visualization and independent interpretation of an image, tracing, or specimen previously or subsequently interpreted by another physician should be documented

Risk of Significant Complications, Morbidity, and/or Mortality

The risk of significant complications, morbidity, and/or mortality is based on the risks associated with the presenting problem, the diagnostic procedure, and the possible management options.

- DG: Comorbidities/underlying disease or other factors that increase the complexity of medical decision making by increasing the risk of complications, morbidity, and/or mortality should be documented
- DG: If a surgical or invasive diagnostic procedure is ordered, planned, or scheduled at the time of the E/M encounter, the type of procedure (e.g., laparoscopy) should be documented
- DG: If a surgical or invasive diagnostic procedure is performed at the time of the E/M encounter, the specific procedure should be documented
- DG: The referral for or decision to perform a surgical or invasive diagnostic procedure on an urgent basis should be documented or implied

The following Table of Risk may be used to help determine whether the risk of significant complications, morbidity, and/or mortality is minimal, low, moderate, or high. Because the determination of risk is complex and not readily quantifiable, the table includes common clinical examples rather than absolute measures of risk. The assessment of risk of the presenting problem is based on the risk related to the disease process anticipated between the present encounter and the next one. The assessment of risk of selecting diagnostic procedures and management options is based on the risk during and immediately following any procedures or treatment. The highest level of risk in any one category (presenting problem, diagnostic procedure, or management options) determines the overall risk.

Table of Risk

Level of Risk	Presenting Problem(s)	Diagnostic Procedure(s) Ordered	Management Options Selected
Minimal	One self-limited or minor problem (e.g., cold, insect bite, tinea corporis)	Laboratory test requiring venipuncture Chest x-rays EKG/EEG Urinalysis Ultrasound (e.g., echocardiography) KOH prep	Rest Gargles Elastic bandages Superficial dressings
Low	Two or more self-limited or minor problems One stable chronic illness (e.g., well controlled hypertension, non-insulin dependent diabetes, cataract, BPH) Acute, uncomplicated illness or injury (e.g., cystitis, allergic rhinitis, simple sprain)	Physiologic tests not under stress (e.g., pulmonary function tests) Non-cardiovascular imaging studies with contrast (e.g., barium enema) Superficial needle biopsies Clinical laboratory tests requiring arterial puncture Skin biopsies	Over-the-counter drugs Minor surgery with no identified risk factors Physical therapy Occupational therapy IV fluids without additives
Moderate	One or more chronic illnesses with mild exacerbation, progression or side effects of treatment Two or more stable chronic illnesses Undiagnosed new problem with uncertain prognosis (e.g., lump in breast) Acute illness with systemic symptoms (e.g., pyelonephritis, pneumonitis, colitis) Acute complicated injury (e.g., head injury with brief loss of consciousness)	Physiologic tests not under stress (e.g., cardiac stress test, fetal contraction stress test) Diagnostic endoscopies with no identified risk factors Deep needle or incisional biopsy Cardiovascular imaging studies with contrast and no identified risk factors (e.g., arteriogram, cardiac catheterization) Obtain fluid from body cavity (e.g., lumbar puncture, thoracentesis, culdocentesis)	Minor surgery with identified risk factors Effective major surgery (open, percutaneous or endoscopic) with no identified risk factors Prescription drug management Therapeutic nuclear medicine IV fluids with additives Closed treatment of fracture or dislocation without manipulation
High	One or more chronic illnesses with severe exacerbation, progression or side effects of treatment Acute/chronic illnesses that may pose a threat to life or bodily function (e.g., multiple trauma, acute MI, pulmonary embolus, severe respiratory distress, progressive severe rheumatoid arthritis, psychiatric illness with potential threat to self or others, peritonitis, acute renal failure An abrupt change in neurologic status (e.g., seizure, TIA, weakness or sensory loss)	Cardiovascular imaging studies with contrast with identified risk factors Cardiac electrophysiological tests Diagnostic endoscopies with identified risk factors Discography	Elective major surgery (open, percutaneous or endoscopic) with identified risk factors Emergency major surgery (open, percutaneous or endoscopic) Parenteral controlled substances Drug therapy requiring intensive monitoring for toxicity Decision not to resuscitate or to de-escalate care because of poor prognosis

D. *Documentation of an Encounter Dominated by Counseling or Coordination of Care*

In the case where counseling and/or coordination of care dominates (more than 50 percent) the physician/patient and/or family encounter (face-to-face time in the office or other outpatient setting or floor-unit time in the hospital or nursing facility), time is considered the key or controlling factor to qualify for a particular level of E/M service.

- DG: If the physician elects to report the level of service based on counseling and/or coordination of care, the total length of time of the encounter (face-to-face or floor time, as appropriate) should be documented and the record should describe the counseling and/or activities to coordinate care

Appendix D — Crosswalk of Deleted Codes

The deleted code crosswalk is meant to be used as a reference tool to find active codes that could be used in place of the deleted code. This will not always be an exact match. Please review the code descriptions and guidelines before selecting a code.

Code	Cross reference
19260	To report, see 21601
19271	To report, see 21602
19272	To report, see 21603
33010	To report, see 33016-33019
33011	To report, see 33016-33019
33015	To report, see 33017-33019
33860	To report, see 33858-33859
33870	To report, see 33871
64402	To report, see 64999
64410	To report, see 64999
64413	To report, see 64999
74241	To report, see 74240
74245	To report, see 74240, 74248
74247	To report, see 74246
74249	To report, see 74246, 74248
74260	To report, see 74251
76930	To report, see 33016-33018
78205	To report, see 78803
78206	To report, see 78803
78320	To report, see 78803
78607	To report, see 78803
78647	To report, see 78803
78710	To report, see 78803
78805	To report, see 78300, 78305-78306, 78315, 78800-78803, 78830-78332
78806	To report, see 78300, 78305-78306, 78315, 78800-78803, 78830-78332
78807	To report, see 78300, 78305-78306, 78315, 78800-78803, 78830-78332
90911	To report, see 90912-90913
92225	To report, see 92201-92202
92226	To report, see 92201-92202
93299	To report, see 93297-93298
95827	To report, see 95705-95707, 95711-95713, 95717-95718
95831	To report, see [97161-97172]
95832	To report, see [97161-97172]
95833	To report, see [97161-97172]
95834	To report, see [97161-97172]
95950	To report, see [95700-95726]
95951	To report, see [95700-95726]
95953	To report, see [95700-95726]
95956	To report, see [95700-95726]
96150	To report, see 96156, 96158-96159
96151	To report, see 96156, 96158-96159
96152	To report, see 96156, 96158-96159
96153	To report, see [96164-96165]
96154	To report, see [96167-96168]
96155	To report, see [96170-9617]
97127	To report, see 97129
98969	To report, see 98970-98972
99444	To report, see [99421-99423]
3045F	To report, see 3051F, 3052F
0249T	To report, see 46948
0254T	To report, see 34717-34718
0399T	To report, see 93356
0081U	To report, see 81552

Appendix E — Resequenced Codes

Code	Reference
10004	See code following 10021.
10005	See code following 10021.
10006	See code following 10021.
10007	See code following 10021.
10008	See code following 10021.
10009	See code following 10021.
10010	See code following 10021.
10011	See code following 10021.
10012	See code following 10021.
11045	See code following 11042.
11046	See code following 11043.
15769	See code following 15770.
20560	See code following 20553.
20561	See code before 20555.
21552	See code following 21555.
21554	See code following 21556.
22858	See code following 22856.
22859	See code following 22854.
23071	See code following 23075.
23073	See code following 23076.
24071	See code following 24075.
24073	See code following 24076.
25071	See code following 25075.
25073	See code following 25076.
26111	See code following 26115.
26113	See code following 26116.
27043	See code following 27047.
27045	See code following 27048.
27059	See code following 27049.
27329	See code following 27360.
27337	See code following 27327.
27339	See code before 27330.
27632	See code following 27618.
27634	See code following 27619.
28039	See code following 28043.
28041	See code following 28045.
28295	See code following 28296.
29914	See code following 29863.
29915	See code following 29863.
29916	See code before 29866.
31253	See code following 31255.
31257	See code following 31255.
31259	See code following 31255.
31551	See code following 31580.
31552	See code following 31580.
31553	See code following 31580.
31554	See code following 31580.
31572	See code following 31578.
31573	See code following 31578.
31574	See code following 31578.

Code	Reference
31651	See code following 31647.
32994	See code following 32998.
33221	See code following 33213.
33227	See code following 33233.
33228	See code following 33233.
33229	See code before 33234.
33230	See code following 33240.
33231	See code before 33241.
33262	See code following 33241.
33263	See code following 33241.
33264	See code before 33243.
33270	See code following 33249.
33271	See code following 33249.
33272	See code following 33249.
33273	See code following 33249.
33274	See code following 33249.
33275	See code following 33249.
33440	See code following 33410.
33962	See code following 33959.
33963	See code following 33959.
33964	See code following 33959.
33965	See code following 33959.
33966	See code following 33959.
33969	See code following 33959.
33984	See code following 33959.
33985	See code following 33959.
33986	See code following 33959.
33987	See code following 33959.
33988	See code following 33959.
33989	See code following 33959.
34717	See code following 34708.
34718	See code following 34709.
34812	See code following 34713.
34820	See code following 34714.
34833	See code following 34714.
34834	See code following 34714.
36465	See code following 36471.
36466	See code following 36471.
36482	See code following 36479.
36483	See code following 36479.
36572	See code following 36569.
36573	See code following 36569.
37246	See code following 37235.
37247	See code following 37235.
37248	See code following 37235.
37249	See code following 37235.
38243	See code following 38241.
43210	See code following 43259.
43211	See code following 43217.
43212	See code following 43217.
43213	See code following 43220.

Code	Reference
43214	See code following 43220.
43233	See code following 43249.
43266	See code following 43255.
43270	See code following 43257.
43274	See code following numeric code 43270.
43275	See code following numeric code 43270.
43276	See code following numeric code 43270.
43277	See code following numeric code 43270.
43278	See code following numeric code 43270.
44381	See code following 44382.
44401	See code following 44392.
45346	See code following 45338.
45388	See code following 45382.
45390	See code following 45392.
45398	See code following 45393.
45399	See code before 45990.
46220	See code before 46230.
46320	See code following 46230.
46945	See code following 46221.
46946	See code following resequenced code 46945.
46947	See code following 46761.
46948	See code before resequenced code 46220.
50430	See code following 50396.
50431	See code following 50396.
50432	See code following 50396.
50433	See code following 50396.
50434	See code following 50396.
50435	See code following 50396.
50436	See code following 50391.
50437	See code following 50391.
51797	See code following 51729.
52356	See code following 52353.
58674	See code before 58541.
62328	See code following 62270.
62329	See code following 62272.
64461	See code following 64484.
64462	See code following 64484.
64463	See code following 64484.
64624	See code following 64610.
64625	See code before 64611.
64633	See code following 64620.
64634	See code following 64620.
64635	See code following 64620.
64636	See code before 64630.
66987	See code following 66982.
66988	See code following 66984.

Code	Reference
67810	See code following 67715.
77085	See code following 77081.
77086	See code before 77084.
77295	See code before 77300.
77385	See code following 77417.
77386	See code following 77417.
77387	See code following 77417.
77424	See code following 77417.
77425	See code following 77417.
78429	See code following 78459.
78430	See code following 78491.
78431	See code following 78492.
78432	See code following 78492.
78433	See code following 78492.
78434	See code following 78492.
78804	See code following 78802.
78830	See code following numeric code 78804.
78831	See code following numeric code 78804.
78832	See code following numeric code 78804.
78835	See code following numeric code 78804.
80081	See code following 80055.
80164	See code following 80201.
80165	See code following 80201.
80171	See code following 80169.
80230	See code following 80173.
80235	See code before 80175.
80280	See code following 80202.
80285	See code before 80203.
80305	See code before 80145.
80306	See code before 80145.
80307	See code before 80145.
80320	See code before 80145.
80321	See code before 80145.
80322	See code before 80145.
80323	See code before 80145.
80324	See code before 80145.
80325	See code before 80145.
80326	See code before 80145.
80327	See code before 80145.
80328	See code before 80145.
80329	See code before 80145.
80330	See code before 80145.
80331	See code before 80145.
80332	See code before 80145.
80333	See code before 80145.
80334	See code before 80145.
80335	See code before 80145.
80336	See code before 80145.
80337	See code before 80145.
80338	See code before 80145.
80339	See code before 80145.
80340	See code before 80145.
80341	See code before 80145.
80342	See code before 80145.
80343	See code before 80145.
80344	See code before 80145.
80345	See code before 80145.
80346	See code before 80145.
80347	See code before 80145.
80348	See code before 80145.
80349	See code before 80145.
80350	See code before 80145.
80351	See code before 80145.
80352	See code before 80145.
80353	See code before 80145.
80354	See code before 80145.
80355	See code before 80145.
80356	See code before 80145.
80357	See code before 80145.
80358	See code before 80145.
80359	See code before 80145.
80360	See code before 80145.
80361	See code before 80145.
80362	See code before 80145.
80363	See code before 80145.
80364	See code before 80145.
80365	See code before 80145.
80366	See code before 80145.
80367	See code before 80145.
80368	See code before 80145.
80369	See code before 80145.
80370	See code before 80145.
80371	See code before 80145.
80372	See code before 80145.
80373	See code before 80145.
80374	See code before 80145.
80375	See code before 80145.
80376	See code before 80145.
80377	See code before 80145.
81105	See code before 81260.
81106	See code before 81260.
81107	See code before 81260.
81108	See code before 81260.
81109	See code before 81260.
81110	See code before 81260.
81111	See code before 81260.
81112	See code before 81260.
81120	See code before 81260.
81121	See code before 81260.
81161	See code following numeric code 81231.
81162	See code following resequenced code 81210.
81163	See code following resequenced code 81210.
81164	See code following resequenced code 81210.
81165	See code following 81212.
81166	See code following 81212.
81167	See code following 81216.
81173	See code following resequenced code 81204.
81174	See code following resequenced code 81204.
81184	See code following resequenced code 81233.
81185	See code following resequenced code 81233.
81186	See code following resequenced code 81233.
81187	See code following resequenced code 81268.
81188	See code following resequenced code 81266.
81189	See code following resequenced code 81266.
81190	See code following resequenced code 81266.
81200	See code before 81175.
81201	See code following numeric code 81174.
81202	See code following numeric code 81174.
81203	See code following numeric code 81174.
81204	See code following numeric code 81174.
81205	See code following numeric code 81210.
81206	See code following numeric code 81210.
81207	See code following numeric code 81210.
81208	See code following numeric code 81210.
81209	See code following numeric code 81210.
81210	See code following numeric code 81210.
81219	See code before 81218.
81227	See code before 81225.
81230	See code following numeric code 81227.
81231	See code following numeric code 81227.
81233	See code following 81217.
81234	See code following numeric code 81231.
81238	See code following 81241.
81239	See code before 81232.
81245	See code following 81242.
81246	See code following 81242.
81250	See code before 81247.
81257	See code following 81254.
81258	See code following 81254.

Code	Reference
81259	See code following 81254.
81261	See code before 81260.
81262	See code before 81260.
81263	See code before 81260.
81264	See code before 81260.
81265	See code following resequenced code 81187.
81266	See code following resequenced code 81187.
81267	See code following 81224.
81268	See code following 81224.
81269	See code following resequenced code 81259.
81271	See code following numeric code 81259.
81274	See code following resequenced code 81271.
81277	See code following 81229.
81283	See code following resequenced code 81121.
81284	See code following numeric code 81246.
81285	See code following numeric code 81246.
81286	See code following numeric code 81246.
81287	See code following resequenced code 81304.
81288	See code following resequenced code 81292.
81289	See code following numeric code 81246.
81291	See code before 81305.
81292	See code before numeric code 81291.
81293	See code before numeric code 81291.
81294	See code before numeric code 81291.
81295	See code before numeric code 81291.
81301	See code following resequenced code 81287.
81302	See code following 81290.
81303	See code following 81290.
81304	See code following 81290.
81306	See code following resequenced code 81312.
81307	See code before 81313.
81308	See code before 81313.
81309	See code following 81314.
81312	See code following numeric code 81312.
81320	See code before 81315.
81324	See code following 81316.
81325	See code following 81316.
81326	See code following 81316.
81332	See code following 81327.
81334	See code following numeric code 81326.
81336	See code following 81329.
81337	See code following 81329.
81343	See code following numeric code 81320.
81344	See code following numeric code 81332.
81345	See code following numeric code 81332.
81361	See code following 81254.
81362	See code following 81254.
81363	See code following 81254.
81364	See code following 81254.
81443	See code following 81422.
81448	See code following 81438.
81479	See code following 81408.
81522	See code following 81518.
82042	See code following 82045.
82652	See code following 82306.
83992	See code following resequenced code 80365.
86152	See code folowing 86147.
86153	See code before 86148.
87623	See code following 87539.
87624	See code following 87539.
87625	See code before 87540.
87806	See code following 87803.
87906	See code following 87901.
87910	See code following 87900.
87912	See code before 87902.
88177	See code following 88173.
88341	See code following 88342.
88350	See code following 88346.
88364	See code following 88365.
88373	See code following 88367.
88374	See code following 88367.
88377	See code following 88369.
90619	See code following 90734.
90620	See code following 90734.
90621	See code following 90734.
90625	See code following 90723.
90630	See code following 90654.
90644	See code following 90732.
90672	See code following 90660.
90673	See code before 90662.
90674	See code following 90661.
90694	See code following 90689.
90750	See code following 90736.
90756	See code following 90661.
92558	See code following 92586.
92597	See code following 92604.
92618	See code following 92605.
92920	See code following 92998.
92921	See code following 92998.
92924	See code following 92998.
92925	See code following 92998.
92928	See code following 92998.
92929	See code following 92998.
92933	See code following 92998.
92934	See code following 92998.
92937	See code following 92998.
92938	See code following 92998.
92941	See code following 92998.
92943	See code following 92998.
92944	See code following 92998.
92973	See code following 92998.
92974	See code following 92998.
92975	See code following 92998.
92977	See code following 92998.
92978	See code following 92998.
92979	See code following 92998.
93260	See code following 93284.
93261	See code following 93289.
93264	See code before 93279.
93356	See code following 93351.
95249	See code following 95250.
95700	See code following 95967.
95705	See code following 95967.
95706	See code following 95967.
95707	See code following 95967.
95708	See code following 95967.
95709	See code following 95967.
95710	See code following 95967.
95711	See code following 95967.
95712	See code following 95967.
95713	See code following 95967.
95714	See code following 95967.
95715	See code following 95967.
95716	See code following 95967.
95717	See code following 95967.
95718	See code following 95967.
95719	See code following 95967.
95720	See code following 95967.
95721	See code following 95967.
95722	See code following 95967.
95723	See code following 95967.
95724	See code following 95967.
95725	See code following 95967.
95726	See code following 95967.
95782	See code following 95811.
95783	See code following 95811.
95800	See code following 95806.
95801	See code following 95806.
95829	See code following 95830.
95836	See code following 95830.
95885	See code following 95872.
95886	See code following 95872.
95887	See code before 95873.
95938	See code following 95926.
95939	See code following 95929.
95940	See code following 95913.
95941	See code following 95913.

Code	Reference
95943	See code following 95924.
95983	See code following 95977.
95984	See code following 95977.
96125	See code following 96105.
96127	See code following 96113.
96164	See code following 96159.
96165	See code following 96159.
96167	See code following 96159.
96168	See code following 96159.
96170	See code following 96159.
96171	See code following 96159.
97151	See code following 96040.
97152	See code following 96040.
97153	See code following 96040.
97154	See code following 96040.
97155	See code following 96040.
97156	See code following 96040.
97157	See code following 96040.
97158	See code following 96040.
97161	See code before 97010.
97162	See code before 97010.
97163	See code before 97010.
97164	See code before 97010.

Code	Reference
97165	See code before 97010.
97166	See code before 97010.
97167	See code before 97010.
97168	See code before 97010.
97169	See code before 97010.
97170	See code before 97010.
97171	See code before 97010.
97172	See code before 97010.
99091	See code following resequenced code 99454.
99177	See code following 99174.
99224	See code following 99220.
99225	See code following 99220.
99226	See code following 99220.
99415	See code following 99359.
99416	See code following 99359.
99421	See code following 99443.
99422	See code following 99443.
99423	See code following 99443.
99451	See code following 99449.
99452	See code following 99449.
99453	See code following 99449.
99454	See code following 99449.

Code	Reference
99457	See code before 99450.
99458	See code before 99450.
99473	See code before 99450.
99474	See code before 99450.
99484	See code following 99498.
99485	See code following 99467.
99486	See code following 99467.
99490	See code before 99487.
99491	See code before 99487.
2033F	See code following 2026F.
3051F	See code following 3044F.
3052F	See code before 3046F.
0253T	See code before 0198T.
0376T	See code following 0191T.
0464T	See code following 0333T.
0488T	See code following 0403T.
0510T	See code following 0335T.
0511T	See code following 0335T.
0512T	See code following 0102T.
0513T	See code following 0102T.
0523T	See code following 0504T.
0563T	See code following 0207T.

Appendix F — Add-on Codes, Optum Modifier 50 Exempt, Modifier 51 Exempt, Optum Modifier 51 Exempt, Modifier 63 Exempt, and Modifier 95 Telemedicine Services

Codes specified as add-on, exempt from modifiers 50, 51 and 63, and modifier 95 (telemedicine services) are listed. The lists are designed to be read left to right rather than vertically.

Add-on Codes

0054T 0055T 0071U 0072U 0073U 0074U 0075U
0076T 0076U 0095T 0098T 0130U 0131U 0132U
0133U 0134U 0135U 0136U 0137U 0138U 0157U
0158U 0159T 0159U 0160U 0161U 0162U 0163T
0164T 0165T 0174T 0189T 0190T 01953 01968
01969 0196T 0205T 0214T 0215T 0217T 0218T
0222T 0229T 0231T 0290T 0346T 0361T 0363T
0365T 0367T 0369T 0374T 0376T 0396T 0397T
0399T 0437T 0439T 0443T 0450T 0466T 0471T
0480T 0482T 0492T 0496T 0513T 0514T 0523T
0560T 0562T 0570T 10004 10006 10008 10010
10012 10036 11001 11008 11045 11046 11047
11101 11103 11105 11107 11201 11732 11922
13102 13122 13133 13153 14302 15003 15005
15101 15111 15116 15121 15131 15136 15151
15152 15156 15157 15201 15221 15241 15261
15272 15274 15276 15278 15772 15774 15777
15787 15847 16036 17003 17312 17314 17315
19001 19082 19084 19086 19126 19282 19284
19286 19288 19294 19297 20700 20701 20702
20703 20704 20705 20930 20931 20932 20933
20934 20936 20937 20938 20939 20985 22103
22116 22208 22216 22226 22328 22512 22515
22527 22534 22552 22585 22614 22632 22634
22840 22841 22842 22843 22844 22845 22846
22847 22848 22853 22854 22858 22859 22868
22870 26125 26861 26863 27358 27692 29826
31627 31632 31633 31637 31649 31651 31654
32501 32506 32507 32667 32668 32674 33141
33225 33257 33258 33259 33367 33368 33369
33419 33508 33517 33518 33519 33521 33522
33523 33530 33572 33768 33866 33884 33924
33929 33987 34709 34711 34713 34714 34715
34716 34717 34808 34812 34813 34820 34833
34834 35306 35390 35400 35500 35572 35600
35681 35682 35683 35685 35686 35697 35700
36218 36227 36228 36248 36474 36476 36479
36483 36907 36908 36909 37185 37186 37222
37223 37232 37233 37234 37235 37237 37239
37247 37249 37252 37253 38102 38746 38747
38900 43273 43283 43338 43635 44015 44121
44128 44139 44203 44213 44701 44955 47001
47542 47543 47544 47550 48400 49326 49327
49412 49435 49568 49905 50606 50705 50706
51797 52442 56606 57267 58110 58611 59525
60512 61316 61517 61610 61611 61612 61641
61642 61651 61781 61782 61783 61797 61799
61800 61864 61868 62148 62160 63035 63043
63044 63048 63057 63066 63076 63078 63082
63086 63088 63091 63103 63295 63308 63621
64421 64462 64480 64484 64491 64492 64494
64495 64634 64636 64643 64645 64727 64778
64783 64787 64832 64837 64859 64872 64874
64876 64901 64902 64913 65757 66990 67225
67320 67331 67332 67334 67335 67340 69990
74248 74301 74713 75565 75774 76125 76802
76810 76812 76814 76937 76979 76983 77001
77002 77003 77063 77293 78020 78434 78496
78730 78835 81266 81416 81426 81536 82952
86826 87187 87503 87904 88155 88177 88185
88311 88314 88332 88334 88341 88350 88364
88369 88373 88388 90461 90472 90474 90785
90833 90836 90838 90840 90863 90913 91013
92547 92608 92618 92621 92627 92921 92925
92929 92934 92938 92944 92973 92974 92978
92979 92998 93320 93321 93325 93352 93356
93462 93463 93464 93563 93564 93565 93566
93567 93568 93571 93572 93592 93609 93613
93621 93622 93623 93655 93657 93662 94645
94729 94781 95079 95873 95874 95885 95886
95887 95940 95941 95962 95967 95975 95979
95984 96113 96121 96131 96133 96137 96139
96159 96165 96168 96171 96361 96366 96367
96368 96370 96371 96375 96376 96411 96415
96417 96423 96570 96571 96934 96935 96936
97130 97546 97598 97811 97814 99100 99116
99135 99140 99153 99157 99292 99354 99355
99356 99357 99359 99415 99416 99458 99467
99486 99489 99494 99498 99602 99607

Optum Modifier 50 Exempt Codes

0214T 0215T 0217T 0218T 15777 20939 34713
34714 34715 34716 34717 34812 34820 34833
34834 35572 36227 36228 49568 63035 63043
63044 64421 64462 64480 64484 64491 64492
64494 64495 64634 64636

AMA Modifier 51 Exempt Codes

20697 20974 20975 44500 61107 93600 93602
93603 93610 93612 93615 93616 93618 94610
95905 99151 99152

Optum Modifier 51 Exempt Codes

90281 90283 90284 90287 90288 90291 90296
90371 90375 90376 90378 90384 90385 90386
90389 90393 90396 90399 90476 90477 90581
90585 90586 90587 90620 90621 90625 90630
90632 90633 90634 90636 90644 90647 90648
90649 90650 90651 90653 90654 90655 90656
90657 90658 90660 90661 90662 90664 90666
90667 90668 90670 90672 90673 90674 90675
90676 90680 90681 90682 90685 90686 90687
90688 90689 90690 90691 90696 90697 90698
90700 90702 90707 90710 90713 90714 90715
90716 90717 90723 90732 90733 90734 90736
90738 90739 90740 90743 90744 90746 90747
90748 90749 90750 90756 97010 97012 97014
97016 97018 97022 97024 97026 97028 97032
97033 97034 97035 97036 97110 97112 97113
97116 97124 97129 97130 97140 97150 97530
97533 97535 97537 97542 97545 97546 97597
97598 97602 97605 97606 97607 97608 97610
97750 97755 97760 97761 97763 99050 99051
99053 99056 99058 99060

Modifier 63 Exempt Codes

30540 30545 31520 33470 33502 33503 33505
33506 33610 33611 33619 33647 33670 33690
33694 33730 33732 33735 33736 33750 33755
33762 33778 33786 33922 33946 33947 33948
33949 36415 36420 36450 36456 36460 36510
36660 39503 43313 43314 43520 43831 44055
44126 44127 44128 46070 46705 46715 46716
46730 46735 46740 46742 46744 47700 47701

49215	49491	49492	49495	49496	49600	49605
49606	49610	49611	53025	54000	54150	54160
63700	63702	63704	63706	65820		

Telemedicine Services Codes

The codes on the following list may be used to report telemedicine services when modifier 95 Synchronous Telemedicine Service Rendered via a Real-Time Interactive Audio and Visual Telecommunications System, is appended.

90791	90792	90832	90833	90834	90836	90837
90838	90845	90846	90847	90863	90951	90952
90954	90955	90957	90958	90960	90961	92227
92228	93228	93229	93268	93270	93271	93272
96040	96116	97802	97803	97804	98960	98961
98962	99201	99202	99203	99204	99205	99212
99213	99214	99215	99231	99232	99233	*99241
*99242	*99243	*99244	*99245	*99251	*99252	*99253
*99254	*99255	99307	99308	99309	99310	99354
99355	99406	99407	99408	99409	99495	99496

* Consultations are noncovered by Medicare

Appendix G — Medicare Internet-only Manuals (IOMs)

The Centers for Medicare and Medicaid Services restructured its paper-based manual system as a web-based system on October 1, 2003. Called the online CMS manual system, it combines all of the various program instructions into internet-only manuals (IOMs), which are used by all CMS programs and contractors. In many instances, the references from the online manuals in appendix G contain a mention of the old paper manuals from which the current information was obtained when the manuals were converted. This information is shown in the header of the text, in the following format, when applicable, as A3-3101, HO-210, and B3-2049. Complete versions of all of the manuals can be found at https://www.cms.gov/Regulations-and-Guidance/Guidance/Manuals/Internet-Only-Manuals-IOMs.html.

Effective with implementation of the IOMs, the former method of publishing program memoranda (PMs) to communicate program instructions was replaced by the following four templates:

- One-time notification
- Manual revisions
- Business requirements
- Confidential requirements

The web-based system has been organized by functional area (e.g., eligibility, entitlement, claims processing, benefit policy, program integrity) in an effort to eliminate redundancy within the manuals, simplify updating, and make CMS program instructions available more quickly. The web-based system contains the functional areas included below:

Pub. 100	Introduction
Pub. 100-01	Medicare General Information, Eligibility, and Entitlement Manual
Pub. 100-02	Medicare Benefit Policy Manual
Pub. 100-03	Medicare National Coverage Determinations (NCD) Manual
Pub. 100-04	Medicare Claims Processing Manual
Pub. 100-05	Medicare Secondary Payer Manual
Pub. 100-06	Medicare Financial Management Manual
Pub. 100-07	State Operations Manual
Pub. 100-08	Medicare Program Integrity Manual
Pub. 100-09	Medicare Contractor Beneficiary and Provider Communications Manual
Pub. 100-10	Quality Improvement Organization Manual
Pub. 100-11	Programs of All-Inclusive Care for the Elderly (PACE) Manual
Pub. 100-12	State Medicaid Manual (under development)
Pub. 100-13	Medicaid State Children's Health Insurance Program (under development)
Pub. 100-14	Medicare ESRD Network Organizations Manual
Pub. 100-15	Medicaid Integrity Program (MIP)
Pub. 100-16	Medicare Managed Care Manual
Pub. 100-17	CMS/Business Partners Systems Security Manual
Pub. 100-18	Medicare Prescription Drug Benefit Manual
Pub. 100-19	Demonstrations
Pub. 100-20	One-Time Notification
Pub. 100-21	Recurring Update Notification
Pub. 100-22	Medicare Quality Reporting Incentive Programs Manual
Pub. 100-24	State Buy-In Manual
Pub. 100-25	Information Security Acceptable Risk Safeguards Manual

A brief description of the Medicare manuals primarily used for *CPC Expert* follows:

The ***National Coverage Determinations Manual*** (NCD), is organized according to categories such as diagnostic services, supplies, and medical procedures. The table of contents lists each category and subject within that category. Revision transmittals identify any new or background material, recap the changes, and provide an effective date for the change.

When complete, the manual will contain two chapters. Chapter 1 currently includes a description of CMS's national coverage determinations. When available, chapter 2 will contain a list of HCPCS codes related to each coverage determination. The manual is organized in accordance with CPT category sequences.

The ***Medicare Benefit Policy Manual*** contains Medicare general coverage instructions that are not national coverage determinations. As a general rule, in the past these instructions have been found in chapter II of the ***Medicare Carriers Manual,*** the ***Medicare Intermediary Manual***, other provider manuals, and program memoranda.

The ***Medicare Claims Processing Manual*** contains instructions for processing claims for contractors and providers.

The ***Medicare Program Integrity Manual*** communicates the priorities and standards for the Medicare integrity programs.

Medicare IOM references

100-01, 3, 20.5

Blood Deductibles (Part A and Part B)

(Rev. 1, 09-11-02)

Program payment may not be made for the first 3 pints of whole blood or equivalent units of packed red cells received under Part A and Part B combined in a calendar year. However, blood processing (e.g., administration, storage) is not subject to the deductible.

The blood deductibles are in addition to any other applicable deductible and coinsurance amounts for which the patient is responsible.

The deductible applies only to the first 3 pints of blood furnished in a calendar year, even if more than one provider furnished blood.

100-01, 5, 70.6

Chiropractors

(Rev. 1, 09-11-02)

A. General

A licensed chiropractor who meets uniform minimum standards (see subsection C) is a physician for specified services. Coverage extends only to treatment by means of manual manipulation of the spine to correct a subluxation demonstrated by X-ray, provided such treatment is legal in the State where performed. All other services furnished or ordered by chiropractors are not covered. An X-ray obtained by a chiropractor for his or her own diagnostic purposes before commencing treatment may suffice for claims documentation purposes. This means that if a chiropractor orders, takes, or interprets an X-ray to demonstrate a subluxation of the spine, the X-ray can be used for claims processing purposes. However, there is no coverage or payment for these services or for any other diagnostic or therapeutic service ordered or furnished by the chiropractor. In addition, in performing manual manipulation of the spine, some chiropractors use manual devices that are hand-held with the thrust of the force of the device being controlled manually. While such manual manipulation may be covered, there is no separate payment permitted for use of this device.

B. Licensure and Authorization to Practice

A chiropractor must be licensed or legally authorized to furnish chiropractic services by the State or jurisdiction in which the services are furnished.

C. Uniform Minimum Standards

I. Prior to July 1, 1974, Chiropractors licensed or authorized to practice prior to July 1, 1974, and those individuals who commenced their studies in a chiropractic college before that date must meet all of the following minimum standards to render payable services under the program:

   a. Preliminary education equal to the requirements for graduation from an accredited high school or other secondary school;

b. Graduation from a college of chiropractic approved by the State's chiropractic examiners that included the completion of a course of study covering a period of not less than 3 school years of 6 months each year in actual continuous attendance covering adequate course of study in the subjects of anatomy, physiology, symptomatology and diagnosis, hygiene and sanitation, chemistry, histology, pathology, and principles and practice of chiropractic, including clinical instruction in vertebral palpation, nerve tracing and adjusting; and

c. Passage of an examination prescribed by the State's chiropractic examiners covering the subjects listed in subsection b.

2. After June 30, 1974 - Individuals commencing their studies in a chiropractic college after June 30, 1974, must meet all of the following additional requirements:

a. Satisfactory completion of 2 years of pre-chiropractic study at the college level;

b. Satisfactory completion of a 4-year course of 8 months each year (instead of a 3-year course of 6 months each year) at a college or school of chiropractic that includes not less than 4,000 hours in the scientific and chiropractic courses specified in subsection1.b, plus courses in the use and effect of X-ray and chiropractic analysis; and

c. The practitioner must be over 21 years of age.

100-02, 1, 90

Termination of Pregnancy

(Rev. 1, 10-01-03) B3-4276.1,.2

Effective for services furnished on or after October 1, 1998, Medicare will cover abortions procedures in the following situations:

1. If the pregnancy is the result of an act or rape or incest; or
2. In the case where a woman suffers from a physical disorder, physical injury, or physical illness, including a life-endangering physical condition caused by the pregnancy itself that would, as certified by a physician, place the woman in danger of death unless an abortion is performed.

NOTE: The "G7" modifier must be used with the following CPT codes in order for these services to be covered when the pregnancy resulted from rape or incest, or the pregnancy is certified by a physician as life threatening to the mother:

59840, 59841, 59850, 59851, 59852, 59855, 59856, 59857, 59866

100-02, 1, 100

Treatment for Infertility

(Rev. 1, 10-01-03) A3-3101.13

Effective for services rendered on or after January 15, 1980, reasonable and necessary services associated with treatment for infertility are covered under Medicare. Like pregnancy (see Sec. 80 above), infertility is a condition sufficiently at variance with the usual state of health to make it appropriate for a person who normally would be expected to be fertile to seek medical consultation and treatment. Contractors should coordinate with QIOs to see that utilization guidelines are established for this treatment if inappropriate utilization or abuse is suspected.

100-02, 11, 20

Renal Dialysis Items and Services

(Rev.199, Issued: 11-14-14-Effective: 01-01-15, Implementation: 01-05-15)

Medicare provides payment under the ESRD PPS for all renal dialysis services for outpatient maintenance dialysis when they are furnished to Medicare ESRD patients for the treatment of ESRD by a Medicare certified ESRD facility or a special purpose dialysis facility. Renal dialysis services are the items and services included under the composite rate and the ESRD-related items and services that were separately paid as of December 31, 2010 that were used for the treatment of ESRD.

Renal dialysis services are furnished in various settings including hospital outpatient ESRD facilities, independent ESRD facilities, or in the patient's home. Renal dialysis items and services furnished at ESRD facilities differ according to the types of patients being treated, the types of equipment and supplies used, the preferences of the treating physician, and the capability and makeup of the staff. Although not all facilities provide an identical range of services, the most common elements of dialysis treatment include:

- Laboratory Tests;
- Drugs and Biologicals;
- Equipment and supplies - dialysis machine use and maintenance;
- Personnel services;
- Administrative services;
- Overhead costs;
- Monitoring access and related declotting or referring the patient, and
- Direct nursing services include registered nurses, licensed practical nurses, technicians, social workers, and dietitians.

100-02, 11, 20.2

Laboratory Services

(Rev. 224, Issued: 06-03-16, Effective: 01-01-16, Implementation: 09-06-16)

All laboratory services furnished to individuals for the treatment of ESRD are included in the ESRD PPS as Part B services and are not paid separately as of January 1, 2011. The laboratory services include but are not limited to:

- Laboratory tests included under the composite rate as of December 31, 2010 (discussed below); and
- Former separately billable Part B laboratory tests that were billed by ESRD facilities and independent laboratories for ESRD patients.

Composite rate laboratory tests are listed in §20.2.E of this chapter. More information regarding composite rate laboratory tests can be found in Pub. 100-4, Medicare Claims Processing Manual, chapter 8, §50.1, §60.1, and §80. As discussed below, composite rate laboratory services should not be reported on claims.

The distinction of what is considered to be a renal dialysis laboratory test is a clinical decision determined by the ESRD patient's ordering practitioner. If a laboratory test is ordered for the treatment of ESRD, then the laboratory test is not paid separately.

Payment for all renal dialysis laboratory tests furnished under the ESRD PPS is made directly to the ESRD facility responsible for the patient's care. The ESRD facility must furnish the laboratory tests directly or under arrangement and report renal dialysis laboratory tests on the ESRD facility claim (with the exception of composite rate laboratory services).

An ESRD facility must report renal dialysis laboratory services on its claims in order for the laboratory tests to be included in the outlier payment calculation. Renal dialysis laboratory services that were or would have been paid separately under Medicare Part B prior to January 1, 2011, are priced for the outlier payment calculation using the Clinical Laboratory Fee Schedule. Further information regarding the outlier policy can be found in §60.D of this chapter.

Certain laboratory services will be subject to Part B consolidated billing requirements and will no longer be separately payable when provided to ESRD beneficiaries by providers other than the renal dialysis facility. The list below includes the renal dialysis laboratory tests that are routinely performed for the treatment of ESRD. Payment for the laboratory tests identified on this list is included in the ESRD PPS. The laboratory tests listed in the table are used to enforce consolidated billing edits to ensure that payment is not made for renal dialysis laboratory tests outside of the ESRD PPS. The list of renal dialysis laboratory tests is not an all-inclusive list. If any laboratory test is ordered for the treatment of ESRD, then the laboratory test is considered to be included in the ESRD PPS and is the responsibility of the ESRD facility. Additional renal dialysis laboratory tests may be added through administrative issuances in the future.

LABS SUBJECT TO ESRD CONSOLIDATED BILLING

CPT/ HCPCS	Short Description
80047	Basic Metabolic Panel (Calcium, ionized)
80048	Basic Metabolic Panel (Calcium, total)
80051	Electrolyte Panel
80053	Comprehensive Metabolic Panel
80061	Lipid Panel
80069	Renal Function Panel
80076	Hepatic Function Panel
82040	Assay of serum albumin
82108	Assay of aluminum
82306	Vitamin d, 25 hydroxy
82310	Assay of calcium
82330	Assay of calcium, Ionized
82374	Assay, blood carbon dioxide
82379	Assay of carnitine
82435	Assay of blood chloride
82565	Assay of creatinine
82570	Assay of urine creatinine
82575	Creatinine clearance test
82607	Vitamin B-12
82652	Vit d 1, 25-dihydroxy
82668	Assay of erythropoietin
82728	Assay of ferritin
82746	Blood folic acid serum
83540	Assay of iron
83550	Iron binding test
83735	Assay of magnesium
83970	Assay of parathormone
84075	Assay alkaline phosphatase
84100	Assay of phosphorus
84132	Assay of serum potassium

CPT/ HCPCS	Short Description
84134	Assay of prealbumin
84155	Assay of protein, serum
84157	Assay of protein by other source
84295	Assay of serum sodium
84466	Assay of transferrin
84520	Assay of urea nitrogen
84540	Assay of urine/urea-n
84545	Urea-N clearance test
85014	Hematocrit
85018	Hemoglobin
85025	Complete (cbc), automated (HgB, Hct, RBC, WBC, and Platelet count) and automated differential WBC count.
85027	Complete (cbc), automated (HgB, Hct, RBC, WBC, and Platelet count)
85041	Automated rbc count
85044	Manual reticulocyte count
85045	Automated reticulocyte count
85046	Reticyte/hgb concentrate
85048	Automated leukocyte count
86704	Hep b core antibody, total
86705	Hep b core antibody, igm
86706	Hep b surface antibody
87040	Blood culture for bacteria
87070	Culture, bacteria, other
87071	Culture bacteri aerobic othr
87073	Culture bacteria anaerobic
87075	Cultr bacteria, except blood
87076	Culture anaerobe ident, each
87077	Culture aerobic identify
87081	Culture screen only
87340	Hepatitis b surface ag, eia
G0306	CBC/diff WBC w/o platelet
G0307	CBC without platelet

A. Automated Multi-Channel Chemistry (AMCC) Tests

During the ESRD PPS transition period (see §70 of this chapter) ESRD facilities are required to report the renal dialysis AMCC tests with the appropriate modifiers (CD, CE, or CF) on their claims for purposes of applying the 50/50 rule under the composite rate portion of the blended payment. Refer to §70.B of this chapter for additional information regarding the composite rate portion of the blended payment during the transition.

The 50/50 rule is necessary for those ESRD facilities that chose to go through the transition period. If the 50/50 rule allows for separate payment, then the laboratory tests are priced using the clinical laboratory fee schedule. Information regarding the 50/50 rule can be found in §20.2.E of this chapter and in Pub. 100-4, Medicare Claims Processing Manual, chapter 16, §40.6.

NOTE: An ESRD facility billing a renal dialysis AMCC test must use the CF modifier when the AMCC is not in the composite rate but is a renal dialysis service. AMCC tests that are furnished to individuals for reasons other than for the treatment of ESRD should be billed with the AY modifier to Medicare directly by the entity furnishing the service with the AY modifier.

B. Laboratory Services Furnished for Reasons Other Than for the Treatment of ESRD

1. **Independent Laboratory**

   A patient's physician or practitioner may order a laboratory test that is included on the list of items and services subject to consolidated billing edits for reasons other than for the treatment of ESRD. When this occurs, the patient's physician or practitioner should notify the independent laboratory or the ESRD facility (with the appropriate clinical laboratory certification in accordance with the Clinical Laboratory Improvement Act) that furnished the laboratory service that the test is not a renal dialysis service and that entity may bill Medicare separately using the AY modifier. The AY modifier serves as an attestation that the item or service is medically necessary for the patient but is not being used for the treatment of ESRD.

2. **Hospital-Based Laboratory**

   Hospital outpatient clinical laboratories furnishing renal dialysis laboratory tests to ESRD patients for reasons other than for the treatment of ESRD may submit a claim for separate payment using the AY modifier. The AY modifier serves as an attestation that the item or service is medically necessary for the patient but is not being used for the treatment of ESRD.

C. Laboratory Services Performed in Emergency Rooms or Emergency Departments

In an emergency room or emergency department, the ordering physician or practitioner may not know at the time the laboratory test is being ordered, if it is being ordered as a renal dialysis service. Consequently, emergency rooms or emergency departments are not required to append an AY modifier to these laboratory tests when submitting claims with dates of service on or after January 1, 2012.

When a renal dialysis laboratory service is furnished to an ESRD patient in an emergency room or emergency department on a different date of service, hospitals can append an ET modifier to the laboratory tests furnished to ESRD patients to indicate that the laboratory test was furnished in conjunction with the emergency visit. Appending the ET modifier indicates that the laboratory service being furnished on a day other than the emergency visit is related to the emergency visit and at the time the ordering physician was unable to determine if the test was ordered for reasons of treating the patient's ESRD.

Allowing laboratory testing to bypass consolidated billing edits in the emergency room or department does not mean that ESRD facilities should send patients to other settings for routine laboratory testing for the purpose of not assuming financial responsibility of renal dialysis items and services. For additional information regarding laboratory services furnished in a variety of settings, see Pub. 100-4, Medicare Claims Processing Manual, chapter 16, §30.3 and §40.6.

D. Hepatitis B Laboratory Services for Transient Patients

Laboratory testing for hepatitis B is a renal dialysis service. Effective January 1, 2011, hepatitis B testing is included in the ESRD PPS and therefore cannot be billed separately to Medicare.

The Conditions for Coverage for ESRD facilities require routine hepatitis B testing (42 CFR §494.30(a)(1)). The ESRD facility is responsible for the payment of the laboratory test, regardless of frequency. If an ESRD patient wishes to travel, the patient's home ESRD facility should have systems in place for communicating hepatitis B test results to the destination ESRD facility.

E. Laboratory Services Included Under Composite Rate

Prior to the implementation of the ESRD PPS, the costs of certain ESRD laboratory services furnished for outpatient maintenance dialysis by either the ESRD facility's staff or an independent laboratory, were included in the composite rate calculations. Therefore, payment for all of these laboratory tests was included in the ESRD facility's composite rate and the tests could not have been billed separately to the Medicare program.

All laboratory services that were included under the composite rate are included under the ESRD PPS unless otherwise specified. Payments for these laboratory tests are included in the ESRD PPS and are not paid separately under the composite rate portion of the blended payment and are not eligible for outlier payments. Therefore, composite rate laboratory services should not be reported on the claim. Laboratory tests included in the composite payment rate are identified below.

1. **Routinely Covered Tests Paid Under Composite Rate**

   The tests listed below are usually performed for dialysis patients and were routinely covered at the frequency specified in the absence of indications to the contrary, (i.e., no documentation of medical necessity was required other than knowledge of the patient's status as an ESRD beneficiary). When any of these tests were performed at a frequency greater than that specified, the additional tests were separately billable and were covered only if they were medically justified by accompanying documentation. A diagnosis of ESRD alone was not sufficient medical evidence to warrant coverage of the additional tests. The nature of the illness or injury (diagnosis, complaint, or symptom) requiring the performance of the test(s) must have been present, along with ICD diagnosis coding, on the claim for payment.

   a. Hemodialysis, IPD, CCPD, and Hemofiltration

      - Per Treatment - All hematocrit, hemoglobin, and clotting time tests furnished incident to dialysis treatments;
      - Weekly - Prothrombin time for patients on anticoagulant therapy and Serum Creatinine;
      - Weekly or Thirteen Per Quarter - BUN;
      - Monthly - Serum Calcium, Serum Potassium, Serum Chloride, CBC, Serum Bicarbonate, Serum Phosphorous, Total Protein, Serum Albumin, Alkaline Phosphatase, aspartate amino transferase (AST) (SGOT) and LDH; and
      - Automated Multi-Channel Chemistry (AMCC) - If an automated battery of tests, such as the SMA-12, is performed and contains most of the tests listed in one of the weekly or monthly categories, it is not necessary to separately identify any tests in the battery that are not listed. Further information concerning automated tests and the "50 percent rule" can be found below and in Pub. 100-4, Medicare Claims Processing Manual, chapter 16, §40.6.1.

   b. CAPD

      - Monthly – BUN, Creatinine, Sodium, Potassium, CO2, Calcium, Magnesium, Phosphate, Total Protein, Albumin, Alkaline Phosphatase, LDH, AST, SGOT, HCT, Hbg, and Dialysate Protein.

   Under the ESRD PPS, frequency requirements do not apply for the purpose of payment. However, laboratory tests should be ordered as necessary and should not be restricted because of financial reasons.

2. **Separately Billable Tests Under the Composite Rate**

   The following list identifies certain separately billable laboratory tests that were covered routinely and without documentation of medical necessity other than knowledge of the patient's status as an ESRD beneficiary, when furnished at specified frequencies. If they were performed at a frequency greater than that specified, they were covered only if accompanied by medical documentation. A diagnosis of ESRD alone was not sufficient documentation. The medical necessity of the test(s), the nature of the illness or injury (diagnosis, complaint or symptom) requiring the performance of the test(s) must have been furnished on claims using the ICD diagnosis coding system.

— Separately Billable Tests for Hemodialysis, IPD, CCPD, and Hemofiltration

  Serum Aluminum - one every 3 months

  Serum Ferritin - one every 3 months

— Separately Billable Tests for CAPD

  WBC, RBC, and Platelet count – One every 3 months

  Residual renal function and 24 hour urine volume – One every 6 months

Under the ESRD PPS frequency requirements do not apply for the purpose of payment. However, laboratory tests should be ordered as necessary and should not be restricted because of financial reasons.

3. **Automated Multi-Channel Chemistry (AMCC) Tests Under the Composite Rate**

Clinical diagnostic laboratory tests that comprise the AMCC (listed in Appendix A and B) could be considered to be composite rate and non-composite rate laboratory services. Composite rate payment was paid by the A/B MAC (A). To determine if separate payment was allowed for non-composite rate tests for a particular date of service, 50 percent or more of the covered tests must be non-composite rate tests. This policy also applies to the composite rate portion of the blended payment during the transition. Beginning January 1, 2014, the 50 percent rule will no longer apply and no separate payment will be made under the composite rate portion of the blended payment.

Medicare applied the following to AMCC tests for ESRD beneficiaries:

— Payment was the lowest rate for services performed by the same provider, for the same beneficiary, for the same date of service.

— The A/B MAC identified, for a particular date of service, the AMCC tests ordered that were included in the composite rate and those that were not included. The composite rate tests were defined for Hemodialysis, IPD, CCPD, and Hemofiltration (see Appendix A) and for CAPD (see Appendix B).

— If 50 percent or more of the covered tests were included under the composite rate payment, then all submitted tests were included within the composite payment. In this case, no separate payment in addition to the composite rate was made for any of the separately billable tests.

— If less than 50 percent of the covered tests were composite rate tests, all AMCC tests submitted for that Date of Service (DOS) were separately payable.

— A non-composite rate test was defined as any test separately payable outside of the composite rate or beyond the normal frequency covered under the composite rate that was reasonable and necessary.

Three pricing modifiers identify the different payment situations for ESRD AMCC tests. The physician who ordered the tests was responsible for identifying the appropriate modifier when ordering the tests.

— CD - AMCC test had been ordered by an ESRD facility or Medicare capitation payment (MCP) physician that was part of the composite rate and was not separately billable

— CE - AMCC test had been ordered by an ESRD facility or MCP physician that was a composite rate test but was beyond the normal frequency covered under the rate and was separately reimbursable based on medical necessity

— CF - AMCC test had been ordered by an ESRD facility or MCP physician that was not part of the composite rate and was separately billable

The ESRD clinical diagnostic laboratory tests identified with modifiers "CD", "CE" or "CF" may not have been billed as organ or disease panels. Effective October 1, 2003, all ESRD clinical diagnostic laboratory tests must be billed individually. See Pub. 100-4, Medicare Claims Processing Manual, chapter 16, §40.6.1, for additional billing and payment instructions as well as examples of the 50/50 rule.

For ESRD dialysis patients, CPT code 82330 Calcium; ionized shall be included in the calculation for the 50/50 rule (Pub. 100-4, Medicare Claims Processing Manual, chapter 16, §40.6.1). When CPT code 82330 is billed as a substitute for CPT code 82310, Calcium; total, it shall be billed with modifier CD or CE. When CPT code 82330 is billed in addition to CPT 82310, it shall be billed with CF modifier.

100-02, 12, 30.1

(Rev.255, Issued: 01-25-19, Effective: 01- 01- 19, Implementation: 02-26-19)

Rules for Payment of CORF Services

The payment basis for CORF services is 80 percent of the lesser of: (1) the actual charge for the service or (2) the physician fee schedule amount for the service when the physician fee schedule establishes a payment amount for such service. Payment for CORF services under the physician fee schedule is made for physical therapy, occupational therapy, speech-language pathology and respiratory therapy services, as well as the nursing and social and/or psychological services, which are a part of, or directly relate to, the rehabilitation plan of treatment.

Payment for covered durable medical equipment, orthotic and prosthetic (DMEPOS) devices and supplies provided by a CORF is based upon: the lesser of 80 percent of actual charges or the payment amount established under the DMEPOS fee schedule; or, the single payment amount established under the DMEPOS competitive bidding program, provided that payment for such an item is not included in the payment amount for other CORF services.

If there is no fee schedule amount for a covered CORF item or service, payment should be based on the lesser of 80 percent of the actual charge for the service provided or an amount determined by the local Medicare contractor.

The following conditions apply to CORF physical therapy, occupational therapy, and speech-language pathology services;

- Claims must contain the required functional reporting. (Reference: Sections 42 CFR 410.105.) Refer to Pub. 100-04, Medicare Claims Processing Manual, chapter 5, section 10.6. NOTE: Functional reporting and documentation requirements are no longer applicable for claims for dates of service on and after January 1, 2019. For more information, refer to subsection F in section 30 above.
- The functional reporting on claims must be consistent with the functional limitations identified as part of the patient's therapy plan of care and expressed as part of the patient's therapy goals; effective for claims with dates of service on and after January, 1, 2013. (Reference: 42 CFR 410.105.) See Pub. 100-04, Medicare Claims Processing Manual, chapter 5, section 10.6. NOTE: Functional reporting and documentation requirements are no longer applicable for claims for dates of service on and after January 1, 2019. For more information, refer to subsection F in section 30 above.
- The National Provider Identifier (NPI) of the certifying physician identified for a CORF physical therapy, occupational therapy, and speech-language pathology plan of treatment must be included on the therapy claim. This requirement is effective for claims with dates of service on or after October 1, 2012. (See Pub. 100-04, Medicare Claims Processing Manual, chapter 5, section 10.3.)

Payment for CORF social and/or psychological services is made under the physician fee schedule only for HCPCS code G0409, as appropriate, and only when billed using revenue codes 0560, 0569, 0910, 0911, 0914 and 0919.

Payment for CORF respiratory therapy services is made under the physician fee schedule when provided by a respiratory therapist as defined at 42CFR485.70(j) and, only to the extent that these services support or are an adjunct to the rehabilitation plan of treatment, when billed using revenue codes 0410, 0412 and 0419. Separate payment is not made for diagnostic tests or for services related to physiologic monitoring services which are bundled into other respiratory therapy services appropriately performed by a respiratory therapist, such as HCPCS codes G0237, G0238 and G0239.

Payment for CORF nursing services is made under the physician fee schedule only when provided by a registered nurse as defined at 42CFR485.70(h) for nursing services only to the extent that these services support or are an adjunct to the rehabilitation plan of treatment. In addition, payment for CORF nursing services is made only when provided by a registered nurse. HCPCS code G0128 is used to bill for these services and only with revenue codes 0550 and 0559.

For specific payment requirements for CORF items and services see Pub. 100-04, Medicare Claims Processing Manual, Chapter 5, Part B Outpatient Rehabilitation and CORF/OPT Services.

100-02, 13, 220

Preventive Health Services

(Rev. 230, Issued: 12-09-16, Effective: 03-09-17, Implementation: 03-09-17)

RHCs and FQHCs are paid for the professional component of allowable preventive services when all of the program requirements are met and frequency limits (where applicable) have not been exceeded. The beneficiary copayment and deductible (where applicable) is waived by the Affordable Care Act for the IPPE and AWV, and for Medicare-covered preventive services recommended by the USPSTF with a grade or A or B.

100-02, 13, 220.1

Preventive Health Services in RHCs

(Rev. 230, Issued: 12-09-16, Effective: 03-09-17, Implementation: 03-09-17)

Influenza (G0008) and Pneumococcal Vaccines (G0009)

Influenza and pneumococcal vaccines and their administration are paid at 100 percent of reasonable cost through the cost report. No visit is billed, and these costs should not be included on the claim. The beneficiary coinsurance and deductible are waived.

Hepatitis B Vaccine (G0010)

Hepatitis B vaccine and its administration is included in the RHC visit and is not separately billable. The cost of the vaccine and its administration can be included in the line item for the otherwise qualifying visit. A visit cannot be billed if vaccine administration is the only service the RHC provides. The beneficiary coinsurance and deductible are waived.

Initial Preventive Physical Exam (G0402)

The IPPE is a face-to-face one-time exam that must occur within the first 12 months following the beneficiary's enrollment. The IPPE can be billed as a stand-alone visit if it is the only medical service provided on that day with an RHC practitioner. If an IPPE visit is furnished on the same day as another billable visit, two visits may be billed. The beneficiary coinsurance and deductible are waived.

Annual Wellness Visit (G0438 and G0439)
The AWV is a personalized face-to-face prevention visit for beneficiaries who are not within the first 12 months of their first Part B coverage period and have not received an IPPE or AWV within the past12 months. The AWV can be billed as a stand-alone visit if it is the only medical service provided on that day with an RHC practitioner. If the AWV is furnished on the same day as another medical visit, it is not a separately billable visit. The beneficiary coinsurance and deductible are waived.

Diabetes Self-Management Training (G0108) and Medical Nutrition Therapy (97802 and 97803)
Diabetes self-management training or medical nutrition therapy provided by a registered dietician or nutritional professional at an RHC may be considered incident to a visit with an RHC practitioner provided all applicable conditions are met. DSMT and MNT are not billable visits in an RHC, although the cost may be allowable on the cost report. RHCs cannot bill a visit for services furnished by registered dieticians or nutritional professionals. However, RHCs are permitted to become certified providers of DSMT services and report the cost of such services on their cost report for inclusion in the computation of their AIR. The beneficiary coinsurance and deductible apply.

Screening Pelvic and Clinical Breast Examination (G0101)
Screening pelvic and clinical breast examination can be billed as a stand-alone visit if it is the only medical service provided on that day with an RHC practitioner. If it is furnished on the same day as another medical visit, it is not a separately billable visit. The beneficiary coinsurance and deductible are waived.

Screening Papanicolaou Smear (Q0091)
Screening Papanicolaou smear can be billed as a stand-alone visit if it is the only medical service provided on that day with an RHC practitioner. If it is furnished on the same day as another medical visit, it is not a separately billable visit. The beneficiary coinsurance and deductible are waived.

Prostate Cancer Screening (G0102)
Prostate cancer screening can be billed as a stand-alone visit if it is the only medical service provided on that day with an RHC practitioner. If it is furnished on the same day as another medical visit, it is not a separately billable visit. The beneficiary coinsurance and deductible apply.

Glaucoma Screening (G0117 and G0118)
Glaucoma screening for high risk patients can be billed as a stand-alone visit if it is the only medical service provided on that day with an RHC practitioner. If it is furnished on the same day as another medical visit, it is not a separately billable visit. The beneficiary coinsurance and deductible apply.

Lung Cancer Screening Using Low Dose Computed Tomography (LDCT) (G0296)
LDCT can be billed as a stand-alone visit if it is the only medical service provided on that day with an RHC practitioner. If it is furnished on the same day as another medical visit, it is not a separately billable visit. The beneficiary coinsurance and deductible are waived.

NOTE: Hepatitis C Screening (GO472) is a technical service only and therefore it is not paid as part of the RHC visit.

100-02, 13, 220.3

Preventive Health Services in FQHCs

(Rev. 230, Issued: 12-09-16, Effective: 03-09-17, Implementation: 03-09-17)

FQHCs must provide preventive health services on site or by arrangement with another provider. These services must be furnished by or under the direct supervision of a physician, NP, PA, CNM, CP, or CSW. Section 330(b)(1)(A)(i)(III) of the Public Health Service (PHS) Act required preventive health services can be found at http://bphc.hrsa.gov/policiesregulations/legislation/index.html, and include:

- prenatal and perinatal services;
- appropriate cancer screening;
- well-child services;
- immunizations against vaccine-preventable diseases;
- screenings for elevated blood lead levels, communicable diseases, and cholesterol;
- pediatric eye, ear, and dental screenings to determine the need for vision and hearing correction and dental care;
- voluntary family planning services; and
- preventive dental services.

NOTE: The cost of providing these services may be included in the FQHC cost report but they do not necessarily qualify as FQHC billable visits or for the waiver of the beneficiary coinsurance.

Influenza (G0008) and Pneumococcal Vaccines (G0009)
Influenza and pneumococcal vaccines and their administration are paid at 100 percent of reasonable cost through the cost report. The cost is included in the cost report and no visit is billed. FQHCs must include these charges on the claim if furnished as part of an encounter. The beneficiary coinsurance is waived.

Hepatitis B Vaccine (G0010)
Hepatitis B vaccine and its administration is included in the FQHC visit and is not separately billable. The cost of the vaccine and its administration can be included in the line item for the otherwise qualifying visit. A visit cannot be billed if vaccine administration is the only service the FQHC provides. The beneficiary coinsurance is waived.

Initial Preventive Physical Exam (G0402)
The IPPE is a one-time exam that must occur within the first 12 months following the beneficiary's enrollment. The IPPE can be billed as a stand-alone visit if it is the only medical service provided on that day with a FQHC practitioner. If an IPPE visit is furnished on the same day as another billable visit, FQHCs may not bill for a separate visit. These FQHCs will have an adjustment of 1.3416 to their PPS rate. The beneficiary coinsurance is waived.

Annual Wellness Visit (G0438 and G0439)
The AWV is a personalized prevention plan for beneficiaries who are not within the first 12 months of their first Part B coverage period and have not received an IPPE or AWV within the past12 months. The AWV can be billed as a stand-alone visit if it is the only medical service provided on that day with a FQHC practitioner. If the AWV is furnished on the same day as another medical visit, it is not a separately billable visit. FQHCs that are authorized to bill under the FQHC PPS will have an adjustment of 1.3416 to their PPS rate. The beneficiary coinsurance is waived.

Diabetes Self-Management Training (G0108) and Medical Nutrition Therapy (97802 and 97803)
DSMT and MNT furnished by certified DSMT and MNT providers are billable visits in FQHCs when they are provided in a one-on-one, face-to-face encounter and all program requirements are met. Other diabetes counseling or medical nutrition services provided by a registered dietician at the FQHC may be considered incident to a visit with a FQHC provider. The beneficiary coinsurance is waived for MNT services and is applicable for DSMT.

DSMT must be furnished by a certified DSMT practitioner, and MNT must be furnished by a registered dietitian or nutrition professional. Program requirements for DSMT services are set forth in 42 CFR 410 Subpart H for DSMT and in Part 410, Subpart G for MNT services, and additional guidance can be found at Pub. 100-02, chapter 15, section 300.

Screening Pelvic and Clinical Breast Examination (G0101)
Screening pelvic and clinical breast examination can be billed as a stand-alone visit if it is the only medical service provided on that day with a FQHC practitioner. If it is furnished on the same day as another medical visit, it is not a separately billable visit. The beneficiary coinsurance is waived.

Screening Papanicolaou Smear (Q0091)
Screening Papanicolaou smear can be billed as a stand-alone visit if it is the only medical service provided on that day with a FQHC practitioner. If it is furnished on the same day as another medical visit, it is not a separately billable visit. The beneficiary coinsurance is waived.

Prostate Cancer Screening (G0102)
Prostate cancer screening can be billed as a stand-alone visit if it is the only medical service provided on that day with a FQHC practitioner. If it is furnished on the same day as another medical visit, it is not a separately billable visit. The beneficiary coinsurance applies.

Glaucoma Screening (G0117 and G0118)
Glaucoma screening for high risk patients can be billed as a stand-alone visit if it is the only medical service provided on that day with a FQHC practitioner. If it is furnished on the same day as another medical visit, it is not a separately billable visit. The beneficiary coinsurance applies.

Lung Cancer Screening Using Low Dose Computed Tomography (LDCT) (G0296)
LDCT can be billed as a stand-alone visit if it is the only medical service provided on that day with a FQHC practitioner. If it is furnished on the same day as another medical visit, it is not a separately billable visit. The beneficiary coinsurance is waived.

NOTE: Hepatitis C Screening (GO472) is a technical service only and therefore not paid as part of the FQHC visit.

100-02, 13, 230

Care Management Services

(Rev. 239, Issued: 01-09-18, Effective: 1-22-18, Implementation: 1-22-18)

Care management services are RHC and FQHC services. Except for TCM services, care management services are paid separately from the RHC AIR or FQHC PPS payment methodology.

100-02, 13, 230.1

Transitional Care Management Services

(Rev. 239, Issued: 01-09-18, Effective: 1-22-18, Implementation: 1-22-18)

Effective January 1, 2013, RHCs and FQHCs are paid for TCM services furnished by an RHC or FQHC practitioner when all TCM requirements are met. TCM services must be furnished within 30 days of the date of the patient's discharge from a hospital (including outpatient observation or partial hospitalization), SNF, or community mental health center.

Communication (direct contact, telephone, or electronic) with the patient or caregiver must commence within 2 business days of discharge, and a face-to-face visit must occur within 14 days of discharge for moderate complexity decision making (CPT code 99495), or within 7 days of discharge for high complexity decision making (CPT code 99496). The TCM visit is billed on the day that the TCM visit takes place, and only one TCM visit may be paid per beneficiary for services furnished during that 30 day post-discharge period. The TCM visit is subject to applicable copayments and deductibles.

TCM services can be billed as a stand-alone visit if it is the only medical service provided on that day with an RHC or FQHC practitioner and it meets the TCM billing requirements. If it is furnished on the same day as another visit, only one visit can be billed. Beginning on January 1, 2017, services furnished by auxiliary personnel incident to a TCM visit may be furnished under general supervision.

100-02, 13, 230.2

General Care Management Services – Chronic Care Management and General Behavioral Health Integration Services

(Rev. 239, Issued: 01-09-18, Effective: 1-22-18, Implementation: 1-22-18)

Chronic Care Management (CCM)

Effective January 1, 2016, RHCs and FQHCs are paid for CCM services when a minimum of 20 minutes of qualifying CCM services during a calendar month is furnished to patients with multiple chronic conditions that are expected to last at least 12 months or until the death of the patient, and that place the patient at significant risk of death, acute exacerbation/decompensation, or functional decline. For CCM services furnished between January 1, 2016, and December 31, 2017, payment is based on the PFS national average non-facility payment rate when CPT code 99490 is billed alone or with other payable services on an RHC or FQHC claim.

CCM Service Requirements

- Structured recording of patient health information using Certified EHR Technology including demographics, problems, medications, and medication allergies that inform the care plan, care coordination, and ongoing clinical care;
- 24/7 access to physicians or other qualified health care professionals or clinical staff including providing patients/caregivers with a means to make contact with health care professionals in the practice to address urgent needs regardless of the time of day or day of week, and continuity of care with a designated member of the care team with whom the patient is able to schedule successive routine appointments;
- Comprehensive care management including systematic assessment of the patient's medical, functional, and psychosocial needs; system-based approaches to ensure timely receipt of all recommended preventive care services; medication reconciliation with review of adherence and potential interactions; and oversight of patient self-management of medications;
- Comprehensive care plan including the creation, revision, and/or monitoring of an electronic care plan based on a physical, mental, cognitive, psychosocial, functional, and environmental (re)assessment and an inventory of resources and supports; a comprehensive care plan for all health issues with particular focus on the chronic conditions being managed;
- Care plan information made available electronically (including fax) in a timely manner within and outside the RHC or FQHC as appropriate and a copy of the plan of care given to the patient and/or caregiver;
- Management of care transitions between and among health care providers and settings, including referrals to other clinicians; follow-up after an emergency department visit; and follow-up after discharges from hospitals, skilled nursing facilities, or other health care facilities; timely creation and exchange/transmit continuity of care document(s) with other practitioners and providers;
- Coordination with home- and community-based clinical service providers, and documentation of communication to and from home- and community-based providers regarding the patient's psychosocial needs and functional deficits in the patient's medical record; and
- Enhanced opportunities for the patient and any caregiver to communicate with the practitioner regarding the patient's care through not only telephone access, but also through the use of secure messaging, Internet, or other asynchronous non-face-to-face consultation methods.

General Behavioral Health Integration (BHI)

General BHI is a team-based, collaborative approach to care that focuses on integrative treatment of patients with primary care and mental or behavioral health conditions. Patients are eligible to receive BHI services if they have one or more new or pre-existing behavioral health or psychiatric conditions being treated by the RHC or FQHC primary care practitioner, including substance use disorders, that, in the clinical judgment of the RHC or FQHC primary care practitioner, warrants BHI services.

General BHI Service Requirements

- An initial assessment and ongoing monitoring using validated clinical rating scales;
- Behavioral health care planning in relation to behavioral/psychiatric health problems, including revision for patients who are not progressing or whose status changes;
- Facilitating and coordinating treatment such as psychotherapy, pharmacotherapy, counseling and/or psychiatric consultation; and
- Continuity of care with a designated member of the care team.

Care Management Payment

Effective January 1, 2018, RHCs and FQHCs are paid for CCM or general BHI services when general care management G code, G0511, is on an RHC or FQHC claim, either alone or with other payable services, for CCM or BHI services furnished on or after January 1, 2018.

A separately billable initiating visit with an RHC or FQHC primary care practitioner (physician, NP, PA, or CNM) is required before care management services can be furnished. This visit can be an E/M, AWV, or IPPE visit, and must occur no more than one-year prior to commencing care management services.

Documentation that the beneficiary has consented to receive CCM or BHI services must be in the beneficiary's medical record before CCM or BHI services are furnished. This should include that the beneficiary has

- Given permission to consult with relevant specialists as needed;
- Been informed that there may be cost-sharing (e.g. deductible and coinsurance in RHCs, and coinsurance in FQHCs) for both in-person and non-face-to-face services that are provided
- Been informed that only one practitioner/facility can furnish and be paid for these services during a calendar month; and
- Been informed that they can stop care management services at any time, effective at the end of the calendar month.

Payment for G0511 is set at the average of the national non-facility PFS payment rate for CPT codes 99490 (30 minutes or more of CCM services), 99487 (60 minutes or more of complex CCM services), and 99484 (20 minutes or more of general behavioral health integration services). This rate is updated annually based on the PFS amounts.

RHCs and FQHCs can bill G0511 when the requirements for either CPT codes 99490, 99487, or 99484 are met. G0511 can be billed alone or in addition to other services furnished during an RHC or FQHC visit. Coinsurance and deductibles are applied as applicable to RHC claims, and coinsurance is applied as applicable to FQHC claims. General Care Management services furnished by auxiliary personnel may be provided under general supervision and the face-to-face requirements are waived.

RHCs and FQHCs may not bill for care management services for a patient if another practitioner or facility has already billed for care management services for the same beneficiary during the same time period. RHCs and FQHCs may not bill for care management and TCM services, or another program that provides additional payment for care management services (outside of the RHC AIR or FQHC PPS payment), for the same beneficiary during the same time period.

100-02, 13, 230.3

Psychiatric Collaborative Care Model (CoCM) Services

(Rev. 239, Issued: 01-09-18, Effective: 1-22-18, Implementation: 1-22-18)

Effective January 1, 2018, RHCs and FQHCs are paid for psychiatric CoCM services when psychiatric CoCM G code, G0512, is on an RHC or FQHC claim, either alone or with other payable services. At least 70 minutes in the first calendar month, and at least 60 minutes in subsequent calendar months, of psychiatric CoCM services must have been furnished in order to bill for this service.

Psychiatric CoCM is a specific model of care provided by a primary care team consisting of a primary care provider and a health care manager who work in collaboration with a psychiatric consultant to integrate primary health care services with care management support for patients receiving behavioral health treatment. It includes regular psychiatric inter-specialty consultation with the primary care team, particularly regarding patients whose conditions are not improving. Patients with mental health, behavioral health, or psychiatric conditions, including substance use disorders, who are being treated by an RHC or FQHC practitioner may be eligible for psychiatric CoCM services, as determined by the RHC or FQHC practitioner.

The psychiatric CoCM team must include the RHC or FQHC practitioner, a behavioral health care manager, and a psychiatric consultant. The primary care team regularly reviews the beneficiary's treatment plan and status with the psychiatric consultant and maintains or adjusts treatment, including referral to behavioral health specialty care, as needed.

RHC or FQHC Practitioner Requirements

The RHC or FQHC practitioner is a primary care physician, NP, PA, or CNM who:

- Directs the behavioral health care manager and any other clinical staff;
- Oversees the beneficiary's care, including prescribing medications, providing treatments for medical conditions, and making referrals to specialty care when needed; and
- Remains involved through ongoing oversight, management, collaboration and reassessment.

Behavioral Health Care Manager Requirements

The behavioral health care manager is a designated individual with formal education or specialized training in behavioral health, including social work, nursing, or psychology, and has a minimum of a bachelor's degree in a behavioral health field (such as in clinical social work or psychology), or is a clinician with behavioral health training, including RNs and LPNs. The behavioral health care manager furnishes both face-to-face and non-face-to-face services under the general supervision of the RHC or FQHC practitioner and may be employed by or working under contract to the RHC or FQHC. The behavioral health care manager:

- Provides assessment and care management services, including the administration of validated rating scales;

- Provides behavioral health care planning in relation to behavioral/psychiatric health problems, including revision for patients who are not progressing or whose status changes;
- Provides brief psychosocial interventions;
- Maintains ongoing collaboration with the RHC or FQHC practitioner;
- Maintains a registry that tracks patient follow-up and progress;
- Acts in consultation with the psychiatric consultant;
- Is available to provide services face-to-face with the beneficiary; and
- Has a continuous relationship with the patient and a collaborative, integrated relationship with the rest of the care team.

Psychiatric Consultant Requirements

The psychiatric consultant is a medical professional trained in psychiatry and qualified to prescribe the full range of medications. The psychiatric consultant is not required to be on site or to have direct contact with the patient and does not prescribe medications or furnish treatment to the beneficiary directly. The psychiatric consultant:

- Participates in regular reviews of the clinical status of patients receiving psychiatric CoCM services;
- Advises the RHC or FQHC practitioner regarding diagnosis and options for resolving issues with beneficiary adherence and tolerance of behavioral health treatment; making adjustments to behavioral health treatment for beneficiaries who are not progressing; managing any negative interactions between beneficiaries' behavioral health and medical treatments; and
- Facilitates referral for direct provision of psychiatric care when clinically indicated.

A separately billable initiating visit with an RHC or FQHC primary care practitioner (physician, NP, PA, or CNM) is required before psychiatric CoCM services can be furnished. This visit can be an E/M, AWV, or IPPE visit, and must occur no more than one-year prior to commencing psychiatric CoCM services.

Documentation that the beneficiary has consented to receive psychiatric CoCM services must be in the beneficiary's medical record before CCM or BHI services are furnished. This should include that the beneficiary has

- Given permission to consult with relevant specialists as needed;
- Been informed that there may be cost-sharing (e.g. deductible and coinsurance in RHCs, and coinsurance in FQHCs) for both in-person and non-face-to-face services that are provided;
- Been informed that only one practitioner/facility can furnish and be paid for these services during a calendar month; and
- Been informed that they can stop care management services at any time, effective at the end of the calendar month.

RHCs and FQHCs can bill G0512 when the requirements for either initial or subsequent psychiatric CoCM services are met. G0512 can be billed alone or in addition to other services furnished during an RHC or FQHC visit. To prevent duplication of payment, this code can only be billed once per month per beneficiary, and cannot be billed if other care management services are billed for the same time period.

Payment for G0512 is set at the average of the national non-facility PFS payment rate for CPT code 99492 (70 minutes or more of initial psychiatric CoCM services) and CPT code 99493 (60 minutes or more of subsequent psychiatric CoCM services). This rate is updated annually based on the PFS amounts. Coinsurance is applied as applicable to FQHC claims, and coinsurance and deductibles are applied as applicable to RHC claims. Psychiatric CoCM services furnished by auxiliary personnel may be provided under general supervision and the face-to-face requirements are waived.

100-02, 15, 20.1

Physician Expense for Surgery, Childbirth, and Treatment for Infertility

(Rev. 1, 10-01-03) B3-2005.l

A. Surgery and Childbirth

Skilled medical management is covered throughout the events of pregnancy, beginning with diagnosis, continuing through delivery and ending after the necessary postnatal care. Similarly, in the event of termination of pregnancy, regardless of whether terminated spontaneously or for therapeutic reasons (i.e., where the life of the mother would be endangered if the fetus were brought to term), the need for skilled medical management and/or medical services is equally important as in those cases carried to full term. After the infant is delivered and is a separate individual, items and services furnished to the infant are not covered on the basis of the mother's eligibility.

Most surgeons and obstetricians bill patients an all-inclusive package charge intended to cover all services associated with the surgical procedure or delivery of the child. All expenses for surgical and obstetrical care, including preoperative/prenatal examinations and tests and post-operative/postnatal services, are considered incurred on the date of surgery or delivery, as appropriate. This policy applies whether the physician bills on a package charge basis, or itemizes the bill separately for these items.

Occasionally, a physician's bill may include charges for additional services not directly related to the surgical procedure or the delivery. Such charges are considered incurred on the date the additional services are furnished.

The above policy applies only where the charges are imposed by one physician or by a clinic on behalf of a group of physicians. Where more than one physician imposes charges for surgical or obstetrical services, all preoperative/prenatal and post-operative/postnatal services performed by the physician who performed the surgery or delivery are considered incurred on the date of the surgery or delivery. Expenses for services rendered by other physicians are considered incurred on the date they were performed.

B. Treatment for Infertility

Reasonable and necessary services associated with treatment for infertility are covered under Medicare. Infertility is a condition sufficiently at variance with the usual state of health to make it appropriate for a person who normally is expected to be fertile to seek medical consultation and treatment.

100-02, 15, 30.4

Optometrist's Services

(Rev. 1, 10-01-03) B3-2020.25

Effective April 1, 1987, a doctor of optometry is considered a physician with respect to all services the optometrist is authorized to perform under State law or regulation. To be covered under Medicare, the services must be medically reasonable and necessary for the diagnosis or treatment of illness or injury, and must meet all applicable coverage requirements. See the Medicare Benefit Policy Manual, Chapter 16, "General Exclusions from Coverage," for exclusions from coverage that apply to vision care services, and the Medicare Claims Processing Manual, Chapter 12, "Physician/Practitioner Billing," for information dealing with payment for items and services furnished by optometrists.

A. FDA Monitored Studies of Intraocular Lenses

Special coverage rules apply to situations in which an ophthalmologist is involved in a Food and Drug Administration (FDA) monitored study of the safety and efficacy of an investigational Intraocular Lens (IOL). The investigation process for IOLs is unique in that there is a core period and an adjunct period. The core study is a traditional, well-controlled clinical investigation with full record keeping and reporting requirements. The adjunct study is essentially an extended distribution phase for lenses in which only limited safety data are compiled. Depending on the lens being evaluated, the adjunct study may be an extension of the core study or may be the only type of investigation to which the lens may be subject.

All eye care services related to the investigation of the IOL must be provided by the investigator (i.e., the implanting ophthalmologist) or another practitioner (including a doctor of optometry) who provides services at the direction or under the supervision of the investigator and who has an agreement with the investigator that information on the patient is given to the investigator so that he or she may report on the patient to the IOL manufacturer. Eye care services furnished by anyone other than the investigator (or a practitioner who assists the investigator, as described in the preceding paragraph) are not covered during the period the IOL is being investigated, unless the services are not related to the investigation.

B. Concurrent Care

Where more than one practitioner furnishes concurrent care, services furnished to a beneficiary by both an ophthalmologist and another physician (including an optometrist) may be recognized for payment if it is determined that each practitioner's services were reasonable and necessary. (See Sec.30.E.)

100-02, 15, 30.5

Chiropractor's Services

(Rev. 23, Issued: 10-08-04, Effective: 10-01-04, Implementation: 10-04-04) B3-2020.26

A chiropractor must be licensed or legally authorized to furnish chiropractic services by the State or jurisdiction in which the services are furnished. In addition, a licensed chiropractor must meet the following uniform minimum standards to be considered a physician for Medicare coverage. Coverage extends only to treatment by means of manual manipulation of the spine to correct a subluxation provided such treatment is legal in the State where performed. All other services furnished or ordered by chiropractors are not covered. If a chiropractor orders, takes, or interprets an x-ray or other diagnostic procedure to demonstrate a subluxation of the spine, the x-ray can be used for documentation. However, there is no coverage or payment for these services or for any other diagnostic or therapeutic service ordered or furnished by the chiropractor. For detailed information on using x-rays to determine subluxation, see Sec.240.1.2. In addition, in performing manual manipulation of the spine, some chiropractors use manual devices that are hand-held with the thrust of the force of the device being controlled manually. While such manual manipulation may be covered, there is no separate payment permitted for use of this device.

A. Uniform Minimum Standards

Prior to July 1, 1974

Chiropractors licensed or authorized to practice prior to July 1, 1974, and those individuals who commenced their studies in a chiropractic college before that date must meet all of the following three minimum standards to render payable services under the program:

- Preliminary education equal to the requirements for graduation from an accredited high school or other secondary school;

- Graduation from a college of chiropractic approved by the State's chiropractic examiners that included the completion of a course of study covering a period of not less than 3 school years of 6 months each year in actual continuous attendance covering adequate course of study in the subjects of anatomy, physiology, symptomatology and diagnosis, hygiene and sanitation, chemistry, histology, pathology, and principles and practice of chiropractic, including clinical instruction in vertebral palpation, nerve tracing, and adjusting; and
- Passage of an examination prescribed by the State's chiropractic examiners covering the subjects listed above.

After June 30, 1974

Individuals commencing their studies in a chiropractic college after June 30, 1974, must meet all of the above three standards and all of the following additional requirements:

- Satisfactory completion of 2 years of pre-chiropractic study at the college level;
- Satisfactory completion of a 4-year course of 8 months each year (instead of a 3-year course of 6 months each year) at a college or school of chiropractic that includes not less than 4,000 hours in the scientific and chiropractic courses specified in the second bullet under "Prior to July 1, 1974" above, plus courses in the use and effect of x-ray and chiropractic analysis; and
- The practitioner must be over 21 years of age.

B. Maintenance Therapy

Under the Medicare program, Chiropractic maintenance therapy is not considered to be medically reasonable or necessary, and is therefore not payable. Maintenance therapy is defined as a treatment plan that seeks to prevent disease, promote health, and prolong and enhance the quality of life; or therapy that is performed to maintain or prevent deterioration of a chronic condition. When further clinical improvement cannot reasonably be expected from continuous ongoing care, and the chiropractic treatment becomes supportive rather than corrective in nature, the treatment is then considered maintenance therapy. For information on how to indicate on a claim a treatment is or is not maintenance, see Sec.240.1.3.

100-02, 15, 50.4.4.2

Immunizations

(Rev. 202, Issued: 12-31-14, Effective: 09-19-14, Imp: 02-02-15)

Vaccinations or inoculations are excluded as immunizations unless they are directly related to the treatment of an injury or direct exposure to a disease or condition, such as anti-rabies treatment, tetanus antitoxin or booster vaccine, botulin antitoxin, antivenin sera, or immune globulin. In the absence of injury or direct exposure, preventive immunization (vaccination or inoculation) against such diseases as smallpox, polio, diphtheria, etc., is not covered. However, pneumococcal, hepatitis B, and influenza virus vaccines are exceptions to this rule. (See items A, B, and C below.) In cases where a vaccination or inoculation is excluded from coverage, related charges are also not covered.

A. Pneumococcal Pneumonia Vaccinations

1. Background and History of Coverage:

   Section 1861(s)(10)(A) of the Social Security Act and regulations at 42 CFR 410.57 authorize Medicare coverage under Part B for pneumococcal vaccine and its administration.

   For services furnished on or after May 1, 1981 through September 18, 2014, the Medicare Part B program covered pneumococcal pneumonia vaccine and its administration when furnished in compliance with any applicable State law by any provider of services or any entity or individual with a supplier number. Coverage included an initial vaccine administered only to persons at high risk of serious pneumococcal disease (including all people 65 and older; immunocompetent adults at increased risk of pneumococcal disease or its complications because of chronic illness; and individuals with compromised immune systems), with revaccination administered only to persons at highest risk of serious pneumococcal infection and those likely to have a rapid decline in pneumococcal antibody levels, provided that at least 5 years had passed since the previous dose of pneumococcal vaccine.

   Those administering the vaccine did not require the patient to present an immunization record prior to administering the pneumococcal vaccine, nor were they compelled to review the patient's complete medical record if it was not available, relying on the patient's verbal history to determine prior vaccination status.

   Effective July 1, 2000, Medicare no longer required for coverage purposes that a doctor of medicine or osteopathy order the vaccine. Therefore, a beneficiary could receive the vaccine upon request without a physician's order and without physician supervision.

2. Coverage Requirements:

   Effective for claims with dates of service on and after September 19, 2014, an initial pneumococcal vaccine may be administered to all Medicare beneficiaries who have never received a pneumococcal vaccination under Medicare Part B. A different, second pneumococcal vaccine may be administered 1 year after the first vaccine was administered (i.e., 11 full months have passed following the month in which the last pneumococcal vaccine was administered).

   Those administering the vaccine should not require the patient to present an immunization record prior to administering the pneumococcal vaccine, nor should they feel compelled to review the patient's complete medical record if it is not available. Instead, provided that the patient is competent, it is acceptable to rely on the patient's verbal history to determine prior vaccination status.

   Medicare does not require for coverage purposes that a doctor of medicine or osteopathy order the vaccine. Therefore, the beneficiary may receive the vaccine upon request without a physician's order and without physician supervision.

B. Hepatitis B Vaccine

Effective for services furnished on or after September 1, 1984, P.L. 98-369 provides coverage under Part B for hepatitis B vaccine and its administration, furnished to a Medicare beneficiary who is at high or intermediate risk of contracting hepatitis B. High-risk groups currently identified include (see exception below):

- ESRD patients;
- Hemophiliacs who receive Factor VIII or IX concentrates;
- Clients of institutions for the mentally retarded;
- Persons who live in the same household as a Hepatitis B Virus (HBV) carrier;
- Homosexual men;
- Illicit injectable drug abusers; and
- Persons diagnosed with diabetes mellitus.

Intermediate risk groups currently identified include:

- Staff in institutions for the mentally retarded; and
- Workers in health care professions who have frequent contact with blood or blood-derived body fluids during routine work.

EXCEPTION: Persons in both of the above-listed groups in paragraph B, would not be considered at high or intermediate risk of contracting hepatitis B, however, if there were laboratory evidence positive for antibodies to hepatitis B. (ESRD patients are routinely tested for hepatitis B antibodies as part of their continuing monitoring and therapy.)

For Medicare program purposes, the vaccine may be administered upon the order of a doctor of medicine or osteopathy, by a doctor of medicine or osteopathy, or by home health agencies, skilled nursing facilities, ESRD facilities, hospital outpatient departments, and persons recognized under the incident to physicians' services provision of law.

A charge separate from the ESRD composite rate will be recognized and paid for administration of the vaccine to ESRD patients.

C. Influenza Virus Vaccine

Effective for services furnished on or after May 1, 1993, the Medicare Part B program covers influenza virus vaccine and its administration when furnished in compliance with any applicable State law by any provider of services or any entity or individual with a supplier number. Typically, these vaccines are administered once a flu season. Medicare does not require, for coverage purposes, that a doctor of medicine or osteopathy order the vaccine. Therefore, the beneficiary may receive the vaccine upon request without a physician's order and without physician supervision.

100-02, 15, 80.1

Clinical Laboratory Services

(Rev. 80; Issued: 11-11-08; Effective: 01-01-03; Implementation: 11-19-07)

Section 1833 and 1861 of the Act provides for payment of clinical laboratory services under Medicare Part B. Clinical laboratory services involve the biological, microbiological, serological, chemical, immunohematological, hematological, biophysical, cytological, pathological, or other examination of materials derived from the human body for the diagnosis, prevention, or treatment of a disease or assessment of a medical condition. Laboratory services must meet all applicable requirements of the Clinical Laboratory Improvement Amendments of 1988 (CLIA), as set forth at 42 CFR part 493. Section 1862(a)(1)(A) of the Act provides that Medicare payment may not be made for services that are not reasonable and necessary. Clinical laboratory services must be ordered and used promptly by the physician who is treating the beneficiary as described in 42 CFR 410.32(a), or by a qualified nonphysician practitioner, as described in 42 CFR 410.32(a)(3).

See section 80.6 of this manual for related physician ordering instructions.

See the Medicare Claims Processing Manual Chapter 16 for related claims processing instructions.

100-02, 15, 80.2

Psychological Tests and Neuropsychological Tests

(Rev. 85, Issued: 02-29-08, Effective: 01-01-06, Implementation: 12-28-06)

Medicare Part B coverage of psychological tests and neuropsychological tests is authorized under section 1861(s)(3) of the Social Security Act. Payment for psychological and neuropsychological tests is authorized under section 1842(b)(2)(A) of the Social Security Act. The payment amounts for the new psychological and neuropsychological tests (CPT codes 96102, 96103, 96119 and 96120) that are effective January 1, 2006, and are billed for tests administered by a technician or a computer reflect a site of service payment differential for the facility and non-facility settings.

Additionally, there is no authorization for payment for diagnostic tests when performed on an "incident to" basis.

Under the diagnostic tests provision, all diagnostic tests are assigned a certain level of supervision. Generally, regulations governing the diagnostic tests provision require that only physicians can provide the assigned level of supervision for diagnostic tests.

However, there is a regulatory exception to the supervision requirement for diagnostic psychological and neuropsychological tests in terms of who can provide the supervision.

That is, regulations allow a clinical psychologist (CP) or a physician to perform the general supervision assigned to diagnostic psychological and neuropsychological tests.

In addition, nonphysician practitioners such as nurse practitioners (NPs), clinical nurse specialists (CNSs) and physician assistants (PAs) who personally perform diagnostic psychological and neuropsychological tests are excluded from having to perform these tests under the general supervision of a physician or a CP. Rather, NPs and CNSs must perform such tests under the requirements of their respective benefit instead of the requirements for diagnostic psychological and neuropsychological tests. Accordingly, NPs and CNSs must perform tests in collaboration (as defined under Medicare law at section 1861(aa)(6) of the Act) with a physician. PAs perform tests under the general supervision of a physician as required for services furnished under the PA benefit.

Furthermore, physical therapists (PTs), occupational therapists (OTs) and speech language pathologists (SLPs) are authorized to bill three test codes as "sometimes therapy" codes. Specifically, CPT codes 96105, 96110 and 96111 may be performed by these therapists. However, when PTs, OTs and SLPs perform these three tests, they must be performed under the general supervision of a physician or a CP.

Who May Bill for Diagnostic Psychological and Neuropsychological Tests CPs - see qualifications under chapter 15, section 160 of the Benefits Policy Manual, Pub. 100-2.

- NPs -to the extent authorized under State scope of practice. See qualifications under chapter 15, section 200 of the Benefits Policy Manual, Pub. 100-2.
- CNSs -to the extent authorized under State scope of practice. See qualifications under chapter 15, section 210 of the Benefits Policy Manual, Pub. 100-2.
- PAs - to the extent authorized under State scope of practice. See qualifications under chapter 15, section 190 of the Benefits Policy Manual, Pub. 100-2.
- Independently Practicing Psychologists (IPPs) PTs, OTs and SLPs - see qualifications under chapter 15, sections 220-230.6 of the Benefits Policy Manual, Pub. 100-2.

Psychological and neuropsychological tests performed by a psychologist (who is not a CP) practicing independently of an institution, agency, or physician's office are covered when a physician orders such tests. An IPP is any psychologist who is licensed or certified to practice psychology in the State or jurisdiction where furnishing services or, if the jurisdiction does not issue licenses, if provided by any practicing psychologist. (It is CMS' understanding that all States, the District of Columbia, and Puerto Rico license psychologists, but that some trust territories do not. Examples of psychologists, other than CPs, whose psychological and neuropsychological tests are covered under the diagnostic tests provision include, but are not limited to, educational psychologists and counseling psychologists.)

The carrier must secure from the appropriate State agency a current listing of psychologists holding the required credentials to determine whether the tests of a particular IPP are covered under Part B in States that have statutory licensure or certification. In States or territories that lack statutory licensing or certification, the carrier checks individual qualifications before provider numbers are issued. Possible reference sources are the national directory of membership of the American Psychological Association, which provides data about the educational background of individuals and indicates which members are board-certified, the records and directories of the State or territorial psychological association, and the National Register of Health Service Providers. If qualification is dependent on a doctoral degree from a currently accredited program, the carrier verifies the date of accreditation of the school involved, since such accreditation is not retroactive. If the listed reference sources do not provide enough information (e.g., the psychologist is not a member of one of these sources), the carrier contacts the psychologist personally for the required information. Generally, carriers maintain a continuing list of psychologists whose qualifications have been verified.

NOTE: When diagnostic psychological tests are performed by a psychologist who is not practicing independently, but is on the staff of an institution, agency, or clinic, that entity bills for the psychological tests.

The carrier considers psychologists as practicing independently when:

- They render services on their own responsibility, free of the administrative and professional control of an employer such as a physician, institution or agency;
- The persons they treat are their own patients; and
- They have the right to bill directly, collect and retain the fee for their services.

A psychologist practicing in an office located in an institution may be considered an independently practicing psychologist when both of the following conditions exist:

- The office is confined to a separately-identified part of the facility which is used solely as the psychologist's office and cannot be construed as extending throughout the entire institution; and
- The psychologist conducts a private practice, i.e., services are rendered to patients from outside the institution as well as to institutional patients.

Payment for Diagnostic Psychological and Neuropsychological Tests

Expenses for diagnostic psychological and neuropsychological tests are not subject to the outpatient mental health treatment limitation, that is, the payment limitation on treatment services for mental, psychoneurotic and personality disorders as authorized under Section 1833(c) of the Act. The payment amount for the new psychological and neuropsychological tests (CPT codes 96102, 96103, 96119 and 96120) that are billed for tests performed by a technician or a computer reflect a site of service payment differential for the facility and non-facility settings. CPs, NPs, CNSs and PAs are required by law to accept assigned payment for psychological and neuropsychological tests. However, while IPPs are not required by law to accept assigned payment for these tests, they must report the name and address of the physician who ordered the test on the claim form when billing for tests.

CPT Codes for Diagnostic Psychological and Neuropsychological Tests

The range of CPT codes used to report psychological and neuropsychological tests is 96101-96120. CPT codes 96101, 96102, 96103, 96105, 96110, and 96111 are appropriate for use when billing for psychological tests. CPT codes 96116, 96118, 96119 and 96120 are appropriate for use when billing for neuropsychological tests.

All of the tests under this CPT code range 96101-96120 are indicated as active codes under the physician fee schedule database and are covered if medically necessary.

Payment and Billing Guidelines for Psychological and Neuropsychological Tests

The technician and computer CPT codes for psychological and neuropsychological tests include practice expense, malpractice expense and professional work relative value units.

Accordingly, CPT psychological test code 96101 should not be paid when billed for the same tests or services performed under psychological test codes 96102 or 96103. CPT neuropsychological test code 96118 should not be paid when billed for the same tests or services performed under neuropsychological test codes 96119 or 96120. However, CPT codes 96101 and 96118 can be paid separately on the rare occasion when billed on the same date of service for different and separate tests from 96102, 96103, 96119 and 96120.

Under the physician fee schedule, there is no payment for services performed by students or trainees. Accordingly, Medicare does not pay for services represented by CPT codes 96102 and 96119 when performed by a student or a trainee. However, the presence of a student or a trainee while the test is being administered does not prevent a physician, CP, IPP, NP, CNS or PA from performing and being paid for the psychological test under 96102 or the neuropsychological test under 96119.

100-02, 15, 80.5.5

Frequency Standards

(Rev.70, Issued: 05-11-07, Effective: 01-01-07, Implementation: 07-02-07)

Medicare pays for a screening BMM once every 2 years (at least 23 months have passed since the month the last covered BMM was performed).

When medically necessary, Medicare may pay for more frequent BMMs. Examples include, but are not limited to, the following medical circumstances:

- Monitoring beneficiaries on long-term glucocorticoid (steroid) therapy of more than 3 months.
- Confirming baseline BMMs to permit monitoring of beneficiaries in the future.

100-02, 15, 150.1

Treatment of Temporomandibular Joint (TMJ) Syndrome

(Rev. 1, 10-01-03)

There are a wide variety of conditions that can be characterized as TMJ, and an equally wide variety of methods for treating these conditions. Many of the procedures fall within the Medicare program's statutory exclusion that prohibits payment for items and services that have not been demonstrated to be reasonable and necessary for the diagnosis and treatment of illness or injury (§1862(a)(1) of the Act). Other services and appliances used to treat TMJ fall within the Medicare program's statutory exclusion at 1862(a)(12), which prohibits payment "for services in connection with the care, treatment, filling, removal, or replacement of teeth or structures directly supporting teeth...." For these reasons, a diagnosis of TMJ on a claim is insufficient. The actual condition or symptom must be determined.

100-02, 15, 160

Clinical Psychologist Services

(Rev. 51, Issued: 06-23-06, Effective: 01-01-05, Implementation: 09-21-06)

A. Clinical Psychologist (CP) Defined

To qualify as a clinical psychologist (CP), a practitioner must meet the following requirements: Hold a doctoral degree in psychology; Be licensed or certified, on the basis of the doctoral degree in psychology, by the State in which he or she practices, at the independent practice level of psychology to furnish diagnostic, assessment, preventive, and therapeutic services directly to individuals.

B. Qualified Clinical Psychologist Services Defined

Effective July 1, 1990, the diagnostic and therapeutic services of CPs and services and supplies furnished incident to such services are covered as the services furnished by a physician or as incident to physician's services are covered. However, the CP must be legally authorized to perform the services under applicable licensure laws of the State in which they are furnished.

C. Types of Clinical Psychologist Services

That May Be Covered Diagnostic and therapeutic services that the CP is legally authorized to perform in accordance with State law and/or regulation. Carriers pay all qualified CPs based on the physician fee schedule for the diagnostic and therapeutic services. (Psychological tests by practitioners who do not meet the requirements for a CP may be covered under the provisions for diagnostic tests as described in Sec. 80.2.

Services and supplies furnished incident to a CP's services are covered if the requirements that apply to services incident to a physician's services, as described in Sec.60 are met. These services must be:

- Mental health services that are commonly furnished in CPs' offices;
- An integral, although incidental, part of professional services performed by the CP;
- Performed under the direct personal supervision of the CP; i.e., the CP must be physically present and immediately available;
- Furnished without charge or included in the CP's bill; and
- Performed by an employee of the CP (or an employee of the legal entity that employs the supervising CP) under the common law control test of the Act, as set forth in 20 CFR 404.1007 and Sec.RS 2101.020 of the Retirement and Survivors Insurance part of the Social Security Program Operations Manual System.
- Diagnostic psychological testing services when furnished under the general supervision of a CP.

Carriers are required to familiarize themselves with appropriate State laws and/or regulations governing a CP's scope of practice.

D. Noncovered Services

The services of CPs are not covered if the service is otherwise excluded from Medicare coverage even though a clinical psychologist is authorized by State law to perform them.

For example, Sec.1862(a)(1)(A) of the Act excludes from coverage services that are not "reasonable and necessary for the diagnosis or treatment of an illness or injury or to improve the functioning of a malformed body member." Therefore, even though the services are authorized by State law, the services of a CP that are determined to be not reasonable and necessary are not covered. Additionally, any therapeutic services that are billed by CPs under CPT psychotherapy codes that include medical evaluation and management services are not covered.

E. Requirement for Consultation

When applying for a Medicare provider number, a CP must submit to the carrier a signed Medicare provider/supplier enrollment form that indicates an agreement to the effect that, contingent upon the patient's consent, the CP will attempt to consult with the patient's attending or primary care physician in accordance with accepted professional ethical norms, taking into consideration patient confidentiality.

If the patient assents to the consultation, the CP must attempt to consult with the patient's physician within a reasonable time after receiving the consent. If the CP's attempts to consult directly with the physician are not successful, the CP must notify the physician within a reasonable time that he or she is furnishing services to the patient. Additionally, the CP must document, in the patient's medical record, the date the patient consented or declined consent to consultations, the date of consultation, or, if attempts to consult did not succeed, that date and manner of notification to the physician.

The only exception to the consultation requirement for CPs is in cases where the patient's primary care or attending physician refers the patient to the CP. Also, neither a CP nor a primary care nor attending physician may bill Medicare or the patient for this required consultation.

F. Outpatient Mental Health Services Limitation

All covered therapeutic services furnished by qualified CPs are subject to the outpatient mental health services limitation in Pub 100-1, Medicare General Information, Eligibility, and Entitlement Manual, Chapter 3, "Deductibles, Coinsurance Amounts, and Payment Limitations," Sec.30, (i.e., only 62 1/2 percent of expenses for these services are considered incurred expenses for Medicare purposes). The limitation does not apply to diagnostic services.

G. Assignment Requirement Assignment iSec. required.

100-02, 15, 170

Clinical Social Worker (CSW) Services

(Rev. 1, 10-01-03) B3-2152

See the Medicare Claims Processing Manual Chapter 12, Physician/Nonphysician Practitioners, §150, "Clinical Social Worker Services," for payment requirements.

A. Clinical Social Worker Defined

Section 1861(hh) of the Act defines a "clinical social worker" as an individual who:

- Possesses a master's or doctor's degree in social work;
- Has performed at least two years of supervised clinical social work; and
- Is licensed or certified as a clinical social worker by the State in which the services are performed; or
- In the case of an individual in a State that does not provide for licensure or certification, has completed at least 2 years or 3,000 hours of post master's degree supervised clinical social work practice under the supervision of a master's level social worker in an appropriate setting such as a hospital, SNF, or clinic.

B. Clinical Social Worker Services Defined

Section 1861(hh)(2) of the Act defines "clinical social worker services" as those services that the CSW is legally authorized to perform under State law (or the State regulatory mechanism provided by State law) of the State in which such services are performed for the diagnosis and treatment of mental illnesses. Services furnished to an inpatient of a hospital or an inpatient of a SNF that the SNF is required to provide as a requirement for participation are not included. The services that are covered are those that are otherwise covered if furnished by a physician or as incident to a physician's professional service.

C. Covered Services

Coverage is limited to the services a CSW is legally authorized to perform in accordance with State law (or State regulatory mechanism established by State law). The services of a CSW may be covered under Part B if they are:

- The type of services that are otherwise covered if furnished by a physician, or as incident to a physician's service. (See §30 for a description of physicians' services and §70 of Pub 100-1, the Medicare General Information, Eligibility, and Entitlement Manual, Chapter 5, for the definition of a physician.);
- Performed by a person who meets the definition of a CSW (See subsection A.); and
- Not otherwise excluded from coverage. Carriers should become familiar with the State law or regulatory mechanism governing a CSW's scope of practice in their service area.

D. Noncovered Services

Services of a CSW are not covered when furnished to inpatients of a hospital or to inpatients of a SNF if the services furnished in the SNF are those that the SNF is required to furnish as a condition of participation in Medicare. In addition, CSW services are not covered if they are otherwise excluded from Medicare coverage even though a CSW is authorized by State law to perform them. For example, the Medicare law excludes from coverage services that are not "reasonable and necessary for the diagnosis or treatment of an illness or injury or to improve the functioning of a malformed body member."

E. Outpatient Mental Health Services Limitation

All covered therapeutic services furnished by qualified CSWs are subject to the outpatient psychiatric services limitation in Pub 100-1, Medicare General Information, Eligibility, and Entitlement Manual, Chapter 3, "Deductibles, Coinsurance Amounts, and Payment Limitations," §30, (i.e., only 62 1/2 percent of expenses for these services are considered incurred expenses for Medicare purposes). The limitation does not apply to diagnostic services.

F. Assignment Requirement

Assignment is required.

100-02, 15, 180

Nurse-Midwife (CNM) Services

(Rev. 1, 10-01-03) B3-2154

A. General

Effective on or after July 1, 1988, the services provided by a certified nurse-midwife or incident to the certified nurse-midwife's services are covered. Payment is made under assignment only. See the Medicare Claims Processing Manual, Chapter 12, "Physician and Nonphysician Practitioners," §130, for payment methodology for nurse midwife services.

B. Certified Nurse-Midwife Defined

A certified nurse-midwife is a registered nurse who has successfully completed a program of study and clinical experience in nurse-midwifery, meeting guidelines prescribed by the Secretary, or who has been certified by an organization recognized by the Secretary. The Secretary has recognized certification by the American College of Nurse-Midwives and State qualifying requirements in those States that specify a program of education and clinical experience for nurse-midwives for these purposes. A nurse-midwife must:

- Be currently licensed to practice in the State as a registered professional nurse; and
- Meet one of the following requirements:
  1. Be legally authorized under State law or regulations to practice as a nurse-midwife and have completed a program of study and clinical experience for nurse-midwives, as specified by the State; or
  2. If the State does not specify a program of study and clinical experience that nurse-midwives must complete to practice in that State, the nurse-midwife must:
     a. Be currently certified as a nurse-midwife by the American College of Nurse-Midwives;
     b. Have satisfactorily completed a formal education program (of at least one academic year) that, upon completion, qualifies the nurse to take the certification examination offered by the American College of Nurse-Midwives; or

c. Have successfully completed a formal education program for preparing registered nurses to furnish gynecological and obstetrical care to women during pregnancy, delivery, and the postpartum period, and care to normal newborns, and have practiced as a nurse-midwife for a total of 12 months during any 18-month period from August 8, 1976, to July 16, 1982.

C. Covered Services

1. General - Effective January 1, 1988, through December 31, 1993, the coverage of nurse-midwife services was restricted to the maternity cycle. The maternity cycle is a period that includes pregnancy, labor, and the immediate postpartum period.

   Beginning with services furnished on or after January 1, 1994, coverage is no longer limited to the maternity cycle. Coverage is available for services furnished by a nurse-midwife that he or she is legally authorized to perform in the State in which the services are furnished and that would otherwise be covered if furnished by a physician, including obstetrical and gynecological services.

2. Incident To- Services and supplies furnished incident to a nurse midwife's service are covered if they would have been covered when furnished incident to the services of a doctor of medicine or osteopathy, as described in §60.

D. Noncovered Services

The services of nurse-midwives are not covered if they are otherwise excluded from Medicare coverage even though a nurse-midwife is authorized by State law to perform them. For example, the Medicare program excludes from coverage routine physical checkups and services that are not reasonable and necessary for the diagnosis or treatment of an illness or injury or to improve the functioning of a malformed body member. Coverage of service to the newborn continues only to the point that the newborn is or would normally be treated medically as a separate individual. Items and services furnished the newborn from that point are not covered on the basis of the mother's eligibility.

E. Relationship With Physician

Most States have licensure and other requirements applicable to nurse-midwives. For example, some require that the nurse-midwife have an arrangement with a physician for the referral of the patient in the event a problem develops that requires medical attention. Others may require that the nurse-midwife function under the general supervision of a physician. Although these and similar State requirements must be met in order for the nurse-midwife to provide Medicare covered care, they have no effect on the nurse-midwife's right to personally bill for and receive direct Medicare payment. That is, billing does not have to flow through a physician or facility. See §60.2 for coverage of services performed by nurse-midwives incident to the service of physicians.

F. Place of Service

There is no restriction on place of service. Therefore, nurse-midwife services are covered if provided in the nurse-midwife's office, in the patient's home, or in a hospital or other facility, such as a clinic or birthing center owned or operated by a nurse-midwife.

G. Assignment Requirement

Assignment is required.

100-02, 15, 220

Coverage of Outpatient Rehabilitation Therapy Services (Physical Therapy, Occupational Therapy, and Speech-Language Pathology Services) Under Medical Insurance

(Rev. 194, Issued: 09-03-14, Effective: Upon Implementation of ICD-10)

A comprehensive knowledge of the policies that apply to therapy services cannot be obtained through manuals alone. The most definitive policies are Local Coverage Determinations found at the Medicare Coverage Database www.cms.hhs.gov/mcd. A list of Medicare contractors is found at the CMS Web site. Specific questions about all Medicare policies should be addressed to the contractors through the contact information supplied on their Web sites. General Medicare questions may be addressed to the Medicare regional officeshttp://www.cms.hhs.gov/RegionalOffices/.

A. Definitions

The following defines terms used in this section and §230:

ACTIVE PARTICIPATION of the clinician in treatment means that the clinician personally furnishes in its entirety at least 1 billable service on at least 1 day of treatment.

ASSESSMENT is separate from evaluation, and is included in services or procedures, (it is not separately payable). The term assessment as used in Medicare manuals related to therapy services is distinguished from language in Current Procedural Terminology (CPT) codes that specify assessment, e.g., 97755, Assistive Technology Assessment, which may be payable). Assessments shall be provided only by clinicians, because assessment requires professional skill to gather data by observation and patient inquiry and may include limited objective testing and measurement to make clinical judgments regarding the patient's condition(s). Assessment determines, e.g., changes in the patient's status since the last visit/treatment day and whether the planned procedure or service should be modified. Based on these assessment data, the professional may make judgments about progress toward goals and/or determine that a more complete evaluation or re-evaluation (see definitions below) is indicated. Routine weekly assessments of expected progression in accordance with the plan are not payable as re-evaluations.

CERTIFICATION is the physician's/nonphysician practitioner's (NPP) approval of the plan of care. Certification requires a dated signature on the plan of care or some other document that indicates approval of the plan of care.

The CLINICIAN is a term used in this manual and in Pub 100-4, chapter 5, section 10 or section 20, to refer to only a physician, nonphysician practitioner or a therapist (but not to an assistant, aide or any other personnel) providing a service within their scope of practice and consistent with state and local law. Clinicians make clinical judgments and are responsible for all services they are permitted to supervise. Services that require the skills of a therapist, may be appropriately furnished by clinicians, that is, by or under the supervision of qualified physicians/NPPs when their scope of practice, state and local laws allow it and their personal professional training is judged by Medicare contractors as sufficient to provide to the beneficiary skills equivalent to a therapist for that service.

COMPLEXITIES are complicating factors that may influence treatment, e.g., they may influence the type, frequency, intensity and/or duration of treatment. Complexities may be represented by diagnoses (ICD codes), by patient factors such as age, severity, acuity, multiple conditions, and motivation, or by the patient's social circumstances such as the support of a significant other or the availability of transportation to therapy.

A DATE may be in any form (written, stamped or electronic). The date may be added to the record in any manner and at any time, as long as the dates are accurate. If they are different, refer to both the date a service was performed and the date the entry to the record was made. For example, if a physician certifies a plan and fails to date it, staff may add "Received Date" in writing or with a stamp. The received date is valid for certification/re-certification purposes. Also, if the physician faxes the referral, certification, or re-certification and forgets to date it, the date that prints out on the fax is valid. If services provided on one date are documented on another date, both dates should be documented.

The EPISODE of Outpatient Therapy – For the purposes of therapy policy, an outpatient therapy episode is defined as the period of time, in calendar days, from the first day the patient is under the care of the clinician (e.g., for evaluation or treatment) for the current condition(s) being treated by one therapy discipline (PT, or OT, or SLP) until the last date of service for that discipline in that setting.

During the episode, the beneficiary may be treated for more than one condition; including conditions with an onset after the episode has begun. For example, a beneficiary receiving PT for a hip fracture who, after the initial treatment session, develops low back pain would also be treated under a PT plan of care for rehabilitation of low back pain. That plan may be modified from the initial plan, or it may be a separate plan specific to the low back pain, but treatment for both conditions concurrently would be considered the same episode of PT treatment. If that same patient developed a swallowing problem during intubation for the hip surgery, the first day of treatment by the SLP would be a new episode of SLP care.

EVALUATION is a separately payable comprehensive service provided by a clinician, as defined above, that requires professional skills to make clinical judgments about conditions for which services are indicated based on objective measurements and subjective evaluations of patient performance and functional abilities. Evaluation is warranted e.g., for a new diagnosis or when a condition is treated in a new setting. These evaluative judgments are essential to development of the plan of care, including goals and the selection of interventions.

FUNCTIONAL REPORTING, which is required on claims for all outpatient therapy services pursuant to 42CFR410.59, 410.60, and 410.62, uses nonpayable G-codes and related modifiers to convey information about the patient's functional status at specified points during therapy. (See Pub 100-4, chapter 5, section 10.6)

RE-EVALUATION provides additional objective information not included in other documentation. Re-evaluation is separately payable and is periodically indicated during an episode of care when the professional assessment of a clinician indicates a significant improvement, or decline, or change in the patient's condition or functional status that was not anticipated in the plan of care. Although some state regulations and state practice acts require re-evaluation at specific times, for Medicare payment, reevaluations must also meet Medicare coverage guidelines. The decision to provide a reevaluation shall be made by a clinician.

INTERVAL of certified treatment (certification interval) consists of 90 calendar days or less, based on an individual's needs. A physician/NPP may certify a plan of care for an interval length that is less than 90 days. There may be more than one certification interval in an episode of care. The certification interval is not the same as a Progress Report period.

MAINTENANCE PROGRAM (MP) means a program established by a therapist that consists of activities and/or mechanisms that will assist a beneficiary in maximizing or maintaining the progress he or she has made during therapy or to prevent or slow further deterioration due to a disease or illness.

NONPHYSICIAN PRACTITIONERS (NPP) means physician assistants, clinical nurse specialists, and nurse practitioners, who may, if state and local laws permit it, and when appropriate rules are followed, provide, certify or supervise therapy services.

PHYSICIAN with respect to outpatient rehabilitation therapy services means a doctor of medicine, osteopathy (including an osteopathic practitioner), podiatric medicine, or optometry (for low vision rehabilitation only). Chiropractors and doctors of dental surgery or dental medicine are not considered physicians for therapy services and may neither refer patients for rehabilitation therapy services nor establish therapy plans of care.

PATIENT, client, resident, and beneficiary are terms used interchangeably to indicate enrolled recipients of Medicare covered services.

PROVIDERS of services are defined in §1861(u) of the Act, 42CFR400.202 and 42CFR485 Subpart H as participating hospitals, critical access hospitals (CAH), skilled nursing facilities (SNF), comprehensive outpatient rehabilitation facilities (CORF), home health agencies (HHA), hospices, participating clinics, rehabilitation agencies or outpatient rehabilitation facilities (ORF). Providers are also defined as public health agencies with agreements only to furnish outpatient therapy services, or community mental health centers with agreements only to furnish partial hospitalization services. To qualify as providers of services, these providers must meet certain conditions enumerated in the law and enter into an agreement with the Secretary in which they agree not to charge any beneficiary for covered services for which the program will pay and to refund any erroneous collections made. Note that the word PROVIDER in sections 220 and 230 is not used to mean a person who provides a service, but is used as in the statute to mean a facility or agency such as rehabilitation agency or home health agency.

QUALIFIED PROFESSIONAL means a physical therapist, occupational therapist, speech-language pathologist, physician, nurse practitioner, clinical nurse specialist, or physician's assistant, who is licensed or certified by the state to furnish therapy services, and who also may appropriately furnish therapy services under Medicare policies. Qualified professional may also include a physical therapist assistant (PTA) or an occupational therapy assistant (OTA) when furnishing services under the supervision of a qualified therapist, who is working within the state scope of practice in the state in which the services are furnished. Assistants are limited in the services they may furnish (see section 230.1 and 230.2) and may not supervise other therapy caregivers.

QUALIFIED PERSONNEL means staff (auxiliary personnel) who have been educated and trained as therapists and qualify to furnish therapy services only under direct supervision incident to a physician or NPP. See §230.5 of this chapter. Qualified personnel may or may not be licensed as therapists but meet all of the requirements for therapists with the exception of licensure.

SIGNATURE means a legible identifier of any type acceptable according to policies in Pub. 100-08, Medicare Program Integrity Manual, chapter 3, §3.3.2.4 concerning signatures.

SUPERVISION LEVELS for outpatient rehabilitation therapy services are the same as those for diagnostic tests defined in 42CFR410.32. Depending on the setting, the levels include personal supervision (in the room), direct supervision (in the office suite), and general supervision (physician/NPP is available but not necessarily on the premises).

SUPPLIERS of therapy services include individual practitioners such as physicians, NPPs, physical therapists and occupational therapists who have Medicare provider numbers. Regulatory references on physical therapists in private practice (PTPPs) and occupational therapists in private practice (OTPPs) are at 42CFR410.60 (C)(1), 485.701-729, and 486.150-163.

THERAPIST refers only to qualified physical therapists, occupational therapists and speech-language pathologists, as defined in §230. Qualifications that define therapists are in §§230.1, 230.2, and 230.3. Skills of a therapist are defined by the scope of practice for therapists in the state).

THERAPY (or outpatient rehabilitation services) includes only outpatient physical therapy (PT), occupational therapy (OT) and speech-language pathology (SLP) services paid using the Medicare Physician Fee Schedule or the same services when provided in hospitals that are exempt from the hospital Outpatient Prospective Payment System and paid on a reasonable cost basis, including critical access hospitals.

Therapy services referred to in this chapter are those skilled services furnished according to the standards and conditions in CMS manuals, (e.g., in this chapter and in Pub. 100-4, Medicare Claims Processing Manual, chapter 5), within their scope of practice by qualified professionals or qualified personnel, as defined in this section, represented by procedures found in the American Medical Association's "Current Procedural Terminology (CPT)." A list of CPT (HCPCS) codes is provided in Pub. 100-4, chapter 5, §20, and in Local Coverage Determinations developed by contractors.

TREATMENT DAY means a single calendar day on which treatment, evaluation and/or reevaluation is provided. There could be multiple visits, treatment sessions/encounters on a treatment day.

VISITS OR TREATMENT SESSIONS begin at the time the patient enters the treatment area (of a building, office, or clinic) and continue until all services (e.g., activities, procedures, services) have been completed for that session and the patient leaves that area to participate in a non-therapy activity. It is likely that not all minutes in the visits/treatment sessions are billable (e.g., rest periods). There may be two treatment sessions in a day, for example, in the morning and afternoon. When there are two visits/ treatment sessions in a day, plans of care indicate treatment amount of twice a day.

B. References

Paper Manuals. The following manuals, now outdated, were resources for the Internet Only Manuals:

- Part A Medicare Intermediary Manual, (Pub. 13)
- Part B Medicare Carrier Manual, (Pub. 14)
- Hospital Manual, (Pub. 10)
- Outpatient Physical Therapy/CORF Manual, (Pub. 9)

Regulation and Statute. The information in this section is based in part on the following current references:

- 42CFR refers to Title 42, Code of Federal Regulation (CFR).
- The Act refers to the Social Security Act.

Internet Only Manuals. Current Policies that concern providers and suppliers of therapy services are located in many places throughout CMS Manuals. Sites that may be of interest include:

- Pub.100-1 GENERAL INFORMATION, ELIGIBILITY, AND ENTITLEMENT
  - — Chapter 1- General Overview
    - 10.1 - Hospital Insurance (Part A) for Inpatient Hospital, Hospice, Home Health and SNF Services - A Brief Description
    - 10.2 - Home Health Services
    - 10.3 - Supplementary Medical Insurance (Part B) - A Brief Description
    - 20.2 - Discrimination Prohibited
- Pub. 100-2, MEDICARE BENEFIT POLICY MANUAL
  - — Ch 6 - Hospital Services Covered Under Part B
    - 10 - Medical and Other Health Services Furnished to Inpatients of Participating Hospitals
    - 20 - Outpatient Hospital Services
    - 20.2 - Outpatient Defined
    - 20.4.1 - Diagnostic Services Defined
    - 70 - Outpatient Hospital Psychiatric Services
  - — Ch 8 - Coverage of Extended Care (SNF) Services Under Hospital Insurance
    - 30.4. - Direct Skilled Rehabilitation Services to Patients
    - 40 - Physician Certification and Recertification for Extended Care Services
    - 50.3 - Physical Therapy, Speech-Language Pathology, and Occupational Therapy Furnished by the Skilled Nursing Facility or by Others Under Arrangements with the Facility and Under Its Supervision
    - 70.3 - Inpatient Physical Therapy, Occupational Therapy, and Speech Pathology Services
  - — Ch 12 - Comprehensive Outpatient Rehabilitation Facility (CORF) Coverage
    - 10 - Comprehensive Outpatient Rehabilitation Facility (CORF) Services Provided by Medicare
    - 20 - Required and Optional CORF Services
    - 20.1 - Required Services
    - 20.2 - Optional CORF Services
    - 30 - Rules for Provision of Services
    - 30.1 - Rules for Payment of CORF Services
    - 40 - Specific CORF Services
    - 40.1 - Physicians' Services
    - 40.2 - Physical Therapy Services
    - 40.3 - Occupational Therapy Services
    - 40.4 – Speech Language Pathology Services
- Pub. 100-3 MEDICARE NATIONAL COVERAGE DETERMINATIONS MANUAL
  - — Part 1
    - 20.10 - Cardiac Rehabilitation Programs
    - 30.1 - Biofeedback Therapy
    - 30.1.1 - Biofeedback Therapy for the Treatment of Urinary Incontinence
    - 50.1 – Speech Generating Devices
    - 50.2 - Electronic Speech Aids
    - 50.4 - Tracheostomy Speaking Valve
  - — Part 2
    - 150.2 - Osteogenic Stimulator
    - 160.7 - Electrical Nerve Stimulators
    - 160.12 - Neuromuscular Electrical Stimulation (NMES)
    - 160.13 - Supplies Used in the Delivery of Transcutaneous Electrical Nerve Stimulation (TENS) and Neuromuscular Electrical Stimulation (NMES)
    - 160.17 - L-Dopa

- Part 3
  - 170.1 - Institutional and Home Care Patient Education Programs
  - 170.2 - Melodic Intonation Therapy
  - 170.3 - Speech Pathology Services for the Treatment of Dysphagia
  - 180 – Nutrition
- Part 4
  - 230.8 - Non-implantable Pelvic Flood Electrical Stimulator
  - 240.7 - Postural Drainage Procedures and Pulmonary Exercises
  - 270.1 -Electrical Stimulation (ES) and Electromagnetic Therapy for the Treatment of Wounds
  - 270.4 - Treatment of Decubitus Ulcers
  - 280.3 - Mobility Assisted Equipment (MAE)
  - 280.4 - Seat Lift
  - 280.13 - Transcutaneous Electrical Nerve Stimulators (TENS)
  - 290.1 - Home Health Visits to A Blind Diabetic
- Pub. 100-08 PROGRAM INTEGRITY MANUAL
  - Chapter 3 - Verifying Potential Errors and Taking Corrective Actions
    - 3.4.1.1 - Linking LCD and NCD ID Numbers to Edits
  - Chapter 13 - Local Coverage Determinations
    - 13.5.1 - Reasonable and Necessary Provisions in LCDs

Specific policies may differ by setting. Other policies concerning therapy services are found in other manuals. When a therapy service policy is specific to a setting, it takes precedence over these general outpatient policies. For special rules on:

- CORFs - See chapter 12 of this manual and also Pub. 100-4, chapter 5;
- SNF - See chapter 8 of this manual and also Pub. 100-4, chapter 6, for SNF claims/billing;
- HHA - See chapter 7 of this manual, and Pub. 100-4, chapter 10;
- GROUP THERAPY AND STUDENTS - See Pub. 100-2, chapter 15, §230;
- ARRANGEMENTS - Pub. 100-1, chapter 5, §10.3;
- COVERAGE is described in the Medicare Program Integrity Manual, Pub. 100-08, chapter 13, §13.5.1; and
- THERAPY CAPS - See Pub. 100-4, chapter 5, §10.2, for a complete description of this financial limitation.

C. General

Therapy services are a covered benefit in §§1861(g), 1861(p), and 1861(ll) of the Act. Therapy services may also be provided incident to the services of a physician/NPP under §§1861(s)(2) and 1862(a)(20) of the Act.

Covered therapy services are furnished by providers, by others under arrangements with and under the supervision of providers, or furnished by suppliers (e.g., physicians, NPP, enrolled therapists), who meet the requirements in Medicare manuals for therapy services.

Where a prospective payment system (PPS) applies, therapy services are paid when services conform to the requirements of that PPS. Reimbursement for therapy provided to Part A inpatients of hospitals or residents of SNFs in covered stays is included in the respective PPS rates.

Payment for therapy provided by an HHA under a plan of treatment is included in the home health PPS rate. Therapy may be billed by an HHA on bill type 34x if there are no home health services billed under a home health plan of care at the same time (e.g., the patient is not homebound), and there is a valid therapy plan of treatment.

In addition to the requirements described in this chapter, the services must be furnished in accordance with health and safety requirements set forth in regulations at 42CFR484, and 42CFR485.

When therapy services may be furnished appropriately in a community pool by a clinician in a physical therapist or occupational therapist private practice, physician office, outpatient hospital, or outpatient SNF, the practice/office or provider shall rent or lease the pool, or a specific portion of the pool. The use of that part of the pool during specified times shall be restricted to the patients of that practice or provider. The written agreement to rent or lease the pool shall be available for review on request. When part of the pool is rented or leased, the agreement shall describe the part of the pool that is used exclusively by the patients of that practice/office or provider and the times that exclusive use applies. Other providers, including rehabilitation agencies (previously referred to as OPTs and ORFs) and CORFs, are subject to the requirements outlined in the respective State Operations Manual regarding rented or leased community pools.

100-02, 15, 220.4

(Rev.255, Issued: 01-25-19, Effective: 01- 01- 19, Implementation: 02-26-19)

Functional Reporting

NOTE: In the calendar year (CY) 2019 Physician Fee Schedule (PFS) final rule, CMS-1693-F, after consideration of stakeholder comments for burden reduction, a review of all of the requirements under section 3005(g) of Middle Class Tax Relief and Jobs Creation Act of 2012 (MCTRJCA), and in light of the statutory amendments to section 1833(g) of the Act, via section 50202 of Bipartisan Budget Act of 2018 to repeal the therapy caps, CMS concluded that continued collection of functional reporting data through the same or reduced format would not yield additional information to inform future analyses or to serve as a basis for reforms to the payment system for therapy services. To reduce the burden of reporting for providers of therapy services, the CY 2019 PFS final rule ended the requirements of reporting the functional limitation nonpayable HCPCS G-codes and severity modifiers on claims for therapy services and the associated documentation requirements in medical records, effective for dates of service on and after January 1, 2019. The rule also revised regulation text at 42 CFR 410.59, 410.60, 410.61, 410.62, 410.105, accordingly.

The instructions below apply only to dates of service when the functional reporting requirements were effective, January 1, 2013 through December 31, 2018.

A. Selecting the G-codes to Use in Functional Reporting.

There are 42 functional G-codes, 14 sets of three codes each, for that can be used in identifying the functional limitation being reported. Six of the G-code sets are generally for PT and OT functional limitations and eight sets of G-codes are for SLP functional limitations. (For a list of these codes and descriptors, see Pub. 100-04, Medicare Claims Processing Manual, chapter 5, section 10.6 F.)

Only one functional limitation shall be reported at a time. Consequently, the clinician must select the G-code set for the functional limitation that most closely relates to the primary functional limitation being treated or the one that is the primary reason for treatment. When the beneficiary has more than one functional limitation, the clinician may need to make a determination as to which functional limitation is primary. In these cases, the clinician may choose the functional limitation that is:

The instructions below apply only to dates of service when the functional reporting requirements were effective, January 1, 2013 through December 31, 2018.

A. Selecting the G-codes to Use in Functional Reporting.

There are 42 functional G-codes, 14 sets of three codes each, for that can be used in identifying the functional limitation being reported. Six of the G-code sets are generally for PT and OT functional limitations and eight sets of G-codes are for SLP functional limitations. (For a list of these codes and descriptors, see Pub. 100-04, Medicare Claims Processing Manual, chapter 5, section 10.6 F.)

Only one functional limitation shall be reported at a time. Consequently, the clinician must select the G-code set for the functional limitation that most closely relates to the primary functional limitation being treated or the one that is the primary reason for treatment. When the beneficiary has more than one functional limitation, the clinician may need to make a determination as to which functional limitation is primary. In these cases, the clinician may choose the functional limitation that is:

- Most clinically relevant to a successful outcome for the beneficiary;
- The one that would yield the quickest and/or greatest functional progress; or
- The one that is the greatest priority for the beneficiary.

In all cases, this primary functional limitation should reflect the predominant limitation that the furnished therapy services are intended to address.

For services typically reported as PT or OT, the clinician reports one of the "Other PT/OT" functional G-codes sets to report when one of the four PT/OT categorical code sets does not describe the beneficiary's functional limitation, as follows:

- a beneficiary's functional limitation that is not defined by one of the four categories;
- a beneficiary whose therapy services are not intended to treat a functional limitation; or
- a beneficiary's functional limitation where an overall, composite, or other score from a functional assessment tool is used and does not clearly represent a functional limitation defined by one of the above four categorical PT/OT code sets.

In addition, the subsequent "Other PT/OT" G-code set is only reported after the primary "Other PT/OT" G-code set has been reported for the beneficiary during the same episode of care.

For services typically reported as SLP services, the clinician uses the "Other SLP" functional G-code to report when the functional limitation being treated is not represented by one of the seven categorical SLP functional measures. In addition, the "Other SLP" G-code set is used to report where an overall, composite, or other score from an assessment tool that does not clearly represent a functional limitation defined by one of the seven categorical SLP measures.

B. Selecting the severity modifiers to use in functional reporting/documenting.

Each G-code requires one of the following severity modifiers. When the clinician reports any of the following a modifier is used to convey the severity of the functional limitation: current status, the goal status and the discharge status.

Modifier	Impairment Limitation Restriction
CH	0 percent impaired, limited or restricted
CI	At least 1 percent but less than 20 percent impaired, limited or restricted
CJ	At least 20 percent but less than 40 percent impaired, limited or restricted
CK	At least 40 percent but less than 60 percent impaired, limited or restricted
CL	At least 60 percent but less than 80 percent impaired, limited or restricted
CM	At least 80 percent but less than 100 percent impaired, limited or restricted
CN	100 percent impaired, limited or restricted

The severity modifier reflects the beneficiary's percentage of functional impairment as determined by the clinician furnishing the therapy services for each functional status: current, goal, or discharge. In selecting the severity modifier, the clinician:

- Uses the severity modifier that reflects the score from a functional assessment tool or other performance measurement instrument, as appropriate.
- Uses his/her clinical judgment to combine the results of multiple measurement tools used during the evaluative process to inform clinical decision making to determine a functional limitation percentage.
- Uses his/her clinical judgment in the assignment of the appropriate modifier.
- Uses the CH modifier to reflect a zero percent impairment when the therapy services being furnished are not intended to treat (or address) a functional limitation.

In some cases the modifier will be the same for current status and goal status. For example: where improvement is expected but it is not expected to be enough to move to another modifier, such as from 10 percent to 15 percent, the same severity modifier would be used in reporting the current and goal status. Also, when the clinician does not expect improvement, such as for individuals receiving maintenance therapy, the modifier used for projected goal status will be the same as the one for current status. In these cases, the discharge status may also include the same modifier.

Therapists must document in the medical record how they made the modifier selection so that the same process can be followed at succeeding assessment intervals.

C. Documentation of G-code and Severity Modifier Selection.

Documentation of the nonpayable G-codes and severity modifiers regarding functional limitations reported on claims must be included in the patient's medical record of therapy services for each required reporting. (See Pub. 100-04, Medicare Claims Processing Manual, chapter 5, section 10.6 for details about the functional reporting requirements on claims for therapy services, including PT, OT, and SLP services furnished in CORFs.)

Documentation of functional reporting in the medical record of therapy services must be completed by the clinician furnishing the therapy services:

- The qualified therapist furnishing the therapy services
- The physician/NPP personally furnishing the therapy services
- The qualified therapist furnishing services incident to the physician/NPP
- The physician/NPP for incident to services furnished by qualified personnel, who are not qualified therapists.

The qualified therapist furnishing the PT, OT, or SLP services in a CORF

A. Selecting the G-codes to Use in Functional Reporting.

There are 42 functional G-codes, 14 sets of three codes each, for that can be used in identifying the functional limitation being reported. Six of the G-code sets are generally for PT and OT functional limitations and eight sets of G-codes are for SLP functional limitations. (For a list of these codes and descriptors, see Pub. 100-04, Medicare Claims Processing Manual, chapter 5, section 10.6 F.)

Only one functional limitation shall be reported at a time. Consequently, the clinician must select the G-code set for the functional limitation that most closely relates to the primary functional limitation being treated or the one that is the primary reason for treatment. When the beneficiary has more than one functional limitation, the clinician may need to make a determination as to which functional limitation is primary. In these cases, the clinician may choose the functional limitation that is:

- Most clinically relevant to a successful outcome for the beneficiary;
- The one that would yield the quickest and/or greatest functional progress; or
- The one that is the greatest priority for the beneficiary.

In all cases, this primary functional limitation should reflect the predominant limitation that the furnished therapy services are intended to address.

For services typically reported as PT or OT, the clinician reports one of the "Other PT/OT" functional G-codes sets to report when one of the four PT/OT categorical code sets does not describe the beneficiary's functional limitation, as follows:

- a beneficiary's functional limitation that is not defined by one of the four categories;
- a beneficiary whose therapy services are not intended to treat a functional limitation; or
- a beneficiary's functional limitation where an overall, composite, or other score from a functional assessment tool is used and does not clearly represent a functional limitation defined by one of the above four categorical PT/OT code sets.

In addition, the subsequent "Other PT/OT" G-code set is only reported after the primary "Other PT/OT" G-code set has been reported for the beneficiary during the same episode of care.

For services typically reported as SLP services, the clinician uses the "Other SLP" functional G-code to report when the functional limitation being treated is not represented by one of the seven categorical SLP functional measures. In addition, the "Other SLP" G-code set is used to report where an overall, composite, or other score from an assessment tool that does not clearly represent a functional limitation defined by one of the seven categorical SLP measures.

B. Selecting the severity modifiers to use in functional reporting/ documenting.

Each G-code requires one of the following severity modifiers. When the clinician reports any of the following a modifier is used to convey the severity of the functional limitation: current status, the goal status and the discharge status.

Modifier	Impairment Limitation Restriction
CH	0 percent impaired, limited or restricted
CI	At least 1 percent but less than 20 percent impaired, limited or restricted
CJ	At least 20 percent but less than 40 percent impaired, limited or restricted
CK	At least 40 percent but less than 60 percent impaired, limited or restricted
CL	At least 60 percent but less than 80 percent impaired, limited or restricted
CM	At least 80 percent but less than 100 percent impaired, limited or restricted
CN	100 percent impaired, limited or restricted

The severity modifier reflects the beneficiary's percentage of functional impairment as determined by the clinician furnishing the therapy services for each functional status: current, goal, or discharge. In selecting the severity modifier, the clinician:

- Uses the severity modifier that reflects the score from a functional assessment tool or other performance measurement instrument, as appropriate.
- Uses his/her clinical judgment to combine the results of multiple measurement tools used during the evaluative process to inform clinical decision making to determine a functional limitation percentage.
- Uses his/her clinical judgment in the assignment of the appropriate modifier.
- Uses the CH modifier to reflect a zero percent impairment when the therapy services being furnished are not intended to treat (or address) a functional limitation.

In some cases the modifier will be the same for current status and goal status. For example: where improvement is expected but it is not expected to be enough to move to another modifier, such as from 10 percent to 15 percent, the same severity modifier would be used in reporting the current and goal status. Also, when the clinician does not expect improvement, such as for individuals receiving maintenance therapy, the modifier used for projected goal status will be the same as the one for current status. In these cases, the discharge status may also include the same modifier.

Therapists must document in the medical record how they made the modifier selection so that the same process can be followed at succeeding assessment intervals.

C. Documentation of G-code and Severity Modifier Selection.

Documentation of the nonpayable G-codes and severity modifiers regarding functional limitations reported on claims must be included in the patient's medical record of therapy services for each required reporting. (See Pub. 100-04, Medicare Claims Processing Manual, chapter 5, section 10.6 for details about the functional reporting requirements on claims for therapy services, including PT, OT, and SLP services furnished in CORFs.)

Documentation of functional reporting in the medical record of therapy services must be completed by the clinician furnishing the therapy services:

- The qualified therapist furnishing the therapy services
- The physician/NPP personally furnishing the therapy services
- The qualified therapist furnishing services incident to the physician/NPP
- The physician/NPP for incident to services furnished by qualified personnel, who are not qualified therapists.

The qualified therapist furnishing the PT, OT, or SLP services in a CORF

100-02, 15, 230

Practice of Physical Therapy, Occupational Therapy, and Speech-Language Pathology

(Rev. 63, Issued: 12-29-06, Effective: 01-01-07, Implementation: on or before 01-29-07)

A. Group Therapy Services.

Contractors pay for outpatient physical therapy services (which includes outpatient speech-language pathology services) and outpatient occupational therapy services provided simultaneously to two or more individuals by a practitioner as group therapy services (97150). The individuals can be, but need not be performing the same activity. The physician or therapist involved in group therapy services must be in constant attendance, but one-on-one patient contact is not required.

B. Therapy Students

1. General

   Only the services of the therapist can be billed and paid under Medicare Part B. The services performed by a student are not reimbursed even if provided under "line of sight" supervision of the therapist; however, the presence of the student "in the room" does not make the service unbillable. Pay for the direct (one-to-one) patient contact services of the physician or therapist provided to Medicare Part B patients. Group therapy services performed by a therapist or physician may be billed when a student is also present "in the room".

EXAMPLES:

Therapists may bill and be paid for the provision of services in the following scenarios:

- The qualified practitioner is present and in the room for the entire session. The student participates in the delivery of services when the qualified practitioner is directing the service, making the skilled judgment, and is responsible for the assessment and treatment.
- The qualified practitioner is present in the room guiding the student in service delivery when the therapy student and the therapy assistant student are participating in the provision of services, and the practitioner is not engaged in treating another patient or doing other tasks at the same time.
- The qualified practitioner is responsible for the services and as such, signs all documentation. (A student may, of course, also sign but it is not necessary since the Part B payment is for the clinician's service, not for the student's services).

2. Therapy Assistants as Clinical Instructors

   Physical therapist assistants and occupational therapy assistants are not precluded from serving as clinical instructors for therapy students, while providing services within their scope of work and performed under the direction and supervision of a licensed physical or occupational therapist to a Medicare beneficiary.

3. Services Provided Under Part A and Part B

   The payment methodologies for Part A and B therapy services rendered by a student are different. Under the MPFS (Medicare Part B), Medicare pays for services provided by physicians and practitioners that are specifically authorized by statute. Students do not meet the definition of practitioners under Medicare Part B. Under SNF PPS, payments are based upon the case mix or Resource Utilization Group (RUG) category that describes the patient. In the rehabilitation groups, the number of therapy minutes delivered to the patient determines the RUG category. Payment levels for each category are based upon the costs of caring for patients in each group rather than providing specific payment for each therapy service as is done in Medicare Part B.

100-02, 15, 230.1

Practice of Physical Therapy

(Rev. 88, Issued: 05-07-08, Effective: 01-01-08, Implementation: 06-09-08)

A. General

Physical therapy services are those services provided within the scope of practice of physical therapists and necessary for the diagnosis and treatment of impairments, functional limitations, disabilities or changes in physical function and health status. (See Pub. 100-3, the Medicare National Coverage Determinations Manual, for specific conditions or services.) For descriptions of aquatic therapy in a community center pool see section 220C of this chapter.

B. Qualified Physical Therapist Defined

Reference: 42CFR484.4

The new personnel qualifications for physical therapists were discussed in the 2008 Physician Fee Schedule. See the Federal Register of November 27, 2007, for the full text. See also the correction notice for this rule, published in the Federal Register on January 15, 2008.

The regulation provides that a qualified physical therapist (PT) is a person who is licensed, if applicable, as a PT by the state in which he or she is practicing unless licensure does not apply, has graduated from an accredited PT education program and passed a national examination approved by the state in which PT services are provided.

The phrase, "by the state in which practicing" includes any authorization to practice provided by the same state in which the service is provided, including temporary licensure, regardless of the location of the entity billing the services. The curriculum accreditation is provided by the Commission on Accreditation in Physical Therapy Education (CAPTE) or, for those who graduated before CAPTE, curriculum approval was provided by the American Physical Therapy Association (APTA). For internationally educated PTs, curricula are approved by a credentials evaluation organization either approved by the APTA or identified in 8 CFR 212.15(e) as it relates to PTs. For example, in 2007, 8 CFR 212.15(e) approved the credentials evaluation provided by the Federation of State Boards of Physical Therapy (FSBPT) and the Foreign Credentialing Commission on Physical Therapy (FCCPT). The requirements above apply to all PTs effective January 1, 2010, if they have not met any of the following requirements prior to January 1, 2010.

Physical therapists whose current license was obtained on or prior to December 31, 2009, qualify to provide PT services to Medicare beneficiaries if they:

- graduated from a CAPTE approved program in PT on or before December 31, 2009 (examination is not required); or,
- graduated on or before December 31, 2009, from a PT program outside the U.S. that is determined to be substantially equivalent to a U.S. program by a credentials evaluating organization approved by either the APTA or identified in 8 CFR 212.15(e) and also passed an examination for PTs approved by the state in which practicing.

  Or, PTs whose current license was obtained before January 1, 2008, may meet the requirements in place on that date (i.e., graduation from a curriculum approved by either the APTA, the Committee on Allied Health Education and Accreditation of the American Medical Association, or both).

  Or, PTs meet the requirements who are currently licensed and were licensed or qualified as a PT on or before December 31, 1977, and had 2 years appropriate experience as a PT, and passed a proficiency examination conducted, approved, or sponsored by the U.S. Public Health Service.

  Or, PTs meet the requirements if they are currently licensed and before January 1, 1966, they were:

  - admitted to membership by the APTA; or
  - admitted to registration by the American Registry of Physical Therapists; or
  - graduated from a 4-year PT curriculum approved by a State Department of Education; or
  - licensed or registered and prior to January 1, 1970, they had 15 years of fulltime experience in PT under the order and direction of attending and referring doctors of medicine or osteopathy.

  Or, PTs meet requirements if they are currently licensed and they were trained outside the U.S. before January 1, 2008, and after 1928 graduated from a PT curriculum approved in the country in which the curriculum was located, if that country had an organization that was a member of the World Confederation for Physical Therapy, and that PT qualified as a member of the organization.

For outpatient PT services that are provided incident to the services of physicians/NPPs, the requirement for PT licensure does not apply; all other personnel qualifications do apply. The qualified personnel providing PT services incident to the services of a physician/NPP must be trained in an accredited PT curriculum. For example, a person who, on or before December 31, 2009, graduated from a PT curriculum accredited by CAPTE, but who has not passed the national examination or obtained a license, could provide Medicare outpatient PT therapy services incident to the services of a physician/NPP if the physician assumes responsibility for the services according to the incident to policies. On or after January 1, 2010, although licensure does not apply, both education and examination requirements that are effective January 1, 2010, apply to qualified personnel who provide PT services incident to the services of a physician/NPP.

C. Services of Physical Therapy Support Personnel

Reference: 42CFR 484.4

Personnel Qualifications. The new personnel qualifications for physical therapist assistants (PTA) were discussed in the 2008 Physician Fee Schedule. See the Federal Register of November 27, 2007, for the full text. See also the correction notice for this rule, published in the Federal Register on January 15, 2008.

The regulation provides that a qualified PTA is a person who is licensed as a PTA unless licensure does not apply, is registered or certified, if applicable, as a PTA by the state in which practicing, and graduated from an approved curriculum for PTAs, and passed a national examination for PTAs. The phrase, "by the state in which practicing" includes any authorization to practice provided by the same state in which the service is provided, including temporary licensure, regardless of the location or the entity billing for the services. Approval for the curriculum is provided by CAPTE or, if internationally or military trained PTAs apply, approval will be through a credentialing body for the curriculum for PTAs identified by either the American Physical Therapy Association or identified in 8 CFR 212.15(e). A national examination for PTAs is, for example the one furnished by the Federation of State Boards of Physical Therapy. These requirements above apply to all PTAs effective January 1, 2010, if they have not met any of the following requirements prior to January 1, 2010.

Those PTAs also qualify who, on or before December 31, 2009, are licensed, registered or certified as a PTA and met one of the two following requirements:

1. Is licensed or otherwise regulated in the state in which practicing; or
2. In states that have no licensure or other regulations, or where licensure does not apply, PTAs have:
   - graduated on or before December 31, 2009, from a 2-year college-level program approved by the APTA or CAPTE; and
   - effective January 1, 2010, those PTAs must have both graduated from a CAPTE approved curriculum and passed a national examination for PTAs; or
   - PTAs may also qualify if they are licensed, registered or certified as a PTA, if applicable and meet requirements in effect before January 1, 2008, that is,
     - they have graduated before January 1, 2008, from a 2 year college level program approved by the APTA; or
     - on or before December 31, 1977, they were licensed or qualified as a PTA and passed a proficiency examination conducted, approved, or sponsored by the U.S. Public Health Service.

Services. The services of PTAs used when providing covered therapy benefits are included as part of the covered service. These services are billed by the supervising physical therapist. PTAs may not provide evaluation services, make clinical judgments or decisions or take responsibility for the service. They act at the direction and under the supervision of the treating physical therapist and in accordance with state laws.

A physical therapist must supervise PTAs. The level and frequency of supervision differs by setting (and by state or local law). General supervision is required for PTAs in all settings except private practice (which requires direct supervision) unless state practice requirements are more stringent, in which case state or local requirements must be followed. See specific settings for details. For example, in clinics, rehabilitation services, either on or off the organization's premises, those services are supervised by a qualified physical therapist who makes an onsite supervisory visit at least once every 30 days or more frequently if required by state or local laws or regulation.

The services of a PTA shall not be billed as services incident to a physician/NPP's service, because they do not meet the qualifications of a therapist.

The cost of supplies (e.g., theraband, hand putty, electrodes) used in furnishing covered therapy care is included in the payment for the HCPCS codes billed by the physical therapist, and are, therefore, not separately billable. Separate coverage and billing provisions apply to items that meet the definition of brace in Sec.130.

Services provided by aides, even if under the supervision of a therapist, are not therapy services and are not covered by Medicare. Although an aide may help the therapist by providing unskilled services, those services that are unskilled are not covered by Medicare and shall be denied as not reasonable and necessary if they are billed as therapy services.

D. Application of Medicare Guidelines to PT Services
This subsection will be used in the future to illustrate the application of the above guidelines to some of the physical therapy modalities and procedures utilized in the treatment of patients.

100-02, 15, 230.2

Practice of Occupational Therapy

(Rev. 88, Issued: 05-07-08, Effective: 01-01-08, Implementation: 06-09-08)

A. General
Occupational therapy services are those services provided within the scope of practice of occupational therapists and necessary for the diagnosis and treatment of impairments, functional disabilities or changes in physical function and health status. (See Pub. 100- 03, the Medicare National Coverage Determinations Manual, for specific conditions or services.)

Occupational therapy is medically prescribed treatment concerned with improving or restoring functions which have been impaired by illness or injury or, where function has been permanently lost or reduced by illness or injury, to improve the individual's ability to perform those tasks required for independent functioning. Such therapy may involve:

- The evaluation, and reevaluation as required, of a patient's level of function by administering diagnostic and prognostic tests;
- The selection and teaching of task-oriented therapeutic activities designed to restore physical function; e.g., use of woodworking activities on an inclined table to restore shoulder, elbow, and wrist range of motion lost as a result of burns;
- The planning, implementing, and supervising of individualized therapeutic activity programs as part of an overall "active treatment" program for a patient with a diagnosed psychiatric illness; e.g., the use of sewing activities which require following a pattern to reduce confusion and restore reality orientation in a schizophrenic patient;
- The planning and implementing of therapeutic tasks and activities to restore sensoryintegrative function; e.g., providing motor and tactile activities to increase sensory input and improve response for a stroke patient with functional loss resulting in a distorted body image;
- The teaching of compensatory technique to improve the level of independence in the activities of daily living, for example:
  - — Teaching a patient who has lost the use of an arm how to pare potatoes and chop vegetables with one hand;
  - — Teaching an upper extremity amputee how to functionally utilize a prosthesis;
  - — Teaching a stroke patient new techniques to enable the patient to perform feeding, dressing, and other activities as independently as possible; or
  - — Teaching a patient with a hip fracture/hip replacement techniques of standing tolerance and balance to enable the patient to perform such functional activities as dressing and homemaking tasks.

  The designing, fabricating, and fitting of orthotics and self-help devices; e.g., making a hand splint for a patient with rheumatoid arthritis to maintain the hand in a functional position or constructing a device which would enable an individual to hold a utensil and feed independently; or Vocational and prevocational assessment and training, subject to the limitations specified in item B below.

  Only a qualified occupational therapist has the knowledge, training, and experience required to evaluate and, as necessary, reevaluate a patient's level of function, determine whether an occupational therapy program could reasonably be expected to improve, restore, or compensate for lost function and, where appropriate, recommend to the physician/NPP a plan of treatment.

B. Qualified Occupational Therapist Defined
Reference: 42CFR484.4 The new personnel qualifications for occupational therapists (OT) were discussed in the 2008 Physician Fee Schedule. See the Federal Register of November 27, 2007, for the full text. See also the correction notice for this rule, published in the Federal Register on January 15, 2008.

The regulation provides that a qualified OT is an individual who is licensed, if licensure applies, or otherwise regulated, if applicable, as an OT by the state in which practicing, and graduated from an accredited education program for OTs, and is eligible to take or has passed the examination for OTs administered by the National Board for Certification in Occupational Therapy, Inc. (NBCOT). The phrase, "by the state in which practicing" includes any authorization to practice provided by the same state in which the service is provided, including temporary licensure, regardless of the location of the entity billing the services. The education program for U.S. trained OTs is accredited by the Accreditation Council for Occupational Therapy Education (ACOTE). The requirements above apply to all OTs effective January 1, 2010, if they have not met any of the following requirements prior to January 1, 2010.

The OTs may also qualify if on or before December 31, 2009:

- they are licensed or otherwise regulated as an OT in the state in which practicing (regardless of the qualifications they met to obtain that licensure or regulation); or
- when licensure or other regulation does not apply, OTs have graduated from an OT education program accredited by ACOTE and are eligible to take, or have successfully completed the NBCOT examination for OTs.

Also, those OTs who met the Medicare requirements for OTs that were in 42CFR484.4 prior to January 1, 2008, qualify to provide OT services for Medicare beneficiaries if:

- on or before January 1, 2008, they graduated an OT program approved jointly by the American Medical Association and the AOTA, or
- they are eligible for the National Registration Examination of AOTA or the National Board for Certification in OT.

Also, they qualify who on or before December 31, 1977, had 2 years of appropriate experience as an occupational therapist, and had achieved a satisfactory grade on a proficiency examination conducted, approved, or sponsored by the U.S. Public Health Service.

Those educated outside the U.S. may meet the same qualifications for domestic trained OTs. For example, they qualify if they were licensed or otherwise regulated by the state in which practicing on or before December 31, 2009. Or they are qualified if they:

- graduated from an OT education program accredited as substantially equivalent to a U.S. OT education program by ACOTE, the World Federation of Occupational Therapists, or a credentialing body approved by AOTA; and
- passed the NBCOT examination for OT; and
- Effective January 1, 2010, are licensed or otherwise regulated, if applicable as an OT by the state in which practicing.

For outpatient OT services that are provided incident to the services of physicians/NPPs, the requirement for OT licensure does not apply; all other personnel qualifications do apply. The qualified personnel providing OT services incident to the services of a physician/NPP must be trained in an accredited OT curriculum. For example, a person who, on or before December 31, 2009, graduated from an OT curriculum accredited by ACOTE and is eligible to take or has successfully completed the entry-level certification examination for OTs developed and administered by NBCOT, could provide Medicare outpatient OT services incident to the services of a physician/NPP if the physician assumes responsibility for the services according to the incident to policies. On or after January 1, 2010, although licensure does not apply, both education and examination requirements that are effective January 1, 2010, apply to qualified personnel who provide OT services incident to the services of a physician/NPP.

C. Services of Occupational Therapy Support Personnel
Reference: 42CFR 484.4

The new personnel qualifications for occupational therapy assistants were discussed in the 2008 Physician Fee Schedule. See the Federal Register of November 27, 2007, for the full text. See also the correction notice for this rule, published in the Federal Register on January 15, 2008.

The regulation provides that an occupational therapy assistant is a person who is licensed, unless licensure does not apply, or otherwise regulated, if applicable, as an OTA by the state in which practicing, and graduated from an OTA education program accredited by ACOTE and is eligible to take or has successfully completed the NBCOT examination for OTAs. The phrase, "by the state in which practicing" includes any authorization to practice provided by the same state in which the service is provided, including temporary licensure, regardless of the location of the entity billing the services.

If the requirements above are not met, an OTA may qualify if, on or before December 31, 2009, the OTA is licensed or otherwise regulated as an OTA, if applicable, by the state in which practicing, or meets any qualifications defined by the state in which practicing.

Or, where licensure or other state regulation does not apply, OTAs may qualify if they have, on or before December 31, 2009:

- completed certification requirements to practice as an OTA established by a credentialing organization approved by AOTA; and
- after January 1, 2010, they have also completed an education program accredited by ACOTE and passed the NBCOT examination for OTAs.

OTAs who qualified under the policies in effect prior to January 1, 2008, continue to qualify to provide OT directed and supervised OTA services to Medicare beneficiaries.

Therefore, OTAs qualify who after December 31, 1977, and on or before December 31, 2007:

- completed certification requirements to practice as an OTA established by a credentialing organization approved by AOTA; or

- completed the requirements to practice as an OTA applicable in the state in which practicing.

Those OTAs who were educated outside the U.S. may meet the same requirements as domestically trained OTAs. Or, if educated outside the U.S. on or after January 1, 2008, they must have graduated from an OTA program accredited as substantially equivalent to OTA entry level education in the U.S. by ACOTE, its successor organization, or the World Federation of Occupational Therapists or a credentialing body approved by AOTA. In addition, they must have passed an exam for OTAs administered by NBCOT.

Services. The services of OTAs used when providing covered therapy benefits are included as part of the covered service. These services are billed by the supervising occupational therapist. OTAs may not provide evaluation services, make clinical judgments or decisions or take responsibility for the service. They act at the direction and under the supervision of the treating occupational therapist and in accordance with state laws.

An occupational therapist must supervise OTAs. The level and frequency of supervision differs by setting (and by state or local law). General supervision is required for OTAs in all settings except private practice (which requires direct supervision) unless state practice requirements are more stringent, in which case state or local requirements must be followed. See specific settings for details. For example, in clinics, rehabilitation agencies, and public health agencies, 42CFR485.713 indicates that when an OTA provides services, either on or off the organization's premises, those services are supervised by a qualified occupational therapist who makes an onsite supervisory visit at least once every 30 days or more frequently if required by state or local laws or regulation.

The services of an OTA shall not be billed as services incident to a physician/NPP's service, because they do not meet the qualifications of a therapist.

The cost of supplies (e.g., looms, ceramic tiles, or leather) used in furnishing covered therapy care is included in the payment for the HCPCS codes billed by the occupational therapist and are, therefore, not separately billable. Separate coverage and billing provisions apply to items that meet the definition of brace in Sec.130 of this manual.

Services provided by aides, even if under the supervision of a therapist, are not therapy services in the outpatient setting and are not covered by Medicare. Although an aide may help the therapist by providing unskilled services, those services that are unskilled are not covered by Medicare and shall be denied as not reasonable and necessary if they are billed as therapy services.

D. Application of Medicare Guidelines to Occupational Therapy Services

Occupational therapy may be required for a patient with a specific diagnosed psychiatric illness. If such services are required, they are covered assuming the coverage criteria are met. However, where an individual's motivational needs are not related to a specific diagnosed psychiatric illness, the meeting of such needs does not usually require an individualized therapeutic program. Such needs can be met through general activity programs or the efforts of other professional personnel involved in the care of the patient. Patient motivation is an appropriate and inherent function of all health disciplines, which is interwoven with other functions performed by such personnel for the patient. Accordingly, since the special skills of an occupational therapist are not required, an occupational therapy program for individuals who do not have a specific diagnosed psychiatric illness is not to be considered reasonable and necessary for the treatment of an illness or injury. Services furnished under such a program are not covered.

Occupational therapy may include vocational and prevocational assessment and training. When services provided by an occupational therapist are related solely to specific employment opportunities, work skills, or work settings, they are not reasonable or necessary for the diagnosis or treatment of an illness or injury and are not covered. However, carriers and intermediaries exercise care in applying this exclusion, because the assessment of level of function and the teaching of compensatory techniques to improve the level of function, especially in activities of daily living, are services which occupational therapists provide for both vocational and nonvocational purposes. For example, an assessment of sitting and standing tolerance might be nonvocational for a mother of young children or a retired individual living alone, but could also be a vocational test for a sales clerk. Training an amputee in the use of prosthesis for telephoning is necessary for everyday activities as well as for employment purposes. Major changes in life style may be mandatory for an individual with a substantial disability. The techniques of adjustment cannot be considered exclusively vocational or nonvocational.

100-02, 15, 230.4

Services Furnished by a Therapist in Private Practice

(Rev. 179, Issued: 01-14-14, Effective: 01-07-14, Implementation: 01-07-14)

A. General

See section 220 of this chapter for definitions. Therapist refers only to a qualified physical therapist, occupational therapist or speech-language pathologist. TPP refers to therapists in private practice (qualified physical therapists, occupational therapists and speech-language pathologists).

In order to qualify to bill Medicare directly as a therapist, each individual must be enrolled as a private practitioner and employed in one of the following practice types: an unincorporated solo practice, unincorporated partnership, unincorporated group practice, physician/NPP group or groups that are not professional corporations, if allowed by state and local law. Physician/NPP group practices may employ TPP if state and local law permits this employee relationship.

For purposes of this provision, a physician/NPP group practice is defined as one or more physicians/NPPs enrolled with Medicare who may bill as one entity. For further details on issues concerning enrollment, see the provider enrollment Web site at www.cms.hhs.gov/MedicareProviderSupEnroll and Pub. 100-08, Medicare Program Integrity Manual, chapter15, section 15.4.4.9.

Private practice also includes therapists who are practicing therapy as employees of another supplier, of a professional corporation or other incorporated therapy practice. Private practice does not include individuals when they are working as employees of an institutional provider.

Services should be furnished in the therapist's or group's office or in the patient's home. The office is defined as the location(s) where the practice is operated, in the state(s) where the therapist (and practice, if applicable) is legally authorized to furnish services, during the hours that the therapist engages in the practice at that location. If services are furnished in a private practice office space, that space shall be owned, leased, or rented by the practice and used for the exclusive purpose of operating the practice. For descriptions of aquatic therapy in a community center pool see section 220C of this chapter.

Therapists in private practice must be approved as meeting certain requirements, but do not execute a formal provider agreement with the Secretary.

If therapists who have their own Medicare National Provider Identifier (NPI) are employed by therapist groups, physician/NPP groups, or groups that are not professional organizations, the requirement that therapy space be owned, leased, or rented may be satisfied by the group that employs the therapist. Each therapist employed by a group should enroll as a TPP.

When therapists with a Medicare NPI provide services in the physician's/NPP's office in which they are employed, and bill using their NPI for each therapy service, then the direct supervision requirement for enrolled staff apply.

When the therapist who has a Medicare NPI is employed in a physician's/NPP's office the services are ordinarily billed as services of the therapist, with the therapist identified on the claim as the supplier of services. However, services of the therapist who has a Medicare NPI may also be billed by the physician/NPP as services incident to the physician's/NPP's service. (See §230.5 for rules related to therapy services incident to a physician.) In that case, the physician/NPP is the supplier of service, the NPI of the supervising physician/NPP is reported on the claim with the service and all the rules for both therapy services and incident to services (§230.5) must be followed.

B. Private Practice Defined

Reference: Federal Register November, 1998, pages 58863-58869; 42CFR 410.38(b), 42CFR410.59, 42CFR410.60, 42CFR410.62

The contractor considers a therapist to be in private practice if the therapist maintains office space at his or her own expense and furnishes services only in that space or the patient's home. Or, a therapist is employed by another supplier and furnishes services in facilities provided at the expense of that supplier.

The therapist need not be in full-time private practice but must be engaged in private practice on a regular basis; i.e., the therapist is recognized as a private practitioner and for that purpose has access to the necessary equipment to provide an adequate program of therapy.

The therapy services must be provided either by or under the direct supervision of the TPP. Each TPP should be enrolled as a Medicare provider. If a therapist is not enrolled, the services of that therapist must be directly supervised by an enrolled therapist. Direct supervision requires that the supervising private practice therapist be present in the office suite at the time the service is performed. These direct supervision requirements apply only in the private practice setting and only for therapists and their assistants. In other outpatient settings, supervision rules differ. The services of support personnel must be included in the therapist's bill. The supporting personnel, including other therapists, must be W-2 or 1099 employees of the TPP or other qualified employer.

Coverage of outpatient therapy under Part B includes the services of a qualified TPP when furnished in the therapist's office or the beneficiary's home. For this purpose, "home" includes an institution that is used as a home, but not a hospital, CAH or SNF, (Federal Register Nov. 2, 1998, pg 58869).

C. Assignment

Reference: Nov. 2, 1998 Federal Register, pg. 58863

See also Pub. 100-4 chapter 1, §30.2.

When physicians, NPPs, or TPPs obtain provider numbers, they have the option of accepting assignment (participating) or not accepting assignment (nonparticipating). In contrast, providers, such as outpatient hospitals, SNFs, rehabilitation agencies, and CORFs, do not have the option. For these providers, assignment is mandatory.

If physicians/NPPs, or TPPs accept assignment (are participating), they must accept the Medicare Physician Fee Schedule amount as payment. Medicare pays 80% and the patient is responsible for 20%. In contrast, if they do not accept assignment, Medicare will only pay 95% of the fee schedule amount. However, when these services are not furnished on an assignment-related basis, the limiting charge applies. (See §1848(g)(2)(c) of the Act.)

NOTE: Services furnished by a therapist in the therapist's office under arrangements with hospitals in rural communities and public health agencies (or services provided in the beneficiary's home under arrangements with a provider of outpatient physical or occupational therapy services) are not covered under this provision. See section 230.6.

100-02, 15, 232

Cardiac Rehabilitation (CR) and Intensive Cardiac Rehabilitation (ICR) Services Furnished On or After January 1, 2010

(Rev. 256, Issued: 02-01-19, Effective: 02-09-18, Implementation: 03-19-19)

Cardiac rehabilitation (CR) services mean a physician-supervised program that furnishes physician prescribed exercise, cardiac risk factor modification, including education, counseling, and behavioral intervention; psychosocial assessment, outcomes assessment, and other items/services as determined by the Secretary under certain conditions. Intensive cardiac rehabilitation (ICR) services mean a physician-supervised program that furnishes the same items/services under the same conditions as a CR program but must also demonstrate, as shown in peer-reviewed published research, that it improves patients' cardiovascular disease through specific outcome measurements described in 42 CFR 410.49(c). Effective January 1, 2010, Medicare Part B pays for CR/ICR programs and related items/services if specific criteria is met by the Medicare beneficiary, the CR/ICR program itself, the setting in which is it administered, and the physician administering the program, as outlined below:

CR/ICR Program Beneficiary Requirements:

Medicare covers CR/ICR program services for beneficiaries who have experienced one or more of the following:

- Acute myocardial infarction within the preceding 12 months;
- Coronary artery bypass surgery;
- Current stable angina pectoris;
- Heart valve repair or replacement;
- Percutaneous transluminal coronary angioplasty (PTCA) or coronary stenting;
- Heart or heart-lung transplant.

For cardiac rehabilitation only: Stable, chronic heart failure defined as patients with left ventricular ejection fraction of 35% or less and New York Heart Association (NYHA) class II to IV symptoms despite being on optimal heart failure therapy for at least 6 weeks. (Effective February 18, 2014.)

Effective February 9, 2018, section 51004 of the Bipartisan Budget Act (BBA) of 2018, Pub. L. No. 115-123 (2018), amended section 1861(eee)(4)(B) of the Social Security Act to expand coverage in an intensive cardiac rehabilitation program to additional conditions:

- Stable, chronic heart failure defined as patients with left ventricular ejection fraction of 35% or less and New York Heart Association (NYHA) class II to IV symptoms despite being on optimal heart failure therapy for at least 6 weeks; or
- Any additional condition for which the Secretary has determined that a cardiac rehabilitation program shall be covered, unless the Secretary determines, using the same process used to determine that the condition is covered for a cardiac rehabilitation program, that such coverage is not supported by the clinical evidence.

NOTE: CMS plans to amend our intensive cardiac rehabilitation regulations specified at 42 CFR 410.49 to reflect this expanded coverage. CMS anticipates that the changes will be included in the 2020 Medicare Physician Fee Schedule notice of proposed rulemaking. However, because the expanded coverage under the statutory change was effective on enactment, expanded coverage for these conditions will be made effective for services furnished on or after February 9, 2018.

CR/ICR Program Component Requirements:

- Physician-prescribed exercise. This physical activity includes aerobic exercise combined with other types of exercise (i.e., strengthening, stretching) as determined to be appropriate for individual patients by a physician each day CR/ICR items/services are furnished.
- Cardiac risk factor modification. This includes education, counseling, and behavioral intervention, tailored to the patients' individual needs.
- Psychosocial assessment. This assessment means an evaluation of an individual's mental and emotional functioning as it relates to the individual's rehabilitation. It should include: (1) an assessment of those aspects of the individual's family and home situation that affects the individual's rehabilitation treatment, and, (2) a psychosocial evaluation of the individual's response to, and rate of progress under, the treatment plan.
- Outcomes assessment. These should include: (i) minimally, assessments from the commencement and conclusion of CR/ICR, based on patient-centered outcomes which must be measured by the physician immediately at the beginning and end of the program, and, (ii) objective clinical measures of the effectiveness of the CR/ICR program for the individual patient, including exercise performance and self-reported measures of exertion and behavior.
- Individualized treatment plan. This plan should be written and tailored to each individual patient and include (i) a description of the individual's diagnosis; (ii) the type, amount, frequency, and duration of the CR/ICR items/services furnished; and (iii) the goals set for the individual under the plan. The individualized treatment plan must be established, reviewed, and signed by a physician every 30 days.

As specified at 42 CFR 410.49(f)(1), CR sessions are limited to a maximum of 2 1-hour sessions per day for up to 36 sessions over up to 36 weeks with the option for an additional 36 sessions over an extended period of time if approved by the contractor under section 1862(a)(1)(A) of the Act. ICR sessions are limited to 72 1-hour sessions (as defined in section 1848(b)(5) of the Act), up to 6 sessions per day, over a period of up to 18 weeks.

CR/ICR Program Setting Requirements:

CR/ICR services must be furnished in a physician's office or a hospital outpatient setting (for ICR, the hospital outpatient setting must provide ICR using an approved ICR program). All settings must have a physician immediately available and accessible for medical consultations and emergencies at all times when items/services are being furnished under the program. This provision is satisfied if the physician meets the requirements for direct supervision of physician office services as specified at 42 CFR 410.26, and for hospital outpatient services as specified at 42 CFR 410.27.

ICR Program Approval Requirements:

All prospective ICR programs must be approved through the national coverage determination (NCD) process. To be approved as an ICR program, it must demonstrate through peer-reviewed, published research that it has accomplished one or more of the following for its patients: (i) positively affected the progression of coronary heart disease, (ii) reduced the need for coronary bypass surgery, or, (iii) reduced the need for percutaneous coronary interventions.

An ICR program must also demonstrate through peer-reviewed, published research that it accomplished a statistically significant reduction in five or more of the following measures for patients from their levels before CR services to after CR services: (i) low density lipoprotein, (ii) triglycerides, (iii) body mass index, (iv) systolic blood pressure, (v) diastolic blood pressure, and (vi) the need for cholesterol, blood pressure, and diabetes medications.

A list of approved ICR programs, identified through the NCD process, will be posted to the CMS Web site and listed in the Federal Register.

Once an ICR program is approved through the NCD process, all prospective ICR sites wishing to furnish ICR items/services via an approved ICR program may enroll with their local contractor to become an ICR program supplier using the designated forms as specified at 42 CFR 424.510, and report specialty code 31 to be identified as an enrolled ICR supplier. For purposes of appealing an adverse determination concerning site approval, an ICR site is considered a supplier (or prospective supplier) as defined in 42 CFR 498.2.

CR/ICR Program Physician Requirements:

Physicians responsible for CR/ICR programs are identified as medical directors who oversee or supervise the CR/ICR program at a particular site. The medical director, in consultation with staff, is involved in directing the progress of individuals in the program. The medical director, as well as physicians acting as the supervising physician, must possess all of the following: (1) expertise in the management of individuals with cardiac pathophysiology, (2) cardiopulmonary training in basic life support or advanced cardiac life support, and (3) licensed to practice medicine in the state in which the CR/ICR program is offered. Direct physician supervision may be provided by a supervising physician or the medical director.

(See Pub. 100-3, Medicare National Coverage Determinations Manual, Chapter 1, Part 1, section 20.10.1, Pub. 100-4, Medicare Claims Processing Manual, Chapter 32, section 140, Pub. 100-08, Medicare Program Integrity Manual, Chapter 15, section 15.4.2.8, for specific claims processing, coding, and billing requirements for CR/ICR program services.)

100-02, 15, 240

Chiropractic Services - General

(Rev. 1, 10-01-03) B3-2250, B3-4118

The term "physician" under Part B includes a chiropractor who meets the specified qualifying requirements set forth in Sec.30.5 but only for treatment by means of manual manipulation of the spine to correct a subluxation.

Effective for claims with dates of services on or after January 1, 2000, an x-ray is not required to demonstrate the subluxation.

Implementation of the chiropractic benefit requires an appreciation of the differences between chiropractic theory and experience and traditional medicine due to fundamental differences regarding etiology and theories of the pathogenesis of disease. Judgments about the reasonableness of chiropractic treatment must be based on the application of chiropractic principles. So that Medicare beneficiaries receive equitable adjudication of claims based on such principles and are not deprived of the benefits intended by the law, carriers may use chiropractic consultation in carrier review of Medicare chiropractic claims.

Payment is based on the physician fee schedule and made to the beneficiary or, on assignment, to the chiropractor.

A. Verification of Chiropractor's Qualifications

Carriers must establish a reference file of chiropractors eligible for payment as physicians under the criteria in Sec.30.1. They pay only chiropractors on file. Information needed to establish such files is furnished by the CMS RO.

The RO is notified by the appropriate State agency which chiropractors are licensed and whether each meets the national uniform standards.

100-02, 15, 240.1.3

Necessity for Treatment

(Rev. 23, Issued: 10-08-04, Effective: 10-01-04, Implementation: 10-04-04)

The patient must have a significant health problem in the form of a neuromusculoskeletal condition necessitating treatment, and the manipulative services rendered must have a direct therapeutic relationship to the patient's condition and provide reasonable expectation of recovery or improvement of function. The patient must have a subluxation of the spine as demonstrated by x-ray or physical exam, as described above.

Most spinal joint problems fall into the following categories:

- Acute subluxation-A patient's condition is considered acute when the patient is being treated for a new injury, identified by x-ray or physical exam as specified above. The result of chiropractic manipulation is expected to be an improvement in, or arrest of progression, of the patient's condition.
- Chronic subluxation-A patient's condition is considered chronic when it is not expected to significantly improve or be resolved with further treatment (as is the case with an acute condition), but where the continued therapy can be expected to result in some functional improvement. Once the clinical status has remained stable for a given condition, without expectation of additional objective clinical improvements, further manipulative treatment is considered maintenance therapy and is not covered.

For Medicare purposes, a chiropractor must place an AT modifier on a claim when providing active/corrective treatment to treat acute or chronic subluxation. However the presence of the AT modifier may not in all instances indicate that the service is reasonable and necessary. As always, contractors may deny if appropriate after medical review.

A. Maintenance Therapy

Maintenance therapy includes services that seek to prevent disease, promote health and prolong and enhance the quality of life, or maintain or prevent deterioration of a chronic condition. When further clinical improvement cannot reasonably be expected from continuous ongoing care, and the chiropractic treatment becomes supportive rather than corrective in nature, the treatment is then considered maintenance therapy. The AT modifier must not be placed on the claim when maintenance therapy has been provided. Claims without the AT modifier will be considered as maintenance therapy and denied. Chiropractors who give or receive from beneficiaries an ABN shall follow the instructions in Pub. 100-4, Medicare Claims Processing Manual, chapter 23, section 20.9.1.1 and include a GA (or in rare instances a GZ) modifier on the claim.

B. Contraindications

Dynamic thrust is the therapeutic force or maneuver delivered by the physician during manipulation in the anatomic region of involvement. A relative contraindication is a condition that adds significant risk of injury to the patient from dynamic thrust, but does not rule out the use of dynamic thrust. The doctor should discuss this risk with the patient and record this in the chart. The following are relative contraindications to dynamic thrust:

- Articular hyper mobility and circumstances where the stability of the joint is uncertain;
- Severe demineralization of bone;
- Benign bone tumors (spine);
- Bleeding disorders and anticoagulant therapy; and
- Radiculopathy with progressive neurological signs.
- Dynamic thrust is absolutely contraindicated near the site of demonstrated subluxation and proposed manipulation in the following:
- Acute arthropathies characterized by acute inflammation and ligamentous laxity and anatomic subluxation or dislocation; including acute rheumatoid arthritis and ankylosing spondylitis;
- Acute fractures and dislocations or healed fractures and dislocations with signs of instability;
- An unstable os odontoideum;
- Malignancies that involve the vertebral column;
- Infection of bones or joints of the vertebral column;
- Signs and symptoms of myelopathy or cauda equina syndrome;
- For cervical spinal manipulations, vertebrobasilar insufficiency syndrome; and
- A significant major artery aneurysm near the proposed manipulation.

100-02, 15, 280.5.1

Advance Care Planning (ACP) Furnished as an Optional Element with an Annual Wellness Visit (AWV) Upon Agreement with the Patient

(Rev. 216 Issued: 12-22-15, Effective: 01-01-16, Implementation: 01-04-16)

Beginning in CY 2016, CMS will treat an AWV and voluntary ACP that are furnished on the same day and by the same provider as a preventive service. Voluntary ACP services, upon agreement with the patient, will be an optional element of the AWV. (See section 1861(hhh)(2)(G) of the Act.) When ACP services are furnished as a part of an AWV, according to sections 1833(a)(1) and 1833(b)(10) of the Act, the coinsurance and deductible are waived.

Voluntary advance care planning means the face-to-face service between a physician (or other qualified health care professional) and the patient discussing advance directives, with or without completing relevant legal forms. An advance directive is a document appointing an agent and/or recording the wishes of a patient pertaining to his/her medical treatment at a future time should he/she lack decisional capacity at that time.

See Pub. 100-04, *Medicare Claims Processing Manual*, chapter 18, section 140.8 for claims processing and billing instructions.

100-02, 15, 290

Foot Care

(Rev. 1, 10-01-03)

A. Treatment of Subluxation of Foot

Subluxations of the foot are defined as partial dislocations or displacements of joint surfaces, tendons ligaments, or muscles of the foot. Surgical or nonsurgical treatments undertaken for the sole purpose of correcting a subluxated structure in the foot as an isolated entity are not covered.

However, medical or surgical treatment of subluxation of the ankle joint (talo crural joint) is covered. In addition, reasonable and necessary medical or surgical services, diagnosis, or treatment for medical conditions that have resulted from or are associated with partial displacement of structures is covered. For example, if a patient has osteoarthritis that has resulted in a partial displacement of joints in the foot, and the primary treatment is for the osteoarthritis, coverage is provided.

B. Exclusions from Coverage

The following foot care services are generally excluded from coverage under both Part A and Part B. (See Sec. 290.F and Sec. 290.G for instructions on applying foot care exclusions.)

1. Treatment of Flat Foot

   The term "flat foot" is defined as a condition in which one or more arches of the foot have flattened out. Services or devices directed toward the care or correction of such conditions, including the prescription of supportive devices, are not covered.

2. Routine Foot Care

   Except as provided above, routine foot care is excluded from coverage. Services that normally are considered routine and not covered by Medicare include the following:

   — The cutting or removal of corns and calluses;

   — The trimming, cutting, clipping, or debriding of nails; and

   — Other hygienic and preventive maintenance care, such as cleaning and soaking the feet, the use of skin creams to maintain skin tone of either ambulatory or bedfast patients, and any other service performed in the absence of localized illness, injury, or symptoms involving the foot.

3. Supportive Devices for Feet Orthopedic shoes and other supportive devices for the feet generally are not covered.

   However, this exclusion does not apply to such a shoe if it is an integral part of a leg brace, and its expense is included as part of the cost of the brace. Also, this exclusion does not apply to therapeutic shoes furnished to diabetics.

C. Exceptions to Routine Foot Care Exclusion

1. Necessary and Integral Part of Otherwise Covered Services

   In certain circumstances, services ordinarily considered to be routine may be covered if they are performed as a necessary and integral part of otherwise covered services, such as diagnosis and treatment of ulcers, wounds, or infections.

2. Treatment of Warts on Foot

   The treatment of warts (including plantar warts) on the foot is covered to the same extent as services provided for the treatment of warts located elsewhere on the body.

3. Presence of Systemic Condition

   The presence of a systemic condition such as metabolic, neurologic, or peripheral vascular disease may require scrupulous foot care by a professional that in the absence of such condition(s) would be considered routine (and, therefore, excluded from coverage). Accordingly, foot care that would otherwise be considered routine may be covered when systemic condition(s) result in severe circulatory embarrassment or areas of diminished sensation in the individual's legs or feet. (See subsection A.)

   In these instances, certain foot care procedures that otherwise are considered routine (e.g., cutting or removing corns and calluses, or trimming, cutting, clipping, or debriding nails) may pose a hazard when performed by a nonprofessional person on patients with such systemic conditions. (See Sec.290.G for procedural instructions.)

4. Mycotic Nails

   In the absence of a systemic condition, treatment of mycotic nails may be covered.

The treatment of mycotic nails for an ambulatory patient is covered only when the physician attending the patient's mycotic condition documents that (1) there is clinical evidence of mycosis of the toenail, and (2) the patient has marked limitation of ambulation, pain, or secondary infection resulting from the thickening and dystrophy of the infected toenail plate.

The treatment of mycotic nails for a nonambulatory patient is covered only when the physician attending the patient's mycotic condition documents that (1) there is clinical evidence of mycosis of the toenail, and (2) the patient suffers from pain or secondary infection resulting from the thickening and dystrophy of the infected toenail plate.

For the purpose of these requirements, documentation means any written information that is required by the carrier in order for services to be covered. Thus, the information submitted with claims must be substantiated by information found in the patient's medical record. Any information, including that contained in a form letter, used for documentation purposes is subject to carrier verification in order to ensure that the information adequately justifies coverage of the treatment of mycotic nails.

D. Systemic Conditions That Might Justify Coverage

Although not intended as a comprehensive list, the following metabolic, neurologic, and peripheral vascular diseases (with synonyms in parentheses) most commonly represent the underlying conditions that might justify coverage for routine foot care.

Diabetes mellitus *

Arteriosclerosis obliterans (A.S.O., arteriosclerosis of the extremities, occlusive peripheral arteriosclerosis)

Buerger's disease (thromboangiitis obliterans)

Chronic thrombophlebitis *

Peripheral neuropathies involving the feet -

- — Associated with malnutrition and vitamin deficiency *
  - Malnutrition (general, pellagra)
  - Alcoholism
  - Malabsorption (celiac disease, tropical sprue)
  - Pernicious anemia Associated with carcinoma *
- — Associated with diabetes mellitus *
- — Associated with drugs and toxins *
- — Associated with multiple sclerosis *
- — Associated with uremia (chronic renal disease) *
- — Associated with traumatic injury
- — Associated with leprosy or neurosyphilis
- — Associated with hereditary disorders
  - Hereditary sensory radicular neuropathy
  - Angiokeratoma corporis diffusum (Fabry's)
  - Amyloid neuropathy

When the patient's condition is one of those designated by an asterisk (*), routine procedures are covered only if the patient is under the active care of a doctor of medicine or osteopathy who documents the condition.

E. Supportive Devices for Feet Orthopedic shoes and other supportive devices for the feet generally are not covered.

However, this exclusion does not apply to such a shoe if it is an integral part of a leg brace, and its expense is included as part of the cost of the brace. Also, this exclusion does not apply to therapeutic shoes furnished to diabetics.

F. Presumption of Coverage

In evaluating whether the routine services can be reimbursed, a presumption of coverage may be made where the evidence available discloses certain physical and/or clinical findings consistent with the diagnosis and indicative of severe peripheral involvement.

For purposes of applying this presumption the following findings are pertinent:

Class A Findings
Nontraumatic amputation of foot or integral skeletal portion thereof.

Class B Findings
Absent posterior tibial pulse;

Advanced trophic changes as: hair growth (decrease or absence) nail changes (thickening) pigmentary changes (discoloration) skin texture (thin, shiny) skin color (rubor or redness) (Three required); and

Absent dorsalis pedis pulse.

Class C Findings
Claudication;

Temperature changes (e.g., cold feet);

Edema;

Paresthesias (abnormal spontaneous sensations in the feet); and

Burning.

The presumption of coverage may be applied when the physician rendering the routine foot care has identified:

1. A Class A finding;
2. Two of the Class B findings; or
3. One Class B and two Class C findings.

Cases evidencing findings falling short of these alternatives may involve podiatric treatment that may constitute covered care and should be reviewed by the intermediary's medical staff and developed as necessary.

For purposes of applying the coverage presumption where the routine services have been rendered by a podiatrist, the contractor may deem the active care requirement met if the claim or other evidence available discloses that the patient has seen an M.D. or D.O. for treatment and/or evaluation of the complicating disease process during the 6-month period prior to the rendition of the routine-type services. The intermediary may also accept the podiatrist's statement that the diagnosing and treating M.D. or D.O. also concurs with the podiatrist's findings as to the severity of the peripheral involvement indicated.

Services ordinarily considered routine might also be covered if they are performed as a necessary and integral part of otherwise covered services, such as diagnosis and treatment of diabetic ulcers, wounds, and infections.

G. Application of Foot Care Exclusions to Physician's Services

The exclusion of foot care is determined by the nature of the service. Thus, payment for an excluded service should be denied whether performed by a podiatrist, osteopath, or a doctor of medicine, and without regard to the difficulty or complexity of the procedure.

When an itemized bill shows both covered services and noncovered services not integrally related to the covered service, the portion of charges attributable to the noncovered services should be denied. (For example, if an itemized bill shows surgery for an ingrown toenail and also removal of calluses not necessary for the performance of toe surgery, any additional charge attributable to removal of the calluses should be denied.) In reviewing claims involving foot care, the carrier should be alert to the following exceptional situations:

1. Payment may be made for incidental noncovered services performed as a necessary and integral part of, and secondary to, a covered procedure. For example, if trimming of toenails is required for application of a cast to a fractured foot, the carrier need not allocate and deny a portion of the charge for the trimming of the nails. However, a separately itemized charge for such excluded service should be disallowed. When the primary procedure is covered the administration of anesthesia necessary for the performance of such procedure is also covered.
2. Payment may be made for initial diagnostic services performed in connection with a specific symptom or complaint if it seems likely that its treatment would be covered even though the resulting diagnosis may be one requiring only noncovered care.

The name of the M.D. or D.O. who diagnosed the complicating condition must be submitted with the claim. In those cases, where active care is required, the approximate date the beneficiary was last seen by such physician must also be indicated.

NOTE: Section 939 of P.L. 96-499 removed "warts" from the routine foot care exclusion effective July 1, 1981.

Relatively few claims for routine-type care are anticipated considering the severity of conditions contemplated as the basis for this exception. Claims for this type of foot care should not be paid in the absence of convincing evidence that nonprofessional performance of the service would have been hazardous for the beneficiary because of an underlying systemic disease. The mere statement of a diagnosis such as those mentioned in Sec.D above does not of itself indicate the severity of the condition. Where development is indicated to verify diagnosis and/or severity the carrier should follow existing claims processing practices, which may include review of carrier's history and medical consultation as well as physician contacts.

The rules in Sec.290.F concerning presumption of coverage also apply.

Codes and policies for routine foot care and supportive devices for the feet are not exclusively for the use of podiatrists. These codes must be used to report foot care services regardless of the specialty of the physician who furnishes the services. Carriers must instruct physicians to use the most appropriate code available when billing for routine foot care.

100-02, 16, 10

General Exclusions From Coverage

(Rev. 1, 10-01-03) A3-3150, HO-260, HHA-232, B3-2300

No payment can be made under either the hospital insurance or supplementary medicalinsurance program for certain items and services, when the following conditions exist:

- Not reasonable and necessary (§20);
- No legal obligation to pay for or provide (§40);
- Paid for by a governmental entity (§50);
- Not provided within United States (§60);
- Resulting from war (§70);

- Personal comfort (§80);
- Routine services and appliances (§90);
- Custodial care (§110);
- Cosmetic surgery (§120);
- Charges by immediate relatives or members of household (§130);
- Dental services (§140);
- Paid or expected to be paid under workers' compensation (§150);
- Nonphysician services provided to a hospital inpatient that were not provided directly or arranged for by the hospital (§170);
- Services Related to and Required as a Result of Services Which are not Covered Under Medicare (§180);
- Excluded foot care services and supportive devices for feet (§30); or
- Excluded investigational devices (See Chapter 14, §30).

100-02, 16, 100

Hearing Aids and Auditory Implants

(Rev. 39; Issued: 11-10-05; Effective: 11-10-05; Implementation: 12-12-05)

Section 1862(a)(7) of the Social Security Act states that no payment may be made under part A or part B for any expenses incurred for items or services "where such expenses are for . . . hearing aids or examinations therefore. . . ." This policy is further reiterated at 42 CFR 411.15(d) which specifically states that "hearing aids or examination for the purpose of prescribing, fitting, or changing hearing aids" are excluded from coverage.

Hearing aids are amplifying devices that compensate for impaired hearing. Hearing aids include air conduction devices that provide acoustic energy to the cochlea via stimulation of the tympanic membrane with amplified sound. They also include bone conduction devices that provide mechanical energy to the cochlea via stimulation of the scalp with amplified mechanical vibration or by direct contact with the tympanic membrane or middle ear ossicles.

Certain devices that produce perception of sound by replacing the function of the middle ear, cochlea or auditory nerve are payable by Medicare as prosthetic devices. These devices are indicated only when hearing aids are medically inappropriate or cannot be utilized due to congenital malformations, chronic disease, severe sensorineural hearing loss or surgery. The following are prosthetic devices:

- Cochlear implants and auditory brainstem implants, i.e., devices that replace the function of cochlear structures or auditory nerve and provide electrical energy to auditory nerve fibers and other neural tissue via implanted electrode arrays.
- Osseointegrated implants, i.e., devices implanted in the skull that replace the function of the middle ear and provide mechanical energy to the cochlea via a mechanical transducer.

Medicare contractors deny payment for an item or service that is associated with any hearing aid as defined above. See Sec.180 for policy for the medically necessary treatment of complications of implantable hearing aids, such as medically necessary removals of implantable hearing aids due to infection.

100-02, 16, 120

Cosmetic Surgery

(Rev. 1, 10-01-03) A3-3160, HO-260.11, B3-2329

Cosmetic surgery or expenses incurred in connection with such surgery is not covered. Cosmetic surgery includes any surgical procedure directed at improving appearance, except when required for the prompt (i.e., as soon as medically feasible) repair of accidental injury or for the improvement of the functioning of a malformed body member. For example, this exclusion does not apply to surgery in connection with treatment of severe burns or repair of the face following a serious automobile accident, or to surgery for therapeutic purposes which coincidentally also serves some cosmetic purpose.

100-02, 16, 180

Services Related to and Required as a Result of Services Which Are Not Covered Under Medicare

(Rev. 1, 10-03-03) B3-2300.1, A3-3101.14, HO-210.12

Medical and hospital services are sometimes required to treat a condition that arises as a result of services that are not covered because they are determined to be not reasonable and necessary or because they are excluded from coverage for other reasons. Services "related to" noncovered services (e.g., cosmetic surgery, noncovered organ transplants, noncovered artificial organ implants, etc.), including services related to follow-up care and complications of noncovered services which require treatment during a hospital stay in which the noncovered service was performed, are not covered services under Medicare. Services "not related to" noncovered services are covered under Medicare. Following are examples of services "related to" and "not related to" noncovered services while the beneficiary is an inpatient:

- A beneficiary was hospitalized for a noncovered service and broke a leg while in the hospital. Services related to care of the broken leg during this stay is a clear example of "not related to" services and are covered under Medicare.
- A beneficiary was admitted to the hospital for covered services, but during the course of hospitalization became a candidate for a noncovered transplant or implant and actually received the transplant or implant during that hospital stay. When the original admission was entirely unrelated to the diagnosis that led to a recommendation for a noncovered transplant or implant, the services related to the admitting condition would be covered.
- A beneficiary was admitted to the hospital for covered services related to a condition which ultimately led to identification of a need for transplant and receipt of a transplant during the same hospital stay. If, on the basis of the nature of the services and a comparison of the date they are received with the date on which the beneficiary is identified as a transplant candidate, the services could reasonably be attributed to preparation for the noncovered transplant, the services would be "related to" noncovered services and would also be noncovered.

Following is an example of services received subsequent to a noncovered inpatient stay:

- After a beneficiary has been discharged from the hospital stay in which the beneficiary received noncovered services, medical and hospital services required to treat a condition or complication that arises as a result of the prior noncovered services may be covered when they are reasonable and necessary in all other respects. Thus, coverage could be provided for subsequent inpatient stays or outpatient treatment ordinarily covered by Medicare, even if the need for treatment arose because of a previous noncovered procedure. Some examples of services that may be found to be covered under this policy are the reversal of intestinal bypass surgery for obesity, repair of complications from transsexual surgery or from cosmetic surgery, removal of a noncovered bladder stimulator, or treatment of any infection at the surgical site of a noncovered transplant that occurred following discharge from the hospital.

However, any subsequent services that could be expected to have been incorporated into a global fee are considered to have been paid in the global fee, and may not be paid again. Thus, where a patient undergoes cosmetic surgery and the treatment regimen calls for a series of postoperative visits to the surgeon for evaluating the patient's progress, these visits are not paid.

100-03, 10.2

NCD for Transcutaneous Electrical Nerve Stimulation (TENS) for Acute Post-Operative Pain (10.2)

(Rev. 173, Issued: 9-4-14, Effective: With Implementation I-10)

Indications and Limitations of Coverage

The use of Transcutaneous Electrical Nerve Stimulation (TENS) for the relief of acute post-operative pain is covered under Medicare. TENS may be covered whether used as an adjunct to the use of drugs, or as an alternative to drugs, in the treatment of acute pain resulting from surgery.

TENS devices, whether durable or disposable, may be used in furnishing this service. When used for the purpose of treating acute post-operative pain, TENS devices are considered supplies. As such they may be hospital supplies furnished inpatients covered under Part A, or supplies incident to a physician's service when furnished in connection with surgery done on an outpatient basis, and covered under Part B.

It is expected that TENS, when used for acute post-operative pain, will be necessary for relatively short periods of time, usually 30 days or less. In cases when TENS is used for longer periods, Medicare Administrative Contractors should attempt to ascertain whether TENS is no longer being used for acute pain but rather for chronic pain, in which case the TENS device may be covered as durable medical equipment as described in §160.27.

Cross-references: Medicare Benefit Policy Manual, Chapter 1, "Inpatient Hospital Services," §40; Medicare Benefit Policy Manual, Chapter 2, "Hospital Services Covered Under Part B," §§20, 20.4, and 80; Medicare Benefit Policy Manual, Chapter 15, "Covered Medical and other Health Services, §110."

100-03, 10.3

NCD for Inpatient Hospital Pain Rehabilitation Programs (10.3)

(Rev. 1, 10-03-03)

Since pain rehabilitation programs of a lesser scope than that described above would raise a question as to whether the program could be provided in a less intensive setting than on an inpatient hospital basis, carefully evaluate such programs to determine whether the program does, in fact, necessitate a hospital level of care. Some pain rehabilitation programs may utilize services and devices which are excluded from coverage, e.g., acupuncture (see 35-8), biofeedback (see 35-27), dorsal column stimulator (see 65-8), and family counseling services (see 35-I4). In determining whether the scope of a pain program does necessitate inpatient hospital care, evaluate only those services and devices which are covered. Although diagnostic tests may be an appropriate part of pain rehabilitation programs, such tests would be covered in an individual case only where they can be reasonably related to a patient's illness, complaint, symptom, or injury and where they do not represent an unnecessary duplication of tests previously performed.

An inpatient program of 4 weeks' duration is generally required to modify pain behavior. After this period it would be expected that any additional rehabilitation services which might be required could be effectively provided on an outpatient basis under an outpatient pain rehabilitation program (see 10.4 of the NCD Manual) or other outpatient program. The first 7-l0 days of such an inpatient program constitute, in effect, an evaluation period. If a patient is unable to adjust to the program within this period, it is generally concluded that it is unlikely that the program will be effective and the patient is discharged from the program. On occasions a program longer than 4 weeks may be required in a particular case. In such a case there should be documentation to substantiate that inpatient care beyond a 4-week period was reasonable and necessary. Similarly, where it appears that a patient participating in a program is being granted frequent outside passes, a question would exist as to whether an inpatient program is reasonable and necessary for the treatment of the patient's condition.

An inpatient hospital stay for the purpose of participating in a pain rehabilitation program would be covered as reasonable and necessary to the treatment of a patient's condition where the pain is attributable to a physical cause, the usual methods of treatment have not been successful in alleviating it, and a significant loss of ability to function independently has resulted from the pain. Chronic pain patients often have psychological problems which accompany or stem from the physical pain and it is appropriate to include psychological treatment in the multidisciplinary approach. However, patients whose pain symptoms result from a mental condition, rather than from any physical cause, generally cannot be succesfully treated in a pain rehabilitation program.

100-03, 10.4

NCD for Outpatient Hospital Pain Rehabilitation Programs (10.4)

(Rev. 173, Issued: 9-4-14, Effective: With Implementation I-10)

Coverage of services furnished under outpatient hospital pain rehabilitation programs, including services furnished in group settings under individualized plans of treatment, is available if the patient's pain is attributable to a physical cause, the usual methods of treatment have not been successful in alleviating it, and a significant loss of ability by the patient to function independently has resulted from the pain. If a patient meets these conditions and the program provides services of the types discussed in §10.3, the services provided under the program may be covered. Non-covered services (e.g., vocational counseling, meals for outpatients, or acupuncture) continue to be excluded from coverage, and A/B Medicare Administrative Contractors would not be precluded from finding, in the case of particular patients, that the pain rehabilitation program is not reasonable and necessary under §1862(a)(1) of the Social Security Act for the treatment of their conditions.

100-03, 10.5

NCD for Autogenous Epidural Blood Graft (10.5)

(Rev. 1, 10-03-03)

Autogenous epidural blood grafts are considered a safe and effective remedy for severe headaches that may occur after performance of spinal anesthesia, spinal taps or myelograms, and are covered.

100-03, 10.6

NCD for Anesthesia in Cardiac Pacemaker Surgery (10.6)

(Rev. 173, Issued: 9-4-14, Effective: With Implementation I-10)

The use of general or monitored anesthesia during transvenous cardiac pacemaker surgery may be reasonable and necessary and therefore covered under Medicare only if adequate documentation of medical necessity is provided on a case-by-case basis. The Medicare Adminstrative Contractor obtains advice from its medical consultants or from appropriate specialty physicians or groups in its locality regarding the adequacy of documentation before deciding whether a particular claim should be covered.

A second type of pacemaker surgery that is sometimes performed involves the use of the thoracic method of implantation which requires open surgery. Where the thoracic method is employed, general anesthesia is always used and should not require special medical documentation.

100-03, 20.2

NCD for Extracranial-Intracranial (EC-IC) Arterial Bypass Surgery (20.2)

(Rev. 1, 10-03-03)

Extracranial-Intracranial (EC-IC) arterial bypass surgery is not a covered procedure when it is performed as a treatment for ischemic cerebrovascular disease of the carotid or middle cerebral arteries which includes the treatment or prevention of strokes. The premise that this procedure which bypasses narrowed arterial segments, improves the blood supply to the brain and reduces the risk of having a stroke has not been demonstrated to be any more effective than no surgical intervention. Accordingly, EC-IC arterial bypass surgery is not considered reasonable and necessary within the meaning of §1862(a)(1) of the Act when it is performed as a treatment for ischemic cerebrovascular disease of the carotid or middle cerebral arteries.

100-03, 20.8.4

Leadless Pacemakers

(Rev. 201, Issued: 07-28-17, Effective: 01-18-18, Implementation: 08-29-17- for MAC local edits; January 2, 2018 - for MCS shared edits)

A. General

The leadless pacemaker eliminates the need for a device pocket and insertion of a pacing lead which are integral elements of traditional pacing systems. The removal of these elements eliminate an important source of complications associated with traditional pacing systems while providing similar benefits. Leadless pacemakers are delivered via catheter to the heart, and function similarly to other transvenous single-chamber ventricular pacemakers.

B. Nationally Covered Indications

Effective January 18, 2017, the Centers for Medicare & Medicaid Services (CMS) covers leadless pacemakers through Coverage with Evidence Development (CED). CMS covers leadless pacemakers when procedures are performed in Food and Drug Administration (FDA) approved studies. CMS also covers, in prospective longitudinal studies, leadless pacemakers that are used in accordance with the FDA approved label for devices that have either:

- an associated ongoing FDA approved post-approval study; or
- completed an FDA post-approval study.

Each study must be approved by CMS and as a fully-described, written part of its protocol, must address the following research questions:

- What are the peri-procedural and post-procedural complications of leadless pacemakers?
- What are the long term outcomes of leadless pacemakers?
- What are the effects of patient characteristics (age, gender, comorbidities) on the use and health effects of leadless pacemakers?

CMS will review studies to determine if they meet the 13 criteria listed below. If CMS determines that they meet these criteria, the study will be posted on CMS' CED website (https://www.cms.gov/Medicare/Coverage/Coverage-with-Evidence-Development/index.html).

a. The principal purpose of the study is to test whether the item or service meaningfully improves health outcomes of affected beneficiaries who are represented by the enrolled subjects.

b. The rationale for the study is well supported by available scientific and medical evidence.

c. The study results are not anticipated to unjustifiably duplicate existing knowledge.

d. The study design is methodologically appropriate and the anticipated number of enrolled subjects is sufficient to answer the research question(s) being asked in the National Coverage Determination.

e. The study is sponsored by an organization or individual capable of completing it successfully.

f. The research study is in compliance with all applicable Federal regulations concerning the protection of human subjects found in the Code of Federal Regulations (CFR) at 45 CFR Part 46. If a study is regulated by the Food and Drug Administration (FDA), it is also in compliance with 21 CFR Parts 50 and 56. In addition, to further enhance the protection of human subjects in studies conducted under CED, the study must provide and obtain meaningful informed consent from patients regarding the risks associated with the study items and/or services, and the use and eventual disposition of the collected data.

g. All aspects of the study are conducted according to appropriate standards of scientific integrity.

h. The study has a written protocol that clearly demonstrates adherence to the standards listed here as Medicare requirements.

i. The study is not designed to exclusively test toxicity or disease pathophysiology in healthy individuals. Such studies may meet this requirement only if the disease or condition being studied is life threatening as defined in 21 CFR §312.81(a) and the patient has no other viable treatment options.

j. The clinical research studies and registries are registered on the www.ClinicalTrials.gov website by the principal sponsor/investigator prior to the enrollment of the first study subject. Registries are also registered in the Agency for Healthcare Research and Quality (AHRQ) Registry of Patient Registries (RoPR).

k. The research study protocol specifies the method and timing of public release of all prespecified outcomes to be measured including release of outcomes if outcomes are negative or study is terminated early. The results must be made public within 12 months of the study's primary completion date, which is the date the final subject had final data collection for the primary endpoint, even if the trial does not achieve its primary aim. The results must include number started/completed, summary results for primary and secondary outcome measures, statistical analyses, and adverse events. Final results must be reported in a publicly accessibly manner; either in a peer-reviewed scientific journal (in print or on-line), in an on-line publicly accessible registry dedicated to the dissemination of clinical trial information such as ClinicalTrials.gov, or in journals willing to publish in abbreviated format (e.g., for studies with negative or incomplete results).

l. The study protocol must explicitly discuss beneficiary subpopulations affected by the item or service under investigation, particularly traditionally underrepresented groups in clinical studies, how the inclusion and exclusion criteria effect enrollment of these populations, and a plan for the retention and reporting of said populations in the trial. If the inclusion and exclusion criteria are expected to have a negative effect on the recruitment or retention of underrepresented populations, the protocol must discuss why these criteria are necessary.

m. The study protocol explicitly discusses how the results are or are not expected to be generalizable to affected beneficiary subpopulations. Separate discussions in the protocol may be necessary for populations eligible for Medicare due to age, disability or Medicaid eligibility.

Consistent with section 1142 of the Act, the Agency for Healthcare Research and Quality (AHRQ) supports clinical research studies that CMS determines meet the above-listed standards and address the above-listed research questions.

All clinical research study protocols must be reviewed and approved by CMS. The principal investigator must submit the complete study protocol, identify the relevant CMS research question(s) that will be addressed and cite the location of the detailed analysis plan for those questions in the protocol, plus provide a statement addressing how the study satisfies each of the standards of scientific integrity (a. through m. listed above), as well as the investigator's contact information, to the address below. The information will be reviewed, and approved studies will be identified on the CMS website.

Director, Coverage and Analysis Group
Re: Leadless Pacemakers CED
Centers for Medicare & Medicaid Services (CMS)
7500 Security Blvd., Mail Stop S3-02-01
Baltimore, MD 21244-1850

Email address for protocol submissions: clinicalstudynotification@cms.hhs.gov

Email subject line: "CED [NCD topic (i.e. Leadless Pacemakers)] [name of sponsor/primary investigator]"

C. Nationally Non-Covered Indications

Leadless pacemakers are non-covered when furnished outside of a CMS approved CED study.

D. Other

NA

100-03, 20.9

Artificial Hearts and Related Devices (Various Effective Dates Below)

(Rev.172, Issued: 08-29-14, Effective:10-30-13, Implementation: 09- 30-14)

A. General

An artificial heart is a biventricular replacement device which requires removal of a substantial part of the native heart, including both ventricles. Removal of this device is not compatible with life, unless the patient has a heart transplant.

B. Nationally Covered Indications

1. Bridge-to-transplant (BTT) (effective for services performed on or after May 1, 2008)

   An artificial heart for bridge-to-transplantation (BTT) is covered when performed under coverage with evidence development (CED) when a clinical study meets all of the criteria listed below. The clinical study must address at least one of the following questions:

   — Were there unique circumstances such as expertise available in a particular facility or an unusual combination of conditions in particular patients that affected their outcomes?

   — What will be the average time to device failure when the device is made available to larger numbers of patients?

   — Do results adequately give a reasonable indication of the full range of outcomes (both positive and negative) that might be expected from more widespread use?

   The clinical study must meet all of the criteria stated in Section D of this policy. The above information should be mailed to: Director, Coverage and Analysis Group, Centers for Medicare & Medicaid Services (CMS), Re: Artificial Heart, Mailstop S3-02-01, 7500 Security Blvd, Baltimore, MD 21244-1850.

   Clinical studies that are determined by CMS to meet the above requirements will be listed on the CMS Web site at: http://www.cms.gov/Medicare/Coverage/Coverage-with-Evidence-Development/Artificial-Hearts.html.

2. Destination therapy (DT) (effective for services performed on or after May 1, 2008)

   An artificial heart for destination therapy (DT) is covered when performed under CED when a clinical study meets all of the criteria listed below. The clinical study must address at least one of the following questions:

   — Were there unique circumstances such as expertise available in a particular facility or an unusual combination of conditions in particular patients that affected their outcomes?

   — What will be the average time to device failure when the device is made available to larger numbers of patients?

   — Do results adequately give a reasonable indication of the full range of outcomes (both positive and negative) that might be expected from more widespread use?

The clinical study must meet all of the criteria stated in Section D of this policy. The above information should be mailed to: Director, Coverage and Analysis Group, Centers for Medicare & Medicaid Services, Re: Artificial Heart, Mailstop S3-02-01, 7500 Security Blvd, Baltimore, MD 21244-1850.

Clinical studies that are determined by CMS to meet the above requirements will be listed on the CMS Web site at: http://www.cms.gov/Medicare/Coverage/Coverage-with-Evidence-Development/Artificial-Hearts.html.

C. Nationally Non-Covered Indications

All other indications for the use of artificial hearts not otherwise listed remain non-covered, except in the context of Category B investigational device exemption clinical trials (42 CFR 405) or as a routine cost in clinical trials defined under section 310.1 of the National Coverage Determinations (NCD) Manual.

D. Other

Clinical study criteria:

- The study must be reviewed and approved by the Food and Drug Administration (FDA).
- The principal purpose of the research study is to test whether a particular intervention potentially improves the participants' health outcomes.
- The research study is well supported by available scientific and medical information, or it is intended to clarify or establish the health outcomes of interventions already in common clinical use.
- The research study does not unjustifiably duplicate existing studies.
- The research study design is appropriate to answer the research question being asked in the study.
- The research study is sponsored by an organization or individual capable of executing the proposed study successfully.
- The research study is in compliance with all applicable Federal regulations concerning the protection of human subjects found at 45 CFR Part 46. If a study is FDA-regulated it also must be in compliance with 21 CFR Parts 50 and 56.
- All aspects of the research study are conducted according to appropriate standards of scientific integrity (see http://www.icmje.org).
- The research study has a written protocol that clearly addresses, or incorporates by reference, the standards listed here as Medicare requirements for CED.
- The clinical research study is not designed to exclusively test toxicity or disease pathophysiology in healthy individuals. Trials of all medical technologies measuring therapeutic outcomes as one of the objectives meet this standard only if the disease or condition being studied is life threatening as defined in 21 CFR §312.81(a) and the patient has no other viable treatment options.
- The clinical research study is registered on the www.ClinicalTrials.gov Web site by the principal sponsor/investigator as demonstrated by having a Clinicaltrials.gov Identifier.
- The research study protocol specifies the method and timing of public release of all pre-specified outcomes to be measured including release of outcomes if outcomes are negative or study is terminated early. The results must be made public within 24 months of the end of data collection. If a report is planned to be published in a peer-reviewed journal, then that initial release may be an abstract that meets the requirements of the International Committee of Medical Journal Editors (ICMJE) (http://www.icmje.org). However a full report of the outcomes must be made public no later than three (3) years after the end of data collection.
- The research study protocol must explicitly discuss subpopulations affected by the treatment under investigation, particularly traditionally under-represented groups in clinical studies, how the inclusion and exclusion criteria effect enrollment of these populations, and a plan for the retention and reporting of said populations in the trial. If the inclusion and exclusion criteria are expected to have a negative effect on the recruitment or retention of under-represented populations, the protocol must discuss why these criteria are necessary.
- The research study protocol explicitly discusses how the results are or are not expected to be generalizable to the Medicare population to infer whether Medicare patients may benefit from the intervention. Separate discussions in the protocol may be necessary for populations eligible for Medicare due to age, disability, or Medicaid eligibility.

Consistent with section 1142 of the Social Security Act (the Act), the Agency for Healthcare Research and Quality (AHRQ) supports clinical research studies that CMS determines meet the above-listed standards and address the above-listed research questions.

The principal investigator of an artificial heart clinical study seeking Medicare payment should submit the following documentation to CMS and should expect to be notified when the CMS review is complete:

- Complete study protocol (must be dated or identified with a version number);
- Protocol summary;
- Statement that the submitted protocol version has been agreed upon by the FDA;

- Statement that the above study standards are met;
- Statement that the study addresses at least one of the above questions related to artificial hearts;
- Complete contact information (phone number, email address, and mailing address); and,
- Clinicaltrials.gov Identifier.

100-03, 20.9.1

Ventricular Assist Devices (Various Effective Dates Below)

(Rev.172, Issued: 08-29-14, Effective: 10-30-13, Implementation: 09- 30-14)

A. General

A ventricular assist device (VAD) is surgically attached to one or both intact ventricles and is used to assist or augment the ability of a damaged or weakened native heart to pump blood. Improvement in the performance of the native heart may allow the device to be removed.

B. Nationally Covered Indications

1. Post-cardiotomy (effective for services performed on or after October 18, 1993) Post-cardiotomy is the period following open-heart surgery. VADs used for support of blood circulation post-cardiotomy are covered only if they have received approval from the Food and Drug Administration (FDA) for that purpose, and the VADs are used according to the FDA-approved labeling instructions.
2. Bridge-to-Transplant (effective for services performed on or after January 22, 1996)

   The VADs used for bridge to transplant are covered only if they have received approval from the FDA for that purpose, and the VADs are used according to FDA-approved labeling instructions. All of the following criteria must be fulfilled in order for Medicare coverage to be provided for a VAD used as a bridge to transplant:

   — The patient is approved for heart transplantation by a Medicare-approved heart transplant center and is active on the Organ Procurement and Transplantation Network (OPTN) heart transplant waitlist.

   — The implanting site, if different than the Medicare-approved transplant center, must receive written permission from the Medicare-approved transplant center under which the patient is listed prior to implantation of the VAD.
3. Destination Therapy (DT) (effective for services performed on or after October 1, 2003)

   Destination therapy (DT) is for patients that require mechanical cardiac support. The VADs used for DT are covered only if they have received approval from the FDA for that purpose.

   Patient Selection (effective November 9, 2010):

   The VADs are covered for patients who have chronic end-stage heart failure (New York Heart Association Class IV end-stage left ventricular failure) who are not candidates for heart transplantation at the time of VAD implant, and meet the following conditions:Have failed to respond to optimal medical management (including beta-blockers and ACE inhibitors if tolerated) for 45 of the last 60 days, or have been balloon pump-dependent for 7 days, or IV inotrope-dependent for 14 days; and,

   — Have a left ventricular ejection fraction (LVEF) <25%; and,

   — Have demonstrated functional limitation with a peak oxygen consumption of =14 ml/kg/min unless balloon pump- or inotrope-dependent or physically unable to perform the test. Facility Criteria (effective October 30, 2013):

   Facilities currently credentialed by the Joint Commission for placement of VADs as DT may continue as Medicare-approved facilities until October 30, 2014. At the conclusion of this transition period, these facilities must be in compliance with the following criteria as determined by a credentialing organization. As of the effective date, new facilities must meet the following criteria as a condition of coverage of this procedure as DT under section 1862(a)(1)(A) of the Social Security Act (the Act):

   Beneficiaries receiving VADs for DT must be managed by an explicitly identified cohesive, multidisciplinary team of medical professionals with the appropriate qualifications, training, and experience. The team embodies collaboration and dedication across medical specialties to offer optimal patient-centered care. Collectively, the team must ensure that patients and caregivers have the knowledge and support necessary to participate in shared decision making and to provide appropriate informed consent. The team members must be based at the facility and must include individuals with experience working with patients before and after placement of a VAD.

   The team must include, at a minimum:

   – At least one physician with cardiothoracic surgery privileges and individual experience implanting at least 10 durable, intracorporeal, left VADs as BTT or DT over the course of the previous 36 months with activity in the last year.

   – At least one cardiologist trained in advanced heart failure with clinical competence in medical and device-based management including VADs, and clinical competence in the management of patients before and after heart transplant.

   – A VAD program coordinator.

   – A social worker.

   – A palliative care specialist. Facilities must be credentialed by an organization approved by the Centers for Medicare & Medicaid Services.

C. Nationally Non-Covered Indications

All other indications for the use of VADs not otherwise listed remain non-covered, except in the context of Category B investigational device exemption clinical trials (42 CFR 405) or as a routine cost in clinical trials defined under section 310.1 of the National Coverage Determinations (NCD) Manual.

D. Other

This policy does not address coverage of VADs for right ventricular support, biventricular support, use in beneficiaries under the age of 18, use in beneficiaries with complex congenital heart disease, or use in beneficiaries with acute heart failure without a history of chronic heart failure. Coverage under section 1862(a)(1)(A) of the Act for VADs in these situations will be made by local Medicare Administrative Contractors within their respective jurisdictions.

100-03, 20.12

NCD for Diagnostic Endocardial Electrical Stimulation (Pacing) (20.12)

(Rev. 1, 10-03-03)

Diagnostic endocardial electrical stimulation (EES), also called programmed electrical stimulation of the heart, is covered under Medicare when used for patients with severe cardiac arrhythmias.

100-03, 20.19

NCD for Ambulatory Blood Pressure Monitoring (20.19)

(Rev. 1, 10-03-03)

ABPM must be performed for at least 24 hours to meet coverage criteria.

ABPM is only covered for those patients with suspected white coat hypertension. Suspected white coat hypertension is defined as

1) office blood pressure > 140/90 mm Hg on at least three separate clinic/office visits with two separate measurements made at each visit;
2) at least two documented blood pressure measurements taken outside the office which are < 140/90 mm Hg; and
3) no evidence of end-organ damage.

The information obtained by ABPM is necessary in order to determine the appropriate management of the patient. ABPM is not covered for any other uses. In the rare circumstance that ABPM needs to be performed more than once in a patient, the qualifying criteria described above must be met for each subsequent ABPM test.

For those patients that undergo ABPM and have an ambulatory blood pressure of < 135/85 with no evidence of end-organ damage, it is likely that their cardiovascular risk is similar to that of normotensives. They should be followed over time. Patients for which ABPM demonstrates a blood pressure of > 135/85 may be at increased cardiovascular risk, and a physician may wish to consider antihypertensive therapy.

100-03, 20.26

NCD for Partial Ventriculectomy (20.26)

(Rev. 1, 10-03-03)

Since the mortality rate is high and there are no published scientific articles or clinical studies regarding partial ventriculectomy, this procedure cannot be considered reasonable and necessary within the meaning of Sec.1862(a)(1) of the Act. Therefore, partial ventriculectomy is not covered by Medicare.

100-03, 20.28

NCD for Therapeutic Embolization (20.28)

(Rev. 1, 10-03-03)

Therapeutic embolization is covered when done for hemorrhage, and for other conditions amenable to treatment by the procedure, when reasonable and necessary for the individual patient. Renal embolization for the treatment of renal adenocarcinoma continues to be covered, effective December 15, 1978, as one type of therapeutic embolization, to:

- Reduce tumor vascularity preoperatively;
- Reduce tumor bulk in inoperable cases; or
- Palliate specific symptoms.

100-03, 20.29

NCD for Hyperbaric Oxygen Therapy (20.29)

(Rev.203, Issued:11-17-17, Effective: 04- 03-17, Implementation: 12-18-17)

A. Covered Conditions

Program reimbursement for HBO therapy will be limited to that which is administered in a chamber (including the one man unit) and is limited to the following conditions:

1. Acute carbon monoxide intoxication,
2. Decompression illness,
3. Gas embolism,
4. Gas gangrene,
5. Acute traumatic peripheral ischemia. HBO therapy is a valuable adjunctive treatment to be used in combination with accepted standard therapeutic measures when loss of function, limb, or life is threatened.
6. Crush injuries and suturing of severed limbs. As in the previous conditions, HBO therapy would be an adjunctive treatment when loss of function, limb, or life is threatened.
7. Progressive necrotizing infections (necrotizing fasciitis),
8. Acute peripheral arterial insufficiency,
9. Preparation and preservation of compromised skin grafts (not for primary management of wounds),
10. Chronic refractory osteomyelitis, unresponsive to conventional medical and surgical management,
11. Osteoradionecrosis as an adjunct to conventional treatment,
12. Soft tissue radionecrosis as an adjunct to conventional treatment,
13. Cyanide poisoning,
14. Actinomycosis, only as an adjunct to conventional therapy when the disease process is refractory to antibiotics and surgical treatment,
14. Diabetic wounds of the lower extremities in patients who meet the following three criteria:
    a. Patient has type I or type II diabetes and has a lower extremity wound that is due to diabetes;
    b. Patient has a wound classified as Wagner grade III or higher; and
    c. Patient has failed an adequate course of standard wound therapy.

The use of HBO therapy is covered as adjunctive therapy only after there are no measurable signs of healing for at least 30 -days of treatment with standard wound therapy and must be used in addition to standard wound care. Standard wound care in patients with diabetic wounds includes: assessment of a patient's vascular status and correction of any vascular problems in the affected limb if possible, optimization of nutritional status, optimization of glucose control, debridement by any means to remove devitalized tissue, maintenance of a clean, moist bed of granulation tissue with appropriate moist dressings, appropriate off-loading, and necessary treatment to resolve any infection that might be present. Failure to respond to standard wound care occurs when there are no measurable signs of healing for at least 30 consecutive days. Wounds must be evaluated at least every 30 days during administration of HBO therapy. Continued treatment with HBO therapy is not covered if measurable signs of healing have not been demonstrated within any 30-day period of treatment.

B. Noncovered Conditions

All other indications not specified under Sec.270.4(A) are not covered under the Medicare program. No program payment may be made for any conditions other than those listed in Sec. 270.4(A).

No program payment may be made for HBO in the treatment of the following conditions:

1. Cutaneous, decubitus, and stasis ulcers.
2. Chronic peripheral vascular insufficiency.
3. Anaerobic septicemia and infection other than clostridial.
4. Skin burns (thermal).
5. Senility.
6. Myocardial infarction.
7. Cardiogenic shock.
8. Sickle cell anemia.
9. Acute thermal and chemical pulmonary damage, i.e., smoke inhalation with pulmonary insufficiency.
10. Acute or chronic cerebral vascular insufficiency.
11. Hepatic necrosis.
12. Aerobic septicemia.
13. Nonvascular causes of chronic brain syndrome (Pick's disease, Alzheimer's disease, Korsakoff's disease).
14. Tetanus.
15. Systemic aerobic infection.
16. Organ transplantation.
17. Organ storage.
18. Pulmonary emphysema.
19. Exceptional blood loss anemia.
20. Multiple Sclerosis.
21. Arthritic Diseases.
22. Acute cerebral edema.

C. Topical Application of Oxygen

This method of administering oxygen does not meet the definition of HBO therapy as stated above. Also, its clinical efficacy has not been established. Therefore, no Medicare reimbursement may be made for the topical application of oxygen.

100-03, 20.30

Microvolt T-Wave Alternans (MTWA)

(Rev. 182, Issued: 05-22-15, Effective: 01-13- 15, Implementation: 06-23-15)

A. General

Microvolt T-wave Alternans (MTWA) testing is a non-invasive diagnostic test that detects minute electrical activity in a portion of the electrocardiogram (ECG) known as the T-wave. MTWA testing has a role in the stratification of patients who may be at risk for sudden cardiac death (SCD) from ventricular arrhythmias.

Within patient groups that may be considered candidates for implantable cardioverter defibrillator (ICD) therapy, a negative MTWA test may be useful in identifying low-risk patients who are unlikely to benefit from, and who may experience worse outcomes from, ICD placement.

Spectral analysis (SA) is a sensitive mathematical method of measuring and comparing time and the ECG signals. It requires specialized propriety electrodes to calculate minute T-wave voltage changes. Software then analyzes these microvolt changes and produces a report to be interpreted by a physician. The Modified Moving Average (MMA) method uses a temporal domain in which T-wave alternans are assessed as a continuous variable along the complete ECG. The MMA method of MTWA testing is performed using standard ambulatory ECG equipment.

B. Nationally Covered Indications

Effective for dates of service on and after March 21, 2006, MTWA diagnostic testing is covered for the evaluation of patients at risk for SCD, only when the SA method is used.

C. Nationally Non-Covered Indications

N/A

D. Other

Effective for dates of service on and after January 21, 2015, Medicare Administrative Contractors (MACs) acting within their respective jurisdictions may determine coverage of MTWA diagnostic testing for the evaluation of patients at risk for SCD using all other methods.

(This NCD last reviewed January 2015.)

100-03, 20.32

Transcatheter Aortic Valve Replacement (TAVR)

(Rev. 147, Issued: 09-24-12, Effective: 05-01-12, Implementation: 01-07-13)

A. General

Transcatheter aortic valve replacement (TAVR - also known as TAVI or transcatheter aortic valve implantation) is used in the treatment of aortic stenosis. A bioprosthetic valve is inserted percutaneously using a catheter and implanted in the orifice of the aortic valve.

B. Nationally Covered Indications

The Centers for Medicare & Medicaid Services (CMS) covers transcatheter aortic valve replacement (TAVR) under Coverage with Evidence Development (CED) with the following conditions:

A. TAVR is covered for the treatment of symptomatic aortic valve stenosis when furnished according to a Food and Drug Administration (FDA)-approved indication and when all of the following conditions are met:
   1. The procedure is furnished with a complete aortic valve and implantation system that has received FDA premarket approval (PMA) for that system's FDA approved indication.
   2. Two cardiac surgeons have independently examined the patient face-to-face and evaluated the patient's suitability for open aortic valve replacement (AVR) surgery; and both surgeons have documented the rationale for their clinical judgment and the rationale is available to the heart team.
   3. The patient (preoperatively and postoperatively) is under the care of a heart team: a cohesive, multi-disciplinary, team of medical professionals. The heart team concept embodies collaboration and dedication across medical specialties to offer optimal patient-centered care.

      TAVR must be furnished in a hospital with the appropriate infrastructure that includes but is not limited to:
      a. On-site heart valve surgery program,
      b. Cardiac catheterization lab or hybrid operating room/catheterization lab equipped with a fixed radiographic imaging system with flat-panel fluoroscopy, offering quality imaging,
      c. Non-invasive imaging such as echocardiography, vascular ultrasound, computed tomography (CT) and magnetic resonance (MR),

d. Sufficient space, in a sterile environment, to accommodate necessary equipment for cases with and without complications,

e. Post-procedure intensive care facility with personnel experienced in managing patients who have undergone open-heart valve procedures,

f. Appropriate volume requirements per the applicable qualifications below.

There are two sets of qualifications; the first set outlined below is for hospital programs and heart teams without previous TAVR experience and the second set is for those with TAVR experience.

Qualifications to begin a TAVR program for hospitals without TAVR experience:

The hospital program must have the following:

a. ≥ 50 total AVRs in the previous year prior to TAVR, including = 10 high-risk patients, and;

b. ≥ 2 physicians with cardiac surgery privileges, and;

c. ≥ 1000 catheterizations per year, including = 400 percutaneous coronary interventions (PCIs) per year.

Qualifications to begin a TAVR program for heart teams without TAVR experience:

The heart team must include:

a. Cardiovascular surgeon with:

   i. ≥ 100 career AVRs including 10 high-risk patients; or,

   ii. ≥ 25 AVRs in one year; or,

   iii. ≥ 50 AVRs in 2 years; and which include at least 20 AVRs in the last year prior to TAVR initiation; and,

b. Interventional cardiologist with:

   i. Professional experience with 100 structural heart disease procedures lifetime; or,

   ii. 30 left-sided structural procedures per year of which 60% should be balloon aortic valvuloplasty (BAV). Atrial septal defect and patent foramen ovale closure are not considered left-sided procedures; and,

c. Additional members of the heart team such as echocardiographers, imaging specialists, heart failure specialists, cardiac anesthesiologists, intensivists, nurses, and social workers; and,

d. Device-specific training as required by the manufacturer.

Qualifications for hospital programs with TAVR experience:

The hospital program must maintain the following:

a. ≥ 20 AVRs per year or = 40 AVRs every 2 years; and,

b. ≥ 2 physicians with cardiac surgery privileges; and,

c. ≥ 1000 catheterizations per year, including = 400 percutaneous coronary interventions (PCIs) per year.

Qualifications for heart teams with TAVR experience:

The heart team must include:

a. cardiovascular surgeon and an interventional cardiologist whose combined experience maintains the following:

   i. ≥ 20 TAVR procedures in the prior year, or,

   ii. ≥ 40 TAVR procedures in the prior 2 years; and,

b. Additional members of the heart team such as echocardiographers, imaging specialists, heart failure specialists, cardiac anesthesiologists, intensivists, nurses, and social workers.

4. The heart team's interventional cardiologist(s) and cardiac surgeon(s) must jointly participate in the intra-operative technical aspects of TAVR.

5. The heart team and hospital are participating in a prospective, national, audited registry that: 1) consecutively enrolls TAVR patients; 2) accepts all manufactured devices; 3) follows the patient for at least one year; and, 4) complies with relevant regulations relating to protecting human research subjects, including 45 CFR Part 46 and 21 CFR Parts 50 & 56. The following outcomes must be tracked by the registry; and the registry must be designed to permit identification and analysis of patient, practitioner and facility level variables that predict each of these outcomes:

   i. Stroke;

   ii. All cause mortality;

   iii. Transient Ischemic Attacks (TIAs);

   iv. Major vascular events;

   v. Acute kidney injury;

   vi. Repeat aortic valve procedures;

   vii. Quality of Life (QoL).

   The registry should collect all data necessary and have a written executable analysis plan in place to address the following questions (to appropriately address some questions, Medicare claims or other outside data may be necessary):

   – When performed outside a controlled clinical study, how do outcomes and adverse events compare to the pivotal clinical studies?

   – How do outcomes and adverse events in subpopulations compare to patients in the pivotal clinical studies?

   – What is the long term (≥ 5 year) durability of the device?

   – What are the long term (≥ 5 year) outcomes and adverse events?

   – How do the demographics of registry patients compare to the pivotal studies?

   Consistent with section 1142 of the Act, the Agency for Healthcare Research and Quality (AHRQ) supports clinical research studies that CMS determines meet the above-listed standards and address the above-listed research questions.

B. TAVR is covered for uses that are not expressly listed as an FDA-approved indication when performed within a clinical study that fulfills all of the following.

1. The heart team's interventional cardiologist(s) and cardiac surgeon(s) must jointly participate in the intra-operative technical aspects of TAVR.

2. As a fully-described, written part of its protocol, the clinical research study must critically evaluate not only each patient's quality of life pre- and post-TAVR (minimum of 1 year), but must also address at least one of the following questions: § What is the incidence of stroke?

   – What is the rate of all cause mortality?

   – What is the incidence of transient ischemic attacks (TIAs)?

   – What is the incidence of major vascular events?

   – What is the incidence of acute kidney injury?

   – What is the incidence of repeat aortic valve procedures?

3. The clinical study must adhere to the following standards of scientific integrity and relevance to the Medicare population:

   a. The principal purpose of the research study is to test whether a particular intervention potentially improves the participants' health outcomes.

   b. The research study is well supported by available scientific and medical information or it is intended to clarify or establish the health outcomes of interventions already in common clinical use.

   c. The research study does not unjustifiably duplicate existing studies.

   d. The research study design is appropriate to answer the research question being asked in the study.

   e. The research study is sponsored by an organization or individual capable of executing the proposed study successfully.

   f. The research study is in compliance with all applicable Federal regulations concerning the protection of human subjects found in the Code of Federal Regulations (CFR) at 45 CFR Part 46. If a study is regulated by the Food and Drug Administration (FDA), it also must be in compliance with 21 CFR Parts 50 and 56. In particular, the informed consent includes a straightforward explanation of the reported increased risks of stroke and vascular complications that have been published for TAVR.

   g. All aspects of the research study are conducted according to appropriate standards of scientific integrity (see http://www.icmje.org).

   h. The research study has a written protocol that clearly addresses, or incorporates by reference, the standards listed as Medicare coverage requirements.

   i. The clinical research study is not designed to exclusively test toxicity or disease pathophysiology in healthy individuals. Trials of all medical technologies measuring therapeutic outcomes as one of the objectives meet this standard only if the disease or condition being studied is life threatening as defined in 21 CFR §312.81(a) and the patient has no other viable treatment options.

   j. The clinical research study is registered on the www.ClinicalTrials.gov website by the principal sponsor/investigator prior to the enrollment of the first study subject.

   k. The research study protocol specifies the method and timing of public release of all pre-specified outcomes to be measured including release of outcomes if outcomes are negative or study is terminated early. The results must be made public within 24 months of the end of data collection. If a report is planned to be published in a peer reviewed journal, then that initial release may be an abstract that meets the requirements of the International Committee of Medical Journal Editors (http://www.icmje.org). However a full report of the outcomes must be made public no later than three (3) years after the end of data collection.

   l. The research study protocol must explicitly discuss subpopulations affected by the treatment under investigation, particularly traditionally underrepresented groups in clinical studies, how the inclusion and exclusion criteria affect enrollment of these populations, and a plan for the retention and reporting of said populations on the trial. If the inclusion and exclusion criteria are expected to have a negative effect on the recruitment or retention of underrepresented populations, the protocol must discuss why these criteria are necessary.

m. The research study protocol explicitly discusses how the results are or are not expected to be generalizable to the Medicare population to infer whether Medicare patients may benefit from the intervention. Separate discussions in the protocol may be necessary for populations eligible for Medicare due to age, disability or Medicaid eligibility. Consistent with section 1142 of the Act, AHRQ supports clinical research studies that CMS determines meet the above-listed standards and address the above-listed research questions.

4. The principal investigator must submit the complete study protocol, identify the relevant CMS research question(s) that will be addressed, and cite the location of the detailed analysis plan for those questions in the protocol, plus provide a statement addressing how the study satisfies each of the standards of scientific integrity (a. through m. listed above), as well as the investigator's contact information, to the address below. The information will be reviewed, and approved studies will be identified on the CMS Website.

Director, Coverage and Analysis Group
Re: TAVR CED
Centers for Medicare & Medicaid Services (CMS)
7500 Security Blvd., Mail Stop S3-02-01
Baltimore, MD 21244-1850

C. Nationally Non-Covered Indications

TAVR is not covered for patients in whom existing co-morbidities would preclude the expected benefit from correction of the aortic stenosis.

D.

NA

(This NCD last reviewed May 2012.)

100-03, 20.34

Percutaneous Left Atrial Appendage Closure (LAAC)

(Rev. 192, Issued: 05-06-16, Effective: 02-08-16, Implementation: 10-03-16)

A. General

Patients with atrial fibrillation (AF), an irregular heartbeat, are at an increased risk of stroke. The left atrial appendage (LAA) is a tubular structure that opens into the left atrium and has been shown to be one potential source for blood clots that can cause strokes. While thinning the blood with anticoagulant medications has been proven to prevent strokes, percutaneous LAA closure (LAAC) has been studied as a non-pharmacologic alternative for patients with AF.

B. Nationally Covered Indications

The Centers for Medicare & Medicaid Services (CMS) covers percutaneous LAAC for non-valvular atrial fibrillation (NVAF) through Coverage with Evidence Development (CED) with the following conditions:

a. LAAC devices are covered when the device has received Food and Drug Administration (FDA) Premarket Approval (PMA) for that device's FDA-approved indication and meet all of the conditions specified below:

The patient must have:

- A CHADS2 score ≥ 2 (Congestive heart failure, Hypertension, Age >75, Diabetes, Stroke/transient ischemia attack/thromboembolism) or CHA2DS2-VASc score ≥ 3 (Congestive heart failure, Hypertension, Age ≥ 65, Diabetes, Stroke/transient ischemia attack/thromboembolism, Vascular disease, Sex category)
- A formal shared decision making interaction with an independent non-interventional physician using an evidence-based decision tool on oral anticoagulation in patients with NVAF prior to LAAC. Additionally, the shared decision making interaction must be documented in the medical record.
- A suitability for short-term warfarin but deemed unable to take long-term oral anticoagulation following the conclusion of shared decision making, as LAAC is only covered as a second line therapy to oral anticoagulants. The patient (preoperatively and postoperatively) is under the care of a cohesive, multidisciplinary team (MDT) of medical professionals. The procedure must be furnished in a hospital with an established structural heart disease (SHD) and/or electrophysiology (EP) program.

The procedure must be performed by an interventional cardiologist(s), electrophysiologist(s), or cardiovascular surgeon (s) that meet the following criteria:

- Has received training prescribed by the manufacturer on the safe and effective use of the device prior to performing LAAC; and,
- Has performed ≥ 25 interventional cardiac procedures that involve transeptal puncture through an intact septum; and,
- Continues to perform ≥ 25 interventional cardiac procedures that involve transeptal puncture through an intact septum, of which at least 12 are LAAC, over a 2-year period.

The patient is enrolled in, and the MDT and hospital must participate in, a prospective, national, audited registry that: 1) consecutively enrolls LAAC patients, and, 2) tracks the following annual outcomes for each patient for a period of at least 4 years from the time of the LAAC:

- Operator-specific complications
- Device-specific complications including device thrombosis
- Stroke, adjudicated, by type
- Transient Ischemic Attack (TIA)
- Systemic embolism
- Death
- Major bleeding, by site and severity

The registry must be designed to permit identification and analysis of patient, practitioner, and facility level factors that predict patient risk for these outcomes. The registry must collect all data necessary to conduct analyses adjusted for relevant confounders, and have a written executable analysis plan in place to address the following questions:

- How do the outcomes listed above compare to outcomes in the pivotal clinical trials in the short term (≤12 months) and in the long term (≥ 4 years)?
- What is the long term (≥ 4 year) durability of the device?
- What are the short term (≤12 months) and the long term (≥4 years) device-specific complications including device thromboses?

To appropriately address some of these questions, Medicare claims or other outside data may be necessary.

Registries must be reviewed and approved by CMS. Potential registry sponsors must submit all registry documentation to CMS for approval, including the written executable analysis plan and auditing plan. CMS will review the qualifications of candidate registries to ensure that the approved registry follows standard data collection practices, and collects data necessary to evaluate the patient outcomes specified above. The registry's national clinical trial number must be recorded on the claim.

Consistent with section 1142 of the Social Security Act (the Act), the Agency for Healthcare Research and Quality (AHRQ) supports clinical research studies that CMS determines address the above-listed research questions and the a-m criteria listed in Section c. of this decision.

All approved registries will be posted on the CED website located at: https://www.cms.gov/Medicare/Coverage/Coverage-with-Evidence-Development/index.html.

b. LAAC is covered for NVAF patients not included in Section a. of this decision when performed within an FDA-approved randomized controlled trial (RCT) if such trials meet the criteria established below:

As a fully-described written part of its protocol, the RCT must critically answer, in comparison to optimal medical therapy, the following questions:

- As a primary endpoint, what is the true incidence of ischemic stroke and systemic embolism?
- As a secondary endpoint, what is cardiovascular mortality and all-cause mortality?

FDA-approved RCTs must be reviewed and approved by CMS. Consistent with section 1142 of the Act, AHRQ supports clinical research studies that CMS determines address the above-listed research questions and the a-m criteria listed in Section c. of this decision.

The principal investigator must submit the complete study protocol, identify the relevant CMS research question(s) that will be addressed, and cite the location of the detailed analysis plan for those questions in the protocol, plus provide a statement addressing how the study satisfies each of the standards of scientific integrity a. through m. listed in section c. of this decision, as well as the investigator's contact information, to the address below.

Director, Coverage and Analysis Group Re: LAAC CED Centers for Medicare & Medicaid Services 7500 Security Blvd., Mail Stop S3-02-01 Baltimore, MD 21244-1850

c. All clinical studies, RCTs and registries submitted for review must adhere to the following standards of scientific integrity and relevance to the Medicare population:

   a. The principal purpose of the study is to test whether the item or service meaningfully improves health outcomes of affected beneficiaries who are represented by the enrolled subjects.

   b. The rationale for the study is well supported by available scientific and medical evidence.

   c. The study results are not anticipated to unjustifiably duplicate existing knowledge.

   d. The study design is methodologically appropriate and the anticipated number of enrolled subjects is sufficient to answer the research question(s) being asked in the National Coverage Determination.

   e. The study is sponsored by an organization or individual capable of completing it successfully.

   f. The research study is in compliance with all applicable Federal regulations concerning the protection of human subjects found in the Code of Federal Regulations (CFR) at 45 CFR Part 46. If a study is regulated by the FDA, it is also in compliance with 21 CFR Parts 50 and 56. In addition, to further enhance the protection of human subjects in studies conducted under CED, the study must provide and obtain meaningful informed consent from patients regarding the risks associated with the study items and/or services, and the use and eventual disposition of the collected data.

g. All aspects of the study are conducted according to appropriate standards of scientific integrity.

h. The study has a written protocol that clearly demonstrates adherence to the standards listed here as Medicare requirements.

i. The study is not designed to exclusively test toxicity or disease pathophysiology in healthy individuals. Such studies may meet this requirement only if the disease or condition being studied is life threatening as defined in 21 CFR §312.81(a) and the patient has no other viable treatment options.

j. The clinical research studies and registries are registered on the www.ClinicalTrials.gov website by the principal sponsor/investigator prior to the enrollment of the first study subject. Registries are also registered in the AHRQ Registry of Patient Registries (RoPR).

k. The research study protocol specifies the method and timing of public release of all prespecified outcomes to be measured including release of outcomes if outcomes are negative or study is terminated early. The results must be made public within 12 months of the study's primary completion date, which is the date the final subject had final data collection for the primary endpoint, even if the trial does not achieve its primary aim. The results must include number started/completed, summary results for primary and secondary outcome measures, statistical analyses, and adverse events. Final results must be reported in a publicly accessibly manner; either in a peer-reviewed scientific journal (in print or on-line), in an on-line publicly accessible registry dedicated to the dissemination of clinical trial information such as ClinicalTrials.gov, or in journals willing to publish in abbreviated format (e.g., for studies with negative or incomplete results).

l. The study protocol must explicitly discuss beneficiary subpopulations affected by the item or service under investigation, particularly traditionally underrepresented groups in clinical studies, how the inclusion and exclusion criteria effect enrollment of these populations, and a plan for the retention and reporting of said populations in the trial. If the inclusion and exclusion criteria are expected to have a negative effect on the recruitment or retention of underrepresented populations, the protocol must discuss why these criteria are necessary.

m. The study protocol explicitly discusses how the results are or are not expected to be generalizable to affected beneficiary subpopulations. Separate discussions in the protocol may be necessary for populations eligible for Medicare due to age, disability, or Medicaid eligibility.

C. Nationally Non-Covered Indications

LAAC is non-covered for the treatment of NVAF when not furnished under CED according to the above-noted criteria.

(This NCD last reviewed February 2016.)

100-03, 20.35

Supervised Exercise Therapy (SET) for Symptomatic Peripheral Artery Disease (PAD)

(Rev. 207, Issued: 05-11-18, Effective: 05-25-17, Implementation: 07-02-18)

A. General

Research has shown supervised exercise therapy (SET) to be an effective, minimally invasive method to alleviate the most common symptom associated with peripheral artery disease (PAD) – intermittent claudication (IC). SET has been shown to be significantly more effective than unsupervised exercise, and could prevent the progression of PAD and lower the risk of cardiovascular events that are prevalent in these patients. SET has also been shown to perform at least as well as more invasive revascularization treatments that are covered by Medicare.

B. Nationally Covered Indications

Effective for services performed on or after May 25, 2017, the Centers for Medicare & Medicaid Services has determined that the evidence is sufficient to cover SET for beneficiaries with IC for the treatment of symptomatic PAD. Up to 36 sessions over a 12-week period are covered if all of the following components of a SET program are met. The SET program must:

- consist of sessions lasting 30-60 minutes comprising a therapeutic exercise-training program for PAD in patients with claudication;
- be conducted in a physician's office;
- be delivered by qualified auxiliary personnel necessary to ensure benefits exceed harms, and who are trained in exercise therapy for PAD; and
- be under the direct supervision of a physician (as defined in 1861(r)(1)), physician assistant, or nurse practitioner/clinical nurse specialist (as identified in 1861(aa)(5)) who must be trained in both basic and advanced life support techniques.

Beneficiaries must have a face-to-face visit with the physician responsible for PAD treatment to obtain the referral for SET. At this visit, the beneficiary must receive information regarding cardiovascular disease and PAD risk factor reduction, which could include education, counseling, behavioral interventions, and outcome assessments.

C. Nationally Non-Covered Indications

SET is non-covered for beneficiaries with absolute contraindications to exercise as determined by their primary physician.

D. Other

Medicare Administrative Contractors (MACs) have the discretion to cover SET beyond the nationally covered 36 sessions over a 12-week period. MACs may cover an additional 36 sessions over an extended period of time. A second referral is required for these additional sessions.

(This NCD last reviewed May 2017.)

100-03, 20.4

Implantable Cardioverter Defibrillators (ICDs)

(Rev.213, Issued: 02-15-19)

A. General

An ICD is an electronic device designed to diagnose and treat life-threatening ventricular tachyarrhythmias.

B. Nationally Covered Indications

Effective for services performed on or after February 15, 2018, CMS has determined that the evidence is sufficient to conclude that the use of ICDs, (also referred to as defibrillators) is reasonable and necessary:

1. Patients with a personal history of sustained Ventricular Tachyarrhythmia (VT) or cardiac arrest due to Ventricular Fibrillation (VF). Patients must have demonstrated: • An episode of sustained VT, either spontaneous or induced by an Electrophysiology (EP) study, not associated with an acute Myocardial Infarction (MI) and not due to a transient or reversible cause; or
   - An episode of cardiac arrest due to VF, not due to a transient or reversible cause.
2. Patients with a prior MI and a measured Left Ventricular Ejection Fraction (LVEF) ≤ 0.30. Patients must not have: • New York Heart Association (NYHA) classification IV heart failure; or,
   - Had a Coronary Artery Bypass Graft (CABG), or Percutaneous Coronary Intervention (PCI) with angioplasty and/or stenting, within the past three (3) months; or,
   - Had an MI within the past 40 days; or,
   - Clinical symptoms and findings that would make them a candidate for coronary revascularization.

   For these patients identified in B2, a formal shared decision making encounter must occur between the patient and a physician (as defined in Section 1861(r)(1) of the Social Security Act (the Act))or qualified non-physician practitioner (meaning a physician assistant, nurse practitioner, or clinical nurse specialist as defined in §1861(aa)(5) of the Act) using an evidence-based decision tool on ICDs prior to initial ICD implantation. The shared decision making encounter may occur at a separate visit.
3. Patients who have severe, ischemic, dilated cardiomyopathy but no personal history of sustained VT or cardiac arrest due to VF, and have NYHA Class II or III heart failure, LVEF < 35%. Additionally, patients must not have: • Had a CABG, or PCI with angioplasty and/or stenting, within the past three (3) months; or,
   - Had an MI within the past 40 days; or,
   - Clinical symptoms and findings that would make them a candidate for coronary revascularization.

   For these patients identified in B3, a formal shared decision making encounter must occur between the patient and a physician (as defined in Section 1861(r)(1) of the Actor qualified non-physician practitioner (meaning a physician assistant, nurse practitioner, or clinical nurse specialist as defined in §1861(aa)(5) of the Act) using an evidence-based decision tool on ICDs prior to initial ICD implantation. The shared decision making encounter may occur at a separate visit.
4. Patients who have severe, non-ischemic, dilated cardiomyopathy but no personal history of cardiac arrest or sustained VT, NYHA Class II or III heart failure, LVEF < 35%, been on optimal medical therapy for at least three (3) months. Additionally, patients must not have: • Had a CABG or PCI with angioplasty and/or stenting, within the past three (3) months; or,
   - Had an MI within the past 40 days; or,
   - Clinical symptoms and findings that would make them a candidate for coronary revascularization.

   For these patients identified in B4, a formal shared decision making encounter must occur between the patient and a physician (as defined in Section 1861(r)(1) of the Act) or qualified non-physician practitioner (meaning a physician assistant, nurse practitioner, or clinical nurse specialist as defined in §1861(aa)(5) of the Act) using an evidence-based decision tool on ICDs prior to initial ICD implantation. The shared decision making encounter may occur at a separate visit.
5. Patients with documented, familial or genetic disorders with a high risk of life-threatening tachyarrhythmias (sustained VT or VF, to include, but not limited to, long QT syndrome or hypertrophic cardiomyopathy.

   For these patients identified in B5, a formal shared decision making encounter must occur between the patient and a physician (as defined in Section 1861(r)(1) of the Act) or qualified non-physician practitioner (meaning a physician assistant, nurse practitioner, or clinical nurse specialist as defined in §1861(aa)(5) of the Act) using an evidence-based decision tool on ICDs prior to initial ICD implantation. The shared decision making encounter may occur at a separate visit.

6. Patients with an existing ICD may receive an ICD replacement if it is required due to the end of battery life, Elective Replacement Indicator (ERI), or device/lead malfunction.

   For each of the six (6) covered indications above, the following additional criteria must also be met:

   1. Patients must be clinically stable (e.g., not in shock, from any etiology);
   2. LVEF must be measured by echocardiography, radionuclide (nuclear medicine) imaging, cardiac Magnetic Resonance Imaging (MRI), or catheter angiography;
   3. Patients must not have:
      - Significant, irreversible brain damage; or,
      - Any disease, other than cardiac disease (e.g., cancer, renal failure, liver failure) associated with a likelihood of survival less than one (1) year; or,
      - Supraventricular tachycardia such as atrial fibrillation with a poorly controlled ventricular rate.

Exceptions to waiting periods for patients that have had a CABG, or PCI with angioplasty and/or stenting, within the past three (3) months, or had an MI within the past 40 days:

Cardiac Pacemakers: Patients who meet all CMS coverage requirements for cardiac pacemakers, and who meet the criteria in this national coverage determination for an ICD, may receive the combined devices in one procedure, at the time the pacemaker is clinically indicated;

Replacement of ICDs: Patients with an existing ICD may receive an ICD replacement if it is required due to the end of battery life, ERI, or device/lead malfunction.

C. Nationally Non-Covered Indications

N/A

D. Other

For patients that are candidates for heart transplantation on the United Network for Organ Sharing (UNOS) transplant list awaiting a donor heart, coverage of ICDs, as with cardiac resynchronization therapy, as a bridge-to-transplant to prolong survival until a donor becomes available, is determined by the local Medicare Administrative Contractors (MACs).

All other indications for ICDs not currently covered in accordance with this decision may be covered under Category B Investigational Device Exemption (IDE) trials (42 CFR 405.201).

(This NCD last reviewed February 2018.)

100-03, 30.3

NCD for Acupuncture (30.3)

(Rev. 1, 10-03-03)

Although acupuncture has been used for thousands of years in China and for decades in parts of Europe, it is a new agent of unknown use and efficacy in the United States. Even in those areas of the world where it has been widely used, its mechanism is not known. Three units of the National Institutes of Health, the National Institute of General Medical Sciences, National Institute of Neurological Diseases and Stroke, and Fogarty International Center have been designed to assess and identify specific opportunities and needs for research attending the use of acupuncture for surgical anesthesia and relief of chronic pain. Until the pending scientific assessment of the technique has been completed and its efficacy has been established, Medicare reimbursement for acupuncture, as an anesthetic or as an analgesic or for other therapeutic purposes, may not be made. Accordingly, acupuncture is not considered reasonable and necessary within the meaning of §1862(a)(1) of the Act.

100-03, 30.3.1

NCD for Acupuncture for Fibromyalgia (30.3.1)

(Rev. 11, 04-16-04)

General

Although acupuncture has been used for thousands of years in China and for decades in parts of Europe, it is still a relatively new agent of unknown use and efficacy in the United States. Even in those areas of the world where it has been widely used, its mechanism is not known. Three units of the National Institutes of Health, the National Institute of General Medical Sciences, National Institute of Neurological Diseases and Stroke, and Fogarty International Center were designated to assess and identify specific opportunities and needs for research attending the use of acupuncture for surgical anesthesia and relief of chronic pain. Following thorough review, and pending completion of the scientific assessment and efficacy of the technique, CMS initially issued a national noncoverage determination for acupuncture in May 1980.

Nationally Covered Indications

Not applicable.

Nationally Noncovered Indications

After careful reconsideration of its initial noncoverage determination for acupuncture, CMS concludes that there is no convincing evidence for the use of acupuncture for pain relief in patients with fibromyalgia. Study design flaws presently prohibit assessing acupuncture's utility for improving health outcomes. Accordingly, CMS determines that acupuncture is not considered reasonable and necessary for the treatment of fibromyalgia within the meaning of §1862(a)(1) of the Social Security Act, and the national noncoverage determination for acupuncture continues.

(This NCD last reviewed April 2004.)

100-03, 30.3.2

NCD for Acupuncture for Osteoarthritis (30.3.2)

(Rev. 11, 04-16-04)

General

Although acupuncture has been used for thousands of years in China and for decades in parts of Europe, it is still a relatively new agent of unknown use and efficacy in the United States. Even in those areas of the world where it has been widely used, its mechanism is not known. Three units of the National Institutes of Health, the National Institute of General Medical Sciences, National Institute of Neurological Diseases and Stroke, and Fogarty International Center were designated to assess and identify specific opportunities and needs for research attending the use of acupuncture for surgical anesthesia and relief of chronic pain. Following thorough review, and pending completion of the scientific assessment and efficacy of the technique, CMS initially issued a national noncoverage determination for acupuncture in May 1980.

Nationally Covered Indications

Not applicable.

Nationally Noncovered Indications

After careful reconsideration of its initial noncoverage determination for acupuncture, CMS concludes that there is no convincing evidence for the use of acupuncture for pain relief in patients with osteoarthritis. Study design flaws presently prohibit assessing acupuncture's utility for improving health outcomes. Accordingly, CMS determines that acupuncture is not considered reasonable and necessary for the treatment of osteoarthritis within the meaning of §1862(a)(1) of the Social Security Act, and the national noncoverage determination for acupuncture continues.

(This NCD last reviewed April 2004.)

100-03, 80.7

NCD for Refractive Keratoplasty (80.7)

(Rev. 1, 10-03-03)

The correction of common refractive errors by eyeglasses, contact lenses or other prosthetic devices is specifically excluded from coverage. The use of radial keratotomy and/or keratoplasty for the purpose of refractive error compensation is considered a substitute or alternative to eye glasses or contact lenses, which are specifically excluded by Sec.1862(a)(7) of the Act (except in certain cases in connection with cataract surgery). In addition, many in the medical community consider such procedures cosmetic surgery, which is excluded by section Sec.1862(a)(10) of the Act. Therefore, radial keratotomy and keratoplasty to treat refractive defects are not covered.

Keratoplasty that treats specific lesions of the cornea, such as phototherapeutic keratectomy that removes scar tissue from the visual field, deals with an abnormality of the eye and is not cosmetic surgery. Such cases may be covered under Sec.1862(a)(1)(A) of the Act.

The use of lasers to treat ophthalmic disease constitutes opthalmalogic surgery. Coverage is restricted to practitioners who have completed an approved training program in ophthalmologic surgery.

100-03, 80.10

NCD for Phaco-Emulsification procedure - cataract extraction (80.10)

(Rev. 1, 10-03-03)

In view of recommendations of authoritative sources in the field of ophthalmology, the subject technique is viewed as an accepted procedure for removal of cataracts. Accordingly, program reimbursement may be made for necessary services furnished in connection with cataract extraction utilizing the phaco-emulsification procedure.

100-03, 80.12

NCD for Intraocular Lenses (IOLs) (80.12)

(Rev. 1, 10-03-03)

Intraocular lens implantation services, as well as the lens itself, may be covered if reasonable and necessary for the individual. Implantation services may include hospital, surgical, and other medical services, including pre-implantation ultrasound (A-scan) eye measurement of one or both eyes.

100-03, 90.2

Next Generation Sequencing (NGS) for Patients with Advanced Cancer

(Rev.215, Issued: 04-10-19)

A. General

Clinical laboratory diagnostic tests can include tests that, for example, predict the risk associated with one or more genetic variations. In addition, in vitro companion diagnostic laboratory tests provide a report of test results of genetic variations and are essential for the safe and effective use of a corresponding therapeutic product. Next Generation Sequencing (NGS) is one technique that can measure one or more genetic variations as a laboratory diagnostic test, such as when used as a companion in vitro diagnostic test.

Patients with cancer can have recurrent, relapsed, refractory, metastatic, and/or advanced stages III or IV of cancer. Clinical studies show that genetic variations in a patient's cancer can, in concert with clinical factors, predict how each individual responds to specific treatments.

In application, a report of results of a diagnostic laboratory test using NGS (i.e., information on the cancer's genetic variations) can contribute to predicting a patient's response to a given drug: good, bad, or none at all. Applications of NGS to predict a patient's response to treatment occurs ideally prior to initiation of such treatment.

B. Nationally Covered Indications

Effective for services performed on or after March 16, 2018, the Centers for Medicare & Medicaid Services (CMS) has determined that Next Generation Sequencing (NGS) as a diagnostic laboratory test is reasonable and necessary and covered nationally, when performed in a Clinical Laboratory Improvement Amendments (CLIA)-certified laboratory, when ordered by a treating physician, and when all of the following requirements are met:

1. Patient has:
   - either recurrent, relapsed, refractory, metastatic, or advanced stage III or IV cancer; and,
   - either not been previously tested using the same NGS test for the same primary diagnosis of cancer, or repeat testing using the same NGS test only when a new primary cancer diagnosis is made by the treating physician; and,
   - decided to seek further cancer treatment (e.g., therapeutic chemotherapy).
2. The diagnostic laboratory test using NGS must have:
   - Food & Drug Administration (FDA) approval or clearance as a companion in vitro diagnostic; and,
   - an FDA-approved or -cleared indication for use in that patient's cancer; and,
   - results provided to the treating physician for management of the patient using a report template to specify treatment options.

C. Nationally Non-Covered

Effective for services performed on or after March 16, 2018, NGS as a diagnostic laboratory test for patients with cancer are non-covered if the cancer patient does not meet the criteria noted in section B.1. above.

D. Other

1. Effective for services performed on or after March 16, 2018, Medicare Administrative Contractors (MACs) may determine coverage of other NGS as a diagnostic laboratory test for patients with cancer only when the test is performed in a CLIA-certified laboratory, ordered by a treating physician, and the patient has:
   - either recurrent, relapsed, refractory, metastatic, or advanced stages III or IV cancer; and,
   - either not been previously tested using the same NGS test for the same primary diagnosis of cancer or repeat testing using the same NGS test was performed only when a new primary cancer diagnosis is made by the treating physician; and,
   - decided to seek further cancer treatment (e.g., therapeutic chemotherapy).

(This NCD last reviewed March 2018.)

ICD-10-CM	ICD-10-CM Code Descriptor 0037U: Effective Date: 04/01/2018
C00.0	Malignant neoplasm of external upper lip
C00.1	Malignant neoplasm of external lower lip Note that claims for F1CDx test 03/16/2018-03/31/2018 will be recognized with NOC/NOS code 81455 coverable under this policy.
C00.2	Malignant neoplasm of external lip, unspecified
C00.3	Malignant neoplasm of upper lip, inner aspect
C00.4	Malignant neoplasm of lower lip, inner aspect
C00.5	Malignant neoplasm of lip, unspecified, inner aspect
C00.6	Malignant neoplasm of commissure of lip, unspecified
C00.8	Malignant neoplasm of overlapping sites of lip
C00.9	Malignant neoplasm of lip, unspecified
C01	Malignant neoplasm of base of tongue
C02.0	Malignant neoplasm of dorsal surface of tongue

ICD-10-CM	ICD-10-CM Code Descriptor 0037U: Effective Date: 04/01/2018
C02.1	Malignant neoplasm of border of tongue
C02.2	Malignant neoplasm of ventral surface of tongue
C02.3	Malignant neoplasm of anterior two-thirds of tongue, part unspecified
C02.4	Malignant neoplasm of lingual tonsil
C02.8	Malignant neoplasm of overlapping sites of tongue
C02.9	Malignant neoplasm of tongue, unspecified
C03.0	Malignant neoplasm of upper gum
C03.1	Malignant neoplasm of lower gum
C03.9	Malignant neoplasm of gum, unspecified
C04.0	Malignant neoplasm of anterior floor of mouth
C04.1	Malignant neoplasm of lateral floor of mouth
C04.8	Malignant neoplasm of overlapping sites of floor of mouth
C04.9	Malignant neoplasm of floor of mouth, unspecified
C05.0	Malignant neoplasm of hard palate
C05.1	Malignant neoplasm of soft palate
C05.2	Malignant neoplasm of uvula
C05.8	Malignant neoplasm of overlapping sites of palate
C05.9	Malignant neoplasm of palate, unspecified
C06.0	Malignant neoplasm of cheek mucosa
C06.1	Malignant neoplasm of vestibule of mouth
C06.2	Malignant neoplasm of retromolar area
C06.80	Malignant neoplasm of overlapping sites of unspecified parts of mouth
C06.89	Malignant neoplasm of overlapping sites of other parts of mouth
C06.9	Malignant neoplasm of mouth, unspecified
C07	Malignant neoplasm of parotid gland
C08.0	Malignant neoplasm of submandibular gland
C08.1	Malignant neoplasm of sublingual gland
C08.9	Malignant neoplasm of major salivary gland, unspecified
C09.0	Malignant neoplasm of tonsillar fossa
C09.1	Malignant neoplasm of tonsillar pillar (anterior) (posterior)
C09.8	Malignant neoplasm of overlapping sites of tonsil
C09.9	Malignant neoplasm of tonsil, unspecified
C10.0	Malignant neoplasm of vallecula
C10.1	Malignant neoplasm of anterior surface of epiglottis
C10.2	Malignant neoplasm of lateral wall of oropharynx
C10.3	Malignant neoplasm of posterior wall of oropharynx
C10.4	Malignant neoplasm of branchial cleft
C10.8	Malignant neoplasm of overlapping sites of oropharynx
C10.9	Malignant neoplasm of oropharynx, unspecified
C11.0	Malignant neoplasm of superior wall of nasopharynx
C11.1	Malignant neoplasm of posterior wall of nasopharynx
C11.2	Malignant neoplasm of lateral wall of nasopharynx
C11.3	Malignant neoplasm of anterior wall of nasopharynx
C11.8	Malignant neoplasm of overlapping sites of nasopharynx
C11.9	Malignant neoplasm of nasopharynx, unspecified
C12	Malignant neoplasm of pyriform sinus
C13.0	Malignant neoplasm of postcricoid region
C13.1	Malignant neoplasm of aryepiglottic fold, hypopharyngeal aspect
C13.2	Malignant neoplasm of posterior wall of hypopharynx
C13.8	Malignant neoplasm of overlapping sites of hypopharynx
C13.9	Malignant neoplasm of hypopharynx, unspecified
C14.0	Malignant neoplasm of pharynx, unspecified
C14.2	Malignant neoplasm of Waldeyer's ring
C14.8	Malignant neoplasm of overlapping sites of lip, oral cavity and pharynx
C15.3	Malignant neoplasm of upper third of esophagus
C15.4	Malignant neoplasm of middle third of esophagus
C15.5	Malignant neoplasm of lower third of esophagus
C15.8	Malignant neoplasm of overlapping sites of esophagus
C15.9	Malignant neoplasm of esophagus, unspecified
C16.0	Malignant neoplasm of cardia
C16.1	Malignant neoplasm of fundus of stomach
C16.2	Malignant neoplasm of body of stomach
C16.3	Malignant neoplasm of pyloric antrum

ICD-10-CM	ICD-10-CM Code Descriptor 0037U: Effective Date: 04/01/2018
C16.4	Malignant neoplasm of pylorus
C16.5	Malignant neoplasm of lesser curvature of stomach, unspecified
C16.6	Malignant neoplasm of greater curvature of stomach, unspecified
C16.8	Malignant neoplasm of overlapping sites of stomach
C16.9	Malignant neoplasm of stomach, unspecified
C17.0	Malignant neoplasm of duodenum
C17.1	Malignant neoplasm of jejunum
C17.2	Malignant neoplasm of ileum
C17.3	Meckel's diverticulum, malignant
C17.8	Malignant neoplasm of overlapping sites of small intestine
C17.9	Malignant neoplasm of small intestine, unspecified
C18.0	Malignant neoplasm of cecum
C18.1	Malignant neoplasm of appendix
C18.2	Malignant neoplasm of ascending colon
C18.3	Malignant neoplasm of hepatic flexure
C18.4	Malignant neoplasm of transverse colon
C18.5	Malignant neoplasm of splenic flexure
C18.6	Malignant neoplasm of descending colon
C18.7	Malignant neoplasm of sigmoid colon
C18.8	Malignant neoplasm of overlapping sites of colon
C18.9	Malignant neoplasm of colon, unspecified
C19	Malignant neoplasm of rectosigmoid junction
C20	Malignant neoplasm of rectum
C21.0	Malignant neoplasm of anus, unspecified
C21.1	Malignant neoplasm of anal canal
C21.2	Malignant neoplasm of cloacogenic zone
C21.8	Malignant neoplasm of overlapping sites of rectum, anus and anal canal
C22.0	Liver cell carcinoma
C22.1	Intrahepatic bile duct carcinoma
C22.2	Hepatoblastoma
C22.3	Angiosarcoma of liver
C22.4	Other sarcomas of liver
C22.7	Other specified carcinomas of liver
C22.8	Malignant neoplasm of liver, primary, unspecified as to type
C22.9	Malignant neoplasm of liver, not specified as primary or secondary
C23	Malignant neoplasm of gallbladder
C24.0	Malignant neoplasm of extrahepatic bile duct
C24.1	Malignant neoplasm of ampulla of Vater
C24.8	Malignant neoplasm of overlapping sites of biliary tract
C24.9	Malignant neoplasm of biliary tract, unspecified
C25.0	Malignant neoplasm of head of pancreas
C25.1	Malignant neoplasm of body of pancreas
C25.2	Malignant neoplasm of tail of pancreas
C25.3	Malignant neoplasm of pancreatic duct
C25.4	Malignant neoplasm of endocrine pancreas
C25.7	Malignant neoplasm of other parts of pancreas
C25.8	Malignant neoplasm of overlapping sites of pancreas
C25.9	Malignant neoplasm of pancreas, unspecified
C26.0	Malignant neoplasm of intestinal tract, part unspecified
C26.1	Malignant neoplasm of spleen
C26.9	Malignant neoplasm of ill-defined sites within the digestive system
C30.0	Malignant neoplasm of nasal cavity
C30.1	Malignant neoplasm of middle ear
C31.0	Malignant neoplasm of maxillary sinus
C31.1	Malignant neoplasm of ethmoidal sinus
C31.2	Malignant neoplasm of frontal sinus
C31.3	Malignant neoplasm of sphenoid sinus
C31.8	Malignant neoplasm of overlapping sites of accessory sinuses
C31.9	Malignant neoplasm of accessory sinus, unspecified
C32.0	Malignant neoplasm of glottis
C32.1	Malignant neoplasm of supraglottis
C32.2	Malignant neoplasm of subglottis
C32.3	Malignant neoplasm of laryngeal cartilage

ICD-10-CM	ICD-10-CM Code Descriptor 0037U: Effective Date: 04/01/2018
C32.8	Malignant neoplasm of overlapping sites of larynx
C32.9	Malignant neoplasm of larynx, unspecified
C33	Malignant neoplasm of trachea
C34.00	Malignant neoplasm of unspecified main bronchus
C34.01	Malignant neoplasm of right main bronchus
C34.02	Malignant neoplasm of left main bronchus
C34.10	Malignant neoplasm of upper lobe, unspecified bronchus or lung
C34.11	Malignant neoplasm of upper lobe, right bronchus or lung
C34.12	Malignant neoplasm of upper lobe, left bronchus or lung
C34.2	Malignant neoplasm of middle lobe, bronchus or lung
C34.30	Malignant neoplasm of lower lobe, unspecified bronchus or lung
C34.31	Malignant neoplasm of lower lobe, right bronchus or lung
C34.32	Malignant neoplasm of lower lobe, left bronchus or lung
C34.80	Malignant neoplasm of overlapping sites of unspecified bronchus and lung
C34.81	Malignant neoplasm of overlapping sites of right bronchus and lung
C34.82	Malignant neoplasm of overlapping sites of left bronchus and lung
C34.90	Malignant neoplasm of unspecified part of unspecified bronchus or lung
C34.91	Malignant neoplasm of unspecified part of right bronchus or lung
C34.92	Malignant neoplasm of unspecified part of left bronchus or lung
C37	Malignant neoplasm of thymus
C38.0	Malignant neoplasm of heart
C38.1	Malignant neoplasm of anterior mediastinum
C38.2	Malignant neoplasm of posterior mediastinum
C38.3	Malignant neoplasm of mediastinum, part unspecified
C38.4	Malignant neoplasm of pleura
C38.8	Malignant neoplasm of overlapping sites of heart, mediastinum and pleura
C39.0	Malignant neoplasm of upper respiratory tract, part unspecified
C39.9	Malignant neoplasm of lower respiratory tract, part unspecified
C40.00	Malignant neoplasm of scapula and long bones of unspecified upper limb
C40.01	Malignant neoplasm of scapula and long bones of right upper limb
C40.02	Malignant neoplasm of scapula and long bones of left upper limb
C40.10	Malignant neoplasm of short bones of unspecified upper limb
C40.11	Malignant neoplasm of short bones of right upper limb
C40.12	Malignant neoplasm of short bones of left upper limb
C40.20	Malignant neoplasm of long bones of unspecified lower limb
C40.21	Malignant neoplasm of long bones of right lower limb
C40.22	Malignant neoplasm of long bones of left lower limb
C40.30	Malignant neoplasm of short bones of unspecified lower limb
C40.31	Malignant neoplasm of short bones of right lower limb
C40.32	Malignant neoplasm of short bones of left lower limb
C40.80	Malignant neoplasm of overlapping sites of bone and articular cartilage of unspecified limb
C40.81	Malignant neoplasm of overlapping sites of bone and articular cartilage of right limb
C40.82	Malignant neoplasm of overlapping sites of bone and articular cartilage of left limb
C40.90	Malignant neoplasm of unspecified bones and articular cartilage of unspecified limb
C40.91	Malignant neoplasm of unspecified bones and articular cartilage of right limb
C40.92	Malignant neoplasm of unspecified bones and articular cartilage of left limb
C41.0	Malignant neoplasm of bones of skull and face
C41.1	Malignant neoplasm of mandible
C41.2	Malignant neoplasm of vertebral column
C41.3	Malignant neoplasm of ribs, sternum and clavicle
C41.4	Malignant neoplasm of pelvic bones, sacrum and coccyx
C41.9	Malignant neoplasm of bone and articular cartilage, unspecified
C43.0	Malignant melanoma of lip
C43.10	Malignant melanoma of unspecified eyelid, including canthus
C43.11	Malignant melanoma of right eyelid, including canthus Expired 9/30/2018

Appendix G — Medicare Internet-only Manuals (IOMs)

ICD-10-CM	ICD-10-CM Code Descriptor 0037U: Effective Date: 04/01/2018
C43.111	Malignant melanoma of right upper eyelid, including canthus Effective 10/1/2018
C43.112	Malignant melanoma of right lower eyelid, including canthus Effective 10/1/2018
C43.12	Malignant melanoma of left eyelid, including canthus Expired 9/30/2018
C43.121	Malignant melanoma of left upper eyelid, including canthus Effective 10/1/2018
C43.122	Malignant melanoma of left lower eyelid, including canthus Effective 10/1/2018
C43.20	Malignant melanoma of unspecified ear and external auricular canal
C43.21	Malignant melanoma of right ear and external auricular canal
C43.22	Malignant melanoma of left ear and external auricular canal
C43.30	Malignant melanoma of unspecified part of face
C43.31	Malignant melanoma of nose
C43.39	Malignant melanoma of other parts of face
C43.4	Malignant melanoma of scalp and neck
C43.51	Malignant melanoma of anal skin
C43.52	Malignant melanoma of skin of breast
C43.59	Malignant melanoma of other part of trunk
C43.60	Malignant melanoma of unspecified upper limb, including shoulder
C43.61	Malignant melanoma of right upper limb, including shoulder
C43.62	Malignant melanoma of left upper limb, including shoulder
C43.70	Malignant melanoma of unspecified lower limb, including hip
C43.71	Malignant melanoma of right lower limb, including hip
C43.72	Malignant melanoma of left lower limb, including hip
C43.8	Malignant melanoma of overlapping sites of skin
C43.9	Malignant melanoma of skin, unspecified
C44.00	Unspecified malignant neoplasm of skin of lip
C44.01	Basal cell carcinoma of skin of lip
C44.02	Squamous cell carcinoma of skin of lip
C44.09	Other specified malignant neoplasm of skin of lip
C44.101	Unspecified malignant neoplasm of skin of unspecified eyelid, including canthus
C44.102	Unspecified malignant neoplasm of skin of right eyelid, including canthus Expired 9/30/2018
C44.1021	Unspecified malignant neoplasm of skin of right upper eyelid, including canthus Effective 10/1/2018
C44.1022	Unspecified malignant neoplasm of skin of right lower eyelid, including canthus Effective 10/1/2018
C44.109	Unspecified malignant neoplasm of skin of left eyelid, including canthus Expired 9/30/2018
C44.1091	Unspecified malignant neoplasm of skin of left upper eyelid, including canthus Effective 10/1/2018
C44.1092	Unspecified malignant neoplasm of skin of left lower eyelid, including canthus Effective 10/1/2018
C44.111	Basal cell carcinoma of skin of unspecified eyelid, including canthus
C44.112	Basal cell carcinoma of skin of right eyelid, including canthus Expired 9/30/2018
C44.1121	Basal cell carcinoma of skin of right upper eyelid, including canthus Effective 10/1/2018
C44.1122	Basal cell carcinoma of skin of right lower eyelid, including canthus Effective 10/1/2018
C44.119	Basal cell carcinoma of skin of left eyelid, including canthus Expired 9/30/2018
C44.1191	Basal cell carcinoma of skin of left upper eyelid, including canthus Effective 10/1/2018
C44.1192	Basal cell carcinoma of skin of left lower eyelid, including canthus Effective 10/1/2018

ICD-10-CM	ICD-10-CM Code Descriptor 0037U: Effective Date: 04/01/2018
C44.121	Squamous cell carcinoma of skin of unspecified eyelid, including canthus
C44.122	Squamous cell carcinoma of skin of right eyelid, including canthus Expired 9/30/2018
C44.1221	Squamous cell carcinoma of skin of right upper eyelid, including canthus Effective 10/1/2018
C44.1222	Squamous cell carcinoma of skin of right lower eyelid, including canthus Effective 10/1/2018
C44.129	Squamous cell carcinoma of skin of left eyelid, including canthus Expired 9/30/2018
C44.1291	Squamous cell carcinoma of skin of left upper eyelid, including canthus Effective 10/1/2018
C44.1292	Squamous cell carcinoma of skin of left lower eyelid, including canthus Effective 10/1/2018
C44.191	Other specified malignant neoplasm of skin of unspecified eyelid, including canthus
C44.192	Other specified malignant neoplasm of skin of right eyelid, including canthus Expired 9/30/2018
C44.1921	Other specified malignant neoplasm of skin of right upper eyelid, including canthus Effective 10/1/2018
C44.1922	Other specified malignant neoplasm of skin of right lower eyelid, including canthus Effective 10/1/2018
C44.199	Other specified malignant neoplasm of skin of left eyelid, including canthus Expired 9/30/2018
C44.1991	Other specified malignant neoplasm of skin of left upper eyelid, including canthus Effective 10/1/2018
C44.1992	Other specified malignant neoplasm of skin of left lower eyelid, including canthus Effective 10/1/2018
C44.201	Unspecified malignant neoplasm of skin of unspecified ear and external auricular canal
C44.202	Unspecified malignant neoplasm of skin of right ear and external auricular canal
C44.209	Unspecified malignant neoplasm of skin of left ear and external auricular canal
C44.211	Basal cell carcinoma of skin of unspecified ear and external auricular canal
C44.212	Basal cell carcinoma of skin of right ear and external auricular canal
C44.219	Basal cell carcinoma of skin of left ear and external auricular canal
C44.221	Squamous cell carcinoma of skin of unspecified ear and external auricular canal
C44.222	Squamous cell carcinoma of skin of right ear and external auricular canal
C44.229	Squamous cell carcinoma of skin of left ear and external auricular canal
C44.291	Other specified malignant neoplasm of skin of unspecified ear and external auricular canal
C44.292	Other specified malignant neoplasm of skin of right ear and external auricular canal
C44.299	Other specified malignant neoplasm of skin of left ear and external auricular canal
C44.300	Unspecified malignant neoplasm of skin of unspecified part of face
C44.301	Unspecified malignant neoplasm of skin of nose
C44.309	Unspecified malignant neoplasm of skin of other parts of face
C44.310	Basal cell carcinoma of skin of unspecified parts of face
C44.311	Basal cell carcinoma of skin of nose
C44.319	Basal cell carcinoma of skin of other parts of face
C44.320	Squamous cell carcinoma of skin of unspecified parts of face
C44.321	Squamous cell carcinoma of skin of nose
C44.329	Squamous cell carcinoma of skin of other parts of face

ICD-10-CM	ICD-10-CM Code Descriptor 0037U: Effective Date: 04/01/2018
C44.390	Other specified malignant neoplasm of skin of unspecified parts of face
C44.391	Other specified malignant neoplasm of skin of nose
C44.399	Other specified malignant neoplasm of skin of other parts of face
C44.40	Unspecified malignant neoplasm of skin of scalp and neck
C44.41	Basal cell carcinoma of skin of scalp and neck
C44.42	Squamous cell carcinoma of skin of scalp and neck
C44.49	Other specified malignant neoplasm of skin of scalp and neck
C44.500	Unspecified malignant neoplasm of anal skin
C44.501	Unspecified malignant neoplasm of skin of breast
C44.509	Unspecified malignant neoplasm of skin of other part of trunk
C44.510	Basal cell carcinoma of anal skin
C44.511	Basal cell carcinoma of skin of breast
C44.519	Basal cell carcinoma of skin of other part of trunk
C44.520	Squamous cell carcinoma of anal skin
C44.521	Squamous cell carcinoma of skin of breast
C44.529	Squamous cell carcinoma of skin of other part of trunk
C44.590	Other specified malignant neoplasm of anal skin
C44.591	Other specified malignant neoplasm of skin of breast
C44.599	Other specified malignant neoplasm of skin of other part of trunk
C44.601	Unspecified malignant neoplasm of skin of unspecified upper limb, including shoulder
C44.602	Unspecified malignant neoplasm of skin of right upper limb, including shoulder
C44.609	Unspecified malignant neoplasm of skin of left upper limb, including shoulder
C44.611	Basal cell carcinoma of skin of unspecified upper limb, including shoulder
C44.612	Basal cell carcinoma of skin of right upper limb, including shoulder
C44.619	Basal cell carcinoma of skin of left upper limb, including shoulder
C44.621	Squamous cell carcinoma of skin of unspecified upper limb, including shoulder
C44.622	Squamous cell carcinoma of skin of right upper limb, including shoulder
C44.629	Squamous cell carcinoma of skin of left upper limb, including shoulder
C44.691	Other specified malignant neoplasm of skin of unspecified upper limb, including shoulder
C44.692	Other specified malignant neoplasm of skin of right upper limb, including shoulder
C44.699	Other specified malignant neoplasm of skin of left upper limb, including shoulder
C44.701	Unspecified malignant neoplasm of skin of unspecified lower limb, including hip
C44.702	Unspecified malignant neoplasm of skin of right lower limb, including hip
C44.709	Unspecified malignant neoplasm of skin of left lower limb, including hip
C44.711	Basal cell carcinoma of skin of unspecified lower limb, including hip
C44.712	Basal cell carcinoma of skin of right lower limb, including hip
C44.719	Basal cell carcinoma of skin of left lower limb, including hip
C44.721	Squamous cell carcinoma of skin of unspecified lower limb, including hip
C44.722	Squamous cell carcinoma of skin of right lower limb, including hip
C44.729	Squamous cell carcinoma of skin of left lower limb, including hip
C44.791	Other specified malignant neoplasm of skin of unspecified lower limb, including hip
C44.792	Other specified malignant neoplasm of skin of right lower limb, including hip
C44.799	Other specified malignant neoplasm of skin of left lower limb, including hip
C44.80	Unspecified malignant neoplasm of overlapping sites of skin
C44.81	Basal cell carcinoma of overlapping sites of skin
C44.82	Squamous cell carcinoma of overlapping sites of skin
C44.89	Other specified malignant neoplasm of overlapping sites of skin
C44.90	Unspecified malignant neoplasm of skin, unspecified
C44.91	Basal cell carcinoma of skin, unspecified
C44.92	Squamous cell carcinoma of skin, unspecified
C44.99	Other specified malignant neoplasm of skin, unspecified

ICD-10-CM	ICD-10-CM Code Descriptor 0037U: Effective Date: 04/01/2018
C45.0	Mesothelioma of pleura
C45.1	Mesothelioma of peritoneum
C45.2	Mesothelioma of pericardium
C45.7	Mesothelioma of other sites
C45.9	Mesothelioma, unspecified
C47.0	Malignant neoplasm of peripheral nerves of head, face and neck
C47.10	Malignant neoplasm of peripheral nerves of unspecified upper limb, including shoulder
C47.11	Malignant neoplasm of peripheral nerves of right upper limb, including shoulder
C47.12	Malignant neoplasm of peripheral nerves of left upper limb, including shoulder
C47.20	Malignant neoplasm of peripheral nerves of unspecified lower limb, including hip
C47.21	Malignant neoplasm of peripheral nerves of right lower limb, including hip
C47.22	Malignant neoplasm of peripheral nerves of left lower limb, including hip
C47.3	Malignant neoplasm of peripheral nerves of thorax
C47.4	Malignant neoplasm of peripheral nerves of abdomen
C47.5	Malignant neoplasm of peripheral nerves of pelvis
C47.6	Malignant neoplasm of peripheral nerves of trunk, unspecified
C47.8	Malignant neoplasm of overlapping sites of peripheral nerves and autonomic nervous system
C47.9	Malignant neoplasm of peripheral nerves and autonomic nervous system, unspecified
C48.0	Malignant neoplasm of retroperitoneum
C48.1	Malignant neoplasm of specified parts of peritoneum
C48.2	Malignant neoplasm of peritoneum, unspecified
C48.8	Malignant neoplasm of overlapping sites of retroperitoneum and peritoneum
C49.0	Malignant neoplasm of connective and soft tissue of head, face and neck
C49.10	Malignant neoplasm of connective and soft tissue of unspecified upper limb, including shoulder
C49.11	Malignant neoplasm of connective and soft tissue of right upper limb, including shoulder
C49.12	Malignant neoplasm of connective and soft tissue of left upper limb, including shoulder
C49.20	Malignant neoplasm of connective and soft tissue of unspecified lower limb, including hip
C49.21	Malignant neoplasm of connective and soft tissue of right lower limb, including hip
C49.22	Malignant neoplasm of connective and soft tissue of left lower limb, including hip
C49.3	Malignant neoplasm of connective and soft tissue of thorax
C49.4	Malignant neoplasm of connective and soft tissue of abdomen
C49.5	Malignant neoplasm of connective and soft tissue of pelvis
C49.6	Malignant neoplasm of connective and soft tissue of trunk, unspecified
C49.8	Malignant neoplasm of overlapping sites of connective and soft tissue
C49.9	Malignant neoplasm of connective and soft tissue, unspecified
C49.A0	Gastrointestinal stromal tumor, unspecified site
C49.A1	Gastrointestinal stromal tumor of esophagus
C49.A2	Gastrointestinal stromal tumor of stomach
C49.A3	Gastrointestinal stromal tumor of small intestine
C49.A4	Gastrointestinal stromal tumor of large intestine
C49.A5	Gastrointestinal stromal tumor of rectum
C49.A9	Gastrointestinal stromal tumor of other sites
C4A.0	Merkel cell carcinoma of lip
C4A.10	Merkel cell carcinoma of unspecified eyelid, including canthus
C4A.11	Merkel cell carcinoma of right eyelid, including canthus Expired 9/30/2018
C4A.111	Merkel cell carcinoma of right upper eyelid, including canthus Effective 10/1/2018
C4A.112	Merkel cell carcinoma of right lower eyelid, including canthus Effective 10/1/2018

Appendix G — Medicare Internet-only Manuals (IOMs)

ICD-10-CM	ICD-10-CM Code Descriptor 0037U: Effective Date: 04/01/2018
C4A.12	Merkel cell carcinoma of left eyelid, including canthus Expired 9/30/2018
C4A.121	Merkel cell carcinoma of left upper eyelid, including canthus Effective 10/1/2018
C4A.122	Merkel cell carcinoma of left lower eyelid, including canthus Effective 10/1/2018
C4A.20	Merkel cell carcinoma of unspecified ear and external auricular canal
C4A.21	Merkel cell carcinoma of right ear and external auricular canal
C4A.22	Merkel cell carcinoma of left ear and external auricular canal
C4A.30	Merkel cell carcinoma of unspecified part of face
C4A.31	Merkel cell carcinoma of nose
C4A.39	Merkel cell carcinoma of other parts of face
C4A.4	Merkel cell carcinoma of scalp and neck
C4A.51	Merkel cell carcinoma of anal skin
C4A.52	Merkel cell carcinoma of skin of breast
C4A.59	Merkel cell carcinoma of other part of trunk
C4A.60	Merkel cell carcinoma of unspecified upper limb, including shoulder
C4A.61	Merkel cell carcinoma of right upper limb, including shoulder
C4A.62	Merkel cell carcinoma of left upper limb, including shoulder
C4A.70	Merkel cell carcinoma of unspecified lower limb, including hip
C4A.71	Merkel cell carcinoma of right lower limb, including hip
C4A.72	Merkel cell carcinoma of left lower limb, including hip
C4A.8	Merkel cell carcinoma of overlapping sites
C4A.9	Merkel cell carcinoma, unspecified
C50.011	Malignant neoplasm of nipple and areola, right female breast
C50.012	Malignant neoplasm of nipple and areola, left female breast
C50.019	Malignant neoplasm of nipple and areola, unspecified female breast
C50.021	Malignant neoplasm of nipple and areola, right male breast
C50.022	Malignant neoplasm of nipple and areola, left male breast
C50.029	Malignant neoplasm of nipple and areola, unspecified male breast
C50.111	Malignant neoplasm of central portion of right female breast
C50.112	Malignant neoplasm of central portion of left female breast
C50.119	Malignant neoplasm of central portion of unspecified female breast
C50.121	Malignant neoplasm of central portion of right male breast
C50.122	Malignant neoplasm of central portion of left male breast
C50.129	Malignant neoplasm of central portion of unspecified male breast
C50.211	Malignant neoplasm of upper-inner quadrant of right female breast
C50.212	Malignant neoplasm of upper-inner quadrant of left female breast
C50.219	Malignant neoplasm of upper-inner quadrant of unspecified female breast
C50.221	Malignant neoplasm of upper-inner quadrant of right male breast
C50.222	Malignant neoplasm of upper-inner quadrant of left male breast
C50.229	Malignant neoplasm of upper-inner quadrant of unspecified male breast
C50.311	Malignant neoplasm of lower-inner quadrant of right female breast
C50.312	Malignant neoplasm of lower-inner quadrant of left female breast
C50.319	Malignant neoplasm of lower-inner quadrant of unspecified female breast
C50.321	Malignant neoplasm of lower-inner quadrant of right male breast
C50.322	Malignant neoplasm of lower-inner quadrant of left male breast
C50.329	Malignant neoplasm of lower-inner quadrant of unspecified male breast
C50.411	Malignant neoplasm of upper-outer quadrant of right female breast
C50.412	Malignant neoplasm of upper-outer quadrant of left female breast
C50.419	Malignant neoplasm of upper-outer quadrant of unspecified female breast
C50.421	Malignant neoplasm of upper-outer quadrant of right male breast
C50.422	Malignant neoplasm of upper-outer quadrant of left male breast
C50.429	Malignant neoplasm of upper-outer quadrant of unspecified male breast
C50.511	Malignant neoplasm of lower-outer quadrant of right female breast
C50.512	Malignant neoplasm of lower-outer quadrant of left female breast
C50.519	Malignant neoplasm of lower-outer quadrant of unspecified female breast
C50.521	Malignant neoplasm of lower-outer quadrant of right male breast

ICD-10-CM	ICD-10-CM Code Descriptor 0037U: Effective Date: 04/01/2018
C50.522	Malignant neoplasm of lower-outer quadrant of left male breast
C50.529	Malignant neoplasm of lower-outer quadrant of unspecified male breast
C50.611	Malignant neoplasm of axillary tail of right female breast
C50.612	Malignant neoplasm of axillary tail of left female breast
C50.619	Malignant neoplasm of axillary tail of unspecified female breast
C50.621	Malignant neoplasm of axillary tail of right male breast
C50.622	Malignant neoplasm of axillary tail of left male breast
C50.629	Malignant neoplasm of axillary tail of unspecified male breast
C50.811	Malignant neoplasm of overlapping sites of right female breast
C50.812	Malignant neoplasm of overlapping sites of left female breast
C50.819	Malignant neoplasm of overlapping sites of unspecified female breast
C50.821	Malignant neoplasm of overlapping sites of right male breast
C50.822	Malignant neoplasm of overlapping sites of left male breast
C50.829	Malignant neoplasm of overlapping sites of unspecified male breast
C50.911	Malignant neoplasm of unspecified site of right female breast
C50.912	Malignant neoplasm of unspecified site of left female breast
C50.919	Malignant neoplasm of unspecified site of unspecified female breast
C50.921	Malignant neoplasm of unspecified site of right male breast
C50.922	Malignant neoplasm of unspecified site of left male breast
C50.929	Malignant neoplasm of unspecified site of unspecified male breast
C51.0	Malignant neoplasm of labium majus
C51.1	Malignant neoplasm of labium minus
C51.2	Malignant neoplasm of clitoris
C51.8	Malignant neoplasm of overlapping sites of vulva
C51.9	Malignant neoplasm of vulva, unspecified
C52	Malignant neoplasm of vagina
C53.0	Malignant neoplasm of endocervix
C53.1	Malignant neoplasm of exocervix
C53.8	Malignant neoplasm of overlapping sites of cervix uteri
C53.9	Malignant neoplasm of cervix uteri, unspecified
C54.0	Malignant neoplasm of isthmus uteri
C54.1	Malignant neoplasm of endometrium
C54.2	Malignant neoplasm of myometrium
C54.3	Malignant neoplasm of fundus uteri
C54.8	Malignant neoplasm of overlapping sites of corpus uteri
C54.9	Malignant neoplasm of corpus uteri, unspecified
C55	Malignant neoplasm of uterus, part unspecified
C56.1	Malignant neoplasm of right ovary
C56.2	Malignant neoplasm of left ovary
C56.9	Malignant neoplasm of unspecified ovary
C57.00	Malignant neoplasm of unspecified fallopian tube
C57.01	Malignant neoplasm of right fallopian tube
C57.02	Malignant neoplasm of left fallopian tube
C57.10	Malignant neoplasm of unspecified broad ligament
C57.11	Malignant neoplasm of right broad ligament
C57.12	Malignant neoplasm of left broad ligament
C57.20	Malignant neoplasm of unspecified round ligament
C57.21	Malignant neoplasm of right round ligament
C57.22	Malignant neoplasm of left round ligament
C57.3	Malignant neoplasm of parametrium
C57.4	Malignant neoplasm of uterine adnexa, unspecified
C57.7	Malignant neoplasm of other specified female genital organs
C57.8	Malignant neoplasm of overlapping sites of female genital organs
C57.9	Malignant neoplasm of female genital organ, unspecified
C58	Malignant neoplasm of placenta
C60.0	Malignant neoplasm of prepuce
C60.1	Malignant neoplasm of glans penis
C60.2	Malignant neoplasm of body of penis
C60.8	Malignant neoplasm of overlapping sites of penis
C60.9	Malignant neoplasm of penis, unspecified
C61	Malignant neoplasm of prostate
C62.00	Malignant neoplasm of unspecified undescended testis
C62.01	Malignant neoplasm of undescended right testis

ICD-10-CM	ICD-10-CM Code Descriptor 0037U: Effective Date: 04/01/2018
C62.02	Malignant neoplasm of undescended left testis
C62.10	Malignant neoplasm of unspecified descended testis
C62.11	Malignant neoplasm of descended right testis
C62.12	Malignant neoplasm of descended left testis
C62.90	Malignant neoplasm of unspecified testis, unspecified whether descended or undescended
C62.91	Malignant neoplasm of right testis, unspecified whether descended or undescended
C62.92	Malignant neoplasm of left testis, unspecified whether descended or undescended
C63.00	Malignant neoplasm of unspecified epididymis
C63.01	Malignant neoplasm of right epididymis
C63.02	Malignant neoplasm of left epididymis
C63.10	Malignant neoplasm of unspecified spermatic cord
C63.11	Malignant neoplasm of right spermatic cord
C63.12	Malignant neoplasm of left spermatic cord
C63.2	Malignant neoplasm of scrotum
C63.7	Malignant neoplasm of other specified male genital organs
C63.8	Malignant neoplasm of overlapping sites of male genital organs
C63.9	Malignant neoplasm of male genital organ, unspecified
C64.1	Malignant neoplasm of right kidney, except renal pelvis
C64.2	Malignant neoplasm of left kidney, except renal pelvis
C64.9	Malignant neoplasm of unspecified kidney, except renal pelvis
C65.1	Malignant neoplasm of right renal pelvis
C65.2	Malignant neoplasm of left renal pelvis
C65.9	Malignant neoplasm of unspecified renal pelvis
C66.1	Malignant neoplasm of right ureter
C66.2	Malignant neoplasm of left ureter
C66.9	Malignant neoplasm of unspecified ureter
C67.0	Malignant neoplasm of trigone of bladder
C67.1	Malignant neoplasm of dome of bladder
C67.2	Malignant neoplasm of lateral wall of bladder
C67.3	Malignant neoplasm of anterior wall of bladder
C67.4	Malignant neoplasm of posterior wall of bladder
C67.5	Malignant neoplasm of bladder neck
C67.6	Malignant neoplasm of ureteric orifice
C67.7	Malignant neoplasm of urachus
C67.8	Malignant neoplasm of overlapping sites of bladder
C67.9	Malignant neoplasm of bladder, unspecified
C68.0	Malignant neoplasm of urethra
C68.1	Malignant neoplasm of paraurethral glands
C68.8	Malignant neoplasm of overlapping sites of urinary organs
C68.9	Malignant neoplasm of urinary organ, unspecified
C69.00	Malignant neoplasm of unspecified conjunctiva
C69.01	Malignant neoplasm of right conjunctiva
C69.02	Malignant neoplasm of left conjunctiva
C69.10	Malignant neoplasm of unspecified cornea
C69.11	Malignant neoplasm of right cornea
C69.12	Malignant neoplasm of left cornea
C69.20	Malignant neoplasm of unspecified retina
C69.21	Malignant neoplasm of right retina
C69.22	Malignant neoplasm of left retina
C69.30	Malignant neoplasm of unspecified choroid
C69.31	Malignant neoplasm of right choroid
C69.32	Malignant neoplasm of left choroid
C69.40	Malignant neoplasm of unspecified ciliary body
C69.41	Malignant neoplasm of right ciliary body
C69.42	Malignant neoplasm of left ciliary body
C69.50	Malignant neoplasm of unspecified lacrimal gland and duct
C69.51	Malignant neoplasm of right lacrimal gland and duct
C69.52	Malignant neoplasm of left lacrimal gland and duct
C69.60	Malignant neoplasm of unspecified orbit
C69.61	Malignant neoplasm of right orbit
C69.62	Malignant neoplasm of left orbit

ICD-10-CM	ICD-10-CM Code Descriptor 0037U: Effective Date: 04/01/2018
C69.80	Malignant neoplasm of overlapping sites of unspecified eye and adnexa
C69.81	Malignant neoplasm of overlapping sites of right eye and adnexa
C69.82	Malignant neoplasm of overlapping sites of left eye and adnexa
C69.90	Malignant neoplasm of unspecified site of unspecified eye
C69.91	Malignant neoplasm of unspecified site of right eye
C69.92	Malignant neoplasm of unspecified site of left eye
C70.0	Malignant neoplasm of cerebral meninges
C70.1	Malignant neoplasm of spinal meninges
C70.9	Malignant neoplasm of meninges, unspecified
C71.0	Malignant neoplasm of cerebrum, except lobes and ventricles
C71.1	Malignant neoplasm of frontal lobe
C71.2	Malignant neoplasm of temporal lobe
C71.3	Malignant neoplasm of parietal lobe
C71.4	Malignant neoplasm of occipital lobe
C71.5	Malignant neoplasm of cerebral ventricle
C71.6	Malignant neoplasm of cerebellum
C71.7	Malignant neoplasm of brain stem
C71.8	Malignant neoplasm of overlapping sites of brain
C71.9	Malignant neoplasm of brain, unspecified
C72.0	Malignant neoplasm of spinal cord
C72.1	Malignant neoplasm of cauda equina
C72.20	Malignant neoplasm of unspecified olfactory nerve
C72.21	Malignant neoplasm of right olfactory nerve
C72.22	Malignant neoplasm of left olfactory nerve
C72.30	Malignant neoplasm of unspecified optic nerve
C72.31	Malignant neoplasm of right optic nerve
C72.32	Malignant neoplasm of left optic nerve
C72.40	Malignant neoplasm of unspecified acoustic nerve
C72.41	Malignant neoplasm of right acoustic nerve
C72.42	Malignant neoplasm of left acoustic nerve
C72.50	Malignant neoplasm of unspecified cranial nerve
C72.59	Malignant neoplasm of other cranial nerves
C72.9	Malignant neoplasm of central nervous system, unspecified
C73	Malignant neoplasm of thyroid gland
C74.00	Malignant neoplasm of cortex of unspecified adrenal gland
C74.01	Malignant neoplasm of cortex of right adrenal gland
C74.02	Malignant neoplasm of cortex of left adrenal gland
C74.10	Malignant neoplasm of medulla of unspecified adrenal gland
C74.11	Malignant neoplasm of medulla of right adrenal gland
C74.12	Malignant neoplasm of medulla of left adrenal gland
C74.90	Malignant neoplasm of unspecified part of unspecified adrenal gland
C74.91	Malignant neoplasm of unspecified part of right adrenal gland
C74.92	Malignant neoplasm of unspecified part of left adrenal gland
C75.0	Malignant neoplasm of parathyroid gland
C75.1	Malignant neoplasm of pituitary gland
C75.2	Malignant neoplasm of craniopharyngeal duct
C75.3	Malignant neoplasm of pineal gland
C75.4	Malignant neoplasm of carotid body
C75.5	Malignant neoplasm of aortic body and other paraganglia
C75.8	Malignant neoplasm with pluriglandular involvement, unspecified
C75.9	Malignant neoplasm of endocrine gland, unspecified
C76.0	Malignant neoplasm of head, face and neck
C76.1	Malignant neoplasm of thorax
C76.2	Malignant neoplasm of abdomen
C76.3	Malignant neoplasm of pelvis
C76.40	Malignant neoplasm of unspecified upper limb
C76.41	Malignant neoplasm of right upper limb
C76.42	Malignant neoplasm of left upper limb
C76.50	Malignant neoplasm of unspecified lower limb
C76.51	Malignant neoplasm of right lower limb
C76.52	Malignant neoplasm of left lower limb
C76.8	Malignant neoplasm of other specified ill-defined sites
C7A.00	Malignant carcinoid tumor of unspecified site

ICD-10-CM	ICD-10-CM Code Descriptor 0037U: Effective Date: 04/01/2018
C7A.010	Malignant carcinoid tumor of the duodenum
C7A.011	Malignant carcinoid tumor of the jejunum
C7A.012	Malignant carcinoid tumor of the ileum
C7A.019	Malignant carcinoid tumor of the small intestine, unspecified portion
C7A.020	Malignant carcinoid tumor of the appendix
C7A.021	Malignant carcinoid tumor of the cecum
C7A.022	Malignant carcinoid tumor of the ascending colon
C7A.023	Malignant carcinoid tumor of the transverse colon
C7A.024	Malignant carcinoid tumor of the descending colon
C7A.025	Malignant carcinoid tumor of the sigmoid colon
C7A.026	Malignant carcinoid tumor of the rectum
C7A.029	Malignant carcinoid tumor of the large intestine, unspecified portion
C7A.090	Malignant carcinoid tumor of the bronchus and lung
C7A.091	Malignant carcinoid tumor of the thymus
C7A.092	Malignant carcinoid tumor of the stomach
C7A.093	Malignant carcinoid tumor of the kidney
C7A.094	Malignant carcinoid tumor of the foregut, unspecified
C7A.095	Malignant carcinoid tumor of the midgut, unspecified
C7A.096	Malignant carcinoid tumor of the hindgut, unspecified
C7A.098	Malignant carcinoid tumors of other sites
C7A.1	Malignant poorly differentiated neuroendocrine tumors
C7A.8	Other malignant neuroendocrine tumors
C80.0	Disseminated malignant neoplasm, unspecified
C80.1	Malignant (primary) neoplasm, unspecified
C80.2	Malignant neoplasm associated with transplanted organ

ICD-10-CM	ICD-10-CM Code Descriptor 0022U: Effective Date: 03/16/2018
C33	Malignant neoplasm of trachea
C34.00	Malignant neoplasm of unspecified main bronchus
C34.01	Malignant neoplasm of right main bronchus
C34.02	Malignant neoplasm of left main bronchus
C34.10	Malignant neoplasm of upper lobe, unspecified bronchus or lung
C34.11	Malignant neoplasm of upper lobe, right bronchus or lung
C34.12	Malignant neoplasm of upper lobe, left bronchus or lung
C34.2	Malignant neoplasm of middle lobe, bronchus or lung
C34.30	Malignant neoplasm of lower lobe, unspecified bronchus or lung
C34.31	Malignant neoplasm of lower lobe, right bronchus or lung
C34.32	Malignant neoplasm of lower lobe, left bronchus or lung
C34.80	Malignant neoplasm of overlapping sites of unspecified bronchus and lung
C34.81	Malignant neoplasm of overlapping sites of right bronchus and lung
C34.82	Malignant neoplasm of overlapping sites of left bronchus and lung
C34.90	Malignant neoplasm of unspecified part of unspecified bronchus or lung
C34.91	Malignant neoplasm of unspecified part of right bronchus or lung
C34.92	Malignant neoplasm of unspecified part of left bronchus or lung

100-03, 100.1

100.1 - Bariatric Surgery for Treatment of Co-Morbid Conditions Related to Morbid Obesity

(Rev.158, Issued: 12-23-13, Effective: 09-24-13, Implementation: 12-17-13)

Please note, sections 40.5, 100.8, 100.11, and 100.14 have been removed from the National Coverage Determination (NCD) Manual and incorporated into NCD 100.1.

A. General

Obesity may be caused by medical conditions such as hypothyroidism, Cushing's disease, and hypothalamic lesions, or can aggravate a number of cardiac and respiratory diseases as well as diabetes and hypertension. Non-surgical services in connection with the treatment of obesity are covered when such services are an integral and necessary part of a course of treatment for one of these medical conditions.

In addition, supplemented fasting is a type of very low calorie weight reduction regimen used to achieve rapid weight loss. The reduced calorie intake is supplemented by a mixture of protein, carbohydrates, vitamins, and minerals. Serious questions exist about the safety of prolonged adherence for 2 months or more to a very low calorie weight reduction regimen as a general treatment for obesity, because of instances of cardiopathology and sudden death, as well as possible loss of body protein.

Bariatric surgery procedures are performed to treat comorbid conditions associated with morbid obesity. Two types of surgical procedures are employed. Malabsorptive procedures divert food from the stomach to a lower part of the digestive tract where the normal mixing of digestive fluids and absorption of nutrients cannot occur. Restrictive procedures restrict the size of the stomach and decrease intake. Surgery can combine both types of procedures.

The following are descriptions of bariatric surgery procedures:

1. Roux-en-Y Gastric Bypass (RYGBP)

   The RYGBP achieves weight loss by gastric restriction and malabsorption. Reduction of the stomach to a small gastric pouch (30 cc) results in feelings of satiety following even small meals. This small pouch is connected to a segment of the jejunum, bypassing the duodenum and very proximal small intestine, thereby reducing absorption. RYGBP procedures can be open or laparoscopic.

2. Biliopancreatic Diversion with Duodenal Switch (BPD/DS) or Gastric Reduction Duodenal Switch (BPD/GRDS)

   The BPD achieves weight loss by gastric restriction and malabsorption. The stomach is partially resected, but the remaining capacity is generous compared to that achieved with RYGBP. As such, patients eat relatively normal-sized meals and do not need to restrict intake radically, since the most proximal areas of the small intestine (i.e., the duodenum and jejunum) are bypassed, and substantial malabsorption occurs. The partial BPD/DS or BPD/GRDS is a variant of the BPD procedure. It involves resection of the greater curvature of the stomach, preservation of the pyloric sphincter, and transection of the duodenum above the ampulla of Vater with a duodeno-ileal anastomosis and a lower ileo-ileal anastomosis. BPD/DS or BPD/GRDS procedures can be open or laparoscopic.

3. Adjustable Gastric Banding (AGB)

   The AGB achieves weight loss by gastric restriction only. A band creating a gastric pouch with a capacity of approximately 15 to 30 cc's encircles the uppermost portion of the stomach. The band is an inflatable doughnut-shaped balloon, the diameter of which can be adjusted in the clinic by adding or removing saline via a port that is positioned beneath the skin. The bands are adjustable, allowing the size of the gastric outlet to be modified as needed, depending on the rate of a patient's weight loss. AGB procedures are laparoscopic only.

4. Sleeve Gastrectomy

   Sleeve gastrectomy is a 70%-80% greater curvature gastrectomy (sleeve resection of the stomach) with continuity of the gastric lesser curve being maintained while simultaneously reducing stomach volume. In the past, sleeve gastrectomy was the first step in a two-stage procedure when performing RYGBP, but more recently has been offered as a stand-alone surgery. Sleeve gastrectomy procedures can be open or laparoscopic.

5. Vertical Gastric Banding (VGB)

   The VGB achieves weight loss by gastric restriction only. The upper part of the stomach is stapled, creating a narrow gastric inlet or pouch that remains connected with the remainder of the stomach. In addition, a non-adjustable band is placed around this new inlet in an attempt to prevent future enlargement of the stoma (opening). As a result, patients experience a sense of fullness after eating small meals. Weight loss from this procedure results entirely from eating less. VGB procedures are essentially no longer performed.

B. Nationally Covered Indications

Effective for services performed on and after February 21, 2006, Open and laparoscopic Roux-en-Y gastric bypass (RYGBP), open and laparoscopic Biliopancreatic Diversion with Duodenal Switch (BPD/DS) or Gastric Reduction Duodenal Switch (BPD/GRDS), and laparoscopic adjustable gastric banding (LAGB) are covered for Medicare beneficiaries who have a body-mass index = 35, have at least one co-morbidity related to obesity, and have been previously unsuccessful with medical treatment for obesity.

Effective for dates of service on and after February 21, 2006, these procedures are only covered when performed at facilities that are: (1) certified by the American College of Surgeons as a Level 1 Bariatric Surgery Center (program standards and requirements in effect on February 15, 2006); or (2) certified by the American Society for Bariatric Surgery as a Bariatric Surgery Center of Excellence (program standards and requirements in effect on February 15, 2006). Effective for dates of service on and after September 24, 2013, facilities are no longer required to be certified.

Effective for services performed on and after February 12, 2009, the Centers for Medicare & Medicaid Services (CMS) determines that Type 2 diabetes mellitus is a co-morbidity for purposes of this NCD.

A list of approved facilities and their approval dates are listed and maintained on the CMS Coverage Web site at http://www.cms.gov/Medicare/Medicare-General-Information/MedicareApprovedFacilitie/Bariatric-Surgery.html, and published in the Federal Register for services provided up to and including date of service September 23, 2013.

C. Nationally Non-Covered Indications

Treatments for obesity alone remain non-covered.

Supplemented fasting is not covered under the Medicare program as a general treatment for obesity (see section D. below for discretionary local coverage).

The following bariatric surgery procedures are non-covered for all Medicare beneficiaries:

- Open adjustable gastric banding;
- Open sleeve gastrectomy;
- Laparoscopic sleeve gastrectomy (prior to June 27, 2012);
- Open and laparoscopic vertical banded gastroplasty;
- Intestinal bypass surgery; and,
- Gastric balloon for treatment of obesity.

D. Other

Effective for services performed on and after June 27, 2012, Medicare Administrative Contractors (MACs) acting within their respective jurisdictions may determine coverage of stand-alone laparoscopic sleeve gastrectomy (LSG) for the treatment of co-morbid conditions related to obesity in Medicare beneficiaries only when all of the following conditions a.-c. are satisfied.

a. The beneficiary has a body-mass index (BMI) = 35 kg/m2,
b. The beneficiary has at least one co-morbidity related to obesity, and,
c. The beneficiary has been previously unsuccessful with medical treatment for obesity.

The determination of coverage for any bariatric surgery procedures that are not specifically identified in an NCD as covered or non-covered, for Medicare beneficiaries who have a body-mass index = 35, have at least one co-morbidity related to obesity, and have been previously unsuccessful with medical treatment for obesity, is left to the local MACs.

Where weight loss is necessary before surgery in order to ameliorate the complications posed by obesity when it coexists with pathological conditions such as cardiac and respiratory diseases, diabetes, or hypertension (and other more conservative techniques to achieve this end are not regarded as appropriate), supplemented fasting with adequate monitoring of the patient is eligible for coverage on a case-by-case basis or pursuant to a local coverage determination. The risks associated with the achievement of rapid weight loss must be carefully balanced against the risk posed by the condition requiring surgical treatment.

100-03, 100.5

NCD for Diagnostic Breath Analyses (100.5)

(Rev. 1, 10-03-03)

The Following Breath Test is Covered:

- Lactose breath hydrogen to detect lactose malabsorption.

The Following Breath Tests are Excluded from Coverage;

- Lactulose breath hydrogen for diagnosing small bowel bacterial overgrowth and measuring small bowel transit time.
- CO2 for diagnosing bile acid malabsorption.
- CO2 for diagnosing fat malabsorption.

100-03, 100.13

NCD for Laparoscopic Cholecystectomy (100.13)

(Rev. 173, Issued: 09-04-14, Effective: Upon Implementation: of ICD-10)

Laparoscopic cholecystectomy is a covered surgical procedure in which a diseased gall bladder is removed through the use of instruments introduced via cannulae, with vision of the operative field maintained by use of a high-resolution television camera-monitor system (video laparoscope). For inpatient claims, use ICD-9-CM code 51.23, Laparoscopic cholecystectomy. For all other claims, use CPT codes 49310 for laparoscopy, surgical; cholecystectomy (any method), and 49311 for laparoscopy, surgical: cholecystectomy with cholangiography.

100-03, 110.1

NCD for Hyperthermia for Treatment of Cancer (110.1)

(Rev. 1, 10-03-03)

Local hyperthermia is covered under Medicare when used in connection with radiation therapy for the treatment of primary or metastatic cutaneous or subcutaneous superficial malignancies. It is not covered when used alone or in connection with chemotherapy.

100-03, 110.2

NCD for Certain Drugs Distributed by the National Cancer Institute (110.2)

(Rev. 173, Issued: 09-04-14, Effective: Upon Implementation: of ICD-10)

Under its Cancer Therapy Evaluation, the Division of Cancer Treatment of the National Cancer Institute (NCI), in cooperation with the Food and Drug Administration, approves and distributes certain drugs for use in treating terminally ill cancer patients. One group of these drugs, designated as Group C drugs, unlike other drugs distributed by the NCI, is not limited to use in clinical trials for the purpose of testing their efficacy. Drugs are classified as Group C drugs only if there is sufficient evidence demonstrating their efficacy within a tumor type and that they can be safely administered.

A physician is eligible to receive Group C drugs from the Divison of Cancer Treatment only if the following requirements are met:

- A physician must be registered with the NCI as an investigator by having completed an FD-Form 1573;
- A written request for the drug, indicating the disease to be treated, must be submitted to the NCI;
- The use of the drug must be limited to indications outlined in the NCI's guidelines; and
- All adverse reactions must be reported to the Investigational Drug Branch of the Division of Cancer Treatment.

In view of these NCI controls on distribution and use of Group C drugs, A/B Medicare Adminstrative Contractors (MACs) may assume, in the absence of evidence to the contrary, that a Group C drug and the related hospital stay are covered if all other applicable coverage requirements are satisfied.

If there is reason to question coverage in a particular case, the matter should be resolved with the assistance of the Quality Improvement Organization (QIO), or if there is none, the assistance of the MAC's medical consultants.

Information regarding those drugs which are classified as Group C drugs may be obtained from:

Chief, Investigational Drug Branch
Cancer Therapy Evaluation Program
Executive Plaza North, Suite 7134
National Cancer Institute
Rockville, Maryland 20852-7426

100-03, 110.4

Extracorporeal Photopheresis

(Rev.143, Issued: 05-18-12, Effective: 04-30-12, Implementation: 10-01-12)

A. General

Extracorporeal photopheresis is a medical procedure in which a patient's white blood cells are exposed first to a drug called 8-methoxypsoralen (8-MOP) and then to ultraviolet A (UVA) light. The procedure starts with the removal of the patient's blood, which is centrifuged to isolate the white blood cells. The drug is typically administered directly to the white blood cells after they have been removed from the patient (referred to as ex vivo administration) but the drug can alternatively be administered directly to the patient before the white blood cells are withdrawn. After UVA light exposure, the treated white blood cells are then re-infused into the patient.

B. Nationally Covered Indications

The Centers for Medicare & Medicaid Services (CMS) has determined that extracorporeal photopheresis is reasonable and necessary under §1862(a)(1)(A) of the Social Security Act (the Act) under the following circumstances:

1. Effective April 8, 1988, Medicare provides coverage for:

   Palliative treatment of skin manifestations of cutaneous T-cell lymphoma that has not responded to other therapy.

2. Effective December 19, 2006, Medicare also provides coverage for:

   Patients with acute cardiac allograft rejection whose disease is refractory to standard immunosuppressive drug treatment; and,

   Patients with chronic graft versus host disease whose disease is refractory to standard immunosuppressive drug treatment.

3. Effective April 30, 2012, Medicare also provides coverage for:

   Extracorporeal photopheresis for the treatment of bronchiolitis obliterans syndrome (BOS) following lung allograft transplantation only when extracorporeal photopheresis is provided under a clinical research study that meets the following conditions:

   The clinical research study meets the requirements specified below to assess the effect of extracorporeal photopheresis for the treatment of BOS following lung allograft transplantation. The clinical study must address one or more aspects of the following question:

   Prospectively, do Medicare beneficiaries who have received lung allografts, developed BOS refractory to standard immunosuppressive therapy, and received extracorporeal photopheresis , experience improved patient-centered health outcomes as indicated by:

   a. improved forced expiratory volume in one second (FEV1);
   b. improved survival after transplant; and/or,
   c. improved quality of life?

   The required clinical study must adhere to the following standards of scientific integrity and relevance to the Medicare population:

   a. The principal purpose of the research study is to test whether extracorporeal photopheresis potentially improves the participants' health outcomes.
   b. The research study is well supported by available scientific and medical information or it is intended to clarify or establish the health outcomes of interventions already in common clinical use.
   c. The research study does not unjustifiably duplicate existing studies.

d. The research study design is appropriate to answer the research question being asked in the study.

e. The research study is sponsored by an organization or individual capable of successfully executing the proposed study.

f. The research study is in compliance with all applicable Federal regulations concerning the protection of human subjects found at 45 CFR Part 46. If a study is regulated by the Food and Drug Administration (FDA), it must also be in compliance with 21 CFR parts 50 and 56.

g. All aspects of the research study are conducted according to appropriate standards of scientific integrity (see http://www.icmje.org).

h. The research study has a written protocol that clearly addresses, or incorporates by reference, the standards listed here as Medicare requirements for coverage with evidence development.

i. The clinical research study is not designed to exclusively test toxicity or disease pathophysiology in healthy individuals. Trials of all medical technologies measuring therapeutic outcomes as one of the objectives meet this standard only if the disease or condition being studied is life threatening as defined in 21 CFR § 312.81(a) and the patient has no other viable treatment options.

j. The clinical research study is registered on the ClinicalTrials.gov website by the principal sponsor/investigator prior to the enrollment of the first study subject.

k. The research study protocol specifies the method and timing of public release of all prespecified outcomes to be measured including release of outcomes if outcomes are negative or study is terminated early. The results must be made public within 24 months of the end of data collection. If a report is planned to be published in a peer-reviewed journal, then that initial release may be an abstract that meets the requirements of the International Committee of Medical Journal Editors (http://www.icmje.org).

l. The research study protocol must explicitly discuss subpopulations affected by the treatment under investigation, particularly traditionally underrepresented groups in clinical studies, how the inclusion and exclusion criteria effect enrollment of these populations, and a plan for the retention and reporting of said populations on the trial. If the inclusion and exclusion criteria are expected to have a negative effect on the recruitment or retention of underrepresented populations, the protocol must discuss why these criteria are necessary.

m. The research study protocol explicitly discusses how the results are or are not expected to be generalizable to the Medicare population to infer whether Medicare patients may benefit from the intervention. Separate discussions in the protocol may be necessary for populations eligible for Medicare due to age, disability or Medicaid eligibility.

Consistent with section 1142 of the Act, the Agency for Healthcare Research and Quality supports clinical research studies that CMS determines meet the above-listed standards and address the above-listed research questions.

Any clinical study under which there is coverage of extracorporeal photopheresis for this indication pursuant to this national coverage determination (NCD) must be approved by April 30, 2014. If there are no approved clinical studies on this date, this NCD will expire and coverage of extracorporeal photopheresis for BOS will revert to the coverage policy in effect prior to the issuance of the final decision memorandum for this NCD.

C. Nationally Non-Covered Indications

All other indications for extracorporeal photopheresis not otherwise indicated above as covered remain non-covered.

D. Other

Claims processing instructions can be found in chapter 32, section 190 of the Medicare Claims Processing Manual.

(This NCD last reviewed April 2012.)

100-03, 110.6

NCD for Scalp Hypothermia During Chemotherapy, to Prevent Hair Loss (110.6)

(Rev. 1, 10-03-03)

While ice-filled bags or bandages or other devices used for scalp hypothermia during chemotherapy may be covered as supplies of the kind commonly furnished without a separate charge, no separate charge for them would be recognized.

100-03, 110.7

NCD for Blood Transfusions (110.7)

(Rev. 1, 10-03-03)

Blood transfusions are used to restore blood volume after hemorrhage, to improve the oxygen carrying capacity of blood in severe anemia, and to combat shock in acute hemolytic anemia.

A. Definitions

1. Homologous Blood Transfusion

   Homologous blood transfusion is the infusion of blood or blood components that have been collected from the general public.

2. Autologous Blood Transfusion

   An autologous blood transfusion is the precollection and subsequent infusion of a patient's own blood.

3. Donor Directed Blood Transfusion

   A donor directed blood transfusion is the infusion of blood or blood components that have been precollected from a specific individual(s) other than the patient and subsequently infused into the specific patient for whom the blood is designated. For example, patient B's brother predeposits his blood for use by patient B during upcoming surgery.

4. Perioperative Blood Salvage

   Perioperative blood salvage is the collection and reinfusion of blood lost during and immediately after surgery.

B. Policy Governing Transfusions

For Medicare coverage purposes, it is important to distinguish between a transfusion itself and preoperative blood services; e.g., collection, processing, storage. Medically necessary transfusion of blood, regardless of the type, may generally be a covered service under both Part A and Part B of Medicare. Coverage does not make a distinction between the transfusion of homologous, autologous, or donor-directed blood. With respect to the coverage of the services associated with the preoperative collection, processing, and storage of autologous and donor-directed blood, the following policies apply.

1. Hospital Part A and B Coverage and Payment

   Under Sec.1862(a)(14) of the Act, non-physician services furnished to hospital patients are covered and paid for as hospital services. As provided in Sec.1886 of the Act, under the prospective [payment system (PPS), the diganosis related group (DRG) payment to the hospital includes all covered blood and blood processing expenses, whether or not the blood is eventually used.

   Under its provider agreement, a hospital is required to furnish or arrange for all covered services furnished to hospital patients. medicare payment is made to the hospital, under PPS or cost reimbursement, for covered inpatient services, and it is intended to reflect payment for all costs of furnishing those services.

2. Nonhospital Part B Coverage

   Under Part B, to be eligible for separate coverage, a service must fit the definition of one of the services authorized by Sec.1832 of the Act. These services are defined in 42 CFR 410.10 and do not include a separate category for a supplier's services associated with blood donation services, either autologous or donor-directed. That is, the collection, processing, and storage of blood for later transfusion into the beneficiary is not recognized as a separate service under Part B. Therefore, there is no avenue through which a blood supplier can receive direct payment under Part B for blood donation services.

C. Perioperative Blood Salvage

When the perioperative blood salvage process is used in surgery on a hospital patient, payment made to the hospital (under PPS or through cost reimbursement) for the procedure in which that process is used is intended to encompass payment for all costs relating to that process.

100-03, 110.8

NCD for Blood Platelet Transfusions (110.8)

(Rev. 1, 10-03-03)

Blood platelet transplants are safe and effective for the correction of thrombocytopenia and other blood defects. It is covered under Medicare when treatment is reasonable and necessary for the individual patient.

100-03, 110.9

NCD for Antigens Prepared for Sublingual Administration (110.9)

(Rev. 1, 10-03-03)

For antigens provided to patients on or after November 17, 1996, Medicare does not cover such antigens if they are to be administered sublingually, i.e., by placing drops under the patient's tongue. This kind of allergy therapy has not been proven to be safe and effective. Antigens are covered only if they are administered by injection.

100-03, 110.12

NCD for Challenge Ingestion Food Testing (110.12)

(Rev. 1, 10-03-03)

This procedure is covered when it is used on an outpatient basis if it is reasonable and necessary for the individual patient.

Challenge ingestion food testing has not been proven to be effective in the diagnosis of rheumatoid arthritis, depression, or respiratory disorders. Accordingly, its use in the diagnosis of these conditions is not reasonable and necessary within the meaning of section 1862(a)(1) of the Medicare law, and no program payment is made for this procedure when it is so used.

100-03, 110.14

NCD for Apheresis (Therapeutic Pheresis) (110.14)

(Rev. 1, 10-03-03)

A. General

Apheresis (also known as pheresis or therapeutic pheresis) is a medical procedure utilizing specialized equipment to remove selected blood constituents (plasma, leukocytes, plataelets, or cells) from whole blood. The remainder is retransfused into the person from whom the blood was taken.

For purposes of Medicare coverage, apheresis is defined as an autologous procedure, i.e., blood is taken from the patient, processed, and returned to the patient as part of a continuous procedure (as distinguished from the procedure in which a patient donates blood preoperatively and is transfused with the donated blood at a later date).

B. Indications

Apheresis is covered for the following indications:

- Plasma exchange for acquired myasthenia gravis;
- Leukapheresis in the treatment of leukemekia
- Plasmapheresis in the treatment of primary macroglobulinemia (Waldenstrom);
- Treatment of hyperglobulinemias, including (but not limited to) multiple myelomas, cryoglobulinemia and hyperviscosity syndromes;
- Plasmapheresis or plasma exchange as a last resort treatment of thromobotic thrombocytopenic purpura (TTP);
- Plasmapheresis or plasma exchange in the last resort treatment of life threatening rheumatoid vasculitis;
- Plasma perfusion of charcoal filters for treatment of pruritis of cholestatic liver disease;
- Plasma exchange in the treatment of Goodpasture's Syndrome;
- Plasma exchange in the treatment of glomerulonephritis associated with antiglomerular basement membrane antibodies and advancing renal failure or pulmonary hemorrhage;
- Treatment of chronic relapsing polyneuropathy for patients with severe or life threatening symptoms who have failed to respond to conventional therapy;
- Treatment of life threatening scleroderma and polymyositis when the patient is unresponsive to conventional therapy;
- Treatment of Guillain-Barre Syndrome; and
- Treatment of last resort for life threatening systemic lupus erythematosus (SLE) when conventional therapy has failed to prevent clinical deterioration.

C. Settings

Apheresis is covered only when performed in a hospital setting (either inpatient or outpatient). or in a nonhospital setting. e.g. physician directed clinic when the following conditions are met:

- A physician (or a number of physicians) is present to perform medical services and to respond to medical emergencies at all times during patient care hours;
- Each patient is under the care of a physician; and
- All nonphysician services are furnished under the direct, personal supervision of a physician.

100-03, 110.16

NCD for Nonselective (Random) Transfusions and Living Related Donor Specific Transfusions (DST) in Kidney Transplantation (110.16)

(Rev. 1, 10-03-03)

These pretransplant transfusions are covered under Medicare without a specific limitation on the number of transfusions, subject to the normal Medicare blood deductible provisions. Where blood is given directly to the transplant patient; e.g., in the case of donor specific transfusions, the blood is considered replaced for purposes of the blood deductible provisions.

100-03, 110.23

Stem Cell Transplantation (Formerly 110.8.1) (Various Effective Dates Below)

(Rev. 193, Issued; 07-01-16, Effective: 01-27-16, Implementation: 10-03-16)

A. General

Stem cell transplantation is a process in which stem cells are harvested from either a patient's (autologous) or donor's (allogeneic) bone marrow or peripheral blood for intravenous infusion. Autologous stem cell transplantation (AuSCT) is a technique for restoring stem cells using the patient's own previously stored cells. AuSCT must be used to effect hematopoietic reconstitution following severely myelotoxic doses of chemotherapy (HDCT) and/or radiotherapy used to treat various malignancies. Allogeneic hematopoietic stem cell transplantation (HSCT) is a procedure in which a portion of a healthy donor's stem cell or bone marrow is obtained and prepared for intravenous infusion. Allogeneic HSCT may be used to restore function in recipients having an inherited or acquired deficiency or defect. Hematopoietic stem cells are multi-potent stem cells that give rise to all the blood cell types; these stem cells form blood and immune cells. A hematopoietic stem cell is a cell isolated from blood or bone marrow that can renew itself, differentiate to a variety of specialized cells, can mobilize out of the bone marrow into circulating blood, and can undergo programmed cell death, called apoptosis - a process by which cells that are unneeded or detrimental will self-destruct.

The Centers for Medicare & Medicaid Services (CMS) is clarifying that bone marrow and peripheral blood stem cell transplantation is a process which includes mobilization, harvesting, and transplant of bone marrow or peripheral blood stem cells and the administration of high dose chemotherapy or radiotherapy prior to the actual transplant. When bone marrow or peripheral blood stem cell transplantation is covered, all necessary steps are included in coverage. When bone marrow or peripheral blood stem cell transplantation is non-covered, none of the steps are covered.

B. Nationally Covered Indications

I. Allogeneic Hematopoietic Stem Cell Transplantation (HSCT)

a) Effective for services performed on or after August 1, 1978, for the treatment of leukemia, leukemia in remission, or aplastic anemia when it is reasonable and necessary,

b) Effective for services performed on or after June 3, 1985, for the treatment of severe combined immunodeficiency disease (SCID) and for the treatment of Wiskott-Aldrich syndrome.

c) Effective for services performed on or after August 4, 2010, for the treatment of Myelodysplastic Syndromes (MDS) pursuant to Coverage with Evidence Development (CED) in the context of a Medicare-approved, prospective clinical study.

MDS refers to a group of diverse blood disorders in which the bone marrow does not produce enough healthy, functioning blood cells. These disorders are varied with regard to clinical characteristics, cytologic and pathologic features, and cytogenetics. The abnormal production of blood cells in the bone marrow leads to low blood cell counts, referred to as cytopenias, which are a hallmark feature of MDS along with a dysplastic and hypercellular-appearing bone marrow

Medicare payment for these beneficiaries will be restricted to patients enrolled in an approved clinical study. In accordance with the Stem Cell Therapeutic and Research Act of 2005 (US Public Law 109-129) a standard dataset is collected for all allogeneic transplant patients in the United States by the Center for International Blood and Marrow Transplant Research. The elements in this dataset, comprised of two mandatory forms plus one additional form, encompass the information we require for a study under CED.

A prospective clinical study seeking Medicare payment for treating a beneficiary with allogeneic HSCT for MDS pursuant to CED must meet one or more aspects of the following questions:

1. Prospectively, compared to Medicare beneficiaries with MDS who do not receive HSCT, do Medicare beneficiaries with MDS who receive HSCT have improved outcomes as indicated by:
   - Relapse-free mortality,
   - progression free survival,
   - relapse, and
   - overall survival?
2. Prospectively, in Medicare beneficiaries with MDS who receive HSCT, how do International Prognostic Scoring System (IPSS) scores, patient age, cytopenias, and comorbidities predict the following outcomes:
   - Relapse-free mortality,
   - progression free survival,
   - relapse, and
   - overall survival?
3. Prospectively, in Medicare beneficiaries with MDS who receive HSCT, what treatment facility characteristics predict meaningful clinical improvement in the following outcomes:
   - Relapse-free mortality,
   - progression free survival,
   - relapse, and
   - overall survival?

In addition, the clinical study must adhere to the following standards of scientific integrity and relevance to the Medicare population:

a. The principal purpose of the research study is to test whether a particular intervention potentially improves the participants' health outcomes.

b. The research study is well supported by available scientific and medical information or it is intended to clarify or establish the health outcomes of interventions already in common clinical use.

c. The research study does not unjustifiably duplicate existing studies.

d. The research study design is appropriate to answer the research question being asked in the study.

e. The research study is sponsored by an organization or individual capable of executing the proposed study successfully.

f. The research study is in compliance with all applicable Federal regulations concerning the protection of human subjects found at 45 CFR Part 46. If a study is regulated by the Food and Drug Administration (FDA), it must be in compliance with 21 CFR parts 50 and 56.

g. All aspects of the research study are conducted according to appropriate standards of scientific integrity (see http://www.icmje.org).

h. The research study has a written protocol that clearly addresses, or incorporates by reference, the standards listed here as Medicare requirements for CED coverage.

i. The clinical research study is not designed to exclusively test toxicity or disease pathophysiology in healthy individuals. Trials of all medical technologies measuring therapeutic outcomes as one of the objectives meet this standard only if the disease or condition being studied is life threatening as defined in 21 CFR §312.81(a) and the patient has no other viable treatment options.

j. The clinical research study is registered on the ClinicalTrials.gov Web site by the principal sponsor/investigator prior to the enrollment of the first study subject.

k. The research study protocol specifies the method and timing of public release of all pre-specified outcomes to be measured including release of outcomes if outcomes are negative or study is terminated early. The results must be made public within 24 months of the end of data collection. If a report is planned to be published in a peer-reviewed journal, then that initial release may be an abstract that meets the requirements of the International Committee of Medical Journal Editors (http://www.icmje.org). However a full report of the outcomes must be made public no later than 3 years after the end of data collection.

l. The research study protocol must explicitly discuss subpopulations affected by the treatment under investigation, particularly traditionally underrepresented groups in clinical studies, how the inclusion and exclusion criteria effect enrollment of these populations, and a plan for the retention and reporting of said populations on the trial. If the inclusion and exclusion criteria are expected to have a negative effect on the recruitment or retention of underrepresented populations, the protocol must discuss why these criteria are necessary.

m. The research study protocol explicitly discusses how the results are or are not expected to be generalizable to the Medicare population to infer whether Medicare patients may benefit from the intervention. Separate discussions in the protocol may be necessary for populations eligible for Medicare due to age, disability or Medicaid eligibility.

Consistent with section 1142 of the Social Security Act, the Agency for Health Research and Quality (AHRQ) supports clinical research studies that CMS determines meet the above-listed standards and address the above-listed research questions.

The clinical research study should also have the following features:

- It should be a prospective, longitudinal study with clinical information from the period before HSCT and short- and long-term follow-up information.
- Outcomes should be measured and compared among pre-specified subgroups within the cohort.
- The study should be powered to make inferences in subgroup analyses.
- Risk stratification methods should be used to control for selection bias. Data elements to be used in risk stratification models should include:

Patient selection:

- Patient Age at diagnosis of MDS and at transplantation
- Date of onset of MDS
- Disease classification (specific MDS subtype at diagnosis prior to preparative/conditioning regimen using World Health Organization (WHO) classifications). Include presence/absence of refractory cytopenias
- Comorbid conditions
- IPSS score (and WHO-adapted Prognostic Scoring System (WPSS) score, if applicable) at diagnosis and prior to transplantation
- Score immediately prior to transplantation and one year post-transplantation
- Disease assessment at diagnosis at start of preparative regimen and last assessment prior to preparative regimen Subtype of MDS (refractory anemia with or without blasts, degree of blasts, etc.)
- Type of preparative/conditioning regimen administered (myeloabalative, non-myeloablative, reduced–intensity conditioning)
- Donor type
- Cell Source

Facilities must submit the required transplant essential data to the Stem Cell Therapeutics Outcomes Database.

d) Effective for claims with dates of service on or after January 27, 2016, allogeneic HSCT for multiple myeloma is covered by Medicare only for beneficiaries with Durie-Salmon Stage II or III multiple myeloma, or International Staging System (ISS) Stage II or Stage III multiple myeloma, and participating in an approved prospective clinical study that meets the criteria below. There must be appropriate statistical techniques to control for selection bias and confounding by age, duration of diagnosis, disease classification, International Myeloma Working Group (IMWG) classification, ISS stage, comorbid conditions, type of preparative/conditioning regimen, graft vs. host disease (GVHD) prophylaxis, donor type and cell source.

A prospective clinical study seeking Medicare coverage for allogeneic HSCT for multiple myeloma pursuant to CED must address the following question:

Compared to patients who do not receive allogeneic HSCT, do Medicare beneficiaries with multiple myeloma who receive allogeneic HSCT have improved outcomes as indicated by:

- Graft vs. host disease (acute and chronic);
- Other transplant-related adverse events;
- Overall survival; and
- (optional) Quality of life?

All CMS-approved clinical studies and registries must adhere to the below listed standards of scientific integrity and relevance to the Medicare population as listed in section g.

e) Effective for claims with dates of service on or after January 27, 2016, allogeneic HSCT for myelofibrosis (MF) is covered by Medicare only for beneficiaries with Dynamic International Prognostic Scoring System (DIPSSplus) intermediate-2 or High primary or secondary MF and participating in an approved prospective clinical study. All Medicare approved studies must use appropriate statistical techniques in the analysis to control for selection bias and potential confounding by age, duration of diagnosis, disease classification, DIPSSplus score, comorbid conditions, type of preparative/conditioning regimen, graft vs. host disease (GVHD) prophylaxis, donor type and cell source.

A prospective clinical study seeking Medicare coverage for allogeneic HSCT for myelofibrosis pursuant to Coverage with Evidence Development (CED) must address the following question:

Compared to patients who do not receive allogeneic HSCT, do Medicare beneficiaries with MF who receive allogeneic HSCT transplantation have improved outcomes as indicated by:

- Graft vs. host disease (acute and chronic);
- Other transplant-related adverse events;
- Overall survival; and
- (optional) Quality of life?

All CMS-approved clinical studies and registries must adhere to the below listed standards of scientific integrity and relevance to the Medicare population as listed in section g.

f) Effective for claims with dates of service on or after January 27, 2016, allogeneic HSCT for sickle cell disease (SCD) is covered by Medicare only for beneficiaries with severe, symptomatic SCD who participate in an approved prospective clinical study.

A prospective clinical study seeking Medicare coverage for allogeneic HSCT for sickle cell disease pursuant to Coverage with Evidence Development (CED) must address the following question:

Compared to patients who do not receive allogeneic HSCT, do Medicare beneficiaries with SCD who receive allogeneic HSCT have improved outcomes as indicated by:

- Graft vs. host disease (acute and chronic),
- Other transplant-related adverse events;
- Overall survival; and
- (optional) Quality of life?

All CMS-approved clinical studies and registries must adhere to the below listed standards of scientific integrity and relevance to the Medicare population listed in section g:

g) All CMS-approved clinical studies and registries in sections d, e and f must adhere to the below listed standards of scientific integrity and relevance to the Medicare population:

   a. The principal purpose of the study is to test whether the item or service meaningfully improves health outcomes of affected beneficiaries who are represented by the enrolled subjects.

   b. The rationale for the study is well supported by available scientific and medical evidence.

   c. The study results are not anticipated to unjustifiably duplicate existing knowledge.

d. The study design is methodologically appropriate and the anticipated number of enrolled subjects is sufficient to answer the research question(s) being asked in the National Coverage Determination.

e. The study is sponsored by an organization or individual capable of completing it successfully.

f. The research study is in compliance with all applicable Federal regulations concerning the protection of human subjects found in the Code of Federal Regulations (CFR) at 45 CFR Part 46. If a study is regulated by the Food and Drug Administration (FDA), it is also in compliance with 21 CFR Parts 50 and 56. In addition, to further enhance the protection of human subjects in studies conducted under CED, the study must provide and obtain meaningful informed consent from patients regarding the risks associated with the study items and/or services, and the use and eventual disposition of the collected data.

g. All aspects of the study are conducted according to appropriate standards of scientific integrity.

h. The study has a written protocol that clearly demonstrates adherence to the standards listed here as Medicare requirements.

i. The study is not designed to exclusively test toxicity or disease pathophysiology in healthy individuals. Such studies may meet this requirement only if the disease or condition being studied is life threatening as defined in 21 CFR §312.81(a) and the patient has no other viable treatment options.

j. The clinical research studies and registries are registered on the www.ClinicalTrials.gov website by the principal sponsor/investigator prior to the enrollment of the first study subject. Registries are also registered in the Agency for Healthcare Quality (AHRQ) Registry of Patient Registries (RoPR).

k. The research study protocol specifies the method and timing of public release of all prespecified outcomes to be measured including release of outcomes if outcomes are negative or study is terminated early. The results must be made public within 12 months of the study's primary completion date, which is the date the final subject had final data collection for the primary endpoint, even if the trial does not achieve its primary aim. The results must include number started/completed, summary results for primary and secondary outcome measures, statistical analyses, and adverse events. Final results must be reported in a publicly accessibly manner; either in a peer-reviewed scientific journal (in print or on-line), in an on-line publicly accessible registry dedicated to the dissemination of clinical trial information such as ClinicalTrials.gov, or in journals willing to publish in abbreviated format (e.g., for studies with negative or incomplete results).

l. The study protocol must explicitly discuss beneficiary subpopulations affected by the item or service under investigation, particularly traditionally underrepresented groups in clinical studies, how the inclusion and exclusion criteria effect enrollment of these populations, and a plan for the retention and reporting of said populations in the trial. If the inclusion and exclusion criteria are expected to have a negative effect on the recruitment or retention of underrepresented populations, the protocol must discuss why these criteria are necessary.

m. The study protocol explicitly discusses how the results are or are not expected to be generalizable to affected beneficiary subpopulations. Separate discussions in the protocol may be necessary for populations eligible for Medicare due to age, disability or Medicaid eligibility.

Consistent with section 1142 of the Act, the Agency for Healthcare Research and Quality (AHRQ) supports clinical research studies that CMS determines meet the above-listed standards and address the above-listed research questions.

II. Autologous Stem Cell Transplantation (AuSCT)

a) Effective for services performed on or after April 28, 1989, AuSCT is considered reasonable and necessary under §l862(a)(1)(A) of the Act for the following conditions and is covered under Medicare for patients with:

1. Acute leukemia in remission who have a high probability of relapse and who have no human leucocyte antigens (HLA)-matched;
2. Resistant non-Hodgkin's lymphomas or those presenting with poor prognostic features following an initial response;
3. Recurrent or refractory neuroblastoma; or,
4. Advanced Hodgkin's disease who have failed conventional therapy and have no HLA-matched donor.

b) Effective October 1, 2000, single AuSCT is only covered for Durie-Salmon Stage II or III patients that fit the following requirements:

- Newly diagnosed or responsive multiple myeloma. This includes those patients with previously untreated disease, those with at least a partial response to prior chemotherapy (defined as a 50% decrease either in measurable paraprotein [serum and/or urine] or in bone marrow infiltration, sustained for at least 1 month), and those in responsive relapse; and
- Adequate cardiac, renal, pulmonary, and hepatic function.

c) Effective for services performed on or after March 15, 2005, when recognized clinical risk factors are employed to select patients for transplantation, high dose melphalan (HDM) together with AuSCT is reasonable and necessary for Medicare beneficiaries of any age group with primary amyloid light chain (AL) amyloidosis who meet the following criteria:

- Amyloid deposition in 2 or fewer organs; and,
- Cardiac left ventricular ejection fraction (EF) greater than 45%.

C. Nationally Non-Covered Indications

I. Allogeneic Hematopoietic Stem Cell Transplantation (HSCT)

Effective for claims with dates of service on or after May 24, 1996, through January 26, 2016, allogeneic HSCT is not covered as treatment for multiple myeloma.

II. Autologous Stem Cell Transplantation (AuSCT)

Insufficient data exist to establish definite conclusions regarding the efficacy of AuSCT for the following conditions:

a) Acute leukemia not in remission;

b) Chronic granulocytic leukemia;

c) Solid tumors (other than neuroblastoma);

d) Up to October 1, 2000, multiple myeloma;

e) Tandem transplantation (multiple rounds of AuSCT) for patients with multiple myeloma;

f) Effective October 1, 2000, non primary AL amyloidosis; and,

g) Effective October 1, 2000, through March 14, 2005, primary AL amyloidosis for Medicare beneficiaries age 64 or older.

In these cases, AuSCT is not considered reasonable and necessary within the meaning of §l862(a)(1)(A) of the Act and is not covered under Medicare.

D. Other

All other indications for stem cell transplantation not otherwise noted above as covered or non-covered remain at local Medicare Administrative Contractor discretion.

(This NCD last reviewed January 2016.)

100-03, 130.1

NCD for Inpatient Hospital Stays for Treatment of Alcoholism (130.1)

(Rev. 1, 10-03-03)

A. Inpatient Hospital Stay for Alcohol Detoxification

Many hospitals provide detoxification services during the more acute stages of alcoholism or alcohol withdrawal. When the high probability or occurrence of medical complications (e.g., delirium, confusion, trauma, or unconsciousness) during detoxification for acute alcoholism or alcohol withdrawal necessitates the constant availability of physicians and/or complex medical equipment found only in the hospital setting, inpatient hospital care during this period is considered reasonable and necessary and is therefore covered under the program. Generally, detoxification can be accomplished within two to three days with an occasional need for up to five days where the patient's condition dictates. This limit (five days) may be extended in an individual case where there is a need for a longer period for detoxification for a particular patient.

In such cases, however, there should be documentation by a physician which substantiates that a longer period of detoxification was reasonable and necessary. When the detoxification needs of an individual no longer require an inpatient hospital setting, coverage should be denied on the basis that inpatient hospital care is not reasonable and necessary as required by §1862(a)(l) of the Social Security Act (the Act). Following detoxification a patient may be transferred to an inpatient rehabilitation unit or discharged to a residential treatment program or outpatient treatment setting.

B. Inpatient Hospital Stay for Alcohol Rehabilitation

Hospitals may also provide structured inpatient alcohol rehabilitation programs to the chronic alcoholic. These programs are composed primarily of coordinated educational and psychotherapeutic services provided on a group basis. Depending on the subject matter, a series of lectures, discussions, films, and group therapy sessions are led by either physicians, psychologists, or alcoholism counselors from the hospital or various outside organizations. In addition, individual psychotherapy and family counseling (see §70.1) may be provided in selected cases. These programs are conducted under the supervision and direction of a physician. Patients may directly enter an inpatient hospital rehabilitation program after having undergone detoxification in the same hospital or in another hospital or may enter an inpatient hospital rehabilitation program without prior hospitalization for detoxification.

Alcohol rehabilitation can be provided in a variety of settings other than the hospital setting. In order for an inpatient hospital stay for alcohol rehabilitation to be covered under Medicare it must be medically necessary for the care to be provided in the inpatient hospital setting rather than in a less costly facility or on an outpatient basis. Inpatient hospital care for receipt of an alcohol rehabilitation program would generally be medically necessary where either (l) there is documentation by the physician that recent alcohol rehabilitation services in a less intensive setting or on an outpatient basis have proven unsuccessful and, as a consequence, the patient requires the supervision and intensity of services which can only be found in the controlled environment of the hospital, or (2) only the hospital environment can assure the medical management or control of the patient's concomitant conditions during the course of alcohol rehabilitation. (However, a patient's concomitant condition may make the use of certain alcohol treatment modalities medically inappropriate.)

In addition, the "active treatment" criteria (see the Medicare Benefit Policy Manual, Chapter 2, "Inpatient Psychiatric Hospital Services," §20) should be applied to psychiatric care in the general hospital as well as to psychiatric care in a psychiatric hospital. Since alcoholism is classifiable as a psychiatric condition the "active treatment" criteria must also be met in order for alcohol rehabilitation services to be covered under Medicare. (Thus, it is the combined need for "active treatment" and for covered care which can only be provided in the inpatient hospital setting, rather than the fact that rehabilitation immediately follows a period of detoxification which provides the basis for coverage of inpatient hospital alcohol rehabilitation programs.)

Generally 16-19 days of rehabilitation services are sufficient to bring a patient to a point where care could be continued in other than an inpatient hospital setting. An inpatient hospital stay for alcohol rehabilitation may be extended beyond this limit in an individual case where a longer period of alcohol rehabilitation is medically necessary. In such cases, however, there should be documentation by a physician which substantiates the need for such care. Where the rehabilitation needs of an individual no longer require an inpatient hospital setting, coverage should be denied on the basis that inpatient hospital care is not reasonable and necessary as required by §1862 (a)(l) of the Act.

Subsequent admissions to the inpatient hospital setting for alcohol rehabilitation follow-up, reinforcement, or "recap" treatments are considered to be readmissions (rather than an extension of the original stay) and must meet the requirements of this section for coverage under Medicare. Prior admissions to the inpatient hospital setting - either in the same hospital or in a different hospital - may be an indication that the "active treatment" requirements are not met (i.e., there is no reasonable expectation of improvement) and the stay should not be covered. Accordingly, there should be documentation to establish that "readmission" to the hospital setting for alcohol rehabilitation services can reasonably be expected to result in improvement of the patient's condition. For example, the documentation should indicate what changes in the patient's medical condition, social or emotional status, or treatment plan make improvement likely, or why the patient's initial hospital treatment was not sufficient.

C. Combined Alcohol Detoxification/Rehabilitation Programs

Medicare Administrative Contractors (MACs) should apply the guidelines in A. and B. above to both phases of a combined inpatient hospital alcohol detoxification/rehabilitation program. Not all patients who require the inpatient hospital setting for detoxification also need the inpatient hospital setting for rehabilitation. (See §130.1 for coverage of outpatient hospital alcohol rehabilitation services.) Where the inpatient hospital setting is medically necessary for both alcohol detoxification and rehabilitation, generally a 3-week period is reasonable and necessary to bring the patient to the point where care can be continued in other than an inpatient hospital setting.

Decisions regarding reasonableness and necessity of treatment, the need for an inpatient hospital level of care, and length of treatment should be made by A/B MAC (A) based on accepted medical practice with the advice of their medical consultant. (In hospitals under PSRO review, PSRO determinations of medical necessity of services and appropriateness of the level of care at which services are provided are binding on A/B MAC (A) for purposes of adjudicating claims for payment.)

100-03, 130.2

NCD for Outpatient Hospital Services for Treatment of Alcoholism (130.2)

(Rev. 1, 10-03-03)

Coverage is available for both diagnostic and therapeutic services furnished for the treatment of alcoholism by the hospital to outpatients subject to the same rules applicable to outpatient hospital services in general. While there is no coverage for day hospitalization programs, per se, individual services which meet the requirements in the Medicare Benefit Policy Manual, Chapter 6, Sec.20 may be covered. (Meals, transportation and recreational and social activities do not fall within the scope of covered outpatient hospital services under Medicare.)

All services must be reasonable and necessary for diagnosis or treatment of the patient's condition (see the Medicare Benefit Policy Manual, chapter 16 Sec.20). Thus, educational services and family counseling would only be covered where they are directly related to treatment of the patient's condition. The frequency of treatment and period of time over which it occurs must also be reasonable and necessary.

100-03, 130.3

NCD for Chemical Aversion Therapy for Treatment of Alcoholism (130.3)

(Rev. 173, Issued: 09-04-14, Effective: Upon Implementation: of ICD-10, Implementation: Upon Implementation of ICD-10)

Chemical aversion therapy is a behavior modification technique that is used in the treatment of alcoholism. Chemical aversion therapy facilitates alcohol abstinence through the development of conditioned aversions to the taste, smell, and sight of alcohol beverages. This is accomplished by repeatedly pairing alcohol with unpleasant symptoms (e.g., nausea) which have been induced by one of several chemical agents. While a number of drugs have been employed in chemical aversion therapy, the three most commonly used are emetine, apomorphine, and lithium. None of the drugs being used, however, have yet been approved by the Food and Drug Administration specifically for use in chemical aversion therapy for alcoholism. Accordingly, when these drugs are being employed in conjunction with this therapy, patients undergoing this treatment need to be kept under medical observation.

Available evidence indicates that chemical aversion therapy may be an effective component of certain alcoholism treatment programs, particularly as part of multi-modality treatment programs which include other behavioral techniques and therapies, such as psychotherapy. Based on this evidence, the Centers for Medicare & Medicaid Services' medical consultants have recommended that chemical aversion therapy be covered under Medicare. However, since chemical aversion therapy is a demanding therapy which may not be appropriate for all Medicare beneficiaries needing treatment for alcoholism, a physician should certify to the appropriateness of chemical aversion therapy in the individual case. Therefore, if chemical aversion therapy for treatment of alcoholism is determined to be reasonable and necessary for an individual patient, it is covered under Medicare.

When it is medically necessary for a patient to receive chemical aversion therapy as a hospital inpatient, coverage for care in that setting is available. (See §130.1 regarding coverage of multi-modality treatment programs.) Follow-up treatments for chemical aversion therapy can generally be provided on an outpatient basis. Thus, where a patient is admitted as an inpatient for receipt of chemical aversion therapy, there must be documentation by the physician of the need in the individual case for the inpatient hospital admission.

Decisions regarding reasonableness and necessity of treatment and the need for an inpatient hospital level of care should be made by the A/B MAC (A) based on accepted medical practice with the advice of their medical consultant. (In hospitals under Quality Improvement Organization (QIO) review, QIO determinations of medical necessity of services and appropriateness of the level of care at which services are provided are binding on the A/B MAC (A) for purposes of adjudicating claims for payment.)

100-03, 140.1

NCD for Abortion (140.1)

(Rev. 48, Issued: 03-17-06; Effective/Implementation Dates: 06-19-06)

Abortions are not covered Medicare procedures except:

1. If the pregnancy is the result of an act of rape or incest; or
2. In the case where a woman suffers from a physical disorder, physical injury, or physical illness, including a life-endangering physical condition caused by or arising from the pregnancy itself, that would, as certified by a physician, place the woman in danger of death unless an abortion is performed.

100-03, 140.2

NCD for Breast Reconstruction Following Mastectomy (140.2)

(Rev. 1, 10-03-03)

CIM 35-47

Reconstruction of the affected and the contralateral unaffected breast following a medically necessary mastectomy is considered a relatively safe and effective noncosmetic procedure. Accordingly, program payment may be made for breast reconstruction surgery following removal of a breast for any medical reason.

Program payment may not be made for breast reconstruction for cosmetic reasons. (Cosmetic surgery is excluded from coverage under Sec.l862(a)(l0) of the Social Security Act.)

100-03, 140.5

NCD for Laser Procedures (140.5)

(Rev. 173, Issued: 09-04-14, Effective: Upon Implementation: of ICD-10)

Medicare recognizes the use of lasers for many medical indications. Procedures performed with lasers are sometimes used in place of more conventional techniques. In the absence of a specific noncoverage instruction, and where a laser has been approved for marketing by the Food and Drug Administration, Medicare Administrative Contractor discretion may be used to determine whether a procedure performed with a laser is reasonable and necessary and, therefore, covered.

The determination of coverage for a procedure performed using a laser is made on the basis that the use of lasers to alter, revise, or destroy tissue is a surgical procedure. Therefore, coverage of laser procedures is restricted to practitioners with training in the surgical management of the disease or condition being treated.

100-03, 150.1

NCD for Manipulation (150.1)

(Rev. 1, 10-03-03)

CIM 35-2

A. Manipulation of the Rib Cage

Manual manipulation of the rib cage contributes to the treatment of respiratory conditions such as bronchitis, emphysema, and asthma as part of a regimen that includes other elements of therapy, and is covered only under such circumstances.

B. Manipulation of the Head

Manipulation of the occipitocervical or temporomandibular regions of the head when indicated for conditions affecting those portions of the head and neck is a covered service.

100-03, 150.2

NCD for Osteogenic Stimulators (150.2)

(Rev. 41, Issued: 06-24-05, Effective: 04-27-05, Implementation: 08-01-05)

Electrical Osteogenic Stimulators

A. General

Electrical stimulation to augment bone repair can be attained either invasively or non-invasively. Invasive devices provide electrical stimulation directly at the fracture site either through percutaneously placed cathodes or by implantation of a coiled cathode wire into the fracture site. The power pack for the latter device is implanted into soft tissue near the fracture site and subcutaneously connected to the cathode, creating a self-contained system with no external components. The power supply for the former device is externally placed and the leads connected to the inserted cathodes. With the non-invasive device, opposing pads, wired to an external power supply, are placed over the cast. An electromagnetic field is created between the pads at the fracture site.

B. Nationally Covered Indications

1. Noninvasive Stimulator.

   The noninvasive stimulator device is covered only for the following indications:

   — Nonunion of long bone fractures;

   — Failed fusion, where a minimum of nine months has elapsed since the last surgery;

   — Congenital pseudarthroses; and

   — Effective July 1, 1996, as an adjunct to spinal fusion surgery for patients at high risk of pseudarthrosis due to previously failed spinal fusion at the same site or for those undergoing multiple level fusion. A multiple level fusion involves 3 or more vertebrae (e.g., L3-L5, L4-S1, etc).

   — Effective September 15, 1980, nonunion of long bone fractures is considered to exist only after 6 or more months have elapsed without healing of the fracture.

   — Effective April 1, 2000, nonunion of long bone fractures is considered to exist only when serial radiographs have confirmed that fracture healing has ceased for 3 or more months prior to starting treatment with the electrical osteogenic stimulator. Serial radiographs must include a minimum of 2 sets of radiographs, each including multiple views of the fracture site, separated by a minimum of 90 days.

2. Invasive (Implantable) Stimulator.

   The invasive stimulator device is covered only for the following indications:

   — Nonunion of long bone fractures

   — Effective July 1, 1996, as an adjunct to spinal fusion surgery for patients at high risk of pseudarthrosis due to previously failed spinal fusion at the same site or for those undergoing multiple level fusion. A multiple level fusion involves 3 or more vertebrae (e.g., L3-5, L4-S1, etc.)

   — Effective September 15, 1980, nonunion of long bone fractures is considered to exist only after 6 or more months have elapsed without healing of the fracture.

   — Effective April 1, 2000, non union of long bone fractures is considered to exist only when serial radiographs have confirmed that fracture healing has ceased for 3 or more months prior to starting treatment with the electrical osteogenic stimulator. Serial radiographs must include a minimum of 2 sets of radiographs, each including multiple views of the fracture site, separated by a minimum of 90 days.

   — Effective for services performed on or after January 1, 2001, ultrasonic osteogenic stimulators are covered as medically reasonable and necessary for the treatment of non-union fractures. In demonstrating nonunion of fractures, we would expect:

   - A minimum of two sets of radiographs obtained prior to starting treatment with the osteogenic stimulator, separated by a minimum of 90 days. Each radiograph must include multiple views of the fracture site accompanied with a written interpretation by a physician stating that there has been no clinically significant evidence of fracture healing between the two sets of radiographs.

   - Indications that the patient failed at least one surgical intervention for the treatment of the fracture.

   — Effective April 27, 2005, upon the recommendation of the ultrasound stimulation for nonunion fracture healing, CMS determins that the evidence is adequate to condlude that noninvasive ultrasound stimulation for the treatment of nonunion bone fractures prior to surfical intervention is reasonable and necessary. In demonstrating non-union fracturs, CMS expects:

   - A minimum of 2 sets of radiographs, obtained prior to starting treating with the osteogenic stimulator, separated by a minimum of 90 days. Each radiograph set must include multiple views of the fracture site accompanied with a written interpretation by a physician stating that there has been no clinically significant evidence of fracture healing between the 2 sets of radiographs.

C. Nationally Non-Covered Indications

Nonunion fractures of the skull, vertebrae and those that are tumor-related are excluded from coverage.

Ultrasonic osteogenic stimulators may not be used concurrently with other non-invasive osteogenic devices.

Ultrasonic osteogenic stimulators for fresh fracturs and delayed unions remain non-covered.

(This NCD last reviewed June 2005)

100-03, 150.7

NCD for Prolotherapy, Joint Sclerotherapy, and Ligamentous Injections with Sclerosing Agents (150.7)

(Rev. 1, 10-03-03)

CIM 35-13

Not Covered

The medical effectiveness of the above therapies has not been verified by scientifically controlled studies. Accordingly, reimbursement for these modalities should be denied on the ground that they are not reasonable and necessary as required by Sec.1862(a)(1) of the Act.

100-03, 150.10

NCD for Lumbar Artificial Disc Replacement (LADR) (150.10)

(Rev. 173, Issued: 09-04-14, Effective: Upon Implementation: of ICD–10)

A. General

The lumbar artificial disc replacement (LADR) is a surgical procedure on the lumbar spine that involves complete removal of the damaged or diseased lumbar intervertebral disc and implantation of an artificial disc. The procedure may be done as an alternative to lumbar spinal fusion and is intended to reduce pain, increase movement at the site of surgery and restore intervertebral disc height. The Food and Drug Administration has approved the use of LADR for spine arthroplasty in skeletally mature patients with degenerative or discogenic disc disease at one level for L3 to S1.

B. Nationally Covered Indications

N/A

C. Nationally Non-Covered Indications

Effective for services performed from May 16, 2006 through August 13, 2007, the Centers for Medicare and Medicaid Services (CMS) has found that LADR with the ChariteTM lumbar artificial disc is not reasonable and necessary for the Medicare population over 60 years of age; therefore, LADR with the ChariteTM lumbar artificial disc is non-covered for Medicare beneficiaries over 60 years of age.

Effective for services performed on or after August 14, 2007, CMS has found that LADR is not reasonable and necessary for the Medicare population over 60 years of age; therefore, LADR is non-covered for Medicare beneficiaries over 60 years of age.

D. Other

For Medicare beneficiaries 60 years of age and younger, there is no national coverage determination for LADR, leaving such determinations to continue to be made by the local Medicare Administrative Contractors.

For dates of service May 16, 2006 through August 13, 2007, Medicare coverage under the investigational device exemption (IDE) for LADR with a disc other than the ChariteTM lumbar disc in eligible clinical trials is not impacted.

100-03, 160.8

NCD for Electroencephalographic (EEG) Monitoring During Surgical Procedures Involving the Cerebral Vasculature (160.8)

(Rev. 48, Issued: 03-17-06; Effective/Implementation Dates: 06-19-06)

CIM 35-57

Electroencephalographic (EEG) monitoring is a safe and reliable technique for the assessment of gross cerebral blood flow during general anesthesia and is covered under Medicare. Very characteristic changes in the EEG occur when cerebral perfusion is inadequate for cerebral function. EEG monitoring as an indirect measure of cerebral perfusion requires the expertise of an electroencephalographer, a neurologist trained in EEG, or an advanced EEG technician for its proper interpretation.

The EEG monitoring may be covered routinely in carotid endarterectomies and in other neurological procedures where cerebral perfusion could be reduced. Such other procedures might include aneurysm surgery where hypotensive anesthesia is used or other cerebral vascular procedures where cerebral blood flow may be interrupted.

100-03, 160.17

NCD for L-DOPA (160.17)

(Rev. 1, 10-03-03)

A. Part A Payment for L-Dopa and Associated Inpatient Hospital Services

A hospital stay and related ancillary services for the administration of L-Dopa are covered if medically required for this purpose. Whether a drug represents an allowable inpatient hospital cost during such stay depends on whether it meets the definition of a drug in Sec.1861(t) of the Act; i.e., on its inclusion in the compendia named in the Act or approval by the hospital's pharmacy and drug therapeutics (P&DT) or equivalent committee. (Levodopa (L-Dopa) has been favorably evaluated for the treatment of Parkinsonism by A.M.A. Drug Evaluations, First Edition 1971, the replacement compendia for "New Drugs.")

Inpatient hospital services are frequently not required in many cases when L-Dopa therapy is initiated. Therefore, determine the medical need for inpatient hospital services on the basis of medical facts in the individual case. It is not necessary to hospitalize the typical, well-functioning, ambulatory Parkinsonian patient who has no concurrent disease at the start of L-Dopa treatment. It is reasonable to provide inpatient hospital services for Parkinsonian patients with concurrent diseases, particularly of the cardiovascular, gastrointestinal, and neuropsychiatric systems. Although many patients require hospitalization for a period of under 2 weeks, a 4-week period of inpatient care is not unreasonable.

Laboratory tests in connection with the administration of L-Dopa - The tests medically warranted in connection with the achievement of optimal dosage and the control of the side effects of L-Dopa include a complete blood count, liver function tests such as SGOT, SGPT, and/or alkaline phosphatase, BUN or creatinine and urinalysis, blood sugar, and electrocardiogram.

Whether or not the patient is hospitalized, laboratory tests in certain cases are reasonable at weekly intervals although some physicians prefer to perform the tests much less frequently.

Physical therapy furnished in connection with administration of L-Dopa - Where, following administration of the drug, the patient experiences a reduction of rigidity which permits the reestablishment of a restorative goal for him/her, physical therapy services required to enable him/her to achieve this goal are payable provided they require the skills of a qualified physical therapist and are furnished by or under the supervision of such a therapist. However, once the individual's restoration potential has been achieved, the services required to maintain him/her at this level do not generally require the skills of a qualified physical therapist. In such situations, the role of the therapist is to evaluate the patient's needs in consultation with his/her physician and design a program of exercise appropriate to the capacity and tolerance of the patient and treatment objectives of the physician, leaving to others the actual carrying out of the program. While the evaluative services rendered by a qualified physical therapist are payable as physical therapy, services furnished by others in connection with the carrying out of the maintenance program established by the therapist are not.

B. Part A Reimbursement for L-Dopa Therapy in SNFs

Initiation of L-Dopa therapy can be appropriately carried out in the SNF setting, applying the same guidelines used for initiation of L-Dopa therapy in the hospital, including the types of patients who should be covered for inpatient services, the role of physical therapy, and the use of laboratory tests. (See subsection A.) Where inpatient care is required and L-Dopa therapy is initiated in the SNF, limit the stay to a maximum of 4 weeks; but in many cases the need may be no longer than 1 or 2 weeks, depending upon the patient's condition. However, where L-Dopa therapy is begun in the hospital and the patient is transferred to an SNF for continuation of the therapy, a combined length of stay in hospital and SNF of no longer than 4 weeks is reasonable (i.e., 1 week hospital stay followed by 3 weeks SNF stay; or 2 weeks hospital stay followed by 2 weeks SNF stay; etc.). Medical need must be demonstrated in cases where the combined length of stay in hospital and SNF is longer than 4 weeks. The choice of hospital or SNF, and the decision regarding the relative length of time spent in each, should be left to the medical judgment of the treating physician.

C. L-Dopa Coverage Under Part B

Part B reimbursement may not be made for the drug L-Dopa since it is a self-administrable drug. However, physician services rendered in connection with its administration and control of its side effects are covered if determined to be reasonable and necessary. Initiation of L-Dopa therapy on an outpatient basis is possible in most cases. Visit frequency ranging from every week to every 2 or 3 months is acceptable. However, after half a year of therapy, visits more frequent than every month would usually not be reasonable.

100-03, 180.1

NCD for Medical Nutrition Therapy (180.1)

(Rev. 1, 10-03-03)

Effective October 1, 2002, basic coverage of MNT for the first year a beneficiary receives MNT with either a diagnosis of renal disease or diabetes as defined at 42 CFR Sec.410.130 is 3 hours. Also effective October 1, 2002, basic coverage in subsequent years for renal disease or diabetes is 2 hours. The dietitian/nutritionist may choose how many units are performed per day as long as all of the other requirements in this NCD and 42 CFR Secs.410.130-410.134 are met. Pursuant to the exception at 42 CFR Sec.410.132(b)(5), additional hours are considered to be medically necessary and covered if the treating physician determines that there is a change in medical condition, diagnosis, or treatment regimen that requires a change in MNT and orders additional hours during that episode of care.

Effective October 1, 2002, if the treating physician determines that receipt of both MNT and DSMT is medically necessary in the same episode of care, Medicare will cover both DSMT and MNT initial and subsequent years without decreasing either benefit as long as DSMT and MNT are not provided on the same date of service. The dietitian/nutritionist may choose how many units are performed per day as long as all of the other requirements in the NCD and 42 CFR Secs.410.130-410.134 are met. Pursuant to the exception at 42 CFR 410.132(b)(5), additional hours are considered to be medically necessary and covered if the treating physician determines that there is a change in medical condition, diagnosis, or treatment regimen that requires a change in MNT and orders additional hours during that episode of care.

100-03, 190.1

NCD for Histocompatibility Testing (190.1)

(Rev. 1, 10-03-03)

This testing is safe and effective when it is performed on patients:

- In preparation for a kidney transplant;
- In preparation for bone marrow transplantation;
- In preparation for blood platelet transfusions (particularly where multiple infusions are involved); or
- Who are suspected of having ankylosing spondylitis.

This testing is covered under Medicare when used for any of the indications listed in A, B, and C and if it is reasonable and necessary for the patient.

It is covered for ankylosing spondylitis in cases where other methods of diagnosis would not be appropriate or have yielded inconclusive results. Request documentation supporting the medical necessity of the test from the physician in all cases where ankylosing spondylitis is indicated as the reason for the test.

100-03, 190.3

NCD for Cytogenetic Studies (190.3)

(Rev. 1, 10-03-03)

Medicare covers these tests when they are reasonable and necessary for the diagnosis or treatment of the following conditions:

- Genetic disorders (e.g., mongolism) in a fetus (See Medicare Benefit Policy Manual, Chapter 15, "Covered medical and Other health Services," Sec. 20.1)
- Failure of sexual development;
- Chronic myelogenous leukemia;
- Acute leukemias lymphoid (FAB L1-L3), myeloid (FAB M0-M7), and unclassified; or
- Mylodysplasia

100-03, 190.8

NCD for Lymphocyte Mitogen Response Assays (190.8)

(Rev. 1, 10-03-03)

It is a covered test under Medicare when it is medically necessary to assess lymphocytic function in diagnosed immunodeficiency diseases and to monitor immunotherapy.

It is not covered when it is used to monitor the treatment of cancer, because its use for that purpose is experimental.

100-03, 190.9

NCD for Serologic Testing for Acquired Immunodeficiency Syndrome (AIDS) (190.9)

(Rev. 1, 10-03-03)

These tests may be covered when performed to help determine a diagnosis for symptomatic patients. They are not covered when furnished as part of a screening program for asymptomatic persons.

Note: Two enzyme-linked immunosorbent assay (ELISA) tests that were conducted on the same specimen must both be positive before Medicare will cover the Western blot test.

100-03, 190.11

NCD for Home Prothrombin Time International Normalized Ratio (INR) Monitoring for Anticoagulation Management (190.11)

(Rev. 90, Issued: 07-25-08, Effective: 03-19-08, Implementation: 08-25-08)

A. General

Use of the International Normalized Ratio (INR) or prothrombin time (PT) - standard measurement for reporting the blood's clotting time) - allows physicians to determine the level of anticoagulation in a patient independent of the laboratory reagents used. The INR is the ratio of the patient's PT (extrinsic or tissue-factor dependent coagulation pathway) compared to the mean PT for a group of normal individuals. Maintaining patients within his/her prescribed therapeutic range minimizes adverse events associated with inadequate or excessive anticoagulation such as serious bleeding or thromboembolic events. Patient self-testing and self-management through the use of a home INR monitor may be used to improve the time in therapeutic rate (TTR) for select groups of patients. Increased TTR leads to improved clinical outcomes and reductions in thromboembolic and hemorrhagic events.

Warfarin (also prescribed under other trade names, e.g., Coumadin(R)) is a self-administered, oral anticoagulant (blood thinner) medication that affects the vitamin K- dependent clotting factors II, VII, IX and X. It is widely used for various medical conditions, and has a narrow therapeutic index, meaning it is a drug with less than a 2-fold difference between median lethal dose and median effective dose. For this reason, since October 4, 2006, it falls under the category of a Food and Drug dministration (FDA) "black-box" drug whose dosage must be closely monitored to avoid serious complications. A PT/INR monitoring system is a portable testing device that includes a finger-stick and an FDA-cleared meter that measures the time it takes for a person's blood plasma to clot.

B. Nationally Covered Indications

For services furnished on or after March 19, 2008, Medicare will cover the use of home PT/INR monitoring for chronic, oral anticoagulation management for patients with mechanical heart valves, chronic atrial fibrillation, or venous thromboembolism (inclusive of deep venous thrombosis and pulmonary embolism) on warfarin. The monitor and the home testing must be prescribed by a treating physician as provided at 42 CFR 410.32(a), and all of the following requirements must be met:

1. The patient must have been anticoagulated for at least 3 months prior to use of the home INR device; and,
2. The patient must undergo a face-to-face educational program on anticoagulation anagement and must have demonstrated the correct use of the device prior to its use in the home; and,
3. The patient continues to correctly use the device in the context of the management of the anticoagulation therapy following the initiation of home monitoring; and,
4. Self-testing with the device should not occur more frequently than once a week.

C. Nationally Non-Covered Indications

N/A

D. Other

1. All other indications for home PT/INR monitoring not indicated as nationally covered above remain at local Medicare contractor discretion.
2. This national coverage determination (NCD) is distinct from, and makes no changes to, the PT clinical laboratory NCD at section 190.17 of Publication 100-3 of the NCD Manual.

100-03, 190.14

NCD for Human Immunodeficiency Virus (HIV) Testing (Diagnosis) (190.14)

(Rev. 113, Issued: 02-19-10, Effective: 12-08-09, Implementation; 07-06-10)

Indications and Limitations of Coverage

Indications

Diagnostic testing to establish HIV infection may be indicated when there is a strong clinical suspicion supported by one or more of the following clinical findings:

- The patient has a documented, otherwise unexplained, AIDS-defining or AIDS-associated opportunistic infection.
- The patient has another documented sexually transmitted disease which identifies significant risk of exposure to HIV and the potential for an early or subclinical infection.
- The patient has documented acute or chronic hepatitis B or C infection that identifies a significant risk of exposure to HIV and the potential for an early or subclinical infection.
- The patient has a documented AIDS-defining or AIDS-associated neoplasm.
- The patient has a documented AIDS-associated neurologic disorder or otherwise unexplained dementia.
- The patient has another documented AIDS-defining clinical condition, or a history of other severe, recurrent, or persistent conditions which suggest an underlying immune deficiency (for example, cutaneous or mucosal disorders).
- The patient has otherwise unexplained generalized signs and symptoms suggestive of a chronic process with an underlying immune deficiency (for example, fever, weight loss, malaise, fatigue, chronic diarrhea, failure to thrive, chronic cough, hemoptysis, shortness of breath, or lymphadenopathy).
- The patient has otherwise unexplained laboratory evidence of a chronic disease process with an underlying immune deficiency (for example, anemia, leukopenia, pancytopenia, lymphopenia, or low CD4+ lymphocyte count).
- The patient has signs and symptoms of acute retroviral syndrome with fever, malaise, lymphadenopathy, and skin rash.
- The patient has documented exposure to blood or body fluids known to be capable of transmitting HIV (for example, needlesticks and other significant blood exposures) and antiviral therapy is initiated or anticipated to be initiated.
- The patient is undergoing treatment for rape. (HIV testing is a part of the rape treatment protocol.)

Limitations

HIV antibody testing in the United States is usually performed using HIV-1 or HIV-½ combination tests. HIV-2 testing is indicated if clinical circumstances suggest HIV-2 is likely (that is, compatible clinical findings and HIV-1 test negative). HIV-2 testing may also be indicated in areas of the country where there is greater prevalence of HIV-2 infections.

The Western Blot test should be performed only after documentation that the initial EIA tests are repeatedly positive or equivocal on a single sample.

- The HIV antigen tests currently have no defined diagnostic usage.
- Direct viral RNA detection may be performed in those situations where serologic testing does not establish a diagnosis but strong clinical suspicion persists (for example, acute retroviral syndrome, nonspecific serologic evidence of HIV, or perinatal HIV infection).
- If initial serologic tests confirm an HIV infection, repeat testing is not indicated.
- If initial serologic tests are HIV EIA negative and there is no indication for confirmation of infection by viral RNA detection, the interval prior to retesting is 3-6 months.
- Testing for evidence of HIV infection using serologic methods may be medically appropriate in situations where there is a risk of exposure to HIV. However, in the absence of a documented AIDS defining or HIV- associated disease, an HIV associated sign or symptom, or documented exposure to a known HIV-infected source, the testing is considered by Medicare to be screening and thus is not covered by Medicare (for example, history of multiple blood component transfusions, exposure to blood or body fluids not resulting in consideration of therapy, history of transplant, history of illicit drug use, multiple sexual partners, same-sex encounters, prostitution, or contact with prostitutes).
- The CPT Editorial Panel has issued a number of codes for infectious agent detection by direct antigen or nucleic acid probe techniques that have not yet been developed or are only being used on an investigational basis. Laboratory providers are advised to remain current on FDA-approval status for these tests.

100-03, 190.15

NCD for Blood Counts (190.15)

(Rev. 17, Issued: 07-02-04) (Effective/Implementation: Not Applicable)

Indications

Indications for a CBC or hemogram include red cell, platelet, and white cell disorders. Examples of these indications are enumerated individually below.

1. Indications for a CBC generally include the evaluation of bone marrow dysfunction as a result of neoplasms, therapeutic agents, exposure to toxic substances, or pregnancy. The CBC is also useful in assessing peripheral destruction of blood cells, suspected bone marrow failure or bone marrow infiltrate, suspected myeloproliferative, myelodysplastic, or lymphoproliferative processes, and immune disorders.
2. Indications for hemogram or CBC related to red cell (RBC) parameters of the hemogram include signs, symptoms, test results, illness, or disease that can be associated with anemia or other red blood cell disorder (e.g., pallor, weakness, fatigue, weight loss, bleeding, acute injury associated with blood loss or suspected blood loss, abnormal menstrual bleeding, hematuria, hematemesis, hematochezia, positive fecal occult blood test, malnutrition, vitamin deficiency, malabsorption, neuropathy, known malignancy, presence of acute or chronic disease that may have associated anemia, coagulation or hemostatic disorders, postural dizziness, syncope, abdominal pain, change in bowel habits, chronic marrow hypoplasia or decreased RBC production, tachycardia, systolic heart murmur, congestive heart failure, dyspnea, angina, nailbed deformities, growth retardation, jaundice, hepatomegaly, splenomegaly, lymphadenopathy, ulcers on the lower extremities).
3. Indications for hemogram or CBC related to red cell (RBC) parameters of the hemogram include signs, symptoms, test results, illness, or disease that can be associated with polycythemia (for example, fever, chills, ruddy skin, conjunctival redness, cough, wheezing, cyanosis, clubbing of the fingers, orthopnea, heart murmur, headache, vague cognitive changes including memory changes, sleep apnea, weakness, pruritus, dizziness, excessive sweating, visual symptoms, weight loss, massive obesity, gastrointestinal bleeding, paresthesias, dyspnea, joint symptoms, epigastric distress, pain and erythema of the fingers or toes, venous or arterial thrombosis, thromboembolism, myocardial infarction, stroke, transient ischemic attacks, congenital heart disease, chronic obstructive pulmonary disease, increased erythropoietin production associated with neoplastic, renal or hepatic disorders, androgen or diuretic use, splenomegaly, hepatomegaly, diastolic hypertension.)
4. Specific indications for CBC with differential count related to the WBC include signs, symptoms, test results, illness, or disease associated with leukemia, infections or inflammatory processes, suspected bone marrow failure or bone marrow infiltrate, suspected myeloproliferative, myelodysplastic or lymphoproliferative disorder, use of drugs that may cause leukopenia, and immune disorders (e.g., fever, chills, sweats, shock, fatigue, malaise, tachycardia, tachypnea, heart murmur, seizures, alterations of consciousness, meningismus, pain such as headache, abdominal pain, arthralgia, odynophagia, or dysuria, redness or swelling of skin, soft tissue bone, or joint, ulcers of the skin or mucous

membranes, gangrene, mucous membrane discharge, bleeding, thrombosis, respiratory failure, pulmonary infiltrate, jaundice, diarrhea, vomiting, hepatomegaly, splenomegaly, lymphadenopathy, opportunistic infection such as oral candidiasis.)

5. Specific indications for CBC related to the platelet count include signs, symptoms, test results, illness, or disease associated with increased or decreased platelet production and destruction, or platelet dysfunction (e.g., gastrointestinal bleeding, genitourinary tract bleeding, bilateral epistaxis, thrombosis, ecchymosis, purpura, jaundice, petechiae, fever, heparin therapy, suspected DIC, shock, pre-eclampsia, neonate with maternal ITP, massive transfusion, recent platelet transfusion, cardiopulmonary bypass, hemolytic uremic syndrome, renal diseases, lymphadenopathy, hepatomegaly, splenomegaly, hypersplenism, neurologic abnormalities, viral or other infection, myeloproliferative, myelodysplastic, or lymphoproliferative disorder, thrombosis, exposure to toxic agents, excessive alcohol ingestion, autoimmune disorders (SLE, RA and other).
6. Indications for hemogram or CBC related to red cell (RBC) parameters of the hemogram include, in addition to those already listed, thalassemia, suspected hemoglobinopathy, lead poisoning, arsenic poisoning, and spherocytosis.
7. Specific indications for CBC with differential count related to the WBC include, in addition to those already listed, storage diseases; mucopolysaccharidoses, and use of drugs that cause leukocytosis such as G-CSF or GM-CSF.
8. Specific indications for CBC related to platelet count include, in addition to those already listed, May-Hegglin syndrome and Wiskott-Aldrich syndrome.

Limitations

1. Testing of patients who are asymptomatic, or who do not have a condition that could be expected to result in a hematological abnormality, is screening and is not a covered service.
2. In some circumstances it may be appropriate to perform only a hemoglobin or hematocrit to assess the oxygen carrying capacity of the blood. When the ordering provider requests only a hemoglobin or hematocrit, the remaining components of the CBC are not covered.
3. When a blood count is performed for an end-stage renal disease (ESRD) patient, and is billed outside the ESRD rate, documentation of the medical necessity for the blood count must be submitted with the claim.
4. In some patients presenting with certain signs, symptoms or diseases, a single CBC may be appropriate. Repeat testing may not be indicated unless abnormal results are found, or unless there is a change in clinical condition. If repeat testing is performed, a more descriptive diagnosis code (e.g., anemia) should be reported to support medical necessity. However, repeat testing may be indicated where results are normal in patients with conditions where there is a continued risk for the development of hematologic abnormality.

100-03, 190.18

Serum Iron Studies

(Rev. 17, Issued: 07-02-04) (Effective/Implementation: Not Applicable)

Indications:

1. Ferritin (82728), iron (83540) and either iron binding capacity (83550) or transferrin (84466) are useful in the differential diagnosis of iron deficiency, anemia, and for iron overload conditions.
   a. The following presentations are examples that may support the use of these studies for evaluating iron deficiency:
      - Certain abnormal blood count values (i.e., decreased mean corpuscular volume (MCV), decreased hemoglobin/hematocrit when the MCV is low or normal, or increased red cell distribution width (RDW) and low or normal MCV);
      - Abnormal appetite (pica);
      - Acute or chronic gastrointestinal blood loss;
      - Hematuria;
      - Menorrhagia;
      - Malabsorption;
      - Status post-gastrectomy;
      - Status post-gastrojejunostomy;
      - Malnutrition;
      - Preoperative autologous blood collection(s);
      - Malignant, chronic inflammatory and infectious conditions associated with anemia which may present in a similar manner to iron deficiency anemia;
      - Following a significant surgical procedure where blood loss had occurred and had not been repaired with adequate iron replacement.
   b. The following presentations are examples that may support the use of these studies for evaluating iron overload:
      - Chronic Hepatitis;
      - Diabetes;
      - Hyperpigmentation of skin;
      - Arthropathy;
      - Cirrhosis;
      - Hypogonadism;
      - Hypopituitarism;
      - Impaired porphyrin metabolism;
      - Heart failure;
      - Multiple transfusions;
      - Sideroblastic anemia;
      - Thalassemia major;
      - Cardiomyopathy, cardiac dysrhythmias and conduction disturbances.
2. Follow-up testing may be appropriate to monitor response to therapy, e.g., oral or parenteral iron, ascorbic acid, and erythropoietin.
3. Iron studies may be appropriate in patients after treatment for other nutritional deficiency anemias, such as folate and vitamin B12, because iron deficiency may not be revealed until such a nutritional deficiency is treated.
4. Serum ferritin may be appropriate for monitoring iron status in patients with chronic renal disease with or without dialysis.
5. Serum iron may also be indicated for evaluation of toxic effects of iron and other metals (e.g., nickel, cadmium, aluminum, lead) whether due to accidental, intentional exposure or metabolic causes.

Limitations:

1. Iron studies should be used to diagnose and manage iron deficiency or iron overload states. These tests are not to be used solely to assess acute phase reactants where disease management will be unchanged. For example, infections and malignancies are associated with elevations in acute phase reactants such as ferritin, and decreases in serum iron concentration, but iron studies would only be medically necessary if results of iron studies might alter the management of the primary diagnosis or might warrant direct treatment of an iron disorder or condition.
2. If a normal serum ferritin level is documented, repeat testing would not ordinarily be medically necessary unless there is a change in the patient's condition, and ferritin assessment is needed for the ongoing management of the patient. For example, a patient presents with new onset insulin-dependent diabetes mellitus and has a serum ferritin level performed for the suspicion of hemochromatosis. If the ferritin level is normal, the repeat ferritin for diabetes mellitus would not be medically necessary.
3. When an End Stage Renal Disease (ESRD) patient is tested for ferritin, testing more frequently than every three months (the frequency authorized by 3167.3, Fiscal Intermediary manual) requires documentation of medical necessity [e.g., other than "Chronic Renal Failure" (ICD-9-CM 585) or "Renal Failure, Unspecified" (ICD-9-CM 586)].
4. It is ordinarily not necessary to measure both transferrin and TIBC at the same time because TIBC is an indirect measure of transferrin. When transferrin is ordered as part of the nutritional assessment for evaluating malnutrition, it is not necessary to order other iron studies unless iron deficiency or iron overload is suspected as well.
5. It is not ordinarily necessary to measure both iron/TIBC (or transferrin) and ferritin in initial patient testing. If clinically indicated after evaluation of the initial iron studies, it may be appropriate to perform additional iron studies either on the initial specimen or on a subsequently obtained specimen. After a diagnosis of iron deficiency or iron overload is established, either iron/TIBC (or transferrin) or ferritin may be medically necessary for monitoring, but not both.
6. It would not ordinarily be considered medically necessary to do a ferritin as a preoperative test except in the presence of anemia or recent autologous blood collections prior to the surgery.

100-03, 190.19

Collagen Crosslinks, Any Method

(Rev. 17, Issued: 07-02-04) (Effective/Implementation: Not Applicable)

Indications:

Generally speaking, collagen crosslink testing is useful mostly in "fast losers" of bone. The age when these bone markers can help direct therapy is often pre-Medicare. By the time a fast loser of bone reaches age 65, she will most likely have been stabilized by appropriate therapy or have lost so much bone mass that further testing is useless. Coverage for bone marker assays may be established, however, for younger Medicare beneficiaries and for those men and women who might become fast losers because of some other therapy such as glucocorticoids. Safeguards should be incorporated to prevent excessive use of tests in patients for whom they have no clinical relevance.

Collagen crosslinks testing is used to:

- Identify individuals with elevated bone resorption, who have osteoporosis in whom response to treatment is being monitored;
- Predict response (as assessed by bone mass measurements) to FDA approved antiresorptive therapy in postmenopausal women; and
- Assess response to treatment of patients with osteoporosis, Paget's disease of the bone, or risk for osteoporosis where treatment may include FDA approved antiresorptive agents, anti-estrogens or selective estrogen receptor moderators.

Limitations:

Because of significant specimen to specimen collagen crosslink physiologic variability (15-20%), current recommendations for appropriate utilization include: one or two base-line assays from specified urine collections on separate days; followed by a repeat assay about three months after starting anti-resorptive therapy; followed by a repeat assay in 12 months after the three-month assay; and thereafter not more than annually, unless there is a change in therapy in which circumstance an additional test may be indicated three months after the initiation of new therapy.

Some collagen crosslink assays may not be appropriate for use in some disorders, according to FDA labeling restrictions.

Note: Scroll down for links to the quarterly Covered Code Lists (including narrative).

100-03, 190.20

NCD for Blood Glucose Testing (190.20)

(Rev. 28, Issued: 02-11-05, Effective: 01-01-05, Implementation: 03-11-05)

Indications:

Blood glucose values are often necessary for the management of patients with diabetes mellitus, where hyperglycemia and hypoglycemia are often present. They are also critical in the determination of control of blood glucose levels in the patient with impaired fasting glucose (FPG 110-125 mg/dL), the patient with insulin resistance syndrome and/or carbohydrate intolerance (excessive rise in glucose following ingestion of glucose or glucose sources of food), in the patient with a hypoglycemia disorder such as nesidioblastosis or insulinoma, and in patients with a catabolic or malnutrition state. In addition to those conditions already listed, glucose testing may be medically necessary in patients with tuberculosis, unexplained chronic or recurrent infections, alcoholism, coronary artery disease (especially in women), or unexplained skin conditions (including pruritis, local skin infections, ulceration and gangrene without an established cause).

Many medical conditions may be a consequence of a sustained elevated or depressed glucose level. These include comas, seizures or epilepsy, confusion, abnormal hunger, abnormal weight loss or gain, and loss of sensation. Evaluation of glucose may also be indicated in patients on medications known to affect carbohydrate metabolism.

Effective January 1, 2005, the Medicare law expanded coverage to diabetic screening services. Some forms of blood glucode testing covered under this national coverage determination may be covered for screening purposes subject to specified frequencies. See 42 CFR 410.18 and section 90, chapter 18 of the Claims Processing Manual, for a full description of this screening benefit.

Limitations:

Frequent home blood glucose testing by diabetic patients should be encouraged. In stable, non-hospitalized patients who are unable or unwilling to do home monitoring, it may be reasonable and necessary to measure quantitative blood glucose up to four times annually.

Depending upon the age of the patient, type of diabetes, degree of control, complications of diabetes, and other co-morbid conditions, more frequent testing than four times annually may be reasonable and necessary.

In some patients presenting with nonspecific signs, symptoms, or diseases not normally associated with disturbances in glucose metabolism, a single blood glucose test may be medically necessary. Repeat testing may not be indicated unless abnormal results are found or unless there is a change in clinical condition. If repeat testing is performed, a specific diagnosis code (e.g., diabetes) should be reported to support medical necessity. However, repeat testing may be indicated where results are normal in patients with conditions where there is a confirmed continuing risk of glucose metabolism abnormality (e.g., monitoring glucocorticoid therapy).

100-03, 190.22

NCD for Thyroid Testing (190.22)

(Rev. 17, Issued: 07-02-04) (Effective/Implementation: Not Applicable)

Indications

Thyroid function tests are used to define hyper function, euthyroidism, or hypofunction of thyroid disease. Thyroid testing may be reasonable and necessary to:

- Distinguish between primary and secondary hypothyroidism;
- Confirm or rule out primary hypothyroidism;
- Monitor thyroid hormone levels (for example, patients with goiter, thyroid nodules, or thyroid cancer);
- Monitor drug therapy in patients with primary hypothyroidism;
- Confirm or rule out primary hyperthyroidism; and
- Monitor therapy in patients with hyperthyroidism.

Thyroid function testing may be medically necessary in patients with disease or neoplasm of the thyroid and other endocrine glands. Thyroid function testing may also be medically necessary in patients with metabolic disorders; malnutrition; hyperlipidemia; certain types of anemia; psychosis and non-psychotic personality disorders; unexplained depression; ophthalmologic disorders; various cardiac arrhythmias; disorders of menstruation; skin conditions; myalgias; and a wide array of signs and symptoms, including alterations in consciousness; malaise; hypothermia; symptoms of the nervous and musculoskeletal system; skin and integumentary system; nutrition and metabolism; cardiovascular; and gastrointestinal system.

It may be medically necessary to do follow-up thyroid testing in patients with a personal history of malignant neoplasm of the endocrine system and in patients on long-term thyroid drug therapy.

Limitations

Testing may be covered up to two times a year in clinically stable patients; more frequent testing may be reasonable and necessary for patients whose thyroid therapy has been altered or in whom symptoms or signs of hyperthyroidism or hypothyroidism are noted.

100-03, 190.23

NCD for Lipid Testing (190.23)

(Rev. 28, Issued: 02-11-05, Effective: 01-01-05, Implementation: 03-11-05)

Indications and Limitations of Coverage

Indications

The medical community recognizes lipid testing as appropriate for evaluating atherosclerotic cardiovascular disease. Conditions in which lipid testing may be indicated include:

- Assessment of patients with atherosclerotic cardiovascular disease.
- Evaluation of primary dyslipidemia.
- Any form of atherosclerotic disease, or any disease leading to the formation of atherosclerotic disease.
- Diagnostic evaluation of diseases associated with altered lipid metabolism, such as: nephrotic syndrome, pancreatitis, hepatic disease, and hypo and hyperthyroidism.
- Secondary dyslipidemia, including diabetes mellitus, disorders of gastrointestinal absorption, chronic renal failure.
- Signs or symptoms of dyslipidemias, such as skin lesions.
- As follow-up to the initial screen for coronary heart disease (total cholesterol + HDL cholesterol) when total cholesterol is determined to be high (>240 mg/dL), or borderline-high (200-240 mg/dL) plus two or more coronary heart disease risk factors, or an HDL cholesterol, <35 mg/dl.

To monitor the progress of patients on anti-lipid dietary management and pharmacologic therapy for the treatment of elevated blood lipid disorders, total cholesterol, HDL cholesterol and LDL cholesterol may be used. Triglycerides may be obtained if this lipid fraction is also elevated or if the patient is put on drugs (for example, thiazide diuretics, beta blockers, estrogens, glucocorticoids, and tamoxifen) which may raise the triglyceride level.

When monitoring long term anti-lipid dietary or pharmacologic therapy and when following patients with borderline high total or LDL cholesterol levels, it may be reasonable to perform the lipid panel annually. A lipid panel at a yearly interval will usually be adequate while measurement of the serum total cholesterol or a measured LDL should suffice for interim visits if the patient does not have hypertriglyceridemia.

Any one component of the panel or a measured LDL may be reasonable and necessary up to six times the first year for monitoring dietary or pharmacologic therapy. More frequent total cholesterol HDL cholesterol, LDL cholesterol and triglyceride testing may be indicated for marked elevations or for changes to anti-lipid therapy due to inadequate initial patient response to dietary or pharmacologic therapy. The LDL cholesterol or total cholesterol may be measured three times yearly after treatment goals have been achieved.

Electrophoretic or other quantitation of lipoproteins may be indicated if the patient has a primary disorder of lipid metabolism.

Effective January 1, 2005, the Medicare law expanded coverage to cardiovascular screening services. Several of the procedures included in this NCD may be covered for screening purposes subject to specified frequencies. See 42 CFR 410.17 and section 100, chapter 18, of the Claims Processing Manual, for a full description of this benefit.

Limitations

Lipid panel and hepatic panel testing may be used for patients with severe psoriasis which has not responded to conventional therapy and for which the retinoid etretinate has been prescribed and who have developed hyperlipidemia or hepatic toxicity. Specific examples include erythrodermia and generalized pustular type and psoriasis associated with arthritis.

Routine screening and prophylactic testing for lipid disorder are not covered by Medicare. While lipid screening may be medically appropriate, Medicare by statute does not pay for it. Lipid testing in asymptomatic individuals is considered to be screening regardless of the presence of other risk factors such as family history, tobacco use, etc.

Once a diagnosis is established, one or several specific tests are usually adequate for monitoring the course of the disease. Less specific diagnoses (for example, other chest pain) alone do not support medical necessity of these tests.

When monitoring long term anti-lipid dietary or pharmacologic therapy and when following patients with borderline high total or LDL cholesterol levels, it is reasonable to perform the lipid panel annually. A lipid panel at a yearly interval will usually be adequate while measurement of the serum total cholesterol or a measured LDL should suffice for interim visits if the patient does not have hypertriglyceridemia.

Any one component of the panel or a measured LDL may be medically necessary up to six times the first year for monitoring dietary or pharmacologic therapy. More frequent total cholesterol HDL cholesterol, LDL cholesterol and triglyceride testing may be indicated for marked elevations or for changes to anti-lipid therapy due to inadequate initial patient response to dietary or pharmacologic therapy. The LDL cholesterol or total cholesterol may be measured three times yearly after treatment goals have been achieved.

If no dietary or pharmacological therapy is advised, monitoring is not necessary.

When evaluating non-specific chronic abnormalities of the liver (for example, elevations of transaminase, alkaline phosphatase, abnormal imaging studies, etc.), a lipid panel would generally not be indicated more than twice per year.

100-03, 190.26

NCD for Carcinoembryonic Antigen (CEA)

(Rev. 17, Issued: 07-02-04)

Carcinoembryonic antigen (CEA) is a protein polysaccharide found in some carcinomas. It is effective as a biochemical marker for monitoring the response of certain malignancies to therapy.

Indications

CEA may be medically necessary for follow-up of patients with colorectal carcinoma. It would however only be medically necessary at treatment decision-making points. In some clinical situations (e.g. adenocarcinoma of the lung, small cell carcinoma of the lung, and some gastrointestinal carcinomas) when a more specific marker is not expressed by the tumor, CEA may be a medically necessary alternative marker for monitoring. Preoperative CEA may also be helpful in determining the post-operative adequacy of surgical resection and subsequent medical management. In general, a single tumor marker will suffice in following patients with colorectal carcinoma or other malignancies that express such tumor markers.

In following patients who have had treatment for colorectal carcinoma, ASCO guideline suggests that if resection of liver metastasis would be indicated, it is recommended that post-operative CEA testing be performed every two to three months in patients with initial stage II or stage III disease for at least two years after diagnosis.

For patients with metastatic solid tumors which express CEA, CEA may be measured at the start of the treatment and with subsequent treatment cycles to assess the tumor's response to therapy.

Limitations:

Serum CEA determinations are generally not indicated more frequently than once per chemotherapy treatment cycle for patients with metastatic solid tumors which express CEA or every two months post-surgical treatment for patients who have had colorectal carcinoma. However, it may be proper to order the test more frequently in certain situations, for example, when there has been a significant change from prior CEA level or a significant change in patient status which could reflect disease progression or recurrence.

Testing with a diagnosis of an in situ carcinoma is not reasonably done more frequently than once, unless the result is abnormal, in which case the test may be repeated once.

100-03, 190.31

NCD for Prostate Specific Antigen (PSA) (190.31)

(Rev. 17, Issued: 07-02-04) (Effective/Implementation: Not Applicable)

Indications:

PSA is of proven value in differentiating benign from malignant disease in men with lower urinary tract signs and symptoms (e.g., hematuria, slow urine stream, hesitancy, urgency, frequency, nocturia and incontinence) as well as with patients with palpably abnormal prostate glands on physician exam, and in patients with other laboratory or imaging studies that suggest the possibility of a malignant prostate disorder. PSA is also a marker used to follow the progress of prostate cancer once a diagnosis has been established, such as in detecting metastatic or persistent disease in patients who may require additional treatment. PSA testing may also be useful in the differential diagnosis of men presenting with as yet undiagnosed disseminated metastatic disease.

Limitations:

Generally, for patients with lower urinary tract signs or symptoms, the test is performed only once per year unless there is a change in the patient's medical condition.

Testing with a diagnosis of in situ carcinoma is not reasonably done more frequently than once, unless the result is abnormal, in which case the test may be repeated once.

100-03, 210.1

NCD for Prostate Cancer Screening Tests (210.1)

(Rev. 48, Issued: 03-17-06; Effective/Implementation Dates: 06-19-06)

Indications and Limitations of Coverage

CIM 50-55

Covered

A. General

Section 4103 of the Balanced Budget Act of 1997 provides for coverage of certain prostate cancer screening tests subject to certain coverage, frequency, and payment limitations. Medicare will cover prostate cancer screening tests/procedures for the early detection of prostate cancer. Coverage of prostate cancer screening tests includes the following procedures furnished to an individual for the early detection of prostate cancer:

- Screening digital rectal examination; and
- Screening prostate specific antigen blood test

B. Screening Digital Rectal Examinations

Screening digital rectal examinations are covered at a frequency of once every 12 months for men who have attained age 50 (at least 11 months have passed following the month in which the last Medicare-covered screening digital rectal examination was performed). Screening digital rectal examination means a clinical examination of an individual's prostate for nodules or other abnormalities of the prostate. This screening must be performed by a doctor of medicine or osteopathy (as defined in §1861(r)(1) of the Act), or by a physician assistant, nurse practitioner, clinical nurse specialist, or certified nurse midwife (as defined in §1861(aa) and §1861(gg) of the Act) who is authorized under State law to perform the examination, fully knowledgeable about the beneficiary's medical condition, and would be responsible for using the results of any examination performed in the overall management of the beneficiary's specific medical problem.

C. Screening Prostate Specific Antigen Tests

Screening prostate specific antigen tests are covered at a frequency of once every 12 months for men who have attained age 50 (at least 11 months have passed following the month in which the last Medicare-covered screening prostate specific antigen test was performed). Screening prostate specific antigen tests (PSA) means a test to detect the marker for adenocarcinoma of prostate. PSA is a reliable immunocytochemical marker for primary and metastatic adenocarcinoma of prostate. This screening must be ordered by the beneficiary's physician or by the beneficiary's physician assistant, nurse practitioner, clinical nurse specialist, or certified nurse midwife (the term "attending physician"; is defined in §1861(r)(1) of the Act to mean a doctor of medicine or osteopathy and the terms ";physician assistant, nurse practitioner, clinical nurse specialist, or certified nurse midwife"; are defined in §1861(aa) and §1861(gg) of the Act) who is fully knowledgeable about the beneficiary's medical condition, and who would be responsible for using the results of any examination (test) performed in the overall management of the beneficiary's specific medical problem.

100-03, 210.2

NCD for Screening Pap Smears and Pelvic Examinations for Early Detection of Cervical or Vaginal Cancer (210.2)

(Rev. 173, Issued: 09-04-14, Effective: Upon Implementation: of ICD–10)

Screening Pap Smear

A screening pap smear and related medically necessary services provided to a woman for the early detection of cervical cancer (including collection of the sample of cells and a physician's interpretation of the test results) and pelvic examination (including clinical breast examination) are covered under Medicare Part B when ordered by a physician (or authorized practitioner) under one of the following conditions:

- She has not had such a test during the preceding two years or is a woman of childbearing age (Â§1861(nn) of the Social Security Act (the Act).
- There is evidence (on the basis of her medical history or other findings) that she is at high risk of developing cervical cancer and her physician (or authorized practitioner) recommends that she have the test performed more frequently than every two years.

High risk factors for cervical and vaginal cancer are:

- Early onset of sexual activity (under 16 years of age)
- Multiple sexual partners (five or more in a lifetime)
- History of sexually transmitted disease (including HIV infection)
- Fewer than three negative or any pap smears within the previous seven years; and
- DES (diethylstilbestrol) - exposed daughters of women who took DES during pregnancy.

NOTE: Claims for pap smears must indicate the beneficiary's low or high risk status by including the appropriate diagnosis code on the line item (Item 24E of the Form CMS-1500).

Definitions

A woman as described in Â§1861(nn) of the Act is a woman who is of childbearing age and has had a pap smear test during any of the preceding 3 years that indicated the presence of cervical or vaginal cancer or other abnormality, or is at high risk of developing cervical or vaginal cancer.

A woman of childbearing age is one who is premenopausal and has been determined by a physician or other qualified practitioner to be of childbearing age, based upon the medical history or other findings.

Other qualified practitioner, as defined in 42 CFR 410.56(a) includes a certified nurse midwife (as defined in Â§1861(gg) of the Act), or a physician assistant, nurse practitioner, or clinical nurse specialist (as defined in Â§1861(aa) of the Act) who is authorized under State law to perform the examination.

Screening Pelvic Examination

Section 4102 of the Balanced Budget Act of 1997 provides for coverage of screening pelvic examinations (including a clinical breast examination) for all female beneficiaries, subject to certain frequency and other limitations. A screening pelvic examination (including a clinical breast examination) should include at least seven of the following eleven elements:

- Inspection and palpation of breasts for masses or lumps, tenderness, symmetry, or nipple discharge.
- Digital rectal examination including sphincter tone, presence of hemorrhoids, and rectal masses. Pelvic examination (with or without specimen collection for smears and cultures) including:
- External genitalia (for example, general appearance, hair distribution, or lesions).
- Urethral meatus (for example, size, location, lesions, or prolapse).
- Urethra (for example, masses, tenderness, or scarring).
- Bladder (for example, fullness, masses, or tenderness).
- Vagina (for example, general appearance, estrogen effect, discharge lesions, pelvic support, cystocele, or rectocele).
- Cervix (for example, general appearance, lesions, or discharge).
- Uterus (for example, size, contour, position, mobility, tenderness, consistency, descent, or support).
- Adnexa/parametria (for example, masses, tenderness, organomegaly, or nodularity).
- Anus and perineum.

This description is from Documentation Guidelines for Evaluation and Management Services, published in May 1997 and was developed by the Centers for Medicare & Medicaid Services and the American Medical Association.

100-03, 210.2.1

Screening for Cervical Cancer with Human Papillomavirus (HPV) Testing (Effective July 9, 2015)

(Rev. 189, Issued: 02-05-16, Effective: 07-05-16; Implementation: 03-07-16 - for non-shared MAC edits; 07-05-16 - CWF analysis and design; 10-03-16 - CWF Coding, Testing and Implementation, MCS, and FISS Implementation; 01-03-17 - Requirement BR9434.04.8.2)

A. General

Medicare covers a screening pelvic examination and Pap test for all female beneficiaries at 12 or 24 month intervals, based on specific risk factors. See 42 C.F.R. §410.56; Medicare National Coverage Determinations Manual, §210.2.1 Current Medicare coverage does not include the HPV testing. Pursuant to §1861(ddd) of the Social Security Act, the Secretary may add coverage of "additional preventive services" if certain statutory requirements are met.

B. Nationally Covered Indications

Effective for services performed on or after July 9, 2015, CMS has determined that the evidence is sufficient to add Human Papillomavirus (HPV) testing once every five years as an additional preventive service benefit under the Medicare program for asymptomatic beneficiaries aged 30 to 65 years in conjunction with the Pap smear test. CMS will cover screening for cervical cancer with the appropriate U.S. Food and Drug Administration (FDA) approved/cleared laboratory tests, used consistent with FDA approved labeling and in compliance with the Clinical Laboratory Improvement Act (CLIA) regulations.

C. Nationally Non-Covered Indications

Unless specifically covered in this NCD, any other NCD, by statute or regulation, preventive services are non-covered by Medicare.

D. Other

(This NCD last reviewed July 2015.)

100-03, 210.4.1

Counseling to Prevent Tobacco Use (Effective August 25, 2010)

(Rev.202, Issued: 08-25-17, Effective: 09-26-17, Implementation: 09- 26-17)

A. General

Tobacco use remains the leading cause of preventable morbidity and mortality in the U.S. and is a major contributor to the nation's increasing medical costs. Despite the growing list of adverse health effects associated with smoking, more than 45 million U.S. adults continue to smoke and approximately 1,200 die prematurely each day from tobacco-related diseases. Annual smoking-attributable expenditures can be measured both in direct medical costs ($96 billion) and in lost productivity ($97 billion), but the results of national surveys have raised concerns that recent declines in smoking prevalence among U.S. adults may have come to an end. According to the U.S. Department of Health and Human Services (DHHS) Public Health Service (PHS) Clinical Practice Guideline on Treating Tobacco Use and Dependence (2008), 4.5 million adults over 65 years of age smoke cigarettes. Even smokers over age 65, however, can benefit greatly from abstinence, and older smokers who quit can reduce their risk of death from coronary heart disease, chronic obstructive lung disease and lung cancer, as well as decrease their risk of osteoporosis.

B. Nationally Covered Indications

Effective for claims with dates of service on or after August 25, 2010, CMS will cover tobacco cessation counseling for outpatient and hospitalized Medicare beneficiaries

1. Who use tobacco, regardless of whether they have signs or symptoms of tobacco-related disease;
2. Who are competent and alert at the time that counseling is provided; and,
3. Whose counseling is furnished by a qualified physician or other Medicare-recognized practitioner.

Intermediate and intensive smoking cessation counseling services will be covered under Medicare Part B when the above conditions of coverage are met, subject to frequency and other limitations. That is, similar to existing tobacco cessation counseling for symptomatic individuals, CMS will allow 2 individual tobacco cessation counseling attempts per 12-month period. Each attempt may include a maximum of 4 intermediate OR intensive sessions, with a total benefit covering up to 8 sessions per 12-month period per Medicare beneficiary who uses tobacco. The practitioner and patient have the flexibility to choose between intermediate (more than 3 minutes but less than 10 minutes), or intensive (more than 10 minutes) cessation counseling sessions for each attempt.

C. Nationally Non-Covered Indications

Inpatient hospital stays with the principal diagnosis of tobacco use disorder are not reasonable and necessary for the effective delivery of tobacco cessation counseling services. Therefore, we will not cover tobacco cessation services if tobacco cessation is the primary reason for the patient's hospital stay.

D. Other

Section 4104 of the Affordable Care Act provided for a waiver of the Medicare coinsurance and Part B deductible requirements for this service effective on or after January 1, 2011. Until that time, this service will continue to be subject to the standard Medicare coinsurance and Part B deductible requirements.

100-03, 220.2

(Rev. 173, Issued: 09-04-14, Effective: Upon Implementation: of ICD-10, Implementation: Upon Implementation of ICD-10)

A. General

1. Method of Operation

    Magnetic Resonance Imaging (MRI), formerly called nuclear magnetic resonance (NMR), is a non-invasive method of graphically representing the distribution of water and other hydrogen-rich molecules in the human body. In contrast to conventional radiographs or computed tomography (CT) scans, in which the image is produced by x-ray beam attenuation by an object, MRI is capable of producing images by several techniques. In fact, various combinations of MRI image production methods may be employed to emphasize particular characteristics of the tissue or body part being examined. The basic elements by which MRI produces an image are the density of hydrogen nuclei in the object being examined, their motion, and the relaxation times, and the period of time required for the nuclei to return to their original states in the main, static magnetic field after being subjected to a brief additional magnetic field. These relaxation times reflect the physical-chemical properties of tissue and the molecular environment of its hydrogen nuclei. Only hydrogen atoms are present in human tissues in sufficient concentration for current use in clinical MRI.

    Magnetic Resonance Angiography (MRA) is a non-invasive diagnostic test that is an application of MRI. By analyzing the amount of energy released from tissues exposed to a strong magnetic field, MRA provides images of normal and diseased blood vessels, as well as visualization and quantification of blood flow through these vessels.

2. General Clinical Utility

    Overall, MRI is a useful diagnostic imaging modality that is capable of demonstrating a wide variety of soft-tissue lesions with contrast resolution equal or superior to CT scanning in various parts of the body.

    Among the advantages of MRI are the absence of ionizing radiation and the ability to achieve high levels of tissue contrast resolution without injected iodinated radiological contrast agents. Recent advances in technology have resulted in development and Food and Drug Administration (FDA) approval of new paramagnetic contrast agents for MRI which allow even better visualization in some instances. Multi-slice imaging and the ability to image in multiple planes, especially sagittal and coronal, have provided flexibility not easily available with other modalities. Because cortical (outer layer) bone and metallic prostheses do not cause distortion of MR images, it has been possible to visualize certain lesions and body regions with greater certainty than has been possible with CT. The use of MRI on certain soft tissue structures for the purpose of detecting disruptive, neoplastic, degenerative, or inflammatory lesions has now become established in medical practice.

    Phase contrast (PC) and time-of-flight (TOF) are some of the available MRA techniques at the time these instructions are being issued. PC measures the difference between the phases of proton spins in tissue and blood and measures both the venous and arterial blood flow at any point in the cardiac cycle. TOF measures the difference between the amount of magnetization of tissue and blood and provides information on the structure of blood vessels, thus indirectly indicating blood flow. Two-dimensional (2D) and three-dimensional (3D) images can be obtained using each method.

Contrast-enhanced MRA (CE-MRA) involves blood flow imaging after the patient receives an intravenous injection of a contrast agent. Gadolinium, a non-ionic element, is the foundation of all contrast agents currently in use. Gadolinium affects the way in which tissues respond to magnetization, resulting in better visualization of structures when compared to un-enhanced studies. Unlike ionic (i.e., iodine-based) contrast agents used in conventional contrast angiography (CA), allergic reactions to gadolinium are extremely rare. Additionally, gadolinium does not cause the kidney failure occasionally seen with ionic contrast agents. Digital subtraction angiography (DSA) is a computer-augmented form of CA that obtains digital blood flow images as contrast agent courses through a blood vessel. The computer "subtracts" bone and other tissue from the image, thereby improving visualization of blood vessels. Physicians elect to use a specific MRA or CA technique based upon clinical information from each patient.

B. Nationally Covered MRI and MRA Indications

1. MRI

   Although several uses of MRI are still considered investigational and some uses are clearly contraindicated (see subsection C), MRI is considered medically efficacious for a number of uses. Use the following descriptions as general guidelines or examples of what may be considered covered rather than as a restrictive list of specific covered indications. Coverage is limited to MRI units that have received FDA premarket approval, and such units must be operated within the parameters specified by the approval. In addition, the services must be reasonable and necessary for the diagnosis or treatment of the specific patient involved.

   a. Effective November 22, 1985, MRI is useful in examining the head, central nervous system, and spine. Multiple sclerosis can be diagnosed with MRI and the contents of the posterior fossa are visible. The inherent tissue contrast resolution of MRI makes it an appropriate standard diagnostic modality for general neuroradiology.

   b. Effective November 22, 1985, MRI can assist in the differential diagnosis of mediastinal and retroperitoneal masses, including abnormalities of the large vessels such as aneurysms and dissection. When a clinical need exists to visualize the parenchyma of solid organs to detect anatomic disruption or neoplasia, this can be accomplished in the liver, urogenital system, adrenals, and pelvic organs without the use of radiological contrast materials. When MRI is considered reasonable and necessary, the use of paramagnetic contrast materials may be covered as part of the study. MRI may also be used to detect and stage pelvic and retroperitoneal neoplasms and to evaluate disorders of cancellous bone and soft tissues. It may also be used in the detection of pericardial thickening. Primary and secondary bone neoplasm and aseptic necrosis can be detected at an early stage and monitored with MRI. Patients with metallic prostheses, especially of the hip, can be imaged in order to detect the early stages of infection of the bone to which the prosthesis is attached.

   c. Effective March 22, 1994, MRI may also be covered to diagnose disc disease without regard to whether radiological imaging has been tried first to diagnose the problem.

   d. Effective March 4, 1991, MRI with gating devices and surface coils, and gating devices that eliminate distorted images caused by cardiac and respiratory movement cycles are now considered state of the art techniques and may be covered. Surface and other specialty coils may also be covered, as they are used routinely for high resolution imaging where small limited regions of the body are studied. They produce high signal-to-noise ratios resulting in images of enhanced anatomic detail.

2. MRA (MRI for Blood Flow)

   Currently covered indications include using MRA for specific conditions to evaluate flow in internal carotid vessels of the head and neck, peripheral arteries of lower extremities, abdomen and pelvis, and the chest. Coverage is limited to MRA units that have received FDA premarket approval, and such units must be operated within the parameters specified by the approval. In addition, the services must be reasonable and necessary for the diagnosis or treatment of the specific patient involved.

   a. Head and Neck

      Effective April 15, 2003, studies have proven that MRA is effective for evaluating flow in internal carotid vessels of the head and neck. However, not all potential applications of MRA have been shown to be reasonable and necessary. All of the following criteria must apply in order for Medicare to provide coverage for MRA of the head and neck:

      - MRA is used to evaluate the carotid arteries, the circle of Willis, the anterior, middle or posterior cerebral arteries, the vertebral or basilar arteries or the venous sinuses;
      - MRA is performed on patients with conditions of the head and neck for which surgery is anticipated and may be found to be appropriate based on the MRA. These conditions include, but are not limited to, tumor, aneurysms, vascular malformations, vascular occlusion or thrombosis.

      Within this broad category of disorders, medical necessity is the underlying determinant of the need for an MRA in specific diseases. The medical records should clearly justify and demonstrate the existence of medical necessity; and

      - MRA and CA are not expected to be performed on the same patient for diagnostic purposes prior to the application of anticipated therapy. Only one of these tests will be covered routinely unless the physician can demonstrate the medical need to perform both tests.

   b. Peripheral Arteries of Lower Extremities

      Effective April 15, 2003, studies have proven that MRA of peripheral arteries is useful in determining the presence and extent of peripheral vascular disease in lower extremities. This procedure is non-invasive and has been shown to find occult vessels in some patients for which those vessels were not apparent when CA was performed. Medicare will cover either MRA or CA to evaluate peripheral arteries of the lower extremities. However, both MRA and CA may be useful in some cases, such as:

      - A patient has had CA and this test was unable to identify a viable run-off vessel for bypass. When exploratory surgery is not believed to be a reasonable medical course of action for this patient, MRA may be performed to identify the viable runoff vessel; or
      - A patient has had MRA, but the results are inconclusive.

   c. Abdomen and Pelvis

      i. Pre-operative Evaluation of Patients Undergoing Elective Abdominal Aortic Aneurysm (AAA) Repair

         Effective July 1, 1999, MRA is covered for pre-operative evaluation of patients undergoing elective AAA repair if the scientific evidence reveals MRA is considered comparable to CA in determining the extent of AAA, as well as in evaluating aortoiliac occlusion disease and renal artery pathology that may be necessary in the surgical planning of AAA repair. These studies also reveal that MRA could provide a net benefit to the patient. If preoperative CA is avoided, then patients are not exposed to the risks associated with invasive procedures, contrast media, end-organ damage, or arterial injury.

      ii. Imaging the Renal Arteries and the Aortoiliac Arteries in the Absence of AAA or Aortic Dissection

         Effective July 1, 2003, MRA coverage is expanded to include imaging the renal arteries and the aortoiliac arteries in the absence of AAA or aortic dissection. MRA should be obtained in those circumstances in which using MRA is expected to avoid obtaining CA, when physician history, physical examination, and standard assessment tools provide insufficient information for patient management, and obtaining an MRA has a high probability of positively affecting patient management. However, CA may be ordered after obtaining the results of an MRA in those rare instances where medical necessity is demonstrated.

   d. Chest

      i. Diagnosis of Pulmonary Embolism

         Current scientific data has shown that diagnostic pulmonary MRAs are improving due to recent developments such as faster imaging capabilities and gadolinium-enhancement. However, these advances in MRA are not significant enough to warrant replacement of pulmonary angiography in the diagnosis of pulmonary embolism for patients who have no contraindication to receiving intravenous iodinated contrast material. Patients who are allergic to iodinated contrast material face a high risk of developing complications if they undergo pulmonary angiography or computed tomography angiography. Therefore, Medicare will cover MRA of the chest for diagnosing a suspected pulmonary embolism when it is contraindicated for the patient to receive intravascular iodinated contrast material.

      ii. Evaluation of Thoracic Aortic Dissection and Aneurysm

         Studies have shown that MRA of the chest has a high level of diagnostic accuracy for pre-operative and post-operative evaluation of aortic dissection of aneurysm. Depending on the clinical presentation, MRA may be used as an alternative to other non-invasive imaging technologies, such as transesophageal echocardiography and CT. Generally, Medicare will provide coverage only for MRA or for CA when used as a diagnostic test. However, if both MRA and CA of the chest are used, the physician must demonstrate the medical need for performing these tests.

         While the intent of this policy is to provide reimbursement for either RA or CA, the Centers for Medicare & Medicaid Services (CMS) is also allowing flexibility for physicians to make appropriate decisions concerning the use of these tests based on the needs of individual patients. CMS anticipates, however, low utilization of the combined use of MRA and CA. As a result, CMS encourages the Medicare Administrative Contractors (MACs) to monitor the use of these tests and, where indicated, require evidence of the need to perform both MRA and CA.

C. Contraindications and Nationally Non-Covered Indications

1. Contraindications

   The MRI is not covered when the following patient-specific contraindications are present:

   MRI is not covered for patients with cardiac pacemakers or with metallic clips on vascular aneurysms unless the Medicare beneficiary meets the provisions of the following exceptions:

   Effective July 7, 2011, the contraindications will not apply to pacemakers when used according to the FDA-approved labeling in an MRI environment, or

Effective February 24, 2011, CMS believes that the evidence is promising although not yet convincing that MRI will improve patient health outcomes if certain safeguards are in place to ensure that the exposure of the device to an MRI environment adversely affects neither the interpretation of the MRI result nor the proper functioning of the implanted device itself. We believe that specific precautions (as listed below) could maximize benefits of MRI exposure for beneficiaries enrolled in clinical trials designed to assess the utility and safety of MRI exposure. Therefore, CMS determines that MRI will be covered by Medicare when provided in a clinical study under section 1862(a)(1)(E) (consistent with section 1142 of the Social Security Act (the Act)) through the Coverage with Study Participation (CSP) form of Coverage with Evidence Development (CED) if the study meets the criteria in each of the three paragraphs below:

The approved prospective clinical study of MRI must, with appropriate methodology, address one or more aspects of the following questions:

1. Do results of MRI in implanted permanent pacemaker (PM)/implantable cardioverter defibrillator (ICD) beneficiaries with implanted cardiac devices affect physician decision making related to:
   a. Clinical management strategy (e.g., in oncology, toward palliative or curative care)?
   b. Planning of treatment interventions?; or
   c. Prevention of unneeded diagnostic studies or interventions, or preventable exposures?
2. Do results of MRI in PM/ICD beneficiaries with implanted cardiac devices affect patient outcomes related to:
   a. Survival?
   b. Quality of life?; or
   c. Adverse events during and after MR scanning?

In addition, the prospective clinical study of MRI must include safety criteria for all participants. Such required safety measures for such studies, as further explained in guidance documents from professional societies must include, but are not limited to:

1. MRI should be done on a case-by-case and site-by-site basis.
2. MRI scan sequences, field intensity, and field(s) of exposure should be selected to minimize risk to the patient while gaining needed diagnostic information for diagnosis or for managing therapy.
3. MRI scanning should be done only if the site is staffed with individuals with the appropriate radiology and cardiology knowledge and expertise on hand.
4. Implanted device patients who are candidates for recruitment for an MRI clinical study should be advised that life-threatening arrhythmias might occur during MRI and serious device malfunction might occur, requiring replacement of the device.
5. Radiology and cardiology personnel and a fully stocked crash cart should be readily available throughout the procedure in case a significant arrhythmia develops during the examination that does not terminate with the cessation of the MRI study. The cardiologist should be familiar with the patient's arrhythmia history and the implanted device. A programmer that can be used to adjust the device as necessary should be readily available.
6. All such patients should be actively monitored for cardiac and respiratory function throughout the examination. At a minimum, ECG and pulse oximetry should be used. Visual and verbal contact with the patient must be maintained throughout the MRI scan. The patient should be instructed to alert the MRI staff on hand to any unusual sensations, pains, or to any problems.
7. At the conclusion of the examination, the cardiologist should examine the device to confirm that the function is consistent with its pre-examination state.
8. Follow-up should include a check of the patient's device at a time remote (1-6 weeks) after the scan to confirm appropriate function.
9. If the implanted device manufacturer has indicated additional safety precautions appropriate for safe MRI performance, these must be included in the study protocol.

   The clinical study must adhere to the following standards of scientific integrity and relevance to the Medicare population:

   a. The principal purpose of the research study is to test whether a particular intervention potentially improves the participants' health outcomes.
   b. The research study is well supported by available scientific and medical information or it is intended to clarify or establish the health outcomes of interventions already in common clinical use.
   c. The research study does not unjustifiably duplicate existing studies.
   d. The research study design is appropriate to answer the research question being asked in the study.
   e. The research study is sponsored by an organization or individual capable of executing the proposed study successfully.
   f. The research study is in compliance with all applicable Federal regulations concerning the protection of human subjects found at 45 CFR Part 46. If a study is regulated by the FDA, it must be in compliance with 21 CFR Parts 50 and 56.
   g. All aspects of the research study are conducted according to appropriate standards of scientific integrity (see http://www.icmje.org).
   h. The research study has a written protocol that clearly addresses, or incorporates by reference, the standards listed here as Medicare requirements for CED coverage.
   i. The clinical research study is not designed to exclusively test toxicity or disease pathophysiology in healthy individuals. Trials of all medical technologies measuring therapeutic outcomes as one of the objectives meet this standard only if the disease or condition being studied is life threatening as defined in 21 CFR §312.81(a) and the patient has no other viable treatment options.
   j. The clinical research study is registered on the www.ClinicalTrials.gov website by the principal sponsor/investigator prior to the enrollment of the first study subject.
   k. The research study protocol specifies the method and timing of public release of all pre-specified outcomes to be measured, including release of outcomes if outcomes are negative or study is terminated early. The results must be made public within 24 months of the end of data collection. If a report is planned to be published in a peer reviewed journal, then that initial release may be an abstract that meets the requirements of the International Committee of Medical Journal Editors (http://www.icmje.org). However, a full report of the outcomes must be made public no later than three (3) years after the end of data collection.
   l. The research study protocol must explicitly discuss subpopulations affected by the treatment under investigation, particularly traditionally underrepresented groups in clinical studies, how the inclusion and exclusion criteria effect enrollment of these populations, and a plan for the retention and reporting of said populations in the trial. If the inclusion and exclusion criteria are expected to have a negative effect on the recruitment or retention of underrepresented populations, the protocol must discuss why these criteria are necessary.
   m. The research study protocol explicitly discusses how the results are or are not expected to be generalizable to the Medicare population to infer whether Medicare patients may benefit from the intervention. Separate discussions in the protocol may be necessary for populations eligible for Medicare due to age, disability, or Medicaid eligibility.

   Consistent with section 1142 of the Act, the Agency for Healthcare Research and Quality supports clinical research studies that CMS determines meet the above-listed standards and address the above-listed research questions.

   - MRI during a viable pregnancy is also contraindicated at this time.
   - The danger inherent in bringing ferromagnetic materials within range of MRI units generally constrains the use of MRI on acutely ill patients requiring life support systems and monitoring devices that employ ferromagnetic materials.
   - In addition, the long imaging time and the enclosed position of the patient may result in claustrophobia, making patients who have a history of claustrophobia unsuitable candidates for MRI procedures.

2. Nationally Non-Covered Indications

   CMS has determined that MRI of cortical bone and calcifications, and procedures involving spatial resolution of bone and calcifications, are not considered reasonable and necessary indications within the meaning of section 1862(a)(1)(A) of the Act, and are therefore non-covered.

D. Other

Effective June 3, 2010, all other uses of MRI or MRA for which CMS has not specifically indicated coverage or non-coverage continue to be eligible for coverage through individual MAC discretion.

100-03, 220.6.9

NCD for PET (FDG) for Refractory Seizures (220.6.9)

(Rev. 120; Issued: 05-06-10; Effective Date: 04-03-09; Implementation Date: 10-30-09)

Beginning July 1, 2001, Medicare covers FDG PET for pre-surgical evaluation for the purpose of localization of a focus of refractory seizure activity.

Limitations: Covered only for pre-surgical evaluation.

Documentation that these conditions are met should be maintained by the referring physician in the beneficiary's medical record, as is normal business practice.

(This NCD last reviewed June 2001.)

100-03, 220.6.17

NCD for Positron Emission Tomography (FDG) for Oncologic Conditions (220.6.17)

(Rev. 173, Issued: 09-04-14, Effective: Upon Implementation: of ICD–10)

A. General

FDG (2-[F18] fluoro-2-deoxy-D-glucose) Positron Emission Tomography (PET) is a minimally-invasive diagnostic imaging procedure used to evaluate glucose metabolism in normal tissue as well as in diseased tissues in conditions such as cancer, ischemic heart disease, and some neurologic disorders. FDG is an injected radionuclide (or radiopharmaceutical) that emits sub-atomic particles, known as positrons, as it decays. FDG PET uses a positron camera (tomograph) to measure the decay of FDG. The rate of FDG decay provides biochemical information on glucose metabolism in the tissue being studied. As malignancies can cause abnormalities of metabolism and blood flow, FDG PET evaluation may indicate the probable presence or absence of a malignancy based upon observed differences in biologic activity compared to adjacent tissues.

The Centers for Medicare and Medicaid Services (CMS) was asked by the National Oncologic PET Registry (NOPR) to reconsider section 220.6 of the National Coverage Determinations (NCD) Manual to end the prospective data collection requirements under Coverage with Evidence Development (CED) across all oncologic indications of FDG PET imaging. The CMS received public input indicating that the current coverage framework of prospective data collection under CED be ended for all oncologic uses of FDG PET imaging.

1. Framework

   Effective for claims with dates of service on and after June 11, 2013, CMS is adopting a coverage framework that ends the prospective data collection requirements by NOPR under CED for all oncologic uses of FDG PET imaging. CMS is making this change for all NCDs that address coverage of FDG PET for oncologic uses addressed in this decision. This decision does not change coverage for any use of PET imaging using radiopharmaceuticals NaF-18 (fluorine-18 labeled sodium fluoride), ammonia N-13, or rubidium-82 (Rb-82).

2. Initial Anti-Tumor Treatment Strategy

   CMS continues to believe that the evidence is adequate to determine that the results of FDG PET imaging are useful in determining the appropriate initial anti-tumor treatment strategy for beneficiaries with suspected cancer and improve health outcomes and thus are reasonable and necessary under §1862(a)(1)(A) of the Social Security Act (the Act).

   Therefore, CMS continues to nationally cover one FDG PET study for beneficiaries who have cancers that are biopsy proven or strongly suspected based on other diagnostic testing when the beneficiary's treating physician determines that the FDG PET study is needed to determine the location and/or extent of the tumor for the following therapeutic purposes related to the initial anti-tumor treatment strategy:

   — To determine whether or not the beneficiary is an appropriate candidate for an invasive diagnostic or therapeutic procedure; or

   — To determine the optimal anatomic location for an invasive procedure; or

   — To determine the anatomic extent of tumor when the recommended antitumor treatment reasonably depends on the extent of the tumor.

   See the table at the end of this section for a synopsis of all nationally covered and noncovered oncologic uses of FDG PET imaging.

   B.1. Initial Anti-Tumor Treatment Strategy Nationally Covered Indications

   a. CMS continues to nationally cover FDG PET imaging for the initial anti-tumor treatment strategy for male and female breast cancer only when used in staging distant metastasis.

   b. CMS continues to nationally cover FDG PET to determine initial anti-tumor treatment strategy for melanoma other than for the evaluation of regional lymph nodes.

   c. CMS continues to nationally cover FDG PET imaging for the detection of pre-treatment metastasis (i.e., staging) in newly diagnosed cervical cancers following conventional imaging.

   C.1. Initial Anti-Tumor Treatment Strategy Nationally Non-Covered Indications

   a. CMS continues to nationally non-cover initial anti-tumor treatment strategy in Medicare beneficiaries who have adenocarcinoma of the prostate.

   b. CMS continues to nationally non-cover FDG PET imaging for diagnosis of breast cancer and initial staging of axillary nodes.

   c. CMS continues to nationally non-cover FDG PET imaging for initial anti-tumor treatment strategy for the evaluation of regional lymph nodes in melanoma.

   d. CMS continues to nationally non-cover FDG PET imaging for the diagnosis of cervical cancer related to initial anti-tumor treatment strategy.

3. Subsequent Anti-Tumor Treatment Strategy

   B.2. Subsequent Anti-Tumor Treatment Strategy Nationally Covered Indications

   Three FDG PET scans are nationally covered when used to guide subsequent management of anti-tumor treatment strategy after completion of initial anti-cancer therapy. Coverage of more than three FDG PET scans to guide subsequent management of anti-tumor treatment strategy after completion of initial anti-cancer therapy shall be determined by the local Medicare Administrative Contractors.

4. Synopsis of Coverage of FDG PET for Oncologic Conditions

   Effective for claims with dates of service on and after June 11, 2013, the chart below summarizes national FDG PET coverage for oncologic conditions:

FDG PET for Cancers Tumor Type	**Initial Treatment Strategy** (formerly "diagnosis" & "staging")	**Subsequent Treatment Strategy** (formerly "restaging" & "monitoring response to treatment"
Colorectal	Cover	Cover
Esophagus	Cover	Cover
Head & Neck (not Thyroid, CNS)	Cover	Cover
Lymphoma	Cover	Cover
Non-Small Cell Lung	Cover	Cover
Ovary	Cover	Cover
Brain	Cover	Cover
Cervix	Cover w/exception*	Cover
Small Cell Lung	Cover	Cover
Soft Tissue Sarcoma	Cover	Cover
Pancreas	Cover	Cover
Testes	Cover	Cover
Prostate	Non-cover	Cover
Thyroid	Cover	Cover
Breast (male and female)	Cover w/exception*	Cover
Melanoma	Cover w/exception*	Cover
All Other Solid Tumors	Cover	Cover
Myeloma	Cover	Cover
All other cancers not listed	Cover	Cover

* Cervix: Nationally non-covered for the initial diagnosis of cervical cancer related to initial anti-tumor treatment strategy. All other indications for initial anti-tumor treatment strategy for cervical cancer are nationally covered.

* Breast: Nationally non-covered for initial diagnosis and/or staging of axillary lymph nodes. Nationally covered for initial staging of metastatic disease. All other indications for initial anti-tumor treatment strategy for breast cancer are nationally covered.

* Melanoma: Nationally non-covered for initial staging of regional lymph nodes. All other indications for initial anti-tumor treatment strategy for melanoma are nationally covered.

D. Other

N/A

100-03, 220.6.19

Positron Emission Tomography NaF-18 (NaF-18 PET) to Identify Bone Metastasis of Cancer (Effective February 26, 2010)

(Rev.119, Issued: 03-26-10, Effective: 02-26-10, Implementation: 07-06-10)

A. General

Positron Emission Tomography (PET) is a non-invasive, diagnostic imaging procedure that assesses the level of metabolic activity and perfusion in various organ systems of the body. A positron camera (tomograph) is used to produce cross-sectional tomographic images, which are obtained from positron-emitting radioactive tracer substances (radiopharmaceuticals) such as F-18 sodium fluoride. NaF-18 PET has been recognized as an excellent technique for imaging areas of altered osteogenic activity in bone. The clinical value of detecting and assessing the initial extent of metastatic cancer in bone is attested by a number of professional guidelines for oncology. Imaging to detect bone metastases is also recommended when a patient, following completion of initial treatment, is symptomatic with bone pain suspicious for metastases from a known primary tumor.

B. Nationally Covered Indications

Effective February 26, 2010, the Centers for Medicare & Medicaid Services (CMS) will cover NaF-18 PET imaging when the beneficiary's treating physician determines that the NaF-18 PET study is needed to inform to inform the initial antitumor treatment strategy or to guide subsequent antitumor treatment strategy after the completion of initial treatment, and when the beneficiary is enrolled in, and the NaF-18 PET provider is participating in, the following type of prospective clinical study:

> A NaF-18 PET clinical study that is designed to collect additional information at the time of the scan to assist in initial antitumor treatment planning or to guide subsequent treatment strategy by the identification, location and quantification of bone metastases in beneficiaries in whom bone metastases are strongly suspected based on clinical symptoms or the results of other diagnostic studies. Qualifying clinical studies must ensure that specific hypotheses are addressed; appropriate data elements are collected; hospitals and providers are qualified to provide the PET scan and interpret the results; participating hospitals and

providers accurately report data on all enrolled patients not included in other qualifying trials through adequate auditing mechanisms; and all patient confidentiality, privacy, and other Federal laws must be followed.

The clinical studies for which Medicare will provide coverage must answer one or more of the following questions:

Prospectively, in Medicare beneficiaries whose treating physician determines that the NaF-18 PET study results are needed to inform the initial antitumor treatment strategy or to guide subsequent antitumor treatment strategy after the completion of initial treatment, does the addition of NaF-18 PET imaging lead to:

- A change in patient management to more appropriate palliative care; or
- A change in patient management to more appropriate curative care; or
- Improved quality of life; or Improved survival?

The study must adhere to the following standards of scientific integrity and relevance to the Medicare population:

a. The principal purpose of the research study is to test whether a particular intervention potentially improves the participants' health outcomes.
b. The research study is well-supported by available scientific and medical information or it is intended to clarify or establish the health outcomes of interventions already in common clinical use.
c. The research study does not unjustifiably duplicate existing studies.
d. The research study design is appropriate to answer the research question being asked in the study.
e. The research study is sponsored by an organization or individual capable of executing the proposed study successfully.
f. The research study is in compliance with all applicable Federal regulations concerning the protection of human subjects found in the Code of Federal Regulations (CFR) at 45 CFR Part 46. If a study is regulated by the Food and Drug Administration (FDA), it also must be in compliance with 21 CFR Parts 50 and 56.
g. All aspects of the research study are conducted according to the appropriate standards of scientific integrity.
h. The research study has a written protocol that clearly addresses, or incorporates by reference, the Medicare standards.
i. The clinical research study is not designed to exclusively test toxicity or disease pathophysiology in healthy individuals. Trials of all medical technologies measuring therapeutic outcomes as one of the objectives meet this standard only if the disease or condition being studied is life-threatening as defined in 21 CFR Sec.312.81(a) and the patient has no other viable treatment options.
j. The clinical research study is registered on the www.ClinicalTrials.gov Web site by the principal sponsor/investigator prior to the enrollment of the first study subject.
k. The research study protocol specifies the method and timing of public release of all pre-specified outcomes to be measured including release of outcomes if outcomes are negative or study is terminated early. The results must be made public within 24 months of the end of data collection. If a report is planned to be published in a peer-reviewed journal, then that initial release may be an abstract that meets the requirements of the International Committee of Medical Journal Editors. However, a full report of the outcomes must be made public no later than three (3) years after the end of data collection.
l. The research study protocol must explicitly discuss subpopulations affected by the treatment under investigation, particularly traditionally underrepresented groups in clinical studies, how the inclusion and exclusion criteria affect enrollment of these populations, and a plan for the retention and reporting of said populations on the trial. If the inclusion and exclusion criteria are expected to have a negative effect on the recruitment or retention of underrepresented populations, the protocol must discuss why these criteria are necessary.
m. The research study protocol explicitly discusses how the results are or are not expected to be generalizable to the Medicare population to infer whether Medicare patients may benefit from the intervention. Separate discussions in the protocol may be necessary for populations eligible for Medicare due to age, disability or Medicaid eligibility.

Consistent with section 1142 of the Social Security Act (the Act), the Agency for Healthcare Research and Quality (AHRQ) supports clinical research studies that the Centers for Medicare and Medicaid Services (CMS) determines meet the above-listed standards and address the above-listed research questions.

C. Nationally Non-Covered Indications

Effective February 26, 2010, CMS determines that the evidence is not sufficient to determine that the results of NaF-18 PET imaging to identify bone metastases improve health outcomes of beneficiaries with cancer and is not reasonable and necessary under Sec.1862(a)(1)(A) of the Act unless it is to inform initial antitumor treatment strategy or to guide subsequent antitumor treatment strategy after completion of initial treatment, and then only under CED. All other uses and clinical indications of NaF-18 PET are nationally non-covered.

D. Other

The only radiopharmaceutical diagnostic imaging agents covered by Medicare for PET cancer imaging are 2-[F-18] Fluoro-D-Glucose (FDG) and NaF-18 (sodium fluoride-18). All other PET radiopharmaceutical diagnostic imaging agents are non-covered for this indication.

(This NCD was last reviewed in February 2010.)

100-03, 220.13

NCD for Percutaneous Image-Guided Breast Biopsy (220.13)

(Rev. 173, Issued: 09-04-14, Effective: Upon Implementation: of ICD–10)

Percutaneous image-guided breast biopsy is a method of obtaining a breast biopsy through a percutaneous incision by employing image guidance systems. Image guidance systems may be either ultrasound or stereotactic.

The Breast Imaging Reporting and Data System (or BIRADS system) employed by the American College of Radiology provides a standardized lexicon with which radiologists may report their interpretation of a mammogram. The BIRADS grading of mammograms is as follows: Grade I-Negative, Grade II-Benign finding, Grade III-Probably benign, Grade IV-Suspicious abnormality, and Grade V-Highly suggestive of malignant neoplasm.

A. Non-Palpable Breast Lesions

Effective January 1, 2003, Medicare covers percutaneous image-guided breast biopsy using stereotactic or ultrasound imaging for a radiographic abnormality that is non-palpable and is graded as a BIRADS III, IV, or V.

B. Palpable Breast Lesions

Effective January 1, 2003, Medicare covers percutaneous image guided breast biopsy using stereotactic or ultrasound imaging for palpable lesions that are difficult to biopsy using palpation alone. Medicare Administrative Contractors have the discretion to decide what types of palpable lesions are difficult to biopsy using palpation.

100-03, 230.1

NCD for Treatment of Kidney Stones (230.1)

(Rev. 1, 10-03-03)

In addition to the traditional surgical/endoscopic techniques for the treatment of kidney stones, the following lithotripsy techniques are also covered for services rendered on or after March I5, I985.

Extracorporeal Shock Wave Lithotripsy.--Extracorporeal Shock Wave Lithotripsy (ESWL) is a non-invasive method of treating kidney stones using a device called a lithotriptor. The lithotriptor uses shock waves generated outside of the body to break up upper urinary tract stones. It focuses the shock waves specifically on stones under X-ray visualization, pulverizing them by repeated shocks. ESWL is covered under Medicare for use in the treatment of upper urinary tract kidney stones.

Percutaneous Lithotripsy.--Percutaneous lithotripsy (or nephrolithotomy) is an invasive method of treating kidney stones by using ultrasound, electrohydraulic or mechanical lithotripsy. A probe is inserted through an incision in the skin directly over the kidney and applied to the stone. A form of lithotripsy is then used to fragment the stone. Mechanical or electrohydraulic lithotripsy may be used as an alternative or adjunct to ultrasonic lithotripsy. Percutaneous lithotripsy of kidney stones by ultrasound or by the related techniques of electrohydraulic or mechanical lithotripsy is covered under Medicare.

The following is covered for services rendered on or after January 16, 1988.

Transurethral Ureteroscopic Lithotripsy.--Transurethral ureteroscopic lithotripsy is a method of fragmenting and removing ureteral and renal stones through a cystoscope. The cystoscope is inserted through the urethra into the bladder. Catheters are passed through the scope into the opening where the ureters enter the bladder. Instruments passed through this opening into the ureters are used to manipulate and ultimately disintegrate stones, using either mechanical crushing, transcystoscopic electrohydraulic shock waves, ultrasound or laser. Transurethral ureteroscopic lithotripsy for the treatment of urinary tract stones of the kidney or ureter is covered under Medicare.

100-03, 230.3

NCD for Sterilization (230.3)

(Rev. 173, Issued: 09-04-14, Effective: Upon Implementation: of ICD-10, Implementation: Upon Implementation of ICD-10)

A. Nationally Covered Conditions

Payment may be made only where sterilization is a necessary part of the treatment of an illness or injury, e.g., removal of a uterus because of a tumor, removal of diseased ovaries.

Sterilization of a mentally challenged beneficiary is covered if it is a necessary part of the treatment of an illness or injury (bilateral oophorectomy or bilateral orchidectomy in a case of cancer of the prostate). The Medicare Administrative Contractor denies claims when the pathological evidence of the necessity to perform any such procedures to treat an illness or injury is absent; and

Monitor such surgeries closely and obtain the information needed to determine whether in fact the surgery was performed as a means of treating an illness or injury or only to achieve sterilization.

B. Nationally Non-Covered Conditions

- Elective hysterectomy, tubal ligation, and vasectomy, if the primary indication for these procedures is sterilization;

- A sterilization that is performed because a physician believes another pregnancy would endanger the overall general health of the woman is not considered to be reasonable and necessary for the diagnosis or treatment of illness or injury within the meaning of §1862(a)(1) of the Social Security Act. The same conclusion would apply where the sterilization is performed only as a measure to prevent the possible development of, or effect on, a mental condition should the individual become pregnant; and sterilization of a mentally retarded person where the purpose is to prevent conception, rather than the treatment of an illness or injury.

100-03, 230.4

NCD for Diagnosis and Treatment of Impotence (230.4)

(Rev. 1, 10-03-03)

Program payment may be made for diagnosis and treatment of sexual impotence. Impotence is a failure of a body part for which the diagnosis, and frequently the treatment, require medical expertise. Depending on the cause of the condition, treatment may be surgical; e.g., implantation of a penile prosthesis, or nonsurgical; e.g., medical or psychotherapeutic treatment. Since causes and, therefore, appropriate treatment vary, if abuse is suspected it may be necessary to request documentation of appropriateness in individual cases. If treatment is furnished to patients (other than hospital inpatients) in connection with a mental condition, apply the psychiatric service limitation described in the Medicare General Information, Eligibility, and Entitlement Manual, Chapter 3.

100-03, 230.10

NCD for Incontinence Control Devices (230.10)

(Rev. 1, 10-03-03)

A - Mechanical/Hydraulic Incontinence Control Devices

Mechanical/hydraulic incontinence control devices are accepted as safe and effective in the management of urinary incontinence in patients with permanent anatomic and neurologic dysfunctions of the bladder. This class of devices achieves control of urination by compression of the urethra. The materials used and the success rate may vary somewhat from device to device. Such a device is covered when its use is reasonable and necessary for the individual patient.

B - Collagen Implant

A collagen implant, which is injected into the submucosal tissues of the urethra and/or the bladder neck and into tissues adjacent to the urethra, is a prosthetic device used in the treatment of stress urinary incontinence resulting from intrinsic sphincter deficiency (ISD). ISD is a cause of stress urinary incontinence in which the urethral sphincter is unable to contract and generate sufficient resistance in the bladder, especially during stress maneuvers.

Prior to collagen implant therapy, a skin test for collagen sensitivity must be administered and evaluated over a 4 week period.

In male patients, the evaluation must include a complete history and physical examination and a simple cystometrogram to determine that the bladder fills and stores properly. The patient then is asked to stand upright with a full bladder and to cough or otherwise exert abdominal pressure on his bladder. If the patient leaks, the diagnosis of ISD is established.

In female patients, the evaluation must include a complete history and physical examination (including a pelvic exam) and a simple cystometrogram to rule out abnormalities of bladder compliance and abnormalities of urethral support. Following that determination, an abdominal leak point pressure (ALLP) test is performed. Leak point pressure, stated in cm H2O, is defined as the intra-abdominal pressure at which leakage occurs from the bladder (around a catheter) when the bladder has been filled with a minimum of 150 cc fluid. If the patient has an ALLP of less than 100 cm H_2O, the diagnosis of ISD is established.

To use a collagen implant, physicians must have urology training in the use of a cystoscope and must complete a collagen implant training program.

Coverage of a collagen implant, and the procedure to inject it, is limited to the following types of patients with stress urinary incontinence due to ISD:

- Male or female patients with congenital sphincter weakness secondary to conditions such as myelomeningocele or epispadias;
- Male or female patients with acquired sphincter weakness secondary to spinal cord lesions;
- Male patients following trauma, including prostatectomy and/or radiation; and
- Female patients without urethral hypermobility and with abdominal leak point pressures of 100 cm H2O or less.

Patients whose incontinence does not improve with 5 injection procedures (5 separate treatment sessions) are considered treatment failures, and no further treatment of urinary incontinence by collagen implant is covered. Patients who have a reoccurrence of incontinence following successful treatment with collagen implants in the past (e.g., 6-12 months previously) may benefit from additional treatment sessions. Coverage of additional sessions may be allowed but must be supported by medical justification.

100-03, 260.1

Adult Liver Transplantation

(Rev.146, Issued: 08-03-12, Effective: 06-21-12, Implementation; 09-04-12)

A. General

Liver transplantation, which is in situ replacement of a patient's liver with a donor liver, in certain circumstances, may be an accepted treatment for patients with end-stage liver disease due to a variety of causes. The procedure is used in selected patients as a treatment for malignancies, including primary liver tumors and certain metastatic tumors, which are typically rare but lethal with very limited treatment options. It has also been used in the treatment of patients with extrahepatic perihilar malignancies. Examples of malignancies include extrahepatic unresectable cholangiocarcinoma (CCA), liver metastases due to a neuroendocrine tumor (NET), and, hemangioendothelioma (HAE). Despite potential short- and long-term complications, transplantation may offer the only chance of cure for selected patients while providing meaningful palliation for some others.

B. Nationally Covered Indications

Effective July 15, 1996, adult liver transplantation when performed on beneficiaries with end- stage liver disease other than hepatitis B or malignancies is covered under Medicare when performed in a facility which is approved by the Centers for Medicare & Medicaid Services (CMS) as meeting institutional coverage criteria.

Effective December 10, 1999, adult liver transplantation when performed on beneficiaries with end-stage liver disease other than malignancies is covered under Medicare when performed in a facility which is approved by CMS as meeting institutional coverage criteria.

Effective September 1, 2001, Medicare covers adult liver transplantation for hepatocellular carcinoma when the following conditions are met:

- The patient is not a candidate for subtotal liver resection;
- The patient's tumor(s) is less than or equal to 5 cm in diameter;
- There is no macrovascular involvement;
- There is no identifiable extrahepatic spread of tumor to surrounding lymph nodes, lungs, abdominal organs or bone; and,
- The transplant is furnished in a facility that is approved by CMS as meeting institutional coverage criteria for liver transplants (see 65 FR 15006).

Effective June 21, 2012, Medicare Adminstrative Contractors acting within their respective jurisdictions may determine coverage of adult liver transplantation for the following malignancies: (1) extrahepatic unresectable cholangiocarcinoma (CCA); (2) liver metastases due to a neuroendocrine tumor (NET); and, (3) hemangioendothelioma (HAE).

1. Follow-Up Care
   Follow-up care or re-transplantation required as a result of a covered liver transplant is covered, provided such services are otherwise reasonable and necessary. Follow-up care is also covered for patients who have been discharged from a hospital after receiving non-covered liver transplant. Coverage for follow-up care is for items and services that are reasonable and necessary as determined by Medicare guidelines.
2. Immunosuppressive Drugs
   See the Medicare Benefit Policy Manual, Chapter 15, "Covered Medical and Other Health Services," §50.5.1 and the Medicare Claims Processing Manual, Chapter 17, "Drugs and Biologicals," §80.3.

C. Nationally Non-Covered Indications

Adult liver transplantation for other malignancies remains excluded from coverage.

D. Other

Coverage of adult liver transplantation is effective as of the date of the facility's approval, but for applications received before July 13, 1991, can be effective as early as March 8, 1990. (See 56 FR 15006 dated April 12, 1991.)

(This NCD last reviewed June 2012.)

100-03, 260.2

NCD for Pediatric Liver Transplantation (260.2)

(Rev. 1, 10-03-03)

Liver transplantation is covered for children (under age 18) with extrahepatic biliary atresia or any other form of end stage liver disease, except that coverage is not provided for children with a malignancy extending beyond the margins of the liver or those with persistent viremia.

Liver transplantation is covered for Medicare beneficiaries when performed in a pediatric hospital that performs pediatric liver transplants if the hospital submits an application which CMS approves documenting that:

- The hospital's pediatric liver transplant program is operated jointly by the hospital and another facility that has been found by CMS to meet the institutional coverage criteria in the "Federal Register" notice of April 12, 1991;
- The unified program shares the same transplant surgeons and quality assurance program (including oversight committee, patient protocol, and patient selection criteria); and
- The hospital is able to provide the specialized facilities, services, and personnel that are required by pediatric liver transplant patients.

100-03, 260.3

NCD for Pancreas Transplants (260.3)

(Rev. 56, Issued: 05-19-06, Effective: 04-26-06, Implementation: 07-03-06)

A. General

Pancreas transplantation is performed to induce an insulin-independent, euglycemic state in diabetic patients. The procedure is generally limited to those patients with severe secondary complications of diabetes, including kidney failure. However, pancreas transplantation is sometimes performed on patients with labile diabetes and hypoglycemic unawareness.

B. Nationally Covered Indications

Effective for services performed on or after July 1, 1999, whole organ pancreas transplantation is nationally covered by Medicare when performed simultaneous with or after a kidney transplant. If the pancreas transplant occurs after the kidney transplant, immunosuppressive therapy begins with the date of discharge from the inpatient stay for the pancreas transplant.

Effective for services performed on or after April 26, 2006, pancreas transplants alone (PA) are reasonable and necessary for Medicare beneficiaries in the following limited circumstances:

1. PA will be limited to those facilities that are Medicare-approved for kidney transplantation. (Approved centers can be found at http://www.cms.hhs.gov/ESRDGeneralInformation/02_Data.asp#TopOfPage
2. Patients must have a diagnosis of type I diabetes:
   - — Patient with diabetes must be beta cell autoantibody positive; or
   - — Patient must demonstrate insulinopenia defined as a fasting C-peptide level that is less than or equal to 110% of the lower limit of normal of the laboratory's measurement method. Fasting C-peptide levels will only be considered valid with a concurrently obtained fasting glucose <225 mg/dL;
3. Patients must have a history of medically-uncontrollable labile (brittle) insulin-dependent diabetes mellitus with documented recurrent, severe, acutely life-threatening metabolic complications that require hospitalization. Aforementioned complications include frequent hypoglycemia unawareness or recurring severe ketoacidosis, or recurring severe hypoglycemic attacks;
4. Patients must have been optimally and intensively managed by an endocrinologist for at least 12 months with the most medically-recognized advanced insulin formulations and delivery systems;
5. Patients must have the emotional and mental capacity to understand the significant risks associated with surgery and to effectively manage the lifelong need for immunosuppression; and,
6. Patients must otherwise be a suitable candidate for transplantation.

C. Nationally Non-Covered Indications

The following procedure is not considered reasonable and necessary within the meaning of section 1862(a)(1)(A) of the Social Security Act:

1. Transplantation of partial pancreatic tissue or islet cells (except in the context of a clinical trial (see section 260.3.1 of the National Coverage Determinations Manual).

D. Other

Not applicable.

(This NCD last reviewed April 2006.)

100-03, 260.5

NCD for Intestinal and Multi-Visceral Transplantation (260.5)

(Rev. 58, Issued: 05-26-06; Effective: 05-11-06; Implementation: 06-26-06)

A. General

Medicare covers intestinal and multi-visceral transplantation for the purpose of restoring intestinal function in patients with irreversible intestinal failure. Intestinal failure is defined as the loss of absorptive capacity of the small bowel secondary to severe primary gastrointestinal disease or surgically induced short bowel syndrome. It may be associated with both mortality and profound morbidity. Multi-visceral transplantation includes organs in the digestive system (stomach, duodenum, pancreas, liver and intestine).

The evidence supports the fact that aged patients generally do not survive as well as younger patients receiving intestinal transplantation. Nonetheless, some older patients who are free from other contraindications have received the procedure and are progressing well, as evidenced by the United Network for Organ Sharing (UNOS) data. Thus, it is not appropriate to include specific exclusions from coverage, such as an age limitation, in the national coverage policy.

B. Nationally Covered Indications

Effective for services performed on or after April 1, 2001, this procedure is covered only when performed for patients who have failed total parenteral nutrition (TPN) and only when performed in centers that meet approval criteria.

1. Failed TPN

   The TPN delivers nutrients intravenously, avoiding the need for absorption through the small bowel. TPN failure includes the following:

   - — Impending or overt liver failure due to TPN induced liver injury. The clinical manifestations include elevated serum bilirubin and/or liver enzymes, splenomegaly, thrombocytopenia, gastroesophageal varices, coagulopathy, stomal bleeding or hepatic fibrosis/cirrhosis.
   - — Thrombosis of the major central venous channels; jugular, subclavian, and femoral veins. Thrombosis of two or more of these vessels is considered a life threatening complication and failure of TPN therapy. The sequelae of central venous thrombosis are lack of access for TPN infusion, fatal sepsis due to infected thrombi, pulmonary embolism, Superior Vena Cava syndrome, or chronic venous insufficiency.
   - — Frequent line infection and sepsis. The development of two or more episodes of systemic sepsis secondary to line infection per year that requires hospitalization indicates failure of TPN therapy. A single episode of line related fungemia, septic shock and/or Acute Respiratory Distress Syndrome are considered indicators of TPN failure.
   - — Frequent episodes of severe dehydration despite intravenous fluid supplement in addition to TPN. Under certain medical conditions such as secretory diarrhea and non-constructable gastrointestinal tract, the loss of the gastrointestinal and pancreatobiliary secretions exceeds the maximum intravenous infusion rates that can be tolerated by the cardiopulmonary system. Frequent episodes of dehydration are deleterious to all body organs particularly kidneys and the central nervous system with the development of multiple kidney stones, renal failure, and permanent brain damage.

2. Approved Transplant Facilities

   Intestinal transplantation is covered by Medicare if performed in an approved facility. The criteria for approval of centers will be based on a volume of 10 intestinal transplants per year with a 1-year actuarial survival of 65 percent using the Kaplan-Meier technique.

C. Nationally Non-covered Indications

All other indications remain non-covered.

D. Other

NA.

(This NCD last reviewed May 2006.)

100-03, 260.9

NCD for Heart Transplants (260.9)

(Rev. 95; Issued: 09-10-08; Effective Date: 05-01-08; Implementation Date: 12-01-08)

A. General

Cardiac transplantation is covered under Medicare when performed in a facility which is approved by Medicare as meeting institutional coverage criteria. (See CMS Ruling 87-1.)

B. Exceptions

In certain limited cases, exceptions to the criteria may be warranted if there is justification and if the facility ensures our objectives of safety and efficacy. Under no circumstances will exceptions be made for facilities whose transplant programs have been in existence for less than two years, and applications from consortia will not be approved.

Although consortium arrangements will not be approved for payment of Medicare heart transplants, consideration will be given to applications from heart transplant facilities that consist of more than one hospital where all of the following conditions exist:

- The hospitals are under the common control or have a formal affiliation arrangement with each other under the auspices of an organization such as a university or a legally-constituted medical research institute; and
- The hospitals share resources by routinely using the same personnel or services in their transplant programs. The sharing of resources must be supported by the submission of operative notes or other information that documents the routine use of the same personnel and services in all of the individual hospitals. At a minimum, shared resources means:
- The individual members of the transplant team, consisting of the cardiac transplant surgeons, cardiologists and pathologists, must practice in all the hospitals and it can be documented that they otherwise function as members of the transplant team;
- The same organ procurement organization, immunology, and tissue-typing services must be used by all the hospitals;
- The hospitals submit, in the manner required (Kaplan-Meier method) their individual and pooled experience and survival data; and
- The hospitals otherwise meet the remaining Medicare criteria for heart transplant facilities; that is, the criteria regarding patient selection, patient management, program commitment, etc.

C. Pediatric Hospitals

Cardiac transplantation is covered for Medicare beneficiaries when performed in a pediatric hospital that performs pediatric heart transplants if the hospital submits an application which CMS approves as documenting that:

- The hospital's pediatric heart transplant program is operated jointly by the hospital and another facility that has been found by CMS to meet the institutional coverage criteria in CMS Ruling 87-1;

- The unified program shares the same transplant surgeons and quality assurance program (including oversight committee, patient protocol, and patient selection criteria); and
- The hospital is able to provide the specialized facilities, services, and personnel that are required by pediatric heart transplant patients.

D. Follow-Up Care
Follow-up care required as a result of a covered heart transplant is covered, provided such services are otherwise reasonable and necessary. Follow-up care is also covered for patients who have been discharged from a hospital after receiving a noncovered heart transplant. Coverage for follow-up care would be for items and services that are reasonable and necessary, as determined by Medicare guidelines. (See the Medicare Benefit Policy Manual, Chapter 16, "General Exclusions from Coverage," Sec.180.)

E. Immunosuppressive Drugs
See the Medicare Claims Processing Manual, Chapter 17, "Drugs and Biologicals," Sec.80.3.1, and Chapter 8, "Outpatient ESRD Hospital, Independent Facility, and Physician/Supplier Claims," Sec.120.1.

F. Artificial Hearts
Medicare does not cover the use of artificial hearts as a permanent replacement for a human heart or as a temporary life-support system until a human heart becomes available for transplant (often referred to as a "bridge to transplant"). Medicare does cover a ventricular assist device (VAD) when used in conjunction with specific criteria listed in Sec.20.9 of the NCD Manual.

100-03, 270.3

NCD for Blood-Derived Products for Chronic Non-Healing Wounds (270.3)

(Rev. 154, Issued: 06-10-13, Effective: 08-02-12, Implementation: 07-01-13)

A. General
Wound healing is a dynamic, interactive process that involves multiple cells and proteins. There are three progressive stages of normal wound healing, and the typical wound healing duration is about 4 weeks. While cutaneous wounds are a disruption of the normal, anatomic structure and function of the skin, subcutaneous wounds involve tissue below the skin's surface. Wounds are categorized as either acute, in where the normal wound healing stages are not yet completed but it is presumed they will be, resulting in orderly and timely wound repair, or chronic, in where a wound has failed to progress through the normal wound healing stages and repair itself within a sufficient time period.

Platelet-rich plasma (PRP) is produced in an autologous or homologous manner. Autologous PRP is comprised of blood from the patient who will ultimately receive the PRP. Alternatively, homologous PRP is derived from blood from multiple donors.

Blood is donated by the patient and centrifuged to produce an autologous gel for treatment of chronic, non-healing cutaneous wounds that persists for 30 days or longer and fail to properly complete the healing process. Autologous blood derived products for chronic, non-healing wounds includes both: (1) platelet derived growth factor (PDGF) products (such as Procuren), and (2) PRP (such as AutoloGel).

The PRP is different from previous products in that it contains whole cells including white cells, red cells, plasma, platelets, fibrinogen, stem cells, macrophages, and fibroblasts.

The PRP is used by physicians in clinical settings in treating chronic, non-healing wounds, open, cutaneous wounds, soft tissue, and bone. Alternatively, PDGF does not contain cells and was previously marketed as a product to be used by patients at home.

B. Nationally Covered Indications
Effective August 2, 2012, upon reconsideration, The Centers for Medicare and Medicaid Services (CMS) has determined that platelet-rich plasma (PRP) – an autologous blood-derived product, will be covered only for the treatment of chronic non-healing diabetic, venous and/or pressure wounds and only when the following conditions are met:

The patient is enrolled in a clinical trial that addresses the following questions using validated and reliable methods of evaluation. Clinical study applications for coverage pursuant to this National coverage Determination (NCD) must be received by August 2, 2014.

The clinical research study must meet the requirements specified below to assess the effect of PRP for the treatment of chronic non-healing diabetic, venous and/or pressure wounds. The clinical study must address:

Prospectively, do Medicare beneficiaries that have chronic non-healing diabetic, venous and/or pressure wounds who receive well-defined optimal usual care along with PRP therapy, experience clinically significant health outcomes compared to patients who receive well-defined optimal usual care for chronic non-healing diabetic, venous and/or pressure wounds as indicated by addressing at least one of the following:

a. Complete wound healing?
b. Ability to return to previous function and resumption of normal activities?
c. Reduction of wound size or healing trajectory which results in the patient's ability to return to previous function and resumption of normal activities?

The required clinical trial of PRP must adhere to the following standards of scientific integrity and relevance to the Medicare population:

a. The principal purpose of the CLINICAL STUDY is to test whether PRP improves the participants' health outcomes.
b. The CLINICAL STUDY is well supported by available scientific and medical information or it is intended to clarify or establish the health outcomes of interventions already in common clinical use.
c. The CLINICAL STUDY does not unjustifiably duplicate existing studies.
d. The CLINICAL STUDY design is appropriate to answer the research question being asked in the study.
e. The CLINICAL STUDY is sponsored by an organization or individual capable of executing the proposed study successfully.
f. The CLINICAL STUDY is in compliance with all applicable Federal regulations concerning the protection of human subjects found at 45 CFR Part 46.
g. All aspects of the CLINICAL STUDY are conducted according to appropriate standards of scientific integrity set by the International Committee of Medical Journal Editors (http://www.icmje.org).
h. The CLINICAL STUDY has a written protocol that clearly addresses, or incorporates by reference, the standards listed here as Medicare requirements for coverage with evidence development (CED).
i. The CLINICAL STUDY is not designed to exclusively test toxicity or disease pathophysiology in healthy individuals. Trials of all medical technologies measuring therapeutic outcomes as one of the objectives meet this standard only if the disease or condition being studied is life threatening as defined in 21 CFR §312.81(a) and the patient has no other viable treatment options.
j. The CLINICAL STUDY is registered on the ClinicalTrials.gov website by the principal sponsor/investigator prior to the enrollment of the first study subject.
k. The CLINICAL STUDY protocol specifies the method and timing of public release of all pre-specified outcomes to be measured including release of outcomes if outcomes are negative or study is terminated early. The results must be made public within 24 months of the end of data collection. If a report is planned to be published in a peer reviewed journal, then that initial release may be an abstract that meets the requirements of the International Committee of Medical Journal Editors (http://www.icmje.org). However a full report of the outcomes must be made public no later than three (3) years after the end of data collection.
l. The CLINICAL STUDY protocol must explicitly discuss subpopulations affected by the treatment under investigation, particularly traditionally underrepresented groups in clinical studies, how the inclusion and exclusion criteria effect enrollment of these populations, and a plan for the retention and reporting of said populations on the trial. If the inclusion and exclusion criteria are expected to have a negative effect on the recruitment or retention of underrepresented populations, the protocol must discuss why these criteria are necessary.
m. The CLINICAL STUDY protocol explicitly discusses how the results are or are not expected to be generalizable to the Medicare population to infer whether Medicare patients may benefit from the intervention. Separate discussions in the protocol may be necessary for populations eligible for Medicare due to age, disability or Medicaid eligibility. Consistent with §1142 of the Social Security Act (the Act), the Agency for Healthcare Research and Quality (AHRQ) supports clinical research studies that CMS determines meet the above-listed standards and address the above-listed research questions.

Any clinical study undertaken pursuant to this NCD must be approved no later than August 2, 2014. If there are no approved clinical studies on or before August 2, 2014, this CED will expire. Any clinical study approved will adhere to the timeframe designated in the approved clinical study protocol.

C. Nationally Non-Covered Indications
1. Effective December 28, 1992, the Centers for Medicare & Medicaid Services (CMS) issued a national non-coverage determination for platelet-derived wound-healing formulas intended to treat patients with chronic, non-healing wounds. This decision was based on a lack of sufficient published data to determine safety and efficacy, and a public health service technology assessment.

100-04, 3, 90.1

Kidney Transplant - General

(Rev.1341, Issued: 09-21-07, Effective: 06-28-07, Implementation: 10-22-07)

A3-3612, HO-E414

A major treatment for patients with ESRD is kidney transplantation. This involves removing a kidney, usually from a living relative of the patient or from an unrelated person who has died, and surgically placing the kidney into the patient. After the beneficiary receives a kidney transplant, Medicare pays the transplant hospital for the transplant and appropriate standard acquisition charges. Special provisions apply to payment. For the list of approved Medicare certified transplant facilities, refer to the following Web site:
http://www.cms.hhs.gov/CertificationandComplianc/20_Transplant.asp#TopOfPage

A transplant hospital may acquire cadaver kidneys by:

- Excising kidneys from cadavers in its own hospital; and

- Arrangements with a freestanding organ procurement organization (OPO) that provides cadaver kidneys to any transplant hospital or by a hospital based OPO.

A transplant hospital that is also a certified organ procurement organization may acquire cadaver kidneys by:

- Having its organ procurement team excise kidneys from cadavers in other hospitals;
- Arrangements with participating community hospitals, whether they excise kidneys on a regular or irregular basis; and
- Arrangements with an organ procurement organization that services the transplant hospital as a member of a network.

When the transplant hospital also excises the cadaver kidney, the cost of the procedure is included in its kidney acquisition costs and is considered in arriving at its standard cadaver kidney acquisition charge. When the transplant hospital excises a kidney to provide another hospital, it may use its standard cadaver kidney acquisition charge or its standard detailed departmental charges to bill that hospital.

When the excising hospital is not a transplant hospital, it bills its customary charges for services used in excising the cadaver kidney to the transplant hospital or organ procurement agency.

If the transplanting hospital's organ procurement team excises the cadaver kidney at another hospital, the cost of operating such a team is included in the transplanting hospital's kidney acquisition costs, along with the reasonable charges billed by the other hospital of its services.

100-04, 3, 90.1.1

The Standard Kidney Acquisition Charge

(Rev. 3030, Issued: 08-22-14, Effective: Upon Implementation of ICD-10)

There are two basic standard charges that must be developed by transplant hospitals from costs expected to be incurred in the acquisition of kidneys:

- The standard charge for acquiring a live donor kidney; and
- The standard charge for acquiring a cadaver kidney.

The standard charge is not a charge representing the acquisition cost of a specific kidney; rather, it is a charge that reflects the average cost associated with each type of kidney acquisition.

When the transplant hospital bills the program for the transplant, it shows its standard kidney acquisition charge on revenue code 081X. Kidney acquisition charges are not considered for the IPPS outlier calculation.

Acquisition services are billed from the excising hospital to the transplant hospital. A billing form is not submitted from the excising hospital to the FI. The transplant hospital keeps an itemized statement that identifies the services furnished, the charges, the person receiving the service (donor/recipient), and whether this is a potential transplant donor or recipient. These charges are reflected in the transplant hospital's kidney acquisition costcenter and are used in determining the hospital's standard charge for acquiring a live donor's kidney or a cadaver's kidney. The standard charge is not a charge representing the acquisition cost of a specific kidney. Rather, it is a charge that reflects the average cost associated with each type of kidney acquisition. Also, it is an all-inclusive charge for all services required in acquisition of a kidney, i.e., tissue typing, post-operative evaluation.

A. Billing For Blood And Tissue Typing of the Transplant Recipient Whether or Not Medicare Entitlement Is Established

Tissue typing and pre-transplant evaluation can be reflected only through the kidney acquisition charge of the hospital where the transplant will take place. The transplant hospital includes in its kidney acquisition cost center the reasonable charges it pays to the independent laboratory or other hospital which typed the potential transplant recipient, either before or after his entitlement. It also includes reasonable charges paid for physician tissue typing services, applicable to live donors and recipients (during the preentitlement period and after entitlement, but prior to hospital admission for transplantation).

B. Billing for Blood and Tissue Typing and Other Pre-Transplant Evaluation of Live Donors

The entitlement date of the beneficiary who will receive the transplant is not a consideration in reimbursing for the services to donors, since no bill is submitted directly to Medicare. All charges for services to donors prior to admission into the hospital for excision are "billed" indirectly to Medicare through the live donor acquisition charge of transplanting hospitals.

C. Billing Donor And Recipient Pre-Transplant Services (Performed by Transplant Hospitals or Other Providers) to the Kidney Acquisition Cost Center

The transplant hospital prepares an itemized statement of the services rendered for submittal to its cost accounting department. Regular Medicare billing forms are not necessary for this purpose, since no bills are submitted to the A/B MAC (A) at this point.

The itemized statement should contain information that identifies the person receiving the service (donor/recipient), the health care insurance number, the service rendered and the charge for the service, as well as a statement as to whether this is a potential transplant donor or recipient. If it is a potential donor, the provider must identify the prospective recipient.

EXAMPLE:

Mary Jones
Health care insurance number
200 Adams St.
Anywhere, MS

Transplant donor evaluation services for recipient:

John Jones
Health care insurance number
200 Adams St.
Anywhere, MS

Services performed in a hospital other than the potential transplant hospital or by an independent laboratory are billed by that facility to the potential transplant hospital. This holds true regardless of where in the United States the service is performed. For example, if the donor services are performed in a Florida hospital and the transplant is to take place in a California hospital, the Florida hospital bills the California hospital (as described in above). The Florida hospital is paid by the California hospital, which recoups the monies through the kidney acquisition cost center.

D. Billing for Cadaveric Donor Services

Normally, various tests are performed to determine the type and suitability of a cadaver kidney. Such tests may be performed by the excising hospital (which may also be a transplant hospital) or an independent laboratory. When the excising-only hospital performs the tests, it includes the related charges on its bill to the transplant hospital or to the organ procurement agency. When the tests are performed by the transplant hospital, it uses the related costs in establishing the standard charge for acquiring the cadaver kidney. The transplant hospital includes the costs and charges in the appropriate departments for final cost settlement purposes. When the tests are performed by an independent laboratory for the excising-only hospital or the transplant hospital, the laboratory bills the hospital that engages its services or the organ procurement agency. The excising-only hospital includes such charges in its charges to the transplant hospital, which then includes the charges in developing its standard charge for acquiring the cadaver kidney. It is the transplant hospitals' responsibility to assure that the independent laboratory does not bill both hospitals. The cost of these services cannot be billed directly to the program, since such tests and other procedures performed on a cadaver are not identifiable to a specific patient.

E. Billing For Physicians' Services Prior to Transplantation

Physicians' services applicable to kidney excisions involving live donors and recipients (during the pre-entitlement period and after entitlement, but prior to entrance into the hospital for transplantation) as well as all physicians' services applicable to cadavers are considered Part A hospital services (kidney acquisition costs).

F. Billing for Physicians' Services After Transplantation

All physicians' services rendered to the living donor and all physicians' services rendered to the transplant recipient are billed to the Medicare program in the same manner as all Medicare Part B services are billed. All donor physicians' services must be billed to the account of the recipient (i.e., the recipient's Medicare number).

G. Billing For Physicians' Renal Transplantation Services

To ensure proper payment when submitting a Part B bill for the renal surgeon's services to the recipient, the appropriate HCPCS codes must be submitted, including HCPCS codes for concurrent surgery, as applicable.

The bill must include all living donor physicians' services, e.g., Revenue Center code 081X.

100-04, 3, 90.1.2

Billing for Kidney Transplant and Acquisition Services

(Rev. 3030, Issued: 8/22/14, Eff. ASC X12: January 1, 2012, I-10: w/Imp I -10, ASC X12: 9/23/2014)

Applicable standard kidney acquisition charges are identified separately by revenue code 0811 (Living Donor Kidney Acquisition) or 0812 (Cadaver Donor Kidney Acquisition). Where interim bills are submitted, the standard acquisition charge appears on the billing form for the period during which the transplant took place. This charge is in addition to the hospital's charges for services rendered directly to the Medicare recipient.

The contractor deducts kidney acquisition charges for PPS hospitals for processing through Pricer. These costs, incurred by approved kidney transplant hospitals, are not included in the kidney transplant prospective payment. They are paid on a reasonable cost basis. Interim payment is paid as a "pass through" item. (See the Provider Reimbursement Manual, Part 1, §2802 B.8.) The contractor includes kidney acquisition charges under the appropriate revenue code in CWF.

Bill Review Procedures

The Medicare Code Editor (MCE) creates a Limited Coverage edit for kidney transplant procedure codes. Where these procedure codes are identified by MCE, the contractor checks the provider number to determine if the provider is an approved transplant center, and checks the effective approval date. The contractor shall also determine if the facility is certified for adults and/or pediatric transplants dependent upon the patient's age. If payment is appropriate (i.e., the center is approved and the service is on or after the approval date) it overrides the limited coverage edit.

100-04, 3, 90.2

Heart Transplants

(Rev. 3030, Issued: 8/22/14, Eff. ASC X12: January 1, 2012, I-10: w/Imp I -10, ASC X12: 9/23/2014)

Cardiac transplantation is covered under Medicare when performed in a facility which is approved by Medicare as meeting institutional coverage criteria. On April 6, 1987, CMS Ruling 87-1, "Criteria for Medicare Coverage of Heart Transplants" was published in the "Federal Register." For Medicare coverage purposes, heart transplants are medically reasonable and necessary when performed in facilities that meet these criteria. If a hospital wishes to bill Medicare for heart transplants, it must submit an application and documentation, showing its ongoing compliance with each criterion.

If a contractor has any questions concerning the effective or approval dates of its hospitals, it should contact its RO.

For a complete list of approved transplant centers, visit:

http://www.cms.hhs.gov/CertificationandComplianc/20_Transplant.asp#TopOfPage

A. Effective Dates

The effective date of coverage for heart transplants performed at facilities applying after July 6, 1987, is the date the facility receives approval as a heart transplant facility. Coverage is effective for discharges October 17, 1986 for facilities that would have qualified and that applied by July 6, 1987. All transplant hospitals will be recertified under the final rule, Federal Register / Vol. 72, No. 61 / Friday, March 30, 2007, / Rules and Regulations.

The CMS informs each hospital of its effective date in an approval letter.

B. Drugs

Medicare Part B covers immunosuppressive drugs following a covered transplant in an approved facility.

C. Noncovered Transplants

Medicare will not cover transplants or re-transplants in facilities that have not been approved as meeting the facility criteria. If a beneficiary is admitted for and receives a heart transplant from a hospital that is not approved, physicians' services, and inpatient services associated with the transplantation procedure are not covered.

If a beneficiary received a heart transplant from a hospital while it was not an approved facility and later requires services as a result of the noncovered transplant, the services are covered when they are reasonable and necessary in all other respects.

D. Charges for Heart Acquisition Services

The excising hospital bills the OPO, who in turn bills the transplant (implant) hospital for applicable services. It should not submit a bill to its contractor. The transplant hospital must keep an itemized statement that identifies the services rendered, the charges, the person receiving the service (donor/recipient), and whether this person is a potential transplant donor or recipient. These charges are reflected in the transplant hospital's heart acquisition cost center and are used in determining its standard charge for acquiring a donor's heart. The standard charge is not a charge representing the acquisition cost of a specific heart; rather, it reflects the average cost associated with each type of heart acquisition. Also, it is an all inclusive charge for all services required in acquisition of a heart, i.e., tissue typing, post-operative evaluation, etc.

E. Bill Review Procedures

The contractor takes the following actions to process heart transplant bills. It may accomplish them manually or modify its MCE and Grouper interface programs to handle the processing.

1. MCE Interface

   The MCE creates a Limited Coverage edit for heart transplant procedure codes. Where these procedure codes are identified by MCE, the contractor checks the provider number to determine if the provider is an approved transplant center, and checks the effective approval date. The contractor shall also determine if the facility is certified for adults and/or pediatric transplants dependent upon the patient's age. If payment is appropriate (i.e., the center is approved and the service is on or after the approval date) it overrides the limited coverage edit.

2. Handling Heart Transplant Billings From Nonapproved Hospitals

   Where a heart transplant and covered services are provided by a nonapproved hospital, the bill data processed through Grouper and Pricer must exclude transplant procedure codes and related charges.

100-04, 3, 90.3

Stem Cell Transplantation

(Rev. 3556, Issued: 07-01-16; Effective: 1-27-16; Implementation: 10-3-16)

A. General

Stem cell transplantation is a process in which stem cells are harvested from either a patient's (autologous) or donor's (allogeneic) bone marrow or peripheral blood for intravenous infusion. Autologous stem cell transplantation (AuSCT) is a technique for restoring stem cells using the patient's own previously stored cells. AuSCTmust be used to effect hematopoietic reconstitution following severely myelotoxic doses of chemotherapy (HDCT) and/or radiotherapy used to treat various malignancies. Allogeneic hematopoietic stem cell transplantation (HSCT) is a procedure in which a portion of a healthy donor's stem cell or bone marrow is obtained and prepared for intravenous infusion. Allogeneic HSCTmay be used to restore function in recipients having an inherited or acquired deficiency or defect. Hematopoietic stem cells are multi-potent stem cells that give rise to all the blood cell types; these stem cells form blood and immune cells. A hematopoietic stem cell is a cell isolated from blood or bone marrow that can renew itself, differentiate to a variety of specialized cells, can mobilize out of the bone marrow into circulating blood, and can undergo programmed cell death, called apoptosis - a process by which cells that are unneeded or detrimental will self-destruct.

The Centers for Medicare & Medicaid Services (CMS) is clarifying that bone marrow and peripheral blood stem cell transplantation is a process which includes mobilization, harvesting, and transplant of bone marrow or peripheral blood stem cells and the administration of high dose chemotherapy or radiotherapy prior to the actual transplant. When bone marrow or peripheral blood stem cell transplantation is covered, all necessary steps are included in coverage. When bone marrow or peripheral blood stem cell transplantation is non-covered, none of the steps are covered.

Allogeneic and autologous stem cell transplants are covered under Medicare for specific diagnoses. Effective October 1, 1990, these cases were assigned to MS-DRG 009, Bone Marrow Transplant.

The A/B MAC (A)'s Medicare Code Editor (MCE) will edit stem cell transplant procedure codes against diagnosis codes to determine which cases meet specified coverage criteria. Cases with a diagnosis code for a covered condition will pass (as covered) the MCE noncovered procedure edit. When a stem cell transplant case is selected for review based on the random selection of beneficiaries, the QIO will review the case on a post-payment basis to assure proper coverage decisions.

Bone marrow transplant codes that are reported with an ICD-9-CM that is "not otherwise specified" are returned to the hospital for a more specific procedure code. ICD-10-PCS codes are more precise and clearly identify autologous and nonautologous stem cells.

The A/B MAC (A) may choose to review if data analysis deems it a priority.

B. Nationally Covered Indications

I. Allogeneic Hematopoietic Stem Cell Transplantation (HSCT)

   a. General

      Allogeneic stem cell transplantation (ICD-9-CM Procedure Codes 41.02, 41.03, 41.05, and 41.08,; ICD-10-PCS codes 30230G1, 30230Y1, 30233G1, 30233Y1, 30240G1, 30240Y1, 30243G1, 30243Y1, 30250G1, 30250Y1, 30253G1, 30253Y1, 30260G1, 30260Y1, 30263G1, and 30263Y1) is a procedure in which a portion of a healthy donor's stem cells are obtained and prepared for intravenous infusion to restore normal hematopoietic function in recipients having an inherited or acquired hematopoietic deficiency or defect. See Pub. 100-03, National Coverage Determinations (NCD) Manual, chapter 1, section 110.23, for further information about this policy, and Pub. 100-04, CPM, chapter 32, section 90, for information on coding.

      Expenses incurred by a donor are a covered benefit to the recipient/beneficiary but, except for physician services, are not paid separately. Services to the donor include physician services, hospital care in connection with screening the stem cell, and ordinary follow-up care.

   b. Covered Conditions

      i. Effective for services performed on or after August 1, 1978: For the treatment of leukemia, leukemia in remission, or aplastic anemia when it is reasonable and necessary;

      ii. Effective for services performed on or after June 3, 1985: For the treatment of severe combined immunodeficiency disease (SCID), and for the treatment of Wiskott-Aldrich syndrome;

      iii. Effective for services performed on or after August 4, 2010: For the treatment of Myelodysplastic Syndromes (MDS) pursuant to Coverage with Evidence Development (CED) in the context of a Medicare-approved, prospective clinical study.

      iv. Effective for claims with dates of service on or after January 27, 2016:

1. Allogeneic HSCT for multiple myeloma is covered by Medicare only for beneficiaries with Durie-Salmon Stage II or III multiple myeloma, or International Staging System (ISS) Stage II or Stage III multiple myeloma, and participating in an approved prospective clinical study.
2. Allogeneic HSCT for myelofibrosis (MF) is covered by Medicare only for beneficiaries with Dynamic International Prognostic Scoring System (DIPSSplus) intermediate-2 or High primary or secondary MF and participating in an approved prospective clinical study.
3. Allogeneic HSCT for sickle cell disease (SCD) is covered by Medicare only for beneficiaries with severe, symptomatic SCD who participate in an approved prospective clinical study.

II. Autologous Stem Cell Transplantation (AuSCT)

   a. General

      Autologous stem cell transplantation (ICD-9-CM Procedure Codes 41.01, 41.04, 41.07, and 41.09; ICD-10-PCS codes 30230AZ, 30230G0, 30230Y0, 30233G0, 30233Y0, 30240G0, 30240Y0, 30243G0, 30243Y0, 30250G0, 30250Y0, 30253G0, 30253Y0, 30260G0, 30260Y0, 30263G0, and 30263Y0) is a technique for restoring stem cells using the patient's own previously stored cells. AuSCT must be used to effect hematopoietic reconstitution following severely myelotoxic doses of chemotherapy (high dose chemotherapy (HDCT)) and/or radiotherapy used to treat various malignancies. Refer to Pub. 100-03, NCD Manual, chapter 1, section 110.23, for further information about this policy, and Pub. 100-04, CPM, chapter 32, section 90, for information on coding.

b. Covered Conditions

1. Effective for services performed on or after April 28, 1989: Acute leukemia in remission who have a high probability of relapse and who have no human leucocyte antigens (HLA)-matched; Resistant non-Hodgkin's lymphomas or those presenting with poor prognostic features following an initial response; Recurrent or refractory neuroblastoma; or, Advanced Hodgkin's disease who have failed conventional therapy and have no HLA-matched donor.
2. Effective for services performed on or after October 1, 2000: Single AuSCT is only covered for Durie-Salmon Stage II or III patients that fit the following requirements:
   - Newly diagnosed or responsive multiple myeloma. This includes those patients with previously untreated disease, those with at least a partial response to prior chemotherapy (defined as a 50% decrease either in measurable paraprotein [serum and/or urine] or in bone marrow infiltration, sustained for at least 1 month), and those in responsive relapse; and
   - Adequate cardiac, renal, pulmonary, and hepatic function.
3. Effective for services performed on or after March 15, 2005: When recognized clinical risk factors are employed to select patients for transplantation, high dose melphalan (HDM) together with AuSCT is reasonable and necessary for Medicare beneficiaries of any age group with primary amyloid light chain (AL) amyloidosis who meet the following criteria:
   - Amyloid deposition in 2 or fewer organs; and,
   - Cardiac left ventricular ejection fraction (EF) greater than 45%.

C. Nationally Non-Covered Indications

I. Allogeneic Hematopoietic Stem Cell Transplantation (HSCT)

Effective for claims with dates of service on or after May 24, 1996, through January 26, 2016, allogeneic HSCT is not covered as treatment for multiple myeloma. Refer to Pub. 100-03, NCD Manual, chapter 1, section 110.23, for further information about this policy, and Pub. 100-04, CPM, chapter 32, section 90, for information on coding.

II. Autologous Stem Cell Transplantation (AuSCT)

Insufficient data exist to establish definite conclusions regarding the efficacy of AuSCT for the following conditions:

a) Acute leukemia not in remission;

b) Chronic granulocytic leukemia;

c) Solid tumors (other than neuroblastoma); Up to October 1, 2000, multiple myeloma;

e) Tandem transplantation (multiple rounds of AuSCT) for patients with multiple myeloma;

f) Effective October 1, 2000, non primary AL amyloidosis; and,

g) Effective October 1, 2000, through March 14, 2005, primary AL amyloidosis for Medicare beneficiaries age 64 or older. In these cases, AuSCT is not considered reasonable and necessary within the meaning of §1862(a)(1)(A) of the Act and is not covered under Medicare. Refer to Pub. 100-03, NCD Manual, chapter 1, section 110.23, for further information about this policy, and Pub. 100-04, CPM, chapter 32, section 90, for information on coding.

D. Other

All other indications for stem cell transplantation not otherwise noted above as covered or non-covered remain at local Medicare Administrative Contractor discretion.

100-04, 3, 90.3.1

Billing for Stem Cell Transplantation

(Rev. 3571, Issued: 07-29-16; Effective: 01-01-17; Implementation; 01-03-17)

A. Billing for Allogeneic Stem Cell Transplants

1. Definition of Acquisition Charges for Allogeneic Stem Cell Transplants

Acquisition charges for allogeneic stem cell transplants include, but are not limited to, charges for the costs of the following services:

- National Marrow Donor Program fees, if applicable, for stem cells from an unrelated donor;
- Tissue typing of donor and recipient;
- Donor evaluation;
- Physician pre-admission/pre-procedure donor evaluation services;
- Costs associated with harvesting procedure (e.g., general routine and special care services, procedure/operating room and other ancillary services, apheresis services, etc.);
- Post-operative/post-procedure evaluation of donor; and
- Preparation and processing of stem cells.

Payment for these acquisition services is included in the MS-DRG payment for the allogeneic stem cell transplant when the transplant occurs in the inpatient setting, and in the OPPS APC payment for the allogeneic stem cell transplant when the transplant occurs in the outpatient setting. The Medicare contractor does not make separate payment for these acquisition services, because hospitals may bill and receive payment only for services provided to the Medicare beneficiary who is the recipient of the stem cell transplant and whose illness is being treated with the stem cell transplant. Unlike the acquisition costs of solid organs for transplant (e.g., hearts and kidneys), which are paid on a reasonable cost basis, acquisition costs for allogeneic stem cells are included in prospective payment.

Acquisition charges for stem cell transplants apply only to allogeneic transplants, for which stem cells are obtained from a donor (other than the recipient himself or herself). Acquisition charges do not apply to autologous transplants (transplanted stem cells are obtained from the recipient himself or herself), because autologous transplants involve services provided to the beneficiary only (and not to a donor), for which the hospital may bill and receive payment (see Pub. 100-04, chapter 4, §231.10 and paragraph B of this section for information regarding billing for autologous stem cell transplants).

2. Billing for Acquisition Services

The hospital bills and shows acquisition charges for allogeneic stem cell transplants based on the status of the patient (i.e., inpatient or outpatient) when the transplant is furnished. See Pub. 100-04, chapter 4, §231.11 for instructions regarding billing for acquisition services for allogeneic stem cell transplants that are performed in the outpatient setting.

When the allogeneic stem cell transplant occurs in the inpatient setting, the hospital identifies stem cell acquisition charges for allogeneic bone marrow/stem cell transplants separately by using revenue code 0815 (Stem Cell Acquisition). Revenue code 0815 charges should include all services required to acquire stem cells from a donor, as defined above.

On the recipient's transplant bill, the hospital reports the acquisition charges, cost report days, and utilization days for the donor's hospital stay (if applicable) and/or charges for other encounters in which the stem cells were obtained from the donor. The donor is covered for medically necessary inpatient hospital days of care or outpatient care provided in connection with the allogeneic stem cell transplant under Part A. Expenses incurred for complications are paid only if they are directly and immediately attributable to the stem cell donation procedure. The hospital reports the acquisition charges on the billing form for the recipient, as described in the first paragraph of this section. It does not charge the donor's days of care against the recipient's utilization record. For cost reporting purposes, it includes the covered donor days and charges as Medicare days and charges.

The transplant hospital keeps an itemized statement that identifies the services furnished, the charges, the person receiving the service (donor/recipient), and whether this is a potential transplant donor or recipient. These charges will be reflected in the transplant hospital's stem cell/bone marrow acquisition cost center. For allogeneic stem cell acquisition services in cases that do not result in transplant, due to death of the intended recipient or other causes, hospitals include the costs associated with the acquisition services on the Medicare cost report.

The hospital shows charges for the transplant itself in revenue center code 0362 or another appropriate cost center. Selection of the cost center is up to the hospital.

B. Billing for Autologous Stem Cell Transplants

The hospital bills and shows all charges for autologous stem cell harvesting, processing, and transplant procedures based on the status of the patient (i.e., inpatient or outpatient) when the services are furnished. It shows charges for the actual transplant, in revenue center code 0362 or another appropriate cost center. ICD-9-CM or ICD-10-PCS codes are used to identify inpatient procedures.

The HCPCS codes describing autologous stem cell harvesting procedures may be billed and are separately payable under the OPPS when provided in the hospital outpatient setting of care. Autologous harvesting procedures are distinct from the acquisition services described in Pub. 100-04, chapter 4, §231.11 and section A. above for allogeneic stem cell transplants, which include services provided when stem cells are obtained from a donor and not from the patient undergoing the stem cell transplant. The HCPCS codes describing autologous stem cell processing procedures also may be billed and are separately payable under the OPPS when provided to hospital outpatients.

Payment for autologous stem cell harvesting procedures performed in the hospital inpatient setting of care, with transplant also occurring in the inpatient setting of care, is included in the MS-DRG payment for the autologous stem cell transplant.

100-04, 3, 90.3.2

Autologous Stem Cell Transplantation (AuSCT)

(Rev. 3030, Issued: 8/22/14, Eff. ASC X12: January 1, 2012, I-10: w/Imp I -10, ASC X12: 9/23/2014)

Autologous Stem Cell Transplantation (AuSCT)

A. General

Autologous stem cell transplantation (AuSCT) (ICD-9-CM procedure code 41.01, 41.04, 41.07, and 41.09 and CPT-4 code 38241) is a technique for restoring stem cells using the patient's own previously stored cells. AuSCT must be used to effect hematopoietic reconstitution following severely myelotoxic doses of chemotherapy (high dose chemotherapy (HDCT)) and/or radiotherapy used to treat various malignancies.

If ICD-9-CM is applicable, use the following Procedure Codes and Descriptions

ICD-9-CM Code	Description
41.01	Autologous bone marrow transplant without purging
41.04	Autologous hematopoietic stem cell transplant without purging
41.07	Autologous hematopoietic stem cell transplant with purging
41.09	Autologous bone marrow transplant with purging

If ICD-10-PCS is applicable, use the following Procedure Codes and Descriptions

ICD-10-PCS Code	Description
30230AZ	Transfusion of Embryonic Stem Cells into Peripheral Vein, Open Approach
30230G0	Transfusion of Autologous Bone Marrow into Peripheral Vein, Open Approach
30230Y0	Transfusion of Autologous Hematopoietic Stem Cells into Peripheral Vein, Open Approach
30233G0	Transfusion of Autologous Bone Marrow into Peripheral Vein, Percutaneous Approach
30233Y0	Transfusion of Autologous Hematopoietic Stem Cells into Peripheral Vein, Percutaneous Approach
30240G0	Transfusion of Autologous Bone Marrow into Central Vein, Open Approach
30240Y0	Transfusion of Autologous Bone Marrow into Central Vein, Open Approach
30243G0	Transfusion of Autologous Bone Marrow into Central Vein, Percutaneous Approach
30243Y0	Transfusion of Autologous Hematopoietic Stem Cells into Central Vein, Percutaneous Approach
30250G0	Transfusion of Autologous Bone Marrow into Peripheral Artery, Open Approach
30250Y0	Transfusion of Autologous Hematopoietic Stem Cells into Peripheral Artery, Open Approach
30253G0	Transfusion of Autologous Bone Marrow into Peripheral Artery, Percutaneous Approach
30253Y0	Transfusion of Autologous Hematopoietic Stem Cells into Peripheral Artery, Percutaneous Approach
30260G0	Transfusion of Autologous Bone Marrow into Central Artery, Open Approach
30260Y0	Transfusion of Autologous Hematopoietic Stem Cells into Central Artery, Open Approach
30263G0	Transfusion of Autologous Bone Marrow into Central Artery, Percutaneous Approach
30263Y0	Transfusion of Autologous Hematopoietic Stem Cells into Central Artery, Percutaneous Approach

B. Covered Conditions

1. Effective for services performed on or after April 28, 1989:

For acute leukemia in remission for patients who have a high probability of relapse and who have no human leucocyte antigens (HLA)-matched the following diagnosis codes are reported:

If ICD-9-CM is applicable, use the following Diagnosis Codes and Descriptions

Diagnosis Code	Description
204.01	Lymphoid leukemia, acute, in remission
205.01	Myeloid leukemia, acute, in remission
206.01	Monocytic leukemia, acute, in remission
207.01	Acute erythremia and erythroleukemia, in remission
208.01	Leukemia of unspecified cell type, acute, in remission

If ICD-10-CM is applicable, use the following Diagnosis Codes and Descriptions

Diagnosis Code	Description
C91.01	Acute lymphoblastic leukemia, in remission
C92.01	Acute myeloblastic leukemia, in remission
C92.41	Acute promyelocytic leukemia, in remission
C92.51	Acute myelomonocytic leukemia, in remission
C92.61	Acute myeloid leukemia with 11q23-abnormality in remission
C92.A1	Acute myeloid leukemia with multilineage dysplasia, in remission
C93.01	Acute monoblastic/monocytic leukemia, in remission
C94.01	Acute erythroid leukemia, in remission
C94.21	Acute megakaryoblastic leukemia, in remission
C94.41	Acute parmyelosis with myelofibrosis, in remission
C95.01	Acute leukemia of unspecified cell type, in remission

For resistant non-Hodgkin's lymphomas (or those presenting with poor prognostic features following an initial response the following diagnosis codes are reported:

If ICD-9-CM is applicable, use the following code ranges:

200.00 - 200.08,

200.10 - 00.18,

200.20 - 200.28,

200.80 - 200.88,

202.00 - 202.08,

202.80 - 202.88, and

202.90 - 202.98.

If ICD-10-CM is applicable use the following code ranges:

C82.00 - C85.29,

C85.80 - C86.6,

C96.4, and

C96.Z - C96.9.

For recurrent or refractory neuroblastoma (see ICD-9-CM Neoplasm by site, malignant for the appropriate diagnosis code)

If ICD-10-CM is applicable the following ranges are reported:

C00 - C96, and

D00 - D09 Resistant non-Hodgkin's lymphomas

For advanced Hodgkin's disease patients who have failed conventional therapy and have no HLA-matched donor the following diagnosis codes are reported:

If ICD-9-CM is applicable, 201.00-201.98.

If ICD-10-CM is applicable, C81.00 – C81.99.

2. Effective for services performed on or after October 1, 2000:

   Durie-Salmon Stage II or III that fit the following requirement are covered: Newly diagnosed or responsive multiple myeloma (if ICD-9-CM is applicable, diagnosis codes 203.00 and 238.6, and, if ICD-10-CM is applicable, diagnosis codes C90.00 and D47.Z9). This includes those patients with previously untreated disease, those with at least a partial response to prior chemotherapy (defined as a 50% decrease either in measurable paraprotein [serum and/or urine] or in bone marrow infiltration, sustained for at least 1 month), and those in responsive relapse, and adequate cardiac, renal, pulmonary, and hepatic function.

3. Effective for Services On or After March 15, 2005

   Effective for services performed on or after March 15, 2005 when recognized clinical risk factors are employed to select patients for transplantation, high-dose melphalan (HDM), together with AuSCT, in treating Medicare beneficiaries of any age group with primary amyloid light-chain (AL) amyloidosis who meet the following criteria:

   Amyloid deposition in 2 or fewer organs; and,

   Cardiac left ventricular ejection fraction (EF) of 45% or greater.

C. Noncovered Conditions

Insufficient data exist to establish definite conclusions regarding the efficacy of autologous stem cell transplantation for the following conditions:

- Acute leukemia not in remission:
  - — If ICD-9-CM is applicable, diagnosis codes 204.00, 205.00, 206.00, 207.00 and 208.00 are noncovered;
  - — If ICD-10-CM is applicable, diagnosis codes C91.00, C92.00, C92.40, C92.50, C92.60, C92.A0, C93.00, C94.00, and C95.00 are noncovered.
- Chronic granulocytic leukemia:
  - — If ICD-9-CM is applicable, diagnosis codes 205.10 and 205.11;
  - — If ICD-10-CM is applicable, diagnosis codes C92.10 and C92.11.
- Solid tumors (other than neuroblastoma):
  - — If ICD-9-CM is applicable, diagnosis codes 140.0-199.1;

— If ICD-10-CM is applicable, diagnosis codes C00.0 - C80.2 and D00.0 - D09.9. Multiple myeloma (ICD-9-CM codes 203.00 and 238.6), through September 30, 2000.

- Tandem transplantation (multiple rounds of autologous stem cell transplantation) for patients with multiple myeloma
  - — If ICD-9-CM is applicable, diagnosis codes 203.00 and 238.6 and,
  - — If ICD-10-CM is applicable, diagnosis codes C90.00 and D47.Z9)
- Non-primary (AL) amyloidosis,
  - — If ICD-9-CM is applicable, diagnosis code 277.3. Effective October 1, 2000; ICD-9-CM code 277.3 was expanded to codes 277.30, 277.31, and 277.39 effective October 1, 2006.
  - — If ICD-10-CM is applicable, diagnosis codes are E85.0 – E85.9. or
- Primary (AL) amyloidosis
  - — If ICD-9-CM is applicable, diagnosis codes 277.30, 277.31, and 277.39 and for Medicare beneficiaries age 64 or older, effective October 1, 2000, through March 14, 2005.
  - — If ICD-10-CM is applicable, diagnosis codes are E85.0 - E85.9.

NOTE: Coverage for conditions other than these specifically designated as covered or non-covered is left to the discretion of the A/B MAC (A).

100-04, 3, 90.3.3

Billing for Stem Cell Transplantation

(Rev. 3030, Issued: 8/22/14, Eff. ASC X12: January 1, 2012, I-10: w/Imp I -10, ASC X12: 9/23/2014)

A. Billing for Allogeneic Stem Cell Transplants

1. Definition of Acquisition Charges for Allogeneic Stem Cell Transplants

   Acquisition charges for allogeneic stem cell transplants include, but are not limited to, charges for the costs of the following services:

   - — National Marrow Donor Program fees, if applicable, for stem cells from an unrelated donor;
   - — Tissue typing of donor and recipient;
   - — Donor evaluation;
   - — Physician pre-admission/pre-procedure donor evaluation services;
   - — Costs associated with harvesting procedure (e.g., general routine and special care services, procedure/operating room and other ancillary services, apheresis services, etc.);
   - — Post-operative/post-procedure evaluation of donor; and
   - — Preparation and processing of stem cells.

   Payment for these acquisition services is included in the MS-DRG payment for the allogeneic stem cell transplant when the transplant occurs in the inpatient setting, and in the OPPS APC payment for the allogeneic stem cell transplant when the transplant occurs in the outpatient setting. The Medicare contractor does not make separate payment for these acquisition services, because hospitals may bill and receive payment only for services provided to the Medicare beneficiary who is the recipient of the stem cell transplant and whose illness is being treated with the stem cell transplant. Unlike the acquisition costs of solid organs for transplant (e.g., hearts and kidneys), which are paid on a reasonable cost basis, acquisition costs for allogeneic stem cells are included in prospective payment.

   Acquisition charges for stem cell transplants apply only to allogeneic transplants, for which stem cells are obtained from a donor (other than the recipient himself or herself). Acquisition charges do not apply to autologous transplants (transplanted stem cells are obtained from the recipient himself or herself), because autologous transplants involve services provided to the beneficiary only (and not to a donor), for which the hospital may bill and receive payment (see Pub. 100-4, chapter 4, §231.10 and paragraph B of this section for information regarding billing for autologous stem cell transplants).

2. Billing for Acquisition Services

   The hospital bills and shows acquisition charges for allogeneic stem cell transplants based on the status of the patient (i.e., inpatient or outpatient) when the transplant is furnished. See Pub. 100-4, chapter 4, §231.11 for instructions regarding billing for acquisition services for allogeneic stem cell transplants that are performed in the outpatient setting.

   When the allogeneic stem cell transplant occurs in the inpatient setting, the hospital identifies stem cell acquisition charges for allogeneic bone marrow/stem cell transplants separately in FL 42 of Form CMS-1450 (or electronic equivalent) by using revenue code 0819 (Other Organ Acquisition). Revenue code 0819 charges should include all services required to acquire stem cells from a donor, as defined above.

   On the recipient's transplant bill, the hospital reports the acquisition charges, cost report days, and utilization days for the donor's hospital stay (if applicable) and/or charges for other encounters in which the stem cells were obtained from the donor. The donor is covered for medically necessary inpatient hospital days of care or outpatient care provided in connection with the allogeneic stem cell transplant under Part A. Expenses incurred for complications are paid only if they are directly and immediately attributable to the stem cell donation procedure. The hospital reports the acquisition charges on the billing form for the recipient, as described in the first paragraph of this section. It does not charge the donor's days of care against the recipient's utilization record. For cost reporting purposes, it includes the covered donor days and charges as Medicare days and charges.

   The transplant hospital keeps an itemized statement that identifies the services furnished, the charges, the person receiving the service (donor/recipient), and whether this is a potential transplant donor or recipient. These charges will be reflected in the transplant hospital's stem cell/bone marrow acquisition cost center. For allogeneic stem cell acquisition services in cases that do not result in transplant, due to death of the intended recipient or other causes, hospitals include the costs associated with the acquisition services on the Medicare cost report.

   The hospital shows charges for the transplant itself in revenue center code 0362 or another appropriate cost center. Selection of the cost center is up to the hospital.

B. Billing for Autologous Stem Cell Transplants

The hospital bills and shows all charges for autologous stem cell harvesting, processing, and transplant procedures based on the status of the patient (i.e., inpatient or outpatient) when the services are furnished. It shows charges for the actual transplant, described by the appropriate ICD-9-CM procedure or CPT codes, in revenue center code 0362 or another appropriate cost center. ICD-9-CM or ICD-10-PCS codes are used to identify inpatient procedures.

The CPT codes describing autologous stem cell harvesting procedures may be billed and are separately payable under the OPPS when provided in the hospital outpatient setting of care. Autologous harvesting procedures are distinct from the acquisition services described in Pub. 100-4, chapter 4, §231.11 and section A. above for allogeneic stem cell transplants, which include services provided when stem cells are obtained from a donor and not from the patient undergoing the stem cell transplant. The CPT codes describing autologous stem cell processing procedures also may be billed and are separately payable under the OPPS when provided to hospital outpatients.

Payment for autologous stem cell harvesting procedures performed in the hospital inpatient setting of care, with transplant also occurring in the inpatient setting of care, is included in the MS-DRG payment for the autologous stem cell transplant.

100-04, 3, 90.4

Liver Transplants

(Rev. 2513, Issued: 08-03-12, Effective: 06-21-12, Implementation: 09-04-12)

A. Background

For Medicare coverage purposes, liver transplants are considered medically reasonable and necessary for specified conditions when performed in facilities that meet specific criteria. Coverage guidelines may be found in Publication 100-3, Section 260.1.

Effective for claims with dates of service June 21, 2012 and later, contractors may, at their discretion cover adult liver transplantation for patients with extrahepatic unresectable cholangiocarcinoma (CCA), (2) liver metastases due to a neuroendocrine tumor (NET) or (3) hemangioendothelimo (HAE) when furnished in an approved Liver Transplant Center (below). All other nationally non-covered malignancies continue to remain nationally non-covered.

To review the current list of approved Liver Transplant Centers, see http://www.cms.hhs.gov/CertificationandComplianc/20_Transplant.asp#TopOfPage

100-04, 3, 90.4.1

Standard Liver Acquisition Charge

(Rev. 1, 10-01-03) A3-3615.1, A3-3615.3

Each transplant facility must develop a standard charge for acquiring a cadaver liver from costs it expects to incur in the acquisition of livers.

This standard charge is not a charge that represents the acquisition cost of a specific liver. Rather, it is a charge that reflects the average cost associated with a liver acquisition.

Services associated with liver acquisition are billed from the organ procurement organization or, in some cases, the excising hospital to the transplant hospital. The excising hospital does not submit a billing form to the FI. The transplant hospital keeps an itemized statement that identifies the services furnished, the charges, the person receiving the service (donor/recipient), and the potential transplant donor. These charges are reflected in the transplant hospital's liver acquisition cost center and are used in determining the hospital's standard charge for acquiring a cadaver's liver. The standard charge is not a charge representing the acquisition cost of a specific liver. Rather, it is a charge that reflects the average cost associated with liver acquisition. Also, it is an all inclusive charge for all services required in acquisition of a liver, e.g., tissue typing, transportation of organ, and surgeons' retrieval fees.

100-04, 3, 90.4.2

Billing for Liver Transplant and Acquisition Services

(Rev. 3030, Issued: 8/22/14, Eff. ASC X12: January 1, 2012, I-10: w/Imp I -10, ASC X12: 9/23/2014)

The inpatient claim is completed in accordance with instructions in chapter 25 for the beneficiary who receives a covered liver transplant. Applicable standard liver acquisition charges are identified separately in FL 42 by revenue code 0817 (Donor-Liver). Where interim bills are submitted, the standard acquisition charge appears on the billing form for the period during which the transplant took place. This charge is in addition to the hospital's charge for services furnished directly to the Medicare recipient.

The contractor deducts liver acquisition charges for IPPS hospitals prior to processing through Pricer. Costs of liver acquisition incurred by approved liver transplant facilities are not included in prospective payment DRG 480 (Liver Transplant). They are paid on a reasonable cost basis. This item is a "pass-through" cost for which interim payments are made. (See the Provider Reimbursement Manual, Part 1, §2802 B.8.) The contractor includes liver acquisition charges under revenue code 0817 in the HUIP record that it sends to CWF and the QIO.

A. Bill Review Procedures

The contractor takes the following actions to process liver transplant bills.

1. Operative Report

   The contractor requires the operative report with all claims for liver transplants, or sends a development request to the hospital for each liver transplant with a diagnosis code for a covered condition.

2. MCE Interface

   The MCE contains a limited coverage edit for liver transplant procedures using ICD-9-CM code 50.59 if ICD-9 is applicable, and, if ICD-10 is applicable, using ICD-10-PCS codes 0FY00Z0, 0FY00Z1, and 0FY00Z2.

   Where a liver transplant procedure code is identified by the MCE, the contractor shall check the provider number and effective date to determine if the provider is an approved liver transplant facility at the time of the transplant, and the contractor shall also determine if the facility is certified for adults and/or pediatric transplants dependent upon the patient's age. If yes, the claim is suspended for review of the operative report to determine whether the beneficiary has at least one of the covered conditions when the diagnosis code is for a covered condition. If payment is appropriate (i.e., the facility is approved, the service is furnished on or after the approval date, and the beneficiary has a covered condition), the contractor sends the claim to Grouper and Pricer.

   If none of the diagnoses codes are for a covered condition, or if the provider is not an approved liver transplant facility, the contractor denies the claim.

   NOTE: Some noncovered conditions are included in the covered diagnostic codes. (The diagnostic codes are broader than the covered conditions. Do not pay for noncovered conditions.

3. Grouper

   If the bill shows a discharge date before March 8, 1990, the liver transplant procedure is not covered. If the discharge date is March 8, 1990 or later, the contractor processes the bill through Grouper and Pricer. If the discharge date is after March 7, 1990, and before October 1, 1990, Grouper assigned CMS DRG 191 or 192. The contractor sent the bill to Pricer with review code 08. Pricer would then overlay CMS DRG 191 or 192 with CMS DRG 480 and the weights and thresholds for CMS DRG 480 to price the bill. If the discharge date is after September 30, 1990, Grouper assigns CMS DRG 480 and Pricer is able to price without using review code 08. If the discharge date is after September 30, 2007, Grouper assigns MS-DRG 005 or 006 (Liver transplant with MCC or Intestinal Transplant or Liver transplant without MCC, respectively) and Pricer is able to price without using review code 08.

4. Liver Transplant Billing From Non-approved Hospitals

   Where a liver transplant and covered services are provided by a non-approved hospital, the bill data processed through Grouper and Pricer must exclude transplant procedure codes and related charges.

   When CMS approves a hospital to furnish liver transplant services, it informs the hospital of the effective date in the approval letter. The contractor will receive a copy of the letter.

100-04, 3, 90.5

Pancreas Transplants Kidney Transplants

(Rev. 3481, Issued: 03-18-16. Effective: 06-20-16, Implementation: 06-20-16)

A. Background

Effective July 1, 1999, Medicare covered pancreas transplantation when performed simultaneously with or following a kidney transplant if ICD-9 is applicable, ICD-9-CM procedure code 55.69. If ICD-10 is applicable, the following ICD-10-PCS codes will be used:

ØTYØØZØ, ØTYØØZ1, ØTYØØZ2, ØTY1ØZØ. ØTY1ØZ1, and ØTY1ØZ2.

Pancreas transplantation is performed to induce an insulin independent, euglycemic state in diabetic patients. The procedure is generally limited to those patients with severe secondary complications of diabetes including kidney failure. However, pancreas transplantation is sometimes performed on patients with labile diabetes and hypoglycemic unawareness.

Medicare has had a policy of not covering pancreas transplantation. The Office of Health Technology Assessment performed an assessment on pancreas-kidney transplantation in 1994. They found reasonable graft survival outcomes for patients receiving either simultaneous pancreas-kidney (SPK) transplantation or pancreas after kidney (PAK) transplantation. For a list of facilities approved to perform SPK or PAK, refer to the following Web site: https://www.cms.gov/Medicare/Provider-Enrollment-and-Certification/CertificationandComplianc/downloads/ApprovedTransplantPrograms.pdf

B. Billing for Pancreas Transplants

There are no special provisions related to managed care participants. Managed care plans are required to provide all Medicare covered services. Medicare does not restrict which hospitals or physicians may perform pancreas transplantation.

The transplant procedure and revenue code 0360 for the operating room are paid under these codes. Procedures must be reported using the current ICD-9-CM procedure codes for pancreas and kidney transplants. Providers must place at least one of the following transplant procedure codes on the claim:

If ICD-9 Is Applicable

52.80 Transplant of pancreas

52.82 Homotransplant of pancreas

The Medicare Code Editor (MCE) has been updated to include 52.80 and 52.82 as limited coverage procedures. The contractor must determine if the facility is approved for the transplant and certified for either pediatric or adult transplants dependent upon the age of the patient.

Effective October 1, 2000, ICD-9-CM code 52.83 was moved in the MCE to non-covered. The contractor must override any deny edit on claims that came in with 52.82 prior to October 1, 2000 and adjust, as 52.82 is the correct code.

If the discharge date is July 1, 1999, or later: the contractor processes the bill through Grouper and Pricer.

If ICD-10 is applicable, the following procedure codes (ICD-10-PCS) are:

ØFYGØZØ Transplantation of Pancreas, Allogeneic, Open Approach

ØFYGØZ1 Transplantation of Pancreas, Syngeneic, Open Approach

Pancreas transplantation is reasonable and necessary for the following diagnosis codes. However, since this is not an all-inclusive list, the contractor is permitted to determine if any additional diagnosis codes will be covered for this procedure.

If ICD-9-CM is applicable, Diabetes Diagnosis Codes and Descriptions

ICD-9-CM Code	Description
250.00	Diabetes mellitus without mention of complication, type II (non-insulin dependent) (NIDDM) (adult onset) or unspecified type, not stated as uncontrolled.
250.01	Diabetes mellitus without mention of complication, type I (insulin dependent) (IDDM) (juvenile), not stated as uncontrolled.
250.02	Diabetes mellitus without mention of complication, type II (non-insulin dependent) (NIDDM) (adult onset) or unspecified type, uncontrolled.
250.03	Diabetes mellitus without mention of complication, type I (insulin dependent) (IDDM) (juvenile), uncontrolled.
250.1X	Diabetes with ketoacidosis
250.2X	Diabetes with hyperosmolarity
250.3X	Diabetes with coma
250.4X	Diabetes with renal manifestations
250.5X	Diabetes with ophthalmic manifestations
250.6X	Diabetes with neurological manifestations
250.7X	Diabetes with peripheral circulatory disorders
250.8X	Diabetes with other specified manifestations
250.9X	Diabetes with unspecified complication

NOTE: X=0-3

If ICD-10-CM is applicable, the diagnosis codes are: E10.10 - E10.9

Hypertensive Renal Diagnosis Codes and Descriptions if ICD-9-CM is applicable :

ICD-9-CM Code	Description
403.01	Malignant hypertensive renal disease, with renal failure
403.11	Benign hypertensive renal disease, with renal failure
403.91	Unspecified hypertensive renal disease, with renal failure
404.02	Malignant hypertensive heart and renal disease, with renal failure
404.03	Malignant hypertensive heart and renal disease, with congestive heart failure or renal failure
404.12	Benign hypertensive heart and renal disease, with renal failure

ICD-9-CM Code	Description
404.13	Benign hypertensive heart and renal disease, with congestive heart failure or renal failure
404.92	Unspecified hypertensive heart and renal disease, with renal failure
404.93	Unspecified hypertensive heart and renal disease, with congestive heart failure or renal failure
585.1–585.6, 585.9	Chronic Renal Failure Code

If ICD-10-CM is applicable, diagnosis codes and descriptions are:

ICD-10-CM code	Description
I12.Ø	Hypertensive chronic kidney disease with stage 5 chronic kidney disease or end stage renal disease
I13.11	Hypertensive heart and chronic kidney disease without heart failure, with stage 5 chronic kidney disease, or end stage renal disease
I13.2	Hypertensive heart and chronic kidney disease with heart failure and with stage 5 chronic kidney disease, or end stage renal disease
N18.1	Chronic kidney disease, stage 1
N18.2	Chronic kidney disease, stage 2 (mild)
N18.3	Chronic kidney disease, stage 3 (moderate)
N18.4	Chronic kidney disease, stage 4 (severe)
N18.5	Chronic kidney disease, stage 5
N18.6	End stage renal disease
N18.9	Chronic kidney disease, unspecified

NOTE: If a patient had a kidney transplant that was successful, the patient no longer has chronic kidney failure, therefore it would be inappropriate for the provider to bill ICD-9-CM codes 585.1 - 585.6, 585.9 or, if ICD-10-CM is applicable, the diagnosis codes N18.1 - N18.9 on such a patient. In these cases one of the following codes should be present on the claim or in the beneficiary's history.

The provider uses the following ICD-9-CM status codes only when a kidney transplant was performed before the pancreas transplant and ICD-9 is applicable:

ICD-9-CM code	Description
V42.0	Organ or tissue replaced by transplant kidney
V43.89	Organ tissue replaced by other means, kidney or pancreas

If ICD-10-CM is applicable, the following ICD-10-CM status codes will be used:

ICD-10-CM code	Description
Z48.22	Encounter for aftercare following kidney transplant
Z94.Ø	Kidney transplant status

NOTE: If a kidney and pancreas transplants are performed simultaneously, the claim should contain a diabetes diagnosis code and a renal failure code or one of the hypertensive renal failure diagnosis codes. The claim should also contain two transplant procedure codes. If the claim is for a pancreas transplant only, the claim should contain a diabetes diagnosis code and a status code to indicate a previous kidney transplant. If the status code is not on the claim for the pancreas transplant, the contractor will search the beneficiary's claim history for a status code indicating a prior kidney transplant.

C. Drugs

If the pancreas transplant occurs after the kidney transplant, immunosuppressive therapy will begin with the date of discharge from the inpatient stay for the pancreas transplant.

D. Charges for Pancreas Acquisition Services

A separate organ acquisition cost center has been established for pancreas transplantation. The Medicare cost report will include a separate line to account for pancreas transplantation costs. The 42 CFR 412.2(e)(4) was changed to include pancreas in the list of organ acquisition costs that are paid on a reasonable cost basis.

Acquisition costs for pancreas transplantation as well as kidney transplants will occur in Revenue Center 081X. The contractor overrides any claims that suspend due to repetition of revenue code 081X on the same claim if the patient had a simultaneous kidney/pancreas transplant. It pays for acquisition costs for both kidney and pancreas organs if transplants are performed simultaneously. It will not pay for more than two organ acquisitions on the same claim.

E. Medicare Summary Notices (MSN) and Remittance Advice Messages

If the provider submits a claim for simultaneous pancreas kidney transplantation or pancreas transplantation following a kidney transplant, and omits one of the appropriate diagnosis/procedure codes, the contractor shall reject the claim.

The following reflects the remittance advice messages and associated codes that will appear when rejecting/denying claims under this policy. This CARC/RARC combination is compliant with CAQH CORE Business Scenario 3.

Group Code: CO

CARC: B15

RARC: N/A

MSN: 16.32

If no evidence of a prior kidney transplant is presented, then the contractor shall deny the claim.

The following reflects the remittance advice messages and associated codes that will appear when rejecting/denying claims under this policy. This CARC/RARC combination is compliant with CAQH CORE Business Scenario 3.

Group Code: CO

CARC: 50

RARC: MA126

MSN: 15.4

100-04, 3, 90.5.1

Pancreas Transplants Alone (PA)

Rev.3481, Issued: 03-18-16. Effective: 06-20-16, Implementation: 06-20-16

A. General

Pancreas transplantation is performed to induce an insulin-independent, euglycemic state in diabetic patients. The procedure is generally limited to those patients with severe secondary complications of diabetes, including kidney failure. However, pancreas transplantation is sometimes performed on patients with labile diabetes and hypoglycemic unawareness. Medicare has had a long-standing policy of not covering pancreas transplantation, as the safety and effectiveness of the procedure had not been demonstrated. The Office of Health Technology Assessment performed an assessment of pancreas-kidney transplantation in 1994. It found reasonable graft survival outcomes for patients receiving either simultaneous pancreas-kidney transplantation or pancreas-after-kidney transplantation.

B. Nationally Covered Indications

CMS determines that whole organ pancreas transplantation will be nationally covered by Medicare when performed simultaneous with or after a kidney transplant. If the pancreas transplant occurs after the kidney transplant, immunosuppressive therapy will begin with the date of discharge from the inpatient stay for the pancreas transplant.

C. Billing and Claims Processing

Contractors shall pay for Pancreas Transplantation Alone (PA) effective for services on or after April 26, 2006 when performed in those facilities that are Medicare-approved for kidney transplantation. Approved facilities are located at the following address: https://www.cms.gov/Medicare/Provider-Enrollment-and-Certification/CertificationandComplianc/downloads/ApprovedTransplantPrograms.pdf

Contractors who receive claims for PA services that were performed in an unapproved facility, should reject such claims. The following reflects the remittance advice messages and associated codes that will appear when rejecting/denying claims under this policy. This CARC/RARC combination is compliant with CAQH CORE Business Scenario 3.

Group Code: CO

CARC: 58

RARC: N/A

MSN: 16.2.

Payment will be made for a PA service performed in an approved facility, and which meets the coverage guidelines mentioned above for beneficiaries with type I diabetes.

All-Inclusive List of Covered Diagnosis Codes for PA if ICD-9-CM is applicable

(NOTE: "X" = 1 and 3 only)

ICD-9-CM code	Description
250.0X	Diabetes mellitus without mention of complication, type I (insulin dependent) (IDDM) (juvenile), not stated as uncontrolled.
250.1X	Diabetes with ketoacidosis
250.2X	Diabetes with hyperosmolarity
250.3X	Diabetes with coma
250.4X	Diabetes with renal manifestations
250.5X	Diabetes with ophthalmic manifestations
250.6X	Diabetes with neurological manifestations
250.7X	Diabetes with peripheral circulatory disorders
250.8X	Diabetes with other specified manifestations
250.9X	Diabetes with unspecified complication

If ICD-10-CM is applicable, the provider uses the following range of ICD-10-CM codes:

E1Ø.1Ø – E1Ø.9.

Procedure Codes

If ICD-9 CM is applicable

52.80 - Transplant of pancreas

52.82 - Homotransplant of pancreas

If ICD-10 is applicable, the provider uses the following ICD-10-PCS codes:

ØFYGØZØ Transplantation of Pancreas, Allogeneic, Open Approach

ØFYGØZ1 Transplantation of Pancreas, Syngeneic, Open Approach

Contractors who receive claims for PA that are not billed using the covered diagnosis/procedure codes listed above shall reject such claims. The MCE edits to ensure that the transplant is covered based on the diagnosis. The MCE also considers ICD-9-CM codes 52.80 and 52.82 and ICD-10-PCS codes ØFYGØZØ and ØFYGØZ1 as limited coverage dependent upon whether the facility is approved to perform the transplant and is certified for the age of the patient.

The following reflects the remittance advice messages and associated codes that will appear when rejecting/denying claims under this policy. This CARC/RARC combination is compliant with CAQH CORE Business Scenario 3.

Group Code: CO

CARC: 50

RARC: N/A

MSN: 15.4

Contractors shall hold the provider liable for denied\rejected claims unless the hospital issues a Hospital Issued Notice of Non-coverage (HINN) or a physician issues an Advanced Beneficiary Notice (ABN) for Part-B for physician services.

D. Charges for Pancreas Alone Acquisition Services

A separate organ acquisition cost center has been established for pancreas transplantation. The Medicare cost report will include a separate line to account for pancreas transplantation costs. The 42 CFR 412.2(e)(4) was changed to include PA in the list of organ acquisition costs that are paid on a reasonable cost basis.

Acquisition costs for PA transplantation are billed in Revenue Code 081X. The contractor removes acquisition charges prior to sending the claims to Pricer so such charges are not included in the outlier calculation.

100-04, 3, 90.6

Intestinal and Multi-Visceral Transplants

(Rev. 3481, Issued: 03-18-16. Effective: 06-20-16, Implementation: 06-20-16)

A. Background

Effective for services on or after April 1, 2001, Medicare covers intestinal and multi-visceral transplantation for the purpose of restoring intestinal function in patients with irreversible intestinal failure. Intestinal failure is defined as the loss of absorptive capacity of the small bowel secondary to severe primary gastrointestinal disease or surgically induced short bowel syndrome. Intestinal failure prevents oral nutrition and may be associated with both mortality and profound morbidity. Multi-Visceral transplantation includes organs in the digestive system (stomach, duodenum, liver, and intestine). See §260.5 of the National Coverage Determinations Manual for further information.

B. Approved Transplant Facilities

Medicare will cover intestinal transplantation if performed in an approved facility. The approved facilities are located at: https://www.cms.gov/Medicare/Provider-Enrollment-and-Certification/CertificationandComplianc/downloads/ApprovedTransplantPrograms.pdf

C. Billing

If ICD-9-CM is applicable, ICD-9-CM procedure code 46.97 is effective for discharges on or after April 1, 2001. If ICD-10 is applicable, the ICD-10-PCS procedure codes are ØDY80ZØ, ØDY80Z1, ØDY80Z2, ØDYEØZØ, ØDYEØZ1, and ØDYEØZ2. The Medicare Code Editor (MCE) lists these codes as limited coverage procedures. The contractor shall override the MCE when this procedure code is listed and the coverage criteria are met in an approved transplant facility, and also determine if the facility is certified for adults and/or pediatric transplants dependent upon the patient's age.

For these procedures where the provider is approved as transplant facility and certified for the adult and/or pediatric population, and the service is performed on or after the transplant approval date, the contractor must suspend the claim for clerical review of the operative report to determine whether the beneficiary has at least one of the covered conditions listed when the diagnosis code is for a covered condition.

This review is not part of the contractor's medical review workload. Instead, the contractor should complete this review as part of its claims processing workload.

If ICD-9-CM is applicable, charges for ICD-9-CM procedure code 46.97, and, if ICD-10 is applicable, the ICD-10-PCS procedure codes ØDY80ZØ, ØDY80Z1, ØDY80Z2, ØDYEØZØ, ØDYEØZ1, or ØDYEØZ2 should be billed under revenue code 0360, Operating Room Services.

For discharge dates on or after October 1, 2001, acquisition charges are billed under revenue code 081X, Organ Acquisition. For discharge dates between April 1, 2001, and September 30, 2001, hospitals were to report the acquisition charges on the claim, but there was no interim pass-through payment made for these costs.

Bill the procedure used to obtain the donor's organ on the same claim, using appropriate ICD procedure codes.

The 11X bill type should be used when billing for intestinal transplants.

Immunosuppressive therapy for intestinal transplantation is covered and should be billed consistent with other organ transplants under the current rules.

If ICD-9-CM is applicable, there is no specific ICD-9-CM diagnosis code for intestinal failure. Diagnosis codes exist to capture the causes of intestinal failure. Some examples of intestinal failure include but are not limited to the following conditions and their associated ICD-9-CM codes:

- Volvulus 560.2,
- Volvulus gastroschisis 756.79, other [congenital] anomalies of abdominal wall,
- Volvulus gastroschisis 569.89, other specified disorders of intestine,
- Necrotizing enterocolitis 777.5, necrotizing enterocolitis in fetus or newborn,
- Necrotizing enterocolitis 014.8, other tuberculosis of intestines, peritoneum, and mesenteric,
- Necrotizing enterocolitis and splanchnic vascular thrombosis 557.0, acute vascular insufficiency of intestine,
- Inflammatory bowel disease 569.9, unspecified disorder of intestine,
- Radiation enteritis 777.5, necrotizing enterocolitis in fetus or newborn, and
- Radiation enteritis 558.1.

If ICD-10-CM is applicable, some diagnosis codes that may be used for intestinal failure are:

- Volvulus K56.2,
- Enteroptosis K63.4,
- Other specified diseases of intestine K63.89,
- Other specified diseases of the digestive system K92.89,
- Postsurgical malabsorption, not elsewhere classified K91.2,
- Other congenital malformations of abdominal wall Q79.59,
- Necrotizing enterocolitis in newborn, unspecified P77.9,
- Stage 1 necrotizing enterocolitis in newborn P77.1,
- Stage 2 necrotizing enterocolitis in newborn P77.2, and
- Stage 3 necrotizing enterocolitis in newborn P77.3

D. Acquisition Costs

A separate organ acquisition cost center was established for acquisition costs incurred on or after October 1, 2001. The Medicare Cost Report will include a separate line to account for these transplantation costs.

For intestinal and multi-visceral transplants performed between April 1, 2001, and October 1, 2001, the DRG payment was payment in full for all hospital services related to this procedure.

E. Medicare Summary Notices (MSN), Remittance Advice Messages, and Notice of Utilization Notices (NOU)

If an intestinal transplant is billed by an unapproved facility after April 1, 2001, the contractor shall deny the claim.

The following reflects the remittance advice messages and associated codes that will appear when rejecting/denying claims under this policy. This CARC/RARC combination is compliant with CAQH CORE Business Scenario 3.

Group Code: CO

CARC: 171

RARC: N/A

MSN: 21.6 or 21.18 or 16.2

100-04, 3, 100.1

Billing for Abortion Services

(Rev. 3481, Issued: 03-18-16. Effective: 06-20-16, Implementation: 06-20-16)

Effective October 1, 1998, abortions are not covered under the Medicare program except for instances where the pregnancy is a result of an act of rape or incest; or the woman suffers from a physical disorder, physical injury, or physical illness, including a life endangering physical condition caused by the pregnancy itself that would, as certified by a physician, place the woman in danger of death unless an abortion is performed.

A. "G" Modifier

The "G7" modifier is defined as "the pregnancy resulted from rape or incest, or pregnancy certified by physician as life threatening."

Beginning July 1, 1999, providers should bill for abortion services using the new Modifier G7. This modifier can be used on claims with dates of services October 1, 1998, and after. CWF will be able to recognize the modifier beginning July 1, 1999.

B. A/B MAC (A) Billing Instructions

1. Hospital Inpatient Billing

Hospitals use bill type 11X. Medicare will pay only when one of the following condition codes is reported:

Condition Code	Description
AA	Abortion Performed due to Rape
AB	Abortion Performed due to Incest
AD	Abortion Performed due to life endangering physical condition

With one of the following:

If ICD-9-CM Is Applicable:

- an appropriate ICD principal diagnosis code that will group to DRG 770 (Abortion W D&C, Aspiration Curettage Or Hysterotomy) or
- an appropriate ICD principal diagnosis code and one of the following ICD-9-CM operating room procedure that will group to DRG 779 (Abortion W/O D&C):69.01, 69.02, 69.51, 74.91.

If ICD-10-CM is applicable, one of the following ICD-10-PCS codes are used:

ICD-10-PCS code	Description
10A07ZZ	Abortion of Products of Conception, Via Natural or Artificial Opening
10A08ZZ	Abortion of Products of Conception, Via Natural or Artificial Opening Endoscopic
10D17ZZ	Extraction of Products of Conception, Retained, Via Natural or Artificial Opening
10D18ZZ	Extraction of Products of Conception, Retained, Via Natural or Artificial Opening Endoscopic
10A07ZZ	Abortion of Products of Conception, Via Natural or Artificial Opening
10A08ZZ	Abortion of Products of Conception, Via Natural or Artificial Opening Endoscopic
10A00ZZ	Abortion of Products of Conception, Open Approach
10A03ZZ	Abortion of Products of Conception, Percutaneous Approach
10A04ZZ	Abortion of Products of Conception, Percutaneous Endoscopic Approach

Providers must use ICD-9-CM codes 69.01 and 69.02 if ICD-9-CM is applicable, or, if ICD-10-CM is applicable, the related 1CD-10-PCS codes to describe exactly the procedure or service performed.

The A/B MAC (A) must manually review claims with the above ICD-9-CM/ICD-10-PCS procedure codes to verify that all of the above conditions are met.

2. Outpatient Billing

   Hospitals will use bill type 13X and 85X. Medicare will pay only if one of the following CPT codes is used with the "G7" modifier.

59840	59851	59856	59841	59852
59857	59850	59855	59866	

C. Common Working File (CWF) Edits

For hospital outpatient claims, CWF will bypass its edits for a managed care beneficiary who is having an abortion outside their plan and the claim is submitted with the "G7" modifier and one of the above CPT codes.

For hospital inpatient claims, CWF will bypass its edits for a managed care beneficiary who is having an abortion outside their plan and the claim is submitted with one of the above inpatient procedure codes.

D. Medicare Summary Notices (MSN)/Explanation of Your Medicare Benefits Remittance Advice Message

If a claim is submitted with one of the above CPT procedure codes but no "G7" modifier, the claim is denied.

The following reflects the remittance advice messages and associated codes that will appear when rejecting/denying claims under this policy. This CARC/RARC combination is compliant with CAQH CORE Business Scenario 3.

Group Code: CO

CARC: 272

RARC: N/A

MSN: 21.21

100-04, 3, 100.6

Inpatient Renal Services

(Rev. 1, 10-01-03) HO-E400

Section 405.103I of Subpart J of Regulation 5 stipulates that only approved hospitals may bill for ESRD services. Hence, to allow hospitals to bill and be reimbursed for inpatient dialysis services furnished under arrangements, both facilities participating in the arrangement must meet the conditions of 405.2120 and 405.2160 of Subpart U of Regulation 5. In order for renal dialysis facilities to have a written arrangement with each other to provide inpatient dialysis care both facilities must meet the minimum utilization rate requirement, i.e., two dialysis stations with a performance capacity of at least four dialysis treatments per week.

Dialysis may be billed by an SNF as a service if: (a) it is provided by a hospital with which the facility has a transfer agreement in effect, and that hospital is approved to provide staff-assisted dialysis for the Medicare program; or (b) it is furnished directly by an SNF meeting all nonhospital maintenance dialysis facility requirements, including minimum utilization requirements. (See 1861(h)(6), 1861(h)(7), title XVIII.)

100-04, 4, 20.6.12

Use of HCPCS Modifier – CT

(Rev. 3425, Issued: 12-18-15, Effective: 01-01-16, Implementation: 01-04-16)

Effective January 1, 2016, the definition of modifier – CT is "Computed tomography services furnished using equipment that does not meet each of the attributes of the National Electrical Manufacturers Association (NEMA) XR-29-2013 standard." This modifier is required to be reported on claims for computed tomography (CT) scans described by applicable HCPCS codes that are furnished on non-NEMA Standard XR-29-2013-compliant equipment. The applicable CT services are identified by HCPCS codes 70450 through 70498; 71250 through 71275; 72125 through 72133; 72191 through 72194; 73200 through 73206; 73700 through 73706; 74150 through 74178; 74261 through 74263; and 75571 through 75574 (and any succeeding codes).

This modifier should not be reported with codes that describe CT scans not listed above.

100-04, 4, 160

Clinic and Emergency Visits

(Rev. 1445, Issued: 02-08-08; Effective: 01-01-08; Implementation: 03-10-08)

CMS has acknowledged from the beginning of the OPPS that CMS believes that CPT Evaluation and Management (E/M) codes were designed to reflect the activities of physicians and do not describe well the range and mix of services provided by hospitals during visits of clinic and emergency department patients. While awaiting the development of a national set of facility-specific codes and guidelines, providers should continue to apply their current internal guidelines to the existing CPT codes. Each hospital's internal guidelines should follow the intent of the CPT code descriptors, in that the guidelines should be designed to reasonably relate the intensity of hospital resources to the different levels of effort represented by the codes. Hospitals should ensure that their guidelines accurately reflect resource distinctions between the five levels of codes.

Effective January 1, 2007, CMS is distinguishing between two types of emergency departments: Type A emergency departments and Type B emergency departments.

A Type A emergency department is defined as an emergency department that is available 24 hours a day, 7 days a week and is either licensed by the State in which it is located under applicable State law as an emergency room or emergency department or it is held out to the public (by name, posted signs, advertising, or other means) as a place that provides care for emergency medical conditions on an urgent basis without requiring a previously scheduled appointment.

A Type B emergency department is defined as an emergency department that meets the definition of a "dedicated emergency department" as defined in 42 CFR 489.24 under the EMTALA regulations. It must meet at least one of the following requirements: (1) It is licensed by the State in which it is located under applicable State law as an emergency room or emergency department; (2) It is held out to the public (by name, posted signs, advertising, or other means) as a place that provides care for emergency medical conditions on an urgent basis without requiring a previously scheduled appointment; or (3) During the calendar year immediately preceding the calendar year in which a determination under 42 CFR 489.24 is being made, based on a representative sample of patient visits that occurred during that calendar year, it provides at least one-third of all of its outpatient visits for the treatment of emergency medical conditions on an urgent basis without requiring a previously scheduled appointment.

Hospitals must bill for visits provided in Type A emergency departments using CPT emergency department E/M codes. Hospitals must bill for visits provided in Type B emergency departments using the G-codes that describe visits provided in Type B emergency departments.

Hospitals that will be billing the new Type B ED visit codes may need to update their internal guidelines to report these codes.

Emergency department and clinic visits are paid in some cases separately and in other cases as part of a composite APC payment. See section 10.2.1 of this chapter for further details.

100-04, 4, 200.1

Billing for Corneal Tissue

(Rev. 3425, Issued: 12-18-15, Effective: 01-01-16, Implementation: 01-04-16)

Corneal tissue will be paid on a cost basis, not under OPPS, only when it is used in a corneal transplant procedure described by one of the following CPT codes: 65710, 65730, 65750, 65755, 65756, 65765, 65767, and any successor code or new code describing a new type of corneal transplant procedure that uses eye banked corneal tissue. In all other procedures cornea tissue is packaged. To receive cost based reimbursement hospitals must bill charges for corneal tissue using HCPCS code V2785.

100-04, 4, 200.3.1

Billing Instructions for IMRT Planning and Delivery

(Rev. 3685, Issued: 12-22-16, Effective: 01-01-17, Implementation: 01-03-17)

Payment for the services identified by CPT codes 77014, 77280, 77285, 77290, 77295, 77306 through 77321, 77331, and 77370 are included in the APC payment for CPT code 77301 (IMRT planning). These codes should not be reported in addition to CPT code 77301 when provided prior to or as part of the development of the IMRT plan. In addition, CPT codes 77280-77290 (simulation-aided field settings) should not be reported for verification of the treatment field during a course of IMRT.

100-04, 4, 200.3.2

Billing for Multi-Source Photon (Cobalt 60-Based) Stereotactic Radiosurgery (SRS) Planning and Delivery

(Rev. 3685, Issued: 12-22-16, Effective: 01-01-17, Implementation: 01-03-17)

Effective for services furnished on or after January 1, 2014, hospitals must report SRS planning and delivery services using only the CPT codes that accurately describe the service furnished. For the delivery services, hospitals must report CPT code 77371, 77372, or 77373.

CPT Code	Long Descriptor
77371	Radiation treatment delivery, stereotactic radiosurgery (srs), complete course of treatment of cranial lesion(s) consisting of 1 session; multi- source cobalt 60 based
77372	Radiation treatment delivery, stereotactic radiosurgery (srs), complete course of treatment of cranial lesion(s) consisting of 1 session; linear accelerator based
77373	Stereotactic body radiation therapy, treatment delivery, per fraction to 1 or more lesions, including image guidance, entire course not to exceed 5 fractions

As instructed in the CY 2014 OPPS/ASC final rule, CPT code 77371 is to be used only for single session cranial SRS cases performed with a Cobalt-60 device, and CPT code 77372 is to be used only for single session cranial SRS cases performed with a linac-based device. The term "cranial" means that the pathological lesion(s) that are the target of the radiation is located in the patient's cranium or head. The term "single session" means that the entire intracranial lesion(s) that comprise the patient's diagnosis are treated in their entirety during a single treatment session on a single day. CPT code 77372 is never to be used for the first fraction or any other fraction of a fractionated SRS treatment. CPT code 77372 is to be used only for single session cranial linac-based SRS treatment. Fractionated SRS treatment is any SRS delivery service requiring more thana single session of SRS treatment for a cranial lesion, up to a total of no more than five fractions, and one to five sessions (but no more than five) for non-cranial lesions. CPT code 77373 is to be used for any fraction (including the first fraction) in any series of fractionated treatments, regardless of the anatomical location of the lesion or lesions being radiated. Fractionated cranial SRS is any cranial SRS that exceeds one treatment session and fractionated non-cranial SRS is any non-cranial SRS, regardless of the number of fractions but never more than five. Therefore, CPT code 77373 is the exclusive code (and the use of no other SRS treatment delivery code is permitted) for any and all fractionated SRS treatment services delivered anywhere in the body, including, but not limited to, the cranium or head. 77372 is not to be used for the first fraction of a fractionated cranial SRS treatment series and must only be used in cranial SRS when there is a single treatment session to treat the patient's entire condition.

In addition, for the planning services, hospitals must report the specific CPT code that accurately describes the service provided. The planning services may include but are not limited to CPT code 77290, 77295, 77300, 77334, or 77370.

CPT Code	Long Descriptor
77290	Therapeutic radiology simulation-aided field setting; complex
77295	Therapeutic radiology simulation-aided field setting; 3-dimensional
77300	Basic radiation dosimetry calculation, central axis depth dose calculation, tdf, nsd, gap calculation, off axis factor, tissue inhomogeneity factors, calculation of non-ionizing radiation surface and depth dose, as required during course of treatment, only when prescribed by the treating physician
77334	Treatment devices, design and construction; complex (irregular blocks, special shields, compensators, wedges, molds or casts)
77370	Special medical radiation physics consultation

Effective for cranial single session stereotactic radiosurgery procedures (CPT code 77371 or 77372) furnished on or after January 1, 2016 until December 31, 2017, costs for certain adjunctive services (e.g., planning and preparation) are not factored into the APC payment rate for APC 5627 (Level 7 Radiation Therapy). Rather, the ten planning and preparation codes listed in table below, will be paid according to their assigned status indicator when furnished 30 days prior or 30 days post SRS treatment delivery.

In addition, hospitals must report modifier "CP" (Adjunctive service related to a procedure assigned to a comprehensive ambulatory payment classification [C-APC] procedure) on TOB 13X claims for any other services (excluding the ten codes in table below) that are adjunctive or related to SRS treatment but billed on a different claim and within either 30 days prior or 30 days after the date of service for either CPT code 77371 (Radiation treatment delivery, stereotactic radiosurgery, complete course of treatment cranial lesion(s) consisting of 1 session; multi-source Cobalt 60-based) or CPT code 77372 (Linear accelerator based). The "CP" modifier need not be reported with the ten planning and preparation CPT codes table below. Adjunctive/related services include but are not necessarily limited to imaging, clinical treatment planning/preparation, and consultations. Any service related to the SRS delivery should have the CP modifier appended. We would not expect the "CP" modifier to be reported with services such as chemotherapy administration as this is considered to be a distinct service that is not directly adjunctive, integral, or dependent on delivery of SRS treatment.

Excluded Planning and Preparation CPT Codes

CPT Code	CY 2017 Short Descriptor	CY 2017 Opps Status Indicator
70551	Mri brain stem w/o dye	Q3
70552	Mri brain stem w/dye	Q3
70553	Mri brain stem w/o & w/dye	Q3
77011	Ct scan for localization	N
77014	Ct scan for therapy guide	N
77280	Set radiation therapy field	S
77285	Set radiation therapy field	S
77290	Set radiation therapy field	S
77295	3-d radiotherapy plan	S
77336	Radiation physics consult	S

100-04, 4, 200.11

Billing Advance Care Planning (ACP) as an Optional Element of an Annual Wellness Visit (AWV)

(Rev. 3739, Issued: 03-17-17, Effective: 01-01-16, Implementation: 06-19-17)

Effective January 1, 2016 payment for the service described by CPT code 99497 (Advance care planning including the explanation and discussion of advance directives such as standard forms (with completion of such forms, when performed), by the physician or other qualified health care professional; first 30 minutes, face-to-face with the patient, family member(s), and/or surrogate) is conditionally packaged under the OPPS and is consequently assigned to a conditionally packaged payment status indicator of "Q1." When this service is furnished with another service paid under the OPPS, payment is packaged; when it is the only service furnished, payment is made separately. CPT code 99498 (Advance care planning including the explanation and discussion of advance directives such as standard forms (with completion of such forms, when performed), by the physician or other qualified health care professional; each additional 30 minutes (List separately in addition to code for primary procedure)) is an add-on code and therefore payment for the service described by this code is unconditionally packaged (assigned status indicator "N") in the OPPS in accordance with 42 CFR 419.2(b)(18).

In addition, for services furnished on or after January 1, 2016, Advance Care Planning (ACP) is treated as a preventive service when furnished with an AWV. The Medicare coinsurance and Part B deductible are waived for ACP when furnished as an optional element of an AWV.

The codes for the optional ACP services furnished as part of an AWV are 99497 (Advance care planning including the explanation and discussion of advance directives such as standard forms (with completion of such forms, when performed), by the physician or other qualified health professional; first 30 minutes, face-to-face with the patient, family member(s) and/or surrogate;) and an add-on code 99498 (each additional 30 minutes (List separately in addition to code for primary procedure)). When ACP services are provided as a part of an AWV, practitioners would report CPT code 99497 (and add-on CPT code 99498 when applicable) for the ACP services in addition to either of the AWV codes (G0438 or G0439).

The deductible and coinsurance for ACP will only be waived when billed on the same day and on the same claim as an AWV (code G0438 or G0439), and must also be furnished by the same provider. Waiver of the deductible and coinsurance for ACP is limited to once per year. Payment for an AWV is limited to once per year. If the AWV billed with ACP is denied for exceeding the once per year limit, the deductible and coinsurance will be applied to the ACP.

Also see Pub. 100-02, Medicare Benefit Policy Manual, chapter 15, section 280.5.1 for more information.

100-04, 4, 231.10

Billing for Autologous Stem Cell Transplants

(Rev.3556, Issued: 07-01-2016; Effective: 1-27-16; Implementation: 10-3-16)

The hospital bills and shows all charges for autologous stem cell harvesting, processing, and transplant procedures based on the status of the patient (i.e., inpatient or outpatient) when the services are furnished. It shows charges for the actual transplant, described by the appropriate ICD procedure or CPT codes in

Revenue Center 0362 (Operating Room Services; Organ Transplant, Other than Kidney) or another appropriate cost center.

The CPT codes describing autologous stem cell harvesting procedures may be billed and are separately payable under the Outpatient Prospective Payment System (OPPS) when provided in the hospital outpatient setting of care. Autologous harvesting procedures are distinct from the acquisition services described in Pub. 100-04, Chapter 3, §90.3.1 and §231.11 of this chapter for allogeneic stem cell transplants, which include services provided when stem cells are obtained from a donor and not from the patient undergoing the stem cell transplant.

The CPT codes describing autologous stem cell processing procedures also may be billed and are separately payable under the OPPS when provided to hospital outpatients.

100-04, 4, 231.11

Billing for Allogeneic Stem Cell Transplants

(Rev. 3571, Issued: 07-29-16, Effective: 01-01-17, Implementation: 01-03-17)

1. Definition of Acquisition Charges for Allogeneic Stem Cell Transplants

Acquisition charges for allogeneic stem cell transplants include, but are not limited to, charges for the costs of the following services:

- National Marrow Donor Program fees, if applicable, for stem cells from an unrelated donor;
- Tissue typing of donor and recipient;
- Donor evaluation;
- Physician pre-procedure donor evaluation services;
- Costs associated with harvesting procedure (e.g., general routine and special care services, procedure/operating room and other ancillary services, apheresis services,etc.);
- Post-operative/post-procedure evaluation of donor; and
- Preparation and processing of stem cells.

Payment for these acquisition services is included in the OPPS C-APC payment for the allogeneic stem cell transplant when the transplant occurs in the hospital outpatient setting, and in the MS-DRG payment for the allogeneic stem cell transplant when the transplant occurs in the inpatient setting. The Medicare contractor does not make separate payment for these acquisition services, because hospitals may bill and receive payment only for services provided to the Medicare beneficiary who is the recipient of the stem cell transplant and whose illness is being treated with the stem cell transplant. Unlike the acquisition costs of solid organs for transplant (e.g., hearts and kidneys), which are paid on a reasonable cost basis, acquisition costs for allogeneic stem cells are included in prospective payment. Recurring update notifications describing changes to and billing instructions for various payment policies implemented in the OPPS are issued annually.

Acquisition charges for stem cell transplants apply only to allogeneic transplants, for which stem cells are obtained from a donor (other than the recipient himself or herself). Acquisition charges do not apply to autologous transplants (transplanted stem cells are obtained from the recipient himself or herself), because autologous transplants involve services provided to the beneficiary only (and not to a donor), for which the hospital may bill and receive payment (see Pub. 100-04, chapter 3, §90.3.1 and §231.10 of this chapter for information regarding billing for autologous stem cell transplants).

2. Billing for Acquisition Services

The hospital bills and shows acquisition charges for allogeneic stem cell transplants based on the status of the patient (i.e., inpatient or outpatient) when the transplant is furnished. See Pub. 100-04, chapter 3, §90.3.1 for instructions regarding billing for acquisition services for allogeneic stem cell transplants that are performed in the inpatient setting.

Effective January 1, 2017, when the allogeneic stem cell transplant occurs in the outpatient setting, the hospital identifies stem cell acquisition charges for allogeneic bone marrow/stem cell transplants separately in FL 42 of Form CMS-1450 (or electronic equivalent) by using revenue code 0815 (Other Organ Acquisition). Revenue code 0815 charges should include all services required to acquire stem cells from a donor, as defined above, and should be reported on the same date of service as the transplant procedure in order to be appropriately packaged for payment purposes.

The transplant hospital keeps an itemized statement that identifies the services furnished, the charges, the person receiving the service (donor/recipient), and whether this is a potential transplant donor or recipient. These charges will be reflected in the transplant hospital's stem cell/bone marrow acquisition cost center. For allogeneic stem cell acquisition services in cases that do not result in transplant, due to death of the intended recipient or other causes, hospitals include the costs associated with the acquisition services on the Medicare cost report.

In the case of an allogeneic transplant in the hospital outpatient setting, the hospital reports the transplant itself with the appropriate CPT code, and a charge under revenue center code 0362 or another appropriate cost center. Selection of the cost center is up to the hospital.

100-04, 4, 250.16

Multiple Procedure Payment Reduction (MPPR) on Certain Diagnostic Imaging Procedures Rendered by Physicians

(Rev. 3578, Issued: 08-05 Effective: 01-01-17, Implementation: 01-03-17)

Diagnostic imaging procedures rendered by a physician that has reassigned their billing rights to a Method II CAH are payable by Medicare when the procedures are eligible and billed on type of bill 85x with revenue code (RC) 096x, 097x and/or 098x.

The MPPR on diagnostic imaging applies when multiple services are furnished by the same physician to the same patient in the same session on the same day. Full payment is made for each service with the highest payment under the MPFS. Effective for dates of services on or after January 1, 2012, payment is made at 75 percent for each subsequent service; and effective for dates of services on or after January 1, 2017, payment is made at 95 percent for each subsequent service.

100-04, 4, 250.18

Incomplete Colonoscopies (Codes 44388, 45378, G0105 and G0121)

(Rev. 4153, Issued: 10-26-18, Effective: 04-01-19, Implementation: 04-01-19)

An incomplete colonoscopy, e.g., the inability to advance the colonoscope to the cecum or colon-small intestine anastomosis due to unforeseen circumstances, is billed and paid using colonoscopy through stoma code 44388, colonoscopy code 45378, and screening colonoscopy codes G0105 and G0121 with modifier "-53." (Code 44388 is valid with modifier 53 beginning January 1, 2016.) The Medicare physician fee schedule database has specific values for codes 44388-53, 45378-53, G0105-53 and G0121-53. An incomplete colonoscopy performed prior to January 1, 2016, is paid at the same rate as a sigmoidoscopy. Beginning January 1, 2016, Medicare will pay for the interrupted colonoscopy at a rate that is calculated using one-half the value of the inputs for the codes.

As such, instruct CAHs that elect Method II payment to use modifier "-53" to identify an incomplete screening colonoscopy (physician professional service(s) billed in revenue code 096X, 097X, and/or 098X).

CAH Method II shall be consistent with the guidelines outlined in PUB. 100-04, chapter 12, section 30.1 and chapter 18, section 60.2.

100-04, 4, 260.1

Special Partial Hospitalization Billing Requirements forHospitals, Community Mental Health Centers, and Critical Access Hospitals

(Rev. 4204, Issued: 01-17-19, Effective: 01-01-19, Implementation: 01-07-19)

Medicare Part B coverage is available for hospital outpatient partial hospitalization services.

A. Billing Requirement

Section 1861 (http://www.socialsecurity.gov/OP_Home/ssact/title18/1800.htm) of the Act defines the services under the partial hospitalization benefit in a hospital.

Section 1866(e)(2) of the Act (http://www.socialsecurity.gov/OP_Home/ssact/title18/1800.htm)recognizes CMHCs as "providers of services" but only for furnishing partial hospitalization services. See §261.1.1 of this chapter for CMHC partial hospitalization bill review directions.

Hospitals and CAHs report condition code 41 in FLs 18-28 (or electronic equivalent) to indicate the claim is for partial hospitalization services. They must also report a revenue code and the charge for each individual covered service furnished. In addition, hospital outpatient departments are required to report HCPCS codes. CAHs are not required to report HCPCS code for this benefit.

Under component billing, hospitals are required to report a revenue code and the charge for each individual covered service furnished under a partial hospitalization program. In addition, hospital outpatient departments are requlred to report HCPCS codes. Component billing assures that only those partial hospitalization services covered under §1861(ff) of the Act are paid by the Medicare program.

Effective January 1, 2017, non-excepted off-campus provider-based departments of a hospital are required to report a "PN" modifier on each claim line for non-excepted items and services. The use of modifier "PN" will trigger a payment rate under the Medicare Physician Fee Schedule. We expect the PN modifier to be reported with each non-excepted item and service including those for which payment will not be adjusted, such as separately payable drugs, clinical laboratory tests, and therapy services.

Excepted off-campus provider-based departments of a hospital must continue to report existing modifier "PO" (Services, procedures and/or surgeries provided at off-campus provider-based outpatient departments) for all excepted items and services furnished. Use of the off-campus PBD modifier became mandatory beginning January 1, 2016.

All hospitals are required to report condition code 41 in FLs 18-28 to indicate the claim is for partial hospitalization services. Hospitals use bill type 13X and CAHs use bill type 85X. The following special procedures apply.

Bills must contain an acceptable revenue code. They are as follows:

Revenue Code	Description
0250	Drugs and Biologicals
043X	Occupational Therapy
0900	Behavioral Health Treatment/Services
0904	Activity Therapy
0910	Psychiatric/Psychological Services (Dates of Service prior to October 16, 2003)
0914	Individual Therapy
0915	Group Therapy
0916	Family Therapy
0918	Behavioral Health/Testing
0942	Education/Training

Psychiatric diagnostic evaluation (no medical services) completed by a non-physician.

*****The definition of code 90792 is as follows:

Psychiatric diagnostic evaluation (with medical services) completed by a physician.

Codes G0129 and G0176 are used only for partial hospitalization programs.

Code G0177 may be used in both partial hospitalization program and outpatient mental health settings.

Revenue code 250 does not require HCPCS coding. However, Medicare does not cover drugs that can be self-administered.

Edit to assure that HCPCS are present when the above revenue codes are billed and that they are valid HCPCS codes. Do not edit for the matching of revenue code to HCPCS.

B. Professional Services

The professional services listed below when provided in all hospital outpatient departments are separately covered and paid as the professional services of physicians and other practitioners. These professional services are unbundled and these practitioners (other than physician assistants (PA) bill the Medicare A/B MAC (B) directly for the professional services furnished to hospital outpatient partial hospitalization patients. The hospital can also serve as a billing agent for these professionals by billing the A/B MAC (B) on their behalf under their billing number for their professional services. The professional services of a PA can be billed to the A/B MAC (B) only by the PAs employer. The employer of a PA may be such entities or individuals as a physician, medical group, professional corporation, hospital, SNF, or nursing facility. For example, if a physician is the employer of the PA and the PA renders services in the hospital, the physician and not the hospital would be responsible for billing the A/B MAC (B) on Form CMS-1500 for the services of the PA. The following direct professional services are unbundled and not paid as partial hospitalization services.

- Physician services that meet the criteria of 42 CFR 415.102, for payment on a fee schedule basis;
- Physician assistant (PA) services as defined in §1861(s)(2)(K)(i) of the Act;
- Nurse practitioner and clinical nurse specialist services, as defined in §1861(s)(2)(K)(ii) of the Act; and
- Clinical psychologist services as defined in §1861(ii) of the Act.

The services of other practitioners (including clinical social workers and occupational therapists), are bundled when furnished to hospital patients, including partial hospitalization patients. The hospital must bill the contractor for such nonphysician practitioner services as partial hospitalization services. Make payment for the services to the hospital.

C. Outpatient Mental Health Treatment Limitation

The outpatient mental health treatment limitation may apply to services to treat mental, psychoneurotic, and

personality disorders when furnished by physicians, clinical psychologists, NPs, CNSs, and PAs to partial hospitalization patients. However, the outpatient mental health treatment limitation does not apply to such mental health treatment services billed to the A/B MAC (A) by a CMHC or hospital outpatient department as partial hospitalization services.

D. Reporting of Service Units

Hospitals report the number of times the service or procedure, as defined by the HCPCS code, was performed. CAHs report the number of times the revenue code visit was performed.

NOTE: Service units are not required to be reported for drugs and biologicals (Revenue Code 250).

E. Line Item Date of Service Reporting

Hospitals other than CAHs are required to report line item dates of service per revenue code line for partial hospitalization claims. This means each service (revenue code) provided must be repeated on a separate line item along with the specific date the service was provided for every occurrence. Line item dates of service are reported in FL 45 "Service Date" (MMDDYY). See §260.5 for a detailed explanation.

F. Payment

Starting in CY 2017 and subsequent years, the payment structure for partial hospitalization services provided in hospital outpatient departments and CMHCs has been reduced from four APCs (two for CMHCs and two for hospital-based PHPs) to a single APC by provider type. Effective January 2, 2017, we are replacing existing CMHC APCs 5851 (Level 1 Partial Hospitalization (3 services)) and 5852 (Level 2 Partial Hospitalization (4 or more services)) with a new CMHC APC 5853 (Partial Hospitalization (3 or More Services Per Day)), and replacing existing hospital-based PHP APCs 5861 (Level 1 Partial Hospitalization (3 services)) and 5862 (Level 2 Partial Hospitalization (4 or more services)) with a new hospital-based PHP APC 5863 (Partial Hospitalization (3 or More Services Per Day)). The following chart displays the CMHC and hospital-based PHPAPCs:

Hospital-Based and Community Mental Health Center PHP APCs CY 2017 APC	Group Title
5853	Partial Hospitalization (3 or more services per day) for CMHCs
5863	Partial Hospitalization (3 or more services per day) for hospital-based PHPs

Apply Part B deductible, if any, and coinsurance.

G. Data for CWF and PS&R

Include revenue codes, HCPCS/CPT codes, units, and covered charges in the financial data section (fields 65a - 65j), as appropriate. Report the billed charges in field 65h, "Charges," of the CWF record.

Include in the financial data portion of the PS&R UNIBILL, revenue codes, HCPCS/CPT codes, units, and charges, as appropriate.

Future updates will be issued in a Recurring Update Notification.

100-04, 4, 260.1.1

Bill Review for Partial Hospitalization Services Provided in Community Mental Health Centers (CMHC)

(Rev. 4204, Issued: 01-17-19, Effective: 01-01-19, Implementation: 01-07-19)

A. General

Medicare Part B coverage for partial hospitalization services provided by CMHCs is available effective for services provided on or after October 1, 1991.

B. Special Requirements

Section 1866(e)(2) (http://www.socialsecurity.gov/OP_Home/ssact/title18/1800.htm) of the Act recognizes CMHCs as "providers of services" but only for furnishing partial hospitalization services. Applicable provider ranges are 1400-1499, 4600-4799, and 4900-4999.

C. Billing Requirements

The CMHCs bill for partial hospitalization services under bill type 76X. The A/B MACs (A) follow bill review instructions in chapter 25 of this manual, except for those listed below.

The acceptable revenue codes are as follows:

Revenue Code	Description
0250	Drugs and Biologicals
043X	Occupational Therapy
0900	Behavioral Health Treatments/Services
0904	Activity Therapy
0910	Psychiatric/Psychological Services (Dates of Service prior to October 16, 2003)
0914	Individual Therapy
0915	Group Therapy
0916	Family Therapy
0918	Behavioral Health/Testing
0942	Education/Training

The A/B MAC(s) (A) edit to assure that HCPCS are present when the above revenue codes are billed and that they are valid HCPCS codes. They do not edit for the matching of revenue codes to HCPCS.

Definitions each of the asterisked HCPCS codes follows:

*The definition of code G0129 is as follows:

Occupational therapy services requiring the skills of a qualified occupational therapist, furnished as a component of a partial hospitalization treatment program, per session (45 minutes or more).

**The definition of code G0176 is as follows:

Activity therapy, such as music, dance, art or play therapies not for recreation, related to the care and treatment of patient's disabling mental health problems, per session (45 minutes or more).

***The definition of code G0177 is as follows:

Training and educational services related to the care and treatment of patient's disabling mental health problems, per session (45 minutes or more).

****The definition of code 90791 is as follows:

Psychiatric diagnostic evaluation (no medical services) completed by a non-physician.

*****The definition of code 90792 is as follows:

Psychiatric diagnostic evaluation (with medical services) completed by a physician.

Codes G0129 and G0176 are used only for partial hospitalization programs.

Code G0177 may be used in both partial hospitalization program and outpatient mental health settings.

Revenue code 0250 does not require HCPCS coding. However, drugs that can be self-administered are not covered by Medicare.

HCPCS includes CPT-4 codes. See the ASC X12 837 institutional claim guide for how to report HCPCS electronically. CMHCs report HCPCS codes on Form CMS-1450 in FL44, "HCPCS/Rates." HCPCS code reporting is effective for claims with dates of service on or after April 1, 2000.

The A/B MACs (A) are to advise their CMHCs of these requirements. CMHCs should complete the remaining items on the claim in accordance with the ASC X12 837 Institutional Claim implementation guide and the Form CMS-1450 instructions in Chapter 25 of this manual.

The professional services listed below are separately covered and are paid as the professional services of physicians and other practitioners. These professional services are unbundled and these practitioners (other than physician assistants (PAs)) bill the A/B MAC (B) directly for the professional services furnished to CMHC partial hospitalization patients. The ASC X12 837 professional claim format or the paper form 1500 is used. The CMHC can also serve as a billing agent for these professionals by billing the A/B MAC (B) on their behalf for their professional services. The professional services of a PA can be billed to the A/B MAC (B) only by the PAs employer. The employer of a PA may be such entities or individuals as a physician, medical group, professional corporation, hospital, SNF, or nursing facility. For example, if a physician is the employer of the PA and the PA renders services in the CMHC, the physician and not the CMHC would be responsible for billing the A/B MAC (B) for the services of the PA.

The following professional services are unbundled and not paid as partial hospitalization services:

- Physician services that meet the criteria of 42 CFR 415.102, for payment on a fee schedule basis;
- PA services, as defined in §1861(s)(2)(K)(i) (http://www.socialsecurity.gov/OP_Home/ssact/title18/1800.htm) of the Act;
- Nurse practitioner and clinical nurse specialist services, as defined in §1861(s)(2)(K)(ii) (http://www.socialsecurity.gov/OP_Home/ssact/title18/1800.htm) of the Act; and,
- Clinical psychologist services, as defined in §1861(ii) (http://www.socialsecurity.gov/OP_Home/ssact/title18/1800.htm) of the Act.

The services of other practitioners (including clinical social workers and occupational therapists) are bundled when furnished to CMHC patients. The CMHC must bill the A/B MAC (A) for such nonphysician practitioner services as partial hospitalization services. The A/B MAC (A) makes payment for the services to the CMHC.

D. Outpatient Mental Health Treatment Limitation

The outpatient mental health treatment limitation may apply to services to treat mental, psychoneurotic, and personality disorders when furnished by physicians, clinical psychologists, NPs, CNSs, and PAs to partial hospitalization patients. However, the outpatient mental health treatment limitation does not apply to such mental health treatment services billed to the A/B MAC (A) as partial hospitalization services.

E. Reporting of Service Units

Visits should no longer be reported as units. Instead, CMHCs report in the field, "Service Units," the number of times the service or procedure, as defined by the HCPCS code, was performed when billing for partial hospitalization services identified by revenue code in subsection C.

EXAMPLE: A beneficiary received psychological testing performed by a physician for a total of 3 hours during one day (HCPCS code 96130, first hour; HCPCS code 96131 for 2 additional hours). The CMHC reports revenue code 0918, HCPCS code 96130, and 1 unit; and a second line on the claim showing revenue code 918, HCPCS code 96131, and 2 units.

When reporting service units for HCPCS codes where the definition of the procedure does not include any reference to time (either minutes, hours or days), CMHCs should not bill for sessions of less than 45 minutes.

The CMHC need not report service units for drugs and biologicals (Revenue Code 0250)

NOTE: Information regarding the Form CMS-1450 form locators that correspond with these fields is found in Chapter 25 of this manual. See the ASC X12 837 Institutional Claim implementation guide for related guidelines for the electronic claim.

F. Line Item Date of Service Reporting

Dates of service per revenue code line for partial hospitalization claims that span two or more dates. This means each service (revenue code) provided must be repeated on a separate line item along with the specific date the service was provided for every occurrence. Line item dates of service are reported in "Service Date". See examples below of reporting line item dates of service. These examples are for group therapy services provided twice during a billing period.

For claims, report as follows:

Revenue Code	HCPCS	Dates of Service	Units	Total Charges
0915	G0176	20090505	1	$80
0915	G0176	20090529	2	$160

NOTE: Information regarding the Form CMS-1450 form locators that correspond with these fields is found in Chapter 25 of this manual. See the ASC X12 837 Institutional Claim Implementation Guide for related guidelines for the electronic claim.

The A/B MACs (A) return to provider claims that span two or more dates if a line item date of service is not entered for each HCPCS code reported or if the line item dates of service reported are outside of the statement covers period. Line item date of service reporting is effective for claims with dates of service on or after June 5, 2000.

G. Payment

Section 1833(a)(2)(B) (http://www.socialsecurity.gov/OP_Home/ssact/title18/1800.htm) of the Act provides the statutory authority governing payment for partial hospitalization services provided by a CMHC. A/B MAC(s) (A) made payment on a reasonable cost basis until OPPS was implemented. The Part B deductible and coinsurance applied.

Payment principles applicable to partial hospitalization services furnished in CMHCs are contained in §2400 of the Medicare Provider Reimbursement Manual.

The A/B MACs (A) make payment on a per diem basis under the hospital outpatient prospective payment system for partial hospitalization services. CMHCs must continue to maintain documentation to support medical necessity of each service provided, including the beginning and ending time.

Effective January 1, 2011, there were four separate APC payment rates for PHP: two for CMHCs (for Level I and Level II services based on only CMHC data) and two for hospital-based PHPs (for Level I and Level II services based on only hospital-based PHP data).

The two CMHC APCS for providing partial hospitalization services were: APC 5851 (Level 1 Partial Hospitalization (3 services)) and APC 5852 (Level 2 Partial Hospitalization (4 or more services)). Effective January 1, 2017, we are combining APCs 5851 and 5852 into one new APC 5853 (Partial Hospitalization (3 or more services) for CMHCs).

Community Mental Health Center PHP APC APC	Group Title
5853	Partial Hospitalization (3 or more services per day) for CMHCs

NOTE: Occupational therapy services provided to partial hospitalization patients are not subject to the prospective payment system for outpatient rehabilitation services, and therefore the financial limitation required under §4541 of the Balanced Budget Act (BBA) does not apply.

H. Medical Review

The A/B MACs (A) follow medical review guidelines in Pub. 100-08, Medicare Program Integrity Manual.

I. Coordination with CWF

See chapter 27 of this manual. All edits for bill type 74X apply, except provider number ranges 4600-4799 are acceptable only for services provided on or after October 1, 1991.

100-04, 4, 290.5.3

Billing and Payment for Observation Services Furnished Beginning January 1, 2016

(Rev. 3425, Issued: 12-18-15, Effective: 01-01-16, Implementation: 01-04-16)

Observation services are reported using HCPCS code G0378 (Hospital observation service, per hour). Beginning January 1, 2008, HCPCS code G0378 for hourly observation services is assigned status indicator N, signifying that its payment is always packaged. No separate payment is made for observation services reported with HCPCS code G0378, and APC 0339 is deleted as of January 1, 2008. In most circumstances, observation services are supportive and ancillary to the other services provided to a patient. Beginning January 1, 2016, in certain circumstances when observation services are billed in conjunction with a clinic visit, Type A emergency department visit (Level 1 through 5), Type B emergency department visit (Level 1 through 5), critical care services, or a direct referral as an integral part of a patient's extended encounter of care, comprehensive payment may be made for all services on the claim including, the entire extended care encounter through comprehensive APC 8011 (Comprehensive Observation Services) when certain criteria are met. For information about comprehensive APCs, see §10.2.3 (Comprehensive APCs) of this chapter.

There is no limitation on diagnosis for payment of APC 8011; however, comprehensive APC payment will not be made when observation services are reported in association with a surgical procedure (T status procedure) or the hours of observation care reported are less than 8. The I/OCE evaluates every claim received to determine if payment through a comprehensive APC is appropriate. If payment through a comprehensive APC is inappropriate, the I/OCE, in conjunction with the Pricer, determines the appropriate status indicator, APC, and payment for every code on a claim.

All of the following requirements must be met in order for a hospital to receive a comprehensive APC payment through the Comprehensive Observation Services APC (APC 8011):

1. Observation Time
   a. Observation time must be documented in the medical record.
   b. Hospital billing for observation services begins at the clock time documented in the patient's medical record, which coincides with the time that observation services are initiated in accordance with a physician's order for observation services.
   c. A beneficiary's time receiving observation services (and hospital billing) ends when all clinical or medical interventions have been completed, including follow-up care furnished by hospital staff and physicians that may take place after a physician has ordered the patient be released or admitted as an inpatient.
   d. The number of units reported with HCPCS code G0378 must equal or exceed 8 hours.
2. Additional Hospital Services
   a. The claim for observation services must include one of the following services in addition to the reported observation services. The additional services listed below must have a line item date of service on the same day or the day before the date reported for observation:
      - A Type A or B emergency department visit (CPT codes 99281 through 99285 or HCPCS codes G0380 through G0384); or
      - A clinic visit (HCPCS code G0463); or
      - Critical care (CPT code 99291); or
      - Direct referral for observation care reported with HCPCS code G0379 (APC 5013) must be reported on the same date of service as the date reported for observation services.
   b. No procedure with a T status indicator or a J1 status indicator can be reported on the claim.
3. Physician Evaluation
   a. The beneficiary must be in the care of a physician during the period of observation, as documented in the medical record by outpatient registration, discharge, and other appropriate progress notes that are timed, written, and signed by the physician.
   b. The medical record must include documentation that the physician explicitly assessed patient risk to determine that the beneficiary would benefit from observation care.

Criteria 1 and 3 related to observation care beginning and ending time and physician evaluation apply regardless of whether the hospital believes that the criteria will be met for payment of the extended encounter through the Comprehensive Observation Services APC (APC 8011).

Only visits, critical care and observation services that are billed on a 13X bill type may be considered for a comprehensive APC payment through the Comprehensive Observation Services APC (APC 8011).

Non-repetitive services provided on the same day as either direct referral for observation care or observation services must be reported on the same claim because the OCE claim-by-claim logic cannot function properly unless all services related to the episode of observation care, including hospital clinic visits, emergency department visits, critical care services, and T status procedures, are reported on the same claim. Additional guidance can be found in chapter 1, section 50.2.2 of this manual.

If a claim for services provided during an extended assessment and management encounter including observation care does not meet all of the requirements listed above, then the usual APC logic will apply to separately payable items and services on the claim; the special logic for direct admission will apply, and payment for the observation care will be packaged into payments for other separately payable services provided to the beneficiary in the same encounter.

100-04, 5, 10

Part B Outpatient Rehabilitation and Comprehensive Outpatient Rehabilitation Facility (CORF) Services - General

(Rev. 3454, Issued: 02-04-16, Effective: 07-01-16, Implementation: 07-05-16)

Language in this section is defined or described in Pub. 100-02, chapter 15, sections 220 and 230.

Section §1834(k)(5) to the Social Security Act (the Act), requires that all claims for outpatient rehabilitation services and comprehensive outpatient rehabilitation facility (CORF) services, be reported using a uniform coding system. The CMS chose HCPCS (Healthcare Common Procedure Coding System) as the coding system to be used for the reporting of these services. This coding requirement is effective for all claims for outpatient rehabilitation services and CORF services submitted on or after April 1, 1998.

The Act also requires payment under a prospective payment system for outpatient rehabilitation services including CORF services. Effective for claims with dates of service on or after January 1, 1999, the Medicare Physician Fee Schedule (MPFS) became the method of payment for outpatient therapy services furnished by:

- Comprehensive outpatient rehabilitation facilities (CORFs);
- Outpatient physical therapy providers (OPTs), also known as rehabilitation agencies;
- Hospitals (to outpatients and inpatients who are not in a covered Part A stay);
- Skilled nursing facilities (SNFs) (to residents not in a covered Part A stay and to nonresidents who receive outpatient rehabilitation services from the SNF); and
- Home health agencies (HHAs) (to individuals who are not homebound or otherwise are not receiving services under a home health plan of care (POC)).

NOTE: No provider or supplier other than the SNF will be paid for therapy services during the time the beneficiary is in a covered SNF Part A stay. For information regarding SNF consolidated billing see chapter 6, section 10 of this manual.

Similarly, under the HH prospective payment system, HHAs are responsible to provide, either directly or under arrangements, all outpatient rehabilitation therapy services to beneficiaries receiving services under a home health POC. No other provider or supplier will be paid for these services during the time the beneficiary is in a covered Part A stay. For information regarding HH consolidated billing see chapter10, section 20 of this manual.

Section 143 of the Medicare Improvements for Patients and Provider's Act of 2008 (MIPPA) authorizes the Centers for Medicare & Medicaid Services (CMS) to enroll speech-language pathologists (SLP) as suppliers of Medicare services and for SLPs to begin billing Medicare for outpatient speech-language pathology services furnished in private practice beginning July 1, 2009. Enrollment will allow SLPs in private practice to bill Medicare and receive direct payment for their services. Previously, the Medicare program could only pay SLP services if an institution, physician or nonphysician practitioner billed them.

In Chapter 23, as part of the CY 2009 Medicare Physician Fee Schedule Database, the descriptor for PC/TC indicator "7", as applied to certain HCPCS/CPT codes, is described as specific to the services of privately practicing therapists. Payment may not be made if the service is provided to either a hospital outpatient or a hospital inpatient by a physical therapist, occupational therapist, or speech-language pathologist in private practice.

The MPFS is used as a method of payment for outpatient rehabilitation services furnished under arrangement with any of these providers.

In addition, the MPFS is used as the payment system for CORF services identified by the HCPCS codes in §20. Assignment is mandatory.

Services that are paid subject to the MPFS are adjusted based on the applicable payment locality. Rehabilitation agencies and CORFs with service locations in different payment localities shall follow the instructions for multiple service locations in chapter 1, section 170.1.1.

The Medicare allowed charge for the services is the lower of the actual charge or the MPFS amount. The Medicare payment for the services is 80 percent of the allowed charge after the Part B deductible is met. Coinsurance is made at 20 percent of the lower of the actual charge or the MPFS amount. The general coinsurance rule (20 percent of the actual charges) does not apply when making payment under the MPFS. This is a final payment.

The MPFS does not apply to outpatient rehabilitation services furnished by critical access hospitals (CAHs) or hospitals in Maryland. CAHs are to be paid on a reasonable cost basis. Maryland hospitals are paid under the Maryland All-Payer Model.

Contractors process outpatient rehabilitation claims from hospitals, including CAHs, SNFs, HHAs, CORFs, outpatient rehabilitation agencies, and outpatient physical therapy providers for which they have received a tie in notice from the Regional Office (RO). These provider types submit their claims to the contractors using the ASC X12 837 institutional claim format or the CMS-1450 paper form when permissible. Contractors also process claims from physicians, certain nonphysician practitioners (NPPs), therapists in private practices (TPPs), (which are limited to physical and occupational therapists, and speech-language pathologists in private practices), and physician-directed clinics that bill for services furnished incident to a physician's service (see Pub. 100-02, Medicare Benefit Policy Manual, chapter 15, for a definition of "incident to"). These provider types submit their claims to the contractor using the ASC X 12 837 professional claim format or the CMS-1500 paper form when permissible.

There are different fee rates for nonfacility and facility services. Chapter 23 describes the differences in these two rates. (See fields 28 and 29 of the record therein described). Facility rates apply to professional services performed in a facility other than the professional's office. Nonfacility rates apply when the service is performed in the professional's office. The nonfacility rate (that is paid when the provider performs the services in its own facility) accommodates overhead and indirect expenses the provider incurs by operating its own facility. Thus it is somewhat higher than the facility rate.

Contractors pay the nonfacility rate on institutional claims for services performed in the provider's facility. Contractors may pay professional claims using the facility or nonfacility rate depending upon where the service is performed (place of service on the claim), and the provider specialty.

Contractors pay the codes in §20 under the MPFS on professional claims regardless of whether they may be considered rehabilitation services. However, contractors must use this list for institutional claims to determine whether to pay under outpatient rehabilitation rules or whether payment rules for other types of service may apply, e.g., OPPS for hospitals, reasonable costs for CAHs.

Note that because a service is considered an outpatient rehabilitation service does not automatically imply payment for that service. Additional criteria, including coverage, plan of care and physician certification must also be met. These criteria are described in Pub. 100-02, Medicare Benefit Policy Manual, chapters 1 and 15.

Payment for rehabilitation services provided to Part A inpatients of hospitals or SNFs is included in the respective PPS rate. Also, for SNFs (but not hospitals), if the beneficiary has Part B, but not Part A coverage (e.g., Part A benefits are exhausted), the SNF must bill for any rehabilitation service.

Payment for rehabilitation therapy services provided by home health agencies under a home health plan of care is included in the home health PPS rate. HHAs may submit bill type 34X and be paid under the MPFS if there are no home health services billed under a home health plan of care at the same time, and there is a valid rehabilitation POC (e.g., the patient is not homebound).

An institutional employer (other than a SNF) of the TPPs, or physician performing outpatient services, (e.g., hospital, CORF, etc.), or a clinic billing on behalf of the physician or therapist may bill the contractor on a professional claim.

The MPFS is the basis of payment for outpatient rehabilitation services furnished by TPPs, physicians, and certain nonphysician practitioners or for diagnostic tests provided incident to the services of such physicians or nonphysician practitioners. (See Pub. 100-02, Medicare Benefit Policy Manual, Chapter 15, for a definition of "incident to, therapist, therapy and related instructions.") Such services are billed to the contractor on the professional claim format. Assignment is mandatory.

The following table identifies the provider and supplier types, and identifies which claim format they may use to submit claims for outpatient therapy services to the contractor.

"Provider/Supplier Service" Type	Format	Bill Type	Comment
Inpatient SNF Part A	Institutional	21X	Included in PPS
Inpatient hospital Part B	Institutional	12X	Hospital may obtain services under arrangements and bill, or rendering provider may bill.
Inpatient SNF Part B (audiology tests are not included)	Institutional	22X	SNF must provide and bill, or obtain under arrangements and bill.
Outpatient hospital	Institutional	13X	Hospital may provide and bill or obtain under arrangements and bill.
Outpatient SNF	Institutional	23X	SNF must provide and bill or obtain under arrangements and bill.
HHA billing for services not rendered under a Part A or Part B home health plan of care, but rendered under a therapy plan of care.	Institutional	34X	Service not under home health plan of care.
Outpatient physical therapy providers (OPTs), also known as rehabilitation agencies	Institutional	74X	Paid MPFS for outpatient rehabilitation services.
Comprehensive Outpatient Rehabilitation Facility (CORF)	Institutional	75X	Paid MPFS for outpatient rehabilitation services and all other services except drugs. Drugs are paid 95% of the AWP.
Physician, NPPs, TPPs, (therapy services in hospital or SNF)	Professional	See Chapter 26 for place of service coding.	Payment may not be made for therapy services to Part A inpatients of hospitals or SNFs, or for Part B SNF residents. **NOTE:** Payment may be made to physicians and NPPs for their professional services defined as "sometimes therapy" (not part of a therapy plan) in certain situations; for example, when furnished to a beneficiary registered as an outpatient of a hospital.
Physician/NPP/TPPs office, or patient's home	Professional	See Chapter 26 for place of service coding.	Paid via MPFS.
Critical Access Hospital - inpatient Part B	Institutional	12X	Rehabilitation services are paid at cost.
Critical Access Hospital – outpatient Part B	Institutional	85X	Rehabilitation services are paid at cost.

For a list of the outpatient rehabilitation HCPCS codes see §20.

If a contractor receives an institutional claim for one of these HCPCS codes with dates of service on or after July 1, 2003, that does not appear on the supplemental file it currently uses to pay the therapy claims, it contacts its professional claims area to obtain the non-facility price in order to pay the claim.

NOTE: The list of codes in §20 contains commonly utilized codes for outpatient rehabilitation services. Contractors may consider other codes on institutional claims for payment under the MPFS as outpatient rehabilitation services to the extent that such codes are determined to be medically reasonable and necessary and could be performed within the scope of practice of the therapist providing the service.

100-04, 5, 10.2

The Financial Limitation Legislation

(Rev. 2073, Issued:10-22-10, Effective: 01-01-11, Implementation: 01-03-11)

A. Legislation on Limitations

The dollar amount of the limitations (caps) on outpatient therapy services is established by statute. The updated amount of the caps is released annually via Recurring Update Notifications and posted on the CMS Website www.cms.gov/TherapyServices, on contractor Websites, and on each beneficiary's Medicare Summary Notice. Medicare contractors shall publish the financial limitation amount in educational articles. It is also available at 1-800-Medicare.

Section 4541(a)(2) of the Balanced Budget Act (BBA) (P.L. 105-33) of 1997, which added §1834(k)(5) to the Act, required payment under a prospective payment system (PPS) for outpatient rehabilitation services (except those furnished by or under arrangements with a hospital). Outpatient rehabilitation services include the following services:

- Physical therapy
- Speech-language pathology; and
- Occupational therapy.

Section 4541(c) of the BBA required application of financial limitations to all outpatient rehabilitation services (except those furnished by or under arrangements with a hospital).

In 1999, an annual per beneficiary limit of $1,500 was applied, including all outpatient physical therapy services and speech-language pathology services. A separate limit applied to all occupational therapy services. The limits were based on incurred expenses and included applicable deductible and coinsurance. The BBA provided that the limits be indexed by the Medicare Economic Index (MEI) each year beginning in 2002.

Since the limitations apply to outpatient services, they do not apply to skilled nursing facility (SNF) residents in a covered Part A stay, including patients occupying swing beds. Rehabilitation services are included within the global Part A per diem payment that the SNF receives under the prospective payment system (PPS) for the covered stay. Also, limitations do not apply to any therapy services covered under prospective payment systems for home health or inpatient hospitals, including critical access hospitals.

The limitation is based on therapy services the Medicare beneficiary receives, not the type of practitioner who provides the service. Physical therapists, speech-language pathologists, and occupational therapists, as well as physicians and certain nonphysician practitioners, could render a therapy service.

B. Moratoria and Exceptions for Therapy Claims

Since the creation of therapy caps, Congress has enacted several moratoria. The Deficit Reduction Act of 2005 directed CMS to develop exceptions to therapy caps for calendar year 2006 and the exceptions have been extended periodically. The cap exception for therapy services billed by outpatient hospitals was part of the original legislation and applies as long as caps are in effect. Exceptions to caps based on the medical necessity of the service are in effect only when Congress legislates the exceptions.

C. Repeal of Original Legislation and Replacement with Thresholds to Ensure Appropriate Therapy.

Section 50202 of the Bipartisan Budget Act of 2018 repeals application of the Medicare outpatient therapy caps but retains the former cap amounts as a threshold of incurred expenses above which claims must include a modifier as a confirmation that services are medically necessary as justified by appropriate documentation in the medical record. This is termed the KX modifier threshold.

Along with this KX modifier threshold, the new law retains the targeted medical review process but at a lower threshold amount of $3,000. For more information about the medical review (MR) threshold see the below section 10.3.4.

100-04, 5, 10.3.2

Exceptions Process

(Rev. 3670, Issued: 12-01-16, Effective: 01-01-17, Implementation: 01-03-17)

An exception may be made when the patient's condition is justified by documentation indicating that the beneficiary requires continued skilled therapy, i.e., therapy beyond the amount payable under the therapy cap, to achieve their prior functional status or maximum expected functional status within a reasonable amount of time.

No special documentation is submitted to the contractor for exceptions. The clinician is responsible for consulting guidance in the Medicare manuals and in the professional literature to determine if the beneficiary may qualify for the exception because documentation justifies medically necessary services above the caps. The clinician's opinion is not binding on the Medicare contractor who makes the final determination concerning whether the claim is payable.

Documentation justifying the services shall be submitted in response to any Additional Documentation Request (ADR) for claims that are selected for medical review. Follow the documentation requirements in Pub. 100-02, chapter 15, section 220.3. If medical records are requested for review, clinicians may include, at their discretion, a summary that specifically addresses the justification for therapy cap exception.

In making a decision about whether to utilize the exception, clinicians shall consider, for example, whether services are appropriate to--

The patient's condition, including the diagnosis, complexities, and severity;

The services provided, including their type, frequency, and duration;

The interaction of current active conditions and complexities that directly and significantly influence the treatment such that it causes services to exceed caps.

In addition, the following should be considered before using the exception process:

1. Exceptions for Evaluation Services

Evaluation. The CMS will accept therapy evaluations from caps after the therapy caps are reached when evaluation is necessary, e.g., to determine if the current status of the beneficiary requires therapy services. For example, the following CPT codes for evaluation procedures may be appropriate:

92521, 92522, 92523, 92524, 92597, 92607, 92608, 92610, 92611, 92612, 92614, 92616, 96105, 96125. 97161, 97162, 97163, 97164, 97165, 97166, 97167, and 97168.

These codes will continue to be reported as outpatient therapy procedures as listed in the Annual Therapy Update for the current year at: http://www.cms.gov/TherapyServices/05_Annual_Therapy_Update.asp#TopOfPage.

They are not diagnostic tests. Definitions of evaluations and documentation are found in Pub. 100-02, chapter 15, sections 220 and 230.

Other Services. There are a number of sources that suggest the amount of certain services that may be typical, either per service, per episode, per condition, or per discipline. For example, see the CSC - Therapy Cap Report, 3/21/2008, and CSC – Therapy Edits Tables 4/14/2008 at www.cms.hhs.gov/TherapyServices (Studies and Reports), or more recent utilization reports. Professional literature and guidelines from professional associations also provide a basis on which to estimate whether the type, frequency, and intensity of services are appropriate to an individual. Clinicians and contractors should utilize available evidence related to the patient's condition to justify provision of medically necessary services to individual beneficiaries, especially when they exceed caps. Contractors shall not limit medically necessary services that are justified by scientific research applicable to the beneficiary. Neither contractors nor clinicians shall utilize professional literature and scientific reports to justify payment for continued services after an individual's goals have been met earlier than is typical. Conversely, professional literature and scientific reports shall not be used as justification to deny payment to patients whose needs are greater than is typical or when the patient's condition is not represented by the literature.

2. Exceptions for Medically Necessary Services

Clinicians may utilize the process for exception for any diagnosis or condition for which they can justify services exceeding the cap. Regardless of the diagnosis or condition, the patient must also meet other requirements for coverage.

Bill the most relevant diagnosis. As always, when billing for therapy services, the diagnosis code that best relates to the reason for the treatment shall be on the claim, unless there is a compelling reason to report another diagnosis code. For example, when a patient with diabetes is being treated with therapy for gait training due to amputation, the preferred diagnosis is abnormality of gait (which characterizes the treatment). Where it is possible in accordance with State and local laws and the contractors' local coverage determinations, avoid using vague or general diagnoses. When a claim includes several types of services, or where the physician/NPP must supply the diagnosis, it may not be possible to use the most relevant therapy diagnosis code in the primary position. In that case, the relevant diagnosis code should, if possible, be on the claim in another position.

Codes representing the medical condition that caused the treatment are used when there is no code representing the treatment. Complicating conditions are preferably used in non-primary positions on the claim and are billed in the primary position only in the rare circumstance that there is no more relevant code.

The condition or complexity that caused treatment to exceed caps must be related to the therapy goals and must either be the condition that is being treated or a complexity that directly **and significantly impacts the rate of recovery of the condition being treated** such that it is appropriate to exceed the caps. Documentation for an exception should indicate how the complexity (or combination of complexities) directly and significantly affects treatment for a therapy condition.

If the contractor has determined that certain codes do not characterize patients who require medically necessary services, providers/suppliers may not use those codes, but must utilize a billable diagnosis code allowed by their contractor to describe the patient's condition. Contractors shall not apply therapy caps to services based on the patient's condition, but only on the medical necessity of the service for the condition. If a service would be payable before the cap is reached and is still medically necessary after the cap is reached, that service is excepted.

Contact your contractor for interpretation if you are not sure that a service is applicable for exception.

It is very important to recognize that most conditions would not ordinarily result in services exceeding the cap. Use the KX modifier only in cases where the condition of the individual patient is such that services are APPROPRIATELY provided in an episode that exceeds the cap. Routine use of the KX modifier for all patients with these conditions will likely show up on data analysis as aberrant and invite inquiry. Be sure that documentation is sufficiently detailed to support the use of the modifier.

In justifying exceptions for therapy caps, clinicians and contractors should not only consider the medical diagnoses and medical complications that might directly and significantly influence the amount of treatment required. Other variables (such as the availability of a caregiver at home) that affect appropriate treatment shall also be considered. Factors that influence the need for treatment should be supportable by published research, clinical guidelines from professional sources, and/or clinical or common sense. See Pub. 100-02, chapter 15, section 220.3 for information related to documentation of the evaluation, and section 220.2 on medical necessity for some factors that complicate treatment.

NOTE: The patient's lack of access to outpatient hospital therapy services alone, when outpatient hospital therapy services are excluded from the limitation, does not justify excepted services. Residents of skilled nursing facilities prevented by consolidated billing from accessing hospital services, debilitated patients for whom transportation to the hospital is a physical hardship, or lack of therapy services at hospitals in the beneficiary's county may or may not qualify as justification for continued services above the caps. The patient's condition and complexities might justify extended services, but their location does not. For dates of service on or after October 1, 2012, therapy services furnished in an outpatient hospital are not excluded from the limitation.

100-04, 5, 10.6

Functional Reporting

(Rev. 3670, Issued: 12-01-16, Effective: 01-01-17, Implementation: 01-03-17)

A. General

Section 3005(g) of the Middle Class Tax Relief and Jobs Creation Act (MCTRJCA) amended Section 1833(g) of the Act to require a claims-based data collection system for outpatient therapy services, including physical therapy (PT), occupational therapy (OT) and speech-language pathology (SLP) services. 42 CFR 410.59, 410.60, 410.61, 410.62 and 410.105 implement this requirement. The system will collect data on beneficiary function during the course of therapy services in order to better understand beneficiary conditions, outcomes, and expenditures.

Beneficiary unction information is reported using 42 nonpayable functional G-codes and seven severity/complexity modifiers on claims for PT, OT, and SLP services. Functional reporting on one functional limitation at a time is required periodically throughout an entire PT, OT, or SLP therapy episode of care.

The nonpayable G-codes and severity modifiers provide information about the beneficiary's functional status at the outset of the therapy episode of care, including projected goal status, at specified points during treatment, and at the time of discharge. These G-codes, along with the associated modifiers, are required at specified intervals on all claims for outpatient therapy services – not just those over the cap.

B. Application of New Coding Requirements

This functional data reporting and collection system is effective for therapy services with dates of service on and after January 1, 2013. A testing period will be in effect from January 1, 2013, until July 1, 2013, to allow providers and practitioners to use the new coding requirements to assure that systems work. Claims for therapy services furnished on and after July 1, 2013, that do not contain the required functional G-code/modifier information will be returned or rejected, as applicable.

C. Services Affected

These requirements apply to all claims for services furnished under the Medicare Part B outpatient therapy benefit and the PT, OT, and SLP services furnished under the CORF benefit. They also apply to the therapy services furnished personally by and incident to the service of a physician or a nonphysician practitioner (NPP), including a nurse practitioner (NP), a certified nurse specialist (CNS), or a physician assistant (PA), as applicable.

D. Providers and Practitioners Affected.

The functional reporting requirements apply to the therapy services furnished by the following providers: hospitals, CAHs, SNFs, CORFs, rehabilitation agencies, and HHAs (when the beneficiary is not under a home health plan of care). It applies to the following practitioners: physical therapists, occupational therapists, and speech-language pathologists in private practice (TPPs), physicians, and NPPs as noted above. The term "clinician" is applied to these practitioners throughout this manual section. (See definition section of Pub. 100-02, chapter 15, section 220.)

E. Function-related G-codes

There are 42 functional G-codes, 14 sets of three codes each. Six of the G-code sets are generally for PT and OT functional limitations and eight sets of G-codes are for SLP functional limitations.

The following G-codes are for functional limitations typically seen in beneficiaries receiving PT or OT services. The first four of these sets describe categories of functional limitations and the final two sets describe "other" functional limitations, which are to be used for functional limitations not described by one of the four categories.

NONPAYABLE G-CODES FOR FUNCTIONAL LIMITATIONS

	Long Descriptor	Short Descriptor
Mobility G-code Set		
G8978	Mobility: walking & moving around functional limitation, current status, at therapy episode outset and at reporting intervals	Mobility current status
G8979	Mobility: walking & moving around functional limitation, projected goal status, at therapy episode outset, at reporting intervals, and at discharge or to end reporting	Mobility goal status
G8980	Mobility: walking & moving around functional limitation, discharge status, at discharge from therapy or to end reporting	Mobility D/C status
Changing & Maintaining Body Position G-code Set		
G8981	Changing & maintaining body position functional limitation, current status, at therapy episode outset and at reporting intervals	Body pos current status
G8982	Changing & maintaining body position functional limitation, projected goal status, at therapy episode outset, at reporting intervals, and at discharge or to end reporting	Body pos goal status
G8983	Changing & maintaining body position functional limitation, discharge status, at discharge from therapy or to end reporting	Body pos D/C status
Carrying, Moving & Handling Objects G-code Set		
G8984	Carrying, moving & handling objects functional limitation, current status, at therapy episode outset and at reporting intervals	Carry current status
G8985	Carrying, moving & handling objects functional limitation, projected goal status, at therapy episode outset, at reporting intervals, and at discharge or to end reporting	Carry goal status
G8986	Carrying, moving & handling objects functional limitation, discharge status, at discharge from therapy or to end reporting	Carry D/C status
Self Care G-code Set		
G8987	Self care functional limitation, current status, at therapy episode outset and at reporting intervals	Self care current status
G8988	Self care functional limitation, projected goal status, at therapy episode outset, at reporting intervals, and at discharge or to end reporting	Self care goal status
G8989	Self care functional limitation, discharge status, at discharge from therapy or to end reporting	Self care D/C status

- The following "other PT/OT" functional G-codes are used to report:
- a beneficiary's functional limitation that is not defined by one of the above four categories;
- a beneficiary whose therapy services are not intended to treat a functional limitation;
- or a beneficiary's functional limitation when an overall, composite or other score from a functional assessment too is used and it does not clearly represent a functional limitation defined by one of the above four code sets.

	Long Descriptor	Short Descriptor
Other PT/OT Primary G-code Set		
G8990	Other physical or occupational therapy primary functional limitation, current status, at therapy episode outset and at reporting intervals	Other PT/OT current status
G8991	Other physical or occupational therapy primary functional limitation, projected goal status, at therapy episode outset, at reporting intervals, and at discharge or to end reporting	Other PT/OT goal status
G8992	Other physical or occupational therapy primary functional limitation, discharge status, at discharge from therapy or to end reporting	Other PT/OT D/C status
Other PT/OT Subsequent G-code Set		
G8993	Other physical or occupational therapy subsequent functional limitation, current status, at therapy episode outset and at reporting intervals	Sub PT/OT current status
G8994	Other physical or occupational therapy subsequent functional limitation, projected goal status, at therapy episode outset, at reporting intervals, and at discharge or to end reporting	Sub PT/OT goal status
G8995	Other physical or occupational subsequent functional limitation, discharge from therapy or end reporting.	Sub PT/OT D/C status

The following G-codes are for functional limitations typically seen in beneficiaries receiving SLP services. Seven are for specific functional communication measures, which are modeled after the National Outcomes Measurement System (NOMS), and one is for any "other" measure not described by one of the other seven.

	Long Descriptor	Short Descriptor
Swallowing G-code Set		
G8996	Swallowing functional limitation, current status, at therapy episode outset and at reporting intervals	Swallow current status
G8997	Swallowing functional limitation, projected goal status, at therapy episode outset, at reporting intervals, and at discharge or to end reporting	Swallow goal status
G8998	Swallowing functional limitation, discharge status, at discharge from therapy or to end reporting	Swallow D/C status
Motor Speech G-code Set (Note: These codes are not sequentially numbered)		
G8999	Motor speech functional limitation, current status, at therapy episode outset and at reporting intervals	Motor speech current status
G9186	Motor speech functional limitation, projected goal status at therapy episode outset, at reporting intervals, and at discharge or to end reporting	Motor speech goal status
G9158	Motor speech functional limitation, discharge status, at discharge from therapy or to end reporting	Motor speech D/C status
Spoken Language Comprehension G-code Set		
G9159	Spoken language comprehension functional limitation, current status, at therapy episode outset and at reporting intervals	Lang comp current status
G9160	Spoken language comprehension functional limitation, projected goal status, at therapy episode outset, at reporting intervals, and at discharge or to end reporting	Lang comp goal status
G9161	Spoken language comprehension functional limitation, discharge status, at discharge from therapy or to end reporting	Lang comp D/C status
Spoken Language Expressive G-code Set		
G9162	Spoken language expression functional limitation, current status, at therapy episode outset and at reporting intervals	Lang express current status
G9163	Spoken language expression functional limitation, projected goal status, at therapy episode outset, at reporting intervals, and at discharge or to end reporting	Lang press goal status
G9164	Spoken language expression functional limitation, discharge status, at discharge from therapy or to end reporting	Lang express D/C status
Attention G-code Set		
G9165	Attention functional limitation, current status, at therapy episode outset and at reporting intervals	Atten current status
G9166	Attention functional limitation, projected goal status, at therapy episode outset, at reporting intervals, and at discharge or to end reporting	Atten goal status

Appendix G — Medicare Internet-only Manuals (IOMs)

	Long Descriptor	Short Descriptor
G9167	Attention functional limitation, discharge status, at discharge from therapy or to end reporting	Atten D/C status
Memory G-code Set		
G9168	Memory functional limitation, current status, at therapy episode outset and at reporting intervals	Memory current status
G9169	Memory functional limitation, projected goal status, at therapy episode outset, at reporting intervals, and at discharge or to end reporting	Memory goal status
G9170	Memory functional limitation, discharge status, at discharge from therapy or to end reporting	Memory D/C status
Voice G-code Set		
G9171	Voice functional limitation, current status, at therapy episode outset and at reporting intervals	Voice current status
G9172	Voice functional limitation, projected goal status, at therapy episode outset, at reporting intervals, and at discharge or to end reporting	Voice goal status
G9173	Voice functional limitation, discharge status, at discharge from therapy or to end reporting	Voice D/C status

The following "other SLP" G-code set is used to report:

- on one of the other eight NOMS-defined functional measures not described by the above code sets; or
- to report an overall, composite or other score from assessment tool that does not clearly represent one of the above seven categorical SLP functional measures.

	Long Descriptor	Short Descriptor
Other Speech Language Pathology G-code Set		
G9174	Other speech language pathology functional limitation, current status, at therapy episode outset and at reporting intervals	Speech lang current status
G9175	Other speech language pathology functional limitation, projected goal status, at therapy episode outset, at reporting intervals, and at discharge or to end reporting	Speech lang goal status
G9176	Other speech language pathology functional limitation, discharge status, at discharge from therapy or to end reporting	Speech lang D/C status

F. Severity/Complexity Modifiers

For each nonpayable functional G-code, one of the modifiers listed below must be used to report the severity/complexity for that functional limitation.

Modifier	Impairment Limitation Restriction
CH	0 percent impaired, limited or restricted
CI	At least 1 percent but less than 20 percent impaired, limited or restricted
CJ	At least 20 percent but less than 40 percent impaired, limited or restricted
CK	At least 40 percent but less than 60 percent impaired, limited or restricted
CL	At least 60 percent but less than 80 percent impaired, limited or restricted
CM	At least 80 percent but less than 100 percent impaired, limited or restricted
CN	100 percent impaired, limited or restricted

The severity modifiers reflect the beneficiary's percentage of functional impairment as determined by the clinician furnishing the therapy services.

G. Required Reporting of Functional G-codes and Severity Modifiers

The functional G-codes and severity modifiers listed above are used in the required reporting on therapy claims at certain specified points during therapy episodes of care. Claims containing these functional G-codes must also contain another billable and separately payable (non-bundled) service. Only one functional limitation shall be reported at a given time for each related therapy plan of care (POC).

Functional reporting using the G-codes and corresponding severity modifiers is required reporting on specified therapy claims. Specifically, they are required on claims:

- At the outset of a therapy episode of care (i.e., on the claim for the date of service (DOS) of the initial therapy service);
- At least once every 10 treatment days, which corresponds with the progress reporting period;
- When an evaluative procedure, including a re-evaluative one, (HCPCS/CPT codes 92521, 92522, 92523, 92524, 92597, 92607, 92608, 92610, 92611, 92612, 92614, 92616, 96105, 96125, 97161, 97162, 97163, 97164, 97165, 97166, 97167, 97168) is furnished and billed;
- At the time of discharge from the therapy episode of care–(i.e., on the date services related to the discharge [progress] report are furnished); and
- At the time reporting of a particular functional limitation is ended in cases where the need for further therapy is necessary.
- At the time reporting is begun for a new or different functional limitation within the same episode of care (i.e., after the reporting of the prior functional limitation is ended)

Functional reporting is required on claims throughout the entire episode of care. When the beneficiary has reached his or her goal or progress has been maximized on the initially selected functional limitation, but the need for treatment continues, reporting is required for a second functional limitation using another set of G-codes. In these situations two or more functional limitations will be reported for a beneficiary during the therapy episode of care. Thus, reporting on more than one functional limitation may be required for some beneficiaries but not simultaneously.

When the beneficiary stops coming to therapy prior to discharge, the clinician should report the functional information on the last claim. If the clinician is unaware that the beneficiary is not returning for therapy until after the last claim is submitted, the clinician cannot report the discharge status.

When functional reporting is required on a claim for therapy services, two G-codes will generally be required.

Two exceptions exist:

1. Therapy services under more than one therapy POC. Claims may contain more than two nonpayable functional G-codes when in cases where a beneficiary receives therapy services under multiple POCs (PT, OT, and/or SLP) from the same therapy provider.
2. One-Time Therapy Visit. When a beneficiary is seen and future therapy services are either not medically indicated or are going to be furnished by another provider, the clinician reports on the claim for the DOS of the visit, all three G-codes in the appropriate code set (current status, goal status and discharge status), along with corresponding severity modifiers. Each reported functional G-code must also contain the following line of service information:
    - Functional severity modifier
    - Therapy modifier indicating the related discipline/POC -- GP, GO or GN -- for PT, OT, and SLP services, respectively
    - Date of the related therapy service
    - Nominal charge, e.g., a penny, for institutional claims submitted to the FIs and A/MACs. For professional claims, a zero charge is acceptable for the service line. If provider billing software requires an amount for professional claims, a nominal charge, e.g., a penny, may be included. Note: The KX modifier is not required on the claim line for nonpayable G-codes, but would be required with the procedure code for medically necessary therapy services furnished once the beneficiary's annual cap has been reached.

The following example demonstrates how the G-codes and modifiers are used. In this example, the clinician determines that the beneficiary's mobility restriction is the most clinically relevant functional limitation and selects the Mobility G-code set (G8978 – G8980) to represent the beneficiary's functional limitation. The clinician also determines the severity/complexity of the beneficiary's functional limitation and selects the appropriate modifier. In this example, the clinician determines that the beneficiary has a 75 percent mobility restriction for which the CL modifier is applicable. The clinician expects that at the end of therapy the beneficiaries will have only a 15 percent mobility restriction for which the CI modifier is applicable. When the beneficiary attains the mobility goal, therapy continues to be medically necessary to addresss a functional limitation for which there is no categorical G-code. The clinician reports this using (G8990 – G8992).

At the outset of therapy. On the DOS for which the initial evaluative procedure is furnished or the initial treatment day of a therapy POC, the claim for the service will also include two G-codes as shown below.

- G8978-CL to report the functional limitation (Mobility with current mobility limitation of "at least 60 percent but less than 80 percent impaired, limited or restricted")
- G8979-CI to report the projected goal for a mobility restriction of "at least 1 percent but less than 20 percent impaired, limited or restricted."

At the end of each progress reporting period. On the claim for the DOS when the services related to the progress report (which must be done at least once each 10 treatment days) are furnished, the clinician will report the same two G-codes but the modifier for the current status may be different.

- G8978 with the appropriate modifier are reported to show the beneficiary's current status as of this DOS. So if thebeneficiary has made no progress, this claim will include G8978-CL. If the beneficiary made progress and now has a mobility restriction of 65 percent CL would still be the appropriate modifier for 65 percent, and G8978-CL would be reported in this case. If the beneficiary now has a mobility restriction of 45 percent, G8978-CK would be reported.
- G8979-CI would be reported to show the projected goal. This severity modifier would not change unless the clinician adjusts the beneficiary's goal. This step is repeated as necessary and clinically appropriate, adjusting the current status modifier used as the beneficiary progresses through therapy.

- At the time the beneficiary is discharged from the therapy episode. The final claim for therapy episode will include two G-codes.
- G8979-CI would be reported to show the projected goal. G8980-CI would be reported if the beneficiary attained the 15 percent mobility goal. Alternatively, if the beneficiary's mobility restriction only reached 25 percent; G8980-CJ would be reported. To end reporting of one functional limitation. As noted above, functional reporting is required to continue throughout the entire episode of care. Accordingly, when further therapy is medically necessary after the beneficiary attains the goal for the first reported functional limitation, the clinician would end reporting of the first functional limitation by using the same G-codes and modifiers that would be used at the time of discharge. Using the mobility example, to end reporting of the mobility functional limitation, G8979-CI and G8980-CI would be reported on the same DOS that coincides with end of that progress reporting period.

To begin reporting of a second functional limitation. At the time reporting is begun for a new and different functional limitation, within the same episode of care (i.e., after the reporting of the prior functional limitation is ended). Reporting on the second functional limitation, however, is not begun until the DOS of the next treatment day -- which is day one of the new progress reporting period. When the next functional limitation to be reported is NOT defined by one of the other three PT/OT categorical codes, the G-code set (G8990 - G8992) for the "other PT/OT primary" functional limitation is used, rather than the G-code set for the "other PT/OT subsequent" because it is the first reported "other PT/OT" functional limitation. This reporting begins on the DOS of the first treatment day following the mobility "discharge" reporting, which is counted as the initial service for the "other PT/OT primary" functional limitation and the first treatment day of the new progress reporting period. In this case, G8990 and G8991, along with the corresponding modifiers, are reported on the claim for therapy services.

The table below illustrates when reporting is required using this example and what G-codes would be used.

Example of Required Reporting

Key: Reporting Period (RP)	**Begin RP #1 for Mobility at Episode Outset**	**End RP#1for Mobility at Progress Report**	**Mobility RP #2 Begins Next Treatment Day**	**End RP#2 for Mobility at Progress Report**	**Mobility RP #3 Begins Next Treatment Day**	**D/C or End Reporting for \Mobility**	**Begin RP #1 for Other PT/OT Primary**
Mobility: Walking & Moving Around							
G8978 – Current Status	X	X		X			
G 8979– Goal Status	X	X		X		X	
G8980 – Discharge Status						X	
Other PT/OT Primary							
G8990 – Current Status							X
G8991 – Goal Status							X
G8992 – Discharge Status							
No Functional Reporting Req'd			X		X		

H. Required Tracking and Documentation of Functional G-codes and Severity Modifiers

The clinician who furnishes the services must not only report the functional information on the therapy claim, but, he/she must track and document the G-codes and severity modifiers used for this reporting in the beneficiary's medical record of therapy services.

For details related to the documentation requirements, refer to Pub. 100-02, Medicare Benefit Policy Manual, chapter 15, section 220.4, - MCTRJCA-required Functional Reporting. For coverage rules related to MCTRJCA and therapy goals, refer to Pub. 100-02: a) for outpatient therapy services, see chapter 15, section 220.1.2 B and b) for instructions specific to PT, OT, and SLP services in the CORF, see chapter 12, section 10.

100-04, 5, 20.2

Reporting of Service Units With HCPCS

(Rev. 3670, Issued: 12-01-16, Effective: 01-01-17, Implementation: 01-03-17)

A. General

Effective with claims submitted on or after April 1, 1998, providers billing on the ASC X12 837 institutional claim format or Form CMS-1450 were required to report the number of units for outpatient rehabilitation services based on the procedure or service, e.g., based on the HCPCS code reported instead of the revenue code. This was already in effect for billing on the Form CMS-1500, and CORFs were required to report their full range of CORF services on the institutional claim. These unit-reporting requirements continue with the standards required for electronically submitting health care claims under the Health Insurance Portability and Accountability Act of 1996 (HIPAA) - the currently adopted version of the ASC X12 837 transaction standards and implementation guides. The Administrative Simplification Compliance Act mandates that claims be sent to Medicare electronically unless certain exceptions are met.

B. Timed and Untimed Codes

When reporting service units for HCPCS codes where the procedure is not defined by a specific timeframe ("untimed" HCPCS), the provider enters "1" in the field labeled units. For timed codes, units are reported based on the number of times the procedure is performed, as described in the HCPCS code definition.

EXAMPLE: A beneficiary received a speech-language pathology evaluation represented by HCPCS "untimed" code 92521. Regardless of the number of minutes spent providing this service only one unit of service is appropriately billed on the same day.

Several CPT codes used for therapy modalities, procedures, and tests and measurements specify that the direct (one on one) time spent in patient contact is 15 minutes. Providers report these "timed" procedure codes for services delivered on any single calendar day using CPT codes and the appropriate number of 15 minute units of service.

EXAMPLE: A beneficiary received a total of 60 minutes of occupational therapy, e.g., HCPCS "timed" code 97530 which is defined in 15 minute units, on a given date of service. The provider would then report 4 units of 97530.

C. Counting Minutes for Timed Codes in 15 Minute Units

When only one service is provided in a day, providers should not bill for services performed for less than 8 minutes. For any single timed CPT code in the same day measured in 15 minute units, providers bill a single 15-minute unit for treatment greater than or equal to 8 minutes through and including 22 minutes. If the duration of a single modality or procedure in a day is greater than or equal to 23 minutes, through and including 37 minutes, then 2 units should be billed. Time intervals for 1 through 8 units are as follows:

Units Number of Minutes

1 unit: ≥ 8 minutes through 22 minutes

2 units:≥ 23 minutes through 37 minutes

3 units:≥ 38 minutes through 52 minutes

4 units:≥ 53 minutes through 67 minutes

5 units:≥ 68 minutes through 82 minutes

6 units:≥ 83 minutes through 97 minutes

7 units:≥ 98 minutes through 112 minutes

8 units:≥ 113 minutes through 127 minutes

The pattern remains the same for treatment times in excess of 2 hours.

If a service represented by a 15 minute timed code is performed in a single day for at least 15 minutes, that service shall be billed for at least one unit. If the service is performed for at least 30 minutes, that service shall be billed for at least two units, etc. It is not appropriate to count all minutes of treatment in a day toward the units for one code if other services were performed for more than 15 minutes. See examples 2 and 3 below.

When more than one service represented by 15 minute timed codes is performed in a single day, the total number of minutes of service (as noted on the chart above) determines the number of timed units billed. See example 1 below.

If any 15 minute timed service that is performed for 7 minutes or less than 7 minutes on the same day as another 15 minute timed service that was also performed for 7 minutes or less and the total time of the two is 8 minutes or greater than 8 minutes, then bill one unit for the service performed for the most minutes. This is correct because the total time is greater than the minimum time for one unit. The same logic is applied when three or more different services are provided for 7 minutes or less than 7 minutes. See example 5 below.

The expectation (based on the work values for these codes) is that a provider's direct patient contact time for each unit will average 15 minutes in length. If a provider has a consistent practice of billing less than 15 minutes for a unit, these situations should be highlighted for review.

If more than one 15 minute timed CPT code is billed during a single calendar day, then the total number of timed units that can be billed is constrained by the total treatment minutes for that day. See all examples below.

Pub. 100-02, Medicare Benefit Policy Manual, Chapter 15, Section 220.3B, Documentation Requirements for Therapy Services, indicates that the amount of time for each specific intervention/modality provided to the patient is not required to be documented in the Treatment Note. However, the total number of timed minutes must be documented. These examples indicate how to count the appropriate number of units for the total therapy minutes provided.

Example 1 –

24 minutes of neuromuscular reeducation, code 97112,

23 minutes of therapeutic exercise, code 97110,

Total timed code treatment time was 47 minutes.

See the chart above. The 47 minutes falls within the range for 3 units = 38 to 52 minutes.

Appropriate billing for 47 minutes is only 3 timed units. Each of the codes is performed for more than 15 minutes, so each shall be billed for at least 1 unit. The correct coding is 2 units of code 97112 and one unit of code 97110, assigning more timed units to the service that took the most time.

Example 2 –

20 minutes of neuromuscular reeducation (97112)

20 minutes therapeutic exercise (97110),

40 Total timed code minutes.

Appropriate billing for 40 minutes is 3 units. Each service was done at least 15 minutes and should be billed for at least one unit, but the total allows 3 units. Since the time for each service is the same, choose either code for 2 units and bill the other for 1 unit. Do not bill 3 units for either one of the codes.

Example 3 –

33 minutes of therapeutic exercise (97110),

7 minutes of manual therapy (97140),

40 Total timed minutes

Appropriate billing for 40 minutes is for 3 units. Bill 2 units of 97110 and 1 unit of 97140. Count the first 30 minutes of 97110 as two full units. Compare the remaining time for 97110 (33-30 = 3 minutes) to the time spent on 97140 (7 minutes) and bill the larger, which is 97140.

Example 4 –

18 minutes of therapeutic exercise (97110),

13 minutes of manual therapy (97140),

10 minutes of gait training (97116),

8 minutes of ultrasound (97035),

49 Total timed minutes

Appropriate billing is for 3 units. Bill the procedures you spent the most time providing. Bill 1 unit each of 97110, 97116, and 97140. You are unable to bill for the ultrasound because the total time of timed units that can be billed is constrained by the total timed code treatment minutes (i.e., you may not bill 4 units for less than 53 minutes regardless of how many services were performed). You would still document the ultrasound in the treatment notes.

Example 5 –

7 minutes of neuromuscular reeducation (97112)

7 minutes therapeutic exercise (97110)

7 minutes manual therapy (97140)

21 Total timed minutes

Appropriate billing is for one unit. The qualified professional (See definition in Pub. 100-02, chapter 15, section 220) shall select one appropriate CPT code (97112, 97110, 97140) to bill since each unit was performed for the same amount of time and only one unit is allowed.

NOTE: The above schedule of times is intended to provide assistance in rounding time into 15-minute increments. It does not imply that any minute until the eighth should be excluded from the total count. The total minutes of active treatment counted for all 15 minute timed codes includes all direct treatment time for the timed codes. Total treatment minutes - including minutes spent providing services represented by untimed codes - are also documented. For documentation in the medical record of the services provided see Pub. 100-02, chapter 15, section 220.3.

D. Specific Limits for HCPCS

The Deficit Reduction Act of 2005, section 5107 requires the implementation of clinically appropriate code edits to eliminate improper payments for outpatient therapy services. The following codes may be billed, when covered, only at or below the number of units indicated on the chart per treatment day. When higher amounts of units are billed than those indicated in the table below, the units on the claim line that exceed the limit shall be denied as medically unnecessary (according to 1862(a)(1)(A)). Denied claims may be appealed and an ABN is appropriate to notify the beneficiary of liability.

This chart does not include all of the codes identified as therapy codes; refer to section 20 of this chapter for further detail on these and other therapy codes. For example, therapy codes called "always therapy" must always be accompanied by therapy modifiers identifying the type of therapy plan of care under which the service is provided.

Use the chart in the following manner:

The codes that are allowed one unit for "Allowed Units" in the chart below may be billed no more than once per provider, per discipline, per date of service, per patient.

The codes allowed 0 units in the column for "Allowed Units", may not be billed under a plan of care indicated by the discipline in that column. Some codes may be billed by one discipline (e.g., PT) and not by others (e.g., OT or SLP).

When physicians/NPPs bill "always therapy" codes they must follow the policies of the type of therapy they are providing e.g., utilize a plan of care, bill with the appropriate therapy modifier (GP, GO, GN), bill the allowed units on the chart below for PT, OT or SLP depending on the plan. A physician/NPP shall not bill an "always therapy" code unless the service is provided under a therapy plan of care. Therefore, NA stands for "Not Applicable" in the chart below.

When a "sometimes therapy" code is billed by a physician/NPP, but as a medical service, and not under a therapy plan of care, the therapy modifier shall not be used, but the number of units billed must not exceed the number of units indicated in the chart below per patient, per provider/supplier, per day.

NOTE: As of April 1, 2017, the chart below uses the CPT Consumer Friendly Code Descriptions which are intended only to assist the reader in identifying the service related to the CPT/HCPCS code. The reader is reminded that these descriptions cannot be used in place of the CPT long descriptions which officially define each of the services. The table below no longer contains a column noting whether a code is "timed" or "untimed" as this notation is not relevant to the number of units allowed per code on claims for the listed therapy services. We note that the official long descriptors for the CPT codes can be found in the latest CPT code book.

CPT/ HCPCS Code	CPT Consumer Friendly Code Descriptions and Claim Line Outlier/Edit Details	PT Allowed Units	OT Allowed Units	SLP Allowed Units	Physician /NPP Not Under Therapy POC
92521	Evaluation of speech fluency	0	0	1	NA
92522	Evaluation of speech sound production	0	0	1	NA
92523	Evaluation of speech sound production with evaluation of language comprehension and expression	0	0	1	NA
92524	Behavioral and qualitative analysis of voice and resonance	0	0	1	NA
92597	Evaluation for use and/or fitting of voice prosthetic device to supplement oral speech	0	0	1	NA
92607	Evaluation of patient with prescription of speech-generating and alternative communication device	0	0	1	NA
92611	Fluoroscopic and video recorded motion evaluation of swallowing function	0	1	1	1
92612	Evaluation and recording of swallowing using an endoscope Evaluation and recording of swallowing using an endoscope	0	1	1	1
92614	Evaluation and recording of voice box sensory function using an endoscope	0	1	1	1
92616	Evaluation and recording of swallowing and voice box sensory function using an endoscope	0	1	1	1
95833	Manual muscle testing of whole body	1	1	0	1
95834	Manual muscle testing of whole body including hands	1	1	0	1
96110	Developmental screening	1	1	1	1
96111	Developmental testing	1	1	1	1
97161	Evaluation of physical therapy, typically 20 minutes	1	0	0	NA
97162	Evaluation of physical therapy, typically 30 minutes	1	0	0	NA
97163	Evaluation of physical therapy, typically 45 minutes	1	0	0	NA
97164	Re-evaluation of physical therapy, typically 20 minutes	1	0	0	NA
97165	Evaluation of occupational therapy, typically 30 minutes	0	1	0	NA
97166	Evaluation of occupational therapy, typically 45 minutes	0	1	0	NA
97167	Evaluation of occupational therapy, typically 60 minutes	0	1	0	NA
97168	Re-evaluation of occupational therapy established plan of care, typically 30 minutes	0	1	0	NA

100-04, 8, 60.4.2

Facility Billing Requirements for ESAs

(Rev.4105, Issued: 08- 03-18, Effective: 01-01-19, Implementation: 01-07-19)

Hematocrit and Hemoglobin Levels

Renal dialysis facilities are required to report hematocrit or hemoglobin levels for their Medicare patients receiving erythropoietin products. Hematocrit levels are reported in value code 49 and reflect the most recent reading taken before the start of the billing period. Hemoglobin readings before the start of the billing period are reported in value code 48.

To report a hemoglobin or hematocrit reading for a new patient on or after January 1, 2006, the provider should report the reading that prompted the treatment of epoetin alfa. The provider may use results documented on form CMS 2728 or the patient's medical records from a transferring facility.

Effective January 1, 2012, ESRD facilities are required to report hematocrit or hemoglobin levels on all ESRD claims. Reporting the value 99.99 is not permitted when billing for an ESA.

The revenue codes for reporting Epoetin Alfa are 0634 and 0635. All other ESAs are reported using revenue code 0636. The HCPCS code for the ESA must be included:

HCPCS	HCPCS Description	Dates of Service
Q4055	Injection, Epoetin Alfa, 1,000 units (for ESRD on Dialysis)	1/1/2004 through 12/31/2005
J0886	Injection, Epoetin Alfa, 1,000 units (for ESRD on Dialysis)	1/1/2006 through 12/31/2006
Q4081	Injection, Epoetin alfa, 100	1/1/2007 through 7/1/2015
Q5105	Injection, epoetin alfa, biosimilar, (Retacrit) (For ESRD on Dialysis), 100 units	7/1/2018 to present

Each administration of an ESA is reported on a separate line item with the units reported used as a multiplier by the dosage description in the HCPCS to arrive at the dosage per administration.

Route of Administration Modifiers

Patients with end stage renal disease (ESRD) receiving administrations of erythropoiesis stimulating agents (ESA) for the treatment of anemia may receive intravenous administration or subcutaneous administrations of the ESA. Effective for claims with dates of services on or after January 1, 2012, all facilities billing for injections of ESA for ESRD beneficiaries must include the modifier JA on the claim to indicate an intravenous administration or modifier JB to indicate a subcutaneous administration. ESRD claims containing ESA administrations that are submitted without the route of administration modifiers will be returned to the provider for correction. Renal dialysis facilities claim including charges for administrations of the ESA by both methods must report separate lines to identify the number of administration provided using each method.

Effective July 1, 2013, providers must identify when a drug is administered via the dialysate by appending the modifier JE (administered via dialysate).

ESA Monitoring Policy Modifiers

Append modifiers ED, EE and GS as applicable, see instructions in section 60.4.1.

Maximum Allowable Administrations

The maximum number of administrations of EPO for a billing cycle is 13 times in 30 days and 14 times in 31 days.

The maximum number of administrations of Aranesp for a billing cycle is 5 times in 30/ 31days.

The maximum number of administrations of Peginesatide is 1 time in 30/ 31days.

100-04, 8, 140.1

Payment for ESRD-Related Services Under the Monthly Capitation Payment (Center Based Patients)

(Rev. 2269, Issued: 08-05-11, Effective: 01-01-11, Implementation: 11-07-11)

Physicians and practitioners managing center based patients on dialysis are paid a monthly rate for most outpatient dialysis-related physician services furnished to a Medicare ESRD beneficiary. The payment amount varies based on the number of visits provided within each month and the age of the ESRD beneficiary. Under this methodology, separate codes are billed for providing one visit per month, two to three visits per month and four or more visits per month. The lowest payment amount applies when a physician provides one visit per month; a higher payment is provided for two to three visits per month. To receive the highest payment amount, a physician or practitioner would have to provide at least four ESRD-related visits per month. The MCP is reported once per month for services performed in an outpatient setting that are related to the patients' ESRD.

The physician or practitioner who provides the complete assessment, establishes the patient's plan of care, and provides the ongoing management is the physician or practitioner who submits the bill for the monthly service.

a. Month defined.

For purposes of billing for physician and practitioner ESRD related services, the term 'month' means a calendar month. The first month the beneficiary begins dialysis treatments is the date the dialysis treatments begin through the end of the calendar month. Thereafter, the term 'month' refers to a calendar month.

b. Determination of the age of beneficiary.

The beneficiary's age at the end of the month is the age of the patient for determining the appropriate age related ESRD-related services code.

c. Qualifying Visits Under the MCP

- General policy.

Visits must be furnished face-to-face by a physician, clinical nurse specialist, nurse practitioner, or physician's assistant.

- Visits furnished by another physician or practitioner (who is not the MCP physician or practitioner).

The MCP physician or practitioner may use other physicians or qualified nonphysician practitioners to provide some of the visits during the month. The MCP physician or practitioner does not have to be present when these other physicians or practitioners provide visits. In this instance, the rules are consistent with the requirements for hospital split/shared evaluation and management visits. The non-MCP physician or practitioner must be a partner, an employee of the same group practice, or an employee of the MCP physician or practitioner. For example, the physician or practitioner furnishing visits under the MCP may be either a W-2 employee or 1099 independent contractor.

When another physician is used to furnish some of the visits during the month, the physician who provides the complete assessment, establishes the patient's plan of care, and provides the ongoing management should bill for the MCP service.

If the nonphysician practitioner is the practitioner who performs the complete assessment and establishes the plan of care, then the MCP service should be billed under the PIN of the clinical nurse specialist, nurse practitioner, or physician assistant.

- Residents, interns and fellows.

Patient visits by residents, interns and fellows enrolled in an approved Medicare graduate medical education (GME) program may be counted towards the MCP visits if the teaching MCP physician is present during the visit.

- Patients designated/admitted as hospital observation status.

ESRD-related visits furnished to patients in hospital observation status that occur on or after January 1, 2005, should be counted for purposes of billing the MCP codes. Visits furnished to patients in hospital observation status are included when submitting MCP claims for ESRD-related services.

- ESRD-related visits furnished to beneficiaries residing in a SNF.

ESRD-related visits furnished to beneficiaries residing in a SNF should be counted for purposes of billing the MCP codes.

- SNF residents admitted as an inpatient.

Inpatient visits are not counted for purposes of the MCP service. If the beneficiary residing in a SNF is admitted to the hospital as an inpatient, the appropriate inpatient visit code should be billed.

- ESRD Related Visits as a Telehealth Service

ESRD-related services with 2 or 3 visits per month and ESRD-related services with 4 or more visits per month may be furnished as a telehealth service. However, at least one visit per month is required in person to examine the vascular access site. A clinical examination of the vascular access site must be furnished face-to-face (not as a telehealth service) by a physician, nurse practitioner or physician's assistant. For more information on how ESRD-related visits may be furnished as a Medicare telehealth service and for general Medicare telehealth policy see Pub. 100-2, Medicare Benefit Policy manual, chapter 15, section 270. For claims processing instructions see Pub. 100-4, Medicare Claims Processing manual chapter 12, section 190.

100-04, 8, 140.1.1

Payment for Managing Patients on Home Dialysis

(Rev. 2269, Issued: 08-05-11, Effective: 01-01-11, Implementation: 11-07-11)

Physicians and practitioners managing ESRD patients who dialyze at home are paid a single monthly rate based on the age of the beneficiary. The MCP physician (or practitioner) must furnish at least one face-to-face patient visit per month for the home dialysis MCP service. Documentation by the MCP physician (or practitioner) should support at least one face-to-face encounter per month with the home dialysis patient. Medicare contractors may waive the requirement for a monthly face-to-face visit for the home dialysis MCP service on a case by case basis, for example, when the nephrologist's notes indicate that the physician actively and adequately managed the care of the home dialysis patient throughout the month. The management of home dialysis patients who remain a home dialysis patient the entire month should be coded using the ESRD-related services for home dialysis patients HCPCS codes.

When another physician is used to furnish some of the visits during the month, the physician who provides the complete assessment, establishes the patient's plan of care, and provides the ongoing management should bill for the MCP service.

If the nonphysician practitioner is the practitioner who performs the complete assessment and establishes the plan of care, then the MCP service should be billed under the PIN of the clinical nurse specialist, nurse practitioner, or physician assistant.

Residents, interns and fellows. Patient visits by residents, interns and fellows enrolled in an approved Medicare graduate medical education (GME) program may be counted towards the MCP visits if the teaching MCP physician is present during the visit.

a. Month defined.

For purposes of billing for physician and practitioner ESRD related services, the term 'month' means a calendar month. The first month the beneficiary begins dialysis treatments is the date the dialysis treatments begin through the end of the calendar month. Thereafter, the term 'month' refers to a calendar month.

b. Qualifying Visits under the MCP

- General policy.

Visits must be furnished face-to-face by a physician, clinical nurse specialist, nurse practitioner, or physician's assistant.

- Visits furnished by another physician or practitioner (who is not the MCP physician or practitioner).

The MCP physician or practitioner may use other physicians or qualified nonphysician practitioners to provide the visit(s) during the month. The MCP physician or practitioner does not have to be present when these other physicians or practitioners provide visit(s). The non-MCP physician or practitioner must be a partner, an employee of the same group practice, or an employee of the MCP physician or practitioner. For example, the physician or practitioner furnishing visits under the MCP may be either a W-2 employee or 1099 independent contractor.

When another physician is used to furnish some of the visits during the month, the physician who provides the complete assessment, establishes the patient's plan of care, and provides the ongoing management should bill for the MCP service.

If the nonphysician practitioner is the practitioner who performs the complete assessment and establishes the plan of care, then the MCP service should be billed under the PIN of the clinical nurse specialist, nurse practitioner, or physician assistant.

- Residents, interns and fellows.

Patient visits by residents, interns and fellows enrolled in an approved Medicare graduate medical education (GME) program may be counted towards the MCP visits if the teaching MCP physician is present during the visit.

100-04, 8, 180

Noninvasive Studies for ESRD Patients - Facility and Physician Services

(Rev. 3650, Issued: 11-10-16, Effective: 02-10-17, Implementation: 02-10-17)

For Medicare coverage of noninvasive vascular studies, see the Medicare Benefit Policy Manual, Chapter 11.

For dialysis to take place there must be a means of access so that the exchange of waste products may occur. As part of the dialysis treatment, ESRD facilities are responsible for monitoring access, and when occlusions occur, either declot the access or refer the patient for appropriate treatment. Procedures associated with monitoring access involve taking venous pressure, aspirating thrombus, observing elevated recirculation time, reduced urea reduction ratios, or collapsed shunt, etc. All such procedures are covered under the composite rate.

ESRD facilities may not monitor access through noninvasive vascular studies such as duplex and Doppler flow scans and bill separately for these procedures. Noninvasive vascular studies are not covered as a separately billable service if used to monitor a patient's vascular access site.

Medicare pays for the technical component of the procedure in the composite payment rate.

Where there are signs and symptoms of vascular access problems, Doppler flow studies may be used as a means to obtain diagnostic information to permit medical intervention to address the problem. Doppler flow studies may be considered medically necessary in the presence of signs or symptoms of possible failure of the ESRD patient's vascular access site, and when the results are used in determining the clinical course of the treatment for the patient.

The only Current Procedural Terminology (CPT) billing code for noninvasive vascular testing of a hemodialysis access site is 93990. A/B MACs (B) must deny separate billing of the technical component of this code if it is performed on any patient for whom the ESRD composite rate for dialysis is being paid, unless there is appropriate medical indication of the need for a Doppler flow study.

When a dialysis patient exhibits signs and symptoms of compromise to the vascular access site, Doppler flow studies may provide diagnostic information that will determine the appropriate medical intervention. Medicare considers a Doppler flow study medically necessary when the beneficiary's dialysis access site manifests signs or symptoms associated with vascular compromise, and when the results of this test are necessary to determine the clinical course of treatment.

Examples supporting the medical necessity for Doppler flow studies include:

a. Elevated dynamic venous pressure >200mm HG when measured during dialysis with the blood pump set on a 200cc/min.,

b. Access recirculation of 12 percent or greater,

c. An otherwise unexplained urea reduction ration <60 oercebtm abd

d. An access with a palpable "water hammer" pulse on examination, (which implies venous outflow obstruction).

Unless the documentation is provided supporting the necessity of more than one study, Medicare will limit payment to either a Doppler flow study or an arteriogram (fistulogram, venogram), but not both.

An example of when both studies may be clinically necessary is when a Doppler flow study demonstrates reduced flow (blood flow rate less than 800cc/min or a decreased flow of 25 percent or greater from previous study) and the physician requires an arteriogram to further define the extent of the problem. The patient's medical record(s) must provide documentation supporting the need for more than one imaging study.

This policy is applicable to claims from ESRD facilities and all other sources, such as independent diagnostic testing facilities, and hospital outpatient departments.

A/B MACs (B) shall develop LMRP for Doppler flow studies if this service meets the criteria listed in the Medicare Program Integrity Manual, Chapter 1. This provides guidance to contractors on the scope, purpose, and meaning of LMRP.

The professional component of the procedure is included in the monthly capitation payment (MCP) (See §140 above.) The professional component should be denied for code 93990 if billed by the MCP physician. Medically necessary services that are included or bundled into the MCP (e.g., test interpretations) are separately payable when furnished by physicians other than the MCP physician.

The contractor shall use the following remittance advice messages and associated codes when rejecting/denying claims under this policy. This CARC/RARC combination is compliant with CAQH CORE Business Scenario Four.

Group Code: CO
CARC: 24
RARC: N/A
MSN:16.32

Billing for monitoring of hemodialysis access using CPT codes for noninvasive vascular studies other than 93990 is considered a misrepresentation of the service actually provided and contractors will consider this action for fraud investigation. They will conduct data analysis on a periodic basis for noninvasive diagnostic studies of the extremities (including CPT codes 93922, 93923, 93924, 93925, 93926, 93930, 93931, 93965, 93970, 93971). Contractors should handle aberrant findings under normal program safeguard processes by taking whatever corrective action is deemed necessary.

100-04, 11, 40.1.3

Independent Attending Physician Services

(Rev. 4280, Issued: 04-19-2019, Effective: 07-21-19, Implementation: 07-21-19)

When hospice coverage is elected, the beneficiary waives all rights to Medicare Part B payments for professional services that are related to the treatment and management of his/her terminal illness during any period his/her hospice benefit election is in force, except for professional services of an independent attending physician, who is not an employee of the designated hospice nor receives compensation from the hospice for those services. For purposes of administering the hospice benefit provisions, an "attending physician" means an individual who:

- Is a doctor of medicine or osteopathy or
- A nurse practitioner (for professional services related to the terminal illness that are furnished on or after December 8, 2003); and
- Is identified by the individual, at the time he/she elects hospice coverage, as having the most significant role in the determination and delivery of their medical care.

Hospices should reiterate with patients that they must not see independent physicians for care related to their terminal illness other than their independent attending physician unless the hospice arranges it.

Even though a beneficiary elects hospice coverage, he/she may designate and use an independent attending physician, who is not employed by nor receives compensation from the hospice for professional services furnished, in addition to the services of hospice-employed physicians. The professional services of an independent attending physician, who may be a nurse practitioner as defined in Chapter 9, that are reasonable and necessary for the treatment and management of a hospice patient's terminal illness are not considered Medicare Part A hospice services.

Where the service is related to the hospice patient's terminal illness but was furnished by someone other than the designated "attending physician" [or a physician substituting for the attending physician]) the physician or other provider must look to the hospice for payment.

Professional services related to the hospice patient's terminal condition that were furnished by an independent attending physician, who may be a nurse practitioner, are billed to the Medicare contractor through Medicare Part B. When the independent attending physician furnishes a terminal illness related service that includes both a professional and technical component (e.g., x-rays), he/she bills the professional component of such services to the Medicare contractor on a professional claim and looks to the hospice for payment for the technical component. Likewise, the independent attending physician, who may be a nurse practitioner, would look to the hospice for payment for terminal illness related services furnished that have no professional component (e.g., clinical lab tests). The remainder of this section explains this in greater detail.

When a Medicare beneficiary elects hospice coverage he/she may designate an attending physician, who may be a nurse practitioner, not employed by the hospice, in addition to receiving care from hospice-employed physicians. The professional services of a non-hospice affiliated attending physician for the treatment and management of a hospice patient's terminal illness are not considered Medicare Part A "hospice services." These independent attending physician services are billed through Medicare Part B to the Medicare contractor, provided they were not furnished under a payment arrangement with the hospice. The independent attending physician codes services with the GV modifier "Attending physician not employed or paid under agreement by the patient's hospice provider" when billing his/her professional services furnished for the treatment and management of a hospice patient's terminal condition. The Medicare contractor makes payment to the independent attending physician or beneficiary, as appropriate, based on the payment and deductible rules applicable to each covered service.

Payments for the services of an independent attending physician are not counted in determining whether the hospice cap amount has been exceeded because Part B services provided by an independent attending physician are not part of the hospice's care.

Services provided by an independent attending physician who may be a nurse practitioner must be coordinated with any direct care services provided by hospice physicians.

Only the direct professional services of an independent attending physician, who may be a nurse practitioner, to a patient may be billed; the costs for services such as lab or x-rays are not to be included in the bill.

If another physician covers for a hospice patient's designated attending physician, the services of the substituting physician are billed by the designated attending physician under the reciprocal or locum tenens billing instructions. In such instances, the attending physician bills using the GV modifier in conjunction with either the Q5 or Q6 modifier.

When services related to a hospice patient's terminal condition are furnished under a payment arrangement with the hospice by the designated attending physician who may be a nurse practitioner (i.e., by a non-independent physician/nurse practitioner), the physician must look to the hospice for payment. In this situation the physicians' services are Part A hospice services and are billed by the hospice to its Medicare contractor.

Medicare contractors must process and pay for covered, medically necessary Part B services that physicians furnish to patients after their hospice benefits are revoked even if the patient remains under the care of the hospice. Such services are billed without the GV or GW modifiers. Make payment based on applicable Medicare payment and deductible rules for each covered service even if the beneficiary continues to be treated by the hospice after hospice benefits are revoked.

The CWF response contains the periods of hospice entitlement. This information is a permanent part of the notice and is furnished on all CWF replies and automatic notices. Medicare contractor use the CWF reply for validating dates of hospice coverage and to research, examine and adjudicate services coded with the GV or GW modifiers.

100-04, 12, 20.4.7

Services That Do Not Meet the National Electrical Manufacturers Association (NEMA) Standard XR-29-2013

(Rev. 3820, Issued: 11-21-17, Effective: 01-01-18, Implementation; 01-02-18)

Several provisions provide for a payment reduction to the technical component (and the technical component of the global fee) for X-rays and imaging services under certain circumstances. Please see Chapter 13, Section 20.2 of this publication for more information.

100-04, 12, 30.1

Digestive System

(Rev. 3368, Issued: 10-09-15, Effective: 01-01-16, Implementation: 01-01-16)

A. Upper Gastrointestinal Endoscopy Including Endoscopic Ultrasound (EUS) (Code 43259)

If the person performing the original diagnostic endoscopy has access to the EUS and the clinical situation requires an EUS, the EUS may be done at the same time. The procedure, diagnostic and EUS, is reported under the same code, CPT 43259. This code conforms to CPT guidelines for the indented codes. The service represented by the indented code, in this case code 43259 for EUS, includes the service represented by the unintended code preceding the list of indented codes. Therefore, when a diagnostic examination of the upper gastrointestinal tract "including esophagus, stomach, and either the duodenum or jejunum as appropriate," includes the use of endoscopic ultrasonography, the service is reported by a single code, namely 43259.

Interpretation, whether by a radiologist or endoscopist, is reported under CPT code 76975-26. These codes may both be reported on the same day.

B. Incomplete Colonoscopies (Codes 44388, 45378, G0105 and G0121)

An incomplete colonoscopy, e.g., the inability to advance the colonoscope to the cecum or colon-small intestine anastomosis due to unforeseen circumstances, is billed and paid using colonoscopy through stoma code 44388, colonoscopy code 45378, and screening colonoscopy codes G0105 and G0121 with modifier "-53." (Code 44388 is valid with modifier 53 beginning January 1, 2016.) The Medicare physician fee schedule database has specific values for codes 44388-53, 45378-53, G0105-53 and G0121-53. An incomplete colonoscopy performed prior to January 1, 2016, is paid at the same rate as a sigmoidoscopy. Beginning January 1, 2016, Medicare will pay for the interrupted colonoscopy at a rate that is calculated using one-half the value of the inputs for the codes.

100-04, 12, 30.6.2

Billing for Medically Necessary Visit on Same Occasion as Preventive Medicine Service

(Rev. 1, 10-01-03)

See Chapter 18 for payment for covered preventive services.

When a physician furnishes a Medicare beneficiary a covered visit at the same place and on the same occasion as a noncovered preventive medicine service (CPT codes 99381- 99397), consider the covered visit to be provided in lieu of a part of the preventive medicine service of equal value to the visit. A preventive medicine service (CPT codes 99381-99397) is a noncovered service. The physician may charge the beneficiary, as a charge for the noncovered remainder of the service, the amount by which the physician's current established charge for the preventive medicine service exceeds his/her current established charge for the covered visit. Pay for the covered visit based on the lesser of the fee schedule amount or the physician's actual charge for the visit. The physician is not required to give the beneficiary written advance notice of noncoverage of the part of the visit that constitutes a routine preventive visit. However, the physician is responsible for notifying the patient in advance of his/her liability for the charges for services that are not medically necessary to treat the illness or injury.

There could be covered and noncovered procedures performed during this encounter (e.g., screening x-ray, EKG, lab tests.). These are considered individually. Those procedures which are for screening for asymptomatic conditions are considered noncovered and, therefore, no payment is made. Those procedures ordered to diagnose or monitor a symptom, medical condition, or treatment are evaluated for medical necessity and, if covered, are paid.

100-04, 12, 30.6.4

Evaluation and Management (E/M) Services Furnished Incident to Physician's Service by Nonphysician Practitioners

(Rev. 1, 10-01-03)

When evaluation and management services are furnished incident to a physician's service by a nonphysician practitioner, the physician may bill the CPT code that describes the evaluation and management service furnished.

When evaluation and management services are furnished incident to a physician's service by a nonphysician employee of the physician, not as part of a physician service, the physician bills code 99211 for the service.

A physician is not precluded from billing under the "incident to" provision for services provided by employees whose services cannot be paid for directly under the Medicare program. Employees of the physician may provide services incident to the physician's service, but the physician alone is permitted to bill Medicare.

Services provided by employees as "incident to" are covered when they meet all the requirements for incident to and are medically necessary for the individual needs of the patient.

100-04, 12, 30.6.7

Payment for Office or Other Outpatient Evaluation and Management (E/M) Visits

(Rev. 3315, Issued: 08-06-15, Effective: 01-01-16, Implementation: 01-04-16)

A. Definition of New Patient for Selection of E/M Visit Code

Interpret the phrase "new patient" to mean a patient who has not received any professional services, i.e., E/M service or other face-to-face service (e.g., surgical procedure) from the physician or physician group practice (same physician specialty) within the previous 3 years. For example, if a professional component of a previous procedure is billed in a 3 year time period, e.g., a lab interpretation is billed and no E/M service or other face-to-face service with the patient is performed, then this patient remains a new patient for the initial visit. An interpretation of a diagnostic test, reading an x-ray or EKG etc., in the absence of an E/M service or other face-to-face service with the patient does not affect the designation of a new patient.

B. Office/Outpatient E/M Visits Provided on Same Day for Unrelated Problems

As for all other E/M services except where specifically noted, the Medicare Administrative Contractors (MACs) may not pay two E/M office visits billed by a physician (or physician of the same specialty from the same group practice) for the same beneficiary on the same day unless the physician documents that the visits were for unrelated problems in the office, off campus-outpatient hospital, or on campus-outpatient hospital setting which could not be provided during the same encounter (e.g., office visit for blood pressure medication evaluation, followed five hours later by a visit for evaluation of leg pain following an accident).

C. Office/Outpatient or Emergency Department E/M Visit on Day of Admission to Nursing Facility

MACs may not pay a physician for an emergency department visit or an office visit and a comprehensive nursing facility assessment on the same day. Bundle E/M visits on the same date provided in sites other than the nursing facility into the initial nursing facility care code when performed on the same date as the nursing facility admission by the same physician.

D. Drug Administration Services and E/M Visits Billed on Same Day of Service

MACs must advise physicians that CPT code 99211 cannot be paid if it is billed with a drug administration service such as a chemotherapy or nonchemotherapy drug infusion code (effective January 1, 2004). This drug administration policy was expanded in the Physician Fee Schedule Final Rule, November 15, 2004, to also include a therapeutic or diagnostic injection code (effective January 1, 2005). Therefore, when a medically necessary, significant and separately identifiable E/M service (which meets a higher complexity level than CPT code 99211) is performed, in addition to one of these drug administration services, the appropriate E/M CPT code should be reported with modifier -25. Documentation should support the level of E/M service billed. For an E/M service provided on the same day, a different diagnosis is not required.

100-04, 12, 30.6.8

Payment for Hospital Observation Services and Observation or Inpatient Care Services (Including Admission and Discharge Services)

(Rev. 2282, Issued: 08-26-11, Effective: 01-01-11, Implementation: 11-28-11)

A. Who May Bill Observation Care Codes

Observation care is a well-defined set of specific, clinically appropriate services, which include ongoing short term treatment, assessment, and reassessment, that are furnished while a decision is being made regarding whether patients will require further treatment as hospital inpatients or if they are able to be discharged from the hospital. Observation services are commonly ordered for patients who present to the emergency department and who then require a significant period of treatment or monitoring in order to make a decision concerning their admission or discharge.

In only rare and exceptional cases do reasonable and necessary outpatient observation services span more than 48 hours. In the majority of cases, the decision whether to discharge a patient from the hospital following resolution of the reason for the observation care or to admit the patient as an inpatient can be made in less than 48 hours, usually in less than 24 hours.

Contractors pay for initial observation care billed by only the physician who ordered hospital outpatient observation services and was responsible for the patient during his/her observation care. A physician who does not have inpatient admitting privileges but who is authorized to furnish hospital outpatient observation services may bill these codes.

For a physician to bill observation care codes, there must be a medical observation record for the patient which contains dated and timed physician's orders regarding the observation services the patient is to receive, nursing notes, and progress notes prepared by the physician while the patient received observation services. This record must be in addition to any record prepared as a result of an emergency department or outpatient clinic encounter.

Payment for an initial observation care code is for all the care rendered by the ordering physician on the date the patient's observation services began. All other physicians who furnish consultations or additional evaluations or services while the patient is receiving hospital outpatient observation services must bill the appropriate outpatient service codes.

For example, if an internist orders observation services and asks another physician to additionally evaluate the patient, only the internist may bill the initial and subsequent observation care codes. The other physician who evaluates the patient must bill the new or established office or other outpatient visit codes as appropriate.

For information regarding hospital billing of observation services, see Chapter 4, §290.

B. Physician Billing for Observation Care Following Initiation of Observation Services

Similar to initial observation codes, payment for a subsequent observation care code is for all the care rendered by the treating physician on the day(s) other than the initial or discharge date. All other physicians who furnish consultations or additional evaluations or services while the patient is receiving hospital outpatient observation services must bill the appropriate outpatient service codes.

When a patient receives observation care for less than 8 hours on the same calendar date, the Initial Observation Care, from CPT code range 99218 – 99220, shall be reported by the physician. The Observation Care Discharge Service, CPT code 99217, shall not be reported for this scenario.

When a patient is admitted for observation care and then is discharged on a different calendar date, the physician shall report Initial Observation Care, from CPT code range 99218 – 99220, and CPT observation care discharge CPT code 99217. On the rare occasion when a patient remains in observation care for 3 days, the physician shall report an initial observation care code (99218-99220) for the first day of observation care, a subsequent observation care code (99224-99226) for the second day of observation care, and an observation care discharge CPT code 99217 for the observation care on the discharge date. When observation care continues beyond 3 days, the physician shall report a subsequent observation care code (99224-99226) for each day between the first day of observation care and the discharge date.

When a patient receives observation care for a minimum of 8 hours, but less than 24 hours, and is discharged on the same calendar date, Observation or Inpatient Care Services (Including Admission and Discharge Services) from CPT code range 99234 – 99236 shall be reported. The observation discharge, CPT code 99217, cannot also be reported for this scenario.

C. Documentation Requirements for Billing Observation or Inpatient Care Services (Including Admission and Discharge Services)

The physician shall satisfy the E/M documentation guidelines for furnishing observation care or inpatient hospital care. In addition to meeting the documentation requirements for history, examination, and medical decision making, documentation in the medical record shall include:

- Documentation stating the stay for observation care or inpatient hospital care involves 8 hours, but less than 24 hours;
- Documentation identifying the billing physician was present and personally performed the services; and
- Documentation identifying the order for observation services, progress notes, and discharge notes were written by the billing physician.

In the rare circumstance when a patient receives observation services for more than 2 calendar dates, the physician shall bill observation services furnished on day(s) other than the initial or discharge date using subsequent observation care codes. The physician may not use the subsequent hospital care codes since the patient is not an inpatient of the hospital.

D. Admission to Inpatient Status Following Observation Care

If the same physician who ordered hospital outpatient observation services also admits the patient to inpatient status before the end of the date on which the patient began receiving hospital outpatient observation services, pay only an initial hospital visit for the evaluation and management services provided on that date. Medicare payment for the initial hospital visit includes all services provided to the patient on the date of admission by that physician, regardless of the site of service. The physician may not bill an initial or subsequent observation care code for services on the date that he or she admits the patient to inpatient status. If the patient is admitted to inpatient status from hospital outpatient observation care subsequent to the date of initiation of observation services, the physician must bill an initial hospital visit for the services provided on that date. The physician may not bill the hospital observation discharge management code (code 99217) or an outpatient/office visit for the care provided while the patient received hospital outpatient observation services on the date of admission to inpatient status.

E. Hospital Observation Services During Global Surgical Period

The global surgical fee includes payment for hospital observation (codes 99217, 99218, 99219, 99220, 99224, 99225, 99226, 99234, 99235, and 99236) services unless the criteria for use of CPT modifiers "-24," "-25," or "-57" are met. Contractors must pay for these services in addition to the global surgical fee only if both of the following requirements are met:

- The hospital observation service meets the criteria needed to justify billing it with CPT modifiers "-24," "-25," or "-57" (decision for major surgery); and
- The hospital observation service furnished by the surgeon meets all of the criteria for the hospital observation code billed.

Examples of the decision for surgery during a hospital observation period are:

- An emergency department physician orders hospital outpatient observation services for a patient with a head injury. A neurosurgeon is called in to evaluate the need for surgery while the patient is receiving observation services and decides that the patient requires surgery. The surgeon would bill a new or established office or other outpatient visit code as appropriate with the "-57" modifier to indicate that the decision for surgery was made during the evaluation. The surgeon must bill the office or other outpatient visit code because the patient receiving hospital outpatient observation services is not an inpatient of the hospital. Only the physician who ordered hospital outpatient observation services may bill for observation care.
- A neurosurgeon orders hospital outpatient observation services for a patient with a head injury. During the observation period, the surgeon makes the decision for surgery. The surgeon would bill the appropriate level of hospital observation code with the "-57" modifier to indicate that the decision for surgery was made while the surgeon was providing hospital observation care.

Examples of hospital observation services during the postoperative period of a surgery are:

- A surgeon orders hospital outpatient observation services for a patient with abdominal pain from a kidney stone on the 80th day following a TURP (performed by that surgeon). The surgeon decides that the patient does not require surgery. The surgeon would bill the observation code with CPT modifier "-24" and documentation to support that the observation services are unrelated to the surgery.
- A surgeon orders hospital outpatient observation services for a patient with abdominal pain on the 80th day following a TURP (performed by that surgeon). While the patient is receiving hospital outpatient observation services, the surgeon decides that the patient requires kidney surgery. The surgeon would bill the observation code with HCPCS modifier "-57" to indicate that the decision for

surgery was made while the patient was receiving hospital outpatient observation services. The subsequent surgical procedure would be reported with modifier "-79."

- A surgeon orders hospital outpatient observation services for a patient with abdominal pain on the 20th day following a resection of the colon (performed by that surgeon). The surgeon determines that the patient requires no further colon surgery and discharges the patient. The surgeon may not bill for the observation services furnished during the global period because they were related to the previous surgery.

An example of a billable hospital observation service on the same day as a procedure is when a physician repairs a laceration of the scalp in the emergency department for a patient with a head injury and then subsequently orders hospital outpatient observation services for that patient. The physician would bill the observation code with a CPT modifier 25 and the procedure code.

100-04, 12, 30.6.9

Payment for Inpatient Hospital Visits - General

(Rev. 2282, Issued: 08-26-11, Effective: 01-01-11, Implementation: 11-28-11)

A. Hospital Visit and Critical Care on Same Day

When a hospital inpatient or office/outpatient evaluation and management service (E/M) are furnished on a calendar date at which time the patient does not require critical care and the patient subsequently requires critical care both the critical Care Services (CPT codes 99291 and 99292) and the previous E/M service may be paid on the same date of service. Hospital emergency department services are not paid for the same date as critical care services when provided by the same physician to the same patient.

During critical care management of a patient those services that do not meet the level of critical care shall be reported using an inpatient hospital care service with CPT Subsequent Hospital Care using a code from CPT code range 99231 – 99233.

Both Initial Hospital Care (CPT codes 99221 – 99223) and Subsequent Hospital Care codes are "per diem" services and may be reported only once per day by the same physician or physicians of the same specialty from the same group practice.

Physicians and qualified nonphysician practitioners (NPPs) are advised to retain documentation for discretionary contractor review should claims be questioned for both hospital care and critical care claims. The retained documentation shall support claims for critical care when the same physician or physicians of the same specialty in a group practice report critical care services for the same patient on the same calendar date as other E/M services.

B. Two Hospital Visits Same Day

Contractors pay a physician for only one hospital visit per day for the same patient, whether the problems seen during the encounters are related or not. The inpatient hospital visit descriptors contain the phrase "per day" which means that the code and the payment established for the code represent all services provided on that date. The physician should select a code that reflects all services provided during the date of the service.

C. Hospital Visits Same Day But by Different Physicians

In a hospital inpatient situation involving one physician covering for another, if physician A sees the patient in the morning and physician B, who is covering for A, sees the same patient in the evening, contractors do not pay physician B for the second visit. The hospital visit descriptors include the phrase "per day" meaning care for the day.

If the physicians are each responsible for a different aspect of the patient's care, pay both visits if the physicians are in different specialties and the visits are billed with different diagnoses. There are circumstances where concurrent care may be billed by physicians of the same specialty.

D. Visits to Patients in Swing Beds

If the inpatient care is being billed by the hospital as inpatient hospital care, the hospital care codes apply. If the inpatient care is being billed by the hospital as nursing facility care, then the nursing facility codes apply.

100-04, 12, 30.6.9.1

Payment for Initial Hospital Care Services and Observation or Inpatient Care Services (Including Admission and Discharge Services)

(Rev. 2282, Issued: 08-26-11, Effective: 01-01-11, Implementation: 11-28-11)

A. Initial Hospital Care From Emergency Room

Contractors pay for an initial hospital care service if a physician sees a patient in the emergency room and decides to admit the person to the hospital. They do not pay for both E/M services. Also, they do not pay for an emergency department visit by the same physician on the same date of service. When the patient is admitted to the hospital via another site of service (e.g., hospital emergency department, physician's office, nursing facility), all services provided by the physician in conjunction with that admission are considered part of the initial hospital care when performed on the same date as the admission.

B. Initial Hospital Care on Day Following Visit

Contractors pay both visits if a patient is seen in the office on one date and admitted to the hospital on the next date, even if fewer than 24 hours has elapsed between the visit and the admission.

C. Initial Hospital Care and Discharge on Same Day

When the patient is admitted to inpatient hospital care for less than 8 hours on the same date, then Initial Hospital Care, from CPT code range 99221 – 99223, shall be reported by the physician. The Hospital Discharge Day Management service, CPT codes 99238 or 99239, shall not be reported for this scenario.

When a patient is admitted to inpatient initial hospital care and then discharged on a different calendar date, the physician shall report an Initial Hospital Care from CPT code range 99221 – 99223 and a Hospital Discharge Day Management service, CPT code 99238 or 99239.

When a patient has been admitted to inpatient hospital care for a minimum of 8 hours but less than 24 hours and discharged on the same calendar date, Observation or Inpatient Hospital Care Services (Including Admission and Discharge Services), from CPT code range 99234 – 99236, shall be reported.

D. Documentation Requirements for Billing Observation or Inpatient Care Services (Including Admission and Discharge Services)

The physician shall satisfy the E/M documentation guidelines for admission to and discharge from inpatient observation or hospital care. In addition to meeting the documentation requirements for history, examination and medical decision making documentation in the medical record shall include:

- Documentation stating the stay for hospital treatment or observation care status involves 8 hours but less than 24 hours;
- Documentation identifying the billing physician was present and personally performed the services; and
- Documentation identifying the admission and discharge notes were written by the billing physician.

E. Physician Services Involving Transfer From One Hospital to Another; Transfer Within Facility to Prospective Payment System (PPS) Exempt Unit of Hospital; Transfer From One Facility to Another Separate Entity Under Same Ownership and/or Part of Same Complex; or Transfer From One Department to Another Within Single Facility

Physicians may bill both the hospital discharge management code and an initial hospital care code when the discharge and admission do not occur on the same day if the transfer is between:

- Different hospitals;
- Different facilities under common ownership which do not have merged records; or
- Between the acute care hospital and a PPS exempt unit within the same hospital when there are no merged records.

In all other transfer circumstances, the physician should bill only the appropriate level of subsequent hospital care for the date of transfer.

F. Initial Hospital Care Service History and Physical That Is Less Than Comprehensive

When a physician performs a visit that meets the definition of a Level 5 office visit several days prior to an admission and on the day of admission performs less than a comprehensive history and physical, he or she should report the office visit that reflects the services furnished and also report the lowest level initial hospital care code (i.e., code 99221) for the initial hospital admission. Contractors pay the office visit as billed and the Level 1 initial hospital care code.

Physicians who provide an initial visit to a patient during inpatient hospital care that meets the minimum key component work and/or medical necessity requirements shall report an initial hospital care code (99221-99223). The principal physician of record shall append modifier "-AI" (Principal Physician of Record) to the claim for the initial hospital care code. This modifier will identify the physician who oversees the patient's care from all other physicians who may be furnishing specialty care.

Physicians may bill initial hospital care service codes (99221-99223), for services that were reported with CPT consultation codes (99241 – 99255) prior to January 1, 2010, when the furnished service and documentation meet the minimum key component work and/or medical necessity requirements. Physicians must meet all the requirements of the initial hospital care codes, including "a detailed or comprehensive history" and "a detailed or comprehensive examination" to report CPT code 99221, which are greater than the requirements for consultation codes 99251 and 99252.

Subsequent hospital care CPT codes 99231 and 99232, respectively, require "a problem focused interval history" and "an expanded problem focused interval history." An E/M service that could be described by CPT consultation code 99251 or 99252 could potentially meet the component work and medical necessity requirements to report 99231 or 99232. Physicians may report a subsequent hospital care CPT code for services that were reported as CPT consultation codes (99241 – 99255) prior to January 1, 2010, where the medical record appropriately demonstrates that the work and medical necessity requirements are met for reporting a subsequent hospital care code (under the level selected), even though the reported code is for the provider's first E/M service to the inpatient during the hospital stay.

Reporting CPT code 99499 (Unlisted evaluation and management service) should be limited to cases where there is no other specific E/M code payable by Medicare that describes that service.

Reporting CPT code 99499 requires submission of medical records and contractor manual medical review of the service prior to payment. Contractors shall expect reporting under these circumstances to be unusual.

G. Initial Hospital Care Visits by Two Different M.D.s or D.O.s When They Are Involved in Same Admission

In the inpatient hospital setting all physicians (and qualified nonphysician practitioners where permitted) who perform an initial evaluation may bill the initial hospital care codes (99221 – 99223) or nursing facility care codes (99304 – 99306). Contractors consider only one M.D. or D.O. to be the principal physician of record (sometimes referred to as the admitting physician.) The principal physician of record is identified in Medicare as the physician who oversees the patient's care from other physicians who may be furnishing specialty care. Only the principal physician of record shall append modifier "-AI" (Principal Physician of Record) in addition to the E/M code. Follow-up visits in the facility setting shall be billed as subsequent hospital care visits and subsequent nursing facility care visits.

100-04, 12, 30.6.9.2

Subsequent Hospital Visit and Hospital Discharge Day Management (Codes 99231–99239)

(Rev. 1460, Issued: 02-22-08, Effective: 04-01-08, Implementation: 04-07-08)

A. Subsequent Hospital Visits During the Global Surgery Period

(Refer to Secs.40-40.4 on global surgery) The Medicare physician fee schedule payment amount for surgical procedures includes all services (e.g., evaluation and management visits) that are part of the global surgery payment; therefore, contractors shall not pay more than that amount when a bill is fragmented for staged procedures.

B. Hospital Discharge Day Management Service Hospital Discharge Day

Management Services, CPT code 99238 or 99239 is a face-to-face evaluation and management (E/M) service between the attending physician and the patient. The E/M discharge day management visit shall be reported for the date of the actual visit by the physician or qualified nonphysician practitioner even if the patient is discharged from the facility on a different calendar date. Only one hospital discharge day management service is payable per patient per hospital stay.

Only the attending physician of record reports the discharge day management service. Physicians or qualified nonphysician practitioners, other than the attending physician, who have been managing concurrent health care problems not primarily managed by the attending physician, and who are not acting on behalf of the attending physician, shall use Subsequent Hospital Care (CPT code range 99231 - 99233) for a final visit.

Medicare pays for the paperwork of patient discharge day management through the pre- and post- service work of an E/M service.

C. Subsequent Hospital Visit and Discharge Management on Same Day

Pay only the hospital discharge management code on the day of discharge (unless it is also the day of admission, in which case, refer to Sec.30.6.9.1 C for the policy on Observation or Inpatient Care Services (Including Admission and Discharge Services CPT Codes 99234 - 99236). Contractors do not pay both a subsequent hospital visit in addition to hospital discharge day management service on the same day by the same physician. Instruct physicians that they may not bill for both a hospital visit and hospital discharge management for the same date of service.

D. Hospital Discharge Management (CPT Codes 99238 and 99239) and Nursing Facility Admission Code When Patient Is Discharged From Hospital and Admitted to Nursing Facility on Same Day

Contractors pay the hospital discharge code (codes 99238 or 99239) in addition to a nursing facility admission code when they are billed by the same physician with the same date of service.

If a surgeon is admitting the patient to the nursing facility due to a condition that is not as a result of the surgery during the postoperative period of a service with the global surgical period, he/she bills for the nursing facility admission and care with a modifier "-24" and provides documentation that the service is unrelated to the surgery (e.g., return of an elderly patient to the nursing facility in which he/she has resided for five years following discharge from the hospital for cholecystectomy).

Contractors do not pay for a nursing facility admission by a surgeon in the postoperative period of a procedure with a global surgical period if the patient's admission to the nursing facility is to receive post operative care related to the surgery (e.g., admission to a nursing facility to receive physical therapy following a hip replacement). Payment for the nursing facility admission and subsequent nursing facility services are included in the global fee and cannot be paid separately.

E. Hospital Discharge Management and Death Pronouncement

Only the physician who personally performs the pronouncement of death shall bill for the face-to-face Hospital Discharge Day Management Service, CPT code 99238 or 99239. The date of the pronouncement shall reflect the calendar date of service on the day it was performed even if the paperwork is delayed to a subsequent date.

100-04, 12, 30.6.10

Consultation Services

(Rev. 2282, Issued: 08-26-11, Effective: 01-01-11, Implementation: 11-28-11)

Consultation Services versus Other Evaluation and Management (E/M) Visits

Effective January 1, 2010, the consultation codes are no longer recognized for Medicare Part B payment. Physicians shall code patient evaluation and management visits with E/M codes that represent where the visit occurs and that identify the complexity of the visit performed.

In the inpatient hospital setting and the nursing facility setting, physicians (and qualified nonphysician practitioners where permitted) may bill the most appropriate initial hospital care code (99221-99223), subsequent hospital care code (99231 and 99232), initial nursing facility care code (99304-99306), or subsequent nursing facility care code (99307-99310) that reflects the services the physician or practitioner furnished. Subsequent hospital care codes could potentially meet the component work and medical necessity requirements to be reported for an E/M service that could be described by CPT consultation code 99251 or 99252. Contractors shall not find fault in cases where the medical record appropriately demonstrates that the work and medical necessity requirements are met for reporting a subsequent hospital care code (under the level selected), even though the reported code is for the provider's first E/M service to the inpatient during the hospital stay. Unlisted evaluation and management service (code 99499) shall only be reported for consultation services when an E/M service that could be described by codes 99251 or 99252 is furnished, and there is no other specific E/M code payable by Medicare that describes that service. Reporting code 99499 requires submission of medical records and contractor manual medical review of the service prior to payment. CMS expects reporting under these circumstances to be unusual. T he principal physician of record is identified in Medicare as the physician who oversees the patient's care from other physicians who may be furnishing specialty care. The principal physician of record shall append modifier "-AI" (Principal Physician of Record), in addition to the E/M code. Follow-up visits in the facility setting shall be billed as subsequent hospital care visits and subsequent nursing facility care visits.

In the CAH setting, those CAHs that use method II shall bill the appropriate new or established visit code for those physician and non-physician practitioners who have reassigned their billing rights, depending on the relationship status between the physician and patient.

In the office or other outpatient setting where an evaluation is performed, physicians and qualified nonphysician practitioners shall use the CPT codes (99201 – 99215) depending on the complexity of the visit and whether the patient is a new or established patient to that physician. All physicians and qualified nonphysician practitioners shall follow the E/M documentation guidelines for all E/M services. These rules are applicable for Medicare secondary payer claims as well as for claims in which Medicare is the primary payer.

100-04, 12, 30.6.11

Emergency Department Visits (Codes 99281–99288)

(Rev. 1875, Issued: 12-14-09, Effective: 01-01-10, Implementation: 01-04-10)

A. Use of Emergency Department Codes by Physicians Not Assigned to Emergency Department

Any physician seeing a patient registered in the emergency department may use emergency department visit codes (for services matching the code description). It is not required that the physician be assigned to the emergency department.

B. Use of Emergency Department Codes In Office

Emergency department coding is not appropriate if the site of service is an office or outpatient setting or any sight of service other than an emergency department. The emergency department codes should only be used if the patient is seen in the emergency department and the services described by the HCPCS code definition are provided. The emergency department is defined as an organized hospital-based facility for the provision of unscheduled or episodic services to patients who present for immediate medical attention.

C. Use of Emergency Department Codes to Bill Nonemergency Services

Services in the emergency department may not be emergencies. However the codes (99281 - 99288) are payable if the described services are provided.

However, if the physician asks the patient to meet him or her in the emergency department as an alternative to the physician's office and the patient is not registered as a patient in the emergency department, the physician should bill the appropriate office/outpatient visit codes. Normally a lower level emergency department code would be reported for a nonemergency condition.

D. Emergency Department or Office/Outpatient Visits on Same Day As Nursing Facility Admission

Emergency department visit provided on the same day as a comprehensive nursing facility assessment are not paid. Payment for evaluation and management services on the same date provided in sites other than the nursing facility are included in the payment for initial nursing facility care when performed on the same date as the nursing facility admission.

E. Physician Billing for Emergency Department Services Provided to Patient by Both Patient's Personal Physician and Emergency Department Physician

If a physician advises his/her own patient to go to an emergency department (ED) of a hospital for care and the physician subsequently is asked by the ED physician to come to the hospital to evaluate the patient and to advise the ED physician as to whether the patient should be admitted to the hospital or be sent home, the physicians should bill as follows:

If the patient is admitted to the hospital by the patient's personal physician, then the patient's regular physician should bill only the appropriate level of the initial hospital care (codes 99221 - 99223) because all evaluation and management services provided by that physician in conjunction with that admission are considered part of the initial hospital care when performed on the same date as the admission. The ED physician who saw the patient in the emergency department should bill the appropriate level of the ED codes.

If the ED physician, based on the advice of the patient's personal physician who came to the emergency department to see the patient, sends the patient home, then the ED physician should bill the appropriate level of emergency department service. The patient's personal physician should also bill the level of emergency department code that describes the service he or she provided in the emergency department. If the patient's personal physician does not come to the hospital to see the patient, but only advises the emergency department physician by telephone, then the patient's personal physician may not bill.

F. Emergency Department Physician Requests Another Physician to See the Patient in Emergency Department or Office/Outpatient Setting

If the emergency department physician requests that another physician evaluate a given patient, the other physician should bill an emergency department visit code. If the patient is admitted to the hospital by the second physician performing the evaluation, he or she should bill an initial hospital care code and not an emergency department visit code.

100-04, 12, 30.6.13

Nursing Facility Services

(Rev. 2282, Issued: 08-26-11, Effective: 01-01-11, Implementation: 11-28-11)

A. Visits to Perform the Initial Comprehensive Assessment and Annual Assessments

The distinction made between the delegation of physician visits and tasks in a skilled nursing facility (SNF) and in a nursing facility (NF) is based on the Medicare Statute. Section 1819 (b) (6) (A) of the Social Security Act (the Act) governs SNFs while section 1919 (b) (6) (A) of the Act governs NFs. For further information refer to Medlearn Matters article number SE0418 at www.cms.hhs.gov/medlearn/matters.

The federally mandated visits in a SNF and NF must be performed by the physician except as otherwise permitted (42 CFR 483.40 (c) (4) and (f)). The principal physician of record must append the modifier "-AI", (Principal Physician of Record), to the initial nursing facility care code. This modifier will identify the physician who oversees the patient's care from other physicians who may be furnishing specialty care. All other physicians or qualified NPPs who perform an initial evaluation in the NF or SNF may bill the initial nursing facility care code. The initial federally mandated visit is defined in S&C-04-08 (see www.cms.hhs.gov/medlearn/matters) as the initial comprehensive visit during which the physician completes a thorough assessment, develops a plan of care, and writes or verifies admitting orders for the nursing facility resident. For Survey and Certification requirements, a visit must occur no later than 30 days after admission.

Further, per the Long Term Care regulations at 42 CFR 483.40 (c) (4) and (e) (2), in a SNF the physician may not delegate a task that the physician must personally perform. Therefore, as stated in S&C-04-08 the physician may not delegate the initial federally mandated comprehensive visit in a SNF.

The only exception, as to who performs the initial visit, relates to the NF setting. In the NF setting, a qualified NPP (i.e., a nurse practitioner (NP), physician assistant (PA), or a clinical nurse specialist (CNS)), who is not employed by the facility, may perform the initial visit when the State law permits. The evaluation and management (E/M) visit shall be within the State scope of practice and licensure requirements where the E/M visit is performed and the requirements for physician collaboration and physician supervision shall be met.

Under Medicare Part B payment policy, other medically necessary E/M visits may be performed and reported prior to and after the initial visit, if the medical needs of the patient require an E/M visit. A qualified NPP may perform medically necessary E/M visits prior to and after the initial visit if all the requirements for collaboration, general physician supervision, licensure, and billing are met.

The CPT Nursing Facility Services codes shall be used with place of service (POS) 31 (SNF) if the patient is in a Part A SNF stay. They shall be used with POS 32 (nursing facility) if the patient does not have Part A SNF benefits or if the patient is in a NF or in a non-covered SNF stay (e.g., there was no preceding 3-day hospital stay). The CPT Nursing Facility code definition also includes POS 54 (Intermediate Care Facility/Mentally Retarded) and POS 56 (Psychiatric Residential Treatment Center). For further guidance on POS codes and associated CPT codes refer to §30.6.14.

Effective January 1, 2006, the Initial Nursing Facility Care codes 99301– 99303 are deleted.

Beginning January 1, 2006, the new CPT codes, Initial Nursing Facility Care, per day, (99304 – 99306) shall be used to report the initial federally mandated visit. Only a physician may report these codes for an initial federally mandated visit performed in a SNF or NF (with the exception of the qualified NPP in the NF setting who is not employed by the facility and when State law permits, as explained above).

A readmission to a SNF or NF shall have the same payment policy requirements as an initial admission in both the SNF and NF settings.

A physician who is employed by the SNF/NF may perform the E/M visits and bill independently to Medicare Part B for payment. An NPP who is employed by the SNF or NF may perform and bill Medicare Part B directly for those services where it is permitted as discussed above. The employer of the PA shall always report the visits performed by the PA. A physician, NP or CNS has the option to bill Medicare directly or to reassign payment for his/her professional service to the facility.

As with all E/M visits for Medicare Part B payment policy, the E/M documentation guidelines apply.

Medically Necessary Visits

Qualified NPPs may perform medically necessary E/M visits prior to and after the physician's initial federally mandated visit in both the SNF and NF. Medically necessary E/M visits for the diagnosis or treatment of an illness or injury or to improve the functioning of a malformed body member are payable under the physician fee schedule under Medicare Part B. A physician or NPP may bill the most appropriate initial nursing facility care code (CPT codes 99304-99306) or subsequent nursing facility care code (CPT codes 99307-99310), even if the E/M service is provided prior to the initial federally mandated visit.

SNF Setting--Place of Service Code 31

Following the initial federally mandated visit by the physician, the physician may delegate alternate federally mandated physician visits to a qualified NPP who meets collaboration and physician supervision requirements and is licensed as such by the State and performing within the scope of practice in that State.

NF Setting--Place of Service Code 32

Per the regulations at 42 CFR 483.40 (f), a qualified NPP, who meets the collaboration and physician supervision requirements, the State scope of practice and licensure requirements, and who is not employed by the NF, may at the option of the State, perform the initial federally mandated visit in a NF, and may perform any other federally mandated physician visit in a NF in addition to performing other medically necessary E/M visits.

Questions pertaining to writing orders or certification and recertification issues in the SNF and NF settings shall be addressed to the appropriate State Survey and Certification Agency departments for clarification.

B. Visits to Comply With Federal Regulations (42 CFR 483.40 (c) (1)) in the SNF and NF

Payment is made under the physician fee schedule by Medicare Part B for federally mandated visits. Following the initial federally mandated visit by the physician or qualified NPP where permitted, payment shall be made for federally mandated visits that monitor and evaluate residents at least once every 30 days for the first 90 days after admission and at least once every 60 days thereafter.

Effective January 1, 2006, the Subsequent Nursing Facility Care, per day, codes 99311– 99313 are deleted.

Beginning January 1, 2006, the new CPT codes, Subsequent Nursing Facility Care, per day, (99307 – 99310) shall be used to report federally mandated physician E/M visits and medically necessary E/M visits.

Carriers shall not pay for more than one E/M visit performed by the physician or qualified NPP for the same patient on the same date of service. The Nursing Facility Services codes represent a "per day" service.

The federally mandated E/M visit may serve also as a medically necessary E/M visit if the situation arises (i.e., the patient has health problems that need attention on the day the scheduled mandated physician E/M visit occurs). The physician/qualified NPP shall bill only one E/M visit.

Beginning January 1, 2006, the new CPT code, Other Nursing Facility Service (99318), may be used to report an annual nursing facility assessment visit on the required schedule of visits on an annual basis. For Medicare Part B payment policy, an annual nursing facility assessment visit code may substitute as meeting one of the federally mandated physician visits if the code requirements for CPT code 99318 are fully met and in lieu of reporting a Subsequent Nursing Facility Care, per day, service (codes 99307 – 99310). It shall not be performed in addition to the required number of federally mandated physician visits. The new CPT annual assessment code does not represent a new benefit service for Medicare Part B physician services.

Qualified NPPs, whether employed or not by the SNF, may perform alternating federally mandated physician visits, at the option of the physician, after the initial federally mandated visit by the physician in a SNF.

Qualified NPPs in the NF setting, who are not employed by the NF and who are working in collaboration with a physician, may perform federally mandated physician visits, at the option of the State.

Medicare Part B payment policy does not pay for additional E/M visits that may be required by State law for a facility admission or for other additional visits to satisfy facility or other administrative purposes. E/M visits, prior to and after the initial federally mandated physician visit, that are reasonable and medically necessary to meet the medical needs of the individual patient (unrelated to any State requirement or administrative purpose) are payable under Medicare Part B.

C. Visits by Qualified Nonphysician Practitioners

All E/M visits shall be within the State scope of practice and licensure requirements where the visit is performed and all the requirements for physician collaboration and physician supervision shall be met when performed and reported by qualified NPPs. General physician supervision and employer billing requirements shall be met for PA services in addition to the PA meeting the State scope of practice and licensure requirements where the E/M visit is performed.

Medically Necessary Visits

Qualified NPPs may perform medically necessary E/M visits prior to and after the physician's initial visit in both the SNF and NF. Medically necessary E/M visits for the diagnosis or treatment of an illness or injury or to improve the functioning of a malformed body member are payable under the physician fee schedule under Medicare Part B. A physician or NPP may bill the most appropriate initial nursing facility care code (CPT codes 99304-99306) or subsequent nursing facility care code (CPT codes 99307-99310), even if the E/M service is provided prior to the initial federally mandated visit.

SNF Setting--Place of Service Code 31

Following the initial federally mandated visit by the physician, the physician may delegate alternate federally mandated physician visits to a qualified NPP who meets collaboration and physician supervision requirements and is licensed as such by the State and performing within the scope of practice in that State.

NF Setting--Place of Service Code 32

Per the regulations at 42 CFR 483.40 (f), a qualified NPP, who meets the collaboration and physician supervision requirements, the State scope of practice and licensure requirements, and who is not employed by the NF, may at the option of the State, perform the initial federally mandated visit in a NF, and may perform any other federally mandated physician visit in a NF in addition to performing other medically necessary E/M visits.

Questions pertaining to writing orders or certification and recertification issues in the SNF and NF settings shall be addressed to the appropriate State Survey and Certification Agency departments for clarification.

D. Medically Complex Care

Payment is made for E/M visits to patients in a SNF who are receiving services for medically complex care upon discharge from an acute care facility when the visits are reasonable and medically necessary and documented in the medical record. Physicians and qualified NPPs shall report initial nursing facility care codes for their first visit with the patient. The principal physician of record must append the modifier "-AI" (Principal Physician of Record), to the initial nursing facility care code when billed to identify the physician who oversees the patient's care from other physicians who may be furnishing specialty care. Follow-up visits shall be billed as subsequent nursing facility care visits.

E. Incident to Services

Where a physician establishes an office in a SNF/NF, the "incident to" services and requirements are confined to this discrete part of the facility designated as his/her office. "Incident to" E/M visits, provided in a facility setting, are not payable under the Physician Fee Schedule for Medicare Part B. Thus, visits performed outside the designated "office" area in the SNF/NF would be subject to the coverage and payment rules applicable to the SNF/NF setting and shall not be reported using the CPT codes for office or other outpatient visits or use place of service code 11.

F. Use of the Prolonged Services Codes and Other Time-Related Services

Beginning January 1, 2008, typical/average time units for E/M visits in the SNF/NF settings are reestablished. Medically necessary prolonged services for E/M visits (codes 99356 and 99357) in a SNF or NF may be billed with the Nursing Facility Services in the code ranges (99304 – 99306, 99307 – 99310 and 99318).

Counseling and Coordination of Care Visits

With the reestablishment of typical/average time units, medically necessary E/M visits for counseling and coordination of care, for Nursing Facility Services in the code ranges (99304 – 99306, 99307 – 99310 and 99318) that are time-based services, may be billed with the appropriate prolonged services codes (99356 and 99357).

G. Multiple Visits

The complexity level of an E/M visit and the CPT code billed must be a covered and medically necessary visit for each patient (refer to §§1862 (a)(1)(A) of the Act). Claims for an unreasonable number of daily E/M visits by the same physician to multiple patients at a facility within a 24-hour period may result in medical review to determine medical necessity for the visits. The E/M visit (Nursing Facility Services) represents a "per day" service per patient as defined by the CPT code. The medical record must be personally documented by the physician or qualified NPP who performed the E/M visit and the documentation shall support the specific level of E/M visit to each individual patient.

H. Split/Shared E/M Visit

A split/shared E/M visit cannot be reported in the SNF/NF setting. A split/shared E/M visit is defined by Medicare Part B payment policy as a medically necessary encounter with a patient where the physician and a qualified NPP each personally perform a substantive portion of an E/M visit face-to-face with the same patient on the same date of service. A substantive portion of an E/M visit involves all or some portion of the history, exam or medical decision making key components of an E/M service. The physician and the qualified NPP must be in the same group practice or be employed by the same employer. The split/shared E/M visit applies only to selected E/M visits and settings (i.e., hospital inpatient, hospital outpatient, hospital observation, emergency department, hospital discharge, office and non facility clinic visits, and prolonged visits associated with these E/M visit codes). The split/shared E/M policy does not apply to critical care services or procedures.

I. SNF/NF Discharge Day Management Service

Medicare Part B payment policy requires a face-to-face visit with the patient provided by the physician or the qualified NPP to meet the SNF/NF discharge day management service as defined by the CPT code. The E/M discharge day management visit shall be reported for the date of the actual visit by the physician or qualified NPP even if the patient is discharged from the facility on a different calendar date. The CPT codes 99315 - 99316 shall be reported for this visit. The Discharge Day Management Service may be reported using CPT code 99315 or 99316, depending on the code requirement, for a patient who has expired, but only if the physician or qualified NPP personally performed the death pronouncement.

100-04, 12, 30.6.14

Home Care and Domiciliary Care Visits (Codes 99324–99350)

(Rev. 775, Issued: 12-02-05, Effective: 01-01-06, Implementation: 01-03-06)

Physician Visits to Patients Residing in Various Places of Service

The American Medical Association's Current Procedural Terminology (CPT) 2006 new patient codes 99324 - 99328 and established patient codes 99334 - 99337(new codes beginning January 2006), for Domiciliary, Rest Home (e.g., Boarding Home), or Custodial Care Services, are used to report evaluation and management (E/M) services to residents residing in a facility which provides room, board, and other personal assistance services, generally on a long-term basis. These CPT codes are used to report E/M services in facilities assigned places of service (POS) codes 13 (Assisted Living Facility), 14 (Group Home), 33 (Custodial Care Facility) and 55 (Residential Substance Abuse Facility). Assisted living facilities may also be known as adult living facilities.

Physicians and qualified nonphysician practitioners (NPPs) furnishing E/M services to residents in a living arrangement described by one of the POS listed above must use the level of service code in the CPT code range 99324 - 99337 to report the service they provide. The CPT codes 99321 - 99333 for Domiciliary, Rest Home (e.g., Boarding Home), or Custodial Care Services are deleted beginning January, 2006.

Beginning in 2006, reasonable and medically necessary, face-to-face, prolonged services, represented by CPT codes 99354 - 99355, may be reported with the appropriate companion E/M codes when a physician or qualified NPP, provides a prolonged service involving direct (face-to-face) patient contact that is beyond the usual E/M visit service for a Domiciliary, Rest Home (e.g., Boarding Home) or Custodial Care Service. All the requirements for prolonged services at Sec.30.6.15.1 must be met.

The CPT codes 99341 through 99350, Home Services codes, are used to report E/M services furnished to a patient residing in his or her own private residence (e.g., private home, apartment, town home) and not residing in any type of congregate/shared facility living arrangement including assisted living facilities and group homes. The Home Services codes apply only to the specific 2-digit POS 12 (Home). Home Services codes may not be used for billing E/M services provided in settings other than in the private residence of an individual as described above.

Beginning in 2006, E/M services provided to patients residing in a Skilled Nursing Facility (SNF) or a Nursing Facility (NF) must be reported using the appropriate CPT level of service code within the range identified for Initial Nursing Facility Care (new CPT codes 99304 - 99306) and Subsequent Nursing Facility Care (new CPT codes 99307 - 99310). Use the CPT code, Other Nursing Facility Services (new CPT code 99318), for an annual nursing facility assessment. Use CPT codes 99315 - 99316 for SNF/NF discharge services. The CPT codes 99301 - 99303 and 99311 - 99313 are deleted beginning January, 2006. The Home Services codes should not be used for these places of service.

The CPT SNF/NF code definition includes intermediate care facilities (ICFs) and long term care facilities (LTCFs). These codes are limited to the specific 2-digit POS 31 (SNF), 32 (Nursing Facility), 54 (Intermediate Care Facility/Mentally Retarded) and 56 (Psychiatric Residential Treatment Center).

The CPT nursing facility codes should be used with POS 31 (SNF) if the patient is in a Part A SNF stay and POS 32 (nursing facility) if the patient does not have Part A SNF benefits. There is no longer a different payment amount for a Part A or Part B benefit period in these POS settings.

100-04, 12, 30.6.14.1

Home Care and Domiciliary Care Visits (Codes 99324–99350)

(Rev. 775, Issued: 12-02-05, Effective: 01-01-06, Implementation: 01-03-06)

Physician Visits to Patients Residing in Various Places of Service

The American Medical Association's Current Procedural Terminology (CPT) 2006 new patient codes 99324 - 99328 and established patient codes 99334 - 99337(new codes beginning January 2006), for Domiciliary, Rest Home (e.g., Boarding Home), or Custodial Care Services, are used to report evaluation and management (E/M) services to residents residing in a facility which provides room, board, and other personal assistance services, generally on a long-term basis. These CPT codes are used to report E/M services in facilities assigned places of service (POS) codes 13 (Assisted Living Facility), 14 (Group Home), 33 (Custodial Care Facility) and 55 (Residential Substance Abuse Facility). Assisted living facilities may also be known as adult living facilities.

Physicians and qualified nonphysician practitioners (NPPs) furnishing E/M services to residents in a living arrangement described by one of the POS listed above must use the level of service code in the CPT code range 99324 - 99337 to report the service they provide. The CPT codes 99321 - 99333 for Domiciliary, Rest Home (e.g., Boarding Home), or Custodial Care Services are deleted beginning January, 2006.

Beginning in 2006, reasonable and medically necessary, face-to-face, prolonged services, represented by CPT codes 99354 - 99355, may be reported with the appropriate companion E/M codes when a physician or qualified NPP, provides a prolonged service involving direct (face-to-face) patient contact that is beyond the usual E/M visit service for a Domiciliary, Rest Home (e.g., Boarding Home) or Custodial Care Service. All the requirements for prolonged services at §30.6.15.1 must be met.

The CPT codes 99341 through 99350, Home Services codes, are used to report E/M services furnished to a patient residing in his or her own private residence (e.g., private home, apartment, town home) and not residing in any type of congregate/shared facility living arrangement including assisted living facilities and group homes. The Home Services codes apply only to the specific 2-digit POS 12 (Home). Home Services codes may not be used for billing E/M services provided in settings other than in the private residence of an individual as described above.

Beginning in 2006, E/M services provided to patients residing in a Skilled Nursing Facility (SNF) or a Nursing Facility (NF) must be reported using the appropriate CPT level of service code within the range identified for Initial Nursing Facility Care (new CPT codes 99304 - 99306) and Subsequent Nursing Facility Care (new CPT codes 99307 - 99310). Use the CPT code, Other Nursing Facility Services (new CPT code 99318), for an annual nursing facility assessment. Use CPT codes 99315 - 99316 for SNF/NF discharge services. The CPT codes 99301 - 99303 and 99311 - 99313 are deleted beginning January, 2006. The Home Services codes should not be used for these places of service.

The CPT SNF/NF code definition includes intermediate care facilities (ICFs) and long term care facilities (LTCFs). These codes are limited to the specific 2-digit POS 31 (SNF), 32 (Nursing Facility), 54 (Intermediate Care Facility/Mentally Retarded) and 56 (Psychiatric Residential Treatment Center).

The CPT nursing facility codes should be used with POS 31 (SNF) if the patient is in a Part A SNF stay and POS 32 (nursing facility) if the patient does not have Part A SNF benefits. There is no longer a different payment amount for a Part A or Part B benefit period in these POS settings.

100-04, 12, 30.6.15.1

Prolonged Services With Direct Face-to-Face Patient Contact Service (ZZZ codes)

(Rev. 2282, Issued: 08-26-11, Effective: 01-01-11, Implementation: 11-28-11)

A. Definition

Prolonged physician services (CPT code 99354) in the office or other outpatient setting with direct face-to-face patient contact which require 1 hour beyond the usual service are payable when billed on the same day by the same physician or qualified nonphysician practitioner (NPP) as the companion evaluation and management codes. The time for usual service refers to the typical/average time units associated with the companion evaluation and management service as noted in the CPT code. Each additional 30 minutes of direct face-to-face patient contact following the first hour of prolonged services may be reported by CPT code 99355.

Prolonged physician services (code 99356) in the inpatient setting, with direct face-to-face patient contact which require 1 hour beyond the usual service are payable when they are billed on the same day by the same physician or qualified NPP as the companion evaluation and management codes. Each additional 30 minutes of direct face-to-face patient contact following the first hour of prolonged services may be reported by CPT code 99357.

Prolonged service of less than 30 minutes total duration on a given date is not separately reported because the work involved is included in the total work of the evaluation and management codes.

Code 99355 or 99357 may be used to report each additional 30 minutes beyond the first hour of prolonged services, based on the place of service. These codes may be used to report the final 15 – 30 minutes of prolonged service on a given date, if not otherwise billed. Prolonged service of less than 15 minutes beyond the first hour or less than 15 minutes beyond the final 30 minutes is not reported separately.

B. Required Companion Codes

- The companion evaluation and management codes for 99354 are the Office or Other Outpatient visit codes (99201 - 99205, 99212 – 99215), the Domiciliary, Rest Home, or Custodial Care Services codes (99324 – 99328, 99334 – 99337), the Home Services codes (99341 - 99345, 99347 – 99350);
- The companion codes for 99355 are 99354 and one of the evaluation and management codes required for 99354 to be used;
- The companion evaluation and management codes for 99356 are the Initial Hospital Care codes and Subsequent Hospital Care codes (99221 - 99223, 99231 – 99233); Nursing Facility Services codes (99304 -99318); or
- The companion codes for 99357 are 99356 and one of the evaluation and management codes required for 99356 to be used.

Prolonged services codes 99354 – 99357 are not paid unless they are accompanied by the companion codes as indicated.

C. Requirement for Physician Presence

Physicians may count only the duration of direct face-to-face contact between the physician and the patient (whether the service was continuous or not) beyond the typical/average time of the visit code billed to determine whether prolonged services can be billed and to determine the prolonged services codes that are allowable. In the case of prolonged office services, time spent by office staff with the patient, or time the patient remains unaccompanied in the office cannot be billed. In the case of prolonged hospital services, time spent reviewing charts or discussion of a patient with house medical staff and not with direct face-to-face contact with the patient, or waiting for test results, for changes in the patient's condition, for end of a therapy, or for use of facilities cannot be billed as prolonged services.

D. Documentation

Documentation is not required to accompany the bill for prolonged services unless the physician has been selected for medical review. Documentation is required in the medical record about the duration and content of the medically necessary evaluation and management service and prolonged services billed. The medical record must be appropriately and sufficiently documented by the physician or qualified NPP to show that the physician or qualified NPP personally furnished the direct face-to-face time with the patient specified in the CPT code definitions. The start and end times of the visit shall be documented in the medical record along with the date of service.

E. Use of the Codes

Prolonged services codes can be billed only if the total duration of the physician or qualified NPP direct face-to-face service (including the visit) equals or exceeds the threshold time for the evaluation and management service the physician or qualified NPP provided (typical/average time associated with the CPT E/M code plus 30 minutes). If the total duration of direct face-to-face time does not equal or exceed the threshold time for the level of evaluation and management service the physician or qualified NPP provided, the physician or qualified NPP may not bill for prolonged services.

F. Threshold Times for Codes 99354 and 99355 (Office or Other Outpatient Setting)

If the total direct face-to-face time equals or exceeds the threshold time for code 99354, but is less than the threshold time for code 99355, the physician should bill the evaluation and management visit code and code 99354. No more than one unit of 99354 is acceptable. If the total direct face-to-face time equals or exceeds the threshold time for code 99355 by no more than 29 minutes, the physician should bill the visit code 99354 and one unit of code 99355. One additional unit of code 99355 is billed for each additional increment of 30 minutes extended duration. Contractors use the following threshold times to determine if the prolonged services codes 99354 and/or 99355 can be billed with the office or other outpatient settings including domiciliary, rest home, or custodial care services and home services codes.

Threshold Time for Prolonged Visit Codes 99354 and/or 99355 Billed with Office/Outpatient Code

Code	Typical Time for Code	Threshold Time to Bill Code 99354	Threshold Time to Bill Codes 99354 and 99355
99201	10	40	85
99202	20	50	95
99203	30	60	105
99204	45	75	120
99205	60	90	135
99212	10	40	85
99213	15	45	90
99214	25	55	100
99215	40	70	115
99324	20	50	95
99325	30	60	105
99326	45	75	120
99327	60	90	135
99328	75	105	150
99334	15	45	90
99335	25	55	100
99336	40	70	115
99337	60	90	135
99341	20	50	95
99342	30	60	105
99343	45	75	120
99344	60	90	135
99345	75	105	150
99347	15	45	90
99348	25	55	100
99349	40	70	115
99350	60	90	135

G. Threshold Times for Codes 99356 and 99357

(Inpatient Setting) If the total direct face-to-face time equals or exceeds the threshold time for code 99356, but is less than the threshold time for code 99357, the physician should bill the visit and code 99356. Contractors do not accept more than one unit of code 99356. If the total direct face-to-face time equals or exceeds the threshold time for code 99356 by no more than 29 minutes, the physician bills the visit code 99356 and one unit of code 99357. One additional unit of code 99357 is billed for each additional increment of 30 minutes extended duration. Contractors use the following threshold times to determine if the prolonged services codes 99356 and/or 99357 can be billed with the inpatient setting codes.

Threshold Time for Prolonged Visit Codes 99356 and/or 99357 Billed with Inpatient Setting Codes Code

Code	Typical Time for Code	Threshold Time to Bill Code 99356	Threshold Time to Bill Codes 99356 and 99357
99221	30	60	105
99222	50	80	125
99223	70	100	145
99231	15	45	90
99232	25	55	100
99233	35	65	110
99304	25	55	100
99305	35	65	110
99306	45	75	120
99307	10	40	85
99308	15	45	90
99309	25	55	100
99310	35	65	110
99318	30	60	10

Add 30 minutes to the threshold time for billing codes 99356 and 99357 to get the threshold time for billing code 99356 and two units of 99357.

H. Prolonged Services Associated With Evaluation and Management Services Based on Counseling and/or Coordination of Care (Time-Based)

When an evaluation and management service is dominated by counseling and/or coordination of care (the counseling and/or coordination of care represents more than 50% of the total time with the patient) in a face-to-face encounter between the physician or qualified NPP and the patient in the office/clinic or the floor time (in the scenario of an inpatient service), then the evaluation and management code is selected based on the typical/average time associated with the code levels. The time approximation must meet or exceed the specific CPT code billed (determined by the typical/average time associated with the evaluation and management code) and should not be "rounded" to the next higher level.

In those evaluation and management services in which the code level is selected based on time, prolonged services may only be reported with the highest code level in that family of codes as the companion code.

I. Examples of Billable Prolonged Services

EXAMPLE 1

A physician performed a visit that met the definition of an office visit code 99213 and the total duration of the direct face-to-face services (including the visit) was 65 minutes. The physician bills code 99213 and one unit of code 99354.

EXAMPLE 2

A physician performed a visit that met the definition of a domiciliary, rest home care visit code 99327 and the total duration of the direct face-to-face contact (including the visit) was 140 minutes. The physician bills codes 99327, 99354, and one unit of code 99355.

EXAMPLE 3

A physician performed an office visit to an established patient that was predominantly counseling, spending 75 minutes (direct face-to-face) with the patient. The physician should report CPT code 99215 and one unit of code 99354.

J. Examples of Nonbillable Prolonged Services

EXAMPLE 1

A physician performed a visit that met the definition of visit code 99212 and the total duration of the direct face-to-face contact (including the visit) was 35 minutes. The physician cannot bill prolonged services because the total duration of direct face-to-face service did not meet the threshold time for billing prolonged services.

EXAMPLE 2

A physician performed a visit that met the definition of code 99213 and, while the patient was in the office receiving treatment for 4 hours, the total duration of the direct face-to-face service of the physician was 40 minutes. The physician cannot bill prolonged services because the total duration of direct face-to-face service did not meet the threshold time for billing prolonged services.

EXAMPLE 3

A physician provided a subsequent office visit that was predominantly counseling, spending 60 minutes (face-to-face) with the patient. The physician cannot code 99214, which has a typical time of 25 minutes, and one unit of code 99354. The physician must bill the highest level code in the code family (99215 which has 40 minutes typical/average time units associated with it). The additional time spent beyond this code is 20 minutes and does not meet the threshold time for billing prolonged services.

100-04, 12, 30.6.15.2

Prolonged Services Without Direct Face-to-Face Patient Contact Service (Codes 99358 - 99359)

(Rev. 3678, Issued: 12-16-16, Effective: 01-01-17, Implementation: 01-03-17)

Until CY 2017, CPT codes 99358 and 99359 were not separately payable and were bundled (included for payment) under the related face-to-face E/M service code. Practitioners were not permitted to bill the patient for services described by CPT codes 99358 and 99359 since they are Medicare covered services and payment was included in the payment for other billable services.

Beginning in CY 2017, CPT codes 99358 and 99359 are separately payable under the physician fee schedule. The CPT prefatory language and reporting rules for these codes apply for Medicare billing. For example, CPT codes 99358 and 99359 cannot be reported during the same service period as complex chronic care management (CCM) services or transitional care management services. They are not reported for time spent in non-face-to-face care described by more specific codes having no upper time limit in the CPT code set. We have posted a file that notes the times assumed to be typical for purposes of PFS rate-setting. That file is available on our website under downloads for our annual regulation at http://www.cms.gov/Medicare/Medicare-Fee-for-Service-Payment/PhysicianFeeSched/PFS-Federal-Regulation-Notices.html. We note that while these typical times are not required to bill the displayed codes, we would expect that only time spent in excess of these times would be reported under CPT codes 99358 and 99359. We note that CPT codes 99358 and 99359 can only be used to report extended qualifying time of the billing physician or other practitioner (not clinical staff). Prolonged services cannot be reported in association with a companion E/M code that also qualifies as the initiating visit for CCM services. Practitioners should instead report the add-on code for CCM initiation, if applicable.

100-04, 12, 30.6.15.3

Physician Standby Service (Code 99360)

(Rev. 1, 10-01-03)

Standby services are not payable to physicians. Physicians may not bill Medicare or beneficiaries for standby services. Payment for standby services is included in the Part A payment to the facility. Such services are a part of hospital costs to provide quality care. If hospitals pay physicians for standby services, such services are part of hospital costs to provide quality care.

100-04, 12, 30.6.17

Physician Management Associated with Superficial Radiation Treatment

(Rev. 4339, Issued: 07-25-19, Effective: 01-01-19, Implementation: 08-27-19)

Evaluation and management codes for levels I through III (99211, 99212, and 99213) may be billed with modifier 25 when performed for the purpose of reporting physician work associated with radiation therapy planning, radiation treatment device construction, and radiation treatment management when performed on the same date of service as superficial radiation treatment delivery. See chapter 13, section 70.2, of this manual for information regarding services bundled into treatment management codes.

100-04, 12, 40.3

Claims Review for Global Surgeries

(Rev. 2997, Issued: 07-25-14, Effective: Upon implementation of ICD-10; 01-01-2012 - ASC X12, Implementation: 08-25-2014 - ASC X12; Upon Implementation of ICD-10)

A. Relationship to Correct Coding Initiative (CCI)

The CCI policy and computer edits allow A/B MACs (B) to detect instances of fragmented billing for certain intra-operative services and other services furnished on the same day as the surgery that are considered to be components of the surgical procedure and, therefore, included in the global surgical fee. When both correct coding and global surgery edits apply to the same claim, A/B MACs (B) first apply the correct coding edits, then, apply the global surgery edits to the correctly coded services.

B. Prepayment Edits to Detect Separate Billing of Services Included in the Global Package

In addition to the correct coding edits, A/B MACs (B) must be capable of detecting certain other services included in the payment for a major or minor surgery or for an endoscopy. On a prepayment basis, A/B MACs (B) identify the services that meet the following conditions:

- Preoperative services that are submitted on the same claim or on a subsequent claim as a surgical procedure; or
- Same day or postoperative services that are submitted on the same claim or on a subsequent claim as a surgical procedure or endoscopy;

  and -

- Services that were furnished within the prescribed global period of the surgical procedure;
- Services that are billed without modifier "-78," "-79," "-24," "25," or "-57" or are billed with modifier "-24" but without the required documentation; and

- Services that are billed with the same provider or group number as the surgical procedure or endoscopy. Also, edit for any visits billed separately during the postoperative period without modifier "-24" by a physician who billed for the postoperative care only with modifier "-55."

A/B MACs (B) use the following evaluation and management codes in establishing edits for visits included in the global package. CPT codes 99241, 99242, 99243, 99244, 99245, 99251, 99252, 99253, 99254, 99255, 99271, 99272, 99273, 99274, and 99275 have been transferred from the excluded category and are now included in the global surgery edits.

Evaluation and Management Codes for A/B MAC (B) Edits

92012	92014	99211	99212	99213	99214	99215
99217	99218	99219	99220	99221	99222	99223
99231	99232	99233	99234	99235	99236	99238
99239	99241	99242	99243	99244	99245	99251
99252	99253	99254	99255	99261	99262	99263
99271	99272	99273	99274	99275	99291	99292
99301	99302	99303	99311	99312	99313	99315
99316	99331	99332	99333	99347	99348	99349
99350	99374	99375	99377	99378		

NOTE: In order for codes 99291 or 99292 to be paid for services furnished during the preoperative or postoperative period, modifier "-25" or "-24," respectively, must be used to indicate that the critical care was unrelated to the specific anatomic injury or general surgical procedure performed.

If a surgeon is admitting a patient to a nursing facility for a condition not related to the global surgical procedure, the physician should bill for the nursing facility admission and care with a "-24" modifier and appropriate documentation. If a surgeon is admitting a patient to a nursing facility and the patient's admission to that facility relates to the global surgical procedure, the nursing facility admission and any services related to the global surgical procedure are included in the global surgery fee.

C. Exclusions from Prepayment Edits

A/B MACs (B) exclude the following services from the prepayment audit process and allow separate payment if all usual requirements are met:

- Services listed in §40.1.B; and
- Services billed with the modifier "-25," "-57," "-58," "-78," or "-79."

Exceptions

See §§40.2.A.8, 40.2.A.9, and 40.4.A for instances where prepayment review is required for modifier "-25." In addition, prepayment review is necessary for CPT codes 90935, 90937, 90945, and 90947 when a visit and modifier "-25" are billed with these services.

Exclude the following codes from the prepayment edits required in §40.3.B.

92002	92004	99201	99202	99203	99204	99205
99281	99282	99283	99284	99285	99321	99322
99323	99341	99342	99343	99344	99345	

100-04, 12, 40.7

Claims for Bilateral Surgeries

(Rev. 1, 10-01-03) B3-4827, B3-15040

A. General

Bilateral surgeries are procedures performed on both sides of the body during the same operative session or on the same day.

The terminology for some procedure codes includes the terms "bilateral" (e.g., code 27395; Lengthening of the hamstring tendon; multiple, bilateral.) or "unilateral or bilateral" (e.g., code 52290; cystourethroscopy; with ureteral meatotomy, unilateral or bilateral). The payment adjustment rules for bilateral surgeries do not apply to procedures identified by CPT as "bilateral" or "unilateral or bilateral" since the fee schedule reflects any additional work required for bilateral surgeries.

Field 22 of the MFSDB indicates whether the payment adjustment rules apply to a surgical procedure.

B. Billing Instructions for Bilateral Surgeries

If a procedure is not identified by its terminology as a bilateral procedure (or unilateral or bilateral), physicians must report the procedure with modifier "-50." They report such procedures as a single line item. (NOTE: This differs from the CPT coding guidelines which indicate that bilateral procedures should be billed as two line items.)

If a procedure is identified by the terminology as bilateral (or unilateral or bilateral), as in codes 27395 and 52290, physicians do not report the procedure with modifier "-50."

C. Claims Processing System Requirements

Carriers must be able to:

1. Identify bilateral surgeries by the presence on the claim form or electronic submission of the "-50" modifier or of the same code on separate lines reported once with modifier "-LT" and once with modifier "-RT";
2. Access Field 34 or 35 of the MFSDB to determine the Medicare payment amount;
3. Access Field 22 of the MFSDB:
   — If Field 22 contains an indicator of "0," "2," or "3," the payment adjustment rules for bilateral surgeries do not apply. Base payment on the lower of the billed amount or 100 percent of the fee schedule amount (Field 34 or 35) unless other payment adjustment rules apply.

   NOTE: Some codes which have a bilateral indicator of "0" in the MFSDB may be performed more than once on a given day. These are services that would never be considered bilateral and thus should not be billed with modifier "-50." Where such a code is billed on multiple line tems or with more than 1 in the units field and carriers have determined that the code may be reported more than once, bypass the "0" bilateral indicator and refer to the multiple surgery field for pricing;

   — If Field 22 contains an indicator of "1," the standard adjustment rules apply. Base payment on the lower of the billed amount or 150 percent of the fee schedule amount (Field 34 or 35). (Multiply the payment amount in Field 34 or 35 for the surgery by 150 percent and round to the nearest cent.)
4. Apply the requirements 40 - 40.4 on global surgeries to bilateral surgeries; and
5. Retain the "-50" modifier in history for any bilateral surgeries paid at the adjusted amount.

   (NOTE: The "-50" modifier is not retained for surgeries which are bilateral by definition such as code 27395.)

100-04, 12, 40.8

Claims for Co-Surgeons and Team Surgeons

(Rev. 3721, Issued: 02-24-17, Effective: 05-25-17, Implementation: 05-25-17)

A. General

Under some circumstances, the individual skills of two or more surgeons are required to perform surgery on the same patient during the same operative session. This may be required because of the complex nature of the procedure(s) and/or the patient's condition.

In these cases, the additional physicians are not acting as assistants-at-surgery.

B. Billing Instructions

The following billing procedures apply when billing for a surgical procedure or procedures that required the use of two surgeons or a team of surgeons:

- If two surgeons (each in a different specialty) are required to perform a specific procedure, each surgeon bills for the procedure with a modifier "-62. " Co-surgery also refers to surgical procedures involving two surgeons performing the parts of the procedure simultaneously, i.e., heart transplant or bilateral knee replacements. Documentation of the medical necessity for two surgeons is required for certain services identified in the MFSDB. (See 40.8.C.5.);
- If a team of surgeons (more than 2 surgeons of different specialties) is required to perform a specific procedure, each surgeon bills for the procedure with a modifier "-66." Field 25 of the MFSDB identifies certain services submitted with a "-66" modifier which must be sufficiently documented to establish that a team was medically necessary. All claims for team surgeons must contain sufficient information to allow pricing "by report."
- If surgeons of different specialties are each performing a different procedure (with specific CPT codes), neither co-surgery nor multiple surgery rules apply (even if the procedures are performed through the same incision). If one of the surgeons performs multiple procedures, the multiple procedure rules apply to that surgeon's services. (See 40.6 for multiple surgery payment rules.)

For co-surgeons (modifier 62), the fee schedule amount applicable to the payment for each co-surgeon is 62.5 percent of the global surgery fee schedule amount. Team surgery (modifier 66) is paid for on a "By Report" basis.

C. Claims Processing System Requirements

Carriers must be able to:

1. Identify a surgical procedure performed by two surgeons or a team of surgeons by the presence on the claim form or electronic submission of the "-62" or "-66" modifier;
2. Access Field 34 or 35 of the MFSDB to determine the fee schedule payment amount for the surgery;
3. Access Field 24 or 25, as appropriate, of the MFSDB. These fields provide guidance on whether two or team surgeons are generally required for the surgical procedure;
4. If the surgery is billed with a "-62" or "-66" modifier and Field 24 or 25 contains an indicator of "0," payment adjustment rules for two or team surgeons do not apply:
   — Carriers pay the first bill submitted, and base payment on the lower of the billed amount or 100 percent of the fee schedule amount (Field 34 or 35) unless other payment adjustment rules apply;

   — Carriers deny bills received subsequently from other physicians and use the appropriate MSN message in 40.8.D. As these are medical necessity denials, the instructions in the Program Integrity Manual regarding denial of unassigned claims for medical necessity are applied;

5. If the surgery is billed with a "-62" modifier and Field 24 contains an indicator of "1," suspend the claim for manual review of any documentation submitted with the claim. If the documentation supports the need for co-surgeons, base payment for each physician on the lower of the billed amount or 62.5 percent of the fee schedule amount (Field 34 or 35);
6. If the surgery is billed with a "-62" modifier and Field 24 contains an indicator of "2," payment rules for two surgeons apply. Carriers base payment for each physician on the lower of the billed amount or 62.5 percent of the fee schedule amount (Field 34 or 35);
7. If the surgery is billed with a "-66" modifier and Field 25 contains an indicator of "1," carriers suspend the claim for manual review. If carriers determine that team surgeons were medically necessary, each physician is paid on a "by report" basis;
8. If the surgery is billed with a "-66" modifier and Field 25 contains an indicator of "2," carriers pay "by report";

   NOTE: A Medicare fee may have been established for some surgical procedures that are billed with the "-66" modifier. In these cases, all physicians on the team must agree on the percentage of the Medicare payment amount each is to receive.

   If carriers receive a bill with a "-66" modifier after carriers have paid one surgeon the full Medicare payment amount (on a bill without the modifier), deny the subsequent claim.
9. Apply the rules global surgical packages to each of the physicians participating in a co- or team surgery; and
10. Retain the "-62" and "-66" modifiers in history for any co- or team surgeries.

D. Beneficiary Liability on Denied Claims for Assistant, Co- surgeon and Team Surgeons

When the procedure is subject to the statutory restriction against payment for assistants-at-surgery, such payment shall be denied.

The following reflects the remittance advice messages and associated codes that will appear when rejecting/denying claims under this policy. This CARC/RARC combination is compliant with CAQH CORE Business Scenario 3.

Group Code: CO
CARC: 54
RARC: N/A
MSN: 15.11

Carriers include the following statement in the MSN:

"You cannot be charged for this service." (Unnumbered add-on message.)

If Field 23 of the MFSDB contains an indicator of "0" or "1" (assistant-at-surgery may not be paid) for procedures CMS has determined that an assistant surgeon is not generally medically necessary.

The following reflects the remittance advice messages and associated codes that will appear when rejecting/denying claims under this policy. This CARC/RARC combination is compliant with CAQH CORE Business Scenario 3.

Group Code: CO
CARC: 54
RARC: N/A
MSN: 15.12

For those procedures with an indicator of "0," the limitation on liability provisions described in Chapter 30 apply to assigned claims. Therefore, carriers include the appropriate limitation of liability language from Chapter 21. For unassigned claims, apply the rules in the Program Integrity Manual concerning denial for medical necessity.

Where payment may not be made for a co- or team surgeon, deny the claim

The following reflects the remittance advice messages and associated codes that will appear when rejecting/denying claims under this policy. This CARC/RARC combination is compliant with CAQH CORE Business Scenario 3.

Group Code: CO
CARC: 54
RARC: N/A
MSN: 15.13

Where payment may not be made for a two surgeons, deny the claim.

The following reflects the remittance advice messages and associated codes that will appear when rejecting/denying claims under this policy. This CARC/RARC combination is compliant with CAQH CORE Business Scenario 3.

Group Code: CO
CARC: 54
RARC: N/A
MSN: 15.12

Also see limitation of liability remittance notice Remittance Advice Remark Code Alert M27 and use when appropriate.

100-04, 12, 50

Payment for Anesthesiology Services

(Rev. 3747; Issued: 04-14-17; Effective: 01-01-17; Implementation: 05-15-17)

A. General Payment Rule

The fee schedule amount for physician anesthesia services furnished is, with the exceptions noted, based on allowable base and time units multiplied by an anesthesia conversion factor specific to that locality. The base unit for each anesthesia procedure is communicated to the A/B MACs by means of the HCPCS file released annually. CMS releases the conversion factor annually. The base units and conversion factor are available on the CMS website at: https://www.cms.gov/Center/Provider-Type/Anesthesiologists-Center.html.

B. Payment at Personally Performed Rate

The A/B MAC must determine the fee schedule payment, recognizing the base unit for the anesthesia code and one time unit per 15 minutes of anesthesia time if:

- The physician personally performed the entire anesthesia service alone;
- The physician is involved with one anesthesia case with a resident, the physician is a teaching physician as defined in §100;
- The physician is involved in the training of physician residents in a single anesthesia case, two concurrent anesthesia cases involving residents or a single anesthesia case involving a resident that is concurrent to another case that meets the requirements for payment at the medically directed rate. The physician meets the teaching physician criteria in §100.1.4;
- The physician is continuously involved in a single case involving a student nurse anesthetist;
- If the physician is involved with a single case with a qualified nonphysician anesthetist (a certified registered nurse anesthetist (CRNA) or an anesthesiologist's assistant)), A/B MACs may pay the physician service and the qualified nonphysician anesthetist service in accordance with the requirements for payment at the medically directed rate;

Or

- The physician and the CRNA (or anesthesiologist's assistant) are involved in one anesthesia case and the services of each are found to be medically necessary. Documentation must be submitted by both the CRNA and the physician to support payment of the full fee for each of the two providers. The physician reports the AA modifier and the CRNA reports the QZ modifier.

C. Payment at the Medically Directed Rate

The A/B MAC determines payment at the medically directed rate for the physician on the basis of 50 percent of the allowance for the service performed by the physician alone. Payment will be made at the medically directed rate if the physician medically directs qualified individuals (all of whom could be CRNAs, anesthesiologists' assistants, interns, residents, or combinations of these individuals) in two, three, or four concurrent cases and the physician performs the followingactivities.

- Performs a pre-anesthetic examination and evaluation;
- Prescribes the anesthesia plan;
- Personally participates in the most demanding procedures in the anesthesia plan, including, if applicable, induction and emergence;
- Ensures that any procedures in the anesthesia plan that he or she does not perform are performed by a qualified individual;
- Monitors the course of anesthesia administration at frequent intervals;
- Remains physically present and available for immediate diagnosis and treatment of emergencies; and
- Provides indicated post-anesthesia care.

The physician must document in the medical record that he or she performed the pre-anesthetic examination and evaluation. Physicians must also document that they provided indicated post-anesthesia care, were present during some portion of the anesthesia monitoring, and were present during the most demanding procedures in the anesthesia plan, including induction and emergence, where indicated.

NOTE: Concurrency refers to to the maximum number of procedures that the physician is medically directing within the context of a single procedure andwhether these other procedures overlap each other. Concurrency is not dependent on each of the cases involving a Medicare patient. For example, if an anesthesiologist medically directs three concurrent procedures, two of which involve non-Medicare patients and the remaining a Medicare patient, this represents three concurrent cases.

The requirements for payment at the medically directed rate also apply to cases involving student nurse anesthetists if the physician medically directs two concurrent cases, with each of the two cases involving a student nurse anesthetist, or the physician directs one case involving a student nurse anesthetist and another involving a qualified individual (for example: CRNA, anesthesiologist's assistant, intern or resident).

The requirements for payment at the medically directed rate do not apply to a single resident case that is concurrent to another anesthesia case paid at the medically directed rate or to two concurrent anesthesia cases involving residents.

If anesthesiologists are in a group practice, one physician member may provide the pre- anesthesia examination and evaluation while another fulfills the other criteria. Similarly, one physician member of the group may provide post-anesthesia care while another member of the group furnishes the other component parts of the anesthesia service. However, the medical record must indicate that the services were furnished by physicians and identify the physicians who furnished them.

A physician who is concurrently furnishing services that meet the requirements for payment at the medically directed rate cannot ordinarily be involved in furnishing additional services to other patients. However, addressing an emergency of short duration in the immediate area, administering an epidural or caudal anesthetic to ease labor pain, periodic (rather than continuous) monitoring of an obstetrical patient, receiving patients entering the operating suite for the next surgery, checking or discharging patients in the recovery room, or handling scheduling matters, do not substantially diminish the scope of control exercised by the physician and do not constitute a separate service for the purpose of determining whether the requirements for payment at the medically directed rate are met.

However, if the physician leaves the immediate area of the operating suite for other than short durations or devotes extensive time to an emergency case or is otherwise not available to respond to the immediate needs of the surgical patients, the physician's services to the surgical patients would not meet the requirements for payment at the medically directed rate. A/B MACs may not make payment under the feeschedule.

D. Payment at Medically Supervised Rate

The A/B MAC may allow only three base units per procedure when the anesthesiologist is involved in furnishing more than four procedures concurrently or is performing other services while directing the concurrent procedures. An additional time unit may be recognized if the physician can document he or she was present atinduction.

E. Billing and Payment for Multiple Anesthesia Procedures

Physicians bill for the anesthesia services associated with multiple bilateral surgeries by reporting the anesthesia procedure with the highest base unit value with the multiple procedure modifier -51. They report the total time for all procedures in the line item with the highest base unit value.

If the same anesthesia CPT code applies to two or more of the surgical procedures, billers enter the anesthesia code with the -51 modifier and the number of surgeries to which the modified CPT code applies.

Payment can be made under the fee schedule for anesthesia services associated with multiple surgical procedures or multiple bilateral procedures. Payment is determined based on the base unit of the anesthesia procedure with the highest base unit value and time units based on the actual anesthesia time of the multiple procedures. See §§40.6-40.7 for billing and claims processing instructions for multiple and bilateral surgeries.

F. Payment for Medical and Surgical Services Furnished in Addition to Anesthesia Procedure

Payment may be made under the fee schedule for specific medical and surgical services furnished by the anesthesiologist as long as these services are reasonable and medically necessary or provided that other rebundling provisions (see §30 and Chapter 23) do not preclude separate payment. These services may be furnished in conjunction with the anesthesia procedure to the patient or may be furnished as single services, e.g., during the day of or the day before the anesthesia service. These services include the insertion of a Swan Ganz catheter, the insertion of central venous pressure lines, emergency intubation, and critical care visits.

G. Anesthesia Time and Calculation of Anesthesia TimeUnits

Anesthesia time is defined as the period during which an anesthesia practitioner is present with the patient. It starts when the anesthesia practitioner begins to prepare the patient for anesthesia services in the operating room or an equivalent area and ends when the anesthesia practitioner is no longer furnishing anesthesia services to the patient, that is, when the patient may be placed safely under postoperative care. Anesthesia time is a continuous time period from the start of anesthesia to the end of an anesthesia service. In counting anesthesia time for services furnished, the anesthesia practitioner can add blocks of time around an interruption in anesthesia time as long as the anesthesia practitioner is furnishing continuous anesthesia care within the time periods around the interruption.

Actual anesthesia time in minutes is reported on the claim. For anesthesia services furnished, the A/B MAC computes time units by dividing reported anesthesia time by 15 minutes. Round the time unit to one decimal place. The A/B MAC does not recognize time units for CPT code 01996 (daily hospital management of epidural or subarachnoid continuous drug administration).

For purposes of this section, anesthesia practitioner means:

- a physician who performs the anesthesia service alone,
- a CRNA who is furnishing services that do not meet the requirements for payment at the medically directed rate,
- a qualified nonphysician anesthetist who is furnishing services that meet the requirements for payment at the medically directed rate.

The physician who medically directs the qualified nonphysician anesthetist would ordinarily report the same time as the qualified nonphysician anesthetist reports for the service.

H. Monitored Anesthesia Care

Monitored anesthesia care involves the intra-operative monitoring by a physician or qualified individual under the medical direction of a physician or of the patient's vital physiological signs in anticipation of the need for administration of general anesthesia or of the development of adverse physiological patient reaction to the surgical procedure. It also includes the performance of a pre-anesthetic examination and evaluation, prescription of the anesthesia care required, administration of any necessary oral or parenteral medications (e.g., atropine, demerol, valium) and provision of indicated postoperative anesthesia care.

The A/B MAC pays for reasonable and medically necessary monitored anesthesia care services on the same basis as other anesthesia services. If the physician personally performs the monitored anesthesia care case, payment is made under the fee schedule using the payment rules for payment at the personally performed rate. If the physician medically directs four or fewer concurrent cases and monitored anesthesia care represents one or more of these concurrentcases, payment is made under the fee schedule using the payment rules for payment at the medically directed rate. Anesthesiologists use the QS modifier to report monitored anesthesia care cases, in addition to reporting the actual anesthesia time and one of the payment modifiers on the claim.

I. Anesthesia Claims Modifiers

Physicians report the appropriate modifier to denote whether the service meets the requirements for payment at the personally performed rate, medically directed rate, or medically supervised rate.

AA Anesthesia Services performed personally by the anesthesiologist

AD Medical Supervision by a physician; more than 4 concurrent anesthesia procedures

G8 Monitored anesthesia care (MAC) for deep complex, complicated, or markedly invasive surgical procedures

G9 Monitored anesthesia care for patient who has a history of severe cardio-pulmonary condition

QK Medical direction of two, three or four concurrent anesthesia procedures involving qualified individuals

QS Monitored anesthesia care service

NOTE: The QS modifier can be used by a physician or a qualified nonphysician anesthetist and is for informational purposes. Providers must report actual anesthesia time and one of the payment modifiers on the claim.

QY Medical direction of one qualified nonphysician anesthetist by an anesthesiologist

GC These services have been performed by a resident under the direction of a teaching physician.

NOTE: The GC modifier is reported by the teaching physician to indicate he/she rendered the service in compliance with the teaching physician requirements in §100 of this chapter. One of the payment modifiers must be used in conjunction with the GC modifier.

The A/B MAC must determine payment for anesthesia in accordance with these instructions. They must be able to determine the uniform base unit that is assigned to the anesthesia code and apply the appropriate reduction where the anesthesia procedure meets the requirements for payment at the medically directed rate. They must also be able to determine the number of anesthesia time units from actual anesthesia time reported on the claim. The A/B MAC must multiply allowable units by the anesthesia-specific conversion factor used to determine fee schedule payment for the payment area.

J. Moderate Sedation Services Furnished in Conjunction with and in Support of Procedural Services

Anesthesia services range in complexity. The continuum of anesthesia services, from least intense to most intense in complexity is as follows: local or topical anesthesia, moderate (conscious) sedation, regional anesthesia and general anesthesia. Moderate sedation is a drug induced depression of consciousness during which the patient responds purposefully to verbal commands, either alone or accompanied by light tactile stimulation. Moderate sedation does not include minimal sedation, deep sedation or monitored anesthesia care.

Practitioners will report the appropriate CPT and/or HCPCS code that describes the moderate sedation services furnished during a patient encounter, which are furnished in conjunction with and in support of a procedural service, consistent with CPT guidance.

Refer to §50 and §140 of this chapter for information regarding reporting of anesthesia services furnished in conjunction with and in support of procedural services.

K. Anesthesia for Diagnostic or Therapeutic Nerve Blocks and Services Lower in Intensity than Moderate Sedation

If the anesthesiologist or CRNA provides anesthesia for diagnostic or therapeutic nerve blocks or injections and a different provider performs the block or injection, then the anesthesiologist or CRNA may report the anesthesia service using the appropriate CPT code consistent with CPT guidance. The service must meet the criteria for monitored anesthesia care as described in this section. If the anesthesiologist or CRNA provides both the anesthesia service and the block or injection, then the anesthesiologist or CRNA may report the anesthesia service and the injection or block. However, the anesthesia service must meet the requirements for moderate sedation and if a lower level complexity anesthesia service is provided, then the moderate sedation code should not be reported.

If the physician performing the medical or surgical procedure also provides a level of anesthesia lower in intensity than moderate sedation, such as a local or topical anesthesia, then the moderate sedation code should not be reported and no separate payment should be allowed by the A/B MAC.

100-04, 12, 100

Teaching Physician Services

(Rev. 811, Issued: 01-13-06, Effective: 01-01-06, Implementation: 02-13-06)

Definitions

For purposes of this section, the following definitions apply.

Resident -An individual who participates in an approved graduate medical education (GME) program or a physician who is not in an approved GME program but who is authorized to practice only in a hospital setting. The term includes interns and fellows in GME programs recognized as approved for purposes of direct GME payments made by the FI. Receiving a staff or faculty appointment or participating in a fellowship does not by itself alter the status of "resident". Additionally, this status remains unaffected regardless of whether a hospital includes the physician in its full time equivalency count of residents.

Student- An individual who participates in an accredited educational program (e.g., a medical school) that is not an approved GME program. A student is never considered to be an intern or a resident. Medicare does not pay for any service furnished by a student. See 100.1.1B for a discussion concerning E/M service documentation performed by students.

Teaching Physician -A physician (other than another resident) who involves residents in the care of his or her patients.

Direct Medical and Surgical Services -Services to individual beneficiaries that are either personally furnished by a physician or furnished by a resident under the supervision of a physician in a teaching hospital making the reasonable cost election for physician services furnished in teaching hospitals. All payments for such services are made by the FI for the hospital.

Teaching Hospital -A hospital engaged in an approved GME residency program in medicine, osteopathy, dentistry, or podiatry.

Teaching Setting -Any provider, hospital-based provider, or nonprovider setting in which Medicare payment for the services of residents is made by the FI under the direct graduate medical education payment methodology or freestanding SNF or HHA in which such payments are made on a reasonable cost basis.

Critical or Key Portion- That part (or parts) of a service that the teaching physician determines is (are) a critical or key portion(s). For purposes of this section, these terms are interchangeable.

Documentation- Notes recorded in the patient's medical records by a resident, and/or teaching physician or others as outlined in the specific situations below regarding the service furnished. Documentation may be dictated and typed or hand-written, or computer-generated and typed or handwritten. Documentation must be dated and include a legible signature or identity. Pursuant to 42 CFR 415.172 (b), documentation must identify, at a minimum, the service furnished, the participation of the teaching physician in providing the service, and whether the teaching physician was physically present. In the context of an electronic medical record, the term 'macro' means a command in a computer or dictation application that automatically generates predetermined text that is not edited by the user.

When using an electronic medical record, it is acceptable for the teaching physician to use a macro as the required personal documentation if the teaching physician adds it personally in a secured (password protected) system. In addition to the teaching physician's macro, either the resident or the teaching physician must provide customized information that is sufficient to support a medical necessity determination. The note in the electronic medical record must sufficiently describe the specific services furnished to the specific patient on the specific date. It is insufficient documentation if both the resident and the teaching physician use macros only.

Physically Present- The teaching physician is located in the same room (or partitioned or curtained area, if the room is subdivided to accommodate multiple patients) as the patient and/or performs a face-to-face service.

100-04, 12, 100.1.1

Evaluation and Management (E/M) Services

(Rev. 4283, Issued: 04- 26-19, Effective: 01-01-19, 07-29-19)

A. General Documentation Requirements

Evaluation and Management (E/M) Services -- For a given encounter, the selection of the appropriate level of E/M service should be determined according to the code definitions in the American Medical Association's Current Procedural Terminology (CPT) book and any applicable documentation guidelines.

For purposes of payment, E/M services billed by teaching physicians require that the medical records must demonstrate:

- That the teaching physician performed the service or was physically present during the key or critical portions of the service when performed by the resident; and
- The participation of the teaching physician in the management of the patient.

The presence of the teaching physician during E/M services may be demonstrated by the notes in the medical records made by physicians, residents, or nurses.

B. E/M Service Documentation Provided By Students

Any contribution and participation of students to the performance of a billable service (other than the review of systems and/or past family/social history which are not separately billable, but are taken as part of an E/M service) must be performed in the physical presence of a teaching physician or physical presence of a resident in a service meeting the requirements set forth in this section for teaching physician billing.

Students may document services in the medical record. However, the teaching physician must verify in the medical record all student documentation or findings, including history, physical exam and/or medical decision making. The teaching physician must personally perform (or re-perform) the physical exam and medical decision making activities of the E/M service being billed, but may verify any student documentation of them in the medical record, rather than re-documenting this work.

C. Exception for E/M Services Furnished in Certain Primary CareCenters

Teaching physicians providing E/M services with a GME program granted a primary care exception may bill Medicare for lower and mid-level E/M services provided by residents. For the E/M codes listed below, teaching physicians may submit claims for services furnished by residents in the absence of a teaching physician:

New Patient	Established Patient
99201	99211
99202	99212
99203	99213

Effective January 1, 2005, the following code is included under the primary care exception: HCPCS code G0402 (Initial preventive physical examination; face-to-face visit services limited to new beneficiary during the first 12 months of Medicare enrollment).

Effective January 1, 2011, the following codes are included under the primary care exception: HCPCS codes G0438 (Annual wellness visit, including personal preventive plan service, first visit) and G0439 (Annual wellness visit, including personal preventive plan service, subsequent visit).

If a service other than those listed above needs to be furnished, then the general teaching physician policy set forth in §100.1 applies. For this exception to apply, a center must attest in writing that all the following conditions are met for a particular residency program. Prior approval is not necessary, but centers exercising the primary care exception must maintain records demonstrating that they qualify for the exception.

The services must be furnished in a center located in the outpatient department of a hospital or another ambulatory care entity in which the time spent by residents in patient care activities is included in determining direct GME payments to a teaching hospital by the hospital's A/B MAC (A). This requirement is not met when the resident is assigned to a physician's office away from the center or makes home visits. In the case of a nonhospital entity, verify with the A/B MAC (A) that the entity meets the requirements of a written agreement between the hospital and the entity set forth at 42 CFR 413.78(e)(3)(ii).

Under this exception, residents providing the billable patient care service without the physical presence of a teaching physician must have completed at least 6 months of a GME approved residency program. Centers must maintain information under the provisions at 42 CFR 413.79(a)(6).

Teaching physicians submitting claims under this exception may not supervise more than four residents at any given time and must direct the care from such proximity as to constitute immediate availability. Teaching physicians may include residents with less than 6 months in a GME approved residency program in the mix of four residents under the teaching physician's supervision. However, the teaching physician must be physically present for the critical or key portions of services furnished by the residents with less than 6 months in a GME approved residency program. That is, the primary care exception does not apply in the case of residents with less than 6 months in a GME approved residency program.

Teaching physicians submitting claims under this exception must:

- Not have other responsibilities (including the supervision of other personnel) at the time the service was provided by the residents;
- Have the primary medical responsibility for patients cared for by the residents;
- Ensure that the care provided was reasonable and necessary;
- Review the care provided by the residents during or immediately after each visit. This must include a review of the patient's medical history, the resident's findings on physical examination, the patient's diagnosis, and treatment plan (i.e., record of tests and therapies); and

Patients under this exception should consider the center to be their primary location for health care services. The residents must be expected to generally provide care to the same group of established patients during their residency training. The types of services furnished by residents under this exception include:

- Acute care for undifferentiated problems or chronic care for ongoing conditions including chronic mental illness;
- Coordination of care furnished by other physicians and providers; and,
- Comprehensive care not limited by organ system or diagnosis.

Residency programs most likely qualifying for this exception include family practice, general internal medicine, geriatric medicine, pediatrics, and obstetrics/gynecology.

Certain GME programs in psychiatry may qualify in special situations such as when the program furnishes

comprehensive care for chronically mentally ill patients. These would be centers in which the range of services the residents are trained to furnish, and actually do furnish, include comprehensive medical care as well as psychiatric care. For example, antibiotics are being prescribed as well as psychotropic drugs.

The patient medical record must document the extent of the teaching physician's participation in the review and direction of the services furnished to each beneficiary. The extent of the teaching physician's participation may be demonstrated by the notes in the medical records made by physicians, residents, or nurses.

100-04, 12, 140.1

Qualified Nonphysician Anesthetists

(Rev. 3747; Issued: 04-14-17; Effective: 01-01-17; Implementation: 05-15-17)

For payment purposes, the term "qualified nonphysician anesthetist" is used to refer to both certified registered nurse anesthetists (CRNAs) and anesthesiologists' assistants unless otherwise separately discussed.

An anesthesiologist's assistant means a person who:

- Works under the direction of an anesthesiologist;
- Is in compliance with all applicable requirements of State law, including any licensure requirements the state imposes on nonphysician anesthetists; and
- Is a graduate of a medical school based anesthesiologist assistant educational program that –
  — Is accredited by the Committee on Allied Health Education and Accreditation;

And

  — Includes approximately two years of specialized basic science and clinical education in anesthesia at a level that builds on a premedical undergraduate science background.

A CRNA is a registered nurse who:

- is licensed as a registered professional nurse by the State in which the nurse practices;
- Meets any licensure requirements the State imposes with respect to nonphysician anesthetists;
- Has graduated from a nurse anesthesia educational program that meets the standards of the Council on Accreditation of Nurse Anesthesia Programs; and
- Meets the following criteria:
  — Has passed a certification examination of the Council on Certification of Nurse Anesthetists or the Council on Recertification of Nurse Anesthetists;

Or

  — Is a graduate of a nurse anesthesia educational program that meets the standards of the Council of Accreditation of Nurse Anesthesia Educational Programs, and within 24 months of graduation, has passed a certification examination of the Council on Certification of Nurse Anesthetists or the Council on Recertification of Nurse Anesthetists.

100-04, 12, 140.2

Entity or Individual to Whom Fee Schedule is Payable for Qualified Nonphysician Anesthetists

(Rev. 3747; Issued: 04-14-17; Effective: 01-01-17; Implementation: 05-15-17)

Payment for the services of a qualified nonphysician anesthetist may be made directly to the qualified nonphysician anesthetist who furnished the anesthesia services or to a hospital, physician, group practice, or ASC with which the qualified nonphysician anesthetist has an employment or contractual relationship.

100-04, 12, 140.3

Anesthesia Fee Schedule Payment for Qualified Nonphysician Anesthetists

(Rev. 3747; Issued: 04-14-17; Effective: 01-01-17; Implementation: 05-15-17)

Payment for the services furnished by qualified nonphysician anesthetists are subject to the usual Part B coinsurance and deductible, and are made only on an assignment basis. The assignment agreed to by the qualified nonphysician anesthetist is binding upon any other person or entity claiming payment for the service. Except for deductible and coinsurance amounts, any person who knowingly and willfully presents or causes to be presented to a Medicare beneficiary a bill or request for payment for services of a qualified nonphysician anesthetist for which payment may be made on an assignment-related basis is subject to civil monetary penalties.

The fee schedule for anesthesia services furnished by qualified nonphysician anesthetists is the least of 80 percent of:

- The actual charge;
- The applicable locality anesthesia conversion factor multiplied by the sum of allowable base and time units.

100-04, 12, 140.3.1

Conversion Factors Used for Qualified Nonphysician Anesthetists

(Rev. 3747; Issued: 04-14-17; Effective: 01-01-17; Implementation: 05-15-17)

The conversion factors applicable to anesthesia services are increased by the update factor used to update physicians' services under the physician fee schedule. They are generally published in November of the year preceding the year in which they apply.

100-04, 12, 140.3.2

Anesthesia Time and Calculation of Anesthesia TimeUnits

(Rev. 3747; Issued: 04-14-17; Effective: 01-01-17; Implementation: 05-15-17)

Anesthesia time means the time during which a qualified nonphysician anesthetist is present with the patient. It starts when the qualified nonphysician anesthetist begins to prepare the patient for anesthesia services in the operating room or an equivalent area and ends when the qualified nonphysician anesthetist is no longer furnishing anesthesia services to the patient, that is, when the patient may be placed safely under postoperative care. Anesthesia time is a continuous time period from the start of anesthesia to the end of an anesthesia service. In counting anesthesia time, the qualified nonphysician anesthetist can add blocks of time around an interruption in anesthesia time as long as the qualified nonphysician anesthetist is furnishing continuous anesthesia care within the time periods around the interruption.

100-04, 12, 140.3.3

Billing Modifiers

(Rev. 3747; Issued: 04-14-17; Effective: 01-01-17; Implementation: 05-15-17)

The following modifiers are used by qualified nonphysician anesthetists when billing for anesthesia services:

- QX – Qualified nonphysician anesthetist service: With medical direction by a physician.
- QZ – CRNA service: Without medical direction by a physician.
- QS – Monitored anesthesia care services
  — **NOTE:** The QS modifier can be used by a physician or a qualified nonphysician anesthetist and is for informational purposes. Providers must report actual anesthesia time and one of the payment modifiers on the claim.

100-04, 12, 140.3.4

General Billing Instructions

(Rev. 3747; Issued: 04-14-17; Effective: 01-01-17; Implementation: 05-15-17)

Claims for reimbursement for qualified nonphysician anesthetist services should be completed in accordance with existing billing instructions for anesthesiologists with the following additions.

- If an employer-physician furnishes concurrent medical direction for a procedure involving CRNAs and the medical direction service is unassigned, the physician should bill on an assigned basis on a separate claim for the qualified nonphysician anesthetist service. If the physician is participating or takes assignment, both services should be billed on one claim but as separate line items.
- All claims forms must have the provider billing number of the qualified nonphysician anesthetist and/or the employer of the qualified nonphysician anesthetist performing the service in either block 24.H of the Form CMS-1500 and/or block 31 as applicable. Verify that the billing number is valid before making payment.

Payments should be calculated in accordance with Medicare payment rules in §140.3. The A/B MAC must institute all necessary payment edits to assure that duplicate payments are not made to physicians for qualified nonphysician anesthetist services or to a qualified nonphysician anesthetist directly for bills submitted on their behalf by qualified billers.

A CRNA is identified on the provider file by specialty code 43. An anesthesiologist's assistant is identified on the provider file by specialty code 32.

100-04, 12, 140.4.1

An Anesthesiologist and Qualified Nonphysician Anesthetist Work Together

(Rev. 3747; Issued: 04-14-17; Effective: 01-01-17; Implementation: 05-15-17)

A/B MACs will distribute educational releases and use other established means to ensure that anesthesiologists understand the requirements for medical direction of qualified nonphysician anesthetists.

A/B MACs will perform reviews of payments for anesthesiology services to identify situations in which an excessive number of concurrent anesthesiology services may have been performed. They will use peer practice and their experience in developing review criteria. They will also periodically review a sample of claims for medical direction of four or fewer concurrent anesthesia procedures. During this process physicians may be requested to submit documentation of the names of procedures performed and the names of the anesthetists medically directed.

Physicians who cannot supply the necessary documentation for the sample claims must submit documentation with all subsequent claims before payment will be made.

100-04, 12, 140.4.2

Qualified Nonphysician Anesthetist and an Anesthesiologist in a Single Anesthesia Procedure

(Rev. 3747; Issued: 04-14-17; Effective: 01-01-17; Implementation: 05-15-17)

Where a single anesthesia procedure involves both a physician medical direction service and the service of the medically directed qualified nonphysician anesthetist, the payment amount for the service of each is 50 percent of the allowance otherwise recognized had the service been furnished by the anesthesiologist alone. For the single medically directed service, the physician will use the QY modifier and the qualified nonphysician anesthetist will use the QX modifier.

In unusual circumstances when it is medically necessary for both the CRNA and the anesthesiologist to be completely and fully involved during a procedure, full payment for the services of each provider is allowed. The physician would report using the AA modifier and the CRNA would report using the QZ modifier. Documentation must be submitted by each provider to support payment of the full fee.

100-04, 12, 140.4.3

Payment for Medical or Surgical Services Furnished by CRNAs

(Rev. 3747; Issued: 04-14-17; Effective: 01-01-17; Implementation: 05-15-17)

Payment shall be made for reasonable and necessary medical or surgical services furnished by CRNAs if they are legally authorized to perform these services in the state in which services are furnished. Payment is determined under the physician fee schedule on the basis of the national physician fee schedule conversion factor, the geographic adjustment factor, and the resource-based relative value units for the medical or surgical service.

100-04, 12, 140.5

Payment for Anesthesia Services Furnished by a Teaching CRNA

(Rev. 3747; Issued: 04-14-17; Effective: 01-01-17; Implementation: 05-15-17)

Payment can be made under Part B to a teaching CRNA who supervises a single case involving a student nurse anesthetist where the CRNA is continuously present. The CRNA reports the service using the QZ modifier. No payment is made under Part B for the service provided by a student nurse anesthetist.

The A/B MAC may allow payment, as follows, if a teaching CRNA is involved in cases with two student nurse anesthetists:

- Recognize the full base units (assigned to the anesthesia code) where the teaching CRNA is present with the student nurse anesthetist throughout pre and post anesthesia care; and
- Recognize the actual time the teaching CRNA is personally present with the student nurse anesthetist. Anesthesia time may be discontinuous. For example, a teaching CRNA is involved in two concurrent cases with student nurse anesthetists. Case 1 runs from 9:00 a.m. to 11:00 a.m. and case 2 runs from 9:45a.m. to 11:30 a.m. The teaching CRNA is present in case 1 from 9:00 a.m. to 9:30 a.m. and from 10:15 a.m. to 10:30 a.m. From 9:45 a.m. to 10:14 a.m. and from 10:31 a.m. to 11:30 a.m., the CRNA is present in case 2. The CRNA may report 45 minutes of anesthesia time for case 1 (i.e., 3 time units) and 88 minutes (i.e., 5.9 units) of anesthesia time for case 2.

The teaching CRNA must document his/her involvement in cases with student nurse anesthetists. The documentation must be sufficient to support the payment of the fee and available for review upon request.

The teaching CRNA (not under the medical direction of a physician), can be paid for his or her involvement in each of two concurrent cases with student nurse anesthetists; allow payment at the regular fee schedule rate. The teaching CRNA reports the anesthesia service using the QZmodifier.

To bill the anesthesia base units, the teaching CRNA must be present with the student nurse anesthetist during pre and post anesthesia care for each of the two cases. To bill anesthesia time for each case, the teaching CRNA must continue to devote his or her time to the two concurrent cases and not be involved in other activities. The teaching CRNA can decide how to allocate his or her time to optimize patient care in the two cases based on the complexity of the anesthesia cases, the experience and skills of the student nurse anesthetists, and the patients' health status and other factors. The teaching CRNA must document his or her involvement in the cases with the student nurse anesthetists.

100-04, 12, 160

Independent Psychologist Services

(Rev. 1, 10-01-03) B3-2150, B3-2070.2

See the Medicare Benefit Policy Manual, Chapter 15, for coverage requirements.

There are a number of types of psychologists. Educational psychologists engage in identifying and treating education-related issues. In contrast, counseling psychologists provide services that include a broader realm including phobias, familial issues, etc.

Psychometrists are psychologists who have been trained to administer and interpret tests.

However, clinical psychologists are defined as a provider of diagnostic and therapeutic services. Because of the differences in services provided, services provided by psychologists who do not provide clinical services are subject to different billing guidelines. One service often provided by nonclinical psychologist is diagnostic testing.

NOTE: Diagnostic psychological testing services performed by persons who meet these requirements are covered as other diagnostic tests. When, however, the psychologist is not practicing independently, but is on the staff of an institution, agency, or clinic, that entity bills for the diagnostic services.

Expenses for such testing are not subject to the payment limitation on treatment for mental, psychoneurotic, and personality disorders. Independent psychologists are not required by law to accept assignment when performing psychological tests. However, regardless of whether the psychologist accepts assignment, he or she must report on the claim form the name and address of the physician who ordered the test.

100-04, 12, 160.1

Payment

(Rev. 1, 10-01-03)

Diagnostic testing services are not subject to the outpatient mental health limitation. Refer to §210, below, for a discussion of the outpatient mental health limitation. The diagnostic testing services performed by a psychologist (who is not a clinical psychologist) practicing independently of an institution, agency, or physician's office are covered as other diagnostic tests if a physician orders such testing. Medicare covers this type of testing as an outpatient service if furnished by any psychologist who is licensed or certified to practice psychology in the State or jurisdiction where he or she is furnishing services or, if the jurisdiction does not issue licenses, if provided by any practicing psychologist. (It is CMS' understanding that all States, the District of Columbia, and Puerto Ricolicense psychologists, but that some trust territories do not. Examples of psychologists, other than clinical psychologists, whose services are covered under this provision include, but are not limited to, educational psychologists and counseling psychologists.)

To determine whether the diagnostic psychological testing services of a particular independent psychologist are covered under Part B in States which have statutory licensure or certification, carriers must secure from the appropriate State agency a current listing of psychologists holding the required credentials. In States or territories which lack statutory licensing and certification, carriers must check individual qualifications as claims are submitted. Possible reference sources are the national directory of membership of the American Psychological Association, which provides data about the educational background of individuals and indicates which members are board-certified, and records and directories of the State or territorial psychological association. If qualification is dependent on a doctoral degree from a currently accredited program, carriers must verify the date of accreditation of the school involved, since such accreditation is not retroactive. If the reference sources listed above do not provide enough information (e.g., the psychologist is not a member of the association), carriers must contact the psychologist personally for the required information. Carriers may wish to maintain a continuing list of psychologists whose qualifications have been verified.

Medicare excludes expenses for diagnostic testing from the payment limitation on treatment for mental/psychoneurotic/personality disorders.

Carriers must identify the independent psychologist's choice whether or not to accept assignment when performing psychological tests.

Carriers must accept an independent psychologist claim only if the psychologist reports the name/UPIN of the physician who ordered a test.

Carriers pay nonparticipating independent psychologists at 95 percent of the physician fee schedule allowed amount.

Carriers pay participating independent psychologists at 100 percent of the physician fee schedule allowed amount. Independent psychologists are identified on the provider file by specialty code 62 and provider type 35.

100-04, 12, 170

Clinical Psychologist Services

(Rev. 1, 10-01-03)

B3-2150 See Medicare Benefit Policy Manual, Chapter 15, for general coverage requirements.

Direct payment may be made under Part B for professional services. However, services furnished incident to the professional services of CPs to hospital patients remain bundled.

Therefore, payment must continue to be made to the hospital (by the FI) for such "incident to" services.

100-04, 12, 180

Care Plan Oversight Services

(Rev. 999, Issued: 07-14-06; Effective: 01-01-05; Implementation: 10-02-06)

The Medicare Benefit Policy Manual, Chapter 15, contains requirements for coverage for medical and other health services including those of physicians and non-physician practitioners.

Care plan oversight (CPO) is the physician supervision of a patient receiving complex and/or multidisciplinary care as part of Medicare-covered services provided by a participating home health agency or Medicare approved hospice.

CPO services require complex or multidisciplinary care modalities involving:

- Regular physician development and/or revision of care plans;
- Review of subsequent reports of patient status;
- Review of related laboratory and other studies;
- Communication with other health professionals not employed in the same practice who are involved in the patient's care;
- Integration of new information into the medical treatment plan; and/or
- Adjustment of medical therapy.

The CPO services require recurrent physician supervision of a patient involving 30 or more minutes of the physician's time per month. Services not countable toward the 30 minutes threshold that must be provided in order to bill for CPO include, but are not limited to:

- Time associated with discussions with the patient, his or her family or friends to adjust medication or treatment;
- Time spent by staff getting or filing charts;
- Travel time; and/or Physician's time spent telephoning prescriptions into the pharmacist unless the telephone conversation involves discussions of pharmaceutical therapies.

Implicit in the concept of CPO is the expectation that the physician has coordinated an aspect of the patient's care with the home health agency or hospice during the month for which CPO services were billed. The physician who bills for CPO must be the same physician who signs the plan of care.

Nurse practitioners, physician assistants, and clinical nurse specialists, practicing within the scope of State law, may bill for care plan oversight. These non-physician practitioners must have been providing ongoing care for the beneficiary through evaluation and management services. These non-physician practitioners may not bill for CPO if they have been involved only with the delivery of the Medicare-covered home health or hospice service.

A. Home Health CPO

Non-physician practitioners can perform CPO only if the physician signing the plan of care provides regular ongoing care under the same plan of care as does the NPP billing for CPO and either:

- The physician and NPP are part of the same group practice; or
- If the NPP is a nurse practitioner or clinical nurse specialist, the physician signing the plan of care also has a collaborative agreement with the NPP; or
- If the NPP is a physician assistant, the physician signing the plan of care is also the physician who provides general supervision of physician assistant services for the practice.

Billing may be made for care plan oversight services furnished by an NPP when:

- The NPP providing the care plan oversight has seen and examined the patient;
- The NPP providing care plan oversight is not functioning as a consultant whose participation is limited to a single medical condition rather than multidisciplinary coordination of care; and
- The NPP providing care plan oversight integrates his or her care with that of the physician who signed the plan of care.

NPPs may not certify the beneficiary for home health care.

B. Hospice CPO

The attending physician or nurse practitioner (who has been designated as the attending physician) may bill for hospice CPO when they are acting as an "attending physician".

An "attending physician" is one who has been identified by the individual, at the time he/she elects hospice coverage, as having the most significant role in the determination and delivery of their medical care. They are not employed nor paid by the hospice. The care plan oversight services are billed using Form CMS-1500 or electronic equivalent.

For additional information on hospice CPO, see Chapter 11, 40.1.3.1 of this manual.

100-04, 12, 180.1

Care Plan Oversight Billing Requirements

(Rev. 999, Issued: 07-14-06; Effective: 01-01-05; Implementation: 10-02-06)

A. Codes for Which Separate Payment May Be Made

Effective January 1, 1995, separate payment may be made for CPO oversight services for 30 minutes or more if the requirements specified in the Medicare Benefits Policy Manual, Chapter 15 are met.

Providers billing for CPO must submit the claim with no other services billed on that claim and may bill only after the end of the month in which the CPO services were rendered. CPO services may not be billed across calendar months and should be submitted (and paid) only for one unit of service.

Physicians may bill and be paid separately for CPO services only if all the criteria in the Medicare Benefit Policy Manual, Chapter 15 are met.

B. Physician Certification and Recertification of Home Health Plans of Care

Effective 2001, two new HCPCS codes for the certification and recertification and development of plans of care for Medicare-covered home health services were created.

See the Medicare General Information, Eligibility, and Entitlement Manual, Pub. 100-1, Chapter 4, "Physician Certification and Recertification of Services," 10-60, and the Medicare Benefit Policy Manual, Pub. 100-2, Chapter 7, "Home Health Services", 30.

The home health agency certification code can be billed only when the patient has not received Medicare-covered home health services for at least 60 days. The home health agency recertification code is used after a patient has received services for at least 60 days (or one certification period) when the physician signs the certification after the initial certification period. The home health agency recertification code will be reported only once every 60 days, except in the rare situation when the patient starts a new episode before 60 days elapses and requires a new plan of care to start a new episode.

C. Provider Number of Home Health Agency (HHA) or Hospice

For claims for CPO submitted on or after January 1, 1997, physicians must enter on the Medicare claim form the 6-character Medicare provider number of the HHA or hospice providing Medicare-covered services to the beneficiary for the period during which CPO services was furnished and for which the physician signed the plan of care. Physicians are responsible for obtaining the HHA or hospice Medicare provider numbers.

Additionally, physicians should provide their UPIN to the HHA or hospice furnishing services to their patient.

NOTE: There is currently no place on the HIPAA standard ASC X12N 837 professional format to specifically include the HHA or hospice provider number required for a care plan oversight claim. For this reason, the requirement to include the HHA or hospice provider number on a care plan oversight claim is temporarily waived until a new version of this electronic standard format is adopted under HIPAA and includes a place to provide the HHA and hospice provider numbers for care plan oversight claims.

100-04, 12, 190.3

List of Medicare Telehealth Services

(Rev. 3476, Issued: 03-11-16, Effective: 01-01-15, Effective: 04-11-16)

The use of a telecommunications system may substitute for an in-person encounter for professional consultations, office visits, office psychiatry services, and a limited number of other physician fee schedule (PFS) services. The various services and corresponding current procedure terminology (CPT) or Healthcare Common Procedure Coding System (HCPCS) codes are listed on the CMS website at www.cms.gov/Medicare/Medicare-General-Information/Telehealth/.

NOTE: Beginning January 1, 2010, CMS eliminated the use of all consultation codes, except for inpatient telehealth consultation G-codes. CMS no longer recognizes office/outpatient or inpatient consultation CPT codes for payment of office/outpatient or inpatient visits. Instead, physicians and practitioners are instructed to bill a new or established patient office/outpatient visit CPT code or appropriate hospital or nursing facility care code, as appropriate to the particular patient, for all office/outpatient or inpatient visits.

100-04, 12, 190.3.4

Payment for ESRD-Related Services as a Telehealth Service

(Rev. 3476, Issued: 03-11-16, Effective: 01-01-15, Effective: 04-11-16)

The ESRD-related services included in the monthly capitation payment (MCP) with 2 or 3 visits per month and ESRD-related services with 4 or more visits per month may be paid as Medicare telehealth services. However, at least 1 visit must be furnished face-to-face "hands on" to examine the vascular access site by a physician, clinical nurse specialist, nurse practitioner, or physician assistant. An interactive audio and video telecommunications system may be used for providing additional visits required under the 2-to-3 visit MCP and the 4-or-more visit MCP. The medical record must indicate that at least one of the visits was furnished face-to-face "hands on" by a physician, clinical nurse specialist, nurse practitioner, or physician assistant.

The MCP physician, for example, the physician or practitioner who is responsible for the complete monthly assessment of the patient and establishes the patient's plan of care, may use other physicians and practitioners to furnish ESRD-related visits through an interactive audio and video telecommunications system. The non-MCP physician or practitioner must have a relationship with the billing physician or practitioner such as a partner, employees of the same group practice or an employee of the MCP physician, for example, the non MCP physician or practitioner is either a W-2 employee or 1099 independent contractor. However, the physician or practitioner who is responsible for the complete monthly assessment and establishes the ESRD beneficiary's plan of care should bill for the MCP in any given month.

Clinical Criteria

The visit, including a clinical examination of the vascular access site, must be conducted face-to-face "hands on" by a physician, clinical nurse specialist, nurse practitioner or physician's assistant. For additional visits, the physician or practitioner at the distant site is required, at a minimum, to use an interactive audio and video telecommunications system that allows the physician or practitioner to provide medical management services for a maintenance dialysis beneficiary. For example, an

ESRD-related visit conducted via telecommunications system must permit the physician or practitioner at the distant site to perform an assessment of whether the dialysis is working effectively and whether the patient is tolerating the procedure well (physiologically and psychologically). During this assessment, the physician or practitioner at the distant site must be able to determine whether alteration in any aspect of the beneficiary's prescription is indicated, due to such changes as the estimate of the patient's dry weight.

100-04, 12, 190.3.5

Payment for Subsequent Hospital Care Services and Subsequent Nursing Facility Care Services as Telehealth Services

(Rev. 3476, Issued: 03-11-16, Effective: 01-01-15, Effective: 04-11-16)

Subsequent hospital care services are limited to one telehealth visit every 3 days. The frequency limit of the benefit is not intended to apply to consulting physicians or practitioners, who should continue to report initial or follow-up inpatient telehealth consultations using the applicable HCPCS G-codes.

Similarly, subsequent nursing facility care services are limited to one telehealth visit every 30 days. Furthermore, subsequent nursing facility care services reported for a Federally-mandated periodic visit under 42 CFR 483.40(c) may not be furnished through telehealth. The frequency limit of the benefit is not intended to apply to consulting physicians or practitioners, who should continue to report initial or follow-up inpatient telehealth consultations using the applicable HCPCS G-codes.

Inpatient telehealth consultations are furnished to beneficiaries in hospitals or skilled nursing facilities via telehealth at the request of the physician of record, the attending physician, or another appropriate source. The physician or practitioner who furnishes the initial inpatient consultation via telehealth cannot be the physician or practitioner of record or the attending physician or practitioner, and the initial inpatient telehealth consultation would be distinct from the care provided by the physician or practitioner of record or the attending physician or practitioner. Counseling and coordination of care with other providers or agencies is included as well, consistent with the nature of the problem(s) and the patient's needs. Initial and follow-up inpatient telehealth consultations are subject to the criteria for inpatient telehealth consultation services, as described in section 190.3 of this chapter.

100-04, 12, 190.3.6

Payment for Diabetes Self-Management Training (DSMT) as a Telehealth Service

(Rev. 3476, Issued: 03-11-16, Effective: 01-01-15, Effective: 04-11-16)

Individual and group DSMT services may be paid as a Medicare telehealth service; however, at least 1 hour of the 10 hour benefit in the year following the initial DSMT service must be furnished in-person to allow for effective injection training. The injection training may be furnished through either individual or group DSMT services. By reporting the –GT or –GQ modifier with HCPCS code G0108 (Diabetes outpatient self-management training services, individual, per 30 minutes) or G0109 (Diabetes outpatient self-management training services, group session (2 or more), per 30 minutes), the distant site practitioner certifies that the beneficiary has received or will receive 1 hour of in-person DSMT services for purposes of injection training during the year following the initial DSMT service.

As specified in 42 CFR 410.141(e) and stated in Pub. 100-02, Medicare Benefit Policy Manual, chapter 15, section 300.2, individual DSMT services may be furnished by a physician, individual, or entity that furnishes other services for which direct Medicare payment may be made and that submits necessary documentation to, and is accredited by, an accreditation organization approved by CMS. However, consistent with the statutory requirements of section 1834(m)(1) of the Act, as provided in 42 CFR 410.78(b)(1) and (b)(2) and stated in section 190.6 of this chapter, Medicare telehealth services, including individual DSMT services furnished as a telehealth service, could only be furnished by a licensed PA, NP, CNS, CNM, clinical psychologist, clinical social worker, or registered dietitian or nutrition professional.

100-04, 12, 190.5

Originating Site Facility Fee Payment Methodology

(Rev. 3476, Issued: 03-11-16, Effective: 01-01-15, Effective: 04-11-16)

1. Originating site defined

The term originating site means the location of an eligible Medicare beneficiary at the time the service being furnished via a telecommunications system occurs. For asynchronous, store and forward telecommunications technologies, an originating site is only a Federal telemedicine demonstration program conducted in Alaska or Hawaii.

2. Facility fee for originating site

The originating site facility fee is a separately billable Part B payment. The contractor pays it outside of other payment methodologies. This fee is subject to post payment verification.

For telehealth services furnished from October 1, 2001, through December 31, 2002, the originating site facility fee was the lesser of $20 or the actual charge. For services furnished on or after January 1 of each subsequent year, the originating site facility fee is updated by the Medicare Economic Index. The updated fee is included in the Medicare Physician Fee Schedule (MPFS) Final Rule, which is published by November 1 prior to the start of the calendar year for which it is effective. The updated fee for each calendar year is also issued annually in a Recurring Update Notification instruction for January of each year.

3. Payment amount:

The originating site facility fee is a separately billable Part B payment. The payment amount to the originating site is the lesser of 80 percent of the actual charge or 80 percent of the originating site facility fee, except CAHs. The beneficiary is responsible for any unmet deductible amount and Medicare coinsurance.

The originating site facility fee payment methodology for each type of facility is clarified below.

Hospital outpatient department. When the originating site is a hospital outpatient department, payment for the originating site facility fee must be made as described above and not under the OPPS. Payment is not based on the OPPS payment methodology.

Hospital inpatient. For hospital inpatients, payment for the originating site facility fee must be made outside the diagnostic related group (DRG) payment, since this is a Part B benefit, similar to other services paid separately from the DRG payment, (e.g., hemophilia blood clotting factor).

Critical access hospitals. When the originating site is a critical access hospital, make payment separately from the cost-based reimbursement methodology. For CAH's, the payment amount is 80 percent of the originating site facility fee.

Federally qualified health centers (FQHCs) and rural health clinics (RHCs). The originating site facility fee for telehealth services is not an FQHC or RHC service. When an FQHC or RHC serves as the originating site, the originating site facility fee must be paid separately from the center or clinic all-inclusive rate.

Physicians' and practitioners' offices. When the originating site is a physician's or practitioner's office, the payment amount, in accordance with the law, is the lesser of 80 percent of the actual charge or 80 percent of the originating site facility fee, regardless of geographic location. The A/B MAC (B) shall not apply the geographic practice cost index (GPCI) to the originating site facility fee. This fee is statutorily set and is not subject to the geographic payment adjustments authorized under the MPFS.

Hospital-based or critical access-hospital based renal dialysis center (or their satellites). When a hospital-based or critical access hospital-based renal dialysis center (or their satellites) serves as the originating site, the originating site facility fee is covered in addition to any composite rate or MCP amount.

Skilled nursing facility (SNF). The originating site facility fee is outside the SNF prospective payment system bundle and, as such, is not subject to SNF consolidated billing. The originating site facility fee is a separately billable Part B payment.

Community Mental Health Center (CMHC). The originating site facility fee is not a partial hospitalization service. The originating site facility fee does not count towards the number of services used to determine payment for partial hospitalization services. The originating site facility fee is not bundled in the per diem payment for partial hospitalization. The originating site facility fee is a separately billable Part B payment.

To receive the originating facility site fee, the provider submits claims with HCPCS code "Q3014, telehealth originating site facility fee"; short description "telehealth facility fee." The type of service for the telehealth originating site facility fee is "9, other items and services." For A/B MAC (B) processed claims, the "office" place of service (code 11) is the only payable setting for code Q3014. There is no participation payment differential for code Q3014. Deductible and coinsurance rules apply to Q3014. By submitting Q3014 HCPCS code, the originating site authenticates they are located in either a rural HPSA or non-MSA county.

This benefit may be billed on bill types 12X, 13X, 22X, 23X, 71X, 72X, 73X, 76X, and 85X. Unless otherwise applicable, report the originating site facility fee under revenue code 078X and include HCPCS code "Q3014, telehealth originating site facility fee."

Hospitals and critical access hospitals bill their A/B/MAC (A) for the originating site facility fee. Telehealth bills originating in inpatient hospitals must be submitted on a 12X TOB using the date of discharge as the line item date of service.

Independent and provider-based RHCs and FQHCs bill the appropriate A/B/MAC (A) using the RHC or FQHC bill type and billing number. HCPCS code Q3014 is the only non-RHC/FQHC service that is billed using the clinic/center bill type and provider number. All RHCs and FQHCs must use revenue code 078X when billing for the originating site facility fee. For all other non-RHC/FQHC services, provider based RHCs and FQHCs must bill using the base provider's bill type and billing number. Independent RHCs and FQHCs must bill the A/B MAC (B) for all other non-RHC/FQHC services. If an RHC/FQHC visit occurs on the same day as a telehealth service, the RHC/FQHC serving as an originating site must bill for HCPCS code Q3014 telehealth originating site facility fee on a separate revenue line from the RHC/FQHC visit using revenue code 078X.

Hospital-based or CAH-based renal dialysis centers (including satellites) bill their A/B/MAC (A) for the originating site facility fee. Telehealth bills originating in renal dialysis centers must be submitted on a 72X TOB. All hospital-based or CAH-based renal dialysis centers (including satellites) must use revenue code 078X when billing for the originating site facility fee. The renal dialysis center serving as an originating site must bill for HCPCS code Q3014, telehealth originating site facility fee, on a separate revenue line from any other services provided to the beneficiary.

Skilled nursing facilities (SNFs) bill their A/B/MAC (A) for the originating site facility fee. Telehealth bills originating in SNFs must be submitted on TOB 22X or 23X. For SNF inpatients in a covered Part A stay, the originating site facility fee must be submitted on a 22X TOB. All SNFs must use revenue code 078X when billing for the originating site facility fee. The SNF serving as an originating site must bill for HCPCS code Q3014, telehealth originating site facility fee, on a separate revenue line from any other services provided to the beneficiary.

Community mental health centers (CMHCs) bill their A/B/MAC (A) for the originating site facility fee. Telehealth bills originating in CMHCs must be submitted on a 76X TOB. All CMHCs must use revenue code 078X when billing for the originating site facility fee. The CMHC serving as an originating site must bill for HCPCS code Q3014, telehealth originating site facility fee, on a separate revenue line from any other services provided to the beneficiary. Note that Q3014 does not count towards the number of services used to determine per diem payments for partial hospitalization services.

The beneficiary is responsible for any unmet deductible amount and Medicare coinsurance.

100-04, 12, 190.6

Payment Methodology for Physician/Practitioner at the Distant Site

(Rev. 3586, Issued: 08-12-16, Effective: 01-01-17, Effective: 01-03-17)

1. Distant Site Defined

The term "distant site" means the site where the physician or practitioner, providing the professional service, is located at the time the service is provided via a telecommunications system.

2. Payment Amount (professional fee)

The payment amount for the professional service provided via a telecommunications system by the physician or practitioner at the distant site is equal to the current fee schedule amount for the service provided at the facility rate. Payment for an office visit, consultation, individual psychotherapy or pharmacologic management via a telecommunications system should be made at the same facility amount as when these services are furnished without the use of a telecommunications system. For Medicare payment to occur, the service must be within a practitioner's scope of practice under State law. The beneficiary is responsible for any unmet deductible amount and applicable coinsurance.

3. Medicare Practitioners Who May Receive Payment at the Distant Site (i.e., at a site other than where beneficiary is)

As a condition of Medicare Part B payment for telehealth services, the physician or practitioner at the distant site must be licensed to provide the service under state law. When the physician or practitioner at the distant site is licensed under state law to provide a covered telehealth service (i.e., professional consultation, office and other outpatient visits, individual psychotherapy, and pharmacologic management) then he or she may bill for and receive payment for this service when delivered via a telecommunications system.

If the physician or practitioner at the distant site is located in a CAH that has elected Method II, and the physician or practitioner has reassigned his/her benefits to the CAH, the CAH bills its regular A/B/MAC (A) for the professional services provided at the distant site via a telecommunications system, in any of the revenue codes 096x, 097x or 098x. All requirements for billing distant site telehealth services apply.

4. Medicare Practitioners Who May Bill for Covered Telehealth Services are Listed Below (subject to State law)

- Physician
- Nurse practitioner
- Physician assistant
- Nurse-midwife
- Clinical nurse specialist
- Clinical psychologist*
- Clinical social worker*
- Registered dietitian or nutrition professional
- Certified registered nurse anesthetist

*Clinical psychologists and clinical social workers cannot bill for psychotherapy services that include medical evaluation and management services under Medicare. These practitioners may not bill or receive payment for the following CPT codes: 90805, 90807, and 90809.

100-04, 12, 190.6.1

Submission of Telehealth Claims for Distant Site Practitioners

(Rev. 3586, Issued: 08-12-16, Effective: 01-01-17, Implementation: 01-03-17)

Claims for telehealth services are submitted to the contractors that process claims for the performing physician/practitioner's service area. Physicians/practitioners submit the appropriate HCPCS procedure code for covered professional telehealth services with place of service code 02 (Telehealth) along with the "GT" modifier ("via interactive audio and video telecommunications system"). By coding and billing the "GT" modifier with a covered telehealth procedure code, the distant site physician/practitioner certifies that the beneficiary was present at an eligible originating site when the telehealth service was furnished. By coding and billing the "GT" modifier with a covered ESRD-related service telehealth code, the distant site physician/practitioner certifies that 1 visit per month was furnished face-to-face "hands on" to examine the vascular access site. Refer to section 190.3.4 of this chapter for the conditions of telehealth payment for ESRD-related services.

In situations where a CAH has elected payment Method II for CAH outpatients, and the practitioner has reassigned his/her benefits to the CAH, A/B/MACs (A) should make payment for telehealth services provided by the physician or practitioner at 80 percent of the MPFS facility amount for the distant site service. In all other cases, except for MNT services as discussed in Section 190.7- A/B MAC (B) Editing of Telehealth Claims, telehealth services provided by the physician or practitioner at the distant site are billed to the A/B/MAC (B).

Physicians and practitioners at the distant site bill their A/B/MAC (B) for covered telehealth services, for example, "99245 GT." Physicians' and practitioners' offices serving as a telehealth originating site bill their A/B/MAC (B) for the originating site facility fee.

100-04, 12, 190.7

A/B MAC (B) Editing of Telehealth Claims

(Rev. 3721, Issued: 02-24-17, Effective: 05-25-17, Implementation: 05-25-17)

Medicare telehealth services (as listed in section 190.3) are billed with either the "GT" or "GQ" modifier. The contractor shall approve covered telehealth services if the physician or practitioner is licensed under State law to provide the service. Contractors must familiarize themselves with licensure provisions of States for which they process claims and disallow telehealth services furnished by physicians or practitioners who are not authorized to furnish the applicable telehealth service under State law. For example, if a nurse practitioner is not licensed to provide individual psychotherapy under State law, he or she would not be permitted to receive payment for individual psychotherapy under Medicare. The contractor shall install edits to ensure that only properly licensed physicians and practitioners are paid for covered telehealth services.

If a contractor receives claims for professional telehealth services coded with the "GQ" modifier (representing "via asynchronous telecommunications system"), it shall approve/pay for these services only if the physician or practitioner is affiliated with a Federal telemedicine demonstration conducted in Alaska or Hawaii. The contractor may require the physician or practitioner at the distant site to document his or her participation in a Federal telemedicine demonstration program conducted in Alaska or Hawaii prior to paying for telehealth services provided via asynchronous, store and forward technologies.

Contractors shall deny telehealth services if the physician or practitioner is not eligible to bill for them.

The following reflects the remittance advice messages and associated codes that will appear when rejecting/denying claims under this policy. This CARC/RARC combination is compliant with CAQH CORE Business Scenario 3.

Group Code: CO
CARC: 185
RARC: N/A
MSN: 21.18

If a service is billed with one of the telehealth modifiers and the procedure code is not designated as a covered telehealth service, the contractor denies the service.

The following reflects the remittance advice messages and associated codes that will appear when rejecting/denying claims under this policy. This CARC/RARC combination is compliant with CAQH CORE Business Scenario 3.

Group Code: CO
CARC: 96
RARC: N776
MSN: 9.4

The only claims from institutional facilities that FIs shall pay for telehealth services at the distant site, except for MNT services, are for physician or practitioner services when the distant site is located in a CAH that has elected Method II, and the physician or practitioner has reassigned his/her benefits to the CAH. The CAH bills its regular FI for the professional services provided at the distant site via a telecommunications system, in any of the revenue codes 096x, 097x or 098x. All requirements for billing distant site telehealth services apply.

Claims from hospitals or CAHs for MNT services are submitted to the hospital's or CAH's regular FI. Payment is based on the non-facility amount on the Medicare Physician Fee Schedule for the particular HCPCS codes.

100-04, 12, 230

Primary Care Incentive Payment Program (PCIP)

(Rev. 2161, Issued: 02-25-11, Effective: 01-01-11- Analysis/04-04-11-Design, Implementation: 01-01-11)

Section 5501(a) of the Affordable Care Act revises Section 1833 of the Social Security Act (the Act) by adding a new paragraph, (x), "Incentive Payments for Primary Care Services." Section 1833(x) of the Act states that in the case of primary care services furnished on or after January 1, 2011, and before January 1, 2016, there shall be a 10 percent incentive payment for such services under Part B when furnished by a primary care practitioner.

Information regarding Primary Care Incentive Payment Program (PCIP) payments made to critical access hospitals (CAHs) paid under the optional method can be found in Pub. 100-4, Chapter 4, §250.12 of this manual.

100-04, 12, 230.1

Definition of Primary Care Practitioners and Primary Care Services

(Rev. 2161, Issued: 02-25-11, Effective: 01-01-11- Analysis/04-04-11-Design, Implementation: 01-01-11)

Primary care practitioners are defined as:

1. A physician who has a primary specialty designation of family medicine, internal medicine, geriatric medicine, or pediatric medicine for whom primary care services accounted for at least 60 percent of the allowed charges under Part B for the practitioner in a prior period as determined appropriate by the Secretary; or
2. A nurse practitioner, clinical nurse specialist, or physician assistant for whom primary care services accounted for at least 60 percent of the allowed charges under Part B for the practitioner in a prior period as determined appropriate by the Secretary.

Primary care services are defined as HCPCS Codes:

1. 99201 through 99215 for new and established patient office or outpatient evaluation and management (E/M) visits;
2. 99304 through 99340 for initial, subsequent, discharge, and other nursing facility E/M services; new and established patient domiciliary, rest home or custodial care E/M services; and domiciliary, rest home or home care plan oversight services; and
3. 99341 through 99350 for new and established patient home E/M visits.

Practitioner Identification

Eligible practitioners will be identified on claims by the National Provider Identifier (NPI) number of the rendering practitioner. If the claim is submitted by a practitioner's group practice, the rendering practitioner's NPI must be included on the line-item for the primary care service and reflect an eligible HCPCS as identified. In order to be eligible for the PCIP, physician assistants, clinical nurse specialists, and nurse practitioners must be billing for their services under their own NPI and not furnishing services incident to physicians' services. Regardless of the specialty area in which they may be practicing, the specific nonphysician practitioners are eligible for the PCIP based on their profession and historical percentage of allowed charges as primary care services that equals or exceeds the 60 percent threshold.

Beginning in calendar year (CY) 2011, primary care practitioners will be identified based on their primary specialty of enrollment in Medicare and percentage of allowed charges for primary care services that equals or exceeds the 60 percent threshold from Medicare claims data 2 years prior to the bonus payment year.

Eligible practitioners for PCIP payments in a given calendar year (CY) will be listed by eligible NPI in the Primary Care Incentive Payment Program Eligibility File, available after January 31, of the payment year on their Medicare contractor's website. Practitioners should contact their contractor with any questions regarding their eligibility for the PCIP.

100-04, 12, 230.2

Coordination with Other Payments

(Rev. 2161, Issued: 02-25-11, Effective: 01-01-11- Analysis/04-04-11-Design, Implementation: 01-01-11)

Section 5501(a)(3) of the Affordable Care Act provides payment under the PCIP as an additional payment amount for specified primary care services without regard to any additional payment for the service under Section 1833(m) of the Act. Therefore, an eligible primary care physician furnishing a primary care service in a health professional shortage area (HPSA) may receive both a HPSA physician bonus payment (as described in the Medicare Claims Processing Manual, Pub. 100-4, Chapter 12, §90.4) under the HPSA physician bonus program and a PCIP incentive payment under the new program beginning in CY 2011.

100-04, 12, 230.3

Claims Processing and Payment

(Rev. 2161, Issued: 02-25-11, Effective: 01-01-11- Analysis/04-04-11-Design, Implementation: 01-01-11)

A. General Overview

Incentive payments will be made on a quarterly basis and shall be equal to 10 percent of the amount paid for such services under the Medicare Physician Fee Schedule (PFS) for those services furnished during the bonus payment year. For information on PCIP payments to CAHs paid under the optional method, see the Medicare Claims Processing Manual, Pub. 100-4, Chapter 4, §250.12.

On an annual basis Medicare contractors shall receive a Primary Care Incentive Payment Program Eligibility File that they shall post to their website. The file will list the NPIs of all practitioners who are eligible to receive PCIP payments for the upcoming CY.

B. Method of Payment

- Calculate and pay qualifying primary care practitioners an additional 10 percent incentive payment;
- Calculate the payment based on the amount actually paid for the services, not the Medicare approved amounts;
- Combine the PCIP incentive payments, when appropriate, with other incentive payments, including the HPSA physician bonus payment, and the HPSA Surgical Incentive Payment Program (HSIP) payment;
- Provide a special remittance form that is forwarded with the incentive payment so that physicians and practitioners can identify which type of incentive payment (HPSA physician and/or PCIP) was paid for which services.
- Practitioners should contact their contractor with any questions regarding PCIP payments.

C. Changes for Contractor Systems

The Medicare Carrier System, (MCS), Common Working File (CWF) and the National Claims History (NCH) shall be modified to accept a new PCIP indicator on the claim line. Once the type of incentive payment has been identified by the shared systems, the shared system shall modify their systems to set the indicator on the claim line as follows:

1 = HPSA;

2 = PSA;

3 = HPSA and PSA;

4 = HSIP;

5 = HPSA and HSIP;

6 = PCIP;

7 = HPSA and PCIP; and

Space = Not Applicable.

The contractor shared system shall send the HIGLAS 810 invoice for incentive payment invoices, including the new PCIP payment. The contractor shall also combine the provider's HPSA physician bonus, physician scarcity (PSA) bonus (if it should become available at a later date), HSIP payment and/or PCIP payment invoice per provider. The contractor shall receive the HIGLAS 835 payment file from HIGLAS showing a single incentive payment per provider.

100-04, 13, 30.1.3.1

A/B MAC (A) Payment for Low Osmolar Contrast Material (LOCM) (Radiology)

(Rev. 3227, Issued: 04-02-15, Effective--multiple effective dates)

The LOCM is paid on a reasonable cost basis when rendered by a SNF to its Part B patients (in addition to payment for the radiology procedure) when it is used in one of the situations listed below.

The following HCPCS are used when billing for LOCM.

HCPCS Code	Description (January 1. 1994, and later)
A4644	Supply of low osmolar contrast material (100-199 mgs of iodine);
A4645	Supply of low osmolar contrast material (200-299 mgs of iodine); or
A4646	Supply of low osmolar contrast material (300-399 mgs of iodine).

When billing for LOCM, SNFs use revenue code 0636. If the SNF charge for the radiology procedure includes a charge for contrast material, the SNF must adjust the charge for the radiology procedure to exclude any amount for the contrast material.

NOTE: LOCM is never billed with revenue code 0255 or as part of the radiology procedure.

The A/B MAC (A) will edit for the intrathecal procedure codes and the following codes to determine if payment for LOCM is to be made. If an intrathecal procedure code is not present, or one of the ICD codes is not present to indicate that a required medical condition is met, the A/B MAC (A) will deny payment for LOCM. In these instances, LOCM is not covered and should not be billed to Medicare.

When LOCM Is Separately Billable and Related Coding Requirements

- In all intrathecal injections. HCPCS codes that indicate intrathecal injections are:

  70010, 70015, 72240, 72255, 72265, 72270, 72285, 72295

  One of these must be included on the claim; or

- In intravenous and intra-arterial injections only when certain medical conditions are present in an outpatient. The SNF must verify the existence of at least one of the following medical conditions, and report the applicable diagnosis code(s) either as a principal diagnosis code or other diagnosis codes on the claim:
  — A history of previous adverse reaction to contrast material. The applicable ICD-9-CM codes are V14.8 and V14.9. The applicable ICD-10-CM codes are Z88.8 and Z88.9. The conditions which should not be considered adverse reactions are a sensation of heat, flushing, or a single episode of nausea or vomiting. If the adverse reaction occurs on that visit with the induction of contrast material, codes describing hives, urticaria, etc. should also be present, as well as a code describing the external cause of injury and poisoning, ICD-9-CM code E947.8. The applicable ICD-10 CM codes are: T50.8X5A Adverse effect of diagnostic agents, initial encounter, T50.8X5S Adverse effect of diagnostic agents, sequela , T50.995A Adverse effect of other drugs, medicaments and biological substances, initial encounter, or

T50.995S Adverse effect of other drugs, medicaments and biological substances, sequela;

— A history or condition of asthma or allergy. The applicable ICD-9-CM codes are V07.1, V14.0 through V14.9, V15.0, 493.00, 493.01, 493.10, 493.11, 493.20, 493.21, 493.90, 493.91, 495.0, 495.1, 495.2, 495.3, 495.4, 495.5, 495.6, 495.7, 495.8, 495.9, 995.0, 995.1, 995.2, and 995.3. The applicable ICD-10-CM codes are in the table below:

ICD-10-CM Codes

J44.0	J44.9	J45.20	J45.22	J45.30	J45.32	J45.40
J45.42	J45.50	J45.52	J45.902	J45.909	J45.998	J67.0
J67.1	JJ67.2	J67.3	J67.4	J67.5	J67.6	J67.7
J67.8	J67.9	J96.00	J96.01	J96.02	J96.90	J96.91
J96.92	T36.0X5A	T36.1X5A	T36.2X5A	T36.3X5A	T36.4X5A	T36.5X5A
T36.6X5A	T36.7X5A	T36.8X5A	T36.95XA	T37.0X5A	T37.1X5A	T37.2X5A
T37.3X5A	T37.8X5A	T37.95XA	T38.0X5A	T38.1X5A	T38.2X5A	T38.3X5A
T38.4X5A	T38.6X5A	T38.7X5A	T38.805A	T38.815A	T38.895A	T38.905A
T38.995A	T39.015A	T39.095A	T39.1X5A	T39.2X5A	T39.2X5A	T39.315A
T39.395A	T39.4X5A	T39.8X5A	T39.95XA	T40.0X5A	T40.1X5A	T40.2X5A
T40.3X5A	T40.4X5A	T40.5X5A	T40.605A	T40.695A	T40.7X5A	T40.8X5A
T40.905A	T40.995A	T41.0X5A	T41.1X5A	T41.205A	T41.295A	T41.3X5A
T41.4X5A	T41.X5A	T41.5X5A	T42.0X5A	T42.1X5A	T42.2X5A	T42.3X5A
T42.4X5A	T42.5X5A	T42.6X5A	427.5XA	428.X5A	T43.015A	T43.025A
T43.1X5A	T43.205A	T43.215A	T43.225A	T43.295A	T43.3X5A	T43.4X5A
T43.505A	T43.595A	T43.605A	T43.615A	T43.625A	T43.635A	T43.695A
T43.8X5A	T43.95XA	T44.0X5A	T44.1X5A	T44.2X5A	T44.3X5A	T44.6X5A
T44.7X5A	T44.8X5A	T44.905A	T44.995A	T45.0X5A	T45.1X5A	T45.2X5A
T45.3X5A	T45.4X5A	T45.515A	T45.525A	T45.605A	T45.615A	T45.625A
T45.695A	T45.7X5A	T45.8X5A	T45.95XA	T46.0X5A	T46.1X5A	T46.2X5A
T46.3X5A	T46.4X5A	T46.5X5A	T46.6X5A	T46.7X5A	T46.8X5A	T46.905A
T46.995A	T47.0X5A	T47.1X5A	T47.2X5A	T47.3X5A	T47.4X5A	T47.5X5A
T47.6X5A	T47.7X5A	T47.8X5A	T47.95XA	T48.0X5A	T48.1X5A	T48.205A
T48.295A	T48.3X5A	T48.4X5A	T48.5X5A	T48.6X5A	T48.905A	T48.995A
T49.0X5A	T49.1X5A	T49.2X5A	T49.3X5A	T49.4X5A	T49.5X5A	T49.6X5A
T49.6X5A	T47.X5A9	T49.8X5A	T49.95XA	T50.0X5A	T50.1X5A	T50.2X5A
T50.3X5A	T50.4X5A	T50.5X5A	T50.6X5A	T50.7X5A	T50.8X5A	T50.905a
T50.995A	T50.A15A	T50.A25A	T50.A95A	T50.B15A	T50.B95A	T50.Z15A
T50.Z95A	T78.2XXA	T78.3XXA	T78.40XA	T78.41XA	T88.52XA	T88.59XA
T88.6XXA	Z51.89	Z88.0	Z88.1	Z88.2	Z88.3	Z88.4
Z88.5	Z88.6	Z88.7	Z88.8	Z88.9	Z91.010	

— Significant cardiac dysfunction including recent or imminent cardiac decompensation, severe arrhythmia, unstable angina pectoris, recent myocardial infarction, and pulmonary hypertension. The applicable ICD-9-CM codes are:

ICD-9-CM

402.00	402.01	402.10	402.11	402.90	402.91	404.00
404.01	404.02	404.03	404.10	404.11	404.12	404.13
404.90	404.91	404.92	404.93	410.00	410.01	410.02
410.10	410.11	410.12	410.20	410.21	410.22	410.30
410.31	410.32	410.40	410.41	410.42	410.50	410.51
410.52	410.60	410.61	410.62	410.70	410.71	410.72
410.80	410.81	410.82	410.90	410.91	410.92	411.1
415.0	416.0	416.1	416.8	416.9	420.0	420.90
420.91	420.99	424.90	424.91	424.99	427.0	427.1
427.2	427.31	427.32	427.41	427.42	427.5	427.60
427.61	427.69	427.81	427.89	427.9	428.0	428.1
428.9	429.0	429.1	429.2	429.3	429.4	429.5
429.6	429.71	429.79	429.81	429.82	429.89	429.9
785.50	785.51	785.59				

— The applicable ICD-10-CM codes are in the table below:

ICD-10-CM Codes

A18.84	I11.0	I11.9	I13.0	I13.10	I13.11	I13.2
I20.0	I21.01	I21.02	I21.09	I21.11	I21.19	I21.21
I21.29	I21.3	I21.4	I22.1	I22.2	I22.8	I23.0
I23.1	I23.2	I23.3	I23.4	I23.5	I23.6	I23.7
I23.8	I25.10	I25.110	I25.700	I25.710	I25.720	I25.730
I25.750	I25.760	I25.790	I26.01	I26.02	I26.09	I27.0
I27.1	I27.2	I27.81	I27.89	I27.9	I30.0	I30.1
I30.8	I30.9	I32	I38	I39	I46.2	I46.8
I46.9	I47.0	I471	I472	I47.9	I48.0	I48.1
I48.1	I48.2	I48.3	I48.4	I48.91	I48.92	I49.01
I49.02	I49.1	I49.2	I49.3	I49.40	I49.49	I49.5
I49.8	I49.9	I50.1	I50.20	I50.21	I50.22	I50.23
I50.30	I50.31	I50.32	I50.33	I50.40	I50.41	I50.42
I50.43	I50.9	I51	I51.0	I51.1	I51.2	I51.3
I51.4	I51.5	I51.7	I51.89	I51.9	I52	I97.0
I97.110	I97.111	I97.120	I97.121	I97.130	I97.131	I97.190
I97.191	M32.11	M32.12	R00.1	R57.0	R57.8	R57.9

— Generalized severe debilitation. The applicable ICD-9-CM codes are: 203.00, 203.01, all codes for diabetes mellitus, 518.81, 585, 586, 799.3, 799.4, and V46.1. The applicable ICD-10-CM codes are: J96.850, J96.00 through J96.02, J96.90 through J96.91, N18.1 through N19, R53.81, R64, and Z99.11 through Z99.12. Or

— Sickle Cell disease. The applicable ICD-9-CM codes are 282.4, 282.60, 282.61, 282.62, 282.63, and 282.69. The applicable ICD-10-CM codes are D56.0 through D56.3, D56.5 through D56.9, D57.00 through D57.1, D57.20, D57.411 through D57.419, and D57.811 through D57.819.

100-04, 13, 40

Magnetic Resonance Imaging (MRI) Procedures

(Rev. 4147, Issued: 10-19-18, Effective: 04- 10-18, Implementation: 12-10-18)

The Centers for Medicare & Medicaid Services (CMS) finds that the non-coverage of magnetic resonance imaging (MRI) for blood flow determination is no longer supported by the available evidence. CMS is removing the phrase "blood flow measurement" and local Medicare contractors will have the discretion to cover (or not cover).

Consult Publication (Pub.) 100-03, National Coverage Determinations (NCD) Manual, chapter 1, section 220.2, for specific coverage and non-coverage indications associated with MRI and MRA (Magnetic Resonance Angiography).

A/B MACs (B) do not make additional payments for three or more MRI sequences. The relative value units (RVUs) reflect payment levels for two sequences.

The technical component (TC) RVUs for MRI procedures that specify "with contrast" include payment for paramagnetic contrast media. A/B MACs (B) do not make separate payment under code A4647.

A diagnostic technique has been developed under which an MRI of the brain or spine is first performed without contrast material, then another MRI is performed with a standard (0.1mmol/kg) dose of contrast material and, based on the need to achieve a better image, a third MRI is performed with an additional double dosage (0.2mmol/kg) of contrast material. When the high-dose contrast technique is utilized, A/B MACs (B):

- Do not pay separately for the contrast material used in the second MRI procedure;
- Pay for the contrast material given for the third MRI procedure through supply code Q9952, the replacement code for A4643, when billed with Current Procedural Terminology (CPT) codes 70553, 72156, 72157, and 72158;
- Do not pay for the third MRI procedure. For example, in the case of an MRI of the brain, if CPT code 70553 (without contrast material, followed by with contrast material(s) and further sequences) is billed, make no payment for CPT code 70551 (without contrast material(s)), the additional procedure given for the purpose of administering the double dosage, furnished during the same session. Medicare does not pay for the third procedure (as distinguished from the contrast material) because the CPT definition of code 70553 includes all further sequences; and
- Do not apply the payment criteria for low osmolar contrast media in §30.1.2 to billings for code Q9952, the replacement code for A4643. Effective January 1, 2008, Q9952 is replaced with A9579.

With the implementation for calendar year 2007 of a bottom-up methodology, which utilizes the direct inputs to determine the practice expense (PE) relative value units (RVUs), the cost of the contrast media is not included in the PE RVUs. Therefore, a separate payment for the contrast media used in various imaging procedures is paid. In addition to the CPT code representing the imaging procedure, separately bill the appropriate HCPCS "Q" code (Q9945 – Q9954; Q9958-Q9964) for the contrast medium utilized in performing the service. Effective January 1, 2008, HCPCS code ranges changed to Q9950-Q9954, Q9958-Q9967.

For claims with dates of service on or after February 24, 2011, through April 9, 2018, Medicare will allow for coverage of MRI for beneficiaries with implanted pacemakers (PMs) or cardioverter defibrillators

(ICDs) for use in an MRI environment in a Medicare-approved clinical study as described in section 220.C.1 of the NCD Manual.

For claims with dates of service on or after July 7, 2011, through April 9, 2018, Medicare will allow for coverage of MRI for beneficiaries with implanted PMs when the PMs are used according to the Food and Drug Administration (FDA)-approved labeling for use in an MRI environment as described in section 220.2.C.1 of the NCD Manual.

For claims with dates of service on or after April 10, 2018, Medicare will allow for coverage for MRIs for beneficiaries with implanted PMs, ICDs, cardiac resynchronization therapy pacemakers (CRT-Ps), or cardiac resynchronization therapy defibrillators (CRT-Ds), both on and off FDA label, for use in an MRI environment as described in section 220.2.B.3 of the NCD Manual. The data collection requirement under coverage with evidence development ceases April 9, 2018.

100-04, 13, 40.1.1

Magnetic Resonance Angiography (MRA) Coverage Summary

(Rev. 2171, Issued: 03-04-11, Effective: 02-24-11, Implementation: 04-04-11)

Section 1861(s)(2)(C) of the Social Security Act provides for coverage of diagnostic testing. Coverage of magnetic resonance angiography (MRA) of the head and neck, and MRA of the peripheral vessels of the lower extremities is limited as described in Publication (Pub.) 100-3, the Medicare National Coverage Determinations (NCD) Manual. This instruction has been revised as of July 1, 2003, based on a determination that coverage is reasonable and necessary in additional circumstances. Under that instruction, MRA is generally covered only to the extent that it is used as a substitute for contrast angiography, except to the extent that there are documented circumstances consistent with that instruction that demonstrates the medical necessity of both tests. Prior to June 3, 2010, there was no coverage of MRA outside of the indications and circumstances described in that instruction.

Effective for claims with dates of service on or after June 3, 2010, contractors have the discretion to cover or not cover all indications of MRA (and magnetic resonance imaging (MRI)) that are not specifically nationally covered or nationally non-covered as stated in section 220.2 of the NCD Manual.

Because the status codes for HCPCS codes 71555, 71555-TC, 71555-26, 74185, 74185-TC, and 74185-26 were changed in the Medicare Physician Fee Schedule Database from 'N' to 'R' on April 1, 1998, any MRA claims with those HCPCS codes with dates of service between April 1, 1998, and June 30, 1999, are to be processed according to the contractor's discretionary authority to determine payment in the absence of national policy.

Effective for claims with dates of service on or after February 24, 201l, Medicare will provide coverage for MRIs for beneficiaries with implanted cardiac pacemakers or implantable cardioverter defibrillators if the beneficiary is enrolled in an approved clinical study under the Coverage with Study Participation form of Coverage with Evidence Development that meets specific criteria per Pub. 100-3, the NCD Manual, chapter 1, section 220.2.C.1

100-04, 13, 40.1.2

HCPCS Coding Requirements

(Rev. 1472, Issued: 03-06-08, Effective: 05-23-07, Implementation: 04-07-08)

Providers must report HCPCS codes when submitting claims for MRA of the chest, abdomen, head, neck or peripheral vessels of lower extremities. The following HCPCS codes should be used to report these services:

MRA of head	70544, 70544-26, 70544-TC
MRA of head	70545, 70545-26, 70545-TC
MRA of head	70546, 70546-26, 70546-TC
MRA of neck	70547, 70547-26, 70547-TC
MRA of neck	70548, 70548-26, 70548-TC
MRA of neck	70549, 70549-26, 70549-TC
MRA of chest	71555, 71555-26, 71555-TC
MRA of pelvis	72198, 72198-26, 72198-TC
MRA of abdomen (dates of service on or after July 1, 2003) – see below.	74185, 74185-26, 74185-TC
MRA of peripheral vessels of lower extremities	73725, 73725-26, 73725-TC

100-04, 13, 60

Positron Emission Tomography (PET) Scans - General Information

(Rev. 1833; Issued: 10-16-09; Effective Date: 04-03-09; Implementation Date: 10-30-09)

Positron emission tomography (PET) is a noninvasive imaging procedure that assesses perfusion and the level of metabolic activity in various organ systems of the human body. A positron camera (tomograph) is used to produce cross-sectional tomographic images which are obtained by detecting radioactivity from a radioactive tracer substance radiopharmaceutical) that emits a radioactive tracer substance (radiopharmaceutical FDG) such as 2 -[F-18] flouro-D-glucose FDG, that is administered intravenously to the patient.

The Medicare National Coverage Determinations (NCD) Manual, Chapter 1, Sec.220.6, contains additional coverage instructions to indicate the conditions under which a PET scan is performed.

A. Definitions

For all uses of PET, excluding Rubidium 82 for perfusion of the heart, myocardial viability and refractory seizures, the following definitions apply:

- **Diagnosis:** PET is covered only in clinical situations in which the PET results may assist in avoiding an invasive diagnostic procedure, or in which the PET results may assist in determining the optimal anatomical location to perform an invasive diagnostic procedure. In general, for most solid tumors, a tissue diagnosis is made prior to the performance of PET scanning. PET scans following a tissue diagnosis are generally performed for the purpose of staging, rather than diagnosis. Therefore, the use of PET in the diagnosis of lymphoma, esophageal and colorectal cancers, as well as in melanoma, should be rare. PET is not covered for other diagnostic uses, and is not covered for screening (testing of patients without specific signs and symptoms of disease).
- **Staging:** PET is covered in clinical situations in which (1) (a) the stage of the cancer remains in doubt after completion of a standard diagnostic workup, including conventional imaging (computed tomography, magnetic resonance imaging, or ultrasound) or, (b) the use of PET would also be considered reasonable and necessary if it could potentially replace one or more conventional imaging studies when it is expected that conventional study information is insufficient for the clinical management of the patient and, (2) clinical management of the patient would differ depending on the stage of the cancer identified.

  NOTE: Effective for services on or after April 3, 2009, the terms "diagnosis" and "staging" will be replaced with "Initial Treatment Strategy." For further information on this new term, refer to Pub. 100-3, NCD Manual, section 220.6.17.
- **Restaging:** PET will be covered for restaging: (1) after the completion of treatment for the purpose of detecting residual disease, (2) for detecting suspected recurrence, or metastasis, (3) to determine the extent of a known recurrence, or (4) if it could potentially replace one or more conventional imaging studies when it is expected that conventional study information is to determine the extent of a known recurrence, or if study information is insufficient for the clinical management of the patient. Restaging applies to testing after a course of treatment is completed and is covered subject to the conditions above.
- **Monitoring:** Use of PET to monitor tumor response to treatment during the planned course of therapy (i.e., when a change in therapy is anticipated).

  NOTE: Effective for services on or after April 3, 2009, the terms "restaging" and "monitoring" will be replaced with "Subsequent Treatment Strategy." For further information on this new term, refer to Pub. 100-3, NCD Manual, section 220.6.17.

B. Limitations

For staging and restaging: PET is covered in either/or both of the following circumstances:

- The stage of the cancer remains in doubt after completion of a standard diagnostic workup, including conventional imaging (computed tomography, magnetic resonance imaging, or ultrasound); and/or
- The clinical management of the patient would differ depending on the stage of the cancer identified. PET will be covered for restaging after the completion of treatment for the purpose of detecting residual disease, for detecting suspected recurrence, or to determine the extent of a known recurrence. Use of PET would also be considered reasonable and necessary if it could potentially replace one or more conventional imaging studies when it is expected that conventional study information is insufficient for the clinical management of the patient.

The PET is not covered for other diagnostic uses, and is not covered for screening (testing of patients without specific symptoms). Use of PET to monitor tumor response during the planned course of therapy (i.e. when no change in therapy is being contemplated) is not covered.

100-04, 13, 60.2

Use of Gamma Cameras and Full Ring and Partial Ring PET Scanners for PET Scans

(Rev. 527, Issued: 04-15-05, Effective: 01-28-05, Implementation: 04-18-05)

See the Medicare NCD Manual, Section 220.6, concerning 2-[F-18] Fluoro-D-Glucose (FDG) PET scanners and details about coverage.

On July 1, 2001, HCPCS codes G0210 - G0230 were added to allow billing for all currently covered indications for FDG PET. Although the codes do not indicate the type of PET scanner, these codes were used until January 1, 2002, by providers to bill for services in a manner consistent with the coverage policy.

Effective January 1, 2002, HCPCS codes G0210 - G0230 were updated with new descriptors to properly reflect the type of PET scanner used. In addition, four new HCPCS codes became effective for dates of service on and after January 1, 2002, (G0231, G0232, G0233, G0234) for covered conditions that may be billed if a gamma camera is used for the PET scan. For services performed from January 1, 2002, through January 27, 2005, providers should bill using the revised HCPCS codes G0210 - G0234.

Beginning January 28, 2005 providers should bill using the appropriate CPT code.

100-04, 13, 60.3

PET Scan Qualifying Conditions and HCPCS Code Chart

(Rev. 527, Issued: 04-15-05, Effective: 01-28-05, Implementation: 04-18-05)

Below is a summary of all covered PET scan conditions, with effective dates.

NOTE: The G codes below except those a # can be used to bill for PET Scan services through January 27, 2005. Effective for dates of service on or after January 28, 2005, providers must bill for PET Scan services using the appropriate CPT codes. See section 60.3.1. The G codes with a # can continue to be used for billing after January 28, 2005 and these remain non-covered by Medicare. (NOTE: PET Scanners must be FDA-approved.)

Conditions	Coverage Effective Date	**** HCPCS/CPT
*Myocardial perfusion imaging (following previous PET G0030-G0047) single study, rest or stress (exercise and/or pharmacologic)	3/14/95	G0030
*Myocardial perfusion imaging (following previous PET G0030-G0047) multiple studies, rest or stress (exercise and/or pharmacologic)	3/14/95	G0031
*Myocardial perfusion imaging (following rest SPECT, 78464); single study, rest or stress (exercise and/or pharmacologic)	3/14/95	G0032
*Myocardial perfusion imaging (following rest SPECT 78464); multiple studies, rest or stress (exercise and/or pharmacologic)	3/14/95	G0033
*Myocardial perfusion (following stress SPECT 78465); single study, rest or stress (exercise and/or pharmacologic)	3/14/95	G0034
*Myocardial Perfusion Imaging (following stress SPECT 78465); multiple studies, rest or stress (exercise and/or pharmacologic)	3/14/95	G0035
*Myocardial Perfusion Imaging (following coronary angiography 93510-93529); single study, rest or stress (exercise and/or pharmacologic)	3/14/95	G0036
*Myocardial Perfusion Imaging, (following coronary angiography), 93510-93529); multiple studies, rest or stress (exercise and/or pharmacologic)	3/14/95	G0037
*Myocardial Perfusion Imaging (following stress planar myocardial perfusion, 78460); single study, rest or stress (exercise and/or pharmacologic)	3/14/95	G0038
*Myocardial Perfusion Imaging (following stress planar myocardial perfusion, 78460); multiple studies, rest or stress (exercise and/or pharmacologic)	3/14/95	G0039
*Myocardial Perfusion Imaging (following stress echocardiogram 93350); single study, rest or stress (exercise and/or pharmacologic)	3/14/95	G0040
*Myocardial Perfusion Imaging (following stress echocardiogram, 93350); multiple studies, rest or stress (exercise and/or pharmacologic)	3/14/95	G0041
*Myocardial Perfusion Imaging (following stress nuclear ventriculogram 78481 or 78483); single study, rest or stress (exercise and/or pharmacologic)	3/14/95	G0042
*Myocardial Perfusion Imaging (following stress nuclear ventriculogram 78481 or 78483); multiple studies, rest or stress (exercise and/or pharmacologic)	3/14/95	G0043
*Myocardial Perfusion Imaging (following stress ECG, 93000); single study, rest or stress (exercise and/or pharmacologic)	3/14/95	G0044
*Myocardial perfusion (following stress ECG, 93000), multiple studies; rest or stress (exercise and/or pharmacologic)	3/14/95	G0045
*Myocardial perfusion (following stress ECG, 93015), single study; rest or stress (exercise and/or pharmacologic)	3/14/95	G0046
*Myocardial perfusion (following stress ECG, 93015); multiple studies, rest or stress (exercise and/or pharmacologic)	3/14/95	G0047
PET imaging regional or whole body; single pulmonary nodule	1/1/98	G0125
Lung cancer, non-small cell (PET imaging whole body) Diagnosis, Initial Staging, Restaging	7/1/01	G0210 G0211 G0212
Colorectal cancer (PET imaging whole body) Diagnosis, Initial Staging, Restaging	7/1/01	G0213 G0214 G0215
Melanoma (PET imaging whole body) Diagnosis, Initial Staging, Restaging	7/1/01	G0216 G0217 G0218
Melanoma for non-covered indications	7/1/01	#G0219
Lymphoma (PET imaging whole body) Diagnosis, Initial Staging, Restaging	7/1/01	G0220 G0221 G0222
Head and neck cancer; excluding thyroid and CNS cancers (PET imaging whole body or regional) Diagnosis, Initial Staging, Restaging	7/1/01	G0223 G0224 G0225
Esophageal cancer (PET imaging whole body) Diagnosis, Initial Staging, Restaging	7/1/01	G0226 G0227 G0228
Metabolic brain imaging for pre-surgical evaluation of refractory seizures	7/1/01	G0229
Metabolic assessment for myocardial viability following inconclusive SPECT study	7/1/01	G0230
Recurrence of colorectal or colorectal metastatic cancer (PET whole body, gamma cameras only)	1/1/02	G0231
Staging and characterization of lymphoma (PET whole body, gamma cameras only)	1/1/02	G0232
Recurrence of melanoma or melanoma metastatic cancer (PET whole body, gamma cameras only)	1/1/02	G0233
Regional or whole body, for solitary pulmonary nodule following CT, or for initial staging of nonsmall cell lung cancer (gamma cameras only)	1/1/02	G0234
Non-Covered Service PET imaging, any site not otherwise specified	1/28/05	#G0235
Non-Covered Service Initial diagnosis of breast cancer and/or surgical planning for breast cancer (e.g., initial staging of axillary lymph nodes), not covered (full- and partialring PET scanners only)	10/1/02	#G0252
Breast cancer, staging/restaging of local regional recurrence or distant metastases, i.e., staging/restaging after or prior to course of treatment (full- and partial-ring PET scanners only)	10/1/02	G0253
Breast cancer, evaluation of responses to treatment, performed during course of treatment (full- and partial-ring PET scanners only)	10/1/02	G0254
Myocardial imaging, positron emission tomography (PET), metabolic evaluation)	10/1/02	78459
Restaging or previously treated thyroid cancer of follicular cell origin following negative I-131 whole body scan (full- and partial-ring PET scanner only)	10/1/03	G0296
Tracer Rubidium**82 (Supply of Radiopharmaceutical Diagnostic Imaging Agent) (This is only billed through Outpatient Perspective Payment System, OPPS.) (Carriers must use HCPCS Code A4641).	10/1/03	Q3000
Supply of Radiopharmaceutical Diagnostic Imaging Agent, Ammonia N-13	01/1/04	A9526
PET imaging, brain imaging for the differential diagnosis of Alzheimer's disease with aberrant features vs. fronto-temporal dementia	09/15/04	Appropriate CPT Code from section 60.3.1
PET Cervical Cancer Staging as adjunct to conventional imaging, other staging, diagnosis, restaging, monitoring	1/28/05	Appropriate CPT Code from section 60.3.1

* NOTE: Carriers must report A4641 for the tracer Rubidium 82 when used with PET scan codes G0030 through G0047 for services performed on or before January 27, 2005

** NOTE: Not FDG PET

*** NOTE: For dates of service October 1, 2003, through December 31, 2003, use temporary code Q4078 for billing this radiopharmaceutical.

100-04, 13, 60.3.1

Appropriate CPT Codes Effective for PET Scans for Services Performed on or After January 28, 2005

(Rev. 1301, Issued: 07-20-07, Effective: 01-28-05 CPT Code 78609/01-01-08 HCPCS Code A4641, Implementation: 01-07-08)

NOTE: All PET scan services require the use of a radiopharmaceutical diagnostic imaging agent (tracer). The applicable tracer code should be billed when billing for a PET scan service. See section 60.3.2 below for applicable tracer codes.

CPT Code	Description
78459	Myocardial imaging, positron emission tomography (PET), metabolic evaluation
78491	Myocardial imaging, positron emission tomography (PET), perfusion, single study at rest or stress
78492	Myocardial imaging, positron emission tomography (PET), perfusion, multiple studies at rest and/or stress
78608	Brain imaging, positron emission tomography (PET); metabolic evaluation
78811	Tumor imaging, positron emission tomography (PET); limited area (eg, chest, head/neck)
78812	Tumor imaging, positron emission tomography (PET); skull base to mid-thigh
78813	Tumor imaging, positron emission tomography (PET); whole body
78814	Tumor imaging, positron emission tomography (PET) with concurrently acquired computed tomography (CT) for attenuation correction and anatomical localization; limited area (eg, chest, head/neck)
78815	Tumor imaging, positron emission tomography (PET) with concurrently acquired computed tomography (CT) for attenuation correction and anatomical localization; skull base to mid-thigh
78816	Tumor imaging, positron emission tomography (PET) with concurrently acquired computed tomography (CT) for attenuation correction and anatomical localization; whole body

100-04, 13, 60.3.2

Tracer Codes Required for Positron Emission Tomography (PET) Scans

(Rev.3911, Issued: 11-09-17, Effective: 01-01-18, Implementation: 12-11-17)

An applicable tracer/radiopharmaceutical code, along with an applicable Current Procedural Technology (CPT) code, is necessary for claims processing of any Positron Emission Tomography (PET) scan services. While there are a number of PET tracers already billable for a diverse number of medical indications, there have been, and may be in the future, additional PET indications that might require a new PET tracer. Under those circumstances, the process to request/approve/implement a new code could be time-intensive. To help alleviate inordinate spans of time between when a national coverage determination is made, or when the Food and Drug Administration (FDA) approves a particular radiopharmaceutical for an oncologic indication already approved by the Centers for Medicare & Medicaid Services (CMS), and when it can be fully implemented via valid claims processing, CMS has created two new PET radiopharmaceutical unclassified tracer codes that can be used temporarily. This time period would be pending the creation/approval/implementation of permanent CPT codes that would later specifically define their function by CMS in official instructions.

Effective with dates of service on or after January 1, 2018, the following Healthcare Common Procedure Coding System (HCPCS) codes shall be used ONLY AS NECESSARY FOR AN INTERIM PERIOD OF TIME under the circumstances explained here. Specifically, there are two circumstances that would warrant use of the below codes: (1) After FDA approval of a PET oncologic indication, or, (2) after CMS approves coverage of a new PET indication, and ONLY if either of those situations requires the use of a dedicated PET radiopharmaceutical/tracer that is currently non-existent. Once permanent replacement codes are officially implemented by CMS, use of the temporary code for that particular indication will simultaneously be discontinued.

NOTE: The following two codes were effective as of January 1, 2017, with the January 2017 quarterly HCPCS update.

A9597 - Positron emission tomography radiopharmaceutical, diagnostic, for tumor identification, not otherwise classified

A9598 - Positron emission tomography radiopharmaceutical, diagnostic, for non-tumor identification, not otherwise classified

Effective for claims with dates of service on and after January 1, 2018, when PET tracer code A9597 or A9598 are present on a claim, that claim must also include:

- an appropriate PET HCPCS code, either 78459, 78491, 78492, 78608, 78811, 78812, 78813, 78814, 78815, or 78816,
- if tumor-related, either the -PI or -PS modifier as appropriate,
- if clinical trial, registry, or study-related outside of NCD220.6.17, PET for Solid Tumors, clinical trial modifier –Q0,
- if clinical trial, registry, or study-related, all claims require the 8-digit clinical trial number,
- if Part A OP and clinical trial, registry, or study-related outside of NCD220.6.17, PET for Solid Tumors, also include condition code 30 and ICD-10 diagnosis Z00.6.

Effective for claims with dates of service on and after January 1, 2018, A/Medicare Administrative Contractors (MACs) shall line-item deny, and B/MACs shall line-item reject, PET claims for A9597 or A9598 that don't include the elements noted above as appropriate.

Contractors shall use the following messaging when line-item denying (Part A) or line-item rejecting (Part B) PET claims containing HCPCS A9597 or A9598:

Remittance Advice Remark Codes (RARC) N386

Claim Adjustment Reason Code (CARC) 50, 96, and/or 119.

Group Code CO (Contractual Obligation) assigning financial liability to the provider (if a claim is received with a GZ modifier indicating no signed ABN is on file).

(The above new verbiage will supersede any existing verbiage in chapter 13, section 60.3.2.)

100-04, 13, 60.12

Coverage for PET Scans for Dementia and Neurodegenerative Diseases

(Rev. 3650, Issued: 11-10-16, Effective: 02-10-17, Implementation: 02-10-17)

Effective for dates of service on or after September 15, 2004, Medicare will cover FDG PET scans for a differential diagnosis of fronto-temporal dementia (FTD) and Alzheimer's disease OR; its use in a CMS-approved practical clinical trial focused on the utility of FDG-PET in the diagnosis or treatment of dementing neurodegenerative diseases. Refer to Pub. 100-03, NCD Manual, section 220.6.13, for complete coverage conditions and clinical trial requirements and section 60.15 of this manual for claims processing information.

A. A/B MAC (A and B) Billing Requirements for PET Scan Claims for FDG-PET for the Differential Diagnosis of Fronto-temporal Dementia and Alzheimer's Disease:

CPT Code for PET Scans for Dementia and Neurodegenerative Diseases

Contractors shall advise providers to use the appropriate CPT code from section 60.3.1 for dementia and neurodegenerative diseases for services performed on or after January 28, 2005.

Diagnosis Codes for PET Scans for Dementia and Neurodegenerative Diseases

The contractor shall ensure one of the following appropriate diagnosis codes is present on claims for PET Scans for AD:

- If ICD-9-CM is applicable, ICD-9 codes are: 290.0, 290.10 - 290.13, 290.20 - 290, 21, 290.3, 331.0, 331.11, 331.19, 331.2, 331.9, 780.93
- If ICD-10-CM is applicable, ICD-10 codes are: F03.90, F03.90 plus F05, G30.9, G31.01, G31.9, R41.2 or R41.3

Medicare contractors shall deny claims when submitted with an appropriate CPT code from section 60.3.1 and with a diagnosis code other than the range of codes listed above.

Medicare contractors shall instruct providers to issue an Advanced Beneficiary Notice to beneficiaries advising them of potential financial liability prior to delivering the service if one of the appropriate diagnosis codes will not be present on the claim.

The contractor shall use the following remittance advice messages and associated codes when rejecting/denying claims under this policy. This CARC/RARC combination is compliant with CAQH CORE Business Scenario Three.

Group Code: PR (if claim is received with a GA modifier) otherwise CO

CARC: 11

RARC: N/A

MSN: 16.48

Provider Documentation Required with the PET Scan Claim

Medicare contractors shall inform providers to ensure the conditions mentioned in the NCD Manual, section 220.6.13, have been met. The information must also be maintained in the beneficiary's medical record:

- Date of onset of symptoms;
    - Diagnosis of clinical syndrome (normal aging, mild cognitive impairment or MCI: mild, moderate, or severe dementia);
    - Mini mental status exam (MMSE) or similar test score;
    - Presumptive cause (possible, probably, uncertain AD);
    - Any neuropsychological testing performed;
    - Results of any structural imaging (MRI, CT) performed;
    - Relevant laboratory tests (B12, thyroid hormone); and,
    - Number and name of prescribed medications.

B. Billing Requirements for Beta Amyloid Positron Emission Tomography (PET) in Dementia and Neurodegenerative Disease:

Effective for claims with dates of service on and after September 27, 2013, Medicare will only allow coverage with evidence development (CED) for Positron Emission Tomography (PET) beta amyloid (also referred to as amyloid-beta (Aβ)) imaging (HCPCS A9586)or (HCPCS A9599) (one PET Aβ scan per patient).

NOTE: Please note that effective January 1, 2014 the following code A9599 will be updated in the IOCE and HCPCS update. This code will be contractor priced.

Medicare Summary Notices, Remittance Advice Remark Codes, and Claim Adjustment Reason Codes

Effective for dates of service on or after September 27, 2013, contractors shall return as unprocessable/return to provider claims for PET Aβ imaging, through CED during a clinical trial, not containing the following:

- Condition code 30, (A/B MAC (A) only)
- Modifier Q0 and/or modifier Q1 as appropriate
- ICD-9 dx code V70.7/ICD-10 dx code Z00.6 (on either the primary/secondary position)
- A PET HCPCS code (78811 or 78814)
- At least, one Dx code from the table below

ICD-9 Codes	Corresponding ICD-10 Codes
290.0 Senile dementia, uncomplicated	F03.90 Unspecified dementia without behavioral disturbance
290.10 Presenile dementia, uncomplicated	F03.90 Unspecified dementia without behavioral disturbance
290.11 Presenile dementia with delirium	F03.90 Unspecified dementia without behavioral disturbance
290.12 Presenile dementia with delusional features	F03.90 Unspecified dementia without behavioral disturbance
290.13 Presenile dementia with depressive features	F03.90 Unspecified dementia without behavioral disturbance
290.20 Senile dementia with delusional features	F03.90 Unspecified dementia without behavioral disturbance
290.21 Senile dementia with depressive features	F03.90 Unspecified dementia without behavioral disturbance
290.3 Senile dementia with delirium	F03.90 Unspecified dementia without behavioral disturbance
290.40 Vascular dementia, uncomplicated	F01.50 Vascular dementia without behavioral disturbance
290.41 Vascular dementia with delirium	F01.51 Vascular dementia with behavioral disturbance
290.42 Vascular dementia with delusions	F01.51 Vascular dementia with behavioral disturbance
290.43 Vascular dementia with depressed mood	F01.51 Vascular dementia with behavioral disturbance
294.10 Dementia in conditions classified elsewhere without behavioral disturbance	F02.80 Dementia in other diseases classified elsewhere without behavioral disturbance
294.11 Dementia in conditions classified elsewhere with behavioral disturbance	F02.81 Dementia in other diseases classified elsewhere with behavioral disturbance
294.20 Dementia, unspecified, without behavioral disturbance	F03.90 Unspecified dementia without behavioral disturbance
294.21 Dementia, unspecified, with behavioral disturbance	F03.91 Unspecified dementia with behavioral disturbance
331.11 Pick's Disease	G31.01 Pick's disease
331.19 Other Frontotemporal dementia	G31.09 Other frontotemporal dementia
331.6 Corticobasal degeneration	G31.85 Corticobasal degeneration
331.82 Dementia with Lewy Bodies	G31.83 Dementia with Lewy bodies
331.83 Mild cognitive impairment, so stated	G31.84 Mild cognitive impairment, so stated
ICD-9 Codes	Corresponding ICD-10 Codes
780.93 Memory Loss	R41.1 Anterograde amnesia
	R41.2 Retrograde amnesia
	R41.3 Other amnesia (Amnesia NOS, Memory loss NOS)
V70.7 Examination for normal comparison or control in clinical	Z00.6 Encounter for examination for normal comparison and control in clinical research program

and

- Aβ HCPCS code A9586 or A9599

The contractor shall use the following remittance advice messages and associated codes when returning claims under this policy. This CARC/RARC combination is compliant with CAQH CORE Business Scenario Two.

Group Code: CO
CARC: 4
RARC: N517, N519
MSN: N/A

Contractors shall line-item deny claims for PET Aβ, HCPCS code A9586 or A9599, where a previous PET Aβ, HCPCS code A9586 or A9599 is paid in history.

The contractor shall use the following remittance advice messages and associated codes when rejecting/denying claims under this policy. This CARC/RARC combination is compliant with CAQH CORE Business Scenario Three.

Group Code: PR (if claim is received with a GA modifier) otherwise CO

CARC: 149
RARC: N587
MSN: 20.12

100-04, 13, 60.13

Billing Requirements for PET Scans for Specific Indications of Cervical Cancer for Services Performed on or After January 28, 2005

(Rev. 1888; Issued: 01-06-10, Effective date: 11-10-09; Implementation Date: 01-04-10)

Contractors shall accept claims for these services with the appropriate CPT code listed in section 60.3.1. Refer to Pub. 100-3, section 220.6.17, for complete coverage guidelines for this new PET oncology indication. The implementation date for these CPT codes will be April 18, 2005. Also see section 60.17, of this chapter for further claims processing instructions for cervical cancer indications.

100-04, 13, 60.15

Billing Requirements for CMS - Approved Clinical Trials and Coverage With Evidence Development Claims for PET Scans for Neurodegenerative Diseases, Previously Specified Cancer Indications, and All Other Cancer Indications Not Previously Specified

(Rev. 3227, Issued: 04-02-15, Multiple effective dates)

A/B MACs (A and B)

Effective for services on or after January 28, 2005, contractors shall accept and pay for claims for Positron Emission Tomography (PET) scans for lung cancer, esophageal cancer, colorectal cancer, lymphoma, melanoma, head & neck cancer, breast cancer, thyroid cancer, soft tissue sarcoma, brain cancer, ovarian cancer, pancreatic cancer, small cell lung cancer, and testicular cancer, as well as for neurodegenerative diseases and all other cancer indications not previously mentioned in this chapter, if these scans were performed as part of a Centers for Medicare & Medicaid (CMS)-approved clinical trial. (See Pub. 100-3, National Coverage Determinations (NCD) Manual, sections 220.6.13 and 220.6.17.)

Contractors shall also be aware that PET scans for all cancers not previously specified at Pub. 100-3, NCD Manual, section 220.6.17, remain nationally non-covered unless performed in conjunction with a CMS-approved clinical trial.

Effective for dates of service on or after June 11, 2013, Medicare has ended the coverage with evidence development (CED) requirement for FDG (2-[F18] fluoro-2-deoxy-D-glucose) PET and PET/computed tomography (CT) and PET/magnetic resonance imaging (MRI) for all oncologic indications contained in section 220.6.17 of the NCD Manual. Modifier -Q0 (Investigational clinical service provided in a clinical research study that is in an approved clinical research study) or -Q1 (routine clinical service provided in a clinical research study that is in an approved clinical research study) is no longer mandatory for these services when performed on or after June 11, 2013.

A/B MACs (B) Only

A/B MACs (B) shall pay claims for PET scans for beneficiaries participating in a CMS-approved clinical trial submitted with an appropriate current procedural terminology (CPT) code from section 60.3.1 of this chapter and modifier Q0/Q1 for services performed on or after January 1, 2008, through June 10, 2013. (NOTE: Modifier QR (Item or service provided in a Medicare specified study) and QA (FDA investigational device exemption) were replaced by modifier Q0 effective January 1, 2008.) Modifier QV (item or service provided as routine care in a Medicare qualifying clinical trial) was replaced by modifier Q1 effective January 1, 2008.) Beginning with services performed on or after June 11, 2013, modifier Q0/Q1 is no longer required for PET FDG services.

A/B MACs (A) Only

In order to pay claims for PET scans on behalf of beneficiaries participating in a CMS-approved clinical trial, A/B MACs (A) require providers to submit claims with, if ICD-9-CM is applicable, ICD-9 code V70.7; if ICD-10-CM is applicable, ICD-10 code Z∅∅.6 in the primary/secondary diagnosis position using the ASC X12 837 institutional claim format or on Form CMS-1450, with the appropriate principal diagnosis code and an appropriate CPT code from section 60.3.1. Effective for PET scan claims for dates of service on or after January 28, 2005, through December 31, 2007, A/B MACs (A) shall accept claims with the QR, QV, or QA modifier on other than inpatient claims. Effective for services on or after January 1, 2008, through June 10, 2013, modifier Q0 replaced the-QR and QA modifier, modifier Q1 replaced the QV modifier. Modifier Q0/Q1 is no longer required for services performed on or after June 11, 2013.

100-04, 13, 60.16

Billing and Coverage Changes for PET Scans Effective for Services on or After April 3, 2009

(Rev. 3650, Issued: 11-10-16, Effective: 02-10-17, Implementation: 02-10-17)

A. Summary of Changes

Effective for services on or after April 3, 2009, Medicare will not cover the use of FDG PET imaging to determine initial treatment strategy in patients with adenocarcinoma of the prostate.

Medicare will also not cover FDG PET imaging for subsequent treatment strategy for tumor types other than breast, cervical, colorectal, esophagus, head and neck (non-CNS/thyroid), lymphoma, melanoma, myeloma, non-small cell lung, and ovarian, unless the FDG PET is provided under the coverage with evidence development (CED) paradigm (billed with modifier -Q0/-Q1, see section 60.15 of this chapter).

Medicare will cover FDG PET imaging for initial treatment strategy for myeloma.

Effective for services performed on or after June 11, 2013, Medicare has ended the CED requirement for FDG PET and PET/CT and PET/MRI for all oncologic indications contained in section 220.6.17 of the NCD Manual. Effective for services on or after June 11, 2013, the Q0/Q1 modifier is no longer required.

Beginning with services performed on or after June 11, 2013, contractors shall pay for up to three (3) FDG PET scans when used to guide subsequent management of anti-tumor treatment strategy (modifier PS) after completion of initial anti-cancer therapy (modifier PI) for the exact same cancer diagnosis.

Coverage of any additional FDG PET scans (that is, beyond 3) used to guide subsequent management of anti-tumor treatment strategy after completion of initial anti-tumor therapy for the same cancer diagnosis will be determined by the A/B MACs (A or B). Claims will include the KX modifier indicating the coverage criteria is met for coverage of four or more FDG PET scans for subsequent treatment strategy for the same cancer diagnosis under this NCD.

A different cancer diagnosis whether submitted with a PI or a PS modifier will begin the count of one initial and three subsequent FDG PET scans not requiring the KX modifier and four or more FDG PET scans for subsequent treatment strategy for the same cancer diagnosis requiring the KX modifier.

NOTE: The presence or absence of an initial treatment strategy claim in a beneficiary's record does not impact the frequency criteria for subsequent treatment strategy claims for the same cancer diagnosis.

NOTE: Providers please refer to the following link for a list of appropriate diagnosis codes, http://cms.gov/medicare/coverage/determinationprocess/downloads/petforsolidtumorsoncologicdxcodesattachment_NCD220_6_17.pdf

For further information regarding the changes in coverage, refer to Pub.100-03, NCD Manual, section 220.6.17.

B. Modifiers for PET Scans

Effective for claims with dates of service on or after April 3, 2009, the following modifiers have been created for use to inform for the initial treatment strategy of biopsy-proven or strongly suspected tumors or subsequent treatment strategy of cancerous tumors:

PI Positron Emission Tomography (PET) or PET/Computed Tomography (CT) to inform the initial treatment strategy of tumors that are biopsy proven or strongly suspected of being cancerous based on other diagnostic testing.

Short descriptor: PET tumor init tx strat

PS Positron Emission Tomography (PET) or PET/Computed Tomography (CT) to inform the subsequent treatment strategy of cancerous tumors when the beneficiary's treatment physician determines that the PET study is needed to inform subsequent anti-tumor strategy.

Short descriptor: PS - PET tumor subsq tx strategy

C. Billing for A/B MACs (A and B)

Effective for claims with dates of service on or after April 3, 2009, contractors shall accept FDG PET claims billed to inform initial treatment strategy with the following CPT codes AND modifier PI: 78608, 78811, 78812, 78813, 78814, 78815, 78816.

Effective for claims with dates of service on or after April 3, 2009, contractors shall accept FDG PET claims with modifier PS for the subsequent treatment strategy for solid tumors using a CPT code above AND a cancer diagnosis code.

Contractors shall also accept FDG PET claims billed to inform initial treatment strategy or subsequent treatment strategy when performed under CED with one of the PET or PET/CT CPT codes above AND modifier PI OR modifier PS AND a cancer diagnosis code AND modifier Q0/Q1. Effective for services performed on or after June 11, 2013, the CED requirement has ended and modifier Q0/Q1, along with condition code 30 (institutional claims only), or ICD-9 code V70.7, (both institutional and practitioner claims) are no longer required.

D. Medicare Summary Notices, Remittance Advice Remark Codes, and Claim Adjustment Reason Codes

Effective for dates of service on or after April 3, 2009, contractors shall return as unprocessable/return to provider claims that do not include the PI modifier with one of the PET/PET/CT CPT codes listed in subsection C. above when billing for the initial treatment strategy for solid tumors in accordance with Pub.100-03, NCD Manual, section 220.6.17.

In addition, contractors shall return as unprocessable/return to provider claims that do not include the PS modifier with one of the CPT codes listed in subsection C. above when billing for the subsequent treatment strategy for solid tumors in accordance with Pub.100-03, NCD Manual, section 220.6.17.

The contractor shall use the following remittance advice messages and associated codes when returning claims under this policy. This CARC/RARC combination is compliant with CAQH CORE Business Scenario Two.

Group Code: CO
CARC: 4
RARC: MA130
MSN: N/A

Effective for claims with dates of service on or after April 3, 2009, through June 10, 2013, contractors shall return as unprocessable/return to provider FDG PET claims billed to inform initial treatment strategy or subsequent treatment strategy when performed under CED without one of the PET/PET/CT CPT codes listed in subsection C. above AND modifier PI OR modifier PS AND a cancer diagnosis code AND modifier Q0/Q1.

The contractor shall use the following remittance advice messages and associated codes when returning claims under this policy. This CARC/RARC combination is compliant with CAQH CORE Business Scenario Two.

Group Code: CO
CARC: 4
RARC: MA130
MSN: N/A

Effective April 3, 2009, contractors shall deny claims with ICD-9/ICD-10 diagnosis code 185/C61 for FDG PET imaging for the initial treatment strategy of patients with adenocarcinoma of the prostate.

For dates of service prior to June 11, 2013, contractors shall also deny claims for FDG PET imaging for subsequent treatment strategy for tumor types other than breast, cervical, colorectal, esophagus, head and neck (non-CNS/thyroid), lymphoma, melanoma, myeloma, non-small cell lung, and ovarian, unless the FDG PET is provided under CED (submitted with the Q0/Q1 modifier) and use the following messages:

The contractor shall use the following remittance advice messages and associated codes when rejecting/denying claims under this policy. This CARC/RARC combination is compliant with CAQH CORE Business Scenario Three.

Group Code: PR (if claim is received with a GA modifier) otherwise CO
CARC: 50
RARC: N/A
MSN: 15.4

Effective for dates of service on or after June 11, 2013, contractors shall use the following messages when denying claims in excess of three for PET FDG scans for subsequent treatment strategy when the KX modifier is not included, identified by CPT codes 78608, 78811, 78812, 78813, 78814, 78815, or 78816, modifier PS, HCPCS A9552, and the same cancer diagnosis code.

The contractor shall use the following remittance advice messages and associated codes when rejecting/denying claims under this policy. This CARC/RARC combination is compliant with CAQH CORE Business Scenario Three.

Group Code: PR (if claim is received with a GA modifier) otherwise CO
CARC: 96
RARC: N435
MSN: 23.17

100-04, 13, 60.17

Billing and Coverage Changes for PET Scans for Cervical Cancer Effective for Services on or After November 10, 2009

(Rev. 3650, Issued: 11-10-16, Effective: 02-10-17, Implementation: 02-10-17)

A. Billing Changes for A/B MACs (A and B)

Effective for claims with dates of service on or after November 10, 2009, contractors shall accept FDG PET oncologic claims billed to inform initial treatment strategy; specifically for staging in beneficiaries who have biopsy-proven cervical cancer when the beneficiary's treating physician determines the FDG PET study is needed to determine the location and/or extent of the tumor as specified in Pub. 100-03, section 220.6.17.

EXCEPTION: CMS continues to non-cover FDG PET for initial diagnosis of cervical cancer related to initial treatment strategy.

NOTE: Effective for claims with dates of service on and after November 10, 2009, the –Q0 modifier is no longer necessary for FDG PET for cervical cancer.

B. Medicare Summary Notices, Remittance Advice Remark Codes, and Claim Adjustment Reason Codes

Additionally, contractors shall return as unprocessable /return to provider for FDG PET for cervical cancer for initial treatment strategy billed without the following: one of the PET/PET/ CT CPT codes listed in 60.16 C above AND modifier PI AND a cervical cancer diagnosis code.

The contractor shall use the following remittance advice messages and associated codes when returning claims under this policy. This CARC/RARC combination is compliant with CAQH CORE Business Scenario Two.

Group Code: CO
CARC: 4
RARC: MA130
MSN: N/A

100-04, 13, 60.18

Billing and Coverage Changes for PET (NaF-18) Scans to Identify Bone Metastasis of Cancer Effective for Claims With Dates of Services on or After February 26, 2010

(Rev. 3650, Issued: 11-10-16, Effective: 02-10-17, Implementation: 02-10-17)

A. Billing Changes for A/B MACs (A and B)

Effective for claims with dates of service on and after February 26, 2010, contractors shall pay for NaF-18 PET oncologic claims to inform of initial treatment strategy (PI) or subsequent treatment strategy (PS) for suspected or biopsy proven bone metastasis ONLY in the context of a clinical study and as specified in Pub. 100-03, section 220.6. All other claims for NaF-18 PET oncology claims remain non-covered.

B. Medicare Summary Notices, Remittance Advice Remark Codes, and Claim Adjustment Reason Codes

Effective for claims with dates of service on or after February 26, 2010, contractors shall return as unprocessable NaF-18 PET oncologic claims billed with modifier TC or globally (for A/B MACs (A) modifier TC or globally does not apply) and HCPCS A9580 to inform the initial treatment strategy or subsequent treatment strategy for bone metastasis that do not include ALL of the following:

- PI or PS modifier AND
- PET or PET/CT CPT code (78811, 78812, 78813, 78814, 78815, 78816) AND
- Cancer diagnosis code AND
- Q0 modifier - Investigational clinical service provided in a clinical research study, are present on the claim.

NOTE: For institutional claims, continue to include ICD-9 diagnosis code V70.7 or ICD-10 diagnosis code Z00.6 and condition code 30 to denote a clinical study.

The contractor shall use the following remittance advice messages and associated codes when returning claims under this policy. This CARC/RARC combination is compliant with CAQH CORE Business Scenario Two.

Group Code: CO
CARC: 4
RARC: MA130
MSN: N/A

Effective for claims with dates of service on or after February 26, 2010, contractors shall accept PET oncologic claims billed with modifier 26 and modifier KX to inform the initial treatment strategy or subsequent treatment strategy for bone metastasis that include the following:

- PI or PS modifier AND
- PET or PET/CT CPT code (78811, 78812, 78813, 78814, 78815, 78816) AND
- Cancer diagnosis code AND
- Q0 modifier - Investigational clinical service provided in a clinical research study, are present on the claim.

NOTE: If modifier KX is present on the professional component service, Contractors shall process the service as PET NaF-18 rather than PET with FDG.

Contractors shall also return as unprocessable NaF-18 PET oncologic professional component claims (i.e., claims billed with modifiers 26 and KX) to inform the initial treatment strategy or subsequent treatment strategy for bone metastasis billed with HCPCS A9580.

The contractor shall use the following remittance advice messages and associated codes when returning claims under this policy. This CARC/RARC combination is compliant with CAQH CORE Business Scenario Two.

Group Code: CO
CARC: 4
RARC: MA130
MSN: N/A

Claim Adjustment Reason Code 97 – The benefit for this service is included in the payment/allowance for another service/procedure that has already been adjudicated.

NOTE: Refer to the 835 Healthcare Policy identification Segment (loop 2110 Service Payment Information REF), if present.

100-04, 13, 70.2

Services Bundled Into Treatment Management Codes

(Rev.4267, Issued: 03-27-19, Effective: 01-01-19, Implementation: 03-25-19)

A/B MACs (B) do not make separate payment for services rendered by the radiation oncologists or in conjunction with radiation therapy.

11920 Tattooing, intradermal introduction of insoluble opaque pigments to correct color defects of skin; 6.0 sq. cm or less
11921 6.11 to 20.0 sq. cm
11922 Each additional 20.0 sq. cm
16000 Initial treatment, first-degree burn, when no more than local treatment is required
16010 Dressings and/or debridement, initial or subsequent; under anesthesia, small
16015 Under anesthesia, medium or large, or with major debridement
16020 Without anesthesia, office or hospital, small
16025 Without anesthesia, medium (e.g., whole face or whole extremity)
16030 Without anesthesia, large (e.g., more than one extremity)
36425 Venipuncture, cut down age 1 or over
53670 Catheterization, urethra; simple
53675 Complicated (may include difficult removal of balloon catheter)
99211 Office or other outpatient visit, established patient; Level I*
99212 Level II*
99213 Level III*
99214 Level IV
99215 Level V
99238 Hospital discharge day management
99281 Emergency department visit, new or established patient; Level I
99282 Level II
99283 Level III
99284 Level IV
99285 Level V
90780 IV Infusion therapy, administered by physician or under direct supervision of physician; up to one hour
90781 Each additional hour, up to 8 hours
90847 Family medical psychotherapy (conjoint psychotherapy) by a physician, with continuing medical diagnostic evaluation, and drug management when indicated
99050 Services requested after office hours in addition to basic service
99052 Services requested between 10:00 PM and 8:00 AM in addition to basic service
99054 Services requested on Sundays and holidays in addition to basic service
99058 Office services provided on an emergency basis
99071 Educational supplies, such as books, tapes, and pamphlets, provided by the physician for the patient's education at cost to physician
99090 Analysis of information data stored in computers (e.g., ECG, blood pressures, hematologic data)
99185 Hypothermia; regional
99371 Telephone call by a physician to patient or for consultation or medical management or for coordinating medical management with other health care professionals; simple or brief (e.g., to report on tests and/or laboratory results, to clarify or alter previous instructions, to integrate new information from other health professionals into the medical treatment plan, or to adjust therapy)
99372 Intermediate (e.g., to provide advice to an established patient on a new problem, to initiate therapy that can be handled by telephone, to discuss test results in detail, to coordinate medical management of a new problem in an established patient, to discuss and evaluate new information and details, or to initiate a new plan of care)
99373 Complex or lengthy (e.g., lengthy counseling session with anxious or distraught patient, detailed or prolonged discussion with family members regarding seriously ill patient, lengthy communication necessary to coordinate complex services or several different health professionals working on different aspects of the total patient care plan)

- Anesthesia (whatever code billed)
- Care of Infected Skin (whatever code billed)
- Checking of Treatment Charts
- Verification of Dosage, As Needed (whatever code billed)
- Continued Patient Evaluation, Examination, Written Progress Notes, As Needed (whatever code billed)
- Final Physical Examination (whatever code billed)
- Medical Prescription Writing (whatever code billed
- Nutritional Counseling (whatever code billed)
- Pain Management (whatever code billed)
- Review & Revision of Treatment Plan (whatever code billed)
- Routine Medical Management of Unrelated Problem (whatever code billed)
- Special Care of Ostomy (whatever code billed)
- Written Reports, Progress Note (whatever code billed)

- Follow-up Examination and Care for 90 Days After Last Treatment (whatever code billed)

*NOTE: May be billed with Radiation Treatment Delivery, superficial and/or ortho voltage, for the purpose of reporting physician services consisting of radiation therapy planning (including, but not limited to clinical treatment planning, isodose planning, physics consultation), radiation treatment device construction, and radiation treatment management when performed on the same date of service as treatment delivery. Billing with modifier 25 may be necessary if National Correct Coding Initiative (NCCI) edits apply.

100-04, 13, 70.4

Clinical Brachytherapy (CPT Codes 77750 - 77799)

(Rev. 1, 10-01-03)

A/B MACs (B) must apply the bundled services policy to procedures in this family of codes other than CPT code 77776. For procedures furnished in settings in which TC payments are made, A/B MACs (B) must pay separately for the expendable source associated with these procedures under CPT code 79900 except in the case of remote after-loading high intensity brachytherapy procedures (CPT codes 77781-77784). In the four codes cited, the expendable source is included in the RVUs for the TC of the procedures.

100-04, 13, 70.5

Radiation Physics Services (CPT Codes 77300 - 77399)

(Rev. 1, 10-01-03)

A/B MACs (B) pay for the PC and TC of CPT codes 77300-77334 and 77399 on the same basis as they pay for radiologic services generally. For professional component billings in all settings, A/B MACs (B) presume that the radiologist participated in the provision of the service, e.g., reviewed/validated the physicist's calculation. CPT codes 77336 and 77370 are technical services only codes that are payable by A/B MACs (B) in settings in which only technical component is are payable.

100-04, 13, 80.1

Physician Presence

(Rev. 1, 10-01-03)

Radiologic supervision and interpretation (S&I) codes are used to describe the personal supervision of the performance of the radiologic portion of a procedure by one or more physicians and the interpretation of the findings. In order to bill for the supervision aspect of the procedure, the physician must be present during its performance. This kind of personal supervision of the performance of the procedure is a service to an individual beneficiary and differs from the type of general supervision of the radiologic procedures performed in a hospital for which FIs pay the costs as physician services to the hospital. The interpretation of the procedure may be performed later by another physician. In situations in which a cardiologist, for example, bills for the supervision (the "S") of the S&I code, and a radiologist bills for the interpretation (the "I") of the code, both physicians should use a "-52" modifier indicating a reduced service, e.g., only one of supervision and/or interpretation. Payment for the fragmented S&I code is no more than if a single physician furnished both aspects of the procedure.

100-04, 13, 80.2

Multiple Procedure Reduction

(Rev. 1, 10-01-03)

A/B MACs (B) make no multiple procedure reductions in the S&I or primary non-radiologic codes in these types of procedures, or in any procedure codes for which the descriptor and RVUs reflect a multiple service reduction. For additional procedure codes that do not reflect such a reduction, A/B MACs (B) apply the multiple procedure reductions.

100-04, 13, 140.1

Payment Methodology and HCPCS Coding

(Rev.4150, Issued: 10-26-2018, Effective: 04-01-19, Implementation: 04-01-19)

A/B MACs (B) pay for BMM procedures based on the Medicare physician fee schedule. Claims from physicians, other practitioners, or suppliers where assignment was not taken are subject to the Medicare limiting charge.

The A/B MACs (A) pay for BMM procedures under the current payment methodologies for radiology services according to the type of provider.

Do not pay BMM procedure claims for dual photon absorptiometry, CPT procedure code 78351.

Deductible and coinsurance do not apply.

Any of the following CPT procedure codes may be used when billing for BMMs through December 31, 2006. All of these codes are bone densitometry measurements except code 76977, which is bone sonometry measurements. CPT procedure codes are applicable to billing A/B MACs (A and B).

76070 76071 76075 76076 76078 76977 78350 G0130

Effective for dates of services on and after January 1, 2007, the following changes apply to BMM:

New 2007 CPT bone mass procedure codes have been assigned for BMM. The following codes will replace current codes, however the CPT descriptors for the services remain the same:

77078 replaces 76070

77079 replaces 76071

77080 replaces 76075

77081 replaces 76076

77083 replaces 76078

Effective for dates of service on and after January 1, 2015, contractors shall pay for bone mass procedure code 77085 (Dual-energy X-ray absorptiometry (DXA), bone density study, 1 or more sites, axial skeleton, (e.g., hips, pelvis, spine), including vertebral fracture assessment.)

Certain BMM tests are covered when used to screen patients for osteoporosis subject to the frequency standards described in chapter 15, section 80.5.5 of the Medicare Benefit Policy Manual.

Contractors will pay claims for screening tests when coded as follows:

Contains CPT procedure code 77078, 77079, 77080, 77081, 77083, 76977 or G0130, and

Contains a valid diagnosis code indicating the reason for the test is postmenopausal female, vertebral fracture, hyperparathyroidism, or steroid therapy. Contractors are to maintain local lists of valid codes for the benefit's screening categories.

Contractors will deny claims for screening tests when coded as follows:

Contains CPT procedure code 77078, 77079, 77081, 77083, 76977 or G0130, but

Does not contain a valid diagnosis code from the local lists of valid diagnosis codes maintained by the contractor for the benefit's screening categories indicating the reason for the test is postmenopausal female, vertebral fracture, hyperparathyroidism, or steroid therapy.

Dual-energy x-ray absorptiometry (axial) tests are covered when used to monitor FDA-approved osteoporosis drug therapy subject to the 2-year frequency standards described in chapter 15, section 80.5.5 of the Medicare Benefit Policy Manual.

Contractors will pay claims for monitoring tests when coded as follows:

Contains CPT procedure code 77080 or 77085, and

Contains 733.00, 733.01, 733.02, 733.03, 733.09, 733.90, or 255.0 as the ICD-9-CM diagnosis code or M81.0, M81.8, M81.6 or M94.9 as the ICD-10-CM diagnosis code.

Contractors will deny claims for monitoring tests when coded as follows:

Contains CPT procedure code 77078, 77079, 77081, 77083, 76977 or G0130, and

Contains 733.00, 733.01, 733.02, 733.03, 733.09, 733.90, or 255.0 as the ICD-9-CM diagnosis code, but

Does not contain a valid ICD-9-CM diagnosis code from the local lists of valid ICD-9-CM diagnosis codes maintained by the contractor for the benefit's screening categories indicating the reason for the test is postmenopausal female, vertebral fracture, hyperparathyroidism, or steroid therapy.

Does not contain a valid ICD-10-CM diagnosis code from the local lists of valid ICD-10-CM diagnosis codes maintained by the contractor for the benefit's screening categories indicating the reason for the test is postmenopausal female, vertebral fracture, hyperparathyroidism, or steroid therapy.

Single photon absorptiometry tests are not covered. Contractors will deny CPT procedure code 78350.

The A/B MACs (A) are billed using the ASC X12 837 institutional claim format or hardcopy Form CMS-1450. The appropriate bill types are: 12X, 13X, 22X, 23X, 34X, 71X (Provider-based and independent), 72X, 77X (Provider-based and freestanding), 83X, and 85X. Effective April 1, 2006, type of bill 14X is for non-patient laboratory specimens and is no longer applicable for bone mass measurements. Information regarding the claim form locators that correspond to the HCPCS/CPT code or Type of Bill are found in chapter 25.

Providers must report HCPCS codes for bone mass measurements under revenue code 320 with number of units and line item dates of service per revenue code line for each bone mass measurement reported.

A/B MACs (B) are billed for bone mass measurement procedures using the ASC X12 837 professional claim format or hardcopy Form CMS-1500.

100-04, 15, 20.4

Ambulance InflationFactor (AIF)

(Rev. 4172, Issued: 11-30-18, Effective: 01-01-19, Implementation: 01-07-19)

Section 1834(l)(3)(B) of the Social Security Act (the Act) provides the basis for an update to the payment limits for ambulance services that is equal to the percentage increase in the consumer price index for all urban consumers (CPI-U) for the 12-month period ending with June of the previous year. Section 3401 of the Affordable Care Act amended Section 1834(l)(3) of the Act to apply a productivity adjustment to this update equal to the 10-year moving average of changes in economy-wide private nonfarm business multi- factor productivity beginning January 1, 2011. The resulting update percentage is referred to as the Ambulance Inflation Factor (AIF). These updated percentages are issued via Recurring Update Notifications.

Part B coinsurance and deductible requirements apply to payments under the ambulance fee schedule. Following is a chart tracking the history of the AIF:

CY	AIF
2003	1.1
2004	2.1
2005	3.3
2006	2.5
2007	4.3
2008	2.7
2009	5.0
2010	0.0
2011	-0.1
2012	2.4
2013	0.8
2014	1.0
2015	1.5
2016	-0.4
2017	0.7
2018	1.1
2019	2.3

100-04, 16, 40.6.1

Automated Multi-Channel Chemistry (AMCC) Tests for ESRD Beneficiaries

(Rev. 3116, Issued: 11-06-14, Effective: 04-01-15, Implementation: 04-06-15)

Instructions for Services Provided on and After January 1, 2011

Section 153b of the MIPPA requires that all ESRD-related laboratory tests must be reported by the ESRD facility whether provided directly or under arrangements with an independent laboratory. When laboratory services are billed by providers other than the ESRD facility and the laboratory test furnished is designated as a laboratory test that is included in the ESRD PPS (ESRD-related), the claim will be rejected or denied. In the event that an ESRD-related laboratory test was furnished to an ESRD beneficiary for reasons other than for the treatment of ESRD, the provider may submit a claim for separate payment using modifier AY. The AY modifier serves as an attestation that the item or service is medically necessary for the dialysis patient but is not being used for the treatment of ESRD. The items and services subject to consolidated billing located on the CMS website includes the list of ESRD-related laboratory tests that are routinely performed for the treatment of ESRD.

For services provided on or after January 1, 2011, the 50/50 rule no longer applies to independent laboratory claims for AMCC tests furnished to ESRD beneficiaries. The 50/50 rule modifiers (CD, CE, and CF) are no longer required for independent laboratories effective for dates of service on and after January 1, 2011. However, for services provided between January 1, 2011 and March 31, 2015, the 50/50 rule modifiers are still required for use by ESRD facilities that are receiving the transitional blended payment amount (the transition ends in CY 2014). For services provided on or after April 1, 2015, the 50/50 rule modifiers are no longer required for use by ESRD facilities.

Effective for dates of service on and after January 1, 2012, contractors shall allow organ disease panel codes (i.e., HCPCS codes 80047, 80048, 80051, 80053, 80061, 80069, and 80076) to be billed by independent laboratories for AMCC panel tests furnished to ESRD eligible beneficiaries if:

- The beneficiary is not receiving dialysis treatment for any reason (e.g., post-transplant beneficiaries), or
- The test is not related to the treatment of ESRD, in which case the supplier would append modifier "AY".

Contractors shall make payment for organ disease panels according to the Clinical Laboratory Fee Schedule and shall apply the normal ESRD PPS editing rules for independent laboratory claims. The aforementioned organ disease panel codes were added to the list of bundled ESRD PPS laboratory tests in January 2012.

Effective for dates of service on and after April 1, 2015, contractors shall allow organ disease panel codes (i.e., HCPCS codes 80047, 80048, 80051, 80053, 80061, 80069, and 80076) to be billed by ESRD facilities for AMCC panel tests furnished to ESRD eligible beneficiaries if:

- These codes best describe the laboratory services provided to the beneficiary, which are paid under the ESRD PPS, or
- The test is not related to the treatment of ESRD, in which case the ESRD facility would append modifier "AY" and the service may be paid separately from the ESRD PPS.

Instructions for Services Provided Prior to January 1, 2011

For claims with dates of service prior to January 1, 2011, Medicare will apply the following rules to Automated Multi-Channel Chemistry (AMCC) tests for ESRD beneficiaries:

- Payment is at the lowest rate for tests performed by the same provider, for the same beneficiary, for the same date of service.
- The facility/laboratory must identify, for a particular date of service, the AMCC tests ordered that are included in the composite rate and those that are not included. See Publication 100-02, Chapter 11, Section 30.2.2 for the chart detailing the composite rate tests for Hemodialysis, Intermittent Peritoneal Dialysis (IPD), Continuous Cycling Peritoneal Dialysis (CCPD), and Hemofiltration as well as a second chart detailing the composite rate tests for Continuous Ambulatory Peritoneal Dialysis (CAPD).
- If 50 percent or more of the covered tests are included under the composite rate payment, then all submitted tests are included within the composite payment. In this case, no separate payment in addition to the composite rate is made for any of the separately billable tests.
- If less than 50 percent of the covered tests are composite rate tests, all AMCC tests submitted for that Date of Service (DOS) for that beneficiary are separately payable.
- A noncomposite rate test is defined as any test separately payable outside of the composite rate or beyond the normal frequency covered under the composite rate that is reasonable and necessary.
- For carrier processed claims, all chemistries ordered for beneficiaries with chronic dialysis for ESRD must be billed individually and must be rejected when billed as a panel.

(See §100.6UH for details regarding pricing modifiers.)

Implementation of this Policy:

ESRD facilities when ordering an ESRD-related AMCC must specify for each test within the AMCC whether the test:

a. Is part of the composite rate and not separately payable;
b. Is a composite rate test but is, on the date of the order, beyond the frequency covered under the composite rate and thus separately payable; or
c. Is not part of the ESRD composite rate and thus separately payable.

Laboratories must:

a. Identify which tests, if any, are not included within the ESRD facility composite rate payment
b. Identify which tests ordered for chronic dialysis for ESRD as follows:
    1) Modifier CD: AMCC Test has been ordered by an ESRD facility or MCP physician that is part of the composite rate and is not separately billable.
    2) Modifier CE: AMCC Test has been ordered by an ESRD facility or MCP physician that is a composite rate test but is beyond the normal frequency covered under the rate and is separately reimbursable based on medical necessity.
    3) Modifier CF: AMCC Test has been ordered by an ESRD facility or MCP physician that is not part of the composite rate and is separately billable.
c. Bill all tests ordered for a chronic dialysis ESRD beneficiary individually and not as a panel.

The shared system must calculate the number of AMCC tests provided for any given date of service. Sum all AMCC tests with a CD modifier and divide the sum of all tests with a CD, CE, and CF modifier for the same beneficiary and provider for any given date of service.

If the result of the calculation for a date of service is 50 percent or greater, do not pay for the tests.

If the result of the calculation for a date of service is less than 50 percent, pay for all of the tests.

For FI processed claims, all tests for a date of service must be billed on the monthly ESRD bill. Providers that submit claims to a FI must send in an adjustment if they identify additional tests that have not been billed.

Carrier standard systems shall adjust the previous claim when the incoming claim for a date of service is compared to a claim on history and the action is adjust payment. Carrier standard systems shall spread the payment amount over each line item on both claims (the claim on history and the incoming claim).

The organ and disease oriented panels (80048, 80051, 80053, and 80076) are subject to the 50 percent rule. However, clinical diagnostic laboratories shall not bill these services as panels, they must be billed individually. Laboratory tests that are not covered under the composite rate and that are furnished to CAPD end stage renal disease (ESRD) patients dialyzing at home are billed in the same way as any other test furnished home patients.

FI Business Requirements for ESRD Reimbursement of AMCC Tests:

Requirement #	Requirements	Responsibility
1.1	The FI shared system must RTP a claim for AMCC tests when a claim for that date of service has already been submitted.	Shared system
1.2	Based upon the presence of the CD, CE and CF payment modifiers, identify the AMCC tests ordered that are included and not included in the composite rate payment.	Shared System
1.3	Based upon the determination of requirement 1.2, if 50 percent or more of the covered tests are included under the composite rate, no separate payment is made.	Shared System
1.4	Based upon the determination of requirement 1.2, if less than 50 percent are covered tests included under the composite rate, all AMCC tests for that date of service are payable.	Shared System
1.5	Effective for claims with dates of service on or after January 1, 2006, include any line items with a modifier 91 used in conjunction with the "CD," "CE," or "CF" modifier in the calculation of the 50/50 rule.	Shared System
1.6	FIs must return any claims for additional tests for any date of service within the billing period when the provider has already submitted a claim. Instruct the provider to adjust the first claim.	FI or Shared System
1.7	After the calculation of the 50/50 rule, services used to determine the payment amount may never exceed 22. Effective for claims with dates of service on or after January 1, 2006, accept all valid line items submitted for the date of service and pay a maximum of the ATP 22 rate.	Shared System

Carrier Business Requirements for ESRD Reimbursement of AMCC Tests:

Requirement #	Requirements	Responsibility
1	The standard systems shall calculate payment at the lowest rate for these automated tests even if reported on separate claims for services performed by the same provider, for the same beneficiary, for the same date of service.	Standard Systems
2	Standard Systems shall identify the AMCC tests ordered that are included and are not included in the composite rate payment based upon the presence of the "CD," "CE" and "CF" modifiers.	Standard Systems
3	Based upon the determination of requirement 2 if 50 percent or more of the covered services are included under the composite rate payment, Standard Systems shall indicate that no separate payment is provided for the services submitted for that date of service.	Standard Systems
4	Based upon the determination of requirement 2 if less than 50 percent are covered services included under the composite rate, Standard Systems shall indicate that all AMCC tests for that date of service are payable under the 50/50 rule.	Standard Systems
5	Effective for claims with dates of service on or after January 1, 2006, include any line items with a modifier 91 used in conjunction with the "CD," "CE," or "CF" modifier in the calculation of the 50/50 rule.	Standard Systems
6	Standard Systems shall adjust the previous claim when the incoming claim is compared to the claim on history and the action is to deny the previous claim. Spread the payment amount over each line item on both claims (the adjusted claim and the incoming claim).	Standard Systems
7	Standard Systems shall spread the adjustment across the incoming claim unless the adjusted amount would exceed the submitted amount of the services on the claim.	Standard System
8	After the calculation of the 50/50 rule, services used to determine the payment amount may never exceed 22. Accept all valid line items for the date of service and pay a maximum of the ATP 22 rate.	Standard Systems

Examples of the Application of the 50/50 Rule

The following examples are to illustrate how claims should be paid. The percentages in the action section represent the number of composite rate tests over the total tests. If this percentage is 50 percent or greater, no payment should be made for the claim.

Example 1:
Provider Name: Jones Hospital
DOS 2/1/02

Claim/Services
82040 Mod CD
82310 Mod CD
82374 Mod CD
82435 Mod CD
82947 Mod CF
84295 Mod CF
82040 Mod CD (Returned as duplicate)
84075 Mod CE
82310 Mod CE
84155 Mod CE

ACTION: 9 services total, 2 non-composite rate tests, 3 composite rate tests beyond the frequency, 4 composite rate tests; 4/9 = 44.4%<50% pay at ATP 09

Example 2:
Provider Name: Bon Secours Renal Facility
DOS 2/15/02

Claim/Services
82040 Mod CE and Mod 91
84450 Mod CE
82310 Mod CE
82247 Mod CF
82465 No modifier present
82565 Mod CE
84550 Mod CF
82040 Mod CD
84075 Mod CE
82435 Mod CE
82550 Mod CF
82947 Mod CF
82977 Mod CF

ACTION: 12 services total, 5 non-composite rate tests, 6 composite rate tests beyond the frequency, 1 composite rate test; 1/12 = 8.3%<50% pay at ATP 12

Example 3:
Provider Name: Sinai Hospital Renal Facility
DOS 4/02/02

Claim/Services
82565 Mod CD
83615 Mod CD
82247 Mod CF
82248 Mod CF
82040 Mod CD
84450 Mod CD
82565 Mod CE
84550 Mod CF
82248 Mod CF (Duplicate

ACTION: 8 services total, 3 non-composite rate tests, 4 composite rate tests, 1 composite rate test beyond the frequency; 4/8 = 50%, therefore no payment is made

Example 4:
Provider Name: Dr. Andrew Ross
DOS 6/01/02

Claim/Services
84460 Mod CF
82247 Mod CF
82248 Mod CF
82040 Mod CD
84075 Mod CD
84450 Mod CD

ACTION: 6 services total, 3 non-composite rate tests and 3 composite rate tests; 3/6 = 50%, therefore no payment

Example 5: (Carrier Processing Example Only)
Payment for first claim, second creates a no payment for either claim
Provider Name: Dr. Andrew Ross
DOS 6/01/06

Claim/Services
84460 Mod CF
82247 Mod CF
82248 Mod CF

ACTION: 3 services total, 3 non-composite rate tests, 0 composite rate tests beyond the frequency, and 0 composite rate tests, 0/3 = 0%, therefore ATP 03

Provider Name: Dr. Andrew Ross
DOS 6/01/06

Claim/Services	82040 Mod CD
	84075 Mod CD
	84450 Mod CD

ACTION: An additional 3 services are billed, 0 non-composite rate tests, 8 composite rate test beyond the frequency, 3 composite rate tests. For both claims there are 6 services total, 3 non-composite rate tests and 3 composite rate tests; 3/6 = 50% U>U 50%, therefore no payment. An overpayment should be recovered for the ATP 03 payment.

100-04, 16, 60.2

Travel Allowance

(Rev. 4199, Issued: 01-11-19, Effective: 01-01-19, Implementation: 02-12-19)

In addition to a specimen collection fee allowed under §60.1, Medicare, under Part B, covers a specimen collection fee and travel allowance for a laboratory technician to draw a specimen from either a nursing home patient or homebound patient under §1833(h)(3) of the Act and payment is made based on the clinical laboratory fee schedule. The travel allowance is intended to cover the estimated travel costs of collecting a specimen and to reflect the technician's salary and travel costs.

The additional allowance can be made only where a specimen collection fee is also payable, i.e., no travel allowance is made where the technician merely performs a messenger service to pick up a specimen drawn by a physician or nursing home personnel. The travel allowance may not be paid to a physician unless the trip to the home, or to the nursing home was solely for the purpose of drawing a specimen. Otherwise travel costs are considered to be associated with the other purposes of the trip.

The travel allowance is not distributed by CMS. Instead, the carrier must calculate the travel allowance for each claim using the following rules for the particular Code. The following HCPCS codes are used for travel allowances:

Per Mile Travel Allowance (P9603)

- The minimum "per mile travel allowance" is $1.03. The per mile travel allowance is to be used in situations where the average trip to patients' homes is longer than 20 miles round trip, and is to be pro-rated in situations where specimens are drawn or picked up from non-Medicare patients in the same trip. - one way, in connection with medically necessary laboratory specimen collection drawn from homebound or nursing home bound patient; prorated miles actually traveled (carrier allowance on per mile basis); or
- The per mile allowance was computed using the Federal mileage rate plus an additional 45 cents a mile to cover the technician's time and travel costs. Contractors have the option of establishing a higher per mile rate in excess of the minimum ($1.03 a mile in CY 2019) if local conditions warrant it. The minimum mileage rate will be reviewed and updated in conjunction with the clinical lab fee schedule as needed. At no time will the laboratory be allowed to bill for more miles than are reasonable or for miles not actually traveled by the laboratory technician.

Example 1: In CY 2019, a laboratory technician travels 60 miles round trip from a lab in a city to a remote rural location, and back to the lab to draw a single Medicare patient's blood. The total reimbursement would be $61.80 (60 miles x $1.03 a mile), plus the specimen collection fee.

Example 2: In CY 2019, a laboratory technician travels 40 miles from the lab to a Medicare patient's home to draw blood, and then travels an additional 10 miles to a non-Medicare patient's home and then travels 30 miles to return to the lab. The total miles traveled would be 80 miles. The claim submitted would be for one half of the miles traveled or $41.20 (40 x $1.03), plus the specimen collection fee.

Flat Rate (P9604)

The CMS will pay a minimum of $10.30 (based on CY 2019) one way flat rate travel allowance. The flat rate travel allowance is to be used in areas where average trips are less than 20 miles round trip. The flat rate travel fee is to be pro-rated for more than one blood drawn at the same address, and for stops at the homes of Medicare and non-Medicare patients. The laboratory does the pro-ration when the claim is submitted based on the number of patients seen on that trip. The specimen collection fee will be paid for each patient encounter.

This rate is based on an assumption that a trip is an average of 15 minutes and up to 10 miles one way. It uses the Federal mileage rate and a laboratory technician's time of $17.66 an hour, including overhead. Contractors have the option of establishing a flat rate in excess of the minimum of $10.00, if local conditions warrant it. The minimum national flat rate will be reviewed and updated in conjunction with the clinical laboratory fee schedule, as necessitated by adjustments in the Federal travel allowance and salaries.

The claimant identifies round trip travel by use of the LR modifier

Example 3: A laboratory technician travels from the laboratory to a single Medicare patient's home and returns to the laboratory without making any other stops. The flat rate would be calculated as follows: 2 x $10.30 for a total trip reimbursement of $20.60, plus the specimen collection fee.

Example 4: A laboratory technician travels from the laboratory to the homes of five patients to draw blood, four of the patients are Medicare patients and one is not. An additional flat rate would be charged to cover the 5 stops and the return trip to the lab (6 x $10.30 = $61.80). Each of the claims submitted would be for $12.36 ($61.80/5 = $12.36). Since one of the patients is non-Medicare, four claims would be submitted for $12.36 each, plus the specimen collection fee for each.

Example 5: A laboratory technician travels from a laboratory to a nursing home and draws blood from 5 patients and returns to the laboratory. Four of the patients are on Medicare and one is not. The $10.30 flat rate is multiplied by two to cover the return trip to the laboratory (2 x $10.30 = $20.60) and then divided by five (1/5 of $20.60 = $4.12). Since one of the patients is non-Medicare, four claims would be submitted for $4.12 each, plus the specimen collection fee.

If a carrier determines that it results in equitable payment, the carrier may extend the former payment allowances for additional travel (such as to a distant rural nursing home) to all circumstances where travel is required. This might be appropriate, for example, if the carrier's former payment allowance was on a per mile basis. Otherwise, it should establish an appropriate allowance and inform the suppliers in its service area. If a carrier decides to establish a new allowance, one method is to consider developing a travel allowance consisting of:

- The current Federal mileage allowance for operating personal automobiles, plus a personnel allowance per mile to cover personnel costs based upon an estimate of average hourly wages and average driving speed.

Carriers must prorate travel allowance amounts claimed by suppliers by the number of patients (including Medicare and non-Medicare patients) from whom specimens were drawn on a given trip.

The carrier may determine that payment in addition to the routine travel allowance determined under this section is appropriate if:

- The patient from whom the specimen must be collected is in a nursing home or is homebound; and
- The clinical laboratory tests are needed on an emergency basis outside the general business hours of the laboratory making the collection.
- Subsequent updated travel allowance amounts will be issued by CMS via Recurring Update Notification (RUN) on an annual basis.

100-04, 16, 70.8

Certificate of Waiver

(Rev. 1652, Issued: 12-19-08, Effective: 01-01-09, Implementation: 01-05-09)

Effective September 1, 1992, all laboratory testing sites (except as provided in 42 CFR 493.3(b)) must have either a CLIA certificate of waiver, certificate for provider-performed microscopy procedures, certificate of registration, certificate of compliance, or certificate of accreditation to legally perform clinical laboratory testing on specimens from individuals in the United States.

The Food and Drug Administration approves CLIA waived tests on a flow basis. The CMS identifies CLIA waived tests by providing an updated list of waived tests to the Medicare contractors on a quarterly basis via a Recurring Update Notification. To be recognized as a waived test, some CLIA waived tests have unique HCPCS procedure codes and some must have a QW modifier included with the HCPCS code.

For a list of specific HCPCS codes subject to CLIA see

http://www.cms.hhs.gov/CLIA/downloads/waivetbl.pdf

100-04, 16, 90.2

Organ or Disease Oriented Panels

(Rev. 4299; Issued: 05-03-19; Effective: 01-01-19; Implementation: 10-07-19)

Prior to January 1, 2018, organ or disease panels must be paid at the lower of the billed charge, the fee amount for the panel, or the sum of the fee amounts for all components. When panels contain one or more automated tests, the A/B MAC (A) or (B) determines the correct price for the panel by comparing the price for the automated profile laboratory tests with the sum of the fee amounts for individual tests. Payment for the total panel may not exceed the sum total of the fee amounts for individual covered tests. All Medicare coverage rules apply.

The Medicare shared systems must calculate the correct payment amount. The CMS furnishes fee prices for each code but the A/B MAC (A) or (B) system must compare individual codes billed with codes and prices for related individual tests. (With each HCPCS update, HCPCS codes are reviewed and the system is updated). Once the codes are identified, A/B MACs (A) and (B) publish panel codes to providers.

The only acceptable Medicare definition for the component tests included in the CPT codes for organ or disease oriented panels is the American Medical Association (AMA) definition of component tests. The CMS will not pay for the panel code unless all of the tests in the definition are performed. If the laboratory has a custom panel that includes other tests, in addition to those in the defined CPT or HCPCS panels, the additional tests, whether on the list of automated tests or not, are billed separately in addition to the CPT or HCPCS panel code.

NOTE: If a laboratory chooses, it can bill each of the component tests of these panels individually, but payment will be based upon the above rules.

Effective for claims with dates of service on or after January 1, 2019, laboratories shall bill the HCPCS panel test code and not unbundle the individual components if all components of the HCPCS panel are performed. Claims will be returned as unprocessable/rejected if the HCPCS panel test code is not billed. Providers and suppliers are required to submit all AMCC laboratory test HCPCS for the same beneficiary, performed on the same date of service on the same claim. This billing policy applies when:

a). Submitting a complete organ disease panel; or

b). Submitting individual component tests of an organ disease panel when all components of the panel were not performed.

TABLE OF CHEMISTRY PANELS

Chemistry	CPT	Hepatic Function Panel 80076	Basic Metabolic Panel (Calcium, ionized) 80047	Basic Metabolic Panel (Calcium, total) 80048	Comprehensive Metabolic Panel 80053	Renal Function Panel 80069	Lipid[1] Panel 80061	Electrolyte Panel 80051
Albumin	82040	X			X	X		
Alkaline phosphatase	84075	X			X			
ALT (SGPT)	84460	X			X			
AST (SGOT)	84450	X			X			
Bilirubin, total	82247	X			X			
Bilirubin, direct	82248	X						
Calcium	82310			X	X	X		
Calcium ionized	82330		X					
Chloride	82435		X	X	X	X		X
Cholesterol	82465						X	
CK, CPK	82550							
CO2 (bicarbonate)	82374		X	X	X	X		X
Creatinine	82565		X	X	X	X		
GGT	82977							
Glucose	82947		X	X	X	X		
LDH	83615							
Phosphorus	84100					X		
Potassium	84132		X	X	X	X		X
Protein	84155	X			X			
Sodium	84295		X	X	X	X		X
Triglycerides	84478						X	
Urea nitrogen (BUN)	84520		X	X	X	X		
Uric Acid	84550							

1 CPT code 83718 is billed with Organ/Disease Panel 80061 but is not included in the AMCC bundling.

100-04, 18, 1.2

Table of Preventive and Screening Services

(Rev. 4150, Issued: 10-26-2018, Effective: 04-01-19, Implementation: 04-01-19)

Service	CPT/ HCPCS	Long Descriptor	USPSTF Rating	Coins./ Deductible
Initial Preventive Physical Examination, IPPE	G0402	Initial preventive physical examination; face to face visits, services limited to new beneficiary during the first 12 months of Medicare enrollment	*Not Rated	WAIVED
	G0403	Electrocardiogram, routine ECG with 12 leads; performed as a screening for the initial preventive physical examination with interpretation and report		Not Waived
	G0404	Electrocardiogram, routine ECG with 12 leads; tracing only, without interpretation and report, performed as a screening for the initial preventive physical examination		Not Waived
	G0405	Electrocardiogram, routine ECG with 12 leads; interpretation and report only, performed as a screening for the initial preventive physical examination		Not Waived
Ultrasound Screening for Abdominal Aortic Aneurysm (AAA) furnished prior to January 1, 2017	G0389	Ultrasound, B-scan and/or real time with image documentation; for abdominal aortic aneurysm (AAA) ultrasound screening	B	WAIVED
Ultrasound Screening for Abdominal Aortic Aneurysm (AAA) services furnished on or after January 1, 2017	76706	Ultrasound, abdominal aorta, real time with image documentation, screening study for abdominal aortic aneurysm (AAA)		WAIVED
Cardio-vascular Disease Screening	80061	Lipid panel	A	WAIVED
	82465	Cholesterol, serum or whole blood, total		WAIVED
	83718	Lipoprotein, direct measurement; high density cholesterol (hdl cholesterol)		WAIVED
	84478	Triglycerides		WAIVED
Diabetes Screening Tests	82947	Glucose; quantitative, blood (except reagent strip)	B	WAIVED
	82950	Glucose; post glucose dose (includes glucose)		WAIVED
	82951	Glucose; tolerance test (gtt), three specimens (includes glucose)	*Not Rated	WAIVED
Diabetes Self-Management Training Services (DSMT)	G0108	Diabetes outpatient self-management training services, individual, per 30 minutes	*Not Rated	Not Waived
	G0109	Diabetes outpatient self-management training services, group session (2 or more), per 30 minutes		Not Waived
Medical Nutrition Therapy (MNT) Services	97802	Medical nutrition therapy; initial assessment and intervention, individual, face-to-face with the patient, each 15 minutes	B	WAIVED
	97803	Medical nutrition therapy; re-assessment and intervention, individual, face-to-face with the patient, each 15 minutes		WAIVED
	97804	Medical nutrition therapy; group (2 or more individual(s)), each 30 minutes		WAIVED
	G0270	Medical nutrition therapy; reassessment and subsequent intervention(s) following second referral in same year for change in diagnosis, medical condition or treatment regimen (including additional hours needed for renal disease), individual, face to face with the patient, each 15 minutes	B	WAIVED
	G0271	Medical nutrition therapy, reassessment and subsequent intervention(s) following second referral in same year for change in diagnosis, medical condition, or treatment regimen (including additional hours needed for renal disease), group (2 or more individuals), each 30 minutes		WAIVED

Service	CPT/ HCPCS	Long Descriptor	USPSTF Rating	Coins./ Deductible
Screening Pap Test	G0123	Screening cytopathology, cervical or vaginal (any reporting system), collected in preservative fluid, automated thin layer preparation, screening by cytotechnologist under physician supervision	A	WAIVED
	G0124	Screening cytopathology, cervical or vaginal (any reporting system), collected in preservative fluid, automated thin layer preparation, requiring interpretation by physician		WAIVED
	G0141	Screening cytopathology smears, cervical or vaginal, performed by automated system, with manual rescreening, requiring interpretation by physician	A	WAIVED
	G0143	Screening cytopathology, cervical or vaginal (any reporting system), collected in preservative fluid, automated thin layer preparation, with manual screening and rescreening by cytotechnologist under physician supervision	A	WAIVED
	G0144	Screening cytopathology, cervical or vaginal (any reporting system), collected in preservative fluid, automated thin layer preparation, with screening by automated system, under physician supervision	A	WAIVED
	G0145	Screening cytopathology, cervical or vaginal (any reporting system), collected in preservative fluid, automated thin layer preparation, with screening by automated system and manual rescreening under physician supervision	A	WAIVED
	G0147	Screening cytopathology smears, cervical or vaginal, performed by automated system under physician supervision	A	WAIVED
	G0148	Screening cytopathology smears, cervical or vaginal, performed by automated system with manual rescreening	A	WAIVED
	P3000	Screening papanicolaou smear, cervical or vaginal, up to three smears, by technician under physician supervision		WAIVED
	P3001	Screening papanicolaou smear, cervical or vaginal, up to three smears, requiring interpretation by physician		WAIVED
	Q0091	Screening papanicolaou smear; obtaining, preparing and conveyance of cervical or vaginal smear to laboratory		WAIVED
Screening Pelvic Exam	G0101	Cervical or vaginal cancer screening; pelvic and clinical breast examination	A	WAIVED
Screening Mammography	77052	Computer-aided detection (computer algorithm analysis of digital image data for lesion detection) with further physician review for interpretation, with or without digitization of film radiographic images; screening mammography (list separately in addition to code for primary procedure)	B	WAIVED
	77057	Screening mammography, bilateral (2-view film study of each breast)	B	WAIVED
	77063	Screening digital breast tomosynthesis, bilateral		WAIVED
Screening Mammography (continued)	77067	Screening mammography, bilateral (2-view study of each breast), including computer-aided detection (CAD) when performed	B	WAIVED
Bone Mass Measurement	G0130	Single energy x-ray absorptiometry (sexa) bone density study, one or more sites; appendicular skeleton (peripheral) (e.g., radius, wrist, heel)	B	WAIVED
	77078	Computed tomography, bone mineral density study, 1 or more sites; axial skeleton (e.g., hips, pelvis, spine)		WAIVED
	77079	Computed tomography, bone mineral density study, 1 or more sites; appendicular skeleton (peripheral) (e.g., radius, wrist, heel)		WAIVED
	77080	Dual-energy x-ray absorptiometry (dxa), bone density study, 1 or more sites; axial skeleton (e.g., hips, pelvis, spine)		WAIVED
	77081	Dual-energy x-ray absorptiometry (dxa), bone density study, 1 or more sites; appendicular skeleton (peripheral) (e.g., radius, wrist, heel)		WAIVED
	77083	Radiographic absorptiometry (e.g., photo densitometry, radiogrammetry), 1 or more sites		WAIVED
	77085	Dual-energy X-ray absorptiometry (DXA), bone density study, 1 or more sites, axial skeleton, (e.g., hips, pelvis, spine), including vertebral fracture assessment.		WAIVED
	76977	Ultrasound bone density measurement and interpretation, peripheral site(s), any method		WAIVED

NOTE: Anesthesia services furnished in conjunction with and in support of a screening colonoscopy are reported with CPT code 00812 and coinsurance and deductible are waived. When a screening colonoscopy becomes a diagnostic colonoscopy, anesthesia services are reported with CPT code 00811 and with the PT modifier; only the deductible is waived.

Coinsurance and deductible are waived for moderate sedation services (reported with G0500 or 99153) when furnished in conjunction with and in support of a screening colonoscopy service and when reported with modifier 33. When a screening colonoscopy becomes a diagnostic colonoscopy, moderate sedation services (G0500 or 99153) are reported with only the PT modifier; only the deductible is waived.

Service	CPT/ HCPCS	Long Descriptor	USPSTF Rating	Coins./ Deductible
Colorectal Cancer Screening	G0104	Colorectal cancer screening; flexible sigmoidoscopy	A	WAIVED
	G0105	Colorectal cancer screening; colonoscopy on individual at high risk		WAIVED
	G0106	Colorectal cancer screenng; alternative to G0104, screening sigmoidoscopy, barium enema	*Not Rated	Coins. Applies & Ded. is waived
	G0120	Colorectal cancer screening; alternative to G0105, screening colonoscopy, barium enema.i		Coins. Applies & Ded. is waived
	G0121	Colorectal cancer screening; colonoscopy on individual not meeting criteria for high risk	A	WAIVED
	82270	Blood, occult, by peroxidase activity (e.g., guaiac), qualitative; feces, consecutive		WAIVED
	G0328	Colorectal cancer screening; fecal occult blood test, immunoassay, 1-3 simultaneous		WAIVED
Prostate Cancer Screening	G0102	Prostate cancer screening; digital rectal examination	D	Not Waived
	G0103	Prostate cancer screening; prostate specific antigen test (PSA)		WAIVED

Service	CPT/ HCPCS	Long Descriptor	USPSTF Rating	Coins./ Deductible
Glaucoma Screening	G0117	Glaucoma screening for high risk patients furnished by an optometrist or ophthalmologist	I	Not Waived
	G0118	Glaucoma screening for high risk patient furnished under the direct supervision of an optometrist or ophthalmologist		Not Waived
Influenza Virus Vaccine	90630	Influenza virus vaccine, quadrivalent (IIV4), split virus, preservative free, for intradermal use	B	WAIVED
	90653	Influenza virus vaccine, inactivated, subunit, adjuvanted, for intramuscular use		WAIVED
	90654	Influenza virus vaccine, split virus, preservative free, for intradermal use, for adults ages 18-64		WAIVED
	90655	Influenza virus vaccine, split virus, preservative free, when administered to children 6-35 months of age, for intramuscular use		WAIVED
	90656	Influenza virus vaccine, split virus, preservative free, when administered to individuals 3 years and older, for intramuscular use		WAIVED
	90657	Influenza virus vaccine, split virus, when administered to children 6- 35 months of age, for intramuscular use		WAIVED
	90658	Influenza virus vaccine, trivalent (IIV3), split virus, 0.5 mL dosage, for intramuscular use		WAIVED
	90660	Influenza virus vaccine, live, for intranasal use		WAIVED
	90661	Influenza virus vaccine, derived from cell cultures, subunit, preservative and antibiotic free, for intramuscular use		WAIVED
	90662	Influenza virus vaccine, split virus, preservative free, enhanced immunogenicity via increased antigen content, for intramuscular use		WAIVED
	90672	Influenza virus vaccine, live, quadrivalent, for intranasal use		WAIVED
	90673	Influenza virus vaccine, trivalent, derived from recombinant DNA (RIV3), hemagglutinin (HA) protein only, preservative and antibiotic free, for intramuscular use		WAIVED
	90674	Influenza virus vaccine, quadrivalent (ccIIV4), derived from cell cultures, subunit, preservative and antibiotic free, 0.5 mL dosage, for intramuscular use		WAIVED
	90682	Influenza virus vaccine, quadrivalent (RIV4), derived from recombinant DNA, hemagglutinin (HA) protein only, preservative and antibiotic free, for intramuscular use		WAIVED
	90685	Influenza virus vaccine, quadrivalent, split virus, preservative free, when administered to children 6- 35 months of age, for intramuscular use		WAIVED

Service	CPT/ HCPCS	Long Descriptor	USPSTF Rating	Coins./ Deductible
Influenza Virus Vaccine (continued)	90686	Influenza virus vaccine, quadrivalent, split virus, preservative free, when administered to individuals 3 years of age and older, for intramuscular use	B	WAIVED
	90687	Influenza virus vaccine, quadrivalent, split virus, when administered to children 6-35 months of age, for intramuscular use		WAIVED
	90688	Influenza virus vaccine, quadrivalent, split virus, when administered to individuals 3 years of age and older, for intramuscular use		WAIVED
	90689	Influenza virus vaccine, quadrivalent (IIV4), inactivated, adjuvanted, preservative free, 0.25 mL dosage, for INtramuscular use		WAIVED
	90756	Influenza virus vaccine, quadrivalent (ccIIV4), derived from cell cultures, subunit, antibiotic free, 0.5mL dosage, for intramuscular use		WAIVED
	G0008	Administration of influenza virus vaccine		WAIVED
Pneumo-coccal Vaccine	90669	Pneumococcal conjugate vaccine, polyvalent, when administered to children younger than 5 years, for intramuscular use		WAIVED
	90670	Pneumococcal conjugate vaccine, 13 valent, for intramuscular use		WAIVED
	90732	Pneumococcal polysaccharide vaccine, 23-valent, adult or immunosuppressed patient dosage, when administered to individuals 2 years or older, for subcutaneous or intramuscular use		WAIVED
	G0009	Administration of pneumococcal vaccine		WAIVED
Hepatitis B Vaccine	90739	Hepatitis B vaccine, adult dosage (2 dose schedule), for intramuscular use	A	WAIVED
	90740	Hepatitis B vaccine, dialysis or immunosuppressed patient dosage (3 dose schedule), for intramuscular use		WAIVED
	90743	Hepatitis B vaccine, adolescent (2 dose schedule), for intramuscular use		WAIVED
	90744	Hepatitis B vaccine, pediatric/adolescent dosage (3 dose schedule), for intramuscular use		WAIVED
	90746	Hepatitis B vaccine, adult dosage, for intramuscular use		WAIVED
	90747	Hepatitis B vaccine, dialysis or immunosuppressed patient dosage (4 dose schedule), for intramuscular use		WAIVED
	G0010	Administration of Hepatitis B vaccine	A	WAIVED
Hepatitis C Virus Screening	G0472	Screening for Hepatitis C antibody	B	WAIVED

Service	CPT/ HCPCS	Long Descriptor	USPSTF Rating	Coins./ Deductible
HIV Screening	G0432	Infectious agent antigen detection by enzyme immunoassay (EIA) technique, qualitative or semi-qualitative, multiple- step method, HIV-1 or HIV-2, screening	A	WAIVED
	G0433	Infectious agent antigen detection by enzyme- linked immunosorbent assay (ELISA) technique, antibody, HIV-1 or HIV-2, screening		WAIVED
	G0435	Infectious agent antigen detection by rapid antibody test of oral mucosa transudate, HIV-1 or HIV- 2 , screening		WAIVED
Smoking Cessation for services furnished prior to October 1, 2016	G0436	Smoking and tobacco cessation counseling visit for the asymptomatic patient; intermediate, greater than 3 minutes, up to 10 minutes	A	WAIVED
	G0437	Smoking and tobacco cessation counseling visit for the asymptomatic patient intensive, greater than 10 minutes		WAIVED
Smoking Cessation for services furnished on or after October 1, 2016	99406	Smoking and tobacco cessation counseling visit for the asymptomatic patient; intermediate, greater than 3 minutes, up to 10 minutes	A	WAIVED
	99407	Smoking and tobacco cessation counseling visit for the asymptomatic patient intensive, greater than 10 minutes		
Annual Wellness Visit	G0438	Annual wellness visit, including PPPS, first visit	*Not Rated	WAIVED
	G0439	Annual wellness visit, including PPPS, subsequent visit		WAIVED
Intensive Behavioral Therapy for Obesity	G0447	Face-to-Face Behavioral Counseling for Obesity, 15 minutes	B	WAIVED
	G0473	Face-to-face behavioral counseling for obesity, group (2-10), 30 minute(s)		
Lung Cancer Screening	G0296	Counseling visit to discuss need for lung cancer screening (LDCT) using low dose CT scan (service is for eligibility determination and shared decision making)	B	WAIVED
	G0297	Low dose CT scan (LDCT) for lung cancer screening		

100-04, 18, 10.2.1

Healthcare Common Procedure Coding System (HCPCS) and Diagnosis Codes

(Rev. 4100, Issued: 08-03-18; Effective: 01-01-19; Implementation: 01-07-19)

Vaccines and their administration are reported using separate codes. The following codes are for reporting the vaccines only.

HCPCS	Definition
90630	Influenza virus vaccine, quadrivalent (IIV4), split virus, preservative free, for intradermal use
90653	Influenza virus vaccine, inactivated, subunit, adjuvanted, for intramuscular use
90654	Influenza virus vaccine, split virus, preservative-free, for intradermal use, for adults ages 18 – 64;
90655	Influenza virus vaccine, split virus, preservative free, for children 6- 35 months of age, for intramuscular use;
90656	Influenza virus vaccine, split virus, preservative free, for use in individuals 3 years and above, for intramuscular use;
90657	Influenza virus vaccine, split virus, for children 6-35 months of age, for intramuscular use;
90658	Influenza virus vaccine, trivalent (IIV3), split virus, 0.5 mL dosage, for intramuscular use
90660	Influenza virus vaccine, live, for intranasal use;
90661	Influenza virus vaccine, derived from cell cultures, subunit, preservative and antibiotic free, for intramuscular use
90662	Influenza virus vaccine, split virus, preservative free, enhanced immunogenicity via increased antigen content, for intramuscular use
90669	Pneumococcal conjugate vaccine, polyvalent, for children under 5 years, for intramuscular use
90670	Pneumococcal conjugate vaccine, 13 valent, for intramuscular use
90672	Influenza virus vaccine, live, quadrivalent, for intranasal use
90673	Influenza virus vaccine, trivalent, derived from recombinant DNA (RIV3), hemagglutinin (HA) protein only, preservative and antibiotic free, for intramuscular use
90674	Influenza virus vaccine, quadrivalent (ccIIV4), derived from cell cultures, subunit, preservative and antibiotic free, 0.5 mL dosage, for intramuscular use
90682	Influenza virus vaccine, quadrivalent (RIV4), derived from recombinant DNA, hemagglutinin (HA) protein only, preservative and antibiotic free, for intramuscular use
90685	Influenza virus vaccine, quadrivalent, split virus, preservative free, when administered to children 6-35 months of age, for intramuscular use
90686	Influenza virus vaccine, quadrivalent, split virus, preservative free, when administered to individuals 3 years of age and older, for intramuscular use
90687	Influenza virus vaccine, quadrivalent, split virus, when administered to children 6-35 months of age, for intramuscular use
90688	Influenza virus vaccine, quadrivalent, split virus, when administered to individuals 3 years of age and older, for intramuscular use
90689	Influenza virus vaccine, quadrivalent (IIV4), inactivated, adjuvanted, preservative free, 0.25mL dosage, for intramuscular use
90732	Pneumococcal polysaccharide vaccine, 23-valent, adult or immunosuppressed patient dosage, for use in individuals 2 years or older, for subcutaneous or intramuscular use;
90739	Hepatitis B vaccine, adult dosage (2 dose schedule), for intramuscular use
90740	Hepatitis B vaccine, dialysis or immunosuppressed patient dosage (3 dose schedule), for intramuscular use;
90743	Hepatitis B vaccine, adolescent (2 dose schedule), for intramuscular use;
90744	Hepatitis B vaccine, pediatric/adolescent dosage (3 dose schedule), for intramuscular use;
90746	Hepatitis B vaccine, adult dosage, for intramuscular use; and
90747	Hepatitis B vaccine, dialysis or immunosuppressed patient dosage (4 dose schedule), for intramuscular use.
90756	Influenza virus vaccine, quadrivalent (ccIIV4), derived from cell cultures, subunit, antibiotic free, 0.5mL dosage, for intramuscular use

The following codes are for reporting administration of the vaccines only. The administration of the vaccines is billed using:

HCPCS	Definition
G0008	Administration of influenza virus vaccine;
G0009	Administration of pneumococcal vaccine; and
*G0010	Administration of hepatitis B vaccine.
*90471	Immunization administration. (For OPPS hospitals billing for the hepatitis B vaccine administration)
*90472	Each additional vaccine. (For OPPS hospitals billing for the hepatitis B vaccine administration)

* **NOTE:** For claims with dates of service prior to January 1, 2006, OPPS and non-OPPS hospitals report G0010 for hepatitis B vaccine administration. For claims with dates of service January 1, 2006 until December 31, 2010, OPPS hospitals report 90471 or 90472 for hepatitis B vaccine administration as appropriate in place of G0010. Beginning January 1, 2011, providers should report G0010 for billing under the OPPS rather than 90471 or 90472 to ensure correct waiver of coinsurance and deductible for the administration of hepatitis B vaccine.

One of the following diagnosis codes must be reported as appropriate. If the sole purpose for the visit is to receive a vaccine or if a vaccine is the only service billed on a claim, the applicable following diagnosis code may be used.

ICD-9-CM Diagnosis Code	Description
V03.82	Pneumococcus
V04.81**	Influenza
V06.6***	Pneumococcus and Influenza
V05.3	Hepatitis B

**Effective for influenza virus claims with dates of service October 1, 2003 and later.

***Effective October 1, 2006, providers may report ICD-9-CM diagnosis code V06.6 on claims for pneumococcus and/or influenza virus vaccines when the purpose of the visit was to receive both vaccines.

NOTE: ICD-10-CM diagnosis code Z23 may be used for an encounter for immunizations effective October 1, 2015, when ICD-10 was implemented.

If a diagnosis code for pneumococcus, hepatitis B, or influenza virus vaccination is not reported on a claim, contractors may not enter the diagnosis on the claim. Contractors must follow current resolution processes for claims with missing diagnosis codes.

If the diagnosis code and the narrative description are correct, but the HCPCS code is incorrect, the A/B MAC (A or B) may correct the HCPCS code and pay the claim. For example, if the reported diagnosis code is V04.81 and the narrative description (if annotated on the claim) says "flu shot" but the HCPCS code is incorrect, contractors may change the HCPCS code and pay for the flu vaccine. Effective October 1, 2006, A/B MACs (B) should follow the instructions in Pub. 100-04, Chapter 1, Section 80.3.2.1.1 (A/B MAC (B) Data Element Requirements) for claims submitted without a HCPCScode.

Claims for hepatitis B vaccinations must report the I.D. Number of the referring physician. In addition, if a doctor of medicine or osteopathy does not order the influenza virus vaccine, the A/B MACs (A) claims require:

- UPIN code SLF000 to be reported on claims submitted prior to May 23, 2008, when Medicare began accepting NPIs, only
- The provider's own NPI to be reported in the NPI field for the attending physician on claims submitted on or after May 23, 2008, when NPI requirements were implemented.

100-04, 18, 10.2.2.1

Payment for Pneumococcal Pneumonia Virus, Influenza Virus, and Hepatitis B Virus Vaccines and Their Administration on Institutional Claims

(Rev. 3754, Issued: 04-21-17; Effective: 07-01-17; Implementation: 07-03-17)

Payment for Vaccines

Payment for these vaccines is as follows:

Facility	Type of Bill	Payment
Hospitals, other than Indian Health Service (IHS) Hospitals and Critical Access Hospitals (CAHs)	012x, 013x	Reasonable cost
IHS Hospitals	012x, 013x, 083x	95% of AWP
IHS CAHs	085x	95% of AWP
CAHs Method I and Method II	085x	Reasonable cost
Skilled Nursing Facilities	022x, 023x	Reasonable cost
Home Health Agencies	034x	Reasonable cost
Hospice	081x, 082x	95% of the AWP
Comprehensive Outpatient Rehabilitation Facilities	075x	95% of the AWP
Independent Renal Dialysis Facilities	072x	95% of the AWP
Hospital-based Renal Dialysis Facilities	072x	Reasonable cost

Payment for Vaccine Administration

Payment for the administration of Influenza Virus and PPV vaccines is as follows:

Facility	Type of Bill	Payment
Hospitals, other than IHS Hospitals and CAHs	012x, 013x	Outpatient Prospective Payment System (OPPS) for hospitals subject to OPPS Reasonable cost for hospitals not subject to OPPS
IHS Hospitals	012x, 013x, 083x	MPFS as indicated in guidelines below.
IHS CAHs	085x	MPFS as indicated in guidelines below.
CAHs Method I and II	085x	Reasonable cost
Skilled Nursing Facilities	022x, 023x	MPFS
Home Health Agencies	034x	OPPS
Hospices	081x, 082x	MPFS
Comprehensive Outpatient Rehabilitation Facilities	075x	MPFS
Independent RDFs	072x	MPFS
Hospital-based RDFs	072x	Reasonable cost

Payment for the administration of Hepatitis B vaccine is as follows:

Facility	Type of Bill	Payment
Hospitals other than IHS hospitals and CAHs	012x, 013x	Outpatient Prospective Payment System (OPPS) for hospitals subject to OPPS Reasonable cost for hospitals not subject to OPPS
IHS Hospitals	012x, 013x, 083x	MPFS
CAHs	085x	Reasonable cost
Method I and II		
IHS CAHs	085x	MPFS
Skilled Nursing Facilities	022x, 023x	MPFS
Home Health Agencies	034x	OPPS
Hospices	081x, 082x	MPFS
Comprehensive Outpatient Rehabilitation Facilities	075x	MPFS
Independent RDFs	072x	MPFS
Hospital-based RDFs	072x	Reasonable cost

100-04, 18, 10.4.1

CWF Edits on A/B MAC (A) Claims

(Rev. 4100, Issued: 08-03-18; Effective: 01-01-19; Implementation: 01-07-19)

In order to prevent duplicate payment by the same A/B MAC (A), CWF edits by line item on the A/B MAC (A) number, the beneficiary Health Insurance Claim (HIC) number, and the date of service, the influenza virus procedure codes 90630, 90653, 90654, 90655, 90656, 90657, 90658, 90660, 90661, 90662, 90672, 90673, 90674, 90682, 90685, 90686, 90687, 90688, 90689, or 90756 and the pneumococcal procedure codes 90669, 90670, or 90732, and the administration codes G0008 or G0009.

If CWF receives a claim with either HCPCS codes 90630, 90653, 90654, 90655, 90656, 90657, 90658, 90658, 90660, 90661, 90662, 90672, 90673, 90674, 90682, 90685, 90686, 90687, 90688, 90689, or 90756 and it already has on record a claim with the same HIC number, same A/B MAC (A) number, same date of service, and any one of those HCPCS codes, the second claim submitted to CWF rejects.

If CWF receives a claim with HCPCS codes 90669, 90670, or 90732 and it already has on record a claim with the same HIC number, same A/B MAC (A) number, same date of service, and the same HCPCS code, the second claim submitted to CWF rejects when all four items match.

If CWF receives a claim with HCPCS administration codes G0008 or G0009 and it already has on record a claim with the same HIC number, same A/B MAC (A) number, same date of service, and same procedure code, CWF rejects the second claim submitted when all four items match.

CWF returns to the A/B MAC (A) a reject code "7262" for this edit. A/B MACs (A) must deny the second claim and use the same messages they currently use for the denial of duplicate claims.

100-04, 18, 10.4.2

CWF Edits on A/B MAC (B) Claims

(Rev. 4100, Issued: 08-03-18; Effective: 01-01-19; Implementation: 01-07-19)

In order to prevent duplicate payment by the same A/B MAC (B), CWF will edit by line item on the A/B MAC (B) number, the HIC number, the date of service, the influenza virus procedure codes 90630, 90653, 90654, 90655, 90656, 90657, 90658, 90660, 90661, 90662, 90672, 90673, 90674, 90682, 90685, 90686, 90687, 90688, 90689, or 90756; the pneumococcal procedure codes 90669, 90670, or 90732; and the administration code G0008 or G0009.

If CWF receives a claim with either HCPCS codes 90630, 90653, 90654, 90655, 90656, 90657, 90658, 90660, 90661, 90662, 90672, 90673, 90674, 90682, 90685, 90686, 90687, 90688, 90689, or 90756 and it already has on record a claim with the same HIC number, same A/B MAC (B) number, same date of service, and any one of those HCPCS codes, the second claim submitted to CWF will reject.

If CWF receives a claim with HCPCS codes 90669, 90670, or 90732 and it already has on record a claim with the same HIC number, same A/B MAC (B) number, same date of service, and the same HCPCS code, the second claim submitted to CWF will reject when all four items match.

If CWF receives a claim with HCPCS administration codes G0008 or G0009 and it already has on record a claim with the same HIC number, same A/B MAC (B) number, same date of service, and same procedure code, CWF will reject the second claim submitted.

CWF will return to the A/B MAC (B) a specific reject code for this edit. A/B MACs (B) must deny the second claim and use the same messages they currently use for the denial of duplicate claims.

In order to prevent duplicate payment by the centralized billing contractor and local A/B MAC (B), CWF will edit by line item for A/B MAC (B) number, same HIC number, same date of service, the influenza virus procedure codes 90630, 90653, 90654, 90655, 90656, 90657, 90658, 90660, 90661, 90662, 90672, 90673, 90674, 90682,

90685, 90686, 90687, 90688, 90689, or 90756; the pneumococcal procedure codes 90669, 90670, or 90732; and the administration code G0008 or G0009.

If CWF receives a claim with either HCPCS codes 90630, 90653, 90654, 90655, 90656, 90657, 90658, 90660, 90661, 90662, 90672, 90673, 90674, 90682, 90685, 90686, 90687, 90688, 90689, or 90756 and it already has on record a claim with a different A/B MAC (B) number, but same HIC number, same date of service, and any one of those same HCPCS codes, the second claim submitted to CWF will reject.

If CWF receives a claim with HCPCS codes 90669, 90670, or 90732 and it already has on record a claim with the same HIC number, different A/B MAC (B) number, same date of service, and the same HCPCS code, the second claim submitted to CWF will reject.

If CWF receives a claim with HCPCS administration codes G0008 or G0009 and it already has on record a claim with a different A/B MAC (B) number, but the same HIC number, same date of service, and same procedure code, CWF will reject the second claim submitted.

CWF will return a specific reject code for this edit. A/B MACs (B) must deny the second claim. For the second edit, the reject code should automatically trigger the following Medicare Summary Notice (MSN) and Remittance Advice (RA) messages.

MSN: 7.2 – "This is a duplicate of a claim processed by another contractor. You should receive a Medicare Summary Notice from them."

Claim Adjustment Reason Code 18 – Exact duplicate claim/service

100-04, 18, 10.4.3

CWF Crossover Edits A/B MAC (B) Claims

(Rev. 4100, Issued: 08-03-18; Effective: 01-01-19; Implementation: 01-07-19)

When CWF receives a claim from the A/B MAC (B), it will review Part B outpatient claims history to verify that a duplicate claim has not already been posted.

CWF will edit on the beneficiary HIC number; the date of service; the influenza virus procedure codes 90630, 90653, 90654, 90655, 90656, 90657, 90658, 90660, 90661, 90662, 90672, 90673, 90674, 90682, 90685, 90686, 90687, 90688, 90689, or 90756; the pneumococcal procedure codes 90669, 90670, or 90732; and the administration code G0008 or G0009.

CWF will return a specific reject code for this edit. A/B MACs (B) must deny the second claim and use the same messages they currently use for the denial of duplicate claims.

100-04, 18, 20.2

HCPCS and Diagnosis Codes for Mammography Services

(Rev. 3844, Issued: 08-18-17, Effective: 01-01-18, Implementation: 01-02-18)

The following HCPCS codes are used to bill for mammography services.

HCPCS Code	Definition
77065* (G0206*)	Diagnostic mammography, including computer-aided detection (CAD) when performed; unilateral
77066* (G0204*)	Diagnostic mammography, including computer-aided detection (CAD) when performed; bilateral
77067* (G0202*)	Screening mammography, bilateral (2-view study of each breast), including computer-aided detection (CAD) when performed
77063**	Screening Breast Tomosynthesis; bilateral (list separately in addition to code for primary procedure).
G0279**	Diagnostic digital breast tomosynthesis, unilateral or bilateral (List separately in addition to code for primary procedure)

* NOTE: For claims with dates of service January 1, 2017 through December 31, 2017 providers report HCPCS codes G0202, G0204, and G0206. For claims with dates of service on or after January 1, 2018 providers report CPT codes 77067, 77066, and 77065 respectively.

** NOTE: HCPCS codes 77063 and G0279 are effective for claims with dates of service on or after January 1, 2015.

New Modifier "-GG": Performance and payment of a screening mammography and diagnostic mammography on same patient same day - This is billed with the Diagnostic Mammography code to show the test changed from a screening test to a diagnostic test. A/B MACs (A) and (B) will pay both the screening and diagnostic mammography tests. This modifier is for tracking purposes only. This applies to claims with dates of service on or after January 1, 2002.

A. Diagnosis for Services On or After January 1, 1998

The BBA of 1997 eliminated payment based on high-risk indicators. However, to ensure proper coding, one of the following diagnosis codes should be reported on screening mammography claims as appropriate:

ICD-9-CM

V76.11 - "Special screening for malignant neoplasm, screening mammogram for high- risk patients" or;

V76.12 - "Special screening for malignant neoplasm, other screening mammography."

ICD-10-CM

Z12.31 - Encounter for screening mammogram for malignant neoplasm of breast.

Beginning October 1, 2003, A/B MACs (B) are not permitted to plug the code for a screening mammography when the screening mammography claim has no diagnosis code. Screening mammography claims with no diagnosis code must be returned as unprocessable for assigned claims. For unassigned claims, deny the claim.

In general, providers report diagnosis codes in accordance with the instructions in the appropriate ASC X12 837 claim technical report 3 (institutional or professional) and the paper claim form instructions found in chapters 25 (institutional) and 26 (professional).

In addition, for institutional claims, providers report diagnosis code V76.11 or V76.12 (ICD-9-CM) or Z12.31 (if ICD-10-CM is applicable) in "Principal Diagnosis Code" if the screening mammography is the only service reported on the claim. If the claim contains other services in addition to the screening mammography, these diagnostic codes V76.11 or V76.12 (ICD-9-CM) or Z12.31 (ICD-10-CM) are reported, as appropriate, in "Other Diagnostic Codes." NOTE: Information regarding the form locator number that corresponds to the principal and other diagnosis codes is found in chapter 25.

A/B MACs (B) receive this diagnosis in field 21 and field 24E with the appropriate pointer code of Form CMS-1500 or in Loop 2300 of ASC- X12 837 professional claim format.

Diagnosis codes for a diagnostic mammography will vary according to diagnosis.

100-04, 18, 20.2.2

Claim Adjustment Reason Codes (CARCs), Remittance Advice Remark Codes (RARCs), Group Codes, and Medicare Summary Notice (MSN) Messages

(Rev. 3844, Issued: 08-18-17, Effective: 01-01-18, Implementation: 01-02-18)

When denying claim lines for HCPCS code 77063 that are not submitted with the diagnosis code V76.11 or V76.12, the contractor shall use the following remittance advice messages and associated codes when rejecting/denying claims under this policy. This CARC/RARC combination is compliant with CAQH CORE Business Scenario Three.

CARC: 167 RARC: N386

MSN: 14.9

Group Code PR (Patient Responsibility) assigning financial responsibility to the beneficiary (if a claim is received with a GA modifier indicating a signed ABN is on file).

Group Code CO (Contractual Obligation) assigning financial liability to the provider (if a claim is received with a GZ modifier indicating no signed ABN is on file).

When denying claim lines for HCPCS code G0279 that are not submitted with HCPCS 77066 or 77065.

100-04, 18, 20.4.1

Rural Health Clinics and Federally Qualified Health Centers

(Rev. 4225, Issues: 02-01-19, Effective: 07-01-19, Implementation: 07-01-19)

A. Provider-Based RHC & FQHC - Technical Component

The technical component of a screening or diagnostic mammography is outside the scope of the RHC/FQHC benefit. In a provider-based RHC or FQHC, the technical component is billed by the base provider to the A/B MAC (A) under bill type 12X, 13X, 22X, 23X or 85X as appropriate using the base provider's outpatient provider number (not the RHC/FQHC provider number). The revenue code for a screening mammography is 0403, and the HCPCS code is 77067*, (G0202)*). The revenue code for a diagnostic mammography is 0401, and the HCPCS codes are 77065* (G0206*), 77066* (G0204*). Payment is based on the payment method for the base provider.

** G0236 is a deleted code after December 31, 2003. Use 76082* for claims with dates of service January 1, 2004 through December 31, 2006, and code 77051 for claims with dates of service January 1, 2007 and later.

* For claims with dates of service January 1, 2017 through December 31, 2017, report CPT codes G0206, G0204, and G0202. For claims with dates of service January 1, 2018 and later, report CPT codes 77065, 77066, and 77067respectively.

B. Independent RHCs and Freestanding FQHCs - Technical Component

The technical component of a screening or diagnostic mammography is outside the scope of the RHC/FQHC benefit. The practitioner that renders the technical service bills their A/B MACs (B) using Form CMS-1500. Payment is based on the MPFS national non- facility rate.

C. Provider-Based RHC & FQHC, Independent RHCs and Freestanding FQHCs - Professional Component

The professional component of a screening or diagnostic mammography is within the scope of the RHC/FQHC benefit and is billed under the RHC AIR or the FQHC PPS payment methodology with revenue code 052X. A/B MACs (A) should assure payment is not made for revenue code 0403 (screening mammography) or 0401 (diagnostic mammography). No payment is made on the line item reporting revenue code 0403.

For claims with dates of service on or after April 1, 2005, RHCs and FQHCs bill the A/B MAC (A) under bill type 71X or 77X for the professional component of a diagnostic mammography. No payment is made for the professional component of a diagnostic mammography unless there is a qualifying visit on the same day. The services should be billed with the appropriate revenue code. HCPCS coding is required for the diagnostic mammography.

100-04, 18, 20.6

Instructions When an Interpretation Results in Additional Films

(Rev. 3844, Issued: 08-18-17, Effective: 01-01-18, Implementation: 01-02-18)

A radiologist who interprets a screening mammography is allowed to order and interpret additional films based on the results of the screening mammogram while a beneficiary is still at the facility for the screening exam. When a radiologist's interpretation results in additional films, Medicare will pay for both the screening and diagnostic mammogram.

A/B MACs (B) Claims

For A/B MACs (B) claims, providers submitting a claim for a screening mammography and a diagnostic mammography for the same patient on the same day, attach modifier "- GG" to the diagnostic mammography. A modifier "-GG" is appended to the claim for the diagnostic mammogram for tracking and data collection purposes. Medicare will reimburse both the screening mammography and the diagnostic mammography.

A/B MAC (A) Claims

A/B MACs (A) require the diagnostic claim be prepared reflecting the diagnostic revenue code (0401) along with HCPCS code 77065*(G0206*), 77066*(G0204*), or G0279 and modifier "-GG" "Performance and payment of a screening mammogram and diagnostic mammogram on the same patient, same day." Reporting of this modifier is needed for data collection purposes. Regular billing instructions remain in place for a screening mammography that does not fit this situation.

Both A/B MACs (A) and (B) systems must accept the GH and GG modifiers where appropriate.

For claims with dates of service prior to January 1, 2017 thru December 31, 2017, providers report CPT codes G0206 and G0204. For claims with dates of service January 1, 2018 and later, providers report CPT codes 77065 and 77066 respectively.

100-04, 18, 60

Colorectal Cancer Screening

(Rev. 3436, Issued: 12-30-15, Effective: 10-09-14, Implementation: 09-08-15 for non-shared MAC edits; 01-04-16 - For all shared system changes.)

See the Medicare Benefit Policy Manual, Chapter 15, and the Medicare National Coverage Determinations (NCD) Manual, Chapter 1, Section 210.3 for Medicare Part B coverage requirements and effective dates of colorectal cancer screening services.

Effective for services furnished on or after January 1, 1998, payment may be made for colorectal cancer screening for the early detection of cancer. For screening colonoscopy services (one of the types of services included in this benefit) prior to July 2001, coverage was limited to high-risk individuals. For services July 1, 2001, and later screening colonoscopies are covered for individuals not at high risk.

The following services are considered colorectal cancer screening services:

- Fecal-occult blood test (FOBT),1-3 simultaneous determinations (guaiac-based);
- Flexible sigmoidoscopy;
- Colonoscopy; and,
- Barium enema

Effective for services on or after January 1, 2004, payment may be made for the following colorectal cancer screening service as an alternative for the guaiac-based FOBT, 1-3 simultaneous determinations:

- Fecal-occult blood test, immunoassay, 1-3 simultaneous determinations

Effective for claims with dates of service on or after October 9, 2014, payment may be made for colorectal cancer screening using the Cologuard™ multitarget stool DNA (sDNA) test:

G0464 (Colorectal cancer screening; stool-based DNA and fecal occult hemoglobin (e.g., KRAS, NDRG4 and BMP3).

Note: HCPCS code G0464 expired on December 31, 2015 and has been replaced in the 2016 Clinical Laboratory Fee Schedule with CPT code 81528, Oncology (colorectal) screening, quantitative real-time target and signal amplification of 10 DNA markers (KRAS mutations, promoter methylation of NDRG4 and BMP3) and fecal hemoglobin, utilizing stool, algorithm reported as a positive or negative result.

100-04, 18, 80.2

A/B Medicare Administrative Contractor (MAC) (B) Billing Requirements

(Rev. 3329, Issued: 08-14-15, Effective: 01-01-12, Implementation: 09-14-15)

Effective for dates of service on and after January 1, 2005, through December 31, 2008, contractors shall recognize the HCPCS codes G0344, G0366, G0367, and G0368 shown above in §80.1 for an IPPE. The type of service (TOS) for each of these codes is as follows:

G0344: TOS = 1

G0366: TOS = 5

G0367: TOS = 5

G0368: TOS = 5

Contractors shall pay physicians or qualified nonphysician practitioners for only one IPPE performed not later than 6 months after the date the individual's first coverage begins under Medicare Part B, but only if that coverage period begins on or after January 1, 2005.

Effective for dates of service on and after January 1, 2009, contractors shall recognize the HCPCS codes G0402, G0403, G0404, and G0405 shown above in §80.1 for an IPPE. The TOS for each of these codes is as follows:

G0402: TOS = 1

G0403: TOS = 5

G0404: TOS = 5

G0405: TOS = 5

Under the MIPPA of 2008, contractors shall pay physicians or qualified nonphysician practitioners for only one IPPE performed not later than 12 months after the date the individual's first coverage begins under Medicare Part B only if that coverage period begins on or after January 1, 2009.

Contractors shall allow payment for a medically necessary Evaluation and Management (E/M) service at the same visit as the IPPE when it is clinically appropriate. Physicians and qualified nonphysician practitioners shall use CPT codes 99201-99215 to report an E/M with CPT modifier 25 to indicate that the E/M is a significant, separately identifiable service from the IPPE code reported (G0344 or G0402, whichever applies based on the date the IPPE is performed). Refer to chapter 12, § 30.6.1.1, of this manual for the physician/practitioner billing correct coding and payment policy regarding E/M services.

If the EKG performed as a component of the IPPE is not performed by the primary physician or qualified NPP during the IPPE visit, another physician or entity may perform and/or interpret the EKG. The referring physician or qualified NPP needs to make sure that the performing physician or entity bills the appropriate G code for the screening EKG, and not a CPT code in the 93000 series. **Both the IPPE and the EKG should be billed in order for the beneficiary to receive the complete IPPE service.** Effective for dates of service on and after January 1, 2009, the screening EKG is optional and is no longer a mandated service of an IPPE if performed as a result of a referral from an IPPE.

Should the same physician or NPP need to perform an additional medically necessary EKG in the 93000 series on the same day as the IPPE, report the appropriate EKG CPT code(s) with modifier 59, indicating that the EKG is a distinct procedural service.

Physicians or qualified nonphysician practitioners shall bill the contractor the appropriate HCPCS codes for IPPE on the Form CMS-1500 claim or an approved electronic format. The HCPCS codes for an IPPE and screening EKG are paid under the Medicare Physician Fee Schedule (MPFS).

See §1.3 of this chapter for waiver of cost sharing requirements of coinsurance, copayment and deductible for furnished preventive services available in Medicare.

100-04, 18, 140.8

Advance Care Planning (ACP) as an Optional Element of an Annual Wellness Visit (AWV)

(Rev. 3428 Issued: 12-22-15, Effective: 01-01-16, Implementation: 01-04-16)

For services furnished on or after January 1, 2016, Advance Care Planning (ACP) is treated as a preventive service when furnished with an AWV. The Medicare coinsurance and Part B deductible are waived for ACP when furnished as an optional element of an AWV.

The codes for the optional ACP services furnished as part of an AWV are 99497 (Advance care planning including the explanation and discussion of advance directives such as standard forms (with completion of such forms, when performed), by the physician or other qualified health professional; first 30 minutes, face-to-face with the patient, family member(s) and/or surrogate;) and an add-on code 99498 (each additional 30 minutes (List separately in addition to code for primary procedure)). When ACP services are provided as a part of an AWV, practitioners would report CPT code 99497 (and add-on CPT code 99498 when applicable) for the ACP services in addition to either of the AWV codes (G0438 or G0439).

The deductible and coinsurance for ACP will only be waived when billed with modifier 33 on the same day and on the same claim as an AWV (code G0438 or G0439), and must also be furnished by the same provider. Waiver of the deductible and coinsurance for ACP is limited to once per year. Payment for an AWV is limited to once per year. If the AWV billed with ACP is denied for exceeding the once per year limit, the deductible and coinsurance will be applied to the ACP.

Also see Pub. 100-02, *Medicare Benefit Policy Manual*, chapter 15, section 280.5.1 for more information.

100-04, 23, 30.2

MPFSDB Record Layout

(Rev. 4298, Issued: 05-03-19, Effective: 01-01-19, Implementation 10-07-19)

The CMS MPFSDB includes the total fee schedule amount, related component parts, and payment policy indicators. The record layout is provided in the Addendum below.

Addendum - MPFSDB File Record Layout and Field Descriptions

(Rev. 4298, Issued: 05-03-19, Effective: 01-01-19, Implementation 10-07-19)

The CMS MPFSDB includes the total fee schedule amount, related component parts, and payment policy indicators. The record layout is provided below. Beginning with the 2019 MPFSDB, and thereafter, the MPFSDB File Record Layout will no longer be revised annually in this section for the sole purpose of changing the calendar year, but will only be revised when there is a change to a field. Previous MPFSDB file layouts (for 2018 and prior) can be found on the CMS web site on the Physician Fee Schedule web page at: https://www.cms.gov/Medicare/Medicare-Fee-for-Service-Payment/PhysicianFeeSched/index.html.

MPFSDB File Layout

HEADER RECORD

FIELD #	DATA ELEMENT NAME	LOCATION	PIC
1	Header ID	1-4	x(4) Value "Head"
2	Header Number	5	x(1)
3	Data Set Name	6-50	x(45)
4	Record Length	51-53	x(3)
5	Filler	54-54	x(1)
6	Block size	55-58	x(4)
7	Filler	59-59	x(1)
8	Number of Records Number does not include this header record.		
	60-69	9(10)	
9	Date Created	70-77	x(8) YYYYMMDD
10	Blanks	78-345	x(268)

DATA RECORD

FIELD # & ITEM	LENGTH & PIC
1 File Year This field displays the effective year of the file.	4 Pic x(4)
2 A/B MAC (B) Number This field represents the 5-digit number assigned to the A/B MAC (B).	5 Pic x(5)
3 Locality This 2-digit code identifies the pricing locality used.	2 Pic x(2)
4 HCPCS Code This field represents the procedure code. Each A/B MAC (B) Current Procedural Terminology (CPT) code (other than codes for Multianalyte Assays with Algorithmic Analyses (MAAA) and Proprietary Laboratory Analyses (PLA)) and alpha-numeric HCPCS codes other than B, C, E, K and L codes will be included. The standard sort for this field is blanks, alpha, and numeric in ascending order. Note: MAAA and PLA are alpha-numeric CPT codes.	5 Pic x(5)
5 Modifier For diagnostic tests, a blank in this field denotes the global service and the following modifiers identify the components: 26 = Professional component TC = Technical component For services other than those with a professional and/or technical component, a blank will appear in this field with one exception: the presence of CPT modifier -53 which indicates that separate Relative Value Units (RVUs) and a fee schedule amount have been established for procedures which the physician terminated before completion. This modifier is used only with colonoscopy through stoma code 44388, colonoscopy code 45378 and screening colonoscopy codes G0105 and G0121. Any other codes billed with modifier -53 are subject to medical review and priced by individual consideration. Modifier-53 = Discontinued Procedure - Under certain circumstances, the physician may elect to terminate a surgical or diagnostic procedure. Due to extenuating circumstances, or those that threaten the well being of the patient, it may be necessary to indicate that a surgical or diagnostic procedure was started but discontinued.	2 Pic x(2)
6 Descriptor This field will include a brief description of each procedure code.	50 Pic x(50)
7 Code Status This 1 position field provides the status of each code under the full fee schedule. Each status code is explained in §30.2.2.	1 Pic x(1)
8 Conversion Factor This field displays the multiplier which transforms relative values into payment amounts. The file will contain the conversion factor for the File Year which will reflect all adjustments.	8 Pic 9(4)v9999
9 Update Factor This update factor has been included in the conversion factor in Field 8.	6 Pic 9(2)v9999
10 Work Relative Value Unit This field displays the unit value for the physician work RVU.	9 Pic 9(7)v99
11 Filler	9 Pic 9(7)v99
12 Malpractice Relative Value Unit This field displays the unit value for the malpractice expense RVU.	9 Pic 9(7)v99
13 Work Geographic Practice Cost Indices (GPCIs) This field displays a work geographic adjustment factor used in computing the fee schedule amount.	5 Pic 99v999
14 Practice Expense GPCI This field displays a practice expense geographic adjustment factor used in computing the fee schedule amount.	5 Pic 99v999
15 Malpractice GPCI This field displays a malpractice expense geographic adjustment factor used in computing the fee schedule amount.	5 Pic 99v999

FIELD # & ITEM	LENGTH & PIC
16 Global Surgery This field provides the postoperative time frames that apply to payment for each surgical procedure or another indicator that describes the applicability of the global concept to the service. 000 = Endoscopic or minor procedure with related preoperative and postoperative relative values on the day of the procedure only included in the fee schedule payment amount; evaluation and management services on the day of the procedure generally not payable. 010 = Minor procedure with preoperative relative values on the day of the procedure and postoperative relative values during a 10-day postoperative period included in the fee schedule amount; evaluation and management services on the day of the procedure and during this 10-day postoperative period generally not payable. 090 = Major surgery with a 1-day preoperative period and 90-day postoperative period included in the fee schedule payment amount. MMM = Maternity codes; usual global period does not apply. XXX = Global concept does not apply. YYY = A/B MAC (B) determines whether global concept applies and establishes postoperative period, if appropriate, at time of pricing. ZZZ = Code related to another service and is always included in the global period of the other service. (Note: Physician work is associated with intra-service time and in some instances the post service time.)	3 Pic x(3)
17 Preoperative Percentage (Modifier 56) This field contains the percentage (shown in decimal format) for the preoperative portion of the global package. For example, 10 percent will be shown as 010000. The total of fields 17, 18, and 19 will usually equal one. Any variance is slight and results from rounding.	6 Pic 9v9(5)
18 Intraoperative Percentage (Modifier 54) This field contains the percentage (shown in decimal format) for the intraoperative portion of the global package including postoperative work in the hospital. For example, 63 percent will be shown as 063000. The total of fields 17, 18, and 19 will usually equal one. Any variance is slight and results from rounding.	6 Pic 9v9(5)
19 Postoperative Percentage (Modifier 55) This field contains the percentage (shown in decimal format) for the postoperative portion of the global package that is provided in the office after discharge from the hospital. For example, 17 percent will be shown as 017000. The total of fields 17, 18, and 19 will usually equal one. Any variance is slight and results from rounding.	6 Pic 9v9(5)

FIELD # & ITEM	LENGTH & PIC
20 Professional Component (PC)/Technical Component (TC) Indicator 0 = Physician service codes: This indicator identifies codes that describe physician services. Examples include visits, consultations, and surgical procedures. The concept of PC/TC does not apply since physician services cannot be split into professional and technical components. Modifiers 26 & TC cannot be used with these codes. The total Relative Value Units (RVUs) include values for physician work, practice expense and malpractice expense. There are some codes with no work RVUs. 1 = Diagnostic tests or radiology services: This indicator identifies codes that describe diagnostic tests, e.g., pulmonary function tests, or therapeutic radiology procedures, e.g., radiation therapy. These codes generally have both a professional and technical component. Modifiers 26 and TC can be used with these codes. The total RVUs for codes reported with a 26 modifier include values for physician work, practice expense, and malpractice expense. The total RVUs for codes reported with a TC modifier include values for practice expense and malpractice expense only. The total RVUs for codes reported without a modifier equals the sum of RVUs for both the professional and technical component. 2 = Professional component only codes: This indicator identifies stand alone codes that describe the physician work portion of selected diagnostic tests for which there is an associated code that describes the technical component of the diagnostic test only and another associated code that describes the global test. An example of a professional component only code is 93010, Electrocardiogram; interpretation and report. Modifiers 26 and TC cannot be used with these codes. The total RVUs for professional component only codes include values for physician work, practice expense, and malpractice expense. 3 = Technical component only codes: This indicator identifies stand alone codes that describe the technical component (i.e., staff and equipment costs) of selected diagnostic tests for which there is an associated code that describes the professional component of the diagnostic tests only. An example of a technical component code is 93005, Electrocardiogram, tracing only, without interpretation and report. It also identifies codes that are covered only as diagnostic tests and therefore do not have a related professional code. Modifiers 26 and TC cannot be used with these codes. The total RVUs for technical component only codes include values for practice expense and malpractice expense only. 4 = Global test only codes: This indicator identifies stand alone codes for which there are associated codes that describe: a) the professional component of the test only and b) the technical component of the test only. Modifiers 26 and TC cannot be used with these codes. The total RVUs for global procedure only codes include values for physician work, practice expense, and malpractice expense. The total RVUs for global procedure only codes equals the sum of the total RVUs for the professional and technical components only codes combined. 5 = Incident to codes: This indicator identifies codes that describe services covered incident to a physicians service when they are provided by auxiliary personnel employed by the physician and working under his or her direct supervision. Payment may not be made by A/B MACs (B) for these services when they are provided to hospital inpatients or patients in a hospital outpatient department. Modifiers 26 and TC cannot be used with these codes. 6 = Laboratory physician interpretation codes: This indicator identifies clinical laboratory codes for which separate payment for interpretations by laboratory physicians may be made. Actual performance of the tests is paid for under the lab fee schedule. Modifier TC cannot be used with these codes. The total RVUs for laboratory physician interpretation codes include values for physician work, practice expense and malpractice expense. 7 = Private practice therapist's service: Payment may not be made if the service is provided to either a hospital outpatient or a hospital inpatient by a physical therapist, occupational therapist, or speech-language pathologist in private practice. 8 = Physician interpretation codes: This indicator identifies the professional component of clinical laboratory codes for which separate payment may be made only if the physician interprets an abnormal smear for hospital inpatient. This applies only to code 85060. No TC billing is recognized because payment for the underlying clinical laboratory test is made to the hospital, generally through the PPS rate. No payment is recognized for code 85060 furnished to hospital outpatients or non-hospital patients. The physician interpretation is paid through the clinical laboratory fee schedule payment for the clinical laboratory test. 9 = Concept of a professional/technical component does not apply.	

FIELD # & ITEM	LENGTH & PIC
21	

Multiple Procedure (Modifier 51)

Indicator indicates which payment adjustment rule for multiple procedures applies to the service.

0 = No payment adjustment rules for multiple procedures apply. If procedure is reported on the same day as another procedure, base payment on the lower of: (a) the actual charge or (b) the fee schedule amount for the procedure.

1 = Standard payment adjustment rules in effect before January 1, 1996, for multiple procedures apply. In the 1996 MPFSDB, this indicator only applies to codes with procedure status of "D." If a procedure is reported on the same day as another procedure with an indicator of 1,2, or 3, rank the procedures by fee schedule amount and apply the appropriate reduction to this code (100 percent, 50 percent, 25 percent, 25 percent, 25 percent, and by report). Base payment on the lower of: (a) the actual charge or (b) the fee schedule amount reduced by the appropriate percentage.

2 = Standard payment adjustment rules for multiple procedures apply. If procedure is reported on the same day as another procedure with an indicator of 1, 2, or 3, rank the procedures by fee schedule amount and apply the appropriate reduction to this code (100 percent, 50 percent, 50 percent, 50 percent, 50 percent, and by report). Base payment on the lower of: (a) the actual charge or (b) the fee schedule amount reduced by the appropriate percentage.

3 = Special rules for multiple endoscopic procedures apply if procedure is billed with another endoscopy in the same family (i.e., another endoscopy that has the same base procedure). The base procedure for each code with this indicator is identified in field 31G.

Apply the multiple endoscopy rules to a family before ranking the family with other procedures performed on the same day (for example, if multiple endoscopies in the same family are reported on the same day as endoscopies in another family or on the same day as a non-endoscopic procedure).

If an endoscopic procedure is reported with only its base procedure, do not pay separately for the base procedure. Payment for the base procedure is included in the payment for the other endoscopy.

4 = Subject to 25% reduction of the TC diagnostic imaging (effective for services January 1, 2006 through June 30, 2010). Subject to 50% reduction of the TC diagnostic imaging (effective for services July 1, 2010 and after). Subject to 25% reduction of the PC of diagnostic imaging (effective for services January 1, 2012 through December 31, 2016). Subject to 5% reduction of the PC of diagnostic imaging (effective for services January 1, 2017 and after).

5 = Subject to 20% reduction of the practice expense component for certain therapy services furnished in office and other non-institutional settings, and 25% reduction of the practice expense component for certain therapy services furnished in institutional settings (effective for services January 1, 2011 and after). Subject to 50% reduction of the practice expense component for certain therapy services furnished in both institutional and non-institutional settings (effective for services April 1, 2013 and after).

6 = Subject to 25% reduction of the TC diagnostic cardiovascular services (effective for services January 1, 2013 and after).

7 = Subject to 20% reduction of the TC diagnostic ophthalmology services (effective for services January 1, 2013 and after).

9 = Concept does not apply.

FIELD # & ITEM	LENGTH & PIC
22	1 Pic (x)1

Bilateral Surgery Indicator (Modifier 50)

This field provides an indicator for services subject to a payment adjustment.

0 = 150 percent payment adjustment for bilateral procedures does not apply. If procedure is reported with modifier -50 or with modifiers RT and LT, base payment for the two sides on the lower of: (a) the total actual charge for both sides or (b) 100 percent of the fee schedule amount for a single code. Example: The fee schedule amount for code XXXXX is $125. The physician reports code XXXXX-LT with an actual charge of $100 and XXXXX-RT with an actual charge of $100.

Payment would be based on the fee schedule amount ($125) since it is lower than the total actual charges for the left and right sides ($200).

The bilateral adjustment is inappropriate for codes in this category because of (a) physiology or anatomy or (b) because the code descriptor specifically states that it is a unilateral procedure and there is an existing code for the bilateral procedure.

1 = 150 percent payment adjustment for bilateral procedures applies. If code is billed with the bilateral modifier or is reported twice on the same day by any other means (e.g., with RT and LT modifiers or with a 2 in the units field), base payment for these codes when reported as bilateral procedures on the lower of: (a) the total actual charge for both sides or (b) 150 percent of the fee schedule amount for a single code.

If code is reported as a bilateral procedure and is reported with other procedure codes on the same day, apply the bilateral adjustment before applying any applicable multiple procedure rules.

2 = 150 percent payment adjustment for bilateral procedure does not apply. RVUs are already based on the procedure being performed as a bilateral procedure. If procedure is reported with modifier -50 or is reported twice on the same day by any other means (e.g., with RT and LT modifiers with a 2 in the units field), base payment for both sides on the lower of (a) the total actual charges by the physician for both sides or (b) 100 percent of the fee schedule amount for a single

1 Pic (x)1 code.

Example: The fee schedule amount for code YYYYY is $125. The physician reports code YYYYY-LT with an actual charge of $100 and YYYYY-RT with an actual charge of $100. Payment would be based on the fee schedule amount ($125) since it is lower than the total actual charges for the left and right sides ($200).

The RVUs are based on a bilateral procedure because: (a) the code descriptor specifically states that the procedure is bilateral; (b) the code descriptor states that the procedure may be performed either unilaterally or bilaterally; or (c) the procedure is usually performed as a bilateral procedure.

3 = The usual payment adjustment for bilateral procedures does not apply. If procedure is reported with modifier -50 or is reported for both sides on the same day by any other means (e.g., with RT and LT modifiers or with a 2 in the units field), base payment for each side or organ or site of a paired organ on the lower of: (a) the actual charge for each side or (b) 100% of the fee schedule amount for each side. If procedure is reported as a bilateral procedure and with other procedure codes on the same day, determine the fee schedule amount for a bilateral procedure before applying any applicable multiple procedure rules.

Services in this category are generally radiology procedures or other diagnostic tests which are not subject to the special payment rules for other bilateral procedures.

9 = Concept does not apply.

FIELD # & ITEM	LENGTH & PIC
23 Assistant at Surgery This field provides an indicator for services where an assistant at surgery is never paid for per IOM. 0 = Payment restriction for assistants at surgery applies to this procedure unless supporting documentation is submitted to establish medical necessity. 1 = Statutory payment restriction for assistants at surgery applies to this procedure. Assistant at surgery may not be paid. 2 = Payment restriction for assistants at surgery does not apply to this procedure. Assistant at surgery may be paid. 9 = Concept does not apply. 24 Co-Surgeons (Modifier 62) This field provides an indicator for services for which two surgeons, each in a different specialty, may be paid. 0 = Co-surgeons not permitted for this procedure. 1 = Co-surgeons could be paid; supporting documentation required to establish medical necessity of two surgeons for the procedure. 2 = Co-surgeons permitted; no documentation required if two specialty requirements are met. 9 = Concept does not apply.	1 Pic (x)1
25 9 Pic 9(7)v99 Team Surgeons (Modifier 66) This field provides an indicator for services for which team surgeons may be paid. 0 = Team surgeons not permitted for this procedure. 1 = Team surgeons could be paid; supporting documentation required to establish medical necessity of a team; pay by report. 2 = Team surgeons permitted; pay by report. 9 = Concept does not apply.	1 Pic (x)1
26 Filler	1 Pic (x)1
27 Site of Service Differential For 1999 and beyond, the site of service differential no longer applies. The following definitions will apply for all years after 1998: 0 = Facility pricing does not apply. 1 = Facility pricing applies. 9 = Concept does not apply. 28 Non-Facility Fee Schedule Amount This field shows the fee schedule amount for the non-facility setting. This amount equals Field 34. Note: Field 33 D indicates if an additional adjustment should be applied to this formula. Non-Facility Pricing Amount for the File Year [(Work RVU * Work GPCI) + (Non-Facility PE RVU * PE GPCI) + (MP RVU * MP GPCI)] * Conversion Factor	1 Pic (x)1
29 Facility Fee Schedule Amount This field shows the fee schedule amount for the facility setting. This amount equals Field 35. Note: Field 33D indicates if an additional adjustment should be applied to this formula. Facility Pricing Amount for the File Year [(Work RVU * Work GPCI) + (Facility PE RVU * PE GPCI) + (MP RVU * MP GPCI)] * Conversion Factor Place of service codes to be used to identify facilities. 02 – Telehealth-Medicare pays telehealth services at the facility rate. 19 – Off Campus-Outpatient Hospital 21 - Inpatient Hospital 22 – On Campus-Outpatient Hospital 23 - Emergency Room - Hospital 24 - Ambulatory Surgical Center – In a Medicare approved ASC, for an approved procedure on the ASC list, Medicare pays the lower facility fee to physicians. Beginning with dates of service January 1, 2008, in a Medicare approved ASC, for procedures NOT on the ASC list of approved procedures, contractors will also pay the lower facility fee to physicians. 26 - Military Treatment Facility 31 - Skilled Nursing Facility 34 - Hospice 41 - Ambulance - Land 42 - Ambulance Air or Water 51 - Inpatient Psychiatric Facility 52 - Psychiatric Facility Partial Hospitalization 53 - Community Mental Health Center 56 - Psychiatric Residential Treatment Facility 61 - Comprehensive Inpatient Rehabilitation Facility	9 Pic 9(7)v99
29A Anti-markup Test Indicator This field providers an indicator for Anti-markup Test HCPCS codes: '1' = Anti-markup Test HCPCS. '9' = Concept does not apply.	1 Pic x
30 Record Effective Date This field identifies the effective date for the MPFSDB record for each HCPCS. The field is in YYYYMMDD format. NOTE: This is not the date the HCPCS code was created. It is the date the code was updated or added to the MPFSDB file for the current file year. This field is set to January 1 for all codes during the annual update process.	8 Pic x(8)
31 Filler	28 Pic x(28)
31EE Reduced therapy fee schedule amount	9Pic(7)v99
31DD Filler	1Pic x(2)
31CC Imaging Cap Indicator A value of "1" means subject to OPPS payment cap determination. A value of "9" means not subject to OPPS payment cap determination.	1Pic x(1)
31BB Non-Facility Imaging Payment Amount	9Pic(7)v99
31AA Facility Imaging Payment Amount	9Pic(7)v99

FIELD # & ITEM	LENGTH & PIC
31A Physician Supervision of Diagnostic Procedures This field is for use in post payment review. 01 = Procedure must be performed under the general supervision of a physician. 02 = Procedure must be performed under the direct supervision of a physician. 03 = Procedure must be performed under the personal supervision of a physician. (Diagnostic imaging procedures performed by a Registered Radiologist Assistant (RRA) who is certified and registered by The American Registry of Radiologic Technologists (ARRT) or a Radiology Practitioner Assistant (RPA) who is certified by the Certification Board for Radiology Practitioner Assistants (CBRPA), and is authorized to furnish the procedure under state law, may be performed under direct supervision.) 04 = Physician supervision policy does not apply when procedure is furnished by a qualified, independent psychologist or a clinical psychologist; otherwise must be performed under the general supervision of a physician. 05 = Not subject to supervision when furnished personally by a qualified audiologist, physician or non physician practitioner. Direct supervision by a physician is required for those parts of the test that may be furnished by a qualified technician when appropriate to the circumstances of the test. 06 = Procedure must be personally performed by a physician or a physical therapist (PT) who is certified by the American Board of Physical Therapy Specialties (ABPTS) as a qualified electrophysiological clinical specialist and is permitted to provide the procedure under State law. Procedure may also be performed by a PT with ABPTS certification without physician supervision. 21 = Procedure may be performed by a technician with certification under general supervision of a physician; otherwise must be performed under direct supervision of a physician. Procedure may also be performed by a PT with ABPTS certification without physician supervision. 22 = May be performed by a technician with on-line real-time contact with physician. 66 = May be personally performed by a physician or by a physical therapist with ABPTS certification and certification in this specific procedure. 6A = Supervision standards for level 66 apply; in addition, the PT with ABPTS certification may personally supervise another PT, but only the PT with ABPTS certification may bill. 77 = Procedure must be performed by a PT with ABPTS 1 Pic x(1) certification (TC & PC) or by a PT without certification under direct supervision of a physician (TC & PC), or by a technician with certification under general supervision of a physician (TC only; PC always physician). 7A = Supervision standards for level 77 apply; in addition, the PT with ABPTS certification may personally supervise another PT, but only the PT with ABPTS certification may bill. 09 = Concept does not apply.	2 Pic x(2)
31B This field has been deleted to allow for the expansion of field 31A.	
31C Facility Setting Practice Expense Relative Value Units	9 Pic(7)v99
31D Non-Facility Setting Practice Expense Relative Value Units	9 Pic(7)v99
31E Filler	9 Pic(7)v99
31F Filler Reserved for future use.	1 Pic x(1)
31G Endoscopic Base Codes	5 Pic x(5)
This field identifies an endoscopic base code for each code with a multiple surgery indicator of 3.	
32A 1996 Transition/Fee Schedule Amount This field is no longer applicable since transitioning ended in 1996. This field will contain a zero.	9 Pic 9(7)v99

FIELD # & ITEM	LENGTH & PIC
32B 1996 Transition/Fee Schedule This field is no longer applicable since transitioning ended in 1996. This field will contain spaces.	1 Pic x(1)
32C 1996 Transition/Fee Schedule Amount When Site or Service Differential Applies This field is no longer applicable since transitioning ended in 1996. This field will contain a zero. 33A Units Payment Rule Indicator Reserved for future use. 9 = Concept does not apply.	9 Pic 9(7)v99
33B Mapping Indicator This field is no longer applicable since transitioning ended in 1996.	1 Pic x(1)
3 Pic x (3)	
This field will contain spaces.	
33C Anti-markup Locality—Informational Use—Locality used for reporting utilization of anti-markup services. NOT FOR A/B MAC (B) USE: These Medicare Advantage encounter pricing localities are for Shared System Maintainer purposes only. The locality values were developed to facilitate centralized processing of encounter data by the Medicare Advantage organizations.	2 Pic x(2)
33D Calculation Flag This field is informational only; the SSMs do not need to add this field. The intent is to assist A/B MACs (B) to understand how the fee schedule amount in fields 28 and 29 are calculated. The MMA mandates an additional adjustment to selected HCPCS codes. A value of "1" indicates an additional fee schedule adjustment of 1.32 in 2004 and 1.03 in 2005. A value of "0" indicates no additional adjustment needed. A value of "2" indicates an additional fee schedule adjustment of 1.05 effective 7/1/2008.	1 Pic x(1)
33 E Diagnostic Imaging Family Indicator For services effective January 1, 2011, and after, family indicators 01 - 11 will not be populated. 01 = Family 1 Ultrasound (Chest/Abdomen/Pelvis – Non Obstetrical 02 = Family 2 CT and CTA (Chest/Thorax/Abd/Pelvis) 03 = Family 3 CT and CTA (Head/Brain/Orbit/Maxillofacial/Neck) 04 = Family 4 MRI and MRA (Chest/Abd/Pelvis) 05 = Family 5 MRI and MRA (Head/Brain/Neck) 06 = Family 6 MRI and MRA (spine) 07 = Family 7 CT (spine) 08 = Family 8 MRI and MRA (lower extremities) 09 = Family 9 CT and CTA (lower extremities) 10 = Family 10 Mr and MRI (upper extremities and joints) 11 = Family 11 CT and CTA (upper extremities) 88 = Subject to the reduction of the TC diagnostic imaging (effective for services January 1, 2011, and after). Subject to the reduction of the PC diagnostic imaging (effective for services January 1, 2012 and after). 99 = Concept Does Not Apply	2Pic x(2)
33F Performance Payment Indicator (For future use) 33G National Level Future Expansion	1 Pic x (1)
34 Non-Facility Fee Schedule Amount This field replicates field 28.	9 Pic 9(7)v99
35 Facility Fee Schedule Amount This field replicates field 29.	9 Pic 9(7)v99
36 Filler	1 Pic x(1)

FIELD # & ITEM	LENGTH & PIC
37 Future Local Level Expansion** The Updated 1992 Transition Amount was previously stored in this field. A/B MACs (B) can continue to maintain the updated transition amount in this field.	7 Pic x(7)
38A Future Local Level Expansion** The adjusted historical payment basis (AHPB) was previously stored in this field. A/B MACs (B) can continue to maintain the AHPB in this field.	7 Pic x(7)
38 B Filler This field was originally established for 15 spaces. Since AHPB data will only use 7 of the 15 spaces, A/B MACs (B) have 8 remaining spaces for their purposes. ** These fields will be appended by each A/B MAC (B) at the local level.	8 Pix x(8)

100-04, 32, 10.1

Ambulatory Blood Pressure Monitoring (ABPM) Billing Requirements

(Rev. 2998, Issued: 07-25-14, Effective: Upon implementation of ICD-10; 01-01-12 - ASC X12, Implementation: 08-25-2014 - ASC X12; Upon Implementation of ICD-10)

A. Coding Applicable to A/B MACs (A and B)

Effective April 1, 2002, a National Coverage Decision was made to allow for Medicare coverage of ABPM for those beneficiaries with suspected "white coat hypertension" (WCH). ABPM involves the use of a non-invasive device, which is used to measure blood pressure in 24-hour cycles. These 24-hour measurements are stored in the device and are later interpreted by a physician. Suspected "WCH" is defined as: (1) Clinic/office blood pressure >140/90 mm Hg on at least three separate clinic/office visits with two separate measurements made at each visit; (2) At least two documented separate blood pressure measurements taken outside the clinic/office which are < 140/90 mm Hg; and (3) No evidence of end-organ damage. ABPM is not covered for any other uses. Coverage policy can be found in Medicare National Coverage Determinations Manual, Chapter 1, Part 1, §20.19. (http://www.cms.hhs.gov/manuals/103_cov_determ/ncd103index.asp).

The ABPM must be performed for at least 24 hours to meet coverage criteria. Payment is not allowed for institutionalized beneficiaries, such as those receiving Medicare covered skilled nursing in a facility. In the rare circumstance that ABPM needs to be performed more than once for a beneficiary, the qualifying criteria described above must be met for each subsequent ABPM test.

Effective dates for applicable Common Procedure Coding System (HCPCS) codes for ABPM for suspected WCH and their covered effective dates are as follows:

HCPCS	Definition	Effective Date
93784	ABPM, utilizing a system such as magnetic tape and/or computer disk, for 24 hours or longer; including recording, scanning analysis, interpretation and report.	04/01/2002
93786	ABPM, utilizing a system such as magnetic tape and/or computer disk, for 24 hours or longer; recording only.	04/01/2002
93788	ABPM, utilizing a system such as magnetic tape and/or computer disk, for 24 hours or longer; scanning analysis with report.	01/01/2004
93790	ABPM, utilizing a system such as magnetic tape and/or computer disk, for 24 hours or longer; physician review with interpretation and report.	04/01/2002

In addition, one of the following diagnosis codes must be present:

	Diagnosis Code	Description
If ICD-9-CM is applicable	796.2	Elevated blood pressure reading without diagnosis of hypertension.
If ICD-10-CM is applicable	RØ3.Ø	Elevated blood pressure reading without diagnosis of hypertension

B. A/B MAC (A) Billing Instructions

The applicable types of bills acceptable when billing for ABPM services are 13X, 23X, 71X, 73X, 75X, and 85X. Chapter 25 of this manual provides general billing instructions that must be followed for bills submitted to A/B MACs (A). The A/B MACs (A) pay for hospital outpatient ABPM services billed on a 13X type of bill with HCPCS 93786 and/or 93788 as follows: (1) Outpatient Prospective Payment System (OPPS) hospitals pay based on the Ambulatory Payment Classification (APC); (2) non-OPPS hospitals (Indian Health Services Hospitals, Hospitals that provide Part B services only, and hospitals located in American Samoa, Guam, Saipan and the Virgin Islands) pay based on reasonable cost, except for Maryland Hospitals which are paid based on a percentage of cost. Effective 4/1/06, type of bill 14X is for non-patient laboratory specimens and is no longer applicable for ABPM.

The A/B MACs (A) pay for comprehensive outpatient rehabilitation facility (CORF) ABPM services billed on a 75x type of bill with HCPCS code 93786 and/or 93788 based on the Medicare Physician Fee Schedule (MPFS) amount for that HCPCS code.

The A/B MACs (A) pay for ABPM services for critical access hospitals (CAHs) billed on a 85x type of bill as follows: (1) for CAHs that elected the Standard Method and billed HCPCS code 93786 and/or 93788, pay based on reasonable cost for that HCPCS code; and (2) for CAHs that elected the Optional Method and billed any combination of HCPCS codes 93786, 93788 and 93790 pay based on reasonable cost for HCPCS 93786 and 93788 and pay 115% of the MPFS amount for HCPCS 93790.

The A/B MACs (A) pay for ABPM services for skilled nursing facility (SNF) outpatients billed on a 23x type of bill with HCPCS code 93786 and/or 93788, based on the MPFS.

The A/B MACs (A) accept independent and provider-based rural health clinic (RHC) bills for visits under the all-inclusive rate when the RHC bills on a 71x type of bill with revenue code 052x for providing the professional component of ABPM services. The A/B MACs (A) should not make a separate payment to a RHC for the professional component of ABPM services in addition to the all-inclusive rate. RHCs are not required to use ABPM HCPCS codes for professional services covered under the all-inclusive rate.

The A/B MACs (A) accept free-standing and provider-based federally qualified health center (FQHC) bills for visits under the all-inclusive rate when the FQHC bills on a 73x type of bill with revenue code 052x for providing the professional component of ABPM services.

The A/B MACs (A) should not make a separate payment to a FQHC for the professional component of ABPM services in addition to the all-inclusive rate. FQHCs are not required to use ABPM HCPCS codes for professional services covered under the all-inclusive rate.

The A/B MACs (A) pay provider-based RHCs/FQHCs for the technical component of ABPM services when billed under the base provider's number using the above requirements for that particular base provider type, i.e., a OPPS hospital based RHC would be paid for the ABPM technical component services under the OPPS using the APC for code 93786 and/or 93788 when billed on a 13x type of bill.

Independent and free-standing RHC/FQHC practitioners are only paid for providing the technical component of ABPM services when billed to the A/B MAC (B) following the MAC's instructions.

C. A/B MAC (B) Claims

A/B MACs (B) pay for ABPM services billed with ICD-9-CM diagnosis code 796.2 (if ICD-9 is applicable) or, if ICD-10 is applicable, ICD-10-CM diagnosis code R03.0 and HCPCS codes 93784 or for any combination of 93786, 93788 and 93790, based on the MPFS for the specific HCPCS code billed.

D. Coinsurance and Deductible

The A/B MACs (A and B) shall apply coinsurance and deductible to payments for ABPM services except for services billed to the A/B MAC (A) by FQHCs. For FQHCs only co-insurance applies.

100-04, 32, 12

Counseling to Prevent Tobacco Use

(Rev.3848, Issued: 08- 25-17, Effective: 09-26-17, Implementation: 09- 26-17)

Background: Effective for services furnished on or after March 22, 2005, a National Coverage Determination (NCD) provided for coverage of smoking and tobacco-use cessation counseling services located at Medicare National Coverage Determinations Manual, Publication 100-03 section 210.4. CMS established a related policy entitled Counseling to Prevent Tobaccos Use at NCD Manual 210.4.1 effective August 25, 2010. However, effective September 30, 2016, the conditions of Medicare Part A and Medicare Part B coverage for smoking and tobacco-use cessation counseling services (210.4) were deleted. The remaining NCD entitled Counseling to Prevent Tobacco Use (210.4.1), remains in effect, along with HCPCS codes 99406 and 99407, specifically payable for counseling to prevent tobacco use effective October 1, 2016.

100-04, 32, 12.1

Counseling to Prevent Tobacco Use HCPCS and Diagnosis Coding

(Rev. 4237, Issued: 02-08- 19, Effective: 03-12- 19, Implementation: 03-12-19)

The following HCPCS codes should be reported when billing for counseling to prevent tobacco use services:

99406 Smoking and tobacco-use cessation counseling visit; intermediate, greater than 3 minutes up to 10 minutes

99407 Smoking and tobacco-use cessation counseling visit; intensive, greater than 10 minutes

Note the above codes were effective for dates of service on or after January 1, 2008, and specifically effective for counseling to prevent tobacco use claims on or after October 1, 2016.

Contractors shall allow payment for a medically necessary E/M service on the same day as the counseling to prevent tobacco use service when it is clinically appropriate. Physicians and qualified non-physician practitioners shall use an appropriate HCPCS code, such as HCPCS 99201– 99215, to report an E/M service with modifier 25 to indicate that the E/M service is a separately identifiable service from 99406 or 99407.

Contractors shall only pay for 8 counseling to prevent tobacco use sessions in a 12-month period. The beneficiary may receive another 8 sessions during a second or subsequent year after 11 full months have passed since the first Medicare covered counseling session was performed. To start the count for the second or subsequent 12-month period, begin with the month after the month in which the first Medicare covered counseling session was performed and count until 11 full months have elapsed.

Claims for counseling to prevent tobacco use services shall be submitted with an appropriate diagnosis code.

NOTE: This decision does not modify existing coverage for minimal cessation counseling (defined as 3 minutes or less in duration) which is already considered to be covered as part of each Evaluation and Management (E/M) visit and is not separately billable.

Claims for counseling to prevent tobacco use services shall be submitted with an applicable diagnosis code:

ICD-9-CM (prior to October 1, 2015)

V15.82, personal history of tobacco use, or

305.1, non-dependent tobacco use disorder

989.84, toxic effect of tobacco

ICD-10-CM (effective October 1, 2015)

F17.210, nicotine dependence, cigarettes, uncomplicated,

F17.211, nicotine dependence, cigarettes, in remission,

F17.213 Nicotine dependence, cigarettes, with withdrawal

F17.218 Nicotine dependence, cigarettes, with other nicotine-induced disorders

F17.219 Nicotine dependence, cigarettes, with unspecified nicotine-induced disorders

F17.220, nicotine dependence, chewing tobacco, uncomplicated,

F17.221, nicotine dependence, chewing tobacco, in remission,

F17.223 Nicotine dependence, chewing tobacco, with withdrawal

F17.228 Nicotine dependence, chewing tobacco, with other nicotine-induced disorders

F17.229 Nicotine dependence, chewing tobacco, with unspecified nicotine-induced disorders

F17.290, nicotine dependence, other tobacco product, uncomplicated,

F17.291, nicotine dependence, other tobacco product, in remission, or

F17.293 Nicotine dependence, other tobacco product, with withdrawal

F17.298 Nicotine dependence, other tobacco product, with other nicotine-induced disorders

F17.299 Nicotine dependence, other tobacco product, with unspecified nicotine-induced disorders

Z87.891, personal history of nicotine dependence, unspecified, uncomplicated.

T65.211A, Toxic effect of chewing tobacco, accidental (unintentional), initial encounter

T65.212A, Toxic effect of chewing tobacco, intentional self-harm, initial encounter

T65.213A, Toxic effect of chewing tobacco, assault, initial encounter

T65.214A, Toxic effect of chewing tobacco, undetermined, initial encounter

T65.221A, Toxic effect of tobacco cigarettes, accidental (unintentional), initial encounter

T65.222A, Toxic effect of tobacco cigarettes, intentional self-harm, initial encounter

T65.223A, Toxic effect of tobacco cigarettes, assault, initial encounter

T65.224A, Toxic effect of tobacco cigarettes, undetermined, initial encounter

T65.291A, Toxic effect of other tobacco and nicotine, accidental (unintentional), initial encounter

T65.292A, Toxic effect of other tobacco and nicotine, intentional self-harm, initial encounter

T65.293A, Toxic effect of other tobacco and nicotine, assault, initial encounter

T65.294A, Toxic effect of other tobacco and nicotine, undetermined, initial encounter

100-04, 32, 30.1

Billing Requirements for HBO Therapy for the Treatment of Diabetic Wounds of the Lower Extremities

(Rev. 2998, Issued: 07-25-14, Effective: Upon implementation of ICD-10; 01-01-12 - ASC X12, Implementation: 08-25-2014 - ASC X12; Upon Implementation of ICD-10)

Hyperbaric Oxygen Therapy is a modality in which the entire body is exposed to oxygen under increased atmospheric pressure. Effective April 1, 2003, a National Coverage Decision expanded the use of HBO therapy to include coverage for the treatment of diabetic wounds of the lower extremities. For specific coverage criteria for HBO Therapy, refer to the National Coverage Determinations Manual, Chapter 1, section 20.29.

NOTE: Topical application of oxygen does not meet the definition of HBO therapy as stated above. Also, its clinical efficacy has not been established. Therefore, no Medicare reimbursement may be made for the topical application of oxygen.

I. Billing Requirements for A/B MACs (A)

Claims for HBO therapy should be submitted using the ASC X12 837 institutional claim format or, in rare cases, on Form CMS-1450.

a. Applicable Bill Types

The applicable hospital bill types are 11X, 13X and 85X.

b. Procedural Coding

99183– Physician attendance and supervision of hyperbaric oxygen therapy, per session.

C1300 – Hyperbaric oxygen under pressure, full body chamber, per 30-minute interval.

NOTE: Code C1300 is not available for use other than in a hospital outpatient department. In skilled nursing facilities (SNFs), HBO therapy is part of the SNF PPS payment for beneficiaries in covered Part A stays.

For hospital inpatients and critical access hospitals (CAHs) not electing Method I, HBO therapy is reported under revenue code 940 without any HCPCS code. For inpatient services, if ICD-9-is applicable, show ICD-9-CM procedure code 93.59. If ICD-10 is applicable, show ICD-10-PCS code 5A05121.

For CAHs electing Method I, HBO therapy is reported under revenue code 940 along with HCPCS code 99183.

c. Payment Requirements for A/B MACs (A)

Payment is as follows:

A/B MAC (A) payment is allowed for HBO therapy for diabetic wounds of the lower extremities when performed as a physician service in a hospital outpatient setting and for inpatients. Payment is allowed for claims with valid diagnosis codes as shown above with dates of service on or after April 1, 2003. Those claims with invalid codes should be denied as not medically necessary.

For hospitals, payment will be based upon the Ambulatory Payment Classification (APC) or the inpatient Diagnosis Related Group (DRG). Deductible and coinsurance apply.

Payment to Critical Access Hospitals (electing Method I) is made under cost reimbursement. For Critical Access Hospitals electing Method II, the technical component is paid under cost reimbursement and the professional component is paid under the Physician Fee Schedule.

II. A/B MAC (B) Billing Requirements

Claims for this service should be submitted using the ASC X12 837 professional claim format or Form CMS-1500.

The following HCPCS code applies:

99183 – Physician attendance and supervision of hyperbaric oxygen therapy, per session.

a. Payment Requirements for A/B MACs (B)

Payment and pricing information will occur through updates to the Medicare Physician Fee Schedule Database (MPFSDB). Pay for this service on the basis of the MPFSDB. Deductible and coinsurance apply. Claims from physicians or other practitioners where assignment was not taken, are subject to the Medicare limiting charge.

III. Medicare Summary Notices (MSNs)

Use the following MSN Messages where appropriate:

In situations where the claim is being denied on the basis that the condition does not meet our coverage requirements, use one of the following MSN Messages:

"Medicare does not pay for this item or service for this condition." (MSN Message 16.48)

The Spanish version of the MSN message should read:

"Medicare no paga por este articulo o servicio para esta afeccion."

In situations where, based on the above utilization policy, medical review of the claim results in a determination that the service is not medically necessary, use the following MSN message:

"The information provided does not support the need for this service or item." (MSN Message 15.4)

The Spanish version of the MSN message should read:

"La informacion proporcionada no confirma la necesidad para este servicio o articulo."

IV. Remittance Advice Notices

Use appropriate existing remittance advice remark codes and claim adjustment reason codes at the line level to express the specific reason if you deny payment for HBO therapy for the treatment of diabetic wounds of lower extremities.

100-04, 32, 60.4.1

Allowable Covered Diagnosis Codes

(Rev. 2998, Issued: 07-25-14, Effective: Upon implementation of ICD-10; 01-01-12 - ASC X12, Implementation: 08-25-2014 - ASC X12; Upon Implementation of ICD-10)

For services furnished on or after July 1, 2002, the applicable ICD-9-CM diagnosis code for this benefit is V43.3, organ or tissue replaced by other means; heart valve.

For services furnished on or after March 19, 2008, the applicable ICD-9-CM diagnosis codes for this benefit are:

- V43.3 (organ or tissue replaced by other means; heart valve),
- 289.81 (primary hypercoagulable state),
- 451.0-451.9 (includes 451.11, 451.19, 451.2, 451.80-451.84, 451.89) (phlebitis & thrombophlebitis),
- 453.0-453.3 (other venous embolism & thrombosis),
- 453.40-453.49 (includes 453.40-453.42, 453.8-453.9) (venous embolism and thrombosis of the deep vessels of the lower extremity, and other specified veins/unspecified sites)
- 415.11-415.12, 415.19 (pulmonary embolism & infarction) or,
- 427.31 (atrial fibrillation (established) (paroxysmal)).

For services furnished on or after the implementation of ICD-10 the applicable ICD-10-CM diagnosis codes for this benefit are:

Heart Valve Replacement

- Z95.2 - Presence of prosthetic heart valve

Primary Hypercoagulable State

ICD-10-CM	Code Description
D68.51	Activated protein C resistance
D68.52	Prothrombin gene mutation
D68.59	Other primary thrombophilia
D68.61	Antiphospholipid syndrome
D68.62	Lupus anticoagulant syndrome

Phlebitis & Thrombophlebitis

ICD-10-CM	Code Description
I8Ø.ØØ	Phlebitis and thrombophlebitis of superficial vessels of unspecified lower extremity
I8Ø.Ø1	Phlebitis and thrombophlebitis of superficial vessels of right lower extremity
I8Ø.Ø2	Phlebitis and thrombophlebitis of superficial vessels of left lower extremity
I8Ø.Ø3	Phlebitis and thrombophlebitis of superficial vessels of lower extremities, bilateral
I8Ø.1Ø	Phlebitis and thrombophlebitis of unspecified femoral vein
I8Ø.11	Phlebitis and thrombophlebitis of right femoral vein
I8Ø.12	Phlebitis and thrombophlebitis of left femoral vein
I8Ø.13	Phlebitis and thrombophlebitis of femoral vein, bilateral
I8Ø.2Ø1	Phlebitis and thrombophlebitis of unspecified deep vessels of right lower extremity
I8Ø.2Ø2	Phlebitis and thrombophlebitis of unspecified deep vessels of left lower extremity
I8Ø.2Ø3	Phlebitis and thrombophlebitis of unspecified deep vessels of lower extremities, bilateral
I8Ø.2Ø9	Phlebitis and thrombophlebitis of unspecified deep vessels of unspecified lower extremity
I8Ø.221	Phlebitis and thrombophlebitis of right popliteal vein
I8Ø.222	Phlebitis and thrombophlebitis of left popliteal vein
I8Ø.223	Phlebitis and thrombophlebitis of popliteal vein, bilateral
I8Ø.229	Phlebitis and thrombophlebitis of unspecified popliteal vein
I8Ø.231	Phlebitis and thrombophlebitis of right tibial vein
I8Ø.232	Phlebitis and thrombophlebitis of left tibial vein
I8Ø.233	Phlebitis and thrombophlebitis of tibial vein, bilateral
I8Ø.239	Phlebitis and thrombophlebitis of unspecified tibial vein
I8Ø.291	Phlebitis and thrombophlebitis of other deep vessels of right lower extremity
I8Ø.292	Phlebitis and thrombophlebitis of other deep vessels of left lower extremity
I8Ø.293	Phlebitis and thrombophlebitis of other deep vessels of lower extremity, bilateral
I8Ø.299	Phlebitis and thrombophlebitis of other deep vessels of unspecified lower extremity
I8Ø.3	Phlebitis and thrombophlebitis of lower extremities, unspecified
I8Ø.211	Phlebitis and thrombophlebitis of right iliac vein
I8Ø.212	Phlebitis and thrombophlebitis of left iliac vein
I8Ø.213	Phlebitis and thrombophlebitis of iliac vein, bilateral
I8Ø.219	Phlebitis and thrombophlebitis of unspecified iliac vein
I8Ø.8	Phlebitis and thrombophlebitis of other sites
I8Ø.9	Phlebitis and thrombophlebitis of unspecified site

Other Venous Embolism & Thrombosis

ICD-10-CM	Code Description
I82.Ø	Budd- Chiari syndrome
I82.1	Thrombophlebitis migrans
I82.211	Chronic embolism and thrombosis of superior vena cava
I82.22Ø	Acute embolism and thrombosis of inferior vena cava
I82.221	Chronic embolism and thrombosis of inferior vena cava
I82.291	Chronic embolism and thrombosis of other thoracic veins
I82.3	Embolism and thrombosis of renal vein

Venous Embolism and thrombosis of the deep vessels of the lower extremity, and other specified veins/unspecified sites

ICD-10-CM	Code Description
I82.4Ø1	Acute embolism and thrombosis of unspecified deep veins of right lower extremity
I82.4Ø2	Acute embolism and thrombosis of unspecified deep veins of left lower extremity
I82.4Ø3	Acute embolism and thrombosis of unspecified deep veins of lower extremity, bilateral
I82.4Ø9	Acute embolism and thrombosis of unspecified deep veins of unspecified lower extremity
I82.411	Acute embolism and thrombosis of right femoral vein
I82.412	Acute embolism and thrombosis of left femoral vein
I82.413	Acute embolism and thrombosis of femoral vein, bilateral
I82.419	Acute embolism and thrombosis of unspecified femoral vein
I82.421	Acute embolism and thrombosis of right iliac vein
I82.422	Acute embolism and thrombosis of left iliac vein
I82.423	Acute embolism and thrombosis of iliac vein, bilateral
I82.429	Acute embolism and thrombosis of unspecified iliac vein
I82.431	Acute embolism and thrombosis of right popliteal vein
I82.432	Acute embolism and thrombosis of left popliteal vein
I82.433	Acute embolism and thrombosis of popliteal vein, bilateral
I82.439	Acute embolism and thrombosis of unspecified popliteal vein
I82.4Y1	Acute embolism and thrombosis of unspecified deep veins of right proximal lower extremity
I82.4Y2	Acute embolism and thrombosis of unspecified deep veins of left proximal lower extremity
I82.4Y3	Acute embolism and thrombosis of unspecified deep veins of proximal lower extremity, bilateral
I82.4Y9	Acute embolism and thrombosis of unspecified deep veins of unspecified proximal lower extremity
I82.441	Acute embolism and thrombosis of right tibial vein
I82.442	Acute embolism and thrombosis of left tibial vein
I82.443	Acute embolism and thrombosis of tibial vein, bilateral
I82.449	Acute embolism and thrombosis of unspecified tibial vein
I82.491	Acute embolism and thrombosis of other specified deep vein of right lower extremity
I82.492	Acute embolism and thrombosis of other specified deep vein of left lower extremity
I82.493	Acute embolism and thrombosis of other specified deep vein of lower extremity, bilateral
I82.499	Acute embolism and thrombosis of other specified deep vein of unspecified lower extremity
I82.4Z1	Acute embolism and thrombosis of unspecified deep veins of right distal lower extremity
I82.4Z2	Acute embolism and thrombosis of unspecified deep veins of left distal lower extremity
I82.4Z3	Acute embolism and thrombosis of unspecified deep veins of distal lower extremity, bilateral
I82.4Z9	Acute embolism and thrombosis of unspecified deep veins of unspecified distal lower extremity
I82.5Ø1	Chronic embolism and thrombosis of unspecified deep veins of right lower extremity

ICD-10-CM	Code Description
I82.5Ø2	Chronic embolism and thrombosis of unspecified deep veins of left lower extremity
I82.5Ø3	Chronic embolism and thrombosis of unspecified deep veins of lower extremity, bilateral
I82.5Ø9	Chronic embolism and thrombosis of unspecified deep veins of unspecified lower extremity
I82.591	Chronic embolism and thrombosis of other specified deep vein of right lower extremity
I82.592	Chronic embolism and thrombosis of other specified deep vein of left lower extremity
I82.593	Chronic embolism and thrombosis of other specified deep vein of lower extremity, bilateral
I82.599	Chronic embolism and thrombosis of other specified deep vein of unspecified lower extremity
I82.511	Chronic embolism and thrombosis of right femoral vein
I82.512	Chronic embolism and thrombosis of left femoral vein
I82.513	Chronic embolism and thrombosis of femoral vein, bilateral
I82.519	Chronic embolism and thrombosis of unspecified femoral vein
I82.521	Chronic embolism and thrombosis of right iliac vein
I82.522	Chronic embolism and thrombosis of left iliac vein
I82.523	Chronic embolism and thrombosis of iliac vein, bilateral
I82.529	Chronic embolism and thrombosis of unspecified iliac vein
I82.531	Chronic embolism and thrombosis of right popliteal vein
I82.532	Chronic embolism and thrombosis of left popliteal vein
I82.533	Chronic embolism and thrombosis of popliteal vein, bilateral
I82.539	Chronic embolism and thrombosis of unspecified popliteal vein
I82.5Y1	Chronic embolism and thrombosis of unspecified deep veins of right proximal lower extremity
I82.5Y2	Chronic embolism and thrombosis of unspecified deep veins of left proximal lower extremity
I82.5Y3	Chronic embolism and thrombosis of unspecified deep veins of proximal lower extremity, bilateral
I82.5Y9	Chronic embolism and thrombosis of unspecified deep veins of unspecified proximal lower extremity
I82.541	Chronic embolism and thrombosis of right tibial vein
I82.542	Chronic embolism and thrombosis of left tibial vein
I82.543	Chronic embolism and thrombosis of tibial vein, bilateral
I82.549	Chronic embolism and thrombosis of unspecified tibial vein
I82.5Z1	Chronic embolism and thrombosis of unspecified deep veins of right distal lower extremity
I82.5Z2	Chronic embolism and thrombosis of unspecified deep veins of left distal lower extremity
I82.5Z3	Chronic embolism and thrombosis of unspecified deep veins of distal lower extremity, bilateral
I82.5Z9	Chronic embolism and thrombosis of unspecified deep veins of unspecified distal lower extremity
I82.611	Acute embolism and thrombosis of superficial veins of right upper extremity
I82.612	Acute embolism and thrombosis of superficial veins of left upper extremity
I82.613	Acute embolism and thrombosis of superficial veins of upper extremity, bilateral
I82.619	Acute embolism and thrombosis of superficial veins of unspecified upper extremity
I82.621	Acute embolism and thrombosis of deep veins of right upper extremity
I82.622	Acute embolism and thrombosis of deep veins of left upper extremity
I82.623	Acute embolism and thrombosis of deep veins of upper extremity, bilateral
I82.629	Acute embolism and thrombosis of deep veins of unspecified upper extremity
I82.6Ø1	Acute embolism and thrombosis of unspecified veins of right upper extremity
I82.6Ø2	Acute embolism and thrombosis of unspecified veins of left upper extremity
I82.6Ø3	Acute embolism and thrombosis of unspecified veins of upper extremity, bilateral
I82.6Ø9	Acute embolism and thrombosis of unspecified veins of unspecified upper extremity
I82.A11	Acute embolism and thrombosis of right axillary vein
I82.A12	Acute embolism and thrombosis of left axillary vein

ICD-10-CM	Code Description
I82.A13	Acute embolism and thrombosis of axillary vein, bilateral
I82.A19	Acute embolism and thrombosis of unspecified axillary vein
I82.A21	Chronic embolism and thrombosis of right axillary vein
I82.A22	Chronic embolism and thrombosis of left axillary vein
I82.A23	Chronic embolism and thrombosis of axillary vein, bilateral
I82.A29	Chronic embolism and thrombosis of unspecified axillary vein
I82.B11	Acute embolism and thrombosis of right subclavian vein
I82.B12	Acute embolism and thrombosis of left subclavian vein
I82.B13	Acute embolism and thrombosis of subclavian vein, bilateral
I82.B19	Acute embolism and thrombosis of unspecified subclavian vein
I82.B21	Chronic embolism and thrombosis of right subclavian vein
I82.B22	Chronic embolism and thrombosis of left subclavian vein
I82.B23	Chronic embolism and thrombosis of subclavian vein, bilateral
I82.B29	Chronic embolism and thrombosis of unspecified subclavian vein
I82.C11	Acute embolism and thrombosis of right internal jugular vein
I82.C12	Acute embolism and thrombosis of left internal jugular vein
I82.C13	Acute embolism and thrombosis of internal jugular vein, bilateral
I82.C19	Acute embolism and thrombosis of unspecified internal jugular vein
I82.C21	Chronic embolism and thrombosis of right internal jugular vein
I82.C22	Chronic embolism and thrombosis of left internal jugular vein
I82.C23	Chronic embolism and thrombosis of internal jugular vein, bilateral
I82.C29	Chronic embolism and thrombosis of unspecified internal jugular vein
I82.21Ø	Acute embolism and thrombosis of superior vena cava
I82.29Ø	Acute embolism and thrombosis of other thoracic veins
I82.7Ø1	Chronic embolism and thrombosis of unspecified veins of right upper extremity
I82.7Ø2	Chronic embolism and thrombosis of unspecified veins of left upper extremity
I82.7Ø3	Chronic embolism and thrombosis of unspecified veins of upper extremity, bilateral
I82.7Ø9	Chronic embolism and thrombosis of unspecified veins of unspecified upper extremity
I82.711	Chronic embolism and thrombosis of superficial veins of right upper extremity
I82.712	Chronic embolism and thrombosis of superficial veins of left upper extremity
I82.713	Chronic embolism and thrombosis of superficial veins of upper extremity, bilateral
I82.719	Chronic embolism and thrombosis of superficial veins of unspecified upper extremity
I82.721	Chronic embolism and thrombosis of deep veins of right upper extremity
I82.722	Chronic embolism and thrombosis of deep veins of left upper extremity
I82.723	Chronic embolism and thrombosis of deep veins of upper extremity, bilateral
I82.729	Chronic embolism and thrombosis of deep veins of unspecified upper extremity
I82.811	Embolism and thrombosis of superficial veins of right lower extremities
I82.812	Embolism and thrombosis of superficial veins of left lower extremities
I82.813	Embolism and thrombosis of superficial veins of lower extremities, bilateral
I82.819	Embolism and thrombosis of superficial veins of unspecified lower extremities
I82.89Ø	Acute embolism and thrombosis of other specified veins
I82.891	Chronic embolism and thrombosis of other specified veins
I82.9Ø	Acute embolism and thrombosis of unspecified vein
I82.91	Chronic embolism and thrombosis of unspecified vein

Pulmonary Embolism & Infarction

ICD-10-CM	Code Description
I26.9Ø	Septic pulmonary embolism without acute cor pulmonale
I26.99	Other pulmonary embolism without acute cor pulmonale
I26.Ø1	Septic pulmonary embolism with acute cor pulmonale
I26.9Ø	Septic pulmonary embolism without acute cor pulmonale
I26.Ø9	Other pulmonary embolism with acute cor pulmonale
I26.99	Other pulmonary embolism without acute cor pulmonale

Atrial Fibrillation

ICD-10-CM	Code Description
I48.Ø	Paroxysmal atrial fibrillation
I48.2	Chronic atrial fibrillation
I48	-91 Unspecified atrial fibrillation Other
I23.6	Thrombosis of atrium, auricular appendage, and ventricle as current complications following acute myocardial infarction
I27.82	Chronic pulmonary embolism
I67.6	Nonpyogenic thrombosis of intracranial venous system
O22.5Ø	Cerebral venous thrombosis in pregnancy, unspecified trimester
O22.51	Cerebral venous thrombosis in pregnancy, first trimester
O22.52	Cerebral venous thrombosis in pregnancy, second trimester
O22.53	Cerebral venous thrombosis in pregnancy, third trimester
O87.3	Cerebral venous thrombosis in the puerperium
Z79.Ø1	Long term (current) use of anticoagulants

Coverage policy can be found in Pub. 100-3, Medicare National Coverage Determinations Manual, Chapter 1, section 190.11 PT/INR. (http://www.cms.hhs.gov/manuals/103_cov_determ/ncd103index.asp

100-04, 32, 60.5.2

Applicable Diagnosis Codes for A/B Macs

(Rev. 2998, Issued: 07-25-14, Effective: Upon implementation of ICD-10; 01-01-12 - ASC X12, Implementation: 08-25-2014 - ASC X12; Upon Implementation of ICD-10)

For services furnished on or after July 1, 2002, the applicable ICD-9-CM diagnosis code for this benefit is V43.3, organ or tissue replaced by other means; heart valve.

For services furnished on or after March 19, 2008, the applicable ICD-9-CM diagnosis codes for this benefit are:

- V43.3 (organ or tissue replaced by other means; heart valve),
- 289.81 (primary hypercoagulable state),
- 451.0-451.9 (includes 451.11, 451.19, 451.2, 451.80-451.84, 451.89) (phlebitis & thrombophlebitis),
- 453.0-453.3 (other venous embolism & thrombosis),
- 453.40-453.49 (includes 453.40-453.42,'453.8-453.9) (venous embolism and thrombosis of the deep vessels of the lower extremity, and other specified veins/unspecified sites)
- 415.11-415.12, 415.19 (pulmonary embolism & infarction) or,
- 427.31 (atrial fibrillation (established) (paroxysmal)).

For services furnished on or after implementation of ICD-10 the applicable ICD-10-CM diagnosis codes for this benefit are:

Heart Valve Replacement

- Z95.2 - Presence of prosthetic heart valve

Primary Hypercoagulable State

ICD-10-CM	Code Description
D68.51	Activated protein C resistance
D68.52	Prothrombin gene mutation
D68.59	Other primary thrombophilia
D68.61	Antiphospholipid syndrome
D68.62	Lupus anticoagulant syndrome

Phlebitis & Thrombophlebitis

ICD-10-CM	Code Description
I8Ø.ØØ	Phlebitis and thrombophlebitis of superficial vessels of unspecified lower extremity
I8Ø.Ø1	Phlebitis and thrombophlebitis of superficial vessels of right lower extremity
I8Ø.Ø2	Phlebitis and thrombophlebitis of superficial vessels of left lower extremity
I8Ø.Ø3	Phlebitis and thrombophlebitis of superficial vessels of lower extremities, bilateral
I8Ø.1Ø	Phlebitis and thrombophlebitis of unspecified femoral vein
I8Ø.11	Phlebitis and thrombophlebitis of right femoral vein
I8Ø.12	Phlebitis and thrombophlebitis of left femoral vein
I8Ø.13	Phlebitis and thrombophlebitis of femoral vein, bilateral
I8Ø.2Ø1	Phlebitis and thrombophlebitis of unspecified deep vessels of right lower extremity
I8Ø.2Ø2	Phlebitis and thrombophlebitis of unspecified deep vessels of left lower extremity
I8Ø.2Ø3	Phlebitis and thrombophlebitis of unspecified deep vessels of lower extremities, bilateral
I8Ø.2Ø9	Phlebitis and thrombophlebitis of unspecified deep vessels of unspecified lower extremity
I8Ø.221	Phlebitis and thrombophlebitis of right popliteal vein
I8Ø.222	Phlebitis and thrombophlebitis of left popliteal vein
I8Ø.223	Phlebitis and thrombophlebitis of popliteal vein, bilateral
I8Ø.229	Phlebitis and thrombophlebitis of unspecified popliteal vein
I8Ø.231	Phlebitis and thrombophlebitis of right tibial vein
I8Ø.232	Phlebitis and thrombophlebitis of left tibial vein
I8Ø.233	Phlebitis and thrombophlebitis of tibial vein, bilateral
I8Ø.239	Phlebitis and thrombophlebitis of unspecified tibial vein
I8Ø.291	Phlebitis and thrombophlebitis of other deep vessels of right lower extremity
I8Ø.292	Phlebitis and thrombophlebitis of other deep vessels of left lower extremity
I8Ø.293	Phlebitis and thrombophlebitis of other deep vessels of lower extremity, bilateral
I8Ø.299	Phlebitis and thrombophlebitis of other deep vessels of unspecified lower extremity
I8Ø.3	Phlebitis and thrombophlebitis of lower extremities, unspecified
I8Ø.211	Phlebitis and thrombophlebitis of right iliac vein
I8Ø.212	Phlebitis and thrombophlebitis of left iliac vein
I8Ø.213	Phlebitis and thrombophlebitis of iliac vein, bilateral
I8Ø.219	Phlebitis and thrombophlebitis of unspecified iliac vein
I8Ø.8	Phlebitis and thrombophlebitis of other sites
I8Ø.9	Phlebitis and thrombophlebitis of unspecified site

Other Venous Embolism & Thrombosis

ICD-10-CM	Code Description
I82.0	Budd- Chiari syndrome
I82.1	Thrombophlebitis migrans
I82.211	Chronic embolism and thrombosis of superior vena cava
I82220	Acute embolism and thrombosis of inferior vena cava
I82.221	Chronic embolism and thrombosis of inferior vena cava
I82.291	Chronic embolism and thrombosis of other thoracic veins
I82.3	Embolism and thrombosis of renal vein

Venous Embolism and thrombosis of the deep vessels of the lower extremity, and other specified veins/unspecified sites

ICD-10-CM	Code Description
I82.4Ø1	Acute embolism and thrombosis of unspecified deep veins of right lower extremity
I82.4Ø2	Acute embolism and thrombosis of unspecified deep veins of left lower extremity
I82.4Ø3	Acute embolism and thrombosis of unspecified deep veins of lower extremity, bilateral
I82. 4Ø9	Acute embolism and thrombosis of unspecified deep veins of unspecified lower extremity
I82.411	Acute embolism and thrombosis of right femoral vein
I82.412	Acute embolism and thrombosis of left femoral vein
I82.413	Acute embolism and thrombosis of femoral vein, bilateral
I82.419	Acute embolism and thrombosis of unspecified femoral vein
I82.421	Acute embolism and thrombosis of right iliac vein
I82.422	Acute embolism and thrombosis of left iliac vein
I82.423	Acute embolism and thrombosis of iliac vein, bilateral
I82.429	Acute embolism and thrombosis of unspecified iliac vein
I82.431	Acute embolism and thrombosis of right popliteal vein
I82.432	Acute embolism and thrombosis of left popliteal vein
I82.433	Acute embolism and thrombosis of popliteal vein, bilateral
I82.439	Acute embolism and thrombosis of unspecified popliteal vein
I82.4Y1	Acute embolism and thrombosis of unspecified deep veins of right proximal lower extremity
I82.4Y2	Acute embolism and thrombosis of unspecified deep veins of left proximal lower extremity
I82.4Y3	Acute embolism and thrombosis of unspecified deep veins of proximal lower extremity, bilateral
I82.4Y9	Acute embolism and thrombosis of unspecified deep veins of unspecified proximal lower extremity
I82.441	Acute embolism and thrombosis of right tibial vein
I82.442	Acute embolism and thrombosis of left tibial vein

ICD-10-CM	Code Description
I82.443	Acute embolism and thrombosis of tibial vein, bilateral
I82.449	Acute embolism and thrombosis of unspecified tibial vein
I82.491	Acute embolism and thrombosis of other specified deep vein of right lower extremity
I82.492	Acute embolism and thrombosis of other specified deep vein of left lower extremity
I82.493	Acute embolism and thrombosis of other specified deep vein of lower extremity, bilateral
I82.499	Acute embolism and thrombosis of other specified deep vein of unspecified lower extremity
I82.4Z1	Acute embolism and thrombosis of unspecified deep veins of right distal lower extremity
I82.4Z2	Acute embolism and thrombosis of unspecified deep veins of left distal lower extremity
I82.4Z3	Acute embolism and thrombosis of unspecified deep veins of distal lower extremity, bilateral
I82.4Z9	Acute embolism and thrombosis of unspecified deep veins of unspecified distal lower extremity
I82.501	Chronic embolism and thrombosis of unspecified deep veins of right lower extremity
I82.502	Chronic embolism and thrombosis of unspecified deep veins of left lower extremity
I82.503	Chronic embolism and thrombosis of unspecified deep veins of lower extremity, bilateral
I82.509	Chronic embolism and thrombosis of unspecified deep veins of unspecified lower extremity
I82.591	Chronic embolism and thrombosis of other specified deep vein of right lower extremity
I82.592	Chronic embolism and thrombosis of other specified deep vein of left lower extremity
I82.593	Chronic embolism and thrombosis of other specified deep vein of lower extremity, bilateral
I82.599	Chronic embolism and thrombosis of other specified deep vein of unspecified lower extremity
I82.511	Chronic embolism and thrombosis of right femoral vein
I82.512	Chronic embolism and thrombosis of left femoral vein
I82.513	Chronic embolism and thrombosis of femoral vein, bilateral
I82.519	Chronic embolism and thrombosis of unspecified femoral vein
I82.521	Chronic embolism and thrombosis of right iliac vein
I82.522	Chronic embolism and thrombosis of left iliac vein
I82.523	Chronic embolism and thrombosis of iliac vein, bilateral
I82.529	Chronic embolism and thrombosis of unspecified iliac vein
I82.531	Chronic embolism and thrombosis of right popliteal vein
I82.532	Chronic embolism and thrombosis of left popliteal vein
I82.533	Chronic embolism and thrombosis of popliteal vein, bilateral
I82.539	Chronic embolism and thrombosis of unspecified popliteal vein
I82.5Y1	Chronic embolism and thrombosis of unspecified deep veins of right proximal lower extremity
I82.5Y2	Chronic embolism and thrombosis of unspecified deep veins of left proximal lower extremity
I82.5Y3	Chronic embolism and thrombosis of unspecified deep veins of proximal lower extremity, bilateral
I82.5Y9	Chronic embolism and thrombosis of unspecified deep veins of unspecified proximal lower extremity
I82.541	Chronic embolism and thrombosis of right tibial vein
I82.42	Chronic embolism and thrombosis of left tibial vein
I82.543	Chronic embolism and thrombosis of tibial vein, bilateral
I82.549	Chronic embolism and thrombosis of unspecified tibial vein
I82.5Z1	Chronic embolism and thrombosis of unspecified deep veins of right distal lower extremity
I82.5Z2	Chronic embolism and thrombosis of unspecified deep veins of left distal lower extremity
I82.5Z3	Chronic embolism and thrombosis of unspecified deep veins of distal lower extremity, bilateral
I82.5Z9	Chronic embolism and thrombosis of unspecified deep veins of unspecified distal lower extremity
I82.611	Acute embolism and thrombosis of superficial veins of right upper extremity
I82.612	Acute embolism and thrombosis of superficial veins of left upper extremity

ICD-10-CM	Code Description
I82.613	Acute embolism and thrombosis of superficial veins of upper extremity, bilateral
I82.619	Acute embolism and thrombosis of superficial veins of unspecified upper extremity
I82.621	Acute embolism and thrombosis of deep veins of right upper extremity
I82.622	Acute embolism and thrombosis of deep veins of left upper extremity
I82.623	Acute embolism and thrombosis of deep veins of upper extremity, bilateral
I82.629	Acute embolism and thrombosis of deep veins of unspecified upper extremity
I82.601	Acute embolism and thrombosis of unspecified veins of right upper extremity
I82.602	Acute embolism and thrombosis of unspecified veins of left upper extremity
I82.603	Acute embolism and thrombosis of unspecified veins of upper extremity, bilateral
I82.609	Acute embolism and thrombosis of unspecified veins of unspecified upper extremity
I82.A11	Acute embolism and thrombosis of right axillary vein
I82.A12	Acute embolism and thrombosis of left axillary vein
I82.A13	Acute embolism and thrombosis of axillary vein, bilateral
I82.A19	Acute embolism and thrombosis of unspecified axillary vein
I82.A21	Chronic embolism and thrombosis of right axillary vein
I82.A22	Chronic embolism and thrombosis of left axillary vein
I82.A23	Chronic embolism and thrombosis of axillary vein, bilateral
I82.A29	Chronic embolism and thrombosis of unspecified axillary vein
I82.B11	Acute embolism and thrombosis of right subclavian vein
I82.B12	Acute embolism and thrombosis of left subclavian vein
I82.B13	Acute embolism and thrombosis of subclavian vein, bilateral
I82.B19	Acute embolism and thrombosis of unspecified subclavian vein
I82.B21	Chronic embolism and thrombosis of right subclavian vein
I82.B22	Chronic embolism and thrombosis of left subclavian vein
I82.B23	Chronic embolism and thrombosis of subclavian vein, bilateral
I82.B29	Chronic embolism and thrombosis of unspecified subclavian vein
I82.C11	Acute embolism and thrombosis of right internal jugular vein
I82.C12	Acute embolism and thrombosis of left internal jugular vein
I82.C13	Acute embolism and thrombosis of internal jugular vein, bilateral
I82.C19	Acute embolism and thrombosis of unspecified internal jugular vein
I82.C21	Chronic embolism and thrombosis of right internal jugular vein
I82.C22	Chronic embolism and thrombosis of left internal jugular vein
I82.C23	Chronic embolism and thrombosis of internal jugular vein, bilateral
I82.C29	Chronic embolism and thrombosis of unspecified internal jugular vein
I82.210	Acute embolism and thrombosis of superior vena cava
I82.290	Acute embolism and thrombosis of other thoracic veins
I82.701	Chronic embolism and thrombosis of unspecified veins of right upper extremity
I82.702	Chronic embolism and thrombosis of unspecified veins of left upper extremity
I82.703	Chronic embolism and thrombosis of unspecified veins of upper extremity, bilateral
I82.709	Chronic embolism and thrombosis of unspecified veins of unspecified upper extremity
I82.711	Chronic embolism and thrombosis of superficial veins of right upper extremity
I82.712	Chronic embolism and thrombosis of superficial veins of left upper extremity
I82.713	Chronic embolism and thrombosis of superficial veins of upper extremity, bilateral
I82.719	Chronic embolism and thrombosis of superficial veins of unspecified upper extremity
I82.721	Chronic embolism and thrombosis of deep veins of right upper extremity
I82.722	Chronic embolism and thrombosis of deep veins of left upper extremity
I82.723	Chronic embolism and thrombosis of deep veins of upper extremity, bilateral
I82.729	Chronic embolism and thrombosis of deep veins of unspecified upper extremity

ICD-10-CM	Code Description
I82.811	Embolism and thrombosis of superficial veins of right lower extremities
I82.812	Embolism and thrombosis of superficial veins of left lower extremities
I82.813	Embolism and thrombosis of superficial veins of lower extremities, bilateral
I82.819	Embolism and thrombosis of superficial veins of unspecified lower extremities
I82.890	Acute embolism and thrombosis of other specified veins
I82.891	Chronic embolism and thrombosis of other specified veins
I82.90	Acute embolism and thrombosis of unspecified vein
I82.91	Chronic embolism and thrombosis of unspecified vein

Pulmonary Embolism & Infarction

ICD-10-CM	Code Description
I26.01	Septic pulmonary embolism with acute cor pulmonale
I26.90	Septic pulmonary embolism without acute cor pulmonale
I26.09	Other pulmonary embolism with acute cor pulmonale
I26.99	Other pulmonary embolism without acute cor pulmonale

Atrial Fibrillation

ICD-10-CM	Code Description
I48.0	Paroxysmal atrial fibrillation
I48.2	Chronic atrial fibrillation
I48.	-91 Unspecified atrial fibrillation Other
I23.6	Thrombosis of atrium, auricular appendage, and ventricle as current complications following acute myocardial infarction
I27.82	Chronic pulmonary embolism
I67.6	Nonpyogenic thrombosis of intracranial venous system
O22.50	Cerebral venous thrombosis in pregnancy, unspecified trimester
O22.51	Cerebral venous thrombosis in pregnancy, first trimester
O22.52	Cerebral venous thrombosis in pregnancy, second trimester
O22.53	Cerebral venous thrombosis in pregnancy, third trimester
O87.3	Cerebral venous thrombosis in the puerperium
Z79.01	Long term (current) use of anticoagulants
Z86.718	Personal history of other venous thrombosis and embolism
Z95.4	Presence of other heart

Coverage policy can be found in Pub. 100-3, Medicare National Coverage Determinations Manual, Chapter 1, section 190.11 PT/INR. (http://www.cms.hhs.gov/manuals/103_cov_determ/ncd103index.asp

100-04, 32, 80.8

CWF Utilization Edits

(Rev. 1742, Issued: 05-22-09, Effective: 06-08-09, Implementation: 06-08-09)

Edit 1

Should CWF receive a claim from an FI for G0245 or G0246 and a second claim from a contractor for either G0245 or G0246 (or vice versa) and they are different dates of service and less than 6 months apart, the second claim will reject. CWF will edit to allow G0245 or G0246 to be paid no more than every 6 months for a particular beneficiary, regardless of who furnished the service. If G0245 has been paid, regardless of whether it was posted as a facility or professional claim, it must be 6 months before G0245 can be paid again or G0246 can be paid. If G0246 has been paid, regardless of whether it was posted as a facility or professional claim, it must be 6 months before G0246 can be paid again or G0245 can be paid. CWF will not impose limits on how many times each code can be paid for a beneficiary as long as there has been 6 months between each service.

The CWF will return a specific reject code for this edit to the contractors and FIs that will be identified in the CWF documentation. Based on the CWF reject code, the contractors and FIs must deny the claims and return the following messages:

> MSN 18.4 -- This service is being denied because it has not been __ months since your last examination of this kind (NOTE: Insert 6 as the appropriate number of months.)
>
> RA claim adjustment reason code 96 - Non-covered charges, along with remark code M86 - Service denied because payment already made for same/similar procedure within set time frame.

Edit 2

The CWF will edit to allow G0247 to pay only if either G0245 or G0246 has been submitted and accepted as payable on the same date of service. CWF will return a specific reject code for this edit to the contractors and FIs that will be identified in the CWF documentation. Based on this reject code, contractors and FIs will deny the claims and return the following messages:

> MSN 21.21 - This service was denied because Medicare only covers this service under certain circumstances.
>
> RA claim adjustment reason code 107 - The related or qualifying claim/service was not identified on this claim.

Edit 3

Once a beneficiary's condition has progressed to the point where routine foot care becomes a covered service, payment will no longer be made for LOPS evaluation and management services. Those services would be considered to be included in the regular exams and treatments afforded to the beneficiary on a routine basis. The physician or provider must then just bill the routine foot care codes, per Pub 100-2, Chapter 15, Sec. 290.

The CWF will edit to reject LOPS codes G0245, G0246, and/or G0247 when on the beneficiary's record it shows that one of the following routine foot care codes were billed and paid within the prior 6 months: 11055, 11056, 11057, 11719, 11720, and/or 11721.

The CWF will return a specific reject code for this edit to the contractors and FIs that will be identified in the CWF documentation. Based on the CWF reject code, the contractors and FIs must deny the claims and return the following messages:

> MSN 21.21 - This service was denied because Medicare only covers this service under certain circumstances.
>
> The RA claim adjustment reason code 96 - Non-covered charges, along with remark code M86 - Service denied because payment already made for same/similar procedure within set time frame.

100-04, 32, 90

Stem Cell Transplantation

(Rev. 3556, Issued: 07-01-2016; Effective: 1-27-16; Implementation: 10-3-16)

A. General

Stem cell transplantation is a process in which stem cells are harvested from either a patient's (autologous) or donor's (allogeneic) bone marrow or peripheral blood for intravenous infusion.

Allogeneic and autologous stem cell transplants are covered under Medicare for specific diagnoses. See Pub. 100-03, National Coverage Determinations Manual, section 110.23, for a complete description of covered and noncovered conditions. For Part A hospital inpatient claims processing instructions, refer to Pub. 100-04, Chapter 3, section 90. The following sections contain claims processing instructions for all other claims.

B. Nationally Covered Indications

I. Allogeneic Hematopoietic Stem Cell Transplantation (HSCT)

HCPCS Code 38240

ICD-9-CM Procedure Codes 41.02, 41.03, 41.05, and 41.08

ICD-10-PCS Procedure Codes 30230G1, 30230Y1, 30233G1, 30233Y1, 30240G1, 30240Y1, 30243G1, 30243Y1, 30250G1, 30250Y1, 30253G1, 30253Y1, 30260G1, 30260Y1, 30263G1, and 30263Y1

a. Effective for services performed on or after August 1, 1978:

    i. For the treatment of leukemia, leukemia in remission (ICD-9-CM codes 204.00 through 208.91; see table below for ICD-10-CM codes)

ICD-10	Description
C91.01	Acute lymphoblastic leukemia, in remission
C91.11	Chronic lymphocytic leukemia of B-cell type in remission
C91.31	Prolymphocytic leukemia of B-cell type, in remission
C91.51	Adult T-cell lymphoma/leukemia (HTLV-1-associated), in remission
C91.61	Prolymphocytic leukemia of T-cell type, in remission
C91.91	Lymphoid leukemia, unspecified, in remission
C91.A1	Mature B-cell leukemia Burkitt-type, in remission
C91.Z1	Other lymphoid leukemia, in remission
C92.01	Acute myeloblastic leukemia, in remission
C92.11	Chronic myeloid leukemia, BCR/ABL-positive, in remission
C92.21	Atypical chronic myeloid leukemia, BCR/ABL-negative, in remission
C92.31	Myeloid sarcoma, in remission
C92.41	Acute promyelocytic leukemia, in remission
C92.51	Acute myelomonocytic leukemia, in remission
C92.61	Acute myeloid leukemia with 11q23-abnormality in remission
C92.91	Myeloid leukemia, unspecified in remission
C92.A1	Acute myeloid leukemia with multilineage dysplasia, in remission
C92.Z1	Other myeloid leukemia, in remission
C93.01	Acute monoblastic/monocytic leukemia, in remission
C93.11	Chronic myelomonocytic leukemia, in remission
C93.31	Juvenile myelomonocytic leukemia, in remission
C93.91	Monocytic leukemia, unspecified in remission

ICD-10	Description
C93.Z1	Other monocytic leukemia, in remission
C94.01	Acute erythroid leukemia, in remission
C94.21	Acute megakaryoblastic leukemia, in remission
C94.31	Mast cell leukemia, in remission
C94.81	Other specified leukemias, in remission
C95.01	Acute leukemia of unspecified cell type, in remission
C95.11	Chronic leukemia of unspecified cell type, in remission
C95.91	Leukemia, unspecified, in remission
D45	Polycythemia vera

ii. For the treatment of aplastic anemia (ICD-9-CM codes 284.0 through 284.9; see table below for ICD-10-CM codes)

ICD-10	Description
D60.0	Chronic acquired pure red cell aplasia
D60.1	Transient acquired pure red cell aplasia
D60.8	Other acquired pure red cell aplasias
D60.9	Acquired pure red cell aplasia, unspecified
D61.01	Constitutional (pure) red blood cell aplasia
D61.09	Other constitutional aplastic anemia
D61.1	Drug-induced aplastic anemia
D61.2	Aplastic anemia due to other external agents
D61.3	Idiopathic aplastic anemia
D61.810	Antineoplastic chemotherapy induced pancytopenia
D61.811	Other drug-induced pancytopenia
D61.818	Other pancytopenia
D61.82	Myelophthisis
D61.89	Other specified aplastic anemias and other bone marrow failure syndromes
D61.9	Aplastic anemia, unspecified

b. Effective for services performed on or after June 3, 1985:

i. For the treatment of severe combined immunodeficiency disease (SCID) (ICD-9-CM code 279.2; ICD-10-CM codes D81.0, D81.1, D81.2, D81.6, D81.7, D81.89, and D81.9). ii. For the treatment of Wiskott-Aldrich syndrome (ICD-9-CM code 279.12; ICD-10-CM code D82.0)

c. Effective for services performed on or after August 4, 2010: For the treatment of Myelodysplastic Syndromes (MDS) (ICD-9-CM codes 238.72, 238.73, 238.74, 238.75 and ICD-10-CM codes D46.A, D46.B, D46.C, D46.0, D46.1, D46.20, D46.21, D46.22, D46.4, D46.9, D46.Z) pursuant to Coverage with Evidence Development (CED) in the context of a Medicare-approved, prospective clinical study. Refer to Pub. 100-03, NCD Manual, chapter 1, section 110.23, for further information about this policy. See section F below for billing instructions.

d. Effective for services performed on or after January 27, 2016:

i. Allogeneic HSCT for multiple myeloma (ICD-10-CM codes C90.00, C90.01, and C90.02) is covered by Medicare only for beneficiaries with Durie-Salmon Stage II or III multiple myeloma, or International Staging System (ISS) Stage II or Stage III multiple myeloma, and participating in an approved prospective clinical study. Refer to Pub. 100-03, NCD Manual, chapter 1, section 110.23, for further information about this policy. See section F below for billing instructions.

ii. Allogeneic HSCT for myelofibrosis (MF) (ICD-10-CM codes C94.40, C94.41, C94.42, D47.4, and D75.81) is covered by Medicare only for beneficiaries with Dynamic International Prognostic Scoring System (DIPSSplus) intermediate-2 or High primary or secondary MF and participating in an approved prospective clinical study. Refer to Pub. 100-03, NCD Manual, chapter 1, section 110.23, for further information about this policy. See section F below for billing instructions.

iii. Allogeneic HSCT for sickle cell disease (SCD) (ICD-10-CM codes D57.00, D57.01, D57.02, D57.1, D57.20, D57.211, D57.212, D57.219, D57.40, D57.411, D57.412, D57.419, D57.80, D57.811, D57.812, and D57.819) is covered by Medicare only for beneficiaries with severe, symptomatic SCD who participate in an approved prospective clinical study. Refer to Pub. 100-03, NCD Manual, chapter 1, section 110.23, for further information about this policy. See section F below for billing instructions.

II. Autologous Stem Cell Transplantation (AuSCT)

HCPCS Code 38241

ICD-9-CM Procedure Codes 41.01, 41.04, 41.07, and 41.09;

ICD-10-PCS Procedure Codes 30230AZ, 30230G0, 30230Y0, 30233G0, 30233Y0, 30240G0, 30240Y0, 30243G0, 30243Y0, 30250G0, 30250Y0, 30253G0, 30253Y0, 30260G0, 30260Y0, 30263G0, and 30263Y0

a. Effective for services performed on or after April 28, 1989: Acute leukemia in remission who have a high probability of relapse and who have no human leucocyte antigens (HLA)-matched (ICD-9-CM codes 204.01, 205.01, 206.01, 207.01, 208.01; ICD-10-CM diagnosis codes C91.01, C92.01, C92,41, C92.51, C92.61, C92.A1, C93.01, C94.01, C94.21, C94.41, C95.01); Resistant non-Hodgkin's lymphomas or those presenting with poor prognostic features following an initial response (ICD-9-CM codes 200.00 - 200.08, 200.10-200.18, 200.20-200.28, 200.80-200.88, 202.00-202.08, 202.80-202.88 or 202.90-202.98; ICD-10-CM diagnosis codes C82.00-C85.29, C85.80-C86.6, C96.4, and C96.Z-C96.9); Recurrent or refractory neuroblastoma (see ICD-9-CM codes Neoplasm by site, malignant for the appropriate diagnosis code; if ICD-10-CM is applicable the following ranges are reported: C00 - C96, and D00 - D09 Resistant non-Hodgkin's lymphomas); or, Advanced Hodgkin's disease who have failed conventional therapy and have no HLA-matched donor (ICD-9-CM codes 201.00 - 201.98; ICD-10-CM codes C81.00 - C81.99).

b. Effective for services performed on or after October 1, 2000: Single AuSCT is only covered for Durie-Salmon Stage II or III multiple myeloma patients (ICD-9-CM codes 203.00 or 238.6; ICD-10-CM codes C90.00, C90.01, C90.02 and D47.Z9) that fit the following requirements:

- Newly diagnosed or responsive multiple myeloma. This includes those patients with previously untreated disease, those with at least a partial response to prior chemotherapy (defined as a 50% decrease either in measurable paraprotein [serum and/or urine] or in bone marrow infiltration, sustained for at least 1 month), and those in responsive relapse; and • Adequate cardiac, renal, pulmonary, and hepatic function.

c. Effective for services performed on or after March 15, 2005: When recognized clinical risk factors are employed to select patients for transplantation, high dose melphalan (HDM) together with AuSCT is reasonable and necessary for Medicare beneficiaries of any age group with primary amyloid light chain (AL) amyloidosis (ICD-9-CM code 277.3 or 277.39) who meet the following criteria:

- Amyloid deposition in 2 or fewer organs; and,
- Cardiac left ventricular ejection fraction (EF) greater than 45%.

ICD-9-CM code	Description	ICD-10-CM code	Description
277.30	Amyloidosis, unspecified	E85.9	Amyloidosis, unspecified
277.39	Other amyloidosis	E85.8	Other amyloidosis
		E85.4	Organ-limited amyloidosis

As the ICD-9-CM codes 277.3, and 277.39 for amyloidosis do not differentiate between primary and non-primary, A/B MACs (B) should perform prepay reviews on all claims with a diagnosis of ICD-9-CM code 277.3 to determine whether payment is appropriate.

If ICD-10-CM is applicable, as the applicable ICD-10 CM codes E85.4, E85.8, and E85.9 for amyloidosis do not differentiate between primary and non-primary, A/B MACs (B) should perform prepay reviews on all claims with a diagnosis of ICD-10-CM code E85.4, E85.8, and E85.9 to determine whether payment is appropriate.

C. Nationally Non-Covered Indications

I. Allogeneic Hematopoietic Stem Cell Transplantation (HSCT)

Effective for claims with dates of service on or after May 24, 1996, through January 27, 2016, allogeneic HSCT is not covered as treatment for multiple myeloma (if ICD-9-CM is applicable, ICD-9-CM code 203.00 and 203.01; or if ICD-10-CM is applicable, ICD-10-CMcodes C90.00, C90.01, C90.02 and D47.Z9).

II. Autologous Stem Cell Transplantation (AuSCT)

AuSCT is not considered reasonable and necessary within the meaning of §l862(a)(1)(A) of the Act and is not covered under Medicare for the following conditions:

a) Acute leukemia not in remission (if ICD-9-CM is applicable, ICD-9-CM codes 204.00, 205.00, 206.00, 207.00 and 208.00; or if ICD-10-CM is applicable, ICD-10-CM codes C91.00, C92.00, C93.00, C94.00, andC95.00)

b) Chronic granulocytic leukemia (if ICD-9-CM is applicable, ICD-9-CM codes 205.10 and 205.11; or if ICD-10-CM is applicable, ICD-10-CM codes C92.10 andC92.11);

c) Solid tumors (other than neuroblastoma) (if ICD-9-CM is applicable, ICD-9-CM codes 140.0 through 199.1; or if ICD-10-CM is applicable, ICD-10-CM codesC00.0 – C80.2 and D00.0 – D09.9);

d) Up to October 1, 2000, multiple myeloma (if ICD-9-CM is applicable, ICD-9-CM code 203.00 and 203.01; or if ICD-10-CM is applicable, ICD-10-CM codes C90.00, C90.01, C90.02 and D47.Z9);

e) Tandem transplantation (multiple rounds of AuSCT) for patients with multiple myeloma (if ICD-9-CM is applicable, ICD-9-CM code 203.00 and 203.01; or if ICD-10-CM is applicable, ICD-10-CM codes C90.00, C90.01, C90.02 and D47.Z9);

f) Effective October 1, 2000, non-primary AL amyloidosis (see table below for applicable ICD codes); and,

Appendix G — Medicare Internet-only Manuals (IOMs)

g) Effective October 1, 2000, through March 14, 2005, primary AL amyloidosis for Medicare beneficiaries age 64 or older (see table below for applicable ICD codes).

ICD-9-CM codes	Description	ICD-10-CM codes	Description
277.30	Amyloidosis, unspecified	E85.9	Amyloidosis, unspecified
277.31	Familial Mediterranean fever	E85.0	Non-neuropathic heredofamilial amyloidosis
277.39	Other amyloidosis	E85.8	Other amyloidosis
		E85.1	Neuropathic heredofamilial amyloidosis
		E85.2	Heredofamilial amyloidosis, unspecified
		E85.3	Secondary systemic amyloidosis
		E85.4	Organ-limited amyloidosis

As the ICD-9-CM code 277.3 and 277.39 for amyloidosis do not differentiate between primary and non-primary, A/B MACs (B) should perform prepay reviews on all claims with a diagnosis of ICD-9-CM code 277.3 and 277.39 to determine whether payment is appropriate.

If ICD-10-CM is applicable, as the applicable ICD-10 CM codes E85.4, E85.8, and E85.9 for amyloidosis do not differentiate between primary and non-primary, A/B MACs (B) should perform prepay reviews on all claims with a diagnosis of ICD-10-CM code E85.4, E85.8, and E85.9 to determine whether payment is appropriate.

D. Other

All other indications for stem cell transplantation not otherwise noted above as covered or non-covered remain at local Medicare Administrative Contractor discretion.

E. Suggested MSN and RA Messages

The contractor shall use an appropriate MSN and RA message such as the following:

MSN - 15.4, The information provided does not support the need for this service or item;

RA - 150, Payment adjusted because the payer deems the information submitted does not support this level of service.

F. Clinical Trials for Allogeneic Hematopoietic Stem Cell Transplantation (HSCT) for Myelodysplastic Syndrome (MDS), Multiple Myeloma, Myelofibrosis (MF), and for Sickle Cell Disease (SCD)

I. Background

Effective for services performed on or after August 4, 2010, contractors shall pay for claims for allogeneic HSCT for the treatment of Myelodysplastic Syndromes (MDS) pursuant to Coverage with Evidence Development (CED) in the context of a Medicare-approved, prospective clinical study.

Effective for services performed on or after January 27, 2016, contractors shall pay for claims for allogeneic HSCT for the treatment of multiple myeloma, myelofibrosis (MF), and for sickle cell disease (SCD) pursuant to CED, in the context of a Medicare-approved, prospective clinical study.

Refer to Pub.100-03, National Coverage Determinations Manual, Chapter 1, section 110.23, for more information about this policy, and Pub. 100-04, Medicare Claims Processing Manual, Chapter 3, section 90.3, for information on inpatient billing of this CED.

II. Adjudication Requirements Payable Conditions. For claims with dates of service on and after August 4, 2010, contractors shall pay for claims for allogeneic HSCT for MDS when the service was provided pursuant to a Medicare-approved clinical study under CED; these services are paid only in the inpatient setting (Type of Bill (TOB) 11X), as outpatient Part B (TOB 13X), and in Method II critical access hospitals (TOB 85X).

Contractors shall require the following coding in order to pay for these claims:

- Existing Medicare-approved clinical trial coding conventions, as required in Pub. 100-04, Medicare Claims Processing Manual, Chapter 32, section 69, and inpatient billing requirements regarding acquisition of stem cells in Pub. 100-04, Medicare Claims Processing Manual, Chapter 3, section 90.3.1.
- If ICD-9-CM is applicable, for Inpatient Hospital Claims: ICD-9-CM procedure codes 41.02, 41.03, 41.05, and 41.08 or,
- If ICD-10-CM is applicable, ICD-10-PCS, procedure codes 30230G1, 30230Y1, 30233G1, 30233Y1, 30240G1, 30240Y1, 30243G1, 30243Y1, 30250G1,30250Y1, 30253G1, 30253Y1, 30260G1, 30260Y1, 30263G1, and 30263Y1
- If Outpatient Hospital or Professional Claims: HCPCS procedure code 38240
- If ICD-9-CM is applicable, ICD-9-CM diagnosis codes 238.72, 238.73, 238.74, 238.75 or,
- If ICD-10-CM is applicable, ICD-10-CM codes D46.A, D46.B, D46.C, D46.0, D46.1, D46.20, D46.21, D46.22, D46.4, D46.9, D46.Z,
- Professional claims only: place of service codes 19, 21, or 22.

Payable Conditions. For claims with dates of service on and after January 27, 2016, contractors shall pay for claims for allogeneic HSCT for multiple myeloma, myelofibrosis (MF), and for sickle cell disease (SCD) when the service was provided pursuant to a Medicare-approved clinical study under CED; these services are paid only in the inpatient setting (Type of Bill (TOB) 11X), as outpatient Part B (TOB 13X), and in Method II critical access hospitals (TOB 85X).

Contractors shall require the following coding in order to pay for these claims:

- Existing Medicare-approved clinical trial coding conventions, as required in Pub. 100-04, Medicare Claims Processing Manual, Chapter 32, section 69, and inpatient billing requirements regarding acquisition of stem cells in Pub. 100-04, Medicare Claims Processing Manual, Chapter 3, section 90.3.1.
- ICD-10-PCS codes 30230G1, 30230Y1, 30233G1, 30233Y1, 30240G1, 30240Y1, 30243G1, 30243Y1, 30250G1, 30250Y1, 30253G1, 30253Y1, 30260G1, 30260Y1, 30263G1, and 30263Y1
- If Outpatient Hospital or Professional Claims: HCPCS procedure code 38240
- ICD-10-CM diagnosis codes C90.00, C90.01, C90.02, C94.40, C94.41, C94.42, D47.4, D75.81, D57.00, D57.01, D57.02, D57.1, D57.20, D57.211, D57.212, D57.219, D57.40, D57.411, D57.412, D57.419, D57.80, D57.811, D57.812, and D57.819
- Professional claims only: place of service codes 19, 21, or 22.

Denials. Contractors shall deny claims failing to meet any of the above criteria. In addition, contractors shall apply the following requirements:

- Providers shall issue a hospital issued notice of non-coverage (HINN) or advance beneficiary notice (ABN) to the beneficiary if the services performed are not provided in accordance with CED.
- Contractors shall deny claims that do not meet the criteria for coverage with the following messages:

CARC 50 - These are non-covered services because this is not deemed a 'medical necessity' by the payer.

NOTE: Refer to the 835 Healthcare Policy Identification Segment (loop 2110 Service Payment Information REF), if present.

RARC N386 - This decision was based on a National Coverage Determination (NCD). An NCD provides a coverage determination as to whether a particular item or service is covered. A copy of this policy is available at http:www.cms.hhs.gov/mcd/search.asp. If you do not have web access, you may contact the contractor to request a copy of the NCD.

Group Code – Patient Responsibility (PR) if HINN/ABN issued, otherwise Contractual Obligation (CO)

MSN 16.77 – This service/item was not covered because it was not provided as part of a qualifying trial/study. (Este servicio/artículo no fue cubierto porque no estaba incluido como parte de un ensayo clínico/estudio calificado.)

MSN 15.20 – The following policies [NCD 110.23] were used when we made this decision. (Las siguientes políticas [NCD 110.23] fueron utilizadas cuando se tomó esta decisión.)

100-04, 32, 90.2

HCPCS and Diagnosis Coding

(Rev. 2998, Issued: 07-25-14, Effective: Upon implementation of ICD-10; 01-01-12 - ASC X12, Implementation: 08-25-2014 - ASC X12; Upon Implementation of ICD-10)

Allogeneic Stem Cell Transplantation

- Effective for services performed on or after August 1, 1978:
  - — For the treatment of leukemia or leukemia in remission, providers shall use ICD-9-CM codes 204.00 through 208.91 and HCPCS code 38240.
  - — For the treatment of aplastic anemia, providers shall use ICD-9-CM codes 284.0 through 284.9 and HCPCS code 38240.
- Effective for services performed on or after June 3, 1985:
  - — For the treatment of severe combined immunodeficiency disease, providers shall use ICD-9-CM code 279.2 and HCPCS code 38240.
  - — For the treatment of Wiskott-Aldrich syndrome, providers shall use ICD-9-CM code 279.12 and HCPCS code 38240.
- Effective for services performed on or after May 24, 1996:
  - — Allogeneic stem cell transplantation, HCPCS code 38240 is not covered as treatment for the diagnosis of multiple myeloma ICD-9-CM codes 203.00 or 203.01.

Autologous Stem Cell Transplantation.--Is covered under the following circumstances effective for services performed on or after April 28, 1989:

- For the treatment of patients with acute leukemia in remission who have a high probability of relapse and who have no human leucocyte antigens (HLA) matched, providers shall use ICD-9-CM code 204.01 lymphoid; ICD-9-CM code 205.01 myeloid; ICD-9-CM code 206.01 monocytic; or ICD-9-CM code 207.01 acute erythremia and erythroleukemia; or ICD-9-CM code 208.01 unspecified cell type and HCPCS code 38241.
- For the treatment of resistant non-Hodgkin's lymphomas for those patients presenting with poor prognostic features following an initial response, providers shall use ICD-9-CM codes 200.00 - 200.08, 200.10-200.18, 200.20-200.28,

200.80-200.88, 202.00-202.08, 202.80-202.88 or 202.90-202.98 and HCPCS code 38241.

- For the treatment of recurrent or refractory neuroblastoma, providers shall use ICD-9-CM codes Neoplasm by site, malignant, the appropriate HCPCS code and HCPCS code 38241.
- For the treatment of advanced Hodgkin's disease for patients who have failed conventional therapy and have no HLA-matched donor, providers shall use ICD-9-CM codes 201.00 - 201.98 and HCPCS code 38241.

Autologous Stem Cell Transplantation.--Is covered under the following circumstances effective for services furnished on or after October 1, 2000:

- For the treatment of multiple myeloma (only for beneficiaries who are less than age 78, have Durie-Salmon stage II or III newly diagnosed or responsive multiple myeloma, and have adequate cardiac, renal, pulmonary and hepatic functioning), providers shall use ICD- 9-CM code 203.00 or 238.6 and HCPCS code 38241.
- For the treatment of recurrent or refractory neuroblastoma, providers shall use appropriate code (see ICD-9-CM neoplasm by site, malignant) and HCPCS code 38241.
- Effective for services performed on or after March 15, 2005, when recognized clinical risk factors are employed to select patients for transplantation, high-dose melphalan (HDM) together with autologous stem cell transplantation (HDM/AuSCT) is reasonable and necessary for Medicare beneficiaries of any age group for the treatment of primary amyloid light chain (AL) amyloidosis, ICD-9-CM code 277.3 who meet the following criteria:
- Amyloid deposition in 2 or fewer organs; and,
- Cardiac left ventricular ejection fraction (EF) greater than 45%.

100-04, 32, 90.2.1

HCPCS and Diagnosis Coding for Stem Cell Transplantation - ICD-10-CM Applicable

(Rev. 2998, Issued: 07-25-14, Effective: Upon implementation of ICD-10; 01-01-12 - ASC X12, Implementation: 08-25-2014 - ASC X12; Upon Implementation of ICD-10)

ICD-10 is applicable to services on and after the implementation of ICD-.

For services provided use the appropriate code from the ICD-10 CM codes in the table below. See §90.2 for a list of covered conditions.

ICD-10	Description
C91.Ø1	Acute lymphoblastic leukemia, in remission
C91.11	Chronic lymphocytic leukemia of B-cell type in remission
C91.31	Prolymphocytic leukemia of B-cell type, in remission
C91.51	Adult T-cell lymphoma/leukemia (HTLV-1-associated), in remission
C91.61	Prolymphocytic leukemia of T-cell type, in remission
C91.91	Lymphoid leukemia, unspecified, in remission
C91.A1	Mature B-cell leukemia Burkitt-type, in remission
C91.Z1	Other lymphoid leukemia, in remission
C92.Ø1	Acute myeloblastic leukemia, in remission
C92.11	Chronic myeloid leukemia, BCR/ABL-positive, in remission
C92.21	Atypical chronic myeloid leukemia, BCR/ABL-negative, in remission
C92.31	Myeloid sarcoma, in remission
C92.41	Acute promyelocytic leukemia, in remission
C92.51	Acute myelomonocytic leukemia, in remission
C92.61	Acute myeloid leukemia with 11q23-abnormality in remission
C92.91	Myeloid leukemia, unspecified in remission
C92.A1	Acute myeloid leukemia with multilineage dysplasia, in remission
C92.Z1	Other myeloid leukemia, in remission
C93.Ø1	Acute monoblastic/monocytic leukemia, in remission
C93.11	Chronic myelomonocytic leukemia, in remission
C93.31	Juvenile myelomonocytic leukemia, in remission
C93.91	Monocytic leukemia, unspecified in remission
C93.91	Monocytic leukemia, unspecified in remission
C93.Z1	Other monocytic leukemia, in remission
C94.Ø1	Acute erythroid leukemia, in remission
C94.21	Acute megakaryoblastic leukemia, in remission
C94.31	Mast cell leukemia, in remission
C94.81	Other specified leukemias, in remission
C95.Ø1	Acute leukemia of unspecified cell type, in remission
C95.11	Chronic leukemia of unspecified cell type, in remission
C95.91	Leukemia, unspecified, in remission
D45	Polycythemia vera
D61.Ø1	Constitutional (pure) red blood cell aplasia
D61.Ø9	Other constitutional aplastic anemia
D82.Ø	Wiskott-Aldrich syndrome
D81.Ø	Severe combined immunodeficiency [SCID] with reticular dysgenesis
D81.1	Severe combined immunodeficiency [SCID] with low T- and B-cell numbers
D81.2	Severe combined immunodeficiency [SCID] with low or normal B-cell numbers
D81.6	Major histocompatibility complex class I deficiency
D81.7	Major histocompatibility complex class II deficiency
D81.89	Other combined immunodeficiencies
D81.9	Combined immunodeficiency, unspecified
D81.2	Severe combined immunodeficiency [SCID] with low or normal B-cell numbers
D81.6	Major histocompatibility complex class I deficiency
D6Ø.Ø	Chronic acquired pure red cell aplasia
D6Ø.1	Transient acquired pure red cell aplasia
D6Ø.8	Other acquired pure red cell aplasias
D6Ø.9	Acquired pure red cell aplasia, unspecified
D61.Ø1	Constitutional (pure) red blood cell aplasia
D61.Ø9	Other constitutional aplastic anemia
D61.1	Drug-induced aplastic anemia
D61.2	Aplastic anemia due to other external agents
D61.3	Idiopathic aplastic anemia
D61.81Ø	Antineoplastic chemotherapy induced pancytopenia
D61.811	Other drug-induced pancytopenia
D61.818	Other pancytopenia
D61.82	Myelophthisis
D61.89	Other specified aplastic anemias and other bone marrow failure syndromes
D61.9	Aplastic anemia, unspecified

- If ICD-10-CM is applicable, the following ranges of ICD-10-CM codes are also covered for AuSCT: Resistant non-Hodgkin's lymphomas, ICD-10-CM diagnosis codes C82.00-C85.29, C85.80-C86.6, C96.4, and C96.Z-C96.9.
- Tandem transplantation (multiple rounds of autologous stem cell transplantation) for patients with multiple myeloma, ICD-10-CM codes C90.00 and D47.Z9

NOTE: The following conditions are not covered:

- Acute leukemia not in remission
- Chronic granulocytic leukemia
- Solid tumors (other than neuroblastoma)
- Multiple myeloma
- For Medicare beneficiaries age 64 or older, all forms of amyloidosis, primary and non-primary
- Non-primary amyloidosis

Also coverage for conditions other than those specifically designated as covered in §90.2 or specifically designated as non-covered in this section or in §90.3will be at the discretion of the individual contractor.

100-04, 32, 90.3

Non-Covered Conditions

(Rev. 2998, Issued: 07-25-14, Effective: Upon implementation of ICD-10; 01-01-12 - ASC X12, Implementation: 08-25-2014 - ASC X12; Upon Implementation of ICD-10)

Autologous stem cell transplantation is not covered for the following conditions:

- Acute leukemia not in remission (If ICD-9-CM is applicable, ICD-9-CM codes 204.00, 205.00, 206.00, 207.00 and 208.00) or (If ICD-10-CM is applicable, ICD-10-CM codes C91.00, C92.00, C93.00, C94.00, and C95.00)
- Chronic granulocytic leukemia (ICD-9-CM codes 205.10 and 205.11 if ICD-9-CM is applicable) or (if ICD-10-CM is applicable, ICD-10-CM codes C92.10 and C92.11);
- Solid tumors (other than neuroblastoma) (ICD-9-CM codes 140.0 through 199.1 if ICD-9-CM is applicable or if ICD-10-CM is applicable, ICD-10-CM codes C00.0 – C80.2 and D00.0 – D09.9.)
- Effective for services rendered on or after May 24, 1996 through September 30, 2000, multiple myeloma (ICD-9-CM code 203.00 and 203.01 if ICD-9-CM is applicable or if ICD-10-CM is applicable, ICD-10-CM codes C90.00 and D47.Z9);
- Effective for services on or after October 1, 2000, through March 14, 2005, for Medicare beneficiaries age 64 or older, all forms of amyloidosis, primary and non-primary
- Effective for services on or after 10/01/00, for all Medicare beneficiaries, non-primary amyloidosis

ICD-9-CM	Description	ICD-10-CM	Description
277.3Ø	Amyloidosis, unspecified	E85.9	Amyloidosis, unspecified
277.31	Familial Mediterranean fever	E85.Ø	Non-neuropathic heredofamilial amyloidosis
277.39	Other amyloidosis	E85.1	Neuropathic heredofamilial amyloidosis
277.39	Other amyloidosis	E85.2	Heredofamilial amyloidosis, unspecified
277.39	Other amyloidosis	E85.3	Secondary systemic amyloidosis
277.39	Other amyloidosis	E85.4	Organ-limited amyloidosis
277.39	Other amyloidosis	E85.8	Other amyloidosis

NOTE: Coverage for conditions other than those specifically designated as covered in 90.2 or 90.2.1 or specifically designated as non-covered in this section will be at the discretion of the individual A/B MAC (B).

100-04, 32, 90.4

Edits

(Rev. 2998, Issued: 07-25-14, Effective: Upon implementation of ICD-10; 01-01-12 - ASC X12, Implementation: 08-25-2014 - ASC X12; Upon Implementation of ICD-10)

NOTE: Coverage for conditions other than those specifically designated as covered in 80.2 or specifically designated as non-covered in this section will be at the discretion of the individual A/B MAC (B).

Appropriate diagnosis to procedure code edits should be implemented for the non-covered conditions and services in 90.2 90.2.1, and 90.3 as applicable.

As the ICD-9-CM code 277.3 for amyloidosis does not differentiate between primary and non-primary, A/B MACs (B) should perform prepay reviews on all claims with a diagnosis of ICD-9-CM code 277.3 and a HCPCS procedure code of 38241 to determine whether payment is appropriate.

If ICD-10-CM is applicable, the applicable ICD-10 CM codes are: E85.Ø, E85.1, E85.2, E85.3, E85.4, E85.8, and E85.9.

100-04, 32, 90.6

Clinical Trials for Allogeneic Hematopoietic Stem Cell Transplantation (HSCT) for Myelodysplastic Syndrome (MDS)

(Rev. 2998, Issued: 07-25-14, Effective: Upon implementation of ICD-10; 01-01-12 - ASC X12, Implementation: 08-25-2014 - ASC X12; Upon Implementation of ICD-10)

A. Background

Myelodysplastic Syndrome (MDS) refers to a group of diverse blood disorders in which the bone marrow does not produce enough healthy, functioning blood cells. These disorders are varied with regard to clinical characteristics, cytologic and pathologic features, and cytogenetics.

On August 4, 2010, the Centers for Medicare & Medicaid Services (CMS) issued a national coverage determination (NCD) stating that CMS believes that the evidence does not demonstrate that the use of allogeneic hematopoietic stem cell transplantation (HSCT) improves health outcomes in Medicare beneficiaries with MDS. Therefore, allogeneic HSCT for MDS is not reasonable and necessary under §1862(a)(1)(A) of the Social Security Act (the Act). However, allogeneic HSCT for MDS is reasonable and necessary under §1862(a)(1)(E) of the Act and therefore covered by Medicare ONLY if provided pursuant to a Medicare-approved clinical study under Coverage with Evidence Development (CED). Refer to Pub.100-3, NCD Manual, Chapter 1, section 110.8.1, for more information about this policy, and Pub. 100-4, MCP Manual, Chapter 3, section 90.3.1, for information on CED.

B. Adjudication Requirements

Payable Conditions. For claims with dates of service on and after August 4, 2010, contractors shall pay for claims for HSCT for MDS when the service was provided pursuant to a Medicare-approved clinical study under CED; these services are paid only in the inpatient setting (Type of Bill (TOB) 11X), as outpatient Part B (TOB 13X), and in Method II critical access hospitals (TOB 85X). Contractors shall require the following coding in order to pay for these claims:

- Existing Medicare-approved clinical trial coding conventions, as required in Pub. 100-4, MCP Manual, Chapter 32, section 69, and inpatient billing requirements regarding acquisition of stem cells in Pub. 100-4, MCP Manual, Chapter 3, section 90.3.3.
- If ICD-9-CM is applicable, for Inpatient Hospital Claims: ICD-9-CM procedure codes 41.02, 41.03, 41.05, and 41.08 or,
- If ICD-10-CM is applicable, ICD-10-PCS, procedure codes 3Ø23ØG1, 3Ø23ØY1, 3Ø23G1, 3Ø233Y1, 3Ø24ØG1, 3Ø24ØY1, 3Ø243G1, 3Ø243Y1, 3Ø25ØG1,3Ø25ØY1, 3Ø253G1, 3Ø253Y1, 3Ø26ØG1, 3Ø26ØY1, 3Ø263G1, and 3Ø263Y1
- If Outpatient Hospital or Professional Claims: HCPCS procedure code 38240
- If ICD-9-CM is applicable, ICD-9-CM diagnosis code 238.75 or If ICD-10-CM is applicable, ICD-10-CM diagnosis codes D46.9, D46.Z, or Z00.6 Professional claims only: place of service codes 21 or 22.

Denials. Contractors shall deny claims failing to meet any of the above criteria. In addition, contractors shall apply the following requirements:

- Providers shall issue a hospital issued notice of non-coverage (HINN) or advance beneficiary notice (ABN) to the beneficiary if the services performed are not provided in accordance with CED.
- Contractors shall deny claims that do not meet the criteria for coverage with the following messages:

  CARC 50 - These are non-covered services because this is not deemed a 'medical necessity' by the payer.

  NOTE: Refer to the 835 Healthcare Policy Identification Segment (loop 2110 Service Payment Information REF), if present.

  RARC N386 - This decision was based on a National Coverage Determination (NCD). An NCD provides a coverage determination as to whether a particular item or service is covered. A copy of this policy is available at http://www.cms.hhs.gov/mcd/search.asp. If you do not have web access, you may contact the contractor to request a copy of the NCD.

  Group Code – Patient Responsibility (PR) if HINN/ABN issued, otherwise Contractual Obligation (CO)

  MSN 16.77 – This service/item was not covered because it was not provided as part of a qualifying trial/study. (Este servicio/artículo no fue cubierto porque no estaba incluido como parte de un ensayo clínico/estudio calificado.)

100-04, 32, 120.2

Coding and General Billing Requirements

(Rev. 1430; Issued: 02-01-08; Effective: 01-01-08; Implementation: 03-03-08)

Physicians and hospitals must report one of the following Current Procedural Terminology (CPT) codes on the claim:

66982 Extracapsular cataract removal with insertion of intraocular lens prosthesis (one stage procedure), manual or mechanical technique (e.g., irrigation and aspiration or phacoemulsification), complex requiring devices or techniques not generally used in routine cataract surgery (e.g., iris expansion device, suture support for intraocular lens, or primary posterior capsulorrhexis) or performed on patients in the amblyogenic development stage.

66983 Intracapsular cataract with insertion of intraocular lens prosthesis (one stage procedure)

66984 Extracapsular cataract removal with insertion of intraocular lens prosthesis (one stage procedure), manual or mechanical technique (e.g., irrigation and aspiration or phacoemulsification)

66985 Insertion of intraocular lens prosthesis (secondary implant), not associated with concurrent cataract extraction

66986 Exchange of intraocular lens

In addition, physicians inserting a P-C IOL or A-C IOL in an office setting may bill code V2632 (posterior chamber intraocular lens) for the IOL. Medicare will make payment for the lens based on reasonable cost for a conventional IOL. Place of Service (POS) = 11.

Effective for dates of service on and after January 1, 2006, physician, hospitals and ASCs may also bill the non-covered charges related to the P-C function of the IOL using HCPCS code V2788. Effective for dates of service on and after January 22, 2007 through January 1, 2008, non-covered charges related to A-C function of the IOL can be billed using HCPCS code V2788. The type of service indicator for the non-covered billed charges is Q. (The type of service is applied by the Medicare carrier and not the provider). Effective for A-C IOL insertion services on or after January 1, 2008, physicians, hospitals and ASCs should use V2787 rather than V2788 to report any additional charges that accrue.

When denying the non-payable charges submitted with V2787 or V2788, contractors shall use an appropriate Medical Summary Notice (MSN) such as 16.10 (Medicare does not pay for this item or service) and an appropriate claim adjustment reason code such as 96 (non-covered charges) for claims submitted with the non-payable charges.

Hospitals and physicians may use the proper CPT code(s) to bill Medicare for evaluation and management services usually associated with services following cataract extraction surgery, if appropriate.

A - Applicable Bill Types

The hospital applicable bill types are 12X, 13X, 83X and 85X.

B - Other Special Requirements for Hospitals

Hospitals shall continue to pay CAHs method 2 claims under current payment methodologies for conditional IOLs.

100-04, 32, 130.1

Billing and Payment Requirements

(Rev. 898, Issued: 03-31-06; Effective/Implementation Dates: 03-31-06)

Effective for dates of service on or after January 1, 2000, use HCPCS code G0166 (External counterpulsation, per session) to report ECP services. The codes for external cardiac assist (92971), ECG rhythm strip and report (93040 or 93041), pulse oximetry (94760 or 94761) and plethysmography (93922 or 93923) or other monitoring tests for examining the effects of this treatment are not clinically necessary with this service and should not be paid on the same day, unless they occur in a clinical setting not connected with the delivery of the ECP. Daily evaluation and management service, e.g., 99201-99205, 99211-99215, 99217-99220, 99241-99245, cannot be billed with the ECP treatments. Any evaluation and management service must be justified with adequate documentation of the medical necessity of the visit. Deductible and coinsurance apply.

100-04, 32, 140.2

Cardiac Rehabilitation Program Services Furnished On or After January 1, 2010

(Rev. 3058, Issued: 08-29-14, Effective: 02-18-14, Implementation: 08-18-14)

As specified at 42 CFR 410.49, Medicare covers cardiac rehabilitation items and services for patients who have experienced one or more of the following:

- An acute myocardial infarction within the preceding 12 months; or
- A coronary artery bypass surgery; or
- Current stable angina pectoris; or
- Heart valve repair or replacement; or
- Percutaneous transluminal coronary angioplasty (PTCA) or coronary stenting; or
- A heart or heart-lung transplant or;
- Stable, chronic heart failure defined as patients with left ventricular ejection fraction of 35% or less and New York Heart Association (NYHA) class II to IV symptoms despite being on optimal heart failure therapy for at least 6 weeks (effective February 18, 2014).

Cardiac rehabilitation programs must include the following components:

- Physician-prescribed exercise each day cardiac rehabilitation items and services are furnished;
- Cardiac risk factor modification, including education, counseling, and behavioral intervention at least once during the program, tailored to patients' individual needs;
- Psychosocial assessment;
- Outcomes assessment; and
- An individualized treatment plan detailing how components are utilized for each patient.

Cardiac rehabilitation items and services must be furnished in a physician's office or a hospital outpatient setting. All settings must have a physician immediately available and accessible for medical consultations and emergencies at all times items and services are being furnished under the program. This provision is satisfied if the physician meets the requirements for the direct supervision of physician's office services as specified at 42 CFR 410.26 and for hospital outpatient therapeutic services as specified at 42 CFR 410.27.

As specified at 42 CFR 410.49(f)(1), cardiac rehabilitation program sessions are limited to a maximum of 2 1-hour sessions per day for up to 36 sessions over up to 36 weeks, with the option for an additional 36 sessions over an extended period of time if approved by the Medicare contractor.

100-04, 32, 140.2.1

Coding Requirements for Cardiac Rehabilitation Services Furnished On or After January 1, 2010

(Rev. 1882, Issued: 12-21-09; Effective Date: 01-01-10; Implementation Date: 01-04-10)

The following are the applicable CPT codes for cardiac rehabilitation services: 93797 - Physician services for outpatient cardiac rehabilitation; without continuous ECG monitoring (per session) and 93798 - Physician services for outpatient cardiac rehabilitation; with continuous ECG monitoring (per session) Effective for dates of service on or after January 1, 2010, hospitals and practitioners may report a maximum of 2 1-hour sessions per day. In order to report one session of cardiac rehabilitation services in a day, the duration of treatment must be at least 31 minutes. Two sessions of cardiac rehabilitation services may only be reported in the same day if the duration of treatment is at least 91 minutes. In other words, the first session would account for 60 minutes and the second session would account for at least 31 minutes if two sessions are reported. If several shorter periods of cardiac rehabilitation services are furnished on a given day, the minutes of service during those periods must be added together for reporting in 1-hour session increments.

Example: If the patient receives 20 minutes of cardiac rehabilitation services in the day, no cardiac rehabilitation session may be reported because less than 31 minutes of services were furnished.

Example: If a patient receives 20 minutes of cardiac rehabilitation services in the morning and 35 minutes of cardiac rehabilitation services in the afternoon of a single day, the hospital or practitioner would report 1 session of cardiac rehabilitation services under 1 unit of the appropriate CPT code for the total duration of 55 minutes of cardiac rehabilitation services on that day.

Example: If the patient receives 70 minutes of cardiac rehabilitation services in the morning and 25 minutes of cardiac rehabilitation services in the afternoon of a single day, the hospital or practitioner would report two sessions of cardiac rehabilitation services under the appropriate CPT code(s) because the total duration of cardiac rehabilitation services on that day of 95 minutes exceeds 90 minutes.

Example: If the patient receives 70 minutes of cardiac rehabilitation services in the morning and 85 minutes of cardiac rehabilitation services in the afternoon of a single day, the hospital or practitioner would report two sessions of cardiac rehabilitation services under the appropriate CPT code(s) for the total duration of cardiac rehabilitation services of 155 minutes. A maximum of two sessions per day may be reported, regardless of the total duration of cardiac rehabilitation services.

100-04, 32, 140.2.2.2

Requirements for CR and ICR Services on Institutional Claims

(Rev. 3084, Issued: 10-03-14, Effective: 05-06-14, Implementation: 11-04-14)

Effective for claims with dates of service on and after January 1, 2010, contractors shall pay for CR and ICR services when submitted on Types of Bill (TOBs) 13X and 85X only. All other TOBs shall be denied.

The following messages shall be used when contractors deny CR and ICR claims for TOBs 13X and 85X:

> Claim Adjustment Reason Code (CARC) 171 – Payment is denied when performed/billed by this type of provider in this type of facility.
>
> Remittance Advice Remark Code (RARC) N428 - Service/procedure not covered when performed in this place of service.
>
> Medicare Summary Notice (MSN) 21.25 - This service was denied because Medicare only covers this service in certain settings.
>
> Group Code PR (Patient Responsibility) – Where a claim is received with the GA modifier indicating that a signed ABN is on file.
>
> Group Code CO (Contractor Responsibility) – Where a claim is received with the GZ modifier indicating that no signed ABN is on file.

100-04, 32, 140.2.2.4

Edits for CR Services Exceeding 36 Sessions

(Rev. 3058, Issued: 08-29-14, Effective: 02-18-14, Implementation: 08-18-14)

Effective for claims with dates of service on or after January 1, 2010, contractors shall deny all claims with HCPCS 93797 and 93798 (both professional and institutional claims) that exceed 36 CR sessions when a KX modifier is not included on the claim line.

The following messages shall be used when contractors deny CR claims that exceed 36 sessions, when a KX modifier is not included on the claim line:

> Claim Adjustment Reason Code (CARC) 119 – Benefit maximum for this period or occurrence has been reached.
>
> RARC N435 - Exceeds number/frequency approved/allowed within time period without support documentation.
>
> MSN 23.17- Medicare won't cover these services because they are not considered medically necessary.
>
> Spanish Version - Medicare no cubrirá estos servicios porque no son considerados necesarios por razones médicas.
>
> Group Code PR (Patient Responsibility) – Where a claim is received with the GA modifier indicating that a signed ABN is on file.
>
> Group Code CO (Contractor Responsibility) – Where a claim is received with the GZ modifier indicating that no signed ABN is on file.

Contractors shall not research and adjust CR claims paid for more than 36 sessions processed prior to the implementation of CWF edits. However, contractors may adjust claims brought to their attention.

100-04, 32, 140.3

Intensive Cardiac Rehabilitation Program Services Furnished On or After January 1, 2010

(Rev. 4222, Issued: 02-01-19, Effective: 02-09-18, Implementation: 03-19-19)

As specified at 42 CFR 410.49, Medicare covers intensive cardiac rehabilitation items and services for patients who have experienced one or more of the following:

- An acute myocardial infarction within the preceding 12 months;
- A coronary artery bypass surgery;
- Current stable angina pectoris;
- Heart valve repair or replacement;
- Percutaneous transluminal coronary angioplasty or coronary stenting;
- A heart or heart-lung transplant.

Effective February 9, 2018, section 51004 of the Bipartisan Budget Act (BBA) of 2018, Pub. L. No. 115-123 (2018), amended section 1861(eee)(4)(B) of the Social Security Act to expand coverage in an intensive cardiac rehabilitation program to additional conditions:

- Stable, chronic heart failure defined as patients with left ventricular ejection fraction of 35% or less and New York Heart Association (NYHA) class II to IV symptoms despite being on optimal heart failure therapy for at least 6 weeks; or
- Any additional condition for which the Secretary has determined that a cardiac rehabilitation program shall be covered, unless the Secretary determines, using the same process used to determine that the condition is covered for a cardiac rehabilitation program, that such coverage is not supported by the clinical evidence.

NOTE: CMS plans to amend our intensive cardiac rehabilitation regulations specified at 42 CFR 410.49 to reflect this expanded coverage. CMS anticipates that the changes will be included in the 2020 Medicare Physician Fee Schedule notice of proposed rulemaking. However, because the expanded coverage under the statutory change was effective on enactment, expanded coverage for these conditions will be made effective for services furnished on or after February 9, 2018.

Intensive cardiac rehabilitation programs must include the following components:

- Physician-prescribed exercise each day cardiac rehabilitation items and services are furnished;
- Cardiac risk factor modification, including education, counseling, and behavioral intervention at least once during the program, tailored to patients' individual needs;
- Psychosocial assessment;
- Outcomes assessment; and,
- An individualized treatment plan detailing how components are utilized for each patient.

Intensive cardiac rehabilitation programs must be approved by Medicare. In order to be approved, a program must demonstrate through peer-reviewed published research that it has accomplished one or more of the following for its patients:

- Positively affected the progression of coronary heart disease;
- Reduced the need for coronary bypass surgery; and,
- Reduced the need for percutaneous coronary interventions.

An intensive cardiac rehabilitation program must also demonstrate through peer-reviewed published research that it accomplished a statistically significant reduction in five or more of the following measures for patients from their levels before cardiac rehabilitation services to after cardiac rehabilitation services:

- Low density lipoprotein;
- Triglycerides;
- Body mass index;
- Systolic blood pressure;
- Diastolic blood pressure; and,
- The need for cholesterol, blood pressure, and diabetes medications.

Intensive cardiac rehabilitation items and services must be furnished in a physician's office or a hospital outpatient setting. All settings must have a physician immediately available and accessible for medical consultations and emergencies at all times items and services are being furnished under the program. This provision is satisfied if the physician meets the requirements for direct supervision of physician office services as specified at 42 CFR 410.26 and for hospital outpatient therapeutic services as specified at 42 CFR 410.27. As specified at 42 CFR 410.49(f)(2), ICR program sessions are limited to 72 1-hour sessions, up to 6 sessions per day, over a period of up to 18 weeks.

100-04, 32, 150.1

Bariatric Surgery for Treatment of Co-Morbid Conditions Related to Morbid Obesity

(Rev. 2841, Issued: 12-23-13, Effective: 09-24-13, Implementation: 12-17-13)

Effective for services on or after February 21, 2006, Medicare has determined that the following bariatric surgery procedures are reasonable and necessary under certain conditions for the treatment of morbid obesity. The patient must have a body-mass index (BMI) =35, have at least one co-morbidity related to obesity, and have been previously unsuccessful with medical treatment for obesity. This medical information must be documented in the patient's medical record. In addition, the procedure must be performed at an approved facility. A list of approved facilities may be found at http://www.cms.gov/Medicare/Medicare-General-Information/MedicareApprovedFacilitie/Bariatric-Surgery.html

Effective for services performed on and after February 12, 2009, Medicare has determined that Type 2 diabetes mellitus is a co-morbidity for purposes of processing bariatric surgery claims.

Effective for dates of service on and after September 24, 2013, the Centers for Medicare & Medicaid Services (CMS) has removed the certified facility requirements for Bariatric Surgery for Treatment of Co-Morbid Conditions Related to Morbid Obesity.

Please note the additional national coverage determinations related to bariatric surgery will be consolidated and subsumed into Publication 100-3, Chapter 1, section 100.1. These include sections 40.5, 100.8, 100.11 and 100.14.

- Open Roux-en-Y gastric bypass (RYGBP)
- Laparoscopic Roux-en-Y gastric bypass (RYGBP)
- Laparoscopic adjustable gastric banding (LAGB)
- Open biliopancreatic diversion with duodenal switch (BPD/DS) or gastric reduction duodenal switch (BPD/GRDS)
- Laparoscopic biliopancreatic diversion with duodenal switch (BPD/DS) or gastric reduction duodenal switch (BPD/GRDS)
- Laparoscopic sleeve gastrectomy (LSG) (Effective June 27, 2012, covered at Medicare Administrative Contractor (MAC) discretion.

100-04, 32, 150.2

HCPCS Procedure Codes for Bariatric Surgery

(Rev. 2641, Issued: 01-29-13, Effective: 06-27-12, Implementation: 02-28-13)

A. Covered HCPCS Procedure Codes

For services on or after February 21, 2006, the following HCPCS procedure codes are covered for bariatric surgery:

43770 Laparoscopy, surgical, gastric restrictive procedure; placement of adjustable gastric band (gastric band and subcutaneous port components).

43644 Laparoscopy, surgical, gastric restrictive procedure; with gastric bypass and Roux-en-Y gastroenterostomy (roux limb 150 cm or less).

43645 Laparoscopy with gastric bypass and small intestine reconstruction to limit absorption. (Do not report 43645 in conjunction with 49320, 43847.)

43845 Gastric restrictive procedure with partial gastrectomy, pylorus-preserving duodenoileostomy and ileoieostomy (50 to 100 cm common channel) to limit absorption (biliopancreatic diversion with duodenal switch).

43846 Gastric restrictive procedure, with gastric bypass for morbid obesity; with short limb (150 cm or less Roux-en-Y gastroenterostomy. (For greater than 150 cm, use 43847.) (For laparoscopic procedure, use 43644.)

43847 With small intestine reconstruction to limit absorption.

43775 Laparoscopy, surgical, gastric restrictive procedure; longitudinal gastrectomy (i.e., sleeve gastrectomy) (Effective June 27, 2012, covered at contractor's discretion.)

B. Noncovered HCPCS Procedure Codes

For services on or after February 21, 2006, the following HCPCS procedure codes are non-covered for bariatric surgery:

43842 Gastric restrictive procedure, without gastric bypass, for morbid obesity; vertical banded gastroplasty.

NOC code 43999 used to bill for:

Laparoscopic vertical banded gastroplasty

Open sleeve gastrectomy

Laparoscopic sleeve gastrectomy (for contractor non-covered instances)

Open adjustable gastric banding

100-04, 32, 150.5

ICD Diagnosis Codes for BMI Greater Than or Equal to 35

(Rev. 2841, Issued: 12-23-13, Effective: 09-24-13, Implementation: 12-17-13)

The following ICD-9 diagnosis codes identify BMI >=35 :

V85.35 - Body Mass Index 35.0-35.9, adult

V85.36 - Body Mass Index 36.0-36.9, adult

V85.37 - Body Mass Index 37.0-37.9, adult

V85.38 - Body Mass Index 38.0-38.9, adult

V85.39 - Body Mass Index 39.0-39.9, adult

V85.41 - Body Mass Index 40.0-44.9, adult

V85.42 - Body Mass Index 45.0-49.9, adult

V85.43 - Body Mass Index 50.0-59.9, adult

V85.44 - Body Mass Index 60.0-69.9, adult

V85.45 - Body Mass Index 70.0 and over, adult

The following ICD-10 diagnosis codes identify BMI >=35:

Z6835 - Body Mass Index 35.0-35.9, adult

Z6836 - Body Mass Index 36.0-36.9, adult.

Z6837 - Body Mass Index 37.0-37.9, adult

Z6838 - Body Mass Index 38.0-38.9, adult

Z6839 - Body Mass Index 39.0-39.9, adult

Z6841 - Body Mass Index 40.0-44.9, adult

Z6842 - Body Mass Index 45.0-49.9, adult

Z6843 - Body Mass Index 50.0-59.9, adult

Z6844 - Body Mass Index 60.0-69.9, adult

Z6845 - Body Mass Index 70.0 and over, adult

100-04, 32, 150.6

Claims Guidance for Payment

(Rev. 2841, Issued: 12-23-13, Effective: 09-24-13, Implementation: 12-17-13)

Covered Bariatric Surgery Procedures for Treatment of Co-Morbid Conditions Related to Morbid Obesity

Contractors shall process covered bariatric surgery claims as follows:

1. Identify bariatric surgery claims.

   Contractors identify inpatient bariatric surgery claims by the presence of ICD-9/ICD-10 diagnosis code 278.01/E66.01as the primary diagnosis (for morbid obesity) and one of the covered ICD-9/ICD-10 procedure codes listed in §150.3.

   Contractors identify practitioner bariatric surgery claims by the presence of ICD-9/ICD-10 diagnosis code 278.01/E66.01 as the primary diagnosis (for morbid obesity) and one of the covered HCPCS procedure codes listed in §150.2.

2. Perform facility certification validation for all bariatric surgery claims on a pre-pay basis up to and including date of service September 23, 2013.

   A list of approved facilities are found at the link noted in section 150.1, section A, above.

3. Review bariatric surgery claims data and determine whether a pre- or post-pay sample of bariatric surgery claims need further review to assure that the beneficiary has a BMI =35 (V85.35-V85.45/Z68.35-Z68.45) (see ICD-10 equivalents above in section 150.5), and at least one co-morbidity related to obesity

   The A/B MAC medical director may define the appropriate method for addressing the obesity-related co-morbid requirement.

   Effective for dates of service on and after September 24, 2013, CMS has removed the certified facility requirements for Bariatric Surgery for Treatment of Co-Morbid Conditions Related to Morbid Obesity.

NOTE: If ICD-9/ICD-10 diagnosis code 278.01/E66.01 is present, but a covered procedure code (listed in §150.2 or §150.3) is/are not present, the claim is not for bariatric surgery and should be processed under normal procedures.

100-04, 32, 161

Intracranial Percutaneous Transluminal Angioplasty (PTA) With Stenting

(Rev. 2998, Issued: 07-25-14, Effective: Upon implementation of ICD-10; 01-01-12 - ASC X12, Implementation: 08-25-2014 - ASC X12; Upon Implementation of ICD-10)

A. Background

In the past, PTA to treat obstructive lesions of the cerebral arteries was non-covered by Medicare because the safety and efficacy of the procedure had not been established. This national coverage determination (NCD) meant that the procedure was also non-covered for beneficiaries participating in Food and Drug Administration (FDA)-approved investigational device exemption (IDE) clinical trials.

B. Policy

On February 9, 2006, a request for reconsideration of this NCD initiated a national coverage analysis. CMS reviewed the evidence and determined that intracranial PTA with stenting is reasonable and necessary under §1862(a)(1)(A) of the Social Security Act for the treatment of cerebral vessels (as specified in The National Coverage Determinations Manual, Chapter 1, part 1, section 20.7) only when furnished in accordance with FDA-approved protocols governing Category B IDE clinical trials. All other indications for intracranial PTA with stenting remain non-covered.

C. Billing

Providers of covered intracranial PTA with stenting shall use Category B IDE billing requirements, as listed above in section 68.4. In addition to these requirements, providers must bill the appropriate procedure and diagnosis codes for the date of service to receive payment. That is, under Part A, providers must bill intracranial PTA using ICD-9-CM procedure codes 00.62 and 00.65, if ICD-9-CM is applicable, or, if ICD-10-PCS is applicable, ICD-10-PCS procedure codes 037G34Z, 037G3DZ, 037G3ZZ, 037G44Z, 037G4DZ, 037G4ZZ, 03CG3ZZ, 057L3DZ, 057L4DZ and 05CL3ZZ. ICD-9-CM diagnosis code 437.0 or ICD-10-CM diagnosis code 167.2applies, depending on the date of service.

Under Part B, providers must bill HCPCS procedure code 37799. If ICD-9-CM is applicable ICD-9-CM diagnosis code 437.0 or if ICD-10-CM is applicable,ICD-10-CM diagnosis code 167.2 applies.

NOTE: ICD- codes are subject to modification. Providers must always ensure they are using the latest and most appropriate codes.

100-04, 32, 190

Billing Requirements for Extracorporeal Photopheresis

(Rev. 3050, Issued: 08-22-14, Effective: 09-23-14, ICD-10: Upon Implementation of ICD-10, Implementation: 09-23-14, ICD-10: Upon Implementation of ICD-10)

Effective for dates of services on and after December 19, 2006, Medicare has expanded coverage for extracorporeal photopheresis for patients with acute cardiac allograft rejection whose disease is refractory to standard immunosuppresive drug treatment and patients with chronic graft versus host disease whose disease is refractory to standard immunosuppresive drug treatment. (See Pub. 100-3, chapter 1, section 110.4, for complete coverage guidelines).

Effective for claims with dates of service on or after April 30, 2012, CMS has expanded coverage for extracorporeal photopheresis for the treatment of BOS following lung allograft transplantation only when extracorporeal photopheresis is provided under a clinical research study that meets specific requirements to assess the effect of extracorporeal photopheresis for the treatment of BOS following lung allograft transplantation. Further coverage criteria is outlined in Publication 100-3, Section 110.4 of the NCD.

100-04, 32, 190.2

Healthcare Common Procedural Coding System (HCPCS), Applicable Diagnosis Codes and Procedure Code

(Rev. 3050, Issued: 08-22-14, Effective: 09-23-14, ICD-10: Upon Implementation of ICD-10, Implementation: 09-23-14, ICD-10: Upon Implementation of ICD-10)

The following HCPCS procedure code is used for billing extracorporeal photopheresis:

- 36522 - Photopheresis, extracorporeal

The following are the applicable ICD-9-CM diagnosis codes for the new expanded coverage:

- 996.83 - Complications of transplanted heart, or,
- 996.85 - Complications of transplanted bone marrow, or,
- 996.88 – Complications of transplanted organ, stem cell

Effective for services for BOS following lung allograft transplantation the following is a list of applicable ICD-9-CM diagnosis codes:

- 996.84 – Complications of transplanted lung
- 491.9 - Unspecified chronic bronchitis
- 491.20 – Obstructive chronic bronchitis without exacerbation
- 491.21 – Obstructive chronic bronchitis with (acute) exacerbation
- 496 – Chronic airway obstruction, not elsewhere classified

The following is the applicable ICD-9-CM procedure code for the new expanded coverage:

- 99.88 - Therapeutic photopheresis

NOTE: Contractors shall edit for an appropriate oncological and autoimmune disorder diagnosis for payment of extracorporeal photopheresis according to the NCD.

Effective for claims with dates of service on or after April 30, 2012, in addition to HCPCS 36522, the following ICD-9-CM codes are applicable for extracorporeal photopheresis for the treatment of BOS following lung allograft transplantation only when extracorporeal photopheresis is provided under a clinical research study as outlined in Section 190 above:

A reference listing of ICD-9 CM and ICD-10-CM coding and descriptions is listed V70.7 below:

ICD9	Long Description	ICD10	ICD10 Description
491.20	Obstructive chronic	J44.9	Chronic obstructive bronchitis without exacerbation pulmonary disease, unspecified
491.21	Obstructive chronic bronchitis with (acute) exacerbation	J44.1	Chronic obstructive pulmonary disease with (acute) exacerbation
491.9	Unspecified chronic bronchitis	J42	Unspecified chronic bronchitis
496	Chronic airway obstruction, not elsewhere classified	J44.9	Chronic obstructive pulmonary disease, unspecified
996.84	Complications of transplanted lung	T86.810	Lung transplant rejection
996.84	Complications of transplanted lung	T86.811	Lung transplant failure
996.84	Complications of transplanted lung	T86.812	Lung transplant infection (not recommended for extracorporeal photopheresis coverage)
996.84	Complications of transplanted lung	T86.818	Other complications of lung transplant
996.84	Complications of transplanted lung	T86.819	Unspecified complication of lung transplant
996.88	Complications of Transplanted organ, Stem cell	T86.5	Complications of Stem Cell Transplant
V70.7	Examination of participant in clinical trial	Z00.6	Encounter for examination for normal comparison and control in clinical research program (needed for CED)

Contractors must also report modifier Q0 - (investigational clinical service provided in a clinical research study that is in an approved research study) or Q1 (routine clinical service provided in a clinical research study that is in an approved clinical research study) as appropriate on these claims. Contractors must use diagnosis code V70.7/Z00.6 and condition code 30 (A/B MAC (A) only), along with value code D4 and the 8-digit clinical identifier number (A/MACs only) for these claims.

100-04, 32, 190.3

Medicare Summary Notices (MSNs), Remittance Advice Remark Codes (RAs) and Claim Adjustment Reason Code

(Rev. 3050, Issued: 08-22-14, Effective: 09-23-14, ICD-10: Upon Implementation of ICD-10, Implementat)

Contractors shall continue to use the appropriate existing messages that they have in place when denying claims submitted that do not meet the Medicare coverage criteria for extracorporeal photopheresis.

Medicare coverage for extracorporeal photopheresis is restricted to the inpatient or outpatient hospital settings specifically for BOS, and not for the other covered diagnosis (including chronic graft versus host disease) which remain covered in the hospital inpatient, hospital outpatient, and non-facility (physician-directed clinic or office settings) settings.

Contractors shall deny claims for extracorporeal photopheresis for BOS when the service is not rendered to an inpatient or outpatient of a hospital, including critical access hospitals using the following codes:

- Claim Adjustment Reason Code (CARC) 96 – Non-covered charge(s). At least one Remark Code must be provided (may be comprised of either the NCPDP Reject Reason [sic] Code, or Remittance Advice Remark Code that is not an ALERT.) NOTE: Refer to the 835 Healthcare Policy Identification Segment (loop 2110 Service Payment Information REF), if present.
- CARC 171 – Payment is denied when performed/billed by this type of provider in this type of facility. NOTE: Refer to the 835 Healthcare Policy Identification Segment (loop 2110 Service Payment Information REF), if present.
- Medicare Summary Notice 16.2 - This service cannot be paid when provided in this location/facility." Spanish translation: "Este servicio no se puede pagar cuando es suministrado en esta sitio/facilidad. (Include either MSN 36.1 or 36.2 dependent on liability.)
- Remittance Advice Remark Code (RARC) N428 – Not covered when performed in this place of service. (A/MACs only) Group Code CO (Contractual Obligations) or PR (Patient Responsibility) dependent on liability.

Contractors shall return to provider/ return as unprocessable claims for BOS containing HCPCS procedure code 36522 along with one of the following ICD-9-CM diagnosis codes: 996.84, 491.9, 491.20, 491.21, and 496 but is missing diagnosis code V70.7 (as primary/secondary diagnosis, institutional only), condition code 30 (institutional claims only), clinical trial modifier Q0/Q1, and value code D4 with an 8-digit clinical trial identifier number (A/MACs only). Use the following messages:

- CARC 4 – The procedure code is inconsistent with the modifier used or a required modifier is missing. NOTE: Refer to the 835 Healthcare Policy Identification Segment (loop 2110 Service Payment Information REF), if present.
- RARC N517 – Resubmit a new claim with the requested information.

100-04, 32, 220.1

220.1 - General

(Rev. 1646, Issued: 12-09-08, Effective: 09-29-08, Implementation: 01-05-09)

Effective for services on or after September 29, 2008, the Center for Medicare & Medicaid Services (CMS) made the decision that Thermal Intradiscal Procedures (TIPS) are not reasonable and necessary for the treatment of low back pain. Therefore, TIPs are non-covered. Refer to Pub.100-3, Medicare National Coverage Determination (NCD) Manual Chapter 1, Part 2, Section 150.11, for further information on the NCD.

100-04, 32, 290.1.1

Coding Requirements for TAVR Services Furnished on or After January 1, 2013

(Rev. 2827. Issued: 11-29-13, Effective: 01-01-14, Implementation: 01-06-14)

Beginning January 1, 2013, the following are the applicable Current Procedural Terminology (CPT) codes for TAVR:

33361 Transcatheter aortic valve replacement (TAVR/TAVI) with prosthetic valve; percutaneous femoral artery approach

33362 Transcatheter aortic valve replacement (TAVR/TAVI) with prosthetic valve; open femoral approach

33363 Transcatheter aortic valve replacement (TAVR/TAVI) with prosthetic valve; open axillary artery approach

33364 Transcatheter aortic valve replacement (TAVR/TAVI) with prosthetic valve; open iliac artery approach

3336 Transcatheter aortic valve replacement (TAVR/TAVI) with prosthetic valve; transaortic approach (e.g., median sternotomy, mediastinotomy)

0318T Transcatheter aortic valve replacement (TAVR/TAVI) with prosthetic valve; transapical approach (e.g., left thoracotomy)

Beginning January 1, 2014, temporary CPT code 0318T above is retired. TAVR claims with dates of service on and after January 1, 2014 shall instead use permanent CPT code:

33366 Transcatheter aortic valve replacement (TAVR/TAVI) with prosthetic valve; transapical exposure (e.g., left thoracotomy)

100-04, 32, 290.2

Claims Processing Requirements for TAVR Services on Professional Claims

(Rev. 2827. Issued: 11-29-13, Effective: 01-01-14, Implementation: 01-06-14)

Place of Service (POS) Professional Claims

Effective for claims with dates of service on and after May 1, 2012, place of service (POS) code 21 shall be used for TAVR services. All other POS codes shall be denied.

The following messages shall be used when Medicare contractors deny TAVR claims for POS:

Claim Adjustment Reason Code (CARC) 58: "Treatment was deemed by the payer to have been rendered in an inappropriate or invalid place of service. NOTE: Refer to the 835 Healthcare Policy Identification Segment (loop 2110 Service Payment Information REF), if present."

Remittance advice remark code (RARC) N428: "Not covered when performed in this place of service."

Medicare Summary Notice (MSN) 21.25: "This service was denied because Medicare only covers this service in certain settings."

Spanish Version: "El servicio fue denegado porque Medicare solamente lo cubre en ciertas situaciones."

Professional Claims Modifier -62

For TAVR claims processed on or after July 1, 2013, contractors shall pay claim lines with 0256T, 0257T, 0258T, 0259T, 33361, 33362, 33363, 33364, 33365 & 0318T only when billed with modifier -62. Claim lines billed without modifier -62 shall be returned as unprocessable.

Beginning January 1, 2014, temporary CPT code 0318T above is retired. TAVR claims with dates of service on and after January 1, 2014 shall instead use permanent CPT code 33366.

The following messages shall be used when Medicare contractors return TAVR claims billed without modifier -62 as unprocessable:

CARC 4: "The procedure code is inconsistent with the modifier used or a required modifier is missing. Note: Refer to the 835 Healthcare Policy Identification Segment (loop 2110 Service Payment Information REF), if present."

RARC N29: "Missing documentation/orders/notes/summary/report/chart."

RARC MA130: "Your claim contains incomplete and/or invalid information, and no appeal rights are afforded because the claim is unprocessable. Please submit a new claim with the complete/correct information."

Professional Claims Modifier -Q0

For claims processed on or after July 1, 2013, contractors shall pay TAVR claim lines for 0256T, 0257T, 0258T, 0259T, 33361, 33362, 33363, 33364, 33365 & 0318T when billed with modifier -Q0. Claim lines billed without modifier -Q0 shall be returned as unprocessable.

Beginning January 1, 2014, temporary CPT code 0318T above is retired. TAVR claims with dates of service on and after January 1, 2014 shall instead use permanent CPT code 33366.

The following messages shall be used when Medicare contractors return TAVR claims billed without modifier -Q0 as unprocessable:

CARC 4: "The procedure code is inconsistent with the modifier used or a required modifier is missing. Note: Refer to the 835 Healthcare Policy Identification Segment (loop 2110 Service Payment Information REF), if present."

RARC N29: "Missing documentation/orders/notes/summary/report/chart."

RARC MA130: "Your claim contains incomplete and/or invalid information, and no appeal rights are afforded because the claim is unprocessable. Please submit a new claim with the complete/correct information."

For claims processed on or after July 1, 2013, contractors shall pay TAVR claim lines for 0256T, 0257T, 0258T, 0259T, 33361, 33362, 33363, 33364, 33365 & 0318T when billed with diagnosis code V70.7 (ICD-10=Z00.6). Claim lines billed without diagnosis code V70.7 (ICD-10=Z00.6) shall be returned as unprocessable.

Beginning January 1, 2014, temporary CPT code 0318T above is retired. TAVR claims with dates of service on and after January 1, 2014 shall instead use permanent CPT code 33366.

The following messages shall be used when Medicare contractors return TAVR claims billed without diagnosis code V70.7 (ICD-10=Z00.6) as unprocessable:

CARC 16: "Claim/service lacks information which is needed for adjudication. At least one Remark Code must be provided (may be comprised of either the NCPDP Reject Reason Code, or Remittance Advice Remark Code that is not an ALERT)."

RARC M76: "Missing/incomplete/invalid diagnosis or condition"

RARC MA130: "Your claim contains incomplete and/or invalid information, and no appeal rights are afforded because the claim is unprocessable. Please submit a new claim with the complete/correct information."

Professional Claims 8-digit ClinicalTrials.gov Identifier Number

For claims processed on or after July 1, 2013, contractors shall pay TAVR claim lines for 0256T, 0257T, 0258T, 0259T, 33361, 33362, 33363, 33364, 33365 & 0318T when billed with the numeric, 8-digit clinicaltrials.gov identifier number preceded by the two alpha characters "CT" when placed in Field 19 of paper Form CMS-1500, or when entered without the "CT" prefix in the electronic 837P in Loop 2300REF02(REF01=P4). Claim lines billed without an 8-digit clinicaltrials.gov identifier number shall be returned as unprocessable.

Beginning January 1, 2014, temporary CPT code 0318T above is retired. TAVR claims with dates of service on and after January 1, 2014 shall instead use permanent CPT code 33366.

The following messages shall be used when Medicare contractors return TAVR claims billed without an 8-digit clinicaltrials.gov identifier number as unprocessable:

CARC 16: "Claim/service lacks information which is needed for adjudication. At least one Remark Code must be provided (may be comprised of either NCPDP Reject Reason Code, or Remittance Advice Remark Code that is not an ALERT)."

RARC MA50: "Missing/incomplete/invalid Investigational Device Exemption number for FDA-approved clinical trial services."

RARC MA130: "Your claim contains incomplete and/or invalid information, and no appeal rights are afforded because the claim is unprocessable. Please submit a new claim with the complete/correct information."

NOTE: Clinicaltrials.gov identifier numbers for TAVR are listed on our website:

(http://www.cms.gov/Medicare/Coverage/Coverage-with-Evidence-Development/Transcatheter-Aortic-Valve-Replacement-TAVR-.html)

100-04, 32, 290.3

Claims Processing Requirements for TAVR Services on Inpatient Hospital Claims

(Rev.2827. Issued: 11-29-13, Effective: 01-01-14, Implementation: 01-06-14)

Inpatient hospitals shall bill for TAVR on an 11X TOB effective for discharges on or after May 1, 2012. Refer to Section 69 of this chapter for further guidance on billing under CED.

Inpatient hospital discharges for TAVR shall be covered when billed with:

- V70.7 and Condition Code 30.
- An 8-digit clinicaltrials.gov identifier number listed on the CMS website (effective July 1, 2013)

Inpatient hospital discharges for TAVR shall be rejected when billed without:

- V70.7 and Condition Code 30.
- An 8-digit clinicaltrials.gov identifier number listed on the CMS website (effective July 1, 2013)

Claims billed by hospitals not participating in the trial/registry shall be rejected with the following messages:

CARC: 50 -These are non-covered services because this is not deemed a "medical necessity" by the payer.

RARC N386 - This decision was based on a National Coverage Determination (NCD). An NCD provides a coverage determination as to whether a particular item or service is covered. A copy of this policy is available at http://www.cms.hhs.gov/mcd/
search.asp. If you do not have web access, you may contact the contractor to request a copy of the NCD.

Group Code –Contractual Obligation (CO)

MSN 16.77 – This service/item was not covered because it was not provided as part of a qualifying trial/study. (Este servicio/artículo no fue cubierto porque no estaba incluido como parte de un ensayo clínico/estudio calificado.)

100-04, 32, 290.4

Claims Processing Requirements for TAVR Services for Medicare Advantage (MA) Plan Participants

(Rev. 3943; Issued: 12-22-17; Effective: 04- 01-15; Implementation: 04-02-18)

MA plans are responsible for payment of TAVR services for MA plan participants. Medicare coverage for TAVR is not included under section 310.1 of the NCD Manual (Routine Costs in Clinical Trials).

100-04, 32, 320.1

Coding Requirements for Artificial Hearts Furnished Before May 1, 2008

(Rev. 3054, Issued: 08-29-14, Effective: 10-30- 13, Implementation: 09-30-14)

Effective for discharges before May 1, 2008, Medicare does not cover the use of artificial hearts, either as a permanent replacement for a human heart or as a temporary life-support system until a human heart becomes available for transplant (often referred to a "bridge to transplant").

100-04, 32, 320.2

Coding Requirements for Artificial Hearts Furnished On or After May 1, 2008

(Rev. 3054, Issued: 08-29-14, Effective: 10-30- 13, Implementation: 09-30-14)

Effective for discharges on or after May 1, 2008, the use of artificial hearts will be covered by Medicare under Coverage with Evidence Development (CED) when beneficiaries are enrolled in a clinical study that meets all of the criteria listed in IOM Pub. 100-3, Medicare NCD Manual, section 20.9.

Claims Coding

For claims with dates of service on or after May 1, 2008, artificial hearts in the context of an approved clinical study for a Category A IDE, refer to section 69 in this manual for more detail on CED billing. Appropriate ICD-10 diagnosis and procedure codes are included below:

ICD-10 Diagnosis Code	Definition	Discharges Effective
I09.81	Rheumatic heart failure	On or After ICD-10 Implementation
I11.0	Hypertensive heart disease with heart failure	
I13.0	Hypertensive heart and chronic kidney disease with heart failure and stage 1 through stage 4 chronic kidney disease, or unspecified chronic kidney disease	
I13.2	Hypertensive heart and chronic kidney disease with heart failure and with stage 5 chronic kidney disease, or end stage renal disease	
I20.0	Unstable angina	
I21.01	ST elevation (STEMI) myocardial infarction involving left main coronary artery	
I21.02	ST elevation (STEMI) myocardial infarction involving left anterior descending coronary artery	
I21.09	ST elevation (STEMI) myocardial infarction involving other coronary artery of anterior wall	
I21.11	ST elevation (STEMI) myocardial infarction involving right coronary artery	
I21.19	ST elevation (STEMI) myocardial infarction involving other coronary artery of inferior wall	
I21.21	ST elevation (STEMI) myocardial infarction involving left circumflex coronary artery	
I21.29	ST elevation (STEMI) myocardial infarction involving other sites	
I21.3	ST elevation (STEMI) myocardial infarction of unspecified site	
I21.4	Non-ST elevation (NSTEMI) myocardial infarction	
I22.0	Subsequent ST elevation (STEMI) myocardial infarction of anterior wall	
I22.1	Subsequent ST elevation (STEMI) myocardial infarction of inferior wall	
I22.2	Subsequent non-ST elevation (NSTEMI) myocardial infarction	
I22.8	Subsequent ST elevation (STEMI) myocardial infarction of other sites	
I22.9	Subsequent ST elevation (STEMI) myocardial infarction of unspecified site	
I24.0	Acute coronary thrombosis not resulting in myocardial infarction	
I24.1	Dressler's syndrome	
I24.8	Other forms of acute ischemic heart disease	
I24.9	Acute ischemic heart disease, unspecified	
I25.10	Atherosclerotic heart disease of native coronary artery without angina pectoris	
I25.110	Atherosclerotic heart disease of native coronary artery with unstable angina pectoris	
I25.111	Atherosclerotic heart disease of native coronary artery with angina pectoris with documented spasm	
I25.118	Atherosclerotic heart disease of native coronary artery with other forms of angina pectoris	
I25.119	Atherosclerotic heart disease of native coronary artery with unspecified angina pectoris	
I25.5	Ischemic cardiomyopathy	
I25.6	Silent myocardial ischemia	

ICD-10 Diagnosis Code	Definition	Discharges Effective
I25.7ØØ	Atherosclerosis of coronary artery bypass graft(s), unspecified, with unstable angina pectoris	On or After ICD-10 Implementation
I25.7Ø1	Atherosclerosis of coronary artery bypass graft(s), unspecified, with angina pectoris with documented spasm	
I25.7Ø8	Atherosclerosis of coronary artery bypass graft(s), unspecified, with other forms of angina pectoris	
I25.7Ø9	Atherosclerosis of coronary artery bypass graft(s), unspecified, with unspecified angina pectoris	
I25.71Ø	Atherosclerosis of autologous vein coronary artery bypass graft(s) with unstable angina pectoris	
I25.711	Atherosclerosis of autologous vein coronary artery bypass graft(s) with angina pectoris with documented spasm	
I25.718	Atherosclerosis of autologous vein coronary artery bypass graft(s) with other forms of angina pectoris	
I25.719	Atherosclerosis of autologous vein coronary artery bypass graft(s) with unspecified angina pectoris	
I25.72Ø	Atherosclerosis of autologous artery coronary artery bypass graft(s) with unstable angina pectoris	
I25.721	Atherosclerosis of autologous artery coronary artery bypass graft(s) with angina pectoris with documented spasm	
I25.728	Atherosclerosis of autologous artery coronary artery bypass graft(s) with other forms of angina pectoris	
I25.729	Atherosclerosis of autologous artery coronary artery bypass graft(s) with unspecified angina pectoris	
I25.73Ø	Atherosclerosis of nonautologous biological coronary artery bypass graft(s) with unstable angina pectoris	
I25.731	Atherosclerosis of nonautologous biological coronary artery bypass graft(s) with angina pectoris with documented spasm	
I25.738	Atherosclerosis of nonautologous biological coronary artery bypass graft(s) with other forms of angina pectoris	
I25.739	Atherosclerosis of nonautologous biological coronary artery bypass graft(s) with unspecified angina pectoris	
I25.75Ø	Atherosclerosis of native coronary artery of transplanted heart with unstable angina	
I25.751	Atherosclerosis of native coronary artery of transplanted heart with angina pectoris with documented spasm	
I25.758	Atherosclerosis of native coronary artery of transplanted heart with other forms of angina pectoris	
I25.759	Atherosclerosis of native coronary artery of transplanted heart with unspecified angina pectoris	
I25.76Ø	Atherosclerosis of bypass graft of coronary artery of transplanted heart with unstable angina	
I25.761	Atherosclerosis of bypass graft of coronary artery of transplanted heart with angina pectoris with documented spasm	
I25.768	Atherosclerosis of bypass graft of coronary artery of transplanted heart with other forms of angina pectoris	
I25.769	Atherosclerosis of bypass graft of coronary artery of transplanted heart with unspecified angina pectoris	
I25.79Ø	Atherosclerosis of other coronary artery bypass graft(s) with unstable angina pectoris	
I25.791	Atherosclerosis of other coronary artery bypass graft(s) with angina pectoris with documented spasm	
I25.798	Atherosclerosis of other coronary artery bypass graft(s) with other forms of angina pectoris	On or After ICD-10 Implementation
I25.799	Atherosclerosis of other coronary artery bypass graft(s) with unspecified angina pectoris	
I25.81Ø	Atherosclerosis of coronary artery bypass graft(s) without angina pectoris	
I25.811	Atherosclerosis of native coronary artery of transplanted heart without angina pectoris	
I25.812	Atherosclerosis of bypass graft of coronary artery of transplanted heart without angina pectoris	
I25.89	Other forms of chronic ischemic heart disease	
I25.9	Chronic ischemic heart disease, unspecified	
I34.Ø	Nonrheumatic mitral (valve) insufficiency	
I34.1	Nonrheumatic mitral (valve) prolapse	
I34.2	Nonrheumatic mitral (valve) stenosis	
I34.8	Other nonrheumatic mitral valve disorders	
I34.9	Nonrheumatic mitral valve disorder, unspecified	
I35.Ø	Nonrheumatic aortic (valve) stenosis	
I35.1	Nonrheumatic aortic (valve) insufficiency	
I35.2	Nonrheumatic aortic (valve) stenosis with insufficiency	
I35.8	Other nonrheumatic aortic valve disorders	
I35.9	Nonrheumatic aortic valve disorder, unspecified	
I36.Ø	Nonrheumatic tricuspid (valve) stenosis	
I36.1	Nonrheumatic tricuspid (valve) insufficiency	
I36.2	Nonrheumatic tricuspid (valve) stenosis with insufficiency	
I36.8	Other nonrheumatic tricuspid valve disorders	
I36.9	Nonrheumatic tricuspid valve disorder, unspecified	
I37.Ø	Nonrheumatic pulmonary valve stenosis	
I37.1	Nonrheumatic pulmonary valve insufficiency	
I37.2	Nonrheumatic pulmonary valve stenosis with insufficiency	
I37.8	Other nonrheumatic pulmonary valve disorders	
I37.9	Nonrheumatic pulmonary valve disorder, unspecified	
I38	Endocarditis, valve unspecified	
I39	Endocarditis and heart valve disorders in diseases classified elsewhere	
I42.Ø	Dilated cardiomyopathy	
I42.2	Other hypertrophic cardiomyopathy	
I42.3	Endomyocardial (eosinophilic) disease	
I42.4	Endocardial fibroelastosis	
I42.5	Other restrictive cardiomyopathy	
I42.6	Alcoholic cardiomyopathy	
I42.7	Cardiomyopathy due to drug and external agent	
I42.8	Other cardiomyopathies	
I42.9	Cardiomyopathy, unspecified	
I43	Cardiomyopathy in diseases classified elsewhere	
I46.2	Cardiac arrest due to underlying cardiac condition	
I46.8	Cardiac arrest due to other underlying condition	
I46.9	Cardiac arrest, cause unspecified	
I47.Ø	Re-entry ventricular arrhythmia	
I47.1	Supraventricular tachycardia	
I47.2	Ventricular tachycardia	
I47.9	Paroxysmal tachycardia, unspecified	
I48.Ø	Atrial fibrillation	
I48.1	Atrial flutter	
I49.Ø1	Ventricular fibrillation	
I49.Ø2	Ventricular flutter	
I49.1	Atrial premature depolarization	

ICD-10 Diagnosis Code	Definition	Discharges Effective
I49.2	Junctional premature depolarization	On or After ICD-10 Implementation
I49.3	Ventricular premature depolarization	
I49.40	Unspecified premature depolarization	
I49.49	Other premature depolarization	
I49.5	Sick sinus syndrome	
I49.8	Other specified cardiac arrhythmias	
I49.9	Cardiac arrhythmia, unspecified	
I50.1	Left ventricular failure	
I50.20	Unspecified systolic (congestive) heart failure	
I50.21	Acute systolic (congestive) heart failure	
I50.22	Chronic systolic (congestive) heart failure	
I50.23	Acute on chronic systolic (congestive) heart failure	
I50.30	Unspecified diastolic (congestive) heart failure	
I50.31	Acute diastolic (congestive) heart failure	
I50.32	Chronic diastolic (congestive) heart failure	
I50.33	Acute on chronic diastolic (congestive) heart failure	
I50.40	Unspecified combined systolic (congestive) and diastolic (congestive) heart failure	
I50.41	Acute combined systolic (congestive) and diastolic (congestive) heart failure	
I50.42	Chronic combined systolic (congestive) and diastolic (congestive) heart failure	
I50.43	Acute on chronic combined systolic (congestive) and diastolic (congestive) heart failure	
I50.9	Heart failure, unspecified	
I51.4	Myocarditis, unspecified	
I51.9	Heart disease, unspecified	
I52	Other heart disorders in diseases classified elsewhere	
I97.0	Postcardiotomy syndrome	
I97.110	Postprocedural cardiac insufficiency following cardiac surgery	
I97.111	Postprocedural cardiac insufficiency following other surgery	
I97.120	Postprocedural cardiac arrest following cardiac surgery	
I97.121	Postprocedural cardiac arrest following other surgery	
I97.130	Postprocedural heart failure following cardiac surgery	
I97.131	Postprocedural heart failure following other surgery	
I97.190	Other postprocedural cardiac functional disturbances following cardiac surgery	
I97.191	Other postprocedural cardiac functional disturbances following other surgery	
I97.710	Intraoperative cardiac arrest during cardiac surgery	
I97.711	Intraoperative cardiac arrest during other surgery	
I97.790	Other intraoperative cardiac functional disturbances during cardiac surgery	
I97.791	Other intraoperative cardiac functional disturbances during other surgery	
I97.88	Other intraoperative complications of the circulatory system, not elsewhere classified	
I97.89	Other postprocedural complications and disorders of the circulatory system, not elsewhere classified	
M32.11	Endocarditis in systemic lupus erythematosus	
O90.89	Other complications of the puerperium, not elsewhere classified	
Q20.0	Common arterial trunk	
Q20.1	Double outlet right ventricle	
Q20.2	Double outlet left ventricle	
Q20.3	Discordant ventriculoarterial connection	
Q20.4	Double inlet ventricle	

ICD-10 Diagnosis Code	Definition	Discharges Effective
Q20.5	Discordant atrioventricular connection	On or After ICD-10 Implementation
Q20.6	Isomerism of atrial appendages	
Q20.8	Other congenital malformations of cardiac chambers and connections	
Q20.9	Congenital malformation of cardiac chambers and connections, unspecified	
Q21.0	Ventricular septal defect	
Q21.1	Atrial septal defect	
Q21.2	Atrioventricular septal defect	
Q21.3	Tetralogy of Fallot	
Q21.4	Aortopulmonary septal defect	
Q21.8	Other congenital malformations of cardiac septa	
Q21.9	Congenital malformation of cardiac septum, unspecified	
Q22.0	Pulmonary valve atresia	
Q22.1	Congenital pulmonary valve stenosis	
Q22.2	Congenital pulmonary valve insufficiency	
Q22.3	Other congenital malformations of pulmonary valve	
Q22.4	Congenital tricuspid stenosis	
Q22.5	Ebstein's anomaly	
Q22.6	Hypoplastic right heart syndrome	
Q22.8	Other congenital malformations of tricuspid valve	
Q22.9	Congenital malformation of tricuspid valve, unspecified	
Q23.0	Congenital stenosis of aortic valve	
Q23.1	Congenital insufficiency of aortic valve	
Q23.2	Congenital mitral stenosis	
Q23.3	Congenital mitral insufficiency	
Q23.4	Hypoplastic left heart syndrome	
Q23.8	Other congenital malformations of aortic and mitral valves	
Q23.9	Congenital malformation of aortic and mitral valves, unspecified	
Q24.0	Dextrocardia	
Q24.1	Levocardia	
Q24.2	Cor triatriatum	
Q24.3	Pulmonary infundibular stenosis	
Q24.4	Congenital subaortic stenosis	
Q24.5	Malformation of coronary vessels	
Q24.6	Congenital heart block	
Q24.8	Other specified congenital malformations of heart	
Q24.9	Congenital malformation of heart, unspecified	
R00.1	Bradycardia, unspecified	
R57.0	Cardiogenic shock	
T82.221A	Breakdown (mechanical) of biological heart valve graft, initial encounter	
T82.222A	Displacement of biological heart valve graft, initial encounter	
T82.223A	Leakage of biological heart valve graft, initial encounter	
T82.228A	Other mechanical complication of biological heart valve graft, initial encounter	
T82.512A	Breakdown (mechanical) of artificial heart, initial encounter	
T82.514A	Breakdown (mechanical) of infusion catheter, initial encounter	
T82.518A	Breakdown (mechanical) of other cardiac and vascular devices and implants, initial encounter	
T82.519A	Breakdown (mechanical) of unspecified cardiac and vascular devices and implants, initial encounter	
T82.522A	Displacement of artificial heart, initial encounter	
T82.524A	Displacement of infusion catheter, initial encounter	

Appendix G — Medicare Internet-only Manuals (IOMs)

ICD-10 Diagnosis Code	Definition	Discharges Effective
T82.528A	Displacement of other cardiac and vascular devices and implants, initial encounter	On or After ICD-10 Implementation
T82.529A	Displacement of unspecified cardiac and vascular devices and implants, initial encounter	On or After ICD-10 Implementation
T82.532A	Leakage of artificial heart, initial encounter	
T82.534A	Leakage of infusion catheter, initial encounter	
T82.538A	Leakage of other cardiac and vascular devices and implants, initial encounter	
T82.539A	Leakage of unspecified cardiac and vascular devices and implants, initial encounter	
T82.592A	Other mechanical complication of artificial heart, initial encounter	
T82.594A	Other mechanical complication of infusion catheter, initial encounter	
T82.598A	Other mechanical complication of other cardiac and vascular devices and implants, initial encounter	
T82.599A	Other mechanical complication of unspecified cardiac and vascular devices and implants, initial encounter	
T86.2Ø	Unspecified complication of heart transplant	
T86.21	Heart transplant rejection	
T86.22	Heart transplant failure	
T86.23	Heart transplant infection	
T86.29Ø	Cardiac allograft vasculopathy	
T86.298	Other complications of heart transplant	
T86.3Ø	Unspecified complication of heart-lung transplant	
T86.31	Heart-lung transplant rejection	
T86.32	Heart-lung transplant failure	
T86.33	Heart-lung transplant infection	
T86.39	Other complications of heart-lung transplant	
Z48.21	Encounter for aftercare following heart transplant	
Z48.28Ø	Encounter for aftercare following heart-lung transplant	
Z94.1	Heart transplant status	
Z94.3	Heart and lungs transplant status	
Z95.9	Presence of cardiac and vascular implant and graft, unspecified	
Q24.Ø	Dextrocardia	
Q24.1	Levocardia	
Q24.2	Cor triatriatum	
Q24.3	Pulmonary infundibular stenosis	
Q24.4	Congenital subaortic stenosis	
Q24.5	Malformation of coronary vessels	
Q24.6	Congenital heart block	
Q24.8	Other specified congenital malformations of heart	
Q24.9	Congenital malformation of heart, unspecified	
RØØ.1	Bradycardia, unspecified	
R57.Ø	Cardiogenic shock	
T82.221A	Breakdown (mechanical) of biological heart valve graft, initial encounter	
T82.222A	Displacement of biological heart valve graft, initial encounter	
T82.223A	Leakage of biological heart valve graft, initial encounter	
T82.228A	Other mechanical complication of biological heart valve graft, initial encounter	
T82.512A	Breakdown (mechanical) of artificial heart, initial encounter	
T82.514A	Breakdown (mechanical) of infusion catheter, initial encounter	
T82.518A	Breakdown (mechanical) of other cardiac and vascular devices and implants, initial encounter	
T82.519A	Breakdown (mechanical) of unspecified cardiac and vascular devices and implants, initial encounter	

ICD-10 Diagnosis Code	Definition	Discharges Effective
T82.522A	Displacement of artificial heart, initial encounter	On or After ICD-10 Implementation
T82.524A	Displacement of infusion catheter, initial encounter	
T82.528A	Displacement of other cardiac and vascular devices and implants, initial encounter	
T82.529A	Displacement of unspecified cardiac and vascular devices and implants, initial encounter	
T82.532A	Leakage of artificial heart, initial encounter	
T82.534A	Leakage of infusion catheter, initial encounter	
T82.538A	Leakage of other cardiac and vascular devices and implants, initial encounter	
T82.539A	Leakage of unspecified cardiac and vascular devices and implants, initial encounter	
T82.592A	Other mechanical complication of artificial heart, initial encounter	
T82.594A	Other mechanical complication of infusion catheter, initial encounter	
T82.598A	Other mechanical complication of other cardiac and vascular devices and implants, initial encounter	
T82.599A	Other mechanical complication of unspecified cardiac and vascular devices and implants, initial encounter	
T86.2Ø	Unspecified complication of heart transplant	
T86.21	Heart transplant rejection	
T86.22	Heart transplant failure	
T86.23	Heart transplant infection	
T86.29Ø	Cardiac allograft vasculopathy	
T86.298	Other complications of heart transplant	
T86.3Ø	Unspecified complication of heart-lung transplant	
T86.31	Heart-lung transplant rejection	
T86.32	Heart-lung transplant failure	
T86.33	Heart-lung transplant infection	
T86.39	Other complications of heart-lung transplant	
Z48.21	Encounter for aftercare following heart transplant	
Z48.28Ø	Encounter for aftercare following heart-lung transplant	
Z94.1	Heart transplant status	
Z94.3	Heart and lungs transplant status	
Z95.9	Presence of cardiac and vascular implant and graft, unspecified	
Ø2RKØJZ	Replacement of Right Ventricle with Synthetic Substitute, Open Approach	
Ø2RLØJZ	Revision of Synthetic Substitute in Heart, Open Approach	
Ø2WAØJZ	Revision of Synthetic Substitute in Heart, Open Approach	

NOTE: Total artificial heart is reported with a "cluster" of 2 codes for open replacement with synthetic substitute of the right and left ventricles- 02RK0JZ + 02RL0JZ

100-04, 32, 320.3

Ventricular Assist Devices

(Rev. 3054, Issued: 08-29-14, Effective: 10-30-13, Implementation: 09-30-14)

Medicare may cover a Ventricular Assist Device (VAD). A VAD is used to assist a damaged or weakened heart in pumping blood. VADs are used as a bridge to a heart transplant, for support of blood circulation post-cardiotomy or destination therapy. Refer to the IOM Pub. 100-3, NCD Manual, section 20.9.1 for coverage criteria.

100-04, 32, 320.3.1

Post-cardiotomy

(Rev. 3054, Issued: 08-29-14, Effective: 10-30-13, Implementation: 09-30-14)

Post-cardiotomy is the period following open-heart surgery. VADs used for support of blood circulation post-cardiotomy are covered only if they have received approval from the Food and Drug Administration (FDA) for that purpose, and the VADs are used according to the FDA-approved labeling instructions.

100-04, 32, 320.3.2

Bridge- to -Transplantation (BTT)

(Rev. 3054, Issued: 08-29-14, Effective: 10-30-13, Implementation: 09-30-14)

Coverage for BTT is restricted to patients listed for heart transplantation. The Centers for Medicare & Medicaid Services (CMS) has clearly identified that the patient must be active on the waitlist maintained by the Organ Procurement and Transplantation Network. CMS has also removed the general time requirement that patients receive a transplant as soon as medically reasonable.

100-04, 32, 370

Microvolt T-wave Alternans (MTWA)

(Rev. 3265, Issued: 05-22-15, Effective: 01-13-15, Implementation: 06-23-15)

On March 21, 2006, the Centers for Medicare & Medicaid Services (CMS) began national coverage of microvolt T-wave Alternans (MTWA) diagnostic testing when it was performed using only the spectral analysis (SA) method for the evaluation of patients at risk for sudden cardiac death (SCD) from ventricular arrhythmias and patients who may be candidates for Medicare coverage of the placement of an implantable cardiac defibrillator (ICD).

Effective for claims with dates of service on and after January 13, 2015, Medicare Administrative Contractors (MACs) may determine coverage of MTWA diagnostic testing when it is performed using methods of analysis other than SA for the evaluation of patients at risk for SCD from ventricular arrhythmias. Further information can be found at Publication 100-3, section 20.30, of the National Coverage Determinations Manual.

100-04, 32, 370.1

Coding and Claims Processing for MTWA

(Rev. 3265, Issued: 05-22-15, Effective: 01-13-15, Implementation: 06-23-15)

Effective for claims with dates of service on and after March 21, 2006, MACs shall accept CPT 93025 (MTWA for assessment of ventricular arrhythmias) for MTWA diagnostic testing for the evaluation of patients at risk for SCD with the SA method of analysis only. All other methods of analysis for MTWA are non-covered.

Effective for claims with dates of service on and after January 13, 2015, MACs shall at their discretion determine coverage for CPT 93025 for MTWA diagnostic testing for the evaluation of patients at risk for SCD with methods of analysis other than SA. The –KX modifier shall be used as an attestation by the practitioner and/or provider of the service that documentation is on file verifying the MTWA was performed using a method of analysis other than SA for the evaluation of patients at risk for SCD from ventricular arrhythmias and that all other NCD criteria was met.

NOTE: The –KX modifier is NOT required on MTWA claims for the evaluation of patients at risk for SCD if the SA analysis method is used.

NOTE: This diagnosis code list/translation was approved by CMS/Coverage. It may or may not be a complete list of covered indications/diagnosis codes that are covered but should serve as a finite starting point.

As this policy indicates, individual A/B MACs within their respective jurisdictions have the discretion to make coverage determinations they deem reasonable and necessary under section 1862(a)1)(A) of the Social Security Act. Therefore, A/B MACs may have additional covered diagnosis codes in their individual policies where contractor discretion is appropriate.

ICD-9 Codes

410.11	Acute myocardial infarction of other anterior wall, initial episode of care
410.11	Acute myocardial infarction of other anterior wall, initial episode of care
410.01	Acute myocardial infarction of anterolateral wall, initial episode of care
410.11	Acute myocardial infarction of other anterior wall, initial episode of care
410.31	Acute myocardial infarction of inferoposterior wall, initial episode of care
410.21	Acute myocardial infarction of inferolateral wall, initial episode of care
410.41	Acute myocardial infarction of other inferior wall, initial episode of care
410.81	Acute myocardial infarction of other specified sites, initial episode of care
410.51	Acute myocardial infarction of other lateral wall, initial episode of care
410.61	True posterior wall infarction, initial episode of care
410.81	Acute myocardial infarction of other specified sites, initial episode of care
410.91	Acute myocardial infarction of unspecified site, initial episode of care
410.71	Subendocardial infarction, initial episode of care
410.01	Acute myocardial infarction of anterolateral wall, initial episode of care
410.11	Acute myocardial infarction of other anterior wall, initial episode of care
410.21	Acute myocardial infarction of inferolateral wall, initial episode of care
410.31	Acute myocardial infarction of inferoposterior wall, initial episode of care
410.41	Acute myocardial infarction of other inferior wall, initial episode of care
410.71	Subendocardial infarction, initial episode of care
410.51	Acute myocardial infarction of other lateral wall, initial episode of care
410.61	True posterior wall infarction, initial episode of care
410.81	Acute myocardial infarction of other specified sites, initial episode of care
410.91	Acute myocardial infarction of unspecified site, initial episode of care
411.89	Other acute and subacute forms of ischemic heart disease, other
411.89	Other acute and subacute forms of ischemic heart disease, other
427.1	Paroxysmal ventricular tachycardia
427.1	Paroxysmal ventricular tachycardia
427.41	Ventricular fibrillation
427.42	Ventricular flutter
780.2	Syncope and collapse
V45.89	Other postprocedural status

ICD- 10 Codes

I21.Ø1	ST elevation (STEMI) myocardial infarction involving left main coronary artery
I21.Ø2	ST elevation (STEMI) myocardial infarction involving left anterior descending coron
I21.Ø9	ST elevation (STEMI) myocardial infarction involving other coronary artery of anteri
I21.Ø9	ST elevation (STEMI) myocardial infarction involving other coronary artery of anteri
I21.11	ST elevation (STEMI) myocardial infarction involving right coronary artery
I21.19	ST elevation (STEMI) myocardial infarction involving other coronary artery of inferi
I21.19	ST elevation (STEMI) myocardial infarction involving other coronary artery of inferi
I21.21	ST elevation (STEMI) myocardial infarction involving left circumflex coronary artery
I21.29	ST elevation (STEMI) myocardial infarction involving other sites
I21.29	ST elevation (STEMI) myocardial infarction involving other sites
I21.29	ST elevation (STEMI) myocardial infarction involving other sites
I21.3	ST elevation (STEMI) myocardial infarction of unspecified site
I21.4	Non-ST elevation (NSTEMI) myocardial infarction
I22.Ø	Subsequent ST elevation (STEMI) myocardial infarction of anterior wall
I22.Ø	Subsequent ST elevation (STEMI) myocardial infarction of anterior wall
I22.1	Subsequent ST elevation (STEMI) myocardial infarction of inferior wall
I22.1	Subsequent ST elevation (STEMI) myocardial infarction of inferior wall
I22.1	Subsequent ST elevation (STEMI) myocardial infarction of inferior wall
I22.2	Subsequent non-ST elevation (NSTEMI) myocardial infarction
I22.8	Subsequent ST elevation (STEMI) myocardial infarction of other sites
I22.8	Subsequent ST elevation (STEMI) myocardial infarction of other sites
I22.8	Subsequent ST elevation (STEMI) myocardial infarction of other sites
I22.9	Subsequent ST elevation (STEMI) myocardial infarction of unspecified site
I24.8	Other forms of acute ischemic heart disease
I24.9	Acute ischemic heart disease, unspecified
I47.Ø	Re-entry ventricular arrhythmia
I47.2	Ventricular tachycardia
I49.Ø1	Ventricular fibrillation
I49.Ø2	Ventricular flutter
R55	Syncope and collapse
Z98.89	Other specified postprocedural states

100-04, 32, 370.2

Messaging for MTWA

(Rev. 3265, Issued: 05-22-15, Effective: 01-13-15, Implementation: 06-23-15)

Effective for claims with dates of service on and after January 13, 2015, MACs shall deny claims for MTWA CPT 93025 with methods of analysis other than SA without modifier -KX using the following messages:

CARC 4: "The procedure code is inconsistent with the modifier used or a required modifier is missing. Note: Refer to the 835 Healthcare Policy Identification Segment (loop 2110 Service Payment Information REF), if present."

RARC N657 – This should be billed with the appropriate code for these services.

Group Code: CO (Contractual Obligation) assigning financial liability to the provider

MSN 15.20 - The following policies [NCD 20.30] were used when we made this decision

Spanish Equivalent - 15.20 - Las siguientes políticas [NCD 20.30] fueron utilizadas cuando se tomó esta decisión.

100-04, 32, 380

Leadless Pacemakers

(Rev. 3815, Issued: 07-28-17, Effective: 01-18-18, Implementation: 08-29-17 - for MAC local edits; January 2, 2018 - for MCS shared edits)

Effective for dates of service on or after January 18, 2017, contractors shall cover leadless pacemakers through Coverage with Evidence Development (CED) when procedures are performed in CMS-approved CED studies. Please refer to the National Coverage Determinations Manual (Publication 100-03, Section 20.8.4) for more information.

100-04, 32, 380.1

Leadless Pacemaker Coding and Billing Requirements for Professional Claims

(Rev. 3815, Issued: 07-28-17, Effective: 01-18-18, Implementation: 08-29-17 - for MAC local edits; January 2, 2018 - for MCS shared edits)

Effective for dates of service on or after January 18, 2017, contractors shall allow the following procedure codes on claims for leadless pacemakers:

0387T Transcatheter insertion or replacement of permanent leadless pacemaker, ventricular

0389T Programming device evaluation (in person) with iterative adjustment of the implantable device to test the function of the device and select optimal permanent programmed values with analysis, review and report, leadless pacemaker system.

0390T Peri-procedural device evaluation (in person) and programming of device system parameters before or after surgery, procedure or test with analysis, review and report, leadless pacemaker system.

0391T Interrogation device evaluation (in person) with analysis, review and report, includes connection, recording and disconnection per patient encounter, leadless pacemaker system.

Effective for dates of service on or after January 18, 2017, contractors shall allow the following ICD-10 diagnosis codes on claims for leadless pacemakers:

Z00.6 – Encounter for examination for normal comparison and control in clinical research program.

100-04, 32, 380.1.1

Leadless Pacemaker Place of Service Restrictions

(Rev. 3815, Issued: 07-28-17, Effective: 01-18-18, Implementation: 08-29-17 - for MAC local edits; January 2, 2018 - for MCS shared edits)

Effective for dates of service on or after January 18, 2017, contractors shall only pay claims for leadless pacemakers when services are provided in one of the following places of service (POS):

POS 06 – Indian Health Service Provider Based Facility

POS 21 – Inpatient Hospital

POS 22 - On Campus-Outpatient Hospital

POS 26 – Military Treatment Facility

100-04, 32, 380.1.2

Leadless Pacemaker Modifier

(Rev. 3815, Issued: 07-28-17, Effective: 01-18-18, Implementation: 08-29-17 - for MAC local edits; January 2, 2018 - for MCS shared edits)

Effective for claims with dates of service on or after January 18, 2017, modifier Q0 – Investigational clinical service provided in a clinical research study that is an approved clinical research study, must also be included.

100-04, 32, 390

Supervised exercise therapy (SET) Symptomatic Peripheral Artery Disease

(Rev. 4049, Issued: 05- 11-18, Effective: 05-25-17, Implementation: 07-02-18)

Effective for claims with dates of service on or after May 25, 2017, the Centers for Medicare and Medicaid Services (CMS) will cover supervised exercise therapy (SET) for beneficiaries with intermittent claudication (IC) for the treatment of symptomatic peripheral artery disease (PAD). Up to 36 sessions over a 12 week period are covered if all of the following components of a SET program are met:

The SET program must:

- consist of sessions lasting 30-60 minutes comprising a therapeutic exercise-training program for PAD in patients with claudication;
- be conducted in a physician's office;
- be delivered by qualified auxiliary personnel necessary to ensure benefits exceed harms, and who are trained in exercise therapy for PAD; and
- be under the direct supervision of a physician (as defined in 1861(r)(1)) of the Social Security Act (the Act)), physician assistant, or nurse practitioner/clinical nurse specialist (as identified in 1861(aa)(5)) of (the Act) who must be trained in both basic and advanced life support techniques.

Beneficiaries must have a face-to-face visit with the physician responsible for PAD treatment to obtain the referral for SET. At this visit, the beneficiary must receive information regarding cardiovascular disease and PAD risk factor reduction, which could include education, counseling, behavioral interventions, and outcome assessments.

SET is non-covered for beneficiaries with absolute contraindications to exercise as determined by their primary attending physician.

Please refer to the National Coverage Determinations Manual (Publication 100-03, Section 20.35) for more information.

100-04, 32, 390.1

General Billing Requirements

(Rev. 4049, Issued: 05- 11-18, Effective: 05-25-17, Implementation: 07-02-18)

Effective for claims with date of services on or after May 25, 2017, contractors shall pay claims for SET for beneficiaries with IC for the treatment of symptomatic PAD, with a referral from the physician responsible for PAD treatment.

Medicare Administrative Contractors (MACs) have the discretion to cover SET beyond 36 sessions over 12 weeks and may cover an additional 36 sessions over an extended period of time. Contractors shall accept the inclusion of the KX modifier on the claim line(s) as an attestation by the provider of the services that documentation is on file verifying that further treatment beyond the 36 sessions of SET over a 12 week period meets the requirements of the medical policy.

100-04, 32, 390.2

Coding Requirements for SET for PAD

(Rev. 4229, Issued: 02-01-19, Effective: 05-25-17, Implementation: 03-19-19)

- CPT 93668 Peripheral arterial disease (PAD) rehabilitation, per session
- ICD-10 Codes

  I70.211 Atherosclerosis of native arteries of extremities with intermittent claudication, right leg

  I70.212 Atherosclerosis of native arteries of extremities with intermittent claudication, left leg

  I70.213 Atherosclerosis of native arteries of extremities with intermittent claudication, bilateral legs

  I70.218 Atherosclerosis of native arteries of extremities with intermittent claudication, other extremity

  I70.311 Atherosclerosis of unspecified type of bypass graft(s) of the extremities with intermittent claudication, right leg

  I70.312 Atherosclerosis of unspecified type of bypass graft(s) of the extremities with intermittent claudication, left leg

  I70.313 Atherosclerosis of unspecified type of bypass graft(s) of the extremities with intermittent claudication, bilateral legs

  I70.318 Atherosclerosis of unspecified type of bypass graft(s) of the extremities with intermittent claudication, other extremity

  I70.411 Atherosclerosis of autologous vein bypass graft(s) of the extremities with intermittent claudication, right leg

  I70.412 Atherosclerosis of autologous vein bypass graft(s) of the extremities with intermittent claudication, left leg

  I70.413 Atherosclerosis of autologous vein bypass graft(s) of the extremities with intermittent claudication, bilateral legs

  I70.418 Atherosclerosis of autologous vein bypass graft(s) of the extremities with intermittent claudication, other extremity

  I70.511 Atherosclerosis of nonautologous biological bypass graft(s) of the extremities with intermittent claudication, right leg

  I70.512 Atherosclerosis of nonautologous biological bypass graft(s) of the extremities with intermittent claudication, left leg

  I70.513 Atherosclerosis of nonautologous biological bypass graft(s) of the extremities with intermittent claudication, bilateral legs

  I70.518 Atherosclerosis of nonautologous biological bypass graft(s) of the extremities with intermittent claudication, other extremity

  I70.611 Atherosclerosis of nonbiological bypass graft(s) of the extremities with intermittent claudication, right leg

  I70.612 Atherosclerosis of nonbiological bypass graft(s) of the extremities with intermittent claudication, left leg

  I70.613 Atherosclerosis of nonbiological bypass graft(s) of the extremities with intermittent claudication, bilateral legs

  I70.618 Atherosclerosis of nonbiological bypass graft(s) of the extremities with intermittent claudication, other extremity

  I70.711 Atherosclerosis of other type of bypass graft(s) of the extremities with intermittent claudication, right leg

I70.712 Atherosclerosis of other type of bypass graft(s) of the extremities with intermittent claudication, left leg

I70.713 Atherosclerosis of other type of bypass graft(s) of the extremities with intermittent claudication, bilateral legs

I70.718 Atherosclerosis of other type of bypass graft(s) of the extremities with intermittent claudication, other extremity

100-04, 32, 390.3

Special Billing Requirements for Institutional Claims

(Rev. 4229, Issued: 02-01-19, Effective: 05-25-17, Implementation: 03-19-19)

Professional claim services for SET are only allowed in place of service (POS) 11. All other POS for SET will be denied. See section 390.4 for hospital outpatient center billing requirements.

100-04, 32, 390.4

Common Working File (CWF) Requirements

(Rev. 4049, Issued: 05- 11-18, Effective: 05-25-17, Implementation: 07-02-18)

Contractors shall pay claims for SET services containing CPT code 93668 on Types of Bill (TOBs) 13X under OPPS and 85X based on reasonable cost.

Contractors shall not pay claims for SET services containing CPT 93668 with revenue codes 096X, 097X, or 098X when billed on TOB 85X Method II.

100-04, 32, 390.5

Common Working File (CWF) Requirements

(Rev. 4229, Issued: 02-01-19, Effective: 05-25-17, Implementation: 03-19-19)

CWF shall create a new edit for CPT 93668 to reject claims when a beneficiary has reached 36 SET sessions within 84 days after the date of the first SET session and the -KX modifier is not included on the claim, or to reject any SET session provided after 84 days from the date of the first session and the -KX modifier is not included on the claim.

CWF shall determine the remaining SET sessions.

The CWF determination, to parallel claims processing, shall include all applicable factors including:

- Beneficiary entitlement status
- Beneficiary claims history
- Utilization rules

CWF shall update the determination when any changes occur to the beneficiary master data or claims data that would result in a change to the calculation.

CWF shall display the remaining SET sessions on all CWF provider query screens.

The Multi-Carrier System Desktop Tool (MCSDT) shall display the remaining SET sessions in a format equivalent to the CWF HIMR screen(s).

100-04, 32, 390.6

Applicable Medicare Summary Notice (MSN), Remittance Advice Remark Codes (RARCs), and Claim Adjustment Reason Code (CARC) Messaging

(Rev. 4229, Issued: 02-01-19, Effective: 05-25-17, Implementation: 03-19-19)

- Effective for claims with dates of service on or after May 25, 2017, contractor shall deny claims for SET in Place of Service (POS) other than 11, office using the following messages:

  Medicare Summary Notice (MSN) 15.20: "The following policies National Coverage Determination 20.35 (NCD) were used when we made this decision." Spanish Version: "Las siguientes políticas NCD 20.35 fueron utilizadas cuando se tomó esta decisión."

  Claim Adjustment Reason Code (CARC) 58: "Treatment was deemed by the payer to have been rendered in an inappropriate or invalid place of service. NOTE: Refer to the 835 Healthcare Policy Identification Segment (loop 2110 Service payment Information REF), if present."

  Remittance Advice Remark Code (RARC) N386: "This decision was based on a NCD 20.35. An NCD provides a coverage determination as to whether a particular item or service is covered. A copy of this policy is available at www.cms.gov/mcd/search.asp. If you do not have web access, you may contact the contractor to request a copy of the NCD."

  Contractors shall use Group CO (Contractual Obligation) assigning financial liability to the provider, if a claim is received with a GZ modifier indicating no signed Advance Beneficiary Notice (ABN) is on file.

- Contractors shall deny claims for SET when services are provided on other than TOBs 13X and 85X using the following messages:

  MSN 15.20: "The following policies NCD 20.35 were used when we made this decision."

  Spanish Version: "Las siguientes políticas NCD 20.35 fueron utilizadas cuando se tomó esta decisión."

  (Part A only) MSN 15.19: "Local Coverage Determinations (LCDs) help Medicare decide what is covered. An LCD was used for your claim. You can compare your case to the LCD, and send information from your doctor if you think it could change our decision. Call 1-800-MEDICARE (1-800-633-4227) for a copy of the LCD."

  Spanish Version: "Las Determinaciones Locales de Cobertura (LCDs en inglés) le ayudan a decidir a Medicare lo que está cubierto. Un LCD se usó para su reclamación. Usted puede comparar su caso con la determinación y enviar información de su médico si piensa que puede cambiar nuestra decisión. Para obtener una copia del LCD, llame al 1-800-MEDICARE (1800-633-4227)."

  CARC 58: "Treatment was deemed by the payer to have been rendered in an inappropriate or invalid place of service. NOTE: Refer to the 835 Healthcare Policy Identification Segment (loop 2110 Service payment Information REF), if present.

  RARC N386: This decision was based on a National Coverage Determination (NCD) 20.35. An NCD provides a coverage determination as to whether a particular item or service is covered. A copy of this policy is available at www.cms.gov/mcd/search.asp. If you do not have web access, you may contact the contractor to request a copy of the NCD.

  Contractors shall use Group Code CO (Contractual Obligation) assigning financial liability to the provider, if a claim is received with a GZ modifier indicating no signed ABN is on file.

  For professional claims only, contractors shall deny line items on claims for SET services performed in POS other than POS 11 and use the following messages:

  MSN 15.20: "The following policies NCD 20.35 were used when we made this decision."

  Spanish Version: "Las siguientes políticas NCD 20.35 fueron utilizadas cuando se tomó esta decisión." CARC 58: "Treatment was deemed by the payer to have been rendered in an inappropriate or invalid place of service. NOTE: Refer to the 835 Healthcare Policy Identification Segment (loop 2110 Service payment Information REF), if present.

  RARC N386: "This decision was based on a National Coverage Determination 20.35 (NCD). An NCD provides a coverage determination as to whether a particular item or service is covered. A copy of this policy is available at www.cms.gov/mcd/search.asp. If you do not have web access, you may contact the contractor to request a copy of the NCD.

  Contractors shall use Group CO (Contractual Obligation) assigning financial liability to the provider, if a claim is received with a GZ modifier indicating no signed ABN is on file.

- Contractors shall deny/reject claim lines for CPT 93668 without one of the diagnosis codes listed in section 390.2 above and use the following messages:

  MSN 15.20: "The following policies NCD 20.35 were used when we made this decision."

  Spanish Version: "Las siguientes políticas NCD 20.35 fueron utilizadas cuando se tomó esta decisión."

  (Part A only) MSN 15.19: "Local Coverage Determinations (LCDs) help Medicare decide what is covered. An LCD was used for your claim. You can compare your case to the LCD, and send information from your doctor if you think it could change our decision. Call 1-800-MEDICARE (1-800-633-4227) for a copy of the LCD".

  Spanish Version: "Las Determinaciones Locales de Cobertura (LCDs en inglés) le ayudan a decidir a Medicare lo que está cubierto. Un LCD se usó para su reclamación. Usted puede comparar su caso con la determinación y enviar información de su médico si piensa que puede cambiar nuestra decisión. Para obtener una copia del LCD, llame al 1-800-MEDICARE (1800-633-4227)."

  CARC 167: "This (these) diagnosis(es) is (are) not covered. Note: Refer to the 835 Healthcare Policy Identification Segment (loop 2110 Service Payment Information REF), if present."

  RARC N386: "This decision was based on a National Coverage Determination (NCD). An NCD provides a coverage determination as to whether a particular item or service is covered. A copy of this policy is available at

  www.cms.gov/mcd/search.asp. If you do not have web access, you may contact the contractor to request a copy of the NCD."

  Contractors shall use Group Code PR (Patient Responsibility) assigning financial liability to the beneficiary if a claim is received with a GA modifier indicating a signed ABN is on file.

  Contractors shall use Group CO (Contractual Obligation) assigning financial liability to the provider, if a claim is received with a GZ modifier indicating no signed ABN is on file.

- Contractors shall reject claims with CPT 93668 which exceed 36 sessions within 84 days from the date of the first session when the -KX modifier is not included on the claim line OR any SET session provided after 84 days from the date of the first session and the -KX modifier is not included on the claim and use the following messages:

CARC 96: "Non-covered charge(s). At least one Remark Code must be provided (may be comprised of either the NCPDP Reject Reason [sic] Code, or Remittance Advice Remark Code that is not an ALERT.) Note: Refer to the 835 Healthcare Policy Identification Segment (loop 2110 Service Payment Information REF), if present."

RARC N640: "Exceeds number/frequency approved/allowed within time period."

Group Code CO (Contractual Obligation) assigning financial liability to the provider (if a claim line-item is received with a GZ modifier indicating no signed ABN is on file and occurrence code 32 is not present).

- Contractors shall deny/reject claim lines with CPT 93668 when 73 sessions have been reached using the following messages:

MSN 15.20: "The following policies NCD 20.35 were used when we made this decision." Spanish Version: "Las siguientes políticas NCD 20.35 fueron utilizadas cuando se tomó esta decisión."

(Part A only) MSN 15.19: "Local Coverage Determinations (LCDs) help Medicare decide what is covered. An LCD was used for your claim. You can compare your case to the LCD, and send information from your doctor if you think it could change our decision. Call 1-800-MEDICARE (1-800-633-4227) for a copy of the LCD".

Spanish Version: "Las Determinaciones Locales de Cobertura (LCDs en inglés) le ayudan a decidir a Medicare lo que está cubierto. Un LCD se usó para su reclamación. Usted puede comparar su caso con la determinación y enviar información de su médico si piensa que puede cambiar nuestra decisión. Para obtener una copia del LCD, llame al 1-800-MEDICARE (1800-633-4227)."

CARC 119: "Benefit maximum for this time period or occurrence has been reached."

RARC N386: "This decision was based on a National Coverage Determination (NCD). An NCD provides a coverage determination as to whether a particular item or service is covered. A copy of this policy is available at www.cms.gov/mcd/search.asp. If you do not have web access, you may contact the contractor to request a copy of the NCD."

Group Code PR (Patient Responsibility) assigning financial responsibility to the beneficiary (if a claim is received with occurrence code 32 with or without a GA modifier or a claim-line is received with a GA modifier indicating a signed ABN is on file)

Group Code CO (Contractual Obligation) assigning financial liability to the provider (if a claim line-item is received with a GZ modifier indicating no signed ABN is on file and occurrence code 32 is not present

- Contractors shall deny claim line-items for SET, CPT 93668, when 73 sessions have been reached with or without the -KX modifier present using the following messages:

MSN 15.20: "The following policies NCD 20.35 were used when we made this decision."

Spanish Version: "Las siguientes políticas NCD 20.35 fueron utilizadas cuando se tomó esta decisión."

(Part A only) MSN 15.19: "Local Coverage Determinations (LCDs) help Medicare decide what is covered. An LCD was used for your claim. You can compare your case to the LCD, and send information from your doctor if you think it could change our decision. Call 1-800-MEDICARE (1-800-633-4227) for a copy of the LCD".

Spanish Version: "Las Determinaciones Locales de Cobertura (LCDs en inglés) le ayudan a decidir a Medicare lo que está cubierto. Un LCD se usó para su reclamación. Usted puede comparar su caso con la determinación y enviar información de su médico si piensa que puede cambiar nuestra decisión. Para obtener una copia del LCD, llame al 1-800- MEDICARE (1800-633-4227)."

CARC 119: "Benefit maximum for this time period or occurrence has been reached."

RARC N386: "This decision was based on a National Coverage Determination (NCD). An NCD provides a coverage determination as to whether a particular item or service is covered. A copy of this policy is available at www.cms.gov/mcd/search.asp. If you do not have web access, you may contact the contractor to request a copy of the NCD."

Group Code PR (Patient Responsibility) assigning financial responsibility to the beneficiary (if a claim is received with occurrence code 32 with or without a GA modifier or a claim-line is received with a GA modifier indicating a signed ABN is on file)

Group Code CO (Contractual Obligation) assigning financial liability to the provider (if a claim line-item is received with a GZ modifier indicating no signed ABN is on file and occurrence code 32 is not present).

100-05, 10.3.2

Exceptions Process

(Rev. 3367 Issued: 10-07-2015, Effective: 01-01-2016, Implementation: 01-04-2016)

An exception may be made when the patient's condition is justified by documentation indicating that the beneficiary requires continued skilled therapy, i.e., therapy beyond the amount payable under the therapy cap, to achieve their prior functional status or maximum expected functional status within a reasonable amount of time.

No special documentation is submitted to the contractor for exceptions. The clinician is responsible for consulting guidance in the Medicare manuals and in the professional literature to determine if the beneficiary may qualify for the exception because documentation justifies medically necessary services above the caps. The clinician's opinion is not binding on the Medicare contractor who makes the final determination concerning whether the claim is payable.

Documentation justifying the services shall be submitted in response to any Additional Documentation Request (ADR) for claims that are selected for medical review. Follow the documentation requirements in Pub. 100-02, chapter 15, section 220.3. If medical records are requested for review, clinicians may include, at their discretion, a summary that specifically addresses the justification for therapy cap exception.

In making a decision about whether to utilize the exception, clinicians shall consider, for example, whether services are appropriate to--

The patient's condition, including the diagnosis, complexities, and severity;

The services provided, including their type, frequency, and duration;

The interaction of current active conditions and complexities that directly and significantly influence the treatment such that it causes services to exceed caps.

In addition, the following should be considered before using the exception process:

1. Exceptions for Evaluation Services

Evaluation. The CMS will except therapy evaluations from caps after the therapy caps are reached when evaluation is necessary, e.g., to determine if the current status of the beneficiary requires therapy services. For example, the following CPT codes for evaluation procedures may be appropriate:

92521, 92522, 92523, 92524, 92597, 92607, 92608, 92610, 92611, 92612, 92614, 92616, 96105, 96125, 97001, 97002, 97003, 97004.

These codes will continue to be reported as outpatient therapy procedures as listed in the Annual Therapy Update for the current year at: http://www.cms.gov/TherapyServices/05_Annual_Therapy_Update.asp#TopOfPage.

They are not diagnostic tests. Definitions of evaluations and documentation are found in Pub. 100-02, chapter 15, sections 220 and 230.

Other Services. There are a number of sources that suggest the amount of certain services that may be typical, either per service, per episode, per condition, or per discipline. For example, see the CSC - Therapy Cap Report, 3/21/2008, and CSC – Therapy Edits Tables 4/14/2008 at www.cms.hhs.gov/TherapyServices (Studies and Reports), or more recent utilization reports. Professional literature and guidelines from professional associations also provide a basis on which to estimate whether the type, frequency, and intensity of services are appropriate to an individual. Clinicians and contractors should utilize available evidence related to the patient's condition to justify provision of medically necessary services to individual beneficiaries, especially when they exceed caps. Contractors shall not limit medically necessary services that are justified by scientific research applicable to the beneficiary. Neither contractors nor clinicians shall utilize professional literature and scientific reports to justify payment for continued services after an individual's goals have been met earlier than is typical. Conversely, professional literature and scientific reports shall not be used as justification to deny payment to patients whose needs are greater than is typical or when the patient's condition is not represented by the literature.

2. Exceptions for Medically Necessary Services

Clinicians may utilize the process for exception for any diagnosis or condition for which they can justify services exceeding the cap. Regardless of the diagnosis or condition, the patient must also meet other requirements for coverage.

Bill the most relevant diagnosis. As always, when billing for therapy services, the diagnosis code that best relates to the reason for the treatment shall be on the claim, unless there is a compelling reason to report another diagnosis code. For example, when a patient with diabetes is being treated with therapy for gait training due to amputation, the preferred diagnosis is abnormality of gait (which characterizes the treatment). Where it is possible in accordance with State and local laws and the contractors' local coverage determinations, avoid using vague or general diagnoses. When a claim includes several types of services, or where the physician/NPP must supply the diagnosis, it may not be possible to use the most relevant therapy diagnosis code in the primary position. In that case, the relevant diagnosis code should, if possible, be on the claim in another position.

Codes representing the medical condition that caused the treatment are used when there is no code representing the treatment. Complicating conditions are preferably used in non-primary positions on the claim and are billed in the primary position only in the rare circumstance that there is no more relevant code.

The condition or complexity that caused treatment to exceed caps must be related to the therapy goals and must either be the condition that is being treated or a complexity that directly and significantly impacts the rate of recovery of the condition being treated such that it is appropriate to exceed the caps. Documentation for an exception should indicate how the complexity (or combination of complexities) directly and significantly affects treatment for a therapy condition.

If the contractor has determined that certain codes do not characterize patients who require medically necessary services, providers/suppliers may not use those codes, but must utilize a billable diagnosis code allowed by their contractor to describe the patient's condition. Contractors shall not apply therapy caps to services based on the patient's condition, but only on the medical necessity of the service for the condition. If a service would be payable before the cap is reached and is still medically necessary after the cap is reached, that service is excepted.

Contact your contractor for interpretation if you are not sure that a service is applicable for exception.

It is very important to recognize that most conditions would not ordinarily result in services exceeding the cap. Use the KX modifier only in cases where the condition of the individual patient is such that services are APPROPRIATELY provided in an episode that exceeds the cap. Routine use of the KX modifier for all patients with these conditions will likely show up on data analysis as aberrant and invite inquiry. Be sure that documentation is sufficiently detailed to support the use of the modifier.

In justifying exceptions for therapy caps, clinicians and contractors should not only consider the medical diagnoses and medical complications that might directly and significantly influence the amount of treatment required. Other variables (such as the availability of a caregiver at home) that affect appropriate treatment shall also be considered. Factors that influence the need for treatment should be supportable by published research, clinical guidelines from professional sources, and/or clinical or common sense. See Pub. 100-02, chapter 15, section 220.3 for information related to documentation of the evaluation, and section 220.2 on medical necessity for some factors that complicate treatment.

NOTE: The patient's lack of access to outpatient hospital therapy services alone, when outpatient hospital therapy services are excluded from the limitation, does not justify excepted services. Residents of skilled nursing facilities prevented by consolidated billing from accessing hospital services, debilitated patients for whom transportation to the hospital is a physical hardship, or lack of therapy services at hospitals in the beneficiary's county may or may not qualify as justification for continued services above the caps. The patient's condition and complexities might justify extended services, but their location does not. For dates of service on or after October 1, 2012, therapy services furnished in an outpatient hospital are not excluded from the limitation.

Appendix H — Quality Payment Program

In 2015, Congress passed the Medicare Access and CHIP Reauthorization Act (MACRA), which included sweeping changes for practitioners who provide services reimbursed under the Medicare physician fee schedule (MPFS). The act focused on repealing the faulty Medicare sustainable growth rate, focusing on quality of patient outcomes, and controlling Medicare spending.

A MACRA final rule in October 2016 established the Quality Payment Program (QPP) that was effective January 1, 2017.

The QPP has two tracks:

- The merit-based incentive payment system (MIPS)
- Alternative payment models (APMs)

MIPS uses the existing quality and value reporting systems—Physician Quality Reporting System (PQRS) (which ends January 1, 2019), Medicare meaningful use (MU), and value-based modifier (VBM) programs—to define certain performance categories that determine an overall score. Eligible clinicians (ECs) can obtain a composite performance score (CPS) of up to 100 points from these weighted performance categories. This performance score then defines the payment adjustments in the second calendar year after the year the score is obtained. For instance, the score obtained for the 2017 performance year is linked to payment for Medicare Part B services in 2019.

The performance categories, along with the weights used to determine the overall score, are:

- Quality
- Advancing care information (previously called meaningful use)
- Clinical practice improvement activities (CPIA)
- Resource use

ECs may also choose to participate in APMs. These payment models, created in conjunction with the clinician community, provide additional incentives to those clinicians in the APM who provide high-quality care as cost-efficiently as possible. APMs can be created around specific clinical conditions, a care episode, or a patient population type. An APM can also be described as a new way of paying the healthcare provider for the care rendered to Medicare patients.

Advanced APMs are a subset of APMs; practices participating in an advanced APM can earn even more incentives because the ECs take on risk related to their patients' outcomes. For calendar years 2019 through 2024, clinicians participating in advanced APMs have the potential to earn an additional 5 percent incentive payment; furthermore, they are exempt from having to participate in MIPS as long as they have sufficiently participated in the advanced APM.

Eligible clinicians have three flexible options for submitting data to the MIPS and a fourth option to join advanced APMs. Under the QPP, providers can receive increased payment by providing high-quality care and by controlling costs. ECs who successfully report determined criteria—defined by the pathway chosen—receive a larger payment depending on how successful they are at meeting performance thresholds. Those who do not participate or who do not fulfill the defined requirements receive a negative penalty; failure to participate in a track in 2020 results in 9 percent payment reduction in 2022.

ECs can receive incentives under the QPP. Once the performance threshold is established, ALL ECs who score above that threshold are eligible to receive a positive payment adjustment. Keep in mind that the key requirement is that an EC **submit data** to avoid the negative payment adjustment and receive the incentives. CMS has redesigned the scoring so that clinicians are able to know how well they are doing in the program, as benchmarks are known in advance of participating.

Proposed 2020 Changes

A number of revisions have been proposed for 2020. As noted earlier, in 2020, the maximum negative payment for payment adjustment is negative 9 percent. The positive payment, not including additional positive payments adjustments for exceptional performance is also up to a 9 percent adjustment. CMS is proposing additions, revisions, and deletions to many of the current reporting measures. Other proposals affecting the MIPS program for 2020 include:

- In the MIPS performance category CMS proposes to reduce the Quality performance category weight from 45 percent to 40 percent and to increase the Cost performance category weight from 15 percent to 20 percent. This is in accordance with CMS's effort to equalize weighting between the Quality and Cost performance categories by 2022 as indicated in MACRA.
- The data completeness requirements for 2020 are proposed to increase to 70 percent of the Quality performance category. This is up from 2019, which had a 60 percent requirement.
- New specialty sets would be added for Speech Language Pathology, Audiology, Clinical Social Work, Chiropractic Medicine, Pulmonology, Nutrition/Dietician, and Endocrinology.
- CMS proposes 10 new episode-based measures and revisions to two current measures (Medicare Spending Per Beneficiary Clinician and Total Per Capita Cost measures) to the Cost performance category.
- In the Improvement Activities performance category, CMS recommends modifying the definition of rural areas, removing the accreditation from criteria for patient-centered medical home designation, and increasing the participation threshold for group reporting from a single clinician to 50 percent of the practice clinicians.

Within the advanced alternative payment models (APMs). CMS has proposed MIPS quality reporting options for APM participants. Previously, CMS has tried to streamline APM participation in MIPS; however, the agency feels that allowing MIPS quality measures reported by the APMs would offer flexibility and improve meaningful measurement.

Appendix I — Medically Unlikely Edits (MUEs)

The Centers for Medicare & Medicaid Services (CMS) began to publish many of the edits used in the medically unlikely edits (MUE) program for the first time effective October 2008. What follows below is a list of the published CPT codes that have MUEs assigned to them and the number of units allowed with each code. CMS publishes the updates on a quarterly basis. Not all MUEs will be published, however. MUEs intended to detect and discourage any questionable payments will not be published as the agency feels the efficacy of these edits would be compromised. CMS added another component to the MUEs—the MUE Adjudication Indicator (MAI). The appropriate MAI can be found in parentheses following the MUE in this table and specify the maximum units of service (UOS) for a CPT/HCPCS code for the service. The MAI designates whether the UOS edit is applied to the line or claim.

The three MAIs are defined as follows:

MAI 1 (Line Edit) This MAI will continue to be adjudicated as the line edit on the claim and is auto-adjudicated by the contractor.

MAI 2 (Date of Service Edit, Policy) This MAI is considered to be the "absolute date of service edit" and is based on policy. The total unit of services (UOS) for that CPT code and that date of service (DOS) are combined for this edit. Medicare contractors are required to review all claims for the same patient, same date of service, and same provider.

MAI 3 (Date of Service Edit: Clinical) This MAI is also a date-of-service edit but is based upon clinical standards. The review takes current and previously submitted claims for the same patient, same date of service, and same provider into account. When medical necessity is clearly documented, the edit may be bypassed or the claim resubmitted.

The quarterly updates are published on the CMS website at http://www.cms.gov/NationalCorrectCodInitEd/MUE.html.

Professional

CPT	MUE
0001U	1(2)
0002M	1(3)
0002U	1(2)
0003M	1(3)
0003U	1(2)
0004M	1(2)
0005U	1(2)
0006M	1(2)
0006U	1(2)
0007M	1(2)
0007U	1(2)
0008U	1(3)
0009M	1(2)
0009U	2(3)
0010U	2(3)
0011M	1(2)
0011U	1(2)
0012M	1(2)
0012U	1(2)
0013M	1(2)
0013U	1(3)
0014U	1(3)
0016U	1(3)
0017U	1(3)
0018U	1(1)
0019U	1(3)
0021U	1(2)
0022U	2(3)
0023U	1(2)
0024U	1(2)
0025U	1(2)
0026U	1(3)
0027U	1(2)
0029U	1(2)
0030U	1(2)
0031U	1(2)
0032U	1(2)
0033U	1(2)
0034U	1(2)
0035U	1(2)
0036U	1(3)
0037U	1(3)
0038U	1(2)
0039U	1(2)

CPT	MUE
0040U	1(2)
0041U	1(2)
0042T	1(3)
0042U	1(2)
0043U	1(2)
0044U	1(2)
0045U	1(3)
0046U	1(3)
0047U	1(3)
0048U	1(3)
0049U	1(3)
0050U	1(3)
0051U	1(2)
0052U	1(2)
0053U	1(3)
0054T	1(3)
0054U	1(2)
0055T	1(3)
0055U	1(2)
0056U	1(3)
0057U	1(3)
0058T	1(2)
0058U	1(2)
0059U	1(2)
0060U	1(2)
0061U	1(2)
0062U	1(2)
0063U	1(2)
0064U	2(3)
0065U	2(3)
0066U	1(3)
0067U	2(3)
0068U	1(3)
0069U	1(3)
0070U	1(2)
0071T	1(2)
0071U	1(2)
0072T	1(2)
0072U	1(2)
0073U	1(2)
0074U	1(2)
0075T	1(2)
0075U	1(2)
0076T	1(2)

CPT	MUE
0076U	1(2)
0077U	2(2)
0078U	1(2)
0079U	0(3)
0080U	1(2)
0081U	1(3)
0082U	1(2)
0083U	1(3)
0085T	0(3)
0095T	1(3)
0098T	2(3)
0100T	1(2)
0101T	1(3)
0102T	2(2)
0106T	4(2)
0107T	4(2)
0108T	4(2)
0109T	4(2)
0110T	4(2)
0111T	1(3)
0126T	1(3)
0163T	1(3)
0164T	4(2)
0165T	4(2)
0174T	1(3)
0175T	1(3)
0184T	1(3)
0191T	2(2)
0198T	2(2)
01996	1(2)
0200T	1(2)
0201T	1(2)
0202T	1(3)
0205T	3(3)
0206T	1(3)
0207T	2(2)
0208T	1(3)
0209T	1(3)
0210T	1(3)
0211T	1(3)
0212T	1(3)
0213T	1(2)
0214T	1(2)
0215T	1(2)

CPT	MUE
0216T	1(2)
0217T	1(2)
0218T	1(2)
0219T	1(2)
0220T	1(2)
0221T	1(2)
0222T	1(3)
0228T	1(2)
0229T	2(3)
0230T	1(2)
0231T	2(3)
0232T	1(3)
0234T	2(2)
0235T	2(3)
0236T	1(2)
0237T	2(3)
0238T	2(3)
0249T	1(2)
0253T	1(3)
0254T	2(2)
0263T	1(3)
0264T	1(3)
0265T	1(3)
0266T	1(2)
0267T	1(3)
0268T	1(3)
0269T	1(2)
0270T	1(3)
0271T	1(3)
0272T	1(3)
0273T	1(3)
0274T	1(2)
0275T	1(2)
0278T	1(3)
0290T	1(3)
0295T	1(2)
0296T	1(2)
0297T	1(2)
0298T	1(2)
0308T	1(3)
0312T	1(3)
0313T	1(3)
0314T	1(3)
0315T	1(3)

CPT	MUE
0316T	1(3)
0317T	1(3)
0329T	1(2)
0330T	1(2)
0331T	1(3)
0332T	1(3)
0333T	1(2)
0335T	2(2)
0338T	1(2)
0339T	1(2)
0341T	1(2)
0342T	1(3)
0345T	1(2)
0347T	1(3)
0348T	1(3)
0349T	1(3)
0350T	1(3)
0351T	5(3)
0352T	5(3)
0353T	2(3)
0354T	2(3)
0355T	1(2)
0356T	4(2)
0357T	1(2)
0358T	1(2)
0362T	8(3)
0373T	24(3)
0375T	1(2)
0376T	2(3)
0377T	1(2)
0378T	1(2)
0379T	1(2)
0380T	1(2)
0381T	1(2)
0382T	1(2)
0383T	1(2)
0384T	1(2)
0385T	1(2)
0386T	1(2)
0394T	2(3)
0395T	2(3)
0396T	2(2)
0397T	1(3)
0398T	1(3)

CPT	MUE
0399T	1(3)
0400T	1(2)
0401T	1(2)
0402T	2(2)
0403T	1(2)
0404T	1(2)
0405T	1(2)
0408T	1(3)
0409T	1(3)
0410T	1(3)
0411T	1(3)
0412T	1(2)
0413T	1(3)
0414T	1(2)
0415T	1(3)
0416T	1(3)
0417T	1(3)
0418T	1(3)
0419T	1(2)
0420T	1(2)
0421T	1(2)
0422T	1(3)
0423T	1(3)
0424T	1(3)
0425T	1(3)
0426T	1(3)
0427T	1(3)
0428T	1(2)
0429T	1(2)
0430T	1(2)
0431T	1(2)
0432T	1(3)
0433T	1(3)
0434T	1(3)
0435T	1(3)
0436T	1(3)
0437T	1(3)
0439T	1(3)
0440T	3(3)
0441T	3(3)
0442T	3(3)
0443T	1(2)
0444T	1(2)
0445T	1(2)

CPT	MUE
0446T	1(3)
0447T	1(3)
0448T	1(3)
0449T	1(2)
0450T	1(3)
0451T	1(3)
0452T	1(3)
0453T	1(3)
0454T	3(3)
0455T	1(3)
0456T	1(3)
0457T	1(3)
0458T	3(3)
0459T	1(3)
0460T	3(3)
0461T	1(3)
0462T	1(2)
0463T	1(2)
0464T	1(2)
0465T	1(3)
0466T	1(3)
0467T	1(3)
0468T	1(3)
0469T	1(2)
0470T	1(2)
0471T	2(1)
0472T	1(2)
0473T	1(2)
0474T	2(2)
0475T	1(3)
0476T	1(3)
0477T	1(3)
0478T	1(3)
0479T	1(2)
0480T	4(1)
0481T	1(3)
0482T	1(3)
0483T	1(2)
0484T	1(2)
0485T	1(2)
0486T	1(2)
0487T	1(3)
0488T	1(2)
0489T	1(2)

CPT	MUE
0490T	1(2)
0491T	1(2)
0492T	4(3)
0493T	1(3)
0494T	1(2)
0495T	1(2)
0496T	4(3)
0497T	1(3)
0498T	1(2)
0499T	1(2)
0500T	1(3)
0501T	1(2)
0502T	1(2)
0503T	1(2)
0504T	1(2)
0505T	1(3)
0506T	1(2)
0507T	1(2)
0508T	1(3)
0509T	1(2)
0510T	1(2)
0511T	1(2)
0512T	1(2)
0513T	2(3)
0514T	2(2)
0515T	1(3)
0516T	1(3)
0517T	1(3)
0518T	1(3)
0519T	1(3)
0520T	1(3)
0521T	1(3)
0522T	1(3)
0523T	1(3)
0524T	3(3)
0525T	1(3)
0526T	1(3)
0527T	1(3)
0528T	1(3)
0529T	1(3)
0530T	1(3)
0531T	1(3)
0532T	1(3)
0533T	1(2)

CPT	MUE	CPT	MUE	CPT	MUE	CPT	MUE	CPT	MUE	CPT	MUE	CPT	MUE	CPT	MUE
0534T	1(2)	11308	2(3)	11922	1(3)	14041	3(3)	15758	2(3)	15956	2(3)	19272	1(3)	20552	1(2)
0535T	1(2)	11310	4(3)	11950	1(2)	14060	2(3)	15760	2(3)	15958	2(3)	19281	1(2)	20553	1(2)
0536T	1(2)	11311	4(3)	11951	1(2)	14061	2(3)	15770	2(3)	15999	1(3)	19282	2(3)	20555	1(3)
0537T	1(2)	11312	3(3)	11952	1(2)	14301	2(3)	15775	1(2)	16000	1(2)	19283	1(2)	20600	6(3)
0538T	1(3)	11313	3(3)	11954	1(3)	14302	8(3)	15776	1(2)	16020	1(3)	19284	2(3)	20604	4(3)
0539T	1(3)	11400	3(3)	11960	2(3)	14350	2(3)	15777	1(3)	16025	1(3)	19285	1(2)	20605	2(3)
0540T	1(3)	11401	3(3)	11970	2(3)	15002	1(2)	15780	1(2)	16030	1(3)	19286	2(3)	20606	2(3)
0541T	1(3)	11402	3(3)	11971	2(3)	15003	60(3)	15781	1(3)	16035	1(2)	19287	1(2)	20610	2(3)
0542T	1(3)	11403	2(3)	11976	1(2)	15004	1(2)	15782	1(3)	16036	8(3)	19288	2(3)	20611	2(3)
10004	3(3)	11404	2(3)	11980	1(2)	15005	19(3)	15783	1(3)	17000	1(2)	19294	2(3)	20612	2(3)
10005	1(2)	11406	2(3)	11981	1(3)	15040	1(2)	15786	1(2)	17003	13(2)	19296	1(3)	20615	1(3)
10006	3(3)	11420	3(3)	11982	1(3)	15050	1(3)	15787	2(3)	17004	1(2)	19297	2(3)	20650	4(3)
10007	1(2)	11421	3(3)	11983	1(3)	15100	1(2)	15788	1(2)	17106	1(2)	19298	1(2)	20660	1(2)
10008	3(3)	11422	3(3)	12001	1(2)	15101	40(3)	15789	1(2)	17107	1(2)	19300	1(2)	20661	1(2)
10009	1(2)	11423	2(3)	12002	1(2)	15110	1(2)	15792	1(3)	17108	1(2)	19301	1(2)	20662	1(2)
10010	3(3)	11424	2(3)	12004	1(2)	15111	5(3)	15793	1(3)	17110	1(2)	19302	1(2)	20663	1(2)
10011	1(2)	11426	2(3)	12005	1(2)	15115	1(2)	15819	1(2)	17111	1(2)	19303	1(2)	20664	1(2)
10012	3(3)	11440	4(3)	12006	1(2)	15116	2(3)	15820	1(2)	17250	4(3)	19304	1(2)	20665	1(2)
10021	1(2)	11441	3(3)	12007	1(2)	15120	1(2)	15821	1(2)	17260	7(3)	19305	1(2)	20670	3(3)
10030	2(3)	11442	3(3)	12011	1(2)	15121	8(3)	15822	1(2)	17261	7(3)	19306	1(2)	20680	3(3)
10035	1(2)	11443	2(3)	12013	1(2)	15130	1(2)	15823	1(2)	17262	6(3)	19307	1(2)	20690	2(3)
10036	2(3)	11444	2(3)	12014	1(2)	15131	2(3)	15824	1(2)	17263	3(3)	19316	1(2)	20692	2(3)
10040	1(2)	11446	2(3)	12015	1(2)	15135	1(2)	15825	1(2)	17264	3(3)	19318	1(2)	20693	2(3)
10060	1(2)	11450	1(2)	12016	1(2)	15136	1(3)	15826	1(2)	17266	2(3)	19324	1(2)	20694	2(3)
10061	1(2)	11451	1(2)	12017	1(2)	15150	1(2)	15828	1(2)	17270	6(3)	19325	1(2)	20696	2(3)
10080	1(3)	11462	1(2)	12018	1(2)	15151	1(2)	15829	1(2)	17271	4(3)	19328	1(2)	20697	4(3)
10081	1(3)	11463	1(2)	12020	2(3)	15152	5(3)	15830	1(2)	17272	5(3)	19330	1(2)	20802	1(2)
10120	3(3)	11470	3(2)	12021	3(3)	15155	1(2)	15832	1(2)	17273	4(3)	19340	1(2)	20805	1(2)
10121	2(3)	11471	2(3)	12031	1(2)	15156	1(2)	15833	1(2)	17274	2(3)	19342	1(2)	20808	1(2)
10140	2(3)	11600	2(3)	12032	1(2)	15157	1(3)	15834	1(2)	17276	2(3)	19350	1(2)	20816	3(3)
10160	3(3)	11601	2(3)	12034	1(2)	15200	1(2)	15835	1(3)	17280	6(3)	19355	1(2)	20822	3(3)
10180	2(3)	11602	3(3)	12035	1(2)	15201	7(3)	15836	1(2)	17281	5(3)	19357	1(2)	20824	1(2)
11000	1(2)	11603	2(3)	12036	1(2)	15220	1(2)	15837	2(3)	17282	4(3)	19361	1(2)	20827	1(2)
11001	1(3)	11604	2(3)	12037	1(2)	15221	9(3)	15838	1(2)	17283	4(3)	19364	1(2)	20838	1(2)
11004	1(2)	11606	2(3)	12041	1(2)	15240	1(2)	15839	2(3)	17284	2(3)	19366	1(2)	20900	2(3)
11005	1(2)	11620	2(3)	12042	1(2)	15241	9(3)	15840	1(3)	17286	2(3)	19367	1(2)	20902	2(3)
11006	1(2)	11621	2(3)	12044	1(2)	15260	1(2)	15841	2(3)	17311	4(3)	19368	1(2)	20910	1(3)
11008	1(2)	11622	2(3)	12045	1(2)	15261	6(3)	15842	2(3)	17312	6(3)	19369	1(2)	20912	1(3)
11010	2(3)	11623	2(3)	12046	1(2)	15271	1(2)	15845	2(3)	17313	3(3)	19370	1(2)	20920	1(3)
11011	2(3)	11624	2(3)	12047	1(2)	15272	3(3)	15847	1(2)	17314	4(3)	19371	1(2)	20922	1(3)
11012	2(3)	11626	2(3)	12051	1(2)	15273	1(2)	15850	0(3)	17315	15(3)	19380	1(2)	20924	2(3)
11042	1(2)	11640	2(3)	12052	1(2)	15274	60(3)	15851	1(2)	17340	1(2)	19396	1(2)	20926	2(3)
11043	1(2)	11641	2(3)	12053	1(2)	15275	1(2)	15852	1(3)	17360	1(2)	19499	1(3)	20930	0(3)
11044	1(2)	11642	3(3)	12054	1(2)	15276	3(2)	15860	1(3)	17380	1(3)	20100	2(3)	20931	1(2)
11045	12(3)	11643	2(3)	12055	1(2)	15277	1(2)	15876	1(2)	17999	1(3)	20101	2(3)	20932	1(3)
11046	10(3)	11644	2(3)	12056	1(2)	15278	15(3)	15877	1(2)	19000	2(3)	20102	3(3)	20933	1(3)
11047	10(3)	11646	2(3)	12057	1(2)	15570	2(3)	15878	1(2)	19001	5(3)	20103	3(3)	20934	1(3)
11055	1(2)	11719	1(2)	13100	1(2)	15572	2(3)	15879	1(2)	19020	2(3)	20150	2(3)	20936	0(3)
11056	1(2)	11720	1(2)	13101	1(2)	15574	2(3)	15920	1(3)	19030	1(2)	20200	2(3)	20937	1(2)
11057	1(2)	11721	1(2)	13102	9(3)	15576	2(3)	15922	1(3)	19081	1(2)	20205	3(3)	20938	1(2)
11102	1(2)	11730	1(2)	13120	1(2)	15600	2(3)	15931	1(3)	19082	2(3)	20206	3(3)	20939	1(3)
11103	6(3)	11732	4(3)	13121	1(2)	15610	2(3)	15933	1(3)	19083	1(2)	20220	3(3)	20950	2(3)
11104	1(2)	11740	2(3)	13122	9(3)	15620	2(3)	15934	1(3)	19084	2(3)	20225	2(3)	20955	1(3)
11105	3(3)	11750	6(3)	13131	1(2)	15630	2(3)	15935	1(3)	19085	1(2)	20240	4(3)	20956	1(3)
11106	1(2)	11755	2(3)	13132	1(2)	15650	1(3)	15936	1(3)	19086	2(3)	20245	3(3)	20957	1(3)
11107	2(3)	11760	4(3)	13133	7(3)	15730	1(3)	15937	1(3)	19100	4(3)	20250	1(3)	20962	1(3)
11200	1(2)	11762	2(3)	13151	1(2)	15731	1(3)	15940	2(3)	19101	3(3)	20251	2(3)	20969	2(3)
11201	0(3)	11765	4(3)	13152	1(2)	15733	2(3)	15941	2(3)	19105	2(3)	20500	2(3)	20970	1(3)
11300	5(3)	11770	1(3)	13153	2(3)	15734	4(3)	15944	2(3)	19110	1(3)	20501	2(3)	20972	2(3)
11301	6(3)	11771	1(3)	13160	2(3)	15736	2(3)	15945	2(3)	19112	2(3)	20520	2(3)	20973	1(2)
11302	4(3)	11772	1(3)	14000	2(3)	15738	3(3)	15946	2(3)	19120	1(2)	20525	4(3)	20974	1(3)
11303	3(3)	11900	1(2)	14001	2(3)	15740	2(3)	15950	2(3)	19125	1(2)	20526	1(2)	20975	1(3)
11305	4(3)	11901	1(2)	14020	2(3)	15750	2(3)	15951	2(3)	19126	3(3)	20527	2(3)	20979	1(3)
11306	4(3)	11920	1(2)	14021	2(3)	15756	2(3)	15952	2(3)	19260	2(3)	20550	5(3)	20982	1(2)
11307	3(3)	11921	1(2)	14040	2(3)	15757	2(3)	15953	2(3)	19271	1(3)	20551	5(3)	20983	1(2)

CPT	MUE
20985	2(3)
20999	1(3)
21010	1(2)
21011	4(3)
21012	3(3)
21013	2(3)
21014	2(3)
21015	1(3)
21016	2(3)
21025	2(3)
21026	2(3)
21029	1(3)
21030	1(3)
21031	2(3)
21032	1(3)
21034	1(3)
21040	2(3)
21044	1(3)
21045	1(3)
21046	2(3)
21047	2(3)
21048	2(3)
21049	1(3)
21050	1(2)
21060	1(2)
21070	1(2)
21073	1(2)
21076	1(2)
21077	1(2)
21079	1(2)
21080	1(2)
21081	1(2)
21082	1(2)
21083	1(2)
21084	1(2)
21085	1(3)
21086	1(2)
21087	1(2)
21088	1(2)
21089	1(3)
21100	1(2)
21110	2(3)
21116	1(2)
21120	1(2)
21121	1(2)
21122	1(2)
21123	1(2)
21125	2(2)
21127	2(3)
21137	1(2)
21138	1(2)
21139	1(2)
21141	1(2)
21142	1(2)
21143	1(2)
21145	1(2)
21146	1(2)
21147	1(2)
21150	1(2)
21151	1(2)
21154	1(2)
21155	1(2)
21159	1(2)
21160	1(2)
21172	1(3)

CPT	MUE
21175	1(2)
21179	1(2)
21180	1(2)
21181	1(3)
21182	1(2)
21183	1(2)
21184	1(2)
21188	1(2)
21193	1(2)
21194	1(2)
21195	1(2)
21196	1(2)
21198	1(3)
21199	1(2)
21206	1(3)
21208	1(3)
21209	1(3)
21210	2(3)
21215	2(3)
21230	2(3)
21235	2(3)
21240	1(2)
21242	1(2)
21243	1(2)
21244	1(2)
21245	2(2)
21246	2(2)
21247	1(2)
21248	2(3)
21249	2(3)
21255	1(2)
21256	1(2)
21260	1(2)
21261	1(2)
21263	1(2)
21267	1(2)
21268	1(2)
21270	1(2)
21275	1(2)
21280	1(2)
21282	1(2)
21295	1(2)
21296	1(2)
21299	1(3)
21310	1(2)
21315	1(2)
21320	1(2)
21325	1(2)
21330	1(2)
21335	1(2)
21336	1(2)
21337	1(2)
21338	1(2)
21339	1(2)
21340	1(2)
21343	1(2)
21344	1(2)
21345	1(2)
21346	1(2)
21347	1(2)
21348	1(2)
21355	1(2)
21356	1(2)
21360	1(2)
21365	1(2)

CPT	MUE
21366	1(2)
21385	1(2)
21386	1(2)
21387	1(2)
21390	1(2)
21395	1(2)
21400	1(2)
21401	1(2)
21406	1(2)
21407	1(2)
21408	1(2)
21421	1(2)
21422	1(2)
21423	1(2)
21431	1(2)
21432	1(2)
21433	1(2)
21435	1(2)
21436	1(2)
21440	2(2)
21445	2(2)
21450	1(2)
21451	1(2)
21452	1(2)
21453	1(2)
21454	1(2)
21461	1(2)
21462	1(2)
21465	1(2)
21470	1(2)
21480	1(2)
21485	1(2)
21490	1(2)
21497	1(2)
21499	1(3)
21501	3(3)
21502	1(3)
21510	1(3)
21550	2(3)
21552	2(3)
21554	2(3)
21555	2(3)
21556	2(3)
21557	1(3)
21558	1(3)
21600	5(3)
21610	1(3)
21615	1(2)
21616	1(2)
21620	1(2)
21627	1(2)
21630	1(2)
21632	1(2)
21685	1(2)
21700	1(2)
21705	1(2)
21720	1(3)
21725	1(3)
21740	1(2)
21742	1(2)
21743	1(2)
21750	1(2)
21811	1(2)
21812	1(2)
21813	1(2)

CPT	MUE
21820	1(2)
21825	1(2)
21899	1(3)
21920	2(3)
21925	2(3)
21930	5(3)
21931	3(3)
21932	2(3)
21933	2(3)
21935	1(3)
21936	1(3)
22010	2(3)
22015	2(3)
22100	1(2)
22101	1(2)
22102	1(2)
22103	3(3)
22110	1(2)
22112	1(2)
22114	1(2)
22116	3(3)
22206	1(2)
22207	1(2)
22208	5(3)
22210	1(2)
22212	1(2)
22214	1(2)
22216	6(3)
22220	1(2)
22222	1(2)
22224	1(2)
22226	4(3)
22310	1(2)
22315	1(2)
22318	1(2)
22319	1(2)
22325	1(2)
22326	1(2)
22327	1(2)
22328	6(3)
22505	1(2)
22510	1(2)
22511	1(2)
22512	3(3)
22513	1(2)
22514	1(2)
22515	4(3)
22526	0(3)
22527	0(3)
22532	1(2)
22533	1(2)
22534	3(3)
22548	1(2)
22551	1(2)
22552	5(3)
22554	1(2)
22556	1(2)
22558	1(2)
22585	5(3)
22586	1(2)
22590	1(2)
22595	1(2)
22600	1(2)
22610	1(2)
22612	1(2)

CPT	MUE
22614	13(3)
22630	1(2)
22632	4(2)
22633	1(2)
22634	4(2)
22800	1(2)
22802	1(2)
22804	1(2)
22808	1(2)
22810	1(2)
22812	1(2)
22818	1(2)
22819	1(2)
22830	1(2)
22840	1(3)
22841	0(3)
22842	1(3)
22843	1(3)
22844	1(3)
22845	1(3)
22846	1(3)
22847	1(3)
22848	1(2)
22849	1(2)
22850	1(2)
22852	1(2)
22853	4(3)
22854	4(3)
22855	1(2)
22856	1(2)
22857	1(2)
22858	1(2)
22859	4(3)
22861	1(2)
22862	1(2)
22864	1(2)
22865	1(2)
22867	1(2)
22868	1(2)
22869	1(2)
22870	1(2)
22899	1(3)
22900	3(3)
22901	2(3)
22902	4(3)
22903	3(3)
22904	1(3)
22905	1(3)
22999	1(3)
23000	1(2)
23020	1(2)
23030	2(3)
23031	1(3)
23035	1(3)
23040	1(2)
23044	1(3)
23065	2(3)
23066	2(3)
23071	2(3)
23073	2(3)
23075	2(3)
23076	2(3)
23077	1(3)
23078	1(3)
23100	1(2)

CPT	MUE
23101	1(3)
23105	1(2)
23106	1(2)
23107	1(2)
23120	1(2)
23125	1(2)
23130	1(2)
23140	1(3)
23145	1(3)
23146	1(3)
23150	1(3)
23155	1(3)
23156	1(3)
23170	1(3)
23172	1(3)
23174	1(3)
23180	1(3)
23182	1(3)
23184	1(3)
23190	1(3)
23195	1(2)
23200	1(3)
23210	1(3)
23220	1(3)
23330	2(3)
23333	1(3)
23334	1(2)
23335	1(2)
23350	1(2)
23395	1(2)
23397	1(3)
23400	1(2)
23405	2(3)
23406	1(3)
23410	1(2)
23412	1(2)
23415	1(2)
23420	1(2)
23430	1(2)
23440	1(2)
23450	1(2)
23455	1(2)
23460	1(2)
23462	1(2)
23465	1(2)
23466	1(2)
23470	1(2)
23472	1(2)
23473	1(2)
23474	1(2)
23480	1(2)
23485	1(2)
23490	1(2)
23491	1(2)
23500	1(2)
23505	1(2)
23515	1(2)
23520	1(2)
23525	1(2)
23530	1(2)
23532	1(2)
23540	1(2)
23545	1(2)
23550	1(2)
23552	1(2)

CPT	MUE
23570	1(2)
23575	1(2)
23585	1(2)
23600	1(2)
23605	1(2)
23615	1(2)
23616	1(2)
23620	1(2)
23625	1(2)
23630	1(2)
23650	1(2)
23655	1(2)
23660	1(2)
23665	1(2)
23670	1(2)
23675	1(2)
23680	1(2)
23700	1(2)
23800	1(2)
23802	1(2)
23900	1(2)
23920	1(2)
23921	1(2)
23929	1(3)
23930	2(3)
23931	2(3)
23935	2(3)
24000	1(2)
24006	1(2)
24065	2(3)
24066	2(3)
24071	2(3)
24073	2(3)
24075	5(3)
24076	4(3)
24077	1(3)
24079	1(3)
24100	1(2)
24101	1(2)
24102	1(2)
24105	1(2)
24110	1(3)
24115	1(3)
24116	1(3)
24120	1(3)
24125	1(3)
24126	1(3)
24130	1(2)
24134	1(3)
24136	1(3)
24138	1(3)
24140	1(3)
24145	1(3)
24147	1(2)
24149	1(2)
24150	1(3)
24152	1(3)
24155	1(2)
24160	1(2)
24164	1(2)
24200	3(3)
24201	3(3)
24220	1(2)
24300	1(2)
24301	2(3)

CPT	MUE
24305	4(3)
24310	2(3)
24320	2(3)
24330	1(3)
24331	1(3)
24332	1(2)
24340	1(2)
24341	2(3)
24342	2(3)
24343	1(2)
24344	1(2)
24345	1(2)
24346	1(2)
24357	1(3)
24358	1(3)
24359	2(3)
24360	1(2)
24361	1(2)
24362	1(2)
24363	1(2)
24365	1(2)
24366	1(2)
24370	1(2)
24371	1(2)
24400	1(3)
24410	1(2)
24420	1(2)
24430	1(3)
24435	1(3)
24470	1(2)
24495	1(2)
24498	1(2)
24500	1(2)
24505	1(2)
24515	1(2)
24516	1(2)
24530	1(2)
24535	1(2)
24538	1(2)
24545	1(2)
24546	1(2)
24560	1(3)
24565	1(3)
24566	1(3)
24575	1(3)
24576	1(3)
24577	1(3)
24579	1(3)
24582	1(3)
24586	1(3)
24587	1(2)
24600	1(2)
24605	1(2)
24615	1(2)
24620	1(2)
24635	1(2)
24640	1(2)
24650	1(2)
24655	1(2)
24665	1(2)
24666	1(2)
24670	1(2)
24675	1(2)
24685	1(2)
24800	1(2)

CPT	MUE
24802	1(2)
24900	1(2)
24920	1(2)
24925	1(2)
24930	1(2)
24931	1(2)
24935	1(2)
24940	1(2)
24999	1(3)
25000	2(3)
25001	1(3)
25020	1(2)
25023	1(2)
25024	1(2)
25025	1(2)
25028	4(3)
25031	2(3)
25035	2(3)
25040	1(3)
25065	2(3)
25066	2(3)
25071	3(3)
25073	2(3)
25075	6(3)
25076	3(3)
25077	1(3)
25078	1(3)
25085	1(2)
25100	1(2)
25101	1(2)
25105	1(2)
25107	1(2)
25109	4(3)
25110	2(3)
25111	1(3)
25112	1(3)
25115	1(3)
25116	1(3)
25118	5(3)
25119	1(2)
25120	1(3)
25125	1(3)
25126	1(3)
25130	1(3)
25135	1(3)
25136	1(3)
25145	1(3)
25150	1(3)
25151	1(3)
25170	1(3)
25210	2(3)
25215	1(2)
25230	1(2)
25240	1(2)
25246	1(2)
25248	3(3)
25250	1(2)
25251	1(2)
25259	1(2)
25260	9(3)
25263	4(3)
25265	4(3)
25270	8(3)
25272	4(3)
25274	4(3)

CPT	MUE
25275	2(3)
25280	9(3)
25290	10(3)
25295	9(3)
25300	1(2)
25301	1(2)
25310	5(3)
25312	4(3)
25315	1(3)
25316	1(3)
25320	1(2)
25332	1(2)
25335	1(2)
25337	1(2)
25350	1(3)
25355	1(3)
25360	1(3)
25365	1(3)
25370	1(2)
25375	1(2)
25390	1(2)
25391	1(2)
25392	1(2)
25393	1(2)
25394	1(3)
25400	1(2)
25405	1(2)
25415	1(2)
25420	1(2)
25425	1(2)
25426	1(2)
25430	1(3)
25431	1(3)
25440	1(2)
25441	1(2)
25442	1(2)
25443	1(2)
25444	1(2)
25445	1(2)
25446	1(2)
25447	4(3)
25449	1(2)
25450	1(2)
25455	1(2)
25490	1(2)
25491	1(2)
25492	1(2)
25500	1(2)
25505	1(2)
25515	1(2)
25520	1(2)
25525	1(2)
25526	1(2)
25530	1(2)
25535	1(2)
25545	1(2)
25560	1(2)
25565	1(2)
25574	1(2)
25575	1(2)
25600	1(2)
25605	1(2)
25606	1(2)
25607	1(2)
25608	1(2)

CPT	MUE
25609	1(2)
25622	1(2)
25624	1(2)
25628	1(2)
25630	1(3)
25635	1(3)
25645	1(3)
25650	1(2)
25651	1(2)
25652	1(2)
25660	1(2)
25670	1(2)
25671	1(2)
25675	1(2)
25676	1(2)
25680	1(2)
25685	1(2)
25690	1(2)
25695	1(2)
25800	1(2)
25805	1(2)
25810	1(2)
25820	1(2)
25825	1(2)
25830	1(2)
25900	1(2)
25905	1(2)
25907	1(2)
25909	1(2)
25915	1(2)
25920	1(2)
25922	1(2)
25924	1(2)
25927	1(2)
25929	1(2)
25931	1(2)
25999	1(3)
26010	2(3)
26011	3(3)
26020	4(3)
26025	1(2)
26030	1(2)
26034	2(3)
26035	1(3)
26037	1(3)
26040	1(2)
26045	1(2)
26055	5(3)
26060	5(3)
26070	2(3)
26075	3(3)
26080	3(3)
26100	1(3)
26105	2(3)
26110	2(3)
26111	4(3)
26113	3(3)
26115	4(3)
26116	2(3)
26117	2(3)
26118	1(3)
26121	1(2)
26123	1(2)
26125	4(3)
26130	1(3)

CPT	MUE
26135	4(3)
26140	2(3)
26145	6(3)
26160	4(3)
26170	4(3)
26180	4(3)
26185	1(3)
26200	2(3)
26205	1(3)
26210	2(3)
26215	2(3)
26230	2(3)
26235	2(3)
26236	2(3)
26250	2(3)
26260	1(3)
26262	1(3)
26320	4(3)
26340	4(3)
26341	2(3)
26350	6(3)
26352	2(3)
26356	4(3)
26357	2(3)
26358	2(3)
26370	3(3)
26372	1(3)
26373	2(3)
26390	2(3)
26392	2(3)
26410	4(3)
26412	3(3)
26415	2(3)
26416	2(3)
26418	4(3)
26420	3(3)
26426	4(3)
26428	2(3)
26432	2(3)
26433	2(3)
26434	2(3)
26437	4(3)
26440	6(3)
26442	5(3)
26445	5(3)
26449	5(3)
26450	6(3)
26455	6(3)
26460	4(3)
26471	4(3)
26474	4(3)
26476	4(3)
26477	2(3)
26478	6(3)
26479	4(3)
26480	4(3)
26483	4(3)
26485	4(3)
26489	2(3)
26490	3(3)
26492	2(3)
26494	1(3)
26496	1(3)
26497	2(3)
26498	1(3)

CPT	MUE
26499	2(3)
26500	3(3)
26502	2(3)
26508	1(2)
26510	4(3)
26516	1(2)
26517	1(2)
26518	1(2)
26520	4(3)
26525	4(3)
26530	4(3)
26531	4(3)
26535	3(3)
26536	4(3)
26540	4(3)
26541	4(3)
26542	4(3)
26545	4(3)
26546	2(3)
26548	3(3)
26550	1(2)
26551	1(2)
26553	1(3)
26554	1(3)
26555	2(3)
26556	2(3)
26560	2(3)
26561	2(3)
26562	2(3)
26565	2(3)
26567	3(3)
26568	2(3)
26580	1(2)
26587	2(3)
26590	2(3)
26591	4(3)
26593	8(3)
26596	1(3)
26600	2(3)
26605	3(3)
26607	2(3)
26608	4(3)
26615	3(3)
26641	1(2)
26645	1(2)
26650	1(2)
26665	1(2)
26670	2(3)
26675	1(3)
26676	2(3)
26685	3(3)
26686	3(3)
26700	2(3)
26705	3(3)
26706	2(3)
26715	3(3)
26720	4(3)
26725	3(3)
26727	3(3)
26735	4(3)
26740	3(3)
26742	3(3)
26746	3(3)
26750	3(3)
26755	2(3)

CPT	MUE
26756	2(3)
26765	3(3)
26770	3(3)
26775	2(3)
26776	4(3)
26785	3(3)
26820	1(2)
26841	1(2)
26842	1(2)
26843	2(3)
26844	2(3)
26850	5(3)
26852	2(3)
26860	1(2)
26861	4(3)
26862	1(2)
26863	2(3)
26910	4(3)
26951	8(3)
26952	4(3)
26989	1(3)
26990	2(3)
26991	1(3)
26992	2(3)
27000	1(3)
27001	1(3)
27003	1(2)
27005	1(2)
27006	1(2)
27025	1(3)
27027	1(2)
27030	1(2)
27033	1(2)
27035	1(2)
27036	1(2)
27040	2(3)
27041	3(3)
27043	2(3)
27045	3(3)
27047	2(3)
27048	2(3)
27049	1(3)
27050	1(2)
27052	1(2)
27054	1(2)
27057	1(2)
27059	1(3)
27060	1(2)
27062	1(2)
27065	1(3)
27066	1(3)
27067	1(3)
27070	1(3)
27071	1(3)
27075	1(3)
27076	1(2)
27077	1(2)
27078	1(2)
27080	1(2)
27086	1(3)
27087	1(3)
27090	1(2)
27091	1(2)
27093	1(2)
27095	1(2)

CPT	MUE
27096	1(2)
27097	1(3)
27098	1(2)
27100	1(2)
27105	1(3)
27110	1(2)
27111	1(2)
27120	1(2)
27122	1(2)
27125	1(2)
27130	1(2)
27132	1(2)
27134	1(2)
27137	1(2)
27138	1(2)
27140	1(2)
27146	1(3)
27147	1(3)
27151	1(3)
27156	1(2)
27158	1(2)
27161	1(2)
27165	1(2)
27170	1(2)
27175	1(2)
27176	1(2)
27177	1(2)
27178	1(2)
27179	1(2)
27181	1(2)
27185	1(2)
27187	1(2)
27197	1(2)
27198	1(2)
27200	1(2)
27202	1(2)
27215	0(3)
27216	0(3)
27217	0(3)
27218	0(3)
27220	1(2)
27222	1(2)
27226	1(2)
27227	1(2)
27228	1(2)
27230	1(2)
27232	1(2)
27235	1(2)
27236	1(2)
27238	1(2)
27240	1(2)
27244	1(2)
27245	1(2)
27246	1(2)
27248	1(2)
27250	1(2)
27252	1(2)
27253	1(2)
27254	1(2)
27256	1(2)
27257	1(2)
27258	1(2)
27259	1(2)
27265	1(2)
27266	1(2)

CPT	MUE
27267	1(2)
27268	1(2)
27269	1(2)
27275	2(2)
27279	1(2)
27280	1(2)
27282	1(2)
27284	1(2)
27286	1(2)
27290	1(2)
27295	1(2)
27299	1(3)
27301	3(3)
27303	2(3)
27305	1(2)
27306	1(2)
27307	1(2)
27310	1(2)
27323	2(3)
27324	3(3)
27325	1(2)
27326	1(2)
27327	5(3)
27328	3(3)
27329	1(3)
27330	1(2)
27331	1(2)
27332	1(2)
27333	1(2)
27334	1(2)
27335	1(2)
27337	3(3)
27339	4(3)
27340	1(2)
27345	1(2)
27347	1(2)
27350	1(2)
27355	1(3)
27356	1(3)
27357	1(3)
27358	1(3)
27360	2(3)
27364	1(3)
27365	1(3)
27369	1(2)
27372	2(3)
27380	1(2)
27381	1(2)
27385	2(3)
27386	2(3)
27390	1(2)
27391	1(2)
27392	1(2)
27393	1(2)
27394	1(2)
27395	1(2)
27396	1(2)
27397	1(2)
27400	1(2)
27403	1(3)
27405	2(2)
27407	2(2)
27409	1(2)
27412	1(2)
27415	1(2)

CPT	MUE
27416	1(2)
27418	1(2)
27420	1(2)
27422	1(2)
27424	1(2)
27425	1(2)
27427	1(2)
27428	1(2)
27429	1(2)
27430	1(2)
27435	1(2)
27437	1(2)
27438	1(2)
27440	1(2)
27441	1(2)
27442	1(2)
27443	1(2)
27445	1(2)
27446	1(2)
27447	1(2)
27448	1(3)
27450	1(3)
27454	1(2)
27455	1(3)
27457	1(3)
27465	1(2)
27466	1(2)
27468	1(2)
27470	1(2)
27472	1(2)
27475	1(2)
27477	1(2)
27479	1(2)
27485	1(2)
27486	1(2)
27487	1(2)
27488	1(2)
27495	1(2)
27496	1(2)
27497	1(2)
27498	1(2)
27499	1(2)
27500	1(2)
27501	1(2)
27502	1(2)
27503	1(2)
27506	1(2)
27507	1(2)
27508	1(2)
27509	1(2)
27510	1(2)
27511	1(2)
27513	1(2)
27514	1(2)
27516	1(2)
27517	1(2)
27519	1(2)
27520	1(2)
27524	1(2)
27530	1(2)
27532	1(2)
27535	1(2)
27536	1(2)
27538	1(2)
27540	1(2)

CPT	MUE
27550	1(2)
27552	1(2)
27556	1(2)
27557	1(2)
27558	1(2)
27560	1(2)
27562	1(2)
27566	1(2)
27570	1(2)
27580	1(2)
27590	1(2)
27591	1(2)
27592	1(2)
27594	1(2)
27596	1(2)
27598	1(2)
27599	1(3)
27600	1(2)
27601	1(2)
27602	1(2)
27603	2(3)
27604	2(3)
27605	1(2)
27606	1(2)
27607	2(3)
27610	1(2)
27612	1(2)
27613	3(3)
27614	3(3)
27615	1(3)
27616	1(3)
27618	3(3)
27619	2(3)
27620	1(2)
27625	1(2)
27626	1(2)
27630	2(3)
27632	3(3)
27634	2(3)
27635	1(3)
27637	1(3)
27638	1(3)
27640	1(3)
27641	1(3)
27645	1(3)
27646	1(3)
27647	1(3)
27648	1(2)
27650	1(2)
27652	1(2)
27654	1(2)
27656	1(3)
27658	2(3)
27659	2(3)
27664	2(3)
27665	2(3)
27675	1(2)
27676	1(2)
27680	2(3)
27681	1(2)
27685	2(3)
27686	3(3)
27687	1(2)
27690	2(3)
27691	2(3)

CPT	MUE
27692	4(3)
27695	1(2)
27696	1(2)
27698	2(2)
27700	1(2)
27702	1(2)
27703	1(2)
27704	1(2)
27705	1(3)
27707	1(3)
27709	1(3)
27712	1(2)
27715	1(2)
27720	1(2)
27722	1(2)
27724	1(2)
27725	1(2)
27726	1(2)
27727	1(2)
27730	1(2)
27732	1(2)
27734	1(2)
27740	1(2)
27742	1(2)
27745	1(2)
27750	1(2)
27752	1(2)
27756	1(2)
27758	1(2)
27759	1(2)
27760	1(2)
27762	1(2)
27766	1(2)
27767	1(2)
27768	1(2)
27769	1(2)
27780	1(2)
27781	1(2)
27784	1(2)
27786	1(2)
27788	1(2)
27792	1(2)
27808	1(2)
27810	1(2)
27814	1(2)
27816	1(2)
27818	1(2)
27822	1(2)
27823	1(2)
27824	1(2)
27825	1(2)
27826	1(2)
27827	1(2)
27828	1(2)
27829	1(2)
27830	1(2)
27831	1(2)
27832	1(2)
27840	1(2)
27842	1(2)
27846	1(2)
27848	1(2)
27860	1(2)
27870	1(2)
27871	1(3)

CPT	MUE
27880	1(2)
27881	1(2)
27882	1(2)
27884	1(2)
27886	1(2)
27888	1(2)
27889	1(2)
27892	1(2)
27893	1(2)
27894	1(2)
27899	1(3)
28001	2(3)
28002	3(3)
28003	2(3)
28005	3(3)
28008	2(3)
28010	4(3)
28011	4(3)
28020	2(3)
28022	3(3)
28024	4(3)
28035	1(2)
28039	2(3)
28041	2(3)
28043	4(3)
28045	4(3)
28046	1(3)
28047	1(3)
28050	2(3)
28052	2(3)
28054	2(3)
28055	1(3)
28060	1(2)
28062	1(2)
28070	2(3)
28072	4(3)
28080	3(3)
28086	2(3)
28088	2(3)
28090	2(3)
28092	2(3)
28100	1(3)
28102	1(3)
28103	1(3)
28104	2(3)
28106	1(3)
28107	1(3)
28108	2(3)
28110	1(2)
28111	1(2)
28112	4(3)
28113	1(2)
28114	1(2)
28116	1(2)
28118	1(2)
28119	1(2)
28120	2(3)
28122	4(3)
28124	4(3)
28126	4(3)
28130	1(2)
28140	3(3)
28150	4(3)
28153	4(3)
28160	5(3)

CPT	MUE
28171	1(3)
28173	2(3)
28175	2(3)
28190	3(3)
28192	2(3)
28193	2(3)
28200	4(3)
28202	2(3)
28208	4(3)
28210	2(3)
28220	1(2)
28222	1(2)
28225	1(2)
28226	1(2)
28230	1(2)
28232	6(3)
28234	6(3)
28238	1(2)
28240	1(2)
28250	1(2)
28260	1(2)
28261	1(3)
28262	1(2)
28264	1(2)
28270	6(3)
28272	6(3)
28280	1(2)
28285	4(3)
28286	1(2)
28288	4(3)
28289	1(2)
28291	1(2)
28292	1(2)
28295	1(2)
28296	1(2)
28297	1(2)
28298	1(2)
28299	1(2)
28300	1(2)
28302	1(2)
28304	1(3)
28305	1(3)
28306	1(2)
28307	1(2)
28308	4(3)
28309	1(2)
28310	1(2)
28312	4(3)
28313	4(3)
28315	1(2)
28320	1(2)
28322	2(3)
28340	2(3)
28341	2(3)
28344	1(2)
28345	2(3)
28360	1(2)
28400	1(2)
28405	1(2)
28406	1(2)
28415	1(2)
28420	1(2)
28430	1(2)
28435	1(2)
28436	1(2)

CPT	MUE
28445	1(2)
28446	1(2)
28450	2(3)
28455	3(3)
28456	2(3)
28465	3(3)
28470	2(3)
28475	5(3)
28476	4(3)
28485	5(3)
28490	1(2)
28495	1(2)
28496	1(2)
28505	1(2)
28510	4(3)
28515	4(3)
28525	4(3)
28530	1(2)
28531	1(2)
28540	1(3)
28545	1(3)
28546	1(3)
28555	1(3)
28570	1(2)
28575	1(2)
28576	1(2)
28585	1(3)
28600	2(3)
28605	2(3)
28606	3(3)
28615	5(3)
28630	2(3)
28635	2(3)
28636	4(3)
28645	4(3)
28660	4(3)
28665	3(3)
28666	4(3)
28675	3(3)
28705	1(2)
28715	1(2)
28725	1(2)
28730	1(2)
28735	1(2)
28737	1(2)
28740	1(2)
28750	1(2)
28755	1(2)
28760	1(2)
28800	1(2)
28805	1(2)
28810	5(3)
28820	6(3)
28825	8(2)
28890	1(2)
28899	1(3)
29000	1(3)
29010	1(3)
29015	1(3)
29035	1(3)
29040	1(3)
29044	1(3)
29046	1(3)
29049	1(3)
29055	1(3)

CPT	MUE
29058	1(3)
29065	1(3)
29075	1(3)
29085	1(3)
29086	2(3)
29105	1(2)
29125	1(2)
29126	1(2)
29130	3(3)
29131	2(3)
29200	1(2)
29240	1(2)
29260	1(3)
29280	2(3)
29305	1(3)
29325	1(3)
29345	1(3)
29355	1(3)
29358	1(3)
29365	1(3)
29405	1(3)
29425	1(3)
29435	1(3)
29440	1(2)
29445	1(3)
29450	1(3)
29505	1(2)
29515	1(2)
29520	1(2)
29530	1(2)
29540	1(2)
29550	1(2)
29580	1(2)
29581	1(2)
29584	1(2)
29700	2(3)
29705	1(3)
29710	1(2)
29720	1(2)
29730	1(3)
29740	1(3)
29750	1(3)
29799	1(3)
29800	1(2)
29804	1(2)
29805	1(2)
29806	1(2)
29807	1(2)
29819	1(2)
29820	1(2)
29821	1(2)
29822	1(2)
29823	1(2)
29824	1(2)
29825	1(2)
29826	1(2)
29827	1(2)
29828	1(2)
29830	1(2)
29834	1(2)
29835	1(2)
29836	1(2)
29837	1(2)
29838	1(2)
29840	1(2)

CPT	MUE
29843	1(2)
29844	1(2)
29845	1(2)
29846	1(2)
29847	1(2)
29848	1(2)
29850	1(2)
29851	1(2)
29855	1(2)
29856	1(2)
29860	1(2)
29861	1(2)
29862	1(2)
29863	1(2)
29866	1(2)
29867	1(2)
29868	1(3)
29870	1(2)
29871	1(2)
29873	1(2)
29874	1(2)
29875	1(2)
29876	1(2)
29877	1(2)
29879	1(2)
29880	1(2)
29881	1(2)
29882	1(2)
29883	1(2)
29884	1(2)
29885	1(2)
29886	1(2)
29887	1(2)
29888	1(2)
29889	1(2)
29891	1(2)
29892	1(2)
29893	1(2)
29894	1(2)
29895	1(2)
29897	1(2)
29898	1(2)
29899	1(2)
29900	2(3)
29901	2(3)
29902	2(3)
29904	1(2)
29905	1(2)
29906	1(2)
29907	1(2)
29914	1(2)
29915	1(2)
29916	1(2)
29999	1(3)
30000	1(3)
30020	1(3)
30100	2(3)
30110	1(2)
30115	1(2)
30117	2(3)
30118	1(3)
30120	1(2)
30124	2(3)
30125	1(3)
30130	1(2)

CPT	MUE	CPT	MUE	CPT	MUE	CPT	MUE	CPT	MUE	CPT	MUE	CPT	MUE	CPT	MUE
30140	1(2)	31241	1(2)	31573	1(2)	31780	1(2)	32650	1(2)	33214	1(3)	33365	1(2)	33536	1(2)
30150	1(2)	31253	1(2)	31574	1(2)	31781	1(2)	32651	1(2)	33215	2(3)	33366	1(3)	33542	1(2)
30160	1(2)	31254	1(2)	31575	1(3)	31785	1(3)	32652	1(2)	33216	1(3)	33367	1(2)	33545	1(2)
30200	1(2)	31255	1(2)	31576	1(3)	31786	1(3)	32653	1(3)	33217	1(3)	33368	1(2)	33548	1(2)
30210	1(3)	31256	1(2)	31577	1(3)	31800	1(3)	32654	1(3)	33218	1(3)	33369	1(2)	33572	3(2)
30220	1(2)	31257	1(2)	31578	1(3)	31805	1(3)	32655	1(3)	33220	1(3)	33390	1(2)	33600	1(3)
30300	1(3)	31259	1(2)	31579	1(2)	31820	1(2)	32656	1(2)	33221	1(3)	33391	1(2)	33602	1(3)
30310	1(3)	31267	1(2)	31580	1(2)	31825	1(2)	32658	1(3)	33222	1(3)	33404	1(2)	33606	1(2)
30320	1(3)	31276	1(2)	31584	1(2)	31830	1(2)	32659	1(2)	33223	1(3)	33405	1(2)	33608	1(2)
30400	1(2)	31287	1(2)	31587	1(2)	31899	1(3)	32661	1(3)	33224	1(3)	33406	1(2)	33610	1(2)
30410	1(2)	31288	1(2)	31590	1(2)	32035	1(2)	32662	1(3)	33225	1(3)	33410	1(2)	33611	1(2)
30420	1(2)	31290	1(2)	31591	1(2)	32036	1(3)	32663	1(3)	33226	1(3)	33411	1(2)	33612	1(2)
30430	1(2)	31291	1(2)	31592	1(2)	32096	1(3)	32664	1(2)	33227	1(3)	33412	1(2)	33615	1(2)
30435	1(2)	31292	1(2)	31599	1(3)	32097	1(3)	32665	1(2)	33228	1(3)	33413	1(2)	33617	1(2)
30450	1(2)	31293	1(2)	31600	1(2)	32098	1(2)	32666	1(3)	33229	1(3)	33414	1(2)	33619	1(2)
30460	1(2)	31294	1(2)	31601	1(2)	32100	1(3)	32667	3(3)	33230	1(3)	33415	1(2)	33620	1(2)
30462	1(2)	31295	1(2)	31603	1(2)	32110	1(3)	32668	2(3)	33231	1(3)	33416	1(2)	33621	1(3)
30465	1(2)	31296	1(2)	31605	1(2)	32120	1(3)	32669	2(3)	33233	1(2)	33417	1(2)	33622	1(2)
30520	1(2)	31297	1(2)	31610	1(2)	32124	1(3)	32670	1(2)	33234	1(2)	33418	1(3)	33641	1(2)
30540	1(2)	31298	1(2)	31611	1(2)	32140	1(3)	32671	1(2)	33235	1(2)	33419	1(2)	33645	1(2)
30545	1(2)	31299	1(3)	31612	1(3)	32141	1(3)	32672	1(3)	33236	1(2)	33420	1(2)	33647	1(2)
30560	1(2)	31300	1(2)	31613	1(2)	32150	1(3)	32673	1(2)	33237	1(2)	33422	1(2)	33660	1(2)
30580	2(3)	31360	1(2)	31614	1(2)	32151	1(3)	32674	1(2)	33238	1(2)	33425	1(2)	33665	1(2)
30600	1(3)	31365	1(2)	31615	1(3)	32160	1(3)	32701	1(2)	33240	1(3)	33426	1(2)	33670	1(2)
30620	1(2)	31367	1(2)	31622	1(3)	32200	2(3)	32800	1(3)	33241	1(2)	33427	1(2)	33675	1(2)
30630	1(2)	31368	1(2)	31623	1(3)	32215	1(2)	32810	1(3)	33243	1(2)	33430	1(2)	33676	1(2)
30801	1(2)	31370	1(2)	31624	1(3)	32220	1(2)	32815	1(3)	33244	1(2)	33440	1(2)	33677	1(2)
30802	1(2)	31375	1(2)	31625	1(2)	32225	1(2)	32820	1(2)	33249	1(3)	33460	1(2)	33681	1(2)
30901	1(3)	31380	1(2)	31626	1(2)	32310	1(3)	32850	1(2)	33250	1(2)	33463	1(2)	33684	1(2)
30903	1(3)	31382	1(2)	31627	1(3)	32320	1(3)	32851	1(2)	33251	1(2)	33464	1(2)	33688	1(2)
30905	1(2)	31390	1(2)	31628	1(2)	32400	2(3)	32852	1(2)	33254	1(2)	33465	1(2)	33690	1(2)
30906	1(3)	31395	1(2)	31629	1(2)	32405	2(3)	32853	1(2)	33255	1(2)	33468	1(2)	33692	1(2)
30915	1(3)	31400	1(3)	31630	1(3)	32440	1(2)	32854	1(2)	33256	1(2)	33470	1(2)	33694	1(2)
30920	1(3)	31420	1(2)	31631	1(2)	32442	1(2)	32855	1(2)	33257	1(2)	33471	1(2)	33697	1(2)
30930	1(2)	31500	2(3)	31632	2(3)	32445	1(2)	32856	1(2)	33258	1(2)	33474	1(2)	33702	1(2)
30999	1(3)	31502	1(3)	31633	2(3)	32480	1(2)	32900	1(2)	33259	1(2)	33475	1(2)	33710	1(2)
31000	1(2)	31505	1(3)	31634	1(3)	32482	1(2)	32905	1(2)	33261	1(2)	33476	1(2)	33720	1(2)
31002	1(2)	31510	1(2)	31635	1(3)	32484	2(3)	32906	1(2)	33262	1(3)	33477	1(2)	33722	1(3)
31020	1(2)	31511	1(3)	31636	1(2)	32486	1(3)	32940	1(3)	33263	1(3)	33478	1(2)	33724	1(2)
31030	1(2)	31512	1(3)	31637	2(3)	32488	1(2)	32960	1(2)	33264	1(3)	33496	1(3)	33726	1(2)
31032	1(2)	31513	1(3)	31638	1(3)	32491	1(2)	32994	1(2)	33265	1(2)	33500	1(3)	33730	1(2)
31040	1(2)	31515	1(3)	31640	1(3)	32501	1(3)	32997	1(2)	33266	1(2)	33501	1(3)	33732	1(2)
31050	1(2)	31520	1(3)	31641	1(3)	32503	1(2)	32998	1(2)	33270	1(3)	33502	1(3)	33735	1(2)
31051	1(2)	31525	1(3)	31643	1(2)	32504	1(2)	32999	1(3)	33271	1(3)	33503	1(3)	33736	1(2)
31070	1(2)	31526	1(3)	31645	1(2)	32505	1(2)	33010	1(2)	33272	1(3)	33504	1(3)	33737	1(2)
31075	1(2)	31527	1(2)	31646	2(3)	32506	3(3)	33011	1(3)	33273	1(3)	33505	1(3)	33750	1(3)
31080	1(2)	31528	1(2)	31647	1(2)	32507	2(3)	33015	1(3)	33274	1(3)	33506	1(3)	33755	1(2)
31081	1(2)	31529	1(3)	31648	1(2)	32540	1(3)	33020	1(3)	33275	1(3)	33507	1(3)	33762	1(2)
31084	1(2)	31530	1(3)	31649	2(3)	32550	2(3)	33025	1(2)	33285	1(3)	33508	1(2)	33764	1(3)
31085	1(2)	31531	1(3)	31651	3(3)	32551	2(3)	33030	1(2)	33286	1(3)	33510	1(2)	33766	1(2)
31086	1(2)	31535	1(3)	31652	1(2)	32552	2(2)	33031	1(2)	33289	1(3)	33511	1(2)	33767	1(2)
31087	1(2)	31536	1(3)	31653	1(2)	32553	1(2)	33050	1(2)	33300	1(3)	33512	1(2)	33768	1(2)
31090	1(2)	31540	1(3)	31654	1(3)	32554	2(3)	33120	1(3)	33305	1(3)	33513	1(2)	33770	1(2)
31200	1(2)	31541	1(3)	31660	1(2)	32555	2(3)	33130	1(3)	33310	1(2)	33514	1(2)	33771	1(2)
31201	1(2)	31545	1(2)	31661	1(2)	32556	2(3)	33140	1(2)	33315	1(2)	33516	1(2)	33774	1(2)
31205	1(2)	31546	1(2)	31717	1(3)	32557	2(3)	33141	1(2)	33320	1(3)	33517	1(2)	33775	1(2)
31225	1(2)	31551	1(2)	31720	1(3)	32560	1(3)	33202	1(2)	33321	1(3)	33518	1(2)	33776	1(2)
31230	1(2)	31552	1(2)	31725	1(3)	32561	1(2)	33203	1(2)	33322	1(3)	33519	1(2)	33777	1(2)
31231	1(2)	31553	1(2)	31730	1(3)	32562	1(2)	33206	1(3)	33330	1(3)	33521	1(2)	33778	1(2)
31233	1(2)	31554	1(2)	31750	1(2)	32601	1(3)	33207	1(3)	33335	1(3)	33522	1(2)	33779	1(2)
31235	1(2)	31560	1(2)	31755	1(2)	32604	1(3)	33208	1(3)	33340	1(2)	33523	1(2)	33780	1(2)
31237	1(2)	31561	1(2)	31760	1(2)	32606	1(3)	33210	1(3)	33361	1(2)	33530	1(2)	33781	1(2)
31238	1(3)	31570	1(2)	31766	1(2)	32607	1(3)	33211	1(3)	33362	1(2)	33533	1(2)	33782	1(2)
31239	1(2)	31571	1(2)	31770	2(3)	32608	1(3)	33212	1(3)	33363	1(2)	33534	1(2)	33783	1(2)
31240	1(2)	31572	1(2)	31775	1(3)	32609	1(3)	33213	1(3)	33364	1(2)	33535	1(2)	33786	1(2)

CPT	MUE	CPT	MUE	CPT	MUE	CPT	MUE	CPT	MUE	CPT	MUE	CPT	MUE	CPT	MUE
33788	1(2)	33968	1(3)	34832	1(2)	35305	1(2)	35642	1(3)	36227	1(3)	36575	2(3)	37195	1(3)
33800	1(2)	33969	1(3)	34833	1(2)	35306	2(3)	35645	1(3)	36228	4(3)	36576	2(3)	37197	2(3)
33802	1(3)	33970	1(3)	34834	1(2)	35311	1(2)	35646	1(3)	36245	6(3)	36578	2(3)	37200	2(3)
33803	1(3)	33971	1(3)	34839	1(2)	35321	1(2)	35647	1(3)	36246	4(3)	36580	2(3)	37211	1(2)
33813	1(2)	33973	1(3)	34841	1(2)	35331	1(2)	35650	1(3)	36247	3(3)	36581	2(3)	37212	1(2)
33814	1(2)	33974	1(3)	34842	1(2)	35341	3(3)	35654	1(3)	36248	6(3)	36582	2(3)	37213	1(2)
33820	1(2)	33975	1(3)	34843	1(2)	35351	1(3)	35656	1(3)	36251	1(3)	36583	2(3)	37214	1(2)
33822	1(2)	33976	1(3)	34844	1(2)	35355	1(2)	35661	1(3)	36252	1(3)	36584	2(3)	37215	1(2)
33824	1(2)	33977	1(3)	34845	1(2)	35361	1(2)	35663	1(3)	36253	1(3)	36585	2(3)	37216	0(3)
33840	1(2)	33978	1(3)	34846	1(2)	35363	1(2)	35665	1(3)	36254	1(3)	36589	2(3)	37217	1(2)
33845	1(2)	33979	1(3)	34847	1(2)	35371	1(2)	35666	2(3)	36260	1(2)	36590	2(3)	37218	1(2)
33851	1(2)	33980	1(3)	34848	1(2)	35372	1(2)	35671	2(3)	36261	1(2)	36591	2(3)	37220	1(2)
33852	1(2)	33981	1(3)	35001	1(2)	35390	1(3)	35681	1(3)	36262	1(2)	36592	1(3)	37221	1(2)
33853	1(2)	33982	1(3)	35002	1(2)	35400	1(3)	35682	1(2)	36299	1(3)	36593	2(3)	37222	2(2)
33860	1(2)	33983	1(3)	35005	1(2)	35500	2(3)	35683	1(2)	36400	1(3)	36595	2(3)	37223	2(2)
33863	1(2)	33984	1(3)	35011	1(2)	35501	1(3)	35685	2(3)	36405	1(3)	36596	2(3)	37224	1(2)
33864	1(2)	33985	1(3)	35013	1(2)	35506	1(3)	35686	1(3)	36406	1(3)	36597	2(3)	37225	1(2)
33866	1(2)	33986	1(3)	35021	1(2)	35508	1(3)	35691	1(3)	36410	3(3)	36598	2(3)	37226	1(2)
33870	1(2)	33987	1(3)	35022	1(2)	35509	1(3)	35693	1(3)	36415	2(3)	36600	4(3)	37227	1(2)
33875	1(2)	33988	1(3)	35045	1(3)	35510	1(3)	35694	1(3)	36416	0(3)	36620	3(3)	37228	1(2)
33877	1(2)	33989	1(3)	35081	1(2)	35511	1(3)	35695	1(3)	36420	2(3)	36625	2(3)	37229	1(2)
33880	1(2)	33990	1(3)	35082	1(2)	35512	1(3)	35697	2(3)	36425	2(3)	36640	1(3)	37230	1(2)
33881	1(2)	33991	1(3)	35091	1(2)	35515	1(3)	35700	2(3)	36430	1(2)	36660	1(3)	37231	1(2)
33883	1(2)	33992	1(2)	35092	1(2)	35516	1(3)	35701	1(2)	36440	1(3)	36680	1(3)	37232	2(3)
33884	2(3)	33993	1(3)	35102	1(2)	35518	1(3)	35721	1(2)	36450	1(3)	36800	1(3)	37233	2(3)
33886	1(2)	33999	1(3)	35103	1(2)	35521	1(3)	35741	1(2)	36455	1(3)	36810	1(3)	37234	2(3)
33889	1(2)	34001	1(3)	35111	1(2)	35522	1(3)	35761	2(3)	36456	1(3)	36815	1(3)	37235	2(3)
33891	1(2)	34051	1(3)	35112	1(2)	35523	1(3)	35800	2(3)	36460	2(3)	36818	1(3)	37236	1(2)
33910	1(3)	34101	1(3)	35121	1(3)	35525	1(3)	35820	2(3)	36465	1(2)	36819	1(3)	37237	2(3)
33915	1(3)	34111	2(3)	35122	1(3)	35526	1(3)	35840	2(3)	36466	1(2)	36820	1(3)	37238	1(2)
33916	1(3)	34151	1(3)	35131	1(2)	35531	1(3)	35860	2(3)	36468	2(3)	36821	2(3)	37239	2(3)
33917	1(2)	34201	1(3)	35132	1(2)	35533	1(3)	35870	1(3)	36470	1(2)	36823	1(3)	37241	2(3)
33920	1(2)	34203	1(2)	35141	1(2)	35535	1(3)	35875	2(3)	36471	1(2)	36825	1(3)	37242	2(3)
33922	1(2)	34401	1(3)	35142	1(2)	35536	1(3)	35876	2(3)	36473	1(3)	36830	2(3)	37243	1(3)
33924	1(2)	34421	1(3)	35151	1(2)	35537	1(3)	35879	2(3)	36474	1(3)	36831	1(3)	37244	2(3)
33925	1(2)	34451	1(3)	35152	1(2)	35538	1(3)	35881	1(3)	36475	1(3)	36832	2(3)	37246	1(2)
33926	1(2)	34471	1(2)	35180	2(3)	35539	1(3)	35883	1(3)	36476	2(3)	36833	1(3)	37247	2(3)
33927	1(3)	34490	1(2)	35182	2(3)	35540	1(3)	35884	1(3)	36478	1(3)	36835	1(3)	37248	1(2)
33928	1(3)	34501	1(2)	35184	2(3)	35556	1(3)	35901	1(3)	36479	2(3)	36838	1(3)	37249	3(3)
33929	1(3)	34502	1(2)	35188	2(3)	35558	1(3)	35903	2(3)	36481	1(3)	36860	2(3)	37252	1(2)
33930	1(2)	34510	2(3)	35189	1(3)	35560	1(3)	35905	1(3)	36482	1(3)	36861	2(3)	37253	5(3)
33933	1(2)	34520	1(3)	35190	2(3)	35563	1(3)	35907	1(3)	36483	2(3)	36901	1(3)	37500	1(3)
33935	1(2)	34530	1(2)	35201	2(3)	35565	1(3)	36000	4(3)	36500	4(3)	36902	1(3)	37501	1(3)
33940	1(2)	34701	1(2)	35206	2(3)	35566	1(3)	36002	2(3)	36510	1(3)	36903	1(3)	37565	1(2)
33944	1(2)	34702	1(2)	35207	3(3)	35570	1(3)	36005	2(3)	36511	1(3)	36904	1(3)	37600	1(3)
33945	1(2)	34703	1(2)	35211	3(3)	35571	1(3)	36010	2(3)	36512	1(3)	36905	1(3)	37605	1(3)
33946	1(2)	34704	1(2)	35216	2(3)	35572	2(3)	36011	4(3)	36513	1(3)	36906	1(3)	37606	1(3)
33947	1(2)	34705	1(2)	35221	3(3)	35583	1(2)	36012	4(3)	36514	1(3)	36907	1(3)	37607	1(3)
33948	1(2)	34706	1(2)	35226	3(3)	35585	2(3)	36013	2(3)	36516	1(3)	36908	1(3)	37609	1(2)
33949	1(2)	34707	1(2)	35231	2(3)	35587	1(3)	36014	2(3)	36522	1(3)	36909	1(3)	37615	2(3)
33951	1(3)	34708	1(2)	35236	2(3)	35600	2(3)	36015	4(3)	36555	2(3)	37140	1(2)	37616	1(3)
33952	1(3)	34709	3(3)	35241	2(3)	35601	1(3)	36100	2(3)	36556	2(3)	37145	1(3)	37617	3(3)
33953	1(3)	34710	1(2)	35246	2(3)	35606	1(3)	36140	3(3)	36557	2(3)	37160	1(3)	37618	2(3)
33954	1(3)	34711	2(3)	35251	2(3)	35612	1(3)	36160	2(3)	36558	2(3)	37180	1(2)	37619	1(2)
33955	1(3)	34712	1(2)	35256	2(3)	35616	1(3)	36200	2(3)	36560	2(3)	37181	1(2)	37650	1(2)
33956	1(3)	34713	1(2)	35261	1(3)	35621	1(3)	36215	6(3)	36561	2(3)	37182	1(2)	37660	1(2)
33957	1(3)	34714	1(2)	35266	2(3)	35623	1(3)	36216	4(3)	36563	1(3)	37183	1(2)	37700	1(2)
33958	1(3)	34715	1(2)	35271	2(3)	35626	3(3)	36217	2(3)	36565	1(3)	37184	1(2)	37718	1(2)
33959	1(3)	34716	1(2)	35276	2(3)	35631	4(3)	36218	6(3)	36566	1(3)	37185	2(3)	37722	1(2)
33962	1(3)	34808	1(3)	35281	2(3)	35632	1(3)	36221	1(3)	36568	2(3)	37186	2(3)	37735	1(2)
33963	1(3)	34812	1(2)	35286	2(3)	35633	1(3)	36222	1(3)	36569	2(3)	37187	1(3)	37760	1(2)
33964	1(3)	34813	1(2)	35301	2(3)	35634	1(3)	36223	1(3)	36570	2(3)	37188	1(3)	37761	1(2)
33965	1(3)	34820	1(2)	35302	1(2)	35636	1(3)	36224	1(3)	36571	2(3)	37191	1(3)	37765	1(2)
33966	1(3)	34830	1(2)	35303	1(2)	35637	1(3)	36225	1(3)	36572	1(3)	37192	1(3)	37766	1(2)
33967	1(3)	34831	1(2)	35304	1(2)	35638	1(3)	36226	1(3)	36573	1(3)	37193	1(3)	37780	1(2)

CPT	MUE
37785	1(2)
37788	1(2)
37790	1(2)
37799	1(3)
38100	1(2)
38101	1(3)
38102	1(2)
38115	1(3)
38120	1(2)
38129	1(3)
38200	1(3)
38204	0(3)
38205	1(3)
38206	1(3)
38207	0(3)
38208	0(3)
38209	0(3)
38210	0(3)
38211	0(3)
38212	0(3)
38213	0(3)
38214	0(3)
38215	0(3)
38220	1(3)
38221	1(3)
38222	1(2)
38230	1(2)
38232	1(2)
38240	1(3)
38241	1(2)
38242	1(2)
38243	1(3)
38300	1(3)
38305	1(3)
38308	1(3)
38380	1(2)
38381	1(2)
38382	1(2)
38500	2(3)
38505	2(3)
38510	1(2)
38520	1(2)
38525	1(2)
38530	1(2)
38531	1(2)
38542	1(2)
38550	1(3)
38555	1(3)
38562	1(2)
38564	1(2)
38570	1(2)
38571	1(2)
38572	1(2)
38573	1(2)
38589	1(3)
38700	1(2)
38720	1(2)
38724	1(2)
38740	1(2)
38745	1(2)
38746	1(2)
38747	1(2)
38760	1(2)
38765	1(2)
38770	1(2)

CPT	MUE
38780	1(2)
38790	1(2)
38792	1(3)
38794	1(2)
38900	1(3)
38999	1(3)
39000	1(2)
39010	1(2)
39200	1(2)
39220	1(2)
39401	1(3)
39402	1(3)
39499	1(3)
39501	1(3)
39503	1(2)
39540	1(2)
39541	1(2)
39545	1(2)
39560	1(3)
39561	1(3)
39599	1(3)
40490	2(3)
40500	2(3)
40510	2(3)
40520	2(3)
40525	2(3)
40527	2(3)
40530	2(3)
40650	2(3)
40652	2(3)
40654	2(3)
40700	1(2)
40701	1(2)
40702	1(2)
40720	1(2)
40761	1(2)
40799	1(3)
40800	2(3)
40801	2(3)
40804	1(3)
40805	2(3)
40806	2(2)
40808	2(3)
40810	2(3)
40812	2(3)
40814	4(3)
40816	2(3)
40818	2(3)
40819	2(2)
40820	2(3)
40830	2(3)
40831	2(3)
40840	1(2)
40842	1(2)
40843	1(2)
40844	1(2)
40845	1(3)
40899	1(3)
41000	1(3)
41005	1(3)
41006	2(3)
41007	2(3)
41008	2(3)
41009	2(3)
41010	1(2)

CPT	MUE
41015	2(3)
41016	1(3)
41017	2(3)
41018	2(3)
41019	1(2)
41100	2(3)
41105	2(3)
41108	2(3)
41110	2(3)
41112	2(3)
41113	2(3)
41114	2(3)
41115	1(2)
41116	2(3)
41120	1(2)
41130	1(2)
41135	1(2)
41140	1(2)
41145	1(2)
41150	1(2)
41153	1(2)
41155	1(2)
41250	2(3)
41251	2(3)
41252	2(3)
41510	1(2)
41512	1(2)
41520	1(3)
41530	1(3)
41599	1(3)
41800	2(3)
41805	1(3)
41806	1(3)
41820	4(2)
41821	2(3)
41822	1(2)
41823	1(2)
41825	2(3)
41826	2(3)
41827	2(3)
41828	4(2)
41830	2(3)
41850	2(3)
41870	2(3)
41872	4(2)
41874	4(2)
41899	1(3)
42000	1(3)
42100	2(3)
42104	2(3)
42106	2(3)
42107	2(3)
42120	1(2)
42140	1(2)
42145	1(2)
42160	1(3)
42180	1(3)
42182	1(3)
42200	1(2)
42205	1(2)
42210	1(2)
42215	1(2)
42220	1(2)
42225	1(2)
42226	1(2)

CPT	MUE
42227	1(2)
42235	1(2)
42260	1(3)
42280	1(2)
42281	1(2)
42299	1(3)
42300	2(3)
42305	2(3)
42310	2(3)
42320	2(3)
42330	1(3)
42335	2(2)
42340	1(2)
42400	2(3)
42405	2(3)
42408	1(3)
42409	1(3)
42410	1(2)
42415	1(2)
42420	1(2)
42425	1(2)
42426	1(2)
42440	1(2)
42450	1(3)
42500	2(3)
42505	2(3)
42507	1(2)
42509	1(2)
42510	1(2)
42550	2(3)
42600	1(3)
42650	2(3)
42660	2(3)
42665	2(3)
42699	1(3)
42700	2(3)
42720	1(3)
42725	1(3)
42800	3(3)
42804	1(3)
42806	1(3)
42808	2(3)
42809	1(3)
42810	1(3)
42815	1(3)
42820	1(2)
42821	1(2)
42825	1(2)
42826	1(2)
42830	1(2)
42831	1(2)
42835	1(2)
42836	1(2)
42842	1(3)
42844	1(3)
42845	1(3)
42860	1(3)
42870	1(3)
42890	1(2)
42892	1(3)
42894	1(3)
42900	1(3)
42950	1(2)
42953	1(3)
42955	1(2)

CPT	MUE
42960	1(3)
42961	1(3)
42962	1(3)
42970	1(3)
42971	1(3)
42972	1(3)
42999	1(3)
43020	1(2)
43030	1(2)
43045	1(2)
43100	1(3)
43101	1(3)
43107	1(2)
43108	1(2)
43112	1(2)
43113	1(2)
43116	1(2)
43117	1(2)
43118	1(2)
43121	1(2)
43122	1(2)
43123	1(2)
43124	1(2)
43130	1(3)
43135	1(3)
43180	1(2)
43191	1(3)
43192	1(3)
43193	1(3)
43194	1(3)
43195	1(3)
43196	1(3)
43197	1(3)
43198	1(3)
43200	1(3)
43201	1(2)
43202	1(2)
43204	1(2)
43205	1(2)
43206	1(2)
43210	1(2)
43211	1(3)
43212	1(3)
43213	1(2)
43214	1(3)
43215	1(3)
43216	1(2)
43217	1(2)
43220	1(3)
43226	1(3)
43227	1(3)
43229	1(3)
43231	1(2)
43232	1(2)
43233	1(3)
43235	1(3)
43236	1(2)
43237	1(2)
43238	1(2)
43239	1(2)
43240	1(2)
43241	1(3)
43242	1(2)
43243	1(2)
43244	1(2)

CPT	MUE
43245	1(2)
43246	1(2)
43247	1(2)
43248	1(3)
43249	1(3)
43250	1(2)
43251	1(2)
43252	1(2)
43253	1(3)
43254	1(3)
43255	2(3)
43257	1(2)
43259	1(2)
43260	1(3)
43261	1(2)
43262	2(2)
43263	1(2)
43264	1(2)
43265	1(2)
43266	1(3)
43270	1(3)
43273	1(2)
43274	2(3)
43275	1(3)
43276	2(3)
43277	3(3)
43278	1(3)
43279	1(2)
43280	1(2)
43281	1(2)
43282	1(2)
43283	1(2)
43284	1(2)
43285	1(2)
43286	1(2)
43287	1(2)
43288	1(2)
43289	1(3)
43300	1(2)
43305	1(2)
43310	1(2)
43312	1(2)
43313	1(2)
43314	1(2)
43320	1(2)
43325	1(2)
43327	1(2)
43328	1(2)
43330	1(2)
43331	1(2)
43332	1(2)
43333	1(2)
43334	1(2)
43335	1(2)
43336	1(2)
43337	1(2)
43338	1(2)
43340	1(2)
43341	1(2)
43351	1(2)
43352	1(2)
43360	1(2)
43361	1(2)
43400	1(2)
43401	1(2)

CPT	MUE
43405	1(2)
43410	1(3)
43415	1(3)
43420	1(3)
43425	1(3)
43450	1(3)
43453	1(3)
43460	1(3)
43496	1(3)
43499	1(3)
43500	1(2)
43501	1(3)
43502	1(2)
43510	1(2)
43520	1(2)
43605	1(2)
43610	2(3)
43611	2(3)
43620	1(2)
43621	1(2)
43622	1(2)
43631	1(2)
43632	1(2)
43633	1(2)
43634	1(2)
43635	1(2)
43640	1(2)
43641	1(2)
43644	1(2)
43645	1(2)
43647	1(2)
43648	1(2)
43651	1(2)
43652	1(2)
43653	1(2)
43659	1(3)
43752	2(3)
43753	1(3)
43754	1(3)
43755	1(3)
43756	1(2)
43757	1(2)
43761	2(3)
43762	2(3)
43763	2(3)
43770	1(2)
43771	1(2)
43772	1(2)
43773	1(2)
43774	1(2)
43775	1(2)
43800	1(2)
43810	1(2)
43820	1(2)
43825	1(2)
43830	1(2)
43831	1(2)
43832	1(2)
43840	2(3)
43842	0(3)
43843	1(2)
43845	1(2)
43846	1(2)
43847	1(2)
43848	1(2)

CPT	MUE
43850	1(2)
43855	1(2)
43860	1(2)
43865	1(2)
43870	1(2)
43880	1(3)
43881	1(3)
43882	1(3)
43886	1(2)
43887	1(2)
43888	1(2)
43999	1(3)
44005	1(2)
44010	1(2)
44015	1(2)
44020	2(3)
44021	1(3)
44025	1(3)
44050	1(2)
44055	1(2)
44100	1(2)
44110	1(2)
44111	1(2)
44120	1(2)
44121	2(3)
44125	1(2)
44126	1(2)
44127	1(2)
44128	2(3)
44130	2(3)
44132	1(2)
44133	1(2)
44135	1(2)
44136	1(2)
44137	1(2)
44139	1(2)
44140	2(3)
44141	1(3)
44143	1(2)
44144	1(3)
44145	1(2)
44146	1(2)
44147	1(3)
44150	1(2)
44151	1(2)
44155	1(2)
44156	1(2)
44157	1(2)
44158	1(2)
44160	1(2)
44180	1(2)
44186	1(2)
44187	1(3)
44188	1(3)
44202	1(2)
44203	2(3)
44204	2(3)
44205	1(2)
44206	1(2)
44207	1(2)
44208	1(2)
44210	1(2)
44211	1(2)
44212	1(2)
44213	1(2)

CPT	MUE
44227	1(3)
44238	1(3)
44300	1(3)
44310	2(3)
44312	1(2)
44314	1(2)
44316	1(2)
44320	1(2)
44322	1(2)
44340	1(2)
44345	1(2)
44346	1(2)
44360	1(3)
44361	1(2)
44363	1(3)
44364	1(2)
44365	1(2)
44366	1(3)
44369	1(2)
44370	1(2)
44372	1(2)
44373	1(2)
44376	1(3)
44377	1(2)
44378	1(3)
44379	1(2)
44380	1(3)
44381	1(3)
44382	1(2)
44384	1(3)
44385	1(3)
44386	1(2)
44388	1(3)
44389	1(2)
44390	1(3)
44391	1(3)
44392	1(2)
44394	1(2)
44401	1(2)
44402	1(3)
44403	1(3)
44404	1(3)
44405	1(3)
44406	1(3)
44407	1(2)
44408	1(3)
44500	1(3)
44602	1(2)
44603	1(2)
44604	1(2)
44605	1(2)
44615	3(3)
44620	2(3)
44625	1(3)
44626	1(3)
44640	2(3)
44650	2(3)
44660	1(3)
44661	1(3)
44680	1(3)
44700	1(2)
44701	1(2)
44705	1(3)
44715	1(2)
44720	2(3)

CPT	MUE
44721	2(3)
44799	1(3)
44800	1(3)
44820	1(3)
44850	1(3)
44899	1(3)
44900	1(2)
44950	1(2)
44955	1(2)
44960	1(2)
44970	1(2)
44979	1(3)
45000	1(3)
45005	1(3)
45020	1(3)
45100	2(3)
45108	1(2)
45110	1(2)
45111	1(2)
45112	1(2)
45113	1(2)
45114	1(2)
45116	1(2)
45119	1(2)
45120	1(2)
45121	1(2)
45123	1(2)
45126	1(2)
45130	1(2)
45135	1(2)
45136	1(2)
45150	1(2)
45160	1(3)
45171	2(3)
45172	2(3)
45190	1(3)
45300	1(3)
45303	1(3)
45305	1(2)
45307	1(3)
45308	1(2)
45309	1(2)
45315	1(2)
45317	1(3)
45320	1(2)
45321	1(2)
45327	1(2)
45330	1(3)
45331	1(2)
45332	1(3)
45333	1(2)
45334	1(3)
45335	1(2)
45337	1(2)
45338	1(2)
45340	1(2)
45341	1(2)
45342	1(2)
45346	1(2)
45347	1(3)
45349	1(3)
45350	1(2)
45378	1(3)
45379	1(3)
45380	1(2)

CPT	MUE
45381	1(2)
45382	1(3)
45384	1(2)
45385	1(2)
45386	1(2)
45388	1(2)
45389	1(3)
45390	1(3)
45391	1(2)
45392	1(2)
45393	1(3)
45395	1(2)
45397	1(2)
45398	1(2)
45399	1(3)
45400	1(2)
45402	1(2)
45499	1(3)
45500	1(2)
45505	1(2)
45520	1(2)
45540	1(2)
45541	1(2)
45550	1(2)
45560	1(2)
45562	1(2)
45563	1(2)
45800	1(3)
45805	1(3)
45820	1(3)
45825	1(3)
45900	1(2)
45905	1(2)
45910	1(2)
45915	1(2)
45990	1(2)
45999	1(3)
46020	2(3)
46030	1(3)
46040	2(3)
46045	2(3)
46050	2(3)
46060	2(3)
46070	1(2)
46080	1(2)
46083	2(3)
46200	1(3)
46220	1(2)
46221	1(2)
46230	1(2)
46250	1(2)
46255	1(2)
46257	1(2)
46258	1(2)
46260	1(2)
46261	1(2)
46262	1(2)
46270	1(3)
46275	1(3)
46280	1(2)
46285	1(3)
46288	1(3)
46320	2(3)
46500	1(2)
46505	1(2)

CPT	MUE
46600	1(3)
46601	1(3)
46604	1(2)
46606	1(2)
46607	1(2)
46608	1(3)
46610	1(2)
46611	1(2)
46612	1(2)
46614	1(3)
46615	1(2)
46700	1(2)
46705	1(2)
46706	1(3)
46707	1(3)
46710	1(3)
46712	1(3)
46715	1(2)
46716	1(2)
46730	1(2)
46735	1(2)
46740	1(2)
46742	1(2)
46744	1(2)
46746	1(2)
46748	1(2)
46750	1(2)
46751	1(2)
46753	1(2)
46754	1(3)
46760	1(2)
46761	1(2)
46900	1(2)
46910	1(2)
46916	1(2)
46917	1(2)
46922	1(2)
46924	1(2)
46930	1(2)
46940	1(2)
46942	1(3)
46945	1(2)
46946	1(2)
46947	1(2)
46999	1(3)
47000	3(3)
47001	3(3)
47010	1(3)
47015	1(2)
47100	3(3)
47120	2(3)
47122	1(2)
47125	1(2)
47130	1(2)
47133	1(2)
47135	1(2)
47140	1(2)
47141	1(2)
47142	1(2)
47143	1(2)
47144	1(2)
47145	1(2)
47146	2(3)
47147	1(3)
47300	2(3)

CPT	MUE
47350	1(3)
47360	1(3)
47361	1(3)
47362	1(3)
47370	1(2)
47371	1(2)
47379	1(3)
47380	1(2)
47381	1(2)
47382	1(2)
47383	1(2)
47399	1(3)
47400	1(3)
47420	1(2)
47425	1(2)
47460	1(2)
47480	1(2)
47490	1(2)
47531	2(3)
47532	1(3)
47533	1(3)
47534	2(3)
47535	1(3)
47536	2(3)
47537	1(3)
47538	2(3)
47539	2(3)
47540	2(3)
47541	1(3)
47542	2(3)
47543	1(3)
47544	1(3)
47550	1(3)
47552	1(3)
47553	1(2)
47554	1(3)
47555	1(2)
47556	1(2)
47562	1(2)
47563	1(2)
47564	1(2)
47570	1(2)
47579	1(3)
47600	1(2)
47605	1(2)
47610	1(2)
47612	1(2)
47620	1(2)
47700	1(2)
47701	1(2)
47711	1(2)
47712	1(2)
47715	1(2)
47720	1(2)
47721	1(2)
47740	1(2)
47741	1(2)
47760	1(2)
47765	1(2)
47780	1(2)
47785	1(2)
47800	1(2)
47801	1(3)
47802	1(2)
47900	1(2)

CPT	MUE
47999	1(3)
48000	1(2)
48001	1(2)
48020	1(3)
48100	1(3)
48102	1(3)
48105	1(2)
48120	1(3)
48140	1(2)
48145	1(2)
48146	1(2)
48148	1(2)
48150	1(2)
48152	1(2)
48153	1(2)
48154	1(2)
48155	1(2)
48160	0(3)
48400	1(3)
48500	1(3)
48510	1(3)
48520	1(3)
48540	1(3)
48545	1(3)
48547	1(2)
48548	1(2)
48550	1(2)
48551	1(2)
48552	2(3)
48554	1(2)
48556	1(2)
48999	1(3)
49000	1(2)
49002	1(3)
49010	1(3)
49020	2(3)
49040	2(3)
49060	2(3)
49062	1(3)
49082	1(3)
49083	2(3)
49084	1(3)
49180	2(3)
49185	2(3)
49203	1(2)
49204	1(2)
49205	1(2)
49215	1(2)
49220	1(2)
49250	1(2)
49255	1(2)
49320	1(3)
49321	1(2)
49322	1(2)
49323	1(2)
49324	1(2)
49325	1(2)
49326	1(2)
49327	1(2)
49329	1(3)
49400	1(3)
49402	1(3)
49405	2(3)
49406	2(3)
49407	1(3)

CPT	MUE
49411	1(2)
49412	1(2)
49418	1(3)
49419	1(2)
49421	1(2)
49422	1(2)
49423	2(3)
49424	3(3)
49425	1(2)
49426	1(3)
49427	1(3)
49428	1(2)
49429	1(2)
49435	1(2)
49436	1(2)
49440	1(3)
49441	1(3)
49442	1(3)
49446	1(2)
49450	1(3)
49451	1(3)
49452	1(3)
49460	1(3)
49465	1(3)
49491	1(2)
49492	1(2)
49495	1(2)
49496	1(2)
49500	1(2)
49501	1(2)
49505	1(2)
49507	1(2)
49520	1(2)
49521	1(2)
49525	1(2)
49540	1(2)
49550	1(2)
49553	1(2)
49555	1(2)
49557	1(2)
49560	2(3)
49561	1(3)
49565	2(3)
49566	2(3)
49568	2(3)
49570	1(3)
49572	1(3)
49580	1(2)
49582	1(2)
49585	1(2)
49587	1(2)
49590	1(2)
49600	1(2)
49605	1(2)
49606	1(2)
49610	1(2)
49611	1(2)
49650	1(2)
49651	1(2)
49652	2(3)
49653	2(3)
49654	1(3)
49655	1(3)
49656	1(3)
49657	1(3)

CPT	MUE
49659	1(3)
49900	1(3)
49904	1(3)
49905	1(3)
49906	1(3)
49999	1(3)
50010	1(2)
50020	1(3)
50040	1(2)
50045	1(2)
50060	1(2)
50065	1(2)
50070	1(2)
50075	1(2)
50080	1(2)
50081	1(2)
50100	1(2)
50120	1(2)
50125	1(2)
50130	1(2)
50135	1(2)
50200	1(3)
50205	1(3)
50220	1(2)
50225	1(2)
50230	1(2)
50234	1(2)
50236	1(2)
50240	1(2)
50250	1(3)
50280	1(2)
50290	1(3)
50300	1(2)
50320	1(2)
50323	1(2)
50325	1(2)
50327	2(3)
50328	1(3)
50329	1(3)
50340	1(2)
50360	1(2)
50365	1(2)
50370	1(2)
50380	1(2)
50382	1(3)
50384	1(3)
50385	1(3)
50386	1(3)
50387	1(3)
50389	1(3)
50390	2(3)
50391	1(3)
50396	1(3)
50400	1(2)
50405	1(2)
50430	2(3)
50431	2(3)
50432	2(3)
50433	2(3)
50434	2(3)
50435	2(3)
50436	1(3)
50437	1(3)
50500	1(3)
50520	1(3)

CPT	MUE
50525	1(3)
50526	1(3)
50540	1(2)
50541	1(2)
50542	1(2)
50543	1(2)
50544	1(2)
50545	1(2)
50546	1(2)
50547	1(2)
50548	1(2)
50549	1(3)
50551	1(3)
50553	1(3)
50555	1(2)
50557	1(2)
50561	1(2)
50562	1(3)
50570	1(3)
50572	1(3)
50574	1(2)
50575	1(2)
50576	1(2)
50580	1(2)
50590	1(2)
50592	1(2)
50593	1(2)
50600	1(3)
50605	1(3)
50606	1(3)
50610	1(2)
50620	1(2)
50630	1(2)
50650	1(2)
50660	1(3)
50684	1(3)
50686	2(3)
50688	2(3)
50690	2(3)
50693	2(3)
50694	2(3)
50695	2(3)
50700	1(2)
50705	2(3)
50706	2(3)
50715	1(2)
50722	1(2)
50725	1(3)
50727	1(3)
50728	1(3)
50740	1(2)
50750	1(2)
50760	1(2)
50770	1(2)
50780	1(2)
50782	1(2)
50783	1(2)
50785	1(2)
50800	1(2)
50810	1(3)
50815	1(2)
50820	1(2)
50825	1(3)
50830	1(3)
50840	1(2)

CPT	MUE
50845	1(2)
50860	1(2)
50900	1(3)
50920	2(3)
50930	2(3)
50940	1(2)
50945	1(2)
50947	1(2)
50948	1(2)
50949	1(3)
50951	1(3)
50953	1(3)
50955	1(2)
50957	1(2)
50961	1(2)
50970	1(3)
50972	1(3)
50974	1(2)
50976	1(2)
50980	1(2)
51020	1(2)
51030	1(2)
51040	1(3)
51045	2(3)
51050	1(3)
51060	1(3)
51065	1(3)
51080	1(3)
51100	1(3)
51101	1(3)
51102	1(3)
51500	1(2)
51520	1(2)
51525	1(2)
51530	1(2)
51535	1(2)
51550	1(2)
51555	1(2)
51565	1(2)
51570	1(2)
51575	1(2)
51580	1(2)
51585	1(2)
51590	1(2)
51595	1(2)
51596	1(2)
51597	1(2)
51600	1(3)
51605	1(3)
51610	1(3)
51700	1(3)
51701	2(3)
51702	2(3)
51703	2(3)
51705	1(3)
51710	1(3)
51715	1(2)
51720	1(3)
51725	1(3)
51726	1(3)
51727	1(3)
51728	1(3)
51729	1(3)
51736	1(3)
51741	1(3)

CPT	MUE
51784	1(3)
51785	1(3)
51792	1(3)
51797	1(3)
51798	1(3)
51800	1(2)
51820	1(2)
51840	1(2)
51841	1(2)
51845	1(2)
51860	1(3)
51865	1(3)
51880	1(2)
51900	1(3)
51920	1(3)
51925	1(2)
51940	1(2)
51960	1(2)
51980	1(2)
51990	1(2)
51992	1(2)
51999	1(3)
52000	1(3)
52001	1(3)
52005	2(3)
52007	1(2)
52010	1(2)
52204	1(2)
52214	1(2)
52224	1(2)
52234	1(2)
52235	1(2)
52240	1(2)
52250	1(2)
52260	1(2)
52265	1(2)
52270	1(2)
52275	1(2)
52276	1(2)
52277	1(2)
52281	1(2)
52282	1(2)
52283	1(2)
52285	1(2)
52287	1(2)
52290	1(2)
52300	1(2)
52301	1(2)
52305	1(2)
52310	1(3)
52315	2(3)
52317	1(3)
52318	1(3)
52320	1(2)
52325	1(3)
52327	1(2)
52330	1(2)
52332	1(2)
52334	1(2)
52341	1(2)
52342	1(2)
52343	1(2)
52344	1(2)
52345	1(2)
52346	1(2)

CPT	MUE
52351	1(3)
52352	1(2)
52353	1(2)
52354	1(3)
52355	1(3)
52356	1(2)
52400	1(2)
52402	1(2)
52441	1(2)
52442	6(3)
52450	1(2)
52500	1(2)
52601	1(2)
52630	1(2)
52640	1(2)
52647	1(2)
52648	1(2)
52649	1(2)
52700	1(3)
53000	1(2)
53010	1(2)
53020	1(2)
53025	1(2)
53040	1(3)
53060	1(3)
53080	1(3)
53085	1(3)
53200	1(3)
53210	1(2)
53215	1(2)
53220	1(3)
53230	1(3)
53235	1(3)
53240	1(3)
53250	1(3)
53260	1(2)
53265	1(3)
53270	1(2)
53275	1(2)
53400	1(2)
53405	1(2)
53410	1(2)
53415	1(2)
53420	1(2)
53425	1(2)
53430	1(2)
53431	1(2)
53440	1(2)
53442	1(2)
53444	1(3)
53445	1(2)
53446	1(2)
53447	1(2)
53448	1(2)
53449	1(2)
53450	1(2)
53460	1(2)
53500	1(2)
53502	1(3)
53505	1(3)
53510	1(3)
53515	1(3)
53520	1(3)
53600	1(3)
53601	1(3)

CPT	MUE
53605	1(3)
53620	1(2)
53621	1(3)
53660	1(2)
53661	1(3)
53665	1(3)
53850	1(2)
53852	1(2)
53854	1(2)
53855	1(2)
53860	1(2)
53899	1(3)
54000	1(2)
54001	1(2)
54015	1(3)
54050	1(2)
54055	1(2)
54056	1(2)
54057	1(2)
54060	1(2)
54065	1(2)
54100	2(3)
54105	2(3)
54110	1(2)
54111	1(2)
54112	1(3)
54115	1(3)
54120	1(2)
54125	1(2)
54130	1(2)
54135	1(2)
54150	1(2)
54160	1(2)
54161	1(2)
54162	1(2)
54163	1(2)
54164	1(2)
54200	1(2)
54205	1(2)
54220	1(3)
54230	1(3)
54231	1(3)
54235	1(3)
54240	1(2)
54250	1(2)
54300	1(2)
54304	1(2)
54308	1(2)
54312	1(2)
54316	1(2)
54318	1(2)
54322	1(2)
54324	1(2)
54326	1(2)
54328	1(2)
54332	1(2)
54336	1(2)
54340	1(2)
54344	1(2)
54348	1(2)
54352	1(2)
54360	1(2)
54380	1(2)
54385	1(2)
54390	1(2)

CPT	MUE
54400	1(2)
54401	1(2)
54405	1(2)
54406	1(2)
54408	1(2)
54410	1(2)
54411	1(2)
54415	1(2)
54416	1(2)
54417	1(2)
54420	1(2)
54430	1(2)
54435	1(2)
54437	1(2)
54438	1(2)
54440	1(2)
54450	1(2)
54500	1(3)
54505	1(3)
54512	1(3)
54520	1(2)
54522	1(2)
54530	1(2)
54535	1(2)
54550	1(2)
54560	1(2)
54600	1(2)
54620	1(2)
54640	1(2)
54650	1(2)
54660	1(2)
54670	1(3)
54680	1(2)
54690	1(2)
54692	1(2)
54699	1(3)
54700	1(3)
54800	1(2)
54830	1(2)
54840	1(2)
54860	1(2)
54861	1(2)
54865	1(3)
54900	1(2)
54901	1(2)
55000	1(3)
55040	1(2)
55041	1(2)
55060	1(2)
55100	2(3)
55110	1(2)
55120	1(3)
55150	1(2)
55175	1(2)
55180	1(2)
55200	1(2)
55250	1(2)
55300	1(2)
55400	1(2)
55500	1(2)
55520	1(2)
55530	1(2)
55535	1(2)
55540	1(2)
55550	1(2)

CPT	MUE
55559	1(3)
55600	1(2)
55605	1(2)
55650	1(2)
55680	1(3)
55700	1(2)
55705	1(2)
55706	1(2)
55720	1(3)
55725	1(3)
55801	1(2)
55810	1(2)
55812	1(2)
55815	1(2)
55821	1(2)
55831	1(2)
55840	1(2)
55842	1(2)
55845	1(2)
55860	1(2)
55862	1(2)
55865	1(2)
55866	1(2)
55870	1(2)
55873	1(2)
55874	1(2)
55875	1(2)
55876	1(2)
55899	1(3)
55920	1(2)
55970	1(2)
55980	1(2)
56405	2(3)
56420	1(3)
56440	1(3)
56441	1(2)
56442	1(2)
56501	1(2)
56515	1(2)
56605	1(2)
56606	6(3)
56620	1(2)
56625	1(2)
56630	1(2)
56631	1(2)
56632	1(2)
56633	1(2)
56634	1(2)
56637	1(2)
56640	1(2)
56700	1(2)
56740	1(3)
56800	1(2)
56805	1(2)
56810	1(2)
56820	1(2)
56821	1(2)
57000	1(3)
57010	1(3)
57020	1(3)
57022	1(3)
57023	1(3)
57061	1(2)
57065	1(2)
57100	2(3)

CPT	MUE
57105	2(3)
57106	1(2)
57107	1(2)
57109	1(2)
57110	1(2)
57111	1(2)
57112	1(2)
57120	1(2)
57130	1(2)
57135	2(3)
57150	1(3)
57155	1(3)
57156	1(3)
57160	1(2)
57170	1(2)
57180	1(3)
57200	1(3)
57210	1(3)
57220	1(2)
57230	1(2)
57240	1(2)
57250	1(2)
57260	1(2)
57265	1(2)
57267	2(3)
57268	1(2)
57270	1(2)
57280	1(2)
57282	1(2)
57283	1(2)
57284	1(2)
57285	1(2)
57287	1(2)
57288	1(2)
57289	1(2)
57291	1(2)
57292	1(2)
57295	1(2)
57296	1(2)
57300	1(3)
57305	1(3)
57307	1(3)
57308	1(3)
57310	1(3)
57311	1(3)
57320	1(3)
57330	1(3)
57335	1(2)
57400	1(2)
57410	1(2)
57415	1(3)
57420	1(3)
57421	1(3)
57423	1(2)
57425	1(2)
57426	1(2)
57452	1(3)
57454	1(3)
57455	1(3)
57456	1(3)
57460	1(3)
57461	1(3)
57500	1(3)
57505	1(3)
57510	1(3)

CPT	MUE
57511	1(3)
57513	1(3)
57520	1(3)
57522	1(3)
57530	1(3)
57531	1(2)
57540	1(2)
57545	1(3)
57550	1(3)
57555	1(2)
57556	1(2)
57558	1(3)
57700	1(3)
57720	1(3)
57800	1(3)
58100	1(3)
58110	1(3)
58120	1(3)
58140	1(3)
58145	1(3)
58146	1(3)
58150	1(3)
58152	1(2)
58180	1(3)
58200	1(2)
58210	1(2)
58240	1(2)
58260	1(3)
58262	1(3)
58263	1(2)
58267	1(2)
58270	1(2)
58275	1(2)
58280	1(2)
58285	1(3)
58290	1(3)
58291	1(2)
58292	1(2)
58293	1(2)
58294	1(2)
58300	0(3)
58301	1(3)
58321	1(2)
58322	1(2)
58323	1(3)
58340	1(3)
58345	1(3)
58346	1(2)
58350	1(2)
58353	1(3)
58356	1(3)
58400	1(3)
58410	1(2)
58520	1(2)
58540	1(3)
58541	1(3)
58542	1(2)
58543	1(3)
58544	1(2)
58545	1(2)
58546	1(2)
58548	1(2)
58550	1(3)
58552	1(3)
58553	1(3)

CPT	MUE
58554	1(2)
58555	1(3)
58558	1(3)
58559	1(3)
58560	1(3)
58561	1(3)
58562	1(3)
58563	1(3)
58565	1(2)
58570	1(3)
58571	1(2)
58572	1(3)
58573	1(2)
58575	1(2)
58578	1(3)
58579	1(3)
58600	1(2)
58605	1(2)
58611	1(2)
58615	1(2)
58660	1(2)
58661	1(2)
58662	1(2)
58670	1(2)
58671	1(2)
58672	1(2)
58673	1(2)
58674	1(2)
58679	1(3)
58700	1(2)
58720	1(2)
58740	1(2)
58750	1(2)
58752	1(2)
58760	1(2)
58770	1(2)
58800	1(2)
58805	1(2)
58820	1(3)
58822	1(3)
58825	1(2)
58900	1(2)
58920	1(2)
58925	1(3)
58940	1(2)
58943	1(2)
58950	1(2)
58951	1(2)
58952	1(2)
58953	1(2)
58954	1(2)
58956	1(2)
58957	1(2)
58958	1(2)
58960	1(2)
58970	1(3)
58974	1(3)
58976	2(3)
58999	1(3)
59000	2(3)
59001	2(3)
59012	2(3)
59015	2(3)
59020	2(3)
59025	2(3)

CPT	MUE
59030	2(3)
59050	2(3)
59051	2(3)
59070	2(3)
59072	2(3)
59074	2(3)
59076	2(3)
59100	1(2)
59120	1(3)
59121	1(3)
59130	1(3)
59135	1(3)
59136	1(3)
59140	1(2)
59150	1(3)
59151	1(3)
59160	1(2)
59200	1(3)
59300	1(2)
59320	1(2)
59325	1(2)
59350	1(2)
59400	1(2)
59409	2(3)
59410	1(2)
59412	1(3)
59414	1(3)
59425	1(2)
59426	1(2)
59430	1(2)
59510	1(2)
59514	1(3)
59515	1(2)
59525	1(2)
59610	1(2)
59612	2(3)
59614	1(2)
59618	1(2)
59620	1(2)
59622	1(2)
59812	1(2)
59820	1(2)
59821	1(2)
59830	1(2)
59840	1(2)
59841	1(2)
59850	1(2)
59851	1(2)
59852	1(2)
59855	1(2)
59856	1(2)
59857	1(2)
59866	1(2)
59870	1(2)
59871	1(2)
59897	1(3)
59898	1(3)
59899	1(3)
60000	1(3)
60100	3(3)
60200	2(3)
60210	1(2)
60212	1(2)
60220	1(3)
60225	1(2)

CPT	MUE
60240	1(2)
60252	1(2)
60254	1(2)
60260	1(2)
60270	1(2)
60271	1(2)
60280	1(3)
60281	1(3)
60300	2(3)
60500	1(2)
60502	1(3)
60505	1(3)
60512	1(3)
60520	1(2)
60521	1(2)
60522	1(2)
60540	1(2)
60545	1(2)
60600	1(3)
60605	1(3)
60650	1(2)
60659	1(3)
60699	1(3)
61000	1(2)
61001	1(2)
61020	2(3)
61026	2(3)
61050	1(3)
61055	1(3)
61070	2(3)
61105	1(3)
61107	1(3)
61108	1(3)
61120	1(3)
61140	1(3)
61150	1(3)
61151	1(3)
61154	1(3)
61156	1(3)
61210	1(3)
61215	1(3)
61250	1(3)
61253	1(3)
61304	1(3)
61305	1(3)
61312	2(3)
61313	2(3)
61314	2(3)
61315	1(3)
61316	1(3)
61320	2(3)
61321	1(3)
61322	1(3)
61323	1(3)
61330	1(2)
61333	1(2)
61340	1(2)
61343	1(2)
61345	1(3)
61450	1(3)
61458	1(2)
61460	1(2)
61500	1(3)
61501	1(3)
61510	1(3)

CPT	MUE
61512	1(3)
61514	2(3)
61516	1(3)
61517	1(3)
61518	1(3)
61519	1(3)
61520	1(3)
61521	1(3)
61522	1(3)
61524	2(3)
61526	1(3)
61530	1(3)
61531	1(2)
61533	2(3)
61534	1(3)
61535	2(3)
61536	1(3)
61537	1(3)
61538	1(2)
61539	1(3)
61540	1(3)
61541	1(2)
61543	1(2)
61544	1(3)
61545	1(2)
61546	1(2)
61548	1(2)
61550	1(2)
61552	1(2)
61556	1(3)
61557	1(2)
61558	1(3)
61559	1(3)
61563	2(3)
61564	1(2)
61566	1(3)
61567	1(2)
61570	1(3)
61571	1(3)
61575	1(2)
61576	1(2)
61580	1(2)
61581	1(2)
61582	1(2)
61583	1(2)
61584	1(2)
61585	1(2)
61586	1(3)
61590	1(2)
61591	1(2)
61592	1(2)
61595	1(2)
61596	1(2)
61597	1(2)
61598	1(3)
61600	1(3)
61601	1(3)
61605	1(3)
61606	1(3)
61607	1(3)
61608	1(3)
61611	1(3)
61613	1(3)
61615	1(3)
61616	1(3)

CPT	MUE
61618	2(3)
61619	2(3)
61623	2(3)
61624	2(3)
61626	2(3)
61630	1(3)
61635	2(3)
61640	0(3)
61641	0(3)
61642	0(3)
61645	1(3)
61650	1(2)
61651	2(2)
61680	1(3)
61682	1(3)
61684	1(3)
61686	1(3)
61690	1(3)
61692	1(3)
61697	2(3)
61698	1(3)
61700	2(3)
61702	1(3)
61703	1(3)
61705	1(3)
61708	1(3)
61710	1(3)
61711	1(3)
61720	1(3)
61735	1(3)
61750	2(3)
61751	2(3)
61760	1(2)
61770	1(2)
61781	1(3)
61782	1(3)
61783	1(3)
61790	1(2)
61791	1(2)
61796	1(2)
61797	4(3)
61798	1(2)
61799	4(3)
61800	1(2)
61850	1(3)
61860	1(3)
61863	1(2)
61864	1(3)
61867	1(2)
61868	2(3)
61870	1(3)
61880	1(2)
61885	1(3)
61886	1(3)
61888	1(3)
62000	1(3)
62005	1(3)
62010	1(3)
62100	1(3)
62115	1(2)
62117	1(2)
62120	1(2)
62121	1(2)
62140	1(3)
62141	1(3)

CPT	MUE
62142	2(3)
62143	2(3)
62145	2(3)
62146	2(3)
62147	1(3)
62148	1(3)
62160	1(3)
62161	1(3)
62162	1(3)
62163	1(3)
62164	1(3)
62165	1(2)
62180	1(3)
62190	1(3)
62192	1(3)
62194	1(3)
62200	1(2)
62201	1(2)
62220	1(3)
62223	1(3)
62225	2(3)
62230	2(3)
62252	2(3)
62256	1(3)
62258	1(3)
62263	1(2)
62264	1(2)
62267	2(3)
62268	1(3)
62269	2(3)
62270	2(3)
62272	1(3)
62273	2(3)
62280	1(3)
62281	1(3)
62282	1(3)
62284	1(3)
62287	1(2)
62290	5(2)
62291	4(3)
62292	1(2)
62294	1(3)
62302	1(3)
62303	1(3)
62304	1(3)
62305	1(3)
62320	1(3)
62321	1(3)
62322	1(3)
62323	1(3)
62324	1(3)
62325	1(3)
62326	1(3)
62327	1(3)
62350	1(3)
62351	1(3)
62355	1(3)
62360	1(2)
62361	1(2)
62362	1(2)
62365	1(2)
62367	1(3)
62368	1(3)
62369	1(3)
62370	1(3)

CPT	MUE
62380	2(3)
63001	1(2)
63003	1(2)
63005	1(2)
63011	1(2)
63012	1(2)
63015	1(2)
63016	1(2)
63017	1(2)
63020	1(2)
63030	1(2)
63035	4(3)
63040	1(2)
63042	1(2)
63043	4(3)
63044	4(2)
63045	1(2)
63046	1(2)
63047	1(2)
63048	5(3)
63050	1(2)
63051	1(2)
63055	1(2)
63056	1(2)
63057	3(3)
63064	1(2)
63066	1(3)
63075	1(2)
63076	3(3)
63077	1(2)
63078	3(3)
63081	1(2)
63082	6(2)
63085	1(2)
63086	2(3)
63087	1(2)
63088	3(3)
63090	1(2)
63091	3(3)
63101	1(2)
63102	1(2)
63103	3(3)
63170	1(3)
63172	1(3)
63173	1(3)
63180	1(2)
63182	1(2)
63185	1(2)
63190	1(2)
63191	1(2)
63194	1(2)
63195	1(2)
63196	1(2)
63197	1(2)
63198	1(2)
63199	1(2)
63200	1(2)
63250	1(3)
63251	1(3)
63252	1(3)
63265	1(3)
63266	1(3)
63267	1(3)
63268	1(3)
63270	1(3)

CPT	MUE	CPT	MUE	CPT	MUE	CPT	MUE	CPT	MUE	CPT	MUE	CPT	MUE	CPT	MUE
63271	1(3)	64447	1(3)	64681	1(2)	64872	1(3)	65756	1(2)	66825	1(2)	67346	1(3)	67999	1(3)
63272	1(3)	64448	1(2)	64702	2(3)	64874	1(3)	65757	1(3)	66830	1(2)	67399	1(3)	68020	1(3)
63273	1(3)	64449	1(2)	64704	4(3)	64876	1(3)	65760	0(3)	66840	1(2)	67400	1(2)	68040	1(2)
63275	1(3)	64450	10(3)	64708	3(3)	64885	1(3)	65765	0(3)	66850	1(2)	67405	1(2)	68100	1(3)
63276	1(3)	64455	1(2)	64712	1(2)	64886	1(3)	65767	0(3)	66852	1(2)	67412	1(2)	68110	1(3)
63277	1(3)	64461	1(2)	64713	1(2)	64890	2(3)	65770	1(2)	66920	1(2)	67413	1(2)	68115	1(3)
63278	1(3)	64462	1(2)	64714	1(2)	64891	2(3)	65771	0(3)	66930	1(2)	67414	1(2)	68130	1(3)
63280	1(3)	64463	1(3)	64716	2(3)	64892	2(3)	65772	1(2)	66940	1(2)	67415	1(3)	68135	1(3)
63281	1(3)	64479	1(2)	64718	1(2)	64893	2(3)	65775	1(2)	66982	1(2)	67420	1(2)	68200	1(3)
63282	1(3)	64480	4(3)	64719	1(2)	64895	2(3)	65778	1(2)	66983	1(2)	67430	1(2)	68320	1(2)
63283	1(3)	64483	1(2)	64721	1(2)	64896	2(3)	65779	1(2)	66984	1(2)	67440	1(2)	68325	1(2)
63285	1(3)	64484	4(3)	64722	4(3)	64897	2(3)	65780	1(2)	66985	1(2)	67445	1(2)	68326	1(2)
63286	1(3)	64486	1(3)	64726	2(3)	64898	2(3)	65781	1(2)	66986	1(2)	67450	1(2)	68328	1(2)
63287	1(3)	64487	1(2)	64727	2(3)	64901	2(3)	65782	1(2)	66990	1(3)	67500	1(3)	68330	1(3)
63290	1(3)	64488	1(3)	64732	1(2)	64902	1(3)	65785	1(2)	66999	1(3)	67505	1(3)	68335	1(3)
63295	1(2)	64489	1(2)	64734	1(2)	64905	1(3)	65800	1(2)	67005	1(2)	67515	1(3)	68340	1(3)
63300	1(2)	64490	1(2)	64736	1(2)	64907	1(3)	65810	1(2)	67010	1(2)	67550	1(2)	68360	1(3)
63301	1(2)	64491	1(2)	64738	1(2)	64910	3(3)	65815	1(3)	67015	1(2)	67560	1(2)	68362	1(3)
63302	1(2)	64492	1(2)	64740	1(2)	64911	2(3)	65820	1(2)	67025	1(2)	67570	1(2)	68371	1(3)
63303	1(2)	64493	1(2)	64742	1(2)	64912	3(3)	65850	1(2)	67027	1(2)	67599	1(3)	68399	1(3)
63304	1(2)	64494	1(2)	64744	1(2)	64913	3(3)	65855	1(2)	67028	1(3)	67700	2(3)	68400	1(2)
63305	1(2)	64495	1(2)	64746	1(2)	64999	1(3)	65860	1(2)	67030	1(2)	67710	1(2)	68420	1(2)
63306	1(2)	64505	1(3)	64755	1(2)	65091	1(2)	65865	1(2)	67031	1(2)	67715	1(3)	68440	2(3)
63307	1(2)	64510	1(3)	64760	1(2)	65093	1(2)	65870	1(2)	67036	1(2)	67800	1(2)	68500	1(2)
63308	3(3)	64517	1(3)	64763	1(2)	65101	1(2)	65875	1(2)	67039	1(2)	67801	1(2)	68505	1(2)
63600	2(3)	64520	1(3)	64766	1(2)	65103	1(2)	65880	1(2)	67040	1(2)	67805	1(2)	68510	1(2)
63610	1(3)	64530	1(3)	64771	2(3)	65105	1(2)	65900	1(3)	67041	1(2)	67808	1(2)	68520	1(2)
63620	1(2)	64553	1(3)	64772	2(3)	65110	1(2)	65920	1(2)	67042	1(2)	67810	2(3)	68525	1(2)
63621	2(2)	64555	2(3)	64774	2(3)	65112	1(2)	65930	1(3)	67043	1(2)	67820	1(2)	68530	1(2)
63650	2(3)	64561	1(3)	64776	1(2)	65114	1(2)	66020	1(3)	67101	1(2)	67825	1(2)	68540	1(2)
63655	1(3)	64566	1(3)	64778	1(3)	65125	1(2)	66030	1(3)	67105	1(2)	67830	1(2)	68550	1(2)
63661	1(2)	64568	1(3)	64782	2(2)	65130	1(2)	66130	1(3)	67107	1(2)	67835	1(2)	68700	1(2)
63662	1(2)	64569	1(3)	64783	2(3)	65135	1(2)	66150	1(2)	67108	1(2)	67840	3(3)	68705	2(3)
63663	1(3)	64570	1(3)	64784	3(3)	65140	1(2)	66155	1(2)	67110	1(2)	67850	3(3)	68720	1(2)
63664	1(3)	64575	2(3)	64786	1(3)	65150	1(2)	66160	1(2)	67113	1(2)	67875	1(2)	68745	1(2)
63685	1(3)	64580	2(3)	64787	4(3)	65155	1(2)	66170	1(2)	67115	1(2)	67880	1(2)	68750	1(2)
63688	1(3)	64581	2(3)	64788	5(3)	65175	1(2)	66172	1(2)	67120	1(2)	67882	1(2)	68760	4(2)
63700	1(3)	64585	2(3)	64790	1(3)	65205	1(3)	66174	1(2)	67121	1(2)	67900	1(2)	68761	4(2)
63702	1(3)	64590	1(3)	64792	2(3)	65210	1(3)	66175	1(2)	67141	1(2)	67901	1(2)	68770	1(3)
63704	1(3)	64595	1(3)	64795	2(3)	65220	1(3)	66179	1(2)	67145	1(2)	67902	1(2)	68801	4(2)
63706	1(3)	64600	2(3)	64802	1(2)	65222	1(3)	66180	1(2)	67208	1(2)	67903	1(2)	68810	1(2)
63707	1(3)	64605	1(2)	64804	1(2)	65235	1(3)	66183	1(3)	67210	1(2)	67904	1(2)	68811	1(2)
63709	1(3)	64610	1(2)	64809	1(2)	65260	1(3)	66184	1(2)	67218	1(2)	67906	1(2)	68815	1(2)
63710	1(3)	64611	1(2)	64818	1(2)	65265	1(3)	66185	1(2)	67220	1(2)	67908	1(2)	68816	1(2)
63740	1(3)	64612	1(2)	64820	4(3)	65270	1(3)	66225	1(2)	67221	1(2)	67909	1(2)	68840	1(2)
63741	1(3)	64615	1(2)	64821	1(2)	65272	1(3)	66250	1(2)	67225	1(2)	67911	2(3)	68850	1(3)
63744	1(3)	64616	1(2)	64822	1(2)	65273	1(3)	66500	1(2)	67227	1(2)	67912	1(2)	68899	1(3)
63746	1(2)	64617	1(2)	64823	1(2)	65275	1(3)	66505	1(2)	67228	1(2)	67914	2(3)	69000	1(3)
64400	4(3)	64620	5(3)	64831	1(2)	65280	1(3)	66600	1(2)	67229	1(2)	67915	2(3)	69005	1(3)
64402	1(3)	64630	1(3)	64832	3(3)	65285	1(3)	66605	1(2)	67250	1(2)	67916	2(3)	69020	1(3)
64405	1(3)	64632	1(2)	64834	1(2)	65286	1(3)	66625	1(2)	67255	1(2)	67917	2(3)	69090	0(3)
64408	1(3)	64633	1(2)	64835	1(2)	65290	1(3)	66630	1(2)	67299	1(3)	67921	2(3)	69100	3(3)
64410	1(3)	64634	4(3)	64836	1(2)	65400	1(3)	66635	1(2)	67311	1(2)	67922	2(3)	69105	1(3)
64413	1(3)	64635	1(2)	64837	2(3)	65410	1(3)	66680	1(2)	67312	1(2)	67923	2(3)	69110	1(2)
64415	1(3)	64636	4(2)	64840	1(2)	65420	1(2)	66682	1(2)	67314	1(2)	67924	2(3)	69120	1(3)
64416	1(2)	64640	5(3)	64856	2(3)	65426	1(2)	66700	1(2)	67316	1(2)	67930	2(3)	69140	1(2)
64417	1(3)	64642	1(2)	64857	2(3)	65430	1(2)	66710	1(2)	67318	1(2)	67935	2(3)	69145	1(3)
64418	1(3)	64643	3(2)	64858	1(2)	65435	1(2)	66711	1(2)	67320	2(3)	67938	2(3)	69150	1(3)
64420	3(3)	64644	1(2)	64859	2(3)	65436	1(2)	66720	1(2)	67331	1(2)	67950	2(2)	69155	1(3)
64421	3(3)	64645	3(2)	64861	1(2)	65450	1(3)	66740	1(2)	67332	1(2)	67961	2(3)	69200	1(2)
64425	1(3)	64646	1(2)	64862	1(2)	65600	1(2)	66761	1(2)	67334	1(2)	67966	2(3)	69205	1(3)
64430	1(3)	64647	1(2)	64864	2(3)	65710	1(2)	66762	1(2)	67335	1(2)	67971	1(2)	69209	1(2)
64435	1(3)	64650	1(2)	64865	1(3)	65730	1(2)	66770	1(3)	67340	2(2)	67973	1(2)	69210	1(2)
64445	1(3)	64653	1(2)	64866	1(3)	65750	1(2)	66820	1(2)	67343	1(2)	67974	1(2)	69220	1(2)
64446	1(2)	64680	1(2)	64868	1(3)	65755	1(2)	66821	1(2)	67345	1(3)	67975	1(2)	69222	1(2)

CPT	MUE
69300	1(2)
69310	1(2)
69320	1(2)
69399	1(3)
69420	1(2)
69421	1(2)
69424	1(2)
69433	1(2)
69436	1(2)
69440	1(2)
69450	1(2)
69501	1(3)
69502	1(2)
69505	1(2)
69511	1(2)
69530	1(2)
69535	1(2)
69540	1(3)
69550	1(3)
69552	1(2)
69554	1(2)
69601	1(2)
69602	1(2)
69603	1(2)
69604	1(2)
69605	1(2)
69610	1(2)
69620	1(2)
69631	1(2)
69632	1(3)
69633	1(2)
69635	1(3)
69636	1(3)
69637	1(3)
69641	1(2)
69642	1(2)
69643	1(2)
69644	1(2)
69645	1(2)
69646	1(2)
69650	1(2)
69660	1(2)
69661	1(2)
69662	1(2)
69666	1(2)
69667	1(2)
69670	1(2)
69676	1(2)
69700	1(3)
69710	0(3)
69711	1(2)
69714	1(2)
69715	1(3)
69717	1(2)
69718	1(2)
69720	1(2)
69725	1(2)
69740	1(2)
69745	1(2)
69799	1(3)
69801	1(3)
69805	1(3)
69806	1(3)
69905	1(2)
69910	1(2)

CPT	MUE
69915	1(3)
69930	1(2)
69949	1(3)
69950	1(2)
69955	1(2)
69960	1(2)
69970	1(3)
69979	1(3)
69990	1(3)
70010	1(3)
70015	1(3)
70030	2(2)
70100	2(3)
70110	2(3)
70120	1(3)
70130	1(3)
70134	1(3)
70140	2(3)
70150	1(3)
70160	1(3)
70170	2(2)
70190	1(2)
70200	2(3)
70210	1(3)
70220	1(3)
70240	1(2)
70250	2(3)
70260	1(3)
70300	1(3)
70310	1(3)
70320	1(3)
70328	1(3)
70330	1(3)
70332	2(3)
70336	1(3)
70350	1(3)
70355	1(3)
70360	2(3)
70370	1(3)
70371	1(2)
70380	2(3)
70390	2(3)
70450	3(3)
70460	1(3)
70470	2(3)
70480	1(3)
70481	1(3)
70482	1(3)
70486	1(3)
70487	1(3)
70488	1(3)
70490	1(3)
70491	1(3)
70492	1(3)
70496	2(3)
70498	2(3)
70540	1(3)
70542	1(3)
70543	1(3)
70544	2(3)
70545	1(3)
70546	1(3)
70547	1(3)
70548	1(3)
70549	1(3)

CPT	MUE
70551	2(3)
70552	2(3)
70553	2(3)
70554	1(3)
70555	1(3)
70557	1(3)
70558	1(3)
70559	1(3)
71045	4(3)
71046	2(3)
71047	1(3)
71048	1(3)
71100	2(3)
71101	2(3)
71110	1(3)
71111	1(3)
71120	1(3)
71130	1(3)
71250	2(3)
71260	2(3)
71270	1(3)
71275	1(3)
71550	1(3)
71551	1(3)
71552	1(3)
71555	1(3)
72020	4(3)
72040	3(3)
72050	1(3)
72052	1(3)
72070	1(3)
72072	1(3)
72074	1(3)
72080	1(3)
72081	1(3)
72082	1(3)
72083	1(3)
72084	1(3)
72100	2(3)
72110	1(3)
72114	1(3)
72120	1(3)
72125	1(3)
72126	1(3)
72127	1(3)
72128	1(3)
72129	1(3)
72130	1(3)
72131	1(3)
72132	1(3)
72133	1(3)
72141	1(3)
72142	1(3)
72146	1(3)
72147	1(3)
72148	1(3)
72149	1(3)
72156	1(3)
72157	1(3)
72158	1(3)
72159	1(3)
72170	2(3)
72190	1(3)
72191	1(3)
72192	1(3)

CPT	MUE
72193	1(3)
72194	1(3)
72195	1(3)
72196	1(3)
72197	1(3)
72198	1(3)
72200	2(3)
72202	1(3)
72220	1(3)
72240	1(2)
72255	1(2)
72265	1(2)
72270	1(2)
72275	1(3)
72285	4(3)
72295	5(3)
73000	2(3)
73010	2(3)
73020	2(3)
73030	4(3)
73040	2(2)
73050	1(3)
73060	2(3)
73070	2(3)
73080	2(3)
73085	2(2)
73090	2(3)
73092	2(3)
73100	2(3)
73110	3(3)
73115	2(2)
73120	2(3)
73130	3(3)
73140	3(3)
73200	2(3)
73201	2(3)
73202	2(3)
73206	2(3)
73218	2(3)
73219	2(3)
73220	2(3)
73221	2(3)
73222	2(3)
73223	2(3)
73225	2(3)
73501	2(3)
73502	2(3)
73503	2(3)
73521	2(3)
73522	2(3)
73523	2(3)
73525	2(2)
73551	2(3)
73552	2(3)
73560	4(3)
73562	3(3)
73564	4(3)
73565	1(3)
73580	2(2)
73590	3(3)
73592	2(3)
73600	2(3)
73610	3(3)
73615	2(2)
73620	2(3)

CPT	MUE
73630	3(3)
73650	2(3)
73660	2(3)
73700	2(3)
73701	2(3)
73702	2(3)
73706	2(3)
73718	2(3)
73719	2(3)
73720	2(3)
73721	3(3)
73722	2(3)
73723	2(3)
73725	2(3)
74018	3(3)
74019	2(3)
74021	2(3)
74022	2(3)
74150	1(3)
74160	1(3)
74170	1(3)
74174	1(3)
74175	1(3)
74176	2(3)
74177	2(3)
74178	1(3)
74181	1(3)
74182	1(3)
74183	1(3)
74185	1(3)
74190	1(3)
74210	1(3)
74220	1(3)
74230	1(3)
74235	1(3)
74240	2(3)
74241	1(3)
74245	1(3)
74246	1(3)
74247	1(3)
74249	1(3)
74250	1(3)
74251	1(3)
74260	1(2)
74261	1(2)
74262	1(2)
74263	0(3)
74270	1(3)
74280	1(3)
74283	1(3)
74290	1(3)
74300	1(3)
74301	1(3)
74328	1(3)
74329	1(3)
74330	1(3)
74340	1(3)
74355	1(3)
74360	1(3)
74363	2(3)
74400	1(3)
74410	1(3)
74415	1(3)
74420	2(3)
74425	2(3)

CPT	MUE
74430	1(3)
74440	1(2)
74445	1(2)
74450	1(3)
74455	1(3)
74470	2(2)
74485	2(3)
74710	1(3)
74712	1(3)
74713	2(3)
74740	1(3)
74742	2(2)
74775	1(2)
75557	1(3)
75559	1(3)
75561	1(3)
75563	1(3)
75565	1(3)
75571	1(3)
75572	1(3)
75573	1(3)
75574	1(3)
75600	1(3)
75605	1(3)
75625	1(3)
75630	1(3)
75635	1(3)
75705	20(3)
75710	2(3)
75716	1(3)
75726	3(3)
75731	1(3)
75733	1(3)
75736	2(3)
75741	1(3)
75743	1(3)
75746	1(3)
75756	2(3)
75774	7(3)
75801	1(3)
75803	1(3)
75805	1(2)
75807	1(2)
75809	1(3)
75810	1(3)
75820	2(3)
75822	1(3)
75825	1(3)
75827	1(3)
75831	1(3)
75833	1(3)
75840	1(3)
75842	1(3)
75860	2(3)
75870	1(3)
75872	1(3)
75880	1(3)
75885	1(3)
75887	1(3)
75889	1(3)
75891	1(3)
75893	2(3)
75894	2(3)
75898	2(3)
75901	1(3)

CPT	MUE
75902	2(3)
75956	1(2)
75957	1(2)
75958	2(3)
75959	1(2)
75970	1(3)
75984	2(3)
75989	2(3)
76000	3(3)
76010	2(3)
76080	3(3)
76098	3(3)
76100	2(3)
76101	1(3)
76102	1(3)
76120	1(3)
76125	1(3)
76140	0(3)
76376	2(3)
76377	2(3)
76380	2(3)
76390	0(3)
76391	1(3)
76496	1(3)
76497	1(3)
76498	1(3)
76499	1(3)
76506	1(2)
76510	2(2)
76511	2(2)
76512	2(2)
76513	2(2)
76514	1(2)
76516	1(2)
76519	2(2)
76529	2(2)
76536	1(3)
76604	1(3)
76641	2(2)
76642	2(2)
76700	1(3)
76705	2(3)
76706	1(2)
76770	1(3)
76775	2(3)
76776	2(3)
76800	1(3)
76801	1(2)
76802	2(3)
76805	1(2)
76810	2(3)
76811	1(2)
76812	2(3)
76813	1(2)
76814	2(3)
76815	1(2)
76816	2(3)
76817	1(3)
76818	2(3)
76819	2(3)
76820	3(3)
76821	2(3)
76825	2(3)
76826	2(3)
76827	2(3)

CPT	MUE
76828	2(3)
76830	1(3)
76831	1(3)
76856	1(3)
76857	1(3)
76870	1(2)
76872	1(3)
76873	1(2)
76881	2(3)
76882	2(3)
76885	1(2)
76886	1(2)
76930	1(3)
76932	1(2)
76936	1(3)
76937	2(3)
76940	1(3)
76941	3(3)
76942	1(3)
76945	1(3)
76946	1(3)
76948	1(2)
76965	2(3)
76970	2(3)
76975	1(3)
76977	1(2)
76978	1(2)
76979	3(3)
76981	1(3)
76982	1(2)
76983	3(3)
76998	1(3)
76999	1(3)
77001	2(3)
77002	1(3)
77003	1(3)
77011	1(3)
77012	1(3)
77013	1(3)
77014	2(3)
77021	1(3)
77022	1(3)
77046	1(2)
77047	1(2)
77048	1(2)
77049	1(2)
77053	2(2)
77054	2(2)
77061	1(2)
77062	1(2)
77063	1(2)
77065	1(2)
77066	1(2)
77067	1(2)
77071	1(3)
77072	1(2)
77073	1(2)
77074	1(2)
77075	1(2)
77076	1(2)
77077	1(2)
77078	1(2)
77080	1(2)
77081	1(2)
77084	1(2)

CPT	MUE
77085	1(2)
77086	1(2)
77261	1(3)
77262	1(3)
77263	1(3)
77280	2(3)
77285	1(3)
77290	1(3)
77293	1(3)
77295	1(3)
77299	1(3)
77300	10(3)
77301	1(3)
77306	1(3)
77307	1(3)
77316	1(3)
77317	1(3)
77318	1(3)
77321	1(2)
77331	3(3)
77332	4(3)
77333	2(3)
77334	10(3)
77336	1(2)
77338	1(3)
77370	1(3)
77371	1(2)
77372	1(2)
77373	1(3)
77385	1(3)
77386	1(3)
77387	1(3)
77399	1(3)
77401	1(2)
77402	2(3)
77407	2(3)
77412	2(3)
77417	1(2)
77423	1(3)
77424	1(2)
77425	1(3)
77427	1(2)
77431	1(2)
77432	1(2)
77435	1(2)
77469	1(2)
77470	1(2)
77499	1(3)
77520	1(3)
77522	1(3)
77523	1(3)
77525	1(3)
77600	1(3)
77605	1(3)
77610	1(3)
77615	1(3)
77620	1(3)
77750	1(3)
77761	1(3)
77762	1(3)
77763	1(3)
77767	2(3)
77768	2(3)
77770	2(3)
77771	2(3)

CPT	MUE
77772	2(3)
77778	1(3)
77789	2(3)
77790	1(3)
77799	1(3)
78012	1(3)
78013	1(3)
78014	1(2)
78015	1(3)
78016	1(3)
78018	1(2)
78020	1(3)
78070	1(2)
78071	1(3)
78072	1(3)
78075	1(2)
78099	1(3)
78102	1(2)
78103	1(2)
78104	1(2)
78110	1(2)
78111	1(2)
78120	1(2)
78121	1(2)
78122	1(2)
78130	1(2)
78135	1(3)
78140	1(3)
78185	1(2)
78191	1(2)
78195	1(2)
78199	1(3)
78201	1(3)
78202	1(3)
78205	1(3)
78206	1(3)
78215	1(3)
78216	1(3)
78226	1(3)
78227	1(3)
78230	1(3)
78231	1(3)
78232	1(3)
78258	1(2)
78261	1(2)
78262	1(2)
78264	1(2)
78265	1(2)
78266	1(2)
78267	1(2)
78268	1(2)
78278	2(3)
78282	1(2)
78290	1(3)
78291	1(3)
78299	1(3)
78300	1(2)
78305	1(2)
78306	1(2)
78315	1(2)
78320	1(2)
78350	0(3)
78351	0(3)
78399	1(3)
78414	1(2)

CPT	MUE
78428	1(3)
78445	1(3)
78451	1(2)
78452	1(2)
78453	1(2)
78454	1(2)
78456	1(3)
78457	1(2)
78458	1(2)
78459	1(3)
78466	1(3)
78468	1(3)
78469	1(3)
78472	1(2)
78473	1(2)
78481	1(2)
78483	1(2)
78491	1(3)
78492	1(2)
78494	1(3)
78496	1(3)
78499	1(3)
78579	1(3)
78580	1(3)
78582	1(3)
78597	1(3)
78598	1(3)
78599	1(3)
78600	1(3)
78601	1(3)
78605	1(3)
78606	1(3)
78607	1(3)
78608	1(3)
78609	0(3)
78610	1(3)
78630	1(3)
78635	1(3)
78645	1(3)
78647	1(3)
78650	1(3)
78660	1(2)
78699	1(3)
78700	1(3)
78701	1(3)
78707	1(2)
78708	1(2)
78709	1(2)
78710	1(3)
78725	1(3)
78730	1(2)
78740	1(2)
78761	1(2)
78799	1(3)
78800	1(2)
78801	1(2)
78802	1(2)
78803	1(2)
78804	1(2)
78805	1(3)
78806	1(2)
78807	1(3)
78808	1(2)
78811	1(2)
78812	1(2)

CPT	MUE
78813	1(2)
78814	1(2)
78815	1(2)
78816	1(2)
78999	1(3)
79005	1(3)
79101	1(3)
79200	1(3)
79300	1(3)
79403	1(3)
79440	1(3)
79445	1(3)
79999	1(3)
80047	2(3)
80048	2(3)
80050	0(3)
80051	2(3)
80053	1(3)
80055	1(3)
80061	1(3)
80069	1(3)
80074	1(2)
80076	1(3)
80081	1(2)
80150	2(3)
80155	1(3)
80156	2(3)
80157	2(3)
80158	1(3)
80159	2(3)
80162	2(3)
80163	1(3)
80164	2(3)
80165	1(3)
80168	2(3)
80169	1(3)
80170	2(3)
80171	1(3)
80173	2(3)
80175	1(3)
80176	1(3)
80177	1(3)
80178	2(3)
80180	1(3)
80183	1(3)
80184	2(3)
80185	2(3)
80186	2(3)
80188	2(3)
80190	2(3)
80192	2(3)
80194	2(3)
80195	2(3)
80197	2(3)
80198	2(3)
80199	1(3)
80200	2(3)
80201	2(3)
80202	2(3)
80203	1(3)
80299	3(3)
80305	1(2)
80306	1(2)
80307	1(2)
80320	1(3)

CPT	MUE
80321	1(3)
80322	1(3)
80323	1(3)
80324	1(3)
80325	1(3)
80326	1(3)
80327	1(3)
80328	1(3)
80329	1(3)
80330	1(3)
80331	1(3)
80332	1(3)
80333	1(3)
80334	1(3)
80335	1(3)
80336	1(3)
80337	1(3)
80338	1(3)
80339	1(3)
80340	1(3)
80341	1(3)
80342	1(3)
80343	1(3)
80344	1(3)
80345	1(3)
80346	1(3)
80347	1(3)
80348	1(3)
80349	1(3)
80350	1(3)
80351	1(3)
80352	1(3)
80353	1(3)
80354	1(3)
80355	1(3)
80356	1(3)
80357	1(3)
80358	1(3)
80359	1(3)
80360	1(3)
80361	1(3)
80362	1(3)
80363	1(3)
80364	1(3)
80365	1(3)
80366	1(3)
80367	1(3)
80368	1(3)
80369	1(3)
80370	1(3)
80371	1(3)
80372	1(3)
80373	1(3)
80374	1(3)
80375	1(3)
80376	1(3)
80377	1(3)
80400	1(3)
80402	1(3)
80406	1(3)
80408	1(3)
80410	1(3)
80412	1(3)
80414	1(3)
80415	1(3)

CPT	MUE
80416	1(3)
80417	1(3)
80418	1(3)
80420	1(2)
80422	1(3)
80424	1(3)
80426	1(3)
80428	1(3)
80430	1(3)
80432	1(3)
80434	1(3)
80435	1(3)
80436	1(3)
80438	1(3)
80439	1(3)
80500	1(3)
80502	1(3)
81000	2(3)
81001	2(3)
81002	2(3)
81003	2(3)
81005	2(3)
81007	1(3)
81015	2(3)
81020	1(3)
81025	1(3)
81050	2(3)
81099	1(3)
81105	1(2)
81106	1(2)
81107	1(2)
81108	1(2)
81109	1(2)
81110	1(2)
81111	1(2)
81112	1(2)
81120	1(3)
81121	1(3)
81161	1(3)
81162	1(2)
81163	1(2)
81164	1(2)
81165	1(2)
81166	1(2)
81167	1(2)
81170	1(2)
81171	1(2)
81172	1(2)
81173	1(2)
81174	1(2)
81175	1(3)
81176	1(3)
81177	1(2)
81178	1(2)
81179	1(2)
81180	1(2)
81181	1(2)
81182	1(2)
81183	1(2)
81184	1(2)
81185	1(2)
81186	1(2)
81187	1(2)
81188	1(2)
81189	1(2)

CPT	MUE
81190	1(2)
81200	1(2)
81201	1(2)
81202	1(3)
81203	1(3)
81204	1(2)
81205	1(3)
81206	1(3)
81207	1(3)
81208	1(3)
81209	1(3)
81210	1(3)
81212	1(2)
81215	1(2)
81216	1(2)
81217	1(2)
81218	1(3)
81219	1(3)
81220	1(3)
81221	1(3)
81222	1(3)
81223	1(2)
81224	1(3)
81225	1(3)
81226	1(3)
81227	1(3)
81228	1(3)
81229	1(3)
81230	1(2)
81231	1(2)
81232	1(2)
81233	1(3)
81234	1(2)
81235	1(3)
81236	1(3)
81237	1(3)
81238	1(2)
81239	1(2)
81240	1(2)
81241	1(2)
81242	1(3)
81243	1(3)
81244	1(3)
81245	1(3)
81246	1(3)
81247	1(2)
81248	1(2)
81249	1(2)
81250	1(3)
81251	1(3)
81252	1(3)
81253	1(3)
81254	1(3)
81255	1(3)
81256	1(2)
81257	1(2)
81258	1(2)
81259	1(2)
81260	1(3)
81261	1(3)
81262	1(3)
81263	1(3)
81264	1(3)
81265	1(3)
81266	2(3)

CPT	MUE
81267	1(3)
81268	4(3)
81269	1(2)
81270	1(2)
81271	1(2)
81272	1(3)
81273	1(3)
81274	1(2)
81275	1(3)
81276	1(3)
81283	1(2)
81284	1(2)
81285	1(2)
81286	1(2)
81287	1(3)
81288	1(3)
81289	1(2)
81290	1(3)
81291	1(3)
81292	1(2)
81293	1(3)
81294	1(3)
81295	1(2)
81296	1(3)
81297	1(3)
81298	1(2)
81299	1(3)
81300	1(3)
81301	1(3)
81302	1(3)
81303	1(3)
81304	1(3)
81305	1(3)
81306	1(2)
81310	1(3)
81311	1(3)
81312	1(2)
81313	1(3)
81314	1(3)
81315	1(3)
81316	1(2)
81317	1(3)
81318	1(3)
81319	1(2)
81320	1(3)
81321	1(3)
81322	1(3)
81323	1(3)
81324	1(3)
81325	1(3)
81326	1(3)
81327	1(2)
81328	1(2)
81329	1(2)
81330	1(3)
81331	1(3)
81332	1(3)
81333	1(2)
81334	1(3)
81335	1(2)
81336	1(2)
81337	1(2)
81340	1(3)
81341	1(3)
81342	1(3)

CPT	MUE
81343	1(2)
81344	1(2)
81345	1(3)
81346	1(2)
81350	1(3)
81355	1(3)
81361	1(2)
81362	1(2)
81363	1(2)
81364	1(2)
81370	1(2)
81371	1(2)
81372	1(2)
81373	2(2)
81374	1(3)
81375	1(2)
81376	5(3)
81377	2(3)
81378	1(2)
81379	1(2)
81380	2(2)
81381	3(3)
81382	6(3)
81383	2(3)
81400	2(3)
81401	2(3)
81402	1(3)
81403	4(3)
81404	5(3)
81405	2(3)
81406	2(3)
81407	1(3)
81408	2(3)
81410	1(2)
81411	1(2)
81412	1(2)
81413	1(2)
81414	1(2)
81415	1(2)
81416	2(3)
81417	1(3)
81420	1(2)
81422	1(2)
81425	1(2)
81426	2(3)
81427	1(3)
81430	1(2)
81431	1(2)
81432	1(2)
81433	1(2)
81434	1(2)
81435	1(2)
81436	1(2)
81437	1(2)
81438	1(2)
81439	1(2)
81440	1(2)
81442	1(2)
81443	1(2)
81445	1(2)
81448	1(2)
81450	1(2)
81455	1(2)
81460	1(2)
81465	1(2)

CPT	MUE
81470	1(2)
81471	1(2)
81479	3(3)
81490	1(2)
81493	1(2)
81500	1(2)
81503	1(2)
81504	1(3)
81506	1(2)
81507	1(2)
81508	1(2)
81509	1(2)
81510	1(2)
81511	1(2)
81512	1(2)
81518	1(3)
81519	1(2)
81520	1(3)
81521	1(3)
81525	1(3)
81528	1(2)
81535	1(2)
81536	11(3)
81538	1(2)
81539	1(2)
81540	1(3)
81541	1(2)
81545	1(3)
81551	1(2)
81595	1(2)
81596	1(2)
81599	1(3)
82009	1(3)
82010	1(3)
82013	1(3)
82016	1(3)
82017	1(3)
82024	4(3)
82030	1(3)
82040	1(3)
82042	2(3)
82043	1(3)
82044	1(3)
82045	1(3)
82075	2(3)
82085	1(3)
82088	2(3)
82103	1(3)
82104	1(2)
82105	1(3)
82106	2(3)
82107	1(3)
82108	1(3)
82120	1(3)
82127	1(3)
82128	2(3)
82131	2(3)
82135	1(3)
82136	2(3)
82139	2(3)
82140	2(3)
82143	2(3)
82150	2(3)
82154	1(3)
82157	1(3)

CPT	MUE
82160	1(3)
82163	1(3)
82164	1(3)
82172	2(3)
82175	2(3)
82180	1(2)
82190	2(3)
82232	2(3)
82239	1(3)
82240	1(3)
82247	2(3)
82248	2(3)
82252	1(3)
82261	1(3)
82270	1(3)
82271	1(3)
82272	1(3)
82274	1(3)
82286	1(3)
82300	1(3)
82306	1(2)
82308	1(3)
82310	2(3)
82330	2(3)
82331	1(3)
82340	1(3)
82355	2(3)
82360	2(3)
82365	2(3)
82370	2(3)
82373	1(3)
82374	1(3)
82375	1(3)
82376	1(3)
82378	1(3)
82379	1(3)
82380	1(3)
82382	1(2)
82383	1(3)
82384	2(3)
82387	1(3)
82390	1(2)
82397	3(3)
82415	1(3)
82435	1(3)
82436	1(3)
82438	1(3)
82441	1(2)
82465	1(3)
82480	2(3)
82482	1(3)
82485	1(3)
82495	1(2)
82507	1(3)
82523	1(3)
82525	2(3)
82528	1(3)
82530	4(3)
82533	5(3)
82540	1(3)
82542	6(3)
82550	3(3)
82552	3(3)
82553	3(3)
82554	1(3)

CPT	MUE
82565	2(3)
82570	3(3)
82575	1(3)
82585	1(2)
82595	1(3)
82600	1(3)
82607	1(2)
82608	1(2)
82610	1(3)
82615	1(3)
82626	1(3)
82627	1(3)
82633	1(3)
82634	1(3)
82638	1(3)
82642	1(2)
82652	1(2)
82656	1(3)
82657	2(3)
82658	2(3)
82664	2(3)
82668	1(3)
82670	2(3)
82671	1(3)
82672	1(3)
82677	1(3)
82679	1(3)
82693	2(3)
82696	1(3)
82705	1(3)
82710	1(3)
82715	3(3)
82725	1(3)
82726	1(3)
82728	1(3)
82731	1(3)
82735	1(3)
82746	1(2)
82747	1(2)
82757	1(2)
82759	1(3)
82760	1(3)
82775	1(3)
82776	1(2)
82777	1(3)
82784	6(3)
82785	1(3)
82787	4(3)
82800	1(3)
82803	2(3)
82805	2(3)
82810	2(3)
82820	1(3)
82930	1(3)
82938	1(3)
82941	1(3)
82943	1(3)
82945	4(3)
82946	1(2)
82947	5(3)
82948	2(3)
82950	3(3)
82951	1(2)
82952	3(3)
82955	1(2)

CPT	MUE
82960	1(2)
82962	2(3)
82963	1(3)
82965	1(3)
82977	1(3)
82978	1(3)
82979	1(3)
82985	1(3)
83001	1(3)
83002	1(3)
83003	5(3)
83006	1(2)
83009	1(3)
83010	1(3)
83012	1(2)
83013	1(3)
83014	1(2)
83015	1(2)
83018	4(3)
83020	2(3)
83021	2(3)
83026	1(3)
83030	1(3)
83033	1(3)
83036	1(2)
83037	1(2)
83045	1(3)
83050	1(3)
83051	1(3)
83060	1(3)
83065	1(2)
83068	1(2)
83069	1(3)
83070	1(2)
83080	2(3)
83088	1(3)
83090	2(3)
83150	1(3)
83491	1(3)
83497	1(3)
83498	2(3)
83500	1(3)
83505	1(3)
83516	4(3)
83518	1(3)
83519	5(3)
83520	8(3)
83525	4(3)
83527	1(3)
83528	1(3)
83540	2(3)
83550	1(3)
83570	1(3)
83582	1(3)
83586	1(3)
83593	1(3)
83605	1(3)
83615	2(3)
83625	1(3)
83630	1(3)
83631	1(3)
83632	1(3)
83633	1(3)
83655	2(3)
83661	3(3)

CPT	MUE
83662	4(3)
83663	3(3)
83664	3(3)
83670	1(3)
83690	2(3)
83695	1(3)
83698	1(3)
83700	1(2)
83701	1(3)
83704	1(3)
83718	1(3)
83719	1(3)
83721	1(3)
83722	1(2)
83727	1(3)
83735	4(3)
83775	1(3)
83785	1(3)
83789	4(3)
83825	2(3)
83835	2(3)
83857	1(3)
83861	2(2)
83864	1(2)
83872	2(3)
83873	1(3)
83874	2(3)
83876	1(3)
83880	1(3)
83883	4(3)
83885	2(3)
83915	1(3)
83916	2(3)
83918	2(3)
83919	1(3)
83921	2(3)
83930	2(3)
83935	2(3)
83937	1(3)
83945	2(3)
83950	1(2)
83951	1(2)
83970	2(3)
83986	2(3)
83987	1(3)
83992	2(3)
83993	1(3)
84030	1(2)
84035	1(2)
84060	1(3)
84066	1(3)
84075	2(3)
84078	1(2)
84080	1(3)
84081	1(3)
84085	1(2)
84087	1(3)
84100	2(3)
84105	1(3)
84106	1(2)
84110	1(3)
84112	1(3)
84119	1(2)
84120	1(3)
84126	1(3)

CPT	MUE
84132	2(3)
84133	2(3)
84134	1(3)
84135	1(3)
84138	1(3)
84140	1(3)
84143	2(3)
84144	1(3)
84145	1(3)
84146	3(3)
84150	2(3)
84152	1(2)
84153	1(2)
84154	1(2)
84155	1(3)
84156	1(3)
84157	2(3)
84160	2(3)
84163	1(3)
84165	1(2)
84166	2(3)
84181	3(3)
84182	6(3)
84202	1(2)
84203	1(2)
84206	1(2)
84207	1(2)
84210	1(3)
84220	1(3)
84228	1(3)
84233	1(3)
84234	1(3)
84235	1(3)
84238	3(3)
84244	2(3)
84252	1(2)
84255	2(3)
84260	1(3)
84270	1(3)
84275	1(3)
84285	1(3)
84295	1(3)
84300	2(3)
84302	1(3)
84305	1(3)
84307	1(3)
84311	2(3)
84315	1(3)
84375	1(3)
84376	1(3)
84377	1(3)
84378	2(3)
84379	1(3)
84392	1(3)
84402	1(3)
84403	2(3)
84410	1(2)
84425	1(2)
84430	1(3)
84431	1(3)
84432	1(2)
84436	1(2)
84437	1(2)
84439	1(2)
84442	1(2)

CPT	MUE
84443	4(2)
84445	1(2)
84446	1(2)
84449	1(3)
84450	1(3)
84460	1(3)
84466	1(3)
84478	1(3)
84479	1(2)
84480	1(2)
84481	1(2)
84482	1(2)
84484	2(3)
84485	1(3)
84488	1(3)
84490	1(2)
84510	1(3)
84512	1(3)
84520	1(3)
84525	1(3)
84540	2(3)
84545	1(3)
84550	1(3)
84560	2(3)
84577	1(3)
84578	1(3)
84580	1(3)
84583	1(3)
84585	1(2)
84586	1(2)
84588	1(3)
84590	1(2)
84591	1(3)
84597	1(3)
84600	2(3)
84620	1(2)
84630	2(3)
84681	1(3)
84702	2(3)
84703	1(3)
84704	1(3)
84830	1(2)
84999	1(3)
85002	1(3)
85004	1(3)
85007	1(3)
85008	1(3)
85009	1(3)
85013	1(3)
85014	2(3)
85018	2(3)
85025	2(3)
85027	2(3)
85032	1(3)
85041	1(3)
85044	1(2)
85045	1(2)
85046	1(2)
85048	2(3)
85049	2(3)
85055	1(3)
85060	1(3)
85097	2(3)
85130	1(3)
85170	1(3)

CPT	MUE	CPT	MUE	CPT	MUE	CPT	MUE	CPT	MUE	CPT	MUE	CPT	MUE	CPT	MUE
85175	1(3)	85612	1(3)	86331	12(3)	86666	4(3)	86813	1(2)	87081	2(3)	87299	1(3)	87525	1(3)
85210	2(3)	85613	3(3)	86332	1(3)	86668	2(3)	86816	1(2)	87084	1(3)	87300	2(3)	87526	1(3)
85220	2(3)	85635	1(3)	86334	2(2)	86671	3(3)	86817	1(2)	87086	3(3)	87301	1(3)	87527	1(3)
85230	2(3)	85651	1(2)	86335	2(3)	86674	3(3)	86821	1(3)	87088	3(3)	87305	1(3)	87528	1(3)
85240	2(3)	85652	1(2)	86336	1(3)	86677	3(3)	86825	1(3)	87101	2(3)	87320	1(3)	87529	2(3)
85244	1(3)	85660	2(3)	86337	1(2)	86682	2(3)	86826	2(3)	87102	4(3)	87324	2(3)	87530	2(3)
85245	2(3)	85670	2(3)	86340	1(2)	86684	2(3)	86828	1(3)	87103	2(3)	87327	1(3)	87531	1(3)
85246	2(3)	85675	1(3)	86341	1(3)	86687	1(3)	86829	1(3)	87106	3(3)	87328	2(3)	87532	1(3)
85247	2(3)	85705	1(3)	86343	1(3)	86688	1(3)	86830	2(3)	87107	4(3)	87329	2(3)	87533	1(3)
85250	2(3)	85730	4(3)	86344	1(2)	86689	2(3)	86831	2(3)	87109	2(3)	87332	1(3)	87534	1(3)
85260	2(3)	85732	4(3)	86352	1(3)	86692	2(3)	86832	2(3)	87110	2(3)	87335	1(3)	87535	1(3)
85270	2(3)	85810	2(3)	86353	7(3)	86694	2(3)	86833	1(3)	87116	2(3)	87336	1(3)	87536	1(3)
85280	2(3)	85999	1(3)	86355	1(2)	86695	2(3)	86834	1(3)	87118	3(3)	87337	1(3)	87537	1(3)
85290	2(3)	86000	6(3)	86356	7(3)	86696	2(3)	86835	1(3)	87140	3(3)	87338	1(3)	87538	1(3)
85291	1(3)	86001	20(3)	86357	1(2)	86698	3(3)	86849	1(3)	87143	2(3)	87339	1(3)	87539	1(3)
85292	1(3)	86005	2(3)	86359	1(2)	86701	1(3)	86850	3(3)	87149	4(3)	87340	1(2)	87540	1(3)
85293	1(3)	86008	20(3)	86360	1(2)	86702	2(3)	86860	2(3)	87150	12(3)	87341	1(2)	87541	1(3)
85300	2(3)	86021	1(2)	86361	1(2)	86703	1(2)	86870	2(3)	87152	1(3)	87350	1(2)	87542	1(3)
85301	1(3)	86022	1(2)	86367	1(3)	86704	1(2)	86880	4(3)	87153	3(3)	87380	1(2)	87550	1(3)
85302	1(3)	86023	3(3)	86376	2(3)	86705	1(2)	86885	2(3)	87158	1(3)	87385	2(3)	87551	2(3)
85303	2(3)	86038	1(3)	86382	3(3)	86706	2(3)	86886	3(3)	87164	2(3)	87389	1(3)	87552	1(3)
85305	2(3)	86039	1(3)	86384	1(3)	86707	1(3)	86890	1(3)	87166	2(3)	87390	1(3)	87555	1(3)
85306	2(3)	86060	1(3)	86386	1(2)	86708	1(2)	86891	1(3)	87168	2(3)	87391	1(3)	87556	1(3)
85307	2(3)	86063	1(3)	86403	2(3)	86709	1(2)	86900	1(3)	87169	2(3)	87400	2(3)	87557	1(3)
85335	2(3)	86077	1(2)	86406	2(3)	86710	4(3)	86901	1(3)	87172	1(3)	87420	1(3)	87560	1(3)
85337	1(3)	86078	1(3)	86430	2(3)	86711	2(3)	86902	6(3)	87176	2(3)	87425	1(3)	87561	1(3)
85345	1(3)	86079	1(3)	86431	2(3)	86713	3(3)	86904	2(3)	87177	3(3)	87427	2(3)	87562	1(3)
85347	3(3)	86140	1(2)	86480	1(3)	86717	8(3)	86905	8(3)	87181	12(3)	87430	1(3)	87580	1(3)
85348	1(3)	86141	1(2)	86481	1(3)	86720	2(3)	86906	1(2)	87184	8(3)	87449	3(3)	87581	1(3)
85360	1(3)	86146	3(3)	86485	1(2)	86723	2(3)	86910	0(3)	87185	4(3)	87450	2(3)	87582	1(3)
85362	2(3)	86147	4(3)	86486	2(3)	86727	2(3)	86911	0(3)	87186	12(3)	87451	2(3)	87590	1(3)
85366	1(3)	86148	3(3)	86490	1(2)	86732	2(3)	86920	9(3)	87187	3(3)	87471	1(3)	87591	3(3)
85370	1(3)	86152	1(3)	86510	1(2)	86735	2(3)	86921	2(3)	87188	6(3)	87472	1(3)	87592	1(3)
85378	1(3)	86153	1(3)	86580	1(2)	86738	2(3)	86922	5(3)	87190	9(3)	87475	1(3)	87623	1(2)
85379	2(3)	86155	1(3)	86590	1(3)	86741	2(3)	86923	10(3)	87197	1(3)	87476	1(3)	87624	1(3)
85380	1(3)	86156	1(2)	86592	2(3)	86744	2(3)	86927	2(3)	87205	3(3)	87480	1(3)	87625	1(3)
85384	2(3)	86157	1(2)	86593	2(3)	86747	2(3)	86930	0(3)	87206	6(3)	87481	5(3)	87631	1(3)
85385	1(3)	86160	4(3)	86602	3(3)	86750	4(3)	86931	1(3)	87207	3(3)	87482	1(3)	87632	1(3)
85390	3(3)	86161	2(3)	86603	2(3)	86753	3(3)	86932	1(3)	87209	4(3)	87483	1(2)	87633	1(3)
85396	1(2)	86162	1(2)	86609	14(3)	86756	2(3)	86940	1(3)	87210	4(3)	87485	1(3)	87634	1(3)
85397	2(3)	86171	2(3)	86611	4(3)	86757	6(3)	86941	1(3)	87220	3(3)	87486	1(3)	87640	1(3)
85400	1(3)	86200	1(3)	86612	2(3)	86759	2(3)	86945	2(3)	87230	2(3)	87487	1(3)	87641	1(3)
85410	1(3)	86215	1(3)	86615	6(3)	86762	2(3)	86950	1(3)	87250	1(3)	87490	1(3)	87650	1(3)
85415	2(3)	86225	1(3)	86617	2(3)	86765	2(3)	86960	1(3)	87252	2(3)	87491	3(3)	87651	1(3)
85420	2(3)	86226	1(3)	86618	2(3)	86768	5(3)	86965	1(3)	87253	2(3)	87492	1(3)	87652	1(3)
85421	1(3)	86235	10(3)	86619	2(3)	86771	2(3)	86970	1(3)	87254	7(3)	87493	2(3)	87653	1(3)
85441	1(2)	86255	5(3)	86622	2(3)	86774	2(3)	86971	1(3)	87255	2(3)	87495	1(3)	87660	1(3)
85445	1(2)	86256	9(3)	86625	1(3)	86777	2(3)	86972	1(3)	87260	1(3)	87496	1(3)	87661	1(3)
85460	1(3)	86277	1(3)	86628	3(3)	86778	2(3)	86975	1(3)	87265	1(3)	87497	2(3)	87662	2(3)
85461	1(2)	86280	1(3)	86631	6(3)	86780	2(3)	86976	1(3)	87267	1(3)	87498	1(3)	87797	3(3)
85475	1(3)	86294	1(3)	86632	3(3)	86784	1(3)	86977	1(3)	87269	1(3)	87500	1(3)	87798	13(3)
85520	1(3)	86300	2(3)	86635	4(3)	86787	2(3)	86978	1(3)	87270	1(3)	87501	1(3)	87799	3(3)
85525	2(3)	86301	1(2)	86638	6(3)	86788	2(3)	86985	1(3)	87271	1(3)	87502	1(3)	87800	2(3)
85530	1(3)	86304	1(2)	86641	2(3)	86789	2(3)	86999	1(3)	87272	1(3)	87503	1(3)	87801	3(3)
85536	1(2)	86305	1(2)	86644	2(3)	86790	4(3)	87003	1(3)	87273	1(3)	87505	1(2)	87802	2(3)
85540	1(2)	86308	1(2)	86645	1(3)	86793	2(3)	87015	3(3)	87274	1(3)	87506	1(2)	87803	3(3)
85547	1(2)	86309	1(2)	86648	2(3)	86794	1(3)	87040	2(3)	87275	1(3)	87507	1(2)	87804	3(3)
85549	1(3)	86310	1(2)	86651	2(3)	86800	1(3)	87045	3(3)	87276	1(3)	87510	1(3)	87806	1(2)
85555	1(2)	86316	2(3)	86652	2(3)	86803	1(3)	87046	6(3)	87278	1(3)	87511	1(3)	87807	2(3)
85557	1(2)	86317	6(3)	86653	2(3)	86804	1(2)	87070	3(3)	87279	1(3)	87512	1(3)	87808	1(3)
85576	7(3)	86318	2(3)	86654	2(3)	86805	2(3)	87071	2(3)	87280	1(3)	87516	1(3)	87809	2(3)
85597	1(3)	86320	1(2)	86658	12(3)	86806	2(3)	87073	2(3)	87281	1(3)	87517	1(3)	87810	2(3)
85598	1(3)	86325	2(3)	86663	2(3)	86807	2(3)	87075	6(3)	87283	1(3)	87520	1(3)	87850	1(3)
85610	4(3)	86327	1(3)	86664	2(3)	86808	1(3)	87076	2(3)	87285	1(3)	87521	1(3)	87880	2(3)
85611	2(3)	86329	3(3)	86665	2(3)	86812	1(2)	87077	4(3)	87290	1(3)	87522	1(3)	87899	4(3)

CPT	MUE	CPT	MUE	CPT	MUE	CPT	MUE	CPT	MUE	CPT	MUE	CPT	MUE	CPT	MUE
87900	1(2)	88235	2(3)	88373	3(3)	90287	0(3)	90687	1(2)	90935	1(3)	92083	1(2)	92538	1(2)
87901	1(2)	88237	4(3)	88374	5(3)	90288	0(3)	90688	1(2)	90937	1(3)	92100	1(2)	92540	1(3)
87902	1(2)	88239	3(3)	88375	1(3)	90291	0(3)	90689	1(2)	90940	1(3)	92132	1(2)	92541	1(3)
87903	1(2)	88240	1(3)	88377	5(3)	90296	1(2)	90690	1(2)	90945	1(3)	92133	1(2)	92542	1(3)
87904	14(3)	88241	3(3)	88380	1(3)	90371	10(3)	90691	1(2)	90947	1(3)	92134	1(2)	92544	1(3)
87905	2(3)	88245	1(2)	88381	1(3)	90375	20(3)	90696	1(2)	90951	1(2)	92136	2(2)	92545	1(3)
87906	2(3)	88248	1(2)	88387	2(3)	90376	20(3)	90697	1(2)	90952	1(2)	92145	1(2)	92546	1(3)
87910	1(3)	88249	1(2)	88388	1(3)	90378	4(3)	90698	1(2)	90953	1(2)	92225	2(2)	92547	1(3)
87912	1(3)	88261	2(3)	88399	1(3)	90384	0(3)	90700	1(2)	90954	1(2)	92226	2(2)	92548	1(3)
87999	1(3)	88262	2(3)	88720	1(3)	90385	1(2)	90702	1(2)	90955	1(2)	92227	1(2)	92550	1(2)
88000	0(3)	88263	1(3)	88738	1(3)	90386	0(3)	90707	1(2)	90956	1(2)	92228	1(2)	92551	0(3)
88005	0(3)	88264	1(3)	88740	1(2)	90389	0(3)	90710	1(2)	90957	1(2)	92230	2(2)	92552	1(2)
88007	0(3)	88267	2(3)	88741	1(2)	90393	1(2)	90713	1(2)	90958	1(2)	92235	1(2)	92553	1(2)
88012	0(3)	88269	2(3)	88749	1(3)	90396	1(2)	90714	1(2)	90959	1(2)	92240	1(2)	92555	1(2)
88014	0(3)	88271	16(3)	89049	1(3)	90399	0(3)	90715	1(2)	90960	1(2)	92242	1(2)	92556	1(2)
88016	0(3)	88272	12(3)	89050	2(3)	90460	9(3)	90716	1(2)	90961	1(2)	92250	1(2)	92557	1(2)
88020	0(3)	88273	3(3)	89051	2(3)	90461	8(3)	90717	1(2)	90962	1(2)	92260	1(2)	92558	0(3)
88025	0(3)	88274	5(3)	89055	2(3)	90471	1(2)	90723	0(3)	90963	1(2)	92265	1(2)	92559	0(3)
88027	0(3)	88275	12(3)	89060	2(3)	90472	8(3)	90732	1(2)	90964	1(2)	92270	1(2)	92560	0(3)
88028	0(3)	88280	1(3)	89125	2(3)	90473	1(2)	90733	1(2)	90965	1(2)	92273	1(2)	92561	1(2)
88029	0(3)	88283	5(3)	89160	1(3)	90474	1(3)	90734	1(2)	90966	1(2)	92274	1(2)	92562	1(2)
88036	0(3)	88285	10(3)	89190	1(3)	90476	1(2)	90736	1(2)	90967	1(2)	92283	1(2)	92563	1(2)
88037	0(3)	88289	1(3)	89220	1(3)	90477	1(2)	90738	1(2)	90968	1(2)	92284	1(2)	92564	1(2)
88040	0(3)	88291	1(3)	89230	1(2)	90581	1(2)	90739	1(2)	90969	1(2)	92285	1(2)	92565	1(2)
88045	0(3)	88299	1(3)	89240	1(3)	90585	1(2)	90740	1(2)	90970	1(2)	92286	1(2)	92567	1(2)
88099	0(3)	88300	4(3)	89250	1(2)	90586	1(2)	90743	1(2)	90989	1(2)	92287	1(2)	92568	1(2)
88104	5(3)	88302	4(3)	89251	1(2)	90587	1(2)	90744	1(2)	90993	1(3)	92310	0(3)	92570	1(2)
88106	5(3)	88304	5(3)	89253	1(3)	90620	1(2)	90746	1(2)	90997	1(3)	92311	1(2)	92571	1(2)
88108	6(3)	88305	16(3)	89254	1(3)	90621	1(2)	90747	1(2)	90999	1(3)	92312	1(2)	92572	1(2)
88112	6(3)	88307	8(3)	89255	1(3)	90625	1(2)	90748	0(3)	91010	1(2)	92313	1(3)	92575	1(2)
88120	2(3)	88309	3(3)	89257	1(3)	90630	1(2)	90749	1(3)	91013	1(3)	92314	0(3)	92576	1(2)
88121	2(3)	88311	4(3)	89258	1(2)	90632	1(2)	90750	1(2)	91020	1(2)	92315	1(2)	92577	1(2)
88125	1(3)	88312	9(3)	89259	1(2)	90633	1(2)	90756	1(2)	91022	1(2)	92316	1(2)	92579	1(2)
88130	1(2)	88313	8(3)	89260	1(2)	90634	1(2)	90785	3(3)	91030	1(2)	92317	1(3)	92582	1(2)
88140	1(2)	88314	6(3)	89261	1(2)	90636	1(2)	90791	1(3)	91034	1(2)	92325	1(3)	92583	1(2)
88141	1(3)	88319	11(3)	89264	1(3)	90644	1(2)	90792	1(3)	91035	1(2)	92326	2(2)	92584	1(2)
88142	1(3)	88321	1(2)	89268	1(2)	90647	1(2)	90832	2(3)	91037	1(2)	92340	0(3)	92585	1(2)
88143	1(3)	88323	1(2)	89272	1(2)	90648	1(2)	90833	2(3)	91038	1(2)	92341	0(3)	92586	1(2)
88147	1(3)	88325	1(2)	89280	1(2)	90649	1(2)	90834	2(3)	91040	1(2)	92342	0(3)	92587	1(2)
88148	1(3)	88329	2(3)	89281	1(2)	90650	1(2)	90836	2(3)	91065	2(2)	92352	0(3)	92588	1(2)
88150	1(3)	88331	11(3)	89290	1(2)	90651	1(2)	90837	2(3)	91110	1(2)	92353	0(3)	92590	0(3)
88152	1(3)	88332	13(3)	89291	1(2)	90653	1(2)	90838	2(3)	91111	1(2)	92354	0(3)	92591	0(3)
88153	1(3)	88333	4(3)	89300	1(2)	90654	1(2)	90839	1(2)	91112	1(3)	92355	0(3)	92592	0(3)
88155	1(3)	88334	5(3)	89310	1(2)	90655	1(2)	90840	3(3)	91117	1(2)	92358	0(3)	92593	0(3)
88160	4(3)	88341	13(3)	89320	1(2)	90656	1(2)	90845	1(2)	91120	1(2)	92370	0(3)	92594	0(3)
88161	4(3)	88342	3(3)	89321	1(2)	90657	1(2)	90846	1(3)	91122	1(2)	92371	0(3)	92595	0(3)
88162	3(3)	88344	6(3)	89322	1(2)	90658	1(2)	90847	1(3)	91132	1(3)	92499	1(3)	92596	1(2)
88164	1(3)	88346	2(3)	89325	1(2)	90660	1(2)	90849	1(3)	91133	1(3)	92502	1(3)	92597	1(3)
88165	1(3)	88348	1(3)	89329	1(2)	90661	1(2)	90853	1(3)	91200	1(2)	92504	1(3)	92601	1(3)
88166	1(3)	88350	8(3)	89330	1(2)	90662	1(2)	90863	1(3)	91299	1(3)	92507	1(3)	92602	1(3)
88167	1(3)	88355	1(3)	89331	1(2)	90664	1(2)	90865	1(3)	92002	1(2)	92508	1(3)	92603	1(3)
88172	5(3)	88356	3(3)	89335	1(3)	90666	1(2)	90867	1(2)	92004	1(2)	92511	1(3)	92604	1(3)
88173	5(3)	88358	2(3)	89337	1(2)	90667	1(2)	90868	1(3)	92012	1(3)	92512	1(2)	92605	0(3)
88174	1(3)	88360	6(3)	89342	1(2)	90668	1(2)	90869	1(3)	92014	1(3)	92516	1(3)	92606	0(3)
88175	1(3)	88361	6(3)	89343	1(2)	90670	1(2)	90870	2(3)	92015	0(3)	92520	1(2)	92607	1(3)
88177	6(3)	88362	1(3)	89344	1(2)	90672	1(2)	90875	0(3)	92018	1(2)	92521	1(2)	92608	4(3)
88182	2(3)	88363	2(3)	89346	1(2)	90673	1(2)	90876	0(3)	92019	1(2)	92522	1(2)	92609	1(3)
88184	2(3)	88364	3(3)	89352	1(2)	90674	1(2)	90880	1(3)	92020	1(2)	92523	1(2)	92610	1(2)
88185	35(3)	88365	4(3)	89353	1(3)	90675	1(2)	90882	0(3)	92025	1(2)	92524	1(2)	92611	1(3)
88187	2(3)	88366	2(3)	89354	1(3)	90676	1(2)	90885	0(3)	92060	1(2)	92526	1(2)	92612	1(3)
88188	2(3)	88367	3(3)	89356	2(3)	90680	1(2)	90887	0(3)	92065	1(2)	92531	0(3)	92613	1(2)
88189	2(3)	88368	3(3)	89398	1(3)	90681	1(2)	90889	0(3)	92071	2(2)	92532	0(3)	92614	1(3)
88199	1(3)	88369	3(3)	90281	0(3)	90682	1(2)	90899	1(3)	92072	1(2)	92533	0(3)	92615	1(2)
88230	2(3)	88371	1(3)	90283	0(3)	90685	1(2)	90901	1(3)	92081	1(2)	92534	0(3)	92616	1(3)
88233	2(3)	88372	1(3)	90284	0(3)	90686	1(2)	90911	1(3)	92082	1(2)	92537	1(2)	92617	1(2)

CPT	MUE
92618	1(3)
92620	1(2)
92621	2(3)
92625	1(2)
92626	1(2)
92627	6(3)
92630	0(3)
92633	0(3)
92640	1(3)
92700	1(3)
92920	3(3)
92921	6(2)
92924	2(3)
92925	6(2)
92928	3(3)
92929	6(2)
92933	2(3)
92934	6(2)
92937	2(3)
92938	6(3)
92941	1(3)
92943	2(3)
92944	3(3)
92950	2(3)
92953	2(3)
92960	2(3)
92961	1(3)
92970	1(3)
92971	1(3)
92973	2(3)
92974	1(3)
92975	1(3)
92977	1(3)
92978	1(3)
92979	2(3)
92986	1(2)
92987	1(2)
92990	1(2)
92992	1(2)
92993	1(2)
92997	1(2)
92998	2(3)
93000	3(3)
93005	3(3)
93010	5(3)
93015	1(3)
93016	1(3)
93017	1(3)
93018	1(3)
93024	1(3)
93025	1(2)
93040	3(3)
93041	2(3)
93042	3(3)
93050	1(3)
93224	1(2)
93225	1(2)
93226	1(2)
93227	1(2)
93228	1(2)
93229	1(2)
93260	1(2)
93261	1(3)
93264	1(2)
93268	1(2)
93270	1(2)
93271	1(2)
93272	1(2)
93278	1(3)
93279	1(3)
93280	1(3)
93281	1(3)
93282	1(3)
93283	1(3)
93284	1(3)
93285	1(3)
93286	2(3)
93287	2(3)
93288	1(3)
93289	1(3)
93290	1(3)
93291	1(3)
93292	1(3)
93293	1(2)
93294	1(2)
93295	1(2)
93296	1(2)
93297	1(2)
93298	1(2)
93299	1(2)
93303	1(3)
93304	1(3)
93306	1(3)
93307	1(3)
93308	1(3)
93312	1(3)
93313	1(3)
93314	1(3)
93315	1(3)
93316	1(3)
93317	1(3)
93318	1(3)
93320	1(3)
93321	1(3)
93325	1(3)
93350	1(2)
93351	1(2)
93352	1(3)
93355	1(3)
93451	1(3)
93452	1(3)
93453	1(3)
93454	1(3)
93455	1(3)
93456	1(3)
93457	1(3)
93458	1(3)
93459	1(3)
93460	1(3)
93461	1(3)
93462	1(3)
93463	1(3)
93464	1(3)
93503	2(3)
93505	1(2)
93530	1(3)
93531	1(3)
93532	1(3)
93533	1(3)
93561	1(3)
93562	1(3)
93563	1(3)
93564	1(3)
93565	1(3)
93566	1(3)
93567	1(3)
93568	1(3)
93571	1(3)
93572	2(3)
93580	1(3)
93581	1(3)
93582	1(2)
93583	1(2)
93590	1(2)
93591	1(2)
93592	2(3)
93600	1(3)
93602	1(3)
93603	1(3)
93609	1(3)
93610	1(3)
93612	1(3)
93613	1(3)
93615	1(3)
93616	1(3)
93618	1(3)
93619	1(3)
93620	1(3)
93621	1(3)
93622	1(3)
93623	1(3)
93624	1(3)
93631	1(3)
93640	1(3)
93641	1(2)
93642	1(3)
93644	1(3)
93650	1(2)
93653	1(3)
93654	1(3)
93655	2(3)
93656	1(3)
93657	1(3)
93660	1(3)
93662	1(3)
93668	1(3)
93701	1(2)
93702	1(2)
93724	1(3)
93740	0(3)
93745	1(2)
93750	4(3)
93770	0(3)
93784	1(2)
93786	1(2)
93788	1(2)
93790	1(2)
93792	1(2)
93793	1(2)
93797	2(2)
93798	2(2)
93799	1(3)
93880	1(3)
93882	1(3)
93886	1(3)
93888	1(3)
93890	1(3)
93892	1(3)
93893	1(3)
93895	1(3)
93922	2(2)
93923	2(2)
93924	1(2)
93925	1(3)
93926	1(3)
93930	1(3)
93931	1(3)
93970	1(3)
93971	1(3)
93975	1(3)
93976	1(3)
93978	1(3)
93979	1(3)
93980	1(3)
93981	1(3)
93990	2(3)
93998	1(3)
94002	1(2)
94003	1(2)
94004	1(2)
94005	0(3)
94010	1(3)
94011	1(3)
94012	1(3)
94013	1(3)
94014	1(2)
94015	1(2)
94016	1(2)
94060	1(3)
94070	1(2)
94150	0(3)
94200	1(3)
94250	1(3)
94375	1(3)
94400	1(3)
94450	1(3)
94452	1(2)
94453	1(2)
94610	2(3)
94617	1(3)
94618	1(3)
94621	1(3)
94640	4(3)
94642	1(3)
94644	1(2)
94645	2(3)
94660	1(2)
94662	1(2)
94664	1(3)
94667	1(2)
94668	2(3)
94669	2(3)
94680	1(3)
94681	1(3)
94690	1(3)
94726	1(3)
94727	1(3)
94728	1(3)
94729	1(3)
94750	1(3)
94760	1(3)
94761	1(2)
94762	1(2)
94770	1(3)
94772	1(2)
94774	1(2)
94775	1(2)
94776	1(2)
94777	1(2)
94780	1(2)
94781	2(3)
94799	1(3)
95004	80(3)
95012	2(3)
95017	27(3)
95018	19(3)
95024	40(3)
95027	90(3)
95028	30(3)
95044	80(3)
95052	20(3)
95056	1(2)
95060	1(2)
95065	1(3)
95070	1(3)
95071	1(2)
95076	1(2)
95079	2(3)
95115	1(2)
95117	1(2)
95120	0(3)
95125	0(3)
95130	0(3)
95131	0(3)
95132	0(3)
95133	0(3)
95134	0(3)
95144	30(3)
95145	10(3)
95146	10(3)
95147	10(3)
95148	10(3)
95149	10(3)
95165	30(3)
95170	10(3)
95180	6(3)
95199	1(3)
95249	1(2)
95250	1(2)
95251	1(2)
95782	1(2)
95783	1(2)
95800	1(2)
95801	1(2)
95803	1(2)
95805	1(2)
95806	1(2)
95807	1(2)
95808	1(2)
95810	1(2)
95811	1(2)
95812	1(3)
95813	1(3)
95816	1(3)
95819	1(3)
95822	1(3)
95824	1(3)
95827	1(2)
95829	1(3)
95830	1(3)
95831	5(2)
95832	1(3)
95833	1(3)
95834	1(3)
95836	1(2)
95851	3(3)
95852	1(3)
95857	1(2)
95860	1(3)
95861	1(3)
95863	1(3)
95864	1(3)
95865	1(3)
95866	1(3)
95867	1(3)
95868	1(3)
95869	1(3)
95870	4(3)
95872	4(3)
95873	1(2)
95874	1(2)
95875	2(3)
95885	4(2)
95886	4(2)
95887	1(2)
95905	2(3)
95907	1(2)
95908	1(2)
95909	1(2)
95910	1(2)
95911	1(2)
95912	1(2)
95913	1(2)
95921	1(3)
95922	1(3)
95923	1(3)
95924	1(3)
95925	1(3)
95926	1(3)
95927	1(3)
95928	1(3)
95929	1(3)
95930	1(3)
95933	1(3)
95937	4(3)
95938	1(3)
95939	1(3)
95940	32(3)
95941	0(3)
95943	1(3)
95950	1(2)
95951	1(2)
95953	1(2)
95954	1(3)
95955	1(3)
95956	1(2)
95957	1(3)
95958	1(3)
95961	1(2)
95962	5(3)
95965	1(3)
95966	1(3)
95967	3(3)
95970	1(3)
95971	1(3)
95972	1(3)
95976	1(3)
95977	1(3)
95980	1(3)
95981	1(3)
95982	1(3)
95983	1(2)
95984	11(3)
95990	1(3)
95991	1(3)
95992	1(2)
95999	1(3)
96000	1(2)
96001	1(2)
96002	1(3)
96003	1(3)
96004	1(2)
96020	1(2)
96040	4(3)
96105	3(3)
96110	3(3)
96112	1(2)
96113	6(3)
96116	1(2)
96121	3(3)
96125	2(3)
96127	2(3)
96130	1(2)
96131	7(3)
96132	1(2)
96133	7(3)
96136	1(2)
96137	11(3)
96138	1(2)
96139	11(3)
96146	1(2)
96150	8(3)
96151	6(3)
96152	6(3)
96153	8(3)
96154	8(3)
96155	0(3)
96160	3(3)
96161	1(3)
96360	1(3)
96361	8(3)
96365	1(3)
96366	8(3)
96367	4(3)
96368	1(2)
96369	1(2)
96370	3(3)
96371	1(3)
96372	4(3)
96373	2(3)
96374	1(3)
96375	6(3)
96376	0(3)
96377	1(3)
96379	1(3)
96401	3(3)
96402	2(3)
96405	1(2)
96406	1(2)
96409	1(3)
96411	3(3)
96413	1(3)
96415	8(3)
96416	1(3)
96417	3(3)
96420	1(3)
96422	2(3)
96423	1(3)
96425	1(3)
96440	1(3)
96446	1(3)
96450	1(3)
96521	2(3)
96522	1(3)
96523	1(3)
96542	1(3)
96549	1(3)
96567	1(3)
96570	1(2)
96571	2(3)
96573	1(2)
96574	1(2)
96900	1(3)
96902	0(3)
96904	1(2)
96910	1(3)
96912	1(3)
96913	1(3)
96920	1(2)
96921	1(2)
96922	1(2)
96931	1(2)
96932	1(2)
96933	1(2)
96934	2(3)
96935	2(3)
96936	2(3)
96999	1(3)
97010	0(3)
97012	1(3)
97014	0(3)
97016	1(3)
97018	1(3)
97022	1(3)
97024	1(3)
97026	1(3)
97028	1(3)
97032	4(3)
97033	4(3)
97034	2(3)
97035	2(3)
97036	3(3)
97039	1(3)
97110	6(3)
97112	4(3)
97113	6(3)
97116	4(3)
97124	4(3)
97127	1(2)
97139	1(3)

CPT	MUE
97140	6(3)
97150	1(3)
97151	8(3)
97152	8(3)
97153	32(3)
97154	12(3)
97155	24(3)
97156	16(3)
97157	16(3)
97158	16(3)
97161	1(2)
97162	1(2)
97163	1(2)
97164	1(2)
97165	1(2)
97166	1(2)
97167	1(2)
97168	1(2)
97169	0(3)
97170	0(3)
97171	0(3)
97172	0(3)
97530	6(3)
97533	4(3)
97535	8(3)
97537	6(3)
97542	8(3)
97545	1(2)
97546	2(3)
97597	1(3)
97598	8(3)
97602	0(3)
97605	1(3)
97606	1(3)
97607	1(3)
97608	1(3)
97610	1(2)
97750	8(3)
97755	8(3)
97760	6(3)
97761	6(3)
97763	6(3)
97799	1(3)
97802	8(3)
97803	8(3)
97804	6(3)
97810	0(3)
97811	0(3)
97813	0(3)
97814	0(3)
98925	1(2)
98926	1(2)
98927	1(2)
98928	1(2)
98929	1(2)
98940	1(2)
98941	1(2)
98942	1(2)
98943	0(3)
98960	0(3)
98961	0(3)
98962	0(3)
98966	0(3)
98967	0(3)
98968	0(3)

CPT	MUE
98969	0(3)
99000	0(3)
99001	0(3)
99002	0(3)
99024	1(3)
99026	0(3)
99027	0(3)
99050	0(3)
99051	0(3)
99053	0(3)
99056	0(3)
99058	0(3)
99060	0(3)
99070	0(3)
99071	0(3)
99075	0(3)
99078	0(3)
99080	0(3)
99082	1(3)
99091	1(2)
99100	1(3)
99116	0(3)
99135	0(3)
99140	0(3)
99151	1(3)
99152	2(3)
99153	9(3)
99155	1(3)
99156	1(3)
99157	6(3)
99170	1(3)
99172	0(3)
99173	0(3)
99174	0(3)
99175	1(3)
99177	1(2)
99183	1(3)
99184	1(2)
99188	1(2)
99190	1(3)
99191	1(3)
99192	1(3)
99195	2(3)
99199	1(3)
99201	1(2)
99202	1(2)
99203	1(2)
99204	1(2)
99205	1(2)
99211	1(3)
99212	2(3)
99213	2(3)
99214	2(3)
99215	1(3)
99217	1(2)
99218	1(2)
99219	1(2)
99220	1(2)
99221	1(3)
99222	1(3)
99223	1(3)
99224	1(2)
99225	1(2)
99226	1(2)
99231	1(3)

CPT	MUE
99232	1(3)
99233	1(3)
99234	1(3)
99235	1(3)
99236	1(3)
99238	1(2)
99239	1(2)
99241	0(3)
99242	0(3)
99243	0(3)
99244	0(3)
99245	0(3)
99251	0(3)
99252	0(3)
99253	0(3)
99254	0(3)
99255	0(3)
99281	1(3)
99282	1(3)
99283	1(3)
99284	1(3)
99285	1(3)
99288	0(3)
99291	1(2)
99292	8(3)
99304	1(2)
99305	1(2)
99306	1(2)
99307	1(2)
99308	1(2)
99309	1(2)
99310	1(2)
99315	1(2)
99316	1(2)
99318	1(2)
99324	1(2)
99325	1(2)
99326	1(2)
99327	1(2)
99328	1(2)
99334	1(3)
99335	1(3)
99336	1(3)
99337	1(3)
99339	0(3)
99340	0(3)
99341	1(2)
99342	1(2)
99343	1(2)
99344	1(2)
99345	1(2)
99347	1(3)
99348	1(3)
99349	1(3)
99350	1(3)
99354	1(2)
99355	4(3)
99356	1(2)
99357	4(3)
99358	1(2)
99359	2(3)
99360	1(3)
99366	0(3)
99367	0(3)
99368	0(3)

CPT	MUE
99374	0(3)
99375	0(3)
99377	0(3)
99378	0(3)
99379	0(3)
99380	0(3)
99381	0(3)
99382	0(3)
99383	0(3)
99384	0(3)
99385	0(3)
99386	0(3)
99387	0(3)
99391	0(3)
99392	0(3)
99393	0(3)
99394	0(3)
99395	0(3)
99396	0(3)
99397	0(3)
99401	0(3)
99402	0(3)
99403	0(3)
99404	0(3)
99406	1(2)
99407	1(2)
99408	0(3)
99409	0(3)
99411	0(3)
99412	0(3)
99415	1(2)
99416	3(3)
99429	0(3)
99441	0(3)
99442	0(3)
99443	0(3)
99444	0(3)
99446	1(2)
99447	1(2)
99448	1(2)
99449	1(2)
99450	0(3)
99451	1(2)
99452	1(2)
99453	1(2)
99454	1(2)
99455	1(3)
99456	1(3)
99457	1(2)
99460	1(2)
99461	1(2)
99462	1(2)
99463	1(2)
99464	1(2)
99465	1(2)
99466	1(2)
99467	4(3)
99468	1(2)
99469	1(2)
99471	1(2)
99472	1(2)
99475	1(2)
99476	1(2)
99477	1(2)
99478	1(2)

CPT	MUE
99479	1(2)
99480	1(2)
99483	1(2)
99484	1(2)
99485	1(3)
99486	4(1)
99487	1(2)
99489	10(3)
99490	1(2)
99491	1(2)
99492	1(2)
99493	1(2)
99494	2(3)
99495	1(2)
99496	1(2)
99497	1(2)
99498	3(3)
99499	1(3)
99500	0(3)
99501	0(3)
99502	0(3)
99503	0(3)
99504	0(3)
99505	0(3)
99506	0(3)
99507	0(3)
99509	0(3)
99510	0(3)
99511	0(3)
99512	0(3)
99600	0(3)
99601	0(3)
99602	0(3)
99605	0(2)
99606	0(3)
99607	0(3)
A0021	0(3)
A0080	0(3)
A0090	0(3)
A0100	0(3)
A0110	0(3)
A0120	0(3)
A0130	0(3)
A0140	0(3)
A0160	0(3)
A0170	0(3)
A0180	0(3)
A0190	0(3)
A0200	0(3)
A0210	0(3)
A0225	0(3)
A0380	0(3)
A0382	0(3)
A0384	0(3)
A0390	0(3)
A0392	0(3)
A0394	0(3)
A0396	0(3)
A0398	0(3)
A0420	0(3)
A0422	0(3)
A0424	0(3)
A0425	250(1)
A0426	2(3)
A0427	2(3)

CPT	MUE
A0428	2(3)
A0429	2(3)
A0430	1(3)
A0431	1(3)
A0432	1(3)
A0433	1(3)
A0434	2(3)
A0435	999(3)
A0436	300(3)
A0888	0(3)
A0998	0(3)
A0999	1(3)
A4206	0(3)
A4207	0(3)
A4208	0(3)
A4209	0(3)
A4210	0(3)
A4211	0(3)
A4212	0(3)
A4213	0(3)
A4215	0(3)
A4216	0(3)
A4217	0(3)
A4218	0(3)
A4220	1(3)
A4221	0(3)
A4222	0(3)
A4223	0(3)
A4224	0(3)
A4225	0(3)
A4230	0(3)
A4231	0(3)
A4232	0(3)
A4233	0(3)
A4234	0(3)
A4235	0(3)
A4236	0(3)
A4244	0(3)
A4245	0(3)
A4246	0(3)
A4247	0(3)
A4248	0(3)
A4250	0(3)
A4252	0(3)
A4253	0(3)
A4255	0(3)
A4256	0(3)
A4257	0(3)
A4258	0(3)
A4259	0(3)
A4261	0(3)
A4262	0(3)
A4263	0(3)
A4264	0(3)
A4265	0(3)
A4266	0(3)
A4267	0(3)
A4268	0(3)
A4269	0(3)
A4270	0(3)
A4280	0(3)
A4281	0(3)
A4282	0(3)
A4283	0(3)
A4284	0(3)

CPT	MUE
A4285	0(3)
A4286	0(3)
A4290	2(3)
A4300	0(3)
A4301	1(2)
A4305	0(3)
A4306	0(3)
A4310	0(3)
A4311	0(3)
A4312	0(3)
A4313	0(3)
A4314	0(3)
A4315	0(3)
A4316	0(3)
A4320	0(3)
A4321	1(3)
A4322	0(3)
A4326	0(3)
A4327	0(3)
A4328	0(3)
A4330	0(3)
A4331	1(3)
A4332	2(3)
A4333	1(3)
A4334	1(3)
A4335	0(3)
A4336	1(3)
A4337	0(3)
A4338	0(3)
A4340	0(3)
A4344	0(3)
A4346	0(3)
A4349	1(3)
A4351	0(3)
A4352	0(3)
A4353	1(3)
A4354	0(3)
A4355	0(3)
A4356	0(3)
A4357	0(3)
A4358	0(3)
A4360	1(3)
A4361	0(3)
A4362	0(3)
A4363	1(3)
A4364	0(3)
A4366	1(3)
A4367	0(3)
A4368	1(3)
A4369	1(3)
A4371	1(3)
A4372	1(3)
A4373	1(3)
A4375	2(3)
A4376	2(3)
A4377	2(3)
A4378	2(3)
A4379	2(3)
A4380	2(3)
A4381	2(3)
A4382	2(3)
A4383	2(3)
A4384	2(3)
A4385	2(3)
A4387	1(3)

CPT	MUE
A4388	1(3)
A4389	2(3)
A4390	1(3)
A4391	1(3)
A4392	2(3)
A4393	1(3)
A4394	1(3)
A4395	3(3)
A4396	2(3)
A4397	0(3)
A4398	0(3)
A4399	0(3)
A4400	0(3)
A4402	0(3)
A4404	0(3)
A4405	1(3)
A4406	1(3)
A4407	2(3)
A4408	1(3)
A4409	1(3)
A4410	2(3)
A4411	1(3)
A4412	1(3)
A4413	2(3)
A4414	1(3)
A4415	1(3)
A4416	2(3)
A4417	2(3)
A4418	2(3)
A4419	2(3)
A4420	1(3)
A4422	7(3)
A4423	2(3)
A4424	1(3)
A4425	1(3)
A4426	2(3)
A4427	1(3)
A4428	1(3)
A4429	2(3)
A4430	1(3)
A4431	1(3)
A4432	2(3)
A4433	1(3)
A4434	1(3)
A4435	2(3)
A4450	0(3)
A4452	0(3)
A4455	0(3)
A4458	0(3)
A4459	0(3)
A4461	2(3)
A4463	0(3)
A4465	0(3)
A4467	0(3)
A4470	0(3)
A4480	0(3)
A4481	0(3)
A4483	0(3)
A4490	0(3)
A4495	0(3)
A4500	0(3)
A4510	0(3)
A4520	0(3)
A4550	0(3)
A4553	0(3)

CPT	MUE	CPT	MUE	CPT	MUE	CPT	MUE	CPT	MUE	CPT	MUE	CPT	MUE	CPT	MUE
A4554	0(3)	A4690	0(3)	A5121	0(3)	A6241	0(3)	A6534	0(3)	A7523	0(3)	A9547	2(3)	B4157	0(3)
A4555	0(3)	A4706	0(3)	A5122	0(3)	A6242	0(3)	A6535	0(3)	A7524	0(3)	A9548	2(3)	B4158	0(3)
A4556	0(3)	A4707	0(3)	A5126	0(3)	A6243	0(3)	A6536	0(3)	A7525	0(3)	A9550	1(3)	B4159	0(3)
A4557	0(3)	A4708	0(3)	A5131	0(3)	A6244	0(3)	A6537	0(3)	A7526	0(3)	A9551	1(3)	B4160	0(3)
A4558	0(3)	A4709	0(3)	A5200	2(3)	A6245	0(3)	A6538	0(3)	A7527	0(3)	A9552	1(3)	B4161	0(3)
A4559	0(3)	A4714	0(3)	A5500	0(3)	A6246	0(3)	A6539	0(3)	A8000	0(3)	A9553	1(3)	B4162	0(3)
A4561	1(3)	A4719	0(3)	A5501	0(3)	A6247	0(3)	A6540	0(3)	A8001	0(3)	A9554	1(3)	B4164	0(3)
A4562	1(3)	A4720	0(3)	A5503	0(3)	A6248	0(3)	A6541	0(3)	A8002	0(3)	A9555	2(3)	B4168	0(3)
A4563	1(2)	A4721	0(3)	A5504	0(3)	A6250	0(3)	A6544	0(3)	A8003	0(3)	A9556	10(3)	B4172	0(3)
A4565	2(3)	A4722	0(3)	A5505	0(3)	A6251	0(3)	A6545	0(3)	A8004	0(3)	A9557	2(3)	B4176	0(3)
A4566	0(3)	A4723	0(3)	A5506	0(3)	A6252	0(3)	A6549	0(3)	A9152	0(3)	A9558	7(3)	B4178	0(3)
A4570	0(3)	A4724	0(3)	A5507	0(3)	A6253	0(3)	A6550	0(3)	A9153	0(3)	A9559	1(3)	B4180	0(3)
A4575	0(3)	A4725	0(3)	A5508	0(3)	A6254	0(3)	A7000	0(3)	A9155	1(3)	A9560	2(3)	B4185	0(3)
A4580	0(3)	A4726	0(3)	A5510	0(3)	A6255	0(3)	A7001	0(3)	A9180	0(3)	A9561	1(3)	B4189	0(3)
A4590	0(3)	A4728	0(3)	A5512	0(3)	A6256	0(3)	A7002	0(3)	A9270	0(3)	A9562	2(3)	B4193	0(3)
A4595	0(3)	A4730	0(3)	A5513	0(3)	A6257	0(3)	A7003	0(3)	A9272	0(3)	A9563	10(3)	B4197	0(3)
A4600	0(3)	A4736	0(3)	A5514	0(3)	A6258	0(3)	A7004	0(3)	A9273	0(3)	A9564	20(3)	B4199	0(3)
A4601	0(3)	A4737	0(3)	A6000	0(3)	A6259	0(3)	A7005	0(3)	A9274	0(3)	A9566	1(3)	B4216	0(3)
A4602	0(3)	A4740	0(3)	A6010	0(3)	A6260	0(3)	A7006	0(3)	A9275	0(3)	A9567	2(3)	B4220	0(3)
A4604	0(3)	A4750	0(3)	A6011	0(3)	A6261	0(3)	A7007	0(3)	A9276	0(3)	A9568	0(3)	B4222	0(3)
A4605	0(3)	A4755	0(3)	A6021	0(3)	A6262	0(3)	A7008	0(3)	A9277	0(3)	A9569	1(3)	B4224	0(3)
A4606	0(3)	A4760	0(3)	A6022	0(3)	A6266	0(3)	A7009	0(3)	A9278	0(3)	A9570	1(3)	B5000	0(3)
A4608	0(3)	A4765	0(3)	A6023	0(3)	A6402	0(3)	A7010	0(3)	A9279	0(3)	A9571	1(3)	B5100	0(3)
A4611	0(3)	A4766	0(3)	A6024	0(3)	A6403	0(3)	A7012	0(3)	A9280	0(3)	A9572	1(3)	B5200	0(3)
A4612	0(3)	A4770	0(3)	A6025	0(3)	A6404	0(3)	A7013	0(3)	A9281	0(3)	A9575	300(3)	B9002	0(3)
A4613	0(3)	A4771	0(3)	A6154	0(3)	A6407	0(3)	A7014	0(3)	A9282	0(3)	A9576	40(3)	B9004	0(3)
A4614	0(3)	A4772	0(3)	A6196	0(3)	A6410	2(3)	A7015	0(3)	A9283	0(3)	A9577	50(3)	B9006	0(3)
A4615	0(3)	A4773	0(3)	A6197	0(3)	A6411	0(3)	A7016	0(3)	A9284	0(3)	A9578	50(3)	B9998	0(3)
A4616	0(3)	A4774	0(3)	A6198	0(3)	A6412	0(3)	A7017	0(3)	A9285	0(3)	A9579	100(3)	B9999	0(3)
A4617	0(3)	A4802	0(3)	A6199	0(3)	A6413	0(3)	A7018	0(3)	A9286	0(3)	A9580	1(3)	C1713	20(3)
A4618	1(3)	A4860	0(3)	A6203	0(3)	A6441	0(3)	A7020	0(3)	A9300	0(3)	A9581	20(3)	C1714	4(3)
A4619	0(3)	A4870	0(3)	A6204	0(3)	A6442	0(3)	A7025	0(3)	A9500	3(3)	A9582	1(3)	C1715	45(3)
A4620	0(3)	A4890	0(3)	A6205	0(3)	A6443	0(3)	A7026	0(3)	A9501	1(3)	A9583	18(3)	C1716	4(3)
A4623	0(3)	A4911	0(3)	A6206	0(3)	A6444	0(3)	A7027	0(3)	A9502	3(3)	A9584	1(3)	C1717	10(3)
A4624	0(3)	A4913	0(3)	A6207	0(3)	A6445	0(3)	A7028	0(3)	A9503	1(3)	A9585	300(3)	C1719	99(3)
A4625	30(3)	A4918	0(3)	A6208	0(3)	A6446	0(3)	A7029	0(3)	A9504	1(3)	A9586	1(3)	C1721	1(3)
A4626	0(3)	A4927	0(3)	A6209	0(3)	A6447	0(3)	A7030	0(3)	A9505	4(3)	A9587	54(3)	C1722	1(3)
A4627	0(3)	A4928	0(3)	A6210	0(3)	A6448	0(3)	A7031	0(3)	A9507	1(3)	A9588	10(3)	C1724	5(3)
A4628	0(3)	A4929	0(3)	A6211	0(3)	A6449	0(3)	A7032	0(3)	A9508	2(3)	A9589	1(3)	C1725	9(3)
A4629	0(3)	A4930	0(3)	A6212	0(3)	A6450	0(3)	A7033	0(3)	A9509	5(3)	A9600	7(3)	C1726	5(3)
A4630	0(3)	A4931	0(3)	A6213	0(3)	A6451	0(3)	A7034	0(3)	A9510	1(3)	A9604	1(3)	C1727	4(3)
A4633	0(3)	A4932	0(3)	A6214	0(3)	A6452	0(3)	A7035	0(3)	A9512	30(3)	A9606	224(3)	C1728	5(3)
A4634	0(3)	A5051	0(3)	A6215	0(3)	A6453	0(3)	A7036	0(3)	A9513	200(3)	A9698	2(3)	C1729	6(3)
A4635	0(3)	A5052	0(3)	A6216	0(3)	A6454	0(3)	A7037	0(3)	A9515	1(3)	A9700	2(3)	C1730	4(3)
A4636	0(3)	A5053	0(3)	A6217	0(3)	A6455	0(3)	A7038	0(3)	A9516	4(3)	A9900	1(3)	C1731	2(3)
A4637	0(3)	A5054	0(3)	A6218	0(3)	A6456	0(3)	A7039	0(3)	A9517	200(3)	A9901	0(3)	C1732	3(3)
A4638	0(3)	A5055	0(3)	A6219	0(3)	A6457	0(3)	A7040	2(3)	A9520	1(3)	A9999	1(3)	C1733	3(3)
A4639	0(3)	A5056	90(3)	A6220	0(3)	A6460	1(1)	A7041	2(3)	A9521	2(3)	B4034	0(3)	C1749	1(3)
A4640	0(3)	A5057	90(3)	A6221	0(3)	A6461	1(1)	A7044	0(3)	A9524	10(3)	B4035	0(3)	C1750	2(3)
A4642	1(3)	A5061	0(3)	A6222	0(3)	A6501	0(3)	A7045	0(3)	A9526	2(3)	B4036	0(3)	C1751	3(3)
A4648	5(3)	A5062	0(3)	A6223	0(3)	A6502	0(3)	A7046	0(3)	A9527	195(3)	B4081	0(3)	C1752	2(3)
A4649	1(3)	A5063	0(3)	A6224	0(3)	A6503	0(3)	A7047	0(3)	A9528	10(3)	B4082	0(3)	C1753	2(3)
A4650	3(3)	A5071	0(3)	A6228	0(3)	A6504	0(3)	A7048	2(3)	A9529	10(3)	B4083	0(3)	C1754	2(3)
A4651	0(3)	A5072	0(3)	A6229	0(3)	A6505	0(3)	A7501	0(3)	A9530	200(3)	B4087	0(3)	C1755	2(3)
A4652	0(3)	A5073	0(3)	A6230	0(3)	A6506	0(3)	A7502	0(3)	A9531	100(3)	B4088	0(3)	C1756	2(3)
A4653	0(3)	A5081	0(3)	A6231	0(3)	A6507	0(3)	A7503	0(3)	A9532	10(3)	B4100	0(3)	C1757	6(3)
A4657	0(3)	A5082	0(3)	A6232	0(3)	A6508	0(3)	A7504	0(3)	A9536	1(3)	B4102	0(3)	C1758	2(3)
A4660	0(3)	A5083	5(3)	A6233	0(3)	A6509	0(3)	A7505	0(3)	A9537	1(3)	B4103	0(3)	C1759	2(3)
A4663	0(3)	A5093	0(3)	A6234	0(3)	A6510	0(3)	A7506	0(3)	A9538	1(3)	B4104	0(3)	C1760	4(3)
A4670	0(3)	A5102	0(3)	A6235	0(3)	A6511	0(3)	A7507	0(3)	A9539	2(3)	B4149	0(3)	C1762	4(3)
A4671	0(3)	A5105	0(3)	A6236	0(3)	A6513	0(3)	A7508	0(3)	A9540	2(3)	B4150	0(3)	C1763	4(3)
A4672	0(3)	A5112	0(3)	A6237	0(3)	A6530	0(3)	A7509	0(3)	A9541	1(3)	B4152	0(3)	C1764	1(3)
A4673	0(3)	A5113	0(3)	A6238	0(3)	A6531	0(3)	A7520	0(3)	A9542	1(3)	B4153	0(3)	C1765	4(3)
A4674	0(3)	A5114	0(3)	A6239	0(3)	A6532	0(3)	A7521	0(3)	A9543	1(3)	B4154	0(3)	C1766	4(3)
A4680	0(3)	A5120	150(3)	A6240	0(3)	A6533	0(3)	A7522	0(3)	A9546	1(3)	B4155	0(3)	C1767	2(3)

CPT	MUE
C1768	3(3)
C1769	9(3)
C1770	3(3)
C1771	1(3)
C1772	1(3)
C1773	3(3)
C1776	10(3)
C1777	2(3)
C1778	4(3)
C1779	2(3)
C1780	2(3)
C1781	4(3)
C1782	1(3)
C1783	2(3)
C1784	2(3)
C1785	1(3)
C1786	1(3)
C1787	2(3)
C1788	2(3)
C1789	2(3)
C1813	1(3)
C1814	2(3)
C1815	1(3)
C1816	2(3)
C1817	1(3)
C1818	2(3)
C1819	4(3)
C1820	2(3)
C1821	4(3)
C1822	1(3)
C1823	1(3)
C1830	2(3)
C1840	1(3)
C1841	1(2)
C1842	1(2)
C1874	5(3)
C1875	4(3)
C1876	5(3)
C1877	5(3)
C1878	2(3)
C1880	2(3)
C1881	2(3)
C1882	1(3)
C1883	4(3)
C1884	4(3)
C1885	2(3)
C1886	1(3)
C1887	7(3)
C1888	2(3)
C1889	1(3)
C1891	1(3)
C1892	6(3)
C1893	6(3)
C1894	6(3)
C1895	2(3)
C1896	2(3)
C1897	2(3)
C1898	2(3)
C1899	2(3)
C1900	1(3)
C2613	2(3)
C2614	3(3)
C2615	2(3)
C2616	1(3)
C2617	4(3)

CPT	MUE
C2618	4(3)
C2619	1(3)
C2620	1(3)
C2621	1(3)
C2622	1(3)
C2623	2(3)
C2624	1(3)
C2625	4(3)
C2626	1(3)
C2627	2(3)
C2628	4(3)
C2629	4(3)
C2630	3(3)
C2631	1(3)
C2634	24(3)
C2635	124(3)
C2636	690(3)
C2637	0(3)
C2638	150(3)
C2639	150(3)
C2640	150(3)
C2641	150(3)
C2642	120(3)
C2643	120(3)
C2644	500(1)
C2645	4608(3)
C5271	1(2)
C5272	3(2)
C5273	1(2)
C5274	35(3)
C5275	1(2)
C5276	3(2)
C5277	1(2)
C5278	15(3)
C8900	1(3)
C8901	1(3)
C8902	1(3)
C8903	1(3)
C8905	1(3)
C8906	1(3)
C8908	1(3)
C8909	1(3)
C8910	1(3)
C8911	1(3)
C8912	1(3)
C8913	1(3)
C8914	1(3)
C8918	1(3)
C8919	1(3)
C8920	1(3)
C8921	1(3)
C8922	1(3)
C8923	1(3)
C8924	1(3)
C8925	1(3)
C8926	1(3)
C8927	1(3)
C8928	1(2)
C8929	1(3)
C8930	1(2)
C8931	1(3)
C8932	1(3)
C8933	1(3)
C8934	2(3)
C8935	2(3)

CPT	MUE
C8936	2(3)
C8937	2(2)
C8957	2(3)
C9035	675(3)
C9036	300(3)
C9037	240(3)
C9038	160(3)
C9039	500(3)
C9040	675(3)
C9041	180(3)
C9043	300(3)
C9044	350(3)
C9045	600(3)
C9046	160(3)
C9113	10(3)
C9132	5500(3)
C9248	25(3)
C9250	1(3)
C9254	400(3)
C9257	5(3)
C9285	2(3)
C9290	266(3)
C9293	700(3)
C9352	3(3)
C9353	4(3)
C9354	300(3)
C9355	3(3)
C9356	125(3)
C9358	800(3)
C9359	30(3)
C9360	300(3)
C9361	10(3)
C9362	60(3)
C9363	500(3)
C9364	600(3)
C9407	15(3)
C9408	510(3)
C9447	1(3)
C9460	1(3)
C9462	600(3)
C9482	150(3)
C9488	20(3)
C9600	3(3)
C9601	2(3)
C9602	2(3)
C9603	2(3)
C9604	2(3)
C9605	2(3)
C9606	1(3)
C9607	1(2)
C9608	2(3)
C9725	1(3)
C9726	2(3)
C9727	1(2)
C9728	1(2)
C9733	1(3)
C9734	1(3)
C9738	1(3)
C9739	1(2)
C9740	1(2)
C9745	2(2)
C9747	1(2)
C9749	1(2)
C9751	1(3)
C9752	1(2)

CPT	MUE
C9753	3(3)
C9754	1(2)
C9755	1(2)
D0150	1(3)
D0240	1(3)
D0250	2(3)
D0270	1(3)
D0272	1(3)
D0274	1(3)
D0277	1(3)
D0412	0(3)
D0416	1(3)
D0431	1(3)
D0460	1(2)
D0484	1(2)
D0485	1(2)
D0601	1(2)
D0602	1(2)
D0603	1(2)
D1510	2(2)
D1516	1(2)
D1517	1(2)
D1520	2(2)
D1526	1(2)
D1527	1(2)
D1550	2(3)
D1575	4(2)
D4260	4(2)
D4263	4(2)
D4264	3(3)
D4270	4(3)
D4273	1(2)
D4277	1(2)
D4278	3(3)
D4355	1(2)
D4381	12(3)
D5282	0(3)
D5283	0(3)
D5876	0(3)
D5911	1(3)
D5912	1(2)
D5983	1(3)
D5984	1(3)
D5985	1(3)
D7111	20(3)
D7140	32(2)
D7210	32(2)
D7220	6(3)
D7230	6(3)
D7240	6(3)
D7241	6(3)
D7250	32(2)
D7260	1(3)
D7261	1(3)
D7283	4(3)
D7288	2(3)
D7321	4(2)
D9110	1(3)
D9130	0(3)
D9230	1(3)
D9248	1(3)
D9613	0(3)
D9930	1(2)
D9944	0(3)
D9945	0(3)

CPT	MUE
D9946	0(3)
D9950	1(3)
D9951	1(3)
D9952	1(3)
D9961	0(3)
D9990	0(3)
E0100	0(3)
E0105	0(3)
E0110	0(3)
E0111	0(3)
E0112	0(3)
E0113	0(3)
E0114	0(3)
E0116	0(3)
E0117	0(3)
E0118	0(3)
E0130	0(3)
E0135	0(3)
E0140	0(3)
E0141	0(3)
E0143	0(3)
E0144	0(3)
E0147	0(3)
E0148	0(3)
E0149	0(3)
E0153	0(3)
E0154	0(3)
E0155	0(3)
E0156	0(3)
E0157	0(3)
E0158	0(3)
E0159	2(2)
E0160	0(3)
E0161	0(3)
E0162	0(3)
E0163	0(3)
E0165	0(3)
E0167	0(3)
E0168	0(3)
E0170	0(3)
E0171	0(3)
E0172	0(3)
E0175	0(3)
E0181	0(3)
E0182	0(3)
E0184	0(3)
E0185	0(3)
E0186	0(3)
E0187	0(3)
E0188	0(3)
E0189	0(3)
E0190	0(3)
E0191	0(3)
E0193	0(3)
E0194	0(3)
E0196	0(3)
E0197	0(3)
E0198	0(3)
E0199	0(3)
E0200	0(3)
E0202	0(3)
E0203	0(3)
E0205	0(3)
E0210	0(3)
E0215	0(3)

CPT	MUE
E0217	0(3)
E0218	0(3)
E0221	0(3)
E0225	0(3)
E0231	0(3)
E0232	0(3)
E0235	0(3)
E0236	0(3)
E0239	0(3)
E0240	0(3)
E0241	0(3)
E0242	0(3)
E0243	0(3)
E0244	0(3)
E0245	0(3)
E0246	0(3)
E0247	0(3)
E0248	0(3)
E0249	0(3)
E0250	0(3)
E0251	0(3)
E0255	0(3)
E0256	0(3)
E0260	0(3)
E0261	0(3)
E0265	0(3)
E0266	0(3)
E0270	0(3)
E0271	0(3)
E0272	0(3)
E0273	0(3)
E0274	0(3)
E0275	0(3)
E0276	0(3)
E0277	0(3)
E0280	0(3)
E0290	0(3)
E0291	0(3)
E0292	0(3)
E0293	0(3)
E0294	0(3)
E0295	0(3)
E0296	0(3)
E0297	0(3)
E0300	0(3)
E0301	0(3)
E0302	0(3)
E0303	0(3)
E0304	0(3)
E0305	0(3)
E0310	0(3)
E0315	0(3)
E0316	0(3)
E0325	0(3)
E0326	0(3)
E0328	0(3)
E0329	0(3)
E0350	0(3)
E0352	0(3)
E0370	0(3)
E0371	0(3)
E0372	0(3)
E0373	0(3)
E0424	0(3)
E0425	0(3)

CPT	MUE
E0430	0(3)
E0431	0(3)
E0433	0(3)
E0434	0(3)
E0435	0(3)
E0439	0(3)
E0440	0(3)
E0441	0(3)
E0442	0(3)
E0443	0(3)
E0444	0(3)
E0445	0(3)
E0446	0(3)
E0447	0(3)
E0455	0(3)
E0457	0(3)
E0459	0(3)
E0462	0(3)
E0465	0(3)
E0466	0(3)
E0467	0(3)
E0470	0(3)
E0471	0(3)
E0472	0(3)
E0480	0(3)
E0481	0(3)
E0482	0(3)
E0483	0(3)
E0484	0(3)
E0485	0(3)
E0486	0(3)
E0487	0(3)
E0500	0(3)
E0550	0(3)
E0555	0(3)
E0560	0(3)
E0561	0(3)
E0562	0(3)
E0565	0(3)
E0570	0(3)
E0572	0(3)
E0574	0(3)
E0575	0(3)
E0580	0(3)
E0585	0(3)
E0600	0(3)
E0601	0(3)
E0602	0(3)
E0603	0(3)
E0604	0(3)
E0605	0(3)
E0606	0(3)
E0607	0(3)
E0610	0(3)
E0615	0(3)
E0616	1(2)
E0617	0(3)
E0618	0(3)
E0619	0(3)
E0620	0(3)
E0621	0(3)
E0625	0(3)
E0627	0(3)
E0629	0(3)
E0630	0(3)

CPT	MUE
E0635	0(3)
E0636	0(3)
E0637	0(3)
E0638	0(3)
E0639	0(3)
E0640	0(3)
E0641	0(3)
E0642	0(3)
E0650	0(3)
E0651	0(3)
E0652	0(3)
E0655	0(3)
E0656	0(3)
E0657	0(3)
E0660	0(3)
E0665	0(3)
E0666	0(3)
E0667	0(3)
E0668	0(3)
E0669	0(3)
E0670	0(3)
E0671	0(3)
E0672	0(3)
E0673	0(3)
E0675	0(3)
E0676	1(3)
E0691	0(3)
E0692	0(3)
E0693	0(3)
E0694	0(3)
E0700	0(3)
E0705	0(3)
E0710	0(3)
E0720	0(3)
E0730	0(3)
E0731	0(3)
E0740	0(3)
E0744	0(3)
E0745	0(3)
E0746	1(3)
E0747	0(3)
E0748	0(3)
E0749	1(3)
E0755	0(3)
E0760	0(3)
E0761	0(3)
E0762	0(3)
E0764	0(3)
E0765	0(3)
E0766	0(3)
E0769	0(3)
E0770	1(3)
E0776	0(3)
E0779	0(3)
E0780	0(3)
E0781	1(2)
E0782	1(2)
E0783	1(2)
E0784	0(3)
E0785	1(2)
E0786	1(2)
E0791	0(3)
E0830	0(3)
E0840	0(3)
E0849	0(3)

CPT	MUE
E0850	0(3)
E0855	0(3)
E0856	0(3)
E0860	0(3)
E0870	0(3)
E0880	0(3)
E0890	0(3)
E0900	0(3)
E0910	0(3)
E0911	0(3)
E0912	0(3)
E0920	0(3)
E0930	0(3)
E0935	0(3)
E0936	0(3)
E0940	0(3)
E0941	0(3)
E0942	0(3)
E0944	0(3)
E0945	0(3)
E0946	0(3)
E0947	0(3)
E0948	0(3)
E0950	0(3)
E0951	0(3)
E0952	0(3)
E0953	0(3)
E0954	0(3)
E0955	0(3)
E0956	0(3)
E0957	0(3)
E0958	0(3)
E0959	0(3)
E0960	0(3)
E0961	0(3)
E0966	0(3)
E0967	0(3)
E0968	0(3)
E0969	0(3)
E0970	0(3)
E0971	0(3)
E0973	0(3)
E0974	0(3)
E0978	0(3)
E0980	0(3)
E0981	0(3)
E0982	0(3)
E0983	0(3)
E0984	0(3)
E0985	0(3)
E0986	0(3)
E0988	0(3)
E0990	0(3)
E0992	0(3)
E0994	0(3)
E0995	0(3)
E1002	0(3)
E1003	0(3)
E1004	0(3)
E1005	0(3)
E1006	0(3)
E1007	0(3)
E1008	0(3)
E1009	0(3)
E1010	0(3)

CPT	MUE
E1011	0(3)
E1012	0(3)
E1014	0(3)
E1015	0(3)
E1016	0(3)
E1017	0(3)
E1018	0(3)
E1020	0(3)
E1028	0(3)
E1029	0(3)
E1030	0(3)
E1031	0(3)
E1035	0(3)
E1036	0(3)
E1037	0(3)
E1038	0(3)
E1039	0(3)
E1050	0(3)
E1060	0(3)
E1070	0(3)
E1083	0(3)
E1084	0(3)
E1085	0(3)
E1086	0(3)
E1087	0(3)
E1088	0(3)
E1089	0(3)
E1090	0(3)
E1092	0(3)
E1093	0(3)
E1100	0(3)
E1110	0(3)
E1130	0(3)
E1140	0(3)
E1150	0(3)
E1160	0(3)
E1161	0(3)
E1170	0(3)
E1171	0(3)
E1172	0(3)
E1180	0(3)
E1190	0(3)
E1195	0(3)
E1200	0(3)
E1220	0(3)
E1221	0(3)
E1222	0(3)
E1223	0(3)
E1224	0(3)
E1225	0(3)
E1226	0(3)
E1227	0(3)
E1228	0(3)
E1229	0(3)
E1230	0(3)
E1231	0(3)
E1232	0(3)
E1233	0(3)
E1234	0(3)
E1235	0(3)
E1236	0(3)
E1237	0(3)
E1238	0(3)
E1239	0(3)
E1240	0(3)

CPT	MUE
E1250	0(3)
E1260	0(3)
E1270	0(3)
E1280	0(3)
E1285	0(3)
E1290	0(3)
E1295	0(3)
E1296	0(3)
E1297	0(3)
E1298	0(3)
E1300	0(3)
E1310	0(3)
E1352	0(3)
E1353	0(3)
E1354	0(3)
E1355	0(3)
E1356	0(3)
E1357	0(3)
E1358	0(3)
E1372	0(3)
E1390	0(3)
E1391	0(3)
E1392	0(3)
E1399	1(3)
E1405	0(3)
E1406	0(3)
E1500	0(3)
E1510	0(3)
E1520	0(3)
E1530	0(3)
E1540	0(3)
E1550	0(3)
E1560	0(3)
E1570	0(3)
E1575	0(3)
E1580	0(3)
E1590	0(3)
E1592	0(3)
E1594	0(3)
E1600	0(3)
E1610	0(3)
E1615	0(3)
E1620	0(3)
E1625	0(3)
E1630	0(3)
E1632	0(3)
E1634	0(3)
E1635	0(3)
E1636	0(3)
E1637	0(3)
E1639	0(3)
E1699	0(3)
E1700	0(3)
E1701	0(3)
E1702	0(3)
E1800	0(3)
E1801	0(3)
E1802	0(3)
E1805	0(3)
E1806	0(3)
E1810	0(3)
E1811	0(3)
E1812	0(3)
E1815	0(3)
E1816	0(3)

CPT	MUE
E1818	0(3)
E1820	0(3)
E1821	0(3)
E1825	0(3)
E1830	0(3)
E1831	0(3)
E1840	0(3)
E1841	0(3)
E1902	0(3)
E2000	0(3)
E2100	0(3)
E2101	0(3)
E2120	0(3)
E2201	0(3)
E2202	0(3)
E2203	0(3)
E2204	0(3)
E2205	0(3)
E2206	0(3)
E2207	0(3)
E2208	0(3)
E2209	0(3)
E2210	0(3)
E2211	0(3)
E2212	0(3)
E2213	0(3)
E2214	0(3)
E2215	0(3)
E2216	0(3)
E2217	0(3)
E2218	0(3)
E2219	0(3)
E2220	0(3)
E2221	0(3)
E2222	0(3)
E2224	0(3)
E2225	0(3)
E2226	0(3)
E2227	0(3)
E2228	0(3)
E2230	0(3)
E2231	0(3)
E2291	1(2)
E2292	1(2)
E2293	1(2)
E2294	1(2)
E2295	0(3)
E2300	0(3)
E2301	0(3)
E2310	0(3)
E2311	0(3)
E2312	0(3)
E2313	0(3)
E2321	0(3)
E2322	0(3)
E2323	0(3)
E2324	0(3)
E2325	0(3)
E2326	0(3)
E2327	0(3)
E2328	0(3)
E2329	0(3)
E2330	0(3)
E2331	0(3)
E2340	0(3)

CPT	MUE
E2341	0(3)
E2342	0(3)
E2343	0(3)
E2351	0(3)
E2358	0(3)
E2359	0(3)
E2360	0(3)
E2361	0(3)
E2362	0(3)
E2363	0(3)
E2364	0(3)
E2365	0(3)
E2366	0(3)
E2367	0(3)
E2368	0(3)
E2369	0(3)
E2370	0(3)
E2371	0(3)
E2372	0(3)
E2373	0(3)
E2374	0(3)
E2375	0(3)
E2376	0(3)
E2377	0(3)
E2378	0(3)
E2381	0(3)
E2382	0(3)
E2383	0(3)
E2384	0(3)
E2385	0(3)
E2386	0(3)
E2387	0(3)
E2388	0(3)
E2389	0(3)
E2390	0(3)
E2391	0(3)
E2392	0(3)
E2394	0(3)
E2395	0(3)
E2396	0(3)
E2397	0(3)
E2402	0(3)
E2500	0(3)
E2502	0(3)
E2504	0(3)
E2506	0(3)
E2508	0(3)
E2510	0(3)
E2511	0(3)
E2512	0(3)
E2599	0(3)
E2601	0(3)
E2602	0(3)
E2603	0(3)
E2604	0(3)
E2605	0(3)
E2606	0(3)
E2607	0(3)
E2608	0(3)
E2609	0(3)
E2610	0(3)
E2611	0(3)
E2612	0(3)
E2613	0(3)
E2614	0(3)

CPT	MUE
E2615	0(3)
E2616	0(3)
E2617	0(3)
E2619	0(3)
E2620	0(3)
E2621	0(3)
E2622	0(3)
E2623	0(3)
E2624	0(3)
E2625	0(3)
E2626	0(3)
E2627	0(3)
E2628	0(3)
E2629	0(3)
E2630	0(3)
E2631	0(3)
E2632	0(3)
E2633	0(3)
E8000	0(3)
E8001	0(3)
E8002	0(3)
G0008	1(2)
G0009	1(2)
G0010	1(3)
G0027	1(2)
G0068	16(3)
G0069	16(3)
G0070	16(3)
G0071	1(3)
G0076	1(3)
G0077	1(3)
G0078	1(3)
G0079	1(3)
G0080	1(3)
G0081	1(3)
G0082	1(3)
G0083	1(3)
G0084	1(3)
G0085	1(3)
G0086	1(3)
G0087	1(3)
G0101	1(2)
G0102	1(2)
G0103	1(2)
G0104	1(2)
G0105	1(2)
G0106	1(2)
G0108	6(3)
G0109	12(3)
G0117	1(2)
G0118	1(2)
G0120	1(2)
G0121	1(2)
G0122	0(3)
G0123	1(3)
G0124	1(3)
G0127	1(2)
G0128	1(3)
G0130	1(2)
G0141	1(3)
G0143	1(3)
G0144	1(3)
G0145	1(3)
G0147	1(3)
G0148	1(3)

CPT	MUE
G0166	2(3)
G0168	2(3)
G0175	1(3)
G0177	0(3)
G0179	1(2)
G0180	1(2)
G0181	1(2)
G0182	1(2)
G0186	1(2)
G0219	0(3)
G0235	1(3)
G0237	8(3)
G0238	8(3)
G0239	1(3)
G0245	1(2)
G0246	1(2)
G0247	1(2)
G0248	1(2)
G0249	3(3)
G0250	1(2)
G0252	0(3)
G0255	0(3)
G0257	0(3)
G0259	2(3)
G0260	2(3)
G0268	1(2)
G0269	0(3)
G0270	8(3)
G0271	4(3)
G0276	1(3)
G0277	5(3)
G0278	1(2)
G0279	1(2)
G0281	1(3)
G0282	0(3)
G0283	1(3)
G0288	1(2)
G0289	1(2)
G0293	1(2)
G0294	1(2)
G0295	0(3)
G0296	1(2)
G0297	1(2)
G0302	1(2)
G0303	1(2)
G0304	1(2)
G0305	1(2)
G0306	1(3)
G0307	1(3)
G0328	1(2)
G0329	1(3)
G0333	0(3)
G0337	1(2)
G0339	1(2)
G0340	1(3)
G0341	1(2)
G0342	1(2)
G0343	1(2)
G0365	2(3)
G0372	1(2)
G0378	0(3)
G0379	0(3)
G0380	0(3)
G0381	0(3)
G0382	0(3)

CPT	MUE
G0383	0(3)
G0384	0(3)
G0390	0(3)
G0396	1(2)
G0397	1(2)
G0398	1(2)
G0399	1(2)
G0400	1(2)
G0402	1(2)
G0403	1(2)
G0404	1(2)
G0405	1(2)
G0406	1(3)
G0407	1(3)
G0408	1(3)
G0410	4(3)
G0411	4(3)
G0412	1(2)
G0413	1(2)
G0414	1(2)
G0415	1(2)
G0416	1(2)
G0420	2(3)
G0421	2(3)
G0422	6(2)
G0423	6(2)
G0424	2(2)
G0425	1(3)
G0426	1(3)
G0427	1(3)
G0428	0(3)
G0429	1(2)
G0432	1(2)
G0433	1(2)
G0435	1(2)
G0438	1(2)
G0439	1(2)
G0442	1(2)
G0443	1(2)
G0444	1(2)
G0445	1(2)
G0446	1(3)
G0448	1(3)
G0451	1(3)
G0452	6(3)
G0453	40(3)
G0454	1(2)
G0455	1(2)
G0458	1(3)
G0459	1(3)
G0460	1(3)
G0463	0(3)
G0466	1(2)
G0467	1(3)
G0468	1(2)
G0469	1(2)
G0470	1(3)
G0471	2(3)
G0472	1(2)
G0473	1(3)
G0475	1(2)
G0476	1(2)
G0480	1(2)
G0481	1(2)
G0482	1(2)

CPT	MUE
G0483	1(2)
G0490	1(3)
G0491	1(3)
G0492	1(3)
G0493	1(3)
G0494	1(3)
G0495	1(3)
G0496	1(3)
G0498	1(2)
G0499	1(2)
G0500	1(3)
G0501	0(3)
G0506	1(2)
G0508	1(2)
G0509	1(2)
G0511	1(2)
G0512	1(2)
G0513	1(2)
G0514	1(1)
G0515	8(3)
G0516	1(2)
G0517	1(2)
G0518	1(2)
G0659	1(2)
G2000	1(3)
G2001	1(3)
G2002	1(3)
G2003	1(3)
G2004	1(3)
G2005	1(3)
G2006	1(3)
G2007	1(3)
G2008	1(3)
G2009	1(3)
G2010	1(3)
G2011	1(2)
G2012	1(3)
G2013	1(3)
G2014	1(3)
G2015	1(3)
G6001	2(3)
G6002	2(3)
G6003	2(3)
G6004	2(3)
G6005	2(3)
G6006	2(3)
G6007	2(3)
G6008	2(3)
G6009	2(3)
G6010	2(3)
G6011	2(3)
G6012	2(3)
G6013	2(3)
G6014	2(3)
G6015	2(3)
G6016	2(3)
G6017	2(3)
G9143	1(2)
G9147	0(3)
G9148	1(3)
G9149	1(3)
G9150	1(3)
G9151	1(3)
G9152	1(3)
G9153	1(3)

CPT	MUE
G9156	1(2)
G9157	1(2)
G9187	1(3)
G9480	1(3)
G9481	1(3)
G9482	1(3)
G9483	1(3)
G9484	1(3)
G9485	1(3)
G9486	1(3)
G9487	1(3)
G9488	1(3)
G9489	1(3)
G9490	1(3)
G9678	1(2)
G9685	1(3)
G9978	1(3)
G9979	1(3)
G9980	1(3)
G9981	1(3)
G9982	1(3)
G9983	1(3)
G9984	1(3)
G9985	1(3)
G9986	1(3)
G9987	1(3)
J0120	1(3)
J0129	100(3)
J0130	4(3)
J0131	400(3)
J0132	12(3)
J0133	1200(3)
J0135	8(3)
J0153	180(3)
J0171	20(3)
J0178	4(3)
J0180	125(3)
J0185	130(3)
J0190	0(3)
J0200	0(3)
J0202	12(3)
J0205	0(3)
J0207	4(3)
J0210	4(3)
J0215	30(3)
J0220	1(3)
J0221	250(3)
J0256	1600(3)
J0257	1400(3)
J0270	32(3)
J0275	1(3)
J0278	15(3)
J0280	7(3)
J0282	5(3)
J0285	5(3)
J0287	50(3)
J0288	0(3)
J0289	50(3)
J0290	24(3)
J0295	12(3)
J0300	8(3)
J0330	10(3)
J0348	200(3)
J0350	0(3)
J0360	2(3)

CPT	MUE
J0364	6(3)
J0365	0(3)
J0380	1(3)
J0390	0(3)
J0395	0(3)
J0400	39(3)
J0401	400(3)
J0456	4(3)
J0461	200(3)
J0470	2(3)
J0475	8(3)
J0476	2(3)
J0480	1(3)
J0485	1500(3)
J0490	160(3)
J0500	4(3)
J0515	3(3)
J0517	30(3)
J0520	0(3)
J0558	24(3)
J0561	24(3)
J0565	200(3)
J0567	300(3)
J0570	4(3)
J0571	0(3)
J0572	0(3)
J0573	0(3)
J0574	0(3)
J0575	0(3)
J0583	250(3)
J0584	90(3)
J0585	600(3)
J0586	300(3)
J0587	300(3)
J0588	600(3)
J0592	6(3)
J0594	320(3)
J0595	8(3)
J0596	840(3)
J0597	250(3)
J0598	100(3)
J0599	900(3)
J0600	3(3)
J0606	150(3)
J0610	15(3)
J0620	1(3)
J0630	1(3)
J0636	100(3)
J0637	20(3)
J0638	150(3)
J0640	24(3)
J0641	1200(3)
J0670	10(3)
J0690	12(3)
J0692	12(3)
J0694	8(3)
J0695	60(3)
J0696	16(3)
J0697	4(3)
J0698	10(3)
J0702	18(3)
J0706	1(3)
J0710	0(3)
J0712	120(3)
J0713	12(3)

CPT	MUE
J0714	4(3)
J0715	0(3)
J0716	4(3)
J0717	400(3)
J0720	15(3)
J0725	10(3)
J0735	50(3)
J0740	2(3)
J0743	16(3)
J0744	6(3)
J0745	2(3)
J0770	5(3)
J0775	180(3)
J0780	4(3)
J0795	100(3)
J0800	3(3)
J0834	3(3)
J0840	6(3)
J0841	20(3)
J0850	9(3)
J0875	300(3)
J0878	1500(3)
J0881	500(3)
J0882	300(3)
J0883	1125(3)
J0884	1125(3)
J0885	60(3)
J0887	360(3)
J0888	360(3)
J0890	0(3)
J0894	100(3)
J0895	12(3)
J0897	120(3)
J0945	4(3)
J1000	1(3)
J1020	8(3)
J1030	8(3)
J1040	4(3)
J1050	1000(3)
J1071	400(3)
J1094	0(3)
J1095	517(1)
J1100	120(3)
J1110	3(3)
J1120	2(3)
J1130	300(3)
J1160	2(3)
J1162	1(3)
J1165	50(3)
J1170	350(3)
J1180	0(3)
J1190	8(3)
J1200	8(3)
J1205	4(3)
J1212	1(3)
J1230	3(3)
J1240	6(3)
J1245	6(3)
J1250	2(3)
J1260	2(3)
J1265	20(3)
J1267	150(3)
J1270	8(3)
J1290	30(3)
J1300	120(3)

CPT	MUE
J1301	60(3)
J1320	0(3)
J1322	150(3)
J1324	108(3)
J1325	1(3)
J1327	1(3)
J1330	1(3)
J1335	2(3)
J1364	2(3)
J1380	4(3)
J1410	4(3)
J1428	450(3)
J1430	10(3)
J1435	1(3)
J1436	0(3)
J1438	2(3)
J1439	750(3)
J1442	1500(3)
J1443	272(3)
J1444	272(3)
J1447	960(3)
J1450	4(3)
J1451	1(3)
J1452	0(3)
J1453	150(3)
J1454	1(3)
J1455	18(3)
J1457	0(3)
J1458	100(3)
J1459	300(3)
J1460	10(2)
J1555	480(3)
J1556	300(3)
J1557	300(3)
J1559	300(3)
J1560	1(2)
J1561	300(3)
J1562	0(3)
J1566	300(3)
J1568	300(3)
J1569	300(3)
J1570	4(3)
J1571	20(3)
J1572	300(3)
J1573	130(3)
J1575	650(3)
J1580	9(3)
J1595	1(3)
J1599	300(3)
J1600	2(3)
J1602	300(3)
J1610	2(3)
J1620	0(3)
J1626	30(3)
J1627	100(3)
J1628	100(3)
J1630	5(3)
J1631	9(3)
J1640	672(3)
J1642	100(3)
J1644	40(3)
J1645	10(3)
J1650	30(3)
J1652	20(3)
J1655	0(3)

CPT	MUE
J1670	1(3)
J1675	0(3)
J1700	0(3)
J1710	0(3)
J1720	10(3)
J1726	28(3)
J1729	25(3)
J1730	0(3)
J1740	3(3)
J1741	8(3)
J1742	2(3)
J1743	66(3)
J1744	30(3)
J1745	150(3)
J1746	200(3)
J1750	45(3)
J1756	500(3)
J1786	680(3)
J1790	2(3)
J1800	6(3)
J1810	0(3)
J1815	8(3)
J1817	0(3)
J1826	1(3)
J1830	1(3)
J1833	372(3)
J1835	0(3)
J1840	3(3)
J1850	4(3)
J1885	8(3)
J1890	0(3)
J1930	120(3)
J1931	377(3)
J1940	6(3)
J1942	1064(3)
J1945	0(3)
J1950	12(3)
J1953	300(3)
J1955	11(3)
J1956	4(3)
J1960	0(3)
J1980	2(3)
J1990	0(3)
J2001	60(3)
J2010	10(3)
J2020	6(3)
J2060	4(3)
J2062	10(3)
J2150	8(3)
J2170	8(3)
J2175	4(3)
J2180	0(3)
J2182	300(3)
J2185	30(3)
J2186	600(3)
J2210	1(3)
J2212	240(3)
J2248	150(3)
J2250	22(3)
J2260	4(3)
J2265	400(3)
J2270	9(3)
J2274	250(3)
J2278	1000(3)
J2280	4(3)

CPT	MUE
J2300	4(3)
J2310	4(3)
J2315	380(3)
J2320	4(3)
J2323	300(3)
J2325	0(3)
J2326	120(3)
J2350	600(3)
J2353	60(3)
J2354	60(3)
J2355	2(3)
J2357	90(3)
J2358	405(3)
J2360	2(3)
J2370	2(3)
J2400	4(3)
J2405	64(3)
J2407	120(3)
J2410	2(3)
J2425	125(3)
J2426	819(3)
J2430	3(3)
J2440	4(3)
J2460	0(3)
J2469	10(3)
J2501	2(3)
J2502	60(3)
J2503	2(3)
J2504	15(3)
J2505	1(3)
J2507	8(3)
J2510	4(3)
J2513	1(3)
J2515	1(3)
J2540	75(3)
J2543	16(3)
J2545	1(3)
J2547	600(3)
J2550	3(3)
J2560	1(3)
J2562	48(3)
J2590	3(3)
J2597	45(3)
J2650	0(3)
J2670	0(3)
J2675	1(3)
J2680	4(3)
J2690	4(3)
J2700	48(3)
J2704	80(3)
J2710	2(3)
J2720	5(3)
J2724	3500(3)
J2725	0(3)
J2730	2(3)
J2760	2(3)
J2765	10(3)
J2770	6(3)
J2778	10(3)
J2780	16(3)
J2783	60(3)
J2785	4(3)
J2786	500(3)
J2787	1(3)
J2788	1(3)

CPT	MUE
J2790	1(3)
J2791	15(3)
J2792	450(3)
J2793	320(3)
J2794	100(3)
J2795	200(3)
J2796	150(3)
J2797	333(3)
J2800	3(3)
J2805	3(3)
J2810	5(3)
J2820	15(3)
J2840	160(3)
J2850	16(3)
J2860	170(3)
J2910	0(3)
J2916	20(3)
J2920	25(3)
J2930	25(3)
J2940	0(3)
J2941	8(3)
J2950	0(3)
J2993	2(3)
J2995	0(3)
J2997	8(3)
J3000	2(3)
J3010	100(3)
J3030	1(3)
J3060	760(3)
J3070	3(3)
J3090	200(3)
J3095	150(3)
J3101	50(3)
J3105	2(3)
J3110	2(3)
J3121	400(3)
J3145	750(3)
J3230	2(3)
J3240	1(3)
J3243	150(3)
J3245	100(3)
J3246	1(3)
J3250	2(3)
J3260	8(3)
J3262	800(3)
J3265	0(3)
J3280	0(3)
J3285	1(3)
J3300	160(3)
J3301	16(3)
J3302	0(3)
J3303	24(3)
J3304	64(2)
J3305	0(3)
J3310	0(3)
J3315	6(3)
J3316	6(3)
J3320	0(3)
J3350	0(3)
J3355	1(3)
J3357	90(3)
J3358	520(3)
J3360	6(3)
J3364	0(3)
J3365	0(3)

CPT	MUE	CPT	MUE	CPT	MUE	CPT	MUE	CPT	MUE	CPT	MUE	CPT	MUE	CPT	MUE
J3370	12(3)	J7207	7500(1)	J7610	0(3)	J8565	0(3)	J9207	90(3)	K0004	0(3)	K0801	0(3)	L0113	0(3)
J3380	300(3)	J7208	12000(1)	J7611	10(3)	J8597	0(3)	J9208	15(3)	K0005	0(3)	K0802	0(3)	L0120	0(3)
J3385	80(3)	J7209	7500(1)	J7612	10(3)	J8600	0(3)	J9209	55(3)	K0006	0(3)	K0806	0(3)	L0130	0(3)
J3396	150(3)	J7210	22000(1)	J7613	10(3)	J8610	0(3)	J9211	6(3)	K0007	0(3)	K0807	0(3)	L0140	0(3)
J3397	600(3)	J7211	22000(1)	J7614	10(3)	J8650	0(3)	J9212	0(3)	K0008	0(3)	K0808	0(3)	L0150	0(3)
J3398	150(2)	J7296	0(3)	J7615	0(3)	J8655	1(3)	J9213	12(3)	K0009	0(3)	K0812	0(3)	L0160	0(3)
J3400	0(3)	J7297	0(3)	J7620	6(3)	J8670	0(3)	J9214	100(3)	K0010	0(3)	K0813	0(3)	L0170	0(3)
J3410	8(3)	J7298	0(3)	J7622	0(3)	J8700	0(3)	J9215	0(3)	K0011	0(3)	K0814	0(3)	L0172	0(3)
J3411	4(3)	J7300	0(3)	J7624	0(3)	J8705	0(3)	J9216	2(3)	K0012	0(3)	K0815	0(3)	L0174	0(3)
J3415	6(3)	J7301	0(3)	J7626	2(3)	J8999	0(3)	J9217	6(3)	K0013	0(3)	K0816	0(3)	L0180	0(3)
J3420	1(3)	J7303	0(3)	J7627	0(3)	J9000	20(3)	J9218	1(3)	K0014	0(3)	K0820	0(3)	L0190	0(3)
J3430	25(3)	J7304	0(3)	J7628	0(3)	J9015	1(3)	J9219	1(3)	K0015	0(3)	K0821	0(3)	L0200	0(3)
J3465	40(3)	J7306	0(3)	J7629	0(3)	J9017	30(3)	J9225	1(3)	K0017	0(3)	K0822	0(3)	L0220	0(3)
J3470	3(3)	J7307	0(3)	J7631	4(3)	J9019	60(3)	J9226	1(3)	K0018	0(3)	K0823	0(3)	L0450	0(3)
J3471	999(2)	J7308	3(3)	J7632	0(3)	J9020	0(3)	J9228	1100(3)	K0019	0(3)	K0824	0(3)	L0452	0(3)
J3472	2(3)	J7309	1(3)	J7633	0(3)	J9022	168(3)	J9229	27(3)	K0020	0(3)	K0825	0(3)	L0454	0(3)
J3473	450(3)	J7310	0(3)	J7634	0(3)	J9023	140(3)	J9230	5(3)	K0037	0(3)	K0826	0(3)	L0455	0(3)
J3475	20(3)	J7311	1(3)	J7635	0(3)	J9025	300(3)	J9245	9(3)	K0038	0(3)	K0827	0(3)	L0456	0(3)
J3480	40(3)	J7312	14(3)	J7636	0(3)	J9027	100(3)	J9250	25(3)	K0039	0(3)	K0828	0(3)	L0457	0(3)
J3485	160(3)	J7313	38(3)	J7637	0(3)	J9030	50(3)	J9260	20(3)	K0040	0(3)	K0829	0(3)	L0458	0(3)
J3486	4(3)	J7315	2(3)	J7638	0(3)	J9032	300(3)	J9261	80(3)	K0041	0(3)	K0830	0(3)	L0460	0(3)
J3489	5(3)	J7316	3(2)	J7639	3(3)	J9033	300(3)	J9262	700(3)	K0042	0(3)	K0831	0(3)	L0462	0(3)
J3520	0(3)	J7318	120(3)	J7640	0(3)	J9034	360(3)	J9263	700(3)	K0043	0(3)	K0835	0(3)	L0464	0(3)
J3530	0(3)	J7320	50(3)	J7641	0(3)	J9035	170(3)	J9264	600(3)	K0044	0(3)	K0836	0(3)	L0466	0(3)
J3535	0(3)	J7321	2(2)	J7642	0(3)	J9036	360(3)	J9266	2(3)	K0045	0(3)	K0837	0(3)	L0467	0(3)
J3570	0(3)	J7322	48(3)	J7643	0(3)	J9039	210(3)	J9267	750(3)	K0046	0(3)	K0838	0(3)	L0468	0(3)
J7030	5(3)	J7323	2(2)	J7644	3(3)	J9040	4(3)	J9268	1(3)	K0047	0(3)	K0839	0(3)	L0469	0(3)
J7040	6(3)	J7324	2(2)	J7645	0(3)	J9041	35(3)	J9270	0(3)	K0050	0(3)	K0840	0(3)	L0470	0(3)
J7042	6(3)	J7325	96(3)	J7647	0(3)	J9042	200(3)	J9271	300(3)	K0051	0(3)	K0841	0(3)	L0472	0(3)
J7050	10(3)	J7326	2(2)	J7648	0(3)	J9043	60(3)	J9280	12(3)	K0052	0(3)	K0842	0(3)	L0480	0(3)
J7060	10(3)	J7327	2(2)	J7649	0(3)	J9044	35(3)	J9285	200(3)	K0053	0(3)	K0843	0(3)	L0482	0(3)
J7070	4(3)	J7328	336(3)	J7650	0(3)	J9045	22(3)	J9293	8(3)	K0056	0(3)	K0848	0(3)	L0484	0(3)
J7100	2(3)	J7329	50(2)	J7657	0(3)	J9047	160(3)	J9295	800(3)	K0065	0(3)	K0849	0(3)	L0486	0(3)
J7110	2(3)	J7330	1(3)	J7658	0(3)	J9050	6(3)	J9299	480(3)	K0069	0(3)	K0850	0(3)	L0488	0(3)
J7120	4(3)	J7336	1120(3)	J7659	0(3)	J9055	120(3)	J9301	100(3)	K0070	0(3)	K0851	0(3)	L0490	0(3)
J7121	4(3)	J7340	1(3)	J7660	0(3)	J9057	60(3)	J9302	200(3)	K0071	0(3)	K0852	0(3)	L0491	0(3)
J7131	500(3)	J7342	10(3)	J7665	0(3)	J9060	24(3)	J9303	90(3)	K0072	0(3)	K0853	0(3)	L0492	0(3)
J7170	1800(3)	J7345	200(3)	J7667	0(3)	J9065	100(3)	J9305	150(3)	K0073	0(3)	K0854	0(3)	L0621	0(3)
J7175	9000(1)	J7500	0(3)	J7668	0(3)	J9070	55(3)	J9306	840(3)	K0077	0(3)	K0855	0(3)	L0622	0(3)
J7177	10500(3)	J7501	1(3)	J7669	0(3)	J9098	5(3)	J9307	60(3)	K0098	0(3)	K0856	0(3)	L0623	0(3)
J7178	7700(1)	J7502	0(3)	J7670	0(3)	J9100	120(3)	J9308	280(3)	K0105	0(3)	K0857	0(3)	L0624	0(3)
J7179	7500(1)	J7503	0(3)	J7674	100(3)	J9120	5(3)	J9311	160(3)	K0108	0(3)	K0858	0(3)	L0625	0(3)
J7180	6000(1)	J7504	15(3)	J7676	0(3)	J9130	24(3)	J9312	150(3)	K0195	0(3)	K0859	0(3)	L0626	0(3)
J7181	3850(1)	J7505	1(3)	J7677	175(3)	J9145	240(3)	J9315	40(3)	K0455	0(3)	K0860	0(3)	L0627	0(3)
J7182	22000(1)	J7507	0(3)	J7680	0(3)	J9150	12(3)	J9320	4(3)	K0462	0(3)	K0861	0(3)	L0628	0(3)
J7183	7500(1)	J7508	0(3)	J7681	0(3)	J9151	10(3)	J9325	400(3)	K0553	0(3)	K0862	0(3)	L0629	0(3)
J7185	22000(1)	J7509	0(3)	J7682	2(3)	J9153	132(3)	J9328	400(3)	K0554	0(3)	K0863	0(3)	L0630	0(3)
J7186	7500(1)	J7510	0(3)	J7683	0(3)	J9155	240(3)	J9330	50(3)	K0602	0(3)	K0864	0(3)	L0631	0(3)
J7187	7500(1)	J7511	9(3)	J7684	0(3)	J9160	7(3)	J9340	4(3)	K0604	0(3)	K0868	0(3)	L0632	0(3)
J7188	22000(1)	J7512	0(3)	J7685	0(3)	J9165	0(3)	J9351	120(3)	K0605	0(3)	K0869	0(3)	L0633	0(3)
J7189	13000(1)	J7513	0(3)	J7686	1(3)	J9171	240(3)	J9352	40(3)	K0606	0(3)	K0870	0(3)	L0634	0(3)
J7190	22000(1)	J7515	0(3)	J7699	1(3)	J9173	150(3)	J9354	600(3)	K0607	0(3)	K0871	0(3)	L0635	0(3)
J7191	0(3)	J7516	1(3)	J7799	2(3)	J9175	10(3)	J9355	105(3)	K0608	0(3)	K0877	0(3)	L0636	0(3)
J7192	22000(1)	J7517	0(3)	J7999	2(3)	J9176	3000(3)	J9356	60(3)	K0609	0(3)	K0878	0(3)	L0637	0(3)
J7193	4000(1)	J7518	0(3)	J8498	0(3)	J9178	150(3)	J9357	4(3)	K0669	0(3)	K0879	0(3)	L0638	0(3)
J7194	9000(1)	J7520	0(3)	J8499	0(3)	J9179	50(3)	J9360	40(3)	K0672	0(3)	K0880	0(3)	L0639	0(3)
J7195	6000(1)	J7525	2(3)	J8501	0(3)	J9181	100(3)	J9370	4(3)	K0730	0(3)	K0884	0(3)	L0640	0(3)
J7196	175(3)	J7527	0(3)	J8510	0(3)	J9185	2(3)	J9371	5(3)	K0733	0(3)	K0885	0(3)	L0641	0(3)
J7197	6300(1)	J7599	1(3)	J8515	0(3)	J9190	20(3)	J9390	36(3)	K0738	0(3)	K0886	0(3)	L0642	0(3)
J7198	6000(1)	J7604	0(3)	J8520	0(3)	J9200	5(3)	J9395	20(3)	K0740	0(3)	K0890	0(3)	L0643	0(3)
J7200	20000(1)	J7605	2(3)	J8521	0(3)	J9201	20(3)	J9400	500(3)	K0743	0(3)	K0891	0(3)	L0648	0(3)
J7201	9000(1)	J7606	2(3)	J8530	0(3)	J9202	3(3)	J9600	4(3)	K0744	0(3)	K0898	1(2)	L0649	0(3)
J7202	11550(1)	J7607	0(3)	J8540	0(3)	J9203	180(3)	K0001	0(3)	K0745	0(3)	K0899	0(3)	L0650	0(3)
J7203	12000(1)	J7608	3(3)	J8560	0(3)	J9205	215(3)	K0002	0(3)	K0746	0(3)	K0900	0(3)	L0651	0(3)
J7205	9750(1)	J7609	0(3)	J8562	0(3)	J9206	42(3)	K0003	0(3)	K0800	0(3)	L0112	0(3)	L0700	0(3)

CPT	MUE
L0710	0(3)
L0810	0(3)
L0820	0(3)
L0830	0(3)
L0859	0(3)
L0861	0(3)
L0970	0(3)
L0972	0(3)
L0974	0(3)
L0976	0(3)
L0978	0(3)
L0980	0(3)
L0982	0(3)
L0984	0(3)
L0999	0(3)
L1000	0(3)
L1001	0(3)
L1005	0(3)
L1010	0(3)
L1020	0(3)
L1025	0(3)
L1030	0(3)
L1040	0(3)
L1050	0(3)
L1060	0(3)
L1070	0(3)
L1080	0(3)
L1085	0(3)
L1090	0(3)
L1100	0(3)
L1110	0(3)
L1120	0(3)
L1200	0(3)
L1210	0(3)
L1220	0(3)
L1230	0(3)
L1240	0(3)
L1250	0(3)
L1260	0(3)
L1270	0(3)
L1280	0(3)
L1290	0(3)
L1300	0(3)
L1310	0(3)
L1499	1(3)
L1600	0(3)
L1610	0(3)
L1620	0(3)
L1630	0(3)
L1640	0(3)
L1650	0(3)
L1652	0(3)
L1660	0(3)
L1680	0(3)
L1685	0(3)
L1686	0(3)
L1690	0(3)
L1700	0(3)
L1710	0(3)
L1720	0(3)
L1730	0(3)
L1755	0(3)
L1810	0(3)
L1812	0(3)
L1820	0(3)

CPT	MUE
L1830	0(3)
L1831	0(3)
L1832	0(3)
L1833	0(3)
L1834	0(3)
L1836	0(3)
L1840	0(3)
L1843	0(3)
L1844	0(3)
L1845	0(3)
L1846	0(3)
L1847	0(3)
L1848	0(3)
L1850	0(3)
L1851	0(3)
L1852	0(3)
L1860	0(3)
L1900	0(3)
L1902	0(3)
L1904	0(3)
L1906	0(3)
L1907	0(3)
L1910	0(3)
L1920	0(3)
L1930	0(3)
L1932	0(3)
L1940	0(3)
L1945	0(3)
L1950	0(3)
L1951	0(3)
L1960	0(3)
L1970	0(3)
L1971	0(3)
L1980	0(3)
L1990	0(3)
L2000	0(3)
L2005	0(3)
L2010	0(3)
L2020	0(3)
L2030	0(3)
L2034	0(3)
L2035	0(3)
L2036	0(3)
L2037	0(3)
L2038	0(3)
L2040	0(3)
L2050	0(3)
L2060	0(3)
L2070	0(3)
L2080	0(3)
L2090	0(3)
L2106	0(3)
L2108	0(3)
L2112	0(3)
L2114	0(3)
L2116	0(3)
L2126	0(3)
L2128	0(3)
L2132	0(3)
L2134	0(3)
L2136	0(3)
L2180	0(3)
L2182	0(3)
L2184	0(3)
L2186	0(3)

CPT	MUE
L2188	0(3)
L2190	0(3)
L2192	0(3)
L2200	0(3)
L2210	0(3)
L2220	0(3)
L2230	0(3)
L2232	0(3)
L2240	0(3)
L2250	0(3)
L2260	0(3)
L2265	0(3)
L2270	0(3)
L2275	0(3)
L2280	0(3)
L2300	0(3)
L2310	0(3)
L2320	0(3)
L2330	0(3)
L2335	0(3)
L2340	0(3)
L2350	0(3)
L2360	0(3)
L2370	0(3)
L2375	0(3)
L2380	0(3)
L2385	0(3)
L2387	0(3)
L2390	0(3)
L2395	0(3)
L2397	0(3)
L2405	0(3)
L2415	0(3)
L2425	0(3)
L2430	0(3)
L2492	0(3)
L2500	0(3)
L2510	0(3)
L2520	0(3)
L2525	0(3)
L2526	0(3)
L2530	0(3)
L2540	0(3)
L2550	0(3)
L2570	0(3)
L2580	0(3)
L2600	0(3)
L2610	0(3)
L2620	0(3)
L2622	0(3)
L2624	0(3)
L2627	0(3)
L2628	0(3)
L2630	0(3)
L2640	0(3)
L2650	0(3)
L2660	0(3)
L2670	0(3)
L2680	0(3)
L2750	0(3)
L2755	0(3)
L2760	0(3)
L2768	0(3)
L2780	0(3)
L2785	0(3)

CPT	MUE
L2795	0(3)
L2800	0(3)
L2810	0(3)
L2820	0(3)
L2830	0(3)
L2840	0(3)
L2850	0(3)
L2861	0(3)
L2999	0(3)
L3000	0(3)
L3001	0(3)
L3002	0(3)
L3003	0(3)
L3010	0(3)
L3020	0(3)
L3030	0(3)
L3031	0(3)
L3040	0(3)
L3050	0(3)
L3060	0(3)
L3070	0(3)
L3080	0(3)
L3090	0(3)
L3100	0(3)
L3140	0(3)
L3150	0(3)
L3160	0(3)
L3170	0(3)
L3201	0(3)
L3202	0(3)
L3203	0(3)
L3204	0(3)
L3206	0(3)
L3207	0(3)
L3208	0(3)
L3209	0(3)
L3211	0(3)
L3212	0(3)
L3213	0(3)
L3214	0(3)
L3215	0(3)
L3216	0(3)
L3217	0(3)
L3219	0(3)
L3221	0(3)
L3222	0(3)
L3224	0(3)
L3225	0(3)
L3230	0(3)
L3250	0(3)
L3251	0(3)
L3252	0(3)
L3253	0(3)
L3254	0(3)
L3255	0(3)
L3257	0(3)
L3260	0(3)
L3265	0(3)
L3300	0(3)
L3310	0(3)
L3320	0(3)
L3330	0(3)
L3332	0(3)
L3334	0(3)
L3340	0(3)

CPT	MUE
L3350	0(3)
L3360	0(3)
L3370	0(3)
L3380	0(3)
L3390	0(3)
L3400	0(3)
L3410	0(3)
L3420	0(3)
L3430	0(3)
L3440	0(3)
L3450	0(3)
L3455	0(3)
L3460	0(3)
L3465	0(3)
L3470	0(3)
L3480	0(3)
L3485	0(3)
L3500	0(3)
L3510	0(3)
L3520	0(3)
L3530	0(3)
L3540	0(3)
L3550	0(3)
L3560	0(3)
L3570	0(3)
L3580	0(3)
L3590	0(3)
L3595	0(3)
L3600	0(3)
L3610	0(3)
L3620	0(3)
L3630	0(3)
L3640	0(3)
L3649	0(3)
L3650	0(3)
L3660	0(3)
L3670	0(3)
L3671	0(3)
L3674	0(3)
L3675	0(3)
L3677	0(3)
L3678	0(3)
L3702	0(3)
L3710	0(3)
L3720	0(3)
L3730	0(3)
L3740	0(3)
L3760	0(3)
L3761	0(3)
L3762	0(3)
L3763	0(3)
L3764	0(3)
L3765	0(3)
L3766	0(3)
L3806	0(3)
L3807	0(3)
L3808	0(3)
L3809	0(3)
L3891	0(3)
L3900	0(3)
L3901	0(3)
L3904	0(3)
L3905	0(3)
L3906	0(3)
L3908	0(3)

CPT	MUE
L3912	0(3)
L3913	0(3)
L3915	0(3)
L3916	0(3)
L3917	0(3)
L3918	0(3)
L3919	0(3)
L3921	0(3)
L3923	0(3)
L3924	0(3)
L3925	0(3)
L3927	0(3)
L3929	0(3)
L3930	0(3)
L3931	0(3)
L3933	0(3)
L3935	0(3)
L3956	0(3)
L3960	0(3)
L3961	0(3)
L3962	0(3)
L3967	0(3)
L3971	0(3)
L3973	0(3)
L3975	0(3)
L3976	0(3)
L3977	0(3)
L3978	0(3)
L3980	0(3)
L3981	0(3)
L3982	0(3)
L3984	0(3)
L3995	0(3)
L3999	0(3)
L4000	0(3)
L4002	0(3)
L4010	0(3)
L4020	0(3)
L4030	0(3)
L4040	0(3)
L4045	0(3)
L4050	0(3)
L4055	0(3)
L4060	0(3)
L4070	0(3)
L4080	0(3)
L4090	0(3)
L4100	0(3)
L4110	0(3)
L4130	0(3)
L4205	0(3)
L4210	0(3)
L4350	0(3)
L4360	0(3)
L4361	0(3)
L4370	0(3)
L4386	0(3)
L4387	0(3)
L4392	0(3)
L4394	0(3)
L4396	0(3)
L4397	0(3)
L4398	0(3)
L4631	0(3)
L5000	0(3)

CPT	MUE
L5010	0(3)
L5020	0(3)
L5050	0(3)
L5060	0(3)
L5100	0(3)
L5105	0(3)
L5150	0(3)
L5160	0(3)
L5200	0(3)
L5210	0(3)
L5220	0(3)
L5230	0(3)
L5250	0(3)
L5270	0(3)
L5280	0(3)
L5301	0(3)
L5312	0(3)
L5321	0(3)
L5331	0(3)
L5341	0(3)
L5400	0(3)
L5410	0(3)
L5420	0(3)
L5430	0(3)
L5450	0(3)
L5460	0(3)
L5500	0(3)
L5505	0(3)
L5510	0(3)
L5520	0(3)
L5530	0(3)
L5535	0(3)
L5540	0(3)
L5560	0(3)
L5570	0(3)
L5580	0(3)
L5585	0(3)
L5590	0(3)
L5595	0(3)
L5600	0(3)
L5610	0(3)
L5611	0(3)
L5613	0(3)
L5614	0(3)
L5616	0(3)
L5617	0(3)
L5618	0(3)
L5620	0(3)
L5622	0(3)
L5624	0(3)
L5626	0(3)
L5628	0(3)
L5629	0(3)
L5630	0(3)
L5631	0(3)
L5632	0(3)
L5634	0(3)
L5636	0(3)
L5637	0(3)
L5638	0(3)
L5639	0(3)
L5640	0(3)
L5642	0(3)
L5643	0(3)
L5644	0(3)

CPT	MUE
L5645	0(3)
L5646	0(3)
L5647	0(3)
L5648	0(3)
L5649	0(3)
L5650	0(3)
L5651	0(3)
L5652	0(3)
L5653	0(3)
L5654	0(3)
L5655	0(3)
L5656	0(3)
L5658	0(3)
L5661	0(3)
L5665	0(3)
L5666	0(3)
L5668	0(3)
L5670	0(3)
L5671	0(3)
L5672	0(3)
L5673	0(3)
L5676	0(3)
L5677	0(3)
L5678	0(3)
L5679	0(3)
L5680	0(3)
L5681	0(3)
L5682	0(3)
L5683	0(3)
L5684	0(3)
L5685	0(3)
L5686	0(3)
L5688	0(3)
L5690	0(3)
L5692	0(3)
L5694	0(3)
L5695	0(3)
L5696	0(3)
L5697	0(3)
L5698	0(3)
L5699	0(3)
L5700	0(3)
L5701	0(3)
L5702	0(3)
L5703	0(3)
L5704	0(3)
L5705	0(3)
L5706	0(3)
L5707	0(3)
L5710	0(3)
L5711	0(3)
L5712	0(3)
L5714	0(3)
L5716	0(3)
L5718	0(3)
L5722	0(3)
L5724	0(3)
L5726	0(3)
L5728	0(3)
L5780	0(3)
L5781	0(3)
L5782	0(3)
L5785	0(3)
L5790	0(3)
L5795	0(3)

CPT	MUE	CPT	MUE	CPT	MUE	CPT	MUE	CPT	MUE	CPT	MUE	CPT	MUE	CPT	MUE
L5810	0(3)	L6300	0(3)	L6692	0(3)	L7400	0(3)	L8605	4(3)	P9022	2(3)	Q0477	1(1)	Q4018	2(3)
L5811	0(3)	L6310	0(3)	L6693	0(3)	L7401	0(3)	L8606	5(3)	P9023	2(3)	Q0478	1(3)	Q4021	2(3)
L5812	0(3)	L6320	0(3)	L6694	0(3)	L7402	0(3)	L8607	20(3)	P9031	12(3)	Q0479	1(3)	Q4025	1(3)
L5814	0(3)	L6350	0(3)	L6695	0(3)	L7403	0(3)	L8609	1(3)	P9032	12(3)	Q0480	1(3)	Q4026	1(3)
L5816	0(3)	L6360	0(3)	L6696	0(3)	L7404	0(3)	L8610	1(3)	P9033	12(3)	Q0481	1(2)	Q4027	1(3)
L5818	0(3)	L6370	0(3)	L6697	0(3)	L7405	0(3)	L8612	1(3)	P9034	2(3)	Q0482	1(3)	Q4028	1(3)
L5822	0(3)	L6380	0(3)	L6698	0(3)	L7499	0(3)	L8613	1(3)	P9035	2(3)	Q0483	1(3)	Q4030	2(3)
L5824	0(3)	L6382	0(3)	L6703	0(3)	L7510	4(3)	L8614	1(3)	P9036	2(3)	Q0484	1(3)	Q4037	2(3)
L5826	0(3)	L6384	0(3)	L6704	0(3)	L7600	0(3)	L8615	2(3)	P9037	2(3)	Q0485	1(3)	Q4042	2(3)
L5828	0(3)	L6386	0(3)	L6706	0(3)	L7700	0(3)	L8616	2(3)	P9038	2(3)	Q0486	1(3)	Q4046	2(3)
L5830	0(3)	L6388	0(3)	L6707	0(3)	L7900	0(3)	L8617	2(3)	P9039	2(3)	Q0487	1(3)	Q4050	2(3)
L5840	0(3)	L6400	0(3)	L6708	0(3)	L7902	0(3)	L8618	2(3)	P9040	3(3)	Q0488	1(3)	Q4051	2(3)
L5845	0(3)	L6450	0(3)	L6709	0(3)	L8000	0(3)	L8619	2(3)	P9041	5(3)	Q0489	1(3)	Q4074	3(3)
L5848	0(3)	L6500	0(3)	L6711	0(3)	L8001	0(3)	L8621	360(3)	P9043	5(3)	Q0490	1(3)	Q4081	100(3)
L5850	0(3)	L6550	0(3)	L6712	0(3)	L8002	0(3)	L8622	2(3)	P9044	10(3)	Q0491	1(3)	Q4103	0(3)
L5855	0(3)	L6570	0(3)	L6713	0(3)	L8010	0(3)	L8625	1(3)	P9045	20(3)	Q0492	1(3)	Q5101	1500(3)
L5856	0(3)	L6580	0(3)	L6714	0(3)	L8015	0(3)	L8627	2(2)	P9046	25(3)	Q0493	1(3)	Q5103	150(3)
L5857	0(3)	L6582	0(3)	L6715	0(3)	L8020	0(3)	L8628	2(2)	P9047	20(3)	Q0494	1(3)	Q5104	150(3)
L5858	0(3)	L6584	0(3)	L6721	0(3)	L8030	0(3)	L8629	2(2)	P9048	1(3)	Q0495	1(3)	Q5105	100(3)
L5859	0(3)	L6586	0(3)	L6722	0(3)	L8031	0(3)	L8631	1(3)	P9050	1(3)	Q0496	1(3)	Q5106	60(3)
L5910	0(3)	L6588	0(3)	L6805	0(3)	L8032	0(3)	L8641	4(3)	P9051	2(3)	Q0497	2(3)	Q5107	170(3)
L5920	0(3)	L6590	0(3)	L6810	0(3)	L8035	0(3)	L8642	2(3)	P9052	2(3)	Q0498	1(3)	Q5108	12(3)
L5925	0(3)	L6600	0(3)	L6880	0(3)	L8039	0(3)	L8658	2(3)	P9053	2(3)	Q0499	1(3)	Q5109	150(3)
L5930	0(3)	L6605	0(3)	L6881	0(3)	L8040	0(3)	L8659	2(3)	P9054	2(3)	Q0501	1(3)	Q5110	1500(3)
L5940	0(3)	L6610	0(3)	L6882	0(3)	L8041	0(3)	L8670	2(3)	P9055	2(3)	Q0502	1(3)	Q5111	12(3)
L5950	0(3)	L6611	0(3)	L6883	0(3)	L8042	0(3)	L8679	1(3)	P9056	2(3)	Q0503	3(3)	Q5112	120(3)
L5960	0(3)	L6615	0(3)	L6884	0(3)	L8043	0(3)	L8681	1(3)	P9057	2(3)	Q0504	1(3)	Q5113	120(3)
L5961	0(3)	L6616	0(3)	L6885	0(3)	L8044	0(3)	L8682	2(3)	P9058	2(3)	Q0506	8(3)	Q5114	120(3)
L5962	0(3)	L6620	0(3)	L6890	0(3)	L8045	0(3)	L8683	1(3)	P9059	2(3)	Q0507	1(3)	Q5115	120(3)
L5964	0(3)	L6621	0(3)	L6895	0(3)	L8046	0(3)	L8684	1(3)	P9060	2(3)	Q0508	4(3)	Q9950	5(3)
L5966	0(3)	L6623	0(3)	L6900	0(3)	L8047	0(3)	L8685	1(3)	P9070	2(3)	Q0509	2(3)	Q9951	0(3)
L5968	0(3)	L6624	0(3)	L6905	0(3)	L8048	1(3)	L8686	2(3)	P9071	2(3)	Q0510	0(3)	Q9953	10(3)
L5969	0(3)	L6625	0(3)	L6910	0(3)	L8049	0(3)	L8687	1(3)	P9073	2(3)	Q0511	0(3)	Q9954	18(3)
L5970	0(3)	L6628	0(3)	L6915	0(3)	L8300	0(3)	L8688	1(3)	P9100	2(3)	Q0512	0(3)	Q9955	0(3)
L5971	0(3)	L6629	0(3)	L6920	0(3)	L8310	0(3)	L8689	1(3)	P9603	300(3)	Q0513	0(3)	Q9956	9(3)
L5972	0(3)	L6630	0(3)	L6925	0(3)	L8320	0(3)	L8690	2(2)	P9604	2(3)	Q0514	0(3)	Q9957	3(3)
L5973	0(3)	L6632	0(3)	L6930	0(3)	L8330	0(3)	L8691	1(3)	P9612	1(3)	Q0515	0(3)	Q9958	300(3)
L5974	0(3)	L6635	0(3)	L6935	0(3)	L8400	0(3)	L8692	0(3)	P9615	1(3)	Q1004	2(2)	Q9959	0(3)
L5975	0(3)	L6637	0(3)	L6940	0(3)	L8410	0(3)	L8693	1(3)	Q0035	1(3)	Q1005	2(2)	Q9960	250(3)
L5976	0(3)	L6638	0(3)	L6945	0(3)	L8415	0(3)	L8694	1(3)	Q0081	1(3)	Q2004	1(3)	Q9961	200(3)
L5978	0(3)	L6640	0(3)	L6950	0(3)	L8417	0(3)	L8695	1(3)	Q0083	1(3)	Q2009	100(3)	Q9962	150(3)
L5979	0(3)	L6641	0(3)	L6955	0(3)	L8420	0(3)	L8696	1(3)	Q0084	1(3)	Q2017	12(3)	Q9963	240(3)
L5980	0(3)	L6642	0(3)	L6960	0(3)	L8430	0(3)	L8701	0(3)	Q0085	1(3)	Q2026	45(3)	Q9964	0(3)
L5981	0(3)	L6645	0(3)	L6965	0(3)	L8435	0(3)	L8702	0(3)	Q0091	1(3)	Q2028	1470(3)	Q9966	250(3)
L5982	0(3)	L6646	0(3)	L6970	0(3)	L8440	0(3)	M0075	0(3)	Q0111	2(3)	Q2034	1(2)	Q9967	300(3)
L5984	0(3)	L6647	0(3)	L6975	0(3)	L8460	0(3)	M0076	0(3)	Q0112	3(3)	Q2035	1(2)	Q9969	3(3)
L5985	0(3)	L6648	0(3)	L7007	0(3)	L8465	0(3)	M0100	0(3)	Q0113	1(3)	Q2036	1(2)	Q9982	1(3)
L5986	0(3)	L6650	0(3)	L7008	0(3)	L8470	0(3)	M0300	0(3)	Q0114	1(3)	Q2037	1(2)	Q9983	1(3)
L5987	0(3)	L6655	0(3)	L7009	0(3)	L8480	0(3)	M0301	0(3)	Q0115	1(3)	Q2038	1(2)	Q9991	1(3)
L5988	0(3)	L6660	0(3)	L7040	0(3)	L8485	0(3)	P2028	1(2)	Q0138	510(3)	Q2039	1(2)	Q9992	1(3)
L5990	0(3)	L6665	0(3)	L7045	0(3)	L8499	1(3)	P2029	1(2)	Q0139	510(3)	Q2043	1(2)	R0070	2(3)
L5999	0(3)	L6670	0(3)	L7170	0(3)	L8500	0(3)	P2031	0(3)	Q0144	0(3)	Q2049	14(3)	R0075	2(3)
L6000	0(3)	L6672	0(3)	L7180	0(3)	L8501	0(3)	P2033	1(2)	Q0161	0(3)	Q2050	14(3)	R0076	1(3)
L6010	0(3)	L6675	0(3)	L7181	0(3)	L8505	0(3)	P2038	1(2)	Q0162	0(3)	Q2052	1(3)	V2020	0(3)
L6020	0(3)	L6676	0(3)	L7185	0(3)	L8507	0(3)	P3000	1(3)	Q0163	0(3)	Q3014	1(3)	V2025	0(3)
L6026	0(3)	L6677	0(3)	L7186	0(3)	L8509	1(3)	P3001	1(3)	Q0164	0(3)	Q3027	30(3)	V2100	0(3)
L6050	0(3)	L6680	0(3)	L7190	0(3)	L8510	0(3)	P7001	0(3)	Q0166	0(3)	Q3028	0(3)	V2101	0(3)
L6055	0(3)	L6682	0(3)	L7191	0(3)	L8511	1(3)	P9010	2(3)	Q0167	0(3)	Q3031	1(3)	V2102	0(3)
L6100	0(3)	L6684	0(3)	L7259	0(3)	L8512	1(3)	P9011	2(3)	Q0169	0(3)	Q4001	1(3)	V2103	0(3)
L6110	0(3)	L6686	0(3)	L7360	0(3)	L8513	1(3)	P9012	8(3)	Q0173	0(3)	Q4002	1(3)	V2104	0(3)
L6120	0(3)	L6687	0(3)	L7362	0(3)	L8514	1(3)	P9016	3(3)	Q0174	0(3)	Q4003	2(3)	V2105	0(3)
L6130	0(3)	L6688	0(3)	L7364	0(3)	L8515	1(3)	P9017	2(3)	Q0175	0(3)	Q4004	2(3)	V2106	0(3)
L6200	0(3)	L6689	0(3)	L7366	0(3)	L8600	2(3)	P9019	2(3)	Q0177	0(3)	Q4012	2(3)	V2107	0(3)
L6205	0(3)	L6690	0(3)	L7367	0(3)	L8603	4(3)	P9020	2(3)	Q0180	0(3)	Q4013	2(3)	V2108	0(3)
L6250	0(3)	L6691	0(3)	L7368	0(3)	L8604	3(3)	P9021	3(3)	Q0181	0(3)	Q4014	2(3)	V2109	0(3)

CPT	MUE
V2110	0(3)
V2111	0(3)
V2112	0(3)
V2113	0(3)
V2114	0(3)
V2115	0(3)
V2118	0(3)
V2121	0(3)
V2199	2(3)
V2200	0(3)
V2201	0(3)
V2202	0(3)
V2203	0(3)
V2204	0(3)
V2205	0(3)
V2206	0(3)
V2207	0(3)
V2208	0(3)
V2209	0(3)
V2210	0(3)
V2211	0(3)
V2212	0(3)
V2213	0(3)
V2214	0(3)

CPT	MUE
V2215	0(3)
V2218	0(3)
V2219	0(3)
V2220	0(3)
V2221	0(3)
V2299	0(3)
V2300	0(3)
V2301	0(3)
V2302	0(3)
V2303	0(3)
V2304	0(3)
V2305	0(3)
V2306	0(3)
V2307	0(3)
V2308	0(3)
V2309	0(3)
V2310	0(3)
V2311	0(3)
V2312	0(3)
V2313	0(3)
V2314	0(3)
V2315	0(3)
V2318	0(3)
V2319	0(3)

CPT	MUE
V2320	0(3)
V2321	0(3)
V2399	0(3)
V2410	0(3)
V2430	0(3)
V2499	2(3)
V2500	0(3)
V2501	0(3)
V2502	0(3)
V2503	0(3)
V2510	0(3)
V2511	0(3)
V2512	0(3)
V2513	0(3)
V2520	2(3)
V2521	2(3)
V2522	2(3)
V2523	2(3)
V2530	0(3)
V2531	0(3)
V2599	2(3)
V2600	0(2)
V2610	0(2)
V2615	0(2)

CPT	MUE
V2623	0(3)
V2624	0(3)
V2625	0(3)
V2626	0(3)
V2627	0(3)
V2628	0(3)
V2629	0(3)
V2630	2(2)
V2631	2(2)
V2632	2(2)
V2700	0(3)
V2702	0(3)
V2710	0(3)
V2715	0(3)
V2718	0(3)
V2730	0(3)
V2744	0(3)
V2745	0(3)
V2750	0(3)
V2755	0(3)
V2756	0(3)
V2760	0(3)
V2761	0(2)
V2762	0(3)

CPT	MUE
V2770	0(3)
V2780	0(3)
V2781	0(2)
V2782	0(3)
V2783	0(3)
V2784	0(3)
V2785	2(2)
V2786	0(3)
V2787	0(3)
V2788	0(3)
V2790	1(3)
V2797	0(3)
V5008	0(3)
V5010	0(3)
V5011	0(3)
V5014	0(3)
V5020	0(3)
V5030	0(3)
V5040	0(3)
V5050	0(3)
V5060	0(3)
V5070	0(3)
V5080	0(3)
V5090	0(3)

CPT	MUE
V5095	0(3)
V5100	0(3)
V5110	0(3)
V5120	0(3)
V5130	0(3)
V5140	0(3)
V5150	0(3)
V5160	0(3)
V5171	0(3)
V5172	0(3)
V5181	0(3)
V5190	0(3)
V5200	0(3)
V5211	0(3)
V5212	0(3)
V5213	0(3)
V5214	0(3)
V5215	0(3)
V5221	0(3)
V5230	0(3)
V5240	0(3)
V5241	0(3)
V5242	0(3)
V5243	0(3)

CPT	MUE
V5244	0(3)
V5245	0(3)
V5246	0(3)
V5247	0(3)
V5248	0(3)
V5249	0(3)
V5250	0(3)
V5251	0(3)
V5252	0(3)
V5253	0(3)
V5254	0(3)
V5255	0(3)
V5256	0(3)
V5257	0(3)
V5258	0(3)
V5259	0(3)
V5260	0(3)
V5261	0(3)
V5262	0(3)
V5263	0(3)
V5264	0(3)
V5265	0(3)
V5266	0(3)
V5267	0(3)

CPT	MUE
V5268	0(3)
V5269	0(3)
V5270	0(3)
V5271	0(3)
V5272	0(3)
V5273	0(3)
V5274	0(3)
V5275	0(3)
V5281	0(3)
V5282	0(3)
V5283	0(3)
V5284	0(3)
V5285	0(3)
V5286	0(3)
V5287	0(3)
V5288	0(3)
V5289	0(3)
V5290	0(3)
V5298	0(3)
V5299	1(3)
V5336	0(3)
V5362	0(3)
V5363	0(3)
V5364	0(3)

OPPS

CPT	MUE
0001U	1(2)
0002M	1(3)
0002U	1(2)
0003M	1(3)
0003U	1(2)
0004M	1(2)
0005U	1(2)
0006M	1(2)
0006U	1(2)
0007M	1(2)
0007U	1(2)
0008U	1(3)
0009M	1(2)
0009U	2(3)
0010U	2(3)
0011M	1(2)
0011U	1(2)
0012M	1(2)
0012U	1(2)
0013M	1(2)
0013U	1(3)
0014U	1(3)
0016U	1(3)
0017U	1(3)
0018U	1(1)
0019U	1(3)
0021U	1(2)
0022U	2(3)
0023U	1(2)
0024U	1(2)
0025U	1(2)
0026U	1(3)
0027U	1(2)
0029U	1(2)
0030U	1(2)
0031U	1(2)
0032U	1(2)
0033U	1(2)
0034U	1(2)
0035U	1(2)
0036U	1(3)
0037U	1(3)
0038U	1(2)
0039U	1(2)
0040U	1(2)
0041U	1(2)
0042T	1(3)
0042U	1(2)
0043U	1(2)
0044U	1(2)
0045U	1(3)
0046U	1(3)
0047U	1(3)
0048U	1(3)
0049U	1(3)
0050U	1(3)
0051U	1(2)
0052U	1(2)
0053U	1(3)
0054T	1(3)
0054U	1(2)
0055T	1(3)
0055U	1(2)
0056U	1(3)

CPT	MUE
0057U	1(3)
0058T	1(2)
0058U	1(2)
0059U	1(2)
0060U	1(2)
0061U	1(2)
0062U	1(2)
0063U	1(2)
0064U	2(3)
0065U	2(3)
0066U	1(3)
0067U	2(3)
0068U	1(3)
0069U	1(3)
0070U	1(2)
0071T	1(2)
0071U	1(2)
0072T	1(2)
0072U	1(2)
0073U	1(2)
0074U	1(2)
0075T	1(2)
0075U	1(2)
0076T	1(2)
0076U	1(2)
0077U	2(2)
0078U	1(2)
0079U	0(3)
0080U	1(2)
0081U	1(3)
0082U	1(2)
0083U	1(3)
0085T	0(3)
0095T	1(3)
0098T	2(3)
0100T	1(2)
0101T	1(3)
0102T	2(2)
0106T	4(2)
0107T	4(2)
0108T	4(2)
0109T	4(2)
0110T	4(2)
0111T	1(3)
0126T	1(3)
0163T	1(3)
0164T	4(2)
0165T	4(2)
0174T	1(3)
0175T	1(3)
0184T	1(3)
0191T	2(2)
0198T	2(2)
01996	1(2)
0200T	1(2)
0201T	1(2)
0202T	1(3)
0205T	3(3)
0206T	1(3)
0207T	2(2)
0208T	1(3)
0209T	1(3)
0210T	1(3)
0211T	1(3)

CPT	MUE
0212T	1(3)
0213T	1(2)
0214T	1(2)
0215T	1(2)
0216T	1(2)
0217T	1(2)
0218T	1(2)
0219T	1(2)
0220T	1(2)
0221T	1(2)
0222T	1(3)
0228T	1(2)
0229T	2(3)
0230T	1(2)
0231T	2(3)
0232T	1(3)
0234T	2(2)
0235T	2(3)
0236T	1(2)
0237T	2(3)
0238T	2(3)
0249T	1(2)
0253T	1(3)
0254T	2(2)
0263T	1(3)
0264T	1(3)
0265T	1(3)
0266T	1(2)
0267T	1(3)
0268T	1(3)
0269T	1(2)
0270T	1(3)
0271T	1(3)
0272T	1(3)
0273T	1(3)
0274T	1(2)
0275T	1(2)
0278T	1(3)
0290T	1(3)
0295T	1(2)
0296T	1(2)
0297T	1(2)
0298T	1(2)
0308T	1(3)
0312T	1(3)
0313T	1(3)
0314T	1(3)
0315T	1(3)
0316T	1(3)
0317T	1(3)
0329T	0(3)
0330T	1(2)
0331T	1(3)
0332T	1(3)
0333T	0(3)
0335T	2(2)
0338T	1(2)
0339T	1(2)
0341T	1(2)
0342T	1(3)
0345T	1(2)
0347T	1(3)
0348T	1(3)
0349T	1(3)

CPT	MUE
0350T	1(3)
0351T	5(3)
0352T	5(3)
0353T	2(3)
0354T	2(3)
0355T	1(2)
0356T	4(2)
0357T	1(2)
0358T	1(2)
0362T	8(3)
0373T	24(3)
0375T	1(2)
0376T	2(3)
0377T	1(2)
0378T	1(2)
0379T	1(2)
0380T	1(2)
0381T	1(2)
0382T	1(2)
0383T	1(2)
0384T	1(2)
0385T	1(2)
0386T	1(2)
0394T	2(3)
0395T	2(3)
0396T	2(2)
0397T	1(3)
0398T	1(3)
0399T	1(3)
0400T	1(2)
0401T	1(2)
0402T	2(2)
0403T	0(3)
0404T	1(2)
0405T	1(2)
0408T	1(3)
0409T	1(3)
0410T	1(3)
0411T	1(3)
0412T	1(2)
0413T	1(3)
0414T	1(2)
0415T	1(3)
0416T	1(3)
0417T	1(3)
0418T	1(3)
0419T	1(2)
0420T	1(2)
0421T	1(2)
0422T	1(3)
0423T	1(3)
0424T	1(3)
0425T	1(3)
0426T	1(3)
0427T	1(3)
0428T	1(2)
0429T	1(2)
0430T	1(2)
0431T	1(2)
0432T	1(3)
0433T	1(3)
0434T	1(3)
0435T	1(3)
0436T	1(3)

CPT	MUE
0437T	1(3)
0439T	1(3)
0440T	3(3)
0441T	3(3)
0442T	3(3)
0443T	1(2)
0444T	1(2)
0445T	1(2)
0446T	1(3)
0447T	1(3)
0448T	1(3)
0449T	1(2)
0450T	1(3)
0451T	1(3)
0452T	1(3)
0453T	1(3)
0454T	3(3)
0455T	1(3)
0456T	1(3)
0457T	1(3)
0458T	3(3)
0459T	1(3)
0460T	3(3)
0461T	1(3)
0462T	1(2)
0463T	1(2)
0464T	1(2)
0465T	1(3)
0466T	1(3)
0467T	1(3)
0468T	1(3)
0469T	1(2)
0470T	1(2)
0471T	2(1)
0472T	1(2)
0473T	1(2)
0474T	2(2)
0475T	1(3)
0476T	1(3)
0477T	1(3)
0478T	1(3)
0479T	1(2)
0480T	4(1)
0481T	1(3)
0482T	1(3)
0483T	1(2)
0484T	1(2)
0485T	1(2)
0486T	1(2)
0487T	1(3)
0488T	1(2)
0489T	1(2)
0490T	1(2)
0491T	1(2)
0492T	4(3)
0493T	1(3)
0494T	1(2)
0495T	1(2)
0496T	4(3)
0497T	1(3)
0498T	1(2)
0499T	1(2)
0500T	1(3)
0501T	1(2)

CPT	MUE
0502T	1(2)
0503T	1(2)
0504T	1(2)
0505T	1(3)
0506T	1(2)
0507T	1(2)
0508T	1(3)
0509T	1(2)
0510T	1(2)
0511T	1(2)
0512T	1(2)
0513T	2(3)
0514T	2(2)
0515T	1(3)
0516T	1(3)
0517T	1(3)
0518T	1(3)
0519T	1(3)
0520T	1(3)
0521T	1(3)
0522T	1(3)
0523T	1(3)
0524T	3(3)
0525T	1(3)
0526T	1(3)
0527T	1(3)
0528T	1(3)
0529T	1(3)
0530T	1(3)
0531T	1(3)
0532T	1(3)
0533T	1(2)
0534T	1(2)
0535T	1(2)
0536T	1(2)
0537T	1(2)
0538T	1(3)
0539T	1(3)
0540T	1(3)
0541T	1(3)
0542T	1(3)
10004	3(3)
10005	1(2)
10006	3(3)
10007	1(2)
10008	3(3)
10009	1(2)
10010	3(3)
10011	1(2)
10012	3(3)
10021	1(2)
10030	2(3)
10035	1(2)
10036	3(3)
10040	1(2)
10060	1(2)
10061	1(2)
10080	1(3)
10081	1(3)
10120	3(3)
10121	2(3)
10140	2(3)
10160	3(3)
10180	2(3)

CPT	MUE
11000	1(2)
11001	1(3)
11004	1(2)
11005	1(2)
11006	1(2)
11008	1(2)
11010	2(3)
11011	2(3)
11012	2(3)
11042	1(2)
11043	1(2)
11044	1(2)
11045	12(3)
11046	4(3)
11047	4(3)
11055	1(2)
11056	1(2)
11057	1(2)
11102	1(2)
11103	6(3)
11104	1(2)
11105	3(3)
11106	1(2)
11107	2(3)
11200	1(2)
11201	0(3)
11300	5(3)
11301	6(3)
11302	4(3)
11303	3(3)
11305	4(3)
11306	4(3)
11307	3(3)
11308	2(3)
11310	4(3)
11311	4(3)
11312	3(3)
11313	3(3)
11400	3(3)
11401	3(3)
11402	3(3)
11403	2(3)
11404	2(3)
11406	2(3)
11420	3(3)
11421	3(3)
11422	3(3)
11423	2(3)
11424	2(3)
11426	2(3)
11440	4(3)
11441	3(3)
11442	3(3)
11443	2(3)
11444	2(3)
11446	2(3)
11450	1(2)
11451	1(2)
11462	1(2)
11463	1(2)
11470	3(2)
11471	2(3)
11600	2(3)
11601	2(3)

CPT	MUE
11602	3(3)
11603	2(3)
11604	2(3)
11606	2(3)
11620	2(3)
11621	2(3)
11622	2(3)
11623	2(3)
11624	2(3)
11626	2(3)
11640	2(3)
11641	2(3)
11642	3(3)
11643	2(3)
11644	2(3)
11646	2(3)
11719	1(2)
11720	1(2)
11721	1(2)
11730	1(2)
11732	4(3)
11740	2(3)
11750	6(3)
11755	2(3)
11760	4(3)
11762	2(3)
11765	4(3)
11770	1(3)
11771	1(3)
11772	1(3)
11900	1(2)
11901	1(2)
11920	1(2)
11921	1(2)
11922	1(3)
11950	1(2)
11951	1(2)
11952	1(2)
11954	1(3)
11960	2(3)
11970	2(3)
11971	2(3)
11976	1(2)
11980	1(2)
11981	1(3)
11982	1(3)
11983	1(3)
12001	1(2)
12002	1(2)
12004	1(2)
12005	1(2)
12006	1(2)
12007	1(2)
12011	1(2)
12013	1(2)
12014	1(2)
12015	1(2)
12016	1(2)
12017	1(2)
12018	1(2)
12020	2(3)
12021	3(3)
12031	1(2)
12032	1(2)

CPT	MUE
12034	1(2)
12035	1(2)
12036	1(2)
12037	1(2)
12041	1(2)
12042	1(2)
12044	1(2)
12045	1(2)
12046	1(2)
12047	1(2)
12051	1(2)
12052	1(2)
12053	1(2)
12054	1(2)
12055	1(2)
12056	1(2)
12057	1(2)
13100	1(2)
13101	1(2)
13102	9(3)
13120	1(2)
13121	1(2)
13122	9(3)
13131	1(2)
13132	1(2)
13133	7(3)
13151	1(2)
13152	1(2)
13153	2(3)
13160	2(3)
14000	2(3)
14001	2(3)
14020	2(3)
14021	2(3)
14040	2(3)
14041	3(3)
14060	2(3)
14061	2(3)
14301	2(3)
14302	8(3)
14350	2(3)
15002	1(2)
15003	9(3)
15004	1(2)
15005	2(3)
15040	1(2)
15050	1(3)
15100	1(2)
15101	9(3)
15110	1(2)
15111	2(3)
15115	1(2)
15116	2(3)
15120	1(2)
15121	5(3)
15130	1(2)
15131	2(3)
15135	1(2)
15136	1(3)
15150	1(2)
15151	1(2)
15152	2(3)
15155	1(2)
15156	1(2)
15157	1(3)

CPT	MUE
15200	1(2)
15201	7(3)
15220	1(2)
15221	9(3)
15240	1(2)
15241	9(3)
15260	1(2)
15261	6(3)
15271	1(2)
15272	3(3)
15273	1(2)
15274	6(3)
15275	1(2)
15276	3(2)
15277	1(2)
15278	3(3)
15570	2(3)
15572	2(3)
15574	2(3)
15576	2(3)
15600	2(3)
15610	2(3)
15620	2(3)
15630	2(3)
15650	1(3)
15730	1(3)
15731	1(3)
15733	2(3)
15734	4(3)
15736	2(3)
15738	3(3)
15740	2(3)
15750	2(3)
15756	2(3)
15757	2(3)
15758	2(3)
15760	2(3)
15770	2(3)
15775	1(2)
15776	1(2)
15777	1(3)
15780	1(2)
15781	1(3)
15782	1(3)
15783	1(3)
15786	1(2)
15787	2(3)
15788	1(2)
15789	1(2)
15792	1(3)
15793	1(3)
15819	1(2)
15820	1(2)
15821	1(2)
15822	1(2)
15823	1(2)
15824	1(2)
15825	1(2)
15826	1(2)
15828	1(2)
15829	1(2)
15830	1(2)
15832	1(2)
15833	1(2)
15834	1(2)

CPT	MUE
15835	1(3)
15836	1(2)
15837	2(3)
15838	1(2)
15839	2(3)
15840	1(3)
15841	2(3)
15842	2(3)
15845	2(3)
15847	1(2)
15850	1(2)
15851	1(2)
15852	1(3)
15860	1(3)
15876	1(2)
15877	1(2)
15878	1(2)
15879	1(2)
15920	1(3)
15922	1(3)
15931	1(3)
15933	1(3)
15934	1(3)
15935	1(3)
15936	1(3)
15937	1(3)
15940	2(3)
15941	2(3)
15944	2(3)
15945	2(3)
15946	2(3)
15950	2(3)
15951	2(3)
15952	2(3)
15953	2(3)
15956	2(3)
15958	2(3)
15999	1(3)
16000	1(2)
16020	1(3)
16025	1(3)
16030	1(3)
16035	1(2)
16036	2(3)
17000	1(2)
17003	13(2)
17004	1(2)
17106	1(2)
17107	1(2)
17108	1(2)
17110	1(2)
17111	1(2)
17250	4(3)
17260	7(3)
17261	7(3)
17262	6(3)
17263	3(3)
17264	3(3)
17266	2(3)
17270	6(3)
17271	4(3)
17272	5(3)
17273	4(3)
17274	2(3)
17276	2(3)

CPT	MUE
17280	6(3)
17281	5(3)
17282	4(3)
17283	4(3)
17284	2(3)
17286	2(3)
17311	4(3)
17312	6(3)
17313	3(3)
17314	4(3)
17315	15(3)
17340	1(2)
17360	1(2)
17380	1(3)
17999	1(3)
19000	2(3)
19001	5(3)
19020	2(3)
19030	1(2)
19081	1(2)
19082	2(3)
19083	1(2)
19084	2(3)
19085	1(2)
19086	2(3)
19100	4(3)
19101	3(3)
19105	2(3)
19110	1(3)
19112	2(3)
19120	1(2)
19125	1(2)
19126	3(3)
19260	2(3)
19271	1(3)
19272	1(3)
19281	1(2)
19282	2(3)
19283	1(2)
19284	2(3)
19285	1(2)
19286	2(3)
19287	1(2)
19288	2(3)
19294	2(3)
19296	1(3)
19297	2(3)
19298	1(2)
19300	1(2)
19301	1(2)
19302	1(2)
19303	1(2)
19304	1(2)
19305	1(2)
19306	1(2)
19307	1(2)
19316	1(2)
19318	1(2)
19324	1(2)
19325	1(2)
19328	1(2)
19330	1(2)
19340	1(2)
19342	1(2)
19350	1(2)

CPT	MUE
19355	1(2)
19357	1(2)
19361	1(2)
19364	1(2)
19366	1(2)
19367	1(2)
19368	1(2)
19369	1(2)
19370	1(2)
19371	1(2)
19380	1(2)
19396	1(2)
19499	1(3)
20100	2(3)
20101	2(3)
20102	3(3)
20103	3(3)
20150	2(3)
20200	2(3)
20205	3(3)
20206	3(3)
20220	3(3)
20225	2(3)
20240	4(3)
20245	3(3)
20250	1(3)
20251	2(3)
20500	2(3)
20501	2(3)
20520	2(3)
20525	4(3)
20526	1(2)
20527	2(3)
20550	5(3)
20551	5(3)
20552	1(2)
20553	1(2)
20555	1(3)
20600	6(3)
20604	4(3)
20605	2(3)
20606	2(3)
20610	2(3)
20611	2(3)
20612	2(3)
20615	1(3)
20650	4(3)
20660	1(2)
20661	1(2)
20662	1(2)
20663	1(2)
20664	1(2)
20665	1(2)
20670	3(3)
20680	3(3)
20690	2(3)
20692	2(3)
20693	2(3)
20694	2(3)
20696	2(3)
20697	4(3)
20802	1(2)
20805	1(2)
20808	1(2)
20816	3(3)

CPT	MUE
20822	3(3)
20824	1(2)
20827	1(2)
20838	1(2)
20900	2(3)
20902	2(3)
20910	1(3)
20912	1(3)
20920	1(3)
20922	1(3)
20924	2(3)
20926	2(3)
20930	1(3)
20931	1(2)
20932	1(3)
20933	1(3)
20934	1(3)
20936	1(3)
20937	1(2)
20938	1(2)
20939	1(3)
20950	2(3)
20955	1(3)
20956	1(3)
20957	1(3)
20962	1(3)
20969	2(3)
20970	1(3)
20972	2(3)
20973	1(2)
20974	1(3)
20975	1(3)
20979	1(3)
20982	1(2)
20983	1(2)
20985	2(3)
20999	1(3)
21010	1(2)
21011	4(3)
21012	3(3)
21013	2(3)
21014	2(3)
21015	1(3)
21016	2(3)
21025	2(3)
21026	2(3)
21029	1(3)
21030	1(3)
21031	2(3)
21032	1(3)
21034	1(3)
21040	2(3)
21044	1(3)
21045	1(3)
21046	2(3)
21047	2(3)
21048	2(3)
21049	1(3)
21050	1(2)
21060	1(2)
21070	1(2)
21073	1(2)
21076	1(2)
21077	1(2)
21079	1(2)

CPT	MUE
21080	1(2)
21081	1(2)
21082	1(2)
21083	1(2)
21084	1(2)
21085	1(3)
21086	1(2)
21087	1(2)
21088	1(2)
21089	1(3)
21100	1(2)
21110	2(3)
21116	1(2)
21120	1(2)
21121	1(2)
21122	1(2)
21123	1(2)
21125	2(2)
21127	2(3)
21137	1(2)
21138	1(2)
21139	1(2)
21141	1(2)
21142	1(2)
21143	1(2)
21145	1(2)
21146	1(2)
21147	1(2)
21150	1(2)
21151	1(2)
21154	1(2)
21155	1(2)
21159	1(2)
21160	1(2)
21172	1(3)
21175	1(2)
21179	1(2)
21180	1(2)
21181	1(3)
21182	1(2)
21183	1(2)
21184	1(2)
21188	1(2)
21193	1(2)
21194	1(2)
21195	1(2)
21196	1(2)
21198	1(3)
21199	1(2)
21206	1(3)
21208	1(3)
21209	1(3)
21210	2(3)
21215	2(3)
21230	2(3)
21235	2(3)
21240	1(2)
21242	1(2)
21243	1(2)
21244	1(2)
21245	2(2)
21246	2(2)
21247	1(2)
21248	2(3)
21249	2(3)

CPT	MUE
21255	1(2)
21256	1(2)
21260	1(2)
21261	1(2)
21263	1(2)
21267	1(2)
21268	1(2)
21270	1(2)
21275	1(2)
21280	1(2)
21282	1(2)
21295	1(2)
21296	1(2)
21299	1(3)
21310	1(2)
21315	1(2)
21320	1(2)
21325	1(2)
21330	1(2)
21335	1(2)
21336	1(2)
21337	1(2)
21338	1(2)
21339	1(2)
21340	1(2)
21343	1(2)
21344	1(2)
21345	1(2)
21346	1(2)
21347	1(2)
21348	1(2)
21355	1(2)
21356	1(2)
21360	1(2)
21365	1(2)
21366	1(2)
21385	1(2)
21386	1(2)
21387	1(2)
21390	1(2)
21395	1(2)
21400	1(2)
21401	1(2)
21406	1(2)
21407	1(2)
21408	1(2)
21421	1(2)
21422	1(2)
21423	1(2)
21431	1(2)
21432	1(2)
21433	1(2)
21435	1(2)
21436	1(2)
21440	2(2)
21445	2(2)
21450	1(2)
21451	1(2)
21452	1(2)
21453	1(2)
21454	1(2)
21461	1(2)
21462	1(2)
21465	1(2)
21470	1(2)

CPT	MUE
21480	1(2)
21485	1(2)
21490	1(2)
21497	1(2)
21499	1(3)
21501	3(3)
21502	1(3)
21510	1(3)
21550	2(3)
21552	2(3)
21554	2(3)
21555	2(3)
21556	2(3)
21557	1(3)
21558	1(3)
21600	5(3)
21610	1(3)
21615	1(2)
21616	1(2)
21620	1(2)
21627	1(2)
21630	1(2)
21632	1(2)
21685	1(2)
21700	1(2)
21705	1(2)
21720	1(3)
21725	1(3)
21740	1(2)
21742	1(2)
21743	1(2)
21750	1(2)
21811	1(2)
21812	1(2)
21813	1(2)
21820	1(2)
21825	1(2)
21899	1(3)
21920	2(3)
21925	2(3)
21930	5(3)
21931	3(3)
21932	2(3)
21933	2(3)
21935	1(3)
21936	1(3)
22010	2(3)
22015	2(3)
22100	1(2)
22101	1(2)
22102	1(2)
22103	3(3)
22110	1(2)
22112	1(2)
22114	1(2)
22116	3(3)
22206	1(2)
22207	1(2)
22208	5(3)
22210	1(2)
22212	1(2)
22214	1(2)
22216	6(3)
22220	1(2)
22222	1(2)

CPT	MUE
22224	1(2)
22226	4(3)
22310	1(2)
22315	1(2)
22318	1(2)
22319	1(2)
22325	1(2)
22326	1(2)
22327	1(2)
22328	6(3)
22505	1(2)
22510	1(2)
22511	1(2)
22512	3(3)
22513	1(2)
22514	1(2)
22515	4(3)
22526	0(3)
22527	0(3)
22532	1(2)
22533	1(2)
22534	3(3)
22548	1(2)
22551	1(2)
22552	5(3)
22554	1(2)
22556	1(2)
22558	1(2)
22585	5(3)
22586	1(2)
22590	1(2)
22595	1(2)
22600	1(2)
22610	1(2)
22612	1(2)
22614	13(3)
22630	1(2)
22632	4(2)
22633	1(2)
22634	4(2)
22800	1(2)
22802	1(2)
22804	1(2)
22808	1(2)
22810	1(2)
22812	1(2)
22818	1(2)
22819	1(2)
22830	1(2)
22840	1(3)
22841	0(3)
22842	1(3)
22843	1(3)
22844	1(3)
22845	1(3)
22846	1(3)
22847	1(3)
22848	1(2)
22849	1(2)
22850	1(2)
22852	1(2)
22853	4(3)
22854	4(3)
22855	1(2)
22856	1(2)

CPT	MUE
22857	1(2)
22858	1(2)
22859	4(3)
22861	1(2)
22862	1(2)
22864	1(2)
22865	1(2)
22867	1(2)
22868	1(2)
22869	1(2)
22870	1(2)
22899	1(3)
22900	3(3)
22901	2(3)
22902	4(3)
22903	3(3)
22904	1(3)
22905	1(3)
22999	1(3)
23000	1(2)
23020	1(2)
23030	2(3)
23031	1(3)
23035	1(3)
23040	1(2)
23044	1(3)
23065	2(3)
23066	2(3)
23071	2(3)
23073	2(3)
23075	2(3)
23076	2(3)
23077	1(3)
23078	1(3)
23100	1(2)
23101	1(3)
23105	1(2)
23106	1(2)
23107	1(2)
23120	1(2)
23125	1(2)
23130	1(2)
23140	1(3)
23145	1(3)
23146	1(3)
23150	1(3)
23155	1(3)
23156	1(3)
23170	1(3)
23172	1(3)
23174	1(3)
23180	1(3)
23182	1(3)
23184	1(3)
23190	1(3)
23195	1(2)
23200	1(3)
23210	1(3)
23220	1(3)
23330	2(3)
23333	1(3)
23334	1(2)
23335	1(2)
23350	1(2)
23395	1(2)

CPT	MUE
23397	1(3)
23400	1(2)
23405	2(3)
23406	1(3)
23410	1(2)
23412	1(2)
23415	1(2)
23420	1(2)
23430	1(2)
23440	1(2)
23450	1(2)
23455	1(2)
23460	1(2)
23462	1(2)
23465	1(2)
23466	1(2)
23470	1(2)
23472	1(2)
23473	1(2)
23474	1(2)
23480	1(2)
23485	1(2)
23490	1(2)
23491	1(2)
23500	1(2)
23505	1(2)
23515	1(2)
23520	1(2)
23525	1(2)
23530	1(2)
23532	1(2)
23540	1(2)
23545	1(2)
23550	1(2)
23552	1(2)
23570	1(2)
23575	1(2)
23585	1(2)
23600	1(2)
23605	1(2)
23615	1(2)
23616	1(2)
23620	1(2)
23625	1(2)
23630	1(2)
23650	1(2)
23655	1(2)
23660	1(2)
23665	1(2)
23670	1(2)
23675	1(2)
23680	1(2)
23700	1(2)
23800	1(2)
23802	1(2)
23900	1(2)
23920	1(2)
23921	1(2)
23929	1(3)
23930	2(3)
23931	2(3)
23935	2(3)
24000	1(2)
24006	1(2)
24065	2(3)

CPT	MUE
24066	2(3)
24071	2(3)
24073	2(3)
24075	5(3)
24076	4(3)
24077	1(3)
24079	1(3)
24100	1(2)
24101	1(2)
24102	1(2)
24105	1(2)
24110	1(3)
24115	1(3)
24116	1(3)
24120	1(3)
24125	1(3)
24126	1(3)
24130	1(2)
24134	1(3)
24136	1(3)
24138	1(3)
24140	1(3)
24145	1(3)
24147	1(2)
24149	1(2)
24150	1(3)
24152	1(3)
24155	1(2)
24160	1(2)
24164	1(2)
24200	3(3)
24201	3(3)
24220	1(2)
24300	1(2)
24301	2(3)
24305	4(3)
24310	2(3)
24320	2(3)
24330	1(3)
24331	1(3)
24332	1(2)
24340	1(2)
24341	2(3)
24342	2(3)
24343	1(2)
24344	1(2)
24345	1(2)
24346	1(2)
24357	1(3)
24358	1(3)
24359	2(3)
24360	1(2)
24361	1(2)
24362	1(2)
24363	1(2)
24365	1(2)
24366	1(2)
24370	1(2)
24371	1(2)
24400	1(3)
24410	1(2)
24420	1(2)
24430	1(3)
24435	1(3)
24470	1(2)

CPT	MUE
24495	1(2)
24498	1(2)
24500	1(2)
24505	1(2)
24515	1(2)
24516	1(2)
24530	1(2)
24535	1(2)
24538	1(2)
24545	1(2)
24546	1(2)
24560	1(3)
24565	1(3)
24566	1(3)
24575	1(3)
24576	1(3)
24577	1(3)
24579	1(3)
24582	1(3)
24586	1(3)
24587	1(2)
24600	1(2)
24605	1(2)
24615	1(2)
24620	1(2)
24635	1(2)
24640	1(2)
24650	1(2)
24655	1(2)
24665	1(2)
24666	1(2)
24670	1(2)
24675	1(2)
24685	1(2)
24800	1(2)
24802	1(2)
24900	1(2)
24920	1(2)
24925	1(2)
24930	1(2)
24931	1(2)
24935	1(2)
24940	1(2)
24999	1(3)
25000	2(3)
25001	1(3)
25020	1(2)
25023	1(2)
25024	1(2)
25025	1(2)
25028	4(3)
25031	2(3)
25035	2(3)
25040	1(3)
25065	2(3)
25066	2(3)
25071	3(3)
25073	2(3)
25075	6(3)
25076	3(3)
25077	1(3)
25078	1(3)
25085	1(2)
25100	1(2)
25101	1(2)

CPT	MUE
25105	1(2)
25107	1(2)
25109	4(3)
25110	2(3)
25111	1(3)
25112	1(3)
25115	1(3)
25116	1(3)
25118	5(3)
25119	1(2)
25120	1(3)
25125	1(3)
25126	1(3)
25130	1(3)
25135	1(3)
25136	1(3)
25145	1(3)
25150	1(3)
25151	1(3)
25170	1(3)
25210	2(3)
25215	1(2)
25230	1(2)
25240	1(2)
25246	1(2)
25248	3(3)
25250	1(2)
25251	1(2)
25259	1(2)
25260	7(3)
25263	4(3)
25265	4(3)
25270	8(3)
25272	4(3)
25274	4(3)
25275	2(3)
25280	9(3)
25290	10(3)
25295	9(3)
25300	1(2)
25301	1(2)
25310	5(3)
25312	4(3)
25315	1(3)
25316	1(3)
25320	1(2)
25332	1(2)
25335	1(2)
25337	1(2)
25350	1(3)
25355	1(3)
25360	1(3)
25365	1(3)
25370	1(2)
25375	1(2)
25390	1(2)
25391	1(2)
25392	1(2)
25393	1(2)
25394	1(3)
25400	1(2)
25405	1(2)
25415	1(2)
25420	1(2)
25425	1(2)

CPT	MUE
25426	1(2)
25430	1(3)
25431	1(3)
25440	1(2)
25441	1(2)
25442	1(2)
25443	1(2)
25444	1(2)
25445	1(2)
25446	1(2)
25447	4(3)
25449	1(2)
25450	1(2)
25455	1(2)
25490	1(2)
25491	1(2)
25492	1(2)
25500	1(2)
25505	1(2)
25515	1(2)
25520	1(2)
25525	1(2)
25526	1(2)
25530	1(2)
25535	1(2)
25545	1(2)
25560	1(2)
25565	1(2)
25574	1(2)
25575	1(2)
25600	1(2)
25605	1(2)
25606	1(2)
25607	1(2)
25608	1(2)
25609	1(2)
25622	1(2)
25624	1(2)
25628	1(2)
25630	1(3)
25635	1(3)
25645	1(3)
25650	1(2)
25651	1(2)
25652	1(2)
25660	1(2)
25670	1(2)
25671	1(2)
25675	1(2)
25676	1(2)
25680	1(2)
25685	1(2)
25690	1(2)
25695	1(2)
25800	1(2)
25805	1(2)
25810	1(2)
25820	1(2)
25825	1(2)
25830	1(2)
25900	1(2)
25905	1(2)
25907	1(2)
25909	1(2)
25915	1(2)

CPT	MUE
25920	1(2)
25922	1(2)
25924	1(2)
25927	1(2)
25929	1(2)
25931	1(2)
25999	1(3)
26010	2(3)
26011	3(3)
26020	4(3)
26025	1(2)
26030	1(2)
26034	2(3)
26035	1(3)
26037	1(3)
26040	1(2)
26045	1(2)
26055	5(3)
26060	5(3)
26070	2(3)
26075	3(3)
26080	3(3)
26100	1(3)
26105	2(3)
26110	2(3)
26111	4(3)
26113	3(3)
26115	4(3)
26116	2(3)
26117	2(3)
26118	1(3)
26121	1(2)
26123	1(2)
26125	4(3)
26130	1(3)
26135	4(3)
26140	2(3)
26145	6(3)
26160	4(3)
26170	4(3)
26180	4(3)
26185	1(3)
26200	2(3)
26205	1(3)
26210	2(3)
26215	2(3)
26230	2(3)
26235	2(3)
26236	2(3)
26250	2(3)
26260	1(3)
26262	1(3)
26320	4(3)
26340	4(3)
26341	2(3)
26350	6(3)
26352	2(3)
26356	4(3)
26357	2(3)
26358	2(3)
26370	3(3)
26372	1(3)
26373	2(3)
26390	2(3)
26392	2(3)

CPT	MUE
26410	4(3)
26412	3(3)
26415	2(3)
26416	2(3)
26418	4(3)
26420	3(3)
26426	4(3)
26428	2(3)
26432	2(3)
26433	2(3)
26434	2(3)
26437	4(3)
26440	6(3)
26442	5(3)
26445	5(3)
26449	5(3)
26450	6(3)
26455	6(3)
26460	4(3)
26471	4(3)
26474	4(3)
26476	4(3)
26477	2(3)
26478	6(3)
26479	4(3)
26480	4(3)
26483	4(3)
26485	4(3)
26489	2(3)
26490	3(3)
26492	2(3)
26494	1(3)
26496	1(3)
26497	2(3)
26498	1(3)
26499	2(3)
26500	3(3)
26502	2(3)
26508	1(2)
26510	4(3)
26516	1(2)
26517	1(2)
26518	1(2)
26520	4(3)
26525	4(3)
26530	4(3)
26531	4(3)
26535	3(3)
26536	4(3)
26540	4(3)
26541	4(3)
26542	4(3)
26545	4(3)
26546	2(3)
26548	3(3)
26550	1(2)
26551	1(2)
26553	1(3)
26554	1(3)
26555	2(3)
26556	2(3)
26560	2(3)
26561	2(3)
26562	2(3)
26565	2(3)

CPT	MUE
26567	3(3)
26568	2(3)
26580	1(2)
26587	2(3)
26590	2(3)
26591	4(3)
26593	8(3)
26596	1(3)
26600	2(3)
26605	3(3)
26607	2(3)
26608	4(3)
26615	3(3)
26641	1(2)
26645	1(2)
26650	1(2)
26665	1(2)
26670	2(3)
26675	1(3)
26676	2(3)
26685	3(3)
26686	3(3)
26700	2(3)
26705	3(3)
26706	2(3)
26715	3(3)
26720	4(3)
26725	3(3)
26727	3(3)
26735	4(3)
26740	3(3)
26742	3(3)
26746	3(3)
26750	3(3)
26755	2(3)
26756	2(3)
26765	3(3)
26770	3(3)
26775	2(3)
26776	4(3)
26785	3(3)
26820	1(2)
26841	1(2)
26842	1(2)
26843	2(3)
26844	2(3)
26850	5(3)
26852	2(3)
26860	1(2)
26861	4(3)
26862	1(2)
26863	2(3)
26910	4(3)
26951	8(3)
26952	4(3)
26989	1(3)
26990	2(3)
26991	1(3)
26992	2(3)
27000	1(3)
27001	1(3)
27003	1(2)
27005	1(2)
27006	1(2)
27025	1(3)

CPT	MUE
27027	1(2)
27030	1(2)
27033	1(2)
27035	1(2)
27036	1(2)
27040	2(3)
27041	3(3)
27043	2(3)
27045	3(3)
27047	2(3)
27048	2(3)
27049	1(3)
27050	1(2)
27052	1(2)
27054	1(2)
27057	1(2)
27059	1(3)
27060	1(2)
27062	1(2)
27065	1(3)
27066	1(3)
27067	1(3)
27070	1(3)
27071	1(3)
27075	1(3)
27076	1(2)
27077	1(2)
27078	1(2)
27080	1(2)
27086	1(3)
27087	1(3)
27090	1(2)
27091	1(2)
27093	1(2)
27095	1(2)
27096	1(2)
27097	1(3)
27098	1(2)
27100	1(2)
27105	1(3)
27110	1(2)
27111	1(2)
27120	1(2)
27122	1(2)
27125	1(2)
27130	1(2)
27132	1(2)
27134	1(2)
27137	1(2)
27138	1(2)
27140	1(2)
27146	1(3)
27147	1(3)
27151	1(3)
27156	1(2)
27158	1(2)
27161	1(2)
27165	1(2)
27170	1(2)
27175	1(2)
27176	1(2)
27177	1(2)
27178	1(2)
27179	1(2)
27181	1(2)

CPT	MUE
27185	1(2)
27187	1(2)
27197	1(2)
27198	1(2)
27200	1(2)
27202	1(2)
27215	0(3)
27216	0(3)
27217	0(3)
27218	0(3)
27220	1(2)
27222	1(2)
27226	1(2)
27227	1(2)
27228	1(2)
27230	1(2)
27232	1(2)
27235	1(2)
27236	1(2)
27238	1(2)
27240	1(2)
27244	1(2)
27245	1(2)
27246	1(2)
27248	1(2)
27250	1(2)
27252	1(2)
27253	1(2)
27254	1(2)
27256	1(2)
27257	1(2)
27258	1(2)
27259	1(2)
27265	1(2)
27266	1(2)
27267	1(2)
27268	1(2)
27269	1(2)
27275	2(2)
27279	1(2)
27280	1(2)
27282	1(2)
27284	1(2)
27286	1(2)
27290	1(2)
27295	1(2)
27299	1(3)
27301	3(3)
27303	2(3)
27305	1(2)
27306	1(2)
27307	1(2)
27310	1(2)
27323	2(3)
27324	3(3)
27325	1(2)
27326	1(2)
27327	5(3)
27328	3(3)
27329	1(3)
27330	1(2)
27331	1(2)
27332	1(2)
27333	1(2)
27334	1(2)

CPT	MUE
27335	1(2)
27337	3(3)
27339	4(3)
27340	1(2)
27345	1(2)
27347	1(2)
27350	1(2)
27355	1(3)
27356	1(3)
27357	1(3)
27358	1(3)
27360	2(3)
27364	1(3)
27365	1(3)
27369	1(2)
27372	2(3)
27380	1(2)
27381	1(2)
27385	2(3)
27386	2(3)
27390	1(2)
27391	1(2)
27392	1(2)
27393	1(2)
27394	1(2)
27395	1(2)
27396	1(2)
27397	1(2)
27400	1(2)
27403	1(3)
27405	2(2)
27407	2(2)
27409	1(2)
27412	1(2)
27415	1(2)
27416	1(2)
27418	1(2)
27420	1(2)
27422	1(2)
27424	1(2)
27425	1(2)
27427	1(2)
27428	1(2)
27429	1(2)
27430	1(2)
27435	1(2)
27437	1(2)
27438	1(2)
27440	1(2)
27441	1(2)
27442	1(2)
27443	1(2)
27445	1(2)
27446	1(2)
27447	1(2)
27448	1(3)
27450	1(3)
27454	1(2)
27455	1(3)
27457	1(3)
27465	1(2)
27466	1(2)
27468	1(2)
27470	1(2)
27472	1(2)

CPT	MUE
27475	1(2)
27477	1(2)
27479	1(2)
27485	1(2)
27486	1(2)
27487	1(2)
27488	1(2)
27495	1(2)
27496	1(2)
27497	1(2)
27498	1(2)
27499	1(2)
27500	1(2)
27501	1(2)
27502	1(2)
27503	1(2)
27506	1(2)
27507	1(2)
27508	1(2)
27509	1(2)
27510	1(2)
27511	1(2)
27513	1(2)
27514	1(2)
27516	1(2)
27517	1(2)
27519	1(2)
27520	1(2)
27524	1(2)
27530	1(2)
27532	1(2)
27535	1(2)
27536	1(2)
27538	1(2)
27540	1(2)
27550	1(2)
27552	1(2)
27556	1(2)
27557	1(2)
27558	1(2)
27560	1(2)
27562	1(2)
27566	1(2)
27570	1(2)
27580	1(2)
27590	1(2)
27591	1(2)
27592	1(2)
27594	1(2)
27596	1(2)
27598	1(2)
27599	1(3)
27600	1(2)
27601	1(2)
27602	1(2)
27603	2(3)
27604	2(3)
27605	1(2)
27606	1(2)
27607	2(3)
27610	1(2)
27612	1(2)
27613	3(3)
27614	3(3)
27615	1(3)

CPT	MUE
27616	1(3)
27618	3(3)
27619	2(3)
27620	1(2)
27625	1(2)
27626	1(2)
27630	2(3)
27632	3(3)
27634	2(3)
27635	1(3)
27637	1(3)
27638	1(3)
27640	1(3)
27641	1(3)
27645	1(3)
27646	1(3)
27647	1(3)
27648	1(2)
27650	1(2)
27652	1(2)
27654	1(2)
27656	1(3)
27658	2(3)
27659	2(3)
27664	2(3)
27665	2(3)
27675	1(2)
27676	1(2)
27680	2(3)
27681	1(2)
27685	2(3)
27686	3(3)
27687	1(2)
27690	2(3)
27691	2(3)
27692	4(3)
27695	1(2)
27696	1(2)
27698	2(2)
27700	1(2)
27702	1(2)
27703	1(2)
27704	1(2)
27705	1(3)
27707	1(3)
27709	1(3)
27712	1(2)
27715	1(2)
27720	1(2)
27722	1(2)
27724	1(2)
27725	1(2)
27726	1(2)
27727	1(2)
27730	1(2)
27732	1(2)
27734	1(2)
27740	1(2)
27742	1(2)
27745	1(2)
27750	1(2)
27752	1(2)
27756	1(2)
27758	1(2)
27759	1(2)

CPT	MUE	CPT	MUE	CPT	MUE	CPT	MUE	CPT	MUE	CPT	MUE	CPT	MUE	CPT	MUE
27760	1(2)	28054	2(3)	28289	1(2)	28615	5(3)	29540	1(2)	29885	1(2)	30905	1(2)	31390	1(2)
27762	1(2)	28055	1(3)	28291	1(2)	28630	2(3)	29550	1(2)	29886	1(2)	30906	1(3)	31395	1(2)
27766	1(2)	28060	1(2)	28292	1(2)	28635	2(3)	29580	1(2)	29887	1(2)	30915	1(3)	31400	1(3)
27767	1(2)	28062	1(2)	28295	1(2)	28636	4(3)	29581	1(2)	29888	1(2)	30920	1(3)	31420	1(2)
27768	1(2)	28070	2(3)	28296	1(2)	28645	4(3)	29584	1(2)	29889	1(2)	30930	1(2)	31500	2(3)
27769	1(2)	28072	4(3)	28297	1(2)	28660	4(3)	29700	2(3)	29891	1(2)	30999	1(3)	31502	1(3)
27780	1(2)	28080	3(3)	28298	1(2)	28665	3(3)	29705	1(3)	29892	1(2)	31000	1(2)	31505	1(3)
27781	1(2)	28086	2(3)	28299	1(2)	28666	4(3)	29710	1(2)	29893	1(2)	31002	1(2)	31510	1(2)
27784	1(2)	28088	2(3)	28300	1(2)	28675	3(3)	29720	1(2)	29894	1(2)	31020	1(2)	31511	1(3)
27786	1(2)	28090	2(3)	28302	1(2)	28705	1(2)	29730	1(3)	29895	1(2)	31030	1(2)	31512	1(3)
27788	1(2)	28092	2(3)	28304	1(3)	28715	1(2)	29740	1(3)	29897	1(2)	31032	1(2)	31513	1(3)
27792	1(2)	28100	1(3)	28305	1(3)	28725	1(2)	29750	1(3)	29898	1(2)	31040	1(2)	31515	1(3)
27808	1(2)	28102	1(3)	28306	1(2)	28730	1(2)	29799	1(3)	29899	1(2)	31050	1(2)	31520	1(3)
27810	1(2)	28103	1(3)	28307	1(2)	28735	1(2)	29800	1(2)	29900	2(3)	31051	1(2)	31525	1(3)
27814	1(2)	28104	2(3)	28308	4(3)	28737	1(2)	29804	1(2)	29901	2(3)	31070	1(2)	31526	1(3)
27816	1(2)	28106	1(3)	28309	1(2)	28740	1(2)	29805	1(2)	29902	2(3)	31075	1(2)	31527	1(2)
27818	1(2)	28107	1(3)	28310	1(2)	28750	1(2)	29806	1(2)	29904	1(2)	31080	1(2)	31528	1(2)
27822	1(2)	28108	2(3)	28312	4(3)	28755	1(2)	29807	1(2)	29905	1(2)	31081	1(2)	31529	1(3)
27823	1(2)	28110	1(2)	28313	4(3)	28760	1(2)	29819	1(2)	29906	1(2)	31084	1(2)	31530	1(3)
27824	1(2)	28111	1(2)	28315	1(2)	28800	1(2)	29820	1(2)	29907	1(2)	31085	1(2)	31531	1(3)
27825	1(2)	28112	4(3)	28320	1(2)	28805	1(2)	29821	1(2)	29914	1(2)	31086	1(2)	31535	1(3)
27826	1(2)	28113	1(2)	28322	2(3)	28810	5(3)	29822	1(2)	29915	1(2)	31087	1(2)	31536	1(3)
27827	1(2)	28114	1(2)	28340	2(3)	28820	6(3)	29823	1(2)	29916	1(2)	31090	1(2)	31540	1(3)
27828	1(2)	28116	1(2)	28341	2(3)	28825	8(2)	29824	1(2)	29999	1(3)	31200	1(2)	31541	1(3)
27829	1(2)	28118	1(2)	28344	1(2)	28890	1(2)	29825	1(2)	30000	1(3)	31201	1(2)	31545	1(2)
27830	1(2)	28119	1(2)	28345	2(3)	28899	1(3)	29826	1(2)	30020	1(3)	31205	1(2)	31546	1(2)
27831	1(2)	28120	2(3)	28360	1(2)	29000	1(3)	29827	1(2)	30100	2(3)	31225	1(2)	31551	1(2)
27832	1(2)	28122	4(3)	28400	1(2)	29010	1(3)	29828	1(2)	30110	1(2)	31230	1(2)	31552	1(2)
27840	1(2)	28124	4(3)	28405	1(2)	29015	1(3)	29830	1(2)	30115	1(2)	31231	1(2)	31553	1(2)
27842	1(2)	28126	4(3)	28406	1(2)	29035	1(3)	29834	1(2)	30117	2(3)	31233	1(2)	31554	1(2)
27846	1(2)	28130	1(2)	28415	1(2)	29040	1(3)	29835	1(2)	30118	1(3)	31235	1(2)	31560	1(2)
27848	1(2)	28140	3(3)	28420	1(2)	29044	1(3)	29836	1(2)	30120	1(2)	31237	1(2)	31561	1(2)
27860	1(2)	28150	4(3)	28430	1(2)	29046	1(3)	29837	1(2)	30124	2(3)	31238	1(3)	31570	1(2)
27870	1(2)	28153	4(3)	28435	1(2)	29049	1(3)	29838	1(2)	30125	1(3)	31239	1(2)	31571	1(2)
27871	1(3)	28160	5(3)	28436	1(2)	29055	1(3)	29840	1(2)	30130	1(2)	31240	1(2)	31572	1(2)
27880	1(2)	28171	1(3)	28445	1(2)	29058	1(3)	29843	1(2)	30140	1(2)	31241	1(2)	31573	1(2)
27881	1(2)	28173	2(3)	28446	1(2)	29065	1(3)	29844	1(2)	30150	1(2)	31253	1(2)	31574	1(2)
27882	1(2)	28175	2(3)	28450	2(3)	29075	1(3)	29845	1(2)	30160	1(2)	31254	1(2)	31575	1(3)
27884	1(2)	28190	3(3)	28455	3(3)	29085	1(3)	29846	1(2)	30200	1(2)	31255	1(2)	31576	1(3)
27886	1(2)	28192	2(3)	28456	2(3)	29086	2(3)	29847	1(2)	30210	1(3)	31256	1(2)	31577	1(3)
27888	1(2)	28193	2(3)	28465	3(3)	29105	1(2)	29848	1(2)	30220	1(2)	31257	1(2)	31578	1(3)
27889	1(2)	28200	4(3)	28470	2(3)	29125	1(2)	29850	1(2)	30300	1(3)	31259	1(2)	31579	1(2)
27892	1(2)	28202	2(3)	28475	5(3)	29126	1(2)	29851	1(2)	30310	1(3)	31267	1(2)	31580	1(2)
27893	1(2)	28208	4(3)	28476	4(3)	29130	3(3)	29855	1(2)	30320	1(3)	31276	1(2)	31584	1(2)
27894	1(2)	28210	2(3)	28485	5(3)	29131	2(3)	29856	1(2)	30400	1(2)	31287	1(2)	31587	1(2)
27899	1(3)	28220	1(2)	28490	1(2)	29200	1(2)	29860	1(2)	30410	1(2)	31288	1(2)	31590	1(2)
28001	2(3)	28222	1(2)	28495	1(2)	29240	1(2)	29861	1(2)	30420	1(2)	31290	1(2)	31591	1(2)
28002	3(3)	28225	1(2)	28496	1(2)	29260	1(3)	29862	1(2)	30430	1(2)	31291	1(2)	31592	1(2)
28003	2(3)	28226	1(2)	28505	1(2)	29280	2(3)	29863	1(2)	30435	1(2)	31292	1(2)	31599	1(3)
28005	3(3)	28230	1(2)	28510	4(3)	29305	1(3)	29866	1(2)	30450	1(2)	31293	1(2)	31600	1(2)
28008	2(3)	28232	6(3)	28515	4(3)	29325	1(3)	29867	1(2)	30460	1(2)	31294	1(2)	31601	1(2)
28010	4(3)	28234	6(3)	28525	4(3)	29345	1(3)	29868	1(3)	30462	1(2)	31295	1(2)	31603	1(2)
28011	4(3)	28238	1(2)	28530	1(2)	29355	1(3)	29870	1(2)	30465	1(2)	31296	1(2)	31605	1(2)
28020	2(3)	28240	1(2)	28531	1(2)	29358	1(3)	29871	1(2)	30520	1(2)	31297	1(2)	31610	1(2)
28022	3(3)	28250	1(2)	28540	1(3)	29365	1(3)	29873	1(2)	30540	1(2)	31298	1(2)	31611	1(2)
28024	4(3)	28260	1(2)	28545	1(3)	29405	1(3)	29874	1(2)	30545	1(2)	31299	1(3)	31612	1(3)
28035	1(2)	28261	1(3)	28546	1(3)	29425	1(3)	29875	1(2)	30560	1(2)	31300	1(2)	31613	1(2)
28039	2(3)	28262	1(2)	28555	1(3)	29435	1(3)	29876	1(2)	30580	2(3)	31360	1(2)	31614	1(2)
28041	2(3)	28264	1(2)	28570	1(2)	29440	1(2)	29877	1(2)	30600	1(3)	31365	1(2)	31615	1(3)
28043	4(3)	28270	6(3)	28575	1(2)	29445	1(3)	29879	1(2)	30620	1(2)	31367	1(2)	31622	1(3)
28045	4(3)	28272	6(3)	28576	1(2)	29450	1(3)	29880	1(2)	30630	1(2)	31368	1(2)	31623	1(3)
28046	1(3)	28280	1(2)	28585	1(3)	29505	1(2)	29881	1(2)	30801	1(2)	31370	1(2)	31624	1(3)
28047	1(3)	28285	4(3)	28600	2(3)	29515	1(2)	29882	1(2)	30802	1(2)	31375	1(2)	31625	1(2)
28050	2(3)	28286	1(2)	28605	2(3)	29520	1(2)	29883	1(2)	30901	1(3)	31380	1(2)	31626	1(2)
28052	2(3)	28288	4(3)	28606	3(3)	29530	1(2)	29884	1(2)	30903	1(3)	31382	1(2)	31627	1(3)

CPT	MUE
31628	1(2)
31629	1(2)
31630	1(3)
31631	1(2)
31632	2(3)
31633	2(3)
31634	1(3)
31635	1(3)
31636	1(2)
31637	2(3)
31638	1(3)
31640	1(3)
31641	1(3)
31643	1(2)
31645	1(2)
31646	2(3)
31647	1(2)
31648	1(2)
31649	2(3)
31651	3(3)
31652	1(2)
31653	1(2)
31654	1(3)
31660	1(2)
31661	1(2)
31717	1(3)
31720	3(3)
31725	1(3)
31730	1(3)
31750	1(2)
31755	1(2)
31760	1(2)
31766	1(2)
31770	2(3)
31775	1(3)
31780	1(2)
31781	1(2)
31785	1(3)
31786	1(3)
31800	1(3)
31805	1(3)
31820	1(2)
31825	1(2)
31830	1(2)
31899	1(3)
32035	1(2)
32036	1(3)
32096	1(3)
32097	1(3)
32098	1(2)
32100	1(3)
32110	1(3)
32120	1(3)
32124	1(3)
32140	1(3)
32141	1(3)
32150	1(3)
32151	1(3)
32160	1(3)
32200	2(3)
32215	1(2)
32220	1(2)
32225	1(2)
32310	1(3)
32320	1(3)

CPT	MUE
32400	2(3)
32405	2(3)
32440	1(2)
32442	1(2)
32445	1(2)
32480	1(2)
32482	1(2)
32484	2(3)
32486	1(3)
32488	1(2)
32491	1(2)
32501	1(3)
32503	1(2)
32504	1(2)
32505	1(2)
32506	3(3)
32507	2(3)
32540	1(3)
32550	2(3)
32551	2(3)
32552	2(2)
32553	1(2)
32554	2(3)
32555	2(3)
32556	2(3)
32557	2(3)
32560	1(3)
32561	1(2)
32562	1(2)
32601	1(3)
32604	1(3)
32606	1(3)
32607	1(3)
32608	1(3)
32609	1(3)
32650	1(2)
32651	1(2)
32652	1(2)
32653	1(3)
32654	1(3)
32655	1(3)
32656	1(2)
32658	1(3)
32659	1(2)
32661	1(3)
32662	1(3)
32663	1(3)
32664	1(2)
32665	1(2)
32666	1(3)
32667	3(3)
32668	2(3)
32669	2(3)
32670	1(2)
32671	1(2)
32672	1(3)
32673	1(2)
32674	1(2)
32701	1(2)
32800	1(3)
32810	1(3)
32815	1(3)
32820	1(2)
32850	1(2)
32851	1(2)

CPT	MUE
32852	1(2)
32853	1(2)
32854	1(2)
32855	1(2)
32856	1(2)
32900	1(2)
32905	1(2)
32906	1(2)
32940	1(3)
32960	1(2)
32994	1(2)
32997	1(2)
32998	1(2)
32999	1(3)
33010	1(2)
33011	1(3)
33015	1(3)
33020	1(3)
33025	1(2)
33030	1(2)
33031	1(2)
33050	1(2)
33120	1(3)
33130	1(3)
33140	1(2)
33141	1(2)
33202	1(2)
33203	1(2)
33206	1(3)
33207	1(3)
33208	1(3)
33210	1(3)
33211	1(3)
33212	1(3)
33213	1(3)
33214	1(3)
33215	2(3)
33216	1(3)
33217	1(3)
33218	1(3)
33220	1(3)
33221	1(3)
33222	1(3)
33223	1(3)
33224	1(3)
33225	1(3)
33226	1(3)
33227	1(3)
33228	1(3)
33229	1(3)
33230	1(3)
33231	1(3)
33233	1(2)
33234	1(2)
33235	1(2)
33236	1(2)
33237	1(2)
33238	1(2)
33240	1(3)
33241	1(2)
33243	1(2)
33244	1(2)
33249	1(3)
33250	1(2)
33251	1(2)

CPT	MUE
33254	1(2)
33255	1(2)
33256	1(2)
33257	1(2)
33258	1(2)
33259	1(2)
33261	1(2)
33262	1(3)
33263	1(3)
33264	1(3)
33265	1(2)
33266	1(2)
33270	1(3)
33271	1(3)
33272	1(3)
33273	1(3)
33274	1(3)
33275	1(3)
33285	1(3)
33286	1(3)
33289	1(3)
33300	1(3)
33305	1(3)
33310	1(2)
33315	1(2)
33320	1(3)
33321	1(3)
33322	1(3)
33330	1(3)
33335	1(3)
33340	1(2)
33361	1(2)
33362	1(2)
33363	1(2)
33364	1(2)
33365	1(2)
33366	1(3)
33367	1(2)
33368	1(2)
33369	1(2)
33390	1(2)
33391	1(2)
33404	1(2)
33405	1(2)
33406	1(2)
33410	1(2)
33411	1(2)
33412	1(2)
33413	1(2)
33414	1(2)
33415	1(2)
33416	1(2)
33417	1(2)
33418	1(3)
33419	1(2)
33420	1(2)
33422	1(2)
33425	1(2)
33426	1(2)
33427	1(2)
33430	1(2)
33440	1(2)
33460	1(2)
33463	1(2)
33464	1(2)

CPT	MUE
33465	1(2)
33468	1(2)
33470	1(2)
33471	1(2)
33474	1(2)
33475	1(2)
33476	1(2)
33477	1(2)
33478	1(2)
33496	1(3)
33500	1(3)
33501	1(3)
33502	1(3)
33503	1(3)
33504	1(3)
33505	1(3)
33506	1(3)
33507	1(3)
33508	1(2)
33510	1(2)
33511	1(2)
33512	1(2)
33513	1(2)
33514	1(2)
33516	1(2)
33517	1(2)
33518	1(2)
33519	1(2)
33521	1(2)
33522	1(2)
33523	1(2)
33530	1(2)
33533	1(2)
33534	1(2)
33535	1(2)
33536	1(2)
33542	1(2)
33545	1(2)
33548	1(2)
33572	3(2)
33600	1(3)
33602	1(3)
33606	1(2)
33608	1(2)
33610	1(2)
33611	1(2)
33612	1(2)
33615	1(2)
33617	1(2)
33619	1(2)
33620	1(2)
33621	1(3)
33622	1(2)
33641	1(2)
33645	1(2)
33647	1(2)
33660	1(2)
33665	1(2)
33670	1(2)
33675	1(2)
33676	1(2)
33677	1(2)
33681	1(2)
33684	1(2)
33688	1(2)

CPT	MUE
33690	1(2)
33692	1(2)
33694	1(2)
33697	1(2)
33702	1(2)
33710	1(2)
33720	1(2)
33722	1(3)
33724	1(2)
33726	1(2)
33730	1(2)
33732	1(2)
33735	1(2)
33736	1(2)
33737	1(2)
33750	1(3)
33755	1(2)
33762	1(2)
33764	1(3)
33766	1(2)
33767	1(2)
33768	1(2)
33770	1(2)
33771	1(2)
33774	1(2)
33775	1(2)
33776	1(2)
33777	1(2)
33778	1(2)
33779	1(2)
33780	1(2)
33781	1(2)
33782	1(2)
33783	1(2)
33786	1(2)
33788	1(2)
33800	1(2)
33802	1(3)
33803	1(3)
33813	1(2)
33814	1(2)
33820	1(2)
33822	1(2)
33824	1(2)
33840	1(2)
33845	1(2)
33851	1(2)
33852	1(2)
33853	1(2)
33860	1(2)
33863	1(2)
33864	1(2)
33866	1(2)
33870	1(2)
33875	1(2)
33877	1(2)
33880	1(2)
33881	1(2)
33883	1(2)
33884	2(3)
33886	1(2)
33889	1(2)
33891	1(2)
33910	1(3)
33915	1(3)

CPT	MUE
33916	1(3)
33917	1(2)
33920	1(2)
33922	1(2)
33924	1(2)
33925	1(2)
33926	1(2)
33927	1(3)
33928	1(3)
33929	1(3)
33930	1(2)
33933	1(2)
33935	1(2)
33940	1(2)
33944	1(2)
33945	1(2)
33946	1(2)
33947	1(2)
33948	1(2)
33949	1(2)
33951	1(3)
33952	1(3)
33953	1(3)
33954	1(3)
33955	1(3)
33956	1(3)
33957	1(3)
33958	1(3)
33959	1(3)
33962	1(3)
33963	1(3)
33964	1(3)
33965	1(3)
33966	1(3)
33967	1(3)
33968	1(3)
33969	1(3)
33970	1(3)
33971	1(3)
33973	1(3)
33974	1(3)
33975	1(3)
33976	1(3)
33977	1(3)
33978	1(3)
33979	1(3)
33980	1(3)
33981	1(3)
33982	1(3)
33983	1(3)
33984	1(3)
33985	1(3)
33986	1(3)
33987	1(3)
33988	1(3)
33989	1(3)
33990	1(3)
33991	1(3)
33992	1(2)
33993	1(3)
33999	1(3)
34001	1(3)
34051	1(3)
34101	1(3)
34111	2(3)

CPT	MUE
34151	1(3)
34201	1(3)
34203	1(2)
34401	1(3)
34421	1(3)
34451	1(3)
34471	1(2)
34490	1(2)
34501	1(2)
34502	1(2)
34510	2(3)
34520	1(3)
34530	1(2)
34701	1(2)
34702	1(2)
34703	1(2)
34704	1(2)
34705	1(2)
34706	1(2)
34707	1(2)
34708	1(2)
34709	3(3)
34710	1(2)
34711	2(3)
34712	1(2)
34713	1(2)
34714	1(2)
34715	1(2)
34716	1(2)
34808	1(3)
34812	1(2)
34813	1(2)
34820	1(2)
34830	1(2)
34831	1(2)
34832	1(2)
34833	1(2)
34834	1(2)
34839	1(2)
34841	1(2)
34842	1(2)
34843	1(2)
34844	1(2)
34845	1(2)
34846	1(2)
34847	1(2)
34848	1(2)
35001	1(2)
35002	1(2)
35005	1(2)
35011	1(2)
35013	1(2)
35021	1(2)
35022	1(2)
35045	1(3)
35081	1(2)
35082	1(2)
35091	1(2)
35092	1(2)
35102	1(2)
35103	1(2)
35111	1(2)
35112	1(2)
35121	1(3)
35122	1(3)

CPT	MUE
35131	1(2)
35132	1(2)
35141	1(2)
35142	1(2)
35151	1(2)
35152	1(2)
35180	2(3)
35182	2(3)
35184	2(3)
35188	2(3)
35189	1(3)
35190	2(3)
35201	2(3)
35206	2(3)
35207	3(3)
35211	3(3)
35216	2(3)
35221	3(3)
35226	3(3)
35231	2(3)
35236	2(3)
35241	2(3)
35246	2(3)
35251	2(3)
35256	2(3)
35261	1(3)
35266	2(3)
35271	2(3)
35276	2(3)
35281	2(3)
35286	2(3)
35301	2(3)
35302	1(2)
35303	1(2)
35304	1(2)
35305	1(2)
35306	2(3)
35311	1(2)
35321	1(2)
35331	1(2)
35341	3(3)
35351	1(3)
35355	1(2)
35361	1(2)
35363	1(2)
35371	1(2)
35372	1(2)
35390	1(3)
35400	1(3)
35500	2(3)
35501	1(3)
35506	1(3)
35508	1(3)
35509	1(3)
35510	1(3)
35511	1(3)
35512	1(3)
35515	1(3)
35516	1(3)
35518	1(3)
35521	1(3)
35522	1(3)
35523	1(3)
35525	1(3)
35526	1(3)

CPT	MUE
35531	1(3)
35533	1(3)
35535	1(3)
35536	1(3)
35537	1(3)
35538	1(3)
35539	1(3)
35540	1(3)
35556	1(3)
35558	1(3)
35560	1(3)
35563	1(3)
35565	1(3)
35566	1(3)
35570	1(3)
35571	1(3)
35572	2(3)
35583	1(2)
35585	2(3)
35587	1(3)
35600	2(3)
35601	1(3)
35606	1(3)
35612	1(3)
35616	1(3)
35621	1(3)
35623	1(3)
35626	3(3)
35631	4(3)
35632	1(3)
35633	1(3)
35634	1(3)
35636	1(3)
35637	1(3)
35638	1(3)
35642	1(3)
35645	1(3)
35646	1(3)
35647	1(3)
35650	1(3)
35654	1(3)
35656	1(3)
35661	1(3)
35663	1(3)
35665	1(3)
35666	2(3)
35671	2(3)
35681	1(3)
35682	1(2)
35683	1(2)
35685	2(3)
35686	1(3)
35691	1(3)
35693	1(3)
35694	1(3)
35695	1(3)
35697	2(3)
35700	2(3)
35701	1(2)
35721	1(2)
35741	1(2)
35761	2(3)
35800	2(3)
35820	2(3)
35840	2(3)

CPT	MUE
35860	2(3)
35870	1(3)
35875	2(3)
35876	2(3)
35879	2(3)
35881	1(3)
35883	1(3)
35884	1(3)
35901	1(3)
35903	2(3)
35905	1(3)
35907	1(3)
36000	4(3)
36002	2(3)
36005	2(3)
36010	2(3)
36011	4(3)
36012	4(3)
36013	2(3)
36014	2(3)
36015	4(3)
36100	2(3)
36140	3(3)
36160	2(3)
36200	2(3)
36215	2(3)
36216	2(3)
36217	2(3)
36218	2(3)
36221	1(3)
36222	1(3)
36223	1(3)
36224	1(3)
36225	1(3)
36226	1(3)
36227	1(3)
36228	2(3)
36245	3(3)
36246	4(3)
36247	2(3)
36248	2(3)
36251	1(3)
36252	1(3)
36253	1(3)
36254	1(3)
36260	1(2)
36261	1(2)
36262	1(2)
36299	1(3)
36400	1(3)
36405	1(3)
36406	1(3)
36410	3(3)
36415	2(3)
36416	6(3)
36420	2(3)
36425	2(3)
36430	1(2)
36440	1(3)
36450	1(3)
36455	1(3)
36456	1(3)
36460	2(3)
36465	1(2)
36466	1(2)

CPT	MUE
36468	2(3)
36470	1(2)
36471	1(2)
36473	1(3)
36474	1(3)
36475	1(3)
36476	2(3)
36478	1(3)
36479	2(3)
36481	1(3)
36482	1(3)
36483	2(3)
36500	4(3)
36510	1(3)
36511	1(3)
36512	1(3)
36513	1(3)
36514	1(3)
36516	1(3)
36522	1(3)
36555	2(3)
36556	2(3)
36557	2(3)
36558	2(3)
36560	2(3)
36561	2(3)
36563	1(3)
36565	1(3)
36566	1(3)
36568	2(3)
36569	2(3)
36570	2(3)
36571	2(3)
36572	1(3)
36573	1(3)
36575	2(3)
36576	2(3)
36578	2(3)
36580	2(3)
36581	2(3)
36582	2(3)
36583	2(3)
36584	2(3)
36585	2(3)
36589	2(3)
36590	2(3)
36591	2(3)
36592	1(3)
36593	2(3)
36595	2(3)
36596	2(3)
36597	2(3)
36598	2(3)
36600	4(3)
36620	3(3)
36625	2(3)
36640	1(3)
36660	1(3)
36680	1(3)
36800	1(3)
36810	1(3)
36815	1(3)
36818	1(3)
36819	1(3)
36820	1(3)

CPT	MUE
36821	2(3)
36823	1(3)
36825	1(3)
36830	2(3)
36831	1(3)
36832	2(3)
36833	1(3)
36835	1(3)
36838	1(3)
36860	2(3)
36861	2(3)
36901	1(3)
36902	1(3)
36903	1(3)
36904	1(3)
36905	1(3)
36906	1(3)
36907	1(3)
36908	1(3)
36909	1(3)
37140	1(2)
37145	1(3)
37160	1(3)
37180	1(2)
37181	1(2)
37182	1(2)
37183	1(2)
37184	1(2)
37185	2(3)
37186	2(3)
37187	1(3)
37188	1(3)
37191	1(3)
37192	1(3)
37193	1(3)
37195	1(3)
37197	2(3)
37200	2(3)
37211	1(2)
37212	1(2)
37213	1(2)
37214	1(2)
37215	1(2)
37216	0(3)
37217	1(2)
37218	1(2)
37220	1(2)
37221	1(2)
37222	2(2)
37223	2(2)
37224	1(2)
37225	1(2)
37226	1(2)
37227	1(2)
37228	1(2)
37229	1(2)
37230	1(2)
37231	1(2)
37232	2(3)
37233	2(3)
37234	2(3)
37235	2(3)
37236	1(2)
37237	2(3)
37238	1(2)

CPT	MUE
37239	2(3)
37241	2(3)
37242	2(3)
37243	1(3)
37244	2(3)
37246	1(2)
37247	2(3)
37248	1(2)
37249	3(3)
37252	1(2)
37253	5(3)
37500	1(3)
37501	1(3)
37565	1(2)
37600	1(3)
37605	1(3)
37606	1(3)
37607	1(3)
37609	1(2)
37615	2(3)
37616	1(3)
37617	3(3)
37618	2(3)
37619	1(2)
37650	1(2)
37660	1(2)
37700	1(2)
37718	1(2)
37722	1(2)
37735	1(2)
37760	1(2)
37761	1(2)
37765	1(2)
37766	1(2)
37780	1(2)
37785	1(2)
37788	1(2)
37790	1(2)
37799	1(3)
38100	1(2)
38101	1(3)
38102	1(2)
38115	1(3)
38120	1(2)
38129	1(3)
38200	1(3)
38204	1(2)
38205	1(3)
38206	1(3)
38207	1(3)
38208	1(3)
38209	1(3)
38210	1(3)
38211	1(3)
38212	1(3)
38213	1(3)
38214	1(3)
38215	1(3)
38220	1(3)
38221	1(3)
38222	1(2)
38230	1(2)
38232	1(2)
38240	1(3)
38241	1(2)

CPT	MUE
38242	1(2)
38243	1(3)
38300	1(3)
38305	1(3)
38308	1(3)
38380	1(2)
38381	1(2)
38382	1(2)
38500	2(3)
38505	2(3)
38510	1(2)
38520	1(2)
38525	1(2)
38530	1(2)
38531	1(2)
38542	1(2)
38550	1(3)
38555	1(3)
38562	1(2)
38564	1(2)
38570	1(2)
38571	1(2)
38572	1(2)
38573	1(2)
38589	1(3)
38700	1(2)
38720	1(2)
38724	1(2)
38740	1(2)
38745	1(2)
38746	1(2)
38747	1(2)
38760	1(2)
38765	1(2)
38770	1(2)
38780	1(2)
38790	1(2)
38792	1(3)
38794	1(2)
38900	1(3)
38999	1(3)
39000	1(2)
39010	1(2)
39200	1(2)
39220	1(2)
39401	1(3)
39402	1(3)
39499	1(3)
39501	1(3)
39503	1(2)
39540	1(2)
39541	1(2)
39545	1(2)
39560	1(3)
39561	1(3)
39599	1(3)
40490	2(3)
40500	2(3)
40510	2(3)
40520	2(3)
40525	2(3)
40527	2(3)
40530	2(3)
40650	2(3)
40652	2(3)

CPT	MUE
40654	2(3)
40700	1(2)
40701	1(2)
40702	1(2)
40720	1(2)
40761	1(2)
40799	1(3)
40800	2(3)
40801	2(3)
40804	1(3)
40805	2(3)
40806	2(2)
40808	2(3)
40810	2(3)
40812	2(3)
40814	4(3)
40816	2(3)
40818	2(3)
40819	2(2)
40820	2(3)
40830	2(3)
40831	2(3)
40840	1(2)
40842	1(2)
40843	1(2)
40844	1(2)
40845	1(3)
40899	1(3)
41000	1(3)
41005	1(3)
41006	2(3)
41007	2(3)
41008	2(3)
41009	2(3)
41010	1(2)
41015	2(3)
41016	1(3)
41017	2(3)
41018	2(3)
41019	1(2)
41100	2(3)
41105	2(3)
41108	2(3)
41110	2(3)
41112	2(3)
41113	2(3)
41114	2(3)
41115	1(2)
41116	2(3)
41120	1(2)
41130	1(2)
41135	1(2)
41140	1(2)
41145	1(2)
41150	1(2)
41153	1(2)
41155	1(2)
41250	2(3)
41251	2(3)
41252	2(3)
41510	1(2)
41512	1(2)
41520	1(3)
41530	1(3)
41599	1(3)

CPT	MUE
41800	2(3)
41805	1(3)
41806	1(3)
41820	4(2)
41821	2(3)
41822	1(2)
41823	1(2)
41825	2(3)
41826	2(3)
41827	2(3)
41828	4(2)
41830	2(3)
41850	2(3)
41870	2(3)
41872	4(2)
41874	4(2)
41899	1(3)
42000	1(3)
42100	2(3)
42104	2(3)
42106	2(3)
42107	2(3)
42120	1(2)
42140	1(2)
42145	1(2)
42160	1(3)
42180	1(3)
42182	1(3)
42200	1(2)
42205	1(2)
42210	1(2)
42215	1(2)
42220	1(2)
42225	1(2)
42226	1(2)
42227	1(2)
42235	1(2)
42260	1(3)
42280	1(2)
42281	1(2)
42299	1(3)
42300	2(3)
42305	2(3)
42310	2(3)
42320	2(3)
42330	1(3)
42335	2(2)
42340	1(2)
42400	2(3)
42405	2(3)
42408	1(3)
42409	1(3)
42410	1(2)
42415	1(2)
42420	1(2)
42425	1(2)
42426	1(2)
42440	1(2)
42450	1(3)
42500	2(3)
42505	2(3)
42507	1(2)
42509	1(2)
42510	1(2)
42550	2(3)

CPT	MUE
42600	1(3)
42650	2(3)
42660	2(3)
42665	2(3)
42699	1(3)
42700	2(3)
42720	1(3)
42725	1(3)
42800	3(3)
42804	1(3)
42806	1(3)
42808	2(3)
42809	1(3)
42810	1(3)
42815	1(3)
42820	1(2)
42821	1(2)
42825	1(2)
42826	1(2)
42830	1(2)
42831	1(2)
42835	1(2)
42836	1(2)
42842	1(3)
42844	1(3)
42845	1(3)
42860	1(3)
42870	1(3)
42890	1(2)
42892	1(3)
42894	1(3)
42900	1(3)
42950	1(2)
42953	1(3)
42955	1(2)
42960	1(3)
42961	1(3)
42962	1(3)
42970	1(3)
42971	1(3)
42972	1(3)
42999	1(3)
43020	1(2)
43030	1(2)
43045	1(2)
43100	1(3)
43101	1(3)
43107	1(2)
43108	1(2)
43112	1(2)
43113	1(2)
43116	1(2)
43117	1(2)
43118	1(2)
43121	1(2)
43122	1(2)
43123	1(2)
43124	1(2)
43130	1(3)
43135	1(3)
43180	1(2)
43191	1(3)
43192	1(3)
43193	1(3)
43194	1(3)

CPT	MUE
43195	1(3)
43196	1(3)
43197	1(3)
43198	1(3)
43200	1(3)
43201	1(2)
43202	1(2)
43204	1(2)
43205	1(2)
43206	1(2)
43210	1(2)
43211	1(3)
43212	1(3)
43213	1(2)
43214	1(3)
43215	1(3)
43216	1(2)
43217	1(2)
43220	1(3)
43226	1(3)
43227	1(3)
43229	1(3)
43231	1(2)
43232	1(2)
43233	1(3)
43235	1(3)
43236	1(2)
43237	1(2)
43238	1(2)
43239	1(2)
43240	1(2)
43241	1(3)
43242	1(2)
43243	1(2)
43244	1(2)
43245	1(2)
43246	1(2)
43247	1(2)
43248	1(3)
43249	1(3)
43250	1(2)
43251	1(2)
43252	1(2)
43253	1(3)
43254	1(3)
43255	2(3)
43257	1(2)
43259	1(2)
43260	1(3)
43261	1(2)
43262	2(2)
43263	1(2)
43264	1(2)
43265	1(2)
43266	1(3)
43270	1(3)
43273	1(2)
43274	2(3)
43275	1(3)
43276	2(3)
43277	3(3)
43278	1(3)
43279	1(2)
43280	1(2)
43281	1(2)

CPT	MUE
43282	1(2)
43283	1(2)
43284	1(2)
43285	1(2)
43286	1(2)
43287	1(2)
43288	1(2)
43289	1(3)
43300	1(2)
43305	1(2)
43310	1(2)
43312	1(2)
43313	1(2)
43314	1(2)
43320	1(2)
43325	1(2)
43327	1(2)
43328	1(2)
43330	1(2)
43331	1(2)
43332	1(2)
43333	1(2)
43334	1(2)
43335	1(2)
43336	1(2)
43337	1(2)
43338	1(2)
43340	1(2)
43341	1(2)
43351	1(2)
43352	1(2)
43360	1(2)
43361	1(2)
43400	1(2)
43401	1(2)
43405	1(2)
43410	1(3)
43415	1(3)
43420	1(3)
43425	1(3)
43450	1(3)
43453	1(3)
43460	1(3)
43496	1(3)
43499	1(3)
43500	1(2)
43501	1(3)
43502	1(2)
43510	1(2)
43520	1(2)
43605	1(2)
43610	2(3)
43611	2(3)
43620	1(2)
43621	1(2)
43622	1(2)
43631	1(2)
43632	1(2)
43633	1(2)
43634	1(2)
43635	1(2)
43640	1(2)
43641	1(2)
43644	1(2)
43645	1(2)

CPT	MUE
43647	1(2)
43648	1(2)
43651	1(2)
43652	1(2)
43653	1(2)
43659	1(3)
43752	2(3)
43753	1(3)
43754	1(3)
43755	1(3)
43756	1(2)
43757	1(2)
43761	2(3)
43762	2(3)
43763	2(3)
43770	1(2)
43771	1(2)
43772	1(2)
43773	1(2)
43774	1(2)
43775	1(2)
43800	1(2)
43810	1(2)
43820	1(2)
43825	1(2)
43830	1(2)
43831	1(2)
43832	1(2)
43840	2(3)
43842	0(3)
43843	1(2)
43845	1(2)
43846	1(2)
43847	1(2)
43848	1(2)
43850	1(2)
43855	1(2)
43860	1(2)
43865	1(2)
43870	1(2)
43880	1(3)
43881	1(3)
43882	1(3)
43886	1(2)
43887	1(2)
43888	1(2)
43999	1(3)
44005	1(2)
44010	1(2)
44015	1(2)
44020	2(3)
44021	1(3)
44025	1(3)
44050	1(2)
44055	1(2)
44100	1(2)
44110	1(2)
44111	1(2)
44120	1(2)
44121	2(3)
44125	1(2)
44126	1(2)
44127	1(2)
44128	2(3)
44130	2(3)

CPT	MUE
44132	1(2)
44133	1(2)
44135	1(2)
44136	1(2)
44137	1(2)
44139	1(2)
44140	2(3)
44141	1(3)
44143	1(2)
44144	1(3)
44145	1(2)
44146	1(2)
44147	1(3)
44150	1(2)
44151	1(2)
44155	1(2)
44156	1(2)
44157	1(2)
44158	1(2)
44160	1(2)
44180	1(2)
44186	1(2)
44187	1(3)
44188	1(3)
44202	1(2)
44203	2(3)
44204	2(3)
44205	1(2)
44206	1(2)
44207	1(2)
44208	1(2)
44210	1(2)
44211	1(2)
44212	1(2)
44213	1(2)
44227	1(3)
44238	1(3)
44300	1(3)
44310	2(3)
44312	1(2)
44314	1(2)
44316	1(2)
44320	1(2)
44322	1(2)
44340	1(2)
44345	1(2)
44346	1(2)
44360	1(3)
44361	1(2)
44363	1(3)
44364	1(2)
44365	1(2)
44366	1(3)
44369	1(2)
44370	1(2)
44372	1(2)
44373	1(2)
44376	1(3)
44377	1(2)
44378	1(3)
44379	1(2)
44380	1(3)
44381	1(3)
44382	1(2)
44384	1(3)

CPT	MUE
44385	1(3)
44386	1(2)
44388	1(3)
44389	1(2)
44390	1(3)
44391	1(3)
44392	1(2)
44394	1(2)
44401	1(2)
44402	1(3)
44403	1(3)
44404	1(3)
44405	1(3)
44406	1(3)
44407	1(2)
44408	1(3)
44500	1(3)
44602	1(2)
44603	1(2)
44604	1(2)
44605	1(2)
44615	3(3)
44620	2(3)
44625	1(3)
44626	1(3)
44640	2(3)
44650	2(3)
44660	1(3)
44661	1(3)
44680	1(3)
44700	1(2)
44701	1(2)
44705	1(3)
44715	1(2)
44720	2(3)
44721	2(3)
44799	1(3)
44800	1(3)
44820	1(3)
44850	1(3)
44899	1(3)
44900	1(2)
44950	1(2)
44955	1(2)
44960	1(2)
44970	1(2)
44979	1(3)
45000	1(3)
45005	1(3)
45020	1(3)
45100	2(3)
45108	1(2)
45110	1(2)
45111	1(2)
45112	1(2)
45113	1(2)
45114	1(2)
45116	1(2)
45119	1(2)
45120	1(2)
45121	1(2)
45123	1(2)
45126	1(2)
45130	1(2)
45135	1(2)

CPT	MUE
45136	1(2)
45150	1(2)
45160	1(3)
45171	2(3)
45172	2(3)
45190	1(3)
45300	1(3)
45303	1(3)
45305	1(2)
45307	1(3)
45308	1(2)
45309	1(2)
45315	1(2)
45317	1(3)
45320	1(2)
45321	1(2)
45327	1(2)
45330	1(3)
45331	1(2)
45332	1(3)
45333	1(2)
45334	1(3)
45335	1(2)
45337	1(2)
45338	1(2)
45340	1(2)
45341	1(2)
45342	1(2)
45346	1(2)
45347	1(3)
45349	1(3)
45350	1(2)
45378	1(3)
45379	1(3)
45380	1(2)
45381	1(2)
45382	1(3)
45384	1(2)
45385	1(2)
45386	1(2)
45388	1(2)
45389	1(3)
45390	1(3)
45391	1(2)
45392	1(2)
45393	1(3)
45395	1(2)
45397	1(2)
45398	1(2)
45399	1(3)
45400	1(2)
45402	1(2)
45499	1(3)
45500	1(2)
45505	1(2)
45520	1(2)
45540	1(2)
45541	1(2)
45550	1(2)
45560	1(2)
45562	1(2)
45563	1(2)
45800	1(3)
45805	1(3)
45820	1(3)

CPT	MUE
45825	1(3)
45900	1(2)
45905	1(2)
45910	1(2)
45915	1(2)
45990	1(2)
45999	1(3)
46020	2(3)
46030	1(3)
46040	2(3)
46045	2(3)
46050	2(3)
46060	2(3)
46070	1(2)
46080	1(2)
46083	2(3)
46200	1(3)
46220	1(2)
46221	1(2)
46230	1(2)
46250	1(2)
46255	1(2)
46257	1(2)
46258	1(2)
46260	1(2)
46261	1(2)
46262	1(2)
46270	1(3)
46275	1(3)
46280	1(2)
46285	1(3)
46288	1(3)
46320	2(3)
46500	1(2)
46505	1(2)
46600	1(3)
46601	1(3)
46604	1(2)
46606	1(2)
46607	1(2)
46608	1(3)
46610	1(2)
46611	1(2)
46612	1(2)
46614	1(3)
46615	1(2)
46700	1(2)
46705	1(2)
46706	1(3)
46707	1(3)
46710	1(3)
46712	1(3)
46715	1(2)
46716	1(2)
46730	1(2)
46735	1(2)
46740	1(2)
46742	1(2)
46744	1(2)
46746	1(2)
46748	1(2)
46750	1(2)
46751	1(2)
46753	1(2)
46754	1(3)

CPT	MUE
46760	1(2)
46761	1(2)
46900	1(2)
46910	1(2)
46916	1(2)
46917	1(2)
46922	1(2)
46924	1(2)
46930	1(2)
46940	1(2)
46942	1(3)
46945	1(2)
46946	1(2)
46947	1(2)
46999	1(3)
47000	3(3)
47001	3(3)
47010	1(3)
47015	1(2)
47100	3(3)
47120	2(3)
47122	1(2)
47125	1(2)
47130	1(2)
47133	1(2)
47135	1(2)
47140	1(2)
47141	1(2)
47142	1(2)
47143	1(2)
47144	1(2)
47145	1(2)
47146	2(3)
47147	1(3)
47300	2(3)
47350	1(3)
47360	1(3)
47361	1(3)
47362	1(3)
47370	1(2)
47371	1(2)
47379	1(3)
47380	1(2)
47381	1(2)
47382	1(2)
47383	1(2)
47399	1(3)
47400	1(3)
47420	1(2)
47425	1(2)
47460	1(2)
47480	1(2)
47490	1(2)
47531	2(3)
47532	1(3)
47533	1(3)
47534	2(3)
47535	1(3)
47536	2(3)
47537	1(3)
47538	2(3)
47539	2(3)
47540	2(3)
47541	1(3)
47542	2(3)

CPT	MUE
47543	1(3)
47544	1(3)
47550	1(3)
47552	1(3)
47553	1(2)
47554	1(3)
47555	1(2)
47556	1(2)
47562	1(2)
47563	1(2)
47564	1(2)
47570	1(2)
47579	1(3)
47600	1(2)
47605	1(2)
47610	1(2)
47612	1(2)
47620	1(2)
47700	1(2)
47701	1(2)
47711	1(2)
47712	1(2)
47715	1(2)
47720	1(2)
47721	1(2)
47740	1(2)
47741	1(2)
47760	1(2)
47765	1(2)
47780	1(2)
47785	1(2)
47800	1(2)
47801	1(3)
47802	1(2)
47900	1(2)
47999	1(3)
48000	1(2)
48001	1(2)
48020	1(3)
48100	1(3)
48102	1(3)
48105	1(2)
48120	1(3)
48140	1(2)
48145	1(2)
48146	1(2)
48148	1(2)
48150	1(2)
48152	1(2)
48153	1(2)
48154	1(2)
48155	1(2)
48160	0(3)
48400	1(3)
48500	1(3)
48510	1(3)
48520	1(3)
48540	1(3)
48545	1(3)
48547	1(2)
48548	1(2)
48550	1(2)
48551	1(2)
48552	2(3)
48554	1(2)

CPT	MUE
48556	1(2)
48999	1(3)
49000	1(2)
49002	1(3)
49010	1(3)
49020	2(3)
49040	2(3)
49060	2(3)
49062	1(3)
49082	1(3)
49083	2(3)
49084	1(3)
49180	2(3)
49185	2(3)
49203	1(2)
49204	1(2)
49205	1(2)
49215	1(2)
49220	1(2)
49250	1(2)
49255	1(2)
49320	1(3)
49321	1(2)
49322	1(2)
49323	1(2)
49324	1(2)
49325	1(2)
49326	1(2)
49327	1(2)
49329	1(3)
49400	1(3)
49402	1(3)
49405	2(3)
49406	2(3)
49407	1(3)
49411	1(2)
49412	1(2)
49418	1(3)
49419	1(2)
49421	1(2)
49422	1(2)
49423	2(3)
49424	3(3)
49425	1(2)
49426	1(3)
49427	1(3)
49428	1(2)
49429	1(2)
49435	1(2)
49436	1(2)
49440	1(3)
49441	1(3)
49442	1(3)
49446	1(2)
49450	1(3)
49451	1(3)
49452	1(3)
49460	1(3)
49465	1(3)
49491	1(2)
49492	1(2)
49495	1(2)
49496	1(2)
49500	1(2)
49501	1(2)

CPT	MUE
49505	1(2)
49507	1(2)
49520	1(2)
49521	1(2)
49525	1(2)
49540	1(2)
49550	1(2)
49553	1(2)
49555	1(2)
49557	1(2)
49560	2(3)
49561	1(3)
49565	2(3)
49566	2(3)
49568	2(3)
49570	1(3)
49572	1(3)
49580	1(2)
49582	1(2)
49585	1(2)
49587	1(2)
49590	1(2)
49600	1(2)
49605	1(2)
49606	1(2)
49610	1(2)
49611	1(2)
49650	1(2)
49651	1(2)
49652	2(3)
49653	2(3)
49654	1(3)
49655	1(3)
49656	1(3)
49657	1(3)
49659	1(3)
49900	1(3)
49904	1(3)
49905	1(3)
49906	1(3)
49999	1(3)
50010	1(2)
50020	1(3)
50040	1(2)
50045	1(2)
50060	1(2)
50065	1(2)
50070	1(2)
50075	1(2)
50080	1(2)
50081	1(2)
50100	1(2)
50120	1(2)
50125	1(2)
50130	1(2)
50135	1(2)
50200	1(3)
50205	1(3)
50220	1(2)
50225	1(2)
50230	1(2)
50234	1(2)
50236	1(2)
50240	1(2)
50250	1(3)

CPT	MUE
50280	1(2)
50290	1(3)
50300	1(2)
50320	1(2)
50323	1(2)
50325	1(2)
50327	2(3)
50328	1(3)
50329	1(3)
50340	1(2)
50360	1(2)
50365	1(2)
50370	1(2)
50380	1(2)
50382	1(3)
50384	1(3)
50385	1(3)
50386	1(3)
50387	1(3)
50389	1(3)
50390	2(3)
50391	1(3)
50396	1(3)
50400	1(2)
50405	1(2)
50430	2(3)
50431	2(3)
50432	2(3)
50433	2(3)
50434	2(3)
50435	2(3)
50436	1(3)
50437	1(3)
50500	1(3)
50520	1(3)
50525	1(3)
50526	1(3)
50540	1(2)
50541	1(2)
50542	1(2)
50543	1(2)
50544	1(2)
50545	1(2)
50546	1(2)
50547	1(2)
50548	1(2)
50549	1(3)
50551	1(3)
50553	1(3)
50555	1(2)
50557	1(2)
50561	1(2)
50562	1(3)
50570	1(3)
50572	1(3)
50574	1(2)
50575	1(2)
50576	1(2)
50580	1(2)
50590	1(2)
50592	1(2)
50593	1(2)
50600	1(3)
50605	1(3)
50606	1(3)

CPT	MUE
50610	1(2)
50620	1(2)
50630	1(2)
50650	1(2)
50660	1(3)
50684	1(3)
50686	2(3)
50688	2(3)
50690	2(3)
50693	2(3)
50694	2(3)
50695	2(3)
50700	1(2)
50705	2(3)
50706	2(3)
50715	1(2)
50722	1(2)
50725	1(3)
50727	1(3)
50728	1(3)
50740	1(2)
50750	1(2)
50760	1(2)
50770	1(2)
50780	1(2)
50782	1(2)
50783	1(2)
50785	1(2)
50800	1(2)
50810	1(3)
50815	1(2)
50820	1(2)
50825	1(3)
50830	1(3)
50840	1(2)
50845	1(2)
50860	1(2)
50900	1(3)
50920	2(3)
50930	2(3)
50940	1(2)
50945	1(2)
50947	1(2)
50948	1(2)
50949	1(3)
50951	1(3)
50953	1(3)
50955	1(2)
50957	1(2)
50961	1(2)
50970	1(3)
50972	1(3)
50974	1(2)
50976	1(2)
50980	1(2)
51020	1(2)
51030	1(2)
51040	1(3)
51045	2(3)
51050	1(3)
51060	1(3)
51065	1(3)
51080	1(3)
51100	1(3)
51101	1(3)

CPT	MUE
51102	1(3)
51500	1(2)
51520	1(2)
51525	1(2)
51530	1(2)
51535	1(2)
51550	1(2)
51555	1(2)
51565	1(2)
51570	1(2)
51575	1(2)
51580	1(2)
51585	1(2)
51590	1(2)
51595	1(2)
51596	1(2)
51597	1(2)
51600	1(3)
51605	1(3)
51610	1(3)
51700	1(3)
51701	2(3)
51702	2(3)
51703	2(3)
51705	2(3)
51710	1(3)
51715	1(2)
51720	1(3)
51725	1(3)
51726	1(3)
51727	1(3)
51728	1(3)
51729	1(3)
51736	1(3)
51741	1(3)
51784	1(3)
51785	1(3)
51792	1(3)
51797	1(3)
51798	1(3)
51800	1(2)
51820	1(2)
51840	1(2)
51841	1(2)
51845	1(2)
51860	1(3)
51865	1(3)
51880	1(2)
51900	1(3)
51920	1(3)
51925	1(2)
51940	1(2)
51960	1(2)
51980	1(2)
51990	1(2)
51992	1(2)
51999	1(3)
52000	1(3)
52001	1(3)
52005	2(3)
52007	1(2)
52010	1(2)
52204	1(2)
52214	1(2)
52224	1(2)

CPT	MUE
52234	1(2)
52235	1(2)
52240	1(2)
52250	1(2)
52260	1(2)
52265	1(2)
52270	1(2)
52275	1(2)
52276	1(2)
52277	1(2)
52281	1(2)
52282	1(2)
52283	1(2)
52285	1(2)
52287	1(2)
52290	1(2)
52300	1(2)
52301	1(2)
52305	1(2)
52310	1(3)
52315	2(3)
52317	1(3)
52318	1(3)
52320	1(2)
52325	1(3)
52327	1(2)
52330	1(2)
52332	1(2)
52334	1(2)
52341	1(2)
52342	1(2)
52343	1(2)
52344	1(2)
52345	1(2)
52346	1(2)
52351	1(3)
52352	1(2)
52353	1(2)
52354	1(3)
52355	1(3)
52356	1(2)
52400	1(2)
52402	1(2)
52441	1(2)
52442	6(3)
52450	1(2)
52500	1(2)
52601	1(2)
52630	1(2)
52640	1(2)
52647	1(2)
52648	1(2)
52649	1(2)
52700	1(3)
53000	1(2)
53010	1(2)
53020	1(2)
53025	1(2)
53040	1(3)
53060	1(3)
53080	1(3)
53085	1(3)
53200	1(3)
53210	1(2)
53215	1(2)
53220	1(3)
53230	1(3)
53235	1(3)
53240	1(3)
53250	1(3)
53260	1(2)
53265	1(3)
53270	1(2)
53275	1(2)
53400	1(2)
53405	1(2)
53410	1(2)
53415	1(2)
53420	1(2)
53425	1(2)
53430	1(2)
53431	1(2)
53440	1(2)
53442	1(2)
53444	1(3)
53445	1(2)
53446	1(2)
53447	1(2)
53448	1(2)
53449	1(2)
53450	1(2)
53460	1(2)
53500	1(2)
53502	1(3)
53505	1(3)
53510	1(3)
53515	1(3)
53520	1(3)
53600	1(3)
53601	1(3)
53605	1(3)
53620	1(2)
53621	1(3)
53660	1(2)
53661	1(3)
53665	1(3)
53850	1(2)
53852	1(2)
53854	1(2)
53855	1(2)
53860	1(2)
53899	1(3)
54000	1(2)
54001	1(2)
54015	1(3)
54050	1(2)
54055	1(2)
54056	1(2)
54057	1(2)
54060	1(2)
54065	1(2)
54100	2(3)
54105	2(3)
54110	1(2)
54111	1(2)
54112	1(3)
54115	1(3)
54120	1(2)
54125	1(2)
54130	1(2)
54135	1(2)
54150	1(2)
54160	1(2)
54161	1(2)
54162	1(2)
54163	1(2)
54164	1(2)
54200	1(2)
54205	1(2)
54220	1(3)
54230	1(3)
54231	1(3)
54235	1(3)
54240	1(2)
54250	1(2)
54300	1(2)
54304	1(2)
54308	1(2)
54312	1(2)
54316	1(2)
54318	1(2)
54322	1(2)
54324	1(2)
54326	1(2)
54328	1(2)
54332	1(2)
54336	1(2)
54340	1(2)
54344	1(2)
54348	1(2)
54352	1(2)
54360	1(2)
54380	1(2)
54385	1(2)
54390	1(2)
54400	1(2)
54401	1(2)
54405	1(2)
54406	1(2)
54408	1(2)
54410	1(2)
54411	1(2)
54415	1(2)
54416	1(2)
54417	1(2)
54420	1(2)
54430	1(2)
54435	1(2)
54437	1(2)
54438	1(2)
54440	1(2)
54450	1(2)
54500	1(3)
54505	1(3)
54512	1(3)
54520	1(2)
54522	1(2)
54530	1(2)
54535	1(2)
54550	1(2)
54560	1(2)
54600	1(2)
54620	1(2)
54640	1(2)
54650	1(2)
54660	1(2)
54670	1(3)
54680	1(2)
54690	1(2)
54692	1(2)
54699	1(3)
54700	1(3)
54800	1(2)
54830	1(2)
54840	1(2)
54860	1(2)
54861	1(2)
54865	1(3)
54900	1(2)
54901	1(2)
55000	1(3)
55040	1(2)
55041	1(2)
55060	1(2)
55100	2(3)
55110	1(2)
55120	1(3)
55150	1(2)
55175	1(2)
55180	1(2)
55200	1(2)
55250	1(2)
55300	1(2)
55400	1(2)
55500	1(2)
55520	1(2)
55530	1(2)
55535	1(2)
55540	1(2)
55550	1(2)
55559	1(3)
55600	1(2)
55605	1(2)
55650	1(2)
55680	1(3)
55700	1(2)
55705	1(2)
55706	1(2)
55720	1(3)
55725	1(3)
55801	1(2)
55810	1(2)
55812	1(2)
55815	1(2)
55821	1(2)
55831	1(2)
55840	1(2)
55842	1(2)
55845	1(2)
55860	1(2)
55862	1(2)
55865	1(2)
55866	1(2)
55870	1(2)
55873	1(2)
55874	1(2)
55875	1(2)
55876	1(2)
55899	1(3)
55920	1(2)
55970	1(2)
55980	1(2)
56405	2(3)
56420	1(3)
56440	1(3)
56441	1(2)
56442	1(2)
56501	1(2)
56515	1(2)
56605	1(2)
56606	6(3)
56620	1(2)
56625	1(2)
56630	1(2)
56631	1(2)
56632	1(2)
56633	1(2)
56634	1(2)
56637	1(2)
56640	1(2)
56700	1(2)
56740	1(3)
56800	1(2)
56805	1(2)
56810	1(2)
56820	1(2)
56821	1(2)
57000	1(3)
57010	1(3)
57020	1(3)
57022	1(3)
57023	1(3)
57061	1(2)
57065	1(2)
57100	2(3)
57105	2(3)
57106	1(2)
57107	1(2)
57109	1(2)
57110	1(2)
57111	1(2)
57112	1(2)
57120	1(2)
57130	1(2)
57135	2(3)
57150	1(3)
57155	1(3)
57156	1(3)
57160	1(2)
57170	1(2)
57180	1(3)
57200	1(3)
57210	1(3)
57220	1(2)
57230	1(2)
57240	1(2)
57250	1(2)
57260	1(2)
57265	1(2)
57267	2(3)
57268	1(2)
57270	1(2)
57280	1(2)
57282	1(2)
57283	1(2)
57284	1(2)
57285	1(2)
57287	1(2)
57288	1(2)
57289	1(2)
57291	1(2)
57292	1(2)
57295	1(2)
57296	1(2)
57300	1(3)
57305	1(3)
57307	1(3)
57308	1(3)
57310	1(3)
57311	1(3)
57320	1(3)
57330	1(3)
57335	1(2)
57400	1(2)
57410	1(2)
57415	1(3)
57420	1(3)
57421	1(3)
57423	1(2)
57425	1(2)
57426	1(2)
57452	1(3)
57454	1(3)
57455	1(3)
57456	1(3)
57460	1(3)
57461	1(3)
57500	1(3)
57505	1(3)
57510	1(3)
57511	1(3)
57513	1(3)
57520	1(3)
57522	1(3)
57530	1(3)
57531	1(2)
57540	1(2)
57545	1(3)
57550	1(3)
57555	1(2)
57556	1(2)
57558	1(3)
57700	1(3)
57720	1(3)
57800	1(3)
58100	1(3)
58110	1(3)
58120	1(3)
58140	1(3)
58145	1(3)
58146	1(3)
58150	1(3)
58152	1(2)
58180	1(3)
58200	1(2)
58210	1(2)
58240	1(2)
58260	1(3)
58262	1(3)
58263	1(2)
58267	1(2)
58270	1(2)
58275	1(2)
58280	1(2)
58285	1(3)
58290	1(3)
58291	1(2)
58292	1(2)
58293	1(2)
58294	1(2)
58300	0(3)
58301	1(3)
58321	1(2)
58322	1(2)
58323	1(3)
58340	1(3)
58345	1(3)
58346	1(2)
58350	1(2)
58353	1(3)
58356	1(3)
58400	1(3)
58410	1(2)
58520	1(2)
58540	1(3)
58541	1(3)
58542	1(2)
58543	1(3)
58544	1(2)
58545	1(2)
58546	1(2)
58548	1(2)
58550	1(3)
58552	1(3)
58553	1(3)
58554	1(2)
58555	1(3)
58558	1(3)
58559	1(3)
58560	1(3)
58561	1(3)
58562	1(3)
58563	1(3)
58565	1(2)
58570	1(3)
58571	1(2)
58572	1(3)
58573	1(2)
58575	1(2)
58578	1(3)
58579	1(3)
58600	1(2)
58605	1(2)
58611	1(2)
58615	1(2)
58660	1(2)
58661	1(2)
58662	1(2)
58670	1(2)
58671	1(2)
58672	1(2)
58673	1(2)
58674	1(2)
58679	1(3)
58700	1(2)
58720	1(2)
58740	1(2)
58750	1(2)
58752	1(2)
58760	1(2)
58770	1(2)
58800	1(2)
58805	1(2)
58820	1(3)
58822	1(3)
58825	1(2)
58900	1(2)
58920	1(2)
58925	1(3)
58940	1(2)
58943	1(2)
58950	1(2)
58951	1(2)
58952	1(2)
58953	1(2)
58954	1(2)
58956	1(2)
58957	1(2)
58958	1(2)
58960	1(2)
58970	1(3)
58974	1(3)
58976	2(3)
58999	1(3)
59000	2(3)
59001	2(3)
59012	2(3)
59015	2(3)
59020	2(3)
59025	2(3)
59030	2(3)
59050	2(3)
59051	2(3)
59070	2(3)
59072	2(3)
59074	2(3)
59076	2(3)
59100	1(2)
59120	1(3)
59121	1(3)
59130	1(3)
59135	1(3)
59136	1(3)
59140	1(2)
59150	1(3)
59151	1(3)
59160	1(2)
59200	1(3)
59300	1(2)
59320	1(2)
59325	1(2)
59350	1(2)
59400	1(2)
59409	2(3)
59410	1(2)
59412	1(3)
59414	1(3)
59425	1(2)
59426	1(2)
59430	1(2)

CPT	MUE
59510	1(2)
59514	1(3)
59515	1(2)
59525	1(2)
59610	1(2)
59612	2(3)
59614	1(2)
59618	1(2)
59620	1(2)
59622	1(2)
59812	1(2)
59820	1(2)
59821	1(2)
59830	1(2)
59840	1(2)
59841	1(2)
59850	1(2)
59851	1(2)
59852	1(2)
59855	1(2)
59856	1(2)
59857	1(2)
59866	1(2)
59870	1(2)
59871	1(2)
59897	1(3)
59898	1(3)
59899	1(3)
60000	1(3)
60100	3(3)
60200	2(3)
60210	1(2)
60212	1(2)
60220	1(3)
60225	1(2)
60240	1(2)
60252	1(2)
60254	1(2)
60260	1(2)
60270	1(2)
60271	1(2)
60280	1(3)
60281	1(3)
60300	2(3)
60500	1(2)
60502	1(3)
60505	1(3)
60512	1(3)
60520	1(2)
60521	1(2)
60522	1(2)
60540	1(2)
60545	1(2)
60600	1(3)
60605	1(3)
60650	1(2)
60659	1(3)
60699	1(3)
61000	1(2)
61001	1(2)
61020	2(3)
61026	2(3)
61050	1(3)
61055	1(3)
61070	2(3)

CPT	MUE
61105	1(3)
61107	1(3)
61108	1(3)
61120	1(3)
61140	1(3)
61150	1(3)
61151	1(3)
61154	1(3)
61156	1(3)
61210	1(3)
61215	1(3)
61250	1(3)
61253	1(3)
61304	1(3)
61305	1(3)
61312	2(3)
61313	2(3)
61314	2(3)
61315	1(3)
61316	1(3)
61320	2(3)
61321	1(3)
61322	1(3)
61323	1(3)
61330	1(2)
61333	1(2)
61340	1(2)
61343	1(2)
61345	1(3)
61450	1(3)
61458	1(2)
61460	1(2)
61500	1(3)
61501	1(3)
61510	1(3)
61512	1(3)
61514	2(3)
61516	1(3)
61517	1(3)
61518	1(3)
61519	1(3)
61520	1(3)
61521	1(3)
61522	1(3)
61524	2(3)
61526	1(3)
61530	1(3)
61531	1(2)
61533	2(3)
61534	1(3)
61535	2(3)
61536	1(3)
61537	1(3)
61538	1(2)
61539	1(3)
61540	1(3)
61541	1(2)
61543	1(2)
61544	1(3)
61545	1(2)
61546	1(2)
61548	1(2)
61550	1(2)
61552	1(2)
61556	1(3)

CPT	MUE
61557	1(2)
61558	1(3)
61559	1(3)
61563	2(3)
61564	1(2)
61566	1(3)
61567	1(2)
61570	1(3)
61571	1(3)
61575	1(2)
61576	1(2)
61580	1(2)
61581	1(2)
61582	1(2)
61583	1(2)
61584	1(2)
61585	1(2)
61586	1(3)
61590	1(2)
61591	1(2)
61592	1(2)
61595	1(2)
61596	1(2)
61597	1(2)
61598	1(3)
61600	1(3)
61601	1(3)
61605	1(3)
61606	1(3)
61607	1(3)
61608	1(3)
61611	1(3)
61613	1(3)
61615	1(3)
61616	1(3)
61618	2(3)
61619	2(3)
61623	2(3)
61624	2(3)
61626	2(3)
61630	1(3)
61635	2(3)
61640	0(3)
61641	0(3)
61642	0(3)
61645	1(3)
61650	1(2)
61651	2(2)
61680	1(3)
61682	1(3)
61684	1(3)
61686	1(3)
61690	1(3)
61692	1(3)
61697	2(3)
61698	1(3)
61700	2(3)
61702	1(3)
61703	1(3)
61705	1(3)
61708	1(3)
61710	1(3)
61711	1(3)
61720	1(3)
61735	1(3)

CPT	MUE
61750	2(3)
61751	2(3)
61760	1(2)
61770	1(2)
61781	1(3)
61782	1(3)
61783	1(3)
61790	1(2)
61791	1(2)
61796	1(2)
61797	4(3)
61798	1(2)
61799	4(3)
61800	1(2)
61850	1(3)
61860	1(3)
61863	1(2)
61864	1(3)
61867	1(2)
61868	2(3)
61870	1(3)
61880	1(2)
61885	1(3)
61886	1(3)
61888	1(3)
62000	1(3)
62005	1(3)
62010	1(3)
62100	1(3)
62115	1(2)
62117	1(2)
62120	1(2)
62121	1(2)
62140	1(3)
62141	1(3)
62142	2(3)
62143	2(3)
62145	2(3)
62146	2(3)
62147	1(3)
62148	1(3)
62160	1(3)
62161	1(3)
62162	1(3)
62163	1(3)
62164	1(3)
62165	1(2)
62180	1(3)
62190	1(3)
62192	1(3)
62194	1(3)
62200	1(2)
62201	1(2)
62220	1(3)
62223	1(3)
62225	2(3)
62230	2(3)
62252	2(3)
62256	1(3)
62258	1(3)
62263	1(2)
62264	1(2)
62267	2(3)
62268	1(3)
62269	2(3)

CPT	MUE
62270	2(3)
62272	2(3)
62273	2(3)
62280	1(3)
62281	1(3)
62282	1(3)
62284	1(3)
62287	1(2)
62290	5(2)
62291	4(3)
62292	1(2)
62294	1(3)
62302	1(3)
62303	1(3)
62304	1(3)
62305	1(3)
62320	1(3)
62321	1(3)
62322	1(3)
62323	1(3)
62324	1(3)
62325	1(3)
62326	1(3)
62327	1(3)
62350	1(3)
62351	1(3)
62355	1(3)
62360	1(2)
62361	1(2)
62362	1(2)
62365	1(2)
62367	1(3)
62368	1(3)
62369	1(3)
62370	1(3)
62380	2(3)
63001	1(2)
63003	1(2)
63005	1(2)
63011	1(2)
63012	1(2)
63015	1(2)
63016	1(2)
63017	1(2)
63020	1(2)
63030	1(2)
63035	4(3)
63040	1(2)
63042	1(2)
63043	4(3)
63044	4(2)
63045	1(2)
63046	1(2)
63047	1(2)
63048	5(3)
63050	1(2)
63051	1(2)
63055	1(2)
63056	1(2)
63057	3(3)
63064	1(2)
63066	1(3)
63075	1(2)
63076	3(3)
63077	1(2)

CPT	MUE
63078	3(3)
63081	1(2)
63082	6(2)
63085	1(2)
63086	2(3)
63087	1(2)
63088	3(3)
63090	1(2)
63091	3(3)
63101	1(2)
63102	1(2)
63103	3(3)
63170	1(3)
63172	1(3)
63173	1(3)
63180	1(2)
63182	1(2)
63185	1(2)
63190	1(2)
63191	1(2)
63194	1(2)
63195	1(2)
63196	1(2)
63197	1(2)
63198	1(2)
63199	1(2)
63200	1(2)
63250	1(3)
63251	1(3)
63252	1(3)
63265	1(3)
63266	1(3)
63267	1(3)
63268	1(3)
63270	1(3)
63271	1(3)
63272	1(3)
63273	1(3)
63275	1(3)
63276	1(3)
63277	1(3)
63278	1(3)
63280	1(3)
63281	1(3)
63282	1(3)
63283	1(3)
63285	1(3)
63286	1(3)
63287	1(3)
63290	1(3)
63295	1(2)
63300	1(2)
63301	1(2)
63302	1(2)
63303	1(2)
63304	1(2)
63305	1(2)
63306	1(2)
63307	1(2)
63308	3(3)
63600	2(3)
63610	1(3)
63620	1(2)
63621	2(2)
63650	2(3)

CPT	MUE
63655	1(3)
63661	1(2)
63662	1(2)
63663	1(3)
63664	1(3)
63685	1(3)
63688	1(3)
63700	1(3)
63702	1(3)
63704	1(3)
63706	1(3)
63707	1(3)
63709	1(3)
63710	1(3)
63740	1(3)
63741	1(3)
63744	1(3)
63746	1(2)
64400	4(3)
64402	1(3)
64405	1(3)
64408	1(3)
64410	1(3)
64413	1(3)
64415	1(3)
64416	1(2)
64417	1(3)
64418	1(3)
64420	3(3)
64421	3(3)
64425	1(3)
64430	1(3)
64435	1(3)
64445	1(3)
64446	1(2)
64447	1(3)
64448	1(2)
64449	1(2)
64450	10(3)
64455	1(2)
64461	1(2)
64462	1(2)
64463	1(3)
64479	1(2)
64480	4(3)
64483	1(2)
64484	4(3)
64486	1(3)
64487	1(2)
64488	1(3)
64489	1(2)
64490	1(2)
64491	1(2)
64492	1(2)
64493	1(2)
64494	1(2)
64495	1(2)
64505	1(3)
64510	1(3)
64517	1(3)
64520	1(3)
64530	1(3)
64553	1(3)
64555	2(3)
64561	1(3)

CPT	MUE
64566	1(3)
64568	1(3)
64569	1(3)
64570	1(3)
64575	2(3)
64580	2(3)
64581	2(3)
64585	2(3)
64590	1(3)
64595	1(3)
64600	2(3)
64605	1(2)
64610	1(2)
64611	1(2)
64612	1(2)
64615	1(2)
64616	1(2)
64617	1(2)
64620	5(3)
64630	1(3)
64632	1(2)
64633	1(2)
64634	4(3)
64635	1(2)
64636	4(2)
64640	5(3)
64642	1(2)
64643	3(2)
64644	1(2)
64645	3(2)
64646	1(2)
64647	1(2)
64650	1(2)
64653	1(2)
64680	1(2)
64681	1(2)
64702	2(3)
64704	4(3)
64708	3(3)
64712	1(2)
64713	1(2)
64714	1(2)
64716	2(3)
64718	1(2)
64719	1(2)
64721	1(2)
64722	4(3)
64726	2(3)
64727	2(3)
64732	1(2)
64734	1(2)
64736	1(2)
64738	1(2)
64740	1(2)
64742	1(2)
64744	1(2)
64746	1(2)
64755	1(2)
64760	1(2)
64763	1(2)
64766	1(2)
64771	2(3)
64772	2(3)
64774	2(3)
64776	1(2)

CPT	MUE
64778	1(3)
64782	2(2)
64783	2(3)
64784	3(3)
64786	1(3)
64787	4(3)
64788	5(3)
64790	1(3)
64792	2(3)
64795	2(3)
64802	1(2)
64804	1(2)
64809	1(2)
64818	1(2)
64820	4(3)
64821	1(2)
64822	1(2)
64823	1(2)
64831	1(2)
64832	3(3)
64834	1(2)
64835	1(2)
64836	1(2)
64837	2(3)
64840	1(2)
64856	2(3)
64857	2(3)
64858	1(2)
64859	2(3)
64861	1(2)
64862	1(2)
64864	2(3)
64865	1(3)
64866	1(3)
64868	1(3)
64872	1(3)
64874	1(3)
64876	1(3)
64885	1(3)
64886	1(3)
64890	2(3)
64891	2(3)
64892	2(3)
64893	2(3)
64895	2(3)
64896	2(3)
64897	2(3)
64898	2(3)
64901	2(3)
64902	1(3)
64905	1(3)
64907	1(3)
64910	3(3)
64911	2(3)
64912	3(3)
64913	3(3)
64999	1(3)
65091	1(2)
65093	1(2)
65101	1(2)
65103	1(2)
65105	1(2)
65110	1(2)
65112	1(2)
65114	1(2)

CPT	MUE
65125	1(2)
65130	1(2)
65135	1(2)
65140	1(2)
65150	1(2)
65155	1(2)
65175	1(2)
65205	1(3)
65210	1(3)
65220	1(3)
65222	1(3)
65235	1(3)
65260	1(3)
65265	1(3)
65270	1(3)
65272	1(3)
65273	1(3)
65275	1(3)
65280	1(3)
65285	1(3)
65286	1(3)
65290	1(3)
65400	1(3)
65410	1(3)
65420	1(2)
65426	1(2)
65430	1(2)
65435	1(2)
65436	1(2)
65450	1(3)
65600	1(2)
65710	1(2)
65730	1(2)
65750	1(2)
65755	1(2)
65756	1(2)
65757	1(3)
65760	0(3)
65765	0(3)
65767	0(3)
65770	1(2)
65771	0(3)
65772	1(2)
65775	1(2)
65778	1(2)
65779	1(2)
65780	1(2)
65781	1(2)
65782	1(2)
65785	1(2)
65800	1(2)
65810	1(2)
65815	1(3)
65820	1(2)
65850	1(2)
65855	1(2)
65860	1(2)
65865	1(2)
65870	1(2)
65875	1(2)
65880	1(2)
65900	1(3)
65920	1(2)
65930	1(3)
66020	1(3)

CPT	MUE
66030	1(3)
66130	1(3)
66150	1(2)
66155	1(2)
66160	1(2)
66170	1(2)
66172	1(2)
66174	1(2)
66175	1(2)
66179	1(2)
66180	1(2)
66183	1(3)
66184	1(2)
66185	1(2)
66225	1(2)
66250	1(2)
66500	1(2)
66505	1(2)
66600	1(2)
66605	1(2)
66625	1(2)
66630	1(2)
66635	1(2)
66680	1(2)
66682	1(2)
66700	1(2)
66710	1(2)
66711	1(2)
66720	1(2)
66740	1(2)
66761	1(2)
66762	1(2)
66770	1(3)
66820	1(2)
66821	1(2)
66825	1(2)
66830	1(2)
66840	1(2)
66850	1(2)
66852	1(2)
66920	1(2)
66930	1(2)
66940	1(2)
66982	1(2)
66983	1(2)
66984	1(2)
66985	1(2)
66986	1(2)
66990	1(3)
66999	1(3)
67005	1(2)
67010	1(2)
67015	1(2)
67025	1(2)
67027	1(2)
67028	1(3)
67030	1(2)
67031	1(2)
67036	1(2)
67039	1(2)
67040	1(2)
67041	1(2)
67042	1(2)
67043	1(2)
67101	1(2)

CPT	MUE
67105	1(2)
67107	1(2)
67108	1(2)
67110	1(2)
67113	1(2)
67115	1(2)
67120	1(2)
67121	1(2)
67141	1(2)
67145	1(2)
67208	1(2)
67210	1(2)
67218	1(2)
67220	1(2)
67221	1(2)
67225	1(2)
67227	1(2)
67228	1(2)
67229	1(2)
67250	1(2)
67255	1(2)
67299	1(3)
67311	1(2)
67312	1(2)
67314	1(2)
67316	1(2)
67318	1(2)
67320	2(3)
67331	1(2)
67332	1(2)
67334	1(2)
67335	1(2)
67340	2(2)
67343	1(2)
67345	1(3)
67346	1(3)
67399	1(3)
67400	1(2)
67405	1(2)
67412	1(2)
67413	1(2)
67414	1(2)
67415	1(3)
67420	1(2)
67430	1(2)
67440	1(2)
67445	1(2)
67450	1(2)
67500	1(3)
67505	1(3)
67515	1(3)
67550	1(2)
67560	1(2)
67570	1(2)
67599	1(3)
67700	2(3)
67710	1(2)
67715	1(3)
67800	1(2)
67801	1(2)
67805	1(2)
67808	1(2)
67810	2(3)
67820	1(2)
67825	1(2)

CPT	MUE
67830	1(2)
67835	1(2)
67840	3(3)
67850	3(3)
67875	1(2)
67880	1(2)
67882	1(2)
67900	1(2)
67901	1(2)
67902	1(2)
67903	1(2)
67904	1(2)
67906	1(2)
67908	1(2)
67909	1(2)
67911	2(3)
67912	1(2)
67914	2(3)
67915	2(3)
67916	2(3)
67917	2(3)
67921	2(3)
67922	2(3)
67923	2(3)
67924	2(3)
67930	2(3)
67935	2(3)
67938	2(3)
67950	2(2)
67961	2(3)
67966	2(3)
67971	1(2)
67973	1(2)
67974	1(2)
67975	1(2)
67999	1(3)
68020	1(3)
68040	1(2)
68100	1(3)
68110	1(3)
68115	1(3)
68130	1(3)
68135	1(3)
68200	1(3)
68320	1(2)
68325	1(2)
68326	1(2)
68328	1(2)
68330	1(3)
68335	1(3)
68340	1(3)
68360	1(3)
68362	1(3)
68371	1(3)
68399	1(3)
68400	1(2)
68420	1(2)
68440	2(3)
68500	1(2)
68505	1(2)
68510	1(2)
68520	1(2)
68525	1(2)
68530	1(2)
68540	1(2)

CPT	MUE
68550	1(2)
68700	1(2)
68705	2(3)
68720	1(2)
68745	1(2)
68750	1(2)
68760	4(2)
68761	4(2)
68770	1(3)
68801	4(2)
68810	1(2)
68811	1(2)
68815	1(2)
68816	1(2)
68840	1(2)
68850	1(3)
68899	1(3)
69000	1(3)
69005	1(3)
69020	1(3)
69090	0(3)
69100	3(3)
69105	1(3)
69110	1(2)
69120	1(3)
69140	1(2)
69145	1(3)
69150	1(3)
69155	1(3)
69200	1(2)
69205	1(3)
69209	1(2)
69210	1(2)
69220	1(2)
69222	1(2)
69300	1(2)
69310	1(2)
69320	1(2)
69399	1(3)
69420	1(2)
69421	1(2)
69424	1(2)
69433	1(2)
69436	1(2)
69440	1(2)
69450	1(2)
69501	1(3)
69502	1(2)
69505	1(2)
69511	1(2)
69530	1(2)
69535	1(2)
69540	1(3)
69550	1(3)
69552	1(2)
69554	1(2)
69601	1(2)
69602	1(2)
69603	1(2)
69604	1(2)
69605	1(2)
69610	1(2)
69620	1(2)
69631	1(2)
69632	1(3)

CPT	MUE
69633	1(2)
69635	1(3)
69636	1(3)
69637	1(3)
69641	1(2)
69642	1(2)
69643	1(2)
69644	1(2)
69645	1(2)
69646	1(2)
69650	1(2)
69660	1(2)
69661	1(2)
69662	1(2)
69666	1(2)
69667	1(2)
69670	1(2)
69676	1(2)
69700	1(3)
69710	0(3)
69711	1(2)
69714	1(2)
69715	1(3)
69717	1(2)
69718	1(2)
69720	1(2)
69725	1(2)
69740	1(2)
69745	1(2)
69799	1(3)
69801	1(3)
69805	1(3)
69806	1(3)
69905	1(2)
69910	1(2)
69915	1(3)
69930	1(2)
69949	1(3)
69950	1(2)
69955	1(2)
69960	1(2)
69970	1(3)
69979	1(3)
69990	1(3)
70010	1(3)
70015	1(3)
70030	2(2)
70100	2(3)
70110	2(3)
70120	1(3)
70130	1(3)
70134	1(3)
70140	2(3)
70150	1(3)
70160	1(3)
70170	2(2)
70190	1(2)
70200	2(3)
70210	1(3)
70220	1(3)
70240	1(2)
70250	2(3)
70260	1(3)
70300	1(3)
70310	1(3)

CPT	MUE
70320	1(3)
70328	1(3)
70330	1(3)
70332	2(3)
70336	1(3)
70350	1(3)
70355	1(3)
70360	2(3)
70370	1(3)
70371	1(2)
70380	2(3)
70390	2(3)
70450	3(3)
70460	1(3)
70470	2(3)
70480	1(3)
70481	1(3)
70482	1(3)
70486	1(3)
70487	1(3)
70488	1(3)
70490	1(3)
70491	1(3)
70492	1(3)
70496	2(3)
70498	2(3)
70540	1(3)
70542	1(3)
70543	1(3)
70544	2(3)
70545	1(3)
70546	1(3)
70547	1(3)
70548	1(3)
70549	1(3)
70551	2(3)
70552	2(3)
70553	2(3)
70554	1(3)
70555	1(3)
70557	1(3)
70558	1(3)
70559	1(3)
71045	4(3)
71046	3(3)
71047	2(3)
71048	1(3)
71100	2(3)
71101	2(3)
71110	1(3)
71111	1(3)
71120	1(3)
71130	1(3)
71250	2(3)
71260	2(3)
71270	1(3)
71275	1(3)
71550	1(3)
71551	1(3)
71552	1(3)
71555	1(3)
72020	4(3)
72040	3(3)
72050	1(3)
72052	1(3)

CPT	MUE
72070	1(3)
72072	1(3)
72074	1(3)
72080	1(3)
72081	1(3)
72082	1(3)
72083	1(3)
72084	1(3)
72100	2(3)
72110	1(3)
72114	1(3)
72120	1(3)
72125	1(3)
72126	1(3)
72127	1(3)
72128	1(3)
72129	1(3)
72130	1(3)
72131	1(3)
72132	1(3)
72133	1(3)
72141	1(3)
72142	1(3)
72146	1(3)
72147	1(3)
72148	1(3)
72149	1(3)
72156	1(3)
72157	1(3)
72158	1(3)
72159	1(3)
72170	2(3)
72190	1(3)
72191	1(3)
72192	1(3)
72193	1(3)
72194	1(3)
72195	1(3)
72196	1(3)
72197	1(3)
72198	1(3)
72200	2(3)
72202	1(3)
72220	1(3)
72240	1(2)
72255	1(2)
72265	1(2)
72270	1(2)
72275	1(3)
72285	4(3)
72295	5(3)
73000	2(3)
73010	2(3)
73020	2(3)
73030	4(3)
73040	2(2)
73050	1(3)
73060	2(3)
73070	2(3)
73080	2(3)
73085	2(2)
73090	2(3)
73092	2(3)
73100	2(3)
73110	3(3)

CPT	MUE
73115	2(2)
73120	2(3)
73130	3(3)
73140	3(3)
73200	2(3)
73201	2(3)
73202	2(3)
73206	2(3)
73218	2(3)
73219	2(3)
73220	2(3)
73221	2(3)
73222	2(3)
73223	2(3)
73225	2(3)
73501	2(3)
73502	2(3)
73503	2(3)
73521	2(3)
73522	2(3)
73523	2(3)
73525	2(2)
73551	2(3)
73552	2(3)
73560	4(3)
73562	3(3)
73564	4(3)
73565	1(3)
73580	2(2)
73590	3(3)
73592	2(3)
73600	2(3)
73610	3(3)
73615	2(2)
73620	2(3)
73630	3(3)
73650	2(3)
73660	2(3)
73700	2(3)
73701	2(3)
73702	2(3)
73706	2(3)
73718	2(3)
73719	2(3)
73720	2(3)
73721	3(3)
73722	2(3)
73723	2(3)
73725	2(3)
74018	3(3)
74019	2(3)
74021	2(3)
74022	2(3)
74150	1(3)
74160	1(3)
74170	1(3)
74174	1(3)
74175	1(3)
74176	2(3)
74177	2(3)
74178	1(3)
74181	1(3)
74182	1(3)
74183	1(3)
74185	1(3)

CPT	MUE
74190	1(3)
74210	1(3)
74220	1(3)
74230	1(3)
74235	1(3)
74240	2(3)
74241	1(3)
74245	1(3)
74246	1(3)
74247	1(3)
74249	1(3)
74250	1(3)
74251	1(3)
74260	1(2)
74261	1(2)
74262	1(2)
74263	0(3)
74270	1(3)
74280	1(3)
74283	1(3)
74290	1(3)
74300	1(3)
74301	1(3)
74328	1(3)
74329	1(3)
74330	1(3)
74340	1(3)
74355	1(3)
74360	1(3)
74363	2(3)
74400	1(3)
74410	1(3)
74415	1(3)
74420	2(3)
74425	2(3)
74430	1(3)
74440	1(2)
74445	1(2)
74450	1(3)
74455	1(3)
74470	2(2)
74485	2(3)
74710	1(3)
74712	1(3)
74713	2(3)
74740	1(3)
74742	2(2)
74775	1(2)
75557	1(3)
75559	1(3)
75561	1(3)
75563	1(3)
75565	1(3)
75571	1(3)
75572	1(3)
75573	1(3)
75574	1(3)
75600	1(3)
75605	1(3)
75625	1(3)
75630	1(3)
75635	1(3)
75705	20(3)
75710	2(3)
75716	1(3)

CPT	MUE
75726	3(3)
75731	1(3)
75733	1(3)
75736	2(3)
75741	1(3)
75743	1(3)
75746	1(3)
75756	2(3)
75774	7(3)
75801	1(3)
75803	1(3)
75805	1(2)
75807	1(2)
75809	1(3)
75810	1(3)
75820	2(3)
75822	1(3)
75825	1(3)
75827	1(3)
75831	1(3)
75833	1(3)
75840	1(3)
75842	1(3)
75860	2(3)
75870	1(3)
75872	1(3)
75880	1(3)
75885	1(3)
75887	1(3)
75889	1(3)
75891	1(3)
75893	2(3)
75894	2(3)
75898	2(3)
75901	1(3)
75902	2(3)
75956	1(2)
75957	1(2)
75958	2(3)
75959	1(2)
75970	1(3)
75984	2(3)
75989	2(3)
76000	3(3)
76010	2(3)
76080	3(3)
76098	3(3)
76100	2(3)
76101	1(3)
76102	1(3)
76120	1(3)
76125	1(3)
76140	0(3)
76376	2(3)
76377	2(3)
76380	2(3)
76390	0(3)
76391	1(3)
76496	1(3)
76497	1(3)
76498	1(3)
76499	1(3)
76506	1(2)
76510	2(2)
76511	2(2)

CPT	MUE
76512	2(2)
76513	2(2)
76514	1(2)
76516	1(2)
76519	1(3)
76529	2(2)
76536	1(3)
76604	1(3)
76641	2(2)
76642	2(2)
76700	1(3)
76705	2(3)
76706	1(2)
76770	1(3)
76775	2(3)
76776	2(3)
76800	1(3)
76801	1(2)
76802	2(3)
76805	1(2)
76810	2(3)
76811	1(2)
76812	2(3)
76813	1(2)
76814	2(3)
76815	1(2)
76816	2(3)
76817	1(3)
76818	2(3)
76819	2(3)
76820	3(3)
76821	2(3)
76825	2(3)
76826	2(3)
76827	2(3)
76828	2(3)
76830	1(3)
76831	1(3)
76856	1(3)
76857	1(3)
76870	1(2)
76872	1(3)
76873	1(2)
76881	2(3)
76882	2(3)
76885	1(2)
76886	1(2)
76930	1(3)
76932	1(2)
76936	1(3)
76937	2(3)
76940	1(3)
76941	3(3)
76942	1(3)
76945	1(3)
76946	1(3)
76948	1(2)
76965	2(3)
76970	2(3)
76975	1(3)
76977	1(2)
76978	1(2)
76979	3(3)
76981	1(3)
76982	1(2)

CPT	MUE
76983	3(3)
76998	1(3)
76999	1(3)
77001	2(3)
77002	1(3)
77003	1(3)
77011	1(3)
77012	1(3)
77013	1(3)
77014	2(3)
77021	1(3)
77022	1(3)
77046	1(2)
77047	1(2)
77048	1(2)
77049	1(2)
77053	2(2)
77054	2(2)
77061	1(2)
77062	1(2)
77063	1(2)
77065	1(2)
77066	1(2)
77067	1(2)
77071	1(3)
77072	1(2)
77073	1(2)
77074	1(2)
77075	1(2)
77076	1(2)
77077	1(2)
77078	1(2)
77080	1(2)
77081	1(2)
77084	1(2)
77085	1(2)
77086	1(2)
77261	1(3)
77262	1(3)
77263	1(3)
77280	2(3)
77285	1(3)
77290	1(3)
77293	1(3)
77295	1(3)
77299	1(3)
77300	10(3)
77301	1(3)
77306	1(3)
77307	1(3)
77316	1(3)
77317	1(3)
77318	1(3)
77321	1(2)
77331	3(3)
77332	4(3)
77333	2(3)
77334	10(3)
77336	1(2)
77338	1(3)
77370	1(3)
77371	1(2)
77372	1(2)
77373	1(3)
77385	2(3)

CPT	MUE
77386	2(3)
77387	2(3)
77399	1(3)
77401	1(2)
77402	2(3)
77407	2(3)
77412	2(3)
77417	1(2)
77423	1(3)
77424	1(2)
77425	1(3)
77427	1(2)
77431	1(2)
77432	1(2)
77435	1(2)
77469	1(2)
77470	1(2)
77499	1(3)
77520	2(3)
77522	2(3)
77523	2(3)
77525	2(3)
77600	1(3)
77605	1(3)
77610	1(3)
77615	1(3)
77620	1(3)
77750	1(3)
77761	1(3)
77762	1(3)
77763	1(3)
77767	2(3)
77768	2(3)
77770	2(3)
77771	2(3)
77772	2(3)
77778	1(3)
77789	2(3)
77790	1(3)
77799	1(3)
78012	1(3)
78013	1(3)
78014	1(2)
78015	1(3)
78016	1(3)
78018	1(2)
78020	1(3)
78070	1(2)
78071	1(3)
78072	1(3)
78075	1(2)
78099	1(3)
78102	1(2)
78103	1(2)
78104	1(2)
78110	1(2)
78111	1(2)
78120	1(2)
78121	1(2)
78122	1(2)
78130	1(2)
78135	1(3)
78140	1(3)
78185	1(2)
78191	1(2)

CPT	MUE
78195	1(2)
78199	1(3)
78201	1(3)
78202	1(3)
78205	1(3)
78206	1(3)
78215	1(3)
78216	1(3)
78226	1(3)
78227	1(3)
78230	1(3)
78231	1(3)
78232	1(3)
78258	1(2)
78261	1(2)
78262	1(2)
78264	1(2)
78265	1(2)
78266	1(2)
78267	1(2)
78268	1(2)
78278	2(3)
78282	1(2)
78290	1(3)
78291	1(3)
78299	1(3)
78300	1(2)
78305	1(2)
78306	1(2)
78315	1(2)
78320	1(2)
78350	0(3)
78351	0(3)
78399	1(3)
78414	1(2)
78428	1(3)
78445	1(3)
78451	1(2)
78452	1(2)
78453	1(2)
78454	1(2)
78456	1(3)
78457	1(2)
78458	1(2)
78459	1(3)
78466	1(3)
78468	1(3)
78469	1(3)
78472	1(2)
78473	1(2)
78481	1(2)
78483	1(2)
78491	1(3)
78492	1(2)
78494	1(3)
78496	1(3)
78499	1(3)
78579	1(3)
78580	1(3)
78582	1(3)
78597	1(3)
78598	1(3)
78599	1(3)
78600	1(3)
78601	1(3)

CPT	MUE
78605	1(3)
78606	1(3)
78607	1(3)
78608	1(3)
78609	0(3)
78610	1(3)
78630	1(3)
78635	1(3)
78645	1(3)
78647	1(3)
78650	1(3)
78660	1(2)
78699	1(3)
78700	1(3)
78701	1(3)
78707	1(2)
78708	1(2)
78709	1(2)
78710	1(3)
78725	1(3)
78730	1(2)
78740	1(2)
78761	1(2)
78799	1(3)
78800	1(2)
78801	1(2)
78802	1(2)
78803	1(2)
78804	1(2)
78805	1(3)
78806	1(2)
78807	1(3)
78808	1(2)
78811	1(2)
78812	1(2)
78813	1(2)
78814	1(2)
78815	1(2)
78816	1(2)
78999	1(3)
79005	1(3)
79101	1(3)
79200	1(3)
79300	1(3)
79403	1(3)
79440	1(3)
79445	1(3)
79999	1(3)
80047	2(3)
80048	2(3)
80050	0(3)
80051	4(3)
80053	1(3)
80055	1(3)
80061	1(3)
80069	1(3)
80074	1(2)
80076	1(3)
80081	1(2)
80150	2(3)
80155	1(3)
80156	2(3)
80157	2(3)
80158	2(3)
80159	2(3)

CPT	MUE
80162	2(3)
80163	1(3)
80164	2(3)
80165	1(3)
80168	2(3)
80169	2(3)
80170	2(3)
80171	1(3)
80173	2(3)
80175	1(3)
80176	1(3)
80177	1(3)
80178	2(3)
80180	1(3)
80183	1(3)
80184	2(3)
80185	2(3)
80186	2(3)
80188	2(3)
80190	2(3)
80192	2(3)
80194	2(3)
80195	2(3)
80197	2(3)
80198	2(3)
80199	1(3)
80200	2(3)
80201	2(3)
80202	2(3)
80203	1(3)
80299	3(3)
80305	1(2)
80306	1(2)
80307	1(2)
80320	2(3)
80321	1(3)
80322	1(3)
80323	1(3)
80324	1(3)
80325	1(3)
80326	1(3)
80327	1(3)
80328	1(3)
80329	2(3)
80330	1(3)
80331	1(3)
80332	1(3)
80333	1(3)
80334	1(3)
80335	1(3)
80336	1(3)
80337	1(3)
80338	1(3)
80339	2(3)
80340	1(3)
80341	1(3)
80342	1(3)
80343	1(3)
80344	1(3)
80345	2(3)
80346	1(3)
80347	1(3)
80348	1(3)
80349	1(3)
80350	1(3)

CPT	MUE
80351	1(3)
80352	1(3)
80353	1(3)
80354	1(3)
80355	1(3)
80356	1(3)
80357	1(3)
80358	1(3)
80359	1(3)
80360	1(3)
80361	2(3)
80362	1(3)
80363	1(3)
80364	1(3)
80365	2(3)
80366	1(3)
80367	1(3)
80368	1(3)
80369	1(3)
80370	1(3)
80371	1(3)
80372	1(3)
80373	1(3)
80374	1(3)
80375	1(3)
80376	1(3)
80377	1(3)
80400	1(3)
80402	1(3)
80406	1(3)
80408	1(3)
80410	1(3)
80412	1(3)
80414	1(3)
80415	1(3)
80416	1(3)
80417	1(3)
80418	1(3)
80420	1(2)
80422	1(3)
80424	1(3)
80426	1(3)
80428	1(3)
80430	1(3)
80432	1(3)
80434	1(3)
80435	1(3)
80436	1(3)
80438	1(3)
80439	1(3)
80500	1(3)
80502	1(3)
81000	2(3)
81001	2(3)
81002	2(3)
81003	2(3)
81005	2(3)
81007	1(3)
81015	2(3)
81020	1(3)
81025	1(3)
81050	2(3)
81099	1(3)
81105	1(2)
81106	1(2)

CPT	MUE
81107	1(2)
81108	1(2)
81109	1(2)
81110	1(2)
81111	1(2)
81112	1(2)
81120	1(3)
81121	1(3)
81161	1(3)
81162	1(2)
81163	1(2)
81164	1(2)
81165	1(2)
81166	1(2)
81167	1(2)
81170	1(2)
81171	1(2)
81172	1(2)
81173	1(2)
81174	1(2)
81175	1(3)
81176	1(3)
81177	1(2)
81178	1(2)
81179	1(2)
81180	1(2)
81181	1(2)
81182	1(2)
81183	1(2)
81184	1(2)
81185	1(2)
81186	1(2)
81187	1(2)
81188	1(2)
81189	1(2)
81190	1(2)
81200	1(2)
81201	1(2)
81202	1(3)
81203	1(3)
81204	1(2)
81205	1(3)
81206	1(3)
81207	1(3)
81208	1(3)
81209	1(3)
81210	1(3)
81212	1(2)
81215	1(2)
81216	1(2)
81217	1(2)
81218	1(3)
81219	1(3)
81220	1(3)
81221	1(3)
81222	1(3)
81223	1(2)
81224	1(3)
81225	1(3)
81226	1(3)
81227	1(3)
81228	1(3)
81229	1(3)
81230	1(2)
81231	1(2)

CPT	MUE
81232	1(2)
81233	1(3)
81234	1(2)
81235	1(3)
81236	1(3)
81237	1(3)
81238	1(2)
81239	1(2)
81240	1(2)
81241	1(2)
81242	1(3)
81243	1(3)
81244	1(3)
81245	1(3)
81246	1(3)
81247	1(2)
81248	1(2)
81249	1(2)
81250	1(3)
81251	1(3)
81252	1(3)
81253	1(3)
81254	1(3)
81255	1(3)
81256	1(2)
81257	1(2)
81258	1(2)
81259	1(2)
81260	1(3)
81261	1(3)
81262	1(3)
81263	1(3)
81264	1(3)
81265	1(3)
81266	2(3)
81267	1(3)
81268	4(3)
81269	1(2)
81270	1(2)
81271	1(2)
81272	1(3)
81273	1(3)
81274	1(2)
81275	1(3)
81276	1(3)
81283	1(2)
81284	1(2)
81285	1(2)
81286	1(2)
81287	1(3)
81288	1(3)
81289	1(2)
81290	1(3)
81291	1(3)
81292	1(2)
81293	1(3)
81294	1(3)
81295	1(2)
81296	1(3)
81297	1(3)
81298	1(2)
81299	1(3)
81300	1(3)
81301	1(3)
81302	1(3)

CPT	MUE
81303	1(3)
81304	1(3)
81305	1(3)
81306	1(2)
81310	1(3)
81311	1(3)
81312	1(2)
81313	1(3)
81314	1(3)
81315	1(3)
81316	1(2)
81317	1(3)
81318	1(3)
81319	1(2)
81320	1(3)
81321	1(3)
81322	1(3)
81323	1(3)
81324	1(3)
81325	1(3)
81326	1(3)
81327	1(2)
81328	1(2)
81329	1(2)
81330	1(3)
81331	1(3)
81332	1(3)
81333	1(2)
81334	1(3)
81335	1(2)
81336	1(2)
81337	1(2)
81340	1(3)
81341	1(3)
81342	1(3)
81343	1(2)
81344	1(2)
81345	1(3)
81346	1(2)
81350	1(3)
81355	1(3)
81361	1(2)
81362	1(2)
81363	1(2)
81364	1(2)
81370	1(2)
81371	1(2)
81372	1(2)
81373	2(2)
81374	1(3)
81375	1(2)
81376	5(3)
81377	2(3)
81378	1(2)
81379	1(2)
81380	2(2)
81381	3(3)
81382	6(3)
81383	2(3)
81400	2(3)
81401	3(3)
81402	1(3)
81403	3(3)
81404	3(3)
81405	2(3)

CPT	MUE
81406	3(3)
81407	1(3)
81408	1(3)
81410	1(2)
81411	1(2)
81412	1(2)
81413	1(2)
81414	1(2)
81415	1(2)
81416	2(3)
81417	1(3)
81420	1(2)
81422	1(2)
81425	1(2)
81426	2(3)
81427	1(3)
81430	1(2)
81431	1(2)
81432	1(2)
81433	1(2)
81434	1(2)
81435	1(2)
81436	1(2)
81437	1(2)
81438	1(2)
81439	1(2)
81440	1(2)
81442	1(2)
81443	1(2)
81445	1(2)
81448	1(2)
81450	1(2)
81455	1(2)
81460	1(2)
81465	1(2)
81470	1(2)
81471	1(2)
81479	3(3)
81490	1(2)
81493	1(2)
81500	1(2)
81503	1(2)
81504	1(3)
81506	1(2)
81507	1(2)
81508	1(2)
81509	1(2)
81510	1(2)
81511	1(2)
81512	1(2)
81518	1(3)
81519	1(2)
81520	1(3)
81521	1(3)
81525	1(3)
81528	1(2)
81535	1(2)
81536	11(3)
81538	1(2)
81539	1(2)
81540	1(3)
81541	1(2)
81545	1(3)
81551	1(2)
81595	1(2)

CPT	MUE
81596	1(2)
81599	1(3)
82009	3(3)
82010	3(3)
82013	1(3)
82016	1(3)
82017	1(3)
82024	4(3)
82030	1(3)
82040	1(3)
82042	2(3)
82043	1(3)
82044	1(3)
82045	1(3)
82075	2(3)
82085	1(3)
82088	2(3)
82103	1(3)
82104	1(2)
82105	1(3)
82106	2(3)
82107	1(3)
82108	1(3)
82120	1(3)
82127	1(3)
82128	2(3)
82131	2(3)
82135	1(3)
82136	2(3)
82139	2(3)
82140	2(3)
82143	2(3)
82150	4(3)
82154	1(3)
82157	1(3)
82160	1(3)
82163	1(3)
82164	1(3)
82172	2(3)
82175	2(3)
82180	1(2)
82190	2(3)
82232	2(3)
82239	1(3)
82240	1(3)
82247	2(3)
82248	2(3)
82252	1(3)
82261	1(3)
82270	1(3)
82271	3(3)
82272	1(3)
82274	1(3)
82286	1(3)
82300	1(3)
82306	1(2)
82308	1(3)
82310	4(3)
82330	4(3)
82331	1(3)
82340	1(3)
82355	2(3)
82360	2(3)
82365	2(3)
82370	2(3)

CPT	MUE	CPT	MUE	CPT	MUE	CPT	MUE	CPT	MUE	CPT	MUE	CPT	MUE	CPT	MUE
82373	1(3)	82710	1(3)	83070	1(2)	83918	2(3)	84238	3(3)	84597	1(3)	85378	2(3)	86153	1(3)
82374	2(3)	82715	3(3)	83080	2(3)	83919	1(3)	84244	2(3)	84600	2(3)	85379	2(3)	86155	1(3)
82375	4(3)	82725	1(3)	83088	1(3)	83921	2(3)	84252	1(2)	84620	1(2)	85380	2(3)	86156	1(2)
82376	2(3)	82726	1(3)	83090	2(3)	83930	2(3)	84255	2(3)	84630	2(3)	85384	2(3)	86157	1(2)
82378	1(3)	82728	1(3)	83150	1(3)	83935	2(3)	84260	1(3)	84681	1(3)	85385	1(3)	86160	4(3)
82379	1(3)	82731	1(3)	83491	1(3)	83937	1(3)	84270	1(3)	84702	2(3)	85390	3(3)	86161	2(3)
82380	1(3)	82735	1(3)	83497	1(3)	83945	2(3)	84275	1(3)	84703	1(3)	85396	1(2)	86162	1(2)
82382	1(2)	82746	1(2)	83498	2(3)	83950	1(2)	84285	1(3)	84704	1(3)	85397	2(3)	86171	2(3)
82383	1(3)	82747	1(2)	83500	1(3)	83951	1(2)	84295	2(3)	84830	1(2)	85400	1(3)	86200	1(3)
82384	2(3)	82757	1(2)	83505	1(3)	83970	4(3)	84300	2(3)	84999	1(3)	85410	1(3)	86215	1(3)
82387	1(3)	82759	1(3)	83516	5(3)	83986	2(3)	84302	1(3)	85002	1(3)	85415	2(3)	86225	1(3)
82390	1(2)	82760	1(3)	83518	1(3)	83987	1(3)	84305	1(3)	85004	2(3)	85420	2(3)	86226	1(3)
82397	4(3)	82775	1(3)	83519	5(3)	83992	2(3)	84307	1(3)	85007	1(3)	85421	1(3)	86235	10(3)
82415	1(3)	82776	1(2)	83520	8(3)	83993	1(3)	84311	2(3)	85008	1(3)	85441	1(2)	86255	5(3)
82435	2(3)	82777	1(3)	83525	4(3)	84030	1(2)	84315	1(3)	85009	1(3)	85445	1(2)	86256	9(3)
82436	1(3)	82784	6(3)	83527	1(3)	84035	1(2)	84375	1(3)	85013	1(3)	85460	1(3)	86277	1(3)
82438	1(3)	82785	1(3)	83528	1(3)	84060	1(3)	84376	1(3)	85014	4(3)	85461	1(2)	86280	1(3)
82441	1(2)	82787	4(3)	83540	2(3)	84066	1(3)	84377	1(3)	85018	4(3)	85475	1(3)	86294	1(3)
82465	1(3)	82800	2(3)	83550	1(3)	84075	2(3)	84378	2(3)	85025	4(3)	85520	3(3)	86300	2(3)
82480	2(3)	82805	3(3)	83570	1(3)	84078	1(2)	84379	1(3)	85027	4(3)	85525	2(3)	86301	1(2)
82482	1(3)	82810	4(3)	83582	1(3)	84080	1(3)	84392	1(3)	85032	2(3)	85530	1(3)	86304	1(2)
82485	1(3)	82820	1(3)	83586	1(3)	84081	1(3)	84402	1(3)	85041	1(3)	85536	1(2)	86305	1(2)
82495	1(2)	82930	1(3)	83593	1(3)	84085	1(2)	84403	2(3)	85044	1(2)	85540	1(2)	86308	1(2)
82507	1(3)	82938	1(3)	83605	2(3)	84087	1(3)	84410	1(2)	85045	1(2)	85547	1(2)	86309	1(2)
82523	1(3)	82941	1(3)	83615	3(3)	84100	2(3)	84425	1(2)	85046	1(2)	85549	1(3)	86310	1(2)
82525	2(3)	82943	1(3)	83625	1(3)	84105	1(3)	84430	1(3)	85048	2(3)	85555	1(2)	86316	2(3)
82528	1(3)	82945	4(3)	83630	1(3)	84106	1(2)	84431	1(3)	85049	2(3)	85557	1(2)	86317	6(3)
82530	4(3)	82946	1(2)	83631	1(3)	84110	1(3)	84432	1(2)	85055	1(3)	85576	7(3)	86318	2(3)
82533	5(3)	82947	5(3)	83632	1(3)	84112	1(3)	84436	1(2)	85060	1(3)	85597	1(3)	86320	1(2)
82540	1(3)	82950	3(3)	83633	1(3)	84119	1(2)	84437	1(2)	85097	2(3)	85598	1(3)	86325	2(3)
82542	6(3)	82951	1(2)	83655	2(3)	84120	1(3)	84439	1(2)	85130	1(3)	85610	4(3)	86327	1(3)
82550	3(3)	82952	3(3)	83661	3(3)	84126	1(3)	84442	1(2)	85170	1(3)	85611	2(3)	86329	3(3)
82552	3(3)	82955	1(2)	83662	4(3)	84132	3(3)	84443	4(2)	85175	1(3)	85612	1(3)	86331	12(3)
82553	3(3)	82960	1(2)	83663	3(3)	84133	2(3)	84445	1(2)	85210	2(3)	85613	3(3)	86332	1(3)
82554	2(3)	82963	1(3)	83664	3(3)	84134	1(3)	84446	1(2)	85220	2(3)	85635	1(3)	86334	2(2)
82565	2(3)	82965	1(3)	83670	1(3)	84135	1(3)	84449	1(3)	85230	2(3)	85651	1(2)	86335	2(3)
82570	3(3)	82977	1(3)	83690	2(3)	84138	1(3)	84450	1(3)	85240	2(3)	85652	1(2)	86336	1(3)
82575	1(3)	82978	1(3)	83695	1(3)	84140	1(3)	84460	1(3)	85244	1(3)	85660	2(3)	86337	1(2)
82585	1(2)	82979	1(3)	83698	1(3)	84143	2(3)	84466	1(3)	85245	2(3)	85670	2(3)	86340	1(2)
82595	1(3)	82985	1(3)	83700	1(2)	84144	1(3)	84478	1(3)	85246	2(3)	85675	1(3)	86341	1(3)
82600	1(3)	83001	1(3)	83701	1(3)	84145	1(3)	84479	1(2)	85247	2(3)	85705	1(3)	86343	1(3)
82607	1(2)	83002	1(3)	83704	1(3)	84146	3(3)	84480	1(2)	85250	2(3)	85730	4(3)	86344	1(2)
82608	1(2)	83003	5(3)	83718	1(3)	84150	2(3)	84481	1(2)	85260	2(3)	85732	4(3)	86352	1(3)
82610	1(3)	83006	1(2)	83719	1(3)	84152	1(2)	84482	1(2)	85270	2(3)	85810	2(3)	86353	7(3)
82615	1(3)	83009	1(3)	83721	1(3)	84153	1(2)	84484	4(3)	85280	2(3)	85999	1(3)	86355	1(2)
82626	1(3)	83010	1(3)	83722	1(2)	84154	1(2)	84485	1(3)	85290	2(3)	86000	6(3)	86356	7(3)
82627	1(3)	83012	1(2)	83727	1(3)	84155	1(3)	84488	1(3)	85291	1(3)	86001	20(3)	86357	1(2)
82633	1(3)	83013	1(3)	83735	4(3)	84156	1(3)	84490	1(2)	85292	1(3)	86005	6(3)	86359	1(2)
82634	1(3)	83014	1(2)	83775	1(3)	84157	2(3)	84510	1(3)	85293	1(3)	86008	20(3)	86360	1(2)
82638	1(3)	83015	1(2)	83785	1(3)	84160	2(3)	84512	3(3)	85300	2(3)	86021	1(2)	86361	1(2)
82642	1(2)	83018	4(3)	83789	4(3)	84163	1(3)	84520	2(3)	85301	1(3)	86022	1(2)	86367	2(3)
82652	1(2)	83020	2(3)	83825	2(3)	84165	1(2)	84525	1(3)	85302	1(3)	86023	3(3)	86376	2(3)
82656	1(3)	83021	2(3)	83835	2(3)	84166	2(3)	84540	2(3)	85303	2(3)	86038	1(3)	86382	3(3)
82657	2(3)	83026	1(3)	83857	1(3)	84181	3(3)	84545	1(3)	85305	2(3)	86039	1(3)	86384	1(3)
82658	2(3)	83030	1(3)	83861	2(2)	84182	6(3)	84550	1(3)	85306	2(3)	86060	1(3)	86386	1(2)
82664	2(3)	83033	1(3)	83864	1(2)	84202	1(2)	84560	2(3)	85307	2(3)	86063	1(3)	86403	3(3)
82668	1(3)	83036	1(2)	83872	2(3)	84203	1(2)	84577	1(3)	85335	2(3)	86077	1(2)	86406	2(3)
82670	2(3)	83037	1(2)	83873	1(3)	84206	1(2)	84578	1(3)	85337	1(3)	86078	1(3)	86430	2(3)
82671	1(3)	83045	1(3)	83874	4(3)	84207	1(2)	84580	1(3)	85345	1(3)	86079	1(3)	86431	2(3)
82672	1(3)	83050	2(3)	83876	1(3)	84210	1(3)	84583	1(3)	85347	9(3)	86140	1(2)	86480	1(3)
82677	1(3)	83051	1(3)	83880	1(3)	84220	1(3)	84585	1(2)	85348	4(3)	86141	1(2)	86481	1(3)
82679	1(3)	83060	1(3)	83883	4(3)	84228	1(3)	84586	1(2)	85360	1(3)	86146	3(3)	86485	1(2)
82693	2(3)	83065	1(2)	83885	2(3)	84233	1(3)	84588	1(3)	85362	2(3)	86147	4(3)	86486	2(3)
82696	1(3)	83068	1(2)	83915	1(3)	84234	1(3)	84590	1(2)	85366	1(3)	86148	3(3)	86490	1(2)
82705	1(3)	83069	1(3)	83916	2(3)	84235	1(3)	84591	1(3)	85370	1(3)	86152	1(3)	86510	1(2)

CPT	MUE	CPT	MUE	CPT	MUE	CPT	MUE	CPT	MUE	CPT	MUE	CPT	MUE	CPT	MUE
86580	1(2)	86738	2(3)	86930	3(3)	87254	10(3)	87493	2(3)	87653	1(3)	88161	4(3)	88342	3(3)
86590	1(3)	86741	2(3)	86931	4(3)	87255	2(3)	87495	1(3)	87660	1(3)	88162	3(3)	88344	6(3)
86592	2(3)	86744	2(3)	86940	3(3)	87260	1(3)	87496	1(3)	87661	1(3)	88164	1(3)	88346	2(3)
86593	2(3)	86747	2(3)	86941	3(3)	87265	1(3)	87497	2(3)	87662	2(3)	88165	1(3)	88348	1(3)
86602	3(3)	86750	4(3)	86945	5(3)	87267	1(3)	87498	1(3)	87797	3(3)	88166	1(3)	88350	8(3)
86603	2(3)	86753	3(3)	86950	1(3)	87269	1(3)	87500	1(3)	87798	21(3)	88167	1(3)	88355	1(3)
86609	14(3)	86756	2(3)	86960	3(3)	87270	1(3)	87501	1(3)	87799	3(3)	88172	7(3)	88356	3(3)
86611	4(3)	86757	6(3)	86965	4(3)	87271	1(3)	87502	1(3)	87800	2(3)	88173	7(3)	88358	2(3)
86612	2(3)	86759	2(3)	86971	6(3)	87272	1(3)	87503	1(3)	87801	3(3)	88174	1(3)	88360	6(3)
86615	6(3)	86762	2(3)	86972	2(3)	87273	1(3)	87505	1(2)	87802	2(3)	88175	1(3)	88361	6(3)
86617	2(3)	86765	2(3)	86975	2(3)	87274	1(3)	87506	1(2)	87803	3(3)	88177	6(3)	88362	1(3)
86618	2(3)	86768	5(3)	86976	2(3)	87275	1(3)	87507	1(2)	87804	3(3)	88182	2(3)	88363	2(3)
86619	2(3)	86771	2(3)	86977	2(3)	87276	1(3)	87510	1(3)	87806	1(2)	88184	2(3)	88364	3(3)
86622	2(3)	86774	2(3)	86999	1(3)	87278	1(3)	87511	1(3)	87807	2(3)	88185	35(3)	88365	4(3)
86625	1(3)	86777	2(3)	87003	1(3)	87279	1(3)	87512	1(3)	87808	1(3)	88187	2(3)	88366	2(3)
86628	3(3)	86778	2(3)	87015	3(3)	87280	1(3)	87516	1(3)	87809	2(3)	88188	2(3)	88367	3(3)
86631	6(3)	86780	2(3)	87045	3(3)	87281	1(3)	87517	1(3)	87810	2(3)	88189	2(3)	88368	3(3)
86632	3(3)	86784	1(3)	87046	6(3)	87283	1(3)	87520	1(3)	87850	1(3)	88199	1(3)	88369	3(3)
86635	4(3)	86787	2(3)	87071	2(3)	87285	1(3)	87521	1(3)	87880	2(3)	88230	2(3)	88371	1(3)
86638	6(3)	86788	2(3)	87073	2(3)	87290	1(3)	87522	1(3)	87899	6(3)	88233	2(3)	88372	1(3)
86641	2(3)	86789	2(3)	87075	6(3)	87299	1(3)	87525	1(3)	87900	1(2)	88235	2(3)	88373	3(3)
86644	2(3)	86790	4(3)	87076	4(3)	87300	2(3)	87526	1(3)	87901	1(2)	88237	4(3)	88374	5(3)
86645	1(3)	86793	2(3)	87077	6(3)	87301	1(3)	87527	1(3)	87902	1(2)	88239	3(3)	88375	1(3)
86648	2(3)	86794	1(3)	87081	4(3)	87305	1(3)	87528	1(3)	87903	1(2)	88240	3(3)	88377	5(3)
86651	2(3)	86800	1(3)	87084	1(3)	87320	1(3)	87529	2(3)	87904	14(3)	88241	3(3)	88380	1(3)
86652	2(3)	86803	1(3)	87086	3(3)	87324	2(3)	87530	2(3)	87905	2(3)	88245	1(2)	88381	1(3)
86653	2(3)	86804	1(2)	87088	3(3)	87327	1(3)	87531	1(3)	87906	2(3)	88248	1(2)	88387	2(3)
86654	2(3)	86805	12(3)	87101	3(3)	87328	2(3)	87532	1(3)	87910	1(3)	88249	1(2)	88388	1(3)
86658	12(3)	86806	2(3)	87102	4(3)	87329	2(3)	87533	1(3)	87912	1(3)	88261	2(3)	88399	1(3)
86663	2(3)	86807	2(3)	87103	2(3)	87332	1(3)	87534	1(3)	87999	1(3)	88262	2(3)	88720	1(3)
86664	2(3)	86808	1(3)	87106	4(3)	87335	1(3)	87535	1(3)	88000	0(3)	88263	1(3)	88738	1(3)
86665	2(3)	86812	1(2)	87107	4(3)	87336	1(3)	87536	1(3)	88005	0(3)	88264	1(3)	88740	1(2)
86666	4(3)	86813	1(2)	87109	2(3)	87337	1(3)	87537	1(3)	88007	0(3)	88267	2(3)	88741	1(2)
86668	2(3)	86816	1(2)	87110	2(3)	87338	1(3)	87538	1(3)	88012	0(3)	88269	2(3)	88749	1(3)
86671	3(3)	86817	1(2)	87118	3(3)	87339	1(3)	87539	1(3)	88014	0(3)	88271	16(3)	89049	1(3)
86674	3(3)	86821	1(3)	87140	3(3)	87340	1(2)	87540	1(3)	88016	0(3)	88272	12(3)	89050	2(3)
86677	3(3)	86825	1(3)	87143	2(3)	87341	1(2)	87541	1(3)	88020	0(3)	88273	3(3)	89051	2(3)
86682	2(3)	86826	8(3)	87149	11(3)	87350	1(2)	87542	1(3)	88025	0(3)	88274	5(3)	89055	2(3)
86684	2(3)	86828	2(3)	87150	12(3)	87380	1(2)	87550	1(3)	88027	0(3)	88275	12(3)	89060	2(3)
86687	1(3)	86829	2(3)	87152	1(3)	87385	2(3)	87551	2(3)	88028	0(3)	88280	1(3)	89125	2(3)
86688	1(3)	86830	2(3)	87153	3(3)	87389	1(3)	87552	1(3)	88029	0(3)	88283	5(3)	89160	1(3)
86689	2(3)	86831	2(3)	87164	2(3)	87390	1(3)	87555	1(3)	88036	0(3)	88285	10(3)	89190	1(3)
86692	2(3)	86832	2(3)	87166	2(3)	87391	1(3)	87556	1(3)	88037	0(3)	88289	1(3)	89220	2(3)
86694	2(3)	86833	1(3)	87168	2(3)	87400	2(3)	87557	1(3)	88040	0(3)	88291	0(3)	89230	1(2)
86695	2(3)	86834	1(3)	87169	2(3)	87420	1(3)	87560	1(3)	88045	0(3)	88299	1(3)	89240	1(3)
86696	2(3)	86835	1(3)	87172	1(3)	87425	1(3)	87561	1(3)	88099	0(3)	88300	4(3)	89250	1(2)
86698	3(3)	86849	1(3)	87176	3(3)	87427	2(3)	87562	1(3)	88104	5(3)	88302	4(3)	89251	1(2)
86701	1(3)	86850	3(3)	87177	3(3)	87430	1(3)	87580	1(3)	88106	5(3)	88304	5(3)	89253	1(3)
86702	2(3)	86860	2(3)	87181	12(3)	87449	3(3)	87581	1(3)	88108	6(3)	88305	16(3)	89254	1(3)
86703	1(2)	86870	6(3)	87184	8(3)	87450	2(3)	87582	1(3)	88112	6(3)	88307	8(3)	89255	1(3)
86704	1(2)	86880	4(3)	87185	4(3)	87451	2(3)	87590	1(3)	88120	2(3)	88309	3(3)	89257	1(3)
86705	1(2)	86885	3(3)	87186	12(3)	87471	1(3)	87591	3(3)	88121	2(3)	88311	4(3)	89258	1(2)
86706	2(3)	86886	3(3)	87187	3(3)	87472	1(3)	87592	1(3)	88125	1(3)	88312	9(3)	89259	1(2)
86707	1(3)	86890	2(3)	87188	14(3)	87475	1(3)	87623	1(2)	88130	1(2)	88313	8(3)	89260	1(2)
86708	1(2)	86891	2(3)	87190	10(3)	87476	1(3)	87624	1(3)	88140	1(2)	88314	6(3)	89261	1(2)
86709	1(2)	86900	3(3)	87197	1(3)	87480	1(3)	87625	1(3)	88141	1(3)	88319	11(3)	89264	1(3)
86710	4(3)	86901	3(3)	87206	6(3)	87481	6(3)	87631	1(3)	88142	1(3)	88321	1(2)	89268	1(2)
86711	2(3)	86902	40(3)	87207	3(3)	87482	1(3)	87632	1(3)	88143	1(3)	88323	1(2)	89272	1(2)
86713	3(3)	86905	28(3)	87209	4(3)	87483	1(2)	87633	1(3)	88147	1(3)	88325	1(2)	89280	1(2)
86717	8(3)	86906	1(2)	87210	4(3)	87485	1(3)	87634	1(3)	88148	1(3)	88329	2(3)	89281	1(2)
86720	2(3)	86910	0(3)	87220	3(3)	87486	1(3)	87640	1(3)	88150	1(3)	88331	11(3)	89290	1(2)
86723	2(3)	86911	0(3)	87230	2(3)	87487	1(3)	87641	1(3)	88152	1(3)	88332	13(3)	89291	1(2)
86727	2(3)	86920	19(3)	87250	1(3)	87490	1(3)	87650	1(3)	88153	1(3)	88333	4(3)	89300	1(2)
86732	2(3)	86922	10(3)	87252	4(3)	87491	3(3)	87651	1(3)	88155	1(3)	88334	5(3)	89310	1(2)
86735	2(3)	86923	10(3)	87253	3(3)	87492	1(3)	87652	1(3)	88160	4(3)	88341	13(3)	89320	1(2)

CPT	MUE	CPT	MUE	CPT	MUE	CPT	MUE	CPT	MUE	CPT	MUE	CPT	MUE	CPT	MUE
89321	1(2)	90657	1(2)	90846	2(3)	91122	1(2)	92371	1(3)	92595	0(3)	93015	1(3)	93452	1(3)
89322	1(2)	90658	1(2)	90847	2(3)	91132	1(3)	92499	1(3)	92596	1(2)	93016	1(3)	93453	1(3)
89325	1(2)	90660	1(2)	90849	2(3)	91133	1(3)	92502	1(3)	92597	1(3)	93017	1(3)	93454	1(3)
89329	1(2)	90661	1(2)	90853	4(3)	91200	1(2)	92504	1(3)	92601	1(3)	93018	1(3)	93455	1(3)
89330	1(2)	90662	1(2)	90863	1(3)	91299	1(3)	92507	1(3)	92602	1(3)	93024	1(3)	93456	1(3)
89331	1(2)	90664	1(2)	90865	1(3)	92002	1(2)	92508	1(3)	92603	1(3)	93025	1(2)	93457	1(3)
89335	1(3)	90666	1(2)	90867	1(2)	92004	1(2)	92511	1(3)	92604	1(3)	93040	3(3)	93458	1(3)
89337	1(2)	90667	1(2)	90868	1(3)	92012	1(3)	92512	1(2)	92605	1(2)	93041	3(3)	93459	1(3)
89342	1(2)	90668	1(2)	90869	1(3)	92014	1(3)	92516	1(3)	92606	1(2)	93042	3(3)	93460	1(3)
89343	1(2)	90670	1(2)	90870	2(3)	92015	0(3)	92520	1(2)	92607	1(3)	93050	1(3)	93461	1(3)
89344	1(2)	90672	1(2)	90875	0(3)	92018	1(2)	92521	1(2)	92608	4(3)	93224	1(2)	93462	1(3)
89346	1(2)	90673	1(2)	90876	0(3)	92019	1(2)	92522	1(2)	92609	1(3)	93225	1(2)	93463	1(3)
89352	1(2)	90674	1(2)	90880	1(3)	92020	1(2)	92523	1(2)	92610	1(2)	93226	1(2)	93464	1(3)
89353	1(3)	90675	1(2)	90882	0(3)	92025	1(2)	92524	1(2)	92611	1(3)	93227	1(2)	93503	2(3)
89354	1(3)	90676	1(2)	90885	1(3)	92060	1(2)	92526	1(2)	92612	1(3)	93228	1(2)	93505	1(2)
89356	2(3)	90680	1(2)	90887	1(3)	92065	1(2)	92531	1(3)	92613	1(2)	93229	1(2)	93530	1(3)
89398	1(3)	90681	1(2)	90889	1(3)	92071	2(2)	92532	1(3)	92614	1(3)	93260	1(2)	93531	1(3)
90281	0(3)	90682	1(2)	90899	1(3)	92072	1(2)	92533	4(2)	92615	1(2)	93261	1(3)	93532	1(3)
90283	0(3)	90685	1(2)	90901	1(3)	92081	1(2)	92534	1(3)	92616	1(3)	93264	1(2)	93533	1(3)
90284	0(3)	90686	1(2)	90911	1(3)	92082	1(2)	92537	1(2)	92617	1(2)	93268	1(2)	93561	1(3)
90287	0(3)	90687	1(2)	90935	1(3)	92083	1(2)	92538	1(2)	92618	1(3)	93270	1(2)	93562	1(3)
90288	0(3)	90688	1(2)	90937	1(3)	92100	1(2)	92540	1(3)	92620	1(2)	93271	1(2)	93563	1(3)
90291	0(3)	90689	1(2)	90940	1(3)	92132	1(2)	92541	1(3)	92621	4(3)	93272	1(2)	93564	1(3)
90296	1(2)	90690	1(2)	90945	1(3)	92133	1(2)	92542	1(3)	92625	1(2)	93278	1(3)	93565	1(3)
90371	10(3)	90691	1(2)	90947	1(3)	92134	1(2)	92544	1(3)	92626	1(2)	93279	1(3)	93566	1(3)
90375	20(3)	90696	1(2)	90951	1(2)	92136	1(3)	92545	1(3)	92627	6(3)	93280	1(3)	93567	1(3)
90376	20(3)	90697	1(2)	90952	1(2)	92145	1(2)	92546	1(3)	92630	0(3)	93281	1(3)	93568	1(3)
90378	4(3)	90698	1(2)	90953	1(2)	92225	2(2)	92547	1(3)	92633	0(3)	93282	1(3)	93571	1(3)
90384	0(3)	90700	1(2)	90954	1(2)	92226	2(2)	92548	1(3)	92640	1(3)	93283	1(3)	93572	2(3)
90385	0(3)	90702	1(2)	90955	1(2)	92227	1(2)	92550	1(2)	92700	1(3)	93284	1(3)	93580	1(3)
90386	0(3)	90707	1(2)	90956	1(2)	92228	1(2)	92551	0(3)	92920	3(3)	93285	1(3)	93581	1(3)
90389	0(3)	90710	1(2)	90957	1(2)	92230	2(2)	92552	1(2)	92921	6(2)	93286	2(3)	93582	1(2)
90393	1(2)	90713	1(2)	90958	1(2)	92235	1(2)	92553	1(2)	92924	2(3)	93287	2(3)	93583	1(2)
90396	1(2)	90714	1(2)	90959	1(2)	92240	1(2)	92555	1(2)	92925	6(2)	93288	1(3)	93590	1(2)
90399	0(3)	90715	1(2)	90960	1(2)	92242	1(2)	92556	1(2)	92928	3(3)	93289	1(3)	93591	1(2)
90460	9(3)	90716	1(2)	90961	1(2)	92250	1(2)	92557	1(2)	92929	6(2)	93290	1(3)	93592	2(3)
90461	8(3)	90717	1(2)	90962	1(2)	92260	1(2)	92558	0(3)	92933	2(3)	93291	1(3)	93600	1(3)
90471	1(2)	90723	0(3)	90963	1(2)	92265	1(2)	92559	0(3)	92934	6(2)	93292	1(3)	93602	1(3)
90472	8(3)	90732	1(2)	90964	1(2)	92270	1(2)	92560	0(3)	92937	2(3)	93293	1(2)	93603	1(3)
90473	1(2)	90733	1(2)	90965	1(2)	92273	1(2)	92561	1(2)	92938	6(3)	93294	1(2)	93609	1(3)
90474	1(3)	90734	1(2)	90966	1(2)	92274	1(2)	92562	1(2)	92941	1(3)	93295	1(2)	93610	1(3)
90476	1(2)	90736	1(2)	90967	1(2)	92283	1(2)	92563	1(2)	92943	2(3)	93296	1(2)	93612	1(3)
90477	1(2)	90738	1(2)	90968	1(2)	92284	1(2)	92564	1(2)	92944	3(3)	93297	1(2)	93613	1(3)
90581	1(2)	90739	1(2)	90969	1(2)	92285	1(2)	92565	1(2)	92950	2(3)	93298	1(2)	93615	1(3)
90585	1(2)	90740	1(2)	90970	1(2)	92286	1(2)	92567	1(2)	92953	2(3)	93299	1(2)	93616	1(3)
90586	1(2)	90743	1(2)	90989	1(2)	92287	1(2)	92568	1(2)	92960	2(3)	93303	1(3)	93618	1(3)
90587	1(2)	90744	1(2)	90993	1(3)	92310	0(3)	92570	1(2)	92961	1(3)	93304	1(3)	93619	1(3)
90620	1(2)	90746	1(2)	90997	1(3)	92311	1(2)	92571	1(2)	92970	1(3)	93306	1(3)	93620	1(3)
90621	1(2)	90747	1(2)	90999	1(3)	92312	1(2)	92572	1(2)	92971	1(3)	93307	1(3)	93621	1(3)
90625	1(2)	90748	0(3)	91010	1(2)	92313	1(3)	92575	1(2)	92973	2(3)	93308	1(3)	93622	1(3)
90630	1(2)	90749	1(3)	91013	1(3)	92314	0(3)	92576	1(2)	92974	1(3)	93312	1(3)	93623	1(3)
90632	1(2)	90750	1(2)	91020	1(2)	92315	1(2)	92577	1(2)	92975	1(3)	93313	1(3)	93624	1(3)
90633	1(2)	90756	1(2)	91022	1(2)	92316	1(2)	92579	1(2)	92977	1(3)	93314	1(3)	93631	1(3)
90634	1(2)	90785	3(3)	91030	1(2)	92317	1(3)	92582	1(2)	92978	1(3)	93315	1(3)	93640	1(3)
90636	1(2)	90791	1(3)	91034	1(2)	92325	1(3)	92583	1(2)	92979	2(3)	93316	1(3)	93641	1(2)
90644	1(2)	90792	2(3)	91035	1(2)	92326	2(2)	92584	1(2)	92986	1(2)	93317	1(3)	93642	1(3)
90647	1(2)	90832	3(3)	91037	1(2)	92340	0(3)	92585	1(2)	92987	1(2)	93318	1(3)	93644	1(3)
90648	1(2)	90833	3(3)	91038	1(2)	92341	0(3)	92586	1(2)	92990	1(2)	93320	1(3)	93650	1(2)
90649	1(2)	90834	3(3)	91040	1(2)	92342	0(3)	92587	1(2)	92992	1(2)	93321	1(3)	93653	1(3)
90650	1(2)	90836	3(3)	91065	2(2)	92352	1(3)	92588	1(2)	92993	1(2)	93325	1(3)	93654	1(3)
90651	1(2)	90837	3(3)	91110	1(2)	92353	1(3)	92590	0(3)	92997	1(2)	93350	1(2)	93655	2(3)
90653	1(2)	90838	3(3)	91111	1(2)	92354	1(3)	92591	0(3)	92998	2(3)	93351	1(2)	93656	1(3)
90654	1(2)	90839	1(2)	91112	1(3)	92355	1(3)	92592	0(3)	93000	3(3)	93352	1(3)	93657	1(3)
90655	1(2)	90840	4(3)	91117	1(2)	92358	1(3)	92593	0(3)	93005	5(3)	93355	1(3)	93660	1(3)
90656	1(2)	90845	1(2)	91120	1(2)	92370	0(3)	92594	0(3)	93010	5(3)	93451	1(3)	93662	1(3)

CPT	MUE
93668	1(3)
93701	1(2)
93702	1(2)
93724	1(3)
93740	1(3)
93745	1(2)
93750	1(3)
93770	1(3)
93784	1(2)
93786	1(2)
93788	1(2)
93790	1(2)
93792	1(2)
93793	1(2)
93797	2(2)
93798	2(2)
93799	1(3)
93880	1(3)
93882	1(3)
93886	1(3)
93888	1(3)
93890	1(3)
93892	1(3)
93893	1(3)
93895	1(3)
93922	2(2)
93923	2(2)
93924	1(2)
93925	1(3)
93926	1(3)
93930	1(3)
93931	1(3)
93970	1(3)
93971	1(3)
93975	1(3)
93976	1(3)
93978	1(3)
93979	1(3)
93980	1(3)
93981	1(3)
93990	2(3)
93998	1(3)
94002	1(2)
94003	1(2)
94004	1(2)
94005	0(3)
94010	1(3)
94011	1(3)
94012	1(3)
94013	1(3)
94014	1(2)
94015	1(2)
94016	1(2)
94060	1(3)
94070	1(2)
94150	2(3)
94200	1(3)
94250	1(3)
94375	1(3)
94400	1(3)
94450	1(3)
94452	1(2)
94453	1(2)
94610	2(3)
94617	1(3)

CPT	MUE
94618	1(3)
94621	1(3)
94640	1(3)
94642	1(3)
94644	1(2)
94645	4(3)
94660	1(2)
94662	1(2)
94664	1(3)
94667	1(2)
94668	5(3)
94669	4(3)
94680	1(3)
94681	1(3)
94690	1(3)
94726	1(3)
94727	1(3)
94728	1(3)
94729	1(3)
94750	1(3)
94760	1(3)
94761	1(2)
94762	1(2)
94770	1(3)
94772	1(2)
94774	1(2)
94775	1(2)
94776	1(2)
94777	1(2)
94780	1(2)
94781	2(3)
94799	1(3)
95004	80(3)
95012	2(3)
95017	27(3)
95018	19(3)
95024	40(3)
95027	90(3)
95028	30(3)
95044	80(3)
95052	20(3)
95056	1(2)
95060	1(2)
95065	1(3)
95070	1(3)
95071	1(2)
95076	1(2)
95079	2(3)
95115	1(2)
95117	1(2)
95120	0(3)
95125	0(3)
95130	0(3)
95131	0(3)
95132	0(3)
95133	0(3)
95134	0(3)
95144	30(3)
95145	10(3)
95146	10(3)
95147	10(3)
95148	10(3)
95149	10(3)
95165	30(3)
95170	10(3)

CPT	MUE
95180	8(3)
95199	1(3)
95249	1(2)
95250	1(2)
95251	1(2)
95782	1(2)
95783	1(2)
95800	1(2)
95801	1(2)
95803	1(2)
95805	1(2)
95806	1(2)
95807	1(2)
95808	1(2)
95810	1(2)
95811	1(2)
95812	1(3)
95813	1(3)
95816	1(3)
95819	1(3)
95822	1(3)
95824	1(3)
95827	1(2)
95829	1(3)
95830	1(3)
95831	5(2)
95832	1(3)
95833	1(3)
95834	1(3)
95836	1(2)
95851	3(3)
95852	1(3)
95857	1(2)
95860	1(3)
95861	1(3)
95863	1(3)
95864	1(3)
95865	1(3)
95866	1(3)
95867	1(3)
95868	1(3)
95869	1(3)
95870	4(3)
95872	4(3)
95873	1(2)
95874	1(2)
95875	2(3)
95885	4(2)
95886	4(2)
95887	1(2)
95905	2(3)
95907	1(2)
95908	1(2)
95909	1(2)
95910	1(2)
95911	1(2)
95912	1(2)
95913	1(2)
95921	1(3)
95922	1(3)
95923	1(3)
95924	1(3)
95925	1(3)
95926	1(3)
95927	1(3)

CPT	MUE
95928	1(3)
95929	1(3)
95930	1(3)
95933	1(3)
95937	4(3)
95938	1(3)
95939	1(3)
95940	20(3)
95941	8(3)
95943	1(3)
95950	1(2)
95951	1(2)
95953	1(2)
95954	1(3)
95955	1(3)
95956	1(2)
95957	1(3)
95958	1(3)
95961	1(2)
95962	3(3)
95965	1(3)
95966	1(3)
95967	3(3)
95970	1(3)
95971	1(3)
95972	1(3)
95976	1(3)
95977	1(3)
95980	1(3)
95981	1(3)
95982	1(3)
95983	1(2)
95984	11(3)
95990	1(3)
95991	1(3)
95992	1(2)
95999	1(3)
96000	1(2)
96001	1(2)
96002	1(3)
96003	1(3)
96004	1(2)
96020	1(2)
96040	4(3)
96105	3(3)
96110	3(3)
96112	1(2)
96113	6(3)
96116	1(2)
96121	3(3)
96125	2(3)
96127	2(3)
96130	1(2)
96131	7(3)
96132	1(2)
96133	7(3)
96136	1(2)
96137	11(3)
96138	1(2)
96139	11(3)
96146	1(2)
96150	8(3)
96151	6(3)
96152	6(3)
96153	12(3)

CPT	MUE
96154	8(3)
96155	0(3)
96160	3(3)
96161	1(3)
96360	2(3)
96361	24(3)
96365	2(3)
96366	24(3)
96367	4(3)
96368	1(2)
96369	1(2)
96370	3(3)
96371	1(3)
96372	5(3)
96373	3(3)
96374	1(3)
96375	6(3)
96376	10(3)
96377	1(3)
96379	2(3)
96401	4(3)
96402	2(3)
96405	1(2)
96406	1(2)
96409	1(3)
96411	3(3)
96413	1(3)
96415	8(3)
96416	1(3)
96417	3(3)
96420	2(3)
96422	2(3)
96423	2(3)
96425	1(3)
96440	1(3)
96446	1(3)
96450	1(3)
96521	2(3)
96522	1(3)
96523	2(3)
96542	1(3)
96549	1(3)
96567	1(3)
96570	1(2)
96571	2(3)
96573	1(2)
96574	1(2)
96900	1(3)
96902	1(3)
96904	1(2)
96910	1(3)
96912	1(3)
96913	1(3)
96920	1(2)
96921	1(2)
96922	1(2)
96931	1(2)
96932	1(2)
96933	1(2)
96934	2(3)
96935	2(3)
96936	2(3)
96999	1(3)
97010	1(3)
97012	1(3)

CPT	MUE
97014	0(3)
97016	1(3)
97018	1(3)
97022	1(3)
97024	1(3)
97026	1(3)
97028	1(3)
97032	4(3)
97033	4(3)
97034	2(3)
97035	2(3)
97036	3(3)
97039	1(3)
97110	8(3)
97112	6(3)
97113	6(3)
97116	4(3)
97124	4(3)
97127	1(2)
97139	1(3)
97140	6(3)
97150	2(3)
97151	8(3)
97152	8(3)
97153	32(3)
97154	12(3)
97155	24(3)
97156	16(3)
97157	16(3)
97158	16(3)
97161	1(2)
97162	1(2)
97163	1(2)
97164	1(2)
97165	1(2)
97166	1(2)
97167	1(2)
97168	1(2)
97169	0(3)
97170	0(3)
97171	0(3)
97172	0(3)
97530	6(3)
97533	4(3)
97535	8(3)
97537	8(3)
97542	8(3)
97545	1(2)
97546	2(3)
97597	1(3)
97598	8(3)
97602	1(3)
97605	1(3)
97606	1(3)
97607	1(3)
97608	1(3)
97610	1(2)
97750	8(3)
97755	8(3)
97760	6(3)
97761	6(3)
97763	6(3)
97799	1(3)
97802	8(3)
97803	8(3)

CPT	MUE
97804	6(3)
97810	0(3)
97811	0(3)
97813	0(3)
97814	0(3)
98925	1(2)
98926	1(2)
98927	1(2)
98928	1(2)
98929	1(2)
98940	1(2)
98941	1(2)
98942	1(2)
98943	0(3)
98960	0(3)
98961	0(3)
98962	0(3)
98966	0(3)
98967	0(3)
98968	0(3)
98969	0(3)
99000	0(3)
99001	0(3)
99002	1(3)
99024	1(3)
99026	0(3)
99027	0(3)
99050	1(3)
99051	1(3)
99053	1(3)
99056	1(3)
99058	1(3)
99060	1(3)
99070	1(3)
99071	1(3)
99075	0(3)
99078	3(3)
99080	1(3)
99082	1(3)
99091	1(2)
99100	1(3)
99116	1(3)
99135	1(3)
99140	2(3)
99151	1(3)
99152	2(3)
99153	12(3)
99155	1(3)
99156	1(3)
99157	6(3)
99170	1(3)
99172	0(3)
99173	0(3)
99174	0(3)
99175	1(3)
99177	1(2)
99183	1(3)
99184	1(2)
99188	1(2)
99190	1(3)
99191	1(3)
99192	1(3)
99195	2(3)
99199	1(3)
99201	1(2)

CPT	MUE
99202	1(2)
99203	1(2)
99204	1(2)
99205	1(2)
99211	2(3)
99212	2(3)
99213	2(3)
99214	2(3)
99215	2(3)
99217	1(2)
99218	1(2)
99219	1(2)
99220	1(2)
99221	0(3)
99222	0(3)
99223	0(3)
99224	1(2)
99225	1(2)
99226	1(2)
99231	0(3)
99232	0(3)
99233	0(3)
99234	1(3)
99235	1(3)
99236	1(3)
99238	0(3)
99239	0(3)
99241	0(3)
99242	0(3)
99243	0(3)
99244	0(3)
99245	0(3)
99251	0(3)
99252	0(3)
99253	0(3)
99254	0(3)
99255	0(3)
99281	2(3)
99282	2(3)
99283	2(3)
99284	2(3)
99285	2(3)
99288	1(3)
99291	1(2)
99292	8(3)
99304	1(2)
99305	1(2)
99306	1(2)
99307	1(2)
99308	1(2)
99309	1(2)
99310	1(2)
99315	1(2)
99316	1(2)
99318	1(2)
99324	1(2)
99325	1(2)
99326	1(2)
99327	1(2)
99328	1(2)
99334	1(3)
99335	1(3)
99336	1(3)
99337	1(3)
99339	1(2)

CPT	MUE
99340	1(2)
99341	1(2)
99342	1(2)
99343	1(2)
99344	1(2)
99345	1(2)
99347	1(3)
99348	1(3)
99349	1(3)
99350	1(3)
99354	1(2)
99355	4(3)
99356	1(2)
99357	1(3)
99358	1(2)
99359	1(3)
99360	1(3)
99366	2(3)
99367	1(3)
99368	2(3)
99374	1(2)
99375	0(3)
99377	1(2)
99378	0(3)
99379	1(2)
99380	1(2)
99381	0(3)
99382	0(3)
99383	0(3)
99384	0(3)
99385	0(3)
99386	0(3)
99387	0(3)
99391	0(3)
99392	0(3)
99393	0(3)
99394	0(3)
99395	0(3)
99396	0(3)
99397	0(3)
99401	0(3)
99402	0(3)
99403	0(3)
99404	0(3)
99406	1(2)
99407	1(2)
99408	0(3)
99409	0(3)
99411	0(3)
99412	0(3)
99415	1(2)
99416	3(3)
99429	0(3)
99441	0(3)
99442	0(3)
99443	0(3)
99444	0(3)
99446	1(2)
99447	1(2)
99448	1(2)
99449	1(2)
99450	0(3)
99451	1(2)
99452	1(2)
99453	1(2)

CPT	MUE
99454	1(2)
99455	1(3)
99456	1(3)
99457	1(2)
99460	1(2)
99461	1(2)
99462	1(2)
99463	1(2)
99464	1(2)
99465	1(2)
99466	1(2)
99467	4(3)
99468	1(2)
99469	1(2)
99471	1(2)
99472	1(2)
99475	1(2)
99476	1(2)
99477	1(2)
99478	1(2)
99479	1(2)
99480	1(2)
99483	1(2)
99484	1(2)
99485	1(3)
99486	4(1)
99487	1(2)
99489	4(3)
99490	1(2)
99491	1(2)
99492	1(2)
99493	1(2)
99494	2(3)
99495	1(2)
99496	1(2)
99497	1(2)
99498	3(3)
99499	1(3)
99500	0(3)
99501	0(3)
99502	0(3)
99503	0(3)
99504	0(3)
99505	0(3)
99506	0(3)
99507	0(3)
99509	0(3)
99510	0(3)
99511	0(3)
99512	0(3)
99600	0(3)
99601	0(3)
99602	0(3)
99605	0(2)
99606	0(3)
99607	0(3)
A0021	0(3)
A0080	0(3)
A0090	0(3)
A0100	0(3)
A0110	0(3)
A0120	0(3)
A0130	0(3)
A0140	0(3)
A0160	0(3)

CPT	MUE
A0170	0(3)
A0180	0(3)
A0190	0(3)
A0200	0(3)
A0210	0(3)
A0225	0(3)
A0380	0(3)
A0382	0(3)
A0384	0(3)
A0390	0(3)
A0392	0(3)
A0394	0(3)
A0396	0(3)
A0398	0(3)
A0420	0(3)
A0422	0(3)
A0424	0(3)
A0425	250(1)
A0426	2(3)
A0427	2(3)
A0428	2(3)
A0429	2(3)
A0430	1(3)
A0431	1(3)
A0432	1(3)
A0433	1(3)
A0434	2(3)
A0435	999(3)
A0436	300(3)
A0888	0(3)
A0998	0(3)
A0999	1(3)
A4206	1(3)
A4207	1(3)
A4208	4(3)
A4209	6(3)
A4210	0(3)
A4211	1(3)
A4212	2(3)
A4213	5(3)
A4215	9(3)
A4216	25(3)
A4217	4(3)
A4218	20(3)
A4220	1(3)
A4221	1(3)
A4222	2(3)
A4223	1(3)
A4224	1(2)
A4225	1(3)
A4230	1(3)
A4231	1(3)
A4232	0(3)
A4233	0(3)
A4234	0(3)
A4235	1(3)
A4236	0(3)
A4244	1(3)
A4245	1(3)
A4246	1(3)
A4247	1(3)
A4248	10(3)
A4250	0(3)
A4252	0(3)
A4253	0(3)

CPT	MUE
A4255	0(3)
A4256	1(3)
A4257	0(3)
A4258	0(3)
A4259	0(3)
A4261	0(3)
A4262	4(2)
A4263	4(2)
A4264	0(3)
A4265	1(3)
A4266	0(3)
A4267	0(3)
A4268	0(3)
A4269	0(3)
A4270	3(3)
A4280	1(3)
A4281	0(3)
A4282	0(3)
A4283	0(3)
A4284	0(3)
A4285	0(3)
A4286	0(3)
A4290	2(3)
A4300	4(3)
A4301	1(2)
A4305	2(3)
A4306	2(3)
A4310	2(3)
A4311	2(3)
A4312	1(3)
A4313	1(3)
A4314	2(3)
A4315	2(3)
A4316	1(3)
A4320	2(3)
A4321	1(3)
A4322	2(3)
A4326	1(3)
A4327	2(3)
A4328	1(3)
A4330	1(3)
A4331	3(3)
A4332	2(3)
A4335	1(3)
A4336	1(3)
A4337	2(3)
A4338	3(3)
A4340	2(3)
A4344	2(3)
A4346	2(3)
A4351	2(3)
A4352	2(3)
A4353	3(3)
A4354	2(3)
A4355	2(3)
A4356	2(3)
A4357	2(3)
A4360	1(3)
A4361	1(3)
A4362	2(3)
A4363	0(3)
A4364	2(3)
A4366	1(3)
A4367	1(3)
A4368	1(3)

CPT	MUE
A4369	1(3)
A4371	1(3)
A4372	1(3)
A4373	1(3)
A4375	2(3)
A4376	2(3)
A4377	2(3)
A4378	2(3)
A4379	2(3)
A4380	2(3)
A4381	2(3)
A4382	2(3)
A4383	2(3)
A4384	2(3)
A4385	2(3)
A4387	1(3)
A4388	1(3)
A4389	2(3)
A4390	1(3)
A4391	1(3)
A4392	2(3)
A4393	1(3)
A4394	1(3)
A4395	3(3)
A4396	2(3)
A4397	1(3)
A4398	2(3)
A4399	1(3)
A4400	1(3)
A4402	1(3)
A4404	1(3)
A4405	1(3)
A4406	1(3)
A4407	2(3)
A4408	1(3)
A4409	1(3)
A4410	2(3)
A4411	1(3)
A4412	1(3)
A4413	2(3)
A4414	1(3)
A4415	1(3)
A4416	2(3)
A4417	2(3)
A4418	2(3)
A4419	2(3)
A4420	1(3)
A4423	2(3)
A4424	1(3)
A4425	1(3)
A4426	2(3)
A4427	1(3)
A4428	1(3)
A4429	2(3)
A4430	1(3)
A4431	1(3)
A4432	2(3)
A4433	1(3)
A4434	1(3)
A4435	2(3)
A4450	20(3)
A4452	4(3)
A4455	1(3)
A4458	1(3)
A4459	1(3)

CPT	MUE
A4461	2(3)
A4463	2(3)
A4465	1(3)
A4467	0(3)
A4470	1(3)
A4480	1(3)
A4481	2(3)
A4483	1(3)
A4490	0(3)
A4495	0(3)
A4500	0(3)
A4510	0(3)
A4520	0(3)
A4550	3(3)
A4553	0(3)
A4554	0(3)
A4555	0(3)
A4556	2(3)
A4557	2(3)
A4558	1(3)
A4559	1(3)
A4561	1(3)
A4562	1(3)
A4563	1(2)
A4565	2(3)
A4566	0(3)
A4570	0(3)
A4575	0(3)
A4580	0(3)
A4590	0(3)
A4595	2(3)
A4600	0(3)
A4601	0(3)
A4602	1(3)
A4604	1(3)
A4605	1(3)
A4606	1(3)
A4608	1(3)
A4611	0(3)
A4612	0(3)
A4613	0(3)
A4614	1(2)
A4615	2(3)
A4616	1(3)
A4617	1(3)
A4618	1(3)
A4619	1(3)
A4620	1(3)
A4623	10(3)
A4624	2(3)
A4625	30(3)
A4626	1(3)
A4627	0(3)
A4628	1(3)
A4629	1(3)
A4630	0(3)
A4633	0(3)
A4634	1(3)
A4635	0(3)
A4636	0(3)
A4637	0(3)
A4638	0(3)
A4639	0(3)
A4640	0(3)
A4642	1(3)

CPT	MUE
A4648	3(3)
A4650	3(3)
A4651	2(3)
A4652	2(3)
A4653	0(3)
A4657	0(3)
A4660	0(3)
A4663	0(3)
A4670	0(3)
A4671	0(3)
A4672	0(3)
A4673	0(3)
A4674	0(3)
A4680	0(3)
A4690	0(3)
A4706	0(3)
A4707	0(3)
A4708	0(3)
A4709	0(3)
A4714	0(3)
A4719	0(3)
A4720	0(3)
A4721	0(3)
A4722	0(3)
A4723	0(3)
A4724	0(3)
A4725	0(3)
A4726	0(3)
A4728	0(3)
A4730	0(3)
A4736	0(3)
A4737	0(3)
A4740	0(3)
A4750	0(3)
A4755	0(3)
A4760	0(3)
A4765	0(3)
A4766	0(3)
A4770	0(3)
A4771	0(3)
A4772	0(3)
A4773	0(3)
A4774	0(3)
A4802	0(3)
A4860	0(3)
A4870	0(3)
A4890	0(3)
A4911	0(3)
A4913	0(3)
A4918	0(3)
A4927	0(3)
A4928	0(3)
A4929	0(3)
A4930	0(3)
A4931	0(3)
A4932	0(3)
A5051	1(3)
A5052	1(3)
A5053	2(3)
A5054	1(3)
A5055	1(3)
A5056	90(3)
A5057	90(3)
A5061	2(3)
A5062	1(3)

CPT	MUE
A5063	1(3)
A5071	2(3)
A5072	1(3)
A5073	1(3)
A5081	2(3)
A5082	1(3)
A5083	5(3)
A5093	2(3)
A5102	1(3)
A5105	1(3)
A5112	2(3)
A5113	0(3)
A5114	0(3)
A5120	150(3)
A5121	1(3)
A5122	1(3)
A5126	2(3)
A5131	1(3)
A5200	2(3)
A5500	0(3)
A5501	0(3)
A5503	0(3)
A5504	0(3)
A5505	0(3)
A5506	0(3)
A5507	0(3)
A5508	0(3)
A5510	0(3)
A5512	0(3)
A5513	0(3)
A5514	0(3)
A6000	0(3)
A6010	3(3)
A6011	20(3)
A6024	1(3)
A6025	4(3)
A6154	1(3)
A6205	1(3)
A6221	9(3)
A6228	2(3)
A6230	1(3)
A6236	1(3)
A6238	3(3)
A6239	1(3)
A6240	2(3)
A6241	1(3)
A6244	1(3)
A6246	3(3)
A6247	2(3)
A6250	1(3)
A6256	3(3)
A6259	3(3)
A6261	3(3)
A6262	3(3)
A6404	2(3)
A6407	4(3)
A6410	2(3)
A6411	2(3)
A6412	2(3)
A6413	0(3)
A6441	8(3)
A6442	8(3)
A6443	8(3)
A6444	4(3)
A6445	8(3)

CPT	MUE
A6446	14(3)
A6447	6(3)
A6448	24(3)
A6449	12(3)
A6450	8(3)
A6451	8(3)
A6452	22(3)
A6453	6(3)
A6454	25(3)
A6455	4(3)
A6456	20(3)
A6457	12(3)
A6460	1(1)
A6461	1(1)
A6501	1(3)
A6502	1(3)
A6503	1(3)
A6504	2(3)
A6505	2(3)
A6506	2(3)
A6507	2(3)
A6508	2(3)
A6509	1(3)
A6510	1(3)
A6511	1(3)
A6513	1(3)
A6530	0(3)
A6531	2(3)
A6532	2(3)
A6533	0(3)
A6534	0(3)
A6535	0(3)
A6536	0(3)
A6537	0(3)
A6538	0(3)
A6539	0(3)
A6540	0(3)
A6541	0(3)
A6544	0(3)
A6545	2(3)
A6549	0(3)
A6550	1(3)
A7000	0(3)
A7001	0(3)
A7002	0(3)
A7003	0(3)
A7004	0(3)
A7005	0(3)
A7006	0(3)
A7007	0(3)
A7008	0(3)
A7009	0(3)
A7010	0(3)
A7012	0(3)
A7013	0(3)
A7014	0(3)
A7015	0(3)
A7016	0(3)
A7017	0(3)
A7018	0(3)
A7020	0(3)
A7025	0(3)
A7026	0(3)
A7027	0(3)
A7028	0(3)
A7029	0(3)
A7030	0(3)
A7031	0(3)
A7032	0(3)
A7033	0(3)
A7034	0(3)
A7035	0(3)
A7036	0(3)
A7037	0(3)
A7038	0(3)
A7039	0(3)
A7040	2(3)
A7041	2(3)
A7044	0(3)
A7045	0(3)
A7046	0(3)
A7047	1(3)
A7048	2(3)
A7501	1(3)
A7502	1(3)
A7503	1(3)
A7504	180(3)
A7505	1(3)
A7506	0(3)
A7507	200(3)
A7508	0(3)
A7509	0(3)
A7520	1(3)
A7521	1(3)
A7522	0(3)
A7523	0(3)
A7524	1(3)
A7525	0(3)
A7526	0(3)
A7527	1(3)
A8000	0(3)
A8001	0(3)
A8002	0(3)
A8003	0(3)
A8004	0(3)
A9152	0(3)
A9153	0(3)
A9155	1(3)
A9180	0(3)
A9270	0(3)
A9272	0(3)
A9273	0(3)
A9274	0(3)
A9275	0(3)
A9276	0(3)
A9277	0(3)
A9278	0(3)
A9279	0(3)
A9280	0(3)
A9281	0(3)
A9282	0(3)
A9283	0(3)
A9284	0(3)
A9285	0(3)
A9286	0(3)
A9300	0(3)
A9500	3(3)
A9501	1(3)
A9502	3(3)
A9503	1(3)
A9504	1(3)
A9505	4(3)
A9507	1(3)
A9508	2(3)
A9509	5(3)
A9510	1(3)
A9512	30(3)
A9513	200(3)
A9515	1(3)
A9516	4(3)
A9517	200(3)
A9520	1(3)
A9521	2(3)
A9524	10(3)
A9526	2(3)
A9527	195(3)
A9528	10(3)
A9529	10(3)
A9530	200(3)
A9531	100(3)
A9532	10(3)
A9536	1(3)
A9537	1(3)
A9538	1(3)
A9539	2(3)
A9540	2(3)
A9541	1(3)
A9542	1(3)
A9543	1(3)
A9546	1(3)
A9547	2(3)
A9548	2(3)
A9550	1(3)
A9551	1(3)
A9552	1(3)
A9553	1(3)
A9554	1(3)
A9555	2(3)
A9556	10(3)
A9557	2(3)
A9558	7(3)
A9559	1(3)
A9560	2(3)
A9561	1(3)
A9562	2(3)
A9563	10(3)
A9564	0(3)
A9566	1(3)
A9567	2(3)
A9568	0(3)
A9569	1(3)
A9570	1(3)
A9571	1(3)
A9572	1(3)
A9575	300(3)
A9576	100(3)
A9577	50(3)
A9578	50(3)
A9579	100(3)
A9580	1(3)
A9581	20(3)
A9582	1(3)
A9583	18(3)
A9584	1(3)
A9585	300(3)
A9586	1(3)
A9587	54(3)
A9588	10(3)
A9589	1(3)
A9600	7(3)
A9604	1(3)
A9606	224(3)
A9698	3(3)
A9700	2(3)
A9900	0(3)
A9901	0(3)
A9999	0(3)
B4034	0(3)
B4035	0(3)
B4036	0(3)
B4081	0(3)
B4082	0(3)
B4083	0(3)
B4087	1(3)
B4088	1(3)
B4100	0(3)
B4102	0(3)
B4103	0(3)
B4104	0(3)
B4149	0(3)
B4150	0(3)
B4152	0(3)
B4153	0(3)
B4154	0(3)
B4155	0(3)
B4157	0(3)
B4158	0(3)
B4159	0(3)
B4160	0(3)
B4161	0(3)
B4162	0(3)
B4164	0(3)
B4168	0(3)
B4172	0(3)
B4176	0(3)
B4178	0(3)
B4180	0(3)
B4185	0(3)
B4189	0(3)
B4193	0(3)
B4197	0(3)
B4199	0(3)
B4216	0(3)
B4220	0(3)
B4222	0(3)
B4224	0(3)
B5000	0(3)
B5100	0(3)
B5200	0(3)
B9002	0(3)
B9004	0(3)
B9006	0(3)
B9998	0(3)
B9999	0(3)
C1713	20(3)
C1714	4(3)
C1715	45(3)
C1716	4(3)
C1717	10(3)
C1719	99(3)
C1721	1(3)
C1722	1(3)
C1724	5(3)
C1725	9(3)
C1726	5(3)
C1727	4(3)
C1728	5(3)
C1729	6(3)
C1730	4(3)
C1731	2(3)
C1732	3(3)
C1733	3(3)
C1749	1(3)
C1750	2(3)
C1751	3(3)
C1752	2(3)
C1753	2(3)
C1754	2(3)
C1755	2(3)
C1756	2(3)
C1757	6(3)
C1758	2(3)
C1759	2(3)
C1760	4(3)
C1762	4(3)
C1763	4(3)
C1764	1(3)
C1765	4(3)
C1766	4(3)
C1767	2(3)
C1768	3(3)
C1769	9(3)
C1770	3(3)
C1771	1(3)
C1772	1(3)
C1773	3(3)
C1776	10(3)
C1777	2(3)
C1778	4(3)
C1779	2(3)
C1780	2(3)
C1781	4(3)
C1782	1(3)
C1783	2(3)
C1784	2(3)
C1785	1(3)
C1786	1(3)
C1787	2(3)
C1788	2(3)
C1789	2(3)
C1813	1(3)
C1814	2(3)
C1815	1(3)
C1816	2(3)
C1817	1(3)
C1818	2(3)
C1819	4(3)
C1820	2(3)
C1821	4(3)
C1822	1(3)
C1823	1(3)
C1830	2(3)
C1840	1(3)
C1841	1(2)
C1842	0(3)
C1874	5(3)
C1875	4(3)
C1876	5(3)
C1877	5(3)
C1878	2(3)
C1880	2(3)
C1881	2(3)
C1882	1(3)
C1883	4(3)
C1884	4(3)
C1885	2(3)
C1886	1(3)
C1887	7(3)
C1888	2(3)
C1889	2(3)
C1891	1(3)
C1892	6(3)
C1893	6(3)
C1894	6(3)
C1895	2(3)
C1896	2(3)
C1897	2(3)
C1898	2(3)
C1899	2(3)
C1900	1(3)
C2613	2(3)
C2614	3(3)
C2615	2(3)
C2616	1(3)
C2617	4(3)
C2618	4(3)
C2619	1(3)
C2620	1(3)
C2621	1(3)
C2622	1(3)
C2623	4(3)
C2624	1(3)
C2625	4(3)
C2626	1(3)
C2627	2(3)
C2628	4(3)
C2629	4(3)
C2630	3(3)
C2631	1(3)
C2634	24(3)
C2635	124(3)
C2636	690(3)
C2637	0(3)
C2638	150(3)
C2639	150(3)
C2640	150(3)
C2641	150(3)
C2642	120(3)
C2643	120(3)
C2644	500(1)
C2645	4608(3)
C5271	1(2)
C5272	3(2)
C5273	1(2)
C5274	35(3)
C5275	1(2)
C5276	3(2)
C5277	1(2)
C5278	15(3)
C8900	1(3)
C8901	1(3)
C8902	1(3)
C8903	1(3)
C8905	1(3)
C8906	1(3)
C8908	1(3)
C8909	1(3)
C8910	1(3)
C8911	1(3)
C8912	1(3)
C8913	1(3)
C8914	1(3)
C8918	1(3)
C8919	1(3)
C8920	1(3)
C8921	1(3)
C8922	1(3)
C8923	1(3)
C8924	1(3)
C8925	1(3)
C8926	1(3)
C8927	1(3)
C8928	1(2)
C8929	1(3)
C8930	1(2)
C8931	1(3)
C8932	1(3)
C8933	1(3)
C8934	2(3)
C8935	2(3)
C8936	2(3)
C8937	2(2)
C8957	2(3)
C9035	675(3)
C9036	300(3)
C9037	240(3)
C9038	160(3)
C9039	500(3)
C9040	675(3)
C9041	180(3)
C9043	600(3)
C9044	350(3)
C9045	600(3)
C9046	160(3)
C9113	10(3)
C9132	5500(3)
C9248	25(3)
C9250	5(3)
C9254	400(3)
C9257	8000(3)
C9285	2(3)
C9290	266(3)
C9293	700(3)
C9352	3(3)
C9353	4(3)
C9354	300(3)
C9355	3(3)
C9356	125(3)
C9358	800(3)
C9359	30(3)
C9360	300(3)
C9361	10(3)
C9362	60(3)
C9363	500(3)
C9364	600(3)
C9407	15(3)
C9408	510(3)
C9447	1(3)
C9460	100(3)
C9462	600(3)
C9482	300(3)
C9488	40(3)
C9600	3(3)
C9601	2(3)
C9602	2(3)
C9603	2(3)
C9604	2(3)
C9605	2(3)
C9606	1(3)
C9607	1(2)
C9608	2(3)
C9725	1(3)
C9726	2(3)
C9727	1(2)
C9728	1(2)
C9733	1(3)
C9734	1(3)
C9738	1(3)
C9739	1(2)
C9740	1(2)
C9745	1(2)
C9747	1(2)
C9749	1(2)
C9751	1(3)
C9752	1(2)
C9753	3(3)
C9754	1(2)
C9755	1(2)
C9898	1(3)
D0150	1(3)
D0240	1(3)
D0250	2(3)
D0270	1(3)
D0272	1(3)
D0274	1(3)
D0277	1(3)
D0412	0(3)
D0416	1(3)
D0431	1(3)
D0460	1(2)
D0484	1(2)
D0485	1(2)
D0601	0(3)
D0602	0(3)
D0603	0(3)
D1510	2(2)
D1516	1(2)
D1517	1(2)
D1520	2(2)
D1526	1(2)
D1527	1(2)
D1550	2(3)
D1575	4(2)
D1999	0(3)
D4260	4(2)
D4263	4(2)
D4264	3(3)
D4270	4(3)
D4273	1(2)
D4277	0(3)

CPT	MUE	CPT	MUE	CPT	MUE	CPT	MUE	CPT	MUE	CPT	MUE	CPT	MUE	CPT	MUE
D4278	0(3)	E0159	0(3)	E0274	0(3)	E0487	0(3)	E0705	1(2)	E0958	0(3)	E1110	0(3)	E1550	0(3)
D4355	1(2)	E0160	0(3)	E0275	0(3)	E0500	0(3)	E0710	0(3)	E0959	2(2)	E1130	0(3)	E1560	0(3)
D4381	12(3)	E0161	0(3)	E0276	0(3)	E0550	0(3)	E0720	0(3)	E0960	0(3)	E1140	0(3)	E1570	0(3)
D5282	0(3)	E0162	0(3)	E0277	0(3)	E0555	0(3)	E0730	0(3)	E0961	2(2)	E1150	0(3)	E1575	0(3)
D5283	0(3)	E0163	0(3)	E0280	0(3)	E0560	0(3)	E0731	0(3)	E0966	1(2)	E1160	0(3)	E1580	0(3)
D5876	0(3)	E0165	0(3)	E0290	0(3)	E0561	0(3)	E0740	0(3)	E0967	0(3)	E1161	0(3)	E1590	0(3)
D5911	1(3)	E0167	0(3)	E0291	0(3)	E0562	0(3)	E0744	0(3)	E0968	0(3)	E1170	0(3)	E1592	0(3)
D5912	1(2)	E0168	0(3)	E0292	0(3)	E0565	0(3)	E0745	0(3)	E0969	0(3)	E1171	0(3)	E1594	0(3)
D5951	0(3)	E0170	0(3)	E0293	0(3)	E0570	0(3)	E0746	1(3)	E0970	0(3)	E1172	0(3)	E1600	0(3)
D5983	1(3)	E0171	0(3)	E0294	0(3)	E0572	0(3)	E0747	0(3)	E0971	2(3)	E1180	0(3)	E1610	0(3)
D5984	1(3)	E0172	0(3)	E0295	0(3)	E0574	0(3)	E0748	0(3)	E0973	2(2)	E1190	0(3)	E1615	0(3)
D5985	1(3)	E0175	0(3)	E0296	0(3)	E0575	0(3)	E0749	1(3)	E0974	2(2)	E1195	0(3)	E1620	0(3)
D6052	0(3)	E0181	0(3)	E0297	0(3)	E0580	0(3)	E0755	0(3)	E0978	1(3)	E1200	0(3)	E1625	0(3)
D7111	20(3)	E0182	0(3)	E0300	0(3)	E0585	0(3)	E0760	0(3)	E0980	0(3)	E1220	0(3)	E1630	0(3)
D7140	32(2)	E0184	0(3)	E0301	0(3)	E0600	0(3)	E0761	0(3)	E0981	0(3)	E1221	0(3)	E1632	0(3)
D7210	32(2)	E0185	0(3)	E0302	0(3)	E0601	0(3)	E0762	1(3)	E0982	0(3)	E1222	0(3)	E1634	0(3)
D7220	6(3)	E0186	0(3)	E0303	0(3)	E0602	0(3)	E0764	0(3)	E0983	0(3)	E1223	0(3)	E1635	0(3)
D7230	6(3)	E0187	0(3)	E0304	0(3)	E0603	0(3)	E0765	0(3)	E0984	0(3)	E1224	0(3)	E1636	0(3)
D7240	6(3)	E0188	0(3)	E0305	0(3)	E0604	0(3)	E0766	0(3)	E0985	0(3)	E1225	0(3)	E1637	0(3)
D7241	6(3)	E0189	0(3)	E0310	0(3)	E0605	0(3)	E0769	0(3)	E0986	0(3)	E1226	1(2)	E1639	0(3)
D7250	32(2)	E0190	0(3)	E0315	0(3)	E0606	0(3)	E0770	1(3)	E0988	0(3)	E1227	0(3)	E1699	1(3)
D7260	1(3)	E0191	0(3)	E0316	0(3)	E0607	0(3)	E0776	0(3)	E0990	2(2)	E1228	0(3)	E1700	0(3)
D7261	1(3)	E0193	0(3)	E0325	0(3)	E0610	0(3)	E0779	0(3)	E0992	1(2)	E1229	0(3)	E1701	0(3)
D7283	4(3)	E0194	0(3)	E0326	0(3)	E0615	0(3)	E0780	0(3)	E0994	0(3)	E1230	0(3)	E1702	0(3)
D7288	2(3)	E0196	0(3)	E0328	0(3)	E0616	1(2)	E0781	0(3)	E0995	2(2)	E1231	0(3)	E1800	0(3)
D7321	4(2)	E0197	0(3)	E0329	0(3)	E0617	0(3)	E0782	1(2)	E1002	0(3)	E1232	0(3)	E1801	0(3)
D9110	1(3)	E0198	0(3)	E0350	0(3)	E0618	0(3)	E0783	1(2)	E1003	0(3)	E1233	0(3)	E1802	0(3)
D9130	0(3)	E0199	0(3)	E0352	0(3)	E0619	0(3)	E0784	0(3)	E1004	0(3)	E1234	0(3)	E1805	0(3)
D9230	1(3)	E0200	0(3)	E0370	0(3)	E0620	0(3)	E0785	1(2)	E1005	0(3)	E1235	0(3)	E1806	0(3)
D9248	1(3)	E0202	0(3)	E0371	0(3)	E0621	0(3)	E0786	1(2)	E1006	0(3)	E1236	0(3)	E1810	0(3)
D9613	0(3)	E0203	0(3)	E0372	0(3)	E0625	0(3)	E0791	0(3)	E1007	0(3)	E1237	0(3)	E1811	0(3)
D9930	1(2)	E0205	0(3)	E0373	0(3)	E0627	0(3)	E0830	0(3)	E1008	0(3)	E1238	0(3)	E1812	0(3)
D9944	2(2)	E0210	0(3)	E0424	0(3)	E0629	0(3)	E0840	0(3)	E1009	0(3)	E1239	0(3)	E1815	0(3)
D9945	2(2)	E0215	0(3)	E0425	0(3)	E0630	0(3)	E0849	0(3)	E1010	0(3)	E1240	0(3)	E1816	0(3)
D9946	2(2)	E0217	0(3)	E0430	0(3)	E0635	0(3)	E0850	0(3)	E1011	0(3)	E1250	0(3)	E1818	0(3)
D9950	1(3)	E0218	0(3)	E0431	0(3)	E0636	0(3)	E0855	0(3)	E1012	0(3)	E1260	0(3)	E1820	0(3)
D9951	1(3)	E0221	0(3)	E0433	0(3)	E0637	0(3)	E0856	0(3)	E1014	0(3)	E1270	0(3)	E1821	0(3)
D9952	1(3)	E0225	0(3)	E0434	0(3)	E0638	0(3)	E0860	0(3)	E1015	0(3)	E1280	0(3)	E1825	0(3)
D9961	0(3)	E0231	0(3)	E0435	0(3)	E0639	0(3)	E0870	0(3)	E1016	0(3)	E1285	0(3)	E1830	0(3)
D9990	0(3)	E0232	0(3)	E0439	0(3)	E0640	0(3)	E0880	0(3)	E1017	0(3)	E1290	0(3)	E1831	0(3)
E0100	0(3)	E0235	0(3)	E0440	0(3)	E0641	0(3)	E0890	0(3)	E1018	0(3)	E1295	0(3)	E1840	0(3)
E0105	0(3)	E0236	0(3)	E0441	0(3)	E0642	0(3)	E0900	0(3)	E1020	0(3)	E1296	0(3)	E1841	0(3)
E0110	0(3)	E0239	0(3)	E0442	0(3)	E0650	0(3)	E0910	0(3)	E1028	0(3)	E1297	0(3)	E1902	0(3)
E0111	0(3)	E0240	0(3)	E0443	0(3)	E0651	0(3)	E0911	0(3)	E1029	0(3)	E1298	0(3)	E2000	0(3)
E0112	0(3)	E0241	0(3)	E0444	0(3)	E0652	0(3)	E0912	0(3)	E1030	0(3)	E1300	0(3)	E2100	0(3)
E0113	0(3)	E0242	0(3)	E0445	0(3)	E0655	0(3)	E0920	0(3)	E1031	0(3)	E1310	0(3)	E2101	0(3)
E0114	0(3)	E0243	0(3)	E0446	0(3)	E0656	0(3)	E0930	0(3)	E1035	0(3)	E1352	0(3)	E2120	0(3)
E0116	0(3)	E0244	0(3)	E0447	0(3)	E0657	0(3)	E0935	0(3)	E1036	0(3)	E1353	0(3)	E2201	0(3)
E0117	0(3)	E0245	0(3)	E0455	0(3)	E0660	0(3)	E0936	0(3)	E1037	0(3)	E1354	0(3)	E2202	0(3)
E0118	0(3)	E0246	0(3)	E0457	0(3)	E0665	0(3)	E0940	0(3)	E1038	0(3)	E1355	0(3)	E2203	0(3)
E0130	0(3)	E0247	0(3)	E0459	0(3)	E0666	0(3)	E0941	0(3)	E1039	0(3)	E1356	0(3)	E2204	0(3)
E0135	0(3)	E0248	0(3)	E0462	0(3)	E0667	0(3)	E0942	0(3)	E1050	0(3)	E1357	0(3)	E2205	0(3)
E0140	0(3)	E0249	0(3)	E0465	0(3)	E0668	0(3)	E0944	0(3)	E1060	0(3)	E1358	0(3)	E2206	0(3)
E0141	0(3)	E0250	0(3)	E0466	0(3)	E0669	0(3)	E0945	0(3)	E1070	0(3)	E1372	0(3)	E2207	0(3)
E0143	0(3)	E0251	0(3)	E0467	0(3)	E0670	0(3)	E0946	0(3)	E1083	0(3)	E1390	0(3)	E2208	0(3)
E0144	0(3)	E0255	0(3)	E0470	0(3)	E0671	0(3)	E0947	0(3)	E1084	0(3)	E1391	0(3)	E2209	0(3)
E0147	0(3)	E0256	0(3)	E0471	0(3)	E0672	0(3)	E0948	0(3)	E1085	0(3)	E1392	0(3)	E2210	0(3)
E0148	0(3)	E0260	0(3)	E0472	0(3)	E0673	0(3)	E0950	0(3)	E1086	0(3)	E1399	0(3)	E2211	0(3)
E0149	0(3)	E0261	0(3)	E0480	0(3)	E0675	0(3)	E0951	0(3)	E1087	0(3)	E1405	0(3)	E2212	0(3)
E0153	0(3)	E0265	0(3)	E0481	0(3)	E0676	1(3)	E0952	0(3)	E1088	0(3)	E1406	0(3)	E2213	0(3)
E0154	0(3)	E0266	0(3)	E0482	0(3)	E0691	0(3)	E0953	0(3)	E1089	0(3)	E1500	0(3)	E2214	0(3)
E0155	0(3)	E0270	0(3)	E0483	0(3)	E0692	0(3)	E0954	0(3)	E1090	0(3)	E1510	0(3)	E2215	0(3)
E0156	0(3)	E0271	0(3)	E0484	0(3)	E0693	0(3)	E0955	0(3)	E1092	0(3)	E1520	0(3)	E2216	0(3)
E0157	0(3)	E0272	0(3)	E0485	0(3)	E0694	0(3)	E0956	0(3)	E1093	0(3)	E1530	0(3)	E2217	0(3)
E0158	0(3)	E0273	0(3)	E0486	0(3)	E0700	0(3)	E0957	0(3)	E1100	0(3)	E1540	0(3)	E2218	0(3)

CPT	MUE
E2219	0(3)
E2220	0(3)
E2221	0(3)
E2222	0(3)
E2224	0(3)
E2225	0(3)
E2226	0(3)
E2227	0(3)
E2228	0(3)
E2230	0(3)
E2231	0(3)
E2291	1(2)
E2292	1(2)
E2293	1(2)
E2294	1(2)
E2295	0(3)
E2300	0(3)
E2301	0(3)
E2310	0(3)
E2311	0(3)
E2312	0(3)
E2313	0(3)
E2321	0(3)
E2322	0(3)
E2323	0(3)
E2324	0(3)
E2325	0(3)
E2326	0(3)
E2327	0(3)
E2328	0(3)
E2329	0(3)
E2330	0(3)
E2331	0(3)
E2340	0(3)
E2341	0(3)
E2342	0(3)
E2343	0(3)
E2351	0(3)
E2358	0(3)
E2359	0(3)
E2360	0(3)
E2361	0(3)
E2362	0(3)
E2363	0(3)
E2364	0(3)
E2365	0(3)
E2366	0(3)
E2367	0(3)
E2368	0(3)
E2369	0(3)
E2370	0(3)
E2371	0(3)
E2372	0(3)
E2373	0(3)
E2374	0(3)
E2375	0(3)
E2376	0(3)
E2377	0(3)
E2378	0(3)
E2381	0(3)
E2382	0(3)
E2383	0(3)
E2384	0(3)
E2385	0(3)
E2386	0(3)

CPT	MUE
E2387	0(3)
E2388	0(3)
E2389	0(3)
E2390	0(3)
E2391	0(3)
E2392	0(3)
E2394	0(3)
E2395	0(3)
E2396	0(3)
E2397	0(3)
E2402	0(3)
E2500	0(3)
E2502	0(3)
E2504	0(3)
E2506	0(3)
E2508	0(3)
E2510	0(3)
E2511	0(3)
E2512	0(3)
E2599	0(3)
E2601	0(3)
E2602	0(3)
E2603	0(3)
E2604	0(3)
E2605	0(3)
E2606	0(3)
E2607	0(3)
E2608	0(3)
E2609	0(3)
E2610	1(3)
E2611	0(3)
E2612	0(3)
E2613	0(3)
E2614	0(3)
E2615	0(3)
E2616	0(3)
E2617	0(3)
E2619	0(3)
E2620	0(3)
E2621	0(3)
E2622	0(3)
E2623	0(3)
E2624	0(3)
E2625	0(3)
E2626	0(3)
E2627	0(3)
E2628	0(3)
E2629	0(3)
E2630	0(3)
E2631	0(3)
E2632	0(3)
E2633	0(3)
E8000	0(3)
E8001	0(3)
E8002	0(3)
G0008	1(2)
G0009	1(2)
G0010	1(3)
G0027	1(2)
G0068	16(3)
G0069	16(3)
G0070	16(3)
G0071	1(3)
G0076	1(3)
G0077	1(3)

CPT	MUE
G0078	1(3)
G0079	1(3)
G0080	1(3)
G0081	1(3)
G0082	1(3)
G0083	1(3)
G0084	1(3)
G0085	1(3)
G0086	1(3)
G0087	1(3)
G0101	1(2)
G0102	1(2)
G0103	1(2)
G0104	1(2)
G0105	1(2)
G0106	1(2)
G0108	8(3)
G0109	12(3)
G0117	1(2)
G0118	1(2)
G0120	1(2)
G0121	1(2)
G0122	0(3)
G0123	1(3)
G0124	1(3)
G0127	1(2)
G0128	1(3)
G0129	6(3)
G0130	1(2)
G0141	1(3)
G0143	1(3)
G0144	1(3)
G0145	1(3)
G0147	1(3)
G0148	1(3)
G0166	2(3)
G0168	2(3)
G0175	1(3)
G0176	5(3)
G0177	5(3)
G0179	1(2)
G0180	1(2)
G0181	1(2)
G0182	1(2)
G0186	1(2)
G0219	0(3)
G0235	1(3)
G0237	8(3)
G0238	8(3)
G0239	2(3)
G0245	1(2)
G0246	1(2)
G0247	1(2)
G0248	1(2)
G0249	3(3)
G0250	1(2)
G0252	0(3)
G0255	0(3)
G0257	1(3)
G0259	2(3)
G0260	2(3)
G0268	1(2)
G0269	2(3)
G0270	8(3)
G0271	4(3)

CPT	MUE
G0276	1(3)
G0277	5(3)
G0278	1(2)
G0279	1(2)
G0281	1(3)
G0282	0(3)
G0283	1(3)
G0288	1(2)
G0289	1(2)
G0293	1(2)
G0294	1(2)
G0295	0(3)
G0296	1(2)
G0297	1(2)
G0302	1(2)
G0303	1(2)
G0304	1(2)
G0305	1(2)
G0306	4(3)
G0307	4(3)
G0328	1(2)
G0329	1(3)
G0333	0(3)
G0337	1(2)
G0339	1(2)
G0340	1(3)
G0341	1(2)
G0342	1(2)
G0343	1(2)
G0365	2(3)
G0372	1(2)
G0379	1(2)
G0380	2(3)
G0381	2(3)
G0382	2(3)
G0383	2(3)
G0384	2(3)
G0390	1(2)
G0396	1(2)
G0397	1(2)
G0398	1(2)
G0399	1(2)
G0400	1(2)
G0402	1(2)
G0403	1(2)
G0404	1(2)
G0405	1(2)
G0406	1(3)
G0407	1(3)
G0408	1(3)
G0410	6(3)
G0411	6(3)
G0412	1(2)
G0413	1(2)
G0414	1(2)
G0415	1(2)
G0416	1(2)
G0420	2(3)
G0421	2(3)
G0422	6(2)
G0423	6(2)
G0424	2(2)
G0425	1(3)
G0426	1(3)
G0427	1(3)

CPT	MUE
G0428	0(3)
G0429	1(2)
G0432	1(2)
G0433	1(2)
G0435	1(2)
G0438	1(2)
G0439	1(2)
G0442	1(2)
G0443	1(2)
G0444	1(2)
G0445	1(2)
G0446	1(3)
G0447	2(3)
G0448	1(3)
G0451	1(3)
G0452	1(3)
G0453	10(3)
G0454	1(2)
G0455	1(2)
G0458	1(3)
G0459	1(3)
G0460	1(3)
G0463	4(3)
G0466	1(2)
G0467	1(3)
G0468	1(2)
G0469	1(2)
G0470	1(3)
G0471	2(3)
G0472	1(2)
G0473	1(3)
G0475	1(2)
G0476	1(2)
G0480	1(2)
G0481	1(2)
G0482	1(2)
G0483	1(2)
G0490	1(3)
G0491	1(3)
G0492	1(3)
G0493	1(3)
G0494	1(3)
G0495	1(3)
G0496	1(3)
G0498	1(2)
G0499	1(2)
G0500	1(3)
G0501	1(3)
G0506	1(2)
G0508	1(2)
G0509	1(2)
G0511	1(2)
G0512	1(2)
G0513	1(2)
G0514	1(1)
G0515	8(3)
G0516	1(2)
G0517	1(2)
G0518	1(2)
G0659	1(2)
G2000	1(3)
G2001	1(3)
G2002	1(3)
G2003	1(3)
G2004	1(3)

CPT	MUE
G2005	1(3)
G2006	1(3)
G2007	1(3)
G2008	1(3)
G2009	1(3)
G2010	0(3)
G2011	1(2)
G2012	0(3)
G2013	1(3)
G2014	1(3)
G2015	1(3)
G6001	2(3)
G6002	2(3)
G6003	2(3)
G6004	2(3)
G6005	2(3)
G6006	2(3)
G6007	2(3)
G6008	2(3)
G6009	2(3)
G6010	2(3)
G6011	2(3)
G6012	2(3)
G6013	2(3)
G6014	2(3)
G6015	2(3)
G6016	2(3)
G6017	2(3)
G9143	1(2)
G9147	0(3)
G9148	0(3)
G9149	0(3)
G9150	0(3)
G9151	0(3)
G9152	0(3)
G9153	0(3)
G9156	1(2)
G9157	1(2)
G9187	0(3)
G9480	1(3)
G9481	2(3)
G9482	2(3)
G9483	2(3)
G9484	2(3)
G9485	2(3)
G9486	2(3)
G9487	2(3)
G9488	2(3)
G9489	2(3)
G9490	2(3)
G9678	1(2)
G9685	0(3)
G9978	2(3)
G9979	2(3)
G9980	2(3)
G9981	2(3)
G9982	2(3)
G9983	2(3)
G9984	2(3)
G9985	2(3)
G9986	2(3)
G9987	2(3)
J0120	1(3)
J0129	100(3)
J0130	6(3)

CPT	MUE
J0131	400(3)
J0132	300(3)
J0133	1200(3)
J0135	8(3)
J0153	180(3)
J0171	120(3)
J0178	4(3)
J0180	140(3)
J0185	130(3)
J0190	0(3)
J0200	0(3)
J0202	12(3)
J0205	0(3)
J0207	4(3)
J0210	16(3)
J0215	0(3)
J0220	20(3)
J0221	300(3)
J0256	1600(3)
J0257	1400(3)
J0270	32(3)
J0275	1(3)
J0278	15(3)
J0280	10(3)
J0282	70(3)
J0285	5(3)
J0287	60(3)
J0288	0(3)
J0289	115(3)
J0290	24(3)
J0295	12(3)
J0300	8(3)
J0330	50(3)
J0348	200(3)
J0350	0(3)
J0360	6(3)
J0364	6(3)
J0365	0(3)
J0380	1(3)
J0390	0(3)
J0395	0(3)
J0400	120(3)
J0401	400(3)
J0456	4(3)
J0461	800(3)
J0470	2(3)
J0475	8(3)
J0476	2(3)
J0480	1(3)
J0485	1500(3)
J0490	160(3)
J0500	4(3)
J0515	6(3)
J0517	30(3)
J0520	0(3)
J0558	24(3)
J0561	24(3)
J0565	200(3)
J0567	300(3)
J0570	4(3)
J0571	0(3)
J0572	0(3)
J0573	0(3)
J0574	0(3)
J0575	0(3)

CPT	MUE
J0583	1250(3)
J0584	90(3)
J0585	600(3)
J0586	300(3)
J0587	300(3)
J0588	600(3)
J0592	12(3)
J0594	320(3)
J0595	12(3)
J0596	840(3)
J0597	250(3)
J0598	100(3)
J0599	900(3)
J0600	3(3)
J0606	150(3)
J0610	15(3)
J0620	1(3)
J0630	8(3)
J0636	100(3)
J0637	20(3)
J0638	150(3)
J0640	24(3)
J0641	1200(3)
J0670	10(3)
J0690	16(3)
J0692	12(3)
J0694	12(3)
J0695	60(3)
J0696	16(3)
J0697	12(3)
J0698	12(3)
J0702	20(3)
J0706	16(3)
J0710	0(3)
J0712	180(3)
J0713	12(3)
J0714	12(3)
J0715	0(3)
J0716	4(1)
J0717	400(3)
J0720	15(3)
J0725	10(3)
J0735	50(3)
J0740	2(3)
J0743	16(3)
J0744	8(3)
J0745	8(3)
J0770	5(3)
J0775	180(3)
J0780	10(3)
J0795	100(3)
J0800	3(3)
J0834	3(3)
J0840	18(3)
J0841	24(3)
J0850	9(3)
J0875	300(3)
J0878	1500(3)
J0881	500(3)
J0882	300(3)
J0883	1250(3)
J0884	1250(3)
J0885	60(3)
J0887	360(3)
J0888	360(3)

CPT	MUE
J0890	0(3)
J0894	100(3)
J0895	12(3)
J0897	120(3)
J0945	4(3)
J1000	1(3)
J1020	8(3)
J1030	8(3)
J1040	4(3)
J1050	1000(3)
J1071	400(3)
J1094	0(3)
J1095	517(1)
J1100	120(3)
J1110	3(3)
J1120	2(3)
J1130	300(3)
J1160	3(3)
J1162	10(3)
J1165	50(3)
J1170	50(3)
J1180	0(3)
J1190	8(3)
J1200	8(3)
J1205	4(3)
J1212	1(3)
J1230	5(3)
J1240	6(3)
J1245	6(3)
J1250	4(3)
J1260	2(3)
J1265	100(3)
J1267	150(3)
J1270	16(3)
J1290	60(3)
J1300	120(3)
J1301	60(3)
J1320	0(3)
J1322	150(3)
J1324	0(3)
J1325	18(3)
J1327	99(3)
J1330	1(3)
J1335	2(3)
J1364	8(3)
J1380	4(3)
J1410	4(3)
J1428	450(3)
J1430	10(3)
J1435	0(3)
J1436	0(3)
J1438	2(3)
J1439	750(3)
J1442	1500(3)
J1443	272(3)
J1444	272(3)
J1447	960(3)
J1450	4(3)
J1451	200(3)
J1452	0(3)
J1453	150(3)
J1454	1(3)
J1455	18(3)
J1457	0(3)
J1458	100(3)

CPT	MUE
J1459	300(3)
J1460	10(2)
J1555	480(3)
J1556	300(3)
J1557	300(3)
J1559	300(3)
J1560	1(2)
J1561	300(3)
J1562	0(3)
J1566	300(3)
J1568	300(3)
J1569	300(3)
J1570	4(3)
J1571	20(3)
J1572	300(3)
J1573	130(3)
J1575	650(3)
J1580	9(3)
J1595	2(3)
J1599	300(3)
J1600	0(3)
J1602	300(3)
J1610	3(3)
J1620	0(3)
J1626	30(3)
J1627	100(3)
J1628	100(3)
J1630	7(3)
J1631	9(3)
J1640	672(3)
J1642	150(3)
J1644	50(3)
J1645	10(3)
J1650	30(3)
J1652	20(3)
J1655	0(3)
J1670	2(3)
J1675	0(3)
J1700	0(3)
J1710	0(3)
J1720	10(3)
J1726	28(3)
J1729	25(3)
J1730	0(3)
J1740	3(3)
J1741	32(3)
J1742	4(3)
J1743	66(3)
J1744	90(3)
J1745	150(3)
J1746	200(3)
J1750	45(3)
J1756	500(3)
J1786	680(3)
J1790	2(3)
J1800	12(3)
J1810	0(3)
J1815	200(3)
J1817	0(3)
J1826	1(3)
J1830	1(3)
J1833	1116(3)
J1835	0(3)
J1840	3(3)
J1850	14(3)

CPT	MUE
J1885	8(3)
J1890	0(3)
J1930	120(3)
J1931	609(3)
J1940	10(3)
J1942	1064(3)
J1945	0(3)
J1950	12(3)
J1953	300(3)
J1955	11(3)
J1956	4(3)
J1960	0(3)
J1980	8(3)
J1990	0(3)
J2001	400(3)
J2010	10(3)
J2020	6(3)
J2060	10(3)
J2062	10(3)
J2150	8(3)
J2170	8(3)
J2175	6(3)
J2180	0(3)
J2182	300(3)
J2185	60(3)
J2186	600(3)
J2210	5(3)
J2212	240(3)
J2248	300(3)
J2250	30(3)
J2260	16(3)
J2265	400(3)
J2270	15(3)
J2274	100(3)
J2278	1000(3)
J2280	8(3)
J2300	10(3)
J2310	10(3)
J2315	380(3)
J2320	4(3)
J2323	300(3)
J2325	34(3)
J2326	120(3)
J2350	600(3)
J2353	60(3)
J2354	60(3)
J2355	2(3)
J2357	90(3)
J2358	405(3)
J2360	3(3)
J2370	30(3)
J2400	4(3)
J2405	64(3)
J2407	120(3)
J2410	2(3)
J2425	125(3)
J2426	819(3)
J2430	3(3)
J2440	4(3)
J2460	0(3)
J2469	10(3)
J2501	25(3)
J2502	60(3)
J2503	2(3)
J2504	15(3)

CPT	MUE
J2505	1(3)
J2507	8(3)
J2510	4(3)
J2513	1(3)
J2515	8(3)
J2540	75(3)
J2543	20(3)
J2545	1(3)
J2547	600(3)
J2550	3(3)
J2560	16(3)
J2562	48(3)
J2590	15(3)
J2597	45(3)
J2650	0(3)
J2670	0(3)
J2675	1(3)
J2680	4(3)
J2690	4(3)
J2700	48(3)
J2704	400(3)
J2710	10(3)
J2720	10(3)
J2724	3500(3)
J2725	0(3)
J2730	2(3)
J2760	2(3)
J2765	18(3)
J2770	7(3)
J2778	10(3)
J2780	16(3)
J2783	60(3)
J2785	4(3)
J2786	500(3)
J2787	1(3)
J2788	1(3)
J2790	3(3)
J2791	15(3)
J2792	450(3)
J2793	320(3)
J2794	100(3)
J2795	2400(3)
J2796	150(3)
J2797	333(3)
J2800	3(3)
J2805	3(3)
J2810	20(3)
J2820	10(3)
J2840	160(3)
J2850	48(3)
J2860	170(3)
J2910	0(3)
J2916	20(3)
J2920	25(3)
J2930	25(3)
J2940	0(3)
J2941	8(3)
J2950	0(3)
J2993	2(3)
J2995	0(3)
J2997	100(3)
J3000	2(3)
J3010	100(3)
J3030	2(3)
J3060	760(3)

CPT	MUE
J3070	3(3)
J3090	200(3)
J3095	150(3)
J3101	50(3)
J3105	4(3)
J3110	2(3)
J3121	400(3)
J3145	750(3)
J3230	6(3)
J3240	1(3)
J3243	200(3)
J3245	0(3)
J3246	100(3)
J3250	4(3)
J3260	12(3)
J3262	800(3)
J3265	0(3)
J3280	0(3)
J3285	9(3)
J3300	160(3)
J3301	16(3)
J3302	0(3)
J3303	24(3)
J3304	64(2)
J3305	0(3)
J3310	0(3)
J3315	6(3)
J3316	6(3)
J3320	0(3)
J3350	0(3)
J3355	0(3)
J3357	90(3)
J3358	520(3)
J3360	6(3)
J3364	0(3)
J3365	0(3)
J3370	12(3)
J3380	300(3)
J3385	80(3)
J3396	150(3)
J3397	600(3)
J3398	150(2)
J3400	0(3)
J3410	16(3)
J3411	8(3)
J3415	6(3)
J3420	1(3)
J3430	50(3)
J3465	120(3)
J3470	3(3)
J3471	999(2)
J3472	2(3)
J3473	450(3)
J3475	80(3)
J3480	200(3)
J3485	160(3)
J3486	4(3)
J3489	5(3)
J3520	0(3)
J3530	0(3)
J3535	0(3)
J3570	0(3)
J7030	20(3)
J7040	12(3)
J7042	12(3)

CPT	MUE
J7050	20(3)
J7060	10(3)
J7070	7(3)
J7100	2(3)
J7110	3(3)
J7120	20(3)
J7121	5(3)
J7131	500(3)
J7170	1800(3)
J7175	9000(1)
J7177	10500(3)
J7178	7700(1)
J7179	9600(1)
J7180	6000(1)
J7181	3850(1)
J7182	22000(1)
J7183	9600(1)
J7185	22000(1)
J7186	9600(1)
J7187	9600(1)
J7188	22000(1)
J7189	26000(1)
J7190	22000(1)
J7191	0(3)
J7192	22000(1)
J7193	20000(1)
J7194	9000(1)
J7195	20000(1)
J7196	0(3)
J7197	6300(1)
J7198	30000(1)
J7200	20000(1)
J7201	9000(1)
J7202	11550(1)
J7203	12000(1)
J7205	9750(1)
J7207	7500(1)
J7208	18000(1)
J7209	7500(1)
J7210	22000(1)
J7211	22000(1)
J7296	0(3)
J7297	0(3)
J7298	0(3)
J7300	0(3)
J7301	0(3)
J7303	0(3)
J7304	0(3)
J7306	0(3)
J7307	0(3)
J7308	3(3)
J7309	1(3)
J7310	0(3)
J7311	1(3)
J7312	14(3)
J7313	38(3)
J7315	2(3)
J7316	3(2)
J7318	120(3)
J7320	50(3)
J7321	2(2)
J7322	48(3)
J7323	2(2)
J7324	2(2)
J7325	96(3)

CPT	MUE
J7326	2(2)
J7327	2(2)
J7328	336(3)
J7329	0(3)
J7330	1(3)
J7336	1120(3)
J7340	1(3)
J7342	10(3)
J7345	200(3)
J7500	15(3)
J7501	8(3)
J7502	60(3)
J7503	120(3)
J7504	15(3)
J7505	1(3)
J7507	40(3)
J7508	300(3)
J7509	60(3)
J7510	60(3)
J7511	9(3)
J7512	300(3)
J7513	0(3)
J7515	90(3)
J7516	4(3)
J7517	16(3)
J7518	12(3)
J7520	40(3)
J7525	2(3)
J7527	20(3)
J7599	1(3)
J7604	0(3)
J7605	0(3)
J7606	0(3)
J7607	0(3)
J7608	0(3)
J7609	0(3)
J7610	0(3)
J7611	0(3)
J7612	0(3)
J7613	0(3)
J7614	0(3)
J7615	0(3)
J7620	0(3)
J7622	0(3)
J7624	0(3)
J7626	0(3)
J7627	0(3)
J7628	0(3)
J7629	0(3)
J7631	0(3)
J7632	0(3)
J7633	0(3)
J7634	0(3)
J7635	0(3)
J7636	0(3)
J7637	0(3)
J7638	0(3)
J7639	0(3)
J7640	0(3)
J7641	0(3)
J7642	0(3)
J7643	0(3)
J7644	0(3)
J7645	0(3)
J7647	0(3)

CPT	MUE
J7648	0(3)
J7649	0(3)
J7650	0(3)
J7657	0(3)
J7658	0(3)
J7659	0(3)
J7660	0(3)
J7665	0(3)
J7667	0(3)
J7668	0(3)
J7669	0(3)
J7670	0(3)
J7674	100(3)
J7676	0(3)
J7677	175(3)
J7680	0(3)
J7681	0(3)
J7682	0(3)
J7683	0(3)
J7684	0(3)
J7685	0(3)
J7686	0(3)
J7699	0(3)
J7799	2(3)
J7999	6(3)
J8498	1(3)
J8499	0(3)
J8501	57(3)
J8510	5(3)
J8515	0(3)
J8520	50(3)
J8521	15(3)
J8530	60(3)
J8540	48(3)
J8560	6(3)
J8562	12(3)
J8565	0(3)
J8597	4(3)
J8600	40(3)
J8610	20(3)
J8650	0(3)
J8655	1(3)
J8670	180(3)
J8700	120(3)
J8705	22(3)
J8999	2(3)
J9000	20(3)
J9015	1(3)
J9017	30(3)
J9019	60(3)
J9020	0(3)
J9022	168(3)
J9023	140(3)
J9025	300(3)
J9027	100(3)
J9030	50(3)
J9032	300(3)
J9033	300(3)
J9034	360(3)
J9035	170(3)
J9036	360(3)
J9039	210(3)
J9040	4(3)
J9041	35(3)
J9042	200(3)

CPT	MUE	CPT	MUE	CPT	MUE	CPT	MUE	CPT	MUE	CPT	MUE	CPT	MUE	CPT	MUE
J9043	60(3)	J9280	12(3)	K0052	0(3)	K0842	0(3)	L0480	1(2)	L1100	2(2)	L1951	2(2)	L2395	4(2)
J9044	35(3)	J9285	200(3)	K0053	0(3)	K0843	0(3)	L0482	1(2)	L1110	2(2)	L1960	2(2)	L2397	4(3)
J9045	22(3)	J9293	8(3)	K0056	0(3)	K0848	0(3)	L0484	1(2)	L1120	3(3)	L1970	2(2)	L2405	4(2)
J9047	160(3)	J9295	800(3)	K0065	0(3)	K0849	0(3)	L0486	1(2)	L1200	1(2)	L1971	2(2)	L2415	4(2)
J9050	6(3)	J9299	480(3)	K0069	0(3)	K0850	0(3)	L0488	1(2)	L1210	2(3)	L1980	2(2)	L2425	4(2)
J9055	120(3)	J9301	100(3)	K0070	0(3)	K0851	0(3)	L0490	1(2)	L1220	1(3)	L1990	2(2)	L2430	4(2)
J9057	60(3)	J9302	200(3)	K0071	0(3)	K0852	0(3)	L0491	1(2)	L1230	1(2)	L2000	2(2)	L2492	4(2)
J9060	24(3)	J9303	90(3)	K0072	0(3)	K0853	0(3)	L0492	1(2)	L1240	1(3)	L2005	2(2)	L2500	2(2)
J9065	100(3)	J9305	150(3)	K0073	0(3)	K0854	0(3)	L0621	1(2)	L1250	2(3)	L2010	2(2)	L2510	2(2)
J9070	55(3)	J9306	840(3)	K0077	0(3)	K0855	0(3)	L0622	1(2)	L1260	1(3)	L2020	2(2)	L2520	2(2)
J9098	5(3)	J9307	80(3)	K0098	0(3)	K0856	0(3)	L0623	1(2)	L1270	3(3)	L2030	2(2)	L2525	2(2)
J9100	120(3)	J9308	280(3)	K0105	0(3)	K0857	0(3)	L0624	1(2)	L1280	2(3)	L2034	2(2)	L2526	2(2)
J9120	5(3)	J9311	160(3)	K0108	0(3)	K0858	0(3)	L0625	1(2)	L1290	2(3)	L2035	2(2)	L2530	2(2)
J9130	24(3)	J9312	150(3)	K0195	0(3)	K0859	0(3)	L0626	1(2)	L1300	1(2)	L2036	2(2)	L2540	2(2)
J9145	240(3)	J9315	40(3)	K0455	0(3)	K0860	0(3)	L0627	1(2)	L1310	1(2)	L2037	2(2)	L2550	2(2)
J9150	12(3)	J9320	4(3)	K0462	0(3)	K0861	0(3)	L0628	1(2)	L1499	1(3)	L2038	2(2)	L2570	2(2)
J9151	0(3)	J9325	400(3)	K0552	0(3)	K0862	0(3)	L0629	1(2)	L1600	1(2)	L2040	1(2)	L2580	2(2)
J9153	132(3)	J9328	400(3)	K0553	0(3)	K0863	0(3)	L0630	1(2)	L1610	1(2)	L2050	1(2)	L2600	2(2)
J9155	240(3)	J9330	50(3)	K0554	0(3)	K0864	0(3)	L0631	1(2)	L1620	1(2)	L2060	1(2)	L2610	2(2)
J9160	0(3)	J9340	4(3)	K0601	0(3)	K0868	0(3)	L0632	1(2)	L1630	1(2)	L2070	1(2)	L2620	2(2)
J9165	0(3)	J9351	120(3)	K0602	0(3)	K0869	0(3)	L0633	1(2)	L1640	1(2)	L2080	1(2)	L2622	2(2)
J9171	240(3)	J9352	40(3)	K0603	0(3)	K0870	0(3)	L0634	1(2)	L1650	1(2)	L2090	1(2)	L2624	2(2)
J9173	150(3)	J9354	600(3)	K0604	0(3)	K0871	0(3)	L0635	1(2)	L1652	1(2)	L2106	2(2)	L2627	1(3)
J9175	10(3)	J9355	105(3)	K0605	0(3)	K0877	0(3)	L0636	1(2)	L1660	1(2)	L2108	2(2)	L2628	1(3)
J9176	3000(3)	J9356	60(3)	K0606	0(3)	K0878	0(3)	L0637	1(2)	L1680	1(2)	L2112	2(2)	L2630	1(2)
J9178	150(3)	J9357	4(3)	K0607	0(3)	K0879	0(3)	L0638	1(2)	L1685	1(2)	L2114	2(2)	L2640	1(2)
J9179	50(3)	J9360	40(3)	K0608	0(3)	K0880	0(3)	L0639	1(2)	L1686	1(3)	L2116	2(2)	L2650	2(3)
J9181	100(3)	J9370	4(3)	K0609	0(3)	K0884	0(3)	L0640	1(2)	L1690	1(2)	L2126	2(2)	L2660	1(3)
J9185	2(3)	J9371	5(3)	K0669	0(3)	K0885	0(3)	L0641	1(2)	L1700	1(2)	L2128	2(2)	L2670	2(3)
J9190	20(3)	J9390	36(3)	K0672	4(3)	K0886	0(3)	L0642	1(2)	L1710	1(2)	L2132	2(2)	L2680	2(3)
J9200	20(3)	J9395	20(3)	K0730	0(3)	K0890	0(3)	L0643	1(2)	L1720	2(2)	L2134	2(2)	L2750	8(3)
J9201	20(3)	J9400	500(3)	K0733	0(3)	K0891	0(3)	L0648	1(2)	L1730	1(2)	L2136	2(2)	L2755	8(3)
J9202	3(3)	J9600	4(3)	K0738	0(3)	K0898	1(2)	L0649	1(2)	L1755	2(2)	L2180	2(2)	L2760	8(2)
J9203	180(3)	K0001	0(3)	K0740	0(3)	K0899	0(3)	L0650	1(2)	L1810	2(2)	L2182	4(2)	L2768	4(2)
J9205	215(3)	K0002	0(3)	K0743	0(3)	K0900	0(3)	L0651	1(2)	L1812	2(2)	L2184	4(2)	L2780	8(3)
J9206	42(3)	K0003	0(3)	K0800	0(3)	L0112	1(2)	L0700	1(2)	L1820	2(2)	L2186	4(2)	L2785	4(2)
J9207	90(3)	K0004	0(3)	K0801	0(3)	L0113	1(2)	L0710	1(2)	L1830	2(2)	L2188	2(2)	L2795	2(2)
J9208	15(3)	K0005	0(3)	K0802	0(3)	L0120	1(2)	L0810	1(2)	L1831	2(2)	L2190	2(2)	L2800	2(2)
J9209	55(3)	K0006	0(3)	K0806	0(3)	L0130	1(2)	L0820	1(2)	L1832	2(2)	L2192	2(2)	L2810	4(2)
J9211	6(3)	K0007	0(3)	K0807	0(3)	L0140	1(2)	L0830	1(2)	L1833	2(2)	L2200	4(2)	L2820	2(3)
J9212	0(3)	K0008	0(3)	K0808	0(3)	L0150	1(2)	L0859	1(2)	L1834	2(2)	L2210	4(2)	L2830	2(3)
J9213	12(3)	K0009	0(3)	K0812	0(3)	L0160	1(2)	L0861	1(2)	L1836	2(2)	L2220	4(2)	L2861	0(3)
J9214	100(3)	K0010	0(3)	K0813	0(3)	L0170	1(2)	L0970	1(2)	L1840	2(2)	L2230	2(2)	L2999	2(3)
J9215	0(3)	K0011	0(3)	K0814	0(3)	L0172	1(2)	L0972	1(2)	L1843	2(2)	L2232	2(2)	L3000	2(3)
J9216	0(3)	K0012	0(3)	K0815	0(3)	L0174	1(2)	L0974	1(2)	L1844	2(2)	L2240	2(2)	L3001	2(3)
J9217	6(3)	K0013	0(3)	K0816	0(3)	L0180	1(2)	L0976	1(2)	L1845	2(2)	L2250	2(2)	L3002	2(3)
J9218	1(3)	K0014	0(3)	K0820	0(3)	L0190	1(2)	L0978	2(3)	L1846	2(2)	L2260	2(2)	L3003	2(3)
J9219	0(3)	K0015	0(3)	K0821	0(3)	L0200	1(2)	L0980	1(2)	L1847	2(2)	L2265	2(2)	L3010	2(3)
J9225	1(3)	K0017	0(3)	K0822	0(3)	L0220	1(3)	L0982	1(3)	L1848	2(2)	L2270	2(3)	L3020	2(3)
J9226	1(3)	K0018	0(3)	K0823	0(3)	L0450	1(2)	L0984	3(3)	L1850	2(2)	L2275	2(3)	L3030	2(3)
J9228	1100(3)	K0019	0(3)	K0824	0(3)	L0452	1(2)	L0999	1(3)	L1851	2(2)	L2280	2(2)	L3031	2(3)
J9229	27(3)	K0020	0(3)	K0825	0(3)	L0454	1(2)	L1000	1(2)	L1852	2(2)	L2300	1(2)	L3040	2(3)
J9230	5(3)	K0037	0(3)	K0826	0(3)	L0455	1(2)	L1001	1(2)	L1860	2(2)	L2310	1(2)	L3050	2(3)
J9245	11(3)	K0038	0(3)	K0827	0(3)	L0456	1(2)	L1005	1(2)	L1900	2(2)	L2320	2(3)	L3060	2(3)
J9250	50(3)	K0039	0(3)	K0828	0(3)	L0457	1(2)	L1010	2(2)	L1902	2(2)	L2330	2(3)	L3070	2(3)
J9260	20(3)	K0040	0(3)	K0829	0(3)	L0458	1(2)	L1020	2(3)	L1904	2(2)	L2335	2(2)	L3080	2(3)
J9261	80(3)	K0041	0(3)	K0830	0(3)	L0460	1(2)	L1025	1(3)	L1906	2(2)	L2340	2(2)	L3090	2(3)
J9262	700(3)	K0042	0(3)	K0831	0(3)	L0462	1(2)	L1030	1(3)	L1907	2(2)	L2350	2(2)	L3100	2(2)
J9263	700(3)	K0043	0(3)	K0835	0(3)	L0464	1(2)	L1040	1(3)	L1910	2(2)	L2360	2(2)	L3140	1(2)
J9264	600(3)	K0044	0(3)	K0836	0(3)	L0466	1(2)	L1050	1(3)	L1920	2(2)	L2370	2(2)	L3150	1(2)
J9266	2(3)	K0045	0(3)	K0837	0(3)	L0467	1(2)	L1060	1(3)	L1930	2(2)	L2375	2(2)	L3160	2(2)
J9267	750(3)	K0046	0(3)	K0838	0(3)	L0468	1(2)	L1070	2(2)	L1932	2(2)	L2380	2(3)	L3170	2(2)
J9268	1(3)	K0047	0(3)	K0839	0(3)	L0469	1(2)	L1080	2(2)	L1940	2(2)	L2385	4(2)	L3201	1(3)
J9270	0(3)	K0050	0(3)	K0840	0(3)	L0470	1(2)	L1085	1(2)	L1945	2(2)	L2387	4(2)	L3202	1(3)
J9271	300(3)	K0051	0(3)	K0841	0(3)	L0472	1(2)	L1090	1(3)	L1950	2(2)	L2390	4(2)	L3203	1(3)

CPT	MUE
L3204	1(3)
L3206	1(3)
L3207	1(3)
L3208	1(3)
L3209	1(3)
L3211	1(3)
L3212	1(3)
L3213	1(3)
L3214	1(3)
L3215	0(3)
L3216	0(3)
L3217	0(3)
L3219	0(3)
L3221	0(3)
L3222	0(3)
L3224	2(2)
L3225	2(2)
L3230	2(2)
L3250	2(2)
L3251	2(2)
L3252	2(2)
L3253	2(2)
L3254	1(3)
L3255	1(3)
L3257	1(3)
L3260	0(3)
L3265	1(3)
L3300	4(3)
L3310	4(3)
L3330	2(2)
L3332	2(2)
L3334	4(3)
L3340	2(2)
L3350	2(2)
L3360	2(2)
L3370	2(2)
L3380	2(2)
L3390	2(2)
L3400	2(2)
L3410	2(2)
L3420	2(2)
L3430	2(2)
L3440	2(2)
L3450	2(2)
L3455	2(2)
L3460	2(2)
L3465	2(2)
L3470	2(2)
L3480	2(2)
L3485	2(2)
L3500	2(2)
L3510	2(2)
L3520	2(2)
L3530	2(2)
L3540	2(2)
L3550	2(2)
L3560	2(2)
L3570	2(2)
L3580	2(2)
L3590	2(2)
L3595	2(2)
L3600	2(2)
L3610	2(2)
L3620	2(2)
L3630	2(2)

CPT	MUE
L3640	1(2)
L3649	2(3)
L3650	1(2)
L3660	1(2)
L3670	1(3)
L3671	1(3)
L3674	1(3)
L3675	1(2)
L3677	1(2)
L3678	1(2)
L3702	2(2)
L3710	2(2)
L3720	2(2)
L3730	2(2)
L3740	2(2)
L3760	2(2)
L3761	2(2)
L3762	2(2)
L3763	2(2)
L3764	2(2)
L3765	2(2)
L3766	2(2)
L3806	2(2)
L3807	2(2)
L3808	2(2)
L3809	2(2)
L3891	0(3)
L3900	2(2)
L3901	2(2)
L3904	2(2)
L3905	2(2)
L3906	2(2)
L3908	2(2)
L3912	2(3)
L3913	2(2)
L3915	2(2)
L3916	2(3)
L3917	2(2)
L3918	2(2)
L3919	2(2)
L3921	2(2)
L3923	2(2)
L3924	2(2)
L3925	4(3)
L3927	4(3)
L3929	2(2)
L3930	2(2)
L3931	2(2)
L3933	3(3)
L3935	3(3)
L3956	4(3)
L3960	1(3)
L3961	1(3)
L3962	1(3)
L3967	1(3)
L3971	1(3)
L3973	1(3)
L3975	1(3)
L3976	1(3)
L3977	1(3)
L3978	1(3)
L3980	2(2)
L3981	2(2)
L3982	2(2)
L3984	2(2)

CPT	MUE
L3999	2(3)
L4000	1(2)
L4002	4(3)
L4010	2(2)
L4020	2(2)
L4030	2(2)
L4040	2(2)
L4045	2(2)
L4050	2(2)
L4055	2(2)
L4060	2(2)
L4070	2(3)
L4080	2(2)
L4090	4(2)
L4100	2(2)
L4110	4(2)
L4130	2(2)
L4205	8(3)
L4210	4(3)
L4350	2(2)
L4360	2(2)
L4361	2(2)
L4370	2(2)
L4386	2(2)
L4387	2(2)
L4392	2(3)
L4394	2(3)
L4396	2(2)
L4397	2(2)
L4398	2(2)
L4631	2(2)
L5000	2(3)
L5010	2(2)
L5020	2(2)
L5050	2(2)
L5060	2(2)
L5100	2(2)
L5105	2(2)
L5150	2(2)
L5160	2(2)
L5200	2(2)
L5210	2(2)
L5220	2(2)
L5230	2(2)
L5250	2(2)
L5270	2(2)
L5280	2(2)
L5301	2(2)
L5312	2(2)
L5321	2(2)
L5331	2(2)
L5341	2(2)
L5400	2(2)
L5410	2(2)
L5420	2(2)
L5430	2(2)
L5450	2(2)
L5460	2(2)
L5500	2(2)
L5505	2(2)
L5510	2(2)
L5520	2(2)
L5530	2(2)
L5535	2(2)
L5540	2(2)

CPT	MUE
L5560	2(2)
L5570	2(2)
L5580	2(2)
L5585	2(2)
L5590	2(2)
L5595	2(2)
L5600	2(2)
L5610	2(2)
L5611	2(2)
L5613	2(2)
L5614	2(2)
L5616	2(2)
L5617	2(3)
L5618	4(3)
L5620	4(3)
L5622	4(3)
L5624	4(3)
L5626	4(3)
L5628	2(3)
L5629	2(2)
L5630	2(2)
L5631	2(2)
L5632	2(2)
L5634	2(2)
L5636	2(2)
L5637	2(2)
L5638	2(2)
L5639	2(2)
L5640	2(2)
L5642	2(2)
L5643	2(2)
L5644	2(2)
L5645	2(2)
L5646	2(2)
L5647	2(2)
L5648	2(2)
L5649	2(2)
L5650	2(2)
L5651	2(2)
L5652	2(2)
L5653	2(2)
L5654	2(2)
L5655	2(2)
L5656	2(2)
L5658	2(2)
L5661	2(2)
L5665	2(2)
L5666	2(2)
L5668	2(2)
L5670	2(2)
L5671	2(2)
L5672	2(2)
L5673	4(3)
L5676	2(2)
L5677	2(2)
L5678	2(2)
L5679	4(3)
L5680	2(2)
L5681	2(2)
L5682	2(2)
L5683	2(2)
L5684	2(3)
L5685	4(3)
L5686	2(2)
L5688	2(3)

CPT	MUE
L5690	2(3)
L5692	2(2)
L5694	2(2)
L5695	2(3)
L5696	2(2)
L5697	2(2)
L5698	2(2)
L5699	2(3)
L5700	2(2)
L5701	2(2)
L5702	2(2)
L5703	2(2)
L5704	2(2)
L5705	2(2)
L5706	2(2)
L5707	2(2)
L5710	2(2)
L5711	2(2)
L5712	2(2)
L5714	2(2)
L5716	2(2)
L5718	2(2)
L5722	2(2)
L5724	2(2)
L5726	2(2)
L5728	2(2)
L5780	2(2)
L5781	2(2)
L5782	2(2)
L5785	2(2)
L5790	2(2)
L5795	2(2)
L5810	2(2)
L5811	2(2)
L5812	2(2)
L5814	2(2)
L5816	2(2)
L5818	2(2)
L5822	2(2)
L5824	2(2)
L5826	2(2)
L5828	2(2)
L5830	2(2)
L5840	2(2)
L5845	2(2)
L5848	2(2)
L5850	2(2)
L5855	2(2)
L5856	2(2)
L5857	2(2)
L5858	2(2)
L5859	2(2)
L5910	2(2)
L5920	2(2)
L5925	2(3)
L5930	2(2)
L5940	2(2)
L5950	2(2)
L5960	2(2)
L5961	1(3)
L5962	2(2)
L5964	2(2)
L5966	2(2)
L5968	2(2)
L5969	0(3)

CPT	MUE
L5970	2(2)
L5971	2(2)
L5972	2(2)
L5973	2(3)
L5974	2(2)
L5975	2(2)
L5976	2(2)
L5978	2(2)
L5979	2(2)
L5980	2(2)
L5981	2(2)
L5982	2(2)
L5984	2(2)
L5985	2(2)
L5986	2(2)
L5987	2(2)
L5988	2(2)
L5990	2(2)
L5999	2(3)
L6000	2(2)
L6010	2(2)
L6020	2(2)
L6026	2(2)
L6050	2(2)
L6055	2(2)
L6100	2(2)
L6110	2(2)
L6120	2(2)
L6130	2(2)
L6200	2(2)
L6205	2(2)
L6250	2(2)
L6300	2(2)
L6310	2(2)
L6320	2(2)
L6350	2(2)
L6360	2(2)
L6370	2(2)
L6380	2(2)
L6382	2(2)
L6384	2(2)
L6386	2(2)
L6388	2(2)
L6400	2(2)
L6450	2(2)
L6500	2(2)
L6550	2(2)
L6570	2(2)
L6580	2(2)
L6582	2(2)
L6584	2(2)
L6586	2(2)
L6588	2(2)
L6590	2(2)
L6600	2(2)
L6605	2(2)
L6610	2(2)
L6611	2(3)
L6615	2(2)
L6616	2(2)
L6620	2(2)
L6621	2(2)
L6623	2(2)
L6624	2(2)
L6625	2(2)

CPT	MUE
L6628	2(2)
L6629	2(2)
L6630	2(2)
L6632	4(3)
L6635	2(2)
L6637	2(2)
L6638	2(2)
L6640	2(2)
L6641	2(3)
L6642	2(3)
L6645	2(2)
L6646	2(2)
L6647	2(2)
L6648	2(2)
L6650	2(2)
L6655	4(3)
L6660	4(3)
L6665	4(3)
L6670	2(2)
L6672	2(2)
L6675	2(2)
L6676	2(2)
L6677	2(2)
L6680	4(3)
L6682	4(3)
L6684	4(3)
L6686	2(2)
L6687	2(2)
L6688	2(2)
L6689	2(2)
L6690	2(2)
L6691	2(3)
L6692	2(3)
L6693	2(2)
L6694	2(3)
L6695	2(3)
L6696	2(2)
L6697	2(2)
L6698	2(2)
L6703	2(2)
L6704	2(2)
L6706	2(2)
L6707	2(2)
L6708	2(2)
L6709	2(2)
L6711	2(2)
L6712	2(2)
L6713	2(2)
L6714	2(2)
L6715	5(3)
L6721	2(2)
L6722	2(2)
L6805	2(2)
L6810	2(3)
L6880	2(2)
L6881	2(2)
L6882	2(2)
L6883	2(2)
L6884	2(2)
L6885	2(2)
L6890	2(3)
L6895	2(3)
L6900	2(2)
L6905	2(2)
L6910	2(2)

CPT	MUE
L6915	2(2)
L6920	2(2)
L6925	2(2)
L6930	2(2)
L6935	2(2)
L6940	2(2)
L6945	2(2)
L6950	2(2)
L6955	2(2)
L6960	2(2)
L6965	2(2)
L6970	2(2)
L6975	2(2)
L7007	2(2)
L7008	2(2)
L7009	2(2)
L7040	2(2)
L7045	2(2)
L7170	2(2)
L7180	2(2)
L7181	2(2)
L7185	2(2)
L7186	2(2)
L7190	2(2)
L7191	2(2)
L7259	2(2)
L7360	1(3)
L7362	1(2)
L7364	1(3)
L7366	1(2)
L7367	2(3)
L7368	1(2)
L7400	2(2)
L7401	2(2)
L7402	2(2)
L7403	2(2)
L7404	2(2)
L7405	2(2)
L7499	2(3)
L7510	4(3)
L7600	0(3)
L7700	2(1)
L7900	0(3)
L7902	0(3)
L8000	6(3)
L8001	4(3)
L8002	4(3)
L8010	4(3)
L8015	4(3)
L8020	4(3)
L8030	2(3)
L8031	2(3)
L8032	2(2)
L8035	2(3)
L8039	2(3)
L8040	1(2)
L8041	1(2)
L8042	2(2)
L8043	1(2)
L8044	1(2)
L8045	2(2)
L8046	1(3)
L8047	1(2)
L8048	1(3)
L8049	6(3)

CPT	MUE
L8300	1(3)
L8310	1(3)
L8320	2(3)
L8330	2(3)
L8400	12(3)
L8410	12(3)
L8415	6(3)
L8417	12(3)
L8420	14(3)
L8430	12(3)
L8435	12(3)
L8440	4(3)
L8460	4(3)
L8465	4(3)
L8470	14(3)
L8480	12(3)
L8485	12(3)
L8499	1(3)
L8500	1(2)
L8501	2(3)
L8507	3(3)
L8509	1(3)
L8510	1(2)
L8511	1(3)
L8512	1(3)
L8513	1(3)
L8514	1(3)
L8515	1(3)
L8600	2(3)
L8603	4(3)
L8604	3(3)
L8605	4(3)
L8606	5(3)
L8607	20(3)
L8609	1(3)
L8610	2(3)
L8612	1(3)
L8613	2(3)
L8614	2(3)
L8615	2(3)
L8616	2(3)
L8617	2(3)
L8618	2(3)
L8619	2(3)
L8621	360(3)
L8622	2(3)
L8625	1(3)
L8627	2(2)
L8628	2(2)
L8629	2(2)
L8631	2(3)
L8641	4(3)
L8642	2(3)
L8658	3(3)
L8659	4(3)
L8670	3(3)
L8679	3(3)
L8680	0(3)
L8681	1(3)
L8682	2(3)
L8683	1(3)

CPT	MUE
L8684	1(3)
L8685	0(3)
L8686	0(3)
L8687	0(3)
L8688	0(3)
L8689	1(3)
L8690	2(2)
L8691	1(3)
L8692	0(3)
L8693	1(3)
L8694	1(3)
L8695	1(3)
L8696	1(3)
L8701	1(3)
L8702	1(3)
M0075	0(3)
M0076	0(3)
M0100	0(3)
M0300	0(3)
M0301	0(3)
P2028	1(2)
P2029	1(2)
P2031	0(3)
P2033	1(2)
P2038	1(2)
P3000	1(3)
P3001	1(3)
P7001	0(3)
P9010	4(3)
P9011	4(3)
P9012	12(3)
P9016	12(3)
P9017	24(3)
P9019	12(3)
P9020	5(3)
P9021	8(3)
P9022	12(3)
P9023	15(3)
P9031	12(3)
P9032	12(3)
P9033	12(3)
P9034	4(3)
P9035	4(3)
P9036	4(3)
P9037	4(3)
P9038	4(3)
P9039	2(3)
P9040	8(3)
P9041	100(3)
P9043	10(3)
P9044	20(3)
P9045	20(3)
P9046	40(3)
P9047	20(3)
P9048	2(3)
P9050	1(3)
P9051	4(3)
P9052	3(3)
P9053	3(3)
P9054	2(3)
P9055	2(3)

CPT	MUE
P9056	3(3)
P9057	4(3)
P9058	4(3)
P9059	15(3)
P9060	4(3)
P9070	15(3)
P9071	15(3)
P9073	4(3)
P9100	12(3)
P9603	100(3)
P9604	2(3)
P9612	1(3)
P9615	1(3)
Q0035	1(3)
Q0081	2(3)
Q0083	2(3)
Q0084	2(3)
Q0085	2(3)
Q0091	1(3)
Q0092	2(3)
Q0111	2(3)
Q0112	3(3)
Q0113	1(3)
Q0114	1(3)
Q0115	1(3)
Q0138	510(3)
Q0139	510(3)
Q0144	0(3)
Q0161	66(3)
Q0162	24(3)
Q0163	6(3)
Q0164	8(3)
Q0166	2(3)
Q0167	108(3)
Q0169	12(3)
Q0173	5(3)
Q0174	0(3)
Q0175	6(3)
Q0177	16(3)
Q0180	1(3)
Q0181	2(3)
Q0477	1(1)
Q0478	1(3)
Q0479	1(3)
Q0480	1(3)
Q0481	1(2)
Q0482	1(3)
Q0483	1(3)
Q0484	1(3)
Q0485	1(3)
Q0486	1(3)
Q0487	1(3)
Q0488	1(3)
Q0489	1(3)
Q0490	1(3)
Q0491	1(3)
Q0492	1(3)
Q0493	1(3)
Q0494	1(3)
Q0495	1(3)
Q0497	2(3)

CPT	MUE
Q0498	1(3)
Q0499	1(3)
Q0501	1(3)
Q0502	1(3)
Q0503	3(3)
Q0504	1(3)
Q0506	8(3)
Q0507	1(3)
Q0508	24(3)
Q0509	2(3)
Q0510	1(2)
Q0511	1(2)
Q0512	4(3)
Q0513	1(2)
Q0514	1(2)
Q0515	0(3)
Q1004	0(3)
Q1005	0(3)
Q2004	1(3)
Q2009	100(3)
Q2017	12(3)
Q2026	0(3)
Q2028	0(3)
Q2034	1(2)
Q2035	1(2)
Q2036	1(2)
Q2037	1(2)
Q2038	1(2)
Q2039	1(2)
Q2043	1(2)
Q2049	0(3)
Q2050	20(3)
Q2052	0(3)
Q3014	2(3)
Q3027	30(3)
Q3028	0(3)
Q3031	1(3)
Q4001	1(3)
Q4002	1(3)
Q4003	2(3)
Q4004	2(3)
Q4012	2(3)
Q4013	2(3)
Q4014	2(3)
Q4018	2(3)
Q4021	2(3)
Q4025	1(3)
Q4026	1(3)
Q4027	1(3)
Q4028	1(3)
Q4030	2(3)
Q4037	2(3)
Q4042	2(3)
Q4046	2(3)
Q4050	2(3)
Q4051	2(3)
Q4074	0(3)
Q4081	400(3)
Q4103	0(3)
Q5101	1500(3)
Q5103	150(3)

CPT	MUE
Q5104	150(3)
Q5105	400(3)
Q5106	60(3)
Q5107	170(3)
Q5108	12(3)
Q5109	150(3)
Q5110	1500(3)
Q5111	12(3)
Q5112	120(3)
Q5113	120(3)
Q5114	120(3)
Q5115	120(3)
Q9950	5(3)
Q9951	0(3)
Q9953	10(3)
Q9954	18(3)
Q9955	0(3)
Q9956	9(3)
Q9957	3(3)
Q9958	600(3)
Q9959	0(3)
Q9960	250(3)
Q9961	200(3)
Q9962	200(3)
Q9963	240(3)
Q9964	0(3)
Q9966	250(3)
Q9967	300(3)
Q9969	3(3)
Q9982	1(3)
Q9983	1(3)
Q9991	1(3)
Q9992	1(3)
R0070	2(3)
R0075	2(3)
R0076	1(3)
V2020	1(3)
V2025	0(3)
V2100	2(3)
V2101	2(3)
V2102	2(3)
V2103	2(3)
V2104	2(3)
V2105	2(3)
V2106	2(3)
V2107	2(3)
V2108	2(3)
V2109	2(3)
V2110	2(3)
V2111	2(3)
V2112	2(3)
V2113	2(3)
V2114	2(3)
V2115	2(3)
V2118	2(3)
V2121	2(3)
V2199	2(3)
V2200	2(3)
V2201	2(3)
V2202	2(3)
V2203	2(3)

CPT	MUE
V2204	2(3)
V2205	2(3)
V2206	2(3)
V2207	2(3)
V2208	2(3)
V2209	2(3)
V2210	2(3)
V2211	2(3)
V2212	2(3)
V2213	2(3)
V2214	2(3)
V2215	2(3)
V2218	2(3)
V2219	2(3)
V2220	2(3)
V2221	2(3)
V2299	2(3)
V2300	2(3)
V2301	2(3)
V2302	2(3)
V2303	2(3)
V2304	2(3)
V2305	2(3)
V2306	2(3)
V2307	2(3)
V2308	2(3)
V2309	2(3)
V2310	2(3)
V2311	2(3)
V2312	2(3)
V2313	2(3)
V2314	2(3)
V2315	2(3)
V2318	2(3)
V2319	2(3)
V2320	2(3)
V2321	2(3)
V2399	2(3)
V2410	2(3)
V2430	2(3)
V2499	2(3)
V2500	2(3)
V2501	2(3)
V2502	2(3)
V2503	2(3)
V2510	2(3)
V2511	2(3)
V2512	2(3)
V2513	2(3)
V2520	2(3)
V2521	2(3)
V2522	2(3)
V2523	2(3)
V2530	2(3)
V2531	2(3)
V2599	2(3)
V2600	0(2)
V2610	0(2)
V2615	0(2)
V2623	2(2)
V2624	2(2)

CPT	MUE
V2625	2(2)
V2626	2(2)
V2627	2(2)
V2628	2(3)
V2629	2(2)
V2630	2(2)
V2631	2(2)
V2632	2(2)
V2700	2(3)
V2702	0(3)
V2710	2(3)
V2715	4(3)
V2718	2(3)
V2730	2(3)
V2744	2(3)
V2745	2(3)
V2750	2(3)
V2755	2(3)
V2756	0(3)
V2760	0(3)
V2761	0(2)
V2762	0(3)
V2770	2(3)
V2780	2(3)
V2781	0(2)
V2782	2(3)
V2783	2(3)
V2784	2(3)
V2785	2(2)
V2786	0(3)
V2787	0(3)
V2788	0(3)
V2790	1(3)
V2797	0(3)
V5008	0(3)
V5010	0(3)
V5011	0(3)
V5014	0(3)
V5020	0(3)
V5030	0(3)
V5040	0(3)
V5050	0(3)
V5060	0(3)
V5070	0(3)
V5080	0(3)
V5090	0(3)
V5095	0(3)
V5100	0(3)
V5110	0(3)
V5120	0(3)
V5130	0(3)
V5140	0(3)
V5150	0(3)
V5160	0(3)
V5171	0(3)
V5172	0(3)
V5181	0(3)
V5190	0(3)
V5200	0(3)
V5211	0(3)
V5212	0(3)

CPT	MUE
V5213	0(3)
V5214	0(3)
V5215	0(3)
V5221	0(3)
V5230	0(3)
V5240	0(3)
V5241	0(3)
V5242	0(3)
V5243	0(3)
V5244	0(3)
V5245	0(3)
V5246	0(3)
V5247	0(3)
V5248	0(3)
V5249	0(3)
V5250	0(3)
V5251	0(3)
V5252	0(3)
V5253	0(3)
V5254	0(3)
V5255	0(3)
V5256	0(3)
V5257	0(3)
V5258	0(3)
V5259	0(3)
V5260	0(3)
V5261	0(3)
V5262	0(3)
V5263	0(3)
V5264	0(3)
V5265	0(3)
V5266	0(3)
V5267	0(3)
V5268	0(3)
V5269	0(3)
V5270	0(3)
V5271	0(3)
V5272	0(3)
V5273	0(3)
V5274	0(3)
V5275	0(3)
V5281	0(3)
V5282	0(3)
V5283	0(3)
V5284	0(3)
V5285	0(3)
V5286	0(3)
V5287	0(3)
V5288	0(3)
V5289	0(3)
V5290	0(3)
V5298	0(3)
V5299	1(3)
V5336	0(3)
V5362	0(3)
V5363	0(3)
V5364	0(3)

Appendix J — Inpatient-Only Procedures

Inpatient Only Procedures—This appendix identifies services with the status indicator C. Medicare will not pay an OPPS hospital or ASC when they are performed on a Medicare patient as an outpatient. Physicians should refer to this list when scheduling Medicare patients for surgical procedures. CMS updates this list quarterly. The following was updated 10/01/2019.

00176 Anesth pharyngeal surgery
00192 Anesth facial bone surgery
00211 Anesth cran surg hematoma
00214 Anesth skull drainage
00215 Anesth skull repair/fract
00474 Anesth surgery of rib
00524 Anesth chest drainage
00540 Anesth chest surgery
00542 Anesthesia removal pleura
00546 Anesth lung chest wall surg
00560 Anesth heart surg w/o pump
00561 Anesth heart surg <1 yr
00562 Anesth hrt surg w/pmp age 1+
00567 Anesth CABG w/pump
00580 Anesth heart/lung transplnt
00604 Anesth sitting procedure
00632 Anesth removal of nerves
0075T Perq stent/chest vert art
0076T S&i stent/chest vert art
00792 Anesth hemorr/excise liver
00794 Anesth pancreas removal
00796 Anesth for liver transplant
00802 Anesth fat layer removal
00844 Anesth pelvis surgery
00846 Anesth hysterectomy
00848 Anesth pelvic organ surg
00864 Anesth removal of bladder
00865 Anesth removal of prostate
00866 Anesth removal of adrenal
00868 Anesth kidney transplant
00882 Anesth major vein ligation
00904 Anesth perineal surgery
00908 Anesth removal of prostate
00932 Anesth amputation of penis
00934 Anesth penis nodes removal
00936 Anesth penis nodes removal
00944 Anesth vaginal hysterectomy
0095T Rmvl artific disc addl crvcl
0098T Rev artific disc addl
01140 Anesth amputation at pelvis
01150 Anesth pelvic tumor surgery
01212 Anesth hip disarticulation
01214 Anesth hip arthroplasty
01232 Anesth amputation of femur
01234 Anesth radical femur surg
01272 Anesth femoral artery surg
01274 Anesth femoral embolectomy
01404 Anesth amputation at knee
01442 Anesth knee artery surg
01444 Anesth knee artery repair
01486 Anesth ankle replacement
01502 Anesth lwr leg embolectomy
01634 Anesth shoulder joint amput
01636 Anesth forequarter amput
01638 Anesth shoulder replacement
0163T Lumb artif diskectomy addl
0164T Remove lumb artif disc addl
01652 Anesth shoulder vessel surg
01654 Anesth shoulder vessel surg
01656 Anesth arm-leg vessel surg
0165T Revise lumb artif disc addl
01756 Anesth radical humerus surg
01990 Support for organ donor
0202T Post vert arthrplst 1 lumbar
0219T Plmt post facet implt cerv
0220T Plmt post facet implt thor
0235T Trluml perip athrc visceral
0254T Evasc rpr iliac art bifur
0345T Transcath mtral vlve repair
0375T Total disc arthrp ant appr
0451T Insj/rplcmt aortic ventr sys
0452T Insj/rplcmt dev vasc seal
0455T Remvl aortic ventr cmpl sys
0456T Remvl aortic dev vasc seal
0459T Relocaj rplcmt aortic ventr
0461T Repos aortic contrpulsj dev
0483T Tmvi percutaneous approach
0484T Tmvi transthoracic exposure
0494T Prep & cannulj cdvr don lung
0495T Mntr cdvr don lng 1st 2 hrs
0496T Mntr cdvr don lng ea addl hr
0543T Ta mv rpr w/artif chord tend
0544T Tcat mv annulus rcnstj
0545T Tcat tv annulus rcnstj
11004 Debride genitalia & perineum
11005 Debride abdom wall
11006 Debride genit/per/abdom wall
11008 Remove mesh from abd wall
15756 Free myo/skin flap microvasc
15757 Free skin flap microvasc
15758 Free fascial flap microvasc
16036 Escharotomy addl incision
19271 Revision of chest wall
19272 Extensive chest wall surgery
19305 Mast radical
19306 Mast rad urban type
19361 Breast reconstr w/lat flap
19364 Breast reconstruction
19367 Breast reconstruction
19368 Breast reconstruction
19369 Breast reconstruction
20661 Application of head brace
20664 Application of halo
20802 Replantation arm complete
20805 Replant forearm complete
20808 Replantation hand complete
20816 Replantation digit complete
20824 Replantation thumb complete
20827 Replantation thumb complete
20838 Replantation foot complete
20955 Fibula bone graft microvasc
20956 Iliac bone graft microvasc
20957 Mt bone graft microvasc
20962 Other bone graft microvasc
20969 Bone/skin graft microvasc
20970 Bone/skin graft iliac crest
21045 Extensive jaw surgery
21141 Lefort i-1 piece w/o graft
21142 Lefort i-2 piece w/o graft
21143 Lefort i-3/> piece w/o graft
21145 Lefort i-1 piece w/ graft
21146 Lefort i-2 piece w/ graft
21147 Lefort i-3/> piece w/ graft
21151 Lefort ii w/bone grafts
21154 Lefort iii w/o lefort i
21155 Lefort iii w/ lefort i
21159 Lefort iii w/fhdw/o lefort i
21160 Lefort iii w/fhd w/ lefort i
21179 Reconstruct entire forehead
21180 Reconstruct entire forehead
21182 Reconstruct cranial bone
21183 Reconstruct cranial bone
21184 Reconstruct cranial bone
21188 Reconstruction of midface
21194 Reconst lwr jaw w/graft
21196 Reconst lwr jaw w/fixation
21247 Reconstruct lower jaw bone
21255 Reconstruct lower jaw bone
21268 Revise eye sockets
21343 Open tx dprsd front sinus fx
21344 Open tx compl front sinus fx
21347 Opn tx nasomax fx multple
21348 Opn tx nasomax fx w/graft
21366 Opn tx complx malar w/grft
21422 Treat mouth roof fracture
21423 Treat mouth roof fracture
21431 Treat craniofacial fracture
21432 Treat craniofacial fracture
21433 Treat craniofacial fracture
21435 Treat craniofacial fracture
21436 Treat craniofacial fracture
21510 Drainage of bone lesion
21615 Removal of rib
21616 Removal of rib and nerves
21620 Partial removal of sternum
21627 Sternal debridement
21630 Extensive sternum surgery
21632 Extensive sternum surgery
21705 Revision of neck muscle/rib

21740 Reconstruction of sternum
21750 Repair of sternum separation
21825 Treat sternum fracture
22010 I&d p-spine c/t/cerv-thor
22015 I&d abscess p-spine l/s/ls
22110 Remove part of neck vertebra
22112 Remove part thorax vertebra
22114 Remove part lumbar vertebra
22116 Remove extra spine segment
22206 Incis spine 3 column thorac
22207 Incis spine 3 column lumbar
22208 Incis spine 3 column adl seg
22210 Incis 1 vertebral seg cerv
22212 Incis 1 vertebral seg thorac
22214 Incis 1 vertebral seg lumbar
22216 Incis addl spine segment
22220 Incis w/discectomy cervical
22222 Incis w/discectomy thoracic
22224 Incis w/discectomy lumbar
22226 Revise extra spine segment
22318 Treat odontoid fx w/o graft
22319 Treat odontoid fx w/graft
22325 Treat spine fracture
22326 Treat neck spine fracture
22327 Treat thorax spine fracture
22328 Treat each add spine fx
22532 Lat thorax spine fusion
22533 Lat lumbar spine fusion
22534 Lat thor/lumb addl seg
22548 Neck spine fusion
22556 Thorax spine fusion
22558 Lumbar spine fusion
22586 Prescrl fuse w/ instr l5-s1
22590 Spine & skull spinal fusion
22595 Neck spinal fusion
22600 Neck spine fusion
22610 Thorax spine fusion
22630 Lumbar spine fusion
22632 Spine fusion extra segment
22633 Lumbar spine fusion combined
22634 Spine fusion extra segment
22800 Post fusion </6 vert seg
22802 Post fusion 7-12 vert seg
22804 Post fusion 13/> vert seg
22808 Ant fusion 2-3 vert seg
22810 Ant fusion 4-7 vert seg
22812 Ant fusion 8/> vert seg
22818 Kyphectomy 1-2 segments
22819 Kyphectomy 3 or more
22830 Exploration of spinal fusion
22841 Insert spine fixation device
22843 Insert spine fixation device
22844 Insert spine fixation device
22846 Insert spine fixation device
22847 Insert spine fixation device
22848 Insert pelv fixation device
22849 Reinsert spinal fixation
22850 Remove spine fixation device
22852 Remove spine fixation device
22855 Remove spine fixation device
22857 Lumbar artif diskectomy
22861 Revise cerv artific disc
22862 Revise lumbar artif disc
22864 Remove cerv artif disc
22865 Remove lumb artif disc
23200 Resect clavicle tumor
23210 Resect scapula tumor
23220 Resect prox humerus tumor
23335 Shoulder prosthesis removal
23472 Reconstruct shoulder joint
23474 Revis reconst shoulder joint
23900 Amputation of arm & girdle
23920 Amputation at shoulder joint
24900 Amputation of upper arm
24920 Amputation of upper arm
24930 Amputation follow-up surgery
24931 Amputate upper arm & implant
24940 Revision of upper arm
25900 Amputation of forearm
25905 Amputation of forearm
25915 Amputation of forearm
25920 Amputate hand at wrist
25924 Amputation follow-up surgery
25927 Amputation of hand
26551 Great toe-hand transfer
26553 Single transfer toe-hand
26554 Double transfer toe-hand
26556 Toe joint transfer
26992 Drainage of bone lesion
27005 Incision of hip tendon
27025 Incision of hip/thigh fascia
27030 Drainage of hip joint
27036 Excision of hip joint/muscle
27054 Removal of hip joint lining
27070 Part remove hip bone super
27071 Part removal hip bone deep
27075 Resect hip tumor
27076 Resect hip tum incl acetabul
27077 Resect hip tum w/innom bone
27078 Rsect hip tum incl femur
27090 Removal of hip prosthesis
27091 Removal of hip prosthesis
27120 Reconstruction of hip socket
27122 Reconstruction of hip socket
27125 Partial hip replacement
27130 Total hip arthroplasty
27132 Total hip arthroplasty
27134 Revise hip joint replacement
27137 Revise hip joint replacement
27138 Revise hip joint replacement
27140 Transplant femur ridge
27146 Incision of hip bone
27147 Revision of hip bone
27151 Incision of hip bones
27156 Revision of hip bones
27158 Revision of pelvis
27161 Incision of neck of femur
27165 Incision/fixation of femur
27170 Repair/graft femur head/neck
27175 Treat slipped epiphysis
27176 Treat slipped epiphysis
27177 Treat slipped epiphysis
27178 Treat slipped epiphysis
27181 Treat slipped epiphysis
27185 Revision of femur epiphysis
27187 Reinforce hip bones
27222 Treat hip socket fracture
27226 Treat hip wall fracture
27227 Treat hip fracture(s)
27228 Treat hip fracture(s)
27232 Treat thigh fracture
27236 Treat thigh fracture
27240 Treat thigh fracture
27244 Treat thigh fracture
27245 Treat thigh fracture
27248 Treat thigh fracture
27253 Treat hip dislocation
27254 Treat hip dislocation
27258 Treat hip dislocation
27259 Treat hip dislocation
27268 Cltx thigh fx w/mnpj
27269 Optx thigh fx
27280 Fusion of sacroiliac joint
27282 Fusion of pubic bones
27284 Fusion of hip joint
27286 Fusion of hip joint
27290 Amputation of leg at hip
27295 Amputation of leg at hip
27303 Drainage of bone lesion
27365 Resect femur/knee tumor
27445 Revision of knee joint
27448 Incision of thigh
27450 Incision of thigh
27454 Realignment of thigh bone
27455 Realignment of knee
27457 Realignment of knee
27465 Shortening of thigh bone
27466 Lengthening of thigh bone
27468 Shorten/lengthen thighs
27470 Repair of thigh
27472 Repair/graft of thigh
27486 Revise/replace knee joint
27487 Revise/replace knee joint
27488 Removal of knee prosthesis
27495 Reinforce thigh
27506 Treatment of thigh fracture
27507 Treatment of thigh fracture
27511 Treatment of thigh fracture
27513 Treatment of thigh fracture
27514 Treatment of thigh fracture
27519 Treat thigh fx growth plate
27535 Treat knee fracture
27536 Treat knee fracture
27540 Treat knee fracture
27556 Treat knee dislocation
27557 Treat knee dislocation
27558 Treat knee dislocation

27580 Fusion of knee
27590 Amputate leg at thigh
27591 Amputate leg at thigh
27592 Amputate leg at thigh
27596 Amputation follow-up surgery
27598 Amputate lower leg at knee
27645 Resect tibia tumor
27646 Resect fibula tumor
27702 Reconstruct ankle joint
27703 Reconstruction ankle joint
27712 Realignment of lower leg
27715 Revision of lower leg
27724 Repair/graft of tibia
27725 Repair of lower leg
27727 Repair of lower leg
27880 Amputation of lower leg
27881 Amputation of lower leg
27882 Amputation of lower leg
27886 Amputation follow-up surgery
27888 Amputation of foot at ankle
28800 Amputation of midfoot
31225 Removal of upper jaw
31230 Removal of upper jaw
31290 Nasal/sinus endoscopy surg
31291 Nasal/sinus endoscopy surg
31360 Removal of larynx
31365 Removal of larynx
31367 Partial removal of larynx
31368 Partial removal of larynx
31370 Partial removal of larynx
31375 Partial removal of larynx
31380 Partial removal of larynx
31382 Partial removal of larynx
31390 Removal of larynx & pharynx
31395 Reconstruct larynx & pharynx
31725 Clearance of airways
31760 Repair of windpipe
31766 Reconstruction of windpipe
31770 Repair/graft of bronchus
31775 Reconstruct bronchus
31780 Reconstruct windpipe
31781 Reconstruct windpipe
31786 Remove windpipe lesion
31800 Repair of windpipe injury
31805 Repair of windpipe injury
32035 Thoracostomy w/rib resection
32036 Thoracostomy w/flap drainage
32096 Open wedge/bx lung infiltr
32097 Open wedge/bx lung nodule
32098 Open biopsy of lung pleura
32100 Exploration of chest
32110 Explore/repair chest
32120 Re-exploration of chest
32124 Explore chest free adhesions
32140 Removal of lung lesion(s)
32141 Remove/treat lung lesions
32150 Removal of lung lesion(s)
32151 Remove lung foreign body
32160 Open chest heart massage
32200 Drain open lung lesion
32215 Treat chest lining
32220 Release of lung
32225 Partial release of lung
32310 Removal of chest lining
32320 Free/remove chest lining
32440 Remove lung pneumonectomy
32442 Sleeve pneumonectomy
32445 Removal of lung extrapleural
32480 Partial removal of lung
32482 Bilobectomy
32484 Segmentectomy
32486 Sleeve lobectomy
32488 Completion pneumonectomy
32491 Lung volume reduction
32501 Repair bronchus add-on
32503 Resect apical lung tumor
32504 Resect apical lung tum/chest
32505 Wedge resect of lung initial
32506 Wedge resect of lung add-on
32507 Wedge resect of lung diag
32540 Removal of lung lesion
32650 Thoracoscopy w/pleurodesis
32651 Thoracoscopy remove cortex
32652 Thoracoscopy rem totl cortex
32653 Thoracoscopy remov fb/fibrin
32654 Thoracoscopy contrl bleeding
32655 Thoracoscopy resect bullae
32656 Thoracoscopy w/pleurectomy
32658 Thoracoscopy w/sac fb remove
32659 Thoracoscopy w/sac drainage
32661 Thoracoscopy w/pericard exc
32662 Thoracoscopy w/mediast exc
32663 Thoracoscopy w/lobectomy
32664 Thoracoscopy w/ th nrv exc
32665 Thoracoscop w/esoph musc exc
32666 Thoracoscopy w/wedge resect
32667 Thoracoscopy w/w resect addl
32668 Thoracoscopy w/w resect diag
32669 Thoracoscopy remove segment
32670 Thoracoscopy bilobectomy
32671 Thoracoscopy pneumonectomy
32672 Thoracoscopy for lvrs
32673 Thoracoscopy w/thymus resect
32674 Thoracoscopy lymph node exc
32800 Repair lung hernia
32810 Close chest after drainage
32815 Close bronchial fistula
32820 Reconstruct injured chest
32850 Donor pneumonectomy
32851 Lung transplant single
32852 Lung transplant with bypass
32853 Lung transplant double
32854 Lung transplant with bypass
32855 Prepare donor lung single
32856 Prepare donor lung double
32900 Removal of rib(s)
32905 Revise & repair chest wall
32906 Revise & repair chest wall
32940 Revision of lung
32997 Total lung lavage
33015 Incision of heart sac
33020 Incision of heart sac
33025 Incision of heart sac
33030 Partial removal of heart sac
33031 Partial removal of heart sac
33050 Resect heart sac lesion
33120 Removal of heart lesion
33130 Removal of heart lesion
33140 Heart revascularize (tmr)
33141 Heart tmr w/other procedure
33202 Insert epicard eltrd open
33203 Insert epicard eltrd endo
33236 Remove electrode/thoracotomy
33237 Remove electrode/thoracotomy
33238 Remove electrode/thoracotomy
33243 Remove eltrd/thoracotomy
33250 Ablate heart dysrhythm focus
33251 Ablate heart dysrhythm focus
33254 Ablate atria lmtd
33255 Ablate atria w/o bypass ext
33256 Ablate atria w/bypass exten
33257 Ablate atria lmtd add-on
33258 Ablate atria x10sv add-on
33259 Ablate atria w/bypass add-on
33261 Ablate heart dysrhythm focus
33265 Ablate atria lmtd endo
33266 Ablate atria x10sv endo
33300 Repair of heart wound
33305 Repair of heart wound
33310 Exploratory heart surgery
33315 Exploratory heart surgery
33320 Repair major blood vessel(s)
33321 Repair major vessel
33322 Repair major blood vessel(s)
33330 Insert major vessel graft
33335 Insert major vessel graft
33340 Perq clsr tcat l atr apndge
33361 Replace aortic valve perq
33362 Replace aortic valve open
33363 Replace aortic valve open
33364 Replace aortic valve open
33365 Replace aortic valve open
33366 Trcath replace aortic valve
33367 Replace aortic valve w/byp
33368 Replace aortic valve w/byp
33369 Replace aortic valve w/byp
33390 Valvuloplasty aortic valve
33391 Valvuloplasty aortic valve
33404 Prepare heart-aorta conduit
33405 Replacement of aortic valve
33406 Replacement of aortic valve
33410 Replacement of aortic valve
33411 Replacement of aortic valve
33412 Replacement of aortic valve
33413 Replacement of aortic valve
33414 Repair of aortic valve
33415 Revision subvalvular tissue

33416 Revise ventricle muscle
33417 Repair of aortic valve
33418 Repair tcat mitral valve
33420 Revision of mitral valve
33422 Revision of mitral valve
33425 Repair of mitral valve
33426 Repair of mitral valve
33427 Repair of mitral valve
33430 Replacement of mitral valve
33440 Rplcmt a-valve tlcj autol pv
33460 Revision of tricuspid valve
33463 Valvuloplasty tricuspid
33464 Valvuloplasty tricuspid
33465 Replace tricuspid valve
33468 Revision of tricuspid valve
33470 Revision of pulmonary valve
33471 Valvotomy pulmonary valve
33474 Revision of pulmonary valve
33475 Replacement pulmonary valve
33476 Revision of heart chamber
33477 Implant tcat pulm vlv perq
33478 Revision of heart chamber
33496 Repair prosth valve clot
33500 Repair heart vessel fistula
33501 Repair heart vessel fistula
33502 Coronary artery correction
33503 Coronary artery graft
33504 Coronary artery graft
33505 Repair artery w/tunnel
33506 Repair artery translocation
33507 Repair art intramural
33510 Cabg vein single
33511 Cabg vein two
33512 Cabg vein three
33513 Cabg vein four
33514 Cabg vein five
33516 Cabg vein six or more
33517 Cabg artery-vein single
33518 Cabg artery-vein two
33519 Cabg artery-vein three
33521 Cabg artery-vein four
33522 Cabg artery-vein five
33523 Cabg art-vein six or more
33530 Coronary artery bypass/reop
33533 Cabg arterial single
33534 Cabg arterial two
33535 Cabg arterial three
33536 Cabg arterial four or more
33542 Removal of heart lesion
33545 Repair of heart damage
33548 Restore/remodel ventricle
33572 Open coronary endarterectomy
33600 Closure of valve
33602 Closure of valve
33606 Anastomosis/artery-aorta
33608 Repair anomaly w/conduit
33610 Repair by enlargement
33611 Repair double ventricle
33612 Repair double ventricle
33615 Repair modified fontan
33617 Repair single ventricle
33619 Repair single ventricle
33620 Apply r&l pulm art bands
33621 Transthor cath for stent
33622 Redo compl cardiac anomaly
33641 Repair heart septum defect
33645 Revision of heart veins
33647 Repair heart septum defects
33660 Repair of heart defects
33665 Repair of heart defects
33670 Repair of heart chambers
33675 Close mult vsd
33676 Close mult vsd w/resection
33677 Cl mult vsd w/rem pul band
33681 Repair heart septum defect
33684 Repair heart septum defect
33688 Repair heart septum defect
33690 Reinforce pulmonary artery
33692 Repair of heart defects
33694 Repair of heart defects
33697 Repair of heart defects
33702 Repair of heart defects
33710 Repair of heart defects
33720 Repair of heart defect
33722 Repair of heart defect
33724 Repair venous anomaly
33726 Repair pul venous stenosis
33730 Repair heart-vein defect(s)
33732 Repair heart-vein defect
33735 Revision of heart chamber
33736 Revision of heart chamber
33737 Revision of heart chamber
33750 Major vessel shunt
33755 Major vessel shunt
33762 Major vessel shunt
33764 Major vessel shunt & graft
33766 Major vessel shunt
33767 Major vessel shunt
33768 Cavopulmonary shunting
33770 Repair great vessels defect
33771 Repair great vessels defect
33774 Repair great vessels defect
33775 Repair great vessels defect
33776 Repair great vessels defect
33777 Repair great vessels defect
33778 Repair great vessels defect
33779 Repair great vessels defect
33780 Repair great vessels defect
33781 Repair great vessels defect
33782 Nikaidoh proc
33783 Nikaidoh proc w/ostia implt
33786 Repair arterial trunk
33788 Revision of pulmonary artery
33800 Aortic suspension
33802 Repair vessel defect
33803 Repair vessel defect
33813 Repair septal defect
33814 Repair septal defect
33820 Revise major vessel
33822 Revise major vessel
33824 Revise major vessel
33840 Remove aorta constriction
33845 Remove aorta constriction
33851 Remove aorta constriction
33852 Repair septal defect
33853 Repair septal defect
33860 Ascending aortic graft
33863 Ascending aortic graft
33864 Ascending aortic graft
33870 Transverse aortic arch graft
33875 Thoracic aortic graft
33877 Thoracoabdominal graft
33880 Endovasc taa repr incl subcl
33881 Endovasc taa repr w/o subcl
33883 Insert endovasc prosth taa
33884 Endovasc prosth taa add-on
33886 Endovasc prosth delayed
33889 Artery transpose/endovas taa
33891 Car-car bp grft/endovas taa
33910 Remove lung artery emboli
33915 Remove lung artery emboli
33916 Surgery of great vessel
33917 Repair pulmonary artery
33920 Repair pulmonary atresia
33922 Transect pulmonary artery
33924 Remove pulmonary shunt
33925 Rpr pul art unifocal w/o cpb
33926 Repr pul art unifocal w/cpb
33927 Impltj tot rplcmt hrt sys
33928 Rmvl & rplcmt tot hrt sys
33929 Rmvl rplcmt hrt sys f/trnspl
33930 Removal of donor heart/lung
33933 Prepare donor heart/lung
33935 Transplantation heart/lung
33940 Removal of donor heart
33944 Prepare donor heart
33945 Transplantation of heart
33946 Ecmo/ecls initiation venous
33947 Ecmo/ecls initiation artery
33948 Ecmo/ecls daily mgmt-venous
33949 Ecmo/ecls daily mgmt artery
33951 Ecmo/ecls insj prph cannula
33952 Ecmo/ecls insj prph cannula
33953 Ecmo/ecls insj prph cannula
33954 Ecmo/ecls insj prph cannula
33955 Ecmo/ecls insj ctr cannula
33956 Ecmo/ecls insj ctr cannula
33957 Ecmo/ecls repos perph cnula
33958 Ecmo/ecls repos perph cnula
33959 Ecmo/ecls repos perph cnula
33962 Ecmo/ecls repos perph cnula
33963 Ecmo/ecls repos perph cnula
33964 Ecmo/ecls repos perph cnula
33965 Ecmo/ecls rmvl perph cannula
33966 Ecmo/ecls rmvl prph cannula
33967 Insert i-aort percut device
33968 Remove aortic assist device

33969 Ecmo/ecls rmvl perph cannula
33970 Aortic circulation assist
33971 Aortic circulation assist
33973 Insert balloon device
33974 Remove intra-aortic balloon
33975 Implant ventricular device
33976 Implant ventricular device
33977 Remove ventricular device
33978 Remove ventricular device
33979 Insert intracorporeal device
33980 Remove intracorporeal device
33981 Replace vad pump ext
33982 Replace vad intra w/o bp
33983 Replace vad intra w/bp
33984 Ecmo/ecls rmvl prph cannula
33985 Ecmo/ecls rmvl ctr cannula
33986 Ecmo/ecls rmvl ctr cannula
33987 Artery expos/graft artery
33988 Insertion of left heart vent
33989 Removal of left heart vent
33990 Insert vad artery access
33991 Insert vad art&vein access
33992 Remove vad different session
33993 Reposition vad diff session
34001 Removal of artery clot
34051 Removal of artery clot
34151 Removal of artery clot
34401 Removal of vein clot
34451 Removal of vein clot
34502 Reconstruct vena cava
34701 Evasc rpr a-ao ndgft
34702 Evasc rpr a-ao ndgft rpt
34703 Evasc rpr a-unilac ndgft
34704 Evasc rpr a-unilac ndgft rpt
34705 Evac rpr a-biiliac ndgft
34706 Evasc rpr a-biiliac rpt
34707 Evasc rpr ilio-iliac ndgft
34708 Evasc rpr ilio-iliac rpt
34709 Plmt xtn prosth evasc rpr
34710 Dlyd plmt xtn prosth 1st vsl
34711 Dlyd plmt xtn prosth ea addl
34712 Tcat dlvr enhncd fixj dev
34808 Endovas iliac a device addon
34812 Xpose for endoprosth femorl
34813 Femoral endovas graft add-on
34820 Xpose for endoprosth iliac
34830 Open aortic tube prosth repr
34831 Open aortoiliac prosth repr
34832 Open aortofemor prosth repr
34833 Xpose for endoprosth iliac
34834 Xpose endoprosth brachial
34841 Endovasc visc aorta 1 graft
34842 Endovasc visc aorta 2 graft
34843 Endovasc visc aorta 3 graft
34844 Endovasc visc aorta 4 graft
34845 Visc & infraren abd 1 prosth
34846 Visc & infraren abd 2 prosth
34847 Visc & infraren abd 3 prosth
34848 Visc & infraren abd 4+ prost
35001 Repair defect of artery
35002 Repair artery rupture neck
35005 Repair defect of artery
35013 Repair artery rupture arm
35021 Repair defect of artery
35022 Repair artery rupture chest
35081 Repair defect of artery
35082 Repair artery rupture aorta
35091 Repair defect of artery
35092 Repair artery rupture aorta
35102 Repair defect of artery
35103 Repair artery rupture aorta
35111 Repair defect of artery
35112 Repair artery rupture spleen
35121 Repair defect of artery
35122 Repair artery rupture belly
35131 Repair defect of artery
35132 Repair artery rupture groin
35141 Repair defect of artery
35142 Repair artery rupture thigh
35151 Repair defect of artery
35152 Repair ruptd popliteal art
35182 Repair blood vessel lesion
35189 Repair blood vessel lesion
35211 Repair blood vessel lesion
35216 Repair blood vessel lesion
35221 Repair blood vessel lesion
35241 Repair blood vessel lesion
35246 Repair blood vessel lesion
35251 Repair blood vessel lesion
35271 Repair blood vessel lesion
35276 Repair blood vessel lesion
35281 Repair blood vessel lesion
35301 Rechanneling of artery
35302 Rechanneling of artery
35303 Rechanneling of artery
35304 Rechanneling of artery
35305 Rechanneling of artery
35306 Rechanneling of artery
35311 Rechanneling of artery
35331 Rechanneling of artery
35341 Rechanneling of artery
35351 Rechanneling of artery
35355 Rechanneling of artery
35361 Rechanneling of artery
35363 Rechanneling of artery
35371 Rechanneling of artery
35372 Rechanneling of artery
35390 Reoperation carotid add-on
35400 Angioscopy
35501 Art byp grft ipsilat carotid
35506 Art byp grft subclav-carotid
35508 Art byp grft carotid-vertbrl
35509 Art byp grft contral carotid
35510 Art byp grft carotid-brchial
35511 Art byp grft subclav-subclav
35512 Art byp grft subclav-brchial
35515 Art byp grft subclav-vertbrl
35516 Art byp grft subclav-axilary
35518 Art byp grft axillary-axilry
35521 Art byp grft axill-femoral
35522 Art byp grft axill-brachial
35523 Art byp grft brchl-ulnr-rdl
35525 Art byp grft brachial-brchl
35526 Art byp grft aor/carot/innom
35531 Art byp grft aorcel/aormesen
35533 Art byp grft axill/fem/fem
35535 Art byp grft hepatorenal
35536 Art byp grft splenorenal
35537 Art byp grft aortoiliac
35538 Art byp grft aortobi-iliac
35539 Art byp grft aortofemoral
35540 Art byp grft aortbifemoral
35556 Art byp grft fem-popliteal
35558 Art byp grft fem-femoral
35560 Art byp grft aortorenal
35563 Art byp grft ilioiliac
35565 Art byp grft iliofemoral
35566 Art byp fem-ant-post tib/prl
35570 Art byp tibial-tib/peroneal
35571 Art byp pop-tibl-prl-other
35583 Vein byp grft fem-popliteal
35585 Vein byp fem-tibial peroneal
35587 Vein byp pop-tibl peroneal
35600 Harvest art for cabg add-on
35601 Art byp common ipsi carotid
35606 Art byp carotid-subclavian
35612 Art byp subclav-subclavian
35616 Art byp subclav-axillary
35621 Art byp axillary-femoral
35623 Art byp axillary-pop-tibial
35626 Art byp aorsubcl/carot/innom
35631 Art byp aor-celiac-msn-renal
35632 Art byp ilio-celiac
35633 Art byp ilio-mesenteric
35634 Art byp iliorenal
35636 Art byp spenorenal
35637 Art byp aortoiliac
35638 Art byp aortobi-iliac
35642 Art byp carotid-vertebral
35645 Art byp subclav-vertebrl
35646 Art byp aortobifemoral
35647 Art byp aortofemoral
35650 Art byp axillary-axillary
35654 Art byp axill-fem-femoral
35656 Art byp femoral-popliteal
35661 Art byp femoral-femoral
35663 Art byp ilioiliac
35665 Art byp iliofemoral
35666 Art byp fem-ant-post tib/prl
35671 Art byp pop-tibl-prl-other
35681 Composite byp grft pros&vein
35682 Composite byp grft 2 veins
35683 Composite byp grft 3/> segmt
35691 Art trnsposj vertbrl carotid
35693 Art trnsposj subclavian
35694 Art trnsposj subclav carotid
35695 Art trnsposj carotid subclav

35697 Reimplant artery each
35700 Reoperation bypass graft
35701 Exploration carotid artery
35721 Exploration femoral artery
35741 Exploration popliteal artery
35800 Explore neck vessels
35820 Explore chest vessels
35840 Explore abdominal vessels
35870 Repair vessel graft defect
35901 Excision graft neck
35905 Excision graft thorax
35907 Excision graft abdomen
36660 Insertion catheter artery
36823 Insertion of cannula(s)
37140 Revision of circulation
37145 Revision of circulation
37160 Revision of circulation
37180 Revision of circulation
37181 Splice spleen/kidney veins
37182 Insert hepatic shunt (tips)
37215 Transcath stent cca w/eps
37217 Stent placemt retro carotid
37218 Stent placemt ante carotid
37616 Ligation of chest artery
37617 Ligation of abdomen artery
37618 Ligation of extremity artery
37660 Revision of major vein
37788 Revascularization penis
38100 Removal of spleen total
38101 Removal of spleen partial
38102 Removal of spleen total
38115 Repair of ruptured spleen
38380 Thoracic duct procedure
38381 Thoracic duct procedure
38382 Thoracic duct procedure
38562 Removal pelvic lymph nodes
38564 Removal abdomen lymph nodes
38724 Removal of lymph nodes neck
38746 Remove thoracic lymph nodes
38747 Remove abdominal lymph nodes
38765 Remove groin lymph nodes
38770 Remove pelvis lymph nodes
38780 Remove abdomen lymph nodes
39000 Exploration of chest
39010 Exploration of chest
39200 Resect mediastinal cyst
39220 Resect mediastinal tumor
39499 Chest procedure
39501 Repair diaphragm laceration
39503 Repair of diaphragm hernia
39540 Repair of diaphragm hernia
39541 Repair of diaphragm hernia
39545 Revision of diaphragm
39560 Resect diaphragm simple
39561 Resect diaphragm complex
39599 Diaphragm surgery procedure
41130 Partial removal of tongue
41135 Tongue and neck surgery
41140 Removal of tongue
41145 Tongue removal neck surgery
41150 Tongue mouth jaw surgery
41153 Tongue mouth neck surgery
41155 Tongue jaw & neck surgery
42426 Excise parotid gland/lesion
42845 Extensive surgery of throat
42894 Revision of pharyngeal walls
42953 Repair throat esophagus
42961 Control throat bleeding
42971 Control nose/throat bleeding
43045 Incision of esophagus
43100 Excision of esophagus lesion
43101 Excision of esophagus lesion
43107 Removal of esophagus
43108 Removal of esophagus
43112 Removal of esophagus
43113 Removal of esophagus
43116 Partial removal of esophagus
43117 Partial removal of esophagus
43118 Partial removal of esophagus
43121 Partial removal of esophagus
43122 Partial removal of esophagus
43123 Partial removal of esophagus
43124 Removal of esophagus
43135 Removal of esophagus pouch
43279 Lap myotomy heller
43283 Lap esoph lengthening
43286 Esphg tot w/laps moblj
43287 Esphg dstl 2/3 w/laps moblj
43288 Esphg thrsc moblj
43300 Repair of esophagus
43305 Repair esophagus and fistula
43310 Repair of esophagus
43312 Repair esophagus and fistula
43313 Esophagoplasty congenital
43314 Tracheo-esophagoplasty cong
43320 Fuse esophagus & stomach
43325 Revise esophagus & stomach
43327 Esoph fundoplasty lap
43328 Esoph fundoplasty thor
43330 Esophagomyotomy abdominal
43331 Esophagomyotomy thoracic
43332 Transab esoph hiat hern rpr
43333 Transab esoph hiat hern rpr
43334 Transthor diaphrag hern rpr
43335 Transthor diaphrag hern rpr
43336 Thorabd diaphr hern repair
43337 Thorabd diaphr hern repair
43338 Esoph lengthening
43340 Fuse esophagus & intestine
43341 Fuse esophagus & intestine
43351 Surgical opening esophagus
43352 Surgical opening esophagus
43360 Gastrointestinal repair
43361 Gastrointestinal repair
43400 Ligate esophagus veins
43401 Esophagus surgery for veins
43405 Ligate/staple esophagus
43410 Repair esophagus wound
43415 Repair esophagus wound
43425 Repair esophagus opening
43460 Pressure treatment esophagus
43496 Free jejunum flap microvasc
43500 Surgical opening of stomach
43501 Surgical repair of stomach
43502 Surgical repair of stomach
43520 Incision of pyloric muscle
43605 Biopsy of stomach
43610 Excision of stomach lesion
43611 Excision of stomach lesion
43620 Removal of stomach
43621 Removal of stomach
43622 Removal of stomach
43631 Removal of stomach partial
43632 Removal of stomach partial
43633 Removal of stomach partial
43634 Removal of stomach partial
43635 Removal of stomach partial
43640 Vagotomy & pylorus repair
43641 Vagotomy & pylorus repair
43644 Lap gastric bypass/roux-en-y
43645 Lap gastr bypass incl smll i
43771 Lap revise gastr adj device
43775 Lap sleeve gastrectomy
43800 Reconstruction of pylorus
43810 Fusion of stomach and bowel
43820 Fusion of stomach and bowel
43825 Fusion of stomach and bowel
43832 Place gastrostomy tube
43840 Repair of stomach lesion
43843 Gastroplasty w/o v-band
43845 Gastroplasty duodenal switch
43846 Gastric bypass for obesity
43847 Gastric bypass incl small i
43848 Revision gastroplasty
43850 Revise stomach-bowel fusion
43855 Revise stomach-bowel fusion
43860 Revise stomach-bowel fusion
43865 Revise stomach-bowel fusion
43880 Repair stomach-bowel fistula
43881 Impl/redo electrd antrum
43882 Revise/remove electrd antrum
44005 Freeing of bowel adhesion
44010 Incision of small bowel
44015 Insert needle cath bowel
44020 Explore small intestine
44021 Decompress small bowel
44025 Incision of large bowel
44050 Reduce bowel obstruction
44055 Correct malrotation of bowel
44110 Excise intestine lesion(s)
44111 Excision of bowel lesion(s)
44120 Removal of small intestine
44121 Removal of small intestine
44125 Removal of small intestine
44126 Enterectomy w/o taper cong
44127 Enterectomy w/taper cong
44128 Enterectomy cong add-on

44130 Bowel to bowel fusion
44132 Enterectomy cadaver donor
44133 Enterectomy live donor
44135 Intestine transplnt cadaver
44136 Intestine transplant live
44137 Remove intestinal allograft
44139 Mobilization of colon
44140 Partial removal of colon
44141 Partial removal of colon
44143 Partial removal of colon
44144 Partial removal of colon
44145 Partial removal of colon
44146 Partial removal of colon
44147 Partial removal of colon
44150 Removal of colon
44151 Removal of colon/ileostomy
44155 Removal of colon/ileostomy
44156 Removal of colon/ileostomy
44157 Colectomy w/ileoanal anast
44158 Colectomy w/neo-rectum pouch
44160 Removal of colon
44187 Lap ileo/jejuno-stomy
44188 Lap colostomy
44202 Lap enterectomy
44203 Lap resect s/intestine addl
44204 Laparo partial colectomy
44205 Lap colectomy part w/ileum
44206 Lap part colectomy w/stoma
44207 L colectomy/coloproctostomy
44208 L colectomy/coloproctostomy
44210 Laparo total proctocolectomy
44211 Lap colectomy w/proctectomy
44212 Laparo total proctocolectomy
44213 Lap mobil splenic fl add-on
44227 Lap close enterostomy
44300 Open bowel to skin
44310 Ileostomy/jejunostomy
44314 Revision of ileostomy
44316 Devise bowel pouch
44320 Colostomy
44322 Colostomy with biopsies
44345 Revision of colostomy
44346 Revision of colostomy
44602 Suture small intestine
44603 Suture small intestine
44604 Suture large intestine
44605 Repair of bowel lesion
44615 Intestinal stricturoplasty
44620 Repair bowel opening
44625 Repair bowel opening
44626 Repair bowel opening
44640 Repair bowel-skin fistula
44650 Repair bowel fistula
44660 Repair bowel-bladder fistula
44661 Repair bowel-bladder fistula
44680 Surgical revision intestine
44700 Suspend bowel w/prosthesis
44715 Prepare donor intestine
44720 Prep donor intestine/venous
44721 Prep donor intestine/artery
44800 Excision of bowel pouch
44820 Excision of mesentery lesion
44850 Repair of mesentery
44899 Bowel surgery procedure
44900 Drain appendix abscess open
44960 Appendectomy
45110 Removal of rectum
45111 Partial removal of rectum
45112 Removal of rectum
45113 Partial proctectomy
45114 Partial removal of rectum
45116 Partial removal of rectum
45119 Remove rectum w/reservoir
45120 Removal of rectum
45121 Removal of rectum and colon
45123 Partial proctectomy
45126 Pelvic exenteration
45130 Excision of rectal prolapse
45135 Excision of rectal prolapse
45136 Excise ileoanal reservior
45395 Lap removal of rectum
45397 Lap remove rectum w/pouch
45400 Laparoscopic proc
45402 Lap proctopexy w/sig resect
45540 Correct rectal prolapse
45550 Repair rectum/remove sigmoid
45562 Exploration/repair of rectum
45563 Exploration/repair of rectum
45800 Repair rect/bladder fistula
45805 Repair fistula w/colostomy
45820 Repair rectourethral fistula
45825 Repair fistula w/colostomy
46705 Repair of anal stricture
46710 Repr per/vag pouch sngl proc
46712 Repr per/vag pouch dbl proc
46715 Rep perf anoper fistu
46716 Rep perf anoper/vestib fistu
46730 Construction of absent anus
46735 Construction of absent anus
46740 Construction of absent anus
46742 Repair of imperforated anus
46744 Repair of cloacal anomaly
46746 Repair of cloacal anomaly
46748 Repair of cloacal anomaly
46751 Repair of anal sphincter
47010 Open drainage liver lesion
47015 Inject/aspirate liver cyst
47100 Wedge biopsy of liver
47120 Partial removal of liver
47122 Extensive removal of liver
47125 Partial removal of liver
47130 Partial removal of liver
47133 Removal of donor liver
47135 Transplantation of liver
47140 Partial removal donor liver
47141 Partial removal donor liver
47142 Partial removal donor liver
47143 Prep donor liver whole
47144 Prep donor liver 3-segment
47145 Prep donor liver lobe split
47146 Prep donor liver/venous
47147 Prep donor liver/arterial
47300 Surgery for liver lesion
47350 Repair liver wound
47360 Repair liver wound
47361 Repair liver wound
47362 Repair liver wound
47380 Open ablate liver tumor rf
47381 Open ablate liver tumor cryo
47400 Incision of liver duct
47420 Incision of bile duct
47425 Incision of bile duct
47460 Incise bile duct sphincter
47480 Incision of gallbladder
47550 Bile duct endoscopy add-on
47570 Laparo cholecystoenterostomy
47600 Removal of gallbladder
47605 Removal of gallbladder
47610 Removal of gallbladder
47612 Removal of gallbladder
47620 Removal of gallbladder
47700 Exploration of bile ducts
47701 Bile duct revision
47711 Excision of bile duct tumor
47712 Excision of bile duct tumor
47715 Excision of bile duct cyst
47720 Fuse gallbladder & bowel
47721 Fuse upper gi structures
47740 Fuse gallbladder & bowel
47741 Fuse gallbladder & bowel
47760 Fuse bile ducts and bowel
47765 Fuse liver ducts & bowel
47780 Fuse bile ducts and bowel
47785 Fuse bile ducts and bowel
47800 Reconstruction of bile ducts
47801 Placement bile duct support
47802 Fuse liver duct & intestine
47900 Suture bile duct injury
48000 Drainage of abdomen
48001 Placement of drain pancreas
48020 Removal of pancreatic stone
48100 Biopsy of pancreas open
48105 Resect/debride pancreas
48120 Removal of pancreas lesion
48140 Partial removal of pancreas
48145 Partial removal of pancreas
48146 Pancreatectomy
48148 Removal of pancreatic duct
48150 Partial removal of pancreas
48152 Pancreatectomy
48153 Pancreatectomy
48154 Pancreatectomy
48155 Removal of pancreas
48400 Injection intraop add-on
48500 Surgery of pancreatic cyst
48510 Drain pancreatic pseudocyst
48520 Fuse pancreas cyst and bowel

48540 Fuse pancreas cyst and bowel
48545 Pancreatorrhaphy
48547 Duodenal exclusion
48548 Fuse pancreas and bowel
48551 Prep donor pancreas
48552 Prep donor pancreas/venous
48554 Transpl allograft pancreas
48556 Removal allograft pancreas
49000 Exploration of abdomen
49002 Reopening of abdomen
49010 Exploration behind abdomen
49020 Drainage abdom abscess open
49040 Drain open abdom abscess
49060 Drain open retroperi abscess
49062 Drain to peritoneal cavity
49203 Exc abd tum 5 cm or less
49204 Exc abd tum over 5 cm
49205 Exc abd tum over 10 cm
49215 Excise sacral spine tumor
49220 Multiple surgery abdomen
49255 Removal of omentum
49412 Ins device for rt guide open
49425 Insert abdomen-venous drain
49428 Ligation of shunt
49605 Repair umbilical lesion
49606 Repair umbilical lesion
49610 Repair umbilical lesion
49611 Repair umbilical lesion
49900 Repair of abdominal wall
49904 Omental flap extra-abdom
49905 Omental flap intra-abdom
49906 Free omental flap microvasc
50010 Exploration of kidney
50040 Drainage of kidney
50045 Exploration of kidney
50060 Removal of kidney stone
50065 Incision of kidney
50070 Incision of kidney
50075 Removal of kidney stone
50100 Revise kidney blood vessels
50120 Exploration of kidney
50125 Explore and drain kidney
50130 Removal of kidney stone
50135 Exploration of kidney
50205 Renal biopsy open
50220 Remove kidney open
50225 Removal kidney open complex
50230 Removal kidney open radical
50234 Removal of kidney & ureter
50236 Removal of kidney & ureter
50240 Partial removal of kidney
50250 Cryoablate renal mass open
50280 Removal of kidney lesion
50290 Removal of kidney lesion
50300 Remove cadaver donor kidney
50320 Remove kidney living donor
50323 Prep cadaver renal allograft
50325 Prep donor renal graft
50327 Prep renal graft/venous
50328 Prep renal graft/arterial
50329 Prep renal graft/ureteral
50340 Removal of kidney
50360 Transplantation of kidney
50365 Transplantation of kidney
50370 Remove transplanted kidney
50380 Reimplantation of kidney
50400 Revision of kidney/ureter
50405 Revision of kidney/ureter
50500 Repair of kidney wound
50520 Close kidney-skin fistula
50525 Close nephrovisceral fistula
50526 Close nephrovisceral fistula
50540 Revision of horseshoe kidney
50545 Laparo radical nephrectomy
50546 Laparoscopic nephrectomy
50547 Laparo removal donor kidney
50548 Laparo remove w/ureter
50600 Exploration of ureter
50605 Insert ureteral support
50610 Removal of ureter stone
50620 Removal of ureter stone
50630 Removal of ureter stone
50650 Removal of ureter
50660 Removal of ureter
50700 Revision of ureter
50715 Release of ureter
50722 Release of ureter
50725 Release/revise ureter
50728 Revise ureter
50740 Fusion of ureter & kidney
50750 Fusion of ureter & kidney
50760 Fusion of ureters
50770 Splicing of ureters
50780 Reimplant ureter in bladder
50782 Reimplant ureter in bladder
50783 Reimplant ureter in bladder
50785 Reimplant ureter in bladder
50800 Implant ureter in bowel
50810 Fusion of ureter & bowel
50815 Urine shunt to intestine
50820 Construct bowel bladder
50825 Construct bowel bladder
50830 Revise urine flow
50840 Replace ureter by bowel
50845 Appendico-vesicostomy
50860 Transplant ureter to skin
50900 Repair of ureter
50920 Closure ureter/skin fistula
50930 Closure ureter/bowel fistula
50940 Release of ureter
51525 Removal of bladder lesion
51530 Removal of bladder lesion
51550 Partial removal of bladder
51555 Partial removal of bladder
51565 Revise bladder & ureter(s)
51570 Removal of bladder
51575 Removal of bladder & nodes
51580 Remove bladder/revise tract
51585 Removal of bladder & nodes
51590 Remove bladder/revise tract
51595 Remove bladder/revise tract
51596 Remove bladder/create pouch
51597 Removal of pelvic structures
51800 Revision of bladder/urethra
51820 Revision of urinary tract
51840 Attach bladder/urethra
51841 Attach bladder/urethra
51865 Repair of bladder wound
51900 Repair bladder/vagina lesion
51920 Close bladder-uterus fistula
51925 Hysterectomy/bladder repair
51940 Correction of bladder defect
51960 Revision of bladder & bowel
51980 Construct bladder opening
53415 Reconstruction of urethra
53448 Remov/replc ur sphinctr comp
54125 Removal of penis
54130 Remove penis & nodes
54135 Remove penis & nodes
54390 Repair penis and bladder
54430 Revision of penis
54438 Replantation of penis
55605 Incise sperm duct pouch
55650 Remove sperm duct pouch
55801 Removal of prostate
55810 Extensive prostate surgery
55812 Extensive prostate surgery
55815 Extensive prostate surgery
55821 Removal of prostate
55831 Removal of prostate
55840 Extensive prostate surgery
55842 Extensive prostate surgery
55845 Extensive prostate surgery
55862 Extensive prostate surgery
55865 Extensive prostate surgery
56630 Extensive vulva surgery
56631 Extensive vulva surgery
56632 Extensive vulva surgery
56633 Extensive vulva surgery
56634 Extensive vulva surgery
56637 Extensive vulva surgery
56640 Extensive vulva surgery
57110 Remove vagina wall complete
57111 Remove vagina tissue compl
57112 Vaginectomy w/nodes compl
57270 Repair of bowel pouch
57280 Suspension of vagina
57296 Revise vag graft open abd
57305 Repair rectum-vagina fistula
57307 Fistula repair & colostomy
57308 Fistula repair transperine
57311 Repair urethrovaginal lesion
57531 Removal of cervix radical
57540 Removal of residual cervix
57545 Remove cervix/repair pelvis
58140 Myomectomy abdom method
58146 Myomectomy abdom complex

58150 Total hysterectomy
58152 Total hysterectomy
58180 Partial hysterectomy
58200 Extensive hysterectomy
58210 Extensive hysterectomy
58240 Removal of pelvis contents
58267 Vag hyst w/urinary repair
58275 Hysterectomy/revise vagina
58280 Hysterectomy/revise vagina
58285 Extensive hysterectomy
58293 Vag hyst w/uro repair compl
58400 Suspension of uterus
58410 Suspension of uterus
58520 Repair of ruptured uterus
58540 Revision of uterus
58548 Lap radical hyst
58575 Laps tot hyst resj mal
58605 Division of fallopian tube
58611 Ligate oviduct(s) add-on
58700 Removal of fallopian tube
58720 Removal of ovary/tube(s)
58740 Adhesiolysis tube ovary
58750 Repair oviduct
58752 Revise ovarian tube(s)
58760 Fimbrioplasty
58822 Drain ovary abscess percut
58825 Transposition ovary(s)
58940 Removal of ovary(s)
58943 Removal of ovary(s)
58950 Resect ovarian malignancy
58951 Resect ovarian malignancy
58952 Resect ovarian malignancy
58953 Tah rad dissect for debulk
58954 Tah rad debulk/lymph remove
58956 Bso omentectomy w/tah
58957 Resect recurrent gyn mal
58958 Resect recur gyn mal w/lym
58960 Exploration of abdomen
59120 Treat ectopic pregnancy
59121 Treat ectopic pregnancy
59130 Treat ectopic pregnancy
59135 Treat ectopic pregnancy
59136 Treat ectopic pregnancy
59140 Treat ectopic pregnancy
59325 Revision of cervix
59350 Repair of uterus
59514 Cesarean delivery only
59525 Remove uterus after cesarean
59620 Attempted vbac delivery only
59830 Treat uterus infection
59850 Abortion
59851 Abortion
59852 Abortion
59855 Abortion
59856 Abortion
59857 Abortion
60254 Extensive thyroid surgery
60270 Removal of thyroid
60505 Explore parathyroid glands
60521 Removal of thymus gland
60522 Removal of thymus gland
60540 Explore adrenal gland
60545 Explore adrenal gland
60600 Remove carotid body lesion
60605 Remove carotid body lesion
60650 Laparoscopy adrenalectomy
61105 Twist drill hole
61107 Drill skull for implantation
61108 Drill skull for drainage
61120 Burr hole for puncture
61140 Pierce skull for biopsy
61150 Pierce skull for drainage
61151 Pierce skull for drainage
61154 Pierce skull & remove clot
61156 Pierce skull for drainage
61210 Pierce skull implant device
61250 Pierce skull & explore
61253 Pierce skull & explore
61304 Open skull for exploration
61305 Open skull for exploration
61312 Open skull for drainage
61313 Open skull for drainage
61314 Open skull for drainage
61315 Open skull for drainage
61316 Implt cran bone flap to abdo
61320 Open skull for drainage
61321 Open skull for drainage
61322 Decompressive craniotomy
61323 Decompressive lobectomy
61332 Explore/biopsy eye socket
61333 Explore orbit/remove lesion
61340 Subtemporal decompression
61343 Incise skull (press relief)
61345 Relieve cranial pressure
61450 Incise skull for surgery
61458 Incise skull for brain wound
61460 Incise skull for surgery
61500 Removal of skull lesion
61501 Remove infected skull bone
61510 Removal of brain lesion
61512 Remove brain lining lesion
61514 Removal of brain abscess
61516 Removal of brain lesion
61517 Implt brain chemotx add-on
61518 Removal of brain lesion
61519 Remove brain lining lesion
61520 Removal of brain lesion
61521 Removal of brain lesion
61522 Removal of brain abscess
61524 Removal of brain lesion
61526 Removal of brain lesion
61530 Removal of brain lesion
61531 Implant brain electrodes
61533 Implant brain electrodes
61534 Removal of brain lesion
61535 Remove brain electrodes
61536 Removal of brain lesion
61537 Removal of brain tissue
61538 Removal of brain tissue
61539 Removal of brain tissue
61540 Removal of brain tissue
61541 Incision of brain tissue
61543 Removal of brain tissue
61544 Remove & treat brain lesion
61545 Excision of brain tumor
61546 Removal of pituitary gland
61548 Removal of pituitary gland
61550 Release of skull seams
61552 Release of skull seams
61556 Incise skull/sutures
61557 Incise skull/sutures
61558 Excision of skull/sutures
61559 Excision of skull/sutures
61563 Excision of skull tumor
61564 Excision of skull tumor
61566 Removal of brain tissue
61567 Incision of brain tissue
61570 Remove foreign body brain
61571 Incise skull for brain wound
61575 Skull base/brainstem surgery
61576 Skull base/brainstem surgery
61580 Craniofacial approach skull
61581 Craniofacial approach skull
61582 Craniofacial approach skull
61583 Craniofacial approach skull
61584 Orbitocranial approach/skull
61585 Orbitocranial approach/skull
61586 Resect nasopharynx skull
61590 Infratemporal approach/skull
61591 Infratemporal approach/skull
61592 Orbitocranial approach/skull
61595 Transtemporal approach/skull
61596 Transcochlear approach/skull
61597 Transcondylar approach/skull
61598 Transpetrosal approach/skull
61600 Resect/excise cranial lesion
61601 Resect/excise cranial lesion
61605 Resect/excise cranial lesion
61606 Resect/excise cranial lesion
61607 Resect/excise cranial lesion
61608 Resect/excise cranial lesion
61611 Transect artery sinus
61613 Remove aneurysm sinus
61615 Resect/excise lesion skull
61616 Resect/excise lesion skull
61618 Repair dura
61619 Repair dura
61624 Transcath occlusion cns
61630 Intracranial angioplasty
61635 Intracran angioplsty w/stent
61645 Perq art m-thrombect &/nfs
61650 Evasc prlng admn rx agnt 1st
61651 Evasc prlng admn rx agnt add
61680 Intracranial vessel surgery
61682 Intracranial vessel surgery
61684 Intracranial vessel surgery
61686 Intracranial vessel surgery

61690 Intracranial vessel surgery
61692 Intracranial vessel surgery
61697 Brain aneurysm repr complx
61698 Brain aneurysm repr complx
61700 Brain aneurysm repr simple
61702 Inner skull vessel surgery
61703 Clamp neck artery
61705 Revise circulation to head
61708 Revise circulation to head
61710 Revise circulation to head
61711 Fusion of skull arteries
61735 Incise skull/brain surgery
61750 Incise skull/brain biopsy
61751 Brain biopsy w/ct/mr guide
61760 Implant brain electrodes
61850 Implant neuroelectrodes
61860 Implant neuroelectrodes
61863 Implant neuroelectrode
61864 Implant neuroelectrde addl
61867 Implant neuroelectrode
61868 Implant neuroelectrde addl
61870 Implant neuroelectrodes
62005 Treat skull fracture
62010 Treatment of head injury
62100 Repair brain fluid leakage
62115 Reduction of skull defect
62117 Reduction of skull defect
62120 Repair skull cavity lesion
62121 Incise skull repair
62140 Repair of skull defect
62141 Repair of skull defect
62142 Remove skull plate/flap
62143 Replace skull plate/flap
62145 Repair of skull & brain
62146 Repair of skull with graft
62147 Repair of skull with graft
62148 Retr bone flap to fix skull
62161 Dissect brain w/scope
62162 Remove colloid cyst w/scope
62163 Zneuroendoscopy w/fb removal
62164 Remove brain tumor w/scope
62165 Remove pituit tumor w/scope
62180 Establish brain cavity shunt
62190 Establish brain cavity shunt
62192 Establish brain cavity shunt
62200 Establish brain cavity shunt
62201 Brain cavity shunt w/scope
62220 Establish brain cavity shunt
62223 Establish brain cavity shunt
62256 Remove brain cavity shunt
62258 Replace brain cavity shunt
63050 Cervical laminoplsty 2/> seg
63051 C-laminoplasty w/graft/plate
63077 Spine disk surgery thorax
63078 Spine disk surgery thorax
63081 Remove vert body dcmprn crvl
63082 Remove vertebral body add-on
63085 Remove vert body dcmprn thrc
63086 Remove vertebral body add-on
63087 Remov vertbr dcmprn thrclmbr
63088 Remove vertebral body add-on
63090 Remove vert body dcmprn lmbr
63091 Remove vertebral body add-on
63101 Remove vert body dcmprn thrc
63102 Remove vert body dcmprn lmbr
63103 Remove vertebral body add-on
63170 Incise spinal cord tract(s)
63172 Drainage of spinal cyst
63173 Drainage of spinal cyst
63180 Revise spinal cord ligaments
63182 Revise spinal cord ligaments
63185 Incise spine nrv half segmnt
63190 Incise spine nrv >2 segmnts
63191 Incise spine accessory nerve
63194 Incise spine & cord cervical
63195 Incise spine & cord thoracic
63196 Incise spine&cord 2 trx crvl
63197 Incise spine&cord 2 trx thrc
63198 Incise spin&cord 2 stgs crvl
63199 Incise spin&cord 2 stgs thrc
63200 Release spinal cord lumbar
63250 Revise spinal cord vsls crvl
63251 Revise spinal cord vsls thrc
63252 Revise spine cord vsl thrlmb
63265 Excise intraspinl lesion crv
63266 Excise intrspinl lesion thrc
63267 Excise intrspinl lesion lmbr
63268 Excise intrspinl lesion scrl
63270 Excise intrspinl lesion crvl
63271 Excise intrspinl lesion thrc
63272 Excise intrspinl lesion lmbr
63273 Excise intrspinl lesion scrl
63275 Bx/exc xdrl spine lesn crvl
63276 Bx/exc xdrl spine lesn thrc
63277 Bx/exc xdrl spine lesn lmbr
63278 Bx/exc xdrl spine lesn scrl
63280 Bx/exc idrl spine lesn crvl
63281 Bx/exc idrl spine lesn thrc
63282 Bx/exc idrl spine lesn lmbr
63283 Bx/exc idrl spine lesn scrl
63285 Bx/exc idrl imed lesn cervl
63286 Bx/exc idrl imed lesn thrc
63287 Bx/exc idrl imed lesn thrlmb
63290 Bx/exc xdrl/idrl lsn any lvl
63295 Repair laminectomy defect
63300 Remove vert xdrl body crvcl
63301 Remove vert xdrl body thrc
63302 Remove vert xdrl body thrlmb
63303 Remov vert xdrl bdy lmbr/sac
63304 Remove vert idrl body crvcl
63305 Remove vert idrl body thrc
63306 Remov vert idrl bdy thrclmbr
63307 Remov vert idrl bdy lmbr/sac
63308 Remove vertebral body add-on
63700 Repair of spinal herniation
63702 Repair of spinal herniation
63704 Repair of spinal herniation
63706 Repair of spinal herniation
63707 Repair spinal fluid leakage
63709 Repair spinal fluid leakage
63710 Graft repair of spine defect
63740 Install spinal shunt
64755 Incision of stomach nerves
64760 Incision of vagus nerve
64809 Remove sympathetic nerves
64818 Remove sympathetic nerves
64866 Fusion of facial/other nerve
64868 Fusion of facial/other nerve
65273 Repair of eye wound
69155 Extensive ear/neck surgery
69535 Remove part of temporal bone
69554 Remove ear lesion
69950 Incise inner ear nerve
75956 Xray endovasc thor ao repr
75957 Xray endovasc thor ao repr
75958 Xray place prox ext thor ao
75959 Xray place dist ext thor ao
92941 Prq card revasc mi 1 vsl
92970 Cardioassist internal
92971 Cardioassist external
92975 Dissolve clot heart vessel
92992 Revision of heart chamber
92993 Revision of heart chamber
93583 Perq transcath septal reduxn
99184 Hypothermia ill neonate
99190 Special pump services
99191 Special pump services
99192 Special pump services
99356 Prolonged service inpatient
99357 Prolonged service inpatient
99462 Sbsq nb em per day hosp
99468 Neonate crit care initial
99469 Neonate crit care subsq
99471 Ped critical care initial
99472 Ped critical care subsq
99475 Ped crit care age 2-5 init
99476 Ped crit care age 2-5 subsq
99477 Init day hosp neonate care
99478 Ic lbw inf < 1500 gm subsq
99479 Ic lbw inf 1500-2500 g subsq
99480 Ic inf pbw 2501-5000 g subsq
C9606 PC H rev ac tot/subtot occl 1 ves
G0341 Percutaneous islet celltrans
G0342 Laparoscopy islet cell trans
G0343 Laparotomy islet cell transp
G0412 Open tx iliac spine uni/bil
G0414 Pelvic ring fx treat int fix
G0415 Open tx post pelvic fxcture

Appendix K — Place of Service and Type of Service

Place-of-Service Codes for Professional Claims

Listed below are place of service codes and descriptions. These codes should be used on professional claims to specify the entity where service(s) were rendered. Check with individual payers (e.g., Medicare, Medicaid, other private insurance) for reimbursement policies regarding these codes. To comment on a code(s) or description(s), please send your request to posinfo@cms.gov.

Code	Name	Description
01	Pharmacy	A facility or location where drugs and other medically related items and services are sold, dispensed, or otherwise provided directly to patients.
02	Telehealth	The location where health services and health related services are provided or received through telecommunication technology.
03	School	A facility whose primary purpose is education.
04	Homeless shelter	A facility or location whose primary purpose is to provide temporary housing to homeless individuals (e.g., emergency shelters, individual or family shelters).
05	Indian Health Service freestanding facility	A facility or location, owned and operated by the Indian Health Service, which provides diagnostic, therapeutic (surgical and non-surgical), and rehabilitation services to American Indians and Alaska natives who do not require hospitalization.
06	Indian Health Service provider-based facility	A facility or location, owned and operated by the Indian Health Service, which provides diagnostic, therapeutic (surgical and nonsurgical), and rehabilitation services rendered by, or under the supervision of, physicians to American Indians and Alaska natives admitted as inpatients or outpatients.
07	Tribal 638 freestanding facility	A facility or location owned and operated by a federally recognized American Indian or Alaska native tribe or tribal organization under a 638 agreement, which provides diagnostic, therapeutic (surgical and nonsurgical), and rehabilitation services to tribal members who do not require hospitalization.
08	Tribal 638 provider-based Facility	A facility or location owned and operated by a federally recognized American Indian or Alaska native tribe or tribal organization under a 638 agreement, which provides diagnostic, therapeutic (surgical and nonsurgical), and rehabilitation services to tribal members admitted as inpatients or outpatients.
09	Prison/correctional facility	A prison, jail, reformatory, work farm, detention center, or any other similar facility maintained by either federal, state or local authorities for the purpose of confinement or rehabilitation of adult or juvenile criminal offenders.
10	Unassigned	N/A
11	Office	Location, other than a hospital, skilled nursing facility (SNF), military treatment facility, community health center, State or local public health clinic, or intermediate care facility (ICF), where the health professional routinely provides health examinations, diagnosis, and treatment of illness or injury on an ambulatory basis.
12	Home	Location, other than a hospital or other facility, where the patient receives care in a private residence.
13	Assisted living facility	Congregate residential facility with self-contained living units providing assessment of each resident's needs and on-site support 24 hours a day, 7 days a week, with the capacity to deliver or arrange for services including some health care and other services.
14	Group home	A residence, with shared living areas, where clients receive supervision and other services such as social and/or behavioral services, custodial service, and minimal services (e.g., medication administration).
15	Mobile unit	A facility/unit that moves from place-to-place equipped to provide preventive, screening, diagnostic, and/or treatment services.
16	Temporary lodging	A short-term accommodation such as a hotel, campground, hostel, cruise ship or resort where the patient receives care, and which is not identified by any other POS code.
17	Walk-in retail health clinic	A walk-in health clinic, other than an office, urgent care facility, pharmacy, or independent clinic and not described by any other place of service code, that is located within a retail operation and provides preventive and primary care services on an ambulatory basis.
18	Place of employment/ worksite	A location, not described by any other POS code, owned or operated by a public or private entity where the patient is employed, and where a health professional provides on-going or episodic occupational medical, therapeutic or rehabilitative services to the individual.
19	Off campus-outpatient hospital	A portion of an off-campus hospital provider based department which provides diagnostic, therapeutic (both surgical and nonsurgical), and rehabilitation services to sick or injured persons who do not require hospitalization or institutionalization.
20	Urgent care facility	Location, distinct from a hospital emergency room, an office, or a clinic, whose purpose is to diagnose and treat illness or injury for unscheduled, ambulatory patients seeking immediate medical attention.

21	Inpatient hospital	A facility, other than psychiatric, which primarily provides diagnostic, therapeutic (both surgical and nonsurgical), and rehabilitation services by, or under, the supervision of physicians to patients admitted for a variety of medical conditions.
22	On campus-outpatient hospital	A portion of a hospital's main campus which provides diagnostic, therapeutic (both surgical and nonsurgical), and rehabilitation services to sick or injured persons who do not require hospitalization or institutionalization.
23	Emergency room—hospital	A portion of a hospital where emergency diagnosis and treatment of illness or injury is provided.
24	Ambulatory surgical center	A freestanding facility, other than a physician's office, where surgical and diagnostic services are provided on an ambulatory basis.
25	Birthing center	A facility, other than a hospital's maternity facilities or a physician's office, which provides a setting for labor, delivery, and immediate post-partum care as well as immediate care of new born infants.
26	Military treatment facility	A medical facility operated by one or more of the uniformed services. Military treatment facility (MTF) also refers to certain former U.S. Public Health Service (USPHS) facilities now designated as uniformed service treatment facilities (USTF).
27-30	Unassigned	N/A
31	Skilled nursing facility	A facility which primarily provides inpatient skilled nursing care and related services to patients who require medical, nursing, or rehabilitative services but does not provide the level of care or treatment available in a hospital.
32	Nursing facility	A facility which primarily provides to residents skilled nursing care and related services for the rehabilitation of injured, disabled, or sick persons, or, on a regular basis, health-related care services above the level of custodial care to individuals other than those with intellectual disabilities.
33	Custodial care facility	A facility which provides room, board, and other personal assistance services, generally on a long-term basis, and which does not include a medical component.
34	Hospice	A facility, other than a patient's home, in which palliative and supportive care for terminally ill patients and their families is provided.
35-40	Unassigned	N/A
41	Ambulance—land	A land vehicle specifically designed, equipped and staffed for lifesaving and transporting the sick or injured.
42	Ambulance—air or water	An air or water vehicle specifically designed, equipped and staffed for lifesaving and transporting the sick or injured.
43-48	Unassigned	N/A
49	Independent clinic	A location, not part of a hospital and not described by any other place-of-service code, that is organized and operated to provide preventive, diagnostic, therapeutic, rehabilitative, or palliative services to outpatients only.
50	Federally qualified health center	A facility located in a medically underserved area that provides Medicare beneficiaries with preventive primary medical care under the general direction of a physician.
51	Inpatient psychiatric facility	A facility that provides inpatient psychiatric services for the diagnosis and treatment of mental illness on a 24-hour basis, by or under the supervision of a physician.
52	Psychiatric facility-partial hospitalization	A facility for the diagnosis and treatment of mental illness that provides a planned therapeutic program for patients who do not require full time hospitalization, but who need broader programs than are possible from outpatient visits to a hospital-based or hospital-affiliated facility.
53	Community mental health center	A facility that provides the following services: outpatient services, including specialized outpatient services for children, the elderly, individuals who are chronically ill, and residents of the CMHC's mental health services area who have been discharged from inpatient treatment at a mental health facility; 24 hour a day emergency care services; day treatment, other partial hospitalization services, or psychosocial rehabilitation services; screening for patients being considered for admission to state mental health facilities to determine the appropriateness of such admission; and consultation and education services.
54	Intermediate care facility/individuals with intellectual disabilities	A facility which primarily provides health-related care and services above the level of custodial care to individuals with Intellectual Disabilities but does not provide the level of care or treatment available in a hospital or SNF.
55	Residential substance abuse treatment facility	A facility which provides treatment for substance (alcohol and drug) abuse to live-in residents who do not require acute medical care. Services include individual and group therapy and counseling, family counseling, laboratory tests, drugs and supplies, psychological testing, and room and board.
56	Psychiatric residential treatment center	A facility or distinct part of a facility for psychiatric care which provides a total 24-hour therapeutically planned and professionally staffed group living and learning environment.
57	Non-residential substance abuse treatment facility	A location which provides treatment for substance (alcohol and drug) abuse on an ambulatory basis. Services include individual and group therapy and counseling, family counseling, laboratory tests, drugs and supplies, and psychological testing.
58-59	Unassigned	N/A

60	Mass immunization center	A location where providers administer pneumococcal pneumonia and influenza virus vaccinations and submit these services as electronic media claims, paper claims, or using the roster billing method. This generally takes place in a mass immunization setting, such as, a public health center, pharmacy, or mall but may include a physician office setting.
61	Comprehensive inpatient rehabilitation facility	A facility that provides comprehensive rehabilitation services under the supervision of a physician to inpatients with physical disabilities. Services include physical therapy, occupational therapy, speech pathology, social or psychological services, and orthotics and prosthetics services.
62	Comprehensive outpatient rehabilitation facility	A facility that provides comprehensive rehabilitation services under the supervision of a physician to outpatients with physical disabilities. Services include physical therapy, occupational therapy, and speech pathology services.
63-64	Unassigned	N/A
65	End-stage renal disease treatment facility	A facility other than a hospital, which provides dialysis treatment, maintenance, and/or training to patients or caregivers on an ambulatory or home-care basis.
66-70	Unassigned	N/A
71	Public health clinic	A facility maintained by either state or local health departments that provides ambulatory primary medical care under the general direction of a physician.
72	Rural health clinic	A certified facility which is located in a rural medically underserved area that provides ambulatory primary medical care under the general direction of a physician.
73-80	Unassigned	N/A
81	Independent laboratory	A laboratory certified to perform diagnostic and/or clinical tests independent of an institution or a physician's office.
82-98	Unassigned	N/A
99	Other place of service	Other place of service not identified above.

Type of Service

Common Working File Type of Service (TOS) Indicators

For submitting a claim to the Common Working File (CWF), use the following table to assign the proper TOS. Some procedures may have more than one applicable TOS. CWF will reject codes with incorrect TOS designations. CWF will produce alerts on codes with incorrect TOS designations.

The only exceptions to this annual update are:

- Surgical services billed for dates of service through December 31, 2007, containing the ASC facility service modifier SG must be reported as TOS F. Effective for services on or after January 1, 2008, the SG modifier is no longer applicable for Medicare services. ASC providers should discontinue applying the SG modifier on ASC facility claims. The indicator F does not appear in the TOS table because its use depends upon claims submitted with POS 24 (ASC facility) from an ASC (specialty 49). This became effective for dates of service January 1, 2008, or after.
- Surgical services billed with an assistant-at-surgery modifier (80-82, AS) must be reported with TOS 8. The 8 indicator does not appear on the TOS table because its use is dependent upon the use of the appropriate modifier. (See Pub. 100-4 *Medicare Claims Processing Manual,* chapter 12, "Physician/Practitioner Billing," for instructions on when assistant-at-surgery is allowable.)
- TOS H appears in the list of descriptors. However, it does not appear in the table. In CWF, "H" is used only as an indicator for hospice. The contractor should not submit TOS H to CWF at this time.
- For outpatient services, when a transfusion medicine code appears on a claim that also contains a blood product, the service is paid under reasonable charge at 80 percent; coinsurance and deductible apply. When transfusion medicine codes are paid under the clinical laboratory fee schedule they are paid at 100 percent; coinsurance and deductible do not apply.

Note: For injection codes with more than one possible TOS designation, use the following guidelines when assigning the TOS:

When the choice is L or 1:

- Use TOS L when the drug is used related to ESRD; or
- Use TOS 1 when the drug is not related to ESRD and is administered in the office.

When the choice is G or 1:

- Use TOS G when the drug is an immunosuppressive drug; or
- Use TOS 1 when the drug is used for other than immunosuppression.

When the choice is P or 1:

- Use TOS P if the drug is administered through durable medical equipment (DME); or
- Use TOS 1 if the drug is administered in the office.

The place of service or diagnosis may be considered when determining the appropriate TOS. The descriptors for each of the TOS codes listed in the annual HCPCS update are:

0	Whole blood
1	Medical care
2	Surgery
3	Consultation
4	Diagnostic radiology
5	Diagnostic laboratory
6	Therapeutic radiology
7	Anesthesia
8	Assistant at surgery
9	Other medical items or services
A	Used DME
B	High risk screening mammography
C	Low risk screening mammography
D	Ambulance
E	Enteral/parenteral nutrients/supplies
F	Ambulatory surgical center (facility usage for surgical services)
G	Immunosuppressive drugs
H	Hospice
J	Diabetic shoes
K	Hearing items and services
L	ESRD supplies
M	Monthly capitation payment for dialysis
N	Kidney donor
P	Lump sum purchase of DME, prosthetics, orthotics
Q	Vision items or services
R	Rental of DME
S	Surgical dressings or other medical supplies
U	Occupational therapy
V	Pneumococcal/flu vaccine
W	Physical therapy

Appendix L — Multianalyte Assays with Algorithmic Analyses

The following tables contain the Administrative Codes for Multianalyte Assays with Algorithmic Analyses (MAAA), category I codes for Administrative Codes for Multianalyte Assays with Algorithmic Analyses (MAAA) and the most current list of Proprietary Laboratory Analysis (PLA) codes.

The following is a list of administrative codes for multianalyte assays with algorithmic analysis (MAAA) procedures that are usually exclusive to one single clinical laboratory or manufacturer. These tests use the results from several different assays, including molecular pathology assays, fluorescent in situ hybridization assays, and nonnucleic acid-based assays (e.g., proteins, polypeptides, lipids, and carbohydrates) to perform an algorithmic analysis that is reported as a numeric score or probability. Although the laboratory report may list results of individual component tests of the MAAAs, these assays are not separately reportable.

The following list includes the proprietary name and clinical laboratory/manufacturer, an alphanumeric code, and the code descriptor.

The format for the code descriptor usually includes:

- Type of disease (e.g., oncology, autoimmune, tissue rejection)
- Chemical(s) analyzed (e.g., DNA, RNA, protein, antibody)
- Number of markers (e.g., number of genes, number of proteins)
- Methodology(s) (e.g., microarray, real-time [RT]-PCR, in situ hybridization [ISH], enzyme linked immunosorbent assays [ELISA])
- Number of functional domains (when indicated)
- Type of specimen (e.g., blood, fresh tissue, formalin-fixed paraffin embedded)
- Type of algorithm result (e.g., prognostic, diagnostic)
- Report (e.g., probability index, risk score)

MAAA procedures with a Category I code are noted on the following list and can also be found in code range 81500–81599 in the pathology and laboratory chapter. If a specific MAAA test does not have a Category I code, it is denoted with a four-digit number and the letter M. Use code 81599 if an MAAA test is not included on the following list or in the Category I codes. The codes on the list are exclusive to the assays identified by proprietary name. Report code 81599 also when an analysis is performed that may possibly fall within a specific descriptor but the proprietary name is not included in the list. The list does not contain all MAAA procedures.

Proprietary Name/Clinical Laboratory/Manufacturer	Code	Descriptor
Administrative Codes for Multianalyte Assays with Algorithmic Analyses (MAAA)		
	0001M (0001M has been deleted. To report, see 81596.)	
ASH FibroSURE™, BioPredictive S.A.S	0002M	Liver disease, 10 biochemical assays (ALT, A2-macroglobulin, apolipoprotein A-1, total bilirubin, GGT, haptoglobin, AST, glucose, total cholesterol, and triglycerides) utilizing serum, prognostic algorithm reported as quantitative scores for fibrosis, steatosis, and alcoholic steatohepatitis (ASH)
NASH FibroSURE™, BioPredictive S.A.S	0003M	Liver disease, 10 biochemical assays (ALT, A2-macroglobulin, apolipoprotein A-1, total bilirubin, GGT, haptoglobin, AST, glucose, total cholesterol, and triglycerides) utilizing serum, prognostic algorithm reported as quantitative scores for fibrosis, steatosis, and nonalcoholic steatohepatitis (NASH)
ScoliScore™ Transgenomic	0004M	Scoliosis, DNA analysis of 53 single nucleotide polymorphisms (SNPs), using saliva, prognostic algorithm reported as a risk score
HeproDX™, GoPath Laboratories, LLC	0006M	Oncology (hepatic), mRNA expression levels of 161 genes, utilizing fresh hepatocellular carcinoma tumor tissue, with alpha-fetoprotein level, algorithm reported as a risk classifier
NETest (Wren Laboratories, LLC)	0007M	Oncology (gastrointestinal neuroendocrine tumors), real-time PCR expression analysis of 51 genes, utilizing whole peripheral blood, algorithm reported as a nomogram of tumor disease index
	0008M (0008M has been deleted. To report, see 81520.)	
	(0009M has been deleted)	
	(0010M has been deleted. To report, see 81539.)	
NeoLAB™ Prostate Liquid Biopsy, NeoGenomics Laboratories	▲ 0011M	Oncology, prostate cancer, mRNA expression assay of 12 genes (10 content and 2 housekeeping), RT-PCR test utilizing blood plasma and urine, algorithms to predict high-grade prostate cancer risk
Cxbladder™ Detect, Pacific Edge Diagnostics USA, Ltd.	0012M	Oncology (urothelial), mRNA, gene expression profiling by real-time quantitative PCR of five genes (*MDK, HOXA13, CDC2 [CDK1], IGFBP5*, and *CXCR2*), utilizing urine, algorithm reported as a risk score for having urothelial carcinoma
Cxbladder™ Monitor, Pacific Edge Diagnostics USA, Ltd.	0013M	Oncology (urothelial), mRNA, gene expression profiling by real-time quantitative PCR of five genes (*MDK, HOXA13, CDC2 [CDK1], IGFBP5*, and *CXCR2*), utilizing urine, algorithm reported as a risk score for having recurrent urothelial carcinoma

Proprietary Name/Clinical Laboratory/Manufacturer	Code	Descriptor
Category I Codes for Multianalyte Assays with Algorithmic Analyses (MAAA)		
Vectra® DA, Crescendo Bioscience, Inc.	81490	Autoimmune (rheumatoid arthritis), analysis of 12 biomarkers using immunoassays, utilizing serum, prognostic algorithm reported as a disease activity score (Do not report 81490 with 86140)
Corus® CAD, CardioDx, Inc.	81493	Coronary artery disease, mRNA, gene expression profiling by real-time RT-PCR of 23 genes, utilizing whole peripheral blood, algorithm reported as a risk score
AlloMap®, CareDx, Inc.	81595	Cardiology (heart transplant), mRNA, gene expression profiling by real-time quantitative PCR of 20 genes (11 content and 9 housekeeping), utilizing subfraction of peripheral blood, algorithm reported as a rejection risk score
Risk of Ovarian Malignancy Algorithm (ROMA)™, Fujirebio Diagnostics	81500	Oncology (ovarian), biochemical assays of two proteins (CA-125 and HE4), utilizing serum, with menopausal status, algorithm reported as a risk score
OVA1™, Vermillion, Inc.	81503	Oncology (ovarian), biochemical assays of five proteins (CA-125, apolipoprotein A1, beta-2 microglobulin, transferrin, and pre-albumin), utilizing serum, algorithm reported as a risk score
Tissue of Origin Test, Kit-FFPE, Cancer Genetics, Inc.	81504	Oncology (tissue of origin), microarray gene expression profiling of >2000 genes, utilizing formalin-fixed paraffin embedded tissue, algorithm reported as tissue similarity scores
PreDx Diabetes Risk Score™, Tethys Clinical Laboratory	81506	Endocrinology (type 2 diabetes), biochemical assays of seven analytes (glucose, HbA1c, insulin, hs-CRP, adiponectin, ferritin, interleukin 2-receptor alpha), utilizing serum or plasma, algorithm reporting a risk score
Harmony™ Prenatal Test, Ariosa Diagnostics	81507	Fetal aneuploidy (trisomy 21, 18, and 13) DNA sequence analysis of selected regions using maternal plasma, algorithm reported as a risk score for each trisomy
No proprietary name and clinical laboratory or manufacturer. Maternal serum screening procedures are performed by many labs and are not exclusive to a single facility.	81508	Fetal congenital abnormalities, biochemical assays of two proteins (PAPP-A, hCG [any form]), utilizing maternal serum, algorithm reported as a risk score
	81509	Fetal congenital abnormalities, biochemical assays of three proteins (PAPP-A, hCG [any form], DIA), utilizing maternal serum, algorithm reported as a risk score
	81510	Fetal congenital abnormalities, biochemical assays of three analytes (AFP, uE3, hCG (any form)), utilizing maternal serum, algorithm reported as a risk score
	81511	Fetal congenital abnormalities, biochemical assays of four analytes (AFP, uE3, hCG (any form), DIA) utilizing maternal serum, algorithm reported as a risk score (may include additional results from previous biochemical testing)
	81512	Fetal congenital abnormalities, biochemical assays of five analytes (AFP, uE3, total hCG, hyperglycosylated hCG, DIA) utilizing maternal serum, algorithm reported as a risk score
Breast Cancer Index, Biotheranostics, Inc	81518	Oncology (breast), mRNA, gene expression profiling by real-time RT-PCR of 11 genes (7 content and 4 housekeeping), utilizing formalin-fixed paraffin-embedded tissue, algorithms reported as percentage risk for metastatic recurrence and likelihood of benefit from extended endocrine therapy
EndoPredict®, Myriad Genetic Laboratories, Inc.	# ● 81522	Oncology (breast), mRNA, gene expression profiling by RT-PCR of 12 genes (8 content and 4 housekeeping), utilizing formalin-fixed paraffin-embedded tissue, algorithm reported as recurrence risk score
Oncotype DX® Genomic Health	81519	Oncology (breast), mRNA, gene expression profiling by real-time RT-PCR of 21 genes, utilizing formalin-fixed paraffin embedded tissue, algorithm reported as recurrence score
Prosigna® Breast Cancer Assay, NanoString Technologies, Inc.	81520	Oncology (breast), mRNA gene expression profiling by hybrid capture of 58 genes (50 content and 8 housekeeping), utilizing formalin-fixed paraffin-embedded tissue, algorithm reported as a recurrence risk score
MammaPrint®, Agendia, Inc.	81521	Oncology (breast), mRNA, microarray gene expression profiling of 70 content genes and 465 housekeeping genes, utilizing fresh frozen or formalin-fixed paraffin-embedded tissue, algorithm reported as index related to risk of distant metastasis
Oncotype DX® Colon Cancer Assay, Genomic Health	81525	Oncology (colon), mRNA, gene expression profiling by real-time RT-PCR of 12 genes (7 content and 5 housekeeping), utilizing formalin-fixed paraffin-embedded tissue, algorithm reported as a recurrence score
Cologuard™, Exact Sciences, Inc.	81528	Oncology (colorectal) screening, quantitative real-time target and signal amplification of 10 DNA markers (KRAS mutations, promoter methylation of NDRG4 and BMP3) and fecal hemoglobin, utilizing stool, algorithm reported as a positive or negative result (Do not report 81528 with 81275, 82274)
ChemoFX®, Helomics, Corp.	81535	Oncology (gynecologic), live tumor cell culture and chemotherapeutic response by DAPI stain and morphology, predictive algorithm reported as a drug response score; first single drug or drug combination
ChemoFX®, Helomics, Corp.	+ 81536	Oncology (gynecologic), live tumor cell culture and chemotherapeutic response by DAPI stain and morphology, predictive algorithm reported as a drug response score; each additional single drug or drug combination (List separately in addition to code for primary procedure) (Code first 81535)

Proprietary Name/Clinical Laboratory/Manufacturer	Code	Descriptor
VeriStrat, Biodesix, Inc.	81538	Oncology (lung), mass spectrometric 8-protein signature, including amyloid A, utilizing serum, prognostic and predictive algorithm reported as good versus poor overall survival
4Kscore test, OPKO Health Inc.	81539	Oncology (high-grade prostate cancer), biochemical assay of four proteins (Total PSA, Free PSA, Intact PSA, and human kallikrein-2 [hK2]), utilizing plasma or serum, prognostic algorithm reported as a probability score
CancerTYPE ID, bioTheranostics, Inc.	81540	Oncology (tumor of unknown origin), mRNA, gene expression profiling by real-time RT-PCR of 92 genes (87 content and 5 housekeeping) to classify tumor into main cancer type and subtype, utilizing formalin-fixed paraffin-embedded tissue, algorithm reported as a probability of a predicted main cancer type and subtype
Prolaris®, Myriad Genetic Laboratories, Inc.	81541	Oncology (prostate), mRNA gene expression profiling by real-time RT-PCR of 46 genes (31 content and 15 housekeeping), utilizing formalin- fixed paraffin-embedded tissue, algorithm reported as a disease-specific mortality risk score
Decipher® Prostate, Decipher® Biosciences	● 81542	Oncology (prostate), mRNA, microarray gene expression profiling of 22 content genes, utilizing formalin-fixed paraffin-embedded tissue, algorithm reported as metastasis risk score
Afirma® Gene Expression Classifier, Veracyte, Inc.	81545	Oncology (thyroid), gene expression analysis of 142 genes, utilizing fine needle aspirate, algorithm reported as a categorical result (eg, benign or suspicious)
ConfirmMDx® for Prostate Cancer, MDxHealth, Inc.	81551	Oncology (prostate), promoter methylation profiling by real-time PCR of 3 genes (GSTP1, APC, RASSF1), utilizing formalin-fixed paraffin-embedded tissue, algorithm reported as a likelihood of prostate cancer detection on repeat biopsy
DecisionDx®-UM test, Castle Biosciences, Inc.	● 81552	Oncology (uveal melanoma), mRNA, gene expression profiling by real-time RT-PCR of 15 genes (12 content and 3 housekeeping), utilizing fine needle aspirate or formalin-fixed paraffin-embedded tissue, algorithm reported as risk of metastasis
HCV FibroSURE™, FibroTest™, BioPredictive S.A.S.	81596	Infectious disease, chronic hepatitis C virus (HCV) infection, six biochemical assays (ALT, A2-macroglobulin, apolipoprotein A-1, total bilirubin, GGT, and haptoglobin) utilizing serum, prognostic algorithm reported as scores for fibrosis and necroinflammatory activity in liver
	81599	Unlisted multianalyte assay with algorithmic analysis
Proprietary Laboratory Analyses (PLA)		
PreciseType® HEA Test, Immucor, Inc.	0001U	Red blood cell antigen typing, DNA, human erythrocyte antigen gene analysis of 35 antigens from 11 blood groups, utilizing whole blood, common RBC alleles reported
PolypDX™, Atlantic Diagnostic Laboratories, LLC, Metabolomic Technologies, Inc.	0002U	Oncology (colorectal), quantitative assessment of three urine metabolites (ascorbic acid, succinic acid and carnitine) by liquid chromatography with tandem mass spectrometry (LC-MS/MS) using multiple reaction monitoring acquisition, algorithm reported as likelihood of adenomatous polyps
Overa (OVA1 Next Generation), Aspira Labs, Inc, Vermillion, Inc.	0003U	Oncology (ovarian) biochemical assays of five proteins (apolipoprotein A-1, CA 125 II, follicle stimulating hormone, human epididymis protein 4, transferrin), utilizing serum, algorithm reported as a likelihood score
	(0004U has been deleted)	
ExosomeDx®, Prostate (IntelliScore), Exosome Diagnostics, Inc, Exosome Diagnostics, Inc	0005U	Oncology (prostate) gene expression profile by real-time RT-PCR of 3 genes (ERG, PCA3, and SPDEF), urine, algorithm reported as risk score
Drug-drug, Drug-substance Identification and Interaction, Aegis Sciences Corporation	0006U	Detection of interacting medications, substances, supplements and foods, 120 or more analytes, definitive chromatography with mass spectrometry, urine, description and severity of each interaction identified, per date of service
ToxProtect, Genotox Laboratories Ltd	0007U	Drug test(s), presumptive, with definitive confirmation of positive results, any number of drug classes, urine, includes specimen verification including DNA authentication in comparison to buccal DNA, per date of service.
AmHPR® H. pylori Antibiotic Resistance Panel, American Molecular Laboratories, Inc.	▲ 0008U	Helicobacter pylori detection and antibiotic resistance, DNA, 16S and 23S rRNA, gyrA, pbp1,rdxA and rpoB, next generation sequencing, formalin-fixed paraffin-embedded or fresh tissue or fecal sample, predictive, reported as positive or negative for resistance to clarithromycin, fluoroquinolones, metronidazole, amoxicillin, tetracycline, and rifabutin
DEPArray™HER2, PacificDx	0009U	Oncology (breast cancer), *ERBB2* (HER2) copy number by FISH, tumor cells from formalin-fixed paraffin-embedded tissue isolated using image-based dielectrophoresis (DEP) sorting, reported as *ERBB2* gene amplified or non-amplified
Bacterial Typing by Whole Genome Sequencing, Mayo Clinic	0010U	Infectious disease (bacterial), strain typing by whole genome sequencing, phylogenetic-based report of strain relatedness, per submitted isolate
Cordant CORE™, Cordant Health Solutions	0011U	Prescription drug monitoring, evaluation of drugs present by LC-MS/MS, using oral fluid, reported as a comparison to an estimated steady-state range, per date of service including all drug compounds and metabolites
MatePair Targeted Rearrangements, Congenital, Mayo Clinic	0012U	Germline disorders, gene rearrangement detection by whole genome next-generation sequencing, DNA, whole blood, report of specific gene rearrangement(s)

Proprietary Name/Clinical Laboratory/Manufacturer	Code	Descriptor
MatePair Targeted Rearrangements, Oncology, Mayo Clinic	0013U	Oncology (solid organ neoplasia), gene rearrangement detection by whole genome next-generation sequencing, DNA, fresh or frozen tissue or cells, report of specific gene rearrangement(s)
MatePair Targeted Rearrangements, Hematologic, Mayo Clinic	0014U	Hematology (hematolymphoid neoplasia), gene rearrangement detection by whole genome next-generation sequencing, DNA, whole blood or bone marrow, report of specific gene
	(0015U has been deleted)	
BCR-ABL1 major and minor breakpoint fusion transcripts, University of Iowa, Department of Pathology, Asuragen	0016U	Oncology (hematolymphoid neoplasia), RNA, BCR/ABL1 major and minor breakpoint fusion transcripts, quantitative PCR amplification, blood or bone marrow, report of fusion not detected or detected with quantitation
JAK2 Mutation, University of Iowa, Department of Pathology	0017U	Oncology (hematolymphoid neoplasia), *JAK2* mutation, DNA, PCR amplification of exons 12-14 and sequence analysis, blood or bone marrow, report of JAK2 mutation not detected or detected
ThyraMIR™, Interpace Diagnostics	0018U	Oncology (thyroid), microRNA profiling by RT-PCR of 10 microRNA sequences, utilizing fine needle aspirate, algorithm reported as a positive or negative result for moderate to high risk of malignancy
OncoTarget/OncoTreat, Columbia University Department of Pathology and Cell Biology, Darwin Health	0019U	Oncology, RNA, gene expression by whole transcriptome sequencing, formalin-fixed paraffin embedded tissue or fresh frozen tissue, predictive algorithm reported as potential targets for therapeutic agents
	(0020U has been deleted)	
Apifiny®, Armune BioScience, Inc	0021U	Oncology (prostate), detection of 8 autoantibodies (ARF 6, NKX3-1, 5'-UTR-BMI1, CEP 164, 3'-UTR-Ropporin, Desmocollin, AURKAIP-1, CSNK2A2), multiplexed immunoassay and flow cytometry serum, algorithm reported as risk score
Oncomine™ Dx Target Test, Thermo Fisher Scientific	0022U	Targeted genomic sequence analysis panel, non-small cell lung neoplasia, DNA and RNA analysis, 23 genes, interrogation for sequence variants and rearrangements, reported as presence/absence of variants and associated therapy(ies) to consider
LeukoStrat® CDx *FLT3* Mutation Assay, LabPMM LLC, an Invivoscribe Technologies, Inc Company, Invivoscribe Technologies, Inc	0023U	Oncology (acute myelogenous leukemia), DNA, genotyping of internal tandem duplication, p.D835, p.I836, using mononuclear cells, reported as detection or non-detection of FLT3 mutation and indication for or against the use of midostaurin
GlycA, Laboratory Corporation of America, Laboratory Corporation of America	0024U	Glycosylated acute phase proteins (GlycA), nuclear magnetic resonance spectroscopy, quantitative
UrSure Tenofovir Quantification Test, Synergy Medical Laboratories, UrSure Inc	0025U	Tenofovir, by liquid chromatography with tandem mass spectrometry (LC-MS/MS), urine, quantitative
Thyroseq Genomic Classifier, CBLPath, Inc, University of Pittsburgh Medical Center	0026U	Oncology (thyroid), DNA and mRNA of 112 genes, next-generation sequencing, fine needle aspirate of thyroid nodule, algorithmic analysis reported as a categorical result ("Positive, high probability of malignancy" or "Negative, low probability of malignancy")
JAK2 Exons 12 to 15 Sequencing, Mayo Clinic, Mayo Clinic	0027U	*JAK2* (Janus kinase 2) (eg, myeloproliferative disorder) gene analysis, targeted sequence analysis exons 12-15
	(0028U has been deleted)	
Focused Pharmacogenomics Panel, Mayo Clinic, Mayo Clinic	0029U	Drug metabolism (adverse drug reactions and drug response), targeted sequence analysis (ie, *CYP1A2, CYP2C19, CYP2C9, CYP2D6, CYP3A4, CYP3A5, CYP4F2, SLCO1B1, VKORC1* and rs12777823)
Warfarin Response Genotype, Mayo Clinic, Mayo Clinic	0030U	Drug metabolism (warfarin drug response), targeted sequence analysis (i.e., *CYP2C9, CYP4F2, VKORC1*, rs12777823)
Cytochrome P450 1A2 Genotype, Mayo Clinic, Mayo Clinic	0031U	*CYP1A2 (cytochrome P450 family 1, subfamily A, member 2)* (eg, drug metabolism) gene analysis, common variants (ie, *1F, *1K, *6, *7)
Catechol-O- Methyltransferase *(COMT)* Genotype, Mayo Clinic, Mayo Clinic	0032U	*COMT (catechol-O-methyltransferase)* (eg, drug metabolism) gene analysis, c.472G>A (rs4680) variant
Serotonin Receptor Genotype *(HTR2A* and *HTR2C)*, Mayo Clinic, Mayo Clinic	0033U	*HTR2A (5-hydroxytryptamine receptor 2A), HTR2C (5-hydroxytryptamine receptor 2C) (eg, citalopram metabolism) gene analysis, common variants* (i.e., *HTR2A* rs7997012 [c.614-2211T>C], *HTR2C* rs3813929 [c.- 759C>T] and rs1414334 [c.551-3008C>G])
Thiopurine Methyltransferase *(TPMT)* and Nudix Hydrolase *(NUDT15)* Genotyping, Mayo Clinic, Mayo Clinic	0034U	*TPMT (thiopurine S-methyltransferase), NUDT15 (nudix hydroxylase 15)* (eg, thiopurine metabolism) gene analysis, common variants (i.e., *TPMT* *2, *3A, *3B, *3C, *4, *5, *6, *8, *12; *NUDT15* *3, *4, *5)
Real-time quaking- induced conversion for prion detection (RT- QuIC), National Prion Disease Pathology Surveillance Center	0035U	Neurology (prion disease), cerebrospinal fluid, detection of prion protein by quaking- induced conformational conversion, qualitative
EXaCT-1 Whole Exome Testing, Lab of Oncology-Molecular Detection, Weill Cornell Medicine-Clinical Genomics Laboratory	0036U	Exome (ie, somatic mutations), paired formalin-fixed paraffin-embedded tumor tissue and normal specimen, sequence analyses
FoundationOne CDx™ (F1CDx), Foundation Medicine, Inc, Foundation Medicine, Inc	0037U	Targeted genomic sequence analysis, solid organ neoplasm, DNA analysis of 324 genes, interrogation for sequence variants, gene copy number amplifications, gene rearrangements, microsatellite instability and tumor mutational burden

Proprietary Name/Clinical Laboratory/Manufacturer	Code	Descriptor
Sensieva ™ Droplet 25OH Vitamin D2/D3 Microvolume LC/MS Assay, InSource Diagnostics, InSource Diagnostics	0038U	Vitamin D, 25 hydroxy D2 and D3, by LC- MS/MS, serum microsample, quantitative
Anti-dsDNA, High Salt/Avidity, University of Washington, Department of Laboratory Medicine, Bio-Rad	0039U	Deoxyribonucleic acid (DNA) antibody, double stranded, high avidity
MRDx BCR-ABL Test, MolecularMD, MolecularMD	0040U	*BCR/ABL1 (t(9;22))* (eg, chronic myelogenous leukemia) translocation analysis, major breakpoint, quantitative
Lyme ImmunoBlot IgM, IGeneX Inc, ID-FISH Technology Inc. (ASR) (Lyme ImmunoBlot IgM Strips Only)	0041U	Borrelia burgdorferi, antibody detection of 5 recombinant protein groups, by immunoblot, IgM
Lyme ImmunoBlot IgG, IGeneX Inc, ID-FISH Technology Inc (ASR) (Lyme ImmunoBlot IgG Strips Only)	0042U	Borrelia burgdorferi, antibody detection of 12 recombinant protein groups, by immunoblot, IgG
Tick-Borne Relapsing Fever (TBRF) Borrelia ImmunoBlots IgM Test, IGeneX Inc, ID-FISH Technology Inc (Provides TBRF ImmunoBlot IgM Strips)	0043U	Tick-borne relapsing fever Borrelia group, antibody detection to 4 recombinant protein groups, by immunoblot, IgM
Tick-Borne Relapsing Fever (TBRF) Borrelia ImmunoBlots IgG Test, IGeneX Inc., ID-FISH Technology Inc (Provides TBRF ImmunoBlot IgG Strips)	0044U	Tick-borne relapsing fever Borrelia group, antibody detection to 4 recombinant protein groups, by immunoblot, IgG
The Oncotype DX® Breast DCIS Score™ Test, Genomic Health, Inc, Genomic Health, Inc	0045U	Oncology (breast ductal carcinoma in situ), mRNA, gene expression profiling by real- time RT-PCR of 12 genes (7 content and 5 housekeeping), utilizing formalin-fixed paraffin-embedded tissue, algorithm reported as recurrence score
FLT3 ITD MRD by NGS, LabPMM LLC, an Invivoscribe Technologies, Inc Company	0046U	*FLT3 (fms-related tyrosine kinase 3)* (eg, acute myeloid leukemia) internal tandem duplication (ITD) variants, quantitative
Oncotype DX Genomic Prostate Score, Genomic Health, Inc, Genomic Health, Inc	0047U	Oncology (prostate), mRNA, gene expression profiling by real-time RT-PCR of 17 genes (12 content and 5 housekeeping), utilizing formalin-fixed paraffin-embedded tissue, algorithm reported as a risk score
MSK-IMPACT (Integrated Mutation Profiling of Actionable Cancer Targets), Memorial Sloan Kettering Cancer Center	0048U	Oncology (solid organ neoplasia), DNA, targeted sequencing of protein-coding exons of 468 cancer-associated genes, including interrogation for somatic mutations and microsatellite instability, matched with normal specimens, utilizing formalin-fixed paraffin-embedded tumor tissue, report of clinically significant mutation(s)
NPM1 MRD by NGS, LabPMM LLC, an Invivoscribe Technologies, Inc Company	0049U	*NPM1 (nucleophosmin)* (eg, acute myeloid leukemia) gene analysis, quantitative
MyAML NGS Panel, LabPMM LLC, an Invivoscribe Technologies, Inc Company	0050U	Targeted genomic sequence analysis panel, acute myelogenous leukemia, DNA analysis, 194 genes, interrogation for sequence variants, copy number variants or rearrangements
UCompliDx, Elite Medical Laboratory Solutions, LLC, Elite Medical Laboratory Solutions, LLC (LDT)	0051U	Prescription drug monitoring, evaluation of drugs present by LC-MS/MS, urine, 31 drug panel, reported as quantitative results, detected or not detected, per date of service
VAP Cholesterol Test, VAP Diagnostics Laboratory, Inc, VAP Diagnostics Laboratory, Inc	0052U	Lipoprotein, blood, high resolution fractionation and quantitation of lipoproteins, including all five major lipoprotein classes and subclasses of HDL, LDL, and VLDL by vertical auto profile ultracentrifugation
Prostate Cancer Risk Panel, Mayo Clinic, Laboratory Developed Test	0053U	Oncology (prostate cancer), FISH analysis of 4 genes (*ASAP1, HDAC9, CHD1 and PTEN*), needle biopsy specimen, algorithm reported as probability of higher tumor grade
AssuranceRx Micro Serum, Firstox Laboratories, LLC, Firstox Laboratories, LLC	0054U	Prescription drug monitoring, 14 or more classes of drugs and substances, definitive tandem mass spectrometry with chromatography, capillary blood, quantitative report with therapeutic and toxic ranges, including steady-state range for the prescribed dose when detected, per date of service
myTAIHEART, TAI Diagnostics, Inc, TAI Diagnostics, Inc	0055U	Cardiology (heart transplant), cell-free DNA, PCR assay of 96 DNA target sequences (94 single nucleotide polymorphism targets and two control targets), plasma
MatePair Acute Myeloid Leukemia Panel, Mayo Clinic, Laboratory Developed Test	0056U	Hematology (acute myelogenous leukemia), DNA, whole genome next-generation sequencing to detect gene rearrangement(s), blood or bone marrow, report of specific gene rearrangement(s)
	(0057U has been deleted)	
Merkel SmT Oncoprotein Antibody Titer, University of Washington, Department of Laboratory Medicine	0058U	Oncology (Merkel cell carcinoma), detection of antibodies to the Merkel cell polyoma virus oncoprotein (small T antigen), serum, quantitative
Merkel Virus VP1 Capsid Antibody, University of Washington, Department of Laboratory Medicine	0059U	Oncology (Merkel cell carcinoma), detection of antibodies to the Merkel cell polyoma virus capsid protein (VP1), serum, reported as positive or negative
Twins Zygosity PLA, Natera, Inc, Natera, Inc	0060U	Twin zygosity, genomic-targeted sequence analysis of chromosome 2, using circulating cell-free fetal DNA in maternal blood
Transcutaneous multispectral measurement of tissue oxygenation and hemoglobin using spatial frequency domain imaging (SFDI), Modulated Imaging, Inc, Modulated Imaging, Inc	0061U	Transcutaneous measurement of five biomarkers (tissue oxygenation [StO2], oxyhemoglobin [ctHbO2], deoxyhemoglobin [ctHbR], papillary and reticular dermal hemoglobin concentrations [ctHb1 and ctHb2]), using spatial frequency domain imaging (SFDI) and multi-spectral analysis

Proprietary Name/Clinical Laboratory/Manufacturer	Code	Descriptor
SLE-key® Rule Out, Veracis Inc, Veracis Inc	● 0062U	Autoimmune (systemic lupus erythematosus), IgG and IgM analysis of 80 biomarkers, utilizing serum, algorithm reported with a risk score
NPDX ASD ADM Panel I, Stemina Biomarker Discovery, Inc, Stemina Biomarker Discovery, Inc d/b/a NeuroPointDX	● 0063U	Neurology (autism), 32 amines by LC-MS/MS, using plasma, algorithm reported as metabolic signature associated with autism spectrum disorder
BioPlex 2200 Syphilis Total & RPR Assay, Bio-Rad Laboratories, Bio-Rad Laboratories	● 0064U	Antibody, Treponema pallidum, total and rapid plasma reagin (RPR), immunoassay, qualitative
BioPlex 2200 RPR Assay, Bio-Rad Laboratories, Bio-Rad Laboratories	● 0065U	Syphilis test, non-treponemal antibody, immunoassay, qualitative (RPR)
PartoSure™ Test, Parsagen Diagnostics, Inc, Parsagen Diagnostics, Inc, a QIAGEN Company	● 0066U	Placental alpha-micro globulin-1 (PAMG-1), immunoassay with direct optical observation, cervico-vaginal fluid, each specimen
BBDRisk Dx™, Silbiotech, Inc, Silbiotech, Inc	● 0067U	Oncology (breast), immunohistochemistry, protein expression profiling of 4 biomarkers (matrix metalloproteinase-1 [MMP-1], carcinoembryonic antigen-related cell adhesion molecule 6 [CEACAM6], hyaluronoglucosaminidase [HYAL1], highly expressed in cancer protein [HEC1]), formalin-fixed paraffin-embedded precancerous breast tissue, algorithm reported as carcinoma risk score
MYCODART Dual Amplification Real Time PCR Panel for 6 Candida species, RealTime Laboratories, Inc, RealTime Laboratories, Inc	● 0068U	Candida species panel *(C. albicans, C. glabrata, C. parapsilosis, C. kruseii, C tropicalis, and C. auris)*, amplified probe technique with qualitative report of the presence or absence of each species
miR-31now™, GoPath Laboratories, GoPath Laboratories	● 0069U	Oncology (colorectal), microRNA, RT-PCR expression profiling of miR-31-3p, formalin-fixed paraffin-embedded tissue, algorithm reported as an expression score
CYP2D6 Common Variants and Copy Number, Mayo Clinic, Laboratory Developed Test	● 0070U	*CYP2D6 (cytochrome P450, family 2, subfamily D, polypeptide 6)* (eg, drug metabolism) gene analysis, common and select rare variants (ie, *2, *3, *4, *4N, *5, *6, *7, *8, *9, *10, *11, *12, *13, *14A, *14B, *15, *17, *29, *35, *36, *41, *57, *61, *63, *68, *83, *xN)
CYP2D6 Full Gene Sequencing, Mayo Clinic, Laboratory Developed Test	+● 0071U	*CYP2D6 (cytochrome P450, family 2, subfamily D, polypeptide 6)* (eg, drug metabolism) gene analysis, full gene sequence (List separately in addition to code for primary procedure)
CYP2D6-2D7 Hybrid Gene Targeted Sequence Analysis, Mayo Clinic, Laboratory Developed Test	+● 0072U	*CYP2D6 (cytochrome P450, family 2, subfamily D, polypeptide 6)* (eg, drug metabolism) gene analysis, targeted sequence analysis (ie, CYP2D6-2D7 hybrid gene) (List separately in addition to code for primary procedure)
CYP2D7-2D6 Hybrid Gene Targeted Sequence Analysis, Mayo Clinic, Laboratory Developed Test	+● 0073U	*CYP2D6 (cytochrome P450, family 2, subfamily D, polypeptide 6)* (eg, drug metabolism) gene analysis, targeted sequence analysis (ie, CYP2D7-2D6 hybrid gene) (List separately in addition to code for primary procedure)
CYP2D7-2D6 trans-duplication/multiplication non-duplicated gene targeted sequence analysis, Mayo Clinic, Laboratory Developed Test	+● 0074U	*CYP2D6 (cytochrome P450, family 2, subfamily D, polypeptide 6)* (eg, drug metabolism) gene analysis, targeted sequence analysis (ie, non-duplicated gene when duplication/multiplication is trans) (List separately in addition to code for primary procedure)
CYP2D6 5' gene duplication/multiplication targeted sequence analysis, Mayo Clinic, Laboratory Developed Test	+● 0075U	*CYP2D6 (cytochrome P450, family 2, subfamily D, polypeptide 6)* (eg, drug metabolism) gene analysis, targeted sequence analysis (ie, 5' gene duplication/multiplication) (List separately in addition to code for primary procedure)
CYP2D6 3' gene duplication/multiplication targeted sequence analysis, Mayo Clinic, Laboratory Developed Test	+● 0076U	*CYP2D6 (cytochrome P450, family 2, subfamily D, polypeptide 6)* (eg, drug metabolism) gene analysis, targeted sequence analysis (ie, 3' gene duplication/multiplication) (List separately in addition to code for primary procedure)
M-Protein Detection and Isotyping by MALDI-TOF Mass Spectrometry, Mayo Clinic, Laboratory Developed Test	● 0077U	Immunoglobulin paraprotein (M-protein), qualitative, immunoprecipitation and mass spectrometry, blood or urine, including isotype
INFINITI® Neural Response Panel, PersonalizeDx Labs, AutoGenomics Inc	● 0078U	Pain management (opioid-use disorder) genotyping panel, 16 common variants (ie, *ABCB1, COMT, DAT1, DBH, DOR, DRD1, DRD2, DRD4, GABA, GAL, HTR2A, HTTLPR, MTHFR, MUOR, OPRK1, OPRM1*), buccal swab or other germline tissue sample, algorithm reported as positive or negative risk of opioid-use disorder
ToxLok™, InSource Diagnostics, InSource Diagnostics	● 0079U	Comparative DNA analysis using multiple selected single-nucleotide polymorphisms (SNPs), urine and buccal DNA, for specimen identity verification
BDX-XL2, Biodesix®, Inc, Biodesix®, Inc	● 0080U	Oncology (lung), mass spectrometric analysis of galectin-3-binding protein and scavenger receptor cysteine-rich type 1 protein M130, with five clinical risk factors (age, smoking status, nodule diameter, nodule-spiculation status and nodule location), utilizing plasma, algorithm reported as a categorical probability of malignancy
	(0081U has been deleted. To report, use 81552)	

Proprietary Name/Clinical Laboratory/Manufacturer	Code	Descriptor
NextGen Precision™ Testing, Precision Diagnostics, Precision Diagnostics LBN Precision Toxicology, LLC	● 0082U	Drug test(s), definitive, 90 or more drugs or substances, definitive chromatography with mass spectrometry, and presumptive, any number of drug classes, by instrument chemistry analyzer (utilizing immunoassay), urine, report of presence or absence of each drug, drug metabolite or substance with description and severity of significant interactions per date of service
Onco4D™, Animated Dynamics, Inc, Animated Dynamics, Inc	● 0083U	Oncology, response to chemotherapy drugs using motility contrast tomography, fresh or frozen tissue, reported as likelihood of sensitivity or resistance to drugs or drug combinations
BLOODchip®, ID CORE XT™, Grifols Diagnostic Solutions Inc	● 0084U	Red blood cell antigen typing, DNA, genotyping of 10 blood groups with phenotype prediction of 37 red blood cell antigens
	(0085U has been deleted)	
Accelerate PhenoTest™ BC kit, Accelerate Diagnostics, Inc	● 0086U	Infectious disease (bacterial and fungal), organism identification, blood culture, using rRNA FISH, 6 or more organism targets, reported as positive or negative with phenotypic minimum inhibitory concentration (MIC)-based antimicrobial susceptibility
Molecular Microscope® MMDx—Heart, Kashi Clinical Laboratories	● 0087U	Cardiology (heart transplant), mRNA gene expression profiling by microarray of 1283 genes, transplant biopsy tissue, allograft rejection and injury algorithm reported as a probability score
Molecular Microscope® MMDx—Kidney, Kashi Clinical Laboratories	● 0088U	Transplantation medicine (kidney allograft rejection), microarray gene expression profiling of 1494 genes, utilizing transplant biopsy tissue, algorithm reported as a probability score for rejection
Pigmented Lesion Assay (PLA), DermTech	● 0089U	Oncology (melanoma), gene expression profiling by RTqPCR, *PRAME* and *LINC00518*, superficial collection using adhesive patch(es)
myPath® Melanoma, Myriad Genetic Laboratories	● 0090U	Oncology (cutaneous melanoma), mRNA gene expression profiling by RT-PCR of 23 genes (14 content and 9 housekeeping), utilizing formalin-fixed paraffin-embedded tissue, algorithm reported as a categorical result (ie, benign, indeterminate, malignant)
FirstSight[CRC], CellMax Life	● 0091U	Oncology (colorectal) screening, cell enumeration of circulating tumor cells, utilizing whole blood, algorithm, for the presence of adenoma or cancer, reported as a positive or negative result
REVEAL Lung Nodule Characterization, MagArray, Inc	● 0092U	Oncology (lung), three protein biomarkers, immunoassay using magnetic nanosensor technology, plasma, algorithm reported as risk score for likelihood of malignancy
ComplyRX, Claro Labs	● 0093U	Prescription drug monitoring, evaluation of 65 common drugs by LC-MS/MS, urine, each drug reported detected or not detected
RCIGM Rapid Whole Genome Sequencing, Rady Children's Institute for Genomic Medicine (RCIGM)	● 0094U	Genome (eg, unexplained constitutional or heritable disorder or syndrome), rapid sequence analysis
Esophageal String Test™ (EST), Cambridge Biomedical, Inc	● 0095U	Inflammation (eosinophilic esophagitis), ELISA analysis of eotaxin-3 *(CCL26 [C-C motif chemokine ligand 26])* and major basic protein *(PRG2 [proteoglycan 2, pro eosinophil major basic protein])*, specimen obtained by swallowed nylon string, algorithm reported as predictive probability index for active eosinophilic esophagitis
HPV, High-Risk, Male Urine, Molecular Testing Labs	● 0096U	Human papillomavirus (HPV), high-risk types (ie, 16, 18, 31, 33, 35, 39, 45, 51, 52, 56, 58, 59, 66, 68), male urine
BioFire® FilmArray® Gastrointestinal (GI) Panel, BioFire® Diagnostics	● 0097U	Gastrointestinal pathogen, multiplex reverse transcription and multiplex amplified probe technique, multiple types or subtypes, 22 targets (Campylobacter [C. jejuni/C. coli/C. upsaliensis], Clostridium difficile [C. difficile] toxin A/B, Plesiomonas shigelloides, Salmonella, Vibrio [V. parahaemolyticus/V. vulnificus/V. cholerae], including specific identification of Vibrio cholerae, Yersinia enterocolitica, Enteroaggregative Escherichia coli [EAEC], Enteropathogenic Escherichia coli [EPEC], Enterotoxigenic Escherichia coli [ETEC] lt/st, Shiga-like toxin-producing Escherichia coli [STEC] stx1/stx2 [including specific identification of the E. coli O157 serogroup within STEC], Shigella/Enteroinvasive Escherichia coli [EIEC], Cryptosporidium, Cyclospora cayetanensis, Entamoeba histolytica, Giardia lamblia [also known as G. intestinalis and G. duodenalis], adenovirus F 40/41, astrovirus, norovirus GI/GII, rotavirus A, sapovirus [Genogroups I, II, IV, and V])

Proprietary Name/Clinical Laboratory/Manufacturer	Code	Descriptor
BioFire® FilmArray® Respiratory Panel (RP) EZ, BioFire® Diagnostics	● 0098U	Respiratory pathogen, multiplex reverse transcription and multiplex amplified probe technique, multiple types or subtypes, 14 targets (adenovirus, coronavirus, human metapneumovirus, influenza A, influenza A subtype H1, influenza A subtype H3, influenza A subtype H1-2009, influenza B, parainfluenza virus, human rhinovirus/enterovirus, respiratory syncytial virus, Bordetella pertussis, Chlamydophila pneumoniae, Mycoplasma pneumoniae)
BioFire® FilmArray® Respiratory Panel (RP), BioFire® Diagnostics	● 0099U	Respiratory pathogen, multiplex reverse transcription and multiplex amplified probe technique, multiple types or subtypes, 20 targets (adenovirus, coronavirus 229E, coronavirus HKU1, coronavirus, coronavirus OC43, human metapneumovirus, influenza A, influenza A subtype, influenza A subtype H3, influenza A subtype H1-2009, influenza, parainfluenza virus, parainfluenza virus 2, parainfluenza virus 3, parainfluenza virus 4, human rhinovirus/enterovirus, respiratory syncytial virus, Bordetella pertussis, Chlamydophila pneumonia, Mycoplasma pneumoniae)
BioFire® FilmArray® Respiratory Panel 2 (RP2), BioFire® Diagnostics	● 0100U	Respiratory pathogen, multiplex reverse transcription and multiplex amplified probe technique, multiple types or subtypes, 21 targets (adenovirus, coronavirus 229E, coronavirus HKU1, coronavirus NL63, coronavirus OC43, human metapneumovirus, human rhinovirus/enterovirus, influenza A, including subtypes H1, H1-2009, and H3, influenza B, parainfluenza virus 1, parainfluenza virus 2, parainfluenza virus 3, parainfluenza virus 4, respiratory syncytial virus, Bordetella parapertussis [IS1001], Bordetella pertussis [ptxP], Chlamydia pneumoniae, Mycoplasma pneumoniae)
ColoNext®, Ambry Genetics®, Ambry Genetics®	● 0101U	Hereditary colon cancer disorders (eg, Lynch syndrome, *PTEN* hamartoma syndrome, Cowden syndrome, familial adenomatosis polyposis), genomic sequence analysis panel utilizing a combination of NGS, Sanger, MLPA, and array CGH, with MRNA analytics to resolve variants of unknown significance when indicated (15 genes [sequencing and deletion/duplication], *EPCAM* and *GREM1* [deletion/duplication only])
BreastNext®, Ambry Genetics®, Ambry Genetics®	● 0102U	Hereditary breast cancer-related disorders (eg, hereditary breast cancer, hereditary ovarian cancer, hereditary endometrial cancer), genomic sequence analysis panel utilizing a combination of NGS, Sanger, MLPA, and array CGH, with MRNA analytics to resolve variants of unknown significance when indicated (17 genes [sequencing and deletion/duplication])
OvaNext®, Ambry Genetics®, Ambry Genetics®	● 0103U	Hereditary ovarian cancer (eg, hereditary ovarian cancer, hereditary endometrial cancer), genomic sequence analysis panel utilizing a combination of NGS, Sanger, MLPA, and array CGH, with MRNA analytics to resolve variants of unknown significance when indicated (24 genes [sequencing and deletion/duplication], *EPCAM* [deletion/duplication only])
	(0104U has been deleted)	
KidneyIntelXT™, RenalytixAI, RenalytixAI	● 0105U	Nephrology (chronic kidney disease), multiplex electrochemiluminescent immunoassay (ECLIA) of tumor necrosis factor receptor 1A, receptor superfamily 2 *(TNFR1, TNFR2)*, and kidney injury molecule-1 (KIM-1) combined with longitudinal clinical data, including *APOL1* genotype if available, and plasma (isolated fresh or frozen), algorithm reported as probability score for rapid kidney function decline (RKFD)
13C-Spirulina Gastric Emptying Breath Test (GEBT), Cairn Diagnostics d/b/a Advanced Breath Diagnostics, LLC, Cairn Diagnostics d/b/a Advanced Breath Diagnostics, LLC	● 0106U	Gastric emptying, serial collection of 7 timed breath specimens, non-radioisotope carbon-13(^{13}C) spirulina substrate, analysis of each specimen by gas isotope ratio mass spectrometry, reported as rate of $^{13}CO_2$ excretion
Singulex Clarity C.diff toxins A/B aAssay, Singulex	● 0107U	Clostridium difficile toxin(s) antigen detection by immunoassay technique, stool, qualitative, multiple-step method
TissueCypher® Barrett's Esophagus Assay, Cernostics, Cernostics	● 0108U	Gastroenterology (Barrett's esophagus), whole slide-digital imaging, including morphometric analysis, computer-assisted quantitative immunolabeling of 9 protein biomarkers (p16, AMACR, p53, CD68, COX-2, CD45RO, HIF1a, HER-2, K20) and morphology, formalin-fixed paraffin-embedded tissue, algorithm reported as risk of progression to high-grade dysplasia or cancer

Proprietary Name/Clinical Laboratory/Manufacturer	Code	Descriptor
MYCODART Dual Amplification Real Time PCR Panel for 4 Aspergillus species, RealTime Laboratories, Inc/MycoDART, Inc	● 0109U	Infectious disease (Aspergillus species), real-time PCR for detection of DNA from 4 species *(A. fumigatus, A. terreus, A. niger,* and *A. flavus)*, blood, lavage fluid, or tissue, qualitative reporting of presence or absence of each species
Oral OncolyticAssuranceRX, Firstox Laboratories, LLC, Firstox Laboratories, LLC	● 0110U	Prescription drug monitoring, one or more oral oncology drug(s) and substances, definitive tandem mass spectrometry with chromatography, serum or plasma from capillary blood or venous blood, quantitative report with steady-state range for the prescribed drug(s) when detected
Praxis(™) Extended RAS Panel, Illumina, Illumina	● 0111U	Oncology (colon cancer), targeted *KRAS* (codons 12, 13, and 61) and *NRAS* (codons 12, 13, and 61) gene analysis utilizing formalin-fixed paraffin-embedded tissue
MicroGenDX qPCR & NGS For Infection, MicroGenDX, MicroGenDX	● 0112U	Infectious agent detection and identification, targeted sequence analysis (16S and 18S rRNA genes) with drug-resistance gene
MiPS (Mi-Prostate Score), MLabs, MLabs	● 0113U	Oncology (prostate), measurement of *PCA3* and *TMPRSS2-ERG* in urine and PSA in serum following prostatic massage, by RNA amplification and fluorescence-based detection, algorithm reported as risk score
EsoGuard™, Lucid Diagnostics, Lucid Diagnostics	● 0114U	Gastroenterology (Barrett's esophagus), *VIM* and *CCNA1* methylation analysis, esophageal cells, algorithm reported as likelihood for Barrett's esophagus
ePlex Respiratory Pathogen (RP) Panel, GenMark Diagnostics, Inc, GenMark Diagnostics, Inc	● 0115U	Respiratory infectious agent detection by nucleic acid (DNA and RNA), 18 viral types and subtypes and 2 bacterial targets, amplified probe technique, including multiplex reverse transcription for RNA targets, each analyte reported as detected or not detected
Snapshot Oral Fluid Compliance, Ethos Laboratories	● 0116U	Prescription drug monitoring, enzyme immunoassay of 35 or more drugs confirmed with LC-MS/MS, oral fluid, algorithm results reported as a patient-compliance measurement with risk of drug to drug interactions for prescribed medications
Foundation PI?, Ethos Laboratories	● 0117U	Pain management, analysis of 11 endogenous analytes (methylmalonic acid, xanthurenic acid, homocysteine, pyroglutamic acid, vanilmandelate, 5-hydroxyindoleacetic acid, hydroxymethylglutarate, ethylmalonate, 3-hydroxypropyl mercapturic acid (3-HPMA), quinolinic acid, kynurenic acid), LC-MS/MS, urine, algorithm reported as a pain-index score with likelihood of atypical biochemical function associated with pain
Viracor TRAC™ dd-cfDNA, Viracor Eurofins, Viracor Eurofins	● 0118U	Transplantation medicine, quantification of donor-derived cell-free DNA using whole genome next-generation sequencing, plasma, reported as percentage of donor-derived cell-free DNA in the total cell-free DNA
MI-HEART Ceramides, Plasma, Mayo Clinic, Laboratory Developed Test	● 0119U	Cardiology, ceramides by liquid chromatography-tandem mass spectrometry, plasma, quantitative report with risk score for major cardiovascular events
Lymph3Cx Lymphoma Molecular Subtyping Assay, Mayo Clinic, Laboratory Developed Test	● 0120U	Oncology (B-cell lymphoma classification), mRNA, gene expression profiling by fluorescent probe hybridization of 58 genes (45 content and 13 housekeeping genes), formalin-fixed paraffin-embedded tissue, algorithm reported as likelihood for primary mediastinal B-cell lymphoma (PMBCL) and diffuse large B-cell lymphoma (DLBCL) with cell of origin subtyping in the latter
Flow Adhesion of Whole Blood on VCAM-1 (FAB-V), Functional Fluidics, Functional Fluidics	● 0121U	Sickle cell disease, microfluidic flow adhesion (VCAM-1), whole blood
Flow Adhesion of Whole Blood to P-SELECTIN (WB-PSEL), Functional Fluidics, Functional Fluidics	● 0122U	Sickle cell disease, microfluidic flow adhesion (P-Selectin), whole blood
Mechanical Fragility, RBC by shear stress profiling and spectral analysis, Functional Fluidics, Functional Fluidics	● 0123U	Mechanical fragility, RBC, shear stress and spectral analysis profiling
First Trimester Screen | Fß?, Eurofins NTD, LLC, Eurofins NTD, LLC	● 0124U	Fetal congenital abnormalities, biochemical assays of 3 analytes (free beta-hCG, PAPP-A, AFP), time-resolved fluorescence immunoassay, maternal dried-blood spot, algorithm reported as risk scores for fetal trisomies 13/18 and 21

Proprietary Name/Clinical Laboratory/Manufacturer	Code	Descriptor
Maternal Fetal Screen | T1?, Eurofins NTD, LLC, Eurofins NTD, LLC	● 0125U	Fetal congenital abnormalities and perinatal complications, biochemical assays of 5 analytes (free beta-hCG, PAPP-A, AFP, placental growth factor, and inhibin-A), time-resolved fluorescence immunoassay, maternal serum, algorithm reported as risk scores for fetal trisomies 13/18, 21, and preeclampsia
Maternal Fetal Screen | T1 + Y Chromosome ?, Eurofins NTD, LLC, Eurofins NTD, LLC	● 0126U	Fetal congenital abnormalities and perinatal complications, biochemical assays of 5 analytes (free beta-hCG, PAPP-A, AFP, placental growth factor, and inhibin-A), time-resolved fluorescence immunoassay, includes qualitative assessment of Y chromosome in cell-free fetal DNA, maternal serum and plasma, predictive algorithm reported as a risk scores for fetal trisomies 13/18, 21, and preeclampsia
Preeclampsia Screen | T1?, Eurofins NTD, LLC, Eurofins NTD, LLC	● 0127U	Obstetrics (preeclampsia), biochemical assays of 3 analytes (PAPP-A, AFP, and placental growth factor), time-resolved fluorescence immunoassay, maternal serum, predictive algorithm reported as a risk score for preeclampsia
Preeclampsia Screen | T1 + Y Chromosome?, Eurofins NTD, LLC, Eurofins NTD, LLC	● 0128U	Obstetrics (preeclampsia), biochemical assays of 3 analytes (PAPP-A, AFP, and placental growth factor), time-resolved fluorescence immunoassay, includes qualitative assessment of Y chromosome in cell-free fetal DNA, maternal serum and plasma, predictive algorithm reported as a risk score for preeclampsia
BRCAplus, Ambry Genetics	● 0129U	Hereditary breast cancer-related disorders (eg, hereditary breast cancer, hereditary ovarian cancer, hereditary endometrial cancer), genomic sequence analysis and deletion/duplication analysis panel *(ATM, BRCA1, BRCA2, CDH1, CHEK2, PALB2, PTEN,* and *TP53)*
+RNAinsight™ for ColoNext®, Ambry Genetics	+● 0130U	Hereditary colon cancer disorders (eg, Lynch syndrome, PTEN hamartoma syndrome, Cowden syndrome, familial adenomatosis polyposis), targeted mRNA sequence analysis panel *(APC, CDH1, CHEK2, MLH1, MSH2, MSH6, MUTYH, PMS2, PTEN,* and *TP53)* (List separately in addition to code for primary procedure)
+RNAinsight™ for BreastNext®, Ambry Genetics	+● 0131U	Hereditary breast cancer-related disorders (eg, hereditary breast cancer, hereditary ovarian cancer, hereditary endometrial cancer), targeted mRNA sequence analysis panel (13 genes) (List separately in addition to code for primary procedure)
+RNAinsight™ for OvaNext®, Ambry Genetics	+● 0132U	Hereditary ovarian cancer-related disorders (eg, hereditary breast cancer, hereditary ovarian cancer, hereditary endometrial cancer), targeted mRNA sequence analysis panel (17 genes) (List separately in addition to code for primary procedure)
+RNAinsight™ for ProstateNext®, Ambry Genetics	+● 0133U	Hereditary prostate cancer-related disorders, targeted mRNA sequence analysis panel (11 genes) (List separately in addition to code for primary procedure)
+RNAinsight™ for CancerNext®, Ambry Genetics	+● 0134U	Hereditary pan cancer (eg, hereditary breast and ovarian cancer, hereditary endometrial cancer, hereditary colorectal cancer), targeted mRNA sequence analysis panel (18 genes) (List separately in addition to code for primary procedure)
+RNAinsight™ for GYNPlus®, Ambry Genetics	+● 0135U	Hereditary gynecological cancer (eg, hereditary breast and ovarian cancer, hereditary endometrial cancer, hereditary colorectal cancer), targeted mRNA sequence analysis panel (12 genes) (List separately in addition to code for primary procedure)
+RNAinsight™ for *ATM*, Ambry Genetics	+● 0136U	*ATM (ataxia telangiectasia mutated)* (eg, ataxia telangiectasia) mRNA sequence analysis (List separately in addition to code for primary procedure)
+RNAinsight™ for *PALB2*, Ambry Genetics	+● 0137U	*PALB2 (partner and localizer of BRCA2)* (eg, breast and pancreatic cancer) mRNA sequence analysis (List separately in addition to code for primary procedure)
+RNAinsight™ for *BRCA1/2*, Ambry Genetics	+● 0138U	*BRCA1 (BRCA1, DNA repair associated), BRCA2 (BRCA2, DNA repair associated)* (eg, hereditary breast and ovarian cancer) mRNA sequence analysis (List separately in addition to code for primary procedure)
NPDX ASD Energy Metabolism, Stemina Biomarker Discovery, Inc, Stemina Biomarker Discovery, Inc.	● 0139U	Neurology (autism spectrum disorder [ASD]), quantitative measurements of 6 central carbon metabolites (ie, α-ketoglutarate, alanine, lactate, phenylalanine, pyruvate, and succinate), LC-MS/MS, plasma, algorithmic analysis with result reported as negative or positive (with metabolic subtypes of ASD)

Proprietary Name/Clinical Laboratory/Manufacturer	Code	Descriptor
ePlex® BCID Fungal Pathogens Panel, GenMark Diagnostics, Inc, GenMark Diagnostics, Inc	● 0140U	Infectious disease (fungi), fungal pathogen identification, DNA (15 fungal targets), blood culture, amplified probe technique, each target reported as detected or not detected
ePlex® BCID Gram-Positive Panel, GenMark Diagnostics, Inc, GenMark Diagnostics, Inc	● 0141U	Infectious disease (bacteria and fungi), gram-positive organism identification and drug resistance element detection, DNA (20 gram-positive bacterial targets, 4 resistance genes, 1 pan gram-negative bacterial target, 1 pan Candida target), blood culture, amplified probe technique, each target reported as detected or not detected
ePlex® BCID Gram-Negative Panel, GenMark Diagnostics, Inc, GenMark Diagnostics, Inc	● 0142U	Infectious disease (bacteria and fungi), gram-negative bacterial identification and drug resistance element detection, DNA (21 gram-negative bacterial targets, 6 resistance genes, 1 pan gram-positive bacterial target, 1 pan Candida target), amplified probe technique, each target reported as detected or not detected
CareViewRx, Newstar Medical Laboratories, LLC, Newstar Medical Laboratories, LLC PsychViewRx Plus analysis by Newstar Medical Laboratories, LLC. To report, see (~0150U)	● 0143U	Drug assay, definitive, 120 or more drugs or metabolites, urine, quantitative liquid chromatography with tandem mass spectrometry (LC-MS/MS) using multiple reaction monitoring (MRM), with drug or metabolite description, comments including sample validation, per date of service
CareViewRx Plus, Newstar Medical Laboratories, LLC, Newstar Medical Laboratories, LLC	● 0144U	Drug assay, definitive, 160 or more drugs or metabolites, urine, quantitative liquid chromatography with tandem mass spectrometry (LC-MS/MS) using multiple reaction monitoring (MRM), with drug or metabolite description, comments including sample validation, per date of service
PainViewRx, Newstar Medical Laboratories, LLC, Newstar Medical Laboratories, LLC	● 0145U	Drug assay, definitive, 65 or more drugs or metabolites, urine, quantitative liquid chromatography with tandem mass spectrometry (LC-MS/MS) using multiple reaction monitoring (MRM), with drug or metabolite description, comments including sample validation, per date of service
PainViewRx Plus, Newstar Medical Laboratories, LLC, Newstar Medical Laboratories, LLC	● 0146U	Drug assay, definitive, 80 or more drugs or metabolites, urine, by quantitative liquid chromatography with tandem mass spectrometry (LC-MS/MS) using multiple reaction monitoring (MRM), with drug or metabolite description, comments including sample validation, per date of service
RiskViewRx, Newstar Medical Laboratories, LLC, Newstar Medical Laboratories, LLC	● 0147U	Drug assay, definitive, 85 or more drugs or metabolites, urine, quantitative liquid chromatography with tandem mass spectrometry (LC-MS/MS) using multiple reaction monitoring (MRM), with drug or metabolite description, comments including sample validation, per date of service
RiskViewRx Plus, Newstar Medical Laboratories, LLC, Newstar Medical Laboratories, LLC	● 0148U	Drug assay, definitive, 100 or more drugs or metabolites, urine, quantitative liquid chromatography with tandem mass spectrometry (LC-MS/MS) using multiple reaction monitoring (MRM), with drug or metabolite description, comments including sample validation, per date of service
PsychViewRx, Newstar Medical Laboratories, LLC, Newstar Medical Laboratories, LLC	● 0149U	Drug assay, definitive, 60 or more drugs or metabolites, urine, quantitative liquid chromatography with tandem mass spectrometry (LC-MS/MS) using multiple reaction monitoring (MRM), with drug or metabolite description, comments including sample validation, per date of service
PsychViewRx Plus, Newstar Medical Laboratories, LLC, Newstar Medical Laboratories, LLC CareViewRx analysis by Newstar Medical Laboratories, LLC. To report, see (~0143U)	● 0150U	Drug assay, definitive, 120 or more drugs or metabolites, urine, quantitative liquid chromatography with tandem mass spectrometry (LC-MS/MS) using multiple reaction monitoring (MRM), with drug or metabolite description, comments including sample validation, per date of service
BioFire® FilmArray® Pneumonia Panel, BioFire® Diagnostics, BioFire® Diagnostics	● 0151U	Infectious disease (bacterial or viral respiratory tract infection), pathogen specific nucleic acid (DNA or RNA), 33 targets, real-time semi-quantitative PCR, bronchoalveolar lavage, sputum, or endotracheal aspirate, detection of 33 organismal and antibiotic resistance genes with limited semi-quantitative results
Karius® Test, Karius Inc, Karius Inc	● 0152U	Infectious disease (bacteria, fungi, parasites, and DNA viruses), DNA, PCR and next-generation sequencing, plasma, detection of >1,000 potential microbial organisms for significant positive pathogens

Proprietary Name/Clinical Laboratory/Manufacturer	Code	Descriptor
Insight TNBCtype™, Insight Molecular Labs	● 0153U	Oncology (breast), mRNA, gene expression profiling by next-generation sequencing of 101 genes, utilizing formalin-fixed paraffin-embedded tissue, algorithm reported as a triple negative breast cancer clinical subtype(s) with information on immune cell involvement
therascreen® *FGFR* RGQ RT-PCR Kit, QIAGEN, QIAGEN GmbH	● 0154U	*FGFR3 (fibroblast growth factor receptor 3)* gene analysis (ie, p.R248C [c.742C>T], p.S249C [c.746C>G], p.G370C [c.1108G>T], p.Y373C [c.1118A>G], FGFR3-TACC3v1, and FGFR3-TACC3v3)
therascreen *PIK3CA* RGQ PCR Kit, QIAGEN, QIAGEN GmbH	● 0155U	*PIK3CA (phosphatidylinositol-4,5-bisphosphate 3-kinase, catalytic subunit alpha)* (eg, breast cancer) gene analysis (ie, p.C420R, p.E542K, p.E545A, p.E545D [g.1635G>T only], p.E545G, p.E545K, p.Q546E, p.Q546R, p.H1047L, p.H1047R, p.H1047Y)
SMASH™, New York Genome Center, Marvel Genomics™	● 0156U	Copy number (eg, intellectual disability, dysmorphology), sequence analysis
CustomNext + RNA: *APC*, Ambry Genetics®, Ambry Genetics®	+● 0157U	*APC (APC regulator of WNT signaling pathway)* (eg, familial adenomatosis polyposis [FAP]) mRNA sequence analysis (List separately in addition to code for primary procedure)
CustomNext + RNA: *MLH1*, Ambry Genetics®, Ambry Genetics®	+● 0158U	*MLH1 (mutL homolog 1)* (eg, hereditary non-polyposis colorectal cancer, Lynch syndrome) mRNA sequence analysis (List separately in addition to code for primary procedure)
CustomNext + RNA: *MSH2*, Ambry Genetics®, Ambry Genetics®	+● 0159U	*MSH2 (mutS homolog 2)* (eg, hereditary colon cancer, Lynch syndrome) mRNA sequence analysis (List separately in addition to code for primary procedure)
CustomNext + RNA: *MSH6*, Ambry Genetics®, Ambry Genetics®	+● 0160U	*MSH6 (mutS homolog 6)* (eg, hereditary colon cancer, Lynch syndrome) mRNA sequence analysis (List separately in addition to code for primary procedure)
CustomNext + RNA: *PMS2*, Ambry Genetics®, Ambry Genetics®	+● 0161U	*PMS2 (PMS1 homolog 2, mismatch repair system component)* (eg, hereditary non-polyposis colorectal cancer, Lynch syndrome) mRNA sequence analysis (List separately in addition to code for primary procedure)
CustomNext + RNA: Lynch *(MLH1, MSH2, MSH6, PMS2)*, Ambry Genetics®, Ambry Genetics®	+● 0162U	Hereditary colon cancer (Lynch syndrome), targeted mRNA sequence analysis panel *(MLH1, MSH2, MSH6, PMS2)* (List separately in addition to code for primary procedure)

Appendix M — Glossary

-centesis. Puncture, as with a needle, trocar, or aspirator; often done for withdrawing fluid from a cavity.

-ectomy. Excision, removal.

-orrhaphy. Suturing.

-ostomy. Indicates a surgically created artificial opening.

-otomy. Making an incision or opening.

-plasty. Indicates surgically formed or molded.

abdominal lymphadenectomy. Surgical removal of the abdominal lymph nodes grouping, with or without para-aortic and vena cava nodes.

ablation. Removal or destruction of a body part or tissue or its function. Ablation may be performed by surgical means, hormones, drugs, radiofrequency, heat, chemical application, or other methods.

abnormal alleles. Form of gene that includes disease-related variations.

absorbable sutures. Strands prepared from collagen or a synthetic polymer and capable of being absorbed by tissue over time. Examples include surgical gut and collagen sutures; or synthetics like polydioxanone (PDS), polyglactin 910 (Vicryl), poliglecaprone 25 (Monocryl), polyglyconate (Maxon), and polyglycolic acid (Dexon).

acetabuloplasty. Surgical repair or reconstruction of the large cup-shaped socket in the hipbone (acetabulum) with which the head of the femur articulates.

Achilles tendon. Tendon attached to the back of the heel bone (calcaneus) that flexes the foot downward.

acromioclavicular joint. Junction between the clavicle and the scapula. The acromion is the projection from the back of the scapula that forms the highest point of the shoulder and connects with the clavicle. Trauma or injury to the acromioclavicular joint is often referred to as a dislocation of the shoulder. This is not correct, however, as a dislocation of the shoulder is a disruption of the glenohumeral joint.

acromionectomy. Surgical treatment for acromioclavicular arthritis in which the distal portion of the acromion process is removed.

acromioplasty. Repair of the part of the shoulder blade that connects to the deltoid muscles and clavicle.

actigraphy. Science of monitoring activity levels, particularly during sleep. In most cases, the patient wears a wristband that records motion while sleeping. The data are recorded, analyzed, and interpreted to study sleep/wake patterns and circadian rhythms.

air conduction. Transportation of sound from the air, through the external auditory canal, to the tympanic membrane and ossicular chain. Air conduction hearing is tested by presenting an acoustic stimulus through earphones or a loudspeaker to the ear.

air puff device. Instrument that measures intraocular pressure by evaluating the force of a reflected amount of air blown against the cornea.

alleles. Form of gene usually arising from a mutation responsible for a hereditary variation.

allogeneic collection. Collection of blood or blood components from one person for the use of another. Allogeneic collection was formerly termed homologous collection.

allograft. Graft from one individual to another of the same species.

amniocentesis. Surgical puncture through the abdominal wall, with a specialized needle and under ultrasonic guidance, into the interior of the pregnant uterus and directly into the amniotic sac to collect fluid for diagnostic analysis or therapeutic reduction of fluid levels.

anastomosis. Surgically created connection between ducts, blood vessels, or bowel segments to allow flow from one to the other.

anesthesia time. Time period factored into anesthesia procedures beginning with the anesthesiologist preparing the patient for surgery and ending when the patient is turned over to the recovery department.

Angelman syndrome. Early childhood emergence of a pattern of interrupted development, stiff, jerky gait, absence or impairment of speech, excessive laughter, and seizures.

angioplasty. Reconstruction or repair of a diseased or damaged blood vessel.

annuloplasty. Surgical plication of weakened tissue of the heart, to improve its muscular function. Annuli are thick, fibrous rings and one is found surrounding each of the cardiac chambers. The atrial and ventricular muscle fibers attach to the annuli. In annuloplasty, weakened annuli may be surgically plicated, or tucked, to improve muscular functions.

anorectal anometry. Measurement of pressure generated by anal sphincter to diagnose incontinence.

anterior chamber lenses. Lenses inserted into the anterior chamber following intracapsular cataract extraction.

applanation tonometer. Instrument that measures intraocular pressure by recording the force required to flatten an area of the cornea.

appropriateness of care. Proper setting of medical care that best meets the patient's care or diagnosis, as defined by a health care plan or other legal entity.

aqueous humor. Fluid within the anterior and posterior chambers of the eye that is continually replenished as it diffuses out into the blood. When the flow of aqueous is blocked, a build-up of fluid in the eye causes increased intraocular pressure and leads to glaucoma and blindness.

arteriogram. Radiograph of arteries.

arteriovenous fistula. Connecting passage between an artery and a vein.

arteriovenous malformation. Connecting passage between an artery and a vein.

arthrotomy. Surgical incision into a joint that may include exploration, drainage, or removal of a foreign body.

ASA. 1) Acetylsalicylic acid. Synonym(s): aspirin. 2) American Society of Anesthesiologists. National organization for anesthesiology that maintains and publishes the guidelines and relative values for anesthesia coding.

aspirate. To withdraw fluid or air from a body cavity by suction.

assay. Chemical analysis of a substance to establish the presence and strength of its components. A therapeutic drug assay is used to determine if a drug is within the expected therapeutic range for a patient.

atrial septal defect. Cardiac anomaly consisting of a patent opening in the atrial septum due to a fusion failure, classified as ostium secundum type, ostium primum defect, or endocardial cushion defect.

attended surveillance. Ability of a technician at a remote surveillance center or location to respond immediately to patient transmissions regarding rhythm or device alerts as they are produced and received at the remote location. These transmissions may originate from wearable or implanted therapy or monitoring devices.

auricle. External ear, which is a single elastic cartilage covered in skin and normal adnexal features (hair follicles, sweat glands, and sebaceous glands), shaped to channel sound waves into the acoustic meatus.

autogenous transplant. Tissue, such as bone, that is harvested from the patient and used for transplantation back into the same patient.

autograft. Any tissue harvested from one anatomical site of a person and grafted to another anatomical site of the same person. Most commonly, blood vessels, skin, tendons, fascia, and bone are used as autografts.

autologous. Tissue, cells, or structure obtained from the same individual.

AVF. Arteriovenous fistula.

AVM. Arteriovenous malformation. Clusters of abnormal blood vessels that grow in the brain comprised of a blood vessel "nidus" or nest through which arteries and veins connect directly without going through the capillaries. As time passes, the nidus may enlarge resulting in the formation of a mass that may bleed. AVMs are more prone to bleeding in patients ages 10 to 55. Once older than age 55, the possibility of bleeding is reduced dramatically.

backbench preparation. Procedures performed on a donor organ following procurement to prepare the organ for transplant into the recipient. Excess fat and other tissue may be removed, the organ may be perfused, and vital arteries may be sized, repaired, or modified to fit the patient. These procedures are done on a back table in the operating room before transplantation can begin.

Bartholin's gland. Mucous-producing gland found in the vestibular bulbs on either side of the vaginal orifice and connected to the mucosal membrane at the opening by a duct.

Bartholin's gland abscess. Pocket of pus and surrounding cellulitis caused by infection of the Bartholin's gland and causing localized swelling and pain in the posterior labia majora that may extend into the lower vagina.

basic value. Relative weighted value based upon the usual anesthesia services and the relative work or cost of the specific anesthesia service assigned to each anesthesia-specific procedure code.

Berman locator. Small, sensitive tool used to detect the location of a metallic foreign body in the eye.

bifurcated. Having two branches or divisions, such as the left pulmonary veins that split off from the left atrium to carry oxygenated blood away from the heart.

Billroth's operation. Anastomosis of the stomach to the duodenum or jejunum.

bioprosthetic heart valve. Replacement cardiac valve made of biological tissue. Allograft, xenograft or engineered tissue.

biopsy. Tissue or fluid removed for diagnostic purposes through analysis of the cells in the biopsy material.

Blalock-Hanlon procedure. Atrial septectomy procedure to allow free mixing of the blood from the right and left atria.

Blalock-Taussig procedure. Anastomosis of the left subclavian artery to the left pulmonary artery or the right subclavian artery to the right pulmonary artery in order to shunt some of the blood flow from the systemic to the pulmonary circulation.

blepharochalasis. Loss of elasticity and relaxation of skin of the eyelid, thickened or indurated skin on the eyelid associated with recurrent episodes of edema, and intracellular atrophy.

blepharoplasty. Plastic surgery of the eyelids to remove excess fat and redundant skin weighting down the lid. The eyelid is pulled tight and sutured to support sagging muscles.

blepharoptosis. Droop or displacement of the upper eyelid, caused by paralysis, muscle problems, or outside mechanical forces.

blepharorrhaphy. Suture of a portion or all of the opposing eyelids to shorten the palpebral fissure or close it entirely.

bone conduction. Transportation of sound through the bones of the skull to the inner ear.

bone mass measurement. Radiologic or radioisotopic procedure or other procedure approved by the FDA for identifying bone mass, detecting bone loss, or determining bone quality. The procedure includes a physician's interpretation of the results. Qualifying individuals must be an estrogen-deficient woman at clinical risk for osteoporosis with vertebral abnormalities.

brachytherapy. Form of radiation therapy in which radioactive pellets or seeds are implanted directly into the tissue being treated to deliver their dose of radiation in a more directed fashion. Brachytherapy provides radiation to the prescribed body area while minimizing exposure to normal tissue.

breakpoint. Point at which a chromosome breaks.

Bristow procedure. Anterior capsulorrhaphy prevents chronic separation of the shoulder. In this procedure, the bone block is affixed to the anterior glenoid rim with a screw.

buccal mucosa. Tissue from the mucous membrane on the inside of the cheek.

bundle of His. Bundle of modified cardiac fibers that begins at the atrioventricular node and passes through the right atrioventricular fibrous ring to the interventricular septum, where it divides into two branches. Bundle of His recordings are taken for intracardiac electrograms.

Caldwell-Luc operation. Intraoral antrostomy approach into the maxillary sinus for the removal of tooth roots or tissue, or for packing the sinus to reduce zygomatic fractures by creating a window above the teeth in the canine fossa area.

canthorrhaphy. Suturing of the palpebral fissure, the juncture between the eyelids, at either end of the eye.

canthotomy. Horizontal incision at the canthus (junction of upper and lower eyelids) to divide the outer canthus and enlarge lid margin separation.

cardio-. Relating to the heart.

cardiopulmonary bypass. Venous blood is diverted to a heart-lung machine, which mechanically pumps and oxygenates the blood temporarily so the heart can be bypassed while an open procedure on the heart or coronary arteries is performed. During bypass, the lungs are deflated and immobile.

cardioverter-defibrillator. Device that uses both low energy cardioversion or defibrillating shocks and antitachycardia pacing to treat ventricular tachycardia or ventricular fibrillation.

care plan oversight services. Physician's ongoing review and revision of a patient's care plan involving complex or multidisciplinary care modalities.

case management services. Physician case management is a process of involving direct patient care as well as coordinating and controlling access to the patient or initiating and/or supervising other necessary health care services.

cataract extraction. Surgical removal of the cataract or cloudy lens. Anterior chamber lenses are inserted in conjunction with intracapsular cataract extraction and posterior chamber lenses are inserted in conjunction with extracapsular cataract extraction.

catheter. Flexible tube inserted into an area of the body for introducing or withdrawing fluid.

Centers for Medicare and Medicaid Services. Federal agency that oversees the administration of the public health programs such as Medicare, Medicaid, and State Children's Insurance Program.

certified nurse midwife. Registered nurse who has successfully completed a program of study and clinical experience or has been certified by a recognized organization for the care of pregnant or delivering patients.

CFR. Code of Federal Regulations.

CGMS. Continuous glucose monitoring system.

CHAMPUS. Civilian Health and Medical Program of the Uniformed Services. See Tricare.

CHAMPVA. Civilian Health and Medical Program of the Department of Veterans Affairs.

chemodenervation. Chemical destruction of nerves. A substance, for example, Botox, is used to temporarily inhibit the transfer of chemicals at the presynaptic membrane, blocking the neuromuscular junctions.

chemoembolization. Administration of chemotherapeutic agents directly to a tumor in combination with the percutaneous administration of an occlusive substance into a vessel to deprive the tumor of its blood supply. This ensures a prolonged level of therapy directed at the tumor. Chemoembolization is primarily being used for cancers of the liver and endocrine system.

chemosurgery. Application of chemical agents to destroy tissue, originally referring to the in situ chemical fixation of premalignant or malignant lesions to facilitate surgical excision.

Chiari osteotomy. Top of the femur is altered to correct a dislocated hip caused by congenital conditions or cerebral palsy. Plate and screws are often used.

chimera. Organ or anatomic structure consisting of tissues of diverse genetic constitution.

choanal atresia. Congenital, membranous, or bony closure of one or both posterior nostrils due to failure of the embryonic bucconasal membrane to rupture and open up the nasal passageway.

chondromalacia. Condition in which the articular cartilage softens, seen in various body sites but most often in the patella, and may be congenital or acquired.

chorionic villus sampling. Aspiration of a placental sample through a catheter, under ultrasonic guidance. The specialized needle is placed transvaginally through the cervix or transabdominally into the uterine cavity.

chronic pain management services. Distinct services frequently performed by anesthesiologists who have additional training in pain management procedures. Pain management services include initial and subsequent evaluation and management (E/M) services, trigger point injections, spine and spinal cord injections, and nerve blocks.

cineplastic amputation. Amputation in which muscles and tendons of the remaining portion of the extremity are arranged so that they may be utilized for motor functions. Following this type of amputation, a specially constructed prosthetic device allows the individual to execute more complex movements because the muscles and tendons are able to communicate independent movements to the device.

circadian. Relating to a cyclic, 24-hour period.

CLIA. Clinical Laboratory Improvement Amendments. Requirements set in 1988, CLIA imposes varying levels of federal regulations on clinical procedures. Few laboratories, including those in physician offices, are exempt. Adopted by Medicare and Medicaid, CLIA regulations redefine laboratory testing in regard to laboratory certification and accreditation, proficiency testing, quality assurance, personnel standards, and program administration.

clinical social worker. Individual who possesses a master's or doctor's degree in social work and, after obtaining the degree, has performed at least two years of supervised clinical social work. A clinical social worker must be licensed by the state or, in the case of states without licensure, must completed at least two years or 3,000 hours of post-master's degree supervised clinical social work practice under the supervision of a master's level social worker.

clinical staff. Someone who works for, or under, the direction of a physician or qualified health care professional and does not bill services separately. The person may be licensed or regulated to help the physician perform specific duties.

clonal. Originating from one cell.

CMS. Centers for Medicare and Medicaid Services. Federal agency that administers the public health programs.

CO_2 laser. Carbon dioxide laser that emits an invisible beam and vaporizes water-rich tissue. The vapor is suctioned from the site.

codons. Series of three adjoining bases in one polynucleotide chain of a DNA or RNA molecule that provides the codes for a specific amino acid.

cognitive. Being aware by drawing from knowledge, such as judgment, reason, perception, and memory.

colostomy. Artificial surgical opening anywhere along the length of the colon to the skin surface for the diversion of feces.

commissurotomy. Surgical division or disruption of any two parts that are joined to form a commissure in order to increase the opening. The procedure most often refers to opening the adherent leaflet bands of fibrous tissue in a stenosed mitral valve.

common variants. Nucleotide sequence differences associated with abnormal gene function. Tests are usually performed in a single series of laboratory testing (in a single, typically multiplex, assay arrangement or using more than one assay to include all variants to be examined). Variants are representative of a mutation that mainly causes a single disease, such as cystic fibrosis. Other uncommon variants could provide additional information. Tests may be performed based on society recommendations and guidelines.

community mental health center. Facility providing outpatient mental health day treatment, assessments, and education as appropriate to community members.

component code. In the National Correct Coding Initiative (NCCI), the column II code that cannot be charged to Medicare when the column I code is reported.

comprehensive code. In the National Correct Coding Initiative (NCCI), the column I code that is reported to Medicare and precludes reporting column II codes.

computerized corneal topography. Digital imaging and analysis by computer of the shape of the corneal.

conjunctiva. Mucous membrane lining of the eyelids and covering of the exposed, anterior sclera.

conjunctivodacryocystostomy. Surgical connection of the lacrimal sac directly to the conjunctival sac.

conjunctivorhinostomy. Correction of an obstruction of the lacrimal canal achieved by suturing the posterior flaps and removing any lacrimal obstruction, preserving the conjunctiva.

constitutional. Cells containing genetic code that may be passed down to future generations. May also be referred to as germline.

consultation. Advice or opinion regarding diagnosis and treatment or determination to accept transfer of care of a patient rendered by a medical professional at the request of the primary care provider.

continuous positive airway pressure device. Pressurized device used to maintain the patient's airway for spontaneous or mechanically aided breathing. Often used for patients with mild to moderate sleep apnea.

core needle biopsy. Large-bore biopsy needle inserted into a mass and a core of tissue is removed for diagnostic study.

corpectomy. Removal of the body of a bone, such as a vertebra.

costochondral. Pertaining to the ribs and the scapula.

COTD. Cardiac output thermodilution. Cardiac output measured by thermodilution method that requires heart catheterization and then injection of a thermal indicator, usually iced saline. A computer calculates the cardiac output using an equation that incorporates body temperature, injectate volume and temperature, time, and other calculated ratios over a denominator of the integral of the change in blood temperature during the cold injection, reflected by the area of the inscribed curve.

CPT. 1) Chest physical therapy. 2) Cold pressor test. 3) Current Procedural Terminology.

craniosynostosis. Congenital condition in which one or more of the cranial sutures fuse prematurely, creating a deformed or aberrant head shape.

craterization. Excision of a portion of bone creating a crater-like depression to facilitate drainage from infected areas of bone.

cricoid. Circular cartilage around the trachea.

CRNA. Certified registered nurse anesthetist. Nurse trained and specializing in the administration of anesthesia.

cryolathe. Tool used for reshaping a button of corneal tissue.

cryosurgery. Application of intense cold, usually produced using liquid nitrogen, to locally freeze diseased or unwanted tissue and induce tissue necrosis without causing harm to adjacent tissue.

CT. Computed tomography.

cutdown. Small, incised opening in the skin to expose a blood vessel, especially over a vein (venous cutdown) to allow venipuncture and permit a needle or cannula to be inserted for the withdrawal of blood or administration of fluids.

cyclophotocoagulation. Procedure done to prevent vision loss from glaucoma in which a neodymium: YAG laser is used to burn and destroy a portion of the ciliary body in order to decrease the amount of aqueous humor being produced in the eye. This procedure is only done when creating a drain for aqueous humor to reduce intraocular pressure would not be successful. Destroying portions of the ciliary body reduces the amount of fluid present in the eye.

cytogenetic studies. Procedures in CPT that are related to the branch of genetics that studies cellular (cyto) structure and function as it relates to heredity (genetics). White blood cells, specifically T-lymphocytes, are the most commonly used specimen for chromosome analysis.

cytogenomic. Chromosomic evaluation using molecular methods.

dacryocystotome. Instrument used for incising the lacrimal duct strictures.

DBS. Deep brain stimulation. Treatment for disabling neurological symptoms associated with diseases including Parkinson's. DBS requires three components: the implanted electrode, extension, and neurostimulator. Electrical impulses are sent from the neurostimulator to the implant to block tremors.

debride. To remove all foreign objects and devitalized or infected tissue from a burn or wound to prevent infection and promote healing.

definitive drug testing. Drug tests used to further analyze or confirm the presence or absence of specific drugs or classes of drugs used by the patient. These tests are able to provide more conclusive information regarding the concentration of the drug and their metabolites. May be used for medical, workplace, or legal purposes.

definitive identification. Identification of microorganisms using additional tests to specify the genus or species (e.g., slide cultures or biochemical panels).

dentoalveolar structure. Area of alveolar bone surrounding the teeth and adjacent tissue.

Department of Health and Human Services. Cabinet department that oversees the operating divisions of the federal government responsible for health and welfare. HHS oversees the Centers for Medicare and Medicaid Services, Food and Drug Administration, Public Health Service, and other such entities.

Department of Justice. Attorneys from the DOJ and the United States Attorney's Office have, under the memorandum of understanding, the same direct access to contractor data and records as the OIG and the Federal Bureau of Investigation (FBI). DOJ is responsible for prosecution of fraud and civil or criminal cases presented.

dermis. Skin layer found under the epidermis that contains a papillary upper layer and the deep reticular layer of collagen, vascular bed, and nerves.

dermis graft. Skin graft that has been separated from the epidermal tissue and the underlying subcutaneous fat, used primarily as a substitute for fascia grafts in plastic surgery.

desensitization. 1) Administration of extracts of allergens periodically to build immunity in the patient. 2) Application of medication to decrease the symptoms, usually pain, associated with a dental condition or disease.

destruction. Ablation or eradication of a structure or tissue.

diabetes outpatient self-management training services. Educational and training services furnished by a certified provider in an outpatient setting. The physician managing the individual's diabetic condition must certify that the services are needed under a comprehensive plan of care and provide the patient with the skills and knowledge necessary for therapeutic program compliance (including skills related to the self-administration of injectable drugs). The provider must meet applicable standards established by the National Diabetes Advisory or be recognized by an organization that represents individuals with diabetes as meeting standards for furnishing the services.

diagnostic procedures. Procedure performed on a patient to obtain information to assess the medical condition of the patient or to identify a disease and to determine the nature and severity of an illness or injury.

dialysis. Artificial filtering of the blood to remove contaminating waste elements and restore normal balance.

diaphragm. 1) Muscular wall separating the thorax and its structures from the abdomen. 2) Flexible disk inserted into the vagina and against the cervix as a method of birth control.

diaphysectomy. Surgical removal of a portion of the shaft of a long bone, often done to facilitate drainage from infected bone.

diathermy. Applying heat to body tissues by various methods for therapeutic treatment or surgical purposes to coagulate and seal tissue.

dilation. Artificial increase in the diameter of an opening or lumen made by medication or by instrumentation.

dissect. Cut apart or separate tissue for surgical purposes or for visual or microscopic study.

DNA. Deoxyribonucleic acid. Chemical containing the genetic information necessary to produce and propagate living organisms. Molecules are comprised of two twisting paired strands, called a double helix.

DNA marker. Specific gene sequence within a chromosome indicating the inheritance of a certain trait.

dorsal. Pertaining to the back or posterior aspect.

drugs and biologicals. Drugs and biologicals included - or approved for inclusion - in the United States Pharmacopoeia, the National Formulary, the United States Homeopathic Pharmacopoeia, in New Drugs or Accepted Dental Remedies, or approved by the pharmacy and drug therapeutics committee of the medical staff of the hospital. Also included are medically accepted and FDA approved drugs used in an anticancer chemotherapeutic regimen. The carrier determines medical acceptance based on supportive clinical evidence.

dual-lead device. Implantable cardiac device (pacemaker or implantable cardioverter-defibrillator [ICD]) in which pacing and sensing components are placed in only two chambers of the heart.

duplex scan. Noninvasive vascular diagnostic technique that uses ultrasonic scanning to identify the pattern and direction of blood flow within arteries or veins displayed in real time images. Duplex scanning combines B-mode two-dimensional pictures of the vessel structure with spectra and/or color flow Doppler mapping or imaging of the blood as it moves through the vessels.

duplication/deletion (DUP/DEL). Term used in molecular testing which examines genomic regions to determine if there are extra chromosomes (duplication) or missing chromosomes (deletions). Normal gene dosage is two copies per cell except for the sex chromosomes which have one per cell.

DuToit staple capsulorrhaphy. Reattachment of the capsule of the shoulder and glenoid labrum to the glenoid lip using staples to anchor the avulsed capsule and glenoid labrum.

Dx. Diagnosis.

DXA. Dual energy x-ray absorptiometry. Radiological technique for bone density measurement using a two-dimensional projection system in which two x-ray beams with different levels of energy are pulsed alternately and the results are given in two scores, reported as standard deviations from peak bone mass density.

dynamic mutation. Unstable or changing polynucleotides resulting in repeats related to genes that can undergo disease-producing increases or decreases in the repeats that differ within tissues or over generations.

ECMO. Extracorporeal membrane oxygenation.

ectropion. Drooping of the lower eyelid away from the eye or outward turning or eversion of the edge of the eyelid, exposing the palpebral conjunctiva and causing irritation.

Eden-Hybinette procedure. Anterior shoulder repair using an anterior bone block to augment the bony anterior glenoid lip.

EDTA. Drug used to inhibit damage to the cornea by collagenase. EDTA is especially effective in alkali burns as it neutralizes soluble alkali, including lye.

effusion. Escape of fluid from within a body cavity.

electrocardiographic rhythm derived. Analysis of data obtained from readings of the heart's electrical activation, including heart rate and rhythm, variability of heart rate, ST analysis, and T-wave alternans. Other data may also be assessed when warranted.

electrocautery. Division or cutting of tissue using high-frequency electrical current to produce heat, which destroys cells.

electrode array. Electronic device containing more than one contact whose function can be adjusted during programming services. Electrodes are specialized for a particular electrochemical reaction that acts as a medium between a body surface and another instrument.

electromyography. Test that measures muscle response to nerve stimulation determining if muscle weakness is present and if it is related to the muscles themselves or a problem with the nerves that supply the muscles.

electrooculogram (EOG). Record of electrical activity associated with eye movements.

electrophysiologic studies. Electrical stimulation and monitoring to diagnose heart conduction abnormalities that predispose patients to bradyarrhythmias and to determine a patient's chance for developing ventricular and supraventricular tachyarrhythmias.

embolization. Placement of a clotting agent, such as a coil, plastic particles, gel, foam, etc., into an area of hemorrhage to stop the bleeding or to block blood flow to a problem area, such as an aneurysm or a tumor.

emergency. Serious medical condition or symptom (including severe pain) resulting from injury, sickness, or mental illness that arises suddenly and requires immediate care and treatment, generally received within 24 hours of onset, to avoid jeopardy to the life, limb, or health of a covered person.

empyema. Accumulation of pus within the respiratory, or pleural, cavity.

EMTALA. Emergency Medical Treatment and Active Labor Act.

end-stage renal disease. Chronic, advanced kidney disease requiring renal dialysis or a kidney transplant to prevent imminent death.

endarterectomy. Removal of the thickened, endothelial lining of a diseased or damaged artery.

endomicroscopy. Diagnostic technology that allows for the examination of tissue at the cellular level during endoscopy. The technology decreases the need for biopsy with histological examination for some types of lesions.

endovascular embolization. Procedure whereby vessels are occluded by a variety of therapeutic substances for the treatment of abnormal blood vessels by inhibiting the flow of blood to a tumor, arteriovenous malformations, lymphatic malformation, and to prevent or stop hemorrhage.

entropion. Inversion of the eyelid, turning the edge in toward the eyeball and causing irritation from contact of the lashes with the surface of the eye.

enucleation. Removal of a growth or organ cleanly so as to extract it in one piece.

epidermis. Outermost, nonvascular layer of skin that contains four to five differentiated layers depending on its body location: stratum corneum, lucidum, granulosum, spinosum, and basale.

epiphysiodesis. Surgical fusion of an epiphysis performed to prematurely stop further bone growth.

escharotomy. Surgical incision into the scab or crust resulting from a severe burn in order to relieve constriction and allow blood flow to the distal unburned tissue.

established patient. 1) Patient who has received professional services in a face-to-face setting within the last three years from the same physician/qualified health care professional or another physician/qualified health care professional of the exact same specialty and subspecialty who belongs to the same group practice. 2) For OPPS hospitals, patient who has been registered as an inpatient or outpatient in a hospital's provider-based clinic or emergency department within the past three years.

evacuation. Removal or purging of waste material.

evaluation and management codes. Assessment and management of a patient's health care.

evaluation and management service components. Key components of history, examination, and medical decision making that are key to selecting the correct E/M codes. Other non-key components include counseling, coordination of care, nature of presenting problem, and time.

event recorder. Portable, ambulatory heart monitor worn by the patient that makes electrocardiographic recordings of the length and frequency of aberrant cardiac rhythm to help diagnose heart conditions and to assess pacemaker functioning or programming.

exenteration. Surgical removal of the entire contents of a body cavity, such as the pelvis or orbit.

exon. One of multiple nucleic acid sequences used to encode information for a gene polypeptide or protein. Exons are separated from other exons by non-protein-coding sequences known as introns.

extended care services. Items and services provided to an inpatient of a skilled nursing facility, including nursing care, physical or occupational therapy, speech pathology, drugs and supplies, and medical social services.

external electrical capacitor device. External electrical stimulation device designed to promote bone healing. This device may also promote neural regeneration, revascularization, epiphyseal growth, and ligament maturation.

external pulsating electromagnetic field. External stimulation device designed to promote bone healing. This device may also promote neural regeneration, revascularization, epiphyseal growth, and ligament maturation.

extracorporeal. Located or taking place outside the body.

Eyre-Brook capsulorrhaphy. Reattachment of the capsule of the shoulder and glenoid labrum to the glenoid lip.

False Claims Act. Governs civil actions for filing false claims. Liability under this act pertains to any person who knowingly presents or causes to be presented a false or fraudulent claim to the government for payment or approval.

fascia. Fibrous sheet or band of tissue that envelops organs, muscles, and groupings of muscles.

fasciectomy. Excision of fascia or strips of fascial tissue.

fasciotomy. Incision or transection of fascial tissue.

fat graft. Graft composed of fatty tissue completely freed from surrounding tissue that is used primarily to fill in depressions.

FDA. Food and Drug Administration. Federal agency responsible for protecting public health by substantiating the safety, efficacy, and security of human and veterinary drugs, biological products, medical devices, national food supply, cosmetics, and items that give off radiation.

filtered speech test. Test most commonly used to identify central auditory dysfunction in which the patient is presented monosyllabic words that are low pass filtered, allowing only the parts of each word below a certain pitch to be presented. A score is given on the number of correct responses. This may be a subset of a standard battery of tests provided during a single encounter.

fissure. Deep furrow, groove, or cleft in tissue structures.

fistulization. Creation of a communication between two structures that were not previously connected.

flexor digitorum profundus tendon. Tendon originating in the proximal forearm and extending to the index finger and wrist. A thickened FDP sheath, usually caused by age, illness, or injury, can fill the carpal canal and lead to impingement of the median nerve.

fluoroscopy. Radiology technique that allows visual examination of part of the body or a function of an organ using a device that projects an x-ray image on a fluorescent screen.

focal length. Distance between the object in focus and the lens.

focused medical review. Process of targeting and directing medical review efforts on Medicare claims where the greatest risk of inappropriate program payment exists. The goal is to reduce the number of noncovered claims or unnecessary services. CMS analyzes national data such as internal billing, utilization, and payment data and provides its findings to the FI. Local medical review policies are developed identifying aberrances, abuse, and overutilized services. Providers are responsible for knowing national Medicare coverage and billing guidelines and local medical review policies, and for determining whether the services provided to Medicare beneficiaries are covered by Medicare.

fragile X syndrome. Intellectual disabilities, enlarged testes, big jaw, high forehead, and long ears in males. In females, fragile X presents with mild intellectual disabilities and heterozygous sexual structures. In some families, males have shown no symptoms but carry the gene.

free flap. Tissue that is completely detached from the donor site and transplanted to the recipient site, receiving its blood supply from capillary ingrowth at the recipient site.

free microvascular flap. Tissue that is completely detached from the donor site following careful dissection and preservation of the blood vessels, then attached to the recipient site with the transferred blood vessels anastomosed to the vessels in the recipient bed.

fulguration. Destruction of living tissue by using sparks from a high-frequency electric current.

gas tamponade. Absorbable gas may be injected to force the retina against the choroid. Common gases include room air, short-acting sulfahexafluoride, intermediate-acting perfluoroethane, or long-acting perfluorooctane.

Gaucher disease. Genetic metabolic disorder in which fat deposits may accumulate in the spleen, liver, lungs, bone marrow, and brain.

gene. Basic unit of heredity that contains nucleic acid. Genes are arranged in different and unique sequences or strings that determine the gene's function. Human genes usually include multiple protein coding regions such as exons separated by introns which are nonprotein coding sections.

genome. Complete set of DNA of an organism. Each cell in the human body is comprised of a complete copy of the approximately three billion DNA base pairs that constitute the human genome.

habilitative services. Procedures or services provided to assist a patient in learning, keeping, and improving new skills needed to perform daily living activities. Habilitative services assist patients in acquiring a skill for the first time.

HCPCS. Healthcare Common Procedure Coding System.

HCPCS Level I. Healthcare Common Procedure Coding System Level I. Numeric coding system used by physicians, facility outpatient departments, and ambulatory surgery centers (ASC) to code ambulatory, laboratory, radiology, and other diagnostic services for Medicare billing. This coding system contains only the American Medical Association's Physicians' Current Procedural Terminology (CPT) codes. The AMA updates codes annually.

HCPCS Level II. Healthcare Common Procedure Coding System Level II. National coding system, developed by CMS, that contains alphanumeric codes for physician and nonphysician services not included in the CPT coding system. HCPCS Level II covers such things as ambulance services, durable medical equipment, and orthotic and prosthetic devices.

HCPCS modifiers. Two-character code (AA-ZZ) that identifies circumstances that alter or enhance the description of a service or supply. They are recognized by carriers nationally and are updated annually by CMS.

Hct. Hematocrit.

health care provider. Entity that administers diagnostic and therapeutic services.

hemilaminectomy. Excision of a portion of the vertebral lamina.

hemodialysis. Cleansing of wastes and contaminating elements from the blood by virtue of different diffusion rates through a semipermeable membrane, which separates blood from a filtration solution that diffuses other elements out of the blood. The blood is slowly filtered extracorporeally through special dialysis equipment and returned to the body. Synonym(s): renal dialysis.

hemodialysis. Cleansing of wastes and contaminating elements from the blood by virtue of different diffusion rates through a semipermeable membrane, which separates blood from a filtration solution that diffuses other elements out of the blood.

hemoperitoneum. Effusion of blood into the peritoneal cavity, the space between the continuous membrane lining the abdominopelvic walls and encasing the visceral organs.

heterograft. Surgical graft of tissue from one animal species to a different animal species. A common type of heterograft is porcine (pig) tissue, used for temporary wound closure.

heterotopic transplant. Tissue transplanted from a different anatomical site for usage as is natural for that tissue, for example, buccal mucosa to a conjunctival site.

HGNC. HUGO gene nomenclature committee.

HGVS. Human genome variation society.

Hickman catheter. Central venous catheter used for long-term delivery of medications, such as antibiotics, nutritional substances, or chemotherapeutic agents.

HLA. Human leukocyte antigen.

home health services. Services furnished to patients in their homes under the care of physicians. These services include part-time or intermittent skilled nursing care, physical therapy, medical social services, medical supplies, and some rehabilitation equipment. Home health supplies and services must be prescribed by a physician, and the beneficiary must be confined at home in order for Medicare to pay the benefits in full.

homograft. Graft from one individual to another of the same species.

hospice care. Items and services provided to a terminally ill individual by a hospice program under a written plan established and periodically reviewed by the individual's attending physician and by the medical director: Nursing care provided by or under the supervision of a registered professional nurse; Physical or occupational therapy or speech-language pathology services; Medical social services under the direction of a physician; Services of a home health aide who has successfully completed a training program; Medical supplies (including drugs and biologicals) and the use of medical appliances; Physicians' services; Short-term inpatient care (including both respite care and procedures necessary for pain control and acute and chronic symptom management) in an inpatient facility on an intermittent basis and not consecutively over longer than five days; Counseling (including dietary counseling) with respect to care of the terminally ill individual and adjustment to his death; Any item or service which is specified in the plan and for which payment may be made.

hospital. Institution that provides, under the supervision of physicians, diagnostic, therapeutic, and rehabilitation services for medical diagnosis, treatment, and care of patients. Hospitals receiving federal funds must maintain clinical records on all patients, provide 24-hour nursing services, and have a discharge planning process in place. The term "hospital" also includes religious nonmedical health care institutions and facilities of 50 beds or less located in rural areas.

HUGO. Human genome organization

IA. Intra-arterial.

ICD. Implantable cardioverter defibrillator.

ICD-10-CM. International Classification of Diseases, 10th Revision, Clinical Modification. Clinical modification of the alphanumeric classification of diseases used by the World Health Organization, already in use in much of the world, and used for mortality reporting in the United States. The implementation date for ICD-10-CM diagnostic coding system to replace ICD-9-CM in the United States was October 1, 2015.

ICD-10-PCS. International Classification of Diseases, 10th Revision, Procedure Coding System. Beginning October 1, 2015, inpatient hospital services and surgical procedures must be coded using ICD-10-PCS codes, replacing ICD-9-CM, Volume 3 for procedures.

ICM. Implantable cardiovascular monitor.

ileostomy. Artificial surgical opening that brings the end of the ileum out through the abdominal wall to the skin surface for the diversion of feces through a stoma.

iliopsoas tendon. Fibrous tissue that connects muscle to bone in the pelvic region, common to the iliacus and psoas major.

ILR. Implantable loop recorder.

IM. 1) Infectious mononucleosis. 2) Internal medicine. 3) Intramuscular.

immunotherapy. Therapeutic use of serum or gamma globulin.

implant. Material or device inserted or placed within the body for therapeutic, reconstructive, or diagnostic purposes.

implantable cardiovascular monitor. Implantable electronic device that stores cardiovascular physiologic data such as intracardiac pressure waveforms collected from internal sensors or data such as weight and blood pressure collected from external sensors. The information stored in these devices is used as an aid in managing patients with heart failure and other cardiac conditions that are non-rhythm related. The data may be transmitted via local telemetry or remotely to a surveillance technician or an internet-based file server.

implantable cardioverter-defibrillator. Implantable electronic cardiac device used to control rhythm abnormalities such as tachycardia, fibrillation, or bradycardia by producing high- or low-energy stimulation and pacemaker functions. It may also have the capability to provide the functions of an implantable loop recorder or implantable cardiovascular monitor.

implantable loop recorder. Implantable electronic cardiac device that constantly monitors and records electrocardiographic rhythm. It may be triggered by the patient when a symptomatic episode occurs or activated automatically by rapid or slow heart rates. This may be the sole purpose of the device or it may be a component of another cardiac device, such as a pacemaker or implantable cardioverter-defibrillator. The data can be transmitted via local telemetry or remotely to a surveillance technician or an internet-based file server.

implantable venous access device. Catheter implanted for continuous access to the venous system for long-term parenteral feeding or for the administration of fluids or medications.

IMRT. Intensity modulated radiation therapy. External beam radiation therapy delivery using computer planning to specify the target dose and to modulate the radiation intensity, usually as a treatment for a malignancy. The delivery system approaches the patient from multiple angles, minimizing damage to normal tissue.

in situ. Located in the natural position or contained within the origin site, not spread into neighboring tissue.

incontinence. Inability to control urination or defecation.

infundibulectomy. Excision of the anterosuperior portion of the right ventricle of the heart.

internal direct current stimulator. Electrostimulation device placed directly into the surgical site designed to promote bone regeneration by encouraging cellular healing response in bone and ligaments.

interrogation device evaluation. Assessment of an implantable cardiac device (pacemaker, cardioverter-defibrillator, cardiovascular monitor, or loop recorder) in which collected data about the patient's heart rate and rhythm, battery and pulse generator function, and any leads or sensors present, are retrieved and evaluated. Determinations regarding device programming and appropriate treatment settings are made based on the findings. CPT provides required components for evaluation of the various types of devices.

intramedullary implants. Nail, rod, or pin placed into the intramedullary canal at the fracture site. Intramedullary implants not only provide a method of aligning the fracture, they also act as a splint and may reduce fracture pain. Implants may be rigid or flexible. Rigid implants are preferred for prophylactic treatment of diseased bone, while flexible implants are preferred for traumatic injuries.

intraocular lens. Artificial lens implanted into the eye to replace a damaged natural lens or cataract.

intravenous. Within a vein or veins.

introducer. Instrument, such as a catheter, needle, or tube, through which another instrument or device is introduced into the body.

intron. Nonprotein section of a gene that separates exons in human genes. Contains vital sequences that allow splicing of exons to produce a functional protein from a gene. Sometimes referred to as intervening sequences (IVS).

IP. 1) Interphalangeal. 2) Intraperitoneal.

irrigation. To wash out or cleanse a body cavity, wound, or tissue with water or other fluid.

Kayser-Fleischer ring. Condition found in Wilson's disease in which deposits of copper cause a pigmented ring around the cornea's outer border in the deep epithelial layers.

keratoprosthesis. Surgical procedure in which the physician creates a new anterior chamber with a plastic optical implant to replace a severely damaged cornea that cannot be repaired.

keratotomy. Surgical incision of the cornea.

krypton laser. Laser light energy that uses ionized krypton by electric current as the active source, has a radiation beam between the visible yellow-red spectrum, and is effective in photocoagulation of retinal bleeding, macular lesions, and vessel aberrations of the choroid.

lacrimal. Tear-producing gland or ducts that provides lubrication and flushing of the eyes and nasal cavities.

lacrimal punctum. Opening of the lacrimal papilla of the eyelid through which tears flow to the canaliculi to the lacrimal sac.

lacrimotome. Knife for cutting the lacrimal sac or duct.

lacrimotomy. Incision of the lacrimal sac or duct.

laparotomy. Incision through the flank or abdomen for therapeutic or diagnostic purposes.

laryngoscopy. Examination of the hypopharynx, larynx, and tongue base with an endoscope.

larynx. Musculocartilaginous structure between the trachea and the pharynx that functions as the valve preventing food and other particles from entering the respiratory tract, as well as the voice mechanism. Also called the voicebox, the larynx is composed of three single cartilages: cricoid, epiglottis, and thyroid; and three paired cartilages: arytenoid, corniculate, and cuneiform.

laser surgery. Use of concentrated, sharply defined light beams to cut, cauterize, coagulate, seal, or vaporize tissue.

LEEP. Loop electrode excision procedure. Biopsy specimen or cone shaped wedge of cervical tissue is removed using a hot cautery wire loop with an electrical current running through it.

levonorgestrel. Drug inhibiting ovulation and preventing sperm from penetrating cervical mucus. It is delivered subcutaneously in polysiloxone capsules. The capsules can be effective for up to five years, and provide a cumulative pregnancy rate of less than 2 percent. The capsules are not biodegradable, and therefore must be removed. Removal is more difficult than insertion of levonorgestrel capsules because fibrosis develops around the capsules. Normal hormonal activity and a return to fertility begins immediately upon removal.

ligament. Band or sheet of fibrous tissue that connects the articular surfaces of bones or supports visceral organs.

ligation. Tying off a blood vessel or duct with a suture or a soft, thin wire.

lymphadenectomy. Dissection of lymph nodes free from the vessels and removal for examination by frozen section in a separate procedure to detect early-stage metastases.

lysis. Destruction, breakdown, dissolution, or decomposition of cells or substances by a specific catalyzing agent.

Magnuson-Stack procedure. Treatment for recurrent anterior dislocation of the shoulder that involves tightening and realigning the subscapularis tendon.

maintenance of wakefulness test. Attended study determining the patient's ability to stay awake.

Manchester operation. Preservation of the uterus following prolapse by amputating the vaginal portion of the cervix, shortening the cardinal ligaments, and performing a colpoperineorrhaphy posteriorly.

mapping. Multidimensional depiction of a tachycardia that identifies its site of origin and its electrical conduction pathway after tachycardia has been induced. The recording is made from multiple catheter sites within the heart, obtaining electrograms simultaneously or sequentially.

marsupialization. Creation of a pouch in surgical treatment of a cyst in which one wall is resected and the remaining cut edges are sutured to adjacent tissue creating an open pouch of the previously enclosed cyst.

mastectomy. Surgical removal of one or both breasts.

McDonald procedure. Polyester tape is placed around the cervix with a running stitch to assist in the prevention of pre-term delivery. Tape is removed at term for vaginal delivery.

MCP. Metacarpophalangeal.

medial. Middle or midline.

mediastinotomy. Incision into the mediastinum for purposes of exploration, foreign body removal, drainage, or biopsy.

medical review. Review by a Medicare administrative contractor, carrier, and/or quality improvement organization (QIO) of services and items provided by physicians, other health care practitioners, and providers of health care services under Medicare. The review determines if the items and services are reasonable and necessary and meet Medicare coverage requirements, whether the quality meets professionally recognized standards of health care, and whether the services are medically appropriate in an inpatient, outpatient, or other setting as supported by documentation.

Medicare contractor. Medicare Part A fiscal intermediary, Medicare Part B carrier, Medicare administrative contractor (MAC), or a durable medical equipment Medicare administrative contractor (DME MAC).

Medicare physician fee schedule. List of payments Medicare allows by procedure or service. Payments may vary through geographic adjustments. The MPFS is based on the resource-based relative value scale (RBRVS). A national total relative value unit (RVU) is given to each procedure (HCPCS Level I CPT, Level II national codes). Each total RVU has three components: physician work, practice expense, and malpractice insurance.

meibomian gland. Sebaceous gland located in the tarsal plates along the eyelid margins that produces the lipid components found in tears.

metabolite. Chemical compound resulting from the natural process of metabolism. In drug testing, the metabolite of the drug may endure in a higher concentration or for a longer duration than the initial "parent" drug.

methylation. Mechanism used to regulate genes and protect DNA from some types of cleavage.

microarray. Small surface onto which multiple specific nucleic acid sequences can be attached to be used for analysis. Microarray may also be known as a gene chip or DNA chip. Tests can be run on the sequences for any variants that may be present.

mitral valve. Valve with two cusps that is between the left atrium and left ventricle of the heart.

moderate sedation. Medically controlled state of depressed consciousness, with or without analgesia, while maintaining the patient's airway, protective reflexes, and ability to respond to stimulation or verbal commands.

Mohs micrographic surgery. Special technique used to treat complex or ill-defined skin cancer and requires a single physician to provide two distinct services. The first service is surgical and involves the destruction of the lesion by a combination of chemosurgery and excision. The second service is that of a pathologist and includes mapping, color coding of specimens, microscopic examination of specimens, and complete histopathologic preparation.

monitored anesthesia care. Sedation, with or without analgesia, used to achieve a medically controlled state of depressed consciousness while maintaining the patient's airway, protective reflexes, and ability to respond to stimulation or verbal commands. In dental conscious sedation, the patient is rendered free of fear, apprehension, and anxiety through the use of pharmacological agents.

monoclonal. Relating to a single clone of cells.

mosaicplasty. Multiple, small grafts composed of bone and cartilage placed to treat osteochondral defects of the knee. The grafts are cylindrical in shape and are placed in corresponding size holes made to the desired depth to fill the defect and allow for a more naturally shaped reconstruction.

multiple sleep latency test (MSLT). Attended study to determine the tendency of the patient to fall asleep.

multiple-lead device. Implantable cardiac device (pacemaker or implantable cardioverter-defibrillator [ICD]) in which pacing and sensing components are placed in at least three chambers of the heart.

Mustard procedure. Corrective measure for transposition of great vessels involves an intra-atrial baffle made of pericardial tissue or synthetic material. The baffle is secured between pulmonary veins and mitral valve and between mitral and tricuspid valves. The baffle directs systemic venous flow into the left ventricle and lungs and pulmonary venous flow into the right ventricle and aorta.

mutation. Alteration in gene function that results in changes to a gene or chromosome. Can cause deficits or disease that can be inherited, can have beneficial effects, or result in no noticeable change.

mutation scanning. Process normally used on multiple polymerase chain reaction (PCR) amplicons to determine DNA sequence variants by differences in characteristics compared to normal. Specific DNA variants can then be studied further.

myotomy. Surgical cutting of a muscle to gain access to underlying tissues or for therapeutic reasons.

myringotomy. Incision in the eardrum done to prevent spontaneous rupture precipitated by fluid pressure build-up behind the tympanic membrane and to prevent stagnant infection and erosion of the ossicles.

nasal polyp. Fleshy outgrowth projecting from the mucous membrane of the nose or nasal sinus cavity that may obstruct ventilation or affect the sense of smell.

nasal sinus. Air-filled cavities in the cranial bones lined with mucous membrane and continuous with the nasal cavity, draining fluids through the nose.

nasogastric tube. Long, hollow, cylindrical catheter made of soft rubber or plastic that is inserted through the nose down into the stomach, and is used for feeding, instilling medication, or withdrawing gastric contents.

nasolacrimal punctum. Opening of the lacrimal duct near the nose.

nasopharynx. Membranous passage above the level of the soft palate.

Nd:YAG laser. Laser light energy that uses an yttrium, aluminum, and garnet crystal doped with neodymium ions as the active source, has a radiation beam nearing the infrared spectrum, and is effective in photocoagulation, photoablation, cataract extraction, and lysis of vitreous strands.

nebulizer. Latin for mist, a device that converts liquid into a fine spray and is commonly used to deliver medicine to the upper respiratory, bronchial, and lung areas.

nerve conduction study. Diagnostic test performed to assess muscle or nerve damage. Nerves are stimulated with electric shocks along the course of the muscle. Sensors are utilized to measure and record nerve functions, including conduction and velocity.

neurectomy. Excision of all or a portion of a nerve.

neuromuscular junction. Nerve synapse at the meeting point between the terminal end of a nerve (motor neuron) and a muscle fiber.

neuropsychological testing. Evaluation of a patient's behavioral abilities wherein a physician or other health care professional administers a series of tests in thinking, reasoning, and judgment.

new patient. Patient who is receiving face-to-face care from a provider/qualified health care professional or another physician/qualified health care professional of the exact same specialty and subspecialty who belongs to the same group practice for the first time in three years. For OPPS hospitals, a patient who has not been registered as an inpatient or outpatient, including off-campus provider based clinic or emergency department, within the past three years.

Niemann-Pick syndrome. Accumulation of phospholipid in histiocytes in the bone marrow, liver, lymph nodes, and spleen, cerebral involvement, and red macular spots similar to Tay-Sachs disease. Most commonly found in Jewish infants.

Nissen fundoplasty. Surgical repair technique that involves the fundus of the stomach being wrapped around the lower end of the esophagus to treat reflux esophagitis.

nonabsorbable sutures. Strands of natural or synthetic material that resist absorption into living tissue and are removed once healing is under way. Nonabsorbable sutures are commonly used to close skin wounds and repair tendons or collagenous tissue.

obturator. Prosthesis used to close an acquired or congenital opening in the palate that aids in speech and chewing.

obturator nerve. Lumbar plexus nerve with anterior and posterior divisions that innervate the adductor muscles (e.g., adductor longus, adductor brevis) of the leg and the skin over the medial area of the thigh or

Appendix M — Glossary

a sacral plexus nerve with anterior and posterior divisions that innervate the superior gemellus muscles.

occult blood test. Chemical or microscopic test to determine the presence of blood in a specimen.

ocular implant. Implant inside muscular cone.

oophorectomy. Surgical removal of all or part of one or both ovaries, either as open procedure or laparoscopically. Menstruation and childbearing ability continues when one ovary is removed.

orthosis. Derived from a Greek word meaning "to make straight," it is an artificial appliance that supports, aligns, or corrects an anatomical deformity or improves the use of a moveable body part. Unlike a prosthesis, an orthotic device is always functional in nature.

osteo-. Having to do with bone.

osteogenesis stimulator. Device used to stimulate the growth of bone by electrical impulses or ultrasound.

osteotomy. Surgical cutting of a bone.

ostomy. Artificial (surgical) opening in the body used for drainage or for delivery of medications or nutrients.

pacemaker. Implantable cardiac device that controls the heart's rhythm and maintains regular beats by artificial electric discharges. This device consists of the pulse generator with a battery and the electrodes, or leads, which are placed in single or dual chambers of the heart, usually transvenously.

palmaris longus tendon. Tendon located in the hand that flexes the wrist joint.

paracentesis. Surgical puncture of a body cavity with a specialized needle or hollow tubing to aspirate fluid for diagnostic or therapeutic reasons.

paratenon graft. Graft composed of the fatty tissue found between a tendon and its sheath.

passive mobilization. Pressure, movement, or pulling of a limb or body part utilizing an apparatus or device.

pedicle flap. Full-thickness skin and subcutaneous tissue for grafting that remains partially attached to the donor site by a pedicle or stem in which the blood vessels supplying the flap remain intact.

Pemberton osteotomy. Osteotomy is performed to position triradiate cartilage as a hinge for rotating the acetabular roof in cases of dysplasia of the hip in children.

penetrance. Being formed by, or pertaining to, a single clone.

percutaneous intradiscal electrothermal annuloplasty. Procedure corrects tears in the vertebral annulus by applying heat to the collagen disc walls percutaneously through a catheter. The heat contracts and thickens the wall, which may contract and close any annular tears.

percutaneous skeletal fixation. Treatment that is neither open nor closed and the injury site is not directly visualized. Fixation devices (pins, screws) are placed through the skin to stabilize the dislocation using x-ray guidance.

pericardium. Thin and slippery case in which the heart lies that is lined with fluid so that the heart is free to pulse and move as it beats.

peripheral arterial tonometry (PAT). Pulsatile volume changes in a digit are measured to determine activity in the sympathetic nervous system for respiratory analysis.

peritoneal. Space between the lining of the abdominal wall, or parietal peritoneum, and the surface layer of the abdominal organs, or visceral peritoneum. It contains a thin, watery fluid that keeps the peritoneal surfaces moist.

peritoneal dialysis. Dialysis that filters waste from blood inside the body using the peritoneum, the natural lining of the abdomen, as the semipermeable membrane across which ultrafiltration is accomplished. A special catheter is inserted into the abdomen and a dialysis solution is drained into the abdomen. This solution extracts fluids and wastes, which are then discarded when the fluid is drained. Various forms of peritoneal dialysis include CAPD, CCPD, and NIDP.

peritoneal effusion. Persistent escape of fluid within the peritoneal cavity.

pessary. Device placed in the vagina to support and reposition a prolapsing or retropositioned uterus, rectum, or vagina.

phacoemulsification. Cataract extraction in which the lens is fragmented by ultrasonic vibrations and simultaneously irrigated and aspirated.

phenotype. Physical expression of a trait or characteristic as determined by an individual's genetic makeup or genotype.

photocoagulation. Application of an intense laser beam of light to disrupt tissue and condense protein material to a residual mass, used especially for treating ocular conditions.

physical status modifiers. Alphanumeric modifier used to identify the patient's health status as it affects the work related to providing the anesthesia service.

physical therapy modality. Therapeutic agent or regimen applied or used to provide appropriate treatment of the musculoskeletal system.

physician. Legally authorized practitioners including a doctor of medicine or osteopathy, a doctor of dental surgery or of dental medicine, a doctor of podiatric medicine, a doctor of optometry, and a chiropractor only with respect to treatment by means of manual manipulation of the spine (to correct a subluxation).

PICC. Peripherally inserted central catheter. PICC is inserted into one of the large veins of the arm and threaded through the vein until the tip sits in a large vein just above the heart.

PKR. Photorefractive therapy. Procedure involving the removal of the surface layer of the cornea (epithelium) by gentle scraping and use of a computer-controlled excimer laser to reshape the stroma.

pleurodesis. Injection of a sclerosing agent into the pleural space for creating adhesions between the parietal and the visceral pleura to treat a collapsed lung caused by air trapped in the pleural cavity, or severe cases of pleural effusion.

plication. Surgical technique involving folding, tucking, or pleating to reduce the size of a hollow structure or organ.

polyclonal. Containing one or more cells.

polymorphism. Genetic variation in the same species that does not harm the gene function or create disease.

polypeptide. Chain of amino acids held together by covalent bonds. Proteins are made up of amino acids.

polysomnography. Test involving monitoring of respiratory, cardiac, muscle, brain, and ocular function during sleep.

Potts-Smith-Gibson procedure. Side-to-side anastomosis of the aorta and left pulmonary artery creating a shunt that enlarges as the child grows.

Prader-Willi syndrome. Rounded face, almond-shaped eyes, strabismus, low forehead, hypogonadism, hypotonia, intellectual disabilities, and an insatiable appetite.

presumptive drug testing. Drug screening tests to identify the presence or absence of drugs in a patient's system. Tests are usually able to identify low concentrations of the drug. These tests may be used for medical, workplace, or legal purposes.

presumptive identification. Identification of microorganisms using media growth, colony morphology, gram stains, or up to three specific tests (e.g., catalase, indole, oxidase, urease).

professional component. Portion of a charge for health care services that represents the physician's (or other practitioner's) work in providing the service, including interpretation and report of the procedure. This component of the service usually is charged for and billed separately from the inpatient hospital charges.

profunda. Denotes a part of a structure that is deeper from the surface of the body than the rest of the structure.

prolonged physician services. Extended pre- or post-service care provided to a patient whose condition requires services beyond the usual.

prostate. Male gland surrounding the bladder neck and urethra that secretes a substance into the seminal fluid.

prosthetic. Device that replaces all or part of an internal body organ or body part, or that replaces part of the function of a permanently inoperable or malfunctioning internal body organ or body part.

provider of services. Institution, individual, or organization that provides health care.

proximal. Located closest to a specified reference point, usually the midline or trunk.

psychiatric hospital. Specialized institution that provides, under the supervision of physicians, services for the diagnosis and treatment of mentally ill persons.

pterygium. Benign, wedge-shaped, conjunctival thickening that advances from the inner corner of the eye toward the cornea.

pterygomaxillary fossa. Wide depression on the external surface of the maxilla above and to the side of the canine tooth socket.

pulmonary artery banding. Surgical constriction of the pulmonary artery to prevent irreversible pulmonary vascular obstructive changes and overflow into the left ventricle.

Putti-Platt procedure. Realignment of the subscapularis tendon to treat recurrent anterior dislocation, thereby partially eliminating external rotation. The anterior capsule is also tightened and reinforced.

pyloroplasty. Enlargement and reconstruction of the lower portion of the stomach opening into the duodenum performed after vagotomy to speed gastric emptying and treat duodenal ulcers.

qualified health care professional. Educated, licensed or certified, and regulated professional operating under a specified scope of practice to provide patient services that are separate and distinct from other clinical staff. Services may be billed independently or under the facility's services.

RAC. Recovery audit contractor. National program using CMS-affiliated contractors to review claims prior to payment as well as for payments on claims already processed, including overpayments and underpayments.

radiation therapy simulation. Radiation therapy simulation. Procedure by which the specific body area to be treated with radiation is defined and marked. A CT scan is performed to define the body contours and these images are used to create a plan customized treatment for the patient, targeting the area to be treated while sparing adjacent tissue. The center of the area to be treated is marked and an immobilization device (e.g., cradle, mold) is created to make sure the patient is in the same position each time for treatment. Complexity of treatment depends on the number of treatment areas and the use of tools to isolate the area of treatment.

radioactive substances. Materials used in the diagnosis and treatment of disease that emit high-speed particles and energy-containing rays.

radiology services. Services that include diagnostic and therapeutic radiology, nuclear medicine, CT scan procedures, magnetic resonance imaging services, ultrasound, and other imaging procedures.

radiotherapy afterloading. Part of the radiation therapy process in which the chemotherapy agent is actually instilled into the tumor area subsequent to surgery and placement of an expandable catheter into the void remaining after tumor excision. The specialized catheter remains in place and the patient may come in for multiple treatments with radioisotope placed to treat the margin of tissue surrounding the excision. After the radiotherapy is completed, the patient returns to have the catheter emptied and removed. This is a new therapy in breast cancer treatment.

Rashkind procedure. Transvenous balloon atrial septectomy or septostomy performed by cardiac catheterization. A balloon catheter is inserted into the heart either to create or enlarge an opening in the interatrial septal wall.

rehabilitation services. Therapy services provided primarily for assisting in a rehabilitation program of evaluation and service including cardiac rehabilitation, medical social services, occupational therapy, physical therapy, respiratory therapy, skilled nursing, speech therapy, psychiatric rehabilitation, and alcohol and substance abuse rehabilitation.

respiratory airflow (ventilation). Assessment of air movement during inhalation and exhalation as measured by nasal pressure sensors and thermistor.

respiratory analysis. Assessment of components of respiration obtained by other methods such as airflow or peripheral arterial tone.

respiratory effort. Measurement of diaphragm and/or intercostal muscle for airflow using transducers to estimate thoracic and abdominal motion.

respiratory movement. Measurement of chest and abdomen movement during respiration.

ribbons. In oncology, small plastic tubes containing radioactive sources for interstitial placement that may be cut into specific lengths tailored to the size of the area receiving ionizing radiation treatment.

Ridell sinusotomy. Frontal sinus tissue is destroyed to eliminate tumors.

RNA. Ribonucleic acid.

rural health clinic. Clinic in an area where there is a shortage of health services staffed by a nurse practitioner, physician assistant, or certified nurse midwife under physician direction that provides routine diagnostic services, including clinical laboratory services, drugs, and biologicals and that has prompt access to additional diagnostic services from facilities meeting federal requirements.

Salter osteotomy. Innominate bone of the hip is cut, removed, and repositioned to repair a congenital dislocation, subluxation, or deformity.

saucerization. Creation of a shallow, saucer-like depression in the bone to facilitate drainage of infected areas.

Schiotz tonometer. Instrument that measures intraocular pressure by recording the depth of an indentation on the cornea by a plunger of known weight.

screening mammography. Radiologic images taken of the female breast for the early detection of breast cancer.

screening pap smear. Diagnostic laboratory test consisting of a routine exfoliative cytology test (Papanicolaou test) provided to a woman for the early detection of cervical or vaginal cancer. The exam includes a clinical breast examination and a physician's interpretation of the results.

seeds. Small (1 mm or less) sources of radioactive material that are permanently placed directly into tumors.

Senning procedure. Flaps of intra-atrial septum and right atrial wall are used to create two interatrial channels to divert the systemic and pulmonary venous circulation.

sensitivity tests. Number of methods of applying selective suspected allergens to the skin or mucous.

sensorineural conduction. Transportation of sound from the cochlea to the acoustic nerve and central auditory pathway to the brain.

sentinel lymph node. First node to which lymph drainage and metastasis from a cancer can occur.

separate procedures. Services commonly carried out as a fundamental part of a total service and, as such, do not usually warrant separate identification. These services are identified in CPT with the parenthetical phrase (separate procedure) at the end of the description and are payable only when performed alone.

septectomy. 1) Surgical removal of all or part of the nasal septum. 2) Submucosal resection of the nasal septum.

Shirodkar procedure. Treatment of an incompetent cervical os by placing nonabsorbent suture material in purse-string sutures as a cerclage to support the cervix.

short tandem repeat (STR). Short sequences of a DNA pattern that are repeated. Can be used as genetic markers for human identity testing.

sialodochoplasty. Surgical repair of a salivary gland duct.

single-lead device. Implantable cardiac device (pacemaker or implantable cardioverter-defibrillator [ICD]) in which pacing and sensing components are placed in only one chamber of the heart.

single-nucleotide polymorphism (SNP). Single nucleotide (A, T, C, or G that is different in a DNA sequence. This difference occurs at a significant frequency in the population.

sinus of Valsalva. Any of three sinuses corresponding to the individual cusps of the aortic valve, located in the most proximal part of the aorta just above the cusps. These structures are contained within the pericardium and appear as distinct but subtle outpouchings or dilations of the aortic wall between each of the semilunar cusps of the valve.

sleep apnea. Intermittent cessation of breathing during sleep that may cause hypoxemia and pulmonary arterial hypertension.

sleep latency. Time period between lying down in bed and the onset of sleep.

sleep staging. Determination of the separate levels of sleep according to physiological measurements.

somatic. 1) Pertaining to the body or trunk. 2) In genetics acquired or occurring after birth.

SPECT. Single photon emission computerized tomography. SPECT images are taken after the injection of a radionuclide using a special camera containing a detector crystal, usually sodium iodide. Images are captured as the gamma radiation from the radionuclide scintillates or gives off its energy in a flash of light when coming in contact with the crystal. This type of imaging is reported for the anatomical area and purpose such as detecting liver function or myocardial perfusion after an ischemic event.

speculoscopy. Viewing the cervix utilizing a magnifier and a special wavelength of light, allowing detection of abnormalities that may not be discovered on a routine Pap smear.

speech-language pathology services. Speech, language, and related function assessment and rehabilitation service furnished by a qualified speech-language pathologist. Audiology services include hearing and balance assessment services furnished by a qualified audiologist. A qualified speech pathologist and audiologist must have a master's or doctoral degree in their respective fields and be licensed to serve in the state. Speech pathologists and audiologists practicing in states without licensure must complete 350 hours of supervised clinical work and perform at least nine months of supervised full-time service after earning their degrees.

sphincteroplasty. Surgical repair done to correct, augment, or improve the muscular function of a sphincter, such as the anus or intestines.

spirometry. Measurement of the lungs' breathing capacity.

splint. Brace or support. 1) dynamic splint: brace that permits movement of an anatomical structure such as a hand, wrist, foot, or other part of the body after surgery or injury. 2) static splint: brace that prevents movement and maintains support and position for an anatomical structure after surgery or injury.

stent. Tube to provide support in a body cavity or lumen.

stereotactic radiosurgery. Delivery of externally-generated ionizing radiation to specific targets for destruction or inactivation. Most often utilized in the treatment of brain or spinal tumors, high-resolution stereotactic imaging is used to identify the target and then deliver the treatment. Computer-assisted planning may also be employed. Simple and complex cranial lesions and spinal lesions are typically treated in a single planning and treatment session, although a maximum of five sessions may be required. No incision is made for stereotactic radiosurgery procedures.

stereotaxis. Three-dimensional method for precisely locating structures.

Stoffel rhizotomy. Nerve roots are sectioned to relieve pain or spastic paralysis.

strabismus. Misalignment of the eyes due to an imbalance in extraocular muscles.

surgical package. Normal, uncomplicated performance of specific surgical services, with the assumption that, on average, all surgical procedures of a given type are similar with respect to skill level, duration, and length of normal follow-up care.

symblepharopterygium. Adhesion in which the eyelid is adhered to the eyeball by a band that resembles a pterygium.

sympathectomy. Surgical interruption or transection of a sympathetic nervous system pathway.

tarso-. 1) Relating to the foot. 2) Relating to the margin of the eyelid.

tarsocheiloplasty. Plastic operation upon the edge of the eyelid for the treatment of trichiasis.

tarsorrhaphy. Suture of a portion or all of the opposing eyelids together for the purpose of shortening the palpebral fissure or closing it entirely.

technical component. Portion of a health care service that identifies the provision of the equipment, supplies, technical personnel, and costs attendant to the performance of the procedure other than the professional services.

tendon. Fibrous tissue that connects muscle to bone, consisting primarily of collagen and containing little vasculature.

tendon allograft. Allografts are tissues obtained from another individual of the same species. Tendon allografts are usually obtained from cadavers and frozen or freeze dried for later use in soft tissue repairs where the physician elects not to obtain an autogenous graft (a graft obtained from the individual on whom the surgery is being performed).

tendon suture material. Tendons are composed of fibrous tissue consisting primarily of collagen and containing few cells or blood vessels. This tissue heals more slowly than tissues with more vascularization. Because of this, tendons are usually repaired with nonabsorbable suture material. Examples include surgical silk, surgical cotton, linen, stainless steel, surgical nylon, polyester fiber, polybutester (Novafil), polyethylene (Dermalene), and polypropylene (Prolene, Surilene).

tendon transplant. Replacement of a tendon with another tendon.

tenon's capsule. Connective tissue that forms the capsule enclosing the posterior eyeball, extending from the conjunctival fornix and continuous with the muscular fascia of the eye.

tenonectomy. Excision of a portion of a tendon to make it shorter.

tenotomy. Cutting into a tendon.

TENS. Transcutaneous electrical nerve stimulator. TENS is applied by placing electrode pads over the area to be stimulated and connecting the electrodes to a transmitter box, which sends a current through the skin to sensory nerve fibers to help decrease pain in that nerve distribution.

tensilon. Edrophonium chloride. Agent used for evaluation and treatment of myasthenia gravis.

terminally ill. Individual whose medical prognosis for life expectancy is six months or less.

tetralogy of Fallot. Specific combination of congenital cardiac defects: obstruction of the right ventricular outflow tract with pulmonary stenosis, interventricular septal defect, malposition of the aorta, overriding the interventricular septum and receiving blood from both the venous and arterial systems, and enlargement of the right ventricle.

therapeutic services. Services performed for treatment of a specific diagnosis. These services include performance of the procedure, various incidental elements, and normal, related follow-up care.

thoracentesis. Surgical puncture of the chest cavity with a specialized needle or hollow tubing to aspirate fluid from within the pleural space for diagnostic or therapeutic reasons.

thoracic lymphadenectomy. Procedure to cut out the lymph nodes near the lungs, around the heart, and behind the trachea.

thoracostomy. Creation of an opening in the chest wall for drainage.

thyroglossal duct. Embryonic duct at the front of the neck, which becomes the pyramidal lobe of the thyroid gland with obliteration of the remaining duct, but may form a cyst or sinus in adulthood if it persists.

total disc arthroplasty with artificial disc. Removal of an intravertebral disc and its replacement with an implant. The implant is an artificial disc consisting of two metal plates with a weight-bearing surface of polyethylene between the plates. The plates are anchored to the vertebral immediately above and below the affected disc.

total shoulder replacement. Prosthetic replacement of the entire shoulder joint, including the humeral head and the glenoid fossa.

trabeculae carneae cordis. Bands of muscular tissue that line the walls of the ventricles in the heart.

trabeculectomy. Surgical incision between the anterior portion of the eye and the canal of Schlemm to drain the aqueous humor.

tracheostomy. Formation of a tracheal opening on the neck surface with tube insertion to allow for respiration in cases of obstruction or decreased patency. A tracheostomy may be planned or performed on an emergency basis for temporary or long-term use.

tracheotomy. Formation of a tracheal opening on the neck surface with tube insertion to allow for respiration in cases of obstruction or decreased patency. A tracheotomy may be planned or performed on an emergency basis for temporary or long-term use.

traction. Drawing out or holding tension on an area by applying a direct therapeutic pulling force.

transcranial magnetic stimulation. Application of electromagnetic energy to the brain through a coil placed on the scalp. The procedure stimulates cortical neurons and is intended to activate and normalize their processes.

transcription. Process by which messenger RNA is synthesized from a DNA template resulting in the transfer of genetic information from the DNA molecule to the messenger RNA.

translocation. Disconnection of all or part of a chromosome that reattaches to another position in the DNA sequence of the same or another chromosome. Often results in a reciprocal exchange of DNA sequences between two differently numbered chromosomes. May or may not result in a clinically significant loss of DNA.

trephine. 1) Specialized round saw for cutting circular holes in bone, especially the skull. 2) Instrument that removes small disc-shaped buttons of corneal tissue for transplanting.

tricuspid atresia. Congenital absence of the valve that may occur with other defects, such as atrial septal defect, pulmonary atresia, and transposition of great vessels.

turbinates. Scroll or shell-shaped elevations from the wall of the nasal cavity, the inferior turbinate being a separate bone, while the superior and middle turbinates are of the ethmoid bone.

tympanic membrane. Thin, sensitive membrane across the entrance to the middle ear that vibrates in response to sound waves, allowing the waves to be transmitted via the ossicular chain to the internal ear.

tympanoplasty. Surgical repair of the structures of the middle ear, including the eardrum and the three small bones, or ossicles.

unlisted procedure. Procedural descriptions used when the overall procedure and outcome of the procedure are not adequately described by an existing procedure code. Such codes are used as a last resort and only when there is not a more appropriate procedure code.

ureterorrhaphy. Surgical repair using sutures to close an open wound or injury of the ureter.

vagotomy. Division of the vagus nerves, interrupting impulses resulting in lower gastric acid production and hastening gastric emptying. Used in the treatment of chronic gastric, pyloric, and duodenal ulcers that can cause severe pain and difficulties in eating and sleeping.

variant. Nucleotide deviation from the normal sequence of a region. Variations are usually either substitutions or deletions. Substitution variations are the result of one nucleotide taking the place of another. A deletion occurs when one or more nucleotides are left out. In some cases, several in a reasonably close proximity on the same chromosome in a DNA strand. These variations result in amino acid changes in the protein made by the gene. However, the term variant does not itself imply a functional change. Intron variations are usually described in one of two ways: 1) the changed nucleotide is defined by a plus or a minus sign indicating the position relative to the first or last nucleotide to the intron, or 2) the second variant description is indicated relative to the last nucleotide of the preceding exon or first nucleotide of the following exon.

vascular family. Group of vessels (family) that branch from the aorta or vena cava. At each branching, the vascular order increases by one. The first order vessel is the primary branch off the aorta or vena cava. The second order vessel branches from the first order, the third order branches from the second order, and any further branching is beyond the third order. For example, for the inferior vena cava, the common iliac artery is a first order vessel. The internal and external iliac arteries are second order vessels, as they each originate from the first order common iliac artery. The external iliac artery extends directly from the common iliac artery and the internal iliac artery bifurcates from the common iliac artery. A third order vessel from the external iliac artery is the inferior epigastric artery and a third order vessel from the internal iliac artery is the obturator artery. Note orders are not always identical bilaterally (e.g., the left common carotid artery is a first order and the right common carotid is a second order. Synonym(s): vascular origins and distributions.

vasectomy. Surgical procedure involving the removal of all or part of the vas deferens, usually performed for sterilization or in conjunction with a prostatectomy.

vena cava interruption. Procedure that places a filter device, called an umbrella or sieve, within the large vein returning deoxygenated blood to the heart to prevent pulmonary embolism caused by clots.

ventricular assist device. Temporary measure used to support the heart by substituting for left and/or right heart function. The device replaces the work of the left and/or right ventricle when a patient has a damaged or weakened heart. A left ventricular assist device (VAD) helps the heart pump blood through the rest of the body. A right VAD helps the heart pump blood to the lungs to become oxygenated again. Catheters are inserted to circulate the blood through external tubing to a pump machine located outside of the body and back to the correct artery.

ventricular septal defect. Congenital cardiac anomaly resulting in a continual opening in the septum between the ventricles that, in severe cases, causes oxygenated blood to flow back into the lungs, resulting in pulmonary hypertension.

vertebral interspace. Non-bony space between two adjacent vertebral bodies that contains the cushioning intervertebral disk.

volar. Palm of the hand (palmar) or sole of the foot (plantar).

Waterston procedure. Type of aortopulmonary shunting done to increase pulmonary blood flow. The ascending aorta is anastomosed to the right pulmonary artery.

Wharton's ducts. Salivary ducts below the mandible.

wick catheter. Device used to monitor interstitial fluid pressure, and sometimes used intraoperatively during fasciotomy procedures to evaluate the effectiveness of the decompression.

wound closure. Closure or repair of a wound created surgically or due to trauma (e.g., laceration). The closure technique depends on the type, site, and depth of the defect. Consideration is also given to cosmetic and functional outcome. A single layer closure involves approximation of the edges of the wound. The second type of closure involves closing the one or more deeper layers of tissue prior to skin closure. The most complex type of closure may include techniques such as debridement or undermining, which involves manipulation of tissue around the wound to allow the skin to cover the wound. The AMA CPT® book defines these as Simple, Intermediate and Complex repair.

xenograft. Tissue that is nonhuman and harvested from one species and grafted to another. Pigskin is the most common xenograft for human skin and is applied to a wound as a temporary closure until a permanent option is performed.

z-plasty. Plastic surgery technique used primarily to release tension or elongate contractured scar tissue in which a Z-shaped incision is made with the middle line of the Z crossing the area of greatest tension. The triangular flaps are then rotated so that they cross the incision line in the opposite direction, creating a reversed Z.

ZPIC. Zone Program Integrity Contractor. CMS contractor that replaced the existing Program Safeguard Contractors (PSC). Contractors are responsible for ensuring the integrity of all Medicare-related claims under Parts A and B (hospital, skilled nursing, home health, provider, and durable medical equipment claims), Part C (Medicare Advantage health plans), Part D (prescription drug plans), and coordination of Medicare-Medicaid data matches (Medi-Medi).

Appendix N — Listing of Sensory, Motor, and Mixed Nerves

This list contains the sensory, motor, and mixed nerves assigned to each nerve conduction study to improve coding accuracy. Each nerve makes up one single unit of service.

Motor Nerves Assigned to Codes 95907-95913

I. Upper extremity, cervical plexus, and brachial plexus motor nerves
   A. Axillary motor nerve to the deltoid
   B. Long thoracic motor nerve to the serratus anterior
   C. Median nerve
      1. Median motor nerve to the abductor pollicis brevis
      2. Median motor nerve, anterior interosseous branch, to the flexor pollicis longus
      3. Median motor nerve, anterior interosseous branch, to the pronator quadratus
      4. Median motor nerve to the first lumbrical
      5. Median motor nerve to the second lumbrical
   D. Musculocutaneous motor nerve to the biceps brachii
   E. Radial nerve
      1. Radial motor nerve to the extensor carpi ulnaris
      2. Radial motor nerve to the extensor digitorum communis
      3. Radial motor nerve to the extensor indicis proprius
      4. Radial motor nerve to the brachioradialis
   F. Suprascapular nerve
      1. Suprascapular motor nerve to the supraspinatus
      2. Suprascapular motor nerve to the infraspinatus
   G. Thoracodorsal motor nerve to the latissimus dorsi
   H. Ulnar nerve
      1. Ulnar motor nerve to the abductor digiti minimi
      2. Ulnar motor nerve to the palmar interosseous
      3. Ulnar motor nerve to the first dorsal interosseous
      4. Ulnar motor nerve to the flexor carpi ulnaris
   I. Other

II. Lower extremity motor nerves
   A. Femoral motor nerve to the quadriceps
      1. Femoral motor nerve to vastus medialis
      2. Femoral motor nerve to vastus lateralis
      3. Femoral motor nerve to vastus intermedialis
      4. Femoral motor nerve to rectus femoris
   B. Ilioinguinal motor nerve
   C. Peroneal (fibular) nerve
      1. Peroneal motor nerve to the extensor digitorum brevis
      2. Peroneal motor nerve to the peroneus brevis
      3. Peroneal motor nerve to the peroneus longus
      4. Peroneal motor nerve to the tibialis anterior
   D. Plantar motor nerve
   E. Sciatic nerve
   F. Tibial nerve
      1. Tibial motor nerve, inferior calcaneal branch, to the abductor digiti minimi
      2. Tibial motor nerve, medial plantar branch, to the abductor hallucis
      3. Tibial motor nerve, lateral plantar branch, to the flexor digiti minimi brevis
   G. Other

III. Cranial nerves and trunk
   A. Cranial nerve VII (facial motor nerve)
      1. Facial nerve to the frontalis
      2. Facial nerve to the nasalis
      3. Facial nerve to the orbicularis oculi
      4. Facial nerve to the orbicularis oris
   B. Cranial nerve XI (spinal accessory motor nerve)
   C. Cranial nerve XII (hypoglossal motor nerve)
   D. Intercostal motor nerve
   E. Phrenic motor nerve to the diaphragm
   F. Recurrent laryngeal nerve
   G. Other

IV. Nerve Roots
   A. Cervical nerve root stimulation
      1. Cervical level 5 (C5)
      2. Cervical level 6 (C6)
      3. Cervical level 7 (C7)
      4. Cervical level 8 (C8)
   B. Thoracic nerve root stimulation
      1. Thoracic level 1 (T1)
      2. Thoracic level 2 (T2)
      3. Thoracic level 3 (T3)
      4. Thoracic level 4 (T4)
      5. Thoracic level 5 (T5)
      6. Thoracic level 6 (T6)
      7. Thoracic level 7 (T7)
      8. Thoracic level 8 (T8)
      9. Thoracic level 9 (T9)
      10. Thoracic level 10 (T10)
      11. Thoracic level 11 (T11)
      12. Thoracic level 12 (T12)
   C. Lumbar nerve root stimulation
      1. Lumbar level 1 (L1)
      2. Lumbar level 2 (L2)
      3. Lumbar level 3 (L3)
      4. Lumbar level 4 (L4)
      5. Lumbar level 5 (L5)
   D. Sacral nerve root stimulation
      1. Sacral level 1 (S1)
      2. Sacral level 2 (S2)
      3. Sacral level 3 (S3)
      4. Sacral level 4 (S4)

Sensory and Mixed Nerves Assigned to Codes 95907–95913

I. Upper extremity sensory and mixed nerves
   A. Lateral antebrachial cutaneous sensory nerve
   B. Medial antebrachial cutaneous sensory nerve
   C. Medial brachial cutaneous sensory nerve
   D. Median nerve
      1. Median sensory nerve to the first digit
      2. Median sensory nerve to the second digit
      3. Median sensory nerve to the third digit
      4. Median sensory nerve to the fourth digit
      5. Median palmar cutaneous sensory nerve
      6. Median palmar mixed nerve
   E. Posterior antebrachial cutaneous sensory nerve
   F. Radial sensory nerve
      1. Radial sensory nerve to the base of the thumb
      2. Radial sensory nerve to digit 1
   G. Ulnar nerve
      1. Ulnar dorsal cutaneous sensory nerve
      2. Ulnar sensory nerve to the fourth digit
      3. Ulnar sensory nerve to the fifth digit
      4. Ulnar palmar mixed nerve
   H. Intercostal sensory nerve
   I. Other

II. Lower extremity sensory and mixed nerves
   A. Lateral femoral cutaneous sensory nerve
   B. Medical calcaneal sensory nerve
   C. Medial femoral cutaneous sensory nerve
   D. Peroneal nerve
      1. Deep peroneal sensory nerve
      2. Superficial peroneal sensory nerve, medial dorsal cutaneous branch
      3. Superficial peroneal sensory nerve, intermediate dorsal cutaneous branch
   E. Posterior femoral cutaneous sensory nerve
   F. Saphenous nerve
      1. Saphenous sensory nerve (distal technique)
      2. Saphenous sensory nerve (proximal technique)
   G. Sural nerve
      1. Sural sensory nerve, lateral dorsal cutaneous branch
      2. Sural sensory nerve
   H. Tibial sensory nerve (digital nerve to toe 1)
   I. Tibial sensory nerve (medial plantar nerve)
   J. Tibial sensory nerve (lateral plantar nerve)
   K. Other

III. Head and trunk sensory nerves
   A. Dorsal nerve of the penis
   B. Greater auricular nerve
   C. Ophthalmic branch of the trigeminal nerve
   D. Pudendal sensory nerve
   E. Suprascapular sensory nerves
   F. Other

In the following table, the reasonable maximum number of studies per diagnostic category is listed that allows for a physician or other qualified health care professional to obtain a diagnosis for 90 percent of patients with that same final diagnosis. The numbers denote the suggested number of studies, although the decision is up to the provider.

Type of Study/Maximum Number of Studies

Indication	Limbs Studied by Needle EMG (95860–95864, 95867–95870, 95885–95887)	Nerve Conduction Studies (Total nerves studied, 95907-95913)	Neuromuscular Junction Testing (Repetitive Stimulation 95937)
Carpal Tunnel (Unilateral)	1	7	—
Carpal Tunnel (Bilateral)	2	10	—
Radiculopathy	2	7	—
Mononeuropathy	1	8	—
Polyneuropathy/Mononeuropathy Multiplex	3	10	—
Myopathy	2	4	2
Motor Neuronopathy (e.g., ALS)	4	6	2
Plexopathy	2	12	—
Neuromuscular Junction	2	4	3
Tarsal Tunnel Syndrome (Unilateral)	1	8	—
Tarsal Tunnel Syndrome (Bilateral)	2	11	—
Weakness, Fatigue, Cramps, or Twitching (Focal)	2	7	2
Weakness, Fatigue, Cramps, or Twitching (General)	4	8	2
Pain, Numbness, or Tingling (Unilateral)	1	9	—
Pain, Numbness, or Tingling (Bilateral)	2	12	—

Appendix O — Vascular Families

This table assumes that the starting point is aortic catheterization. This categorization would not be accurate if, for instance, a femoral or carotid artery were catheterized with the blood's flow. The names of the arteries appearing in bold face type in the following table indicate those arteries that are most often the subject of arteriographic procedures.

Arterial Vascular Family

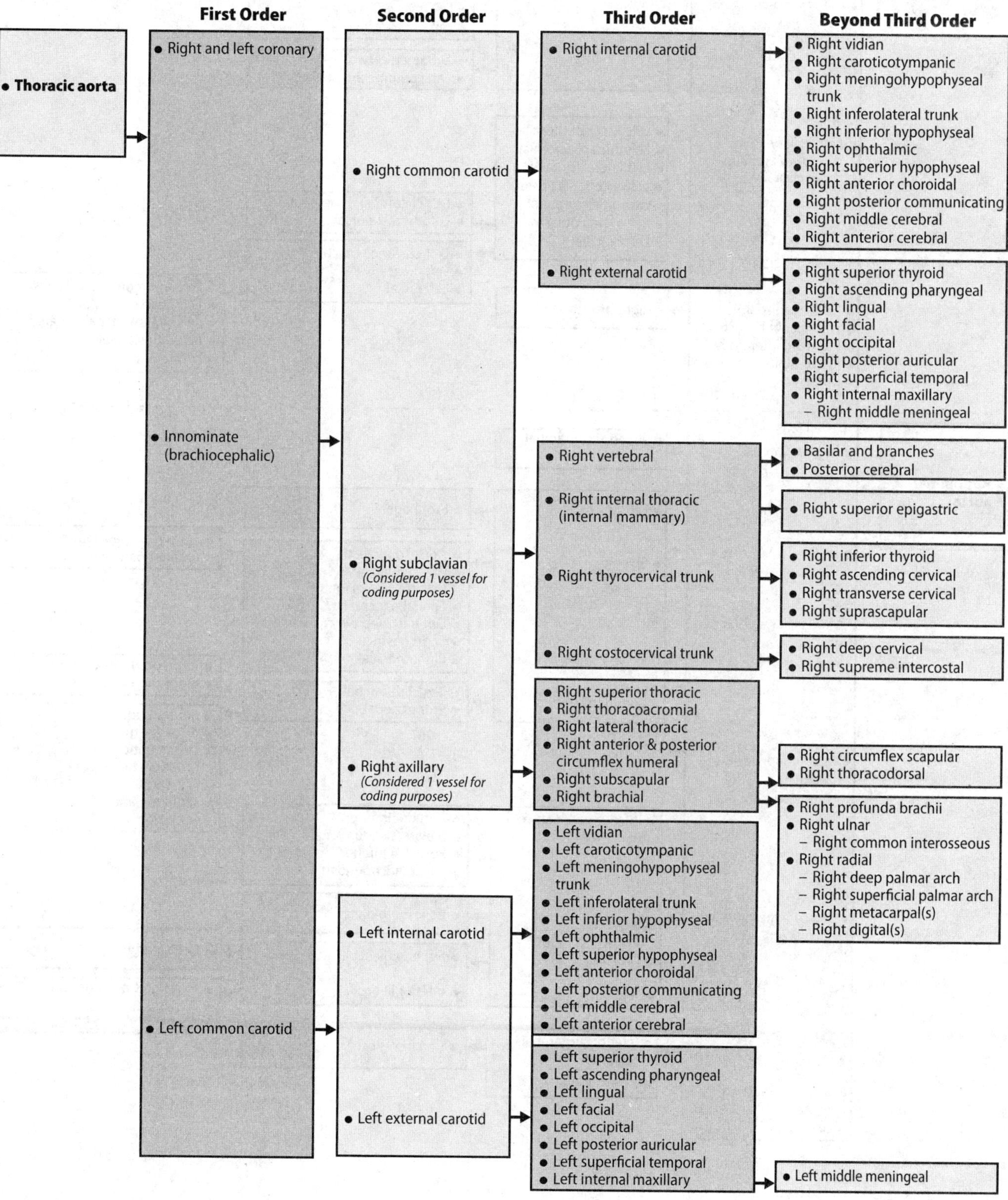

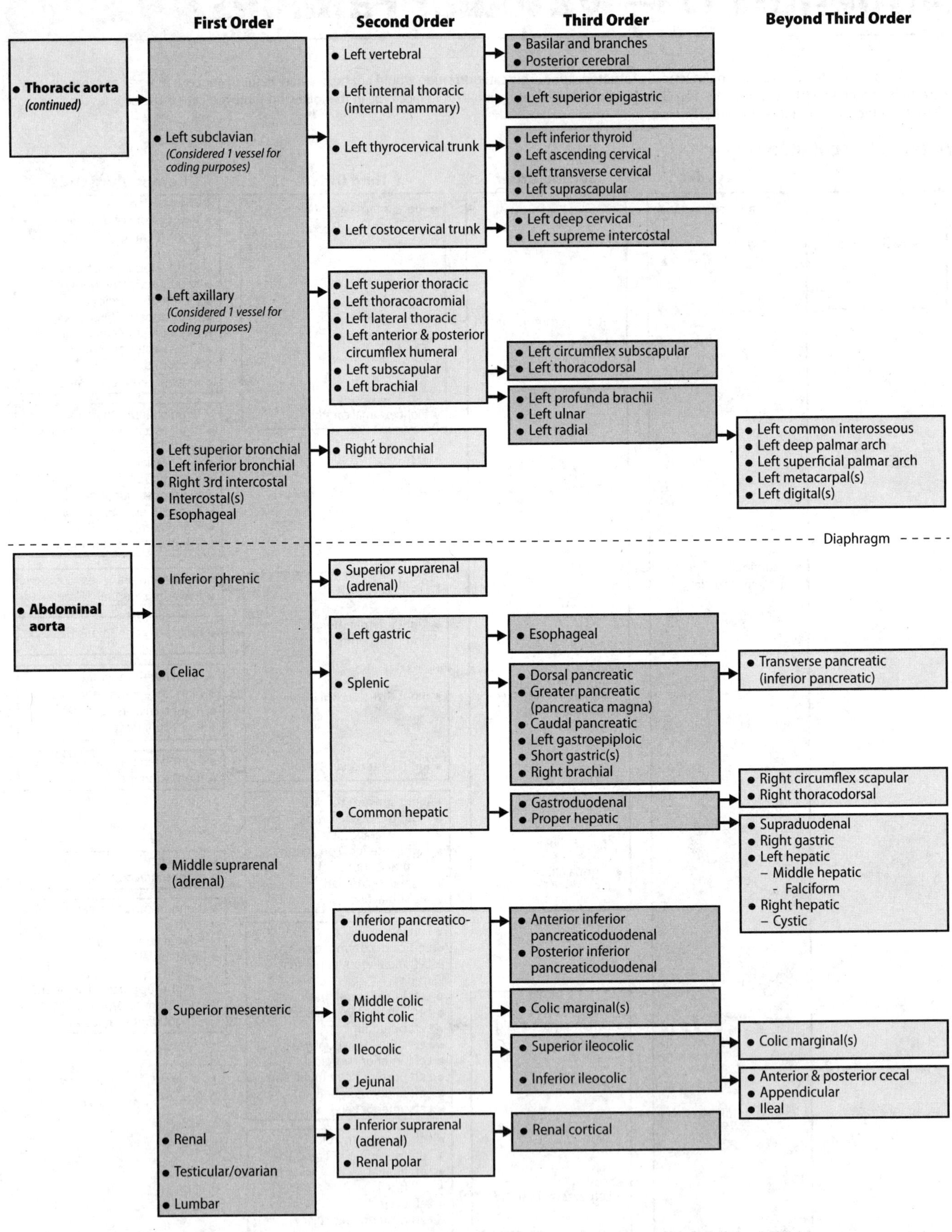
First Order
Second Order
Third Order
Beyond Third Order
• Thoracic aorta (continued)
• Left subclavian (Considered 1 vessel for coding purposes)
• Left vertebral
• Basilar and branches
• Posterior cerebral
• Left internal thoracic (internal mammary)
• Left superior epigastric
• Left thyrocervical trunk
• Left inferior thyroid
• Left ascending cervical
• Left transverse cervical
• Left suprascapular
• Left costocervical trunk
• Left deep cervical
• Left supreme intercostal
• Left axillary (Considered 1 vessel for coding purposes)
• Left superior thoracic
• Left thoracoacromial
• Left lateral thoracic
• Left anterior & posterior circumflex humeral
• Left subscapular
• Left brachial
• Left circumflex subscapular
• Left thoracodorsal
• Left profunda brachii
• Left ulnar
• Left radial
• Left common interosseous
• Left deep palmar arch
• Left superficial palmar arch
• Left metacarpal(s)
• Left digital(s)
• Left superior bronchial
• Left inferior bronchial
• Right 3rd intercostal
• Intercostal(s)
• Esophageal
• Right bronchial
Diaphragm
• Abdominal aorta
• Inferior phrenic
• Superior suprarenal (adrenal)
• Celiac
• Left gastric
• Esophageal
• Splenic
• Dorsal pancreatic
• Greater pancreatic (pancreatica magna)
• Caudal pancreatic
• Left gastroepiploic
• Short gastric(s)
• Right brachial
• Transverse pancreatic (inferior pancreatic)
• Common hepatic
• Gastroduodenal
• Proper hepatic
• Right circumflex scapular
• Right thoracodorsal
• Supraduodenal
• Right gastric
• Left hepatic
– Middle hepatic
- Falciform
• Right hepatic
– Cystic
• Middle suprarenal (adrenal)
• Superior mesenteric
• Inferior pancreaticoduodenal
• Anterior inferior pancreaticoduodenal
• Posterior inferior pancreaticoduodenal
• Middle colic
• Right colic
• Colic marginal(s)
• Ileocolic
• Superior ileocolic
• Colic marginal(s)
• Inferior ileocolic
• Anterior & posterior cecal
• Appendicular
• Ileal
• Jejunal
• Renal
• Inferior suprarenal (adrenal)
• Renal polar
• Renal cortical
• Testicular/ovarian
• Lumbar

- **Abdominal aorta** *(continued)*
  - First Order: Inferior mesenteric
    - Second Order: Left colic; Sigmoid; Superior rectal
      - Third Order: Ascending left colic; Ascending left colic
        - Beyond Third Order: Colic marginal(s)
  - First Order: Middle (median) sacral
  - First Order: Common iliac
    - Second Order: Internal iliac
      - Third Order: Posterior division
        - Beyond Third Order: Iliolumbar; Lateral sacral; Superior gluteal
      - Third Order: Anterior division
        - Beyond Third Order: Obturator; Umbilical (– Superior vesical); Uterine; Vaginal; Inferior vesical; Middle rectal (– Prostate); Internal pudendal (– Inferior rectal); Inferior gluteal
    - Second Order: External iliac *(Considered 1 vessel for coding purposes)*
      - Third Order: Deep circumflex iliac; Inferior epigastric
        - Beyond Third Order: Cremasteric
    - Second Order: Common femoral *(Considered 1 vessel for coding purposes)*
      - Third Order: Profunda femoris; Deep external pudendal; Superficial external pudendal; Superficial femoral *(Considered 1 vessel for coding purposes)*; Popliteal *(Considered 1 vessel for coding purposes)*
        - Beyond Third Order: Medial femoral circumflex; Lateral femoral circumflex
        - Beyond Third Order: Geniculate; Anterior tibial; Posterior tibial; Peroneal; Pedal arch; Digital(s)

Venous Vascular Family

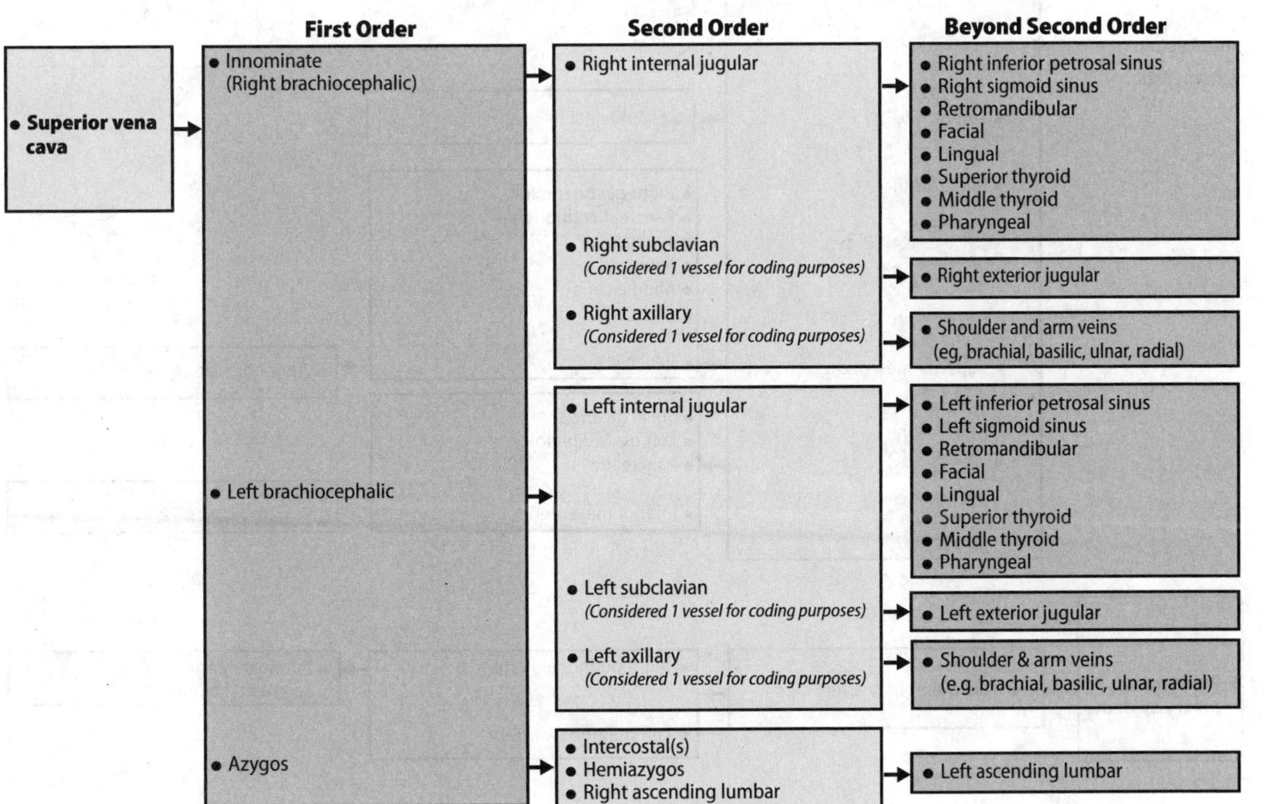

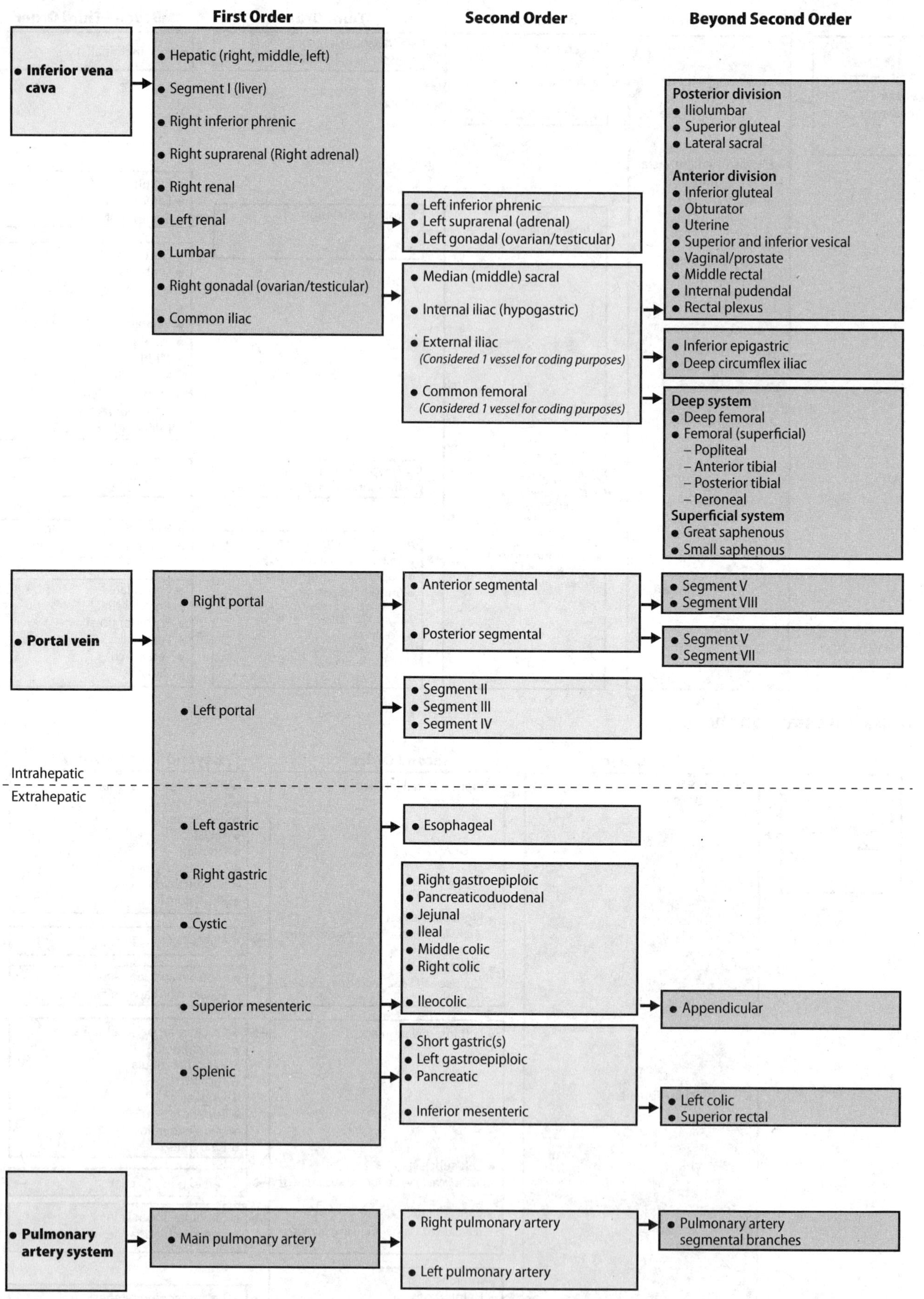
First Order
Second Order
Beyond Second Order
• Inferior vena cava
• Hepatic (right, middle, left)
• Segment I (liver)
• Right inferior phrenic
• Right suprarenal (Right adrenal)
• Right renal
• Left renal
• Lumbar
• Right gonadal (ovarian/testicular)
• Common iliac
• Left inferior phrenic
• Left suprarenal (adrenal)
• Left gonadal (ovarian/testicular)
• Median (middle) sacral
• Internal iliac (hypogastric)
• External iliac
(Considered 1 vessel for coding purposes)
• Common femoral
(Considered 1 vessel for coding purposes)
Posterior division
• Iliolumbar
• Superior gluteal
• Lateral sacral
Anterior division
• Inferior gluteal
• Obturator
• Uterine
• Superior and inferior vesical
• Vaginal/prostate
• Middle rectal
• Internal pudendal
• Rectal plexus
• Inferior epigastric
• Deep circumflex iliac
Deep system
• Deep femoral
• Femoral (superficial)
– Popliteal
– Anterior tibial
– Posterior tibial
– Peroneal
Superficial system
• Great saphenous
• Small saphenous
• Portal vein
• Right portal
• Left portal
• Anterior segmental
• Posterior segmental
• Segment V
• Segment VIII
• Segment V
• Segment VII
• Segment II
• Segment III
• Segment IV
Intrahepatic
Extrahepatic
• Left gastric
• Right gastric
• Cystic
• Superior mesenteric
• Splenic
• Esophageal
• Right gastroepiploic
• Pancreaticoduodenal
• Jejunal
• Ileal
• Middle colic
• Right colic
• Ileocolic
• Appendicular
• Short gastric(s)
• Left gastroepiploic
• Pancreatic
• Inferior mesenteric
• Left colic
• Superior rectal
• Pulmonary artery system
• Main pulmonary artery
• Right pulmonary artery
• Left pulmonary artery
• Pulmonary artery segmental branches

Appendix P — Interventional Radiology Illustrations

Internal Carotid and Vertebral Arterial Anatomy

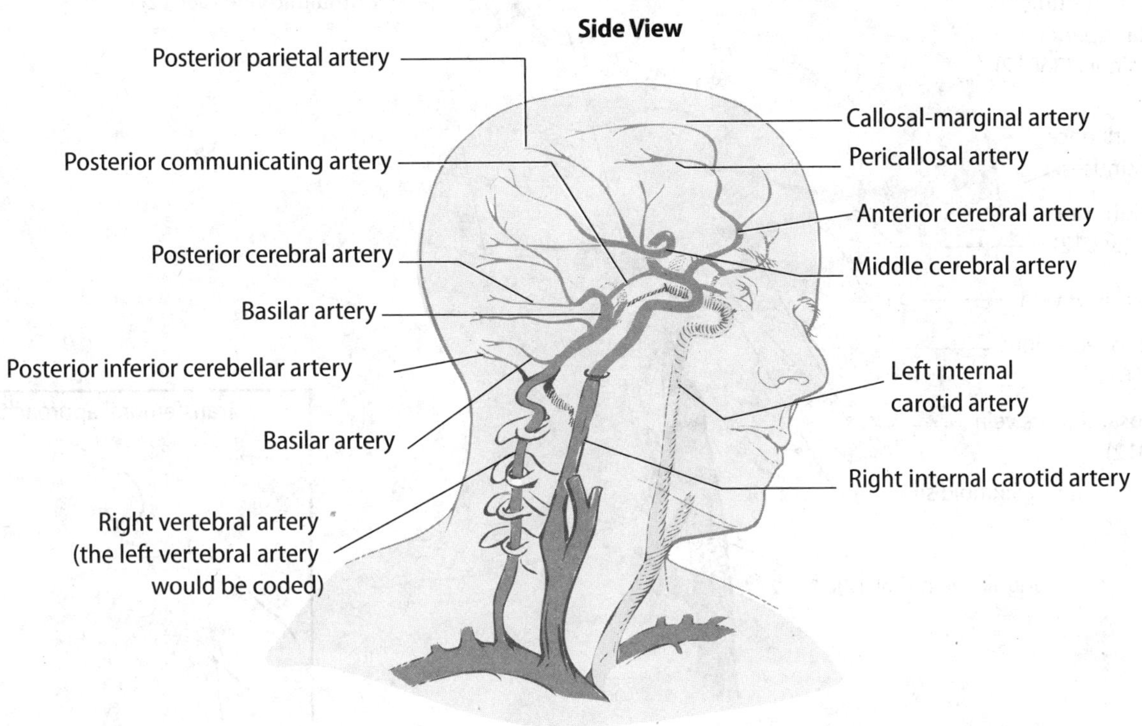

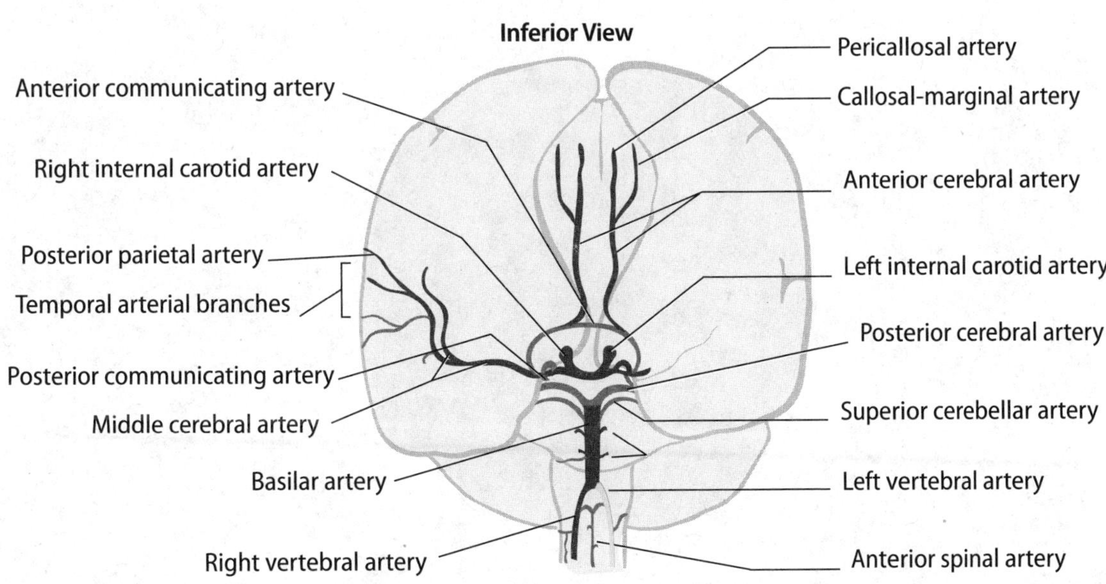

Cerebral Venous Anatomy

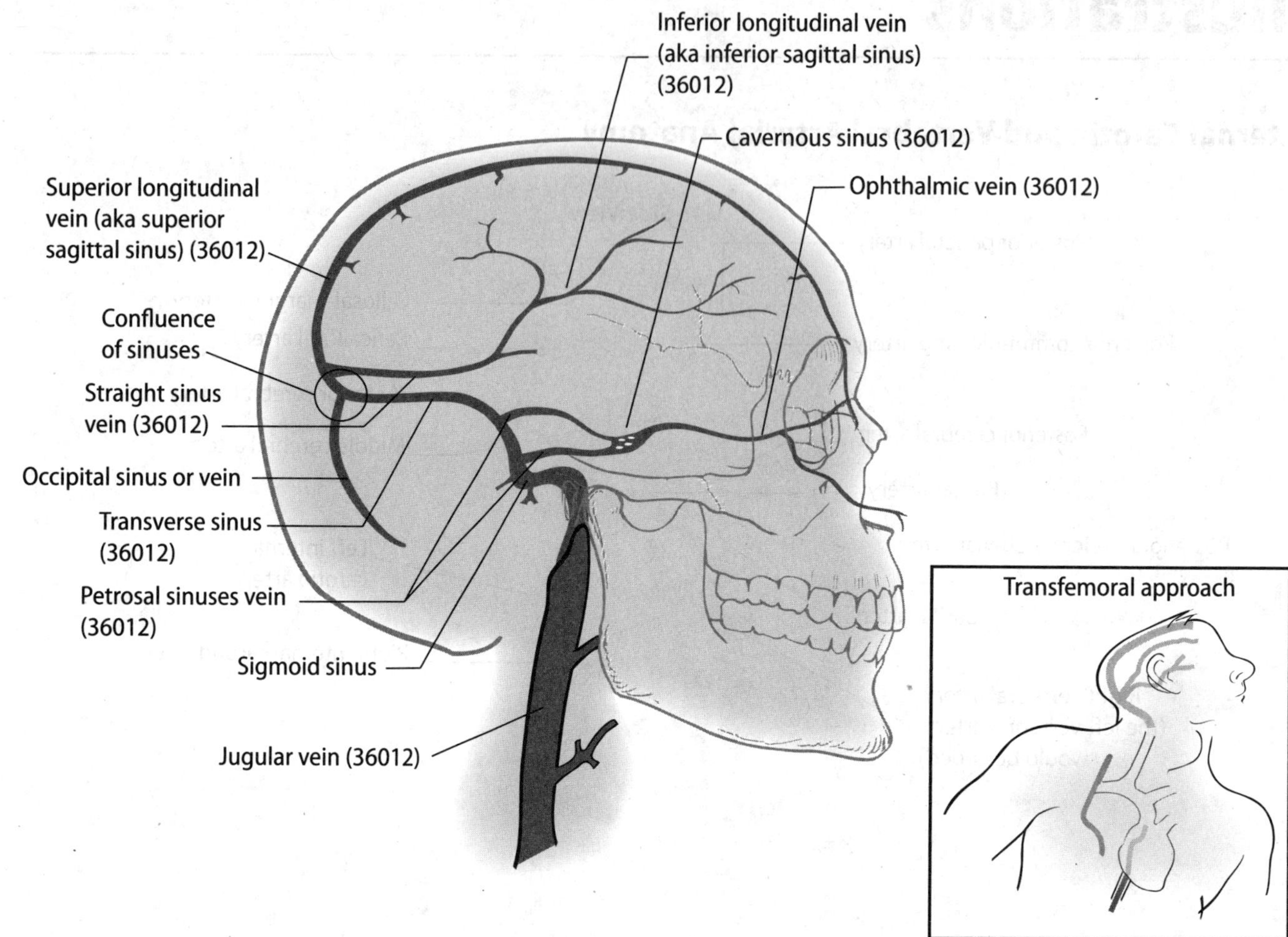

Normal Aortic Arch and Branch Anatomy—Transfemoral Approach

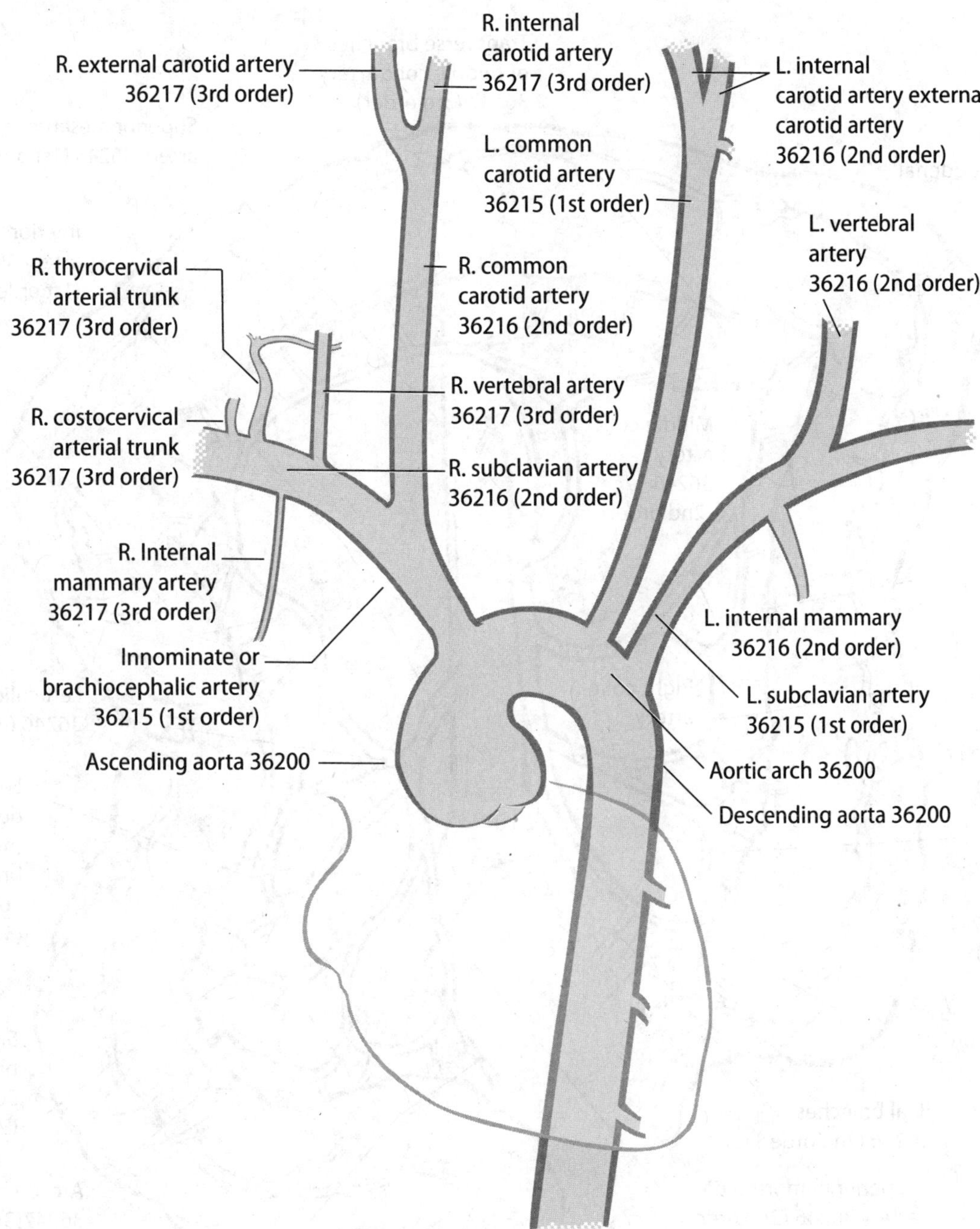

Superior and Inferior Mesenteric Arteries and Branches

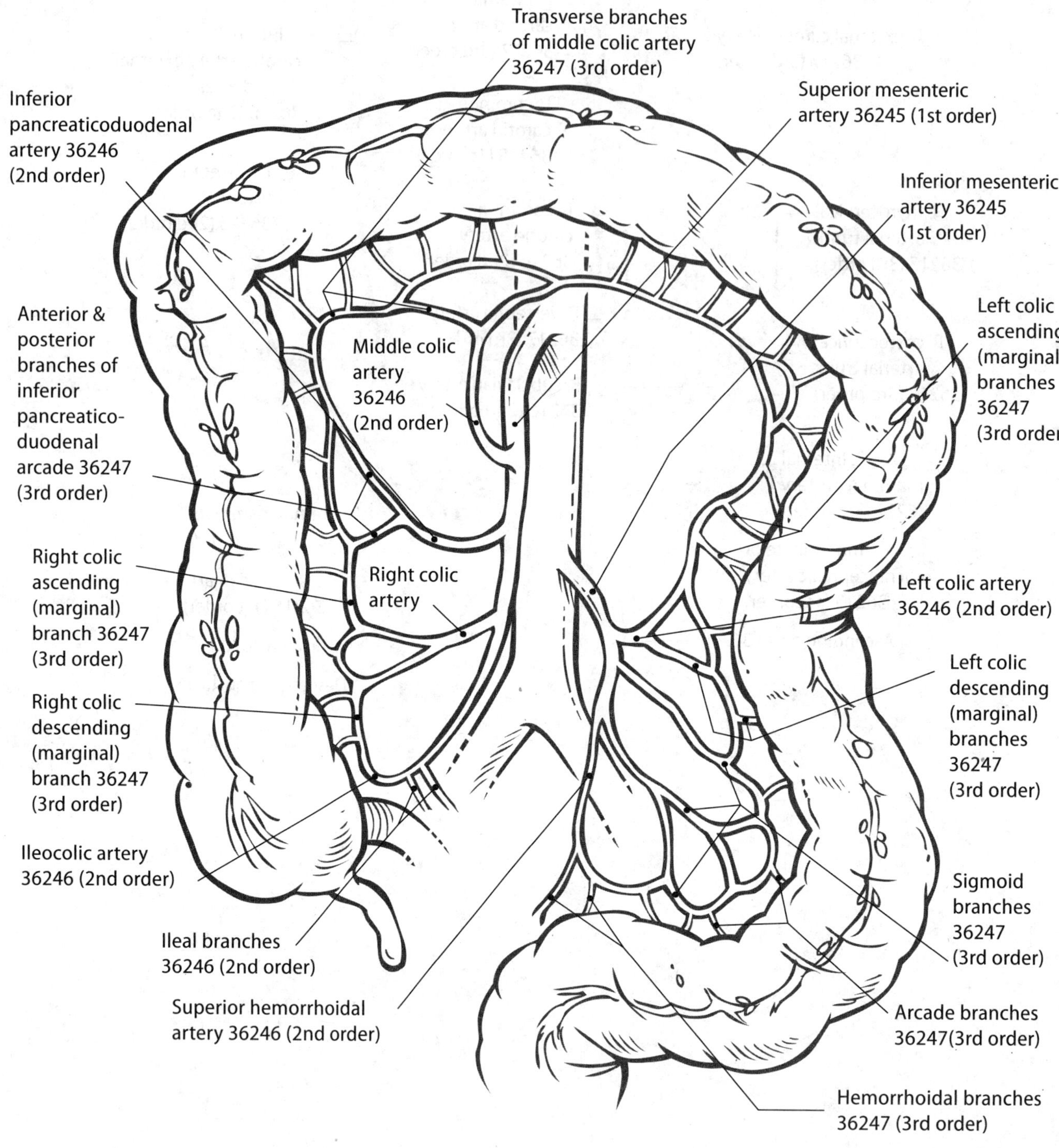

Renal Artery Anatomy—Femoral Approach

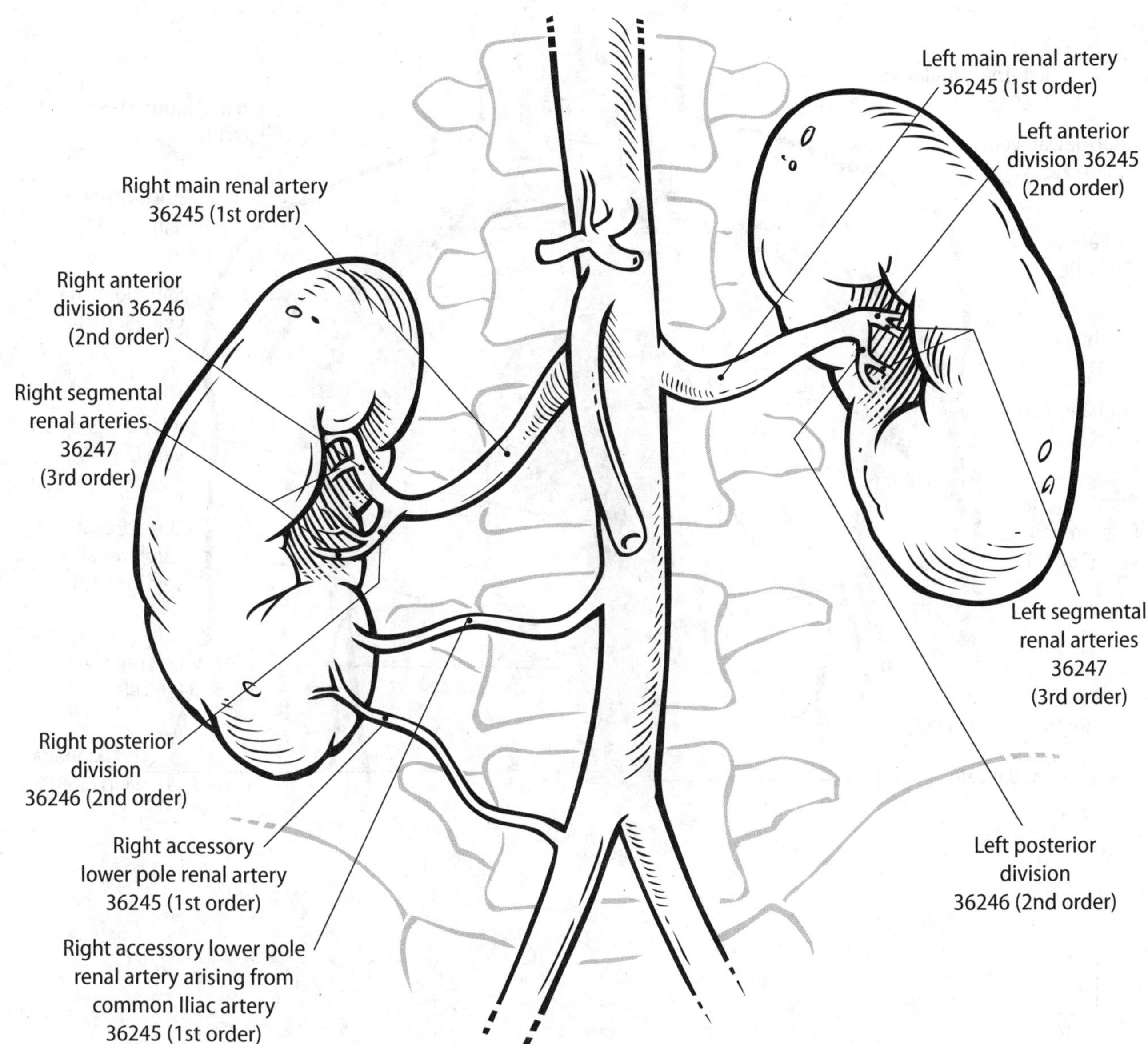

Central Venous Anatomy

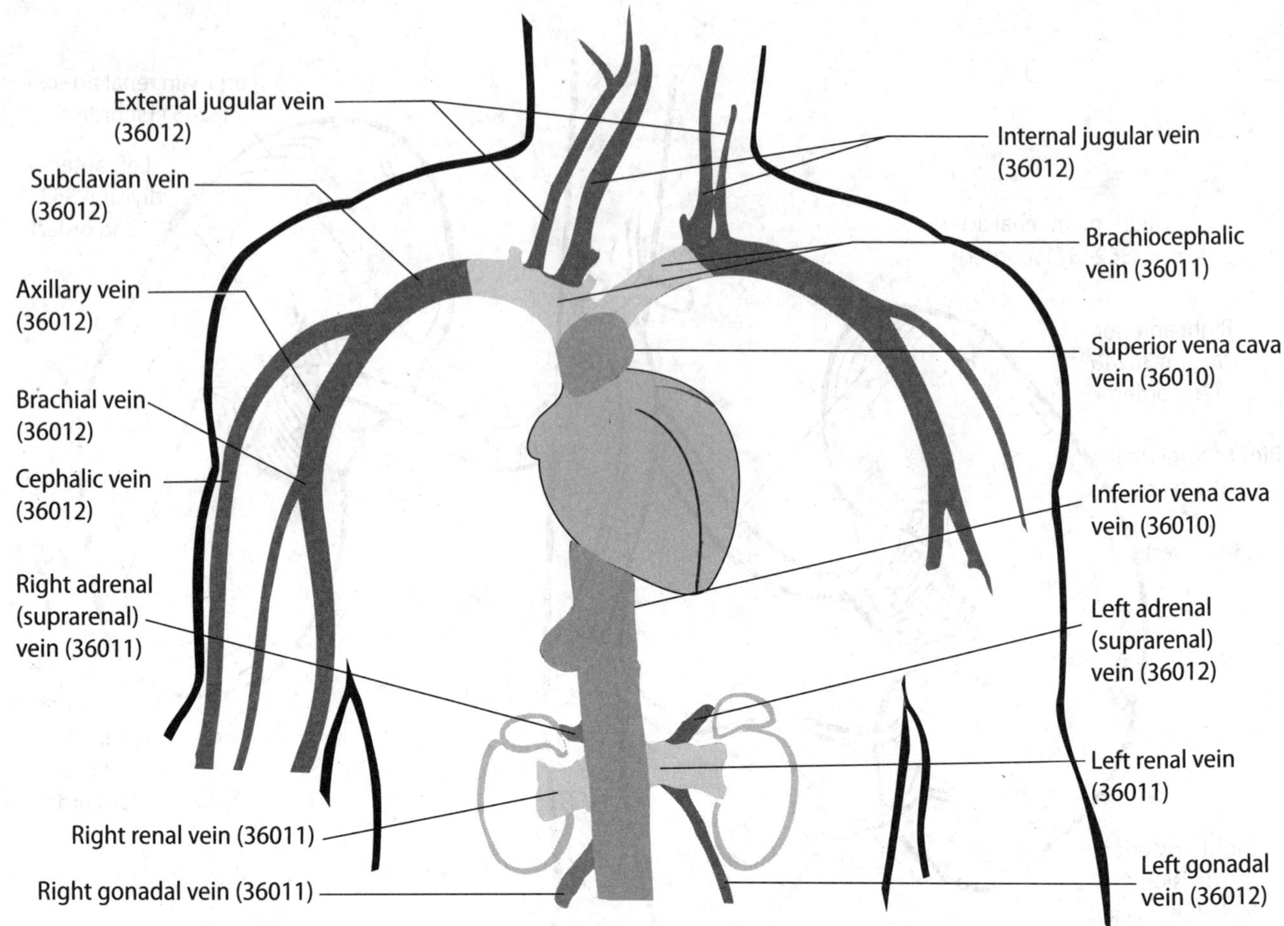

Portal System (Arterial)

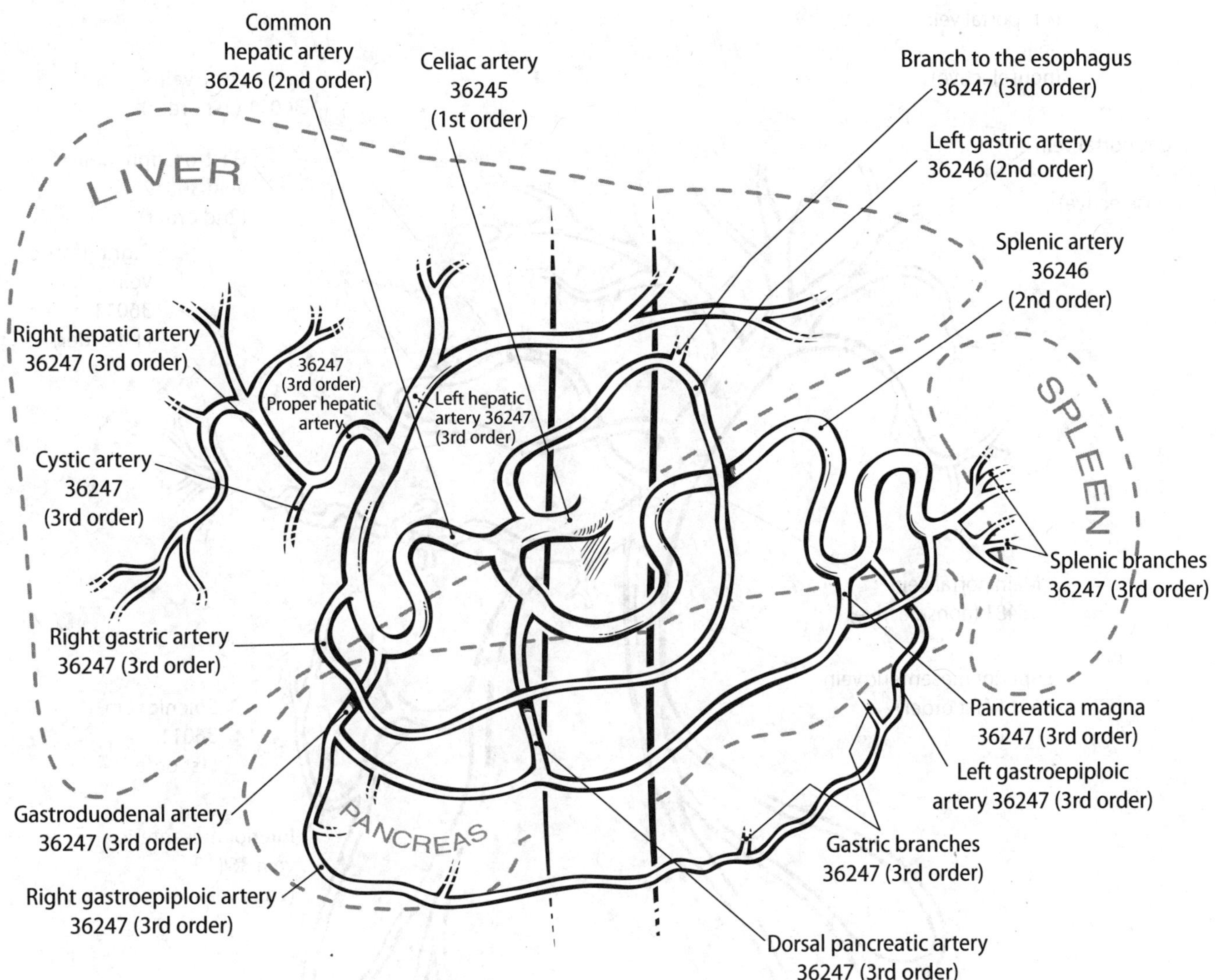

Portal System (Venous)

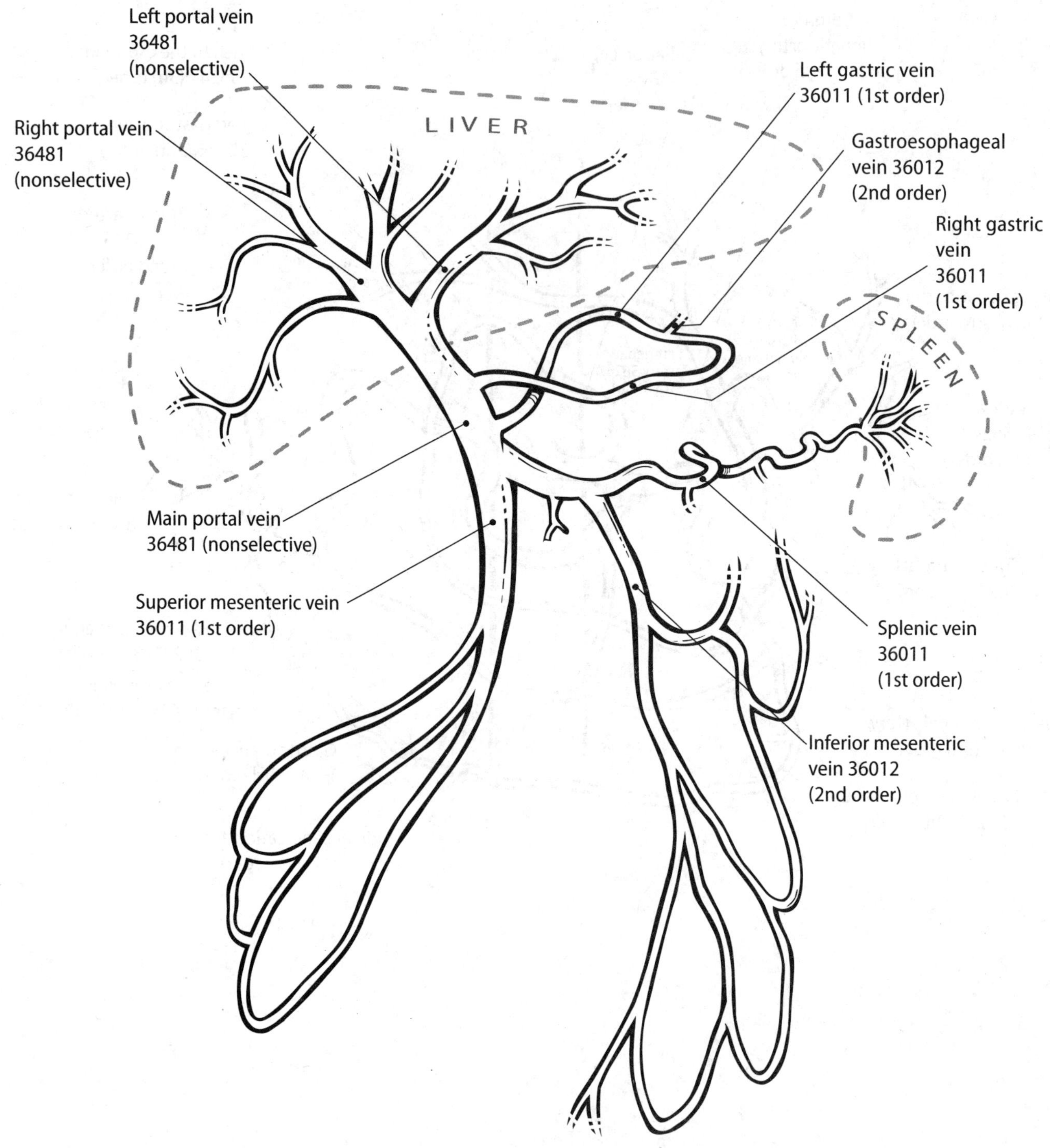

Pulmonary Artery Angiography

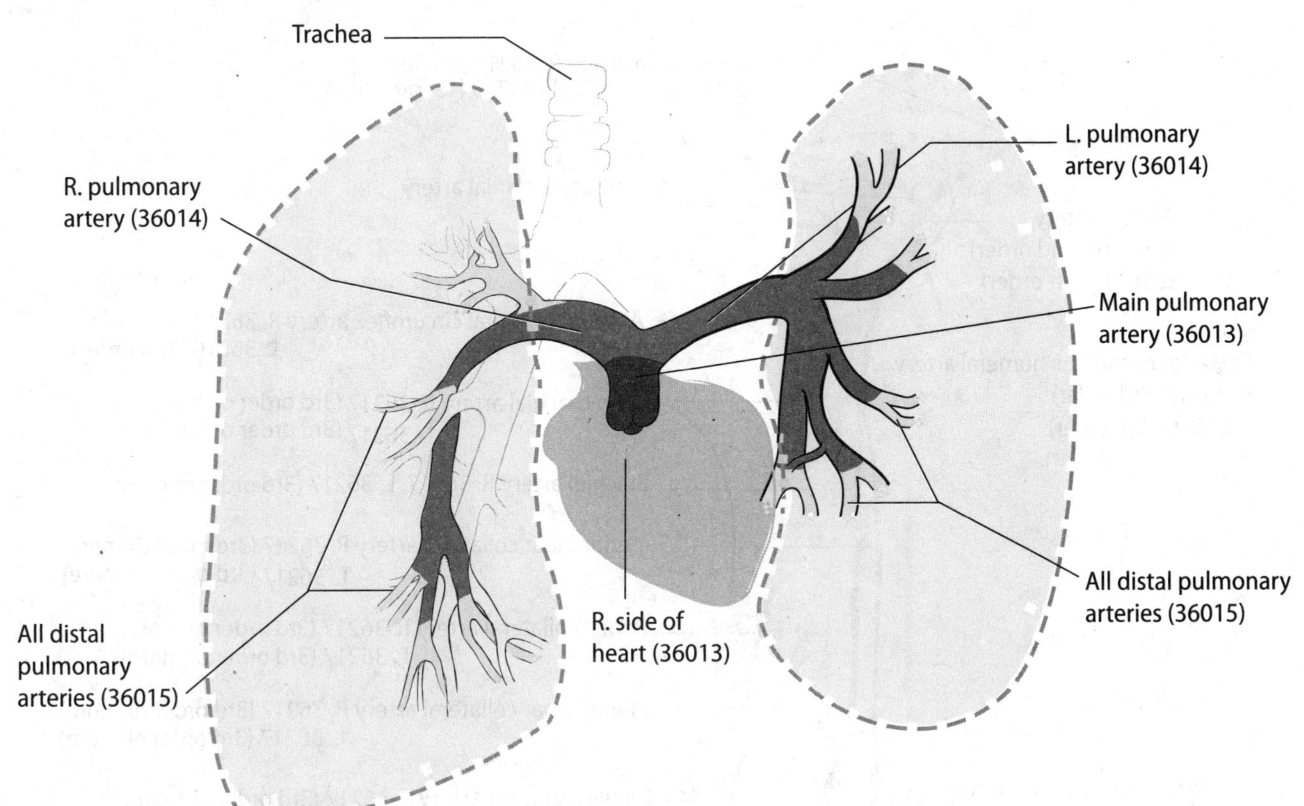

Upper Extremity Arterial Anatomy—Transfemoral or Contralateral Approach

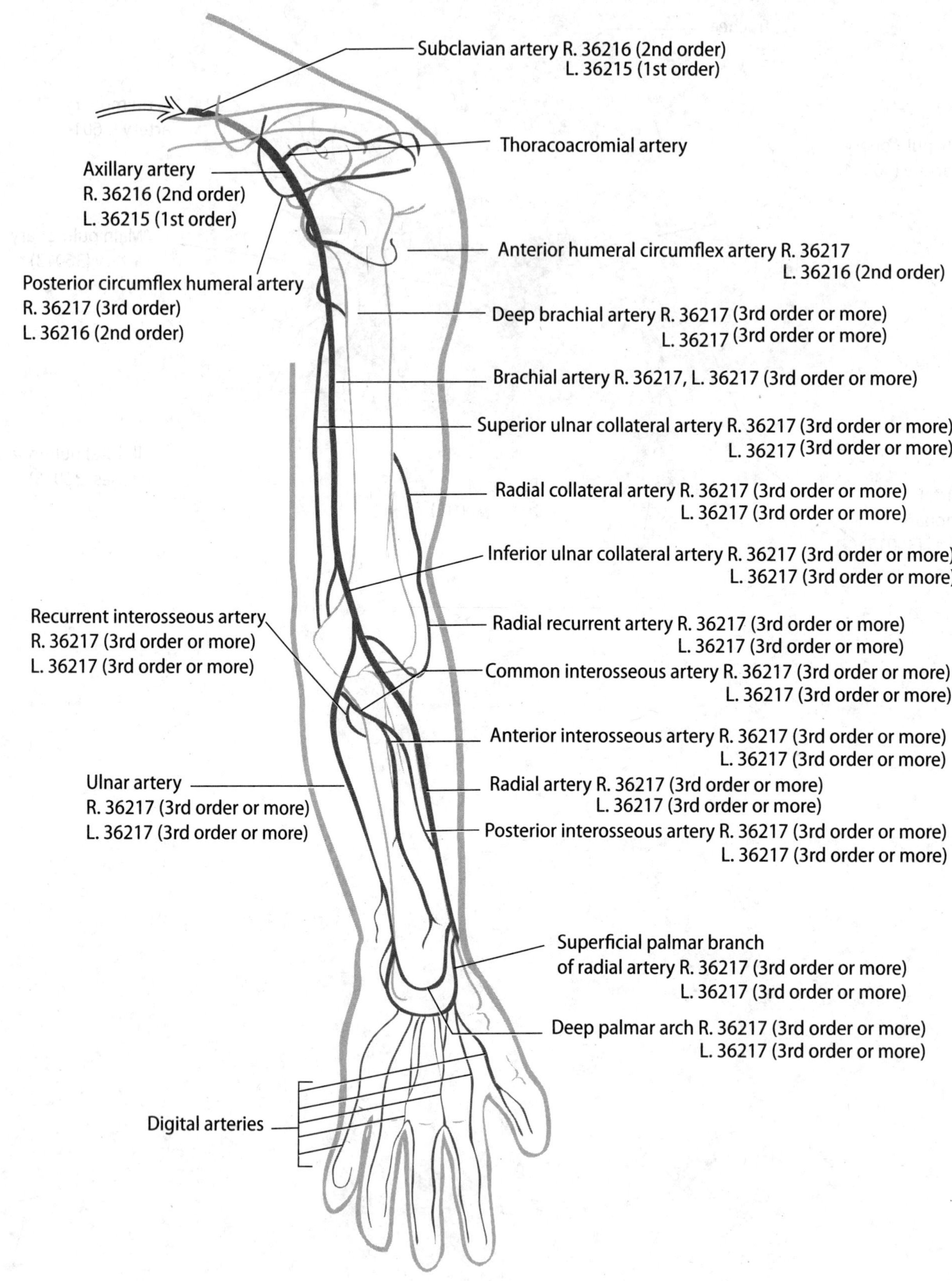

Lower Extremity Arterial Anatomy—Contralateral, Axillary or Brachial Approach

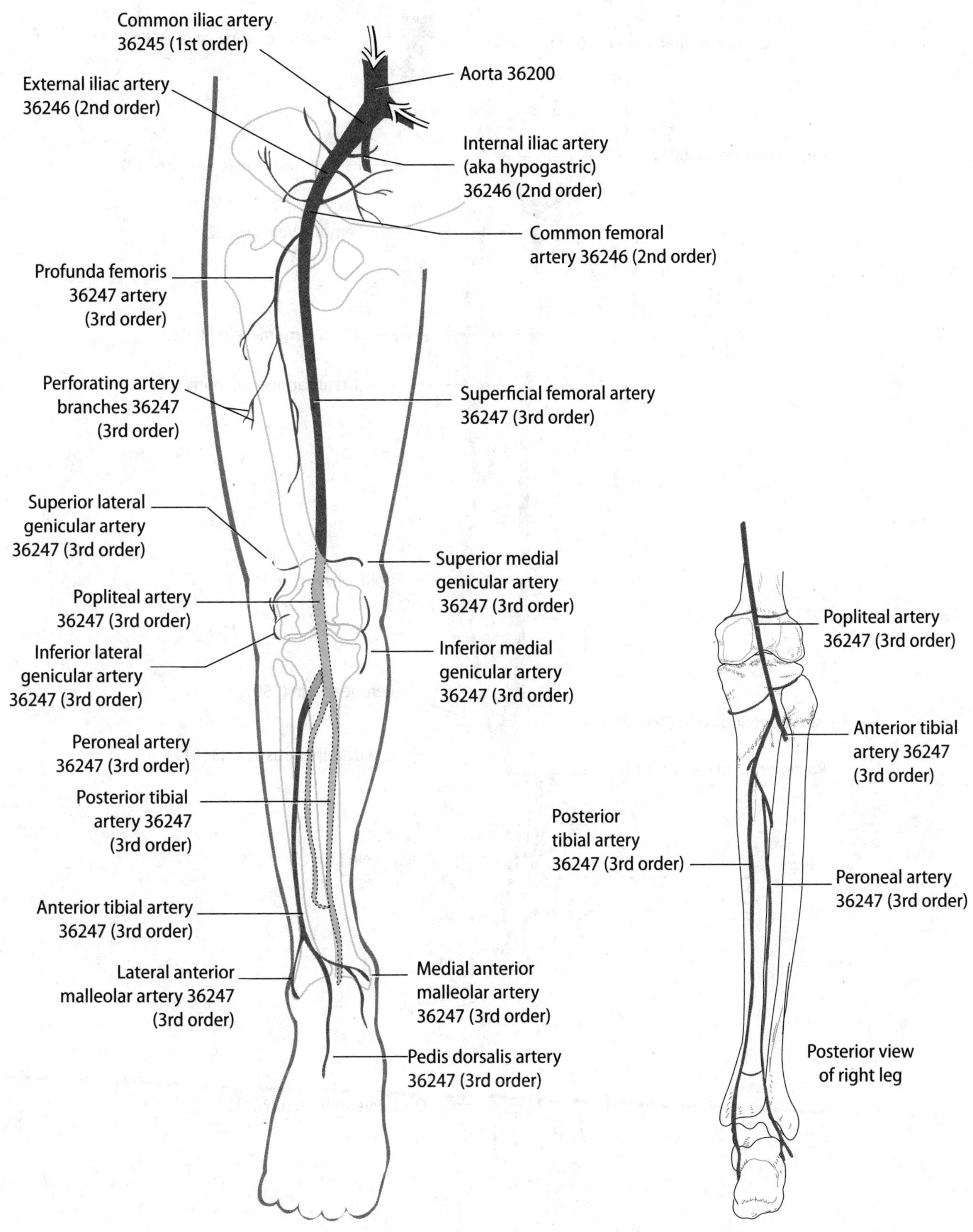

Lower Extremity Venous Anatomy

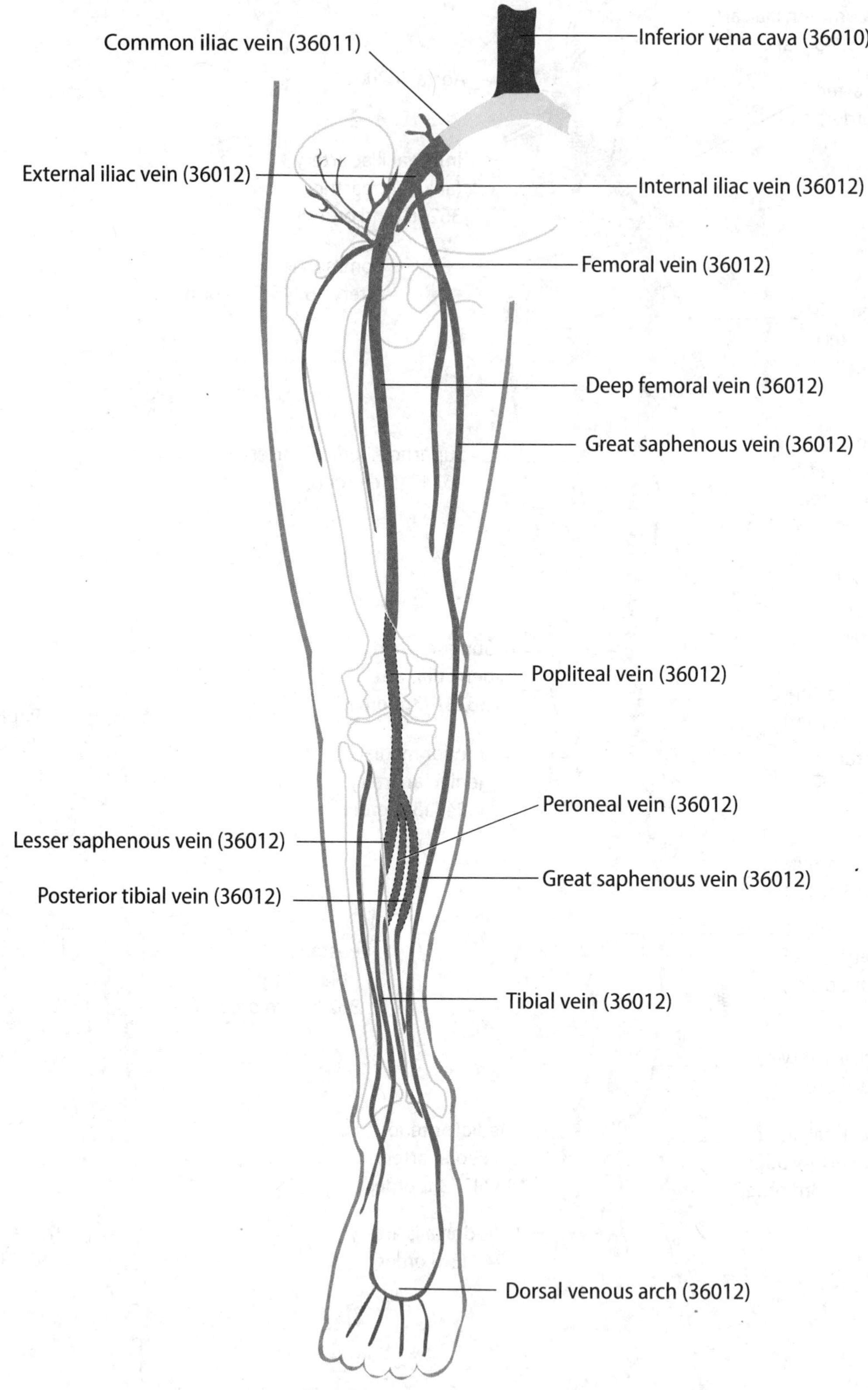

Coronary Arteries Anterior View

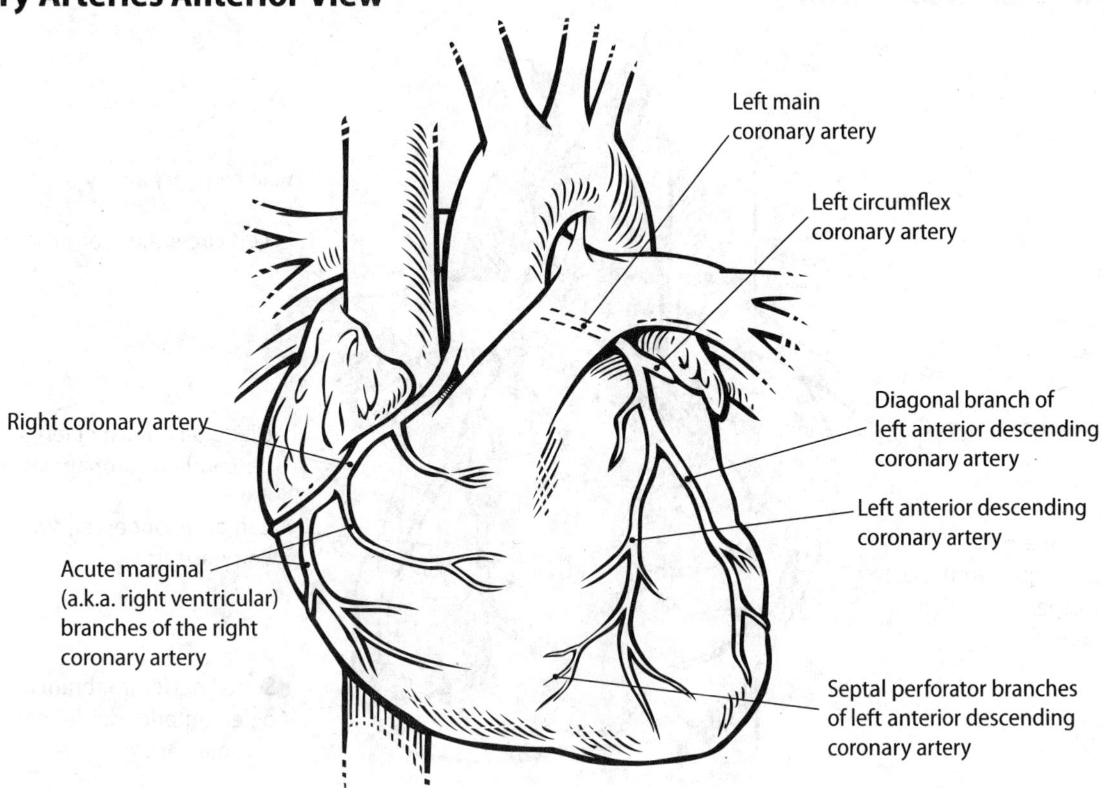

Left Heart Catheterization

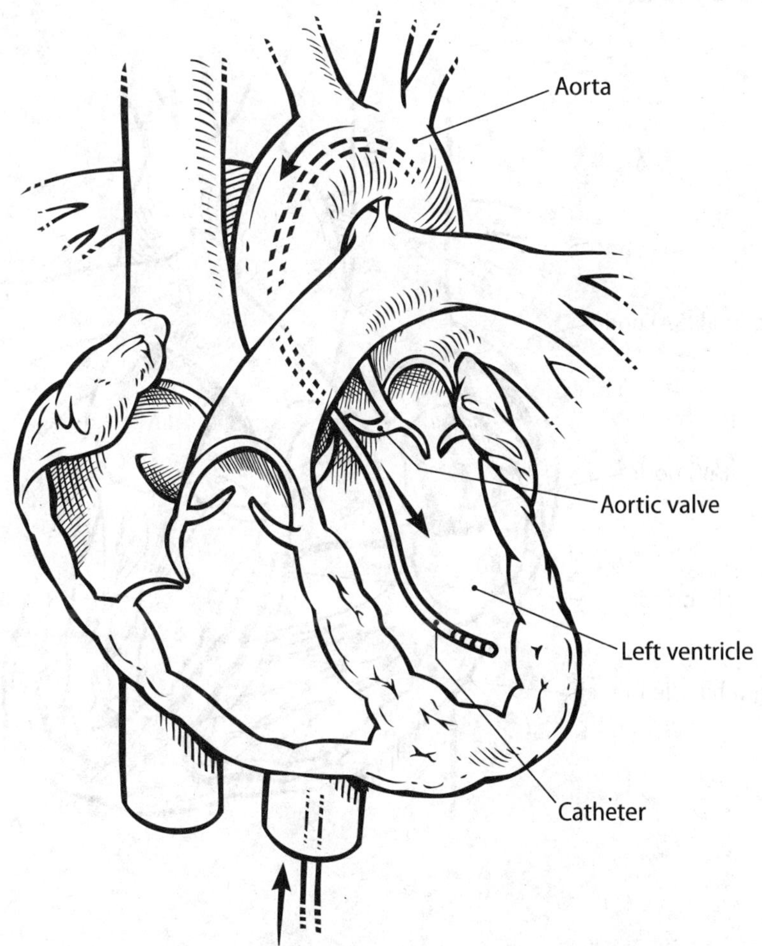

Right Heart Catheterization

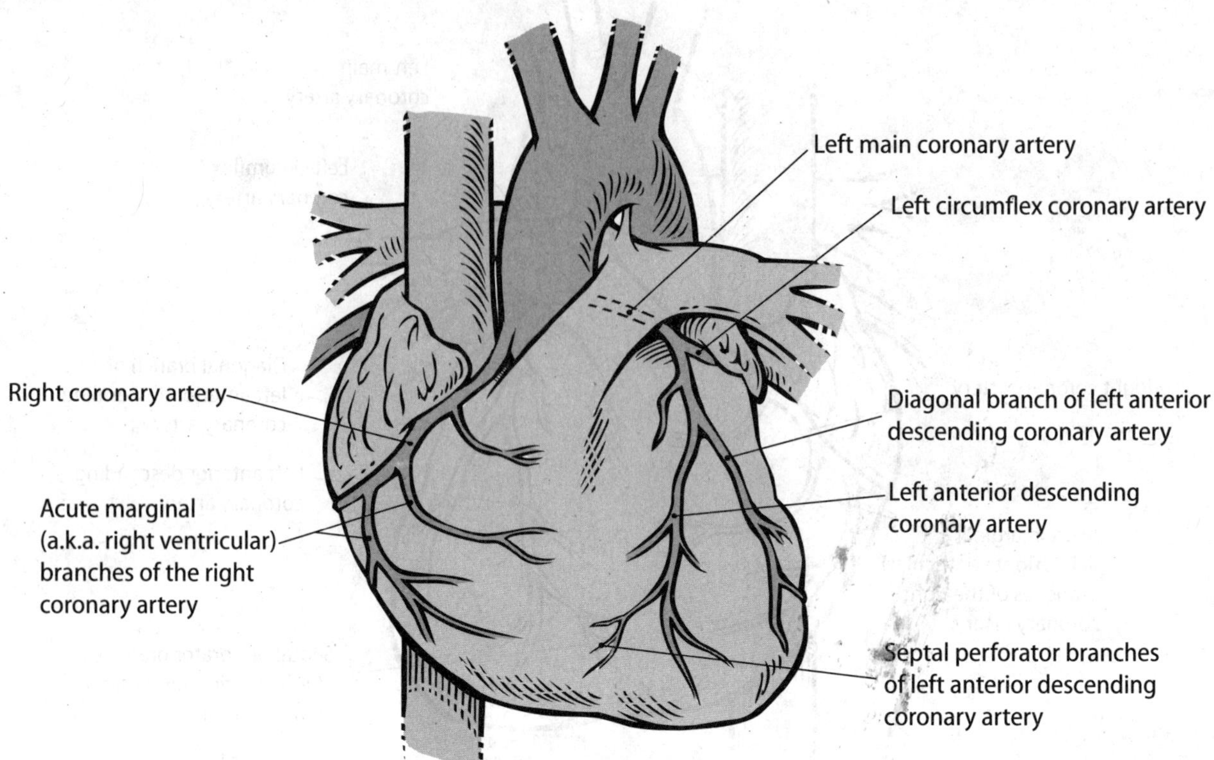

Heart Conduction System

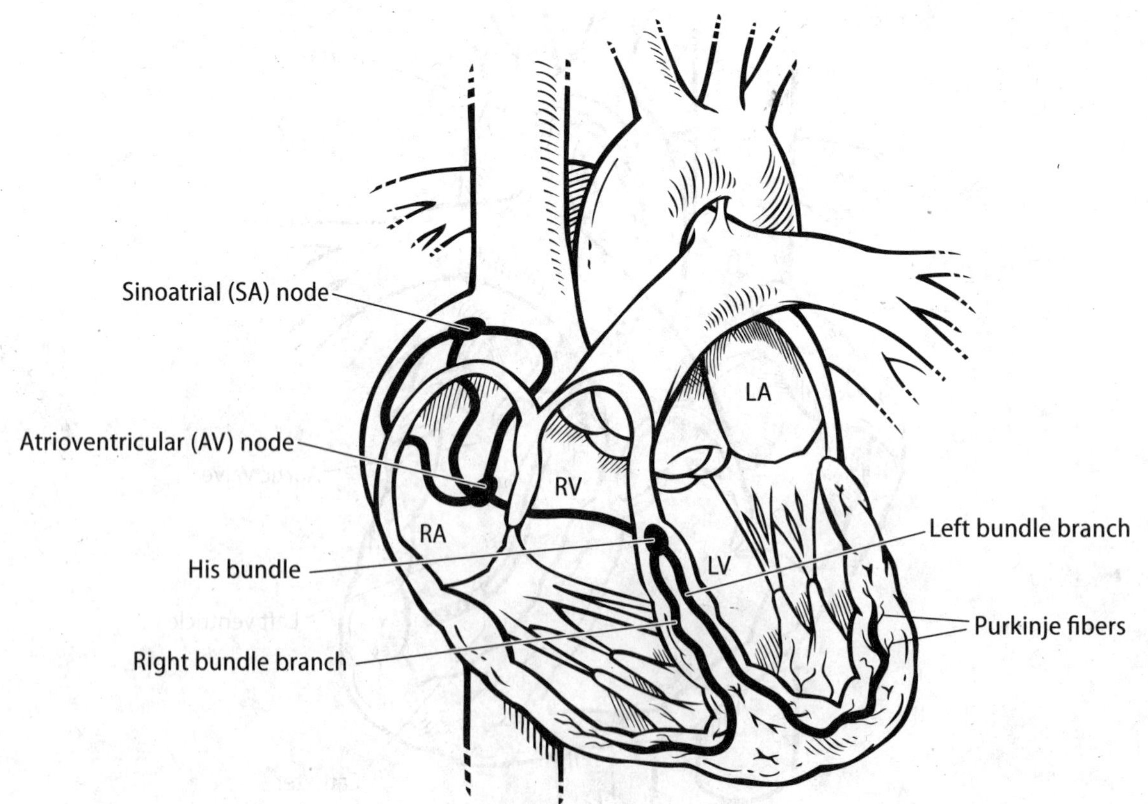